2/29/88

6 45

GERALD E. SWANSON, M.D.
9601 UPTON ROAD
MINNEAPOLIS, MN 55431
TELE: 881-6869

CURRENT THERAPY IN INTERNAL MEDICINE - 2

Current Therapy Series

Bayless:
Current Therapy in Gastroenterology and Liver Disease
Bayless, Brain, Cherniack:
Current Therapy in Internal Medicine
Brain, Carbone:
Current Therapy in Hematology-Oncology
Callaham:
Current Therapy in Emergency Medicine
Cameron:
Current Surgical Therapy
Charles:
Current Therapy in Obstetrics
Cherniack:
Current Therapy of Respiratory Disease
Dubovsky, Shore:
Current Therapy in Psychiatry
Ernst, Stanley:
Current Therapy in Vascular Surgery
Fazio:
Current Therapy in Colon and Rectal Surgery
Foley, Payne:
Current Therapy of Pain
Fortuin:
Current Therapy in Cardiovascular Disease
Garcia, Mastroianni, Amelar, Dubin:
Current Therapy of Infertility
Garcia, Mikuta, Rosenblum:
Current Therapy in Surgical Gynecology
Gates:
Current Therapy in Otolaryngology—Head and Neck Surgery
Glassock:
Current Therapy in Nephrology and Hypertension
Grillo, Austen, Wilkins, Mathisen, Vlahakes:
Current Therapy in Cardiothoracic Surgery
Jeejeebhoy:
Current Therapy in Nutrition
Johnson:
Current Therapy in Neurologic Disease
Kass, Platt:
Current Therapy in Infectious Disease
Krieger, Bardin:
Current Therapy in Endocrinology and Metabolism
Lichtenstein, Fauci:
Current Therapy in Allergy, Immunology and Rheumatology
Long:
Current Therapy in Neurological Surgery
Marsh:
Current Therapy in Plastic and Reconstructive Surgery
McGinty, Jackson:
Current Therapy in Orthopaedic Surgery
Nelson:
Current Therapy in Neonatal-Perinatal Medicine
Nelson:
Current Therapy in Pediatric Infectious Disease
Parrillo:
Current Therapy in Critical Care Medicine
Provost, Farmer:
Current Therapy in Dermatology
Resnick, Kursh:
Current Therapy in Genitourinary Surgery
Rogers:
Current Practice of Anesthesiology
Spaeth:
Current Ophthalmic Surgery
Trunkey, Lewis:
Current Therapy of Trauma
Welsh, Torg, Shephard:
Current Therapy in Sports Medicine

CURRENT THERAPY IN INTERNAL MEDICINE - 2

THEODORE M. BAYLESS, M.D.
Professor of Medicine
The Johns Hopkins University
School of Medicine
Medical Director, Meyerhoff Digestive Disease–
Inflammatory Bowel Disease Center
Baltimore, Maryland

MICHAEL C. BRAIN, D.M.
Professor of Medicine
McMaster University Faculty of Health Sciences
Hamilton, Ontario, Canada

REUBEN M. CHERNIACK, M.D.
Department of Medicine
The National Jewish Center
for Immunology and Respiratory Disease
Professor, Department of Medicine
University of Colorado
School of Medicine
Denver, Colorado

1987
B.C. DECKER INC • Toronto • Philadelphia

Publisher

B.C. Decker Inc.
3228 South Service Road
Burlington, Ontario L7N 3H8

B.C. Decker Inc.
P.O. Box 30246
Philadelphia, Pennsylvania 19103

Sales and Distribution

United States and Possessions
The C.V. Mosby Company
11830 Westline Industrial Drive
Saint Louis, Missouri 63146

Canada
The C.V. Mosby Company, Ltd.
5240 Finch Avenue East, Unit No. 1
Scarborough, Ontario M1S 4P2

United Kingdom, Europe and the Middle East
Blackwell Scientific Publications, Ltd.
Osney Mead, Oxford OX2 OEL, England

Australia
CBS Publishing Australia Pty. Limited
9 Waltham Street
Artarmon, N.S.W. 2064
Australia

Japan
Igaku-Shoin Ltd.
Tokyo International P.O. Box 5063
1-28-36 Hongo, Bunkyo-ku, Tokyo 113, Japan

Asia
CBS Publishing Asia Limited
10/F, Inter-Continental Plaza
Tsim Sha Tsui East
Kowloon, Hong Kong

Current Therapy in Internal Medicine - 2 ISBN 0–941158–69–1

Library of Congress catalog card number: 83-73070

10 9 8 7 6 5 4 3 2 1

ASSOCIATE EDITORS

ASSOCIATE EDITORS

PREFACE

Although there are a number of excellent textbooks of internal medicine, most are designed to provide information on etiology, pathophysiologic presentation, and differential diagnosis, as well as general statements on treatment; often, the therapy section includes a well-referenced literature review. However, the reader is apt to be left without the specific information he needs for his patient's problem, and he may even wonder if the author of the textbook chapter has had to make very many patient-care decisions.

We learned that practitioners of internal medicine appreciate direct and specific opinions on the important, and at times controversial, areas of therapeutics that we included in the first edition of *Current Therapy in Internal Medicine*. More than 300 physicians described their mode of therapy for a specific disease or management problem, as if they were providing a consultation. Those selected were involved in patient care as well as teaching and research, their critical approach to decision making being seasoned by several years of patient-care experience.

For this second edition, we have enlisted new authors for every topic. They are the same type of clinically active experts as authors they are replacing. We really have a new book. The authors of this second edition represent over 100 medical schools in the United States, Canada, and other countries and thus provide a broad view of medical care practices. The editors and coeditors have been trained in internal medicine and represent 15 areas of the specialty, including infectious disease, immunology, rheumatology, allergy, dermatology, hematology, oncology, gastroenterology, liver disease, metabolism, endocrinology, pulmonary disease, nephrology, cardiovascular disorders, and neurology.

How were the subjects chosen? Is this the "core" of internal medicine? It is difficult to define which are the most "important" diseases. We have selected relatively common disorders in which some type of therapeutic decision is needed. Controversial issues have been included; areas of consensus have, at times, been omitted. Some topics covered in the first edition have been omitted and new ones, perhaps reflecting new investigative advances, have been added. The subjects are balanced between common diseases and less frequent disorders which present difficult therapeutic dilemmas.

Additional subjects are included in a series of 10 subspecialty "Current Therapy" books that are being published in 1986 and 1987. The chapters in *Current Therapy in Internal Medicine* represent about one-third of the chapters in the series. It is clear that changes in therapy in internal medicine occur frequently. This was the motivation for this second edition. Future editions, utilizing new authors, are planned at 2-year intervals to meet this continuing need for revision. Comments from the readers to the editors, coeditors, or publisher will help to ensure that this series meets the needs of the practicing internist.

The editors and coeditors gratefully acknowledge the clearly written contributions of the authors who have shared their "methods" with us. The publisher, Brian Decker, has had a clear and well organized view of the role of the consultant as a writer of therapeutic recommendations. We are most appreciative of his aid and advice.

It is impossible to compensate authors adequately for their contributed chapters. In lieu of disbursing hundreds of small honoraria to our authors, we feel a consolidated contribution to the American College of Physicians would produce greater benefit. For each edition of CTIM, then, we are donating not less than $2500 to the Educational Development Fund of the College. The funds will be applied at the discretion of the officers of the College.

The Editors

CONTRIBUTORS

STEPHEN C. ACHUFF, M.D.

Associate Professor of Medicine; Attending Staff, The Johns Hopkins Medical Institutes, Baltimore, Maryland
Unstable Angina Pectoris

RODNEY D. ADAM, M.D.

Fellow, Section of Infectious Disease, Department of Internal Medicine, University of Arizona College of Medicine, Tucson, Arizona
Chronic Mucocutaneous Candidiasis

GAIL K. ADLER, M.D., Ph.D.

Clinical Research Fellow in Medicine, Harvard Medical School and Brigham and Women's Hospital; Associate, Howard Hughes Medical Institute, Boston, Massachusetts
Primary Aldosteronism
Mineralocorticoid Hypertension

SHARON G. ADLER, M.D.

Assistant Professor of Medicine, Division of Nephrology, Department of Medicine, Harbor-UCLA Medical Center, Torrance, California
Mesangial Proliferative Glomerulonephritis

MAHMOUD A. M. ALI, M.D., Ph.D., F.R.C.P.(C)

Professor, Pathology and Medicine, McMaster University School of Medicine; Head of Service, Hematology-Oncology, St. Joseph's Hospital, Hamilton, Ontario, Canada
Iron Deficiency Anemia

NANCY BATES ALLEN, M.D.

Assistant Professor of Medicine, Duke University Medical Center, Durham, North Carolina
Wegener's Granulomatosis

STEVEN G. ALSIP, M.D.

Assistant Professor of Medicine, Division of Infectious Diseases and Allergy, University of South Alabama College of Medicine, Mobile, Alabama
Endocarditis Caused by Gram-Positive Organisms

THOMAS F. ANDERSON, M.D.

Associate Professor, Department of Dermatology, University of Michigan Medical School; Attending Staff, University of Michigan Hospitals, Veterans Administration Medical Center, Ann Arbor, Michigan
Psoriasis

GERALD S. ARBUS, M.D., F.R.C.P.(C)

Associate Professor, University of Toronto Faculty of Medicine; Chief, Division of Nephrology, The Hospital for Sick Children, Toronto, Ontario, Canada
Focal Segmental Glomerulosclerosis

ALLEN A. ARIEFF, M.D.

Chief, Division of Nephrology, San Francisco Veterans Administration Medical Center, San Francisco, California
Hypernatremia in the Adult

RONALD A. ARKY, M.D.

Charles S. Davidson Professor of Medicine, Harvard Medical School at Mount Auburn Hospital; Chief of Medicine, Mount Auburn Hospital, Cambridge, Massachusetts
Functional and Reactive Hypoglycemia

ENRICO ASCER, M.D.

Assistant Professor of Surgery, Albert Einstein College of Medicine; Vascular Surgeon in Charge, North Central Bronx Hospital; Head, Surgical Vascular Laboratory, Montefiore Medical Center, New York, New York
Abdominal Aortic Aneurysm

ROBERT R. BAHNSON, MD.

Assistant Professor of Surgery (Urology), Washington University School of Medicine; Assistant Urologic Surgeon, Barnes Hospital, St. Louis, Missouri
Obstructive Uropathy

WILLIAM C. BAILEY, M.D.

Professor of Medicine, University of Alabama School of Medicine; Associate Chief of Staff for Education, Veterans Administration Medical Center, Birmingham, Alabama
Mycobacterium Kansaii Infection

H. W. GORDON BAKER, M.D., Ph.D., F.R.A.C.P.

Senior Research Fellow, Medical Research Center, Prince Henry's Hospital and Howard Florey Institute of Experimental Physiology and Medicine, Melbourne, Victoria, Australia
Male Infertility of Undetermined Etiology

GARY J. BALADY, M.D.

Assistant Professor of Medicine, Boston University School of Medicine; Director, Cardiac Rehabilitation, University Hospital-Boston University Medical Center, Boston, Massachusetts
Rehabilitation After Myocardial Infarction

ROBERT W. BALOH, M.D.

Professor, Department of Neurology, UCLA School of Medicine, Los Angeles, California
Vertigo

PETER A. BANKS, M.D.

Associate Professor of Medicine, Tufts University School of Medicine, Lecturer in Medicine, Harvard Medical School; Chief of Gastroenterology, Saint Elizabeth's Hospital, Boston, Massachusetts
Acute Pancreatitis: Medical Considerations

ROBERT A. BARBEE, M.D.

Professor of Medicine, Division of Respiratory Sciences, University of Arizona College of Medicine; Director, Chest Allergy Clinic, University Medical Center, Tucson, Arizona
Coccidioidomycosis

DAVID W. BARNES, M.D.

Associate in Medicine, Division of Infectious Diseases, University of Alabama School of Medicine, Birmingham, Alabama
Herpes Simplex

JOHN G. BARTLETT, M.D.

Professor of Medicine, The Johns Hopkins Medical Institutions, Baltimore, Maryland
Pulmonary Infection Involving Aerobic Gram-Positive Cocci

KENNETH L. BAUGHMAN, M.D.

Associate Professor of Medicine, Attending Staff, The Johns Hopkins Medical Institutes, Baltimore, Maryland
Dilated Cardiomyopathy

REUBEN BAUMAL, M.D., Ph.D., F.R.C.P.(C)

Associate Professor, University of Toronto, Faculty of Medicine; Staff Pathologist, The Hospital for Sick Children, Toronto, Ontario, Canada
Focal Segmental Glomerulosclerosis

NORMAN H. BELL, M.D.

Professor of Medicine and Pharmacology, Medical University of South Carolina College of Medicine; Medical Investigator, Veterans Administration Medical Center, Charleston, South Carolina
Hypocalcemia

SETH F. BERKLEY, M.D.

Respiratory and Special Pathogens Epidemiology Branch, Division of Bacterial Diseases, Centers for Disease Control, Atlanta, Georgia
Toxic Shock Syndrome

ROBERT O. BERKSETH, M.D.

Assistant Professor of Medicine, University of Minnesota Medical School; Assistant Professor of Medicine, Division of Nephrology, Hennepin County Medical Center Minneapolis, Minnesota
Dialytic Management of Acute Renal Failure

RAMÓN H. BERMÚDEZ, M.D., F.A.C.P.

Associate Professor of Medicine, University of Puerto Rico School of Medicine; Chief, Infectious Disease Section, Veterans Administration Medical Center, San Juan, Puerto Rico
Infection Caused by Intestinal Helminths

DAVID R. BICKERS, M.D.

Professor and Chairman, Department of Dermatology, Case Western Reserve University School of Medicine; Chief of Dermatology, Veterans Administration Medical Center, Cleveland, Ohio
Porphyrias

LAURENCE M. BLENDIS, M.D., F.R.C.P., F.R.C.P.(C)

Professor of Medicine, University of Toronto Faculty of Medicine; Senior Staff Physician and Service Chief, General Medical Floor, Toronto General Hospital, Toronto, Ontario, Canada
Portosystemic Encephalopathy

CLARA D. BLOOMFIELD, M.D.

Professor of Medicine, Section of Medical Oncology, University of Minnesota School of Medicine, Minneapolis, Minnesota
Acute Myelocytic Leukemia in Adults

DAVID S. BLUMENTHAL, M.D.

Assistant Professor of Medicine, Cornell University Medical College; Assistant Attending Physician, The New York Hospital, New York, New York
Acute Pulmonary Edema

GERALD P. BODEY, M.D., F.A.C.P., F.A.C.C.P., F.R.S.M., F.R.S.H.

Professor of Medicine, Baylor College of Medicine; Internist, The University of Texas System Cancer Center, M.D. Anderson Hospital and Tumor Institute, Houston, Texas
Solid Tumor and Associated Infection

FRANK G. BOINEAU M.D.

Associate Professor of Pediatrics, Tulane University School of Medicine; Head, Section of Pediatric Nephrology, Tulane University Medical Center, New Orleans, Louisiana
Poststreptococcal Glomerulonephritis

WAYNE A. BORDER

Professor of Medicine and Chief, Division of Nephrology, University of Utah Health Sciences Center; Director, Kolff Dialysis Center, Salt Lake City, Utah
Acute Hypersensitivity Interstitial Nephritis

DONALD L. BORNSTEIN, M.D.

Associate Professor of Medicine; Chief, Infectious Disease Section, State University of New York Health Sciences Center, Syracuse, New York
Tetanus

WALTER G. BRADLEY, M.D, F.R.C.P.

Professor and Chairman, Department of Neurology, University of Vermont College of Medicine, Burlington, Vermont
Polymyositis and Dermatomyositis

BEN V. BRANSCOMB, M.D., F.A.C.P., F.C.C.P.

The Alabama Professor of Medicine in Emphysema and Respiratory Diseases, Division of Pulmonary and Critical Care Medicine, University of Alabama Medical Center, Birmingham, Alabama
Lung Abscess

WILLIAM E. BRAUN, M.D.

Director, Histocompatibility and Immunogenetics Laboratory and Consultant in Transplantation, Cleveland Clinic Foundation, Cleveland, Ohio
Renal Allograft Rejection

MARTIN L. BRECHER, M.D.

Assistant Professor of Pediatrics, State University of New York School of Medicine; Clinician II, Roswell Park Memorial Institute, Buffalo, New York
Acute Lymphoblastic Leukemia in Childhood

HENRY BREM, M.D.

Assistant Professor of Neurosurgery, Ophthalmology and Oncology, The Johns Hopkins University School of Medicine; Attending Neurosurgeon, The Johns Hopkins Hospital, Baltimore, Maryland
Glioma

JOEL G. BREMAN, M.D., D.T.P.H.

Chief, Malaria Control Activity, Division of Parasitic Diseases, Center for Infectious Diseases, Centers for Disease Control, Atlanta, Georgia
Malaria

WILLIAM J. BREMNER, M.D.., Ph.D.

Associate Professor of Medicine, University of Washington School of Medicine; Chief, Endocrinology Section, Veterans Administration Medical Center, Seattle, Washington
Hypogonadism: Androgen Therapy

JOHN C.M. BRUST, M.D.

Professor of Clinical Neurology, Columbia University College of Physicians and Surgeons; Director, Department of Neurology, Harlem Hospital Center and Attending in Neurology, The Presbyterian Hospital, New York, New York
Drug Abuse: Overdose and Withdrawal

DAVID BUCHHOLZ, M.D., A.C.P.

Assistant Professor of Neurology, The Johns Hopkins University School of Medicine; Director, Neurological Consultation Clinic, The Johns Hopkins Hospital, Baltimore, Maryland
Sleep Disorders

REBECCA H. BUCKLEY, M.D.

J. B. Sidbury Professor of Pediatrics and Professor of Immunology, Duke University School of Medicine; Chief, Division of Allergy and Immunology, Department of Pediatrics, Duke University Medical Center, Durham, North Carolina
Common Variable Immunodeficiency

JAMES F. BURDICK, M.D.

Associate Professor of Surgery, Department of Surgery; Director, Transplant Service, Department of Surgery, The Johns Hopkins Medical Institutions, Baltimore, Maryland
Arterial Occlusive Disease

RICHARD J. BURNS, M.B., F.R.A.C.P., F.R.C.P.(Lond)

Associate Professor of Medicine, Flinders University of South Australia; Senior Director of Neurology, Flinders Medical Center, Bedford Park, South Australia
Temporal Arteritis and Cerebral Vasculitis

GEORGE F. CAHILL Jr., M.D.

Professor of Medicine, Harvard Medical School; Director of Research, Howard Hughes Medical Institute and Senior Physician, Brigham and Women's Hospital, Boston, Massachusetts
Hyperosmolar Nonketotic Coma

JEFFREY P. CALLEN, M.D., F.A.C.P.

Associate Professor of Medicine (Dermatology). University of Louisville School of Medicine; Chief of Dermatology, Louisville Veterans Administration Medical Center, Louisville, Kentucky
Erythema Nodosum

J. STEWART CAMERON, M.D.

Professor of Renal Medicine and Director, Clinical Science Laboratories, Guy's Campus, United Medical and Dental Schools of Guy's and St. Thomas's Hospitals; Honorary Consultant Renal Physician, Guy's Hospital, London, England
Schönlein-Henoch Purpura

VITO M. CAMPESE, M.D.

Professor of Medicine, University of Southern California School of Medicine, Los Angeles, California
Individualized Care in Mild Essential Hypertension

STEPHEN V. CANTRILL, M.D., F.A.C.E.P.

Assistant Clinical Professor of Emergency Medicine, Oregon Health Sciences Center, Portland, Oregon; Attending Staff Physician, Emergency Medical Services, Denver General Hospital, Denver, Colorado
Coma

PAUL P. CARBONE, M.D.

Professor and Chairman, Department of Human Oncology, University of Wisconsin Medical School; Director, University of Wisconsin Clinical Cancer Center, Madison, Wisconsin
Hodgkin's Disease

BAYARD D. CATHERWOOD, M.D.

Assistant Professor of Medicine, University of California School of Medicine; Clinical Investigator, Veterans Administration Hospital, San Diego, California
Hypercalcemia

DAVID A. CHAD, M.D.

Associate Professor, Department of Neurology, University of Massachusetts, Medical Center, Worcester, Massachusetts
Bell's Palsy

KANU CHATTERJEE, M.B., F.R.C.P.

Professor of Medicine, L. Stern Professor of Cardiology, University of California School of Medicine; Director, Cardiac Care Unit and Associate Chief, Cardiovascular Division, Department of Medicine, University of California, Moffitt-Long Hospitals, San Francisco, California
Hypotension and Shock Following Myocardial Infarction

VICTOR CHERNICK, M.D.

Professor of Pediatrics, Associate Dean, Research and Graduate Studies, University of Manitoba Faculty of Medicine; Chief, Pediatric Pulmonary Section, Children's Hospital, Winnipeg, Manitoba, Canada
Acute Upper Airway Infection

NICHOLAS P. CHRISTY, M.D.

Professor of Medicine, State University of New York, Downstate Medical Center College of Medicine; Chief of Staff, Veterans Administration Medical Center, Brooklyn, New York
Principles of Systemic Corticosteroid Therapy in Nonendocrine Disease
Corticosteroid Withdrawal

E. LESLIE CHUSID, M.D., F.C.C.P., F.A.C.P. (Deceased)

Former Associate Clinical Professor of Medicine, Mount Sinai School of Medicine of the City University of New York; Former Director, Respiratory Care Services, Mount Sinai Medical Center, New York, New York
Loeffler's Syndrome

DENNIS L. CITRIN, M.B., Ch.B., Ph.D.

Associate Professor of Medicine, Northwestern University Medical School, Chicago, Illinois
Carcinoma of the Prostate

CHRISTOPHER M. CLARK, M.D.

Assistant Professor, Neurology, Duke University Medical School, Durham, North Carolina
Polymyositis

TIMOTHY J. H. CLARK, B. Sc., M.D., F.R.C.P.

Professor of Thoracic Medicine, United Medical and Dental Schools of Guy's and St. Thomas's Hospitals; Physician, Brompton Hospital, London, England
Chronic Asthma

JOHN N. CLASSEN, M.D.

Associate Professor of Surgery, The Johns Hopkins Medical Institutions; Consulting Surgeon, Union Memorial Hospital and Greater Baltimore Medical Center, Baltimore, Maryland
Postphlebitic Syndrome

RALPH V. CLAYMAN, M.D.

Associate Professor of Surgery (Urology), Washington University School of Medicine; Associate Urologic Surgeon, Barnes Hospital, St. Louis, Missouri
Obstructive Uropathy

C. GLENN COBBS, M.D.

Professor of Medicine and Director, Division of Infectious Diseases, The University of Alabama School of Medicine, Birmingham, Alabama
Endocarditis Caused by Gram-Positive Organisms

CECIL H. COGGINS, M.D.

Associate Professor of Medicine, Harvard Medical School; Clinical Director, Renal Unit, Massachusetts General Hospital, Boston, Massachusetts
Membranous Nephropathy

ARTHUR H. COHEN, M.D.

Professor of Pathology and Medicine, UCLA School of Medicine; Staff, Department of Pathology and Medicine, Harbor-UCLA Medical Center, Torrance, California
Mesangial Proliferative Glomerulonephritis

SIDNEY COHEN, M.D.

T. Grier Miller Professor of Medicine, Gastrointestinal Section–Department of Medicine, University of Pennsylvania School of Medicine; Chief, Gastrointestinal Section, Hospital of the University of Pennsylvania, Philadelphia, Pennsylvania
Diffuse Esophageal Spasm and Related Disorders

ALASTAIR M. CONNELL, M.D.

Professor of Internal Medicine, Virginia Commonwealth University Medical College of Virginia; Vice President for Health Sciences, Virginia Commonwealth University Richmond, Virginia
Constipation

BERNARD A. COOPER, M.D.

Professor, Departments of Medicine and Physiology; Director, Division of Hematology, Royal Victoria Hospital, Montreal, Quebec, Canada
Megaloblastic Anemia

JAMES J. CORBETT, M.D.

Professor of Neurology and Ophthalmology, University of Iowa School of Medicine; Staff, University of Iowa Hospitals and Clinics, Iowa City, Iowa
Pseudotumor Cerebri

WILLIAM G. COUSER, M.D.

Professor of Medicine and Head, Division of Nephrology, University of Washington School of Medicine, Seattle, Washington,
Idiopathic Rapidly Progressive Glomerulonephritis

DONALD E. CRAVEN, M.D.

Associate Professor of Medicine, Boston University School of Medicine; Hospital Epidemiologist, Department of Medicine, Division of Infectious Diseases, Boston City Hospital, Boston, Massachusetts
Gram-Negative Bacteremia

MICHAEL D. CRESSMAN, D.O.

Assistant Staff, Research Institute and the Department of Hypertension and Nephrology, The Cleveland Clinic Foundation, Cleveland, Ohio
Pheochromocytoma

DONALD J. DALESSIO, M.D.

Chairman, Department of Medicine, Scripps Clinic and Research Foundation, La Jolla; Clinical Professor of Neurology, University of California School of Medicine, San Diego, California
Trigeminal and Glossopharyngeal Neuralgia

GIUSEPPE D'AMICO, M.D.

Professor of Medicine, University of Milan; Head, Division of Nephrology, S. Carlo Borromeo Hospital, Milan, Italy
IgA Nephropathy (Berger's Disease).

GABRIEL M. DANOVITCH, M.D.

Associate Professor of Medicine, and Director of Clinical Nephrology and Renal Transplantation, UCLA School of Medicine, Los Angeles, California
Principles of Management of the Nephrotic Syndrome
Diuretic Use in Edematous and Nonedematous States

DAVID R. DANTZKER, M.D.

Professor of Internal Medicine, University of Texas Medical School; Director, Division of Pulmonary Medicine, University of Texas Health Science Center, Houston, Texas

Cor Pulmonale

TERRY F. DAVIES, M.D., M.R.C.P.

Associate Professor of Medicine, Mount Sinai School of Medicine, New York, New York

Thyroiditis

GERALD S. DAVIS, M.D.

Professor, Department of Medicine, University of Vermont College of Medicine; Director, Pulmonary Medicine Division, Medical Center Hospital of Vermont, Burlington, Vermont

Idiopathic Pulmonary Fibrosis

HUGH L. DAVIS, M.D., F.A.C.P.

Professor of Medicine, University of Wisconsin Medical School, Madison, Section Head, Hematology–Oncology, Department of Medicine, Mount Sinai Medical Center, Milwaukee, Wisconsin

Endocrine Therapy of Breast Cancer

LEONARD J. DEFTOS, M.D.

Professor of Medicine, University of California School of Medicine, Chief, Endocrine Section, Veterans Administration Hospital, San Diego, California

Hypercalcemia

VINCENT A. DE LEO, M.D.

Assistant Professor of Dermatology, Columbia University College of Physicians and Surgeons; Assistant Attending Dermatologist, Presbyterian Hospital, New York, New York

Photoallergic Dermatitis

ALBERT A. DEL NEGRO, M.D., F.A.C.C.

Assistant Professor of Medicine, Georgetown University School of Medicine, Staff Physician, Veterans Medical Center, Washington, D.C.

Supraventricular Tachycardia

GREGORY J. DEL ZOPPO, M.D.

Senior Research Associate, Department of Basic and Clinical Research, Scripps Clinic and Research Foundation, La Jolla, California

Thrombotic Thrombocytopenic Purpura

HENRY B. DINSDALE, M.D., F.R.C.P.(C), F.A.C.P.

Professor and Head, Department of Medicine, Queen's University Faculty of Medicine; Physician-in-Chief, Kingston General Hospital and Hotel Dieu Hospital, Kingston, Ontario, Canada

Hypertensive Encephalopathy

JOHN W. DOBBINS, M.D

Associate Professor of Medicine, Yale University School of Medicine; Attending Physician, Yale-New Haven Hospital, and Consultant, West Haven Veterans Administration Hospital, New Haven, Connecticut

Hyperoxaluria and Nephrolithiasis

RALPH R. DOBELBOWER Jr., M.D., Ph.D

Associate Professor and Director, Division of Radiation Oncology, Medical College of Ohio, Toledo, Ohio

Pancreatic Cancer

ROBERT M. DOROGHAZI, M.D.

Cardiologist, The Boone Clinic, Columbia, Missouri

Aortic Dissection

NEIL J. DOUGLAS, M.B., Ch.B., M.D., F.R.C.P. (Edin)

Senior Lecturer in Respiratory Medicine and Medicine, University of Edinburgh; Honorary Consultant Physician, City Hospital, Edinburgh, Scotland

Sleep Disordered Breathing

DAVID A. DRACHMAN, M.D.

Professor and Chairman, Department of Neurology, University of Massachusetts Medical Center Worcester, Massachusetts

Bell's Palsy

STEPHEN C. DRESKIN, M.D., Ph.D.

Medical Staff Fellow, Bacterial Diseases Section, Laboratory of Clinical Investigation, National Institute of Allergy and Infectious Diseases, National Institutes of Health, Bethesda, Maryland

Hyperimmunoglobulin E and Recurrent Infection (Job's) Syndrome

HOWARD M. DRUCE, M.D.

Assistant Professor, Division of Allergy and Immunology. Saint Louis University School of Medicine, Saint Louis, Missouri

Allergic Rhinitis

THOMAS DuBOSE Jr., M.D.

Professor of Medicine, Physiology and Biophysics and Division Chief, Nephrology, University of Texas Medical School, Galveston, Texas
Metabolic Acidosis

HERBERT L. DUPONT, M.D.

Professor of Medicine and Director, Program in Infectious Diseases and Clinical Microbiology, University of Texas Medical School, Houston, Texas
Infectious Diarrhea: A Patient Outside the United States

MICHAEL P. EARNEST, M.D.

Associate Professor of Neurology and Preventive Medicine, University of Colorado School of Medicine; Director of Neurology, Denver General Hospital, Denver, Colorado
Coma

THEODORE C. EICKHOFF, M.D.

Professor of Medicine, University of Colorado School of Medicine; Director of Internal Medicine, Presbyterian-St. Luke's Medical Center, Denver, Colorado
Mycoplasmal Pulmonary Infection

LAWRENCE H. EINHORN, M.D.

Professor of Medicine, Indiana University School of Medicine; Director of Clinical Oncology, Indiana University Hospital, Indianapolis, Indiana
Testicular Cancer

HANS EINSTEIN, M.D.

Professor of Clinical Medicine, University of Southern California School of Medicine; Medical Director, Barlow Hospital, Los Angeles, California
Histoplasmosis

ERNST EPSTEIN, M.D.

Clinical Associate Professor of Dermatology, University of California School of Medicine, San Francisco; Private Practice, San Mateo, California
Contact Dermatitis

DAVID S. ETTINGER, M.D.

Associate Professor, Department of Oncology and Medicine, The Johns Hopkins University School of Medicine, Baltimore, Maryland
Chemotherapy in Lung Cancer

STEFAN S. FAJANS, M.D.

Professor of Internal Medicine, University of Michigan Medical School; Chief, Division of Endocrinology and Metabolism and Director, Michigan Diabetes Research and Training Center, Ann Arbor, Michigan
The Adult Diabetic Patient

ARTHUR M. FELDMAN, M.D. Ph.D.

Fellow in Cardiology, The Johns Hopkins Medical Institutions, Baltimore, Maryland
Dilated Cardiomyopathy

M. IRENÉ FERRER, M.D.

Professor of Clinical Medicine, College of Physicians and Surgeons, Columbia University; Director, Electro-Cardiographic Laboratory, Columbia-Presbyterian Medical Center, New York, New York
Sinus Node Dysfunction

LEON G. FINE, M.B., Ch.B., F.R.C.P, F.A.C.P.

Professor of Medicine and Chief, Division of Nephrology, UCLA School of Medicine; Attending Physician, UCLA Medical Center, Los Angles, California
Hyperkalemia

GUY P. FIOCCO, M.D.

Fellow, Division of Allergy, University of Virginia School of Medicine, Charlottesville, Virginia
Asthma in Adults

JAMES E. FISH, M.D.

Professor of Medicine; Director, Division of Pulmonary Diseases, Jefferson Medical College of Thomas Jefferson University, Philadelphia, Pennsylvania
Status Asthmaticus
Extrinsic Allergic Alveolitis

RICHARD I. FISHER, M.D.

Professor of Medicine, Loyola University of Chicago Stritch School of Medicine; Chief of Hematology-Oncology, Loyola University Medical Center, Maywood, Illinois
NonHodgkin's Disease: Unfavorable Lymphomas

ROBERT FISHER, M.D., Ph.D

Assistant Professor of Neurology, The Johns Hopkins University School of Medicine; Attending Neurologist, The Johns Hopkins Hospital, Baltimore, Maryland
Complex Partial Epilepsy

LAWRENCE M. FISHMAN, M.D.

Professor of Medicine, University of Miami School of Medicine; Chief, Endocrinology Section and Associate Chief of Staff, Research, Miami Veterans Administration Medical Center, Miami, Flordia
Cushing's Syndrome

THOMAS B. FITZPATRICK, M.D.

Professor and Chairman, Department of Dermatology, Harvard Medical School; Chief, Dermatology Service, Massachusetts General Hospital, Boston, Massachusetts
Primary Malignant Melanoma

C. RICHARD FLEMING, M.D.

Associate Professor of Medicine, Mayo Medical School; Consultant in Gastroenterology, Mayo Clinic, Rochester, Minnesota
Parenteral Nutrition

DAVID C. FLENLEY, Ph.D., F.R.C.P., F.R.C.P.(Edin)

Professor of Respiratory Medicine, University of Edinburgh; Honorary Consultant Physician, City Hospital, Edinburgh, Scotland
Sleep Disordered Breathing

ROSS D. FLETCHER, M.D., F.A.C.C.

Associate Professor, Internal Medicine, Georgetown University Medical Center; Chief, Cardiology Section, Veterans Medical Center, Washington, D.C.
Supraventricular Tachycardia

MARY E. FONTANA, M.D.

Associate Professor of Medicine, Division of Cardiology, The Ohio State University, Columbus, Ohio
Calcific Aortic Stenosis

NICHOLAS J. FORTUIN, M.D.

Professor of Medicine, The Johns Hopkins Medical Institutions, Baltimore, Maryland
Stable Angina Pectoris

DANIEL W. FOSTER, M.D.

Professor of Internal Medicine, University of Texas Southwestern Medical School, Dallas, Texas
Diabetic Ketoacidosis

MICHAEL M. FRANK, M.D.

Chief, Laboratory of Clinical Investigation and Clinical Director, National Institute of Allergy and Infectious Disease, National Institutes of Health, Bethesda, Maryland
Hereditary Angioedema

STANLEY S. FRANKLIN, M.D.

Professor of Medicine, UCLA School of Medicine; Director of Hypertension, Divison of Nephrology, UCLA Center for Health Sciences, Los Angeles, California
Hypertensive Emergencies and Urgencies

ARNOLD I. FREEMAN, M.D.

Professor of Pediatrics, State University of New York School of Medicine; Chief, Department of Pediatrics, Roswell Park Memorial Institute, Buffalo, New York
Acute Lymphoblastic Leukemia in Childhood

RUTH K. FREINKEL, M.D.

Professor of Dermatology, Northwestern University Medical School, Chicago, Illinois
Acne Vulgaris

JACOB K. FRENKEL, M.D., Ph.D.

Professor of Pathology and Oncology, University of Kansas School of Medicine; Staff, University of Kansas Medical Center, Kansas City, Kansas
Toxoplasmosis

GERALD H. FRIEDLAND, M.D.

Associate Professor of Medicine, Albert Einstein College of Medicine; Director, Medical Service, Montefiore Medical Center, Bronx, New York
Acquired Immunodeficiency Syndrome

ALVIN E. FRIEDMAN-KIEN, M.D.

Associate Professor of Dermatology and Microbiology, New York University School of Medicine, New York, New York
Kaposi's Sarcoma

LAWRENCE A. FROHMAN, M.D.

Professor of Medicine, University of Cincinnati College of Medicine; Director, Division of Endocrinology and Metabolism, University of Cincinnati Medical Center, Cincinnati, Ohio
Acromegaly

HANS FROMM, M.D.

Professor of Medicine, George Washington University School of Medicine and Health Sciences; Director, Division of Gastroenterology, George Washington University Medical Center, Washington, D. C.
Colelithiasis

JACK D. FULMER, M.D.

Professor of Medicine, University of Alabama School of Medicine, Divison of Pulmonary and Critical Care Medicine, Veterans Administration Medical Center, Birmingham, Alabama

Collagen Vascular Lung Disorders

ANTHONY J. FURLAN, M.D.

Assistant Clinical Professor Case Western Reserve University School of Medicine; Director, Cerebrovascular Program, Cleveland Clinic Foundation, Cleveland Ohio

Transient Ischemic Attack

PATRICIA A. GABOW, M.D.

Associate Professor, Department of Medicine, University of Colorado School of Medicine; Director Department of Medicine, Denver General Hospital, Denver, Colorado

Cystic Diseases of the Kidney

J. LESTER GABRILOVE, M.D.

Baumritter Professor of Medicine, Mount Sinai School of Medicine; Attending Physician and Chief of the Endocrine Clinic; The Mount Sinai Hospital, New York, New York

Adrenocortical Insufficiency

STANLEY P. GALANT, M.D.

Clinical Professor of Pediatrics and Acting Director, Pediatric Allergy-Immunology, University of California School of Medicine, Irvine, California

Food Allergy in Adults

JOHN H. GALLA, M.D.

Professor of Medicine, University of Alabama School of Medicine; Attending Physician, University of Alabama Hospital, Birmingham, Alabama

Metabolic Alkalosis

JOHN I. GALLIN, M.D.

Chief, Bacterial Diseases Section, Laboratory of Clinical Investigation, National Institute of Allergy and Infectious Diseases, National Institutes of Health, Bethesda, Maryland

Hyperimmunoglobulin E and Recurrent Infection (Job's) Syndrome

JERRY D. GARDNER, M.D.

Chief, Digestive Diseases Branch, National Institute of Arthritis, Diabetes, Digestive and Kidney Diseases, Bethesda, Maryland

Gastrinoma

MARC B. GARNICK, M.D.

Assistant Professor of Medicine, Harvard Medical School; Assistant Physician, Dana-Farber Cancer Institute and Associate Physician, Brigham and Women's Hospital, Boston, Massachusetts

Renal Complications of Cancer

ABRAHAM GENECIN, M.D.

Associate Professor of Medicine; Physician, The Johns Hopkins Medical Institutions, Baltimore, Maryland

Noncardiac Surgery in the Patient with Heart Disease

W. LANCE GEORGE, M.D.

Associate Professor of Medicine, UCLA School of Medicine; Assistant Chief, Infectious Disease Section, Wadsworth Division, West Los Angeles Veterans Administration Medical Center, Los Angeles, California

Crepitus and Gangrene

DEREK G. GIBSON, M.B., F.R.C.P.

Consultant Cardiologist, Brompton Hospital, London, England

Aortic Regurgitation

RAY W. GIFFORD Jr., M.D.

Senior Vice-Chairman, Division of Medicine and Senior Physician, Department of Hypertension and Nephrology, The Cleveland Clinic Foundation, Cleveland, Ohio

Pheochromocytoma

ALAN R. GILES, M.D., F.R.C.P.(C)

Associate Professor, Departments of Pathology and Medicine, Queen's University Faculty of Medicine; Director, Blood Bank and Hemostasis Laboratory, Kingston General Hospital, Kingston, Ontario, Canada

Vitamin K-Dependent Coagulation Factor Deficiency States

DAVID W. GOLDE, M.D.

Professor of Medicine; Chief, Division of Haematology-Oncology, UCLA School of Medicine, Los Angeles, California

Hairy-Cell Leukemia

JOHN M. GOLDMAN, D.M., F.R.C.P.

Senior Lecturer, Royal Postgraduate Medical School; Honorary Consultant Physician, Hammersmith Hospital, London, England

Chronic Granulocytic Leukemia

EDWARD C. GORDON-SMITH, M.D., M.Sc., F.R.C.P.

Reader in Haematology, Royal Postgraduate Medical School; Internal Medicine and Haematology Consultant, Hammersmith Hospital, London, England
Aplastic Anemia and Allied Disorders

PETER D. GOREVIC, M.D.

Associate Professor of Medicine and Pathology, State University of New York, Stony Brook, New York
Amyloidosis

JEAN L. GREM, M.D.

Clinical Fellow, Department of Human Oncology, University of Wisconsin Hospitals, Madison, Wisconsin
Chemotherapy in Breast Cancer

DIANE E. GRIFFIN, M.D., Ph.D.

Professor of Medicine and Neurology, The Johns Hopkins University School of Medicine; Active Staff, The Johns Hopkins Hospital, Baltimore, Maryland
Herpes Zoster

JAMES GROTTA, M.D.

Associate Professor, University of Texas Health Science Center, Houston, Texas
Embolic Strokes of Cardiac Origin

SCOTT M. GRUNDY, M.D., Ph.D.

Professor of Internal Medicine and Biochemistry, University of Texas Southwestern Medical School; Director, Center for Human Nutrition, University of Texas Health Science Center, Dallas, Texas
Hyperlipidemia

RICHARD L. GUERRANT, M.D.

Professor of Medicine, Division of Geographic Medicine, Department of Internal Medicine, University of Virginia School of Medicine, Charlottesville, Virginia
Infectious Diarrhea: A Patient in the United States

EUGEN HALAR, M.D.

Associate Professor, Department of Rehabilitation Medicine, University of Washington School of Medicine; Chief, Rehabilitation Medicine Service, Veterans Administration Medical Center, Seattle, Washington
Diabetic Neuropathy

DANIEL G. HALLER, M.D.

Assistant Professor of Medicine, University of Pennsylvania School of Medicine, Philadelphia, Pennsylvania
Gastric Cancer

JEFFREY B. HALTER, M.D.

Professor of Internal Medicine, University of Michigan Medical School; Chief, Division of Geriatric Medicine, Turner Geriatric Clinic, Ann Arbor, Michigan
Diabetic Neuropathy

STEPHEN B. HANAUER, M.D.

Assistant Professor of Medicine, Section of Gastroenterology, University of Chicago Medical Center, Chicago, Illinois
Crohn's Disease of the Small Bowel

LEONARD C. HARBER, M.D.

Professor and Chairman, Department of Dermatology, Columbia University College of Physicians and Surgeons, New York, New York
Photoallergic Dermatitis

LAURENCE A. HARKER, M.D.

Member, Department of Basic and Clinical Research; Director, Roon Research Center for Arteriosclerosis and Thrombosis, Scripps Clinic and Research Foundation, La Jolla, California
Thrombotic Thrombocytopenic Purpura

W. PROCTOR HARVEY, M.D.

Professor of Medicine, Division of Cardiology, Georgetown University Medical Center, Washington, D.C.
Mitral Valve Prolapse

ROBERT C. HASTINGS, M.D., Ph.D.

Adjunct Professor of Pharmacology and Clinical Professor of Medicine, Tulane University School of Medicine, New Orleans; Chief, Laboratory Research Branch, National Hansen's Disease Center, Carville, Louisiana
Leprosy

GEORGE B. HAYCOCK, M.B., B.Chir., F.R.C.P., D.C.H.

Consultant Pediatric Nephrologist, Guy's Hospital, London, England
Schönlein-Henoch Purpura

LOUIS A. HEALEY, M.D.

Clinical Professor of Medicine, University of Washington School of Medicine; Rheumatologist, Mason Clinic, Seattle, Washington
Temporal Arteritis

I. CRAIG HENDERSON, M.D.

Associate Professor of Medicine, Harvard Medical School; Director, Breast Evaluation Center, Division of Medical Oncology, Dana-Farber Cancer Institute, Boston, Massachusetts

Hypercalcemia of Malignant Disease

THOMAS R. HENDRIX, M.D.

Moses and Helen Golden Paulson Professor of Gastroenterology, The Johns Hopkins University School of Medicine, Baltimore, Maryland

Gastroesophageal Reflux: Medical Treatment

H. FRANKLIN HERLONG, M.D.

Associate Professor of Medicine, The Johns Hopkins University School of Medicine, Baltimore, Maryland

Hepatorenal Syndrome and Ascites

JOHN D. HINES, M.D., F.A.C.P.

Professor of Medicine, Case Western Reserve University School of Medicine; Director of Medical Oncology, Cleveland Metropolitan General Hospital, Cleveland, Ohio

Refractory Anemias

BASIL I. HIRSCHOWITZ, B.Sc., M.B., B.Ch., M.D., F.A.C.P., F.R.C.P.E., F.R.C.P.

Professor of Medicine, Professor of Physiology and Biophysics, and Director, Division of Gastroenterology, Department of Medicine, University of Alabama School of Medicine; Consultant, Birmingham Veterans Administration Hospital, Birmingham, Alabama

Duodenal Ulcer

JOHN E. HODGKIN, M.D.

Clinical Professor of Medicine, University of California School of Medicine, Davis, Medical Director, Center for Health Promotion and Rehabilitation, St. Helena Hospital, St. Helena, California

Pulmonary Rehabilitation

DIETER F. HOELZER, M.D.

Professor of Internal Medicine; Chief of Department of Hematology, Johann Wolfgang Goethe University, Frankfurt, West Germany

Acute Lymphoblastic Leukemia in Adults

PHILIP C. HOPEWELL, M.D.

Associate Professor, University of California School of Medicine; Chest Service, San Francisco General Hospital, San Francisco, California

Tuberculosis

SIMON HORENSTEIN, M.D.

Professor of Neurology, St. Louis University School of Medicine; Director, Neurological Rehabilitation Unit of St. Louis University at Bethesda General Hospital and Chief, Neurological Service, St. Louis Veterans Administration Hospital, St. Louis, Missouri

Cervical Spondylosis

RICHARD HORTON, M.D.

Professor of Medicine and Chief, Endocrine and Metabolism Section, Department of Medicine, University of Southern California School of Medicine, Los Angeles, California

Hirsutism

MELVIN HORWITH, M.D.

Professor of Clinical Medicine, Cornell University Medical College; Attending Physician (Endocrinology), The New York Hospital-Cornell Medical Center, New York, New York

Paget's Disease of Bone

JOHN M. HOWARD, M.D.

Professor of Surgery, Department of Surgery, Medical College of Ohio, Toledo, Ohio

Pancreatic Cancer

STEVEN J. HUBER, Ph.D.

Research Associate, Department of Neurology, The Ohio State University College of Medicine, Columbus, Ohio

Essential Tremor

J. CLARK HUFF, M.D.

Associate Professor, Departments of Dermatology and Medicine, University of Colorado School of Medicine, Denver, Colorado

Erythema Multiforme

ALAN HULL, M.D.

Clinical Professor, University of Texas health Science Center Southwestern Medical School Director, Dallas Transplant Institute, Dallas Nephrology Associates, Dallas, Texas

Hemodialysis

THOMAS M. HYERS, M.D.

Professor of Internal Medicine, Saint Louis University School of Medicine; Director, Division of Pulmonary Diseases, Saint Louis University Medical Center, Saint Louis, Missouri

Pulmonary Embolism

SIDNEY H. INGBAR, M.D.

William Bosworth Castle Professor of Medicine, Harvard Medical School; Chief, Division of Endocrinology and Metabolism, Beth Israel Hospital, Boston, Massachusetts
Hyperthyroidism in Graves' Disease

GEORGE G. JACKSON, M.D.

Keeton Professor of Medicine and Chief, Section of Infectious Diseases, University of Illinois College of Medicine, Chicago, Illinois
Viral Respiratory Disease

PAUL H. JACOBS, M.D.

Professor, Department of Dermatology, Stanford University School of Medicine; Director, Dermatology Clinic and Superficial Mycoses Laboratory, Stanford, California
Dermatophytosis

ROBERT P. JACOBS, M.D.

Chairman, Department of Medicine, Jeanes Hospital and Fox Chase Cancer Center, Philadelphia, Pennsylvania
Reiter's Syndrome
Ankylosing Spondylitis

D. GERAINT JAMES, M.A., M.D.(Cantab), F.R.C.P.(Lond), L.L.D.(Hon)

Dean and Senior Physician, Royal Northern Hospital, London, England
Sarcoidosis

ROBERT T. JENSEN, M.D.

Senior Investigator Digestive Diseases Branch, National Institute of Arthritis, Diabetes, Digestive and Kidney Diseases, National Institutes of Health, Bethesda, Maryland
Gastrinoma

RICHARD T. JOHNSON, M.D.

Eisenhower Professor of Neurology and Professor of Microbiology and Neuroscience, The Johns Hopkins University School of Medicine; Neurologist, The Johns Hopkins Hospital, Baltimore, Maryland
Viral Encephalitis

JAMES H. JOHNSTON, M.D.

Clinical Associate Professor of Medicine, University of Mississippi School of Medicine; Staff Physician, Saint Dominic Hospital and Baptist Medical Center, Jackson, Mississippi
Lower Gastrointestinal Bleeding

C. RONALD KAHN, M.D.

Professor of Medicine, Harvard Medical School; Director, Elliott P. Joslin Research Laboratory, Joslin Diabetes Center and Chief, Division of Diabetes and Metabolism, Brigham and Women's Hospital, Boston, Massachusetts
Insulin Allergy and Insulin Resistance

MICHAEL A. KALINER, M.D.

Head, Allergic Diseases Section, Laboratory of Clinical Investigation, National Institute of Allergy and Infectious Diseases, Bethesda, Maryland
Allergic Rhinitis

DON W. KANNANGARA, M.D., Ph.D.

Assistant Professor of Medicine, Division of Infectious Diseases and Clinical Microbiology, Hahnemann Medical College and Hospital, Philadelphia, Pennsylvania
Bacterial Arthritis

BARRY H. KAPLAN, M.D., Ph.D.

Associate Clinical Professor, Albert Einstein College of Medicine, Bronx, New York
Chemotherapy in Head and Neck Cancer

BERNARD S. KAPLAN, M.B, B.Ch., F.C.P.(S.A.)

Associate Professor of Pediatrics, McGill University Faculty of Medicine; Director of Nephrology, The Montreal Children's Hospital, Montreal, Quebec, Canada
Hemolytic-Uremic Syndrome

NORMAN M. KAPLAN, M.D.

Professor of Internal Medicine, University of Texas Health Science Center Southwestern Medical School; Attending Staff, Parkland Hospital, Dallas, Texas
Mild Hypertension: New Strategies in Therapy

SELNA L. KAPLAN, M.D., Ph.D.

Professor of Pediatrics and Director, Pediatric Endocrine Unit, University of California School of Medicine, San Francisco, California
Short Stature

ELAINE M. KAPTEIN, M.D., F.A.C.P.

Associate Professor of Medicine, University of Southern California School of Medicine and Los Angeles County-Medical Center, Los Angeles, California
Renal Osteodystrophy

LISSA KAPUST, M.S.W.

Senior Social Worker, Behavioral Neurology Unit, Beth Israel Hospital, Boston, Massachusetts
Alzheimer's Disease

ADOLF W. KARCHMER, M.D.

Associate Professor of Medicine, Harvard Medical School; Chief, Infectious Disease Section, New England Deaconess Hospital, Boston, Massachusetts
Prosthetic Valve Endocarditis

ADRIAN I. KATZ, M.D., F.A.C.P.

Professor of Medicine, The University of Chicago Pritzker School of Medicine; Attending Physician, University of Chicago Medical Center, Chicago, Illinois
Hypertension in Pregnancy

JOHN I. KENNEDY, M.D.

Associate in Medicine, Division of Pulmonary and Critical Care Medicine, University of Alabama; Veterans Administration Medical Center, Birmingham, Alabama
Collagen Vascular Lung Disorders

GERALD R. KERBY, M.D.

Professor of Medicine, Division of Pulmonary and Critical Care Medicine, University of Kansas School of Medicine; Staff Physician, University of Kansas Medical Center, Kansas City, Kansas
Pleural Effusion

CRAIG M. KESSLER, M.D.

Associate Professor of Medicine, Division of Hematology-Oncology and, Director, Coagulation Laboratories, George Washington University School of Medicine, Washington, D.C.
Acute Thrombophlebitis

JOHN G. KIRBY, M.B., M.R.C.P.I., F.R.C.P.(C)

Clinical Fellow, Firestone Regional Chest and Allergy Unit, St. Joseph's Hospital and Chedoke-McMaster Hospitals, McMaster University Medical Center Division, Hamilton, Ontario, Canada
Bronchiectasis

J. PHILIP KISTLER, M.D.

Associate Professor of Neurology, Harvard Medical School; Associate Neurologist, Massachusetts General Hospital, Boston, Massachusetts
Atherothrombotic Cerebral Vascular Disease

RAYMOND N. KJELLBERG, M.D.

Associate Clinical Professor of Surgery, Harvard Medical School; Visiting Neurosurgeon, Department of Neurosurgery, Massachusetts General Hospital, Boston, Massachusetts
Nonfunctioning Pituitary Adenoma

CARL M. KJELLSTRAND, M.D., F.A.C.P.

Professor of Medicine and Surgery, University of Minnesota Medical School, Minnesota, Minneapolis, Chief, Division of Nephrology, Karolinska Hospital, Stockholm, Sweden
Dialytic Management of Acute Renal Failure

SAULO KLAHR, M.D.

Professor of Medicine and Director, Renal Division, Washington University School of Medicine; Physician, Barnes Hospital, St. Louis, Missouri
Obstructive Uropathy

JEROME O. KLEIN, M.D.

Professor of Pediatrics, Boston University School of Medicine; Director, Division of Pediatric Infectious Diseases, Boston City Hospital, Boston, Massachusetts
Childhood Immunization

BERNARD KLIMAN, M.D.

Associate Professor of Medicine, Harvard Medical School; Associate Physician, Department of Medicine, Endocrine Unit, Massachusetts General Hospital, Boston, Massachusetts
Nonfunctioning Pituitary Adenoma

RAYMOND S. KOFF, M.D.

Professor of Medicine, Boston University School of Medicine; Chief, Hepatology Sections, Boston University Medical Center and Veterans Administration Medical Center, Boston, Massachusetts
Chronic Hepatitis

JOEL D. KOPPLE, M.D.

Professor of Medicine and Public Health, UCLA Schools of Medicine and Public Health, Los Angeles; Chief, Division of Nephrology and Hypertension, Harbor-UCLA Medical Center, Torrance, California
Acute Renal Failure: Conservative Nondialytic Management
Chronic Renal Failure: Nutritional and Nondialytic Management

ROBERT L. KRIGEL, M.D.

Director of Hematology, Fox Chase Cancer Center, Philadelphia, Pennsylvania
Kaposi's Sarcoma

MEIR H. KRYGER, M.D., F.R.C.P.(C)

Associate Professor of Medicine and Director, Sleep Laboratory, University of Manitoba Faculty of Medicine, Winnipeg, Manitoba, Canada
Upper Airway Obstruction

IRA KURTZ, M.D., F.R.C.P. (C)

Assistant Professor of Medicine, Division of Nephrology, UCLA School of Medicine; Attending Physician, UCLA Medical Center, Los Angeles, California
Hyperkalemia

NEIL A. KURTZMAN, M.D., F.A.C.P.

Arnett Professor of Medicine, Professor of Physiology and Chairman, Department of Internal Medicine, Texas Tech University Health Sciences Center; Attending in Nephrology, Lubbock General Hospital, Lubbock, Texas
Mixed Acid-Base Disturbances

ROBERT A. KYLE, M.D.

William H. Donner Professor of Medicine and Laboratory Medicine, Mayo Medical School; Consultant, Division of Hematology and Internal Medicine, Mayo Clinic and Mayo Foundation, Rochester, Minnesota
Multiple Myeloma and Related Monoclonal Gammopathy

EDWARD C. LaCAVA, M.D.

Senior Fellow in Endocrinology-Metabolism, Department of Medicine, University of Washington School of Medicine; Staff, Department of Medicine, Veterans Administration Medical Center, Seattle, Washington
Diabetic Neuropathy

CHARLES R. LAMBERT, M.D. Ph.D

Fellow in Cardiovascular Medicine, University of Florida, Gainesville, Florida
Coronary Artery Spasm

BARRY C. LAMKIN, M.D.

Assistant Professor of Dermatology, Case Western Reserve University School of Medicine; Assistant Chief of Dermatology, Veterans Administration Medical Center, Cleveland, Ohio
Porphyrias

JAMES W. LANCE, M.D., F.R.C.P. (Lond), F.R.A.C.P. F.A.A.

Professor of Neurology, University of New South Wales: Chairman, Department of Neurology, The Prince Henry and Prince of Wales Hospitals, Sydney, Australia
Migraine and Cluster Headache

JACK L. LEFROCK, M.D.

Scientific Director, Therapeutic Research Institute Inc., Sarasota, Florida
Bacterial Osteomyelitis
Bacterial Arthritis

A. MARTIN LERNER, M.D.

Clinical Professor of Medicine, Wayne State University, Detroit, Michigan
Endocarditis Caused by Gram-Negative Organisms and Fungi

E. CARWILE LEROY, M.D.

Professor of Medicine and Director, Division of Rheumatology, Medical University of South Carolina College of Medicine, Charleston, South Carolina
Systemic Sclerosis (Scleroderma)

ROLAND A. LEVANDOWSKI, M.D.

Assistant Professor of Medicine, University of Illinois College of Medicine, Chicago, Illinois
Viral Respiratory Disease

HOWARD LEVENTHAL, Ph.D.

Professor of Psychology, University of Wisconsin Medical School; Associate, Wisconsin Clinical Cancer Center, Madison, Wisconsin
Communicating with the Patient Receiving Chemotherapy

ALLAN B. LEVIN, M.D.

Associate Professor of Neurological Surgery, University of Wisconsin Medical School, Madison, Wisconsin
Pain Control in the Cancer Patient

HENRY LEVISON, M.B., F.R.C.P.(C)

Professor of Pediatrics, University of Toronto Faculty of Medicine; Head, Department of Respiratory Medicine, The Hospital for Sick Children, Toronto, Ontario, Canada
Cystic Fibrosis

RICHARD P. LEWIS, M.D.

Professor of Medicine and Director, Division of Cardiology, The Ohio State University College of Medicine, Columbus, Ohio
Calcific Aortic Stenosis

JOHN E. LEWY, M.D.

Professor of Pediatrics, Tulane University School of Medicine; Chairman, Department of Pediatrics, Tulane University Medical Center, New Orleans, Louisiana
Poststreptococcal Glomerulonephritis

ABRAHAM N. LIEBERMAN, M.D.

Professor of Neurology, New York University School of Medicine, New York, New York
Parkinson's Disease

MARSHALL D. LINDHEIMER, M.D., F.A.C.P.

Professor of Medicine and Obstetrics and Gynecology, University of Chicago Pritzker School of Medicine; Attending Physician, University of Chicago Hospitals and Clinics and Director, Medical High Risk Clinic, Chicago Lying-In Hospital, Chicago, Illinois
Hypertension in Pregnancy

ROBERT LINDSAY, M.B., Ch.B., Ph.D., M.R.C.P.

Professor of Clinical Medicine, Columbia University College of Physicians and Surgeons, New York; Research Director and Director of Internal Medicine, Helen Hayes Hospital, Haverstraw, New York
Osteoporosis

PETER E. LIPSKY, M.D.

Professor of Internal Medicine and Microbiology, University of Texas Southwestern Medical School; Chief of Rheumatic Diseases Unit, Director of the Harold C. Simmons Arthritis Research Center, Attending Physician, Parkland Memorial Hospital and Director, Parkland Memorial Hospital Arthritis Outpatient Clinic, Dallas, Texas
Rheumatoid Arthritis

WILLIAM J. LITCHY, M.D.

Instructor in Neurology, Mayo Medical School; Consultant, Department of Neurology, Mayo Clinic and Mayo Foundation, Rochester, Minnesota
Motor Neuron Disease

ROGER LOBO, M.D.

Associate Professor and Chief, Reproductive Endocrinology, Department of Obsterics and Gynecology, University of Southern California School of Medicine, Los Angeles, California
Hirsutism

PATRICK J. LOEHRER Sr., M.D.

Assistant Professor of Medicine, Section of Hematology–Oncology, Indiana University School of Medicine, Indianapolis, Indiana
Testicular Cancer

DAN L. LONGO, M.D.

Head, Experimental Immunology Section, Medicine Branch, National Cancer Institutes, Bethesda, Maryland
NonHodgkin's Disease: Unfavorable Lymphomas

CHARLES L. LOPRINZI, M.D.

Instructor, Department of Human Oncology, University of Wisconsin Medical School, Madison, Wisconsin
Hodgkin's Disease

JOHN M. LUCE, M.D.

Assistant Professor of Medicine and Anesthesia, University of California School of Medicine; Associate Director, Medical-Surgical Intensive Care Unit, San Fransisco General Hospital, San Francisco, California
Acute Respiratory Distress Syndrome

ROBERT G. LUKE, M.B., Ch.B., F.R.C.P.

Professor of Medicine and Director, Division of Nephrology and Nephrology Research and Training Center, University of Alabama School of Medicine; Physician, University of Alabama Medical Center, Birmingham, Alabama
Metabolic Alkalosis

RAYMOND MACIEWICZ, M.D., Ph.D.

Assistant Professor of Neurology (Neuroscience), Harvard Medical School; Assistant Neurologist, Massachusetts General Hospital, Boston, Massachusetts.
Principles of Pain Management

IAN MacLUSKY, M.B., B.S., F.R.C.P.(C)

Assistant Professor, Division of Chest Medicine, Department of Pediatrics, University of Toronto Faculty of Medicine; Staff Physician, Hospital for Sick Children, Toronto, Ontario, Canada
Cystic Fibrosis

HOWARD I. MAIBACH, M.D.

Professor of Dermatology, University of California School of Medicine, San Francisco, California
Contact Dermatitis

MAURO MALAVOLTI, M.D.

Visiting Assistant Professor, George Washington University School of Medicine and Health Sciences, Washington, D.C.
Cholelithiasis

ELLIOTT L. MANCALL, M.D.

Professor and Chairman, Department of Neurology, Hahnemann University School of Medicine, Philadelphia, Pennsylvania
Alcohol Intoxication and Withdrawal

SIMEON MARGOLIS, M.D., Ph.D.

Professor of Medicine and Biological Chemistry, The Johns Hopkins University School of Medicine; Active Staff, The Johns Hopkins Hospital, Baltimore, Maryland
Food Fads and Alternatives

LAURI E. MARKOWITZ, M.D.

Respiratory and Special Pathogens, Epidemiology Branch, Bacterial Diseases Division, Centers for Disease Control, Atlanta, Georgia
Lyme Disease

RICHARD J. MARTIN, M.D.

Associate Professor of Medicine, University of Colorado Health Sciences Center; Staff Physician, National Jewish Center for Immunology and Respiratory Medicine, Denver, Colorado
Pulmonary Alveolar Proteinosis

SHAUL G. MASSRY, M.D.

Professor of Medicine, University of Southern California School of Medicine, Los Angeles County-Medical Center, Los Angeles, California
Renal Osteodystrophy

LUIGI MASTROIANNI Jr., M.D.

William Goodell Professor and Chairman, Department of Obstetrics and Gynecology, University of Pennsylvania School of Medicine; Chief of Obstetrics and Gynecology, Hospital of the University of Pennsylvania, Pittsburgh, Pennsylvania
Menopause

ALVIN M. MATSUMOTO, M.D.

Assistant Professor of Medicine, University of Washington School of Medicine; Research Associate, Veterans Administration Medical Center, Seattle, Washington
Hypogonadism: Androgen Therapy

KENNETH H. MAYER, M.D.

Assistant Professor of Medicine, Brown University Program in Medicine, Providence; Head, Division of Infectious Diseases, Memorial Hospital, Pawtucket, Rhode Island
Infection Associated with Hematologic Malignancy

MORTON H. MAXWELL, M.D.

Clinical Professor of Medicine, UCLA School of Medicine, Los Angeles, California
Renovascular Hypertension

JUSTIN C. McARTHUR M.B., B.S.

Assistant Professor of Neurology, The Johns Hopkins University School of Medicine; Co-Director, The Johns Hopkins University Multiple Sclerosis Program, Baltimore, Maryland
Multiple Sclerosis

WILLIAM R. McCABE, M.D.

Professor of Medicine and Microbiology and Director, Division of Infectious Diseases, Boston University School of Medicine; Director, Maxwell Finland Laboratory, Boston City Hospital, Boston, Massachusetts
Gram-Negative Bacteremia

RICHARD W. McCALLUM, M.D., F.A.C.P., F.R.A.C.P. (Austral), F.A.C.G.

Professor of Medicine, University of Virginia School of Medicine; Chief, Division of Gastroenterology, University of Virginia Medical Center, Charlottesville, Virginia
Functional Disorders of the Upper Gastrointestinal Tract

DAVID A. McCARRON, M.D.

Professor of Medicine, Associate Head, Division of Nephrology and Hypertension and Director, Oregon Hypertension Program, The Oregon Health Sciences University, Portland, Oregon
Nonpharmacologic Treatment of Essential Hypertension

E. R. McFADDEN Jr., M.D.

Professor of Medicine, Case Western Reserve University School of Medicine; Director, Asthma and Allergic Disease Center, University Hospitals, Cleveland, Ohio
Exercise-Induced Asthma, Urticaria, and Anaphylaxis

JAMES G. McLEOD, M.B., B.S., D.Phil.(Oron), F.R.C.P., F.R.A.C.P.

Bushell Professor of Neurology, University of Sydney; Head, Department of Neurology, Royal Prince Alfred Hospital, Sydney, Australia
Chronic Noninflammatory Peripheral Neuropathy

ROBERT McMILLAN, M.D.

Director, Weingart Center for Bone Marrow Transplantation; Member, Department of Basic and Clinical Research, Scripps Clinic and Research Foundation, La Jolla, California
Chronic Immune Thrombocytopenic Purpura

TYRONE R. MELVIN, M.D.

Instructor, University of Minnesota Medical School, Minneapolis, Minnesota
Idiopathic Nephrotic Syndrome: Minimal Change Disease

JACK MENDELSON, M.D., M.S., F.R.C.P.(C)

Professor of Medicine and Microbiology, McGill University Faculty of Medicine; Senior Physician, Sir Mortimer B. Davis–Jewish General Hospital, Montreal, Quebec, Canada
Aseptic Meningitis

MAREK-MARSEL MESULAM, M.D.

Professor of Neurology, Harvard Medical School; Director, Division of Neuroscience and Behavioral Neurology, Beth Israel Hospital, Boston, Massachusetts
Alzheimer's Disease

JOEL D. MEYERS, M.D.

Associate Professor of Medicine, Divisions of Infectious Diseases and Oncology, Department of Medicine, University of Washington School of Medicine; Associate Member and Head, Program in Infectious Diseases and Clinical Virology, Fred Hutchinson Cancer Research Center, Seattle, Washington
Viral Infections in the Compromised Host

ALFRED F. MICHAEL, M.D.

Regents Professor, Department of Pediatrics and Laboratory Medicine and Pathology, University of Minnesota School of Medicine, Minneapolis, Minnesota
Idiopathic Nephrotic Syndrome: Minimal Change Disease

DANIEL R. MISHELL Jr., M.D.

Chairman and Professor, Department of Obstetrics and Gynecology, University of Southern California School of Medicine; Chief of Professional Services, Women's Hospital, USC–LAC Medical Center, Los Angeles, California
Oral Steroid Contraceptives

KARL E. MISULIS, M.D., Ph.D.

Assistant Professor of Neurology, Vanderbilt University School of Medicine; Attending Physician (Neurology), Vanderbilt University Hospital, Nashville, Tennessee
Neoplastic Spinal Cord Compression and Carcinomatous Meningitis

MACK C. MITCHELL, M.D.

Assistant Professor of Medicine, The Johns Hopkins University School of Medicine; Active Staff Physician, The Johns Hopkins Hospital, Baltimore, Maryland
Drug-Induced Liver Damage

ABDOLGHADER MOLAVI, M.D.

Associate Professor of Medicine, Hahnemann University School of Medicine, Philadelphia, Pennsylvania
Bacterial Osteomyelitis

HAMILTON MOSES III, M.D.

Associate Professor of Neurology and Deputy Director, Department of Neurology, The Johns Hopkins Hospital, Baltimore, Maryland
Normal Pressure Hydrocephalus

ARTHUR J. MOSS, M.D., F.A.C.C.

Clinical Professor of Medicine, University of Rochester School of Medicine and Dentistry; Attending Staff Physician, The Strong Memorial Hospital, Rochester, New York
Arrhythmias and Conduction Disturbances Complicating Myocardial Infarction

LENNART MUCKE, M.D.

Clinical Fellow in Neurology, Harvard Medical School and Massachusetts General Hospital, Boston, Massachusetts
Principles of Pain Management

DONALD W. MULDER, M.D.

Emeritus Professor of Neurology, Mayo Medical School; Emeritus Consultant, Department of Neurology, Mayo Clinic and Mayo Foundation, Rochester, Minnesota
Motor Neuron Disease

SCOTT MURPHY, M.D.

Professor of Medicine, Cardeza Foundation for Hematologic Research and Department of Medicine, Jefferson Medical College of Thomas Jefferson University, Philadelphia, Pennsylvania
Polycythemia Vera

BRADFORD A. NAVIA, M.D.

Instructor, Cornell University Medical College; Fellow, Memorial Sloan-Kettering Cancer Center, New York, New York
Neurological Dysfunction in Acquired Immunodeficiency Syndrome

MICHAEL T. NEWHOUSE, M.D., M.Sc., F.R.C.P.(C), F.A.C.P.

Head, Firestone Regional Chest and Allergy Unit, St. Joseph's Hospital and Chedoke-McMaster Hospitals, McMaster University Medical Center Division, Hamilton, Ontario, Canada
Bronchiectasis

GARY A. NEWMAN, M.D.

Assistant Clinical Professor of Medicine, Jefferson Medical College of Thomas Jefferson University; Consultant Gastroenterologist, Lankenau Hospital, Philadelphia, Pennsylvania
Functional Disorders of the Upper Gastrointestinal Tract

M. BROOKE NICOTRA, M.D., F.A.C.P., F.C.C.P.

Professor of Clinical Medicine and Chief of Pulmonary Disease, University of Texas Health Center, Tyler, Texas
Thoracic Actinomycosis

ALLEN R. NISSENSON, M.D.

Associate Professor of Medicine, UCLA School of Medicine; Director, Dialysis Program, UCLA Medical Center, Los Angeles, California
Peritoneal Dialysis

REX F. OCHI, M.D.

Senior Fellow in Medicine and Nephrology, Division of Nephrology, University of Washington School of Medicine, Seattle, Washington
Idiopathic Rapidly Progressive Glomerulonephritis

MICHAEL J. O'CONNELL, M.D.

Associate Professor of Oncology, Mayo Medical School; Consultant, Division of Medical Oncology, Mayo Clinic, Rochester, Minnesota
Favorable NonHodgkin's Lymphomas

J. DESMOND O'DUFFY, M.B.

Professor of Medicine, Mayo Medical School; Consultant in Medicine, Mayo Clinic, Rochester, Minnesota
Behçet's Syndrome

MICHAEL N. OXMAN, M.D.

Professor of Medicine and Pathology, University of California School of Medicine, San Diego; Chief, Infectious Diseases Section, San Diego Veterans Administration Medical Center, La Jolla, California
Antiviral Chemotherapy

MILTON PACKER, M.D.

Associate Professor of Medicine, Cardiology and Clinical Pharmacology, Mount Sinai School of Medicine; Director, Coronary Care Units, Cardiovascular Training Program, Mount Sinai Medical Center, New York, New York
Chronic Congestive Heart Failure

CHARLES Y.C. PAK, M.D.

Professor of Internal Medicine, University of Texas Health Science Center Southwestern Medical School, Dallas, Texas
Urolithiasis: Calcium Stones

THOMAS PARKER III, B.S., M.D.

Clinical Professor, University of Texas Health Science Center Southwestern Medical School; Medical Director, Dallas Kidney Disease Center and Southwestern Dialysis Center, Dallas Nephrology Associates, Dallas, Texas
Hemodialysis

ALAN G. PALESTINE, M.D.

Staff Ophthalmologist, National Eye Institute, National Institutes of Health, Bethesda, Maryland
Autoimmune Uveitis

HANS PASTERKAMP, M.D.

Assistant Professor of Pediatrics, University of Manitoba Faculty of Medicine and Children's Hospital, Winnipeg, Manitoba, Canada
Acute Upper Airway Infection

GEORGE W. PAULSON, M.D.

Professor and Chairman, Department of Neurology, Ohio State University College of Medicine, Columbus, Ohio
Essential Tremor

TIMOTHY A. PEDLEY, M.D.

Professor and Vice-Chairman, Department of Neurology, Columbia University College of Physicians and Surgeons; Director, Clinical Neurophysiology Laboratories, Columbia-Presbyterian Medical Center and Attending Neurologist, The Neurological Institute at Columbia-Presbyterian Medical Center, New York, New York
Focal and Generalized Seizures

JAMES E. PENNINGTON, M.D.

Associate Professor of Medicine, Harvard Medical School; Physician, Brigham and Women's Hospital, Boston, Massachusetts
Organ Transplantation and Associated Infection

CARL J. PEPINE, M.D.

Professor of Medicine and Associate Director, Division of Cardiovascular Medicine, University of Florida; Chief of Cardiology, Veterans Administration Medical Center, Gainesville, Florida
Coronary Artery Spasm

MARK A. PEPPERCORN, M.D.

Associate Professor of Medicine, Harvard Medical School; Director of Gastroenterology Clinic, Beth Israel Hospital, Boston, Massachusetts
Ulcerative Colitis and Proctitis

ROGELIO J. PEREZ-PADILLA, M.D.

National Institute of Cardiology, Ignacio Chavez, Cardiopulmonary Department, Mexico City, Mexico
Upper Airway Obstruction

JAY A. PERMAN, M.D.

Associate Professor of Pediatrics, The Johns Hopkins University School of Medicine; Director, Pediatric Gastroenterology and Nutrition, The Johns Hopkins Children's Center, Baltimore, Maryland
Carbohydrate Malabsorption

STEPHEN P. PETERS, M.D., Ph.D.

Assistant Professor of Medicine, Divisions of Immunology and Respiratory Medicine, The Johns Hopkins University School of Medicine, Baltimore, Maryland
Systemic Anaphylaxis

ESKILD A. PETERSEN, M.D.

Associate Professor, Department of Internal Medicine, University of Arizona College of Medicine; Chief, Section of Infectious Disease, University of Arizona Health Sciences Center, Tucson, Arizona
Chronic Mucocutaneous Candidiasis

MARTA PETERSEN, M.D.

Resident in Dermatology, Department of Dermatology, University of North Carolina School of Medicine, Chapel Hill, North Carolina
Dermatitis Herpetiformis

L. CREED PETTIGREW, M.D.

Assistant Professor, Department of Neurology, University of Texas Medical School, Houston, Texas
Embolic Strokes of Cardiac Origin

THOMAS L. PETTY, M.D.

Professor of Medicine and Anesthesiology, University of Colorado Health Sciences Center; Director, Webb-Waring Lung Institute, Denver, Colorado
Chronic Bronchitis

J. LOREN PITCHER, M.D., F.A.C.P.

Professor of Medicine, Associate Dean for Clinical Affairs and Medical Director, University of New Mexico School of Medicine and University of New Mexico Hospital, Albuquerque, New Mexico
Acute Upper Gastrointestinal Bleeding

AUBREY PITT, M.D., F.R.A.C.P., F.A.C.C.

Associate Professor of Medicine, Monash University; Director, Cardiology Service, Alfred Hospital, Melbourne, Australia
Uncomplicated Myocardial Infarction

HENRY A. PITT, M.D.

Associate Professor of Surgery, The Johns Hopkins University School of Medicine; Attending Staff, The Johns Hopkins Hospital, Baltimore, Maryland
Acute Cholecystitis

RICHARD PLATT, M.D.

Assistant Professor of Medicine, Harvard Medical School; Associate Hospital Epidemiologist, Brigham and Women's Hospital and Hospital Epidemiologist, New England Deaconess Hospital, Boston, Massachusetts
Adult Immunization

THOMAS A. E. PLATTS-MILLS, M.D., Ph.D.

Professor of Medicine, Division of Allergy, University of Virginia School of Medicine, Charlottesville, Virginia
Asthma in Adults

ALAN L. PLUMMER, M.D.

Associate Professor of Medicine (Pulmonary Diseases), Emory University School of Medicine, Atlanta, Georgia
Acute Respiratory Failure in Asthma

RONALD J. POLINSKY, M.D.

Chief, Clinical Neuropharmacology Section, Medical Neurology Branch, National Institutes of Health, Bethesda, Maryland
Orthostatic Hypotension

DANIEL PORTE Jr., M.D.

Professor of Medicine and Director, Diabetes Research Center, University of Washington; Chief, Division of Endocrinology–Metabolism and Associate Chief of Staff for Research, Veterans Administration Medical Center, Seattle, Washington,
Diabetic Neuropathy

THOMAS POZEFSKY, M.D.

Assistant Professor of Medicine, The Johns Hopkins Medical Institutions, Baltimore, Maryland
Obesity

RICHARD W. PRICE, M.D.

Associate Professor of Neurology, Cornell University Medical College; Associate Attending Neurologist, Memorial Sloan-Kettering Cancer Center, New York, New York
Neurological Dysfunction in Acquired Immunodeficiency Syndrome

THOMAS C. QUINN, M.D.

Associate Professor of Medicine, The Johns Hopkins University School of Medicine, Baltimore, Maryland; Senior Investigator, Laboratory of Immunoregulation, National Institute of Allergy and Infectious Diseases, National Institutes of Health, Bethesda, Maryland
Infection Other Than AIDS in Homosexual Men

KANTI R. RAI, M.D.

Professor of Medicine, State University of New York School of Medicine, Stony Brook; Chief, Division of Hematology-Oncology, Long Island Jewish Medical Center, New Hyde Park, New York
Chronic Lymphocytic Leukemia

LAWRENCE I. RAND, M.D.

Director of Research, William P. Beetham Eye Unit, Joslin Diabetes Center, Boston, Massachusetts
Diabetic Retinopathy

JAMES E. RASMUSSEN, M.D.

Professor of Dermatology and Pediatrics, University of Michigan Medical School; Chief of Clinic, Department of Dermatology, University of Michigan Hospitals, Ann Arbor, Michigan
Atopic Dermatitis

WILLIAM J. RAVICH, M.D.

Assistant Professor in Medicine, Gastroenterology Division and Clinical Director, The Swallowing Center, The Johns Hopkins University School of Medicine; Director, Gastrointestinal Laboratory and Endoscopy Unit, The Johns Hopkins Hospital, Baltimore, Maryland
Pharyngeal Dysphagia

ANTHONY S. REBUCK, M.D., F.C.C.P., F.A.C.P.

Professor of Medicine, University of Toronto Faculty of Medicine; Head, Respiratory Division, Toronto Western Hospital, Toronto, Ontario, Canada
Acute Respiratory Failure in Chronic Obstructive Pulmonary Disease

ANDREW J. REES, M.B., M.Sc., F.R.C.P.

Senior Lecturer, Royal Postgraduate Medical School; Consultant Physician, Hammersmith Hospital, London, England
Goodpasture's Syndrome

SAMUEL REFETOFF, M.D.

Professor of Medicine and Pediatrics, University of Chicago Pritzker School of Medicine, Chicago, Illinois
Primary Hypothyroidism

MORRIS REICHLIN, M.D.

Professor and Chief, Combined Immunology Section, Department of Medicine, University of Oklahoma College of Medicine, Oklahoma City, Oklahoma
Mixed Connective Tissue Disease

ARTHUR L. REINGOLD, M.D.

Assistant Branch Chief, Respiratory and Special Pathogens Epidemiology Branch, Division of Bacterial Disease, Centers for Disease Control, Atlanta, Georgia
Toxic Shock Syndrome

MILAGROS P. REYES, M.D.

Associate Professor of Medicine, Wayne State University; Chief, Section of Infectious Diseases, Hutzel Hospital, Detroit, Michigan
Endocarditis Caused by Gram-Negative Organisms and Fungi

HERBERT Y. REYNOLDS, M.D.

Professor of Internal Medicine and Head, Pulmonary Section, Yale University School of Medicine, New Haven, Connecticut
Aerobic Gram-Negative Pneumonia

EVERETT R. RHOADES, M.D., F.A.C.P.

Director, Indian Health Service, United States Public Health Service, Rockville, Maryland
Pulmonary Nocardiosis

RICHARD E. RIESELBACH, M.D.

Professor and Chairman, Department of Medicine, Milwaukee Clinical Campus, University of Wisconsin Medical School, Madison; Physician-in-Chief, Department of Medicine, Mount Sinai Medical Center, Milwaukee, Wisconsin
Renal Complications of Cancer

JACK E. RIGGS, M.D.

Associate Professor of Neurology and Medicine, West Virginia University School of Medicine; Attending Neurologist, West Virginia University Medical Center, Morgantown, West Virginia
Periodic Paralysis

MANUEL RIVERA, M.D., F.A.C.P., F.C.C.P.

Associate Professor of Clinical Medicine, Pulmonary Section, The University of Texas Health Center, Tyler, Texas
Thoracic Actinomycosis

RICHARD B. ROBERTS, M.D.

Professor of Medicine, Cornell University Medical College; Attending Physician, New York Hospital, New York, New York
Bacterial Meningitis in Adults

GARY L. ROBERTSON, M.D.

Professor of Medicine, Division of Endocrinology, University of Chicago Pritzker School of Medicine, Chicago, Illinois
Diabetes Insipidus

CHARLES A. ROBINSON, M.D.

Adjunct Assistant Member, Scripps Clinic and Research Foundation, La Jolla, California
Systemic Lupus Erythematosus

RICHARD W. ROBINSON, M.D.

Instructor in Medicine, Pulmonary Division, M. S. Hershey Medical Center of the Pennsylvania State University, Hershey, Pennsylvania
Obesity Hypoventilation Syndrome

DAN M. RODEN, M.D.

Associate Professor of Medicine and Pharmacology, Vanderbilt University School of Medicine, Nashville, Tennessee
Ventricular Tachycardia: Drug Therapy

ROY S. ROGERS III, M.D.

Professor of Dermatology, Mayo Medical School, Rochester, Minnesota
Recurrent Aphthous Stomatitis

JAE KYU ROH, M.D.

Assistant Professor, Department of Neurology, College of Medicine, Seoul National University; Assistant Professor in Neurology, Seoul National University Hospital, Seoul, Korea
Atherothrombotic Cerebral Vascular Disease

ROLANDO H. ROLANDELLI, M.D.

Research Associate, Harrison Department of Surgical Research, University of Pennsylvania School of Medicine; Fellow Nutrition and Metabolism, Philadelphia Veterans Administration Medical Center, Philadelphia, Pennsylvania
Enteral Feeding: Liquid Formula Diets

JOHN A. ROMANKIEWICZ, Pharm.D.

President, Scientific Therapeutics Information, Fort Lee, New Jersey
Bacterial Meningitis in Adults

JOHN L. ROMBEAU, M.D., F.A.C.S.

Assistant Professor of Surgery, University of Pennsylvania School of Medicine; Director of Nutritional Support Service, Veterans Administration Medical Center, Philadelphia, Pennsylvania
Enteral Feeding: Liquid Formula Diets

ALLAN R. RONALD, M.D., F.R.C.P.(C), F.A.C.P.

Professor and Head, Department of Medicine, University of Manitoba Faculty of Medicine, Winnipeg, Manitoba, Canada
Anaerobic Bacterial Pulmonary Infection

ALLAN H. ROPPER, M.D.

Associate Professor of Neurology, Harvard Medical School; Director, Neurological-Neurosurgical Intensive Care Unit, Massachusetts General Hospital, Boston, Massachusetts
Cerebral Hemorrhage

BURTON D. ROSE, M.D.

Associate Professor of Medicine, Harvard Medical School; Director, Clinical Nephrology, Brigham and Women's Hospital, Boston, Massachusetts
Hyponatremia

LANNY J. ROSENWASSER, M.D.

Associate Professor of Medicine, Tufts University School of Medicine; Physician, Allergy Service, New England Medical Center Hospital, Boston, Massachusetts
Systemic Vasculitis

JOEL J. ROSLYN, M.D.

Assistant Professor of Surgery, University of California School of Medicine, UCLA Medical Center, Los Angeles, California
Acute Cholecystitis

EDWARD A. ROSS, M.D.

Assistant Professor of Medicine and Director, University of California, Irvine-Long Beach Veterans Administration Medical Program, Irvine, California
Peritoneal Dialysis

MARY E. RUBENIS, B.S.

Senior Research Associate, University of Illinois College of Medicine, Chicago, Illinois
Viral Respiratory Disease

LEWIS J. RUBIN, M.D.

Associate Professor of Medicine and Head, Division of Pulmonary Medicine, University of Maryland School of Medicine, Baltimore, Maryland
Primary Pulmonary Hypertension

ALEXANDER P. RUGGIERI, M.D.

Fellow, Division of Rheumatology, Medical University of South Carolina College of Medicine, Charleston, South Carolina
Systemic Sclerosis (Scleroderma)

JOHN D. RYBOCK, M.D.

Assistant Professor of Neurological Surgery, The Johns Hopkins University School of Medicine, Baltimore, Maryland
Acute Back Pain and Disc Herniation

SANDRA SABATINI, M.D., Ph.D.

Professor of Internal Medicine and Physiology, Texas Tech University Health Science Center; Attending in Nephrology, Lubbock General Hospital, Lubbock, Texas
Mixed Acid-Base Disturbances

STEVEN A. SAHN, M.D.

Professor of Medicine and Director, Division of Pulmonary and Critical Care Medicine, Medical University of South Carolina College of Medicine, Charleston, South Carolina
Empyema

HERBERT A. SALTZMAN M.D.

Professor of Medicine, Duke University Medical Center, Durham, North Carolina
Wegener's Granulomatosis

ROBERT A. SANDHAUS, M.D., Ph.D.

Assistant Professor of Medicine (Pulmonary), University of Colorado School of Medicine; Staff Physician, Pulmonary Medicine, National Jewish Center for Immunology and Respiratory Medicine, Denver, Colorado
Alpha$_1$-Proteinase Inhibitor Deficiency

JAY P. SANFORD, M.D.

Professor of Medicine and Dean, F. Edward Hébert School of Medicine, Uniformed Services University of the Health Sciences; Attending Physician, Walter Reed Army Medical Center, Naval Hospital, Bethesda, Maryland
Nosocomial Pulmonary Infection

GEORGE W. SANTOS, M.D.

Professor of Oncology and Medicine, The Johns Hopkins Medical Institutions, Baltimore, Maryland
Bone Marrow Transplantation

DAVID H. SARNE, M.D.

Assistant Professor of Medicine, University of Chicago Pritzker School of Medicine, Chicago, Illinois
Primary Hypothyroidism

MARIA C. SAVOIA, M.D.

Assistant Adjunct Professor of Medicine, University of California School of Medicine, San Diego; Assistant Chief, Medical Services, San Diego Veterans Administration Medical Center, La Jolla, California
Antiviral Chemotherapy

PERITZ SCHEINBERG, M.D.

Professor and Chairman, Department of Neurology, University of Miami School of Medicine, Miami, Florida
Syncope

LEONARD SCHERLIS, M.D.

Professor, Department of Medicine, University of Maryland Medical School; Attending Physician, University of Maryland Hospital, Baltimore, Maryland
Atrioventricular Block and Implantation of Permanent Cardiac Pacemakers

ROBERT C. SCHLANT, M.D.

Professor of Medicine and Director, Division of Cardiology, Emory University School of Medicine, Atlanta, Georgia
Mitral Regurgitation

ALAN D. SCHREIBER, M.D.

Professor of Medicine, University of Pennsylvania School of Medicine, Philadelphia, Pennsylvania
Autoimmune Hemolytic Anemia

MARVIN M. SCHUSTER, M.D.

Professor of Medicine and Psychiatry, The Johns Hopkins University School of Medicine; Director, Division of Digestive Diseases, Francis Scott Key Medical Center, Baltimore, Maryland
Irritable Bowel Syndrome

LEONARD B. SEEFF, M.D.

Professor of Medicine, Georgetown University School of Medicine, Chief, Gastroenterology-Hepatology Section, Veterans Administration Medical Center, Washington, D.C.
Acute Viral Hepatitis

ARTHUR SELZER, M.D.

Clinical Professor of Medicine, University of California, Clinical Professor Emeritus, Stanford University; Cardiologist, Pacific Presbyterian Medical Center, San Francisco, California
Mitral Stenosis

GRAHAM R. SERJEANT, C.M.G., M.D., F.R.C.P.

Director MIC Laboratories (Jamaica), University of West Indies, Jamaica, West Indies
Sickle Cell Disease

KAREN S. SERVILLA, M.D.

Instructor, Division of Nephrology and Nephrology Director of Transplantation, University of Utah Health Sciences Center, Salt Lake City, Utah
Acute Hypersensitivity Interstitial Nephritis

MARJORIE E. SEYBOLD, M.D.

Professor of Neurosciences and Ophthalmology, University of California School of Medicine; Staff Neurologist, Veterans Administration Medical Center, San Diego, California
Myasthenia Gravis

RALPH SHABETAI, M.D.

Professor of Medicine, University of California, San Diego, School of Medicine, La Jolla, California
Cardiac Tamponade

GERARD J. SHEEHAN, M.B., M.R.C.P.I.

Fellow in Infectious Diseases and Critical Care, University of Manitoba Faculty of Medicine, Winnipeg, Manitoba
Anaerobic Bacterial Pulmonary Infection

DAVID H. SHEPP, M.D.

Senior Fellow in Medicine, University of Washington School of Medicine; Fred Hutchinson Cancer Research Center, Seattle, Washington
Viral Infections in the Compromised Host

KATSUTARO SHIMAOKA, M.D.

Research Professor, Department of Medicine, State University of New York School of Medicine; Associate Chief, Clinical Pharmacology and Therapeutics, Roswell Park Memorial Institute, Buffalo, New York
Thyroid Cancer

CATHY A. SILA, M.D.

Cerebrovascular Disease Research Fellow, Cleveland Clinic Foundation, Cleveland, Ohio
Transient Ischemic Attack

PAUL A. SILVER, M.D.

Assistant Professor, Departments of Mental Health Sciences and Neurology, Hahnemann University School of Medicine; Attending Psychiatrist, Division of Liaison Psychiatry and Psychosomatic Medicine, Hahnemann University Hospital, Philadelphia, Pennsylvania
Alcohol Intoxication and Withdrawal

RONALD A. SIMON, M.D.

Clinical Member, Department of Basic and Clinical Research, Division of Allergy and Immunology, Scripps Clinic and Research Foundation, La Jolla, California
Sulfite-Induced Asthma

MEHRSHEED SINAKI, M.D.

Associate Professor of Physical Medicine and Rehabilitation, Mayo Medical School; Consultant, Department of Physical Medicine and Rehabilitation, Mayo Clinic and Mayo Foundation, Rochester, Minnesota
Motor Neuron Disease

ROLAND T. SKEEL, M.D.

Professor of Medicine and Chief, Division of Hematology–Oncology, Medical College of Ohio, Toledo, Ohio
Chemotherapy in Head and Neck Cancer

EVE ELIZABETH SLATER, M.D.

Associate Professor of Medicine, Columbia University College of Physicians and Surgeons and Senior Director, Biochemical Endocrinology at Merck Sharp & Dohme Research Laboratories, Rahway, New Jersey; Associate Attending Physician, Columbia Presbyterian Hospital, New York, New York
Aortic Dissection

ARTHUR S. SLUTSKY, M.D.

Associate Professor of Medicine, University of Toronto Faculty of Medicine; Staff Physician, Mount Sinai Hospital, Toronto, Ontario, Canada
Acute Respiratory Failure in Chronic Obstructive Pulmonary Disease

BRUCE R. SMITH, Pharm.D.

Therapeutic Research Institute Inc., Sarasota, Florida
Bacterial Osteomyelitis

NEAL A. SNYDER

Attending Staff, San Francisco Veterans Administration, Medical Center, San Francisco, California
Hypernatremia in the Adult

ARTHUR J. SOBER, M.D.

Associate Professor of Dermatology, Harvard Medical School; Associate Dermatologist, Massachusetts General Hospital, Boston, Massachusetts
Primary Malignant Melanoma

DAVID H. SPODICK, M.D., D.Sc.

Professor of Medicine, University of Massachusetts Medical School, Worcester and Lecturer in Medicine, Tufts University School of Medicine, and Lecturer in Medicine, Boston University School of Medicine; Cardiologist, St. Vincent Hospital, Attending Cardiologist, University of Massachusetts School of Medicine, Worcester, Clinical Associate in Medicine, Boston City Hospital, Boston Massachusetts
Acute and Recurrent Pericarditis

SUBRAMANIAM SRIRAM, M.D.

Assistant Professor of Neurology, University of Vermont College of Medicine, Burlington, Vermont
Polymyositis and Dermatomyositis

ALLEN C. STEERE, M.D.

Associate Professor of Medicine, Yale University School of Medicine, New Haven, Connecticut
Lyme Disease

NEAL H. STEIGBIGEL, M.D.

Professor of Medicine, Albert Einstein College of Medicine; Head, Division of Infectious Diseases, Montefiore Medical Center, Bronx, New York
Acquired Immunodeficiency Syndrome

DONALD D. STEVENSON, M.D.

Clinical Member, Division of Allergy and Immunology, Scripps Clinic and Research Foundation, La Jolla, California
Sulfite-Induced Asthma

DAVID H. P. STREETEN, M.B., D. Phil., F.R.C.P.

Professor of Medicine and Head, Section of Endocrinology, State University of New York Upstate Medical Center; Attending in Medicine, State University Hospital, Consultant in Medicine, Veterans Administration, Crouse-Irving Memorial, and St. Joseph's Hospitals, Syracuse, New York
Idiopathic Edema

TIMOTHY J. SULLIVAN, M.D.

Associate Professor of Internal Medicine and Microbiology, University of Texas Southwestern Medical School; Head of Allergy and Immunology, Parkland Memorial Hospital, Dallas, Texas
Penicillin Allergy

ALAN G. SUNSHINE, M.D.

Fellow in Gastroenterology, Hospital of the University of Pennsylvania, Philadelphia, Pennsylvania
Diffuse Esophageal Spasm and Related Disorders

BERNARD TABATZNIK, M.D., F.R.C.P.

Assistant Professor of Medicine, The Johns Hopkins Medical Institutions: Chief, Cardiology Department, North Charles General Hospital, Baltimore, Maryland
Atrial and Ventricular Ectopic Beats

NORMAN TALAL, M.D.

Professor of Medicine and Microbiology, University of Texas Medical School at San Antonio; Chief, Clinical Immunology Section, Audie L. Murphy Memorial Veterans Administration Hospital, San Antonio, Texas
Sjögren's Syndrome

ENG M. TAN, M.D.

Member, Scripps Clinic and Research Foundation, La Jolla, California
Systemic Lupus Erythematosus

RICHARD L. TANNEN, M.D.

Professor of Medicine and Director, Nephrology Division, University of Michigan Medical Center, Ann Arbor, Michigan
Hypokalemia

VINCENT A. TARASKA, M.D., F.R.C.P.(C), F.A.C.P., F.C.C.P.

Assistant Professor, University of Manitoba Faculty of Medicine; Consultant in Pulmonary Medicine, Health Sciences Center, St. Boniface General, Misericordia, and Municipal Hospitals, Winnipeg, Manitoba
Drug-Induced Lung Disease

ROBERT M. TATE, M.D.

Assistant Professor of Medicine, Division of Pulmonary Sciences, University of Colorado Health Sciences Center, Denver, Colarado
Spontaneous Pneumothorax

CATHERINE S. THOMPSON, M.D.

Assistant Professor, Department of Internal Medicine, Divison of Nephrology, University of Texas Medical School; Attending Physician, Hermann Hospital, Houston, Texas
Acute and Chronic Hyperuricemic Nephropathy

PETER D. THOMSON, M.B., B.Ch., F.C.P. (S.A.)

Senior Lecturer, University of Witwatersrand; Director, Renal Unit, University Hospital, Johannesburg, South Africa
Hemolytic-Uremic Syndrome

MICHAEL O. THORNER, M.B., F.R.C.P.

Professor of Medicine and Director, Clinical Research Center, University of Virginia School of Medicine, Charlottesville, Virgina
Prolactinoma

ROBERT R. TIGHT, M.D.

Associate Professor of Medicine, University of North Dakota School of Medicine; Chief, Infectious Diseases, Fargo Veterans Administration Hospital, Fargo, North Dakota
Syphilis

MARCIA G. TONNESEN, M.D.

Assistant Professor of Dermatology, University of Colorado School of Medicine; Chief, Dermatology Service, Veterans Administration Medical Center, Denver, Colorado
Erythema Multiforme

DOUGLASS C. TORMEY, M.D., Ph.D.

Professor of Human Oncology and Medicine, Departments of Human Oncology and Medicine, University of Wisconsin Medical School, Madison, Wisconsin
Chemotherapy in Breast Cancer

PHILLIP P. TOSKES, M.D.

Professor of Medicine, University of Florida College of Medicine; Director, Division of Gastroenterology, Hepatology and Nutrition, University of Florida College of Medicine and Veterans Administration Medical Center, Gainesville, Florida
Chronic Pancreatitis: Exocrine and Endocrine Insufficiencies

PHILIP TROEN, M.D.

Professor and Vice-Chairman, Department of Medicine, University of Pittsburgh School of Medicine; Physician-in-Chief, Montefiore Hospital, Pittsburgh, Pennsylvania
Hypogonadotropic Hypogonadism: Gonadotropin Therapy

TADAHIRO TSUBAKIO, M.D.

Research Fellow, Department of Basic and Clinical Research, Scripps Clinic and Research Foundation, La Jolla, California
Chronic Immune Thrombocytopenic Purpura

DENNY L. TUFFANELLI, M.D.

Clincal Professor of Dermatology, University of California School of Medicine, San Francisco, California
Pemphigus and Pemphigoid

PHILIP A. TUMULTY, M.D.

David J. Carver Professor Emeritus of Medicine, The Johns Hopkins Hospital, Baltimore, Maryland
Functional Illness

ALEXANDER G. G. TURPIE, M.B., Ch.B., F.R.C.P., F.A.C.P., F.R.C.P.(C)

Professor of Medicine, McMaster University School of Medicine; Internist, Hamilton General Hospital, Hamilton, Ontario, Canada
Venous Thromboembolism

KENNETH L. TYLER, M.D.

Assistant Professor of Neurology, Instructor of Microbiology and Molecular Genetics, Harvard Medical School; Clinical Assistant in Neurology, Massachusetts General Hospital, Boston, Massachusetts
Localized Infection of the Central Nervous System

JOHN P. UTZ, M.D.

Professor of Medicine, Georgetown University School of Medicine, Washington, D.C.
Blastomycosis

JUDITH L. VAITUKAITIS, M.D.

Professor of Medicine and Physiology, Boston University School of Medicine; Head, Section of Endocrinology and Metabolism, Boston City Hospital, Boston, Massachusetts
Principles of Estrogen Therapy

MARTIN D. VALENTINE, M.D.

Associate Professor of Medicine, The Johns Hopkins University School of Medicine; Clinical Director, Johns Hopkins University Center for Allergic Diseases at Good Samaritan Hospital, Baltimore, Maryland
Chronic Urticaria

PAUL P. VAN ARSDEL Jr., M.D.

Professor of Medicine and Head, Allergy Section, University of Washington School of Medicine; Attending Physician and Chief-of-Staff, University Hospital, Seattle, Washington
Drug Reactions

CURTIS F. VEAL Jr., M.D.

Associate in Medicine, Division of Pulmonary and Critical Care Medicine, The University of Alabama, Birmingham, Alabama
Mycobacterium Kansasii Infection

V. V. VEDANARAYANAN, M.D.

Research Fellow, Nephrology Service, McGill University Faculty of Medicine and Montreal Children's Hospital Research Institute, Montreal, Quebec, Canada
Hemolytic-Uremic Syndrome

FRANK J. VEITH, M.D.

Professor of Surgery, Albert Einstein College of Medicine; Chief of Vascular Surgery, Montefiore Medical Center, Albert Einstein College of Surgery, New York, New York
Abdominal Aortic Aneurysm

JOHANNES D. VELDHUIS, M.D.

Associate Professor of Internal Medicine, Division of Endocrinology and Metabolism, University of Virginia Medical School, Charlottesville, Virginia
Hypopituitarism

GIANCARLO VIBERTI, M.D., M.R.C.P.

Senior Lecturer, United Medical and Dental Schools of Guy's and St. Thomas's Hospitals, Guy's Campus; Honorary Consultant, Guy's Hospital, London, England
Strategies for Preventive Treatment of Renal Failure in Diabetes

NICHOLAS A. VICK, M.D.

Professor of Neurology, Northwestern University Medical School, Chicago; Head, Division of Neurology, Evanston Hospital, Evanston, Illinois
Metastasis to the Brain

MAURICE VICTOR, M.D.

Professor of Medicine (Neurology), Dartmouth Medical School, Hanover, New Hampshire; Distinguished Physician, Veterans Administration Medical Center, White River Junction, Vermont
Wernicke's Encephalopathy and Other Alcoholic Nutritional Disorders

JOHN J. VOORHEES, M.D.

Professor and Chairman, Department of Dermatology, The University of Michigan Medical School; Attending Staff, University of Michigan Hospitals, Veterans Administration Medical Center, Ann Arbor, Michigan
Psoriasis

BURTON A. WAISBREN, B.S., M.S., M.D., F.A.C.P., F.A.S.I.D.

Director, Waisbren Clinic and Clinical Cell Biology Laboratory, Milwaukee, Wisconsin
Sinusitis

PAUL G. WALFISH, M.D., F.R.C.P.(C), F.A.C.P.

Professor of Medicine and Pediatrics, University of Toronto Faculty of Medicine; Senior Attending Physician, Department of Medicine and Director, Division of Endocrinology and Metabolism, Mount Sinai Hospital, Toronto, Ontario, Canada
Single Thyroid Nodule

ABRAHAM U. WAKS, M.D.

Assistant Clinical Professor of Medicine, UCLA School of Medicine, Los Angeles, California
Renovascular Hypertension

IRWIN R. WALKER, M.B., B.S., F.R.A.C.P., F.R.C.P.(C)

Associate Professor, Departments of Medicine and Pathology, McMaster University School of Medicine; Director, Hamilton-Niagara Regional Hemophilia Clinic, Hamilton, Ontario, Canada
Hemophilia

RICHARD J. WALLACE Jr., M.D., F.A.C.P., F.C.C.P.

Associate Professor of Research and Clinical Medicine; Chief, Department of Microbiology, The University of Texas Health Center, Tyler, Texas
Thoracic Actinomycosis

PETER D. WALZER, M.D.

Professor of Medicine, University of Cincinnati College of Medicine; Chief, Infectious Diseases, Cincinnati Veterans Administration Medical Center, Cincinnati, Ohio
Pneumocystosis

RICHARD R. P. WARNER, M.D.

Associate Clinical Professor of Medicine, Mount Sinai School of Medicine of the City University of New York; Associate Attending Physician of Medicine (Gastroenterology), The Mount Sinai Hospital; Attending Physician-in-Chief, Gastroenterology and Joint Diseases, North General Hospital, New York, New York
Carcinoid Tumors

JOHN W. WARREN, M.D.

Associate Professor of Medicine, Division of Infectious Diseases, University of Maryland School of Medicine: Attending Physician, University of Maryland Hospital and Psychiatric Institute, Baltimore, Maryland
Catheter-Associated Urinary Tract Infection

LEONARD WARTOFSKY, M.S., M.D., F.A.C.P.

Professor of Medicine, Uniformed Services University of the Health Sciences, Bethesda, Maryland: Colonel, United States Army Medical Department, Walter Reed Army Medical Center, Washington, D.C.
Diffuse Nontoxic and Multinodular Goiter

THOMAS L. WATT, M.D.

Head, Section of Dermatology, Eastern Maine Medical Center, Bangor, Maine
Warts

JEROME D. WAYE, M.D.

Clinical Professor of Medicine, Mount Sinai School of Medicine of the City University of New York; Chief, Gastrointestinal Endoscopy Unit, Mount Sinai Hospital and Lenox Hill Hospital, New York, New York
Polyps of the Colon

CYNTHIA S. WEIKEL, M.D.

Assistant Professor of Medicine, Division of Geographic Medicine, Department of Internal Medicine, University of Virginia School of Medicine, Charlottesville, Virginia
Infectious Diarrhea: A Patient in the United States

DONALD A. WEINER, M.D.

Associate Professor of Medicine, Boston University School of Medicine; Director, Heart Station, University Hospital, Boston, Massachusetts
Rehabilitation After Myocardial Infarction

EDWARD WEINMAN, M.D.

Professor and Director, Division of Nephrology, University of Texas Medical School; Attending Physician and Director, Nephrology Division, Hermann Hospital, Houston, Texas
Acute and Chronic Hyperuricemic Nephropathy

SANDRA WEINTRAUB, Ph.D.

Instructor of Neurology (Neuropsychology), Harvard Medical School; Head of Neuropsychology, Behavioral Neurology Unit, Beth Israel Hospital, Boston, Massachusetts
Alzheimer's Disease

HARVEY J. WEISS, M.D.

Professor of Medicine, Columbia University College of Physicians and Surgeons; Director, Division of Hematology–Oncology, St. Lukes-Roosevelt Hospital Center (Roosevelt Site), New York, New York
Von Willebrand's Disease

NED M. WEISS, M.D.

Fellow, Division of Endocrinology, Department of Medicine, University of Chicago Pritzker School of Medicine, Chicago, Illinois
Diabetes Insipidus

THOMAS L. WENGER, M.D., F.A.C.C.

Adjunct Assistant Professor of Medicine, Duke University Medical Center, Durham; Head, Department of Medical Sciences, Burroughs Wellcome Company, Research Triangle Park, North Carolina
Digitalis Toxicity

CLARK D. WEST, M.D.

Professor, Department of Pediatrics, University of Cincinnati College of Medicine; Director, Division of Nephrology, Children's Hospital Medical Center, Cincinnati, Ohio
Membranoproliferative Glomerulonephritis

GORDON WETHERLEY-MEIN, B.A., M.D. (Cantab), F.R.C.P. (Lond), F.R.C.Path. (U.K.)

Emeritus Professor of Haematology, University of London; Consulting Haematologist, St. Thomas's Hospital and Wolfson Research Fellow, Royal College of Physicians, London, England
Erythrocytosis

RICHARD J. WHITLEY, M.D.

Professor of Pediatrics and Microbiology, University of Alabama School of Medicine, Birmingham, Alabama
Herpes Simplex

E. DOUGLAS WIGLE, M.D., F.R.C.P.(C), F.A.C.P., F.A.C.C.

Professor, Department of Medicine, Faculty of Medicine University of Toronto; Director, Division of Cardiology, Toronto General Hospital, Toronto, Ontario, Canada
Hypertrophic Cardiomyopathy

FREDRICK M. WIGLEY, M.D.

Assistant Professor of Medicine, The Johns Hopkins University School of Medicine; Attending Staff, Baltimore City Hospitals, Baltimore, Maryland
Raynaud's Phenomenon

SUSAN WILANSKY, M.D., F.R.C.P.(C)

Lecturer, Department of Medicine, University of Toronto; Clinical Associate, Division of Cardiology, Toronto General Hospital, Toronto, Ontario, Canada
Hypertrophic Cardiomyopathy

RONALD G. WILEY, M.D., Ph.D.

Assistant Professor of Neurology and Instructor in Pharmacology, Vanderbilt University School of Medicine; Staff Neurologist, Nashville Veterans Administration Medical Center and Consultant in Neuro-Oncology, Vanderbilt University Hospital, Nashville, Tennessee
Neoplastic Spinal Cord Compression and Carcinomatous Meningitis

GORDON H. WILLIAMS, M.D.

Professor of Medicine, Harvard Medical School; Director,, Endocrine-Hypertension Unit, Brigham and Women's Hospital, Boston, Massachusetts
Primary Aldosteronism
Mineralocorticoid Hypertension

STEPHEN J. WINTERS, M.D.

Associate Professor, University of Pittsburgh School of Medicine; Attending Staff, Division of Endocrinology and Metabolism, Montefiore Hospital, Pittsburgh, Pennsylvania
Hypogonadotropic Hypogonadism: Gonadotropin Therapy

BRUCE U. WINTROUB, M.D.

Associate Professor and Vice-Chairman, Department of Dermatology, University of California School of Medicine, San Francisco, California
Pemphigus and Pemphigoid

SHELDON M. WOLFF, M.D.

Endicott Professor and Chairman, Department of Medicine, Tufts University School of Medicine; Physician-in-Chief, New England Medical Center Hospital, Boston, Massachusetts
Systemic Vasculitis

JERRY S. WOLINSKY, M.D.

Professor, Department of Neurology, University of Texas Health Science Center Houston, Texas
Acute Inflammatory Polyneuropathy

FRANK M. YATSU, M.D.

Professor and Chairman, Department of Neurology, University of Texas Medical School, Houston, Texas
Embolic Strokes of Cardiac Origin

THOMAS T. YOSHIKAWA, M.D.

Professor, Department of Internal Medicine, UCLA School of Medicine; Chief, Division of Geriatric Medicine and Clinical Director of Geriatric Research, Education and Cinical Center, West Los Angeles Veterans Administration Medical Center, Los Angeles, California
Cellulitis and Soft Tissue Infection

EDWARD J. YOUNG, M.D.

Associate Professor of Medicine, Microbiology and Immunology, Baylor College of Medicine; Chief of Staff, The Veterans Administration Medical Center, Houston, Texas
Human Brucellosis

LOWELL S. YOUNG, M.D.

Professor of Medicine, Division of Infectious Diseases, UCLA School of Medicine, Los Angles, California
Bacterial and Fungal Infection in the Compromised Host

ROBERT C. YOUNG, M.D.

Chief, Medicine Branch, National Cancer Institute, Bethesda, Maryland,
NonHodgkin's Disease: Unfavorable Lymphomas

TSAI-FAN YU, B.A., M.D.

Research Professor of Medicine, Emeritus, Mount Sinai School of Medicine, New York, New York
Gout

VICTOR L. YU, M.D., F.A.C.P.

Associate Professor of Medicine, University of Pittsburgh School of Medicine; Chief, Infectious Disease Section, Veterans Administration Medical Center, Pittsburgh, Pennsylvania
Legionellosis

JOHN W. YUNGINGER, M.D.

Professor of Pediatrics and Associate Professor of Medicine, Mayo Medical School; Consultant in Pediatrics and Internal Medicine (Allergy), Mayo Clinic and Foundation, Rochester, Minnesota
Insect Sting Allergy in Adults

STEPHEN H. ZINNER, M.D.

Professor of Medicine, Brown University Program in Medicine; Director, Division of Infectious Diseases, Roger Williams General Hospital, Providence, Rhode Island
Infection Associated with Hematologic Malignancy

ALVIN M. ZFASS, M.D.

Professor of Medicine, Director of Endoscopy, Medical College of Virgina of Virginia Commonwealth University, Richmond, Virginia
Constipation

JOHN J. ZONE, M.D.

Associate Professor of Medicine, Division of Dermatology, Department of Medicine, University of Utah School of Medicine, Salt Lake City, Utah
Dermatitis Herpetiformis

CLIFFORD W. ZWILLICH, M.D.

Professor of Medicine; Chief, Pulmonary Division of the Department of Medicine; M.S. Hershey Medical Center of the Pennsylvania State University, Hershey, Pennsylvania
Obesity Hypoventilation Syndrome

CONTENTS

INFECTIOUS DISEASES

Hematologic Diseases

Neoplastic Disorders

ENDOCRINE AND METABOLIC DISORDERS

CARDIOVASCULAR DISEASES

HYPERTENSION AND RENAL DISEASES

Neurologic Diseases

IMMUNE AND ALLERGIC DISORDERS

ASTHMA IN ADULTS

THOMAS A. E. PLATTS-MILLS, M.D., Ph.D.
GUY P. FIOCCO, M.D.

The definition of asthma is airway obstruction which varies with time, either spontaneously or in response to treatment. The symptoms include coughing, increased secretions, a sense of difficulty breathing, and chest tightness or chest pain. In addition, many patients become frightened both during attacks and also when they feel an attack is starting. The importance of this is that fear can exacerbate both the symptoms and the airway obstruction. Certainly, there is a tendency for attacks of asthma that are initially mild to progress rapidly to severe obstruction. While the symptoms are caused by bronchospasm, most patients with chronic or recurrent asthma have nonspecific bronchial hyper-reactivity which can be demonstrated when they have normal spirometry. This underlying hyper-reactivity is the hallmark of the disease. Exposure to irritating pollutants, viral infections, or specific allergens may lead to inflammation and epithelial damage which, in turn, may cause or increase bronchial reactivity. In attempting to identify the etiology of the disease, one must consider not only what events trigger acute attacks, but also which factors may be contributing to the underlying bronchial reactivity. The patients tend only to recognize short-term trigger factors, and when asked about the cause of their attacks, they describe exercise, emotional factors, infections, and cold air. Only in a minority of cases do patients recognize allergen exposure as an important precipitant of attacks. Nonetheless, many of the patients are allergic as judged by skin tests and RAST assays. In recent years, it has become clear that allergens can be and perhaps often are an important contributing cause of chronic bronchial hyper-reactivity.

In considering the management of an asthmatic patient, it is worth dividing treatment into 3 categories, although in practice there may be great overlap among the 3 phases.

1. Management of the acute or severe attack which is primarily pharmacologic but may be unsuccessful if the patient's anxiety is not relieved at the same time.
2. A long-term plan for the patient to cope with his symptoms with an adequate supply of medicines. This requires considerable education both about the drugs and also about the indications for various types of treatment.
3. Finally, in any patient who is having severe trouble requiring continuous medication or repeated emergency room visits, an attempt should be made to identify and treat or avoid any relevant allergic component.

We do not have a very clear understanding of the inflammatory events involved in bronchial hyper-reactivity, and we do not understand the physical basis for many of the symptoms that patients feel. Not surprisingly, patients vary in their responses to different drugs. Although there are relatively few drugs which are widely used, there are many different, sometimes unexpected, drugs which appear to benefit individual patients. The management of chronic severe asthma requires great flexibility in adjusting both pharmacologic, allergic, and psychologic approaches. No simple regimen will adequately treat more than a few of the severe cases.

ASSESSMENT

While the assessment of patients with severe asthma may need to be extensive, there is a tendency to restrict the work-up of mild cases. It is always important to establish the diagnosis, and even when the history is very clear, it is much better to have documented evidence of reversible airway obstruction, that is, peak flow or FEV_1 records. In patients whose attacks have not been documented, it may be necessary to demonstrate bronchial hyper-reactivity by methacoline, histamine, cold air, or exercise challenge tests.

Initial assessment should encompass a full history including an allergic history. The history should record treatment the patient has received for other conditions as well as asthma. In particular, it is important to know about β-adrenergic blocking drugs, which can exacerbate asthma; aspirin, which can exacerbate or cause asthma in a minority of cases; and other nonsteroidal anti-inflammatory drugs. Occasional patients present with recurrent wheezing secondary to inhaling regurgitated food because of a hiatal hernia, and this should be considered in taking the history. Assessment of sputum for eosinophils may be useful in patients in whom the diagnosis is in doubt, particularly in older patients with only partially reversible airway obstruction.

The major forms of treatment will be discussed separately, and finally, a brief outline of our policy for severe attacks, exercise, and long-term management will be given.

INHALED β_2 AGONISTS

It is now generally accepted that the primary adrenergic receptor that stimulates relaxation of bronchial smooth muscle is a β_2 receptor. For a given bronchodilator effect, both epinephrine and nonselective β agonists have more stimulant effect on the heart than the ''selective'' β_2 agonists. Furthermore, when given as tablets, all the β_2 selective agonists can produce a sensation of shaking or agitation, and this effect is much less marked with the inhaled route. Thus, selective β_2 agonists, either in a pressurized inhaler or nebulized, are becoming not only the first line of treatment for mild asthma but are also replacing epinephrine injections as the initial management of acute asthma in the emergency room.

The β_2 agonists available include albuterol, metaproterenol, and terbutaline. In addition, the β-selective catecholamine isoetharine is used. All are available as tablets or pressurized aerosols (inhaler), while in the United States, only metaproterenol, terbutaline, and isoetharine are currently available for use in a nebulizer. These agents need to reach the large to medium bronchi to be effective, and the difference between the 2 methods of delivery largely depends on individual skill and, possibly, local anatomy. Although many patients report that their β_2 agonist inhaler has stopped working, these patients have usually not exhausted their receptors, since either nebulized or intravenous agonist will still be effective. The great advantages of the inhalers are that they are small, relatively easy to use, and, in most cases, effective. The advantages of using the nebulizer are: (1) no skill in timing the puff is required, (2) the treatment takes longer (10 minutes) and has more tendency to calm the patient down, and (3) repeated breathing over a period of time allows agonist to enter the lungs as they dilate. Recently, several different types of ''spacers'' have been introduced to help patients inhale β_2 agonists from inhalers. Many of these are too large for a pocket and therefore lose some of the advantages of an inhaler. Furthermore, they have been shown to increase deposition in the lung by only 7 percent; however, they may be very helpful in patients who have great difficulty timing their inhalers. They certainly illustrate the importance of careful instruction and observation of patients in the use of all inhalers.

None of the β_2 agonists is fully selective, so they are all potentially cardiotoxic; indeed, tachycardia is commonly reported with albuterol tablets. Nonetheless, with the present generation of inhaled β_2 agonists, it has proved difficult to identify a dangerous upper dose in short-term use. Many patients take grossly excessive numbers of puffs with increasingly little benefit, but it is very unusual for them to suffer severe side effects. There are animal experiments which show that the combination of high-dose adrenergic agonist and theophylline can cause myocardial damage and dangerous arrhythmia. However, there is no clear evidence that this occurs in man, and direct studies on theophylline combined with β_2 selective agonists have not revealed evidence for increase in arrhythmia. Thus, it appears that inhaled β_2 agonists have a wide safety margin in normal use and that patients can be encouraged to use them either ''as needed'' or as regular treatment, 2 puffs 3 or 4 times a day.

THEOPHYLLINE

The effectiveness of theophylline compounds in relieving bronchospasm has been recognized for many years. Although the mechanism remains in doubt, the effect of high-dose intravenous aminophylline can be very rapid. The mechanism of action of theophyllines remains in doubt. While high-dose intravenous aminophylline can have a rapid bronchodilator effect, it seems that continuous low-dose aminophylline may act in a different way to reduce the frequency of attacks of bronchospasm. Oral aminophylline tends to cause gastric irritation, which limited its use until the introduction of delayed release preparations of theophylline. It has now become common practice to use oral treatment to maintain a blood level within a close range, from 5 to 10 μg/ml to 20 μg/ml. While this approach is effective for many cases, there are major objections, which are listed below, to this being seen as the only way to use theophylline.

1. There is no evidence for a lower limit to the therapeutic range and many patients gain considerable benefit when their blood level is well below 10 μg/ml. There is no indication for increasing theophylline treatment just because the blood level is low. Furthermore, theophylline has additive effects with adrenergic agonists when serum levels are below the "therapeutic range".
2. The upper limit for a safe blood theophylline level (20 μg/ml) is the concentration that avoids or minimizes serious risks of cardiotoxicity or convulsions. Nonetheless, patients may have side effects of theophylline when in the therapeutic range. Most commonly, nausea, a sense of anxiety, or malaise may occur at blood levels as low as 5 μg/ml. In children, learning difficulty can occur in the "therapeutic range"; the adult equivalent of learning difficulty is not well defined!
3. The metabolism of theophylline is altered by a wide variety of factors—including concomitant use of other drugs, infection, acidosis, and smoking—posing definite hazards to maintaining continuous high levels of theophylline. It is important to remember that some over-the-counter asthma medicines contain 100 mg of theophylline, and patients may inadvertently add to their total theophylline intake.

Recently, several so-called 24-hour theophylline preparations have been introduced with recommendations for large (> 600 mg) daily doses. At present, it seems unwise to use single doses as high as this because absorption can be variable, giving rise to unacceptably high peak levels. It is also not clear that these preparations can maintain levels over 24 hours. In addition, we have not been impressed that once a day dosage leads to better patient compliance in asthmatics.

Our present policy is to use delayed release theophylline, 200 to 300 mg 2 or 3 times daily, in conjunction with inhaled β-agonists. One serum theophylline measurement should be adequate. Only in rare cases is it necessary to push the dosage higher or to carry out repeated serum theophylline levels. One tablet of delayed release theophylline (200 to 300 mg) at night either regularly or occasionally at the discretion of the patient is also a useful treatment for nocturnal symptoms.

CROMOLYN SODIUM

Cromolyn, or disodium cromoglycate, was introduced about 15 years ago as an agent that would control mediator release from mast cells and, therefore, be useful in allergic asthma. Since that time, we have come to realize that we do not fully understand its mode of action, and it may well act by some more general mechanism to stabilize membranes. Thus, cromolyn will not only inhibit allergen-induced bronchospasm but may also be effective in inhibiting exercise or cold-air-induced bronchospasm. Cromolyn has not been shown to have any bronchodilator effect and cannot be used to treat acute bronchospasm. It may be very effective as a regular prophylactic treatment in moderate cases of allergic or nonallergic asthma in which symptoms are not adequately controlled by β_2 agonist inhalers. Cromolyn is supplied either as powder in capsules for use in a "Spinhaler" or as nebulizer solution. In Europe, cromolyn is also available in a pressurized inhaler which delivers 2-mg doses. This does not work as well as the 20-mg capsules via the Spinhaler. The nebulizer fluid avoids some of the irritant effects of the inhaled powder but is much slower to use and is not portable. The great majority of patients using cromolyn should take 1 or 2 capsules by Spinhaler 3 times daily. The timing of doses is not critical, so that generally the Spinhaler need not be taken to school or work.

A really important feature of cromolyn is that it has negligible side effects; thus, no acute effects of overdosage or cumulative effects from long-term use have been described. Many patients have difficulty using spinhalers and need to be instructed carefully. Some patients cough when they inhale the particles and may find it easier to take cromolyn 5 or 10 minutes after a β_2 agonist. Occasional patients react acutely to cromolyn with flushing or even bronchospasm. This effect, which may be related to the lactose used in the capsules in the United States, is rare.

INHALED STEROIDS

Inhaled steroids, like cromolyn, have no rapid effect on acute bronchospasm and are used either continuously or in short courses in the management of chronic or seasonal asthma. Several different steroids are available as pressurized inhalers. Most information is available about beclomethasone dipropionate. This drug is poorly absorbed from local surfaces and generally has no significant effect on adrenal function. However, in high doses, inhaled steroids can delay recovery of adrenal function after withdrawal of oral steroids. Thus, their systemic effects cannot be ignored. When initially introduced, the locally active steroids gave rise to many problems with *Candida* infection in the throat. This problem can usually be resolved by rinsing the throat after each inhalation of steroid. It has not been shown that inhaled steroids cause *Candida* infection in the lungs. However, it is worth screening for *Candida* in the sputum of patients who are not doing well and are producing sputum. We have seen patients who improved after stopping inhaled steroids, as if they were having a direct or indirect irritant effect. Surprisingly, the dilated blood vessels and mild bleeding which are very common with beclomethasone in the nose have not proven to be a problem in the lungs. Despite some worries about lung development in children, very little evidence that inhaled steroids cause structural changes in the lung has appeared, and it is unlikely that long-term use of inhaled beclomethasone has harmful effects on the adult lung. With inhaled beclomethasone dipropionate, there is no clearly defined upper limit to dosage. However, using more than 4 puffs 4 times daily represents a significant dose of Freon gas, which may well be an irritant. In Europe, beclomethasone is available in a 5 times stronger form (250 μg per puff). The indications for this higher dosage are not yet clear.

SYSTEMIC STEROIDS

Systemic steroids are a major part of the treatment of severe acute asthma attacks. Although there is little evidence to support the optimal dose or preparation, experience suggests they should be given in large doses—300 mg of hydrocortisone IV every 6 hours, or 60 mg of prednisone orally per day, to any patient with uncontrolled bronchospasm. The regimens for this acute use vary from a single day to one month, with the rate of dose reduction varying depending on the conditions and the objective. Some patients find that they can control their symptoms if they use 20 mg of prednisone for 1 day and increase their regular treatment at the same time. On the other hand, allergic patients who require hospitalization during the grass or ragweed pollen season may require prednisone, 10 to 15 mg per day for 6 weeks, until the season is over. In a patient who has not previously had a severe attack, it is also wise to continue steroid courses for at least 2 weeks after the acute phase so that a treatment regimen (cromolyn, beclomethasone, theophylline, and so on) can be established. Often, patients with asthma of recent onset are given a short course of steroids (e.g., 4 days) and then return to the emergency room within 2 weeks. In addition, although skin testing should not be carried out while the patient has severe bronchospasm, it can be done while he is still receiving steroids. The results of these tests may be helpful in giving advice regarding avoidance measures before steroid treatment is reduced. The reasons for avoiding long-term steroids are well known. Asthmatic patients can suffer very badly from long-term steroid use because weight gain, rib fractures, loss of vertebral height due to osteoporosis, mental changes, and muscle weakness all make it more difficult to cope with attacks of breathlessness. None of this would be a problem if steroids were not such an effective treatment. In our opinion, very few young asthmatic adults require continuous oral steroids. Furthermore, almost all allergic patients can be maintained without continuous oral steroids by using aggressive avoidance measures and standard pharmacological management with or without desensitization. Thus, the major group in which long-term oral steroids are necessary is late-onset nonallergic patients, the group most prone to the development of osteoporosis. Nonetheless, some of the patients respond very well to steroids and are not controlled adequately by other treatment. It is important to remember that when Rackeman first described "intrinsic" asthma, he described a disease that was often rapidly fatal, and the main change in prognosis came with the introduction of oral steroids. Some of these patients require high-dose steroids for 1 or 2 years, but after that, many will be able to reduce the dose gradually to under 10 mg per day, at which dose it may be necessary and/or safe to continue for 5 years or more.

Various tricks may prove helpful in reducing steroid doses. The most commonly used is alternate-day therapy. Our experience is that day-to-day differences of greater than 10 mg are difficult to tolerate in patients with truly steroid-dependent asthma. However, alternating doses of 10 mg and 15 mg, and so on, may be helpful during withdrawal. In patients who have been on steroids for a long time, withdrawal below 10 mg must be carried out very slowly: Reduce by 1 mg per day each month or alternate months. The macrolide antibiotic troleandomycin (TAO) has been recommended as a steroid sparing agent, but it works only with methylprednisolone. TAO has been shown to delay metabolism of methylprednisolone as well as other drugs, including theophylline. It has been estimated that TAO can increase the resulting dose of methylprednisolone by as much as threefold. In addition, TAO can cause serious liver toxicity. Thus, while TAO may be useful if used to withdraw steroids completely, it often represents simply an increased dose of steroid with consequent increased steroid side effects.

In conclusion, steroids should be used freely in short courses, that is, up to 1 month, for patients with acute symptoms. Oral steroids should be used for long periods only if full doses of other medicines have failed to control symptoms and full consideration of allergens or other causes of the disease has not helped.

ALLERGIC MANAGEMENT OF ASTHMA

There are great differences of opinion about the role that allergens play in asthma and about the stage in the disease when allergic assessment should be undertaken. Our rule of thumb is that anyone who requires continuous treatment, high-dose theophylline, or has had more than one emergency room visit should definitely be assessed. There is certainly no excuse for using long courses of systemic steroids without considering the cause of the disease. Allergic management consists of 4 phases: allergic history, skin testing with or without radioallergosorbent testing, education (including advice on avoidance), and finally, consideration of desensitization.

We find that there are great advantages to discussing causes of the disease with patients because they often have their own ideas, correct or not, which need to be brought out. Secondly, some patients are really helped by the demonstration of skin sensitivity, both in terms of demystifying the disease and also to make them think about avoidance measures. Avoidance measures are very largely concerned with houses, because this is usually the largest source of protein inhalation and, unlike the outside air, can be influenced by the patient. There are several different groups of allergens that may be helped by avoidance measures in the house.

1. *Pets.* Animal dander accumulates in houses over a prolonged period and will take several weeks to eliminate after the cat or dog is removed. Although it is difficult to persuade patients to get rid of animals, it may be possible to move the pet into the garage or restrict its range in the house. Dogs kept outside and allowed into the house occasionally do not appear to be an important cause of sensitization or symptoms. Attempting to treat cat allergic patients who allow cats in their bedrooms is very frustrating.
2. *Dust Mites.* In the United States, the prevalence of dust mite allergy in asthma is still in doubt. However, there is good evidence that dust mite allergy is of major importance on the West Coast, Hawaii, the Gulf Coast, Atlanta, and much of the Southeast and is probably relevant in all areas where there are more than 6 humid months in the year. Mites grow well only with a relative humidity of greater than 55 percent. "Avoidance" of mites involves 4 principles. First, remove reservoirs for mite growth, namely, cover mattresses, remove fitted carpets, and upholstered furniture from bedrooms. Second, keep relative humidity below 50 percent if possible, that is, humidifiers in the winter should be run at a maximum of 40 percent relative humidity, and tightly sealed houses should be aired regularly. Third, wash bedding in a hot cycle; cool cycle washing or dry cleaning of bedding does not kill mites. Fourth, wear a simple mask at times when dust is being disturbed and for 10 minutes afterward to allow large particles to settle.
3. *Fungi.* The role of indoor fungal allergens in asthma is, if anything, more difficult to assess than that for mites. However, many of the measures suggested for mites are helpful. In addition, windows, shower curtains, and indoor plants are important sites for fungal growth. It is technically possible to do spore counts inside houses but they are not freely available. Therefore, in general it is not possible to define what species or quantities of spores are present in a particular house.
4. *Cockroaches.* In some houses, and particularly apartment blocks, very large numbers of cockroaches are present. In addition, in some areas, especially large cities, skin sensitivity to cockroach allergen extracts is common among asthmatics. While it may be difficult to kill cockroaches in an apartment, it is not very difficult to keep a house clear of cockroaches by using chemical sprays, traps, baking soda, ultrasound, and so on. Care must be taken when using chemical sprays because they may prove to be an irritant to asthmatic patients.
5. *House Dust.* Most of the allergens in house dust are produced in the house, and the important treatment is to reduce sites of production and reservoirs. For these allergens, air filtration can play only a limited role. However, outdoor pollen and fungal spores can enter houses and contribute to house dust. These allergens can be effectively eliminated from houses by good quality filters on the air coming into an air conditioning system. Window fans without filters are a very effective method for bringing pollen into a house. Patients often ask about electrostatic precipitation, and occasionally report benefit from these devices; however, these do not reduce the quantity of allergen in a house and are able to affect only the small quantities of allergen that remain airborne.

DESENSITIZATION TREATMENT

Although desensitization treatment is considered controversial by some authors, it is very widely used and some patients show very gratifying improvement. It is unlikely that it will have any effect in nonallergic patients. If patients are exposed to very large quantities of cat dander or dust mite allergen at home, it is difficult to establish desensitization treatment. Thus, desensitization should always be accompanied by a program of education about avoidance, as well as continuing pharmacologic management.

Extracts of several hundred different allergens are available for desensitization treatment; only a small number are used in any quantity. The most widely used extract is house dust (which is used for, perhaps, 1 million patients in the United States), prepared from vacuum cleaner dust. The extracts are unstandardized and probably contain a random mixture of dust mite, cockroach, and fungal allergens, together with small quantities of pollen and animal dander allergens. The alternative is to use a mixture of the allergens relevant to each patient. Most experienced allergists believe that mixtures of a limited number of extracts do work. Although the experimental evidence on the use of mixtures of allergens to treat asthma is poor, this reflects more the complexity of the situation rather than clear evidence that mixtures do not work.

At present, we recommend desensitization to approximately one-quarter of our allergic asthmatics; most of the others are adequately controlled by a combination of avoidance and pharmacologic treatment.

OTHER TREATMENT

It is well established that opiate and barbiturate sedatives are dangerous to asthmatic patients. However, sedatives such as diazepam can be used with caution, and codeine may be useful as an antitussive. Alternatively, a small dose of promethazine, for example, 12.5 mg, at night may be very helpful both as a sedative and an antitussive. Promethazine is an antihistamine but has marked anticholinergic effects as well, and it may well be the anticholinergic effects that are helpful. On the other hand, all antihistamines should be used with caution in asthma because they may exacerbate mucous plugging.

Atropine, Atropine Methonitrate, and Glycopyrrolate

Atropine and atropine-like agents, for example, stramonium cigarettes, have been used to treat asthma for thousands of years. The use of atropine is entirely logical if a contributing mechanism of bronchospasm is increased activity in parasympathetic fibers to bronchial smooth muscle. The benefits of anticholinergic agents in acute asthma may vary markedly among individuals. The use of atropine has been limited by autonomic side effects. Several anticholinergic agents now undergoing trials in the United States offer greater bronchodilator properties than atropine at doses that avoid severe side effects, for example, glycopyrrolate, 0.8 mg in 4 ml saline *bid* by nebulizer. The role that these agents will have in chronic management of asthma remains unclear.

Aspirin

Aspirin (and other nonsteroidal anti-inflammatory drugs) has profound effects on prostaglandin and leukotriene metabolism which are dosage dependent and differ from one individual to another. Furthermore, the effect of aspirin may vary from time to time. It is well established that aspirin causes severe asthma attacks in some patients. Although these attacks may have the appearance of anaphylaxis, true IgE mediated allergy to contaminants in aspirin is very rare. There is also a group of asthmatic patients who experience significant but subclinical decline in their pulmonary function (FEV_1) with aspirin ingestion. The presence of nasal polyps in asthmatics should alert one to the increased possibility of aspirin sensitivity. On the other hand, many asthmatic patients use aspirin for headaches and find that aspirin *improves* their bronchospasm. Policy in relation to aspirin sensitivity varies from establishing a complete salicylate-free diet which is occasionally helpful, to attempting aspirin desensitization. However, starting "aspirin desensitization" in patients who experience bronchospasm with aspirin is dangerous and should be attempted only in the hospital with full resuscitation facilities available.

EXERCISE INDUCED ASTHMA

Exercise that increases ventilation can result in increased bronchospasm in patients with asthma. The mechanism for this is probably respiratory heat exchange in the trachea and large bronchi secondary to evaporation of water. It follows that breathing fully humidified air or swimming will not induce bronchospasm. Furthermore, the colder, and thus drier, the air is, the less increase in ventilation is necessary to induce bronchospasm. In children and young adults, avoiding exercise because of the fear of inducing bronchospasm often leads to a progressive downward cycle in which reduced "fitness", invalidism, and increased exposure to household allergens may all play a role. While it has been difficult to prove that exercise is directly beneficial to asthmatic patients, it is a common observation that patients have less trouble with their disease if they maintain a high level of activity. It is therefore important to provide adequate medication. Both inhaled β_2 agonists and cromolyn are effective in reducing exercise induced bronchospasm. Two capsules of cromolyn 15 minutes prior to exercise and/or 2 puffs of albuterol 5 minutes before exercise may be helpful. In addition, it is possible to take extra inhaled β_2 agonist during an intermittent sport, such as basketball. There is no satisfactory answer to the problem of pollen allergic patients who are liable to increase allergen exposure by running; masks are usually not acceptable. In some cases, masks or scarves may serve to increase the humidity of the inspired air, but this is usually unacceptable to the patient.

EMERGENCY

The Management of Asthma

The management of severe, prolonged asthma in the hospital requires extensive supportive therapy and difficult decisions about when to consider artificial ventilation. Here we are merely outlining an approach to be used in an emergency room or office (Table 1).

Parenteral use of sympathomimetics, epinephrine in particular, has been the mainstay of therapy. It has now been adequately demonstrated that inhaled β agonists are quite effective for first-line treatment. They will replace epinephrine because of their advantage of decreased systemic toxicity. These inhaled agents are easy to administer and their prolonged duration of

TABLE 1 Emergency Treatment of Asthma

1. Nebulized bronchodilator (0.3 ml Alupent in 4 ml saline) (or SC epinephrine, 0.3 ml of 1:1000). Repeated 2 or 3 times at 30-min intervals.
2. Aminophylline IV, 250-mg bolus then 0.4 mg/kg/h (blood level within 12 hours)
3. Steroids IV (or oral); 300 mg hydrocortisone IV every 6 hours if severe or no improvement within 3 hours
4. Assess need for admission

Additional: Humidified oxygen, rehydration
Plan for continuing treatment and follow-up
Plan for further investigation

therapy (approximately 10 minutes) may offer steady reassurance. Pressure delivery systems (IPPB) are clearly not necessary and may create additional danger for the patient, contributing to hyperinflation and the risk of pneumothorax.

Aminophylline should be added next. While it is not the most effective single drug therapy, it does promote further bronchodilation when combined with a β agonist. The combination also permits lower doses of each drug, thus minimizing toxicity. In any patient who has not received an oral preparation of a methylxanthine in the previous 24 hours, a loading bolus of 5 to 6 mg per kilogram of body weight should be given. When there is any doubt of prior intake, this dose must be adjusted downward or eliminated entirely. A maintenance infusion of aminophylline should be continued at an hourly rate which will take into account factors that decrease clearance of the drug, such as liver disease, advanced age, or congestive heart failure. Liberal hydration is important, since fluid depletion is common and contributes to inspissation of secretions. Humidified nasal oxygen generally improves the sensation of dyspnea. Steroids, because of their delayed onset of action, should be considered early. The toxicity of a single dose of hydrocortisone is minimal compared with the potential benefit that will be derived if the attack persists. In addition, no further doses need be given if improvement is seen early. Acute bronchospasm is heightened by anxiety and reassurance is an important aspect of emergency room treatment.

Several articles have suggested that the need for admission can be predicted when the patient enters the emergency room. However, these studies were generally retrospective and self-fulfilling. Prospective studies using an "index" have not been so successful. Admission has to be considered in any patient who fails to improve after 2 hours of appropriate treatment. The important features to be considered include $FEV_1 < 50$ percent predicted, peak flow < 150 L/min, tachycardia > 110, continued use of accessory muscles, abnormal blood gases, and the patient's sense of dyspnea or anxiety. All these factors require adjustment for individual cases, and it is not possible to apply fixed criteria to patients who do not have fully reversible airway obstruction.

Hospital Management

Most patients will respond within 24 hours to the regimen established in the emergency room, that is, nebulized bronchodilator every 4 hours; intravenous aminophylline, 0.4 or 0.5 mg/kg/hr; and intravenous hydrocortisone, 300 mg every 6 hours. Steroids may need to be continued for as long as 2 weeks to break some attacks. Procedures such as bronchial lavage and inhaled atropine, 1 to 2 mg every 6 hours by nebulizer may have a place in treatment of persistent severe asthma, but their role is not established. Intubation and artificial ventilation is only rarely required and is essentially a treatment for patients who are making inadequate respiratory effort with persistent or progressive hypoxia and hypercapnia. Any patient who continues to have severe obstruction—peak flow < 100, persistent tachycardia, and abnormal blood gases—requires very close observation and may well require intensive care.

CHRONIC MANAGEMENT

First Line. β_2 Agonist inhaler to be used either as necessary or 1 or 2 puffs 3 times daily and as necessary.

Second Line. Either regular use of cromolyn Spinhaler, 1 capsule 3 times daily; or beclomethasone dipropionate inhaler, 1 or 2 puffs 3 times daily; or long-acting theophylline, 300 mg 2 or 3 times daily or just at night.

Third Line. Add other second-line drug and increase doses progressively: first, β_2 agonist up to 2 puffs every 4 hours, or convert to nebulizer treatment at home; second, cromolyn increase to 2 capsules 4 times a day; third, beclomethasone up to 3 puffs 4 times a day; fourth, theophylline increase only if blood level < 10 μg/ml. If a patient requires this level of therapy, he should definitely be assessed for an allergic contribution to his asthma.

Fourth Line. Oral steroids, intermittent courses of 1 to 2 weeks or prolonged therapy.

CONCLUSIONS

Despite dramatic improvements in the drugs available to manage asthma, it is not clear that either the morbidity or mortality of the disease has been reduced. This may partly reflect the large number of patients who do not receive regular medical attention. Alternatively, it has been suggested that there has been an increase in asthma due to increased additives in diet or increased inhalant allergens in houses with fitted carpets (e.g., mites). The long-term objectives of treatment is to maintain the patient without symptoms and, if possible, with bronchial reactivity reduced to a level where severe attacks of bronchospasm are less likely. Many different treatments can achieve this control in some patients, including steroids, cromolyn, allergen avoidance, desensitization, and theophylline. Of these, theophylline and steroids have the most marked side effects. The route pursued in any particular patient will depend on his previous response to treatment, the severity of his disease, the family's ability to change their home conditions, as well as the known risks or toxicity of the treatments and the personal preference of the physician.

STATUS ASTHMATICUS

JAMES E. FISH, M.D.

Status asthmaticus has been broadly defined as a severe exacerbation of asthma refractory to medical therapy. In this context, the term refractory is used in a relative rather than an absolute sense, for in most cases the management of status asthmaticus has a successful outcome. Indeed, the mortality rate in patients hospitalized with severe asthma is estimated to be as low as 1 percent. Despite a low inpatient mortality rate, asthma remains accountable for the deaths of approximately 3000 patients each year in this country alone. What is particularly regrettable about this alarming statistic is the fact that avoidable factors are identified as responsible for the events leading up to a majority of these deaths. Among these factors are failure on the part of patients to comply with recommended therapy or to seek medical help early in the course of an exacerbation, as well as failure on the part of physicians to recognize the severity of an episode or to provide adequate treatment. Though numerous definitions have been applied to status asthmaticus, we refer to it in this discussion as severe and persistent asthma that requires prolonged and intense inpatient therapy because of failure to respond to outpatient or emergency room treatment. Because the need for hospitalization is usually established in the emergency room, it is worth reviewing those factors that are considered important in assessing the severity of an episode as well as what, in our view, constitutes an adequate therapeutic trial in the outpatient setting.

The initial clinical evaluation should include, in addition to the usual vital signs and physical examination, an assessment of accessory muscle use and general level of difficulty in breathing as well as a measurement of the degree of pulsus paradoxus. Measurements of the one-second forced expired volume (FEV_1), or peak expiratory flow rate (PEFR), and arterial blood gases should be determined to assess the level of impairment of mechanical lung function and gas exchange. Serial determinations of the latter tests are of particular value, since they provide an objective means of monitoring the response to therapy. In our experience, these objective measurements are far more reliable indicators of progress or deterioration than clinical signs and symptoms, since there is frequently a poor correlation between the level of physiologic impairment and clinical variables. The following findings are indicative of a severe and potentially fatal episode of asthma demanding immediate aggressive therapy: (1) altered mental status; (2) elevation in arterial Pco_2 (3) significant hypoxemia ($Po_2 \leq 65$ mmHg); (4) FEV_1 <25 percent of the predicted value or PEFR <150 L/min; (5) pulsus paradoxus >18 mmHg; and (6) history of previous or recurrent episodes of status asthmaticus.

Once it is established that a patient has severe asthma, aggressive therapy should begin immediately. The reversibility of an episode and the need for hospitalization are determined on the basis of the early response to this initial treatment effort. Our practice is to administer inhaled or injected sympathomimetic agents as the first line of therapy. Isoproterenol is given by inhalation as 0.5 cc of 0.5 percent solution (2.5 mg) diluted in 2 cc normal saline using a hand-held wet nebulizer every 20 minutes for 3 separate doses. If the patient is unable to use the nebulizer effectively, we give epinephrine (0.3 cc of 1:1000 dilution) by subcutaneous injection every 20 minutes for three consecutive doses. After this regimen, the patient is reevaluated clinically and by spirometry. Those showing symptomatic improvement with an increase in the FEV_1 to within 40 percent of the predicted value will generally continue to improve, provided aggressive therapy is continued in the outpatient setting. Those failing to demonstrate clinical improvement with an increase in FEV_1 to within 40 percent of predicted value are considered refractory and in need of hospitalization for an intensified and extended treatment regimen as well as for close observation in the case of further deterioration and acute respiratory failure.

The principal agents used in chemotherapy for status asthmaticus fall into three major drug classes: sympathomimetics, methylxanthines, and corticosteroids. While these same medications are commonly used for outpatient management of asthma, their usage in status asthmaticus differs chiefly in terms of dose, frequency, and route of administration. Sympathomimetic agents and methylxanthines are generally viewed as bronchodilators, and as such benefit the patient by reducing airway smooth muscle constriction. Experimental evidence indicates, however, that these agents may also contribute to the therapeutic process by facilitating mobilization of secretions and by inhibiting release of inflammatory mediators that promote edema of airways and cause smooth muscle contraction. Although the precise mechanism of corticosteroid action is unknown, steroids are generally thought to reduce the inflammatory component of airway obstruction, and there is evidence that they may also enhance the effect of sympathomimetic drugs.

Some authors have stated that patients with status asthmaticus are by definition refractory to sympathomimetic drugs and that continued use of these agents in this setting is either controversial or unsound. While repeated administration of beta-adrenergic agents may result in a decrease in receptor activity in some experimental systems, there is no evidence that significant drug tolerance develops at the clinical level with regard to bronchodilator activity. It is our view that sympathomimetic agents are central to proper management of status asthmaticus, and failure to use them in this condition is unsound practice. Because of worsening symptoms, most patients admit to using inhaled or oral sympathomimetic bronchodilators with increasing frequency before coming to the hospital. Thus, it is conceivable that at the time of admission these patients have already achieved maximum bronchodilatation in terms of attainable smooth muscle relaxation. The lack of an immediate response to sympathomimetics in this situation should suggest that the predominant elements of obstruction at the time are related to other pathophysiologic processes, such as mucous accumulation and mucosal edema; it should not suggest drug tolerance. Continued use of these agents is strongly recommended, not only as a means of maintaining and promoting further smooth muscle relaxation, but also because these drugs may inhibit mediator release and enhance mucociliary clearance mechanisms.

We have found that isoproterenol in a dose of 2.5 mg by aerosol can be administered hourly for several hours after the initial three treatments in young and otherwise healthy adult asthmatics. Thereafter, the interval between treatments should be extended to 3 to 4 hours. If pulmonary function fails to improve after the first 24 hours of therapy, the initial regimen may be gradually increased from 2.5 mg up to 5 mg by aerosol, as long as the heart rate does not exceed 150/min. Alternatively, metaproterenol inhalant solution (5%) may be given as 0.3 ml in 2.5 ml saline every 2 hours for a period of 24 hours or longer. The most common side effects from nebulized sympathomimetics are palpitations, nervousness, nausea, headache, and tremor. We have found extrasystoles to be uncommon, and in general, the cardiovascular complications are minimal in relation to the benefits achieved. Indeed, overall improvement in airway function may lead to a reduction in patient stress with a lowering of the heart rate and blood pressure.

Methylxanthines have been used in the treatment of asthma for well over a half century and remain a critical element in successful management. The major effect of methylxanthines is bronchodilatation through relaxation of airway smooth muscle, although there is evidence that theophylline can also increase mucociliary transport mechanisms and hence facilitate mobilization of secretions. Moreover, recent work has shown that aminophylline can increase diaphragmatic strength and suppress muscle fatigue in patients with airway obstruction. This latter effect may very well be an important component of the overall benefit of aminophylline therapy, especially in the patient at risk of developing acute respiratory failure from fatigue. Theophylline itself is relatively insoluble in aqueous solution and is therefore administered as the ethylenediamine salt, aminophylline, which contains 80 percent theophylline by weight.

Our approach is first to administer a loading dose of 5.6 mg/kg by intravenous bolus over a 20-minute interval. In patients already taking theophylline-containing compounds as outpatients, the loading dose is reduced by one-half. This is followed by a maintenance dose of 0.6 mg/kg/hr given by continuous intravenous infusion. It should be noted that the preceding maintenance dose has been calculated to achieve therapeutic levels in otherwise healthy adults under the age of 50 years. In older patients we use a continuous infusion of 0.4 mg/kg/hr and in patients with congestive heart failure or liver dysfunction we reduce the maintenance infusion rate to 0.2 to 0.3 mg/kg/hr. These maintenance dosage schedules are recommended only as general guidelines, since there is considerably interpatient variability in theophylline metabolism; subsequent modifications in dose may be required based on serum theophylline levels. Our pratice is to obtain theophylline levels approximately 6 to 8 hours after the initial infusion to verify that excess levels have not been achieved. Further adjustments in dose should be made to achieve equilibrium blood levels between 15 and 20 μg/ml within the first 24 hours. Because of dose-dependent changes in pharmacokinetics, incremental changes in the theophylline infusion rate should be made cautiously to avoid toxicity. Our approach is to increase the infusion rate by an increment of 0.1 mg/kg/hr until the desired blood level is attained. Nausea and vomiting are reported to be among the leading manifestations of theophylline toxicity. We have found that irritability, restlessness, and headache are also early manifestations. When these occur, the theophylline level should be documented and the maintenance infusion rate should be decreased to avoid more serious toxic effects, including hallucinations, convulsions, and life-threatening arrhythmias.

In our experience, successful management almost always requires the use of corticosteroids. Controlled studies have shown that patients who fail to demonstrate a rapid response to sympathomimetics in the emergency room also tend to respond poorly to continued sympathomimetic and aminophylline therapy over the next 24 hours unless they are treated concomitantly with corticosteriods. It is important to remember that the therapeutic effects of steroids are not immediate; rather, the response is slow, often taking as long as 6 to 8 hours to achieve an appreciable effect. Accordingly, we recommend strongly that steroid therapy not be delayed. It should be started as soon as refractoriness to sympathomimetics and the need for hospitalization are recognized. Delays in the start of this therapy will not only place the patient in jeopardy by prolonging the risks of status asthmaticus, but it may also unnecessarily prolong the duration of inpatient management.

The recommended corticosteroid doses for status asthmaticus are largely empiric, since controlled studies to establish optimal doses have not been carried out. Most dose regimens recommended in the literature have proven efficacious, though it is not known whether lower doses would be equally effective. It is our practice to administer methylprednisolone, 40 to 60 mg every 6 hours IV. Alternatively, hydrocortisone, 100 to 200 mg every 4 hours IV is equally effective, but it produces more sodium retention and potassium excretion. The acute toxicity of these high doses, except for potassium wasting with hydrocrotisone, is generally no greater than that observed with substantially smaller doses, so it is our policy to be aggressive in the use of steroids in patients with potentially life-threatening asthma.

Most patients will begin to show definite signs of clinical recovery within 24 to 48 hours after the above treatment regimen has been instituted. It should be anticipated, however, that occasionally a patient will fail to show signs of satisfactory progress over this interval. In these instances, we merely recommend perseverance with the same intensive measures for a more prolonged interval. In these relatively resistant patients, we have found that aerosolized atropine is sometimes helpful, although there are no controlled clinical trials that establish the therapeutic value of this approach. As a parasympatholytic agent, atropine is capable of reducing that component of bronchoconstriction due to vagal stimulation. Atropine is also a potent inhibitor of exocrine gland function, but earlier concerns that it could produce a "drying effect" and increase the risk of retained secretions are probably exaggerated. Most evidence indicates that anticholinergic therapy has no significant effect on sputum volume or viscosity when used in the treatment of asthma. Our current practice is to administer 1 mg of atropine sulfate in 1 ml saline every 4 to 6 hours, alternating with either isoproterenol or metaproterenol nebulization. Side effects of therapy include dryness of mouth, thirst, tachycardia, and mydriasis. It should also be noted that anticholinergic drugs are contraindicated in patients with glaucoma, especially narrow-angle glaucoma, and they may cause urinary retention in patients with prostatic hypertrophy.

As indicated earlier, we strongly urge that objective measurements of gas exchange and lung mechanics be used to monitor the response to therapy. For example, if on initial examination the patient is found to have carbon dioxide retention and acute respiratory failure, serial blood gas determinations will be necessary for proper management. Patients with significant hypoxemia (Po_2 <65 mmHg) are routinely given low-flow oxygen by nasal cannula, and subsequent blood gas determinations are made if there are signs of further deterioration. We routinely measure the FEV_1 or PEFR in all patients undergoing treatment for severe asthma and use serial measurements to monitor the response to therapy. In severely obstructed and distressed patients, the latter measurements of forced expiration may be difficult to obtain, but as recovery begins most patients are able to perform the required forced expiratory maneuvers satisfactorily.

In general, we begin to taper therapy when patients show objective signs of functional improvement. For example, when the FEV_1 returns to approximately 50 percent of the expected value, intravenous therapy is discontinued and the patient is placed on an oral regimen of 60 mg of prednisone or its equivalent as a single daily dose. At that time the patient is also switched from intravenous aminophylline to a long-acting theophylline preparation. Aggressive therapy with inhaled sympathomimetics is continued, however. Care must be taken to ensure that adequate theophylline levels are maintained when switching from the parenteral to the oral route. Further tapering of oral corticosteroids is carried out according to the needs and response of the patient. Other medications that the patient may have been taking prior to the severe episode, such as cromolyn sodium or topical corticosteroids, may be reinstituted as the dose of prednisone is tapered below 40 mg per day.

Not infrequently, we encounter asthmatic patients who even at their very best have significant impairment of lung function due to a seemingly irreversible component of their disease. When these patients experience severe acute exacerbations, we apply the same aggressive treatment measures described above. Tapering of medications after signs of clinical improvement, however, is done much more cautiously. In general, we tend to continue aggressive inpatient therapy until the FEV_1 improves to the highest attainable level.

A number of ancillary measures have been applied in the management of status asthmaticus, and while most of these procedures are of questionable value as standard treatment measures, some have merit in specific clinical situations. Antibiotic therapy, for example, is indicated when there is reasonable clinical evidence of bacterial infection. Though it was once common practice to use antibiotics routinely in status asthmaticus, it is now known that bacterial infection is a rare precipitating factor. We use a broad-spectrum antibiotic, such as ampicillin, erythromycin, or trimethoprim sulfamethoxazole, if the patient presents with clinical or laboratory signs of bacterial infection. These include spiking fever, purulent sputum, or an infiltrate on the chest radiograph. It should be noted that eosinophils can impart the characteristic discoloration of sputum purulence, so it is important to establish by appropriate microscopic examination that discoloration is due to a predominance of polymorphonuclear leukocytes. In our experience, sputum cultures are rarely helpful, and these are not performed unless the patient has signs of sepsis or there is a defined infiltrate on the chest radiograph.

In general, we have found no use for intermittent positive pressure breathing (IPPB) or chest physiotherapy in patients with status asthmaticus. The administration of IPPB therapy with saline alone may increase bronchospasm as well as compromise cardiac output and risk barotrauma due to high inflation pressure. Moreover, there is no evidence that IPPB offers advantages over simple hand-held wet nebulizers for delivering aerosolized bronchodilators. Chest physiotherapy is poorly tolerated by exhausted and distressed patients during the acute phases of an episode and may only serve to cause further distress and anxiety. On the other hand, physical measures, such as chest clapping and vibration, may be life-saving procedures in the event of mucus impaction of a major airway, an uncommon but serious complication of asthma. Signs of mucus impaction of a major airway include a sudden increase in work of breathing, rapid deterioration in gas exchange, and lobar atelectasis on the chest radiograph. If physical measures are unsuccessful, fiberoptic bronchoscopy may be indicated to remove a mucus impaction.

A number of measures have also been promoted as being useful for mobilizing respiratory secretions. Maintaining a normal state of hydration is important in the overall care of the asthmatic patient, but there is no evidence that "pushing fluids" or overhydration facilitates transport of secretions. Likewise, there is no firm evidence that expectorants or mucolytic agents that decrease mucus viscoelasticity aid in the recovery process. Mucolytic agents, such as N-acetylcystine, can be irritating to the airways and because of their unpleasant smell they may produce nausea and vomiting.

It should be emphasized that the use of sedatives has no place in the treatment of status asthmaticus. The anxiety and distress experienced by patients are a consequence of the increased work of breathing imposed by obstructed airways and are best treated by relief of obstruction. Sedatives can blunt respiratory responsiveness and lead to alveolar hypoventilation and acute respiratory failure.

The indications for mechanical ventilatory support in status asthmaticus include progressive or unremitting hypercarbia and severe deterioration in mental status. In our experience, the need for mechanical assistance is rare if the treatment measures described above are administered in aggressive and timely fashion. If therapy is adequate, hypercarbia rarely develops in patients with initial P_{CO_2} levels less than 35 mmHg. Moreover, mild to moderate elevations in P_{CO_2} frequently normalize in the early stages of treatment. Mechanical ventilatory support and its attendant complications can therefore be avoided in patients with hypercarbia if they are alert, show good respiratory effort, and the response to therapy is carefully monitored by serial arterial blood gases. The major complications of mechanical ventilation in severe asthma are related to the high inflation pressures needed to overcome the resistive and elastic load imposed by obstructed airways in an already overdistended lung. These include pneumothorax, pneumomediastinum, and hypotension. The risk of these complications can be minimized by adjusting the ventilator settings so that adequate alveolar ventilation is achieved at the lowest possible inflation pressure. In this case, adequate alveolar ventilation does not imply achieving normal P_{CO_2} levels; rather, the goal is to maintain adequate oxygenation and to prevent more severe hypercarbia and acidosis. In patients with an arterial blood pH less than 7.29, sodium bicarbonate may be administered in a dose of 44 mEq at 30-minute intervals until the pH is above 7.30. It is not necessary, however, to restore pH to a normal value.

If mechanical ventilatory support is required, intubation should be performed with the largest endotracheal tube that can be inserted safely to minimize expiratory resistance and to facilitate suctioning of the airway. The respiratory rate should be adjusted to as slow a rate as possible to allow sufficient time for the expiratory phase of the respiratory cycle and to avoid further air trapping. If sedation is required to control agitation, tachypnea, and dissynchronous breathing while the patient is on ventilatory assistance, diazepam is preferred to morphine, since the latter has histamine-releasing properties. Pancuronium bromide in combination with diazepam is recommended if it is necessary to paralyze the patient completely.

Although this discussion has focused primarily on management of the acute phase of status asthmaticus, the importance of treatment during the recovery phase must also be stressed. The underlying pathologic processes that initially contribute to a severe exacerbation generally require an extended period of treatment for complete resolution. In the early stages of recovery, patients frequently manifest wide swings in clinical and physiologic status, suffering persistent cough and intermittent episodes of bronchospasm as signs that the underlying inflammatory component of the disease, though resolving, is still present. During the recovery phase, we monitor the FEV_1 daily and continue aggressive therapy with maximum doses of bronchodilators and oral corticosteriods until bronchospastic episodes are completely controlled and the FEV_1 is at or near the highest achievable level. Successful management of status asthmaticus does not end at the time of hospital discharge. Most patients will require continued aggressive therapy, including steroids, for a variable interval after discharge to complete the recovery process. While the risks associated with high-dose medications, especially corticosteroids, must always be borne in mind, it is emphasized that early withdrawal of drug therapy is one of the more common causes of readmission for status asthmaticus.

FOOD ALLERGY IN ADULTS

STANLEY P. GALANT, M.D.

Few areas in medicine are associated with as much controversy as food allergy. A comprehensive report by the NIAID task force, entitled *Adverse Reactions to Foods*, has been recently published and is a major contribution in this regard. Although adverse reactions to foods are thought to be common in the adult population, the incidence of true food allergy is estimated at 0.1 percent. Nonetheless, food-induced reactions comprise an important medical problem which must be dealt with by the practicing clinician. Review of the current pertinent literature provides several important concepts which should be considered in managing the patient with an adverse reaction to foods.

Food allergy tends to decrease with age, so that adults have a lower incidence than children. Furthermore, food allergy may also diminish with continued avoidance of the food allergen. Most reactions to foods are not immunologically mediated. The term *food allergy* should be reserved only for those reactions which can be shown to have an immunologic basis. Foods can also cause symptoms by pharmacologic and metabolic pathways and they can contain toxins. Examples are shown in Table 1. These nonimmunologic reactions should be called *food intolerance* to distinguish their mechanism of action. Clinical manifestations, however, can be very similar in these two broad categories, a basis for much of the existing confusion.

The diagnosis of food allergy requires two criteria. First, the suspected food should reproducibly induce allergic-type symptoms. These include, in approximate order of decreasing frequency, gastrointestinal (vomiting, diarrhea, abdominal pain), dermatologic (eczema, urticaria), and respiratory (rhinorrhea, bronchospasm) symptoms, and rarely, anaphylaxis. Vague symptoms, such as headache, tension, fatigue, and depression, have no proven association with food allergy, although symptoms—particularly headache—may be exacerbated by certain foods by other mechanisms. Second, an immunologic mechanism must be demonstrated, usually by skin test or radioallergosorbent test (RAST), for specific IgE antibodies. Proof of other immunologic mechanisms (immune complexes or cell-mediated immunity) could also fulfill their criterion. Gluten-induced enteropathy and dermatitis herpetiformis may be examples of several of these immunologic mechanisms. These concepts will be explored in more detail below.

TABLE 1 Important Causes of Food Intolerance

Additives and Contaminants
Dyes
Tartrazine
Flavorings and preservatives
Nitrites and nitrates
Monosodium glutamate
Sulfiting agents
Sodium benzoate
Toxins
Histamine intoxication — scombroid fish (tuna and mackerel)
Endogenous Pharmacologic Agents
Caffeine
Theobromine
Histamine
Tyramine
Phenylethylamine
Alcohol
Enzyme Deficiency
Lactase deficiency

TABLE 2 Food Groups of Allergenic Importance

Plant (Families)	
Citrus — oranges, lemons, grapefruit	
Cola nut — chocolate, cola	
Gourd — melons, cucumbers, squash, pumpkin	
Grass — corn, wheat, rye, oats, rice	
Laurel — cinnamon, bay leaf	
Lily — onion, garlic, asparagus	
Mustard — cabbage, broccoli, mustard, cauliflower, brussel sprout	
Nightshade — tomato, potato	
Pea — peanuts, peas, beans (including soybean, alfalfa, clover, licorice)	
Pepper — black pepper	
Plum — plums, peaches, apricots, almonds	
Rose — strawberry, raspberry	
Sunflower — lettuce, artichoke, sunflower	
Animal (Listed by phylum, family or class as appropriate)	
Mollusks — abalone, clams, oysters, scallops, mussels	Shellfish
Crustaceans — shrimp, lobster, crab	Shellfish
Fish (common families) — flounder, halibut, cod, trout, tuna, salmon (bony fish)	
Birds — turkey, chicken, duck (including egg)	
Mammals — cow, goat, sheep, pig (including milk)	

Source: Adapted from Speer, 1973

DIAGNOSIS

Elimination Diets

Using the diagnostic criteria described for food allergy, several approaches have been employed. First, one must reproducibly demonstrate that elimination of the suspected food results in termination of symptoms and challenge in exacerbation. Selection of the appropriate food for testing requires detective work. A careful history of frequently eaten foods, including hidden foods which may not be suspected (such as egg in mayonnaise), and symptom pattern may reveal a cause-and-effect relationship, particularly if reactions occur within 2 hours after ingestion. Details regarding quantity and food preparation (for example, cooked or uncooked) and other factors, including potential relationship to exercise, concomitant respiratory infection, or pollen season, should be noted.

Knowledge of major food families is important, since cross-reactivity within botanical groups, for example, can occur, and this may suggest a particular food (for example, peanut and other legumes) (Table 2). If symptoms occur infrequently, a food diary over a suitable time period may be useful. Foods eaten on days when symptoms occur should be compared with foods eaten on asymptomatic days. Foods suspected by these techniques are then eliminated for 2 to 3 weeks. A detailed list of foods to avoid, including hidden foods and those permitted, is provided and explained in detail. A medication and symptom score should be kept for this elimination period and compared with a baseline period of approximately 1 to 2 weeks before the elimination diet is started. If significant improvement occurs (≥ 50 percent reduction in symptoms and medication requirements) during the elimination phase, foods are reintroduced singly at 5- to 7-day intervals and exacerbation evaluated. This should be repeated at least once to demonstrate reproducibility. If no improvement occurs or the results are equivocal, and elimination has been adequate, a regular diet is restored, and symptoms and medication scores again compared, since a combination of foods (assuming more than one food is involved) rather than a single food could cause symptoms. Foods known to cause anaphylactic reactions are not tested in this manner.

Reactions occurring up to 2 hours after ingestion are very suggestive of an IgE allergic reaction. However, foods may cause symptoms after 2 hours, and perhaps up to 2 days after ingestion. These "delayed onset" food reactions are thought to be mediated by immune complexes or cell-mediated immunity where an immunologic mechanism could be demonstrated. In this type of reaction, the patient is often unaware of which foods are involved.

Selection of an appropriate elimination diet is based on the probability that frequently implicated foods may be causative in these cases. In most centers, these foods include cow's milk, egg, wheat, corn, fish, pork, citrus, tomatoes, and legumes. Our basic elimination diet, which avoids these foods, is shown in Table 3. In a particularly difficult or severe case, we have used an elemental diet, such as Vivonex, with success. The duration of these elimination diets is generally 2 to 3 weeks, if possible. If no significant improvement occurs within this period, one can reasonably assume that foods are not a major cause of the allergic manifestations. Food challenges are carried out as described above, with each single food group at 5- to 7-day intervals, in conjunction with clinical monitoring. Although very laborious, this is the most useful method currently available for suspected food allergy.

More recently, the use of a double-blind technique with dried food in gelatin capsules has been shown to trace allergy objectively to several foods in an experimental setting. Foods selected for study generally are reported to cause symptoms within 2 hours of ingestion and give positive prick skin tests. This method remains experimental, with few studies in the adult population. It may prove useful if history, skin tests, and elimination diet fail to result in a diagnosis.

TABLE 3 Basic Elimination Diet

Food and Beverages Allowed	
Meat and Poultry	Beef, lamb, chicken, turkey (no hens)
Vegetables	Carrots, squash, potato, sweet potato, cauliflower, lettuce, beets, broccoli, celery
Fruit	Fresh, frozen, or water-packed apples, pears, bananas, plums, peaches, apricots
Grains	Tapioca, potato flour, arrowroot, buckwheat, rice
Eliminate	
All foods not listed above, including coffee, tea, soft drinks, chewing gum, toothpaste, vitamins	

Immunologic Testing

Skin Testing. The usefulness of skin testing for food allergy remains controversial. However, the prick-puncture method with potent (1:20 weight per volume) food antigen would appear useful for two reasons. First, a positive response (wheal ≥ 3 mm above control) suggests an individual is atopic, and therefore, the symptoms may be caused by allergy. Second, the demonstration of specific IgE in the skin, particularly to nuts, egg, milk, soy, and fish, may be clinically relevant, and helps select foods for the elimination diet. It should be emphasized that diagnosis of food allergy requires both the demonstration of symptoms with food challenge and a positive skin test to that allergen. Intradermal skin testing is not recommended, since specificity appears too low to be clinically useful, and in some cases, it may be dangerous. In the absence of demonstrable IgE antibodies, the diagnosis of allergy would require other immunologic mechanisms, such as the presence of specific immune complexes or cell-mediated immune reaction to clinically relevant food allergens.

In Vitro Testing. There is little indication for *in vitro* testing for the presence of IgE antibodies by RAST, ELISA, or basophil histamine release techniques in most cases of food allergy. Skin tests are more sensitive, more rapid, less expensive, and the selection of allergen greater than with RAST, for example. The latter might be useful in those cases in which anaphylaxis might occur with skin testing, or the patient has extensive eczema, and in which avoidance of antihistamines might be difficult.

Controversial techniques for the diagnosis of food allergy, including leukocyte cytotoxic test and food antigen provocation by sublingual, intracutaneous, or subcutaneous routes, have been reviewed by the American Academy of Allergy. From existing studies, they have concluded that these techniques have not been proven effective. Until well-controlled studies have demonstrated their validity, they remain of questionable value.

THERAPY

Avoidance

As is true for all allergen-induced processes, avoidance of known allergens is fundamental. In this regard, a list of specific foods to avoid and those which can be eaten is critical for each patient. Patients should be careful when eating out, and must learn to read labels for foods to which they are particularly sensitive. However, many patients may be able to tolerate small quantities of these foods, particularly if they have been avoided for some time. Patients will frequently establish their tolerance to each food and adhere to it. Even if the patient is quite sensitive, careful reintroduction under the physician's guidance should be tried after a 6- to 12-month period of avoidance. Food challenges should be tried only in the doctor's office, if previous reactions were severe. Rotating foods every 3 to 5 days may be useful to decrease the likelihood of developing new allergies to foods or redeveloping old ones. Any elimination diet should be palatable and nutritionally adequate. If this proves difficult in patients with multiple allergies, a dietitian can prove useful in planning nutritious, attractive menus, even with a rather limited selection of foods.

Pharamacologic Therapy

Although food avoidance is usually effective when completely implemented, there are situations in which drugs may be a necessary adjunct. Examples include acute anaphylaxis and atopic symptoms such as asthma and chronic urticaria. Furthermore, preventive agents may be potentially useful.

Patients who experience anaphylactic reactions must be taught to use epinephrine and to take H_1 antihistamines at the first sign of a reaction. The use of preloaded syringes designed to deliver multiple set doses of epinephrine (0.3 ml per dose) (ANA-Kit, Hollister-Stier Laboratories) can be lifesaving. An antihistamine is also provided in the kit. An epinephrine autoinjector (EpiPen, Center Laboratories) also delivers 0.3 ml per dose and may make injections easier for the patient. These agents must be carried at all times. The treatment of atopic symptoms is symptomatic and does not differ from inhaled-induced disease.

Disodium cromoglycate (DSC) is a unique preventive drug which inhibits mast cell degranulation if administered before allergen challenge. Several clinical studies support the view that an adequate dosage of DSC can prevent the clinical manifestations of IgE mediated food allergy. However, the appropriate dosage and proper timing before feeding remain to be determined. Furthermore, the nonlactose preparation for oral usage is not yet commercially available. Therefore, the role of DSC in preventing food allergy remains to be established. Ketotifen, a drug with both antihistaminic and antianaphylactic properties, also shows promise in inhibiting IgE mediated food reactions, but more controlled studies are necessary to determine its clinical usefulness.

Immunotherapy

There are no controlled studies showing the efficacy of classic immunotherapy with food antigens as there are with inhalant allergy. Furthermore, oral desensitization and sublingual and subcutaneous neutralization techniques have not been shown effective to date. Therefore, these modalities cannot be recommended for the treatment of food allergy.

SULFITE-INDUCED ASTHMA

DONALD D. STEVENSON, M.D.
RONALD A. SIMON, M.D.

Sulfites, in the form of sodium and potassium salts, free sulfite ions (water-soluble form), and sulfur dioxide (gaseous form) are ubiquitous in the human environment. Sulfites are widely used in the food, beverage, and pharmaceutical industries as fresheners, antioxidants, and preservatives. Sulfur dioxide SO_2 is produced when sulfur-containing petroleum products are burned. Dietary protein contains small amounts of sulfur in certain amino acids, and these, as well as endogenous proteins, are metabolized to sulfites, then sulfates, where they are excreted in the urine.

Using double blind challenge procedures, we reported in October 1981 that ingested sulfite salts produced asthmatic attacks in selected asthmatic subjects. This finding has been confirmed by others. Since these original observations, the following facts have emerged:

1. Only a small number of asthmatics give a history of severe asthma while eating restaurant meals. In such individuals, double blind placebo controlled sulfite challenges, with dosages of potassium metabisulfite between 5 and 50 mg, stimulate asthmatic attacks.
2. Approximately 5 to 10 percent of all asthmatics develop asthma 10 to 15 minutes after ingesting sulfite salts in dosages between 50 and 200 mg.
3. All asthmatics wheeze after inhalation of SO_2 in 1 to 5 ppm concentrations.
4. A few asthmatics experience bronchoconstriction, rather than bronchodilation, after inhaling β-agonist solutions which contain sulfites.
5. Rarely, asthmatics develop asthma and even shock after injections of sulfite-containing pharmaceutical solutions.
6. Except for one reported case of anaphylaxis associated with angioedema, and isolated reports of urticaria associated with sulfite ingestion, sulfites have not been proven to adversely affect other patient populations. Generalized cutaneous flushing does occur during severe asthmatic reactions to sulfites. Normal individuals, ingesting huge doses of sulfites, may experience nausea, flushing, diapheresis, and headache.

PATHOPHYSIOLOGY

Inhalation of SO_2 stimulates afferent parasympathetic tracheobronchial receptors, which induces cholinergic reflex asthma. Inhalation of pharmaceutic solutions that contain sulfites generates SO_2 during aerosolization. However, since asthmatic reactions occur following the ingestion of sulfites contained in capsules, SO_2 inhalation is excluded as the potential mechanism in the pathogenesis of all oral sulfite-provoked asthmatic attacks. Presumably, soluble sulfites travel to bronchial tissues via the bloodstream.

Sulfite oxidase is an essential oxidative enzyme in the conversion of active sulfite to inactive sulfate. In severely sensitive asthmatics a relative deficiency of this enzyme has been identified in many of the patients studied. A hypothetical mechanism to explain sulfite sensitivity is that ingested sulfite loads are normally cleared by sulfite oxidase in normal individuals and nonsulfite-sensitive asthmatics. If an individual is partially deficient in the oxidative enzyme and also has asthma (cholinergic sensitivity), sulfite loads, presented to the bronchial tissue, activate cholinergic afferent receptors. Most sulfite-sensitive subjects have negative skin tests to sulfite solutions. However, 2 patients (one asthmatic) have been reported to have positive skin tests. Therefore, the possibility of an IgE mediated mechanism cannot be completely excluded in all such patients.

CLINICAL PROFILES OF SULFITE-SENSITIVE ASTHMATICS

Two profiles have been observed in asthmatics who are sensitive to sulfite by oral challenge.

Severe Group

Severely sulfite-sensitive patients give a history of severe asthma, with or without shock and flushing, while eating a meal in a restaurant or after drinking wine or beer. The reaction is dose dependent. In the laboratory, 1 to 50 mg of sulfite salts in capsules or a solution, when swallowed, will produce a fall in FEV_1 values greater than or equal to 25 percent 10 to 15 minutes later. Restaurant meals may contain up to 400 mg of sulfite. Deaths in restaurants may, on occasion, be due to this reaction. The number of patients who are highly sensitive is relatively small, with approximately 40 having been identified and reported in the literature. This subgroup of asthmatics have severe corticosteroid-dependent asthma even when they are avoiding ingested sulfites. Smog and other inhaled sources of SO_2 stimulate increased asthma. Such patients have vasomotor rhinitis, low serum IgE levels, and largely negative wheal and flare cutaneous responses to injected allergen extracts including foods. In a study from Australia, a few sulfite-sensitive asthmatics were reported to be cross-sensitive to aspirin, tartrazine, and monosodium glutamate. We have not been able to document such cross-sensitivities in the sulfite-sensitive asthmatics studied at the Scripps Clinic.

Moderate Group

During capsule sulfite challenges, approximately 5 to 10 percent of adult asthmatic patients develop mild to moderate bronchospasm 10 to 20 minutes after ingesting 50 to 200 mg of sulfite salts. This group appears to be less sensitive than the severe group (larger provoking dose and smaller fall in FEV_1) and generally does not experience flush or shock when exposed to larger doses of sulfites found in restaurant meals.

Other than having asthma, these patients do not exhibit any distinguishing characteristics. Some do recall mild asthma after ingesting wine or beer or while eating in a restaurant. However, in many the signs of asthma are mild enough to be either ignored or treated with a sympathomimetic inhaler in the restaurant. The connection between ingestion of sulfites and onset of asthma activity is only infrequently observed. Recently, asthmatics have been identified who react only to sulfites swished in the mouth as solutions and do not react to ingestion of capsules.

Reactors to Sulfites in the Pharmaceuticals

Sulfites are widely used as antioxidants by the pharmaceutical industry. At the same time we reported on asthmatics with sensitivity to ingested sulfites, investigators in Australia found asthmatics sensitive to sulfites in medications delivered parenterally. Since that report, an additional patient has been described with severe asthma and respiratory insufficiency following the intravenous administration of metachlopramide (Reglan). Table 1 contains a partial list of medications that contain sulfites. Of particular interest to physicians who care for asthmatics are a number of commonly used bronchodilator solutions, which are discussed below. Sulfites are also contained

TABLE 1 Partial List of Medications Containing Sulfites

Type of Agent	*Common Names*
Bronchodilator solutions	Bronkosol, Alupent, Isuprel, Metaprel, Vaponefrin
Epinephrine	Adrenalin
Local anesthetics	Xylocaine (lidocaine), Novocain (procaine)
Corticosteroids	Decadron, Hydrocortone (Hydrocortisone), Celestone
Antibiotics	Garamycin (gentamicin), Amikin (amikacin), Nebcin (tobramycin)
Analgesics	Demerol
Antishock	Intropin (dopamine), Aramine (metaraminol), Levophed
Eye drops	Pred Mild, Pred Forte, sulfacetamide, prednisolone, dexamethasone
Solutions for total nutrition and dialysis, Thorazine, others	

in medications, such as epinephrine and local anesthetics, which are administered subcutaneously, and a number of intravenous preparations, including corticosteroids (Decadron and Celestone), antibiotics, antiarrhythmic medications, and others. A serious problem occurs if a sulfite-sensitive asthmatic is found in shock and given one of the pressors listed in Table 1.

In double blind, placebo-controlled provocation challenges, we have found that the inhalation of sulfite solutions produces reactions in all subjects with ingested sulfite sensitivity. The dose of sulfite required to produce reactions by inhalation was a mere fraction of the oral provoking dose and significantly less than the levels of sulfites found in the usual doses of preparations such as Bronkosol and Isuprel solutions. Alupent solution in multidose vials contains only 0.1 mg per milliliter of sulfite, which is below the threshold of all sulfite-sensitive asthmatics which we have tested. However, this may not be the case for the 2 reported sulfite-sensitive asthmatics with paradoxic responses to inhaled β-agonist solutions.

We have not been able to provoke bronchospasm in sulfite-sensitive asthmatics when sulfite is administered subcutaneously. This may be because the oral provoking dose is usually not achieved during subcutaneous challenges, owing to local discomfort at the site of the injection. Some of our extremely sulfite-sensitive patients have reached or exceeded their oral provoking dose by subcutaneous administration and experienced only mild reactions; others experienced no adverse effects. Therefore, the levels of sulfites contained in the usual doses of epinephrine and local anesthetics (1 mg/ml), when injected subcutaneously into sulfite-sensitive asthmatics, have not provoked bronchospasm.

Although not tested, the levels of sulfites found in intravenous medications are likely to be major problems for many sulfite-sensitive asthmatics based on studies in the literature. Since we estimate that approximately 5 to 10 percent of the asthmatic population is sulfite sensitive, such asthmatics and their physicians must carefully examine the content of all medications which might be administered. It should also be noted that sulfites are not found in the metered dose inhalers that asthmatics routinely use. Likewise, we are not aware of sulfites being used to preserve oral pharmaceutical preparations (tablets and capsules) such as theophylline, β-agonists or antihistamines/decongestants.

Inhalation Reactors to Sulfites

A specific profile for this group of asthmatics does not exist, and indeed, the criteria for inclusion in this group have not been satisfactorily defined. Since all asthmatics are sensitive to inhalation of SO_2 in 1 to 5 ppm concentrations, and since aerosolization of many standard β-agonist solutions produces up to 5 to 10 ppm SO_2, it is likely that all asthmatics undergo stimulation of cholinergic afferent tracheobronchial receptors during inhalation of isoproterenol, isoetharine, metaproterenol, and epinephrine. However, despite stimulation of afferent cholinergic fibers and activation of the entire cholinergic reflex arc, bronchospasm is usually prevented by the simultaneous inhalation of potent β-agonists. Thus, adverse effects are rarely observed. In fact, solutions of β-agonists produce bronchodilatation in both sulfite-sensitive and sulfite-insensitive asthmatics. Interestingly, an asthmatic reaction induced by oral challenge with sulfite can be routinely reversed with solutions of isoetharine containing sulfite. There are 2 reported cases of asthmatics who had paradoxic responses to inhaled β-agonist solutions that contained sulfites. These patients appeared to have exquisite sensitivity to inhaled sulfites or SO_2, perhaps overriding the bronchodilatory effects of the associated β-agonist.

Treatment of Sulfite-Induced Asthmatic Attacks

Asthmatic and even systemic anaphylactoid events produced by sulfites are remarkably responsive to intervention with standard adrenergic bronchodilators. Whether by inhalation or injection, β-agonists reverse the reaction within minutes after intervention in most instances. It seems prudent to use sulfite-free pharmaceuticals whenever possible. For example, metaproterenol solutions are now available in single-dose vials without sulfites. Terbutaline is also available in single-dose vials which do not contain sulfites, and can be safely used for subcutaneous or inhalation treatment. For known sensitive restaurant reactors ($K_2S_2O_5$ ingestion of 1–50 mg) it is prudent to teach self injection of epinephrine (or Epi-pen) or terbutaline.

If treatment with sulfite-free β-agonists is ineffective in reversing what is alleged to be a sulfite-provoked asthma attack, the astute clinician should suspect that another stimulus to asthma may be in effect. For instance, aspirin-induced asthmatic reactions are relatively resistant to adrenergic drugs. Standard measures for treatment of unresponsive asthma should be employed, including oxygen fluids, theophylline, and intravenous methylprednisolone. If shock is present, avoid pressors with sulfite preservatives, such as dopamine (Intropin) or metaraminol (Aramine).

PREVENTION OF SULFITE-INDUCED ASTHMA

As stated earlier, withholding sulfites from these patients does not induce remission of their asthma. Therefore, standard treatment of the underlying asthmatic condition continues to be important. Most of the patients with severe sulfite sensitivity (reacting to oral dosages of 1 to 50 mg) require continuous systemic corticosteroid treatment.

Nevertheless, reduction in exposure to inhaled, ingested, and injected SO_2 and sulfite salts might improve the course of asthma in sulfite-sensitive asthmatics. Avoiding inhaled SO_2, including sulfite solutions, may have advantages for all asthmatics; however, dietary avoidance of sulfites by ''insensitive'' asthmatics is of doubtful value. Therefore, the first task is identification of sulfite sensitivity. Some propose challenging all new asthmatics with sulfites. Others feel that only those with a ''restaurant asthma'' history should undergo challenge. Since some patients are unaware of their sulfite sensitivity, any chronic asthmatic may be a candidate for diagnostic challenge testing. Table 2 contains details of our current screening challenge procedure and Table 3 contains details of our double blind challenge procedure.

For those asthmatics who are sensitive to ingestion of sulfites, dietary avoidance of sulfites is prudent. Unfortunately, at the time this chapter was written, the Food and Drug Administration has not moved toward either disclosure or banning of sulfites in foods and drinks. Obviously, from the standpoint of the afflicted patient, banning sulfites, except for use in avoidable products, such as wine and beer, would be preferable. Disclosure is a much more difficult task, since sulfites can be added anywhere in the food chain. Accountability and enforcement might be impractical even if labeling were required by law.

Table 4 contains a list of foods which are likely to be contaminated with sulfites. Avoidance of these foods can reduce dietary sulfites to levels between 1 and 10 mg per day. Further, more rigid restriction of dietary sulfites can be maintained by eating health foods and natural farm fresh fruits and vegetables, and by avoiding restaurants, cafeterias, and even many hospital dietary services.

TABLE 2 Potassium Metabisulfite Oral Challenge: Open Screening Procedure

	Solution*	Capsule†
Sulfite doses:	1, 5, 10, 25, 50	100, 200 mg

1. Challenges are performed when asthma is stable. Usual medications, except antihistamine, β-agonists, and cromolyn, are taken. FEV_1 value at least 70% of predicted or best prior value. Absolute lowest value for an adult is 1.5 L.
2. Sulfite dosages and interval between challenges can be individualized at the discretion of the physician.
3. Interval between challenge dosages is 20 minutes. FEV_1 value obtained, and if stable, next dosage administered.
4. Positive challenge is a fall in FEV_1 value equal to or greater than 25% from baseline value. Reverse reaction with Alupent solution (in single-dose vials) or Terbutaline (inhalation).
5. A "positive" open challenge should be repeated after 48 hours using the "double blind" protocol.

* Potassium metabisulfite (USP $K_2S_2O_5$) can be obtained from Mallinckrodt Chemical Company, St. Louis, MO. As stated earlier, the FDA considers this salt to be "harmless and safe." Dissolve 1 mg/ml, 5 mg/ml, etc., in water and add to 2–4 oz of fresh or additive-free lemonade. The solution is held in the mouth, swished from side to side, for 30 seconds, and swallowed.

† Opaque capsules are filled with $K_2S_2O_5$ salt by a pharmacist and placed in labeled bottles, 100 mg/capsule, 200 mg/capsule. Shelf life has not been determined but we have found capsules filled over a year which induce reactions.

TABLE 3 Potassium Metabisulfite Oral Challenges: Double Blind Procedure

	capsules† / solution
Sulfite doses:	1, 5, 10, 25, 50, 100, 200 mg.

1. Double blind challenge conducted if screening challenge is positive or for research purposes.
2. Provoking dose from positive screening challenge selected. If dose given as a solution, both capsule and solution challenge are suggested to differentiate potential routes of provocation for sulfite sensitivity (sublingual vs. G1).
3. Procedure:
   a) Capsule: Two placebo capsules and one $K_2S_2O_5$ capsule (provoking dosage) selected by unblinded nurse and labeled #1, #2, #3. "Blinded" nurse and physician administer test. FEV_1 should fall by 25% after administration of capsule containing $K_2S_2O_5$.
   b) Solution: If provoking dosage between 1 and 50 mg (solution), a positive challenge may have resulted from sublingual absorption or by SO_2 inhalation. Therefore, if capsule challenge for dosage 1–50 mg is negative, repeat double blind using three solutions, 2 of which are without $K_2S_2O_5$.

† Opaque capsules are filled with $K_2S_2O_5$ salt containing 1, 5, 10, 25, 50, 100 and 200 mg.

Blocking studies in sulfite-sensitive asthma are currently under investigation. Compounds such as atropine, cromolyn, doxepin and cyanocobalamin (vitamin B_{12}) have been shown to effectively block induced asthma after provocation with sulfites in many sulfite-sensitive asthmatics. Long-term treatment with these drugs has not been thoroughly studied. Atropine is likely to be effective by blocking cholinergic pathways. The mechanism for cromolyn blockade is un-

TABLE 4 Partial List of Foodstuffs to which Sulfites (Metabisulfite) are Added

In Food Purchased (Grocery Stores)
- Beer
- Wine
- Shrimp and other seafoods*
- Dried fruits*
- Some fresh fruits*
- Some fresh vegetables*
- Potato chips

In Restaurants†
- Salads, particularly lettuce
- Potatoes — chips, fries, salads, any peeled
- Guacamole
- Wine
- Beer
- Seafoods

* Wash thoroughly before eating

† Enquire from manager whether or not preservative, crisper, sulfite solutions/sprays are used in his/her restaurant *and* whether they prepare (cut, slice) their own produce, especially lettuce and potatoes.

Manager may not be aware that sulfites were added to foods and drinks earlier in the food distribution chain.

known. Whether doxepin works via antihistamine or anticholinergic mechanisms is unclear. Vitamin B_{12} probably is a nonspecific catalyst of oxidation of sulfites to inactive sulfate. Many of our sulfite-sensitive asthmatics have low levels of the enzyme sulfite oxidase, which normally converts active sulfite into inactive sulfate.

Inhalation of Sulfites

Air pollution control measures will be necessary if SO_2 in ambient air will be reduced or eliminated. Some patients, afflicted with this syndrome, must leave air-polluted cities and live in less densely populated areas.

Inhaled bronchodilators, which are currently free of sulfites, are metaproterenol (single-dose vials) and terbutaline. It seems likely that other manufacturers will find ways to eliminate sulfites from inhaled bronchodilators.

Parenteral Injection of Sulfites

Injectable sulfite-free antiasthma preparations include terbutaline, methylprednisolone, and aminophylline.

EXERCISE-INDUCED ASTHMA, URTICARIA, AND ANAPHYLAXIS

E.R. McFADDEN Jr., M.D.

Since the concept of continuing physical fitness has gained popularity in America, a number of nontraumatic exercise-related syndromes have begun to be recognized in medical practice. The most common of these is exercise-induced asthma, but others, such as exercise-induced anaphylaxis and urticaria, are also assuming clinical importance. This chapter will deal with the current therapeutic modalities of each.

EXERCISE-INDUCED ASTHMA

One of the most ubiquitous triggers of bronchial asthma is physical exertion, so the phenomenon of exercise-induced asthma is frequently encountered. Exercise-induced asthma is not a disease, nor an isolated disorder in its own right. The term is actually a misnomer, for exercise does not cause asthma. Rather, physical exertion is but one of many stimuli that can evoke acute airway obstruction in asthmatic individuals. Occasionally, exercise-induced bronchospasm can be the presenting or sole manifestation of asthma, but generally, with the passage of time, other stimuli also become apparent. Typically, this aspect of the asthmatic diathesis is most commonly found in children and young adults because of their high level of physical activity, but it can occur in any age group.

Occasionally, exercise-induced asthma may be so severe that it dominates the entire clinical picture. Usually, however, it is more of a nuisance, and although the attacks can be quite severe under certain circumstances, they are transitory, and spontaneous recovery is the rule. The significance of this problem is that it affects the quality of the patients' life styles by materially interfering with their ability to engage in physical activity.

Generally, the patient with exercise-induced asthma develops the classic signs of airflow obstruction (namely, wheezing, dyspnea, and cough) at the end of exercise simultaneously with the onset of the changes in lung function, and so the diagnosis can frequently be made historically. It should be noted, however, that this is not always the case. Some individuals may complain only of cough following exertion, or dyspnea that is disproportionate to the physical task performed. The correct diagnosis can thus be overlooked. In these circumstances, some clinicians feel that any patient with exercise-related symptoms should be challenged in the laboratory before the complaints are dismissed or ascribed to some other source. Exercise-induced changes in lung function can also occur in some individuals with atopic histories but with no other stigmata of asthma, as well as in first-degree relatives of asthmatics who are otherwise asymptomatic.

The object of therapy is prophylaxis. In the past some physicians have instructed their patients to avoid all strenuous activity, while others have cautioned moderation and only forbade certain exercise tasks (such as running or cycling) or competitive athletics. While avoidance may work well for allergens, this strategy is unwise with regard to exercise, particularly when applied to children, because it sets the individual apart from his peers and invites the generation of unnecessary internal and external psychologic and psychosocial pressures. In addition, this approach does not offer any remedy for the random, unexpected bouts of exertion, such as having to run for a bus or up a flight of stairs, that are part of daily life. Because of these considerations, the mainstay of treatment is pharmacologic intervention. In general, with the exception of the glucocorticoids, all of the drugs that are useful in the management of the other facets of the asthmatic diathesis are useful here as well. Not all agents are equally effective, however, and in the past there has been considerable controversy as to which is best.

Recent insights into the pathogenesis of exercise-induced asthma have cleared up much of the previous confusion, and most authorities would now agree that the treatment of choice for this condition is the use of inhaled agents, such as the sympathomimetics and cromolyn. The advantages of the β-adrenergic agonists are that they are quite successful in both relieving an established attack of exercise-induced airway obstruction and in preventing its occurrence when the drug is administered shortly before undertaking exercise. β_2 selective compounds, such as salbutamol, terbutaline, and fenoterol, have rapid onsets of action, can be used on an as-needed basis, and can completely block exercise-induced asthma from developing for 4 or more hours. Cromolyn sodium also acts rapidly, but its effect is of shorter duration, lasting only 2 to 3 hours. Unlike the sympathomimetics, pretreatment with cromolyn does not abolish the changes in lung function, but rather attenuates the postobstructive response so that the patient's symptoms are ameliorated. In contrast to its prophylactic effect, this drug has no influence on established, or developing, airway obstruction, so it cannot be used for treatment of the patient's problem once it has begun.

In treating exercise-induced asthma, it is important to remember that the degree of exercise required to induce discomfort in a given patient varies as a function of the underlying airway lability, which in turn is a function of the activity of the disease process. Hence, the choice of drugs and doses to be employed should be made on an individual basis with those factors in mind. In most clinical situations, one can typically begin treatment with an inhaled β_2 agonist, such as salbutamol, and have the patient use it prior to undertaking the physical activity that produces his symptoms. (If the patient is unwilling, or unable, to use a β-stimulant, cromolyn sodium can be substituted.) When exercise is the predominant feature of the illness, there is no need to institute treatment on a regularly scheduled basis and the adrenergic agonist or cromolyn can be employed strictly as needed. For example, for scheduled activities such as a gym class or other exercise program, the inhalation of 2 puffs of salbutamol, or its equivalent, or ingestion of a single capsule of cromolyn, 10 to 15 minutes before starting exercise will generally suffice to keep the patient symptom free. To prevent the obstructive consequences of unscheduled physical activities, heavy reliance is placed on sympathomimetic aerosols because of their rapidity of onset. If, however, airway lability is high so that drug consumption is excessive (that is exceeding 20 to 30 puffs of β-agonist during waking hours), or if the patient's exercise component is but one of many triggers producing his complaints, it is helpful to begin with cromolyn sodium, or add it to the patient's existing regimen. The rationale for this approach is that one can use this drug to treat the exercise component and reduce the underlying airway reactivity simultaneously. To be successful, cromolyn must be taken on a regular basis (4 times daily) as well as before exercise. A short but intense course of glucocorticoids (40 to 60 mg daily tapering to zero over 12 to 16 days) can also be helpful in these circumstances. Like cromolyn, the glucocorticoids will reduce the underlying airway reactivity and so make the exercise component easier to manage. Unlike cromolyn, however, steroids do not influence the exercise response per se. When the airway lability is controlled, single drug therapy can then be resumed on an as-needed basis.

Both chromolyn and inhaled β-agonists are extremely well tolerated and the sympathomimetics produce few side effects by this route of administration. There have been no clinicaly significant instances of tolerance, or lack of effectiveness, reported with prolonged use of either class of drugs, and no cumulative untoward effects with continued use have been observed. Hence, this form of therapy is extremely safe.

In patients who cannot effectively use a metered dose inhaler, such as small children or individuals with physical impairments, other delivery systems, such as rotohalers or spacers, can be employed. These devices obviate the need for coordinating the activation of the cannister with the respiratory maneuvers necessary to deposit the drug in the airways, and as such, are valuable adjuncts. Alternatively, sympathomimetics can be administered orally. This form of therapy, although effective, has several disadvantages that limit its utility. The prime difficulty is the uncertainty surrounding the coordination of the onset of exercise with the peak absorption of the drug used. The second problem is that this route of administration increases the side effects encountered, particularly tremor and palpitations.

The other classes of bronchodilators that can inhibit exercise-induced asthma are the methylxanthines and anticholinergics. Initially, because of the use of low dose in some studies, there was controversy over whether theophylline and its congeners really prevented postexertional bronchospasm. However, it is now clear that the degree of inhibition that develops directly relates to the serum theophylline concentrations achieved. Although the methylxanthines are not as potent bronchodilators as the sympathomimetics, the chief disadvantage with this class of drugs is that they must be given orally, so their effectiveness varies as a function of the quantity absorbed and the time prior to exercise that they are administered. It remains to be determined if these disadvantages can be overcome with the use of daily or twice daily sustained release compounds.

The effect of atropine and similar parasympatholytics on exercise-induced bronchospasm is less uniform than that of the other drugs. This class of compounds tends to work only in selected individuals and so tends to be used only when all else fails.

There is a significant interaction between the strength of the stimulus in exercise-induced asthma and the protection offered by medications. None of the available agents abolishes, in an all-or-none fashion, the bronchoconstriction that develops after exertion; rather, they produce a parallel displacement of the stimulus-response relationship to the right such that the beneficial consequence of any given drug can be overcome by increasing the stimulus. For example, the airway obstruction that follows exercise tasks with low levels of ventilation, such as walking or slow jogging, will be totally abolished with a sympathomimetic. However, this protective effect can be overcome, and the patient's symptoms return, when he performs more strenuous tasks, or when the temperature and/or humidity of the inspired air is lowered. Hence, a treatment schedule that permits a person with asthma to walk briskly on spring or summer days without difficulty can become ineffective in protecting him from exercise tasks that require high ventilations in frigid environments, such as ice skating, ice hockey, or cross-country skiing. This phenomenon, when present, can be abolished by giving more β-agonist (for example, 4 puffs) or by using a combination of agents, such as an inhaled β-agonist and cromolyn before exercise. The latter approach frequently works quite well in athletes or in others who wish to perform strenuous types of physical exertion.

In rare circumstances it may be necessary to evaluate objectively the effectiveness of various therapeutic modalities by reproducing the patient's complaints in the laboratory with an exercise or other form of thermal challenge. In this fashion, one can systematically examine the protective effect offered by each class of drugs alone or in combination, and so design a program to meet the patient's specific needs.

EXERCISE-INDUCED ANAPHYLAXIS

Exercise-induced anaphylaxis is a condition of unknown origin and prevalence characterized by the development of cutaneous erythema and urticaria, vascular collapse, and upper respiratory tract obstruction during or following strenuous physical exertion. In many instances, the patient's signs and symptoms are accentuated by exercising in a warm environment and/or by exercising postprandially. An important, and poorly understood, aspect of his syndrome is its episodic nature. Attacks do not occur with each exercise experience, and it has proven difficult to reproduce the syndrome in the laboratory.

Since the etiologic agent is unknown, treatment is nonspecific and directed toward the reversal of symptoms and, where possible, prophylaxis. The syncope and vascular collapse are treated with epinephrine and fluid replacement much the same as in antigen-induced anaphylaxis. Like other forms of anaphylaxis, persistent hypotension requires aggressive therapy in an appropriately staffed and equipped facility, such as an emergency room. Although respiratory symptoms of wheezing and choking are frequent, life-threatening laryngeal edema or acute severe respiratory dysfunction has not been reported. These complaints respond to epinephrine and antihistamines. Systemic antihistamines, with or without epinephrine, reduce the erythema, urticaria and angioedema and their associated symptoms once they have developed. However, when given over time, or before exercise, antihistamines have not been found to prevent attacks, although they may modify their severity.

Prevention of acute episodes is considered to be the best form of therapy. Although no controlled trials exist, anecdotal information suggests that this can be achieved by limitation of the severity of the exertion, avoidance of contributory factors, such as exercising after meals or in a hot humid environment, and cessation of the exercise program at the appearance of prodromal signs, such as generalized pruritus and/or urticaria. Total avoidance of all exercise activity does not seem warranted at the present time, since there is no evidence yet that continued exercise leads to serious medical illness.

CHOLINERGIC URTICARIA

Another form of urticarial reaction that can develop with exercise is cholinergic urticaria. This condition is a generalized heat urticaria that consists of tiny pruritic wheals surrounded by large areas of erythema which occasionally become confluent. In addition to exercise, symptoms will also occur with fever and following a hot bath or shower. Typically the only complaint that the patient experiences with exercise is intense itching, but occasionally wheezing and dyspnea will occur. Syncope is very rare.

In approximately 50 percent of affected individuals the urticaria can be prevented with 25 mg of Atarax given 4 times daily. This drug can also be given prophylactically 45 minutes before commencing exercise or showering. In the remainder of patients, another antihistamine may afford relief; one should try more than one type before abandoning this treatment. If this approach is unsuccessful, both H_1 and H_2 blockers can be administered simultaneously. Use of the new tricyclic antidepressant, Sinequan, is also said to be efficacious in patients resistant to Atarax. The pulmonary complaints, when present, can readily be prevented or reversed with an inhaled sympathomimetic.

INSECT STING ALLERGY IN ADULTS

JOHN W. YUNGINGER, M.D.

Successful long-term management of insect sting–sensitive patients depends on identification of the culprit insect, proper classification of the sting reaction, and knowledge of the natural history of insect sting allergy.

THE INSECTS

Stinging insects are members of the order *Hymenoptera*, which includes bees, wasps, yellow jackets, hornets, and fire ants. Only about one-third of sting victims can reliably identify the insect responsible for their sting, so that some rudimentary knowledge of entomology will aid the clinician in correctly identifying the culprit insect.

Honeybees are common throughout the United States; they are mild-mannered insects which usually will not sting unless their hive is disturbed or unless stepped or sat upon. The honeybee sting is barbed and usually remains embedded in the sting victim. Honeybee venom is bacteriostatic, so it is unusual for honeybee stings to become secondarily infected. Bumblebees are large, noisy, slow-flying insects which rarely cause sting reactions, except in small children who capture them from flowers or in farmers who disturb their ground nests during plowing or mowing.

Wasps, yellow jackets, and hornets are collectively referred to as vespids. Paper wasps are widely distributed throughout the United States, building open aerial nests under the overhangs of homes or outbuildings or in barn rafters. The coloration of paper wasps varies widely in different geographic areas, ranging from gray to yellow to reddish-orange. Yellow jackets are ill-tempered, ground-nesting insects that often sting without provocation. They will frequently nest in cracks in sidewalks or in the foundations of buildings. Yellow jackets are scavengers, often feeding in garbage cans in picnic areas or on fallen rotting fruit in orchards. Consequently, cellulitis is occasionally seen following yellow jacket stings. Hornets build aerial nests which resemble Japanese lanterns, usually located on the overhangs of buildings or in hedges or shrubs. Hornets are of two types; the white-faced hornet (American hornet, bald-faced hornet) and the yellow hornet (European hornet).

Fire ants are particularly widespread along the southern Atlantic coast and the Gulf of Mexico, building dirt mounds about one or two feet in height. They frequently anchor themselves by their mandibles when stinging, leaving a semicircular row of vesicles at the sting site.

CLASSIFICATION OF STING REACTIONS

Reactions to insect stings are conveniently divided into immediate (2 to 4 hours) or delayed (after 4 hours), depending on the time elapsed between the sting and the development of signs or symptoms.

Immediate reactions are in turn divided into local, large local, systemic, and toxic reactions. Local reactions are normal and consist of transient pain, erythema, and swelling at the sting site. Large local reactions are more extensive, often involving swelling and erythema of most of an extremity; however, by definition, all signs and symptoms are contiguous with the sting site. Systemic reactions are generalized and involve signs or symptoms at a site or sites remote from the sting site. For example, a sting on the forehead resulting in angioedema of the eyelids would be classified as a local or large local reaction, whereas a sting on the foot resulting in angioedema of the eyelids would be considered a systemic reaction. Systemic reactions may involve generalized urticaria and pruritus, cutaneous or laryngeal edema, bronchospasm, or vascular collapse. There are IgE mediated reactions which may be life-threatening if pulmonary or cardiovascular symptoms predominate. Toxic reactions may occur after a person receives multiple stings within a short period of time. The signs and symptoms are identical to those of systemic reactions, but in this case the symptoms are produced by exogenous vasoactive amines delivered in the venom, rather than by endogenous vasoactive materials released as a consequence of venom allergen-IgE antibody interaction on mast cell surfaces.

Delayed reactions may take several clinical forms, including serum sickness–like reactions, transverse myelitis, or myocarditis. Many large local reactions attain maximal size 12 to 24 hours after the sting. Honeybee stings are occasionally followed by an influenza-like syndrome involving fever, myalgia, and shaking chills 8 to 24 hours after the sting. The pathophysiology of most delayed reactions is unclear; immunologic mechanisms may not be involved. Delayed reactions are rarely life-threatening.

TREATMENT OF ACUTE REACTIONS

Local reactions require no therapy. Large local reactions are frequently treated with antihistamines or short courses of oral glucocorticoids. Although such therapy poses little risk to most patients, these medications are prescribed more by reflex action than as a result of any scientific documentation of efficacy in the medical literature.

The treatment of systemic reactions is in essence the treatment of anaphylaxis. For severe reactions, maintenance of the airway and administration of oxygen become the primary goals. Epinephrine is the drug of choice in most instances, unless the patient has a history of moderate to severe cardiovascular disease. There is a deplorable tendency for emergency room personnel to withhold administration of epinephrine unless the patient is experiencing bronchospasm or cardiovascular collapse. Epinephrine is a much more efficient drug for rapid relief of generalized urticaria and pruritus than is an antihistamine; the latter medication can be used in conjunction with epinephrine, however. The usual dose of epinephrine in adults is 0.3 ml of the 1:1000 concentration subcutaneously. This dose can be repeated at 15 to 20 minute intervals if necessary. Larger doses are not usually more effective and are often associated with uncomfortable side effects, such as tremors, nausea, and vomiting. Patients who are receiving beta-blocking agents, such as propranolol, may be refractory to the usual doses of epinephrine. Although the effect of epinephrine is quite rapid, the duration of action is brief. If there has been a beneficial response to epinephrine, a long-acting preparation, such as Susphrine should be administered prior to dismissing the patient. Theophylline, glucocorticoids, pressor agents, or intravenous colloid solutions are occasionally required for management of more severe reactions. Overnight hospitalization is indicated for patients with refractory hypotension, ventricular arrhythmias, coexisting cardiovascular disease, or patients who live at some distance from medical facilities.

Finally, patients who sustain generalized sting reactions should be provided with an epinephrine-containing emergency kit and instructed in its use. The commercially available kits include the Ana-Kit (Hollister-Stier Laboratories) and the Epi-Pen and Epi-Pen Jr. (Center Laboratories). The former contains a syringe containing two 0.5-ml doses of aqueous epinephrine (1:1000), along with chewable antihistamine tablets, alcohol wipes, and a string tourniquet; the patient is required to self-inject the epinephrine. The latter kit contains a single 0.3-ml dose of aqueous epinephrine (1:1000 for the Epi-Pen; 1:-2000 for the Epi-Pen Jr.). Each Epi-Pen unit contains a pressure-sensitive spring-loaded device which automatically makes the needle puncture and injects the medication. The Ana-Kit is less expensive, but the Epi-Pen may be attractive to those patients who do not feel comfortable with the self-injection technique. Epinephrine-containing kits should be carried by sting-sensitive persons during the local insect "season". Patients should be reassured that exposure of the kits to ambient temperatures will not destroy the effectiveness of the epinephrine. Exposure to sunlight is more deleterious to the drug than is exposure to ambient temperatures. The epinephrine kits should be inspected frequently and replaced at the end of the expiration date shown on the label or if they acquire a pinkish-tan discoloration.

DIAGNOSTIC EVALUATIONS IN STING-SENSITIVE PATIENTS

Diagnostic evaluations for sting sensitivity are indicated only for patients with histories of systemic reactions. IgE antibodies to insect venoms may be measured by skin testing or by in vitro immunoassay or leukocyte histamine release procedures.

Skin Tests

Honeybee, wasp, yellow jacket, yellow hornet, and white-faced hornet venoms are marketed commercially by two firms in the United States. The venoms should be diluted in special albumin-containing diluent to prevent adsorption of the venom to the inside of the glass vials. Initial scratch or puncture tests are placed at venom concentrations of 1 μg/ml. If these screening tests are negative, intradermal tests using venom concentrations between 1 ng/ml and 1 μg/ml may be placed. A significant positive skin test is a wheal at least 5 to 10 mm in diameter with at least 11 to 20 mm of erythema, measured 15 minutes after intradermal injection of 0.05 ml of the diluted venom. Irritant positive reactions may be produced in nonsensitive persons at test concentrations exceeding 1 μg/ml. Particular attention should be paid to the recommended dating period for the venom skin test materials. The nanogram per milliter concentrations should be replaced on a daily basis and the microgram per milliliter concentrations on a monthly basis. Finally, positive and negative control tests with histamine phosphate and diluent, respectively, should be placed at the same time as the venom skin tests.

Measurement of Venom-Specific IgE Antibodies

Radioimmunoassays and enzyme immunoassays are available commercially for in vitro measurement of specific IgE antibody. However, elevated IgE antibody levels are seen in only 80 percent of persons who have significant positive venom skin tests. Moreover, there is no correlation between the magnitude of the IgE antibody level and the degree of clinical sensitivity of the patient as assessed by deliberate sting challenges. Consequently, skin testing is the preferred diagnostic procedure at present. The decision whether to administer or withhold venom immunotherapy can almost always be made on the basis of the clinical history and the venom skin test results.

Venom-Induced Leukocyte Histamine Release

This diagnostic test is available in only a few centers.

INDICATIONS FOR VENOM IMMUNOTHERAPY

The medical indications for venom immunotherapy are outlined in Table 1. Venom immunotherapy is indicated only for adults who have clinical histories of systemic reactions following stings and who have positive venom skin tests. It was formerly believed that such individuals were at 100 percent risk of systemic reactions with future stings; some patients are still mistakenly advised that future stings will be fatal unless venom immunotherapy is received. In fact, in the absence of venom immunotherapy, such adults are

TABLE 1 Indications for Venom Immunotherapy in Adults

Classification of Sting Reaction by History	*Venom Skin Test*	*Venom Immunotherapy*
Local	Not indicated	No
Large local	Not indicated	No
Systemic	Positive	Yes
	Negative	No
Toxic	Not indicated	No
Delayed	Not indicated	No

at approximately 60 percent risk of repeat systemic reactions with subsequent stings. Venom immunotherapy will reduce this risk to approximately 2 percent. However, nonmedical considerations are often important in an individual's decision to accept or decline immunotherapy. The cost of treatment should be discussed with the patient, along with the time commitment required. In addition, patients residing at some distance from medical centers must frequently depend on primary care physicians for administration of immunotherapy; occasionally, physicians refuse to administer venom injections and the patient winds up being caught in the middle. Although it is not possible to quantitate the "mental wear and tear" experienced by sting-sensitive persons and their family members (for example, fear of repeat stings, maintaining an awareness of insects, alterations in occupational or leisure pursuits), the physician should attempt to assess the degree of such mental wear and tear in each individual situation. Because the risk of systemic reactions to venom immunotherapy is greater during the build-up stage than during the maintenance stage, we usually defer venom immunotherapy in pregnant females until after delivery. For females who are tolerating maintenance venom immunotherapy and become pregnant, however, there is no reason to alter the injection schedules or to discontinue treatment. Finally, it is currently appropriate to discuss venom immunotherapy as a control measure and not as a cure. Although some individuals have been able to discontinue venom immunotherapy after a few years of treatment without a return of sensitivity, the frequency with which this occurs and the underlying mechanisms are not known at present.

TECHNIQUE OF VENOM IMMUNOTHERAPY

Venoms for immunotherapy, as well as 0.03 percent albumin-containing diluent, are available from two manufacturers (Albay, Hollister-Stier Laboratories; Pharmalgen, Pharmacia Laboratories). The United States Food and Drug Administration requires that venoms be standardized based on their hyaluronidase content; consequently, venom preparations from the two commercial suppliers are quite similar in allergenic potency. For physicians who treat several insect sting–sensitive persons it is usually easier and more economical to work with stock solutions, rather than with separate solutions for each individual patient. Venoms from honeybee, wasp, yellow jacket, yellow hornet, and white-faced hornet are available separately in 500 μg lyophilized quantities. A "mixed vespid" preparation containing 500 μg each of yellow jacket, yellow hornet, and white-faced hornet venom is also available. These vials are reconstituted with the albumin-containing diluent to produce stock solutions of 100 μg/ml (300 μg/ml for mixed vespid venom). Two tenfold dilutions for immunotherapy are made from this stock solution. The 100 μg/ml and 300 μg/ml solutions retain their potency for at least 6 months at 4°C. The more dilute solutions should be replaced at monthly intervals.

Patients are usually treated with all venoms to which they show significant positive skin tests. There is a good deal of cross-allergenicity among vespid venoms, and patients will frequently exhibit positive skin tests to all vespid venoms following a single vespid sting. Unless the identity of the culprit insect can be confirmed with certainty, however, it is prudent in such a case to treat with all vespid venoms producing positive skin tests.

The dosage schedule employed for venom immunotherapy in our clinic is shown in Table 2. It is similar to the dosage schedule suggested in the Albay package insert and involves one injection per patient visit. The dosage schedule in the Pharmalgen package recommends from 1 to 3 injections at 30-minute intervals during each patient visit. With the latter schedule patients can reach the 100 μg maintenance dose in approximately 6 weeks. However, many patients are not able to spend up to 90 minutes per treatment session and find the single injection schedule to be preferable. With the schedule shown in Table 2, injections may be given once, twice, or thrice weekly.

Venom injections are given subcutaneously with disposable tuberculin syringes in the outer midportion of the upper arm. Patients should be observed in the office for 30 minutes after the injection; most serious reactions to injections occur during this time interval. If patients are receiving more than one venom, we administer each venom as a separate injection in a different site; persons receiving the mixed vespid venom receive one injection, however. If a patient shows large local or systemic reactions to venom therapy, the venom responsible for the reaction can be identified more easily if the injections are separated. Subsequently, the dosage of each venom can be adjusted independently. When the patients reach maintenance dose (100 μg), the interval between injections is lengthened to 4 weeks, and separate injections are then combined into a single injection. After 6 months of maintenance immunotherapy, the interval between injections is lengthened to 6 weeks.

Transient local reactions at the venom injection site can be expected. These involve erythema, itching, and swelling, which appear during the first 30 minutes and may last several hours. Occasionally, these local reactions may be several centimeters in diameter

TABLE 2 Dosage Schedules for Hymenoptera Venom Immunotherapy

	Individual Venoms			*Mixed Vespid Venom*		
Dose No.	*Volume (ml)*	*Concentration* (μg/ml)	*Dose* (μg)	*Volume (ml)*	*Concentration* (μg/ml)	*Dose* (μg)
1	0.05	1	0.05	0.05	3	0.15
2	0.10	1	0.10	0.10	3	0.30
3	0.20	1	0.20	0.20	3	0.60
4	0.40	1	0.40	0.40	3	1.2
5	0.70	1	0.70	0.70	3	2.1
6	0.05	10	0.50	0.05	30	1.5
7	0.10	10	1.0	0.10	30	3.0
8	0.20	10	2.0	0.20	30	6.0
9	0.40	10	4.0	0.40	30	12
10	0.70	10	7.0	0.70	30	21
11	0.05	100	5.0	0.05	300	15
12	0.10	100	10	0.10	300	30
13	0.20	100	20	0.20	300	60
14	0.40	100	40	0.40	300	120
15	0.60	100	60	0.60	300	180
16	0.80	100	80	0.80	300	240
17	1.00	100	100	1.00	300	300

and involve most of the upper arm. These reactions occur most frequently at delivered venom doses between 10 and 30 μg, and they tend to disappear when the venom doses exceed 60 μg. The local reactions may be treated with oral antihistamines and/or glucocorticoids, but it is usually best to continue advancing the dosage administered. Conversely, the dosage should be reduced if systemic reactions (scattered urticaria or wheezing) occur after venom injections. The signs and symptoms experienced during a systemic reaction tend to be stereotyped for a given individual; this is frequently helpful in assessing reactions to immunotherapy. We discourage patients from premedicating themselves with antihistamines or glucocorticoids prior to reporting for venom injections; such therapy may obscure useful signs and symptoms of venom overdose. Personnel administering venom injections should routinely inquire about medication intake by patients. If large local or systemic reactions occur repeatedly, various strategies can be tried, including (1) increasing the frequency of injections from once weekly to twice weekly; (2) splitting the desired dose into 2 or 3 portions and administering each portion at 30-minute intervals; or (3) increasing the total volume in which the desired dose is delivered, by adding extra diluent to the syringe.

MONITORING PATIENTS RECEIVING VENOM IMMUNOTHERAPY

Patients receiving venom immunotherapy may be skin tested with venoms at annual or biannual intervals. However, the majority of patients will continue to show significant positive venom skin tests despite being able to tolerate repeat insect stings. Therefore, venom immunotherapy does not produce true desensitization in the majority of cases. In a minority of patients venom skin tests will revert to negative within 2 to 4 years after venom immunotherapy is begun. In such instances it is reasonable to consider discontinuation of immunotherapy. Relatively small numbers of such patients have been followed up, however, and a definitive recommendation cannot be made at this time.

Immunoassays for measuring serum IgE and IgG antibodies to venoms are available from several reference laboratories. IgE antibody levels usually rise following institution of venom immunotherapy, then gradually decline; the IgE antibody levels do not usually fall into the normal or negative range, however. IgG antibody levels usually rise following venom immunotherapy, plateau after the patient reaches maintenance dose, and decline slightly with time thereafter.

Some authorities recommend that IgE and IgG antibody levels be routinely monitored after the patient reaches maintenance dose and at annual intervals thereafter. Although there may be merit to measuring venom-specific antibody levels for research purposes, the clinical relevance of the data obtained has not been demonstrated conclusively. IgG antibody levels have been studied in groups of patients who were either immunotherapy successes or immunotherapy failures. Although the mean IgG antibody was higher in the immunotherapy success group, there was much overlap in individual IgG antibody levels between the immunotherapy success and immunotherapy failure groups. There were patients with low IgG antibody levels who tolerated insect stings with no difficulty, and a few patients with high IgG antibody levels who continued to show generalized reactions following insect stings. Therefore, if such IgE and IgG specific antibody levels are monitored, the physician should realize that what is being measured is the immune response to venom immunotherapy, rather than a parameter which will predict with certainty the clinical outcome of the patient's next Hymenoptera sting. In addition to immunologic factors, there are probably biochemical, physiologic, and psychologic factors which are also important in determining the patient's clinical response to insect stings.

Deliberate insect sting challenges under carefully controlled conditions represent the most unambiguous test of the clinical efficacy of venom immunotherapy. Such challenges pose patient risks, however, and are available at only a few research centers.

FUTURE AREAS OF INVESTIGATION

Although venom immunotherapy is remarkedly effective in providing clinical immunity to Hymenoptera stings, there are several unanswered questions concerning insect sting allergy. Efforts are underway to identify subgroups of sting-sensitive patients in whom venom immunotherapy may not be warranted. Considerable work is required to determine whether there is a minimal or optimal length of time that venom immunotherapy should be given. Finally, development of new treatment regimens utilizing modified venom extracts may permit clinical immunity to be achieved with fewer side effects and fewer total injections.

Supported in part by a U.S. Public Health Service Grant (AI-21398) and by the Mayo Foundation.

ALLERGIC RHINITIS

HOWARD M. DRUCE, M.D.
MICHAEL A. KALINER, M.D.

Allergic rhinitis is recognized as a constellation of symptoms caused by exposure to inhaled allergens. These symptoms include rhinorrhea in which a clear fluid is produced, sneezing, nasal obstruction, and itching in the nose and adjacent mucous membranes. Increased nasal secretion often leads to a postnasal drip that stimulates the cough reflex, an occurrence more likely to develop at night because of the difficulty in clearing secretions in a prone position. Patients may also complain of symptoms related to the paranasal sinuses (headache, facial pressure, or congestion), middle ear (pressure, itching, or popping), and eyes (redness, discharge, itching), and of generalized fatigue and malaise.

Proper treatment of allergic rhinitis requires some understanding of its pathophysiology. Exposure to allergens (most commonly dust, pollens, molds, or animal emanations) leads to the formation of IgE antibody and to the sensitization of mast cells found in the mucous membrane of the nose. Subsequent exposure to the sensitizing antigen causes the mast cells to release a number of chemicals, known as the mediators of allergy, that produce all the symptoms of the disease. Although a great number of mediators are released by mast cells, only a few are relevant to our current understanding of allergic rhinitis. Table 1 presents the putative mediators responsible for the major events involved in allergic rhinitis.

MANAGEMENT

Treatment depends on the severity and duration of the symptoms and which of the symptom predominates. Once the identity of the allergen has been confirmed by history and skin test results, the best treatment is avoidance. Such an approach may be feasible in some cases (as in the removal of a feather pillow or a pet from the bedroom), but generally it is not possible when the case involves seasonal aeroallergens. However, some relief may be obtained by filtering the air in the house, office, or car. We also recommend air conditioning, perhaps augmented by an electrostatic precipitator or a high-efficiency particulate air filter. Among the many other methods of avoiding aeroallergens, we suggest use of nuisance masks to filter pollen from the air when outside and avoidance of the outdoors at peak pollenation times (early morning, especially on sunny, windy days).

Environmental Control

In patients who are sensitive to dust and mold, environmental control is especially recommended to reduce the patient's exposure to such elements. The bedroom should be the key target of attention; some useful measures include removal of heavy drapes, old furniture, rugs, and potted plants. Pillows should be made of nonallergenic material, and the mattress and box springs should be totally enclosed in a dust-proof encasement. Particular attention should be paid to air filtration and humidification in homes heated with forced hot air.

TABLE 1 Allergic Rhinitis: Major Symptoms and Responsible Mediators

Pathologic Event	*Symptoms Elicited*	*Mediator(s) Responsible*
Pruritus	Tickling, palatal "clicking"	Histamine (H_1 receptor), prostaglandins
Mucosal edema	Nasal obstruction	Histamine (H_1), eicosanoids, kinins
Sneezing	Sneezing and the irrepressible feeling of the need to sneeze	Histamine (H_1), eicosanoids
Mucus secretion	Runny nose, postnasal drip	Histamine ($H_1 \pm H_2$), eicosanoids, muscarinic discharge
Late-phase allergic reactions	Congestion, nasal hyperirritability	Inflammatory factors, eicosanoids, chemotactic factors

Antihistamines

Pharmacotherapy should be tailored to the predominant symptoms. Short-lived, acute, intermittent symptoms such as itching, sneezing, and rhinorrhea are frequently related to histamine release and generally respond to oral H_1-antihistamines such as the alkylamine chlorpheniramine maleate USP, 4 mg three times a day. The sedation that is associated with antihistamine treatment may be avoided by starting at a subtherapeutic dose (e.g., 2 mg at bedtime) and then gradually (over a 10- to 15-day period) increasing the amount until the full therapeutic dose is achieved.

There are six classes of H_1-receptor antagonists available, each effective at preventing H_1-mediated actions. The limiting side effects are usually drowsiness or loss of mental acuity. Nonsedating antihistamines are now obtainable in the United States. Terfenadine is the first such agent to be introduced and has been demonstrated to be effective in allergic rhinitis. Currently, alkylamines such as chlorpheniramine combine efficacy with the least detrimental side effects; thus, we recommend starting with this agent.

Oral Decongestants

When nasal blockage is prominent, an oral decongestent such as pseudoephedrine hydrochloride (60 mg three times a day) may be used, either separately or in combination with an antihistamine. We have successfully used long-acting antihistamine-decongestant formulations such as Trinalin or Isoclor (both administered in one-tablet doses, twice a day), but many other effective preparations are available.

Topical Decongestants

The use of topical nasal decongestants should be discouraged except in isolated episodes as they tend to cause major side effects. Application of alpha-adrenergic agonists to the mucosa causes the constriction of blood vessels and the resolution of edema that leads to decongestion. However, as the effect dissipates, patients often experience rebound congestion more severe than the pretreatment symptoms. Moreover, reapplication of decongestants leads to tachyphylaxis, requiring increasing frequency of reapplication. Finally, the mucosa becomes inflamed and irritated, a condition known as rhinitis medicamentosa, the treatment of which is to taper the decongestants while starting topical corticosteroids. Thus, topical decongestants are used sparingly and never for more than 3 days out of 7.

Topical Corticosteroids

Topical nasal steroids affect neither immediate allergic reactions nor the nasal response to histamine or muscarinic agonists. However, nasal steroids are extremely useful in treating allergic rhinitis, probably because they prevent or reverse late-phase allergic reactions (by inhibiting the inflammation that is the major pathologic event in these reactions); they also reduce mucus secretion, reduce vascular permeability (and thus, congestion), and prevent eicosanoid formation. Our experience has been that the combination of regular topical nasal steroids with an acceptable antihistamine is exceedingly well tolerated by patients and reduces or abolishes all the symptoms associated with allergic rhinitis.

Three preparations of nasal steroids are available, and each is effective. Nasalide (flunisolide, 0.25 mg per milliliter; used as a starting dose of two sprays twice a day) has the advantages of twice daily administration and approval for use in children. The major disadvantage is a peculiar burning sensation induced by the vehicle propylene glycol, which some subjects cannot tolerate. However, because of the superior design of the applicator and the clear-cut effectiveness of the product, we encourage the patients to apply a saline spray before using the Nasalide in order to reduce the burning sensation. Generally, the uncomfortable side effects diminish within a few days after starting this drug.

Beclomethasone diproprionate (Vancenase or Beconase; starting dose, one spray four times a day) is another effective nasal steroid that is pharmacologically equivalent to flunisolide. However, the drug is expelled from the metered-dose applicator with such force that some patients resist using it; in addition, much of the agent passes beyond the nasal cavity to the pharynx. Despite the poor dispensing mechanism, beclomethasone does not cause a burning sensation and is effective in the treatment of allergic rhinitis.

Both flunisolide and beclomethasone act topically, and although they are absorbed on swallowing, both have minimal systemic effects at the recommended doses. Dexamethasone sodium phosphate (Decadron Turbinaire) is a very potent nasal steroid that is indicated in severe cases of allergic rhinitis, in sinusitis, and in rhinitis medicamentosa. However, if used excessively, this agent can cause adrenal suppression and systemic effets. The usual dosage is two sprays (100 μg per spray) three times a day, which is then tapered gradually over a month to one spray into each nostril once or twice a day. Caution should be advised in using this agent for more than 24 sprays per day.

Monilial pharyngitis, a minor complication of nasal steroid use, is seen only rarely. It is not a limiting complication and can be prevented by drinking some water after each application of the steroids.

Disodium Cromoglycate

Disodium cromoglycate is now available as a nasal formulation (Nasalcrom). This preparation, which is dispensed by a hand-activated pump, is not only effective in treating allergic rhinitis, but is well tolerated. This drug acts by stabilizing mast cells and therefore prevents mediator release. However, effective management requires four to six treatments per day, and many patients fail to follow this regimen. Because disodium cromoglycate acts prophylactically, it would be useful to give patients an initial trial course. For those who cannot comply with the regimen or who fail to respond, the medication should be switched to nasal steroids plus antihistamines. Alternatively, the combination of Nasalcrom and nasal steroids is also effective and causes no systemic symptoms.

We suggest that patients with clear-cut seasonal allergies start using flunisolide or cromoglycate on a regular basis, starting several weeks before the predicted onset of symptoms and continuing until the end of the season. Patients with perennial symptoms should take the medication continuously.

Patients whose symptoms are well controlled on either nasal steroids or nasal cromoglycate, but who have short periods of breakthrough at the height of the season, may be managed in several ways. The dosage of the same medication may be increased, or a short course of nasal dexamethasone can be substituted. Some patients may require short courses of oral steroids, especially when they have systemic effects. A course of prednisone begun at 40 mg daily and tapered rapidly over 1 to 2 weeks is preferable to intramuscular or intraturbinate injections of long-acting steroids.

Immunotherapy

We reserve immunotherapy (allergy desensitization) for patients who have had an adequate trial of pharmacotherapy (generally over two seasons) without adequate relief or for patients in whom medications with alpha-adrenergic properties are contraindicated (hypertension, glaucoma). Patients such as airline pilots or military personnel, whose activities require a high degree of alertness, are also candidates for early immunotherapy. We counsel patients that immunotherapy may not be curative, but, if given appropriately, has a good likelihood of substantially reducing their need for other medication. An immunotherapy prescription is individually formulated on the basis of the patient's positive reactions to skin tests with clinically relevant aeroallergens.

The desensitization regimen is carried out on a year-round basis, building up to the highest tolerated maintenance dose (ideally, a 0.5-ml injection of a 1:50 to 1:200 dilution, weight by volume). Within 6 months to a year, the subject reaches a weekly maintenance dose that usually results in a substantial reduction in symptoms. Thereafter, the dosage should be evaluated every 6 months, at which time the interval between maintenance injections can be increased to 2, 3 and then 4 weeks. Subjects may continue on monthly injections, or after 3 years, a trial of discontinuing desensitization may be attempted. Findings from many studies suggest that some beneficial actions persist for some time after injections are stopped. About 85 percent of allergic rhinitis subjects treated for pollen or dust allergies with high-dose immunotherapy may be expected to improve, as reflected in a reduction in both symptoms and need for drugs. Because of the risk of anaphylaxis, we insist that all injections, both induction and maintenance doses, be administered under the supervision of a physician trained and equipped to provide immediate resuscitation. In case there are any reactions to treatment, patients should be required to wait in the doctor's office for 20 minutes after each injection. Patients should also be taught to recognize the local and systemic side effects of immunotherapy.

Allergic rhinitis is an exceptionally common disease (about 15% of Americans), and the current regimens generally lead to acceptable control in the overwhelming majority of patients. Although this disease has always been regarded as unimportant by many physicians, allergy sufferers are gratifying patients to treat because the symptoms are so bothersome and the available therapy is so effective in reducing them.

SUGGESTED READING

Kaliner M. The mechanisms of action of corticosteroids. J Allergy Clin Immunol In press.

Kniker WT (ed). Allergic and Immunologic Aspects of Ear, Nose and Throat Disease. Part 1: The Nose and Sinuses. Kenilworth, NJ: Schering Corp, 1984.

Metcalfe DD, Kaliner M, Donlon MA. The mast cell. CRC Crit Rev Immunol 1981; 3:27–74.

Mullarkey MF. The classification of nasal disease: an opinion. J Allergy Clin Immunol 1981; 67:251–252.

Norman, PS. Review of nasal therapy: Update. J Allergy Clin Immunol 1983; 72:421–432.

PENICILLIN ALLERGY

TIMOTHY J. SULLIVAN, M.D.

Benzylpenicillin G, semisynthetic penicillins, and cephalosporins constitute an extremely important class of antibiotics, the beta-lactam antibiotics. Each member of the class contains an unstable beta-lactam ring. These agents act by acylating the active sites of bacterial enzymes involved in cell wall synthesis. Approximately 5 percent of the molecules administered to humans become covalently bound to human proteins. Conjugation is predominantly in the penicilloyl configuration, but several other covalently coupled forms occur. These are called the major and minor determinants respectively. Therapeutic preparations of beta-lactam drugs also contain drug polymers and Penicillium mold proteins heavily substituted with beta-lactam determinants.

As one would predict, most patients make brisk immune responses to beta-lactam determinants during and after a course of therapy. Fortunately a minority of patients display clinically detectable immunopathologic disorders (Table 1). Among patients with no an-

TABLE 1 Beta-Lactam Drug-Induced Immunopathologic Reactions

Immune Effector System	*Clinical Manifestations*
IgE	Anaphylaxis Urticaria Angioedema
IgM/IgG	Hemolytic anemia Thrombocytopenia Serum Sickness
Cellular Immunity	Contact sensitivity
Uncertain Mechanisms	Drug fever Interstitial nephritis Toxic epidermal necrolysis Macular cutaneous eruptions

tecedent history of beta-lactam drug allergy, approximately 2 percent experience an allergic reaction during a course of beta-lactam drug therapy. Approximately 25 percent of these reactions occur within 48 hours of beginning therapy, often the result of unrecognized prior IgE sensitization; the other 75 percent of reactions occur during therapy and usually reflect new immune responses.

IgE-mediated reactions are by far the most common immunopathologic reactions to beta-lactam drugs. Anaphylaxis may occur in the first hours of therapy but has not been reported once an uninterrupted course of therapy is in progress. Pruritic cutaneous eruptions, urticaria, and angioedema are much more common manifestations of IgE-mediated reactions than anaphylaxis and can occur at any time during a course of therapy. Pruritic rashes that occur after the completion of a course of therapy are often associated with serum sickness reactions.

High-dose beta-lactam drug therapy (e.g., 10 million units of penicillin per day) leads to dense haptenation of formed elements in the blood. Often the patients' red blood cells are direct Coombs positive (IgG), red cell survival is decreased, and reticulocyte counts are increased. Usually no anemia occurs, but occasionally brisk hemolysis and progressive anemia are observed. Discontinuation of the drug and transfusion may be necessary. Fatal or near-fatal anemias have been reported to develop within four days of the onset of hemolysis. Rarely, IgM-mediated hemolysis occurs, even on low oral doses of beta-lactam drugs. Other formed elements in the blood may be depleted by similar mechanisms, but this is much less common than red cell destruction.

Serum sickness reactions (fever, rash, arthralgias, arthritis) may be triggered by beta-lactam drug therapy. Though seldom as severe as reactions induced by heteroantisera, these reactions can induce significant morbidity and may pose difficult diagnostic challenges in patients apparently recovering from an infection. These immune complex reactions typically appear 7 to 14 days into therapy and may even begin after the termination of therapy.

Contact sensitivity reactions induced by beta-lactam drugs are an occupational hazard for medical personnel, particularly nurses, and may affect pharmacists, individuals administering such drugs to small children, or people involved in the manufacture of these agents.

A variety of other reactions have been associated with beta-lactam drug therapy (Table 1). In some reactions, such as drug fever, the causal association is likely but the mechanism is obscure. In other reactions, such as macular cutaneous eruptions, even the causal role of the drug is uncertain.

DIAGNOSIS OF BETA-LACTAM DRUG ALLERGY

When patients are evaluated during or just after a possible allergic reaction to a beta-lactam drug, the role of the drug can be established with more certainty than when attempts are made at retrospective analysis months or years later. The temporal relationship of drug therapy to the onset of the reaction, the other illnesses present in the patient, other medications being administered (possible alternative explanations or agents such as antihistamines that might alter expression of the reaction), and the effect of discontinuation of the beta-lactam drug are important considerations. If the nature of the reaction suggests an IgE mechanism, skin tests or Radio allergo sorbent tests (RAST) described below may be informative. Tests to detect IgG or IgM that agglutinates or lyses penicillin-treated red blood cells (but not normal red cells) are widely available and are quite useful in the assessment of immune hemolytic anemia that occurs during high-dose enicillin therapy. Serum sickness reactions are associated with: elevated plasma C4a and C3a anaphylatoxin levels (assays commercially available); initially low then, days later, high erythrocyte sedimentation rates; and increased total serum IgE compared to before or after the reaction. Since most patients express IgG and sometimes IgM to beta-lactam determinants, and since free antibody may be low in serum sickness, these values are of little value in assessing the cause of serum sickness. Patch tests can detect contact sensitivity to beta-lactam drugs, but topical application may induce IgE to the drug determinants. Patch testing should be used only when resolution of important problems cannot be achieved by alternative approaches.

The combination of careful history, physical examination, and selected laboratory studies usually defines the nature of the reaction and the role of the beta-lactam drug.

Assessment of Current Allergic Status

When patients are evaluated long after an apparent allergic reaction, the accuracy of the patient's recollections is reduced, relevant laboratory data may not have been obtained, and records may be incomplete or inaccessible. Since most serious or fatal allergic reactions to beta-lactam drugs occur in subjects who have never had clinically detectable prior allergic reactions, a negative history of drug allergy is a dangerously flawed parameter for estimating current allergic status. Presumably these patients were sensitized by their last exposure to beta-lactam drugs. Nevertheless, patients with histories of beta-lactam drug allergy are at increased risk of recurrent reactions upon reexposure to the drugs. Contact sensitivity appears to be the most predictably recurrent reaction based on history alone; serum sickness and hemolytic anemia are the least likely reactions, and IgE-mediated reactions are intermediate between these poles. Patients who have experienced serum sickness reactions to beta-lactam drugs often express persistent IgE to these drugs; such patients are at increased risk of anaphylaxis on reexposure to beta-lactam drugs.

Measurements of serum IgG or IgM to beta-lactam determinants seem to have little value for predicting susceptibility to any form of allergic reaction. Lymphocyte transformation studies also have limited predictive value. Assessment of the presence of specific IgE by skin tests or in vitro methods is valuable for estimating the likelihood of anaphylaxis, urticaria, or angioedema.

Skin Testing to Detect IgE to Beta-Lactam Drugs

Immediate wheal and flare skin tests with penicillin reagents have proven very useful for detecting patients with, or without, IgE sensitivity to penicillin. Penicillin-induced anaphylaxis has not been reported in a penicillin skin test-negative patient. Urticarial reactions occur within 48 hours of the onset of penicillin therapy in approximately 1 percent of patients who have histories of penicillin allergy but negative skin tests. Thus, the likelihood of a serious allergic reaction is virtually nil in skin test-negative patients.

Limited studies of the effect of full-dose parenteral penicillin therapy of penicillin skin test-positive patients have shown that approximately two-thirds of such patients will have acute allergic reactions. Skin tests accurately demonstrate the presence or absence of specific IgE, but positive tests identify some patients who will not have a clinical allergic reaction on any given day. In this sense, penicillin skin testing is associated with few clinical false negatives, but approximately one-third clinical false positives.

Skin tests must be performed with several reagents to reliably detect the full range of possible IgE specificities. Control tests with diluent (to detect dermographism or other nonspecific problems) and with histamine (to detect the presence of antihistaminic drugs that can lead to false negative tests) are very important. Commercial Pre-Pen (Kremers-Urban) used according to the manufacturers' recommendations, commercial benzylpenicillin G (or other beta-lactam drug) diluted to 5000 U/ml or 3.3 mg/ml, and penicilloic acid (the alkaline hydrolysis product of benzylpenicillin G) at 3.3 mg/ml are used for penicillin skin tests.

Prick tests are performed with each of the reagents; if the results are negative, intradermal tests are performed. A positive prick test is one in which a wheal appears at the test site but not at the diluent control site 15 minutes after antigen presentation, or a wheal appears which has a diameter at least 2 mm larger than a control wheal. A positive intradermal test is a wheal at least 2 mm larger than the response to diluent measured 15 minutes after the injections.

Positive penicillin skin tests are complicated by systemic allergic reactions in approximately 1 percent of cases. While these reactions usually are restricted to mild pruritus or urticaria and require no therapy, serious allergic reactions can occur. Penicillin skin testing should be performed in settings that include prompt access to physicians capable of managing anaphylaxis and immediate access to the full range of medications and equipment that are needed to treat anaphylaxis.

Skin tests are usually positive during acute IgE-mediated allergic reactions and can be very helpful in sorting out the role of beta-lactam drugs. Immediate skin tests also are usually positive during penicillin-induced serum sickness. However, as many as one-third of patients have negative skin tests during or just after an acute reaction. Often these subjects are skin test-positive 3 months later. A negative skin test during or just after a clinical reaction does not carry the same significance as a negative skin test in patients assessed months or years after a clinical reaction.

In Vitro Methods for the Detection of IgE to Beta-Lactam Drugs

Solid phase assays for antigen-specific IgE, such as the RAST, have been developed to detect IgE to the penicilloyl determinant. These assays can detect IgE in the serum of 60 to 95 percent of patients who have positive penicilloyl (Pre-Pen) skin tests. No proven in vitro tests are available for detecting IgE to minor determinants. The predictive value of a positive penicilloyl RAST appears to be similar to that for a positive skin test. A negative RAST has little predictive value since minor determinants are not assessed, and not all patients with IgE to the penicilloyl determinants are detected. These limitations coupled with the substantial time required to obtain the results have relegated the in vitro methods to secondary roles, for example when skin tests cannot be performed immediately because of the presence of antihistamines.

MANAGEMENT OF PATIENTS WITH BETA-LACTAM DRUG ALLERGY

Effective alternative antibiotics are usually available for patients with histories of beta-lactam drug allergy. If alternative drugs fail, induce unacceptable side effects, or are for any reason clearly less desirable than a beta-lactam drug, relative risks should be weighed. A history highly suggestive of drug-induced exfoliative dermatitis or the Stevens-Johnson syndrome would present a nearly absolute contraindication to their use. The risk of recurrent serum sickness or hemolytic anemia is difficult to predict. The risk of an IgE-mediated reaction can be estimated with some precision as described above.

Crossreactions Among Beta-Lactam Drugs

Studies of IgE antibodies to benzylpenicillin G, semisynthetic penicillins, and cephalosporins have shown that crossreactions are readily detectable in approximately 80 percent of samples. When patients with positive penicillin skin tests are skin tested with unmodified cephalothin (3.3 mg/ml or less) unequivocally positive wheal and flare responses occur in approximately 50 percent of subjects. Fatal anaphylaxis has been reported on several occasions when cephalosporins were given to penicillin-allergic patients. Immunologic crossreactions are common; clinical crossreactions are observed regularly, but the absolute risk of a clinical crossreaction is not known. A patient allergic to one beta-lactam drug should be considered at increased risk of anaphylaxis to any other beta-lactam drug.

Risk Factors for Allergic Reactions

In addition to the immunologic and historical considerations summarized above, several other factors influence the risk of a serious or fatal reaction. Although children can die from anaphylaxis, the response appears to be less common in children and the case/fatality rate appears to be much lower than in adults. Oral drugs are much safer than parenteral; only 6 deaths from oral beta-lactam drug induced anaphylaxis have been reported. While anaphylaxis seems to be no more common in asthmatics than in other patients, asthmatics are twice as likely to die of anaphylaxis. High-dose drug therapy increases the risk of serum sickness, hemolytic anemia, drug fever, and interstitial nephritis.

Patients receiving beta-adrenergic blocking agents are at increased risk of clinical IgE-mediated reactions. The anaphylaxis they experience tends to be more severe and more prolonged. Treatment is enfeebled to a degree, particularly if the physician does not realize that the patient is receiving beta-adrenergic drug therapy and that beta-adrenergic agonists are not likely to have an effect.

Patients who have IgE to minor determinants may have an increased risk of anaphylaxis, compared to patients with IgE restricted to the penicilloyl determinant. The patients' underlying and concurrent illnesses, medications, and other general medical factors may contribute important forces that could influence the expression or impact of an allergic reaction.

Desensitization of Patients with IgE to Beta-Lactam Drugs

The risk of a clinically detectable allergic reaction if full-dose penicillin is given to a skin test-positive patient is approximately 67 percent. The risk of an anaphylactic reaction is approximately 7 percent of all reactions. The risk that an anaphylactic reaction will be fatal is approximately 5 percent among properly treated patients.

These considerations lead to the expectation that approximately 0.2 percent or 1 in 430 of allergic subjects given full-dose parenteral therapy would experience fatal anaphylaxis. Occasionally, patients develop infections in which the risk of not using a beta-lactam drug appears greater than the risk of using the drug.

Desensitization protocols appear to reduce the risk of anaphylaxis markedly, thereby increasing the number of situations in which the value of beta-lactam therapy outweighs expected risks of allergic complications. Some cases of endocarditis, osteomyelitis, Pseudomonas infections, brain abscess, meningitis, infections in neutropenic patients, and other serious or refractory infections fall into this category. When alternative approaches fail or predictably have little likelihood of success, desensitization should be considered. Central nervous system syphilis has not been proven treatable by agents other than the beta-lactam drugs. Treatment of syphilis in pregnancy with alternative drugs fails to cure as many as one-third of fetuses, while penicillin is uniformly effective. Over half of the unsuccessfully treated babies die or are seriously injured. Since the risks associated with desensitization increasingly appear low, the kinds of infections considered appropriate for desensitization and beta-lactam therapy are expanding.

Assessment of patients for possible desensitization includes demonstration of the presence of IgE to beta-lactam determinants and consideration of alternative therapies and risk factors. Any remediable risk factors should be corrected. Asthma should be under optimal control. Beta-adrenergic blocking drugs usually can be stopped abruptly and replaced by agents such as nifedipine if the dose is 40 mg per day or less. Patients on higher doses can usually tolerate cutting the dose in half on the first day and deleting the drug on the second day, while alternative drugs are introduced.

General desensitization procedures include discussions with the patient, family, and involved physicians to generate informed consent, attention to risk factors, and a careful assessment of the patient's baseline clinical state; ECG and spirometry are usually performed. Intravenous access is established. When possible, desensitization is performed early in the day to permit optimal access to support personnel and facilities. No antiallergic premedication is used under most circumstances because this approach is likely to mask early minor signs of an allergic reaction without certainty of suppressing severe manifestations. Experience to date supports the notion that premedication is not necessary and is undesirable in most circumstances. A physician should be in attendance or immediately available at all times. Vital signs, spirometry if possible, and clinical status should be assessed regularly throughout the procedure and during the first 12 hours of full-dose therapy.

Oral and Parenteral Desensitization Protocols. Specific desensitization protocols can be based on oral or parenteral presentation of initial doses. Published experience with oral desensitization of a total of 72 penicillin-allergic patients indicates that the likelihood of a systemic allergic reaction is low; no reactions involving the cardiovascular or respiratory systems have been detected. Table 2 summarizes a typical oral desensitization protocol. Initial doses can be guided by skin test results. If the patient has tolerated skin tests with the concentrated reagents (approximately 100 U delivered), desensitization can begin at 100 U. Exquisitely sensitive patients can usually be started at 0.1 U. Doses are doubled every 15 minutes if no reaction occurs. If a reaction appears, the nature and intensity of the response determine the change, if any, in the protocol. Mild reactions such as pruritus or a small number of urticariae may not require adjustments in the protocol or treatment. More pronounced cutaneous reactions can be partially suppressed (e.g., 25 mg diphenhydramine IV in an adult) while the procedure continues on schedule. More serious reactions may require repetition of lower doses, increased intervals between doses, or even cessation of the protocol. To date, no need to alter the oral procedure has been reported.

The first oral doses and the first parenteral doses are periods of particular risk. Monitoring of the patients should be intensified at these times. The patients should be observed carefully for at least 12 hours after the first oral dose.

The oral method is preferred when penicillin was the original immunologic stimulus, or when the agent to be used comes in an oral form. When IgE has been elicited by semisynthetic penicillins or cephalosporins, the antibodies may not react with penicillin, and attempts at desensitization with penicillin may not be successful. To avoid this pitfall, a parenteral desensitization method is used when the IgE antibodies were provoked by an agent other than penicillin and the agent needed for therapy is not available in an oral form.

As presented in Table 3, increasing doses of the agent required for therapy are injected subcutaneously in an extremity. Systemic allergic reactions, including responses in the respiratory and cardiovascular systems, may occur during parenteral desensitization. Patients' symptoms, vital signs, airway function, and skin should be followed with particular care. A physician should be present at all times. Some preparations may cause discomfort when given subcutaneously in higher concentrations. Local anesthetics can be mixed with the beta-lactam drugs if necessary, but the compatibility of these agents has not been fully assessed. Adjustments are more likely to be needed with the parenteral protocol than with the oral protocol. If mild reactions occur, the last tolerated dose is repeated and the protocol is resumed. The degree and nature of reactions will dictate repetition of doses, increased intervals between doses, or cessation of the protocol.

Assessing the Safety of Desensitization. Efficacy and safety of desensitization are becoming known with increasing accuracy. All of the reported desensitization procedures, oral or parenteral, performed on skin test-positive allergic patients have led to full-dose therapy. Oral desensitization has never been

TABLE 2 Oral Desensitization Protocol

Step*	*Phenoxymethyl Penicillin (U/ml)*	*Amount (ml)*	*Dose (U)*	*Cumulative Dosage (U)*
1	1000	0.1	100	100
2	1000	0.2	200	300
3	1000	0.4	400	700
4	1000	0.8	800	1500
5	1000	1.6	1600	3100
6	1000	3.2	3200	6300
7	1000	6.4	6400	12,700
8	10,000	1.2	12,000	24,700
9	10,000	2.4	24,000	48,700
10	10,000	4.8	48,000	96,700
11	80,000	1.0	80,000	176,700
12	80,000	2.0	160,000	336,700
13	80,000	4.0	320,000	656,700
14	80,000	8.0	640,000	1,296,700
	Observe patient for 30 min			
	Change to Benzylpenicillin G		*IV*	
15	500,000 U/ml	0.25	125,000	
16	500,000	0.50	250,000	
17	500,000	1.0	500,000	
18	500,000	2.25	1,125,000	

*Interval between steps, 15 min.

TABLE 3 Parenteral Desensitization Protocol

Step*	*Concentration of β-Lactam Drug*	*Amount*	*Dose*	*Cumulative Dosage (mg)*
1	0.1 mg/ml	0.10 ml SQ	0.01 mg	.01
2	0.1	0.20	0.02	.03
3	0.1	0.40	0.04	.07
4	0.1	0.80	0.08	.15
5	1	0.15	0.15	.30
6	1	0.30	0.3	.60
7	1	0.60	0.6	1.2
8	10	0.10	1	2.2
9	10	0.20	2	4.2
10	10	0.40	4	8.2
11	10	0.80	8	16.2
12	100	0.15	15	31.2
13	100	0.30	30	61.2
14	100	0.60	60	121.2
15	1000	0.10	100	221.2
16	1000	0.20	200	421.2
17	1000	0.40	400	821.2
18	1000	0.50	500	1321.2
		Observe patient for 30 min		
19	1000	IV	0.5 g	1821.2
20	1000	IV	1.5 g	3321.2

*Interval between steps, 15 min.

associated with anaphylaxis, but approximately one-third of the patients experience cutaneous pruritus or urticaria at some point in their therapy. Parenteral desensitization may lead to serious allergic reactions, but these reactions have resolved, and successful introduction of full-dose therapy has been accomplished in all reported cases. Approximately two-thirds of patients undergoing parenteral desensitization will have a detectable IgE-mediated reaction at some time in their course of desensitization and therapy.

To date 13 penicillin-allergic pregnant women with serious infections have been desensitized by the oral method. No extracutaneous reactions have occurred, but one-third experienced pruritus or urticaria. Pregnant women appear to be at no greater or lesser risk of complications of desensitization than nonpregnant patients.

Patients with cystic fibrosis and other illnesses that lead to recurrent need for semisynthetic penicillins and cephalosporins are often sensitized by these agents. In most instances, parenteral desensitization with the agent needed for the current infection appears to be the approach most likely to succeed. Patients who can be treated with agents that come in an oral form should receive oral desensitization.

Published evidence indicates that the desensitization procedure permits beta-lactam drug therapy with a much reduced risk of serious clinical reactions. Studies of a small number of patients indicate that the mechanism of desensitization is at least in part, antigen-specific mast cell desensitization.

DRUG REACTIONS

PAUL P. VAN ARSDEL Jr., M.D.

The drug reactions to be discussed here are those that are allergic and those that mimic allergic reactions but are really toxic or pharmacologic actions. The allergic reaction, being dependent on an acquired immunologic response, develops only after several days of drug exposure, often related to some uneventful exposure on an earlier occasion, whereas drugs that mimic allergic reactions do so promptly after treatment is started. Because of the special issues involved in the analysis of drug reactions, it is appropriate to put more emphasis on prevention in this chapter than in others, and this will be presented before the discussion of therapy.

PREVENTION

The incidence of adverse reactions can be reduced in general by limiting the use of drugs to essential indications. In hospitals, at least, the more drugs a patient is given, thee greater the chance of an adverse reaction, allergic or otherwise. In a few instances, severe reactions can be prevented by routine pretreatment skin testing. This should be standard practice before giving any protein or large polypeptide agent, such as horse serum antitoxin. A prick test is done with a 1:10 dilution of the serum. If the reaction is negative in 10 minutes (wheal diameter less than 3 mm larger than control), an intradermal test is done with the 1:10 dilution and then with the undiluted serum. A negative intradermal test is one that is less than 5 mm in diameter.

Routine premedication of all patients before treatment has not proved to be practicable. For example, its use before administering a radiographic contrast medium has largely been abandoned. One exception is premedication in preparation for chymopapain injection to lyse a herniated vertebral disc. This became standard procedure among those licensed to do the procedure before the efficacy of skin testing could be established. According to a nationally generated protocol, the procedure is to be preceded by treatment with diphenhydramine (Benadryl), cimetidine (Tagamet), and a glucocorticoid to reduce the frequency and severity of anaphylaxis from chymopapain. However, because of unanticipated severe toxic effects observed elsewhere that are not affected by this premedication, the procedure is no longer being done at this institution.

The most effective way to prevent allergic reactions is to take a careful history. A positive history must be critical and selective. For example, a history of atopic allergic disease per se is not a significant factor, whereas a history of a previous drug reaction usually is. For most practical purposes, this means a history of a reaction to a drug that is immunochemically or pharmacologically similar to the one being considered for treatment. However, one should be especially careful in selecting and prescribing any drug to someone who gives a history of reacting to numerous different drugs, whatever the mechanism.

Although the history is most important in identifying potential drug risks and is obviously important for medicolegal reasons, it can also result in the labeling of some people as allergic who actually are not. For example, careful questioning may establish that a patient was treated with ampicillin without a problem years after the penicillin reaction of record. Some reactions, notably nausea, headaches, and local pain and swelling after injections may be recorded inappropriately as allergic. The reactions associated with underlying illnesses may be blamed on one or more drugs being used for treatment. Noteworthy examples are the Jarisch-Herxheimer reaction, and urticaria and other skin rashes that may occur during acute viral infections and during the treatment of bacterial endocarditis. Somewhat different is the ampicillin-"induced" maculopapular skin rash (especially during infectious mononucleosis), which cannot be reproduced with that drug after the patient recovers from the illness.

The Patient With A Positive History

In any hospital, patients with a label of drug allergy in their records greatly outnumber those who actually have an allergic drug reaction while in the hospital. This section will be devoted to the proper approach to such a patient who should be treated with the suspected drug. Figure 1 is a diagram depicting this approach.

Alternative Drugs. If a drug of a different structure than that of the suspect drug is available and effective, it should be used. The risk of reacting to the alternative drug must also be considered. For example, vancomycin and the aminoglycoside drugs are alternates to beta-lactam antibiotics, but are substantially more toxic. Thus, it might be prudent to select a cephalosporin as an alternate for treatment of someone thought to be allergic to the penicillins, despite the small risk of cross-sensitivity. In contrast to the usual rule to select a chemically different drug, it is appropriate to select a chemically *similar* drug, sodium salicylate, for analgesic use in aspirin-sensitive patients. These patients tend to react to drugs that share aspirin's property of inhibiting prostaglandin synthesis, but are of different chemical structure.

Immunologic Testing. To confirm or rule out an IgE antibody-mediated allergic drug reaction, the skin test is necessary and sufficient if the appropriate antigen is used. It is sufficient because it recognizes the same sensitivity as do the in vitro methods, namely, the serum radioallergosorbent test (RAST) or its enzyme indicator relative (ELISA), and the antigen-induced basophil histamine release reaction; the last being primarily a research procedure. The skin test is also quicker, cheaper, and more sensitive than the others. Appropriate antigens are xenogeneic sera, immunizing biologicals, enzymes, insulin, and any other agent with a molecular weight large enough for it to act as a complete antigen. Reliable testing reagents are available for testing only for the penicillins among the conventional low-molecular-weight drugs (see chapter on *Penicillin Allergy*). Routine testing for horse serum sensitivity has been

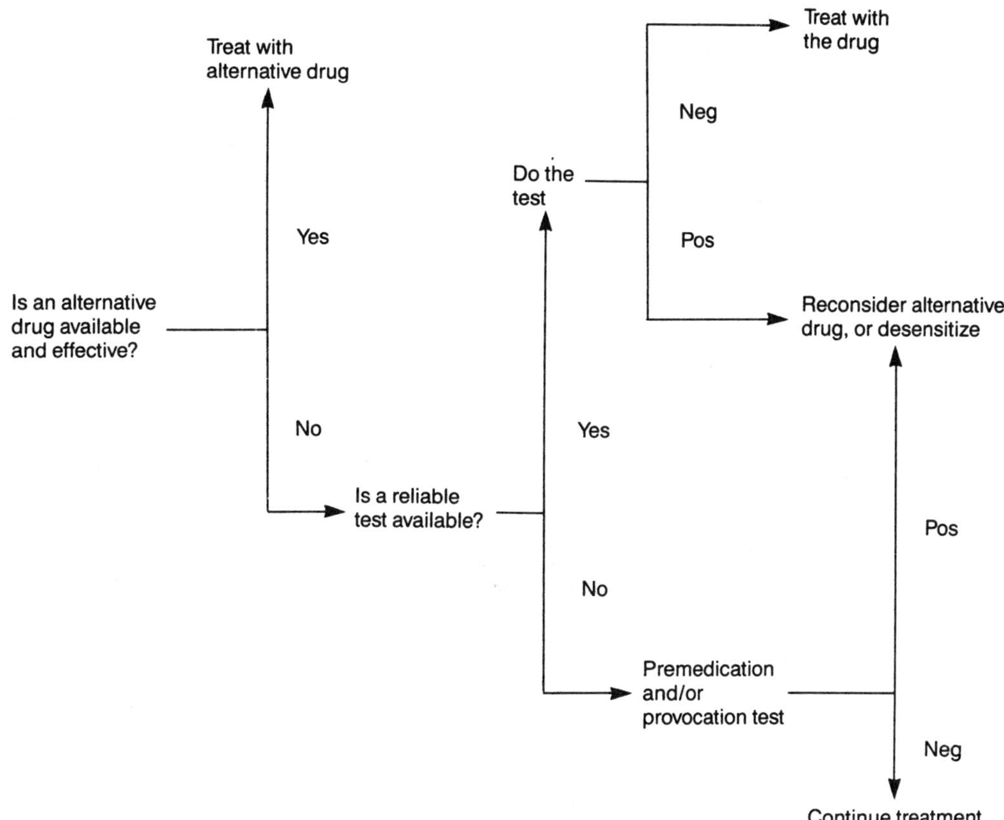

Figure 1 Decision tree demonstrating work-up of patient with positive drug allergy history

discussed. When evaluating someone with a positive history or someone about to receive another macromolecule such as an injected enzyme about which little clinical experience has accumulated, testing should begin with a 1:1000, rather than a 1:10, dilution. It is prudent to start with a 1:100,000 dilution if severe anaphylaxis followed previous use of the suspect agent. Whatever the starting dilution, the first test should be a prick test; intradermal testing is appropriate at tenfold increments thereafter.

Skin testing to local anesthetics, whatever the chemical structure, is an effective way to exclude allergy to these substances, which is extremely rare. Each anesthetic to be tested is obtained epinephrine-free and is diluted 1:10 and 1:100. The patient is tested with the 1:100 dilution with a prick test first, then an intradermal test. If no reaction to either of these tests occurs within 15 minutes, an intradermal test is done with the 1:10, then the undiluted, solution. As a final precaution, a 0.5 ml test dose can be given subcutaneously or into the area to be anesthetized.

The *patch test* is used to establish or rule out the cause of drug-induced allergic eczematous contact dermatitis. It is a T-cell-mediated skin reaction. The suspect drug, in an appropriate vehicle, is applied to the skin under an occlusive adhesive patch. An erythematous pruritic vesicular reaction develops in 48 to 72 hours if that drug was responsible. This is essentially a controlled provocation test (to be discussed).

Provocation Testing. The only completely reliable test for drug sensitivity is to give the drug again, under controlled conditions. If the symptoms and signs recur (as in the patch test example above), the diagnosis is established. When the diagnosis is probable, but the offending drug is in doubt and the reaction is benign or can be contained, challenge is justified, as with the patch test for contact dermatitis, the fixed drug eruption, and uncomplicated drug fever. When the diagnosis of sensitivity is extremely unlikely and the drug is clearly the preferred one, challenge is also justified (this is, in effect, what we do with local anesthetic testing). When the diagnosis is possible, but the reaction is potentially serious or even lethal, challenge is rarely justified. In intermediate situations, careful challenge testing of a drug that is the best choice for diagnosis or treatment may be essential. The first dose given should be 1 percent of the therapeutic dose; if no reaction occurs, 10 percent and the full dose should be given at 15- to 60-minute intervals (depending on the route of administration). This can be expedited if the patient is protected beforehand with appropriate medication (to be described).

Premedication. Antihistaminic, adrenergic, or anti-inflammatory drugs have been used for many years to prevent possible reactions from antituberculosis medication; intramuscular, intra-articular, and allergen immunotherapy injections; or transfusion of blood products. Routine premedication before chymopapain injections has been discussed. Nowhere else has premedication of patients with a positive reaction history been so well evaluated as in those who have had previous radiographic contrast medium reactions. Such patients can be protected from a serious reaction by premedication with oral prednisone, 50 mg *q6h* for three doses, followed by intramuscular diphenhydramine (Benadryl), 50 mg, and subcutaneous ephedrine, 25 mg, one hour before the procedure. As with any challenge procedure, suitable emergency resuscitative equipment should be within reach.

Desensitization. The strategies of careful gradual challenge testing and of premedication can also be applied to desensitization of the sensitive patient. Desensitization of the patient who is sensitive to a xenogeneic serum, as confirmed by a positive skin test, is begun by subcutaneous injection of 0.1 ml of the dilution that gave the smallest positive skin reaction. The dose is doubled every 15 minutes until 1 ml of the undiluted serum has been given. This dose is then given intramuscularly, and then the full dose is given. If any symptom of a reaction appears, the next injection is postponed until it subsides.

Well-defined protocols have also been developed for desensitization to insulin, a rare event since human insulin has become generally available, and to penicillin (see chapter on *Penicillin Allergy).*

Patients who are hyperreactive to aspirin and the other nonsteroidal anti-inflammatory drugs can be desensitized if there is a strong need for treatment with one of these drugs. Since most of these patients are asthmatic, before desensitization is begun the patient should be given intensive antiasthmatic therapy to bring ventilatory function as close to normal as possible. With regular monitoring of ventilatory function, aspirin is given by mouth, starting with 10 mg, and doubling the dose every 3 hours until the full dose is reached. If symptoms develop at any point or the ventilatory function drops more than 20 percent, the reaction should be allowed to subside; then the same dose that provoked it should be given again. Usually the reaction does not recur. To maintain tolerance, which extends to all nonsteroidal anti-inflammatory drugs, the patient must take one of these drugs every day.

TREATMENT

Reactions that are thought to be allergic are listed in Table 1. Their clinical features will not be discussed except as they determine the type of treatment needed. In general, if a reaction develops, treatment with the suspected drug or drugs should be stopped unless, in the physician's judgment, the need for treatment is greater than the risk of the reaction, and its symptoms can be controlled. Stopping treatment is the only necessary step for nonpruritic skin rashes, drug fever, and most reactions involving the major organ systems.

Treatment of Pruritus

Urticaria and other pruritic skin rashes are treated with hydroxyzine, 25 to 100 mg by mouth (Atarax)

TABLE 1 Classification of Drug Reactions

Mast cell-mediated reactions
Systemic anaphylaxis
Urticaria and angioedema
Some pruritic maculopapular eruptions
Serum sickness (in part)
Anaphylactoid (nonimmunologic)
T-lymphocyte-mediated reactions
Allergic eczematous contact dermatitis
Photodermatitis
Other cutaneous reactions (mechanism uncertain)
Maculopapular or exanthematous
Fixed eruptions
Toxic epidermal necrolysis
Drug fever
Systemic lupus erythematosus and other autoimmune reactions
Organ systems reactions
Blood
eosinophilia, hemolytic anemia, thrombocytopenia, granulocytopenia
Lung
Liver
Kidney
Reactions with inconsistent drug associations
Erythema multiforme
Exfoliative dermatitis
Vasculitis

or intramuscularly (Vistaril). Treatment can be repeated every 6 to 8 hours as needed until the eruption subsides. Alternative drugs are diphenhydramine (Benadryl), 25 to 100 mg, and cyproheptadine (Periactin), 4 to 8 mg. The main side effect of treatment is drowsiness, not usually a problem with the hospitalized patient, but any ambulatory patient should be warned about the risk of operating a motor vehicle or other machinery while taking one of these drugs. Skin testing for IgE-mediated sensitivity cannot be performed for at least 72 hours after the last dose of hydroxyzine and 48 hours after the last dose of the others.

If the foregoing treatment is inadequate, one might consider adding the H_2 antihistamine, cimetidine, or substituting the tricyclic antihistamine, doxepin, but the reaction is more likely to resolve if oral prednisone, 40 mg daily, is given and rapidly tapered to zero when the reaction subsides.

Glucocorticoid Treatment

Severe reactions should be treated with oral prednisone or intravenous methylprednisolone from the start. These include urticaria, serum sickness, contact dermatitis, erythema multiforme, and exfoliative dermatitis—such therapy may also hasten recovery from pulmonary, hepatic, and hematologic reactions. Toxic epidermal necrolysis, vasculitis, and interstitial nephritis do not usually respond to glucocorticoid treatment, but it may still be appropriate to use it for a few days.

Treatment of Pain

Pain may be a prominent symptom with some reactions. The arthralgias of serum sickness and systemic lupus erythematosus, and cutaneous pain in vasculitis and some cases of urticaria can be treated with a nonsteroidal anti-inflammatory agent such as indomethacin (Indocin), 25 to 50 mg *q8h*. If this is inadequate, prednisone treatment should be initiated.

Treatment of Anaphylaxis

The treatment is summarized in Table 2 according to the usual sequence of events. Shock and/or upper airway obstruction are the most likely causes of death, and so vital signs and adequacy of respiration should be carefully followed from the onset of the reaction.

As indicated in Table 2, epinephrine is effective in alleviating most of the features of anaphylaxis and should be given promptly; 0.3 to 0.5 mg in a 1:1000 concentration should be given subcutaneously immediately. If the offending agent (an allergenic extract is a good example) was given into an extremity, the injection site should be infiltrated with another 0.2 mg and a tourniquet placed above it. This usually is sufficient to prevent progression of the reaction.

Hypotension. If the patient is hypotensive (systolic pressure less than 60 mm), an intravenous

TABLE 2 Summary Outline of Treatment Anaphylaxis

General
Epinephrine
Tourniquet (when physically possible)
Rapidly progressing symptoms
Intravenous line, dextrose, in 0.5 normal saline
Oxygen and emergency equipment on hand
Hypotension
Epinephrine, slow intravenous, large volumes of dextrose in 0.5 normal saline
ECG monitor
Monitor central venous pressure
Vasopressor drug (?)
Upper airway obstruction
Epinephrine
Diphenhydramine
Oxygen
Endotrachial intubation or tracheostomy
Lower airway obstruction
Epinephrine, isoproterenol
Oxygen
Aminophylline, intravenous
Prepare for treatment of respiratory failure
Cardiac problems
ECG monitor for dysrhythmias
Monitor pulmonary artery wedge pressure
Isoproterenol for cardiogenic shock
Late reactions
Observe and monitor as necessary for 12 hours
Glucocorticoid therapy

line must be placed and a crystalloid solution such as 5 percent dextrose in 0.5 normal saline infused rapidly. Three to four liters of fluid may need to be infused to restore plasma volume. Epinephrine is then infused through a side line at a dilution high enough (e.g., 1:100,000) to allow delivery of the drug at a rate of about 5 to 10 μg/minute, with continuous ECG monitoring for arrhythmias. Anaphylaxis may occur in a patient who has been taking a beta-adrenergic blocking drug. In such a patient, epinephrine resistance may be overcome by increasing the dose, but this maneuver demands careful monitoring for side effects. Ancillary intravenous treatment with both the H_1 antihistamine diphenhydramine (Benadryl), 100 mg, and the H_2 antihistamine cimetidine (Tagamet), 300 mg, may be advisable.

If the blood pressure remains low in the face of a rising central venous pressure, cardiogenic shock may be developed (to be discussed).

Upper Airway Obstruction. Hoarseness, stridor, or the use of accessory respiratory muscles should alert the observer to the possibility of obstructing angioedema. If this happens, diphenhydramine (Benadryl), 100 mg, should be given intravenously in addition to epinephrine, which can be given subcutaneously every 20 minutes. If a No. 6 or No. 7 endotracheal tube cannot be inserted, one must be prepared to perform a tracheostomy or cricothyroid membrane puncture. Oxygen must be provided.

Lower Airway Obstruction. All patients should be examined for symptoms and signs of asthma; those who develop lower airway obstruction usually have a history of asthma. If symptoms of asthma appear despite the epinephrine given earlier aminophylline should be given intravenously, 6 mg/kg over 20 minutes, followed by another 3 mg/kg if necessary. If the symptoms have not subsided, the drug should be continued in a constant infusion of 0.5 mg/kg/hour, adjusted to maintain the blood level at 10 to 20 μg/ml. If toxic symptoms or signs appear (nausea, cardiac dysrhythmia), the infusion should be stopped until they subside. If the patient also is hypotensive, the aminophylline dose should be reduced by 50 percent.

Cardiac Problems. Dysrhythmias may develop from a combination of factors such as drugs, anaphylactogenic mediators, and hypoxia. If a dysrhythmia develops, it is treated by conventional methods that need not be described here. If hypotension persists despite epinephrine infusion and fluid replacement, the patient is usually maximally vasoconstricted and adding treatment with an alpha-adrenergic vasopressor drug will serve no useful purpose. Usually, pressure monitoring reveals a reduced cardiac output, which should be treated with isoproterenol (Isuprel), 1 to 5 μg/minute intravenously, with continuous ECG monitoring. Serving also as a bronchodilator, this drug has a modest advantage over the alternative drugs dopamine and dobutamine.

Prevention of Late Reactions. The acute and potentially life-threatening reactions usually resolve within an hour. A resurgence of the reaction, less serious, but still uncomfortable, may appear 4 to 10 hours later. This may be prevented by giving methylprednisolone (Solu-Medrol), 40 mg intravenously, after all other treatment has been started. This, or 40 mg prednisone by mouth, can be given again 6 hours later.

If no new symptoms develop within 12 hours of the onset, it is unlikely that any will appear later.

SYSTEMIC ANAPHYLAXIS

STEPHEN P. PETERS, M.D., Ph.D.

Anaphylaxis is a generalized reaction to a foreign substance. In this discussion, the term *anaphylaxis* will be used to denote a *clinical syndrome* rather than to imply any series of pathologic events in the production of this syndrome. Commonly, the term anaphylaxis implies a generalized reaction involving an *IgE mediated mechanism*. The term *anaphylactoid* has been used to describe a similar clinical syndrome not initiated by IgE mediated events. The use of the term anaphylaxis for the clinical syndrome without implying anything about pathophysiologic mechanism, as used here, obviates the need for the use of terms such as anaphylactoid. This chapter discusses the following aspects of systemic anaphylaxis: causes, symptoms and diagnosis, treatment, and prevention.

As shown in Table 1, the causes of systemic anaphylaxis are numerous. In the typical IgE mediated event, exposure of an individual to a foreign substance elicits the production of IgE antibody, which becomes bound to high-affinity receptors on mast cells and basophils. Reexposure of the individual to the same substance results in cross-linking of IgE receptors on the surface of these cells and the release of potent inflammatory mediators, including histamine, sulfidopeptide leukotrienes (slow-reacting substance of anaphylaxis), lysosomal hydrolases and other hydrolytic enzymes, and prostaglandin D_2 (from mast cells), as well as other potent mediators. Numerous drugs, particularly of the antibiotic class acting as haptens, such as penicillins and cephalosporins, have been documented to cause anaphylactic reactions. Proteins and foods are other common offenders. The release of mast cell and basophil mediators with secondary stimulation of other cells produces profound physiologic effects and initiates events which result in the syndrome of anaphylaxis. High levels of plasma his-

TABLE 1 Causes of Systemic Anaphylaxis

IgE-Mediated
Antibiotics
Penicillins
Cephalosporins
Tetracyclines
Vancomycin
Nitrofurantoin
Amphoterocin B
Other Therapeutic Agents
Streptokinase
Hydrocortisone
Methylprednisolone
Local anesthetics — some reactions
Muscle relaxants — some reactions
Thiopental
Allergen Extracts
Proteins
Hymenoptera Venom
Antilymphocyte globulin
Insulin
Chymopapain
Seminal plasma
Foods
Milk
Egg white
Shellfish
Fish
Nuts
Chocolate
Histamine Releasing Agents
Radiocontrast Media
Opiates
Dextran
Curare
d-Tubocurarine
Polymyxin B
Iron Dextran (?)
Immune Complex or Complement Mediated
Whole blood
Plasma
Immunoglobulin
Cryoprecipitate
Others
Aspirin
Nonsteroidal anti-inflammatory agents
Benzoates
Exercise
Exercise and food
Idiopathic

Source: Abridged and modified from Wasserman SI, Anaphylaxis, In Middleton, E. Jr, et al eds: *Allergy, Principles and Practice,* 2nd/Ed. St. Louis: CV Mosby, 1983, p. 690.

tamine, as well as abnormalities of complement and clotting proteins, have all been described during human anaphylaxis.

Anaphylactic episodes also apparently result from the direct effect of foreign substances on mast cells and basophils, as in the case of reactions to radiocontrast media, as well as in other physiologic events involving immune complex or complement-mediated injury. In addition, the mechanism by which agents such as aspirin and nonsteroidal anti-inflammatory agents provoke systemic reactions has not been determined. In any event, the clinical consequences of anaphylaxis from any of these mechanisms tend to be similar.

SYMPTOMS AND DIAGNOSIS OF ANAPHYLAXIS

Most instances of anaphylaxis are preceded by a well-documented exposure to a foreign substance, for example, a drug, food, or toxin. Parenteral administration of the agent is more likely to be associated with more severe systemic reactions than oral or topical administration. Symptoms usually occur within minutes of exposure and commonly involve the skin, respiratory tract, and/or cardiovascular system (Table 2). Less commonly, the gastrointestinal or genitourinary tract may be involved.

The most common dermatologic manifestations of anaphylaxis are pruritus with associated urticarial lesions; less commonly, angioedema occurs and, in rare instances, may lead to respiratory compromise. These dermatologic manifestations are usually self-limited and typically resolve within 48 hours.

There are two types of respiratory symptoms: laryngeal and upper airway edema or bronchospasm, either of which may be life threatening. In addition, mucus hypersecretion is also seen in systemic anaphylaxis. Upper airway edema or bronchospasm are among the most dramatic manifestations of anaphylaxis, and both require aggressive therapy.

The cardiovascular manifestations of acute anaphylaxis include hypotension, shock, and cardiac arrhythmias. These symptoms appear to result primarily

TABLE 2 Symptoms of Anaphylaxis

Common
Dermatologic
Pruritus
Urticaria
Angioedema
Respiratory
Laryngeal and upper airway edema*
Bronchospasm*
Mucus hypersecretion
Cardiovascular
Hypotension
Shock*
Cardiac arrythmias*
Uncommon
Gastrointestinal
Nausea
Vomiting
Diarrhea
Intestinal cramps
Genitourinary
Urinary urgency
Uterine cramps

Source: Modified from Patterson, R. and Valentine, M.: Anaphylaxis and related allergic emergencies, JAMA 248:2635, 1982

*Indicates a severe reaction which may be life-threatening

from a decrease in blood return to the heart, secondary to either peripheral venous dilation and/or transudation of fluid into extravascular spaces. Primary cardiac malfunction does not appear to be a frequent occurrence and usually results from decreased perfusion of the coronary arteries. Similarly, cardiac arrhythmias appear to result from decreased coronary perfusion rather than from primary cardiac dysfunction.

The less common manifestations of anaphylaxis, particularly gastrointestinal symptoms, are more often seen after oral ingestion of the provocative agent.

The diagnosis of anaphylaxis is usually a straightforward one. Exposure of an individual to the provocative agent is followed, usually within minutes, by some of the symptoms listed in Table 2. Although isolated dermatologic, respiratory, or cardiovascular symptoms may occur, the syndrome of anaphylaxis often involves multiple organ systems. A combination of dermatologic and respiratory or cardiovascular symptoms after appropriate exposure virtually establishes diagnosis.

Problems in establishing the diagnosis may occur when exposure has not been noted or remembered or when an isolated organ system, such as the cardiovascular or gastrointestinal system, is the only target organ. For example, hypotension occurring as an anaphylactic reaction without concomitant dermatologic or respiratory symptoms may be confused with hypotension secondary to a vasovagal reaction or associated with shock from other causes, such as sepsis or myocardial infarction. However, the cause of hypotension in those circumstances is usually readily apparent.

Although many different combinations of symptoms are possible in a given individual the same pattern of symptoms tends to repeat in a given patient. A tendency toward more severe symptoms with repeated exposure to the initiating agent, particularly involving the respiratory or cardiovascular system, is an ominous sign.

TREATMENT

Since the manifestations of systemic anaphylaxis can vary markedly from a minor generalized skin rash to profound shock with cardiovascular and respiratory failure, the therapy of systemic anaphylaxis needs to be highly individualized. In addition, since the drug of choice for anaphylaxis, epinephrine, may be associated with significant morbidity in elderly persons or in persons with underlying cardiovascular or cerebrovascular disease, potential serious side effects of therapy must be kept in mind when attending such patients. Clearly, the approach to an elderly patient with severe underlying cardiovascular disease who presents with a minor pruritic urticarial reaction after a radiocontrast study would be much different from therapy for a healthy 30-year-old man who presents with cardiovascular collapse after an insect sting. The treatment of anaphylaxis is outlined in Table 3.

Initial Therapy

First, the airway should be stabilized. If symptoms of upper airway edema or obstruction develop (hoarseness, stridor, sensation of upper airway closing), endotracheal intubation by the transoral or transnasal approach should be accomplished. Depending upon the degree of upper airway narrowing, the use of a small endotracheal tube (for example, a size 6 or 7 tube in an adult patient) may be needed. If endotracheal intubation is impossible, puncture of the cricothyroid membrane with a large bore needle and jet ventilation (in facilities with experience with that technique), intubation through an incision in the cricothyroid membrane, or emergency tracheostomy may be required.

The drug of choice for systemic anaphylaxis is epinephrine: 0.3 to 0.5 cc of a 1:1000 solution of aqueous epinephrine should be given subcutaneously. This same dose may be repeated every 15 to 20 minutes if needed.

Venous access should be obtained, preferably with an 18-guage or larger catheter. This site can be used for volume replacement and for intravenous medications.

Finally, if applicable, a tourniquet should be placed above the site of injection or sting to reduce systemic absorption of the provocative agent. The tourniquet should be loosened every 5 minutes.

If symptoms of a severe reaction occur, such as laryngeal or upper airway edema or significant bronchospasm or any cardiovascular symptoms, the patient should be admitted to a hospital and placed in a monitored setting. In any event, the vital signs should be monitored frequently, initially at least every 15 minutes.

Shock

If the patient presents with significant hypotension, he should be placed in a recumbent position with the legs elevated. Rapid infusion of normal saline should be begun; up to 1 liter may be required every 20 minutes or so in severe cases. After several liters of crystalloid solution have been infused, some physicians find the use of colloid solution of albumin or 5 percent plasma protein fraction is also useful. Although large volumes of rapidly infused crystalloid and colloid may precipitate congestive heart failure or pulmonary edema in susceptible patients, that complication is not usually seen in episodes of systemic anaphylaxis. This is probably due, at least in part, to the profound peripheral vasodilation and perhaps transudation of fluid which occur in this setting. However, either one of these complications is certainly possible in any individual with underlying cardiac dysfunction.

If symptoms of hypotension are relatively unresponsive to even large volumes (several liters) of crystalloid solution plus colloid supplementation, in addition to subcutaneous epinephrine as described above, epinephrine, 1 to 3 cc of a 1:10,000 aqueous solution, can be given slowly intravenously, or a continuous infusion of epinephrine can be started (1 ml of 1:1000 or 10 ml of 1:10,000 diluted in 500 ml of D_5W and infused at 0.5 to 5 μg/min; 1 ml/min = 2 μg/min.) As noted above, epinephrine is the drug of choice for this syndrome, and the actions of intravenously administered epinephrine are more rapid and greater than those of subcutaneous epinephrine. It should be remembered that intraveous epinephrine has been associated with significant complications in elderly patients or patients with underlying cerebrovascular or cardiovascular disease and that such conditions should be kept in mind when a decision to use intravenous epinephrine is made.

Many physicians have had more experience using continuous infusions of norepinephrine or dopamine in the setting of persistent hypotension than in the use of intravenous epinephrine. Therefore, hypotension not responding to subcutaneous epinephrine, elevation of the legs, and rapid infusion of crystalloid and colloid solutions can be treated with a continuous infusion of norephinephrine or dopamine, as shown in Table 3. Norepinephrine has the advantage of acting primarily to cause peripheral vasoconstriction, which seems to be a major cause of the hypotension seen in anaphylaxis. In addition to causing peripheral vasoconstriction at high doses, dopamine, at low doses, can also increase myocardial contractility and renal blood flow. In patients who require infusion of these potent vascoconstrictors, monitoring of central venous pressure or pulmonary arterial and capillary wedge pressure, in order to estimate left ventricular filling pressure, is often indicated. The use of a flow-directed pulmonary catheter can be very useful in a patient with underlying cardiac dysfunction in whom the risk of congestive heart failure or pulmonary edema is greater.

Cardiac arrythmias may be related to either anaphylaxis or treatment. If anaphylaxis related, standard antiarrythmic therapy is used. If treatment related (for example, from epinephrine), changing the rate of drug infusion or switching to an alternative agent is usually effective.

Bronchospasm

If significant bronchospasm develops, supplemental oxygen should be given to maintain hemoglobin saturation (that is, $Po_2 \geq 60$ mmHg). In practice, highflow oxygen by nasal cannula (5 L/min) or face mask (40 to 60 percent O_2) is usually begun, and the Po_2 is usually maintained in the 80 to 100 mmHg range.

If bronchospasm is severe, a combination of therapeutic agents is usually required. "Severe" episodes of bronchoconstriction are often associated with one or more of the following: pulsus paradoxus ≥ 18 mmHg, $FEV_1 \leq 1.0$ L, peak flow ≤ 200 L/min., $Pco_2 \geq 42$ mmHg. If the patient has not been receiving a maintenance aminophylline preparation, a loading dose of aminophylline should be given (6 mg/kg IV over 10 to 20 minutes). If the patient has been taking aminophylline, a maximum of one-half of the above loading dose may be given, depending upon the maintenance dose taken by the patient, recent serum theophylline levels, and the time since the last dose. If in doubt, the serum theophylline level should be checked. Maintenance aminophylline dosages range from approximately 0.3 to 0.9 mg/kg/hr IV. In patients in whom hepatic dysfunction or congestive heart failure is present, the hepatic metabolism of aminophylline is slowed, and a lower maintenance dosage is required. Conversely, in patients with a rapid hepatic metabolism, as in cigarette smokers, maintenance dosages toward the high end of the range are often required. Note that aminophylline can interact with other drugs, such as cimetidine, to increase the serum concentration of aminophylline. If prolonged therapy with this agent is required (more than 12 hours), serum aminophylline levels should be checked.

Aminophylline should be supplemented by an inhaled beta-adrenergic agonist every 2 to 4 hours. Any of the standard beta-agonists is appropriate, given either by nebulization or by a hand-held inhaler. In patients in whom significant respiratory distress is present, the use of terbutaline, 0.25 mg (0.25 cc of a 1 mg/ml solution) can be injected subcutaneously, with a second dose administered in 15 to 30 minutes if needed. This subcutaneously administered terbutaline often allows time for intravenous aminophylline and inhaled beta-agonists to begin to take effect.

These measures should ordinarily not take the place of the initial subcutaneous doses of epinephrine, which also will provide significant relief from bronchospasm. In addition, if the episode of anaphylaxis has been severe, or if the bronchospasm has been severe or longstanding, the use of corticosteroids as described in Table 3, is also indicated.

Symptoms of mild bronchospasm can often be treated with only an inhaled beta-adrenergic agonist.

Improvement in the patient with bronchospasm can be documented by observing a decrease in pulsus paradoxus or an increase in pulmonary flow rate, as measured by a spirometer or a peak flow meter.

Urticaria or Angioedema

Urticaria or angioedema is treated with H_1 antihistamines, diphenhydramine, or hydroxyzine in doses of 25 to 50 mg IM or PO every 6 to 8 hours, as needed. In addition, although not of proven benefit in this situation, H_2 antihistamines, such as cimetidine, may also be added. The combination of H_1 and H_2 antihistamines has tended to be superior to H_1 antihistamine alone in cases of chronic urticaria. If a patient presents only with urticaria, antihistamines may be used alone, while the patient is carefully observed for other signs that would signify a more severe reaction. Angioedema that affects the airway should be treated more vigorously as described above in the section Initial Therapy.

TABLE 3 Treatment of Systemic Anaphylaxis

Initial Therapy

Stabilize the airway. If symptoms of upper airway edema or obstruction develop, endotracheal intubation by the transoral or transnasal approach (preferably), or possibly puncture of the cricothyroid membrane or emergency tracheostomy may be required.

Epinephrine, 0.3–0.5 cc of aqueous 1:1,000 dilution. The same dose may be repeated every 15–20 minutes if needed.

Obtain venous access (18 gauge or larger catheter, if possible) for:
Volume replacement
Intravenous medications

If any symptoms of a severe reaction occur (respiratory — laryngeal or upper airway edema or significant bronchospasm; cardiac — hypotension, shock, or cardiac arrhythmias), the patient should be admitted to a hospital and placed in a monitored setting.

Record vital signs frequently in any event (initially, at least every 15 minutes).

If applicable, place a tourniquet above the site of injection or sting to reduce systemic absorption of the agent. Loosen every 5 minutes.

For Shock

Place the patient in a recumbent position. Elevate the legs.

Rapidly infuse normal saline (up to 1 L of saline every 20 minutes or so may be required) or solutions of colloid (albumin or 5% plasma protein fraction).

Epinephrine, 1–3 cc of aqueous 1:10,000 dilution, can be given slowly iv for persistent or recurrent symptoms. Or a continuous infusion of epinephrine can be started, 1 ml of 1:1,000 or 10 ml of 1:10,000 diluted in 500 ml of D_5W and infused at 0.5–5 μg/min; 1 ml/min = 2 μg/min. Weigh the risk versus any possible benefit.

For hypotension not responding to the above measures, continuous infusion of one of the following may be needed:
Norepinephrine, 4–8 mg (1 or 2 ampules) in 1,000 ml of D_5W, $D_5$1/2NS, or D_5NS titrated to maintain systolic blood pressure in the 80–100 mm Hg range. (Maintenance doses of 0.5–3.0 cc per minute are often needed.)
Dopamine, beginning with 1–5 μg/kg/min to maintain systolic blood pressure in the 80–100 mm Hg range.

The goal of therapy is to maintain adequate cerebral, cardiac, and renal perfusion. The blood pressure required to do this may vary in different patients, based on their preanaphylaxis baseline blood pressure. In addition, severely ill or fragile patients may benefit from measurement of central venous pressure or pulmonary arterial and capillary wedge pressures with a flow-directed pulmonary catheter.

For Bronchospasm

Give supplemental oxygen to maintain hemoglobin saturation ($\geq$ 90% saturated), $PO_2 \geq 60$ mm Hg. (To provide a margin of safety, PO_2 should preferably be in the 80–100 mm Hg range.) Five liters of O_2 by nasal cannula or 40–60% O_2 by face mask can be started initially.

If Severe:

Aminophylline, 6 mg/kg iv over 20–30 minutes (if patient has *not* been taking aminophylline regularly); a maximum of half the above loading dose may be given if the patient has been taking aminophylline, depending upon the severity of the symptoms and the time since last dose. If in doubt, a serum theophylline level should be obtained. Maintenance aminophylline doses range from 0.3–0.9 mg/kg/hour iv (toward the low end of the range if the patient has hepatic dysfunction, has congestive heart failure, is taking medication that can increase serum aminophylline level (such as cimetidine), or is elderly; toward the high end of the range if the patient is likely to have increased hepatic metabolism, as in a cigarette smoker).

Inhaled β-adrenergic agonist every 2–4 hours:
Metaproterenol, 0.3 cc of a 5% solution in 2.5 cc of normal saline by nebulizer
or
Metaproterenol inhaler, 2 puffs

Table 3 continues

Miscellaneous

If a severe reaction has occurred or prolonged therapy has been required, blood should be sent for hemogram and electrolyte tests and, if indicated, for arterial blood gas and theophylline measurements. A chest radiograph or electrocardiogram may also be indicated, depending on the nature of the symptoms. Finally, the use of systemic corticosteroids in high doses, as described in Table 3, may prevent the late recrudescence of symptoms.

As noted at the end of Table 3, complications from either the anaphylactic episode itself or from the therapy for anaphylaxis may be severe, and treatment should be individualized to the patient, based on any underlying medical conditions and the severity of the episode.

PREVENTION OF ANAPHYLAXIS

The primary goal of the treatment of anaphylaxis is prevention (Table 4). This goal may be approached by taking a thorough medical history and by avoiding agents historically associated with systemic reactions. If specific skin testing is available for an agent (for example, hymenoptera venom or penicillin), it can be performed to document the risk of anaphylaxis. In certain cases, immunotherapy may be useful. Such therapy has been most effective in cases of individuals undergoing anaphylaxis to specific insect stings (see chapters on *Insect Sting Allergy in Adults*). In addition, if it is absolutely necessary to use a specific drug (for example, penicillin, insulin) in the face of a history of a prior systemic reaction or a positive skin test, desensitization can be attempted.

TABLE 3 Treatment of Systemic Anaphylaxis (Continued)

or

Albuterol inhaler, 2 puffs

If necessary, terbutaline, 0.25 mg (0.25 cc of 1 mg/ml solution) may be injected subcutaneously; a second dose may be administered in 15–30 minutes, with the total not to exceed 0.5 mg in a 4-hour period.

Corticosteroids should be added as described below if significant symptoms persist after 1–2 hours of vigorous therapy.

If Mild:

Inhaled β-adrenergic agonist as described above may be sufficient.

For Urticaria or Angioedema

H_1 antihistamines, diphenhydramine, or hydroxyzine, 25–50 mg im or po every 6–8 hours as needed.

Although not proven to be of benefit in this situation, H_2 blockers, such as cimetidine, 300 mg po or iv every 6 hours, may be added.

Miscellaneous

If prolonged therapy has been required, send blood for hemogram and electrolytes and, if indicated, arterial blood gases and theophylline level.

If indicated:

Chest radiograph (e.g., poorly responsive bronchospasm or localized abnormality on examination)

Electrocardiogram (e.g., chest pain, cardiac arrythmia)

Although not proven effective, corticosteroids have been suggested to be of value in preventing the late recurrence of symptoms:

Hydrocortisone, 250 mg iv every 6 hours for 4 doses,

or

Methylprednisolone or prednisone in equivalent doses

Possible Complications

From Anaphylaxis

Persistent hypotension leading to myocardial infarction, cerebral ischemia, renal failure

Respiratory failure with or without upper airway obstruction

Death

From Therapy

From epinephrine, norepinephrine, or dopamine

Hypertension leading to myocardial infarction, cerebrovascular accident, or other vascular complications

Cardiac arrythmias

Tissue necrosis (should solutions extravasate into extravascular tissues)

From vigorous iv fluid therapy

Congestive heart failure

Pulmonary edema

From Aminophylline

GI distress

Cardiac arrythmias

Seizures

From β-agonists

Nervousness, tremor

Cardiac arrythmias

TABLE 4 Prevention of Anaphylaxis

Take a thorough medical history.

Avoid the use of agents historically associated with systemic reactions. Use alternative agents.

If treatment with a specific drug is highly desirable (for example, penicillin) and accurate skin tests are available, perform skin testing.

If it is absolutely necessary to use a specific drug in the face of a history of a prior systemic reaction and/or positive skin test, (e.g., penicillin, insulin), desensitization can be attempted.

Administer the drug by oral rather than parenteral means, if possible.

Observe the patient for at least 30 minutes following administration of any drug.

Premedication may be useful in certain conditions. For example, in a patient with a history of a reaction to radiocontrast dyes in whom repeat examination is necessary, prednisone, three 50-mg oral doses at 6-hour intervals, with the last dose 1 hour before the procedure, plus diphenhydramine, 50–100 mg im 1 hour before the procedure, has been suggested to be effective.

In patients with a history of idiopathic anaphylaxis or severe reactions and in whom complete elimination of the inciting agent cannot be obtained, use of an epinephrine autoinjector or similar device, after exposure to an inciting agent but before arrival at a medical facility, may be beneficial.

Because parenteral administration of agents is often associated with a higher incidence of anaphylaxis than administration by other routes, the oral route should be chosen, if possible. After administration of any drug, the patient should be observed for at least 30 minutes. In certain conditions, premedication may be useful. For example, in a patient with a history of reaction to radiocontrast dyes and for whom repeat examination is necessary, prednisone, 3 50-mg oral doses at 6-hour intervals, with the last dose 1 hour before the procedure, plus diphenhydramine, 50 to 100 mg IM 1 hour before the procedure, has been suggested to be effective. Finally, in a patient with a history of idiopathic anaphylaxis or severe reactions in whom complete elimination of the inciting agent cannot be achieved, use of an epinephrine autoinjector or a similar device, after exposure to an inciting agent but before arrival at a medical facility, may be beneficial.

Publication No. 585 from the O'Neill Research Laboratories at The Good Samaritan Hospital, 5601 Loch Raven Boulevard, Baltimore, MD, 21239. Supported by grants HL01034 and AI20136 from the Department of Health and Human Services, Bethesda, Maryland. We wish to thank Mrs. Carol Dankelman for assistance in the preparation of the manuscript, and Diane Peters, R.N., and Howard Freeland, M.D., for reviewing the manuscript.

HEREDITARY ANGIOEDEMA

MICHAEL M. FRANK, M.D.

Hereditary angioedema (HAE) is characterized by recurrent attacks of edema of subcutaneous and submucosal tissues. It particularly affects the extremities and the mucosa of the gastrointestinal tract. Typically, attacks have a duration of 1 to 4 days and are harmless, although when they involve the bowel wall they usually induce severe abdominal pain. Occasionally attacks affect subcutaneous and submucosal tissue in the region of the upper airway. In this case they may be associated with respiratory obstruction and asphyxiation. Attacks are sporadic, but in some patients they may be induced by emotional stress or physical trauma. Although attacks usually begin in childhood, they seldom become severe until the time of puberty. This disease is strongly influenced by hormonal factors, as will be discussed in detail.

HAE is associated with depressed functional activity of the serum regulatory protein, the C1 esterase inhibitor, one of the early acting components of the classic complement pathway. This protein also serves as an inhibitor of all of the Hageman factor-dependent mediator pathways, including the kinin-generating, fibrinolytic, and intrinsic clotting pathways. It is believed that unregulated activation of one or more of these pathways leads to the formation or release of mediators that induce vessel leakage or angioedema in the area in which they are generated.

Not all patients with hereditary angioedema require therapy. Many patients have an attack frequency of less than one or two per month. We do not treat patients with an attack frequency of less than one per month unless there are extenuating circumstances. Moreover, we do not treat patients unless the attacks are having a major effect on their life-style. Specifically, we never treat the biochemical indices of hereditary angioedema and almost never treat patients to prevent the possibility of a life-threatening attack. Very few patients have either had multiple life-threatening attacks or are so emotionally disturbed at having seen members of their family die of airway attacks that chronic therapy is appropriate, but this is distinctly unusual. In every case I know, an understanding of the disease and access to adequate medical care can prevent the considerable mortality reported in the past, even in the absence of specific drug administration.

The therapy of HAE can be divided into three phases: (1) treatment of acute attacks, (2) short-term therapy to prevent anticipated attacks, as in patients undergoing dental manipulations, and (3) long-term preventive therapy. Of these, the first phase is the only one that is unsatisfactory at present.

Treatment of acute attacks. Angioedema attacks that involve the extremities are inconvenient but self-limited and usually do not require specific therapy. Abdominal attacks, although painful, require only supportive treatment. If pain is severe, the limited but early use of narcotics is indicated. Many patients report that a single dose of narcotic early in an attack may abort the attack, and I routinely try this approach to therapy. We have also been able to abort attacks with repeated doses of epinephrine 1:1000. It should be kept clearly in mind that narcotic addiction is one of the major problems associated with therapy in these frequently emotionally unstable patients. Often there is no objective evidence to support a patient's claim of severe abdominal pain, and for this reason the use of narcotics should be kept under careful control. Like peripheral attacks, abdominal attacks of angioedema are self-limited and are not associated with bowel rupture. I know of only one case of angioedema leading to volvulus and bowel necrosis. In some cases patients with abdominal attacks may have severe vomiting and/or diarrhea, and appropriate use of intravenous fluids is essential. These patients are often considered candidates for exploratory laporotomy, but this should be resisted. However, if they have fever, leukocytosis, an elevated sedimentation rate, or other unusual features of abdominal HAE, they should be carefully reevaluated to determine whether angioedema of the bowel is truly the cause of their abdominal pain.

On occasion, these patients have attacks involving the airway. This represents a true medical emergency, since these attacks respond poorly to administration of epinephrine, antihistamines, or glucocorticoids and may lead to rapid airway compromise. Airway compromise is usually preceded by a change in the tone of the voice, suggesting edema of the vocal cord area, and difficulty in swallowing secretions. When a patient is seen complaining of angioedema of the airway, an ENT evaluation is essential. If there are no medical contraindications to its use, we use repeated doses of subcutaneous epinephrine (0.2 to 0.3 ml of a 1:1000 dilution) plus antihistamines and a rapidly acting glucocorticoid (Solu-Cortif). In my experience with these drugs, only the first is associated with even a modest improvement in a fairly high percentage of patients. However, because the question has not been examined in detail, I use all three. Certainly, the sedative effect of the antihistamine may be helpful.

In general no airway encroachment should be taken lightly. Nevertheless the aggressiveness of the approach to therapy should be tempered by considerations of the course of an attack. Attacks usually become gradually more extensive and severe for 1 to 2 days and then resolve by 3 or 4 days after onset. Thus, a patient seen with moderate pharyngeal swelling 2 days into an attack should be treated less aggressively than the same patient seen 4 hours into an upper airway attack. Following the aforementioned routine measures, the patient is observed for several hours. If the attack is clearly not progressing, no further therapy is indicated. If the attack is still causing potentially dangerous airway involvement, the patient is admitted to the hospital, and intravenous use of epsilon aminocaproic acid is begun. This drug clearly decreases propagation of swelling. However, our studies suggest that it may not be effective for as long as 48 hours from the onset of therapy. Again, the point is not formally proved; however, the patient may still have a problem 48 hours into therapy and, if there is no medical contraindication to a plasmin inhibitor, we believe that the drug should be administered. We use 8 g intravenously in the first 4 hours and 16 g per day until the attack is over. It is clear that none of the aforementioned agents can be expected to produce rapid resolution of the attacks. We have shown that dramatic resolution can be anticipated following intravenous administration of partially purified C1 esterase inhibitor, the functionally deficient protein in these patients. Infusion of the equivalent of 1000 ml of serum C1 esterase inhibitor will reproducibly terminate attacks within minutes to hours. Unfortunately, this material remains an investigational drug and is not yet available for distribution. There is much anecdotal evidence that fresh frozen plasma will provide relief of attacks, and there is one paper in the literature to support this contention. However, the report in the literature is inadequate to prove efficacy. At least one senior individual responsible for many of these patients claims to have seen attacks become worse, as one rapidly infuses substrate for the complement system present in the fresh plasma at the same time one is infusing C1 esterase inhibitor. Thus, at present, use of fresh frozen plasma cannot be recommended.

If one confronts a potentially life-threatening attack of angioedema and either the patient has not responded to the available agents or the severity of the attack is such that there is not time to evaluate the response thoroughly, attention is turned to preservation of the airway. Tracheostomy has been used in this situation, but we prefer to attempt nasotracheal intubation in an operating room, with a staff prepared to perform a tracheostomy if intubation fails. Although trauma clearly precipitates attacks, in our hands placement of the nasotracheal tube has not led to extension of the edema distal to the tube. The tube remains in place until the attack has subsided. We have had one patient who insisted on placement of a permanent tracheostomy with a plug which he finds affords him complete peace of mind. Given the results of long-term therapy now available, this approach should not be required.

Short-term Therapy When an Attack is Anticipated. Patients with hereditary angioedema often require major dental work. Dental manipulation, particularly associated with traction on the gums and injection of an anesthetic into the gums, often precipitates an attack. Similarly, such patients may require endoscopy, which may precipitate an attack involving the airway. Such attacks can be completely prevented by the infusion of 2 units of fresh frozen plasma during an acute attack, as mentioned—when a patient is depleted of complement components—there appears to be no danger of angioedema being precipitated by fresh frozen plasma when the patient is free of symptoms. We do not infuse the plasma immediately prior to surgery because we prefer to give the 100,000 dalton C1 esterase inhibitor protein time to leave the intravascular space and penetrate into the tissues to be most effective. Nevertheless, we have no clear evidence to support this delay between the time of fresh frozen plasma administration and the traumatic event. Obviously, the infusion of fresh frozen plasma carries with it the danger of inducing hepatitis. We believe the benefits outweigh the risks in this situation, since in our hands no patient who had received fresh frozen plasma prior to a surgical or dental procedure has had any major problems with his angioedema. We believe the patient should be treated to prevent attacks in all major surgical procedures, even though most surgery is not regularly attended by HAE attacks. In some situations chronic suppressive medication can be used to cover patients in the situations just outlined. We believe that when medications are used, proper blood studies should be performed to determine that the patient's C1 inhibitor and C4 have returned to normal levels before the surgical procedure is undertaken. In many cases chronic medication lessens the frequency of attacks, but does not decrease them to zero. Obviously this is not optimal if trauma to the airway is anticipated.

Long-term Preventive Therapy. At present, long-term preventive therapy is satisfactory for most patients. Two classes of drugs can be used for prevention. The most effective agents are the androgens and androgen derivatives. Oral methyltestosterone was the first androgen shown to be effective in HAE, and it remains a drug of choice in men because of high efficacy, low cost, and long experience showing minimal toxicity. We start at 10 mg PO *tid* and gradually decrease the dose after the disease is brought under control. The major danger associated with its use is that of cholestatic jaundice, and liver function should be watched. Methyltestosterone cannot be used in women.

It is important to point out that many women have increased attacks of angioedema while taking estrogen-containing birth control tablets. It is often the case that discontinuation of these birth control tablets is all that is required for therapy in this patient group. In general, estrogen-like drugs increase the frequency of attacks and androgen-like drugs, and progesterone to a lesser extent, have a tendency to decrease attack frequency.

We have had a considerable experience with an attenuated androgen, danazol. In most patients, this drug causes total cessation of attacks. In many patients it completely corrects the biochemical abnormality associated with depressed C1 esterase inhibitor levels. Presumably, it does so by inducing synthesis of C1 esterase inhibitor by hepatocytes. Patients with hereditary angioedema are heterozygous for the deficiency state. They have one normal and one abnormal gene. On danazol therapy, the normal gene is induced to make sufficient product to counteract the genetic deficiency. Other androgens have a tendency to do this as well, but do so less effectively, and the C1 esterase inhibitor level does not return to normal. Danazol has a relatively low incidence of toxicity and is the least masculinizing of all the available androgens in general use. Its major disadvantage is high cost. As with all of the androgens, the use of danazol is associated with weight gain in the majority of patients, usually averaging 8 to 10 pounds. This is associated with an increase in appetite, and the patients who can limit their diet can avoid this complication. Other major side-effects include menometrorrhagia in about one-third of patients. About one-quarter of patients have headaches (mild to moderate), myalgias, or muscle cramps. Less frequently encountered are hirsutism, voice deepening, alopecia, acne, amenorrhea, hot flashes, and altered libido. Of considerable importance is the fact that some patients develop microscopic hematuria, which seems to be associated with a mild inflammation of the bladder. Thus far, in no case has this progressed to fibrosis of the bladder, but consideration should be given to changing drugs when this occurs. Some patients note anxiety, tremulousness, or dizziness on this drug. In fact, all of the androgens can produce similar side-effects. Myalgias and muscle cramps appear to be particularly common in patients with HAE regardless of the type of therapy. The reason for this muscle abnormality in HAE is unknown. In a very limited number of patients, danazol has induced a mild increase in SGOT or SGPT, but has not induced cholestatic jaundice, a common complication of other androgens. In our patient group the drug is started at 600 mg per day and the dosage is gradually decreased. Some patients find relief of symptoms on as little as 50 mg of danazol every other day; however, this is totally unpredictable from patient to patient. In general the patient's drug is decreased gradually until the lowest possible level that is useful in controlling the patient's disease is achieved.

Other androgens are useful in the treatment of hereditary angioedema. Stanazolol is one of the analogous androgens with relatively little masculinizing activity that markedly decreases the incidence of attacks in most patients. In our experience, as well as in published experience of others, attacks continue to occur. However, the severity and frequency are decreased. Oxymetholone and fluoxymesterone can both be used in women and provide long-term relief with relatively few side-effects. The stanazolol dose is approximately 2 to 4 mg per day and oxymetholone about 15 mg per day. In each case, drug dose is gradually lowered until the patient starts to experience symptoms.

Some patients, particularly those with lymphoid malignancies or with ongoing complement activation associated with collagen-vascular diseases, have an HAE-like picture that appears to occur because of increased utilization of normally synthesized C1 esterase inhibitor. It is important to emphasize that the aforementioned drugs have been effective in treating this acquired form of C1 esterase inhibitor deficiency as well as the hereditary form. In general, they are not effective in treatment of angioedema unassociated with depletion of the C1 esterase inhibitor.

The second main group of drugs useful in HAE are the antifibrinolytic agents. Most commonly used has been epsilon aminocaproic acid (AMI-CAR). There is some experience in this country with tranexamic acid, a drug that is considerably more potent, but was removed from the market because of disturbing animal toxicity studies. In double-blind studies we have shown that epsilon aminocaproic acid controls attacks of hereditary angioedema. Unlike the androgens, it does so without altering levels of either C1 esterase inhibitor or complement components. It appears to work by decreasing attack propagation rather than by decreasing attack frequency. Thus patients feel as if they are having the onset of typical attacks of angioedema, but the attacks are greatly decreased in severity. Epsilon aminocaproic acid has to be used in moderate dosage to ameliorate symptoms; the average patient requires 7 or 8 g per day for relief. Nevertheless, the drug is effective and should be considered for therapy. Epsilon aminocaproic acid acts as a potent plasmin inhibitor, although some studies suggest that at the doses used in hereditary angioedema, this is not its mechanism of action. It is obviously not a drug that one would use in any situation where there was a predisposition to thrombosis. Also, it is a drug that could be very dangerous if a patient receiving it were to have myocardial infarct or a cerebral vascular accident. Because it is less effective than the androgens and potentially much more toxic, it is clearly a second-line drug. As with androgens, epsilon aminocaproic acid may cause marked muscle toxicity with muscle pains and/or elevated serum levels of CPK and aldolase. The reasons for this are unknown, but if it occurs, the drug should be immediately discontinued.

It is rare that a child with hereditary angioedema requires therapy and, in fact, we try not to treat children. Nevertheless, if therapy is required in a child, epsilon aminocaproic acid is the drug of choice because it does not affect normal gonadal development.

Patients with hereditary angioedema sometimes have abdominal discomfort that cannot be brought under control with either androgens or antifibrinolytic agents. Endoscopy may reveal that these patients have gastric ulcerations. In such cases, cimetidine is often used. We have found that cimetidine may increase attack frequency in a small percentage of patients with angioedema, presumably by interfering with the function of the administered androgenic agents. We have had considerably more success using renididine in this patient subpopulation.

In general, the vast majority of patients with hereditary angioedema can be controlled following these general principles of drug therapy. Nevertheless, therapy requires considerable attention to detail and careful follow-up, both for signs of toxicity and for signs of other medical problems.

SYSTEMIC LUPUS ERYTHEMATOSUS

CHARLES A. ROBINSON, M.D.
ENG M. TAN, M.D.

Management of patients with systemic lupus erythematosus (SLE) must be highly individualized. Since the disorder cannot be "cured", the goal of therapy is to alleviate symptoms and to suppress abnormalities which are indicative of ongoing injury to vital organs, such as increasing proteinuria and/or declining creatinine clearance in a patient with lupus nephritis. It must also be emphasized that a diagnosis of SLE per se does not always warrant aggressive therapy with potentially toxic medications, since many patients who are diagnosed with the help of sophisticated serologic laboratory tests currently available will have mild disease that is not complicated by major organ system involvement. Those patients who occupy the mild end of the broad spectrum of SLE may be managed very conservatively, with little medication. There is also a misconception that remains all too prevalent among the lay public and physicians with little personal experience with SLE that the disease is usually progressive and devastating and will invariably be complicated by renal failure, infection, or central nervous system involvement. Such misconceptions should be laid to rest because, in many instances, SLE is diagnosed at a stage showing relatively minor systemic complications. Many such patients can be managed very well with little restriction of their daily activities and long life expectancies.

This is publication 3736BCR from the Scripps Clinic and Research Foundation and is supported in part by NIH grants AI10386 and AM32063.

LABORATORY TESTS FOR DIAGNOSIS AND MANAGEMENT OF SLE

Although this is not a treatise on diagnosis, in a disease such as SLE, diagnosis and management are intricately intertwined, so it is necessary to mention a few highlights. Those laboratory tests that are useful in both diagnosis and management are described in Table 1. In all instances, laboratory tests should be guides and not the descriptors of management. Simple

TABLE 1 Laboratory Tests Useful in Diagnosis and Management of SLE

Diagnosis	*Management*
CBC (especially Hct/Hgb, WBC platelets)	Hct/HGB, WBC, platelets
ESR	ESR
Urinalysis (especially 24-hr proteinuria)	24-hr proteinuria
L.E. cells	Not demonstrated
Biologically false-positive STS	Not demonstrated
Total ANA (quantitative)	In some patients
Anti-native DNA	Anti-native DNA
Other antibodies (anti-histone, Sm)	Not demonstrated
Immune complexes	In some patients
Evidence for complement activiation (CH_{50}, C4d/C4 ratio)	In some patients

and routine laboratory tests, such as the complete blood count, erythrocyte sedimentation rate (ESR), and 24-hour urine protein test, are excellent adjuncts to the management of the patient. In general, these tests should be obtained every 2 to 3 months, and when deviations from the norm are observed, they should be performed even more regularly to determine if a trend is developing. There are some tests which are useful in diagnosis but their usefulness in management has not been demonstrated. Among the immunologic tests, antibody to native DNA has been particularly useful as a guide to the management of renal disease. In some patients, but certainly not in all, other studies, such as the total antinuclear antibody (ANA), measurement of immune complexes, and evidence of complement activation, may be useful as additional guides to management regimens.

A SYSTEM FOR MANAGEMENT OF SLE

General Measures

The institution of general measures for the treatment of patients with SLE is extremely important and cannot be overemphasized (Table 2). The outcome in this disease will generally be best when both the physician and the patient are well educated in the various manifestations of the disease and when a compliant patient and a committed, understanding physician form a management partnership. In this respect, patient education is of paramount importance. Some of this patient education should come from the physician, but a large part can be borne by a nurse who is informed about the disease. The second general measure, and very much related to patient education, is the need for emotional support in the form of family counseling and participation in patient self-help groups. Such self-help groups as well as materials for patient and family education about the disease can be obtained from a number of sources, including the following:

TABLE 2 A System for Management of SLE

General Measures	*Specific Treatments*
Patient education	Aspirin and/or nonsteroidal anti-inflammatory drugs
Emotional support (family counselling, lupus societies)	Antimalarial drugs
Rest	Corticosteroids (topical, systemic, intra-articular)
Sun avoidance	Immunosuppressive drugs Continuous vs pulse therapy Single agent vs combination chemotherapy
Adequate nutrition	Apheresis (plasmapheresis, lymphapheresis, cryopheresis)
Physical and occupational therapy	Total lymphoid irradiation

The Arthritis Foundation Medical Information Series
Arthritis Foundation
1314 Spring Street N.W.
Atlanta, GA 30309

Lupus Erythematosus: A Handbook for Physicians, Patients and Their Families
Lupus Foundation of America, Inc.
11673 Holly Springs Drive
St. Louis, MO 63141

Information for Patients with Lupus Erythematosus
The American Lupus Society
4126 Pacific Coast Highway
Torrance, CA 90505

In many cities and towns throughout the country, there are chapters of these health agencies which conduct programs to help patients with lupus and their families.

Rest is often overlooked as an important component of therapy in patients with SLE. To control an exacerbation it may be important for the patient to seek a leave of absence from work for periods of weeks to months. In addition, at least 7 to 8 hours of sleep every night and avoidance of stressful work conditions can be of enormous value to the patient.

Photosensitivity is a feature of SLE in approximately 20 to 25 percent of patients. Although not all patients with SLE manifest sun sensitivity, it is prudent to caution all patients to avoid excessive exposure to sunlight. This entails the use of sunscreen ointments or creams, wide-brimmed hats and long sleeves, and avoidance of peak sunlight hours during the midday period.

While research in mouse models of SLE suggests that certain dietary modifications, primarily those involving prostaglandin precursors (fatty acids), may modify the clinical course and histologic findings in lupus, no specific dietary recommendations can be made to human patients at this time, other than to encourage a wholesome, well-balanced diet and the maintenance of ideal body weight. However, patients who are being treated with high doses of corticosteroids (40 mg and above) should be instructed in a sodium-restricted diet (2 g salt) and a restricted calorie (1800) diet. This dietary regimen will help to reduce fluid retention and obesity. Finally, physical and occupational therapy are also important. These adjunct therapies frequently help the patient adjust to and accept the chronicity of the disease process.

Specific Treatments

Arthralgia, arthritis, myalgia, and fever are symptoms of SLE that may, in many instances, be successfully managed with aspirin and other nonsteroidal anti-inflammatory drugs (NSAIDs) alone. In patients who fail to respond to or are intolerant of aspirin, a variety of other medications are available (Table 3). There are no adequate studies regarding the efficacy of one agent versus another and virtually all of the NSAIDs have been utilized successfully. NSAIDs may impair glomerular filtration in patients with compromised renal blood flow or preexisting renal insufficiency, and their use should be avoided in such situations.

Antimalarial compounds have been used successfully, particularly in the treatment of SLE with predominant skin lesions. In the United States, hydroxychloroquine is used most commonly. An antimalarial agent is often used in conjunction with corticosteroids, and it has been the experience of some investigators that this type of combination therapy may have a steroid-sparing effect. Unfortunately, the usefulness of antimalarials in manifestations of SLE other than skin involvement has not been systematically tested in controlled clinical trials. A major concern with hydroxychloroquine is the development of retinal pigmentation, and patients receiving such treatment should have systematic fundoscopic examinations every 6 to 8 months. The risk of retinopathy is related to the daily and cumulative dosage. Hydroxychloroquine in dosages of 200 mg per day, which is standard maintenance therapy, does not appear to be associated with an appreciable incidence of retinal toxicity.

Systemic corticosteroid therapy is virtually always necessary in patients with the more severe manifestations of SLE. Patients in this category are those whose arthritis, arthralgias, and myalgias do not respond to NSAIDs; those who have involvement of other organ systems, such as the kidney and central and peripheral nervous systems; and those with hematologic disorders, serositis, and so on. Prednisone and prednisolone are the most commonly used preparations because of their low cost, short half-lives, and the lack of evidence that other, more expensive corticosteroid preparations have any distinct advantages. Major flares of SLE are best treated by prompt institution of high-dose corticosteroids, such as 60 to 80 mg of prednisone daily in divided doses (every 6 hours). As a general rule, when the clinical situation warrants the initiation of high-dose steroid therapy, the high dosage will have to be maintained for at least 3 to 4 weeks to gain control of the disease. Once an acceptable clinical response has been achieved and the patient's condition has been stabilized, the steroid dose should be gradually tapered. The goal of therapy is to lower the corticosteroid dosage gradually and continuously without allowing major signs or symptoms of active disease to emerge. The most common error made is to taper the dosage too rapidly. When a patient's disease is well controlled, the dose may be lowered by 5 mg every 2 weeks until a ''moderate'' dose (30 to 40 mg) has been reached. Subsequent tapering should be more gradual, with decrements of 5 mg every 3 to 4 weeks until a dose of 20 to 25 mg daily has been achieved. At this point, it is often possible and desirable to consolidate the dose into a single morning dose. Dose reductions from the 20 to 25 mg range should be in decrements of 2.5 mg every 2 to 4 weeks until the lowest daily maintenance dose is achieved without any recurrence of significant symptoms. In the optimal situation, the disease might be under control with alternate-day steroid therapy, but we have found that—unlike corticosteroid therapy for patients with asthma—it has rarely been successful in the treatment of SLE.

There have been reports recently of the successful use of high-dose (pulse) intravenous corticosteroids (for example 1 g of methylprednisolone intravenously at weekly intervals for 3 to 4 weeks). The results have not been uniformly favorable. The major rationales for the use of pulse steroid therapy are that it may be more effective and that the administration of extremely high doses may be lifesaving in severe conditions, such as central nervous system involvement or active lupus nephritis. High-dose pulse therapy with corticosteroids should be reserved for the unusual situation.

The potential adverse effects of corticosteroids include Cushingoid facies, redistribution of body fat from the extremities to the abdomen and central portions of the trunk, acne, cataracts, thinning of the skin and capillary fragility leading to easy bruising, fluid retention, hypertension, diabetes mellitus, agitation, depression, avascular necrosis, osteopenia, and immunosuppression. Patients must be informed of side effects that may occur but must also be reassured regarding the reversibility of most of the adverse side

TABLE 3 Nonsteroidal Anti-Inflammatory Drugs Which May Be Used for Treatment of SLE

Drug		*Usual Dose Range*
Generic	*Brand Name*	*Anti-inflammatory*
Ibuprofen	Motrin, Rufen, Advil 200, 400 600 mg	400–600 mg *tid–qid*
Naproxen	Naprosyn 250, 375, 500 mg	250–500 mg *bid–tid*
Sulindac	Clinoril 150, 200 mg	150–200 mg *bid*
Piroxicam	Feldene 10, 20 mg	20 mg *qd*
Indomethacin	Indocin 25, 50, 75 mg (SR)	25–50 mg *tid–qid* 75 mg (SR) *qd–bid*
Tolmetin	Tolectin 200, 400 mg	400 mg *tid–qid*
Meclofenamate	Meclomen 50, 100 mg	100 mg *tid–qid*
Salsalate	Disalcid 500, 750 mg	1–1.5 gm *bid*
Diflunisal	Dolobid 500 mg	500 mg *bid*
ASA	Numerous preparations 325, 500, 650, 975 mg	650–975 mg every 4–6 hrs
Zero order Release ASA	Zorprin 800 mg	1600 mg *bid*

effects. Although the side effects are many, they can be diminished by the simple procedures mentioned before, including restriction of salt and caloric intake. Because corticosteroid therapy continues to be the mainstay of treatment for SLE, the benefits of such therapy should be discussed with the patient and an attempt must be made to dispel any distorted fears that the patient may have learned by hearsay.

There have been numerous trials and many reports regarding the use of immunosuppressive medications, such as azathioprine, cyclophosphamide, methotrexate, and chlormbucil, in SLE. The indications for their usage and their therapeutic efficacy remain controversial. Most trials have focused on the efficacy of immunosuppressive agents in lupus nephritis, and in lupus complicated by central nervous system disease. It appears that both azathioprine and cyclophosphamide in conjunction with corticosteroids are more effective in some cases of lupus nephritis than corticosteroids alone. In general, doses of azathioprine and cyclophosphamide are in the range of 2 mg per kilogram of body weight. However, when control of the disease process has been effected, the objective is to reduce the dose to 1 mg per kilogram of body weight or less. Immunosuppressive medications with corticosteroids should be administered only by physicians experienced in their use or with the counsel of such physicians.

Plasmapheresis, lymphapheresis, lymphaplasmapheresis and cryopheresis have all been utilized in treating various manifestations of SLE. There are reports of the use of apheresis in lupus nephritis, central nervous system lupus, thrombocytopenia, hemolytic anemia, and severe vasculitis. While there are many reports of the successful use of apheresis, there are also some reports which raise questions concerning its efficacy. Undoubtedly, there are some patients who have benefited from apheresis, including those with severe central nervous system involvement and rapidly progressive nephritis. The clinical effects of apheresis are very unpredictable and clinical improvement has generally not been sustained beyond a period of weeks, or at most, months. There is a clear need to identify those factors related to the efficacy of this treatment modality. When these factors have been identified, the rationale for assigning patients to this form of treatment will be more firmly established.

Total lymph node irradiation has been introduced recently as a treatment modality for SLE. This type of treatment is available at only a few medical centers in the country. A limited number of clinical trials have been performed in severe, refractory SLE. Again, the outcome has been variable, and until more data are available, lymph node irradiation should be done only in the context of well-designed studies conducted by major research centers.

RHEUMATOID ARTHRITIS

PETER E. LIPSKY, M.D.

Rheumatoid arthritis is a chronic inflammatory disease of unknown origin whose natural history can be quite variable and unpredictable. In most individuals, the inflammatory process is mild to moderate or intermittent. There is therefore little potential for permanent damage to articular structures and, as a result, only minimal deformity or loss of function. In some patients the rheumatoid process may be a much more aggressively destructive one, resulting in considerable damage to articular structures with subsequent deformity and loss of function. In others, extra-articular manifestations, such as vasculitis or the leukopenia of Felty's syndrome, may present additional life-threatening problems. Finally, in patients with longstanding disease, the deformities themselves may cause symptoms even in the absence of active inflammation. Thus, rheumatoid arthritis presents a variety of therapeutic challenges in different patients. Moreover, the natural history of the disease may lead to new therapeutic problems at different stages of its evolution in the same patient. Therefore, no single stereotypical therapy can be advocated for all patients because each may present with a unique constellation of disease-related problems at different times during the course of the disease. Rather, the disease manifestations of the individual patient dictate the appropriate therapeutic intervention.

Many patients with rheumatoid arthritis experience fluctuations of disease activity. As many as 15 percent may have complete remissions of disease activity after an initial period of active inflammation. The majority of patients manifest more chronic courses with alternating exacerbations and remissions of various durations. Only about 10 to 15 percent of all patients experience chronic unremitting courses with progressive deformity and functional disability. Since it is nearly impossible to predict disease outcome or therapeutic response to a given medication at the time a patient first presents with rheumatoid arthritis, it is essential to monitor the progress of the patient closely to ensure that appropriate and timely therapeutic interventions are undertaken, and that unsuccessful approaches are abandoned as the patient's course dictates.

The cause of rheumatoid arthritis is unknown. Thus, all therapeutic interventions are palliative, relieving the signs and symptoms of the disease, but not curing it. The various therapies employed are directed at nonspecific suppression of the inflammatory process in the hope not only of ameliorating symptoms but also of preventing progressive damage to articular structures. A number of diverse therapeutic modalities have been used in the management of rheumatoid arthritis in the hope of achieving these goals.

THERAPEUTIC MODALITIES USED IN THE MANAGEMENT OF RHEUMATOID ARTHRITIS

Management of patients with rheumatoid arthritis involves an interdisciplinary approach that attempts to address the various problems of these individuals (Table 1). General supportive measures may be appropriate for all patients with rheumatoid arthritis. These include counseling to help cope with a chronic, painful, and potentially disabling disease; appropriate vocational training for persons whose condition compromises their capacity to support themselves; and instruction in the use of various physical aids that may help accomplish activities of daily living.

A variety of physical therapy modalities may be useful in decreasing the symptoms of rheumatoid inflammation. Rest ameliorates symptoms of rheumatoid arthritis and can be an important component of the total therapeutic program. In addition, splinting to reduce unwanted motion of individual inflamed joints may be useful in some patients. However, rest or splinting to the point of disuse or complete dependence is to be avoided. Exercise directed at maintaining muscle strength and joint mobility without exacerbating joint inflammation is also an important part of the therapeutic regimen. Isometric exercises to maintain muscle strength and passive range of motion exercises may thus be useful adjunctive therapies. Finally, a variety of orthotic devices can be very helpful in supporting and aligning deformed joints to reduce pain and improve function.

Medical management of rheumatoid arthritis involves two general approaches. The first is the use of aspirin and other nonsteroidal anti-inflammatory drugs (NSAIDs), simple analgesics, and glucocorticoids to control the symptoms and signs of the local inflammatory process. These agents are rapidly effective in mitigating signs and symptoms, but appear to exert little or no effect on the progression of the disease. A second group of drugs includes a variety of agents that have been classified as disease modifying drugs (DMDs) and the immunosuppressive drugs. These agents possess minimal nonspecific anti-inflammatory or analgesic activity and are slowly active, meaning that many months of therapy may be necessary to achieve responses. These agents, however, appear to have the capacity to modify the course of the disease and to slow its progress in some patients.

Surgery plays a role in the management of patients with severely damaged joints. Although arthroplasties are done on shoulders, elbows, wrists, and ankles, the most successful procedures are carried out on hips and knees. Multiple joint replacements have resulted in functional improvement in some patients. To be successful, the patients must be highly motivated because of the rigorous rehabilitation required. Realistic goals of these procedures are relief of pain and modest functional improvement. Reconstructive hand surgery may lead to cosmetic improvement, although functional benefit is often equivocal. Surgical synovectomy is not often done because of the lack of long-term benefit and the loss of joint motion that results. However, arthroscopic synovectomy may be useful in patients with persistent monoarthritis of the knee. In addition, early tenosynovectomy may be useful in preventing tendon rupture.

A number of experimental approaches have been employed to treat rheumatoid arthritis, as shown in Table 1. Although some of these show potential for ameliorating the disease process, none has been shown to be a safe and cost-effective way to treat rheumatoid arthritis.

Finally, a variety of other approaches have been claimed to be effective in treating rheumatoid arthritis, including diets, plant and animal extracts, vaccines, hormones, and topical preparations of various sorts. Many of these are costly and none has been shown to be effective. Moreover, some may have unsuspected toxicity and may also have the disadvantage of leading the patient to discontinue traditional therapies.

TABLE 1 Management of Rheumatoid Arthritis

1. *General*
   - Counseling
   - Vocational training
   - Physical aids
2. *Physical modalities*
   - Rest/exercise
   - Physical therapy
   - Splinting, orthotics
3. *Medical management*
   - Symptomatic therapy
     - Nonsteroidal anti-inflammatory drugs
     - Analgesics
     - Corticosteroids (systemic, local)
   - Disease suppressive therapy
     - Disease-modifying drugs (gold compounds, antimalarials, D-penicillamine)
     - Immunosuppressives/antimetabolites (azathioprine, cyclophosphamide, methotrexate)
4. *Surgery*
   - Synovectomy
   - Resection/arthroplasty
   - Joint replacement, prosthetic arthroplasty
   - Nerve release
5. *Experimental*
   - Total lympoid irradiation
   - Apheresis: plasma, lymphocyte, combination

MEDICAL MANAGEMENT OF RHEUMATOID ARTHRITIS

Nonsteroidal Anti-Inflammatory Drugs

Besides aspirin, there are now several additional NSAIDs available to treat rheumatoid arthritis. As indicated in Table 2, each of these drugs shares with aspirin a number of properties that appear to explain its effectiveness in rheumatoid arthritis. Each of these drugs has been shown to be as effective as aspirin in the treatment of rheumatoid arthritis and in general to be associated with a lower incidence of gastrointestinal intolerance than aspirin. None of the newer NSAIDs appears to exhibit significant therapeutic advantages over the other available agents. In addition, there appears to be no consistent advantage of any of the newer agents over the others with respect to the incidence or severity of toxic manifestations.

From a clinical point of view, the major difference in the newer NSAIDs is the pharmacologic half-life, and thus the frequency with which they must be given to achieve comparable clinical efficacy. The frequencies vary from the four times per day dosage schedule of ibuprofen, fenoprofen, and meclofenamate, through the twice per day schedule for naproxen and sulindac, to the single daily dosage of piroxicam. When convenience of administration is a major issue, the agents given once or twice daily may be advantageous. A possible disadvantage of such preparations, however, is loss of dosage flexibility. Since an individual's symptoms may vary during the day, shorter-acting agents may provide the opportunity to tailor therapy to the individual patient's needs. Thus, for example, a patient with marked morning stiffness may benefit from a large dose of a NSAID at night.

As a result of the capacity of these agents to block the activity of the enzyme cyclooxygenase and therefore the production of prostaglandins, prostacyclin, and thromboxane from a variety of tissues, they all exhibit analgesic, anti-inflammatory, and antipyretic properties. Analgesia seems to be achieved with lower doses of these agents than is necessary to effect suppression of inflammation. Thus, it is important to differentiate patients whose primary problem is pain without inflammation from those experiencing pain in the context of active inflammation, because the former individuals may be adequately treated with lower doses of medication. Discriminating patients requiring mostly analgesia from those who would also benefit from an anti-inflammatory effect is especially important because lower dose NSAID therapy appears to be associated with a decreased incidence of toxicity. These agents are all associated with a wide spectrum of toxic side effects. Some are related to inhibition of cyclooxygenase activity while a variety of others, such as rash, liver function abnormalities, and bone marrow depression, may not be.

Traditionally, aspirin has been advocated as the initial therapy for patients with rheumatoid arthritis, because of its efficacy and low cost. None of the newer NSAIDs has been shown convincingly to be more effecive than aspirin and each costs more. However, aspirin therapy has a number of disadvantages, including its inconvenience, toxicity, and capricious absorption. Standard aspirin preparations require administration every 4 hours to achieve an anti-inflammatory effect. Enteric-coated, longer-acting aspirin preparations are available, but their cost is significantly greater and their absorption somewhat more erratic. In general, aspirin therapy is associated with considerably more gastrointestinal toxicity than therapy with the newer NSAIDs. Such toxicity can be diminished by the use of enteric-coated preparations, but again, there are the problems of cost and unpredictable absorption. The possibility of erratic absorption can be dealt with by measuring blood salicylate levels, but this adds to the overall cost of therapy. These considerations have led many rheumatologists to advocate the use of one of the newer NSAIDs as the drug of first choice in patients with rheumatoid arthritis.

TABLE 2 Properties of Nonsteroidal Anti-Inflammatory Drugs

Drugs
Aspirin, fenoprofen, ibuprofen, indomethacin, naproxen, meclofenamate, piroxicam, sulindac, tolmetin
Mechanism of action
Inhibition of cyclooxygenase activity
Clinical effects
Anti-inflammatory
Analgesic
Antipyretic
Toxicity
Related to cyclooxygenase inhibition
Increased bleeding time
Gastric irritation
Azotemia secondary to decreased renal blood flow
Allergic rhinitis and asthma
Miscellaneous

One important feature to consider when treating patients with NSAIDs is the unpredictability of the response of an individual patient. In large trials, it appears that individual patients may respond differently to the various NSAIDs. When serum drug levels become available and can be monitored, this variability in responsiveness may be lessened. In view of the idiosyncratic nature of the response to these agents, it has become the practice to treat patients sequentially with one NSAID after another until a satisfactory response is obtained. Each drug must be given a fair trial before its efficacy is judged. This may require 2 to 4 weeks of maximal dose therapy. There appears to be no rationale for the use of combination NSAIDs as opposed to maximal dosage with a single compound.

Disease Modifying Drugs

Clinical experience has delineated a number of agents that appear to have the capacity to alter the course of rheumatoid arthritis (Table 3). In practice,

TABLE 3 Properties of Disease Modifying Drugs

1. *Agents*
   - Antimalarials (hydroxychloroquine)
   - Gold compounds
     - Intramuscular: gold sodium thiomalate, gold thioglucose
     - Oral: auranofin
   - D-penicillamine
2. *Clinical effects*
   - Minimal nonspecific anti-inflammatory effects
   - Delayed onset of action
   - Disease-modifying
     - Clinical
     - Serologic
     - ? Radiographic
3. *Expectation of therapy*
   - Improvement: about 2/3
   - Remissions: rare
   - Toxicity: 20–40%
   - Long-term outcome: unknown
4. *Putative mechanism of action*
   - Alteration of macrophage function: gold compounds, antimalarials
   - Alteration of T cell function: D-penicillamine

these agents share a number of characteristics. They exert minimal direct nonspecific anti-inflammatory or analgesic effects and therefore NSAIDs must be continued during their administration, except in the few cases in which true remissions are induced with disease modifying drug (DMD) therapy. The appearance of benefit from DMD therapy is usually delayed. Weeks or months of treatment may be necessary before an impact on disease activity becomes apparent. As many as two-thirds of patients develop some clinical improvement as a result of therapy with any of these agents, although the induction of true remissions is rare. In addition to clinical improvement, there is frequently an improvement in serologic parameters of disease activity. Thus, titers of rheumatoid factor and the erythrocyte sedimentation rate frequently decline as a result of therapy. Despite this, there is scant evidence to support the conclusion that DMDs actually retard the development of bone erosions or facilitate their healing. The mechanism by which these agents are effective remains speculative, although it has been suggested that they function as immunosuppressive agents, altering the function of specific cell types involved in propagating rheumatoid inflammation.

Each of these drugs is associated with considerable toxicity and careful patient monitoring is therefore necessary (Table 4). Auranofin, a new disease modifying drug, has been developed and should soon be available for use. Auranofin is an orally absorbable gold compound that appears to have many of the clinical characteristics of the other drugs of this group. The major toxic effects appear to be diarrhea, abdominal cramping, and rash.

The DMD of first choice remains controversial. Although it is generally believed that gold compounds and D-penicillamine are more effective than antimalarials, trials comparing the efficacy of these various agents have failed to demonstrate a consistent advantage of one over another. The toxicity of the various agents thus becomes important in determining the drug of first choice. Antimalarial therapy appears to be associated with a somewhat lower incidence of serious toxicity. Although early trials suggested that antimalarials induced a significant incidence of ocular toxicity, more recent trials have indicated that the daily administration of less than 6.5 mg/kg of hydroxychloroquine (Plaquenil) poses minimal risk of ocular toxicity. In view of its relative safety and fairly comparable efficacy, hydroxychloroquine is often used as the DMD of first choice.

It is important to note that failure to respond or the development of toxicity to one DMD does not preclude responsiveness to another agent. Thus, for example, the percentages of patients who fail to respond to gold compounds but respond to D-penicillamine and of patients who respond to this agent when it is administered as the initial DMD are similar. It is therefore reasonable to administer these drugs in a sequential fashion. Therapy with a given agent is discontinued when serious toxicity has developed or when an adequate trial has demonstrated lack of efficacy. When gold therapy is employed, 6 months or longer may be necessary to complete the "loading" phase of treatment before therapeutic efficacy can be evaluated. Treatment with D-penicillamine may re-

TABLE 4 Disease Modifying Drugs: Guide to Therapy

	Hydroxychloroquine	*Oral Gold*	*Intramuscular Gold*	*D-penicillamine*
Administration	$<$ 6.5 mg/kg/day	3 mg twice daily	50 mg per week loading → 1 gram total, then taper to 50 mg per month	250 mg per day on empty stomach; increase daily dose by 250 mg every 3 months; maximum 1 gm/day
Major toxicity	Ocular	Rash, diarrhea	Rash, thrombocytopenia, granulocytopenia, proteinuria	Rash, gastrointestinal intolerance, proteinuria, thrombocytopenia, granulocytopenia
Precautions	Ophthalmologic examination every 6 months	?	CBC, platelet count, urinalysis before each injection	CBC, platelet count, urinalysis every 2 weeks × 6 months; then every month

quire 9 months of slowly increasing daily dosage (to 750 to 1000 mg per day) before the scope of the therapeutic response can be evaluated. When evaluating the response to therapy, it is important to keep in mind that DMDs exert their effects on the underlying inflammatory process and therapeutic effect should be gauged accordingly. It would be anticipated that morning stiffness and pain and functional impairment secondary to inflammation might be improved by DMD therapy, whereas symptoms secondary to cartilage damage, deformity, and abnormal alignment would not. DMDs are not curative, and therefore flares of activity can be expected, usually within 3 months of the discontinuation of therapy.

Immunosuppressive Drugs

Azathioprine and cyclophosphamide have both been shown to be effective in the treatment of rheumatoid arthritis and to exert therapeutic effects that are similar to the DMDs, but neither has been shown to be more effective than these agents. Because they are not superior to the DMDs and because of the potential toxic effects of long-term administration, including bone marrow depression and the possibility of the development of malignant neoplasms with cyclophosphamide, these drugs are reserved for patients who have clearly failed to improve after therapy with DMDs. On occasion, extra-articular disease, such as rheumatoid vasculitis, may require immunosuppressive therapy.

Recent experience has suggested that methotrexate, a folic acid antagonist, may be useful in the treatment of rheumatoid arthritis. A variety of low-dose regimens have been employed. One popular regimen involves the use of 3 doses of 2.5 mg orally at 12-hour intervals once a week. Although methotrexate appears to be effective, as many as 20 percent of treated patients may develop liver function abnormalities. Thus, the place of this drug in the therapy of rheumatoid arthritis remains uncertain.

APPROACH TO THE PATIENT WITH RHEUMATOID ARTHRITIS

The most important decision concerning the treatment of patients with rheumatoid arthritis involves the identification of individuals who require DMD therapy and the appropriate time to initiate such therapy (Table 5). At the time of diagnosis, it is difficult to predict the natural history of an individual patient's illness. Therefore, the usual approach is to attempt to alleviate the patient's symptoms with NSAIDs. The major reason to delay more definitive therapy is the possibility that a spontaneous remission will occur. Moreover, since the DMDs are potentially toxic and not universally effective, it does not seem reasonable to begin one of them when a natural remission is still a possibility. As the disease process continues, the likelihood of a spontaneous remission decreases. At some time during the disease course of most individuals, the possibility of initiating DMD therapy is entertained. With aggressive disease, this might occur sooner, often within three months of disease onset, whereas with more indolent disease, smoldering activity may not necessitate such therapy for many years. The development of bone erosions or evidence of cartilage loss on x-ray is clear-cut evidence of the destructive potential of the inflammatory process and indicates the need for DMD therapy. The other indications are much more subjective. Thus, the decision to begin DMD therapy requires careful monitoring of joint swelling and functional activity as well as an understanding of the patient's expectations of therapy and pain tolerance. In this setting, the fully informed patient must play an active role in the decision to begin DMD therapy after careful review of the therapeutic and toxic potential of the various drugs.

TABLE 5 Decision-Making in Rheumatoid Arthritis

1. Reasons to delay therapy with a disease-modifying drug
   - Delay in confirming diagnosis
   - Possibility of spontaneous remission
   - Toxicity
   - Lack of predicatable efficacy
2. Indications for disease-modifying drugs
   - Bone erosions, cartilage loss
   - Failure to respond to NSAIDs
     - Persistent swelling of multiple joints
     - Unrelenting pain
     - Curtailment of activity

If patients respond to a DMD, therapy is continued with careful monitoring to avoid toxicity. Occasionally, the drug dosage may have to be increased to treat exacerbations that may occur during therapy. In addition, as a response to a DMD is achieved, NSAID therapy may be diminished and occasionally discontinued. Even with successful therapy, local injection of glucocorticoids may be necessary to diminish inflammation that may persist in a limited number of joints. Surgery may be necessary to relieve pain or diminish the functional impairment secondary to deformity.

If the patient does not respond after a reasonable trial, a second disease modifying drug is begun. Only when these agents have proven unhelpful or unacceptably toxic, or when extra-articular manifestations, such as vasculitis, develop, should immunosuppressive agents or experimental procedures be considered.

Occasionally a patient's disease defies all forms of medical therapy. Even after such patients develop a number of joint deformities, function may be restored and pain alleviated with total joint replacement.

CONCLUSIONS

In the absence of a better understanding of the origin of rheumatoid arthritis, therapy remains empiric. Of all the therapeutic modalities available, none is either curative or completely effective. By close monitoring of the patient, however, and by developing a unique treatment plan directed toward the specific disease manifestations of the individual, some amelioration of symptoms can usually be achieved.

REITER'S SYNDROME

ROBERT P. JACOBS, M.D.

Reiter's syndrome (RS), initially described as an uncommon medical curiosity, is now recognized as one of the most common forms of arthritis in young adults. The clinical spectrum of RS is no longer limited to the classic triad of arthritis, urethritis, and conjunctivitis, but has expanded to include all of the clinical features of the spondyloarthropathies (Table 1). Despite significant advances in our understanding of the disease, RS continues to be underdiagnosed because of misconceptions regarding disease prevalence, the diversity of clinical manifestations, and the variability of disease presentation and course (Table 2). Thus, the first objective in developing a comprehensive treatment program is to generate an awareness and understanding of this common disease by physicians and patients.

The classic triad includes the three most common clinical manifestations of RS, but they are not always present in all patients. The concept of "incomplete" RS has evolved to accommodate those patients with musculoskeletal manifestations that suggest a diagnosis of RS, but who do not present with or develop conjunctivitis and urethritis. A subcommittee of the American Rheumatism Association proposed as criteria for the diagnosis of RS the presence of peripheral arthritis for more than one month in association with urethritis or cervicitis. While each of these diagnostic concepts of RS encompasses a majority of patients with the disease, they exclude many patients, including those with predominant mucocutaneous lesions, and must be applied carefully in the clinical setting.

TABLE 1 Clinical Manifestations of Reiter's Syndrome

Musculoskeletal	Peripheral oligoarthritis Sacroiliitis Spondylitis Inflammatory enthesopathy
Ocular	Conjunctivitis Iritis
Mucous Membrane	Oral ulcers Urethritis Cervicitis Cystitis
Skin and Nails	Keratodermia blenorrhagica Circinate balanitis Psoriasiform nail lesions
Cardiac	Pericarditis Conduction abnormalities Aortic regurgitation
Pulmonary	Pleurisy Apical fibrocavitary lesion

TABLE 2 Reiter's Syndrome: Sources of Confusion

Prevalence of the disease
Spectrum of clinical manifestations
Classic triad
"Incomplete" Reiter's syndrome
Diagnostic criteria
Females with Reiter's syndrome
Natural history of disease
Infectious etiology
HLA-B27

In addition to the expanded clinical spectrum of disease, our understanding of other important clinical features of RS has been changing. RS has been considered a disease affecting predominantly males. My experience with RS includes a significant number of females with what many would call atypical or seronegative (rheumatoid factor negative) rheumatoid arthritis. In addition to having musculoskeletal manifestations characteristic of the spondyloarthropathies, including asymmetric oligoarthritis affecting primarily lower extremity joints, these women have the same spectrum of extraskeletal manifestations as males with RS. Thus, careful clinical evaluation and follow-up with special attention to the distribution of musculoskeletal and extraskeletal manifestations will usually allow a definite diagnosis of RS to be established in males and females.

Our understanding of the natural history of RS has also been changing. RS has been described as an acute, self-limited disease. While many patients do have an acute illness that undergoes spontaneous remission, the majority of patients with RS have a chronic disease characterized by intermittent or persistent symptoms. The most common chronic disease manifestation is arthritis, but iritis, urethritis, or skin disease may also occur.

A second objective that I would like to identify before discussing a treatment program is that physicians develop an understanding of current theories of disease etiology and pathogenesis. These theories have generated such confusion and misconceptions among patients with RS that we must be able to address them with authority. RS serves as the prototype for diseases that result from an interaction between environmental and host factors. The environmental factors that "trigger" RS include many gram-negative enteric pathogens, including *Shigella, Salmonella, Yersinia*, and *Campylobacter*, and may include several genitourinary pathogens, including *Chlamydia, Ureaplasma*, and *Mycoplasma*. There is little doubt that RS is "triggered" by infections with several enteric pathogens, thus the designation epidemic, or postdysenteric, RS. There is reason to doubt whether all cases of endemic RS are, in fact, acquired by sexual contact and triggered by genitourinary pathogens, since the genitourinary manifestations of the disease may appear in individuals who have not been sexually active or in whom the disease follows an enteric infection. Furthermore, an antecedent infectious "trigger" cannot be identified in all patients with RS. However, the social stigma of a potentially chronic disease that might have been initiated by a sexually acquired infection makes this a most important topic.

The other component of disease pathogenesis that affects treatment is the striking association of RS and the other spondyloarthropathies with HLA-B27. It appears that up to 20 percent of HLA-B27 positive patients who develop an enteric or genitourinary infection with one of the implicated organisms will develop RS. Thus, HLA-B27 does promote disease susceptibility. However, the mechanisms whereby one patient with this genetic marker remains free of disease, another develops all of the clinical manifestations of RS, another reactive arthritis (i.e., postinfectious arthritis without extraskeletal manifestations), and another ankylosing spondylitis unrelated to an identifiable infectious disease, remain unknown. These genetic aspects of the disease will invariably generate questions that must be addressed in developing a treatment program.

TREATMENT

Patient Education

The initial step in the management of all chronic rheumatic diseases is patient education. It is imperative that patients be informed about their disease, its clinical manifestations and natural history, current concepts of disease pathogenesis, the genetic implications of the disease, and our therapeutic expectations. The goals of patient education are to develop an understanding of the disease that allows patients to participate in treatment decisions and address or correct misconceptions about the disease or its treatment.

Patients must understand the multisystem nature of RS even though we cannot yet provide a scientific basis for its diverse clinical manifestations. They must understand the variability and unpredictability of the disease course. The inflammatory nature of the disease must be understood if we are to expect patients to adhere to a chronic anti-inflammatory drug regimen. Theories of disease pathogenesis will require careful explanation if the stigma of a chronic disease triggered by a sexually acquired infection is to be avoided. Finally, the role of HLA-B27 in disease pathogenesis will demand a thoughtful discussion. I do not consider RS, with or without the HLA-B27 marker, a reason to modify family planning.

Physical Therapy

The role of physical therapy in the management of RS will depend on the nature and severity of musculoskeletal involvement. Patients with acute arthritis should be encouraged to rest involved joints and participate in an exercise program as inflammatory symptoms subside. All patients with chronic joint disease should be regular participants in a physical therapy program. For a more detailed discussion of physical therapy, see the chapter on *Ankylosing Spondylitis*.

Local (Lesional) Therapy

Many of the clinical manifestations of RS can be managed with local or lesional therapy. Because local therapy often minimizes the risk of systemic drug toxicity, appropriate clinical manifestations should be identified and so treated.

Musculoskeletal. While most of the musculoskeletal manifestations of RS will require systemic anti-inflammatory drug therapy, some may be amenable to local therapeutic measures. The inflammatory enthesopathies, such as Achilles tendinitis, can be effectively treated by local infiltration with a depot corticosteroid preparation mixed with a local anesthetic. Calcaneal periostitis can also be treated with local injection therapy, but might respond to physical measures such as a heel cup or a sponge rubber donut. Other enthesopathic features, such as chest wall or pelvic pain, might respond to physical therapy modalities, including heat, ultrasound, and electrical stimulation, but often require nonsteroidal anti-inflammatory drugs (NSAIDs).

The intra-articular injection of depot corticosteroids is often useful in the management of pauciarticular disease that has not responded adequately to NSAIDs. It does not appear that the arthritis of RS responds as dramatically to such treatment as does the arthritis of rheumatoid arthritis, nor is the duration of action in RS as prolonged, but is often a useful adjunct to systemic therapy.

Ocular. The conjunctivitis of RS is often asymptomatic and therefore does not require therapy. Symptomatic conjunctivitis and iritis require treatment with topical steroids and should be monitored by an ophthalmologist. Iritis, refractory to topical steroid therapy, requires treatment with intralesional or systemic corticosteroids.

Mucous membranes. Oral lesions rarely require even topical therapy. The major concern regarding genitourinary lesions is whether they require systemic antibiotic therapy.

Skin and nails. The psoriasiform skin and nail lesions of RS often require no therapy, because of their minor or transient nature. Topical steroids are required by many patients and provide effective therapy. Rarely, patients require systemic therapy for skin and nail lesions.

Cardiac. Pericarditis and conduction abnormalities occur during the acute phase of RS and require systemic anti-inflammatory therapy. Late in the course of disease, cardiac conduction abnormalities and aortic regurgitation develop in a small percentage of patients with RS. These lesions appear to represent fibrotic replacement of the elastic tissues in the interventricular septum and aortic root, respectively. Decisions regarding pacemaker insertion or aortic valve replacement are made using conventional criteria under the supervision of a cardiologist.

Pulmonary. The major reason to recognize the pulmonary apical fibrocavitary lesion seen in the spondyloarthropathies is so that unnecessary medical or surgical therapy can be avoided. On occasion, the cavity will contain a mycetoma, a complication that does require medical or surgical intervention.

Systemic Drug Therapy

Therapy with NSAIDs. The majority of patients with RS will require systemic therapy, usually directed at the musculoskeletal manifestations of the disease. Most patients will respond to one of the NSAIDs (Table 3), thus a rational approach to their use must be developed. It must be stated that none of these agents have been formally evaluated in RS, nor have they been approved for use in the treatment of this disease by the Food and Drug Administration. Regardless, there is a general consensus that patients with RS respond better to indomethacin and phenylbutazone than to aspirin or the other NSAIDs. The relative efficacy of the NSAIDs is only one factor that must be considered in developing a treatment program.

Several factors must be considered in choosing the NSAIDs with which to initiate treatment in patients with RS: number of involved joints, intensity of symptoms, associated constitutional symptoms, dosage regimen of the drug, cost of the drug, efficacy of the drug, and toxicity of the drug. Those factors relating to disease severity reflect the urgency with which therapy with indomethacin or phenylbutazone must be initiated versus the opportunity to evaluate the efficacy of drugs with lesser toxicity. Those factors relating to drug dosage, cost, and efficacy indicate the likelihood of patient compliance with the prescribed regimen. I do not feel compelled to initiate therapy with indomethacin or phenylbutazone except in patients with extremely active disease. A rational approach to drug selection is indicated in Figure 1.

The key to therapy with NSAIDs is the continuous administration of an effective dose of drug for a minimum of 7 to 10 days before considering any therapeutic change. Certainly, drug intolerance or worsening symptoms are reasons to modify the drug regimen. Patients who do not tolerate or respond to the initial agent must be reassured that a drug that is both tolerated and effective is eventually identified in most patients. If a decision is made to start with indomethacin, it should be given in a dose of 100 to 150 mg daily in 3 or 4 divided doses. If this regimen proves ineffective, the dose can be increased to 200 mg daily, although this dose is frequently accompanied by headaches and other neurologic symptoms. If indomethacin is either not effective or not tolerated, a decision must be made about switching to phenylbutazone or one of the other NSAIDs, a decision based on the intensity of the disease and the relative toxicities of these drugs.

Toxicity of NSAIDs. It appears that the therapeutic action and many of the toxic manifestations of the NSAIDs (Table 4) are related to their ability to inhibit cyclooxygenase, the enzyme that catalyzes the initial step in the synthesis of the prostaglandins. Furthermore, with the exception of indomethacin and

TABLE 3 Nonsteroidal Anti-Inflammatory Drugs

Generic Drug Name	*Commonly Used Drug Regimens*	*Maximum Total Daily Dose*
Aspirin	*bid*[1]*–qid*	Variable[2]
Fenoprofen calcium	*tid–qid*	2,400 mg
Ibuprofen	*tid–qid*	3,200 mg
Indomethacin	*tid–qid*[3]	200 mg
Meclofenemate sodium	*tid–qid*	400 mg
Naproxen sodium	*bid–tid*	1,500 mg
Phenylbutazone	*tid–qid*	400 mg
Piroxicam	*od*	20 mg
Sulindac	*bid*	400 mg
Tolmetin sodium	*tid–qid*	1,600 mg

[1]Some new aspirin formulations recommend a bid regimen, although aspirin is usually prescribed as a qid regimen.

[2]Maximum aspirin dose is based on an optimal serum salicylate level of 20–25 mg%.

[3]Some patients require only a single hs dose of indomethacin (see text).

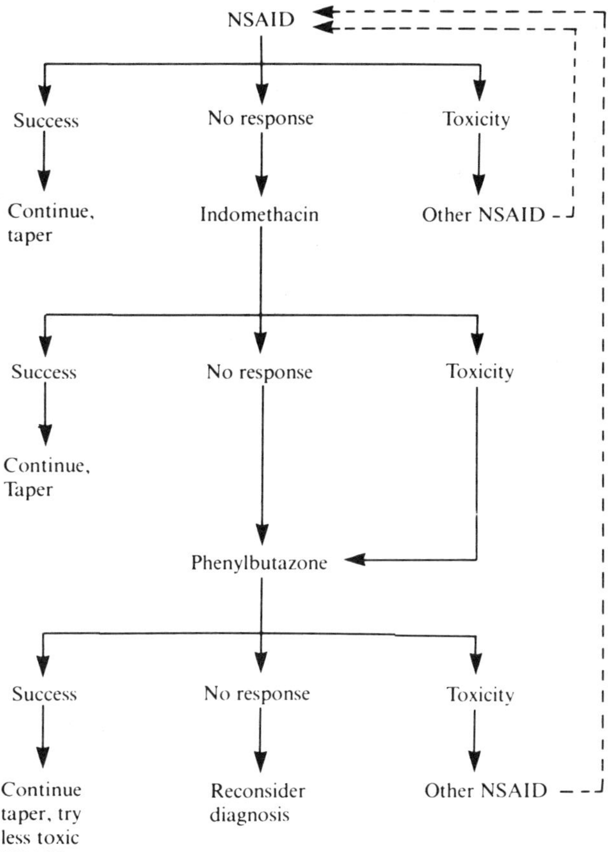

Figure 1 Treatment of RS with NSAID.

TABLE 4 Toxicity of NSAIDs

General	Aspirin "allergy" syndrome Hypersensitivity reactions
Gastrointestinal	Dyspepsia, gastritis, bleeding, gastric erosions, gastric ulcers, diarrhea, constipation
Hematologic	Inhibit platelet function Aplastic anemia Agranulocytosis
Renal	Azotemia Interstitial Nephritis Sodium retension
Cardiovascular	Hypertension
Neurologic	Lethargy, depression Headache
Special senses	Optic neuritis Tinnitus

phenylbutazone, the toxicity of the different NSAIDs is similar and does not currently provide a basis for drug selection. Thus, all of the NSAIDs are contraindicated in patients with a history of aspirin "allergy," the syndrome characterized by aspirin-induced asthma, angioedema, and nasal polyposis. The most common toxic effect of all the NSAIDs is gastrointestinal irritation, including erosions, bleeding, and gastric ulceration. While the effect of aspirin on platelet function is irreversible, the new NSAIDs inhibit platelet function reversibly and only in the presence of active drug. All of the NSAIDs, with the possible exception of sulindac, inhibit renal plasma flow; thus, in the face of a contracted intravascular volume or intrinsic renal disease, these drugs can cause or worsen azotemia. Many of the new NSAIDs have resulted in interstitial nephritis, a toxic manifestation not generally associated with aspirin. All of the NSAIDs facilitate sodium retention and must be monitored carefully in patients with hypertension.

While all of the NSAIDs are associated with neurologic toxicity, including depression and mental status changes, these side effects are most prominent with indomethacin. In addition, indomethacin often produces intense headaches thought to be vascular in origin and related to the imidazole ring structure of the drug which simulates histamine. Reversible optic neuritis is another neurologic toxicity most strongly associated with indomethacin.

Bone marrow suppression is most strongly associated with phenylbutazone, hence the concern about unnecessary use of this drug. Aplastic anemia is a dose-related toxic manifestation which has occurred primarily in the elderly who have been treated inappropriately with phenylbutazone for osteoarthritis. Of greater concern in the population with RS is agranulocytosis, an idiosyncratic toxic manifestation that occurs after a few weeks of therapy. Thus, patients who receive phenylbutazone must be monitored carefully for bone marrow suppression as well as for the other toxic manifestations of the NSAIDs.

Antibiotic Therapy. Because RS is often triggered by an identifiable infection, it seems reasonable to consider treatment with antibiotics. However, there are no data to indicate that RS is caused by persistence of the triggering microorganism or that antibiotic therapy has an effect on the acute illness or chronic phase of the disease. Therefore, antibiotics should be used only to treat identifiable infections according to standard infectious disease criteria. For example, the treatment of nongonococcal urethritis with tetracycline is most appropriate. In addition, barrier methods of contraception seem most appropriate for patients with any signs of genitourinary inflammation or those whose disease appears to be triggered by sexual activity.

Chronic Therapy. The majority of patients with RS will achieve a reasonable symptomatic response to one of the NSAIDs. The goals of chronic therapy will then be to restore optimal function and modify the NSAID regimen to minimize toxicity. Restoration of optimal function requires a careful clinical evaluation by the physician and physical therapist and the implementation of an appropriate exercise program. Modification of the NSAID regimen will be designed primarily to wean the patient from phenylbutazone or indomethacin to potentially safer NSAIDs. The pattern of responsiveness to the different NSAIDs should be recorded, since many patients will have recurrent musculoskeletal symptoms.

Other Drugs. A variable number of patients with RS will be refractory to the available NSAIDs, including phenylbutazone, have unacceptable disease activity on optimal therapy, or show clinical and radiologic signs of progressive joint destruction. Such patients clearly warrant additional therapy, but there are no data to guide us in this difficult decision. Systemic corticosteroids are said to be relatively ineffective in RS, thus they are traditionally not recommended. I utilize systemic corticosteroids only if the intensity of inflammatory or constitutional symptoms precludes an acceptable level of function. I will limit the dose to 5 to 10 mg of prednisone daily and proceed with another drug.

The traditional remission-inducing drugs used in rheumatoid arthritis, including antimalarials, gold, and D-penicillamine, have not been studied in RS. Because these drugs appear to be effective in patients with atypical or seronegative rheumatoid arthritis, some of whom actually have RS, I use them in the treatment of selected patients with chronic, refractory disease.

An alternative approach to the management of refractory disease is to recognize the clinical similarities between RS and psoriatic arthritis and proceed immediately with methotrexate therapy. Because of the age of the RS population and the potential gonadal toxicity of the drug, I usually defer methotrexate therapy until the traditional remission-inducing agents have been exhausted. I attempt to avoid the use of azathioprine or other cytotoxic drugs, because the potential oncogenicity of these agents does not seem warranted in the young population with RS.

SJÖGREN'S SYNDROME

NORMAN TALAL, M.D.

Sjögren's syndrome is a chronic inflammatory and autoimmune disease in which the salivary and lacrimal glands undergo progressive destruction by lymphocytes and plasma cells, resulting in decreased production of saliva and tears. The term *autoimmune exocrinopathy* has been introduced. The spectrum of this illness includes a primary form (sicca complex), a secondary form accompanying rheumatoid arthritis (or occasionally another connective tissue disease), and a form characterized mainly by lymphoproliferation of either a benign infiltrative or a malignant nature. Females are involved ten times more often than males.

The main clinical manifestations of the sicca complex are keratoconjunctivitis sicca (dry eyes), xerostomia (dry mouth), and recurrent episodes of often painful major salivary gland enlargement. Involvement of the exocrine glands of the respiratory tract may lead to persistent hoarseness, chronic nonproductive cough, and/or an increased incidence of respiratory tract infections. Gastrointestinal tract involvement may lead to dysphagia and/or atrophic gastritis. Desiccation of the vagina may result in dyspareunia and pruritus.

GENERAL THERAPEUTIC CONSIDERATIONS

Patients with Sjögren's syndrome should be seen regularly by a rheumatologist, an ophthalmologist, and a dentist. They need to be followed closely for significant functional deterioration, superimposed signs of disease complications, or significant changes in the course of the disease. For example, regular outpatient visits with serial observations of pertinent laboratory parameters may allow for the early diagnosis of extraglandular complications or malignancy.

Sjögren's syndrome is often a neglected disease, so much so that the patients themselves have formed a self-help organization called "The Moisture Seekers." The physician must remember that there is nothing minor about the symptoms of dry eyes and dry mouth. A patient of mine once wrote that "Sjögren's is misery," and so it often seems to the sufferer.

TREATMENT OF THE GLANDULAR DISEASE

Ophthalmologic Keratoconjunctivitis Sicca

The patient with keratoconjunctivitis sicca (KCS) may notice accumulation of thick, ropy secretions along the inner canthus owing to a decreased tear film and an abnormal mucus component. Related complaints include erythema, photosensitivity, eye fatigue, decreased visual acuity, and the sensation of a "film" across the field of vision. Desiccation can cause small superficial erosions of the corneal epithelium. Slit-lamp examination may reveal filamentary keratitis (filaments of corneal epithelium and debris) in severe cases. Conjunctivitis caused by *Staphyloccus aureus* is a complication.

The low level of humidity in air-conditioned environments may make these symptoms worse. Similar problems arise in windy or dry climates. Cigarette smoking and drugs with anticholinergic side effects may also increase symptoms. The most frequently implicated drugs are phenothiazines, tricyclic antidepressants, antispasmodics, and anti-Parkinsonian and decongestant medications. Many of these are available over the counter.

The mainstay of treatment for dry eyes is lubrication through the use of artifical tear drops, which can be used as often as necessary (generally every 1 to 3 hours). A variety of such drops is readily available without prescription, differing primarily in viscosity and preservative. The thicker, more viscous drops require less frequent application, although they can cause blurring and leave a residue on the lashes. Many patients will prefer the thinner drops which require more frequent applications. Patients generally test several different preparations to determine which one is best for them. An apparent failure to respond to artifical tears may actually reflect eye irritation resulting from the topical application of preservatives such as benzalkonium chloride, chlorobutanol, or thimerosal. Also available are lubricating ointments, which may produce significant blurring and are best used at night to provide protection over a longer period.

More recently, a slow release tear has been marketed under the trade name Lacrisert (Merck, Sharp and Dohme). It is a polymer of hydroxypropyl cellulose and comes as a cylinder which is inserted every 6 to 12 hours below the inferior tarsal margin. It absorbs the tears, slowly dissolves, and releases polymer. It is particularly useful in those patients who otherwise would use tear substitutes as frequently as every 15 minutes.

Other steps can be taken to preserve tears if tear substitutes are insufficient to control symptoms. Water tight swimmer's goggles can be very helpful in creating a moist chamber effect by preventing evaporation. They also protect against wind and dust particles. The same effect can be achieved with ordinary food plastic wrap taped over the eyes. Commercial "bubble" bandages are also available.

Soft contact lenses may also help to protect the cornea, especially when filaments are a problem. However, the lenses themselves require wetting and the patients must be followed very carefully, because there is an increased risk of infection. Such lenses are invaluable in the management of corneal ulcers which can arise as a complication of KCS.

Punctal occlusion is another method of conserving the few tears that patients produce. This procedure should be considered only in severe cases when there seems little likelihood of spontaneous increase in tear flow. Stents have been devised as a nonsurgical means of occlusion; this is a good way to predict the success of surgical occlusion.

Autonomic stimulation of tear flow has been relatively neglected as a form of therapy because the eye drops have generally worked well. Sympathomimetics and parasympathomimetics, especially the muscarinics, serve to stimulate tear flow. Pilocarpine taken orally has been reported as successful, as has bromhexine.

In patients with a relative excess of mucin production and formation of filaments, a mucolytic agent such as acetylcysteine has been found useful. However, other investigators have failed to confirm this.

Topical steroid use for the corneal ulcers of Sjögren's syndrome was associated with a worsening clinical course and is not recommended.

Two new approaches to topical therapy have recently been suggested. One is the use of dilute sodium hyaluronate. This compound has recently been approved for intraocular surgery, and the authors recommend a 10% diluted solution for topical use. Another group of investigators has developed a procedure for taking the patient's own serum and using this as an artificial tear. Both of these possibilities are somewhat tedious and need further study before final recommendations can be made.

Salivary

Xerostomia is often the initial symptom of Sjögren's syndrome. However, it is a common and subjective clinical complaint with a large variety of etiologies including emotional factors, sialodochitis, chronic sialadenitis, various drugs already listed, irradiation, and dehydration. It is best considered a relatively nonspecific finding requiring further evaluation by careful history, physical examination, and often labial salivary gland biopsy to confirm the presence of significant lymphocytic infiltrates attaining a focus score compatible with autoimmune exocrinopathy (Sjögren's syndrome).

Complaints resulting from dryness of the mouth are varied. The "cracker sign" describes the difficulties encountered in trying to eat dry foods without sufficient lubrication. A positive "cracker sign" is almost diagnostic of true Sjögren's syndrome. Many subjects require frequent ingestion of liquids. They may resort to carrying water bottles or candy in purse or pocket. Additional features include oral soreness, adherence of food to buccal surfaces, fissuring of the tongue, and dysphagia. Angular cheilitis resulting from superimposed candidiasis may occur. Patients may lose the ability to discriminate foods on the basis of taste and smell. Dental caries are accelerated. The parotid gland enlarges in many patients secondary to cellular infiltration and ductal obstruction. Usually asymptomatic and self-limited, the enlargement can be recurrent and associated with pain or erythema. Because of the potential risk of malignancy, ionizing irradiation of the parotid glands is not recommended.

Treatment of xerostomia associated with Sjögren's syndrome is difficult. No single highly effective method is currently available, and most efforts are aimed only at palliation. Before any treatment program is started, it is important to identify contributing factors, such as mouth breathing, heavy smoking, and drugs with anticholinergic side effects which further decrease salivary flow. Simulation of salivary flow by sucrose-free, highly flavored lozenges or chewing gums, use of lemon-flavored drinks, and dietary counseling to avoid particularly dry foods may also be of assistance. Most patients discover that it is helpful to carry water, sugarless lemon drops, or chewing gum. These must be sugar-free because of the risk of rampant dental caries. Fluids ad libitum should be utilized for all meals and snacks, which should also begin and finish with highly flavored substances which tend to stimulate salivary flow. The consumption of large amounts of water during the day, while symptomatically helpful, may produce nocturia that interrupts sleep patterns and leads to fatigue.

Artificial saliva substitutes offer some additional palliation. Mucin-containing saliva substitutes seem to be more effective than substitutes based on carboxymethyl cellulose or polyethylene oxide. Mucins tend to protect against desiccation, provide for lubrication and cleaning, and appear to have some antimicrobial effect. Saliva substitutes should, however, be utilized sparingly with only the minimum volume necessary for oral lubrication. This usually consists of no more than 2 ml before and after meals, at bedtime, and following oral hygiene. The material can also be applied to any removable intraoral appliance to facilitate more sustained release.

Topical or oral treatment with stannous fluoride enhances dental mineralization and retards damage to tooth surfaces. In cases of rapidly progressive dental disease, the fluoride can be directly applied to the teeth from plastic trays that are used at night. The latter method may be inconvenient but provides better exposure at gingival margins to the fluoride.

Increased salivary flow rates may be induced by potassium iodide or parasympathomimetic agents, such as pilocarpine or neostigmine, systemically or as a mouthwash. Varying degrees of success have been noted. A new battery-powered electronic device for stimulating salivary flow has recently been developed and is currently under study. Bromhexine, a synthetic alkaloid originally used as a mucolytic agent in cough syrups, has been tried in Scandinavia with reported success.

Increased moisture to the upper airways by use of normal saline sprays and humidifiers at night may reduce respiratory symptoms and alleviate mouth breathing. In some cases, nasal irrigation with normal saline proves helpful.

Vaginal dryness is treated with lubricants such as K-Y jelly, and dry skin with moisturizing lotions.

TREATMENT OF EXTRAGLANDULAR DISEASE

Systemic corticosteroids and immunosuppressive drugs are used only to treat potentially life-threatening disease, often involving the lung or kidney. They are not recommended for the treatment of dry eyes and dry mouth.

A diffuse interstitial pneumonitis resulting from lymphocytic infiltration and fibrosis may cause severe exertional dyspnea. Obstructive disease (in the absence of smoking) may result from lymphocytic infiltration surrounding small airways. Pulmonary function tests should be performed and monitored twice yearly to determine the extent of functional impairment. Lung biopsy should be performed before treatment is started. There is a better chance for therapeutic success if a highly cellular infiltrate is found. Conversely, one may decide against treatment if only scar tissue is present on lung biopsy.

Treatment is usually initiated with corticosteroids in the range of 0.5 to 1.0 mg/kg daily. As the patient improves, the dose can be tapered to a maintenance level 50 percent of the starting dose. If there is no apparent responses within 3 to 6 months, steroids should be discontinued and a trial of cyclophosphamide considered. A range of 100 to 150 mg per day is a good starting dose. Cyclophosphamide has succeeded when other immunosuppresive drugs have failed. Although the risk of lymphoma is an important theoretical consideration, in my personal experience, it has not appeared in patients with Sjögren's syndrome treated with cyclophosphamide.

The most common renal abnormalities in Sjögren's syndrome involve the tubules, particularly overt or latent renal tubular acidosis. Steroids have generally been of little value, whereas treatment with cyclophosphamide has been successful. Peripheral and cranial neuropathy has been associated with vasculitis involving the vasa nervorum. Although there are few data concerning the treatment of this complication, bolus cyclophosphamide in a dose of 0.5 to 0.75 g/m^2 may be of benefit.

The incidence of lymphoma is increased 44-fold in Sjögren's syndrome. Pseudomalignant or malignant lymphoprofileration may be present initially or may develop later in the illness. Most lymphomas belong to the B-cell lineage, although the histologic appearance is variable. A diminution of previously elevated immunoglobulins and loss of autoantibodies may precede a malignant transformation. Pseudolymphoma is an intermediate stage in this transition from benign to malignant lymphoproliferation.

The distinction between lymphoma and pseudolymphoma may be difficult even in the hands of highly experienced and expert pathologists. Some patients with pseudolymphoma may not require treatment if there is no functional compromise. If there is, treatment of pseudolymphoma with corticosteroids or cyclophosphamide is often successful. Treatment of lymphoma and decisions regarding chemotherapy and/or radiation therapy should be guided by experienced oncologists. In general, these lesions are highly refractory to treatment.

USE OF NONSTEROIDAL AGENTS AND OTHER MEDICATIONS IN SJÖGREN'S SYNDROME

Treatment of secondary Sjögren's syndrome is usually directed at the associated disease. The treatment of rheumatoid arthritis or systemic lupus erythematosis is not altered because of the concomitant presence of Sjögren's syndrome. The sicca complex is generally milder and managed as already discussed. Arthralgias or myalgias are managed with salicylates or nonsteroidal anti-inflammatory drugs.

These studies were supported in part by the General Medicine Research Service of the Veterans Administration.

ANKYLOSING SPONDYLITIS

ROBERT P. JACOBS, M.D.

Ankylosing spondylitis (AS) is a common inflammatory arthropathy characterized by prominent axial skeletal involvement, variable degrees of peripheral joint disease, and inflammatory enthesopathies. While AS is associated with several extraskeletal manifestations (Table 1) that allow it to serve as the prototype for the spondyloarthropathies (Table 2), the musculoskeletal manifestations of the disease are the major focus of therapeutic intervention and deserve elaboration.

The axial skeletal disease of AS is a symmetric, ascending, inflammatory process that always involves the sacroiliac joints and often involves higher levels of spines. Sacroiliitis results in gluteal pain that often

TABLE 1 Clinical Manifestations of Ankylosing Spondylitis

Musculoskeletal	Sacroiliitis Spondylitis Peripheral oligoarthritis Inflammatory enthesopathy
Ocular	Iritis
Cardiac	Pericarditis Conduction defects Aortic regurgitation
Pulmonary	Pleurisy Apical fibrocavitary lesion

radiates into one or both thighs and can be confused with lumbar disc disease and other causes of low back pain. Lumbar spine involvement is associated with pain and stiffness in the low back that is characterized by a diurnal pattern typical of inflammatory joint disease: Symptoms are maximal in the morning, decrease with mild activity, and increase toward the end of the day or at night. Involvement of the spine is associated with a loss of normal mobility that can serve as both a diagnostic clue and parameter with which to monitor therapy. In the thoracic spine, involvement of the costovertebral joints accounts for the limitation in chest expansion seen commonly in AS. In addition to restricting spinal mobility, the inflammatory component of AS results in changes in the configuration of the spine. Disease in the lumbar and cervical spines results in a loss of the normal lordosis, while disease in the thoracic spine results in an accentuated kyphosis, thus resulting in the characteristic kyphotic posture of the untreated patient with AS.

A majority of patients with AS will have peripheral joint disease. The most commonly affected peripheral joints are the hips and shoulders, often designated the root joints. The hips are a frequent site of destructive joint disease that may require orthopaedic surgical intervention. In addition, patients with AS have peripheral joint involvement typical of that seen in the other spondyloarthropathies and characterized by asymmetric oligoarthritis affecting primarily lower extremity joints.

Another musculoskeletal feature of AS, also typical of that seen in the spondyloarthropathies, is the frequent occurrence of inflammatory enthesopathies. This refers to inflammatory lesions at entheses, or sites of attachment of ligaments and tendons to bone; they include Achilles tendinitis, plantar fasciitis, adductor and abductor tendinitis of the hips, and chest wall pain associated with inflammation at insertions of the intercostal muscles.

AS serves as the prototype for a diverse group of disorders now called the spondyloarthropathies (see Table 2). This group of diseases is characterized by varying combinations of the musculoskeletal features described above and a broad spectrum of extraskeletal manifestations, including involvement of the eyes, mucous membranes, genitourinary system, integument, heart, and lungs. For a more detailed discussion of the extraskeletal manifestations of the spondyloarthropathies, see the chapter on Reiter's syndrome. The spondyloarthropathies have generated much confusion, because of the extensive clinical overlap among the members of the group. However, it is an important clinical concept, because it emphasizes the presence of inflammatory disease of the spine in multiple clinical settings.

TABLE 2 Spondyloarthropathies

Ankylosing spondylitis
Reiter's syndrome
Reactive arthritis
Psoriatic arthritis
Arthropathy of inflammatory bowel disease
Juvenile chronic polyarthritis
Whipple's disease

The striking association of HLA-B27 with AS and the other spondyloarthropathies has had a profound impact on our understanding of this disease group. This association has provided objective scientific data with which to explain the clustering of these diseases with overlapping clinical features. It provided a scientific basis with which to explore the pathogenesis of these disorders. Finally, it provided an epidemiologic marker with which to study the prevalence and natural history of these diseases.

The epidemiologic data are most revealing, because they indicate that AS is much more common than expected, especially in females, and can be diagnosed in up to 20 percent of the HLA-B27 positive population. Since HLA-B27 is found in 6 to 8 percent of white Americans, the prevalence of AS is as high as 1.2 to 1.6 percent of the population. Based on our clinical experience, two conclusions can be drawn: First, there must be a large population with AS who have few, if any, symptoms; second, as a corollary, traditional teaching about AS must be based on those patients with disease severe enough to warrant medical evaluation and treatment.

The clinical heterogeneity of AS makes it difficult to describe the typical disease course and prognosis for a given individual. The presence of HLA-B27 does not appear to correlate with disease severity, nor do other laboratory parameters of disease activity. Extraskeletal manifestations do not predict disease outcome, although cardiopulmonary manifestations reflect disease of long duration. It does appear that patients who maintain spinal mobility during the first ten years of disease are unlikely to show disease progression late in the course of the illness. While the prevalence of AS in women remains to be determined, it does appear that the axial skeletal disease in women is less severe than it is in men. Finally, there are data that suggest that survival of patients with AS is shorter than for control populations, with death occurring from cardiovascular events that do not appear to be related specifically to known disease manifestations.

TREATMENT

The treatment of AS requires a thorough knowledge of the disease. The patient population is usually young, eager to eturn to normal activity, and reluctant to adhere to a rigorous medical regimen. Perhaps it is the youthful nature of the patient population, with the attendant difficulty in evaluating symptoms and subtle physical findings, that results so commonly in a delayed diagnosis.

Patient Education

The management of all chronic diseases is facilitated by patient education. The goals of this aspect of a comprehensive treatment program are to educate the patient about the disease, develop a conceptual framework on which to build a treatment program, and anticipate or correct any misconceptions regarding the disease or treatment.

Patients must understand the chronic inflammatory nature of AS if they are to be expected to adhere to a continuous regimen of anti-inflammatory drugs. A more difficult task is to explain the concept of a multisystem disease when we do not yet understand the biochemical or immunologic basis for the different lesions. Disease course and outcome should be discussed to emphasize the need to adhere to a continuous treatment program and avoid certain activities that might have a deleterious effect on disease outcome. Smoking should be forbidden in patients with a disorder associated with restrictive and fibrocavitary lung disease. While the majority of patients with AS maintain gainful employment, job modification may be required owing to possible limitations imposed by the disease.

Finally, the genetic implications of HLA-B27 deserve careful and thoughtful discussion. Many patients will know that AS is a genetically determined disease, but few understand the distinction between genetic transmission and genetic susceptibility. The most pressing question posed by most patients is whether the disease will be passed on to their children. Explaining that only 50 percent of the children of an HLA-B27 positive heterozygote will carry the marker, that a maximum of 20 percent of HLA-B27 positive individuals will develop disease, that the disease shows marked variability in severity, and that the majority of patients with AS lead active and productive lives is usually sufficient to address parental guilt and fears. I do not consider the presence of AS, with or without the HLA-B27 marker, a reason to modify family planning.

Physical Therapy

All patients with AS should be regular participants in a physical therapy program. As with all forms of chronic arthritis, physical therapy will consist of a balanced program of rest and exercise. The program for the patient with AS will, of course, focus on axial skeletal disease with an emphasis on posture.

Rest is important for all forms of arthritis, especially at times when there is active inflammation. The patient with AS will often notice an increase in morning stiffness, musculoskeletal pain, and fatigability when there has been inadequate rest. As simple as it may seem, rest for the patient with AS is a subject that deserves careful discussion and explicit instructions. A major concern relates to poor posture while in bed, because of an improper sleeping position, inadequate mattress, or too many pillows. The patient with AS must be instructed to sleep in a supine position with the axial skeleton maintained in a normal erect configuration. Patients with active disease often find the fetal position more comfortable. A soft mattress promotes lumbar flexion and pillows force the neck into flexion. Thus, we must identify these postural inadequacies of bed rest and utilize time in bed to correct the natural tendency of the disease to produce forward flexion of the spine.

An exercise program is required by all patients to maintain mobility and promote proper axial skeletal alignment. I suggest that all patients with AS undergo a complete evaluation by a physical therapist and return for regular annual assessments. The patient and therapist might find that physical modalities, including heat and ultrasound, are effective during the acute, inflammatory phase of the illness. While there are no data to support the role of exercise in AS, anecdotal observations of patients who have required spinal immobilization and patients who have not adhered to prescribed exercise programs convince me that regular exercise is associated with greater mobility late in the course of the disease. Exercises must emphasize mobility of all spinal segments, including the costovertebral joints and the root joints. The exercise program must also emphasize posture, with most exercises directed at spinal extension. Finally, patients with restricted chest expansion must be instructed on diaphragmatic breathing exercise.

Anti-Inflammatory Drugs

The mainstays of drug therapy for AS are the nonsteroidal anti-inflammatory drugs (NSAIDs). These drugs are usually quite effective in minimizing or eliminating symptoms and promoting greater or normal spinal mobility in the acute, inflammatory phase of the disease. Therapeutic benefit can be measured both by the patient's subjective clinical response and such objective parameters as cervical spine range of motion, occiput-to-wall distance, chest expansion, lumbosacral spine mobility (e.g., modified Schober test), and finger-to-floor distance. While there are no data to indicate that therapy with NSAIDs alters the long-term course of the disease, it is my opinion that the proper use of these drugs, in conjunction with a regular program of physical therapy, does promote and maintain spinal mobility and alignment. They do not, however, appear to affect the course of destructive root joint disease.

While all of the NSAIDs have measurable therapeutic efficacy in AS, there are data that support the clinical impression that indomethacin and phenylbutazone are more efficacious than aspirin. This has prompted several clinical investigators to recommend initiating therapy for AS with indomethacin. I do not feel so constrained in my therapeutic options for this disease (Fig. 1), and I suggest that the initial thera-

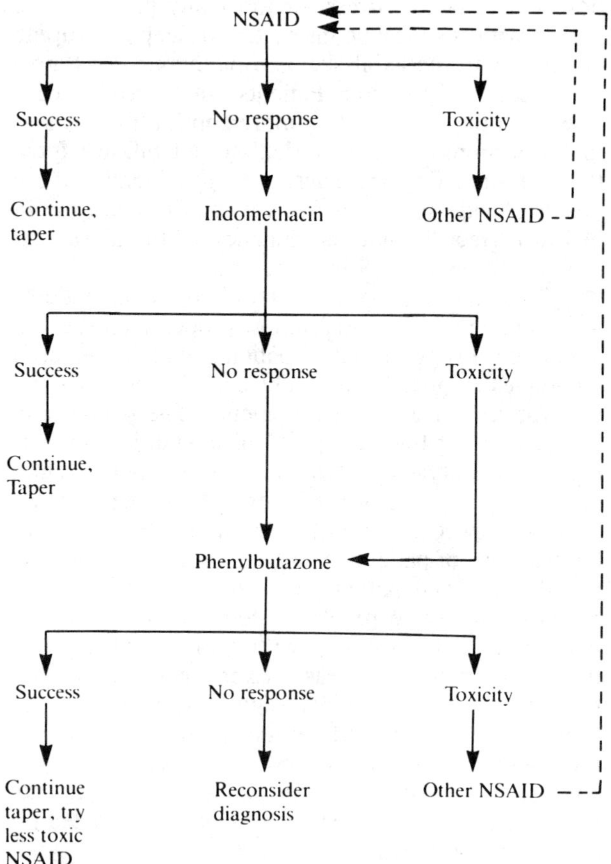

Figure 1 Treatment of RS with NSAID.

TABLE 3 Nonsteroidal Anti-Inflammatory Drugs

Generic Drug Name	*Commonly Used Drug Regimens*	*Maximum Total Daily Dose*
Aspirin	*bid*[1]*–qid*	Variable[2]
Fenoprofen calcium	*tid–qid*	2,400 mg
Ibuprofen	*tid–qid*	3,200 mg
Indomethacin	*tid–qid*[3]	200 mg
Meclofenemate sodium	*tid–qid*	400 mg
Naproxen sodium	*bid–tid*	1,500 mg
Phenylbutazone	*tid–qid*	400 mg
Piroxicam	*od*	20 mg
Sulindac	*bid*	400 mg
Tolmetin sodium	*tid–qid*	1,600 mg

[1]Some new aspirin formulations recommend a bid regimen, although aspirin is usually prescribed as a qid regimen.

[2]Maximum aspirin dose is based on an optimal serum salicylate level of 20–25 mg%.

[3]Some patients require only a single hs dose of indomethacin (see text).

peutic agent be selected on the basis of personal experience, special properties of the drug, and disease activity.

The key to treatment of AS with NSAIDs is the continuous administration of effective therapeutic doses of these agents. The number of NSAIDs available is large and expanding, an indication that no one of these agents is universally effective and tolerated. To maximize compliance, therefore, such factors as frequency of drug administration, cost, and drug toxicity must be considered in our therapeutic recommendations. The frequency of drug administration, an important factor in compliance, varies from a single daily dose (piroxicam) to 4 daily doses (Table 3). Indomethacin and several new aspirin formulations are available as slow or sustained release preparations that offer the advantage of less frequent drug administration. For a detailed discussion of the toxicity of NSAIDs, see the chapter on Reiter's syndrome.

As was made clear by recent epidemiologic studies, many patients with AS do not appear to require therapy. Patients with mild disease associated with nocturnal discomfort, mild morning stiffness, and minimal or no limitation of spinal mobility may respond nicely to a single dose of indomethacin (25 to 50 mg or 75 mg of the sustained release preparation) administered at bed time. A majority of patients with AS who present for evaluation and treatment will, however, require a more intensive drug regimen (see Fig. 1). I prefer to initiate therapy with one of the NSAIDs that can be administered as a *bid* or *tid* regimen to maximize compliance. I do not feel compelled to initiate therapy with indomethacin, but will do so in patients with severe pain or other evidence of considerable disease activity. Patients must take these medications as directed for a minimum of 7 to 10 days before making a preliminary assessment of therapeutic benefit. Maximal therapeutic response often requires several weeks of continuous therapy. If the initial drug is effective, but not tolerated, another NSAID, including aspirin, should be selected. Patients must be reassured that it is not uncommon for a given individual to have problems with several NSAIDs before one is found tht is both effective and tolerated.

If the initial drug is ineffective at maximal therapeutic doses, therapy with indomethacin should be started. If therapy with indomethacin is effective, but not tolerated, another NSAID should be selected. Because therapy with indomethacin is often limited by headache and other neurologic symptoms, I will often turn to tolmetin sodium or sulindac, which do not commonly result in such side effects. If, after an adequate therapeutic trial, indomethacin is found to be ineffective, treatment with phenylbutazone is begun.

If treatment with phenylbutazone is effective, but not tolerated, all of the other NSAIDs must be evaluated for therapeutic efficacy. If treatment with phenylbutazone is effective, the dose should be lowered gradually and periodic attempts made to wean the patient to indomethacin or one of the other NSAIDs with less potential toxicity. If treatment with phenylbutazone is ineffective, the diagnosis of AS should be questioned and the patient reevaluated.

The woman with AS who is contemplating pregnancy presents a difficult therapeutic dilemma. Unlike rheumatoid arthritis, AS does not tend to go into remission during pregnancy. Therefore, pregnant women with symptomatic AS may require treatment with drugs that have not been shown to be safe during pregnancy, although they have not been associated with fetal abnormalities. I do encourage pregnant women with AS to continue treatment with one of the NSAIDs if their symptoms so dictate.

Other Drugs

Corticosteroids. The corticosteroids play little or no role in the treatment of AS. Because patients usually respond well to one of the NSAIDs, the risk of chronic corticosteroid therapy is not warranted. Furthermore, patients with AS do not appear to respond as dramatically to corticosteroids as do patients with rheumatoid arthritis. The local injection of corticosteroids into refractory peripheral joint or enthesopathic lesions may be effective, but is required only rarely.

Immunosuppressives. The traditional remission-inducing drugs used in rheumatoid arthritis, including antimalarials, gold, and D-penicillamine, have never been adequately evaluated in AS, although limited experience suggests that they are not effective. Methotrexate does appear to be efficacious in AS, especially when it occurs in the setting of psoriasis. Therefore, in patients with AS refractory to all of the NSAIDs, a carefully monitored trial of methotrexate is reasonable.

Irradiation. Any discussion of treatment of AS would not be complete without some comment about irradiation therapy. This treatment modality was utilized before the introduction of the vast array of NSAIDs that have been shown to be so very effective in AS. While irradiation therapy did provide temporary symptomatic relief, the ultimate recurrence of active disease and association of this treatment modality with leukemia and aplastic anemia have largely relegated it to the rank of medical antiquity.

Surgical Therapy. There are several aspects of surgical therapy of AS that are relevant to this review. First, there is the concept that patients with AS should be mobilized as soon as possible following any surgical procedure. The most common surgical procedure required by patients with AS for treatment of their disease is total hip replacement. Early mobilization and a regular physical therapy program are essential to the success of this procedure. One complication of the procedure seen commonly in patients with AS is heterotopic bone formation. There are data to suggest that a perioperative course of diphosphonates decreases the frequency and intensity of this complication, but further study is required.

The ankylosed spine is a potential site of fracture following minor injuries. Thus, patients with AS who sustain trauma must be evaluated carefully for evidence of a neurologic deficit. Localized pain following trauma must be evaluated by radiologic and radionuclide studies in search of a nondisplaced fracture or spondylodiscitis.

Lastly, the severely kyphotic patient with AS whose field of vision is limited to the area about his feet might require more aggressive surgical approaches. Much of the problem might be corrected by aggressive physical therapy designed to restore hip extension or total hip replacements. Prism glasses can expand the field of vision. The rare patient, however, may be a candidate for a spinal osteotomy designed to correct the kyphotic deformity resulting from the unimpeded progression of the disease.

MIXED CONNECTIVE TISSUE DISEASE

MORRIS REICHLIN, M.D.

Mixed connective tissue disease (MCTD) was described in the early 1970s by Sharp and associates as an overlap syndrome with features of systemic lupus erythematosus, polymyositis, and scleroderma. The clinical picture of patients was quite pleomorphic, with variable numbers of features of each of the constituent dieases. No fixed clinical criteria for disease definition have been set. The consistent unifying feature of the syndrome was serologic: high titers of antibody to the nuclear RNAprotein antigen, now known to be composed of U1 RNA and 7 proteins comprising an RNAprotein particle with antigenicity residing in several of the polypeptides. Controversy has surrounded the definition and even the existence of this syndrome, but that is not to be the focus of this chapter. Something must be said about disease definition so that one knows for which patients the described treatments are being recommended. For the purpose of this chapter, mixed connective tissue disease is defined primarily by the serologic criterion of antibodies to the nuclear RNP antigen accompanied by features of one or more of the following diseases: systemic lupus erythematosus (SLE), scleroderma, and polymyositis. In that vein, my approach to these patients has been to follow the empirically developed guidelines for the treatment of the constituent diseases that comprise the syndrome. The independent value of defining the disease is in the determination of the specific antibody which carries with it a somewhat more benign prognosis than that of the average patient with any of the three constituent diseases under discussion. If one is dealing with a disease with a benign prognosis, one should be more reserved in utilizing aggressive treatment, but as in all such matters some patients could present with what appears to be a serious complication. In any case, certain of the constituent complications generally require therapy for their resolution, which usually consists of systemic corticosteroids. Table 1 lists the various features of the three constituent diseases which compromise MCTD. They are listed for the first eight manifestations in order of increasing gravity, and therefore the applied therapies are more powerful and concomitantly more dangerous. On the right side of the table in shorthand terms are the suggested therapies.

ARTHRITIS

The first manifestation to be considered is arthritis. Arthritis is extremely common in patients with MCTD, it occurs in 80 to 90 percent of patients. In general, the arthritis is indistinguishable from that which occurs in SLE. It is a rheumatoid-like arthritis in distribution and in character except that the arthritis is largely nondestructive, nonerosive, and tends accordingly to be nondeforming. The frequency of distribution is very similar to that in rheumatoid arthritis, and involvement of the hands and feet is most common, followed by involvement of the wrists, elbows, shoulders, knees, ankles, and hips. Treatment is in every way similar to that of the rheumatoid patient with nonerosive, nondestructive disease. That is, one applies a program of physical therapy, rest, and one of the nonsteroidal anti-inflammatory drugs or aspirin. I do not use Motrin in these patients since a number of patients with SLE have developed aseptic meningitis while receiving this agent. The response is usually similar to that seen in rheumatoid disease, with between a half and two-thirds of the patients responding quite promptly after such therapy and requiring nothing else for this particular manifestation of the disease. It is my experience and that of others that one frequently has problems (perhaps with as many as a third of the patients) with a chemically manifest hepatitis with the use of aspirin. This is quite unfortunate in some cases, since a number of the patients who have chemical hepatitis have responded quite well to the aspirin. On the other hand, it is prudent to discontinue the aspirin under these circumstances. Although I know of no long-term follow-up of such patients in whom the use of aspirin has been continued, clearly this would constitute an experiment which would be very difficult to justify, since there are other agents that are generally quite effective even if considerably more expensive. There is a small proportion of patients with antibodies to nuclear RNP who develop an erosive destructive arthritis which is, in my experience, always rheumatoid factor positive. I approach these patients with exactly the same philosophy as I do patients with erosive, destructive rheumatoid arthritis. The first agent I use in such patients is Plaquenil, and I employ it in doses of 2 200-mg tablets a day with ophthalmologic monitoring every 6 months. If retinal problems occur, the drug must be discontinued. This must now be very rare. If patients respond within the first 2 to 3 months, I reduce the dosage to 1 tablet a day and sustain that for an indefinite period of time. On the other hand, I do not give up on the prospect for success with Plaquenil until patients have been on 2 tablets a day for a minimum of 5 to 6 months. If Plaquenil fails, I then use penicillamine in a manner entirely analogous to that employed for rheumatoid arthritis. I prefer penicillamine to gold because of convenience and a personal impression that allergic reactions to gold are somewhat more frequent than those to penicillamine in lupus patients. I have deliberately not used gold in such patients but have had a number of patients referred to me with severe gold reactions who turned out to be antinuclear RNP positive polyarthritis patients. Obviously, a great deal of patient selection is involved in such observations, but they do influence one's behavior. If penicillamine fails after an appropriate period of treatment, usually not less than 6 months and after having achieved a total dose of 750 mg per day, one is faced with the same difficult situation that is faced in rheumatoid arthritis patients who fail both conservative therapy and remittive drug therapy. At this point I favor the use of Imuran in the same doses recommended for rheumatoid arthritis. This is some dosage between 1 and 2 mg/kg/day to induce a remission and then some lesser dosage for maintenance to be determined empirically by the clinical response. Other modalities for progressive destructive arthritis in such patients are completely empiric and there is very little experience with them.

TABLE 1

Arthritis	Nonsteroidal anti-inflammatory drugs, aspirin
Erosive arthritis	Remittive agents, Plaquenil penicillamine, Imuran
Dermatitis	Local steroids, sun avoidance, sunscreens, antimalarials for extensive disease
Raynaud's phenomenon	Cold avoidance Minipres, nifedipine
Pleuritis, pericarditis, peritonitis	Nonsteroidal anti-inflammatory drugs, if uncomplicated, steroids if accompanied by fever, general systemic signs and symptoms
Hemolytic anemia, thrombocytopenia	Steroids
Nephritis	Same as in lupus, depends on lesion, extent of disease
Central nervous system disease	Steroids
Polymyositis	Steroids
Scleroderma involvement	same approach as in scleroderma, penicillamine may be useful in rapidly progressive skin disease, may prevent internal organ involvement. Steroids may be useful in inflammatory lung disease.

DERMATITIS

Treatment of dermatitis is, in my experience, identical to that for the various forms of dermatitis in lupus patients. Indeed, the skin lesions are completely indistinguishable from those in lupus patients. Guidelines are very similar in terms of approach and management. When photosensitivity accompanies the development and perpetuation of the lesions, the usual precautions should be taken for sun avoidance with appropriate hats, clothing, and the use of sunscreens. I have encouraged my patients, even when they are not demonstrably photosensitive, to take at least reasonable precautions—hats and medium levels of sun block—if they are going to be exposed to the sun. On the other hand, for patients who are very photosensitive and who must occasionally go into the sun there are now very effective sun blocks, and any one of those with a rating of 15 is usually sufficient. For acute and intermittent erythematous eruptions, the use of local steroids is usually effective. There are various grades of creams that can be used, but simple 1 percent hydrocortisone creams at the outset are usually effective. However, creams with triamcinolone are used in more difficult cases. Simple local measures usually are adequate in less severe cases. When skin disease is more widespread, as in the variant known as subacute cutaneous lupus (which also occurs in patients with antinuclear RNP, although not nearly as frequently as in patients with antibodies to Ro/SSA), the use of Plaquenil is very effective and only rarely fails to control such lesions. The mode of administration is entirely similar to that used for the erosive polyarthritis as described above.

Clearly, some patients with difficult and progressive arthritis and widespread dermatitis may be well controlled with the single drug Plaquenil. In my experience, few patients have skin disease so difficult to control that systemic steroids are either warranted or necessary. However, this occasionally occurs and steroids are then used in whatever doses are necessary to control the skin disease. One generally treats for a relatively short period of time to bring the skin lesions under control, that is, with 1 mg/kg/day for a week to 10 days, followed by a sharp reduction in dosage until the dose is found which controls the skin disease. The exception to this is the rare patient who has widespread vasculitic lesions of the skin. In such patients steroids in whatever dose is required are effective. One begins with 1 mg/kg/day to bring the lesions under control and then determine the minimal dose required to control that aspect of the disease.

RAYNAUD'S PHENOMENON

The cardinal principle of management is cold avoidance and appropriate clothing at the time of year when this becomes a problem. Bothersome as it may be for people who are particularly sensitive, gloves should be worn when cold things are removed from the refrigerator or when it is necessary to handle cold objects. Many drugs have been used in the treatment of Raynaud's phenomenon and most are disappointing, although all have been said to be effective at one time or another in individual patients. These include phenoxybenzamine, guanethidine, methyldopa, and reserpine. I no longer use any of these drugs in the management of Raynaud's phenomenon and in difficult situations with particular patients I now first use nifedipine in dosages of 10 mg 3 times a day, increased to 20 mg *tid* if necessary. If nifedipine is ineffective, Minipress is my next choice. Minipress in dosages of 1 mg *tid* increased to 2 or 3 mg *tid*, may be used depending on the response. The first 1-mg tablet of Minipress should be taken at night by the few patients who experience syncope as a reaction to the drug. I find nifedipine particularly useful and have noted rapid healing of small skin lesions resulting from vasoconstriction in patients with Raynaud's phenomenon. I am confident that this drug—like all the others—is not uniformly effective, but it is probably one of the better agents to have been developed in recent years for the treatment of Raynaud's phenomenon in this and other clinical settings.

SEROSITIS

Serositis comprises mainly pleuritis and pericarditis and rarely peritonitis, in order of decreasing frequency of occurrence. I will focus on the first two. They are quite common in patients with this form of lupus or overlap syndrome, and the pleuritis occurs in 50 to 60 percent of such patients, roughly half of these patients also have pericarditis. A number of patients will have isolated pericarditis. In the usual situation involving pleuritis, the decision regarding the mode of treatment depends largely on the clinical setting. If it is an isolated phenomenon, with pleural pain and minimal effusion without other signs of systemic illness, nonsteroidal anti-inflammatory drugs can be quite effective. I usually use Indocin in doses of 50 mg *tid* for the first 2 days or until symptoms are brought under control; the dosage is then reduced to 25 mg 3 times a day. If the pleuritis is accompanied by other signs of systemic disease and the patients are ill with fever, gastrointestinal symptoms, and so on, I consider this an indication for systemic steroids. They should be used for as short a period of time as is necessary to bring these symptoms under control. One may start with 1 mg/kg/day until the signs and symptoms of pleuritis are controlled, the appetite improves, and the patient is afebrile. Thereafter, the steroids are rapidly tapered to whatever dosage is required to maintain the patient in an asymptomatic state. When pleuritis is accompanied by significant fluid accumulation, steroids are almost always necessary for resolution.A similar approach to that for pleuritis is possible with pericarditis. However, I have seen 2 patients with antinuclear RNP alone who presented with cardiac tamponade related to pericarditis and required pericardiocentesis for improvement of their cardiovascular status. Patients are then treated with steroids in a manner and dosage similar to what has been described for the treatment of pleuritis accompanied by fluid in the pleural cavity and/or systemic signs and symptoms.

HEMATOLOGIC INVOLVEMENT

Hematologic complications are common in MCTD. A patient may have hemolytic anemia, thrombocytopenia, or leukopenia. It is an error to consider leukopenia an indication for therapy of any type. It is extremely common, and although the granulocyte and/or the lymphocyte count—both of which are usually depressed—do rise with steroid treatment, I have followed patients with low white counts for many years who do not seem to have unusual problems with infection and are best left alone. On the other hand, Coombs' positive hemolytic anemia with a hemoglobin count of less than 10.0 g/dl in females or less than 12 g/dl in males is to me an indication for steroid treatment. The approach to this, as well as to platelet counts less than 100,000 mm^3, is in all respects similar to the recommendations made for autoimmune hemolytic anemia on the one had, or idiopathic thrombocytopenic purpura on the other. In both instances steroids are the mainstay of treatment and are used—as they are for the other manifestations—at a level of 1 mg/kg/day until there is normalization of either the hematocrit or the platelet count; in some instances normalization may occur within a few days; especially of the platelet count. However, in both instances I have sustained the dosage of medication at the mg/kg level for a minimum of 3 to 4 weeks before beginning a reduction to the lowest dose that will sustain the hemoglobin or platelet count in the normal range. Blockade of the reticuloendothelial system and loss of rapid destruction of red cells or platelets, which is characteristic of both of these syndromes, probably occurs in a few days. On the other hand, it has been shown in autoimmune hemolytic anemia that several weeks are required to reduce effectively the production of autoantibody which is ultimately responsible for the shortened life span of red cells, and presumably similar considerations would apply in idiopathic thrombocytopenic purpura.

RENAL AND CENTRAL NERVOUS SYSTEM INVOLVEMENT

I come now to two manifestations which are only rarely found in patients with the overlap under discussion with antibodies to nuclear RNP, and so I will discuss them only briefly. One is glomerulonephritis, and the other is various forms of central nervous system (CNS) disease, such as generalized seizures, psychosis, and other CNS manifestations, such as stroke, transverse myelitis, or an encephalitis-like picture with coma. Serious renal and CNS diseases are very rare in my experience in patients who truly only have antibodies to nuclear RNP. I hold the view that this syndrome is a variant of lupus with a certain coincident expression of the other two diseases in question (scleroderma and myositis). The issue of the precise serologic definition of these patients is an essential part of the initial evaluation of the patient. Lupus patients who have only antibodies to nuclear RNP rarely, if ever, develop nephritis or CNS diseases. However, patients with antibodies to nuclear RNP which is accompanied by antibodies to either single-stranded DNA or to the Ro/SSA antigen which are not detected in routine laboratory examinations frequently develop nephritis. In my opinion, much of the literature about glomerulopathies and CNS disease in MCTD is probably confounded by incomplete serologic studies which have ignored antibodies to single-stranded DNA and the Ro/SSA antigen. Other antibodies that occur with a lesser but definable frequency and are often missed in routine laboratory examination are low leels of antibodies to Sm and native DNA, and patients with such serologic profiles have, in my experience, the same morbidity from nephritis and CNS disease as any other lupus patient. So the precise serologic definition is, I believe, the key to the frequency of appreciation of these complications in MCTD. If MCTD is defined by antibodies to nuclear RNAprotein alone, then serious nephritis and CNS disease are rare. There is one manifestation in the nervous system which has been frequently described in patients of this type, and that is trigeminal neuropathy, or tic douloureux, which does indeed occur with some real, but as yet undetermined, frequency. The management of this problem is not defined but steroids may not be an effective approach.

The next manifestation of the disease to consider is polymyositis. I refer the reader to the chapter on dermatomyositis for details, because the treatments for dermatomyositis and polymyositis are indistinguishable. The mainstay of treatment of polymyositis when significant weakness is present is corticosteroids. Steroids are used at an initial dosage of 1 mg/kg/day. Higher doses are rarely required for a good clinical effect, although divided doses (20 mg *tid*) may be used for the first week or two in acutely ill or profoundly weak patients. Two guidelines are followed to assess the efficacy of the treatment: the myogenic enzymes which appear in serum and the clinical assessment of strength, including creatinine phosphokinase, or CPK, which is by far the most important, and under certain circumstances, aldolase, LDH, and SGOT, all of which appear in the serum in polymyositis. A rare patient in whom the clinical picture is clear-cut and serum enzymes are normal will show an elevation of the urinary creatine. In the most favorable clinical situations, reduction in serum myogenic enzymes and increased strength occur simultaneously at similar rates. If maximal strength is regained and the serum enzymes return to normal, the dose of corticosteroids may be reduced over a period of 6 to 8 weeks until 20 mg per day is reached, and thereafter the dose may be reduced 10 percent per week until the steroids are no longer given, if there is no flare of the disease. The preferred drug for treatment is prednisone. Triamcinolone preparations should be avoided, since there seems to be an increased incidence of steroid myopathy with the use of that particular steroid preparation. As with all steroid usage, an ulcer regimen should be instituted when the dose of prednisone exceeds 20 mg per day. It is my clinical impression that patients with polymyositis and antibodies to nuclear RNP are more responsive to steroids and are more frequently capable of sustaining a remission in the absence of steroids than patients with polymyositis with other serologic markers. Most patients with polymyositis and antinuclear RNP also have features of lupus and are only rarely encountered as polymyositis alone. Should steroid therapy fail, other drugs used are methotrexate or Imuran.

Finally, the management of the scleroderma type manifestations of the disease is perhaps the most difficult part of the treatment of this overlap syndrome. Because no effective proven treatment of the scleroderma process is available, there are no specific therapies to describe. I do not use steroids for the treatment of the hand swelling or for skin thickening in such patients. There is no evidence that steroids alter the ultimate outcome but they do expose the patients to risks. There are several other manifestations of the scleroderma aspect of the disease in these patients which merit comment. One is the rapid development of skin disease, the second is pulmonary fibrosis, and the third is the late development of pulmonary vascular lesions with pulmonary hypertension and right-sided heart failure. The latter complication is rare, occurs 10 to 30 years after onset of the skin disease, and is extremely serious, since there is no known effective treatment. Rapid progression of skin disease in general is associated with a poor prognosis in scleroderma because of concomitant internal organ involvement, and demonstrably falling pulmonary function with x-ray findings of infiltration is also an area of concern to the physician.

SKIN DISEASE

For the first manifestation of skin diseases, empiric treatment given by most physicians is penicillamine, based on the retrospective studies of the Pittsburgh group which showed some decrease in the expected frequency of internal organ complications in patients whose scleroderma was treated with penicillamine. The penicillamine is used in similar fashion to that described for rheumatoid arthritis. One begins with one 250-mg tablet per day and maintains that for 2 months. Barring any adverse effects, the drug is raised to 500 mg a day for 2 months and ultimately to a maximum of 750 mg per day. I have not yet encountered a patient with antibodies to nuclear RNP whose skin disease was so widespread and rapidly progressive as to warrant the use of penicillamine.

PULMONARY DISEASE

A number of patients do develop pulmonary infiltrative disease, and here again we are in a gray zone. My procedure is as follows: Two examinations that are made if one is concerned about the activity of the pulmonary disease are pulmonary lavage to look for neutrophils and gallium scanning to look for increased uptake in the lung as a manifestation of inflammation. If the pulmonary lavage contains more than 10 percent neutrophils and the patients are not smokers and are found to have a positive gallium scan, I use prednisone in a dosage of 1 mg/kg/day for a period of a month and then repeat the lavage and the gallium scan. If there has been a favorable effect as reflected by these tests, the prednisone can be reduced and the examinations can be repeated at some less frequent interval. The other manifestations of the disease, such as calcinosis, telangiectasias, the skin hardening per se, gastrointestinal involvement, and so on, are not to my knowledge responsive to any specific treatment. Certain maneuvers are useful in the management of specific complications, such as esophageal reflux and the malabsorption of the sclerodermatous bowel, which is frequently due to bacterial overgrowth. The latter may respond to antibiotic treatment, but for these specific situations there are no general systemic treatments that are of proven value. I should say that in my experience almost all patients with scleroderma features with antinuclear RNP have a limited form of the disease known as the CREST syndrome. These patients have calcinosis, Raynaud's phenomenon, esophageal motility disturbances, and telangiectasias but do not in general have widespread skin involvement or internal extensive organ involvement. The usual form of the disease is therefore a limited, extremely chronic one in which late complications may include proliferative endarteritic lesions of the pulmonary vasculature and biliary cirrhosis for which no treatments are known to be effective.

There is no overall treatment for mixed connective tissue disease. Treatment is tailored to the manifestations of the individual constituent diseases. The overall prognosis of these patients tends to be good, and a conservative stance is warranted except in certain specific clinical circumstances in which more aggressive treatments are indicated.

SYSTEMIC VASCULITIS

LANNY J. ROSENWASSER, M.D.
SHELDON M. WOLFF, M.D.

Vasculitis is defined as inflammation and necrosis of blood vessels. Inflammation can occur in association with many clinical conditions. Vasculitis may be the primary manifestation of a number of diseases or it may be a relatively minor secondary component of other illnesses. Historically, many of the early descriptions of the vasculitic syndromes focused on pathologic factors, such as size, location, and type of blood vessel involved, as well as on the histopathologic findings to identify the various vasculitic processes. It is now clear, however, that any size, location, and type of blood vessel may be involved in the inflammatory process and that damage to and necrosis of any vessel in any organ system may be seen.

It is generally accepted that immune mechanisms probably play the key role in the pathogenesis of vasculitis regardless of the type of syndrome or associated disease. Although the exact pathogenesis of most forms of vasculitis have not yet been elucidated, treatment strategies aimed at modifying the immune response by means of immunosuppressive agents such as cytotoxic drugs as well as glucocorticoids have emerged. In particular, several of the most severe necrotizing vasculitides, such as Wegener's granulomatosis and the polyarteritis nodosa group, have been shown to be highly responsive to such therapy. However, before one can apply a therapeutic protocol to a patient with vasculitis, it is necessary to appreciate the need to categorize as well as possible the particular vasculitic syndrome with which one is dealing. This is particularly true in terms of assessing the extent of major organ system involvement.

This report will briefly distinguish among the vasculitic syndromes, provide general guidelines for the treatment of these disorders, and describe in some detail the mechanism of action, dosage regimen, and side effects of the major modalities used in the treatment of the systemic necrotizing vasculitides.

CATEGORIZATION OF THE VASCULITIC SYNDROMES

The vasculitic disorders can be classified into 4 major groups: the hypersensitivity vasculitides, the polyarteritis group of systemic necrotizing vasculitis, the granulomatous vasculitides, and other miscellaneous vasculitic syndromes, as presented in Table 1.

TABLE 1 Classification of the Vasculitides

Hypersensitivity Vasculitides
- Serum sickness and drug reactions
- Henoch-Schönlein purpura
- Vasculitis associated with connective tissue disease
- Vasculitis associated with essential mixed cryoglobulinemia
- Vasculitis associated with other primary disorders, including neoplasia

Polyarteritis Nodosa Group
- Classic polyarterisis nodosa
- Allergic granulomatosis and angiitis (Churg-Strauss syndrome)
- Overlap syndrome

Granulomatous Vasculitides
- Wegener's granulomatosis
- Lymphomatoid granulomatosis
- Giant cell arteritides
  - Temporal arteritis
  - Takayasu's arteritis

Other Syndromes
- Erythema nodosum
- Kawasaki's disease
- Behcet's disease
- Buerger's disease
- Erythema elevatum diutinum

Hypersensitivity Vasculitis

Hypersensitivity vasculitis is characterized by fibrinoid necrosis of small vessels predominantly postcapillary venules with a pleomorphic cellular infiltrate in and around the vessel walls. Such histopathologic changes are usually described as leukocytoclastic vasculitis. Commonly, the skin of the feet and lower legs is the major site of involvement, although other organ systems can be affected. Administration of exogenous heterologous proteins, serum sickness, and some drug reactions are associated with hypersensitivity vasculitis, as are collagen vascular diseases, neoplasia, mixed essential cryoglobulinemia, and Henoch-Schönlein purpura.

Polyarteritis Nodosa Group

Classic polyarteritis nodosa is characterized by segmental vascular lesions in different stages of evolution along medium-sized muscular arteries, particularly at branch points. Fibrinoid necrosis of blood vessel walls with aneurysm formation or nodules is noted. This disorder shows a predilection for renal or visceral arteries with relative sparing of the pulmonary and splenic arterioles and other small vessels, although involvement of the smaller arteriole beds is not known. Further definition of the polyarteritis nodosa group came with the description of the syndrome of allergic granulomatosis and angiitis by Churg and Strauss. The pattern of vascular damage seen in allergic granulomatosis is similar to that seen in polyarteritis nodosa, with sequential fibrinoid necrosis of the muscular arteries and aneurysm formation. However, patients with allergic granulomatosis differ from those with polyarteritis nodosa in having a history of atopy or asthma. Allergic granulomatosis is also distinctive in the involvement of the pulmonary arteries as well as in the appearance of eosinophilic infiltrates and granulomas in the vessel walls and tissues. Once these two syndromes were established it became clear that some of the cases of vasculitis in this category included components of both the classic polyarteritis nodosa and allergic granulomatosis and angiitis. This overlap disorder has been termed the systemic necrotizing vasculitis overlap syndrome. It is classified within the polyarteritis nodosa group.

Granulomatous Vasculitides

Wegener's granulomatosis is characterized by granulomatous necrotizing vasculitis of the upper and lower respiratory tracts with varying degrees of renal involvement (85 to 90% of patients). Limited forms of Wegener's granulomatosis without overt involvement of the kidney have been identified. It should be emphasized that all vessels and organ systems can be and often are involved in Wegener's granulomatosis.

Lymphomatoid granulomatosis has clinical and pathologic similarities to Wegener's granulomatosis. However, lymphomatoid granulomatosis is characterized by an angiocentric and angiodestructive vasculitis. It affects primarily the lungs, but also is characterized by infiltrates in other organ systems. In the lung the infiltrate is bronchocentric. The cellular infiltrate demonstrates considerable cellular pleomorphism and atypism. In a significant number of patients (up to 45%) lymphomatoid granulomatosis progresses to a fatal neoplastic lymphoproliferative process with destruction of blood vessels due to overgrowth of lymphoid tissue.

The giant cell arteritides, temporal arteritis and Takayasu's arteritis or aortic arch syndrome, are panarteritides affecting medium-sized or large arteries. Infiltration with mononuclear cells, giant cell formation, and fragmentation of the internal elastic lamina are classically seen. Temporal arteritis predominantly affects elderly females. It is characterized by a wide variety of presenting symptoms ranging from nonspecific malaise to sudden blindness. Some patients have a polymyalgia syndrome. Most patients have a high blood sedimentation rate and are often anemic. Characteristically, branches of the extracranial carotid arteries are affected.

Takayasu's arteritis occurs most often in young women, particularly those of Japanese extraction. The clinical manifestations include constitutional symptoms often associated with inflammation and localized problems related to alterations in blood flow to large organs or to whole extremities. The pathologic findings are similar to those of temporal arteritis, but Takayasu's arteritis shows a predilection for the aortic arch and its branches.

Miscellaneous Vasculitic Syndromes

Many other vasculitic syndromes have been described which warrant separate consideration. Among these are Behçet's syndrome, thromboangiitis obliterans, Kawasaki's disease, the mucocutaneous lymphnode syndrome, Cogan's syndrome, erythema nodosum, and erythema elevatum diutinum. Detailed accounts of the characteristics, pathology, and treatment of these syndromes are beyond the scope of this review.

APPROACH TO THE THERAPY OF SYSTEMIC VASCULITIS

Table 2 provides some overall guidelines for the treatment of vasculitic syndromes. It is critical to evaluate completely a patient with suspected vasculitis to ascertain the full scope and impact of the clinicopathologic process. Once an adequate base of clinical, laboratory, and pathologic information has been obtained, it is possible to make a specific diagnosis and to classify an individual case within the spectrum of the vasculitides. From this base, a rationale for therapy and systemic treatment can then be formulated. One or more treatment approaches may be appropriate depending on the specific clinical circumstances. Obtaining baseline objective data allows one to follow the course of the disease and the effect of therapy.

Elimination of the Offending Agent

In some cases of vasculitis the disease process can be modified if the offending antigen or agent is identified and eliminated. This is most likely to be applicable in cases of hypersensitivity vasculitis in which drugs, environmental agents, or other antigens should be considered as potential sources for the hypersensitivity. As might be expected, this diverse group of vasculitides responds differently to therapeutic maneuvers. Some cases of hypersensitivity vasculitis respond merely to the elimination of the offending antigen, whereas other cases may require corticosteroids even after the offending antigen has been eliminated. Still other cases may resolve completely without therapeutic intervention of any sort.

If modification of the patient's environment or removal of the offending drug or toxin does produce clinical improvement, a presumptive diagnosis can be made and the putative offending agent should be avoided in the future. However, if no offending agent can be identified, other therapeutic approaches may need to be taken.

TABLE 2 Guidelines for Therapy

Obtain comprehensive base of clinical, laboratory, and pathologic data to make appropriate and specific diagnosis and to establish objective baseline data to follow effect of therapy.

Identify and remove offending antigen or agent, if applicable.
Treat primary disease associated with vasculitis (for example, lymphoma).
Treat primary vasculitic process:
- Anti-inflammatory agents
  - (steroids, colchicine, nonsteroidal anti-inflammatory drugs)
- Immunosuppressive agents
  - (steroids, cytotoxic drugs)
- Elimination of immune complexes (plasmapheresis)

Treatment of the Primary Disease

Vasculitides can be associated with many primary illnesses and conditions, including rheumatic and connective tissue diseases, neoplasia, infectious diseases and inflammatory bowel diseases. When a vasculitis is secondary to an underlying illness, vasculitis often will improve as the primary disease is treated; however, when the vasculitis is a major contributor to morbidity, treatment may have to be directed toward the vasculitis per se regardless of the associated or underlying condition.

Treatment of the Vasculitic Process

In the majority of cases, treatment strategy should be directed against the primary vasculitic process. Such strategies generally fall into 4 categories. First, suppression of the inflammatory response may be of benefit in certain situations (for example, erythema nodosum); therefore, treatment with agents such as nonsteroidal anti-inflammatory agents should be considered. Second, suppression of the immune response may be necessary. Immunosuppression may be achieved with either steroids or cytotoxic drugs such as cyclophosphamide or azathioprine. Next, elimination of circulating immune complexes may be considered if such immune complexes can be demonstrated. Newer modalities of treatment, such as plasmapheresis and lymphapheresis, may be of benefit at this clinical juncture. Finally, newer approaches to the typical therapies outlined above—such as "bolus" corticosteroid and/or cytotoxic drug therapy, in which very high doses of drug are given over a short period of time—are beginning to be used in the treatment of many immunlogic disorders, including the vasculitides. However, these latter forms of therapy have not been proved to be efficacious in patients with vasculitis.

Duration of Therapy

The duration of therapy for vasculitis depends entirely on the type and severity of the underlying vasculitis. For example, in hypersensitivity vasculitis, which is sometimes self-limited, a brief course of corticosteroid therapy may be all that is necessary. In other more serious vasculitides, such as Wegener's granulomatosis or polyarteritis nodosa, prolonged therapy with powerful cytotoxic drugs continuing for 1 year after remission is often required to induce sustained remissions.

MAJOR AGENTS FOR THE TREATMENT OF THE VASCULITIDES

Corticosteroids

Corticosteroids have been used in the treatment of virtually all of the vasculitides. They are the treatment of choice in many patients with hypersensitivity vasculitis. For the most part, corticosteroids are the mainstay of therapy for both giant cell arteritides and are associated with dramatic responses in most patients with temporal arteritis. These agents are also useful as adjunctive therapy in the initial treatment of patients with severe Wegener's granulomatosis, polyarteritis nodosa, systemic necrotizing vasculitis, and lymphomatoid granulomatosis. Both Wegener's granulomatosis and, to a lesser extent, lymphomatoid granulomatosis respond dramatically to a combination of daily cytotoxic and corticosteroid therapy, particularly with cyclophosphamide and prednisone. Cytotoxic drugs alone can be therapeutically effective in Wegener's granulomatosis, although we prefer the combination of cytotoxic drug and prednisone. In contrast, there is no evidence that long-term outcome in Wegener's granulomatosis is altered by corticosteroids alone.

At the dosages usually employed in treating the vasculitides, corticosteroid agents exert both anti-inflammatory and immunosuppressive effects. Steroids have many profound effects on polymorphonuclear leukocyte function both in vivo and in vitro and they induce immunosuppression presumably via multiple effects on both T- and B-lymphocytes and macrophages. A single pharmacologic dose of steroids produces significant lymphopenia and monocytopenia by redistributing lymphocytes and monocytes out of the circulating pool and into the bone marrow. They also inhibit monocyte chemotaxis and bactericidal activity. T cells appear to be more susceptible to the inhibitory effects of steroids than B cells, and helper T cell subpopulations appear to be more susceptible than suppressor T cells.

Corticosteroids may be given in a variety of dosage schedules. The concept of steroid effect may be helpful in selecting the most appropriate regimen. An increase in steroid effect is paralleled by an increase in the degree of immunosuppression, anti-inflammatory activity, and hypothalamic pituitary adrenal suppression, as well as by an increase in the frequency and severity of other associated side effects. Multiple factors, including the preparation of agent used, the half-life of the agent, the total dose received, the frequency of administration, and the overall duration of therapy, contribute to the steroid effect. Increasing the amount of drug in a given dose increases the steroid effect. Within a specific time period, increasing the frequency of administration increases not only the steroid effect but also the risk of potential side effects. Thus, 10 mg of prednisone given 4 times daily has a greater steroid effect than 40 mg once a day, which has a greater effect than 80 mg given every other day. In other words, although the total daily dose of these 3 regimens is the same, the steroid effects are quite different. The duration of therapy is also of major importance. Administering high doses of steroids over a long period is certainly undesirable because of the greater potential for adverse side effects. The benefits of alternate-day steroid therapy must be emphasized. It must also be emphasized, however, that in most, if not all, inflammatory diseases, around the clock administration of steroids is required at least initially to suppress inflammation. After an appropriate period, attempts should be made to convert the schedule to an alternate-day regimen. Employing alternate-day steroid therapy with the proper steroid preparation provides significant anti-inflammatory effects while minimizing side effects such as hypothalamic pituitary adrenal suppression or increased risk of infection.

Another steroid regimen that has attracted interest is the pulse steroid method in which basically 1 g of methylprednisone is given intravenously on a daily basis for 3 or 4 days. This method was first used in the treatment of renal allograft rejection, Goodpasture's syndrome, and rapidly progressive glomerulonephritis. Pulse therapy is now being used in patients with vasculitic syndromes and rheumatic diseases as well as those with systemic lupus erythematosus. However, the efficacy of "bolus" therapy in patients with vasculitis is not well established at present and awaits further evaluation. Nonetheless, since the side effects of 1 to 3 days of bolus corticosteroid administration are minimal, it may not be unreasonable to employ this regimen during the first few days of treatment of a life-threatening fulminant vasculitic syndrome.

Cytotoxic Drugs

Cytotoxic drugs were initially developed for treatment of neoplastic diseases; however, their immunosuppressive actions led to their use in a number of inflammatory diseases. Several classes of cytotoxic drugs have been used in the vasculitides.

Cyclophosphamide, an alkylating agent, is the primary cytotoxic drug used in the treatment of vasculitic diseases. Cyclophosphamide is inert and must be metabolized to active derivatives by the liver. When used chronically in low daily doses that avoid granulocytopenia, cyclophosphamide produces an immunosuppressive effect without a substantial anti-inflammatory effect. This agent alters the circulating pool of mononuclear cells. Cyclophosphamide therapy diminishes both the number and functional capabilities of T cells, B cells, and monocytes. Established delayed hypersensitivity responses generally are unaltered, but both humoral and delayed immune responses to newly administered antigens are suppressed.

In animal models, specific immune tolerance can be achieved with cyclophosphamide therapy. Recently, it has been reported that chronic low-dose cyclophosphamide therapy can have an effect on in vitro T and B cell responses. Cyclophosphamide is the treatment of choice of Wegener's granulomatosis, the polyarteritis nodosa group of systemic necrotizing vasculitis (when resistant to steroids), and in patients with lymphomatoid granulomatosis. Daily low-dose cytotoxic drug therapy usually given with a corticosteroid can induce dramatic remissions in some patients with vasculitis who have failed to respond to or have proven resistant to steroid therapy alone. In addition, there have been anecdotal reports of the efficacy of cyclophosphamide in Behçet's syndrome as well as in patients with hypersensitivity vasculitis who have significant major organ involvement. Other anecdotal reports, in which patients with mixed essential cryoglobulinemia and/or Henoch-Schönlein purpura responded to a trial of cytotoxic agents, have been published. In most cases, cyclophosphamide therapy is begun at a dosage of 2 mg per kilogram of body weight per day. It takes 12 to 14 days for cyclophosphamide to exert its immunosuppressive effects, so the drug is initially given in conjunction with corticosteroids. The corticosteroids are initially given on an around-the-clock schedule with a dose every 6 hours. Once the patient has become stable, corticosteroid dosage is gradually tapered to an alternate-day schedule, generally within the first 2 to 3 months of therapy.

The side effects of daily low-dose cyclophosphamide therapy include bone marrow suppression with leukopenia. Accordingly, after the initial induction therapy, adjustments in the cyclophosphamide dose are made in accordance with peripheral leukocyte counts. In general, the white blood cell count should be maintained above the level of 3500 mm^3. Since the effects of cyclophosphamide on white cell count are not manifested until 5 to 7 days after a dose is given, it is mandatory for white counts to be followed very closely when therapy is initiated or when the white cell count drops precipitously. Once the patient is stable, the white counts may be measured once every 1 to 2 weeks. To prevent the possible development of cyclophosphamide hermorrhagic cystitis, patients receiving the drug should be urged to stay well hydrated. Gonadal dysfunction with premature ovarian failure and azoospermia may also occur during cyclophosphamide therapy. Therefore, the option of depositing sperm in a sperm bank should be discussed with young men who receive cyclophosphamide. Lymphomas and leukemia have been reported in patients with vasculitis who have received long-term cyclophosphamide therapy. Some alopecia and gastrointestinal distress, such as nausea and vomiting, can also be associated with cyclophosphamide therapy. Finally, patients who have received cyclophosphamide run a small but definite risk of developing pulmonary and bladder fibrosis which may occur even years after the treatment. Other cytotoxic drugs have been used to treat the vasculitides. For example, chlorambucil is another alkylating agent that has been used in the treatment of Wegener's granulomatosis.

Azathioprine, an imidazole derivative of 6-mercaptopurine which blocks the intraconversion of nucleotides, is also immunosuppressive. However, azathioprine is not as effective as cyclophosphamide in inducing remissions in patients with Wegener's granulomatosis. For young patients whose future reproductive capacity is a consideration, azathioprine may be a reasonable therapeutic choice.

Recently, bolus cyclophosphamide, 0.5 to 0.75 g/m^2 of body surface, has been employed with and without plasmapheresis in certain inflammatory illnesses. It has recently been reported that in clinical trials of bolus cyclophosphamide in patients with systemic lupus erythematosis, such treatment had an influence on the course of nephritis associated with the disease. However, such bolus cyclophosphamide therapy has not been used in controlled trials for the various vasculitic syndromes, and it is generally felt that intravenous bolus cyclophosphamide therapy is less effective in inducing remissions in such patients. It is not known whether intravenous bolus cyclophosphamide therapy may be effective on an intermittent basis to maintain remissions that have been induced by other more standard regimens. It is also unclear whether plasmapheresis and lymphapheresis are going to be significant adjuncts in the therapy of systemic vasculitis. In general, this approach has not been effective in inducing and maintaining remissions in the severe vasculitic syndromes in the few uncontrolled anecdotal reports which have appeared in the literature. However, a few of our patients with polyarteritis nodosa, hypersensitivity vasculitis, and Wegener's granulomatosis appear to have had some response to plasma exchange that was incorporated in the more standard therapeutic approaches to their diseases. More information will be required before a full evaluation of these modalities as treatment for vasculitis can be judged.

CONCLUSIONS

Establishing an accurate diagnosis when possible is a useful prerequisite for the effective treatment of vasculitis. Cytotoxic drugs and adrenal corticosteroids have been successfully used in the treatment of some of the systemic necrotizing vasculitides and have induced a high percentage of remissions.

TEMPORAL ARTERITIS

LOUIS A. HEALEY, M.D.

Temporal arteritis (giant cell arteritis, cranial arteritis) is a form of vasculitis that is seen in patients over the age of 50, almost all of whom are Caucasian. The inflammation has a predilection for the arteries of head and neck, but nearly any medium-sized or larger artery, including the aorta and its primary branches, may be affected. The inflammation seems to parallel the distribution of the internal elastic lamina throughout the arterial system, with the result that stroke, coronary occlusion, and renal failure are rare. Manifestations depend on the particular artery involved. They include the classic headache which led to the name temporal arteritis, and the most serious complication, sudden unilateral blindness from occlusion of posterior ciliary branches of the ophthalmic artery. Transient diplopia may be due to paralysis of an extraocular muscle when its nutrient vessels are involved, and the pathognomonic pain with chewing (jaw claudication) stems from inflammatory swelling occluding the lumen of the facial artery. Diagnosis is suspected by recognition of typical symptoms in an older patient, further confirmed by finding a very rapid erythrocyte sedimentation rate and documented by temporal artery biopsy showing the typical inflammation. At times systemic manifestations, such as anemia, fever, malaise, anorexia, weight loss, and abnormal liver functions tests, particularly the alkaline phosphatase, may dominate the picture which has then been called occult giant cell arteritis. Recognition is more difficult. The rapid erythrocyte sedimentation rate (ESR) may provide the clue leading to diagnostic biopsy.

A temporal artery biopsy should be obtained in all patients suspected of the diagnosis, even in those in whom it seems certain. Response to steroid treatment is not that specific, and histologic diagnosis is often important later in the course of the disease when the clinical response is less than perfect, the ESR is still elevated, and the patient is facing the complications of prolonged steroid treatment. This is especially true if the physician treating the patient is not the one who made the initial diagnosis. The lesions in giant cell arteritis involve the arteries in interrupted or "skip" fashion so the diagnosis may be missed even if a long segment of artery is excised and examined thoroughly. If the biopsy is normal but the clinical picture strongly suggests the diagnosis, it may be necessary to try a course of steroid therapy while recognizing that this is a less satisfactory situation.

Corticosteroid drugs rapidly suppress the inflammation of giant cell arteritis. It is generally accepted that a high dose (50 mg of prednisone or equivalent daily) is required to prevent the appearance of blindness, which follows occlusion of the posterior ciliary branches and is almost always irreversible. While headache and other symptoms respond to low doses (5 to 15 mg prednisone daily), vision may still be lost. Since the minimal dose sufficient to control inflammation and prevent blindness is not known, it is best to start at 50 mg. Since most patients who lose vision do so either before treatment is started or in the first week of therapy, treatment should be started as soon as the diagnosis of temporal arteritis is strongly suspected, rather than wait for a biopsy to be performed and interpreted. The histologic picture can still be recognized without difficulty after one week of steroid treatment, or even longer.

The drug can be administered orally as a 50-mg tablet each morning. Response is rapid and initial improvement is expected within 24 hours. I have not found it necessary or beneficial to use parenteral steroids, higher doses, or divided doses. If the biopsy is positive (or if the clinical evidence is overwhelming in the face of a negative biopsy), I recommend that the initial daily dose of 50 mg be continued for an arbitrary period of one month, even though the patient is asymptomatic. This schedule has proved effective in controlling the inflammation, preventing vision loss, and reducing the likelihood of subsequent recurrence of inflammation. With this dose, clinical improvement is paralleled by correction of anemia and return of the sedimentation rate and alkaline phosphatase to normal. After one month, the daily dose is tapered fairly rapidly to 20 mg. There are various schedules to accomplish this, but a decrement of 10 mg in the daily dose at monthly intervals is one satisfactory method. Then the dose is lowered more slowly, either 2.5 or 5 mg/month, aiming for a maintenance level of 5 mg/day.

In my experience, it is most important to follow the patient's symptoms, and not the ESR, as the guide to decreasing the dose. Although the ESR does fall in response to initial therapy, there is often a subsequent rebound that is not accompanied by a flare of the disease. As the dose is tapered, the focus is on the patient's symptoms, specifically those that suggest cranial arteritis: head pain or tenderness, transient vision loss, diplopia, or jaw claudication. Treating the ESR leads to steroid doses that inevitably cause toxicity, particularly osteoporosis. Although in rare instances blindness has occurred in patients receiving high-dose steroid treatment, this has been within the first week or two and not subsequently. Exacerbations in the late stages, when the steroid dose has been reduced too rapidly or discontinued too soon, have been those of polymyalgia rheumatica.

Most patients require 5 mg a day for one year and some have to continue the steroid even longer. Fortunately, even elderly patients tolerate 5 mg indefinitely without toxicity. The only way to determine whether the disease has run its course is to stop treatment and observe for a possible recurrence of polymyalgia. Alternate-day steroid treatment is not recommended for initial suppression of inflammation. When the inflammation has been suppressed, it may be tried in lieu of the 5-mg daily dose recommended. Even with the program outlined, osteoporosis is still a risk for these older patients, so that daily calcium, weekly vitamin D supplements, and estrogen replacement are advisable. Following the program of 50 mg prednisone daily for an initial month, "resistant" temporal arteritis, as indicated by symptoms rather than by the ESR, has not been encountered, and medications such as cyclophosphamide or azathioprine are not recommended.

In patients with polymyalgia alone, and no symptoms of temporal arteritis, the chance of finding arteritis on temporal artery biopsy is 10 to 15 percent. Most patients with "pure polymyalgia" do not ever show symptoms of cranial arteritis. For this reason, I do not recommend that all patients with polymyalgia have a biopsy or receive high-dose steroid. Symptoms of polymyalgia respond rapidly to 10 to 15 mg prednisone as the initial daily dose. This is then rapidly tapered to 5 mg and continued for at least one year. The majority of patients require this low dose for even longer periods. These patients, too, are instructed to report immediately any symptom which suggests cranial arteritis.

AUTOIMMUNE UVEITIS

ALAN G. PALESTINE, M.D.

Prior to the initiation of therapy for an intraocular inflammatory process (uveitis), it is important to differentiate between diseases of an autoimmune or presumed autoimmune origin and those clearly due to an infectious or neoplastic process, such as toxoplasmosis, tuberculosis, or reticulum cell sarcoma. Although most cases of intraocular inflammatory disease are not produced by active infection, uveitis due to an infectious agent can often be treated with appropriate specific agents. It is therefore imperative to attempt to exclude an infectious agent prior to the initiation of therapy.

Therapy for uveitis should be directed toward treating the active inflammation to prevent sequelae such as glaucoma, cataract, and irreversible retinal damage. The type of therapy is in part dictated by its effectiveness in treating the inflammation balanced against the ocular and sytemic side effects of therapy. The goal of therapy is to control the inflammation as rapidly as possible in patients with acute disease and to prevent recurrent flareups in patients with chronic disease.

CORTICOSTEROID THERAPY

The cornerstone of therapy in patients with uveitis is corticosteroids. Although a systemic immunologic abnormality may be present, in most patients with uveitis the severe inflammation is localized only to the eye. It may be located in the anterior or posterior portions of the eye and may be unilateral or bilateral. To provide optimal control of the inflammation and to minimize the side effects, there are three routes available for administration of corticosteroids in ocular disease, topical, periocular, and systemic. The choice of steroid preparation is influenced by the anatomic location and the severity of the inflammation. The use of steroid therapy for uveitis is empiric; however, the theoretical considerations for its use are similar to those in other autoimmune diseases. Steroids may alter both ocular and systemic immunologic factors, such as the distribution of lymphocyte subsets, the functions of granulocytes and monocytes, and the permeability of cellular membrane and vascular networks.

Topical Steroid Therapy

Topical steroids are used to treat uveitis involving the anterior segment of the eye. I primarily utilize drops. Although ointments are available, ocular penetration from the ointment vehicle may be variable. Topically applied steroids penetrate the cornea and enter the anterior chamber but have little effect on inflammation posterior to the lens. The advantage of topical therapy is its application directly to the inflamed eye, thereby minimizing systemic toxicity. It is important to monitor the clinical progress and alter the therapy appropriately to minimize the amount of steroid used. Many of the side effects of topical steroids are proportional to the total amount of steroid.

Cycloplegic agents are a useful adjunct in the treatment of anterior segment inflammation. The addition of cycloplegia makes the patient more comfortable, and the concomitant mydriasis decreases the incidence of posterior synechiae and pupillary block glaucoma. For cycloplegia I use 2% homatropine or 1% cyclopentolate once or twice a day, depending on the severity of the inflammation. If maximal cycloplegia is needed, 1 percent atropine 3 times a day is best.

Topical steroid therapy should be instituted as soon as the diagnosis of iritis or iridocyclitis of noninfectious origin has been made. I begin with one drop of 1% prednisolone acetate suspension every 1 or 2 hours while awake. Although this has been found to enter the eye in somewhat higher concentrations than prednisolone phosphate, I have not found a significant practical difference. If the patient has preexisting glaucoma or has a history of steroid-induced glaucoma and the uveitis is mild, I will use 0.1% fluorometholone. This agent has a lower incidence of secondary steroid-induced glaucoma; however, it also appears to have less anti-inflammatory activity. When using topical steroid therapy, it is important to monitor the disease activity. If hourly topical therapy has not begun to improve the inflammation in 3 to 4 days, I will usually add periocular steroids in acute uveitis. If the patient begins to improve, the steroids may be slowly tapered. Abrupt cessation will frequently exacerbate the uveitis. My schedule for tapering is to reduce therapy from every 2 hours to every 3 hours and then to 4 times a day. I will then decrease the number of drops by one daily each week and stop therapy after the patient has been using one drop a day for 5 to 7 days. If the uveitis reactivates at this point, I will repeat the therapy but will go from one drop daily of 1% prednisolone to 3 or 4 drops of 0.125% prednisolone daily and taper this over 3 to 4 weeks. Some patients have chronic inflammation that can be controlled only with long-term therapy. The rate of secondary complications clearly increases in this situation.

There are no absolute contraindications to topical steroids. However, if active herpes simplex keratitis is present, antiviral therapy, such as topical trifluorothymidine, must be used. Topical steroids may cause cataracts, or secondary glaucoma, and increase the incidence of viral, bacterial, and fungal corneal infection. The first two complications are also complications of the underlying uveitis. Steroid induced glaucoma does not usually appear until 2 or 3 weeks of therapy. However, the severity of the inflammation frequently necessitates continuation of therapy and medical or surgical treatment of the glaucoma. Cataracts are an unavoidable complication of long-term steroid therapy. The initiation of topical steroid therapy should not begin before the patient's risk factors, for example glaucoma and cataract, are weighed against the benefit of therapy.

Although topical steroid are systemically absorbed, it is highly unlikely that systemic side effects will occur from these drugs in the adult. Systemic absorption and side effects can occur from topical cycloplegics. One drop of 1% atropine contains approximately 0.5 mg of atropine, and if this is given 3 times a day in both eyes to a child, a systemic overdose can occur.

Periocular Steroid Therapy

I utilize this route of administration in patients with anterior inflammation who have failed to respond to topical therapy or in patients with uniocular intermediate uveitis, such as pars planitis, complicated by cystoid macular edema. High and prolonged steroid concentrations may be delivered using this method. The systemic side effects of steroids can be minimized with this method and compliance is assured. The injection may be given more anteriorly or more posteriorly, depending on the site of the inflammation. Injections may be repeated as frequently as needed, although after 30 or 40 injections, the orbital tissue becomes fibrotic and the injection becomes more difficult.

Both soluble and depot steroid preparations are available. I primarily use soluble preparations, such as 2 mg dexamethasone phosphate. The soluble preparation produces an initial high concentration in the ocular tissues and is rarely associated with secondary glaucoma. It is important to inject the steroid near the globe, rather than in the orbital tissue. I utilize a 25 gauge needle inserted into the fornix. I will use depot steroid preparations when the patient has shown a clear response to soluble injections and does not develop elevated intraocular pressure.

Complications of periocular steroids include steroid induced glaucoma, fibrosis of the orbit and extraocular muscles leading to limitation of gaze, and perforation of the globe. This last is infrequent; however, if perforation occurs with a depot preparation, the prognosis for the eye is poor. If steroid glaucoma occurs with a depot preparation, it may be necessary to excise the remaining depot material. Depot steroids have also rarely caused retinal arterial emboli if injected into an orbital vessel. The use of periocular steroids is contraindicated in scleritis because it may increase melting leading to perforation. It is also contraindicated in any infectious ocular disease unless appropriate antibiotic therapy has been initiated. Properly used, however, this mode of administration is extremely useful and may avoid the initiation of systemic therapy for a uniocular problem.

Systemic Steroids

In general, I reserve the use of systemic steroids for patients with bilateral uveitis in whom vision is decreased in both eyes as a result of the inflammatory disease. A course of systemic steroids is sometimes appropriate in unilateral disease; however, the risks of long-term systemic therapy must be weighed against the visual loss. It may be difficult to discontinue the steroids once they are begun, and over several years the patient may tolerate a decrease in vision in one eye better than the side effects of oral steroids.

I begin with 60 to 80 mg (1 to 2 mg/kg) of prednisone daily by mouth in an attempt to control the acute disease. If there is no response in 2 weeks, I will increase the dose to 100 mg daily. Although some patients may respond to doses of 150 mg daily, their disease reactivates as the dosage is reduced. As the inflammation subsides, I begin to taper the prednisone, using visual acuity and inflammatory activity to assess the effect of the drug. I will initially taper at a rate of 10 mg per week until the dosage reaches 20 mg daily. However, if the patient's disease flares, I will increase the dose and taper more slowly. Once at 20 mg daily, I taper at 5 mg per week to 5 mg daily and then use 5 mg every other day for 2 weeks. If the patient initially responded to prednisone but cannot be weaned, I will try to institute alternate day therapy. I will then attempt to taper this at 5 mg every 2 weeks until a minimal dose is reached. Some patients cannot be controlled on alternate day therapy. The goal is to control the inflammation and preserve the vision while the disease runs it course, often over 20 or more years. One must clearly weigh the relative risks and benefits.

Most patients with chronic uveitis are systemically healthy and will tolerate oral steroids well. It is important to be aware of the medical history, since diabetes, peptic ulcer, hypertension, osteoporosis, and tuberculosis are some of the relative contraindications. The systemic complications of long-term oral steroid therapy are well known and include weight gain, diabetes mellitus, hypertension, osteoporosis and psychosis. Of these, osteoporosis is the most indolent. Ocular complications include glaucoma and cataract formation, especially with long-term therapy.

NONSTEROIDAL MEDICAL THERAPY

For patients who fail to respond to the regimen described above, several other options are available. Immunosuppression by a cytotoxic agent can be extremely effective in selected patients. The alkylating agents chlorambucil and cyclophosphamide are the most widely utilized. Nonsteroidal drugs, such as indomethacin or ibuprofen, may be tried; however, in my experience these are rarely effective in uveitis. Lastly we have utilized cyclosporine in selected patients over the past 3 years as an alternate to immunosuppressive agents.

Systemic Alkylating Agents

I will consider the use of chlorambucil or cyclophosphamide in those patients who have clearly failed to respond to systemic steroids or who have intolerable side effects. Often, the patient will tolerate these drugs in combination with low-dose prednisone. Some patients may respond to one drug but not the other. If such therapy is begun, the physician should seek the help of an internist if he or she is not familiar with these drugs. The patient should be evaluated systemically and all possible side effects, including the risk of neoplasm, must be discussed.

Oral chlorambucil is begun at a dose of 2 mg daily and is increased every 2 to 3 weeks until an effect is noted or side effects occur. The usual therapeutic dose is 6 to 10 mg daily. The dosage of cyclophosphamide is 1 to 2 mg/kg daily; it is decreased as the patient's peripheral leukocyte count decreases. The patient's hematologic profile must be monitored frequently. If there is no response or the response is suboptimal, I do not feel that the potential side effects warrant continuation of therapy. The peripheral leukocyte count should be maintained at approximately 3500 to 4000/mm^3. If there is a good response, it is reasonable to treat the patient for six months and then withdraw the drug. If the disease again flares, therapy is restarted.

Systemic Cyclosporine Therapy

I have used this drug on an investigational basis in patients who have failed to improve with systemic steroids and/or cytotoxic agents. Cyclosporine does not suppress the entire immune system or cause leukopenia; rather, it specifically affects T cell function. I begin therapy at a dosage of 10 mg/kg daily. If there is no response in 7 to 10 days, I increase the dose to 12.5 or 15 mg/kg. If there is improvement in 2 months I will continue therapy, otherwise I will discontinue it.

The dose of cyclosporine must be adjusted according to its side effects. Dose related nephrotoxicity is the most common serious side effect. If the creatinine clearance decreases more than 50 percent, I begin to decrease the dose by 100 to 200 mg increments. The serum creatinine begins to improve in 2 to 3 weeks and the patient's ocular disease and renal function are titrated. Hepatic toxicity is less common, but if it occurs, the dose is decreased. We do not usually adjust the dosage of cyclosporine for other side effects unless the patient is uncomfortable.

If the patient has an initial favorable response to cyclosporine, then develops toxicity, and, when the dose is lowered, the uveitis reactivates, we have found that 10 to 15 mg of oral prednisone daily can be added and will be effective where 80 mg daily had failed.

Preexisting renal disease or hypertension will worsen on cyclosporine and these constitute at least relative contraindications. Previous malignancy is an absolute contraindication at this time.

The side effects of cyclosporine include nephrotoxicity, hypertension, hepatic toxicity, gingivitis, hirsutism, paresthesias and hyperesthesia, tremor, epigastric distress, and mild anemia. Although this drug is still investigational, the initial results are promising and the long-term side effects appear to be well tolerated. Periodically I will attempt to discontinue therapy to ensure that continued therapy is warranted.

SURGICAL APPROACHES

Patients with pars planitis who have neovascularization of the pars plana may be successfully treated with cryopexy. I use a single freeze-thaw technique only where new vessels can be seen.

There are no surgical techniques to control uveitis, but many of the complications of uveitis are treated surgically, including cataract, glaucoma, and vitreous problems. Ideally, the inflammation should be well controlled prior to surgery. I will usually begin 1 mg/kg prednisone orally 3 days prior to surgery to prevent a postoperative flare-up. Although the risks of ocular surgery in the eyes of these patients is higher than in normal eyes, most can undergo surgery safely.

COMMON VARIABLE IMMUNODEFICIENCY

REBECCA H. BUCKLEY, M.D.

Common variable immunodeficiency is a term which encompasses three different categories in the latest revision of the World Health Organization primary immunodeficiency diseases classification. The categories share the feature of profound hypogammaglobulinemia despite normal or low numbers of surface-immunoglobulin–bearing B-lymphocytes. They are based on different presumed underlying causes, one thought to be due to intrinsic abnormalities in B-lymphocytes which lead to failure of normal differentiation; one thought to be secondary to immunoregulatory disorders of T cells; and the other considered to be due to autoantibodies to T or B cells. Terms formerly used to refer to defects in these categories include idiopathic late-onset (or "acquired") hypogammaglobulinemia and congenital non x-linked or sporadic hypogammaglobulinemia. Although these defects have been considered to be acquired, there are few documentations of true "acquisitions" of immunoglobulin deficiency, and considerable evidence has been presented to support the view that genetic mechanisms are involved. These defects are distinct from x-linked agammaglobulinemia, which is characterized by a near absence of blood B cells and normal numbers of bone marrow pre-B cells; however, the immunoglobulin deficiency can be just as profound in common variable immunodeficiency as in that defect. Males and females are equally affected. Common variable immunodeficiency disorders are also to be distinguished from hypogammaglobulinemia due to transcobalamin II deficiency (correctable by intramuscular B_{12} injections); from that due to protein-losing states; and from that secondary to multiple myeloma or chronic lymphocytic leukemia. In protein-losing enteropathy or states of renal protein loss, antibody synthesis proceeds normally, so that replacement therapy is not indicated. Indeed, attempts at replacement are usually futile, as the IgG administered is also lost.

Because they lack the major heat-stable opsonin of body fluids, patients with common variable immunodeficiency are susceptible to infections with high-grade extracellular encapsulated bacterial pathogens. Most commonly, these include *Hemophilus influenzae, Streptococcus pneumoniae*, Group A streptococci, or *Staphylococcus aureus*. A majority of such patients have histories of chronic or recurrent pyogenic infections involving the upper and lower respiratory tracts. Bronchiectasis develops in approximately one-third, often before diagnosis of the immunodeficiency is made. Septicemia and meningitis are also problems prior to initiation of replacement therapy. Much less frequently, patients with common variable immunodeficiency have had pulmonary infections with mycobacterial, fungal, and parasitic (for example, *Pneumocystis carinii*) agents. In addition, there is a high incidence of gastrointestinal problems in patients with these defects. These include (1) diarrhea secondary to infestation with *Giardia lamblia*, bacterial overgrowth, lactose or gluten intolerance, steatorrhea, or autoantibodies against gut epithelial antigens; (2) pernicious anemia, usually associated with atrophic gastritis, achlorhydria, and absence of intrinsic factor; and (3) gallbladder disease, such as cholelithiasis or cholangitis. The pernicious anemia may occur at any age and is not associated with easily demonstrable antibodies to parietal cells or to intrinsic factor. The diarrhea is often accompanied by jejunal villous atrophy and/or nodular follicular lymphoid hyperplasia of the bowel.

Lymphoid hyperplasia is also manifest as splenomegaly, which occurs in 25 to 30 percent of such patients and can result in hematologic evidence of hypersplenism. Pseudolymphoma and lymphoid interstitial pneumonia are also relatively common, and, as with other primary immunodeficiency disorders, there is a high incidence of lymphoreticular malignancy. Finally, because of the tendency of such patients to develop autoimmune reactions, there is an increased incidence of arthritis, thyroid disease, alopecia areata, and keratoconjunctivitis sicca.

THERAPEUTIC APPROACHES

In the past, therapeutic modalities have consisted primarily of intramuscular immune serum globulin (ISG) replacement and antimicrobial therapy. However, during the past two decades, intravenous infusions of whole normal plasma and various experimentally modified Cohn fraction II preparations have been tried as alternatives. Nevertheless, until 1981, only ISG for intramuscular use was available commercially. With the marketing of one form of immune globulin intravenous (IGIV) preparation in that year and of another form more recently, major changes have occurred in gamma globulin replacement therapy. There undoubtedly will be other revisions as additional preparations become available and as the body of information concerning optimal use of IGIV grows.

Intramuscular ISG

Intramuscular ISG is prepared from outdated blood bank or volunteer plasma by the alcohol salt fractionation method of Cohn and is supplied in solutions containing 14.5 to 16.5 g/100 ml of IgG. Although the latter constitutes 95 to 99 percent of the protein, varying quantities of IgA, IgM, IgD, albumin, B1C, and transferrin are also present. The small quantities of immunoglobulin other than IgG are probably inconsequential from a beneficial clinical standpoint. However, patients with selective IgA deficiency or common variable immunodeficiency who have anti-IgA antibodies may have life-threatening anaphylactic reactions to the IgA present in most ISG preparations. Neither hepatitis nor the acquired immunodeficiency syndrome (AIDS) has been transmitted by ISG injections, suggesting either that the antibodies present in such preparations protect against these diseases or that the responsible agents are eliminated by the separation procedures. Such preparations have been shown to aggregate and fragment and, as a consequence, to demonstrate anticomplementary activity which can cause anaphylactoid reactions if they are given intravenously. The half-life of IgG in such preparations ranges from 17.5 to 22.1 days, with a mean of 19.8 days in normal subjects. It is usually longer in agammaglobulinemic subjects, although the presence of active bacterial infection may result in a shortening of the half-life in such patients.

There are a number of problems with intramuscular ISG therapy: (1) the quantity that can be administered is limited by the muscle mass available, (2) such injections are painful, (3) there can be local digestion by muscle enzymes, (4) abscess formation and sciatic nerve injury have been reported, and (5) anaphylactoid reactions can occur if the intravascular space is inadvertently entered. For all of these reasons, there have been major efforts to develop alternatives, including plasma therapy and various IGIV preparations.

Normal Human Plasma

There are several reasons why normal human plasma could be ideal therapy for severe humoral immunodeficiency diseases: first, antibodies of all five immunoglobulin classes can be provided in significant quantities; second, such intravenous infusions are far less painful than intramuscular ISG injections and thus have greater patient acceptability; third, adverse reactions are few; and finally, higher serum immunoglobulin concentrations can be more readily achieved than with intramuscular ISG injections. Ten milliliters of plasma per kilogram of body weight provides approximately 100 mg/kg of IgG. Moreover, the donor can be immunized to provide higher titers of some antibodies than can be achieved with pooled gamma globulin. The disadvantages include the following: (1) There is potential danger of transmitting hepatitis B, non-A, non-B hepatitis, or the acquired immunodeficiency syndrome (AIDS); (2) an available regular donor is required, as random blood bank plasma increases these risks; (3) it provides a narrower range of antibody specificities, since it is derived from a single donor; (4) there is risk of graft-versus-host (GVH) disease in infants with severe T cell defects from immunocompetent cells in the plasma; (5) volume overload can be a problem in some patients, and (6) it is inconvenient or impractical to perform plasmapheresis on a regular basis in some clinical settings. The risk of hepatitis B or AIDS can be greatly reduced by careful donor selection, but non-A, non-B hepatitis remains an uncontrollable risk. The danger of GVH can be avoided either by carefully removing all cellular elements, by freezing the plasma, or by irradiating it sufficiently (with 5000 rads) to destroy the GVH potential of the immunocompetent cells.

Immune Globulin Intravenous Preparations

In my opinion, IGIV preparations clearly constitute the preferred form of therapy. There are several advantages to the administration of gamma globulin by the intravenous route: (1) much larger doses can be given than would be possible by the intramuscular route, (2) the action is more rapid, (3) there is no loss due to local proteolysis, and (4) the therapy is far less painful. There has been considerable interest for over two decades in the development of gamma globulin preparations free of aggregates and anticomplementary activity so that they can be given safely by the intravenous route, and several approaches have been tried. These include physical removal of high molecular weight aggregates by ultracentrifugation or gel filtration; treatment of the preparations with proteolytic enzymes; treatment with certain chemicals that affect specific sites on the gamma globulin molecule or with sulfhydryl bond reducing agents; and incubation of these preparations at a low pH for varying periods of time. A gamma globulin preparation (Gamimune, Cutter) rendered free of anticomplementary activity by treatment with dithiothreitol, a sulfhydryl bond reducing agent, followed by alkylation with iodacetamide, contains IgG with the sedimentation characteristics and antibody potency of that in the untreated material, with the four chains of the molecule held together by noncovalent forces. However, the Fc function may not be entirely normal in this preparation, molecules of the IgG_3 subclass are not determinable, and the half-life is slightly shortened. In contrast, a second preparation now commercially available (Sandoglobulin, Sandoz) prepared by treatment at pH 4 and with a minimal quantity of pepsin (1:10,000) has normal quantities of all four IgG subclasses, normal Fc function, and a normal half-life.

Fourteen IGIV preparations were investigated by Romer and associates in studies comparing protein composition, antibody titers, undesirable contaminants, Fc function, and anticomplementariness. The preparations met the criterion recommended by the World Health Organization that they be derived from a pool of at least 1000 donors to ensure consistency of antibodies in the preparation from batch to batch. All four IgG subclasses were present in normal quantity only in the nonmodified and nonenzymatically degraded preparations. Antiviral and antibacterial antibodies were comparable in all of the preparations except for anti-HBs activity, which exhibited considerable variability. Enzymatically and chemically treated products were devoid of the capacity to fix complement, and the chemically treated preparations bound irregularly to *Staphylococcus* protein A, suggesting altered Fc function. Only the pH 4 and albumin stabilized preparations lacked spontaneous complement-activating properties yet retained normal complement-fixing and Fc functions.

Several of these preparations have been tested in carefully supervised clinical trials. I have personally evaluated four of these and all appear to be clinically effective. However, the only preparation that has undergone a controlled clinical trial to evaluate efficacy is Gamimune. Nevertheless, it appears that a number of IGIV preparations will prove to be both safe and efficacious.

Antimicrobial and Other Nonspecific Therapy

Probably because it is impossible to replace the major host defense component of external secretions, secretory IgA, a majority of patients with common variable immunodeficiency experience chronic or recurrent infections of mucous membrane surfaces (ears, sinuses, lungs, gastrointestinal tract) despite gamma globulin therapy. Even if enriched preparations of IgA were to become available for intramuscular or intravenous administration, the body has no mechanism for transporting IgA molecules from those compartments onto mucous membrane surfaces. Complications of chronic upper and lower respiratory tract infections, such as sinusitis and bronchiectasis, and chronic diarrhea account for most of the morbidity seen in these conditions. Thus, antibiotic therapy is frequently required for control of such infections. Because of a predominance of *H. influenzae* organisms in sputum and other external secretions of such patients, antimicrobials effective against these organisms are preferred. I find ampicillin (or amoxicillin) or trimethoprim and sulfamethoxazole to be effective in most patients. These antibiotics are used either for specific infections at full therapeutic dosage or chronically at lower doses in patients with bronchiectasis or persistent pyogenic infections. If used chronically, I find it helpful to rotate between the two types of antibiotics, usually on a monthly or bimonthly basis. It is important to emphasize that they are given *in addition to* gamma globulin replacement. For those patients who become infected with β-lactamase positive *H. influenzae*, cefaclor (Ceclor) may be given. However, I have found chloromycetin to be the most effective drug in that situation, particularly if the patient shows signs of acute or progressive chronic infection, despite use of the first two mentioned antimicrobials. Ampicillin or amoxicillin is preferable to trimethoprim and sulfamethoxazole if there is concurrent infection with *S. pneumoniae* or Group A β-hemolytic streptococcal organisms. Tetracycline is not very useful for chronic therapy in these patients. Staphylococcal infections are less common; cultures are helpful in alerting to a need for antistaphylococcal agents. Percussion and postural drainage on a twice daily basis are also helpful adjuncts to therapy in patients with bronchiectasis. Occasionally patients with common variable immunodeficiency may develop interstitial pneumonia due to *P. carinii*. This is prevented by chronic therapy with trimethoprim and sulfamethoxazole. If it does occur, it usually responds to high-dose therapy with that agent or to pentamidine isethionate. Patients with these defects may also develop tuberculosis or fungal infections of the lung, but these are far less common than those due to high-grade bacterial pathogens. Nevertheless, opportunistic infections should be suspected in patients with these defects who do not respond to the agents just listed.

Patients with chronic diarrhea may also benefit from antibiotic therapy, particularly when they have persistent infections with *Salmonella* or *Shigella*, but also occasionally when they have an overgrowth of normal intestinal organisms. Most commonly, however, their diarrhea is associated with *G. lamblia* infestation. The latter should be treated with quinacrine HCl (Atabrine) at a dosage of 6 mg/kg/day, not to exceed 300 mg per day, in 3 divided doses orally for 5 days. Alternatively, (as a second choice), metronidazole (Flagyl) may be used in 3 divided doses totaling 15 mg/kd/day (not to exceed 750 mg) for 5 days.

For those patients with pernicious anemia, lifetime therapy with parenteral vitamin B_{12} is usually required.

DOSAGE OF GAMMA GLOBULIN

For the past 32 years, the recommended dose of ISG for the treatment of humoral immunodeficiency has been 100 mg/kg/month (0.6 to 0.7 ml/kg/month), after a loading dose of 2 to 3 times that amount. Those doses necessarily required the administration of large volumes by the intramuscular route, resulting in great discomfort to the recipient. It is well to point out that the doses recommended were selected empirically. Although Janeway and Rosen reported that the 100 mg/kg/month dose resulted in serum levels of approximately 200 mg/dl soon after administration in most of their patients, in my experience IgG concentrations are much lower than this for most of the month. Mean trough serum IgG concentrations of my agammaglobulinemic patients treated with that dose of ISG were generally less than 100 mg/dl, and peak concentrations did not exceed 150 mg/dl. More importantly, there was wide variation from patient to patient in serum IgG concentrations achieved, despite administration of a uniform per kilogram dose. These shortcomings pointed up the pressing need for investigations to determine optimal dosage. Because of volume limitations with intramuscular ISG therapy, however, new dosing is being investigated almost entirely with IGIV preparations. Work to date indicates that there is considerable variability in the half-life of IgG from patient to patient, suggesting that a uniform dose is inappropriate. In studies I did in which 400 mg/kg/month of IGIV was given to a number of patients with common variable immunodeficiency, most had trough serum IgG concentrations of 200 to 400 mg/dl 4 weeks later. It is entirely possible that controlled studies will show dosages of this magnitude to be far more appropriate. However, it is again important to emphasize that the ideal dose is not known and that, in all likelihood, it will not be a uniform one for all patients. In patients with severe or chronic bacterial infections, even higher doses may be needed.

ADVERSE EFFECTS OF GAMMA GLOBULIN THERAPY

Adverse Effects of Intramuscular ISG and Normal Human Plasma Therapy

Adverse effects of therapy with intramuscular ISG and normal human plasma are summarized above under the discussion of ISG and plasma therapy.

Adverse Reactions to IGIV

Reactions to intravenous infusions of unmodified ISG have been known for some time to be more frequent and more severe in patients with antibody deficiency syndromes or with acute infections than in normal individuals, for reasons which are not clear. The same is true with the new IGIV preparations, but fortunately, the overall frequency is much lower. It has been postulated that these reactions are secondary to inflammatory reactions caused by the union of antibodies with free antigen in the patient's circulation, since they occur most frequently in newly treated, infected, or infrequently and inadequately treated patients. Symptoms and signs of such reactions most often include back or abdominal pain, nausea, and vomiting within the first 30 minutes; and chills, fever, and fatigue beginning at the end of the infusion and continuing for several hours afterward. Most of these adverse effects can be prevented by slowing the initial rate of infusion and/or by pretreatment with aspirin. The frequency and severity of these reactions diminish after infection, particularly of the lungs, has been brought under control and IGIV has been given regularly for a few months. Based on the experience with high-dose gamma globulin treatment in idiopathic thrombocytopenic purpura, there appear to be few or no adverse effects from doses as high as 500 mg/kg/day given on 5 successive days. True anaphylactic or anaphylactoid reactions have been rare with any of the IGIV preparations evaluated thus far, except in patients with anti-IgA antibodies.

Adverse Effects of Gamma Globulin Therapy in Patients with Anti-IgA Antibodies

As already noted, systemic anaphylactic reactions to ISG, plasma, and IGIV have been noted in patients with common variable agammaglobulinemia who have antibodies to IgA. Symptoms are those of a classic IgE-mediated anaphylactic reaction, in contrast to those observed with IGIV in patients without anti-IgA antibodies. They appear from seconds to minutes to several hours after the injections and include one or more of the following: flushing, facial swelling, dyspnea, cyanosis, anxiety, nausea, vomiting, malaise, hypotension, loss of consciousness, and death. The treatment of such reactions is the immediate administration of epinephrine, oxygen, antihistamines, and intravenous steroids.

I have evaluated and treated three patients with common variable agammaglobulinemia who have had anaphylactic reactions to IgA and who have high titers of class-specific anti-IgA antibodies. Initially, I used IgA-deficient plasma provided from clinically normal donors by the American Red Cross. However, one patient developed non-A, non-B hepatitis while receiving such infusions. It is important to point out that all gamma globulin preparations except DEAE Sephadex-adsorbed, albumin-stabilized preparations contain 100 μg/ml IgA or more. I have used one of the latter preparations (which contain approximately 4–6 μg IgA/ml) successfully in the treatment of these 3 patients with common variable immunodeficiency who have had near fatal anaphylactic reactions to intramuscular gamma globulin, plasma infections, and/or Gamimune. The unusual feature of these patients is that, although they had no detectable serum IgA, they also had very low concentrations of IgG and IgM, yet were still able to produce anti-IgA antibodies. These experiences clearly indicated that anti-IgA antibodies may exist in immunodeficient patients other than those with typical selective IgA deficiency. Thus, it is imperative that this possibility be investigated prior to beginning replacement therapy in any patient with absent serum IgA, even though concentrations of the other two classes may be abnormally low.

HYPERIMMUNOGLOBULIN E AND RECURRENT INFECTION (JOB'S) SYNDROME

STEPHEN C. DRESKIN, M.D., Ph.D.
JOHN I. GALLIN, M.D.

The hyperimmunoglobulin E and recurrent infection (Job's) syndrome (HIE) is a complex disorder characterized by onset early in life, markedly elevated serum IgE, recurrent serious infections of the skin and sinopulmonary tract, and low-grade eosinophilia. A number of immunologic abnormalities have been identified including the presence of anti-*Staphylococcus aureus* IgE, anti-*Candida albicans* IgE, a deficit of salivary total IgA, deficits of both serum and salivary anti-*S. aureus* IgA, a neutrophil chemotactic defect, and abnormal T-cell number and function.

S. aureus is the most common pathogen, accounting for approximately 60 percent of all infections in patients followed at the National Institutes of Health. *Hemophilus influenzae* is recovered in approximately 10 percent of all infectious episodes. In addition, approximately 50 percent of our patients have chronic mucocutaneous candidiasis. Important but infrequent pathogens include *Streptococcus pneumoniae, Pseudomonas aeruginosa, Klebsiella pneumoniae, Cryptococcus neoformans,* and *Aspergillus fumigatus*. The subcutaneous abcesses almost invariably contain *S. aureus*, either as a pure culture or in conjunction with common organisms such as β-hemolytic streptococcus or *E. coli*.

The most frequent single type of infection is the subcutaneous abscess (20% of all infectious episodes), and *S. aureus* "cold" abscesses are typical in HIE. These "cold" abscesses are notable in that the classic signs and symptoms of inflammation (heat, redness, and pain) are often muted, but this is not a universal finding. Responses to infection in any organ may be depressed, with the host reaction being similar to that seen in neutropenia or in patients receiving high-dose steroids, except that septicemia and central nervous system infections are exceptionally rare. Seventy-five percent of all infections involve organs in which secretory IgA is thought to play an important role in host defense. These sites include the oropharynx and related lymph nodes, the salivary glands, the gingiva, the sinuses, the middle ear, the lungs, and the vagina. At these sites approximately 50 percent of all infections in our series were due to *S. aureus*, and approximately 20 percent were due to *H. influenzae*. It is of interest that a deficiency of antistaphylococcal IgA has recently been recognized in these patients.

Noninfectious clinical problems encountered occasionally in our patients include diffuse pruritic dermatitis (this is not a typical eczematoid dermatitis, although it can be similar), asthma, psychosis, recurrent keratoconjunctivitis, episodic asymmetric noninflammatory oligo-articular arthritis, and severe scoliosis. Other investigators have reported cranial synostosis, osteoporosis, and osteogenesis imperfecta tarda.

THERAPEUTIC ALTERNATIVES

There are three therapeutic approaches to HIE. The first is therapy with conventional drugs, including early intervention with antibiotic therapy of acute infections, antibiotic prophylaxis to avoid acute infections, continuous antimycotic therapy to control mucocutaneous candidiasis, and topical steroids plus antihistamines to treat pruritic dermatitis. The second is a surgical appoach to achieve adequate drainage of subcutaneous abscesses, to resect pulmonary abscesses, to remove persistent pneumatoceles which may expand and compromise lung function, and to remove bronchopleural fistulas that may develop. Another purpose of surgical therapy in some patients is to correct severe scoliosis which may further compromise lung function. Finally, a number of unproved drug therapies directed toward stimulation of immune function have been tried in patients with HIE.

PREFERRED APPROACH

Diagnosis

Diagnosis of an acute infection in HIE is often delayed as these patients have a subdued inflammatory response. Thus, careful evaluation of minor complaints is mandatory, especially with regard to the lungs, where *S. aureus* pneumonia with abscess formation may evolve with minimal early symptoms. As in normal hosts, one must first identify the presence of an infection and its site, attempt to determine the bacteriologic diagnosis, establish drainage if there is localized pus, and institute appropriate antibiotic therapy (Table 1). Since patients with HIE have a defective immune system, we administer antibiotic therapy in higher doses and for a more extended duration than in patients without an underlying immunologic deficit.

Subcutaneous Abscesses

Subcutaneous abscesses generally develop slowly and, at the time of presentation to the physician, frequently have been present for 5 to 10 days. Typically the abscess is minimally red, warm, or tender and may measure 1 to 2 cm or more in diameter; abscesses occasionally are hot and tender. The latter ''hot'' abscesses tend to be polymicrobial. The important points of proper treatment include bacteriologic diagnosis, appropriate antibiotics, and extensive incision with adequate drainage. Pending identification of the pathogen(s), we initiate therapy with a penicillinase-resistant penicillin and an aminoglycoside such as gentamicin (see Table 1). The surgical approach should be tempered by the knowledge that the extent of infected tissue is almost always larger than it appears. Frequently, drainage is maintained for prolonged periods (3 to 4 weeks), and parenteral antibiotic therapy is continued during that time. These general principles of aggressive management are also applied to other abscesses such as sialitis and lymphadenitis. Exceptions are otitis media and sinusitis, which can frequently be treated empirically with oral dicloxacillin. However, two cases of chronic recurrent otitis media have led to chronic mastoiditis and mastoidectomy.

Pulmonary Infections

The lungs are frequent sites of infection and can be the source of great morbidity. For a patient presenting with mild pulmonary complaints (even without a fever), a chest roentgenogram, CBC with differential, and sputum Gram's stain and culture are mandatory. An erythrocyte sedimentation rate (ESR) can be quite useful when baseline values are known but near normal values are frequently seen in conjunction with a significant infection. Often it is difficult to rule out a localized pneumonitis in a patient with chronic pulmonary scarring. In these cases we act conservatively and institute treatment for pneumonia. Initial drug therapy, which is chosen on the basis of sputum Gram's stain, includes an aminoglycoside (gentamicin or tobramycin) and a penicillinase-resistant penicillin if gram-positive cocci (presumably *S. aureus*) are seen and chloramphenicol if pleomorphic gram-negative rods (presumably *H. influenzae*) are apparent. If the Gram's stain is equivocal, antistaphylococcal therapy plus an aminoglycoside should be instituted initially pending bacteriologic results. If *H. influenzae* sensitive to ampicillin is present, obviously chloramphenicol should be discontinued and ampicillin substituted. Intravenous antibiotics (see Table 1) are continued for at least 2 weeks and are followed by 2 weeks of oral antibiotics. Owing to the abnormal inflammatory response in HIE, radiographic abnormalities often lag behind a clinically significant infection and patients without abnormal

TABLE 1 Antibiotics and Dosages Used in the Treatment of Infections Commonly Encountered in HIE

Group	*Drug*	*Adult Dose*	*Pediatric Dose*
Penicillinase-resistant penicillins	Nafcillin	1–1.5 g q4h IV	100–200 mg/kg/d, divided, q4h IV
	Methicillin	1–2 g q4h IV	200–400 mg/kg/d, divided, q4h IV
	Oxacillin	1 g q4h IV	100–400 mg/kg/d, divided, q4h IV
	Dicloxacillin	500 mg q6h PO	25—50 mg/kg/d, divided, q6h PO
Aminoglycosides	Gentamicin	3–5 mg/kg/d, divided, q8h IV	5 mg/kg/d, divided, q8h IV
	Tobramycin	3–5 mg/kg/d, divided, q8h IV	5 mg/kg/d, divided, q8h IV
Cephalosporins	Cephalothin	1–2 g q6h IV	80–160 mg/kg/d, divided, q4h IV
	Cefamandole	1–2 g q4–6h IV	50–150 mg/kg/d, divided, q4h IV
	Cephalexin	250–500 mg q6h PO	25–50 mg/kg/d, divided, q6h PO
Miscellaneous	Vancomycin	500 mg q6h IV	40 mg/kg/d, divided, q6h IV
	Ampicillin	1–2 g q4h IV	200–400 mg/kg/d, divided, q4h IV
	Chloramphenicol	50 mg/kg/d, divided, q6h IV	50–100 mg/kg/d, divided 6qh IV
	Clindamycin	450–900 mg 6qh IV	10–20 mg/kg/d, divided, q6h IV
Antifungals	Amphotericin B	1 mg/kg/d, single dose IV	0.5–1.0 mg/kg/d, single dose, IV
	Ketoconazole	200 mg/day, single dose PO	

chest roentgenograms are also treated aggressively. Thus, we treat patients who have apparent acute bronchitis with parenteral antibiotics for 1 to 2 weeks, followed by 2 weeks of oral antibiotic therapy. The purpose of this aggressive approach is to avoid the occurrence or the worsening of bronchiectasis. Patients who are infected with *S. aureus* and allergic to penicillin can often be treated with a cephalosporin (e.g., cephalothin) recognizing the possibility of cross-sensitivity between these classes of antibiotics. Further alternatives include vancomycin, clindamycin, and erythromycin. Methicillin-resistant *S. aureus* infections are treated with vancomycin. For *H. influenzae* infections, cephamandole can be administered to patients with adverse reactions to chloramphenicol.

If a pulmonary abscess is present, surgical intervention is required. The persistence of an enlarging or recurringly infected pneumatocele or the presence of a bronchopleural fistula following resolution of *S. aureus* pneumonia is also an indication for surgical resection. Severe scoliosis, especially in children, may develop following chest surgery and further compromise lung function. Periodic pulmonary function tests are useful to monitor pulmonary status.

Mucocutaneous Candidiasis

Chronic mucocutaneous candidiasis has been a major cosmetic problem in HIE independent of the frequency of concurrent antibiotic therapy and has responded well to chronic oral administration of ketoconazole. Oral thrush, episodic candida vaginitis, and onychomycosis occur, especially in patients not taking ketoconazole. Candida esophagitis has not been a major problem in our patients. Serious fungal infections are rarely seen in HIE although isolated cases of cryptococcal esophagitis, cryptococcal meningitis, and mediastinal candida granuloma have been reported. These illnesses require treatment with intravenous amphotericin B. A case of pulmonary aspergillosis also has been reported.

Other sites

Two other types of infection that deserve mention are cellulitis and osteomyelitis, both of which can occur as a complication of paronychia. Osteomyelitis has also been seen in the mandible underlying an apical tooth abscess. Since bacteriologic diagnosis is not certain in most of these cases, treatment has included parenteral antistaphylococcal therapy (usually nafcillin) with addition of an aminoglycoside (usually gentamicin). For cellulitis, parenteral treatment of 2 weeks' duration is followed by 2 weeks of oral antistaphylococcal antibiotics. For osteomyelitis, parenteral treatment is given for 6 to 8 weeks, followed by 6 months of oral antistaphylococcal antibiotics.

Prophylaxis

Long-term management of patients with HIE includes a thoughtful approach to prevention of recurrent infections. Chronic therapy with ketoconazole has been shown to alleviate mucocutaneous candidiasis and to be generally free of side effects. Five of our eleven patients with classic presentations of HIE are currently taking this medication with excellent results. Specific prophylaxis for *S. aureus* infections is a more controversial topic. There are some reports that continuous treatment with trimethoprim-sulfamethoxazole (one single strength tablet, *bid*) is efficacious and other reports that continuous dicloxacillin therapy (250 mg *bid*) minimizes staphylococcal infection. However, we have had 2 patients develop new *S. aureus* infections while receiving antistaphylococcal chemotherapy. One of these patients was receiving intravenous medication. Several patients are doing well without continuous prophylaxis. Thus, while prophylactic antibiotics are not effective in all patients, they may be beneficial in selected cases. Clearly, a prospective double-blind study is needed to determine the risks and benefits of this approach. We have two patients who are not candidates for antibacterial prophylaxis. One is intolerant of all available oral antistaphylococcal drugs. The other has had recurrent infections with a methicillin-resistant *S. aureus*. These patients are followed extremely closely.

Prophylactic antibiotics are used routinely in patients with phagocytic functional defects prior to dental and elective surgical procedures. We generally administer oxacillin 2 g IV (adult) or 200 mg/kg (child) 30 to 60 minutes before and 8 and 16 hours following such procedures. Other antistaphylococcal antibiotics are substituted as circumstances dictate (see Table 1).

Pruritic Dermatitis

Pruritic dermatitis is frequently a major problem in HIE. Most patients gain acceptable relief with topical steroid and oral antihistamines (H_1 blockade) such as hydroxyzine and Benadryl. Cimetidine (H_2 blockade) in addition to H_1 blockade may afford further relief. A rare patient may require a brief pulse of prednisone (3 days of 40 to 60 mg daily with rapid taper over 7 to 10 days). However, we strive to avoid the use of oral steroids in these patients. Topical steroid therapy can be optimized by careful attention to the patient's need for the drying aspect of creams and/or the lubricating quality of an ointment. Frequent (*tid* or *qid*) applications of topical preparations of triamcinolone 0.025% or triamcinolone 0.1% are usually sufficient for the treatment of pruritic dermatitis in HIE. However, these preparations should not be used continuously on the face or in the groin as thinning of the skin can occur. For these sites, a 1% hydrocortisone preparation should be used routinely; in rare instances, stronger preparations may be necessary to gain control. The combination of iodochlorhydroxyquin and hydrocortisone (Vioform-Hydrocortisone) has been especially effective for rashes with strong impetiginous features. Other topical antibacterial agents tend to be irritating. Baths in dilute solutions of Hebeclens, pHisoHex, or Betadine can be beneficial for some patients. However, any of these topical agents may exacerbate the dermatitis in sensitive patients. Chronic use of iodine-containing topical agents can precipitate thyrotoxicosis. Several patients experience exacerbations of their dermatitis during the summer months. In this setting, air conditioning can provide a useful adjunct to medical management.

Dental Care

Patients with HIE have an increased incidence of oral ulcerations and gingivitis. In addition, we have seen osteomyelitis secondary to a tooth abcess. Therefore, rigorous oral hygiene, including twice-daily tooth brushing with a paste composed of 3% hydrogen peroxide and baking soda is recommended. A thorough dental examination is performed twice yearly.

Immunomodulators

Therapy with immunomodulators, whose efficacies remain unproved, has become popular during the last decade. Levamisole (an anthelmintic) was shown to normalize in vitro neutrophil chemotaxis in HIE and was claimed anecdotally to help several patients. Unfortunately, this drug was found to be inferior to placebo in a double-blind randomized clinical trial. Transfer factor (an incompletely defined substance derived from mononuclear cell cultures) has been used in HIE with anecdotal reports of clinical efficacy. However, transfer factor has not been tested in a rigorous fashion in this disease, and in one patient recurrent therapy with high-dose transfer factor led to further immunosuppression. Therefore, transfer factor has generally fallen from favor. High-dose ascorbic acid therapy (8 to 10 g daily) has been reported to correct the in vitro chemotactic defect in some patients with the Chediak-Higashi syndrome and may help some patients with HIE, but this application has not been adequately tested. Gammaglobulin therapy has also been ineffective in HIE. This early clinical observation has been strengthened by a recent report of normal levels of anti-*S. aureus* IgG and elevated levels of anti-*S. aureus* IgM in this syndrome. A marked deficit of anti-*S. aureus* IgA has also been reported. However, this is not an indication for parenteral immunoglobulin therapy as parenterally administered IgA does not enter the secretions.

Finally, based on the presence of high levels of IgE, on reports that histamine interferes with leukocyte function in vitro, and on the finding of elevated plasma histamine values in some patients with HIE, antihistamine therapy (combination of H_1 and H_2 blockade) has been proposed, and anecdotal reports of clinical efficacy have appeared. However, elevated histamine levels (plasma or urine) are not the rule in HIE and, when present, are not clearly related to episodes of infection. Nonetheless, it is possible that tissue histamine levels may be elevated sufficiently to interfere with leukocyte function without causing a detectable rise in plasma or urinary histamine values. Thus, antihistamine therapy must be considered of unproved benefit. If cimetidine is used in HIE, its effect on the metabolism of other drugs (e.g., theophylline) must be considered.

COMPLICATIONS OF THERAPY

Complications of therapy are an important consideration. A devastating problem in HIE is loss of pulmonary function following lobectomy. This is unavoidable except, perhaps, in new patients, in whom vigorous aggressive diagnosis and treatment of the initial case of staphylococcal pneumonia is possible. The decision to undertake surgical correction of scoliosis may be mitigated in a patient with a propensity toward cutaneous or subcutaneous *S. aureus* infections. This is especially true in a patient who suffers recurrent infections near the operative field (i.e., the back) or in an area that would be obscured by a total body cast.

Reactions to antibiotics represent the largest category of adverse effects, but in our experience most have been minor and restricted to maculopapular rashes and gastrointestinal disturbances. We have seen isolated instances of leukopenia secondary to trimethoprim-sulfamethoxazole, hepatitis following nafcillin, and pseudomembranous colitis following clindamycin. One patient has had repeated infections with a methicillin-resistant *S. aureus*. Although we have not seen life-threatening IgE-mediated reactions to either penicillin or cephalosporins and have not seen agranulocytosis following chloramphenicol or the Stevens-Johnson syndrome following sulfa administration, these potentially serious complications of antibiotic therapy must not be forgotten. Ketoconazole has been well tolerated by our patients and we have not had to discontinue therapy for any reason. However, common side effects include nausea, vomiting, abdominal pain, and pruritis. In addition, transient asymptomatic elevation of serum transaminases or alkaline phosphatase may occur at any time during treatment. Clinically important hepatitis can occur, particularly during the first few months of therapy, but generally resolves after discontinuation of the drug. Ketoconzaole should be withheld if pregnancy is anticipated.

AMYLOIDOSIS

PETER D. GOREVIC, M.D.

Progress in our understanding of the biochemistry and pathogenesis of the amyloid diseases has not been matched by major therapeutic breakthroughs. The main impact of these studies has been in the refinement of diagnostic techniques for the distinction of the various conditions associated with tissue deposition of amyloid fibrils, and the development of a working nomenclature for their classification (Table 1). Assessment of therapeutic response from historical controls is particularly difficult, as the spectrum of amyloidosis seen in clinical practice is changing. Successive clinical series since the beginning of this century have recorded a progressive decline in secondary (AA) amyloidosis. As many as 80 percent of patients now seen in some large referral centers have amyloidosis due to monoclonal immunoglobulin light chain deposition (AL). Furthermore, heredofamilial and age-associated amyloidoses have emerged as increasingly important disease entities. It should also be appreciated that the clinical course of amyloidosis is quite variable, depending on etiology, host factors, organ systems, and number of organs involved, so that therapeutic nihilism is never warranted.

GENERAL APPROACH TO THERAPY

An outline of a general approach to therapy in amyloidosis is found in Table 2. Commitment to treatment should be preceded by firm tissue diagnosis. Accessible sites for the diagnosis of systemic amyloidosis include abdominal fat pad aspiration or rectal biopsy, and these may yield positive results in as many as 60 to 80 percent of cases. The latter may

TABLE 1 Nomenclature

	Tissue		*Serum*
Type	*Fibril Subunit Protein*		*Amyloid-Related Protein*
Primary			
Myeloma-associated	AL		SAL
Secondary			
Familial Mediterranean fever (FMF)	AA		$SAA_{1,2}$, etc.
Familial amyloid			
Polyneuropathy (FAP) Type I	AP_p		Prealbumin *(transthyretin)*
Diffuse ventricular "senile" cardiac amyloidosis	ASc_1		
Medullary carcinoma thyroid	AE_T		Calcitonin
P-Component	AP	=	SAP

Key: AL = immunoglobulin light chain-derived; AA = Amyloid A protein; AF_p = familial amyloid, prealbumin subunit; AE_T = endocrine, thyrocalcitonin subunit; AP = SAP = serum and tissue forms of P-component appear to be identical to each other; $SAA_{1,2}$, etc. = SAA isotypes.

TABLE 2 General Approach with Amyloidosis

Establish the diagnosis
- Standard screen for Congo Red birefringence
- Characteristic fibrils by electron microscopy
- P-component ? a marker for systemic, as well as some localized, forms of amyloidosis
- Screen AA by permanganate washout
- Immunoperoxidase or immunofluorescence studies with monospecific antisera
  - Anti-AA protein
  - Anti-prealbumin (transthyretin)
  - Anti kappa/lambda
  - ? Anti P-component (AP/SAP)
  - ? Anti V_L subgroup specific
  - Other
- Biochemical studies

Work-up and treat any plasma cell dyscrasia (AL amyloid)
- Immunoelectrophoresis of

	For:
Serum	Monoclonal gammopathy
Urine (50–100 × concentrated if minimal proteinuria or if serum is negative)	Free light chains ($\lambda > \kappa$)
	IgD
	? Polymers

- Bone marrow aspiration(s) and biopsy(ies)
- Bone survey, biopsy other organs as indicated
- Myeloma, primary amyloidosis
  - Melphalan, 0.25 mg/kg/day × 7 days
  - Prednisone, 0.8 mg/kg in 4 divided doses Q 4–6 weeks
- Macroglobulinemia/μ HCD
  - Chlorambucil, 0.1–0.2 mg/kg/day
- Plasmacytomas: surgery, irradiation, melphalan/prednisone
- Alternative: cyclophosphamide, 100–150 mg/day
- Colchicine, 0.5–0.6 mg po bid-tid may be added to each of the above regimens if there are no contraindications. The exact dose is adjusted to tolerance i.e., diarrhea

Eliminate or reduce any inflammatory process (AA amyloid)
- Antibiosis (endocarditis, tuberculosis, osteomyelitis)
- Anti inflammatory agents
  - Inhibition synthesis/biologic effects interleukin I
  - Inhibition SAA synthesis (colchicine)
  - Inhibition of prostaglandin synthesis (?DMSO, other)
- Surgery
  - Tumor (e.g., hypernephroma)
  - Organ (e.g., colectomy in granulomatous colitis)

Identify and treat any underlying neoplastic state
- Hypernephroma, Hodgkin's disease (AA)
- Immunocyte-derived (AL)
- APUD neoplasm (e.g., AE_T)

Suppress the synthesis of precursor proteins
- Chemotherapy (AL/?AA)
- Colchicine (AA ? AL)

Remove or alter precursor (AL)
- ?Plasmapheresis
- ?Depolymerization
- ?Immunoabsorption
- ?Anti–idiotope antibodies

Interfere with tissue factors
- ?Binding to P-component/ground substance(s)
- ?Correct defective enzymatic cleavage of precursor (AA)
- ?Enhance resorption (immunopotentiation)

Dissociate fibrils
- DMSO (AA, AL, ?prealbumin)
- ? D-penicillamine

be performed under direct visualization or via a small bowel biopsy capsule with a short suction wire. These peripheral sites cannot substitute for major organ biopsy (endomyocardial, renal, hepatic, small bowel, and so on), should the diagnosis be in question. Resort to the latter, however, should be preceded by evaluation for associated clotting abnormalities, and tempered by reports in the literature of an increased incidence of bleeding of amyloid-infiltrated organs following biopsy.

Biopsy tissue is processed for immunohistologic studies, electron microscopy, and, if sufficient material is available, biochemical studies.

In some large series of patients with AL amyloidosis, as many as 80 to 90 percent have been found to have a monoclonal protein (intact immunoglobulin and/or light chain) in serum and/or urine. Only 20 percent of these patients have clear-cut multiple myeloma by bone marrow examination, gammopathy, and/or the presence of osteolytic bone lesions. A detailed immunoelectrophoretic evaluation for monoclonal light chains, both as a myeloma protein and free in urine and serum, is an essential part of the work-up.

The decision to treat this group of patients is based on the 5-month median survival of those with myeloma and 13-month median survival of those without myeloma, as well as on the fact that no instance of spontaneous remission of established AL amyloid has yet been recorded. Rationale for the use of combination chemotherapy consisting of intermittent melphalan and prednisone (see Table 2 for specific regimen) is based on the low toxicity of this regimen, its proven efficacy in myeloma, and 8 case reports now in the literature of long-term (up to 70 months) survivals in patients with AL amyloid treated with these drugs. Combination chemotherapy appears to be particularly useful for reducing massive proteinuria in some patients; however, in a controlled study involving 55 patients, no overall improvement in survival from placebo-treated controls was found. Thus, at best, this treatment should be considered palliative. Further caveats include: 1) the development of rapidly fatal acute granulocytic or myelomonocytic leukemia 2 to 5 years later in some patients treated with alkylating agents; 2) the fact that this regimen has not been shown to be effective in azotemic patients; 3) the observation that progression of tissue amyloid can be demonstrated by serial biopsies in spite of good clinical responses; and 4) the existence of an older literature that suggests that steroids may in fact accelerate the progression of amyloidosis.

Use of colchicine for the treatment of amyloidosis is based on the proven efficacy of this drug in attenuating murine AA amyloidosis. In vitro studies indicate that colchicine suppresses the secretion of serum amyloid A protein (SAA) from hepatocytes, and one report has noted less immunoglobulin production by myeloma cells in culture. Paracelsus' prediction that Colchicum autumnale might be the key to longevity has been verified in a large cohort of familial Mediterranean fever (FMF) patients treated with colchicine administered 2 or 3 times daily since 1972. Whereas 10 to 15 new cases of AA amyloidosis could be expected per year among this patient population based on historical controls, none has been seen in patients adhering to this prophylactic regimen (1 to 2 mg per day). Preliminary results at 3 years of a second large group of patients with established amyloidosis receiving colchicine also suggest a striking improvement in survival by comparison with historical controls. Aside from occasional hypersensitivity reactions and the need to titrate against gasrointestinal side effects (diarrhea, nausea, vomiting, abdominal pain), toxicity is rarely encountered. The known ability of this drug to block cell division in metaphase has not been reflected in any detectable abnormalities on detailed karyotype analysis, or in evidence of increased teratogenicity among the offspring of pregnant patients brought to term. The use of colchicine in AL amyloidosis, however, is still problematic, and it is currently being examined in a controlled study. It is relatively contraindicated in patients with ulcer disease or gastrointestinal amyloid involvement (malabsorption, diarrhea, obstruction), but has been introduced for long-term use in most patients without adverse effects.

One case report of long-term survival in a patient with amyloidosis secondary to rheumatoid arthritis included a short course of D-penicillamine. However, there is as yet no evidence that this agent affects amyloid fibrils in vitro or has any impact on the course of murine AA amyloidosis. Unpublished results from one amyloid referral clinic have not shown any impact on survival when this drug is used alone for the treatment of amyloidosis.

Consideration may be given to the use of other cytotoxic agents, both as primary treatment and in the patient failing on, or unable to tolerate, melphalan-prednisone. Chlorambucil would be appropriate therapy for the unusual patient with amyloidosis associated with macroglobulinemia or μ-heavy chain disease. In this setting, it can be given as gradually increased low-dose (10 mg per day) maintenance therapy, often combined with prednisone (10 mg per day), or as a high-dose intermittent pulse regimen. Low-dose chlorambucil has also been used for the treatment of renal manifestations of AA amyloidosis in uncontrolled series of children with juvenile chronic polyarthritis in England and Finland. Patients with AL amyloidosis may be treated with maintenance oral cyclophosphamide (100 to 150 mg per day) if melphalan-prednisone is poorly tolerated. There is as yet no experience with 3- or 4-drug regimens (that is, the M2 protocol), and their use is hardly justified in view of the major toxicities involved and poor quality of life of many patients with severe systemic amyloidosis.

Establishing the diagnosis of AA amyloid is important, because much evidence suggests that treatment of the underlying inflammatory disease may have a significant impact on amyloid deposition. Most remissions described to date have occurred in patients with AA amyloidosis, and this form often proves to be more indolent than the AL variety. AA protein has been identified in amyloid occurring in association with various chronic infectious and inflammatory diseases, in at least two forms of heredofamilial amyloidosis (FMF and the Muckle-Wells syndrome), and in amyloid complicating Hodgkin's disease, hypernephromas, and other solid neoplasms. We have also seen patients labeled "primary" in whom it has been possible to identify AA protein biochemically or immunohistologically in tissue deposits. Regression of amyloid may occur following treatment of the underlying infectious process or surgical extirpation of tumors, and has been reported following colectomy for amyloid complicating granulomatous ileocolitis. Patients in whom AA protein can be demonstrated are now routinely put on colchicine.

Localized amyloid may occur in association with both primary and metastatic lesions of amine precursor uptake and decarboxylation (APUD) neoplasms, such as medullary carcinoma of the thyroid. In the latter instance, the major fibril subunit protein has been shown to be a form of calcitonin, which can be demonstrated in amyloid immunohistologically using monospecific antisera to this protein. Therapy here is directed to the underlying neoplasm and consists mainly of surgical removal (namely, total thyroidectomy).

Dimethylsulfoxide (DMSO) has been used in four uncontrolled series from the United States, the Netherlands, Japan, and Israel, involving patients with AL, AA, and prealbumin-related hereditary amyloidosis. In each series, prolonged therapy, usually longer than six months, was required for effect, and many patients did not respond to treatment. Nevertheless, in some instances, striking improvements in neurologic deficits, renal impairment, and proteinuria, macroglossia, or cardiac function were seen. The drug has been administered orally, rectally, topically, and even intravenously. Orally, it is given as a 10 percent solution in fruit juice, usually in divided doses before meals. It is started at an initial dose of 2 to 3 ml and increased gradually to as much as 15 ml (15 mg) daily. The only major side effect is a persistent intense garlicky odor, a feature which may render the patient a social outcast and which effectively precludes any double-blind studies. In vitro studies in AL and prealbumin-related amyloid have suggested that DMSO is capable of dissociating fibrils to subunit proteins, and the appearance of material with AA reactivity in the urine of FMF amyloid patients and casein amyloidotic mice treated with the drug appears to substantiate this concept. Nevertheless, the poor correlation between clinical responses obtained and actual lysis of existing amyloid deposits has suggested that other mechanisms may be operative, notably a direct anti-inflammatory effect of the drug. It should be stressed that DMSO is licensed only for topical use in the treatment of interstitial cystitis because of the development of cataracts in experimental animals, and it should be used only on an investigational basis with material rigorously checked by the manufacturer for contaminants.

THERAPY DIRECTED TO SPECIFIC ORGAN SYSTEMS

An appreciation of the various clinical syndromes which may present in a patient with amyloidosis is an essential part of patient management and education (Table 3). Whereas AA and AL amyloid may overlap in the liver, spleen, kidney, heart, or gut, direct involvement of joints or nervous system or the appearance of acquired factor X deficiency is not seen in AA amyloidosis; specifically, amyloid arthropathy or factor X deficiency should suggest AL amyloid. Prealbumin-related "senile" amyloidosis may involve both heart and lungs, the former often complicated by arrhythmias or heart block and the latter usually being asymptomatic. Overdosage and toxicity due to digitalis sensitivity, volume depletion in a patient with severe orthostatic hypotension also being treated with diuretics, multiple hemostatic abnormalities, rare cases of adrenal insufficiency due to amyloid infiltration, and secondary immunodeficiency due to hypoglobulinemia, immunosuppression, or functional hyposplenism present potentially remediable complications of disease. Treatment of other syndromes, such as intractable heart failure, orthostatic hypotension, intestinal and neurologic involvement, remains largely supportive and often unsatisfying.

Renal involvement accounts for about 10 percent of mortalities in some recent series and ranks behind cardiac amyloid and underlying disease as a cause of death. This reflects: a) the fact that renal involvement may be present and remain asymptomatic for many years; b) renal involvement may respond to various treatment modalities in the face of ongoing tissue deposition; and c) the availability of hemodialysis and transplantation as potential therapies. However, dialysis is often difficult owing to problems of vascular access, and may be complicated by severe orthostatic hypotension or heart failure. Transplants may develop recurrence of amyloid in the allograft. Deaths in this group are due mainly to complications of transplantation and not to amyloid replacement of other organs. In both the dialyzed and transplanted patients, long-term survival does not match that of patients with renal failure due to more common diseases.

ASSESSMENT OF THERAPY

There is no currently available method that adequately assesses response to therapy, or that provides a good measure of the existing load of silent deposits in liver, spleen, blood vessels, and so on at the onset of treatment. Clinical assessment should include the degree of organomegaly (macroglossia, physical examination, scans) or functional disturbances (neuropathy, malabsorption). Patients with AL amyloid may

TABLE 3 Aspects of Therapy Directed to Specific Organ Systems in Amyloidosis

Organ System	*Manifestation*	*Treatment*	*Comment*
Renal	Nephrotic syndrome	Salt restriction Loop diuretics Chemotherapy	Poor correlation with the extent of amyloid on biopsy
	Renal failure	Diet Electrolytes	Hypertension < 30% Few reports of response to chemotherapy in azotemic patients
		Hemodialysis Transplantation	Access difficulties Experience primarily in AA-FMF Amyloid may recur in the allograft
	Nephrogenic Diabetes insipidus		Rare
	Fanconi's syndrome	Treat underlying disease	Multiple myeloma Bence Jones proteinuria ($\kappa > \lambda$) Kidneys free; amyloid in other organs
	Renal vein thrombosis	Hydration Anticoagulation	
Cardiac	Congestive heart failure	Salt restriction Diuretics Digitalis	AL > ASc > AA Often intractable Follow decreasing EKG voltage, 2D echocardiogram Care re: digitalis sensitivity
	Heart block Sick sinus syndrome Arrhythmias	Antiarrhythmics Pacemaker placement	ASc
	Coronary insufficiency	Antianginal medications Treat infarction	Pseudoanteroseptal infarcts on EKG
Vascular	Orthostatic hypotension	Treat volume depletion Avoid rapid postural changes *Mild:* Antigravity stockings *Moderate:* 9 α fluorohydro-cortisone (Florinef)–NaCl with K supplementation *Severe:* Oral sympathomimetics Ephedrine Hydroxyamphetamine ? Indocin	AL May make dialysis more difficult
	Claudication syndromes		
Gastrointestinal	Prepyloric obstruction Linitis plastica	Small feedings	
	Pseudo-obstruction	Suction	Decreased motor activity

Table 3 continues

show disappearance of monoclonal protein from serum and/or urine, as well as loss of plasmacytosis or frank myeloma on follow-up bone marrow examinations. Renal amyloid may be monitored by serial determinations of the amount of proteinuria, serum albumin, azotemia or glomerular filtration rate. However, repeat biopsy may be necessary to assess any impact on tissue deposition. A poor response to therapy may reflect loss of normal tissue, secondary fibrosis due to replacement by amyloid, or redistribution of amyloid deposits to other organs.

Cardiac amyloid presents a particularly difficult and important problem. Some indication of the presence and extent of disease may be obtained by serial evaluations of ECG voltage (looking for a progressive decrease) and by M-mode and two-dimensional (2D) echocardiographic measurements of ventricular wall thickness. Technetium-99m pyrophosphate scanning, which appears to localize to calcium in amyloid deposits, has also been advocated for the detection of cardiac amyloid. These methods are inexact, are not predictive of rhythm disturbances or vascular compromise, and do not distinguish between AL and "senile" cardiomyopathy. Serial endomyocardial biopsies, as have been utilized in inflammatory cardiomyopathies, may provide an alternative means to follow treatment, but little information is yet available in this regard.

FUTURE THERAPIES

The emergence of prealbumin-related amyloidosis has focused attention on the identification of variant molecules, which may be purified in the future and characterized from small serum or tissue samples. Prealbumin levels in blood often appear to be low, both in patients with some polyneuropathy syndromes and their affected relatives; this may also prove to have some diagnostic utility. Other approaches to serodiagnosis may lie in the identification of specific SAA isotypes, only some of which may

TABLE 3 Aspects of Therapy Directed to Specific Organ Systems in Amyloidosis (Continued)

Organ System	*Manifestation*	*Treatment*	*Comment*
	Malabsorption	Treat bacterial overgrowth	
		Diet	
	Perforation		
Hepatic	Hepatomegaly		Care re: biopsy
	Obstructive jaundice		Rare
			Poor prognosis
	Portal hypertension		Rare
Oral	Macroglossia	Maintain airway	AL
	Sjögren's syndrome	Artificial tears	AL
Nervous system	Peripheral neuropathy	Analgesics	± Autonomic
	Carpal tunnel syndrome	Surgical release	AL, AF
	Hemorrhagic angiopathy		Gamma-trace protein
	Amyloidomas	Surgical excision	Mass lesions
	Alzheimer's disease/ senile dementia		AS_B
Respiratory	Amyloidomas (extramedullary plasmacytomas)	Surgical excision Irradiation	AL
	Diffuse infiltration	Bronchoscopic curettage	
Adrenal	Insufficiency	Replacement Therapy	Rare
			Loss of edema in a patient with known nephrotic syndrome
Joints	Rheumatoidlike arthropathy	Nonsteroidals	AL
		?Prednisone	$\kappa > \lambda$
Blood (clotting factor abnormalities)	Bleeding		AL
	Vitamin K — dependent factors	Vitamin K_1	Due to liver disease or malabsorption
	X > IX, VII, II	Fresh-frozen plasma	Rarely effective if associated fibrinolysis
		Epsilon amino caproic acid	
		Prednisone	
		Splenectomy	Usually splenomegaly on scan
Eye	Vitreous opacities	Vitrectomy	AL, AF
			May recur
	Lattice corneal Dystrophies	Keratoplasty	May recur in allograft
Skin	Petechiae/ecchymoses		
	Papules/nodules	Tread underlying disease	—
	Scleroderma-like Alopecia		
	Pigmentary changes		
	Bullous eruptions		

deposit in tissue to give amyloid, or the use of group-specific anti-V_L antisera that may identify monoclonal light chain fragments circulating in blood; serial measurements might then provide accurate measures of the response to treatment. An alternative approach to the definition of abnormal light chain fragments may be provided by biosynthetic studies of bone marrow aspirates, even in patients without demonstrable serum or urinary monoclonal light chains, looking for aberrant immunoglobulin production in short-term labeling experiments. The rapid (hours) turnover and predominantly renal excretion of light chains make it unlikely that plasma exchange would have a significant impact on the course of AL amyloidosis. Extracorporeal immunoabsorption of blood with, or direct intravascular administration of, anti-idiotype antibodies specific for the patients' own AL subunit protein may provide an alternative approach to reducing the serum load of the putative precursor. Lastly, the possibility remains that in some instances amyloidosis is the consequence of faulty degradation of normal proteins, or abnormal binding to tissue factors, and that a therapy might be designed that specifically corrects or interferes with these pathogenic abnormalities.

SKIN DISEASES

CHRONIC URTICARIA

MARTIN D. VALENTINE, M.D.

Although many patients with urticaria or "hives" come to an allergist expecting to be told the cause of their problem, most of the easy diagnoses have been made by the patient's primary physician without need for consultation. When a thoughtful evaluation fails to reveal a specific cause and when hives recur for more than six weeks, the condition is designated "chronic idiopathic urticaria." Continued physician observation of such patients occasionally will yield a clue as to etiology, but this is the exception rather than the rule, and the physician's role is to provide the therapeutic support that enables the patient to reduce symptoms to a manageable minimum while awaiting a spontaneous regression. Because chronic urticaria may adopt a cyclic pattern and usually regresses spontaneously, sometimes to recur at a later date, what sometimes appears to be a therapeutic triumph may actually turn out to be the natural course of the disease. Although chronic urticaria is usually confined to the skin, mucosal and visceral symptoms occasionally occur, requiring separate therapeutic consideration as noted below.

Histamine is generally considered to be the primary mediator in most cases of chronic urticaria; thus, antihistamines taken systemically are the mainstay of therapy. Topical antihistamines or other agents are rarely helpful, although certain general measures relating to skin care may help the patient feel more comfortable. These include avoidance of conditions that heat the skin, such as hot baths or showers; heavy bed clothing; and other items, such as chili peppers, spicy foods, and systemic ethyl alcohol, which result in cutaneous vasodilatation and increased susceptibility to urticaria. Clothing should be loose, comfortable, and no heavier than necessary for comfort. Skin dryness will exacerbate pruritus and should be prevented with moisturizing lotions or creams.

Most H-1 histamine antagonists also cause drowsiness. Some physicians feel that this is a desirable adjunct of an agent used for treating urticaria, but I disagree. The antihistamine that produces maximal effect in the skin with minimal sedation would be the agent of choice; several H-1 antagonists purported to lack central nervous system activity are currently awaiting Food and Drug Administration approval. A wide variety of H-1 antagonists are currently available, including enthanolamine derivatives, ethylenediamine derivatives, and alkylamines. Although some patients will do well on these drugs, I find hydroxyzine and cyproheptadine generally superior to the other agents. The phenothiazine drugs are generally avoided because of the side effects associated with this family of compounds, although one might consider their use in a patient in whom other H-1 antihistamines have failed. Because of inherent differences in the pharmacology of hydroxyzine and cyproheptadine, their use will be considered separately. Antihistamines work better when taken regularly in a prophylactic regimen; when taken after hives appear, they may relieve itching but will not reverse already visible lesions.

HYDROXYZINE

This drug is available as the pamoate (Vistaril and generic equivalents) and the hydrochloride (Atarax, Durrax, and generic equivalents). Either form may be used, both having inherently long durations of action when administered orally. The hydrochloride is available in smaller oral dosage forms, 10 mg being the smallest tablet dose available for the hydrochloride and 25 mg being the smallest capsule dose available of the pamoate. Both are available as liquids. Either form is relatively contraindicated in early pregnancy because hydroxyzine has caused fetal abnormalities in rats when given in doses substantially above the human therapeutic range. Drowsiness may occur with hydroxyzine, although the duration of sedation with this drug seems to be far shorter than its duration of effect in the skin. Although most people tolerate 10 mg orally 3 to 4 times per day without drowsiness, some patients find this dose to have sedative properties; for such patients, an attempt may be made to give the entire day's dose at bedtime. Some particularly sensitive patients may do well with as small a dose as 10 mg at bedtime, although this will be the exception. As a rule, most patients improve with 20 to 40 mg daily, and some patients will tolerate—and require—100 to 200 mg (rarely more) per 24 hours. Sedation is common but not universal with the higher doses. In patients for whom hydroxyzine does not seem to be therapeutically successful, I will try cyproheptadine.

CYPROHEPTADINE

In addition to being an antihistamine, this drug is also a serotonin antagonist whose nonapproved uses include prophylaxis for vascular headaches and maintenance therapy in certain patients with Cushing's syndrome. Although drowsiness is the major side effect associated with cyproheptadine, increased appetite or weight gain has also been associated with its use, and at one time it was approved for use as an appetite stimulating agent in children. In addition, I have found an occasional patient to experience otherwise unexplainable emotional depression while using this drug. It is not as inherently long acting as hydroxyzine and thus does not lend itself to single bedtime dosing. However, drowsiness does appear to be minimized if the drug is begun at a low dose and gradually increased. In practice, I suggest beginning with 2 mg twice a day, making incremental increases at 2 to 3 day intervals or as tolerated by the patient. After 2 mg *bid*, the next doses are 2 mg *tid*; 4 mg *bid*; 4 mg *tid*; to a maximum of 4 mg *qid*.

COMBINATION THERAPY AND H-2 ANTAGONISTS

A single H-1 antagonist may be insufficient in the management of patients with chronic urticaria. Although some advocate combinations of two or more H-1 antagonists, I feel that other measures are more suitable. I would first consider maintaining the chosen dosage of the H-1 antagonist, for example, hydroxyzine or cyproheptadine, and then adding an H-2 antagonist, such as cimetidine or ranitidine. Some patients apparently respond to the combination of H-1 and H-2 antagonists with resolution of their urticaria. It is usually the case, however, that the patient who responds favorably to the addition of the H-2 antagonist is the patient who has already responded partially to administration of the H-1 antagonist. Certain patients may respond partially to the combination of H-1 and H-2 antagonist and still need additional therapy. Although steroid therapy may be considered for such patients, I would first consider adding the agent ephedrine sulfate, 25 mg 3 to 4 times daily. The combination of α-adrenergic, β_1, and β_2 activities may all be useful adjuncts in the patient with urticaria. Some authorities have favored β_2 agonists based on the inhibitory effects such agents have on mediator release, but I feel that such selective agents are less likely to be useful than the combination of alpha and mixed-beta effects of ephedrine.

TRICYCLICS

It is known that drugs belonging to the tricyclic antidepressant family have very great affinity for H-1 receptors in certain binding assays in vitro. This has led to therapeutic trials in patients with chronic urticaria; some successes have been reported. In addition to H-1 antagonism, some of the tricyclics, such as doxepin, have significant anti-H-2 activity. A trial of doxepin may be warranted if a single conventional H-1 antagonist is ineffectual in patients with chronic urticaria.

CORTICOSTEROIDS

A minority of patients cannot be managed adequately even with a combination of H-1 and H-2 antagonists with ephedrine. In such patients, it may be necessary to resort to systemic corticosteroids. In cases of chronic urticaria one must keep in mind that, since the condition may persist for months or even years, if steroids are employed, they may be necessary—with their attendant potential for side effects—for that period of time as well. In general, the rules for the use of steroids in urticaria are the same as they would be for asthma: One should use an agent that is short acting to avoid suppression of the pituitary-hypothalamic-adrenal axis, and should use the agent initially in a dose sufficient to suppress symptoms completely and taper it fairly rapidly until it can be determined what dose is necessary to achieve satisfactory suppression of symptoms. A subgroup of the physical urticarias known as delayed pressure urticaria often responds poorly, if at all, to antihistamines and often requires steroid therapy. However, in this entity, the nonsteroidal anti-inflammatory agents may have a beneficial therapeutic effect and should be tried before steroids. Some clinicians feel that the nonsteroidal anti-inflammatory agents are relatively contraindicated in chronic urticaria of the usual variety, however, and routinely advise against their use even if specific sensitivity to the drug in question is not suspected.

DRUGS NOT INDICATED

Patients with inherited or acquired deficiency of the inhibitor of Cl do not have urticaria but are susceptible to attacks of cutaneous and mucosal angioedema which do not respond to epinephrine, antihistamines, or corticosteroids. In these syndromes, confirmed by the appropriate immunochemical studies, various anabolic steroids (''impeded androgens'') help prevent attacks by promoting biosynthesis of normal Cl inhibitor protein. Such therapy is *not* indicated in chronic idiopathic urticaria for two reasons: No benefit has been shown, and the anabolic steroids are hepatotoxic and may be tumorigenic.

ACUTE EXACERBATIONS

Occasionally the patient with chronic urticaria may experience an acute exacerbation requiring urgent treatment because a previously effective drug regimen has failed. Acute intervention may also be requested by a patient when urticaria involves an area which results in transient disfigurement, such as the lip or eyelid, causing embarrassment or social inability to continue normal activities. In such situations, 0.3 mg (0.3 cc of 1:1000 solution) of aqueous epinephrine by subcutaneous injection is often rapidly effective in reversing cutaneous lesions. Mucosal urticaria or angioedema may also require and benefit from such intervention to prevent airway compromise. Visceral urticaria can produce pain in the gut; esophageal lesions may produce pain which mimics angina but which is rapidly relieved with epinephrine.

SYSTEMIC SCLEROSIS (SCLERODERMA)

ALEXANDER P. RUGGIERI, M.D.
E. CARWILE LEROY, M.D.

Scleroderma, whose hallmark is thickening and induration of skin, is characterized by excessive synthesis and deposition of connective tissue matrix. Rampant fibrosis is not confined to skin alone but involves other major organ systems, including muscle, heart, lung, kidney, and intestine, as the term *systemic sclerosis* implies. The variability in extent, severity, and rapidity of progression among patients with systemic sclerosis identifies scleroderma not as a single clinical entity but rather as a clinical spectrum.

Diffuse generalized systemic sclerosis, because of the serious clinical implications, is the most important form of scleroderma for the practitioner to recognize. A minority of patients can be identified as being in this most serious subgroup, which is characterized by widespread skin involvement, including the trunk,and by potentially life-threatening visceral involvement in the first few years following symptom onset. A second widely recognized subgroup within this spectrum is characterized by limited cutaneous involvement and has been identified by the acronym "CREST" syndrome (calcinosis, Raynaud's phenomenon, esophageal dysfunction, sclerodactyly, and telangiectasias). This subgroup of patients has restricted cutaneous involvement, a slow evolution, and often subclinical visceral involvement in the first decade, which may become clinically significant and even be fatal in later decades (especially pulmonary hypertension). Serologically, patients with CREST are identified by a high frequency of circulating antibodies to the centromeric region of metaphase chromosomes (anticentromere antibody).

The clinical spectrum of systemic sclerosis is further broadened by the often simultaneous appearance of features of other rheumatic diseases (rheumatoid arthritis, systemic lupus erythematosus, and polymyositis). These patients, sometimes classified as having mixed or undifferentiated connective tissue syndromes (MCTD, UCTS), nevertheless face the same clinical consequences of scleroderma patients without overlap features.

Variability, complexity, and overlapping features of rheumatic diseases make attempts to formulate general treatment and management approaches for scleroderma difficult. Many therapies, including surgical procedures, dietary interventions, hormones, vitamins, and drugs, have been proposed. Most have not withstood the tests of time and controlled trial. To date, there is no specific treatment or combination of treatments that uniformly halts the destructive fibrosis that leads to disfigurement and organ failure in systemic sclerosis. Established, advanced fibrosis in any tissue is essentially irreversible. Nevertheless, the therapeutic approach to systemic sclerosis is not a nihilistic one; many therapies and interventions exist that can potentially alter the course of individual organ involvement and improve the quality of life for individual patients.

Current treatment can be classified into two categories: (1) agents or measures whose actions or effects are aimed at arresting the pathogenic process (presumptive remittive therapies), and (2) agents or measures aimed at reducing organ failure (supportive therapy). Definite therapeutic benefit has been difficult to demonstrate for the former category, owing to absence of widely accepted criteria for improvement, the heterogeneity of populations of scleroderma patients, and the tendency of the disease to demonstrate different stages of activity over time. A future remittive agent will most likely exert its effect early in the course of the disease.

REMITTIVE THERAPIES

Distinct vascular and microvascular abnormalities associated with excessive synthesis and deposition of collagenous matrix are the prominent histopathologic features of scleroderma. A distinct proliferative lesion of the small arteries and alterations in the endothelial lining of blood vessels have been demonstrated in scleroderma patients. Nailfold capillary microscopy has identified distinctive capillary lesions that correlate with disease activity. In vitro studies have demonstrated both an endothelial cell cytotoxic factor in scleroderma serum and evidence for enhanced platelet activation in the earlier stages of the disease. These observations and the prevalent vasospastic component of the disease have inspired intervention aimed at preserving small vessel integrity. Dipyridamole, a pyrimidopyrimidine compound, initially introduced as a coronary vasodilator, subsequently has been shown to have significant vasodilating antiplatelet actions in vitro and in vivo. In high doses, partial inhibition of platelet aggregation, adhesion, and prolongation of platelet survival have been observed. Purported mechanisms include elevation of intracellular cyclic AMP by inhibition of phosphodiesterase, synergism with the antiplatelet effects of prostacyclin, inhibition of adenosine uptake by platelets and by endothelial cells, and potentiation of the inhibitory effect of adenosine on ADP-induced platelet aggregation. Aspirin is an antiplatelet agent by irreversible inhibition of platelet cyclooxygenase in the generation of the proaggregatory substance thromboxane A_2. Aspirin and dipyridamole have been employed together in our clinic in scleroderma patients with early disease who show evidence of enhanced platelet activation (B thromboglobulin levels, increased platelet aggregate ratios). Complete return to normal levels of tests for endothelial injury and concomitant platelet activation have yet to be achieved. Evidence for effects of a remittive nature must await carefully designed controlled clinical trials by several independent clinics.

We use these agents in patients with early disease in whom factors indicative of enhanced platelet activation can be identified. Dipyridamole, 400 to 600 mg, is administered in 4 divided doses daily. Aspirin, 325 mg, is administered once every third day, taking advantage of the faster regeneration of active endothelial cyclooxygenase, an enzyme also inhibited by aspirin and responsible for the synthesis of prostacyclin, a prostaglandin with potent antiaggregatory and vasodilating actions. Side effects of these agents are minor and include dizziness, nausea and dyspepsia which remit promptly upon discontinuation of therapy. These agents are perhaps as safe as any medications currently administered to scleroderma patients.

Vascular and microvascular injury precede and likely herald the generalized fibrosis that dominates scleroderma's clinicopathologic picture. Two agents have been used in scleroderma patients in hopes of arresting the relentless fibrotic replacement and degeneration of critical tissues. These agents are accepted by some as having therapeutic benefit and are actively used in some centers.

D-penicillamine (D-3 mercaptovaline, D-Pen) is known to inhibit the cross-linking of lysine residues in collagen in vitro. This effect is particularly pronounced in the maturation of type I collagen (principal skin collagen), where the enzymatic aldol condensation of allysine residues is important for fibril formation. Observations in patients with Wilson's disease receiving D-penicillamine for prolonged periods revealed thinning of skin and an increase in soluble dermal collagen in skin biopsy tissue. This dermolathyrogenic effect of D-penicillamine formed the basis for its trial in the treatment of scleroderma.

Assessment of the efficacy of D-penicillamine in scleroderma patients has been largely retrospective. Claims of skin softening and a modest increase in 5-year survival have been made in patients with scleroderma receiving 500 to 1500 mg of D-Pen per day over a 10-year period. Criticisms of the trials of D-Pen in scleroderma have focused on problems inherent in retrospective studies in general, the lack of generally accepted objective parameters precisely defining visceral involvement and disease progression, the variable expression of the disease in any given patient, and the tendency for skin to soften spontaneously in many patients over time regardless of therapy. A disturbing array of toxic and untoward effects associated with D-Pen administration further clouds its use. Bone marrow suppression is the most serious. Leukopenia, thrombocytopenia and aplastic anemia have all been reported. Complete blood counts must be obtained at frequent intervals (every 2 weeks for the first 6 months and then every month for the duration of therapy). Proteinuria has been encountered in up to 20 percent of patients receiving D-penicillamine. Its administration can be associated with nephrotic syndrome and may mask recognition of early renal involvement in systemic sclerosis. A period of up to one year may be required before urinary abnormalities clear. Urinalyses must be performed at frequent intervals, along with hematologic studies. Other reported side effects include fever, pulmonary syndromes, autoimmune syndromes (Goodpasture's syndrome, myasthenia gravis, polymyositis, pemphigus, systemic lupus erythematosus, and Sjögren's syndrome), nausea, vomiting, anorexia, dysgeusia, and oral mucosal ulceration. Reinstitution of a therapy of questionable efficacy after a serious side effect occurs is an option viewed with reluctance by most clinicians, and so it should be in scleroderma patients treated with D-Pen. The lack of proven efficacy and the risk of serious side effects that may complicate and add to the afflictions faced by patients with systemic sclerosis leave us unethusiastic about the use of D-Pen, unless the presence of an overlapping condition (such as rheumatoid arthritis) warrants it.

Colchicine is another agent with potential antifibrotic effect. In vitro, colchicine is known to bind to microtubules and interfere with exocytosis, a process whereby collagen synthesizing cells release procollagen for extracellular processing and fibril maturation. Studies showing therapeutic benefit of colchicine in scleroderma have not been confirmed by other clinics. Nevertheless, the impact of long-term administration of colchicine in scleroderma is unknown. Its minimal and reversible side effects (gastrointestinal upset, diarrhea) in the doses employed (0.6 mg orally twice daily) permit continued observation and use. However, we do not routinely use colchicine in our scleroderma patients. Evidence of significant small bowel involvement (diarrhea, malabsorption, hypomotility) constitutes an absolute contraindication for its use.

Despite strong evidence of an immunologic element in the pathogenesis of systemic sclerosis, it remains one of the few immunologically mediated rheumatic diseases in which a clear role for immunosuppressive and cytotxic agents remains to be defined. General use of corticosteroids in scleroderma has produced disappointing, if not deleterious, results. Experience with cytotoxic drugs has been meager, and broad guidelines for their use in patients with systemic sclerosis are difficult to determine. Nonetheless, their short-term use in subgroups of patients with prominent inflammatory features and manifestations overlapping other rheumatic diseases is proposed; one such subgroup is patients with rapidly progressive disease and prominent pulmonary parenchymal inflammation. If the experience in patients with idiopathic interstitial pulmonary fibrosis can be extrapolated to scleroderma patients with pulmonary involvement, identification of an early inflammatory stage with potential reversibility provides a rationale for intervention with immunosuppressive agents. The techniques of bronchalveolar lavage and gallium scanning help identify such patients. Because pulmonary involvement contributes significantly to scleroderma mortality, patients with evidence of early active pulmonary involvement are treated with tapering doses of corticosteriods (prednisone, 1 to 2 mg/kg/day for 60 to 90 days). If available techniques reveal continued inflammation (neutrophils), we recommend cyclophosphamide (Cytoxan, 2 to 3 mg/kg/day). Duration of treatment should depend on the clinical response and the appearance of significant bone marrow suppression (leukopenia, anemia, thrombocytopenia) that often accompanies use of this agent. Complete blood counts and pulmonary function studies should be performed serially (at least monthly) to monitor the response to therapy. Clear understanding on the part of the patient and family of the potential risks and comittment to frequent follow-up visits that attend use of these agents should be gained before embarking on such treatment. Such potentially lethal therapy should be reserved for patients with objective evidence of significant involvement of lung parenchyma.

SUPPORTIVE MEASURES

Skin

Skin involvement in scleroderma evolves through three stages: an early edematous phase, indurative phase, and atrophic phase, often with skin softening and thickening. Skin involvement contributes little to mortality and morbidity but takes a psychologic toll on the patient by serving as an inescapable reminder of his or her affliction. Many agents, including salicylates, nonsteroidal anti-inflammatory drugs, glucocorticoids, corticotropin, EDTA, relaxin, tocapherol (vitamin E), epsilon aminocaproic acid (EACA), triiodothyronine (T3), potassium para-aminobenzoic acid (Potaba), dimethyl sulfoxide (DMSO), have been used without reproducible success in an attempt to halt or reverse skin thickening and tightening. The most valuable intervention for skin involvement in systemic sclerosis is prevention. Creams, lotions, soaps, and bath oils that combat dryness should be used liberally. Avoidance of activities and exposures that may irritate or injure skin, and use of protective coverings (e.g., gloves) are helpful. Regular movement and local massage assist in maintaining pliability and circulation in the skin.

A troublesome consequence of the dermal vascular insufficiency inherent in the disease is the appearance of skin ulcerations, particularly on the distal digits and malleolar and olecranon prominences. Considerable necrotic and infected tissue is often present. Skillful debridement, use of bactericidal cleansing agents, protective dressings, immobilization, and systemic antibiotics are important adjuncts to measures aimed at enhancing nutrient vascular flow (see below). Major surgical intervention (amputations) should be reserved for cases of deep-rooted infection (wet gangrene, osteomyelitis) resistant to medical measures.

RAYNAUD'S PHENOMENON AND PERIPHERAL VASCULAR INSUFFICIENCY

In addition to measures aimed at conserving core body temperature, many vasodilators are used to reverse or prevent episodic exaggerated peripheral vasospasm seen in many patients with systemic sclerosis. The most recent class of agents is calcium channel blockers. Nifedipine, with the strongest direct peripheral vasodilating capability, has been used most, with mixed results. The initial dosage is 10 mg orally 3 times daily, which can be increased to 40 mg every 8 hours. Limiting side effects are postural hypotension, edema, and exacerbation of pre-existing esophageal reflux due to further lowering of lower esophageal sphincter pressure. Nifedipine inhibits transmembrane calcium influx into smooth muscle, a process upon which the contractile mechanism depends. In cardiac muscle, the anticalcium influx action leads to negative inotropic and chronotropic actions. Alternative agents (diltiazam and verapamil) can be tried when postural hypotension limits nifedipine use in Raynaud's phenomenon.

Other vasodilating agents are used in Raynaud's phenomenon, including reserpine (0.25 mg per day orally), which depletes body stores of serotonin and catecholamine; phenoxybenzamine, an α-adrenergic blocking agent (10 to 20 mg 3 times daily); α-methyldopa (0.5 to 2 g per day in divided doses), which inhibits the synthesis of catecholamines via depressed aromatic L-amino acid decarboxylase; guanethidine (up to 50 mg per day), which selectively blocks sympathetic tone by preventing release of norepinephrine at sympathetic neuroeffector junctions and depletes tissue stores of catecholamines; and prozocin, a postsynaptic α-adrenoceptor blocker. Generally speaking, success with these agents is greatest in milder cases of scleroderma associated with Raynaud's phenomenon and in idiopathic Raynaud's phenomenon.

Measures for acute, severe digital ischemia with threatened digital necrosis include intra-arterial reserpine (1 mg bolus) and/or stellate ganglion block. These measures usually are temporary but can provide relief of severe peripheral vasospasm for weeks. Local application of nitroglycerin paste can be helpful in acute cases. Surgical sympathectomy is now widely regarded as an intervention with no benefit in scleroderma-associated or idiopathic Raynaud's phenomenon.

Gastrointestinal

Esophageal dysmotility is the most prevalent gastrointestinal expression of systemic sclerosis. Clinically, it is manifested as dysphagia, reflux peptic esophagitis, and stricture. Both conservative and pharmacologic measures can lessen the frequent esophageal symptoms of patients with systemic sclerosis. Dysphagia is managed by careful mastication and by choosing foods whose consistency promotes easy passage. In severe cases, bethanechol or metoclopromide, motility enhancing agents of uncertain therapeutic effect in systemic sclerosis, may be tried. Pyrosis from reflux of gastric contents can be approached conservatively by reducing the volume of food ingested, avoiding postprandial recumbency, and elevating the head of the bed during sleep. For patients suffering from Sjögren's syndrome, liberal sour-candy sucking helps to generate saliva, which, when swallowed helps to buffer intraluminal esophageal pH. Round-the-clock regimens of antacids (2 hours after meals and at bedtime) can be helpful. In severe cases, histamine-2 receptor blocking agents (cimetidine, ranitidine) can be employed. These agents have side effects (bone marrow suppression, pharmacokinetic interactions with other drugs, dementia, and gynecomastia) that are more prevalent during long-term administration. Sucralfate, a sulfated disaccharide-aluminum complex, minimally absorbed by the gastrointestinal tract which acts as a protective resin by binding to exudative, proteinaceous surfaces and acids, has been shown to promote healing of duodenal ulcers and gastritis. An anecdotally reported but widely appreciated therapeutic effect of the oral suspension form of sucralfate in reflux esophagitis awaits clinical trial and general application in scleroderma populations.

Malabsorption is the hallmark of small intestinal involvement in systemic sclerosis. Causative factors include mucosal atrophy and intestinal hypomotility with resultant bacterial overgrowth. Malabsorption is treated with oral antibiotics, since there is no agent or measure to restore motility or to reverse mucosal atrophy. Severe malnutrition and debilitation secondary to chronic malabsorption are treated with intravenous hyperalimentation.

Large bowel involvement is expressed as chronic constipation and obstipation. Stool softeners and routine laxatives are generally adequate therapy. Agents that depress bowel motility (e.g., narcotics) should be avoided, as they can lead to severe high fecal impactions requiring surgical extrusion.

Cardiopulmonary

Few, if any, therapeutic interventions exist for established pulmonary fibrosis. Pulmonary hypertension is the most serious sequela of interstitial fibrosis. Many agents (hydroalazine, nifedipine, nitroglycerin, isoproterenol) have been used in pulmonary hypertension but results are erratic. Hemodynamic proof of efficacy should be obtained in each patient before an agent is administered chronically. Alleviation of arterial hypoxia with chronic oxygen administration helps to lower pulmonary artery pressure and may improve function. Cor pulmonale which results from chronic pulmonary hypertension is largely untreatable aside from maintaining optimal fluid status and filling pressures. Digitalis and diuretics should be used judiciously, particularly when pericardial effusion is present, because of the association with renal complications. Newer, highly sensitive techniques have detected cardiac microcirculatory abnormalities in most patients with diffuse generalized scleroderma. The management of symptoms of coronary insufficiency in scleroderma patients is the same as in any other patient. Because of the strong microvascular component in their disease, scleroderma patients are poor candidates for coronary bypass procedures.

Pericarditis with pericardial effusion is common in scleroderma and may respond to cautious diuresis, corticosteroids, and/or pericardial window procedures if hemodynamically significant. There is a strong correlation between the presence of pericardial effusion and the emergence of renal failure in scleroderma.

Renal

Renal involvement in systemic sclerosis previously carried a grim prognosis. However, recently, greater recognition of the risk factors for scleroderma renal disease (proteinuria, hypertension, microangiopathic hemolytic anemia, and pericardial effusion), including hyperreninemia, have allowed earlier diagnosis and newer, more rational, approaches to treatment, with dramatic results. Control of blood pressure with the wide array of available vasodilators has preserved and improved renal function in many patients. Captopril, an inhibitor of the angiotensin-converting enzyme, is considered the drug of choice in treating hypertension in the setting of renal involvement. The earlier captopril therapy is instituted in the setting of renal insufficiency, the greater the chance of restoration of lost function. Dialysis can be lifesaving once uremia has ensued and can allow returns after months to years of self-sustaining renal function in some patients. Renal transplantation has been performed with limited success. Some reports exist of recurrence of histopathologic features of scleroderma kidney in allografts, although these features are difficult to distinguish from those of chronic allograft rejection.

Musculoskeletal

Systemic sclerosis can be accompanied by diffuse arthralgias, but true inflammatory joint involvement is unusual. Musculoskeletal pain can be treated with salicylates or other nonsteroidal anti-inflammatory agents. Exercise and musculoskeletal conditioning help prevent flexion contractures and maintain muscle strength. The inflammatory myopathy that accompanies systemic sclerosis (documented by elevated serum creatine phosphokinase and inflammatory changes on muscle biopsy) can be treated with corticosteroids and cytotoxic agents when indicated, as in other patients with myositis.

Psychologic

As with any chronic illness, psychologic factors have considerable influence on the course of the disease and response to therapy. The layman's interpretation of available information on systemic sclerosis often leaves the patient with considerable fear and anxiety. The physician must be supportive and tolerant as he or she helps the patient through the various psychologic stages that ultimately lead to acceptance of the disease. The variable expression of systemic sclerosis should be emphasized and the good prognosis of the CREST variant stressed. When patients have finally come to grips with their affliction, they can be invaluable partners in the general therapeutic approach. Psychophysiologic factors play a role in many aspects of the disease and have formed a basis for trials of biofeedback therapy in Raynaud's phenomenon. Patients find satisfaction in therapeutic measures in which they play an active role. Organizations such as the Arthritis Foundation, and the Scleroderma Foundation provide literature on research efforts directed at scleroderma, which patients find comforting.

POLYMYOSITIS AND DERMATOMYOSITIS

SUBRAMANIAM SRIRAM, M.D.
WALTER G. BRADLEY, M.D., F.R.C.P.

Polymyositis (PM) and dermatomyositis (DM) comprise a heterogeneous group of inflammatory disorders of the skeletal muscle. This complex (PM and DM) may occur alone or may be associated with systemic autoimmune disorders, such as rheumatoid arthritis, systemic lupus erythematosus, and scleroderma. The PM-DM complex is also associated with systemic malignancies. The childhood form of polymyositis is clinically different in that systemic vasculitis, especially vasculitis involving the gastrointestinal tract, is quite common. No single criterion is sufficient to make the diagnosis of PM-DM. The diagnosis is usually made from a composite of clinical findings, elevated creatine kinase (CK) levels in the serum, electromyogram showing increased insertional activity and myopathic potentials, and muscle biopsy evidence of interstitial and perivascular inflammatory cell infiltration and fiber necrosis. PM-DM is a treatable form of muscle disorder, hence this disease should be differentiated from other myopathies and the hereditary muscular dystrophies that are largely untreatable.

THERAPEUTIC RATIONALE

PM-DM have a number of clinical associations which are important to seek. Almost every patient with dermatomyositis over the age of 60 has an underlying neoplasm, and the frequency is almost as high in those with polymyositis in this age group. In younger patients, about a third have a collagen vascular disorder which may require treatment on its own, and conveys a poor prognosis. A moderate proportion of patients have positive toxoplasma titers, and a very small number have evidence of acute toxoplasma infection requiring treatment.

Although the etiologic agent of the PM-DM complex is not known in the vast majority of cases, there is sufficient evidence to suggest that there is an underlying autoimmune process. Since the antigen(s) involved in the autoimmune process are unknown, broad-spectrum immunosuppression with corticosteroids and cytotoxic agents has been used in the treatment. The treatment strategies for the adult and childhood forms of the disease are identical, although the use of cytotoxic therapy in childhood requires greater justification because of the genetic and gonadal damage, and potential long-term predilection for the development of lymphoid malignancies. Two issues complicate treatment of PM-DM. First, the natural history of the untreated disease is not adequately known. Second, there has been no long-term prospective double-blind trial of the various regimens now employed. Thus, it is impossible to prove the efficacy of these regimens in causing remissions or halting the progression of the disease. In spite of these drawbacks, we are convinced of the efficacy of corticosteroids and cytotoxic agents in the treatment of this disease. Even those clinicians who express skepticism about corticosteroids use a regimen similar to that described below.

CORTICOSTEROIDS

Corticosteroids form the mainstay of the therapeutic regimen and prednisone is the drug of first choice. Treatment is begun with a single morning dose of 1.5 mg/kg/body weight. Single daily or alternate daily dosage appears to cause fewer side effects than divided daily doses. Larger doses or divided dose schedules may be given to patients with extreme weakness, systemic toxicity, or those in respiratory distress. The clinical state, that is, the muscle strength, serum CK levels, and erythrocyte sedimentation rate (where appropriate) should be monitored biweekly during the first 8 weeks and then at monthly intervals thereafter. The Medical Research Council (MRC) scale of grading muscle strength should be used. 0, no movement of muscle groups; 1, flicker of movement; 2, movement with gravity eliminated; 3, movement against gravity but not against resistance; 4, movement against resistance; and 5, normal. The serum CK level is generally reduced following initiation of corticosteroid therapy. The mechanism of this reduction is unclear, but a similar reduction occurs in muscular dystrophies treated with corticosteroids, though no therapeutic benefit occurs in these cases. However, the CK is a useful monitor of disease activity in patients who have become stabilized on a dose of corticosteroids. If these patients deteriorate clinically with an increasing CK, then they have suffered a relapse. Thus, the CK should be measured serially in patients undergoing treatment. Most patients begin to show clinical and biochemical improvement within 2 to 12 weeks, depending upon chronicity. Occasionally 4 to 6 months of high-dose corticosteroids are necessary before improvement becomes apparent. Prolonged high-dose corticosteroids therapy almost invariably causes Cushingoid side effects. Interestingly, some patients with florid inflammatory disease do not develop such side effects and behave almost as though there were an increased metabolism of corticosteroids. It is difficult to know when a patient should be classified as being "corticosteroid unresponsive," for even after 6 months of treatment, reduction in dosage in such patients often results in further deteririation. Antacids and potassium supplement should be used in patients taking corticosteroids. Histamine H_2 blockers such as cimetidine may be required. Supplemental calcium (0.5 gm calcium per day) and vitamin D (50,000 units biweekly) are given concomitantly to retard corticosteroid-induced osteoporosis. Careful watch should be kept on the blood pressure, blood sugar, and potential infections,and in the long term on cataracts and osteoporosis.

As soon as clinical improvement allows, that is as soon as the patient appears to have reached a plateau in improvement, the dose of prednisone can be gradually reduced while the muscle strength and serum CK are continually being monitored. In view of the reduced side effects and the lack of suppression of the hypothalamic-pituitary-adrenal (HPA) axis, it is preferable to change the patient from a single daily dose to an every other day regimen. However, there have been no clinical studies comparing the effects of daily and alternate-day dosage in the management of the PM-DM complex. An effective way to convert to an alternate-day therapy is to double the daily corticosteroid dose on the first day and then to reduce the dose on the alternate day. An example of such conversion in a patient receiving 40 mg of prednisone daily for 6 months would be: first week, 80-40-80-35-80-30-80; second week, 25-80-20-15-80-10; third week, 80-7.5-80-5-80-2.5-80-0. The rapidity with which these changes can be made depends on the duration of the therapy prior to switching to alternate-day dose and on the adequacy of control of the underlying disease activity. When the alternate-day regimen has been established, cautious reduction of the total corticosteroid dose is continued in an attempt to use the least dose that will effectively suppress the spontaneously fluctuating levels of polymyositis.

All the well-known side effects of long-term corticosteroid therapy are seen in patients with PM-DM receiving prednisone. These occur in roughly 16 to 22 percent of patients and are fatal in 1 to 3 percent. Corticosteroid myopathy of some degree occurs in almost all patients receiving high-dose prednisone. A negative nitrogen balance and type 2 muscle fiber atrophy are universal findings in such patients. An increase of muscle weakness in patients previously stabilized by corticosteroid therapy poses a difficult diagnostic problem: Is the weakness due to increased myositic activity or to corticosteroid myopathy? The latter should be considered when a patient on long-term high-dose corticosteroid therapy begins to deteriorate without a concomitant rise in serum CK. The diagnosis can be arrived at clinically by reducing the dose of prednisone. If the deterioration results from increased myositic activity, muscle weakness and serum CK will increase. If corticosteroid myopathy is the main problem, then muscle weakness will improve with reduction in dosage. The diagnosis of corticosteroid myopathy may be supported by the finding of a normal serum CK level and a muscle biopsy showing no inflammation but only type 2 fiber atrophy. It seems likely that in most patients with active myositis treated with prednisone, there is a balance between weakness due to myositis and that due to corticosteroid myopathy.

If relapse occurs the dose of prednisone is raised usually to half the difference between the current dosage and the maximal effective dosage, and continued until control is achieved. About 75 percent of patients can stop therapy within 5 years of the onset, though evidence of disease activity continues in the remainder who require continuing corticosteroid therapy. High pulse corticosteroids, such as 1 to 1.5 gm of intravenous methylprednisolone, have been used for a few patients, although this therapy remains experimental.

CYTOTOXIC IMMUNOSUPPRESSIVE THERAPY

Cytotoxic immunosuppressant drugs have been used for "corticosteroid saving effects." They were originally used for patients with corticosteroid failure, but recent evidence indicates that they are best given early in the disease at the same time as corticosteroids are initiated. Our experience indicates that patients with disease that is more severe and of longer duration benefit when they begin to receive corticosteroids and a cytotoxic immunosuppressant simultaneously. We have treated a few patients with cytotoxic agents alone and find them to be relatively ineffective unless they are combined with corticosteroids. There are no clearly established guidelines for the choice of cytotoxic agents. Cycle specific agents, such as azathioprine, and phase specific agents, such as methotrexate, have been used. It is currently uncertain whether treatment should aim at reducing a specific T cell subset, and whether blood level of that subset has any relevance to the myositis. Our experience indicates that it is necessary to reduce the total blood lymphocyte count to 750 to 900/mm^3, while keeping the other formed elements of the blood normal. We adjust the dose depending upon blood counts; the frequency with which blood counts are obtained relates to which drug is being used.

METHOTREXATE

This folic acid analog, which binds to the naturally occurring enzyme dihydrofolate reductase with a far greater affinity than the natural substrate dihydrofolic acid, prevents the synthesis of thymidine and hence DNA. Methotrexate is given in weekly intravenous injections with a starting dose of 10 to 15 mg. Weekly blood counts and liver enzymes are measured (SGOT, SGPT, and alkaline phosphate) and the patient examined for stomatitis, sore throat, and skin rash. The dose is gradually increased to 30 to 50 mg weekly (0.5 to 0.8 mg/kg/body weight). After several weeks (16 to 20 w) of such therapy, and with concomitant improvement in clinical symptoms, the dose is spread out to biweekly, triweekly, or monthly intervals. If sustained clinical improvement is present the dose can eventually be stopped. Oral methotrexate has been used in some cases.

AZATHIOPRINE

This purine analog is converted in vivo to 6-mercaptopurine where it inhibits purine biosynthesis. Azathioprine is administered orally at a dose of 1.5 to 2.5 mg/kg/body weight. The clinical response takes longer to become apparent than with methotrexate, and an adequate therapeutic trial may require at least 6 to 9 months. Serial hemograms (at 1- to 3-week intervals) should be carried out. Liver function tests and chest x-rays are required at intervals (about 3 monthly) because of the potential risk of hepatitis and pulmonary fibrosis. Development of malignancy (usually a lymphoma) in PM-DM patients receiving cytotoxic immunosuppressive therapy is a possibility, although one which we have never observed.

CYCLOPHOSPHAMIDE

Oral treatment with cyclophosphamide, 1.5 to 2.5 mg/kg/day in divided doses, is more rapidly effective than azathioprine. It appears to have a greater toxic effect upon B cells. Though more toxicity has been reported with this drug than with azathioprine, when the dosage is regulated to reduce the total lymphocyte count to 750 to 900/mm^3 with weekly blood counts, we have rarely seen more than slight hair loss. We have not seen the hemorrhagic cystitis which has been reported with high dosages.

Chlorambucil has been used in severe refractory cases, although its toxicity appears to exceed that of other agents.

Nonsteroidal anti-inflammatory agents have no effect on the myositis. They may occasionally be used to treat the arthralgias and nonspecific aches seen in patients with mild PM-DM and rheumatologic conditions not requiring corticosteroid therapy.

PLASMAPHERESIS

Though there are some reports of beneficial effects of plasmapheresis in PM-DM, our experience with 6 patients with a variety of different types of myositis, including one associated with systemic lupus erythematosus, failed to show any benefit.

PHYSICAL THERAPY

Along with immunosuppressive therapy, physical therapy should form a part of the therapeutic regimen. During the acute stage of severe inflammation passive range of motion to prevent soft tissue contractures should be carried out twice daily, but active motion should be discouraged. During recovery or when acute inflammation is not so severe, activity is encouraged. Occupational therapy should be used to help functions that are permanently lost. Aids and appliances, including orthoses and wheelchairs, can be of great help. Patients with weakness of pharyngeal muscles should be followed closely for aspiration. If swallowing difficulty persists, feeding should be done via nasogastric tube.

PROGNOSIS

Although there is considerable difference in the overall prognosis of patients with treated PM-DM at different centers, certain general prognositc features are apparent. In patients with PM-DM associated with systemic malignancy the prognosis is governed by the progression of the tumor. Such patients have the highest mortality. Adults fare worse than children and blacks do worse than whites. Patients with disease involving pharyngeal muscles have a higher morbidity from aspiration pneumonia. Patients with cardiac involvement (usually manifesting as congestive cardiac failure) generally have a worse prognosis. PM-DM are a group of treatable diseases with a large degree of morbidity and mortality, both from disease and, to some extent, from therapy. However, it is justified to describe then as "curable" in a fairly large number of cases. It is, therefore, important to make a proper diagnosis and to treat patients vigorously and as early as possible.

ATOPIC DERMATITIS

JAMES E. RASMUSSEN, M.D.

Atopic dermatitis is not easy to treat. It has a wide variety of clinical manifestations ranging from dry, xerotic skin to the wet, oozing, acute form of eczema which is frequently secondarily infected. In addition, there is a chronic recalcitrant component of lichenification. Patients of all ages can be affected, which further complicates therapy, since drugs useful in adults may be too irritating or cause too much trouble with percutaneous absorption to be safely used in infants and children. Finally, the disease can present on any part of the body with the exception of mucous membranes. Treatment that is quite suitable for the hands and feet would be inappropriate for the more sensitive flexural areas and may produce unpleasant side effects in these intertriginous areas as well as on the face and near mucous membranes.

There is no one therapy that is appropriate for all stages of the disease at every age and part of the body. Consequently, many physicians have a tendency to regionalize therapy with one medication for the face and other for the scalp and a third for the rest of the body. If these multiple treatments are further compounded by attempts to manipulate the diet, environment, bathing habits, exposure to pets, and skin irritability, the plethora of therapeutic modalities will frequently overwhelm the patient's or parent's ability to comply.

It is far better to begin with what I consider basic therapy that will suffice for 75 percent of all patients with atopic dermatitis, adding to or modifying this regimen only if the treatment is not satisfactory. Basic therapy usually consists of a simple lubricant, such as Eucerin or Nivea, applied as often during the day as needed, as well as an intermediate strength topical steroid (triamcinolone 0.1%) applied no more than twice a day. If one insists that these two modalities be followed faithfully and resists the urge to add 5 or 10 other items, most patients will do quite well. I often see patients returning to my practice with their disease unchanged from the initial visit and the skin extremly dry. I do not add other forms of therapy, but insist that the patients obtain satisfactory lubrication before moving on to other, more difficult forms of therapy. If the skin is not well hydrated, it is unlikely that atopic dermatitis will change significantly.

GENERAL THERAPY

Treatment of Xerosis

Most patients with atopic dermatitis have "dry" skin and need to use lubricants. In some, the xerosis is confined to the areas of inflammation such as cheeks, antecubital, and popliteal fossa. In others, the xerosis extends far beyond areas involved with typical atopic dermatitis, and in some patients it takes the form of ichthyosis vulgaris. The dryness is much worse in the winter time and may become less apparent or even completely disappear in the warm, humid summer months. Lubricants can be divided empirically into two groups: lipids and water binders.

Lipids. Lipids is a generic term for most cream and ointment lubricants. The heavier the lubricant, the more effectively it will fight dryness. Unfortunately, heavier lubricants rub in quite poorly, particularly in the colder winter months, and are less cosmetically acceptable as patients age. There are many to choose from, but I prefer Eucerin (approximately 50 percent water, 50 percent petrolatum), Nivea (a somewhat lighter cream), and Vaseline (petrolatum). The least expensive lubricant is Crisco solid vegetable shortening ("the white cream in the blue tub"). Crisco is available for about a $1.00 per pound, which is approximately one-fifth to one-tenth the cost of other commercial lubricants. Liquid lubricants such as Keri lotion, Vaseline Intensive Care hand lotion, and so on, are much less able to lubricate dry skin and require much more frequent applications.

Water Binders. Many small molecules bind water hydroscopically and consequently may make useful lubricants. Urea, citric acid, lactic acid, and salicylic acid can all be used in relatively low concentrations as lubricants in patients who do not like the frequent use of very greasy medications. Unfortunately, many of these are somewhat irritating to patients with atopic dermatitis.

Bath oils are another means of lubricating the skin. They have two principal problems. They make both the patients and the tub slippery. For the stable adult with atopic dermatitis, they pose relatively little hazard, but children and senior citizens may find themselves falling in the tub or slipping out of their parent's hands. Consequently I rarely use bath oils in the bath, but usually advise application after bathing if the patient cares to use them. Room humidifiers are not particularly effective during the winter and are unnecessary during the summer. It is possible to raise humidity substantially in the winter, but this usually produces fogging of windows and the effects last only while the patient is confined to one room of the house. They do have a strong psychologic appeal to parents, however.

Avoid Irritation

The skin of patients with atopic dermatitis is easily irritated because it is dry and inflamed. In addition, atopics have a wide variety of abnormal physiologic functions of the skin, such as decreased sweating and abnormal vascular responses, which make them quite susceptible to environmental problems. Patients with atopic dermatitis are commonly stated to be "allergic" to wool, but this is rarely the case. They are, however, very easily irritated by rough woolen fabrics, and the inherent softness of cotton makes it the fabric of choice.

Atopics do worse in a cold, dry climate and many spontaneously improve during the spring and summer. Excessive heat and perspiration often produce severe pruritus, however. Although not everyone is fortunate enough to live in an ideal locale, I rarely suggest that patients move purely for the management of atopic dermatitis. Frequently, while the climate may agree with them, they may develop other problems, such as asthma or hay fever due to pollens. Atopics should not be ecounraged to participate in strenuous exercise during warm, humid weather. Most patients with atopic dermatitis can tolerate water without irritation, so that an excellent outdoor playtime activity for young children is swimming or wading.

Harsh soaps should be avoided at all costs. If the patient does not experience pain or irritation when bathing, this should be done on a daily basis. Mild soaps, such as Dove, Camay, Tone, or the more expensive "hypoallergenic" soaps, such as Nivea and Oilatum, should be used to wash the affected areas. Immediately after leaving the bath, the patient's skin should be heavily lubricated, as the relief associated with exposure to water is quite temporary, and flares of itching are commonly associated with the subsequent evaporation.

SPECIFIC THERAPY

Topical Corticosteroids

No other drugs are more important in the management of patient than topical corticosteroids. The choice of drug should depend upon extent of disease, severity, site, and cost. In general,it is best to use intermediate strength corticosteroids for initial therapy in most areas of the body. I prefer 0.1 to 0.025% triamcinolone (generic or Aristocort or Kenalog). Other useful choices are Synalar, Cordran, and Westcort. As the disease responds, milder strength corticosteroids are frequently effective. Milder corticosteroids are most appropriate for prolonged use in intertriginous areas, the genitalia, and the face. Here I prefer 1.0 to 2.50% hydrocortisone (generic or Synacort, Cort-Dome, Nutracort, and others). When lichenification is a main component of the eczema, or when the disease is located primarily in acral areas, hydrocortisone is not usually strong enough to achieve a satisfactory effect. In these situations, much more potent corticosteroids can be used safely for short periods of time (up to 2 weeks), and here my choices are primarly brand name items (Topicort, Lidex, Valisone, and others).

Topical corticosteroids should never be applied more than twice a day. More frequent application is not directly related to an increase in efficacy, but it does substantially increase the cost of these medications. The treating physician should recognize that atopic dermatitis is a widespread and chronic disease. Consequently, prescribing corticosteroids in 15 or 30-gram tubes is not appropriate unless the areas affected are limited to such sites as the hands or the feet. Corticosteroids should usually be prescribed in bulk quantities, such as $^1/_2$- to 1-pound containers. While these cost more initially, the cost per gram of steroid is substantially less. Most pharmacies do not carry these bulk sizes but will do so if requested.

Corticosteroids come in many different vehicles: gels, lotions, creams, and ointments. The appropriate choice will depend upon the state of the skin, the site to be treated, and the season of the year. Ointments are much more lubricating than lotions or gels. For general all-around use, however, I usually prefer creams, since they are suitable in almost all sites and during all seasons of the year. Parents and patients should be cautioned that the steroid by itself should never be used to achieve lubrication. As noted, the corticosteroid should not usually be applied more than twice a day, whereas lubricants may need to be applied 4 times a day or more.

Corticosteroids are much more effective when applied under moist occlusive dressings. In addition, this type of dressing usually soothes the inflamed skin of patients with atopic dermatitis, dries up the weeping exudative lesions, and helps remove superficial crusts. Consequently, I usually begin therapy with a thin film of a corticosteroid covered with a reasonably heavy lubricant. The patient is then put into a pair of long-sleeved wet pajamas, covered with a plastic sauna-suit (exercise suit). These are commonly available in adult sizes in many sporting goods stores. Children's sizes are much more difficult to come by, and frequently the physician must resort to a sweat suit, warm-up jersey, or several extra pairs of dry pajamas as a substitute. This wet dressing is kept on for several hours, once to 3 times per day. Immediately upon removing the sauna suit or wet pajamas, the patient must be thoroughly lubricated to prevent the retained moisture from evaporating. Wet pajamas alone produce a substantial amount of heat loss, so the room temperature must be much warmer than usual or the patient will begin shivering. Steroids should not be occluded for more than 5 to 10 days, since atrophy may result.

Antipruritics

Systemically administered antihistamines also play an important role in reducing inflammation and scratching of patients with atopic eczema. Hydroxyzine (Atarax, Vistaril) is my drug of choice, since in many studies it has proved to be a more potent antihistamine than other commercial brands. The dose will vary depending upon the age of the patient and tolerance to the effects of the drug, but usually ranges from 1 to 3 mg/kg/day. Twice that dose can be taken safely if the patient exhibits tolerance, which usually occurs the longer the medication has been used. I generally reserve these antipruritic medications for nighttime use because of the problem of rapid tolerance when they are used 4 times daily. H_2 blockers (cimetidine) should not be used routinely in the management of atopic dermatitis.

At times it may be appropriate to use other topical antipruritic agents, such as Pramosone or Sarna. In some patients they are remarkably effective.

In my experience, cromolyn (sodium cromoglycate) is of little value in the oral or topical management of patients with atopic dermatitis. Several studies have shown that patients with food hypersensitivity may have a somewhat increased tolerance to oral allergens when using cromolyn, but this drug has little direct effect on the skin disease. In addition, it is not available in a form suitable for topical administration.

Coal Tar

Topical application of coal tar is one of the oldest means of treating atopic dermatitis. It still has a place when topical corticosteroids are not completely effective. There are many different forms of coal tar, and the interested physician should appreciate that several can produce substantial irritation of atopic skin, particularly those contained in a gel vehicle (Estar, PsoriGel). Atopics respond better to coal tar in cream or ointment preparations, such as 10% liquor carbonis detergens in water-washable base, 2% crude coal tar in petrolatum, or some of the commercially available tar creams and oil (T-derm, Fototar, Balnetar, and many others). Tars are quite messy to use and produce substantial staining of clothing and bedding; consequently, they are best used at night and washed off in the morning. In addition, coal tars are moderate photosensitizers and should never be used immediately before exposure to high-intensity ultraviolet lights, such as the sun. Tars are somewhat irritating to mucous membranes and intertriginous areas, so they should be used with caution in and around these areas. They can occasionally produce a mild bacterial or sterile folliculitis which usually takes the form of an acneiform eruption or small boils. This usually responds to topical or systemic antibiotics and rarely poses a serious threat in the management of the patient.

Ultraviolet Light

Natural or artificial ultraviolet (UV) light has become an increasingly important modality in the management of chronic, unresponsive atopic dermatitis. Ultra violet B (UVB), as opposed to UVA or UVC, is the preferred wave length, primarily because it is readily accessible in most phototherapy centers. Most departments of dermatology and many physical therapy units will have UVB light units. When not available, home units may be appropriate. These units are available in a wide variety of styles at prices ranging from about $700 to $15,000. Light therapy should be given on a regular basis, at least 3 to 4 times a week, to achieve maximum effectiveness. Its onset of action is slow and most patients do not notice any beneficial response during the first 4 to 6 weeks. Light therapy is not completely effective when used alone and must always be accompanied by topical corticosteroids. The mechanism of action of UV light is not known but probably depends in part on depletion of Langerhans' cells in the epidermis as well as on the nonspecific effect referred to as "hardening." Hardened skin is less easily irritated by a variety of stimuli.

ANTIBIOTICS AND ANTISEPTICS

Investigations have shown that the involved skin of patients with atopic dermatitis has substantially abnormal microflora. Large numbers of coagulase-positive *Staphylococcus aureus* reside in both the wet, weeping areas and the dryer, lichenified sites. Quantitative microbiologic studies frequently show counts of 10^5 and 10^6 organisms per square centimeter. At times the skin of patients with atopic dermatitis appears overtly infected, although cellulitis and sepsis are uncommon. Several groups of investigators have shown that patients with atopic dermatitis have high levels of antistaphylococcal IgE. They postulate that antistaphylococcal IgE binds to bacterial cell products, which in turn release histamine from mast cells. They believe that this cycle is an important factor in the chronic itching that is the main symptom of this disorder.

Consequently, there have been many attempts at degerming the skin of atopics. Topical corticosteroid-antibiotic combinations are effective in reducing the carriage count of *S. aureus*. Unfortunately the antibiotic most commonly used, neomycin, is a moderate allergic sensitizer and frequently produces neomycin-resistant staphylococci. Therefore I believe that corticosteroid-antibiotic combinations should never be used in the routine management of patients with atopic dermatitis. Several double-blind studies have shown that the addition of the antibiotic to the corticosteroid cream does nothing to increase the effectiveness of the corticosteroid when used alone. Routine use of antibacterial soaps such as Hibiclens, Betadine, or Dial can be helpful in the management of selected patients with recalcitrant atopic dermatitis. These soaps are more drying than the ones mentioned above, and when used, extra attention must be paid to lubrication and corticosteroids.

An English group has evaluated the use of a miconazole-hydrocortisone combination. Miconazole is a potent antifungal agent available in this country as Monistat-Derm. Miconazole is also an excellent broad-spectrum antibacterial agent. The English study clearly showed that a miconazole-hydrocortisone combination produced substantial results in about 80 percent of patients who had been unresponsive to other corticosteroids. This was not a controlled study, however, and its results must be interpreted with caution. In addition, miconazole is a relatively expensive topical preparation whose cost may limit its usefulness in patients with widespread disease. Nevertheless it may be an appropriate modality to try in smaller areas of the body when other forms of therapy have not been effective.

Systemic antibiotics may also have a role in the short-term management of patients with atopic dermatitis, whether they appear clinically infected or not.

Most staphylococci are still sensitive to erythromycin and this is the drug of choice for patients with atopic eczema. I normally use 15 to 25 mg/kg in divided daily doses for 2 to 4 weeks. Erythromycin is always used in conjunction with topical corticosteroids. Since many patients with atopic eczema also have asthma, it is important for the prescribing physician to appreciate the interaction between erythromycin and theophylline. Several studies in children and adults using different erythromycin salts have all shown an adverse affect upon the metabolism of theophylline. Erythromycin decreases theophylline secretion by about 25 percent accompanied by a concomitant rise in serum theophylline levels. This can occasionally produce signs and symptoms of theophylline toxicity.

ALLERGY THERAPY

The role of food allergy in atopic dermatitis continues to be controversial. There is an increasing amount of recently introduced evidence suggesting that dietary manipulation may be productive in selected groups of patients. These same studies have also pointed out, however, that histories of food sensitivities as well as scratch tests are notoriously unreliable in documenting clinically important allergic skin disease related to oral allergens. Careful challenge studies seem to be the only appropriate means of eliciting the cause and effect relationship. The most common offending allergens appear to be wheat, milk, nuts, eggs, and dyes, with many patients manifesting multiple hypersensitivities.

Before dietary management has begun, the patient or parent must be given thorough instructions and lists of foods that cannot be eaten as well as acceptable substitutes. Simply telling a parent to avoid eggs, milk, wheat, and nuts will be completely unproductive, since they will not know how to eliminate these products or where to find substitutes. In addition, the physician should appreciate that most food hypersensitivity is a relatively short-term problem. Results of follow-up challenge studies show that most patients lose their hypersensitivities after the first few years of life. Those that persist, however, usually remain indefinitely.

Finally, the interested physican should realize the great hardship that substantial dietary modifications impose upon family life. You must be able to provide them positive support by means of handouts, counseling with dietitians, lists of stores that carry acceptable food substitutes, and so on. Even with this support, compliance with major dietary manipulations is very poor. Several studies have suggested that fewer than 50 percent of the patients maintained dietary modifications for more than 3 to 6 months. This will be particularly true if the diet imposes a substantial economic burden on the household.

Other groups of authors have looked, not at the therapy of established atopic dermatitis, but at its prevention via modification of maternal and infant feeding habits. The studies here are also controversial and no clear pattern has emerged. It would seem prudent, however, to suggest that parents of atopic patients delay the introduction of potentially allergic foods for as long as is nutritionally possible (6 months). Breast feeding should be encouraged in this population, and at the same time the diet of the mother should also be regulated to keep potential allergens from appearing in her breast milk. At no time, however, should the general nutrition of the infant suffer because of the possibility of development of asthma, eczema, and so on.

One of the most rapidly emerging areas in allergy management of asthma patients with atopic dermatitis focuses on the role of mites as potential allergens. The common house dust mite has been shown to play a role in the cutaneous symptoms of affected patients and may explain why many patients who do well in the hospital have a disease flare when returning home to crawl and sit on the carpet. An occasional patient may benefit from substantial environmental modification in which all the carpets are removed from the house and the floors are covered with linoleum or some other easily cleaned surface.

TREATMENT OF COMPLICATIONS

The most substantial complication that any patient with atopic eczema can suffer is infection with herpes simplex. This infection spreads rapidly in atopic patients and can be very difficult to distinguish from acute weeping eczema. The presence of multiple small vesicles is very suggestive of this disorder, which can produce substantial morbidity, but fortunately is usually not fatal. With the advent of newer oral, intravenous, and topical antiviral agents, it becomes increasingly important to establish the diagnosis with certainty. A Tzanck test is a rapid, clinically reliable tool to evaluate the presence of herpes. Viral cultures are also appropriate, although they take from 1 to 3 days and are not available except in large institutions.

Chronic and recurrent infections can be seen in the hyperimmunoglobulin E syndrome (Job's syndrome), which fortunately is uncommon in the atopic population. Appropriate management will probably consist of referral to a specialist in immunology. Repeat cultures and sensitivities are important to identify the causative organism and suggest an appropriate antibiotic.

CONTACT DERMATITIS

ERNST EPSTEIN, M.D.
HOWARD I. MAIBACH, M.D.

Treatment of contact dermatitis requires two completely separate maneuvers: prevention of further contact with the cause and suppression of the skin eruption. In order to prevent future contact with the offending agent, the cause must be identified. Identifying the cause of contact dermatitis may be straightforward as in the case of poison ivy/poison oak contact dermatitis with its typical streaks and patches of acute vesiculating dermatitis in someone who has had brush exposure. On the other hand, finding the cause(s) in the case of industrial contact dermatitis can be an extremely difficult and tedious task requiring sophisticated patch testing and a knowledge of industrial processes and allergens. Active treatment of dermatitis is important since dermatitis has a tendency to persist, and, once initiated, it tends to continue on its own even though the originating cause has been eliminated.

The treatment of dermatitis varies according to the severity of the eruption, not its cause. *Systemic and topical therapy of dermatoses are similar when the stages of the rash are similar*. Consequently, contact dermatitis from poison oak or poison ivy is treated in the same manner as an equally severe rash caused by benzocaine in a topical anesthetic ointment. Chronic lichenified dermatoses are treated similarly whether they represent a hand dermatitis in a mason caused by allergy to chrome in cement or a foot dermatitis caused by rubber compounds in shoes.

PRINCIPLES OF SYSTEMIC TREATMENT

Corticosteroids

Corticosteroids are the only systemic anti-inflammatory agents effective in treating dermatitis. They have revolutionized the treatment of severe contact dermatitis. Adequate doses of systemic corticoids will produce symptomatic improvement in acute dermatitis in 6 to 12 hours. In the pre-corticosteroid era, poison ivy and poison oak contact dermatitis in North America often resulted in severe, blistering eruptions that produced misery for weeks. These horrors are a thing of the past. If a patient with acute contact dermatitis fails to improve within 24 hours after starting systemic corticosteroids, the dose is too low or the diagnosis is in error.

Prednisone by mouth is the corticosteroid of choice and can usually be given as a single morning dose. Prednisone is a short-acting corticosteroid; therefore, very severe dermatoses may require splitting the daily prednisone ration into morning and evening doses. A useful schedule for moderately severe poison ivy/poison oak contact dermatitis is described in Table 1. Very severe cases require more corticoid; this need can be satisfied by initiating treatment with 100 to 200 mg prednisone daily and tapering by 20 to 40 mg per day to a level of 60 mg daily; thereafter follow the schedule in Table 1.

Even very severe contact dermatitis can usually be controlled within 14 days of initiating systemic corticosteroids. While poison ivy/poison oak contact dermatitis tends to linger and usually requires 7 to 14 days, or even longer, of systemic corticoids, other types of acute contact dermatitis often subside with a brief course of prednisone in a dosage of 60 mg, 40 mg, and 20 mg per day for a total of 3 days. Systemic corticoids produce rapid improvement in severe disease, whereas topical corticoids do not. The aim is to shift as soon as possible from systemic to topical corticosteroids. Systemic corticosteroids are used to reduce edema and inflammation sufficiently for topical corticosteroids to be effective. If oral corticoid therapy is required for more than 3 weeks, the treating physician should consider dermatologic consultation and patch testing.

Prednisone and prednisolone are the systemic corticosteroids of choice. Other steroids cost more and have the distinct disadvantage of being long-acting. Injectible, repository corticosteroids are rarely indicated for systemic therapy because of the difficulty in ascertaining drug release. Short courses of systemic corticosteroids are remarkably safe. Peptic ulceration, diabetes, and hypertension require caution in using even short-term systemic corticosteroids. The side effects of short courses of corticosteroids are few and consist mainly of weight gain, gastrointestinal distress, and mood changes. Mild mood changes, usually jitteriness and insomnia, are fairly common with short-term, high-dose corticosteroid therapy. If the insomnia and nervousness are annoying, low doses of a tranquilizer such as hydroxyzine (25–50 mg), promethazine (12.5–25 mg), or diazepam (5–10 mg) at bedtime are helpful. Avoid barbiturates. On rare occasions, systemic corticosteroids produce severe mood changes, particularly depression. If this occurs, discontinue the drug and consider hospitalizing the patient.

TABLE 1 Schedule for Treating Moderately Severe Contact Dermatitis with Prednisone Tablets as a Single Morning Dose

Day	*Prednisone (mg)*	*Dose (No. of 20-mg Tablets)*
1	80	4
2	70	3½
3	60	3
4	50	2½
5	40	2
6	40	2
7	30	1½
8	30	1½
9	20	1
10	20	1
11	10	½
12	10	½
13	0	0

Other Systemic Agents

Only corticosteroids suppress dermatitis; consequently, we do not use antihistamines, aspirin, or nonsteroidal anti-inflammatory agents. Despite their widespread use, antihistamines do not suppress contact dermatitis. Their sedating effect may lessen patient discomfort; however, it is preferable to make the patient comfortable by suppressing the dermatitis with specific therapy rather than by depressing his sensorium. Occasionally, when there is much discomfort and anxiety, mild sedatives may be helpful. We prefer hydroxyzine, promethazine, or diazepam. Avoid barbiturates.

PRINCIPLES OF TOPICAL THERAPY

Topical therapy has a dual role: it delivers active agents to the skin, and it has nonspecific debriding, soothing, and lubricating actions. Considering these two effects separately removes much of the mystique surrounding topical therapy. Our discussion will be limited to corticosteroids, since they have rendered older ''antidermatitic'' agents largely obsolete. It is best to avoid topical antibiotics (e.g., neomycin, bacitracin) or other antimicrobials such as iodochlorhydroxyquin (Vioform) in treating dermatitis. If secondary infection is present or suspected, a systemic antibiotic such as erythromycin is superior to a topical antibiotic.

Topical Corticosteroids

Topical corticosteroids are usually prescribed as commercially prepared formulations. Remember that they are only effective in the less severe and less acute stages of contact dermatitis. The confusing array of different corticosteroids in a variety of vehicles renders the choice difficult. Topical corticosteroid preparations differ markedly in potency depending on the type of corticosteroid, the concentration, and the vehicle. By restricting your prescriptions to only two topical corticoids, you can cut through the bewildering array of available compounds and achieve good results. Both triamcinolone acetonide and hydrocortisone are available as inexpensive generic drugs and in plain petrolatum as well as cream formulations. The rules are simple: use 0.1% triamcinolone acetonide for the more severe dermatoses, 0.025% triamcinolone for mild to moderately severe rashes, and 2.5% and 1% hydrocortisone for milder dermatoses. These two corticoids provide effective, economical, and rational topical therapy for your patients.

How to Use Topical Corticosteroids

1. Become familiar with a few topical corticosteroids and stick to them.
2. Use the least potent corticosteroid necessary.
3. When using potent corticosteroids, two applications daily are enough. There appears to be little additional corticosteroid effect gained by using a topical corticosteroid more than once or twice a day.
4. Creams and ointment formulations are usually best. Many of the newer corticosteroid gels, solutions, or sprays contain vehicles that may irritate. They are best avoided unless a special location (e.g., hairy areas) makes them the vehicle of choice. Some of the newer cream formulations contain large amounts of propylene glycol and may irritate.

Precautions

Highly potent topical corticosteroids can produce many cutaneous side effects. Most common are atrophy, especially in flexural or skin fold areas, and a rosacea-like dermatitis on the face. Highly potent topical corticosteroids should be used only when needed and for the shortest time possible. Shift to low- or intermediate-potency corticosteroids when the acute phase is over. Remember: 1% hydrocortisone can be used anywhere with almost no cutaneous side effects.

Systemic effects from absorption of topical corticosteroids are possible. In adults, this is rarely a clinical problem with the preparations available in the United States. Exceptions are, (1) when high potency corticosteroids are applied to extensive areas of dermatitis, and (2) if occlusion is used to increase the effectiveness of a corticoid. Occlusion with impermeable plastic films significantly increases corticosteroid potency, absorption, and cutaneous side effects.

Nonspecific Aspects of Topical Therapy

Topical agents may be used for their nonspecific effects, for example, soaks to remove crusts. The nonspecific effects of the cream or ointment base used to deliver a specific topical agent (i.e., corticosteroid) to the skin are often overlooked. A soothing and lubricating effect is desired. The wrong vehicle may aggravate the skin condition and seriously interfere with the effectiveness of the corticosteroid. The nonspecific effects of topical therapy must be appropriate for the stage of dermatitis. Table 2 provides instructions for the appropriate vehicle for each stage of dermatitis. The ground rule in using topical agents is not to irritate the skin.

The Appropriate Vehicle

In general, appropriate vehicles for treating acute dermatoses with crusting and vesiculation are soaks and compresses, while chronic lichenified scaling dermatoses benefit from the lubricating effect of greasy ointments. Creams and cream lotions* are appropriate for acute and subacute dermatoses.

---

*There are two types of lotion. Shake lotions are a mixture of powder and water; calamine lotion is an example. Cream lotions are oil-in-water emulsions. Shake lotions leave a messy residue on the skin and are obsolete.

TABLE 2 Treatment of Contact Dermatitis

Acute (Severe) Dermatitis
- Systemic Treatment
  1. Corticosteroids by mouth, perferably prednisone.
  2. A 10- to 14-day course of systemic corticosteroids usually suffices.
  3. Start with enough corticosteroid; i.e., 60–100 mg prednisone the first day.
- Topical Treatment
  1. Nonspecific soothing compresses or baths with water or aluminum acetate solution (Burow's solution) or dilute vinegar (have the patient add two tablespoons of white vinegar to a quart of water) — a very effective, underused treatment.*
  2. Skin may get too dry; if so, lubricate with a water washable cream
  3. Corticosteroids are wasted, since they don't penetrate the inflamed skin. Don't use them at this point. In severe dermatitis topical therapy is only a minor adjunct, since systemic corticosteroids are doing the real work.

Subacute (Moderate) Dermatitis
- Systemic Treatment
  1. Usually none.
  2. Sometimes low-dose prednisone, once daily or every other day, will be required.
- Topical Treatment
  1. Specific
     - A potent corticosteroid applied sparingly twice daily.
     - Cream or ointment corticosteroid preferred.
     - If skin is dry, use greasy corticosteroid ointment at bedtime.
  2. Nonspecific
     - At this stage lubrication is needed; use cream or greasy ointment corticosteroids.
     - Soaks or compresses are not indicated.
     - Avoid shake lotions, e.g., calamine lotion. They only dry out the skin.

Chronic Dermatitis
- Systemic Treatment
  1. None necessary.
- Topical Treatment
  1. Specific
     - Low, medium, or high potency corticosteroid depending on degree of lichenification (thickening).
     - Corticosteroid in a cream or ointment (petrolatum) vehicle. Greasy ointments are preferable, especially at night.
     - Use potent corticosteroid only once or twice daily.
     - Occlusion overnight with plastic film enhances corticosteroid effect; use on stubborn, severely lichenified dermatoses.
     - Caution: Potent corticosteroids can cause skin thinning and other serious skin side effects. Since the face and skinfold areas are especially vulnerable, avoid anything stronger than 1% hydrocortisone in these regions.
  2. Nonspecific
     - Skin lubrication with nonspecific emollient.
     - Lubricant should be used thinly and frequently.
     - White petrolatum is best lubricant. Used very sparingly, it is cosmetically acceptable.

*Should be called water therapy, since it is the water that is important; additives are mainly of psychologic significance. In oozing and crusted dermatoses, water both debrides and soothes. Let the patient decide the temperature; some get most relief with cold water, others prefer their water therapy hot. When the rash is extensive, showers or baths are the most convenient form of water therapy.

Aggravation Caused by Irritating Topicals

Avoiding an irritating topical medicament is more difficult. It is usually evident to clinicians, although not always to patients, that strong remedies such as undecylenic acid creams and Whitfield's ointment may be suitable for athlete's foot but will aggravate contact dermatitis. Not so well known is the fact that many corticosteroid vehicles as well as skin lubricants are irritating. Emulsifying agents or solvents (e.g., propylene glycol) are the usual offenders. Many of the new high-potency topical corticosteroids contain large amounts of propylene glycol to solubilize the corticoid. The irritant effects of propylene glycol are variable and subtle.

The more acute the dermatitis, the greater the likelihood of irritation from surfactant, emulsifying, or solvent components of the vehicle. The newer gel or solution formulations of topical corticosteroids usually contain high concentrations of solvents and should be used with particular caution. Frequently, vehicle irritation manifests itself only by deterioration of the dermatitis. When irritation or sensitivity to the vehicle is suspected, the best strategy is to switch to a corticoid suspended in white petrolatum.

Many of the widely used, heavily advertised over-the-counter skin lubricants are significantly irritating. Caution patients not to use these preparations. White petrolatum is the cheapest bland lubricant, but some patients find it messy. Commercial water-washable cream bases similar to hydrophilic ointment (USP) are good alternatives for something less greasy. Some of these are mildly irritating.

Aggravation Caused by Allergy to a Topical Medicament

Allergy to a topical remedy occasionally aggravates a dermatitis. Topical medicaments cause irritant dermatitis far more often than allergic contact dermatitis. When topical medicaments produce allergic contact dermatitis, it is usually to a nonessential additive such as neomycin, benzocaine, or an antihistamine. Allergy to a preservative, such as the parabens, is a rare event.

Practical Advice: What to Use and When

Table 2 summarizes systemic and topical therapy for dermatitis. It is traditional to classify the severity of a skin eruption as acute, subacute, or chronic, even though these terms incorporate the dual concepts of severity and duration. Systemic corticosteroids are often indicated for acute dermatitis. Rarely are they needed for subacute or chronic eruptions. Topical therapy is used for all three grades of severity, although topical corticosteroids are not of value in acute dermatitis since they do not penetrate severely swollen and blistered skin. In treating dermatitis, decide whether it is acute, subacute, or chronic; then proceed as outlined in Table 2.

SUMMARY OF TOPICAL THERAPY

Proper topical therapy is decisive in healing contact dermatitis. Here are some guidelines to ensure that the treatment will help rather than hinder healing.

1. Tell the patient not to apply anything to his rash except water and what you have prescribed.
2. Provide the patient with specific written instructions. These are not a substitute for, but an addition to, the physician's verbal instructions.
3. Limit yourself to prescribing a few topical corticoids and one or two lubricants which you have found rarely irritate.
4. White petrolatum is the blandest ointment base and rarely irritates. When used sparingly at bedtime it is acceptable to most patients and can be used on subacute and chronic dermatoses. The two recommended corticoids, hydrocortisone and triamcinolone acetonide, are commercially available suspended in white petrolatum.
5. Avoid producing allergic contact dermatitis to a topical medicament. Do not use topical neomycin, benzocaine, antihistamines, and other well-known offenders; they are of no value and may cause trouble. Use a plain corticosteroid topically.
6. If the dermatitis is infected, use a systemic antibiotic, such as erythromycin or a semisynthetic penicillin, by mouth rather than a topical antibiotic. In those rare situations where a topical antibiotic is indicated, use one that is nonsensitizing, such as tetracycline or erythromycin.
7. Be alert. If a dermatitis fails to improve, consider the possibility of irritation or allergy to a topical agent. A useful maneuver if you are concerned about the safety of the topical regimen is to change to a corticosteroid in a plain white petrolatum base.

PEMPHIGUS AND PEMPHIGOID

BRUCE U. WINTROUB, M.D.
DENNY L. TUFFANELLI, M.D.

PEMPHIGUS

The term pemphigus describes a group of intraepidermal bullous diseases, including vulgaris, foliaceous, and erythematosus. The formerly lethal disease pemphigus vulgaris is the most common of these disorders and is characterized by the formation of suprabasilar intraepidermal blisters, mucous membrane lesions, circulating antibodies against an intercellular epidermal antigen, and deposition of antibody between epidermal cells. In contrast, pemphigus foliaceous is a more benign disorder in which blisters occur high in the epidermis, in the presence of circulating and deposited autoantibodies directed at an intercellular epidermal antigen in the upper layers of the epidermis. Pemphigus erythematosus is a variant of pemphigus foliaceous in which features of lupus erythematosus are present. Another variant of pemphigus foliaceous is Brazilian pemphigus, an endemic arthropod-born infectious disease. This section describes our approach to the therapy of pemphigus vulgaris and will only briefly address the treatment of less common and less severe forms of pemphigus.

Therapy

The initial goal of therapy is to stop blister formation and permit healing of previously formed lesions. When this is achieved, therapy is reduced to the lowest level required to maintain a clinical remission. Therapy is discontinued when circulating autoantibodies are no longer detectable.

Our primary therapeutic program is based on the use of systemic corticosteroids for initial disease control in all patients. To control disease or minimize steroid dose, immunosuppressive agents or sulfones may be employed as secondary agents in some patients. After the diagnosis of pemphigus vulgaris is made, patients begin to receive prednisone (or its equivalent), 20 to 150 mg per day in divided dosages depending on disease severity. Therapeutic response is based on clinical evaluation of patients for active blister formation and clearing of existing lesions. If blistering has diminished, the prednisone dose is reduced by approximately 10 mg per week. Over the next few weeks, the patient is changed to 30 mg prednisone every other day, and if possible, gradually reduced to an every-other-day dosage of 15 mg.

Patients who do not respond to adequate dosages of prednisone after 6 to 8 weeks are treated in the following manner. Prednisone dose is maintained, and Imuran (100 to 150 mg per day) or methotrexate (25 to 50 mg IM per week) is begun. Although we rarely employ cyclophosphamide (100 mg per day), it has been used by others. Patients are monitored for clinical response and drug side effects, and when blistering has ceased, the corticosteroid dose is rapidly reduced as described above. In older individuals in whom the concomitant use of steroids and immunosuppressive drugs may be difficult, dapsone (50 to 100 mg per day) may be employed in place of immunosuppressive agents.

If the patients remain free of active disease for approximately 8 weeks on either of these regimens, serum is analyzed by indirect immunofluorescence for titer of pemphigus autoantibodies. If autoantibodies are not detected, therapy can be discontinued. Prednisone may be further reduced at a rate of 2.5 mg per week. If the patient is receiving an immunosuppressive, it may be tapered over a 1- to 2-month period before discontinuation of the steroids. If autoantibodies are detected therapy may be continued but reduced to the lowest clinically tolerated dose. Dosages are increased only on the basis of clinical reactivation of disease.

Two additional therapeutic modalities have been used to treat pemphigus vulgaris: gold and plasmapheresis. Because gold therapy has been successfully used to treat rheumatoid arthritis and may decrease serum rheumatoid factor levels, it has been employed to treat pemphigus vulgaris. We have not used gold often, but if it is given intramuscularly in weekly 25- to 50-mg doses until a total of 1500 mg is administered, a therapeutic effect may be detected. Patients treated with gold have achieved clinical and serologic remissions. Plasmapheresis to remove pemphigus antibody has also been used to treat pemphigus patients who are poorly controlled on prednisone and/or immunosuppressives. However, a therapeutic benefit has not been demonstrated in all patients, and one needs to give steroids and immunosuppressives to prevent rebound antibody synthesis. Additional complications include immunosuppression due to removal of immunoglobulins and a depletive coagulopathy. For these reasons, plasmapheresis is not recommended for routine treatment.

Outcome and Complications

Prior to the use of corticosteroids, pemphigus vulgaris was a lethal disease and at least 50 percent of patients died from infection or fluid and electrolyte imbalance within 12 months after the initial diagnosis. At present, pemphigus mortality is only 8 to 10 percent and the major causes of death in treated patients are complications of high doses of corticosteroids and immunosuppressive therapy or both. Following successful treatment, 30 to 40 percent of pemphigus patients remain in clinical remission, off all therapy.

Controversies

Two controversies should be noted in a discussion of pemphigus therapy: the necessity of initial massive high-dose steroids, and use of immunofluorescence testing to monitor therapy. When first employed in pemphigus therapy, corticosteroids were used in a therapeutic regimen which began at 80 mg of prednisone daily. If the patient did not improve after 2 to 3 weeks, the steroid dose was doubled; this procedure was repeated until clinical response was observed, and it was not uncommon to treat pemphigus patients with extraordinarily high steroid doses. The use of immunosuppressives and the successful results of less aggressive regimens make this approach unnecessary.

Since there is a rough correlation between the extent of clinical disease and the serum pemphigus antibody titer, many clinicians utilize the titer of pemphigus autoantibodies to monitor therapy. We have achieved excellent clinical results through treatment of the patient rather than antibody titer. Therefore, we utilize the relatively expensive immunofluorescent tests for diagnosis and during consideration of discontinuation of therapy in clinically well controlled patients. It is certainly reasonable to discontinue therapy in asymptomatic patients in whom pemphigus autoantibodies are not detectable.

Precautions

Because pemphigus patients are often middle-aged or elderly, steroid and immunosuppressive therapy must be instituted after a thorough evaluation. History and physical evidence of duodenal ulcers, diabetes, hypertension, osteoporosis, tuberculosis, and cataracts must be sought. If there is a history of tuberculosis and a positive skin test, isoniazid therapy (200 mg per day) is appropriate. Patients receiving immunosuppressive agents or sulfones should be followed for appropriate complications with complete blood count, differential, platelet count, urinalysis, and appropriate blood chemistries. As gold is not without complications, patients should be monitored for thrombocytopenia, bone marrow suppression, hematuria, and dermatitis.

Treatment of Pemphigus Foliaceous

Pemphigus foliaceous is a relatively benign, often self-limited disorder. Therefore, therapy need not be as aggressive as in pemphigus vulgaris. Patients are usually treated with corticosteroids, and therapy is begun at 40 to 60 mg of prednisone per day. The disorder is often controlled in 2 to 3 weeks, so steroid dosages are rapidly tapered to every other day and maintained until autoantibodies are not detected. In our experience, the use of adjunctive drugs, including immunosuppressives, is rarely necessary.

BULLOUS PEMPHIGOID

Bullous pemphigoid is a benign, self-limited, inflammatory blistering disease of the elderly. Blisters are tense and frequently localized to the axillary and inguinal skin, and patients experience severe pruritus. The pathologic site of blister formation is the dermal epidermal junction, and the inflammatory infiltrate is characterized by the perivascular presence of mononuclear cells and striking intravascular and basement membrane zone accumulation of eosinophils. Immunopathologic studies have shown invariable deposition of the third component of complement, and frequent linear deposition of IgG at the dermal-epidermal junction. In addition, 75 to 80 percent of patients have serum antibodies directed at an antigen in the laminae lucida of the skin basement membrane.

Therapy

The initial goal in treatment of bullous pemphigoid is to control itching and reduce blister formation to a level consistent with individual patient comfort. It must be stressed that bullous pemphigoid is self-limited and that complete suppression of blister formation is not necessary for management of symptoms. After symptoms are controlled and blistering diminished to tolerable levels, therapy is reduced to the lowest level required to maintain patient comfort. Therapy is discontinued when blister formation ceases.

Systemic steroids are used for initial control of disease in almost all patients. After the diagnosis of bullous pemphigoid is made, patients begin to receive prednisone (or its equivalent), 40 to 60 mg per day in a single morning dose. Therapeutic response is based on clinical evaluation of control of itching and reduction of cutaneous inflammation. After 2 to 3 weeks, 70 to 80 percent of patients show dramatic response, and prednisone is reduced to 30 mg per day by weekly reduction of daily dose by 10 mg. Over the next 2 to 3 weeks, prednisone dosage is further reduced to 30 mg every other day. Finally, dosage is dropped weekly by 5 mg every other day until the lowest amount of prednisone consistent with therapeutic goals is reached.

Patients who do not respond to prednisone after 6 to 8 weeks are treated in the following manner. Prednisone dose is maintained, and Imuran (100 to 150 mg per day) is begun. When clinical response is noted, prednisone and Imuran are tapered as described above until the patient is maintained on steroids alone. As many individuals with bullous pemphigoid are elderly, dapsone (50 to 100 mg per day) is frequently employed rather than Imuran. If there are strong contraindications to steroid use (such as severe osteoporosis, difficult diabetes, or hypertension) initial disease control with dapsone alone may be attempted. In addition to Imuran, some clinicians have employed weekly doses of methotrexate (25 to 50 mg IM); however, we have little experience with this agent.

Outcome

Following successful therapy, the overwhelming majority of patients with bullous pemphigoid go into complete clinical remission. The majority of patients require 4 to 6 months of therapy and the recurrence rate is 10 to 20 percent. The major complications of bullous pemphigoid treatment are those induced by steroid treatment of the elderly. These include diabetes, hypertension, gastrointestinal bleeding, and compression fractures of the spine secondary to osteoporosis.

Controversies

Some clinicians initially treat patients with low-dose corticosteroids equivalent to prednisone 20 to 30 mg per day, and low dose immunosuppressives. It is thought that this approach minimizes steroid side effects. The majority of patients rapidly respond to a short course of steroids which may be quickly tapered to low-dose, alternate-day medication. Therefore, we use the latter approach and thus avoid toxicity induced by immunosuppressive agents.

Therapy for Localized Pemphigoid and Benign Mucous Membrane Pemphigoid

Patients with mild bullous pemphigoid, often localized to the lower extremities, are infrequently encountered. Such patients may respond to saline or aluminum subacetate wet dressings or to topical fluorinated steroids applied 2 to 4 times a day. Systemic steroids may be avoided in these patients.

Benign mucous membrane pemphigoid (cicatricial pemphigoid) is primarily an ophthalmologic disease with histopathologic and immunopathologic similarity to bullous pemphigoid. It may proceed to blindness and has been treated with systemic steroids alone or in combination with a variety of immunosuppressive agents. While some clinicians have reported that cyclophosphamide (50 to 100 mg per day) may be successfully used, in our experience this agent has not been useful.

ERYTHEMA MULTIFORME

MARCIA G. TONNESEN, M.D.
J. CLARK HUFF, M.D.

Erythema multiforme (EM) is an acute, self-limited inflammatory disorder of the skin and mucous membranes, characterized by distinctive target (iris) lesions, a tendency for recurrence, and certain histopathologic changes. The two major clinical subsets of EM have been designated as EM minor and EM major.

EM minor is a relatively mild cutaneous illness which is frequently recurrent. The typical clinical picture is the sudden onset of a symmetric erythematous eruption with a predilection for the extensor aspects of the extremities. Mucosal involvement, when present, is usually limited to the oral cavity. Skin lesions begin as fixed erythematous macules, develop into edematous papules, and may progress to become bullous. At least some of the lesions evolve with concentric zones of color change to form characteristic

Supported by NIH grant 5 RO1 AI 1663T and the Veterans Administration.

target lesions. Individual lesions, usually symptomless but occasionally associated with burning or itching, appear in successive crops which may coalesce, and then resolve within 2 to 4 weeks, leaving residual postinflammatory hyperpigmentation. Most, if not all, cases of classic EM minor are associated with herpes simplex virus and typically occur 7 to 10 days after the appearance of a recurrent herpes simplex lesion.

EM major, also known as Stevens-Johnson syndrome, is a severe mucocutaneous illness characterized by involvement of two or more mucosal surfaces and associated constitutional symptoms, including fever and malaise. Skin lesions evolve with concentric color changes and central blister formation and may progress to widespread epidermal necrosis (toxic epidermal necrolysis), with a mortality rate approaching 50 percent. Painful mucosal erosions result in a foul-smelling mouth, typical hemorrhagic crusting of the lips, and decreased oral intake. Ocular involvement may produce an exudative conjunctivitis with residual scarring and lash and lacrimal abnormalities. Permanent visual impairment may occur in 10 to 20 percent of cases. Mycoplasma pneumoniae infections and certain drugs, particularly the sulfonamides, are important and well-documented etiologic factors in EM major.

THERAPEUTIC APPROACH

Successful therapeutic intervention in EM is hindered by the fact that specific pathogenic mechanisms of tissue injury have not yet been defined. In addition, no controlled studies have been performed to evaluate the effectiveness of any form of treatment in EM. A rational approach to therapy should be based on careful consideration of suspected etiologic factors, clinical characteristics—including extent and severity of mucocutaneous lesions and patient discomfort—and potential complications.

Elimination of any identified or presumed precipitating factors is of prime importance. In drug-associated EM, withdrawal and future avoidance of the drug is mandatory. In mycoplasma-associated EM, treatment of the respiratory infection is recommended. In herpes-associated EM minor, antiviral drugs hold therapeutic promise for the future; however, currently there is little evidence that antiviral therapy affects the course of the disease. Measures should be taken to attempt to decrease the frequency of recurrences of herpes simplex infections to lessen the likelihood of subsequent episodes of EM.

Since no specific treatment is currently available for EM, optimal therapy should combine symptomatic and supportive measures with observation for and treatment of associated complications (Tables 1 and 2). Recommended therapy includes antihistamines and baths to decrease pruritus, analgesics to relieve pain, hydration to maintain fluid balance, wet compresses to cleanse and debride crusted erosions, and good oral hygiene to minimize infection and discomfort. In severe EM major, early consultation with an ophthalmologist and a burn surgeon may be crucial to decrease morbidity and mortality.

Preferred Therapeutic Modalities

EM Minor

Patient Education. Patients should be reassured regarding the usual benign, self-limited course and educated regarding the frequent association of EM minor with recurrent herpes simplex viral infections.

Symptomatic Measures. For pruritic or painful skin lesions, systemic antihistamines (hydroxyzine hydrochloride, 25 to 50 mg *qid* or diphenhydramine hydrochloride, 50 mg *qid*) or analgesics (aspirin, 600 mg *qid* or acetaminophen, 650 mg *qid*) may provide symptomatic relief.

Skin Care. For bullous or crusted erosive skin lesions, mild drying, debridement, and cleansing can be achieved with open wet compresses of tepid water or aluminum acetate (Burow's solution diluted 1:20, or Domeboro tablet dissolved in 1 pint of water) applied for 30 minutes *qid*. Lesions should be observed for signs of secondary infection, cultured when indicated, and treatment initiated with the appropriate systemic antibiotic. Erythromycin, 250 mg *qid* is a

TABLE 1 Therapy For EM Minor

Patient Education	
Emphasize:	Self-limited course
	Association with recurrent herpes simplex infections
Symptomatic Measures	
Antipruritics:	Hydroxyzine HC1, 25–50 mg *qid* or
	Diphenhydramine HC1, 50 mg *qid*
Analgesics:	Aspirin, 600 mg *qid* or
	Acetaminophen, 650 mg *qid*
Skin Care	
To dry, debride and cleanse:	Open wet compresses of tepid water or aluminum acetate (Burow's solution) for 30 min *qid*
To soothe and cleanse:	Baths in tepid water for 30 min *tid*
Mouth Care	
To debride and cleanse:	Hydrogen peroxide (1.5%) mouthwash *q2h*
	Glycerin swabs for teeth
To relieve discomfort:	Topical anesthetic, such as:
	Dyclonine
	Viscous lidocaine
	Kaopectate/diphenhydramine
To maintain hydration and nutrition:	Liquid or soft diet
To treat infection:	Erythromycin, 250 mg *qid* or
	Pencillin, 250 mg *qid* for 10 days
Preventive Measures	
To decrease herpes simplex recurrences:	
Avoid sun:	Sunscreens (SPF 15)
	Sunstick
	Protective clothing
	Remain indoors 10:00 A.M.–2:00 P.M.
Minimize stress	
Future role for antiviral agents?	
Contraindication	
Do not use topical or systemic glucocorticosteroids in herpes-associated EM	

good first choice pending culture results. Frequent bathing (30 minutes *tid*) in lukewarm to cool water has a soothing antipruritic effect as well as serving to cleanse the skin lesions and minimize secondary infection.

Mouth Care. When extensive painful mouth lesions are present, good oral hygiene is critical to minimize infection and discomfort. Hydrogen peroxide (1.5%) mouthwash every 2 hours provides gentle debridement. Glycerin swabs can be used to clean the teeth with a minimum of trauma. Topical anesthetics such as dyclonine, viscous lidocaine, or a 1:1 mixture of Kaopectate and elixir of diphenhydramine used as a mouthwash will provide relief from painful erosions. A liquid or soft diet is usually better tolerated and therefore contributes to the maintenance of hydration and nutrition. When oral lesions are extensive, purulent, foul-smelling, and associated with tender cervical lymphadenopathy, systemic therapy with penicillin or erythromycin, 1 g per day for 10 days, is appropriate to combat secondary bacterial infection.

TABLE 2 Therapy For EM Major

Patient Education
- Emphasize: Self-limited, potentially severe course
  - Association with *Mycoplasma* infections and drugs

Elimination of Etiologic Factors
- *Mycoplasma* infection: Erythromycin, 250–500 mg *qid* or Tetracycline, 250–500 mg *qid*
- Drug: Immediate withdrawal and future avoidance

Supportive Care
- Hospitalization often necessary
- To maintain hydration and nutrition: IV fluids, tube feedings

Symptomatic Measures
- Antipruritics: Hydroxyzine HCl, 25–50 mg *qid* or Diphenhydramine HCl, 50 mg *qid*
- Analgesics/Antipyretics: Aspirin, 600 mg *qid* or Acetaminophen, 650 mg *qid*

Skin Care
- To dry, debride and cleanse: Open wet compresses of tepid water or aluminum acetate (Burow's solution) for 30 min qid
- To soothe and cleanse: Baths in tepid water for 30 min tid

Mouth Care
- To debride and cleanse: Hydrogen peroxide (1.5%) mouthwash *q2h*
  - Glycerin swabs for teeth
- To relieve discomfort: Topical anesthetic, such as:
  - Dyclonine
  - Viscous lidocaine
  - Kaopectate/diphenhydramine
- To treat infection: Erythromycin, 250 mg *qid* or Tetracycline, 250 mg *qid* for 10 days

Eye Care
- Careful monitoring and early consultation with ophthalmologist

Reduction of Morbidity and Mortality
- For progressive disease: Prednisone 1–2 mg/kg/day
- For extensive involvement: (≥ 30% total body surface area): Early referral to burn surgeon
- Measures to guard against infection:
  - Discontinue prednisone
  - Limit antibiotic use to culture proven infections
  - Minimize indwelling lines and catheters
  - Aggressively treat sepsis if it occurs
- Supportive care: Continuous rotational bed
  - Respiratory therapy
  - IV fluids and tube feedings
- Skin care: Gentle debridement followed by biologic dressing

Preventive Measures. Because of the common etiologic association between recurrent herpes simplex infections and EM minor, measures that attempt to prevent recurrences of herpes simplex may lessen the frequency of subsequent episodes of EM. Avoidance of sun exposure through the use of sunscreens (SPF 15), sunsticks (sunscreen-containing chapstick), and protective clothing, and by minimizing sun exposure from 10:00 a.m. to 2:00 p.m. (the peak period for UVB) may reduce ultraviolet light–induced herpes simplex recurrences on sun-exposed skin. Attempts should be made to minimize stress, a well-known precipitating factor in recurrent herpes simplex. Antiviral drugs hold promise for the future. Thus far, topical antiviral preparations have not been clearly shown to prevent or abort recurrent herpes simplex infections. Oral acyclovir has not yet been evaluated in a controlled study for its ability to decrease episodes of herpes-associated EM minor.

Contraindication. The routine use of systemic glucocorticosteroid therapy in herpes-associated EM minor is inadvisable. Steroid therapy has never been proven to be effective and may actually be detrimental in the treatment of EM minor. Systemic steroid therapy might diminish the host's ability to control the herpes simplex virus, resulting in either persistent viral infection or increased frequency of recurrent infections, associated with an atypical form of EM characterized by persistent skin lesions and large annular or arciform plaques. Topical steroid therapy is of little benefit in the treatment of EM.

EM Major

Because of the extensive epidermal and mucosal necrosis which can occur in EM major, careful monitoring is critical, hospitalization is often required, and supportive care is usually necessary.

Patient Education. Patients should be advised that the course is self-limited but potentially severe and educated regarding the frequent association of EM major with mycoplasma infection or drugs.

Elimination of Etiologic Factors. If M. pneumoniae infection is diagnosed or strongly suspected, systemic treatment should be initiated with erythromycin or tetracycline, 1 to 2 g per day. Any suspected or unnecessary drug should be withdrawn and avoided in the future. In particular, no drugs associated with EM major (especially sulfonamides and penicillins) should be used to treat any manifestation of the EM syndrome.

Supportive Care. Hospitalization is often advisable, and intravenous fluid therapy and tube feedings may be necessary to maintain hydration and nutrition.

Symptomatic Measures. As described in EM minor, systemic antipruritics and analgesics are useful to alleviate itching and pain.

Skin Care. For discrete bullous or crusted erosive skin lesions, the conservative therapy outlined for EM minor should be adequate. However, when lesions progress to extensive tissue necrosis with as much as 30 percent total body surface area involved, surgical intervention and transfer to a burn unit are advisable (see below).

Mouth Care. The therapeutic measures described for mouth lesions in EM minor apply to EM major as well. EM major patients often have more extensive oral involvement, however, and may be unable to eat or drink despite the use of topical anesthetics, thus necessitating intravenous fluids and tube feedings.

Eye Care. Because of the potential for long-term sequelae resulting in visual loss, careful monitoring of eye involvement is mandatory and early consultation with, and continuing care by, an ophthalmologist are strongly recommended. Suggested therapeutic measures might include irrigation and compresses to cleanse the eye, lysis of adhesions, and instillation of topical steroids and topical antibiotics when indicated.

Reduction of Morbidity and Mortality. Indication for the use of systemic glucocorticosteroids in EM major is still a controversial issue, since no controlled studies have been conducted to document their efficacy. However, because EM major can progress to widespread epidermal necrosis with a mortality rate as high as 50 percent, early use of systemic steroids in the progressive phase of the disease process in an attempt to decrease the extent of tissue damage is probably appropriate. High-dose therapy (prednisone, 1 to 2 mg/kg/day) should be initiated during the stage of extension of lesions, with gradual tapering during the 2 to 3-week healing phase. If extensive, advanced tissue necrosis occurs or is already evident (approaching 30 percent total body surface area involvement), immediate transfer of the patient to a burn unit under the care of a surgical burn specialist is strongly advocated. Therapeutic recommendations in the surgical literature consist of (1) measures to guard against iatrogenic infection, including withdrawal from prednisone, limitation of antibiotic use to specific culture-proven infections, avoidance of indwelling lines and catheters whenever possible, and aggressive treatment of sepsis if it occurs; (2) supportive care consisting of use of a continuous rotational bed, respiratory therapy, intravenous fluid therapy, and tube feedings; and (3) skin care with emphasis on early gentle debridement followed by application of a biologic dressing to protect the denuded dermis from desiccation and to facilitate rapid re-epithelialization. Reduced mortality has been reported with the use of allografts and porcine xenografts.

THERAPEUTIC OUTCOME

Both EM minor and EM major are self-limited disorders which can be expected to resolve within 4 to 6 weeks. If the disease persists longer than 6 to 8 weeks the diagnosis of EM should be questioned and alternative diagnoses investigated.

CHRONIC MUCOCUTANEOUS CANDIDIASIS

RODNEY D. ADAM, M.D.
ESKILD A. PETERSEN, M.D.

Candida is a part of the normal flora of the oral mucosa, the gastrointestinal tract, and the skin. Clinical candidal disease is often seen when the ecologic balance is upset by intrinsic or extrinsic manipulations. Thus, antibacterial chemotherapy frequently results in candidal proliferation and disease. Contrary to the transient nature of such infections are the persistent and recurrent infections of the skin, mucous membrane, and/or nails with *Candida* in patients with chronic mucocutaneous candidiasis (CMC). CMC is not a single clinical entity but a collection of related syndromes (Table 1), and it therefore includes both patients who have limited local disease and patients with extensive cutaneous (candida granuloma) or mucous involvement. Patients with CMC do not generally suffer from invasive candidiasis. An exception to this is patients with severe underlying diseases such as the acquired immunodeficiency syndrome (AIDS) or hematologic malignancy.

Numerous immunologic defects have been noted in patients with CMC. Cell-mediated immunity is most frequently impaired, with patients failing to show de-

TABLE 1 Spectrum of Chronic Mucocutaneous Candidiasis

Type	*Age of Onset*	*Associated Pathology*
Chronic oral candidiasis	Any	Acquired immune deficiency syndrome
Chronic candidiasis with endocrinopathy	Childhood	Polyglandular failure (adrenal, thyroid, parathyroid, ovaries, pernicious anemia)
Chronic mucocutaneous localized candidiasis	Childhood	None
Chronic diffuse candidiasis	Childhood	None
Chronic candidiasis thymoma	Adulthood	Thymoma, myasthenia

layed skin test hypersensitivity reactions to Candida antigens. In addition, peripheral blood leukocytes from such patients show impaired proliferative responses and lymphokine production when they are exposed to Candida antigen in vitro. Other immunologic abnormalities seen in some CMC patients include deficient secretory IgA, abnormal complement system, and impaired macrophage/monocyte function.

Certain patients with CMC need close observation, among them children, in whom particular attention should be paid to the development of concomitant polyendocrine failure—including hypofunction of the adrenal, thyroid, and parathyroid glands—ovarian failure, and pernicious anemia. Children from a family with a history of CMC and polyendocrinopathy are at special risk. Also, those patients in whom one endocrine deficiency has been identified must be monitored for the development of other endocrine failures. If CMC occurs in a patient older than 35 years, there should be high suspicion of a thymoma. Finally, chronic oral candidiasis in an adult male might well be the first symptom of AIDS, particularly if the individual falls into one of the well-defined risk categories.

TREATMENT

Treatment is directed toward correcting the underlying endocrine or immunologic condition of the CMC and eradicating or controlling the infection. Many antifungal compounds are now available for treatment of the infectious component.

Imidazole Compounds

Ketoconazole

Ketoconazole was first studied 5 years ago in patients with CMC and is now the treatment of choice in such patients. Ketoconazole is toxic to fungal plasma membranes because it inhibits ergosterol synthesis. The usual dosage is 100 mg daily for small children and 200 mg in adults, given as a single oral dose. Some patients with severe manifestations of CMC might need 600 mg daily. The drug has a very high patient acceptance rate but is not without side effects. The continuous use of ketoconazole for years in patients with either CMC or coccidioidomycosis has revealed that the drug is not as innocuous as was originally thought. The principal side effects include nausea and vomiting with the higher dosages, drug-induced hepatitis occurring in about 1 of 10,000 patients, and elevation of SGOT and SGPT in 10 to 15 percent of patients. Ketoconazole hepatitis is the most severe side effect and its occurrence cannot be predicted. Ketoconazole influences sterol hormone metabolism in both men and women. In men it transiently decreases testosterone levels and displaces testosterone and estradiol from their respective serum carrier proteins. Gynecomastia is seen in up to 8 percent of men taking ketoconazole, and patients have also been noted to have impotence and azoospermia associated with the low testosterone levels. In women, menstrual irregularity is not uncommon and often must be controlled with concomitant oral contraceptive administration. Ketoconazole blunts the cortisol response to adrenocorticotropic hormone stimulation, but no known cases of Addison's disease have so far been associated with its use. Thus, the endocrine effects seen in CMC patients treated with ketoconazole might be confusing because many of these patients are already at risk for developing polyendocrinopathy spontaneously.

In CMC patients, ketoconazole predictably clears oral lesions within a week, skin lesions within 2 to 4 weeks, and nails within 3 months. Ketoconazole often provides an added benefit to patients with CMC, because many of them have associated dermatophytosis that also responds well to this antifungal compound. We treat CMC patients with ketoconazole until all signs of candidal infection have cleared. However, the majority of patients in whom treatment has been stopped have had recurrence of their candidiasis. We handle such relapses on an individual basis, trying to find the maintenance dosage of ketoconazole that will keep them from having symptomatic candidiasis. In some patients this means half a tablet (100 mg) every other day; in others, ketoconazole is taken only during menstruation. Some patients with CMC need substantially higher daily doses of ketoconazole than initially used to control their clinical symptoms. An investigator with a great deal of personal experience with CMC has had several patients who were treated with ketoconazole from whom he has isolated *Candida* organisms that, when tested in several different laboratories, have shown a higher resistance pattern to ketoconazole than have other *Candida* strains. At present, it is not known whether this indicates the development of ketoconazole resistance or superinfection with a new ketoconazole-resistant strain. Extrapolating from our experiences with other antifungal and antibacterial agents, we would say this most likely reflects a drug-selected resistant mutant of the original infecting strain. At present, this is not a major clinical problem but could conceivably become so in the future.

Other Imidazoles

Two other imidazole compounds are currently available: clotrimazole and miconazole. Several other imidazoles are presently in phase 2 or 3 trial. Most of these have better in vitro activity against *Candida* than ketoconazole.

Clotrimazole is available as creams, vaginal suppositories, and oral troches. Clotrimazole troches (10 mg) 5 times daily are very effective in controlling oral manifestations of candidiasis and equal ketoconazole in patient acceptance for treatment of the oral infection.

Miconazole is available in creams, sprays, suppositories, and for intravenous use. The topical preparations are acceptable where such application is indicated. In contrast, the intravenous form is time-consuming to administer and associated with numerous side effects. In our opinion, systemic miconazole has no role in the treatment of mucocutaneous or invasive candidiasis.

Polyene Antibiotics

Amphotericin B

Amphotericin B inhibits fungi by binding to sterols and creating channels in the plasma membrane where leakage of cell products can occurs. The molecular weight for amphotericin B is high, the drug is relatively insoluble in aqueous media, and it is available only in a colloidal suspension. A quite high level of toxicity is associated with its systemic use. From our extensive experience with the use of amphotericin B intravenously, we have developed a treatment protocol that differs from the 4 to 6-hour regimens most frequently advocated.

Dosages. Our method includes the following specifics: All patients are premedicated with an antihistamine and acetaminophen 15 minutes before the intravenous infusion is started. The first dose of amphotericin B is 5 mg, diluted in 50 ml of 5 percent dextrose in water with 1000 units of heparin and 25 mg of hydrocortisone, given over half an hour. Temperature, pulse, and blood pressure are monitored and recorded every half hour a total of four times. The second dose is 0.3 mg/kg diluted 1:5 or 1:10 in 5% dextrose in water, likewise with 1000 units of heparin and 25 mg of hydrocortisone added to the bottle. The third and subsequent dosages are 0.7 mg/kg, not to exceed a total dosage of 50 mg, and are likewise diluted 1:5 or 1:10 in 5% dextrose in water with heparin and hydrocortisone added. The amphotericin B is then administered on a Monday/Wednesday/Friday schedule in the outpatient clinic. All doses are administered over a 1-hour period. Most of our patients show greater tolerance to these faster infusions. In addition, our protocol with the faster infusions allows the patients to continue their daily routine when they can be treated in an outpatient setting for a total of 1 to 1/2 hours and not have to spend an entire day in the hospital. For patients with major cardiac problems, we slow the infusion rate to 4 hours. Additionally, we ensure that each patient is treated with the same lot of amphotericin B during the treatment course. The total dose needed for treatment of CMC is less than that for most other fungal diseases, such as coccidioidomycosis. In general, dosages between 500 mg and 1 g total seem to be sufficient to clear the skin and mucous membrane lesions. During the treatment, the patients renal functions are monitored weekly by serum creatinine, blood urea, and potassium measurements. A complete blood count with differential is also done weekly. A flow sheet containing information on treatment given and reactions seen is kept in the front of the patient's chart.

Side Effects. The side effects of amphotericin B administration are many. Nearly every patient will have an episode of shaking chills and fever during the treatment course. We handle this problem by changing the premedication and particularly the interval between the premedication and the intravenous drug administration. In addition, the use of meperidine intravenously early during the chill most often will abate the symptoms.

Systemic Effects. Some degree of azotemia is seen in all patients. Azotemia reaches a plateau during treatment at a level determined by the daily dosage, and all patients will have some degree of reduced glomerular filtration rate. However, the actual increase in the serum creatinine level observed during the treatment period does not indicate the level of permanent damage that can be expected after the treatment has been concluded. We keep the serum creatinine below 3.5 during the treatment period to reduce the nausea and emesis associated with such azotemia. Other side effects include development of hypokalemia, for which supplemental potassium is given. Renal acidosis often occurs but rarely needs specific interaction. A weight loss of 5 to 6 kg is common. Other side effects frequently encountered include anemia and phlebitis.

Amphotericin B is a very effective drug in clearing the skin and mucous membrane lesions of patients with CMC. However, patients with CMC most often relapse within a few months after treatment. Therefore, amphotericin B with its many side effects should be reserved for those patients with severe and potentially invasive disease.

Nystatin

Nystatin, like amphotericin B, is also a polyene antifungal agent. It is available as a cream or ointment for cutaneous disease, as a suspension for oropharyngeal candidiasis, and as a suppository for vaginal infection. Nystatin is the least effect of the preparations available, and we have found that it is not effective in patients who have a significant amount of candidiasis. Therefore, nystatin is reserved for mild cases of oral candidiasis.

5-Flucytosine

Flucytosine is a fluorinated pyrimidine that acts by conversion into 5-fluorouracil by susceptible fungi, thereby halting their DNA synthesis. It is absorbed very well orally and excreted renally. The usual dose is 150 mg/kg per day given every 6 hours. The drug is very active against susceptible organisms. Unfortunately, it is not uncommon that *Candida albicans* has primary resistance to 5-flucytosine or that resistance develops during treatment. There are many toxicities associated with 5-flucytosine, including bone marrow depression, nausea, vomiting, diarrhea, elevated liver enzymes, and occasionally central nervous system side effects. Most of these side effects, however, are seen when 5-flucytosine is given concomitantly with amphotericin B. This impairs renal function and thus elevates the concentration of 5-flucytosine unless the 5-flucytosine dose is corrected. We monitor our patients by obtaining frequent serum levels of 5-flucytosine using a high pressure liquid chromatography assay developed by Dr. Findley at our clinical laboratory at the Arizona Health Sciences Center. This method is very sensitive, reproducible, and not affected by the presence of other antifungal drugs in the serum, such as amphotericin B. We keep our patients' 5-flucytosine level at 50 to 75 μg/ml and thereby preclude most of the side effects associated with 5-flucytosine.

Reconstitution Therapy

The high incidence of relapse with candidiasis after antifungal treatment, together with the findings that CMC patients commonly have associated immune deficiencies, has fostered a great deal of interest in developing relevant immunotherapy. Transfer factor is an experimental immune therapy that has been best evaluated in the many studies conducted by C. Kirkpatrick at the National Jewish Hospital in Denver. Transfer factor obtained from *Candida*-sensitive donors protracts the duration of remission when administered to CMC patients following completed antifungal therapy. Likewise, there is an association between the development of *Candida*-specific immune parameters in the patients and the likelihood that remission will be seen in those patients. Transfer factor thus appears to play a beneficial role in patients with CMC. However, because of the cost of production of transfer factor, as well as the uncertainty of its method of action, it is reserved for only a few patients a the present time. What role, if any, other immune modulatory approaches have, such as the administration of gamma interferon or interleukin-2 in patients with CMC, is not yet known, and only controlled trials will provide this information.

CONCLUSIONS

Management of patients with CMC includes following them closely for signs of the development of associated endocrinopathies or underlying immune deficiency. The current treatment is chiefly directed toward keeping the infection under control rather than eradicating it. Ketoconazole is the best currently available drug and is very well accepted by patients, but it is not free of side effects. Both better antifungal drugs and immune therapeutical procedures are needed to improve the treatment of patients with CMC.

ACNE VULGARIS

RUTH K. FREINKEL, M.D.

Although almost everyone has acne vulgaris at some time, expression of the clinical picture and the course are extremely variable. The various types of lesions (comedones, papules, pustules, nodules, cysts) may be present alone or in combination. The entire acne area (face, neck, upper trunk) may be involved or just one part. Onset may be at puberty or much later in the late teens or early twenties. The disease may be present for a few years or may endure into midlife. The course may be progressive in its evolution or undergo cycles of exacerbation and remission. Inevitably, however, acne resolves spontaneously, leaving in its wake scars, which do not necessarily correlate with the severity of the preceding lesions. Resolution of acne does not appear to be accompanied by any changes in the known pathogenic factors such as hormonal stimulation, levels of sebum production, or follicular bacterial population.

Despite the unpredictability of the clinical picture, basic factors impinging upon pathogenesis are quite well understood. Acne is an inflammatory process centering upon those pilosebaceous organs of the face, neck, and upper trunk in which the patulous ducts of very large sebaceous glands open into the follicular canal of small, relatively inactive hairs. Two necessary but insufficient factors impinge upon this anatomic site in the production of acne lesions. One is the production of large amounts of sebum by the sebaceous gland under stimulation by androgens. The presence of sebum allows colonizaiton of the lower pilosebaceous follicle by microaerobic *Propionibacterium acnes*. Accompanying these changes is the development of the primary lesion of acne: abnormal keratinization of the follicle resulting in obstruction of the duct. Although the precise cause of the dyskeratosis remains unknown, once the flow of sebum is obstructed, both comedones and inflammatory lesions are triggered by bacterial products such as lytic enzymes and their products—specifically, those of the action of bacterial lipases on sebum lipids. The inflammatory response is not directed against *P. acnes* initially. However, when follicular rupture occurs it is followed by a chronic granulomatous response involving the contents of the follicle, including both bacteria and cellular debris. This process produces chronic, often self-perpetuating, nodules and cysts.

The above considerations provide the basis for principles of therapy in acne vulgaris.

1. Since there is, to date, no cure of the primary causes, treatment can only be suppressive until the disease resolves spontaneously.
2. In most cases of acne, excepting the most severe ones, suppression of the inflammatory reaction suffices to produce clinical remission, and, in mild cases, relieving follicular obstruction (comedolysis) may be all that is needed.

3. The unpredictability of the extent and course dictates that treatment be tailored to fit the clinical picture presented by each patient at various points in time.
4. Direct delivery of pharmacologic agents to the skin (i.e., topical applications) is preferable to systemic therapy if the efficacy is equivalent.
5. Acne usually occurs in otherwise healthy young people, and the treatment should not produce iatrogenic diseases.

Using these principles, it is possible to plan effective therapeutic regimens employing currently available agents which (*1*) alleviate blockage of the follicle, (*2*) decrease the follicular population of *P. acnes*, and (*3*) suppress sebum production.

THERAPY

Comedolytic Agents

Vitamin A and its analogues, the retinoids, reverse the follicular hyperkeratosis and thus act as comedolytic agents. Vitamin A acid is the topically active form, and 13-*cis* retinoic acid is the agent used for oral administration. The latter has profound effects on the skin. In addition to comedolysis, it suppresses sebum production and hair growth, and increases skin fragility. It appears to cure severe nodulocystic acne, but ordinary acne recurs after treatment is stopped.

Anti-Inflammatory Agents

A variety of nonspecific and specific topical antimicrobial agents provide effective treatment for mild to moderate inflammatory acne. Lotions containing broad-spectrum antibiotics and formulations containing benzoyl peroxide are the most effective preparations. The latter are available in many nonprescription preparations as are a number of less effective antiseptic creams, lotions, and gels. Systemic administration of broad-spectrum antibiotics tends to be more effective and may afford direct inhibition of chemotaxis in addition to antimicrobial actions. The anti-inflammatory effects of glucocorticoids may be employed advantageously in intralesional injections of chronic nodules and cysts. However, both topically applied and systemically administered fluorinated glucocorticoids are acnegenic and are rarely indicated for the treatment of acne.

Suppression of Sebum Production

Cyclic administration of estrogen-progestin combinations (oral contraceptive agents) induces suppression of sebum production and ameliorates acne. This effect is due to suppression of ovarian function and to some peripheral competition with the actions of androgens on the sebaceous gland. If excess production of adrenal androgens has been documented to provide a major source of androgenic hormones in female patients, oral contraceptives may not suffice. In these cases, low suppressive doses of glucocorticoids with or without oral contraceptives may provide relief for patients with otherwise recalcitrant nodular cystic acne.

Other Modalities

Although moderate attention to normal hygiene need not be discouraged, there is no evidence that cleansing the skin improves acne. On the other hand, cosmetics containing oil, including moisturizing lotions, are comedogenic and should be avoided. Ultraviolet light, either in the form of natural sunlight or artificial ultraviolet radiation, appears to be beneficial. Dietary factors do not have a consistent, documented role in acne, and dietary injunctions should not be imposed.

DOSAGES AND COMPLICATIONS

Vitamin A acid (isotretinoin) in strengths of 0.01 to 0.05 percent in lotions, gels, or creams is usually applied once a day. Irritating effects can be minimized by starting at a low concentration every other day; creams are less irritating than gels at the same concentration. Because topical isotretinoin has been reported to promote ultraviolet-induced skin cancer in animals, it is reasonable to limit its use during heavy sun exposure.

Oral administration of 13-*cis* retinoic acid in doses ranging from 0.1 to 2 mg per kilogram per day is effective in most patients in the range of 0.5 to 1.0 mg per kilogram. Courses of treatment for 4 months are followed by a rest period of several months or longer until the disease recurs. Because of the potentially serious adverse reactions, this drug should be reserved for patients with severe, nodular, recalcitrant cystic acne who have reached sexual maturity. Most patients experience dryness of the mouth, lips, and eyes at higher doses. Nausea, fatigue, myalgias, arthralgias, and alopecia are not uncommon. Serious effects include hyperostosis of bones, calcification of spinal ligaments, and early closure of the epiphysis. 13-*cis* retinoic acid is teratogenic, and severe congenital anomalies occur with alarming frequency when the drug is administered to pregnant women. Therefore, the drug should not be administered to women in the childbearing age in the absence of documented compliance with the most effective methods of birth control. Its use is not recommended as a substitute for other treatment.

Topical preparations of erythromycin, tetracycline, and clindamycin are available as 1 to 2 percent solutions and are applied one to two times daily. They appear to be safe and moderately effective especially when used in conjunction with other topical preparations.

Benzoyl peroxide in concentrations of 2.5 to 10 percent is formulated in lotions, gels, and creams. Irritating effects parallel therapeutic effects and occur least often with lotions and most frequently with gels; however, the irritation decreases with prolonged use, and a regimen of gradual increases in concentration and more efficient vehicles is advisable.

Broad-spectrum antibiotics administered orally remain the mainstay of acne therapy. Tetracycline is the first drug of choice, followed by erythromycin and minocycline.

Most patients respond to moderate or low doses of tetracycline or erythromycin. Treatment may be begun with as little as 500 mg given in a single dose, although large or heavy patients may require 750 mg divided into two doses. It is important to instruct patients to take the drugs on an empty stomach; tetracycline should always be taken at least 1.5 hours after or before ingestion of milk or milk products to insure good absorption. There is no need to prime the patient with a large dose of 1,000 mg per day; although this may slightly accelerate a favorable response, it has the disadvantage of increasing the appearance of gastrointestinal adverse effects and vaginal candidiasis. If response is not satisfactory after 4 weeks, the dose may be increased. Maximal improvement usually requires 2 to 3 months of treatment with the initial dose. After that time, patients can often be maintained on as little as 250 mg given daily or every other day. Treatment should be continued while the disease is active, although rest periods of 2 to 3 months each year are advisable.

Bacterial resistance often develops after prolonged administration of a given antibiotic and requires change to a different agent. In this situation, minocycline (starting at 100 mg per day) is very useful; minocycline is perhaps more effective than either tetracycline or erythromycin, but its use is limited because of its far greater costliness. Trimethoprim-sulfamethoxazole given once a day is also helpful for short-term use when other antibiotics fail or cannot be tolerated.

Gastrointestinal effects are common with all broad-spectrum antibiotics. They should not be ignored because of the danger of pseudomembranous colitis. Vaginitis due to candida albicans is a frequent complication and may prevent the use of oral antibiotics. Tetracyclines can cause phototoxicity and patients need to be careful to avoid excessive sun exposure. Tetracycline should never be used in pregnant women and should be discontinued several months prior to efforts to conceive since the drug deposits in fetal bones and teeth. In addition to other side effects, minocycline causes reversible vestibular dysfunction and may cause hyperpigmentation.

Oral contraceptives are helpful in women when other agents fail to control the disease. Those with very low estrogen content may not be as effective, and, occasionally, sebotrophic effects of certain progestins may worsen acne. In addition, the many other complications of cyclic hormone therapy interdicts their use as a routine treatment for acne, and risk-benefit ratios should be carefully considered before instituting their use.

PSORIASIS

THOMAS F. ANDERSON, M.D.
JOHN J. VOORHEES, M.D.

Psoriasis is a common, chronic heritable skin condition characterized by abnormal proliferation and differentiation of the epidermis in association with an exaggerated inflammation. Clinical involvement can vary from small guttate erythematous papules with little scale in a generalized distribution to well demarcated erythematous plaques with an adherent and flaking, silvery-white scale confined to the extensor surfaces. Macerated fissures in the intertriginous areas or severe scalp and nail involvement can also be seen. Psoriasis patients can also present with a generalized exfoliative erythroderma or pustular psoriasis.

Psoriasis involving the scalp, genitalia, or nail bed and matrix are all treated differently. Thus, treatment for psoriasis must be multifocal and individually designed. Other aspects necessary to consider in the design of appropriate therapy include the patient's physical or emotional state, sophistication, and expectations. The practical limitations of each therapy, including cost, constraints of the therapeutic setting, requirements for patient travel, time off work, compliance, and reliability must also be weighed.

In general, patients with psoriasis can be classified into three major groups based upon severity; mild, moderate, and severe. Mild disease can usually be managed with a combination of bland emollients, keratolytic therapy, or corticosteroids. Moderately severe disease usually requires the addition of tar or anthralin products and possibly ultraviolet light therapy. Severe disease may require all of the preceding in a hospital setting or systemic alternatives such as antimetabolites or psoralen and ultraviolet-A (PUVA) therapy. Experimental therapy with retinoids or other agents can also be considered.

TREATMENT

Bland Emollients

Perhaps the most inexpensive and widely used treatment for psoriasis is the frequent and liberal application of occlusive emollients such as Vaseline Petroleum Jelly, Eucerin, mineral oil, and Lubriderm. These oleaginous substances form a protective coating over the skin. Patients with active psoriasis often form new plaques in the exact sites of cutaneous injury. Emollients may work in part by decreasing this "Koebner phenomenon" by decreasing dry skin and excoriations. They also increase the hydration of the diseased psoriatic stratum corneum, thus facilitating the removal of the excess scale. Mild psoriatic plaques may stabilize then even regress (with decreased mitosis) with continued use of these moisturizing, occlusive emollients as the sole form of therapy.

Keratolytic Therapy

In addition to occlusive emollients, plastic occlusive dressings (such as Saran Wrap, plastic gloves, or total body vinyl suits) have been shown to be useful in the treatment of hyperkeratotic psoriasis. Plastic occlusion not only softens and hydrates the horny layer but also increases the cutaneous penetration of topical drugs. One risk of plastic dressings and occlusive ointments is the overgrowth of cutaneous bacteria with resulting folliculitis or maceration. Therefore, occlusive dressings are generally used only intermittently for 2- to 4-hour periods or, at most, overnight.

Chemical keratolytic agents are also useful in helping to remove excessive hyperkeratosis of the palms and soles or recalcitrant psoriatic plaques elsewhere on the body. Urea in a 20 to 40 percent concentration or salicylic acid in a 2 to 6 percent concentration are the most common agents used. Ammoniated mercury at a 5 percent concentration has been recommended for scalp psoriasis. Its use has been limited, however, by reports of renal tubular damage and allergic hypersensitivity with chronic use.

Propylene glycol solutions at a concentration by volume of 40 to 60 percent in water are particularly effective in removing thick scale when used under moist plastic occlusion. A commonly prescribed preparation, Keralyt, is a combination of 6 percent salicylic acid in a 60 percent propylene glycol gel. This can be applied to thickened areas such as the palms and soles, followed by the application of damp cotton gloves or stockings. Large plastic gloves, booties, or Saran Wrap sheets are then worn with tape at the wrists and ankles, forming a watertight but not constricting seal. After a 3- to 4-hour period during the day or overnight, this plastic dressing is removed and excess keratin atraumatically scraped away with a washcloth, a polyester fiber sponge (Buf-Puf) or an abrasive tool such as a pumice stone. Occlusive ointments must be applied immediately after this procedure to avoid desiccation of the remaining stratum corneum and the development of painful fissures. If a superficial erosion or painful fissure does occur, the area must be protected with an emollient or zinc oxide paste prior to any further treatment.

Urea at a 20 to 40 percent concentration in hydrophilic petrolatum breaks hydrogen bonds in epidermal keratin and can be used as an alternative to Keralyt in this procedure.

Corticosteroids

Topical glucocorticosteroids are perhaps the most commonly prescribed treatment for psoriasis. These agents are vasoconstrictive, anti-inflammatory, and antimitotic; although expensive, they are generally nonstaining and may only need to be applied once per day to once per week in individual cases. Ointment bases, although messy, are generally more effective than creams, especially when treating thick, hyperkeratotic psoriatic areas such as elbows and knees. Hairy areas are best treated with creams or lotions; solutions, gels, and sprays are the easiest preparations to apply to the scalp. Corticosteroid solutions are helpful in treating psoriasis of the ear canal and fingernails.

After the initial use of a high-potency corticosteroid to bring about fast resolution, the potency and frequency of application of these products are gradually reduced in order to prevent adverse cutaneous side effects such as striae, atrophy, telangiectasia, purpura, and acneiform eruptions. Glaucoma or cataracts may result from the chronic application of corticosteroids close to the eyes. Corticosteroid therapy, when combined with plastic occlusive dressings, can be complicated by hypertension, glucosuria in diabetic patients, glaucoma, and pustular psoriasis exacerbation after withdrawal. Continued use of topical corticosteroids is often associated with a loss of their effectiveness. A rebound phenomenon may follow precipitous discontinuation of corticosteroids. Considering the expense, side effects, and loss of effectiveness over time, topical corticosteroids are best used for short periods (less than 3 weeks) for mild psoriasis and never as the sole therapy for psoriasis.

We do not recommend the use of systemic corticosteroids in the treatment of psoriasis. However, intralesional corticosteroids can be a valuable treatment adjunct with a minimum of side effects. Small doses of highly insoluble forms of triamcinolone (such as Kenalog) can be injected into recalcitrant psoriatic plaques up to a total dose of 20 mg without any evidence of systemic effect. One milligram (0.1–0.4 cc) of triamcinolone acetonide injected from a concentration of 2.5 to 10.0 mg per milliliter into any one treatment site may result in a prolonged resolution of a psoriatic papule or plaque, lasting for weeks to months. The use of a 30-gauge needle or a mechanical or air-powered hypodermic gun may be helpful to reduce the amount of discomfort in treating isolated sites, e.g., scalp or fingernail, or recalcitrant plaque psoriasis. Side effects of intralesional corticosteroids include the development of sterile abscess or cellulitis, pain, atrophy, hyper- and hypopigmentation, and telangiectasia. Tachyphylaxis and rebound worsening appear to be less evident with the intralesional dosage route. Many of these side effects are only temporary if care is taken to use the lowest possible dose and to avoid reinjection at the same site for 4 to 6 weeks.

Tar Products

A wide variety of products containing derivatives of crude or refined coal tar are available for the treatment of psoriasis. Although the mechanism of action of tar products is unknown, these agents have been shown to suppress DNA synthesis when applied to mouse skin. Adverse reactions to tar therapy include folliculitis, photosensitivity, and allergic hypersensitivity, not to mention the noxious odor and staining properties of these agents. Animal and epidemiologic studies suggest that tar products may be carcinogens; however, a recent 25-year follow-up study of psoriatics treated with coal tar showed no increase in the incidence of cutaneous or internal malignancy.

Crude coal tar in a 1 to 5 percent concentration may be incorporated into zinc oxide paste, Aquaphor, or washable petrolatum to treat large, thick psoriatic plaques. Tar products should not be applied to intertriginous or hairy areas or under moist plastic occlusion, in order to avoid primary irritation and folliculitis. A less irritating alcohol extract of tar, liquor carbonis detergens (LCD), is commonly used in a 10 percent concentration in hydrophilic creams or lotions for generalized acute guttate psoriasis. Tar extracts formulated in creams or gels such as Fototar, Estar, or Psoragel, have recently been developed for outpatient use and for treatment of the scalp. These preparations are less messy and wash off easily. Although these agents decrease the incidence of staining and folliculitis, the gels tend to desiccate the skin, and they produce a burning sensation upon application. A wide variety of tar-based shampoos and bath and body oils are available without prescription.

Anthralin Products

Anthralin, which is a synthetic replacement for the naturally occurring antipsoriatic agent, chrysarobin, appears to improve psoriasis through a variety of actions. Like tar, it is antimitotic but it also may inhibit the production of a variety of mediators of inflammation. Unfortunately, it is a potent cutaneous irritant and is more likely than tar to stain the skin and clothing. It should be avoided in acute inflammatory psoriasis, flexural areas, and on the face. Accidental contact with the eyes may produce a severe chemical conjunctivitis.

Anthralin is generally compounded in a 0.1 to 2.0 percent concentration in a stiff zinc oxide paste, usually with the addition of salicylic acid in a 0.2 to 4.0 percent concentration as a stabilizing agent. Patients are treated with the lowest concentration initially, gradually raising the strength every few days until either the desired response or irritation occurs. A thick coating of paste must be applied carefully so as to cover only the psoriatic plaques. To prevent irritation and "koebnerization" of the surrounding skin, the plaques are often ringed with a protective coat of petrolatum or plain zinc oxide paste. The anthralin-covered plaques may then be dusted with talc and covered with tube gauze or stockingette bandages for 4- to 12-hour periods. Mineral oil, often with an added emulsifying agent such as 5 percent sodium lauryl sulfate, is then used to remove the paste prior to the next application. Anthralin has also been incorporated into ointments and liquid waxes at lower concentrations for extensive guttate psoriasis and scalp therapy. Staining and irritation can be lessened by using low concentrations of anthralin for long periods of time or high concentrations for short periods (under an hour).

Response to anthralin can be measured by the degree to which the psoriatic plaque acquires the anthralin stain and the amount of desquamation and thinning of the plaque that occurs with continued use. As the plaque thins, lesser concentrations of anthralin or shorter application periods must be utilized to prevent painful, edematous responses and potential koebnerization. Often the concomitant use of low-potency corticosteroids can blunt this irritant effect.

Ultraviolet Light Therapy

Sunlight and artificially produced mid-range "erythemogenic" ultraviolet irradiation (UVB) is an effective antipsoriatic therapy, presumably acting by directly suppressing DNA synthesis. Ultraviolet light damages epidermal DNA, thus producing nuclear photoproducts that must be repaired before further mitosis. This suppression of DNA synthesis is enhanced by anthralin and coal-tar products. Titrated exposures of increasing doses of ultraviolet light can be delivered to the skin through a template with a series of small openings. In this manner, the dose of ultraviolet light necessary to produce a minimum degree of erythema (minimal erythema dose) can be delineated. Starting at a dose just below that necessary to produce erythema, daily treatments are delivered gradually by raising the time of exposure by approximately 10 to 50 percent until minimum erythema is maintained approximately 6 to 24 hours after phototherapy. Twenty to 40 exposures are generally necessary in order to obtain the best results. The end point of treatment is the gradual desquamation and thinning of individual psoriatic plaques in association with a gradual diminution of the erythema within the psoriatic plaque. If the capillary refill time after compression of the treated psoriatic plaque approximates that of the surrounding uninvolved skin, ultraviolet light phototherapy may be discontinued or reduced to once or twice a week as maintenance therapy.

Side effects of ultraviolet phototherapy include acute sunburn-like responses, ranging from erythema and swelling to tenderness and blisters. These are usually prevented by careful monitoring of dosage and reduction of therapy when desquamation of the uninvolved "tanned" skin takes place. The face, breasts, axillae, popliteal fossae, and genitalia are areas that tend to sunburn more easily than other areas and may require a double layer of cloth shielding or UVB sunscreening agents during all or part of the phototherapy exposures. Psoriasis can be exacerbated by too much ultraviolet light (as a Koebner phenomenon), and leg edema is a common side effect. Acute exacerbation of concomitant light-sensitive disorders such as bullous pemphigoid, herpes simplex, and polymorphous light eruption may also occur. Acute painful exposure keratitis and chronic cataract formation can be prevented by wearing ultraviolet light-opaque sunglasses or goggles with each exposure.

Chronic side effects of phototherapy include xerosis, pruritus, premature aging, actinic damage to the skin, freckling, and hyperpigmentation. Further experimental evidence suggests that ultraviolet light with or without coal tar produces a cutaneous immunosuppression and is carcinogenic. However, experience suggests that the incidence of cancer in psoriatic patients treated with phototherapy is not significantly greater than in the general population.

Hospital Treatment

For moderately severe to severe psoriatic patients who are undergoing an acute, generalized eruptive flare of psoriasis or who are suffering with greater than 20 percent body surface area involvement, or who are disabled by their disease (such as palm and sole involvement), hospitalization for a combination of all of the previously described treatments is the treatment of choice. For the first 3 days of hospitalization, we apply a potent topical steroid twice daily to the entire body, excluding the scalp, face, axillae, and groin. Patients are then instructed to wear soft cotton pajamas that have been slightly moistened in tepid water and that which are then covered with a plastic vinyl "sauna suit." If the palms and soles are involved, dampened cotton gloves and socks are placed on the hands and feet, followed by plastic gloves and booties. This total body occlusive corticosteroid therapy should be applied for 4-hour periods twice daily for the first 3 days of hospitalization. This cutaneous corticosteroid "burst" is sufficient to lessen the degree of erythema and edema, as well as to remove psoriatic scale with few local or systemic complications. Total body occlusive steroids should be avoided or used with caution in patients with diabetes, cardiovascular disease or heat intolerance. Between application of the corticosteroids and moist occlusive dressings, patients apply a thick coat of moisturizing emollient such as Eucerin or hydrophilic petrolatum with 20 percent water.

After the last occlusive dressing is applied, the patient is asked to apply a coal tar preparation over the entire body, sparing the face and intertriginous areas. The choice of this tar preparation is based on the patient's previous history, experience with tar products, and seasonal considerations. If the patient gives a strong history of allergic sensitivity to tar or shows an adverse reaction to a test dose, tar products are not used. However, the majority of patients are able to tolerate a tar cream such as Fototar or 10 percent LCD in a water-washable base in the summer months and a 2 percent crude coal tar in washable yellow petrolatum in the winter months. Patients who are prone to develop folliculitis are treated with tar gel products such as Estar or Psoragel. A thin coat of tar is applied initially for 4 hours and gradually increased to continuously as tolerated. This tar preparation is removed in a shower or bath just prior to phototherapy treatments.

Ultraviolet light phototherapy is begun within 24 to 48 hours after hospitalization. The first dose is set at 80 percent of the minimum erythema dose obtained by phototesting and subsequent doses are raised by 10 to 50 percent, based on the patient's history of sun sensitivity and the physical examination. Very fair patients are raised by 10-percent increments and blacks by 50 percent increments, for example. The ultraviolet light dosage is raised daily until the patients exhibit a minimum degree of erythema that lasts from 6 to 24 hours. If patients do not become pink by 6 hours, a second phototherapy treatment is given, consisting of an additional 5 to 25 percent increase. If a patient exhibits more than a minimum erythema, the next phototherapy dose is either held constant, lowered, or postponed as the clinical situation dictates. Any areas that the patient points out as being "sunburned" are shielded from further phototherapy until all tenderness has abated and then gradually reexposed to lower doses of ultraviolet light. Once the psoriatic lesions are entirely flat, ultraviolet light exposures are held constant until the patient is discharged.

Ultraviolet phototherapy is given in a fluorescent tube phototherapy cabinet to the entire body, with recalcitrant plaques on the elbows, knees, palms, and soles given extra isolated phototherapy exposure utilizing a portable hot quartz mercury vapor lamp. Patients are monitored closely for evidence of generalized desquamation. When generalized desquamation appears, the ultraviolet light dose is dropped by 50 percent in an attempt to avoid painful sunburn responses.

For large recalcitrant plaques, anthralin paste is applied as previously described after the daily phototherapy treatments for a maximum of 4 hours after each exposure. Plaques not responding to this regimen may also be injected with 5 mg per milliliter triamcinolone acetonide to a maximum of 20 mg total body dose as needed. Recalcitrant lesions on the palms and soles may be treated with keratolytics as previously described; intertriginous fissuring often responds to a mixture of 1 percent hydrocortisone with 25,000 units per milliliter of nystatin in Cetaphil or Wise's shake lotion.

Scalp psoriasis is treated with a topical corticosteroid gel or solution such as Topsyn, Valisone, or Synalar. This is followed by the application of a thick coat of Baker's P & S scalp oil if there is a lot of hyperkeratotic scale in the scalp. The scalp is then covered with a moist gauze turban that is covered with a plastic Saran Wrap occlusive dressing. This dressing remains in place for 4 hours or overnight, after which the scalp is shampooed with a tar shampoo such as T-gel, Zetar, or 10 percent LCD in a mild shampoo base. After shampooing, the topical corticosteroid is then reapplied to the scalp without occlusion. This occlusive therapy is continued for the first 3 or 4 days of hospitalization and then tapered gradually to daily tar shampoos followed by a weak topical steroid solution or gel without occlusion. As the activity of the scalp disease dictates, this treatment is tapered every other day or less, as tolerated. Recalcitrant scalp disease is occasionally treated with an anthralin or tar pomade gel or cream applied for 10 to 30 minutes prior to shampooing. Nail psoriasis is treated with a combination of surgical management, keratolytic therapy with 20 to 40 percent urea under occulsion, corticosteroids or 5-fluorouracil applied daily without occlusion.

Patients are treated in the hospital until virtually all the psoriasis is flat and showing evidence of slow capillary refill. It is our experience that the less psoriasis at discharge, the longer the clinical remission. Patients are discharged from the hospital using only emollients and tar shampoos if they are completely free of psoriatic disease. If there is residual psoriasis, patients continue to use tar medications (such as Estar or T-derm oil) or anthralin products (such as low-dose Anthraderm or Drithocreme) for a few hours each day on an outpatient basis, in addition to bland emollients. Depending on the amount of psoriasis and the disease activity, patients may also be placed on maintenance outpatient phototherapy once or twice weekly at a dose of ultraviolet light equal to the last phototherapy dose in the hospital. These phototherapy treatments are tapered over a period of a few months and eventually stopped unless the patient's condition worsens. Patients generally can go for months or even years controlling their disease with emollients, keratolytics, and an occasional corticosteroid product before further aggressive therapy is needed.

If patients develop painful chemical irritation from anthralin or tar or a sunburn response from ultraviolet light, a moderate strength corticosteroid is sometimes used for one or two applications to help decrease inflammation and avoid a Koebner response. Pruritus following phototherapy treatments or tar therapy are treated with Atarax, 10 to 25 mg every 6 to 8 hours, and topical counterirritants such as 0.5 percent menthol and 1 percent phenol in Cetaphil lotion. Staining of the skin from anthralin can be removed by using a few daily applications of a keratolytic such as Keralyt.

Systemic Therapy

The rare patients who respond poorly to this regimen, require multiple hospitalizations (with only partial improvement), and continue to be disabled by their disease are candidates for psoralen photochemotherapy or systemic antimitabolte therapy. Psoralen photochemotherapy is administered, as described by the guidelines published in the Journal of the American Academy of Dermatology 1979; 1:106, giving 0.6 mg per kilogram of methoxsalen twice weekly 2 hours prior to graduated exposure to long-wave ultraviolet light type A. Alternatively, methotrexate 15 to 30 mg can be given orally or intramuscularly as a single dose on a weekly basis following the guidelines published in the Journal of the American Academy of Dermatology 1982; 6:145. Experimental therapy with systemic retinoids, nonsteroidal anti-inflammatory drugs, and other agents may be considered. Patients who require methotrexate, psoralen photochemotherapy, or experimental approaches are a small minority; a vast majority of patients can be easily and well managed with the treatment plan described herein.

DERMATITIS HERPETIFORMIS

JOHN J. ZONE, M.D.
MARTA PETERSEN, M.D.

The single greatest source of error in the treatment of dermatitis herpetiformis (DH) is incorrect diagnosis. There are three basic criteria for the diagnosis of DH, and at least two of these should be fulfilled before embarking on any treatment program:

1. Clinical characteristics consisting of involvement of extensor surfaces with a pruritic papulovesicular eruption.
2. Histologic changes in involved skin including vesicle formation at the dermal-epidermal junction and infiltration of dermal papillary tips with neutrophils.
3. The immunopathologic findings of granular or linear IgA at the dermal-epidermal junction on direct immunofluorescence (DIF) of perilesional and/or uninvolved skin.

Clinical response of a dermatitis to dapsone is not considered adequate for the diagnosis of DH since several dapsone-responsive dermatoses have been described. Indeed, clinical trials of dapsone or gluten-free diet for presumptive DH without fulfilling at least two of the aforementioned criteria should be frowned upon, and may be associated with considerable side effects and inconvenience.

The histologic findings mentioned are characteristic although some confusion with vesicular pemphigoid may exist. Histologic patterns do not differentiate between linear and granular IgA and therefore give no insight into the possible efficacy of gluten-free diet (GFD) therapy.

Immunopathologic diagnosis can provide insight into therapy since granular IgA is known to be associated with response to a gluten-free diet and linear IgA may not be associated with gluten sensitivity. Data on the effectiveness of GFD in linear IgA disease are lacking. Extremely rarely (less than 5 percent of cases), patients who fulfill the first two criteria for the disease have been reported to have negative DIF; we consider such cases to be a research curiosity. In our hands, the main cause of negative DIF is biopsying involved skin. It is believed that the inflammatory infiltrate destroys immunoreactants when vesicles are produced. We recommend biopsying perilesional skin (erythema without papules or vesicles). If a negative DIF biopsy is obtained on initial sampling, the immunopathologist should be encouraged to do multiple sections throughout the biopsy, since IgA has been reported to be irregularly present within biopsies. If the specimen is still negative and DH continues to be a serious clinical consideration, a repeat specimen, preferably fresh tissue not immersed in transport medium, should be obtained. IgA deposition has been reported to vary from biopsy to biopsy within the same individual, and the transport medium has been reported on rare occasions to affect IgA positivity. If the DIF is still negative, alternative clinical diagnoses should be considered. Alternative diagnoses are likely if the first two diagnostic criteria are not strictly fulfilled.

Many laboratories offer special transport medium and mail service for the processing of DIF biopsies. Care should be taken to use fresh transport medium (<2–3 months old). Formalin used for routine histology is unacceptable for DIF.

Although at least 80 percent of DH patients demonstrate some degree of histologic small bowel abnormality similar to that seen in gluten sensitive enteropathy (GSE), small-bowel biopsy is not recommended for the routine diagnosis of DH. The severity of the small bowel abnormality does not correlate with response of skin disease to a GFD. Ten to 20 percent of DH patients have significant symptoms of malabsorption. In this group, small bowel biopsy may be helpful to confirm the abnormality, and provide reassurance for both the patient and physician during long-term gluten-free diet therapy.

Both DH and GSE are associated with HLA B8 and DR3 genotype in more than 90 percent of cases, but routine HLA typing in the non-research setting offers little diagnostic advantage.

TREATMENT

Therapeutic Alternatives

Dapsone is the drug of choice in the therapy of DH and is currently the only drug approved by the U.S. Food and Drug Administration for use in this disease. In our experience, it is extremely effective in controlling symptoms. Diasone is metabolized to dapsone but is less well absorbed and offers no advantage. Sulfapyridine, 1 to 4 grams daily, is effective in many cases. However, sulfapyridine may not completely control symptoms at any dosage level and, for uncertain reasons, may be totally ineffective in some cases. Sulfapyridine does not produce significant hemolytic anemia, peripheral neuropathy or psychosis as has been reported with dapsone. Patients with allergic reactions to dapsone may take sulfapyridine. Patients taking sulfapyridine are subject to the known complications and side effects of therapy with other sulfa drugs including nephrolithiasis. Risk of nephrolithiasis may be minimized by adequate fluid intake and alkalinization of the urine.

A variety of other therapies have been described, including colchicine, cholestyramine, pyribenzamine, indomethacin, nicotinic acid and sodium chromalyn. Our experience with these treatments is limited to two or three cases in each instance and occurred in the treatment of patients with severe disease and significant complications of dapsone. In these circumstances, these treatments were subjectively judged to be only minimally effective.

Topical steroid application is generally inadequate when used alone for control of DH symptoms. However, potent steroids in gel form may provide relief of occasional lesions that develop on otherwise adequate dapsone or gluten-free diet therapy. This allows patients to treat lesions without increasing the dosage of dapsone.

Intake of large amounts of inorganic iodide is known to exacerbate symptoms and rare patients have been reported to improve on low iodide diets. However, this is not a mainstay of treatment and need only be considered if patients are consuming excessive iodide in the form of vitamin pills, kelp, or seafood. Likewise, some patients have reported exacerbation with thyroid hormone replacement therapy and thyrotoxicosis. In such cases, excessive thyroid replacement should be avoided and thyrotoxicosis treated appropriately.

Preferred Approach

After the diagnosis is confirmed by the preceeding criteria, the management alternatives should be explained to the patient and he or she should participate in decision making. It is likely that the disease will be lifelong, although severity may wax and wane and remissions may occur in 10 to 20 percent of DH patients. The management alternatives are:

1. Treatment with dapsone which will adequately suppresses (but does not cure) the disease. Dapsone treatment requires continued monitoring and uncommonly may be associated with significant side effects.
2. Treatment with a gluten-free diet. Initial supression of symptoms with dapsone is usually necessary when this treatment is chosen.
3. No treatment. This has been chosen by occasional patients with minimal disease severity.

The exact mechanism of action of dapsone is unknown, but its effectiveness in a variety of neutrophilic dermatoses suggests a mechanism related to neutrophil function or chemotaxis. Inhibition of myeloperoxidase-mediated iodination and chemotaxis to specific agents have been described in vitro. Dapsone serves only to suppress disease activity and recurrence of symptoms occurs within 24 to 72 hours of discontinuing therapy. Dapsone has no effect on the intestinal abnormality or on cutaneous IgA deposition.

Dapsone is available in 25 mg and 100 mg tablets. Initial treatment with 50 mg dapsone by mouth daily usually improves symptoms within 24 to 48 hours in adults. Correspondingly smaller doses should be used in children. When taken daily, dapsone levels reach a steady state within 7 days. Maintenance therapy is then adjusted on a weekly basis to maintain adequate suppression of symptoms; the average maintenance dose is 100 to 200 mg daily. Occasional new lesions (2–3 per week) are to be expected and are not an indication for altering daily dosage. Minor fluctuations in disease severity do occur and are probably related to oral gluten intake. Outbreak of facial and scalp lesions while on otherwise adequate treatment is not uncommon. The authors have found no good method for preventing such situations and increases in dapsone dosage seem to have no effect. Breaking the vesicles followed by application of a potent steroid gel may help healing.

Dapsone exhibits good bioavailability, with absorption being unaffected by presumed GSE. There is wide variation in serum concentration of dapsone and monoacetyl dapsone among individuals, and consequently there is little value in measuring serum dapsone as a guide to therapeutic management. Acetylator phenotype is unrelated to dapsone dose requirement. Although there is wide variability in the half-life of dapsone (10–50 hours), the vast majority of patients are best managed on a single daily dose.

Hemolysis is the most common side effect of treatment. Dapsone is a strong oxidizer and produces a dose-related oxidant stress on normal aging red cells. It may produce severe hemolysis in patients with glucose-6-phosphate dehydrogenase (G-6-PD) deficiency. Blacks and Caucasions of southern Mediterranean origin should be screened for G-6-PD deficiency before dapsone therapy is instituted. If there is concern about cardiac complications from moderate degrees of hemolysis, the physician should start with smaller doses (25 mg daily) and titrate the dosage carefully. Initial reduction of hemoglobin by 2 to 3 grams is common, but subsequent partial compensation by reticulocytosis is the rule.

Methemoglobinemia is seldom a severe problem, but may be tolerated poorly in patients with G-6-PD deficiency, methemoglobin reductase deficiency, or cardiopulmonary decompensation. Methemoglobinemia is usually less than 15 percent, but at higher doses of dapsone (>200 milligrams), symptoms of methemoglobinemia (weakness, headaches, and tachycardia) may become problematic even in normal individuals. Methemoglobinemia may be reversed with methylene blue but this is rarely necessary except in cases of accidental overdosage.

Other dose-related side effects that are rare in doses of less than 200 mg daily include toxic hepatitis, cholestatic jaundice, psychosis, and either motor or sensory peripheral neuropathy. Hypoalbuminemia may occur after chronic use. Carcinogenicity of dapsone has been reported in mice and rats but has not been documented in humans.

An infectious mononucleosis syndrome with fever and lymphadenopathy occurs rarely but may be severe. Deaths from agranulocytosis and aplastic anemia associated with the use of dapsone have been reported. This usually occurs within the first 2 to 12 weeks, and necessitates close observation of blood counts during that period. Idiosyncratic cutaneous reactions that demand discontinuation of the drug include exfoliative dermatitis, erythema multiforme, erythema nodosum, and urticaria.

Since DH affects women of childbearing age, the possible teratogenicity of dapsone is important. Available data are inconclusive, but would suggest that dapsone is safe during pregnancy. Our recommendation for dealing with this is adherence to a strict gluten-free diet, preferably for 6 to 12 months before conception, in the hope of eliminating the need for dapsone during pregnancy. If this is unsuccessful, the patient must participate in further decision making. Discontinuation of dapsone produces rapid exacerbation of vesicles and severe pruritus. However, these symptoms are not life-threatening, and the patient may choose to tolerate the symptoms rather than undertake the risk of a possible teratogenic effect. If the patient prefers the potential risk of dapsone to uncontrolled symptoms, then it would seem prudent to encourage strict adherence to a gluten-free diet and to undertake therapy with the minimum amount of dapsone necessary to control severe symptoms. Dapsone is secreted in breast milk and produces hemolytic anemia in infants; consequently, patients taking dapsone should be discouraged from breastfeeding.

Severe side effects or complications from dapsone therapy are best managed by discontinuing the drug and treating with sulfapyridine and/or a gluten-free diet. Strict adherence to a gluten-free diet should produce improvement of clinical symptoms and a decrease in dapsone requirement in the majority of patients with DH. The advantages of gluten restriction include a reduction of dapsone dosage and its attendant complications, improvement of gastrointestinal symptoms (which range from crampy pain to overt diarrhea), and a therapy aimed at the cause rather than the symptoms of the disease. Additional incentive for gluten-free diet therapy is provided by the fact that patients with DH are known to have an increased incidence of malignancy, particularly lymphoma. Although the data are inconclusive, the incidence of malignancy may be lower when a strict gluten-free diet is maintained. Complete control on a gluten-free diet obviates the need for the hemotologic follow-up which will be outlined. Disadvantages of gluten-free diet therapy include inconvenience and a diet that some patients may find unappetizing. It must be stressed that the patient should actively participate in the decision regarding starting a gluten-free diet. Individual patients vary in their willingness to take medications or adhere to diets over a prolonged period of time. A knowledgeable dermatologist should present the details of alternative forms of therapy. If a gluten-free diet is chosen, consultation with a dietitian is a necessity and strict adherence to the diet for a 1-year trial period should be stressed. A gluten-free diet may clear all skin symptoms, but it is not curative, and resumption of a regular diet produces recurrence of skin disease in weeks to months. Patients should be informed that up to one-third of cases do not respond to gluten restriction. It is not possible to predict with certainty which patients will respond to a gluten-free diet. However, it is currently believed that patients showing linear IgA on direct immunofluorescence do not have gluten-sensitive enteropathy, and therefore are less likely to respond to a gluten-free diet than those patients with granular IgA on biopsy.

Recommendations for the follow-up of patients on dapsone are as follows:

1. Baseline complete blood count (CBC) and liver function tests should be obtained. G-6-PD level should be determined prior to initiating therapy in Asians, Blacks, or those of southern Mediterranean descent.
2. CBC should be checked weekly for the first month, monthly for the next 5 months, and semiannually thereafter.

3. Chemistry profile should be checked at 6 months and then annually to monitor for possible hepatotoxicity, changes in renal function, and hypoalbuminemia.
4. Patients should be made aware of potential hemolytic anemia and the blue-gray discoloration associated with methemoglobinemia in order to avoid undue alarm on the part of the patient or other physicians treating the patient.

Clinical management of therapeutic response should stress maintenance on the smallest dose of dapsone necessary to control disease. Occasional new lesions (2 to 3 per week) are to be expected on an optimal dapsone dose and are not an indication for altering drug dosage. Spontaneous remissions are unusual in our experience, but such remissions will become obvious if the dapsone dose is minimized to allow occasional new lesions. Patients controlled on a strict gluten-free diet usually have recurrence of disease in 2 weeks to 6 months after reinstitution of a regular diet. However, rare spontaneous remissions may also occur in this group and patients should be offered the alternative of a regular diet to evaluate this possibility.

Pros and Cons of Treatment

Rare patients with mild disease may elect no treatment. There seems to be little harm to this choice except for the discomfort and possible increased risk of lymphoma. Patients electing treatment should understand that the need for therapy is usually lifelong. Patient education and participation in decision making is essential for management and compliance. The combination of a compliant patient and a skillful physician can provide excellent relief of symptoms with minimal complications in a disease that is otherwise extremely uncomfortable.

In our opinion, the best and safest treatment is the initial control of symptoms with dapsone and a gluten-free diet with subsequent tapering of dapsone and maintenance on a gluten-free diet.

KAPOSI'S SARCOMA

ROBERT L. KRIGEL, M.D.
ALVIN E. FRIEDMAN-KIEN, M.D.

Since its initial description by Moriz Kaposi in 1872, Kaposi's sarcoma has remained a fascinating curiosity as a rare and unusual tumor which typically runs a benign and indolent course. Most of the cases have been seen in Europe and North America and have occurred predominantly in elderly white men (in the fifth to eighth decade of life) of Italian or eastern European Jewish origin. The male-to-female ratio is 10 to 15:1. It is occasionally late in the course of the disease that systemic or disseminated manifestations may appear.

In the 1950s new interest developed in this disease with the recognition that Kaposi's sarcoma also occurred with high incidence among blacks in an endemic belt located across equatorial Africa. It is now recognized as the second most common malignant tumor in Uganda, with approximately 9 percent of all tumors reported in males being Kaposi's sarcoma. In Africa, the disease is seen primarily among young black men (male-to-female ratio 17:1) but remains extremely uncommon among whites or Asians inhabiting the same regions. Patients with African Kaposi's sarcoma often present with clinical findings that both closely resemble and differ from the classic manifestations usually seen in Europe and North America. Although a benign nodular form of the disease is the type most frequently seen, a more florid and locally aggressive form has been observed with local invasion of subcutaneous tissue and bone. A systemic and fulminant lymphadenopathic form of Kaposi's sarcoma, usually without skin involvement, is also seen among prepubescent African children between 2 and 15 years of age (male-to-female ratio 3:1).

In the early 1970s it was recognized that patients with systemic lupus erythematosus or renal transplants receiving long-term immunosuppressive therapy had an increased incidence of Kaposi's sarcoma. A number of renal allograft recipients receiving prednisone and azathioprine developed Kaposi's sarcoma within 3 to 53 months after the onset of treatment. Most of the transplant patients have been young, with an average age of 42 (range 23 to 59) years at the time of transplantation. Although the tumor in such iatrogenically immunosuppressed individuals often remained localized, widespread dissemination and visceral involvement were not uncommon. Some of these medically induced immunosuppressed patients have experienced a regression of their tumor when the immunosuppressive drug regimen was either discontinued or modified.

In the spring of 1981 the Acquired Immunodeficiency Syndrome (AIDS) was first recognized as a new and epidemic disease which has rapidly increased to become a major worldwide public health concern. The term "AIDS" has been proposed by the Center for Disease Control (CDC) to describe the recent occurrence of virally-induced, profound, acquired disorder of cell-mediated immunity. This virus is variously referred to as human T-cell lymphotrophic virus, type 3 (HTLV-III), lymphadenopathic virus (LAV), AIDS-related virus (ARV), and most recently as human immunodeficiency virus (HIV). It predisposes the afflicted host to a wide variety of unusual and often lethal opportunistic infections such as *Pneumocystis carinii* pneumonia, *Mycobacterium avium* intracellulare, intracerebral toxoplasmosis, and others. About 25 percent of all AIDS patients have also developed a disseminated form of Kaposi's sarcoma, and a few have other tumors such as high-grade malignant lymphomas or primary central nervous system lymphomas. This type of Kaposi's sarcoma is called epidemic Kaposi's sarcoma in order to distinguish it from the classic variety seen in elderly Europeans and North Americans. The cases have occurred primarily among sexually active homosexual or bisexual men between the ages of 20 and 64, with a mean age of about 38. AIDS has also been observed among intravenous drug users, hemophiliacs who received lyophilized factor VIII clotting concentrates, transfusion recipients, sexual partners of AIDS patients, and children born to parents with HTLV-III/LAV infection. The common thread of viral transmission is through blood or semen.

Among the cases of epidemic Kaposi's sarcoma studied at New York University Medical Center, 80 percent of those patients who did not present with a prior or coexistent opportunistic infection were still alive after 1 year. Of those who developed an opportunistic infection, either prior to or coexistent with the diagnosis of epidemic Kaposi's sarcoma, only 30 percent were alive at 1 year, suggesting that the cause of death in these individuals was not the tumor, but the opportunistic infections to which they were susceptible.

The salient characteristics of these different forms of Kaposi's sarcoma are summarized in Table 1.

CLASSIC KAPOSI'S SARCOMA

Classic Kaposi's sarcoma is most often a relatively benign, indolent disease. Patients may survive for 15 years or more after disease onset with the cause of death usually unrelated to the tumor. Patients usually present with asymptomatic, brownish-red to purple or blue patch, plaque, or nodular skin lesions, located on the lower extremities, including the soles of the feet. Other anatomic sites are occasionally involved. Initially the disease may be limited to a single or a few discrete lesions which range in size from a few millimeters to several centimeters in diameter. Lesions tend to slowly increase in size, and those that occur in a localized cluster often coalesce with time.

Although new lesions tend to occur near the original tumor site, they may appear at any time or on any part of the body, such as the upper extremities, the head and neck, or the trunk. Lesions that persist for prolonged periods often become hyperpigmented, especially in darker complexioned individuals. As the disease progresses, the untreated tumors may increase considerably in size and may become fungated and ulcerated. Chronic venous stasis and lymphedema of the involved extremity frequently complicate the prolonged clinical course.

The erratic progression of this tumor has always raised doubts as to the overall therapeutic efficacy from the various modalities, especially when symptoms were not present. In fact, it is far from clear whether treatment of classic Kaposi's sarcoma halts the spread of the disease. It is certain that it may result in a decreased tumor volume, in reduction of discomfort associated with edematous and tumorous extremities, in control of bleeding or symptoms associated with cutaneous, mucosal, or visceral lesions, and rarely, in promoting the healing of bone lesions. There is no data, however, that treatment improves survival.

Small lesions of classic Kaposi's sarcoma may be satisfactorily treated by electrodesiccation and curettage or by surgical excision; however, the tumor is relatively sensitive to local radiation therapy, which is the most frequent and successful treatment employed. Excellent palliation has been achieved with doses not much higher than 2,000 rad. Most of this experience was obtained in cutaneous disease of early isolated macules and papules. Radiation has only rarely been utilized for the treatment of painful bony involvement or localized visceral disease. Large confluent areas of disease have been considered less radiosensitive, and in the presence of moderate edema, complications are frequently encountered. Local complications also occur because of repeated doses for recurrences within previously irradiated areas.

The technique of irradiation usually involves a field that covers the entire distal involved extremity, in 300

TABLE 1 Comparison of Variants of Kaposi's Sarcoma

Type	*Population*	*Clinical Characteristics*	*Course*
Classic	Older Jewish and Italian men	Usually confined to lower extremities, often with venous stasis and lymphedema; late widespread cutaneous and visceral involvement	Indolent; survival 10–15 years; associated with other malignancies in 37%
	Iatrogenically immunosuppressed patients	May be localized to skin or widespread with systemic involvement	Can be indolent or rapidly progressive; may regress when immunosuppressive therapy is changed
African	Young black men	Localized; large exophytic tumors or invasive to underlying bone	Slowly progressive and fatal over 5–8 years
	Children	Generalized lymphadenopathy; rarely involving the skin	Rapidly progressive; fatal within 2 to 3 years
Epidemic	Primarily homosexual men; AIDS	Disseminated mucocutaneous lesions often involving lymph nodes and visceral organs, esp. gastrointestinal tract and lungs	Fulminant, less than 20% survival at 2 years if associated with opportunistic infection

rad fractions or greater, with additional spot radiation to areas of recurrence or only partial regression. Treatment should penetrate beyond cutaneous areas and therefore usually requires supervoltage equipment. Recurrences that are localized to skin can be treated with electron beam therapy. With these techniques, local control has been achieved in more than 35 percent of cases.

In widespread disease, systemic chemotherapy has achieved some beneficial effects. The most commonly used chemotherapeutic agent has been vinblastine, with response rates of 90 to 95 percent. Response durations rarely exceed one year, and a positive effect on survival has not been documented.

EPIDEMIC KAPOSI'S SARCOMA

The mucocutaneous clinical manifestations of epidemic Kaposi's sarcoma are much more varied than that seen in the classic type or African type of this neoplasm. The lesions usually are not localized to the lower extremities as is the case in the classic variety of the disease. Rather, the lesions may appear any place on the lower or upper extremities, the trunk, the genitals, and the face. Particularly common sites are the occipital region of skin behind the ears and the ear lobes themselves. Oropharyngeal lesions on the mucosa are frequently seen on the hard or soft palate. These lesions are usually flat, but may be plaque-like and even nodular and are lavender to blue.

It is not uncommon to find epidemic Kaposi's sarcoma lesions not only on the skin, but simultaneously dispersed throughout the oral mucosa, esophagus, and gastrointestinal tract, usually detectable by endoscopy and colonoscopy. All lesions, cutaneous and visceral, have a tendency to coalesce when they occur in multiple numbers in the same area.

In order to account for this variety of presentations, we have proposed a classification schema that subdivides the presentations of both the epidemic and classic forms of Kaposi's sarcoma as shown in Table 2. Stage I represents the usual Kaposi's sarcoma type seen in elderly patients; stage II represents the African-type Kaposi's sarcoma when locally invasive; stages III and IV stratify the disseminated Kaposi's sarcoma seen primarily in homosexual males, with stage III defined as generalized cutaneous and/or lymph node involvement, and stage IV being visceral involvement. Each stage is further subtyped as to the absence or presence of fever (unrelated to an identifiable source of infection) and/or weight loss (10 percent or more), subtypes A and B respectively.

TABLE 2 Staging System of Kaposi's Sarcoma

Stage I	Cutaneous, locally indolent
Stage II	Cutaneous, locally aggressive with or without regional lymph nodes
Stage III	Generalized cutaneous and/or lymph node involvement
Stage IV	Visceral
Subtypes	
A.	No systemic signs or symptoms.
B.	Systemic signs: 10% weight loss or fever greater than 100°F orally unrelated to an identifiable source of infection lasting more than 2 weeks.

This staging system creates four distinct groups in terms of overall survival in epidemic Kaposi's sarcoma. Patients who present with a coexistent or prior opportunistic infection have a median survival of 8 months with only 30 percent surviving at 12 months. Patients without an opportunistic infection but with B symptoms have a median survival of 14 months with 60 percent surviving at 12 months. Patients without either a coexistent opportunistic infection or B symptoms fall into two categories. Patients with cutaneous disease only or cutaneous and lymph node involvement have a 90 percent survival at 12 months and a 60 percent survival at 24 months. This is in contrast to patients with any visceral involvement in whom survival at 24 months is only 40 percent. Thus, the clinical prognostic factors in epidemic Kaposi's sarcoma consist of: (1)a prior or coexistent opportunistic infection, (2)systemic symptoms, (3)extent of disease, and (4)visceral involvement.

Laboratory parameters indicative of the underlying immunodeficiency have also been correlated with survival. These factors have included the absolute number of helper T-cells, the helper: suppressor T-cell ratio, beta-2 microglobulin, and the presence of an acid-labile alpha interferon. There is a significant correlation between the clinical presentation and the measures of the underlying immunodeficiency.

In general, patients with epidemic Kaposi's sarcoma should be treated on an investigational protocol whenever possible. Current National Cancer Institute sponsored therapies, however, have focused primarily on the underlying HTLV-III/LAV viral infection that has led to the immunodeficiency. Studies with two of these agents, suramin and HPA-23, showed in vivo inhibition of virus replication. However, no change in ultimate survival was seen. The results of studies with two newer agents, ribavirin and azidothymidine (AZT) are still pending. It is hoped that if the underlying viral infection can be controlled, then the immune system can restore itself. However, even if these therapies are successful, combination therapy using an antiviral agent, a potential immune enhancer, and an antitumor agent may be necessary.

These antitumor agents have consisted primarily of standard chemotherapy drugs, used either singly or in combination and the alpha-interferons. Chemotherapy has been used cautiously in epidemic Kaposi's sarcoma because of its potential to worsen the already profoundly depressed immunologic status of the patient. Single agent chemotherapies have included vinblastine, vincristine, bleomycin, etoposide (VP-16), and doxorubicin (Adriamycin). Combination chemotherapy regimens have employed bleomycin in conjunction with vincristine, vinblastine, or etoposide. Methotrexate has also been used in conjunction with vinblastine, and the combination of doxorubicin, bleomycin, and vinblastine has been used with a high degree of efficacy, but with an increased in-

TABLE 3 Chemotherapies of Kaposi's Sarcoma

Agent	*Schedule*
Vinblastine	4–6 mg/m² q 1–2 weeks
Vincristine	1.4 mg/m² (max 2 mg) q 1–2 weeks
Bleomycin	10–15 units q 2 weeks
Etoposide (VP-16)	150 mg/m² × 3 days q 4 weeks
Adriamycin	10–20 mg weekly
Alpha interferons	30 × 10⁶ units/m² t.i.w.

cidence of opportunistic infections. These treatments are summarized in Table 3.

Biologic response modifiers have also been used. The largest experience has been with the alpha-interferons, which as single agents appear to be comparable to the single agent chemotherapies. Studies have also been performed which combine alpha-interferon with either vinblastine or etoposide. In general, single agents, whether chemotherapy or alpha-interferon, appear to have a high response rate in patients with relatively early stage disease (60 to 80 percent response rate). However, in patients with more advanced disease their efficacy is quite low (10 to 20 percent response rate). Combination therapies, however, have a much better response rate in patients with more advanced disease or with the poor prognostic signs of a prior opportunistic infection or B symptoms.

Clinical studies have also been performed using gamma-interferon, interleukin-2, plasmapheresis, TP 5, thymic hormones, and isoprinosine. Overall, these agents have had no significant antitumor effects nor consistent improvements in the underlying immune deficiency.

As in the classic variety, however, there is no evidence that any treatment prolongs survival in epidemic Kaposi's sarcoma. Overall prognosis is dictated by stage and the presence or absence of fever or an opportunistic infection. Chemotherapy serves only to control a neoplastic manifestation of the underlying immunodeficiency.

TABLE 4 Treatment of Kaposi's Sarcoma

Extent of Disease	*Preferred Treatment*
Localized	Surgical excision or radiation therapy
Disseminated cutaneous and/or lymphadenopathic	Observe until progression, then alpha interferon and/or single-agent chemotherapy
Disseminated with visceral involvement, prior opportunistic infection, or B symptoms	Combination chemotherapy

Current treatment guidelines are summarized in Table 4. Patients with relatively early-stage disease can be observed until there is definite progression. At that point, treatment is initiated with single-agent chemotherapy or alpha-interferon. Patients failing one or more treatment trials and patients with aggressive, extensive visceral disease are given combination chemotherapy.

Until recently Kaposi's sarcoma was a rare and unusual neoplasm. Since July 1981, however, an epidemic of over 25,000 cases of AIDS has been reported to the CDC, 25 percent of whom have had Kaposi's sarcoma. Unlike classic Kaposi's sarcoma, with its relatively benign and indolent course, epidemic Kaposi's sarcoma often runs a fulminant course.

Unfortunately, treatment has demonstrated no effect on overall survival for both classic and epidemic Kaposi's sarcoma. Surgical excision and radiation therapy control local problems in patients with limited disease. Chemotherapy provides effective palliation in patients with progressive, disseminated disease. Future efforts are being directed to modulating immune function either alone or in combination with chemotherapy as well as with treatment of the underlying HTLV-III/LAV infection.

PRIMARY MALIGNANT MELANOMA

THOMAS B. FITZPATRICK, M.D.
ARTHUR J. SOBER, M.D.

Primary malignant melanoma of the skin is the leading cause of death of all diseases arising in the skin. At present, surgical excision of early lesions is the only therapy that can increase survival. Therefore, it is essential that the physician approaching the management of a suspicious primary melanoma should follow an accepted surgical protocol, as is outlined in this chapter. Of greatest importance in the management of cutaneous melanoma, once melanoma is suspected, is the establishment of a complete and accurate diagnosis.

TYPE OF BIOPSY

Total excisional biopsy with narrow margins is the procedure of choice, since it provides the complete specimen for the pathologist to study, and if the lesion is benign, definitive therapy has been accomplished. There is no evidence that incisional or punch biopsies reduce survival, and these procedures are currently being performed when the lesions are large and/or located in cosmetically sensitive areas. If punch or incisional biopsy is performed, the area to select for biopsy should be the thickest (most elevated) area for a palpable lesion or the darkest area for a flat one. Punch or incisional biopsy, while usually adequate to establish whether the lesion is malignant, is not sufficient to determine prognosis, since other portions of the tumor may be more invasive. Since therapy is currently based on the anticipated prognosis, final judgement and therapeutic recommendations are deferred until the complete specimen has been removed. Serial sections every 1 to 2 mm throughout the tumor are examined, as is each margin. The pathologist can then report tumor type and level of invasion, thickness, whether regression is present (i.e., the tumor may have been thicker at some point), presence of ulceration, mitotic rate, and whether margins are involved with tumor.

INTERPRETATION OF BIOPSY

If there is any doubt histopathologically about the nature of the tumor, referral for a second opinion by a pathologist highly experienced in the diagnosis of melanoma and its variants is recommended. Such a consultation would be especially useful when the histopathologic diagnosis of melanoma has been made in a non-congenital lesion in a child under 10 years of age. Suspicion should be raised that the "melanoma" might be a Spitz nevus and a second opinion obtained. In addition, if there is a discrepancy between the clinical impression and the histopathologic diagnosis, a second histopathologic opinion is also recommended (i.e., a benign-appearing lesion with a surprise malignant diagnosis or, conversely, a highly suspicious lesion clinically with a benign histopathologic diagnosis).

INFORMING THE PATIENT

The diagnosis, prognosis, and recommended therapy are discussed thoroughly with the patient. Sufficient time is allowed to answer all the patient's questions, and the patient is invited to call the physician should additional questions arise or if any material that has been discussed previously seems unclear upon rethinking. If the patient has a highly favorable prognosis, he is so informed in an attempt to lessen the undue worry that patients develop once the diagnosis of "melanoma" has been made. For patients who request additional information on melanoma, we suggest that they read the most current literature, since the concepts and outcome of melanoma have been changing rapidly. We direct patients to recent reviews on the subject.

THERAPY OF THE PRIMARY TUMOR

Once the diagnosis has been established, appropriate techniques can be selected to eliminate the primary tumor. Table 1 presents the initial work-up prior to definitive treatment. At present, the treatment of primary melanoma of skin is surgical. Surgical margins are in the process of being narrowed from 5 cm, which has been the traditional margin. Nearly all patients with 5-cm excision margins require skin grafts for closure. We are, at present, recommending 1.5-cm margins for primary tumors <0.85 millimeters thick, and 3.0-cm margins for all others (Table 2). These margins allow for primary closure in most instances. If the lesion has been previously removed by excisional biopsy, the margins are taken from the surgical scar. Flaps can be used for closure when appropriate. Efforts are made to preserve vital structures. For example, if the removal of an eye would be required to achieve a 3-cm margin for a cutaneous melanoma adjacent to the eye, a somewhat smaller margin would be taken to preserve the eye. From studies to date, these somewhat smaller margins do not seem to adversely affect ultimate survival.

TABLE 1 Initial Work-up

History
- Lesion—changes such as color, border, growth, and bleeding
- Past history or family history of melanoma or dysplastic nevi, or congenital nevi
- Other symptoms, which might suggest disseminated disease, i.e., bone pain, CNS symptoms; if so, appropriate scans and blood tests are ordered.

Physical examination
- Primary lesion
- General skin examination including scalp and mucous membranes
  - Other suspicious pigmented lesion (second primary or dysplastic nevus)
  - Palpation for intracutaneous and subcutaneous metastases
  - Wood's light examination for suspected hypopigmentation around the primary or at distant sites
- General physical examination
  - Palpation of regional and distant nodal areas
  - Palpation of abdominal viscera; if abnormal, appropriate scans and blood tests are ordered

Biopsy
- Review of biopsy by reference pathologist, if necessary

Discuss results with patient
- Diagnosis
- Prognosis
- Therapy recommended
- Family screening
- Moderation of solar exposure; use of sunscreens

Additional laboratory tests as indicated
- Routine studies for low-risk primary tumors include only the hospital requirements for surgery, i.e., chest roentgenogram, routine blood work, urinalysis
- For high-risk disease, the studies ordered are guided by the symptoms and findings

Definitive therapy

TABLE 2 Excisions and Margins

Advantage of wide local excision (5-cm margin)
- Local recurrence is rarely seen

Disadvantages of 5-cm margin
- Usually requires grafting for closure
- Healing may be delayed
- Donor site needed
- Requires inpatient hospital treatment

Advantages of conservative excision margin (1.5- or 3-cm margin)
- Primary closure usually possible
- Cosmetically less debilitating
- May be done on an outpatient basis

Disadvantage of conservative margin
- May have higher local recurrence rate

Elective Nodal Dissection (nodes clinically negative) for Clinical Stage I Patients

Elective regional lymph node dissection (ERND) is a controversial procedure which at various reputable melanoma centers is always performed, sometimes performed, or never performed, depending on the conviction of the individual surgeon. Our recommendations, at present, fall on the middle ground. We use the following factors in the selection of patients for elective nodal dissection: age, tumor type, location, tumor thickness, and patient's preference.

The Patient's Age. In the very old or in patients in poor health who are likely to die from other diseases, ERND is not performed.

Tumor Type. ERND is not performed in patients with lentigo maligna melanoma in the absence of clinically suspicious regional nodes.

Location of Tumor ERND is *not* performed if the lymph node drainage is not clearly directed to a single nodal area. In ambiguous situations, especially on the torso, we have utilized technetium lymphoscintigraphy (isotope is injected into the primary tumor site and the potential lymph node drainage basins scanned). The finding of multiple drainage pathways would eliminate ERND from considerations.

Primary Tumor Thickness. The likelihood of microscopic tumor deposits in the regional nodes increases with increasing primary tumor thickness. Below a certain thickness, the frequency of micrometastasis is insufficient to justify elective dissection. Above a certain thickness, the frequency of death from hematologic metastasis is so high that regional nodal control does not appear to be beneficial. At present, our surgeons consider ERND for tumors thicker than 1.70 to 2.00 mm. These dissections involve removal of the inguinal nodes (superficial groin dissection) and not the iliacs (radical or deep groin dissection) (Tables 3 and 4).

TABLE 3 Elective Regional Lymph Node Dissection

Advantages
Control of disease in regional nodes
May improve survival
Has prognostic value (i.e., can be used to "stage" the disease)
Disadvantages
If drainage is ambiguous, wrong site may be dissected
Edema of extremity
Longer hospitalization and expense
May not affect survival
May be unnecessary if metastases have not reached the nodal area

TABLE 4 Superficial vs. Deep ERND

Superficial ERND
Less morbidity than deep
Few, if any, survivors if deep nodes involved
Deep (radical) ERND
Involvement of nodes indicates an adverse prognosis
May occasionally be curative

The Patient's Preference. The patient's desires are also weighed as a factor in the decision, since we believe that the procedure is controversial. The potential risks and benefits from ERND are explained in detail to each patient for whom we feel ERND might be beneficial, and the decision to do ERND becomes a joint one. Patients in our experience seem to fall into two groups. The first group wishes to do *only* those procedures of *proved* benefit; the second group will consider *any* procedure that *might* be of benefit to them. In centers where ongoing adjuvant therapy trials are being performed, ERND is an important procedure in the staging of patients and is needed to ensure comparability of the randomized groups. Whether ERND will prove ultimately to be of benefit will depend on adequate *prospective, randomized* trials containing sufficient numbers of comparable patients in each group.

Therapeutic Nodal Dissection

Therapeutic nodal dissections are recommended to achieve *local* tumor control when gross metastases are present in a nodal area. The 5-year survival of this group is about 30 percent. The 10-year survival is unfortunately much lower.

ADJUVANT THERAPY FOR HIGH-RISK PATIENTS

Adjuvant therapy is at present considered for patients who are clinically disease-free, but who are at high risk for the development of recurrent or disseminated disease (Table 5). These would include patients with high-risk primary tumors, patients with local recurrence or intransit metastases, patients who have undergone removal of involved lymph nodes, or patients who have had excision of isolated distant metastases. After several years of BCG-DTIC combination therapy, which appeared promising at our institution but has not appeared beneficial in trials at other institutions, we are currently seeking a more promising therapy. At present, we can determine who *might* benefit from such therapies, but are unaware of any that are of proved benefit.

TABLE 5 Adjuvant Therapy for High-Risk Disease

Advantages
May potentially destroy low volumes of tumor cells to delay or prevent metastases in high-risk patients
Known high risk of recurrence and death in certain patients with conventional therapy alone
Occasional patient may undergo a prolonged remission
Disadvantages
None has been proved beneficial
Side-effects of treatment
Some therapies could result in enhanced tumor spread

TREATMENT OF DISSEMINATED DISEASE

Nearly all patients with disseminated disease die of metastatic melanoma regardless of treatment. We suggest that all these patients be entered into an ongoing treatment protocol so that more successful therapies can be developed. The benchmark drug, DTIC, produces clinical responses in about 20 percent of cases, but complete responses are seen in less than 5 percent and these are usually of brief duration. Response rates appear higher for cutaneous, nodal, and pulmonary sites of metastases than for hepatic, central nervous system, and bony areas. The current treatment ongoing in our institution involves the use of cis-platinum, vinblastine, and DTIC in combination. Chemotherapy protocols change frequently, and oncologic consultation is recommended for each patient with metastatic disease.

Radiation therapy has been used in the palliative treatment of central nervous system and bony metastases with some short-term benefit.

FOLLOW-UP

Patients are seen at 3-month intervals for 2 years, 6-month intervals for 3 subsequent years, and annually thereafter. Patients with thin primary lesions (<.85 millimeter) and no dysplastic nevi clinically may be seen after the initial follow-up visit at 6- to 12-month intervals, since they are highly unlikely to develop recurrent disease.

On the other end of the spectrum of disease, patients with multiple moderately-to-severely atypical dysplastic nevi should be followed at 3- or 4-month intervals even beyond 2 years because of the relatively higher risk of developing a second primary tumor. These patients are followed closely with the use of Polaroid prints and 35-mm color slides. Any changing lesions or highly suspicious ones are candidates for removal and histopathologic evaluation. At each follow-up visit, the following areas are probed: (1) *History* is taken of any new persisting symptoms referrable to general health, bone pain, central nervous system complaint, any "lump or bump," and any changing lesions. (2) *Physical* (the patient is completely undressed at each visit) *palpation* of the entire skin surface is performed for intracutaneous and subcutaneous disease (including the scalp), the surgical scars are examined for adequacy of healing and evidence of recurrent disease, and the skin is examined for a second primary (including scalp and mucous membrane). The patient's pigmented lesions are compared with photos and slides from previous visits. Areas of the lymph nodes and abdominal viscera are palpated. (3) Any new pigmented lesions of interest are photographed. (4) The patient is cautioned about excessive solar exposure and advised to routinely use a sun screen and never to sunbathe. (5) The patient is advised to have all first-degree family members (siblings, children, parents) examined because of the familial tendency of melanoma formation. (6) *Each* patient is told at *each* visit to report any change or new symptom that persists for more than 2 weeks and that is either alarming or unexplained to their primary physician or to us directly, and not to wait until the regularly scheduled visit, so that undue delay is avoided if important changes develop. (7) The patient is given a return appointment before leaving. Patients who fail to return for subsequent appointments are rescheduled for return appointments. (8) The only routine laboratory test is an annual chest roentgenogram unless the patient is on an adjuvant therapy protocol. Other laboratory tests or scans are performed as indicated by clinical symptoms and findings.

RECURRENT APHTHOUS STOMATITIS

ROY S. ROGERS III, M.D.

Recurrent aphthous stomatitis is not a disease *sui generis* but rather a mucosal manifestation of a variety of conditions characterized by aphthous ulcers of the mucosa. Thus, underlying conditions may be identified in approximately 20 percent of patients (Table 1). In assessing a patient with recurrent aphthous stomatitis, it is incumbent upon the clinician to exclude underlying conditions. Unfortunately, in 80 percent of patients their disease remains idiopathic. This represents a challenge to clinical investigation.

BEHÇET'S SYNDROME

Behçet's syndrome is characterized by recurrent oral ulcers, recurrent genital ulcers, and recurrent ocular inflammation. This condition is discussed in more detail in the chapter entitled *Behçet's Syndrome*.

TABLE 1 Conditions Associated with Recurrent Aphthous Stomatitis

Condition	*% of Population*
Behçet's syndrome	1
Severe aphthosis	2
Menstrually related	2
Inflammatory bowel disease	1
Gluten-sensitive enteropathy	2
Hematinic deficiencies	12
Idiopathic	80
	100

FORMES FRUSTES OF BEHÇET'S SYNDROME AND/OR SEVERE APHTHOSIS

Some patients suffer recurrent oral ulcers with occasional genital ulcerations of an aphthous nature. Few of them develop the full-blown Behçet's syndrome, although their disease activity may be intense and more continuous than intermittent. Likewise, some patients with aphthous ulcers limited to the oral mucosa have severe and frequent episodes, sometimes even continuous disease activity with new lesions developing as old ones heal. These patients do not respond to the usual therapeutic approaches and may require aggressive therapy.

Among the therapeutic alternatives are dapsone, colchicine, thalidomide, and other nonsteroidal anti-inflammatory agents. Dapsone may act on the function of the polymorphonuclear leukocyte or monocyte. The treatment course would be similar to that used to treat dermatitis herpetiformis (see chapter entitled *Dermatitis Herpetiformis*). Colchicine is an anti-inflammatory agent that perturbs spindle function and may act on polymorphonuclear leukocytes or migrating inflammatory cells or the release of prostaglandins. The dosage is 0.6 mg daily for one week, b.i.d. for the second week, then t.i.d. until a remission is achieved. The dose is tapered to the lowest dose that maintains a remission. Colchicine is a toxic drug, particularly to the gastrointestinal tract,and causes such side-effects as nausea, vomiting, diarrhea, and abdominal pain. Both dapsone and colchicine should ameliorate the disease activity in 4 to 6 weeks. If a beneficial effect is noted, chronic administration, as for dermatitis herpetiformis or gout, may be considered. If no therapeutic benefit is noted in 4 to 6 weeks, the trial may be abandoned.

Thalidomide is a potentially highly toxic drug that appears to possess anti-inflammatory activity. Teratogenicity and peripheral neuropathy are two of its major potential complications. Some patients with severe aphthosis have responded to doses of 100 to 200 mg per day. Use of thalidomide in women of child-bearing age requires extremely careful discussion and consideration. Other nonsteroidal anti-inflammatory agents such as indomethacin may be tried.

Some patients require intermittent systemic prednisone therapy. For long-standing severe episodes, doses in the range of 1 mg per kilogram per day are necessary to abort the disease activity and induce a remission. This regimen should be tapered over a 3- to 6-week period and discontinued. For shorter, less severe episodes a 2- to 3-week course of systemic corticosteroids, starting with doses of 0.5 to 0.75 mg per kilogram per day, may be effective. Systemic corticosteroid use should remain intermittent and treat disabling and severe episodes as necessary.

None of these therapeutic approaches induces a long-term remission. Therefore, the clinician must be cautious and observe the patient for side-effects of long-term drug administration.

MENSTRUALLY RELATED APHTHOUS STOMATITIS

Some women describe a flare of lesions in the premenstrual phase of the menstrual cycle. These patients respond to the administration of estrogen-dominated oral contraceptives such as Ovulen. A period of 3 to 6 months may be necessary to note the beneficial effect of the anovulatory agent. The mechanism of action is obscure, although estrogen promotes mucosal hyperkeratosis, which may protect against trauma.

INFLAMMATORY BOWEL DISEASE

Crohn's disease and ulcerative colitis are associated with recurrent aphthous stomatitis. Indeed, oral aphthous ulcers may presage a flare of the bowel disease. The aphthous stomatitis tends to improve with improvement of the underlying condition.

GLUTEN-SENSITIVE ENTEROPATHY

Patients with gluten sensitivity often are afflicted with recurrent aphthous stomatitis. As the bowel disease improves with gluten restriction, so do the oral aphthous ulcers. Some patients with no evidence of gluten-sensitive enteropathy note a marked dimunition of aphthous ulcer activity on a gluten-free diet.

HEMATINIC DEFICIENCIES

According to some investigators, as many as one in six patients with oral aphthous ulcers have a deficiency of vitamin B_{12}, folate, or iron, or a combination of two or three of these hematinic agents. Replacement of the deficiency yields a remission or marked decrease in disease activity in the large majority of patients. This process takes 1 to 3 months. Vitamin B_{12} deficiency should be confirmed by appropriate testing. Doses are standard replacement doses. Our studies indicate that our patient population is as likely to be as deficient as are the British populations studied.

ZINC DEFICIENCY

We have not confirmed a zinc-deficient subpopulation among sufferers of recurrent aphthous stomatitis.

IDIOPATHIC RECURRENT APHTHOUS STOMATITIS

The vast majority of patients who suffer from recurrent aphthous ulcerations have few episodes of short duration. The etiology remains obscure. Symptomatic therapy includes viscous lidocaine suspension to anesthetize the mucosa. This may be used before meals and at bedtime. Topical local anesthetics such as Diclone may be applied throughout the day to alleviate pain.

Proprietary, over-the-counter preparations such as Cank-Aid are also helpful in alleviating symptoms. A warm saline mouthwash (1 teaspoon salt to 1 pint water) may be salutary.

In view of the putative immunologic mechanism involved in the pathogenesis of recurrent aphthous stomatitis, the application of topical corticosteroids may ameliorate or abort early lesions. Potent fluorinated corticosteroids in ointment, cream, or gel bases are applied to early lesions every 1 to 2 hours while the patient is awake. Once the ulcer is fully developed, application of topical corticosteroids should be discontinued, as they may retard wound healing. Symptomatic measures are then used.

Some episodes are aborted by topical application of caustics such as silver nitrate. These medicaments provide pain relief and convert the lesion to a burn wound.

Topical or systemic antibiotics may improve individual episodes. For the herpetiform variant of recurrent aphthous stomatitis, tetracycline may be administered. Double-blind studies have failed to demonstrate efficacy.

COMMENTS

Spontaneous long-term remission may be anticipated in the majority of patients with the minor and herpetiform variants. Major aphthous ulcers tend to be a more chronic problem. Most therapeutic trials are characterized by a study population that is heterogeneous and not divided into the aforementioned subsets. Therefore, studies are difficult to perform and interpret. Nonetheless, numerous double-blind studies have been conducted, and the vast majority have failed to demonstrate efficacy of various therapeutic trials. This points out the need for the clinician to evaluate the patient with recurrent aphthous stomatitis with respect to classification into one of the subsets.

In treating recurrent aphthous stomatitis, therapeutic nihilism is not appropriate as long as it is tempered with the cautious use of the large therapeutic armamentarium just described.

BEHCET'S SYNDROME

J. DESMOND O'DUFFY, M.B.

Behçet's syndrome is an idiopathic chronic and relapsing disorder that may have seven cardinal features: aphthous ulcerations of the buccal mucosa, ulcerations of genital mucosa, uveitis, cutaneous vasculitis, synovitis, meningitis usually with meningoencephalitis, and large-vessel inflammation, i.e., phlebitis or arteritis. Typically the diagnosis is secure if aphthous oral lesions coexist with at least two other features, and provided mimicking disorders are excluded. The mimics include Crohn's disease of the colon, hypereosinophilic syndrome, herpes simplex, and cicatricial pemphigoid.

The diagnosis is clinical as there is no pathognomonic test. Skin hyperergy, manifested as pustule formation at sites of skin trauma, is infrequently seen in these patients. "Incomplete forms" of Behçet's syndrome may be considered if recurrent oral aphthous ulcers exist along with one other feature. Purists would require pathologic evidence of inflammatory cells in the eye, cerebrospinal fluid or arterial wall before accepting a diagnosis. The entity "aphthous stomatitis et vulvitis", although chronic, may be self-limited and should not be labeled "Behçet's syndrome." Vasculitis is the cause of the most serious phases. Untreated vasculitis leads to retinal infarction, encephalopathy, and the life-threatening large-vessel occlusions and ruptures. Laboratory abnormalities include elevated acute phase reactants and circulating immune complexes in active phases of the disease.

THERAPEUTIC ALTERNATIVES

There is no alternative to a team approach in the management of Behçet's syndrome. The specialists consulting on an individual patient may include an ophthalmologist, neurologist, vascular radiologist, dermatologist, rheumatologist, and surgeon. No treatment is curative and all treatments are empiric. However, since accumulations of inflammatory cells, specifically lymphocytes and plasma cells, are at the sites of mucosal, synovial, and vasculitic pathology, it is logical that agents reducing the number or activity of such cells might be used.

Treatment for mucosal ulcers, cutaneous vasculitis, and synovitis need not be as drastic as the treatment for posterior uveitis, meningoencephalitis, and large-vessel arteritis. The most effective therapy is the alkylating drug chlorambucil. However, since the mean age at diagnosis is 30 years, the liberal use of chlorambucil cannot be justified. Instead, treatment is tailored to the type and severity of organ involvement.

Oral Ulcers

Multiple painful aphthous ulcers are clearly visible in an individual patient roughly 50 percent of the time. Patients will not treat minor ulcers as they heal spontaneously in several days. More severe crops of ulcers may be treated with 2 percent viscous Xylocaine or, preferably, by topical corticosteroids. The most popular are Kenalog in Orabase (0.1 percent triamcinolone in a paste of gelatin, pectin, carboxymethyl cellulose sodium in Plastabase) and Topsyn gel (Fluocinonide=0.05 percent).

Tetracycline suspension diluted to a mouthwash is probably ineffective. Topical corticosteroids are most useful if applied early to the lesions and up to four times a day, after meals and at bedtime. Patients complain that all topical agents wash off in the mouth. For severe oral aphthosis that interferes with sleep or nutrition, prednisone, 20 to 40 mg per day, is required to prevent or ameliorate the ulcers.

Genital Ulcers

Fortunately, the numbers and frequency of vulvar ulcers are much less than that of oral ones. Here topical corticosteroids are more beneficial. Early herpes simplex lesions are to be distinguished from aphthae as clustered vesicles, and should not be treated with steroids. In the few women or men having such frequent and disabling genital ulcers that sexual intercourse is impossible, oral prednisone, 20 to 40 mg per day, may be given initially and the dose then tapered.

Uveitis

Hypopyon is pus in the anterior chamber of the eye and is now seldom seen in Behçet's disease because of modern treatment. Cells in the anterior chamber seen on slit-lamp biomicroscopy constitute anterior uveitis, and cells in the vitreous chamber signify posterior uveitis. Anterior uveitis may be successfully treated with topical corticosteroid drops such as 1 percent Pred Forte (prednisolone acetate ophthalmic suspension). Posterior uveitis with associated retinal disease has been treated with oral corticosteroids or with subtenon corticosteroid injections, but these are only temporarily or partly supressive. As retinal vasculitis usually results in progressive loss of vision it must be treated vigorously. Therefore, if the patient has unilateral or bilateral posterior uveitis the treatment of choice is chlorambucil, 0.1 mg per kilogram per day. The nonsteroidal anti-inflammatory drugs and colchicine 1.0 mg daily have been advocated, but in my opinion are not useful in uveitis.

Arthritis and Cutaneous Vasculitis

Both of these manifestations usually respond promptly and completely to prednisone, 20 to 60 mg per day. When the inflammation subsides, the dosage is reduced. Although alternate-day prednisone is less toxic and suppresses endogenous cortisol secretion less than daily or split-dose treatments, the latter two forms are more effective. A crude guideline to prednisone tapering is to reduce by 5 to 10 percent every 1 to 2 weeks. Some patients require lengthy treatment with low-dose prednisone, e.g., 5 to 10 mg for prolonged freedom from arthritis or erythema nodosum. Attempts to reduce prednisone further can be successful if 1-mg tablets are used and slowly tapered. Nonsteroidal anti-inflammatory drugs, such as aspirin 4 g per day or indomethacin 100 mg per day, are useful, especially when prednisone is being withdrawn, but like colchicine are disappointing.

Meningoencephalitis

Meningitis is usually manifested as headache, fever, and nuchal rigidity and responds, at least temporarily, to prednisone in a starting dose of 30 to 60 mg per day. Unfortunately, in only a few patients is the meningitis self-limited. Most meningitis patients have or will experience encephalopathy. The cerebrospinal fluid (CSF) cell count exceeds 5 per cubic millimeter, and there is a modest increase in protein. Sudden focal neurologic deficits, typically hemipareses, imply encephalopathy, in which case chlorambucil, 0.1 mg per kilogram per day, is begun. If the patient is seen during an episode, concurrent prednisone, 60 mg per day, is used, but if the patient is seen in the interim between focal neurologic deficits and with a normal CSF, chlorambucil alone is sufficient to prevent recurrences. Tapering of prednisone should be delayed until 2 to 3 months after chlorambucil is begun.

Large-Vessel Arteritis

This phase of Behçet's disease is the most treacherous as the patient can present with such diverse symptoms as myocardial infarction from coronary arteritis or hemoptysis from pulmonary artery-bronchial fistulas or rupture of an aneurysm anywhere. Such patients may die suddenly. However, if diagnosis is made promptly, typically by arteriography, it seems reasonable to try to avert further disasters by using prednisone, 60 mg, along with chlorambucil, 0.1 mg per kilogram per day. Aneurysmectomy, thrombectomy and other emergency operations have been lifesaving in a few patients.

Phlebitis

Superficial phlebitis is often the pathology of "cutaneous nodules" in Behçet's disease and responds to prednisone or, less thoroughly, to indomethacin. Although much has been written of a "hypercoagulable state" in the phlebitis of Behçet's disease, the clotting factors that are elevated merely represent acute-phase reactants signaling inflammation. In the few patients who have profound recurrences of lower extremity phlebitis, anticoagulation with heparin or Coumadin has been ineffective. In them, treatment with prolonged prednisone has been necessary, and in our limited experience, chlorambucil can prevent recurrences.

The syndrome of intracranial venous sinus occlusion is emerging as a complication of Behçet's disease. These patients present with chronic headache, often with papilledema and visual obscurations. A noninvasive diagnostic technique is digital subtraction angiography. In intracranial hypertension, CSF pressures in the region of 300 to 450 mm are recorded at lumbar puncture. A course of prednisone 30 to 60 mg per day can result in lysis of the clot. When occlusion is irreversible, relief of symptoms and signs may require shunting of CSF via a lumboperitoneal shunt.

Other Manifestations

If Crohn's disease of the colon is excluded by barium enema and/or colonoscopy with biopsy, Behçet's disease of the large intestine may be accountable for discrete "aphthous" ulcers if other diagnostic criteria coexist. There is no evidence that corticosteroids or Azulfidine heals these ulcers. When perforation occurs it is almost always in the right side of the colon or cecum. A surgeon who has compiled the entire Japanese experience with this dramatic complication suggests resection of diseased bowel with ileotransverse colostomy. Other serious but rare events in Behçet's disease are glomerulonephritis, aortic valvular insufficiency, and pericarditis. It is not possible to speculate whether these events are better treated with prednisone or alkylation since they are rare.

PREFERRED APPROACH

The patient is thoroughly interviewed and examined in order to establish the diagnosis, rule out mimics, and estimate the current activity of disease. Laboratory studies are a poor guide to treatment. Mucosal ulcers are treated symptomatically with topical corticosteroids, synovitis and cutaneous vasculitis with medium-dose prednisone, and active posterior uveitis or meningoencephalitis are treated with chlorambucil. The patient may be reluctant to embark on toxic oral compounds and often requires a period of education. Contact with other Behçet's disease patients is possible through the American Behçet's Foundation (421 SW 21 Avenue, Rochester, Minn 55902).

Corticosteroids

Among this group of 21-carbon anti-inflammatory immunosuppressive steroid molecules, prednisone, which has a keto group at the 11 position, is favored. Oral prednisone requires hepatic activation to prednisolone for effectiveness. Topical applications of corticosteroids are particularly effective in anterior uveitis as the concentration gradient of the molecules drives them into the anterior chamber. Posterior to the lens, topical therapy is not generally useful. Prednisolone acetate suspension (Pred Forte), given hourly as drops, is most effective, but can elevate intraocular pressures, which are monitored by ophthalmology visits. As rebound inflammation is likely with cessation of this treatment, reduction in dosage must be gradual. Other complications of topical corticosteroid drops are eye infections and cataract.

As little corticosteroid reaches the posterior uvea, in posterior uveitis, prednisone is given orally, 40 to 60 mg per day in single or divided doses. Ophthalmologists give 40 to 60 mg per day in single or divided doses, often punctuated by periocular injections of dexamethasone sodium phosphate, 4 mg per milliliter. Despite corticosteroids, posterior uveitis of Behçet's disease usually remains active and vision may be lost.

Oral prednisone given chronically in doses greater than 10 mg per day has a host of well-known side effects. These include hypertension, diabetes mellitus, osteopenia, avascular necrosis, cataract, susceptibility to infection, Cushingoid fat deposition, and susceptibility to bacterial, fungal, and viral infections. Initial doses for mucosal, cutaneous, and articular inflammation are 20 to 40 mg per day, but 60 to 80 mg per day for meningoencephalitis and large-vessel vasculitis. Since there is a lag period of 4 to 8 weeks for immunosuppression by chlorambucil, it is reasonable to begin high-dose prednisone along with chlorambucil when meningoencephalitis or major arteritis is diagnosed. With posterior uveitis, which may smolder along for months before lasting damage is done, it may be argued that systemic prednisone can be avoided because chlorambucil is effective.

The liaison between the patient's primary specialist, e.g., a rheumatologist, and the ophthalmologist or neurologist provides these advantages over solo physician care of the patient: (1) documentation of visual acuity scores and uveitis activity; (2) documentation of diminished CSF pleocytosis and neurologic status; and (3) management of complications. Thus, women on high-dose prednisone are given oral calcium supplements, e.g., calcium carbonate, 1,500 mg daily, and, if postmenopausal, conjugated estrogens such as Premarin 1.25 mg daily 25 days per month. When the disease is controlled, prednisone is reduced, as already described. As alternate-day prednisone has not been proved as effective as daily therapy, it should only be used in the final tapering phases of withdrawal.

Chlorambucil

Chlorambucil is a bifunctional alkylating agent that is structurally related to nitrogen mustard. It exerts a stronger effect on lymphopoiesis than on the production of other bone marrow cellular elements. It is not known whether its antilymphocyte action is the prime site in Behçet's disease. Like other alkylating agents that are useful in various idiopathic "lymphocytic" diseases, it cross-links with host DNA and impairs division of diverse cells. Therein may lie its toxicity.

Chlorambucil is made up in 2-mg size tablets, and the starting dose in posterior uveitis, meningoencephalitis, and other life-threatening phases of Behçet's syndrome is 0.1 mg per kilogram per day. A few patients may require 0.2 mg per kilogram per day, but bone marrow toxicity is more likely at this dosage. Most fertile women become amenorrheic on 0.1 mg per kilogram per day if taken beyond 1 year. The dose is usually 4 to 8 mg per day and can be given in one daily bolus. Arrest of uveitis and meningoencephalitis is usually evident at 3 to 4 months, and then reduction of the dose by 25 to 33 percent is begun. Since a few patients given chlorambucil alone will experience continued eye or CNS lesions for some weeks, some prefer to use prednisone for the first 3 months. This decision is controversial and must be guided by the severity of the disease. In uveitis chlorambucil alone is best.

Complete blood counts, with particular attention to

leukocytes and platelets, are necessary every 2 weeks for 2 to 3 months and then monthly even as chlorambucil dosage is reduced. Chlorambucil is withheld if leukocytes are less than 3,000 per cubic millimeter or platelets less than 100,000 per cubic millimeter. The drug is cautiously restarted at a lower dose when these values are exceeded. Some patients cannot tolerate continuation of effective dosage. Fertile women beginning chlorambucil should be using birth control to prevent conception of a defective fetus. Pneumonia vaccine should be given before treatment is begun, and annual influenza vaccine is advised. Most patients have their disease controlled in 3 to 6 months, and after successive tapering many are able to discontinue chlorambucil after 1 to 2 years. Some require prolonged (up to 5 years) low dosage, i.e., 2 mg per day or q.o.d. Surveillance for the development of malignant disease, especially acute myelogenous leukemia, requires that prolonged leukopenia be avoided. Relapses of eye or brain disease when the patient is off treatment can be effectively treated.

Women in the childbearing years, and men, are warned that life-long infertility can result.

UNPROVEN THERAPIES

The list of unproven remedies is long and includes transfusions of blood or plasma, vitamins, antimalarials, transfer factor, colchicine, nonsteroidal anti-inflammatory drugs, levamisole, fibrinolytic therapy with phenformin and estradiol, azathioprine, cyclophosphamide, methotrexate, Dapsone, and thalidomide. Thalidomide is usually quickly effective in mucocutaneous phases but has not been proved to suppress ocular or neurologic disease. The early results of Cyclosporin in Behçet's uveitis are encouraging. However, relapses promptly punctuate the cessation of therapy, and renal impairment is a regular result of chronic therapy, at doses of 5 to 10 mg per kilogram per day.

PROS AND CONS OF TREATMENT

Only one study using a double-blind controlled agent has been reported, and that was a negative study of colchicine. Empiric and controlled trials of newer agents such as thalidomide and Cyclosporine are under way. When the disease is mild, empiricism is to be encouraged, but for the three serious manifestations aggressive therapy is reasonable. This guideline holds for posterior uveitis, meningoencephalitis, and major artery involvement.

The patient, typically a young woman already with loss of some vision or a focal neurologic deficit, is faced with the risk of blindness or death from ineffective treatment as compared with the risk of dangerous cytotoxic therapy. Prospective long-term surveillance of chlorambucil-treated patients is necessary. Even more necessary is the development of rational, safer, and more effective regimens.

RAYNAUD'S PHENOMENON

FREDRICK M. WIGLEY, M.D.

Raynaud's phenomenon is characterized by episodes of vasospasm of the vessels of the digits of the hands and feet in response to both cold and emotion. The precapillary vasoconstriction is manifested by cutaneous pallor followed by cyanosis and then, on recovery, rubor secondary to hyperemia. The initial phase of pallor may be transient and often is not observed by the patient. Cyanosis persists until rewarming, following which a period of approximately 15 minutes passes before a gradual return to normal color. Attacks may begin in one or more fingers, but typically spread to the other digits symmetrically and bilaterally. During the phase of pallor and cyanosis, patients may experience a feeling of pins and needles, blunting of normal sensation, and cold damp skin. Occasionally episodes are painful, particularly if the attack is prolonged or a continuous cold exposure is present. Other peripheral parts of the body may be involved, including the tips of the ears, nose, areas of the face, or the nipples.

CLASSIFICATION

Raynaud's phenomenon may occur as the sole clinical problem (Raynaud's disease, idiopathic Raynaud's, primary Raynaud's), or in association with another process (Table 1). Approximately 40 percent of patients presenting to an internist have a defined secondary cause, the most common being a connective tissue disease. Disturbances of neurovascular supply, proximal vascular lesions, hemotologic disorders, exposure to vibratory tools, certain vasoactive drugs, and a variety of miscellaneous disorders need to be carefully considered in the differential diagnosis. Obviously, management of a treatable secondary process may improve or eliminate the Raynaud's episodes.

Primary Raynaud's phenomenon is seen more commonly in young females who are otherwise healthy. Symptoms are limited to bilateral symmetrical Raynaud's phenomenon, which is rarely severe. Digital pitting or superficial ulceration of the fingertips with sclerodactyly may complicate the course in 10 to 15 percent of these patients. An interval of many years from the onset of Raynaud's phenomenon may pass before signs and symptoms of a connective tissue disease emerge. This is estimated to occur in 4 to 20 percent of patients who initially were

TABLE 1 Classification of Raynaud's Phenomenon

A. Primary: Raynaud's disease (idiopathic)
B. Secondary:
  1. Connective tissue diseases
    a. Systemic sclerosis (90%)
    b. Systemic lupus erythematosis (20%)
    c. "Mixed connective tissue disease" (75%)
    d. Dermatomyositis (20%)
    e. Rheumatoid arthritis (10%)
  2. Neurovascular compression
    a. Thoracic outlet syndrome
    b. Carpal tunnel syndrome
  3. Arterial disease
    a. Noninflammatory lesions
    b. Arteritis
  4. Hematologic disorders
    a. Paraproteins
    b. Cryoglobulins
    c. Polycythemia
    d. Hyperviscosity
  5. Occupational
    a. Vibratory tools (white finger syndrome)
    b. Polyvinyl chloride exposure
  6. Drugs
    a. Ergotamine
    b. Beta-adrenergic blockade
    c. Sympathomimetic agents
  7. Other
    a. Primary pulmonary hypertension (30%)
    b. Migraine headache (10%)
    c. Reflex sympathetic dystrophy

thought to have benign primary Raynaud's phenomenon. Frank ulceration, distal digital amputation, and scleroderma with loss of hand function occur primarily in patients with an underlying connective tissue disease such as systemic sclerosis.

MANAGEMENT

In the majority of patients, the management (Table 2) of Raynaud's phenomenon is simple and rarely requires drugs, particularly in cases of the uncomplicated primary or idiopathic variety. Patients with Raynaud's phenomenon are a heterogeneous group with different responses to a given treatment program. Patients with scleroderma, for example, usually have structural abnormalities of the digital vessels as well as a noncompliant overlying skin, both making their response to treatment less successful than that of patients with primary Raynaud's phenomenon. In addition, the pathogenesis of Raynaud's phenomenon is incompletely understood, and consequently no ideal treatment has been found. It is clear that both cold and emotion are major factors that trigger and propagate an attack, and therefore management begins with avoidance of cold and emotional turmoil.

Education and *reassurance* reduce inappropriate anxiety and eliminate misconceptions regarding this condition. Informing the patient of its nature, significance, and precipitating factors often reduces the number and intensity of attacks without the use of other treatment modalities. Following an initial evaluation, the patient can be instructed to maintain a diary of the circumstances that precipitate an attack, the length of attack, and the factors that end the episodes. A review of the diary with the patient serves as a means to define the intensity and character of their afflication. Allied health professionals can help by gathering information pertaining to the patient's current psychosocial situation and by providing support and education. Patients who clearly define emotional upset as a causative factor benefit a great deal from non-drug support that involves physician and family. Stressful situations should be reduced in the home and at work. Psychotherapy in the form of biofeedback or behavioral adaptation has been advocated by some and may be helpful in the subgroup of anxious patients with mild-to-moderate uncomplicated Raynaud's phenomenon. Sedative medications are usually not necessary and have no direct effect on the peripheral vasculature.

Cold is the most common and intense factor that triggers attacks of Raynaud's phenomenon. Patients note that attacks are precipitated by rapidly changing temperatures such as walking into an air-conditioned room, placing their hand into the refrigerator, and walking past open freezers in markets. Patients should be instructed to avoid cold exposure and to dress warmly when it is necessary to go into the cold. Loose-fitting clothing is most effective. It is important to keep the whole body warm, not just the hands and feet. Raynaud's episodes can be precipitated by a general body chill, such as one induced by an ice pack placed on the neck, even if the hands are warm. Mittens are better than fingered gloves. Daily activities can be adjusted to avoid the cold. For example, another family member may do the frozen food shopping. A phone call to an employer may be helpful to adjust working temperatures or to move the patient from an outdoor to an indoor position during the winter months. Moving to a warm climate usually is not necessary, nor is it totally effective, because of the many sources of cold exposure in our daily lives.

There is increasing evidence that cold adaptation occurs both in normal individuals and in patients with Raynaud's phenomenon. Graded exposure to cold has been suggested as a form of treatment, but its efficacy has not

TABLE 2 Management of Raynaud's Phenomenon—Non-Drug Modalities

Education and reassurance
  Establish precipitating factors
  Emotional support
  Behavior adaptation

Avoid cold
  Warm, loose-fitting garments
  Keep the whole body warm
  Adjust life style
  Rewarm quickly

Discontinue
  Vasoconstrictive agents
  Ergot
  Beta-blockers
  Smoking
  Birth control pills

been proved and the methodology is unclear. Gentle and rapid warming of the extremities is an effective means of reversing the cold-induced vasospasm. Patients discover that running warm (not hot) water over their digits or placing their hands close to their bodies will end an attack. Prolonged vasospasm should be avoided because abnormal nutritional blood flow may result in ischemic changes. Patients should, therefore, be encouraged to end attacks by rewarming whenever possible.

Drug Treatment

Patients with mild, noncomplicated Raynaud's phenomenon are more likely to respond to vasodilators, but should be treated with non-drug modalities. Repeated painful attacks (greater than once daily), digital ulceration, or cutaneous changes such as early sclerodactyly warrant consideration for drug intervention. Patients with systemic sclerosis usually have severe Raynaud's phenomenon which needs drug treatment. Drugs that potentially cause vasoconstriction should be discontinued. Ergot-containing compounds used in the treatment of migraine headaches can cause Raynaud's phenomenon and should be avoided. In addition, beta-blocking agents have been reported to cause or aggravate Raynaud's phenomenon. Birth control pills have been suspected, but not proven, as an aggravating factor in the condition, perhaps secondary to increasing fibrinogen levels. Attempts to avoid birth control pills are prudent if practical. Smoking should be stopped because of the proven reflex vasoconstriction caused by nicotine. Sympathomimetic drugs are best avoided.

Drug treatment of Raynaud's phenomenon has been notoriously disappointing, probably because the pathogenesis of this condition is incompletely understood. Various types of drugs have been used that either directly or indirectly cause peripheral vascular dilatation (Table 3). Unfortunately, only a few of these agents have been critically studied in appropriate blinded placebo-controlled trials. In addition, drug toxicity frequently limits the use of a potent vasodilator. It is important to carefully review reports of an effective agent in the treatment of Raynaud's phenomenon because episodes are seasonal and highly variable. Studies need to be placebo-controlled and done in the winter months with measurements of both subjective and objective responses.

TABLE 3 Vasodilators Used in Raynaud's Phenomenon

Alpha-adrenergic receptor blocking agents
Tolazoline
Phenoxybenzamine
Prazosin
Adrenergic neuronal blocking agents
Reserpine
Guanethidine
Methyldopa
Beta-receptor stimulus
Isoxsuprine
Terbutaline
Direct smooth muscle relaxants
Papaverine
Nitrates (topical)
Griseofulvin
Naftidrofuryl oxalate
Calcium-channel blockers

Both oral and intra-arterial reserpine have been suggested as treatment for Raynaud's phenomenon because of its ability to deplete norepinephrine from sympathetic nerve terminals. Oral reserpine is not effective and often leads to significant side-effects. Recent controlled studies have shown that intra-arterial reserpine is no more effective than a saline placebo in both short- and long-term follow-up. Reserpine and other adrenergic neuronal blocking agents should not be used in the treatment of this condition.

Potent vascular alpha-receptor blockers have been used alone or in combination with adrenergic neuronal blocking agents. Phenoxybenzamine and guanethidine have been reported to result in symptomatic relief, but no controlled studies have been done. Significant side-effects, including postural hypotension, reflex tachycardia, nasal congestion, impotency, lassitude, and incontinence, have made these unproven drugs impractical. Prazosin, a specific adrenergic alpha$_1$-receptor antagonist, has been reported to reduce the number of attacks in 5 of 7 patients with primary Raynaud's phenomenon at a low dose (1 mg twice daily). However, during 2 months of treatment with the highest dose tolerated (2 to 8 mg daily), the clinical improvement tended to vanish. In addition, intolerance to the drug made many patients discontinue the drug. This study confirms an anecdotal experience that over time prazosin is generally ineffective or poorly tolerated.

Although most direct smooth muscle relaxants and beta-receptor stimulants have not been effective, the development of drugs that interfere with the entry of calcium into vascular smooth muscle has led to a new exciting approach to the treatment of Raynaud's phenomenon. These calcium-channel blockers have been shown to relax vascular smooth muscle, thus reducing peripheral vascular resistance and increasing peripheral blood flow. Three prospective controlled double-blind studies using nifedipine have demonstrated subjective improvement in 60 percent of patients and a significant reduction in the number of daily attacks. Cold-provoked Raynaud's phenomenon in the laboratory, however, could not be blocked. One recent study has shown that nifedipine was not significantly different from placebo, thus suggesting that further studies are needed. No long-term studies have been done, nor has the ideal dose schedule been determined. There is a great deal of variability in individual responses that cannot be clinically predicted. Patients with primary Raynaud's phenomenon may respond better than patients with systemic sclerosis. Hypotension, dizziness, headache, disorientation, peripheral edema, and aggravation of reflux are problematic side-effects and may occur more frequently in patients with Raynaud's phenomenon than in other patient groups. These drugs should be avoided in the pregnant patient, a significant problem in that affected patients are commonly young women of childbearing age.

Many calcium-channel blockers will be introduced and they may not all be as effective as nifedipine. Verapamil has been carefully studied; it was not effective and significant cardiac arrhythmias occurred. Diltiazem has been reported to be as effective as nifedipine, but further studies are needed to confirm this observation. Nifedipine is a reasonable first choice to use in the subgroup of patients with problematic Raynaud's phenomenon. A 10 mg test dose should be given while the patient is in the doctor's office so that vital signs can be monitored for 1 to 2 hours following the dose. If no hypotension or other problems occur, treatment with 10 mg t.i.d. is started, and a careful diary is kept by the patient to document response. A maximum dose of 30 mg t.i.d. has been used. One can expect a good response in some patients, manifested by a decrease in the number and intensity of daily attacks. The response may be transient and careful follow-up is most important. The medication should not be used in the summer months unless recurrent attacks are documented.

A number of experimental agents are being studied (Table 4). Intravenous prostaglandins (PGE_1, Prostacyclin) have been reported effective, but are not available in oral preparations. Thromboxane synthetase inhibitors have been proposed to inhibit the production of platelet-derived thromboxanes, which are potent vasoconstrictors. One such thromboxane synthetase inhibitor, dazoxiben, has been studied and shown to be no better than placebo. Other more potent selective thromboxane inhibitors need to be investigated. Ketanserin, a serotonin receptor inhibitor, is now under study, and preliminary studies suggest that vasospasm and Raynaud's phenomenon are effectively reversed. Plasmapheresis, fibrinolytic agents, and dextran infusion have been reported effective, but are both unproven and impractical modalities of treatment.

TABLE 4 New Agents in the Treatment of Raynaud's Phenomenon

Prostaglandins
PGE_1
Prostacyclin
Thromboxane synthetase inhibitors
Serotonin receptor inhibitor
Ketanserin
Plasmapheresis
Fibrinolytic agents
Stanozolol
Captopril
Dextran infusion

Surgical Treatment

Surgical sympathectomy was once popular for the treatment of Raynaud's phenomenon, but was disappointing in that improvement was only transient, and the condition returned with the same intensity in a relatively short period. Neither the extent of ganglionectomy nor preganglionic surgery has improved the results. Surgical morbidity and significant postural hypotension have been reported. Digital sympathectomy has recently been reported as a successful mode of treatment, but no control studies have been done. Sympathectomy has been largely abandoned and should only be considered for short-term relief of an intractable course complicated by digital ulceration that has failed medical treatment. Local digital block has been used for transient acute effects in patients with digital tissue compromise. Local debridement and antibiotic treatment may be necessary if ischemic ulceration becomes secondarily infected. Whirlpool treatments have proved the most effective method of ulcer care.

ERYTHEMA NODOSUM

JEFFREY P. CALLEN, M.D., F.A.C.P.

Erythema nodosum (EN) is an inflammatory cutaneous reaction that should alert the clinician to the possibility of an underlying associated condition. EN is clinically characterized by erythematous, tender nodules most commonly on the anterior tibial surface. It is usually an acute self-resolving process, but in an occasional patient the condition is chronic or recurrent. Histologically, EN is considered to be a septal panniculitis, but the histopathology varies, depending on the timing of the biopsy in the progression of the lesion. Biopsy of early lesions is predominantly neutrophilic, but later mononuclear cells predominate, and the lesions can eventually become granulomatous. Although vascular damage is said not to be a primary event, some cases of EN have been associated with circulating immune complexes.

The diagnosis of EN is made on the basis of the clinical findings, but other causes of panniculitis should always be considered. Clinically, EN is more frequent in females (3:1) and usually occurs in young individuals (<40 years of age). Although these painful, red nodules are usually on the anterior lower legs, they can occur on any area of the body. Often there are associated arthralgias and occasionally arthritis. Fever and malaise also frequently accompany this cutaneous disorder. The lesions resolve with a bruised appearance and heal without scarring. They usually do not ulcerate. Other causes of tender nodules include cutaneous polyarteritis nodosa (which is a vasculitis) and the lobular panniculitides such as subcutaneous fat necrosis of the newborn, poststeroid panniculitis, sclerema neonatorum, erythema induratum, pancreatic fat necrosis, lupus panniculitis, and Weber-

Christian disease. In most of the other panniculitides, the histopathologic features allow the physician to distinguish them from EN.

Since erythema nodosum is a reactive process (probably a hypersensitivity phenomenon), therapy is dependent upon the cause or associated condition. Listed in Table 1 are conditions that have been regularly associated with EN. In only 50 to 75 percent of patients with EN will a cause be evident. In my experience, in only 10 percent of the cases seen in the dermatologist's office or dermatology clinic do we find a cause. This seems to be owing to selection of the patients in that emergency medical physicians, family practitioners, internists, gynecologists, and other specialists recognize EN and evaluate the patients. Thus, the dermatologist's group of patients is selected, and those with obvious etiologies have been removed.

Multiple infectious agents have been associated with the development of EN. Prior to the advent of prophylactic chemotherapy for tuberculosis, this myobacterial infection accounted for a large proportion of cases. Recent streptococcal upper respiratory tract infection is probably the most common associated infection. Erythema nodosum leprosum (ENL) is a reaction that is specific for leprosy (see chapter on leprosy). In the Southwest United States, the endemic area for coccidioidomycosis, this agent accounts for many cases of EN. Other fungal infections, both deep and superficial mycoses, have also been reported to occur with EN. Viral infections have been reported in conjunction with EN. It is unclear whether therapy of the infectious agents will always result in resolution of the EN. In many cases the EN is self-limited, as is the infection. For example, EN with coccidiodomycosis is a good prognostic sign, indicative of host response to the infection. Thus, as the host localizes the fungal infection, the EN resolves.

EN has been associated with many ingestants, including various therapeutic agents. A potential problem in therapy occurs when the EN begins during drug therapy for an infection that could cause the skin reaction also. In this case, it may be best to attempt an alternate treatment of the infection. Another interesting phenomenon is the occurrence of EN with bromide or iodide-containing compounds, since potassium iodide is now considered an agent useful in the therapy of EN. Birth control pills can cause EN and may be related to recurrent attacks. These agents prevent pregnancy by hormonally inducing a "pseudo-pregnant" state. EN that occurs in pregnant women will recur when the birth control pill is used.

TABLE 1 Etiologic Associations of Erythema Nodosum

Idiopathic
Sarcoidosis
Inflammatory bowel disease
Infections
- Bacterial (streptococcal, TB, leprosy)
- Fungal (deep and superficial)
- Viral (EB virus, hepatitis)
- Chlamydia

Drugs
- Birth control pills
- Antibiotics
- Sulfonamides
- Bromides, iodides

Pregnancy
Behçet's syndrome
Miscellaneous—Hodgkin's, leukemia, acne fulminans, yersinosis, collagen vascular diseases

Sarcoidosis is one systemic disease that may account for up to 25 percent of EN patients. EN in patients with sarcoidosis is associated with bilateral hilar adenopathy (BHA), anterior uveitis, and arthritis. This tetrad is known as Lofgren's syndrome and is a benign form of sarcoidosis, since less than 90 percent of the cases resolve spontaneously. Similarly, it has been shown that the presence of asymptomatic BHA with EN is pathognomonic for sarcoidosis, and nodal biopsy is not necessary. Recently, many authors have evaluated EN patients with serum angiotensin-converting enzyme levels (ACE) in an attempt to diagnose early sarcoidosis. Usually during the EN episode, the ACE level is normal, but within 3 to 4 months the ACE becomes elevated. Despite this elevation of the ACE level, persistent and progressive sarcoidosis does not seem to occur clinically in these patients.

EN has been reported in conjunction with inflammatory bowel disease (IBD), particularly regional enteritis and its variant, Crohn's disease. Ulcerative colitis has also been reported with EN, but accounts for a lower number of cases. The diagnosis of IBD has almost always been made prior to the EN episode, but usually the episode occurs concurrent with active bowel disease. Possibly this occurrence with active bowel disease is related to bacterial antigens that may penetrate the inflamed bowel more easily.

A host of other disorders have been associated with EN. Behçet's syndrome is worthy of brief mention, since it can have EN-like lesions as part of its presentation. Usually these nodules are attributable to a vasculitic type of hypersensitivity phenomenon often related to pathergy (occurrence of a lesion in a site of injury). I believe that EN is not associated with Behçet's. Summarizing the list of causes, one must consider the following major categories: infections of all types, drug and other ingestants, sarcoidosis, and inflammatory bowel disease. If one considers these and rules them out, we can usually consider the case to be idiopathic.

THERAPEUTIC INTERVENTIONS

Therapy of EN can be as simple as removal of an offending ingestant or treatment of a causative infection or it may be extremely difficult. Thorough evaluation of each case is necessary prior to treatment. Listed in Table 2 are the suggested options for the therapy of EN which includes bed rest, nonsteroidal anti-inflammatory agents, colchicine, potassium iodide (SSKI), and systemic corticosteroids.

A thorough evaluation of the patient with EN includes a careful history, physical examination, and appropriate laboratory tests. Included in the history should be an

TABLE 2 Therapeutic Options for Erythema Nodosum

"Non-treatment"
Removal of a causative factor
Treatment of an associated disorder
Bed rest, elevation of part
Nonsteroidal anti-inflammatory agents
Aspirin
Indomethacin
Naproxen
Ibuprofen
Colchicine
Systemic corticosteroids

evaluation of recent infections, travel history, history of ingestants, the presence of bowel disease, and ownership of animals. Associated symptoms, such as arthritis or uveitis, should also be evaluated. As a minimum, laboratory evaluation should include a PPD skin test, a chest roentgenogram, a throat culture, and an ASO titer. Other serologic tests may be ordered under appropriate circumstances. I do not recommend a serum ACE level, since it may be normal in the face of acute sarcoidosis.

After a thorough evaluation has failed to demonstrate a treatable cause or associated condition, therapy may become necessary. In many patients the condition resolves without specific therapy, but I generally recommend bed rest and aspirin in all patients. When EN does not respond to these conservative measures, I generally try a nonsteroidal anti-inflammatory drug (NSAID). Indomethacin, 25 to 50 mg by mouth three to four times daily, has been reported to be effective in EN. I have treated only about 10 patients with this agent, and in only 3 did it seem to have a beneficial effect. Indomethacin is an inhibitor of prostaglandin synthesis, and through this action it may be effective. It is not without toxicity, in particular at higher doses, which can cause symptoms referable to the gastrointestinal tract and even GI bleeding. Another NSAID that has been reported to be useful is naproxen. I have had no experience with this agent.

Recently, I became intrigued with the use of colchicine, which inhibits the expression of the inflammatory reaction by blocking lysosomal release, decreasing phagocytosis, and inhibiting the release of mediators such as histamines. Two of our patients who were given 0.6 mg of colchicine twice daily had total and rapid resolution of their skin lesions. Colchicine can cause nausea, diarrhea, and headaches. Its chronic use has been associated with toxic myopathy and agranulocytosis, among other symptoms.

Potassium iodide (SSKI) can be given to patients with EN. I have not seen a patient in whom I was convinced that the SSKI was effective. Potassium iodide is given in a dose of 300 mg orally three times daily. SSKI is said to have a rapid effect in EN, but even in the literature, the response occurs in only 75 percent of the patients.

Usually, corticosteroids are the last line of therapy. They should not be used in a patient with an infectious etiology of EN. They are effective in doses as low as 20 mg prednisone every other day. I generally treat with a short course in the form of a 14- to 21-day burst of oral prednisone. In patients with chronic or recurrent EN, corticosteroids may be necessary on a regular basis.

Thus, in summary, EN is a hypersensitivity phenomenon related to many "causes." Since each causative factor implies a different therapy, a thorough evaluation is undertaken before specific therapy. Therapy beyond the conservative measures of rest and elevation consists of an anti-inflammatory agent. Most cases resolve, but chronic EN remains a therapeutic challenge.

PHOTOALLERGIC DERMATITIS

VINCENT A. DE LEO, M.D.
LEONARD C. HARBER, M.D.

Photoallergic dermatitis represents an immunologic response of the delayed-hypersensitivity type elicited by ultraviolet radiation. The role of light is to photochemically alter the haptinic group in the induction process. The remainder of the induction process is similar to that necessary for the development of ordinary allergic contact dermatitis.

Listed in Table 1 are the major common chemical agents responsible for photoallergic dermatitis. These agents usually cause photodermatitis following exposure by topical application. In contrast, photosensitization to systemic agents most frequently results in phototoxicity, but not photoallergy. The "action spectra" of most of the photoallergic agents falls within the UVA range (320 to 400 nm).

Classically, the clinical response to agents responsible for photoallergic contact dermatitis is erythematous and papulovesicular; histologically, it is characterized by a spongiotic dermatitis. The papules and vesicles that initially develop are replaced in chronic cases by scaling, lichenification, excoriation, and hyperpigmentation of light-exposed areas. Histologic examination of the chronic phase is nonspecific, demonstrating acanthosis, vascular dilation, and a perivascular (predominantly mononuclear) infiltrate. Individuals who are immunologically photosensitized react to radiation that can penetrate window glass.

Although a number of "idiopathic" entities have been included in the grouping "photoallergic dermatitis" (Table 2), it is currently thought that the vast majority of these cases are initiated by allergic reaction (probably T-cell-mediated) to the combination of an exogenous agent and light. Most patients with photoallergic contact dermatitis are "transient reactors" who have no dermatologic difficulty after the offending agent is removed. However, a small percentage of patients, "persistent light reactors," continue to react to light for many years after all known chemical exposure has ceased. With few exceptions, the action spectra of these reactions are also in the UVA and visible light ranges (320 to 700 nm). In addition, some of the patients develop an erythematous reaction clinically and an abnormal histopathologic response to exceedingly low doses of UVB (290 to 320 nm).

TABLE 1 Photoallergenic Drugs and Chemicals

Halogenated salicylanilides
Tetrachlorosalicylanilide
Tribromosalicylanilide
Dibromosalicylanilide
Trichlorocarbanilide
Bithionol
Antifungal agents
Multifungin
Fentichlor
Jadit
Phenothiazines
Chlorpromazine
Promethazine
Sulfonamides
Sunscreens
PABA esters
Digalloyl trioleate
Whiteners
Stilbenes
Fragrances
Musk ambrette
Methylcoumarin

THERAPY

The therapeutic approach to patients with a photoallergic contact dermatitis is basically three fold: (1) avoidance of the initiating agent, (2) protection from light exposure, and (3) symptomatic therapy for dermatitis.

Avoidance of Sensitizing Agents

Avoidance of the offending agent, of course, requires identification of that agent. This necessitates an extensive chemical exposure history, phototesting, and photopatch testing. Procedures for phototesting and photopatch testing are outlined in the following section.

Photopatch Testing

Photopatch testing, a confirmatory test for diagnosing photoallergic contact dermatitis, is relatively simple and can be performed in the dermatologist's office with relatively little difficulty. The equipment needed to perform photopatch tests is an artificial light source with a spectral irradiance in the UVA ranges. Selected examples of these light sources are listed in Table 3. Those most suitable for photopatch testing in a doctor's office are the hot quartz mercury vapor lamp, "black light" fluorescent tubes, or a high-intensity specialized Wood's light (Blak-Ray).

Before performing the photopatch test, the physician must select the suspected photoallergic chemicals to be

TABLE 2 Working Classification of Photoallergic Dermatitis

Condition	Example	*Response*				Mechanism	Other Features
		Photopatch + UVA	*UVB*	*UVA*	*Visible*		
1. Localized transient photoallergy		+	–	–	–		
2. Localized specific persistence of photosensitivity	Fentichlor	+ + +	0	+ + +	0	Reaction to photoallergen at site of repetitive photoallergic reactions (light-exposed areas)	Classic photoallergic (T-cell) reaction with photoantigen "trapped" in skin; lasts for months to years
3. Classic generalized "persistent light" reactivity	Halogenated salicylanilides	+ + +	+ + +	0	0	Autophotosensitization (carrier protein?)	Persists for years
3a. Atypic generalized persistent light reactivity	Halogenated salicylanilides	+ + +	+ + +	+	0	Unknown	Persists for years
4. Polyvalent light sensitivity with persistent photosensitivity	No known agent	0	+ + +	+ + +	+ + +	Unknown	Persists for years
5. Actinic reticuloid	No known agent	0	+ + +	+ + +	+ + +	Unknown	Related to lymphomas?
6. Chronic photosensitizing eczema	No known agent	0	+ + +	0	0	Unknown	Persists for years

0 = normal response
\+ = abnormal response

TABLE 3 Light Sources Used in Photopatch Testing

Light Source	*Comment*
Sun	Excellent, but unpredictable and hard to standardize
Carbon arc	Good, but requires close monitoring
Fluorescent tubes:	
Sunlamp	Erythema spectrum essentially UVB
Blacklight	Good, inexpensive source of UVA
Solar simulator	Small field size permits irradiation of only one site; expensive; research tool
Hanovia hot quartz*	Simple and effective with appropriate filter
Krohmayer contact	Simple and effective with appropriate filter
Cold quartz	Ineffective; emission in short ultraviolet (primarily UVC)
Wood's light (ordinary)	Ineffective; low intensity of radiation (UVA)
Wood's light (Blak-Ray)	Simple, inexpensive, effective

* Recommended for office use.

studied. In our experience, a "screening battery" of several chemicals has proved helpful (Table 4). This selection may be modified by information supplied in the patient's history.

Each chemical to be tested should ideally be incorporated into petrolatum at a concentration of 1 percent. The chemical is then applied to two patches delineated by Aluma-test or Band-Aid squares; the patches are applied to symmetrical sites on lesion-free areas of the interscapular or lower lumbar regions of the back, as in ordinary patch test procedures. Photopatch testing is unique, however, in that each chemical is applied in duplicate. One set of the duplicate patches eventually is irradiated with UVA light, whereas the unirradiated set serves as a control.

After the chemicals have been applied, the two sets of patches are covered with light-opaque material. This is important because even trace amounts of light may yield false-positive test results in the photosensitive patient. After 48 hours, one set of patches is uncovered, and each site is evaluated for any visible reaction. A positive test indicates the presence of either an "ordinary" allergic contact dermatitis or a primary irritant reaction to the applied chemical. After the uncovered sites are evaluated, they are irradiated with 5 to 15 J/M^2 of UVA, which can be administered most conveniently by either a bank of multiple fluorescent blacklight lamps or a hot quartz high-pressure mercury vapor lamp with a 3 mm window glass filter. It is important that the entire body of the patient be protected from inadvertent light exposure.

When irradiation has been completed, the irradiated photopatch test sites are recovered again with light-opaque material. Both sets of patches are then left in place for an additional 48 hours. At that time (96 hours after the original application of the chemicals), both sets are uncovered and evaluated according to the protocol presented in Table 5. If the irradiated site shows a positive reaction and the nonirradiated site shows a negative one, contact photoallergy is present. If both sites show equally positive reactions, contact allergy is present.

It is possible, in some cases of allergic contact photosensitivity, to reduce the time of the photopatch test procedure. One set of patches can be uncovered and irradiated 24 hours after application. However, this procedure may yield an excessive number of false negative tests (a possible exception is 6-methylcoumarin).

In accordance with recent recommendations of the North American Contact Dermatitis Group regarding "ordinary" contact dermatitis, our group has evaluated and recommends the use of the Aluminum Patch Test (AL-Test) for photopatch testing. The photopatch material is a cellulose disc applied to thin aluminum foil coated with polyethylene. The aluminum test units come in prepackaged rolls of one thousand, from which the required number can be easily removed. After the patch test material is applied to a disc, the disc itself is held in place by a water-resistant tape, such as Blenderm (3M) or Dermicel (Johnson & Johnson). Aqueous gentian violet is recommended for delineation of sites irradiated with UVA at the time of the first evaluation. It is essential that all the test sites (irradiated and unirradiated) be protected from light. Materials available for covering photopatch test sites include Webril or cotton fabric, aluminum foil, various types of adhesive tape, and blotter paper.

It should be emphasized that photopatch testing is not an innocuous procedure. Some hazards and complications associated with it are outlined in Table 6. It should also be noted that 4$^+$ reactions (see Table 6) may be manifested as marked vesiculations causing extreme discomfort. Photopatch testing should be avoided in patients with acute dermatitis, since false-positive reactions may result from the "hyperirritability" of the entire skin surface.

These diagnostic tests are useful for identifying only agents responsible for topically induced photoallergic dermatitis; the identification of a systemically encountered photosensitizer is based primarily on history.

Once identified, exposure to the photosensitizing agent must be eliminated. It is crucial to acquaint the patient with a list of related agents that may produce cross-photosensitivity reactions, and obviously these cross-reactive substances must be avoided. This is particularly important when the salicylanilides and phenothiazines are

TABLE 4 Photopatch Test Tray*

Tetrachlorocarbanilide 1%
3′, 5′, Dibromosalicylanilide 1%
4′, 5′, Dibromosalicylanilide 1%
Bithionol 1%
Tribromosalicylanilide 1%
Sandalwood oil 1%
Dowicide-32 1%
Fluorophene 1%
Hexachlorophene 1%
Para-aminobenzoic acid 10%
6-Methylcoumarin 5%
Musk ambrette 5%

* Petrolatum is the recommended vehicle for the chemicals listed.

implicated. When topical therapeutic or cosmetic agents are involved, the patient should be given a list of generic and proprietary names of nonsensitizing substitutes.

Protection Against Light

The avoidance of sunlight must often be extended beyond the period of acute dermatitis because excretion of the photosensitizing chemical from the skin may be delayed. In severe cases, confinement of the patient in a darkened room for several days may speed recovery. Window glass usually does not protect against phototoxic contact or photoallergic contact reactions because wavelengths greater than 320 nm are readily transmitted. When the action spectrum of a photosensitizer is below 320 nm, ordinary window glass (3 mm thick) usually affords protection.

Patients with a photosensitivity dermatitis may obtain protection from adequate clothing. Closely woven brown, orange, and red fabrics are best. White shirting becomes much more permeable to erythema-producing radiation when wet with water or perspiration.

Repeated short exposures to sun have occasionally been of aid in "densensitizing" individuals. Such densensitization is probably nonimmunologic and is attributable to increased melanin formation and thickening of the horny layer; it is known that dark-skinned individuals are less apt to have photosensitizing reaction than are fair-skinned people.

Use of Sunscreening Agents

Sunscreening agents are of two main varieties—chemical and physical. Chemical sunscreens, which can absorb specific photons of light, include para-aminobenzoic acid and its esters, the benzophenones, digalloyl trioleate, and the cinnamates. These agents may occasionally cause ordinary allergic contact dermatitis and, more rarely, produce photoallergic contact dermatitis. Since their major protection is to wavelengths below 320 nm, they afford little protection to patients responding to longer wavelengths.

Physical sunscreens form an opaque barrier to all photons of solar radiation without absorbing such rays. These agents do not produce allergic or photoallergic reactions. They contain opaque powders, such as titanium oxide, kaolin, zinc oxide, or talc. The opacity of these powders protects against UVA radiation, but may not be as cosmetically acceptable as sunscreens that are invisible. They may occasionally be so occlusive as to produce miliaria.

TABLE 5 Interpretation of Photopatch Tests

*Reading at Irradiated Site**		*Reading at Nonirradiated Site**	*Interpretation*
0		0	Normal
1-4+		0	Contact photoallergy
1-4+	=	1-4+	Contact allergy alone
1-4+	>	1-3+	Contact photoallergy and contact allergy

* Evaluations are scored 1 through 4 as described by the North American Contact Dermatitis Group.

TABLE 6 Hazards and Complications of Photopatch Testing

- Inadvertent sensitization to photopatch test materials
- Mechanical or radiation injury owing to improper use of light sources
- False-positive and false-negative tests owing to selection of inappropriate type or amount of light
- Undue discomfort at patch test sites and "flares" at previously involved sites
- Inaccurate interpretation of phototest data
- Masked photopatch reaction

Symptomatic Therapy

Once the photosensitizing chemical is eliminated, and if the patient is vigorously protected from ultraviolet radiation, most reactions will abate.

Individuals with severe erythema and edema may obtain relief with ice cold compresses of Burow's solution diluted 1:10. It is often beneficial to superimpose upon these compresses a thin layer of petrolatum to prevent excessive drying.

Emollients in a water-in-oil base soften the scaling of the chronic eruptions. Systemic antihistamines may alleviate pruritus but do not affect the lesions. Usually, their contribution is related to their soporific effect. Corticosteroids, particularly topical and on occasion systemic, are often necessary to achieve relief of symptoms. Fluorinated corticosteroid creams may initially be applied three to four times each day. When symptomatology requires more aggressive therapy, a daily oral dose of adrenocorticosteroids such as prednisone, 30 to 60 mg, is often associated with amelioration of signs and symptoms in 1 or 2 days. Fortunately, when the eruption is transient and exposure to the photoallergen is removed, the steroids can be tapered in a relatively short period of time.

PERSISTENT REACTIONS

A more difficult therapeutic problem is appropriate management of the persistent light reactor. These patients are often severely disabled and venture outdoors only at night. Hospitalization is strongly suggested and usually required. Since avoidance of the allergen is not possible, the prevention of exposure to ultraviolet light is mandatory. Replacement of fluorescent tubes with incandescent light bulbs in some cases is helpful. Topical sunscreens offer some benefit, specifically PABA (UVB) and benzophenones that screen UVA. In addition, light-opaque agents such as titanium dioxide should be used. Beta carotene and PUVA (oral psoralen and ultraviolet light) may be of benefit in selected cases.

In patients with persistent light reactions, the chronicity of the disease may obscure other problems. These individuals often have severe mental depression because of their inability to participate in the normal world of daylight. The clinician must be aware that many of these patients may also have contact sensitivities to other common allergens, and further studies for allergens may be required during the course of managing their disease. A rare entity, actinic reticuloid, may mimic persistent light reactions clinically. Characteristically, the biopsy shows changes consistent with lymphoma. In our experience, the development of true lymphoma has not occurred. As with any chronic dermatosis, it is important that the plan of therapy for persistent light reactors recognizes the need for protracted treatment. The use of long term steroid therapy, hospitalizations, and experimental treatments are often required.

PORPHYRIAS

BARRY C. LAMKIN, M.D.
DAVID R. BICKERS, M.D.

The porphyrias are a fascinating group of clinically diverse diseases linked by one common thread—all are the result of an aberration in the normal process of heme synthesis in the bone marrow or the liver. Currently at least eight distinct porphyrias are recognized: erythropoietic porphyria (EP), erythropoietic protoporphyria (EPP), erythropoietic coproporphyria (EC), porphyria cutanea tarda (PCT), acute intermittent porphyria (AIP), variegate porphyria (VP), hereditary coproporphyria (HP), and hepatoerythropoietic porphyria (HEP). No uniformly satisfactory treatment is as yet available for EP, EC, or HEP, and they will therefore not be discussed further.

ERYTHROPOIETIC PROTOPORPHYRIA

Erythropoietic protoporphyria (EPP) is inherited as an autosomal dominant trait and is usually characterized by the onset in early childhood of acute photosensitivity manifested by burning, stinging, and/or itching of sun-exposed skin, usually within only 5 to 10 minutes of sun exposure. An apparently small percentage (5 percent) of patients with EPP also manifest significant liver disease, which may result in terminal hepatic failure. Therapeutic alternatives include avoidance of sun exposure, use of topical sunscreens, systemic antimalarials, cholestyramine, vitamin E, vitamin C, or beta-carotene.

The preferred approach for the treatment of patients with EPP is the oral administration of beta-carotene, a doublet of vitamin A. The mechanism of action of beta-carotene is not precisely understood, but it is known to be an effective singlet oxygen quencher and a free radical trap. These moieties are generated by the interaction of light (primarily, but not exclusively, at wavelengths of the Soret band, around 400 to 410 nm) with protoporphyrin, which is present in increased concentrations in the skin of patients with EPP. Despite some absorbance around 400 nm, the drug does not appear to function as a "sunscreen" in the way that topical sunscreens do. Once the diagnosis of EPP has been confirmed by the patient's clinical features and by appropriate biochemical test procedures, treatment with beta-carotene can be initiated. First, however, both the patient and the patient's parents must be made aware of the role of sunlight in the dermatologic manipulation of the disease and admonished to wear protective clothing insofar as it is possible. Beta-carotene (Solatene) is usually administered in doses of 60 to 180 mg (two to six 30-mg capsules) per day orally. However, the dose must be adjusted, depending on serum carotene levels. These levels should be monitored and the dose adjusted to maintain serum concentrations in the range of 600 to 800 μg per 100 milliliters. When administered in this fashion, the drug is remarkably well tolerated with no recognized systemic toxicity. The most common undesirable side-effect of beta-carotene is a visible yellow-orange coloration of the skin, which is almost universal at therapeutic levels. This yellowing is particularly prominent in areas where the stratum corneum is thickest (e.g., palms and soles). The yellow color is the result of carotene deposition in the skin and is associated with no known toxicity other than this cosmetic effect. Less frequent adverse effects include diarrhea in a small number of patients and orange or rusty discoloration of feces. Unless the patient finds the yellowing of the skin intolerable cosmetically, none of these changes is an indication for discontinuing the medication. No other complications of beta-carotene therapy have yet been identified.

Maximum effectiveness of beta-carotene may not be observed until 1 to 3 months after initiation of treatment. Its primary beneficial effect is the prevention or alleviation of cutaneous photosensitivity (i.e., burning, stinging, itching, erythema, urticaria, and subsequent scarring). Most patients with EPP observe a significant increase in their tolerance to sunlight while receiving beta-carotene. In assessing the therapeutic response to the drug, it must be remembered that the medication is effective only for the cutaneous photosensitivity of EPP and has no effect on the primary biochemical defect or on the hepatic abnormalities associated with the disease. Therefore, if a patient with EPP who is receiving beta-carotene develops clinical and biochemical evidence of hepatic failure, this is in no way related to or alleviated by the drug. Such patients require intensive supportive care. In a few individuals who developed hepatic failure, some clinical and biochemical improvement occurred following the combined oral administration of the anionic resin cholestyramine (12 g per day in divided doses) and the antioxidant vitamin E (100 units daily). No unequivocally effective treatment, however, is currently available for EPP patients who develop hepatic failure.

PORPHYRIA CUTANEA TARDA

Porphyria cutanea tarda (PCT) is characterized by the presence of increased skin fragility and blisters with subsequent scarring on sun-exposed skin. Milia, hypertrichosis, hyperpigmentation, and sclerodermoid changes of the skin may also be present. Facial plethora with polycythemia may also occur. Various drugs and environmental chemicals may incite or exacerbate PCT. Prominent among these are ethanol, estrogens, and chlorinated hydrocarbons. Hepatic iron overload is a major finding in PCT.

The therapeutic alternatives available for patients with PCT include removal of the inciting agents, administration of iron chelators, metabolic alkalinization of the urine to increase porphyrin excretion, oral administration of cholestyramine or antimalarial drugs, and phlebotomy. Of these alternatives, the most effective measures in our experience are avoidance of inciting factors, phlebotomy, and orally administered antimalarials.

The first step in evaluating a patient with PCT is to actively search for possible etiologic factors. As previously mentioned, estrogens and ethanol are the most commonly recognized agents, although induction or exacerbation of PCT may occur as the result of industrial exposure to chlorinated hydrocarbons such as hexachlorobenzene and chlorinated phenols. The simple avoidance of these factors alone often results in significant reversal of the symptoms. This improvement may be very slow, however, and for most patients more aggressive therapy is usually required. Even in these instances, avoidance of the inciting or exacerbating factors generally enhances the effectiveness of whatever therapy is selected.

In our experience, the preferred therapeutic approach for most patients with PCT is phlebotomy. The mechanism of action of phlebotomy therapy for PCT remains unclear and is the source of some controversy. One proposed mechanism is the depletion of the excessive hepatic iron stores, that are characteristically present in the large majority of patients with PCT. The iron overload is thought to be important in the pathogenesis of the increased hepatic porphyrinogenesis of PCT. It is also possible that affected individuals carry some as yet undefined substance in their serum that can augment hepatic porphyrin production and that is depleted by phlebotomy.

Once the diagnosis of PCT has been established by clinical and biochemical findings and once the hematologic status of the patient has been defined, phlebotomy therapy can be instituted. In general, this consists of the removal of 500 ml of whole blood every 7 to 14 days until the hemoglobin decreases to 10 to 11 g per 100 milliliters or until serum levels decline to 50 to 60 μg per 100 milliliters. Alternatively, 24-hour urinary porphyrin levels may be followed to monitor therapy, but these tests generally are not as readily available or as convenient for the patient as periodic hemoglobin or serum iron determinations. The number of phlebotomies required to induce clinical remission varies considerably among patients but, in our experience, has generally ranged from 3 to 12. The phlebotomies can usually be performed by a local blood bank or similar service, but if this is not available or convenient, the procedure can readily be done in the dermatologist's office with plastic blood drawing bags.

The side-effects of phlebotomy therapy are generally minimal and are well tolerated. An occasional patient may notice moderate fatigue and/or weakness, but this usually resolves rapidly as the hemoglobin levels gradually rise. Complications of phlebotomy treatment are also uncommon. If the patient has coexistent myocardial disease, angina may be induced or exacerbated by phlebotomy. There are also patients with PCT and coexistent disorders such as systemic lupus erythematosus or chronic renal failure in that anemia rather than polycythemia occurs. These individuals therefore cannot tolerate phlebotomy, and an alternative approach would include the use of one of the antimalarial drugs (to be discussed).

In assessing the therapeutic response to phlebotomy, it is important to remember (and to reassure the patient) that biochemical and clinical improvement does not ensue until a variable time after treatment is inaugurated. Urinary porphyrin levels generally return to normal 6 to 18 months following treatment. Clinically, the easy bruisability and blistering are the first cutaneous changes to improve, followed (generally by several weeks) by reduction in skin fragility. The facial hypertrichosis resolves more slowly over a period of months, and the scleroderma-like changes frequently do not resolve, although in some patients even these may improve slowly over a period of years. Following the initial course of phlebotomies, patients with PCT generally remain in remission for variable periods. About 5 to 10 percent of treated patients relapse within one year, but the usual length of remission ranges from 6 months to more than 8 years without further treatment. Remission times tend to be shorter for patients with continued exposure to estrogens, ethanol, or other inciting factors. Should the disease become active, the patient usually responds again to another course of phlebotomy therapy.

It should be remembered that it is not necessary (or desirable) to wait for the reappearance of the clinical signs and symptoms of PCT before reinstituting treatment. Serum iron and/or urinary porphyrin levels may be followed semiannually and treatment initiated if these begin to rise (this often precedes the development of clinical signs and symptoms). Thus, when serum iron rises above 60 μg per 100 milliliters or urinary porphyrins rise above 500 μg per 24 hours, phlebotomy can be reinstituted. Generally one or two phlebotomies are sufficient to again reduce iron and/or porphyrin levels, and the patient remains symptom-free. It should be noted that urinary porphyrins can fluctuate significantly from day to day, so that if this method is used to monitor therapy, an isolated abnormally high reading may not necessarily mean that repeat phlebotomy is required. If there is a persistent increase in urinary porphyrin excretion, however, phlebotomy should be restarted.

As mentioned, certain patients with PCT who suffer from angina pectoris or anemia from coexistent diseases cannot tolerate phlebotomy. For these individuals, the antimalarial drugs (chloroquine, [Aralen], from or hydroxychloroquine /Plaquenil/ are the preferred treatment. Since the incidence of side-effects, particularly retinopathy (to be discussed), is reported to be lower with hydrozycloroquine than with chloroquine, we generally prefer the former agent. The mechanism of action of these drugs in PCT is unclear. Both have been shown to form water-soluble drug-porphyrin complexes in the liver, which are readily removed from the liver and excreted in the urine. The subsequent lowering of hepatic porphyrin concentrations is accompanied by clinical improvement. It has also been suggested that these drugs enhance iron excretion from the liver, resulting in reduced hepatic iron stores.

Selection of the proper dosage of either chloroquine or hydroxychloroquine in PCT patients is critical. If given the "usual" dose (250 to 500 mg per day of chloroquine or 200 to 400 mg per day of hydroxychloroquine), relatively large quantities of hepatic porphyrins are solubilized and excreted in the urine. This acute increase in the mobilization of hepatic porphyrin is usually accompanied by signs and symptoms including fever; abdominal pain; markedly elevated SGOT, SGPT, and bilirubin; and histologic evidence of hepatocellular necrosis. In lower doses, however, the enhanced porphyrin release occurs more gradually, and there is little or no hepatotoxicity. We have used very low doses (i.e., 125 mg chloroquine or 100 mg hydroxychloroquine two to three times weekly) with minimal or no side-effects.

When beginning therapy with either of these agents, the following program is suggested. Baseline 24-hour urinary porphyrin levels, serum hepatic transaminases (SGOT, SGPT), and an ophthalmologic exam (to be discussed) should be obtained. A single "test dose" of either 125 mg chloroquine or 100 mg hydroxychloroquine is then given, and serum transaminases and urinary porphyrin determinations are repeated one week later. If there are no significant clinical symptoms or abnormalities in the liver function tests, the medications are administered at this same dose twice weekly. Serum transaminases and urinary porphyrins are then monitored monthly, and the medication is continued until 24-hour urinary uroporphyrin excretion is less than 500 μg .This generally requires 6 tgo 12 months. It may be necessary in some patinets to tincrease the dosage to 250 mg chloroquine or 200 mg hydroxychloroquine twice weekly to achieve clinical and biochemical remission. If the response to therapy is slow, it is also possible to gradually increase both the dose and the frequency of the medication as hepatic stores are depleted. For example, if necessary, the dose can be increased to 200 mg hydroxychloroquine three times weekly after one month (monitoring urinary porphyrins and serum transaminases), to 300 mg after another month and, if necessary, to as much as 400 mg daily over the next several months. Whenever adjustments in dosage are necessary, however, the urinary porphyrins and serum transaminases must be closely followed to avoid excessive increments in porphyrin excretion and subsequent hepatocellular damage.

Once remission is achieved, the drug may be discontinued and the patient will remain symptom-free for variable periods ranging from several months to, occasionally as long as 4 years. If the disease exacerbates, the drugs may be administered again using the same regimen.

Side-effects and complications of antimalarial therapy are generally minimal when the drugs are used in the manner outlined. As already discussed, it is essential to monitor the patient for incipient hepatotoxicity. An occasional patient may notice mild to moderate nausea, but this rarely necessitates discontinuation of the drug. Ocular toxicity, especially retinal damage, may occur with prolonged high-dose antimalarial administration. This appears to be attributable to a particular affinity of these drugs for pigmented tissue. At the doses recommended for PCT, retinal damage has not, to our knowledge, been reported and the risk is presumably low. Nonetheless, it seems prudent to have the patient examined every 6 to 12 months while on therapy by an ophthalmologist thoroughly familiar with the ocular changes that can be evoked by antimalarial drugs. Also, since chloroquine is generally thought to be more likely to cause retinopathy, we prefer to use hydroxychloroquine in our patients. It should be noted that, contrary to popular belief, patients with G-6-PD deficiency do not appear to be at an increased risk for hemolysis while taking chloroquine or hydroxychloroquine. Consequently, patients receiving these drugs do not require screening for G-6-PD deficiency.

ACUTE HEPATIC PORPHYRIAS

The acute hepatic porphyrias include acute intermittent porphyria (AIP), variegate porphyria (VP), and hereditary coproporphyria (HC) and are characterized by recurrent acute episodes of abdominal pain, muscle weakness, tachycardia, fever, and neuropsychiatric symptoms. These may occur spontaneously or following exposure to inciting factors such as drugs and diet. In addition, VP and, rarely, HC may demonstrate cutaneous changes indistinguishable from those seen in PCT.

The therapeutic alternatives available for the treatment of attacks of acute porphyria include avoidance of inciting factors, glucose loading, and hematin infusions. In addition, the need for skilled supportive nursing care for those patients with severe attacks, frequently in an intensive care setting, cannot be overemphasized. The cutaneous changes seen in many patients with VP and occasional patients with HC unfortunately have not, in our experience, responded consistently to any currently available form of treatment.

Perhaps the simplest known method of alleviating an acute attack of hepatic porphyria is glucose loading. The exact mechanism of action of glucose loading is not currently understood, but there is evidence that high levels of glucose may reduce the inducibility of delta-aminolevulinic acid synthetase (ALAS), which is the rate-limiting enzyme for hepatic heme synthesis and which is greatly increased during acute attacks of these diseases. High doses of 300 to 500 g of glucose daily may be required to abort an acute attack. If the episode is mild and gastrointestinal symptoms permit, it may be possible to supply sufficient glucose by oral administration. For more severe attacks or if there is considerable nausea and vomiting, it may be necessary to use parenteral glucose. If solutions of concentrations greater than 5 percent glucose are needed, it is usually necessary to infuse the solutions through a large indwelling catheter or central venous line to avoid vascular complications, particularly phlebitis and sclerosis. If this precaution is taken, side-effects are generally minimal, provided the patient is not diabetic.

If patients cannot tolerate or do not respond to glucose loading, hematin infusion is thought to be helpful in some patients. Hematin is a structural analogue of heme with iron present in the oxidized (Fe^{+3}) rather than reduced (Fe^{+2}) form. Hematin may be obtained from commercial sources or prepared from outdated human blood. It has been found effective in a number of patients who were unresponsive or only partially responsive to glucose loading. Its mechanism of action is presumed to relate to feedback inhibition ALAS activity. As a result, there is a reduction in the concentration of aminolevulinic acid (ALA) and porphobilinogen (PBG), the porphyrin precursors felt to be important in the pathogenesis of acute attacks of porphyria.

Hematin is administered intravenously, generally in doses of approximately 3 mg per kilogram body weight per day. Solutions consisting of 2 mg hematin per milliliter saline are used and administered over a 10 to 15 minute period into a running infusion of normal saline. The duration of therapy is determined by clinical symptoms. The treatment is generally well tolerated in terms of side-effects or complications, although chemical phlebitis at the site of infusion may often occur.

Assessment of the therapeutic response is based on a combination of objective and subjective findings. Objectively, the hypertension and tachycardia that generally accompany the acute attacks of porphyria improve following the initiation of hematin therapy. Commonly, the blood pressure improves before the tachycardia, usually within 24 to 36 hours. Subjectively, patients notice improvement in abdominal pain, nausea, weakness, parathesias and other symptoms associated with these attacks. Biochemically, marked reduction of urinary ALA and PBG excretion occurs within 2 to 3 days of initiation of hematin therapy. Once the acute symptoms and signs have subsided, hematin may be discontinued. The patient must, of course, be admonished to scrupulously avoid inciting factors, including offending medications and excessively low carbohydrate intake.

In summary, the treatment of the porphyrias is designed either to alter the production of heme pathway intermediates that evoke clinical signs and symptoms or to interfere with the toxic effects of the intermediates themselves. In the future, as our knowledge concerning the pathogenesis of these diseases increases, more specific treatment methods should become available.

DERMATOPHYTOSIS

PAUL H. JACOBS, M.D.

Before treating a dermatophytosis, the physician must consider:

1. Area of involvement. Obviously tinea capitis and tinea corporis are different, yet both may be attributable to the same organism.
2. The etiologic agent. It is important to culture and identify the organism, since the susceptibility to antifungal medication varies with respect to the etiologic agent.
3. The type of infection. A *Trichophyton rubrum* or an *Epidermophyton floccosum* infection of the feet may be eczematous in nature or may be very dry.
4. The patient's susceptibility. Finally, the diabetic or the patient who is immunosuppressed may present with a different clinical picture and also be quite resistant to therapy.

TINEA CAPITIS

Tinea capitis is usually attributable to *Trichophyton tonsurans*. *Microsporum canis* follows as the next most common etiologic agent. *Trichophyton tonsurans* responds best to ketoconazole, 200 mg each morning for the adult. For children the dosage is 3.3 mg per kilogram. The patient should take the medicine each morning with breakfast. Gastric acidity is required for absorption, and if the patient is achlorhydric, the 200-mg tablet should be dissolved first in 4 ml of aqueous solution of 0.2 N hydrochloric acid. The patient then dilutes this with a glass of fruit juice and drinks the mixture with a straw. As an alternative the tablet can be dissolved in fruit juice. Immediately afterward the patient drinks a glass of water to prevent damage to the enamel of the teeth. Patients who are receiving cimetidine therapy must take the cimetidine 2 hours after the ketoconazole. I usually treat these patients for a 3-month period. Instructions in the drug package insert should be followed with respect to ordering the liver function tests, since rare cases of idiosyncratic hepatitis have been reported, the incidence being approximately 1:15,000 patients.

If the tinea capitis is attributable to *Microsporum canis*, I prefer griseofulvin at double the amount recommended in the Physicians' Desk Reference. As with ketoconazole, patients receiving griseofulvin should be monitored as recommended in the drug package insert. If there is no response after 1 month, I treat with ketoconazole as already described. If there is improvement, the griseofulvin should be continued for at least 3 months. At this time the patient should be Woods lamp negative and have a negative Potassium Hydroxide direct preparation (KOH) and culture. Neither griseofulvin nor ketoconazole has had dosages established for children under age 2. Neither drug should be used in the pregnant female or nursing mother to treat dermatophyte infections.

For both forms of tinea capitis, my patients are instructed to shampoo each morning. This rids the scalp of scales and weakened hairs so that the infection does not spread to others. I also recommend that an oil be applied after the shampoo, again so that spores and scales are not as likely to be spread to others. Do not allow others in the family to use the patient's towels, combs, or other toilet articles.

Public Health and school nurses involved in the care of these youngsters should be notified if an anthropophilic variety is identified. If the tinea capitis is attributable to *Microsporum canis*, the physician should also suggest that a veterinarian check household pets since *Microsporum canis* is a zoophilic organism.

TINEA CORPORIS

Tinea corporis, if treated at early onset when only a few lesions are present, responds to the imidazole topical preparations, ciclopirox olamine, or haloprogin. It should be applied twice daily. It is important to have the patient apply these topical drugs beyond the margin of the lesion because mycelia may be found 8 to 10 cm beyond the periphery of the lesion. Usually a 1- to 2-month period of treatment is required.

For the chronic generalized dry type infection with *Trichophyton rubrum*, ketoconazole is my drug of choice, since about one-fourth of these patients either are resistant to griseofulvin or do not respond to treatment with griseofulvin even at high doses. These patients usually are clear after 2 months of treatment with 200 mg ketoconazole daily. To date, development of fungi resistant to ketoconazole has not occurred. After clearing, I prescribe a single dose of 400 mg of ketoconazole to be taken every 2 weeks to prevent reinfection. One should follow the same precautions as stated for tinea capitis with respect to liver function tests.

TINEA CRURIS

Tinea cruris responds to the topical imidazoles, or ciclopirox olamine, or haloprogrin if the preparation is applied twice daily. In addition, the area should be kept dry by using a powder such as methyl cellulose and by the wearing of loose cotton underclothes. After clearing, the use of tolnaftate powder each morning prevents reinfection. If the tinea cruris is of the eczematous type, the patient should first be treated with soothing soaks with Domeboro solution on a twice-daily basis prior to applying the antifungals and the powder. In addition, I prescribe a 10-day course of erythromycin, 500 mg b.i.d., to clear the impetiginization usually present. A topical steroid cream or lotion applied twice daily for 1 week, in addition to the fungicidal preparation, stops the itching and clears the lesion more rapidly.

TINEA PEDIS

Tinea pedis of the eczematous type can be treated in much the same way as the eczematous form of tinea cruris. Again, after the condition clears, it is useful to apply tolnaftate powder each morning to prevent reinfection.

Patients with tinea pedis of the chronic dry-moccasin type or the patient with the two-foot-one-hand type of *Trichophyton rubrum* infection may be resistant to therapy. My best results are achieved with a triple therapeutic approach: (1) ketoconazole, 200 mg each morning, (2) topical application of an imidazole antifungal preparation each morning, and (3) topical application of Whitfield's ointment each night. The combination of these three medicaments yields a high cure rate. Reinfection may be prevented with a single 400-mg dose of ketoconazole every 2 weeks.

TINEA UNGUIUM

Tinea unguium is a difficult disease to cure and it is even more difficult to prevent a recurrence. It is my practice to prescribe 200 mg of ketoconazole daily for 3 months. At the same time I apply an occlusive dressing with 40 percent urea cream to the infected nail, as reported by Farber and South in Cutis 1980; 25:609–612. After 7 to 10 days, the dressing is removed and the diseased portion of the nails is avulsed. In a few patients it is necessary to reapply the dressing and urea cream for a second week to avulse all of the diseased portion of the nail. After the chemical avulsion I prescribe application of an imidazole antifungal each morning to be followed that evening by application of 5 percent thymol in absolute ethyl alcohol. This regimen is continued for a 3-month period. At the end of the 3 months I discontinue all treatment except the ketoconazole, which I prescribe in a dosage of 400 mg every 2 weeks in the hope of preventing reinfections. When tonails are involved, the prognosis for cure is guarded. I usually recommend that patients learn to live with this condition.

TINEA FACEI

Tinea facei is difficult to diagnose because it can mimic so many other diseases such as impetigo, contact dermatitis, granuloma annulare, and even discoid lupus erythematosus and polymorphic light eruption. It is essential that first the diagnosis be confirmed by positive KOH preparation for dermatophyte and hyphae, and preferably by culture. The lesions usually respond to the same therapy used for early-stage tinea corporis. The patient should be cautioned against applying topical antifungal near the eyes. If an extensive or severe infection is present, oral griseofulvin therapy should be instituted.

KERION

Kerion of the scalp should be treated with either griseofulvin, if caused by *Microsporum canis*, or ketoconazole, if caused by *Trichophyton tonsurans*. In addition, a broad-spectrum antibiotic such as oral erythromycin should be given to control the bacteria that are invariably present. A short course of prednisone should also be given to stop the allergic reaction that is taking place and prevent further damage to the hair follicles. Response is usually fairly rapid, and after a 2- to 3-week period, only the oral antifungal drug needs to be continued for the full 3-month period. At 3 months, if examination of hairs is negative, the oral antifungal drug can be discontinued. Again, daily shampoo of the scalp should be prescribed to prevent spread of the disease to others.

MAJOCCHI'S GRANULOMA

Majocchi's granuloma, which is usually attributable to *trichophyton rubrum*, responds to treatment with ketoconazole, 200 mg daily for 2 months.

COMPROMISED HOSTS

The physician must be especially alert to fungal infections in the immunosuppressed patient. Treatment can be given for the type of infection, as already described, but may have to be continued for a longer period of time than recommended.

LEPROSY

ROBERT C. HASTINGS, M.D., Ph.D.

Leprosy (Hansen's disease) is a chronic infectious disease of man caused by *Mycobacterium leprae* and affects some 12 million persons worldwide. The usual clinical manifestations leading to diagnosis are dermatologic lesions of various sorts, neurologic deficits, and acute inflammatory manifestations of hypersensitivity to antigens of *M. leprae*, the so-called lepra reactions. Host-parasite relationships in leprosy are complex and dynamic. Rational therapy begins with an accurate diagnosis of the leprosy itself and an evaluation of these host-parasite relationships, which involves determining the position of a given patient within the spectrum of leprosy, i.e., that patient's classification. Well-localized leprosy with competent cell-mediated immunity and very few *M. leprae* is called tuberculoid disease. Widely disseminated, anergic disease is called lepromatous leprosy. Forms of leprosy between these two extremes are called borderline types. Borderline disease is conventionally subdivided into borderline-tuberculoid, midborderline, and borderline-lepromatous. The very early form of the disease, before full definition of the relative balance between bacterial proliferation and cell-mediated immunity, is called indeterminate leprosy.

The medical therapy of leprosy is designed to render *M. leprae* incapable of multiplication, eliminating the patient's infectivity, and allowing the body to clear the bacilli. A significant and important part of the medical therapy of leprosy is the control of hypersensitivity reactions to antigens of *M. leprae*, i.e., lepra reactions that occur in 25 to 50 percent of patients. Antibacterial chemotherapy is further complicated by the ability of leprosy bacilli to persist for years in a presumably metabolically inactive condition (so-called persisters), an overall generation time on the order of 12 to 15 days, and the propensity of the bacilli to develop resistance to commonly used drugs.

THERAPEUTIC ALTERNATIVES

Current recommendations regarding the antibacterial treatment of leprosy are changing. There is at present considerable disagreement as to the optimum treatment advisable. The controversy stems principally from choices as to the number of drugs to be utilized and the duration of therapy. The more conservative approach is the utilization of a single drug, dapsone, in the treatment of all forms of leprosy. In this approach the duration of therapy is determined by the type of disease. Indeterminate cases are treated until 3 years after their disease is clinically inactive, at which point they are tested for cell-mediated immunity to *M. leprae*; if the immunity is present, treatment is discontinued. If cell-mediated immunity to *M. leprae* is lacking, such patients have no alternative under this type of thinking but to continue dapsone for life. If the patient has tuberculoid leprosy, therapy is generally continued until 3 years after the disease becomes clinically inactive and then discontinued. In borderline disease, in general, treatment is continued until at least 5 years after the disease has become clinically inactive and then may be discontinued if cell-mediated immunity to *M. leprae* is present. If cell-mediated immunity to *M. leprae* is absent, therapy is continued for life. In lepromatous patients, therapy is advisable for life under the conservative approach.

In the last several years, more and more emphasis has been placed on combination therapy for leprosy. This is based on the analogy to tuberculosis and the recognition of strains of *M. leprae* that are resistant to various drugs. In order to minimize the emergence of such resistant strains, as many as four drugs are advocated by some groups for lepromatous disease and as many as three drugs for tuberculoid disease. Again by analogy to short-course chemotherapy of tuberculosis, this school of thought advocates continuing therapy for a finite period of time and then discontinuing it in all cases. Current recommendations from this school of thought are as short as 6 months for tuberculoid and indeterminate cases and as short as 2 years for borderline and lepromatous patients. A variety of doses and dosing intervals have been recommended, commonly based on practical considerations in field leprosy control programs and in efforts to minimize noncompliance.

AVAILABLE DRUGS

Dapsone

Dapsone, or 4,4″-diaminodiphenyl sulfone, is the oldest and most widely used antileprosy drug. A derivative, glucosulphone or Promin, was first used in the treatment of leprosy in man in 1941 and constituted the first reliable antileprosy treatment. Dapsone, like the sulfonamides, is an analog of p-aminobenzoic acid (PABA) and acts in a sulfonamide-like fashion to inhibit the de novo synthesis of folic acid by *M. leprae* by inhibiting dihydropteroate synthetase. The drug is bacteriostatic because of this mechanism of action. Dapsone is given orally in an adult dose of 100 mg daily for normal-sized individuals (1 to 2 mg per kilogram). The half-life of dapsone in plasma is quite variable, 10 to 50 hours, with a mean of approximately 28 hours. Thus, daily dosing is adequate.

On a weight basis, dapsone is more toxic than the sulfonamides. The most common side-effect is gastric intolerance, which usually consists of mild nausea in occasional patients. Other side-effects of dapsone are rare with the usual therapeutic doses used in leprosy. These include headaches, hepatitis (rare), peripheral neuropathy (rare), and drug sensitivity. In patients with G-6-PD deficiency, normal doses of dapsone can induce a significant hemolytic anemia. In high doses, the drug may induce a hemolytic anemia, methemaglobinemia, and cyanosis. Dapsone should be given in maximum subtoxic doses in order to minimize the possibility of leprosy bacilli developing dapsone resistance.

Rifampin

Rifampin is a synthetic derivative of rifamycin B produced by *Streptomyces mediterranei*. Rifampin inhibits bacterial transcription. It inhibits RNA synthesis by inactivating DNA-dependent RNA polymerase. Rifampin is administered for leprosy in a variety of regimens, but the most common regimen in the United States is daily doses of 600 mg for adults. The half-life of the drug in normal individuals is approximately 3 hours. During the first 2 weeks of continuous therapy there is a progressive shortening of the half-life by approximately 40 percent, owing to enhanced biliary excretion of the compound. Rifampin is bactericidal for *M. leprae* and thus can be used in a variety of intermittent or once-monthly regimens. It should be noted that, for practical purposes, a leprosy patient's response to therapy is not hastened by the bactericidal nature of rifampin's action. However, there is some evidence that the patient becomes noninfectious somewhat more rapidly on rifampin.

Adverse reactions to rifampin are strikingly different, depending on whether the drug is administered on a daily basis or administered intermittently. Side-effects attributable to rifampin occur in 1 to 10 percent of patients when the drug is taken daily. These reactions are usually minor, consisting of cutaneous, gastrointestinal, and hepatic reactions that are usually reversible and usually do not interfere with therapy. On the other hand, when intermittent regimens are used, antibodies to rifampin commonly develop, and 15 to 25 percent of patients develop influenza-like symptoms consisting of fever, headache, dizziness, and bone pain. The two most life-threatening adverse reactions to rifampin are thrombocytopenia and renal insufficiency. Generally, once monthly administration of rifampin, as advocated in some anti-leprosy regimens, reportedly avoids these serious manifestations. Patients should be informed that this drug imparts an orange-yellow color to urine, feces, sweat, tears, and saliva that is harmless. Hepatic reactions usually consist of minor elevations in serum transaminases and occur in less than 10 percent of patients receiving rifampin alone. Mild degrees of transaminase elevations usually subside despite continuous drug administration. When rifampin is administered with ethionamide, overt liver damage occurs in up to 15 percent of patients. For this reason this combination is not recommended in the treatment of leprosy. Rifampin induces hepatic drug-metabolizing enzymes and may have clinically significant drug interactions with warfarin type anticoagulants, oral contraceptives, methadone, oral hypoglycemics, and digitalis derivatives.

Clofazimine

Clofazimine is a phenazine derivative that has been used in the treatment of leprosy since 1962. The drug is available only on an experimental basis in the United States. The mechanism of the antibacterial effect of clofazimine is not known with certainty. The drug binds to DNA and may interfere with the replication of bacterial DNA. It is the only antileprosy drug that has both antibacterial and anti-inflammatory activities. The mechanism of its anti-inflammatory action is not known with certainty. The drug accumulates in cells of the reticuloendothelial system and eventually induces blockade of the reticuloendothelial system. Clofazimine is administered orally and is approximately 70 percent absorbed from the small bowel. The drug is soluble in fat and is stored to some extent in adipose tissues. High concentrations of the drug are found in organs of the reticuloendothelial system, e.g., liver, spleen, and lymph nodes. It is not metabolized to a significant degree.

In order to obtain anti-inflammatory effects, the drug must be administered in a dosage of 100 mg three times daily. The anti-inflammatory effect is usually apparent within 30 days. The dose-limiting toxicity is deposition of drug crystals in the small bowel and mesenteric lymph nodes, and results in peri-umbilical cramping, diarrhea, nausea, vomiting, and weight loss. This potentially fatal toxicity is reversible upon discontinuance of the drug. Doses on the order of 100 mg three times daily are not recommended for longer than 6 months because of this small bowel toxicity. For antibacterial effects, the dose of clofazimine ranges from 50 to 100 mg daily. Although considerable quantities of clofazimine accumulate in the body, this regimen is usually tolerated indefinitely. A variety of intermittent dosing schedules have been recommended, but proof of adequate tissue antibacterial effects is lacking.

Clofazimine universally produces a dose-related skin pigmentation ranging from an initial pinkish-red pigmentation to a bluish-black coloration on long-term, high-dose therapy. Additionally, there is some degree of hypermelanosis resulting in increased pigmentation of the skin owing to increased melanin production in sun-exposed areas. The other major toxicity involves the gastrointestinal tract, as mentioned earlier. In addition to skin pigmentation, the drug causes pigmentation of the conjunctiva and reddish coloration of urine, stools, sputum, and sweat. Skin lesions of leprosy are selectively pigmented by the drug, sometimes resulting in a blotchy, cosmetically unacceptable pigmentation. The drug induces dryness of the skin which may progress to typical ichthyosis.

Ethionamide

Ethionamide and its analog, prothionamide, have been shown to have antileprosy activity. Technically ethionamide, like rifampin, is experimental in the treatment of leprosy in the United States. Prothionamide is not available in the United States. There is cross-resistance between ethionamide and the thioureas and thiosemicarbazones, e.g., thiacetazone, indicating that these compounds probably share a common mechanism of action. Theories as to the mechanism of action of ethionamide include inhibition of mycolic acid synthesis and effects on dehydrogenase systems. Ethionamide is bactericidal against *M. leprae*, but less so than rifampin. A dose of 250 to 500 mg daily is usually used to treat adult leprosy patients. If the drug has to be used with daily rifampin, a dose of 250 mg daily is used because of the dangers of hepatotoxicity. In other combinations, e.g., with clofazimine or dapsone, 500 mg daily is used. The principal side-effects of ethionamide are gastrointestinal disturbances in the form of anorexia, nausea, and vomiting. These effects are thought to be mediated by direct central nervous system action of the drug. Hepatitis has been observed in approximately 5 percent of patients treated with the drug, being more common in patients with concomitant diabetes mellitus or preexisting hepatic disease. Hepatotoxicity is monitored with serum transaminases similar to rifampin.

Thalidomide

Thalidomide has been used in the treatment of lepra reactions of the erythema nodosum leprosum (ENL) type since 1965. It is available on an experimental basis in the United States. It has no antibacterial activity against *M. leprae* and is used solely for the treatment of ENL. Thalidomide acts in ENL to inhibit the de novo synthesis of IgM type antibodies, which are presumably involved in the pathogenesis of ENL. The drug also inhibits the chemotaxis of neutrophils. Thalidomide is administered for the initial control of ENL in doses of 100 mg four times daily. Within 48 hours the ENL reaction is usually under control and the dose is then lowered to a maintenance level of 50 to 100 mg daily.

Embryopathy is virtually universal if thalidomide is taken by a pregnant woman between 35 and 50 days after the last normal menstrual period. Thalidomide characteristically causes bony abnormalities, with phocomelia being the characteristic deformity. The only other side-effect of significance is a rare peripheral neuropathy occurring in patients taking the drug on a regular basis for long periods of time. This neuropathy occurs in less than 1 percent of leprosy patients.

MANAGEMENT

The management of leprosy is complex. The disease is chronic and management is a multifaceted process designed to render the patient noninfectious, prevent bacterial multiplication, manage so-called lepra reactions, rehabilitate, and prevent further deformity owing to preexisting or ongoing dermatologic, ophthalmologic, or neurologic processes.

The antibacterial chemotherapy of leprosy, considered alone, is relatively straightforward. Newly diagnosed lepromatous patients harbor up to 10^{13} organisms, of which perhaps 2 percent are typically viable. This population of *M. leprae* may contain mutants that are resistant to dapsone (primary dapsone resistance), the frequency of which is not clear. In the United States, probably 5 percent or less of new patients harbor primary dapsone-resistant *M. leprae*. Primary resistance has not been described for rifampin, clofazimine, or ethionamide.

Variable numbers of treated patients develop drug-resistant bacilli during therapy. This secondary resistance has been described for all four antileprosy drugs. It occurs commonly with dapsone, rarely with rifampin and ethionamide, and only a single case has been described

TABLE 1 The Chemotherapy of Leprosy Patients Harboring Sulfone Sensitive Organisms

Type of Disease	*Drug*	*Duration of Therapy*
Indeterminate	Dapsone, 100 mg daily + rifampin 600 mg daily	Rifampin + dapsone for first 6 months, then dapsone alone until 3 years after the disease becomes clinically inactive.
Tuberculoid	Dapsone, 100 mg daily + rifampin 600 mg daily	Rifampin + dapsone for first 6 months, then dapsone alone until 3 years after the disease becomes clinically inactive.
Borderline-tuberculoid	Dapsone, 100 mg daily + rifampin 600 mg daily	Rifampin + dapsone for first 6 months, then dapsone alone until 5 years after the disease becomes clinically inactive.
Mid-borderline	Dapsone, 100 mg daily + rifampin 600 mg daily	Rifampin + dapsone for 2 years, then dapsone alone for life.
Borderline-lepromatous	Dapsone, 100 mg daily + rifampin 600 mg daily	Rifampin + dapsone for 2 years, then dapsone alone for life.
Lepromatous	Dapsone, 100 mg daily + rifampin 600 mg daily	Rifampin + dapsone for 2 years, then dapsone alone for life.

TABLE 2 The Chemotherapy of Leprosy Patients Harboring Sulfone Resistant Organisms

Type of Disease	*Drug*	*Duration of Therapy*
Indeterminate	Rifampin 600 mg daily + clofazimine, 50–100 mg daily	Rifampin + clofazimine for first 6 months, then clofazimine alone until 3 years after the disease becomes clinically inactive.
Tuberculoid	Rifampin 600 mg daily + clofazimine, 50–100 mg daily	Rifampin + clofazimine for first 6 months, then clofazimine alone until 3 years after the disease becomes clinically inactive.
Borderline-tuberculoid	Rifampin 600 mg daily + clofazimine, 50–100 mg daily	Rifampin + clofazimine for first 6 months, then clofazimine alone until 5 years after the disease becomes clinically inactive.
Mid-borderline	Rifampin 600 mg daily + clofazimine, 50–100 mg daily	Rifampin + clofazimine for 2 years, then clofazimine alone for life.
Borderline-lepromatous	Rifampin 600 mg daily + clofazimine, 50–100 mg daily	Rifampin + clofazimine for 2 years, then clofazimine alone for life.
Lepromatous	Rifampin 600 mg daily + clofazimine, 50–100 mg daily	Rifampin + clofazimine for 2 years, then clofazimine alone for life.

with secondary resistance to clofazimine. Virtually all cases of secondary resistance have arisen in patients treated with monotherapy. For this reason, combination therapy is recommended at least for patients harboring large numbers of *M. leprae* (borderline and lepromatous cases). The major problems in chemotherapy are compliance and the development of secondary resistance. Drug toxicities in the recommended combinations are relatively uncommon.

Approximately 50 percent of treated patients develop so-called lepra reactions. These reactions account for the majority of the ultimate deformities among leprosy patients and need to be treated promptly and effectively to prevent deformity. These are two types of reactions, depending on the immune status of the patient. In patients with effective cell-mediated immunity, delayed hypersensitivity reactions to antigens of *M. leprae* can develop, thereby leading to so-called reversal reactions. These reactions may occur in borderline and tuberculoid patients and principally consist of acute inflammation of preexisting skin lesions and the exacerbation of the development of neuritis. These must be managed with systemic corticosteroids to prevent irreversible nerve damage. In patients lacking effective cell-mediated immunity to *M. leprae*, an antigen-antibody type (multifocal Arthus type) hypersensitivity may develop, called erythema nodosum leprosum. This is characterized by the appearance of crops of new, erythematous, tender, skin nodules with many other complications of an acute nature, such as acute iritis, neuritis, orchitis, and lymphadenitis. The management of ENL reactions requires prompt intervention to reverse acute neuritis, for example, with systemic corticosteroids. Thalidomide is effective within 48 hours and clofazimine in doses of 300 mg daily is effective within 30 days. The initial corticosteroid dose required to control acute reactional neuritis in leprosy may be on the order of 80 mg of prednisone daily. Once the neuritis is brought under control, the dose may then be tapered to maintenance doses, which are the minimum necessary to control the neuritis. A variety of local measures are necessary to control involvement of the anterior third of the eye by lepromatous disease.

A host of preventive and curative measures are necessary to avoid deformity, ulcerations, and misuse of insensitive limbs as a result of preexisting leprous neuritis. These include such measures as special shoes, training in the case of insensitive limbs, tendon transfers for preexisting motor paralyses of the hands and feet, and plastic surgery for preexisting lagophthalmos. Details of these measures are outside the scope of the present chapter.

Response to chemotherapy is gauged by clinical changes in skin, eye, and peripheral nerve lesions (differentiating reactional from progressive changes, and both from trophic changes), measurements of bacterial density, and bacterial morphology on slit skin scrapings, and histopathologic changes on serial skin biopsies. Clearing of acid-fast bacilli is a function of cell-mediated immunity and not primarily chemotherapy. On any effective antibacterial regimen, acid-fast bacilli are cleared from lepromatous patients, for example, at the same rate with a half-life of approximately 250 days.

For the patient who is harboring sulfone-sensitive organisms, the current recommended antibacterial regimens are given in Table 1. For the patient who harbors sulfone resistant organisms, the current recommended regimens are given in Table 2. For practical purposes, sulfone resistant disease is only a problem in borderline to lepromatous leprosy.

WARTS

THOMAS L. WATT, M.D.

Warts are infectious, intraepidermal tumors of the skin and mucous membranes caused by the human papilloma virus (HPV). Formerly, the clinical variants were presumed to be caused by a single, species specific, intracellular, DNA virus. However, recent evidence proves that there are at least two dozen types of HPV and that the clinical manifestations are dictated in part by the regional anatomy of the skin involved and in part by the viral type.

Some of the important clinical variants to be considered are:

A. Comon Wart (Verruca Vulgaris)—(HPV types 1,2,4).
B. Plantar Wart (Verruca Plantaris)—(HPV types 1,2,4).
C. Flat Wart (Verruca Plan)—(HPV types 3,5).
D. Filiform and Digitate Warts—(HPV types 1,2,3).
E. Venereal Wart (Condyloma Accuminata)—(HPV types 7,8,etc).
F. Epidermodysplasia Verruciformis—(HPV types 3,5).
G. Special Situations.

These morphologic variants may be seen in varying numbers exclusively or in combination. Diagnosis is made by clinical observation. Rarely is biopsy necessary.

Skillful management of wart patients is largely dependent upon the proper selection of the treatment modality considering:

1. The age and occupation of the patient;
2. The morphologic type, location and number of lesions;
3. The duration and previous treatment of the disease.

Other factors that sometimes influence selection of therapy and prognosis are pregnancy, hyperhidrosis, atopy, and immunologic deficiency disorders including patients undergoing organ transplants.

The therapist must be ever mindful that warts are in fact benign. Although a nuisance and at times painful, symptoms are rarely debilitating and the lesions are usually self-limited. A study done in the early 1960s on 1,000 institutionalized children indicates that two-thirds of the warts disappear spontaneously over a two year period. An appreciation for the natural history of warts should curb our therapeutic zeal. Treatment must be humane and should minimize pain and permanent scarring.

Often the push for immediate cure comes from a well meaning, but misinformed patient, relative, or friend. This underscores the need to manage the patient and family as well as the disease. This can best be done by a forthright discussion of the cause and natural history of the disease and an understandable outline of alternatives, goals and prognosis of therapy. Sometimes reassurance alone is all that the patient requires. Do not feel obligated to cure every wart.

The power of suggestion and the placebo effect of therapy are powerful allies estimated to influence the response rate in up to 40 percent of wart patients. The placebo effect must be exploited in our treatment of patients and particularly when dealing with children and when relying on more conservative modalities. This can best be done by approaching the patient with an attitude of friendliness, confidence, enthusiasm, and tenacity.

A discussion of wart therapy is not complete without mention of immunity. Clearly immune factors, even if poorly understood, are operative in our patients. Modern therapy should be directed at manipulation of these factors through the reduction of viral load, release of intracellular particles, and local irritation or sensitization. Development of the immune response by B and T lymphocytes triggers spontaneous resolution and therapeutic victories. The lack or delay of the immune response results in conditions such as Epidermodysplasia Verruciformis and therapeutic misadventures.

The outline of treatment that follows is arranged according to morphologic type, number of lesions, and my therapeutic preferences listed in order. It is not intended to be all inclusive. Methods less widely used but deemed effective are listed in the category, Special Situations. For the sake of brevity, each treatment is discussed once when first listed in the outline and mentioned by name only thereafter.

COMMON WARTS

Solitary Lesions

Preferred Treatment

Light Electrodesiccation and Curettage Under Local Anesthesia. This destructive method eliminates viral particles along with tumor mass and reduces focus of infection, but does little to stimulate immune factors. The technique is to trim surrounding callous, lightly electrodesiccate (monopolar current) the wart until softened, and thoroughly curette it away with appropriate-sized dermal curettes. Hemostasis is obtained by pressure and the application of saturated Trichloracetic Acid (Mallinckrodt, Inc., St. Louis, MO 63147) with a Q-tip, followed immediately by neutralization with 70 percent isopropyl alcohol. A Band-aid is applied. Postoperative instructions are for removal of the Band-aid the following day and the application of Polysporin ointment and Band-aids as necessary.

Alternative Treatment

Cryosurgery. Cold injury results in rupture of cells and release of viral particles for exposure to immune factors and the shed of wart mass through blistering. The technique is to trim away callous and dry scale. Then a proctoscopic swab is trimmed to an appropriate size, saturated with liquid nitrogen, and applied directly to the wart under mild pressure for 10 to 15 seconds or until the frost ball extends 1 to 2 mm beyond the visible margin of the wart (I prefer a cryoswab over cryospray). This is done without anesthesia and with the patient in a prone position to avoid a vasovagal reaction. The patient is retreated 2 to 3 weeks later if necessary. The time interval is crucial, as shown by Bunney and her British colleagues. Postoperative care is minimal, but the patient is advised to puncture blisters extending beyond the treated areas, and especialy over joints or pressure areas. Seventy percent isopropyl alcohol on a swab can be applied to ruptured blisters once daily until healing occurs.

Keratolytics. These chemicals are corrosive in action and presumed to destroy and eliminate viral particles by shedding in addition to stimulating immune reaction. A selection of one of the following is made: (1) 10 to 20 percent salicylic acid compounded in flexible collodion (2) Duofilm (16.7 percent salicylic acid and 16.7 percent lactic acid in flexible collodion packaged by Stiefel Laboratories, Inc.), or (3) Lester Bienvenue's Formula:

Podophyllin resin 3
Trichloracetic acid 3
Salicylic acid 3
Acetone 2
Flexible collodion qs ad 30

Bienvenue's Formula is highly irritative and should be used only on stubborn lesions away from tender skin. The technique is to instruct the patient to soak the affected area nightly for 5 minutes in warm water and dry thoroughly. The residual crust and scale are trimmed off, and one or two drops of the selected liquid are applied to the wart using an applicator rod or toothpick. The material is permitted to dry and a Band-aid is applied. This is done until the wart drops off. Care must be exercised to keep the acid material off normal skin. Fingernail polish remover can be used to remove any amount that is accidentally applied to normal skin. Treatment should be temporarily discontinued when the wart becomes sore or inflamed.

Multiple Lesions

Preferred Treatment

Cryosurgery, the preferred treatment, has already been discussed.

Alternative Treatment

Keratolytics. The combined use of cryosurgery and Duofilm was found by Bunney and associates to increase the response rate from 67 to 78 percent at 12 weeks.

Light Electrodesiccation and Curettage. This treatment should be used for specific, symptomatic lesions, and its wholesale use on large numbers of warts or in areas where scarring is of concern is not justified.

PLANTAR WARTS

Solitary Lesions

Preferred Treatment

Aseptic Necrosis. The following is an adaptation of a technique developed by Dr. Otis Jillson. It results in an inflammatory and a presumed immunologic response. It is used when there are one or two warts on the same sole, without anesthesia, and with the patient in a prone position. The callous is carefully trimmed away. The lesion is stippled with a sharpened toothpick immersed in saturated solution of Trichloracetic Acid. A drop of a compound containing 20 percent salicylic acid and 20 percent linseed oil in a compound tincture of benzoin is then applied to the wart, a form-fitted 40 percent salicylic acid plaster (Mediplast, Beiersdorf, Inc., South

Norwalk, CT) is applied, and the area firmly taped with a waterproof adhesive tape. The patient is instructed to reinforce the tape if it loosens, to keep the foot dry (cover in shower with a plastic bag), to call if undue pain develops, and to return to the office in 10 days. At this time the sterile abscess is unroofed and dead wart carefully trimmed away without anesthesia. If a sterile abscess has not developed, the compounded podophyllin and a 40 percent salicylic acid plaster are reapplied. Almost always, aseptic necrosis develops, and after debridement the patient is instructed to soak the foot daily in warm soapy water, to apply Polysporin ointment, and to cover the wound with Band-aids until healed, usually for 2 to 3 weeks. There is some pain associated with this treatment, but it is surprisingly well tolerated. In experienced hands the method is highly successful and with a very low recurrence rate, suggesting development of natural immunity.

Alternative Treatment

Cantharidin. This naturally occurring extract from blister beetles has an effect similar to cold injury. Two popular products containing this vesicant are Cantharone (Seres Laboratories) and Verrusol (C & M Pharmacal). I prefer Verrusol. The technique is as follows: (1) pare away the callous with the patient in a prone position, (2) carefully apply the compound to the wart, keeping it off the surrounding normal skin (to reduce marginal spread), and (3) allow the material to dry and cover it with waterproof adhesive tape. The patient is instructed to leave the tape in place 24 hours or until the development of pain, whereupon the dressing is removed and the foot is soaked in warm soapy water. The patient returns in 10 days for debridement and reapplication if necessary. This treatment is most useful in children because the discomfort in the office is less than with the Jillson technique. However, the disadvantages are lower cure rate and hence the need for more treatments and the occasional development of marginal extension (doughnut wart).

Keratolytics. These have already been discussed.

Blunt Dissection or Enucleation. This treatment, a variation of curettage, works by removal of the wart and viral load. It is carried out under local anesthesia. No electrosurgery is used. The callous is carefully trimmed away and the wart is avulsed or enucleated, using special instruments such as the Ulbrich curette (purchased through Robbins Instrument Co.). The wound margins are beveled with fine scissors. Hemostasis is obtained with firm pressure followed by application of Gelfoam Powder (The Upjohn Co.) or Monsel's solution. Postoperative treatment is the same as with electrodesiccation and curettage. However, the total avoidance of electrosurgery minimizes scar formation. The disadvantage of the technique is the need for local anesthesia, and it is more painful than and has a lower cure rate than Jillson's aseptic necrosis technique in my hands.

X-ray Therapy. The one-dose technique of Pipkin (Pipkin, Lehmann and Ressman, South Med J 1949;43:193-202, is a painless treatment with a high cure rate. However, it is mandatory that the therapist be thoroughly familiar with the use of the x-ray unit and shielding procedures and that the dosage schedule be adhered to strictly. Furthermore, the treatment should be limited to warts less than 1 cm in size, and the quality of x-ray should be limited to so-called superficial x-ray (unfiltered, 60–80 KV, HVL 0.7 mm A1). Its effects are destructive, but scarring is negligible if the correct dosage is administered.

Cryosurgery. This treatment, already discussed, should be reserved for only small or relatively superficial lesions.

Adjunctive Treatment. Foot padding, such as corn pads and shoe inserts of foam rubber, should be employed to alleviate discomfort from pressure when lesions are painful.

Few Lesions

Preferred Treatment

Keratolytics, the preferred treatment, have already been discussed.

Alternative Treatment

Formalin Ointment. Formaldehyde is virucidal, corrosive, and irritating. It appears to stimulate natural immunity. The technique is to apply form-fitted 40 percent salicylic acid plasters to the warts and to cover these with firmly placed waterproof adhesive tape. The plasters are removed 3 to 5 days later at home, and the soggy keratinous debris trimmed away. Then treatment begins with nightly soaks in warm water followed by the application of a compounded cream containing 20 percent formalin in Aquaphor with Q-tips. The warts are covered with Saran wrap, which is taped in place with Blenderm tape (3-M Co.). The callous is trimmed with razor blades every fifth day. The patient returns one month later for review.

Fowler's Solution (Liquor Potassium Arsenite). Topically applied arsenite destroys the wart's blood supply and induces aseptic necrosis. The solution is applied in the same manner as formalin ointment. This treatment causes aseptic necrosis in 4 to 6 weeks and is relatively painless and highly successful. The difficulty is obtaining the material.

Multiple Lesions (And Mosaic Warts)

Preferred Treatment

Dilute Formalin Foot Soaks. The procedure is to apply 40 percent salicylic acid plasters in the office. Three to 5 days later the patient removes the plasters, trims away the soggy keratinous debris, and begins nightly 30-minute soaks in 5 percent formaldehyde solution. The solution is best premixed by the pharmacy. The patient selects a flat-bottomed container of sufficient size to immerse the involved areas, being certain to keep the solution off the dorsal foot and other areas (to minimize sensitization to formaldehyde). If painful fissures develop, treatment is temporarily discontinued and petroleum jelly is applied to fissures before and after soaking as necessary. Usually after 2 to 4 weeks of treatment, significant dryness and scaling develop, and shortly thereafter warts begin to dry up and fall out. The advantage of this technique is that it is usually painless, and it is highly effective with a low recurrence rate. Its disadvantages are: (1) it is time-consuming, (2) it requires patient diligence, and (3) it is potentially skin-sensitizing.

Alternative Treatment

Formaldehyde Ointment. This treatment has already been discussed.

Glutaraldehyde Solution. This material has effects similar to those of formaldehyde. A compound containing 10 percent glutaraldehyde, 2.3 percent sodium bicarbonate, and 0.2 percent Tween-80 is painted on warts twice daily. The callous and dead warts are trimmed every 3 to 5 days. This treatment is easier to use but less effective than dilute formalin soaks. The compound is unstable and must be replaced every 4 weeks.

Forty percent Salicylic Acid Plasters. The plasters are applied weekly after paring and stippling the warts with a saturated solution of Trichloracetic Acid as tolerated. The plasters are left in place until the following treatment. Usually six to ten treatments are necessary.

FLAT WARTS

Few Lesions

Preferred Treatment

Light Cryosurgery (liquid nitrogen). This procedure, already discussed, frequently requires repetition.

Alternative Treatment

Light Electrodesiccation Without Curettage. Curettage increases risk of scarring without effectively increasing the cure rate.

Saturated Solution of Potassium Iodide (SSKI). This is applied topically.

Multiple Lesions

Preferred Treatment

Light Cryosurgery (liquid nitrogen). An acne spray or carbon dioxide slush is used repeatedly at weekly intervals. (Cryosurgery has already been discussed.)

Alternative Treatment

Light Electrodesiccation at Weekly Intervals Without Curettage.

Saturated Solution of Potassium Iodide (SSKI). This is applied topically twice daily.

Vleminckx Solution Hot Packs. These are applied every other night. Vlem Dome packets may be used and the solution saved and reheated.

One Percent Tannic Acid and Two Percent Salicylic Acid Compounded in Bay Rum (Formula of Rees B Rees). This is applied twice daily.

Five percent Efudex solution (5-Fluorouracil). This is applied twice daily to lesions.

Oral Aquasol-A. A daily dose of 75,000 to 100,000 IU is given for one month in conjunction with other treatments.

No Shaving. When the patient's beard area is not responding to treatment, refraining from shaving for 3 to 6 months often ends the dilemma.

FILIFORM AND DIGITATE WARTS

Few Lesions

The *preferred treatment* is light electrodesiccation without curettage, already discussed.

The *alternative treatment* is (1) cryosurgery, or (2) topical SSKI, also already discussed.

Multiple Lesions

The *preferred treatment* is light electrodesiccation without curettage, already discussed.

The *alternative treatment* is (1) cryosurgery, or (2) topical SSKI, or (3) Vleminckx's solution, or (4) no shaving, also already discussed.

VENEREAL WARTS

Few Lesions

Preferred Treatment

Podophyllin. This naturally occurring cytotoxic agent arrests cellular mitosis in metaphase. Its effectiveness is limited to venereal warts and lesions in moist or macerated areas. Initiated as 20 percent podophyllin in compound tincture of benzoin applied every 5 to 7 days, the material is carefully applied to warts, permitted to dry, and is covered with Zeasorb powder or gauze to minimize spread to normal skin. The material is removed with soap and water 6 to 10 hours after application. In resistant cases, a preparation containing 40 percent podophyllin and 10 percent salicylic acid compounded in compound tincture of benzoin is substituted. These materials are not to be used on a pregnant woman.

Alternative Treatment

Saturated Trichloracetic Acid. The material is highly caustic and is cautiously applied with a toothpick or Q-tip directly to warts and immediately neutralized with

70 percent isopropyl alcohol. It can be used in conjunction with podophyllin on stubborn recurrent lesions and is particularly useful on the nonmoist penile shaft.

Cryosurgery (liquid nitrogen). This has already been discussed.

Electrodesiccation With and Without Curettage. This has already been discussed.

Multiple Lesions

Preferred Treatment

Podophyllin, already discussed, is the preferred treatment.

Alternative Treatment

Cryosurgery. This method has already been discussed.

Electrodesiccation With Curettage. This method has been discussed.

Domeboro Solution Compresses Followed by the Application of One Percent Vioform Cream. This is a useful measure for the pregnant woman. It has a drying and soothing effect.

Triple Sulfa Vaginal Cream. This is used in conjunction with other measures when the vagina is infected. This empirical treatment works.

Proctoscopic Examination and Electrosurgery. This technique is used when indicated for perianal warts.

EPIDERMODYSPLASIA VERRUCIFORMIS

Symptomatic or troublesome lesions are best eradicated with either electrosurgery and curettage or cryosurgery. Biopsy and surgical removal are necessary for lesions suspected of undergoing malignant degeneration.

SPECIAL SITUATIONS

Paronychial or Subungual Warts

Preferred Treatment

Litt Taping Method. The technique is reported by Jerome Z. Litt in Cutis 1978; 22:673. It involves an elaborate taping procedure and is especially effective for children. An adaptation is to have the mother apply Castellani's paint to the wart prior to taping.

Alternative Treatment

Alternatives are (1) cryosurgery, (2) cantharidin, and (3) blunt dissection or enucleation, all of which have been discussed.

Lush Wart Growth in Interdigital Spaces in Association with Hyperhidrosis.

Preferred Treatment

Use of Drysol solution in association with keratolytics or Fowler's solution has been discussed.

Alternative Treatment

Technique Developed by Dr. Kenneth Burdick. Nightly foot soaks in warm soapy water, followed by debridement and then the cautious application of a compounded solution containing 20 percent podophyllin and 20 percent linseed oil in compound tincture of benzoin under occlusion of waterproof tape or Saran wrap. This is a highly irritating treatment and requires close supervision for debridement and encouragement, but when effective, it works rapidly.

Cryosurgery. This technique, already discussed, may be combined with Burdick's technique.

Giant Condyloma and Verrucous Carcinoma of the Genitals and Soles

These conditions are treacherous and require the attention of specialized surgeons.

The Desperate Patient with Warts Resistant to All Usual Treatments

These patients are probably best managed by doctors with specialized interests. Treatment with hypnosis, 5-FU, intralesional Bleomycin, sensitization induction to DCNB or poison ivy extract, and interferon are all worth consideration.

INFECTIOUS DISEASES

ANTIVIRAL CHEMOTHERAPY

MARIA C. SAVOIA, M.D.
MICHAEL N. OXMAN, M.D.

Until recently, chapters on antiviral chemotherapy were missing from major textbooks of medicine and even from major texts on infectious diseases. Our traditional approach to the control of viral diseases has been to prevent infection either by limiting exposure or by immunization, techniques of unquestionable merit and unparalleled cost-effectiveness. When virus infections did occur, few if any therapeutic options were available. The recent development of effective antiviral agents has altered this situation. Many compounds are being developed that take advantage of virus-specific metabolic reactions to inhibit virus replication selectively without significant toxicity for host cells. Five antiviral drugs with proven efficacy and acceptable therapeutic to toxic ratios have already been licensed for use in the United States, and many additional agents are currently being evaluated.

While vaccines that prevent infection will continue to be our most important and cost-effective weapons in the battle against viral diseases, physicians will now also have access to an ever-increasing array of therapeutic agents. This chapter is concerned primarily with antiviral agents that are currently approved for use in the United States, but investigational agents and indications for use that are likely to gain such approval are also considered. Guidelines for the use of these agents are summarized in Table 1.

Readers of this chapter should keep in mind the following general principles:

1. *Use of any antiviral agent requires a specific virologic diagnosis.* More than 500 different viruses—belonging to at least 17 distinct virus families—cause disease in humans. Since individual antiviral agents rely for their selective antiviral activity upon virus-specific metabolic reactions that are often unique to individual viruses or virus families, the choice of an appropriate antiviral agent requires a specific virologic diagnosis. Clinical diagnosis is often unreliable because many different viruses may cause the same clinical syndrome. Fortunately, rapid progress is being made in the development and application of laboratory techniques for the quick and accurate diagnosis of viral infections. Physicians should soon be able to obtain reliable diagnostic information early enough to permit the effective utilization of available antiviral agents.

2. *Most viral infections are acute and self-limited.* In many cases, peak virus multiplication and dissemination occur late in the incubation period and rapidly diminish after the onset of symptoms. Since most antiviral agents act by inhibiting virus multiplication, they can only be effective if administered at a time when progression of disease is dependent upon continuing virus replication. In general, this means that antiviral therapy must be initiated very early in the course of the disease. Moreover, the natural history of the untreated infection and the status of host-defense mechanisms are important considerations in selecting patients who might benefit from antiviral therapy. For example, in immunologically normal patients with recurrent mucocutaneous herpes simplex, host defenses rapidly terminate virus replication and lesions quickly resolve without treatment, whereas in immunocompromised patients, lesions may progress and virus multiplication may continue at high levels for many weeks. Clearly, an agent that inhibits herpes simplex virus replication will have a much greater impact on the course of the disease in immunocompromised patients.

3. *Antiviral agents should be reserved for situations in which clinical benefit has been demonstrated.* Anecdotal experience, case reports, and uncontrolled trials often lead to false impressions of clinical efficacy and can encourage both physicians and patients to use ineffective and harmful remedies. In most virus diseases, the effica-

TABLE 1 Indications for the Use of Available Antiviral Agents

Indication	*Antiviral Agent*	*Route*	*Dose*	*Comments*
Treatment of influenza A virus infection	Amantadine	Oral	Adults: 100–200 mg/day (see text) for 5–7 days; children ≤9 years: 4.4–8.8 mg/kg/day for 5–7 days not to exceed 150 mg/day)*	Normal persons >65 years of age should receive 100 mg/day
Prophylaxis against influenza A virus infection	Amantadine	Oral	Adults: 100–200 mg/day (see text); children ≤9 years: 4.4–8.8 mg/kg/day (not to exceed 150 mg/day)*	Should be continued for the duration of the epidemic *or* for 2 weeks in conjunction with influenza vaccination (until vaccine-induced immunity develops); normal persons >65 years of age should receive 100 mg/day
Treatment of herpes simplex virus (HSV) encephalitis†	Acyclovir	IV	10 mg/kg (1 hour infusion) every 8 hours for 10 days‡	Recent comparative studies demonstrate that although IV vidarabine (15 mg/kg by continuous infusion over 12 hours each day for 10 days) is effective, morbidity and mortality are significantly lower in patients treated with acyclovir than with vidarabine
Treatment of neonatal herpes	Vidarabine	IV	30 mg/kg/day (continuous infusion over 12 hours) for 10 days§	Efficacy of vidarabine is established; vidarabine and acyclovir currently being compared in controlled clinical trials
	or			
	Acyclovir	IV	10 mg/kg (1 hour infusion) each 8 hours for 10 days‡	
Treatment of mucocutaneous herpes simplex in immunocompromised hosts	Acyclovir	IV	250 mg/M² (1 hour infusion) every 8 hours for 7 days‡	Choice of topical, oral, or intravenous preparation depends upon clinical severity and setting; topical acyclovir is appropriate only when it can be applied to all lesions; it does not affect untreated lesions or systemic symptoms
	or			
	Acyclovir	Oral	200 mg 5 times/day for 10 days	
	or			
	Acyclovir	Topical	5% ointment; 4–6 applications/day for 7 days or until healed	
Prophylaxis against mucocutaneous herpes simplex during periods of intense immunosuppression	Acyclovir	Oral	200 mg 4 times/day‖	Oral therapy most convenient; lesions recur when therapy stops
	or			
	Acyclovir	IV	250 mg/M² every 8 hours or 5 mg/kg every 12 hours (1 hour infusion)‡	Lesions recur when therapy stops
Treatment of initial genital HSV infections	Acyclovir	Oral	200 mg 5 times/day for 10 days‖	Drug of choice in most clinical settings; treatment has no effect on subsequent recurrence rates
	or			
	Acyclovir	IV	5 mg/kg (1 hour infusion) each 8 hours for 5–7 days‡	When severity of infection merits hospitalization, or with neurologic or other visceral complications
	or			
	Acyclovir	Topical	5% ointment, 4–6 applications/day for 7–14 days	May cause stinging on contact; does not affect constitutional symptoms, new lesion formation, or untreated sites of infection
Treatment of recurrent genital herpes#	Acyclovir	Oral	200 mg 5 times/day for 5 days‖	No effect on subsequent recurrence rates; efficacy greater if used early in attack
Prophylaxis against frequently recurring genital herpes#	Acyclovir	Oral	200 mg 3 times/day for up to 6 months‖	May promote emergence of resistance; occasional "breakthrough" attacks and/or asymptomatic virus shedding during treatment; not recommended for periods exceeding 6 months
Treatment of HSV keratitis	Trifluridine	Topical	One drop of 0.1% ophthalmic solution every 2 hours while awake (up to 9 drops/day)	3% acyclovir ointment (ophthalmic) is equal or superior to idoxuridine, vidarabine and trifluridine for treatment of HSV keratitis, but is not available in the United States
	or			
	Vidarabine	Topical	One-half-inch ribbon of 3% ophthalmic ointment 5 times/day	
	or			

Table 1 Continued

TABLE 1 Indications for the Use of Available Aniviral Agents *(Continued)*

Indication	*Antiviral Agent*	*Route*	*Dose*	*Comments*
	Idoxuridine	Topical	One-half-inch ribbon of 0.5% ophthalmic ointment 5 times/day	
Treatment of varicella in immunocompromised hosts	Acyclovir	IV	500 mg/M² (1 hour infusion) every 8 hours for 7 days‡	In the absence of comparative data, acyclovir is preferred because of its ease of administration and lower toxicity
	or			
	Vidarabine	IV	10 mg/kg/day (continuous infusion over 12 hours) for 5 days§	
Treatment of severe localized or disseminated herpes zoster in immunocompromised hosts	Acyclovir	IV	500 mg/M² or 5–10 mg/kg (1 hour infusion) every 8 hours for 5–7 days‡	Comparative trials in severe localized and disseminated herpes zoster are underway; pending results, acyclovir is preferred because of its ease of administration and lower toxicity
	or			
	Vidarabine	IV	10 mg/kg/day (continuous infusion over 12 hours) for 5–7 days§	

* Dosage adjustment required in patients with renal insufficiency (see Table 2).
† Brain biopsy is required to rule out other diagnoses that require different modalities of therapy.
‡ Dosage adjustment required in patients with renal insufficiency (see Table 3).
§ In patients with severe renal insufficiency (creatinine clearance ≤10 ml/minute/1.73M²), the dose should be reduced by 25%.
‖ In patients with severe renal insufficiency (creatinine clearance ≤10 ml/minute/1.73M²), the dose should be reduced to 200 mg every 12 hours.
Appropriate only for carefully selected patients.

cy and toxicity of an antiviral agent can be evaluated only by randomized, double-blind, placebo-controlled studies involving proven cases.

4. *The indiscriminate use of antiviral agents will hasten the emergence of resistant viruses*. Just as the use of antibiotics has led to the emergence of antibiotic-resistant bacteria, resistance to antiviral agents will develop with their widespread use. Although the clinical importance of this phenomenon may not become apparent for some time, antiviral agents should be used judiciously to minimize the selection of resistant viruses.

AGENTS USEFUL IN THE TREATMENT OF RESPIRATORY VIRUS INFECTIONS

Amantadine (1-adamantanamine hydrochloride)

In 1966, amantadine (Symmetrel), a symmetric tricyclic amine, became the first antiviral agent licensed for systemic use by the U.S. Food and Drug Administration (FDA). Amantadine specifically inhibits the multiplication of influenza A viruses and is clinically effective in the prophylaxis and treatment of influenza A virus infections. Its efficacy is strictly limited to influenza A virus strains. Although its mechanism of action is not precisely known, amantadine acts at an early stage of virus replication; it appears to prevent the uncoating of the viral genome that normally follows attachment and penetration of the virus into the host cell.

Many clinical trials have demonstrated that administration of amantadine within 24 to 48 hours after the onset of symptoms of naturally occurring or experimentally induced influenza A virus infection shortens the duration of illness; fever and systemic symptoms resolve in approximately half the time in treated patients. Subtle abnormalities in peripheral airway function also resolve more quickly in patients with uncomplicated influenza A who are treated with amantadine. However, the efficacy of amantadine in treating or preventing pneumonia due to influenza A virus has not yet been established. Therapeutic responses have also been demonstrated in patients with uncomplicated influenza A treated with aerosolized amantadine—a cumbersome method of delivery, but one that produces higher concentrations of amantadine in respiratory secretions than does oral administration.

Administered prophylactically, amantadine has about the same efficacy as vaccination in preventing influenza A virus infection (50% to 90%). Amantadine recipients who do develop influenza A have milder illnesses.

Pharmacology and Toxicology

Amantadine, which is available in capsules and syrup, is well absorbed following oral administration. The usual dosage for both treatment and prophylaxis is 200 mg per day in healthy adults and 4.4 to 8.8 mg per kilogram per day in children up to 9 years of age. These dosages produce plasma concentrations that average 0.6 to 0.8 μg per milliliter, two- to fourfold higher than the concentration required to inhibit most strains of influenza A virus in vitro. The concentration of amantadine in respiratory tissues and secretions appears to equal or exceed that in the plasma.

Amantadine is excreted unmetabolized in the urine, with a mean plasma half-life of 12 to 18 hours in healthy adults. Plasma half-life increases in elderly individuals and in patients with impaired renal function, necessitating dosage adjustment (Table 2). Orally administered amantadine at dosages of 6 mg per kilogram per day in children and 200 mg per day in healthy adults is generally well tolerated.

TABLE 2 Dosage Adjustment for Oral Amantadine in Patients with Impaired Renal Function

Creatinine Clearance (ml/minute/1.73M²	*Suggested Oral Maintenance Regimen After 200 mg (100 mg BID) on the First Day*
≥ 80	100 mg BID
60–80	100 mg BID alternating with 100 mg daily
40–60	100 mg daily
30–40	200 mg (100 mg BID) twice weekly
20–30	100 mg 3 times each week
10–20	200 mg (100 mg BID) alternating with 100 mg every 7 days
< 10	100 mg every 7 days

Note: Modified from Horadan et al. Ann Intern Med 1981; 94:454–458.

No serious hepatic, hematopoietic, or renal toxicity has been documented. Adverse effects appear to correlate with plasma levels of amantadine and to be limited, with few exceptions, to minor gastrointestinal and central nervous system symptoms that disappear when the drug is discontinued. Complaints such as nausea, loss of appetite, nervousness, insomnia, difficulty in concentrating, drowsiness, lightheadedness, confusion, and mildly diminished intellectual and motor function have been noted in 1 to 10 percent of previously healthy recipients of amantadine, but their incidence in many studies has not differed significantly in amantadine and placebo recipients.

Symptoms of central nervous system toxicity have been observed in up to 20 percent of elderly patients receiving amantadine, probably reflecting higher plasma levels associated with age-related decreases in glomerular filtration rate. Symptoms frequently resolve despite continued administration of the drug, and they may often be avoided by giving amantadine at bedtime rather than in the morning or by administering one-half of the daily dose each 12 hours. Since recent studies indicate that 100 mg per day of amantadine may be just as effective as 200 mg per day, the use of the lower dosage is recommended for prophylaxis in elderly patients.

High doses of amantadine are teratogenic in certain laboratory animals, and thus amantadine is not considered safe for use during pregnancy.

Recommended Usage

Because amantadine is not effective against other agents that may be responsible for flu-like symptoms, including influenza B viruses, its use should be reserved for situations in which infection with an influenza A virus is proven or probable. Thus, amantadine usage is only appropriate when epidemiologic and virologic evidence indicates that influenza A virus infection is prevalent in the community.

Prophylactic administration of amantadine is recommended for individuals at increased risk of complications from influenza A who have not been vaccinated against the prevalent virus strain(s) or who may be expected to have responded poorly to vaccination (e.g., immunocompromised patients). The target population of high-risk individuals includes elderly persons (65 or more years of age), especially those in nursing homes and other institutions; hospitalized patients; and children and adults with underlying pulmonary, cardiovascular, neuromuscular or immunodeficiency disorders. Additional recommended recipients include unvaccinated children and adults with other chronic diseases and malignancies; unvaccinated physicians, nurses, and other health care workers who have extensive contact with high-risk patients; unvaccinated household and institutional contacts of persons with influenza A; and unvaccinated persons who provide essential community services. Prophylaxis should begin as soon as influenza A is identified in the community and must be continued throughout the period of its prevalence (usually 4 to 8 weeks). Influenza vaccine should be administered simultaneously with the initiation of amantadine prophylaxis in unvaccinated individuals. This will provide protection against influenza B as well as influenza A and, in most recipients, reduce the required duration of amantadine administration to 10 to 14 days (i.e., until vaccine-induced immunity develops). Amantadine prophylaxis may also be used as a supplement to vaccination for better protection in immunodeficient and debilitated patients.

Treatment with amantadine is appropriate for patients at increased risk (see above) who develop an illness compatible with influenza during a period of known or suspected influenza A virus activity in the community. Treatment should be initiated as soon as possible (preferably within 48 hours of onset) and continued until 48 hours after the resolution of signs and symptoms. Though its efficacy in this setting remains to be established, it is also reasonable to administer amantadine to patients with life-threatening influenza A virus pneumonia.

Rimantadine (α-methyl-1-adamantanemethylamine hydrochloride)

Rimantadine, a structural analogue of amantadine, has been shown to be effective in the prophylaxis and treatment of infections caused by influenza A viruses. Though similar in their mechanism of action and spectrum of antiviral activity, amantadine and rimantadine differ in several respects. Rimantadine is not as well absorbed as amantadine when given orally, but its plasma half-life is nearly twice as long. Less than 10 percent of the administered dose of rimantidine is recovered unchanged in the urine (versus more than 90% with amantadine), and elevated plasma levels are less of a problem in elderly patients and patients with renal insufficiency. When given in equal doses, both drugs are almost equally effective, but rimantadine is associated with fewer central nervous system adverse effects, probably reflecting lower plasma concentrations. Rimantadine, like amantadine, is successful in reducing the symptoms of illness even when it is not successful in preventing infection. Rimantadine is not yet approved for general use by the FDA.

Ribavirin (1-β-D-ribofuranosyl-1,2,4-triazole-3-carboxamide)

Ribavirin (Virazole) is a synthetic guanosine analogue that inhibits the in vitro replication of a wide range of RNA and DNA viruses. Its mechanism of action is not well understood, but it appears to interfere with the synthesis of messenger RNA. The effect of orally administered ribavirin on influenza A and B virus infections has been evaluated in several clinical trials, and no consistent prophylactic or therapeutic efficacy has been documented. Aerosolized ribavirin has been shown to reduce the severity of illness and virus shedding in young adults with naturally acquired influenza A and B virus infections and in infants hospitalized with respiratory syncytial virus bronchiolitis and pneumonia. The need for prolonged periods of aerosol treatment (from 12 to 20 hours per day for 3 to 6 days) is a disadvantage. Parenteral ribavirin is currently also being evaluated in the treatment of bunyavirus and arenavirus infections (including Lassa fever) and in patients infected with the human retrovirus responsible for the acquired immune deficiency syndrome (AIDS).

Oral ribavirin may cause reversible increases in serum bilirubin, serum iron, and uric acid concentrations, as well as reticulocytosis after cessation of therapy. Aerosolized ribavirin may cause conjunctival injection, but it is generally well tolerated. It has recently been approved by the FDA for treatment of infants hospitalized with bronchiolitis and pneumonia caused by influenza and respiratory syncytial virus.

AGENTS USEFUL IN THE TREATMENT OF HERPESVIRUS INFECTIONS

Acyclovir (9-[2-hydroxyethoxymethyl]guanine)

Acyclovir (Zovirax) is an acyclic purine nucleoside analogue that is useful in the treatment of infections caused by herpes simplex virus types 1 and 2 (HSV-1 and HSV-2) and varicella-zoster virus (VZV). It is a safe and effective drug because it is phosphorylated selectively by a virus-specific thymidine kinase and thus concentrated in infected cells. Cellular enzymes convert acyclovir monophosphate to acyclovir triphosphate, which interferes with viral DNA synthesis by selectively inhibiting viral DNA polymerase. Some acyclovir is also incorporated into viral DNA, where it acts as a chain terminator.

Of the five human herpesviruses, HSV-1, HSV-2, and VZV are sensitive to acyclovir because they encode their own thymidine kinase and possess a sensitive DNA polymerase. In vitro, most strains of HSV-1 are inhibited by acyclovir at concentrations of 0.2 μg per milliliter or less, most strains of HSV-2 by concentrations of 0.4 μg per milliliter or less, and most strains of VZV by concentrations of 2 μg per milliliter or less.

Acyclovir also exhibits some activity against Epstein-Barr virus (EBV), which lacks thymidine kinase but possesses a very sensitive DNA polymerase. This indicates that acyclovir can be phosphorylated to some extent by cellular thymidine kinases and that some acyclovir triphosphate is formed in uninfected cells.

Unfortunately, acyclovir is not useful in the treatment of infections caused by cytomegalovirus (CMV), another member of the herpesvirus family that lacks thymidine kinase, presumably because CMV DNA polymerase is not inhibited by the low concentrations of acyclovir triphosphate formed in the absence of a viral thymidine kinase.

Pharmacology and Toxicology

Acyclovir is available in the United States in intravenous, oral, and topical forms. After intravenous infusion of 5 mg per kilogram every 8 hours, peak and trough plasma concentrations average 9.8 μg per milliliter and 0.7 μg per milliliter, respectively. The concentration of acyclovir in cerebrospinal fluid is approximately one-half of the plasma concentration. Only 15 to 30 percent of an oral dose of acyclovir is absorbed, with bioavailability decreasing slightly with increasing oral doses in the 200- to 600-mg range. Steady-state peak concentrations of acyclovir average 1.4 μg per milliliter in adults given 200 mg orally five times a day. Percutaneous absorption of acyclovir ointment (5% acyclovir in a polyethylene glycol base) is low. Excretion of acyclovir occurs both by glomerular filtration and tubular secretion, with an average plasma half-life of 2.9 hours in normal adults. Sixty to 90 percent of an administered dose may be recovered unmetabolized in the urine. Dosage adjustments are therefore required in patients with diminished renal function (see Table 3).

Acyclovir has been associated with relatively few adverse effects. Phlebitis may occur with extravasation of intravenous acyclovir. When given in high doses (more than 5 mg per kilogram every 8 hours) intravenously, acyclovir has been associated with reversible renal dysfunction in a small percentage of patients, probably due to deposition of acyclovir crystals in renal tubules. Preexisting renal insufficiency, dehydration, and rapid infusion appear to be risk factors. Encepalopathic changes, manifested by lethargy, obtundation, tremors, hallucinations, delirium, seizures, and coma, have been observed in approximately 1 percent of acyclovir recipients, but these have generally resolved following cessation of treat-

TABLE 3 Dosage Adjustment for Intravenous Acyclovir in Patients with Impaired Renal Function

Creatinine Clearance (ml/minute/1.73M²)	*Percentage of Standard Dose*	*Dosing Interval (Hours)*
> 50	100	8
25–50	100	12
10–25	100	24
0–10*	50	24

* Administered after hemodialysis.

ment. Oral acyclovir is generally very well tolerated. It is infrequently associated with nausea and headache. Topical acyclovir may cause transient burning when applied to active genital lesions. Acyclovir is not teratogenic in animals, but safety in human pregnancy has not been established. The safety of chronic administration of acyclovir for prolonged periods in reproductively active young adults also remains to be determined.

Herpes Simplex Virus Infections

All three forms of acyclovir have demonstrated efficacy in the treatment of at least some infections caused by HSV-1 and HSV-2. However, the magnitude of clinical benefit varies with the natural history of the untreated infection, the acyclovir preparation, and the status of the host's defenses. Because of its more reliable absorption and the higher plasma levels achieved, intravenous acyclovir is preferred whenever the severity of the disease warrants hospitalization.

Herpes Simplex Encephalitis. Two recent randomized studies comparing the efficacy of intravenous acyclovir (30 mg per kilogram per day) and vidarabine (15 mg per kilogram per day) in patients with herpes simplex encephalitis (HSE) have demonstrated the superiority of acyclovir. Mortality, expected to exceed 70 percent without treatment, was reduced to approximately 24 percent in recipients of acyclovir compared with 52 percent in vidarabine recipients. In addition, the proportion of the survivors who returned to normal life was twice as high among recipients of acyclovir as among vidarabine recipients. With either drug, the outcome was best in patients treated early, (i.e., before they had lapsed into semicoma or coma). These data indicate that intravenous acyclovir is now the treatment of choice for HSE.

The safety and ease of administration of acyclovir and the importance of early treatment have led some physicians to treat patients on the basis of a presumptive diagnosis of HSE without confirming the diagnosis by brain biopsy. This approach is dangerous because nearly two-thirds of patients begun on therapy on the basis of a presumptive diagnosis of HSE prove on brain biopsy not to have this disease, and nearly one-third of these biopsy-negative patients have an alternative diagnosis revealed by the brain biopsy that requires another form of therapy. The morbidity and mortality resulting from failure to recognize and treat other treatable diseases are far greater than the morbidity and mortality of brain biopsy. Acyclovir treatment may be initiated prior to brain biopsy, but this crucial diagnostic procedure should not be delayed.

Neonatal Herpes. Like HSE, neonatal herpes is a disease with high morbidity and mortality. Efficacy has already been demonstrated for vidarabine (see below), and a trial comparing intravenous acyclovir with vidarabine is nearing completion.

Mucocutaneous Herpes Simplex in Immunocompromised Hosts. In immunocompromised hosts, mucocutaneous HSV infections are characterized by persistent progressive lesions and prolonged virus replication. Several controlled trials have demonstrated that intravenous acyclovir (5 mg per kilogram or 250 mg per square meter each 8 hours for 7 days) markedly reduces the duration of virus shedding, decreases pain, and accelerates healing of mucocutaneous HSV infections in organ allograft recipients and other immunocompromised patients. Uncontrolled trials indicate that oral acyclovir (200 mg five times daily) is also effective. Topical acyclovir (5% acyclovir in polyethylene glycol ointment administered six times daily) has been shown to accelerate the healing of cutaneous lesions in immunocompromised patients with mucocutaneous HSV-1 infections when the lesions are accessible to therapy.

Prophylactic administration of intravenous acyclovir (250 mg per square meter each 8 hours beginning before immunosuppressive therapy) has been shown to prevent reactivation of latent HSV infections in seropostive patients undergoing bone marrow transplantation and remission induction chemotherapy for acute leukemia. Comparable results have been obtained with oral acyclovir (200 mg every 6 hours). Unfortunately, prophylaxis with acyclovir does not eliminate latent HSV infection, and the majority of these patients develop symptomatic HSV infections after acyclovir is stopped.

Genital Herpes. Primary genital herpes is usually more severe than recurrent infection; most patients experience fever, headache, malaise and myalgia, new lesions continue to appear for a week or more, virus shedding continues well into the second week, and complete healing may take several weeks. In patients with first episodes of genital herpes severe enough to warrant hospitalization, intravenous acyclovir (5 mg per kilogram every 8 hours for 5 days) has been shown to reduce the duration of virus shedding, new vesicle formation, local and constitutional symptoms, and time of healing when compared with placebo. Oral acyclovir (200 mg five times daily for 10 days) was similarly effective in outpatients with primary genital herpes. Topical acyclovir (5% acyclovir in polyethylene glycol ointment applied four times daily for 7 days) reduces the duration of virus shedding and shortens the clinical course of local disease in patients with primary genital herpes. However, in contrast to oral and intravenous acyclovir, topical acyclovir does not decrease formation of new lesions or reduce the duration of dysuria, vaginal discharge, or constitutional symptoms. Oral acyclovir is the treatment of choice for most patients with primary genital HSV infections.

Oral and topical acyclovir have been evaluated by means of double-blind, placebo-controlled studies for the treatment of recurrent genital herpes, a self-limited disease of variable but generally mild severity in immunologically normal adults. Therapy with oral acyclovir (200 mg five times daily for 5 days) is associated with statistically significant decreases in the duration of virus shedding, new lesion formation, and time to healing, especially when treatment is begun early. Actual clinical benefits are modest in most patients because of the short duration of the illness even without treatment. Oral acyclovir is useful in some patients whose episodes of recurrent genital herpes are particularly severe or frequent, especially when prodromal symptoms permit treatment to be initiated before the development of vesicular lesions. However, the expense, potential adverse effects, and possible selection and transmission of acyclovir-resistant HSV mutants should discourage the indiscriminate use of oral acyclovir. Topical acyclovir offers no significant clinical benefit to normal hosts with recurrent genital herpes.

Daily prophylactic administration of oral acyclovir (200 mg three to five times daily) to immunocompetent patients with frequently recurring genital herpes has been shown to markedly reduce the frequency and severity of recurrences. Once the drug is stopped, however, recurrences resume, and there is some suggestion that the first recurrence following a period of acyclovir suppression may occur more quickly and be somewhat more severe than that in placebo recipients.

Neuronal HSV latency appears to be established early in the course of primary HSV infections, probably before the onset of symptoms. Once established, latent HSV infection is not abolished by prolonged treatment with intravenous or oral acyclovir. Thus, treatment of primary or recurrent episodes of genital herpes does not appear to affect the rate of subsequent recurrences. Genital herpes invariably recurs when treatment is stopped, even after prolonged and successful suppression with daily acyclovir. Chronic administration of acyclovir has also been associated with the emergence of acyclovir-resistant mutants of HSV. The clinical significance of these mutants, many of which may have reduced virulence, remains to be determined.

Herpes Labialis. Controlled trials of topical acyclovir (either 5% or 10% acyclovir in polyethylene glycol ointment) have failed to demonstrate any clinical benefit for normal hosts with recurrent herpes labialis.

Ocular HSV Infections. Topical acyclovir (3% ophthalmic ointment) is probably the most effective treatment for primary keratoconjunctivitis and recurrent epithelial keratitis caused by HSV. Deep infections, such as stromal disease or uveitis, respond poorly to topical acyclovir or any other topical antiviral agent. Acyclovir ointment is well tolerated. A small proportion of patients develop punctate keratopathy, a problem that also occurs in patients treated with other topical antiviral agents. The ophthalmic preparation of acyclovir is not available in the United States.

Other HSV Infections. Eczema herpeticum, HSV-infected burns, herpetic whitlow, and complications of primary oropharyngeal or genital HSV infections that appear to involve continued viral replication (e.g., cutaneous dissemination, HSV meningitis, sacral radiculopathy) should probably be treated with intravenous (5 mg per kilogram or 250 mg per square meter every 8 hours) or oral (200 mg five times daily) acyclovir for 5 to 10 days. This recommendation is not based upon the results of placebo-controlled clinical trials (which have yet to be carried out), but represents the authors' opinion.

Varicella-Zoster Virus Infections

Varicella. Though generally benign in normal children, varicella may be severe and life-threatening in immunocompromised children and adults. Intravenous acyclovir (500 mg per square meter each 8 hours for 7 days) has been shown to markedly reduce the frequency of visceral complications in immunocompromised children with varicella. Vidarabine is also effective in this setting (see below). Until the results of studies directly comparing the two agents are available, we prefer to use acyclovir because of its lower toxicity and ease of administration.

Herpes Zoster (Shingles). A randomized, double-blind, placebo-controlled clinical trial has demonstrated that intravenous acyclovir (500 mg per square meter each 8 hours for 7 days) shortens the period of virus shedding, decreases acute pain, and reduces the incidence of visceral and progressive cutaneous dissemination in immunocompromised patients with acute herpes zoster. These results are similar to those obtained with intravenous vidarabine (see below) and a direct comparison of the two drugs is currently underway. Until results are available, we prefer to use acyclovir because of its lower toxicity and ease of administration.

In normal hosts with herpes zoster, intravenous acyclovir (either 5 mg per kilogram or 500 mg per square meter each 8 hours for 5 days), if administered within 72 to 96 hours of onset, has been shown to shorten the period of virus shedding and new vesicle formation, accelerate healing, and decrease acute pain. However, there was no effect upon the incidence of postherpetic neuralgia, the most troublesome complication of herpes zoster in the normal host. Thus, in uncomplicated herpes zoster in normal hosts, the inconvenience and expense of intravenous acyclovir treatment appear to outweigh its clinical benefits. A placebo-controlled trial of high-dose oral acyclovir, with and without prednisone, is currently underway in elderly patients with herpes zoster.

Other Herpesviruses

Even at doses high enough to cause some bone marrow and neurologic toxicity, intravenous acyclovir has shown no clinical benefit in immunocompromised patients with cytomegalovirus (CMV) infections.

Intravenous acyclovir has been administered to patients with a variety of Epstein-Barr virus (EBV) associated diseases. Despite transient suppression of EBV shedding, intravenous acyclovir has not been observed to alter significantly the clinical course of the disease in patients with severe infectious mononucleosis. There have been anecdotal reports of transient remissions following treatment with acyclovir in immunocompromised patients with EBV-associated lymphoproliferative disorders, including EBV-associated B-cell lymphomas. However, beneficial effects have generally been transient and their relationship to acyclovir therapy unproven, and other similar patients treated with acyclovir have failed to respond. Controlled trials of acyclovir in normal hosts with infectious mononucleosis are currently underway.

Vidarabine (9-β-D-arabinofuranosyladenine, adenine arabinoside, ara-A)

Vidarabine (Vira-A), an analogue of adenine deoxyriboside, was the first drug licensed by the FDA for systemic treatment of herpesvirus infections. It is available in the United States as an intravenous preparation and as a 3 percent ophthalmic ointment. Its mechanism of action is not completely understood, but it is phosphorylated by cellular enzymes to vidarabine triphosphate, which competitively inhibits herpesvirus DNA polymerase to a greater extent than cellular DNA polymerases. It also acts as a chain terminator and is incorporated into both viral and cellular DNA. Vidarabine inhibits the in vitro replication of HSV-1, HSV-2, VZV, and EBV, but has variable activity against CMV. Vidarabine's water solubility is low (0.45 mg per milliliter at 25 °C), and thus it must be administered in dilute solutions by slow intravenous infusion. The large volumes of fluid required may complicate treatment of patients who ordinarily require fluid restriction or who have herpes simplex encephalitis.

Following intravenous administration, vidarabine is rapidly deaminated to hypoxanthine arabinoside (ara-Hx), which has only 2 to 3 percent of the antiviral activity of vidarabine. Approximately one-half of the total daily dose of vidarabine is excreted in the urine as ara-Hx and 1 to 3 percent as vidarabine. Dosage adjustment is necessary in renal failure. Dose-related gastrointestinal toxicity is common, manifested by anorexia, nausea, vomiting, and diarrhea and/or weight loss. High doses may be associated with megaloblastic changes in the bone marrow and sometimes with anemia, leukopenia, or thrombocytopenia. Thrombophlebitis at the infusion site, the syndrome of inappropriate secretion of antidiuretic hormone, and rash have also been reported. Tremor, myoclonus, ataxia, alterations in mental status, pain syndromes, and, rarely, seizures and coma have been reported during vidarabine therapy and occur more frequently in the presence of preexisting renal or hepatic insufficieny or with concomitant administration of interferon or, possibly, allopurinol. Vidarabine is oncogenic, mutagenic, and teratogenic in some experiental systems, and its systemic use should be reserved for the treatment of serious infections.

A number of randomized, double-blind, placebo-controlled studies have documented the therapeutic efficacy of vidarabine in severe HSV and VZV infections. In such a study, intravenous vidarabine (15 mg per kilogram per day for 10 days) was shown to decrease mortality in patients with biopsy-proven herpes simplex encephalitis from 70 percent in placebo recipients to 40 percent, with the most favorable outcomes observed in young patients treated early, before the onset of semicoma or coma. At the same dose, intravenous vidarabine reduced the mortality in newborns with disseminated and localized central nervous system HSV infections from 74 to 38 percent. Intravenous acyclovir has now supplanted vidarabine for the treatment of HSE and the two drugs are being compared for treatment of neonatal herpes.

Intravenous vidarabine (10 mg per kilogram per day for 5 days) significantly decreased new vesicle formation, fever, and the incidence of visceral complications in immunocompromised patients with varicella. In immunocompromised patients with herpes zoster, intravenous vidarabine administered within 72 hours of onset of rash reduced new vesicle formation, cutaneous and visceral dissemination, and central nervous system complications. Vidarabine also appeared to reduce the duration of acute pain and postherpetic neuralgia. Intravenous vidarabine and acyclovir are currently being compared in immunocompromised patients with VZV infection.

Intravenous vidarabine, especially when administered in conjunction with interferon, reduces hepatitis B virus replication in patients with chronic active hepatitis B. However, the long-term effect on clinical outcome remains to be determined.

Topical vidarabine (3% ophthalmic ointment) is effective treatment for HSV keratoconjunctivitis and is less allergenic than idoxuridine. Topical vidarabine is of no benefit in the treatment of genital or oral HSV infections.

Idoxuridine (5-iodo-2′-deoxyuridine, IDU, IUdR)

Idoxuridine (Stoxil, Dendrid, Herplex) is an iodinated thymidine analogue that inhibits viral DNA synthesis and is incorporated into both viral and cellular DNA. Idoxuridine was administered intravenously in early attempts to treat HSE, but a randomized, double-blind, placebo-controlled study revealed that the drug was ineffective and, in addition, caused life-threatening hematopoietic toxicity. In the United States, idoxuridine is approved only for the topical treatment of HSV keratitis, and a 0.5 percent ophthalmic ointment is available. Resistance to the antiviral effect of IDU may develop during treatment. Adverse reactions include pruritus, pain, inflammation, and edema of the eye or lids as well as rare allergic reactions.

Trifluridine (5-trifluoromethyl-2-′-deoxyuridine trifluorothymidine)

Trifluridine (Viroptic) is an analogue of deoxythymidine, that also inhibits viral DNA synthesis. Viral thymidine kinase is not necessary for its action, and thus it is active against thymidine kinase–negative strains of HSV that are resistant to acyclovir. Its usefulness as an antiviral agent is limited to the topical treatment of ocular HSV infections because of unacceptable toxicity with systemic administration. It is available as a 1 percent ophthalmic solution. Clinical trials suggest that its efficacy is superior to that of idoxuridine and comparable to that of vidarabine. Patients who have not responded to the other topical antivirals may respond to trifluridine. Adverse reactions include stinging upon instillation, palpebral edema, and, rarely, superficial punctate or epithelial keratopathy and hypersensitivity reactions.

NEW ANTIVIRAL AGENTS

At present, a number of promising new antiviral agents are under investigation. These include bromovinyl-deoxyuridine (BVDU), which is highly active against VZV and HSV-1; acyclic nucleosides like 9-(1,3-dihydroxy-2-propoxymethyl) guanine (DHPG), which may be effective in CMV infections; 2-fluoro-arabinosylnucleosides (FIAC, FIAU, FMAU), with in vitro activity similar to that of acyclovir; arildone, a phenoxyl diketone with in vitro activity against a variety of DNA and RNA viruses; phosphonoacetic acid and phosphonoformic acid, which inhibit HSV DNA polymerase; benzimidazole derivatives, which inhibit picornavirus replication; and 3′-azido-3′ deoxythymidine, which inhibits the retrovirus responsible for AIDS. Human interferons have already been shown to have therapeutic efficacy in severe human papillomavirus infections, HSV keratitis, respiratory virus infections, varicella and herpes zoster in immunocompromised patients, and chronic hepatitis B virus infections. The therapeutic efficacy of various human interferon preparations (alone or in combination with other antiviral agents) is currently under active investigation in patients with a variety of viral and neoplastic diseases.

USE OF UNPROVEN THERAPIES

Over the years, many forms of therapy have been advocated for various virus infections, especially infections for which no treatment of proven efficacy was readily available. Nowhere is this more obvious than in recurrent genital herpes. Unfortunately, the remarkable variability in the natural history of recurrent genital herpes, as well as most other viral infections, renders completely uninterpretable data from uncontrolled trials and anecdotal case reports. When unproven forms of therapy, such as 2-deoxy-D-glucose, L-lysine, photodynamic inactivation with neutral red or proflavine and light, topical idoxuridine, topical vidarabine, ether, levamisole, BCG vaccine, or multiple smallpox vaccinations have been carefully evaluated with randomized, placebo-controlled clinical trials, they have been found to be ineffective. Many have actually been harmful. Thus, it is imperative that physicians avoid exposing their patients to the hazards and expense of any form of therapy until its safety and efficacy have been demonstrated by means of randomized, placebo-controlled studies involving adequate numbers of proven cases.

CHILDHOOD IMMUNIZATION

JEROME O. KLEIN, M.D.

Immunization for children can be divided according to products recommended for all children and products recommended for special children or special situations. Seven products are considered routine immunization; these include diphtheria and tetanus toxoids and pertussis whole cell vaccine; measles, mumps, and rubella live vaccines; and oral poliovirus vaccine. Special products include influenza virus vaccine, pneumococcal, meningococcal and *Hemophilus influenzae* type B polysaccharride vaccines, bacille Calmette-Guerin (BCG), hepatitis B vaccine, and live rabies vaccine. Immune globulins are available for prevention and treatment of measles, hepatitis A and B, varicella-zoster, rabies, and tetanus.

Recommendations for immunization in the United States are provided by the Committee on Infectious Diseases of the American Academy of Pediatrics (AAP) and published in the Report of the Committee (revised every 3 to 4 years) and the Advisory Committee on Immunization Practices of the United States Public Health Service, published in the *Morbidity and Mortality Weekly Report* (MMWR). In most circumstances the recommendations of the two groups coincide. Current recommendations for immunization of adults (18 years of age and older) are provided in a recent MMWR supplement (September 28, 1984; vol. 33, no. 1S).

RECOMMENDATIONS FOR IMMUNIZATION OF NORMAL INFANTS AND CHILDREN

The schedule recommended by the AAP and ACIP for active immunization of normal infants and children is provided in Table 1.

TABLE 1 Recommended Schedule for Active Immunization of Normal Infants and Children

Recommended Age	*Vaccine*	*Comments*
2 months	DTP; OPV	Can be initiated earlier in areas of high endemicity
4 months	DTP; OPV	
6 months	DTP; (OPV)	OPV optional for areas where polio may be imported
15 months	MMR	
18 months	DTP; OPV	
4–6 years	DTP; OPV	Up to the 7th birthday
14–16 years	Td	Adult tetanus toxoid (full dose); diphtheria toxoid (reduced dose); repeat every 10 years

Abbreviations: DTP = diphtheria, tetanus, pertussis; OPV = oral poliovirus vaccine; MMR = measles, mumps, rubella; Td = tetanus, diphtheria.

Diphtheria and Tetanus Toxoids and Pertussis Vaccine (DTP)

The primary series of DTP is given at 2, 4, 6, and 18 months, with a booster administered between 4 and 6 years. The primary series of DTP is carried out up to the seventh birthday. After the seventh birthday primary immunization should consist of adult-type tetanus toxoid and reduced dose of diphtheria toxoid (Td). A lapse in the schedule does not require restarting the schedule; subsequent doses are given at the recommended time intervals. Although the optimal age for beginning immunization in infants who are born prematurely is unknown, available data suggest that DTP can be administered at the same chronologic age to premature as to term infants.

The preferred site of administration for DTP and other products administered by the intramuscular route is the anterolateral aspect of the upper thigh (preferred in infants because it is the largest muscle mass) and the deltoid muscle of the upper arm (appropriate for most older children). For routine usage, the buttocks should be avoided as a site for injection. Large volumes may require use of the buttocks; the site should be the upper outer mass of the gluteus maximus to avoid injury to the sciatic nerve.

Approximately one-half of children who receive DTP vaccine have local (tenderness, pain) and systemic (fever, irritability) adverse effects; seizures occur, with or without fever, in approximately one in 2,000 children who receive DTP, and brain damage has been identified 1 year later at a frequency of one in 310,000 doses. These effects are associated with the whole-cell pertussis component of the vaccine. Most public health experts agree that, on balance, the benefits of pertussis vaccine far outweigh the risks and it should be administered as part of the routine schedule. However, concern about toxicity of whole-cell pertussis vaccine has led to reconsideration of contraindications of its use in children. Deferral of DTP is recommended for children who have previously had convulsions (febrile or nonfebrile) until it can be determined whether an evolving neurologic disorder is present. If an evolving disorder is identified, infants or children should be given DT rather than DTP. Pertussis vaccine is also contraindicated if the child has a history of severe reaction following a prior dose (usually within 48 hours). Severe reactions include shock, collapse, persistent screaming episodes, temperature of 40.5 °C (105 °F) or greater, alterations of consciousness, generalized or local neurologic signs, or systemic allergic reactions.

Measles, Mumps, and Rubella Live Vaccines (MMR)

Live attenuated vaccines for measles, mumps, and rubella are administered in a combined vaccine. Single vaccines are also available for special use. A single dose of MMR provides durable protection with minimal side effects when administered at 15 months of age. Reimmunization is not recommended except for children who received immunization at earlier age (under 12 months for measles vaccine), with other products (killed measles vaccine), or in modified dosage or form (administered with gamma globulin).

Rubella vaccine results in viremia and infection of the placenta and fetus, but available data indicate vaccine virus is not a teratogen. Use of rubella vaccine is encouraged for susceptible nonpregnant women in the childbearing age group.

Immunization after exposure to disease may be of value for measles, but not for mumps or rubella. Measles virus vaccine administered as late as 5 days after exposure is protective in a majority of individuals. Administration of immune globulin is preferred for infants 12 months of age and younger who are exposed to measles because of the chance of vaccine failure in this age group.

Oral Poliovirus Vaccine (OPV) and Inactivated Poliovirus Vaccine (IPV)

OPV is administered at ages 2, 4, 18 months, and 4 and 6 years of age. In areas where exposure to wild virus is possible (some of the states in the Southwest), an additional dose at 6 months is recommended.

Paralytic poliomyelitis has resulted from administration of live vaccine to children with immune defects. Live virus vaccines, including OPV, should not be administered to children with known or suspected immunodeficiency. Because the vaccine virus is excreted by the vaccinee and may infect contacts, the live vaccine should not be used in families with a member who is immunodeficient. Inactivated poliovirus vaccine (IPV) should be used in children with immune defects and members of their households.

Routine immunization against poliovirus is not recommended for susceptible adults. For parents or travelers who may be exposed to wild or vaccine virus, IPV should be administered. The primary series of IPV consists of four doses; the first three may be given at the same time as DTP (in a separate syringe); the fourth dose is given 6 to 12 months after the third or on entry to school for children.

VACCINES FOR SPECIAL CHILDREN OR SPECIAL CIRCUMSTANCES

Hepatitis B Vaccine for Prevention of Perinatal Infection

Mothers who are hepatitis B antigen (HBsAg)–positive may infect their newborn infant. The initial infection is usually asymptomatic, but about 25 percent of infant carriers may ultimately develop chronic active hepatitis, cirrhosis, and, possibly, primary hepatocellular carcinoma. The severity and chronicity of the disease warrant protection of any infant born to a mother who is hepatitis B antigen–positive. The recommended schedule combines hepatitis B immune globulin (HBIg) and hepatitis B vaccine. HBIg, 0.5 ml intramuscularly, is administered as soon after birth as possible. The vaccine, 0.5 ml intramuscularly, is given before the infant leaves the hospital or within 1 week after birth and at 1 and 6 months of age. The first dose of vaccine may be given at the same time as HBIg at a separate site.

Pneumococcal Vaccine

A 23-valent polysaccharide vaccine against disease due to *Streptococcus pneumoniae* was licensed in the United States in 1983, replacing the 14-valent vaccine introduced in 1977. Although the vaccine contains serotypes responsible for most pneumococcal disease in children, the immune response to most types for children under 2 years of age is limited. Because of the lack of immunogenicity, the vaccine is not recommended for infants. The vaccine should be used for children 2 years of age and older who are at increased risk for pneumococcal disease; these include children with anatomic or functional asplenia, those with sickle cell disease, nephrotic syndrome, cerebrospinal fluid leaks, and conditions associated with immunosuppression. The vaccine may have some value in prevention of recurrent episodes of otitis media in the older children. Duration of immunity is uncertain; until data are available, reimmunization is not recommended.

Meningococcal Vaccine

A polysaccharide vaccine for groups A, C, Y and W-135 is now available as a quadrivalent product. Group A vaccine produces satisfactory immune response in infants as young as 5 months, but the other group polysaccharides are poor immunogens for infants younger than 18 months of age. Immunity is group-specific, and protective levels of antibody are achieved in 1 week. The duration of immunity is uncertain, but is estimated to be 1 to 3 years. Group B meningococcus is the most prevalent group in the United States today; the polysaccharide is a poor immunogen and does not elicit protective antibody. Current indications in children older than 18 months of age (or younger if disease due to group A is to be prevented) include control of epidemic disease, use for travelers to endemic or epidemic areas, and prolonged prophylaxis for household contacts (because one-half the secondary family cases occur more than 5 days after the primary case).

Hemophilus Influenzae Type B Vaccine

A polysaccharide vaccine against invasive disease caused by *H. influenzae* type B was introduced in the spring of 1985 in the United States. Infants under 18 months of age respond infrequently and with less antibody than do older children. The efficacy of the vaccine was documented in a clinical trial in Finland: the protective efficacy of the vaccine was 90 percent in children 18 to 71 months of age; the vaccine was not effective in children under 18 months of age. Current recommendations for vaccine use include immunization of all children at 24 months of age; optional immunization of children 18 to 23 months of age who are known to be at high risk, including those with sickle cell disease, asplenia, malignancies associated with immunosuppression, and children who attend day-care facilities; and usage in children not previously immunized between 24 months and 59 months of age. New vaccines with improved immunogenicity for children under 18 months of age, including *H. influenzae* type B polysaccharide–protein conjugate vaccines, are now in clinical trial.

Influenza Vaccine

Influenza is a mild illness in most children, and, therefore, there is no basis for routine immunization. Annual immunization with current influenza vaccines is recommended for children with chronic disorders of the cardiovascular or pulmonary systems that are severe enough to have required regular follow-ups or hospitalization during previous years. If the physician believes the child would be harmed if infected, influenza vaccine should be used. Current influenza vaccines are prepared in eggs and contain trace amounts of egg antigens. Children known to be allergic to eggs should not receive influenza vaccine.

Bacille Calmette-Guerin (BCG)

Selective usage of BCG vaccine may be of value in infants and children: those in a household with repeated exposure to patients with infectious tuberculosis; and those in groups with excessive rates of new infection and for whom usual medical care is not feasible. BCG should not be given during INH administration since multiplication of the bacillus is inhibited by the drug. Skin test with purified protein derivative is done 2 months after vaccination; if skin test is negative, BCG is repeated.

Rabies Vaccine

Human diploid cell vaccine (HDCV) and human rabies immune globulin (HRIg) are recommended following bite by a wild animal of a species known to carry the virus (skunk, fox, coyote, raccoon, bat, and other carnivores) unless the animal is proved to be virus-negative by laboratory test. HDCV and HRIg are also recommended if a domestic animal—dog or cat is known or suspected to be rabid. If the animal's health is unknown or the animal has escaped, consultation with a local public health official is important to provide information on the risk of rabies in the area.

Human Immune Globulin

Immune globulin (Ig) is prepared from pooled serum of adults. Ig is of value for prophylaxis against hepatitis A and measles. Special preparations of high-titer immune globulin are available for prevention or treatment of disease due to varicella, hepatitis B, rabies, and tetanus.

Dosage schedules for immune and hyperimmune globulins are given in Table 2. Immune globulins are administered intramuscularly; 1 to 5 ml are administered at one site, depending on the size of the muscle mass.

Ig can be administered to susceptible children who are exposed to measles and is effective for prevention or modification of disease. Ig should be administered to children during the first year of life, to older children who have been exposed for more than 5 days (too late for use of vaccine), and to immunocompromised children. Vaccine should be given 3 or more months after administration of Ig to immunocompetent children.

Ig is recommended for prevention of hepatitis A in households and day care centers. Ig should be administered to all household contacts of a clinical case. If a case of hepatitis A occurs in a child or member of the staff of a day care center or in the households of two or more attendees, Ig should be given to children and staff of the center. Exposure in schools is not a reason for administration of Ig.

Hepatitis B immune globulin is administered to infants of mothers who are HBsAG-positive and to children or adults who are exposed to infected blood.

Varicella-zoster immune globulin should be used for immunocompromised children, for newborns of mothers with peripartum varicella (within 5 days before and 48 hours after delivery) and for premature infants with significant postnatal exposure.

Human rabies hyperimmune globulin should be administered with rabies vaccine (except for those who have been previously immunized). It provides antibody until the initial doses of vaccine have stimulated an immune response. Vaccine and human rabies hyperimmune globulin are administered via the intramuscular route in different sites. If feasible, one-half the dose of human rabies hyperimmune globulin is infiltrated in the area of the wound and one-half, intramuscularly.

Human tetanus immune globulin is indicated for patients whose tetanus toxoid immunization is unknown, those who have received an incomplete series of toxoid immunizations, and those whose wound is older than 24 hours.

TABLE 2 Dosage Schedules for Immune Globulins for Prevention and Treatment of Disease

Agent	*Condition*	*Preparation*	*Dose*
Measles	Normal children	Ig	0.25 ml/kg
	Immunodeficient children	Ig	0.5 ml/kg
Hepatitis A	Household contacts	Ig	0.02 ml/kg
	Day care contacts	Ig	0.02 ml/kg
Hepatitis B	Newborn infants	HBIg	0.5 ml
	Exposure to infected blood	HBIg	0.06 ml/kg
Varicella	Immunodeficient children	VZIg	125 units/10 kg
	Newborn infants	VZIg	125 units
Rabies	Postexposure	HRIg	20 IU/kg; ½ dose IM ½ dose at wound
Tetanus	Postexposure	HTIg	250–500 units IM

Abbreviations: Ig = immune globulin; HBIg = hepatitis B immune globulin; VZIg = varicella-zoster immune globulin; HRIg = human rabies hyperimmune globulin; HTIg = human tetanus immune globulin.

ADULT IMMUNIZATION

RICHARD PLATT, M.D.

The indications for immunization of adults include a number of factors—principally, the individual's age, prior immunization history, exposures to specific pathogens, underlying health problems and availability of newly developed vaccines. The table lists vaccines and immune globulins that are currently available and recommended for use under appropriate circumstances in adults. Most of these preparations are discussed in the separate chapters in this book that address these diseases.

The Advisory Committee on Immunization Practice (ACIP) provides periodic recommendations for use of these agents. These are published as they are developed in *Morbidity and Mortality Weekly Reports*, available from the National Technical Information Service and also from several private publishers. In addition, the American College of Physicians has recently published a *Guide for Adult Immunization*. This guide provides recommendations for adults of different ages, special groups such as pregnant women, health care personnel, day care workers, and homosexually active men, immunologically compromised hosts, and travelers. It also provides discussions of specific vaccines. Single copies may be obtained for $10.00 from the American College of Physicians, Adult Immunization, P.O. Box 7777–R0325, Philadelphia, PA 19175.

Four vaccines merit broad use in various age groups of the general population.

TETANUS/DIPHTHERIA

Tetanus/diphtheria toxoids, provided as a single preparation, should be used for all individuals. For adults the Td (tetanus toxoid) preparation should be used. This contains less diphtheria toxoid than DT, which, along with DPT (diphtheria, pertussis, and tetanus) is routinely used for children. Most young adults have been immunized against tetanus, but a substantial proportion of those over 60 years of age do not have antibody. Individuals who are not known to have completed a three-dose primary immunization series should receive three 0.5-ml doses of Td. The second dose should be given 4 weeks after the first; the third should be given 6 to 12 months after the second. Additional doses should be given approximately every 10 years. The mid-decade birthdays (25, 35, 45 years, etc.) have been suggested as reminders for giving these booster doses.

For postexposure prophylaxis, for instance after wounds, no antitetanus therapy is indicated if the individual has completed a primary immunization course or had received a booster within the preceding 5 years (10 years for a minor wound). If longer intervals have occurred, Td should be given. Therapy should be given as soon as possible after injury occurs. Those who have not completed a primary series should begin one. In addition, individuals who have not completed a primary series should ordinarily receive tetanus immune globulin. The dose of immune globulin depends on the severity of the wound. Tetanus toxoid and tetanus immune globulin should be given at separate sites using different syringes. Adsorbed rather than fluid toxoid should be used if immune globulin is used.

MEASLES/MUMPS/RUBELLA

These are attenuated live virus preparations. They are available singly and in combination. A single dose of each or of the combination is sufficient. Administration of these vaccines to individuals who are immune is not associated with significant adverse effects. Measles and mumps vaccines should not be given to individuals who are allergic to eggs. None of these vaccines should be given to immunocompromised individuals.

Rubella

The principal reason for rubella vaccination is prevention of congenital rubella. Nonpregnant women of childbearing age who do not have documentation of prior vaccination or serologic evidence of immunity should be immunized. Although the risks of vaccination during pregnancy are not known to be great, women should be counseled not to become pregnant within 3 months after immunization. In general, the trivalent preparation should be used for rubella immunization unless the individual is known to be immune to measles and mumps or is allergic to eggs. Rubella immunization should not be given less than 14 days before immune globulin, or within 6 weeks after.

Transient arthralgias or arthritis occur after immunization in a substantial minority of susceptible individuals. This is believed to be a manifestation of mild infection. Other adverse effects, including frank arthritis, have been reported extremely rarely.

Measles

Measles vaccine is indicated for individuals born after 1956 who are not known to be immune. Immunity is likely if live virus vaccine was given after the first birthday or if clinical measles was diagnosed by a physician. In part because the U.S. national measles eradication program has reduced the occurrence of natural measles, the existing cohort of unimmunized young adults has provided a new focus for outbreaks, a number of which have occurred on college campuses in recent years.

Postexposure immunization is most likely to be effective if given within 72 hours. Immune globulin may also be used within 6 days to attentuate or possibly prevent infection, especially for individuals who cannot receive the vaccine.

Individuals who are allergic to eggs should not receive measles vaccine. The principal adverse reactions, occurring in 5 to 15 percent of recipients, are fever, usually lasting 1 to 2 days, and rash. Adverse reactions, including local reactions, are commoner among individuals who have received killed measles vaccine (no longer available).

Mumps

Most adults are immune to mumps virus; however, adults who are suspected to be susceptible should be immunized. The vaccine should not be used for individuals with allergy to eggs. The same time frame before and after immune globulin should be observed as the rubella vaccine.

TABLE 1 Diseases in Adults for Which Immunoprophylaxis Is Available

Cholera
Hepatitis A (immune serum [gamma] globulin)
Hepatitis B (vaccine and immune globulin)
Influenza
Measles (vaccine and immune serum [gamma] globulin)
Meningococcal disease
Mumps
Plague
Pneumococcal pneumonia
Poliomyelitis
Rabies (vaccine and immune globulin)
Rubella
Tetanus (toxoid and immune globulin)
Tuberculosis (BCG)
Typhoid fever
Varicella-Zoster (immune globulin)
Yellow fever

Notes: 1. Except for the preparations discussed in the text, the use of specific agents should be reserved for individuals who are at special risk.
2. The efficacy of some of these, e.g., BCG, and cholera and typhoid vaccines, is either not proved or known to be modest.

INFLUENZA

Influenza vaccine is recommended for all individuals over 65 years of age and for younger individuals with serious underlying diseases or for those who have a substantial occupational exposure, such as health care workers. The vaccine is a killed virus preparation that is not contraindicated in immunosuppressed individuals. The vaccine is reformulated each year to include virus strains that are believed likely to be prevalent during the ensuing season. Vaccination should be repeated each year, during the autumn or early winter.

The vaccine should not be given to individuals with allergy to eggs. Adverse effects include usually mild local reactions and rare constitutional symptoms.

PNEUMOCOCCAL PNEUMONIA

Pneumococcal vaccine contains antigens for the 23 commonest types of pneumococcus. It is indicated for essentially the same individuals who should receive influenza vaccine, except for health care workers. If possible, it should be administered before splenectomy.

Mild local and systemic side effects occur infrequently. Neither allergy to egg nor immunosuppression are contraindications to immunization. The vaccine should be given only once. Unlike the other vaccines discussed here, revaccination is contraindicated at present. A summary of the contents of this chapter is provided in Table 1.

TOXIC SHOCK SYNDROME

SETH F. BERKLEY, M.D.
ARTHUR L. REINGOLD, M.D.

Although sporadic case reports of an illness resembling toxic shock syndrome (TSS) have appeared in the medical literature for years, only recently has a distinct clinical syndrome been defined. TSS is a multisystem illness associated with infection by or carriage of *Staphylococcus aureus*. Most reported cases have occurred in young menstruating women and have been associated with the use of tampons; however, it is clear that TSS can occur in a wide variety of clinical settings in individuals of both sexes and all age groups.

EPIDEMIOLOGY AND PATHOGENESIS

Cases of TSS have been found throughout the United States as well as in Europe, Asia, and Africa. As of June, 1985 more than 2,800 cases of TSS had been reported in the United States, including 122 (4%) with a fatal outcome. Although most of these cases (80%) have been in menstruating women, cases not associated with menstruation have assumed a more prominent position recently. Menstrual cases have been reported overwhelmingly in young (15 to 25 years of age) white women who use tampons. In rare instances, menstrual TSS may occur in the absence of tampon use; however, the risk of developing menstrual TSS is significantly increased in tampon users and may depend on the brand, absorbency, and chemical composition of the tampon used. Although the over all incidence of TSS is not known, the estimated incidence of menstrual TSS in the United States is five to ten cases per 100,000 menstruating women per year.

Nonmenstrual TSS can be seen in association with any of the myriad infections caused by *S. aureus*. It has been reported in both males and females in the pediatric to geriatric age groups. TSS has been associated with *S. aureus* surgical wound infections and has occurred in postpartum women with staphylococcal infections of the vagina, the breast, and cesarean section wounds. In addition, TSS has been observed in patients with primary and secondary *S. aureus* infections of skin, bone, joints, and blood. TSS has also occurred in women in association with the use of barrier-contraceptive methods such as diaphragms and contraceptive sponges.

The pathogenesis of TSS has been a subject of extensive study and is believed to be toxin-mediated. Most *S. aureus* strains recovered from patients with TSS produce a previously undescribed exoprotein, now designated toxic shock syndrome toxin-1 (TSST-1). In addition, it has been demonstrated that most patients with TSS lack antibody against TSST-1 at the onset of illness. However, the *S. aureus* strains from TSS patients also exhibit a wide range of other reasonably distinctive characteristics, and a substantial minority of such strains, particularly those from nonmenstrual cases, do not seem to make TSST-1. Thus, the exact role of TSST-1 in the pathogenesis of TSS and the possible importance of other bacterial products remain to be determined.

CLINICAL MANIFESTATIONS AND DIAGNOSIS

Because there is no currently accepted diagnostic test for TSS that is both sensitive and specific, the diagnosis remains a clinical one, based on the presence of a constellation of clinical findings. The current case definition (Table 1), although quite specific, detects only the severe form of the disease and potentially excludes milder or atypical clinical presentations. The Centers for Disease Control (CDC) defines a case as one with all four of the major criteria (fever, hypotension, rash, and subsequent desquamation), involvement of three or more organ systems, and absence of evidence of a more likely etiology. Fatal cases in which death occurs before desquamation would have been expected are also considered to have met the case definition. It is important to note that recovery

TABLE 1 Case Definition of Toxic Shock Syndrome

Fever: temperature ≥38.9°C (102°F)

Rash: diffuse macular erythroderma

Desquamation: 1–2 weeks after onset, particularly of palms and soles

Hypotension: systolic blood pressure ≤90 mm Hg for adults or below fifth percentile by age for children younger than 16 years of age; orthostatic drop in diastolic blood pressure ≥15 mm Hg from lying to sitting; orthostatic syncope; or orthostatic dizziness

Multisystem involvement, defined as three or more of the following:
- Gastrointestinal: vomiting or diarrhea at onset
- Muscular: severe myalgia or CPK level at least twice the upper limit of normal for laboratory
- Mucous membranous: vaginal, oropharyngeal, or conjunctival hyperemia
- Renal: BUN or creatinine at least twice the upper limit of normal for laboratory or urinary sediment with pyuria (≥5 leukocytes per high-power field) in the absence of urinary tract infection
- Hepatic: total bilirubin, SGOT, SGPT at least twice the upper limit of normal for laboratory
- Hematologic: platelets ≤100,000/mm³
- Central nervous system: disorientation or alterations in consciousness without focal neurologic signs when fever and hypotension are absent

Negative results on the following tests, if obtained:
- Blood, throat, or cerebrospinal fluid cultures (cultures may be positive for *Staphylococcus aureus*)
- Rise in titer to *Rickettsia rickettsii* (Rocky Mountain spotted fever), *Leptospira*, or rubeola virus

SGOT denotes serum aspartate transaminase; SGPT denotes serum alanine transaminase.

of *S. aureus* from a body site is not a criterion required for diagnosis, although if searched for, the presence of *S. aureus* infection can usually be documented with proper culturing techniques.

TSS typically presents in an acute fashion with fever, chills, malaise, and myalgias. These symptoms progress over the course of 24 to 48 hours along with headache, sore throat, nausea, vomiting, diarrhea, and abdominal pain. The rash usually appears 2 to 3 days after the onset of symptoms and is classically described as a diffuse, macular erythroderma (sunburn-like) involving the face, trunk, and extremities. However, the rash, which blanches with pressure, can be focal (limited to the face, extremities, or perineal region), subtle, or transient, and has been mistaken for the flush that sometimes accompanies fever.

Untreated, the illness usually progresses. Vomiting, diarrhea, increased insensible losses due to fever, and poor fluid intake all lead to dehydration, which contributes to the development of hypotension. Although initially manifested as orthostatic dizziness or lightheadedness, increasing hypotension may result in syncope and, in later stages, progress to shock. During this period the patient is extremely ill, and alteration in consciousness, such as confusion, delirium, or combativeness, can be seen. Other signs and symptoms seen during the acute illness include abdominal pain and muscle tenderness; hyperemia of the conjunctivae, throat, and vagina; a strawberry tongue; vaginal discharge; arthralgias; and edema of the hands and feet.

Patients who survive undergo generalized or focal desquamation 1 to 2 weeks after the beginning of their illness. The desquamation is usually most prominent over the hands and feet, where it is often full thickness, and less prominent over the face and trunk, where it usually more superficial. One to 3 months after recovery, reversible loss of fingernails and toenails and thinning of the hair are commonly seen.

COMPLICATIONS

Complications seen in TSS relate to the severity of the illness, and patients who do not receive prompt medical attention and appropriate treatment develop life-threatening, occasionally irreversible complications. Acute respiratory distress syndrome (ARDS) and refractory hypotension, the most commonly reported severe complications, are usually present and are major contributors to the outcome in fatal cases. Renal failure, which is usually due to acute tubular necrosis resulting from hypoperfusion or, occasionally, from myoglobinuria, is almost always reversible. Disseminated intravascular coagulation, profound hypocalcemia with resultant tetany, and myocardial dysfunction are among the other reported complications of TSS and should be watched for in the severely ill patient.

LABORATORY FINDINGS

Laboratory test abnormalities reflect the multiorgan involvement characteristic of the disease, and the magnitude of these abnormalities corresponds with the clinical severity of disease. Abnormalities in renal function are manifested by sterile pyuria and elevated creatinine and blood urea nitrogen (BUN). Hematologic abnormalities commonly seen include normochromic normocytic anemia, leukocytosis, lymphopenia, and thrombocytopenia with recovery thrombocytosis. Involvement of the skeletal muscles can produce an elevated creatine phosphokinase (CPK) level, and, when muscle involvement is severe, myoglobinemia, myoglobinuria, and resulting renal failure can occur. Additional laboratory abnormalities include hypocalcemia which can be profound, hypokalemia, hypophosphatemia, hyperamylasemia, and coagulation abnormalities consistent with disseminated intravascular coagulation. In severely ill patients, metabolic acidosis and hypoxemia may also be present.

Although the case definition of TSS does not require that *S. aureus* infection or colonization be demonstrated, most patients for whom appropriate cultures are performed before antibiotic therapy is initiated will be found to be culture-positive. The most common sites of *S. aureus* infection in TSS patients include the vagina, cutaneous and subcutaneous lesions, and surgical wounds. *S. aureus* bacteremia can be present but is uncommon.

DIFFERENTIAL DIAGNOSIS

The differential diagnosis depends in part on the patient's age and sex, the clinical setting, the predominant signs and symptoms, and even the geographic region in which the illness occurs (Table 2). For example, cases in children in which sore throat, fever, and rash are the predominant findings may be misdiagnosed as scarlet fever, whereas cases in young women in which vomiting, diarrhea, abdominal pain and tenderness, and fever predominate may be misdiagnosed as appendicitis or pelvic inflammatory disease. Postoperative TSS, on the other hand, can be difficult to distinguish from gram-negative bacterial sepsis or an adverse drug reaction. Aside from the common misdiagnoses listed, cases of TSS have been misdiagnosed as an astoundingly wide range of other diseases. However, by obtaining a careful history and physical examination in combination with appropriate laboratory tests, one can usually distinguish between TSS and other illnesses.

THERAPY

All patients should be examined carefully for sites of possible *S. aureus* infection, such as cutaneous and subcutaneous focal lesions. Surgical wounds, if present, should receive special attention. Most cases of postoperative TSS occur in the absence of obvious local signs of infection of the surgical wound, despite cultural documentation of the presence of *S. aureus*. Thus, any surgical wound, even if grossly uninfected, should be closely examined and probably explored. Any focal infection, such as an abscess, should be adequately drained. A careful pelvic examination should be performed on all female patients; any foreign bodies in the vagina, such as tampons, diaphragms, or contraceptive sponges, should be removed and cultured. Care should be taken to avoid leaving any fragments of tampons or contraceptive sponges in the vagina. Cultures of blood, the oropharynx, the vagina, and any focal lesions should be obtained. Some clinicians have recommended saline or povidone-iodine irrigation of any wound present or douching of the vagina on the possibility that this may remove organisms and preformed toxins not yet absorbed; this is of unproven benefit, but unlikely to be harmful.

The therapy of TSS is primarily supportive. The first priority is hemodynamic stability. Patients can have prodigious fluid requirements during the first 24 to 48 hours of their illness, sometimes in the range of 10 to 20 L per day. Initially, attempts should be made to treat hypotension with intravenous crystalloid, such as normal saline, rather than pressors because relative volume depletion is usually present. Vasopressor therapy should be used only if fluid replacement alone fails to achieve adequate blood pressure and urine output.

Moderately to severely ill patients with TSS should be treated intially in an intensive care unit or other setting where they can be monitored closely. Good urine output should be maintained (greater than 25 ml per hour), and careful attention should be paid to records of fluid input and output, since fluid overload commonly occurs. In severely ill patients, monitoring of the central venous pressure, pulmonary capillary wedge pressure, and arterial pressure may be required for optimal management.

Although antimicrobial therapy has not been shown to affect the course of the acute illness, it has been shown to reduce the frequency of recurrent episodes. All patients suspected of having TSS should be treated with parenteral antimicrobial therapy effective against *S. aureus*, such as a penicillinase-resistant penicillin (e.g., nafcillin 1 g IV every 4 hours) or, if penicillin-allergic, with a cephalosporin that has antistaphylococcal activity or with vancomycin. In addition, if gram-negative sepsis cannot be ruled out, the addition of an aminoglycoside until blood culture results are available may be prudent. Parenteral antimicrobial therapy should be continued until the patient is stable and afebrile. The benefit of additional oral antimicrobial therapy after this time is unproven, but many physicians use oral therapy to complete a 10 to 14-day course of treatment.

TABLE 2 Differential Diagnosis of Toxic Shock Syndrome

All Patients	*Infants*	*Postpartum Women*	*Women of Reproductive Age*
Scarlet fever	Kawasaki syndrome	Endometritis	Pelvic inflammatory disease
Drug reaction	Staphylococcal scalded-skin syndrome	Septic pelvic thrombophlebitis	
Sepsis		Septic abortion	
Appendicitis			
Leptospirosis			
Viral illness with exanthem (measles, etc.)			
Rocky Mountain spotted fever			

Although commonly used, high-dose corticosteroid therapy is of unproved benefit in TSS. On the basis of evidence from a retrospective analysis of a limited number of cases, some experts recommend giving methylprednisolone (10 to 20 mg per kg every 6 to 8 hours) for the first 2 to 3 days of illness to patients who are hypotensive; such therapy should be considered for critically ill patients, but is probably unnecessary for most patients.

The outpatient treatment of suspected mild cases of TSS is an unexplored area. Removal of any intravaginal foreign bodies, maintenance of good fluid intake, and administration of oral antibiotics effective against *S. aureus* would be reasonable therapy for patients with mild illness, but there is no published information on this point, and the efficacy of oral antibiotics in eradicating *S. aureus* from the vagina is unknown.

PREVENTION

It is unclear why there has been a recent upsurge in the number of cases of TSS. Until more is understood about the nature of the disease and its relationship to menstruation and tampons, patient education remains the mainstay of prevention. Women need to be aware of the symptoms of TSS and, at the first sign of any of these symtoms, should remove tampons and seek medical assistance.

The risk of developing menstrual TSS, even among tampon users, is low. Women who have not had TSS and who wish to reduce that already-low risk even further can do so by not using tampons. For women who wish to continue using tampons, evidence suggests that they can partially reduce their risk of developing menstrual TSS by using tampons intermittently with napkins or pads and/or by using tampons of the lowest absorbency compatible with their needs. There is no evidence to suggest that more frequent changing of tampons will prevent TSS.

Women who have had menstrual TSS are at risk of having recurrent episodes with subsequent menstrual periods. They should be advised not to use tampons. Women who receive effective antistaphylococcal therapy and who do not resume tampon use have the lowest risk of recurrences (approximately 5% or less).

The value of vaginal cultures in defining those at risk of developing a first episode of TSS is unknown. There is, at present, no indication for performing such cultures for healthy women. The value of follow-up vaginal cultures in women who have had TSS is also unknown. Similarly, although the level of serum antibodies against TSST-1 can be measured, the use of this test to screen women cannot be recommended at this time.

INFECTION ASSOCIATED WITH HEMATOLOGIC MALIGNANCY

KENNETH H. MAYER, M.D.
STEPHEN H. ZINNER, M.D.

DIAGNOSTIC CONSIDERATIONS

Improvements in the care of patients with malignancy range from blood component replacement therapy and bone marrow transplantation to new, intensive chemotherapeutic multidrug protocols. However, patients with hematologic malignancies often die from infection. The frequency of infectious complications in these patients is due to several factors; (*1*) the intrinsic immunosuppression of the underlying process; (*2*) intensive cancer chemotherapy; and (*3*) the increased survival time of patients successfully treated with these regimens.

Certain malignancies and treatments are associated wtih a high likelihood of specific infectious problems (Table 1). For example, *Listeria monocytogenes* is more likely to be implicated in meningitis in patients with lymphomas than in patients with leukemias. The likely pathogens that infect these patients are often a function of specific defects in host defense mechanisms that are associated with the underlying disease (Table 2). Nonetheless, an empiric therapeutic approach based on the probabilities of a specific infection must be tempered by the clinical awareness of the complicated histories of these patients.

For example, a patient with acute myelocytic leukemia may be predisposed to bacterial infection at the time of induction of chemotherapy because of a lack of functional granulocytes but then, after remission, specific cytotoxic chemotherapy and corticosteroids may predispose to infections associated with impaired cellular and humoral immunity.

Integrity of the skin and mucosa is critical to host defense in patients with malignancies. The tissue disruption caused by direct extension or metastasis is more often a problem for patients with solid tumors, but mucosal lesions are not uncommon in patients with leukemias. Nosocomial infections are abetted by procedures that violate the normal barriers, such as the placement of intravenous and urinary catheters or endotracheal tubes, as well as by hyperalimentation and decubitus ulcers. Bacterial pathogens, particularly staphylococci that colonize the skin or aerobic gram-negative bacilli in the gut are the most frequent causes of nosocomial infection.

Polymorphonuclear leukocytes are the most important cellular defense against bacterial and fungal infections. The incidence of infection increases in linear fashion

TABLE 1 Bacterial Pathogens and Hematologic Malignancies

Pathogen	*Acute Leukemia (ALL, AML)*	*Chronic Lymphocytic Leukemia*	*Hodgkin's and Other Lymphomas*	*Multiple Myeloma*
Staphylococci	+	0	+	+
Pneumococci	0	+	+	++
Listeria	0	0	++	0
Enterobacteriaceae	++	+	++	++
Pseudomonas	++	0	+	+
Salmonella	+	0	++	0
Anaerobes	0	0	+	0
M. tuberculosis	+	0	+	0
Nocardia	+	+	++	0

Note: 0=no specific association; +=definite association; ++=frequent association.

TABLE 2 Defects in Host Defenses in Patients with Hematologic Malignancies

	Humoral Immunity	*Cell-Mediated Immunity*	*Granulocyte Number or Function*	*Mechanical Barriers*
Neoplasms*				
Acute myelocytic leukemia	0	+	++	+
Chronic myelocytic leukemia	0	0	0	0
Acute lymphocytic leukemia	0	+	++	+
Chronic lymphocytic leukemia	++	+	0	0
Multiple myeloma	++	0	0	0
Hodgkin's disease: stage I	0	0	0	0
stage II-IV	0	++	0	0
Non-Hodgkin's lymphoma	0	++	0	+
Therapy				
Radiation	0	0	+	+
Steroids	0	++	+	0
Cytotoxic	+	+	++	+
Other factors				
Malnutrition	+	+	0	0
Surgery	0	+	0	++
Hyperalimentation	0	0	+	++
Foreign bodies (e.g., IV lines, catheters)	0	0	0	++

Note: 0=no specific association; +=definite association; ++=frequent association.
* Defects at time of diagnosis, before intervention.

as the neutrophil count falls to fewer than 1,000 cells per cubic millimeter, and infection occurs in more than 50 percent of patients once the white blood cell count has fallen to less than 500 cells per cubic millimeter.

In patients with malignancy, neutropenia may be due to neoplastic infiltration of the bone marrow or to the use of cytostatic agents and marrow irradiation. The underlying illness, as well as cytotoxic chemotherapy, corticosteroids, and radiation, may impair neutrophil function, as may the hypophosphatemia occasionally seen with intravenous hyperalimentation.

Neutropenic patients frequently develop fever. Although temperature elevations may be due to the underlying disease process, several studies have reported that bacteremia is present in approximately 20 percent of these febrile episodes and that other microbiologically documented infections account for another 20 percent. Proven infections and probable infections occur in an additional 40 percent of these patients. Thus, in the majority of neutropenic patients, the presence of fever indicates the presence of infection.

The major pathogens responsible for infection in febrile neutropenic patients include *Staphylococcus aureus, Staphylococcus epidermidis, Pseudomonas aeruginosa, Escherichia coli*, and *Klebsiella pneumoniae*. The presence of fever (higher than 38.5 °C) justifies the empiric use of antibiotics appropriately selected for activity against these organisms (see below and Table 3).

Intact humoral immunity is important for the production of antibodies that potentiate bacterial phagocytosis.

TABLE 3 Useful Antibiotic Combinations for Empiric Therapy of Febrile Neutropenic Patients

1.	A Penicillin	*or*	A Cephalosporin	*or*	A Carbapenem	*plus*	An Aminoglycoside
	Carbenicillin 30 g/day Ticarcillin 18 g/day Timentin 18 g/day Azlocillin 18 g/day Piperacillin 18 g/day Mezlocillin 18 g/day		Cefazolin 6 g/day Cefotaxime 6–12 g/day Ceftizoxime 6–12 g/day Moxalactam 6–12 g/day Cefoperazone 4–6 g/day Ceftazidime* 6–12 g/day		Imipenem* 4 g/day		Amikacin 15 mg/kg/day Gentamicin 5 mg/kg/day Tobramycin 5 mg/kg/day Netilmicin 5 mg/kg/day
				or	A Monobactam Aztreonam 4–8 g/day		
2.	*or*	Double Beta-Lactam Combinations (in doses noted above)					
	Piperacillin Mezlocillin Azlocillin Ticarcillin	*plus*	Moxalactam or Ceftazidime*				

Note: Choice of regimen should be based on local susceptibility data.
* May be useful as a single agent in patients with moderate or predictably short-term granulocytopenia.

Deficits in this limb of the immune response are seen commonly in multiple myeloma and the lymphomas. Splenic infiltration with malignant cells and splenectomy for staging of the disease result in impaired production of opsonizing antibodies, a factor that may predispose to overwhelming infection with *S. pneumoniae, Hemophilus influenzae*, and other encapsulated bacteria. Cytotoxic chemotherapy as well as the malnutrition associated with malignancy may also impair antibody synthesis.

Lymphocytes and macrophages are critical for appropriate immune responses to challenge intracellular organisms—including viruses and protozoa—and intracellular bacteria such as *Salmonella* species, mycobacteria, and *Listeria monocytogenes*. Impairment of cellular immunity occurs in patients with lymphoreticular malignancies and those who receive corticosteroid therapy.

SIGNS AND SYMPTOMS OF INFECTION

Many of the usual hallmarks of infection are not present in these compromised patients. Some malignant processes may themselves mimic infection. Some patients with malignancies may not be febrile when infected; this is especially so in elderly patients.

A careful history and physical examination are critical to establish prompt and appropriate diagnosis of infection even though some or all of the usual clinical signs of infection such as warmth, tenderness, swelling, or erythema might be lacking. Similarly, patients with pneumonia and severe neutropenia may not demonstrate a pulmonary infiltrate on chest roentgenogram until several days after the onset of the infection. Also, iatrogenic foci such as indwelling venous and urinary catheters may be responsible for bacteremia with a minimal local response.

Alimentary tract symptoms of painful perioral ulcerations, enteritis, or proctalgia may indicate the presence of infection with mouth or gut flora and the attendant risk of bacteremia. Rectal fissures and perirectal abscesses may be present with minimal symptoms or clinical findings. Dysphagia should prompt a search for candidal or herpetic esophagitis.

Although some pathogens have predilections for certain sites, the specific infecting organism often cannot be predicted. The depression of host immunity in these patients is such that proper management mandates appropriate cultures and prompt empiric therapy. Occult diagnostic clues may be present in the retina, skin, sinuses, lymph nodes, rectum, and pelvis.

Pulmonary infiltrates in these patients are a special problem, since it is often impossible to make an etiologic diagnosis from the nonspecific signs and symptoms. These patients may be febrile, tachypneic, and hypoxic and usually need prompt diagnosis and therapy. Several organisms may be present simultaneously, including *Pneumocystis carinii*, cytomegalovirus, *Nocardia asteroides, Aspergillus* species, and/or *Candida* species, necessitating prompt bronchoscopy or other invasive procedures for biopsy and culture, although concomitant thrombocytopenia may make such diagnostic procedures hazardous.

Neutropenic patients with profound (fewer than 100 granulocytes per cubic millimeter) and persistent granulocytopenia are at particular risk of gram-negative rod bacteremia. This complication is especially likely when high fever, low platelet count and hypotension are present, although fever alone may indicate bacteremia with these organisms. Because of the high mortality associated with gram-negative rod bacteremia in neutropenic patients, treatment with appropriate antibiotics should be initiated empirically and promptly.

THERAPEUTIC APPROACH

The febrile neutropenic patient represents a particular clinical challenge: the antibiotics selected should provide adequate bactericidal activity against the many different possible pathogens. Cultures of blood, urine, and cerebrospinal fluid (if indicated) should be obtained promptly. Any other obvious foci, such as pus from any inflamed site, swab of an inflamed pharynx, purulent sputum, or drainage fluid should be examined microscopically and cultured.

In the absence of a noninfectious cause of fever such as transfusions or a fever-producing drug, antibiotics should be started immediately. A wide range of antibiotics is available for use as empiric therapy in febrile neutropenic patients. Although single, broad-spectrum antibiotics have been advocated by some, patients with profound and persistent granulocytopenia should be treated with a combination of antibiotics.

Several combinations available can be used in empiric therapy of febrile neutropenic patients (see Table 3). These combinations should provide high serum bactericidal activity and be synergistic in their activity against the common infecting organisms. There is no single drug combination of choice. We recommend the use of a beta-lactam agent (e.g., azlocillin,mezlocillin, or piperacillin) plus an aminoglycoside (e.g., amikacin or other). Local antibiotic susceptibility patterns should determine the precise choice. Double beta-lactam combinations, such as piperacillin or azlocillin plus moxalactam, have been used with some success and these regimens avoid aminoglycoside-associated nephrotoxicity and ototoxicity. All of these drugs should be administered intravenously at their maximal dosage.

The precise choice of the aminoglycoside utilized depends on the local antibiotic susceptibility patterns. Gentamicin, tobramycin, or netilmicin are closely equivalent where aminoglycoside resistance is not common. Since amikacin is less likely to be inactivated by bacterial enzymes than other drugs, it is preferable in institutions with significant aminoglycoside resistance. Aminoglycosides are rapidly bactericidal and are active against most aerobic gram-negative bacilli, including *P. aeruginosa*.

The choice of beta-lactam drug in combination therapy is somewhat wider with the availability of extended-spectrum penicillins (carbenicillin, ticarcillin, azlocillin, mezlocillin, piperacillin), the monobactams (aztreonam), and the newer cephalosporins (cefotaxime, cefoperazone, moxalactam, ceftizoxime, ceftazidime) and carbapenems (imipenem). Timentin, a combination of ticarcillin and the beta-lactamase inhibitor clavulanic acid, may also be useful in this setting.

Most studies comparing various antibiotic combinations have shown equivalent efficacy in febrile neutropenic patients, with response rates approaching 80 percent. Poorer prognosis is likely in profoundly neutropenic patients, especially if infected with organisms susceptible to only one agent in the combination.

A recent multi-institution international study has reported that azlocillin plus amikacin was more effective in single gram-negative rod bacteremia than was cefotaxime plus amikacin when the infecting organisms were sensitive to both drugs in the combination. Azlocillin plus amikacin was also more effective than ticarcillin plus amikacin against ticarcillin-resistant organisms.

Once antibiotics have been instituted empirically, they should be continued for 4 days before reevaluating therapy (Fig. 1). If the patient defervesces, whether or not an organism has been identified, therapy should be con-

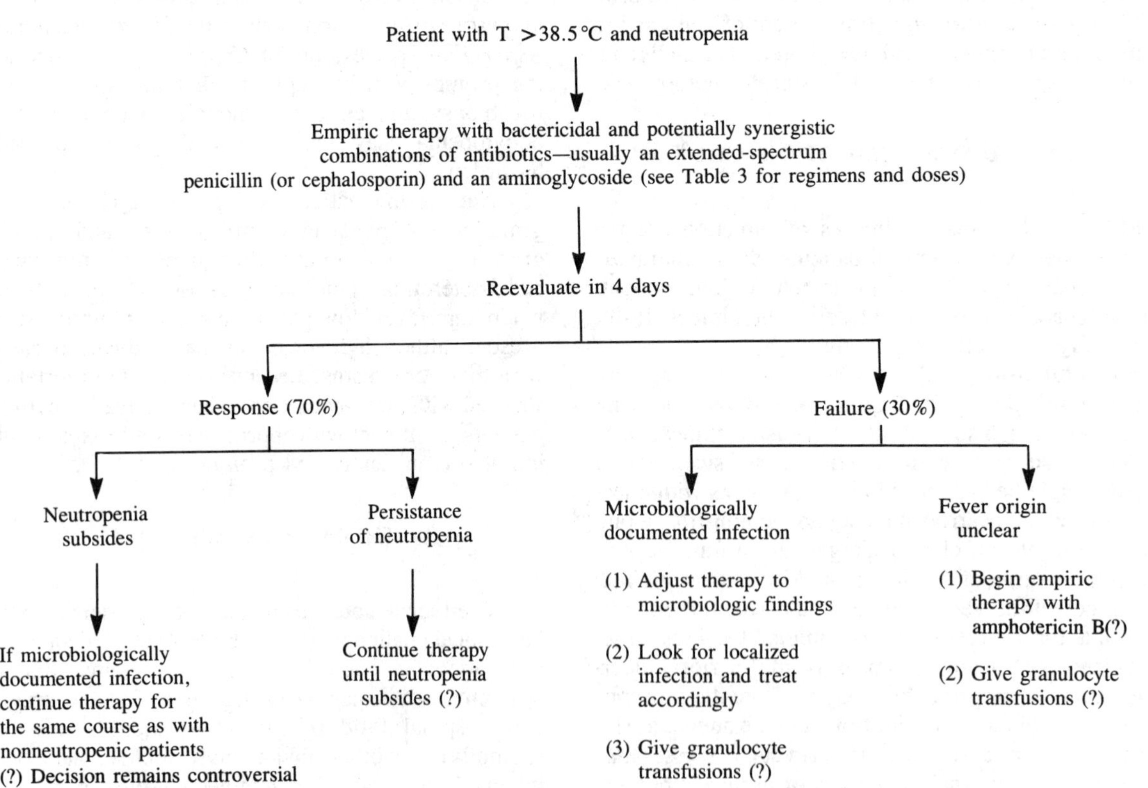

Figure 1 Algorithm for the management of febrile, neutropenic patients with hematologic malignancies.

tinued for an additional 5 to 7 days or until the granulocyte count has exceeded 500 cells per cubic millimeter (this policy remains somewhat controversial). If the patient remains febrile with a microbiologically documented infection, antibiotics may need to be added or changed, localized infections should be sought and drained, and consideration should be given to granulocyte transfusions.

The patient who remains febrile with a presumed but undiagnosed infection is at high risk of fungal infection. Neutropenic patients who succumb to infection have a high frequency of autopsy-proved disseminated fungal infection. Therefore, although it has not been definitively proved, empiric antifungal therapy with amphotericin B should be considered in neutropenic patients with persistent fever (about 4 days) of unknown origin.

Candida and *Aspergillus* infections are the commonest fungal infections in patients with hematologic malignancies. Diagnosis is often difficult and may require biopsy of infected tissue (lung, esophagus, liver). Serologic diagnosis is not always possible, but new techniques for detecting circulating fungal antigens are being introduced. Cryptococcal meningitis is not uncommon in patients with lymphomas and requires examination of cerebrospinal fluid to find the organism on smear (India ink or Gram stain) or in culture. Cryptococcal antigen can be detected in CSF, blood, or urine.

Amphotericin B remains the drug of choice for disseminated fungal infections in the neutropenic patient. It is given intravenously in large volumes of dextrose and water at a dose of 0.7 to 1.0 mg per kilogram per day. We usually begin therapy with a test dose of 1 mg, followed by 5- to 10-mg increments daily or larger increments (e.g., 20 mg) every other day, if tolerated by the patient. 5-Fluorocytosine is useful in combination with amphotericin B in the treatment of cryptococcal meningitis and some candidal infections and allows lower doses of the latter drug. Although useful in localized candidal infections, ketoconazole has not proved useful in disseminated candidal infections or in aspergillus or mucor infections.

Viral infections may cause serious morbidity in patients with hematologic malignancies. Varicella-zoster virus and herpes simplex virus may produce local or disseminated infection. Acyclovir (Zovirax) is useful in decreasing the time required for healing and in decreasing viral shedding. It may prevent dissemination to vital organs. Adenosine arabinoside (Vidarabine) is also useful. Disseminated cytomegaloviral (CMV) and Epstein-Barr viral infections are more refractory to therapy, although interferon has been used with some success in patients with CMV infection.

Specific therapy is necessary for optimal control of infections due to protozoa. *Pneumocystis carinii* pneumonia is treated with trimethoprim-sulfamethoxazole intravenously (20 mg per kilogram per day trimethoprim; 100 mg per kilogram per day sulfamethoxazole) or with pentamidine isethionate (4 mg of base per kilogram per day). *Toxoplasma gondii* meningoencephalitis is best treated with pyrimethamine (25 mg per day after 100 mg loading dose) and sulfamethoxazole (4 to 6 g per day, depending on size of patient and severity of infection).

PREVENTION OF INFECTION IN PATIENTS WITH HEMATOLOGIC MALIGNANCIES

Careful attention to handwashing is one of the most effective methods of prevention of infection. Simple reverse isolation methods have not been proved effective in these patients, although laminar air flow isolation has been useful. Patients who undergo bone marrow transplantation are often treated within these units.

Several approaches to decreasing the bacterial load in the gut have been suggested to minimize dissemination of gram-negative bacilli from this site. None of these regimens has been accepted universally, but it is clear that some form of gut decontamination is important in these patients. Vancomycin (250 mg), gentamicin (200 mg), and nystatin (1.6 million units) given every 4 to 6 hours is useful as an oral nonabsorbable combination to reduce the number of sensitive enteric organisms from the stool. Patient compliance is often poor, as these drugs produce nausea, vomiting, and diarrhea.

Oral trimethoprim-sulfamethoxazole (160 mg and 800 mg, respectively, twice a day) has been studied extensively and shown to reduce bacteremia and infections in neutropenic patients with lymphomas, solid tumors, and lymphocytic leukemias. However, this regimen has not always been successful in patients with acute nonlymphocytic leukemias and we do not use it. Trimethoprim-sulfamethoxazole is effective prophylaxis against *Pneumocystis carinii* pneumonia.

The use of combinations of a variety of antibiotics has been suggested to decontaminate the gut flora selectively to prevent virulent enteric pathogens from proliferating (colonization resistance). This effect is presumably due to the persistence of the anaerobic flora. Agents such as colistin (100 mg every 6 hours), trimethoprim-sulfamethoxazole (160 mg/800 mg twice a day), and nalidixic acid (2 g every 6 hours), titrated to remove enteric pathogens, have been used with some success.

Additional measures to prevent infection include a diet of cooked food that eliminates bacteria-rich foods such as salads and raw fruits, judicious use of intravenous and urinary catheters, and the use of topical antibacterial agents as bathing agents, mouthwashes, and douches. Vaccination against pneumococcal pneumonia and influenza should be used in periods of remission.

SOLID TUMOR AND ASSOCIATED INFECTION

GERALD P. BODEY, M.D., F.A.C.P., F.A.C.C.P., F.R.S.M., F.R.S.H.

Although it is recognized that infection is a common complication in patients with hematologic malignancies, it is not generally appreciated that infection is the proximate cause of death in 50 percent of patients with solid tumors. The discovery of curative chemotherapy for some malignancies has led to the use of more intensive regimens. Consequently, the frequency of infection is increasing in these patients. The spectrum of infection is also changing; some organisms that had been associated with infection in patients with hematologic malignancies are now causing infections in patients with solid tumors.

CONSIDERATIONS IN EVALUATING FEBRILE CANCER PATIENTS

Patients with solid tumors who develop fever fall into one of the following three categories: patients with neutropenia or other impaired host defense mechanisms, patients who are acutely ill and have an obvious site of infection, and patients with prolonged fever and no obvious site of infection. Table 1 lists important factors that must be considered when evaluating the cancer patient who presents with fever. By considering these factors, the physician is able to place the patient into the appropriate category.

Neutropenia is a common factor predisposing to infections, although solid tumors seldom cause neutropenia except when they involve the bone marrow. However, many patients are treated with myelosuppressive antitumor agents. Indeed, the use of chemotherapy as an adjuvant to surgery or radiation is gaining increasing acceptance as more effective regimens are discovered. Since the neutrophil is a primary defense against invasion and dissemination of infection, the neutropenic patient is at high risk of developing infection. Both the frequency and severity of infection are related to the degree and duration of neutropenia. Other deficiencies in host defense mechanisms are more often associated with hematologic malignancies. Nevertheless, deficiencies in cellular immunity and immunoglobulin production may result from cancer chemotherapy, malnutrition, or advanced malignant disease.

The type and stage of malignancy impact on the risk of infectious complications. Bronchogenic carcinoma frequently causes bronchial obstruction leading to pneumonia. Since this malignancy is particularly associated with smoking, many patients also have bronchitis and emphysema. Gynecologic cancers are often treated with radiotherapy, which may lead to infectious complications in the abdomen and pelvis. Large, ulcerated breast tumors may not be resectable and become superinfected.

In addition to causing myelosuppression and immunosuppression, antitumor agents have other effects that may predispose to fever and infection. Drugs such as adriamycin, nitrogen mustard, and vincristine are sclerosing agents and cause thrombophlebitis. Busulfan, mitomycin C, and methotrexate may cause pulmonary infiltrates that resemble an infection. Adrenal corticosteroids are often administered as specific or supportive therapy. They are used to reduce intracranial pressure in patients with primary or metastatic brain tumors. Unfortunately, they adversely affect many host defenses against all types of infection.

The management of malignant disease often requires the insertion of foreign bodies. Patients with genitourinary tumors may require urinary catheters, splints, or external drainage. Patients with central nervous system tumors may require ventricular shunts or Ommaya reservoirs for therapy. Vascular catheters are frequently inserted to facilitate the administration of chemotherapeutic agents or nutritional supplements.

Pneumonia and bacteremia are the predominant infections in patients with solid tumors. However, specific predisposing factors associated with certain tumors may be of critical importance. For example, pneumonia is especially prevalent among patients with head and neck or lung cancers. Abdominal or pelvic abscesses are frequent in patients with gynecologic malignancies, especially if they have received radiotherapy. Since the neutrophil is the primary defense against dissemination of infection, bacteremia is especially common among these patients. Superinfection of necrotic breast tumors is a serious problem and may serve as a focus for dissemination when the patient develops neutropenia following chemotherapy. Most cases of meningitis not associated with prosthetic devices occurring in patients with solid tumors are associated with head and neck malignancies or surgical procedures.

Taking into consideration those predisposing factors applicable to the patient helps the physician to focus on those organisms most likely to cause infection (Table 2). Unfortunately, this is not an infallible guide and broad-spectrum coverage must be provided in most instances if the infecting organism has not been identified at the onset of therapy. However, the application of this knowledge will ensure adequate antibiotic coverage against the like-

TABLE 1 Factors to Consider in Assessing Fever in Cancer Patients

Duration of fever
Neutrophil count
Type of malignancy
Type of antitumor therapy
Administration of adrenal corticosteroids
Other deficient host-defense mechanisms
Presence of foreign body
Hospital- or community-acquired fever
Assessment of patient's condition

TABLE 2 Organisms Likely to Cause Infection Related to Predisposing Factors

Factor	*Organisms*
Neutropenia	*P. aeruginosa*, other gram-negative bacilli, *S. aureus*, fungi
Hospital-acquired	*P. aeruginosa, S. aureus,* other gram-negative bacilli
Lung, head, and neck cancer	*M. tuberculosis*, bacterial pneumonia, and lung abscess
Gastrointestinal, gynecologic cancer	Polymicrobial bacteremia, mixed aerobic and anaerobic abscesses
Parenteral hyperalimentation	*Candida, Torulopsis*
Intravenous catheters	*S. epidermidis, S. aureus, Acinetobacter,* skin organisms, gram-negative bacilli
Ventricular catheters, Ommaya shunts	*S. epidermidis, S. aureus,* gram-negative bacilli
Adrenal corticosteroids	*Candida, Aspergillus*
Impaired cellular immunity	*Listeria, M. tuberculosis, Cryptococcus, Nocardia*

liest infecting organisms. For example, if a patient is neutropenic, the likeliest causes of infection are gram-negative bacilli and *Staphylococcus aureus*. If the patient also has an indwelling intravenous catheter, *Staphylococcus epidermidis* and other skin organisms may be the cause. Pseudomonas infection is especially frequent among neutropenic patients. Patients with prolonged neutropenia are susceptible to fungal infection, especially if they have prior bacterial infection or have received adrenal corticosteroid therapy.

It is important to differentiate between nosocomial and community-acquired infection, since the causative organisms are likely to be different. However, since cancer patients require repeated hospitalizations their infections may be caused by nosocomial pathogens even if onset occurs when the patient is at home. For example, only 19 percent of 410 cases of pseudomonas bacteremia in cancer patients developed when the patients were in the community. However, 34 percent of these latter patients had been discharged from the hospital within the preceding 2-week period. Hence, patients may become colonized while in the hospital, but develop infection after they have returned home.

Although certain organisms are most apt to cause infection, it is important to recognize that these patients may become infected by an extensive array of organisms, especially if they are treated with chemotherapy. Cryptococcal meningitis and disseminated nocardiosis have been found in patients with carcinoma of the breast. Cytomegaloviral infection and legionella pneumonia have occurred in patients with lung cancer and disseminated candidiasis in patients with gynecologic malignancies. *Clostridium difficile* colitis has been described in patients who received cancer chemotherapy but no antibiotics. Hence, one must be aware of the wide variety of possible infecting organisms when approaching the diagnosis and therapy of these patients.

MANAGEMENT OF FEBRILE CANCER PATIENTS

Patients with Neutropenia

The principles that should be applied in the management of febrile neutropenic patients are listed in Table 3. Patients who are neutropenic require immediate attention and prompt antibiotic therapy. The patient should be given a careful physical examination, but it is important to recognize that the classic signs and symptoms of infection are frequently absent in neutropenic patients. Judgement alone is not a reliable prognosticator for the presence of infection in these patients. In one study, infection was found to be present in 28 percent of patients who were initially considered by the examining physician to have fever due to noninfectious causes.

Since untreated infection disseminates rapidly and may be fatal, these patients require prompt antibiotic therapy. Appropriate cultures should be performed immediately, but other diagnostic procedures should be delayed until antibiotic therapy is initiated. In the absence of localized signs of infection, significant fever is a temperature of 101 °F (38.5 °C) if not associated with the administration of pyrogenic substances such as blood transfusions or immunotherapy. If the patient does not appear acutely ill, it is appropriate to collect the necessary specimens for cultures and observe the patient for a few hours. However, if fever persists after 2 to 3 hours, a second blood sample should be collected, and antibiotic therapy should be instituted. Patients who have developed fever after administration of pyrogenic substances should also be considered for antibiotic therapy if they do not begin to defervesce after several hours.

In general, beta-lactam antibiotics are preferred for the treatment of infections in neutropenic patients. If the organism is susceptible, these antibiotics are effective even in patients with severe neutropenia. They are relatively nontoxic and can be administered at high doses to ensure

TABLE 3 Principles Governing the Treatment of Fever in Patients with Neutropenia

- Classic signs and symptoms of infection are often absent; thus, many patients have "fever of unknown origin"
- Untreated infection can disseminate rapidly and terminate fatally; hence, antibiotic therapy must be instituted promptly
- Majority of acute infections are caused by gram-negative bacilli
- Organisms generally considered nonpathogenic can cause serious infection in these patients
- Initial antibiotic selection should be influenced by susceptibility patterns within the hospital
- A single antibiotic is unlikely to provide optimal coverage
- Some antibiotics are suboptimal in neutropenic patients
- Schedule of antibiotic administration may be of importance

adequate serum concentrations. Other proven effective antibiotics in neutropenic patients are vancomycin and the combination trimethoprim-sulfamethoxazole. Unfortunately, although the aminoglycosides have a broad spectrum of activity against most gram-negative bacilli, they are much less effective in neutropenic patients and should not be relied upon as single agents. Furthermore, neutropenic patients have repeated infections and often require prolonged antibiotic therapy, both factors that increase the likelihood of aminoglycoside-induced nephrotoxicity.

At the present time, no single antibiotic provides adequate coverage alone as initial therapy in neutropenic patients. The combination of an antipseudomonal penicillin (ticarcillin, 4 g over 2 hours every 4 hours; piperacillin, 3 g over 2 hours every 4 hours) and an aminoglycoside (gentamicin or tobramycin, 5 mg per kilogram per day, or amikacin, 15 mg per kilogram per day in divided doses every 6 to 8 hours) is usually chosen. However, equally acceptable regimens include a broad-spectrum cephalosporin (cefoperazone, 2 to 3 g every 6 to 8 hours or moxalactam, 2 g every 4 hours) plus an aminoglycoside, an antipseudomonal penicillin plus trimethoprim-sulfamethoxazole, or an antipseudomonal penicillin plus a broad-spectrum cephalosporin. Patients who receive cefoperazone or moxalactam should also be given vitamin K routinely, especially if they have thrombocytopenia. Therapy should subsequently be altered on the basis of the results of cultures from the site of infection. If the infection is believed to be related to an intravascular catheter, vancomycin (500 mg every 6 hours) provides reliable coverage against all of the gram-positive organisms likely to cause these infections. If abdominal symptoms are present, anaerobic coverage should be included.

Patients with Normal or Elevated Neutrophil Counts

Patients with normal or elevated neutrophil counts can be divided into two categories on the basis of the duration of fever and the physical examination (Fig. 1). If the patient has fever of short duration, appears to be acutely ill, or has leukocytosis or an apparent site of infection, appropriate cultures should be performed expeditiously, and the patient should be treated with antibiotics. Table 4 lists some of the possible antibiotic regimens based upon the site of infection. It is recognized that some of these regimens have not been widely utilized, but they are appropriate in these patients when consideration is given to those organisms most likely causing the infection. Every effort should be made to relieve obstruction or provide adequate drainage of abscesses, since these types of infection are not likely to resolve with antibiotics alone.

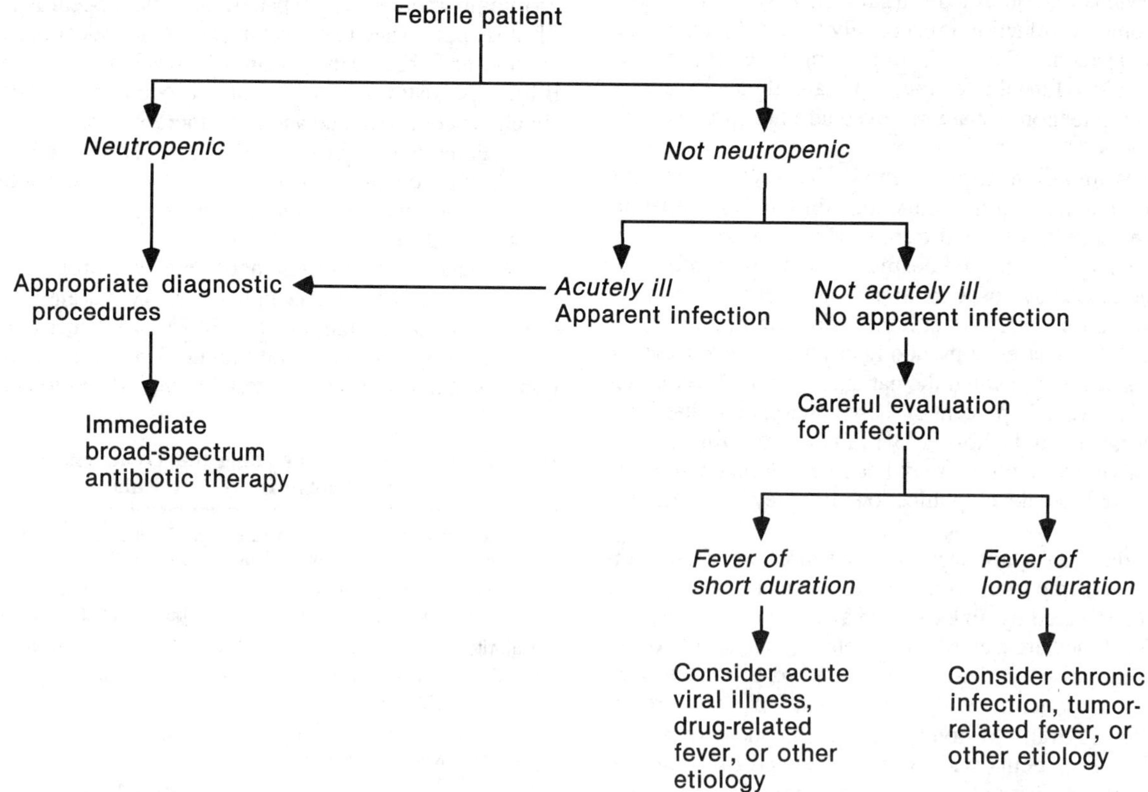

Figure 1 Approach to the febrile cancer patient.

TABLE 4 Initial Antibiotic Combination for Patients with Adequate Neutrophils Based Upon Site of Infection

Site (type)	*Antibiotic Combination*	*Predominant Organisms*
Catheter-related	Antistaphylococcal penicillin* plus aminoglycoside‡	*S. aureus, S. epidermidis,* JK diphtheroids, gram-negative bacilli
Skin and soft tissue	Antistaphylococcal penicillin* or cephalosporin† plus aminoglycoside‡	*S. aureus,* gram-negative bacilli
Pneumonia	Broad-spectrum penicillin or cephalosporin† plus aminoglycoside‡	Usually gram-negative bacilli, including *P. aeruginosa*
Aspiration pneumonia	Penicillin G or clindamycin plus aminoglycoside‡	Mouth flora, anaerobes, gram-negative bacilli
Abdominal or pelvic	Clindamycin or metronidazole plus aminoglycoside‡ or cephalosporin† or trimethoprim-sulfamethoxazole	Multiple organisms
Meningitis	Cefotaxime, moxalactam, or trimethoprim-sulfamethoxazole plus vancomycin or antistaphylococcal penicillin,* if catheter-related	*S. epidermidis, S. aureus,* gram-negative bacilli

* We believe that oxacillin or nafacillin are most appropriate. Vancomycin should be substituted in hospitals where there is a high frequency of infections caused by other gram-positive organisms.
† In immunosuppressed patients we prefer broad-spectrum cephalosporins (cefotaxime, ceftizoxime, cefoperazone, moxalactam) unless in vitro susceptibility testing indicates that the less expensive cephalosporins are as active.
‡ We believe that for routine use gentamicin, tobramycin, amikacin, and netilmicin are equivalent, unless in vitro susceptibility testing indicates otherwise.

If the patient has a normal neutrophil count (or, occasionally, leukocytosis), does not appear ill, and has had fever for several weeks, there is a good possibility that the fever is tumor-induced. Fever is especially likely to occur in patients with hepatoma, renal cell carcinoma, and some sarcomas. Although the mechanism for most tumor-related fever remains unknown, it may be due to tissue necrosis or tumor emboli. Intermittent fever may be caused by antitumor agents such as arabinosylcytosine and bleomycin. Fever is usually intermittent because therapy is usually administered in short courses at several-week intervals. It must be remembered that prolonged fever may be due to chronic infections such as tuberculosis, histoplasmosis, or cytomegaloviral infection, and occasional patients have occult abscesses. A detailed description of the work-up of these patients is beyond the scope of this chapter, but would depend upon a careful history and physical examination. Antibiotic therapy should not be given on an empiric basis to most of these patients.

PREVENTION OF INFECTION

Antibiotic prophylaxis has become an accepted practice for patients with acute leukemia. However, its role in patients with solid tumors is more controversial. Most of the latter patients do not experience severe or prolonged neutropenia; hence, their risk of infection is not very great. There are some patients who develop repeated infection whenever their neutrophil count decreases because they have, for example, persistent localized infection or chronic bronchitis or obstruction. Many of these patients will benefit from the prophylactic administration of trimethoprim-sulfamethoxazole. However, the majority of solid tumor patients do not require infection prophylaxis. They are likely to benefit from the immunity afforded by pneumococcal and influenza vaccines. These vaccines should be administered as far removed from chemotherapy as possible in order to achieve the maximum possible antibody response.

BACTERIAL AND FUNGAL INFECTION IN THE COMPROMISED HOST

LOWELL S. YOUNG, M.D.

The great majority of deaths in immunocompromised patients, particularly those with hematologic malignancy, are caused by bacterial and fungal infections.

Some important epidemiologic trends have occurred during the last decade. Overall, aerobic gram-negative bacilli still cause most serious infections, but there have been interesting changes in disease incidence. Early in the post antimicrobial era, coagulase-positive and penicillin-resistant Staphylococcus aureus infections were prominent in many centers treating patients with hematologic malignancy. With the advent of penicillinase-stable antistaphylococcal penicillins the number of Staphylococcus aureus infections declined in neutropenic patients. Most recently, strains that are methicillin-resistant have appeared sporadically. *Staphylococcus epidermidis*, an organism commonly found on skin, causes serious septicemias. This organism, previously considered avirulent and coagulase-negative, is often resistant to beta lactam agents. Its role as a cause of serious morbidity and mortality seems related to the widespread use of longterm intravascular catheters of the Hickman or Broviac type. Other important gram-positive infections are caused by pneumococci and enterococci.

TREATMENT OF BACTERIAL INFECTIONS

Approach to the Patient

Most antimicrobial therapy, whether given to a patient with neoplastic disease or other serious underlying disorders, is started before the infecting pathogen is known. The likelihood of selecting more specific treatment is increased if preliminary information is obtained from positive blood or infected body fluid cultures, or when rapid diagnostic techniques make selecting specific therapy early in the course of treatment possible. Table 1 is a summary of recommended therapy for established gram-positive and gram-negative bacterial infections when the infecting agent is known. The following three tables summarize recommended doses of commonly used antipseudomonal penicillins (Table 2), aminoglycosides (Table 3), and the newer so-called third generation cephalosporins and related compounds (Table 4). Serious bacterial infections in patients with hematologic malignancy will be treated with one or possibly two agents belonging to these categories of drugs. Not mentioned in these tables are the standard penicillin preparations (benzyl penicillin G) and the antistaphylococcal penicillinase-stable penicillins. For infections caused by such agents as beta hemolytic streptococci or *Streptococcus pneumoniae*, either penicillin G, ampicillin, or the broad spectrum penicillins summarized in Table 2 will be sufficient, but penicillin G or ampicillin are preferred because they cost less. Among the antistaphylococcal agents, the penicillinase-stable penicillins (methicillin, oxacillin, nafcillin) are probably all equally effective, but concern about the relatively greater nephrotoxic potential of methicillin has led to a preference for oxacillin or nafcillin in most situations. Systemic and central nervous system infections due to *Listeria monocytogenes* are probably best treated with large doses of ampicillin (~150 to 200 mg/kg/day *q4h*). The antipseudomonal penicillins lack activity against coagulase-positive penicillinase-producing staphylococci. This is the most compelling reason why these agents would never be used alone as initial therapy in the seriously ill patient unless the physician is confident that he is treating a susceptible organism.

TABLE 1 Recommended Therapy for Established Gram-Positive and Gram-Negative Bacteria

	Agent(s)
Gram-Positive	
Clostridium difficile	vancomycin
Corynebacterium sp.	vancomycin ± Rifampin
Enterococcus	ampicillin or penicillin G plus gentamicin
Listeria monocytogenes	ampicillin
Nocardia asteroides	sulfonamide ± trimethoprim
Staphylococcus aureus	oxacillin (nafcillin), vancomycin
Staphylococcus epidermidis	vancomycin ± rifampin
Streptococcus pyogenes	penicillin, erythromycin
Streptococcus pneumoniae	penicillin, cephalosporin
Gram-Negative	
Acinetobacter sp.	amikacin
Bacteroides sp.	metronidazole, clindamycin
Enteric Bacteria *(E. Coli, Enterobacter Klebsiella, Serratia, Proteus)*	aminoglycoside, 3rd generation cephalosporin
Legionella sp.	erythromycin, rifampin
P. Aeruginosa	aminoglycoside + antipseudomonal penicillin
Providencia	amikacin
Salmonella	chloramphenicol, ampicillin
Shigella	trimethoprim/sulfamethoxazole

TABLE 2 Antipseudomonal Penicillins: Dosage and Comments

Agent	*Dosage* (all q4h)*	*Comments*
Azlocillin	30 mg/kg	Potent antipseudomonal
Carbenicillin	70 mg/kg	High sodium content, electrolyte abnormalities
Mezlocillin	30 mg/kg	Some Klebsiella activity
Piperacillin	30 mg/kg	Potent antipseudomonal some Klebsiella activity
Ticarcillin	40 mg/kg	~2X more potent than carbenicillin

* May be preferable to dose using body surface area nomogram.

TABLE 3 Aminoglycosides: Dosage and Comment

Agent	*Dose* (all q8h)*	*Comment*
Amikacin	5–7.5 mg/kg	Most resistant to enzymatic inactivation
Gentamicin	1.5–1.7 mg/kg	Least expensive but resistance increasing
Netilmicin	1.7–2 mg/kg	May be less ototoxic
Tobramycin	1.5–1.7 mg/kg	Most active vs. *P. aeruginosa*

* Dosing by body surface area nomogram advisable in children and in adults with weight loss. For gentamicin and tobramycin a loading dose 25% of higher dose is recommended.

There has been great interest shown in the third generation cephalosporins. Some commonly used agents that are placed in this group are technically not cephalosporins (e.g., moxalactam). The major compounds that are licensed, or likely to become clinically available, are summarized in Table 4 with comments relating to their use in immunocompromised patients. These agents have broadened activity against gram-negative rods and have longer half-life than first generation compounds, but they are relatively less active against *S. aureus* and pneumococci than "first generation" agents. Like other cephalosporins they are totally without activity against enterococcus and *L. monocytogenes*.

TABLE 4 Third Generation Cephalosporins and Related Compounds

Agent	*Protein Binding (%)*	*Peak Serum levels (μg/ml) after 1 g IV*	*Half-Life (Hours)*	*Comments*
Aztreonam	60	50	2	No activity vs. gram-positive organisms
Cefmenoxime	77	40	1	Weak antipseudomonal activity
Cefotaxime	38	40	1.1	Good CNS penetration but weak antipseudomonal activity
Cefoperazone	90	125	2.1	Primary excretion is biliary with little dose adjustment in renal failure
Cefsulodin	30	65	1.6	Primarily antipseudomonal activity
Ceftazidime	20	70	1.9	Potent antipseudomonal activity
Ceftizoxime	30	75	1.4	Potent gram-negative activity except for Pseudomonas
Ceftriaxone	85	140	8.0	Very long half life, good CNS penetration but poor antipseudomonal activity
Moxalactam	50	60	2.3	Best anaerobe coverage but associated with coagulopathy

It has generally been assumed that cephalosporin agents are nontoxic; clearly, agents such as cephaloridine, which belong to the first generation, are nephrotoxic. Serious concerns have been raised about the ability of third generation compounds to trigger disulfiram reactions and bleeding. Caution should be exercised in using these drugs in patients with severe hepatic disease, thrombocytopenia, or a suspected gastrointestinal lesion that may predispose to bleeding.

Aminoglycoside Therapy

The aminoglycosides, in order of their clinical introduction include gentamicin, tobramycin, amikacin and netilmicin. They are rapidly bactericidal, cover most clinically important gram-negative rods and *S. aureus*, and are potentially toxic to the 8th nerve and to renal function. Amikacin is the most stable agent against enzymatic activation. Susceptibility of organisms to gentamicin and tobramycin is generally similar, except that tobramycin is relatively more active versus *P. aeruginosa*. In some institutions resistance to gentamicin among pseudomonads, Enterobacter species, and Serratia strains is high (>15%) and may necessitate the use of agents such as amikacin. When organisms are equally susceptible to all aminoglycosides there is little evidence that one agent is therapeutically superior to another when used in appropriate dosage. Comments about each of these aminoglycoside compounds and recommendations for total daily dosages are summarized in Table 3. Careful monitoring of doses, renal function, and measurement of blood levels is advised in seriously ill patients.

Other Antimicrobial Agents of Value

Erythromycin is the agent of choice if Legionella pneumonia is suspected or documented. It should be given parenterally in a daily dose of 50 mg/kg. Rifampin is a potent antistaphylococcal agent and in combination may potentiate the antistaphylococcal activity of vancomycin or penicillin. Trimethoprim sulfamethoxazole is available in both oral and parenteral forms and has been widely used to treat Pneumocystis carinii pneumonia, but it also inhibits most gram-negative rods except *P. aeruginosa*. This drug may occasionally be effective against bacteria that are resistant to both aminoglycosides and to third generation cephalosporins. Vancomycin is an agent that has had an inconsistent reputation. Vancomycin is not the agent of first choice in the therapy of staphylococcal or enterococcal infection, but it is an appropriate and reliable substitute in patients who cannot receive beta lactam agents. Moreover, it is probably the therapy of choice for treating S. epidermidis infections as well as infections caused by corynebacteria. (The recommended adult dosage is 0.5 g/day *q6h*.)

Recommendations for Empiric Antibacterial Therapy

If patients are neutropenic (granulocyte count <500 mm^3) or severely immunosuppressed the regimen of choice is an aminoglycoside plus an antipseudomonal penicillin like ticarcillin, azlocillin, or piperacillin. Regimens of antipseudomonal penicillins plus aminoglycosides are effective against enterococci and have sufficient central nervous system penetration to treat pneumococcal disease, meningococcal disease and L. monocytogenes meningitis. For therapy of staphylococcal infection, these regimens appear to offer initial coverage against coagulase-positive *S. aureus* although aminoglycoside resistant *Staphylococcus aureus* strains are occasionally encountered. A cephalosporin-like agent (e.g., cefoperazone, ceftazidine, or moxalactam) is a suitable alternative, but both penicillins and cephalosporins are ineffective against *S. epidermidis*. However, bloodstream infections caused by *S. epidermis* are not rapidly progressive, and regimens of aminoglycosides plus antipseudomonal beta lactam agents are probably sufficient to "hold" the patient until more specific therapy can be initiated. In a newer alternative to aminoglycoside-containing regimens, a cephalosporin-like cefotaxime is used with an antipseudomonal penicillin

TABLE 5 Doses of Antifungal Drugs

Agent	*Dose*	*Comments*
Amphotericin B	0.7 mg/kg/day IV to 1–3 g	See text for escalating dosage to desired maintenance dose. No dose adjustment in renal failure. Use with flucytosine for cryptococcosis, possibly candidiasis
Flucytosine	150–200 mg/kg/day PO in four divided doses	Except for urinary tract infections combine with 0.3 mg/kg/day IV amphotericin B to treat yeasts
Ketoconazole	200–600 mg/day PO	Give once or twice a day with acidic drink and avoid concommitant antacids
Miconazole	400–600 mg IV *q6h*	Probably only active vs. yeasts; many side effects
Nystatin	0.4–6 million units PO *qid* as suspension or troche (suppository)	Topical use only as there is no systemic absorption

such as piperacillin. This alternative may be considered for patients in renal failure (particularly elderly patients) or for individuals with significant hearing loss. For non-neutropenic patients, a broad-spectrum cephalosporin may suffice. Use of more than two initial agents does not seem indicated.

TREATMENT OF FUNGAL INFECTIONS

The biggest problem encountered in treating fungal infections is establishing an accurate diagnosis to serve as the impetus for treatment. Many systemic fungal infections, particularly systemic candidiasis and aspergillosis, go undiagnosed in the compromised host until autopsy. Clues to an underlying deep mycotic infection include: (a) new pulmonary infiltrates or cavities in patients receiving broad antibacterial coverage; (b) persistent high fever and liver function abnormalities in the face of antibacterial treatment; (c) funguria or renal failure in the noncatheterized patient; (d) severe dysphagia in the patient with thrush (usually esophageal candidiasis).

Table 5 summarizes the available antifungal agents, recommended doses, and comments relating to their use. Antifungal therapy in the mid-1980s represents a rather simple clinical proposition: amphotericin B is the only agent that is predictably effective against most of the important opportunistic fungal pathogens, but it often causes renal insufficiency and electrolyte abnormalities, as well as a variety of unpleasant side effects. Treatment should begin with a 1 mg test dose in D_5W (never saline) infused over 2 to 3 hours. Alternatively, 5 mg of amphotericin B is combined with 300 to 400 ml of D_5W, and approximately $^1/_4$ of that dose is infused over the first 2 to 3 hours. If that dose is well tolerated, the remainder of the infusion can be given. The goal in the seriously ill patient is to give approximately 20 mg in the first 24 hours. Increments can be approximately 5 mg per day, with the target a dose of 0.7 mg/kg/day. Patients often develop tolerance to the side effects of amphotericin B and can therefore accept increasingly larger doses of the drug. After the maximally tolerated dose is reached, therapy on an every second day basis or 3 days/week is feasible. A commonly advocated goal of amphotericin therapy is a total dose of 2 g, but lower doses can be used (0.5 g) when one is treating esophageal candidiasis. This lower total dose may be considered if fungemia is related to the removal of a vascular catheter.

In one specific situation, cryptococcal meningitis, the combination of flucytosine and amphotericin B has been quite effective. It has permitted a reduction in the total dosage of amphotericin B and has resulted in an impressively low incidence of relapsed infection. The dose of flucytosine is 150 mg/kg in 4 divided doses, PO. A clinical trial comparing regular dose amphotericin B with a combination of 0.3 mg/kg of amphotericin B plus 150 to 200 mg/kg of flucytosine for six weeks in cryptococcal meningitis showed similar clinical results, even though a significant number of patients could not be continued on flucytosine because of drug toxicity.

Ketoconazole is an imidazole whose primary advantage is oral administration. It is active against some Candida species, *Coccidioides immitis, Histoplasma capsulatum, Blastomyces dermatitis,* and possibly *C. neoformans*, but is usually without effect against Aspergillus, Mucor species, and Torulopsia glabrata (*Candida glabrata*). Its major use is in treating oral candidiasis, but it is wise to avoid the use of ketoconazole in systemic fungal infections in patients with persistent, severe immunologic defects.

Antifungal agents such as nystatin and clotrimazole are used topically. Amphotericin and miconazole may also be administered via bladder irrigation. However, bladder candidiasis is a relatively minor problem; the major concern is that candiduria is a manifestation of upper urinary tract disease rather than being localized to the bladder. If upper tract disease is detected, systemic amphotericin B is necessary.

VIRAL INFECTIONS IN THE COMPROMISED HOST

DAVID H. SHEPP, M.D.
JOEL D. MEYERS, M.D.

Infection is widely recognized as a critical determinant of outcome in patients with cancer, and successful management of malignant disease requires an aggressive diagnostic and therapeutic approach to infectious complications. Physicians caring for immunosuppressed patients commonly employ such an approach to bacterial and fungal infection, but only recently has similar emphasis been placed on viral diseases. Viruses causing infection with greater frequency or severity in this population are shown in Table 1. These viruses assume a greater prominence in immunosuppressed patients in two ways. DNA viruses establish latency after primary infection and reactivate during periods of immunosuppression. Cell-mediated immunity appears most critical for maintenance of latency and for successful control of infection, and both the underlying disease and immunosuppressive therapy may produce defects in cellular immunity. Other viral infections are important because of increased exposure during hospitalization and therapy. These viruses may be either blood-borne or transmitted during hospital outbreaks.

TABLE 1 Causes of Viral Infection in the Immunosuppressed Host

	*Type and Frequency of Infection**	
	Primary Infection	*Reactivation Infection*
DNA viruses		
Herpesviruses		
Herpes simplex virus (HSV), types I–II	+	+++
Varicella-zoster virus (VZV)	++	++
Cytomegalovirus (CMV)	++	+++
Epstein-Barr virus (EBV)	?++	?+++
Adenovirus	?+	?++
Hepatitis B	++	+
Papova viruses		
JC virus, BK virus	?+	++
Vaccinia	rare	—
RNA viruses		
Paramyxoviruses		
Measles	rare	—
Respiratory Syncytial Virus (RSV)	?+	—
Orthomyxoviruses		
Influenza	?+	—
Enteroviruses (picorna)		
Poliovirus (vaccine strains)	rare	—
Coxsackie	?+	—
Uncharacterized Viruses		
Non-A, Non-B (NANB) hepatitis	++	?

*+++ = common; ++ = occasional, + = unusual

HERPES SIMPLEX TYPES I AND II

Although these viruses differ in epidemiology, genetic make-up, and clinical expression, they may be considered together. Both are common pathogens acquired from intimate contact with the secretions of infected individuals. After primary oropharyngeal or genital infection, herpes simplex virus (HSV) usually establishes latency in the trigeminal or sacral nerve ganglia and may reactivate periodically causing labial ("cold sores") or genital lesions. In immunosuppressed patients, infection results almost exclusively from reactivation; nosocomial transmission rarely occurs, and primary infection via the usual routes (e.g., sexual contact) is less likely. Recurrences may be triggered by chemotherapy, radiation, underlying disease, or other clinical events such as fever or sepsis. Serum antibody to HSV is a marker of prior infection and serves to identify those at high risk for reactivation, although antibody acquired from transfusions can produce a false-positive result.

Recurrences are common, occurring in 60 to 80 percent of seropositive patients undergoing induction therapy for leukemia or marrow transplantation, usually within the first 2 to 3 weeks of treatment. Clinical manifestations vary from asymptomatic shedding to severe ulceration of the mouth, face, or genitalia. Many patients have only intraoral lesions, which may be incorrectly attributed to chemotherapy or other infectious agents. Complications of infection include inoculation of eye, genitalia, rectum, or other skin sites, or contiguous spread from the oropharynx to the esophagus, trachea, or lung. Rarely, dissemination to visceral organs may occur. HSV encephalitis in the absence of disseminated disease does not appear to be more frequent in the immunocompromised host.

None of these syndromes has a unique clinical presentation, and specific virologic evidence of infection should be sought. HSV infection can be easily confirmed by culture of vesicular fluid or ulcer scrapings. Rapid diagnosis may be accomplished by immunofluorescence performed on lesion smears or biopsy material and is particularly useful in differentiating HSV from varicella zoster virus. Esophagitis due to HSV requires endoscopy to distinguish it from other causes of esophagitis. The clinical presentation of HSV pneumonia is also nonspecific. Focal infiltrates are most common, but diffuse pneumonia occasionally occurs. Endotracheal intubation and aspiration of oropharyngeal secretions are risk factors for HSV pneumonia. The diagnosis should be suspected in the seropositive patient with HSV recovered from endotracheal aspirate or sputum cytology showing typical inclusions, but definitive diagnosis requires open lung biopsy. In both esophagitis and pneumonia, typical oral herpetic lesions are commonly absent.

Treatment

Both oral and intravenous acyclovir are effective for treatment of HSV infection (Table 2). All patients with moderate or severe HSV disease should be considered for treatment. Acyclovir treatment reduces viral shedding, relieves pain, and speeds healing. The drug has no effect on latency and recurrences are likely. Acyclovir is primarily excreted in the urine, and the dose must be adjusted in renal insufficiency. Nephrotoxicity may occur with higher doses of acyclovir, but is rare during treatment of HSV infection. Uncommon side effects include phlebitis of peripheral infusion sites, nausea, or rash. Central nervous system symptoms are rare and reversible. Five percent acyclovir ointment for topical use may be beneficial in milder cases, but therapy with oral acyclovir is preferable. Although more than 90 percent of patients are culture-negative after 7 days of therapy, longer courses may benefit some who remain virus-positive. Emergence of acyclovir-resistant virus during therapy has been documented and may account for some therapeutic failures. Fortunately, resistant viruses appear to be no more virulent and perhaps less so than sensitive strains.

Acyclovir prophylaxis is an alternative to treatment in patients at high risk for HSV reactivation. Prophylaxis reduces the problem of rapid recurrence after brief therapeutic acyclovir courses, and may also be preferable for limiting the development of resistance. At present only seropositive marrow transplant recipients and patients undergoing leukemic induction therapy have been shown to benefit from prophylaxis, but any seropositive patient with severe, prolonged immunosuppression may be considered. Recommended prophylactic regimens are included in Table 2.

TABLE 2 Regimens for Antiviral Chemotherapy

Mucocutaneous HSV Infection*	
Treatment:	Acyclovir 250 mg/m² IV *q8h* for 7 days OR Acyclovir 400 mg PO† 4–5 times daily for 7–10 days OR Acyclovir 5% ointment to affected areas *q4h* for 7–10 days
Prophylaxis:	Acyclovir 250 mg/m² *q12h* beginning with cytotoxic therapy and continuing until: (1) 30 days after marrow transplant, or (2) resolution of neutropenia after leukemic induction therapy OR Acyclovir 400 mg PO 4–5 times daily for the same period indicated above
VZV Infection	
Treatment:	Acyclovir 500 mg/m² IV *q8h* for 7 days OR Vidarabine 10 mg/kg/day IV over 12 hours once daily for 7 days with infusion concentration not > 0.5 μg/ml

*For treatment of visceral or disseminated HSV infection, only the intravenous regimen (250 mg/m² *q8h*) can be recommended at this time. The acyclovir dose of 500 mg/m² *q8h* is currently being tested for treatment of HSV encephalitis in normal persons.

†Oral acyclovir was not yet licensed in the United States or Canada at the time of writing.

There are no other antiviral agents currently available which are effective for mucocutaneous HSV infection. Despite its apparent efficacy in HSV encephalitis, vidarabine (adenine arabinoside) is not clinically useful for mucocutaneous HSV infection in the immunocompromised host.

VARICELLA ZOSTER VIRUS

Varicella zoster virus (VZV) causes varicella (chicken pox) as a primary infection in susceptible children or adults. Varicella is highly contagious from 2 or more days before the onset of rash until all skin lesions have crusted. A dermatomal eruption (herpes zoster or shingles) occurs when virus latent in the dorsal root ganglia reactivates due to waning immunity associated with advancing age, immunosuppressive illness, or treatment. Varicella is generally a benign disease in normal children, but may be a severe illness in children with hematologic malignant disease. Visceral dissemination occurs in as many as one-third of cases, most often as pneumonia, hepatitis, or encephalitis. Other complications include pancreatitis, arthritis, orchitis, uveitis, and coagulopathy. Mortality is approximately 7 percent. In contrast, herpes zoster is a self-limited infection in the majority of cancer patients. However, patients with more profound degrees of immunosuppression may develop severe dermatomal disease or viremia with cutaneous dissemination of the rash. In disseminated zoster the same visceral complications noted in varicella may occur. Additional complications of zoster are related to damage to that portion of the nervous system affected by virus reactivation. These include postherpetic neuralgia, blindness due to uveitis and contralateral hemiplegia in trigeminal zoster, deafness and vertigo with eighth cranial nerve disease, peripheral motor neuropathy, and paraparesis due to transverse myelitis.

Some immunosuppressed patients with evidence of prior varicella develop a disseminated rash without initial dermatomal disease. These infections may represent recurrent disease (i.e., atypical zoster) with dissemination from a clinically inapparent dermatome. Alternately, epidemiologic data suggest that some of these cases represent true instances of reinfection.

Certain patients at high risk for zoster have been identified. About 25 percent of patients with Hodgkin's disease, 30 to 40 percent of marrow transplant recipients, and 8 to 12 percent of those receiving aggressive chemotherapy for solid tumors or leukemic induction develop zoster. Cutaneous dissemination occurs in up to 30 percent. The occurrence of zoster in an otherwise normal individual is not a marker for occult malignancy.

VZV infection often can be diagnosed on clinical grounds, but many cases have an atypical presentation which may delay diagnosis. For both epidemiologic and therapeutic reasons, early diagnosis is desirable, and therefore laboratory confirmation should be attempted if the diagnosis is uncertain. Infected cells obtained by vigorous swabbing of the unroofed vesicle can be examined by immunofluorescence, providing same-day diagnosis and distinguishing VZV from HSV. Serology is not useful in the diagnosis of acute VZV infection.

Patients with suspected varicella or zoster who require hospitalization should be placed in strict isolation to avoid nosocomial transmission of infection. Hospital staff caring for the patient should have a clear history or serologic evidence of prior varicella. Immunosuppressed individuals with close contact with the index case should be considered for immunoprophylaxis with varicella zoster immune globulin (VZIG). Guidelines for use of VZIG have been published. When given promptly following exposure, VZIG attenuates or prevents the clinical manifestations of varicella.

Treatment

Both acyclovir and vidarabine (adenine arabinoside, Ara-A) are effective for treatment of VZV infection. The major benefit is a significant reduction in the risk of cutaneous or visceral dissemination. Improvement in local parameters of infection such as pain, viral shedding, and new lesion formation is more rapid, althhough the incidence of postherpetic neuralgia is not reduced by therapy with either drug. Recurrent VZV infection, unusual after untreated disease, may occasionally occur within days to months after completion of antiviral therapy.

Patients at high risk of complications of VZV infection should be hospitalized for intravenous therapy with either acyclovir or vidarabine. Included are patients with hematologic malignant disease with varicella as well as patients with cutaneous or visceral dissemination of zoster. In addition, patients with marrow transplants, Hodgkin's disease, or other acute hematologic malignant disease in relapse who have localized zoster should be considered for treatment to prevent dissemination.

Renal toxicity may occur in up to 15 percent of patients receiving intravenous acyclovir for VZV infection, and serum creatinine should be monitored. Toxicity appears to be related to poor solubility in the urine and may be minimized by using supplemental hydration and a one-hour infusion time. In mild cases of renal insufficiency, acyclovir need not be discontinued. The toxicity of vidarabine includes gastrointestinal upset (nausea, vomiting, or diarrhea in 15 to 24%) and mild elevations of serum transaminases. Neurologic toxicity consisting of tremor, myoclonus, confusion, or seizures and hematologic toxicity may occur, but usually in patients with renal insufficiency or at doses higher than those recommended here. For this reason and because pharmacokinetics in renal failure have not been adequately studied, vidarabine should be used cautiously or not at all in patients with renal insufficiency. Oral acyclovir may provide effective outpatient therapy for many patients, including those with a lower risk of complications. However, VZV is 5- to 20-fold less sensitive to acyclovir in vitro than is HSV, and oral therapy cannot be recommended until the appropriate regimen has been defined.

Prevention of varicella by means of live-attenuated varicella vaccine has been studied in both normal and immunocompromised children. Preliminary results suggest that the vaccine can induce immunity with minimal risk of vaccine-related varicella, but a longer period of observation is needed to establish the durability of such immunity. Zoster due to the vaccine strain has occurred, but the frequency and severity of zoster after vaccination are not known.

CYTOMEGALOVIRUS

Like the other herpesviruses, cytomegalovirus (CMV) commonly infects normal individuals. Primary infection is usually asymptomatic, although "heterophil-negative" mononucleosis may occur. Although the site of subsequent CMV latency is not known, epidemiologic data linking acquisition of primary CMV infection to transfusion of leukocyte-containing blood products suggest that a peripheral blood leukocyte may be one cell that harbors latent CMV. In patients with no prior infection, CMV is often acquired from blood products. Other nosocomial transmission appears to be rare. Patients with previous infection, as indicated by the presence of antibody to CMV, commonly have reactivation of latent virus in association with immunosuppression.

Clinically severe CMV disease is confined almost exclusively to patients with significant deficiencies of cell-mediated immunity, particularly neonates, patients with AIDS, and organ transplant recipients. CMV disease may occur in patients with lymphoma or leukemia, but appears to be less common. Clinical syndromes associated with CMV include fever, neutropenia, hepatitis, myalgias and arthralgias, or retinitis. Enteritis may occur anywhere throughout the gastrointestinal tract, but most often causes ulcerative esophagogastritis or cecal lesions which may bleed. Atypical lymphocytosis may not occur. Pneumonia is the most serious complication of CMV infection, occurring most commonly after organ allografting. CMV is also associated with an increased frequency of coinfection with bacterial, fungal, and protozoan pathogens, possibly because it may cause transient neutropenia and produces both functional and quantitative changes in lymphocyte subpopulations.

Rapid noninvasive diagnostic methods for CMV are needed. Viral isolation from throat or urine usually requires 2 to 6 weeks, and isolation alone does not prove that CMV is etiologic since asymptomatic shedding is common. Viremia can be documented by culturing peripheral blood buffy coat, but many viremic patients are asymptomatic. Diagnosis of CMV enteritis or pneumonia can be accomplished by finding characteristic cytology in endoscopic or surgical biopsies. Immunofluorescence may show the presence of CMV when characteristic inclusions are not present. Open lung biopsy remains the procedure of choice for diagnosis of CMV pneumonia.

Effective therapy for serious CMV infection is not available at present. Vidarabine, acyclovir, and various alpha-interferon preparations have been used without consistent benefit. However, prevention of CMV disease in certain high-risk groups may be possible. Seronegative marrow transplant recipients may have the risk of infection or its severity diminished by prophylactic administration of high-titer CMV immune plasma or globulin. Prevention of transfusion-associated infection through use of blood products donated only by CMV seronegative donors has been effective for neonates and cardiac transplant patients. However, passive immunization and use of screened blood products are beneficial only for those lacking serologic evidence of prior CMV infection.

EPSTEIN-BARR VIRUS

When compared to the other herpesviruses, relatively little is known about the epidemiology and pathogenicity of Epstein-Barr virus (EBV) in immunosuppressed patients. More than 90 percent of normal adults have serologic evidence of past EBV infection. Many primary infections are asymptomatic, although some individuals develop the mononucleosis syndrome. Intermittent shedding of EBV from the oropharynx appears to be common in normal individuals and is even more so in immunosuppressed patients. Serologic studies in such patients usually reveal high IgG antibody titers to EBV viral capsid antigen and early antigen, but generally lower titers to EBV nuclear antigen than are seen in normals. Heterophil antibodies and EBV-specific IgM are not found. Clinical syndromes such as fever, neutropenia, and pneumonia may correlate with EBV reactivation in some immunosuppressed patients. EBV is associated with both Burkitt's lymphoma and nasopharyngeal carcinoma. In addition, some immunosuppressed patients with defective T-cell function, including those with congenital immune deficiencies and organ transplant recipients, may be vulnerable to uncontrolled B-cell proliferation during active EBV infection, which may terminate in malignant lymphoma.

Acyclovir is active against EBV in vitro, although the mechanism of activity is not known. A few cases of EBV-related lymphoproliferation appear to have improved with acyclovir when used prior to transition to lymphoma. However, general usage of acyclovir for treatment of EBV infection cannot be recommended at this time.

ADENOVIRUS

This DNA virus recently has gained attention as a serious pathogen in the immunocompromised host, causing respiratory (bronchitis and pneumonia) or urinary (hemorrhagic cystitis and nephritis) infection, gastroenteritis, and disseminated disease. Respiratory infection typically presents with cough, hypoxia, and interstitial infiltrates and is clinically indistinguishable from other respiratory infections. Urinary infection may cause gross or microscopic hematuria, which may be incorrectly attributed to chemotherapeutic agents. Adenovirus has also been associated with gastrointestinal ulceration or diarrhea. Disseminated infection involves any or all of the foregoing features as well as hepatitis.

The source of adenovirus infection in immunocompromised patients is not fully understood. Adenovirus may be capable of latent or persistent infection and, like other DNA viruses, may reactivate periodically. Alternately, adenovirus may be transmitted nosocomially, but data regarding clustering of cases are few. Adenovirus can be recovered from throat, urine, or rectal specimens. As with other viruses, isolation does not always imply disease, and asymptomatic infection is common. Definitive diagnosis requires culture and histologic examination of tissue (lung, liver, kidney biopsies). Serologic confirmation may be helpful in some patients. There is no treatment currently known for adenovirus infection.

VIRAL HEPATITIS

Despite improved methods for screening blood donors, hepatitis still occurs in up to 7 percent of all recipients of transfusions; 10 percent of all cases are due to hepatitis B virus. Among patients undergoing induction therapy for acute leukemia, hepatitis B develops in about 6 percent. Host immune response is an important determinant of the course of infection in both normal and immunosuppressed patients. Hepatic necrosis results from the inflammatory response of the host immune system rather than from viral lysis of hepatocytes. Recovery is indicated by the loss of circulating hepatitis B surface antigen (HBsAg) and the development of antibody to it (anti-HBs), and is associated with immunity. In 20 to 80 percent of immunosuppressed patients, as well as 5 to 10 percent of apparently normal individuals, this process fails, and chronic infection with persistent circulating HBsAg ensues. Chronic infection appears more likely in patients with ongoing immunosuppression, such as organ transplant recipients, than in those with cyclic immunosuppression related to chemotherapy. Patients who are chronically infected before immunosuppressive therapy may develop serologic evidence of increased viral replication during treatment, but clinically severe hepatitis is unusual.

Rarely is a specific agent other than hepatitis B virus found as the cause of post-transfusion hepatitis, and the remaining 90 percent of cases are classified as non-A, non-B (NANB) hepatitis. Although the causes of NANB hepatitis have not been identified, studies in experimentally infected animals suggest that at least two viruses are involved. Up to two-thirds of patients who achieve remission after induction therapy for acute leukemia develop a picture compatible with NANB hepatitis. Symptoms of hepatitis and jaundice occur in more than half the patients, suggesting that infection is more severe than in normal individuals. Chronic infection with fluctuating transaminase elevations is a common sequela in both immunosuppressed and normal patients. Symptoms, progressive liver dysfunction, and "aggressive" histology on liver biopsy are unusual. Conflicting data exist about whether NANB hepatitis prolongs duration of remission of leukemia.

Diagnosis of hepatitis B is made by detection of HBsAg in serum. Detection of anti-HBs is a reliable sign of immunity only when passive acquisition from recent blood transfusions can be excluded. Diagnosis of NANB hepatitis is made on clinical grounds, although liver biopsy is often supportive.

Prevention of hepatitis B depends primarily on application of sensitive screening tests for HBsAg for blood donors and avoidance of paid donations. Administration of hepatitis B vaccine early in the course of treatment is logical in selected chronic conditions associated with large transfusion requirements (e.g., chronic anemias), but is less practical when acute intensive blood product support is needed. Patient-to-patient spread occurs uncommonly with hepatitis B or NANB. Blood precautions are appropriate for all patients with suspected hepatitis, but other isolation procedures are unnecessary. Therapy of acute hepatitis B is supportive and antiviral therapy of chronic infection is not yet of proven value. There are currently no practical methods to prevent or treat NANB hepatitis.

UNUSUAL VIRAL INFECTIONS

Papova viruses are small DNA viruses which are excreted with increased frequency during immunosuppression. JC or BK virus may be detected in the urine of immunosuppressed patients, and although clinical disease is rare, nephritis and renal failure have been described. Serologic studies suggest that infection with these viruses is common in normal persons, and these viruses probably reactivate from a latent focus during immunosuppression. Progressive multifocal leukoencephalopathy (PML) is a rare demyelinating disease of the central nervous system occurring in severely immunosuppressed patients and characterized by waxing and waning neurologic status. PML is ultimately fatal over 3 to 6 months. JC virus and a virus resembling the simian virus SV-40 have been identified in the brain of PML patients. Human papova viruses also cause the common wart.

Disseminated vaccinia infection can result from administration of smallpox vaccine to an immunosuppressed patient. Since smallpox has been eradicated worldwide, vaccination should no longer be used. Measles can be severe in the immunocompromised host, but with the widespread use of measles vaccine in the United States and Canada this infection has become uncommon. Immune serum globulin may attenuate measles in the exposed patient. As a live-virus vaccine, measles vaccine should not be used in immunosuppressed patients. Increased frequency or severity of disease due to influenza, respiratory syncytial virus, or other respiratory viruses may occur especially in immunosuppressed pediatric patients; ribavirin has been used as an investigational agent in the treatment of these infections.

Live-attenuated polio vaccine can produce paralytic disease in immunosuppressed patients and virus can be transmitted from person to person. Inactivated vaccine provides excellent protection against wild-type poliovirus and is preferable in all situations in which vaccination of immunosuppressed patients or their household contacts is otherwise indicated. Finally, coxsackie A virus has been linked to outbreaks of diarrhea in marrow transplant patients, but its role otherwise, except as a sporadic pathogen in immunosuppressed patients, is unknown.

ORGAN TRANSPLANTATION AND ASSOCIATED INFECTION

JAMES E. PENNINGTON, M.D.

Infections, in some cases life-threatening, remain one of the commonest complications associated with organ transplantation. There exists considerable variation in the risk for infection among various types of organ transplant recipients. Although infections occurred in up to 70 percent of renal transplant recipients in the 1960s, the modified and reduced immunosuppressive regimens used following renal transplantation during the past decade have been associated with marked reductions in opportunistic infections. In sharp contrast are bone marrow transplant recipients, in whom infection remains one of the leading causes of fatality. This is, of course, related to the more intensive immunosuppressive chemotherapy employed for bone marrow transplantation and to the fact that myelosuppression is commoner among these patients. Although less common, heart, heart-lung, and liver transplantation procedures are increasing in frequency. The immunosuppressing regimens used for these patients are somewhat more intensive than those used for renal transplant recipients. It is not surprising, therefore, that infectious complications continue to be a relatively common problem among this latter group of patients.

Regardless of which organ is transplanted, the major goal of immunosuppressing regimens is to impair normal function of the lymphocyte-directed cellular immune system. Accordingly, opportunistic infections, for which cell-mediated immune protection is essential, occur with particular frequency among organ transplant recipients. Members of the herpesvirus group, especially cytomegalovirus (CMV), herpes simplex, and Epstein-Barr virus (EBV), are quite common. In addition, Listeria, Nocardia, *Pneumocystis carinii*, Cryptococcus, and *Legionella* species are notable for their frequency.

Somewhat overlooked, however, are the more mundane, yet extremely common, bacterial pathogens causing urinary tract and skin infections. In one recent report, 98 percent of all infections occurring in renal transplantation patients during the first 6 months after transplantation were bacterial in etiology. Nearly one-half of these infections originated in the urinary tract, and no fatalities were reported.

Finally, there have been efforts to correlate frequency and types of infection with specific immunosuppressive agents. For example, an increased risk of *Pneumocystis carinii* pneumonia has been described recently among renal transplant recipients treated with cyclosporine rather than azathioprine. It is the author's view, however, that the major predictor for infection among organ transplant recipients is the intensity of immunosuppression rather than the specific agent. Unfortunately, until more experience is gained with such new agents as cyclosporine or anti-T-cell monoclonal antibodies, the ability to gauge intensity of immunosuppression will be less than precise.

As is common among other groups of immunocompromised patients, the organs at greatest risk for infection among transplantation patients are those most extensively exposed to environmental microorganisms. Thus, mucocutaneous surfaces, the respiratory tract, and the urinary tract are the organs most frequently involved with infection. Somewhat in contrast to patients with hematologic malignancies, but like patients with the acquired immunodeficiency syndrome, the central nervous system is a relatively common site of infection in transplant recipients. Finally, hepatic functional abnormalities are exceedingly common among all types of transplantation patients. Deciphering infectious versus noninfectious etiologies (e.g., azathioprine hepatitis, graft-versus-host disease, veno-occlusive disease, radiation hepatitis) for hepatic dysfunction is exceedingly difficult. Confounding this difficulty is the apparent frequency among transplant recipients of non-A, non-B hepatitis, for which diagnostic serology does not yet exist.

TEMPORAL PATTERN OF INFECTIONS

Renal Transplant Recipients

A temporal pattern exists for infectious complications among renal transplant recipients (Table 1). During the early postoperative period, surgical wound infections, urinary tract infections associated with bladder catheterization, and mucocutaneous herpes simplex infections due to reactivation of endogenous virus are most frequent. Thirty days after transplantation, cytomegaloviral infections of the lung, liver, and bone marrow become the predominant infectious disease. *Pneumocystis carinii* pneumonia also may occur during this period. It is also during this period that rejection-associated fever is most frequent. Differentiation of rejection fever from occult infection may be quite difficult. Recent evidence suggests that occult Epstein-Barr viral infection also may account for cryptic fever during this period. Although the first 3 to 4 months after transplantation is the time of greatest risk for infection, later infections may occur. Cryptococcal pneumonia and meningitis, herpes zoster, and severe pneumococcal infections are notable for their late occurrence.

Bone Marrow Transplant Recipients

The first 4 months following transplantation is the period of highest risk for infection for marrow recipients (Table 2). The greatest difficulties often occur during the period in which marrow recipients are intensely myelosup-

TABLE 1 Temporal Patterns of Infection in Renal Transplantation Patients

Time (days) After Transplant	*Usual Infections*
1–30	Herpes simplex (mucocutaneous) Bacteria (urinary tract, surgical wound IV sites)
30–90	Cytomegalovirus (lung, liver, marrow) *Candida* (mucocutaneous, esophagus, urinary tract) *Pneumocystis* (lungs) *Nocardia* (lungs, brain) *Legionella* species (lungs) *Aspergillus* (lungs, CNS) *Mycobacteria* (lungs, CNS) *Listeria* (CNS) Epstein-Barr virus (liver, occult fever)
>90	*Cryptococcus* (lungs, CNS) Mycobacteria (lungs, CNS) Pneumococcus (lungs, bacteremia)

TABLE 2 Temporal Patterns of Infection in Bone Marrow Transplantation Patients

Time (days) After Transplant	*Usual Infections*
1–30	Gram-negative bacilli (blood, lungs, skin) *Staphylococcus aureus* and *Staphylococcus epidermidis* (blood, skin) Herpes simplex (mucocutaneous, esophagus, trachea, lungs) *Candida* (mucocutaneous, esophagus, disseminated)
30–90*	*Aspergillus* (lungs) *Candida* (as above) Cytomegalovirus (lungs, disseminated)
>90	Herpes zoster (skin, disseminated)

* *Pneumocystis carinii* pneumonia is rarely encountered if patients receive prophylactic TMP/SMZ.

pressed. This is generally the initial 20 to 40 days after the transplantation. The clinical approach to fever during this period resembles closely that described for febrile neutropenic patients with hematologic malignancies. Thus, empiric antibiotics are used routinely for fever and are designed to offer coverage for aerobic gram-negative bacilli. Suspicion of skin- or intravascular-cannula-related sepsis also requires coverage for *Staphylococcus aureus* and *Staphylococcus epidermidis*. In persistently febrile neutropenic patients who do not respond to empiric antibacterial agents, an empiric trial of amphotericin B may be warranted. Mucocutaneous herpes simplex is another common problem during this early posttransplantation period. Intravenous acyclovir is useful in treating such patients. Furthermore, recent investigations suggest that intravenous or oral acyclovir may be useful as prophylaxis against early herpes simplex infections in marrow recipients. Since this approach also appears to retard the development of antiherpes immunity, and since these are as yet investigational, indications for acyclovir prophylaxis cannot be routinely recommended at this time.

The later phase of infections among marrow recipients is remarkable for the high incidence of life-threatening cytomegaloviral pneumonias. To date, there is no specific therapy for CMV infection. DHPG (2′-NDG) is an investigational agent closely related to acyclovir that shows some promise in treating CMV. Also, investigational studies suggest that CMV antisera may be effective as prophylaxis in seronegative patients. At present, however, severe CMV pneumonias are one of the most serious problems among marrow transplant recipients. The routine use of prophylactic trimethoprim-sulfamethoxazole among marrow recipients has greatly reduced the incidence of *Pneumocystis carinii* pneumonias. There is presently no U.S. Food and Drug Administration indication for gamma globulin prophylaxis in these patients.

Other Transplant Groups

By and large, heart and liver transplant recipients most closely resemble renal transplant recipients in the types and times of infectious complications. Naturally, the specific surgical procedures involved increase the incidence of thoracic and pulmonary infections (heart) or intra-abdominal infections (liver) among these patients. Although some have reported a particularly high incidence of nocardial and mycobacterial infections among heart transplant recipients, this experience may be regional.

CLINICAL APPROACH TO INFECTIONS

The diagnostic, therapeutic, and prophylactic approaches for the usual infectious diseases encountered among transplantation patients are presented in Table 3. In Figures 1 and 2, management schemes for two common clinical infectious syndromes (fever with no source and fever with new lung infiltrate) are presented. It should be noted that in Figure 2 an alternative to the early invasive diagnostic procedure (i.e., empiric antibiotic trial) is listed. My strong preference, however, is to obtain a diagnostic specimen (lung biopsy or bronchoscopic lavage specimen) as early as possible (within 24 to 36 hours) in these patients, regardless of the infiltrate pattern. This approach will provide critically important information to guide therapy and will circumvent the common situation in which a patient fails the initial empiric treatment, but by that time has clinically deteriorated and is no longer a surgical, or even bronchoscopic, candidate. As far as

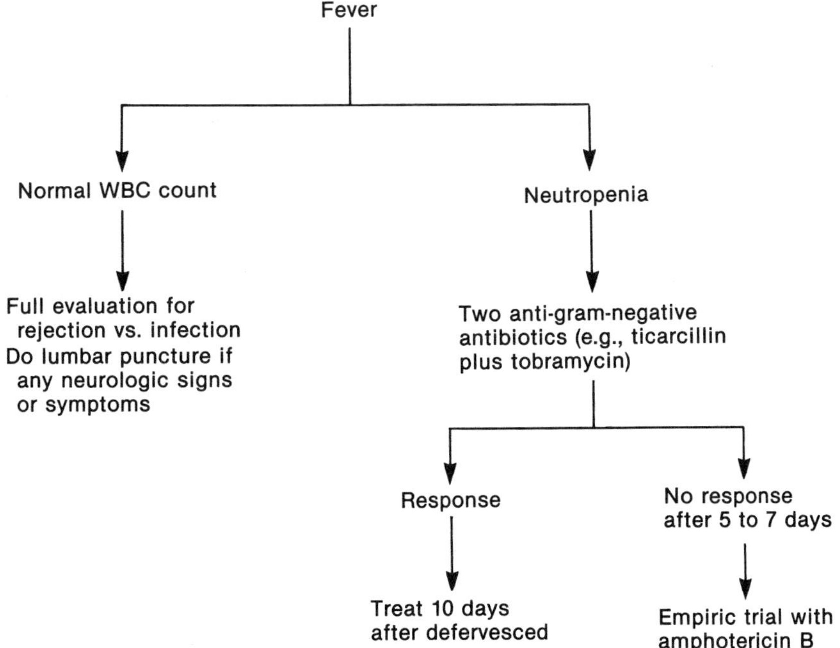

Figure 1 Fever with no apparent source and negative blood cultures.

TABLE 3 Diagnosis, Treatment, and Prophylaxis of Specific Infections in Transplantation Patients

Type of Infection	*Usual Sites*	*Diagnostic Procedures*	*Treatment*	*Prophylaxis*
Bacterial				
Usual (e.g., staphylococci, streptococci, gram-negative bacilli)	Urine Skin Lungs Blood	Cultures and Gram stains of appropriate specimens	Indicated antibiotics	Oral TMP/SMZ (1 single-strength tablet daily) for patients with recurrent urinary tract infections "Pneumococcal vaccine"
Legionella species	Lungs	Culture on charcoal yeast extract medium (sputum, transtracheal aspirate, lung biopsy, blood) Direct fluorescent antibody stains (sputum, tracheal aspirate, lung tissue) Indirect fluorescent antibody titers	Erythromycin, either 1 g IV, q6h or 500 mg PO QID (plus rifampin, 600 mg/day, if needed, on the basis of severity of illness)	None
Listeria monocytogenes	CNS Blood	Gram stains, cultures	Ampicillin IV, 2–3 g (depending on severity of illness) q4h (plus gentamicin if blood culture is positive); duration of treatment: until positive response	None
Viral				
Cytomegalovirus	Lungs Liver Retina	Complement fixation titer Culture of urine, buffy coat, lung tissue Monoclonal antibody stain of lung tissue (frozen sections) DNA hybridization of lung tissue specimen	None currently available (DHPG, investigational)	CMV antisera for seronegative bone marrow recipients (investigational) Alpha-interferon in renal transplant recipients (investigational)
Herpes simplex	Skin Mucosa CNS Lungs	Tzanck preparations (not specific for simplex) Cultures of lesions or tissues Immunofluorescent staining	Acyclovir, 6 mg/kg IV, q8h for 5 days; topical may be effective in renal transplant patients. Oral useful in mildly immunosuppressed patients (investigational)	Intravenous or oral acyclovir in bone marrow recipients (investigational)
Herpes zoster	Skin Lungs Liver	Tzanck preparations (not specific for zoster) Cultures of lesions or tissues Immunofluorescent staining	Acyclovir, 12 mg/kg IV, q8h for 5 days (reduce in patients with renal impairment)	None
Epstein-Barr virus	Liver	Serology only	None currently available	Alpha-interferon in renal transplant recipients (investigational)
Hepatitis B virus	Liver	Serology only	None currently available	Vaccine not used routinely
Fungal				
Cryptococcus	Lungs CNS Skin	Latex agglutination for antigen (serum and CSF) Cultures, India ink (CSF), cytology (CSF)	Amphotericin B 0.3 mg/kg/day plus 5-fluorocytosine (5-FC) 150 mg/kg/day (reduce 5-FC for renal insufficiency)	None
Candida	Skin Mucosa Urinary tract Blood	Cultures, gram-stained smears (Serum candida antigen, investigational)	Mucocutaneous infections: ketoconazole, 200–600 mg (depending on severity of infection) orally per day in a single dose Urinary tract: bladder irrigation with amphotericin B 50 mg/day, if catheter is in place. Oral 5-FC, 50–100 mg/kg/day (depending on severity of infection) in 4 divided doses if not catheterized; *note:* ketoconazole is not well excreted in urine Systemic infection: amphotericin B 0.6 mg/kg/day	Nystatin (oral); ketoconazole 200–400 mg/day (depending on degree of immunosuppression)
Aspergillus	Lungs CNS	Cultures, histology	Amphotericin B 0.6 mg/kg/day	None
Nocardia	Lungs CNS Skin	Cultures, acid-fast stains, Gram stains	Sulfadiazine 8–12 g/day (depending on severity of infection) in 4 divided doses; often required for several months	None

Table 3 *Continued*

TABLE 3 Diagnosis, Treatment, and Prophylaxis of Specific Infections in Transplantation Patients (Continued)

Type of Infection	*Usual Sites*	*Diagnostic Procedures*	*Treatment*	*Prophylaxis*
Mycobacteria				
M. tuberculosis	Lungs CNS	Cultures, acid-fast stains	INH 300 mg/day plus rifampin 600 mg/day plus ethambutol 15 mg/kg/day (see other sections)	INH 300 mg daily for known positive skin reactors, indefinitely
M. avium-M. intracellulare	Lungs Marrow	Cultures, acid-fast stains	Ansamycin plus clofazamine (both investigational but can be obtained) (sensitivities of other agents, unpredictable, and must be carefully monitored)	None
Parasitic				
Pneumocystis carinii	Lungs	Lung biopsy	TMP/SMZ IV (20 mg/kg/day of TMP component; reduce for renal failure) Switch to pentamidine 4 mg/kg/day IM if no response after 4 days of TMP/SMZ	TMP/SMZ double-strength tablet (160 mg TMP and 800 mg SMZ) twice per day
Toxoplasma gondii	Brain Liver Lungs	Indirect immunofluorescent antibody (IgM)	Pyrimethamine 25 mg every other day to 50 mg/day every day plus sulfadiazine 6–8 g/day (depending on severity of infection) plus folinic acid 10 mg/day	None

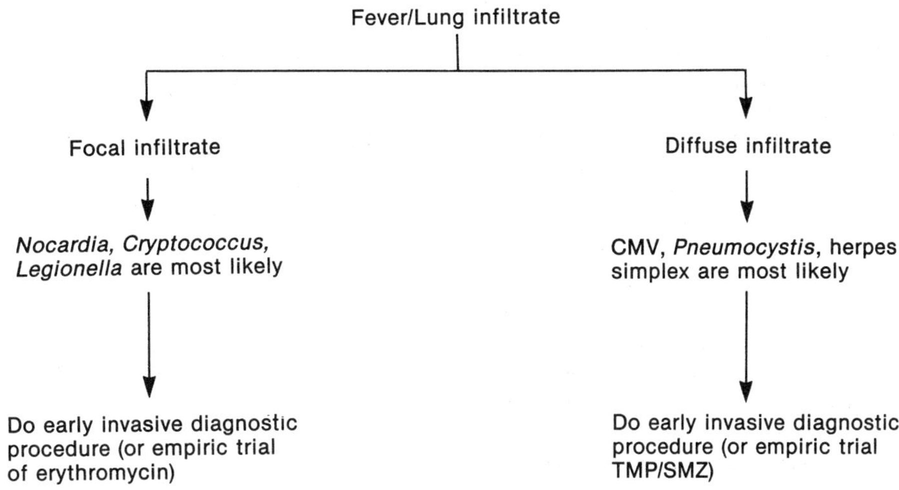

Figure 2 Fever and new lung infiltrate in transplantation patient without purulent sputum and with normal white cell counts. If patient is neutropenic, then gram-negative bacillary pneumonia or invasive aspergillus infection (both present with focal patterns) are also possibilities.

which invasive diagnostic procedure to use, this decision must be individualized. The following factors influence this choice: (1) Tempo of illness. For rapidly advancing pneumonia, only one chance is likely. Thus, open lung biopsy is the procedure of choice (fewest false-negatives). For less acute processes, fiberoptic bronchoscopic biopsy (yield around 50%) can be used first, then followed by open lung biopsy if no diagnosis is obtained. (2) Type of lesion. Peripheral cavitary lesions are particularly amenable to transthoracic thin-needle aspirates, and diffuse infiltrates are particularly poor lesions to approach with this procedure. (3) Bleeding status. For uremic or thrombocytopenic patients, open lung biopsy provides the best hemostasis. (4) Local expertise and experience.

ACQUIRED IMMUNODEFICIENCY SYNDROME

NEAL H. STEIGBIGEL, M.D.
GERALD H. FRIEDLAND, M.D.

DEFINITION, PATHOGENESIS, AND CLINICAL DESCRIPTION

Acquired immunodeficiency syndrome (AIDS) is an infectious disease caused by the retrovirus, human T-cell lymphotropic virus-III/lymphadenopathy-associated virus (HTLV-III/LAV). The disease, AIDS, represents the full-blown clinical manifestation of this viral infection; however, it appears that not all individuals infected with HTLV-III/LAV will develop AIDS. AIDS is primarily defined by the clinical criteria listed in Table 1. These clinical manifestations are largely the result of the lymphotropism of the virus for the T-helper-cell, resulting in dysfunction and premature death of a cell central to the immune system. The grave immune deficiency that results from loss of T-helper-cell function leads to a variety of life-threatening opportunistic infections and sometimes to particular autoimmune disorders, such as thrombocytopenia, or to several types of malignancy (including Kaposi's sarcoma and B-cell lymphomas). The latter may be the result of unregulated replication of potentially oncogenic viruses (possibly cytomegalovirus and Epstein-Barr virus) in a severely immunosuppressed host. Infection with HTLV-III/LAV per se may sometimes be associated with an infectious mononucleosis-like syndrome or aseptic meningitis several weeks after presumed inoculation. In addition, HTLV-III/LAV is particularly neurotropic. A large proportion of patients with AIDS develop dementia months to years after initial infection. This dementia is associated with the presence of HTLV-III/LAV in the brain.

There is a clinical-pathological continuum between asymptomatic infection with HTLV-III/LAV and the full-blown disease, AIDS. The latter must currently be considered an ultimately fatal condition with death caused by major opportunistic infections, malignancy, or inanition within 1 year in about 50 percent and within 2 years in about 80 percent of patients. Intermediate clinical manifestations of the infection include chronic generalized lymphadenopathy (nodes 1 cm or more in size in at least two extrainguinal areas) (lymphadenopathy syndrome, LAS) and a complex (AIDS-related complex, ARC) that may include chronic lymphadenopathy, fever, weight loss, and unexplained oropharyngeal candidiasis. Unexplained oral candidiasis is defined as that which occurs in individuals who have not received antibiotics within 1 month or corticosteroid treatment and who do not have an apparent condition, such as diabetes mellitus, known to be associated with candidiasis. When the manifestations progress to include a particular major opportunistic infection or other conditions listed in Table 1, the condition is defined as AIDS (with the grave prognosis already noted). About 5 to 10 percent of individuals in high-risk groups who have evidence of infection (as indicated by the presence of serum antibodies to HTLV-III/LAV) followed for 2 to 3 years have developed AIDS and 20 to 25 percent, ARC. About 15 to 20 percent of individuals with ARC followed over 2 to 3 years have developed AIDS. High-risk individuals who manifest unexplained oral candidiasis have a particularly high rate of developing AIDS.

TABLE 1 Case Definition of AIDS

Standard definition: The presence of a disease at least moderately indicative of underlying cellular immunodeficiency occurring in a previously healthy individual without a known cause for immunodeficiency; these diseases include

- Opportunistic infections
  - Protozoal or helminthic
    - *Pneumocystis carinii* pneumonia
    - Toxoplasmosis (CNS or pulmonary)
    - Cryptosporidiosis (causing diarrhea >1 month)
    - Strongyloidiasis (pulmonary or disseminated)
  - Fungal
    - Esophageal candidiasis
    - Cryptococcosis (CNS or disseminated)
  - Bacterial
    - "Atypical" mycobacteriosis (disseminated)
  - Viral
    - Cytomegaloviral infection (pulmonary, GI, or CNS)
    - Herpes simplex (mucocutaneous persisting >1 month)
    - Progressive multifocal leukoencephalopathy
- Malignancies
  - Kaposi's sarcoma in persons <60 years
  - Lymphoma limited to brain

Supplementary definition (utilizes results of testing for serum antibodies or culture of HTLV-III/LAV)

- In the absence of the above diseases, any of the following is considered indicative of AIDS if the patient has a positive serologic test or virologic documentation of HTLV-III/LAV infection
  - Disseminated histoplasmosis
  - Isosporiasis (causing diarrhea >1 month)
  - Bronchial or pulmonary candidiasis
  - Non-Hodgkin's lymphoma of high grade pathologic type and of B-cell or unknown immunologic phenotype
  - Kaposi's sarcoma in patients 60 years of age or older
- In the absence of opportunistic infection, a histologically confirmed diagnosis of chronic lymphoid interstitial pneumonia in a child under 13 years of age will be considered as indicating AIDS unless tests for HTLV-III/LAV are negative
- Patients will be excluded from case definition if they have a negative result on testing for serum antibody to HTLV-III/LAV, have no other type of HTLV-III/LAV test with a positive result, and do not have a low number of T-helper lymphocytes or a low ratio of T-helper to T-suppressor lymphocytes

Note: Modified from CDC surveillance definition. MMWR 1982; 31:507–514 and MMWR 1985; 34:373–375.

EPIDEMIOLOGY

Transmission of this retroviral infection appears to require the inoculation of infected body fluids, particularly blood or semen. Therefore, intimate contact between an infected individual and a susceptible person is required for transmission. HTLV-III/LAV can be present in saliva and tears, but there has as yet been no evidence that these fluids play a role in transmission of infection. Therefore, those at high risk for the infection as well as the disease have been sexually active male homosexuals, needle-sharing intravenous drug abusers, recipients of blood transfusions or hemophiliacs, infants born of mothers at high risk, and heterosexual partners of those in high-risk groups. There is as yet no evidence that casual contact with infected individuals may transmit HTLV-III/LAV infection or disease. The incubation period ranges from months to several years. The disease may be transmitted by individuals infected with HTLV-III/LAV who are asymptomatic. Laboratory tests with high sensitivity and specificity have been developed for detecting serum antibodies to HTLV-III/LAV. The vast majority of individuals with tests confirmed as demonstrating such antibodies have been shown to carry viable HTLV-III/LAV in their blood, regardless of their clinical status. They are, therefore, potentially infectious. Individuals in high-risk groups who do not demonstrate serum antibodies will only occasionally harbor HTLV-III/LAV in their blood.

ASSOCIATED LABORATORY FINDINGS IN PATIENTS WITH AIDS

In addition to the presence of HTLV-III/LAV as well as viral-specific antibodies in the blood, the following laboratory abnormalities are usually found in patients with AIDS: leukopenia, lymphopenia, polyclonal increase in immunoglobulins—especially of the IgG and IgA classes—decreased numbers of T-helper lymphocytes, decreased ratio of T-helper to T-suppressor lymphocytes, and cutaneous anergy to antigens of the delayed hypersensitivity type. AIDS patients often have a mild to moderate anemia and sometimes have thrombocytopenia.

MANAGEMENT OF OPPORTUNISTIC INFECTIONS IN PATIENTS WITH AIDS

As yet there is no specific effective therapy for AIDS per se. Antiviral therapy directed at HTLV-III/LAV may become available in the future. Such antiviral agents will probably need to penetrate the central nervous system, which often harbors HTLV-III/LAV. Antiviral therapy will likely require prolonged or even life-long administration. Specific antiviral therapy may need to be combined with agents directed at repairing the immune defects of AIDS. However, no agent has yet been established as an effective immunomodulating agent in AIDS.

In the meantime, our therapy for AIDS is palliative, but it often prolongs life with some reasonable quality. This therapy consists of important supportive measures and specific and effective therapy for the opportunistic infections and, in some cases, for the malignancies that are part of the natural history of this illness.

Most of the opportunistic infections developing in patients with AIDS are caused by ubiquitous organisms of "low virulence," which are known to establish latent infections in normal individuals. These endogenous pathogens become activated to produce disease when there is severe depression of cell-mediated immunity. Following effective treatment of such infections in AIDS, there tends to be a high relapse rate, probably associated with reactivation of residual organisms that cannot be entirely eliminated by either the treatment or the poor cellular defense mechanisms in these patients. True reinfection is also a possibility. Therefore, antimicrobial therapy of such infections must often be prolonged and relapse may be diminished by the use of long-term (indefinite) suppressive therapy following the initial, intensive treatment period. The symptoms, signs, and laboratory abnormalities of these infections—especially when manifest in the lungs and central nervous system—can be too nonspecific to allow an accurate diagnosis unless biopsy and culture of abnormal tissue are undertaken. This principle cannot be overemphasized for proper management of these patients. Our treatment regimens for these infections are outlined in Table 2.

In addition to the infections due to low-virulence organisms (*Pneumocystis carinii, Mycobacterium avium–Mycobacterium intracellulare*, herpes simplex virus, *Toxoplasma gondii, Cryptococcus neoformans*, cytomegalovirus, *Cryptosporidium*) we have also observed life-threatening infections caused by classic virulent pyogenic bacteria (especially, *Streptococcus pneumoniae, Hemophilus influenzae* type b, *Staphylococcus aureus*, and *Salmonella* species) in some AIDS patients.

The commonly encountered opportunistic infections in patients with AIDS often present with characteristic clinical pictures, although etiologic diagnosis should be confirmed with appropriate laboratory or biopsy studies. *P. carinii* pneumonia is the commonest major opportunistic infecton in patients with AIDS and is often the first to occur. Dyspnea and nonproductive cough are characteristic symptoms, often associated wth interstitial pulmonary infiltrates. Diagnosis should be established by bronchoscopy with transbronchial biopsy or examintion of material obtained by bronchial lavage. When the chest roentgenogram is not characteristic, justification for the biopsy may be established by demonstrating either a substantial decrease in arterial oxygen tension with exercise or diffuse uptake of gallium by lung scan. Rapid assessment of biopsy material for *P. carinii* may be obtained by examination of "touch preps" of biopsy material stained by the Giemsa method.

Cytomegaloviral infections are often manifest as chorioretinitis, pneumonitis (sometimes together with *P. carinii*), esophagitis, enteritis, colitis (often showing ulcerated mucosa with characteristic intranuclear and intracytoplasmic inclusions of epithelial cells) or adrenal gland involvement (sometimes with adrenal insufficien-

TABLE 2 Therapy of Opportunistic Infections in AIDS

Organ System and Infection	*Drug*	*Usual Dose and Route in Adults*	*Duration of Therapy**	*Comments*
Skin, mucous membranes				
Herpes simplex	Acyclovir	200–400 mg PO q4–6h† *or* 5 mg/kg IV q8h†	7 days 7 days	Repeat with recurrences
Severe or disseminated herpes zoster	Acyclovir	200–800 mg PO q4–6h† *or* 5 mg/kg IV q8h†	7 days 7 days	
Pulmonary				
Pneumocystis carinii pneumonia	Trimethoprim (TMP)/ sulfamethoxazole (SMZ)	5 mg/kg TMP/ 25 mg/kg SMZ IV q6h†	21 days	After treatment consider initiating suppressive therapy with either TMP/SMZ one double-strength tablet BID twice weekly, or Fansidar (sulfadoxine and pyrimethamine) one tablet weekly
	or Pentamidine isethionate	4 mg/kg/day slowly IV (over 1h) or IM	21 days	
Gastrointestinal				
Oropharyngeal candidiasis	Ketoconazole	200 mg PO daily		Treatment usually required indefinitely
	or Nystatin oral suspension	5 ml "swish and swallow" q4–6h		
	or Clotrimazole troches	One troche 5 × daily		
Candida esophagitis	Ketoconazole	200 mg PO daily or BID		Treatment with ketoconazole usually required indefinitely
	or Amphotericin B	0.6 mg/kg IV daily†	10 days	
Cryptosporidiosis	Spiramycin (?)‡	1 g PO q6h	14 days	Spiramycin therapy of questionable efficacy; opiates and hyperalimentation are palliative
Neurologic				
Toxoplasma gondii encephalitis	Pyrimethamine	75 mg PO on first day, then 25 mg PO daily		Continue indefinitely because of high relapse rate
	and Trisulfapyrimidines	1.0–1.5 g PO q6h		
	and Folinic acid	10 mg PO daily		Folinic acid prevents bone marrow depression from pyrimethamine
Cryptococcal meningitis or other forms of dissemination	Amphotericin B *or*	0.5–0.6 mg/kg IV daily†	Administer total of about 2 g over about 8 weeks	High relapse rate suggests the initiation of suppressive therapy, 25 mg IV twice weekly, after initial therapy
	Amphotericin B *and* Flucytosine	0.3–0.4 mg/kg IV daily† 35 mg/kg PO QID†	6 weeks	Flucytosine often poorly tolerated and should generally not be used in renal failure without determination of blood levels
Systemic infections				
Disseminated *M. avium-M. intracellulare* infection	Isoniazid	300 mg PO daily	Indefinite	Therapy of questionable benefit;§ duration of therapy uncertain
	plus Ansamycin‖	150 mg PO daily		
	plus Clofazamine#	200 mg PO daily		
	plus Ethambutol	15 mg/kg PO daily		
Disseminated cytomegaloviral infection	DHPG**	2.5–5 mg/kg IV q8h†	14 days	Investigational drugs; efficacy under study
	or BW B759U**	2.5 mg/kg IV q8h†	14 days	

* Duration of therapy is not clearly established.
† Dose should be modified with renal insufficiency.
‡ Available as Rovamycin from Poulenc in Canada.
§ Efficacy currently under investigation.
‖ Available from the Centers for Disease Control, Atlanta, Georgia.
\# Available from Ciba-Geigy Pharmaceuticals Company, Summit, New Jersey.
** Investigational acyclic nucleotides available as DHPG (from Syntex, Inc., Palo Alta, California) or as BW B759U (from Burroughs Wellcome, Research, Triangle Park, North Carolina).

cy). Herpes simplex infections are often prolonged and severe, with painful ulcerations of the oropharynx, genitalia, perianal region, and rectum.

M. avium–M. intracellulare infections are frequent and associated with the presence of organisms in the blood, liver, spleen, and bone marrow. Noncaseating granuloma may be found in the liver (often with high levels of serum alkaline phosphatase) or bone marrow. The contribution of this infection to morbidity (fever, inanition) and mortality in these patients is difficult to assess, as multiple opportunistic infections are often present simultaneously. Pulmonary tuberculosis and occasionally disseminated tuberculosis may be encountered. As yet, the duration of treatment for tuberculosis in patients with AIDS is uncertain.

Cryptosporidium may produce enteritis with prolonged, profuse, and debilitating diarrhea. Infections due to *Cryptosporidium,* herpes simplex, and cytomegalovirus are more frequent in patients with AIDS who are male homosexuals compared with those in the heterosexual, intravenous drug-abuser group.

Toxoplasmosis of the central nervous system in patients with AIDS commonly presents as mass lesions in the brain (well-visualized on CT scan, especially in conjunction with use of contrast dye) producing seizures, focal neurologic signs, and altered consciousness. Serologic testing is often not helpful in diagnosis, but brain biopsy utilizing proper staining techniques usually establishes the etiology.

Cryptococcal meningitis also occurs frequently and is usually associated with headaches, nausea and vomiting, and changes in mental status and vision. In these patients the diagnosis is most efficiently made by assaying for the cryptococcal antigen in the cerebrospinal fluid by the latex agglutination technique. Other forms of cryptococcal dissemination are encountered, including involvement of lungs, bone marrow, and spleen. Other neurologic syndromes noted in patients with AIDS include frequent ataxia and progressive dementia, probably due to HTLV-III/LAV infection of brain; and progressive multifocal leukoencephalopathy, a demyelinating disorder characterized by focal weakness, seizures, and changes in mental status and caused by certain strains of papovavirus for which there is no established therapy.

Oropharyngeal candidiasis occurs very frequently in patients with AIDS. Candida infection may involve the esophagus, with resulting dysphagia. Endoscopy readily establishes the diagnosis.

Patients with AIDS often demonstrate adverse reactions to drugs. This is particularly encountered in the treatment of *P. carinii* pneumonia. About two-thirds of AIDS patients treated with trimethoprim-sulfamethoxazole (TMP/SMZ) for this infection will develop rash, leukopenia, or other side effects. Pentamidine therapy is often complicated by hypoglycemia, hyperglycemia, and nephrotoxicity. Both drugs are about equally effective,and there appears to be no advantage to combination therapy that might increase side effects. TMP/SMZ is usually used first; if there is no clinical improvement in 5 to 7 days, pentamidine is substituted. When pentamidine is used because of adverse effects from the use of TMP/SMZ, the clinical response to the former is often satisfactory. However, when the switch is made because of inadequate clinical improvement with TMP/SMZ therapy, the mortality despite pentamidine therapy is very high. Respiratory support is often needed for these patients, but those who require endotracheal intubation have a high mortality, reflecting the far-advanced stage of their respiratory infection and poor host defenses. Recurrence of *Pneumocystis* pneumonia is noted in 20 to 25 percent of AIDS patients. For this reason, the duration of the treatment with TMP/SMZ or pentamidine has not yet been clearly established. Although not yet proved as efficacious by controlled trials, we suggest that indefinite suppression of residual *P. carinii* infection be attempted after initial treatment by the continued use of TMP/SMZ or Fansidar (sulfadoxine and pyrimethamine) in patients who can tolerate these drugs (Table 2).

SUPPORTIVE THERAPY

Appropriate supportive therapy can significantly increase the quality of life of patients with AIDS. Treatment of pain with analgesics and of diarrhea with opiates is often indicated. Maintenance of reasonable nutrition through dietary counseling and high protein, high caloric supplementation is helpful. Emotional support, financial aid, and the provision of medical and personal services and entitlements are essential for the patient with AIDS. These services generally must be facilitated by trained social workers, mental health workers, and also by referral to community groups offering support services. Well-supervised group therapy can provide critical emotional support to selected patients. Finally, avoidance of lifestyle practices that might result in acquisition of new infections should be encouraged.

A discussion of the management of the malignant tumors that occur in AIDS is beyond the scope of this article. However, it should be mentioned that the clinical manifestations of disseminated Kaposi's sarcoma that occur in these patients may mimic those of certain opportunistic infections when there is involvement of lymph nodes, lungs, or gastrointestinal tract by the tumor. Regarding therapy, the use of recombinant alpha-interferon has been associated with temporary remission of Kaposi's sarcoma in some AIDS patients. Local radiation of tumor masses is occasionally indicated.

PREVENTION OF AIDS

The development of a safe and effective vaccine for HTLV-III/LAV infection is a long-range goal. For the present, advice to the general population must focus on sensible behavior modification, namely, warnings concerning the dangers of intravenous drug abuse (particularly needle sharing and the use of unsterile equipment) and promiscuous sexual behavior are indicated. The use of condoms might limit the transmission of infection during sexual intercourse, but is as yet of unproven efficacy. Sexual partners who are in high-risk groups for development of AIDS are a potential danger for HTLV-III/LAV transmission. These include prostitutes, who are often intravenous drug abusers. A number of practices should diminish the frequency of AIDS developing in blood transfusion recipients and hemophiliacs. These include the screening of blood for HTLV-III/LAV antibodies at blood banks (begun in 1985); the continued policy of requesting that high-risk individuals not donate blood; and the development of new practices to inactivate any potentially contaminating HTLV-III/LAV in certain blood fraction products.

Individuals who are already infected with HTLV-III/LAV must be carefully counseled. The ultimate prognosis for an asymptomatic infected individual is unknown. Discussions need to be supportive and compassionate, but also forthright concerning the potential for transmission of infection to sexual partners or, in the case of intravenous drug abusers, to potential needle sharers. Infected individuals must not donate blood, other body fluids, or organs for transplantation.

Finally, neither health care workers (except possibly for rare victims of needle-sticks) nor household contacts of AIDS patients (except for their sexual partners or children born of infected mothers) appear to be at increased risk for developing HTLV-III/LAV infection. Reassurance to these groups will help in the care of patients with AIDS.

INFECTION OTHER THAN AIDS IN HOMOSEXUAL MEN

THOMAS C. QUINN, M.D.

The recognition of the acquired immunodeficiency syndrome (AIDS) as a sexually transmitted disease primarily among homosexual men focused attention on the health care problems of the gay community. Compared with heterosexual men, homosexual men experience greater prevalence rates of gonorrhoea, syphilis, anal warts, hepatitis B infection, and cytomegaloviral infection. Certain enteric diseases, including giardiasis, amebiasis, shigellosis, campylobacteriosis, and salmonellosis, are also endemic and sexually transmitted among homosexual men. The other sexually transmitted infections such as herpes, chlamydial infections, genital warts, chancroid, lymphogranuloma venereum, and granuloma inguinale also occur frequently among homosexual men. In contrast to heterosexuals, homosexuals have many of these infections in nongenital sites such as the mouth, pharynx, intestine, and anorectum. Indeed, many of these infections—hepatitis A, hepatitis B, cytomegalovirus, and secondary syphilis—present with systemic signs of disease.

Because of the magnitude and complexity of these problems and the potential for transmission to other individuals, physicians and public health officials need to be aware of the epidemiology, etiology, and clinical manifestations of these infections. Although the immunosuppresive effects of these infections are not fully realized, indirectly they may have an effect on increasing susceptibility to the etiologic agent of AIDS, HTLV-III.

EPIDEMIOLOGY

There are several factors responsible for the high prevalence rates of these infections. Homosexuality per se is not a major risk factor, but, rather, the promiscuous life style that is practiced by many homosexual men is a predominant factor. A moderately sexually active man not uncommonly has relations with 100 or more men per year. Anonymity of sexual contact exacerbates the risk and complicates contact tracing and prevention of reinfection.

Asymptomatic carriage of sexually transmitted pathogens is a common problem among homosexual men. Urethral, pharyngeal, and anorectal asymptomatic infection with *Neisseria gonorrhoeae, Chlamydia, Treponema,* and enteric organisms—such as *Campylobacter, Entamoeba histolytica* and *Giardia*—occur frequently and must be sought. This carriage state represents a human reservoir of the infection, and this state plus promiscuity are primarily responsible for the continued transmission of these pathogens.

Another major risk factor for increased infection among homosexual men is the frequent practice of sexual activity allowing for infection in nongenital sites, such as anal intercourse, anilingus, and fellatio following anal intercourse. These practices are primarily responsible for the transmission of eneteric pathogens, including hepatitis viruses, in this population. Anorectal infections with the conventional venereal pathogens is caused by rectal intercourse. The role of fomite transmission, such as may occur with the shared use of unsterilized equipment for rectal douching and colonic irrigation in gay houses, remains unknown, although an outbreak of amebiasis has been traced to such use of unsterile equipment.

SCREENING EXAMINATION

Certain sociologic factors must be taken into consideration when obtaining a history from a sexually active homosexual. Preference of sexual partners, number of sexual partners, types of sexual practices, illness of sexual partners, and the past history of sexually transmitted diseases must be assessed and incorporated into the medical evaluation of each patient. A medical history should attempt to differentiate between clinical syndromes that might suggest one or more etiologic infectious agents, since homosexual men are frequently exposed to multiple pathogens.

After the sexual and medical history is obtained, a detailed physical examination with anoscopy should be performed on all high-risk patients. Since many of these individuals are at high risk for AIDS as well as other sexually transmitted pathogens, the physical examination must be complete and include examination of the skin, lymph nodes, oral cavity, abdomen, genitalia—for urethral discharge or genital ulcers—and a complete inspection of the perianal area and anal canal, including digital rectal examination and anoscopy.

Initial screening tests for symptomatic homosexual men should include a urethral and rectal Gram stain for the evaluation of polymorphonuclear leukocytes (PMNs) and intracellular gram-negative cocci indicating infection with *N. gonorrhoeae*. Serologic tests for syphilis, darkfield examination, and Tzanck preparation of any external ulcerations should be performed to rule out syphilis and herpes simplex viral infection. Routine cultures of the pharynx, urethra, and rectum for *N. gonorrhoeae* should be performed. At this point, if any of the screening tests are positive, specific therapy may be instituted (Table 1) and sexual contacts examined for the presence of each particular infection. I recommend a rectal Gram stain for all homosexual men whether symptomatic or not. If symptoms persist following treatment, or if the aforementioned screening tests are negative, more extensive examination and cultures should be performed, including sigmoidoscopy, rectal biopsy, lymph node aspiration, or skin biopsy, as indicated.

URETHRITIS

The etiology of urethritis differs in homosexual and heterosexual men; gonococcal urethritis is more frequent than nongonococcal urethritis (NGU) in homosexual men, whereas heterosexual men have predominantly NGU. In addition, although 40 percent of heterosexual men with NGU have *Chlamydia trachomatis* urethral infection, only 10 to 20 percent of homosexual men with NGU have *Chlamydia* present. *Chlamydia* is also the major cause of postgonococcal urethritis (PGU) in heterosexual men, whereas *Chlamydia* is rarely present among homosexual men with PGU. Indeed, the etiology of NGU and PGU in gay men is unknown at present, but pathogens other than *N. gonorrhoeae* and *Chlamydia* that should be included in the differential diagnosis include *Ureaplasma urealyticum, Trichomonas*, herpes simplex virus, and *N. meningitidis*.

Gonococcal urethritis is usually symptomatic, with asymtomatic urethral infection occurring in less than 5 percent of infected individuals. However, asymptomatic infections accumulate in the population and therefore may account for a higher proportion of cases in a prevalence survey. In contrast, pharyngeal and anorectal infection is frequently asymptomatic in more than 50 percent of cases. The incubation period is 2 to 5 days after contact, and the symptoms may vary from a thin mucoid discharge to grossly purulent discharge in the case of urethral infection. Meatal irritation, dysuria, and frequency are com-

TABLE 1 Treatment of Sexually Transmitted Diseases Commonly Seen In Homosexual Men

Specific Infection	*Recommended Treatment*	*Alternative*
Neisseria gonorrhoeae		
Rectal or urethral infection	APPG* 4.8 million units IM plus probenecid 1.0 g PO	Spectinomycin 2.0 g IM
Pharyngeal infection	APPG* 4.8 million units IM plus probenecid 1.0 g PO	Trimethoprim-sulfamethoxazole (80 mg/400 mg) nine tabs PO daily for 5 days
Chlamydia trachomatis		
Non-LGV serovars	Tetracycline 500 mg PO 4 times a day for 7 days	Erythromycin 500 mg PO 4 times a day for 7 days
LGV serovars	Tetracycline 500 mg PO 4 times a day for 21 days	Erythromycin 500 mg PO 4 times a day for 21 days
Treponema pallidum† 1′, 2′ early latent (<1 yr)	Benzathine penicillin G 2.4 million units IM	Tetracycline 500 mg PO 4 times a day for 15 days
Herpes simplex virus	Acyclovir ointment 5% 6 times a day for 7 days	Supportive therapy
Hemophilus ducreyi (chancroid)	Erythromycin 500 mg PO 4 times a day for 14 days	Trimethoprim-sulfamethoxazole double strength tab (160 mg/800 mg) 2 times a day for 14 days
C. granulomatous (donovanosis)	Tetracycline 500 mg PO 4 times a day for 14–21 days	Ampicillin 500 mg PO 4 times a day for 14–21 days, depending on response
Condyloma accuminata	Podophyllin 25% to lesion every other day	Cryotherapy Surgery
Scabies, pediculosis	Lindane (1%) lotion or shampoo	

* APPG=aqueous procaine penicillin G.

** See elsewhere in this volume for a discussion on treatment of latent and neurosyphilis.

mon complaints. If symptoms are ignored or the infection is only partially treated, it can persist in an asymptomatic or moderately symptomatic state, and can eventually spread to produce complications, including epididymitis, prostatitis, and, rarely, disseminated gonococcal infection (DGI). NGU is also frequently symptomatic, although the symptoms are usually milder than those observed in gonococcal urethritis. The discharge is not as purulent, and there may be only a slight mucoid discharge. Other symptoms include dysuria and pruritus. Epididymitis is a complication of untreated NGU.

The diagnosis of gonococcal urethritis is established by the demonstration of gram-negative diplococci within neutrophils in a Gram stain of the urethral discharge. This diagnosis is then confirmed by the isolation of *N. gonorrhoeae* by culture. The diagnosis of NGU is made when five or more leukocytes per 1,000× magnification are present on Gram stain of the urethra and no gram-negative diplococci are present within the PMNs.

Treatment should be instituted on the basis of the gram-stained urethral smear. Gonococcal urethritis is treated with 4.8 million units of aqueous procaine penicillin G, preceded by 1 g probenecid. Tetracycline, 500 mg orally four times per day for 7 days, is recommended for the treatment of NGU. Persistence of symptoms following treatment usually represents reinfection, antibiotic resistance in the case of penicillinase-producing *N. gonorrhoeae*, poor patient compliance in the case of oral antibiotics, or the emergence of postgonococcal urethritis (PGU). Reinfection is ascertained by history and the failure to treat sexual partners. Penicillinase-producing *N. gonorrhoeae* is confirmed in the laboratory, and treatment consists of spectinomycin, 2 g intramuscularly. Like NGU, PGU is less frequent in homosexual men than in heterosexual men. Cultures for *Chlamydia* and *Ureaplasma*, etiologic agents of PGU, are not routinely available. Empiric therapy, which is usually successful, consists of tetracycline, 500 mg four times per day orally.

ANOGENITAL SKIN LESIONS

Anogenital skin lesions may be classified as ulcerative or nonulcerative. The etiology and incidence of ulcerative lesions vary greatly in different parts of the world and among different populations. Ulcerative lesions most commonly seen in homosexual men include herpes simplex viral infection, syphilis, and less frequently, lymphogranuloma venereum (LGV), chancroid, and donovanosis (granuloma inguinale). Nonulcerative lesions include condyloma accuminata, condyloma lata of secondary syphilis, scabies, genital warts, and molluscum contagiosum. Other sexually transmitted infections may manifest systemically as dermatologic lesions, and these include secondary syphilis, hepatitis, disseminated cytomegalovirus, and disseminated gonococcal infections.

The occurrence of syphilis in homosexual men is responsible for more than 50 percent of all the reported cases in the United States. Although the manifestations of syphilis are the same in homosexual men as in heterosexual men and women, anal and oral chancres are more common in homosexual men and frequently missed by the physician. Since primary chancres are not frequently detected in homosexual men, the lesions of secondary syphilis, such as condyloma lata, maculopapular rash, proctitis, or rectal masses, are frequently identified as the common manifestations of syphilis in homosexual men. Consequently, in order to identify syphilis at an earlier stage in this population, frequent serologic testing for syphilis should be performed in all homosexually active men every 6 months. The other clinical manifestations, diagnosis and treatment of syphilis are discussed in more detail elsewhere in this volume.

Herpes simplex viral infections also occur commonly in homosexual men. Vesicular lesions are usually apparent on the genitalia, the perianal area, and in the oral cavity. The primary infection is usually accompanied by fewer than 10 to 20 vesicles and, sometimes, by a single, painful, shallow ulcer known as herpetic chancre. Urethral infection may present with dysuria and a urethral discharge. The vesicles are present for 3 to 5 days before rupturing to form small, nonindurated ulcers. The primary infection may be accompanied by inguinal pain, lymphadenopathy, and constitutional symptoms such as fever, malaise, and headache. Recurrent attacks occur in about two-thirds of all cases and are usually restricted to a small area for a shorter period of time (10 days).

Diagnosis of herpes simplex viral infection is made by demonstration of the characteristic multinucleated giant cell on a Tzanck smear. The diagnosis is confirmed by isolation of the virus in culture. Treatment has typically been supportive, consisting of analgesics, sitz baths, and stool softeners in the case of anorectal herpes. Recently, acyclovir, an antiherpes drug, has been developed for the treatment of primary herpes infection and is available in intravenous, ointment, and oral forms. Although acyclovir may be beneficial in primary herpes, it does not appear to be significantly effective in recurrent disease, except when taken orally as suppressive therapy. Other aspects of diagnosis and treatment of herpes infection are described in more detail elsewhere in this volume.

Genital ulcers may be secondary to lymphogranuloma venereum (LGV), due to an invasive serovar of *C. trachomatis*. After an incubation period of 1 to 3 weeks, a small painless ulceration may appear at the site of inoculation. This heals spontaneously within several days and is followed by prominent inguinal lymphadenopathy. The adenopathy is unilateral in two-thirds of cases and bilateral in the remainder. These nodes progressively enlarge over a month and eventually become fluctuant and are frequently referred to as bubos. If therapy is delayed, the overlying skin becomes inflamed, and draining fistulas may appear. Systemic symptoms of fever, myalgias, and malaise are common. Late complications, such as anorectal strictures or ulcerative colitis, may occur in neglected cases.

The diagnosis of LGV is dependent on the ability to culture the virus from the infected site. LGV infection can also be confirmed by the demonstration of systemic antibodies to LGV at a titer of greater than 1:256; this will differentiate between LGV and non-LGV infections. Tetracycline is the treatment of choice, 500 mg orally four times a day for 3 weeks. Fluctuant bubos in LGV should be aspirated as needed to prevent spontaneous rupture. As with other STDs, examination and treatment of sexual partners is indicated.

Chancroid, caused by *Hemophilus ducreyi*, causes small painful ulcerations. These ulcerations are usually associated with unilateral, tender, fluctuant inguinal adenopathy. Differential diagnosis includes herpes, primary syphilis, granuloma inguinale, and LGV. The diagnosis is made by culturing the edge of the ulcer or lymph node aspirate on supplemented chocolate agar. Treatment of choice is trimethoprim-sulfamethoxazole, one double-strength table twice daily for 10 days or until the ulcer and lymphadenopathy resolve. Alternative treatment is erythromycin, 500 mg orally four times daily. Fluctuant nodes should be aspirated as needed in order to minimize the risk of spontaneous rupture.

Granuloma inguinale or donovanosis is an infection due to *Calymmatobacterium granulomatis*. Most cases of donovanosis in the United States have been identified in homosexual men. After 1 to 4 weeks of incubation, a beefy, granulomatous ulcer with elevated borders develops in the genitalia or anorectal area. Lymphadenopathy is uncommon, but the surrounding induration can extend into the inguinal area, resulting in an "pseudobubo." The lesion resembles squamous cell carcinoma, which may also complicate long-standing cases, emphasizing the need for biopsy in uncertain cases. Diagnosis is made by a Wright or Giemsa stain of the scraping of the ulcer bed. The presence of blue-black bipolar-staining bacilli in the cytoplasm of large mononuclear cells is diagnostic. The treatment is tetracycline, 500 mg four times daily until the lesion has healed completely. For treatment failures, ampicillin 500 mg four times daily, streptomycin 1.0 g twice daily, gentamicin 1 mg per kilogram twice daily, or chloramphenicol, 500 mg four times daily, have all been advocated.

Condyloma accuminata or anogenital warts are caused by human papilloma viruses. These pink or brown cauliflower-like lesions appear on the glans penis, perineum, and anorectal regions. The lesions may be mildly pruritic, but otherwise cause few symptoms. The highly infectious condyloma accuminata of secondary syphilis need to be differentiated from these warts; this is accomplished by performing darkfield microscopy for spirochetes and on the basis of the flat characteristic appearance of the warts. Therapy varies according to the site of involvement. For external genital and perianal warts, an application of 25 percent podophyllin in compound tincture of benzoin is advocated. For anorectal or oral warts, cryotherapy, electrocauterization or surgery is recommended.

Molluscum contagiosum presents as a flesh-colored, 2 to 5 mm, frequently umbilicated papule; it is caused by a pox virus. A cheesy material can often be expressed from the center of the lesion, and multiple lesions are common. Diagnosis is made by the clinical appearance, which is highly suggestive. Confirmation can be obtained by biopsy or examination of the expressed caseous material, which reveals molluscum bodies (basophilic cytoplasmic inclusions filled with the virium). Treatment consists of removal of the caseous center by pressure after nicking the center with a scalpel or needle. Spontaneous resolution occurs in most cases. Podophyllin 20 percent compound or cryotherapy with liquid nitrogen can be used in resistant cases.

Ectoparasites such as lice (pediculosis) and mites (scabies) are seen more frequently in heterosexuals than in homosexuals. The primary symptom of pediculosis is itching, primarily in the genital area, although any hairy part of the body can be involved. Close examination of the infected area show nits attached one-half to 1 inch from the base of the hair shaft. Scabies is often characterized by pruritis, which is typically worse at night. The lesions are symetric and consist of pathognomonic burrows made by the female. The burrows vary from 1 mm to 10 mm in length and are commonly seen in men in interdigital web spaces of the hand, wrist, elbow, beltline, penis, and scrotum. Gamma benzene hexochloride (lindane) is the treatment of choice for both infections. The medication for pediculosis is applied as a shampoo that can be washed off in 4 minutes. For scabies, a 1 percent lotion or cream is applied to the body from the neck down and washed off the next day. A single application is usually effective for scabies, whereas a second application 1 week later may be necessary for pediculosis.

HEPATITIS

Hepatitis A or B can be sexually transmitted and are frequent infections seen in homosexual men. The risk of developing hepatitis B infection has been shown to exceed 20 percent annually among seronegative homosexual men attending clinics for sexually transmitted diseases. It is estimated that the annual infection rate for hepatitis A is comparable to that observed for hepatitis B infection. Other infections commonly seen in homosexual men that may also manifest as hepatitis include cytomegaloviral infection, Epstein-Barr viral infection, and secondary syphilis. Indeed, more than 95 percent of homosexual men will become seropositive for cytomegalovirus and Epstein-Barr virus. The clinical spectrum of acute hepatitis in homosexual men is similar to that seen in any other group of healthy individuals and ranges from totally asymptomatic and anicteric (50%) to icteric, symptomatic disease (45%) and to severe fulminant disease (5%). The clinical presentation and diagnosis of viral hepatitis is discussed in greater detail in a separate chapter.

Immune serum globulin is recommended for any persons reporting sexual contact within the prior 2 weeks with an individual having a known case of hepatitis A and for persons reporting contact with viral hepatitis of unknown etiology. Immune serum globulin has been shown to be effective in preventing overt hepatitis A viral infection in 80 to 90 percent of persons treated either before or within 2 weeks of intimate contact. The dose is 0.02 ml per kilogram intramuscularly. Presently, there are no studies that demonstrate the efficacy of immune serum globulin prophylaxis in the prevention of non-A, non-B hepatitis in sexual contacts of recently infected homosexual men. When there has been sexual contact with an individual with recent hepatitis B infection, hyperimmune hepatitis B immune globulin (HBIg) is recommended, 0.06 ml per kilogram intramuscularly, as soon after exposure as possible. The dose should be repeated in 1 month.

Hepatitis B vaccine (Merck Sharp & Dohme; Heptavax B vaccine) has recently been developed and is effective in providing a high rate of protection (at least 92%) in persons receiving three vaccinations of 20 μg (1 ml) each over a 6-month period. Due to the high rate of hepatitis B infection, vaccination is recommended for all seronegative homosexual men and sexual contacts of recently infected individuals. In general, if sexual contact has occurred with a person with evidence of a recent hepatitis B infection, the sexual contact should be given passive prophylaxis with HBIg, followed by a vaccination with Heptavax B. These individuals need to be counseled that they still may acquire the disease and that they should refrain from sexual activity until they are HBsAg-negative and HBsAB-positive by serotesting.

INTESTINAL INFECTIONS

Due to the sexual practices that involve fecal or rectal contamination (anilingus, anal intercourse, or fellatio following anal intercourse), homosexual men are particularly susceptible to sexually transmitted gastrointestinal infections. Although many of these infections are polymicrobial and asymptomatic, a systematic approach to diagnosis that incorporates sexual history, symptoms and findings on physical examination, anoscopy, mucosal biopsy, and screening tests should guide the clinician in the selection of specific diagnostic tests and appropriate antimicrobial therapy. A flow chart is shown in Figure 1 that outlines the steps required in the evaluation of a homosexual man with intestinal symptoms.

If the patient is asymptomatic, he should be carefully screened by culture and serologic tests for rectal and pharyngeal gonorrhea and syphilis. About two-thirds of persons with rectal or pharyngeal gonorrhea will be asymptomatic, whereas others will have symptoms consisting of mild proctitis or pharyngitis, respectively. In the case of pharyngeal infection, symptoms can include a sore throat, and on oral examination, the pharynx may appear erythematous or completely normal. In the case of rectal infection, symptoms may include constipation, anorectal discomfort, tenesmus, and a mucopurulent discharge. On anoscopy, the mucosa may appear normal or slightly erythematous in the distal 5 to 10 cm of the rectum. Complications such as fistula formation, perirectal abscess, rectal stricture, and disseminated gonococcal infection have been reported. Diagnosis is based on the identification of intracellular gram-negative diplococci within polymorphonuclear leukocytes on Gram stain of the pharyngeal or rectal mucosa, particularly in symptomatic individuals, and diagnosis is confirmed by culture of *N. gonorrhoeae*. The sensitivity of Gram stain compared with culture is about 50 percent in infections of the rectum or pharynx. Treatment of both rectal and pharyngeal gonorrhea is presented in Table 1.

Anorectal or oral syphilis is commonly asymptomatic and presents as a painless chancre. Darkfield examination is often inadequate since nonpathogenic treponemes are often present within the gastrointestinal tract and may be misdiagnosed for *Treponema pallidum*. Therefore, diagnosis is frequently dependent on the demonstration of seropositivity. A further discussion on diagnosis and treatment of syphilis is presented elsewhere in this volume.

In homosexual men with gastrointestinal symptoms, the presence of anorectal pain and a mucopurulent or bloody discharge suggests proctitis or proctocolitis. Proctitis is commonly associated with tenesmus and constipation, whereas proctocolitis is more often associated with diarrhea. In both, anoscopy usually shows the presence of friability, mucus, and pus, which should be sampled for microbiologic studies and Gram stain. Most cases of proctitis are due to *N. gonorrhoeae*, herpes simplex virus, *C. trachomatis*, or primary or secondary syphilis. Rectal infection with *Chlamydia* is indistinguishable from rectal gonorrhea. Symptoms are often absent or mild. Infection with *C. trachomatis* of the LGV serovar is more pathogenic and often associated with systemic symptoms. Rectal involvement may be characterized by severe anorectal pain, bloody mucopurulent discharge, and tenesmus. LGV infection of the rectum may present as acute ulcerative proctocolitis with evidence of granuloma formation on biopsy specimens. Sigmoidoscopy often reveals diffuse friability in the rectum, with discrete ulcerations occasionally extending to the descending colon. Strictures and fistulas may be prominent, and these can often be misdiagnosed clinically for Crohn's disease or carcinoma of the rectum. Diagnosis of chlamydial proctitis or proctocolitis is made by isolation of *C. trachomatis* in culture. The new rapid diagnostic tests for *C. trachomatis* have not been very helpful for detecting rectal infection. Treatment for chlamydial infection consists of tetracycline, 500 mg four times a day orally for 1 week for non-LGV infections and up to 3 to 4 weeks for LGV infections, depending on response.

Herpes infection in homosexual men can often involve the rectum, the perianal area, the oral cavity, and/or the pharynx. Symptoms of anorectal herpes include localized pain, constipation, rectal discharge, hematochezia, fever, chills, malaise, and headache. Neurologic symptoms include paresthesias, dysesthesias, neuralgia, difficulty with micturition, impotence, and severe constipation. Diagnosis of anorectal HSV infection is based on the clinical appearance of herpetic vesicles or ulcerations—interally, externally, or both—and on the recovery of herpes in culture. Treatment is supportive with use of analgesics, sitz baths, and stool softeners. Acyclovir has not been adequately tested for the treatment of anorectal herpes.

Proctocolitis or colitis reflects more extensive inflammation involving the rectum and colon and is usually caused by enteric pathogens such as *Campylobacter*,

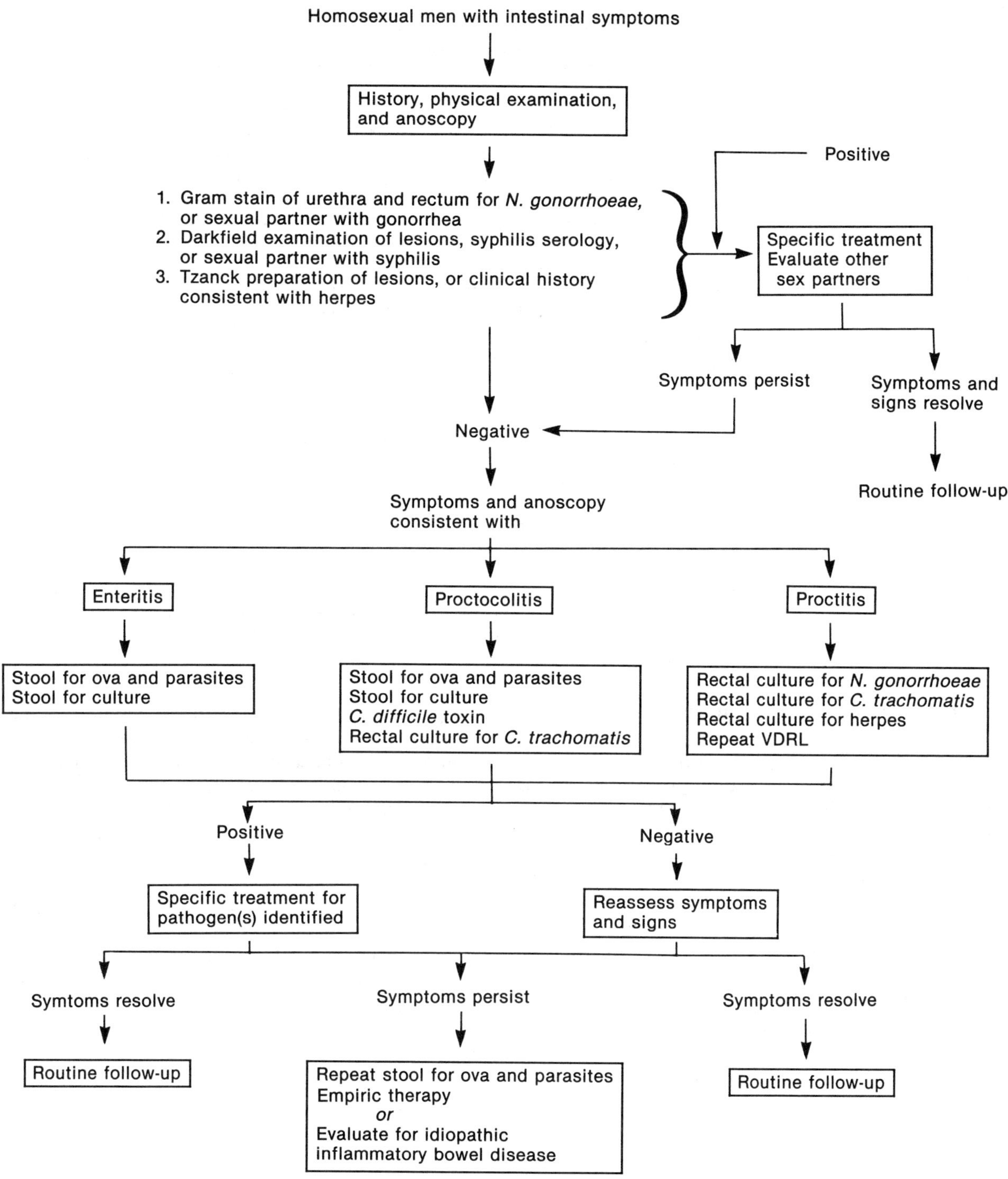

Figure 1 Evaluation of homosexual men with intestinal or anorectal symptoms.

Shigella, Salmonella, E. histolytica, and *C. trachomatis* of the LGV serovar. A history of recent antibiotic use should suggest evaluation for *Clostridium difficile* infection. Treatment regimens are outlined in Table 2 for infections with these pathogens.

The occurrence of diarrhea and abdominal bloating or cramping, without anorectal symptoms, in association with normal anoscopy and sigmoidoscopy, is consistent with inflammation of the small intestine or enteritis. In homosexual men, enteritis limited to the small intestine is often attributable to *Giardia lamblia*, but *Campylobacter, Shigella, E. histolytica,* and *Cryptosporidium* can produce enterocolitis with or without lesions involving the distal colon or rectum. Diagnosis of these pathogens is made by a stool culture for enteric pathogens and stool examination for ova and parasites. Therapeutic options

TABLE 2 Treatment of Enteric Infections Commonly Seen in Homosexual Men

Specific Infection	*Recommended Treatment*	*Alternative*
Entamoeba histolytica	Metronidazole 750 mg PO 3 times a day for 10 days	Diiodohydroxyquine 650 mg PO 3 times a day for 20 days
Giardia lamblia	Metronidazole 250 mg PO 3 times a day for 7 days	Quinacrine hydrochloride 100 mg PO 3 times a day for 7 days
Shigella species	Trimethoprim-sulfamethoxazole (160 mg/800 mg) PO twice a day for 7 days	Ampicillin 500 mg PO 4 times a day for 7 days
Campylobacter species	Erythromycin 500 mg PO 4 times a day for 7 days	Tetracycline 500 mg PO 4 times a day for 7 days
Salmonella species	Antibiotics not recommended except for severe, bacteremic cases	Chloramphenicol 500 mg IV q6h for 10 days; ampicillin 1 g IV q4h for 10 days; trimethoprim-sulfamethoxazole 2 tabs q12h for 10 days (these are therapeutically equivalent regimens)
Cryptosporidium species	Supportive, fluid therapy; spiramycin* 1.0 g PO 4 times a day	
Isospora belli	Supportive, fluid therapy; spiramycin* 1.0 g PO 4 times a day	

* Cryptosporidia and isospora infections do not require treatment in immunocompetent patients. Spiramycin recommended for infections in AIDS patients only. Treat until there is a response and then for an additional week.

for proctocolitis and enteritis are varied and will be influenced by the cause (bacterial or protozoan), by local differences in the prevalence of enteric pathogens, by the patterns of antimicrobial susceptibility of these pathogens, and by the availability of timely microbiologic diagnostic support.

The etiologic diagnosis of proctitis, proctocolitis, and enteritis in homosexual men is compounded by the frequency of mixed infections. It is not uncommon that a homosexual man with one infection will later be found to have additional pathogens present. Symptoms will frequently persist despite adequate treatment of a documented infection. Reinfection, poor compliance, antimicrobial resistance, or the presence of multiple infections may be responsible for persistence of symptoms. Therefore, repeat evaluations or empiric therapy based on signs and symptoms of clinical syndrome may be warranted. Since all of the agents discussed above are sexually transmitted, appropriate treatment of sexual partners is indicated to prevent reinfection and to reduce community spread of these pathogens. Homosexually active men should also be counseled that oral-anal sex with multiple male partners is associated with a high risk of intestinal infection. Furthermore, the presence of intestinal rectal symptoms should lead to medical consultation and cessation of sexual contact until a specific diagnosis is made, therapy is given, and cure is documented.

SINUSITIS

BURTON A. WAISBREN, B.S., M.S., M.D, F.A.C.P., F.A.S.I.D.

The striking feature of my reflection of 30 years of seeing and treating sinusitis is the dichotomy between what I have read and what I have seen in my office. This presentation will concentrate on the latter.

INITIAL DIAGNOSIS AND TREATMENT

Lucy Freeman, in an enjoyable book entitled *Flight from Fear* (delightful for those who do not suffer from sinus trouble), emphasized many years ago that hostility is an important cause of sinus trouble. At the first interview, facing up to this possibility with the patient is as important a maneuver as any other. It may take months of psychiatric care to achieve acceptance on the part of both the patient and the doctor that sinusitis is a psychiatric problem; this etiologic factor must always be kept in mind and attempts made to deal with it.

The second immediate maneuver for the physician is to inquire into the use, and usually the overuse, of decongestants. I believe that these should seldom, if ever, be used. However, the first few days without them are painful for the patient who gives them up, and the patient must be warned of this fact.

The third maneuver is saline lavage performed with an ear syringe filled with warm saline (a pinch of salt in a glass of water). If used three times a day for several days this procedure usually heals the mucosa that has been battered by the decongestant, allows its swelling to subside, and, most important, allows drainage to begin.

Fourth, the patients should be taught to breathe steam after each lavage, perhaps by putting a towel over the head, bending over the wash basin, and turning on hot water while inhaling the steam. They then may find it advantageous to put hot moist towels over the face for 10–15 minutes.

This approach to sinus complaints will, in my experience, resolve the great majority of such problems providing the patient can be made to acknowledge psychological as well as the addictive aspects of the nasal decongestants. However, when the problem is recurrent, I often add tetracycline, 500 mg three times a day for 4 days, to the steam lavage and instruct the patient to start the entire program as soon as the congestion, headache, and sore face that signal an attack of sinus trouble begin. Tetracycline is not indicated if the patient is hypersensitive to it or if the organism is resistant; in the latter case the choice of antibiotic should be based on the results of in vitro studies.

With the knowledge that this five-pronged approach will solve the vast majority of sinus problems, let us consider the type of case that might drive a physician to a reference book of this sort. What pathologic processes or deficiencies can lead to chronic recurrent sinusitis? These will be listed in the order in which they should be ruled out, but not necessarily in their order of recurrence. Here, again, the proposed system is the one I use in my clinical practice.

ETIOLOGIC CONSIDERATIONS AND DIAGNOSTIC WORK-UP

Culturing the nasal secretions is rarely of help, since one rarely cultures known pathogens. The one exception to this is when a pure culture of coagulase-positive staphylococci is obtained on repeated cultures. In this case specific, intense treatment of the staphylococcus is in order. I never use a single agent to treat a serious staphylococcal infection because when this organism is recalcitrant or in an inaccessible place, one ought to try to attack it not only at its cell membranes, but at its ribosomal apparatus as well. For this, oxacillin and lincomycin, given in divided doses of 1.5 g per day for 10 days, are an easily tolerated and safe regimen.

Quantitative immunoglobulins should be studied next. Intractable sinusitis is the usual presenting symptom of immunoglobulin A deficiency, which is the most common immunodeficiency disease. The lack of secretory immunoglobulin A (IgA) causes inability of mucous membranes to protect themselves adequately, and the sinuses are particularly vulnerable.

A second immunologic deficiency disease that might be the cause, particularly of staphylococcal sinusities, is Job's disease, which should be ruled out by an IgE determination and, if available, a polymorphonuclear movement study.

A third immune disease to be sought in difficult cases is granulomatous disease of children, or even adults, in which case tests of polymorphonuclear function show abnormalities. In the case of either Job's disease or granulomatous disease, treatment of the sinusitis depends on control of the underlying immune deficiency with long-term antibiotic and immunomodulation therapy.

Roentgenograms of the sinuses are indicated in all cases of intractable sinusitis, and they occasionally reveal cysts, tumors, or other indications for surgery. However, any type of surgical intervention in sinusitis, whether local lavage or the notorious Caldwell-Luc operation, is usually counterproductive.

Bone scans, on the other hand, are often useful, since they may reveal osteomyelitis of the temporal or maxillary bones, in which case intensive, long-term treatment for this disease is indicated. By the same token, indium scans are helpful because they may reveal a drainable abscess requiring surgery.

A nasal smear may often be helpful in formulating a therapeutic program for sinusitis. If the smear reveals only eosinophils, one would tend to be more aggressive in searching for an allergic cause for the disease.

Additional features of the patient's history to be considered on the initial contact are history of aspirin sensitivity; presence of nasal polyps, bronchitis, asthma, smoking, recurrent boils, recurrent pneumonia; and in this day and age, life style.

Nasal polyps are not an unusual accompaniment to chronic sinusitis and must always be considered. As an internist I have never been able to get a good look into the nasal cavity and suggest that this should be done by an expert. When one finds nasal polyps, aspirin sensitivity should be considered. The patient may have to give up aspirin entirely and even may need to search out a salicylate-free diet. When one finds polyps, asthma often is a factor as well and, in fact, may be the problem that needs the most attention. The treatment of nasal polyps with beclomethasone nasal spray 42 μg per metered spray has been a major development in the control of this condition, and since it has been used the necessity for "scooping out' nasal polyps at frequent intervals seems to have decreased.

OTHER ETIOLOGIES

When one arrives at the point where hostility, drainage, moderate antibiotic use, nasal polyps, aspirin sensitivity, asthma, and immune deficiency have been considered and treated or ruled out, five other possibilities must be considered if symptoms persist. These are fungal infection, bronchiectasis, cystic fibrosis, a tumor, or mixed bacterial infection with anaerobes.

Although one should try to obtain an accurate culture of the sinus secretions, it is often necessary to treat empirically with a combination of antibiotics that will destroy anaerobes and attack resistant bacteria at more than one metabolic site. For this I suggest a combination of chloramphenicol 2 grams per day, lincomycin 1.5 grams per day, and Flagyl 1 gram per day with 10 ml of gamma globulin given as a potentiator. Others may desire to use more conservative and traditional antibiotic combinations.

When one orders cultures for fungi, it should always be remembered that *Actinomyces* is an anaerobic fungus and that blastomycosis is usually best diagnosed by biopsy. Of course, mucomycosis must always be considered as a cause of chronic invading sinusitis in diabetic patients. Blastomycosis and mucomycosis respond to amphotericin B total dose of 1.5 grams; a daily dose of 5 to 20 mg can be increased from 5 mg per day by 5-mg increments to 20 mg per day, provided the patient's blood urea nitrogen level does not become elevated. This is continued until the patient gets a total dose of 1.5 grams. Of course, penicillin is the drug of choice for actinomycosis. Penicillin G 10 million units IV per day for 1 month will cure actinomycosis. It can be given on an outpatient basis via a subclavian catheter left in place. Treatment should be prolonged in these cases for at least a month.

The diagnosis of cystic fibrosis, even in young adults, or of bronchiectasis should be relatively easy if one thinks of them.

Tumors of the sinuses are not rare and they should always be sought in problem cases. The computed tomographic scan will prove a valuable tool when it is added to the more traditional roentgenograms and bone scans. Wegener's granulomatosis is the most common tumor of the sinuses, but the literature abounds with case reports of neoplasms of various other types. The tissue diagnosis in these cases will direct treatment.

Finally, in addition to the immunologic work-up mentioned in the beginning of this paper, in today's society the advent of intractable sinusitis is not infrequently the first manifestation of an acquired immune deficiency (AIDS). As is becoming well known, AIDS is best diagnosed by the test for HTV-III and by T-cell subsets, which should show a deficiency of helper T-cells. Beta-2-microglobulin, for some reason, is also markedly elevated in this disease.

INFECTIOUS DIARRHEA: A PATIENT IN THE UNITED STATES

CYNTHIA S. WEIKEL, M.D.
RICHARD L. GUERRANT, M.D.

Acute infectious diarrhea is a common problem affecting people of all ages throughout the world. In addition to being a major cause of mortality in crowded, tropical, developing areas, it remains second only to the common cold as a cause of morbidity in the United States. In suburban homes, enteric illnesses affect each person from one to three times each year, with the highest rates among young children and those most closely exposed to young children. In contrast to the summer or rainy season peaks of diarrhea in tropical areas, the predominant season of diarrhea in the United States, as in most developed, temperate areas, is in the winter months, with a lesser peak in the late summer months.

PATHOGENESIS OF INFECTION

Microbial Virulence Factors and Host Defenses

Certain microbial virulence and host-defense factors (Table 1) guide the practitioner's approach to the diagnosis and management of infectious diarrhea. As most enteric infections are acquired either directly or indirectly via the fecal-oral route, the characteristic infectious dose of different microorganisms influences the epidemiologic setting of infection. For example, organisms such as *Shigella* and amebic and giardial cysts are readily transmitted (low infectious dose), which accounts for their frequent spread by close interpersonal contact, as in day care centers or among promiscuous gay males. In contrast, the infectious dose of 10^5 organisms or greater required for *Salmonella, Vibrio*, enterotoxigenic *Escherichia coli*, and others is responsible for the more typical association of these organisms with food or waterborne outbreaks.

Recent advances in our understanding of microbial virulence factors have provided new concepts regarding what constitutes an enteric pathogen. For example, *E. coli* may be a harmless component of the normal flora, enteroadherent (resulting in destruction of the brush border and diarrheal illness), enterotoxin-producing (causing

TABLE 1 Factors Guiding Approach to Diagnosis and Management of Infectious Diarrhea

Host Defenses	*versus*	*Microbial Virulence Factors*
Hygiene		Infectious dose
Gastric acid		Adherence
Mucus		Enterotoxins
Immunity (especially IgA)		Cytotoxins
Motility		Invasiveness
Flora		

cholera-like diarrhea), or capable of mucosal invasion (resulting in Shigella-like dysentery), all depending on whether specific virulence plasmids are present at a given time in a particular strain. Consequent limitations on the diagnostic usefulness of taxonomic identification of agents without attention to specific virulence traits are obvious. Even among parasitic pathogens such as *Entamoeba histolytica*, recent developments are now clarifying that certain strains appear to be potentially invasive and others are not, possibly related to certain zymodeme (enzyme) markers.

Alteration of several host factors is recognized to predispose to a number of enteric infections. Diminished gastric acidity and, possibly, mucus production may decrease the infectious dose (e.g., of *Salmonella*) required for illness. Hypogammaglobulinemia (especially selective IgA immunodeficiency) is associated with an increased incidence of enteric infections, particularly giardiasis. Disturbance of normal motility of the gut (e.g., as in diabetes mellitus) may predispose to bacterial overgrowth and altered enteric microflora. Antibiotics routinely alter enteric microflora and may establish an ecologic niche for enteric pathogens such as *Clostridium difficile* or *Salmonella*.

Characterization of Diarrheal Illness

It is useful and significant to consider two basic types of acute infectious diarrhea (Table 2). The noninflammatory diarrheas are much commoner than the inflammatory types and arise either from the action of an enterotoxin or from a selective functional impairment that results in net fluid and electrolyte secretion, usually in the upper small bowel. Etiologic agents of noninflammatory watery diarrhea include *Vibrio cholerae*, enterotoxigenic *E. coli* (ETEC), enteropathogenic *E. coli* (EPEC), rotaviruses, Norwalk-like viruses *Giardia lamblia*, and *Cryptosporidium*. With these etiologies, gross blood and pus as well as microscopic evidence of fecal leukocytes are usually absent. In contrast, inflammatory diarrhea usually results from a more distal invasive process, usually in the colon, which causes a dysenteric syndrome with sheets of fecal polymorphonuclear leukocytes on methylene blue examination. Characteristic pathogens that cause inflammatory diarrhea include nontyphi *Salmonella* species, *Shigella, Campylobacter jejuni, Clostridium difficile* (which may also be associated with noninflammatory "antibiotic-associated" diarrhea), and *Yersinia enterocolitica* (certain serotypes). Although amebic dysentery may be characteristically bloody, fecal leukocytes are often pyknotic or absent, perhaps because of the cytocidal effect of this protozoan parasite.

TABLE 2 Two Types of Infectious Diarrhea

	Noninflammatory	*Inflammatory*
Mechanism	Enterotoxin or reduced absorptive surface	Mucosal invasion
Characteristic location	Small bowel	Colon
Type of diarrhea	Watery	Dysenteric
Presumptive diagnosis	No fecal WBC	Sheets of fecal PMNs
Examples	*V. cholerae* ETEC, EPEC Rotaviruses Norwalk-like viruses *G. lamblia* *Strongyloides* *Cryptosporidium*	*Salmonella* *Shigella* *C. jejuni* *C. difficile* *Y. enterocolitica* *Vibrio* species *E. histolytica** ? *Aeromonas*

* Although an invasive pathogen, *E. histolytica* may be associated with only pyknotic or absent fecal leukocytes. However, blood in the stool is characteristic.

EPIDEMIOLOGY AND DIFFERENTIAL DIAGNOSIS

The list of recognized enteric pathogens has expanded rapidly in the last decade (Table 3). The goal must be to determine the likeliest pathogen on the basis of frequency of occurrence, age of the patient, season of the year, and epidemiologic setting—including travel, sexual history, and food exposures. The differential diagnosis as it relates to a specific epidemiologic setting is summarized in Tables 3 to 6. Particular consideration should be given to the evaluation for potentially treatable pathogens.

Most community-acquired diarrheal illness still remains unexplained. Overall, viruses probably cause most acute, self-limited diarrhea. The major viral causes of enteritis—rotaviruses (especially in children younger than 2 years of age) and Norwalk-like viruses—predominate

TABLE 3 Etiologic Agents of Acute Diarrhea

Bacterial	ETEC EPEC *Campylobacter* (*C. jejuni* and campylobacter-like organisms) *Salmonella* *Shigella* *C. difficile* EIEC *Y. enterocolitica* *Vibrio* species *Aeromonas* *M. avium — M. intracellulare** *Plesiomonas*†
Viral	Rotaviruses Norwalk-like agents Cytomegalovirus* Adenovirus* Coxsackievirus*
Parasitic	*G. lamblia* *Cryptosporidium*‡ *Strongyloides*‡ *E. histolytica*

* Primarily seen in immunodeficient hosts, including AIDS patients and bone marrow transplant recipients.
† Rare cause of diarrhea; the role of antibiotics in therapy is unclear.
‡ Occurs in both immunocompetent and immunodeficient hosts; strikingly severe illnesses may occur in the latter (e.g., 17 liters of stool/day with *Cryptosporidium* or hyperinfection syndrome with *Strongyloides*).

during winter months, whereas the bacterial and certain parasitic pathogens predominate in the summer and fall months. Although most infectious agents cause diarrhea throughout life, rotaviruses typically cause sporadic and, occasionally, epidemic, illness primarily in children younger than 2 years of age. Diarrhea may last 5 to 8 days and may cause significant dehydration. Although immunity develops in the vast majority of the population, mild illnesses with abdominal cramping and mild diarrhea have been associated with rotaviral infection in close, adult family contacts of infected young children. In contrast, Norwalk-like agents are the leading cause of brief (24 to 48 hours) epidemic gastroenteritis and cause disease primarily in adults.

Travel to a tropical developing area is an important historical point to elicit. Short-lived noninflammatory diarrhea in this setting is most likely due to enterotoxigenic *E. coli*. In contrast, certain parasitic infections—in particular, those due to *Giardia, Cryptosporidium*, and *Stronglyoides stercoralis*—may cause more prolonged noninflammatory diarrhea and/or upper abdominal discomfort. The more serious problem of inflammatory diarrhea in this setting raises a spectrum of possibilities including *C. jejuni, Salmonella, Shigella,* enteroinvasive *E. coli* (EIEC) and *E. histolytica*. In addition, travel within the United States may pose certain risks for diarrheal disease. Both *G. lamblia* and *C. jejuni* infections have been reported among hikers or campers drinking unpurified stream water.

Homosexual men provide an important challenge to the diagnostic skills of the clinician. The potential etiologies for intestinal illness are protean and, more significantly, may be multiple in 20 percent or more of patients (Table 4; also see Infections Other Than AIDS Commonly Found in Homosexual Men). Initial evaluation should include rectal Gram stain to evaluate for gonorrhea (gram-negative diplococci are seen in only about 50 percent of culture-positive cases) and anoscopy to identify lesions suitable for darkfield examination and consistent with primary or secondary syphilis. Anorectal herpes simplex viral (HSV) infection is frequently a distinctive syndrome characterized by severe anorectal pain, constitutional symptoms, inguinal lymphadenopathy, and neurologic signs such as difficulty urinating and sacral paresthesias. If these diagnoses cannot be made or the patient has symptoms consistent with enteritis, sigmoidoscopy should be done. This will enable additional specimens for culture to be taken and identify whether the rectal pathology extends beyond 15 cm, which would necessitate further evaluation (e.g., stool cultures and examination for parasites or ova).

Day care centers are an additional epidemiologic setting associated with multiple diarrheal pathogens (Table 5). To date, most outbreaks of diarrhea in day care centers have been associated with *Shigella* or *Giardia* and person-to-person transmission of organisms with a low infectious inoculum (10^1–10^2 bacteria or cysts, respectively). In contrast to shigella infections, which occur in children of all ages, both rotaviral and giardial infections appear to occur primarily in children younger than age 3 who are not toilet trained. Furthermore, outbreaks of diarrhea in day care centers are associated with significant secondary attack rates (10% to 30% in most studies) in the children's families.

Food poisoning is an important, but underestimated, public health problem, with more than 200 reported etiologies. Bacterial contamination of food accounts for more than 90 percent of the total cases in outbreaks where an etiology is determined. However, a specific etiology is identified in only 40 percent of outbreaks. An "outbreak" is defined by the Centers for Disease Control as an incident in which two or more persons experience a similar illness after ingestion of a food epidemiologically implicated as the source of the illness. There are two exceptions: a single case of botulism or chemical poisoning is considered an outbreak.

For convenience in diagnosis, food-poisoning syndromes are best categorized into four groups (Table 6). *Staphylococcus aureus* is the prototypic etiology of short-lived (less than 24 hours) upper gastrointestinal illness due to ingestion of preformed toxin where nausea and vomiting predominate and fever occurs in less than 25 percent of cases. In contrast, ingestion of toxigenic *Clostridium perfringens* results in an illness dominated by noninflammatory diarrhea and abdominal cramps where nausea, vomiting, and fever are uncommon. The commonest recognized cause of food poisoning, *Salmonella*, and other pathogens causing primarily distal ileal and colonic disease, result in inflammatory diarrhea, with polymorphonuclear leukocytes on stool examination with methylene blue.

Recognition of botulism, ciguatera, and certain shellfish poisoning is particularly critical because of the poten-

TABLE 4 Intestinal Infections in Homosexual Men

Proctitis	*Neisseria gonorrhoeae* Herpes simplex virus (mostly type 2) *Chlamydia trachomatis* (non-LGV serotypes) *Treponema pallidum*
Proctocolitis*	*Campylobacter* species† *Shigella flexneri* *C. trachomatis* (LGV serotype) E. histolytica C. difficile
Enteritis‡	*G. lamblia*

* Abnormalities in rectal mucosa extend beyond 15 cm on sigmoidoscopic examination.
† Includes *C. jejuni, fetus*, and campylobacter-like organisms.
‡ Normal sigmoidoscopic examination.

TABLE 5 Pathogens Associated with Outbreaks of Diarrhea in Day Care Centers

Bacterial	*Shigella* *Campylobacter* *C. difficile*
Protozoal	*G. lamblia* *Cryptosporidium*
Viral	Rotavirus

TABLE 6 Food-Poisoning Syndromes

Pathogen	*Source*	*Incubation Time*
Upper gastrointestinal illness (nausea and vomiting predominate)		
*S. aureus**	Meat, poultry, potato and egg salads, cream-filled pastries	1–6 hrs
Bacillus cereus	Rice	1–6 hrs
Heavy metal (Ca, Zn, Cd, Sn)	Acidic or carbonated beverages in rusty or galvanized containers	5 min–2 hrs
Upper small bowel illnesses (noninflammatory diarrhea predominates)		
C. perfringens†	Beef, poultry, ham, lobster	6–24 hrs
B. cereus	Meat, vegetables	6–24 hrs
Distal, ileal, and colonic invasive diseases (inflammatory diarrhea predominates)		
Nontyphoidal *Salmonella*‡ species	Meat, poultry, eggs, fish, salads	6–48 hrs
Shigella species	Waterborne; fish, mixed salads	16–72 hrs
C. jejuni	Poultry, raw milk, waterborne	16–48 hrs
V. parahemolyticus and noncholerae vibrios	Raw or uncooked seafood, waterborne	Usually 24 hrs (range 4–92 hrs)
Y. enterocolitica	Meat, dairy products, waterborne	16–48 hrs
Neurologic disease, usually with gastrointestinal symptoms		
C. botulinium	Usually homemade canned foods; bean or potato salad, meat pies; commercially canned food	6 hrs–8 days; usually 12–36 hrs
Fish poisoning§		
(1) Scombroid	Scombroid fish (tuna including commercially canned; mackeral, bonito, skipjack); dolphin Hawaii/California	1 hr–24 hrs; usually <12 hrs
(2) Ciguatera	Grouper, amberjack, barracuda, red snapper Hawaii/Florida	1 hr–24 hrs; usually <30 min
Shellfish poisoning§ ("red tide")	Bivalve mollusks (mussels, clams, oysters, scallops)	5 min–4 hrs; usually <30 min
Mushroom poisoning	"Wild" mushrooms	Median onset, 2 hrs–12 hrs
(1) Immediate (median onset, 2 hrs): prognosis good; multiple manifestations including gastroenteritis, acute psychosis, parasympathetic hyperactivity and reactions similar to alcohol intoxication or disulfiram use		
(2) Delayed (median onset, 12 hrs): prognosis poor; triphasic illness: phase 1, gastrointestinal illness occasionally with bloody diarrhea; phase 2, occurs 2–3 days later, symptom-free but deterioration of hepatic and renal function; phase 3, hepatorenal failure		

* Commonest cause of food poisoning with an incubation period less than 6 hours.
† Commonest cause of food poisoning with an incubation period of 6 to 24 hours.
‡ The most commonly reported cause of foodborne outbreaks.
§ Fish and shellfish poisoning account for approximately one-half of all food poisonings of chemical etiology.

tial for these illnesses to progress to paralysis and respiratory arrest. Shellfish poisoning may be paralytic (associated with ingestion of bivalve mollusks of New England, Alaska, or the West Coast) or neurotoxic and less serious (associated with shellfish from the Florida coastal region). All of the paralytic illnesses may be accompanied by gastrointestinal symptoms including nausea, vomiting, diarrhea, and abdominal cramps. Notably, patients ingesting the neurotoxin(s) of *Clostridium botulinum* will usually develop a symmetrical, descending paralysis with diplopia, ptosis, dysphonia, and, ultimately, respiratory arrest. Distinguishing features of ciguatera poisoning include paresthesias and shooting muscle and dental pains. The features of paralytic shellfish poisoning overlap with those already mentioned, but the implicated food is distinct. In contrast, the nonfatal scombroid fish poisoning results in a histamine-like reaction (flushing, lip swelling, urticaria, dizziness, pruritis) and symptoms of gastroenteritis.

A recent history of antibiotic use should increase the clinician's suspicion of antibiotic-associated diarrhea due to *C. difficile* It is important to note that 25 percent of cases begin up to 6 weeks after antibiotics have been discontinued. Fecal leukocytes are detectable in more than one-half of these patients, and fever and abdominal tenderness or pain may be marked.

Immunocompromised patients are prone to develop diarrheal illness with both common and uncommon pathogens, which, on occasion, leads to serious systemic illness. Table 3 lists pathogens strongly associated with diarrhea in immunodeficient hosts. Important examples of pathogens causing systemic illness following initial gastrointestinal disease include *Campylobacter fetus* subspecies *fetus, Y. enterocolitica* (e.g., causing hepatic abscess seen primarily in diabetics and patients with iron overload), *Mycobacterium avium intracellulare* (in particular in AIDS patients), nontyphoidal *Salmonella* species (associated with AIDS and lymphoreticular malignancies), cytomegalovirus, and *S. stercoralis* (syndrome of hyperinfection associated with sepsis due to multiple gram-negative rods; pulmonary infiltrates; and, on occasion, meningitis). In contrast, pasteurized milk products contaminated with *Listeria monocytogenes* may lead to systemic infection without gastrointestinal symptoms. Due to the frequent use of antibiotics in this patient population, antibiotic-associated diarrhea caused by *C. difficile* must be considered in the differential diagnosis. In addition, infections with *G. lamblia* or *Cryptosporidium* may be severe and prolonged in patients with hypogammaglobulinemia. Last, chemotherapeutic agents (e.g., methotrexate, cyclophosphamide, *cis*-platinum, vincristine) must be considered as potential noninfectious etiologies of gastrointestinal disease in the immunodeficient host. Of note, are reports suggesting an association between certain chemotherapeutic agents (i.e., methotrexate) and *C. difficile* disease, although a more significant factor is probably the frequent use of antibiotics in this patient population.

DIAGNOSIS AND MANAGEMENT

As shown in Figure 1, a careful history should be taken for fever, bloody diarrhea, tenesmus, and abdominal pain. In addition, a careful epidemiologic history for recent travel, sexual preference, exposure to day care centers, recent foods (e.g., seafood), outbreaks of gastrointestinal illness among others known to the patient, antibiotic use, and conditions associated with immunocompromise must be obtained.

Stool Cultures and Special Examination Procedures

The first decision after obtaining the history and physical examination is whether to get a fecal specimen. Fortunately, several clues can be helpful in selecting those specimens likeliest to yield a useful result. If any epidemiologic or historical features suggestive of an inflammatory diarrhea are elicited, a fecal specimen (obtained in a cup is preferable to a rectal swab) may be useful for both gross and microscopic examination. The presence of blood or leukocytes suggests pathogens associated with an inflammatory process (Table 2) and is important for both therapeutic and epidemiologic reasons. In addition, parasites that may cause acute diarrhea—*G. lamblia, E. histolytica*, or *S. stercoralis*—may be seen in these intial wet-mount preparations. Unfortunately, swab specimens or specimens obtained after any barium radiographic procedures are often falsely negative.

With the burgeoning number of recognized potentially infectious agents that may cause diarrhea, indiscriminate culture and examination of stool specimens for all potential pathogens has become prohibitive. However, if there is a significant history of fever, bloody diarrhea, tenesmus, or abdominal pain or if there are sheets of polymorphonuclear leukocytes on microscopic examination, it is certainly appropriate to culture for *C. jejuni, Salmonella, Shigella*, and, possibly, the recently increasingly appreciated *Aeromonas* species. *Salmonella* and *Shigella* require the standard selective media, whereas *C. jejuni* and *Aeromonas* require special blood agar plates with selective antibiotics.

Special studies for additional agents are dictated by the particular epidemiologic or clinical setting. For example, if unexplained abdominal pain or fever persists, cultures with cold enrichment should be requested for *Y. enterocolitica*. If there is chronic diarrhea beyond 10 days or weight loss, special stains and concentration should be done for *G. lamblia, Cryptosporidium*, and *S. stercoralis* and quantitative cultures of the small bowel

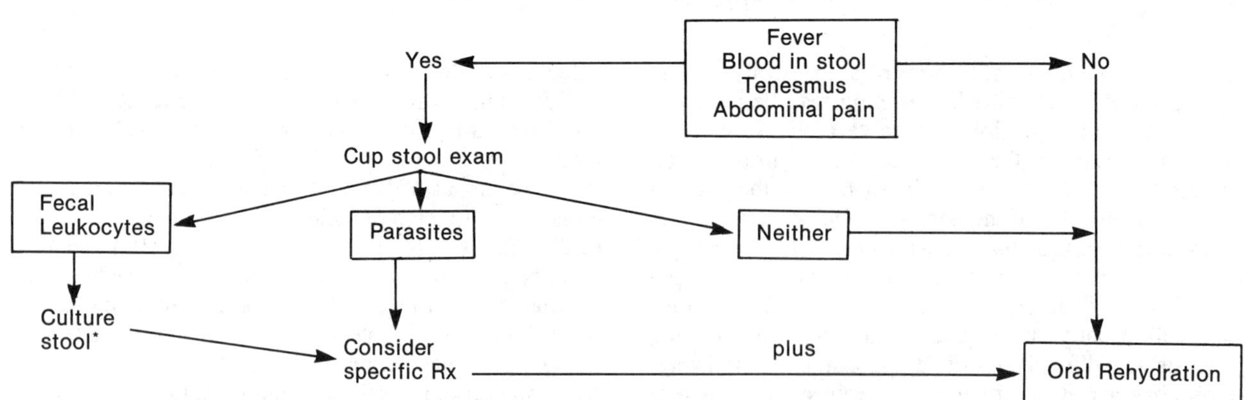

Figure 1 Initial evaluation and management of diarrhea. * Usually for *Salmonella, Shigella*, and *Campylobacter* unless epidemiologic history indicates additional examinations (see text).

for bacterial overgrowth should be considered. Occasionally, small bowel biopsy to identify *Giardia, Cryptosporidium* or pathologic changes consistent with gluten enteropathy, or Whipple's disease may be necessary.

If there is unexplained bloody diarrhea, stool should be examined for *E. histolytica*. If there is seafood or coastal exposure, a special laboratory request for culture for *Vibrio (parahemolyticus, cholerae*, and others) on thiosulfate citrate bile salt sucrose (TCBS) agar should be made. If there has been recent antibiotic use, sigmoidoscopy should be performed to document pseudomembranes (although some patients may have only more proximal colonic involvement), and antibiotics should be discontinued if at all possible. If diarrhea persists or the diagnosis remains unclear, culture for *C. difficile*, or, better yet, direct assay of stool for specifically neutralizable *C. difficile* cytotoxin using culture cells should be obtained.

In the case of suspected food or waterborne outbreaks, the public health department and, possibly, the Centers for Disease Control (in the case of botulism) should be promptly notified, and a food-specific attack rate for the common meal eaten by the affected individuals can be calculated. To be incriminated, a food must have a statistically significantly higher attack rate for those who ate it than those who did not, and almost all of those ill must have eaten the incriminated food. From this information, an incubation period should be estimated and may be diagnostically helpful, as discussed previously.

In the case of diarrhea or rectal symptoms in sexually promiscuous homosexual men, anoscopy and/or sigmoidoscopy may be helpful.

As shown in Table 4, the extent of anatomic involvement is helpful in determining the appropriate pathogens to consider and, thus, the diagnostic tests to be ordered. In the immunocompromised host with diarrheal disease, among other etiologies, one should consider auramine and modified acid-fast stain of stool for detection of *M. avium intracellulare* and *Cryptosporidium*. Furthermore, diagnosis of a specific etiology in immunocompromised patients may require biopsy of the small bowel or colon.

The documentation of rotaviral infection by use of the commercially available rotazyme test is usually not necessary or important in sporadic cases unless the patient is admitted to a hospital ward that requires isolation of rotavirus-infected children or unless this documentation is helpful in excluding other diagnostic possibilities. Likewise, the need to explore specifically for enterotoxins, invasiveness, and cytotoxins, or to serotype *E. coli* is unusual and not required for appropriate fluid management in most cases. Unexplained bloody diarrhea may warrant serotyping of *E. coli* for possible 0157 strains that have increasingly been associated with bloody diarrhea and hemolytic-uremic syndrome in children. Current techniques for identification of Norwalk-like viral agents require either immune electronmicroscopy with acute and convalescent sera or radioimmunoassay, a technique that is not widely available.

Therapy

The cornerstone of therapy for all forms of diarrheal illness is fluid and electrolyte replacement. In the vast majority of patients, this is best accomplished by oral rehydration. Table 7 describes the composition and ingredients required per liter of water in the simple oral rehydration solution recommended by the World Health Organization. Furthermore, temporary elimination of milk products from the diet should be recommended. During acute diarrhea, deficiency of lactase in the intestinal epithelial cell brush border may develop and prevent normal absorption of milk products, with a resulting osmotic effect that aggravates the illness. Despite the overall success of oral rehydration, some patients—particularly the very young, the elderly, and those with protracted vomiting or high fever—will require hospitalization and intravenous hydration.

The differentiation of diarrhea as inflammatory—by the fecal leukocyte examination—is critical both to determining the appropriate diagnostic evaluation and to the institution of therapy. In addition to oral fluids, noninflammatory diarrhea may be treated with absorbents such as kaolin plus pectin (Kaopectate), which serve only to change the consistency of the stools, antimotility agents (e.g., diphenoxylate, paregoric) or bismuth subsalicylate (Pepto-Bismol). In general, we discourage the use of antimotility agents because they occasionally increase toxicity and may precipitate toxic megacolon, particularly in patients with inflammatory diarrhea. Similarly, although large doses of bismuth subsalicylate (30 ml or 2 tablespoons orally every 30 minutes for eight doses) have been shown to be beneficial in diarrhea due to enterotoxigenic *E. coli* and, possibly, Norwalk-like viruses, the usefulness of this therapy in diarrhea of other etiologies is unknown.

Antimicrobial agents are indicated in certain bacterial and parasitic enteric infections (Table 8). In patients with high fever, moderate-to-severe abdominal pain and cramping, and/or bloody diarrhea with fecal leukocytes, initial evaluation—including a wet mount to identify the trophozoites of *E. histolytica* and darkfield examination for the darting motility or stool Gram stain (using carbolfuchsin instead of safranin counterstain) for the characteristic "seagull-appearing" gram-negative rods of

TABLE 7 Oral Rehydration Solution Recommended by the World Health Organization

Composition (mmol)		*Ingredients per liter (1.05 quart) of Water*	
Na^+	90	NaCl (salt)	3.5 g (¾ tsp)
Cl^-	80	$NaHCO_3$ (baking soda)	2.5 g (1 tsp)
K^+	20	KCl	1.5 g (1 cup orange juice or 2 bananas)
HCO_3^-	30		
Glucose	110	Sugar	40 g (4 tbsp)

TABLE 8 Treatment of Specific Diarrheal Diseases

Pathogen	Recommended Therapy*	Alternative Therapy*
Bacterial		
S. dysenteriae, S. flexneri	Trimethoprim 160 mg + sulfamethoxazole 800 mg PO bid × 3–5 days (1 double-strength tablet bid)	Tetracycline 2.5 g PO once *or* Ampicillin 500 mg PO qid × 3–5 days†
Nontyphoidal *Salmonella*‡ (extraintestinal only)	Trimethoprim 160 mg + sulfamethoxazole 800 mg PO bid × 2 weeks§	Ampicillin 2 g IV q4h × 2 weeks‖ *or* Chloramphenicol 50 mg/kg/day in 4 divided doses PO or IV × 2 weeks
C. jejuni	Erythromycin 250 mg PO qid × 5 days#	Gentamicin 3–5 mg/kg/day in 3 divided doses IV × 7–10 days**
C. difficile	Vancomycin 125–500 mg PO qid × 10 days	Metronidazole 250 mg PO qid ×10 days
Y. enterocolitica (extraintestinal)	Gentamicin 5 mg/kg/day given in 3 divided doses IV × 7–10 days *or* Trimethoprim-sulfamethoxazole	Cefotaxime 12 g/day IV given in divided doses q4h
Enterotoxigenic *E. coli*	Trimethoprim 160 mg + sulfamethoxazole 800 mg PO bid × 3–5 days	Ampicillin 500 mg PO qid × 3–5 days *or* Doxycycline 100 mg PO bid × 3–5 days
Parasitic		
G. lamblia	Quinacrine 100 mg PO tid × 7 days	Metronidazole†† 250 mg PO tid × 7–10 days *or* Furazolidone 100 mg PO qid × 7 days
E. histolytica	Metronidazole 750 mg PO tid × 5–10 days *plus* diloxanide furoate 500 mg PO tid × 10 days *or* Diiodohydroxyquin 650 mg PO tid × 21 days	Tetracycline 250 mg PO qid × 15 days *plus* chloroquine (base) 600 mg, 300 mg, then 150 mg PO tid × 14 days
S. stercoralis	Thiabendazole 25 mg/kg bid × 2 days	NA‡‡

* Dosages are for adults unless otherwise specified.
† Sensitivity testing must be done. Ampicillin-resistant strains are common. Do not use amoxicillin.
‡ Antibiotics for simple salmonella gastroenteritis may prolong carriage of the organism or increase the relapse rate.
§ Drug for IV therapy is not known. Serious gram-negative infections have been treated successfully with TMP/SMZ at dosages of 5–10 mg/kg/day (for the trimethoprim component) given in divided doses q8h.
‖ Sensitivity testing must be done.
\# Treatment has been shown to eradicate *C. jejuni* from the stool and perhaps to decrease the chance of relapse, but has not been shown to consistently alter the duration of symptoms.
** Reserved for bacteremic disease, which is seen primarily with *C. fetus* subspecies *fetus*.
†† Metronidazole has not been approved in the United States for therapy for giardiasis.
‡‡ NA = Not available.

C. jejuni—should be done. If these suggest *E. histolytica* or *C. jejuni* infection, specific theray may be instituted (Table 8). It should be noted that therapy for documented *C. jejuni* infections has not been shown to shorten the course of the illness, but does eradicate the organism from the stool and may decrease the incidence of relapses. If one suspects the diagnosis of shigellosis, therapy with trimethoprim-sulfamethoxazole may be prescribed. Of note, gastroenteritis due to nontyphoidal salmonellae may be associated with fecal leukocytes, and antibacterial therapy has been associated with increasing the risk of symptomatic and bacteriologic relapse and prolonged fecal carriage of *Salmonella* species. If antibiotic-associated *C. difficile* disease is suspected, antibiotics should be discontinued. If the disease persists or worsens, therapy with vancomycin or metronidazole should be considered. *Y. enterocolitica* usually causes a self-limited illness that requires therapy only if systemic complications occur.

The commonest cause of noninflammatory diarrhea among international travelers is enterotoxigenic *E. coli*. Although we do not advocate prophylactic antibiotics to prevent diarrheal disease during international travel, individuals developing noninflammatory diarrhea in this setting or upon returning to the United States may be treated with trimethoprim-sulfamethoxazole, which has been shown in a controlled treatment trial to shorten the duration of illness. The therapy for the common parasitic infections is listed in Table 8.

INFECTIOUS DIARRHEA: A PATIENT OUTSIDE THE UNITED STATES

HERBERT L. DuPONT, M.D.

Approximately 40 percent of persons traveling from a low-risk area, such as the United States, Canada, and northwestern Europe, to an area of high risk for acquiring diarrhea, which includes Latin America, southern and Southeast Asia, and Africa, develop diarrhea. The magnitude of the problem reflects the local rate of endemicity of diarrhea. Food and, to a lesser degree, water are the responsible vehicles of transmission. Bacterial agents cause approximately 80 percent of the illness, which explains the beneficial effect of antimicrobial agents in both the prevention and therapy of travelers' diarrhea.

For the average traveler to a high-risk area, exercising care about where and what one eats and drinks and being prepared to treat the illness should it occur represent the optimal approach. Eating at better restaurants (particularly if a local person can vouch for their safety) and selecting only steaming hot food, citrus fruits, bread, and bottled beverages will reduce the risk. For a select group of travelers, chemoprophylaxis is a useful way to prevent travelers' diarrhea (Fig. 1 and Table 1) Chemoprophylaxis is reasonable for the person on a critically important mission or for the person who is either more susceptible to diarrhea or to more serious effects of associated dehydration. This latter group should include patients with achlorhydria, those having had gastric resection, and anyone taking regular antacid therapy (i.e., cimetidine). The shorter the visit, the more reasonable the use of chemoprophylaxis. Stays of less than 1 week are the most appropriate for using this approach, and chemoprophylaxis probably should not be employed if a stay in a high-risk area exceeds 2 weeks. To prevent illness (rather than merely delaying it) the drugs should be started on the day of travel and continued for 1 to 2 days after return to the country of origin. Trimethoprim-sulfamethoxazole (TMP/SMZ) and doxycycline are both effective if used in areas where bacterial enteropathogens are susceptible. Bismuth subsalicylate (Pepto-Bismol) probably is not quite as effective, but it offers some advantages. Problems with the antimicrobial agents include development of rash (5%), sensitivity to sun in persons taking doxycycline, development of resistance of the in-

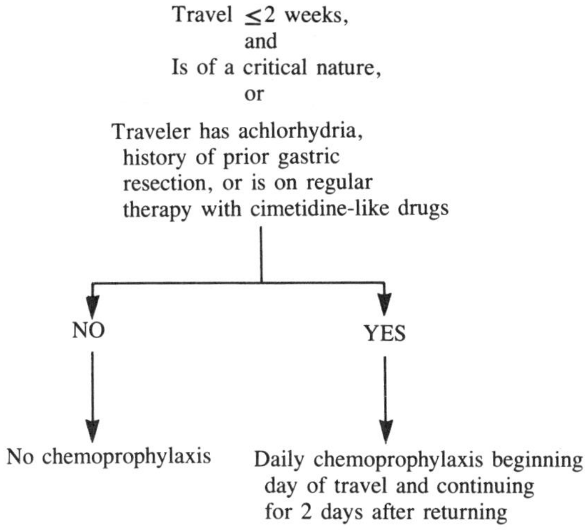

Travel ≤2 weeks,
and
Is of a critical nature,
or
Traveler has achlorhydria, history of prior gastric resection, or is on regular therapy with cimetidine-like drugs

NO → No chemoprophylaxis

YES → Daily chemoprophylaxis beginning day of travel and continuing for 2 days after returning

Figure 1 Indications for chemoprophylaxis for selected persons traveling from low- (United States, Canada, northwestern Europe) to high-risk areas (Latin America, southern and southeast Asia, Africa).

TABLE 1 Chemoprophylaxis of Travelers' Diarrhea

	Drugs	*Daily Dosage**
First choice:	trimethoprim-sulfamethoxazole (TMP/SMZ)	1 double-strength tablet (160 mg TMP/800 mg SMZ) once daily
Alternatives:	doxycycline;	100 mg once daily
	bismuth subsalicylate tablets†	2 tablets chewed thoroughly and swallowed 4 × day

* Dosages are for older children and adults.
† Pepto-Bismol.

TABLE 2 Indications for Empiric Therapy of Travelers' Diarrhea

Mild illness (≤3 unformed stools/day) with little or no associated symptomatology	Fluids only
Moderate illness (3–5 unformed stools/day) without fever, dysentery (bloody stools), or disabling associated symptoms	Symptomatic treatment (loperamide or bismuth subsalicylate*)
Severe illness (≥6 unformed stools) or diarrhea with fever, dysentery or disabling associated symptoms	Antimicrobial therapy with or without symptomatic treatment (TMP/SMZ or furazolidone)

* Pepto-Bismol.

TABLE 3 Therapy of Travelers' Diarrhea: Drugs and Dosage for Older Children and Adults

Drugs	*Dosage*
Loperamide	2 capsules initially, followed by 1 capsule after each unformed stool, not to exceed 8 capsules/day
Bismuth subsalicylate (Pepto-Bismol)	30 ml each 30 minutes × 8 doses (one 8-ounce bottle over 3.5 hours)
Trimethoprim-sulfamethoxazole	One double-strength tablet (160 mg TMP/800 mg SMZ) twice a day × 3–5 days
Furazolidone	100 mg four times/day × 5 days

testinal flora during drug administration, and more severe but less frequent adverse effects.

In treating the acute diarrhea of travelers to tropical areas, it is reasonable to base drug selection on the affected person's symptoms (Tables 2 and 3). Patients with any form of diarrhea should be encouraged to keep up with fluid and salt losses by drinking liquids, augmented by saltine crackers if necessary. Mild diarrhea with few other symptoms need be treated with no more than fluids. For diarrhea of moderate severity, a drug acting nonspecifically probably represents optimal therapy. Loperamide is probably the most effective drug available of those acting symptomatically. Bismuth subsalicylate (Pepto-Bismol), somewhat less active, reduces the diarrhea by about 50 percent. Antimicrobial agents should be reserved for those with more significant illness. This includes those not improved by symptomatic therapy, as well as any persons with more intense diarrhea (6 or more unformed stools per 24 hours), or if there is fever or dysentery (bloody stools), or if associated symptoms (nausea, abdominal pain, and cramps) are disabling. TMP/SMZ is the optimal drug to treat moderate to severe illness. The major treatable agents that would not respond to the combination drug are *Campylobacter* and *Giardia* (together responsible for about 5% of illness). The response to furazolidone therapy is not as rapid as it is for TMP/SMZ, but the drug has a broader spectrum of activity and includes the two organisms not responsive to TMP/SMZ. Travelers going to tropical areas from industrialized regions probably should go armed with a small supply of the two types of drugs used to treat moderate or severe illness.

INFECTION CAUSED BY INTESTINAL HELMINTHS

RAMÓN H. BERMÚDEZ, M.D., F.A.C.P.

The majority of human infections caused by worms are associated with the gastrointestinal tract or liver. These multicellular organisms may parasitize the lumen of the gut, the biliary tract, or the portal venous system, but in some circumstances, tissue invasion may occur as well. Intestinal helminthic infections may be asymptomatic; disease manifestations may, however, be localized to the gastrointestinal tract or there may be more systemic clinical features. Because of their worldwide prevalence, intestinal helminthic infections cause considerable morbidity and mortality. For the purpose of this discussion, worm infections are divided according to their human anatomic habitat and to their general taxonomic features (Table 1).

EPIDEMIOLOGY

Intestinal helminths cause common infections in many parts of the world. Although their prevalence has decreased in the developed countries, they still constitute a reason for concern, particularly in the immunocompromised host. Worm infections in general are characterized by a complex host-parasite relationship. Intestinal worms vary in size from 1 cm to several meters, and their life cycle may require more than one host. Parasitic worms do not multiply within humans; an increase in worm load within a specific individual must, therefore, be the result of further exposure to the infective stage. This general rule applies to all worm infections discussed except strongyloidiasis and echinococcosis; in these infections, massive parasite loads may develop in humans because of special worm characteristics.

Most infected individuals harbor a low worm burden and only a small proportion acquire serious infections. Although there is no satisfactory explanation for this peculiar epidemiologic pattern of worm infections, it is of major clinical and therapeutic significance; pathologic changes and disease due to helminths have been shown to correlate with intensity of worm loads, and low helminth burden has been shown to result in little or no clinically significant disease. These epidemiologic features, which have only recently been fully appreciated, are now being used as the basis for planning strategies for control of worm infections in general.

TABLE 1 Major Intestinal Helminths in Humans

Final Habitat in Humans	*Type and Species*	
Small intestine	Nematodes	*Ascaris lumbricoides*
		Ancylostoma duodenale
		Necator americanus
		Strongyloides stercoralis
	Cestodes	*Taenia saginata*
		Taenia solium
		Diphyllobothrium latum
		Hymenolepsis nana
	Trematodes	*Fasciolopsis buski*
Large intestine	Nematodes	*Trichuris trichiura*
		Enterobius vermicularis
Liver	Nematodes	*Toxocara canis*
		Toxocara cati
	Trematodes	*Clonorchis sinensis*
		Fasciola hepatica
		Opisthorchis viverrini
	Cestodes	*Echinococcus granulosis*
Portal venous system	Trematodes	*Schistosoma mansoni*
		Schistosoma japonicum

CLINICAL PRESENTATIONS AND DIFFERENTIAL DIAGNOSES

Worm infections of the gastrointestinal tract and liver may result in local, distant, or systemic clinical manifestations. Such a protean nature poses a major problem in making an etiologic diagnosis. Symptomatic patients with any of the several intestinal helminths may complain of abdominal pain or diarrhea, whereas organomegaly, ascites, or jaundice are the common features of hepatic disease. Furthermore, distant or systemic manifestations or both may occur in some intestinal worm infections such as epilepsy in cystiscercosis or vitamin B_{12} deficiency in diphyllobothriasis. In spite of these common clinical presentations, recognizing certain clinical associations, obtaining careful geographic history, and performing the correct diagnostic procedures should be of considerable help in diagnosing a specific worm infection.

Most intestinal helminthiases are diagnosed by examination of stools for parasite eggs, larvae, or segments. It is essential that a close coordination between patient, physician, and laboratory personnel be established to obtain appropriate samples and perform the necessary examinations. This is particularly important because the routine stool examination procedures may be grossly inadequate. For example, testing fecal material for *Enterobious vermicularis* eggs is commonly unrewarding; the infection is diagnosed by obtaining samples from the perianal region. It may also be necessary to use special procedures to examine stools for *S. stercoralis* larvae or for cestode segments. Additional diagnostic procedures, such as duodenal aspiration or serology, may be helpful in achieving the correct diagnosis, and others, such as hepatic or intestinal biopsy, are rarely if ever needed.

Peripheral blood eosinophilia may be a useful clinical sign suggesting worm infections. Eosinophilia is defined as total cell count in peripheral blood of more than 350 per cubic millimeter. These or higher levels of eosinophilia have consistently been reported in indviduals with tissue-migrating worm infections. In contrast, worms that parasitize the gut lumen (for example, *Ascaris lumbricoides* and hookworms) are associated with eosinophilia only during their migratory phase in the lungs. Furthermore, in some intestinal worm infections, such as strongyloidiasis and visceral larva migrans, tissue invasion is a common feature; in these situations, peripheral blood, as well as tissue eosinophilia, is marked. Eosinophilia also occurs in association with worm infections of hepatic parenchyma and not the biliary tract. In *Fasciola hepatica* infection, eosinophilia may be noted during larval penetration of the hepatic capsule and migration into the parenchyma, but it decreases when the parasites reach their final habitat in the bile canaliculi.

THERAPY

Treatment of intestinal helminthic infections should take into consideration several important principles. Because most worm infections are asymptomatic and because worms do not multiply within the human host, chemotherapy may not be needed in lightly infected individuals with no clinical disease and no opportunity for reinfection. Chemotherapy, if effective, will markedly reduce worm burden; this also may be associated with recovery from clinical features of disease. Exceptions are particularly relevant in some intestinal worm infections; hookworm anemia necessitates additional iron therapy and diphyllobothriasis-associated pernicious anemia is corrected only by vitamin B_{12} administration. Furthermore, removal of worms may not necessarily result in control of clinical disease; this is especially the case with the chronic permanent pathologic sequelae seen in disease with *Schistosoma mansoni* or *japonica*. Management of some worm infections should therefore be designed after careful evaluation; chemotherapy still plays a central role, but other modalities, either medical or surgical, may be needed.

The objectives in treating an individual patient with a specific worm infection are different from those in effect when chemotherapy is used to control these infections in endemic areas. Although eradication of infection is a feasible goal when treating an individual patient, significant reduction of intensity of infection in selected populations may be the strategy for control in endemic areas, particularly in those areas with limited resources.

The following section deals with chemotherapy of the various intestine-related worm infections. A deliberate attempt was made to select only one effective chemotherapeutic agent. Alternative therapy has been included in the tables presented. Most of these agents have been introduced over the last decade or so. They are administered orally, mainly in single doses or short courses, and have proven efficacy and safety. There are no absolute or relative contraindications to the use of any of the chemotherapeutic agents recommended. Their adverse effects are relatively minor and do not usually require interruption of therapy.

Intestinal Round Worms (Nematodes)

The drug of choice for treatment of ascariasis, hookworm infection and trichuriasis is mebendazole. For these three infections, mebendazole is administered orally, 100 mg twice daily for 3 days. Similar doses are used in children more than 2 years of age. In ascariasis, patients thought to have intestinal or biliary obstruction should receive piperazine citrate because of its relaxing effect on worm musculature. Piperazine citrate is given orally, 75 mg per kilogram per day for 2 days.

Strongyloidiasis in immunocompetent hosts of all ages can easily be treated with oral thiabendazole, 25 mg per kilogram twice daily for 2 days. For the hyperinfection syndrome seen in immunocompromised individuals, strongyloidiasis treatment is much more complex. Thiabendazole should be administered in similar doses, but for 10 days. The serious sequelae of the hyperinfection syndrome are usually due to bacterial infections and associated compromise of cardiopulmonary function. Ap-

TABLE 2 Diagnosis and Treatment of Infections Due to Intestinal Nematodes (round worms)

					Drug of Choice		*Alternative Regimen*	
Infecting Organism	*Diagnostic Stage*	*Specimen*	*Diagnostic Test (Routine)*	*Diagnostic Test (Specialized)*	*Generic (Trade) Name*	*Usual Dose and Route*	*Generic (Trade) Name*	*Usual Dose and Route*
Ascaris lumbricoides (ascariasis)	Egg Larvae Adult worm	Stool Sputum Stool	O & P Examine visually	Direct wet smear Serology	Mebendazole (Vermox)	100 mg PO bid × 3 days	Pyrantel pamoate (Antiminth) Piperazine citrate (Antepar) Levimazole (Ketrex)	11 mg/kg single dose PO (maximum 1 g) 75 mg/kg/day × 2 4 mg/kg PO
Ancylostoma duodenale (ancylostomiasis)	Egg Larvae	Stool Stool	O & P O & P	Baerman Harada-Mori Petri dish	Mebendazole (Vermox)	100 mg PO bid × 3 days	Bephemium hydroxy-naphthoate Pyrantel pamoate	5 g (2.5 g of base) PO bid × 3 days 10 mg/kg/day PO × 3
Necator americanus (hookworm infection)	Egg Larvae	Stool Stool	O & P O & P	Baerman Harada-Mori Petri dish	Mebendazole (Vermox)	100 mg PO bid × 3 days *or* 1.0 g single dose PO	Pyrantel pamoate Thiabendazole (Mintezol)	11 mg/kg single dose PO × 3 days 25 mg/kg PO bid × 2 days (maximum 3 g/day)
Strongyloides stercoralis (strongyloidiasis)	Egg Larvae	Duodernal material Stool	 O & P	Enterotest Duodenal aspirate or drainage Serology	Thiabendazole (Mintezol)	25 mg/kg PO bid × 2 days	Pyrantel pamoate	11 mg/kg single dose PO; repeat every 6 weeks × 2
Trichuris trichiura (whipworm infection)	Egg Adult worm	Stool Stool	O & P O & P		Mebendazole (Vermox)	100 mg PO tid × 3 days Repeat 2 courses if necessary	Hexylresorcinol	500 ml of 0.2% solution Retention enema (30 min)
Enterobius vermicularis (pinworm infection)	Egg Adult worm	Anal impression Smear Stool/tape	Scotch tape Smear Smear		Pyrantel pamoate (Antiminth, Combatrin)	11 mg/kg single dose PO Repeat q6 weeks × 2	Mebendazole (Vermox) Pyrivinium pamoate (Povan, Vamquin)	100 mg single dose PO 5 mg/kg single dose PO (maximum 350 mg, repeat after 2 weeks)
Cutaneous *Larva migrans* (creeping eruption)	Larvae	Skin	Biopsy	Serology	Thiabendazole (Mintezol)	25 mg/kg PO bid × 5 days; repeat in 2days if active lesions persist	Thiabendazole (Mintezol)	Topical application
Visceral *Larva migrans* (toxocariasis, *Toxocara* species) *Capillaria heptica*	Larvae	Tissue	Biopsy	Serology	Thiabendazole (Mintezol)	25 mg/kg PO bid until symptoms subside or toxicity precludes further treatment (7–28 days)	Diethylcarbamazine (DEC, Hetrazan)	5 mg/kg/day PO for 3 weeks

TABLE 3 Diagnosis and Treatment of Infections Due to Cestodes

Infecting Organism	Diagnostic Stage	Specimen	Diagnostic Test (Routine)	Diagnostic Test (Specialized)	Drug of Choice: Generic (Trade) Name	Drug of Choice: Usual Dose and Route	Alternative Regimen: Generic (Trade) Name	Alternative Regimen: Usual Dose and Route
Diphyllobotrium latum (fish tapeworm)	Gravid proglottid	Stool	Visual ID	None	Niclosamide (Niclocide, Cestocide, Yomesan)	1.0 g (2 tablets) PO, chewed, then 1 hr later 1.0 g (2 tablets) more = 2 g	Paromomycin	1.0 g PO q15min × 4 doses
	Egg	Stool	O & P				Praziquantel	10 mg/kg PO single dose
Taenia saginata (beef tapeworm)	Gravid proglottid	Stool	India ink injection		Niclosamide (Niclocide, Cestocide, Yomesan)	1.0 g (2 tablets) PO, chewed, then 1 hr later 1.0 g (2 tablets) more = 2 g	Paromomycin	1.0 g PO q15min × 4 doses
	Egg	Stool	O & P	Scotch tape swab			Praziquantel	10 mg/kg PO single dose
Dipylidium caninum (dog tapeworm)	Gravid proglottid	Stool	Visual ID	None	Niclosamide (Niclocide, Cestocide, Yomesan)	1.0 g (2 tablets) PO chewed, then 1 hr later 1.0 g (2 tablets) more = 2 g	Paromoycin	1.0 g PO q15min × 4 doses
	Egg packet	Stool	O & P					
Hymenollepsis nana (dwarf tapeworm)	Egg	Stool	O & P	None	Niclosamide (Niclocide, Cestocide, Yomesan)	2 g daily = 5 days	Paromomycin	45 mg/kg/day PO single dose × 7
							Praziquantel	25 mg/kg PO × 7 days
Taenia solium (pork tapeworm)	Gravid proglottid	Stool	India ink injection		Niclosamide (Niclocide, Cestocide, Yomesan)	1.0 g (1 tablets) PO chewed, then 1 hr later 1.0 g (2 tablets) more = 2 g	Paromomycin	1.0 g PO q15min × 4 doses
	Egg	Stool	O & P				Praziquantel	10 mg/kg PO single dose
							Mebendazole (Vermox)	100 mg PO bid × 3 days
Cysticercosis	Larvae	Subcutaneous nodules; brain cysts	Biopsy	Serology	Praziquantel (Biltricide)	20 mg/kg PO tid × 10 days	Surgical resection	
					Prednisone	10 mg PO tid start 1 day before, through 3 days		
Echinococcus granulosus and *multilocularis*	Hydatid Sand	Hydatid Fluid	Sedimentation or centrifugation of fluid	Squash prep Serology	Mebendazole (Vermox)	40 mg/kg/day PO × 3 mo up to 14 g; in multilocular cysts: Rx may be continued for 3 years with decreased symptoms, but larvae still viable	Complete surgical excision of unilocular cyst	

TABLE 4 Diagnosis and Treatment of Infections Due to Trematodes (Flukes)

					Drug of Choice		*Alternative Regimen*	
Infecting Organism	*Diagnostic Stage*	*Specimen*	*Diagnostic Test (Routine)*	*Diagnostic Test (Specialized)*	*Generic (Trade) Name*	*Usual Dose and Route*	*Generic (Trade) Name*	*Usual Dose and Route*
Clonorchis sinensis (liver fluke)	Egg	Stool Duodenal material	O & P Wet preparation	None Entero test	Praziquantel (Biltricide)	25 mg/kg PO tid × 1 day	None	
Heterophyes heterophyes (intestinal fluke)	Egg	Stool	O & P	None	Praziquantel (Biltricide)	25 mg/kg PO tid × 1 day	Tetrachloroethylene	0.12 ml/kg PO (maximum, 5 ml)
Metagonimus yokogawai (intestinal fluke)	Egg	Stool	O & P	None	Praziquantel (Biltricide)	25 mg/kg PO tid × 1 day	Tetrachloroethylene	0.12 ml/kg PO (maximum, 5 ml)
Opisthorchis viverrini (liver fluke)	Egg	Stool Duodenal material	O & P Wet preparation	None Entero test	Praziquantel (Biltricide)	25 mg/kg PO tid × 1 day	None	
Fasciola hepatica (sheep liver fluke)	Egg	Stool	O & P	Serology	Praziquantel (Biltricide)	25 mg/kg PO tid × 1 day	Bithionol (Actamer, Bitin)	50 mg/kg PO every other day × 15 doses
Paragonimus westermani (lung fluke)	Egg	Stool	O & P Sputum concentrate	Serology	Praziquantel (Biltricide)	25 mg/kg PO tid × 1 day	Bithionol (Actamer, Bitin)	50 mg/kg PO every other day × 15 doses
Schistosoma haematobium (genitourinary bilharziasis)	Egg	Urine Collection between 10 AM & 2 PM at 24 °C	Urine sedimentation concentrate	Membrane filtration Hatching test Serology	Metrifonate (Bilarcil)	10 mg/kg PO q2–4 weeks (maximum 3 doses)	Praziquantel (Biltricide) Niridazole (Ambilhar) Lucanthone (Miracil D)	20 mg/kg PO tid in 1 day (not <4 hrs or >6 hrs between doses 25 mg/kg PO daily × 7 days 20 mg/kg PO × 8–20 days
Fasciola buski	Egg	Stool	O & P	None	Praziquantel (Biltricide)	25 mg/kg PO tid × 1 day	Tetrachloroethylene (NEMA worm capsule, veterinary)	0.12 ml/kg PO (maximum, 5 ml single dose)
Schistosoma mansoni (intestinal bilharziasis)	Egg	Stool	O & P	Tissue from sigmoidoscopy Hatching test Serology	Oxamniquine (Vansil)	15 mg/kg once (western hemisphere) 15 mg/kg PO bid × 2 days (Africa-Middle East	Praziquantel (Biltricide)	20 mg/kg PO tid in 1 day (not <4 hrs or >6 hrs between doses)
Schistosoma japonicum (oriental schistosomiasis)	Egg	Stool	O & P	Tissue from sigmoidoscopy Hatching test Serology	Praziquantel (Biltricide)	20 mg/kg PO tid in one day	Niridazole (Ambilhar)	25 mg/kg PO daily × 10 days (maximum 1.5 g)

propriate antibiotics, medical management, and reduction of immunosuppressive therapy are essential elements in the treatment of this syndrome (Table 2 illustrates the diagnosis and treatment of these infections).

Intestinal Tapeworms (Cestodes)

Individuals with any of the four common tapeworm infections (*Taenia saginata, Taenia solium, Diphyllobothrium latum* and *Hymenolepsis nana*) are treated with niclosamide. It is administered orally in a single 2-g dose that must be chewed thoroughly. The niclosamide dose for children is 0.5 g for those weighing 11 to 34 kg and 1 g for those above 34 kg. When niclosamide is given to children, the tablets should be crushed to a fine powder and mixed with a small amount of water. In *H. nana* infection, the same dose of niclosamide is recommended for a course of 5 days.

Recently, mebendazole and praziquantel have been shown to be effective against *T. solium* and may be used as alternative drugs (Table 3 presents the diagnosis and management of cestode infections).

Intestinal Flukes (Trematodes)

Praziquantel is currently the drug of choice for treatment of *Fasciolopsis buski* infection. It is administered orally, 25 mg per kilogram three doses a day. This results in elimination of most parasites. Similar doses are used in children. Praziquantel has become the drug of choice for most of the infections due to intestinal trematodes.

Liver Flukes (Trematodes)

Praziquantel is also the drug of choice for treatment of *Clonorchis sinensis, F. hepatica*, and *Opsthorches viverrini* infections. It is used in the same dosage as described for intestinal flukes.

Liver Cestodes

Echinococcus granulosis cysts in the liver are the most common clinical feature of this infection. In many cases cysts are found on routine abdominal roentgenographic examination. Calcified, small, or asymptomatic cysts are better left alone. A trial of mebendazole may be given. Large, or symptomatic cysts, on the other hand, necessitate surgical intervention; cysts contents must be killed by hypertonic saline before their removal either by marsupialization or partial hepatectomy.

Blood Flukes

Oxamniquine is the current drug of choice for treatment of schistosomiasis mansoni. It is administered as a single oral dose of 20 mg per kilogram. The same dose is used for children.

For individuals infected with *S. mansoni* in Africa, a higher dose of 60 mg per kilogram may be required. For *S. japonicum* infection, praziquantel is the currently recommended drug. It is given orally, 20 mg per kilogram three times a day in one day. Praziquantel is also effective against other human schistosomes (*S. mansoni* and *S. haematobia,* see Table 4 for details). Chemotherapy for schistosomiasis mansoni or japonica may, in addition to eliminating worms, also result in regression of disease (hepatosplenomegaly) or arrest its development. This is particularly true if chemotherapy is given to infected children. Once the chronic fibro-obstructive sequelae have developed, chemotherapy results in little clinical improvement. These patients need medical management of complications such as esophageal varices, hematemesis, and ascites.

BACTERIAL MENINGITIS IN ADULTS

RICHARD B. ROBERTS, M.D.
JOHN A. ROMANKIEWICZ, Pharm.D.

Bacterial meningitis is a serious, life-threatening infection. It is a medical emergency that necessitates early recognition and institution of appropriate supportive and antimicrobial therapy. The reported annual incidence in the United States is 2.9 cases per 100,000 population, although this figure reflects gross underreporting, and the true incidence is probably closer to 10 cases per 10,000. *Hemophilus influenzae, Neisseria meningitidis,* and *Streptococcus pneumoniae* are responsible for the majority of these infections, although defects in nonimmunologic and immunologic host defenses predispose patients to meningitis due to other bacterial pathogens.

The clinical presentations of bacterial meningitis are quite similar regardless of the causative organism. Clinicians must rely on age of the patient, the epidemiologic and clinical setting, and, most important, the isolation and identification of the causative agent in order to direct appropriate antimicrobial therapy. Deficiencies, however, exist in our current therapeutic approach to patients with bacterial meningitis, including both host and drug factors. Examples of the former include the immunocompromised host and inadequate host-defense mechanisms of the central nervous system. Factors that limit the usefulness of antimicrobial agents include penetration into the cerebrospinal fluid (CSF) following systemic therapy, development of resistance by many bacteria, necessity for bactericidal (not bacteriostatic) antibiotics, and the low therapeutic index of aminoglycosides. The development of the new beta-lactam antibiotics, however, provides agents that possess a wide spectrum of gram-negative activity, are bactericidal, and achieve adequate concentrations in spinal fluid following parenteral therapy.

PREDISPOSING FACTORS AND MICROBIOLOGY

Patient Age

Hemophilus influenzae, N. meningitidis, and *S. pneumoniae* account for more than 80 percent of bacterial meningitis in children and adults; the former two are commonest in young children and the latter, in adults. As shown in Table 1, the relative frequency of bacteria associated with meningitis depends in part on the patient's age and underlying condition. Thus, *S. pneumoniae* accounts for one-third to one-half of adult cases, followed in decreasing order of frequency *N. meningitidis* (10% to 30%), staphylococci (5% to 15%), and *Listeria monocytogenes* (5%). Gram-negative bacilli and *H. influenzae*, the commonest pathogens in neonates and children respectively, account for only 1 percent each in the adult population.

Impaired Host Defenses

The bacteria associated with meningitis in patients with impaired immunologic host-defense mechanisms are shown in Table 2. The encapsulated bacteria *H. influenzae, N. meningitidis*, and *S. pneumoniae* are most frequently associated with B-cell deficiencies such as are seen in thymoma with agammaglobulinemia, Bruton-type agammaglobulinemia, and multiple myeloma. Other impaired immunologic host-defense mechanisms that result in a predisposition for meningitis due to encapsulated bacteria are sickle cell disease, functional asplenia, and splenectomy. In addition, deficiencies in the latter components of the complement cascade impair the direct serum bactericidal activity against the pathogenic *Neisseriae* including *N. meningitidis. L. monocytogenes* and *Mycobacterium tuberculosis*, two intracellular pathogens that require an intact cell-mediated immune system for control and eradication, are frequent bacterial pathogens in T-cell deficiencies, such as in patients with underlying lymphoma, Hodgkin's disease, or in those receiving immunosuppressive therapy.

Anatomical Defects

Patients who have anatomical defects with direct communication to the subarachnoid space are also at high risk for developing bacterial meningitis. These defects may be congenitally acquired, as occurs with spina bifida and meningomyelocele, or as a result of accidental or surgical trauma. As shown in Table 3, the pathogens responsible for meningitis in these patients are normal flora of the skin (i.e., *Staphylococcus aureus* and *Staphylococcus epidermidis* or gram-negative bacilli) or of the upper respiratory tract (i.e., encapsulated bacteria). In the latter case, patients may have spinal fluid leakage resulting in CSF rhinorrhea and multiple episodes of encapsulated bacterial meningitis.

PATHOGENESIS AND ROUTES OF INFECTION

A description of the anatomy of the meninges and the formation of CSF is beyond the scope of this discussion. The following factors bear directly on the susceptibility and response to infection. The inadequate host defense mechanisms of the central nervous system are reflected in the CSF and most likely play a role in the pathogenesis of bacterial meningitis. Reduced immunoglobulin and complement levels have been noted in normal and infected CSF, accounting for the impaired phagocytic activity necessary in host defense against encapsulated bacteria.

TABLE 1 Bacterial Causes (%) of Meningitis in Different Age Groups

Neonate (under 2 months)	*Children (2 months to 15 years)*	*Adults (over 15 years)*
Gram-negative bacilli (55%–60%)	*H. influenzae* (35%–45%)	*S. pneumoniae* (30%–50%)
(*E. coli, Klebsiella* species)	*N. meningitidis* (30%–40%)	*N. meningitidis* (10%–30%)
Group B streptococci (10%–25%)	*S. pneumoniae* (10%–20%)	*S. aureus, S. epidermidis* (5%–15%)
L. monocytogenes (2%–10%)	*S. aureus, S. epidermidis*	*L. monocytogenes* (5%)
S. aureus, S. epidermidis (5%)	Gram-negative bacilli	*H. influenzae* (1%)
S. pneumoniae		Gram-negative bacilli (1%)
N. meningitidis		Group B streptococci
H. influenzae		
Group A streptococci		

Note: Incidence is in decreasing order of frequency.

TABLE 2 Bacterial Meningitis Associated With Impaired Host-Defense Mechanisms

B-cell deficiency
S. pneumoniae
H. influenzae
N. meningitidis
T-cell deficiency
L. monocytogenes
M. tuberculosis

A diminished polymorphonuclear leukocyte (PMN) response, as reflected in the low ratio of PMNs to bacteria in infected CSF, also contributes to impaired phagocytosis.

Bacteria gain access to the meninges either by direct extension from a contiguous site of infection or via the blood that can carry bacteria to the brain from remote sites of infection. Direct extension may result from infected structures of the upper respiratory tract such as in otitis media, mastoiditis, or sinusitis. Anatomical defects permitting communication of the subarachnoid space with either the nasopharynx or skin also predispose patients to bacterial meningitis. As noted above, such defects may be congenital (i.e., associated with meningomyelocele or spina bifida) or from accidental and surgical trauma.

The bloodstream is the usual route by which bacteria reach the meninges. The initial infected site for bacteremia is often the respiratory tract. It is assumed that bacteria that colonize and infect the respiratory tract may have a predilection for the central nervous system (tissue tropism), although data to support this hypothesis are lacking.

DIAGNOSIS

Clinical Evaluation

Patients with bacterial meningitis present with symptoms and signs related to their systemic illness, the initial focus of infection, and the central nervous system. The relative frequency of symptoms and neurologic signs in bacterial meningitis are listed in Table 4. The duration of systemic symptoms such as fever, chills, headache, and vomiting is often short, i.e., 24 to 48 hours. Changes in mentation—from lethargy, confusion, and disorientation to coma—may progress rapidly and help to distinguish bacterial from viral meningitis; this progression is usually not seen in viral meningitis. Alteration of mental status implies some process other than pure meningitis, e.g., increased intracranial pressure, cortical vein thrombosis, or encephalitis. Evidence of meningeal irritation, either by stiffness of the neck or positive neurologic signs, is observed in the majority of patients. These signs and symptoms may be absent in neonates and the elderly. The clinical diagnosis of bacterial meningitis may be difficult in patients with already altered mental status.

TABLE 3 Bacterial Meningitis Associated With Anatomical Defects

Congenital defects
S. aureus
S. epidermidis
Gram-negative bacilli
Acquired defects
Communication with nasopharynx
S. pneumoniae
H. influenzae
N. meningitidis
Communication with skin
S. aureus
S. epidermidis
Gram-negative bacilli

Upper respiratory tract infections, such as pharyngitis, otitis media, and sinusitis, may occur in more than 50 percent of patients presenting with bacterial meningitis. On physical examination, patients are usually febrile, with evidence of meningeal irritation. Except for changes in mental status (e.g., impaired alertness, confusion, convulsions), the neurologic examination may be unrevealing. Increased intracranial pressure should be suspected in the presence of papilledema. A careful physical examination for extra-central nervous system sites of infection, including parameningeal structures, should always be performed.

In addition to a detailed clinical history and physical examination in patients suspected of having bacterial meningitis, important information may be obtained from a careful evaluation of the clinical and epidemiologic setting. Information regarding age, season of the year, family illness, medications, underlying illnesses, and recent travel may be helpful in indicating specific exposures or specific complications of underlying illnesses.

Laboratory Evaluation

Examination of the CSF is the single most important laboratory test in patients with bacterial meningitis. Obtaining CSF requires an invasive procedure (lumbar punc-

TABLE 4 Frequency (%) of Symptoms and Signs of Bacterial Meningitis

Symptoms	*Neurologic Signs*
Fever (45%–85%)	Nuchal rigidity (11%–50%)
Chills (3%–38%)	Kernig's and Brudzinski's signs (81%)
Headache (25%–47%)	
Vomiting (25%–70%)	Coma (30%)
Confusion (37%–56%)	Neurologic abnormalities (25%)
Seizures (40%)	
Photophobia (0%–4%)	

ture) that can be associated with certain complications (iatrogenic meningitis, paraspinal hematoma). A careful lumbar puncture should be performed, especially in patients with evidence of increased intracranial pressure and thrombocytopenia. If the procedure has to be delayed to evaluate or treat these parameters, empiric antimicrobial therapy should be instituted. The CSF should be handled expeditiously and appropriate studies be performed immediately. Red blood cells and PMNs lyse when CSF is left standing, and fastidious encapsulated bacteria cannot be isolated unless directly inoculated on appropriate laboratory media. Laboratory studies that should be performed on all CSF specimens include the following: (*1*) appearance of CSF and opening pressure, (*2*) presence of red and white blood cells, (*3*) protein and glucose determinations with simultaneous blood glucose (the CSF should be at least two-thirds the blood glucose), (*4*) Gram stain (positive in 70% to 80% of patients) and acid-fast stain, and (*5*) appropriate cultures. As a guideline, the laboratory results of these CSF parameters for different causes of meningitis are shown in Table 5.

Other tests, if indicated, include serologic evidence for neurosyphilis, viral isolation and serology, India ink stain, antigen detection, cultures for fungi, and cytology for malignant cells. The laboratory tests that are currently available to demonstrate the etiology of bacterial meningitis are listed in Table 6. In addition to demonstrating bacteria by stain, Quellung reaction, and culture, specific bacterial antigens may be detected by use of counterimmunoelectrophoresis or latex-agglutination techniques. Nonspecific tests reported by some to be helpful, but which are not readily available, include limulus lysate gelation for endotoxin and lactic acid, lactate dehydrogenase (LDH) isoenzymes, and C-reactive protein determinations. We do not use these latter tests routinely.

Antimicrobial therapy administered prior to the first CSF examination will result in alterations of total leukocyte and differential counts in addition to negative Gram stains and cultures. Because of these findings, patients who have received antibiotics prior to diagnosis usually receive a full 14-day course of antimicrobial therapy. In patients with early viral (aseptic) meningitis, the total and differential counts may be consistent with bacterial meningitis. Repeat CSF examination within 6 to 12 hours may demonstrate a differential count with increased numbers of mononuclear cells, and antimicrobial therapy can be withheld in such patients.

Other laboratory tests that should be performed in patients with suspected meningitis include cultures of blood and other clinically indicated specimens and x-ray studies of the chest, mastoids, and sinuses to identify an initial source of infection.

Complications

The early- and late-onset complications that may be observed in patients with bacterial meningitis are listed in Table 7. An appreciation of these complications is critical in the management and follow-up of these patients. Many of the early complications seen during the initial hospitalization are related to the severity of the systemic illness and include upper gastrointestinal hemorrhage, vasculitis with digital gangrene, herpes labialis, shock, acute respiratory distress syndrome (ARDS), disseminated intravascular coagulation (DIC), and inappropriate antidiuretic hormone (ADH) secretion with hyponatremia.

Early-onset neurologic complications include generalized seizures, cerebellar or temporal lobe herniation secondary to increased intracranial pressure, transient focal signs secondary to superficial cortical vein thrombosis, and sterile subdural effusions. The latter is more commonly recognized in neonates prior to closure of the fontanelle and may be the cause of persistent fever or seizure activity. Diagnostic aspiration is recommended both to relieve pressure and to ensure sterility of the effusion.

Late-onset complications are predominantly neurologic and include perceptual learning defects, mental retardation, seizure disorders, deafness, motor deficits, and hydrocephalus. The latter complication most commonly follows basilar granulomatous meningitis due to tuberculosis or the systemic mycoses.

THERAPEUTIC CONSIDERATIONS

General Supportive Measures

All patients with bacterial meningitis should be hospitalized and isolated for respiratory pathogens for the first 48 hours until the etiologic agent is identified. Intensive care is mandatory, and the following emergency measures should be instituted: (*1*) if needed, establish-

TABLE 5 Cerebrospinal Fluid Profile in Meningitis

	Leukocytes			
	Total No. (cells/mm³)	*Morphology*	*Protein (μl = <45 mg%)*	*Sugar (μl = >⅔ of serum glucose)*
Bacterial	>200	PMN	Increased	Decreased
Viral	<200	Mononuclear	Normal	Normal
Fungal	<200	Mononuclear	Increased	Decreased
Carcinomatous	<200	Malignant cells	Increased	Decreased

TABLE 6 Diagnostic Laboratory Tests of Cerebrospinal Fluid in Bacterial Meningitis

Demonstration of bacteria
Gram-stain, acid-fast bacilli (AFB) stain
Quellung reaction
Culture
Detection of specific bacterial antigens
Counterimmunoelectrophoresis (CIE)
Latex agglutination

ment of a patent airway to prevent aspiration and maintain adequate ventilation, especially in comatose patients; (*2*) maintenance of intravenous access for adequate hydration and various therapeutic drugs; (*3*) monitoring vital signs and maintenance of systolic blood pressure above 90 mm Hg. Caution must be exercised in the administration of intravenous fluids so that congestive heart failure and pulmonary edema are not precipitated by overhydration. Overhydration may also increase the likelihood of cerebral edema, resulting in cranial nerve palsy or respiratory arrest from herniation of the temporal lobe and cerebellum, respectively. Administration of mannitol (1 to 2 g per kilogram as a 15% to 20% solution given over 30 to 60 minutes intravenously) and subsequent diuresis may decrease intracranial pressure due to cerebral edema.

Anticonvulsants should be used to control seizures, but should not be given prophylactically because they may interfere with the monitoring of mental status. Although there is some controversy involved, steroids are generally contraindicated in patients with bacterial meningitis except when acute hydrocephalus due to basilar meningitis is strongly suspected.

Disseminated intravascular coagulation (DIC) may complicate any cause of bacterial meningitis, but is most commonly seen in patients with meningococcal or pneumococcal (with asplenia) meningitis. DIC may be suspected clinically when petechiae and bleeding at needle puncture sites are observed. Measures of coagulation should be obtained immediately and depleted clotting factors replaced. The beneficial role of heparin has not been substantiated, although it is recommended by most hematologists. Full-dose intravenous heparin is initiated by pump: 5,000 units initially, followed by 1,000 units every hour. Response to heparin therapy is determined by the normalization of depleted clotting factors and reduction of fibrinogen levels. The platelet count and prothrombin time are unreliable because the former may also be reduced because of bone marrow suppression from infection and the latter, elevated because of heparin therapy. It has been reported that because DIC in these patients is endotoxin-mediated, efforts to remove endotoxin by plasmaphoresis or to neutralize it by immunotherapy has met with some clinical success. At present, we have not routinely used these methods.

Antimicrobial Therapy

The properties of an ideal antimicrobial agent for bacterial meningitis include: (*1*) bactericidal activity, (*2*) high therapeutic to toxic ratio, and (*3*) sufficient CSF penetration to achieve levels at least several times the minimum bactericidal concentration (MBC) against the infecting bacteria.

CSF Penetration

The determinants of CSF penetration of an antimicrobial agent include the degree of inflammation of the meninges and the physical properties of the drug, including protein binding, ionization, lipid solubility, and carrier transport. Nearly all large molecules are excluded from the CSF; any bound portion of a drug would also be excluded because only free drug crosses the choroid plexus. Drugs that are salts are highly ionized and, therefore, lipid insoluble. The ability of a drug to pass through the choroidal cells is a function of its lipid solubility at body pH. Drug concentration is also dependent on its elimination or removal from the CSF. The recognized mechanisms of drug removal include bulk (mass) flow of CSF, diffusion of lipid soluble substances, and an active transport system, especially for ionized drugs, through the arachnoid villi. Inflammation of the meninges increases capillary permeability and, thereby, enhances drug entry and inhibits active transport out of the CSF, thus increasing the CSF concentration.

The penetration of various antimicrobial agents into the CSF in the presence and absence of inflamed meninges is outlined in Table 8. Data concerning the CSF penetration of various agents are often from single case reports and determined by different methods. Recent studies with animal models have been useful, although the extrapolation of these data to humans is always questionable. In general, CSF penetration increases with inflammation of the meninges, although conflicting results have been reported correlating CSF penetration with in-

TABLE 7 Complications of Bacterial Meningitis

Early-onset
Gastrointestinal hemorrhage—stress ulcer
Vasculitis with distal digital gangrene
Herpes labialis
Congestive heart failure
Shock
Acute respiratory distress syndrome
Disseminated intravascular coagulation
Inappropriate antidiuretic hormone (ADH) secretion with hyponatremia
Neurologic
Generalized seizures
Cerebellar or temporal lobe herniation
Transient focal signs due to cortical vein thrombosis
Subdural effusions
Late-onset (neurologic)
Perceptual learning deficits
Mental retardation
Seizure disorder
Deafness
Motor deficit
Hydrocephalus

TABLE 8 Penetration of Antibiotics into Cerebrospinal Fluid

Good With or Without Inflammation	*Good With Inflammation*	*Unreliable Even With Inflammation*	*No Passage*
Sulfisoxazole	Penicillins	Cephalothin and other	Polymyxin B
Sulfadiazine	Penicillin G	first-generation	Colistin
Trimethoprim-sulfamethoxazole	Ampicillin	cephalosporins	Bacitracin
Chloramphenicol	Carbenicillin	Cefamandole	
Metronidazole	Ticarcillin	Cefoxitin	
Isoniazid	Methicillin	Tetracycline	
Ethionamide	Oxacillin	Clindamycin	
Cycloserine	Nafcillin	Erythromycin	
Flucytosine	Vancomycin	Aminoglycosides	
	New beta-lactams	Gentamicin	
	Cefotaxime	Tobramycin	
	Moxalactam	Amikacin	
	Cefoperazone	Netilmicin	
	Ceftizoxime	Amphotericin B	
	Rifampin		
	Ethambutol		

creased leukocytes or protein in the CSF. The range of drug concentrations in the CSF of patients with meningitis is shown in Table 9.

Bactericidal Activity

Ideally, an antibiotic should be bactericidal against the infecting bacteria. Chloramphenicol is bactericidal against the encapsulated bacteria *H. influenzae*, *N. meningitidis*, and *S. pneumoniae* and is effective in bacterial meningitis caused by these bacteria. However, chloramphenicol is bacteriostatic against the aerobic gram-negative bacilli (MIC, 2 to 6 μg per milliliter; MBC, more than 60 μg per milliliter) and is not generally effective as a single agent in gram-negative bacillary (GNB) meningitis. Emergence of resistance to chloramphenicol has also been documented during therapy. Furthermore, experimental in vitro studies have shown that the combination of chloramphenicol and gentamicin is antagonistic, suggesting that a "static-cidal" drug combination may not be optimal for the treatment of bacterial meningitis. Similar antagonistic results were previously observed in patients with pneumococcal meningitis who received penicillin and tetracycline.

Drug Toxicity

The aminoglycosides have a low therapeutic index and their dose-related ototoxicity and nephrotoxicity preclude achieving CSF levels many times the MBC of gram-negative bacilli following parenteral administration.

Route of Administration

To achieve adequate CSF concentrations, antimicrobial agents must be given by the intravenous route. Because of the unidirectional flow of CSF, adequate ventricular drug levels cannot be obtained following intrathecal administration by the lumbar route. For drugs

TABLE 9 Range of Drug Concentrations in Patients With Bacterial Meningitis

Drug	*Range of CSF Concentration (μg/ml)*	*Percentage of Serum Concentration*
Penicillin	1.0–10	--
Ampicillin	3.0–28	11–65
Methicillin	1.3–2.8	8–23
Nafcillin	2.7–9.8	14–30
Chloramphenicol	10–20	40–50
Gentamicin	0.2–3.0	10–30
Cephalothin	0.5–3.0	4–10
New beta-lactams (cefotaxime, moxalactam, cefoperazone, ceftizoxime)	5.0–30	15–45
Trimethoprim-	0.2–2.35	52–233
sulfamethoxazole	5.0–35	35–90
Metronidazole	12–27	100

that do not adequately enter the CSF after intravenous administration (i.e., aminoglycosides), intraventricular injection may be required. This has been especially true in GNB meningitis because ventriculitis occurs in 70 percent of patients. Unfortunately, intraventricular administration of the aminoglycosides has been associated with local tissue injury and panencephalopathy following repeated injections. Antibiotics can also be delivered into the ventricles by an Ommaya or Rickham reservoir; however, this requires an invasive neurosurgical procedure that is sometimes associated with complications. Intrathecal antibiotics are given (at dosages listed in Table 10) in 3 to 5 ml of nonpreservative 5% dextrose in water or normal saline. Cefotaxime, because of its activity against GNB and excellent penetration into CSF following intravenous administration, is now the preferred agent in meningitis caused by susceptible GNB.

Suspected Pathogen and Susceptibility

In addition to the pharmacologic properties and toxicity of the antimicrobial agent, the suspected pathogen and its susceptibility must be considered in the choice of an antimicrobial agent. As described above, the pathogen may be suspected on the basis of the patient's age and underlying condition and the clinical setting and epidemiologic factors, but is confirmed only by isolation from the CSF or blood. Over the past several years, emergence of resistance of many of the pathogens responsible for bacterial meningitis has been noted, including ampicillin-resistant *H. influenzae*, multiply resistant *S. pneumoniae*, and ampicillin-resistant *Escherichia coli*.

The antimicrobial agents commonly used for treatment of bacterial meningitis and their unique properties include the following:

Penicillin G penetrates inflamed meninges and achieves CSF concentrations well above the MBC of susceptible organisms. It is the drug of choice for pneumococcal and meningococcal meningitis.

Ampicillin penetrates inflamed meninges slightly better than does penicillin G and is bactericidal against not only pneumococci and meningococci but also group B streptococci and *L. monocytogenes*. Emergence of resistance of *H. influenzae* and *E. coli* has limited its usefulness in infections due to these pathogens.

Chloramphenicol is bactericidal and effective as alternate therapy in *H. influenzae*, meningococcal, and pneumococcal meningitis. Less than 1 percent of *H. influenzae* isolates and multiply resistant pneumococci have been resistant to chloramphenicol. Chloramphenicol is bacteriostatic against enteric gram-negative bacteria.

Aminoglycosides do not achieve adequate CSF concentrations, are less active at the lowered pH of inflamed tissues and fluids, and have a low therapeutic index, limiting their usefulness in GNB meningitis. Their only role at the present time is in multiple resistant nosocomial GNB meningitis in which intraventricular administration may be necessary to achieve bacteriologic cure.

New beta-lactams (cefotaxime, moxalactam, cefoperazone, ceftizoxime) achieve excellent CSF levels 50 to 1,000 times the MBC of most susceptible bacteria. Because of their extended half-lives, high serum levels, and possible CSF accumulation, a steady state is reached in the CSF that persists between doses. These agents are active against ampicillin-sensitive and -resistant *H. influenzae*, meningococci, penicillin-sensitive pneumococci, and most Enterobacteriaceae, including *E. coli* and *Klebsiella* species. *Pseudomonas* strains are variable in their sensitivity, and *Acinetobacter* species and *L. monocytogenes* are resistant to the new beta-lactams. It is not recommended that one of these be used as a single agent for empiric therapy. Cefotaxime is our first choice among these agents; it has been used to successfully treat GNB meningitis. Cefoperazone is not approved for this use and reported data are based only on in vitro studies. Moxalactam is not used to treat pneumococcal meningitis.

The CSF penetration of the first- (cephalothin, cefazolin) and second- (cefamandole, cefoxitin) generation cephalosporins is unreliable, and these agents should not be used in bacterial meningitis. Pneumococcal and *H. influenzae* meningitis have developed in patients receiving cephalothin and cefamandole, respectively.

Wide-spectrum penicillins (azlocillin, mezlocillin, piperacillin) have been used to treat meningitis in only a limited number of patients. Although there is evidence that they penetrate inflamed meninges, none is approved for use in the treatment of meningitis.

Initial Therapy

The agents chosen for initial therapy of bacterial meningitis prior to the isolation of the pathogen should be based on the patient's age and the clinical setting and include either ampicillin (12 g per day) or penicillin G (24 million units per day). Alternative choices are either chloramphenicol (4 g per day) or cefotaxime (12 g per day). Drug therapy specifically directed against the causative organism should be instituted when identification and antimicrobial sensitivity are known. The primary and alternative antimicrobial regimens are listed in Table 10.

Duration of Therapy and Monitoring

The duration of parenteral antimicrobial therapy of uncomplicated bacterial meningitis is 2 weeks. Daily monitoring for the complications outlined in Table 7 should be performed. Repeat lumbar punctures should be performed only in the case of suspected complications or emergent resistance.

PROPHYLAXIS

Antimicrobial Prophylaxis

The risk that close contacts of patients with meningococcal meningitis will develop clinical disease is 500 to 600 times that of noncontacts in endemic disease situations and 15,000 times that of noncontacts in epidemic disease. Recent studies suggest that close contacts younger than the age of 4 years of patients with *H. influenzae* have an increased risk of 200 to 400 times normal. Close contacts include immediate family members, children in day care centers, and hospital personnel who have had intimate contact (i.e., mouth-to-mouth resuscitation) with the patient's respiratory secretions. Since most secondary cases in susceptible close contacts occur within 48 to 72 hours, antimicrobial prophylaxis should be given to contacts immediately upon recognition of the index case. For meningococcal prophylaxis, oral rifampin (600 mg twice daily) for 2 days is recommended. Sulfisoxazole (500 mg twice daily) for 2 days or minocycline (150 mg twice daily) for 4 days may be given if the isolate is known to be sensitive to sulfadiazine in the former case or if patients are allergic to rifampin. If the organism is resistant to sulfisoxazole, minocycline may be used; minocycline,

TABLE 10 Antibiotic Therapy for Bacterial Meningitis in Adults

	Preferred Therapy		*Alternative Therapy*		
Organism	*Antibiotic*	*Dosage/24 hours*	*Antibiotic*	*Dosage/24 hours*	*Adjunctive Therapy*
Gram-positive					
Pneumococcus	Penicillin G	24 million units IV	Chloramphenicol *or* New beta-lactam *except* moxalactam	4 g IV 12 g IV	
Multiply resistant	Vancomycin	2 g IV			Vancomycin 2–5 mg (IT)‡
Group A and B *Streptococcus*	Penicillin G	24 million units IV			
S. faecalis	Ampicillin	12 g IV	Vancomycin	2 g IV	
S. aureus	Nafcillin	12 g IV	Vancomycin	2 g IV	
Methicillin resistant *S. aureus*	Vancomycin	2 g IV			Vancomycin 2–5 mg IT
L. monocytogenes	Ampicillin	12 g IV	Trimethoprim-sulfamethoxazole	12 ampules IV	Gentamicin 3–5 mg/kg IV
Gram-negative					
H. influenzae	Ampicillin	12 g IV	New beta-lactams*	12 g IV	
Ampicillin resistant *H. influenzae*	Chloramphenicol	4 g IV	New beta-lactams*	12 g IV	
Meningococcus	Penicillin G	24 million units IV	Chloramphenicol New beta-lactams*	4 g IV 12 g IV	
Aerobic gram-negative bacilli					
Enterobacteriaceae	New beta-lactams*	12 g IV			
Pseudomonas	New beta-lactams* *or* Carbenicillin *plus* Aminoglycoside†	12 g IV 30–40 g IV IV			Aminoglycoside† (2–5 mg) intraventricularly

* Preferred beta-lactam is cefotaxime 2 g q4h IV; others, on the basis of in vitro sensitivity, are moxalactam, or ceftizoxime 3 g q6h.
† Choice of aminoglycoside based on in vitro sensitivity: gentamicin and tobramycin 4–6 mg/kg IV and amikacin 15 mg/kg IV.
‡ IT = intrathecal

however, has been associated with a high incidence of vestibular reactions. For *H. influenzae* prophylaxis, oral rifampin, 20 mg per kilogram per day for 4 days, is recommended for close contacts under 4 years of age.

Immunoprophylaxis

At the present time a tetravalent meningococcal polysaccharide vaccine (groups A, C, Y, W-135) and a 23-valent pneumococcal polysaccharide vaccine (Danish types 1, 2, 3, 4, 5, 8, 9N, 12F, 14, 17, 19F, 20, 22F, 23F, 6B, 10A, 11A, 7F, 15B, 18C, 19A, 9V, 33F) are available for clinical use. Indications for meningococcal immunoprophylaxis include routine prophylaxis in military training installations, outbreaks in civilian closed-population groups, individuals traveling to foreign countries where disease is epidemic, and as an adjunct to antibiotic prophylaxis for family and day care center contacts. Such prophylaxis is effective because 30 percent to 40 percent of secondary disease occurs more than 5 days after exposure to the index case. The frequency and severity of pneumococcal meningitis is increased in patients with splenic dysfunction and asplenia, (i.e., children with sickle cell disease), and indications for pneumococcal immunoprophylaxis include these patients as well. Unfortunately, the bacterial polysaccharide vaccines are not regularly immunogenic in children under 2 years of age, and other forms of prophylaxis are necessary for that age group.

A type B *H. influenzae* vaccine has recently been approved for the following high risk patients: (1) all children at 24 months of age; (2) children at 18 months of age, particularly those with underlying conditions, (e.g., sickle cell disease, primary antibody deficiency) or attendees of day care facilities under 5 years of age. These latter children may require revaccination within 18 months to ensure adequate protection.

ASEPTIC MENINGITIS

JACK MENDELSON, M.D., M.S., F.R.C.P.C.(C)

Aseptic meningitis and atypical pneumonia are analagous conditions, for they both refer to infectious processes where the "usual" bacteria (in meningitis these include *Streptococcus pneumoniae, Neisseria meningitidis,* and *Hemophilus influenzae*) are not cultured from fluids from the infected site in a patient not on antibiotic therapy. The diagnosis and management of aseptic meningitis presents one of the more difficult problems in infectious diseases, because, on the one hand, cases caused by viruses generally have no available specific therapy, and on the other, failure to adequately treat a partially treated bacterial meningitis may have devastating consequences.

Patients who have received only a day or two of oral antibiotics usually do not present a great problem, since bacterial meningitis is not often masked in this situation. Thus, cultures are usually positive, and patients should be treated with appropriate antibiotics. However, patients who received small amounts of antibiotics before admission should not automatically be treated, but, rather, should be observed only if they are not toxic and if the cerebrospinal fluid findings are compatible with an aseptic process; however, should the condition deteriorate or changes occur in the CSF that suggest a bacterial etiology, therapy should be instituted even if the cultures remain negative.

At times it is difficult to be certain that one is actually dealing with meningitis; the classic nuchal rigidity may not be dramatic, and headache may be the most prominent complaint. A rapid onset of symptoms usually suggests a viral etiology, whereas a prolonged history and gradual onset support other etiologies such as tuberculosis, brain abscess, or cryptococcal disease. Once a diagnosis of possible meningitis is entertained, then one must be certain that it is safe to perform a lumbar puncture (LP) based on normal funduscopic examination and absence of signs and symptoms of greatly increased intracranial pressure. Examination of CSF is one of the most critical facets in the work-up of the patient.

Meningitis is an inflammation of the meninges, and the symptoms usually include headache, stiff neck, and fever. Once cerebral function becomes impaired—as manifested by progression to coma, impairment of sensorium, or onset of focal neurologic symptoms—the patient must be subjected to other procedures such as CT scan, electroencephalogram, brain scan, and possible brain biopsy if herpes simplex encephalitis is considered.

No strict guidelines can be given regarding the CSF findings in aseptic meningitis. Naturally, no bacteria are noted on Gram stain of the fluid, and routine bacteriologic cultures are negative. The number of leukocytes found can vary tremendously from as few as 10 to 20 to thousands per cubic millimeter. The demonstration of neutrophils does not necessarily suggest a bacterial etiology since these cells are found at an early stage in viral meningitis. Elevated levels of CSF protein are almost inevitable, but the degree of elevation generally does not suggest any particular group of pathogens. In viral meningitis the CSF glucose levels are usually not depressed, as is often the situation with bacterial meningitis, but, here again, there are exceptions: mumps and lymphocytic choriomeningitic (LCM) infections may present with low CSF glucose levels.

Let us imagine, then, a patient who presents with headache, fever, stiff neck, and modest pleocytosis with 200 white blood cells per cubic millimeter, 75 percent of which are neutrophils. If one is faced with this problem early in the course of the patient's disease, then most often one is dealing with a viral process, particularly if the patient is not very toxic and has received no previous antibiotics. Antibiotics may be withheld, but the patient must be kept under close observation. If the patient deteriorates clinically, a repeat LP should be performed for analysis, and the decision to treat with antibiotics will depend on changes in the CSF, such as an increase in numbers of neutrophils, a lowering of the CSF glucose levels, and an elevation in the protein level. Assuming that the Gram stain is still negative for microorganisms, latex agglutination assays for pneumococcal, meningococcal, or haemophilus antigens may be performed; the latex tests are more sensitive and rapid than counterimmunoelectrophoresis (CIE), where false-negative results are frequent. Once antibiotic therapy has been instituted, the patient should receive a full course of antimicrobial treatment, even if the latex test is negative. Other ancillary tests (other than microbiologic cultures) may be necessary in order to solve this difficult clinical problem. Acute and convalescent serum determinations are not helpful in clarifying the situation early on. CIE or latex agglutination tests (as noted above) may be helpful in the diagnosis of a partially treated pneumococcal, meningococcal, or hemophilus meningitis. A positive limulus lysate test on CSF may indicate a gram-negative meningitis and has its greatest usefulness in two clinical situations. The first is in the neonatal period and the second is in the post-craniotomy patient. A positive CSF VDRL test would suggest syphilis. Recently, a CSF latex agglutination test for cryptococcal meningitis has proved to be an extremely useful diagnostic procedure. Myelography (not CT scan) may aid in the diagnosis of an epidural abscess, whereas CT or a brain scan are of great value in the demonstration of an early brain abscess (see chapter *Localized Infection of the Central Nervous System*).

Epidemiologic and clinical clues are extremely important areas of information in solving the problem of the etiology of an aseptic meningitis and must be sought early on in the work-up of the patient. Enteroviruses and mumps infect mainly children, and herpes simplex and LCM are more often infections of adults. Laboratory workers acquire LCM infections, whereas veterinarians and farmers develop leptospirosis. Enteroviral meningitis, Lyme disease, and leptospirosis occur mainly in summer and late autumn; mumps occurs from January to May. Varicella, herpes simplex, tuberculosis, brain abscess,

TABLE 1 Epidemiology, Diagnosis, and Treatment of Aseptic Meningitis

Etiology of Disease	*Epidemiologic and Clinical Clues*	*CSF Characteristics*	*Ancillary Tests*	*Treatment*
Enterovirus (polio, rare)	1. Mainly children, young adults; rare >40 yrs 2. Late summer, early autumn	1. PMNs, then lymphocytes (20-2,000/mm³) 2. Glucose normal 3. Protein ↑ (rarely >100 mg%)	1. Viral culture 2. Serology only if virus isolated	----
Mumps	1. 90% of disease occurs in children <14 yrs 2. January to May 3. Parotitis and/or orchitis usually present	1. PMNs, then lymphocytes (20-2,000/mm³) 2. Glucose normal (low in up to 30%) 3. Protein ↑ (rarely >70 mg%)	1. Viral culture 2. Serology	----
Herpes simplex (type 1 or 2)	1. Usually adults 2. May progress to encephalitis 3. No seasonal variation 4. May occur in association with genital herpes	1. PMNs, then lymphocytes 2. Glucose normal 3. Protein ↑ 4. May see RBCs	1. Viral isolation from CSF rare 2. Serology	ARA-A?
Varicella-zoster	1. Varicella rash 2. Shingles	1. As for enteroviruses	1. Viral isolation from vesicle on skin 2. Serology	----
Lymphocytic choriomeningitis	1. Mainly young adults 2. Laboratory workers handling mice, hamsters, etc. 3. Fall, winter and spring 4. Occasional associated arthritis, parotitis, orchitis	1. Lymphocytes (may be >2,000/mm³) 2. Glucose may be ↓ (25%) 3. Protein ↑ (average, 100 mg%)	1. Viral isolation from CSF 2. Serology	----
Partially treated meningitis	1. History: antibiotic use 2. Rash (meningococcal) 3. Childhood (*H. influenza*) 4. Otitis, sinusitis mastoiditis (*S. pneumoniae*)	1. Gram stain (+) in 60% 2. PMNs >1,200/mm³ 3. Glucose <30 mg% 4. Protein >150 mg%	1. Culture (may be negative) 2. CIE* not very sensitive (pneumococcus, *H. influenzae*) 3. Latex agglutination (sensitive and rapid) 4. Lactic acid >35 mg% 5. Limulus lysate test (for gram-negative organisms) 6. CSF amino acid levels	1. *S. pneumoniae*: penicillin G, 2 million units IV q2h × 10–14 days 2. *N. meningitides*: as above, but treat for at least 5 days after patient becomes afebrile 3. *H. influenzae*: ampicillin 300 mg/kg/day IV q4h plus chloramphenicol 100 mg/kg/day IV q6h until sensitivities available (alternate regimens include cotrimoxazole, moxalactam)
M. tuberculosis	1. Subacute or chronic 2. Evidence of miliary TB 3. In U.S. mainly in adults, elderly 4. Cranial nerve palsies	1. Acid-fast stain often negative (75%) 2. PMNs, then mononuclears (100–500/mm³) 3. Glucose ↓ (25 mg% = mean) 4. Protein ↑ (30 mg% = mean)	1. Culture-positive approx. 60% (send large volumes of CSF for culture)	1. INH† 300 mg daily 2. Rifampin 600 mg daily 3. Ethambutol 15 mg/kg/day; Treat for 18–24 months

* CIE = counter immunoelectrophoresis (latex agglutination preferred)
† INH = isoniazid

Table 1 *Continued*

TABLE 1 Epidemiology, Diagnosis, and Treatment of Aseptic Meningitis *(Continued)*

Etiology of Disease	*Epidemiologic and Clinical Clues*	*CSF Characteristics*	*Ancillary Tests*	*Treatment*
Spinal epidural abscess	1. Back pain, leg pain 2. May be postoperative (back surgery) 3. Evidence of vertebral osteomyelitis 4. Mostly males 5. Deficits in motor, sensory, or sphincter function	As those found in aseptic meningitis syndrome	Myelography (not CT scan)	1. Immediate surgery, and cloxacillin 2 g IV q4h for 4 weeks at least 2. (*S. aureus* is pathogen in 90% of cases)
Brain abscess	1. Presence of bronchiectasis, lung abscess 2. Poor dental hygiene 3. Congenital heart disease 4. Seizures 5. Focal neurologic findings 6. Usually males	LP may be dangerous and is not advised because of the possibility of herniation	1. CT scan 2. Brain Scan 3. Aspiration or excision	1. Surgery (usually aspiration or excision) 2. Based on bacteriologic results: Penicillin G 2 million units IV q2h for 6–8 weeks *or* Chloramphenicol 1 g IV q4h for 6–8 weeks *or* Metronidazole 15 mg/kg infused IV over 1 hour followed by 7.5 mg/kg infused over 1 hour IV q6h for 6–8 weeks
Secondary syphilis	1. Rare (2% of cases) 2. May be male homosexual 3. Rash (including palms and soles) 4. Mucous membrane lesions 5. Lymphadenopathy 6. Usually subacute	1. Lymphocytes 2. Glucose normal 3. Protein ↑	1. VDRL 2. FTA-abs‡ 3. CSF darkfield	Benzathine penicillin G 2.4 million units IM once
Leptospirosis	1. Usually young adult male 2. Summer and early fall 3. Indirect contact with infected animal's urine via water, soil 4. Occupational exposure (veterinarians, farmers) 5. History of camping, swimming 6. Uveitis in 2% 7. Headache very intense	1. PMNs, then mononuclears 2. Protein normal to 300 mg% 3. Glucose normal	1. Agglutination tests (≥1:100) 2. Isolation of organism from blood, CSF, or urine using Fletcher's medium, EMJH, and Tween 80 albumin medium 3. Hamster inoculation	Treat within first 4 days: Penicillin G 1 million units IV q6h for 1 week
Lyme disease (*Borrelia* species)	1. Most cases in U.S. Northeast (but not all) 2. Classic rash, erythema chronicum migrans	1. Lymphocytes (25–450/mm³) 2. Glucose normal	1. IFA test§	Early manifestations: tetracycline 500 mg PO QID for 10 days

‡ FTA-abs = fluorescent treponemal antibody absorption test
§ IFA = indirect fluorescent antibody

Table 1 *Continued*

TABLE 1 Epidemiology, Diagnosis, and Treatment of Aseptic Meningitis *(Continued)*

Etiology of Disease	*Epidemiologic and Clinical Clues*	*CSF Characteristics*	*Ancillary Tests*	*Treatment*
	3. Arthritis 4. Cardiac arrythmias 5. Summer or early fall 6. Tick bite (recalled by only 20%)	3. Protein normal		
Cryptococcus neoformans	1. Half of patients may be on steroids, and/or have lymphoreticular malignancies 2. Indolent onset 3. Symptoms may wax and wane 4. Minimal nuchal rigidity 5. 20% have cranial nerve palsies	1. Mainly lymphocytes (40–400/mm³) 2. Glucose ↓ in 50% 3. Protein ↑	1. Culture 2. India ink stain 3. Latex agglutination test on CSF	1. Amphotericin B 0.3 mg/kg/day IV for 6 weeks *and* 2. Flucytosine 37.5 mg/kg PO q6h for 6 weeks
Coccidioido-mycosis	1. Occurs in 7 southwestern U.S. states or after travel to area 2. May occur more often in Immunosuppressed patients, Pregnant females, Filipinos, Hispanics, Blacks 3. Usually within 6 months after primary pulmonary infection 4. Signs of meningeal irritation usually absent 5. Cranial nerve palsies	1. Mainly lymphocytes (<500/mm³) 2. Glucose ↓ 3. Protein ↑ 4. May see eosinophils	1. Culture 2. CSF, CF[ll] titres ↑ in 95% 3. Blood CF tests	1. Intrathecal amphotericin B beginning with 0.025 mg and increasing to 0.5 mg if tolerated; administer thrice weekly for 3 months, then twice weekly for 2 months tapering to once every 1–6 weeks; treat until CSF has been normal for 1 year *and* 2. Amphotericin B IV to a total of 1 g (for other system involvement, which is common with meningitis) *or* 3. Miconazole therapy still experimental

[ll] CF = complement fixation

syphilis, and cryptococcosis know no season.

The methods of diagnosis of the latter conditions noted above vary tremendously. Enteroviral, mumps, and LCM infections are diagnosed by the isolation of the virus from spinal fluid. Leptospires may be isolated from the spinal fluid during the first 10 days of the disease and from the urine later on by the use of special media (e.g., Fletcher's) that are not readily available in most laboratories. A darkfield examination of the spinal fluid may reveal the spirochetes. Finally, serologic testing, e.g., slide agglutination, is a useful screening procedure for leptospirosis. For Lyme disease, it is much more difficult to visualize organisms directly in the CSF. Antibody titer tests are more widely used, but the presence of the characteristic rash is most useful in confirming the diagnosis (see chapter *Lyme Disease*).

Various other historical, epidemiologic, and clinical clues may be helpful. Recent travel to the northeastern United States may suggest Lyme disease, particularly if a rash is present, whereas coccidioidomycosis enters the differential if someone has been to one of the seven southwestern states, especially if the patient is immunosuppressed, pregnant, Hispanic, black, or Filipino. Of utmost importance, as noted above, is the history of recent antibiotic administration; without such information it may be impossible to exclude a bacteriologic etiology and necessitate antibiotic therapy. Leg and back pain, particularly in a male who has had recent back surgery, suggests a spinal epidural abscess, and focal neurologic findings (also more frequent in males) may be a manifestation of brain abscess.

Immunosuppressed patients are more predisposed to cryptococcal and tuberculous meningitis. These patients generally have a history of more chronic onset of disease. In the case of cryptococcal meningitis the patients, besides possibly being immunosuppressed, may have evidence of cryptococcal disease elsewhere and should have an India ink or latex agglutination test performed on the spinal fluid. The latex test is very sensitive and is widely used. If one suspects tuberculosis, particularly if the patient is immunosuppressed or has a history of tuberculosis or evidence of pulmonary tuberculosis, acid-fast stains of spinal fluid should be done. These are rarely rewarding, and even cultures may be negative. Once the decision to treat has been made on the basis of the above considerations, antituberculous therapy should be continued even if cultures remain negative.

Many of the aspects relating to the diagnosis and management of aseptic meningitis have been discussed above. As well, specific therapy is outlined when indicated (See Table 1). The clinician faced with the difficult problem of aseptic meningitis will be better able to approach it in a more rewarding manner using all the clinical information that is available.

LOCALIZED INFECTION OF THE CENTRAL NERVOUS SYSTEM

KENNETH L. TYLER, M.D.

Localized infections of the central nervous system (CNS) produce a wide variety of clinical signs and symptoms. Diagnosis of these infections often requires the use and interpretation of specialized diagnostic techniques including computerized tomography (CT scan) and cerebral angiography. Successful therapy depends on a combination of prompt and aggressive medical management and the use of appropriate neurosurgical intervention. Because of the unique features of each type of infection, they are each discussed separately in terms of etiology, pathogenesis, clinical features, laboratory and diagnostic studies, and treatment.

Other CNS infections including bacterial meningitis, aseptic meningitis, and viral encephalitis are discussed in separate chapters as are specific infections such as tuberculosis, syphilis, and certain parasitic diseases.

CEREBRAL SUBDURAL EMPYEMA

Subdural empyema (SDE) can be defined as a collection of pus in the preformed space between the cranial dural and arachnoid membranes. Spinal subdural empyema is a rare form of localized infection of the spinal cord and is discussed separately.

Etiology

Infection of the paranasal sinuses is now the most frequent antecedent to SDE (70% of cases). In most cases, the frontal sinuses are involved, but SDE may follow maxillary sinusitis, and sphenoidal sinusitis may precede SDE in the area of the sella turcica (perihypophyseal abscess). SDE usually follows acute rather than chronic sinusitis. In the preantibiotic era, otitic infections were a common antecedent to SDE, but they now account for less than 30 percent of cases; in these cases, SDE often follows an acute exacerbation of chronic otitis. Unusual antecedents of SDE include secondary infection of a subdural hematoma, cranial osteomyelitis, extension through a dural fistula of an epidural abscess, septic thrombophlebitis of the cerebral veins or sinuses, and metastatic spread from a distant primary site of infection. Chronic septic labyrinthitis or petrous apicitis are rare cases of SDE in the posterior fossa. In children, subdural empyema may develop during the course of acute meningitis.

Pathogenesis

Otogenic infections can spread to the subdural space by direct erosion through the adjacent bone of the tegmen tympani and the underlying dura. Infection usually spreads along the tentorium to the falx, and may extend into the posterior fossa or laterally over the temporal lobe. Patients with sinusitis may develop septic thrombophlebitis of the mucosal veins, with subsequent spread of infection to the dural veins and venous sinuses, resulting in SDE. SDE may also result from direct extension of infection from the sinuses to the subdural space. In these cases, there is often pathologic evidence of osteomyelitis of the adjacent bone. When associated paranasal sinusitis is present, infection of the subdural space often originates near the frontal pole of the skull and then extends posteriorly.

Clinical Features

The clinical features of SDE are due to *(1)* signs and symptoms of any antecedent local infection (e.g., sinusitis or otitis), *(2)* signs and symptoms of increased intracranial pressure, and *(3)* signs and symptoms of focal neurological dysfunction. Local pain referred to the region of an infected ear or sinus is quite common. Typically, there is also pain and tenderness over the brow or between the

Dr. Tyler is supported by a physician-scientist award from the National Institute of Allergy and Infectious Diseases, by a fellowship grant from the Muscular Dystrophy Association, and by a grant from the William P. Anderson Foundation.

eyes that is exacerbated by percussion of the involved sinus. Orbital swelling and mild proptosis frequently occur and presumably reflect infection involving the orbital veins. Scalp swelling or cellulitis, if present, should suggest the possibility of an associated extradural abscess or of cranial osteomyelitis.

General signs and symptoms include the almost invariable presence of fever, severe headache, and nuchal rigidity. Nausea and vomiting accompany the headache in one-half to two-thirds of cases. Patients generally appear to be severely ill. A change in the level of consciousness occurs with progression of the illness. Early on, patients often seem to be sleepy, confused, or inattentive. With further disease progression, they become somnolent, stuporous, and ultimately comatose. Patients with increased intracranial pressure may develop bradycardia, systolic hypertension, and Cheyne-Stokes breathing. Papilloedema is uncommon, and when it appears, there is usually coexisting sinus thrombosis.

Within a few days of the onset of illness, a wide variety of focal signs and symptoms appear. Contralateral hemiparesis or hemiplegia is the commonest focal symptom and eventually develops in almost all patients. Weakness is typically maximal in the face and arm (faciobrachial paresis). The deep tendon reflexes may either be increased or diminished, but the ipsilateral plantar response is usually extensor. Bilaterally upgoing toes should suggest the possibility of transtentorial herniation with compression of the brain stem.

Many patients develop a paresis or palsy of conjugate gaze toward the side opposite the lesion. In more obvious cases, this may result in a resting deviation of the eyes toward the side of the lesion.

Close to 50 percent of patients with SDE will develop seizures. Commonly, focal motor or Jacksonian seizures will antedate more generalized convulsions. Status epilepticus can occur.

Aphasia occurs in many patients with SDE, involving the dominant (typically left) hemisphere. These patients often make naming errors (anomic aphasia), although the full syndrome of either Broca's or, less commonly, Wernicke's aphasia may be seen.

Laboratory and Diagnostic Studies

Computed cranial tomography (CT scanning) has become the cornerstone of diagnosis of SDE. The CT scan is abnormal in virtually all cases. Typically, there is a crescent-shaped region of decreased attenuation between the inner table of the skull and the cerebral cortex. Midline structures are displaced away from the side of the SDE, and there is typically compression of the ipsilateral lateral ventricle. Contrast injection often produces irregular enhancement of the peripheral margin of the SDE. In cases of intrafalcial empyema, there is a lucent area running sagittally between the cerebral hemispheres.

In doubtful cases, cerebral angiography may prove valuable. The angiogram typically shows a displacement of vessels away from the inner skull table, suggesting the presence of an extra-axial avascular mass. Particular attention should be paid to the position of the meningeal arteries and the dural sinuses. Displacement of these structures away from the inner skull table suggests extradural, rather than subdural, location of a mass. In the rare cases of intrafalcial empyema, the proximal branches of the anterior cerebral artery are displaced contralaterally and the distal branches ipsilaterally. This results in distinctive S-shaped configuration of the anterior cerebral artery.

Routine radiographic studies are often of value in identifying the presence of sinusitis, mastoiditis, or cranial osteomyelitis. The CT scan may also provide evidence suggesting sinusitis or mastoiditis.

The EEG (electroencephalogram) is rarely of significant diagnostic value. The EEG may show decreased voltage and slow waves on the side of the SDE.

Lumbar puncture (LP) should be avoided in cases of suspected SDE. The LP rarely adds important diagnostic information and can result in cerebral herniation in patients with increased intracranial pressure. When CSF has been obtained in cases of SDE, the findings are quite variable. The CSF pressure is increased in about 70 percent of cases. Pleocytosis is seen in almost all patients, but the cell count varies from 15 to 1,000 cells. In patients with cell counts greater than 1,000, the possibility of rupture of the SDE into the subarachnoid space should be considered. In infants this number of cells suggests that SDE may have resulted as a complication of acute meningitis. The cells may be either predominantly polymorphonuclear leukocytes (PMNs) (60% of cases) or predominantly lymphocytes (40%). The protein is typically elevated, but rarely more than 200 mg per deciliter. The glucose is normal. Organisms are not seen and CSF cultures are negative unless there is an associated meningitis.

Pathology

A detailed discussion of the pathology of SDE is beyond the scope of this chapter. On gross examination, the subdural exudate usually covers a large part of one cerebral hemisphere. The empyema does not "wall off," and there is no evidence of a limiting membrane surrounding the exudate. Underneath the SDE, the brain is almost always depressed, and there is often evidence of an underlying purulent subarachnoid exudate and thrombosis and/or thrombophlebitis of the subarachnoid veins. Microscopic studies show evidence of infiltration of the dura with inflammatory cells, typically PMNs. The inner surface of the dura is lined with a PMN exudate. The outer layer of the cerebral cortex and subcortical white matter often show evidence of necrosis.

Infecting Agents

The commonest organisms isolated from SDE are aerobic and anaerobic streptococci and *Staphylococcus aureus*. Gram-negative organisms (*Escherichia coli, Pro-*

teus species, *Klebsiella* species, *Pseudomonas* species) may be found in cases that follow otitis or mastoiditis but are rare following paranasal sinusitis. Anaerobic bacteria are often present and may be overlooked unless special culture techniques are utilized.

Therapy

SDE is a fulminating and often life-threatening intracranial infection. Definitive therapy must be initiated without delay. Once the diagnosis is confirmed, operative drainage should be performed urgently. Drainage can be done through burr holes or following craniectomy. In most cases, a surgical approach directed toward the lateral frontal region results in the best drainage of the SDE. Obviously, the surgical approach should be modified according to the best available information on the location of the SDE. Local instillation of penicillin or other antibacterial agents may be helpful and is favored by some neurosurgeons. Surgical therapy should be combined with high doses of parenteral antibiotics in all cases. The combination of (doses are for adults with normal renal function) nafcillin, 2 g intravenously every 4 hours, or oxacillin, 2 g intravenously every 4 hours (these are therapeutically equivalent), and chloramphenicol, 1.5 g intravenously every 6 hours, usually provides satisfactory initial coverage until culture results are available. If the patient is penicillin allergic, vancomycin, 500 mg intravenously every 6 hours may be used in place of oxacillin or nafcillin.

Anticonvulsants are administered for treatment of seizures, and osmotic agents are used, when necessary, to control increased intracranial pressure.

CEREBRAL EPIDURAL ABSCESS

Etiology and Pathogenesis

Epidural abscess (EA) is the rarest of the localized intracranial suppurative infections. Pus collects between the external layer of the dura and the inner table of the skull. EA is typically associated with an overlying focal cranial osteomyelitis. Infection often spreads across the dura through the emissary veins and produces a subdural empyema as well. EA may follow localized infections of the middle ear or paranasal sinuses. EA may also follow either accidental or surgical penetration of the cranial bones. Implanted foreign bodies (dural grafts, tantalum implants, ventricular shunts, Crutchfield tongs) that penetrate the calvarium may become infected and result in the development of EA. Rare causes of EA include spread of septic dural sinus thrombosis (e.g., infectious cavernous sinus thrombosis), spread of a subdural empyema through a dural fistula, and metastatic spread of infection from a distant site.

Clinical Features

The clinical features of EA do not differ significantly from those described for subdural empyema, and distinction between these two conditions on purely clinical grounds may be difficult. Typically, signs and symptoms of a local infection, such as sinusitis or mastoiditis, are followed by severe generalized headache and high fever. With large abscesses there may be progressive alteration in mental status and focal neurologic signs. In these cases, contralateral hemiparesis is particularly common. Smaller abscesses may produce an isolated contralateral monoparesis. Focal motor convulsions occur with frequency and may generalize. An epidural empyema situated near the petrous pyramid may produce ipsilateral facial pain and sensory loss combined with diplopia due to an ipsilateral lateral rectus palsy (Gradenigo's syndrome).

Laboratory and Diagnostic Studies

The CT scan has become the primary diagnostic study for the diagnosis of EA. The typical picture is one of an extracerebral zone of low density. Evidence of sinusitis or osteomyelitis may be seen. Contrast enhancement of the outer margin of the EA is commonly found. Mass effect—including a contralateral shift of midline structures and compression of the ipsilateral lateral ventricle—is usually seen. It may be impossible to differentiate SDE and EA on CT scan.

The typical angiographic features of an epidural mass lesion were discussed in the section on SDE.

Conventional radiographic or polytomographic studies may help suggest the diagnosis of EA by demonstrating the presence of mastoid or paranasal sinus infection or by showing evidence of cranial osteomyelitis.

Lumbar puncture rarely adds valuable diagnostic information and may result in the development of herniation. When CSF has been examined, it typically shows a mild to moderate pleocytosis in which PMNs or lymphocytes may predominate. The protein is almost invariably elevated. The CSF pressure may be normal or elevated. The CSF glucose levels are normal and organisms are not seen or cultured.

Pathology

Extradural empyemas are often small and circumscribed, although large lesions are occasionally seen. Pus is found between the outer surface of the dura and the inner table of the skull. The dura itself often shows evidence of inflammation. In autopsy studies, an associated subdural empyema is found in up to 80 percent of cases, and an associated brain abscess in 15 to 20 percent.

Infecting Agents

The major infecting agents are similar to those responsible for subdural empyema.

Treatment

Optimal treatment of EA requires the combination of surgical debridement and drainage with parenteral antibiotic therapy. Infected bone should be removed, and the abscess should be drained as completely as possible. Antibiotic therapy is similar to that for SDE and should be modified as indicated by operative cultures.

BRAIN ABSCESS

Etiology

Brain abscesses usually arise from direct extension of infection from contiguous sites (e.g., middle ear, paranasal sinuses), from metastatic spread of distant infections, or from either accidental or surgically induced cranial trauma. Even after careful consideration of each of these possibilities, about 15 to 25 percent of intracranial abscesses are idiopathic in nature.

The two major sources of direct spread of infection are the middle ear/mastoid region and the paranasal sinuses. Otogenic abscesses result when infection in the middle ear erodes through the tegmen tympani or tegmen mastoideum. Spread via the lateral or other sinuses may provide an additional route. Chronic otitis, rather than acute disease, is usually the antecedent infection. Frequently, there is a history of an acute exacerbation of chronic otitis immediately preceding the first symptoms of the brain abscess. In adults otogenic abscesses most commonly occur in the temporal lobe, followed by the cerebellum. In children, a higher percentage of otogenic abscesses are cerebellar. As a corollary to this rule, an otogenic source should always be suspected when an abscess is found in the temporal lobe or cerebellum. The abscesses following infection of the frontal or ethmoid sinuses are commonly located in the frontal lobes. Sphenoidal sinusitis may result in frontal lobe, temporal lobe, or even intrasellar abscesses.

Hematogenous dissemination of infection accounts for about 25 percent of all brain abscesses. In about 20 percent of these cases, multiple abscesses are present. The most frequent site of primary infection is the lung. A wide variety of pulmonary infections including lung abscesses, pneumonia, empyema, and bronchiectasis may predispose to brain abscess development. There is also a higher-than-expected incidence of brain abscesses in patients with cystic fibrosis and pulmonary arteriovenous fistulas (e.g., Osler-Weber-Rendu syndrome). Pulmonary alveolar proteinosis predisposes patients to nocardial brain abscesses. Certain cardiac diseases also predispose to the development of brain abscess. Patients with cyanotic congenital heart disease and a right-to-left shunt are at particular risk. Bacterial endocarditis only rarely results in the production of macroabscesses (more than 1 cm diameter) in the brain, although microabscesses (less than 1 cm) are quite common. A variety of other primary infections including peritonsillar abscess, odontogenic abscess, abdominal infections, and infected intrauterine devices account for occasional cases of metastatic brain abscess. Heroin addicts and other intravenous drug abusers also appear to be at higher risk for developing brain abscesses.

Traumatic brain abscesses may be delayed for years or even decades after the acute trauma. Retained bone or metallic fragments seem to increase the risk.

Clinical Features

The signs and symptoms of brain abscess are produced by the primary infection, if one is present, by the focal effects of the brain abscess on the CNS, and by increased intracranial pressure.

General symptoms include fever, chills, and malaise. Fever is more commonly present in acute cases and much less frequent in chronic ones. In most instances the fever appears to be due to the primary infection (e.g., otitis or sinusitis), rather then to the brain abscess. Since fever is only present in about 40 percent of patients and is often low-grade, its absence does not exclude the diagnosis. Signs of increased intracranial pressure can include headache, nausea and vomiting, and alteration in mental status.

Headache may be either generalized or focal and is present in 50 to 70 percent of cases. Its absence does not exclude the diagnosis of brain abscess. Papilloedema has been reported in 25 to 50 percent of patients, but it may be a late finding. Paralysis of one or both VIth cranial nerves may result from increased intracranial pressure. Alterations in mental status—ranging from lethargy to stupor or even coma—are found in 50 to 70 percent of patients. Nuchal rigidity occurs in 20 to 50 percent of patients. Seizures may be focal or generalized and occur in about one-third of cases.

A wide variety of focal neurologic signs can occur and may provide a clue to localization. Hemiparesis occurs in about 50 percent of patients, and abnormalities of the visual fields in 5 to 20 percent. Frontal lobe abscesses may produce deterioration in memory function and attention. Temporal lobe abscesses may result in aphasia, hemiparesis, and superior quadrantopsia. Abscesses in the cerebellum often produce suboccipital headache, which radiates to the neck and interscapular area. Signs of cerebellar dysfunction may be subtle and can include incoordination, ataxia, hypotonia, conjugate gaze palsies, and nystagmus.

Laboratory and Diagnostic Studies

The peripheral white blood cell count is above 10,000 per cubic millimeter in about 50 percent of patients, but exceeds 20,000 in only 10 percent. The ESR is increased in about 75 percent of patients and may be a helpful clue in differentiating brain abscess from other mass lesions.

Of the neurodiagnostic tests, the CT scan is unequivocally the most important aid in diagnosis. It permits accurate localization of the abscess, evaluation of its size, and delineation of associated edema and mass effect. The CT scan identifies virtually 100 percent of cases of brain abscesses. The abscess appears as a mass lesion, often with a central lucent zone and a surrounding area of edema. Contrast enhancement is seen as a rim of increased density around the abscess periphery. The development of this pattern of ring enhancement has been attributed to the vascularity of the abscess capsule. Early in its natural history, an abscess appears as a zone of hypodensity without a clear capsule (cerebritis). After 3 to 6 weeks, ring enhancement is seen on CT scan, and after this point, the abscess becomes well demarcated. It is important to remember that ring-enhancing lesions are also produced by primary and metastatic tumors and, occasionally, by hematomas and hemorrhagic infarcts. The visualization on CT scan of septae inside the lesion and of ependymal or meningeal enhancement favors the diagnosis of an abscess.

Angiography is rarely used today to identify or localize brain abscesses. The usual finding is one of an avascular mass, although an area of increased vascularity corresponding to the abscess capsule may be seen. Angiography is reasonably sensitive in localizing abscesses in the temporal lobe, but frontal and parietal abscesses may be missed. The angiogram does not usually allow a precise etiologic diagnosis to be made, but simply identifies the presence of a mass lesion.

The EEG is no longer a primary diagnostic tool in cases of suspected brain abscess. It is abnormal in 75 to 90 percent of cases of supratentorial brain abscesses. The findings may include focal high amplitude slow (delta) waves, epileptiform discharges, or asymmetric fast activity.

Lumbar puncture should be avoided in cases of suspected brain abscess. The LP rarely adds useful diagnostic information, and it may result in abrupt neurologic deterioration or death. This type of deterioration occurs in up to one-third of patients within 24 to 48 hours of an LP. Reported CSF results generally include increased intracranial pressure, a pleocytosis (more than 10 cells per cubic millimeter) in 70 percent, and an elevated protein in two-thirds of cases. Cell counts of about 10,000 should raise the possibility that ventricular extension has occurred. Cell counts tend to be higher before the abscess is encapsulated and in abscesses located near the ventricles or subarachnoid space. The glucose levels are normal and cultures are negative unless there is an associated meningitis.

Infecting Agents

The bacteriology of brain abscesses is extremely variable. The most frequently isolated organisms are *S. aureus*, aerobic and anaerobic streptococci, *Streptococcus pneumoniae, Bacteroides* species, and gram-negative bacteria. Reports of isolation of a large number of other organisms have appeared. *Listeria monocytogenes* is an important pathogen in immunosuppressed patients. *Clostridia* species and *S. aureus* are often found in post-traumatic abscesses. Multiple pathogens are found in 20 to 30 percent of cases. The reported incidence of anaerobic organisms varies widely and probably depends on the techniques used to culture specimens.

Therapy

The optimal approach to the treatment of brain abscesses is combined medical and neurosurgical therapy. The choice of optimal antibiotic therapy depends on the causative organisms. Every attempt should be made to obtain an aspirate of the abscess material for aerobic, anaerobic, and special cultures. Frequently, a sterotactic aspiration under CT guidance is possible.

Prior to identification of the causative organism(s), empiric antibiotic therapy of abscesses associated with paranasal sinusitis should include intravenous penicillin G, 2 million units every 2 hours, plus chloramphenicol, 1.5 g every 6 hours. Nafcillin or oxacillin, 2 g every 4 hours intravenously, should be substituted for penicillin in abscesses of metastatic or traumatic etiology.

Therapy should be continued for a minimum of 4 weeks or until follow-up CT scans demonstrate resolution of the abscess. Several new agents including moxalactam, TMP/SMZ, and metronidazole may prove to be valuable adjuncts to therapy in specific situations.

There remains controversy over the optimal form of surgical therapy for brain abscess. Some neurosurgeons favor repeated aspirations of the abscess, whereas others feel that total excision is the treatment of choice. In general, definitive therapy involves total excision, although careful consideration of both options should be made for each case in consultation with the neurosurgical staff.

In addition to antibiotic therapy, the use of prophylactic anticonvulsants is warranted in most cases due to the high incidence of seizures. Either diphenylhydantoin (300 mg per day after an initial loading dose of 1 g in divided doses) or carbamazepine (200 mg twice a day increasing in 200-mg increments every 2 days to 200 mg four times per day) are suitable anticonvulsants. Doses should be adjusted to maintain therapeutic blood levels. (Diphenylhydantoin, 10 to 20 μg per deciliter; carbamazepine, 8 to 12 μg per deciliter). Osmotic agents may be required to control increased intracranial pressure. Steroids should be avoided whenever possible as they may inhibit antibiotic penetration into the abscess cavity.

Medical therapy alone is generally not advisable in the treatment of brain abscess. It should be considered only in cases of small abscesses (less than 2.5 cm diameter) with poorly developed or absent capsules.

THROMBOPHLEBITIS OF THE INTRACRANIAL VEINS AND SINUSES

Etiology and Pathogenesis

The etiology of dural sinus or cerebral vein infections varies according to the sinus or vein involved. Infective thrombosis most commonly involves the lateral, cavernous, and petrous sinsues. The superior sagittal sinus (SSS) and straight sinus are more commonly the site of noninfective thrombotic processes.

Lateral Sinus Etiology

The lateral sinus includes the transverse and sigmoid sinuses and terminates at the level of the jugular bulb. In many individuals one of the paired lateral sinuses, typically the right, is dominant. The lateral sinus lies in close relation to the middle ear and mastoid bone. Infection that spreads to the sinus commonly begins as mastoiditis or otitis media. A more unusual cause of lateral sinus infection is retrograde spread, via the jugular vein, of infections in the neck or pharynx (e.g., pharyngitis, adenitis, cellulitis, boils).

Clinical Features

Patients with suppurative lateral sinus thrombosis have fever and chills. Septicemia occurs in about 50 percent of cases. Septic emboli to the lungs, joints, or skin can occur. Local signs include retroauricular pain and pain on tilting or rotation of the neck. A firm cord (the jugular vein) may be felt along the anterior border of the sternocleidomastoid muscle. Involvement of the emissary veins results in swelling, erythema, and venous enlargement behind the ear, over the inion, and in the upper neck. If infection involves the dominant sinus signs of increased intracranial pressure including headache, nausea and vomiting occur. Papilloedema is present in 50 percent of cases. The presence of papilloedema or other signs of increased intracranial pressure should suggest the possibility that the contralateral sinus is hypoplastic or that infection has spread to the torcular or superior sagittal sinus. Unilateral papilloedema is usually indicative of spread of infection to the ipsilateral cavernous sinus.

Cranial nerve involvement commonly occurs. Involvement of the Vth and VIth nerves (Gradenigo's syndrome) results from petrous apicitis or disease in the inferior petrosal sinus. Sixth cranial nerve involvement can also result from increased intracranial pressure. The clinical findings in Gradeningo's syndrome include facial pain and hypesthesia and diplopia due to lateral rectus muscle palsy. Spread of infection to the jugular bulb can result in paralysis of the IXth, Xth, and XIth cranial nerves (Vernet's syndrome). Symptoms include hoarseness and dysphagia. There is usually a diminished gag reflex, poor palatal movement on one side, and decreased sensation in the peritonsillar area. Weakness of the ipsilateral sternocleidomastoid muscle and trapezius can occur. Ipsilateral tongue weakness may result from involvement of the XIIth nerve in the hypoglossal canal.

Focal CNS symptoms are uncommon with lateral sinus infection and usually indicate dissemination of infection. Involvement of the inferior anastomotic vein of Labbé can result in contralateral hemiparesis, aphasia, visual field abnormalities, and focal or generalized seizures.

Cavernous Sinus Etiology

Infection of the cavernous sinus (CS) generally occurs via one of three routes. Localized infections in the orbit, paranasal sinuses, or upper half of the face can spread to the CS from the ophthalmic veins. Infections near the teeth, tonsils, or jaw can produce sphenoid sinus infection with subsequent spread to the CS. Finally, ear infections or lateral sinus infections can spread to the CS by way of the petrosal sinuses. Although most cases of CS infection begin unilaterally, they quickly become bilateral because of the interconnection of the two CSs through the circular sinus.

Clinical Features

The onset of CS infection is abrupt, and most patients are acutely ill with high fever. Local signs and symptoms include eye pain, photophobia, proptosis, corneal clouding, orbital swelling and edema, and chemosis of the eyelid and conjunctiva. Cyanosis of the upper face, including the eyelids and the root of the nose, may be seen.

Cranial nerve palsies are invariably found and produce progressive external ophthalmoplegia. The VIth cranial nerve is usually involved initially, with subsequent involvement of the IIIrd and IVth nerves. The first division, and less commonly the second division, of the Vth (trigeminal) nerve can be involved producing facial pain, paresthesias or hypesthesia, and a diminished corneal reflex. Papilloedema results from impaired venous return. Disease of the optic nerve may result in decreased visual acuity and the appearance of scotomas. The pupils may be increased or decreased in size and are commonly sluggish or unreactive.

Superior Sagittal Sinus Etiology

As indicated earlier, septic thrombosis of the superior sagittal sinus (SSS) is far less common than noninfectious thrombosis. Infection of the SSS may result from nasal infections or infections of the paranasal sinuses. Infection may also spread directly through a contaminated compound skull fracture, or from a subdural empyema, epidural abscess, or meningitis. Metastatic infection from a distant primary site and retrograde spread of infection from tributary dural venous sinuses are often causes of SSS infection.

Clinical Features

Patients generally present with headache, fever, and signs of increased intracranial pressure. Edema of the forehead and scalp may result from involvement of emissary veins.

Focal CNS symptoms include paresis of one or both legs, cortical sensory loss, and unilateral seizures. Focal motor seizures or Jacksonian seizures are particularly common. When hemiparesis is present, the face is often relatively spared, and the weakness is more pronounced in the legs than in the arms. Many of the focal CNS signs and symptoms reflect thrombosis of cortical veins with subsequent hemorrhagic cortical infarction rather than SSS involvement per se.

Diagnosis of Intracranial Thrombophlebitis

The diagnosis usually depends on a high index of clinical suspicion. The CT scan is often helpful in excluding other causes of intracranial suppuration (e.g., brain abscess). The finding on CT scan of single or multiple hemorrhagic cortical infarctions, especially in the parasagittal area, may suggest cortical vein thrombosis. In some cases a high density serpiginous cord—representing a thrombosed cortical vein—can be seen on nonenhanced scans. This sign is virtually pathognomonic of cerebral vein thrombosis. With SSS occlusion, there may be contrast enhancement of the outer margin of the sinus and a hypodense center (''empty delta'' sign).

The most informative test is cerebral angiography. The venous sinuses and cortical veins are well visualized in the late or delayed phases of a cerebral angiogram. Signs of venous sinus occlusion include absent filling, filling defects, dilation or tortuousity of veins, slow venous filling, and reversal of the direction of venous flow. The major venous sinuses are extremely well visualized by digital subtraction angiograhy. In centers where this test is available, it often replaces conventional angiography as the diagnostic procedure of choice.

Lumbar puncture should only be performed if there are no signs of increased intracranial pressure. The spinal fluid usually shows a mild to moderate lymphocytic pleocytosis and a normal or slightly elevated protein. The presence of xanthochromia or frank hemorrhage is indicative of cortical vein thrombosis. The glucose is normal and cultures are sterile unless there is an associated meningitis. Manometric studies are not reliable. The Queckenstedt and Toby-Ayer tests of spinal fluid manometrics are only rarely performed but may be valuable in specific situations.

Therapy

Appropriate therapy consists of antibiotics and, in many cases, neurosurgical intervention. Empiric antibiotic therapy is directed toward adequate coverage of aerobic and anaerobic streptococci, *S. aureus*, and *S. pneumoniae*, and assorted anaerobes. Gram-negative organisms may be important in certain situations, especially with otogenic infections. Fungal infection (mucormycosis) is a special problem in diabetics. Empiric therapy should consist of nafcillin or oxacillin, 2 g intravenously every 4 hours, plus chloramphenicol, 1.5 g intravenously every 6 hours. Nafcillin and oxacillin are therapeutically equivalent.

Surgery should be performed if there is evidence of localized infection (e.g., osteomyelitis, mastoiditis, sinusitis). The roles of thrombectomy or of ligation of infected sinuses or of the jugular vein have not been established, and these procedures should not be routinely performed. The use of anticoagulants is also controversial. These agents should not be used if there is evidence of cortical vein thrombosis or hemorrhagic infarction. Anticoagulants may be of value for patients who develop progressive sinus thrombosis or episodes of septic embolization. Intracranial hypertension may require the use of osmotic agents or ventricular shunting procedures. Anticonvulsants are not used prophylactically, but are required in patients who develop focal or generalized seizures, especially in the setting of cortical vein thrombosis.

INTRACEREBRAL MYCOTIC ANEURYSMS

Etiology and Pathogenesis

Mycotic aneurysms are a rare complication of bacterial endocarditis and occur in less than 5 percent of cases. They constitute about 5 percent of all intracranial aneurysms. In acute bacterial endocarditis (e.g., due to *S. aureus*), mycotic aneurysms tend to develop early in the course of infection, whereas in subacute endocarditis (e.g., due to viridans streptococci), they characteristically appear late. Dissemination of infection to a site of arterial damage may produce a mycotic aneurysm even when bacterial endocarditis is not present.

The pathogenesis of these aneurysms remains unclear. In most cases, septic embolization to the vasa vasorum appears to be the inciting factor. In other cases septic intraluminal arterial emboli appear to produce an endarteritis that subsequently spreads outward through the vessel wall. Spread of infection from contiguous areas to adjacent arteries may be a third mechanism of pathogenesis.

Mycotic aneurysms are solitary in 80 percent of cases and multiple in 20 percent. They tend to involve vessels near their branching points. The distal portion of the middle cerebral artery is probably the most commonly involved site.

Clinical Features

In many cases, mycotic aneurysms, like congenital berry aneurysms, appear to be asymptomatic unless they leak or rupture. Some patients develop severe, unremitting, localized headache. When this symptom develops in a patient with known bacterial endocarditis, aneurysm should be strongly suspected. Many patients will have evidence of cerebral embolization in the period immediately preceding the development of a mycotic aneurysm. Patients with endocarditis who develop focal CNS findings should have a CT scan, followed in most cases by a lumbar puncture. An aseptic CSF pattern (lymphocytic pleocytosis, normal or elevated protein levels, normal glucose level) is usually indicative of embolism, brain abscess, or mycotic aneurysm. The first two possibilities can usually be excluded on the basis of the history and the results of the CT scan. A hemorrhagic spinal fluid (more than 200 red blood cells per cubic millimeter in all tubes after a nontraumatic LP) should always suggest mycotic aneurysm.

Diagnostic Studies

Patients who develop severe and persistent focal headache in the setting of endocarditis should undergo cerebral angiography. Patients with endocarditis and hemorrhagic spinal fluid or evidence of intracerebral hemorrhage by CT should also undergo angiography. Angiography remains the definitive diagnostic test for identification of mycotic aneurysms. However, small aneurysms may be missed. Improved techniques for digital subtraction angiography will make this test increasingly valuable in the future. Due to the incidence of multiple aneurysms (about 20%), injection of both carotid arteries is advisable. Mycotic aneurysms of the posterior circulation are rare. A vertebral injection is probably not routinely required and should be used only when indicated by the clinical situation or when visualization of the carotid circulation does not reveal an aneurysm. Subtraction and magnification views are essential. Patients with an intracerebral hematoma who have a negative angiogram during the acute stage should have the test repeated after the mass effect of the hematoma has resolved. The small size of aneurysms makes CT of limited value in direct diagnosis. The CT scan may be helpful in excluding other diagnoses (e.g., abscess, infarct) or in indirectly suggesting mycotic aneurysm by demonstrating intracerebral or subarachnoid blood.

The mortality of patients with endocarditis and a ruptured mycotic aneurysm exceeds 80 percent. The goal must be to identify patients with unruptured aneurysms and treat them aggressively. Controversy exists about the appropriate role of antibiotic therapy alone in the treatment of mycotic aneurysms. Antibiotic therapy alone results in resolution of almost 50 percent of recognized peripheral mycotic aneurysms. The mortality rate in patients treated with medical therapy is about 15 percent, although mild to moderate neurologic deficits are seen in 25 to 50 percent of survivors. Patients treated medically should have follow-up angiography on a weekly or biweekly basis. If there is an increase in aneurysm size, any evidence of bleeding, or no decrease in aneurysm size over 4 to 6 weeks, then surgery should be performed. The choice of antibiotics depends on isolation of the etiologic agent from the bloodstream or other sites (e.g., embolic material). Regimens for staphylococci and streptococci are listed below.

Streptococcal Endocarditis and Mycotic Aneurysm

Aqueous penicillin G, 2 million units intravenously every 2 hours, plus streptomycin, 0.5 g intramuscularly every 12 hours. These doses should be modified once organism sensitivities are available. Toxicity may require alteration of the streptomycin dose or dosing interval. Therapy should be continued for a minimum of 4 to 6 weeks. If the aneurysm is decreasing in size but has not resolved, therapy should be continued and a decision about surgical therapy made.

Staphylococcal Endocarditis and Mycotic Aneurysm

Nafcillin or oxacillin, 2 g intravenously every 4 hours (for penicillin allergic patients: vancomycin, 500 mg intravenously every 6 hours). Nafcillin and oxacillin are therapeutically equivalent. Duration of therapy is as noted above.

LOCALIZED INFECTIONS OF THE SPINAL CORD

Localized infections of the spinal cord can be classified according to their anatomic location as epidural, subdural, or intraspinal. Epidural abscesses are considerably more frequent than are either subdural or intraspinal infections. Localized infections of the spinal cord are medical and neurosurgical emergencies that require rapid institution of appropriate therapy. Therapeutic delay often results in tragic sequelae for the patient, including permanent paraplegia or quadriplegia and even death.

Pathogenesis

The possible routes of initiation of localized infections of the spinal cord include *(1)* direct extension from contiguous infection (e.g., vertebral osteomyelitis, perinephric or retroperitoneal abscess); *(2)* hematogenous spread from a distant site of infection; *(3)* introduction of infected material (e.g., following knife or gunshot injury, lumbar puncture, operation. In rare cases ("primary"), none of the factors noted above can be identified. Metastatic infection probably accounts for 50 percent of cases of epidural and intraspinal abscess and an even higher percentage of cases of spinal subdural empyema. The primary infection can be in the skin (furunculosis, carbuncles, cellulitis), the lungs (pneumonia, empyema, bronchiectasis), the heart (endocarditis), the genitourinary system (prostatic abscess, purulent cystitis), or the oropharynx (retropharyngeal or tonsillary abscess, dental abscess). Septic abortion may be a site of primary infection in pregnant women.

Clinical Features

Distinction between epidural and subdural infections can rarely be made clinically. These infections appear to occur with increased frequency in immunosuppressed patients, diabetics, and intravenous drug abusers. The initial symptom is usually severe, localized pain, typically in the back. In cases of epidural empyema, pain is increased by percussion or local pressure. Patients with subdural empyema or intraspinal abscess frequently do not have percussion tenderness. With both epi- or subdural infection, patients typically hold the spine rigid and try to avoid any undue motion. At this stage, patients are usually acutely ill. Fever is almost invariably present, and there may be chills or rigors. Headache and meningeal signs are also commonly present. Most patients have radicular pains involving the chest or, less commonly, the arms or legs. Symptoms are followed quickly (in 24 to 48 hours) by signs of an acute transverse spinal cord lesion. Patients develop flaccid paraplegia (or quadriplegia), loss of reflexes, a sensory level, and sphincter disturbances. Babinski's sign is present bilaterally. Flaccidity may subsequently evolve into spasticity with hyperactive reflexes once the period of "spinal shock" is over.

Some patients, especially those whose infection is caused by fungi or mycobacteria (see below), follow a slower ("chronic") course, which can mimic other extradural compressive lesions such as tumors.

Most cases of intraspinal abscesses present with a clinical picture similar to that of epidural or subdural lesions. Constitutional symptoms such as fever, malaise, rigors are followed by back pain with or without meningeal symptoms. Within hours to days, there is paraplegia (flaccid, arreflexic), anesthesia with a sensory level, and disorder of bowel and bladder function. Specific signs pointing to an intramedullary lesion (e.g., dissociated sensory loss, sacral sparing) are frequently obscured by the rapid progression of the illness.

Pathology

A complete discussion of pathology is beyond the scope of this chapter. Most epidural and subdural infections are located posterior (dorsal) to the spinal cord. Infections are more common in the thoracic region, although cervical, and less commonly, lumbar, sacral, or cauda equina lesions occur. In most cases of epidural abscess, the infection extends for several (e.g., three to six) cord segments. Subdural empyema may be present at multiple levels. Intraspinal abscesses are typically located centrally in the cord or in the region of the posterior horns. They are most common in the cervical region and may extend into the brainstem. Abscesses are usually single, but multiple abscesses are not rare. The abscess size is quite variable, from microscopic to the entire length of the cord. Most lesions extend for at least five segments. These abscesses rarely encapsulate.

Infecting Agents

The commonest cause of acute localized spinal infections are bacteria. Cases of chronic epidural abscess are frequently due to mycobacteria, actinomyces, and fungi (blastomycosis, cryptococcosis, aspergillosis, nocardiosis) and, occasionally, result from other agents (e.g., *Echinococcus*). Of the bacterial agents, *S. aureus* is clearly the most frequently encountered and is responsible for one-half to two-thirds of all cases of localized spinal infection. *Staphylococcus* should be particularly suspected in patients with a history of antecedent trauma or skin infection. Streptococci and pneumococci may be encountered in patients with primary pulmonary infections. In intravenous drug abusers and patients with antecedent genitourinary infections, gram-negative organisms (*Escherichia coli, Pseudomonas Aeruginosa, Serratia marcescens, Enterobacter cloacae, Proteus* species) are commonly found.

Laboratory Tests

Patients with acute localized spinal infections will almost invariably have a leukocytosis and an elevated erythrocyte sedimentation rate. Radiographs of the spine are often normal, but may show evidence of localized osteomyelitis with bony destruction and disk-space narrowing. Blood cultures are positive in up to 50 percent of cases. Myelography remains the definitive diagnostic procedure and should be performed immediately in all systemically ill patients who develop severe back pain, radicular symptoms, or signs of spinal cord compression. Ideally, metrizamide myelography should be combined with CT scan of the spine for the best delineation of the lesion. Cervical puncture should be performed for introduction of dye to diminish the risk of entering the abscess if it is located in the lumbar area. In almost all cases of epidural infection or subdural infection, myelography will demonstrate either a complete (80%) or partial (20%) block to the flow of dye. An attempt should be made to define the upper and lower extent of the lesion. CT scan, even without the addition of dye into the subarachnoid space, will often demonstrate an epidural abscess. Patients with intraspinal abscess will commonly have swelling of the spinal cord seen by myelography or CT. In some cases the swelling is severe enough to result in either partial or complete CSF block.

Lumbar puncture is best deferred until the time of myelography. The CSF in patients with acute epidural or subdural infection usually has a polymorphonuclear pleocytosis (50 to 500 cells), an elevated level of protein, and a normal level of glucose. In patients with epidural abscess, the CSF culture is positive in approximately 20 percent. If the CSF pleocytosis is excessive and the glucose is depressed, a concomitant spinal meningitis is usually present. Patients with chronic infections may only have an elevated CSF protein. In cases of suspected epidural abscess, the LP needle should be advanced slowly and aspirated frequently. If frank pus is withdrawn, the procedure should be terminated to avoid introducing infection into the subdural or subarachnoid space.

Therapy

Once a localized spinal infection has been diagnosed and localized, a bilateral exploratory laminectomy should be performed immediately. In cases of intraspinal abscess puncture or incision of the cord and aspiration to evacuate pus should be done. In patients with epidural infection, care should be taken to avoid opening the spinal dura. Aspiration of pus should probably be followed by local antibiotic irrigation (e.g.,bacitracin, 50,000 units per 50 milliliters of normal saline). Drains should be placed between the epidural space and the skin surface. Material obtained at operation should be sent for aerobic and anaerobic bacterial culture and for fungal and mycobacterial culture in all chronic cases. Pathologic material should be examined microscopically for bacteria, mycobacteria, fungi, and for the presence of granulomas. Gram stain, Ziehl-Neelson stain, and other appropriate stains should be performed immediately on some of the available material.

Definitive antibiotic therapy should be based on cultures obtained at operation. Initial antibiotic therapy should be instituted as soon as the diagnosis is suspected. Because of the high frequency of *S. aureus* infections, a semisynthetic penicillin in high doses should be used, e.g., nafcillin sodium, 2 g every 4 hours, intravenously, or (therapeutically equivalent) oxacillin sodium, 2 g every 4 hours, intravenously (alternate therapy if patient is penicillin-allergic: vancomycin hydrochloride, 500 mg every 6 hours intravenously).

In drug addicts or patients with preexisting genitourinary disease, an aminoglycoside should be added, e.g., tobramycin sulfate or gentamicin sulfate, 1.5 mg per kilogram every 8 hours intravenously (4.5 mg per kilogram per day). Serum levels should be monitored. Subsequent doses adjustments should be made on the basis of drug levels. Dose reduction is invariably required in patients with renal insufficiency. Infection caused by tuberculosis should be treated with triple therapy (isoniazid, ethambutol, rifampin, or streptomycin). Amphotericin B or miconazole with or without fluorouracil should be used for fungal infections.

SYPHILIS

ROBERT R. TIGHT, M.D.

Syphilis is an infectious disease of great chronicity caused by *Treponema pallidum*. It is systemic from the outset, usually sexually transmitted, capable of involving practically every organ and system of the body and of mimicking a large number of other disease entities, and is distinguished by florid manifestations in some cases and years of completely asymptomatic latency in others.

ETIOLOGY

Certain characteristics of *Treponema pallidum* have diagnostic and therapeutic relevance. The delicate spiral-shaped organism is relatively thin (0.25 μ) and is not stained readily by ordinary laboratory methods necessitating indirect, darkfield microscopy for optimal visualization in the outpatient setting. *T. pallidum* cannot at present be cultured in vitro. Thus, less direct serologic methods are usually needed for diagnosis. *T. pallidum* is exquisitely sensitive to penicillin (and many other antibiotics), for which the minimal inhibitory concentration is less than 0.03 units per milliliter. To date, there has been no evidence of increasing antibiotic resistance as has occurred with *Neisseria gonorrhoeae*. Finally, *T. pallidum* multiplies much more slowly than many pathogenic bacteria, having a generation time of about 30 to 33 hours early in the course of infection and longer after the development of (partial) host immunity. This is thought to account for the relatively prolonged duration of therapy needed for the cure of syphilis. It appears that treponemacidal serum penicillin levels must be present for at least 1 to 2 days to cure incubating syphilis, for at least 7 days to cure early syphilis, and for at least 3 weeks to cure infections of more than 1 year's duration. This is sometimes referred to as the time-dose relationship in syphilis therapy, that is, low doses of penicillin are adequate, but only if continuously present for a relatively prolonged duration.

CLINICALLY USEFUL CLASSIFICATIONS OF SYPHILIS

Three different ways of classifying syphilis are shown in Table 1. The second is particularly important epidemiologically and therapeutically, since only early syphilis is considered infectious (with a few exceptions, e.g., pregnant females) and late syphilis requires a longer duration of therapy. Some authorities define early syphilis as syphilis of either less than 2 or less than 4 years' duration; I prefer to define early syphilis as being of less than 1 years' duration. It is important to emphasize that when syphilis is clinically latent, a reactive serologic test for syphilis (STS) is, by definition, the only indication of disease.

CLINICAL MANIFESTATIONS OF SYPHILIS

T. pallidum is capable of penetrating intact mucous membranes and cracked or abraded skin. Within a few hours after infection, spread to regional lymph nodes occurs, followed by bacteremic dissemination to metastatic systemic foci, long before the appearance of a chancre. An incubation period averaging about 3 weeks and varying inversely with the treponemal inoculum is followed by the appearance of the primary lesion of syphilis, the chancre. This is a painless shallow ulcer at the site of inoculation, genital or extragenital, and is accompanied by firm, nonsuppurative, nontender regional (typically

TABLE 1 Classifications of Syphilis

1.	Primary:	chancre at site of *T. pallidum* invasion
	Secondary:	mucocutaneous, hepatitis, meningitis, others
	Tertiary:	CNS, cardiovascular, gummatous, other
	Congenital:	early ($\leq$2 years of life), late
	Incubating:	very early syphilis prior to development of a chancre or reactive serologic test for syphilis
2.	Early: (infectious)	infection with *T. pallidum* of less than 1 year (including primary, secondary, incubating, early latent)
	Late:	infection of more than 1 year's duration (includes tertiary, asymptomatic neurosyphilis, late latent)
3.	Latent:	only evidence of syphilis is reactive treponemal STS
	Active:	primary, secondary, tertiary, or congenital

bilateral inguinal) lymphadenopathy. Chancres heal spontaneously in a few weeks even without therapy.

Several weeks to several months later, secondary syphilis may ensue or the disease may remain latent. Secondary syphilis is characterized by highly variable mucocutaneous and systemic findings, including nonpruritic macules on the palmar and plantar skin and elsewhere, highly infectious mucous membrane lesions (mucous patches, condyloma lata), generalized lymphadenopathy, anorexia, fever, aseptic meningitis, hepatitis, nephrotic syndrome, and others. Relapses of secondary syphilis may occur; these generally become progressively milder clinically and usually cease within the first year after infection.

Following the secondary syphilis stage, a period of latency develops, which probably is lifelong in the majority of patients, even without specific antibiotic therapy. However, a minority, perhaps 30 percent, of untreated patients may develop central nervous system, cardiovascular, or gummatous tertiary syphilis.

Classic neurologic syndromes include general paresis and tabes dorsalis. In recent years, cases of classic neurosyphilis have become quite uncommon, presumably due to the widespread use of antibiotics. The Argyll-Robertson pupil—an irregular pupil that does not react to light but does accommodate—is virtually pathognomonic of tertiary syphilis, but is rarely seen now.

In addition, the entity of asymptomatic neurosyphilis is often a clinical concern. Such patients may have nonspecific or no clinical symptoms. The only evidence of neurosyphilis may be a positive serum and cerebrospinal fluid (CSF) serologic test for syphilis (STS) together with CSF pleocytosis and elevation of CSF protein.

Cardiovascular syphilis typically is manifested by development of aneurysmal dilatation of the ascending aorta, resulting in aortic valvular insufficiency. The most significant morbidity and mortality attributable to syphilis is related to cardiovascular and central nervous system syphilis.

The essential lesion of late benign syphilis is the gumma. Gummas result from hypersensitivity reactions, are characterized by granulomatous inflammation with central necrosis, and occur in any organ (and hence are not always "benign"), most commonly in skin, bone, and the liver.

Congenital syphilis, consisting of early and late stages much like those of acquired syphilis, occurs if an untreated mother with syphilis transmits the infection transplacentally to the fetus. In general, the longer the duration of untreated infection in the mother, the less likely the fetus will be infected. The spectrum of illness ranges from a fulminating fetal congenital syphilis to an uninfected child.

EPIDEMIOLOGIC CONSIDERATIONS

Most new cases of syphilis are seen in sexually active persons between the ages of 15 and 30 years. In recent years in the United States, nearly half the cases of early syphilis have occurred in homosexual men. Because of the wide variety of clinical manifestations of syphilis, diagnostic studies are indicated in any sexually active patient with findings consistent with syphilis or suggestive of any sexually transmitted disease (STD) or with a history of contact to a patient with syphilis.

DIFFERENTIAL DIAGNOSIS

Differential diagnosis of primary syphilis includes several other causes of ulcerative genital lesions including trauma, chancroid, lymphogranuloma venereum, and genital herpes simplex virus (HSV) infections. Genital HSV infections are currently much commoner than syphilitic chancres. The situation is further complicated by the possibility that syphilis may coexist with other ulcerative genital lesions and/or other STDs. Any newly developed oral, anal, or genital ulcer in a sexually active person requires that the diagnosis of syphilis be considered and diagnostic studies done.

The differential diagnosis of secondary syphilis is varied, but the diagnosis can be confirmed readily because the STS is virtually always reactive in secondary syphilis. Thus, the main requirement is an appropriate index of suspicion of the diagnosis. Any sexually active patient, especially a male homosexual with new skin lesions, constitutional symptoms, or an undiagnosed illness, should have an STS.

The differential diagnosis of late syphilis most importantly includes cardiovascular diseases resulting in aortic valvular insufficiency and ascending aortic aneurysm and causes of neurologic illness such as the stroke syndrome, seizure disorders, and dementia. Diagnostic studies should be undertaken in any patient with compatible cardiovascular or neurologic illness or possible gummatous lesions for which an alternative etiology is not clearly established. Since nontreponemal STS may be nonreactive in some cases of late syphilis, STS utilizing treponemal antigens (see below) are needed and should be ordered for any patient suspected of having late syphilis, even if a screening, nontreponemal STS is nonreactive.

Syphilis acquired during pregnancy may be subclinical in the mother while frequently causing severe fetal infection. Thus, routine STS at the time of the first prenatal visit is justified in pregnant females. In high-risk patients, an STS should be repeated in the third trimester. In addition, if manifestations of early syphilis develop in pregnancy, prompt diagnostic studies are imperative. Adequate treatment of the mother before the 16th week of pregnancy should prevent fetal damage. Treatment after that time should minimize the damage.

DIAGNOSIS OF SYPHILIS

The diagnosis of syphilis may be made by darkfield (DF) microscopy or serologically. *T. pallidum* may be demonstrated by DF microscopy of an appropriate cutaneous lesion, such as the chancre of primary syphilis or condyloma of secondary syphilis, and is identified by its characteristic morphology and motility. This requires some experience in interpretation since saprophytic nonpathogenic spirochetes morphologically similar to *T. pallidum* may also inhabit moist genital regions and the mouth. Thus, great care must be exercised in interpretation of DF preparations from oral or cervical lesions. Unfortunately, DF microscopy by an experienced microscopist often is not readily available.

There are two main types of STS: nontreponemal tests, such as the Rapid Plasma Reagin (RPR) card test and the Venereal Disease Research Laboratory (VDRL) test; and treponemal tests such as the fluorescent treponemal antibody absorption (FTA-ABS) test or the microhemagglutination test for *T. pallidum* antibodies (MHA-TP, TPHA). Nontreponemal tests utilize a nonspecific (cardiolipin) antigen extracted from beef heart and are technically simple and inexpensive, but have higher incidences of false-positive and false-negative results than treponemal tests. The treponemal tests are more demanding technically (particularly the FTA-ABS test) and more expensive, but utilize specific antigenic material derived from *T. pallidum*. They are more sensitive and specific, though false-positive reactions may occur in pregnancy and collagen-vascular disorders, and false-negative results may occur, particularly in very early syphilis. Nontreponemal tests generally are used for screening purposes and for treatment follow-up. Treponemal tests are used to confirm the diagnosis of syphilis (e.g., +VDRL, +FTA-ABS), to define a ''biologic false-positive'' nontreponemal STS (e.g., +RPR, −FTA-ABS), or in circumstances where a nontreponemal test is thought to be falsely negative, such as in suspected late syphilis. Treponemal tests tend to remain positive for life regardless of therapy, generally are not quantitated (i.e., titered), and are not useful for follow-up purposes or for assessing adequacy of therapy.

The FTA-ABS, MHA-TP, and RPR tests have not been standardized for testing CSF. The laboratory diagnosis of neurosyphilis is most clear in the setting of a reactive serum treponemal STS, CSF pleocytosis, elevated CSF protein, and a reactive CSF VDRL. Occasionally, the situation is not so clear. Nonreactive CSF test results with nontreponemal STS were well known in a small minority, perhaps 10 percent, of patients with classic neurosyphilis. Whether or not CSF FTA-ABS testing would improve sensitivity of CSF serologic testing has not been determined. Thus routine FTA-ABS testing of CSF is not currently recommended. However, in unusual, carefully selected cases (such as in the evaluation of a patient with an undiagnosed neurologic disorder compatible with neurosyphilis, a reactive serum FTA-ABS, and a nonreactive CSF VDRL), the CSF FTA-ABS test might be worth performing, particularly if a decision to hospitalize for intravenous therapy was a consideration. Consultation with an STD or infectious diseases specialist would probably be appropriate in such cases.

A suggested approach for the use of DF microscopy and STS in primary and secondary syphilis is as follows:

Suspected primary syphilis. Perform DF examination if facilities are available. Consider lesion nonsyphilitic only if three daily DF examinations are negative and nontreponemal STS is persistently negative for a month. If DF is positive, diagnose and treat primary syphilis. Obtain nontreponemal STS. If positive, confirm with serum FTA-ABS test. Otherwise, do not use FTA-ABS test in suspected primary syphilis. A negative nontreponemal STS should be repeated in 1 week and, if still negative, 1 month after the first STS. Unless DF microscopy is positive, a negative nontreponemal test after a month excludes the diagnosis. Most (more than 70%) DF-positive patients with primary syphilis have a reactive STS, but a few—if treated very early—may never develop a reactive STS.

Suspected secondary syphilis. Obtain nontreponemal STS. If positive, confirm with a treponemal STS. If nontreponemal STS is negative the diagnosis of secondary syphilis, for practical purposes, is excluded.

The diagnosis of tertiary syphilis is made in patients with clinical findings suggestive of central nervous system or cardiovascular syphilis or a gumma who have a positive serum treponemal STS with or without a positive serum nontreponemal STS. Most, but not all, patients with tertiary syphilis have a reactive serum nontreponemal STS. Patients with no clinical findings of syphilis, but with a reactive treponemal STS, such as elective surgical patients found to have a reactive screening STS, need to have asymptomatic neurosyphilis carefully excluded. Diagnosis of neurosyphilis should be confirmed, in most cases, with a CSF VDRL. As noted above, the FTA-ABS test should not be done routinely on CSF, but might be considered in carefully selected problem cases after consultation with a specialist.

THERAPY OF SYPHILIS

Penicillin is the drug of choice for syphilis therapy. Suggested treatment regimens are summarized in Table 2. Patients with penicillin allergy should be treated with tetracycline. Pregnant women and children under the age of 8 years with congenital or acquired syphilis who are allergic to penicillin should be treated with erythromy-

TABLE 2 Treatment of Syphilis

Stage of Syphilis	*Patients Without Penicillin Allergy*	*Penicillin-Allergic Patients*
Possible incubating* (epidemiologic treatment)	Benzathine penicillin G (BPG) 2.4 million units IM	----
Primary, secondary, or early latent	BPG 2.4 million units IM	Tetracycline HCl 2.0 g/day × 15 days or erythromycin base or stearate 2.0 g/day × 15 days
Late latent or latent of uncertain duration	CSF normal: BPG 2.4 million units weekly for 3 doses CSF abnormal: treat as neurosyphilis	Treat as neurosyphilis
Late neurosyphilis	Aqueous crystalline penicillin G (ACPG), 4 million units IV every 4 hours × 10 days followed by BPG 2.4 million units IM weekly for 3 doses *or* Aqueous procaine penicillin G (APPG) 2.4 million units IM daily plus probenecid 500 mg PO 4 times/day, both for 10 days, followed by BPG 2.4 million units IM weekly for 3 doses *or* BPG 2.4 million units IM weekly for 3 doses	Tetracycline HCl 2.0 g daily for 30 days
Congenital (treat all neonates with either proved or suspected congenital syphilis)	Symptomatic infants or asymptomatic infants with abnormal CSF: ACPG 25,000 units/kg IM or IV every 12 hours (i.e., 50,000 units/kg/day) for at least 10 days *or* APPG 50,000 units/kg IM daily for at least 10 days *or* Asymptomatic infants with normal CSF: BPG 50,000 units IM in a single dose	Antibiotics other than penicillin should not be used to treat neonates; after the neonatal period, penicillin-allergic patients less than 8 years of age should receive erythromycin in individualized doses, not to exceed daily adult doses, for 30 days; more than 8 years of age, treat with tetracycline in individualized doses, not to exceed daily adult doses, for 30 days
Syphilis in pregnancy	Penicillin, use dosage schedules appropriate for stage of syphilis as recommended for treatment of nonpregnant patients (see above)	Erythromycin stearate or base 2.0 g/day × 15 (early syphilis, and also treat infant with penicillin) or 30 (late syphilis) days

Note: Source: derived from Centers for Disease Control *STD Treatment Guidelines*, revised 1982.
* Patients exposed to infectious syphilis and felt to be at high risk of developing syphilis.

cin. Patients treated with tetracycline or erythromycin should receive particularly close follow-up since the efficacy of these drugs in syphilis therapy is not well established. There have been a few reports of infants born with congenital syphilis to mothers treated for syphilis during pregnancy with erythromycin.

ADDITIONAL THERAPEUTIC CONSIDERATIONS

There is some difference of opinion regarding the management of patients with neurosyphilis. Although treatment with benzathine penicillin, as outlined in Table 2, probably is effective in many cases of neurosyphilis, some clinicians prefer to hospitalize patients with neurosyphilis for treatment with 4 million units of aqueous crystalline penicillin G given intravenously every 4 hours each day for 10 days.

Treatment of primary and secondary syphilis with penicillin may be followed by a Jarisch-Herxheimer reaction, characterized by chills, fever, myalgia, headache, and other constitutional symptoms. This reaction is not to be confused with an allergic reaction to penicillin. Patients should be forewarned of this reaction, which is best managed with bedrest and aspirin or acetaminophen.

Patients may contract syphilis and another STD (e.g., gonorrhea) with a shorter incubation time than syphilis. These patients often seek medical evaluation while syphilis is still incubating. The effect on incubating syphilis of treatment for other STDs is therefore of interest. The penicillin regimen currently recommended for gonorrhea therapy has been shown to eradicate incubating syphilis. Spectinomycin, as used for gonorrhea therapy, and metronidazole, as used for treating vaginitis, are considered ineffective therapy for incubating syphilis, on the basis of experimental studies. All other regimens (ampicillin, amoxicillin, tetracycline, doxycycline) currently recommended for gonorrhea therapy and tetracycline regimens recommended for therapy of nongonococcal urethritis and lymphogranuloma venereum probably eradicate incubating syphilis, though this is unproved.

FOLLOW-UP AND RETREATMENT OF SYPHILIS

Quantitative nontreponemal STS results are of value in the follow-up of patients treated for syphilis. A decreasing titer or a stable, low titer typically follows satisfactory therapy. Most patients treated for primary syphilis experience reversion of nontreponemal STS to nonreactive within 12 months following treatment. Reversion takes longer after treatment for reinfection, secondary, or early latent syphilis, but usually occurs within 24 months. After treatment for late syphilis, reversion occurs in some cases, whereas a stable, low titer, so-called serofast syphilis, is the result in other patients. A rising titer (fourfold or more) suggests reinfection or inadequacy of therapy. It is worth pointing out that RPR titers typically are reactive to one or two dilutions higher than VDRL titers. Thus, the same test should be used in following up patients treated for syphilis in order to avoid misdiagnosing relapse or reinfection (as might occur, for example, if a VDRL test is done at the time of diagnosis but follow-up is with RPR tests).

All patients with early syphilis and congenital syphilis should be encouraged to return for repeat quantitative nontreponemal STS 3, 6, and 12 months after treatment. Patients with syphilis for more than 1 year's duration should also have a nontreponemal STS 24 months after treatment. Careful follow-up serologic testing is particularly important in patients treated with antibiotics other than penicillin. Examination of CSF should be planned as part of the last follow-up visit after treatment with alternative antibiotics. All patients with neurosyphilis should be carefully followed up with serologic testing for at least 3 years. Such patients should also be reevaluated clinically at 6 month intervals. Repeat CSF examinations should be considered at these times, unless the spinal fluid becomes completely normal with respect to VDRL testing, protein, and white cell count.

Retreatment should be considered when clinical signs or symptoms of syphilis recur or fail to resolve with therapy, when an increasing (fourfold or greater) titer of a nontreponemal STS occurs, or when an initially high-titer nontreponemal STS fails to decrease at least fourfold after a year. The possibility of reinfection should always be considered when retreating patients with early syphilis. A CSF examination should be performed before retreatment unless reinfection and a diagnosis of early syphilis can be established.

As with any STD, it is imperative for public health and disease control purposes that contacts be identified and treated. Thus, the assistance of public health authorities needs to be requested whenever syphilis is diagnosed. Such cooperation is essential for breaking the chain of infection. It may, for example, be possible to identify persons exposed to syphilis in the incubating stage, before symptoms develop. These individuals should be offered "epidemiologic" treatment even though perhaps only 20 to 30 percent of them have actually contracted the disease.

CELLULITIS AND SOFT TISSUE INFECTION

THOMAS T. YOSHIKAWA, M.D.

Infections of the skin and soft tissue may involve all layers of the integument, fascia, and muscle and may be complicated by necrosis or sepsis. This discussion will be limited to infections involving the skin that are not usually associated with crepitus and gangrene: impetigo, erysipelas, cellulitis, folliculitis, furuncle, and carbuncle.

Several general principles should be considered when managing patients with these particular dermatologic infections:

1. Determine clinically whether the patient can be managed as an outpatient or requires hospitalization. Factors that weigh in favor of inpatient therapy include the presence of systemic toxicity (e.g., fever, chills); the presence of significant underlying conditions such as insulin-dependent diabetes mellitus, neutropenia, or immunosuppression; involvement of the facial region, hands, or adjacent joint space; and the presence of surrounding edema or cutaneous necrosis.
2. Most of these skin infections are caused by group A beta-hemolytic streptococci and/or coagulase-positive *Staphylococcus aureus*.
3. Most strains of *S. aureus* produce penicillinase (i.e., are penicillin-resistant), and therefore this bacterium is best treated with a beta-lactamase-resistant antibiotic.

IMPETIGO

Impetigo is the commonest cutaneous bacterial infection. It presents clinically as two distinct types—crusted impetigo and bullous impetigo.

Crusted Impetigo

This form of impetigo occurs predominantly in preschool-aged children, with a peak seasonal incidence in the late summer and early fall. The commonest etiology is group A beta-hemolytic streptococci with *S. aureus* coisolated in 50 to 60 percent of patients. However, it is thought that the role of *S. aureus* under these circumstances is a subsidiary one. *S. aureus* may be isolated alone in crusted impetigo in 5 to 10 percent of cases. The lesion of crusted impetigo is an inflammation of the superficial skin layer between the stratum corneum and stratum granulosum.

The cutaneous lesions begin as small, thin-roofed vesicles that rapidly become pustular and easily rupture. The purulent drainage then dries, leaving a thick, soft, honey-colored crust. The lesion may vary in size from 1 to 3 cm and may be spread to other parts of the body by autoinoculation. The extremities and face are most commonly infected. The lesions are painless and heal without scarring. Regional lymphadenopathy commonly occurs, but systemic symptoms are generally absent.

The diagnosis is made clinically and generally is not difficult. Early vesicles or weeping lesions can be gram-stained or cultured, but this is not necessary in most patients unless staphylococci are suspected or the initial antibiotic therapy fails.

The treatment of choice for streptococcal impetigo is penicillin. Either oral or intramuscular preparations can be prescribed. Phenoxymethyl penicillin should be given orally for 10 days in doses of 50 mg per kilogram per day (in four equal doses) and 2 g per day (in four equal doses) to children and adults, respectively. Benzathine penicillin as a single intramuscular injection may be given as an alternative drug. The doses for children and adults are 50,000 units per kilogram and 2.4 million units, respectively. Patients allergic to penicillin should be treated with oral erythromycin (50 mg per kilogram per day, divided in four equal doses, for children; 2 g per day, in four equal doses, for adults). Topical treatment using warm soap and water compresses is valuable in removing crusts, debris, and dirt.

Bullous Impetigo

Bullous impetigo occurs less frequently than crusted impetigo. Newborn and older children are particularly susceptible. The infection is caused by *S. aureus*, which liberates a toxin, epidermolysin. These strains generally belong to *S. aureus* phage group II and can cause staphylococcal scalded-skin syndrome. The histopathology of bullous impetigo is similar to that for crusted impetigo.

The lesion of bullous impetigo starts as a vesicle that rapidly evolves to a bulla, 2 to 5 cm in diameter. The bulla is flaccid and has no peripheral erythema. It generally ruptures, leaving a raw, red base, which will eventually dry and form a thin, light brown, lacquer-like crust. Systemic symptoms are generally absent.

The diagnosis of bullous impetigo is made clinically by its typical appearance. *S. aureus* may be isolated from the lesions by culture.

Treatment should be initiated with an oral penicillinase-resistant penicillin, i.e., cloxacillin or dicloxacillin, for 10 days. The doses of cloxacillin or dicloxacillin for children are 50 mg per kilogram per day (not to exceed the adult dose) and 25 mg per kilogram per day, both given in four equally divided doses. Adults should receive 2 g of cloxacillin or 1 g of dicloxacillin in four equally divided doses daily.

ERYSIPELAS

Erysipelas is a relatively uncommon cutaneous infection that occurs in the very young, the elderly, the debilitated, and individuals with chronic ulcers or lymphedema of the skin. Although it is a form of cellulitis, the distinct characteristics of erysipelas warrant a separate discussion.

The etiology of erysipelas is almost always group A beta-hemolytic streptococci. Group B streptococci may be isolated in newborns with this infection. Occasionally, other streptococci or, rarely, *S. aureus* may cause erysipelas. The histopathology of the skin shows intense edema, vascular dilation, abundant streptococci in tissue spaces and lymphatic channels, and leukocytic cellular infiltration. The dermis is primarily involved, with the epidermis only secondarily affected.

The cutaneous lesion of erysipelas is characteristically on the face, but may also be found on the scalp, extremities, and abdominal wall (especially with neonates with umbilical stump infections). The dermopathy is an erythematous, hot, raised (edema), indurated, tender, circumscribed lesion with a distinct advancing and elevated border. The margins are often irregular and serpiginous. Occasionally, vesicles and bullae develop. Patients are generally systemically ill with fever, chills, malaise, and headache.

Erysipelas is diagnosed by the typical clinical features of the lesion in association with constitutional symptoms. Patients may have bacteremia, and, therefore, blood cultures should be obtained. Culture of the skin, including the advancing edge, is of little microbiologic value and is not recommended. A brisk leukocytosis is common.

All patients should be hospitalized, and treatment should be begun with intravenous aqueous penicillin G. Children should receive 25,000 units per kilogram of penicillin per day in four divided doses, and adults should be treated with 8 million units per day in four divided doses. After the patient clinically improves, oral phenoxymethyl penicillin may be prescribed (dose is the same as for impetigo) to complete a 10-day treatment course. Patients with serious penicillin allergy may be treated with parenteral clindamycin (children, 20 mg per kilogram per day in three divided doses; adults, 1,800 mg per kilogram per day in three divided doses or vancomycin (children, 30 mg per kilogram per day in four divided doses; adults, 2 g per day in four divided doses).

CELLULITIS

Cellulitis is an acute inflammatory lesion of the skin that initially involves the epidermis and dermis and later spreads to the deeper subcutaneous tissues. It can occur in all age groups and usually is antedated by some type of skin injury, trauma, or decubitus ulcer.

The etiology of cellulitis is most frequently group A beta-hemolytic streptococci or *S. aureus*. However, in neonates or young children, group B streptococci or *Hemophilus influenzae*, respectively, may also be a cause of this infection. In leukopenic immunocompromised patients, gram-negative bacilli, especially *Pseudomonas aeruginosa*, should be considered as a potential etiology of cellulitis. With long-standing decubitus or diabetic ulcers, anaerobic bacteria, including *Bacteroides fragilis*, may be associated with cellulitis.

Cellulitis is typically erythematous, tender, warm and edematous. The borders are not elevated or sharply defined. Lymphangitic spread may occur proximally; tender, regional lymphadenopathy is found in one-half of the patients. Local abscesses with tissue necrosis may develop. The infection may occur anywhere on the body, but common sites are the extremities, sacrum, and surgical wound. Depending on the severity of the cellulitis or the patient's underlying illness, systemic symptoms—including shock, fever, chills, delirium, malaise, or weakness—may be prominent.

The diagnosis of cellulitis is not difficult and is based on its appearance. Patients who are otherwise healthy and do not have clinical features requiring hospitalization do not require special diagnostic studies. However, inpatients should have blood cultures performed, open wounds or drainage cultured and gram-stained, and the leading edge of the cellulitis aspirated for microbiologic studies.

Outpatient treatment for cellulitis should be with cloxacillin or dicloxacillin (see Impetigo section for doses) for 10 days. Patients with serious penicillin allergies may be treated with oral clindamycin (children, 10 mg per kilogram per day in four divided doses; adults, 600 mg per day in four divided doses) or erythromycin (see Impetigo section for doses). In young children, *H. influenzae* should be considered as a possible etiology if therapy with cloxacillin or dicloxacillin fails to result in clinical improvement or if the cellulitis involves the facial region and the child is ill. The antibiotic recommended for serious *H. influenzae* infection is chloramphenicol, 75 to 100 mg per kilogram per day in four divided doses. If the organism is ampicillin-sensitive, the drug may be given in doses of 200 mg per kilogram per day in six divided doses. Immunocompromised patients with cellulitis should be hospitalized and empirically treated with combination chemotherapy chosen from an aminoglycoside, broad-spectrum penicillin (e.g., piperacillin), or cephalosporin. Patients thought to have anaerobic bacteria (particularly *B. fragilis*) as a component of the cellulitis require therapy with such parenteral antibiotics as clindamycin, metronidazole, chloramphenicol, or cefoxitin.

FOLLICULITIS

Folliculitis is an infection within hair follicles. Damage or traction of the hair, maceration or occlusion of the skin, blockage of a pilosebaceous unit, or exposure to certain chemicals predisposes to folliculitis. The pyoderma may be superficial or deep.

The etiology of folliculitis is usually *S. aureus*, but occasionally streptococci and gram-negative bacilli may be causative. With superficial folliculitis there is an acute inflammatory reaction in the follicle area. With more chronic and deep folliculitis, lymphocytes, plasma cells, granulomatous reaction, destruction of sebaceous gland, or fibrosis may occur.

The skin lesion begins as a small pustule near the hair-follicle opening and is associated with redness and mild tenderness. Crusting forms later as the pustule ages or ruptures. Deep folliculitis is associated with greater inflammatory reaction. Folliculitis occurs in hairy parts of the body, i.e., face, scalp, axilla, groin, and thigh. A form of deep folliculitis of the bearded area is called sycosis barbae.

Therapy is primarily topical care. Cleansing of the involved skin with hexachlorophene-containing soaps is generally adequate for most cases of folliculitis. Occasionally, antibiotics (e.g., cloxacillin or dicloxacillin) may be needed for extensive or deep lesions.

FURUNCLE AND CARBUNCLE

A furuncle (''boil'') is caused by perifolliculitis progressing to a localized abscess of the skin and subcutaneous tissue. A carbuncle is a larger furuncle or several interconnecting furuncles located in deep tissues. Furunculosis occurs frequently in persons with nasal carriage of staphylococci, severe acne, blood dyscrasias, defect in neutrophil function, diabetes mellitus, and immunoglobulinopathy and in patients on corticosteroid therapy. However, most cases of furuncles or recurrent furunculosis occur in healthy persons.

The etiology of furuncles and carbuncles is usually *S. aureus*, although streptococci and, rarely, gram-

TABLE 1 Summary of Cellulitis and Soft Tissue Infection

Type of Infection	*Skin Involvement*	*Etiology*	*Clinical Characteristics*	*Site of Infection*	*Treatment*
Crusted impetigo	Epidermis	Streptococci	Vesiculae; pustules; yellow-brown crusts	Face; extremities	Oral penicillin
Bullous impetigo	Epidermis	Staphylococci	Bullae; raw base	Extremities; trunk	Oral cloxacillin or dicloxacillin
Erysipelas	Epidermis; dermis	Streptococci	Red, hot, tender plaque with elevated borders	Face; extremities	Hospitalization; parenteral penicillin
Cellulitis	Epidermis; dermis; subcutaneous	Streptococci; staphylococci; others	Red, warm, tender, with irregular, flat borders	Anywhere	Oral cloxacillin or dicloxacillin; hospitalization in select patients
Folliculitis	Epidermis; dermis	Staphylococci	Inflammation near hair follicle	Head, neck, groin, axilla, thigh	Local compresses
Furuncle and carbuncle	Epidermis; dermis; subcutaneous	Staphylococci	Abscess around follicle	Same as folliculitis	Local compresses; oral cloxacillin or dicloxacillin; hospitalize select patients, drainage of large lesions

negative bacilli have been isolated from these lesions. The lesion is an abscess consisting of neutrophils and staphylococci in the vicinity of the hair follicles. There is tissue necrosis and perivascular infiltrate. The abscess and inflammatory reaction infiltrate the subcutaneous tissue. With carbuncles, there are multiple abscesses that may coalesce or remain interconnected by channels; these may then drain through the skin. Surrounding cellulitis generally accompanies furuncles and carbuncles. Healing may leave scarring.

Furuncles occur most commonly in the same areas as folliculitis, i.e., head, neck, face, perineum, thigh, axilla, and groin. Carbuncles are found in the back of the neck, shoulders, buttocks, and thighs. Furuncles begin as a small, painful induration of the skin and subcutaneous tissue adjacent to a hair follicle. The lesion enlarges and becomes red, elevated, and more painful. Fluctuance develops and the lesion may rupture spontaneously because of central necrosis. Pain relief occurs immediately and healing is rapid. If the lesion progresses without rupture, then fever, chills, malaise, extensive cellulitis, and carbuncle formation are common complications.

Diagnosis of furuncles and carbuncles is not difficult. Large lesions can be drained for therapeutic reasons and the fluid collected for Gram stain and culture. Patients with systemic symptoms or carbuncles should have blood specimens drawn for culture.

For small furuncles, local warm compresses may be sufficient to promote healing and spontaneous drainage. Patients with facial lesions, significant cellulitis, carbuncles, or systemic symptoms require systemic antibiotics. If patients are deemed appropriate for outpatient therapy, cloxacillin or dicloxacillin (see Impetigo section for doses) is the drug of choice for 10 days. Patients allergic to penicillin may be given erythromycin or clindamycin. Severely ill patients require parenteral antibiotics, e.g., nafcillin, oxacillin, methicillin, or first-generation cephalosporins (dose of 200 mg per kilogram per day in six divided doses for children and adults), bed rest, and surgical drainage (when lesions mature and localize).

Patients with recurrent furuncles should be advised on good skin hygiene and avoidance of trauma; early therapy should be initiated at the first sign of a recurrence. Evaluation of the patient for nasal carriage of *S. aureus* is epidemiologically important, but recent approaches to eliminate the organism permanently have been unsuccessful. Tests to uncover any underlying predisposing factors (e.g., diabetes) may be unrewarding.

For a summary of treatment and characteristics of cellulitis and soft tissue infections see Table 1.

CREPITUS AND GANGRENE

W. LANCE GEORGE, M.D.

The presence of gas in or necrosis of the soft tissues during infection is a relatively common phenomenon; when present, these findings require that the clinician decide whether the disease process is one of several potentially rapidly fatal entities that require emergency medical and surgical management. The presence of gas or of tissue necrosis should suggest that anaerobes are likely to be involved.

Crepitation is a crackling sensation noted upon palpation of soft tissues that contain entrapped gas and is a distinctly uncommon finding. Gas in soft tissue is usually evident on radiographs of the affected area before being detectable on physical examination. The presence of gas in tissues is due to either metabolic production of various gases by bacteria; to mechanical introduction during debridement, irrigation, or surgery; or to accidental injection of air under pressure into the tissues. *Gangrene* simply means "death of the tissue." Although certain potentially lethal anaerobic infections may actually cause tissue necrosis or gangrene, there is a marked propensity for anaerobes (usually in association with facultative or aerobic bacteria) to infect previously devitalized tissue.

A variety of soft tissue infections are associated with either crepitations or gangrene and are listed in Table 1. Although all of these infections may be extremely serious and require aggressive debridement, those that require the most urgent management and have the poorest prognosis are necrotizing fasciitis, Fournier's gangrene, clostridial myonecrosis, and synergistic nonclostridial anaerobic myonecrosis.

NOMA

Noma is a rarely seen, spontaneous, progressive gangrene involving mucous membranes or mucocutaneous orifices that appears to be due to anaerobic bacteria. Major

TABLE 1 Soft Tissue Infections Often Associated with Crepitations or Gangrene

Noma (cancrum oris)
Bacterial synergistic gangrene
Anaerobic cellulitis, gas abscess, and clostridial cellulitis*
Necrotizing fasciitis†
Fournier's gangrene†
Clostridial myonecrosis (gas gangrene)†
Streptococcal myonecrosis
Synergistic nonclostridial anaerobic myonecrosis (synergistic necrotizing cellulitis)†
Infected vascular gangrene*
Miscellaneous other infections involving anaerobes

* Indicates that abundant gas is usually present in the soft tissue early in disease.
† Indicates that the infection may have a rapidly lethal course.

predisposing factors are severe malnutrition and poor oral hygiene. Treatment with high doses of penicillin G (approximately 20 million units per day) is the therapy of choice.

BACTERIAL SYNERGISTIC GANGRENE

This chronic gangrene of the skin and superficial subcutaneous fat usually follows an operation (particularly one involving the abdomen or chest) and is characterized by extreme pain and redness, swelling, and tenderness of the wound. There is little systemic toxicity. Within several days the central area becomes purplish and then frankly gangrenous. There is slow, progressive enlargement of the lesion, such that there may be a central area of granulation tissue surrounded by gangrenous skin. The infection classically involves *Staphylococcus aureus* and a microaerophilic *Streptococcus*; however, facultative gram-negative bacilli, particularly *Proteus*, can also be involved. Treatment consists of debridement of devitalized tissue and antimicrobial therapy, the type of which depends on the organisms isolated.

ANAEROBIC CELLULITIS

Although the term *anaerobic cellulitis* is not properly descriptive—the process is more than just a cellulitis—the appellation persists in common usage. It is synonymous with *gas abscess* and is sometimes known as *clostridial cellulitis*, although the clinical picture for that condition is not necessarily different from those involving non-spore-forming anaerobes. The process involves the epifascial, retroperitoneal, or other connective tissues of the extremities, perineum, abdominal wall, buttock, hip, thorax, or neck. The lesion may exhibit necrotizing features and may spread rapidly but does not usually do so.

Pathologically, the lesion is basically a wet inflammation of the subcutaneous tissues that progresses to necrosis with crepitation within 2 to 5 days of onset; muscle involvement is nil. Pain may be the first symptom, but it is mild; subsequently, there is swelling of the overlying skin, and there may be erythema as well. Tenderness may develop, and soon crepitation becomes evident. Gas is commonly detected by palpation or by radiography; it is important to keep in mind, however, that the extent of infection cannot be judged by the extent of crepitation. Examination of the wound (if it has not been incised previously) at the time of surgery will, in most instances, reveal a foul odor, gas, and variable quantities of pus, along with shreds of devitalized soft tissues. The wound may be lined with a shaggy, gray-white pseudomembrane.

A variety of anaerobic bacteria, including clostridia on occasion, have been recovered from this type of process. The majority of anaerobes recovered are gram-positive cocci and *Bacteroides* species. Coliform bacilli, streptococci, and staphylococci may also be present. Debridement of devitalized tissue and initial empiric antimicrobial therapy are indicated.

NECROTIZING FASCIITIS

This acute, potentially life-threatening condition commonly originates in musculoskeletal wounds, but may also appear in an operative wound or even after trivial injury. A pathognomonic feature is subcutaneous and fascial necrosis, with undermining of the skin. There is sudden onset of pain and swelling; within 24 hours there may be considerable subcutaneous phlegmon, usually with cutaneous erythema or cellulitis. Blue-to-brown ecchymotic skin discoloration commonly develops, and pain is gradually replaced by numbness or anesthesia as a result of compression and destruction of cutaneous nerves at their site of passage through the edematous fascia. Fluid-filled vesicles later appear in the area of cellulitis, following which, the skin becomes necrotic. Local edema is present in most patients and may be massive. The extensive subcutaneous and fascial necrosis can be demonstrated by passing a sterile instrument along the tissue plane just superficial to the deep fascia; this cannot be done in ordinary cellulitis. Soft tissue gas is usually present, but may be demonstrable only on radiographs. This disease is a mixed infection that usually involves anaerobes (*Bacteroides* and *Peptostreptococcus* species), *S. aureus*, streptococci, and aerobic or facultative gram-negative bacilli.

Therapy is by emergency radical surgical debridement of all devitalized tissues; empiric broad-spectrum antimicrobial therapy is indicated.

FOURNIER'S GANGRENE

This is a life-threatening, necrotizing infection that begins in the scrotum or perineum and then spreads along fascial planes to involve the perineum, penis, abdominal wall, and thighs. It is a syndrome with variable involvement of deeper structures. Most cases represent a form of necrotizing fasciitis, but some are in the category of anaerobic cellulitis. On occasion, muscle may be involved also. Treatment involves emergency radical debridement and initial empiric broad-spectrum antimicrobial therapy directed against anaerobes and facultative bacteria.

CLOSTRIDIAL MYONECROSIS

Clostridial myonecrosis (gas gangrene) is a rapidly advancing, and sometimes rapidly lethal, infection that typically manifests with the sudden appearance of pain in a wound. Major predisposing causes of clostridial myonecrosis are extensive laceration or devitalization of muscles (particularly large muscle groups of the extremities), impairment of the blood supply to a limb or muscle group, contamination by foreign bodies, and delay in prompt surgical management of such injuries. Compound fractures predispose to gas gangrene because of the damage to muscles and their blood supply and, frequently, contamination of the wound. Surgery involving the gallbladder or bowel and surgery or manipulation of the upper female genital tract may precede clostridial myonecrosis of the abdominal wall and uterus, respectively. In addition, a number of cases have been reported to be associated with injections of various types. "Spontaneous" clostridial myonecrosis often involves *Clostridium septicum* and usually develops as a consequence of hematogenous seeding of a muscle or muscle group. This association is highly suggestive of an underlying colonic malignancy or other colonic disease.

Soon after the onset of pain, there is localized swelling, edema, and a thin, hemorrhagic exudate. Classically, a marked rise in the pulse rate—out of proportion to the slight elevation of temperature—is noted. The edematous area is very tender; the skin is tense and white, often with areas of blue discoloration. The swelling, edema, and toxemia increase rapidly, the serous discharge becomes more profuse, the skin becomes more dusky or bronzed, and bullae filled with dark red or purplish fluid often appear. Gas is usually present, but is not abundant in the early stages.

Certain peculiar mental changes have been described; these may consist of intellectual clarity with a full appreciation of the gravity of the disease, such that there is a profound terror or sense of impending doom. The toxic delirium may precede any visible changes in the wound.

The involvement of the underlying muscle is much more marked than is the skin involvement; although gas is usually present, it is not a prominent feature early in the course of infection. Changes in the muscle may be noted only at operation; hence it is imperative that prompt surgical exploration be carried out whenever gas gangrene is a clinical consideration. Early changes in the muscle consist primarily of edema and pallor, but later there is change in the color of the muscle, its blood supply is lost, contractility disappears, and gas may be demonstrable. In later stages of muscle involvement, there is progressive reddening, purple mottling, and change to a pasty or mucoid consistency of the muscle; eventually the muscle becomes diffusely gangrenous and even liquefied. Jaundice is rarely seen in clostridial myonecrosis of wounds, in contrast to uterine infection; when it does appear, it is associated with clostridial bacteremia and intravascular hemolysis. The most frequent causes of civilian clostridial myonecrosis are *Clostridium perfringens, Clostridium novyi*, and *C. septicum*; 80 to 95 percent of cases are caused by *C. perfringens*.

Diagnosis

The diagnosis of clostridial myonecrosis is made clinically. Detection of clostridia in a wound is not in itself of diagnostic value, because up to 88 percent of traumatic wounds may become colonized with clostridia in the absence of infection. In cases of myonecrosis, microscopic examination of muscle fragments or exudate may reveal clostridia, usually as large, gram-positive bacilli with square ends and no spores. Radiographs taken at intervals may help to detect early or incipient gas gangrene.

There are no satisfactory laboratory tests for diagnosis of gas gangrene, and one should not lose valuable time awaiting results of diagnostic tests. Rapid spread of the infection may occur within 2 to 4 hours, and irreversible changes may develop extremely rapidly. Accordingly, immediate surgical exploration is indicated when there is clinical suspicion of the possibility of clostridial myonecrosis.

Treatment

The cornerstone of treatment is early and radical surgical debridement of all involved tissues. This will often mean amputation in the case of myonecrosis in an extremity. Reoperation may be often necessary to ensure viability of the remaining tissues. Antibiotic therapy should include high doses of penicillin G (approximately 20 million units per day if renal function is normal). Either chloramphenicol or metronidazole is an acceptable substitute in the patient with a history of an anaphylactic-type reaction to penicillin. Hyperbaric oxygen is not of clear value, but should be considered in the desperate case or when complete resection of infected tissues is not possible (as in involvement of paravertebral muscles). It may also help to demarcate the area of disease and thus facilitate amputation at an appropriate level. Therapy with antitoxin (where it is still available) has not been shown to be beneficial and poses significant risks, because it is a horse-serum preparation.

STREPTOCOCCAL MYONECROSIS

Myositis or myonecrosis may also be caused by organisms other than clostridia, particularly the streptococci. Streptococcal myonecrosis is a fairly uncommon infection that may closely resemble clostridial myonecrosis, but has a less acute course. The incubation period is usually 3 to 4 days, and the presenting signs are swelling, edema, and a purulent or seropurulent wound exudate. Pain comes later in the course of illness (a distinct difference from gas gangrene), but may then be severe. Once pain becomes established as a symptom the progress of the illness is relatively rapid, although not so rapid as with clostridial myonecrosis. Gas is present both inter- and intramuscularly, but is not extensive. Involved muscles are at first pale and soft and later become bright red, with typical regular purple barring. Subsequently, the muscles become dark purple, swollen, friable, and, eventually, gangrenous. There is a peculiar sour odor to both the wound and to the large quantities of seropurulent discharge.

Patients with fatal disease die after one week or longer; toxemia, disorientation or mild delirium, and shock are preterminal events. Although the condition is often called anaerobic streptococcal myonecrosis, the anaerobic streptococci are almost always found in association with other organisms, particularly *Streptococcus pyogenes* and *S. aureus*. The character and course of the disease depend to some extent on the nature of the infecting organisms.

Management requires adequate incision, drainage and debridement of infected tissues, and high-dose penicillin G therapy plus the use of an antistaphylococcal agent if indicated.

SYNERGISTIC NONCLOSTRIDIAL ANAEROBIC MYONECROSIS

Another infection involving muscle has been described by various names, including synergistic necrotizing cellulitis, gram-negative anaerobic cutaneous gangrene, and necrotizing cutaneous myositis. A more appropriate name might be synergistic nonclostridial anaerobic myonecrosis, because this is a highly virulent soft tissue infection involving skin, subcutaneous tissue, fascia, and muscle; this infection occurs predominantly in the lower extremities and perineal areas.

Unique to this infection are discrete, large areas of blue-gray necrotic skin separated by areas of normal skin, with much more extensive involvement of underlying tissues than is evidenced upon superficial examination. There is extensive confluent necrotic liquefaction or dry gangrene of underlying muscle and fascia and subcutaneous tissues. Foul-smelling "dishwater" pus may drain from skin ulcers. Although severe systemic toxicity is usual and may appear suddently, there is usually extensive local necrosis before systemic toxicity occurs; there is also exquisite local tenderness and severe pain. Gas formation, present in 25 percent of cases, is usually not pronounced. Three-fourths of patients have diabetes mellitus; other associated or predisposing factors include advanced age, renal disease, and either obesity or malnutrition. The infecting flora includes aerobic or facultative gram-negative bacilli, anaerobic streptococci, and *Bacteroides*; there is a high incidence (approximately 30%) of bacteremia involving both anaerobes and nonanaerobes. Therapy requires emergency radical debridement and appropriate antimicrobial agents. Best results are seen in patients in whom amputation of the infected area is possible. Mortality is as high as 75 percent.

INFECTED VASCULAR GANGRENE

Infected vascular gangrene is another condition in which both soft tissue gas and gangrene may commonly be found. In this situation the muscle, and frequently the entire limb, has already died as a result of circulatory insufficiency, and the bacteria act primarily as saprophytes. There is little tendency for them to spread beyond the dead tissue into intact, healthy muscle, and there is seldom acute toxemia. There may be an extremely foul odor and considerable gas production, but little systemic toxicity. However, if neglected, infection may spread proximally, and various serious complications may develop. Therapy obviously consists of amputation of the affected extremity; antimicrobial therapy is indicated to protect the patient from bacteremia or proximal spread of the infection.

ANTIMICROBIAL THERAPY

Appropriate antimicrobial therapy of the above infections requires both an appreciation that they are usually polymicrobial and a knowledge of the infecting flora. Initial (empiric) therapy should be selected to cover organisms that are likely to be present; Gram stain of the exudate or infected material usually provides excellent information in this regard. Culture for anaerobes and nonanaerobes is always indicated for evaluation of the types of infection being considered here.

As mentioned above, penicillin G (approximately 20 million units per day—less if renal function is impaired) is the drug of choice for treatment of serious clostridial infections. Chloramphenicol (maximum, 2 g per day in divided doses), clindamycin (maximum, 2.4 g per day in divided doses), and metronidazole (maximum, 30 mg per kilogram per day in divided doses) have traditionally been the agents most active against all anaerobic pathogens; the dosage of these may need to be reduced if hepatic function is impaired. Because a low incidence (approximately 5%) of clindamycin-resistant *Bacteroides fragilis* has recently been noted in many centers, this agent should probably not be used to treat potentially life-threatening infections involving *B. fragilis* unless susceptibility of the isolate to clindamycin has been demonstrated by the laboratory. When either clindamycin or metronidazole is given for a serious or life-threatening anaerobic infection, penicillin should also be administered to ensure adequate coverage of fastidious microaerophilic streptococci and anaerobic gram-positive cocci. Whenever facultative (enteric or coliform) or aerobic gram-negative bacilli are suspected, an aminoglycoside should be administered. Antistaphylococcal therapy (e.g., nafcillin or oxacillin, 9 g per day in divided doses) may also be indicated on occasion. Therapy should, of course, be revised as results of culture and susceptibility testing become available.

BACTERIAL OSTEOMYELITIS

JACK L. LEFROCK, M.D.
BRUCE R. SMITH, Pharm. D.
ABDOLGHADER MOLAVI, M.D.

Osteomyelitis continues to pose both diagnostic and therapeutic dilemmas for the clinician, despite recent advances in radionuclide imaging, surgical techniques, and antimicrobial therapy. Intravenous drug abuse, radiation therapy for cancer, and newer orthopaedic procedures, such as total joint replacements, bone-grafting, and reconstructive surgery, have broadened the scope of this disease.

Osteomyelitis is an inflammatory process in bone and bone marrow. It is caused most often by pyogenic bacteria but may be caused by other microorganisms including mycobacteria and fungi. Osteomyelitis may be classified on the basis of its pathogenesis as of either hematogenous origin or contiguous focus (with or without peripheral vascular disease) (Table 1). These in turn may be classified as either acute or chronic forms of the disease.

In the past, osteomyelitis usually resulted from hematogenous spread of bacteria to bone and was mostly seen in children with *Staphylococcus aureus* as the causative agent in 80 to 90 percent of the cases. However, in recent years the disease has changed. Hematogenous osteomyelitis is decreasing in frequency while contiguous osteomyelitis and osteomyelitis in association with peripheral vascular disease is increasing. In addition to these changes, there also has been a shift in the age distribution to older patients as well as increasing frequency of unusual bacterial causes, including gram-negative bacilli, anaerobes, and mixed organisms.

HEMATOGENOUS OSTEOMYELITIS

This is generally caused by a single organism, with *S. aureus* being responsible for the majority of cases. However, the type of organism may vary with the age of the patient (Table 2). This disease generally occurs in children younger than 12 years, teenagers, and young adults who participate in strenuous physical activities. Bone infection follows bacteremia. The metaphyseal ends of long bones are the most frequent sites of involvement in children and the diaphysis of the long bones in adults.

S. aureus may also cause spinal osteomyelitis with paravertebral abscess formation. This syndrome generally occurs in older men who have had urinary tract manipulation and infection and in drug addicts.

CONTIGUOUS OSTEOMYELITIS

This type is secondary to an adjacent area of infection, as in postoperative infections, direct inoculation from trauma, or extension from an area of soft tissue infection. In contrast to hematogenous osteomyelitis, more than one pathogen is often isolated from the infected bone. *S. aureus* is the most commonly isolated pathogen, but aerobic gram-negative rods and anaerobes also are often isolated. In this form of osteomyelitis, one often finds bone necrosis, compromised soft tissue, and loss of bone stability, which make this type more difficult to treat than acute hematogenous osteomyelitis.

OSTEOMYELITIS ASSOCIATED WITH VASCULAR INSUFFICIENCY

This infection usually develops in a diabetic as an extension of a local infection either from cellulitis or a trophic skin ulcer. The small bones of the feet, generally the

TABLE 1 Classification of Osteomyelitis and Associated Features

	Hematogenous	Secondary to Contiguous Focus of Infection	Due to vascular Insufficiency
Age distribution	1–20 and >50 years	25–50 years	≥50 years
Usual bones involved	Long bones, vertebrae	Long bones	Small bones of feet
Microbiology	Usually monomicrobial: *Staphylococcus aureus*, *Streptococcus* (group B) Gram-negative bacilli (*Hemophilus influenzae*)	Usually mixed infections: *Staphylococcus aureus* and *epidermidis*, gram-negative bacilli	Usually polymicrobial: *Staphylococcus aureus* and *epidermidis*, gram-negative bacilli Anaerobes
Associated factors	Trauma, bacteremia, IV drug abuse	Trauma and surgery, soft tissue infections, radiation therapy	Diabetes mellitus, peripheral vascular disease
Clinical features	Fever, local tension and swelling	Fever, swelling and erythema	Fever, swelling, ulceration and drainage

TABLE 2 Osteomyelitis: Commonly Isolated Organisms

Hematogenous osteomyelitis
- Infants <1 year
  - Group G *Streptococcus*
  - *Staphylococcus aureus*
  - *Escherichia coli*
- Children 1–16 years
  - *Staphylococcus aureus*
  - Group A *Streptococcus*
  - *Hemophilus influenzae*
- Adults >16 years
  - *Staphylococcus aureus*
  - *Staphylococcus epidermidis*
  - Gram-negative bacilli
    - *Pseudomonas aeruginosa*
    - *Serratia marcescens*
    - *Escherichia coli*

Contiguous focus osteomyelitis (polymicrobic infection) all ages
- *Staphylococcus aureus*
- *Staphylococcus epidermidis*
- Group A *Streptococcus*
- Enterococcus
- Gram-negative bacilli
- Anaerobes

metatarsals and phalanges, are involved. These patients have impaired local inflammatory response that predisposes the involved tissues to infection and necrosis. Multiple aerobic and/or anaerobic pathogens often can be isolated from the infected bone.

CHRONIC OSTEOMYELITIS

Both of the above types of osteomyelitis can become chronic. There are no exact criteria as to when acute osteomyelitis becomes chronic.

DIAGNOSIS

In addition to the historical data and physical findings, cultures of infected material and hematologic and radiographic studies are helpful in making a clinical and etiologic diagnosis.

Blood cultures should be performed for all patients with suspected osteomyelitis. Approximately 50 percent of patients with acute hematogenous osteomyelitis will have positive blood cultures. Leukocytosis may occur with white cell counts exceeding 20,000 per cubic millimeter. However, normal or only slightly elevated WBC counts are not uncommon. The erythrocyte sedimentation rate (ESR) may be normal early in the disease, but usually increases with the duration of illness.

Radiographic changes are often difficult to interpret. Bone density must change at least 50 percent to be detected radiologically. Thus, there may be no definable radiologic changes in osteomyelitis for the first 10 to 14 days in spite of bone destruction or periosteal new bone formation. The initial radiologic findings may be simply soft tissue swelling and/or subperiosteal elevation. Roentgenograms may give misleading information in up to 16 percent of patients and are of no diagnostic value in an additional 23 percent of patients with osteomyelitis. Lytic changes are not seen until 2 to 6 weeks after the onset of disease. Sclerotic changes of periosteal new bone formation (involucrum) denote a more chronic process.

On the other hand, changes are seen on bone scintography as early as 24 hours after the onset of symptoms because of increased bone blood flow and early bone reaction. However, not all patients with acute osteomyelitis have abnormal bone scans. There are reports of normal bone scans, or "subtle" or "cold" defects. In some situations gallium scan shows increased uptake in areas of polymorphonuclear leukocyte infiltration. However, gallium scan does not show bone detail well so it is often difficult to distinguish between bone and soft tissue inflammation. Scanning the infected area with gallium 48 hours after injection and comparing with a ^{99m}Tc bone scan helps resolve this problem. Computed tomography (CT) is useful in identifying areas of dead bone (sequestrum). However, CT cannot be utilized when metal is present in or near the area of bone infection because of the scatter effect, with resultant loss of image resolution. Radiographic follow-up is important in assessing the effectiveness of drug therapy and the need for surgical intervention.

The bacteriologic diagnosis of osteomyelitis rests on isolation of the pathogenic bacteria from the bone or the blood. In chronic osteomyelitis, sinus tract cultures are not reliable in predicting which organism(s) will be isolated from the infected bone because there is a poor correlation between these cultures and those done on bone biopsy material. Bone biopsy specimens should be carefully cultured and stained for aerobes, anaerobes, mycobacteria, and fungi. The biopsied material should also be submitted for histopathologic evaluation.

THERAPY FOR HEMATOGENOUS OSTEOMYELITIS

In acute hematogenous osteomyelitis, a prolonged course of antimicrobial therapy (4 to 6 weeks). with a bactericidal agent should be directed toward specific causative bacteria isolated by bone biopsy and culture. Therapy based upon wound swab cultures of skin and skin structures above the infected bone is often inappropriate. These cultures usually reflect bacterial colonization without accurately identifying the organism in the underlying bone itself. Only the isolation of *S. aureus* from deep wound culture has correlated with its presence in bone.

Oral therapy has been used successfully after 2 weeks of parenteral therapy in the treatment of pediatric osteomyelitis. This method of therapy should be entertained where there is good laboratory backup and close patient monitoring to ensure compliance. Patients casually treated with oral antibiotics often receive inadequate dosage and inadequate monitoring, resulting in a failure rate of 19 percent. For successful therapy, the orally administered antibiotic should be monitored by the measurement of serum bactericidal activity against the causative pathogen. A peak bactericidal dilution of at least 1:8 or greater should be maintained. In children, this form of therapy offers advantages in convenience, comfort and cost. We treat adults with 6 weeks of intravenous therapy, and children, with 2 weeks of intravenous therapy followed by 4 weeks of oral therapy.

TREATMENT OF CHRONIC OSTEOMYELITIS

Chronic osteomyelitis secondary to surgery, trauma, or contiguous focal infection must be approached with combined medical and surgical therapy. Debridement should be done as soon as possible to remove all necrotic bone and sequestra. Abscesses or fistulous tracts must be eliminated. Material obtained at the time of surgery should be cultured for aerobes and anaerobes. Internal fixation devices, plates, pins, and screws should be removed. If bone stabilization is required, an external fixation device can be utilized. The wound may have to be debrided every 48 to 72 hours until all nonviable tissue has been removed.

Antimicrobial therapy should be initiated as early as possible, should be directed specifically against the offending pathogen(s), and should be administered intravenously in high doses for 6 weeks after the last debridement. Antimicrobial therapy prior to the time when debridement cultures are obtained should consist of broad-spectrum antibiotics to cover both aerobes and anaerobes. It is advisable to give antibiotics prior to debridement in order to reduce cellulitis or soft tissue swelling and reduce the risk of bacteremia.

THERAPY IN GENERAL

The consequences of inadequate therapy can be grave and lifelong. Knowing the types of organisms producing the osteomyelitis should lead to the use of a specific bactericidal agent except when multiple organisms are involved. Blind therapy is dangerous. Empiric choice of a narrow-spectrum agent not effective against the organism(s) within the bone may lead to treatment failure and chronic relapses. On the other hand, empiric broad-spectrum therapy may unnecessarily expose the patient to excessive or potentially toxic antimicrobial therapy and also inflate the cost of treatment.

The agents chosen for use should be demonstrated to be effective against the organism isolated from bone by in vitro sensitivity tests, such as the minimum inhibitory concentration (MIC) and minimum bactericidal concentration (MBC). Disk sensitivities have been used as the basis of therapy, but disks contain concentrations of drugs in excess of those achievable in bone, and results may not be directly applicable to the clinical situation. The antimicrobial agent chosen should penetrate the involved bone in concentrations greater than those required to be active against the organisms.

Soft tissue swelling, periosteal thickening, and periosteal elevation are the earliest changes but are subtle and may be missed. Lytic changes are not seen until 2 to 6 weeks after the onset of disease. Sclerotic changes of periosteal new bone formation (involvarum) denotes a longer process. Radionucleotide scanning (technetium plus gallium or indium) are most helpful in the course of acute

TABLE 3 Antibiotic Therapy for Osteomyelitis in Adults

Organism	*Antibiotics of First Choice**	*Alternative Antibiotics**
Staphylococcus aureus	Nafcillin or oxacillin 2 g q6h	Clindamycin 600 mg q8h, vancomycin 500 mg q6h, cefazolin 1 g q8h
Staphylococcus epidermidis	Nafcillin or oxacillin 2 g q6h	Vancomycin 500 mg q6h, cefazolin 1 g q8h
Non-enterococcal *Streptococcus*	Penicillin G 3 million units q6h	Clindamycin 600 mg q8h, cefazolin 1 g q8h
Enterococcal *Streptococcus*	Ampicillin 2 g q6h *plus* gentamicin 5 mg/kg per day q8h	Vancomycin 500 mg q6h *plus* gentamicin 5 mg/kg per day q12h
Enterobacter species	Cefotaxime 2 g q8h *plus* gentamicin 5 mg/kg per day q8h	Ceftazidime *or* ceftizoxime 2 g q8h *plus* gentamicin 5 mg/kg per day q12h
Escherichia coli	Ampicillin 2 g q6h	Cefazolin 1 g q8h, cefuroxime 1.5 g q8h
Proteus mirabilis	Ampicillin 2 g q6h	Cefazolin 1 g q8h, cefuroxime 1 g q8h
Proteus vulgaris *Providencia rettgeri* *Morganella morganii*	Cefotaxime 2 g q8h Ceftazidime 2 g q8h Ceftazidime 2 g q8h	Cefuroxime 1.5 g q8h, ceftizoxime 2 g q8h
Serratia marcescens	Cefotaxime 2 g q8h	Ceftazidime *or* ceftizoxime 2 g q8h, mezlocillin *or* piperacillin 4 g q6h, *plus* gentamicin 5 mg/kg per day q12h
Pseudomonas aeruginosa	Azlocillin 4 g q6h *or* piperacillin 3 g q4h *plus* tobramycin 5 mg/kg per day q8h (in order of choice)	Ceftazidime 2 g q8h *plus* tobramycin 5 mg/kg per day q12h
Bacteroides species	Clindamycin 900 mg q8h IV	Metronidazole 500 mg q8h, cefoxitin 2 g q6h

* Administered intravenously.

disease prior to the development of radiologic changes. Positive scans may be seen as early as 24 hours after the onset of symptoms. CT is useful to identify areas of dead bone (sequestrum).

The bacteriologic diagnosis of osteomyelitis rests on the isolation of the pathogenic bacteria from the bone or the blood. In chronic osteomyelitis, sinus tract cultures are not reliable for predicting which organism(s) will be isolated from the infected bone. There is a poor correlation between sinus tract cultures with bone biopsy cultures. Bone biopsy material should be carefully cultured and stained for aerobes, anaerobes, mycobacterium and fungus. The bone should also be submitted for histopathological evaluation.

Antimicrobial therapy should be initiated as early as possible, should be directed specifically against the offending pathogen(s), and should be administered intravenously in high doses for 4 to 6 weeks. Surgical intervention, in the form of bone debridement, is usually required in addition to antibiotics in the therapy of osteomyelitis arising from a contiguous focus of infection, diabetic ulcers, and peripheral vascular disease. In addition, combination intravenous and oral antimicrobial therapy may need to be given for 3 to 6 months in forms of osteomyelitis where extensive bony changes and tissue damage have occurred.

The antimicrobial agent(s) chosen for use should be demonstrated effective against the organism isolated from bone by in vitro sensitivity tests—MIC and MBC. It is best to choose an antibiotic or antibiotic combination that has a low ratio of MIC to MBC relative to its expected serum concentration. We prefer the antibiotic chosen to be able to obtain serum levels at least eight times the MIC. Table 3 outlines the choice of antibiotics for the therapy of bacterial osteomyelitis in adults.

BACTERIAL ARTHRITIS

JACK L. LEFROCK, M.D.
DON W. KANNANGARA, M.D., Ph.D.

Bacterial arthritis is an inflammation of the joint space, synovial fluid, synovium, and articular cartilage caused by a variety of microorganisms. The process is generally acute and constitutes a medical emergency; if untreated for even 24 to 48 hours, permanent joint damage may result. The vast majority of episodes are caused by the common pyogenic bacteria, including *Staphylococcus aureus, Streptococcus* species, *Hemophilus influenzae,* and *Neisseria gonorrhoeae*. The aerobic gram-negative bacilli and anaerobes account for additional cases.

There are three modes by which a joint space may be seeded. For both children and adults, the commonest cause is hematogenous. Roughly 50 percent of patients with septic arthritis will have concomitant postive blood cultures. A primary source, such as otitis, endocarditis, and so on, should be sought. A small percentage of cases will be the result of direct inoculation of the joint space, either accidentally (atypical mycobacteria, actinomyces) or iatrogenically (arthrocentesis, instillation of corticosteroids). Rarely, septic arthritis may result from spread of contiguous infection (*Mycobacterium tuberculosis*).

Once the synovium is seeded, the resulting inflammatory reaction may result in rapid destruction of the articular cartilage. Since this cartilage is avascular and unable to regenerate, permanent damage results.

The specific etiologic agent in any given patient can be anticipated by identifying the patient's age, host factors and presence of prior disease (Table 1).

Patients with chronic underlying diseases, especially those with cirrhosis and diabetes mellitus, have impaired phagocytic defenses, more frequent bacteremias, and consequently a higher incidence of septic arthritis. The importance of underlying joint diseases, for example, rheumatoid arthritis or degenerative joint disease, cannot be overemphasized. Septic arthritis in patients with underlying chronic arthritis is often subacute and may mimic a flare-up in the underlying disease. Aspiration without culture and Gram stain of the material amounts to negligence. Septic arthritis in patients with rheumatoid arthritis is caused by *S. aureus* in 80 percent of cases.

Nearly half of the cases of septic arthritis in adults involve the knee joints, followed in descending order of frequency by hip, shoulder, elbow, sternoclavicular joint, ankle, sacroiliac joint, and small joints of the hands and feet. Monoarticular arthritis is most common when the infecting agent is *S. aureus*, whereas with *N. gonorrhoeae*, polyarticular involvement is usual.

Joints involved in acute pyogenic arthritis are usually warm, tender, erythematous, and associated with general constitutional symptoms, such as malaise and fever. Roentgenographically, the joint capsule may be distended with fluid, accompanied by soft tissue swelling; less

TABLE 1 Causative Organism in Septic Arthritis by Age in Years (Percentages)

	2	*2–15*	*16–50*	*>50*
Staphylococcus aureus	35	50	15	75
Streptococcus hemolyticus	15	20	5	5
Streptococcus pneumoniae	10	10	—	5
Hemophilus influenzae	35	2	—	—
Neisseria gonorrhoeae	—	5	75	—
Other	5	13	5	15

commonly, destructive changes in the bony structures will be evident. The latter may occur with pyogenic arthritis in which there has been delay in diagnosis or in mycobacterial infections or when infections complicate rheumatoid arthritis.

DIAGNOSIS

The diagnosis is established by examination and culture of synovial fluid. A positive Gram stain or culture is generally specific. Prior antibiotic therapy may result in a negative culture or Gram stain. It is important to do a Gram stain, acid-fast stain if the Gram stain is negative, and culture. Synovial fluid is analyzed for total and differential leukocyte count, crystals, glucose, and mucin clot (Table 2). Other parameters include protein, complement, pH, color, and turbidity. However, there is significant overlap of all these findings among different types of inflammatory arthritis, for example, septic, rheumatoid, gouty, and pseudogouty. In septic arthritis, the leukocyte count is usually greater than 50,000 per cubic millimeter with more than 90 percent of the cells being polymorphonuclear leukocytes. The glucose is less than 60 percent of simultaneous serum glocuse, mucin clot is poor, and protein is greater than 3 g. The appearance is cloudy or turbid with a yellow to green hue.

Roentgenograms taken in the first 7 to 10 days of infections are of little diagnostic help because they show only distention of the joint capsule and periarticular swelling. Initial films should nevertheless be obtained, because septic arthritis may be a consequence of preexisting osteomyelitis, which would be revealed on x-ray. Follow-up films are important in evaluating the extent of articular damage.

Skin lesions, particularly those that can be aspirated

TABLE 2 Initial Synovial Fluid Findings in Infectious Arthritis

Disease	*Mucin Clot*	*White Cell Count/mm³*	*Cell Type*	*Synovial Fluid—Blood:Glucose Ratio*	*Stained Smear**	*Culture*
None	Good	200–600	Mononuclear	0.8–1.0	–	–
Acute bacterial arthritis	Poor	10,000–>100,000	>90% polymorphonuclear	<0.5	+	+
Fungal arthritis†	Good-Poor	3,000–30,000	>70% polymorphonuclear	0.5–1.0	±	+
Tuberculous arthritis	Fair-Poor	10,000–20,000	50%–70% polymorphonuclear	≤0.5	±	+

* Gram stain for bacteria; potassium hydroxide (KOH) wet mounts for fungi; Ziehl-Neelsen stain for mycobacteria
† Based on a small number of analyses reported in the literature

TABLE 3 Choice of Antibiotics in Therapy of Septic Arthritis

Organism	*Drugs of First Choice*	*Alternative Drug*
Neisseria gonorrhoeae	Penicillin G, 2 million units IV q4h for 3 days, followed by penicillin V, 500 mg orally qid for 4 days	Cefotaxime, 1 g IV q4h for 1 week Cefoxitin, 2 g IV q6h for 1 week Doxycycline, 100 mg IV q12h for 1 week
Staphylococcus aureus	Nafcillin, 2 g IV q4h for 4 weeks	Oxacillin, 2 g IV q4h for 4 weeks Cephalothin, 2 g IV q4h for 4 weeks Vancomycin, 500 mg IV q6h for 4 weeks
Streptococcus pneumoniae, Streptococcus pyogenes	Penicillin G, 2 million units IV q6h for 2 weeks	Cefazolin, 1 g IV q8h for 2 weeks Vancomycin, 500 mg IV q6h for 2 weeks
Hemophilus influenzae	Ampicillin, 1 g IV q4h for 2 weeks	Cefotaxime, 2 g IV q4h for 2 weeks Cefamandole, 2 g IV q6h for 2 weeks Chloramphenicol, 1 g IV q6h for 2 weeks Cefuroxime 1.5 g IV q8h for 2 weeks
Presumed pygenic arthritis with no organism recovered	Nafcillin, 2 g IV q4h plus gentamicin, 3–5 mg/kg per day in divided doses q8h for 2 weeks	Cephalothin, 2 g IV q4h *or* vancomycin, 500 mg IV q6h plus an aminoglycoside, e.g., gentamicin, 3–5 mg/kg per day IV in divided doses q8h for 2 weeks
Escherichia coli, Proteus mirabilis	Ampicillin, 1 g IV q4h plus gentamicin, 3–5 mg/kg per day in divided doses q8h for 2 weeks	Cefazolin, 2 g IV q8h for 2 weeks Mezlocillin, 3 g IV q4h for 2 weeks Cefuroxime, 1.5 g IV q8h for 2 weeks Ceftriaxone, 1 g IV q24h for 2 weeks
Pseudomonas aeruginosa	Ticarcillin, 3 g IV q4h plus gentamicin 3–5 mg/kg per day in divided doses q8h for 3 weeks	Other anti-*Pseudomonas* penicillin, e.g., piperacillin or azlocillin, 3 g IV q4h plus an aminoglycoside, e.g., gentamicin, 3–5 mg/kg per day in divided doses q8h or amikacin, 15 mg/kg per day in divided doses q8h for 3 weeks Ceftazidime, 2 g IV q8h for 3 weeks

Note: The recommended durations are only approximate. The exact duration of therapy should be determined by the clinical response.

and examined on Gram-stained smears, can provide a clue as to the presence of bacteremia (meningococcal, gonococcal, or staphylococcal) and indicate a specific organism.

TREATMENT

Successful management consists of three elements: prompt diagnosis, appropriate antimicrobial therapy, and drainage of the joint space. Delaying therapy more than 7 days commonly results in incomplete recovery.

Antimicrobial Therapy

Selection of antibiotics is initially determined by the clinical setting, age of the patient, and results of the Gram stain of the joint fluid. Selection may later be modified based on bacteria isolated and their antibiotic susceptibility (Table 3). Parenteral antibiotics reach adequate levels in the joint fluid and intra-articular injection of antibiotics is not indicated for therapy of bacterial arthritis. In fact, intra-articular antibiotics may produce a chemical synovitis. The duration of parenteral antibiotics is generally 14 days or longer, the only exception being gonococcal arthritis, in which the organisms are usually very sensitive and 7 days will suffice. However, when the organism is difficult to eradicate (such as *S. aureus* or gram-negative bacilli) parenteral treatment should be given for 4 weeks.

Joint Drainage

The joint should be aspirated by needle as often as required to remove pus which contains enzymes that destroy cartilage. Repeated aspiration may be required for 7 to 10 days. Indications for open surgical drainage are (1) hip infections; (2) presence of loculations (incompletely removed by aspiration especially when *S. aureus* is the pathogen); and (3) persistently high neutrophil counts (>25,000 per cubic millimeter) in the joint fluid or positive cultures despite appropriate antibiotic treatment and multiple closed aspirations.

After open drainage the wound should be allowed to heal by secondary closure, and antibiotics are continued for 1 week after the procedure.

Other Measures

Weight bearing should be avoided until all signs of inflammation subside. The joint should be maintained in the position of maximal function but strict immobilization is not required. Once the joint is pain free, initially passive and subsequently active exercises are instituted. Weight bearing is allowed when all signs of inflammation have resolved and no effusion is present. Residual problems, such as limitation of movement, difficulty in ambulation, or shortening of an extremity, may occur in a few patients. Appropriate orthopedic measures or rehabilitation medicine is required in such cases. Chronic indolent forms of arthritis may need synovectomy in addition to chemotherapy to eliminate the infection.

TETANUS

DONALD L. BORNSTEIN, M.D.

Tetanus, a potentially lethal neurotoxic illness characterized by intense muscular spasm and rigidity, is caused by the action of tetanospasmin, a potent neurotoxin released by *Clostridium tetani*. Spores of this organism are ubiquitous in soils and dust and can be introduced into the body by major trauma or by trivial or even inapparent penetrations of the skin. The disease is totally preventable by active immunization, and in the United States fewer than 100 cases have been reported annually for the last decade. However, tetanus is still rampant in developing countries, and it is estimated to cause from 160,000 to 900,000 deaths per year, primarily in newborns (tetanus neonatorum) whose mothers have not been immunized.

PATHOGENESIS

C. tetani is an obligate anaerobe and will not germinate after introduction in the human body unless there is accompanying tissue necrosis, anoxia, foreign material, or microorganisms. Spores have lain dormant months to years after the initial seeding only to be reactivated by trauma or surgery (latent tetanus). When conditions permit germination of the spores, tetanospasmin, a 150,000-dalton neurotoxin is released into the local tissues, where it is picked up by lymphatics and carried into the circulation. The toxin binds to motor nerve endings in local and distant muscle fibers and ascends within the axon or perineural sheath to the neuronal cell body in the spinal cord or the brain stem. There it blocks synaptic transmission of motor inhibitory stimuli from interneurons, which are required for coordination of agonistic and antigonistic signals into purposeful motor activity. The toxin appears able to ascend along sympathetic nerve fibers as well. It is no longer believed that the toxin reaches the CNS directly from the bloodstream or that the toxin exerts a significant direct effect on acetylcholine release at the neuromuscular junction. Like strychnine, tetanospasmin blocks inhibitory regulation of motor neurons; does not stimulate excitation directly.

The wounds that introduce tetanal spores are usually minor and occur around the home or in the garden. They include splinters, thornpricks, minor burns, abrasions, scratched dermatitis, and, especially in older persons, contaminated varicose ulcers, as well as sealed puncture wounds, crush injuries, major lacerations, gun-shot wounds, open fractures, and other major trauma accompanied by soil contamination—the so-called tetanus-prone wounds. Drug addiction has caused serious cases of tetanus, especially among "skin-poppers" who use subcutaneous rather than intravenous injection. In the United States, more than two-thirds of cases occur in persons over 50 years of age. In other parts of the world the umbilical stump, the postpartum uterus, and the middle ear (chronic otitis media with perforation of the tympanic membrane) represent major portals of entry. In more than 25 percent of cases in the United States, no wound or site of entry can be identified by examination or by history, which indicates how little inflammation or necrosis is required for the production of lethal amounts of this deadly toxin.

CLINICAL PRESENTATION

The first manifestations of tetanus appear from 3 days to 3 weeks after a known injury, usually between the fifth and tenth day. The commonest presenting symptom is tightness in jaw and facial muscles and in the neck, with or without malaise, headache, or other systemic complaints. Over the next 36 to 72 hours, these symptoms progress to trismus (spasm of the masseters, which prevents opening the mouth), spasm of the facial muscles, which produces a characteristic grimacing facies (risus sardonicus), pain and dysfunction on swallowing, and pain and spasm in the neck and back. In another day or two, the back and trunk muscles and the extremities are tense, rigid, extended, and the abdomen is board-like. Waves of uncoordinated tonic spasms follow, accompanied by great pain and anxiety, causing opisthotonos, an arching of the spine due to extensor spasm severe enough to fracture vertebvral bodies and to tear abdominal muscle fibers. Bowel and bladder function are impaired; swallowing is impossible; laryngeal spasm can occur. The unsedated patient is in terror of the recurrent spasms, exhausted, perspiring excessively, calling out in pain, unable to take fluids or nutrition, and; most important, in danger of asphyxia and anoxia because of aspiration, immobility, rigidity of the chest wall, constriction of the airway, and the more frequent spasms that cause long apneic periods. In the more severe cases, marked sympathetic overactivity is seen, with tachyarrhythmias, hyperthermia, hypertensive episodes, and sometimes refractory hypotension.

In most cases, symptoms and signs reach a plateau after the first 5 days or so and persist at that level until the effects of the fixed neurotoxin wear off, which usually takes from 4 to 6 weeks. Tetanus leaves no permanent neural injury, and if the serious complications accompanying 3 to 6 weeks of intensive hospital care are avoided, full recovery can be expected.

Trismus is an early and almost invariable finding (more than 90% of cases) because toxin carried to myoneural junctions in the masseters has a much shorter intra-axonal path to the CNS than is true for muscles of the arms or legs. Short incubation periods (fewer than 7 days) and rapid development from first symptoms to the first major spasms (less than 3 days) correlate with more severe illness and more complications.

More than 90 percent of cases seen in the United States are generalized. There are a few patients who have partial immunity or have a minor intoxication whose symptoms are limited to rigidity and spasm of the muscles around the site of injury. These patients with local tetanus generally do well, but the disease can become generalized later in its course if not recognized and treated effectively. Another group of patients acquire tetanus after an injury to the head, face, or neck or from a chronic eardrum perforation. In these cases the incubation period is short because the path to the CNS is shorter than from an extremity. Cephalic tetanus has a poorer prognosis, in part from a delay in recognition. Cranial nerve involvement is commonly seen along with trismus.

DIAGNOSIS

There is no laboratory test or pathologic finding that can establish the diagnosis of tetanus; diagnosis rests purely on clinical grounds. It is possible to recover spores of *C. tetani* from wounds in patients without the disease, and organisms are recovered from debrided wounds in only about 30 percent of cases. The clinical diagnosis is distinctive and, except in the earliest stages or in unusual mild cases in persons with partial immunity, is readily distinguishable from other causes of muscular rigidity and spasms. The differential diagnosis of trismus as an isolated finding includes local pathology such as dental abscess, subluxation of the temporomandibular joint, retropharyngeal abscess, and mumps. Painful spasms similar to those in tetanus are seen in strychnine poisoning, but here the muscles are relaxed and not rigid between spasm. There has been some confusion with patients receiving phenothiazine drugs, who may be somewhat rigid, but these patients tend to be dystonic to some degree, have a history of drug ingestion, and their muscular symptoms are rapidly reversible with diphenhydramine, 50 mg intravenously. Hysterical reactions can easily be distinguished by the lack of generalized rigidity, trismus, or true spasms.

TREATMENT

The goals of therapy are twofold: to neutralize unbound toxin while removing any residual nidus of *C. tetani* and to provide optimal physiologic support until the effects of the bound toxin dissipate. The first goal is easily accomplished; the second poses major problems for even the most skilled hospitals and intensive care facilities.

When the diagnosis of tetanus is first made, the patient should be transferred to an intensive care unit with full facilities for cardiovascular and pulmonary monitoring and ventilatory support because the disease progresses rapidly from the initial presentation and emergency intervention may be required.

Human tetanus immune globulin (TIG) should be administered, 3000 units intramuscularly, in several sites; infiltration of a portion of the TIG around the wound of entry is recommended for a particularly contaminated wound. It is customary to begin penicillin G (1 million units intravenously every 4 hours). If a site of entry is found, it should be thoroughly debrided 30 minutes or more after antitoxin has been injected, cultured, and left open. Manipulation may release more toxin into the blood, so it is important to wait until TIG is absorbed into the circulation. Penicillin should be continued for 7 days, if no site can be identified for debridement, to prevent further germination of *C. tetani*. Cefazolin, 1.0 g every 8 hours intravenously, or tetracycline, 0.5 g orally, every 6 hours can be used for those with hypersensitivity to penicillin. Antibiotics alone provide little protection from tetanus, however.

Since a lethal dose of tetanus toxin is much smaller than an immunizing dose, clinical tetanus does not confer protective immunity. It is therefore important to administer a first dose of alum-adsorbed tetanus toxoid, at a different site from the TIG. When the patient is ready to leave the hospital, the first booster dose is administered, and arrangements should be made for a second booster dose 6 months later.

The major cause of death in tetanus is respiratory compromise and failure. The chest wall is fixed and rigid, with low compliance and poor respiratory excursions. Recurrent spasms of chest wall, pharyngeal muscles, or the larynx can produce long apneic periods and hypoxia. Impaired swallowing and deep sedation lead to aspiration of mouth contents and risk of aspiration pneumonia. Immobility and prolonged bed rest favor atelectasis. The result is alveolar hypoventilation, hypoxemia, and respiratory acidosis.

At the first clinical or laboratory signs of respiratory compromise, a cuffed endotracheal tube or, preferably, a tracheostomy tube should be placed, with the patient under appropriate sedation and general anesthesia. This will protect against the dangers of laryngeal spasm and of aspiration and allow for effective suctioning. For most patients who require intubation the duration of need is such that an endotracheal tube would have to be replaced by a tracheostomy tube in any case. Because of the spasticity of the chest wall, protecting the patency of the airway may not be enough, and ventilating the lungs mechanically will be necessary. The stiffness of the chest usually requires total paralysis of skeletal muscle for adequate ventilator function. Paralysis is effected with the nondepolarizing neuromuscular blocker D-tubocurarine by intravenous drip or intramuscularly, about 15 mg per hour. This regimen—paralysis and mechanical ventilation—is the most effective and successful for serious cases, but carries with it grave monitoring responsibilities to ensure that the paralyzed patient is never accidentally disconnected from the respirator, an accident that would cause fatal or crippling anoxic brain damage. In addition, the quality of the nursing care, and especially of tracheostomy care, will determine the course of the recovery in most cases.

The patient will require medication to relieve anxiety, rigidity, and painful spasms, since these patients are mentally alert. Diazepam in the form of a continuous intravenous drip or intermittent intravenous bolus (5 to 20 mg every 3 to 4 hours, as required) has proved to be effective for these problems and for preventing the nightmares that paralyzed but inadequately sedated patients can suffer after recovery. Diazepam is very irritative if it infiltrates; only a secure intravenous line should be used. Painful spasms may require more powerful analgesia, and narcotics may be required. Chlorpromazine is sometimes helpful for its calmative effects, and it is sometimes alternated with diazepam, at doses of 25 to 50 mg (as required) every 6 hours intravenously or intramuscularly. Short-acting barbiturates such as pentobarbital, 50 mg to 100 mg intramuscularly every 6 hours, are generally used for sedation in addition to diazepam. The choice of sedatives and muscle relaxants will depend upon the overall strategy for dealing with respiratory support. If paralysis and ventilator support are required, as in most cases today, these choices may be less critical than when total control of spasm depends on these drugs. It is also important to limit unnecessary stimuli to the patient since minor stimulation can trigger a painful spasm in a lightly sedated patient.

With good control of ventilation and spasm by paralysis and sedation, successful management of the patient rests on avoiding the complications that attend immobility and paralysis in an intensive care setting for the 3- to 6-week period that will pass before the effects of tetanus toxin wear off adequately to allow a simpler regimen. Dedicated nursing care is required to prevent serious decubitus ulcers, atelectasis, contractures, infections around infusion sites, and to keep the tracheostomy stoma clean and the airway clear. Many complications known to occur in such patients can be prevented or recognized and treated promptly. Low-dose heparin is often used to prevent pulmonary embolism; it is appropriate especially in obese or elderly patients (5,000 units every 12 hours by deep subcutaneous injection with a 25-gauge needle using concentrated [10,000 units per milliliter] heparin). Antacids may prevent stress ulcers; daily weighings can help assess fluid losses (which are always much greater than is appreciated) thus avoiding a dangerous degree of hypovolemia; and enteral feeding via a nasogastric tube—or, if necessary, a gastrostomy or jejunostomy tube—can prevent the severe catabolic state and wasting that can otherwise occur. Frequent chest roentgenograms and urine examinations can help detect urinary tract and pulmonary infections at an early stage.

Autonomic dysregulation, a hallmark of the most serious cases, represents the major complication of tetanus after ventilation has been secured. Beginning about 7 to 10 days after admission, or sometimes even earlier, there are episodes of sympathetic hyperactivity with marked and rapid swings of blood pressure, signs of myocardial irritability, hyperthermia, and profuse sweating. Refractory hypotension, bradycardia and cardiac arrest are late and ominous signs. Propanolol (10 mg orally every 3 to 6 hours) or other beta-blockers can control the tachycardia and some other catechol effects. The hypertension may on occasion require phentolamine; the hypotension may respond to stimulating the patient and correcting for hypovolemia. Some patients have had several episodes of cardiac arrest and resuscitation. Aggressive cardiovascular monitoring is required to guide management.

Untreated, more than 80 percent of patients would die; overall, our mortality rates are about 40 percent. In intensive care units, however, this can be reduced to about 10 percent. The role for intrathecal human TIG in severe cases has been claimed, but not substantiated as yet. Hyperbaric oxygen, once advocated by some, is clearly useless and dangerous in this disease.

PREVENTION

Immunization prevents this lethal disease. Cases occur only in unimmunized or partially immunized persons. Yet despite the safety and the wide availability of tetanus toxoid, recent surveys in the United States reveal that 11 percent of young adults and 49 percent to 60 percent of persons over the age of 60 years lack protective levels of antibody. After an immunizing series of three DPT injections in infancy and a booster dose of DPT at age one and on entering school, a booster dose of tetanus toxoid should be administered every 10 years, at age 15, 25, 35, and so on. Since immunity to diphtheria is lost over time, the recommended form of tetanus toxoid for adults (Td) contains a small amount of diphtheria toxoid (2 flocculation units) as well. Whenever a patient is seen with a puncture wound or other penetrating wound or laceration and the possibility of introduction of tetanus spores is considered, the history of the patient's tetanus immunization must be carefully reviewed. If an immunizing course of three injections of toxoid has been received, as in persons with U.S. military service or with childhood immunizations, and if the last booster dose has been administered within 10 years, no further immunization is necessary for minor wounds. If the last booster dose was received within 5 years, no further toxoid is required for major wounds. Since a booster dose of toxoid is innocuous except in the very rare patient with marked hypersensitivity to previous toxoid doses, in most emergency rooms the practice is to boost for minor wounds and for major wounds if the interval since the previous booster dose has been 5 years or 1 year, respectively, although this is probably not necessary.

Persons with a wound who have not been immunized, or whose immunization history is partial or uncertain, require three doses of toxoid, the second following in a month and the third in 6 to 12 months. Since the first injection of Td will not offer protection for the current wound, passive immunization with TIG is additionally required for anything other than innocent, clean, minor wounds. The usual dose is 250 units intramuscularly, but for more serious tetanus-prone wounds, 500 units or as much as 1,000 units are sometimes used, depending on the severity of the wound. Arrangements to complete the immunization series should be made at this time. Infants born of unimmunized mothers should also receive a dose of TIG to prevent the rare and avoidable cases of tetanus neonatorum.

GRAM-NEGATIVE BACTEREMIA

DONALD E. CRAVEN, M.D.
WILLIAM R. McCABE, M.D.

Gram-negative bacteremia is defined as the isolation of gram-negative bacilli from blood cultures. This term is usually reserved for bacteremia caused by members of the families Enterobacteriaceae and Pseudomonadaceae; *Salmonella* and *Hemophilus* species are not included. By comparison, *gram-negative sepsis* is a term often used to describe a clinical condition characterized by fever, chills, and impaired tissue perfusion, irrespective of whether bacteremia has been documented.

Gram-negative bacteremia was uncommon in the preantibiotic era, but since 1950 it has become one of the commonest infectious disease problems in medical centers throughout the United States. An incidence of bacteremia as high as one episode per 100 hospital admissions has been reported in university teaching hospitals, but lower rates have been reported from smaller community hospitals. Common etiologic agents include *Escherichia coli*, species of *Klebsiella, Enterobacter, Serratia, Proteus*, and *Bacteroides*, as well as *Pseudomonas aeruginosa*. Fifteen to 20 percent of gram-negative bacteremias are mixed or polymicrobial. Fatality rates for gram-negative bacteremia vary depending on the patient's underlying disease, but overall fatality rates are in the range of 25 percent.

EPIDEMIOLOGY

Gram-negative bacillemia may be categorized as hospital-acquired (nosocomial), or community-acquired. Community-acquired bacteremia usually originates from the genitourinary or gastrointestinal tracts and is frequently caused by *E. coli* sensitive to many antibiotics. Some "community-acquired" bacteremias, acquired during earlier hospitalization or during residence in nursing homes, may be caused by bacteria that are more antibiotic resistant. Hospital-acquired infections that account for approximately 75 percent of cases, may originate from the urinary tract, gastrointestinal tract, respiratory tract, skin, or mucous membranes. Nosocomial bacteremia may be associated with prior surgery or the use of invasive devices and are generally caused by more antibiotic-resistant species of bacteria.

The increasing frequency of gram-negative bacteremia over the last three decades can be attributed to several factors. Enteric gram-negative bacilli are relatively avirulent and have limited invasive capacity in the normal host, but they comprise the major aerobic flora of the gastrointestinal and female urogenital tract and readily colonize the hospital environment. Nosocomial gram-negative bacilli are known for antibiotic resistance. *P. aeruginosa* is inherently resistant to many antibiotics, whereas other species of gram-negative bacilli acquire antimicrobial resistance from plasmids or R-factors. Plasmids are extrachromosomal fragments of DNA that may rapidly transmit resistance to several antibiotics. Gram-negative bacilli resistant to multiple antimicrobial agents are a continuous problem in hospitals.

The increasing incidence of gram-negative bacteremia over the last 30 years also reflects changes in medical management and the hospital population (Table 1). Patients are older and often have chronic disease. Radical surgery, immunosuppressive therapy, and extensive use of devices that violate natural host barriers have become an integral part of modern medical management.

TABLE 1 Factors that Predispose to Development of Gram-Negative Bacteremia

Underlying host diseases
Diabetes mellitus
Cancer
Congestive heart failure
Hepatic disease
Renal failure
Granulocytopenia
Thermal injury
Devices
Intravascular catheters (peripheral, central, tunneled, and arterial)
Indwelling bladder catheter
Tracheostomy
Endotracheal tube
Nebulization equipment
Prosthetic devices
Treatment Factors
Surgery
Steroids
Cytotoxic drugs
Irradiation

CLINICAL MANIFESTATIONS

The clinical manifestations of gram-negative bacteremia are protean and may vary from fulminant and lethal disease to infections that may go unrecognized for days. Clinical findings suggestive of gram-negative bacteremia are shown in Table 2. Many of these symptoms and clinical signs are nonspecific. Therefore, it is imperative to maintain a high index of suspicion and draw blood for cultures whenever bacteremia is suspected. The classic triad of shaking chills, high fever, and hypotension occurs only in approximately one-third of patients. Fever, although a nonspecific sign, is usually present unless the patient is elderly, uremic, or receiving treatment with corticosteroids. In patients with leukemia, gastrointestinal disease, or those who have had genitourinary tract manipulation, fever may be the only indication of bacteremia.

Approximately 40 to 50 percent of patients with bacteremia develop shock—defined as a decrease in blood pressure to 90/60 mm Hg or less. Shock usually occurs 4 to 10 hours after the initial signs of bacteremia caused by gram-negative bacilli. Because of the high frequency of shock associated with gram-negative bacteremia, it is essential that the etiology of any episode of shock be clearly elucidated and the possibility of bacteremia considered. The combination of hyperpnea, tachypnea, and respiratory alkalosis in the absence of pulmonary abnormalities is an important early clinical sign of bacteremia. In elderly patients, unexplained oliguria, increased confusion, or stupor also may be the only signs of sepsis.

Leukocytosis is common, although some patients may manifest normal or low leukocyte counts. Gram-negative bacteremia is a frequent complication of antineoplastic chemotherapy producing granulocytopenia (less than 1,000 neutrophils per cubic millimeter). Neutropenia secondary to bacteremia is an infrequent consequence in patients with normal hematopoietic function. Mild to

TABLE 2 Clinical Manifestations of Gram-Negative Bacteremia

Fever, chills, hypotension
Fever alone (in a patient with a malignancy, hematologic disorder, urinary tract disease, or intravenous or urinary tract catheters)
Hypotension*
Tachypnea, hyperpnea, and respiratory alkalosis*
Change in mental status (confusion, stupor, agitation)*
Oliguria or anuria*
Acidosis*
Hypothermia*
Thrombocytopenia*
Disseminated intravascular coagulation*
Adult respiratory distress syndrome*
Evidence of a urinary tract or pulmonary infection

* Without an alternative cause.

moderate thrombocytopenia occurs in about 70 percent of patients. Disseminated intravascular coagulation (DIC), characterized by decreased levels of clotting factors II, V, and VIII, together with hypofibrinogenemia, thrombocytopenia and circulating fibrin split products is found in approximately 12 percent of patients but only about one-fourth of these patients exhibit clinical manifestations attributable to DIC.

PATHOPHYSIOLOGY

Endotoxin, or lipopolysaccharide (LPS), a major constituent of the gram-negative cell envelope, is generally thought to initiate the changes observed during bacteremia. However, several careful experimental and clinical studies have indicated that factors other than free endotoxin liberated from the bacterial cell wall contribute to the manifestations of such infections. Irrespective of the role of endotoxin, a variety of vasoactive materials have been implicated as potential mediators of the circulatory changes observed in bacteremic shock. These include endogenous pyrogen (interleukin-1), Hageman factor, plasmin, complement components, kinins, serotonin, histamine, prostaglandins, endorphins, and catecholamines (epinephrine and norepinephrine). However, precise delineation of their role in human disease is limited by the lack of definitive data.

Available evidence suggests that the activation of the coagulation, fibrinolysis, kinin, and complement systems may contribute to the hemodynamic and other pathophysiologic alterations seen in gram-negative bacteremia. Activation of Hageman factor (Factor XII) by either intact bacilli or endotoxin results in sequential activation of the intrinsic coagulation system and the conversion of plasminogen to plasmin. Circulating gram-negative bacilli, endotoxin, and plasmin are all capable of activating the complement system through the classical or alternate (properedin) pathways. Anaphylatoxins (C3a and C5a) cause peripheral vasodilation and increased vascular permeability. Plasmin and activated Hageman factor also activate the kinin pathway, resulting in vascular permeability and early peripheral vasodilatation in shock. Bradykinin, in turn, increases the release of prostaglandins PGE2 and PGF2.

More recent studies have suggested that prostaglandins and endorphins may contribute to the pathogenesis of septic sock. Endotoxin may also release prostaglandins, prostacycline, or thromboxane. Inhibitors of prostaglandin synthesis such as ibuprofen and indomethacin have ameliorated endotoxin-induced hypotension in experimental animals. One uncontrolled clinical study of patients in shock reported improvement in blood pressure following the intravenous administration of 1.2 mg of the endorphin inhibitor naloxone, but a recent, randomized, placebo-controlled clinical study of patients in septic shock at our institution was unable to confirm any beneficial effect of naloxone in septic shock.

Shock in patients with gram-negative bacteremia is associated with a sevenfold increase in fatality. Therefore, goals for treating patients with gram-negative bacteremia include early diagnosis and therapy to prevent shock and rapid correction of any hemodynamic alterations that occur.

Two types of hemodynamic alterations have been noted in patients with gram-negative bacteremia. ''Warm shock'' is characterized by evidence of a hyperdynamic circulation. Increased cardiac output with decreased peripheral resistance is characteristically associated with a high or normal central venous pressure, hyperventilation, and lactate accumulation in the initial phase of sepsis. Patients in ''cold shock'' are usually pale, cyanotic, and have cold and clammy extremities. Cold shock tends to occur late in the course of septic shock. Physiologic alterations in cold shock include decreased cardiac output, increased peripheral vascular resistance associated with decreased central venous pressure, hyperventilation, and lactate accumulation. Respiratory alkalosis usually occurs early and may evolve to a metabolic acidosis, which carries a poorer prognosis.

ANTIBIOTIC TREATMENT

Due to the nature of the disease, therapy for gram-negative bacteremia is usually initiated before the etiologic agent and antibiotic sensitiviities are known. Initial treatment should be based on the type of infection (community-acquired or nosocomial), the probable site of infection, and the bacterial flora residing at that site. Basic principles of management include prompt recognition of the clinical signs and symptoms of bacteremia and identification of the source of infection. Blood cultures, gram stains, and cultures of infected sites should be performed to identify the etiologic agent and determine antibiotic sensitivity. Fluids, oxygen, and adequate doses of an appropriate antibiotic should be administered promptly. In addition, management of complications such as shock, hypoxia, and hemorrhage is of paramount importance. Any abscess should be drained and infected foreign bodies removed as soon as possible.

Once the source of infection is identified, appropriate antimicrobial therapy designed to cover all the pathogenic flora at that site should be instituted (Table 3). Aminoglycosides, such as gentamicin, tobramycin, or amikacin have a broad spectrum of activity against aerobic gram-negative bacilli, including *P. aeruginosa*. The type of aminoglycoside selected (Table 4) will depend on the condition of the patient, the type and location of infection, and the specific antibiotic resistance pattern of the hospital flora. At Boston City Hospital we presently recommend gentamicin for initial coverage of gram-negative rods because it is less expensive and the number of gentamicin-resistant gram-negative bacilli is low. Initial therapy with tobramycin or amikacin may be more appropriate in other hospitals, depending on the general patterns of bacterial resistance. Doses of aminoglycosides should be altered for patients with renal failure and blood levels should be monitored in individuals who have impaired renal function, no response to therapy, or in whom

TABLE 3 The Choice of Antibiotics for Suspected Gram-Negative Bacteremia by Site of Infection

Site of Infection	*Likely Etiologic Agent*	*Initial Antibiotic of Choice*
Urinary tract (community-acquired)	*E. coli* *K. pneumoniae* *P. mirabilis*	Aminoglycoside* *or* Cefoxitin†‡
Urinary tract (hospital-acquired)	*K. pneumoniae* *Proteus* species *P. aeruginosa*	Aminoglycoside* *or* Cefoxitin‡ *or* Third-generation cephalosporin‡
Gastrointestinal tract		
Bowel	*E. coli* *Bacteroides* species *K. pneumoniae* *Proteus* species *P. aeruginosa*	Aminoglycoside* *plus* Clindamycin *or* Cefoxitin
Biliary tract	*E. coli* *K. pneumoniae* *Proteus* species	Aminoglycoside* *plus* Ampicillin
Reproductive tract	*E. coli* *K. pneumoniae* *Bacteroides* species	Aminoglycoside* *plus* Clindamycin *or* Cefoxitin alone
Respiratory tract (patient with tracheostomy or endotracheal tube)	*P. aeruginosa* *Acinetobacter* species *Serratia* species *E. coli* *K. pneumoniae*	Aminoglycoside* *or* Aminoglycoside* *plus either* Carbenicillin§ *or* Cefoxitin‡ *or* Third-generation cephalosporin‡

Aspiration (in hospital)	*E. coli* *Bacteroides* species *Fusobacterium* species *K. pneumoniae* *Acinetobacter* species *Serratia* species	Aminoglycoside* *plus* Penicillin *or* Clindamycin
Decubitus ulcers	*E. coli* *Bacteroides* species *K. pneumoniae* *Proteus* species *P. aeruginosa* *Enterobacter* species	Aminoglycoside* *plus* Clindamycin *or* Cefoxitin *or* Third-generation cephalosporin‡
Burns	*P. aeruginosa* *Enterobacter* species	Aminoglycoside* *or* Aminoglycoside* *plus* Carbenicillin§
Intravascular device	*P. aeruginosa* *Acinetobacter* species *Serratia* species	Aminoglycoside* *or* Cefoxitin *or* Third-generation cephalosporin‡
Neutropenic patient (<100 PMN/mm^3)	*E. coli* *Klebsiella* species *P. aeruginosa*	Aminoglycoside* *plus* Carbenicillin§

* Because of their toxicity, aminoglycosides may soon be replaced by newer agents such as aztreonam or Imipenem-cilastatin. An initial loading dose for amikacin = 8 mg/kg, gentamicin = 2 mg/kg, or tobramycin = 2 mg/kg. Modify dosage in patients with renal insufficiency. Revaluate antibiotic regimen after culture and sensitivity data are available and treat with least toxic drug to which the organism is sensitive.

† Patients having a recent hospitalization, indwelling bladder catheters, or residents of nursing homes should initially receive an aminoglycoside.

‡ If the organism is sensitive. Resistant nosocomial gram-negative bacilli or *P. aeruginosa* bacteremia should be treated with an aminoglycoside. Third-generation cephalosporins include cefotaxime, cefoperazone, ceftazidine, moxalactam, ceftriaxone.

§ Ticarcillin, mezlocillin, azlocillin, or piperacillin may be used interchangeably with carbenicillin. Monitor bleeding parameters when these agents are used.

TABLE 4 Antibiotics Frequently Prescribed for the Treatment of Gram-Negative Rod Bacteremia

Antibiotic	*Dose**	*Comments*
Aminoglycosides		
Gentamicin	1.7 mg/kg IM or IV q8h	Aminoglycosides have excellent spectrum against aerobic gram-negative bacilli, including *P. aeruginosa*
Tobramycin	1.7 mg/kg IM or IV q8h	
Amikacin	7.5 mg/kg IM or IV q12h	
Extended-spectrum penicillins		
Carbenicillin	5 g IV q4h	Useful in combination with an aminoglycoside for treating *P. aeruginosa* bacteremia or for treating patients with neutropenia
Ticarcillin	3 g IV q4h	
Piperacillin	3 g IV q4h	
Mezlocillin	3 g IV q4h	
Azlocillin	3 g IV q4h	
Cephalosporins		
First-generation		
Cephalothin	2 g IV q4h	Activity limited to *E. coli, K. pneumoniae*, and *P. mirabilus*; should should not be used unless sensitivity of organism is known
Cefazolin	2 g IV q8h	
Cephradine	2 g IV q6h	
Cephapirin	2 g IV q4h	
Second-generation		
Cefoxitin	2 g IV q4h	Cefoxitin provides good coverage against *B. fragilis* and most aerobic gram-negative bacilli except *P. aeruginosa*
Cefamandole	2 g IV q4h	
Third-generation		
Moxalactam	4 g IV q8h	Third-generation cephalosporins have limited activity against *P. aeruginosa*; bleeding is a reported adverse effect of moxalactam that is corrected by the use of vitamin K
Cefotaxime	2 g IV q4h	
Cefoperazone	3 g IV q6h	
Ceftriaxone	1 g IV q12h	
Other beta-lactams		
Imipenem-cilastatin	500 mg of each drug IV q6h	Good coverage for aerobic gram-negative bacilli and *B. fragilis*
Monobactams		
Aztreoman	2 g IV q8h	Good coverage for aerobic gram-negative bacilli
Trimethoprim-Sulfamethoxazole	2 ampules IV q8h	Effective against many resistant nosocomial gram-negative bacilli

* Doses are the maximum for patients with bacteremia and normal renal flow. Doses should be adjusted after organism and antibiotic activity are known or if patient has impaired renal function.

long-term therapy is required. Because of their well-known ototoxicity and nephrotoxicity, aminoglycosides may soon be replaced by newer less toxic antibiotics such as aztreonam or imipenem-cilastatin. A cephalosporin is also less nephrotoxic than an aminoglycoside and may be used if the organism is sensitive.

Infections originating from the gastrointestinal tract or the female reproductive tract may involve aerobic gram-negative bacilli and anaerobic organisms such as *Bacteroides fragilis*. For this reason, combinations of antibiotics such as an aminoglycoside (chosen as indicated above) and clindamycin would be indicated for initial therapy.

A cephalosporin may be used for initial therapy only if the organism is likely to be susceptible. First-generation cephalosporins—such as cephalothin, cephapirin, or cephradine—have activity against community strains of *E. coli, Klebsiella pneumoniae*, and *Proteus mirabilis*, but some strains are resistant and activity is lacking against many of the nosocomial gram-negative bacilli making this group of agents inappropriate for initial therapy of suspected gram-negative bacteremia. Second-generation cephalosporins, such as cefoxitin, have a greater spectrum of activity against aerobic gram-negative bacilli. Cefoxitin also has activity against *B. fragilis*, but second-generation cephalosporins have no activity against *P. aeruginosa*. Third-generation cephalosporins—such as moxalactam, cefotaxime, ceftriaxone, ceftazidime, and cefoperazone—have activity against a variety of enteric gram-negative bacilli including some activity against *P. aeruginosa*. These antibiotics have a high therapeutic-toxicity ratio and serum blood levels do not need to be monitored. Consequently, they are easier to use and are less toxic than aminoglycosides for patients with impaired renal function.

Extended-spectrum penicillins—such as ticarcillin, carbenicillin, azlocillin, mezlocillin, and piperacillin—are generally used in combination with an aminoglycoside for treating patients with neutropenia or serious infections caused by *P. aeruginosa*. It should be emphasized that once the sensitivities of the offending organism are known, the least toxic and least expensive antibiotic to which the organism is sensitive should be prescribed. The duration of therapy depends on the source of infection. In general, antibiotics should be continued for a minimum of five afebrile days or longer if a local source of infecton persists.

MANAGEMENT OF SHOCK

Shock is the most frequent complicaton of gram-negative bacteremia. Optimal care requires the prompt institution of appropriate antibiotics as well as maintenance of an adequate intravascular volume. A central venous pressure (CVP) catheter or a Swan-Ganz catheter inserted to measure pulmonary artery wedge pressure (PAWP) are valuable aids for monitoring intravascular fluid expansion. Furthermore, an indwelling bladder catheter (using sterile precautions and a closed drainage system) is usually inserted to measure urinary output and renal perfusion.

Initially fluid (5% dextrose in normal saline) should be infused at a rate of 10 to 20 ml per minute for 10 to 15 minutes. If the CVP or PAWP do not increase by a level of 5 cm of water or 2 mm Hg, respectively, further fluid should be administered. If the need for further fluid volume is established, either colloid or crystalloid may be used at a rate of 10 to 20 ml per minute. Signs of fluid overload and cardiac decompensation include a sudden progressive increase in the CVP of more than 5 cm of water, a CVP of more than 12 to 14 cm of water, or an increase of PAWP of more than 8 mm Hg or an absolute level of more than 20 mm Hg.

If volume expansion does not produce prompt improvement, vasoactive agents should be added to increase cardiac output further. Dopamine is usually given by constant infusion in a dose of 2 to 20 μg per kilogram per minute. If there is no response to dopamine, isoproterenol in a dose of 2 to 8 μg per minute or dobutamine in a dose of 2 to 15 μg per kilogram per minute should be instituted to enhance cardiac output and increase urine output.

The role of corticosteroids in the treatment of shock caused by gram-negative bacilli remains controversial. Based on the available data, we do not recommend the use of steroids for patients in shock. If they are used, doses equivalent to 2 g of methylprednisolone should be administered within the first 24 hours of shock. Although some experts recommend the use of naloxone, a beta-endorphin antagonist for the treatment of septic shock, data from a randomized, placebo-controlled trial at our institution indicate that naloxone (1.2 mg IV) was no more effective than placebo.

Clinical evidence of disseminated intravascular coagulation (DIC) occurs in less than 5 percent of patients with gram-negative bacteremia, and these patients are invariably in shock. Heparin has been suggested for treatment, but enthusiasm for heparin therapy must be tempered by evidence that such treatment failed to reduce fatalities in either experimental models or humans despite improvement in coagulation factors. For treatment of DIC, we suggest that maximal efforts be directed at replacing blood products and reversing the cause of shock.

Hypoxia occurs frequently in septic shock, and monitoring of arterial blood gases is essential to maintain proper tissue oxygenation. Patients who develop adult respiratory distress syndrome (ARDS) often require mechanical ventilation with a volume-cycled ventilator. Patients who have a progressive decrease in their arterial PaO_2 despite the use of increasing oxygen concentrations, may benefit from positive end expiratory pressure (PEEP).

Oliguric renal failure is another complication of septic shock. If the urine flow is less than 30 ml per hour, the patient should be treated with an intravenous infusion of 12.5 g of mannitol over 5 minutes. If there is no response, this dose should be repeated in 2 hours. Individuals failing to respond to mannitol can be given furosemide (240 mg) intravenously.

IMMUNIZATION AND PREVENTION

The search for an effective vaccine against gram-negative bacteremia has been limited by the large number of organisms causing disease. However, it is now known that gram-negative bacilli share common antigens present in the core region of the lipopolysaccharide. Although there is no program for actively vaccinating individuals at risk for gram-negative bacteremia, vaccination of individuals with rough bacterial mutants containing these core antigens is being evaluated, and hyperimmune serum obtained from patients following immunization has been shown to significantly increase the survival rates of patients in septic shock compared with a control group of patients given preimmune serum. Although more research is needed, there appears to be a role for immunotherapy in the treatment of gram-negative sepsis.

In the meantime, major efforts should be directed at preventing gram-negative bacteremia. Since the majority of gram-negative bacteremias are nosocomial in origin, the use of proper handwashing along with careful evaluation of the need for and care of invasive devices such as the indwelling bladder catheter, endotracheal tube, central venous and intravenous catheters will reduce the frequency of local infections and subsequent bacteremia. Additional measures should include the rational use of antibiotics and the appropriate collection and feedback of surveillance data used to monitor nosocomial infection.

HUMAN BRUCELLOSIS

EDWARD J. YOUNG, M.D.

Brucellosis, a disease of animals transmissible to humans (zoonosis), remains an important human health problem, especially in countries where brucellosis in domestic animals has not been controlled or eradicated. Epidemiologic studies have shown that man's risk of contracting brucellosis is closely linked to his methods of animal husbandry, standards of hygiene, and food habits. Since human infection usually occurs from direct contact with infected animals, certain occupations present an increased risk of exposure; these include farmers, veterinarians, abattoir workers, and laboratory personnel. Although a history of animal contact should always be sought, clinicians must also be aware that brucellosis can be transmitted by ingestion of unpasteurized milk or other dairy products, such as cheese that is prepared from "raw" milk. Human-to-human transmission of brucellosis is rare, associated with blood or bone marrow transfusions from infected donors.

PATHOGENESIS

Among the six recognized species in the genus *Brucella*, four are known to cause human disease: *B. abortus* (cattle), *B. melitensis* (goats and sheep) *B. suis* (swine), and *B. canis* (dogs). Animal studies suggest that *B. melitensis* and *B. suis* are the most virulent, but specific virulence factors are poorly understood. The *Brucella* are facultative intracellular bacteria that have the capacity to survive and even multiply within phagocytic cells of the host. Normal human serum and polymorphonuclear leukocytes have a limited ability to kill *Brucella*; macrophages of the reticuloendothelial system (RES) "activated" by specifically sensitized thymus-derived lymphocytes appear to be the principal defense against *Brucella* and other facultative intracellular pathogens. It has even been suggested that intracellular survival may aid in the spread of *Brucella* throughout the body and may protect the bacteria against antimicrobial agents.

CLINICAL MANIFESTATIONS AND COMPLICATIONS

The spectrum of human brucellosis ranges from subclinical (detected by specific antibodies or skin test reactivity in the absence of a known overt infection) to chronic infection characterized by recurrent symptoms over many years. The incubation period varies from weeks to months, and the onset of symptoms is insidious in approximately one-half of cases and acute in the remainder. Patients often have multiple nonspecific complaints, notably, lethargy, body aches, fever, sweats, anorexia, fatigue, and depression. Because there is often a paucity of physical findings, these symptoms may be considered psychosomatic. If empiric antibiotic treatment is given with a penicillin or oral cephalosporin, symptoms may abate, only to recur, since these drugs have little clinical efficacy.

Since *Brucella* localize in tissues rich in elements of the RES, involvement of lymph nodes, spleen, liver, bones, and the genitourinary system is common. Mild lymphadenopathy may be the only physical abnormality in many cases; the spleen may also be enlarged, perhaps more commonly in cases due to *B. abortus*. The liver is probably involved initially in all cases, although icteric hepatitis is rare. Often patients have only mild or no abnormalities demonstrable by hepatic cell function tests, despite the demonstration of lesions on hepatic biopsy. Noncaseating hepatic granulomas, indistinguishable from sarcoid, are characteristic of infection due to *B. abortus*, and diffuse hepatic inflammation with focal microabscesses is often found in infection caused by *B. melitensis*; however, disease caused by the two species is difficult to distinguish clinically.

Skeletal involvement—most often in the spine (60% in the lumbosacral regions)—is frequent in brucellosis. Brucellar spondylitis begins in the intervertebral disk and spreads to contiguous vertebral bodies producing osteomyelitis occasionally with paravertebral abscesses. Inflammation results in narrowing of the intervertebral foramen, causing irritation to dorsal nerve roots. Sacroiliitis is reported to be the commonest joint involvement, occurring alone or in combination with other joints in some 15 percent of cases.

Genitourinary complications occur in up to 20 percent of men infected with *Brucella*, notably, involvement of the testes and epididymis. Pyelonephritis and prostatitis have been reported infrequently. Although abortion is common in animals infected with *Brucella* (due to massive growth of bacteria in placental tissues rich in the growth stimulant erythritol), there is little evidence that *Brucella* causes reproductive failures in humans. Abortion can occur in pregnant women in the course of acute bacteremic brucellosis, but this is not unique to *Brucella*.

DIAGNOSIS

Routine laboratory studies, like physical findings, are few and nonspecific. The white blood count is generally normal or low, and granulocytopenia is commoner than lymphopenia. Blood coagulation abnormalities have been attributed to disseminated intravascular coagulation (DIC), and, rarely, erythrophagocytosis is present in the bone marrow. The diagnosis of human brucellosis rests with isolation of the organism from the blood, bone marrow, or other tissues. One caveat relative to blood cultures in brucellosis is the slow growth of the bacteria in artificial media. If brucellosis is suspected, the laboratory should be instructed to observe routine blood cultures for a minimum of 4 weeks before assuming that they are negative.

In the absence of a positive culture, the diagnosis rests with the demonstration of a rise in specific antibodies. A variety of serologic tests have been employed to diagnose human brucellosis; however, the standard tube agglutination (STA), 2-mercaptoethanol (2-ME) agglutination, and complement fixation (CF) tests are the most useful. The STA test measures total agglutinating immunoglobulins (IgM plus IgG), whereas the 2-ME test measures only IgG (2-ME-resistant) agglutinins. Both IgM and IgG antibodies rise in acute brucellosis, but titers of IgG agglutinins disappear or decrease with treatment and recovery, and low levels of IgM antibodies may persist for many years. This observation is useful in distinguishing chronic brucellosis, relapse, or reinfection, in which IgG antibodies are often elevated and are resistant to treatment with 2-mercaptoethanol. Antigen prepared from *B. abortus* is routinely used in these tests, since cross-reactions between the three major species is sufficient to detect infection due to all but *B. canis*. Caution is advised in interpreting low levels of *Brucella* agglutinins (less than 1:160), especially in patients previously immunized or infected with cholera, tularemia, or *Yersinia enterocolitica* serotype 9. A variety of impure and nonstandardized antigens have been employed in the past to test type IV immune responses to *Brucella*; however, skin tests are not useful in the clinical diagnosis of human brucellosis.

TREATMENT

The evidence for subclinical brucellosis suggests that the body may be capable of recovery from infection without specific chemotherapy; however, the practice of prescribing empiric antibiotics for a variety of nonspecific symptoms precludes the assumption that all such cases were untreated. In fact, the literature is replete with reports of spontaneous, often sudden, recovery from brucellosis without specific treatment. Nevertheless, most authorities agree that antibiotics shorten the course of infection as well as reduce the incidence of complications, some of which may be life threatening.

Sulfadiazine and streptomycin were the first antibiotics used to treat human brucellosis, but the toxicity associated with this combination soon led to the discovery that tetracycline provided an effective and less toxic alternative. In vitro the majority of *Brucella* strains are inhibited by concentrations of tetracycline from 0.1 to 0.5 μg per millimeter, but the drug is not bactericidal. Oral tetracycline (250 mg four times daily) for a minimum of 21 days is adequate theray for uncomplicated cases of brucellosis. Oral doxycycline or minocycline (100 mg twice daily) produces comparable results and may be tolerated better, but is more expensive. Although some studies have reported in vitro synergy between tetracycline and streptomycin, conflicting results have been obtained in clinical studies regarding the incidence of relapses between single versus combination drug therapy. Regardless, most authorities recommend treating seriously ill patients or cases complicated by deep tissue involvement (arthritis, osteomyelitis, among others) with a combination of oral tetracycline for 6 weeks plus intramuscular or intravenous streptomycin (1 to 2 g daily) for the first 1 or 2 weeks. Gentamicin is more active in vitro than streptomycin, but no controlled comparative study using different aminoglycosides in human brucellosis has been reported. The ability of trimethoprim-sulfamethoxazole (TMP/SMZ) to penetrate into cells suggests that this drug combination might be useful for the treatment of human brucellosis. The in vitro sensitivity of TMP/SMZ against *Brucella* ranges from 0.39 to 6.25 μg per millileter (some strains may be higher), and several uncontrolled studies have indicated that it is a reasonable alternative therapy. Since the tetracyclines may cause irreversible staining of deciduous teeth, TMP/SMZ is particularly useful for treating brucellosis in children, and the relapse rate is reportedly less than 5 percent. The usual dose of TMP/SMZ (combination containing 80 mg trimethoprim and 400 mg sulfamethoxazole) is four tablets daily in adults or two tablets daily in children administered for 6 to 12 weeks, depending on response.

Rifampin is another drug with promise in the treatment of human brucellosis. *Brucella* are inhibited in vitro at concentrations of rifampin between 0.15 and 2.5 μg per millileter, and the drug is bactericidal at concentrations approximately four times the MIC. Unfortunately, rifampin-resistant variants are produced in vitro which suggests that it should not be used as single-drug therapy. Several uncontrolled studies using rifampin have reported encouraging results, but it is still too soon to know what role this agent has in the treatment of human brucellosis.

Other drugs such as erythromycin and chloramphenicol have been used to treat brucellosis, but they are less active in vitro than tetracycline, show variable effects against different strains of *Brucella*, and are not recommended alternatives. The penicillins, including ureidopenicillins, and first- or second-generation cephalosporins have little activity against *Brucella* and appear to be ineffective clinically. Some new beta-lactam antibiotics such as thienamycin and moxalactam are effective in vitro against some strains of *Brucella* but are unproved clinically.

Complications of brucellosis, such as meningitis and endocarditis, that require a bactericidal antibiotic remain a difficult problem. Tetracycline penetrates the blood-brain barrier but is only bacteriostatic; aminoglycosides do not penetrate the blood-brain barrier well when given intravenously. Moxalactam and some other new beta-lactam antibiotics achieve adequate CSF levels after intravenous injection, and are useful in treating some gram-negative meningitis without the need for intrathechal or intraventricular administration. Rifampin also enters the CSF in adequate concentrations, and we have successfully treated one case of meningoencephalitis caused by *B. suis* with moxalactam and rifampin after treatment with tetracycline plus streptomycin failed to sterilize the CSF. Additional experience will be required with these agents before a definitive recommendation can be made.

Endocarditis is another rare, but usually fatal, complication of human brucellosis. Most authorities recommend surgical replacement of the infected valve in addition to antibiotics in order to achieve a cure of *Brucella* endocarditis. In order to determine the optimal antibiotic treatment of specific complications, in vitro studies using newer antibiotics may be useful.

CHRONIC BRUCELLOSIS

Perhaps no aspect of human brucellosis is more controversial or difficult to treat than so called chronic brucellosis. This is, in part, due to the disagreement over what constitutes chronicity in a disease that has an insidious onset, extending over many months in half of the cases. If one defines chronic brucellosis as that of patients complaining of ill health for more than a year after the initial diagnosis, then some proportion will represent treatment failures with relapsing infection, and another portion will be patients with an identifiable focus of infection, such as an abscess in the liver, spleen, or other tissue. The majority, however, appear to be patients with no evidence of active disease, but who, after prolonged illness, ascribe all nonspecific symptoms (lethargy, depression, headache, body aches) to the persistence of brucellosis. These patients may have low levels of 2-ME-sensitive (IgM) agglutinins in their serum, which tempts clinicians to retreat with antibiotics. However, residual antibodies are not unusual in the course of adequately treated infection because polysaccharide antigens are very slowly metabolized by the body. Such patients may benefit from assurance, but are more often refractory to all attempted therapy.

LYME DISEASE

LAURI E. MARKOWITZ, M.D.
ALLEN C. STEERE, M.D.

Lyme disease is a systemic, tick-borne spirochetal disease with protean manifestations, including rheumatic, neurologic, cardiac, and dermatologic abnormalities. The best clinical marker for the disease is the initial skin lesion, erythema chronicum migrans (ECM), that occurs at the site of the tick bite. ECM was first reported in Europe in 1910, and the first case of ECM acquired in the United States was reported in 1970. However, it was not until 1975 that investigation of a cluster of cases of arthritis in Lyme, Connecticut, led to the description of the full clinical spectrum of what is now known as Lyme disease. Through subsequent studies, *Ixodes dammini* and *Ixodes pacificus* were identified as the principal vectors of Lyme disease in the United States. In 1981, the etiologic agent of the disease was identified, a previously unrecognized spirochete. This spirochete has been referred to as the Lyme disease spirochete or the *Ixodes dammini* spirochete, but has now been classified taxonomically as a *Borrelia* and named *Borrelia burgdorferi*.

EPIDEMIOLOGY

Lyme disease has been recognized in three major areas in the United States: the coastal areas of the Northeast (Connecticut, Delaware, Maryland, Massachusetts, New Jersey, New York, Rhode Island, and Pennsylvania); the Midwest, (Minnesota and Wisconsin); and the West (California, Oregon, Utah, and Nevada). These areas correspond to the range of *I. dammini* in the Northeast and Midwest and of *I. pacificus* in the West. However, sporadic cases have been reported from states outside the known range of these ticks, including Arkansas, Florida, Georgia, Indiana, Kentucky, Montana, North Carolina, Tennessee, Texas, and Virginia. The occurrence of these cases suggests that there are vectors other than *I. dammini* and *I. pacificus* and/or that these ticks may be spreading to new areas. Recently, *B. burgdorferi* has also been recovered from *Amblyomma americanum* and *Dermacentor variabilis*, suggesting that these ticks may be vectors for Lyme disease. In Europe, where *I. ricinus* is the vector, Lyme disease is known to occur in almost all countries on the continent. The illness has also been reported in Australia, but the vector there is unknown.

The peak incidence of Lyme disease is during the summer months. In more than 80 percent of cases, the patients have onsets in May through August. All age groups have been affected. In 1980, 226 cases were reported to the Centers for Disease Control and in 1982, 487 cases were reported. It is unclear to what extent the increase in reported cases is a result of increased awareness of the disease rather than a true increase in incidence.

CLINICAL MANIFESTATIONS

The manifestations of Lyme disease have been divided into three stages that may overlap or occur alone. During the first stage of Lyme disease, most patients have ECM and constitutional symptoms. ECM occurs at the site of a tick bite after an incubation period of 3 to 32 days (median, 7 days). The skin lesion begins as a red macule or papule that expands to form an annular erythema as large as 70 cm in diameter (median, 15 cm). As it expands, the center of the lesion often clears. Lesions may appear on any part of the body, and multiple lesions occur in about 50 percent of patients (Fig. 1). The lesions are usually not painful, but some patients describe them as burning or pruritic. Atypical ECM may lack central clearing or have a vesicular center. Other cutaneous manifestations have also been reported including localized or generalized urticaria, diffuse erythema, and malar rash. The dermatologic manifestations last for a median of 3 weeks (range, 1 day to 14 months). In untreated patients, skin involvement may recur.

A wide range of symptoms may accompany the skin lesions, including fatigue, headache, stiff neck, chills, sore

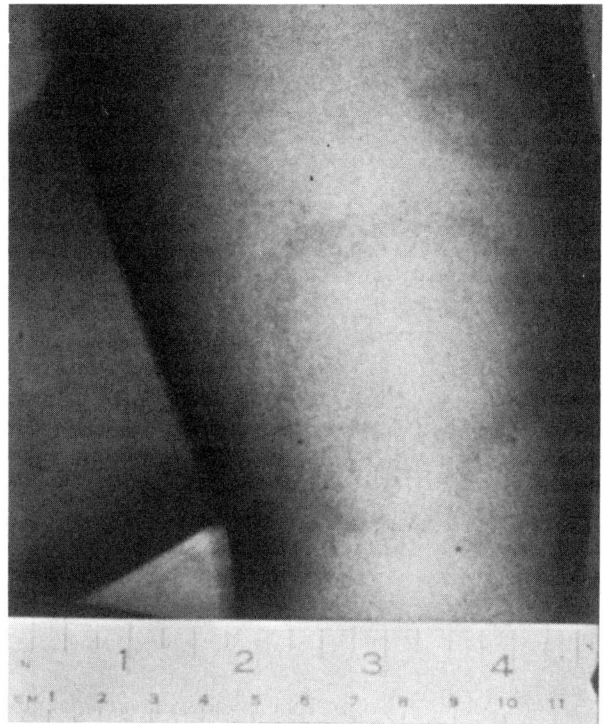

Figure 1 Secondary annular skin lesions of Lyme disease showing the cleared center of the expanded lesions.

throat, arthralgia, myalgia, abdominal pain, nausea, and vomiting. On physical examination, fever and regional lymphadenopathy are the commonest findings. Some patients have generalized lymphadenopathy or splenomegaly. These signs and symptoms are typically intermittent and changing. During early Lyme disease, laboratory findings include an elevated sedimentation rate (50% of patients), elevated white blood cell counts (10% of patients), elevated total serum IgM (33% of patients), and abnormal hepatic function tests (20% of patients). Complement levels are usually normal, and tests for both antinuclear antibody and rheumatoid factor are almost always negative.

Several weeks to months later, approximately 15 percent of untreated patients develop frank neurologic abnormalitis (stage 2) including aseptic meningitis, encephalitis, cranial neuritis, motor and sensory radiculoneuritis, mononeuritis multiplex, or myelitis. The most frequent neurologic presentations are aseptic meningitis, Bell's palsy (which may be bilateral), or radiculoneuritis. While the cerebrospinal fluid may be normal during the first 1 to 2 weeks of illness, most of these patients develop a predominately lymphocytic pleocytosis (40 to 450 cells per cubic millimeter), sometimes accompanied by an elevated protein or a slightly decreased glucose. Multiple neurologic abnormalities can be present simultaneously or, as with all manifestations of Lyme disease, the manifestations may be intermittent and fluctuating. They typically last for months and then resolve, but chronic neurologic involvement may occur later.

Also during stage 2, approximately 8 percent of patients develop cardiac complications, which include conduction abnormalities, myopericarditis, cardiomegaly, and left ventricular dysfunction. Electrocardiographic abnormalities include varying degrees of atrioventricular block, and diffuse T-wave and ST-T segment changes. In patients with atrioventricular block, progression from first to third degree may be rapid. Radionucleotide angiography reveals depressed left ventricular ejection fractions in some patients. Cardiac abnormalities last from 3 days to 6 weeks; they may recur.

Weeks to years after the tick bite or ECM about 60 percent of untreated patients develop arthritis (stage 3), which typically occurs in brief, intermittent attacks for several years. The arthritis can be mono-, oligo-, or polyarticular and typically affects large joints, particularly the knee. However, any joint in the body may be involved. The synovial fluid typically shows evidence of moderate inflammation (2,000 to 100,000 cells per cubic millimeter) with a predominance of neutrophils. Synovial fluid complement levels are normal or slightly reduced. In approximately 10 percent of patients, the arthritis becomes chronic, with pannus formation and cartilage erosion, resembling the process seen in rheumatoid arthritis.

Although the three stages of Lyme disease usually occur separately, it is important to emphasize that they may overlap or occur together. Incomplete pictures are also common. Some patients have only ECM. Others lack this lesion, and in such cases, neurologic, cardiac, or arthritic manifestations may be the presenting features of the illness.

PATHOGENESIS

After inoculation by the tick, *B. burgdorferi* may migrate outward in the skin and produce the enlarging ECM lesion. The organism may also disseminate in the blood to almost any site early in the disease. Spirochetes have been isolated from blood as well as from ECM lesions. Most of the manifestations of stages 2 and 3 Lyme disease, initially thought to be immune mediated, are now thought to be due to tissue invasion by the spirochete. *B. burgdorferi* has been isolated from cerebrospinal fluid several months after disease onset and has been seen in the synovium. The efficacy of antibiotic therapy in patients with these manifestations also suggests spirochetes are alive late in the illness.

DIAGNOSIS

In endemic areas the diagnosis of stage 1 Lyme disease can usually be made on clinical grounds if the characteristic ECM lesion is present. Because the tick vector is tiny, most patients do not give a history of a tick bite. Later in the illness, a history of preceding ECM may be helpful, but some patients lack such a history. If confusion exists in diagnosis, laboratory tests can be used to confirm the clinical suspicion of Lyme disease. Examination and culture of blood, skin, and CSF, if positive for spirochetes, are definitive; at present, these are low-yield procedures. Serologic tests (immunofluoresence assay or enzyme-linked immunosorbent assay) are the most practical diagnostic aid. In stage 1 Lyme disease, these

TABLE 1 Suggested Antibiotic Therapy for Lyme Disease

Stage of Disease	Treatment: Adults	Treatment: Children
ECM (stage 1)	Tetracycline 250 mg PO qid for 10–20 days	Penicillin V 50 mg/kg/d in divided doses for 10–20 days
	Alternatives	
	Penicillin V 500 mg PO qid for 10–20 days Erythromycin 250 mg PO qid for 10–20 days	Erythromycin 30 mg/kg/d in divided doses for 10–20 days
Neurologic (stage 2)	Penicillin G 20 million units/d IV for 10 days	Penicillin G, 300,000 units/kg/d IV for 10 days
Arthritic (stage 3)	Penicillin G 20 million units/d IV for at least 10 days *or* Benzathine penicillin 2.4 million units/week IM × 3	Penicillin G 300,000 units/kg/d IV for at least 10 days

tests have low sensitivity. Only 50 percent of patients with only ECM have elevated antibody titers. However, almost all patients with later manifestations of Lyme disease have elevated titers. Antibody to *B. burgdorferi* cross reacts with other spirochetes, and patients with syphilis may have false-positive Lyme serologic tests. Similarly, patients with Lyme disease may rarely have a false-positive RPR. However, patients with Lyme disease can be distinguished from those with syphilis by the VDRL and MHA-TP tests, which are negative in patients with Lyme disease.

TREATMENT

The treatment of Lyme disease has evolved over the past several years as understanding of the illness has advanced. Before identification of the etiologic agent, studies suggested that antimicrobial treatment was effective for stage 1 Lyme disease. Trials of antimicrobial therapy were then undertaken for both late neurologic and arthritic complications. Antimicrobials are now recommended for treatment of all manifestations of Lyme disease (Table 1).

For patients with stage 1 Lyme disease, tetracycline 250 mg four times per day for 10 to 20 days is the treatment of choice. Penicillin V 500 mg four times per day and erythromycin 250 mg four times per day for 10 to 20 days are alternative treatments. For children less than 8 years of age, penicillin V, 50 mg per kilogram per day (not less than 1 g and not more than 2 g) in divided doses for 10 to 20 days is recommended. All three antimicrobials effectively treat ECM and usually prevent the late complications of the disease. About 15 percent of patients develop an intensification of symptoms (Jarisch-Herxheimer-like reaction) within 24 hours of antimicrobial therapy. A second course of antimicrobials should be given to patients who do not respond to the initial course or for those with recurrent symptoms.

For patients with neurologic complications or who develop them after treatment of early Lyme disease, intravenous penicillin G, 20 million units per day in six divided doses (penicillin G, 300,000 units per kilogram per day in children) is effective therapy. Although meningitic and sensory symptoms often improve quickly, 6 to 8 weeks are often required for the resolution of motor deficits. For patients with arthritis, this intravenous regimen, as well as intramuscular benzathine penicillin, 2.4 million units per week for 3 weeks, are sometimes effective. Although systematic trials have not been undertaken for patients with cardiac complications, antimicrobials should be used for these manifestations as well. Patients with a PR interval greater than 0.30 seconds should be admitted to the hospital for observation because of the risk of progression to higher grade AV block. If high-grade block develops, temporary pacing may be necessary.

The role of corticosteroids in the treatment of any stage or manifestation of Lyme disease appears limited. It is possible that corticosteroids may have some role in patients with Bell's palsy if they are seen within 24 hours of onset and in patients with complete heart block or congestive heart failure if they do not improve on antimicrobial therapy alone within 24 hours.

Prevention

Protective clothing and/or insect repellents may offer some protection against tick bites for those engaged in outdoor activities in endemic areas.

HERPES SIMPLEX

RICHARD J. WHITLEY, M.D.
DAVID W. BARNES, M.D.

Of the recent advances in antiviral therapy, the treatment of herpes simplex virus (HSV) infections has provided the most gratifying results. In the early 1960s, effective topical antiviral therapy for the management of herpes simplex keratoconjunctivitis was introduced. A decade later significant advances were achieved in the treatment of life-threatening herpes simplex encephalitis and neonatal herpes. More recently, with the development of acyclovir, mucocutaneous HSV infections have become treatable. HSV infections of the skin are among the most common diseases of humans. The successful treatment of cutaneous herpex simplex virus infections has been predicated, in large part, upon the physician's ability to diagnose these infections rapidly because of clinically apparent and characteristic skin lesions. A broad spectrum of infection with HSV exists, ranging from totally asymptomatic or benign nuisance infections, such as recurrent labial or genital herpes, to those that are life-threatening, such as herpes simplex encephalitis or neonatal herpes simplex virus infections. With most clinical therapeutics, successful therapy is facilitated by prompt and accurate diagnosis. Treatment of viral infections is no exception. A delay in diagnosis, particularly when organs such as the brain are involved, only leads to progressive disease and poor therapeutic outcome. Similarly, successful therapy of primary genital infections is most beneficial when drug is administered within a few days of the onset of clinical symptoms and signs.

The propensity for HSV infections to be more severe during symptomatic primary disease or when occurring in the immuncompromised host provides a broader therapeutic window for evaluation of antiviral efficacy than with recurrent infection. As with other antimicrobials, the definition of a therapeutic index or ratio of efficacy to toxicity must balance recommendations for application of antivirals to human disease. In defining the numerator of the therapeutic index, efficacy must equate with an enhanced clinical effect beyond that of simply promoting cessation of viral excretion. Similarly, assessment of toxicity must consider both acute laboratory and clinical aberrations associated with the administration of the medication and the long-term consequences of the administration of these drugs. For example, nucleoside analogues must be assessed for potential mutagenicity and teratogenicity, particularly if therapy is to be administered for long periods. Furthermore, the potential for the development of viral resistance must be included in the risk-to-benefit ratio for any treatment modality.

This chapter focuses on the current application of antiviral therapies in the treatment of HSV infections. Each disease state is considered separately; the importance of prompt and accurate diagnosis is emphasized. Although a number of unproven or investigational antiviral agents have potential uses in therapy for herpesvirus infections, they will not be addressed in this summary.

HERPES SIMPLEX ENCEPHALITIS

Herpes simplex encephalitis (HSE) is the commonest cause of sporadic, fatal encephalitis in the United States, with an estimated annual incidence of approximately one in 500,000 individuals. Patients with HSE have clinical evidence of an acute febrile encephalopathy, signs of temporal lobe involvement with disordered mentation, seizures, evidence of localized central nervous system disease by diagnostic studies (brain scan, computerized tomography, and/or electroencephalography), and cerebrospinal fluid findings compatible with viral encephalitis. Even in the presence of these clinical findings, establishment of a diagnosis of HSE is particularly problematic. The only unequivocal method by which the diagnosis of HSE can be confirmed is by brain biopsy. As shown in Figure 1, a logical approach to the evaluation of individuals who present with evidence of localization by neurodiagnostic assessment is the performance of brain biopsy with detailed tissue examination. Such an approach will lead to confirmation of HSV infection of the brain by rapid diagnostic tests and isolation of virus in culture and, of equal importance, to the prompt and expeditious diagnosis of diseases that may mimic herpes simplex encephalitis (Table 1). Complications from the biopsy procedure itself and the likelihood of obtaining a false-negative result for virus are exceedingly small. It should be emphasized that if the patient does not have evidence of a focal encephalitic process, the probability of HSE is very low.

Historically, double-blinded, placebo-controlled studies of vidarabine therapy have demonstrated a reduced mortality in treatment of HSE. Mortality in placebo recipients is 70 percent, with 11 percent of survivors, or 2.5 percent of patients overall, returning to normal function. Vidarabine therapy decreases mortality to 40 percent 6 months after onset of disease. Twenty percent of patients overall return to normal function. These data led to the licensure of vidarabine for the treatment of HSE at a dosage of 15 mg per kilogram per day given intravenously over 12 hours for 10 to 14 days. However, recent data indicate that acyclovir is superior to vidarabine for the treatment of HSE. A further reduction in mortality rate—to 20 percent 6 months after the onset of treatment—has been demonstrated. Normalcy is achieved in 30 to 56 percent of patients six months after treatment. Thus, acyclovir is now the treatment of choice for HSE.

These studies were supported in part by contract No. 1-AI-12667 from the Development and Applications Branch of the National Institute of Allergy and Infectious Diseases, grant NCI-13148 from the National Cancer Institute, and grant RR-032 from the Division of Research Resources.

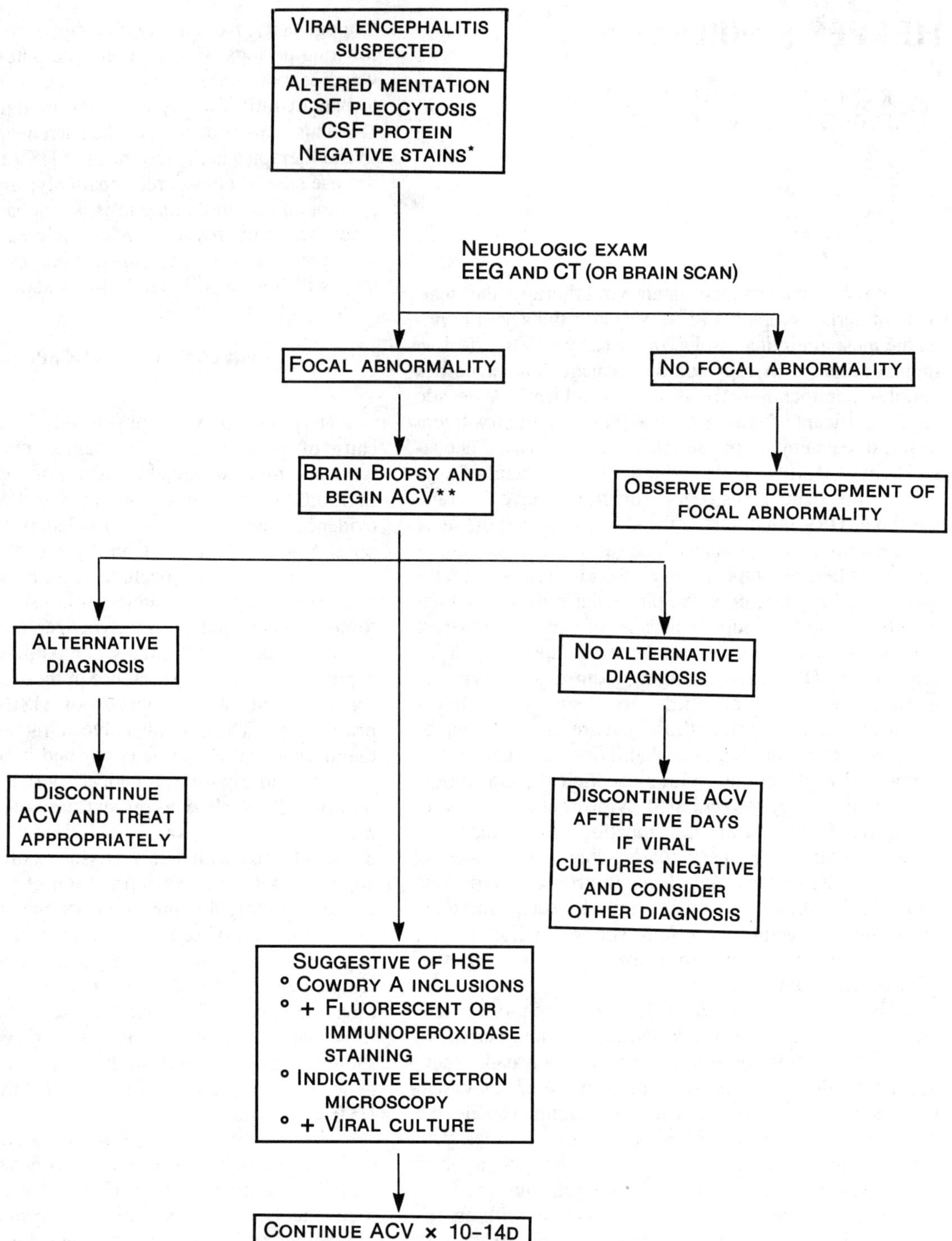

Figure 1 Suggested evaluation and therapy for herpes simplex encephalitis. * = gram, AFB, and India ink stains; ** = 10 mg per kilogram IV every 8 hours.

TABLE 1 Diseases That May Mimic Herpes Simplex Encephalitis

Disease	*No. of Cases in Series*
Vascular disease	8
Coxsackievirus encephalitis	4
Bacterial abscess	3
Mumps encephalitis	3
Cryptococcus infection	2
Subacute sclerosing panencephalitis	2
St. Louis encephalitis	2
Tumor	2
Postinfluenza encephalitis	2
Epstein-Barr virus encephalitis	2
Reye's syndrome	1
Toxic encephalopathy	1
Toxoplasma gondii infection	1
Tuberculosis	1
Lymphocytic choriomeningitis	1
Total	32

Note: Adapted from Whitley RJ, et al. N Engl J Med 1981; 304:313–8. Used with permission.

As shown in Table 2, the dosage of acyclovir is 10 mg per kilogram administered every 8 hours for a period of 10 days. It should be noted that in adults simple meningeal involvement with HSV, which occurs frequently with severe primary mucocutaneous disease, is like other viral meningitides in that it is a self-limited process and requires no specific therapy.

NEONATAL HERPES SIMPLEX

After first being reported in the mid-1930s, neonatal HSV infection has attracted increasing attention because of its association with genital herpes and its life-threatening nature with a known propensity for causing long-term morbidity. Neonatal HSV infection occurs at an estimated frequency of one in 3,000 to one in 15,000 live births per year. Without therapy, the disease will disseminate widely in more than 80 percent of cases. Multiple organ involvement and localized central nervous system disease have mortality rates of 80 percent and 50 percent, respectively. With severe disease, survivors rarely escape significant neurologic impairment without therapy. As many as 30 percent of babies with localized neonatal HSV infection of the skin, eye, and/or mouth—although not at risk for mortality—can have evidence of neurologic impairment on follow-up.

Important observations which suggest a diagnosis of neonatal HSV infection are viral excretion from the maternal genital tract, a maternal history or a sexual partner with genital herpes, the inability to grow bacteria from cerebrospinal fluid or blood cultures of an infant with suspected meningitis or encephalitis, characteristic findings on electroencephalogram or CT scan, and progressively increasing levels of cerebrospinal fluid protein in the presence of clinical deterioration. Confirmation of the diagnosis remains dependent upon the isolation of HSV from vesicles, the hallmark of infection in these children. Cutaneous vesicles appear in clusters as small as one millimeter in diameter and evolve through phases of clear vesicular fluid to pustulation and, ultimately, scabbing. It is important that only 70 to 80 percent of children have evidence of skin vesicles with neonatal infection. The remaining 20 to 30 percent will either excrete virus from the oropharynx or have evidence of brain involvement, which may be misdiagnosed as bacterial infection. In such situations, cultures of cerebrospinal fluid and even brain biopsy may be indicated to establish the diagnosis unequivocally. Serial serologic assessment is of limited value for establishment of the diagnosis in the early phases of disease.

Any neonate with HSV infection, including those with disease confined to the skin, should be treated. At the present time, approved therapy is vidarabine at a dosage of 30 mg per kilogram per day administered intravenously over 12 hours at a concentration of 0.5 mg per milliliter of intravenous fluid. Therapy should be continued for 10 days. Even with adequate therapy, recurrent skin vesicles will appear in virtually every child within 2 to 3 months following the completion of treatment. The recurrence of skin vesicles is not an indication for retreatment unless associated with systemic disease. Eventually the results of ongoing clinical trials comparing vidarabine versus acyclovir therapy for neonatal herpes infections may lead to changes in the recommended therapy.

OCULAR INFECTION

Herpes simplex infection of the eye is recognized as one of the commonest infectious causes of blindness in the United States. Of all modalities of herpesviral therapy available to date, the earliest benefits were achieved with topical therapy of herpes simplex keratoconjunctivitis. A persistent problem encountered with topical therapy—as well as for other modalities of therapy—is the propensity for recurrences even with successful initial treatment. Idoxuridine, trifluorothymidine, and vidarabine all can abort individual attacks with varying but acceptable degrees of toxicity. The most pronounced toxicity is local allergic reaction to idoxuridine. For optimal diagnosis and therapy, care of HSV infections of the eye should be provided by a qualified ophthalmologist. The concomitant prescribing of corticosteroids with antiviral therapy should only be undertaken by physicians experienced in the management of herpes simplex keratoconjunctivitis. The drug of choice at the present time for the treatment of this disease appears to be trifluorothymidine.

TABLE 2 U.S. Food and Drug Administration Approved Antiviral Modalities for Herpes Simplex Virus (HSV) Infections

Antiviral	Formulation	Indication	Dosage Administration	Some Reported Side Effects
5-iodo-2′-deoxyuridine (Idoxuridine, IDU, Stoxil)	Topical ophthalmic 0.1% solution or 0.5% ointment	HSV keratitis	Solution: 1 gtt q1h while awake and q4h at night; ointment: q4h while awake	Contact dermatitis, pruritis, tearing, viral resistance
9-β-D-arabinofuranosyladenine (vidarabine, adenine arabinoside, ara-A, Vira-A)	Topical ophthalmic 3% ointment	HSV keratitis	q4h while awake and qhs	Contact dermatitis, pruritis, tearing, viral resistance
	Intravenous	HSV encephalitis	15 mg/kg/day IV; dilute to 0.5 mg/ml and administer over 12h × 14 days	Nausea and vomiting, diarrhea, megaloblastosis, tremors, myoclonus, seizures
	Intravenous	Neonatal herpes	30 mg/kg/day IV; dilute to 0.5 mg/ml and administer over 12h × 14 days	Elevated SGOT; allopurinol is a relative contraindication-accumulation of toxic metabolites; viral resistance (decreased dose necessary in renal impairment)
2′-deoxy-5-(trifluoromethyl) uridine (TFT, Viroptic)	Topical ophthalmic 1% solution	HSV keratitis	1 gtt q2h × 7 days 1 gtt q4h × 7 days (do not exceed 21 days therapy)	Contact dermatitis, pruritis, tearing, viral resistance
9-[(2-hydroxyethoxy) methyl] guanine (Acyclovir, ACV, Zovirax)	Topical ointment 5%	Primary genital or mucocutaneous HSV	Cover lesions q3h while awake and qhs × 7 days	Drug sensitization, viral resistance
	Oral capsule 200 mg	Primary genital HSV Suppressive therapy with recurrences >6 times/year	1 cap PO q4h while awake × 10 days 1 cap PO q8h for <6 months*	Vomiting, nausea, headache, ? decreased spermiogenesis, viral resistance
	Intravenous	Primary genital HSV and immunocompromised patients with primary or recurrent disease†	Adults: 5 mg/kg IV over 1h q8h × 7 days; children (<12 yrs), 750 mg/m²/day as above	Elevated BUN, nausea, viral resistance, headache, thrombophlebitis (with IV formulation) (decreased dose necessary in renal impairment)
	Intravenous	HSV encephalitis	Adults: 10 mg/kg IV over 1h q8h × 10 days; children (<12 yrs), 1,200 mg/m²/day as above	

* Another option is intermittent therapy initiated by the patient while in the prodromal stage of a recurrent episode and continued for 5 days. Dose is the same as primary infection.
† Oral therapy may be appropriate in some instances.

MUCOCUTANEOUS HERPES SIMPLEX

Herpes simplex labial and genital infections have been a major focus of antiviral research in the United States. Significant advances in the treatment of human HSV infections from a therapeutic and suppressive standpoint have been achieved in this area. At the present time, the management of these infections is dependent in large part upon host immune status (normal or immunocompromised) and the nature of the infection (primary or recurrent). Aside from the classic clinical presentation of vesicular/ulcerative lesions, the standard of diagnosis is the isolation of virus in tissue culture. Evidence of cytopathic effect in tissue culture usually occurs within 48 to 72 hours. More rapid diagnostic techniques have included lesion scrapings followed by staining with monoclonal antibodies, although these techniques may lack sensitivity and specificity. Humoral antibodies to HSV, types 1 and 2 are common, even in persons without clinical disease, and are of limited diagnostic usefulness.

As shown in Figure 2, there is no established or approved therapy for primary herpes simplex gingivostomatitis or recurrent herpes simplex labialis in the normal host. By contrast, in the immunocompromised host who suffers from recurrent orolabial HSV infections, three preparations of acyclovir—topical, oral, and intravenous—have all been shown to be useful. At the present time the topical and intravenous formulations of acyclovir are approved by the U.S. Food and Drug Administration for treatment of labial lesions, progressive stomatitis, and cutaneous disease in the immunocompromised patients. The appropriate dosage regimens for utilization of these compounds in each circumstance appear in Table 2. The recent licensure of the oral formulation of acyclovir should provide an effective therapy for HSV infections in immunocompromised patients who are not systemically ill. Intravenous

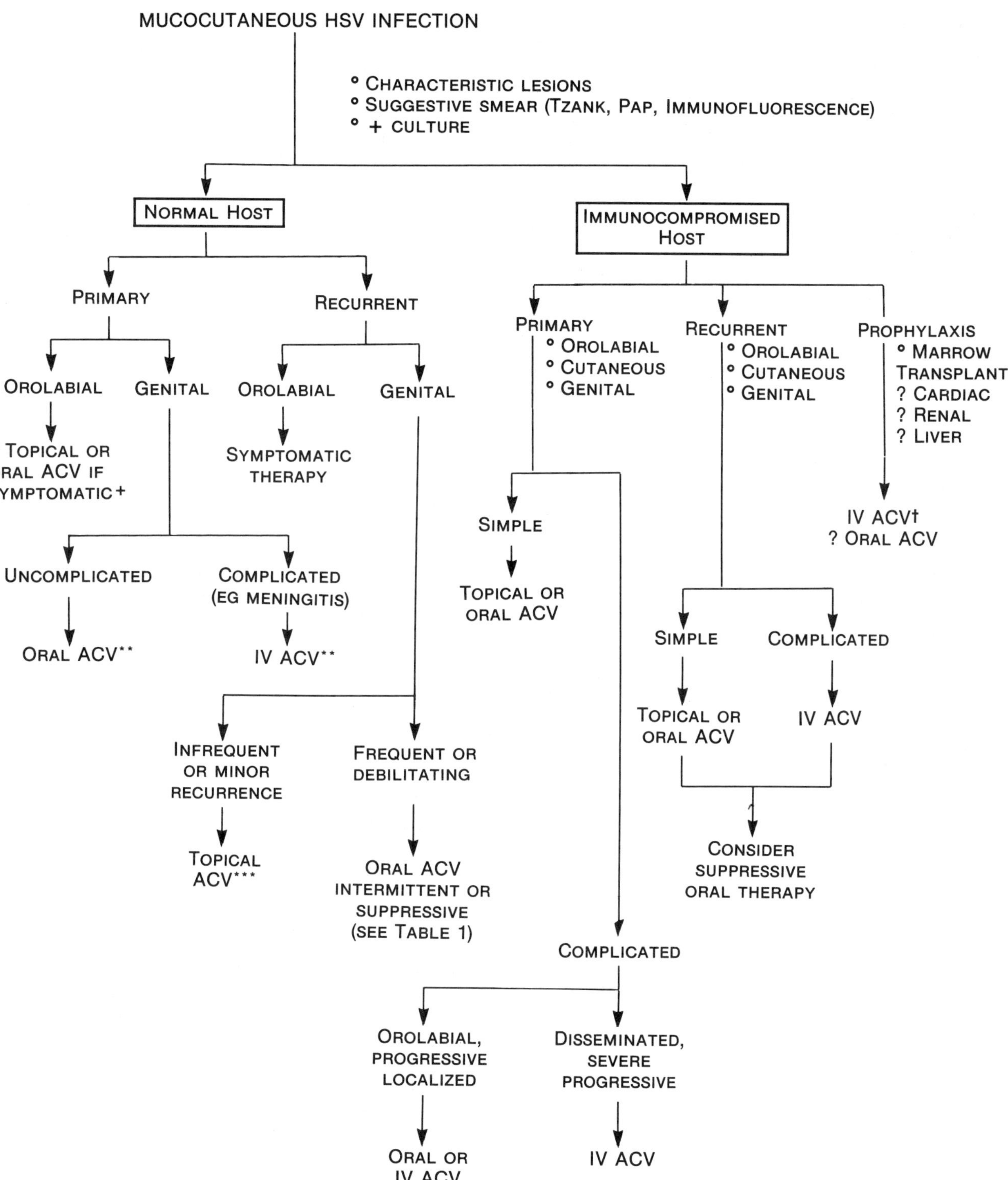

Figure 2 Therapeutic approaches to mucocutaneous herpes simplex virus infections. * = 200 mg PO five times per day for 10 days; ** = 5 mg per kilogram IV every 8 hours for 10 days; *** = 5 percent ointment applied every 3 to 4 hours (initiated during prodrome if recurrent); + = not of proven efficacy; † = 5 mg per kilogram IV every 8 to 12 hours while susceptible.

vidarabine appears to be of limited utility in the treatment of mucocutaneous HSV infections in immunocompromised patients and is not recommended.

The management of genital HSV infections has undergone even more striking advances. Following the demonstration that topical acyclovir accelerated viral clearance and decreased clinical symptomatology in primary genital HSV infections by 24 to 48 hours, further therapeutic advances were achieved with both the intravenous and oral formulations of acyclovir. Although intravenous acyclovir has demonstrated efficacy in the treatment of primary genital herpes infections, its cost as well as the requirement for hospitalization for drug administration restrict this form of therapy to particularly severe cases. The recent licensure of the oral formulation of acyclovir may offer a more efficacious and cost effective treatment for primary genital HSV infections. Significant reductions in the duration of viral shedding, the time to healing, and the duration and severity of the clinical symptoms comparable to those seen with intravenous acyclovir can be achieved with oral therapy. The drug can be administered to the patient in an ambulatory setting, avoiding the expense of hospitalization and the hazards of intravenous therapy.

The effect of acyclovir in the treatment of recurrent episodes of genital HSV infection is less marked. Topical acyclovir, when applied very early in the course of a recurrence, may be of some benefit in decreasing the duration of viral shedding. The effect of topical therapy on the events of healing is minor, but greater benefit may be achieved by beginning application of the ointment during the prodromal phase of a recurrence rather than waiting for lesions to appear. Such an approach has not been proved efficacious. Oral acyclovir has been shown to be effective in shortening the clinical course of recurrent genital herpes simplex infections, but has no significant effect on the frequency of recurrences when taken intermittently. Recent trials have shown that continuous administration of oral acyclovir is effective in suppressing attacks in patients with frequent recurrences. However, discontinuation of suppressive therapy results in the recurrence of disease, with an attack frequency no different from that prior to therapy. The adverse effects of long-term acyclovir administration are not yet known, and caution should be used in prescribing this drug on a continuous-use basis. The use of systemic (oral or intravenous) acyclovir should be avoided in pregnancy because of the potential for adverse effects on the fetus. If therapy is indicated in this setting, topical acyclovir should be used. In addition, acyclovir-resistant herpes simplex viruses have been found in clinical isolates even without prior exposure to drug. Several studies have demonstrated the emergence of acyclovir-resistant herpes simplex virus during acyclovir therapy, but the clinical significance of this observation is unknown. With cessation of acyclovir therapy, there is reversion to acyclovir sensitivity in most cases, perhaps because of reduced pathogenicity of the resistant strain. Thus, intermittent therapy may be perferrable to chronic continuous therapy in the management of recurrent genital herpes.

Acyclovir has also been shown to be effective in the suppression and treatment of recurrent HSV infections in immuncompromised patients. These infections can be particularly troublesome in those patients with hematologic malignancies as well as those on high doses of immunosuppressive agents or with defects in cellular immunity. Oral prophylactic therapy may offer such patients with persistent or recurrent mucocutaneous herpes simplex infections effective outpatient therapy. Intravenous and oral acyclovir prophylaxis have been used successfully in patients undergoing bone marrow transplantation while awaiting marrow recovery.

VISCERAL INVOLVEMENT

Visceral disease associated with HSV infection is generally encountered in two circumstances: newborns with disseminated involvement and immunocompromised hosts, particularly organ transplant recipients. In these individuals, the most common visceral HSV complications include esophagitis, hepatitis, and pneumonitis. Although no controlled data exist to substantiate the clinical utility of therapy in these situations, a reasonable choice for severe or life-threatening disease is the administration of acyclovir, at the dosages indicated in Table 1.

Diagnosis of visceral complications can be difficult and is achieved by isolation of virus from biopsy material (lung, liver, or esophagus). Confirmation of HSV infection can be made in culture either by monoclonal staining of cellular debris or the cell sheet, immunoperoxidase staining, or antigen detection using a variety of procedures. It does not appear that vidarabine is useful in the management of these infections.

CONCLUSIONS

Antiviral therapy has been shown to be effective for many herpes simplex virus infections, particularly those of the genital tract, in the immunocompromised host, and neonatal and encephalitic diseases. However, recurrences cannot be prevented with existing modalities of therapy, even when therapy is administered shortly after the onset of primary infection. This observation is true for all antiviral medicines presently in use. As with other forms of antimicrobial therapy, continual monitoring for potential toxicity is imperative, particularly in the setting of chronic therapy. The evolution of antiviral therapy over the last decade has allowed us to successfully manage severe and life-threatening HSV infections and has allowed for control, albeit not yet optimal, of less severe yet psychologically debilitating mucocutaneous infections. Such advances will provide a foundation for developments in antiviral therapy that will lead to the discovery of more effective drugs and the prevention of recurrent disease.

MALARIA

JOEL G. BREMAN, M.D., D.T.P.H.

Human malaria is a protozoal infection with any of four species of the genus *Plasmodium (P. falciparum, P. vivax, P. malariae, P. ovale)*. An acute infection typically manifests fever, chills, shivering, sweats, and malaise; severe attacks, usually caused by *P. falciparum*, may lead to convulsions, loss of consciousness, and death if the illness is not diagnosed and treated promptly.

The disease is endemic throughout the tropical developing countries in Central and South America, Haiti, the Dominican Republic, Africa, the Middle East, the Indian subcontinent, Asia and Oceania. Although about 7 to 11 million cases are reported to the World Health Organization (WHO) each year, the actual number is at least 20 times greater, because of incomplete reporting. In the United States, where the disease was eradicated in the 1950s, 1,013 cases of malaria were reported in 1984. As in previous years, about one-third of these cases were in U.S. citizens who were infected during travel abroad. From 1966 to 1984, 70 deaths due to malaria were reported in the United States, and 92 percent of these were due to *P. falciparum*.

LIFE CYCLE OF *PLASMODIUM*

A description of the natural cycle of malaria is important to understand the basis of diagnosis, treatment, and prevention. The infected female mosquito injects malaria sporozoites as it feeds, and within 30 minutes these enter hepatocytes (exoerythrocytic stage). After parasitic maturation (primary tissue schizogony), that takes 7 to 15 days, the merozoites rupture from an hepatic cell containing a mature schizontand enter red blood cells (RBCs) beginning the erythrocytic schizogonic cycle. The parasites again mature in the RBCs, become schizonts, containing daughter blood-stage merozoites. The infected RBCs rupture, and the blood stage cycle is continued, with the invasion of other RBCs by merozoites. Most of the blood-stage parasites are asexual, but some parasites differentiate into gametocytes. These sexual forms, when ingested by the feeding mosquito, develop into oocysts in the gut of the mosquito, then into sporozoites, allowing the transmission cycle to begin once again when the mosquito takes another blood meal.

P. vivax and *P. ovale* are relapsing species, meaning that some of the sporozoites may become hypnozoites, or dormant forms in the liver, with the potential to complete development and initiate renewed cycles of RBC infection months or even years later. Parasite density in RBCs may be at very low levels for prolonged periods due to partial immunity of the host, use of incompletely effective drugs or both. Recrudescences are renewed manifestations of an infection due to survival of the erythrocytic forms of the parasite; infectin with *P. falciparum* and *P. malariae* is the commonest cause of recrudescences.

DIAGNOSIS

The individual with malaria almost always reports fever lasting for one or more days; other symptoms are those resembling influenza—chills, sweating, headache, muscle pain, and malaise. In infants the classic signs and symptoms may not be present; there may only be irritability, lethargy, and decreased appetite. Cerebral malaria is the most severe complication. Malaria can cause adult respiratory distress syndrome (ARDS), renal failure, hemolytic anemia, and hypoglycemia in addition to central nervous system complications. A positive blood smear is necessary to confirm the diagnosis.

Patients with malaria have almost always been to malarious areas recently or have had the disease before. This information should be actively sought by the clinician. In nonendemic areas the clinician should ask the patient's residence and travel history and determine which antimalarial drugs, if any, have been taken for prevention. In endemic areas any patient with a febrile illness should be suspected of having malaria. The areas of the world with endemic malaria have not changed greatly over the past 25 years (Fig. 1).

Malaria can also be transmitted by RBC-containing products, either via blood transfusions or from shared needles and syringes of drug abusers; transfusion malaria occurs fewer than nine times per year in the United States. Congenital malaria, also a rare event, occurs when the newborn is inoculated with RBC-containing parasites from the infected mother during delivery. In general, the incubation period for transfusion malaria is about 10 days for *P. falciparum*, for *P. vivax* usually about 16 days, and for *P. malariae* 40 days or longer.

P. falciparum, P. vivax, and *P. ovale* have been called tertian malarias because the paroxysms of fever and chills were first described as occurring at approximately 48-hour intervals; *P. malariae* is a quartan (72-hour) parasite. The intervals reflect the asexual parasite cycle in the blood, and symptoms occur when the merozoite-laden RBCs rupture. Cyclical fevers may not be common, particularly in patients with *P. falciparum* malaria, because parasite development may be asynchronous.

The definitive diagnosis of malaria is made by detecting malaria parasites in a blood smear that is properly taken, stained and examined. A thick and thin blood film should be taken at the time the disease is suspected, and Giemsa stain should be used. The thick film should be examined first, since low-density infections will be more easily detected here; on a thick film, about 40 times the blood volume is represented per microscopic field than on a thin blood smear. The thin smear is used to identify the species of parasite. The distinction between *P. falciparum* and other *Plasmodium* species is important because special treatment may be required, particularly for drug-resistant strains. A quantitative estimation of the parasitemia should be done to follow the clearance of the

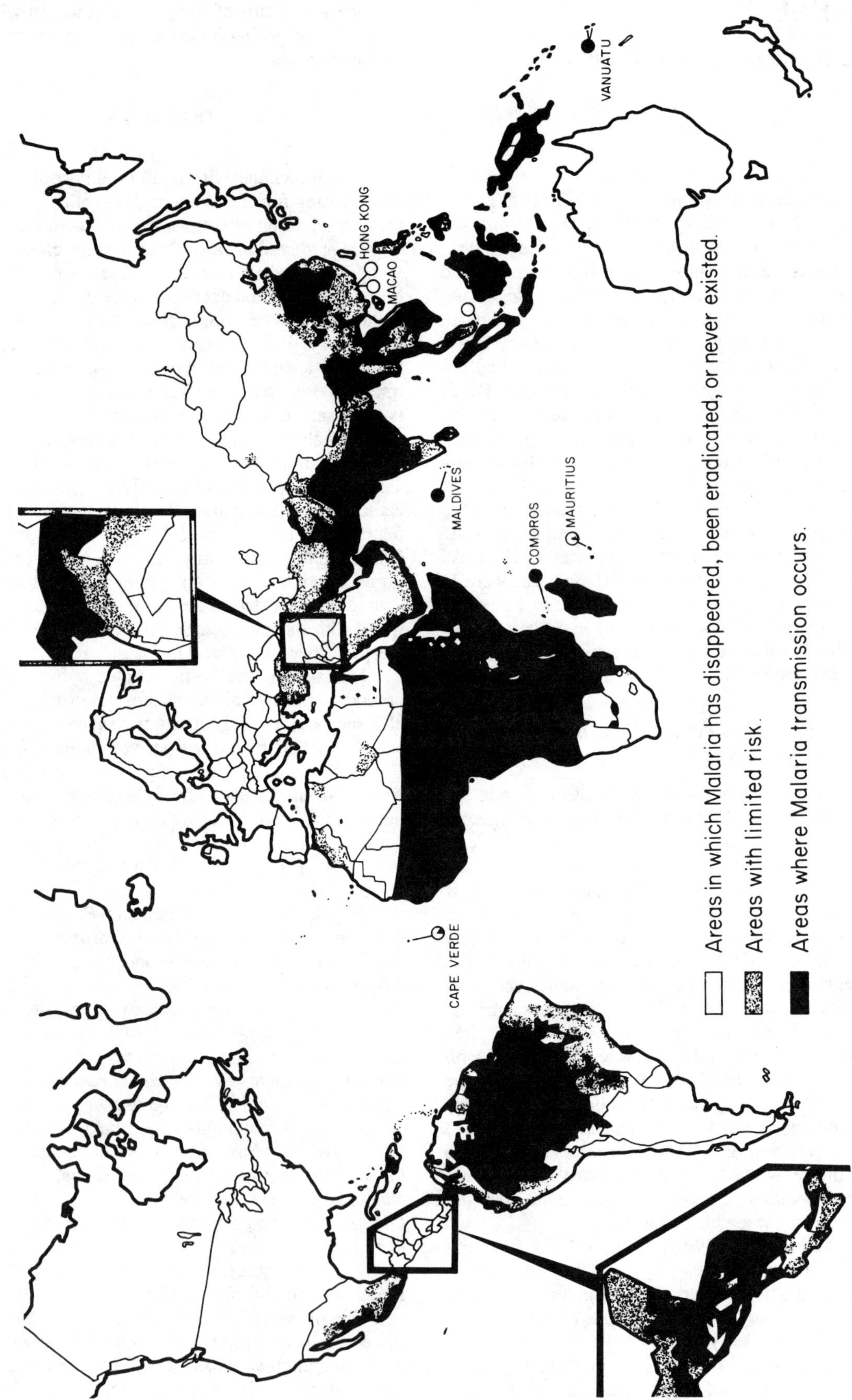

Figure 1 Areas of the world with endemic malaria.

infection after treatment begins. The percentage of RBCs parasitized can be made by estimating the number of RBCs with parasites in a representative thin blood film. If malaria is highly suspected, and the initial blood smear is negative, several repeat blood smears should be taken at 12 hour intervals and examined carefully. Gametocytes of *P. falciparum* can be observed in the blood for weeks after treatment begins, and their presence does not reflect treatment failure.

Serologic testing for immunofluorescent antibodies is useful in diagnosing a prior malaria infection in donors of blood products given to patients with transfusion-induced malaria. Serologic methods are not very useful in diagnosing an acute attack of malaria.

TREATMENT

Prompt diagnosis and effective treatment are key to a rapid recovery from malaria. Objectives of treatment are rapid elimination of parasitemia and prevention of complications due to malaria. The critical factors in determining treatment are the clinical status of the patient, species of parasite present, and the geographic origin and the potential for drug-resistance if the infecting species is *P. falciparum*. Strains of chloroquine-resistant *P. falciparum* (CRPF) are now found in Africa, Asia, and South America (Table 1). They appear to be extending geographically, particularly in Africa where the phenomenon was first reported there in 1978.

TABLE 1 Areas with Reported Chloroquine-Resistant *Plasmodium falciparum*, November 1985

Africa	*Asia*
Angola	Burma
Burundi	China (Hainan Island and southern provinces)
Cameroons	Indonesia
Central African Republic	Kampuchea
Comoros	Laos
Congo	Malaysia
Gabon	Philippines (Luzon, Basilan, Mindoro, Palawan Mindanao Islands, and Sulu Archipelago)
Kenya	Thailand
Madagascar	Vietnam
Malawi	
Mozambique	*Indian Subcontinent*
Namibia	Bangladesh (north and east)
Rwanda	India (Orissa, Assam, Uttar Pradesh, Andhra Pradesh, Madhya Pradesh)
Sudan (northern provinces)	Pakistan (Rawalpindi, Punjab)
Tanzania	Sri Lanka
Uganda	
Zaire	*Oceania*
Zambia (northeastern)	Papua New Guinea
Zimbabwe	Solomon Islands
South America	Vanuatu
Bolivia	
Brazil	
Colombia	
Ecuador	
French Guyana	
Guyana	
Panama (east of the Canal Zone including the San Blas Islands)	
Peru (northern provinces)	
Surinam	
Venezuela	

Note: In some countries relatively few sites have been sampled.

Drugs used clinically are directed toward the asexual parasite within RBCs. These include the 4-aminoquinolines (i.e., chloroquine and amodiaquine), the cinchona alkaloids (i.e., quinine and quinidine), the combination of pyrimethamine and sulfadoxine (Fansidar), and the tetracyclines. Antimalarial drugs and dose schedules for treating mild and severe malaria are shown in Table 2. For *P. falciparum* infections acquired in areas where CRPF exists, patients should be treated with quinine and either Fansidar (25 mg of pyrimethamine and 500 mg of sulfadoxine per tablet) or tetracycline. Parenteral quinine should be given if a patient has had vomiting or manifestations of cerebral malaria, such as obtundation or convulsions. In general, the parenteral route should also be used for nonimmune patients (persons living outside of endemic areas) having greater than about 5 percent parasitemia (about 250,000 parasites per cubic millimeter of blood). Nonimmune and comatose individuals with greater than 10 percent of RBCs parasitized are candidates for exchange blood transfusions. Very rapid recovery has occurred in some critically ill patients with high parasite levels where exchange transfusion was initiated soon after diagnosis was made.

Quinine, given by intravenous infusion to a severely ill (often unconscious) patient over 4 hours, is recommended to assure close regulation of the amount of drug given and absorbed. In the United States, parenteral quinine is only available from the Malaria Branch, Centers for Disease Control, Atlanta, Georgia 30333; telephone 404–452–4046 (nights, weekends: 404-329-2888). Recently, studies in Thailand has shown that quinidine, a diastereoisomer of quinine, may be more effective than quinine when administered intravenously to patients with *P. falciparum* malaria.

Patients with cerebral malaria must have airway maintenance, tracheal suction, and other care to assure that aspiration and bacterial pneumonia do not occur. Convulsions may be due to high fever or to hypoglycemia; depending on the cause, an anticonvulsant or glucose infusion is given. Dexamethasone is not advised for patients with cerebral malaria, because controlled trials have indicated that the drug was associated with prolonged unconsciousness, increased gastrointestinal bleeding, and sepsis. Since cerebral edema is not usually part of the pathologic process in cerebral malaria, tissue diuretics such as urea and mannitol are not advised.

Salt and water loss—associated with high temperature, sweating, and decreased fluid intake—leads to oliguria. In general, fluid and electrolyte replacement will be sufficient to restore hypovolemia and renal function. Diuretics, such as furosemide, should be considered when a rise in blood urea nitrogen and creatinine occurs. Renal dialysis may be required if the patient does not respond.

Red blood cells or whole blood may be given slowly (to limit the danger of pulmonary edema) when severe anemia develops. Platelet transfusions are generally not needed, since the platelet count returns to normal rapidly with treatment.

TABLE 2 Drugs of Choice for the Treatment of Active Malaria Infections

Clinical Setting	*Drug(s) of Choice**	*Dosage†*
Uncomplicated attacks of all species of malaria EXCEPT *P. falciparum* acquired in areas of chloroquine resistance	Chloroquine phosphate (Aralen)	10 mg base/kg (up to maximum of 600 mg base), then 5 mg base/kg (maximum of 300 mg base for follow-up doses) 6 hr later, then 5 mg base/kg per day for 2 days
Uncomplicated attacks of *P. falciparum* acquired in areas of chloroquine resistance	Quinine sulfate	25 mg/kg per day in 3 divided doses for 3 days (maximum of 650 mg/dose)
	plus	
	Pyrimethamine/sulfadoxine (Fansidar)‡	2–11 months; ¼ tablet 1–3 years: ½ tablet 4–8 years: 1 tablet 9–14 years: 2 tablets >14 years: 3 tablets Above as a single dose
	or	
	Quinine sulfate	Same as above
	plus	
	Tetracycline§	5 mg/kg qid for 7 days (maximum of 250 mg/dose)
Severe illness, due to *P. falciparum*; oral therapy cannot be administered for any reason	Quinine dihydrochloride‖	25 mg/kg per day: administer half of dose in a 4-hr IV infusion of 500 ml of 5% glucose and 1 N saline solution, plasma, or dextran; then give the other half 6–8 hr later in the same volume over the same time if oral therapy still cannot be started (maximum dosage: 1,800 mg per day); continue q8h for 3 days of treatment; adjust volume of fluids for pediatric patients.
	plus	
	Pyrimethamine/sulfadoxine or tetracycline, as above, after IV quinine completed	
After treatment of acute attack of *P. vivax* or *P. ovale* to prevent further relapses ("radical cure")	Primaquine phosphate#	0.3 mg base/kg per day for 14 days (maximum dose: 15 mg base/day)

* Consult experts, including the Malaria Branch of the Centers for Diseases Control, Atlanta, Georgia 30333, (404–452–4046; nights, weekends, 404–329–2888), for information regarding alternative regimens.

† Dosages are oral unless otherwise stated.

‡ Fansidar should not be given to persons with known allergy to sulfonamides or pyrimethamine.

§ For the treatment of malaria, the U.S. Food and Drug Administration (FDA) considers tetracycline an investigational drug. Tetracycline has been shown to be effective in the treatment of *F. falciparum* strains resistant to Fansidar and acquired in Southeast Asia. Physicians must weigh the benefit of tetracycline therapy against the possibility of known adverse effects in children under 8 years of age.

‖ In the United States, quinine for parenteral use is available from the Malaria Branch of the Centers for Disease Control. Intravenous administration of quinine can produce arrhythmias and hypotension, and should be given slowly. Constant monitoring of the pulse and blood pressure is recommended. Oral quinine sulfate should be substituted as soon as possible, accompanied by the other drugs recommended for an uncomplicated attack.

\# As primaquine may cause severe hemolysis in persons with a G6PD deficiency, this trait should be tested for before this drug is given. Congenital malaria and transfusion malaria do not require treatment with primaquine.

Pulmonary edema may develop in severely ill patients who have very high parasite counts or who are pregnant, as well as in those who are given excess fluids, blood transfusions, or who have oliguria. Treatment includes sitting the patient up, giving oxygen, diuretics, venesection, and positive end expiratory ventilation.

Hypoglycemia is a recently recognized complication of severe malaria, particularly cerebral malaria. Persons receiving quinine may develop severe hypoglycemia from the hyperinsulinemia effect of this drug; these effects may occur even with continuous infusions of glucose. Patients with malaria and deepening coma or seizures should be assessed for hypoglycemia and treated for this condition until laboratory studies indicate otherwise.

As with many infections during pregnancy, *P. falciparum* malaria can be life threatening to the mother and the fetus; abortion, stillbirth, and an infant with low birth weight can result from malaria. The effect on the fetuses of primagravidae are more severe than on those of multigravidae. The potential risks of using quinine in pregnant women with severe malaria are far outweighed by the need for prompt treatment of these patients. Hypoglycemia and anemia need to be assessed carefully in pregnant women with malaria.

PREVENTION OF MALARIA

The major dilemma in the prevention of malaria is the continuing spread of drug-resistant strains of *P. falciparum*. While most persons can be protected with available drugs, 100 percent assurance of prevention is not possible. Hence, travelers must understand these issues before departure.

Travelers going to malarious areas are strongly advised to take preventive drugs, even if their visit is as brief

TABLE 3 Drugs Used in the Prophylaxis and Presumptive Treatment of Malaria Acquired in Areas with CRPF

	Routine Prophylaxis		*Presumptive Treatment§*	
Drug	*Adult Dose*	*Pediatric Dose*	*Adult Dose*	*Pediatric Dose*
Chloroquine phosphate (Aralen)	300 mg base (500 mg salt) orally once a week	5 mg/kg base (8.3 mg/kg salt) orally once a week, up to maximum adult dose of 300 mg base	Chloroquine is not recommended for the presumptive treatment of malaria acquired in areas of known chloroquine resistance	
Amodiaquine (Camoquin, Flavoquine)*	400 mg base (520 mg salt) orally once a week	7 mg/kg base (9 mg/kg salt) orally once a week, up to maximum adult dose of 400 mg base	Amodiaquine is not recommended for the presumptive treatment of malaria acquired in areas of known chloroquine resistance	
Pyrimethamine-sulfadoxine (Fansidar)†	1 tablet (25 mg pyrimethamine and 500 mg sulfadoxine) orally once a week	2–11 months: ⅛ tab/wk 1–3 years: ¼ tab/wk 4–8 years: ½ tab/wk 9–14 years: ¾ tab/wk >14 years: 1 tab/wk	3 tablets (75 mg pyrimethamine and 1,500 mg sulfadoxine) orally as a single dose	2–11 months: ¼ tab 1–3 years: ½ tab 4–8 years: 1 tab 9–14 years: 2 tabs >14 years: 3 tabs As a single dose
Doxycycline‡	100 mg orally once a day	>8 years of age: 2 mg/kg per day orally, up to adult dose of 100 mg/day	Tetracyclines are not recommended for the presumptive treatment of malaria	

* Unavailable in the United States, but widely available overseas.
† The use of Fansidar is contraindicated in persons with histories of sulfonamide or pyrimethamine intolerance, in pregnancy at term, and in infants under 2 months of age. Physicians who prescribe the drug to be used as presumptive treatment in the event of a febrile illness when professional medical care is not readily available should ensure that such prescriptions are clearly labeled with instructions to be followed in the event of a febrile illness. If used as weekly prophylaxis, travelers should be advised to discontinue the use of the drug immediately in the event of a possible adverse effect, especially if any mucocutaneous signs or symptoms develop.
‡ The use of doxycycline is contraindicated in pregnancy and children under 8 years of age. The FDA considers the use of tetracyclines as antimalarials to be investigational. Physicians who prescribe doxycycline as malaria chemoprophylaxis should advise their patients to limit direct exposure to the sun to minimize the possibility of a photosensitivity reaction.
§ Not confirmed by blood slide.

as an airport stopover. Factors to consider before advising or taking antimalarial drugs include the area to be visited, the predominance of *P. vivax* or *P. falciparum*, the presence of chloroquine-resistant strains of *P. falciparum*, the length and intensity of exposure to infected *Anopheles* mosquitoes, the traveler's history of drug allergy or intolerance, and the pregnancy status of women.

In most areas of the world, malaria transmission in urban areas is much less intense than in rural zones; in some cities, particularly in malarious Asian and South American countries, malaria transmission is limited or nonexistent. *P. vivax* is the most prominent species in most malarious Asian and Central and South American countries, and all *P. vivax* strains are sensitive to chloroquine. The major risk areas for getting severe CRPF malaria are in East and Central Africa, although CRPF strains do exist in South America and Asia.

Table 3 lists the drugs used in the prophylaxis and presumptive treatment of malaria acquired in areas with CRPF. Those travelers spending 3 weeks or less in areas with CRPF are advised to take chloroquine weekly. In addition, they should take along a treatment dose of Fansidar (Table 3) to use in case they develop symptoms and cannot get medical assistance and a slide-confirmed diagnosis. Those with a history of sulfonamide or pyrimethamine allergy should not take this drug.

Fansidar can be considered for persons with prolonged or intense exposure to malaria in areas of CRPF transmission. Physicians who advise these travelers and expatriate residents must assess individual living conditions, availability of local medical care, and the local malarial transmission pattern. Fansidar has recently been associated with erythema multiforma, Stevens-Johnson syndrome, and toxic epidermal necrolysis in persons taking the drug to prevent malaria. Several deaths have occurred, presumably as a result of sulfonamide allergy. Fansidar should be stopped immediately if a reaction occurs; mucocutaneous signs or symptoms such as pruritus, erythema, rash, orogenital lesions, or pharyngitis are indicative of such a reaction. In case of febrile illness during or after the trip , professional care should be sought promptly and a blood smear taken. If such care is not available, the treatment dose of Fansidar should be taken and follow-up care obtained as soon as possible. Alternates to chloroquine and Fansidar are amodiaquine (like chloroquine, a 4-aminoquinoline compound), which is currently not available in the United States but appears to be more effective than chloroquine in areas with CRPF, and tetracycline, for which limited therapeutic studies indicated effectiveness against CRPF. Tetracyclines should not be used in pregnant women or in children younger than 8 years of age. Some persons taking tetracyclines may develop a sunburn-like rash due to photosensitivity. A sun screen should be used when tetracyclines are taken. Other drugs are available throughout the world as preventives against malaria. However, they cannot be recommended because their efficacy is not proved or they are not yet licensed or available in the United States.

Primaquine, an 8-aminoquinoline, is effective against the hepatic phase of the parasite. Some populations of Africa, Mediterranean, Middle Eastern or southeast Asian origin have glucose-6-phosphate dehydrogenase (G6PD) deficiency and may develop hemolysis after taking primaquine; therefore a test for this trait should be done before the drug is given. Primaquine is used for radical cure of patients with a relapsing form of malaria (*P. vivax* or *P. ovale*) and is used as terminal prophylaxis in areas where prolonged exposure to these parasites may have occurred (Table 2). Peace Corps volunteers, missionaries, or others living in areas with relapsing forms are at higher risk. In general, most individuals taking short trips to malarious areas are not candidates for primaquine unless they develop a relapsing form of malaria after returning home.

Travelers should make strong efforts to reduce exposure with mosquitoes. These measures include screening of windows and doors, use of mosquito nets, application of insect repellants containing high concentrations of N,N-diethylmetatoluamide and wearing clothes that cover most of the body, particularly at dawn and dusk. It is also useful to carry a spray for flying insects to use in living and sleeping quarters during night hours.

TOXOPLASMOSIS

JACOB K. FRENKEL, M.D., Ph.D.

Toxoplasma infection occurs worldwide in animals and humans. Asymptomatic acute infection is common, and persistent, chronic latent infection usually follows. The disease, toxoplasmosis, may occur during the acute, subacute, or chronic phase of infection, including congenital infection and recrudescence of a chronic latent infection.

THE ORGANISM

Toxoplasma gondii is a tissue protozoan that occurs in three forms. Tachyzoites are actively multiplying in tissues and lead to most cell and tissue destruction during acute infection. Bradyzoites are slowly multiplying or resting forms causing chronic infection. They are present in cysts in many tissues such as brain, muscle, and retina. Usually bradyzoites give rise to few lesions except when cysts rupture in the retina. Cysts maintain the chronic infection in animals and are important sources of infection for cats—the final host and source of all toxoplasmosis. The sporozoites within oocysts are the resistant infectious stage; they are eliminated in the feces by cats that have eaten bradyzoites.

TRANSMISSION

Humans are infected mainly from oocysts or tissue cysts (Fig. 1). Oocysts come from soil contaminated with cat feces. Most cats get infected from meat, birds, or mice. In the United States, transmission occurs mainly during adulthood and is probably related to meat ingestion. Tissue cysts infect people who eat undercooked meat, mainly pork and mutton. Infection, documented by seroconversion, occurs at a rate of 0.5 to 1 percent per year in the United States. In many developing countries, close to 50 percent of children become infected from oocysts. If a pregnant woman contracts infections, her fetus may be infected in utero, and congenital toxoplasmosis may result. This devastating disease entity should be considered preventable.

CLINICAL ILLNESS

The clinical spectrum of toxoplasmosis includes acute acquired, congenital, ocular, and recrudescent toxoplasmosis.

Acute Acquired Toxoplasmosis

Following an incubation period of 1 to 3 weeks, a febrile illness develops in an estimated 10 to 20 percent of primary infections, irrespective of infecting stage. Signs and symptoms may include headache, myalgia, stiff neck, anorexia, maculopapular rash (sparing palms and soles), arthralgia, signs of hepatitis, and, sometimes, hepatomegaly. Lymphadenopathy is common and appears simultaneously with other signs and symptoms, or it may be the first sign, persisting for weeks or months. Atypical lymphocytes are commonly present in the peripheral blood. Signs of myocarditis, hepatitis, pneumonitis, pericarditis, polymyositis, or meningoencephalitis occur occasionally, singly, or in combination. Retinochoroiditis may follow.

Toxoplasmosis in Pregnant Women

Toxoplasmosis acquired during pregnancy is symptomatic in only 10 to 20 percent of pregnant women. However, the fetus is at risk whether or not symptoms are present. Congenital infections are rare but severe when transmitted in the first and second trimesters and more frequent but less severe in the third trimester.

Congenital Toxoplasmosis

Four patterns of congenital toxoplasmosis can be distinguished: 1. The asymptomatic infection is commonest

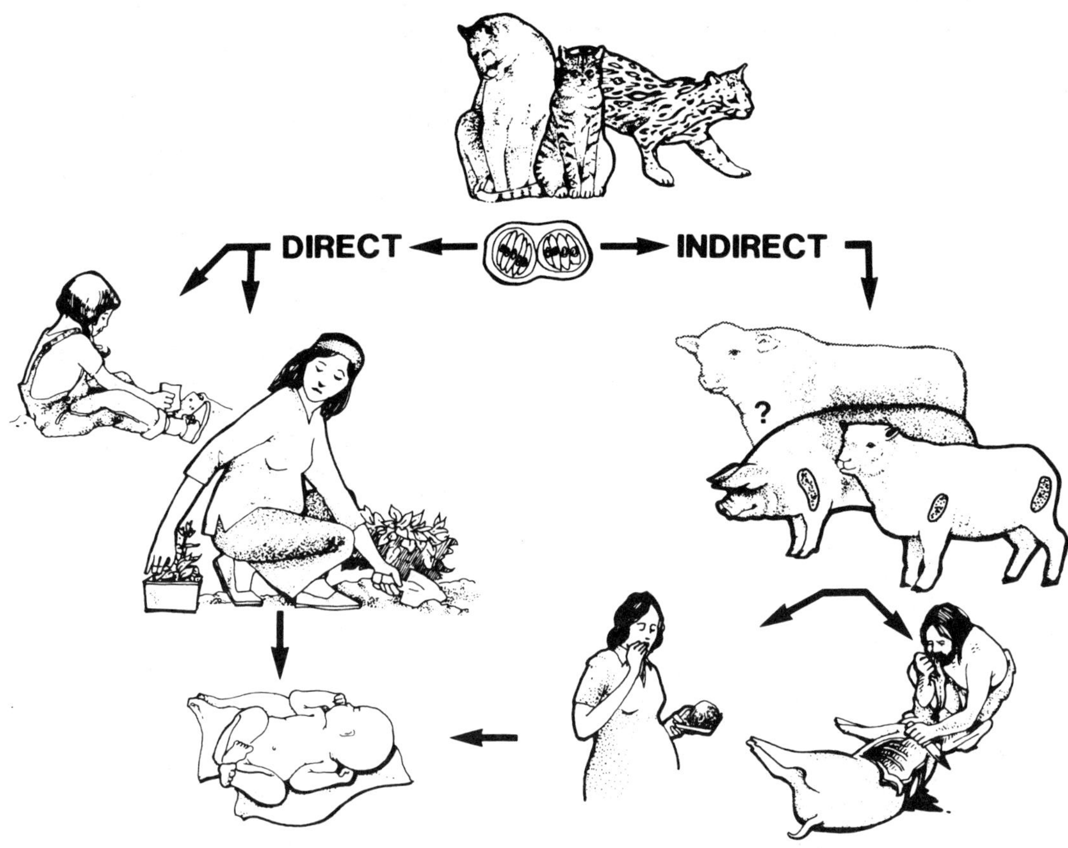

Figure 1 Transmission of *Toxoplasma* to humans.

and usually follows transmission in the third trimester. 2. A mild form, characterized by gestational prematurity, intrauterine growth retardation, abnormal spinal fluid, and failure to thrive. 3. Severe generalized toxoplasmosis, accompanied by one or several of the following: splenomegaly, jaundice, fever, anemia, thrombocytopenia, hepatomegaly, splenomegaly, lymphadenopathy, pneumonia, myocarditis, and a petechial rash. 4. Severe neurologic toxoplasmosis, characterized by convulsions, nystagmus, fever or hypothermia, retinochoroiditis, anemia, intracerebral calcifications, internal hydrocephalus, microencephaly, strabismus, trophic cataracts, glaucoma, optic atrophy, deafness, psychomotor retardation, abnormal spinal fluid findings (including xanthochromia), elevated protein levels (grams percent in the ventricular fluid), and mononuclear pleocytosis.

Transitional forms occur; retinochoroiditis especially may also be present in the third pattern, and it may follow many years after the first and second patterns.

Ocular Toxoplasmosis

Ocular toxoplasmosis is usually an isolated manifestation of chronic latent toxoplasmosis in children or adults. Retinochoroiditis may occur as a single episode or recurrently in the same eye, without generalized symptoms, local pain, or changes in the blood levels of antibody. The acute lesions consist of a focus of retinal necrosis with fuzzy borders accompanied by a cellular exudate in the vitreous that often obscures the lesions and vision in general. The lesion and the vitreous exudate usually start to clear after 2 to 3 weeks. Visual acuity may return to normal if the lesion was distant from the macula. The retinal lesion becomes hyperpigmented. Smoldering lesions with exacerbations have been described. Progressive lesions may result in blindness and glaucoma.

Toxoplasmosis in the Immunocompromised Patient

Two patterns are seen: recrudescent chronic infection and severe primary infection.

Relapsing chronic infection is most commonly manifested as encephalitis; this is characteristically focal and stimulates an abscess or tumor, but can also be multicentric. CT scans may show one or more ring-shaped lesions. Retinochoroiditis, myocarditis, and pneumonia occur less commonly. Most of these patients receive immunosuppressive drugs for a lymphoreticular or other neoplasm or to support an organ transplant; others are immunosuppressed by HTLV-3 that destroys T lymphocytes, resulting in acquired immunodeficiency syndrome.

A severe primary infection may have been acquired

from a transplanted heart or kidney, or it may have been contracted accidentally. Because of the impaired immunity, the primary infection may last longer, and may be more severe.

DIAGNOSIS

Identification of the Organism

Histologic Examination

Biopsy diagnosis may be useful when one or several enlarged lymph nodes are present, preceded or accompanied by fever. Toxoplasmic lymphadenopathy can be differentiated from a lymphoma by the presence of normal architecture, reticular cell hyperplasia, prominent histiocytic infiltration of germinal centers, and by slight periadenitis; however necrosis or Reed-Sternberg cells are absent. Very few Toxoplasma organisms, usually in cysts, may be found in serial sections.

Brain biopsy—used to differentiate a variety of infections, tumors, and vascular phenomena—may demonstrate large numbers of tachyzoites or a few cysts with much necrosis and inflammation. To differentiate between tachzyoites and nuclear debris, an immunoperoxidase stain can be used.

Isolation of Toxoplasma

Inoculation of mice, hamsters, or cell cultures can be attempted with biopsy, placental, or autopsy material in order to enhance the sensitivity and specificity of the histologic examination. In addition, blood, spinal, and ventricular fluids can be used in patients with generalized or neurologic symptoms. Recovery of toxoplasma from blood, placenta, or body fluids generally indicates active infection, whereas isolation from tissues may indicate active or chronic infection. These can generally be differentiated by the histologic picture.

Serologic Diagnosis

Rising antibody titers in the acute infection have been traditionally used to support the diagnosis of clinical toxoplasmosis. However, in immunosuppressed patients, antibody responses cannot be relied upon: it is here that demonstration of the organisms with tissue destruction or demonstration of antigen in the blood is most helpful.

Five types of serologic tests are available for the diagnosis of toxoplasmosis. Usefulness depends on both availability and reliability of the tests. Often kits are used that embody unrealistic assumptions of useful titers and size of test run. Most laboratories will run only occasional specimens and will need more control material than is generally supplied. The laboratory performing the tests must use adequate quality controls.

1. The Sabin-Feldman dye test (DT) is based on antibody-complement-mediated lysis of *Toxoplasma*. Although this is the standard test, it is performed by only a few laboratories in the United States because it requires living *Toxoplasma* and complement from normal human plasma. It measures total antibody.
2. The indirect fluorescent antibody test (IFAT) is the next most useful test, giving results similar to those obtained with the DT. Its drawback is the need for appropriate antisera (separate for humans and mice) and a fluorescent microscope. If antihuman globulin is used, it measures the total antibody. With antihuman IgG, the IgG fraction can be categorized.
3. The indirect hemagglutination test (IHA) is available in kit form and is attractive because of its simplicity. Its drawback is the lack of sensitivity of the antigen usually used, so that it is not dependable for diagnosis of early acute infection nor for congenital toxoplasmosis.
4. The IgM fluorescent antibody test (IgM-IFA), like IFAT, measures, by means of antihuman IgM serum, the binding of IgM antibody in the patient's serum to killed *Toxoplasma* organisms on a slide. This test was designed to distinguish active infection in babies from passively transferred maternal IgG antibody. The large IgM molecule is not transferred past the intact placenta, and in case of a leak, IgM quickly disappears, since it has a half-life of only 3 to 5 days. This test, however, gives false-positive results in the presence of antinuclear antibody and rheumatoid factor and false-negative results when a large quantity of IgG is present in the baby's serum and competes with IgM.
5. IgM capture tests are designed to capture the IgM in the patient's serum and to determine whether this IgM contains antibody to toxoplasma. These capture tests avoid the false-positive and false-negative reactions mentioned above for IgM-IFA. These tests are performed in several laboratories, and at least one kit by Litton has reached the U.S. market. The IgM capture tests give higher titers than the conventional IgM-IFA tests, and the antibody persists longer—perhaps 2 to 3 years.

Strategy of Serologic Diagnosis

When seeking to link an acute illness to *Toxoplasma*, it is important to distinguish preexisting antibody due to a remote infection or passively transferred antibody (acquired by transfusion or in utero, which decays 10-fold every 3 months) from antibody related to the illness. In the United States, DT, IFA, or IHA titers of 1:1,000 suggest acute infection. In areas where such titers are common in a normal population, stable high titers can not be interpreted, but IgM titers correlate with acute or recent infection. The algorithms, Figures 2 to 6, illustrate the sequence of steps and the considerations applied to acute infection (Fig. 2), encephalitis (Fig. 3), retinochoroiditis (Fig. 4), neonatal illness (Fig. 5), suspicion of infection in a pregnant woman (Fig. 6), and the use of IgM antibody titers to analyze the meaning of antibody present in the IgG fraction (Fig. 7).

Serologic diagnosis is generally based on the demonstration of a 4-fold rise in IgG antibody titers between two specimens compared in the same test run. Elevated IgM titers are presumptive evidence of recent infection; conventional IgM-IFA titers persist 6 to 10 months, but with the capture techniques, 2 years or longer.

In immunosuppressed patients, IgG antibody, if present, is interpreted as usual; however, negative titers do not exclude toxoplasmosis. Histologic diagnosis is useful. A test for antigenemia has been developed that appears promising for the rapid diagnosis of acute infection. However, it is not generally available.

Differential Diagnosis

The signs and symptoms of toxoplasmosis are usually so nonspecific that the etiology is not suspected. Most illnesses are mild and they are often not recorded. In a small outbreak in Atlanta, days absent from work or from school were not ascertained, and none of the five students in the New York "hamburger epidemic" became ill enough to be incapacitated. However, patients have been seen with fevers of up to 39.5 °C and malaise lasting for 2 months, sometimes with sore throat and myalgia suggesting infectious mononucleosis or cytomegaloviral infection, which must be excluded. The persistent lymphadenopathy, sometimes with splenomegaly and a

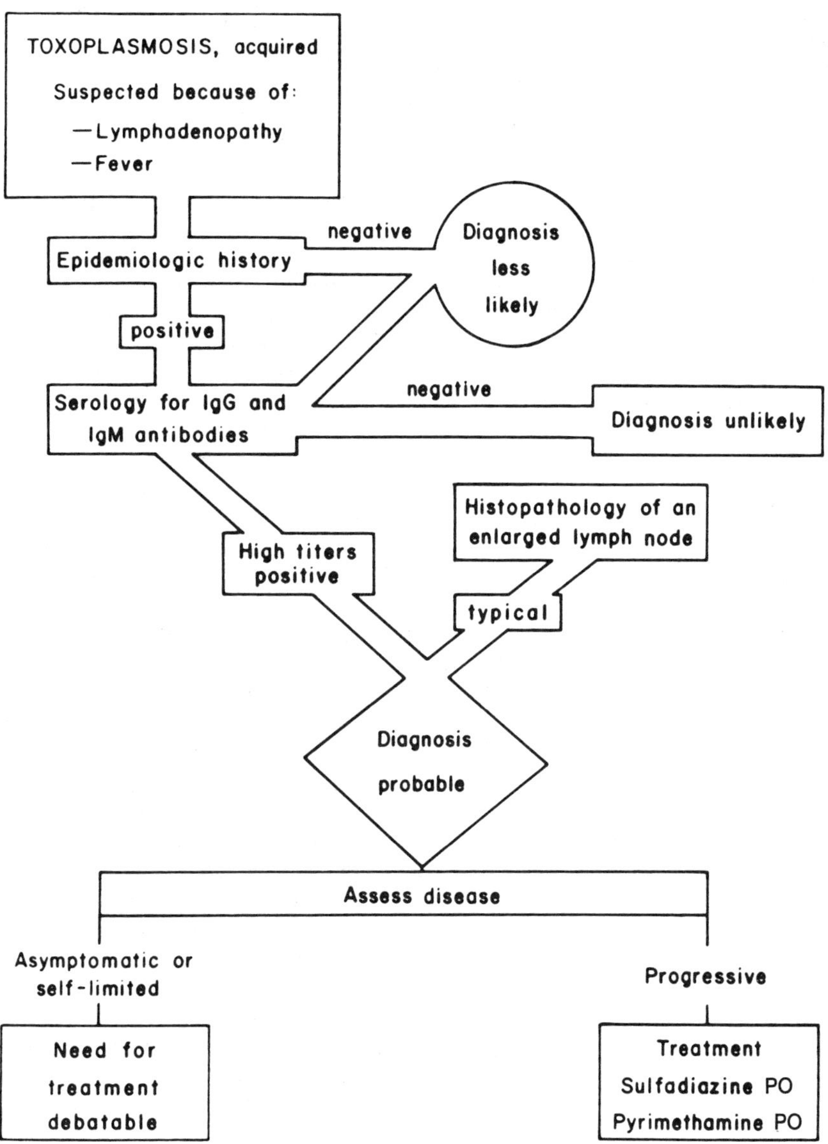

Figure 2 Evaluation of suspected acute toxoplasmosis and lymphadenopathy. (Modified from Mahmond AAF and Warren KS. Toxoplasmosis. J Inf Dis 1977; 135:493)

Coombs' test–negative hemolytic anemia may suggest a lymphoma; lymph node biopsy is diagnositic. The algorithms (Figs. 2 to 6) outline diagnostic steps and considerations to follow with several presenting symptoms.

Isolated anterior segment inflammation in the eye is not likely to be due to toxoplasmosis. The differential diagnosis includes cytomegaloviral infection, syphilis, brucellosis, leptospirosis, tuberculosis, visceral larva migrans, and retinoblastoma; all of these entities should also be considered in the presence of retinochoroiditis.

TREATMENT

Indications for treatment are: diagnosed clinical illness (Figs. 2 and 3), active lesions in the eye (Fig. 4), congenital infection, whether the infant is symptomatic or not (Fig. 5), and signs and symptoms compatible with toxoplasmosis in immunosuppressed patients (Fig. 3). Treatment of a pregnant woman infected during pregnancy is controversial (Fig. 6). The presence of a high antibody titer is not an indication for treatment.

Therapeutic Agents

The most effective treatment for toxoplasmosis employs sulfadiazine together with pyrimethamine (Daraprim, Chloridin, Malocide) because the individual inhibitory effects of each drug become synergistic when used together.

Sulfadiazine (SD, or sulfamerazine, sulfamethazine, sulfapyrazine, sulfalene, sulfadoxine, trisulfapyrimidine) is given in doses of 100 mg per kilogram up to 4 g per day in two to four divided doses. The half-life of sulfadiazine is about 10 to 12 hours. Tablets, liquid oral, and parenteral forms of sulfadiazine are available.

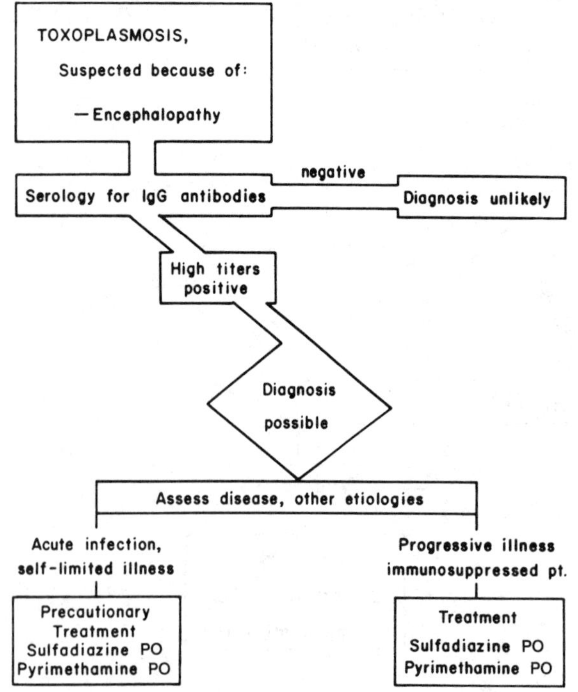

Figure 3 Evaluation of suspected toxoplasmic encephalopathy.

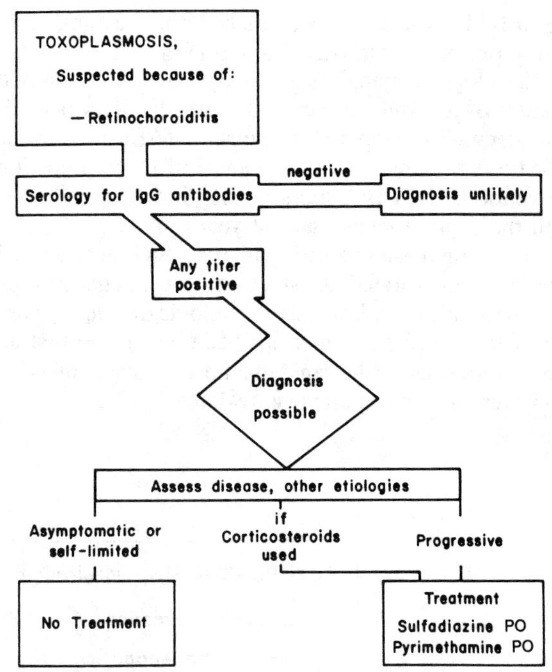

Figure 4 Evaluation of suspected toxoplasmic retinochoroiditis.

Pyrimethamine (PYR) is given in doses of 40 mg per square meter or 1 mg per kilogram for the first 3 days, followed by 15 mg per square meter or 0.3 mg per kilogram daily. The half-life of pyrimethamine is 4 to 5 days. Tablets of 25 mg are the only form available.

Because these drugs are folinic acid antagonists, they may impair platelet and white blood cell production. Counts of platelets and leukocytes should be performed twice weekly. If platelets decline below 100,000 per cubic millimeter, folinic acid (calcium leucovorin), 3 to 10 mg daily, is given either orally or subcutaneously; it is available as 5 and 25 mg tablets and in 3 and 5 mg ampules and 50 mg vials. When folinic acid is not available, 5 to 10 g of fresh yeast (such as Fleischman's, Red Star) daily can be substituted (100 mg for children). It is mixed with food or tomato juice to disguise the taste. These antagonists do not impair the chemotherapeutic effect of the drugs. When platelet counts are not feasible, 5 g of yeast should be given daily.

Toxicity effects of sulfonamides include rashes, the Stevens-Johnson syndrome, crystalluria, hematuria, vasculitis, and hemolytic anemia with deficiency of glucose-6-phosphate dehydrogenase.

Duration of treatment depends on subsidence of signs and symptoms, and immunity can be assumed to have been acquired. If the patient appears to be immunologically competent, treatment for approximately twice the time necessary for disappearance of signs and symptoms is suggested. In an immunosuppressed patient, a period of treatment may need to be followed by

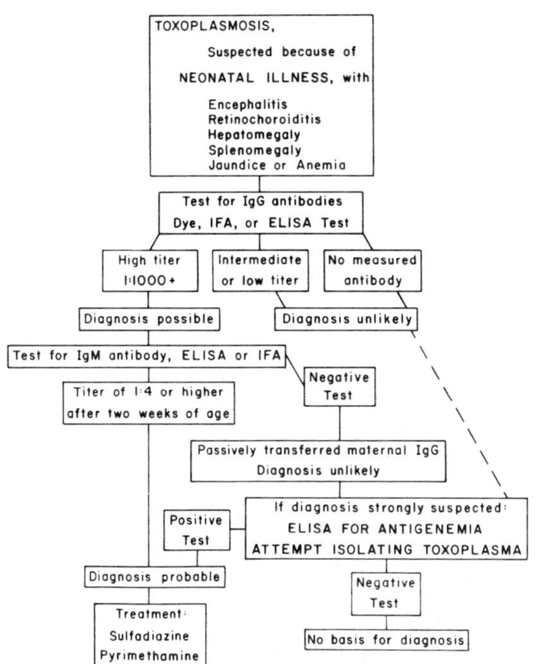

Figure 5 Evaluation of suspected neonatal toxoplasmosis.

chemoprophylaxis until a reasonable immunocompetence appears to have been achieved. Long-term chemoprophylaxis can be conducted with SD alone, 4 to 6 g daily in divided doses.

Other Antitoxoplasmic Agents

Effectiveness has only been shown for the first drug of the sulfamethoxazole-trimethoprim combination. Although synergism was shown in vitro, this combination was less effective than SD-PYR. Clindamycin is effective against *Toxoplasma*. However, it does not penetrate well into the central nervous system, and with its potential enteric side effects, it should be used only under circumstances where SD-PYR toxicity appears unmanageable. Fetal blood levels were about 50 percent of maternal blood levels. Spiramycin, chemically related to erythromycin, is not generally available in the United States; however, it can be obtained from the U.S. Food and Drug Administration (telephone 301-443-4310). It has been used in Europe to treat pregnant women and babies. Although it reaches sufficient concentrations in the placenta, its passage into the fetus appears insufficient for therapeutic effects.

Anti-Inflammatory Treatments with Corticosteroids

The anti-inflammatory effects are useful to moderate manifestation of delayed type hypersensitivity with focal retinochoroiditis in or adjacent to the macula or the optic nerve. Because anti-inflammatory doses are also immunosuppressive, corticosteroids should be used together with the sulfadiazine-pyrimethamine combination. Prednisone, 50 to 100 mg per day (1 to 1.5 mg per kilogram or 10 to 20 replacement doses) are given orally in two divided doses daily until the acute inflammation begins to subside, which usually takes 5 to 10 days, and it is then tapered to zero while the SD-PYR is continued. The corticosteroids should not be injected periocularly.

Therapy of Specific Clinical Illness

Generalized Acute Toxoplasmosis

Diagnosis and treatment is outlined in Figure 2. Defervescence and improvement of signs, symptoms, and abnormal laboratory tests usually occur promptly, and treatment for an additional week appears sufficient. If manifestations recur, treatment can be resumed.

Immunosuppressed Patients

Diagnosis and treatment are as outlined in Figure 3. Because multiple infections may be present, therapeutic response should be measured by regression of toxoplasmic lesions; e.g., in the brain. Sulfadiazine-pyrimethamine treatments should extend approximately a month beyond clinical improvement. Because treatment does not usually eradicate the infection and immunity may not be sufficient to contain it, sulfadiazine prophylaxis should be continued indefinitely until the immune status has improved, as after remission of the underlying neoplasm or stabilization of the graft. The sulfadiazine or combined treatment with pyrimethamine would be also effective prophylaxis against pneumocystosis.

The sulfadoxine-pyrimethamine combination (Fansidar) should be more effective against both toxoplasmosis and pneumocystis infections than sulfamethoxazole-trimethoprim.

Toxoplasmosis in the Pregnant Woman

Diagnostic and management considerations are outlined in Figure 6. If an infection was presumably acquired in first trimester, the chances of severe lesions of the fetus are great, and therapeutic abortion should be considered. The possibility of a severely damaged baby will often extend this consideration into the second trimester. Because pyrimethamine can be teratogenic, it should not be given in the first or second trimester. However, treatment with SD alone, which passes into the fetus, is a reasonable alternative in the second trimester. In the third trimester, when the risk of lesions is less, the possibility of toxic effects of SD-PYR can be controlled with folinic acid and yeast. Once diagnosed, treatment should extend throughout pregnancy until the status of the baby can be evaluated after birth. No controlled studies have been published concerning this treatment.

Clindamycin passes the placenta and fetal blood levels are about half the maternal levels. It could reasonably

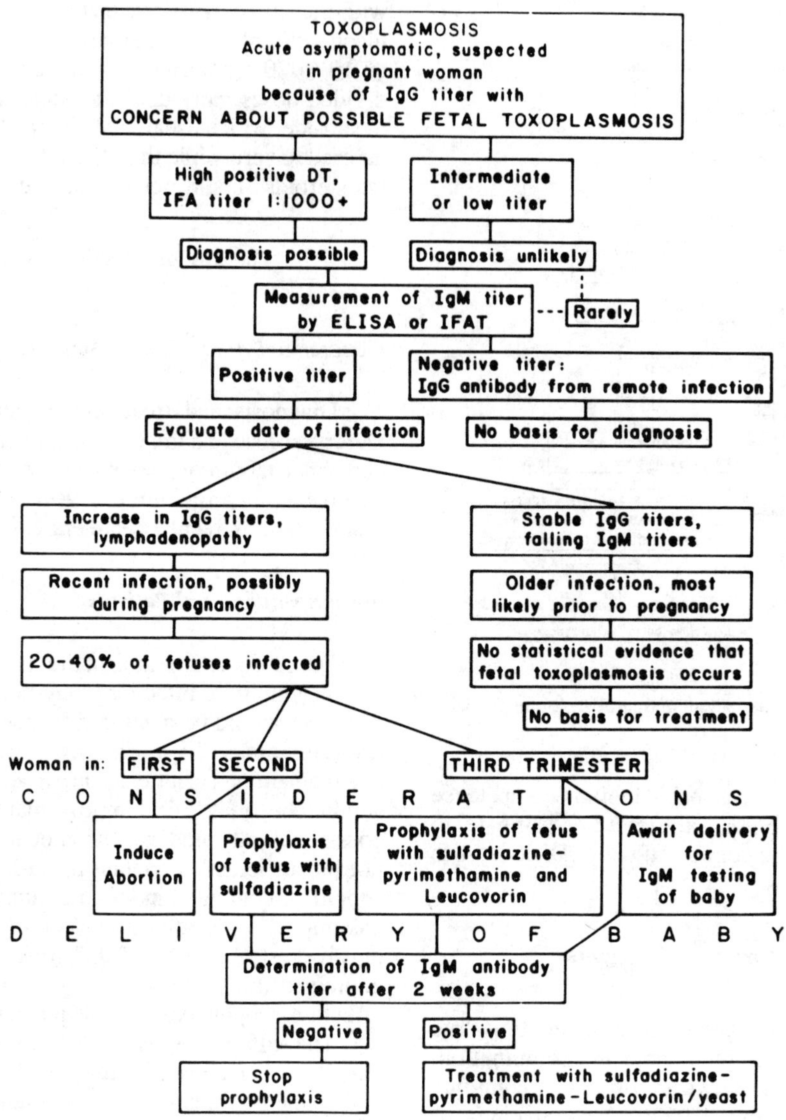

Figure 6 Evaluation of suspected toxoplasmosis in a pregnant woman.

be used if SD–PYR are not tolerated, keeping in mind its poor penetration into brain end eye and its side effects.

Spiramycin, by concentrating in the placenta, can be expected to diminish the chance of fetal infection; however, it is not effective once infection has passed into the fetus.

Congenital Toxoplasmosis

Figure 5 outlines the diagnostic considerations. Diagnosis depends on finding *Toxoplasma* antibody in the IgM fraction, which, because of its size, is not passively acquired. Because antibody in the IgG fraction is quantitatively transferred from mother to fetus it does not aid in the diagnosis or exclusion of fetal infection. IgM antibody can be measured at birth. However, occasionally a placental leak and mixing of maternal and fetal blood occurs, in which case maternal IgM decays, with a half-life of 4 to 5 days; hence the need to check a positive finding after 2 weeks. The conventional IgM antibody tests may be negative because of competition with IgG for the antigen sites; therefore, a test based on the IgM capture technique is preferred.

Treatment for congenital toxoplasmosis should be started, at least with SD alone, when suspicion is strong, if serologic testing takes more than 24 hours. Once the diagnosis is confirmed, treatment with SD–PYR should be initiated and extended for at least 4 to 8 weeks beyond resolution of manifestation of illness. This diminishes the number of organisms and provides time for the immune potential of the newborn baby to mature. After 3 to 6 months, treatment can be given intermittently for 1 month followed by no treatment for another month, or prophylaxis can be maintained with SD alone. Duration of treatment is controversial. Some treat arbitrarily for

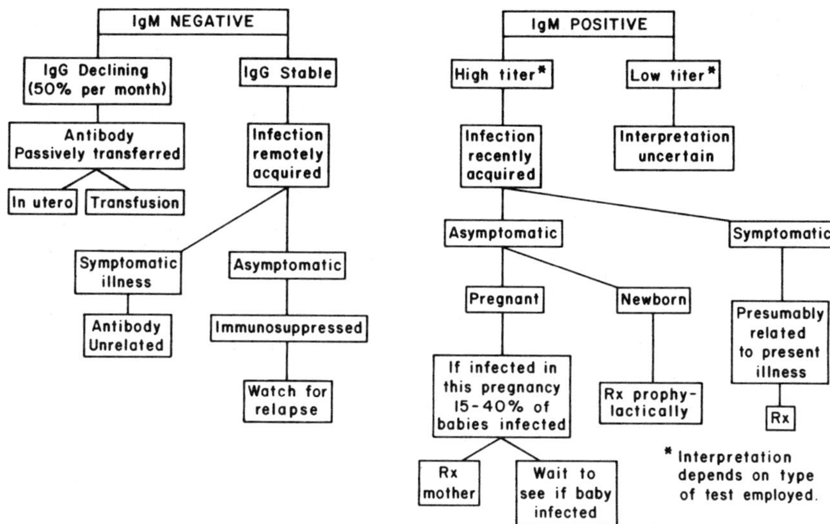

Figure 7 Analyzing IgG antibody to *Toxoplasma* with the IgM technique.

1 year. However, the decisive criterion is the ability to mount a sufficient cellular immunity to contain the chronic infection, and this may be reached earlier. The objective is to prevent all possible cell destruction of nonregenerating brain and retinal tissues while avoiding unnecessary and costly treatment. Treatment with SD–PYR—alternating with SD only or nontreatment—for periods of 1 month appears preferable to monthly treatments with SD–PYR alternating with spiramycin, as is practiced sometimes in Europe.

Ocular Toxoplasmosis

Diagnostic and treatment considerations are outlined in Figure 4. The mere presence of *Toxoplasma* antibody in the IgG fraction indicates that *Toxoplasma* may be the etiology of a retinal lesion. Until CMV, herpes, and other causes of retinitis can be diagnosed and treated, it does not seem imperative to confirm a specific diagnosis. (This could be accomplished by simultaneous measurement of antibody in the aqueous of the anterior chamber and the serum and comparing the antibody ratios for each of the several agents.) Treatment with SD–PYR should be started as soon as possible in patients with periodic relapses without waiting for an appointment with the physician because of the risk of irreparable retinal damage. Oral anti-inflammatory corticosteroid treatment may be added for lesions involving or adjacent to the macula or optic nerve, but they should not be given without drugs that inhibit *Toxoplasma*. The anti-inflammatory corticosteroids should be tapered as soon as the vitreous inflammation begins to subside and should be stopped while the SD–PYR medication is continued for a total of approximately 4 to 8 weeks.

Clindamycin has been used orally or by periocular injection for retinochoroiditis refractory to SD–PYR. If this treatment is successful, it would suggest another etiology rather than drug-resistant *Toxoplasma*. No control studies employing either regimen have been published.

PREVENTION

Toxoplasma oocysts remain viable in moist and shaded soil for a year or longer. Oocysts are ingested by geophagia, whether compulsive (pica) or inadvertent. Hands should be washed after contact with soil potentially contaminated with cat feces. Oocysts are destroyed by exposure to heat over 60 °C, but chemical disinfectants are not effective.

Tissue cysts that have persisted for months or years in the animal remain viable in pork, mutton, and other meats for days at room or refrigerator temperatures. Most of the organisms are destroyed when meat is frozen and thawed, but they are destroyed more effectively by heating to 60 °C, as indicated by a change in color of the meat. Hands should be washed after contact with raw meat. Soap and water, alcohol, and chemical disinfectants inactivate bradyzoites from tissues cysts on the skin. Prevention of toxoplasma infection is most important during pregancy and early childhood, and in immunosuppressed patients, when the consequences of infection tend to be more serious. The admonition to wash hands after contact with cats, soil, and raw meat, and before eating or touching the face and to cook meat thoroughly should be incorporated into the general instructions for pregnant women. Work gloves should be used when handling soil potentially contaminated by cat feces. Because infection of older children, especially young girls, is of value for immunization and the risk of appreciable illness is small, prevention becomes less important in this group. The possibility of a vaccine to protect women during pregnancy is under investigation.

Because toxoplasma cysts are often present in the heart, transplant recipients should be serologically screened and, if negative, the donor should also be screened. If a donor is positive and the recipient negative, toxoplasma infection should be expected and managed by treatment. Once a vaccine is available, negative recipients could be immunized 2 to 4 weeks prior to transplantation.

CATHETER-ASSOCIATED URINARY TRACT INFECTION

JOHN W. WARREN, M.D.

Much of the clinical and research attention directed at catheter-associated bacteriuria has been directed toward the catheter as a means of entry for organisms into the urinary tract. The catheter may, however, play other roles in the development and maintenance of bacteriuria. The catheter and the intravesical balloon may, through mechanical and/or chemical factors, cause erosion and inflammation of the urethral and bladder mucosa. Additionally, the presence of the catheter may cause bacterial adherence properties of uroepithelial cells to change. Once bacteriuria has developed, the catheter acts as a foreign body at the site of infection, thus diminishing the clearance of the infecting organisms. The lumen of the catheter, via the accumulation of adherent organisms and of encrustations formed of other urinary constituents, may become a microenvironment for these organisms, thus allowing them a continuous access to the urinary tract itself. Furthermore, these encrustations may cause a partial or complete obstruction of urine flow, converting an asymptomatic bacteriuria into a symptomatic one and, perhaps, into bacteremia. Finally, the catheter may obstruct periurethral structures with complications of prostatic and epididymal infections.

Although there are many indications for placement of a tube into the urinary bladder to drain urine, the four main indications are (*1*) hemodynamic monitoring of acutely ill patients; (*2*) pelvic or abdominal surgery; (*3*) bladder outlet obstruction; and (*4*) urinary incontinence.

The first two, output measurement and pelvic or abdominal surgery, almost always involve short-term use. The third, bladder outlet obstruction, usually requires transient use if the obstruction can be corrected. The fourth, the management of incontinence, may also be a temporary indication, e.g., for the patient undergoing anesthesia. These temporary indications appear to be commonest for patients in acute care hospitals where the mean and median duration of catheterization is 2 to 4 days. About 10 percent of patients are catheterized during their hospital stay and 10 to 20 percent of catheterized patients become bacteriuric. Although only 1 to 2 percent of these bacteriuric catheterized patients develop bacteremia, the large number of catheterized patients means that the instrumented urinary tract is the most frequent source of gram-negative rod bacteremia in hospitalized patients.

Because the risk of bacteriuria is 5 to 10 percent per day once a urethral catheter is in place, the majority of patients with a catheter in place for 30 days or more are bacteriuric, usually with several organisms. Although difficult to document through published accounts, the main indications for long-term urinary catheterization (30 days or more) are (*1*) bladder outlet obstruction that cannot be corrected by surgery and (*2*) incontinence of urine. The latter is probably the commoner indication. These patients, in whom catheters may be in place for months and years, generally reside in chronic care facilities such as nursing homes.

Evidence is developing that a subtle but important distinction should be made between management techniques for short-term and long-term catheters. The goal of medical management of the patient with a short-term catheter is to postpone the development of bacteriuria. The long-term catheterized patient is almost always bacteriuric, and the goal of medical care might be best termed the prevention of complications of bacteriuria.

DIAGNOSIS OF INFECTION

Many studies of catheter-associated urinary tract infections have required a minimum of 100,000 colony forming units (CFU) per milliliter of urine aspirated from the distal catheter to establish a diagnosis. However, some investigators have arbitrarily selected lower concentrations. Recent studies have suggested that the majority of organisms initially present in catheter urine in concentrations of even 100 CFU per milliliter or less will, over succeeding days, reach concentrations of at least 100,000 CFU per milliliter. This suggests, at least for patients catheterized for only several days, that organisms present even in small numbers in catheter urine represent actual residence in the urine and not contamination. This understanding may or may not have impact upon therapeutic decisions, but is of epidemiologic assistance in dating the incidence of bacteriuric episodes.

But does the presence of an organism in urine aspirated from the distal catheter mean that the organism is present in the bladder as well? Recent studies have found that the majority of bacterial species isolated from catheter urine were also isolated from bladder urine, obtained either by suprapubic aspiration or by removal of the old catheter and insertion of a new one. However, in some patients, a bacterial species was found in catheter urine but not in bladder urine, and in other patients, catheter urine contained the same species of bacteria, but at higher concentrations, than bladder urine. These findings suggest that the most accurate practical means of assessing the presence of bacteria in bladder urine of a catheterized patient is to culture urine draining from a newly replaced catheter. Otherwise, an assessment of isolates obtained from urine aspirated through an indwelling catheter, particularly one in place for a long period, should be viewed only as an approximation of the microbiologic status of bladder urine.

SHORT-TERM CATHETERIZATION

Prevention

Because of the frequency of catheter use and of associated bacteriuria, many efforts have been directed towards prevention or, more accurately, posponement of bacteriuria. By far the most important modification of the venerable catheter has been the closed system, one in which the catheter and collecting tube empty into a receptacle in such a way that urine is always contained within a lumen and protected from the possibly contaminated environment. Although no well-designed controlled trial comparing open with closed catheter systems has been reported, the closed system appears to be associated with a much lower incidence of bacteriuria and has become the standard of care.

Nevertheless, bacteriuria remains the most frequent complication of the use of even closed-system urethral catheters. The risk of bacteriuria is directly associated with female gender, age, duration of catheterization, and presence of periurethral colonization with gram-negative bacteria or enterococci. There are three possible routes of entry for bacteria into the catheter lumen and/or bladder. One route is that by which the catheter acts as a foreign body traversing the urethra from its external orifice to the interior of the bladder. Organisms in the periurethral area may move along the mucous sheath between the catheter's exterior surface and the urethral mucosa and enter the bladder directly. If a closed catheter system is used and maintained well, this route may be the commonest. Other means of bacterial entry involve breaking the integrity of the closed catheter system, either at the disconnectable junction between the catheter and the collection tube or by contamination of the collection bag.

Understanding these origins of catheter-associated bacteriuria has led to several modifications of the closed catheter system in an attempt to prevent or postpone bacteriuria. Only two types of modification appear to be useful. The first is simply a strict adherence to maintaining a closed catheter system, for instance, by the use of a catheter-collection tube junction, which is difficult or impossible to disconnect. The other practice resulting in a lower incidence of bacteriuria has been the use of systemic antibiotics. However, antimicrobial use is associated only with postponement, and the eventual bacteriuria is commonly caused by organisms resistant to the antibiotic used.

Most of the modifications that have been attempted, but that have not reliably reduced the incidence of bacteriuria, include localized use of antiseptics or antimicrobial agents. These ineffective uses of antibacterial substances have included applications to the periurethral area, lubrication for the catheter, impregnation or coating of the catheter, irrigation continuously or periodically of the catheter, and instillation into the collection bag.

Undoubtedly the most effective means of preventing catheter-associated bacteriuria is by preventing the use of the catheter itself. Careful assessment of the patient's needs may reveal that the catheter may not be necessary at all or, if deemed so, for only a short duration. Furthermore, alternatives to indwelling urethral catheters that are dictated by the indications for catheterization are available. For patients with bladder outlet obstruction, intermittent catheterization is a possible alternative. For patients in whom urinary retention is not a problem, condom catheters in males and incontinence clothing in females and males may be used. Suprapubic catheters have been used in gynecologic, urologic, and other types of pelvic or abdominal surgery. None of these alternatives have been well studied in prospective, randomized, controlled trials.

Treatment

Once a urethral catheter is in place, the techniques noted above are only means by which catheter-associated bacteriuria can be postponed. Consequently, given the 5 to 10 percent daily incidence of bacteriuria, some patients catheterized for even short periods will become bacteriuric. I have rarely been compelled to treat patients as long as they remain catheterized and asymptomatic. However, because a recent study has reported excess mortality related to catheter-associated bacteriuria which could not be explained by other confounding factors this posture may have to be modified as further data are developed. Until that time, I suggest that patients with catheter-associated bacteriuria, while asymptomatic and still catheterized, not be treated with antibiotics. However, if the patient becomes symptomatic with fever and/or signs of bacteremia, I would treat as outlined in the chapter on bacteremia, even while the patient has a catheter still in place. Similarly, for the occasional patient with lower abdominal pain or other symptoms suggestive of symptomatic lower urinary tract infection, I recommend treatment with an oral antibiotic active in vitro against the bacteriuric organisms and in doses as outlined in the chapter on urinary tract infections.

I would not, however, treat the asymptomatic catheterized bacteriuric patient. If one would not treat such an infection even if identified, then why identify it? In other words, why culture the urine of patients with indwelling catheters if no action is to be taken on the basis of the results? Although this is a reasonable course for many patients, I believe a urine culture should be performed in several instances. The first is the case of the patient who is to undergo urologic surgery. Because such surgery is associated with a risk of bacteremia with the urinary tract as the source, I believe that most bacteriuric patients should be treated for the bacteriuria before and during the procedure. Second, I recommend once or twice a week surveillance urine cultures of catheterized patients in intensive care units. This will allow the early identification and possible control of an antibiotic-resistant organism that could be transmitted to other patients. Third, I recommend the culture of catheter urine of all patients immediately prior to removal of the catheter. If this culture has organisms in any concentration, I recommend a follow-up urine culture of the now noncatheterized patient within the next week. Although some patients will clear their bacteriuria once the catheter is removed, others will not. I recommend treatment of the latter group if follow-up cultures reveal bacteriuria.

LONG-TERM CATHETERIZATION

The indications for long-term catheterization (30 days or more) are usually either chronic urinary incontinence or urinary retention that is not correctable by surgery. Patients with these problems commonly reside in nursing homes or other chronic care facilities, and relatively little attention has been directed towards this type of associated bacteriuria. Because most long-term catheters in use are closed drainage systems like those used in acute care hospitals, the assumption has been made that many aspects of epidemiology, transmission, and pathogenesis of catheter-associated urinary tract infections are similar to those in the patient with the better-studied short-term catheter. However, two differences are quite clear. The first is that the types of organisms causing bacteriuria in long-term catheterized patients include unfamiliar uropathogens such as *Providencia stuartii, Providencia rettgeri, Morganella morganii*, as well as the better known *Escherichia coli, Proteus mirabilis, Pseudomonas aeruginosa*, and enterococcus. The second is that complications in addition to fever, acute pyelonephritis, and bacteremia occur. These include local periurinary infections such as urethritis, periurethral abscess, epididymitis, prostatitis, prostatic abscess, perivesical abscess, and perinephric abscess as well as complications of a more chronic nature such as urinary tract stones, vesicoureteral reflux, chronic tubulointerstitial nephritis, and renal failure. Much of this information is derived from studies of patients with spinal injuries. Whether one can extrapolate to the less well-studied but larger population of aged long-term catheterized patients is unclear.

Because preventive techniques only postpone but do not actually prevent bacteriuria, virtually all patients catheterized for long periods of time are bacteriuric. Indeed, most such patients have a polymicrobial bacteriuria with a variety of aerobic gram-negative rods and gram-positive cocci. Consequently, in addition to establishing and maintaining appropriate catheter hygiene in the care of these patients, the medical community should devote attention towards preventing the complications of the omnipresent and usually polymicrobial bacteriuria.

However, guidelines for the management of catheterized patients with bacteriuria have not been well developed. Antibiotics active in vitro against the organism(s) present can be expected to eradicate three-fourths of these organisms. However, reinfection commonly occurs, often with organisms resistant to the antibiotics used.

Methenamine preparations have been widely used in chronically catheterized patients, but are ineffective. This conclusion is based not only upon clinical studies but also upon the understanding that methenamine must be hydrolyzed to formaldehyde in order to be effective. At least 60 minutes of exposure to an acidic urine is necessary for the accumulation of a formaldehyde concentration high enough to inhibit bacterial growth. Urine constantly draining through an unobstructed catheter does not accumulate in the bladder for a sufficiently long period to allow an adequate concentration of formaldehyde to form. Nevertheless, several studies have indicated that although bacteriuria per se was not affected, catheterized patients receiving methenamine tended to have lower incidences of symptomatic urinary tract infections, perhaps associated with lower incidences of catheter obstructions. This intriguing finding may not be due to antimicrobial activity of methanamine, but, rather, to a biochemical alteration of salt solubility in the urine.

Another practice that may prevent catheter obstruction and the subsequent development of symptomatic urinary tract infection is periodic irrigation of the catheter. However, because such irrigation jeopardizes the closed nature of the present catheter systems, this procedure should not be practiced until appropriate trials are performed.

Perhaps even more for patients with indications for long-term urine drainage assistance, alternatives to urethral catheters should be sought. The incontinent patient can be managed with condom catheters or diapers. The probable advantage in the lower incidence of bacteriuria and its complication must be balanced against greater nursing effort and potential for skin breakdown. For the patient with urinary retention, suprapubic or intermittent methods of catheterization are available. These alternatives to long-term catheterization require appropriate controlled trials to evaluate acute and chronic complications, mortality, patient comfort, nursing acceptance, and medical cost.

HEMATOLOGIC DISEASES

APLASTIC ANEMIA AND ALLIED DISORDERS

EDWARD C. GORDON-SMITH, M.D., M.Sc., F.R.C.P.

In this chapter the treatment of a variety of disorders, loosely grouped under the heading of "aplastic anemia", is considered. The term "aplastic anemia" is used to mean idiosyncratic, acquired aplastic anemia which may follow exposure to certain drugs, chemicals, or viruses. Hereditary aplastic anemias include two well characterized disorders, Fanconi's anemia and dyskeratosis congenita, as well as some poorly characterized anomalies. Pure red cell aplasia may be acquired or congenital and refers to the erythroblastopenic anemias. The term "congenital hypoplastic anemia", usually used to describe the congenital form of this disorder (Diamond-Blackfan syndrome), is misleading, since the pathogenesis and natural history of the pure red cell aplasia is quite distinct from other types of true aplastic anemia.

ACQUIRED APLASTIC ANEMIA

Acquired aplastic anemia is a relatively rare disorder with an incidence of approximately 13 per million per annum in Europe and North America, though it may be higher in the Far East and in other countries where drugs such as chloramphenicol are widely used. Because it is so rare, treatment is difficult since management requires considerable patience and enthusiasm on the part of both the physician and the patient; the former may have little experience with it, and the latter has never heard of it. The first step in treatment is a careful explanation of the disease, its prolonged course, and its dangers. The usual first reaction of patients and relatives on hearing the diagnosis is relief that the disease is not acute leukemia, but the prognosis for aplastic anemia is certainly worse than for acute lymphoblastic leukemia, and probably worse than for acute myeloid leukemia. On the other hand, aplastic anemia is a deficiency disorder, brought about solely by the failure of hemopoietic stem-cell proliferation, so that the proliferative problems of the leukemias do not occur. Systemic symptoms directly caused by the disease are absent, and although the patient is pancytopenic with a hypoplastic marrow, he may feel completely well and thus not appreciate the dangers of the disease.

Treatment of the patient with aplastic anemia is considered in two distinct parts. The first part concerns replacement therapy or support in the form of blood product transfusion and prevention or treatment of infection; the second concerns ways in which recovery of bone marrow function is accelerated.

Spontaneous remission of aplastic anemia occurs in perhaps as many as 20 percent of patients, and it is not known whether all patients have the capacity to recover if they are kept alive long enough, or whether in some cases the damage to the marrow is irreversible. In any case, it is important to support the patient by careful attention to detail and by anticipating and preventing major problems.

Severe Aplastic Anemia

It is possible to differentiate a group of aplastic anemia patients with a particularly bad prognosis. Many attempts have been made to define the poor prognosis group precisely, but a simple definition seems to be most useful and workable. Severe aplastic anemia defines those patients with pancytopenia with less than

400/mm^3 neutrophils, less than 20,000/mm^3 platelets, less than 0.2 percent reticuloyctes, and a marrow with more than 80 percent of remaining cells nonmyeloid (or at least 3 of the 4 above). These patients have about a 1 in 10 chance of being alive at one year, even with major support. Experience would suggest that the most significant cell line is the granulocytic, and that patients who have even a few neutrophils > 200/mm^3 fare much better than those with none < 100/mm^3. This probably reflects the impossibility of providing granulocyte replacement, but also emphasizes the importance of infection as the main cause of death.

Support Therapy for Aplastic Anemia

It is essential to achieve a stable healthy state before commencing the chosen method of definitive treatment to induce remission of aplastic anemia. The various means to achieve this are considered separately, but in practice, all measures are instituted simultaneously.

Red Cell Transfusion

Most patients at presentation are anemic and require red cell transfusions. In the past, the hemoglobin of patients with aplastic anemia was kept low, < 7 g/dl, in order to provide a large drive for hemopoiesis, but with no clinical evidence to prove this theory, patients are now transfused according to their clinical needs. Red cell transfusions do have special dangers however. Hemorrhage, including fatal cerebral hemorrhage, is more frequent during or just after red cell transfusions than during nontransfused periods in the thrombocytopenic patient. This is related to a fall in platelet count during transfusion of red cells that may be simply a dilutional effect or may be caused by minor degrees of immune complex formation. Whatever the cause it is important to give platelet transfusions at the same time as, or immediately after, red cell transfusions, especially if the platelet count is < 20,000/m^3 before starting.

Problems with iron overload are rare in aplastic anemia. If the patient runs into problems, it is usually after some years of tranfusion therapy and indicates a relatively good prognosis. Chelation therapy need not be started during the first year of treatment.

Transfusion reactions occur with the same frequency in aplastic anemia patients as in other chronically transfused patients, and it may be necessary to use white-cell-poor blood. There are two special features of aplastic anemia which may indicate its use. The first is the emergence of clones of red cells with the characteristics of paroxysmal nocturnal hemoglobinuria (PNH). About 15 percent of patients with aplasia who survive more than three months develop PNH clones at some time. White-cell-poor blood may be necessary to avoid hemolysis in these patients. The second indication for the use of white-cell-poor blood from the beginning is the development of antiplatelet antibodies. There is some indication that these antibodies may be avoided or delayed by giving white-cell-depleted blood products.

Platelet Transfusion

There is no consensus on how platelet transfusions should be used in aplastic anemia. The nature of the disease means that the patient will require such transfusions for a prolonged period of time (unless ''cured'' by bone marrow transplantation or immunosuppression). Antiplatelet antibodies, either anti-HLA or specifically antiplatelet, will develop in the majority (about 60%) of patients after a variable period of time, and support will become difficult. It would be ideal to give only HLA-matched, white-cell-free platelets when clinically indicated, but the availability of such platelets is limited. Furthermore, clinical indications for platelet transfusion are vague. Warning signs include the development of buccal and/or retinal hemorrhages, sudden spread of petechial hemorrhages, and the need for red cell transfusions. Infected patients are much more likely to bleed than uninfected patients. Unfortunately, fatal cerebal hemorrhage may occur without any of these prodromes.

At the opposite end of the therapeutic spectrum is the use of random donor platelets on a prophylactic basis with the introduction of HLA-compatible platelets when required. Several points indicate that this approach may be acceptable. A substantial minority of patients does not develop significant resistance to platelet transfusions. Even if some resistance does develop and platelet increments become poor, bleeding may be arrested by platelet transfusions. I use platelet transfusions routinely with red cell transfusions, give prophylatic transfusion two or three times weekly to out-patients whose platelet count is <20,000/mm^3, and modify this only when the patient is hospitalized and can be very closely observed. Death from cerebral hemorrhage has become rare, except in patients with uncontrollable sepsis.

Granulocyte Transfusions

Prophylactic granulocyte transfusions are not used in the treatment of aplastic anemia. Therapeutic transfusions are given in desperate situations, and certainly with localized infections they may have some beneficial effects. In general, if granuloycte transfusions are required in the support of patients with aplastic anemia, infections are out of control, and intensive granulocyte support for at least four days is required to achieve remission of infection.

Prevention of Infection

Patients with aplastic anemia present a special problem in the prevention of infection. Unlike leukemia, neutropenia is likely to be prolonged for months or even years. If the neutrophil count is very low (< 100/mm^3) it is doubtful that it is ever possible to eradicate an infection. Fungal infections are particularly intransigent. Sources of infection may be endogenous, from the gastrointestinal tract, skin, or upper respiratory passages, or may be exogenous. The exogenous infections are mainly Pseudomonas, Klebsiella or Aspergillus, but each hospital will have its own special problems.

Isolation

Patients with severe aplastic anemia should always be managed in isolation. Minimal requirements include an adequate isolation room and strict attention to details of reverse barrier nursing. Very strict regimes for hand-washing by all staff who enter the room, particularly if they are likely to touch intravenous lines, is essential. It is preferable to have some form of filtered air (laminar air flow is the most effective) to exclude Aspergillus and other fungal pathogens.

Decontamination

Both the patient and the environment should be rid of potential pathogens from the outset. Unfortunately, there is no way to achieve complete bacterial sterilization of the patient short of autoclaving, so a compromise has to be made. Potential pathogens of the gastrointestinal tract are mainly aerobic bacteria and *Candida*. Fatal anaerobic infections are rare. Nonabsorbable antibiotics are given from the outset. A suitable regime consists of nystatin suspension, 500,000 U *q6h*, amphotericin tablets 100 mg *q6h* amphotericin lozenges as much as tolerated, chlorhexidine mouth wash after food, framycetin 500 mg *q6h*, colistin 1.5×10^6 U *q6h* (doses for adults). Food should be freshly cooked and of low bacterial content (sterilized food is difficult to obtain and is unpalatable). The major problem with this regime is patient compliance, and considerable tact and sympathy from nursing staff and relatives are necessary to obtain a satisfactory result. A similar result is achieved by using cotrimoxazole (Bactrim) instead of framycetin and colistin, but cotrimoxazole has a significant marrow suppressive effect and at least initially the nonabsorbable antibiotics are preferred. Cotrimoxazole does prevent *Pneumocystis carinii* infections, and if this is a particular local problem, cyotrimoxazole should be used. Chlorhexidine skin lotion, chlorhexidine baths and antibacterial creams are used for skin and orifice decontamination. Particular care must be taken during insertion of intravenous lines and major procedures (such as the insertion of Hickman catheters) should be accompanied by intravenous vancomycin (500 mg given slowly over 30 mins *q6h* for 24 hours) to prevent *Staphylococcus epidermidis* infection.

Such measures are readily introduced when the patient is hospitalized. The chronic nature of the disease and the psychologic stresses on the patient mean that considerable treatment has to be continued on an out-patient basis. If patient compliance is good, the oral regimes are continued and the patient is advised to keep to a diet of freshly cooked food, and to avoid high bacterial foods such as salads, cooked meats, and fruit. Help from a dietitian is always welcome. Close social contact with people and animals is discouraged, but pets should not be banished from a home, particularly when children are the sufferers. Although cats and dogs are potential transmitters of pathogens, such transfers seem to be very rare and the emotional support of a pet may be very great.

Treatment of Infection

Once an infection is identified, or presumed because of fever, treatment must be started promptly. As with other causes of neutropenia, rapidly fatal gram negative sepsis is most likely if the neutrophil count is less than 100/mm^3. The antibiotic regime chosen should have a broad spectrum of effect, including antibacterial action against *Pseudomonas* and *Klebsiella*. The regimes most favoured are a β-lactam antibiotic with an aminoglycoside, or a third generation cephalosporin on its own. The antibiotics should be started as soon as the appropriate samples for identification of the pathogen have been taken. If a particular organism is isolated, the antibiotics are changed appropriately.

The main problems in the treatment of aplastic anemia are how long to continue with antibiotics, and what to do if the fever does not respond. With very low neutrophil counts it is difficult, if not impossible, to eradicate infection. Even if fever responds promptly and a sensitive organism is isolated, recurrence of infection is common after the antibiotics are stopped. The compromise is to treat the infection as for bacterial endocarditis and continue treatment for three weeks minimum, although this is not always possible in practice. The major toxicity is the nephrotoxicity of the aminoglycosides, and careful monitoring of antibiotic levels for therapeutic and toxic actions is needed. A degree of hypokalemia is usual, and potassium supplements may be required.

If the fever fails to respond to treatment, and no pathogen is isolated, fungal infection should be suspected. Aspergillus infections are the most lethal, and are relatively common in patients with aplastic anemia of some duration who have had multiple antibiotics. Aspergillus infection of the sinuses is particularly distressing and difficult to treat. Amphotericin still seems to be the most effective antifungal agent. It is given intravenously in high dosage (> 0.6 mg/kg) from the outset (after a test dose has been given). Major side effects are nephrotoxicity (which may be minimized by a high urine output) and hypokalemia. Fevers and rashes are common early in the course of treatment; they may resolve spontaneously or respond to hydrocortisone. Again there are major problems with duration of therapy. For proven fungal infections, at least six weeks treatment is needed.

Definitive Treatment for Aplastic Anemia

There are two main therapies which offer some hope of cure or remission in aplastic anemia: bone marrow transplantation or immunosuppressive therapy with antilymphocyte (antithymocyte) globulin. Anabolic steroids have a dubious role in the management of acquired aplastic anemia.

Bone marrow transplantation

For patients < 40 years of age who have severe aplastic anemia and an HLA-identical sibling willing to act as donor, bone marrow transplantation is the first treatment choice. At presentation, all patients are assessed on the basis of age and severity of disease as possible candidates, and HLA-typing is obtained on all family members as soon as possible. If a suitable donor is available, transplantation should be carried out as soon as possible, which usually means 1 to 2 months after diagnosis. Early transplantation minimizes the risk of rejection which is exacerbated by large numbers of transfusions, and the patient is usually in good clinical condition and uninfected at the time of transplantation. Although transfusions have been implicated in graft failure following bone marrow transplantation, it is more important to have a stable transfused patient than a sick, untransfused one.

The details of bone marrow transplantation are discussed elsewhere in this book. For patients with aplastic anemia, the main problem has been graft failure, but an immunosuppressive regime of cyclophosphamide 50 mg/kg per day for 4 days coupled with cyclosporin given for 12 months post transplant achieves a better than 95 percent engraftment and an overall survival of more than 75 percent. Cyclosporin is started the day before the donor bone marrow is infused. Dosage schedules vary. We have used 12.5 mg/kg twice daily by mouth for 4 days and then reduced the dose to 6.25 mg twice daily, modifying the dose according to renal function studies. The drug has considerable renal toxicity and is difficult to use safely. There are fewer problems with pneumonitis in transplants for aplastic anemia (where total body irradiation is not required) than in transplants for leukemia, and severe chronic graft-versus-host disease is reduced in the cyclosporin-treated patients. Unfortunately, T-cell depletion of donor marrow (which reduces the risk of acute graft-versus-host disease) greatly increases the risk of graft failure in aplastic patients. At the present time it is probably better to transplant without T-cell depletion for severe aplastic anemia when an HLA-identical family donor is available.

Transplantation from donors other than matched family members is experimental and should not be considered except for patients who have failed all other treatment, and only then after detailed discussion and in specialist centers.

Immunuosuppressive Treatment

It is now apparent that immunosuppressive treatment with antilymphocyte (antithymocyte) globulin, first introduced by Professor Georges Mathé in Paris, is of benefit in some patients with aplastic anemia.

Sources of Antilymphocyte Globulin. Antilymphocyte globulin (ALG) is prepared by immunizing an appropriate animal with human lymphocytes and absorbing the serum with various human cells and tissues to obtain some degree of specificity. Generally an attempt is made to obtain anti-T-cell specificity, and the resulting product is known as antithymocyte globulin (ATG). ATG implies a degree of specificity which may not be warranted, and ALG is preferred here. Commercial sources employ horses, rabbits, or goats as the immunized animal, and lymphocytes from the thoracic duct or a surgically removed thymus as the immunogen. It is interesting that Mathé's original preparation used peripheral blood lymphocytes. It is possible, though not in any way proven, that ALGs from different sources have different potency. Historically ALG has been combined with anabolic steroids, but there is no evidence that the latter are necessary to achieve remission.

Administration of ALG. ALG is irritative and sclerosing to veins and should be given through a long intravenous line, preferably into the central veins. It contains foreign protein and an anaphylactic reaction is a possibility, so a test dose is mandatory. Unfortunately, skin-testing material from the appropriate animal is not usually available, and it is not possible to skin-test with ALG itself, because it always produces a marked local reaction. A dilution of the recommended full dose, 10 mg ALG in 100 ml of saline, should be given intravenously over 1 hour. A physician should be in attendance throughout with hydrocortisone, piriton and epinephrine instantly available in case an anaphylactic reaction occurs. The first signs of such a reaction are peripheral and circumoral paresthesias, edema of the lips, tongue, and pharynx, bronchospasm, and loss of bowel control. Intravenous hydrocortisone and piriton usually abrogate the attack but epinephrine may be needed. (So far we have seen 1 case of anaphylaxis in more than 150 cases treated with horse ALG, in a patient who received a second course). If the test dose provokes no major reaction, the full dose is given the same or following day.

Dose and Duration of ALG Therapy. There is no standard schedule for the administration of ALG, nor for the duration of therapy. The initial European trials used a 5-day course of ALG but subsequent trials have used up to 8 days. The dose of ALG also varies according to the biologic potency of the material; the suppliers of the selected product will advise on dosage schedules. There is some evidence that higher doses with more lymphocyte-depleting effect, are more effective than lower doses. Numerous controlled trials are currently in progress in different countries to define the optimum schedules so, unless a center is involved in such a trial, a regime based on some previous experience should be used. One such regime is the use of horse ALG (Merieux, France or Upjohn, USA). The Merieux product is given at a dosage of $1^1/_2$ vials per 10 kg body weight in 500 ml of saline over 6 hours by continuous intravenous infusion (appropriate volume adjustments are made for children).

In some centers the same dose is continued for 5 days. I measure the lymphocyte count the following morning, and if it has not been reduced to < 100/mm^3 I increase the dose to 2 vials per 10 kg. Providing reactions to the ALG are tolerated, further increases are made over the next three days.

Toxicity of ALG. There are three main difficulties in the administration of ALG. First, most ALGs have antiplatelet and antigranulocyte activity. Platelet transfusions should be given before and after ALG administration but not during the infusion. The neutropenia produced varies according to the type of ALG used, but it may be marked and prolonged. Extra care to avoid infection is required. The second problem is the immediate reactions which arise during infusion. Fever and skin rashes are common, particularly during the first and second infusion. They usually respond to intravenous hydrocortisone; some schedules use corticosteroids routinely with ALG (see below). The third problem is the development of serum sickness 7 to 10 days after the ALG is given. Fever, joint pains that may be very severe, and skin rash occur. Fortunately, renal impairment caused by the immune complexes seems to be very rare. Again, the problem may be overcome with corticosteroids, initially IV hydrocortisone, followed by prednisone, 40 mg/day PO. The corticosteroids have to be continued for at least seven days; the serum sickness returns if they are stopped too early. Short-acting steroids should be avoided unless given regularly throughout the day.

Anabolic Steroids

The use of anabolic steroids in the treatment of aplastic anemia has a long history, dating back to their use in childhood aplasias by Shahidi and Diamond in 1959. Used alone in high dosage, they increase the hemoglobin and often the platelet and white cell counts in Fanconi's anemia, and in some patients with nonsevere aplastic anemia. There is no evidence that they increase the remission rate in severe aplastic anemia but traditionally anabolic steroids have been combined with ALG therapy in Europe. Several controlled trials are under way to test their efficacy; the first report published suggests that they do not improve the remission rate achieved with ALG. If anabolic steroids are used serious side effects occur when high doses are given. I employ oxymetholone 2.5 mg/kg/day, starting the day after ALG finished and continue it for three months. The dose is modified if liver function tests become abnormal. At the end of three months the patient is reassessed. If there is evidence of a positive response anabolic steroids are continued for a further three months and then slowly reduced to stop by the end of one year. Although there is no evidence to support their use in achieving remission, some patients relapse when anabolic steroids are withdrawn. Serious hepatotoxicity does occur if the anabolic steroids are continued beyond 12 months with the resulting development of peliosis hepatis and hepatocellular carcinoma. Other problems include virilization and fluid retention. Prostatic hypertrophy may be a problem in older men and gynecomastia is troublesome in some males.

Corticosteroids

Corticosteroids in conventional doses (40–80 mg prednisone daily) have no effect in severe aplastic anemia and may increase infection rates. The only exception to this is when acute lymphoblastic leukemia presents as aplastic anemia in children. The aplasia of acute lymphoblastic leukemia responds to corticosteroids with leukemia appearing some weeks later. It has been suggested that corticosteroids be used as a diagnostic trial. The aplasia remits even if steroids are not given. Low-dose steroids have been used to decrease capillary fragility in severely thrombocytopenic patients, although the evidence of success is slim. High dose methylprednisone (HDMP) starting at 20 mg/kg/day and decreased over a period of 30 days, given by intravenous bolus injections, has produced similar remission rates to ALG. The toxicity is considerable. Diabetes may be induced, convulsions may occur, and there is a marked increase in the risk of infection. Recently it has been suggested that HDMP combined with ALG will produce higher remission rates than either agent alone. Again, trial results are awaited to see if this claim is substantiated. The toxic effects of the combined regime are considerable with increased infection rate being the most marked. Medium dose corticosteroids, about 40 mg prednisone daily, given during ALG administration and for 2 weeks after (to cover serum sickness) seems a reasonable compromise for centers not involved in clinical trials.

Results of ALG Therapy. Published results of remission rates of aplastic anemia following ALG therapy vary from 40 percent to > 80 percent. Remission may be defined as independence from transfusion support. Normalization of blood counts occurs rarely. Remission is slow. A median time to transfusion independence is from 3 to 6 months in different series. Responders often show a transient rise in granulocyte count in the two weeks following ALG. Patients who do not respond at all within 6 weeks are unlikely to respond. Patients with severe aplastic anemia respond less often than those with some preservation of marrow function. In my experience approximately 40 percent of patients with severe aplasia respond to the first course of ALG, and 80 percent of those with less severe disease are alive at one year. Age does not seem to be a prognostic factor. Patients with long-standing disease do not respond as well as those with newly diagnosed aplasia. Early treatment seems sensible.

Relapse is not uncommon (possibly 10–20%) and ALG does not eradicate the instability of the marrow even in responders. PNH clones arise, and in 2 out of 60 of our patients severe hemolytic PNH with an active marrow developed. A second course of ALG may be given, either using a second animal source to avoid reactions, or after careful testing, when there is no reaction, with the same source. About 25 percent of nonresponders to a first course respond to a second. The rate of remission is higher in those who responded to the first course but then relapsed.

HEREDITARY APLASTIC ANEMIAS

Fanconi's Anemia

Fanconi's anemia is inherited as an autosomal recessive disorder. It is characterized by skeletal abnormalities, particularly of the hands and forearms, skin changes with areas of pigmentation and depigmentation, renal anomalies, and low birth weight with poor growth. The underlying abnormality is apparently a failure of DNA repair, and cytogenetics reveal multiple chromatid breaks of a nonspecific nature. Hematologically the children are normal at birth, but pancytopenia develops progressively at some future time. Usually, patients develop the first evidence of marrow failure between 5 and 10 years of age, but there is wide variation, possibly indicating heterogeneity of the genetic abnormality. Within families, affected children tend to develop pancytopenia at about the same age. Heterozygotes are apparently normal. Death occurs in the majority of patients from bone marrow failure, transformation to acute myeloid leukemia, or as a result of treatment. There is an increase in the incidence of solid tumors, particularly of the gastrointestinal tract. A few patients have relatively benign disease, and some patients remit at puberty, but usually there is progressive deterioration over a few years.

Treatment relies on anabolic steroids, support, and bone marrow transplantation. The problems of support are similar to those for acquired aplastic anemia and are not considered here.

Anabolic Steroids

Fanconi's anemia responds to anabolic steroids, at least temporarily. When the patient becomes asymptomatic, anabolic steroids are instituted at high dose until a response occurs. Oxymetholone 2.5 mg/kg/day (or its equivalent using another preparation) is suitable. As soon as a response is seen, the dose is reduced until the minimum required to maintain the response is reached. Many centers also given an alternate day low-dose corticosteroid at the same time. The side effects of this treatment are miserable: virilization is unpleasant, especially in girls; behavioral changes including hyperactivity and aggression are common; acne is a potential source of infection and distress; hepatoxicity is a major complication with the eventual development of hepatocellular carcinoma and/or peliosis hepatis. The treatment does not modify the likelihood of acute leukemia or solid tumors. Some of the cosmetic side effects may be modified by treatment, using depilatory creams for hirsutism and clindamycin, 1 percent in alcohol lotion to minimize acne. The unpleasantness of these side effects has to be weighed against the induction of transfusion-free remission which may last several years.

Bone Marrow Transplantation

Patients with Fanconi's anemia may be transplanted from HLA-compatible family donors with the establishment of stable grafts and normal blood counts. The skin and mucous membranes in these patients seem to be markedly sensitive to high-dose cyclophosphamide with a severe exfoliative rash, often complicated by superficial *Candida* infections. Patients may be successfully grafted using cyclophosphamide 50 mg/kg/day for 4 days an immunosuppression but the regime developed by Professor Elianne Gluckman in Paris appears to be less toxic and achieves good results. This immunosuppressive regime consists of cyclophosphamide 5 mg/kg/day for 4 days, followed by total body irradiation of 5 Gy in a single dose (or 2 Gy 3 times in two days). The patients receive immunosuppression post graft with either cyclosporin or methotrexate.

When a sibling donor is found to be HLA-identical it is important to conduct chromosome studies to make sure that the donor does not also have Fanconi's anemia.

The success rate for bone marrow transplantation is approximately 80 percent, but the exclusion of some donors, because they also have the disease, means that the proportion of affected children with a suitable family donor is lower than for the acquired aplastic anemias. In this group of patients it is worthwhile trying to identify a phenotypically-identical volunteer donor, particularly since the graft may be carried out with T-cell depletion with subsequent successful growth, because large numbers of marrow cells may be collected from an adult donor for the child recipient. The use of anabolic steroids may buy time for a thorough search to be conducted. There is no information on the use of HLA-mismatched family donors in Fanconi's anemia.

Dyskeratosis Congenita

This rare inherited disorder causes pancytopenia due to marrow failure, but the pancytopenia develops later than Fanconi's anemia—usually in the third or fourth decade. Nearly all patients are male. The characteristic features are dystrophic nails and changes in pigmentation of the skin with a reticulin pattern of hyperpigmentation, but also areas of depigmentation. Leukoplakia of the buccal mucosa is common. Chromosomal studies are normal.

The only definitive treatment is bone marrow transplantation, but these patients are not sensitive to alkylating agents, and cyclophosphamide is used as for acquired aplastic anemia.

Other Congenital Aplastic Anemias

Rarely, babies present at birth with pancytopenia and skeletal abnormalities that do not conform to those seen in Fanconi's anemia. Chromosomal studies are normal. These children may respond to corticosteroid therapy, and may require a very small, nontoxic dose of corticosteroid to maintain a normal blood count. In this respect they behave like congenital pure red cell aplasia patients, but differ in the pancytopenia and hypocellular marrow.

PURE RED CELL APLASIA

Pure red cell aplasia (PRCA) refers to a group of disorders characterized by failure of red cell production caused by a failure of proliferation of red cell precursors. There is anemia with reticulocytopenia, usually total absence of reticulocytes, and either absent erythroid precursors in the marrow, or arrest of erythropoiesis at a proerythroblastic stage. Granulocytic and megakaryocytic maturation and differentiation are normal. The disorder may be congenital or acquired.

Acquired Pure Red Cell Aplasias

There are two main groups of acquired PRCA, transient or prolonged. The transient erythroblastic anemia of childhood is the result of inhibition of erythropoiesis by viruses (the parvovirus is the best characterized). Symptoms develop mainly in children with hemolytic anemia and, as the disease is transient, no treatment other than transfusion, if indicated, is needed. Recovery occurs as antibodies to the virus develop.

Acquired PRCA of the prolonged type arises without any associated disorder, or occurs in association with different manifestations of an autoimmune disorder including thymoma, acquired hypogammaglobulinemia, systemic lupus erythematosus, x-linked lymphoproliferative disease or multiple autoantibodies (which may occasionally include a positive direct antiglobulin test). It has also been seen following exposure to drugs (e.g., penicillamine) and in association with lymphoma. There is evidence that many cases of acquired PRCA are caused by an immune process, but specific and universal factors have not been identified.

Treatment includes management of associated disorders with corticosteroids or other immunosuppressive agents and red cell transfusions.

The initial approach uses corticosteroids in high dosage to assess the probability of response to immunosuppression. For at least a week, 5 mg/kg/day of methylprednisolone are given in two doses 12 hrs apart, and the bone marrow is examined at the end of that time to assess response. If there is a response the dose of steroids may be reduced promptly to 0.5 mg/kg/day, and then gradually reduced to find the minimum dose which permits normal erythropoiesis. Alternate day therapy may minimize side effects. Care and patience have to be exercised during reduction of steroids, because relapse may occur if they are discontinued too quickly, and it may be difficult, if not impossible, to achieve a second remission. If the dose of corticosteroid which maintains remission is unacceptably high, azathioprine or cyclophosphamide are added with subsequent reduction in steroid dose.

Patients who do not respond to corticosteroids present a problem. All patients with PRCA are investigated for the presence of humoral or cellular immune reactions against red cell precursors; most patients whose in vitro tests produce clear evidence of immune disorder respond to steroids. Antilymphocyte globulin has produced remissions when corticosteroids have failed and may be tried without anabolic steroids. Cyclophosphamide, 150 mg daily (for adults) for 6 months or more, may also be followed by remission but carries its own toxicity and mutagenic potential. Care has to be taken to avoid further marrow depression. Rational treatment, or avoidance of ineffective treatment, will only be possible when more accurate tests of immune mechanisms are available.

When patients fail to respond to treatment, red cell transfusion with chelation therapy is the only approach. The same principles apply for PRCA although iron overload is slightly less likely to occur than in thalassemia, since iron absorption from the gastrointestinal tract is reduced. Unexplained enlargement of the spleen may cause increasing transfusion requirements. Splenectomy is indicated in these patients and response to immunosuppression has been reported after splenectomy when there was no response before.

Congenital Pure Red Cell Aplasia

Congenital PRCA (Diamond-Blackfan syndrome) presents at birth or in the first few months of life with erythroblastopenic anemia. Triphalangeal thumbs may be present, but the babies usually display no abnormalities apart from pallor. Most patients respond to corticosteroids which are given as soon as the diagnosis is made, initially in high dose (1–2 mg prednisone/kg/day) to obtain the maximum resonse. This high dose should not be continued beyond three weeks if there is no response. When a reticulocyte response is established, the dose of steroid is reduced steadily, and an alternate day regime is introduced as soon as possible. The intermittent administration of steroid permits better growth than daily doses. It may be possible to reduce the frequency of steroid administration even further to reduce side effects. The way in which corticosteroids produce a remission in congenital PRCA is not known. Azathioprine does not seem to produce a steroid-sparing effect in congenital PRCA.

Nonresponders will require lifelong transfusions

and iron chelation therapy. As with acquired PRCA, the spleen may enlarge, in which case it is removed and the patient receives suitable therapy post splenectomy to prevent overwhelming pneumococcal sepsis. Sometimes splenectomy is followed by remision. If a matched family donor is available, bone marrow transplantation is considered for tranfusion-dependent infants.

MEGALOBLASTIC ANEMIA

BERNARD A. COOPER, M.D.

Megaloblastic anemia is characterized by megaloblastic morphology in bone marrow smears, caused by either (1) relatively specific and undefined defects in nucleotide metabolism induced by antimetabolites or deficiency of certain coenzymes, or (2) equally undefined metabolic abnormalities in erythroid precursors in some clonal hematologic diseases, such as the leukemias. Although morphologic features in peripheral blood (such as macrocytosis or multilobed neutrophils) and some biochemical abnormalities (such as elevations of levels of iron or LDH in serum, abnormal deoxyuridine suppression test in stimulated lymphocytes, methylmalonate excretion in urine, or low levels of folate or vitamin B_{12} in serum or blood) correlate with megaloblastic morphology, they do not invariably predict it.

DIAGNOSIS

The effectiveness of therapy is often determined by how effectively diagnostic procedures are selected when the patient is first seen. Initial examination should include detailed history for evidence of nutritional deficiency, intestinal disease, dysphagia, ingestion of antimetabolic drugs, alcohol, or other medications which might predispose to deficiency, and previous episodes of anemia and their response to therapy. Careful examination may reveal evidence of weight loss, hepatic cirrhosis, reflex changes, loss of vibration sense, glossitis, or petechiae and/or ecchymosis. Blood samples should be taken for determinations of levels of vitamin B_{12} and folate in serum and of erythrocyte folate. The former utilizes serum from clotted blood, and commercially available vacutainers (red top) are appropriate. The latter requires unclotted blood and should be taken into either EDTA (purple top vacutainer) or citrate (blue top). Routine hematologic studies including reticulocyte count, platelet count, and peripheral smear are required, and prothrombin time determination may aid in recognition of intestinal malabsorption.

Bone marrow aspiration should be performed before therapy is instituted. For most cases, aspiration and smear are adequate, and biopsy is not required.

GENERAL THERAPY

Anemia. If life-threatening, anemia should be treated by blood transfusion sufficient to provide adequate peripheral oxygenation and cardiac function. Patients seeking medical aid because of anemia often do so because the reflex increase of cardiac output caused by the anemia exceeds the capacity of their myocardium. In such cases, cardiac failure responds to transfusion of a single unit of packed erythrocytes, together with appropriate therapy for cardiac failure. Cardiac failure responds to diuretic therapy, and so in the uncomplicated patient, furosamide, 20 mg, should be injected as transfusion is begun or as soon as the patient is seen. Further diuretic therapy should be selected on the basis of central venous pressure observation and standard clinical criteria.

Leukopenia. Seldom is leukopenia of sufficient degree to cause susceptibility to infection.

Thrombocytopenia. Occasionally thrombocytopenia may cause life-threatening hemorrhage. Although in uncomplicated megaloblastic anemia, it usually is associated with severe anemia, it may appear without anemia, and its cause may thus be obscure. Severe thrombocytopenia with evidence of petechiae and ecchymoses or bleeding should be treated with platelet transfusion.

Other Somatic Manifestations. These include glossitis, dysphagia, anorexia, diminished levels of circulating immunoglobulins, and decreased lymphocyte reactivity; they are probably never dangerous and require no specific therapy.

Severe Psychologic Depression. This has been described in association with pernicious anemia and possibly with folate deficiency. There is evidence that the depressive features are corrected when diagnosis is made and may thus be reactive. Specific therapy is thus not required. For serious depression, sedation and antidepressive therapy are identical with those used in depressive disorders of other etiologies. The organic brain syndrome and loss of intellectual function associated with deficiency of vitamin B_{12} respond only to replacement therapy with vitamin B_{12}.

SPECIFIC THERAPY

Clinical Situation I

In this case bone marrow is megaloblastic, with macrogranulocytes present, and clinical examination is consistent with nutritional megaloblastic anemia. Based on clinical information and the presence or absence of neurologic signs or symptoms, a presumptive diagnosis of deficiency of vitamin B_{12} or folate is made.

If the anemia is presumed to be the result of vitamin B_{12} deficiency, treatment consists of subcutaneous injections of vitamin B_{12} (cyanocobalamin), 5 μg per day for 2 days, followed by 100 μg per day if patient is in hospital, or weekly if not.

If the presumption is that the anemia is due to folate deficiency, treatment consists of oral folic acid as follows: 200 μg per day for 2 days followed by 2 mg per day for 1 week.

Monitoring Response

The classic *reticulocyte response* to therapy may be monitored, and some response will be observed, even if anemia is partially corrected by transfusion. *Neutrophil count* increases by the third or fourth day following initiation of therapy, simultaneously with the earliest increase of reticulocytes. *Serum iron*, if elevated, decreases to deficient levels within 24 hours of initiation of specific therapy, and erythropoiesis in the *bone marrow* becomes morphologically normoblastic within 48 hours of initiation of appropriate therapy (macrogranulocytosis persists for 10 to 14 days). If response is not observed in the peripheral blood, demonstration of conversion to normoblastic bone marrow morphology confirms the selection of correct therapy. It is well established that infection and iron deficiency obscure response to therapy in the peripheral blood, but do not prevent conversion of bone marrow to normoblastic.

Follow-Up Therapy

One week after the first injection of 100 μg of vitamin B_{12}, vitamin B_{12} absorption should be tested by the *Schilling test* if deficiency of vitamin B_{12} has been confirmed. If deficiency of vitamin B_{12} is confirmed by serum level and malabsorption of the vitamin confirmed by the Schilling test, therapy should be continued for life with 100 μg of vitamin B_{12} monthly. If vitamin B_{12} malabsorption is shown to be due to lack of intrinsic factor by correction of absorption with a source of intrinsic factor, no further investigation is required. If intestinal malabsorption is suggested by the Schilling test, and the reliability of the test used is confirmed, further investigation is required, but therapy should be continued as above. If blind loop syndrome is recognized, surgical correction is required if vitamin B_{12} injections are to be discontinued. Antibiotic therapy produces only a transient improvement in malabsorption of vitamin B_{12} caused by bacterial infestation of segments of the small bowel.

Clinical Situation II

In this case bone marrow is megaloblastoid, and macrogranulocytes usually are not observed. Deficiency of vitamin B_{12} or folate is clinically improbable.

Atypical morphology in bone marrow usually is not caused by nutritional deficiency, and so specific therapy may be withheld until investigation suggests the presence of deficiency of vitamin B_{12} or folate. A few cases of sideroblastic anemia with megaloblastic changes have responded to large doses of pyridoxine (100 mg per day by mouth) or other nutrients (viz, thiamine), and a few cases have been corrected by discontinuing drugs usually considered innocuous (e.g., analgesics), but most of these are caused either by antimetabolic drugs or by stem cell defects, some of which terminate as acute leukemia.

General therapy should be instituted depending on the clinical situation. Anemia and thrombocytopenia, which may threaten survival, should be treated as already described. In the absence of exposure to antimetabolites, no effective therapy is available for these conditions. Diagnosis must thus be precise and nutritional causes must be excluded. Most observers verify that the cause is not nutritional deficiency by *therapeutic trial* of vitamin B_{12} and folate over several weeks. Although it is possible that treatment with these vitamins may augment the development of early neoplastic disease, the evidence for this is weak, and so such therapeutic trials should not be withheld. A normal *deoxyuridine suppression test* on cells obtained from a bone marrow aspirate also may be used as strong evidence against nutritional deficiency as cause of the megaloblastic morphology.

Treatment consists of the following:

1. Manage life-threatening anemia or thrombocytopenia as above.
2. Exclude nutritional deficiency by either (a) treating with vitamin B_{12} and folate in the doses listed above, and verifying the persistence of megaloblastoid morphology in bone marrow after 3 days, or of failure of hematocytopenias to improve over 2 to 3 weeks, or (b) doing a deoxyuridine suppression test on cells obtained from a bone marrow aspirate and demonstrating that this is normal.
3. Exclude the taking of antimetabolic drugs, especially those with antifolate activity.

If evidence is obtained that the patient has taken a drug known to interfere with intracellular metabolism, this usually should be discontinued. Following discontinuation of some antimetabolites such as 6-mercaptopurine, megaloblastoid features may persist for several weeks with only very slow correction of hematocytopenia. There is no evidence that administration of purines, amino acids, or other nutrients will accelerate the correction of these drug-related diseases except that megaloblastic features and hematocytopenia induced by folate antagonists will respond to administration of folates. Included in this category are: methotrexate, trimethoprim (often administered with sulfonamide), pyrizinamide and certain other antimalarials, triampterin, and a variety of antineoplastic agents that are modifications of methotrexate.

Treatment includes discontinuation of the drug and treatment with either folic acid, 5 mg per day by mouth, or a reduced (tetrahydro-) folate (folinic acid) which may be administered orally at 3 mg/day or by injection at similar dose. It is apparent that in patients receiving large doses of antifols for treatment of neoplastic disease, the usual therapeutic considerations for these are required, including monitoring of plasma methotrexate level and therapy with folinic acid until plasma level approaches 0.1 micromolar (10^{-6}M).In situations in which antifol therapy should not be discontinued (e.g., high-dose trimethoprim-sulfonamide treatment of Pneumocystis infection), treatment with folic acid, 5 mg per day for 3 to 4 days, should revert the megaloblastic change without neutralizing the beneficial effects of the antimicrobial therapy because most organisms inhibited by this type of preparation do not effectively accumulate folate. Following initial therapy of the anemia, however, it probably is prudent to limit daily folic acid intake to 200 to 500 μg per day, a dose that should prevent megaloblastic anemia without affecting antimicrobial activity.

Most megaloblastoid anemias without macrogranulocytes in the bone marrow and in which bone marrow morphology is not typical of megaloblastic change are due to clonal diseases of the bone marrow and may terminate as acute leukemia. Megaloblastic morphology is also observed in some congenital and acquired aplastic anemias. Macrocytosis in peripheral blood and neutropenia and thrombocytopenia often coexist. In a minority of these, bone marrow morphology is typically megaloblastic, and their differentiation from nutritional anemias is more difficult. Bone marrow biopsy in these cases often reveals hypoplasia with islands of erythroid hyperplasia in contrast to the generalized hyperplasia in classic megaloblastic anemia.

NUTRITIONAL MEGALOBLASTIC ANEMIA: ADDITIONAL OBSERVATIONS

Treatment with Large Doses of Vitamin B_{12} and Folate

Patients deficient in either vitamin will respond to such therapy. The availability of assays for vitamin B_{12} and folate in blood make therapeutic trials rarely useful. Most patients with pure deficiency of folate do not respond to usual doses of vitamin B_{12}, although in some, reticulocytosis is observed. Although all patients with pure deficiency of vitamin B_{12} show some hematologic response to large doses of folic acid, conversion of the bone marrow to normoblastic by folic acid alone is probably not complete. Complete conversion of bone marrow to normoblastic after therapy with one or the other vitamin thus is reasonable evidence that deficiency was caused by that vitamin. The latter is little justification for single therapy, however, since second bone marrow aspirations, although useful, are rarely performed in practice.

The major justification for treating with small doses of a single vitamin relates to possible dangers of too rapid conversion of bone marrow to normoblastic. Sudden death has occurred during therapy of pernicious anemia—especially in patients with severe anemia. Some of these have been ascribed to severe hypokalemia, relatively refractory to prophylaxis with potassium supplements, and more severe in severely anemic patients with thrombocytopenia and neutropenia. Thrombotic and embolic episodes have also been reported in patients treated for megaloblastic anemia with large doses of vitamins. It is not known whether these catastrophic episodes during therapy are caused by abrupt conversion of megaloblastic to normoblastic bone marrow with arrest of potassium leak from cells, changes of lipids in the plasma, thrombocytosis, correction of platelet defects observed in megaloblastic anemia, or another cause.

It has been demonstrated that single doses of vitamin B_{12} in excess of 80 μg will completely convert megaloblastic bone marrow to normoblastic with correction of the anemia, whereas single doses less than 15 μg never completely correct the abnormality.

Because of the possibility that abrupt conversion of megaloblastic to normoblastic maturation may be dangerous, and the observations that the rate of correction of anemia is not significantly decreased by treating with small doses of the deficient vitamin, it would seem prudent to initiate therapy with small doses of vitamin B_{12} or folate, which would convert megaloblastic to normoblastic maturation over 3 to 4 days. This can be accomplished with the treatment regimen recommended above, which is best applied using single nutrients for therapy. It must be emphasized, however, that the advantage of this approach has not been tested.

Vitamin B_{12} Absorption Test (Schilling Test) as Initial Therapy

Flushing of radioactivity into the urine in this test requires injection of 1000 μg (1mg) of vitamin B_{12}. As indicated above, it is possible that this may be dangerous. Such an approach may also produce erroneous data with misdiagnosis and inappropriate duration of therapy. A proportion of patients with megaloblastic anemia due to deficiency of vitamin B_{12} or folate develop transient malabsorption of vitamin B_{12}, which is corrected after therapy. Although this correction may occasionally be delayed for several weeks, it probably is corrected in most subjects over one cycle of intestinal epithelial cells—about 3 days. A patient might thus have transient malabsorption of vitamin B_{12} secondary to folate deficiency, with malabsorption observed in the first stage of the test, and with apparent correction with intrinsic factor in a later test because of correction of the intestinal defect by therapy. In tests of vitamin B_{12} absorption using simultaneous administration of free and IF-bound vitamin B_{12}, an intestinal malabsorption pattern is observed. Thus, it is recommended that replacement therapy should be continued for at least 3 to 4 days before absorption of vitamin B_{12} is tested.

Repletion of Stores of the Deficient Vitamin

Vitamin B_{12} stores in the liver are repleted slowly following depletion, and may require many months to reach normal levels. The anemia caused by deficiency of vitamin B_{12} does not respond to therapy more quickly when large doses are administered—maximum rate of hemoglobin rise being achieved by 2 to 5 μg of vitamin B_{12} per day. Patients treated with larger doses of vitamin B_{12} (e.g., 30 to 100 μg per month by injection) require longer to relapse when therapy is discontinued than do patients treated with smaller doses (e.g., 20 μg/month). The benefit of the slower relapse is unknown.

There is no evidence that injections given more frequently produce better health, although many patients insist that they feel fatigued immediately before their next injection. There is no evidence that this represents deficiency of vitamin B_{12}, as serum levels are not depleted, and stores remain high. It is the impression of most physicians that these symptoms are psychologic.

Folate stores are small and are depleted to levels associated with megaloblastic anemia within 4 months of stopping folate intake. There is thus no benefit to treating with more folate than is required to correct clinical and chemical manifestations of deficiency.

Treatment of Patients with Subacute Combined Degeneration of the Spinal Cord

Neurologic lesions similar to human subacute combined degeneration of the spinal cord have been produced in monkeys and bats made deficient in vitamin B_{12} or treated with nitrous oxide. In these animals, folate supplementation appears to aggravate the lesions, and methionine supplementation appears to prevent them. Clinical studies appear to indicate that small doses of vitamin B_{12} arrest neurologic disease in pernicious anemia, and neither clinical studies nor animal experiments have demonstrated benefit with larger doses of vitamin B_{12}. Single injections of vitamin B_{12} of less than 50 to 100 μg do not increase spinal fluid cobalamin level within a few hours of injection, and this might support use of large doses of vitamin B_{12} in neurologic disease. Despite this indirect evidence, treatment with standard doses of vitamin B_{12}, as described above, should be considered adequate.

Situations in which cyanocobalamin or folic acid, the standard vitamin B_{12} and folate preparations available commercially, are not the best forms of vitamin therapy.

In nutritional anemia in adults, the aforementioned commercial forms of vitamin B_{12} and folate are adequate and probably represent the preferred therapy because of their stability and purity. Although the frequency of injections of vitamin B_{12} required to maintain normal levels of serum vitamin B_{12} is less when hydroxocobalamin is used, the trivial clinical advantage is probably offset by the periodic development of antibodies against hydroxocobalamin during such therapy. Because reduced folates are transported 100 times better into most mammalian cells than is folic acid, reduced folate is preferable to folic acid when counteracting antifols, and so folinic acid is used routinely.

In infants and children with inherited intracellular defects of folate or cobalamin metabolism, the inherited defect may prevent optimal utilization of these forms of the vitamins. In children with intracellular defects of cobalamin metabolism, treatment with hydroxocobalamin is more effective than that with cyanocobalamin, and treatment usually requires large doses (500 to 1000 μg/d) of this material. In children with deficiency of transcobalamin 2, either cobalamin may be used, but because cyanocobalamin is more effectively absorbed when fed, these children usually are maintained on oral cyanocobalamin (500 μg, 2 to 7 times per week). In children with defective intracellular folate enzymes (e.g., 5 to 10 methylene tetrahydro folate reductase), folinic acid probably represents better therapy than does folic acid, but optimal therapy would be provided by injections of 5-methyl tetrahydrofolate, if available. Such children also should receive methionine supplements. Note that such children usually do not have megaloblastic anemia.

In inherited metabolic defects, efficacy of therapy should be monitored by disappearance of homocystinuria or methyl malonic aciduria, and by restoration of normal levels of plasma methionine.

IRON DEFICIENCY ANEMIA

MAHMOUD A.M. ALI, M.D., Ph.D., F.R.C.P.(C)

IRON METABOLISM

Although iron deficiency is the most common cause of hypochromic anemia, iron therapy should not be given without knowledge of the status of the iron stores. The body of a normal person contains 4 g of iron, and this amount is distributed as follows:

Nonheme iron	
Ferritin and hemosiderin (storage iron in the liver, spleen, and bone marrow)	— 20%
Transferrin (transport iron)	— 0.01%
Heme iron	
Hemoglobin (in the circulating red cells)	— 70%
Myoglobin (in muscles)	— 5%
Respiratory enzymes in the tissues	— 5%

The iron in the stores is normally divided equally between ferritin and hemosiderin. Ferritin is a soluble complex made of a core of inorganic salts, probably in the form of ferric hydroxide and ferric phosphate, surrounded by a shell of protein. When the ferritin aggregates and denatures, it forms an insoluble compound, hemosiderin. The proportion of hemosiderin increases as the amount of storage iron enlarges. Although the amount of transport iron is small (only 3 to 4 mg of iron is present in the plasma at any one time), the importance of this fraction is out of proportion to its size. Iron in the plasma is the sole link between the sites of iron metabolism in the body. The main traffic is made up of the return of iron, derived from red cells at the end of their life span in the reticuloendothelial system, back to the bone marrow for reincorporation into new red cells. It is normal for the plasma transferrin to be one-third to two-thirds saturated. The extent to which it could combine further with iron is called the unsaturated iron-binding capacity. The level of plasma iron tends to vary considerably with the time of the day, so that in the morning the level is usually higher than the evening value by 25 percent, and it is usually lower in women than in men.

The degree to which the transferrin is saturated with iron influences its function. In order for the developing red cells to wrest the iron from transferrin effectively, its saturation must be above 30 percent. Below that figure, the iron uptake by the developing red cells becomes reduced. However, if the percentage saturation is above 60 percent, the iron begins to be deposited in parenchymal tissue and hemosiderosis may develop, leading to tissue damage, particularly of the heart, liver, and pancreas. The most important factor increasing iron absorption is a raised rate of erythropoiesis and increased plasma iron turnover. Diminished iron stores also tend to increase iron absorption, as well as tissue hypoxia. Whenever there is defective hemoglobin synthesis which is not due to iron deficiency, excess iron accumulates in the reticuloendothelial system, eventually causing tissue damage.

Unnecessary iron therapy and blood transfusion therefore increase the risk of iron overload. The plasma iron is reduced when the body iron stores become exhausted. It is also low in many chronic illnesses unassociated with iron deficiency. The serum iron binding capacity is helpful to distinguish the two conditions, since it is elevated in iron deficiency, but depressed in the anemia of chronic disease. Serum ferritin is more specific in assessing the size of the iron stores.

INCIDENCE

In many parts of the world, 3 to 15 percent of men and 25 to 50 percent of women have hypochromic anemia, and in more than 90 percent of both groups, the cause of the anemia is iron deficiency. The incidence in Canada is similar to that in Britain and the United States—about 3 percent in men and 25 percent in women. Provided iron stores and iron loss were normal, absence of iron from the diet would not lead to anemia until after 5 years in men and 3 years in women of child-bearing age.

Iron loss, therefore, implies blood loss, and the common causes of iron loss in their approximate order of frequency are: (1) menstruation and menorrhagia, (2) peptic ulcer and hiatus hernia, (3) hemorrhoids, (4) gastrointestinal neoplasm, and (5) esophageal varices.

Specific consideration should be given to exclude these causes in patients with documented iron deficiency anemia. Although iron loss is the principal cause of iron deficiency, a low iron content of the diet and possible malabsorption should not be ignored in the diagnosis, as they occasionally cause or contribute to iron deficiency, particularly in patients with borderline iron balance. Women in the child-bearing age are in a precarious iron balance, which can be easily precipitated into negative iron balance by poor diet or by pregnancy and lactation. In adolescent girls, in addition to menstruation, there is the factor of growth which may account for the frequency of iron deficiency in this group. In Canada and the United States, the amount of iron ingested seems to be proportional to the calorie intake. Therefore, an adequate, well-balanced diet of 2000 calories/day should provide about 15 mg of iron daily, which is adequate for maintaining iron balance. The role of gastric achlorhydria in producing iron deficiency has probably been exaggerated, and isotope experiments do not suggest that gastric acidity appreciably influences food iron absorption. Cereals, by virtue of their phytic acid content, which binds iron strongly, may prevent iron absorption in the gut and may play a significant role in producing iron deficiency in communities where cereal intake is very high.

PRESENTATION

Affected patients are most commonly women between the ages of 20 and 50, but in the ages below 10 and above 50, both sexes are equally affected. The sequence of events in iron deficiency is first depletion of iron stores, followed after a varied period of time by anemia. Whether iron depletion without anemia produces symptoms is a controversial issue, and symptoms of anemia are unlikely unless the hemoglobin has fallen below 11 g/dl in women and 13 g/dl in men. On examination, the patients may or may not appear anemic. There may be brittle nails and koilonychia, which may be easier felt than seen. Atrophy of the papillae of the tongue, particularly at the edges, is common in long-standing iron deficiency. Symptoms and signs attributable to the cause of the anemia may be more disturbing to the patient than the anemia itself.

The diagnosis of iron deficiency is not complete without a diagnosis of its cause. In men, gastrointestinal disase should be excluded, and in women, a gynecologic evaluation is essential. It should be emphasized that blood loss in the stools may be intermittent, and tests have to be repeated before a negative result is accepted.

MANAGEMENT

The response of iron deficiency to iron therapy is specific, and if facilities for determining the cause of the anemia are not available and the possibility of hemorrhage or neoplasm has been excluded, it is reasonable to diagnose the disease by a therapeutic trial. No diagnostic confusion will arise from treating an anemia with iron only, but failure to respond to treatment should lead to further investigation. However, it cannot be too strongly stressed that administration of preparations containing multiple hematinics is irrational, unscientific, expensive, and more than likely to be followed by a diagnostic and therapeutic muddle.

The use of iron in medicine dates from several centuries before Christ, when water in which metal weapons were allowed to rust was recognized as a source of strength. Iron fillings were used by Sydenham to treat chlorosis with some success. Today, a vast collection of different iron compounds are available for use, but only a few of these have any particular advantages. Whatever preparation is used, the maximal response to treatment (1.5 g/dl/week) is obtained when 35 mg of iron is absorbed daily. Whenever possible, an oral preparation should be given. Since iron absorption is increased in iron deficiency, it can be reckoned that 30 percent of the dose administered by mouth will be absorbed. Therefore, a daily oral dose, which will provide between 100 and 150 mg of elemental iron, will suffice to provide the patient with adequate therapy. There is no advantage in using higher doses, which are likely to lead to gastrointestinal disturbances.

Available oral iron preparations include:

1. Ferrous sulfate, in the usual dosage of a 300-mg tablet 3 times a day, provides 180 mg of elemental iron daily. This dose should be more than adequate to result in rapid correction of iron deficiency anemia after a latent period of 10 to 14 days. There is no evidence that any other oral preparation results in a more rapid or satisfactory response than ferrous sulfate when administered in equivalent dosage. Ferrous sulfate is regarded by many authorities in the field of iron metabolism as the standard with which other iron preparations are compared. It is the most widely used and least expensive of the preparations. It is marketed under Feosal, Ironate, Irosul.
2. Ferrous gluconate provides 35 mg elemental iron per tablet.
3. Ferrous fumarate provides 60 mg elemental iron per tablet.
4. Ferrous ammonium sulfate mixture for adults provides 40 mg iron per 4 ml, and for infants 20 mg per 4 ml.

Certain side effects are commonly experienced by patients taking iron orally. They are mainly gastrointestinal and consist of nausea, indigestion, diarrhea, and constipation. It is difficult to assess the cause of this intolerance; however, when the side effects appear to be related to iron intake, they can often be minimized by reducing the dose by one-third or one-half, and subsequently increasing the dose gradually to the maximum tolerated.

The prophylactic administration of iron compounds to pregnant mothers is now an established practice, and it is an important means of preventing the iron deficiency that frequently complicates pregnancy.

It should be emphasized again that the majority of patients with iron deficiency anemia should be treated by the oral route, because when properly given, this therapy is well tolerated, effective, and inexpensive. There are circumstances under which it may be necessary to resort to parenteral iron therapy. This should only be used (1) if the patients are unable, or think they are unable, to tolerate oral iron therapy; (2) in patients with chronic ulcerative colitis or regional enteritis, who are better treated parenterally because of the risk of activating their gastrointestinal disease; and (3) in cases of severe malabsorption.

Suitable parenteral preparations include iron dextran complex (Imferon) for intramuscular or intravenous administration and iron sorbital-citric acid complex (Jectofer) for intramuscular administration only. One milliliter of either preparation provides 50 mg of elemental iron, and the recommended dose is 100 mg every other day.

It is preferable to use intramuscular forms of parenteral iron because they are less likely to have severe toxic effects, although they produce staining of the skin, which may be avoided by employing the Z technique of intramuscular injection. Intravenous iron injection may produce vascular collapse if injected too rapidly, and total anaphylactic reactions have been reported. It can cause severe cellulitis if the preparation escapes from the vein. In a small number of patients, an acute arthralgia with fever, resembling serum sickness, may be precipitated by intravenous iron. In view of these complications, if iron has to be administered parenterally, the intramuscular route is strongly recommended. Intravenous iron should only be given in exceptional circumstances when intramuscular iron cannot be administered owing to inadequate muscle mass for injection, and after the patient provides signed informed consent with respect to the risks and complications.

A reticulocyte response is expected between 4 and 7 days after starting treatment, and a rise in hemoglobin after 10 days. The duration of treatment should be extended for 4 to 6 months after the restoration of normal hemoglobin level to replace the exhausted iron stores. Serum ferritin level can be used to monitor the iron level in the stores, and oral iron can be continued until the serum ferritin level is in the normal range.

Failure of hypochromic anemia to respond to iron suggests one of the following causes: (1) continued bleeding, (2) associated hematinic deficiency, i.e., folic acid, (3) coincidental chronic infection or disorders that might interfere with iron utilization, i.e., metastatic carcinoma, collagen disease, and renal or liver disease, and (4) misdiagnosis, i.e., other causes for hypochromic anemia.

The prognosis of iron deficiency anemia depends on its origin. Provided it has no malignant source, the outlook is excellent, so long as the primary cause of iron loss can be corrected. If iron loss continues, relapse is likely to occur, but can often be prevented by repeated prophylactic administration of iron, provided the loss is not too great.

REFRACTORY ANEMIAS

JOHN D. HINES, M.D., F.A.C.P.

The refractory anemias represent a continuum of hematologic disorders ranging from the hereditary and acquired sideroblastic anemias to the refractory anemias with and without excess blasts (RAEB). For clarity of presentation and diagnostic and therapeutic implications, these disorders will be considered separately.

SIDEROBLASTIC ANEMIAS

The sideroblastic anemias (SA) are a heterogeneous group of disorders characterized by the following features: (1) dimorphic or predominantly hypochromic anemia, (2) hyperferremia, usually associated with increased tissue iron overload, (3) bone marrow abnormalities, which include erythroid hyperplasia and, to a varying degree, abnormal erythroid nuclear maturation associated with defective hemoglobinization and, most importantly, the presence of increased number of "ringed" and partially "ringed" sideroblasts on the iron-stained marrow. Table 1 illustrates my classification based on known associated or pathogenetic factors germane to the etiology of these anemias.

Hereditary Sideroblastic Anemia

This condition has been well documented and reported in over 100 families in North America, Europe, the Middle East, and Japan. In the vast majority of cases, the mode of inheritance has been X-linked recessive. However, in several selected family studies it has been demonstrated to be autosomal recessive. In the majority of cases of sex-linked hereditary sideroblastic anemia, only the males are affected and fulfill the diagnostic characteristics of this disorder. However, in recent years it has been more widely appreciated that the female carrier state, although usually asymptomatic with mild or no anemia, is at risk for significant tissue iron overload during adult life.

The affected males represent a relatively heterogeneous group of patients with anemia ranging from mild to severe in degree, and in some cases presenting only with hyperferremia. In spite of this heterogeneity of clinical expression, all anemic patients have hypochromic and microcytic erythrocyte indices (in contrast to the acquired cases) and the erythrocyte size (MCV) correlates directly with the degree of anemia. The morphology of the bone marrow "ringed" sideroblasts in hereditary sideroblastic anemia differs from that in acquired cases in that "ringed" sideroblasts occur only in the late (nondividing) adult erythroid precursors. Most experimental evidence continues to implicate a primary defect in the early stages of heme biosynthesis. The clinical course in these congenitally sideroblastic patients ranges from death in infancy in some to remarkably good survival in others. Often the diagnosis may not be made until adult life. Because

TABLE 1 Classification of the Sideroblastic Anemias

I. Hereditary
  A. X-linked (majority)
  B. Autosomal recessive (rare)

II. Acquired
  A. Primary idiopathic
  B. Secondary
    1. Associated with drugs and chemicals
      a. Ethanol abuse
      b. Antituberculous drugs (isoniazid, cycloserine, Pyrazinamide)
      c. Lead
      d. Chloramphenicol
    2. Proceding or following malignant disease
      a. Myeloma and lymphoma
      b. Acute lymphoblastic and myelogenous leukemia
      c. Chronic and acute myelofibrosis
      d. Aplastic anemia
      e. Chronic lymphocytic and monocytic leukemia
    3. Associated with nonmalignant diseases
      a. Rheumatoid arthritis
      b. Systemic lupus erythematosus
      c. Autoimmune hemolytic anemia
    4. Post bone marrow transplantation (for leukemia or aplastic anemia)

many of these patients exhibit a favorable response to pyridoxine, this should be considered as the primary treatment modality. Most responsive patients require pharmacologic doses ranging from 200 to 300 mg orally per day, and hematologic responses may not occur promptly but may take several months. An equally important consideration in both the affected patients and the female carrier of the trait is prevention of the tissue iron overload that ultimately occurs with time. Serum iron and ferritin levels are sometimes useful in assessing these patients for tissue iron overload. Newer methodology utilizing the magnetic susceptibility properties of ferric storage iron in the liver permits accurate quantitative estimation of hepatic iron stores utilizing a superconducting quantum-interference device which obviates liver biopsy. Nonanemic patients with this hereditary form of sideroblastic anemia should undergo serial phlebotomy until serum ferritin values stabilize under 200 μg/dl. With the current improvements in technology, anemic patients should be considered candidates for long-term desferrioxamine therapy. A smaller selected group of these patients exhibit hematologic responses to the coenzyme form of pyridoxine, pyridoxal–5′–phosphate (PLP), and not to pyridoxine itself. This can easily be administered as a subcutaneous injection of 50 to 100 mg given four times daily for a trial period of 2 weeks. If a therapeutic response ensues, the patient may be maintained on as little as 100 mg thrice weekly.

Acquired Sideroblastic Anemias

Patients with acquired sideroblastic anemia represent the most heterogeneous group of sideroblastic patients in several aspects. The degree of anemia may range from mild to severe. The other major clinical manifestations of the disease relate in large part to the degree of tissue iron overload. The peripheral blood smear is typically dimorphic with both macrocytic and microcytic hypochromic red cells present. Characteristically the MCV is high-normal or frankly elevated. In the bone marrow, "ringed" sideroblasts occur at all stages of erythroid maturation and are usually present in 30 to 85 percent of all erythroid precursors. Essentially, two etiologically unrelated forms of acquired sideroblastic anemia occur. In the first group of patients, no associated or causal factor(s) can be identified. These patients are considered to have the so-called *idiopathic* form of the disease; they tend to be in the older age groups, and diagnosis is usually made after age 50. The disease is often chronic and indolent for many years. Mild-to-moderate degrees of thrombocytopenia and/or leukopenia occur infrequently. In most published series the ultimate progression to acute leukemia occurs in less than 15 percent of patients. Treatment of this group of sideroblastic patients is generally unsatisfactory, and the clinician is ultimately forced to resort to chronic packed erythrocyte transfusions to maintain a hemoglobin between 8 and 10 g/dl. A small but significant subset of patients exhibit a hematologic response to pharmacologic doses of pyridoxine with or without added folic acid, also in pharmacologic doses (5 mg daily). In rare instances, therapy with subcutaneous pyridoxal–5′–phosphate (50 to 100 mg four times/day × 14 days) has achieved significant hematologic responses, some being maintained for months with a maintenance regimen of PLP, 100 mg thrice weekly. Also rare are a limited number of patients who respond to both oral pyridoxine (150 to 300 mg/day) and oral 1–tryptophan, 750 mg daily. Unfortunately there are no predictive laboratory studies that will permit selection of potentially responsive patients for any of these treatment regimens. As was emphasized for the congenital sideroblastic patients and carriers, aggressive attempts to prevent or delay the inexorable morbid tissue iron overload should strongly be considered in all patients. This can be done either by periodic phlebotomy or by the use of continuous subcutaneous desferrioxamine therapy. It is worth noting that the marrow abnormalities persist in nearly all patients despite the documentation of a modest or good hematologic response to the aforementioned regimens. To date I have documented reversal of hepatic tissue iron overload and hepatic fibrosis in two pyridoxine-responsive patients who underwent phlebotomy every week (or two) for periods of 13 and 16 months respectively. Hepatic function, which was initially perturbed, returned to normal in both patients after the tissue iron burden had been relieved. Both patients had restoration of normal hemoglobin and hematocrit levels following pyridoxine administration, and significant numbers (>50 percent) of persisting ringed sideroblasts remained in marrow specimens of both patients until multiple phlebotomies had effected a normal hepatic iron store, as documented by liver biopsy. At that time, the number of marrow "ringed" sideroblasts had diminished to 2 percent and 5 percent respectively. Although still somewhat abnormal, this represented a dramatic morphologic improvement in the nuclear maturation and the marrow iron stores, and a return to nearly normal the number of sideroblasts in these two adult patients.

In the second subgroup of patients with acquired sideroblastic anemia, the disease is considered to be secondary to or associated with (1) certain pharmacologic agents, or (2) excessive ethanol abuse, or (3) certain nonmalignant and malignant disorders of the hemopoietic system (see Table 1).

The cases that occur in association with drug or ethanol ingestion will spontaneously revert to a normal or nonsideroblastic state when the offending agent(s) are discontinued. When the causative agent is isoniazid or another antituberculous drug, the sideroblastic bone marrow abnormalities can usually be prevented by concomitant administration of pharmacologic amounts of oral pyridoxine daily (150 mg/day).

The small but well-documented group of patients

who have or eventually develop a hematologic picture consistent with sideroblastic anemia may have any of a number of documented hematologic malignant diseases, which include multilple myeloma, acute nonlymphocytic leukemia, chronic monocytic and lymphocytic leukemia, Hodgkins and nonHodgkins lymphoma, and chronic and acute forms of myelofibrosis. There is a nearly uniform lack of hematologic response to pyridoxine and other vitamin analogs within this patient group, and transfusion dependency inevitably ensues. However, several patients have now been described with chronic refractory sideroblastic anemia which evolved into acute nonlymphocytic leukemia. Interestingly, although complete hematologic bone remission of the leukemia followed the use of combined anthracycline and cytosine arabinoside therapy, the marrow sideroblastic abnormality and transfusion dependence remained unaltered. The remission durations were predictably brief (<4 mos).

In another group of patients, the coexistence of sideroblastic anemia and autoimmune diseases (rheumatoid arthritis, systemic lupus erythematosus, and autoimmune hemolytic anemia) has been documented. Remission of the autoimmune disorders, whether spontaneous or medically induced, was usually associated with partial or complete disappearance of the marrow sideroblastic abnormalities as well as the anemia.

Finally, with the advent of bone marrow allografting for aplastic anemia and acute leukemia, it is not surprising to find that a small group of patients who achieve successful marrow engraftment have developed bone marrow sideroblastic abnormalities. Whether this is due to host or allograft clonal abnormalities, to the drugs utilized to prevent graft-vs-host disease, or a combination of all events remains unanswered. Of some interest, however, was a recent report which documented definitive hematologic responses to pyridoxine in two such patients following successful engraftment for acute nonlymphocytic leukemia during first remission.

REFRACTORY ANEMIA WITH OR WITHOUT EXCESS BLASTS

These patients with refractory anemia are generally distinct from the aforementioned patients with sideroblastic anemia. These patients have a dysmyelopoietic syndrome characterized by refractory cytopenia of one or more cell lines associated with a cellular to hypercellular marrow with few (≤5 percent) if any ringed sideroblasts. Two broad and heterogeneous groups of patients have emerged from most reported series.

The first consists of patients with so-called "refractory anemia with excess blasts" (RAEB) also designated "preleukemia". The bone marrow morphology in this group of patients is characterized by increased marrow cellularity with relative erythroid hypoplasia. However, dyserythropoietic changes are readily recognized. In addition, there are characteristically 10 to 30 percent myeloblasts and/or abnormal promyelocytes present in aspirated marrow specimens. When performed, cytogenic marrow studies have yielded a high percentage of abnormal karyotype patterns, usually of the C and G groups. Most investigators consider this subset of patients to be "preleukemic", and 30 to 45 percent of patients develop overt leukemia, with a median survival of 15 to 30 months. A substantial percentage of this group of patients succumb to such complications as bleeding secondary to thrombocytopenia and neutropenia-related infections prior to evolution to overt acute leukemia. Previous efforts to treat either the preleukemic syndrome or the leukemic phase of these disorders with chemotherapy have been singularly unsuccessful, and no standard therapeutic regimen has existed. Recently, however, a number of investigators have re-explored the utility of intermittent or continuous infusion of low-dose (20 mg/m^2 per day for 21 days) cytosine arabinoside (Ara-C) in patients during the preleukemic phase of their disease. The rationale for this dose and schedule of drug is largely based on osbervations suggesting that Ara-C in sublethal doses can result in the induction of terminal differentiation in human myeloid leukemic cells in vitro. The preliminary results from a number of centers have been encouraging, with a dramatic decrease in blood component transfusion requirement occurring in as many as 60 percent of patients during the preleukemic state. This treatment regimen is associated with significant myelosuppression in the majority of patients, usually evident by day 14 to 18 irrespective of the route of administration. Hospitalization with platelet and often antimicrobial support is mandated in many of the patients so treated. Several large cooperative trials of this regimen are currently under way in order to more precisely define the response, toxicity, and survival in larger numbers of patients. It must be emphasized that the mechanism(s) by which low-dose infusions of Ara-C induced responses in patients with preleukemia (myelodysplasia) or even in acute leukemia is unclear at present. Moreover, it has not yet been ascertained whether maintenance therapy in responsive patients has any role in subsequent patient management.

The second and equally (if not more) heterogeneous group of patients comprising this latter subset of patients are those with refractory anemia and additional cytopenias who exhibit cellular marrows with dyserythropoiesis and dysmyelopoiesis, but with only a small percentage of ringed sideroblasts or no ringed sideroblasts in the marrow specimens. Characteristically, these patients' marrows contain <10 percent myeloblasts and abnormal promyelocytes, a feature that distinguishes them from the preceding groups of patients. The majority of these refractory anemic patients present in older age groups (>60 years), and the clinical course is intermediate between that of patients with acquired idiopathic sideroblastic anemia and that of patients with preleukemia. The median survival in most reported series ranges from 35 to 60 months, and the risk of evolution into an acute leukemic state is approximately 10 to 15 percent. Therapy in this patient group with refractory anemia is usually limited to red cell transfusion support. Anecdotally, in some series there appears to be a higher risk factor for eventual development of acute leukemia in patients with the most aggressive transfusion requirement and coexisting thrombocytopenia. However, this has not been corroborated in any large series of such patients. Future therapeutic studies within this heterogeneous patient group will focus on efforts to alter the marrow maturation by use of agents such as the low-dose Ara-C schedule already discussed and probably the use of other agents such as cis-retinoic acid (or analogs). Thus far we have observed two gratifying hematologic responses in two of three such patients using Ara-C, 10 mg/m^2 subcutaneously every 12 hours for 21 days. All 3 patients were >68 years of age and each patient exhibited marked dyserythropoiesis, between 5 and 8 percent ringed sideroblasts, and <10 percent myeloblasts and abnormal promyelocytes. All three were transfusion-dependent for >6 months. Two of the three responsive patients have maintained transfusion-free status for 6 and 8 months respectively after one single 21–day course of therapy. The third patient died of infectious complications before completing the 21–day regimen.

AUTOIMMUNE HEMOLYTIC ANEMIA

ALAN D. SCHREIBER, M.D.

The autoimmune hemolytic anemias are a group of disorders in which individuals produce antibodies directed against one of their own erythrocyte membrane antigens. The erythrocyte survival of these antibody-coated cells is decreased, accounting for the hemolysis. The most effective way to approach autoimmune hemolytic anemia is to determine which class of antibody is responsible for the hemolysis. In general, there are two major classes of antierythrocyte antibodies that produce hemolysis in man: IgG and IgM. The pattern of red blood cell clearance, the site of organ sequestration, the response to therapy, and the prognosis all relate to the class of antierythrocyte antibody involved. We will deal with these two different classes of antibody sequentially. In this article, we will discuss primarily immune hemolytic anemia caused by antierythrocyte antibodies of the IgG class (warm reacting).

IgM-INDUCED IMMUNE HEMOLYTIC ANEMIA

Autoimmune hemolytic anemia caused by IgM antibody in humans is generally restricted to the clinical entity termed cold hemagglutinin disease. Cold hemagglutinin disease is almost always caused by an IgM antibody, and most IgM autoantibodies in humans are cold agglutinins. This disease is most commonly associated with an underlying mycoplasmal infection, particularly mycoplasmal pneumonia. It may also occur with other infections, such as infectious mononucleosis. Cold hemagglutinin disease (IgM-induced immune hemolytic anemia) can also be seen with an underlying immunoproliferative disorder, such as chronic lymphocytic leukemia, nonHodgkin's lymphoma, or systemic lupus erythematosus. This disease may also occur without an apparent underlying infection or immunoproliferative disorder, in which case it is termed idiopathic cold hemagglutinin disease. The disease may be chronic, and the IgM protein may tend toward homogeneity and even be monoclonal. When this is the case, one should suspect an underlying immunoproliferative disorder, and the prognosis is adversely affected.

The IgM antibody is usually directed against the I antigen on the erythrocyte membrane. IgM antibody is efficient in agglutinating erythrocytes. The cold agglutinin titer represents the least dilution of patient plasma or serum capable of agglutinating human red blood cells in the cold. In most patients with hemolysis, the cold agglutinin titer is greater than 1:1000.

As in all patients with autoimmune hemolytic anemia, erythrocyte survival is generally proportional to the amount of antibody on the erythrocyte surface. In cold hemagglutinin disease, the extent of hemolysis is largely due to (1) titer of antibody (cold agglutinin titer), (2) thermal amplitude of the IgM antibody (the highest temperature at which the antibody is active), and (3) the level of the circulating control proteins of the C3b inactivator system. Hemolysis is complement-dependent and the IgM-coated erythrocytes are cleared primarily by the macrophage C3b receptors in the liver. The IgM-coated erythrocytes become C3b-coated via classic complement pathway activation.

IgG-INDUCED IMMUNE HEMOLYTIC ANEMIA

In this type of autoimmune hemolytic anemia, the antibodies are of the IgG class, and the antigen to which the antibody is directed is usually an Rh erythrocyte antigen. The antibody has its maximal activity at 37°C, and this entity has been called warm antibody hemolytic anemia. IgG-induced immune hemolytic anemia most often occurs without an apparent underlying disease (idiopathic type); however, it may also occur with an underlying immunoproliferative disorder, such as chronic lymphocytic leukemia, nonHodgkin's lymphoma, or systemic lupus erythematosus. The signs and symptoms are those of anemia in general. The diagnosis is established by directly observing the erythrocyte surface for the presence of cell surface proteins.

Present on macrophages within the reticuloendothelial system are receptors not only for C3b, but for IgG as well. These are termed Fc receptors. The macrophage Fc (IgG) receptor can detect IgG-coated erythrocytes, bind them, make them spherical, or phagocytose them in the absence of C3b. However, once C3b is placed on the erythrocyte surface, through complement activation, erythrocyte clearance is further accelerated. Thus, IgG-coated red cells are progressively cleared from the circulation by macrophages possessing an Fc (IgG) receptor. Hemolysis is almost always extravascular, and these IgG-coated cells are cleared predominantly in the spleen.

THERAPEUTIC MEASURES

In many patients with IgG- or IgM-induced immune hemolytic anemia, no therapeutic intervention is necessary, since the hemolysis may be mild. If an underlying disease is present, control of this disease often brings the hemolytic anemia under control as well. However, if the patient has significant anemia secondary to hemolysis, therapeutic intervention is necessary.

Corticosteroids. Patients with IgG-induced immune hemolytic anemia respond, in general, to corticosteroid therapy in dosages $\geq$ 40 mg of prednisone a day. Corticosteroids work in IgG-induced hemolytic anemia by three basic mechanisms. First, they decrease the production of the abnormal IgG antibody. This is the most common effect and produces a gradual increase in hemoglobin within 2 to 5 weeks. Second, corticosteroids have in several cases been demonstrated to cause elution of IgG antibody off the erythrocyte surface, improving the red blood cell survival. This is probably an uncommon effect of corticosteroid therapy. Third, corticosteroids have been shown in vitro and in vivo to interfere with the macrophage Fc (IgG) and C3b receptors responsible for the erythrocyte destruction in this disease. This effect may be rapid and may be responsible for the rise in hemoglobin noted, in some patients, to occur with 1 to 4 days of corticosteroid therapy. This effect of corticosteroids causes an improvement in erythrocyte survival despite the continued presence of IgG and C3b on the erythrocyte surface.

Once a therapeutic response is achieved, tapering of corticosteroids should be begun. However, this may take several months. Alternate-day corticosteroid therapy can be considered during this time, or until the patient's hematologic picture stabilizes.

Since corticosteroids may improve erythrocyte survival by interfering with macrophage detection of antibody- and complement-coated erythrocytes, the patient's Coombs' test may remain positive in the face of an improved erythrocyte survival. Thus, some patients may continue to improve hematologically despite a persistently positive Coombs' test.

Approximately 80 percent of patients have an initial response to high-dose corticosteroids. Nevertheless, only 20 to 30 percent have a sustained response off therapy. Several patients have control of their hemolytic process on low- to medium-dose corticosteroid therapy or on alternate day steroid therapy. For the patients who are steroid-dependent, the initial and long-term side effects of steroids must be considered. These include gastritis, peptic ulcer disease, emotional lability, exacerbation of diabetes and hypertension, electrolyte imbalance, increased appetite and weight gain, moonlike faces, osteoporosis, myopathy, and increased susceptibility to infection. The severity of these side effects relates to both duration of therapy and the dosage. Splenectomy is recommended for patients who are steroid-unresponsive or require > 10 to 20 mg/day or 20 to 25 mg every other day for maintenance. Each patient requires individual evaluation of underlying disease, surgical risk, extent of anemia, and steroid intolerance. In some patients the presence of a mild hemolytic anemia may be preferable to splenectomy or other modes of therapy. The initial goal of therapy is to return the patient to near-normal hematologic values with corticosteroid therapy while producing minimal toxicity. Alternate-day corticosteroids are worthy of consideration in many patients. Their efficacy is not generally appreciated.

Splenectomy. The reticuloendothelial system of the spleen with its resident macrophages is the major site for sequestration of IgG-coated blood cells. This appears to be due to the unique circulatory system in the spleen whereby hemoconcentration occurs in the splenic cords. This results in intimate contact between macrophages (with their membrane Fc [IgG] receptors) and IgG-coated blood cells in the presence of a minimal amount of circulating plasma IgG; plasma IgG competitively inhibits the macrophage Fc (IgG) receptor binding of IgG-coated cells. Thus, the spleen is usually the major site of red cell sequestration in AIHA, with the liver accounting for a variable degree of red cell destruction.

Removal of the major site of red cell destruction is an effectively therapeutic strategy in IgG-induced immune hemolytic anemia. The response rate to splenectomy is approximately 50 to 70 percent; however, the vast majority of the responses are partial remissions. The partial remissions are often quite helpful in that they result in a lessening of the hemolytic rate, with a rise in the hemoglobin value. Splenectomy usually results in a reduction in the amount of corticosteroids needed to control the hemolytic anemia. Patients who are unresponsive to corticosteroids, those who require moderate-to-high maintenance doses of corticosteroids, or those who have developed corticosteroid intolerance are generally candidates for splenectomy. ^{51}Cr-labeled red cell kinetic studies are probably not beneficial, since the procedure is time-consuming, expensive, and not a reliable indicator of response to splenectomy.

Splenectomy is effective in IgG-induced hemolytic anemia because the cells are cleared primarily in the spleen. In addition, it has been shown that splenectomy can decrease the production of the IgG antierythrocyte antibody, as the spleen represents a large B cell pool. Patients in whom splenectomy fails are probably those with very high concentrations of IgG on the erythrocyte surface in whom the liver plays a more prominent role in clearance.

The side effects of splenectomy vary greatly from institution to institution. I have generally attempted to identify one or two surgical colleagues who carry out most of the splenectomies on our patient population. This experience enhances both the surgical procedures (speed and safety) and the postoperative follow-up. The morbidity of the procedure includes postoperative thromboses and infection, both above and below the diaphragm. The risk of morbidity and mortality is enhanced in older patients, in those with related underlying disease (benign or malignant immunoproliferative disorder) and in those with unrelated medical problems. Thus, consideration of the benefit-versus-risk factors needs to be applied to each patient. Adults who undergo splenectomy may, in rare instances, have a propensity toward life-threatening infection, particularly with pneumococcus. For this reason, I generally immunize patients with Pneumovax some weeks prior to elective splenectomy in an effort to reduce this long-term complication.

Immunosuppressive Agents. Several chemotherapeutic agents with known immunosuppressive effects have been used in the treatment of immune hemolytic anemia. The drugs most commonly used include the thiopurines (6-mercaptopurine, azathioprine, and thioguanine) and alkylating agents (cyclosphosphamide and chlorambucil). Immunosuppressive therapy may be effective for treating patients with IgG-induced immune hemolytic anemia when patients are refractory to steroids or splenectomy. Immunosuppressive agents work by decreasing the production of antibody, and therefore it generally takes at least 2 weeks before any therapeutic result is observed.

Patients are selected for immunosuppressive therapy because they have a clinically unacceptable degree of hemolytic anemia resistant to corticosteroid and splenectomy treatment. Alternatively, they may be corticosteroid-resistant or -intolerant and a poor surgical risk. Clinical benefit has been noted in about 50 percent of patients. A reasonable trial is about 3 to 4 months, and if no beneficial effect is noted, therapy is discontinued. If clinical benefit occurs, one can maintain the dose level for a total of 6 months and then taper dosage over several months. During therapy, patients are instructed to maintain a high fluid intake to reduce the incidence of chemical cystitis seen with cyclophosphamide and the need to have weekly blood counts to monitor bone marrow suppression, which can be seen with any of these immunosuppressive drugs. The dosage of drug should be adjusted to maintain the leukocyte count >2000, granulocytes count >1000, and the platelet count >50,000 to 100,000.

Cyclophosphamide is usually well tolerated, but a variety of side effects may occur, including bone marrow suppression (primarily leukopenia), hemorrhagic cystitis, nausea, partial alopecia, amenorrhea, and impaired spermatogenesis. The use of alkylating agents may also have a long-term potential for increasing the incidence of malignancy, particularly acute leukemia. These side effects require that the clinical indications for an immunosuppressive drug, particularly an alkylating agent, be strong and that patient exposure to the drug be limited.

Transfusion Therapy. The majority of patients with autoimmune hemolytic anemia do not require transfusion therapy because the anemia has occurred gradually and physiologic compensation has occurred. However, occasional patients experience acute and/or severe anemia and require transfusions for support until other treatment modalities reduce the hemolysis. Transfusion therapy is complicated by the fact that the blood bank may be unable to find any "compatible" blood. This is due to the fact that the autoantibody is directed to a component of the Rh locus which is present on the erythrocytes of essentially all potential donors, regardless of Rh subtype. The usual recommendation is for the blood bank to identify the most compatible units of blood of the patient's own major blood group and Rh types. Using this approach, it is unlikely that the donor blood will have a dramatically shortened red blood cell survival.

The goal of transfusion therapy is to prevent any serious complications due to the anemia. These include angina, congestive heart failure, and central nervous system symptoms of hypoxia (e.g., syncope, lightheadedness, impairment of mental acuity). In addition, if the patient is experiencing blood loss, transfusion is required. Usually, the slow infusion of 1 to 2 units of packed red cells improves the clinical status of the patient. Elderly patients especially need to be monitored for circulatory overload and for transfusion reactions. The latter are unlikely to be serious since hemolysis is usually extravascular. In the rare patient with little or no response to steroids and a continuing need for transfusions because of serious side effects of anemia over the first 4 to 6 days of therapy, an early decision for splenectomy may be necessary.

Miscellaneous Therapy. Plasmapheresis has been used in patients with severe IgG-induced immune hemolytic anemia, but has met with limited success, possibly because more than half of the IgG is extravascular and the plasma contains only small amounts of the antibody (most of the antibody being on the red blood cell surface).

Other measures that have been used effectively in some patients with IgG-induced immune hemolysis are vincristine, vinblastine infusions, and hormonal therapy. The most exciting development in hormonal therapy is the recent success of the synthetic androgen, danazol. Because of its limited side effects (limited masculinizing effects, mild weight gain), danazol may become an attractive alternative to corticosteroid therapy in some patients with IgG-induced immune hemolytic anemia. The effect of these agents in IgM-induced hemolysis is untested.

HEMOLYTIC-UREMIC SYNDROME

V.V. VEDANARAYANAN, M.D.,
PETER D. THOMSON, M.B., B.Ch., F.C.P.(S.A.)
BERNARD S. KAPLAN, M.B., B.Ch., F.C.P.(S.A.)

Although the cause of the hemolytic-uremic syndrome (HUS) usually is not determined, a number of etiologic factors have been found including Shigella, pneumonococcal and *E coli* infections, hereditary factors, oral contraceptives, and cyclosporin A. The more commonly occurring "idiopathic form" has an excellent prognosis, but patients with variant forms (e.g., HUS associated with pregnancy) may have a less favorable outcome. Following the realization that different forms of HUS may not have the same etiology and pathogenesis, the need for different specific lines of therapy is being appreciated. Early detection of cases who fare poorly and the use of specific therapeutic measures to correct underlying causes could improve the outcome in these patients. In this article, we describe our experience in the treatment of HUS and discuss the use of newer forms of treatment.

INITIAL EVALUATION AND RESUSCITATION

The more frequently encountered idiopathic form of HUS usually occurs in children under 3 years of age, has a seasonal occurrence, and has a prodrome of diarrhea and/or vomiting followed by sudden onset of acute renal failure, thrombocytopenia, and hemolytic anemia with fragmented erythrocytes. The majority of mildly affected patients do not have anuria but can have combinations of oliguria, hypertension, and seizures. Patients who are severely affected can be moribund and need urgent management of shock, acidosis, and electrolyte disturbances. Despite intravascular hemolysis and acute renal failure, hyperkalemia is uncommon. It is important to identify patients who have a severe form of the disease as they have increased morbidity and mortality. About 15 percent of patients seen by us had a poor prognosis with respect to the ultimate outcome in renal function. The following clinical clues may be associated with a poor outcome: (1) older age at onset, especially adults, (2) nondiarrheal prodrome, (3) familial involvement suggestive of an autosomal recessive or dominant trait, (4) association with pregnancy, (5) sporadic occurrence, (6) association with Shigella dysentery, and (7) association with pneumococcal infection.

GENERAL MEASURES

Once the diagnosis of HUS has been suspected, the patient is admitted for careful monitoring of neurologic status, measurement of urinary output, and frequent recording of blood pressure. Table 1 outlines the treatment approach to HUS. A careful record is maintained of fluid input, urine output, and body weight. BUN, serum creatinine, and serum electrolyte concentrations are measured frequently. If the patient is not dehydrated or edematous, the fluid intake is initially restricted to 5 percent dextrose in water to replace insensible losses. Gastrointestinal losses are estimated and corrected with an equal volume of fluid containing 40 to 50 mEq/L sodium and 30 mEq/L potassium if urine output is adequate. Dehydrated patients are appropriately corrected and then restricted to replacement of insensible losses. Intake of potassium, sodium, and phosphate is withheld during the initial period of the illness. The hemoglobin concentration and platelet count are determined about twice a day. A coagulogram is not essential in every case as a disturbance in coagulation is rarely encountered.

Deterioration in neurologic status, reduction in urine volume, or abdominal tenderness is an indication for reviewing the case and considering additional therapy. The illness in mildly affected cases usually lasts 7 to 10 days. Recovery is heralded by an increase in urine output, a stable hemoglobin concentration, an increase in the platelet count, and a general feeling of well-being. Table 2 lists the potential complications of HUS syndrome.

CORRECTION OF ANEMIA

The anemia is mainly caused by a microangiopathic intravascular process. In HUS associated with pneumococcal infection, hemolysis is the result of immune mechanisms in which IgM antibodies react with the Thomsen-Friedenreich (T-F) cryptantigen exposed by neuraminidase.

Transfusions of fresh packed cells are given in a dose of 10 ml/kg body weight and repeated as often

TABLE 1 Treatment of Hemolytic-Uremic Syndrome

Form	*Treatment*
Mild form	Maintenance of fluid and electrolyte balance; careful packed RBC transfusion to correct anemia; adequate nutrition; careful clinical monitoring
Severe form	Early dialysis (anuria > 24 hours)
Subgroups	
Neuraminidase- and Shigella-associated	Parenteral antibiotics for infective agent; ? anticoagulants;* same regimen as for mild forms
Sporadic forms Prostacyclin-deficient With platelet-aggregating factors Familial forms	FFP, 20 ml/kg infusion for 3 days; if no response or if there is deterioration, plasmapheresis plus regimen for mild forms
With endothelial toxin With hypocomplementemia and C3Nef	Plasmapheresis; dialysis
Recurrent forms	Plasmapheresis weekly 24 times over a year

* Many cases with shigellosis and pneumococcal sepsis have features of DIC, but no studies have been done.

TABLE 2 Complications of Hemolytic-Uremic Syndrome

Acute
Fluid and electrolytes
Overhydration
Hyponatremia
Metabolic acidosis
Hyperphosphatemia
Hypokalemia
Metabolic alkalosis
Hyperkalemia (rarely)
Hypocalcemia
Neurologic
Acute cerebral edema
Hemiplegia
Generalized seizures
Focal seizures
Severe hypertension
Cardiovascular
Congestive heart failure
Arrhythmia
Acute pulmonary edema
Myocardial involvement
Infections
Insulin-dependent diabetes mellitus
Gut
Severe pseudomembranous colitis
Gangrene of the gut
Chronic
Renal
Chronic renal failure
Abnormal urinary sediment
Tubular hyperkalemia
Concentrating defect
Hypertension
Persistent neurologic sequelae
Type I diabetes mellitus
Recurrences

as required to maintain the hemoglobin concentration around 9 g/dl. Fresh red blood cell transfusions are recommended because changes in red blood cells during storage may make them more susceptible to hemolysis.

Overzealous use of blood transfusions causes an increase in intravascular volume which can result in severe hypertension. Increasing blood pressure or fluid overload are indications for stopping the transfusion and for intravenous furosemide, provided the patient is not anuric. If there is no response or if the patient is anuric, rapidly acting vasodilators (e.g., nitroprusside, hydralazine, diazoxide) are given intravenously.

THROMBOCYTOPENIA

Extramedullary factors causing thrombocytopenia include localized intravascular coagulation, microangiopathy, and platelet aggregation in microvessels. The circulating platelets are functionally defective, demonstrate reduced aggregation in vitro, and are depleted of intracellular granular contents. Bleeding is unusual and the thrombocytopenia does not correlate with the severity of the disease.

There is no specific treatment for the thrombocytopenia. In the rare event of bleeding into an organ, platelet concentrate should be infused.

ACUTE RENAL FAILURE

The involvement of the kidney in HUS is variable. Whereas in some patients an abnormal urinary sediment is the only evidence of renal involvement, others can have oliguric or anuric acute renal failure. The mainstay of treatment is control of fluid and electrolyte balance and dialysis when indicated.

In mildly affected cases who have a normal or slightly reduced urine output, monitoring of fluid input and output is all that is required. Administration of sodium, potassium, and phosphate is avoided until renal function is improving.

Dialysis

The roles of dialysis are corrective and supportive. Excess fluid can be removed, and electrolyte and acid-base disturbances can be corrected. Removal of uric acid and phosphate possibly reduces secondary renal damage. Dialysis may remove an antifibrinolytic factor and, theoretically, toxins causing HUS. More fluid can be given during dialysis so that an adequate caloric intake can be achieved without the risk of volume overload.

Cases with anuria for over 24 hours should be dialyzed whether or not they have other indications such as fluid overload, electrolyte disturbance, or acidosis. We prefer peritoneal dialysis in children because of the difficulty of obtaining vascular access for hemodialysis in young infants. It is our practice to start dialysis as early as possible in severely affected patients and to continue until renal function recovers. We now insert a Tenckhoff catheter ab initio and this allows for more protracted dialysis, if required.

Studies in South Africa showed that early dialysis in anuric cases dramatically reduced the acute mortality rate. Since then, early dialysis has been done in all patients who presented with oligoanuria or other features of severe involvement. Complications of dialysis are uncommon except for peritonitis which occurs less often since the more routine use of the Tenckhoff catheter.

HYPERTENSION

The hypertension is mainly the result of fluid overload. Most of our patients who developed hypertension did so after blood transfusions. The role of hyperreninemia is unclear because many are hyperreninemic whether volume is expanded, depleted, or normal. Patients with predominantly glomerular arteriolar injury are more likely to have severe hypertension. Acute severe hypertension must be treated with drugs given intravenously. An intravenous nitroprusside infusion given at a rate of 3 μg/kg/min (range 0.5 μg–8.0 μg/kg/min) is reliable and acts rapidly. Its effect disappears within a few minutes of its cessation, and the rate of its administration can be titrated against the blood pressure response. Prostacyclin (PgI_2) can be as effective as nitroprusside in reducing blood pressure. Its onset of action is as rapid as that of nitroprusside, but it is much safer because the effect levels off once a normal blood pressure is reached.

Oral antihypertensives can be given as soon as the patient can take them. Propranolol is used with or without hydralazine. Alpha-methyldopa or captopril is indicated if the hypertension is difficult to control. Most patients who become hypertensive require short-term treatment, but some may need prolonged treatment. A number of severely affected patients have had prolonged hypertension after recovery from the acute illness.

NEUROLOGIC INVOLVEMENT

Central nervous system complications occur as a result of cerebral edema, microthrombi, or hyponatremia. Generalized seizures are the more usual presenting feature, but signs of diffuse or focal neurologic involvement can be seen.

Cerebral edema is the result of electrolyte, fluid, and acid-base disturbances compounded by severe anemia and hypoxia. It can be impossible to differentiate between edema and microthrombi without a CT scan. Treatment of edema can aggravate cerebral damage when microthrombi are the cause of the neurologic deficits.

Causes of cerebral edema are identified and corrected if possible. Mannitol is indicated if the patient is not anuric. Cerebral microthrombi may be an indication for fresh plasma infusions or plasmapheresis.

FRESH FROZEN PLASMA INFUSION AND PLASMAPHERESIS

A decreased ability of plasma to stimulate prostaglandin synthesis has been found in some patients with noninfantile, nonepidemic HUS. A variety of changes have been found: deficiency of the factors required for PGI_2 production or the presence of a PGI_2 inhibitor. Patients with a deficient factor have responded to fresh plasma infusion. Those with a plasma inhibitor to prostacyclin synthesis and/or platelet aggregating factors do not respond well to plasma infusion, but may improve following plasmapheresis. Fresh plasma infusion should be considered in all cases presenting with atypical features, as well as relapsing forms, and those with an inherited form of HUS. These patients tend to do poorly with supportive treatment alone, and many develop progressive deterioration in renal function, severe hypertension, and multisystem involvement. A treatment schedule consists of infusion of fresh frozen plasma in a volume of 20 ml/kg/day for 3 consecutive days. Dialysis should be started if there are signs of volume expansion. Lack of a response after three infusions or the presence of circulating inhibitors to PgI_2 production or the presence of platelet-aggregating factors are all indications for plasmapheresis. An exchange is done daily for 5 days with a plasma protein fraction (PPF) in a volume twice that of the blood volume. After each exchange, 10 ml/kg of FFP are given to correct resultant deficiencies in clotting factors. During this procedure, the patient must be monitored for signs of fluid overload, and if this occurs, the excess fluid must be removed by dialysis. In a patient with recurrent HUS, plasma exchanges can be done weekly for a year. There are no controlled studies assessing these regimens, although many patients seem to do well with them.

ANTICOAGULANTS, ANTIPLATELET AGENTS, FIBRINOLYTIC THERAPY

Treatment with combinations of heparin, aspirin, dipyridamole, streptokinase, and urokinase has been attempted often in a noncontrolled manner and without demonstrating improvement in mortality or morbidity in the acute stage of the disease.

PgI_2 has been infused on the premise that there is a deficiency of prostacyclin, but its value cannot be assessed.

PROGNOSIS

We classify patients as severely or mildly affected on the basis of whether or not there is anuria for over 24 hours. Some patients who initially appear to be mildly affected tend to have a progressive course with oliguria, hypertension, and/or seizures. Irrespective of the initial presentation, these cases must be evaluated daily as the severity of the disease can change from one day to another. In general, however, the severity of the disease declares itself in the first few days after admission.

The epidemic idiopathic form of HUS in childhood has an excellent prognosis. One hundred percent of mildly affected cases recover with excellent renal function. A younger age, presentation in summer, diarrheal prodrome, and dialysis are associated with good prognosis. The severely affected cases fare less well compared to those who are mildly affected. However, the immediate survival has been improved a great deal by early dialysis and good supportive care. In our experience, the acute mortality in this group has decreased from 72 percent to less than 5 percent. End-stage renal disease and persistent hypertension develop in some.

The progressive form of HUS has a very poor prognosis. Despite dialysis and supportive care, the majority develop end-stage renal disease and persistent hypertension.

Persistent neurologic sequelae are rare, and even in those with severe CNS involvement, the majority recover completely. Cardiac dysfunction, type I diabetes mellitus, and gastrointestinal abnormalities can also occur.

Recovery of renal function can be delayed in some patients: there are well-documented reports of patients whose renal function improved after many months of dialysis and then rapidly became nearly normal. Some HUS patients have persistent urinary sediment abnormalities, slightly elevated BUN, a defect in urine concentration, and tubular hyperkalemia for varying periods of time.

OUR EXPERIENCE

Our experience is based on treatment of HUS in three different areas of the world: The Montreal Children's Hospital, Quebec, Canada; Transvaal Memorial Hospital, South Africa; and All India Institute of Medical Sciences, India. We have found that early dialysis of severe cases is the only therapeutic intervention that has made an important difference in the prognosis.

In 1971, we reported our experience of treating 67 cases of HUS in South Africa. There were 39 cases with mild involvement, and the remainder were severely affected. Whereas there were no deaths in the mildly involved group, 72 percent (20 of 28) severely affected cases died. When the treatment of severely affected cases was analyzed, a striking difference was seen between the early dialyzed cases and those dialyzed late in the course of the disease. The mortality rate was 28 percent (2 of 7 cases) in those dialyzed early versus 85 percent (18 of 21 patients) in those dialyzed late. Four of 8 patients treated with heparin died.

In 1976, we published the results of treatment of 44 consecutive cases seen between 1969 and 1975 in Johannesburg. As a result of the institution of early dialysis in severely affected patients, the mortality rate had decreased from 77 percent to 10 percent (2 of 19) in this group. There have been no further deaths reported in 90 patients treated in Johannesburg since 1975.

In a recent analysis of a long-term follow-up study of these cases in Johannesburg, South Africa, we noted that end-stage renal disease and persistent hypertension occur in an important number of cases. End-stage renal disease developed in 5 of 47 severely affected patients, and 9 had persistent hypertension. Six patients with end-stage renal disease were transplanted, and in four of them, the graft is functioning well (followed for 0.5 to 5 years).

Over the last decade, we have managed 35 cases of HUS at The Montreal Children's Hospital. These patients comprise a much more heterogeneous group. Three patients were siblings with an autosomal recessive form of HUS, 2 patients had recurrent episodes, one had HUS followed by ITP, and HUS was associated with acute glomerulonephritis in one case. All of the 23 mildly affected children survived without residual sequelae; 2 of 6 severely affected cases and the three siblings with familial HUS died. No long-term sequelae were seen in the remainder.

In North India (All India Institute of Medical Sciences, New Delhi), we managed patients with HUS associated with bacterial dysentery (V.V. Vedanarayanan) over a period of 18 months. Ten cases of HUS were treated. Eight patients died during the acute phase, 40 percent of deaths (3 of 8) occurring within 24 hours of admission. Circulatory imbalance, acidosis, electrolyte disturbance (hyponatremia), and malnutrition were frequent findings, and 40 percent of these cases had coagulation disturbance suggestive of disseminated intravascular coagulation. The two cases who survived had normal renal function 6 months after recovery.

SICKLE CELL DISEASE

GRAHAM R. SERJEANT, C.M.G., M.D., F.R.C.P.

The term sickle cell disease covers a broad spectrum of conditions and includes four principal genotypes; homozygous sickle cell (SS) disease, sickle cell-hemoglobin C (SC) disease, sickle cell-β^+ (S β^+) thalassemia and sickle cell-β° (S β°) thalassemia. In addition there are rare forms of sickle cell disease such as sickle cell-hemoglobin D Punjab disease and sickle cell-hemoglobin O Arab disease. The sickle cell trait is not a form of sickle cell disease, and people with this genotype are healthy but may pass on the abnormal gene to their children.

The frequency of these conditions at birth is determined by the frequency of the individual genes. In Jamaica, the sickle cell trait occurs in 10 percent of the population, the SC trait in 3.5 percent, the Sβ^+ thalassemia trait in 1 percent and the sβ° thalassemia trait in 0.5 percent. At birth, SS disease occurs in nearly 4 per 1000 births, SC disease in 2 per 1000 births, Sβ^+ thalassemia once in every 3000 births and Sβ° thalassemia once in every 6000 births. The prevalence of these conditions in older populations will be influenced by their relative mortalities which are highest in SS disease and Sβ° thalassemia and lowest in SC disease and Sβ^+ thalassemia.

The pathophysiology of sickle cell disease is common to all genotypes and results from the tendency of hemoglobin S (HbS) to polymerize within red cells increasing the mean cell hemoglobin concentration and decreasing their ability to be deformed. These changes produce different red cell morphologies in the different genotypes. SS disease is characterized by intravascular sickling and the formation of irreversibly sickled cells and SC disease by a population of small dense cells. All conditions manifest increased red cell destruction and a tendency for less deformed cells to occlude blood vessels.

EFFECTS OF RAPID HEMOLYSIS IN ANEMIA

Steady State

The steady state hemoglobin levels vary in the different genotypes the normal range being, in SS disease (6 to 9 g/dl), SC disease (12 to 16 g/dl), Sβ^+ thalassemia (10 to 14 g/dl), and Sβ° thalassemia (6 to 10 g/dl). Clearly only SS disease and Sβ° thalassemia have consistently anemic hemoglobin levels. However, even these two conditions do not normally present the symptoms of anemia because a markedly reduced oxygen affinity compensates for the decreased hematocrit. Furthermore, the lowest hematocrit levels are associated with the greatest shift in the oxygen affinity curve. The steady state hemoglobin level in these conditions is therefore already adjusted to maintain oxygen delivery satisfactorily, and no purpose is served (in terms of oxygen delivery) by transfusing patients at their steady state hemoglobin level.

There are, however, a variety of conditions when hemoglobin levels fall below steady state values and symptoms may result.

Acute Splenic Sequestration

In this dramatic and serious complication, sudden splenic enlargement filters off circulating red cells; the patient sometimes dies from acute anemia and circulatory failure. It is a pediatric manifestation occurring most commonly between 6 months and 2 years. Since the patient is too young to complain, the presenting symptom is sudden extreme pallor. The etiology is unknown, so attacks cannot be prevented. Treatment consists of early diagnosis and immediate transfusion. Attacks may recur, but repeated attacks can be prevented by splenectomy. This is usually performed after the second attack, but is generally performed after the first attack in poor socio-economic circumstances. Occasionally chronic transfusion programs are proposed to prevent attacks, but these are logistically complex, expensive, have to be stopped some time, and are not a realistic alternative, certainly in the Third World. Early diagnosis is essential, and parental education may assist in this.

Hypersplenism

Sustained splenic enlargment and red cell sequestration may be associated with chronic and markedly increased marrow activity in hypersplenism. Hemoglobin levels are maintained usually in the 3 to 6 g/dl range with reticuloycte counts of 15 to 40 percent and mean red cell survival below 4 days. This is achieved by marked marrow expansion and hyperactivity, and a high energy cost which impairs growth and development. Infrequently hypersplenism may resolve spontaneously, but it is currently impossible to predict those in which this will occur. Otherwise splenectomy should be performed and is consistently followed by dramatic hematologic improvement. Following splenectomy for either hypersplenism or acute splenic sequestration, it is essential to provide the most comprehensive cover against postsplenectomy infection. In Jamaica, parenteral prophylactic penicillin is used for a minimum of three years with pneumococcal and hemophilus influenzae B vaccines.

Aplastic Crisis

This is a clearly defined syndrome with temporary but total arrest of erythropoietic maturation, rapid fall in hemoglobin (1 g per day), and absence of reticulocytes from the peripheral blood. Recovery is spontaneous if the patient survives acute anemia. Treatment is transfusion and the clinical course is so predictable that it is frequently performed on an outpatient basis in Jamaica. Recent evidence suggests that most, if not all, attacks are associated with infections by parvovirus, which raises the possibility of a protective vaccine.

Hypoplastic Episodes

The active marrow is readily suppressed by infections or metabolic disturbances with the result that the hemoglobin level falls below steady state values. The reticulocyte count also falls but not to zero, differentiating hypoplastic episodes from the aplastic crisis. Treatment is for the underlying condition, although transfusion may be necessary to raise the hemoglobin level quickly.

Megaloblastic Change

The accelerated red cell turnover increases the requirement for folic acid. It is customary to give folic acid supplementation, although whether this is needed depends upon the relationship of demand and dietary supply. Requirements are greatest during rapid growth in infancy, adolescence, and pregnancy, and supplementation at these times is logical. It is doubtful whether it is necessary at other times.

Renal Failure

Chronic renal failure is common especially among patients with SS disease over the age of 40 years. It is clinically insidious, and is often only recognized by a slow progressive fall in hemoglobin level, with reticulocyte counts below normal for the patient. The renal pathology is rarely reversible, and treatment is palliative with maintenance of hemoglobin levels in the low normal range (5 to 7 g/dl). Chronic hemodialysis may improve well-being and decrease transfusion requirements; renal transplantation may be considered if nonrenal pathology is minimal.

EFFECTS OF RAPID HEMOLYSIS IN GALLSTONES AND CHOLECYSTECTOMY

Rapid red cell destruction and high bilirubin excretion results in a high prevalence of gallstones. These are generally asymptomatic, but elective cholecystectomy is often advocated. In Jamaican experience, obstruction of the common bile duct is unusual, acute cholecystitis rare, and malignant change in the gall bladder undescribed. The clinical features of patients with gallstones are not obviously different from those without, and prophylactic cholecystectomy does not seem justified.

PRESUMED VASO-OCCLUSIVE EPISODES

Many of the complications of sickle cell disease are caused by, or have an element of, tissue necrosis from presumed vaso-occlusion by cells less readily deformed. These episodes may affect the bones, lungs, brain, eyes, corpora cavernosa of the penis, skin, spleen, or uterus.

Bones

Dactylitis

Dactylitis, or the hand-foot syndrome, is an early form of bone marrow necrosis affecting the small bones of the hands and feet. It is a pediatric manifestation, and its principal importance is that it is frequently the first manifestation of sickle cell disease, and so brings the disease to medical attention. Attacks resolve spontaneously, may be recurrent, and rarely leave permanent bone damage. The only treatment necessary is analgesia, although occasionally marked swelling and fever may indicate salmonella septicemia and osteomyelitis. This complication is more frequent than realized, and it may be wise to perform blood cultures in episodes of dactylitis.

Painful Crisis

The painful crisis is the adult counterpart of dactylitis and results from bone marrow necrosis in the juxta-articular areas of the long bones. The inflammatory response to the necrotic marrow causes extreme pain. Attacks may be precipitated by cold, infection, pregnancy, stress, exercise, or psychologic factors. Known precipitating factors should be avoided and infection treated. Treatment of the established painful crisis requires analgesia, rehydration, and reassurance. Patients may think they are going to die in attacks and reassurance is very important. Analgesia should be the minimal amount required to control the pain, and is frequently rendered more effective by reassurance and rehydration. Addictive preparations may cause serious problems if used for a recurrent problem like painful crisis. During painful crises, negative fluid balance may occur because of fever, reduced oral consumption, and continued urinary losses. Dehydration may aggravate painful crises, so fluid balance must be maintained by large volumes orally or intravenously if the patient is vomiting or cannot cooperate. No antisickling agents have been shown to be unequivocally effective in the painful crisis. Rarely, blood transfusion may assist the resolution of severe persistent pain.

Avascular Necrosis of the Femoral Head

Bone marrow necrosis within the femoral head may damage and soften the bone, and continued weight bearing leads to crushing and damage of the articular surface. If diagnosed before deformity occurs, avoidance of weight bearing (bed rest with traction followed by knee or hip casts to maintain joints in flexion) may allow the femoral head to heal normally. Continued destruction leads to permanent damage and deformity. Occasionally the pain resolves leaving a damaged but functional hip. Continued pain and destruction may need reparative surgery; total hip replacement is generally the most effective solution.

Avascular necrosis may also affect the humeral head, but because of the lack of weight bearing, persistent pain and deformity are unusual. Rarely shoulder replacement has been considered justified to relieve pain and limitation of movement.

Osteomyelitis

Osteomyelitis, particularly with salmonella organisms, occurs as a secondary infection of necrotic bones and this diagnosis should be considered in patients with systemic symptoms, marked swelling, fever, or gross radiologic change. Treatment requires suitable antibiotics (ampicillin, chloramphenicol) for periods of at least 6 to 8 weeks, and occasionally surgical drainage of pus or removal of dead bone.

Acute Chest Syndrome

The acute chest syndrome presents with pleuritic symptoms, and may result from pneumonia, pulmonary embolism, or stasis of sickled cells in pulmonary vessels. The differential diagnosis is complex and often impossible, although pneumonia is considered more likely in young patients. Treatment consists of broad-spectrum antibiotics and rehydration. Oxygen may be necessary to improve arterial oxygen tensions, and exchange transfusion occasionally produces dramatic clearing of signs in severely ill patients.

Brain

Vaso-occlusion affecting the brain may be devastating and most frequently presents as hemiplegia with large vessel involvement on cerebral angiography. Risk factors are unknown except for a low HbF level, and episodes tend to be recurrent especially within 3 years of the first attack. Chronic transfusion therapy appears to prevent recurrences but further episodes are common if transfusion therapy is stopped after 1 to 2 years. Many problems attend chronic transfusion programs including the development of antibodies to red cell antigens, venous access, iron load, and when to stop. It may be feasible in North American and European centers, but is unlikely to be achievable in a Third World context. Furthermore, these efforts are only directed at prevention of recurrence; prevention of the first episode is not yet possible.

Eyes

Retinal infarcts lead to a series of retinal vascular changes culminating in the development of proliferative retinopathy. This may cause transient visual impairment from vitreous hemorrhage or permanent visual impairment from retinal detachment. Treatment has been directed at attempting to close the arterial supply of the lesions of proliferative retinopathy, rendering these lesions avascular and less likely to cause complications. Direct attack on the artery by argon laser was followed by a high frequency of retinal tears, and use of the xenon arc commonly produced choroidal neovascularization. Currently trials are underway on the use of limited scatter photocoagulation, to destroy the retina in the area of these lesions, in the hope of removing the stimulus to new vessel formation. Preliminary results suggest that the scatter method is frequently successful in small lesions, but the feeder vessel technique may be necessary in large lesions. Prospective examinations of young patients may allow all lesions to be treated at an early stage.

Priapism

Occlusion of drainage of the corpora cavernosa results in sustained painful erections or priapism. Attacks may be short-lived or stuttering (1 to 6 hours) and major (>24 hours). Stuttering attacks frequently precede major episodes. Uncontrolled observations suggest that stilbestrol 5 mg daily may abort the pattern of stuttering attacks and a controlled trial is underway. Major attacks of priapism require pain relief and detumescence. This is most readily achieved by creating a simple shunt between the corpus spongiosum and the corpora cavernosa on both sides. Permanent impotence has commonly followed major attacks because the vascular system is no longer capable of maintaining an erection. The use of penile prostheses has successfully managed this problem.

Chronic Leg Ulceration

Lesions around the medial and lateral malleoli are common in Jamaican patients affecting, at some time, three-quarters of the adult population. Approximately half are spontaneous (presumed skin infarction) and half traumatic, the incidence of the latter lesions being reduced by proper footwear. The lesions are frequently infected, may last 10 to 15 years; current treatment is unsatisfactory.

The role of antibiotics is unclear although they are used in the case of cellulitis surrounding the ulcer, or when a dirty ulcer is associated with inguinal lymphadenopathy. A trial of topical antibiotic mixture containing bacitracin, polymyxin B, and neomycin suggested a beneficial effect, but is still under analysis. Necrotic debris and fibrous tissue may impede healing and may be treated by chemical or surgical debridement. Oral supplementation with zinc sulphate 200 mg *tid* was followed by a significant increase in healing. Skin grafting procedures are disappointing with a high recurrence rate, but may have a valuable psychologic effect. Complete bed rest is universally beneficial but often impractical. The role of transfusion is unknown. In Jamaica, twice daily dressings with weak antiseptic solutions, chemical debridement with hydrogen peroxide or papain, and oral zinc sulphate are used, and meet with modest success.

The Spleen and Infection

Continued vaso-occlusion results in destruction of the splenic vasculature, functional asplenia, and eventually a fibrous splenic atrophy. Splenic function is lost early in life with a resulting susceptibility to overwhelming infections, especially pneumococcus infections. Prevention of pneumococcal septicemia and meningitis has been proposed by pneumococcal vaccines, or by prophylactic penicillin. A Jamaican trial comparing the efficacy of 14 valent pneumococcal vaccine given at age 6 months, with monthly injections of long-acting penicillin, noted many septicemias in the vaccine-treated group (vaccine breakthroughs), but none in those treated with penicillin. However, cessation of penicillin was followed by a cluster of pneumococcal events, suggesting that effective penicillin coverage had inhibited the acquisition of natural immunity. The pneumococcal vaccine may be effective in older children, but since the highest risk period for pneumococcal septicemias in SS disease is the first 3 years of life, it appears that little protection is conferred by the existing vaccine during that critical period. Logically penicillin coverage should be continued until pneumococcal vaccines are capable of conferring some protection.

Pregnancy

An increased prevalence of abortions, stillbirths, and low birth weight babies occurs in mothers with SS disease. Regular antenatal care is essential, and supplementation with folic acid and iron is usual for the duration of the pregnancy. There is an increased prevalence of the acute chest syndrome and of painful crisis which should be treated accordingly. Delivery should be by the normal vaginal route unless there are obstetric contraindications. Prophylactic transfusion therapy has been proposed but not subjected to controlled trial, and is not unequivocally beneficial.

Patients desiring contraception should be given the most effective methods. The risks of pregnancy (although small) are of a totally different order from the theoretical risks associated with contraception. The pill, depot preparations of medroxyprogesterone acetate, and the intrauterine device are all used in Jamaica. A controlled trial of medroxyprogesterone acetate indicated a number of hematologic and clinical benefits. Patients should not be condemned to the less effective diaphragm or condom methods. If they have completed their family, patients should be offered tubal ligation as a safe permanent form of contraception.

Growth

Physical and sexual development are frequently retarded in SS disease. The mechanisms are not understood, and there is no effective or rational therapy at the present time. However, patients should be reassured that such retardation is normal for children with sickle cell disease, and that they will develop satisfactorily but at a later age than normal children.

Anesthesia and Surgery

Necessary surgery is occasionally deferred in patients with sickle cell disease because of doubts about the risks posed by anesthesia and surgery. These are minimal with modern medical management, and surgery is frequently performed in Jamaica at steady state hemoglobin levels with replacement of only blood lost at surgery.

SICKLE CELL CLINICS

It is vital that patients with sickle cell disease be monitored regularly by medical advisors experienced with management of sickle cell disease and knowledgeable of the patient's steady state characteristics.

ERYTHROCYTOSIS

GORDON WETHERLEY-MEIN, B.A., M.D. (Cantab), F.R.C.P. (Lond), F.R.C.Path. (U.K.)

In the present context erythrocytosis is defined as any situation in which there is either an *absolute* increase in the cell count above the individual's predicted normal value, a *relative* increase due to a decrease in plasma volume (PV) associated with a normal red cell count, or an *apparent* increase due to a high normal red cell count—either alone or in association with a low normal plasma volume.

In practice it is more convenient to speak in terms of the venous hematocrit or packed cell volume (PCV) rather than of the red cell count, and to use the more familiar term "polycythemia" to describe most of the various forms of erythrocytosis.

CLASSIFICATION

Since the treatment may vary according to the type of polycythemia, some classification which leads to a working diagnosis is necessary for discussion of appropriate therapy. It is hoped that the classification presented in Table 1, although arbitrary, is self-explanatory, and the nature of the individual forms of

TABLE 1 The Erythrocytoses (Polycythemias)

Designation	*Red Cell Mass*	*Plasma Volume*	*Packed Cell Volume*	*Mechanism*
Absolute	Increased	Normal	50–>60%	Primary: polycythemia vera Secondary: 1) Hypoxic a. High altitude b. Cardiac c. Pulmonary d. High O_2 affinity hemoglobin e. Red cell diaphorase deficiency 2) Inappropriate erythropoietin production (renal and other tumours)
Relative (low plasma volume)	Normal	Decreased	50–58%	Acute fluid loss Diuretics Idiopathic (synonyms: pseudo-polycythemia stress polycythemia Gaisböck's disease)
Apparent	High normal	Normal or decreased	52–54%	

polycythemia will be considered briefly when their treatment is discussed.

DIAGNOSIS

Obviously, correct diagnosis is the basis for correct treatment, but it is inappropriate to discuss diagnostic procedures in detail here, although a brief comment on the method of classification is necessary. The criteria for diagnosing absolute, relative, or apparent polycythemia are arbitrary, but do provide, at least temporarily, a working basis. Given the patient's actual red cell mass (ARCM) and plasma volume (PV)—estimated by a reliable technique such as the simultaneous ^{51}Cr and ^{125}I–albumin method—it is preferable to compare these figures with the individual's mean normal predicted values (MNRCM and MNPV) rather than by the ml/kg expression. These mean normal values can easily be calculated from the Nadler height and weight formula for prediction of normal blood volume (PBV) as follows:

1. PBV = $(366.9\ h^3) + (32.19\ w) + 604.1$ ml for males
   PBV = $(356.1\ h^3) + (33.08\ w) + 183.3$ ml for females

   where h = height in m and w = weight in kg
2. Then MNRCM = PBV $\times$ 0.91 $\times$ 0.47 for males
   MNRCM = PBV $\times$ 0.91 $\times$ 0.43 for females

where PBV = mean normal predicted blood volume.

3. Mean normal predicted plasma volume (MNPV) = PBV − MNRCM ml.

This method is preferable to the ml/kg expression and gives equivalent values to those derived from the surface area or lean body mass methods. If the ARCM exceeds the MNRCM by 25 percent a diagnosis of absolute polycythemia can be made with confidence. If the APV is more than 15 percent below the MNPV, in association with normal ARCM, a relative (low plasma volume) polycythemia is diagnosed. With elevated PCV, but ARCM and APV within these limits, it is reasonable to diagnose apparent polycythemia. It is probably wise to investigate all patients, male and female, with resting PCV levels of 51 percent (0.51) and above. This is because the main determinant of symptoms, morbidity, and mortality is the PCV and, as will be discussed, there is evidence to suggest that PCV values within what is commonly regarded as the high *normal* range are associated with increased morbidity, usually due to occlusive vascular lesions (OVL), particularly in hypertensive patients over 50, in whom there is usually coincident atheroma.

Apart from the clinical history, physical findings, and standard peripheral blood count, the optimal range of investigations includes measurement of red cell mass and plasma volume, neutrophil alkaline phosphatase, arterial PO_2 and PCO_2, carbonmonoxyhemoglobin in smokers, oxygen dissociation curve (P50), and exclusion of renal lesions by ultrasound or pyelography. Although whole blood viscosity and cerebral blood flow are important in the pathogenesis of symptoms, morbidity, and mortality, it is unnecessary to measure them in clinical practice, since they are almost directly proportional to the PCV, and any plasma contribution can be assessed by measurement of total protein, albumin, globulin and, if indicated, immunoglobulin. Erythropoietin assays and CFU-e results are, at present, too inconsistent to be of value in the individual patient.

MORBIDITY AND MORTALITY

If the polycythemias were not associated with a remarkably high incidence of transient, severe, or fatal occlusive vascular lesions, it would not be much of an exaggeration to say that they would be, clinically, almost negligible conditions requiring no treatment. Of course this is not so. Transient ischemic attacks, strokes, retinal vein thrombosis, coronary occlusion, and mesenteric and deep vein thrombosis are recognized complications. In one series of primary, untreated polycythemias (PRV), 50 percent died of OVL's—mainly stroke—within 18 months, and in another series, more than 80 percent had some form of trivial or severe OVL during and after treatment. Similar risks occur in the other forms of polycythemia considered here, though some hypoxic polycythemias may be less affected. There is a close relationship between PCV level and incidence of OVL. There is, similarly, a close relationship between rising PCV, whole blood viscosity (which increases), and cerebral blood flow (which falls, except in some hypoxic states). Although cerebral blood flow is determined predominantly by oxygen delivery to the brain, rather than by whole blood viscosity, this is rather an academic point, for it can be assumed that flow and viscosity can make their own contributions to the pathogenesis of OVL in the brain and other areas—particularly if associated with arterial disease and hypertension—with smoking possibly operating as a quite independent factor.

TREATMENT

From what has already been said in relation to symptoms, morbidity, and mortality, it is clear that the object of treatment is to reduce PCV to an "optimal" level. It is necessary to decide what the optimal level is. In all forms of polycythemia (the hypoxic forms are to some extent an exception and are to be discussed), there is evidence, derived from a number of completely different approaches, that although the incidence of cerebral OVL is obviously greatest at the highest PCV levels, e.g., 60 percent plus (0.60+), there is an increased incidence of stroke and subclinical cerebral microscopic infarction when the PCV is at the upper end of the traditionally normal range (50 to 52 percent, 0.50 to 0.52). This is supported by evidence that cerebral flow decreases and whole blood viscosity increases as the PCV moves up from 45 percent (0.45) to 52 percent (0.52) and above. Therefore, except possibly in some hypoxic patients, if a decision is made to treat, the therapeutic objective should be a PCV of 45 percent (0.45) or less.

Against this background it is possible to consider the treatment of the individual types of polycythemias shown in Table 1.

ABSOLUTE POLYCYTHEMIAS

The absolute polycythemias may be primary or secondary. *Primary polycythemia* is considered elsewhere in this work (see chapter entitled *Polycythemia Vera*).

Secondary Polycythemias

Hypoxic Group

Altitude polycythemia is not a common clinical problem. Acute occlusive vascular lesions do occur, and doctors on high altitude expeditions consider them to be as serious as acute mountain sickness. Suggested management can only be speculative without data on cerebral blood flow, oxygen delivery, and measured exercise tolerance. It is possible that the high hemoglobin values achieved (18 g/dl+) are not a beneficial adaptation, and slow acclimatization and the use of oxygen rather than venesection seem, at present, to constitute the most sensible compromise.

Cardiac polycythemia, most commonly due to congenital anomalies, is obviously best treated by surgical correction. The operative procedure and immediate postoperative state are improved—in terms of coagulation defects, operative blood loss, and oxygen debt—by reduction of PCV by repeated small volume venesections. PCV values of 60 percent plus (0.60+) are unlikely to be advantageous, but the level to which they should be reduced is certainly above the low "normal" range, and the "optimal" PCV level (50 percent [0.50] to 54 percent [0.54]) is based on empiric observation of the individual patient. Similar comments apply to patients in whom surgical correction is impossible, and there is no doubt that many patients so treated experience considerable subjective improvement. Although there is a shortage of objective measurements in this area, there is evidence of increased effective cardiac output, tissue oxygen uptake, and measured exercise capacity.

Pulmonary polycythemia is often regarded as an advantageous compensation. It is likely that the erythropoietin response was evolved to respond to the hypoxia of acute blood loss, rather than to hypoxic pulmonary or cyanotic cardiac disease, and the high PCV levels often observed in lung disease are usually a recognizably disadvantageous "overswing". Studies on such patients before and after venesection show subjective improvement in terms of dyspnea, fatigue, and stamina, as well as some objective evidence of increase in measured exercise tolerance, systemic blood flow, and vascular resistance. Cerebral blood flow is decreased, but without treatment the reduction is less at equivalent PCV levels than in the nonhypoxic polycythemias. This may explain why the incidence of cerebral OVL may be lower in this form of polycythemia than in the nonhypoxic types. It is nevertheless an important complication. In one series of patients with pulmonary hypoxic polycythemia, death was due to OVL in 14 percent of cases; in another series, 11 percent of patients had nonfatal OVL.

Therefore, on all accounts, this form of polycythemia should be treated by reduction of high PCV (55 percent [0.55] and above), preferably by careful, small, repeated (350 ml) venesections. Larger isovolemic exchange, using 4 percent dextran in saline or a similar plasma expander, carries risks and is rarely justified. The danger of disease transmission suggests that plasma itself should not be used for replacement.

Limited objective measurements indicate that the optimal PCV is around the 50 percent (0.50) level and that further reduction produces no further improvement. In practice, empiric clinical observation of the individual patient is probably the best method of deciding when the optimal PCV has been reached.

High oxygen affinity hemoglobinopathies (e.g., San Diego, Yakima) are relatively uncommon. In families studied, the PCVs are generally not higher than about 55 percent (0.55), and there is the expected increase in whole blood viscosity. However, the admittedly small number of studies of cerebral blood flow show that these subjects have higher than normal flow rates, supporting the view that oxygen delivery is the major determinant of flow. Even in the elderly, there is as yet no evidence of an increased incidence of cerebral OVL, and usually the patients are asymptomatic and not improved by venesection. On present evidence they should, therefore, be observed and *not treated.*

Diaphorase deficiency responds to specific therapy and rarely requires venesection.

Inappropriate Erythropoietin Group

Most commonly due to renal lesions such as carcinoma of the kidney, renal artery stenosis, and currently the post-transplant syndrome, these polycythemias have symptomatology and risk of OVL which are closely related to the PCV level. In most cases, the treatment of the polycythemia is by surgical correction or, in the case of post-transplant syndrome, by time. In all cases, however, the PCV should be reduced by venesection to around the 45 percent (0.45) level to reduce the risk of OVL and to prevent operative and postoperative complications, which include abnormal bleeding or thrombosis.

With inoperable lesions the PCV should be reduced to, and maintained around, the optimal level of 45 percent (0.45) by a longer-term venesection regimen.

Idiopathic Erythrocytosis

This is defined by a raised PCV associated with an absolutely increased red cell mass, the cause of which cannot be found after adequate investigation. Although the condition is sometimes called "benign" erythrocytosis, ther term "idiopathic" is preferable because in a number of these patients the erythrocytosis eventually undergoes transition to unequivocal primary paolycythemia (PRV), and all are at the same risk of OVL as are patients with primary polycythemia. Treatment therefore consists of venesection to the optimal maintained PCV—about 45 percent (0.45). The patient should continue to be observed for evidence of transition to primary polycythemia (splenomegaly, leukocytosis, increased leukocyte alkaline phosphatase, and thrombocythemia) and treated accordingly—one option being continued control of PCV by venesection rather than by chemotherapy or ^{32}P, using intermittent chemotherapy to control unacceptable thrombocythemia.

Smoking has more widespread implications than its usually modest effect on PCV level and will be discussed under *General Points in Treatment.*

RELATIVE (LOW PLASMA VOLUME) POLYCHTHEMIA

Acute fluid loss, if untreated, can result in occlusive vascular lesions (OVL).

Diuretics in relation to the polycythemias will be discussed under *General Points in Treatment.*

Idiopathic (low plasma volume) polycythemia is an elevation of the PCV due to a reduction of plasma volume below 15 percent of the patient's normal predicted value, in association with a normal red cell mass. The term "idiopathic" is preferred to "stress", "pseudo-polycythemia", "spurious polycythemia", Gaisböck's disease, and other terms, since they cause confusion and the cause *is* unknown. It is probably not primarily a hematologic disorder, but the result of some abnormality of plasma volume control. However, it does carry a risk of OVL equal to that of the absolute nonhypoxic polycythemias at equivalent PCV levels. Treatment regimens that directly attempt to raise the plasma volume (e.g., fludrocortisone, fluid infusion) are ineffective. Surprisingly, venesection to about 45 percent (0.45) produces not only the transient fall in PCV that might be expected from the different rates of renewal of red cells and plasma, but also a longer-lasting effect, often maintainable by an acceptably infrequent venesection regimen. This suggests that this treatment may, in some way, modify the aberrant plasma control mechanism.

APPARENT POLYCYTHEMIAS

The patient with apparent polycythemia usually has a resting PCV of not more than 54 percent (0.54), with red cell mass and plasma volume within the individual's predicted normal ranges (see Table 1). Some authors have called them "the physiological variants", whereas others deny that the group exists at all. In clinical practice, however, they are not an uncommon finding and, irrespective of cause or nature, require attention because (1) PCV in the 50 to 54 percent range may carry a risk of OVL, and (2) any patient who eventually develops some type of unequivocal polycythemia must pass through this "apparent" phase.

The indications for treatment are not clear and a research unit of the Royal College of Physicians (London) is now engaged in a prospective study of this group. In practice, there is strong argument for reducing, by venesection, a PCV of 50 percent or more in individual patients with hypertension or a history of occlusive vascular lesions, particularly when they are over age 50. At present it remains a matter of clinical judgment to decide between observation and treatment. Until the matter is objectively resolved, there is no case for embarkation on the massive, routine venesection program that would be necessary to treat all members of this group.

GENERAL POINTS IN TREATMENT

Venesection Regimens

In patients with nonhypoxic polycythemia in whom it is intended to reduce the PCV to around the 45 percent (0.45) level, 450-ml venesections two to three times weekly will effect this within 3 to 4 weeks without side effects. In pulmonary and cardiac hypoxia the approach should be more cautious with, in adults, clinically monitored venesection of 200 to 300 ml once weekly. Isovolemia, large-volume exchange is rarely necessary and can carry unacceptable risk. Exchange using cell-separator equipment is never necessary.

Careful follow-up is necessary, the frequency depending on the rate of rise of the PCV of the individual patient. The frequency of follow-up required may be as often as 10 times a year, though it is often less. This may seem tedious to patient and doctor, but there is little point in embarking on a treatment regimen if, for 50 percent of the time, the PCV is allowed to run at an unacceptably high level.

Chemotherapy and ^{32}P

While there is continuing debate on, and study of, the role of these forms of treatment in primary polycythemias (PRV), they have no place in the treatment of the group considered here. This is because of the now-established risk of inducing acute leukemia.

Iron Deficiency

Patients on a long-term venesection regimen invariably develop laboratory evidence of iron deficiency, reflected by microcytosis, some hypochromia, absent marrow iron and typical serum iron findings. Surprisingly, they rarely develop subjective or clinical evidence of iron deficiency. It has been suggested that iron-deficient red cells increase whole blood viscosity, but it is now established that this is not the case. Therefore, in the overwhelming majority of patients, iron therapy is unnecessary. Indeed, the induced iron deficiency is probably a factor in controlling unwanted rise in PCV, and administration of iron invariably produces a rapid rise, so that the natural temptation to prescribe it should be resisted. In the rare patient who does develop unacceptable glossitis, angular stomatitis, or "somatic" fatigue, an attempt should be made to strike the difficult balance between continued venesection and careful iron therapy.

Diuretics

Treatment with diuretics probably has an unjustified reputation for inducing relative (low plasma volume) polycythemia. In practice it usually produces a transient rise of no more than about 2 percent in the PCV (e.g., 48 to 50 percent or 0.45 to 0.50), often with subsequent reversion. There is no case for withholding diuretic therapy in the polycythemic patient if, for example, it is considered essential to the management of hypertension. It is better to continue with diuresis and venesect as required.

Smoking

In heavy smokers carbonmonoxyhemoglobin levels up to 11 percent may occur. This in itself may induce some degree of hypoxic polycythemia, but in addition there is evidence that smoking may independently contribute to the development of occlusive vascular lesions. The obvious treatment is to encourage abstinence. This is not always successful, and in persistent smokers, a PCV raised above 52 percent—whether due to smoking alone or to some unrelated cause—should be reduced by venesection.

POLYCYTHEMIA VERA

SCOTT MURPHY, M.D.

Polycythemia vera may have a highly variable clinical picture. It typically appears in the late middle age as a proliferation of all three cell lines of the marrow and is associated with splenomegaly. If inadequately treated, patients may experience thrombotic complications of the arterial and venous circulation as well as pathologic hemorrhage from the gastrointestinal tract and at the time of surgery. On the other hand, the proliferation of one cell lie may predominate, leading to variation in the clinical picture and necessitating appropriate therapy. In the late stages of this chronic illness, the proliferative phase may become spent, resulting eventually in the syndrome of postpolycythemic myeloid metaplasia or myelofibrosis. At this stage, the clinical problems are often anemia, thrombocytopenia, and the complications of massive splenomegaly. Unique manifestations of the disease which require attention are pruritus and hyperuricemia with symptoms of gout.

THERAPEUTIC ALTERNATIVES

There are both mechanical and pharmacologic approaches to the control of the proliferating tissue. An elevated hematocrit may be controlled by phlebotomy with removal of 250 to 500 ml of blood. In an acutely symptomatic patient with thrombocytosis, platelets may be removed on an emergency basis by thrombocytopheresis, using a variety of continuous flow and semicontinuous flow devices such as the Haemonetics Model 30 Cell processor, the Fenwal CS-3000 Cell Separator, or the IBM Blood Processor 2997. Finally, an enlarged spleen that is producing mechanical symptoms, anemia, thrombocytopenia or a combination thereof may be removed surgically.

Many drugs are effective in suppressing marrow proliferation. Since so many are effective, the choice among them is based not on efficacy alone, but on potential for short- and long-term complications. Radioactive phosphorus (^{32}P) essentially irradiates the bone marrow by lodging in marrow tissue and bone after injection. Although the mechanism of action is quite complex, alkylating agents act by cross-linking DNA, leading to permanent DNA damage. Effective drugs in this class are busulfan, melphalan, and chlorambucil. Antimetabolites, such as hydroxyurea, which acts by inhibition of ribonucleotide reductase, are also effective.

Supported in part by United States Public Health Service Grant CA 10728 from the National Cancer Institute to the Polycythemia Vera Study Group

Based on the assumption that thrombotic complications are related to inadequate control of platelet proliferation, drugs directed against platelet function have been employed. Chief among these have been aspirin and dipyridamole (Persantine). Aspirin acts by blocking the platelet enzyme, cyclo-oxygenase. This enzyme catalyzes the production of cyclic endoperoxides and thromboxane A_2, which induce platelet aggregation and vasoconstriction. The mechanism of action of Persantine is uncertain.

Drug therapy of pruritus in this disease is generally unsatisfactory. Cimetidine has been used most recently.

PREFERRED APPROACH

The therapeutic approach depends on several factors: the acute or chronic nature of the presentation, the presence or absence of symptoms, the patient's age, history of prior thrombotic or hemorrhagic manifestations, the cell line or lines predominantly involved, and, most importantly, the stage or phase of the disease.

Proliferative Phase—General Treatment

The patient may present as a medical emergency with severe symptoms secondary to an elevated hematocrit and expansion of the red cell mass. He should be "decompressed" by daily removal of 500 ml of blood until the hematocrit is below 50 percent. Phlebotomies may have to be smaller in volume or less frequent if the patient develops hypotensive symptoms secondary to a rapid reduction of blood volume. If emergency surgery is required, it is probably more important to control the hematocrit than the blood volume, in which case each phlebotomy may be accompanied by an infusion of an equal volume of albumin and electrolyte. Once acute "decompression" has been achieved, one may decide to use phlebotomy as the only mode of therapy. If so, phlebotomies should be continued on a weekly basis as needed to keep the hematocrit below 43 percent. This figure is controversial since many hematologists have been satisfied with a higher level. However, treatment with phlebotomy alone has been associated with an excess incidence of thrombotic complications. This may have been due to inadequate control of blood viscosity at higher hematocrits, since the iron-deficient red cell may be less pliable than normal. If myelosuppression is used, the range of 43 to 47 percent is probably acceptable. The choice between phlebotomy alone and myelosuppression will be discussed.

Patients with thrombocytosis may have alarming symptoms of central nervous system ischemia or peripheral extremity ischemia suggesting impending gangrene. They should be treated by plateletpheresis with return to them of their red cells and plasma. An eight-unit exchange should yield a one-third reduction of the total body platelet mass. Therefore, such an exchange, repeated on 3 or 4 consecutive days, should lower the platelet count satisfactorily as chemotherapy produces myelosuppression. This suggested dose of pheresis is simply a guideline, and therapy should be monitored with frequent platelet counts. Patients with symptomatology severe enough to require plateletpheresis should be treated with myelosuppression to control the platelet count.

As already implied, decision-making is more difficult in the patient whose hematocrit has been controlled by phlebotomy. Repeated phlebotomy produces iron deficiency which inhibits erythropoiesis. Therefore, the frequency of required phlebotomy decreases as time passes. Patients with clear-cut ischemic symptoms consistent with the effect of thrombocytosis and patients with anorexia, weight loss, sweating, and pain consistent with the effect of splenic enlargement should be treated with myelosuppression. The patient who is asymptomatic on phlebotomy therapy presents a difficult problem since, as will be discussed, the long-term effects of myelosuppression can be disastrous. However, patients treated with phlebotomy alone have an excess incidence of thrombotic complications, which are most pronounced in patients over 70 years of age and in patients who have had prior thrombotic events. These patients should be treated with myelosuppression. Young patients without symptoms or histories of thrombosis should be treated with phlebotomy alone.

Special Situations in the Proliferative Phase

Thrombocytosis

Many patients whose hematocrits have been controlled by phlebotomy will be left with an elevated platelet count, often in excess of $1{,}000{,}000/mm^3$. The patient may be asymptomatic or have only nonspecific, subjective symptoms such as headache, paresthesias, or visual disturbances. Some hematologists recommend the use of agents directed against platelet function, such as aspirin and Persantine, in these cases. However, aspirin increases the incidence of gastrointestinal hemorrhage when used in standard doses (600 to 900 mg daily), and there is no documentation that it reduces the incidence of thrombosis. It is preferable to do nothing.

On the other hand, there are patients who have persistent, clear-cut manifestations of microvascular occlusion, such as burning pain in the feet, hands, and digits, sometimes associated with pallor, erythema, or cyanosis. Patients often discover for themselves that aspirin (300 to 600 mg daily) controls these symptoms to a large extent. Reduction of platelet count with myelosuppression also generally controls these symptoms and is recommended. Aspirin can be continued until this occurs.

Erythemia

Patients with polycythemia vera have a panmyelosis with splenomegaly, leukocytosis, and thrombocytosis accompanying the increase in red cell mass. Occasionally, patients have only an increase in red cell mass and no discernible etiology for this. There is little known about the natural history of these patients, particularly their susceptibility to thrombotic complications. Perhaps they would do well with no therapy. However, it seems sensible to treat with phlebotomy, which is essentially risk-free, and to withhold myelosuppression even in the elderly patient.

Pruritus

Generalized pruritus, particularly severe after bathing, is seen in approximately 40 percent of these patients. It is generally mild and often improved by phlebotomy and/or myelosuppressive therapy. However, it may be persistent and incapacitating even after control of marrow proliferation and return of the blood counts to normal levels. Therapy is generally difficult, but cimetidine, 300 mg by mouth four times daily, may be effective.

Gout

Clinical complications of gout are more common in patients with polycythemia vera than in the general population, and an elevated uric acid is found in 40 percent of patients. In patients with elevated uric acid levels, allopurinol, 300 mg by mouth daily, should be administered to reduce the incidence of gouty complications.

The Spent Phase

As the years go by, the need for phlebotomy and myelosuppression gradually lessens and often ceases. In approximately 20 percent of patients, this spent phase progresses into the syndrome of postpolycythemic myeloid metaplasia characterized by marked splenomegaly in combination with varying degrees of anemia and thrombocytopenia. The major decision at this stage is whether or not to remove the spleen. Splenectomy is most helpful when the spleen is producing mechanical symptoms simply because of its size, when there is symptomatic thrombycytopenia, or when the anemia has a major hemolytic component as judged by a $_{51}Cr$ red cell survival study or by an excessive transfusion requirement (more than two units of blood every 2 to 3 weeks). Splenectomy has risks in addition to those associated with any major abdominal surgery. The major concern is postsplenectomy thrombocytosis, which may be extreme and difficult to control. In general, it is unwise to perform a splenectomy unless the platelet count is below the normal range. If it is not, one should consider a period of myelosuppression before the procedure.

Practical Considerations in Myelosuppression

Many agents are available to produce myelosuppression. Of these, three are most useful in polycythemia vera: hydroxyurea, busulfan, and radioactive phosphorus (^{32}P). Each may be used in conjunction with or after reduction of the hematocrit by phlebotomy.

Hydroxyurea

This is the drug of choice for the patient who is available for frequent monitoring of blood counts and who can be relied on to be compliant. The initial dose is 15 to 20 mg per kilogram of body weight per day, with modifications in increments of 5 mg per kilogram per day, downward for white count under 3500 per mm^3 or platelet count under 150,000 per mm^3, upward for inadequate reduction of hematocrit or platelet count. The optimal result is to achieve hematocrit less than 47 and platelet count less than 600,000 per mm^3. It is often necesary to accept leukopenia (3500 to 5000 per mm^3) and occasionally necessary to use supplemental phlebotomy to achieve this goal. In some patients, the platelet count cannot be reduced below 600,000 per mm^3 without lowering the white count below 3500 per mm^3. If the platelet count ranges from 600,000 to 1,000,000 per mm^3, this is an acceptable result.

If the drug is discontinued, unmaintained remissions are extremely short with rebound thrombocytosis frequently occurring in 7 to 10 days. This requirement for continuous therapy and the frequency of significant leukopenia necessitates frequent patient visits and blood counts, at least bimonthly for the first 3 months and monthly thereafter. Thus, the drug is unsuitable for the unreliable patient. Patients who have achieved a good response without supplemental phlebotomy after 6 weeks of therapy always have depleted marrow iron stores because of previous phlebotomies. A cautious trial of iron replacement, ferrous sulfate, 300 mg by mouth twice daily, may be given for the next 6 months to reduce possible complications of long-term iron deficiency. Many patients continue in a good response while others have an increase in hematocrit which cannot be controlled by increasing the hydroxyurea dose without unacceptable leukopenia. In the latter patients, supplemental phlebotomy should be used and chronic absence of iron stores accepted.

At least two-thirds of previously untreated patients have a good response with this regimen. Improvement in the blood counts is generally associated with shrinkage of the spleen, if enlarged, and at least some alleviation of pruritus. Continuing response is expected if the drug dosage is maintained. At intervals of 2 to 3 years, the drug may be stopped to assess the activity of the disease. In some patients, the blood counts remain stable, but in most, the drug has to be resumed.

Busulfan

Some patients treated with hydroxyurea have inadequate control of thrombocytosis and splenomegaly when doses producing leukopenia are used. Busulfan is a satisfactory drug for these patients. The dose is 4 mg per day by mouth for 1 to 2 months. Blood counts should be checked every 2 weeks at least. In the thrombocytotic patients, the drug should be stopped when the platelet count falls below 300,000 to 400,000 per mm^3. This generally occurs before there is a substantial fall in the white count. The goal in these patients should be to control the platelet count and spleen size. Supplemental phlebotomy may be used as needed.

In most patients, this course of treatment allows disease control for many months or years without further drug therapy. The patient should be followed at monthly intervals with phlebotomy as needed to maintain the hematocrit in the range of 43 to 47 percent. If thrombocytosis or splenomegaly recurs, an additional course of busulfan therapy may be given.

Radioactive Phosphorus (^{32}P)

^{32}P is the ideal form of therapy for the unreliable patient who requires myelosuppression; 2.3 mCi/m^2 is given intravenously and the dose is not to exceed 5 mCi. In the majority of patients, normalization of the hematologic picture and spleen size will occur over 2 to 3 months. A second smaller dose of 2 to 3 mCi may be required at 3 or 4 months to bring the disease under complete control. Remission frequently lasts 6 to 24 months or even longer. Follow-up visits are required only every 2 to 3 months.

Immediated Side Effects

With all three myelosuppressive drugs, the major immediate side effects are leukopenia and thrombocytopenia, which are reversible. A major advantage for hydroxyurea is that hematologic toxicity generally reverses itself within 1 to 2 weeks after the drug is discontinued. This is not the case for busulfan and ^{32}P. Although cytopenias generally last for only 3 or 4 weeks, busulfan-induced pancytopenia can persist for many months. Furthermore, chronic busulfan administration has been associated with irreversible pulmonary fibrosis. These are two of the reasons for choosing hydroxyurea as the first-line drug.

The control of myelopoiesis with hydroxyurea is associated with a reduction in the number of red cells produced and an increase in their size. Thus, the mean corpuscular volume (MCV) may be strikingly elevated to the range, 120 to 130μ^3. This is not associated with significant clinical complications.

Long-term Complications of Treatment

Treatment with alkylating agents and radiation is associated with secondary malignant disease of rapidly proliferating tissue, such as the bone marrow and gastrointestinal tract, beginning approximately 3 years after the onset of treatment. The frequency of such secondary malignant disease undoubtedly varies with the alkylating agent used and the schedule of administration. For example, brief exposures to an alkylating agent followed by long rest periods may be less mutagenic than continuous low-dose exposure. Hydroxyurea has not yet been associated with secondary malignant disease or other long-term complications. This is the major reason for choosing it as the first-line drug.

Pros and Cons of Treatment

In polycythemia vera, the hematocrit must be controlled to 43 percent or less if phlebotomy alone is used and to 43 to 47 percent if myelosuppression is used. Phlebotomy alone is associated with an increased risk for thrombotic complications, and myelosuppression would be recommended for all patients were it not for long-term complications. Such complications are definitely established for alkylating agents and radioactive phosphorus. One hopes that they will not be seen with long-term use of hydroxyurea, but the number of patients treated for long periods of time is still relatively small. Thus, phlebotomy alone is recommended for young patients without history of thrombosis who are asymptomatic after control of hematocrit.

CHRONIC GRANULOCYTIC LEUKEMIA

JOHN M. GOLDMAN, D.M., F.R.C.P.

Chronic granulocytic leukemia comprises about 20 percent of all cases of leukemia in the western world. Its overall incidence seems to be remarkably constant worldwide. The majority of patients present themselves with symptoms related to anemia, splenomegaly, or bleeding, but in increasing numbers of patients, the diagnosis is made before the onset of symptoms—leukocytosis is recognized as a result of a routine blood test for totally unrelated reasons.

When diagnosed the disease is usually in the "chronic" or "stable" phase without a major excess of blast cells in the blood or marrow. The median duration of this chronic phase (CP) is about 45 months, but individual patients may die within a few short months of diagnosis or may on occasion survive with little evidence of disease evolution for 10 or more years. Death when it occurs is usually due to rapid or insidious onset of blastic transformation (BT), in which phase immature blast cells predominate in the marrow and blood and the patient becomes unduly susceptible to infection associated with absolute granulocytopenia and to bleeding due to thrombocytopenia. In recent years clinicians have come to recognize in some patients a phase of the disease intermediate between stable CP and overt BT. This so-called accelerated phase (AP) is characterized by increasing thrombocytosis or thrombocytopenia, marked basophilia, an excess of blast cells that falls short of BT, fever, or a series of other features that indicate that the disease is evolving. In a minority of patients, the marrow shows steadily increasing fibrosis with peripheral pancytopenia, but some of these patients also ultimately experience a blastic phase of their disease.

INITIAL EVALUATION

Some patients are already aware of the diagnosis when first referred to a hematologist. However, it is probably advisable for the hematologist to obtain a history and to perform the physical examination before broaching the subject of diagnosis. He or she can then arrange for appropriate blood tests with a comment such as "Let us see whether your blood really is abnormal. Incidentally, what did your family doctor tell you about the results?" this is an important opportunity for the patient to reveal what he or she knows and to express any anxieties. The hematologist should not at this stage accept as accurate the referring physician's diagnosis; indeed, the intelligent patient expects the hematologist to form an independent opinion. Though strictly speaking a diagnosis of CGL can in almost all cases be made with confidence after examination of the peripheral blood film, it is good practice to carry out bone marrow aspiration and biopsy to confirm the myeloid hyperplasia with loss of marrow fat spaces. Moreover, cytogenetic analysis to detect the Philadelphia (Ph^1) chromosome is more reliable with marrow cells than with blood cells, and it is important to quantitate the degree of marrow fibrosis at diagnosis; this can only be done with an adequate bone marrow biopsy.

Once the diagnosis of Ph^1-positive CGL is confirmed, the nature of the disease should be explained to the patient and the overall therapeutic strategy discussed. Since there is no convincing evidence that to maintain the leukocyte count within the normal range prolongs the duration of the CP or of survival, the objectives of treatment in CP are simply to alleviate symptoms or to delay their onset. Thus the asymptomatic patient with a leukocyte count $<100,000/mm^3$ does not require urgent treatment. For patients with counts between 100,000 and $200,000/mm^3$, treatment within a few weeks of diagnosis is desirable to prevent symptoms, and for patients with count $>200,000/mm^3$, almost all of whom have symptoms related to anemia and/or splenomegaly, treatment should be started as soon as possible. If the leukocyte count is relatively low and it is feasible to delay chemotherapy, the reasoning should be explained carefully to the patient. There are a few patients who undoubtedly feel happier with their leukocyte counts strictly within the normal range, and chemotherapy need not necessarily be withheld from these patients.

Until recently it was our normal practice, before initiating chemotherapy with cytotoxic drugs, to subject a newly diagnosed patient to leukapheresis on the continuous flow blood cell separator with subsequent cryopreservation of blood-derived hemopoietic stem cells. These stem cells can be stored in liquid nitrogen for as many years as may be necessary and then used as autografts in the management of BT. Because the results of this approach to treatment are relatively unimpressive (to be discussed), we no longer routinely cryopreserve stem cells from all patients. An alternative approach, also not necessarily essential, would be to harvest hemopoietic stem cell from the patient's bone marrow. However, blood-derived stem cells are easier to collect and function as well as marrow cells as autografts in CGL.

Soon after diagnosis, the possibility of treatment by bone marrow transplantation (BMT) should be raised with the patient, who often has already himself wondered whether it was applicable in this case. For the present, one can immediately say that the procedure is too hazardous to consider in patients older than 50 or for those who lack HLA-identical brothers or sisters as donors. However, the situation may change if the present attempts to prevent graft-versus-host disease (GVHD) with ex vivo T-lymphocyte depletion with monoclonal antibodies are successful. For the younger patient, therefore, one may make arrangements as possible for HLA trying of all available siblings and perhaps other close family members. It is usually technically impossible to type the patient before the leukocyte count is restored to normal. Discussion of the details of BMT can await the identification of a suitable related donor.

CHOICE OF PRIMARY THERAPY

Between 1902 and 1954, newly diagnosed patients were routinely treated by radiotherapy. Originally radiotherapy was administered to the whole body from an external beam or by injection of ^{32}P; subsequently irradiation of the enlarged spleen was found to be equally effective in alleviating symptoms, reducing the size of the spleen and restoring the blood count to normal. In the last thirty years, patients in most centers have been treated at diagnosis with cytotoxic drugs, usually busulfan. In practice there is little to choose between busulfan, hydroxyurea, and dibromomannitol, and it seems reasonable to try to tailor the choice of drug and of dosage to the individual patient.

Busulfan

Busulfan (Myleran) is an alkylating agent first introduced into clinical practice in 1955. It was rapidly apparent that in comparison with other alkylating agents it acted with some selectivity on the myeloid series in blood and marrow and could rapidly restore the blood to complete normality. The appearance of the marrow, however, usually was little changed. It was also apparent that overdosage with busulfan produced aplasia of the bone marrow that could be prolonged and also fatal. It was thus recommended that treatment should begin with 6 mg (or perhaps 8 mg) daily and that the leukocyte count should be monitored closely, at intervals initially not greater than 7 days. If then the rate of fall of the leukocyte count was plotted on semi-log graph paper, dosage could be reduced or stopped before onset of pancytopenia. In practice it is a good rule to stop treatment when the leukocyte count has fallen to 20,000/mm^3 whereafter the count will continue to fall and may stabilize in the normal range. The very rare patient who is hypersensitive to standard doses of busulfan may enter a phase of aplasia within a few weeks of diagnosis; such patients may be detected by observing a very steep initial rate of fall of the leukocyte count soon after starting treatment.

Once the leukocyte count has fallen below 20,000/mm^3 the hemoglobin should have risen substantially, the spleen should have shrunk in size, and the patient should at this stage be totally free of symptoms. There are two approaches to further treatment. One may continue with busulfan at low dosage (e.g., 2 mg three times weekly), or one may stop busulfan completely and observe the patient. At least in the initial phase of treatment the latter course is preferable because it permits the hematologist to assess the duration of hematologic control induced by a single course of chemotherapy. This may in fact vary from a few weeks to two or more years. There is evidence that patients with long periods of hematologic normality may fare better than average whereas patients with a relatively large requirement for treatment during the first year after diagnosis may not reach the median survival time for CGL.

An alternative method of using busulfan is to administer single large doses of 50 or 100 mg. Thereafter the nadir of the leukocyte count is achieved after about 3 weeks, and a further dose can be given then or later according to the blood count. This method gives rather erratic control of the leukocyte count, but is advantageous in that the patient does not have to take daily drugs and the risk of accidental overdosage is greatly reduced.

Busulfan is routinely administered by mouth. Absorption from the gastrointestinal tract is almost complete. In standard dosage it causes no immediate side effects. However, it renders both sexes infertile in a dose-dependent manner. Women should be warned that their menstrual periods will probably cease permanently after treatment for weeks or months, and they may experience menopausal symptoms; men will become permanently azoospermic. Other side effects are less predictable. Some patients become increasingly pigmented after several years of treatment with busulfan. A syndrome superficially resembling Addison's disease and a progressive pulmonary fibrosis with cough and fever, designated "busulfan lung," occur in rare instances.

Hydroxyurea

The precise mode of action of hydroxyurea is unknown, but it probably acts by inhibiting ribonucleotide reductase, an enzyme required for de nova synthesis of deoxynucleotides. It thus blocks DNA synthesis and causes accumulation of cells in the S-phase of the cell cycle. It may be administered to the patient with a high leukocyte count at a starting dose of 2.0 g/day for 1 to 4 weeks, after which time the dose can be adjusted to maintain the leukocyte count in the normal range. The hematologic response to hydroxyurea is very different from that to busulfan. Hydroxyurea has little delayed effect, and the leukocyte count rises rapidly after the drug is stopped or dosage reduced. For this reason one can safely continue treatment until the leukocyte count is normal, and treatment, perhaps at reduced level, must be maintained indefinitely.

Hydroxyurea is relatively free of side effects. Some patients experience gastrointestinal disturbance with nausea and perhaps vomiting. The drug may also cause headaches. The drug causes megaloblastic change in the marrow, but the prolonged marrow hypoplasia that may follow overdosage with busulfan has not been reported after treatment with hydroxyurea.

Dibromomannitol

Dibromomannitol (Myelobromol) was developed in Hungary in 1961. (Although available in Europe it is not currently approved for use in North America.) It is brominated polyhydric alcohol, thought to represent a transitional form between alkylating agents and antimetabolites. The drug is usually administered at a dose of 250 to 850 mg daily, but clinical and hematologic responses are relatively slow. It may cause thrombocytopenia and gastrointestinal disturbances.

MANAGEMENT OF ACCELERATED PHASE DISEASE

The management of the patient in AP must be individualized. For example, the patient with increasing splenomegaly may benefit from splenectomy or splenic irradiation; splenectomy may be particularly valuable for the patient with splenomegaly and thrombocytopenia and/or anemia. A rising leukocyte or platelet count resistant to busulfan or to hydroxyurea may be held in check for a period by a combination of two cytotoxic drugs, such as busulfan and 6-thioguanine or hydroxyurea and 6-thioguanine. If the platelet count exceeds 1,000,000/mm^3, it may be expedient to treat the patient with antiplatelet agents, such as aspirin or dipyridamole. A low-grade fever, for which no infectious cause can be found, may also be a manifestation of acceleration and may respond to a change in schedule of cytotoxic drugs.

MANAGEMENT OF TRANSFORMATION

Once the disease has entered a phase of frank BT, the patient's life is usually measured in months. However, it has become clear that the response to chemotherapy depends to some extent on the phenotypic characteristics of the predominating population of blast cells. Thus blast cells in BT may manifest myeloblastic, monocytic, erythroblastic, megakaryoblastic, or lymphoid features or blast cells reflecting a number of these lineages may coexist, a so-called mixed transformation. A series of cell marker studies should therefore be performed when BT is diagnosed.

The majority of patients, perhaps 60 percent, undergo myeloid transformations. Treatment with increased dosages of single agents, such as busulfan, hydroxyurea, or 6-thioguanine, is often effective in reducing the blast-cell count, but the platelet counts usually fall also, often precipitously. An alternative approach is to treat the patient with drugs suitable for acute myeloid leukemia, for example a 5- or 7-day course incorporating daunorubicin, cytosine arabinoside, and 6-thioguanine. Such treatment reliably reduces the blast cell numbers in the blood and marrow, but CP hemopoiesis, constituting a form of remission, only follows in 10 to 20 percent of cases. More frequently the blast cell number rises again after a few days or weeks, or the patient remains in an aplastic phase until death from infection or hemorrhage.

A smaller portion of patients in BT, perhaps 25 percent, have blast cells with the phenotypic characteristics of pre-B lymphoblasts. The cells are typically positive for common ALL antigen and terminal deoxynucleotidyl transferase (TdT). The majority of these patients with lymphoid transformations respond to treatment with vincristine and corticosteroids. It is thus reasonable to treat all patients newly diagnosed in BT with vincristine (e.g., 1.4 mg/m^2 IV weekly for 2 or 3 doses) together with prednisolone (e.g., 100 mg daily for 2 weeks) while awaiting the results of marker studies, unless the transformation is unequivocally myeloid on morphologic grounds and also negative for TdT.

The patient with lymphoid BT who is successfully restored to CP hemopoiesis by chemotherapy will relapse in BT within a few months unless further chemotherapy is administered. The simplest approach to "maintenance" is to use the favored local protocol for maintaining adult acute lymphoblastic leukemia, which typically incorporates oral methotrexate and 6-mercaptopurine with spaced "reinductions" with vincristine, steroids, and an anthracycline. Because there is a substantial risk of neuroleukemia in these patients in second CP after lymphoid BT, prophylaxis with intrathecal methotrexate (e.g., 6 or 8 lumbar punctures with 10 or 12.5 mg methotrexate at weekly intervals) should be undertaken. Additional cranial irradiation (18 or 24 Gy) should also be considered if the "remission" appears durable.

If stem cells were cryopreserved at diagnosis, the patient may be treated by high-dose chemotherapy followed by autografting. A second CP is thereby predictably achieved in almost all cases, but its duration is short, averaging 3 to 4 months. The median duration of survival from autografting is about 6 months (range 1 to 30 months). The optimal drug schedule before autografting is not established; one could use a 5- or 7-day course of drugs appropriate to the treatment of acute myeloid leukemia or perhaps melphalan or cyclophosphamide at high dosage (e.g., 120 mg/m^2 or 4 g/m^2 respectively).

PLACE OF ALLOGENEIC BONE MARROW TRANSPLANTATION

The decision to recommend treatment of a patient with CGL by bone marrow transplantation must depend on consideration of the perceived risks of the procedure balanced against the likelihood of cure if the transplant is technically successful. At the time of this writing it appears that the risk of death due to the transplant, resulting mainly from graft-versus-host disease and associated complications, or from pneumonitis attributable in part to pulmonary irradiation or to cytomegalovirus infection, is about 20 percent. It is somewhat lower in younger patients and somewhat higher in patients aged 30 to 45. On the other hand, the risk of leukemic relapse seems definitely to be related to the phase of the disease at the time of BMT. Patients in CP appear to have an actuarial risk of relapsing (assuming they do not first die of other causes) of less than 10 percent during the first 3 years following BMT; the corresponding figures for patients transplanted in AP and in BT are about 45 percent and 60 percent respectively.

It thus seems reasonable to recommend allogeneic BMT to the younger patient with CGL while he or she remains in the CP of the disease provided he or she has an HLA-identical sibling donor. This means in practice that BMT should ideally be carried out within a few months, certainly within one year, of diagnosis. There will undoubtedly be patients whose life span is shortened as a result of a failed transplant, but one may hope that for the majority who survive the procedure, survival will be prolonged and a proportion may prove to have been cured. Because of the protracted natural history of CGL, 5 or perhaps 10 years must still elapse before the true cure rate after BMT can be predicted with any accuracy.

CHRONIC LYMPHOCYTIC LEUKEMIA

KANTI R. RAI, M.D.

The most common type of leukemia found in a population aged 50 years and over is chronic lymphocytic leukemia (CLL). The classical form of CLL is of the B-cell type (B-CLL); only about 5 percent of cases manifest as the T-cell type of CLL or as prolymphocytic leukemia. These two latter variants exhibit certain phenotypic and morphologic characteristics, and they are generally less responsive to therapy. However, there are no therapeutic approaches for these variants that are distinct from those applied in B-CLL. This discussion focuses upon management of patients with B-CLL. As is the case with many other malignancies, approach to treatment differs considerably in different centers. The treatment plan practiced in my clinic is detailed in this chapter.

OBSERVATION PHASE

It is our practice not to institute any cytotoxic therapy immediately upon making a diagnosis of CLL. A period of observation after diagnosis is advisable to determine if any treatment is indicated.

Clinical Staging of Chronic Lymphocytic Leukemia

It is first necessary to establish the clinical stage of a patient newly diagnosed as having CLL. The criteria of staging are given as follows:

Stage 0. This stage presents with lymphocytes only in the peripheral blood and the bone marrow. Although an absolute lymphocyte count of 5,000 per mm^3 is an acceptable definition of lymphocytosis in peripheral blood, in most instances this count is over 15,000. Bone marrow aspirate must show more than or equal to 30 percent of mature appearing lymphocytes upon differential count of all nucleated cells, or a biopsy specimen must show lymphocytic infiltration.

Stage I. This stage exhibits lymphocytosis with evidence of enlarged lymph nodes.

Stage II. This stage exhibits lymphocytosis with evidence of enlargment of the spleen and/or the liver. As well, lymph nodes may or may not be enlarged.

Stage III. Stage III is characterized by lymphocytosis with anemia (hemoglobin <11 g percent). The nodes, spleen, and liver may or may not be enlarged.

Stage IV. This stage exhibits lymphocytosis with thrombocytopenia (platelets $<100{,}000$ per mm^3). Anemia and enlargement of nodes, spleen, and liver may or may not be present.

After the clinical stage is determined, I try to find out if symptoms (e.g., weight loss, night sweats, fever, increased susceptibility to infections, and weakness) are present. In addition, blood counts are serially monitored at intervals of 2 to 4 weeks.

INDICATIONS FOR THERAPEUTIC INTERVENTION

After an observation period of about 4 to 6 months, during which time the patient is seen regularly in the clinic, a decision is made about whether therapeutic intervention is necessary. I use the following indications as guidelines and institute therapy, if any one of these is present:

- Progressive disease-related symptoms.
- Evidence of progressive marrow failure (i.e., worsening anemia, thrombocytopenia, and recurrent sepsis associated with granulocytopenia).
- Autoimmune hemolytic anemia or immune thrombocytopenia.
- Massive splenomegaly with or without evidence of hypersplenism.
- "Bulky" disease as evidenced by large lymphoid masses.
- Progressive hyperlymphocytosis. The rate of increase of blood lymphocyte count is a more persuasive indicator than is the absolute number.

I generally do not withhold therapy when the count is greater than 200,000 per mm^3. Leukostasis, which is associated with a high leukocyte count in other leukemias, is seldom encountered in CLL.

On rare occasion, however, the patient is markedly symptomatic at the time of initial diagnosis of CLL. It may not be advisable to withhold therapy under such a circumstance. I do not go through an observation period, but institute therapy immediately in these patients.

THERAPEUTIC PLAN FOR SPECIFIC INDICATIONS

Progressive Disease-Related Symptoms

Usually such symptoms are controlled with chlorambucil and prednisone. I prefer to give intermittent bursts of treatment at intervals of 3 to 4 weeks rather than to treat by continuous daily regimens throughout the month. Chlorambucil is given, 0.6 mg per kilogram by mouth in a single dose on day 1, day 28, and so forth. Prednisone is given, 0.5 mg per kilogram by mouth in one dose daily for 7 days (days 1 through 7) in each monthly cycle. Concomitantly, allopurinol, 300 mg daily by mouth, is prescribed for 7 days of each cycle. Usually, symptoms (e.g., weakness, night sweats, fever, etc.) are controlled within 6 to 8 months after institution of therapy when such therapy may be discontinued and the observation phase resumed.

Evidence of Progressive Marrow Failure

This is treated in the same manner as detailed above, that is to say by intermittent chlorambucil and prednisone.

Autoimmune Hemolytic Anemia or Immune Thrombocytopenia

Prednisone alone is given for these complications. Prednisone is started at 0.8 mg per kilogram per day by mouth for 2 weeks and if the anemia or the thrombocytopenia has started to improve, the prednisone dose is reduced by 50 percent at each 2-week interval for an overall continuous therapy of 6 weeks' duration. Thereafter, prednisone may be given for 1 week every month at 0.5 mg per kilogram per day for an additional 4 to 6 month period.

It should be emphasized that patients with CLL are generally elderly people with a somewhat higher incidence of diabetes mellitus. Therefore, special attention must be given to control hyperglycemia, which may be exaggerated with prednisone therapy.

Massive Splenomegaly With or Without Evidence of Hypersplenism

Radiation therapy of the spleen is our first choice of treatment. Usually total doses between 250 and 1,000 rads, delivered in 5 to 10 fractions, are adequate to reduce spleen size and control hypersplenism. However, if there is inadequate control with radiation therapy or the spleen again enlarges to significant proportions and hypersplenism remains a major problem, splenectomy is advisable. Even elderly patients with good cardiopulmonary status withstand this surgery without undue morbidity. However, it should be noted that if massive splenomegaly is not a solitary feature of a patient's disease, chemotherapy should be the initial therapeutic choice. If hypersplenism and splenomegaly persist after an adequate trial, splenic irradiation or splenectomy should be considered.

"Bulky" Disease of Large Lymphoid Masses

Most often chlorambucil therapy (without prednisone) at the dosage already detailed is adequate to reduce the size of large lymphoid masses. Such therapy is usually necessary for a period of 1 to 2 years on an intermittent monthly schedule. However, if the lymphoid masses are not generalized, but are present at only one or two sites or such masses are causing, or likely to cause, symptoms by pressing upon adjacent vital organs (e.g., on a bronchus or the superior vena cava), local irradiation therapy is recommended. The total dose necessary under these circumstances ranges between 500 to 1,500 rads delivered in 5 to 15 fractions.

Progressive Hyperlymphocytosis

Usually chlorambucil at the dosage already detailed is adequate to reduce the blood lymphocyte count. If resources are available, it is recommended that leukapheresis be the first step in therapy when the starting blood count is in excess of 600,000 per mm^3; chlorambucil therapy is initiated immediately after 3 to 4 treatments on a cell-separator machine. Side effects of chlorambucil are usually mild nausea and minimal suppression of bone marrow function.

THERAPEUTIC GUIDELINES BASED ON CLINICAL STAGING

Stage 0. Patients in this stage are generally without any symptoms and no cytotoxic agent is prescribed. However, they should be seen in the clinic at intervals of 1 to 3 months. Median life expectancy is in excess of 12 years.

Stages I and II. Stages I and II are asymptomatic and there is no evidence that cytotoxic therapy is necessary or beneficial in these patients. I continue to observe these patients at monthly intervals. The median life expectancy of these patients ranges between 6 and 8 years and is probably not changed with therapy.

Stages I and II. Stages I and II are symptomatic and I recommend chlorambucil for these patients on an intermittent, monthly schedule at the dosage already detailed. The median life expectancy of these patients ranges between 3 and 5 years. It is not yet known whether therapy increases life expectancy.

Stages III and IV. Patients in these stages have a median life expectancy of 1.5 years. I give chlorambucil and prednisone to these patients as per the dosage already detailed. The therapeutic objective is to achieve a partial or a complete remission. Usually it takes 8 to 10 months of therapy to achieve a partial remission. Patients achieving either a complete or a partial remission have prolongation of median survival time to about 5 years, whereas those patients achieving less than a partial remission have a 1.5-year median survival.

Alternative to Chlorambucil

I use cyclophosphamide in lieu of chlorambucil if the patient cannot tolerate the latter drug or is no longer showing a satisfactory response to it. Cyclophosphamide is administered by mouth or by intravenous injection. The dose of cyclophosphamide, on intermittent schedule, is 200 mg per meter squared per day by mouth for 5 days in cycles that repeat at 3-week intervals or 750 mg per meter squared on day 1 by intravenous injection every 3 weeks. Toxicity of this drug consists of controllable nausea and vomiting, hair loss, bone marrow suppression, and chemical cystitis.

Second-Line Therapy

When single-agent therapy (chlorambucil or cyclophosphamide) with or without prednisone fails to control CLL-related problems, we resort to combination chemotherapy. These are combinations that are usually administered in treatment of non-Hodgkins lymphoma or multiple myeloma, e.g., cyclophosphamide, vincristine and prednisone (COP), COP with doxorubicin (CHOP) and COP with bisnitrosourea (BCNU) and alkeran (M-2 protocol). The dosages utilized in each drug combination are decided upon after considering each patient's bone marrow reserve, previous exposure and level of tolerance of cytotoxic therapy, and the overall medical status.

Assessment of Therapeutic Response

I define a complete remission (CR) when there are no symptoms, no abnormal findings on physical examination, and hemogram and bone marrow reveal normal values. If all these criteria are fulfilled, but serum immunoglobulin levels are still lower than normal, or there is persistence of increased B-lymphocytes, I would rate such a response as CR. Achievement of even such a CR is a rather unusual occurrence in CLL, and it is my belief that our target must be to increase the incidence of CR according to this clinical definition before we can aim to achieve a CR which would include normalization of immune function and lymphocyte subpopulations ratios as well. A partial remission (PR) is defined as a 50 to 75 percent decrease in absolute lymphocyte count in peripheral blood, hemoglobin more than 11 g percent, platelets more than 100,000 per mm^3 or improvement in these values by 50 to 75 percent of their deviation from normal and decrease in palpable lymph nodes and spleen by at least 50 percent.

SUPPORTIVE THERAPY

In order to control signs and symptoms of anemia, transfusion of packed red cells is given as supportive therapy. Transfusions of platelets and granulocytes are rarely given in CLL. Intramuscular injection of 5 to 10 ml of gammaglobulin is given at intervals of 2 to 4 weeks to those patients who have marked hypogammaglobulinemia associated with recurrent bacterial infections. High-dose gammaglobulin therapy by intravenous route, 400 mg per kilogram body weight every 21 days, may be of benefit to these patients. There are no contraindications to give pneumococcal vaccine or flu vaccine, but the usefulness of such vaccines is in doubt in patients with CLL. Analogs of androgens have been effective on a few occasions by stimulating erythropoiesis in patients with significant anemia. However, such a therapy may be associated with adverse side effects of hepatotoxicity, fluid retention, exacerbation of symptoms of prostatic hypertrophy in men, and masculinizing effects in women.

TERMINAL PHASE OF CLL

In CLL, death occurs most often from infectious complications secondary to disease-induced or therapy-induced neutropenia and immunodeficiency. These complications are especially difficult to control in advanced stages of CLL. Prolymphocytoid transformation is frequently recognized towards the end of the clinical course of CLL when lymphocyte morphology is reviewed periodically. Less frequently, a diffuse large cell lymphoma supervenes as a terminal stage of CLL. Such cases receive aggressive chemotherapy generally used in high grade lymphoma, but there is little evidence that any regimen is effective in prolonging life. Even less frequently, CLL transforms into acute myelocytic leukemia, which is also refractory to intensive therapy that is currently used successfully in de novo acute leukemia.

Acknowledgement: Supported by grants from Helena Rubinstein Foundation, Rosenstiel Foundation, Doyle Dane Bernbach, Mr. Ned Doyle, National Leukemia Foundation, United Leukemia Fund, and Wayne Goldsmith Leukemia Fund.

ACUTE LYMPHOBLASTIC LEUKEMIA IN CHILDHOOD

ARNOLD I. FREEMAN, M.D.
MARTIN L. BRECHER, M.D.

Acute lymphoblastic leukemia accounts for approximately 80 percent of childhood leukemia, and the ensuing discussion will deal solely with this entity. Acute myelocytic leukemia, also seen in childhood, is similar to that seen in adult life and may be found in another chapter in this book.

CLASSIFICATION

A classification of various subtypes of acute lymphoblastic leukemia (ALL) is essential to the individualization of treatment for subgroups of patients, i.e., all patients may not require extremely intensive therapy, and the toxicity from such an approach may outweigh the benefits; conversely, inadequate therapy may lead to early relapse and death.

Morphology

Morphologically, ALL is divided into three groups, according to the combined French, American, and British (FAB) classification (Table 1).

Immune Phenotype

ALL has also been divided into several groups according to immunologic heritage:

Null cell ALL—accounts for 2/3 of patients (approximately 10% of these are negative for common ALL antigen-CALLa)

Pre-B-cell—15–20%
B-cell—<1%
T-cell—15–20%

PROGNOSTIC FACTORS

A number of presenting features exert prognostic significance, the best known being age and white blood cell count (WBC). In addition, race, immune phenotype, hemoglobin, FAB classification, sex, liver and spleen size, central nervous system (CNS) disease, and chromosome findings are of considerable importance. Many of these features may be interrelated, as in the case of the teenage boy presenting with a very high WBC, a large mediastinal mass, and T-cell markers; such a youngster has a very poor prognosis.

Age

Children who are 2 to 9 years of age have the best prognosis. Infants less than one year of age have a poor prognosis and an increased predisposition to be CALLa-negative. With increasing age over 10 years, patients have an increasingly worse prognosis, i.e., teenagers older than 15 years of age have a worse outlook than those aged 10 to 15.

White Blood Count

Patients with a high WBC at presentation have a worse prognosis, and survival is inversely related to the height of the WBC.

TABLE 1 FAB Classification of Acute Lymphoblastic Leukemia

Cytologic Features	L_1	L_2	L_3
Cell size	Small cells predominate	Large, heterogeneous	Large and homogeneous
Nuclear chromatin	Homogeneous in any one case	Variable-heterogeneous in any one case	Finely stippled and homogeneous
Nuclear shape	Regular, occasional clefting or indentation	Irregular, clefting and indentation common	Regular-oval to round
Nucleoli	Not visible or small and inconspicuous	One or more present, often large	Prominent, one of more vesicular
Amount of cytoplasm	Scanty	Variable, often moderately abundant	Moderately abundant
Basophilia of cytoplasm	Slight or moderate, rarely intense	Variable, deep in some	Very deep
Cytoplasmic vacuolation	Variable	Variable	Often prominent

L_1, the most common type (84%) seen in childhood, has the best prognosis; L_3 (1%) has Burkitt's-like morphology and a very dismal outlook, whereas L_2 (14%), with somewhat larger cells than L_1, has been claimed by some investigators to fall intermediate to prognosis.

Immune Phenotype

Patients with T-cell leukemia have a worse prognosis than patients with null cell disease. These patients have a lower induction rate into complete remission and a shorter duration of complete remission. This group of patients also has a greater tendency for extramedullary relapse, especially in the CNS and testes.

Patients with B-cell leukemia are rare and have a dreadful prognosis with a median survival of less than one year.

The pre-B immune phenotype has the same excellent induction rate (95%) as their null cell counterparts, but they experience a greater incidence of systemic and CNS relapse than patients with null cell leukemia.

Chromosomes

Patients whose lymphoblasts are hyperdiploid have a better prognosis than patients whose leukemic cells are pseudodiploid or hypodiploid. Translocation is also associated with a worse prognosis.

TREATMENT

General Considerations

A cancer theoretically may arise from a single cell transforming into a cancer cell. Tumor growth then follows the Gompertzian curve. A 1-cm mass has already passed through 30 doublings. Thus, all cancers when diagnosed are relatively far advanced biologically, even though they may be recognized early in their clinical disease. A child presenting with ALL harbors from 10^{11} to 10^{12} leukemic cells (10^{12} cell has been estimated to weigh approximately 1 kg).

A chemotherapeutic eradication of cancer cells follows first-order kinetics, i.e., a constant percentage rather than a constant number of cells is killed by a couple of drugs. Vincristine and prednisone can reduce the leukemic burden from 10^{12} to 10^{8} by killing 99.99 percent of these cells, and this results in a complete remission. Cure probably requires eradication of every last leukemic cell.

The cell cycle is defined as the interval between the mitosis and the midpoint of the subsequent mitosis in one or both daughter cells. The cycle is subdivided into four phases. The G_1 phase is the first phase during which cells synthesize ribonucleic acid (RNA), enzymes, and proteins in preparation for deoxyribonucleic acid (DNA) synthesis. The G_1 phase is the most variable in time; slowly growing populations contain cells that have long G_1 periods. The S phase is the period during which the DNA replicates and chromosomal proteins are laid down on the newly synthesized DNA. The G_2 phase is the interval between the completion of DNA synthesis and mitosis. In this period, the substrates necessary for the two daughter cells are produced. The M phase is the period of mitosis. In any tumor cell population, some cells are cycling continuously while others may be in the G_0 or resting state. Cells in the G_0 phase, although not actively proliferating, have the potential to re-enter the proliferating pool and cell cycle.

Certain anti-leukemic drugs such as methotrexate, an antimetabolite, require the cell to be synthesizing DNA to exert its cytotoxic effect, whereas vincristine exerts its effect in mitosis. These agents are termed "cell cycle specific" agents. Other agents, such as the alkylating agents, have the ability to destroy leukemic cells whether they are passing through cycle or not; these are termed "non cell cycle specific" agents.

Up to 60 percent of nonchemotherapeutic drugs can influence the action and/or toxicity of chemotherapeutic drugs. For example, methotrexate is 60 percent bound to albumin, but weak acids such as aspirin can free methotrexate from its binding sites, thus increasing its bioavailability.

Drug Resistance

At present, the most prevalent theory is that when a cancer is large enough to be diagnosed, resistant clones are already present. These resistant clones may then be "selected" by a drug as the sensitive cells are eliminated. As a result, the tumor will regrow from cells of the resistant clone. The probability of resistant clones increases parallel with the size of the tumor. Unfortunately, human cancers are biologically far-advanced by the time of diagnosis. There is, therefore, a high likelihood of the presence of resistant cells to any given agent at the time of diagnosis.

Alternating cycles of different effective groups of agents which are non-cross-resistant and equally effective may avoid the problem of emerging resistant cell lines and increase the likelihood of tumor eradication.

TREATMENT OF NEWLY DIAGNOSED ALL

This discussion will not encompass the general support for the child with acute leukemia, which includes the fluid and electrolyte problems and the care of the neutropenic febrile patient.

Induction

The induction phase converts florid disease into complete remission when there is no longer clinically detectable leukemia. When prednisone and vincristine are used, the median time to remission is slightly less than 4 weeks. During this time, the leukemia cell burden declines from approximately 10^{11} or 10^{12} to 10^{8} or less.

The induction agents commonly employed are steroids, vincristine, and L-asparaginase. Initially, L-asparaginase was utilized daily, generally for a 10-day course near the end of the induction program. More recently it has been employed earlier in induction; furthermore, it appears logical to employ L-asparaginase twice weekly, since a single injection of this drug depletes L-Asparagine in the serum for approximately 5 days. It has been our practice to avoid the anthracycline antibiotics (daunomycin and Adriamycin) in standard-risk patients (except in patients with T-cell or B-cell immune phenotype) because they have not been proved to increase the induction rate or the duration of complete remission in this group of patients and because of the potential long-term cardiotoxicity.

Intrathecal chemotherapy should be started during the induction phase. It has been our practice to delay intrathecal chemotherapy for one week from the onset of therapy because of (1) the theoretical risk of introducing leukemic cells into the cerebral spinal fluid (CSF) with a bloody tap if a lumbar puncture is performed on the first day when there are generally large numbers of circulating blasts, and (2) the large number of procedures done on the first day and the attendant pain and emotional turmoil.

The induction rates in standard-risk patients are higher than in increased-risk patients. In Cancer and Leukemia Group B (CALGB) study 7611 of ALL, 96 percent of the standard-risk patients achieved a complete remission (CR), whereas only 88 percent of the increased-risk patients achieved a complete remission.

Slow Inducers and Induction Failures

It has been reported that children who did not achieve a complete remission by week 4 fared significantly worse than those who did, even if they were later "pushed" into complete remission with further therapy. This has also been our experience. Therefore, these patients should be regarded as an extremely poor-risk group even if they eventually achieve complete remission. The use of very aggressive regimens following induction should be explored. Bone marrow transplantation should also be considered as an alternative.

CNS Phase

CNS "prophylaxis" is very important in the overall management of children with ALL, since without this, over half the children would develop overt CNS leukemia, which confers a much poorer chance for survival. Specific CNS therapy with intrathecal and/or cranial radiation therapy (CRT) to the CNS is needed because of the blood-brain barrier (BBB), which excludes most of the effective agents from the CNS. From this vantage point, in 1968 investigators at St. Jude's instituted therapy with 2400 rads of CRT and intrathecal methotrexate, which successfully reduced the incidence of CNS leukemia to less than 10 percent and raised the cure rate to 50 percent. At the same time, investigators in CALGB, in two separate studies, employed a limited number of doses of intrathecal methotrexate alone as CNS prophylaxis and also observed a reduced incidence of CNS leukemia, but not as effectively as CRT plus intrathecal methotrexate.

Recently, Bleyer et al showed that administering intrathecal methotrexate on the basis of CNS volume (which relates to the age of the patient) rather than body surface area was a more rational technique and resulted in less CNS relapse.

CRT plus intrathecal methotrexate became the most commonly employed form of CNS prophylaxis, but within one decade, it became obvious that significant irreversible toxicities occurred secondary to CRT, particularly loss of IQ and learning deficits and reduced school performance. In the 1970's the Pediatric Oncology Group (POG) investigated the use of repetitive intrathecal chemotherapeutic drugs to prevent CNS leukemia (intrathecal methotrexate, Ara-C, and hydrocortisone). Data from POG showed absolutely no difference in the incidence of CNS leukemia or overall CR rate when CRT was compared with repetitive intrathecal chemotherapy. Here the overall incidence of CNS relapse as the first site of failure, with intrathecal chemotherapeutic drugs alone or with CRT and intrathecal chemotherapeutic drugs, was approximately 10 percent. In an attempt to reduce CNS toxicity, Children's Cancer Study Group (CCSG) reduced the dose of CRT to 1800 rads. Results with 1800 rads were equal to those with 2400 rads.

A pilot study at Roswell Park Memorial Institute employed intermediate dose methotrexate (IDM) at 500 mg/m^2 to determine whether IDM could penetrate into the CSF and simultaneously intensify treatment systemically. The pharmacologic basis for the use of IDM was information showing that intravenous methotrexate at 500 mg/m^2 resulted in methotrexate levels of 10^{-7} in the CSF and 10^{-5} in the serum.

In addition to methotrexate, other drugs possess the ability to cross the blood-brain barrier and provide sanctuary therapy along with simultaneous systemic intensification. Ara-C, when administered at 100 mg/m^2 by continuous infusion, results in a ratio of CSF-to-plasma Ara-C of 1:4. Ara-C given at high doses (3 g/m^2 every 12 hours) results in high levels in the CSF and obviates administration of Ara-C via the intrathecal route. Several studies have now shown that high-dose Ara-C alone or followed by L-asparaginase cleared the CSF of leukemic cells.

Sanctuary, Intensification, or Consolidation Therapy

The objective of this phase is to eliminate or at least further decrease the leukemic burden and to simultaneously penetrate sanctuaries and eliminate nests of leukemic cells in these sanctuaries.

In a national study (CALGB), the duration of hematologic remission was statistically superior for standard-risk patients who received IDM on three occasions when compared to those who received CRT. Furthermore, testicular relapse also was statistically less frequent in patients who received IDM.

Furthermore, when the IDM was further intensified to six courses, increased-risk patients who received the six courses had a significantly superior duration of CR when compared in a retrospective analysis to those patients who received only three courses of IDM. This was due to greater systemic protection against hematologic relapse.

Recently it has been shown that continuing L-asparaginase during the first 6 months of treatment has improved the cure rate in children with ALL.

The West Germans employed a very intensive drug consolidation phase for several months. The results of their study showed a 78 percent CR for patients with standard, intermediate, and poor prognoses and demonstrated superior results when retrospectively compared to their prior study.

Preliminary results employing VM-26 and Ara-C as intensification in increased-risk patients also are suggestive of improvement in CR duration.

Thus, it appears that early intensification will play an expanded role in future studies of ALL.

Maintenance

The concept of maintenance therapy arose when patients with ALL were randomized either to receive or not to receive 6-mercaptopurine (6-MP) maintenance therapy following induction with prednisone and 6-MP. Patients who continued daily oral 6-MP following induction had a considerably longer duration of remission than those who received induction therapy only, and it became common practice to add maintenance therapy. The term "maintenance" and the concepts that it evokes are now likely to be counterproductive. It is unlikely that total cell kill is best achieved by administering relatively low-dose oral chemotherapy for 3 years. If the goal is eradication of all leukemic cells, alternating intensive cycles of different efficaceous agents appears to be a logical technique for destroying these blasts and avoiding resistance. Most current protocols do not adhere to such a formula. Various large studies have tested maintenance for periods of 2 to 7 years; currently, a period of 3 years is most commonly employed. The most critical time in therapy appears to be the first 6 months to one year. If aggressive high-dose therapy cannot eradicate all leukemic cells by this time, it seems unlikely that relatively low-dose oral therapy for 2 to 3 years can achieve this goal.

Following cessation of therapy at 3 years, the overall relapse rate is approximately 25 percent. It occurs most frequently in the first year, becomes progressively less common until the fourth year, after which it is very rare. When relapse does occur, it occurs in the bone marrow in 80 percent of patients. However, it is logical that the type and intensity of treatment will influence the relapse rate as well as the pattern of relapse following cessation of treatment.

SUMMATION AND RECOMMENDATIONS FOR THE TREATMENT OF FIRST-LINE PATIENTS

This treatment program (Fig. 1) is a reasonable approach for standard-risk patients and some increased-risk patients with ALL, i.e., patients from 1 through 14 years of age with a WBC up to 50,000/mm^3. Patients with T-cell markers and B-cell markers should also be excluded from this regimen. Note that dexamethasone is used in place of prednisone; this is due to the fact that recent data demonstrates superiority in CNS protection with this agent as compared with prednisone. L-asparaginase is utilized twice weekly during induction. The intensification/sanctuary phase employs IDM at 1 g/m^2 on six occasions. This is employed because IDM given on six occasions was superior to IDM given on three occasions. L-asparaginase is given the day after methotrexate because of potential synergistic effect with methotrexate and because even when given without methotrexate during the first 6 months of treatment, it has improved the duration of complete remission. L-asparaginase is administered intramuscularly since there is a much lower incidence of anaphylaxis ($<1\%$) when it is given

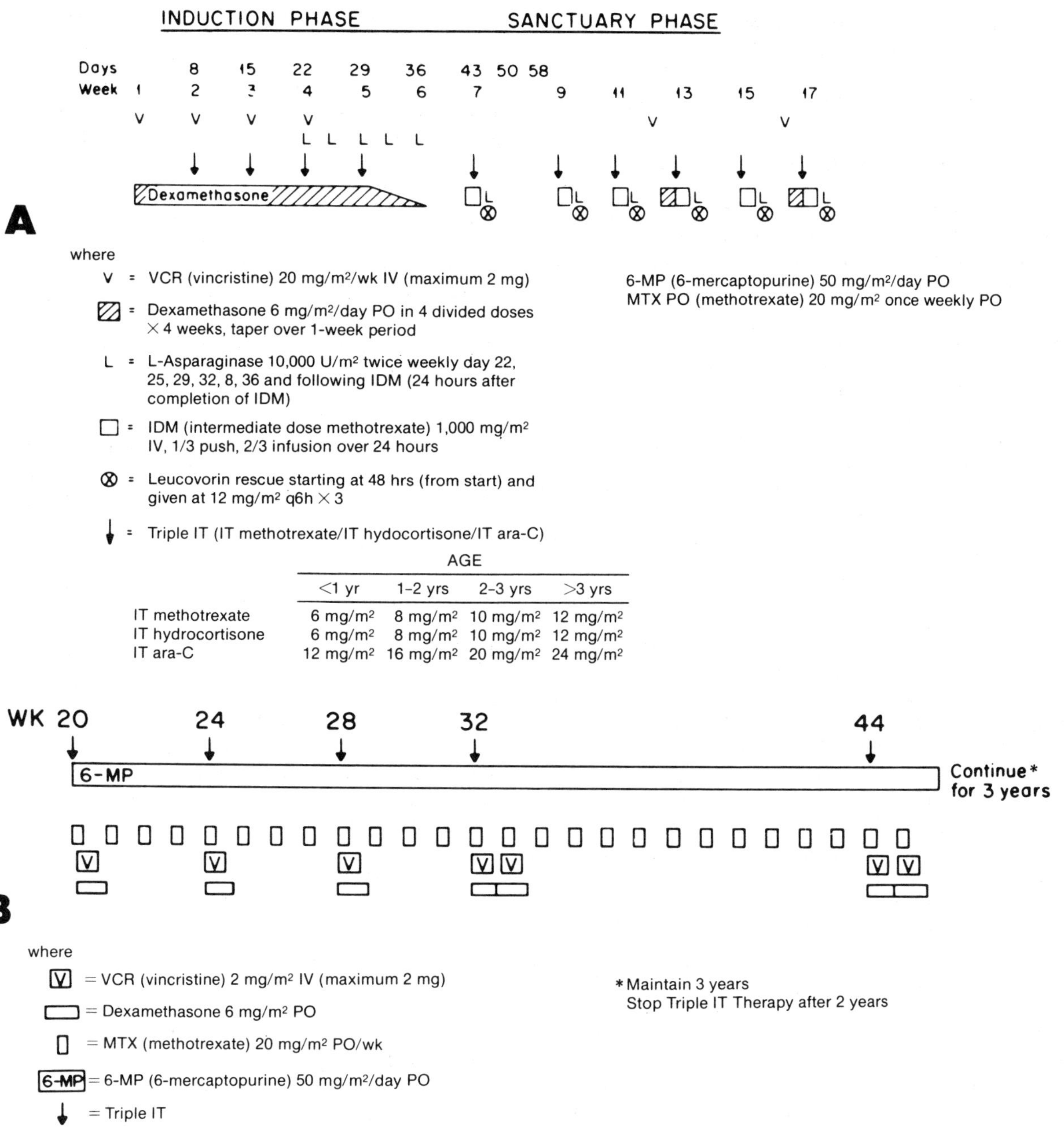

Figure 1 *A*, Induction phase and intensification phase suggested as a reasonable approach for standard-risk patients with ALL. *B*, Continuation phase for these standard-risk patients.

via this route instead of intravenously. However, when intramuscular L-asparaginase is utilized, delayed anaphylaxis may occur. Therefore it has been our practice to observe these patients for 5 to 6 hours following intramuscular administration.

The amount of leucovorin neutralization is also limited because of theoretical risks that excessive leucovorin may make the leukemic cells more resistant to subsequent doses of methotrexate.

Triple intrathecal chemotherapy is employed. Methotrexate should be administered at doses recommended by Bleyer:

Age	<1 yr	1–2 yrs	2–3 yrs	>3 yrs
MTX dose	6 mg	8 mg	10 mg	12 mg

An equivalent dose of hydrocortisone and double the dose of Ara-C should be used. Basing intrathecal dosing on age rather than body surface area is logical because the volume of the CSF is more closely related to the age and is not direclty related to the body surface area.

Intrathecal chemotherapy should be maintained periodically for one to two years. We do not employ CRT in this group of patients because such treatment has demonstrated results equal to CRT plus intrathecal methotrexate and because CRT has resulted in mild global learning deficits, declines in school performance, and loss of approximately 10 to 12 IQ points.

TREATMENT OF HIGH-RISK ALL

The treatment of acute leukemia is changing so quickly that it is difficult to recommend an easy recipe for the best treatment of high-risk patients. In general, these patients should receive a much more intensive regimen than standard-risk ALL patients. Regimens utilizing the intensity of those used for acute myuelocytic leukemia (AML) are indicated.

An induction attempt with steroid, vincristine, and L-asparaginase still appears logical, and 75 to 90 percent of patients will achieve a complete remission with this program. Some investigators advocate the routine use of an anthracyline antibiotic (daunomycin or Adriamycin for induction) in this group of patients. I would suggest that if the bone marrow on day 21 still shows greater than 5 percent blasts, daunomycin at 45 mg/m^2 daily × 3 should then be added. Following successful induction, intensive systemic therapy should be given for 3 to 6 months. During this time, intrathecal chemotherapy should also be given with each intensification course or at least monthly. Intensification may be administered with high-dose cyclical therapy. Cycles of IDM–L-asparaginase and high-dose Ara-C–L-asparaginase may be used. In addition, a course of continuous infusion Ara-C at 100 mg/m^2 for 7 days, 3 days with daunomycin, may be given. We have also administered high-dose cyclophosphamide to these patients during intensification. These regimens (except IDM–L-asparaginase) are extremely ablative to the bone marrow, and these patients must be monitored very closely. Patients become profoundly neutropenic, and in the large majority of cases, they become febrile, frequently due to serious infections. Therefore, it is recommended that only centers with the facilities, manpower, and expertise to support such patients should embark on this type of regimen. Furthermore, these treatments should be administered according to a rigidly controlled protocol.

Following the intensive phase, patients can receive CRT of 1800 rads plus limultaneous intrathecal chemotherapy. They then may be maintained with the standard regimen of daily oral 6-MP, weekly oral methotrexate, and weekly pulses of steroid and vincristine for a total of 2 years of therapy. Note that the patients are "front-loaded" with intensive chemotherapy prior to CRT to enable these drugs to be delivered because bone marrow relapse is a much greater problem than CNS relapse, and because they are "covered" with intrathecal chemotherapy during this time frame. There is also some evidence that the risks of toxicity to the brain are substantially less when intensive high-dose therapy, which crosses into the CNS, is given prior to CRT rather than following CRT.

BONE MARROW TRANSPLANTATION

It has been our practice to recommend tranplantation only for patients with ALL who have relapsed and then achieved a CR, i.e., we do not transplant patients on their initial presentation; this holds even for high-risk patients. However, standard chemotherapy following a bone marrow relapse results in a cure rate that approaches zero, whereas approximately one-fourth of such children with ALL who have a successful allogeneic bone marrow transplant can be cured of their disease following their first bone marrow relapse.

Following bone marrow transplantation in ALL, unlike AML, leukemic relapse is the major cause of failure.

In AML it has been shown that there is a graft-versus-leukemic effect resulting in an improved cure rate for patients who developed limited graft-versus-host disease. Unfortunately it is not possible to orchestrate therapy so that a limited graft-versus-host reaction occurs.

Another major defect with allogeneic transplants is the fact that only in approximately one-third of the cases is there a histocompatibility leukocyte antigen (HLA) identical donor.

RELAPSE

Although relapse of any type remains an ominous event, it no longer is universally fatal. Furthermore, major survival patterns have emerged, depending on the type and timing of relapse.

Relapse Following the Prescribed Completion of Therapy

Approximately 20 to 25 percent of patients who have successfully completed 3 years of CR will relapse after therapy has been electively discontinued. Relapse occurs in the first 4 years, the majority occurring in the first year. Approximately 75 to 80 percent of these relapses occur in the bone marrow, although CNS relapses and increasing numbers of testicular relapses have also been reported in recent years.

In patients being retreated a second time after cessation of therapy, the success rate is approximately 30 percent. The salvage rate appears higher in patients who have extramedullary relapse.

Patients should receive CNS prophylaxis again during retreatment. In children who have had prior CNS radiation, radiation should not be included a second time because of CNS toxicity.

It appears reasonable to regard these as high-risk patients and to give them intensive treatment. However, they may tolerate chemotherapy less well than a newly diagnosed patient and therefore must be monitored accordingly. It also appears reasonable to introduce new effective agents in their retreatment program.

If the relapse is an isolated CNS relapse and the patient has not received prior CRT, CRT therapy should be given following "front-loading" with intensive treatment and intrathecal chemotherapy.

Relapse While Receiving Therapy

Bone Marrow Relapse

To date, bone marrow relapse during chemotherapy has had a disastrous outcome; virtually all patient die of leukemia if they receive conventional therapy. The only notable exception to this occurs in children who achieve a CR and then successfully undergo transplantation. Nonetheless, this group of patients still has a high induction rate. Induction rates of 90 to 95 percent have been achieved by treatment with prednisone, vincristine, L-asparaginase, and daunomycin.

Although remission is readily induced, it is of short duration. Median remission durations of 5 or 6 months are usual.

Among the most successful regimens are a modified Capizzi regimen utilizing vincristine, IDM, and L-asparaginase every 10 to 14 days. Here the reported duration of CR is approximately one year. We are currently exploring whether alternating this regimen with high-dose Ara-C followed by L-asparaginase will extend the duration of remission.

Isolated CNS Relapse

It has been demonstrated that triple intrathecal therapy (methotrexate, Ara-C, and hydrocortisone), when given as maintenance following initial clearing of the CSF, resulted in significant prolongation of CNS remission.

Willoughby observed that radiation therapy to the CNS axis, following clearing of the CSF with intrathecal drugs, resulted in a low salvage rate. More recently, other investigators have shown a successful salvage of approximately 30 percent following CNS relapse. In these latter studies, systemic reintensification, including the use of new drugs, was utilized along with specific CNS therapy.

Thus we would recommend clearing of CSF with triple intrathecal chemotherapy and with systemic reinduction and intensification. New effective agents should be introduced. Of particular benefit may be agents that cross well into the CSF, such as high-dose Ara-C. Following this, cranial or craniospinal radiation may be employed. After radiation, a less vigorous chemotherapy schedule may be carried out. Current data indicate that 2 years of systemic treatment probably should be administered after an isolated relapse.

Testicular Relapse

Isolated testicular relapse may occur while the patient is on chemotherapeutic drugs or following the completion of the maintenance program. Males with T-cell leukemia and/or high WBC count are more likely to experience a testicular relapse. The type of systemic therapy employed plays an important role in the incidence of testicular relapse. The use of IDM has significantly reduced the frequency of testicular involvement.

Patients relapsing early during therapy have a poor prognosis, whereas the success rate is high in patients relapsing after the completion of therapy.

Isolated testicular relapse may foreshadow a bone marrow relapse since the leukemic recurrence frequently extends beyond the testicles. Therapy should be designed accordingly. This means that, in addition to radiation to the testes, systemic reinduction therapy must be employed, and several doses of intrathecal chemotherapy are also recommended.

For patients developing testicular relapse while receiving chemotherapy, it appears logical to switch drugs, as would be done with a bone marrow relapse.

LATE CNS TOXICITY

CNS toxicity, in particular, has been of great concern. Although some early reports suggested that CRT did not interfere with CNS function more extensive recent articles have clearly shown adverse effects.

We evaluated 106 children entered into three CALGB studies who had been randomized to receive intrathecal methotrexate alone, intrathecal methotrexate plus CRT, or intrathecal methotrexate plus IDM. In this study, children who received CRT scored consistently lower in verbal IQ, performance IQ, and full-scale IQ.

The drop in IQ among the radiated group was approximately 12 points. Children who received CRT also scored lower on WRAT tests—a measure of school performance. There were no differences between children who received IDM plus intrathecal methotrexate and those who received intrathecal methotrexate alone; that is; IDM given on three occasions was not appreciably toxic.

ACUTE MYELOCYTIC LEUKEMIA IN ADULTS

CLARA D. BLOOMFIELD, M.D.

Impressive advances in the treatment of adults with acute myelocytic leukemia (AML) have occurred during the last ten years. We have progressed from an era of palliation with only modest benefit from treatment to an era in which significant and increasing numbers of patients appear to be cured. Indeed, it is now possible to achieve complete remission rates of about 80 percent, median durations of remission of more than two years, and 5-year disease-free survival rates of more than 15 percent. The achievement of these encouraging results, however, remains difficult and depends on considerable therapeutic expertise and often extensive support facilities. Patients who wish definitive therapy are best treated in specialized leukemia centers where the necessary diagnostic expertise (e.g., cytologic, cytochemical, cytogenetic, surface marker) and supportive care capabilities exist, and where a multidisciplinary team of physicians, nurses, pharmacists, and other paramedical personnel thoroughly experienced in the management of leukemia are found.

Treatment of AML may be divided into several phases: initial evaluation, induction of remission, consolidation (or intensification) and maintenance of remission, and the management of relapse. Each of these will be considered in turn.

INITIAL EVALUATION

The patient with suspected acute leukemia must be rapidly and thoroughly evaluated since the results of the initial work-up will dictate the therapeutic approach. Optimal results are usually achieved only when the initial approach is correct; salvage therapy rarely results in long-term, disease-free survival. Speed in evaluation is important because the prompt recognition and appropriate treatment of some emergencies that may exist at the time of diagnosis will save many patients from an early death and allow them to survive long enough to receive an adequate trial of definitive chemotherapy.

Appropriate therapy depends on precise subclassification of the leukemia utilizing cytologic, cytochemical, and cytogenetic techniques to evaluate leukemic cells in the bone marrow and blood. Discussion of subclassification is beyond the scope of this article. However, the heterogeneity of AML is increasingly clear, as is the importance of this heterogeneity in selecting therapy. AML must as a minimum be classified using the cytologic and cytochemical criteria of the French-American British (FAB) classification. Cytogenetic findings (e.g., the presence of "t[15;17]" -5 or 5q-, 11q abnormalities, rearrangements of 16q22) are also now beginning to influence the choice of therapy, and in the near future the surface marker type may also be important.

In addition to special studies to subclassify the leukemia, initial evaluation should include a history and physical examination. Careful evaluation of the rectal area for signs of perirectal abscesses or cellulitis is indicated, but we avoid a digital examination, as well as pelvic examinations in women, because of the problems with precipitating significant perineal infections. Baseline laboratory studies should include complete blood counts (hemoglobin, leukocyte count, platelet count, differential, reticulocyte count), posterior iliac crest bone marrow aspirate and biopsy, coagulation studies (prothrombin time, partial thromboplastin time, thrombin time, factor V, fibrin degradation products, fibrinogen), serum electrolytes, calcium, PO_4, uric acid, glucose, liver function tests, renal function testsd, blood gases, posteroanterior and lateral chest roentgenograms, and electrocardiogram. Abnormalities in any of these tests must be considered when initiating induction treatment. Finally, all patients must be carefully evaluated for infection and appropriate treatment undertaken.

INDUCTION OF REMISSION

Chemotherapy

The single most important factor in survival of patients with AML is achieving a complete remission. This is defined as a normocellular bone marrow with less than 5 percent myeloblasts, no evidence of leukemic blasts, normal hematologic parameters, and no signs or symptoms of leukemia. Anything less than a complete remission is of limited benefit.

We attempt curative induction chemotherapy in all adults with AML whose underlying medical condition is satisfactory and who give informed consent. Once the diagnosis of AML is unequivocal, based on results of the battery of tests just mentioned, and any acute medical emergencies are treated, we immediately initiate therapy. We are currently studying the benefit of early curative treatment, even in patients with smoldering leukemia or treatment-induced leukemia (that occurring following chemotherapy or radiotherapy for other disorders). It is already clear that these latter diseases are heterogeneous, and some patients will achieve prolonged complete remissions with the early initiation of therapy.

The treatment of AML remains experimental. Most induction regimens include daunorubicin and continuous infusion of cytosine arabinoside. Which regimen is best for which type of patient and which patient requires an approach different from any current therapies is still being defined. I will discuss our present therapeutic approach, but it is important to emphasize that this is not necessarily the best approach. It is most important that each center use only regimens with which it has considerable familiarity, because each regimen has different toxicities, and in the initial use of any regimen, a certain number of preventable induction deaths will occur.

For adult patients of all ages, with all types of AML, we initiate treatment with daunorubicin, 45 mg/m^2/day IV on days 1 through 3, and cytosine arabinoside, 200 mg/m^2/day by continuous infusion on days 1 through 7. Patients with acute promyelocytic leukemia (M3) also receive continuous infusion of low-dose heparin, large numbers of platelet transfusions, and cryoprecipitate and fresh frozen plasma as required. Bone marrow aspiration and trephine biopsy are performed at 14 days following initiation of therapy. If there are >5 percent leukemic cells and >15 percent cellularity, a second induction cycle is given using the same regimen as initially administerd, except that the cytosine arabinoside is given for only 5 days and daunorubicin for only 2 days. If the day 14 marrow shows aplasis or severe hypoplasia and/or contains <5 percent leukemic cells, the marrow aspirate and biopsy are repeated on day 21. Treatment decisions are based on the day 21 marrow in the same manner as for the day 14 marrow. It is important to remember that the recovering phase of a marrow may be characterized by an "overshoot myeloblastosis", which is not indicative of recurrent or persistent leukemia. A high index of suspicion and serial bone marrow examinations will aid in differentiating between normal immature myeloid cells and recrudescent leukemia.

Most patients who achieve complete remission do so with one cycle of treatment and have adequate marrow regeneration by day 28. Any patient who fails to achieve a complete remission after two courses of the initial regimen is switched to another regimen. For most patients we switch to a high-dose cytosine arabinoside regimen of 3 g/m^2 IV every 12 hours for 6 days. If the patient fails to achieve a complete remission after one cycle of this, we change induction regimens again. If the patient has M3 or erythroleukemia (M6), we use a regimen of daunorubicin, 1 mg/kg/day IV for 5 days, and prednisone, 60 mg PO daily for 5 days. If the patient has a monocytic component to his leukemia, we utilize a regimen that includes VP16–213. If there is not a monocytic component, we utilize a regimen which includes M–AMSA.

Second and subsequent induction regimens are initiated only when medically significant problems (e.g., infections, renal failure) resulting from prior therapy have resolved and the leukocyte count is approaching 1000/mm^3. The exact timing of treatment remains part of the "art" of managing acute leukemia. The early use of alternate regimens increases the number of patients who will achieve complete remission and decreases the frequency of infection and other complications resulting from prolonged aplasia secondary to chemotherapy to which the patient will not respond.

Supportive Treatment

Ancillary supportive treatment is most important to the success of induction therapy. Ancillary treatment is primarily focused on supporting the patient through the period of thrombocytopenia and granulocytopenia induced by chemotherapy. During this period, the patient is at high risk for hemorrhagic and infectious complications, and capabilities for supporting the patient for an extended period must be available. Some of our routine supportive and protectile measures are listed in Table 1.

The incidence of thrombocytopenic hemorrhage as a cause of death during induction chemotherapy has been markedly reduced by the use of platelet transfusions. During febrile periods and the use of drugs that interfere with platelet function, such as the semisynthetic penicillins, platelet supplementation is usually required to prevent bleeding. For patients who become refractory to random donor platelets, the use of single donor or HLA-matched platelets obtained by plateletpheresis may be necessary. In general, attempts should be made to maintain a platelet count greater than 20,000/mm^3 during induction therapy.

Although significant improvements have been

TABLE 1 Partial Listing of Routine Orders and Precautions for Adults with AML Undergoing Induction Chemotherapy

Routine Nursing Orders
- Vital signs (BP, Temp, Pulse) q4h
- Weight b.i.d.; furosemide (Lasix) for weight gain of ≥ 1 kg
- Hemastix: All urine
- Guaiac: All stools and emesis
- Leukemic diet: No pepper, no spicy food, no uncooked vegetables, no fruits unless peeled, 3 g sodium
- Change IV tubing every 48 hours

Routine Medications
- Diotyl sodium sulfosuccinate (Colace), 100 mg PO *bid*
- Trimethoprim-sulfamethoxazole (Septra), two PO *bid*
- Nystatin (Mycostatin), 10 ml swish and swallow *qid*
- Nystatin (Mycostatin) tablets, 2 million units PO *qid*
- Allopurinol, 300 mg PO daily
- Vitamin K, 25 mg IV daily × 3, then 10 mg IV daily

For Temperature > 101F. Following Cultures
- Cephalothin, 4 g IV q6h
- Ticarcillin, 3 g IV q4h
- Tobramycin, 1 mg/kg IV q8h
- Serum creatinine and potassium must be checked daily for patients on these antibiotics. Hold tobramycin for any increase in creatinine. Potassium supplementation up to 200 mEq per day is frequently required.

Routine Precautions
- Reverse protection isolation
- No rectal temperatures, enemas, or suppositories
- No live plants in room
- No humidifiers
- No IM/SQ injections
- No straight-edge razors
- No aspirin or harsh laxatives

made in the prevention, diagnosis, and treatment of infections, infectious complictaions remain the major cause of death during induction chemotherapy. The severe neutropenia and the alterations in the immune system induced by the intensive chemotherapy predispose the patient to infection. Nearly all patients become febrile during the induction period; however, documented infections can be found in only 50 percent. The early empiric institution of broad-spectrum antibiotics, after an appropriate diagnostic evaluation for a source of infection, had been credited with salvaging 70 percent of patients who previously would have died.

A combination of antibiotics, including an aminoglycoside (tobramycin or gentamicin) and a semisynthetic penicillin (ticarcillin or carbenicillin), should be instituted at the appearance of any fever not associated with transfusion of a blood product. Cephalosporins are frequently a valuable addition to the broad-spectrum coverage. Other antibiotics should be added for specific indications. Antibiotics should be continued until the patient is no longer neutropenic, regardless of whether a specific source for the fever can be found.

Fungal infections play an important role in the cause of fevers in the granulocytopenic patient. Frequent evidence of fungal infections at autopsy and the difficulty in making the diagnosis ante mortem have led to the empiric use of amphotericin B in patients who remain febrile or who have a secondary temperature spike while on antibiotics.

The transfusion of granulocytes may benefit neutropenic patients who have bacterial sepsis. Other indications for granulocyte transfusions have not been proved, and a recent study has demonstrated that the prophylactic use of granulocytes may be dangerous. Moreover, there have been reports of patients dying shortly after a granulocyte transfusion when concurrently being treated with amphotericin B. The cautious use of granulocytes can be recommended only for neutropenic patients with documented bacterial septicemias not responding to antibiotics.

Prophylactic oral nonabsorbable antibiotics and trimethoprim-sulfamethoxazole (Septra) have been successfully used to reduce the incidence of infections in patients undergoing induction therapy. Septra is generally better tolerated and less costly than regimens that include oral nonabsorbable antibiotics such as neomycin, vancomycin, and gentamicin. However, patients may demonstrate delayed marrow regeneration from Septra. For patients with Septra-related toxicity we usually use naladixic acid instead. The use of laminar airflow rooms in conjunction with oral nonabsorbable antibiotics and skin decontamination appears to significantly reduce the incidence of serious infections; however, this has improved the remission induction rate in only a few series. A private room, reverse isolation, and most importantly meticulous attention to good hygiene by the patient and staff are usually adequate for patient management during the period of granulocytopenia.

Right atrial catheters (Hickman/Broviac) have greatly increased patient comfort and have proved extremely beneficial for patients with poor venous access. These Silastic catheters should be placed under sterile conditions via cutdown on the cephalic vein or, in children, a branch of the facial vein. The Dacron cuff placed in the subcutaneous channel, the long distance between the exit site and the vascular channel, and the meticulous attention to sterile technique in the placement of and maintenance of the catheter contribute to a low incidence of complications. The design of the catheter allows for both administration of products and venous blood sampling. Strict observation of sterile technique is required to prevent catheter-associated sepsis, but the catheter can often be maintained for periods of many months.

Other supportive measures that are needed for an occasional patient include renal dialysis for acute renal failure and neurosurgical support for evacuation of subdural hematomas or for the placement of Ommaya reservoirs for the prolonged administration of intrathecal antifungal, antibacterial, or antileukemic therapy. These extraordinary procedures may be extremely beneficial for selected patients.

Specific Therapeutic Problems

Hyperleukocytosis. Patients with leukocyte counts of more than 100,000/mm^3 frequently have problems associated with leukostasis. Most serious is rupture of cerebral or pulmonary capillaries. Initial treatment should be directed toward rapidly lowering the number of circulating blasts. Immediate leukopheresis is an easy and effective means of accomplishing this. Definitive induction treatment must be initiated at the completion of the procedure. Alternatively, cranial irradiation may be given with hydroxyurea, 3 g/m^2 orally. Leukopheresis has the advantage of more rapidly reducing the leukocyte count and of eliminating the problems with disseminatd intravascular coagulation and metabolic abnormalities associated with chemotherapy-induced massive tumor lysis.

Disseminated Intravascular Coagulation (DIC). Almost all patients with M3 leukemia, and some with other types of AML, develop consumption coagulopathy and are at high risk of life-threatening hemorrhage. Since laboratory evidence of this complication often is obtained prior to actual bleeding, all AML patients should, at diagnosis and for the first 3 days following initiation of induction chemotherapy, have a complete evaluation of the coagulation profile. We treat the DIC with continuous infusion heparin (10 units/kg/hour) when the fibrin degradation products are greater than 100 μg/ml and the fibrinogen level is low, the prothrombin time is prolonged, or the factor V level is <50 percent. In the presence of DIC we also use vigorous platelet support (8 to 16 units per day), regardless of the platelet count, and cryoprecipitate to maintain a normal fibrinogen level.

CONSOLIDATION AND MAINTENANCE OF REMISSION

Once a complete remission is obtained, most patients will relapse within 2 to 10 months unless something is done to prolong the remission state. Both consolidation and maintenance chemotherapy may prolong remissions.

Intensive consolidation therapy shortly after achieving complete remission currently appears to offer the greatest chance of prolonged disease-free survival in AML. The best consolidation treatment is unknown, but in younger adults (less than 30 years of age) 5-year disease-free survival in 45 to 50 percent of patients has been reported following high-dose chemotherapy, total body irradiation, and allogeneic bone marrow transplantation. In a small series studied at Vanderbilt and Washington University, as many as 50 percent of patients up to the age of 60 years have been reported to continue more than 2 years disease-free after 1 or 2 cycles of intensive consolidation with 6 days of cytosine arabinoside, 3 g/m^2 IV every 12 hours, followed by 3 days of daunorubicin, 30 mg/m^2/day. Other groups are currently exploring other intensive chemotherapy regimens. In general, readministration of the same or less intensive treatment used in induction has not resulted in a significant prolongation of remission duration.

A variety of low-dose maintenance regimens have been used. In many series these have prolonged the median remission duration by a number of months; however, they do not appear to signficantly increse the fraction of cured patients. If intensive consolidation is not to be utilized, we recommend a relatively nontoxic outpatient maintenance regimen such as 6-thioguanine, 2 mg/kg orally on 4 successive days of each week, followed by cytosine arabinoside, 1.5 mg/kg IM on the fifth day. Drug doses are adjusted to keep the leukocyte count between 2000 and $3000/mm^3$ and the platelet count above $100,000/mm^3$. With this regimen it is important to maintain the weekly administration of the drugs even if the doses are substantially reduced. In addition, the cytosine arabinoside must be given intramuscularly, not intravenously. An advantage of this maintenance regimen is that it minimizes the time the patient spends in the hospital while in remission. Patients are taught to administer their cytosine arabinoside at home, and they are seen in clinic for blood counts at 4- to 6-week intervals. Bone marrow examinations must be done at 2- to 3-month intervals during the first 3 years of maintenance therapy. The length of time that maintenance therapy should be administered is not known. We currently continue weekly 6-thioguanine and cytosine arabinoside for 5 years in the absence of significant hepatic toxicity or marrow aplasia.

REINDUCTION THERAPY

To date the majority of patients who achieve a complete remission eventually relapse. Over 50 percent of patients can achieve a second complete remission using the same agents to which they originally responded or by adding new antileukemic drugs to the previously effective treatment regimen. The exact choice of the reinduction regimen depends on the difficulty of the initial remission induction, the length of the prior complete remission, and the type of consolidation and maintenance therapy administered. For patients under the age of 40 who achieve a second remission, bone marrow transplantation should be considered if a donor is available.

MENINGEAL LEUKEMIA

Central nervous system (CNS) involvement by leukemic blasts is not common in AML. It has been reported most frequently in patients whose leukemia has a monocytic component, in those with a rearrangement of chromosome 16 at q22, and in those with hyperleukocytosis. Consequently, we give prophylactic cranial irradiation and intrathecal cytosine arabinoside to patients with M4 and M5 leukemias and those with leukocyte counts greater than $100,000/mm^3$. If prophylactic CNS treatment is not given, these patients should be monitored with monthly cerebral spinal fluid examinations. The results of treatment of asymptomatic meningeal leukemia are better than those of overt CNS leukemia. Either can be successfully treated with cranial irradiation and intrathecal methotrexate or cytosine arabinoside.

LONG-TERM SURVIVAL

The advances in the treatment of AML have resulted in increasing numbers of long-term survivors. In 1967, a worldwide survey suggested that less than 1 percent of adults with AML ever survived more than 5 years. Today 20 to 25 percent of patients achieving complete remission are alive without evidence of disease more than 5 years after diagnosis. Many of these patients have been off chemotherapy for years. How many of these patients are actually cured is not known, since late relapses have been reported.

Risk factor analysis has suggested that patients whose leukemia arises after previous cytotoxic therapy or marrow failure syndromes, patients who have a large tumor load as reflected by a high initial leukcyte count or lactic dehydrogenase (LDH) level, patients with monocytic subtypes of AML, and patients with specific chromosome abnormalities (e.g., abnormalities in 11q, -5 or 5q-) often do not do well with standard chemotherapy approaches. Such patients should be considered early in their course for bone marrow transplantation if an HLA/MLC-matched donor is available.

ACUTE LYMPHOBLASTIC LEUKEMIA IN ADULTS

DIETER F. HOELZER, M.D.

Treatment of acute lymphoblastic leukemia (ALL) has been improved substantially in recent years. After induction therapy, complete remission rates of 70 to 80 percent with disease-free survival of more than 30 percent at five years are realistic achievements. Prospective therapeutic trials in adult ALL with uniform diagnostic procedures, intensified therapy, and a large number of patients have enabled us to define prognostic factors, resulting in risk-adapted therapy and more precise indications for bone marrow transplantation. Several problems related to the improvement of the cure rates remain unsolved, such as further intensification of therapy (carefully weighed against the increased risk of toxicity), the best modality for prophylactic central nervous system (CNS) treatment (with or without cranial irradiation), and the optimal duration of maintenance therapy. To answer such questions, it is important to include adult patients with acute lymphoblastic leukemia in studies whenever possible. Improved remission rates have been achieved by intensifying treatment regimens with increased toxicity. Patients should therefore be treated in hospitals by trained staff who react quickly to complications which may occur.

DIAGNOSIS AND IMMUNOLOGIC CLASSIFICATION

Examination of bone marrow aspirates and blood smears confirms the diagnosis. The first bone marrow aspirates should be used for morphology, cytochemistry, immunologic phenotyping, and cytogenetic analysis. Blast cells in ALL are stained with Wright's or Wright's/Giemsa stain and are classified as L1, L2, or L3 according to the FAB classification. The definitive cytochemical reactions are periodic acid-Schiff (PAS) and acid phosphatase. However, approximately one-quarter of the immunologically-defined ALL subtypes, common-ALL (c-ALL), T-ALL, and null-ALL (here defined as being negative for T-cell and B-cell markers and for c-ALL antigen), are PAS-negative and, in contrast, a small percentage of PAS-positive ALL remains immunologically unclassifiable. A focal acid phosphatase reaction suggests T-ALL, but one-third of the immunologically defined T-ALL is negative for acid phosphatase; occasionally positive reactions are seen in other subtypes. Immunologic phenotyping is thus a diagnostic necessity, especially for B-ALL where a different therapeutic regimen is used. The presence of the enzyme terminal deoxynucleotidyl-transferase should also be assessed for confirmation of the diagnosis of ALL.

Cytogenetic analysis of bone marrow cells (or peripheral blood cells when the leukemia blast cell content is high) is desirable since cytogenetic abnormalities, most often the Ph^1 chromosome, are an adverse prognostic sign for a lengthy duration of disease-free survival. Flow cytophotometry is also a new prognostic tool.

Lumbar puncture is obligatory before therapy in order to determine whether or not the central nervous system is involved, and is omitted only when there is a high danger of bleeding due to a very low platelet count. When the leukocyte count in the spinal fluid is at borderline levels, or the morphology is inconclusive, demonstration of an immunologically defined monoclonality often confirms a decision of CNS involvement.

INITIAL COMPLICATIONS AND SUPPORTIVE THERAPY

Most of the patients present with indirect signs of leukemia such as infection, bleeding, anemia, and metabolic disorders rather than with symptoms due to leukemic cell infiltration. Treatment of initial complications and prophylaxis for complications expected during cytostatic therapy must be started immediately. In only a few cases is the leukemic process so far advanced that immediate treatment of the leukemia is necessary.

The most frequent metabolic abnormality is hyperuricemia, which further increases during therapy and exacerbates cell destruction. Patients should receive Allopurinol to reduce the formation of uric acid and avoid the danger of urate nephropathy. Allopurinol should be given at a dose of 100 mg *q8h* which may be increased to 600 mg per day if high leukocyte counts or organomegaly persist. Allopurinol has to be discontinued when 6-mercaptopurine is given or the dosage of the latter must be reduced. Allopurinol can cause skin rashes but rarely causes severe allergic reactions.

Sufficient fluid intake to guarantee urine production of at least 100 ml/hour throughout induction therapy reduces the danger of uric acid formation. This may require parenteral fluid administration when the patient's oral intake is inadequate because of nausea or difficulty in swallowing. If the venous system does not offer easy access, a Hickman catheter is advantageous when anticipating 8 weeks of induction therapy and is useful when part of the therapy is carried out on an outpatient basis.

Approximately one-third of adult ALL patients present with infection and bleeding, which are major problems in the management of the disease. Bleeding is ususally due to thrombocytopenia, but hyperleukocytosis and plasma clotting deficiencies may exacerbate it. In a small proportion of patients the fibrinogen level is below 100 mg/ml which is probably due to impaired synthesis of clotting factors in an infiltrated liver. Disseminated intravascular coagulation is rarely observed at diagnosis. Leukostatic hemorrhages caused by leukocyte aggregation and infiltration of small vessel walls are most severe in the brain, especially in patients with high leukocyte counts. Cautious reduction of the leukocytes may, but cannot always, prevent fatal complications. In thrombocytopenia, platelets should be transferred when the platelet count falls below 20,000/mm^3 and/or for bleeding. Four to six platelet packs should be given daily until bleeding stops.

Fever or infection present at the time of admission is mainly caused by severe granulocytopenia (granulocyte count below 500/mm^3) but may also be due to immunologic deficiencies or mucosal lesions. Careful physical examination, chest roentgenogram, and cultures of blood, urine, sputum, and other sites of suspected infection are necessary. In patients with severe infection, broad spectrum antibiotics should be given immediately even before the results of cultures are available. For patients with no fever or infection, prophylactic treatment with co-trimoxazole should be initiated prior to cytostatic treatment. Co-trimoxazole in combination with prophylactic polymyxin B and amphothericin B treatment, apparently prevented severe infection in half of the patients in a large ALL multicenter trial.

Prophylactic measures including the regular use of mouth wash, careful disinfection of the anogenital region, general body hygiene, sufficient fluid intake, and regular intake of Allopurinol and co-trimoxazole, are some of the measures that the patient should be motivated to actively contribute to the treatment of his disease.

REMISSION INDUCTION THERAPY

Exact diagnosis and management of initial complications are the prerequisites of cytostatic therapy. Patients with the immunologic subtypes c-ALL, T-ALL, or null-ALL are, in most regimens, initially treated with a combination of vincristine, prednisone, anthracyclines, and L-asparaginase. For B-ALL, a different regimen which includes initial cyclophosphamide is recommended. In patients with a large leukemic cell mass and an especially high leukocyte count (>25,000/mm^3), cell reduction with a cautious pretherapy should be started (Table 1). Extreme leukocytosis (>100,000/mm^3) can best be managed with leukapheresis; however, the technical facilities and experience are not often available. The induction therapy administered during the first four weeks is shown in Table 2.

TABLE 1 Pretherapy for Patients with a Large Leukemic Mass and a High Leucocyte Count

Drug	*Dosage*	*Day*
Vincristine	0.75 mg/m^2	1
Prednisone	30 mg/m^2	1–7

TABLE 2 Phase 1 of ALL Induction Therapy

Drug	*Dosage*	*Days*
Vincristine	1.5 mg/m^2 IV maximal single dose 2 mg	1, 8, 15, 22
Prednisone	60 mg/m^2 PO	1–28
Daunorubicine	25 mg/m^2 IV	1, 8, 15, 22
L-asparaginase	5000 U/m^2 IV	15–28

To further reduce the leukemic cell burden and to avoid the early development of resistant clones, a second course of induction therapy follows. Patients who have already reached complete remission after the first four weeks will benefit most from this second course of therapy. For the remaining patients with partial remission or failure, this will provide a chance to enter complete remission. The second phase of induction therapy includes three other cytostatic drugs, together with CNS prophylaxis with cranial irradiation and intrathecal methotrexate (Table 3).

This part of induction therapy can be started immediately after phase 1 but often a pause of about a week is needed to allow granulocytes and platelets to recover to values of 1500/mm^3 and over 100,000/mm^3 respectively.

With this induction regimen an overall complete remission rate of 70 to 80 percent can be achieved. Nearly all of the patients with T-ALL will already have achieved complete remission after the first four weeks of therapy, while some patients with c-ALL and a substantial proportion with null-ALL need the second phase to enter complete remission. In contrast to earlier findings, it now seems that with this and other intensified regimens, initial parameters such as advanced age, CNS involvement, or a high leukocyte count have no adverse influence on the complete remission rate.

Central Nervous System (CNS) Prophylaxis

CNS prophylaxis consists of 2,400 rads cranial irradiation and intrathecal methotrexate, 10 mg/m^2 (maximum single dose 15 mg), once weekly, for four weeks, and is given during phase 2 if complete remission is achieved during phase 1. When complete remission is delayed until completion of phase 2, CNS prophylaxis is given immediately thereafter. In patients with evidence of involvement of the CNS at

TABLE 3 Phase 2 of ALL Induction Therapy

Drug	*Dosage*
Cyclophosphamide	650 mg/m^2 IV every 2 weeks × 3 doses
Cytosine arabinoside	75 mg/m^2/day IV for 4 consecutive days of each week for 4 weeks
6-Mercaptopurine	60 mg/m^2 PO daily for 4 weeks
Methotrexate	10 mg/m^2 intrathecally (maximal single dose 15 mg)
CNS irradiation	24 Gy

presentation, the radiation dose is increased to 3,000 rads, the field extended to include the spinal column, and the irradiation and intrathecal methotrexate are given in phase 1.

CONSOLIDATION THERAPY

Current concepts of ALL therapy try to improve remission quality by further eradication of leukemic cells with a consolidation therapy. This can be achieved either by repeated cycles of alternating drug combinations, as in the very successful L10/L10M protocol of the Memorial Sloan Kettering Cancer Center, or in a single intensified consolidation course given three months after complete remission. Patients should receive a consolidation therapy with drugs similar to those given in induction therapy (Table 4).

Induction therapy requires at least eight weeks and consolidation therapy six weeks. An attempt therefore must be made to carry out as much of the treatment as possible on an outpatient basis. This can be done in the interval between phase 1 and phase 2 of induction therapy, in the intervals between the 4-day courses of cytosine-arabinoside and during most of the consolidation therapy.

TOXIC SIDE EFFECTS OF INDUCTION THERAPY

When this protocol was used in a large multicenter trial with nearly 400 patients, it became apparent that in phase 1 of therapy the time and dose schedule for prednisone, vincristine, and daunorubicin could almost always be adhered to. L-asparaginase had to be discontinued in nearly one-third of the patients (usually after 10 days) because of reduced fibrinogen levels (below 100 mg%) despite replacement or because of rare complications such as pancreatitis, severe hyperglycemia, or allergic reactions. The second phase of induction therapy is much more toxic with respect to the severity of thrombocytopenia and granulocytopenia. Therefore individually adjusted therapy is necessary in two-thirds of the patients. A postponement of the drug should first be tried; the next alternative is a reduction in dosage before omitting the drug altogether.

Although the second phase of induction therapy is more toxic, severe or fatal complications occur almost exclusively during the first weeks or even days. Bleeding is the most severe complication within the first fortnight, and severe infections are observed throughout the whole induction regimen. Initially bacterial or viral infections are predominant but later, fungal infections, usually candidiasis and occasionally aspergillosis, become a major problem.

Moderate and severe neurotoxicity due to vincristine will be observed in about one-tenth of the patients. Vincristine administration is usually possible in induction therapy but dose reduction or omission of vincristine may be required in the consolidation therapy. Hepatotoxicity is also a complication, mainly in the induction therapy, and is most probably attributable to L-asparaginase. Thus, discontinuation of L-asparaginase and reduction of further cytostatic therapy may be necessary.

TABLE 4 Consolidation Therapy for ALL Patients

Drug	*Dosage*
Part 1*	
Dexamethasone	10 mg/m^2 PO daily for 4 weeks
Vincristine	1.5 mg/m^2 IV (maximal single dose 2 mg) once/week for 4 weeks
Adriamycin	25 mg/m^2 IV once/week for 4 weeks
Part 2	
Cyclophosphamide	650 mg/m^2 IV in a single dose
Cytosine arabinoside	75 mg/m^2 IV for 4 consecutive days of each week for 4 weeks
Thioguanine	60 mg/m^2/day PO for 2 weeks

*A second course of L-asparaginase is not given here since anaphylactic reactions might be expected.

MAINTENANCE THERAPY

In the interval between the end of induction and the beginning of consolidation therapy, and after consolidation therapy, patients should have maintenance therapy (Table 5).

Dosages should be adjusted so that granulocyte levels remain above 1500/mm^3 and platelet counts above 100,000/mm^3. Occasionally hepatotoxicity or reduced creatine clearance also makes a lowering of dose or discontinuation of therapy necessary. This maintenance treatment should be continued for two years. It seems justified to stop at this time since 90 percent of relapses occur during the first two years, and it is questionable whether later occurrence of leukemia can be avoided by a continuation of therapy.

INDUCTION AND CONSOLIDATION THERAPY FOR B-ALL

Experience with treatment of B-ALL in adults up to now has been disappointing. A new protocol with intensive cycles of therapy within the first half year seems promising for B-ALL in children, and is under study for the treatment of adult B-ALL. Patients with a large tumor mass immediately receive the pretherapy shown in Table 6.

Because of the rapid progress of the disease, induction therapy, consisting of alternating cycles 1 and 2, should follow immediately (Table 7).

Prophylactic CNS irradiation should be carried

TABLE 5 Maintenance Therapy for ALL Patients

Drug	*Dosage*
6-Mercaptopurine	60 mg/m^2 PO daily
Methotrexate	20 mg/m^2 PO weekly

TABLE 6 Pretherapy for B-ALL Patients

Drug	*Dosage*	*Days*
Cyclophosphamide	200 mg/m² IV	1–5
Prednisone	0-5–1 mg/kg PO	1–5

out after cycle 2. Four additional alternating cycles should then be administered if possible. Further maintenance is not necessary if complete remission can be achieved after the first courses of induction therapy.

IMMUNOLOGIC SUBTYPES

By membrane and cytoplasmic analysis for immunoglobulin, T-cell antigens and c-ALL antigens, adult ALL can be roughly divided into subtypes with the following frequency distribution: c-ALL 50 to 60 percent (including pre B-ALL), T-ALL 20 percent, null-ALL 25 percent, B-ALL 1 to 2 percent, mixed leukemia 1 to 2 percent (blast cells cALLA$^+$ reacting with antigranulocyte globulin and/or having myeloperoxidase).

The null-ALL subtype can be further subdivided by use of monoclonal antibodies and only a small fraction (about 5%) will remain without any lineage specificity. In these cases, as in patients with mixed leukemia, it is an open question whether the therapeutic regimen for ALL or for ANLL will be better; however, patients should be treated uniformly in order to garner information.

As in childhood ALL, c-ALL is the most frequent subtype; however, prognosis is poorer than for children.

TABLE 7 Induction Therapy for B-ALL Patients

Drug	*Dosage*	*Route*	*Day(s)*
Prednisone	60 mg/m²	PO	every day from commencement of Cycle 1 to the end of Cycle 2
Cycle 1			
Methotrexate	12 mg	intrathecally	1
Methotrexate	500 mg/m²	24-hr infusion*†	1
Cyclophosphamide	200 mg/m²	IV or PO	1–5
VM-26	165 mg/m²	1-hour infusion	5
Cytosine arabinoside	300 mg/m²	1-hour infusion	5
Cycle 2 (begins 14 days after cycle 1 ends)			
Methotrexate	12 mg/m²	intrathecally	1
Methotrexate	500 mg/m²	24-hour infusion*†	1
Cyclophosphamide	200 mg/m²	IV or PO	1–5
Adriamycin	50 mg/m²	IV	5

*1/10 as bolus injection, then 9/10 as an infusion over 24 hours with 3000 ml/m² (if possible). Forced diuresis with 1 mg/kg furosemide after 6 and 12 hours. Urine pH should be above 7.2.

†With leucovorin-rescue (12 mg/m² IM) at 36, 48, and 54 hrs after commencement of methotrexate infusion.

For T-ALL, the outcome has dramatically changed. This subtype, often associated with a high leukocyte count, mediastinal tumor, extramedullary involvement, and rapid progression, formerly had a poor prognosis. With the therapy protocol set out here and also with other intensified schemes such as the L10/L10M protocol, it probably has the best prognosis, with an actuarial disease-free survival at 5 years of about 50 percent. It must be noted that most ALL patients with mediastinal tumor belong to the T-ALL phenotype although occasionally other subtypes are found in these patients.

B-ALL, the least frequently found subtype, is characterized by rapid proliferation, frequent CNS involvement, and massive lymph node enlargement. In this subtype, the very poor prognosis is also changing when the B-ALL protocol is used in childhood ALL and it might also be promising for adult ALL.

PROGNOSTIC FACTORS

Evaluation of prognostic factors and consequent definition of risk groups is urgently needed in adult ALL in order to have a basis for alternative therapeutic approaches, such as bone marrow transplantation or intensification of cytostatic therapy. Recent reports of larger studies with intensified induction and consolidation therapy are increasingly consistent regarding risk factors for adult ALL which affect the length of remission duration (Table 8).

The same induction and consolidation therapy is used for both low- and high-risk adult ALL patients although there is a clear contrast in outcome. Low-risk patients (i.e., those without any of the risk factors) form about one-third of adult ALL patients and may show encouraging treatment results with 50 percent or more disease-free survival with the best current therapy protocols. This figure is too low to permit a reduction in the intensity of the induction regimen. Low-risk patients in first remission are not candidates for bone marrow transplantation.

Patients having one or more of the risk factors belong to the high risk group, with a continuous complete remission rate of about 20 percent at 5 years. In these patients, a further intensification of chemotherapy with additional consolidation cycles is under investigation at present. For high-risk patients, a bone

TABLE 8 Prognostic Factors Affecting Remission Duration

Low risk factors
Time to achieve complete remission ≤ 4 weeks
Initial leukocyte count ≤ 30,000/mm³
Age ≤ 35 years
Immunologic subtype c-ALL or T-ALL
High risk factors
Time to achieve complete remission > 4 weeks
Initial leukocyte count > 30,000/mm³
Age > 35 years
Immunologic subtype null-ALL or B-ALL
Philadelphia chromosome positive

marrow transplantation in first remission is recommended.

RELAPSE SITES

Unfortunately, half or more of ALL patients have a recurrence of leukemia, usually within approximately 2 years of successful induction therapy. The site of relapse is most frequently the bone marrow. Isolated CNS relapse is still a major obstacle and occurs in about 10 percent of patients, whether the CNS prophylaxis consists of cranial irradiation and intrathecal methotrexate, or of high dose methotrexate without cranial irradiation.

Other relapse sites, such as lymph nodes, mediastinum, skin, or testes are not frequent but are preferentially seen in T-ALL and null-ALL patients. The very low incidence of testicular relapse in adult ALL after intensified therapeutic regimens does not warrant prophylactic treatment of the testes.

RELAPSE THERAPY

The outcome for relapse in adult ALL patients is still very poor. With the above induction regimens, a complete remission rate of up to 60 percent can be achieved, depending on how long after remission the relapse occurs. However, the remission duration is only 3 to 6 months and long-term prospects are poor, with a continuous complete remission rate of less than 10 percent after 2 years. Readministering induction therapy might be one approach; another is the use of the B-ALL protocol which includes VM 26 and high-dose methotrexate. Alternatively, protocols with new strategies, such as high-dose cytosine arabinoside or new drugs are justified because of the very poor prognosis for these patients. Bone marrow transplantation in these relapse patients should be carried out whenever possible.

HAIRY-CELL LEUKEMIA

DAVID W. GOLDE, M.D.

Hairy-cell leukemia is a well-defined lymphoproliferative disorder characterized by splenomegaly, pancytopenia, and morphologically typical neoplastic cells in the blood and bone marrow. The disease usually represents a monoclonal proliferation of neoplastic B-lymphocytes, but T-lymphocytic forms of the disease have also been reported. Patients often are referred to the hematologist because of abnormalities noted on routine blood tests or because of symptoms associated with splenomegaly or with intercurrent infection. Diagnosis usually is not difficult when there is pancytopenia circulating tartrate-resistant acid phosphatase-positive hairy cells, nonaspirable bone marrow, and splenomegaly without lymphadenopathy. The disease, however, has a spectrum of presentations and may be confused with other lymphoproliferative disorders, monocytic leukemia, and even aplastic anemia.

In many patients, the diagnosis is made incidentally during routine medical examination or in the course of investigation of symptoms unrelated to hairy-cell leukemia. In these patients, we follow a policy of observation for several months to determine the rate of progression of the disease. If there is no substantial hematopoietic compromise, increasing splenomegaly, or other complications of hairy-cell leukemia, we advise no specific therapy. Generally, hairy-cell leukemia should be treated only when there is advancing splenomegaly, significant cytopenia, or other evidence of progressive infiltrative disease. Although there have been no controlled trials of any therapeutic modality in hairy-cell leukemia, splenectomy is the initial treatment of choice for patients who require treatment.

When there is increasing anemia, thrombocytopenia, or granulocytopenia, we move to splenectomy without waiting for complications or allowing the patient's overall condition to deteriorate. Similarly, if the patient has massive splenomegaly and significant hematopoietic compromise, we do not observe for progression but advise immediate splenectomy. It is not certain whether there is a relationship between spleen size and response to splenectomy; however, we perform splenectomy on all patients with progressive disease irrespective of the spleen size. Splenectomy usually leads to hematologic improvement and a "good response" (hemoglobin above 11 g/dl; neutrophils greater than 1000/μl.; platelets greater than 100,000/μl.) is seen in approximately 50 percent of patients. In general, splenectomy is well tolerated by patients of all ages; however, a high degree of vigilance for infection should be maintained in the perioperative period since these paitents usually have impaired defenses. The incidence of infection generally decreases after splenectomy and the platelet count almost invariably rises. Platelet function (which may be abnormal before splenectomy) usually returns to normal, suggesting that passage of platelets through the involved spleen leads to some degree of degranulation and platelet dysfunction. In patients who have an absolute contraindication to splenectomy, we would recommend treatment with an experimental protocol using alpha-interferon (to be discussed). We do not recommend splenic irradiation as it is often ineffective and usually dangerous. Likewise, glucocorticoids are contraindicated as primary therapy in this disease, but they may be used in treating vasculitis or other autoimmune phenomena. Patients routinely treated with corticosteroids have not had a good outcome, and they have a marked increase in the incidence of opportunistic infections.

Patients with progressive disease after splenectomy present a major therapeutic problem. At present, there is no best approach and many alternatives are available. The recent report of dramatic responses to natural interferon (3×10^6 u/day) in this disease suggests that experimental therapy with interferon may prove to be the best treatment. Good responses to recombinant interferon have also been observed. Since interferon is relatively safe to use, it should be offered on an experimental basis to patients with progressive disease following splenectomy. It is possible that if the efficacy of interferon in hairy-cell leukemia is confirmed, it will be the treatment of choice. Other low-toxicity approaches to therapy have included androgens, lithium, and leukapheresis. Leukapheresis has not been generally useful although some patients have improvement in their blood count when treated with androgen and lithium chloride. The androgen we use is oxymethalone (50 mg *tid*), and lithium is usually given as lithium carbonate starting with a dose of 300 mg *tid* aiming for a serum lithium level of about 1 mEq/Liter. Administration of these agents does require careful monitoring as serious side effects can occur.

Cytotoxic therapy is dangerous in patients with hairy-cell leukemia, but low-dose chlorambucil (2 to 4 mg/day) has yielded gratifying results in some patients with progressive disease following splenectomy. Patients with high white cell counts tend to respond better, and treatment should be continued for at least 6 months. Therapy with alkylating agents, however, is difficult because of an increased incidence of infectious complications, and there is risk of later development of acute leukemia. There has been relatively little experience with ablative chemotherapy in hairy-cell leukemia, and any approach of this nature must be considered highly experimental. Treatment with regimens used in adult acute leukemia may lead to complete or partial remission, but such treatment should be considered only for patients who have failed other available therapy. The successful treatment of a patient with hairy-cell leukemia by ablative chemoradiotherapy and bone marow transplantation from an identical twin has provided important biologic insights into this disease. Based on this single experience, it is clear that the disease can be eradicated by high-dose chemoradiotherapy; however, an alternate source of hematopoietic cells is necessary. Obviously, while twin transplantation will have little application in the general therapy of hairy-cell leukemia, it will stimulate experimental approaches involving allogeneic transplantation in very advanced hairy-cell leukemia in young patients who have HLA-matched donors.

The prognosis of patients with hairy-cell leukemia seems to be steadily improving, and every center has many long-term survivors with stable disease. The median survival time for a group of 71 patients studied at three large institutions was 70 months, and we suspect that the prognosis will improve with more accurate diagnosis and better management. The major problem with regard to morbidity and mortality in hairy-cell leukemia is infection. Patients with hairy-cell leukemia are often immunocompromised, functionally asplenic, and have overall decreased host defense because of granulocytopenia and monocytopenia. They are prone to the development of serious infections with common pyogenic organisms as well as many opportunistic infections of a special nature. A high degree of vigilance must be maintained with regard to infections in these patients. For example, minor areas of folliculitis may spread rapidly and lead to sepsis, and other types of minor skin infection (e.g., paronychia) may prove serious. Fever must be investigated quickly and thoroughly, and appropriate antibiotic therapy initiated at the first sign of infection and before culture results are available. Patients must be informed of the danger of infection and report fever or other signs of infection promptly. Minor skin infection should be treated with antibiotics with good antistaphylococcal coverage (oxacillin, dicloxacillin), and patients with high fever or pneumonitis should be admitted to hospital. Pyogenic sepsis is a frequent cause of death in these patients, and initial therapy before blood culture results are available should include an aminoglycoside and semisynthetic penicillin or third-generation cephalosporin. Pneumonitis may be due to the usual pyogenic organisms; however, Legionella pneumonitis is particularly severe in these patients, and therefore we normally add intravenous erythromycin to our usual coverage antibiotics when pneumonitis is observed on chest roentgenogram. It can be difficult to document Legionella infection because of problems with culturing the organism and the fluorescent antibody test may be unreliable. We therefore normally continue intravenous erythromycin for 2 weeks in hospitalized patient, and give oral erythromycin subsequently. Pneumocystis infection is very rare in hairy-cell leukemia unless the patient is treated with glucocorticoids, and therefore we do not routinely treat with trimethoprim/sulfamethoxazole. Since atypical *Mycobacterium* and *Mycobacterium tuberculosis* occur with considerable frequency in these patients, diagnosis should be actively pursued and treatment should be vigorous. Perirectal infections are particularly severe in patients with hairy-cell leukemia and often lead to sepsis. Early intervention with high-dose combination antibiotic therapy is the approach of choice. Toxoplasmosis, deep mycosis, and nocardiosis are also seen in hairy cell patients. We give pneumococcal vaccine to all patients; however, there is no information regarding its effectiveness.

Autoimmune disease may occur at some point in

almost 30 percent of patients with hairy-cell leukemia. This is usually manifested as a skin vasculitis, but can also occur as vasculitis involving the lungs and the bowel. In rare instances it appears as a full-blown syndrome of polyarteritis nodosa. In many of these patients, serum immune complexes are markedly elevated. Autoimmune manifestations are usually easily controlled by short courses of glucocorticoids in relatively low dose (20 to 40 mg/day for 7 to 10 days) or by low doses of alkylating agent (2 to 4 mg chlorambucil as intermittent therapy for 7 to 10 days). Progressive infiltration of nonhematopoietic tissue by hairy cells is rarely seen. Although portal triads in the liver usually contain hairy cells, massive liver infiltration is rare. Bone involvement, however, does occur and may take the form of lytic lesions or involvement of the femoral necks. Radiation therapy is the treatment of choice for bony disease.

With appropriate diagnosis and therapy, the prognosis in hairy-cell leukemia should improve progressively and long-term survival may be expected in many patients. Overtreatment of patients with indolent disease should be avoided and infections should be promptly identified and treated. Newer therapeutic approaches, such as the use of interferon and perhaps other nontoxic biologic products, may lead to long-term control even in patients with progressive disease.

BONE MARROW TRANSPLANTATION

GEORGE W. SANTOS, M.D.

In general bone marrow transplantation should be considered only when there is a possibility of cure in otherwise incurable diseases. The rationale for use in malignant disease is to provide a "rescue" from potentially lethal hematopoietic toxicity of a cytoreductive treatment regimen designed to completely destroy residual tumor cells. The rationale for its use in aplastic anemia is to provide the affected individual with normal hematopoietic stem cells that will restore the individual to normal health.

MARROW DONOR

Marrow for transplantation may come from an HLA-matched family member (allogeneic donor, usually a sib), from a monozygotic twin (syngeneic), or from the patient (autologous).

The major immunologic barrier to transplantation is determined by the major histocompatibility complex, a linear array of genes located on human chromosome 6. Within this complex of genetic material, a series of alleles exist at the loci A, B, C, and Dr, and can be identified serologically by typing (microcytotoxicity testing) the lymphocytes of the patient and the family. In addition, a fifth locus, the D locus, is closely associated with Dr and may be identified by determining reactivity (nonidentity) or nonreactivity (identity) in one-way mixed lymphocyte cultures in vitro. In simple terms, all these laboratory tests are designed to identify the two paternal and two maternal chromosomes (haplotypes) and their inheritance within the family. Thus, after the typing is finished, a genetic analysis can be made by inspection of the data. Individuals sharing the same haplotypes are said to be genotypically HLA-identical. These individuals differ in terms of minor histocompatibility determinants since their inheritance of other genetic material is not identical. Herein when we consider allogeneic donors they will be genotypically HLA-identical sibs, although in certain situations "mismatched" donors and even unrelated donors may be used.

Since the genes that determine the major blood group antigens are not located on chromosome 6, a situation may arise in which a patient with blood group O has an allogeneic donor who is blood group A, B, or AB. Currently this poses no problem since one may simply centrifuge the collected marrow to remove the mismatched erythrocytes. This is routinely done on our unit and in no way have the results differed therapeutically from situations in which donors with ABO-compatible marrow were used.

The term syngeneic is used when the marrow donor is a monozygotic twin. When the patient serves as his own donor, the term autologous is employed. In these situations, the marrow cells share all the genetic materials of the recipient, and the expected hazards as well as possible therapeutic effects of allogeneic marrow transplantation are absent.

The risks of being a donor are primarily the risks of anesthesia and, when currently analyzed, appear to be less than 0.1 percent. In a number of situations, however, there is a psychologic risk, namely, if the patient does not do well, the donor may generate self-guilt and may feel "left out" or not considered by the rest of the family while the patient is undergoing the transplant. Therefore, it is wise to have conversations with the donor to explain that if anything goes wrong, it is not related to failure on the donor's part.

Marrow is collected in heparinized syringes under general anesthesia from the posterior iliac crests in the amount of 10 to 20 ml/kg, and marrow is then

Supported by PHS Grants CA-15396 and CAO-06973 awarded by the National Cancer Institute, DHHS.

passed through screens of decreasing mesh size and finally transferred to an empty blood bag. The marrow is then immediately brought to the patient and infused intravenously without an in-line filter.

PREPARATIVE REGIMENS

In order for a marrow graft to be successful, the patient should receive therapy that is myeloablative in order to destroy defective or malignant cells and thus make "space". In addition, where allogeneic marrow transplants are concerned, the regimen must supply enough immunosuppression to overcome graft rejection. Commonly used regimens include cyclophosphamide alone or in combination with total body irradiation or busulfan. All of the regimens produce marrow aplasia for 14 to 21 days. Other undesired side effects are often troublesome, but are manageable by experienced teams.

For acute nonlymphocytic leukemia we prepare the patient for transplantation with oral busulfan, given in divided doses over a 4-day period for a total dose of 16 mg/kg. This is followed by intravenous cyclophosphamide in a daily dose of 50 mg/kg for four consecutive daily doses (total dose 200 mg/kg). Patients with acute lymphocytic leukemia are prepared with intravenous cyclophosphamide in a daily dose of 50 mg/kg for 4 consecutive days (total dose of 200 mg/kg) followed by low-dose rate total body irradiation of 300 rads/day for four consecutive daily doses (lungs shielded for third dose). Patients with non-Hodgkin's lymphoma receive treatment similar to that employed in acute lymphocytic leukemia, except that the radiation is hyperfractionated, and boost doses are given to areas of bulky disease. Our preparative regimen for chronic myelogenous leukemia is similar to that used by others and consists of intravenous cyclophosphamide given in two consecutive daily doses of 60 mg/kg. This is followed by 300 rads/day of total body irradiation for four consecutive daily doses (lungs shielded for the third dose).

SUPPORTIVE CARE

Successful marrow transplantation is a major team effort which requires an expert and well-integrated team composed of dedicated physicians, physicians' assistants, nurses, nutritionists, and others. In addition, a sophisticated blood support system to provide platelet, granulocyte, and red cell transfusions is essential. Furthermore, considerable experience is necessary to diagnose and treat the infectious episodes that plague many of the patients in aplasia. Careful attention to nutrition, particularly in the use of intravenous alimentation, is required. All blood products require prior exposure to 1500 to 3000 rads in order that lymphocytes contained in the transfused blood products will not cause graft-versus-host disease in the recipient.

CURRENT CLINICAL RESULTS

The therapeutic results of allogeneic transplants have been encouraging, especially in patients with acute leukemia in remission, chronic myelogenous leukemia in the chronic phase, and lymphoma. Long-term remissions and possible cures have been reported in 50 percent or more of such patients.

In general, the best clinical results are obtained in the younger patients (i.e., 20 years and younger) and when the disease is in the earliest part of its evolution (i.e., acute leukemia in first remission and chronic myelogenous leukemia in the chronic rather than the accelerated or blast crisis phase). It is important that the decision for transplantation be made soon after the diagnosis, and a therapeutic plan should be outlined.

At present, the cure of severe aplastic anemia may approach 70 to 80 percent with allogeneic transplantation, especially when performed early in the disease and ideally before transfusions are given (since transfusion may increase the likelihood of rejection episodes in severe aplastic anemia). Again, the best clinical results are seen in the younger patients.

One should seriously consider using an identical twin donor, if such exists, in cases of various malignant tumors and aplastic anemia. Under these conditions, marrow transplants for diseases such as acute leukemia in remission, chronic myelogenous leukemia in the chronic phase, and lymphoma may provide 50 to 70 percent long-term disease-free survivals and a high percentage of potential cures.

Autologous marrow transplantation is an area of growing interest and may eventually have wider applications in the treatment of malignant tumors. Early results appear to be promising in the treatment of acute leukemias and especially the lymphomas, in which a remission marrow is "purged" of putative tumor cells by chemotherapeutic agents or through the use of monoclonal antibodies directed against antigens on the occult tumor cells.

COMPLICATIONS OF MARROW TRANSPLANTS

Leukemic relapse following allogeneic marrow transplantation does not appear to be a major problem for patients in first remission, but remains a problem in second-remission patients with the use of certain preparative regimens other than those employed by our group. However, a high rate of relapse is the major problem associated with syngeneic and autologous transplantation.

Nevertheless, the most serious complications are seen following allogeneic marrow transplantation. These are viral infections in the form of gastroenteritis and interstitial pneumonitis as well as acute and chronic graft-versus-host disease.

During the first month following transplantation,

patients are highly susceptible to bacterial infections, particularly those gram-negative in origin. Patients in "good" clinical condition (i.e., in remission) are able to weather this period much better than the "end-stage" patients. The appropriate use of some of the newer antibiotics, isolation procedures, and judicious use of granulocyte transfusions have markedly decreased the severity of these complications (unless accompanied by severe acute graft-versus-host disease). Currently, mortality from bacterial infection is less than 5 percent in our center.

Following marrow transplantation, there is a severe combined immune deficiency which, in its gradual repair, mimics that expected in a recapitulation of ontogeny. It is therefore not surprising that these patients are, for a variable length of time, susceptible to life-threatening fungal (i.e., candidiasis, aspergillosis), protozoan (*Pneumocystis carinii*), and viral (herpes simplex, cytomegalovirus and varicella-zoster) infections. Despite the use of amphotericin B, fungal infections account for 5 percent of deaths. The problem of *Pneumocystis carinii* has largely been eliminated with the use of trimethoprim-sulfamethoxazole. Similarly, the morbidity and mortality from herpes simplex and herpes zoster infections have been markedly decreased with the use of the antiviral agent, acylovir. Interstitial pneumonitis, associated with cytomegalovirus in 60 percent of the cases, remains a particularly serious problem in most transplant centers. The incidence of interstitial pneumonitis in allogeneic transplants is 30 to 50 percent in various centers, with a case-fatality rate of 60 to 80 percent. Although prevention of this highly fatal infection is under intense investigation in a number of laboratories and centers, no ideal solution has yet been reached. Recent reports that prophylactic treatment of patients with cytomegalovirus hyperimmune globulin can prevent cytomegalovirus infection after marrow transplantation have been encouraging.

Acute graft-versus-host disease remains a major cause of morbidity and mortality following allogeneic marrow transplantation, despite the use of genotypically HLA-identical sib donors and post-transplant immunosuppression with methotrexate or cyclosphosphamide. This iatrogenic disease shows a varied clinical spectrum ranging from a mild skin rash to severe involvement of the skin, gut, liver, and bronchial mucosa. Depending on its severity, it is associated with profound immunodeficiency and susceptibility to opportunistic infections. Severe acute graft-versus-host disease may occur in 30 to 50 percent of patients, with a mortality of 30 to 60 percent of those affected. Treatment of this disease with steroids or antithymocyte globulin, although partially successful, is far from satisfactory. Some improvement has occurred with the institution of intravenous cyclosporine. A more promising approach is being evaluated at several centers in which an attempt is made to rid the marrow inoculum of the post-thymic T-cells, which initiate acute graft-versus-host disease. A variety of physical, immunologic (i.e., monoclonal antibodies), and pharmacologic methods are being actively pursued. At the moment, there is no clear-cut published series of patients in whom graft-versus-host disease is routinely prevented by these means.

A chronic form of graft-versus-host disease has been recognized in 25 to 40 percent of patients undergoing allogeneic marrow transplantation. The disease is polymorphic and has a number of clinical manifestations similar to the collagen vascular disorders: dyspigmentation, scleroderma-like lesions of the skin, mucositis, malabsorption, and pulmonary insufficiency. Chronic graft-versus-host disease appears to represent a severe imbalance of humoral and cellular immunity without the fine control that regulates an immune response. Mortality in this disease used to be as high as 80 percent, primarily because of the associated immunodeficiency and death due to gram-positive organisms. Currently this mortality has been reduced to about 10 percent as a result of empiric treatment with corticosteroids and azathioprine under trimethoprim-sulfamethoxazole prophylaxis.

DECISIONS RELATED TO TRANSPLANTATION

The decision to perform marrow transplantation depends on the disease being considered, the age of the patient, possible alternative therapy, and finally a personal decision of the patient.

Severe aplastic anemia under supportive care with and without androgen therapy is seldom cured. A patient so managed may show a 2-year survival of approximately 20 percent. Allogeneic or syngeneic marrow transplantation offers the possibility of cure in 50 to 70 percent of patients under the age of 35. Immunosuppressive therapy with antithymocyte globulin may improve the manifestations of severe aplastic anemia in about 40 percent and perhaps cure 20 percent of the patients. Since patients with no or minimal transfusions before the transplant have a much better course, I recommend tissue typing studies soon after diagnosis for patients 35 years of age and younger. The decision whether to perform the transplantation should then be made fairly quickly. In patients 35 years of age and older, one might consider the alternative possibility of immunosuppressive therapy. Clearly, if a hematologically normal identical twin is available as a donor, this should be considered for such patients under the age of 55.

In general, patients with acute leukemia in second or subsequent remission have marrow transplantation as their only hope of cure. Patients 20 years old or less may expect at least a 50 to 60 percent long-term disease-free survival and probable cure in a majority of cases. Patients aged 30 to 40 may expect about a 20 to 35 percent cure rate. In general, it is our policy to consider patients for transplantation somewhere between 4 and 6 weeks after obtaining a complete remission.

Because of the excellent therapeutic results with

acute lymphocytic leukemia in children who have good prognostic factors, marrow transplantation should be reserved until these patients have relapsed and then attained a second remission. It is suggested, and is currently under study in a number of centers, that children with poor prognostic factors for long-term disease-free survival and adults with acute lymphocytic leukemia should at least be considered for marrow transplantation in first remission since, with the exception of one report in the literature, a 2-year disease-free survival of greater than 20 percent is seldom seen following chemotherapy alone in these groups.

Marrow transplantation in acute nonlymphocytic leukemia in first remission may result in a long-term disease-free survival in 50 to 70 percent of patients. Somewhat similar results have been published from a single institution for chemotherapy in patients under the age of 20. Most chemotherapy series, however, do not report such a therapeutic result in the younger patients, and therefore marrow transplantation should at least be considered as a treatment option for these younger patients. In general, patients between the ages of 30 and 40 show only about a 30 percent long-term disease-free survival with marrow transplantation. Since this is not much better than results reported with chemotherapy alone, the decision to undergo transplantation is much more difficult and in part depends on the "track record" of the particular chemotherapy protocol that the patient had or is receiving. In general, patients in other than first remission are not curable with chemotherapy. Such patients under the age of 40 should be considered for allogeneic marrow transplantation.

Allogeneic marrow transplantation in chronic myelogenous leukemia has resulted in a 50 to 60 percent 2- to 3-year disease-free (absence of Ph^1 chromosome) survival in a number of centers. This treatment offers the only potential cure for this disease at the moment. The decision whether to transplant in this disease during the chronic phase is most difficult. Patients in the accelerated phase do less well with transplantation and do very poorly when transplanted in blast crisis. Patients with CML in the chronic phase treated more conservatively may experience a 15 percent mortality in the first year after diagnosis, but there is a 25 percent mortality of the remaining patients each subsequent year. Death is usually associated with blast crisis. Unfortunately, the accelerated phase of the disease may be quite short before blast crisis appears, and operationally there is no real warning as to when the patient will go into blast crisis. When transplantation is considered in the chronic phase, one must realize that the mortality in the first year is higher for those undergoing transplant than for those treated conservatively. By the end of the second and third year, however, the results are in favor of the transplanted patient. This, then, is a very personal decision of the well-informed and intelligent patient. The question posed is this: does the patient wish to take the significant chance of dying in the first several months after transplantation in order to be offered a potential cure of his or her disease? Although in chronic myelogenous leukemia the decision for transplantation is most difficult, it similarly presents a dilemma in acute leukemias, particularly in those patients considering transplantation while in their first remission.

Patients with non-Hodgkin's lymphoma who fail primary first-line therapy are usually not curable, although some subsets of this disease may have a relatively prolonged survival. We believe that patients with poor-risk non-Hodgkin's lymphoma should be offered allogeneic transplantation after they fail first-line cytoreductive therapy and not much later in their course. Current series of such patients are small in number with inadequate follow-up, but projections suggest that 30 to 50 percent of such patients may be curable with allogeneic marrow transplantation.

The immediate mortality associated with syngeneic and autologous transplantation in hematologic malignant disease is very low (5%). Relapse of the disease, however, presents a problem. Since we do not believe that transplantation accelerates the time to relapse, such patients should be considered for transplantation very early in the course of their disease.

Marrow transplantation is under very active and intense investigation in a number of centers around the world. It seems reasonable, therefore, to expect that therapeutic results will only continue to improve.

MULTIPLE MYELOMA AND RELATED MONOCLONAL GAMMOPATHY

ROBERT A. KYLE, M.D.

Multiple myeloma (plasma cell myeloma, myelomatosis, or Kahler's disease) is a malignant disease of plasma cells that typically involves the bone marrow, but often involves other tissue as well. The "myeloma cell" is an immature and atypical neoplastic plasma cell. Multiple myeloma may be regarded as a neoplastic proliferation of a single line of plasma cells engaged in the production of a specific protein. This protein is monoclonal—one class of heavy chains (γ, α, δ, or ϵ) and one type of light chain (κ or λ)—and is often referred to as "M" (monoclonal or myeloma) protein.

The presence of bone pain, fatigue, and an elevated erythrocyte sedimentation rate is suggestive of multiple myeloma. Other findings suggestive of myeloma include multiple osteolytic lesions, pathologic fracture, bone tumors, osteoporosis, hypercalcemia, azotemia, cryoglobulinemia, pyroglobulinemia, hyperglobulinemia, Bence Jones proteinuria, protein electrophoretic abnormalities, and evidence of bleeding or recurrent infections.

If multiple myeloma is suspected, the patient should have—in addition to a complete history and physical examination—determinations of hemoglobin or hematocrit and of leukocyte, differential, and platelet counts; measurements of serum creatinine, calcium, phosphorus, alkaline phosphatase, and uric acid; roentgenographic survey of bones, including humeri and femurs (bone scans with technietium-99m are inferior to conventional roentgenograms, but CT scans may reveal lytic lesions when roentgenograms are negative); serum protein electrophoresis, quantitation of immunoglobulins, immunoelectrophoresis or immunofixation, and tests for cryoglobulins and viscosity if the M-spike is large or symptoms of hyperviscosity exist; bone marrow aspiration and biopsy; routine urinalysis; and electrophoresis, immunoelectrophoresis, and immunofixation of an adequately concentrated aliquot from a 24-hour urine specimen.

Minimal criteria for diagnosis include a bone marrow specimen that contains more than 10 percent abnormal, immature, and atypical plasma cells or histologic proof of an extramedullary plasmacytoma and at least one of the following: M-protein in the serum, M-protein in the urine, or osteolytic lesions. Because marrow involvement may be focal rather than diffuse, repeated bone marrow aspirations and biopsies may be necessary. Connective tissue diseases, chronic infections, carcinoma, lymphoma, and leukemia may simulate some of the characteristics of myeloma and should be excluded unless other features make the diagnosis of multiple myeloma clear.

One must identify patients with monoclonal gammopathy of undetermined significance (benign monoclonal gammopathy), which is characterized by an M-protein of <3 g/dl in the serum, fewer than 5 percent marrow plasma cells, absence of anemia or osteolytic bone lesions, normal serum albumin, and either no M-protein or small amounts of M-protein in the urine—and no evidence of progression for at least 5 years of observation. Smoldering multiple myeloma also must be excluded. In this entity, the patient has an M-protein of >3 g/dl in the serum and >10 percent atypical plasma cells in the bone marrow, in contrast to patient with monoclonal gammopathy of undetermined significance. In addition, the patient frequently has a small amount of M-protein in the urine and a reduction of uninvolved immunoglobulins in the serum. However, anemia, renal insufficiency, and skeletal lesions do not develop and the patient remains stable. A plasma cell labeling index using tritiated thymidine is helpful in differentiating patients with monoclonal gammopathy of undetermined significance and smoldering myeloma from those with multiple myeloma. Careful follow-up is the rule, and the patient should not be treated unless progression occurs. It should be emphasized that clinically overt disease will develop during follow-up of most patients who fulfill the criteria for the diagnosis of multiple myeloma. Because multiple myeloma is not a curable condition, treatment shold be delayed until the patient develops evidence of progression or becomes symptomatic or until treatment is needed to prevent or delay complications.

SPECIFIC THERAPY

Chemotherapy

Chemotherapy is the most effective initial treatment for multiple myeloma. The use of melphalan (L-phenylalanine mustard, L-sarcolysine, Alkeran) and prednisone constitutes a standard approach and produces objective response in approximately 60 percent of patients. I prefer a combination of melphalan in a daily dosage of 0.15 mg/kg orally plus prednisone, 15 mg four times daily, for a 7-day period. The patient should eat a bland diet, avoid caffeine-containing products, and take antacids while on prednisone therapy. The leukocyte and platelet counts should be determined at 3- and 6-week intervals after the initiation of therapy. If the counts have not decreased, the daily dose of melphalan should be increased by 2 mg daily for the next 7-day course; some patients do not adequately absorb melphalan, and some can tolerate more than 200 mg of melphalan during the 7-day course. If the counts are low at 6 weeks, chemotherapy should be delayed and the counts repeated at weekly intervals. If the leukocyte and platelet counts remain low or if the counts obtained at 3 weeks are low, the next 7-day course of melphalan should be reduced accordingly. In the presence of renal insufficiency, the initial dose of melphalan should be modestly reduced (approximately 25 percent) and then increased if possible for the next course. The dose of melphalan should be calculated on the basis of the patient's ideal body weight. The dose of prednisone rarely needs to be reduced. In a few patients, the abrupt cessation of prednisone therapy at 7 days is associated with weakness, fatigue, and generalized aching, and in these patients, the prednisone dosage should be reduced gradually to zero during a 3- to 4-day period. The patient should be given melphalan for at least three courses before its use is discontinued, unless therapy causes significant toxic reactions or the disease progresses rapidly despite clearly adequate therapy. Maximal improvement may not be achieved for several months.

Melphalan also may be given in a daily oral dosage of 0.05 mg/kg after recovery of the leukocyte and platelet counts from an initial 7-day course of melphalan and prednisone. The leukocyte and platelet counts are determined every 2 weeks, and the dose of melphalan is adjusted to keep the leukocyte count near

3000/mm^3 and the platelet count between 100,000 and 150,000/mm^3.

Alternative Chemotherapy

Cyclophosphamide (Cytoxan) may be given in a daily oral dose of 2 mg/kg or intravenously in a dose of 15 mg/kg every 4 weeks. The patient should drink enough fluids so that 3 liters of urine are produced daily, because hemorrhagic cystitis or interstitial fibrosis of the bladder may occur. If the patient is resistant to melphalan, the likelihood of an objective response to cyclophosphamide is small.

Carmustine (BCNU) in a dose of 150 mg/m^2 intravenously every 6 weeks or lomustine (CCNU) in a dose of 100 mg/m^2 orally every 6 weeks also may be used as initial therapeutic agents, but they are generally inferior to melphalan.

A combination of melphalan, cyclophosphamide, carmustine, and prednisone has been reported to be superior to a combination of melphalan and prednisone for poor-risk patients with myeloma, but this has been refuted by other investigators.

The M-2 protocol, which combines melphalan, prednisone, carmustine, vincristine, and prednisone, has been reported to produce benefit in over 80 percent of patients. In a prospective randomized trial comparing the M-2 protocol with only melphalan and prednisone, patients on the M-2 protocol had a higher response rate, but the survival was not different in the two groups.

Duration of Chemotherapy

The duration of chemotherapy is controversial. Cessation of chemotherapy after 1 to 2 years usually results in relapse, and response to retreatment may be less frequent and of shorter duration than that after initial chemotherapy. However, continued chemotherapy may lead to refractory anemia or acute leukemia. Chromosome studies of the bone marrow in patients in whom pancytopenia develops may be useful in detecting patients with a myelodysplastic syndrome. The actuarial incidence of acute nonlymphocytic leukemia is approximately 5 percent at 5 years. A reasonable approach is to continue chemotherapy for 2 years and then to discontinue treatment if the patient has had a satisfactory response. The patient must then be followed up closely for evidence of relapse.

Therapy of Resistant Disease

Some patients with multiple myeloma do not respond to melphalan or cyclophosphamide, and others who do respond eventually become resistant to those agents. In these cases, a combination of carmustine (30 mg/m^2), doxorubicin (30 mg/m^2), and vincristine (2 mg) is given intravenously on day 1, and prednisone (15 mg) is given four times daily for 5 days. This regimen, repeated every 4 weeks, has produced some benefit in 40 percent of patients. The doses of carmustine and doxorubicin can be increased in 10-mg increments every 4 weeks if leukopenia or thrombocytopenia does not develop.

A combination of vincristine (0.4 mg per day) and doxorubicin (9 mg/m^2 per day), both given intravenously continuously for 4 days, plus dexamethasone (40 mg per day for 4 days and repeated every 8 days for three courses), produced objective responses in three-fourths of patients with myeloma who were resistant to melphalan. The cycle was repeated every 25 days.

Vindesine, cisplatin, chlorozotocin, M-AmSA (amsacrine), hexamethylmelamine, and deoxycoformycin (Pentostatin) have all been tried, but with little success. High-dose intravenous melphalan (100 to 140 mg/m^2) has been reported to produce objective responses, but cytopenia has been prominent.

Time-sequential chemotherapeutic regimens may be useful. Some patients with refractory myeloma respond to doxorubicin, carmustine, vincristine, and prednisone after synchronization with hydroxyurea. Occasionally, the use of vincristine every 9 days has been useful. The administration of doxorubicin 9 days after large intravenous doses of cyclophosphamide has also been reported to be of benefit.

Interferon has had considerable notice in both the lay and the medical press. However, enthusiasm in the lay media has far excceeded the reports of benefit in myeloma. Objective improvement has been reported for a minority of patients and is usually of short duration. Side effects are troublesome and include fever, chills, severe malaise, anorexia, loss of weight, leukopenia, and thrombocytopenia.

Bone marrow transplantation from identical twins has produced objective benefit, but multiple myeloma often recurs. Allogeneic bone marrow transplants have been performed in a few patients, but the results have been equivocal. Autologous bone marrow transplantation may prove useful if the myeloma cells can be removed from the marrow. Utilization of an idiotypic antibody to the tumor cells or an antibody to a myeloma-associated antigen may be useful in the future.

The development of a soft agar colony-forming assay for human myeloma stem cells has presented an opportunity for the in vitro prediction of drug sensitivity. With this system, the sensitivity of myeloma cells in the bone marrow has been tested by exposure to pharmacologically achievable concentrations of various chemotherapeutic agents. The assay appears to be more accurate in determining the resistance of a drug than in predicting whether a drug will be effective. However, only a minority of tumor cells will grow satisfactorily, and much needs to be done with this assay.

Radiation Therapy

Radiation is not effective as the only therapy for multiple myeloma because it is a generalized disease.

Radiation should not be given unless pain is severe and focal and does not respond to analgesics and chemotherapy. Palliative radiation in a dosage of 2000 to 2500 rads usually relieves the local pain, but the patient frequently experiences pain at another site. Although radiation may be repeated, it ultimately is limited by the development of leukopenia or thrombocytopenia, which in turn restricts the use of chemotherapy. If given, radiation therapy should be completed 3 weeks before chemotherapy is begun. Leukocyte and platelet counts should be measured before chemotherapy is started because the myelosuppressive effects of radiation and chemotherapy are cumulative. Thus, the role of radiation in multiple myeloma is limited.

Total bone marrow irradiation or hemibody irradiation has been used in a few patients with multiple myeloma, but benefit has been limited and side effects have been considerable.

Criteria for Response

Criteria for response to therapy include (1) decrease of serum M-protein by 50 percent or more, (2) decrease of urinary M-protein by 50 percent or more if initial value was 1.0 g/24 hr or more, (3) increase of hemoglobin concentration by 2.0 g/dl from an initial value of <11.0 g/dl without transfusion, (4) decrease of plasma cells in bone marrow by 50 percent or more, and (5) recalcification of skeletal lesions and absence of new bone lesions.

THERAPY OF SPECIAL PROBLEMS

Hypercalcemia

Hypercalcemia occurs in one-third of patients with multiple myeloma and must be suspected in the presence of anorexia, nausea, vomiting, polyuria, increased constipation, weakness, confusion, stupor, or coma. When hypercalcemia is symptomatic, treatment is urgent because renal insufficiency commonly occurs. Because dehydration frequently accompanies hypercalcemia, the patient should be hydrated. Isotonic saline is the agent of choice because sodium promotes the renal excretion of calcium. After hydration has been achieved, furosemide (Lasix), 40 mg every 4 hours, may be helpful. During diuretic therapy, the electrolytes must be monitored closely. In addition to hydration, prednisone in an initial dose of 25 mg four times daily should be given. This dosage must be reduced when the serum calcium level decreases and should be discontinued as quickly as possible. Hydrocortisone sodium succinate (Solu-Cortef) or methylprednisolone sodium succinate (Solu-Medrol) in equivalent doses may be used if the patient is unable to take prednisone orally. If these measures fail, mithramycin should be given intravenously in a dose of 25 μg/kg. Its effect is produced within 24 to 48 hours, but hypercalcemia often recurs after 2 or 3 days. A qualitative or quantitative platelet abnormality also may develop, further demonstrating that mithramycin has its shortcomings. Calcitonin has been used with some success. Hemodialysis utilizing a low calcium dialysate may be useful. If hypercalcemia recurs after an initial response, inorganic phosphate (Neutra-Phos) may be given on an outpatient basis. It must not be given if renal insufficiency or hyperphosphatemia is present. A dose of 150 ml orally four times daily (2.0 g of phosphorus daily) is usually effective. Since prolonged bed rest often contributes to hypercalcemia, patients with myeloma should be encouraged to be as active as possible.

Renal Insufficiency

More than 50 percent of patients with myeloma will suffer renal insufficiency. Hypercalcemia, protein casts in the proximal and distal tubules (myeloma kidney), hyperuricemia, deposition of amyloid, pyelonephritis, and infiltration of the kidney with plasma cells may all have roles in causing renal insufficiency. Maintaining a urinary output of 3 liters daily will reduce the likelihood of myeloma kidney.

If hyperuricemia occurs, allopurinol, 300 mg daily, provides effective therapy. If the patient is allergic to this agent, sodium bicarbonate, 0.6 to 0.9 g three or four times daily, and acetazolamide (Diamox), 250 mg at bedtime, can adequately alkalinize the urine. Oral tricitrates (Polycitra) also may be used.

Intravenous pyelography can precipitate renal insufficiency, but it can be performed with little risk if dehydration is avoided. Dehydration should be avoided in preparing the patient for a barium enema. Acute renal failure must be recognized and treated promptly with alkalinization and maintenance of fluid and electrolyte balance. If renal failure does not respond to conservative measures, hemodialysis is indicated. Patients with acute renal failure often respond, but if renal failure persists, long-term hemodialysis is successful in prolonging the patient's life. Acute renal failure also may be benefited by total plasma exchange (aggressive plasmapheresis). Renal transplantation for myeloma kidney has been followed by prolonged survival.

Infections

Bacterial infections are more common in patients with myeloma than in the normal population. Gram-negative organisms are as common as gram-positive infections. The frequency of such infections is related to a deficiency of normal immunoglobulins, impairment of antibody response, reduction of delayed hypersensitivity, reduction in numbers and activity of neutrophils, and, in some instances, depression of reticuloendothelial function. Significant fever is an indication for appropriate cultures, chest roentgenograms, and consideration of the use of broad-spectrum antibiotics. The selection of antibiotics can be made more specific once the results of cultures are known. The use of gentamicin in multiple myeloma must be carefully monitored because large decreases in renal function may occur. Injection of γ-globulin for prevention of infections has been ineffective. In the event of recurrent gram-positive bacterial infections, penicillin is useful prophylactically. Although antibody response is impaired in myeloma, pneumococcal vaccine should be given every 5 years.

Anemia

Anemia occurs eventually in almost every patient with myeloma. The anemia in myeloma is due mainly to an inadequate production of red cells by the bone marrow, but mild shortening of red cell survival, iron deficiency, and extravascular loss of blood also may have a significant influence. Increase of plasma volume from the osmotic effect of the monoclonal protein may produce hypervolemia and spuriously lower the hemoglobin or hemaocrit levels. Thus, significant anemia may be indicated by the hemoglobin value when the red cell mass is only slightly reduced. Transfusions with packed red cells remain the cornerstone of treatment, but successful therapy of the primary disease may restore erythropoiesis. A hemoglobin level of 8 to 10 g/dl is adequate unless there is symptomatic coronary artery disease or cerebrovascular insufficiency. Androgens such as fluoxymesterone (Halotestin), 10 mg three times daily, or testosterone enanthate (Delatestryl), 400 mg intramuscularly every 4 weeks, or oxymetholone (Anadrol), 50 mg three times daily, may be beneficial in some patients.

Skeletal Lesions

Bone lesions constitute a major problem. Although such lesions have been reported to heal with chemotherapy, the results are disappointing. Frequently, a brace or supporting garment is helpful, but avoidance of trauma is more important because even mild stress may result in multiple fractures. Nevertheless, the patient should be encouraged to be as active as possible because confinement to bed increases demineralization of the skeleton. Analgesics should be given to control the pain so that the patient can be ambulatory. Acetaminophen or aspirin should be given to control the pain so that the patient can be ambulatory. Acetaminophen or aspirin should be given initially, and if ineffective, codeine may be added. If these are ineffective, levorphanol or methadone may be used. Physical therapy also may be beneficial. Fixation of long-bone fractures or impending fracture with an intramedullary rod and methacrylate has given very satisfactory results. Sodium fluoride, calcium supplemention, vitamin D, and diphosphonates may prove to be of value in the future.

Hyperviscosity

The symptoms of hyperviscosity include oronasal bleeding, blurred vision, neurologic symptoms, and congestive heart failure. Many patients have symptoms when the relative serum viscosity reaches 4 to 5 centipoise (normal <1.8), but the relationship between serum viscosity and clinical manifestations is not precise. Hyperviscosity is more common in IgA myeloma than in IgG myeloma. Vigorous plasmapheresis with a cell separator will relieve the symptoms of hyperviscosity, but treatment with alkylating agents is necessary for long-term benefit.

Neurologic Complications

For the patient with multiple myeloma who states that his legs are weak or that he has difficulty in voiding or defecating, the possibility of extradural myeloma and spinal cord compression must be considered. The sudden onset of severe thoracic pain or the presence of a paraspinal mass also suggests the possibility of spinal cord compression. If any of these occurs, neurosurgical consultation is urgently needed and myelography is essential. Radiation therapy in a dose of approximately 3000 rads is beneficial. Dexamethasone (Decadron) should be administered daily during radiation therapy in order to reduce the edema. If the neurologic deficit worsens during radiation, one must proceed with surgical decompression followed by radiation therapy.

Psychologic Factors

Any patient with a serious disease such as multiple myeloma has psychologic problems and needs substantial, continuing emotional support. The approach must be positive. The physician must have confidence in his ability to cope with the patient's problems, and the patient should be able to sense this confidence. Potential benefits of therapy should be emphasized. It reassures the patient to know that some persons survive for 10 years or more. It is vital that the physician caring for patients with myeloma have the interest and capacity to deal with incurable disease over a span of months to years with assurance, sympathy, and resourcefulness.

VARIANTS OF MULTIPLE MYELOMA

Plasma Cell Leukemia

In plasma cell leukemia, there are more than 20 percent plasma cells in the peripheral blood and an absolute plasma cell content of at least $2000/mm^3$. Plasma cell leukemia may present as a terminal event of multiple myeloma, but more commonly it appears as the initial manifestation. The patient with de novo plasma cell leukemia should be given melphalan and prednisone on the same schedule as is the patient with multiple myeloma. If the patient does not respond or if he responds and then relapses, a combination of carmustine, doxorubicin, vincristine, and prednisone is given.

Solitary Plasmacytoma of Bone

The diagnosis of solitary plasmacytoma of bone depends on histologic proof of a plasma cell tumor without other evidence of multiple myeloma. Treatment of solitary plasmacytoma consists of radiation in the range of 4000 rads. There is no evidence that surgical removal of the plasmacytoma is superior to radiation. Electrophoresis and immunoelectrophoresis of the serum and urine are useful in following the course of a patient who has solitary plasmacytoma because most patients develop multiple myeloma during follow-up.

Extramedullary Plasmacytoma

These plasma cell tumors frequently involve the upper respiratory tract, but may develop in the gastrointestinal tract, lymph nodes, or other tissues. If there is no evidence of multiple myeloma, the patient should be treated with tumoricidal radiation in a dosage of 4000 rads. Occurrence usuallly involves extramedullary sites, and the development of multiple myeloma is infrequent.

HEMOPHILIA

IRWIN R. WALKER, M.B., B.S., F.R.A.C.P., F.R.C.P.(C)

Hemophilia is an X–linked recessive bleeding disorder resulting from a deficiency of either factor VIII (hemophilia A) or factor IX (hemophilia B or Christmas disease). Hemophilia A and B are clinically indistinguishable one from the other; however, they are treated differently. Together they affect about 15 males per 100,000 population, with hemophilia A being five times more common than hemophilia B.

The severity of the disorder correlates with the factor level. Severe hemophiliacs have factor levels of less than 1 percent of normal; they bleed an average of 25 times per year and most of these bleeds are spontaneous. Two-thirds of these are hemarthroses. Moderate hemophiliacs have factor levels of 1 to 5 percent, they bleed about 5 times per year, and most of these episodes are induced by trauma or vigorous activity. Mild hemophiliacs have factor levels between 5 and 50 percent; they rarely bleed spontaneously, most bleeds being related to trauma or surgery. Female carriers often have mildly depressed factor levels and may bleed excessively with surgery.

Bleeding in hemophiliacs is occasionally life-threatening, but the most common clinical problems result from repeated hemarthroses, which account for two-thirds of all bleeds. Repeated hemarthroses lead initially to synovitis, then to damage to cartilage and bone (hemophilic arthropathy), and ultimately to severe forms of osteoarthritis and complete joint destruction.

Inhibitors develop in 7 percent of all factor VIII deficient hemophiliacs, but rarely in factor IX deficient subjects. The inhibitors neutralize the coagulation factors in blood products, thus compromising or even completely preventing any response.

AIMS OF THERAPY

Cessation of Acute Hemorrhage. This is achieved by the prompt infusion of appropriate blood products in quantities to sufficiently elevate factor levels. The infusion is repeated at appropriate intervals until satisfactory resolution of bleeding and hematoma is obtained. Ancillary measures such as physiotherapy, splinting and analgesic administration are often necessary when moderate and severe hemoarthrosis occurs. Prompt therapy usually results in rapid relief of pain, restoration of function, maintenance of muscle tone, and minimal morbidity. This approach appreciably delays and reduces chronic joint destruction but probably does not totally prevent it.

Prevention of Spontaneous Bleeding. This ideal is sometimes attempted by the prophylactic administration of blood products. This approach is limited by the inconvenience of frequent intravenous injections (average 150 infusions per year compared with 40 per year for episodic therapy), by the availability and expense of the blood products, and by the risk of complications, particularly hepatitis, but possibly acquired immunodeficiency syndrome (AIDS) as well. Prophylactic therapy is usually reserved for hemophiliacs who are having more than an average number of bleeds, who are consuming large amounts of blood products, who are having repetitive bleeding into single joints (target joints), whose hemorrhages are causing excessive disability, and who have had a life-threatening bleed. Intracranial bleeding which is unprovoked by obvious trauma often recurs and prophylactic therapy is usually advisable in these cases.

Prophylactic therapy usually reduces the number of hemorrhages, but whether prophylactic therapy using currently accepted dosages can prevent joint damage is unknown. Joint damage tends to be progressive, and any attempt to prevent this by prophylactic therapy would need to be started at an early age.

BLOOD PRODUCTS

Factor VIII is available both as factor VIII concentrate and as cryoprecipitate. Factor VIII concentrate is a purified lyophilized (freeze-dried) preparation which is stable for about one year at 4°C and for about 6 months at room temperature. The exact periods for each vial are specified in the manufacturer's instructions. The concentrate is the most convenient preparation, but it is manufactured from large pools of donors and carries a risk of hepatitis. Cryoprecipitate is a crude preparation which contains fibrinogen and other plasma proteins in addition to factor VIII. It is simple and inexpensive to prepare, and there is a lower risk of hepatitis, but it is stable only when frozen and is therefore less convenient to store and administer. Each bag of cryoprecipitate is prepared from one unit of whole blood and contains approximately 80 units of factor VIII clotting activity and 250 mg fibrinogen in 5 to 10 ml of plasma.

Factor IX concentrate is a lyophilized preparation which also contains the other vitamin K dependent clotting factors (II, VII, and X). There is a high risk of hepatitis especially for nonimmune individuals.

Calculation of Dosage

Clotting activity is expressed in units. One unit is that amount present in 1 ml of fresh plasma pooled from several donors; 1000 ml of plasma therefore contains 1000 units of both factor VIII and factor IX. Average levels of these factors in the plasma of normal subjects is 1 unit/ml with a range of 0.50 to 1.50 units/ml. Traditionally this has been expressed as a mean of 100 percent with a range of 50 to 150 percent.

The rise in factor level in response to the infusion of blood product depends on the dose and volume of distribution. Factor IX has a significant extravascular distribution, and the rise in level will be smaller than that following the same number of units of factor VIII, which is distributed in the vascular volume alone. The formulas for estimating dosages of factor VIII and IX are as follows:

1. 1 unit of factor VIII infused/kg body weight yields a 2 percent rise in plasma VIII level.
2. 1 unit of factor IX infused/kg body weight yields a 1 percent rise in plasma IX level.

To achieve a 50 percent rise in a 70–kg man would require $50 \div 2 \times 70$ kg = 1750 units of factor VIII or 50×70 kg = 3500 units of factor IX. To achieve the same levels with fresh frozen plasma would require 1750 ml and 3500 ml respectively, an impossible task when the need for speed and repeated infusions is taken into account. The number of units in a bottle of concentrate is stated on the label; the number of units of factor VIII in a bag of cryoprecipitate is approximately 80 units, though this may vary widely with each bag.

The frequency of dosage depends on the plasma half-life of the factor; this is 8 to 12 hours for factor VIII and 24 hours for factor IX. To maintain a given factor level (1) administer enough to double the desired level; (2) repeat half this dose every 12 hours in the case of factor VIII, 24 hours for factor IX; and (3) check the estimated level by factor assays every day or two. The dosage intervals should be shortened in life-threatening or in limb-threatening circumstances.

SPECIFIC MANAGEMENT

Acute Hemorrhage. Therapy early in the course of bleeding will minimze the risk of serious complications and disruption of normal activities. However, the diagnosis of bleeding may at times be in doubt, and the physician will be faced with the dilemma of whether or not to administer blood products. The relative risk of a single infusion of blood products is negligible in severe hemophiliacs, most of whom will already have received hundreds of such infusions. In such subjects, *"When in doubt, infuse"*. Attempts to confirm the presence of bleeding should follow therapy—not precede it. Unless the diagnosis of the bleeding disorder is in doubt, measurement of baseline factor levels prior to therapy is unnecessary and delays treatment. Hemophiliacs usually carry documentation of their diagnosis and are experienced in detecting early hemarthrosis even before it is detectable by a physician.

Subjects with mild and moderate hemophilia, most of whom receive infrequent infusions of blood products, undergo a greater risk of developing hepatitis from a single infusion of blood products than do severe hemophiliacs, most of whom have received hundreds or even thousands of such infusions and have either already contracted hepatitis or are partially immune. Measures to decrease the likelihood of hepatitis in moderately or mildly affected subjects should be considered (see Side Effects of Therapy).

Hemorrhages are classified as minor, moderate, and major (Table 1).

Minor bleeds (e.g., are hemarthroses with less than 30 percent loss of range of motion) are treated with factor VIII to attain factor levels of 30 percent, after which restoration of function usually occurs within 24 hours and repeat infusions are unnecessary.

Moderate bleeding (e.g., severe joint or muscle bleeds; bleeds into neck, tongue, or pharynx; gastrointestinal bleeding; head trauma without neurologic defect) is treated by infusion to attain factor levels of 50 percent, and then infusion is repeated until adequate restoration of function has occurred. It is wise to administer the factor therapy prior to physiotherapy.

Major bleeding is that which is threatening to life

TABLE 1 Summary of Initial Doses of Replacement Products

Severity of Bleeding	*Recommended Factor Level (%)*	*Dose of Factor VIII* (μ/kg)*	*Dose of Factor IX† (μ/kg)*
Mild‡	30	15	30
Early joint or muscle bleeding			
Epistaxis			
Dental bleeding			
Persistent hematuria			
Moderate‡	50	25	50
Major joint bleeding			
Muscle bleeding			
Neck, tongue, pharynx bleeding			
Gastrointestinal bleeding			
Suspected abdominal bleeding			
Head trauma without neurologic deficit			
Major§	75–100	40–50	75–100
Intracranial bleeding			
Surgery			
Compartment syndrome			
Major trauma			

* Subsequent doses of factor VIII are given every 8–12 hrs.

† Subsequent doses of factor IX are given every 18–24 hrs.

‡ Duration of therapy is determined by time to adequate resolution.

§ Duration of therapy is for minimum of one week but often several weeks.

or limb (e.g., bleeding into the central nervous system, bleeding involving peripheral nerves, and compartment syndromes). An initial infusion to attain 75 to 100 percent of clotting activity is followed by repeat infusion at frequent intervals (e.g., at 6 to 8 hours for factor VIII, 12 hours for factor IX) to maintain factor levels at greater than 50 percent. In this situation therapy should be monitored by factor levels.

Major Surgery. For elective surgery a test should be carried out for the presence of an inhibitor and a preoperative infusion should result in a factor level of 75 to 100 percent confirmed by factor assay. Failure of factor levels to rise as expected raises the possibility of an inhibitor even though the inhibitor assay has been negative. Dosages are repeated as for major bleeding, and infusions should be continued for the period of risk, usually 7 to 10 days. An infusion should be administered prior to the removal of sutures.

Dental Surgery. As with other surgery, this requires factor levels of 75 to 100 percent prior to the procedure. Antifibrinolytic therapy with epsilon-aminocaproic acid (EACA) or tranexamic acid is commenced immediately and continued by the oral route for 7 to 10 days. Tranexamic acid is usually tolerated better than EACA. Blood products are administered only if bleeding occurs. Note that antifibrinolytic therapy is not useful for situations other than dental work.

INHIBITORS

These develop in 10 to 15 percent of severe factor VIII deficient hemophiliacs, in less than 5 percent of moderately or mildly affected subjects, and only rarely in those with factor IX deficiency. Factor VIII inhibitors neutralize administered factor VIII, thus compromising or even completely preventing any response. Therapy of hemorrhage in affected subjects is most unsatisfactory. Bleeding that seems innocuous can progress and become life-threatening or limb-threatening despite prompt therapy. Management should include consultation with those experienced in treating such patients, usually hematologists at a Comprehensive Hemophilia Center (to be discussed). Assay for inhibitors should be performed annually in severe factor VIII deficient subjects and, in addition, prior to surgery and whenever response to factor VIII therapy seems inadequate. In addition, prior to surgery, factor assay should be performed to ensure that the response to an infusion has been as expected.

Following infusion of factor VIII to subjects with an inhibitor, there will be an anamnestic rise in the titer of the inhibitor in 80 percent of cases (high responder). If factor VIII therapy is then withheld, the level of the inhibitor often falls to low levels over a period of many weeks or months. At that time, the infusion of massive amounts of factor VIII may result in therapeutic levels of factor VIII in the blood until an anamnestic rise in the inhibitor level occurs once again, usually after a period of 24 to 72 hours. In 20 percent of cases the titer is low and does not rise subsequent to the infusion of factor VIII (low responder). However, the behavior of the inhibitor may vary at different times in the same subject.

Factor VIII therapy is reserved for those subjects whose inhibitor level has not previously been rising in response to Factor VIII infusions and in any subject whose inhibitor level is low, e.g., less than 20 Bethesda units, when bleeding is of a life-threatening or limb-threatening degree. Massive doses, e.g., 100 units/kg, may be required in order to attain a measurable level of factor VIII and plasma levels should be assayed following infusion. A response is unlikely when the inhibitor level is greater than 30 Bethseda units. Below this level a trial infusion is recommended if bleeding is of major magnitude. Factor VIII of porcine origin is used in the presence of bleeding when the inhibitor does not cross-react with it in vitro. Good clinical responses to this product occur when measurable levels of factor VIII are attainable. To lower the level of the inhibitor, plasmaphoresis should be considered if time and facilities permit.

Factor IX concentrate contains activities, probably activated clotting factors and phospholipid, which bypass factor VIII in the coagulation cascade. Factor IX concentrate is used when the inhibitor titer is high or if the titer is low but bleeding is not life-threatening. Activated factor IX preparations (Autoplex and FEIBA) may not be more effective than standard products and their use is limited by expense. Use of these products should be considered after lack of response to standard factor IX preparations. In general, response of bleeding to factor IX concentrate in subjects with inhibitors is much less likely than response to factor VIII in subjects without an inhibitor. Following hemarthrosis in a subject with an inhibitor, a prompt response is seen in only 50% of cases following factor IX concentrate compared with over 90% of subjects without an inhibitor who are given factor VIII concentrate.

Therapy for the individual bleeding episode depends therefore on the severity of the bleeding and the level and previous behavior of the inhibitor. The recommended approach is summarized in Table 2. The therapy of hemorrhage in the presence of inhibitors is marked by both uncertainty and controversy, and the recommendations in Table 2 should be taken only as a general guide.

SIDE EFFECTS OF THERAPY

Transmission of hepatitis to regularly transfused hemophiliacs probably occurs universally, and 60 percent of severe hemophiliacs have abnormal liver function. At any one time, 60 percent of patients have raised serum transaminases, 80 percent have antibodies to hepatitis B virus, and 5 percent have detectable hepatitis B antigen. Liver biopsy usually demonstrates either chronic active hepatitis or chronic persistent hepatitis. Chronic hepatitis is probably a result not only of hepatitis B virus but also of other viruses (e.g., non–A, non–B hepatitis, CMV). The prognosis is unknown; occasionally cirrhosis with portal hypertension is documented, but many cases remain compensated over long periods of time without the development of cirrhosis. Acute hepatitis is recognized in only a minority of hemophiliacs. Reduction of therapy is not an acceptable solution; mild and moderate hemophiliacs who consume blood products far less often than severe hemophilacs also have an appreciable incidence of chronic hepatitis. Furthermore, withholding therapy will increase the complications from bleeding. The elimination of hepatitis is not possible at the present time. Patients having no detectable hepatitis B antigen or antibody in the serum should receive hepatitis B vaccine. Cryoprecipitate should be used in preference to factor VIII concentrate in factor VIII deficient subjects who are infrequently transfused and should be considered in newly diagnosed cases as an attempt to delay this inevitable complication. In mild and moderate hemophilia A the use of blood products may be avoided by the use of desmopressin acetate (DDAVP; 1–deamino–8–d–arginine vasopressin) which causes rapid and clinically useful rises of factor VIII. Such responses occur in most mildly affected individuals and some moderately affected ones also. All mildly and moderately affected subjects should receive a trial injection to gauge response. In factor IX deficient subjects, plasma might substitute for factor IX concentrate in some circumstances, particularly if plasmapheresis, which will increase the dose of plasma that can be administered, is available.

Acquired immunodeficiency syndrome (AIDS) has occurred in a number of hemophiliacs, and blood products may be directly or indirectly responsible. At present, information is scarce, and the risks of untreated hemorrhage are greater than the risk of acquiring AIDS. No modifications to therapeutic recommendations can be made at the present time.

Allergic reactions occur in occasional patients receiving cryoprecipitate. These reactions usually are manifested as urticaria, pruritus, or low-grade fever. Anaphylactic reactions are rare. Allergic reactions following concentrate are by contrast infrequent and mild; a change to a different lot number is rarely followed by another reaction. Reactions requiring treatment usually resolve rapidly with antihistamines; adrenaline is reserved for anaphylactic reactions. The risk of allergic reactions can be decreased by a slower rate of infusion of the blood product.

Hemolytic anemia may occur following the infusion of large doses of concentrate. Hemolysis occurs only in those subjects with type A or B red cells and is a result of high titers of anti–A or anti–B antibodies in the concentrate. This side effect is uncommon and resolves spontaneously, but blood transfusion may be necessary, in which case type O red cells should be given.

The development of *inhibitors* may be related to exposure of blood products containing factor VIII. However, it is not related to the frequency or intensity of exposure. There may be a familial predisposition to this complication.

Factor IX concentrate predisposes to *thrombosis*, usually of the deep leg veins. Thrombosis is uncommon except following infusion of large doses of con-

TABLE 2 Treatment of Hemorrhages in the Presence of Inhibitors

Inhibitor Type	*Bleeding Severity*	*Product*	*Dosage and Frequency*
High responder	Minor or moderate	Factor IX concentrate	75 μ/kg q. 12 h.
High responder low titer	Major	Factor VIII concentrate (human or porcine)	50–100 μ/kg
High responder high titer	Major	Factor IX cncentrate	75–100 μ/kg *q6h*. < 48 h.
Low responder	Any severity	Factor VIII concentrate (human)	To maintain Factor VIII at appropriate level

centrate as happens in association with surgery, and it is predisposed to by hepatic dysfunction. When considering surgery in factor IX deficient subjects, this complication should be taken into account.

SELF-INFUSION PROGRAMS

Hemophiliacs who bleed frequently are not satisfactorily treated in hospitals. Hospital-based therapy is frequently delayed or omitted altogether, and there is an unsatisfactory disruption to daily life. Hemophiliacs who self-administer their therapy become more motivated, have less absenteeism from work and school, and maintain self-esteem. A self-infusion program is less costly to both the health care system and the hemophiliac. Self-infusion programs are usually organized through Comprehensive Hemophilia Centers (to be discussed). When hemophiliacs are on such a program, contact with physicians naturally decreases markedly. Monitoring is essential to ensure that recommendations are being followed, that the recommendations are effective, and that the hemophiliac knows when he must consult his physician.

OTHER THERAPIES

Pain relief for acute hemorrhages or occasional arthritic pain can be achieved with acetaminophen alone or in combination with codeine. Aspirin is contraindicated because of its adverse effects on platelet function. Nonsteroidal anti-inflammatory drugs are frequently prescribed for arthritic pain. The effects on platelet function appear not to be clinically significant, and the frequency of bleeding does not increase. However, gastric ulceration with hemorrhage may still occur on rare occasions as in nonhemophiliac subjects. Surgery for the hemophiliac joint is most commonly either synovectomy or arthroplasty. Synovectomy is usually successful in reducing or eliminating the frequency of bleeding, but its performance must be weighed against the loss of range of movement that sometimes occurs and the prolonged rehabilitation that is required. Arthroplasty is performed in cases of advanced arthritis. There is a high rate of success in the relief of pain, but the performance of this operation must be weighed against a number of drawbacks, which include the limited life span of artificial joints and the prolonged postoperative rehabilitation.

COMPREHENSIVE HEMOPHILIA CENTERS

Although hemophilia is a rare disease, its impact on health services is great. The potential for disability resulting in unemployment, absenteeism from school, and the need for social services is high. The provision of blood products is very expensive, and all the plasma from all blood donations may be insufficient to meet a national need. Finally, the skills required to manage many of the medical and surgical problems are beyond the experience of all but a few medical practitioners. Comprehensive Hemophilia Centers, which exist in most developed countries, concentrate the skills and experience. They provide an advisory service, they organize self-infusion programs, and they monitor the utilization of blood products, the correctness and effectiveness of treatment programs, and the social adjustment of the individual. Genetic testing and counseling services are provided, and major surgery is usually carried out at these centers. The centers coordinate their efforts with the primary care physicians and other providers of care. All hemophiliacs should be evaluated by a team from such a center at least once each year.

VON WILLEBRAND'S DISEASE

HARVEY J. WEISS, M.D.

DESCRIPTION OF THE DISORDER

Von Willebrand's disease is an autosomally transmitted disorder of hemostasis due to the deficiency of a protein, the von Willebrand factor, which is synthesized in endothelial cells and megakaryocytes. This protein circulates in plasma as a series of multimers with molecular weights ranging from 1 to 20 million daltons and has two major biologic activities. First, it is necessary for platelets to function normally during primary hemostasis, and its diminished plasma level accounts for the prolonged bleeding time in von Willebrand's disease. Second, the von Willebrand factor somehow controls the plasma level of another protein (possessing factor VIII coagulant activity) whose synthesis is controlled by a gene located on the X-chromosome. Thus, the plasma levels of factor VIII coagulant activity, (VIII:C, also known as the antihemophilic factor, AHF) is diminished in both hemophilia and von Willebrand's disease, but for different reasons. Currently, the von Willebrand factor and antihemophilic factor are both thought to be part of a complex of two proteins (the factor VIII complex), and the von Willebrand factor component of this complex is sometimes referred to as FVIII/VWF. A useful measurement of FVIII/VWF is to assay it by immunologic methods, and the property detected by these methods is designated as FVIII-related antigen (VIIIR:Ag). Clinically, some patients with von Willebrand's disease are relatively severe bleeders (generally those with marked deficiencies of VIIIR:Ag and VIII:C); others, with type I von Willebrand's disease, have less pronounced abnormalities of the FVIII complex and may only bleed excessively in association with trauma or surgical procedures. In another type of von Willebrand's disease (type II), the higher-molecular-weight multimers of FVIII/VWF are absent in the plasma.

THERAPEUTIC AGENTS AVAILABLE

At present, therapy is directed at shortening the bleeding time and increasing the plasma levels of FVIII/VWF and VIII:C during active bleeding or in association with surgical procedures when excessive bleeding may be anticipated.

Transfusion of Plasma or Cryoprecipitate Containing FVIII/VWF and VIII:C

Since both proteins are found in plasma, transfusions of freshly prepared or fresh frozen plasma were used initially to control bleeding. This form of therapy has been superseded by the use of cryoprecipitate, which contains both FVIII/VWF and VIII:C. Cryoprecipitate is generally prepared by freezing a unit (approximately 200 ml) of freshly prepared platelet-poor plasma at −70°C and then allowing the unit to thaw at 4°C. Under these conditions, a small amount of the plasma proteins (including fibrinogen, FVIII/VWF, and VIII:C) remain as a precipitate and, after centrifugation and separation of the thawed plasma, the cryoprecipitate can be stored at −70°C. When needed, the cryoprecipitate is dissolved by incubation (generally 30 min) at 37°C. When administered to a patient with severe von Willebrand's disease (VIIIR:Ag <1 U/dl, VIII:C <3 U/dl), the initial increase in both VIIIR:Ag and VIII:C is in proportion to the amounts contained in the transfused material. In general, a single transfusion of 10 units of cryoprecipitate (e.g., the cryoprecipitate obtained from 10 units, or about 2000 ml, of plasma) can be expected to increase the VIIIR:Ag and VIII:C levels in plasma to about 30 to 50 U/dl in a 70-kg adult. The VIIIR:Ag level in the plasma then declines, with a half-life of approximately 10 to 12 hours. For reasons not entirely clear, the VIII:C level does not decline, but instead continues to increase. The peak plasma level of VIII:C (generally 60 to 100 U per dl) is generally reached in 4 to 6 hours, and normal levels may persist for 24 hours. A correction of the bleeding may also be expected after transfusion of cryoprecipitate. The degree of shortening is unpredictable and is generally observed one hour after transfusion, although occasionally the maximal shortening is observed after 2 to 4 hours. Twenty-four hours after transfusion, the bleeding time has usually returned to pretreatment values.

The specific use of cryoprecipitate in managing patients with von Willebrand's disease will be discussed later. In general, the use of ABO-compatible cryoprecipitate is preferable, although not mandatory in emergency situations. Some patients may experience allergic reactions to cryoprecipitate, which may be attenuated by prior administration of 50 mg of Benadryl (diphenhydramine) or other suitable antihistaminic agents. Occasionally, and unpredictably, more severe anaphylaxis with subglottal edema may occur. Patients receiving cryoprecipitate are also at risk for contracting transfusion-related hepatitis and, in theory, might be at some small risk for developing acquired immunodeficiency syndrome (AIDS), although at this writing no such cases of the latter have been reported.

1-Desamino-8-D-Arginine Vasopressin (DDAVP)

DDAVP is an analog of vasopressin which has been shown to increase the levels of both VIIIR:Ag and VIII:C in normal subjects two- to fourfold, probably by stimulating the release of FVIII/VWF from endothelial cells. DDAVP can also increase the levels of VIIIR:Ag and VIII:C and shorten the bleeding time for 4 to 6 hours in patients with type I von Willebrand's disease. No measurable increases of the FVIII complex, or shortening of the bleeding time, is observed in patients with severe von Willebrand's disease (VIIIR:Ag <1 and VIII:C <3 U/dl), and in type II von Willebrand's disease the bleeding time may not be corrected even when normal levels of VIIIR:Ag are achieved, although VIII:C may be restored to normal. DDAVP may be administered by either the intranasal or intravenous route. The usual intranasal dose is 4 μg/kg. More predictable increases in the FVIII complex can be achieved by intravenous administration of DDAVP, at a dose of 0.4 μg/kg given over 30 minutes. No serious side effects have been reported, but some facial flushing during and immediately after transfusion may occur.

Antifibrinolytic Agents

Agents that inhibit fibrinolysis (such as epsilon-aminocaproic acid [EACA]) do not specifically increase the levels of the FVIII complex in patients with von Willebrand's disease. However, by inhibiting normal fibrinolysis, they may favorably effect hemostasis (particularly in patients with mild von Willebrand's disease), but careful clinical studies with these agents are lacking.

Other Agents

There is no evidence that agents such as corticosteroids, Premarin, or bioflavinoids are useful. Although most of the commercially available factor VIII concentrates used for treating hemophilia also increase the VIII:C and VIIIR:Ag levels in von Willebrand's disease, most of these fractions do not shorten the bleeding time. In addition, the use of these products in North America for treating hemophiliacs has been associated with the development of AIDS. At present, there is no indication that platelet transfusions are useful in von Willebrand's disease (although platelets do contain FVIII/VWF in their granules).

MANAGEMENT OF PATIENTS

In general, the approach to therapy should take into consideration the severity of the disease, as assessed by levels of VIIIR:Ag and VIII:C, and by the patient's previous history of spontaneous and surgery-related bleeding. Drugs that contain aspirin or other cyclo-oxygenase inhibitors should be avoided; acetaminophen may be used for mild analgesia. As a general rule, cryoprecipitate should be used as sparingly as possible to avoid the complications described previously. Below are some guidelines for commonly encountered situations.

Dental Procedures

In patients with mild von Willebrand's disease (by both laboratory and clinical criteria) it is probably best to avoid the use of cryoprecipitate for tooth extractions or minor gingival surgery. Adequate hemostasis in these patients can generally be achieved by the use of local measures and may be enhanced by administering EACA (4 g *qid* for 2 days). Recent reports indicate that DDAVP can raise VIIIR:Ag and VIII:C levels in patients with type I von Willebrand's disease (already discussed), and this agent has been used successfully to manage patients undergoing dental procedures when excessive bleeding is anticipated (for example, multiple extractions of third molar teeth and extensive gingival surgery). Patients with severe von Willebrand's disease undergoing extensive dental procedures, such as those already mentioned, should receive cryoprecipitate, 10 units 3 to 4 hours prior to the procedure, in order to take advantage of the "secondary increase" in VIII:C levels that usually occurs.

Other Surgical Procedures

For surgical procedures in which major bleeding is anticipated, all patients with severe von Willebrand's disease should receive cryoprecipitate. As already described, 10 units should be given preoperatively (a transfusion 8 to 12 hours preoperatively will usually "prime" the VIII:C level), followed by 10 units at the time of surgery. Following extensive surgical procedures, a further transfusion of 10 units of cryoprecipitate, 6 to 12 hours postoperatively, is usually indicated. The patient's clinical course usually determines the need for further transfusions. Unfortunately, measurements of the plasma VIII:C and VIIIR:Ag levels are not always reliable indicators of the need for more therapy (the bleeding time, for example, may not always be corrected to the extent predicted by the VIIIR:Ag level). When clinically indicated, cryoprecipitate (10 to 20 units every 8 to 12 hours) should be administered as required to obtain adequate hemostasis.

Patients with milder forms of von Willebrand's disease who undergo major surgical procedures may be treated with 10 units of cryoprecipitate 2 to 4 hours preoperatively, with subsequent therapy determined by the clinical course. The use of DDAVP as adjunctive therapy may also be considered and, if the VIIIR:Ag, VIII:C, and bleeding time values can be corrected, the use of DDAVP alone may be considered, although there is considerably less experience with this approach.

Other Clinical Situations

The treatment of acute bleeding episodes should be similar to that described above for major surgery. The therapy of patients who develop gastrointestinal bleeding may be particularly frustrating for both patient and physician. Frequently, bleeding occurs from blood vessels that have undergone angiodysplastic changes, and these may occur at multiple sites in the gastrointestinal tract. The requirements for cryoprecipitate must be determined entirely by the patient's clinical response and occasionally it may be necessary to administer 10 to 20 units three to five times per week before gastrointestinal bleeding stops. Recently, the fulgurization of these lesions under direct endoscopic vision by means of laser therapy has been successful in some patients. Surgical resection should be considered only when there is some assurance that the lesions are entirely localized to one segment of the bowel and when the aforementioned forms of therapy have been unsuccessful in controlling bleeding.

Obstetric and Gynecologic Bleeding

For unknown reasons, the VIII:C and VIIIR:Ag levels generally increase in pregnant patients with mild type I von Willebrand's disease. These levels should be followed carefully and, if the bleeding time is normal at the time of delivery, cryoprecipitate need not be given. However, 10 units should be kept at hand in the unlikely event that excessive postpartum bleeding occurs. In contrast, it would be prudent to administer cryoprecipitate at delivery to all patients with severe von Willebrand's disease. Menorrhagia is a frequent symptom in patients with severe forms of von Willebrand's disease and is usually treated with drugs to suppress ovulation.

VITAMIN K-DEPENDENT COAGULATION FACTOR DEFICIENCY STATES

ALAN R. GILES, M.D., F.R.C.P.(C)

Vitamin K plays an essential cofactor role in the synthesis of a number of unique proteins, all of which may be identified by the presence of γ-carboxyglutamic acid residues, which are responsible for calcium ion binding. Four of these proteins are essential zymogens in the coagulation cascade and are collectively known as the prothrombin complex. These are factor II (prothrombin), factor VII (proconvertin), factor IX (Christmas factor), and factor X (Stuart-Prower factor). Qualitative or quantitative deficiencies of these factors are associated with a more or less severe bleeding disorder, as will be discussed. Of the remaining vitamin K-dependent proteins, protein C has recently received particular attention as current experimental data suggest that it is a significantly important physiologic anticoagulant and promoter of fibrinolytic activity. The former activity is exerted by its potent ability to inactivate the critical cofactors V and VIII:C. Deficiencies of protein C appear to be associated with a thrombotic tendency. The roles of the remaining K-dependent proteins in normal physiology are still under evaluation. In this chapter, an overview of the treatment of the deficiency states of vitamin K-dependent proteins as they relate to hemostasis will be given. Although rapid progress may be expected in the area of protein C deficiency, this review is confined to deficiencies of the prothrombin complex.

GENERAL CONSIDERATIONS IN THERAPY

Bleeding may occur as a result of isolated or multiple deficiencies of the prothrombin complex. The former usually occur as a result of congenital deficiency, whereas the latter usually represent an acquired deficiency state resulting from vitamin K deficiency or generalized impairment of hepatic synthesis. The rational use of available therapies requires that, wherever possible, the precise deficiency should be established by both appropriate coagulation tests and consideration of the patient's personal and family history. Therapy is also dictated by the relative urgency of the clinical situation. Life-threatening bleeding, actual or potential, requires the immediate replacement of the deficient clotting factor(s). Non-life-threatening deficiency states or prophylactic considerations may be handled by appropriate attention to the underlying mechanism responsible for the disorder.

BLOOD PRODUCTS

The use of blood products is required when immediate replacement is essential in order to correct life-threatening bleeding or when there is impairment of synthesis despite adequate availability of vitamin K.

Single Donor Plasma

Single donor plasma is available as fresh frozen plasma (FFP) from most blood transfusion agencies throughout the world. Each pack represents the plasma prepared by simple separation techniques from a single donation of blood from one normal individual. The plasma is usually frozen within 6 hours of collection and has a volume of 200 to 250 ml. As the plasma has been collected from normal individuals, it is assumed by international convention that it contains 1.0 unit/ml of all coagulation factors including the temperature-labile factors V and VIII:C. Stored at −30° C, a shelf life of one year can be expected, although this may vary due to differing regulations in the countries concerned.

The plasma is prepared for administration by thawing in a 37° C waterbath with regular agitation. Most agencies provide ABO, but not rhesus, grouping of availble plasma. Cross-matching is not required, but plasma infused should be compatible with the recipient as shown in Table 1.

As all factors are provided, FFP is particularly useful when the precise nature of the coagulation factor deficiency is unknown. However, its use in established deficiencies of the prothrombin complex is wasteful because it is a valuable source of factors V and VIII:C, which are not required in this condition. Some transfusion agencies provide single-donor plasma which, although collected and separated in an identical fashion to FFP, is either not frozen or not frozen within the required interval to protect the labile clotting factors V and VIII:C. Such plasma may be stored for as long as 4 weeks at 4° C without any loss of potency of the K-dependent clotting factors. Plasma frozen within 6 to 24 hours retains full potency for as long as 5 years stored at −20° C or lower. The former has the advantage of being ready for immediate use, i.e., transfusion, as defrosting is not required.

When large increments of clotting factor activity are required, the need for relatively large-volume infusions may result in volume overload, particularly in patients with compromised cardiovascular or renal function. This volume overload is the principal dis-

TABLE 1 ABO Blood Group

Recipients	*Donor*
O	O,A,B,AB
A	A,AB
B	B,AB
AB	AB

advantage of the use of single-donor plasma replacement.

Prothrombin Complex Concentrates (Factor IX Concentrates)

Concentrates of the prothrombin complex (PCC) are generally available from either commercial or federally funded agencies. In almost all cases, the final product is lyophilized (freeze-dried) and must be reconstituted with water for injection prior to infusion. PCC were primarily developed as replacement therapy for congenital factor IX deficiency (Christmas disease), and assay data on factor IX content only is provided. However, most products contain equivalent amounts of factors II (prothrombin) and X. The content of factor VII may vary considerably. Some products are known to be factor VII-depleted, and this information is provided on the product insert by the manufacturer. Other products may have extremely variable amounts of factor VII from one manufacturing lot to another, and this is not always recognized in the information provided with the product. It is recommended that the product be assayed prior to use and the in vivo recovery of the transfused material determined in order to confirm the precise factor VII content.

The advantages of the use of PCC are that relatively large amounts of clotting factors can be given in very small volumes. Precise volumes cannot be specified as the number of units per vial may vary from one lot of a product to another. As a rough guide, approximately 100 ml of reconstituted material will elevate factor IX activity by 50 percent in a 70-kg patient.

Activated Prothrombin Complex Concentrates

These concentrates have been developed specifically for the treatment of patients with acquired inhibitors to factor VIII:C (hemophilia A). Their use will be more fully described in the chapter entitled *Hemophilia*. Although extremely rare, patients with Christmas disease (factor IX deficiency) may also acquire antibodies to factor IX following replacement therapy. The use of activated PCC has been advocated in such patients, but their role requires further clinical evaluation.

Adverse Effects of Blood Products

A risk associated with all blood products is the transmission of infective disorders. Most agencies screen blood donors for the presence of hepatitis B surface antigen (HBsAg). Although this minimizes the risk, approximately 0.5 to 1 percent of all recipients still develop this infection. The risk increases in direct proportion to the number of donors to which the recipient is exposed. Consequently, this is much higher following the use of PCC when the donor plasma pool may consist of many thousands of donor units of plasma. This factor should be borne in mind when considering the relative advantages and disadvantages of using concentrates over simple plasma infusion. Of great concern at present is the risk of contracting non-A/non-B hepatitis, or AIDS (acquired immunodeficiency syndrome). In the case of the former, failure to identify the agent or agents responsible precludes an effective screening program, and non-A/non-B hepatitis probably accounts for at least 90 percen of all post-transfusional hepatitis observed at the present time. The risk of acquiring AIDS, although minimal, is of obvious major concern in view of the high mortality rate in patients acquiring this condition. Again, due consideration should be given to these risk factors in reaching decisions as to the therapeutic options available.

In addition to the above, disseminated intravascular coagulation (DIC) and thromboembolic disorders are a significant risk with all varieties of PCC. This appears to relate to the presence of activated clotting factors and coagulant-active phospholipid in these products. Patients with relative or absolute hepatic insufficiency appear to be at high risk owing to the compromise of normal clearance and inhibitory mechanisms required for neutralizing inappropriately activated clotting factors. Antithrombin III deficiency appears to be of particular importance in this respect. Consequently, the use of these products in neonates and patients with liver disease is relatively contraindicated.

VITAMIN K PREPARATIONS

When time permits, vitamin K may be administered to patients who have an acquired deficiency due to its relative or absolute nonavailability. The ability of individual patients to respond will depend on the liver's ability to synthesize the appropriate clotting factors. Even when there is significant hepatic impairment, vitamin K deficiency may coexist and represent the principal contributor to the deficiency state.

Vitamin K is a fat-soluble vitamin and must, therefore, either be administered systemically or provided in an alternative water-soluble form.

Phytonadione (Synthetic Vitamin K_1)

This synthetic vitamin has the same physiologic activity as natural vitamin K_1. It is provided as a solution for injection. It should be protected from light and not frozen, as both conditions modify the product's activity. It may be administered by subcutaneous, intramuscular (IM), or intravenous injection (IV). Used prophylactically, e.g., for prevention of hemolytic disease of the newborn, it may be given intramuscularly. It should *not* be given intramuscularly to patients with an established bleeding tendency. Intramuscular injections are contraindicated in such patients because of the risk of developing hematomas. Moreover, confinement of the drug at the site of the hematoma may result in unpredictable absorption characteristics and result in the unnecessary administration of further therapy. Intravenous administration produces rapid correction of the deficiency, but a few patients may demonstrate adverse effects when the drug is administered by this route. In some cases, these may be severe and even life-threatening. The reaction is anaphylactoid in type, i.e., it is not a true anaphylactic reaction because it may be encountered after the first administration of the drug and does not appear to be associated with the development of IgE antibodies. The clinical consequences, however, are similar to those of a true anaphylactic reaction. The following protocol is recommended for IV administration when oral therapy (to be discussed) is impracticable or rapid correction of the deficiency is required: 10 mg vitamin K_1 is diluted in 50 ml of an appropriate IV fluid (the drug is compatible with most standard IV solutions). An IV infusion should be established at a rate of 5 ml/minute, using the same IV solution as that used as the diluent. The diluted vitamin K_1 should be placed in an auxillary IV administration set on a "Y" to the main IV line. Approximately 1 ml of the diluted vitamin K_1 should be allowed to run into the main line; this infusion is then stopped but the main infusion is continued. During the next 15 minutes, the patient should be observed for adverse effects by close monitoring of vital signs. If no untoward effect is noted, the auxiliary line is opened and the balance of the vitamin K_1 run in over 30 minutes. In my experience, patients who are likely to develop severe adverse reactions usually show evidence of this by developing tachycardia or a temperature spike after the dose is given. Vitamin K_1 should *never* be given by a rapid, direct intravenous injection.

Menadiol Sodium Diphosphate (Synkavite)

Menadiol sodium diphosphate is a synthetic water-soluble derivative of menadione (vitamin K_3) to which it is converted in vivo. The product is available in tablet and parenteral form. The facility and safety of oral administration makes it the vitamin K replacement therapy of choice in non-life-threatening situations. The parenteral form may also be given orally to patients restricted to fluids only. It is very rapidly absorbed from the GI tract, and the activity observed approaches that achieved by parenteral therapy.

INDIVIDUAL DEFICIENCY STATES

From the previous description of available therapies, it should be clear that the treatment may be optimized by defining first the precise nature of the coagulation disorder and, second, the level of urgency and/or need for restoring the levels of the clotting factor or clotting factors concerned. In consideration of the latter, the risks of the alternative therapies available must be set against the specific benefits expected.

Congenital Deficiencies

Congenital deficiencies of the vitamin K-dependent clotting factors are very rare, with the most common, factor IX deficiency (Christmas disease), affecting 1 in 80,000 to 100,000 of the North American male population. In all cases, active treatment associated with either bleeding or its prevention requires the administration of blood products containing the appropriate clotting factors. In addition, certain general principles of management should be adopted and are more fully described in the chapter entitled *Hemophilia*.

In designing a protocol for replacement therapy, the minimum hemostatic level of each coagulation factor required must be considered together with information relating to the kinetics of each clotting factor in vivo.

Factor II (Prothrombin) Deficiency

Levels of 10 to 15 percent appear to be adequate for normal physical activity, but the requirement is increased during trauma or when surgery is indicated. The precise level depends on the degree of trauma or type of surgery and the physical location of the possible bleeding site. For example, bleeding in the region of the head or neck requires more aggressive therapy than a hemarthrosis. Levels of 50 percent would appear adequate for the former and 20 to 30 percent for the latter. In vivo recovery data suggest that the infusion of 1 unit of factor II/kg body weight would elevate the circulating level by 1 percent or 0.01 unit/ml. The precise dose may then be calculated on the basis of the clinical need, as described above. Current information suggests an in vivo half-life of approximately 48 hours, and consequently, daily infusions are adequate to maintain the chosen hemostatic level. The replacement product used may be either single-donor plasma or PCC. The former has the advantage of reduced risk of hepatitis, but the disadvantage of requiring large infusion volumes. The latter is circumvented by the use of PCC, but this benefit must be set against the increased risks of transmission of infections and thrombogenicity.

Factor VII

Patients with factor VII deficiency should be carefully evaluated with regard to a previous history of bleeding. Some controversy exists whether patients with this extremely rare congenital disorder of coagulation out of necessity will have a severe bleeding tendency despite very low levels of factor VII. Some patients may have no previous history of bleeding. Such patients may require little or no replacement therapy. In others, a severe bleeding tendency is recorded. The reasons for this discrepancy remain unclear. It would appear, however, that relatively minor elevations of factor VII activity (5 to 10%) will control spontaneous bleeding even in patients who do bleed. Similarly, 10 to 20 percent appears to be adequate for major surgery or bleeding. Although the reported half-life of factor VII is relatively short (6 to 7 hours), daily infusions of 10 units/kg body weight appears to be adequate in most situations. This can be relatively easily achieved with the use of single-donor plasma. If PCC treatment is required, the previous reservations with regard to factor VII content of available preparations should be noted. As before, the relatively greater risks associated with these preparations should also be considered.

Factor X Deficiency

Fifteen to 20 percent of factor X activity appears to be satisfactory in controlling minor bleeding and 20 to 30 percent in the case of major bleeding or surgery. Consequently, 15 to 30 units/kg body weight provides the appropriate cover, and its half-life of approximately 32 to 48 hours results in the requirement for daily infusion. In most patients, adequate responses may be obtained using single-donor plasma. Alternatively, PCC may be considered subject to the previously stated reservations with regard to risk.

Factor IX Deficiency

The treatment of factor IX deficiency or Christmas disease is included in the chapter entitled *Hemophilia*. The use of PCC is widely advocated as the most convenient and effective available treatment, particularly for home therapy. The use of activated prothrombin complex concentrates in patients unfortunate enough to develop inhibitors to factor IX requires further clinical evaluation.

ACQUIRED DEFICIENCY STATES

This group of hemostatic disorders usually presents as a multiple clotting factor deficiency. The precipitating mechanism is either a relative or absolute unavailability of vitamin K and/or a failure in hepatic synthesis due to liver disease. Occasionally, an apparently discrete acquired factor VII deficiency state may occur. Patients presenting with acute severe congestive cardiac failure may demonstrate a prolongation of the prothrombin time, which can subsequently be related to decreased factor VII levels. This presumably relates to impaired hepatic synthesis of the prothrombin complex secondary to congestive failure, with factor VII demonstrating the major effect due to its short half-life. The deficiency usually corrects quickly following successful treatment of the primary condition. Very rarely, discrete deficiencies may occur due to the development of autoantibodies to one or more of the prothrombin complex.

Vitamin K Deficiency

Bleeding due to vitamin K deficiency is not uncommon in modern hospital practice, particularly in intensive care units where poor nutritional status may be exacerbated by broad-spectrum antibiotic therapy. Such patients should receive prophylactic vitamin K orally, 5 to 10 mg *bid*. When oral administration is compromised, the intramuscular route should be given, provided the patient does not have a manifest bleeding tendency. When bleeding is occurring, vitamin K should be administered orally whenever possible or intravenously when indicated, according to the guidelines previously described.

Oral Anticoagulant Therapy

The oral anticoagulants are competitive antagonists of vitamin K_1. Reversal of anticoagulant therapy may be required either in an overdosage situation or when surgical intervention is required in an anticoagulated patient, e.g., correction of a malseated prosthetic heart valve. Minimal overdosage situations are best handled by withdrawal of anticoagulant therapy, but due consideration should be given to the slope of the rise in prothrombin time over the period of previous observation. When bleeding is occurring or can be anticipated, a more aggressive approach to therapy is indicated. The options lie between the administration of vitamin K or blood product replacement. Most patients with normal hepatic function demonstrate a significant response 3 to 4 hours following the administration of 10 mg of vitamin K_1 IV. In some patients, the effect may be even more rapid, whereas in others, usually as a consequence of coexistent liver disease, up to 12 hours may be required before an optimal response is recorded. When a shorter response time is required, replacement therapy with single donor plasma or PCC is indicated. In my experience, the use of single-donor plasma is often precluded out of concern for volume overload, particularly in the decompensating cardiac patient. Consequently, despite the acknowledged risk of treatment, the use of PCC probably represents the optimum approach. Since the half-life of vitamin K is shorter than that of Coumadin, the prothrombin time often lengthens again after 24 hours if further vitamin K supplementation is not given. In patients who require reanticoagulation, it is not unusual for some temporary "resistance" to be encountered when Coumadin therapy is restarted. Such patients should be anticoagulated with heparin during the period following vitamin K correction.

Liver Disease

Since all the K-dependent clotting factors are synthesized in the liver, it is not unusual for liver disease to be complicated by deficiencies of the prothrombin complex. Unfortunately, the currently available therapeutic options are very limited. Although the clotting factor deficiency is primarily a disorder of synthesis, the possibility of coexistent vitamin K deficiency should not be forgotten because many of these patients are of poor nutritional status and have frequently been treated with broad-spectrum antibiotics as part of the regimen instituted in the management of hepatic failure. Vitamin K should be given orally at a dose of 10 mg/day for 3 days. If no response occurs after this period, there is little point in continuing therapy. In acute life-threatening bleeding situations, vitamin K_1 should be administered IV following the protocol previously described. If no response occurs following IV therapy, further doses should not be administered.

Correction of the clotting factor deficiency by replacement therapy is extremely difficult. Theoretically, the use of PCC should represent the most ideal approach. Unfortunately, this is contraindicated in the light of significant thrombogenicity in such patients. The use of single-donor plasma is logistically difficult owing to the large volumes required to attain significant increments in clotting factor activity. It is unusual to detect any change in the prothrombin time despite the infusion of large volumes of plasma. Nonetheless, a clinical effect in terms of control of bleeding is sometimes observed despite the failure to document this by laboratory testing. There would appear to be a clear need for the development of a PCC preparation with reduced thrombogenicity for the treatment of this commonly encountered clinical problem.

VENOUS THROMBOEMBOLISM

ALEXANDER G.G. TURPIE, M.B., Ch.B., F.R.C.P., F.A.C.P., F.R.C.P.(C)

Venous thrombosis and pulmonary embolism may occur in symptomatic outpatients or as a common and serious complication in hospitalized patients. In the majority of patients, venous thrombosis in the lower limbs begins in the veins of the calf and remains localized producing few, if any, symptoms and no significant longterm consequences. In approximately half of these patients, pulmonary emboli occur, but these are usually small and well tolerated. In approximately 20 percent of patients with calf vein thrombosis, the thrombi extend into the popliteal and more proximal veins and in approximately 40 percent of these patients, pulmonary emboli develop that may lead to a fatal outcome. Calf vein thrombi often resolve, but once there has been extension into the more proximal vessels, complete resolution is less likely. Nearly two thirds of these patients have residual thrombosis and loss of venous function that produces altered venous return and some of the manifestations of the postphlebitic syndrome. In patients with symptomatic pulmonary embolism, fatal recurrence is likely in approximately 20 percent of untreated patients. In almost all of these, death is from recurrence, and at autopsy there is evidence of prior emboli in more than 75 percent of patients.

Since progression and embolization occur rapidly and unpredictably, it is imperative that all patients with confirmed venous thromboembolic disease receive prompt antithrombotic therapy. When this therapy is given, the outlook for survival and complete recovery is excellent. In patients treated with heparin for deep vein thrombosis, progression or embolization occurs in less than 5 percent of patients, and in patients with pulmonary embolism, the recurrence rate is less than 5 percent with a very low mortality rate. Even in patients with massive embolism and shock the mortality rate is less than 20 percent after treatment.

Safe effective methods of prophylaxis against venous thrombosis are available and should be used in high-risk patients to prevent death and morbidity from venous thromboembolism. Prophylaxis is more cost-effective than treating the established event.

TREATMENT OF VENOUS THROMBOEMBOLISM

The approach to antithrombotic therapy in venous thromboembolic disease involves the use of anticoagulants. Heparin is the only drug that has been established to predictively arrest active thrombosis. Following a primary course of treatment with heparin, the majority of patients with thromboembolic diseases require a period of secondary prophylaxis using an oral anticoagulant. In selected patients, thrombolytic therapy may be used to accelerate the rate of removal of the thrombotic or embolic obstruction (e.g., rare patients with hypotension or shock from obstruction of venous return from iliac or femoral thrombi, or patients with hypotension from massive pulmonary embolism). Venous thrombosis is treated surgically with thrombectomy and pulmonary embolism with pulmonary embolectomy. In addition, procedures such as plication or the use of vena caval clips designed to reduce the vena cava lumen, or an intraluminal filter device to prevent embolization may be used.

Heparin

Heparin is the treatment of choice in patients with acute venous thrombosis or pulmonary embolism because it is both effective and relatively safe. Heparin is a polydispersed mucopolysaccharide with a variable molecular weight ranging from 500 to 16,000 daltons with a mean of 14,300 daltons. The anticoagulant activity of heparin is influenced by its molecular weight, its degree of n-sulphation and the sequence of the saccharide units. The anticoagulant activity of heparin resides in approximately one-third of the molecules of USP heparin and the fraction of each molecule most active in terms of antithrombin III-binding is the fraction representing less than 10 percent of its bulk. There is a close relationship between the affinity of heparin to antithrombin III and its anticoagulant properties. Heparin's anticoagulant action occurs as a result of combining heparin with antithrombin III to inhibit thrombin, and a number of activated clotting factors including Xa, IXa, XIa, and XIIa. Heparin has also been shown to combine with heparin cofactor II to provide an additional antithrombin effect. Following intravenous injection, heparin distributes throughout the plasma volume and is cleared with a halflife that varies considerably between individuals. In plasma, heparin is completely bound to proteins. After a single intravenous injection, there is initial rapid disappearance of approximately 40 percent of the injected heparin within 5 minutes, followed by a more gradual clearance with mean halflife of 60 minutes in normal individuals. The rapid clearance is probably due to the absorption of heparin onto endothelial cells and its diffusion into the extravascular tissues. The slower clearance is due to elimination of heparin from plasma by an unknown mechanism. It has been demonstrated that the clearance of heparin is more rapid in patients with pulmonary embolism than in those with venous thrombosis, but the mechanism for this is not understood.

Heparin Therapy

Heparin in therapeutic doses is usually given by continuous or intermittent intravenous injections but can also be given subcutaneously. It is usual to start with an intravenous bolus of 5000–7500 units; this anticoagulates the vast majority of patients. The halflife of heparin is 1 to 2 hours and in the majority of patients, the bolus has cleared in 4 hours. If heparin is administered by continuous intravenous infusion, approximately 30,000 units per day are sufficient to produce an adequate anticoagulant response in most patients. If heparin is given by intermittent intravenous injection, approximately 5000–10,000 units every 4 to 6 hours are required. Recent evidence shows that heparin may be given by subcutaneous injection in doses of 10,000–15,000 units every 12 hours which maintain the blood levels at therapeutic concentrations throughout the 24 hour period.

Monitoring Heparin Therapy

The response of most patients to heparin falls within a predictable range; however, approximately 15–25 percent of patients either have an inadequate or excessive response to heparin. Clinical evidence indicates that patients most likely to have recurrent thromboembolism are those who are inadequately anticoagulated. Patients who are excessively anticoagulated have an increased incidence of bleeding. Therefore, it is desirable to monitor their anticoagulant response by means of one of the clotting tests that are affected by heparin. The choice is usually based on local preference, but it is essential that the test chosen, detects therapeutic levels of heparin and has a reasonable linear response curve. With an appropriately sensitive test, it is possible, soon after starting heparin therapy, to document that anticoagulation has been achieved. The tests used to monitor heparin therapy are the whole blood clotting time, activated partial thromboplastin time, and more recently, plasma heparin levels. The thrombin clotting time and the prothrombin time are less useful tests.

A recommended method for monitoring continuous intravenous heparin therapy is to perform the activated partial thromboplastin time (PTT) 4 to 6 hours after the initial intravenous bolus, and then, on a daily basis to ensure that an adequate heparin response is obtained. Sufficient heparin is administered for 24 hours to maintain the PTT at $1^1/_2$–2 times the preheparin control value. This anticoagulant response is equivalent to 0.3–0.4 units of heparin/ml of plasma using protamine sulphate titration. If the PTT response is above the therapeutic range, the dose of heparin is reduced by 2000–4000 units for 24 hours depending on the degree of prolongation and the test is repeated 4 to 6 hours later. If the test result of the PTT is below the therapeutic range, the 24 hour intravenous dose is augmented by 2000–4000 units for 24 hours. If the PTT shows no or very little prolongation, an addition 2000–5000 unit bolus of heparin is given. After 72 hours, the dose of heparin usually stabilizes with good control of the PTT. To control therapeutic-dose subcutaneous heparin, the PTT is performed at the midinterval between the 12-hourly doses, and increments or decrements are made in the dose according to the result of the PTT.

Duration of Heparin Therapy

The precise duration of treatment with heparin is difficult to define, but the objective is to maintain full anticoagulation until active thrombosis is arrested and the thrombi are firmly attached to the vessel wall. This requires a minimum of 5 days and may take 8 to 10 days to occur. Based on this fact and on retrospective data that recurrence is less likely with heparin therapy than with warfarin therapy, most authorities recommend the use of heparin for 7 to 10 days followed by secondary prophylaxis with warfarin.

Complications of Heparin

Several complications have been reported with heparin therapy, including hemorrhage, hypersensitivity reactions, thrombocytopenia and osteoporosis. Bleeding is the most important complication that occurs in 5–10 percent of patients. It is particularly likely to occur in patients with an underlying hemostatic defect, patients treated with aspirin, and patients exposed to recent surgery or trauma. There is some evidence that the risk of bleeding increases with the dose of heparin, and in patients at high risk, the use of intermittent intravenous injections is probably associated with a higher risk of bleeding than is the continuous infusion of the drug.

Heparin-induced thrombocytopenia has been reported with varying frequency but probably occurs in less than 4 percent of patients. It is more common in patients receiving beef lung heparin than in those receiving porcine gut heparin. Thrombocytopenia associated with arterial thromboembolism is a rare complication of heparin therapy. This is a life-threatening complication that usually occurs about 10 days after starting heparin therapy. Patients develop multiple arterial occlusion which often involves larger arteries (even the aorta). This complication requires that heparin therapy be discontinued and an alternative form of antithrombotic therapy be instituted (such as therapy with one of the new low-molecular weight fractions of heparin that have recently been introduced). There is recent evidence that heparin-induced thrombocytopenia is caused by an immune mechanism.

Hypersensitivity is uncommon, but does occur and ranges between cutaneous urticaria and anaphylaxis. The mechanism of hypersensitivity is not understood. Osteoporosis occurs rarely in patients who receive heparin longer than 6 months; they usually present with spontaneous fractures of the vertebrae or ribs. Alopecia has also been reported.

Treatment of Hemorrhage Associated With Heparin Therapy

The bleeding complications of heparin can be prevented by careful attention to the dosage. However, if bleeding occurs, heparin should be stopped, and if rapid reversal is required, the use of protamine sulphate, which combines with and inactivates heparin, is indicated. The approximate neutralizing dose depends upon the estimated amount of heparin in the circulation; 1 mg of protamine sulphate for each 100 units of heparin should be given. Because of the rapid clearance of heparin from the circulation, it is seldom necessary to give more than 50–75 mg of protamine sulphate. Because patients occasionally become hypotensive in response to protamine sulphate, it should be injected slowly over a 10–30 minute period. Protamine sulphate may be repeated since it is cleared rapidly from the blood. After subcutaneous heparin, protamine sulphate should be given in a dose equivalent to 50 percent of the last heparin dose.

Secondary Prophylaxis

After the primary treatment of the thromboembolic episode (usually 7 to 10 days of heparin), patients require 3 to 6 months of secondary prophylaxis with oral anticoagulants or adjusted-dose subcutaneous heparin. Oral anticoagulants should be started 5 to 6 days before heparin therapy is discontinued and maintain for 3 to 6 months. The dose of anticoagulants is monitored by the prothrombin time maintained in a therapeutic range depending upon the test and the reagent used.

Oral Anticoagulant Therapy

The coumadins and the indanedione derivatives produce indirect anticoagulant effect by antagonizing the effect of vitamin K, inhibiting its effect on the hepatic synthesis of coagulation factors II, VII, IX, and X. Oral anticoagulant therapy leads to synthesis of biologically inactive forms of these clotting proteins. The anticoagulant effect of these drugs occurs only after the normal clotting factors are cleared from the circulation. Thus the peak inhibitory effect on the synthesis of biologically active vitamin K-dependent clotting factors takes place 36 to 72 hours after drug administration. With a 40 mg loading dose, factor VII levels usually fall rapidly to $<$ 20 percent of normal, and sometimes $<$ 10 percent of normal, for as long as 3 to 4 days. In some patients, however, suppression of factor VII to this level is seen within 24 hours. Sick patients with impaired liver functions or reduced vitamin K stores are particularly susceptible to large loading doses. Equilibrium levels of factors II, IX, and X are not reached until about one week after initiation of therapy. The use of a small loading dose and an initial daily dose tends to avoid overdosage, especially in patients who are sensitive to warfarin, so this is the preferred approach. Recent randomized trials have demonstrated that warfarin sodium therapy is effective in the long-term treatment of patients with venous thromboembolism. The rate of recurrent venous thromboembolism is reduced to less than 2 percent during long-term therapy with warfarin sodium.

For standard secondary prophylaxis, warfarin sodium is administered in an initial dose of 10 mg/day for the first 2 days, and the daily dose is then adjusted according to the prothrombin time. Heparin therapy is discontinued on the fourth or fifth day and the prothrombin time is prolonged into the therapeutic range, which varies depending on the test and the prothrombin reagent used. There is evidence that when using rabbit brain thromboplastin, the conventional therapeutic range of 24 to 26 weeks results in administering too high a dose; the prothrombin time should be maintained between 16 and 18 seconds. The use of human brain thromboplastin, which is more sensitive to changes in coagulation factors, may allow more accurate control of the oral anticoagulant dose. There is experimental evidence that the maximal antithrombotic effect of oral anticoagulant therapy is delayed for as long as 5 days, even though the anticoagulant effect, reflected by an increase in the prothrombin time (due mainly to a fall in factor VII), may be evident within 2 to 3 days. For this reason, it is important to overlap oral anticoagulant therapy with heparin therapy for 4 to 5 days, even though the prothrombin time may be prolonged into the therapeutic range after 2 to 3 days. Once the patient's condition is stable, the prothrombin time is monitored every 2 to 3 weeks throughout the course of oral anticoagulant therapy. However, if there are factors that can produce an unpredictable response to warfarin (e.g., concomittant drug therapy), the prothrombin time is monitored more frequently to minimize the risk of complications.

Complications of Oral Anticoagulant Therapy

The major side effect of oral anticoagulants is bleeding. Bleeding during well-controlled oral anticoagulant therapy is usually secondary to surgery, other forms of trauma, or local lesions, such as peptic ulcer or carcinoma. Spontaneous bleeding occurs if oral anticoagulants are given in excessive doses and results in marked prolongation of the prothrombin time; this bleeding may be severe and even life-threatening.

The nonhemorrhagic side effects of oral anticoagulants differ when the coumadin derivatives (e.g., warfarin sodium) or indanedione are administered. Nonhemorrhagic side effects of coumadins are uncommon. These include skin necrosis, dermatitis, and a syndrome of painful blue toes. The nonhemorrhagic side effects occur more frequently with the indanedione derivatives. Hypersensitivity reactions have been reported to occur in 1–3 percent of patients receiving indanedione derivatives; these include rash, fever, hepatitis, leukopenia, renal failure and diarrhea, and they are sometimes fatal. In many patients the indanedione derivatives also produce red discoloration of the urine that is sometimes confused with hematuria.

Since the nonhemorrhagic side effects of the coumadins are very uncommon, these agents are the oral anticoagulants of choice.

Oral anticoagulants cross the placenta and cause fetal malformations when used in the first trimester. This complication has been reported with both warfarin and phenindione. Characteristic stippling of the vertebral and tarsal bones sometimes associated with nasal hypoplasia may occur. Microcephaly, blindness, and mental retardation have also been described. Oral anticoagulants are also secreted in the milk of nursing mothers, but it is debatable whether the prothrombin time is significantly altered in breast-fed infants, even when mothers receive full therapeutic doses. Thus, the use of these agents while a mother is breast feeding is controversial.

Drug Interaction

Oral anticoagulant therapy is influenced by many factors that may dramatically alter the response of the patient. The most important interaction is produced by concomittant drug therapy. Many drugs interact with oral anticoagulants and produce either a prolongation or reduction in the anticoagulant effect. The most important of these are barbiturates, phenylbutazone, sulphinpyrazone, large doses of aspirin, anabolic steroids, trimethorprim sulfamethoxale (Septra, Bactrim), sulfonamides and cimetidine. Antibiotic drugs appear to affect oral anticoagulants only if dietary sources of vitamin K are reduced (e.g., in patients on intravenous therapy). The mechanisms of the drug interactions are complex and include reducing absorption of vitamin K (e.g., nortriptyline), reducing binding of anticoagulants to albumin which results in an increase in concentration of a pharmacologically active unbound drug (e.g., sulfonamide, phenylbutazone, chloralhydrate), and altering the rate of inactivation of coumadin by the hepatic microsomal oxidizing systems (e.g., barbiturates, glutethamide, rifampicin). Other mechanisms include (1) increasing the rate by which drugs are inactivated to enhance rapid disappearance and reduce the anticoagulant effect (e.g., allopurinol), (2) increasing the rate of synthesis of the vitamin K-dependent clotting factors to produce a relative resistance to the effect of oral anticoagulants (e.g., estrogens), and (3) increasing the rate of metabolism of the vitamin K-dependent clotting factors to enhance the effect of oral anticoagulants (e.g., thyroxin). Drugs may also potentiate the effect of oral anticoagulants on hemostatic mechanisms by imparing platelet function (e.g., aspirin, phenylbutazone).

Special care should be taken to adjust the dose of oral anticoagulant therapy during the time that other drugs are being taken to minimize the risk of inadequate anticoagulant control.

Antidote to Oral Anticoagulants

The antidote to the vitamin K antagonists is vitamin K_1. If excessive prolongation of the prothrombin time occurs, the treatment depends on the degree of prolongation of the prothrombin time and whether or not the patient is bleeding. If the prolongation is mild, $<$ 3 times the control value, and the patient is not bleeding, no specific treatment is necessary other than discontinuing the warfarin until the prothrombin time returns to the therapeutic range. With more marked prolongation in patients who are not bleeding, treatment with small doses of vitamin K_1 given either orally or by subcutaneous injection (2.5–5 mg) could be considered. With very marked prolongation of the prothrombin time, particularly in a patient who is either at risk of or is actively bleeding, vitamin K_1 should be given. If vitamin K_1 is given intravenously, this must be done cautiously in order to obviate an anaphylactoid reaction (which has occurred in rare cases). Reported side effects include flushing, dizziness, tachycardia, hypotension, dyspnea, and sweating. The risk of anaphylactoid reaction can be reduced by giving vitamin K_1 well diluted in a soluset at a rate no faster than 1 mg/min. However, when possible, it is preferable to administer vitamin K_1 subcutaneously to minimize the risk of serious adverse reactions. In most patients, K_1 produces a demonstrable effect on the prothrombin time within 3 to 4 hours and corrects the prolonged prothrombin time within 6 to 8 hours. Because the halflife of vitamin K_1 is less than that of warfarin sodium, a repeat course of vitamin K_1 may be necessary. If bleeding is very severe and life-threatening, vitamin K_1 therapy can be supplemented by using concentrates of coagulation factors II, VII, IX and X.

Anticoagulant Therapy During Pregnancy

Anticoagulant therapy is indicated in all patients with venous thromboembolism during pregnancy. The initial phase of treatment is with full therapeutic dose heparin, and is identical for that described for the management of nonpregnant patients. There is, however, a controversy as to the optimal method of secondary prophylaxis. The recommended approach is to use long-term adjusted-dose subcutaneous heparin on an out-patient basis. Heparin does not cross the placental barrier so there is no risk of hemorrhage in the fetus. The use of warfarin for secondary prophylaxis during pregnancy is not recommended because of the possible teratogenic effects, and because it crosses the placental barrier with possible risk of hemorrhage in the fetus. Since the patient remains at high risk of recurrence throughout pregnancy, heparin should be continued past the early postpartum period. Heparin is continued until labor begins, interrupted until 6 to 8 hours postpartum and resumed for a minimum of 5 to 7 days. The patient is then switched to coumadin for 6 to 8 weeks or continued on subcutaneous heparin.

Thrombolytic Therapy

The frequency of recurrent clinically suspected venous thromboembolism is very low during anticoagulant therapy, and this remains the treatment of choice in the majority of patients with venous thromboembolism. Anticoagulant therapy is not ideal, however, because it does not induce thrombolysis. Therefore, it does not eliminate an important potential source for subsequent embolization, nor alleviate hemodynamic disturbance associated with major pulmonary embolism nor does it prevent damage to the deep venous system, which predisposes to the postphlebitic syndrome. Thus, although anticoagulant therapy is effective in reducing the important immediate complications of venous thromboembolism, it may be relatively ineffective in preventing some of the late sequelae.

For these reasons, thrombolytic therapy is recommended in selected patients with acute massive venous thrombosis or massive pulmonary embolism. Thrombolytic therapy has a number of potential advantages. These include (1) lysis of the thrombi and emboli with restoration of the circulation to normal, (2) rapid reduction of hemodynamic disturbances, (3) reduction or prevention of venous valve damage, (4) potential prevention of the post-phlebitic syndrome, and (5) prevention or reduction of damage to the pulmonary vascular bed, reducing the likelihood of chronic thromboembolic pulmonary hypertension.

There are two major classes of thrombolytic drugs, the plasminogen activators, which convert plasminogen to plasmin, and the proteolytic enzymes, plasmin and brinase, which hydrolyze fibrin directly. Only the plasminogen activators have undergone extensive clinical testing. There are two chemically and pharmacologically distinct plasminogen activators available commercially. These are streptokinase and urokinase. Streptokinase is a thrombolytic agent that combines with plasminogen producing a confirmational change that exposes an active site, which in turn converts noncomplex plasminogen to plasmin by proteolytic cleavage. Streptokinase is cleared relatively rapidly from the circulation and has a halflife of approximately 90 minutes. Streptokinase is a product of hemolytic streptococci and is antigenic in man and stimulates the production of neutralizing antibodies. Urokinase is a naturally occurring human activator of plasminogen. It is present in human urine and is produced by renal parenchymal cells and possibly by cells lying in the urinary tract. Urokinase is non-antigenic in man, and therefore does not stimulate the formation of neutralizing antibodies. Both streptokinase and urokinase have been used extensively in humans for the treatment of thromboembolic disease. A major advance in the field of thrombolysis is the development of fibrin-specific thrombolytic agents including acylated streptokinase/plasminogen complex and tissue plasminogen activator, which is isolated from melanoma cell culture supernate or by recombinant DNA technology. These latter agents have yet to be evaluated clinically.

Thrombolytic therapy has been evaluated in the treatment of pulmonary embolism and in deep vein thrombosis. Two large-scale multicenter trials have demonstrated that the use of thrombolytic therapy for pulmonary embolism produces more rapid lysis of the emboli than heparin although this benefit on mortality has not been demonstrated. However, thrombolytic therapy would appear to be particularly useful in patients with massive pulmonary embolism, in patients with cardiac or pulmonary disease, or in patients in whom even a small or moderate embolus may be life-threatening. Thrombolytic therapy has been evaluated in a number of small studies of deep vein thrombosis. Thrombolytic therapy has been shown to produce greater lysis of deep vein thrombi than heparin, but whether or not thrombolytic therapy produces the frequency of the postphlebitic syndrome has not been established. Thrombolytic therapy has, however, great potential in the management of acute massive deep vein thrombosis.

Thrombolytic therapy should not be administered before objective evidence of venous thromboembolic disease has been established. When the decision is made that thrombolytic therapy is indicated, contraindications to therapy including active internal bleeding, recent cerebrovascular accident or other intracranial disease, recent surgery, recent trauma, and severe arterial hypertension should be sought. Other contraindications to thrombolytic therapy include: recent minor trauma, cardiopulmonary resuscitation, possibility of a left ventricular mural thrombosis, bacterial endocarditis, severe hepatorenal disease, pregnancy, elderly patients, and patients with diabetic hemorrhagic retinopathy. Either urokinase or streptokinase may be used, depending upon the availability. Although streptokinase is reported to produce a greater instance of pyrogenic and allergic reactions, there is no convincing evidence that either drug is superior to the other. Streptokinase is more readily available and is less expensive.

Prior to the commencement of thrombolytic therapy, a baseline prothrombin time, partial thromboplastin time, thrombin clotting time, platelet count, baseline hemoglobin, and hematocrit determination should be obtained. To minimize the risk of bleeding, invasive arterial procedures, such as measurement of blood gases, should be avoided and venepunctures should be kept to an absolute minimum. If arterial blood samples are required, blood is taken from the radial artery and local compression is maintained for at least 20 minutes. The effect of thrombolytic therapy can be monitored by tests such as the thrombin time or euglobulin lysis time, to establish the presence of a systemic thrombolytic state; there is no evidence that these tests predict clinical efficacy or reduce bleeding complications.

Streptokinase should be given in a loading dose of 250,000 units given over 30 minutes. This will neutralize naturally occurring antibodies in the majority of patients. Streptokinase should then be continued by intravenous infusion of 100,000–200,000/hr. Streptokinase therapy is monitored by carrying out a thrombin clotting time approximately 2 hours after the onset of the loading dose and adjusting the dose of the infusion accordingly. Once the thrombolytic treatment is established, the thrombin time should be repeated at 4-hourly intervals. If the thrombin time remains 2–5 times the control value, no change in dose is required. Tests of fibrinolytic activity such as euglobulin lysis time can be performed if available, but they are not necessary. Urokinase should be given in a loading dose of 4400 U/kg with a maintenance dose of 4400 U/kg/hr.

The duration of thrombolytic therapy varies with the condition being treated. In most cases of pulmonary embolism, maximum effect is seen after 12 to 24 hours of therapy. In deep vein thrombosis, however, a longer period of treatment is usually necessary (a minimum of 48 hours which may be extended to 72 hours). Thrombotic and embolic lesions are more susceptible to lysis when they are new, and patients should be selected with lesions considered to be more than 72 hours old.

The major complication of thrombolytic therapy is hemorrhage which occurs with considerably greater frequency with this therapy than with heparin therapy. Bleeding is directly related to areas of trauma, and therefore, is most likely to occur in patients with recent surgery or other forms of vascular trauma. Bleeding may be prevented by careful selection of patients, rigorous attention to limiting vascular invasion, and careful application of pressure dressings over areas of vessel injury. Once bleeding has started, local measures such as pressure may arrest the hemorrhage but if bleeding is severe, it is usually necessary to discontinue treatment. Since the plasma halflife of both streptokinase and urokinase is short, the fibrinolytic effect disappears within 30 to 60 minutes after stopping treatment. In the occasional patient, rapid reversal of fibrinolytic activity is necessary and can be accomplished by the use of epsilon-aminocaproic acid. The anticoagulant effects of thrombolytic therapy can be reversed by the administration of plasma or fibrinogen. If bleeding is severe, whole blood transfusion may be required.

Thrombolytic therapy for venous thromboembolic disease should be followed by full-dose intravenous heparin therapy and the usual course of secondary prophylaxis with oral anticoagulants.

Surgical Treatment of Venous Thromboembolism

Although the management of venous thromboembolism is almost always medical, there are a number of surgical procedures which may be indicated in some patients for the management of deep vein thrombosis and pulmonary embolism. Originally, thrombectomy was used in the management of venous thrombosis but this technique has been all but abandoned because rethrombosis almost always occurred.

In patients with deep vein thrombosis in whom anticoagulant therapy has failed or in whom there is an absolute contraindication, surgical procedures designed to reduce the lumen of the inferior vena cava are available. These include caval ligation, the insertion of various devices to plicate the cava and the insertion via the jugular or the femoral vein of a nonthrombogenic filter into the inferior vena cava below the level of the renal veins. These procedures are designed to prevent recurrent emboli but the indications for these procedures occur infrequently.

For pulmonary embolism, pulmonary embolectomy using cardiopulmonary bypass has been used. This procedure is done as a last result for patients with massive embolism who are in shock or who have a cardiac arrest while being adequately treated. Although embolectomy may be life-saving, few patients survive long enough to reach the operating room.

CHRONIC IMMUNE THROMBOCYTOPENIC PURPURA

TADAHIRO TSUBAKIO, M.D.
ROBERT MCMILLAN, M.D.

Idiopathic (immune) thrombocytopenic purpura (ITP) is a common immune disorder due to the binding of a circulating antiplatelet factor to the patient's platelets that results in platelet destruction by the reticuloendothelial system. It can be subdivided into two major types: acute ITP, a self-limited disorder most common in children and usually occurring 1 to 6 weeks after a viral illness, and chronic ITP, a disorder of more insidious onset which occurs most commonly in women between the ages of 20 and 40. The patients usually present with isolated thrombocytopenia and a bone marrow aspirate showing normal or increased numbers of megakaryocytes. These diseases are diagnoses of exclusion since other types of immune thrombocytopenia, particularly those due to drug-dependent antibodies or isoantibodies or those related to other disease (e.g., systemic lupus erythematosus), can closely mimic the clinical picture of ITP. Significant hepatosplenomegaly or adenopathy suggests another etiology.

Patients with thrombocytopenia may manifest bruising or petechiae (dry purpura) or may bleed from mucosal surfaces (wet purpura). Mucosal bleeding, particularly from the gastrointestinal or genitourinary tract, suggests extremely low platelet counts and the danger of central nervous system (CNS) bleeding. Platelet counts greater than 50,000/mm^3 are rarely associated with symptoms. Purpura with minor trauma is common with platelet counts of 30,000 to 50,000/mm^3; spontaneous bruising occurs with counts of less than 30,000/mm^3. Serious mucosal bleeding and CNS bleeding are rare in patients with ITP unless the platelet count is less than 5000 to 10,000/mm^3. Initial therapeutic approaches should be aimed at attaining a complete remission (normal platelet counts on no therapy). In patients treated unsuccessfully with corticosteroids and splenectomy, the aim should be the achievement of "safe platelet counts" (above 20,000/mm^3). Therapeutic approaches have been divided into emergency and specific therapy. Emergency therapy is designed to provide the physician with time to allow specific types of treatment to become effective.

EMERGENCY THERAPY

Patients who have active bleeding from mucosal surfaces (except menstrual bleeding) are at risk for CNS bleeding, and for this reason they should be hospitalized and specific therapy should be started immediately.

Platelet Transfusion

If the patient's platelet count is extremely low (less than 10,000/mm^3) and mucosal bleeding is severe from the upper respiratory tract or the gastrointestinal tract or the genitourinary tract, platelet transfusions (6 to 8 units of random platelets per transfusion) should be given as often as needed (e.g., q.4 to 6h) to control hemorrhage. Although the transfused platelets are destroyed rapidly and do not affect the patient's count, they protect against catastrophic bleeding until the more specific forms of therapy become effective.

Gammaglobulin

High-dose intravenous gammaglobulin (0.4 g/kg/d, IV daily for 5 days) may be used as emergency therapy, since an increase in the platelet count and a reduced bleeding tendency often occur early after this treatment.

Plasmapheresis

Plasma exchange (3-liter exchange daily for 3 to 5 days) may also be used, although this is technically more difficult in the severely thrombocytopenic patient.

Splenectomy

Either of these latter treatments should allow time for specific therapeutic manipulations to increase the platelet count. However, if hemorrhage remains uncontrollable despite these measures, emergency splenectomy should be performed.

SPECIFIC THERAPY

The types of specific therapy are described in the order in which we would advise their use. This order has been advised on the basis of either their relative effectiveness or lack of dangerous side effects. Other physicians may differ in their opinions concerning the order of therapy. Table 1 summarizes these recommendations as well as the common side effects.

Corticosteroids

In patients with chronic ITP, prednisone (1 mg/kg/d or the therapeutic equivalent) is started at the time of diagnosis. Most patients respond within 1 or 2 weeks by a rise in the platelet count. If the platelet count becomes normal, the dose is maintained for 1 or 2 additional weeks and then tapered as follows: 10 mg/week until the dosage reaches 0.5 mg/kg and then 5 mg/week thereafter. A complete remission is rare

TABLE 1 Summary of Therapy for Chronic ITP

Therapy	*Dose*	*Onset of Response*	*Common Side Effects*
Gamma globulin	0.4 g/kg/d × 5	5–10 days	Headache, fever
Corticosteroids (prednisone)	60–100 mg PO daily	7–10 days	Hypokalemia, gastric irritation, sodium and fluid retention (hypertension, congestive failure), weight gain, myopathy, psychosis, adrenal suppression, susceptibility to infection
Splenectomy	—	7–10 days	Overwhelming sepsis (rare)
Colchicine	0.6–1.2 mg PO q. 6 h.	2–8 wks	Nausea, vomiting, diarrhea
Danazol	200 mg PO q.i.d.	1–6 wks	Fluid retention, weight gain, masculinizing and hypoestrogen symptoms, liver toxicity
Vincristine	1–2 mg IV weekly	7–10 days	Neuropathy, constipation, alopecia, cellulitis
Vinblastine	5–10 mg IV weekly	7–10 days	Leukopenia, alopecia, cellulitis, neuropathy (less common than with vincristine)
Cyclophosphamide	50–200 mg PO daily	2–6 wks	Cytopenia, hemorrhagic cystitis, GI symptoms, alopecia, gonadal suppression, malignant disease*
Azathioprine	100–400 mg PO daily	2–12 mos	Cytopenia, GI symptoms, malignant disease*

* Acute leukemia, lymphoproliferative disorders, or solid tumors have occurred in patients receiving these drugs for prolonged periods.

(10 to 15 percent of patients), and most patients become thrombocytopenic as the steroids are tapered.

In patients on high doses of steroids, the serum potassium should be monitored weekly, and they should be observed for signs of gastric irritation and the onset of mental symptoms (steroid psychosis), which may be severe. Antacids one hour after meals and at bedtime are suggested.

If a complete remission does not occur with corticosteroids, splenectomy is usually recommended in adults, although some physicians would give a short therapeutic trial of vincristine (1 mg/week for 4 weeks) prior to surgery to see if a complete remission can be obtained.

In children with acute ITP, most clinicians do not advise corticosteroids, since they do not shorten the duration of thrombocytopenia or improve survival. However, some physicians may use these agents in doses of 1 mg/kg during the first 2 to 4 weeks for their possible effect on capillary integrity. Recently, intravenous gamma globulin (see above) has been found useful as a temporizing measure to control the platelet count in patients with acute ITP until spontaneous remission occurs.

Splenectomy

About 70 percent of patients with chronic ITP achieve a complete remission and an additional 10 percent attain "safe platelet counts" after splenectomy. An increase in the platelet count after splenectomy occurs within hours and usually peaks within 2 weeks. A complete remission is more likely in patients who respond to corticosteroids, have recent onset of their disease, attain platelet counts above 500,000/mm^3 after surgery, or are less than 60 years of age. If a complete remission does not occur, the presence of an accessory spleen should be ruled out (technetium scan), although this is extremely uncommon. Patients who do not respond to splenectomy should receive a second trial of corticosteroids (see above) to see whether "safe counts" can be achieved with doses of prednisone (5 to 10 mg/d) that are acceptable for long-term administration. In children, splenectomy should be postponed, if possible, until at least the age of 6 years because of the risk of overwhelming septicemia in children without a spleen. Pneumococcal vaccine should be administered to all patients who undergo splenectomy, preferably prior to surgery.

THERAPY OF PATIENTS REFRACTORY TO CORTICOSTEROIDS AND SPLENECTOMY

Additional therapy is required in patients who fail to respond to corticosteroids and splenectomy and who are unable to maintain "safe platelet counts" (greater than 20,000/mm^3) on acceptable doses of corticosteroids. The agents listed below should be tried in the order in which they are listed. Usually these agents are added to moderate doses of corticosteroids (e.g., 30 to 40 mg prednisone), and then if a response occurs, the corticosteroids are tapered. Initially, patients should be followed at weekly intervals with complete blood counts.

Vinca Alkaloids

Initially vincristine (1 to 2 mg IV every 7 days for 4 to 6 weeks) is suggested. A response usually occurs within 7 to 10 days, but in most patients thrombocytopenia reappears within 2 to 3 weeks. Occasionally, long-term complete remissions are obtained, but this is uncommon. In some patients, an acceptable platelet count can be maintained with intermittent infrequent therapy with vincristine, but if frequent doses are required, peripheral neuropathy usually occurs. Vinblastine (5 to 10 mg IV/week) may be equally useful in some patients, and this agent carries a low risk of peripheral neuropathy. Some physicians believe that if these vinca alkaloids are infused over a period of 6 hours, they are more effective.

Colchicine

This agent, which is used primarily for the treatment of gout, has been reported to give a positive effect in approximately 25 percent of refractory patients. Dosage is limited by the onset of gastrointestinal side effects (diarrhea). The suggested dosage is 0.6 to 1.2 mg PO 4 times daily. A therapeutic trial of 1 to 2 months should be given, if possible.

Danazol

This modified androgen is given in a dosage of 200 mg PO 2 to 4 times daily. Responses are noted within 1 to 6 weeks and often require the simultaneous use of corticosteroids. Preliminary reports suggest that approximately 50 percent of refractory ITP patients will have a beneficial effect. If no improvement is noted within 2 months, it is unlikely to occur.

Cyclophosphamide

This chemotherapeutic agent should be given at doses of 50 to 200 mg/day PO or 0.5 to 1.0 g IV every 3 to 4 weeks. A response usually occurs within 2 to 6 weeks, and complete unmaintained remissions have been reported in 25 to 40 percent of patients with refractory chronic ITP. If normal platelet counts are achieved, treatment is continued for 4 to 6 additional weeks and then discontinued. While being treated with cytoxan, patients should drink at least 2 liters of fluid daily to prevent cystitis, and their blood count should be monitored at least once a week for neutropenia. If relapse should occur, the risk of using additional courses of cyclophosphamide (small risk of developing acute leukemia) must be weighed against the benefit achieved with the drug, the severity of the patient's thrombocytopenia, and the availability of alternative therapy.

Azathioprine

This is the safest immunosuppressive agent for long-term maintenance therapy. Daily doses of 1 to 4 mg/kg are given initially, and then the dosage is tapered to maintain safe platelet counts. A response occurs slowly over 3 to 12 months, and complete remissions are unusual. Neutropenia occurs at higher doses.

THERAPY DURING PREGNANCY

Since the IgG antiplatelet antibody in ITP crosses the placenta, the infant is at risk for thrombocytopenia. Corticosteroid therapy is indicated if the mother has marked thrombocytopenia, but unless the situation is life-threatening, additional therapy (splenectomy, immunosuppressants) should be withheld until after delivery.

Therapy may be required to protect the child at the time of delivery. It is suggested that the mother receive corticosteroids (30 to 40 mg daily) during the last 3 or 4 weeks of pregnancy, regardless of her platelet count. There is evidence that this prevents severe thrombocytopenia in the child. At the time of delivery, the major risk to the infant is CNS bleeding during vaginal delivery. Cesarean section theoretically reduces this risk. At the time of delivery, a scalp vein platelet count should be performed on the infant as soon as the maternal membranes have ruptured. Capillary tubes containing EDTA instead of heparin should be used to collect the specimen, since heparinized tubes allow clumping of the platelets. Vaginal delivery is considered safe if the fetal count is greater than 50,000/mm^3. Prompt cesarean section is indicated if the fetal count is less than 50,000/mm^3. The child's platelet count should be monitored for at least one week, since delayed thrombocytopenia may occur. If significant thrombocytopenia develops in the infant after delivery, corticosteroids (hydrocortisone 10 mg IM every 12 hours, followed 2 or 3 days later by oral prednisone 1 to 2 mg/kg/day) should be given until the platelet count becomes normal. If thrombocytopenia is severe, platelet transfusions can usually maintain the infant until the maternal antibody clears from the child's circulation. Exchange transfusion is almost never indicated in this situation.

THERAPY FOR CNS BLEEDING

If central nervous system bleeding is suspected (usually in children with chronic ITP), a CAT scan of the head should be obtained to localize the site of bleeding. If posterior compartment bleeding is noted, emergency splenectomy followed by a craniotomy should be performed. If the bleeding is in the hemispheric regions, the necessity for surgery depends on the patient's neurologic status and response to specific therapy for thrombocytopenia.

THROMBOTIC THROMBOCYTOPENIC PURPURA

GREGORY J. DEL ZOPPO, M.D.
LAURENCE A. HARKER, M.D.

Thrombotic thrombocytopenic purpura (TTP) is a heterogeneous disorder characterized by the pentad of thrombocytopenic purpura, microangiopathic hemolytic anemia, renal dysfunction, a spectrum of fluctuating neurologic abnormalities, and fever. The variable neurologic findings may include headache, paresthesias, hemiparesis, hemisensory defects, aphasia, and coma. In addition, myocardial ischemia has been reported. Characteristic laboratory abnormalities include anemia with red cell fragmentation and nucleated red cells, decreased red cell life span, thrombocytopenia with a decreased platelet survival time, and increased fibrin degradation products with a relatively normal fibrinogen turnover. Prothrombin and partial thromboplastin times are normal in 90 percent of patients, whereas reticulocytosis, an elevated serum lactate dehydrogenase (LDH), and unconjugated hyperbilirubinemia are nearly always present. Proteinuria, hematuria, or an increased BUN indicates renal involvement. TTP represents a spectrum of clinical and laboratory findings from mild symptoms with thrombocytopenia to severe disease with a fatal outcome.

The etiology and pathogenesis of TTP are unknown. However, the presence of hyaline occlusion of arterioles and capillaries by platelet-fibrin microthrombi suggests that vascular injury may be central. Proposed etiologies include the presence of a platelet-aggregating factor; the absence of an inhibitor of the platelet-aggregating factor; toxic, infectious, or immune-mediated endothelial injury; diminished endothelial prostacyclin (PGI_2) production, or other abnormalities of small blood vessels. Gingival, bone marrow, and lymph node biopsies may demonstrate microthrombotic lesions; occlusion of small vessels may also occur in the myocardium, brain, and abdominal viscera. However, the presence of these histologic thrombotic lesions is not pathognomonic for TTP.

TTP may occur as an isolated condition or in association with other disorders. It has been reported in association with infectious mononucleosis, influenza vaccination, *Mycoplasma pneumoniae* infections, acute pancreatitis, pregnancy, eclampsia, autoimmune disorders (e.g., systemic lupus erythematosus, polyarteritis nodosa, and Sjögren's syndrome), circulating immune complexes, oral contraceptives, penicillin and penicillamine, dysfibrinogenemia, or cirrhosis. The multiplicity of disorders associated with TTP implies that multiple pathophysiologic processes may lead to peripheral platelet thrombus formation in arterioles, platelet consumption, and erythrocyte fragmentation. While primary endothelial cell damage with subsequent platelet thrombus formation may account for most of the clinical features of the syndrome, the nature of the mechanism leading to endothelial injury remains unknown.

The prognosis of TTP is poor, with mortality particularly high during pregnancy. Increased BUN and creatinine are significant indications of a poor outcome. The reported remission rates for TTP have improved, approaching 60 to 80 percent with current combinations of therapeutic measures. Because the pathogenetic process of TTP remains undefined and may be multifactorial, a successful rational therapeutic approach based on a single etiologic mechanism has not been developed. Therefore, empiric therapy is directed to stabilizing the hematologic abnormalities and to altering the presumed underlying process(es). Clinical improvement is accompanied by an increase in platelet count, decrease in serum LDH, and resolution of the microangiopathic hemolytic anemia.

INITIAL THERAPY

Treatment has included transfusions of red cells and platelets, plasma infusion, exchange transfusion with plasma, antiplatelet agents, immunosuppressive agents, hemodialysis, anticoagulants, thrombolytic agents, and splenectomy. Therapeutic efficacy is judged from anecdotal reports and retrospective series. No prospective controlled trials of any of these approaches are available.

Transfusions. Management of severe or symptomatic anemia requires the transfusion of packed red cells. Type-specific random donor platelet transfusions have also been used initially, but such transfusions are generally not beneficial because of the rapid platelet consumption and decreased platelet survival. Indeed, platelet transfusions may exacerbate the clinical picture by fueling intra-arterial platelet-mediated thrombosis. Therefore, platelet transfusions are not recommended unless life-threatening hemorrhage develops. Alternatively, plasma infusions or plasma exchange transfusions may effect an improvement in platelet count and produce clinical remission in some patients.

Plasma Infusions. The possible presence of circulating toxic substances or immune complexes and early limited experience with whole blood transfusions have prompted the use of plasma exchange transfusions. Plasma infusions have been reported to induce remission in 60 to 70 percent of patients. This

Supported in part by Grant 1 PO HL31950 of the National Institutes of Health, and by the Roon Research Center for Arteriosclerosis and Thrombosis.

effect is consistent with the notion that plasma infusions may provide a "plasma factor" deficient in TTP patients. Serial infusions of fresh frozen plasma are generally initiated immediately upon diagnosis. A clinical response with a significant increase in the platelet count should be expected within 48 to 72 hours following the infusion of 6 to 8 units of fresh frozen plasma per day. However, there is little relationship among disease severity, volume of plasma infused, and degree of clinical response. For example, remission may be achieved with as little as 2 units infused, and relapse may occur despite continued plasma administration or upon discontinuation of the infusions. In the latter case, reinstitution of plasma infusions with continued maintenance therapy may be necessary. Maintenance infusions should be continued until relapse or remission in the absence of infusions can be documented. The limitations of this approach are confined to (1) patients for whom a plasma volume load is a hazard, (2) the time necessary to effect a clinical response, or (3) lack of response. The risk of transfusion-related hepatitis is not a contraindication, as these patients are invariably very ill.

Plasma Exchange Transfusions. In patients who fail to respond to plasma infusions within 48 hours or in patients with limited capacity to tolerate a large plasma infusion volume, exchange transfusion with 2 to 3 liters of fresh frozen plasma should be initiated. This may be accomplished by daily plasmapheresis and replacement with an equal volume of fresh frozen plasma. Response rates of 80 percent have been reported. Exchange transfusions should be continued until a clinical remission is achieved. Antiplatelet and immunosuppressive agents are usually employed as adjunctive therapy. Since few patients are treated with plasma infusions or plasma exchange transfusions alone, the inherent efficacy of these measures is not entirely clear.

Antiplatelet Agents. The finding of disseminated arteriolar microthrombi in TTP has prompted the use of agents that prevent platelet-dependent aggregation and thrombus formation. The combination *aspirin/dipyridamole* has induced remission when administered alone or in combination with other modalities, as noted in individual case reports. Aspirin and dipyridamole doses ranging from 0.1 to 3.6 g per day and 0.15 to 1.6 g per day, respectively, have been employed with varying clinical responses. In some patients aspirin/dipyridamole alone may have induced a clinical remission. Despite conflicting data, antiplatelet agents are thought to play a salutary role and are generally recommended when the diagnosis is suspect. However, they are usually combined with plasma infusion or exchange therapy when TTP is confirmed. Doses recommended are aspirin, 325 mg, and dipyridamole, 75 mg, given together as a combination every 8 hours. *Sulfinpyrazone* (200 mg *q6h*) has been used together with, or as a substitute for, either aspirin or dipyridamole. It is unclear whether this agent is a suitable alternative for, or an additive to, combination aspirin/dipyridamole.

Dextran infusions (250 to 500 ml *q12h*) have been used to inhibit platelet function in the initial treatment of TTP. Because many of the patients reported also received corticosteroids and/or splenectomy, a beneficial outcome cannot necessarily be attributed to dextran alone. Nevertheless, remission has been achieved in some patients receiving corticosteroids and dextran 70. With the more widespread use of oral antiplatelet agents, dextran infusions have been used less frequently. Serious bleeding may develop in patients receiving large amounts of dextran.

Intravenous infusion of *prostacyclin* (PGI_2) has been recommended for occasional patients who are therapeutic failures with plasma infusion/plasmapheresis and other antiplatelet agents. Decreased vascular PGI_2 production with regional platelet aggregation secondary to the absence of a PGI_2 stimulatory factor or stabilizing factor has been postulated as an explanation for the prothrombotic basis of TTP. Clinical experience to support this approach is not convincing, particularly with regard to short-term PGI_2 infusions. Several reports of long-term infusions in refractory patients may have demonstrated efficacy. An initial PGI_2 infusion dose rate of 4 $ng \cdot kg^{-1} \cdot min^{-1}$ for 24 hours, with dose escalation at hourly intervals thereafter, has been reported in one successful outcome. Continuation of the infusions for as long as 3 weeks has been reported. PGI_2 infusions require assiduous monitoring for diastolic hypotension and tachycardia, particularly at high dose rates. Unfortunately, PGI_2 has usually been administered in combination with one or several other modalities, so that no firm conclusions regarding its contribution can be drawn.

Other approaches that modify platelet function by manipulating the vascular PGI_2-platelet thromboxane A_2 axis have not been used in TTP. The role of a more stable analog of prostacyclin, thromboxane synthetase inhibitors, or thromboxane receptor inhibitors remains to be defined.

Immunosuppressive Agents. One rationale for the use of systemic corticosteroids is that TTP may represent the clinical equivalent of the generalized Schwartzman reaction. Few reports support the use of corticosteroids alone, and the role of this approach remains uncertain. Patients in whom antiplatelet antibodies can be demonstrated may have additional justification for corticosteroid therapy. Clinical response has been reported in 67 percent of TTP patients receiving high-dose corticosteroids and combination antiplatelet agents, with or without dextran, heparin, or splenectomy. However, there is little support for the use of corticosteroid therapy alone.

Although other immunosuppressive agents such as vincristine, azathioprine, and 6-mercaptopurine have been employed in TTP, in general, there is little evidence to support their use alone.

Splenectomy. Despite earlier enthusiasm, there appears in retrospective studies to be little evidence that splenectomy offers any survival advantage. Therefore, the added risk of splenectomy is not justified theoretically. It is possible that the benefit noted with splenectomy in early reports was related to the volume of plasma and blood transfused at operation. One retrospective series has reported a 67 percent disease-free survival with splenectomy, corticosteroids, and dextran 70. In general, however, splenectomy is not used.

Anticoagulants. Heparin and warfarin are contraindicated in TTP because full-dose anticoagulation with heparin has been associated with increased mortality.

Thrombolytic Agents. There is no evidence to support the use of streptokinase or urokinase in TTP, and there are significant theoretical risks associated with this approach.

MAINTENANCE THERAPY

Maintenance therapy with aspirin/dipyridamole may be appropriate as it may prevent relapse in certain patients. Doses should be those used during initial therapy. Plasma infusions have also been required in some patients. Unfortunately, there are no prospectively controlled comparisons to verify either approach.

A THERAPEUTIC APPROACH

At present, the treatment of TTP reflects the bias of the physician based on a combination of personal experience and current anecdotal information. The following recommendations should be taken in this light. In patients in whom the diagnosis is suspect, therapy with aspirin/dipyridamole and high-dose prednisone should be initiated. If the patient deteriorates or no improvement is noted within 24 to 48 hours and the diagnosis is certain, serial infusion of 6 to 8 units of fresh frozen plasma should be added as tolerated by the patient's plasma volume status. In nonresponding patients and those unable to tolerate volume infusion, plasmapheresis with plasma exchange transfusion of one plasma volume equivalent per day is appropriate. Exchange transfusion should be performed daily as tolerated for 2 weeks and thereafter as necessary. Whole blood exchange transfusion may be substituted if plasmapheresis is not available; however the latter is preferable. Should a combination of plasma exchange transfusion, antiplatelet agents, and corticosteroids fail to lead to clinical improvement, immunosuppressive agents may replace corticosteroids. Finally, in patients refractory to the aforementioned maneuvers, dextran therapy or PGI_2 infusion may be considered. Splenectomy, anticoagulants, and thrombolytic agents are not recommended in the management of TTP because of their lack of efficacy and their hazard. Once remission is achieved, maintenance therapy with antiplatelet agents may be necessary. Long-term intermittent plasma infusions may be required in some patients. Multicenter prospective clinical trials that test regimens containing the most potentially successful approaches should be conducted.

NEOPLASTIC DISORDERS

HODGKIN'S DISEASE

CHARLES L. LOPRINZI, M.D.
PAUL P. CARBONE, M.D.

Hodgkin's disease has been intensely investigated since Thomas Hodgkin's original paper in 1832. Major advances during the last few decades have taken this disease from an almost uniformly fatal one to one that is now frequently cured. For the most part, this success is the result of good clinical trials and the development of effective radiation therapy and combination chemotherapy. The success seen in Hodgkin's disease has produced a goal that researchers are trying to emulate in other malignant diseases.

INCIDENCE AND ETIOLOGY

Hodgkin's disease occurs in a bimodal age distribution with peaks occurring in young adults and after age 50. Males and females are equally affected in the younger age group, in which there is a predominance of the nodular sclerosis type of histology. There is an overabundance of males in the older age group along with an increased proportion of mixed cellularity and lymphocyte-depleted histologic patterns.

Extensive work in searching for the etiology of Hodgkin's disease has been done. Epidemiologic studies have suggested a role for genetic factors, environmental factors, and infectious agents. Both defective host immune systems and hydantoin drugs have been implicated. Despite the aforementioned leads, and decades of research, the etiology of Hodgkin's disease remains unclear.

PRESENTATION AND DIAGNOSIS

Hodgkin's disease most commonly presents as a progressive, painless lymph node mass in the neck or axilla. The mass usually has been present for weeks to months. Some patients present with mediastinal disease apparent on chest roentgenograms. Localized inguinal or abdominal presentations are unusual. Occasionally, constitutional symptoms, including night sweats, fever, weight loss, and pruritus, are the presenting complaints of a patient with Hodgkin's disease. Rarely the disease presents with the superior vena cava syndrome, renal failure, bowel obstruction, bone pain, or a painful spleen. Neurologic symptoms are infrequently seen except late in the course of the disease, when spinal cord compression may occur.

Histologic tissue examination is required before Hodgkin's disease can be definitively diagnosed. This diagnosis requires the presence of characteristic giant cells, Reed-Sternberg cells, in an appropriate cellular and architectural background. Reed-Sternberg cells are mono- or binucleated cells which probably originate from a histiocyte. They, by themselves, are not specific for Hodgkin's disease and can be seen in patients with a wide variety of benign or malignant diseases. Based on histologic criteria, Hodgkin's disease is routinely subdivided according to the Rye modification of the Lukes and Butler classification (Table 1). These subdivisions have been correlated with the patient's age, the disease stage, and the prognosis.

TABLE 1 Histologic Subclassification of Hodgkin's Disease

	Incidence (%)
Lymphocyte predominant	10–15
Mixed cellularity	20–40
Nodular sclerosis	20–50
Lymphocyte depleted	5–15

STAGING

Staging procedures are done to determine the therapy and evaluate the prognosis of individual patients with Hodgkin's disease. The Ann Arbor staging classification is routinely used (Table 2). This classification is based on the anatomic areas of disease as opposed to the bulk of disease. A patient's stage can be defined as either clinical (from information obtained from the initial biopsy and subsequent noninvasive studies; CS) or pathologic (following results of laporotomy and/or other tissue biopsy procedures; PS). Following complete pathologic staging, 10 to 15 percent of patients are stage I; 35 to 46 percent, stage II; 25 to 40 percent, stage III; and 10 to 15 percent, stage IV.

In addition to defining the areas of disease involvement, the Ann Arbor classification segregates patients based on certain systemic symptoms. Patients with night sweats, unexplained fever >38°C, or unexplained weight loss of more than 10 percent of their body weight during the previous 6 months are classified as B; those without such symptoms are classified as A. Less commonly seen systemic symptoms which do not result in a B classification include pruritus, malaise, and alcohol-related pain. Systemic symptoms usually correlate with the extent of disease; less than 10 percent of stage I patients have B symptoms as opposed to more than 70 percent of stage IV patients.

A good history and physical examination should be the initial step in evaluating disease extent in a patient with Hodgkin's disease. Other recommended tests include a complete blood count including platelets, serum chemistries, a PA and lateral chest roentgenogram, a bipedal lymphangiogram, and an abdominal computerized tomographic scan. The latter two tests are complementary to each other and if one is normal, the other should be obtained. A computerized tomographic scan may detect visceral disease or enlarged nodes that are not seen by lymphangiography. A lymphangiogram, on the other hand, may reveal abnormal nodal architecture in relatively small lymph nodes and may be a more economical method of following abdominal lymph nodes during and following therapy. Other tests, such as bone scans, bone surveys, gallium scans, intravenous pyelograms, and chest tomograms, should be done in selected cases as directed by abnormalities on the routine screening tests. Additional tests that may be abnormal in patients with Hodgkin's disease include sedimentation rates, serum copper levels, and serum ceruloplasmin levels; the utility of these tests is less clear.

TABLE 2 Stages of Hodgkin's disease

Stage	*Criteria*
I	Involvement of a single lymph node region (I) or of a single extralymphatic organ or site (I_E).
II	Involvement of two or more lymph node regions on the same side of the diaphragm (II) or localized involvement of an extralymphatic organ or site and of one or more lymph node regions on the same side of the diaphragm (II_E).
III	Involvement of lymph node regions on both sides of the diaphragm (III), which may include involvement of the spleen (III_S) or localized involvement of an extralymphatic organ or site (III_E) or both (III_{SE}).
IV	Diffuse or disseminated involvement of one or more extralymphatic organs or tissues, with or without associated lymph node involvement.
	Each case is subclassified as:
	A Without B symptoms.
	B Presence of unexplained fever above 38°C, night sweats, and/or unexplained weight loss of more than 10% of body weight in the preceding 6 months.

Bone marrow involvement is frequently found in advanced cases, but is rarely seen in patients who otherwise have CSI or II disease. Percutaneous bone marrow biopsies should be obtained in patients with B symptoms and/or stage III-IV disease. In patients with early clinical stage Hodgkin's disease, some physicians bypass this procedure and, instead, opt for an open bone marrow biopsy at the time of a staging laporotomy.

In the past, extensive information concerning the pathophysiology of Hodgkin's disease was gleaned through routine use of staging laparotomies in research centers. Currently, staging laparotomies should be done when their results will influence the therapeutic approach. Staging laparotomies are not necessary in patients with clinical or pathologic stage IIIB or IV, as they require systemic chemotherapy. Many oncologists recommend staging laparotomies primarily in patients with clinical stages IB, IIA, IIB, or IIIA. Patients with disease confined to the mediastinum after extensive clinical staging and those with CS IA disease in the axilla or high cervical nodes rarely have abdominal disease; laparotomies may not be necessary in these patients.

Staging laparotomies should be performed by an experienced surgeon. It is advantageous for the surgeon to preoperatively discuss each individual case with the medical oncologist, radiation oncologist, and radiologist. During the procedure, the abdomen must be thoroughly explored. A splenectomy and multiple liver biopsies should be done. Lymph node biopsies are obtained from the major lymph node chains and from any suspicious-appearing areas seen at surgery or identified by preoperative radiologic tests (e.g., lymphangiogram). Radiopaque clips, preferably ones that do not interfere with future computerized tomographic scans (e.g., titanium), may help to define radiation therapy ports; they are often placed to locate the splenic pedicle, the ovaries, and other important disease sites. Open bone marrow biopsies are often obtained, and oophoropexies, for preservation of ovarian function, are performed in selected cases.

Staging laparotomies are associated with less than a 1 percent mortality and about a 15 percent perisurgical morbidity incidence. Respiratory complications make them less safe in patients with large mediastinal masses. Long-term complications can also occur. Despite pneumovax immunization, splenectomized patients are at increased risk of life-threatening infections with encapsulated bacteria. In addition, splenectomized patients have elevated platelet counts and may be predisposed to accelerated atherosclerotic vascular disease.

THERAPY AND PROGNOSIS

The therapy of Hodgkin's disease is based on clinical and pathologic staging. Early stage disease is treated with radiation therapy using megavoltage beam energies obtained with ^{60}Co teletherapy or a linear accelerator. Radiation therapy is designed to treat areas of known disease plus contiguous lymph node regions. Between 4000 and 4500 rads are delivered to areas of gross disease; slightly lower doses are used for contiguous lymph node regions. Typical radiation therapy fields include the mantle (cervical, supraclavicular, infraclavicular, axillary, mediastinal, and hilar lymph nodes); spade (para-aortic nodes and spleen or splenic pedicle); and inverted Y (spade plus the iliac and femoral lymph nodes). Total nodal irradiation (TNI) refers to the combination of the mantle and inverted Y fields, whereas subtotal nodal irradiation (STNI) refers to the combination of the mantle and spade fields.

Patients with stage I-II disease are treated with STNI, TNI, or involved field radiation depending on disease site, presence or absence of B symptoms, and histologic subclassification. Up to 75 percent of stage IB-IIB and 85 percent of stage IA-IIA patients can be cured with radiation therapy alone. Patients who develop recurrent disease following radiation therapy often can be effectively treated and cured with salvage chemotherapy.

Bulky clinical stage II mediastinal disease (involving more than a third of the width of the chest cavity as seen on a PA chest film) is a special problem. A pretreatment staging laparotomy is associated with an untoward incidence of respiratory complications. At times, these patients are initially treated with shrinking radiation fields. If, after a few weeks, the mass has appropriately diminished, a staging laparotomy can be safely done to evaluate infradiaphragmatic disease. In other cases, initial combination chemotherapy is utilized with follow-up radiation to the original areas of bulky disease.

Stage IIIA Hodgkin's disease has been subdivided (in different manners by various study groups) to further define disease extent and determine appropriate therapy. One manner is defined by the number of splenic tumor nodules, another by the location of disease below the diaphragm, i.e., upper abdominal disease only ($IIIA_1$) versus involvement of para-aortic, iliac, or mesenteric nodes ($IIIA_2$).

Patients with stage $IIIA_1$ disease are routinely treated with TNI. The therapy of stage $IIIA_2$ disease is more controversial. One option is to treat these patients with initial TNI and use combination chemotherapy only for patients who experience relapse. This spares a number of patients from the increased risk of sterility and acute leukemia associated with alkylating agent chemotherapy. The other option is to initially employ combination chemotherapy with or without radiation therapy. Some authors believe that combined modality treatment increases the cure rate of patients with stage $IIIA_2$ disease; the long-term results from prospective studies, however, are pending.

As already mentioned, the prognosis of stage III Hodgkin's disease depends on the extent of disease involvement. With current therapeutic modalities, 60 to 80 percent of all stage IIIA patients survive ten or more years after their initial diagnosis.

Patients with stage IIIB or IV Hodgkin's disease are rarely cured with radiation alone and are thus treated with combination chemotherapy. A number of effective regimens have been developed (Table 3). MOPP, developed at the National Cancer Institute in the 1960s, causes complete remissions in 70 to 80 percent of patients with advanced disease. Approximately half of these remissions are durable and presumably represent cures. MOPP therapy is responsible for a number of acute and chronic toxicities; the most notable of the chronic toxicities are germ cell sterility and second malignant tumors. A randomized Eastern Cooperative Oncology Group trial compared MOPP and BCVPP. BCVPP had similar antitumor efficacy with a decreased incidence of acute toxicity. ABVD is a regimen initially developed in Italy for MOPP-resistant patients. Following promising results in these patients, it showed comparable remission rates and durations to MOPP as initial therapy for advanced Hodgkin's disease. More recent studies reveal promising early data in patients treated with alternating cycles of MOPP and ABVD. To date, it appears that ABVD does not have the leukemogenic potential of MOPP. The long-term follow-up of ABVD-treated patients, however, is important with respect to possible doxorubicin-related cardiac dysfunction and bleomycin-related pulmonary toxicity. A number of

TABLE 3 Effective Combination Chemotherapy Regimens for Patients with Advanced Hodgkin's Disease

Acronym	*Drugs*	*Doses**
MOPP	Nitrogen mustard	6 mg/m² IV days 1, 8
	Vincristine	1.4 mg/m² IV days 1, 8†
	Procarbazine	100 mg/m² PO days 1–14
	Prednisone	40 mg/m² PO days 1–14‡
BCVPP	BCNU	100 mg/m² IV day 1
	Cyclophosphamide	600 mg/m² IV day 1
	Vinblastine	5 mg/m² IV day 1
	Procarbazine	100 mg/m² PO days 1–10
	Prednisone	60 mg/m² PO days 1–10
ABVD	Doxorubicin	25 mg/m² IV days 1, 15
	Bleomycin	10 mg/m² IV days 1, 15
	Vinblastine	6 mg/m² IV days 1, 15
	Dacarbazine	375 mg/m² IV days 1, 15

* 28-day cycles
† 2 mg maximum dose
‡ Cycles one and four only

other, less thoroughly studied, combination chemotherapy regimens have also shown curative potential in advanced Hodgkin's disease. Most of the chemotherapy regimens are given for at least six cycles, with at least two cycles given after a complete remission is achieved. Prolonged maintenance therapy does not appear beneficial.

In some institutions, stage IIIB and IV patients are treated with radiotherapy in addition to combination chemotherapy. The use of combined-modality therapy to treat such patients has not, so far, been adequately compared to chemotherapy alone. Ongoing trials are looking at this comparison. In addition to the early data derived from these trials, long-term data will be important with respect to toxicities such as acute leukemia, non-Hodgkin's lymphomas, solid tumors, and cardiac toxicity.

Many patients who relapse following initial therapy for Hodgkin's disease are still cured with salvage therapy. Patients who relapse following radiation therapy for early-stage disease may actually have a better complete response rate and survival following MOPP than do those patients who initially present with advanced disease. Patients who suffer relapse following initial chemotherapy do not have as good a prognosis. Nonetheless, therapy with an alternative non-cross-resistant regimen may result in prolonged disease-free survival in a minority of such patients.

Patients who do not obtain prolonged complete remissions following primary or salvage therapy usually die from their disease. A minority of them, however, can be effectively palliated for long periods of time with individual chemotherapeutic drugs.

FUTURE DIRECTIONS

Ongoing research is aimed at improving the successes already accomplished in Hodgkin's disease. As most patients with early-stage disease can currently be cured, the present focus is on those with advanced or recurrent disease. Trials using alternating, non-cross-resistant, combination chemotherapy regimens and others looking at the combination of chemotherapy and radiation therapy for advanced-stage disease are in progress. Both the early antitumor data and the acute and late toxicity results will be important in determining the most effective available therapy. As with other malignant conditions, determination of the disease etiology and implementation of effective disease prevention would be ideal.

FAVORABLE NONHODGKIN'S LYMPHOMAS

MICHAEL J. O'CONNELL, M.D.

It has long been recognized clinically that malignant nonHodgkin's lymphomas exhibit a marked spectrum of biologic aggressiveness. The nodular (follicular) lymphomas as a group tend to follow a more indolent clinical course than the more aggressive lymphomas, which typically display a diffuse growth pattern within affected tissues. Nodular poorly differentiated lymphocytic lymphoma (NPDL) frequently and nodular mixed lymphoma (NM) somewhat less commonly remain indolent for months or years without causing significant clinical symptoms. Nodular histiocytic (NH) lymphoma is usually a more virulent disorder with shorter symptom-free periods following diagnosis and a less favorable response to conservative chemotherapy, and it generally is not included in the favorable category. Diffuse well-differentiated lymphocytic lymphomaa (DWDL) is frequently very indolent clinically and is also considered a favorable histologic subtype. This discussion will focus on treatment strategies for patients with NPDL, NM, and DWDL malignant lymphomas.

CLINICAL EVALUATION OF THE PATIENT WITH FAVORABLE LYMPHOMA

Before the optimal lymphoma treatment strategy can be selected for an individual patient, certain aspects of the clinical presentation must be addressed:

Does the Patient Have Disease Amenable to Cure with Radiation Therapy? The vast majority of patients with favorable lymphomas present with widespread nodal disease and frequently have bone marrow and/or visceral involvement. However, a small minority may have limited nodal or extranodal disease on one side of the diaphragm which can be cured with radiation therapy. Because of the high incidence of occult abdominal lymphoma in spite of negative clinical staging among patients with these histologic subtypes, staging laparotomy and splenectomy should be considered as a potential component of this aggressive approach in highly selected cases.

Is the Patient in Imminent Danger of Developing a Severe or Life-threatening Complication? Bulky mediastinal or retroperitoneal adenopathy producing bronchial or ureteral obstruction and epidural lymphoma causing spinal cord compression are examples of complications that can occur and may be managed effectively with radiation therapy. Cytopenias due to bone marrow involvement are uncommon at the time of initial diagnosis, but if present, they indicate the need for systemic therapy to prevent bleeding or infections.

Does the Patient Have Significant Symptoms Related to the Malignant Lymphoma? The classic systemic symptoms of weight loss, fever, and sweats or other constitutional symptoms may occur in patients with histologically favorable lymphoma. These patients require early treatment, respond more poorly to chemotherapy, and have shortened survival. More intensive combination chemotherapy (to be discussed) may be appropriate in these patients with clinically aggressive disease in spite of favorable histology.

Is There Evidence of Progressive Symptoms or Enlargement of Lymphomatous Masses? Significant tumor-related symptoms or rapidly enlarging tumor masses indicate the need for early treatment regardless of histology. However, many patients with favorable lymphomas are entirely symptom-free. Such individuals commonly have disseminated adenopathy with frequent involvement of the bone marrow. In the absence of bulky nodal disease, which could produce obstructive tracheobronchial or urinary tract complications, it is entirely reasonable to observe these patients without treatment to determine the pace of their disease. The initial follow-up observation should be made in 4 to 6 weeks to ascertain that the lymphoma is not clinically aggressive. If no symptoms hav developed and there has been no growth in nodes or lymphomatous masses, the patient can then be observed at 2- to 3-month intervals. In carefully selected cases, these patients may remain symptom-free for 2 to 3 years, and a minority may be clinically stable beyond 5 years without treatment. Overall, DWDL lymphoma tends to be most indolent, with NPDL lymphoma intermediate, and NM lymphoma least likely to remain indolent for years without therapy.

The advantages of expectant observation in asymptomatic patients with indolent disease are apparent: The patient is spared the toxicity, inconvenience, expense, and risk of chemotherapy until symptoms or tumor progression warrant intervention. Although excellent tumor responses are seen in the vast majority of patients, there is no evidence that chemotherapy can cure these disorders, and therefore chemotherapy should currently be viewed as a palliative treatment modality for patients with favorable lymphoma. On the other hand, if these patients are not carefully followed, they may develop severe or life-threatening complications which could be prevented by treatment. In addition, *complete* response rates to chemotherapy in patients with favorable lymphomas have been higher in asymptomatic patients (60 to 70 percent) compared to those with systemic symptoms (35 to 50 percent), suggesting that early treatment with chemotherapy in the asymptomatic patient might result in higher complete tumor regression rates. In the absence of prospective, controlled observations, however, careful follow-up without early treatment remains an entirely reasonable approach for carefully selected patients who can be reliably monitored. Randomized clinical trials are currently in progress to determine the effect on survival, if any, of early systemic therapy in patients with indolent lymphomas.

Does the Patient Have Intercurrent Medical Problems which Would Have Impact on Treatment Selection? Many patients with favorable lymphomas are elderly and subject to a wide variety of complicating medical disorders. Given the relatively favorable prognosis of these lymphomas and their propensity to respond to moderate doses of local radiotherapy and low-dose, relatively nontoxic chemotherapy, elderly or medically infirm patients may be best served by a conservative treatment approach aimed primarily at palliating specific lymphoma-related symptoms.

RADIATION THERAPY

The favorable lymphomas frequently respond to moderate doses of radiation (3000 to 4000 rads over 4 weeks) with excellent local tumor control. Complications such as obstructive uropathy, tracheobronchial obstruction, spinal cord compression, central nervous system involvement, and other symptoms due to local tumor growth may be effectively palliated with radiation therapy. Curative radiation therapy may be considered for a highly select minority of patients with localized disease following thorough staging.

CHEMOTHERAPY

The favorable lymphomas are usually highly sensitive to cytotoxic chemotherapy. Objective tumor responses are anticipated in more than 90 percent of patients. However, although tumor responses may last an average of 3 or more years following initiation of chemotherapy, with 20 to 30 percent of responses continuing beyond 5 years, there is no "plateau" in long-term disease-free survival which would document curability of these tumors, as has been seen in Hodgkin's disease and diffuse large cell (histiocytic) lymphoma.

Shrinkage of tumor may occur gradually over many months when alkylating agents such as chlorambucil or cyclophosphamide are used in low daily doses by oral route of administration. Symptomatic patients with clinically aggressive disease, who require more rapid tumor response, should receive higher intermittent doses of intravenous chemotherapy. Regardless of the chemotherapy regiment, treatment should be continued until maximal tumor response has been observed. This typically requires 6 to 12 months of therapy, although some favorable lymphomas require more prolonged treatment exposure to reach maximal cytoreduction. Since there is no evidence that chronic maintenance chemotherapy can improve survival, it is not recommended except in patients demonstrated to require continuous chemotherapy to control symptomatic lymphoma.

There is no evidence from controlled clinical trials that intensive combination chemotherapy results in improved response rates or survival compared to more

TABLE 1 Chemotherapy Regimens for Treatment of Favorable Lymphomas

	Drug	Dose	Route	Schedule
Conservative				
CP regimen	Cyclophosphamide	600 mg/m^2	IV	Days 1, 8
	Prednisone	100 mg/m^2	PO	Days 1–5
	(Retreatment interval—28 days)			
Chlorambucil		3–6 mg/m^2	PO	Daily
Intensive				
COPA	Cyclophosphamide	600 mg/m^2	IV	Day 1
	Vincristine	1.2 mg/m^2 (2.0 mg max. dose)	IV	Day 1
	Doxorubicin	50 mg/m^2	IV	Day 1
	Prednisone	100 mg/m^2	PO	Days 1–5
	(Retreatment interval—21 days)			
BCVP	BCNU (Carmustine)	60 mg/m^2	IV	Day 1
	Cyclophosphamide	1000 mg/m^2	IV	Day 1
	Vincristine	1.2 mg/m^2 (2.0 mg max. dose)	IV	Day 1
	Prednisone	100 mg/m^2	PO	Days 1–5
	(Retreatment interval—21 days)			
BAP	BCNU (Carmustine)	60 mg/m^2	IV	Day 1
	Doxorubicin	60 mg/m^2	IV	Day 1
	Prednisone	100 mg/m^2	PO	Days 1–5
	(Retreatment interval—21 days)			

conservative chemotherapy in patients with favorable lymphomas, and intensive chemotherapy is certainly more toxic. My personal preference for the patient with progressive favorable lymphoma who requires systemic treatment is to initiate therapy with intravenous cyclophosphamide and oral prednisone (CP regimen) and to intensify therapy by adding additional agents such as doxorubicin plus vincristine (COPA regimen) or BCNU (carmustine) plus vincristine (BCVP regimen) only if satisfactory tumor response is not observe (Table 1). Oral chlorambucil is a reasonable alternative to CP in patients with relatively indolent disease who have poor venous access or other complicating conditions that would make frequent intravenous injections difficult.

If the response duration resulting from a particular chemotherapy regimen is relatively long (e.g., greater than one year) and the treatment is well tolerated, the patient may experience another clinically useful tumor response following reinduction with the same regimen. A variety of palliative commercially available drug combinations (e.g., the BAP regimen) or experimental chemotherapeutic agents may be employed for the symptomatic patient who becomes refractory to first-line chemotherapy, although there is currently no preferred ''salvage'' regimen.

NONHODGKIN'S DISEASE: UNFAVORABLE LYMPHOMAS

ROBERT C. YOUNG, M.D.
RICHARD I. FISHER, M.D.
DAN L. LONGO, M.D.

The past decade has witnessed a major change in the therapeutic approach to the diffuse aggressive lymphomas, and with this change has come a substantial change in the prognosis of patients with this family of diseases. It was once popular to divide the nonHodgkin's lymphomas into two broad groups, the nodular or indolent varieties and the diffuse aggressive lymphomas. Although historically this was valid and it remains valid for the selection of therapeutic approaches, it is now clear that current therapies offer a much higher probability of cure in the diffuse aggressive lymphomas than in the nodular varieties. The probability of remaining alive and free of disease at 10 years is now much better for the diffuse lymphomas than for the so-called indolent lymphomas. It is remarkable when one considers the dramatic change in prognosis which has occurred over the past decade.

Even 10 years ago, the terminology of diffuse aggressive lymphomas was apt. These lymphomas have a more aggressive natural history. They are high growth fraction tumors with a rapid doubling time, and complete remission rates with single-agent chemotherapy were reported to be 5 percent. Even with early combination chemotherapy regimens, complete remission rates were approximately half of those seen in nodular disease, and median survivals were consistently 1 year or less. Salvage chemotherapy after initial relapse was, and still is, rarely successful.

Our initial efforts with combination chemotherapy in patients with advanced-stage (stage III and IV) diffuse histiocytic lymphoma began with the combination chemotherapy regimens MOPP and C-MOPP and were reported in the early 1970's. The regimen included cyclophosphamide (650 mg/m^2 given intravenously on days 1 and 8), vincristine (1.4 mg/m^2 given intravenously on days 1 and 8), procarbazine (100 mg/m^2 PO for 14 days), and prednisone (40 mg/m^2 PO for 14 days). After 2 weeks of therapy, the patients received no further treatment for the next 2 weeks, and then the monthly cycles were repeated for six or more cycles until a complete remission was achieved, which was documented by careful restaging.

Forty-one percent of patients treated with C-MOPP achieved complete remission, and 37 percent were alive and free of disease with no maintenance chemotherapy at 5 years. This study demonstrated that, while less than half the patients entered a complete remission, those successfully treated had a very high potential for sustained disease-free survival off all therapy and were potentially cured. Relapses were uncommon, and when they occurred it was generally within the first 18 months after completing therapy. Once the curability of this disease had been demonstrated, all investigators felt challenged to increase the complete remission rate and, more importantly, to increase the number of patients remaining disease-free off chemotherapy.

Subsequent studies by our group and others in the mid-1970's introduced two new active agents, Adriamycin and bleomycin, into induction regimes for this disease. While the initial complete remission rate in BACOP (cyclophosphamide, 650 mg/m^2, Adriamycin, 25 mg/m^2, and vincristine, 1.4 mg/m^2, given intravenously on days 1 and 8; bleomycin, 5 U/m^2 intravenously on days 15 and 22; and prednisone, 60 mg/m^2 orally on days 15 through 29) was satisfactory (48%), at 5-year follow-up only 40 percent of all patients treated were surviving free of disease off all therapy. Because the complete remission rates of these two regimens (C-MOPP and BACOP) were similar, as were the overall sustained disease-free survivals, we attempted to analyze the groups for prognostic factors which would allow careful comparison of the two patient groups. Stage IV disease, bone marrow involvement, gastrointestinal involvement, a tumor mass greater than 10 cm in diameter in a single location, and an LDH > 250 were all found to be poor prognostic factors. In contrast to each of these clinical factors which provide highly significant prognostic information ($p < 0.001$), the division of patients into diffuse mixed, histiocytic, or undifferentiated lymphoma categories did not provide significant information about their prognosis ($p = 0.27$). In addition, it proved difficult for expert hematopathologists, even at the same institution, to consistently separate diffuse mixed, diffuse histiocytic, and diffuse undifferentiated nonHodgkin's lymphoma. Therefore, the term "diffuse aggressive lymphomas" has been used and seems appropriate.

These studies and several from other institutions, including the Dana Farber Institute, Cornell University, and the University of Chicago, established (1) that complete remission rates after careful staging correlated closely with long-term disease-free survival; (2) that roughly 30 to 40 percent of the entire population was already curable with combination regimens; and (3) that there were still subsets of patients (i.e., those with bone marrow, GI, and huge masses) which possessed a low (14%) probability of achieving a complete remission with existing therapies. The challenge was then to increase the overall complete remission (CR) rate and especialy improve the CR rate in poor prognostic categories, while not compromising the long-term survivals achieved. Furthermore, despite the good survival rates of patients achieving a CR, the median survival of all patients remained at less than one year (11.2 months).

In 1977 we began a new approach to the treatment of advanced diffuse aggressive lymphomas. This program alternated a flexible number of cycles of one combination chemotherapy regimen with a flexible number of cycles of a second chemotherapy regimen composed of different drugs. This non-cross-resistant combination approach was designed after the Goldie-Coldman somatic mutation model of tumor cell drug resistance, which suggests that the use of multiple non-cross-resistant chemotherapeutic agents would maximize the potential for tumor eradication since this approach would have the highest likelihood of preventing the growth of tumor clones that might be resistant to one or more drugs. Patients initially received a new drug combination termed ProMACE (prednisone, methotrexate, Adriamycin, cyclophosphamide, and the epipodophyllotoxin VP-16), then MOPP (nitrogen mustard, Oncovin, procarbazine, and prednisone), and finally late intensification with ProMACE. The number of cycles of each phase of treatment was determined by the patient's rate of tumor response, i.e., patients were treated with the alternate chemotherapy regimen whenever clinical measurements of tumor size revealed that the rate of tumor response had decreased. This was based on the rationale that a reduction in the rate of tumor response indicated either a reduced rate of cell kill and/or growth of cells that were resistant to the chemotherapy being used at that time.

In the ProMACE regimen, VP-16, 120 mg/m^2, cyclophosphamide, 650 mg/m^2, and Adriamycin (doxorubicin), 25 mg/m^2 are administered intravenously on days 1 and 8. Methotrexate, 1.5 g/m^2, is given intravenously as a 12-hour infusion on day 14 and followed by leucovorin, 50 mg/m^2 intravenously *q6h* for 5 doses, beginning 24 hours after the initiation of the methotrexate infusion. All patients received intravenous hydration at a rate of 3000 ml/m^2/24 hours from 12 hours prior to the methotrexate infusion until the completion of leucovorin rescue. Sodium bicarbonate was added to the intravenous fluids as needed in order to maintain urinary pH > 7.0. The serum methotrexate level was determined 48 hours after the initiation of the methotrexate infusion. If the 48-hour level was $< 5 \times 10^{-7}$ M, the patient was discharged; if the level was $\geq 5 \times 10^{-7}$ M, intravenous hydration, alkalinization, and leucovorin rescue were continued until the serum methotrexate was $< 5 \times 10^{-7}$ M. Prednisone, 60 mg/m^2, was given orally every day for the first 14 days of the cycle. No cytotoxic drugs were administered from days 15 to 28. A complete cycle of ProMACE chemotherapy lasted 28 days. MOPP chemotherapy was administered in the usual manner, but included prednisone in every cycle.

The doses of chemotherapy administered during each cycle were reduced according to a sliding scale based on the patient's white blood cell and platelet count.

One month after the completion of all therapy, patients considered to be in CR by clinical criteria were re-evaluated for evidence of residual tumor by repetition of any previously abnormal staging studies, including appropriate biopsies. Only patients with no evidence of residual disease were designated to be in C.R.

Fifty-five of the 74 patients (74%) achieved a complete remission as documented at a restaging evaluation. Complete remission rates were also analyzed according to factors known to influence the prognosis of patients with diffuse aggressive lymphomas. Complete remissions were achieved in 66 percent of stage IV patients, 50 percent of those with bone marrow involvement, and 64 percent of patients with gastrointestinal masses. Thus, the most dramatic change in complete remission rate made by the ProMACE-MOPP regimen affected the group with the worst prognosis.

Essentially all patients who achieved a complete remission required six or nine cycles of chemotherapy. Patients appeared to enter a complete clinical remission throughout the three phases of their therapy. Forty-five percent of the complete responders entered complete clinical remission during the ProMACE induction, 27 percent during MOPP consolidation, and 15 percent during late intensification. The durability of these CRs appears to be very good. Eighteen percent of the complete responders have relapsed.

The survival of all 79 patients treated with ProMACE-MOPP chemotherapy is shown in Figure 1. Median survival has not been reached. Actuarial analysis predicts that median survival will be in excess of 4 years, with 65 percent of all patients alive at that time. As expected, the prolonged survival observed in the entire population is a function of the survival of the complete responders. Eighty-two percent of the complete responders are predicted to be alive at 4 years, whereas only 10 percent of partial responders and none of the nonresponders survive 2 years.

Dose-limiting toxicity for the ProMACE-MOPP chemotherapy regimen was myelosuppression. Eighty-five percent of patients demonstrated a nadir white blood cell count of less than 1500 at some time during

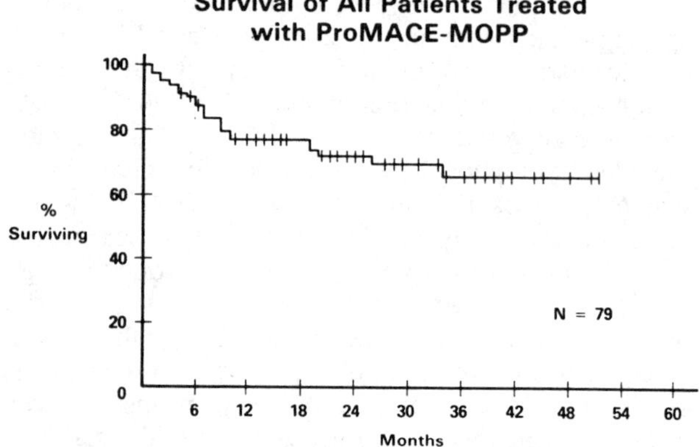

Figure 1 Overall survival for all patients treated with ProMACE-MOPP.

their therapy. Fevers of unknown origin, which require empiric therapy with multiple broad-spectrum antibiotics, occurred in 72/491 (15%) cycles. Eight of 79 patients (10%) died of sepsis while leukopenic.

Platelet toxicity was less severe than white cell toxicity. However, at some time during their therapy, 34 percent of patients developed a platelet count of less than 50,000. In addition, severe mucositis was observed at some time during treatment in 12/79 (15%) patients.

The median follow-up for this study now exceeds 40 months and the fact that 2 years of disease-free survival has been tantamount to cure in previous studies suggests that approximately 75 percent of the complete responders will be cured. The comparison between the survival of advanced diffuse aggressive lymphoma patients treated with ProMACE-MOPP and our previous C-MOPP and BACOP regimens is shown in Figure 2. In these trials and in the other studies listed in Table 1, there is no evidence that maintenance therapy is effective in improving disease-free or overall survival to any significant degree.

Comparisons of the ProMACE-MOPP regimen with other published regimens is shown in Table 1. It is apparent that the latter four regimens have an expected cure rate that substantially exceeds previous trials.

Probably the most commonly utilized chemotherapy in the United States for the treatment of diffuse lymphomas is the CHOP regimen (cyclophosphamide, Adriamycin, vincristine, and prednisone). CR rates have varied in previous CHOP studies, depending on whether restaging of all previously involved sites was performed. In more recent studies, the CR rates were 51 to 58 percent; yet even with pathologic restaging, 30 to 50 percent of the complete responders had already relapsed by 2 years, and relapses have occurred 5 years after treatment. Thus, approximtely 30 percent of all patients would be expected to have long-term disease-free survival.

The newer regimens—M-BACOD, COMLA, COP-BLAM, and ProMACE-MOPP—appear to induce durable CRs (although it is too early to evaluate

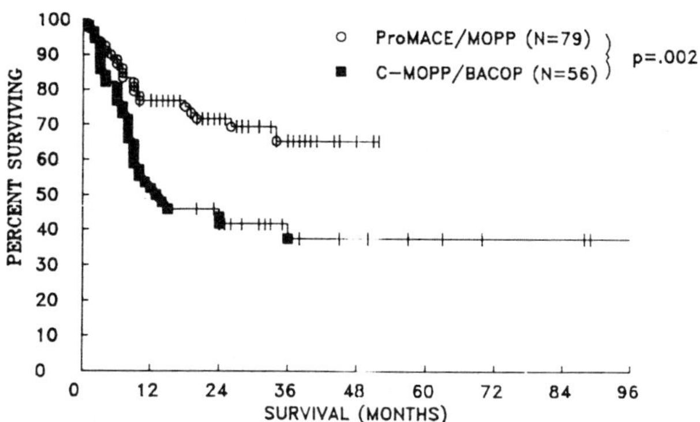

Figure 2 Overall survival of all patients with diffuse aggressive lymphomas treated with either the ProMACE-MOPP or C-MOPP/BACOP regimens.

COP-BLAM fully). Only 17 percent of COP-BLAM-induced CRs have relapsed at 23 months; 26 perent of M-BACOD-induced CRs and 18 percent of ProMACE-MOPP-induced CRs have relapsed at 3-year follow-up.

Unfortunately, these recent advances in the treatment of diffuse aggressive lymphoma have not been accomplished without a price, and 5 to 10 percent of patients die from treatment-related causes. In addition, the regimens are complicated and not easily applied to non-research hospitals or to an office practice setting. The high-dose methotrexate used in several of these regimens frequently required in-hospital administration and careful pharmacologic monitoring.

As a result of these limitations of the ProMACE-MOPP regimen, the newest NCI study is a prospective randomized comparison of two regimens, ProMACE (day 1)-MOPP (day 8) (with methotrexate given at a dose of 500 mg/m^2 rather than the original 1.5 g/m^2) and ProMACE-CytaBOM (a regimen which combines ProMACE [cyclophosphamide, Adriamycin, VP-16, and prednisone on day 1] with cytaBOM [cytarabine, bleomycin, vincristine, and methotrexate 120 mg/m^2] on day 8). Both these regimens were designed to allow outpatient administration and to eliminate the need for hospitalization related to methotrexate administration. At present, 89 patients have been entered on trial, and 33 on ProMACE-MOPP and 35 on ProMACE-CytaBOM have completed therapy. Preliminary results indicate a CR rate of 70 percent for ProMACE-MOPP and 80 percent for ProMACE-CytaBOM. Although it is much too early for definitive conclusions, both regimens appear to be very effective, and the septic death rate has been significantly reduced (4.3%). Both regimens can be safely administered largely on an outpatient basis. However, there were seven biopsy-proved and four clinically suspected cases of *Pneumocystis carinii* pneumonia in the group of patients treated with ProMACE-CytaBOM. Since this observation, all patients on this regimen receive prophylactic therapy with trimethoprim-sulfamethoxazole during induction therapy. Since the introduction of this antibiotic prophylaxis, there have been no additional cases of Pneumocystis in patients treated with ProMACE-CytaBOM. The reason for this peculiar susceptibility to this infectious complication is unknown.

TABLE 1 Regimens for Advanced Aggressive Diffuse Lymphomas

Regimen (Institution)	*Patient No.*	*Path. CR*	*Long-Term Survivors*
MOPP/C-MOPP (NCI)	24	45%	37%
BACOP (NCI)	32	46%	40%
CHOP (SWOG)	112	58%	<30%
COMLA (Chicago)	42	55%	<48%
M-BACOD (Dana Farber)	101	72%	59%
COP-BLAM (Cornell)	33	73%	Not Available
ProMACE-MOPP (NCI)	79	74%	65%

The success of aggressive combination chemotherapy in advanced disease has led to the consideration of its use in clinically staged patients with early (stage I and II) disease. Prior to the routine introduction of staging laparotomies, patients with clinical stage I diffuse lymphoma had approximately a 50 percent 5-year disease-free survival with involved field or extended field irradiation. Careful surgical staging improved the 5-year survival, but only 70 to 80 percent of patient achieved long-term disease-free survival even with comprehensive surgical staging. Furthermore, the morbidity of staging laparotomy in patients with nonHodgkin's lymphoma is significant and produces a delay in initiation of therapy and added expense. These observations have led to the application of combination chemotherapy to patients with earlier stages of diffuse lymphoma. A recent study from the University of Arizona reported 45 patients with clinical stage I and II disease treated with CHOP combination chemotherapy alone (28 patients) or CHOP followed by involved-field radiation (17 patients). The chemotherapy group achieved a 100 percent complete response rate and only five patients (18%) relapsed, all within the first 18 months. There was no significant difference between the chemotherapy alone and the combined modality approach, and the overall survival is 93 percent with a median follow-up over 3 years. A second and similar study from Japan has demonstrated similar results.

The current NCI study also attempts to avoid both the morbidity and treatment delay associated with staging laparotomy in such patients. After clinical staging, all stage I diffuse lymphoma patients receive combination chemotherapy with modified ProMACE-MOPP. After completion of combination chemotherapy, involved field irradiation is used to maximze the prevention of any local recurrence. In the present study, the monthly cycles of both the ProMACE regimen and the MOPP regimen, which have been highly effective in advanced disease, are combined so that the patients are treated with all eight drugs during the first month. Doses of myelosuppressive drugs have been reduced to 75 percent of the original ProMACE-MOPP combination so that all chemotherapy can be given in the outpatient clinic and nadir white blood counts above 2000 are achieved, thereby minimizing significant septic complications. In the first 80 cycles of chemotherapy completed, there have been no bleeding episodes, only one episode of leukopenic fever requiring hospitalization, and no septic deaths. Patient numbers are too small and follow-up too short to make any firm conclusions about this approach at present, although the overall experience now with the approach of clinical staging, bypassing laparotomy and going directly to combination chemotherapy in such patients, appears to produce excellent results.

ENDOCRINE THERAPY OF BREAST CANCER

HUGH L. DAVIS, M.D., F.A.C.P.

In at least 50 percent of cases, the patient fails primary treatment for breast cancer within 10 years. When surgery and/or radiation therapy is the sole primary treatment, 25 to 30 percent of node-negative patients (stage I) and 75 percent of node-positive patients (stage II) can be expected to have a recurrence over the 10 years following mastectomy. Increasing tumor size and number of metastatic axillary nodes portend higher rates of recurrence, and patients with four or more positive nodes show a recurrence rate of greater than, or equal to, 85 percent. The majority (80 to 90 percent) of recurrences occur over the first 5 years, but recurrences may occur decades after primary treatment.

Once breast cancer recurs, it is eventually fatal in all but a small minority of patients, and the goal of therapy is palliation and high-quality prolongation of useful life for those afflicted.

Endocrine therapy (hormonal manipulation) has been utilized to provide this palliation since the report of the first successful therapeutic oophorectomy by Beatson in 1896. In 1984, the clinician is presented with a wide variety of therapeutic options: ablative endocrine surgery, additive hormonal therapy, antiestrogens, and medical adrenalectomy, as well as highly effective combination chemotherapy. The selection of patients for initial and subsequent endocrine manipulations versus cytotoxic chemotherapy can now be based on knowledge of the patient's hormone receptor status as well as the clinical variables, reflecting the tempo of progress of the metastatic disease and ongoing assessment of the tumor burden and the host response.

DETECTION OF RECURRENT BREAST CANCER

Following mastectomy, the patient should be followed at 3–month intervals for 3 to 5 years and at 6–month intervals thereafter for life. The first recurrence occurs in skin and regional lymph nodes in 20 to 30 percent, in bone in approximately 40 percent, and in lungs or pleura in 20 to 25 percent of cases. In the remaining cases, sites of recurrence include liver, central nervous system, peritoneum, bone marrow, or multiple sites. The majority of recurrences can be detected by history and physical examination. Periodic blood chemical surveys, including LDH and alkaline phosphatase determinations, are widely utilized, and chest roentgenograms at 3– to 6-month intervals will detect asymptomatic pleural and pulmonary metastases. Skeletal scintograms in the asymptomatic patient probably are not cost-effective, but any musculoskeletal complaints *must* be promptly investigated by isotope bone scanning and radiographs of painful areas or areas demonstrating uptake on scan. Areas of suspected metastases should be histologically confirmed whenever possible to avoid confusion with the many nonmalignant conditions mimicking metastatic cancer and for biochemical analysis of estrogen and progesterone recepter status. It is likewise assumed that all patients will have receptor analysis performed on their previous primary tumors as well, as this is critical information for prognosis and prediction of later utility of endocrine manipulation if recurrence occurs.

ASSESSMENT OF TUMOR BURDEN

After recurrence is detected, it is critical to assess the number of sites and extent of metastases. A full work-up should be performed including:

1. Chest roentgenogram.
2. Isotope scanning.
3. Careful examination of blood for anemia and other cytopenias and the presence of nucleated red blood cells or young white cells (metamyelocytes, myelocytes), suggesting bone marrow involvement.
4. Baseline calcium, phosphorus.
5. Baseline renal function.
6. Serum enzymes; alkaline phosphatase, LDH, SGOT, and, if necessary, 5′ nucleotidase or gamma glutamyl transpeptidase.

In addition to this basic work-up, isotope liver scanning or computed tomography should be used to evaluate hepatomegaly or abnormal hepatic enzyme tests. Any hematologic abnormalities encountered should be investigated by bone marrow biopsy and aspiration. Computed tomography of the brain and lumbar puncture should be reserved for symptomatic patients with suspicion of brain or leptomeningeal lesions, which are uncommon as initial recurrences.

ONCOLOGIC EMERGENCIES: CRITICAL SITES OF METASTASES

Prior to a decision regarding initial systemic management, effective local therapy must be given if the following urgent situations occur at presentation:

1. Osseous metastases in weight-bearing areas where pathologic fracture or spinal cord compression may rapidly occur. Prompt radiation therapy and/or prophylactic orthopedic stabilization must be considered.
2. Central nervous system involvement. Major neurologic deficit due to parenchymal brain metastases should be averted by treatment of cerebral edema with dexamethasone and prompt radiation therapy.
3. Hypercalcemia at presentation. This rare initial presentation occurs in the setting of widespread osteolytic bone metastases. Prompt treatment (discussed elsewhere in this volume) must be instituted to prevent death from coma, cardiac arrest, or renal failure.

SELECTION OF INITIAL SYSTEMIC THERAPY

The dilemma confronting the clinician at this point is whether to offer combination chemotherapy with a high (50 to 75 percent) probability of initial response in most patients or to offer endocrine manipulation, which produces a consistently lower response rate of 30 percent in *unselected* patients. Careful case selection provides the answer to this therapeutic question and allows the properly evaluated patient a 50 to 70 percent chance of response to initial endocrine therapy, with cytotoxic chemotherapy reserved for failure and specific indications.

ESTROGEN AND PROGESTERONE RECEPTOR STATUS

Steroid hormones (estrogens, progestins, androgens, corticoids) require cytoplasmic hormone receptor with high specific steroid binding for their action on the hormone-dependent target tissue of the host, including the breast, uterus, and prostate. The complex series of events includes binding to the cytoplasmic receptor, translocation to the nucleus, and binding to the DNA–chromatin where the receptor hormone complex directs transcriptional events resulting in specific protein production, maturation, and carefully orchestrated cell proliferation. Estrogen receptors were first demonstrated in human breast cancer specimens in 1970 and progesterone receptors subsequently. Estrogen/progesterone receptor determinations are now widely available in commercial and research laboratories in the United States.

The determination of estrogen and progesterone receptors is the major variable affecting response to endocrine treatment. Table 1 is a summary of the average distribution of estrogen receptors (ER) and progesterone receptors (PgR) in tumor specimens and the probability of overall response to endocrine maneuvers. Before the demonstration of progesterone receptors, 55 to 60 percent of ER–positive patients were demonstrated to respond to ablative and additive therapies, and now with the various subsets of ER and PgR, the highest response rates are seen with ER/PgR–positive patients (up to 81 percent), intermediate rates with ER^+/PgR^- and ER^-/PgR^+ patients, and very few responses in the ER^-/PgR^- setting. This low response rate may reflect tumor cell heterogeneity, which has been demonstrated experimentally and clinically, reflecting a mixture consisting of a dominant receptor negative population and a lesser population of ER–positive clones. The determination of hormone receptors is complex, and tissue must be promptly frozen, as the receptor proteins are heat-labile and rapidly denaturate. Thus the small proportion of responding patients may be the consequence of processing and technical difficulties (false negatives).

The most widely used assay is the Dextran-Charcoal method. Results are reported in femtomoles (10^{-15}M) per milligram of cytosol protein. Values of less than 3 are clearly negative, values of 3 to 9 are borderline, and values greater than 10 are positive. The research method of sucrose density gradient ultracentrafugeration give sedimentation constant information. The active receptor is 8S for estrogen receptor determinations, and patients with predominantly 4S constants are less likely to respond to encodrine therapy. ER values by Dextran-Charcoal assay of greater than 100 are associated with the highest proportion of PgR positivity and the highest response rates. Estrogen receptor studies on primary tumors are concordant with those subsequently obtained on metastases in 80 to 85 percent of cases. When they are discordant, the most commonly observed difference is

TABLE 1 Estrogen and Progesterone Receptors: Overall Distribution and Probability of Response to Endocrine Therapy

Subsets	*Distribution (%)*	*% Response to Endocrine Therapy**
ER + /PgR +	35	75–80
ER + /PgR −	30	30
ER − /PgR +	3–9	30–45
ER − /PgR −	30–50†	<10 to any maneuver

ER = Estrogen Receptor (± positive/negative assay)
PgR = Progesterone Receptor (± positive/negative assay)
* Endocrine therapy includes oophorectomy, adrenalectomy, hypophysectomy, additive hormone therapy, and antiestrogens.
† Variation with age, with patients less than 35 having the highest percent of ER/PgR-negative; up to 70 percent in some series.

an ER^+ primary and an ER^- metastasis. ER/PgR content varies with age. The young (less than 35) premenopausal patient is most likely to be receptor-negative. With advancing age, the proportion of receptor-positive patients increases, and up to 85 percent of elderly (greater than 75) patients are receptor-positive. Exposure to additive hormone therapy or antiestrogens results in an overall decline of receptor content, even to the extent of receptor negativity. This may result from elimination of positive clones or from hormonal interference with receptor production. The clinician must interpret low value cautiously in the face of ongoing or recent hormonal treatment, as secondary responses to different endocrine therapy are frequently observed.

CLINICAL VARIABLES GUIDING THE SELECTION OF INITIAL THERAPY

Prior to the availability of receptor determinations, several clinical variables were useful in selecting patients for initial endocrine therapy versus chemotherapy. They remain useful parameters, particularly when the receptor status of the primary or metastatic tumor is unknown. They relate to the biologic aggressiveness of the disease and are shown in Table 2. When the tumor is receptor-negative, chemotherapy is almost always indicated as initial therapy, even when the clinical situation is favorable (unless the receptor determination is of doubtful accuracy). When combined with receptor information, however, the majority of receptor-positive patients fit in with the clinical variables of relatively indolent disease: longer disease-free intervals, smaller tumor burdens, and overall longer life expectancies. Thus the most difficult decisions are in the ER-status unknown, ER^+, or ER^+ PgR^+ patient with unfavorable clinical characteristics. The response to endocrine therapy is slower than that seen with combination chemotherapy; it may take 3 months or more for the patient to respond. I address this question by attempting to project the status of the patient in 3 months if she does *not* respond to endocrine therapy. If the tumor burden is significant, if visceral sites are extensively involved, or if the appearance of metastases is rapidly progressive, I believe that combination chemotherapy is superior with greater probabilities of rapid response. Endocrine therapy can be offered later, and response rates are not significantly compromised.

INITIAL AND SEQUENTIAL ENDOCRINE THERAPY

Table 3 outlines my therapy preference for sequential management of recurrent breast cancer in receptor-positive or receptor-unknown patients. Note that secondary endocrine therapies are offered only to patients who have responded well to the previous therapy. Initial failure (lack of any objective signs of response or very transient or "mixed" responses) requires that chemotherapy be instituted without delay for maximal therapeutic benefit. Similarly, in patients whose relapse is in critical sites (e.g., extensive liver or lung involvement), I prefer to use cytotoxic combination chemotherapy without delay. Table 4 gives guidelines for evaluations of useful therapeutic response. Patients showing stability of lesions and a good performance status are continued on therapy until progression is clearly evident objectively or by increasing symptoms of disease.

PREMENOPAUSAL PATIENTS

Surgical oophorectomy remains the standard for initial therapy; radiation castration is reserved for patients who cannot tolerate surgery. A number of clinical trials have explored chemotherapy alone, chemotherapy immediately following oophorectomy, or the antiestrogen tamoxifen as an alternative. The results are mixed. Although initial response rates to chemotherapy and/or oophorectomy are higher in unselected cases, the results at 2 to 3 years are similar after the inevitable eventual relapse following oophorectomy (12– to 18–month median duration of response). There are two alternatives for secondary

TABLE 2 Clinical Variables Influencing Selection of Initial Therapy*

Clinical Variables	*Favor Endocrine Therapy*	*Favor Chemotherapy*
Disease-free interval (DFI) from primary to metastases	>2 years	<2 years
Age in relation to menopause	Premenopausal >35 yrs. Postmenopausal >5 yrs.	<35 years Perimenopausal (1–5 yrs. postmenopausal)
Dominant site of metastases	Soft tissue, bone, minor visceral site (e.g., nodular lung)	Visceral sites, extensive liver, brain
Number of metastatic sites	One or two	>2
Extent of involvement	Minimal or extensive bone, soft tissue, minimal visceral involvement	Extensive visceral
Performance status	Fully ambulatory	Nonambulatory

*Assumes receptor status known

"Favorable" Er negative patients usually receive chemotherapy. Receptor "unknown" patients are best selected by "Favorable" vs "Unfavorable", clinical characteristics. (table headings above)

TABLE 3 Sequential Endocrine Therapy: ER-Positive or Unknown*

First Recurrence	Preferred Therapy	Alternative
Premenopausal patients	Oophorectomy—surgical	Radiation oophorectomy
Relapse after response	Tamoxifen	Major endocrine ablation; hypophysectomy preferred
Relapse after response	Megesterol acetate or medical adrenalectomy with aminoglutethimide plus hydrocortisone	Tamoxifen
Relapse after response	Chemotherapy; occasionally megestrol or aminoglutethimide plus hydrocortisone	Chemotherapy; occasionally androgens
Postmenopausal patients (>5 years postmenopausal)		
First recurrence	Tamoxifen	Stilbestrol (DES)
Relapse after response	Megestrol acetate	Aminoglutethimide plus hydrocortisone
Relapse after response	Aminoglutethimide plus hydrocortisone	Androgens

* For initial failures of initial or secondary therapy or patients who relapse in unfavorable sites or rapidly progressive disease, proceed without delay to chemotherapy.

TABLE 4 Modified Criteria of Response in Advanced Breast Cancer

Objective response	Measurable disease in soft tissue, lymph nodes, liver, lungs.
Complete response	All evidence of disease gone.
Partial response	Greater than 50% reduction in the surface area of *all* measurable disease—no new lesions may appear. Reduction of sum of liver measurements below costal margin by greater than 30%. Bone lesions must remain stable or show healing.
Stable disease	Lesser degrees of response or no change.
Progression	Appearance of any new lesions. Increase in area of any lesion by 25% (may require 50% in small [<2 cm] lesions).
Special Consideration in Response and Progression	
Bone metastases	Recalcification of osteolytic lesions, relief of bone pain. Temporary increase in bone alkaline phosphatase followed by decrease may indicate response before radiographic changes. Appearance of new blastic lesions may indicate response of subclinical disease if not associated with pain or progression elsewhere.
Biochemical parameters	Reduction of abnormal hepatic enzymes, resolution of hematologic abnormalities, >50% reduction of CEA levels if elevated.
Subjective parameters	Pain relief, weight gain, improved performance.

therapy: the medical course, utilizing tamoxifen (which I prefer), or medical adrenalectomy with aminoglutethimide plus hydrocortisone or dexamethasone, which is promising (but remains investigational), or the surgical courses, which offers hypophysectomy or adrenalectomy as secondary therapy to oophorectomy responders. Tamoxifen has few side effects and is useful as secondary therapy, with a variable response duration of 10 to 12 months for the 40 to 50 percent that respond. The major endocrine ablative procedures, hypophysectomy and adrenalectomy, have produced a 40 to 50 percent response rate overall in prior oophorectomy responders. The necessity for case selection for these major procedures excludes patients with unfavorable sites and extent of disease, and the high reported rates partially reflect case selection. The overall duration of response has averaged 18 to 20 months for hypophysectomy and 15 months for adrenalectomy. These procedures are used less often in clinical practice because of the availability of tamoxifen, megesterol, and the promise of medical adrenalectomy. Nevertheless, indolent disease in prior oophorectomy responders responds well, and I would be more enthusiastic about offering tarnssphenoidal hypophysectomy to such patients if the surgical enthusiasm were higher. It clearly is an excellent alternative to tamoxifen. With advancing disease at the second and subsequent relapse, response rates to endocrine therapy drop to 30 percent or less. My preference at this point is to use megesterol acetate, as it is well tolerated and anabolic. Androgens in this setting produce disappointingly low response rates when used alone (10 to 15 percent).

The proper sequence in the premenopausal patient still remains empirical, and secondary and tertiary therapies share the problems encountered in the postmenopausal group. Active clinical investigation of chemotherapy plus endocrine therapy with oophorectomy or tamoxifen is ongoing, and surgical oophorectomy may well be reserved for the patients with the lowest tumor burden in the future. Clearly, medical adrenalectomy has promise and, when FDA approval is complete, may well be the secondary therapy of choice.

PERI– AND POSTMENOPAUSAL PATIENTS

The perimenopausal period (up to 5 years after the last menstrual period) has been regarded as a period of low response rates to endocrine therapy. It is now known that the majority of such patients are hormone receptor-negative, which accounts for this observation. The subset that is receptor-positive can be handled as postmenopausal. The receptor-unknown group is better handled by initial chemotherapy in my experience.

For the patient more than 5 years postmenopausal who is hormone receptor-positive or who is receptor-unknown with favorable clinical characteristics, antiestrogens, estrogens, and progestins give equivalent response rates and durations in similar patients, that is, patients balanced for tumor burden, receptor content, and rate of disease progression. The choice of agents is based on tolerance of treatment and the severity and incidence of adverse effects. Androgens are also effective, but consistently less so than estrogens or antiestrogens as initial therapy. My preference, shared by the majority of oncologists, is to use tamoxifen as initial treatment largely because of excellent patient acceptance. For responding patients who later fail to respond, megesterol acetate is an excellent second-line therapy. Third-line endocrine therapy choices include androgens or medical adrenalectomy with aminoglutethimide plus hydrocortisone. Rapid progression at any step along this sequence is an indication for chemotherapy.

Table 5 lists the dose and schedules of the commonly used agents, and Table 6 lists the pros and cons for selection based on incidence and severity of adverse reactions.

TABLE 5 Dose and Schedule of Endocrine Agents

Class	*Agent/Dose Plus Schedule*
Estrogens	Diethylstilbestrol (DES) 5 mg *tid* PO Conjugated estrogen 5–10 mg *tid* PO Ethinyl-estradiol 1 mg *tid* PO
Androgens	Fluoxymesterone 10 mg *bid* PO Testosterone propionate 100 mg IM 3 × weekly
Progestins	Megestrol acetate 40 mg PO *qid* Medroxyprogesterone 100 mg *qid* PO or 200 mg − 1.5 g IM daily to biweekly
Antiestrogens	Tamoxifen 10 mg *bid* PO or 20 mg m^2 PO *bid* × 7–14 days then 10–20 mg *bid* PO
Glucocorticoids	Prednisone 40–60 mg PO daily, taper to lowest dose possible: 60–80 mg PO daily for hypercalcemia—short course. Dexamethasone 4–10 mg IV IM or PO *q6h* for cerebral edema
Replacement therapy after adrenalectomy	Cortisone acetate 12.5 mg *bid* to *qid* or hydrocortisone 20–40 mg in divided dosage. Fluorohydrocortisone 0.1 mg daily of every other day
Replacement therapy after hypophysectomy	Hydrocortisone 20–40 mg day in divided dosage; thyroid replacement
Medical adrenalectomy	Aminoglutethimide 250 mg PO *tid* plus hydrocortisone 40 mg day in divided doses Fluorohydrocortisone 0.1 mg every other day, or daily if evidence of salt wasting

SPECIAL CONSIDERATIONS

The Use of Corticosteroids. Corticosteroids were commonly used as palliative therapy after failure of sequential endocrine treatment. Brief (6 to 8 months) subjective responses were seen frequently, but objective response occurred in only 10 percent. At times this therapy remains useful for the terminal patient, starting with 40 to 60 mg of prednisone per day and tapering the dose rapidly to that which continues to provide symptomatic benefit.

Cerebral edema from brain metastases and spinal cord compression are usually effectively relieved by dexamethasone, 4 to 10 mg IV or orally every 6 hours allowing time for radiation therapy to reduce the tumor burden in these sites.

Corticosteroids are useful in hypercalcemia of breast cancer due to osteolytic metastases, restoring calcium levels to normal in 7 to 10 days in 70 percent of instances, and may be used in conjunction with saline hydration and diuresis. The slow onset of action may be troublesome, and most oncologists depend on more rapidly acting measures such as mithramycin.

Exacerbation of Symptoms (Flare) and Hormone-Induced Hypercalcemia. An acute exacerbation of bone pain or soft tissue pain is seen early in all trials of additive and antiestrogen therapy in a minority of patients. With symptomatic treatment this subsides in 1 or 2 weeks and may be associated with subsequent objective response. The current practice is to continue the hormonal agent while awaiting subsidence of the exacerbation. True tumor stimulation with explosive progression is rarely encountered, perhaps in only 1 to 2 percent of trials. Hypercalcemia, occurring in 2 to 10 days after initiation of endocrine therapy, has been encountered in 5 to 10 percent of trials with estrogen, androgens, progestins, and antiestrogens. If hypercalcemia is mild it may be treated with hydration, diuresis, ambulation, and at times the addition of corticosteroids or a single dose of mithramycin. This is an unpredictable complication and persistent levels over 12 mg/dl or acute rises to 14 mg/dl or greater may threaten renal function or even life. Patients should be appraised of the symptoms of hypercalcemia and frequently observed during the initial weeks of an endocrine trial if they have bone metastases. I routinely monitor serum calcium determinators weekly for the first 3 weeks in the presence of bone metastases. This includes patients following oophorectomy or major endocrine ablative surgery.

If the calcium levels do not fall with aggressive therapy, the offending agents must be stopped and alternative therapy instituted. Switching to another agent of endocrine ablative surgery has been tried and at times has been successful; consider chemotherapy when in doubt.

Hormone Withdrawal Regression. This curious phenomenon has been noted principally with estrogen (30 percent) and tamoxifen and less often with androgens and progestins. It is seen in responding pa-

TABLE 6 Selection of Endocrine Therapy Based on Adverse Reactions*

Class	*Agents*	*Adverse Reactions*	*Benefits*
Estrogens	Diethylstilbestrol (DES); other estrogens	Nausea in 50% Vomiting in 25% Edema in 50% Vaginal bleeding in 15% Potential for congestive heart failure and thromboembolic phenomena†	Inexpensive. Rate and duration of response equivalent to other agents in postmenopausal patients
Adrogens	Fluoxymesterone	Virilization, hepatic toxicity, erythrocytosis	Anabolic, said to promote bone healing, relief of anemia
Progestins	Megestrol acetate Medroxyprogesterone	Excessive weight gain	Relative freedom from gastrointestinal side effects, equivalent response rates as secondary therapy
Antiestrogens	Tamoxifen	Low incidence of side effects, principally hot flashes, occasionally depression, mild leukopenia, thrombocytopenia in 10%	Rate and duration of response similar to DES, excellent therapeutic index, excellent agent for initial therapy
Glucocorticoids	Prednisone and other agents	Usual dose/duration dependent adverse reactions	Palliation in end-stage disease, adjunct to treatment of hypercalemia
Medical adrenal inhibition	Aminoglutethimide Hydrocortisone	Investigational; somnolence ataxia, skin rashes rare, pancytopenia	Equivalent to surgical adrenalectomy in suitable candidates; attractive second-line therapy
Surgical ablation	Adrenalectomy	Requires glucocorticoid and mineral corticoid replacement, surgical complications, poor stress tolerance	Rarely used; medical adrenalectomy equivalent or superior
	Transsphenoidal hypophysectomy	May develop diabetes insipidus, permanently reduced stress tolerance; thyroid replacement required	Easier to manage than adrenalectomy, mineral corticoid replacement unnecessary

* All endocrine therapies have been associated with early hypercalcemia and the temporary "flare" of symptoms, especially bone pain.

† Although DES and other estrogens have been associated most frequently with thromboembolism, occasionally thromboembolic episodes have been associated with other agents; the cause and effect relationship remains uncertain.

tients who subsequently fail and relapse. Discontinuing the agent and observing the patient may lead to a new regression of disease for up to 6 to 12 months. Upon relapse the agent can be re-introduced and a new regression obtained. I have seen as many as four such serial responses in an occasional patient. Because of this, most clinical trials require cessation of endocrine therapy and 4 weeks of observation with continued progression before instituting the study therapy.

NEW DEVELOPMENTS: INVESTIGATION APPROACHES

Medical Adrenalectomy with Aminoglutethimide. This agent, originally introduced as an anticonvulsant, inhibits the conversion of cholesterol to delta–5–pregnanalone and is theoretically able to suppress all steroid hormone synthesis. In practice this agent is given with hydrocortisone to suppress the rebound rise in ACTH that occurs. Probably the most important additional action is to inhibit the peripheral conversion of adrenal and ovarian androstenedione to estrone. The results are equivalent to surgical adrenalectomy and better tolerated. The agent is marketed as Cytadren for the treatment of ectopic Cushing's syndrome and some cases of adrenal hyperplasia. When this agent receives FDA approval for treatment of metastatic breast cancer, it may rank with megesterol as the preferred second-line therapy in postmenopausal patients and also have a prominent role in secondary therapy of initially premenopausal patients.

Combined Endocrine Therapy and Chemotherapy. The majority of studies of combined oophorectomy and chemotherapy show a higher response rate than that of oophorectomy alone. This effect is most marked early, and the survival curves merge after 2 or 3 years. Then the combined approach is not clearly superior to sequential oophorectomy with chemotherapy promptly initiated upon failure.

Combinations of tamoxifen or DES with active multiagent chemotherapy are likewise under investigation. For indolent disease in postmenopausal patients, the sequential approach may be superior. For more aggressive disease, a role may emerge with continued trials. Whenever possible, I try to enter such patients in a clinical trial. The use of combined chemohormonal therapy cannot be recommended as routine practice at this time.

Adjuvant Endocrine Therapy. Early trials utilizing radiation castration demonstrated a prolongation of the disease-free interval in the early period (1 to 4 years) of observation. Since this did not persist, the method fell into disfavor. Long follow-up in a Canadian trial combining radiation castration with low-dose (7.5 mg per day) prednisone for adrenal suppression continues to show superior survival for the subset of premenopausal patients 45 to 50 years of age.

At this time a number of trials of adjuvant endocrine therapy are ongoing, but it is too early for results to permit a definitive conclusion. These trials include tamoxifen alone in pre– and postmenopausal patients and tamoxifen plus low-dose prednisone in postmenopausal women. An additional major effort combining tamoxifen with chemotherapy is in progress. Preliminary results suggest superior results in terms of disease-free interval in postmenopausal receptor-positive patients, with less or no effect in the premenopausal subset.

It will be several years before conclusions are definitive. The clinician today has the opportunity to refer patients to or directly participate in these important trials. There is not enough evidence to recommend wide application in clinical practice.

CHEMOTHERAPY IN BREAST CANCER

JEAN L. GREM, M.D.
DOUGLASS C. TORMEY, M.D., Ph.D.

Chemotherapy is currently being used in the treatment of breast cancer as an adjuvant to primary local-regional therapy as well as in metastatic disease. This discussion will deal separately with the use of systemic chemotherapy in four general clinical settings: (1) adjuvant therapy for "early disease"; (2) combined modality approaches for locally advanced breast cancer; (3) local-regional recurrence; and (4) metastatic disease.

ADJUVANT THERAPY

Although conventional surgical therapy and minimal breast surgery combined with radiotherapy appear to provide effective local-regional control of breast cancer, the majority of patients with positive axillary nodes or primary tumor with an estrogen receptor negative status are destined to develop systemic relapse within 10 years of primary therapy. For this reason, there has been intense interest in the use of adjuvant chemotherapy in an effort to eradicate occult systemic metastases.

Data from several large surgical adjuvant clinical trials have demonstrated that 6 to 24 months of adjuvant chemotherapy with L-phenylalanine mustard (L-Pam), cyclophosphamide plus methotrexate and fluorouracil (CMF), cyclophosphamide plus methotrexate plus fluorouracil plus prednisone with or without tamoxifen (CMFP, CMFPT), or CMFP plus vincristine (CMFVP) provides an improved relapse-free interval and survival advantage in premenopausal patients with 1 to 3 axillary nodes positive. In premenopausal patients with more than three nodes positive, polychemotherapy can improve the relapse-free interval, although this has not always translated into an improved survival. There does not currently appear to be any added benefit of continuing therapy beyond 6 months with the combination therapy regimens; however, this is still under investigation. Current recommendations would be to use 12 months of one of the combination chemotherapy regimens.

The benefit of adjuvant chemotherapy in high-risk postmenopausal patients is less clear. Trials from several groups comparing chemotherapy to observation alone have shown no difference in survival between the treatment versus observation groups. An early advantage in time to relapse was noted in the treatment groups, but this advantage disappeared by 3 years.

Another trial, however, demonstrated an improved relapse-free survival and overall survival in postmenopausal patients treated with CMFVP compared to L-PAM. This study did not include an observation-only control arm. Retrospective analysis of one trial suggests an improvement in the relapse-free interval and a survival advantage in postmenopausal patients who received over 85 percent of their calculated chemotherapy dose. Until the issue is clarified, the use of adjuvant chemotherapy in postmenopausal patients would best be employed in the setting of a controlled clinical trial. Similarly, the benefit of adding a hormonal agent such as tamoxifen to adjuvant chemotherapy regimens is controversial and should currently be reserved for controlled clinical investigations.

LOCALLY ADVANCED THERAPY

The optimal therapy of locally advanced breast cancer (stage III) has yet to be determined. This group of patients has a poor prognosis by virtue of a high likelihood of local-regional recurrence when treated by surgery or radiation therapy alone and a high probability of distant relapse within the first three years of primary treatment. The use of aggressive combined modality therapy has been associated with improved local-regional control and a delay in the appearance of distant metastases. The systemic therapy regimens usually employed have been Adriamycin plus vincristine (AV), CMF, CMFP, or cyclophosphamide plus Adriamycin plus fluorouracil (CAF).

Patients with technically resectable disease should undergo surgical extirpation of the primary tumor. Radiation therapy should then be delivered to the breast and regional lymph node areas (45 to 50 Gy). If the breast was not removed in toto, this should be followed by an electron boost or interstitial implant to deliver an additional 10 to 15 Gy to the primary tumor site. Experience from several centers indicates that patients undergoing excisional biopsy of gross disease have better local tumor control than patients having diagnostic biopsies. Local tumor control is improved with increasing radiation dose, the best results being achieved with total dosages above 60 Gy. The addition of systemic therapy appears to improve the local-regional response and the time to relapse.

If the primary tumor is not technically resectable, one approach is to utilize systemic therapy as the initial therapy. If the tumor responds to treatment, surgery and/or radiation therapy can then be employed with an improved chance for local control. If there is no response to systemic therapy, radiation therapy should be initiated.

Despite the improved local control and relapse-free interval with the use of combined modality therapy, the 5-year survival remains disappointing at less than 20 percent. It is unclear whether these combined modality approaches improve overall survival. Nevertheless, they are important for providing local-regional control. Further clinical trials are necessary to define the proper sequencing of local-regional therapy and systemic therapy.

MANAGEMENT OF LOCAL-REGIONAL RECURRENCE

Increasing primary tumor size and increasing number of involved axillary nodes are the major prognostic indicators of a local-regional recurrence. The pattern of recurrence is in part defined by the primary procedure, and the management of local recurrence will vary depending on the primary treatment.

Local-regional recurrence in the scar or chest wall after a modified radical mastectomy is optimally treated by excisional biopsy followed by total field radiation with a boost to the site of recurrence. In-breast recurrence in a patient with prior partial mastectomy and radiotherapy should be treated by a total mastectomy and axillary node dissection (if not done previously). The role of chemotherapy in this setting still needs to be defined in the context of a randomized clinical trial.

Axillary or supraclavicular nodal recurrence in a patient with prior mastectomy or prior breast-conserving surgery can be managed by axillary resection or supraclavicular node excision. Radiotherapy to the nodal area of recurrence and to the regional nodes at risk should be administered if not given previously. The presence of nodal involvement portends a very high risk of systemic relapse. Systemic combination chemotherapy, with or without the addition of a hormonal agent such as tamoxifen for estrogen receptor positive patients, may be employed. The impact of systemic therapy upon either time to second recurrence or survival is not yet known, and the optimal regimen has not yet been determined.

TREATMENT OF METASTATIC DISEASE

Although patients who develop disseminated breast cancer will ultimately die from their disease, significant palliation of symptoms and prolongation of survival can be achieved with the use of combination chemotherapy. Chemotherapy is warranted for metastatic disease in the following situations: (1) estrogen and progesterone receptor negative status; (2) short disease-free interval of less than 5 years from the time of primary therapy; (3) failure to respond to prior hormonal manipulation; (4) liver involvement, particularly if hepatomegaly is present and there is jaundice or elevated liver enzymes; (5) pulmonary involvement, particularly if there is lymphangitic disease, >4 pulmonary nodules, nodules >2.0 cm in size, or a malignant pleural effusion; (6) malignant ascites; or (7) bone marrow involvement with anemia, leukopenia, or thrombocytopenia. A combination of several drugs is superior to a single agent in terms of the frequency of response. A number of combination regimens have been demonstrated to induce regression of breast cancer metastases. Several of the more commonly used chemotherapy regimens are outlined in Table 1.

Doxorubicin (Adriamycin)-containing regimens (CAF, AV) have been shown to produce response rates of 50 to 80 percent and are superior to non-Adriamycin-containing regimens with respect to duration of disease control. A survival advantage over non-Adriamycin-containing regimens has been demonstrated in some studies. The morbidity is greater with Adriamycin-based regimens.

Alternative regimens include CMF, CMF plus prednisone, and CMFVP. The addition of prednisone to CMF results in improved duration of remission and improved survival. In addition, hematologic toxicity is reduced, permitting delivery of more of the target dose.

Although there are a number of clinical trials which are investigating the role of chemohormonal therapy for metastatic breast cancer, no survival advantage has been demonstrated for simultaneous chemohormonal therapy versus sequential administration of hormonal agents at the time of relapse. The monthly rotating administration of non-cross-resistant combination chemotherapy with fixed crossover to the alternate regimen is being evaluated in clinical trials. To date, this rotating approach has been advantageous over a sequential approach only if the regimens are nearly equivalent and non-cross-resistant (for example, CMF and AV). If either regimen is known to be superior, the rotating therapy is equivalent to using only the more effective of the two regimens (for example, rotating CMFP/AV is equivalent to CMFP alone).

Salvage therapy for patients who fail first-line agents has generally been disappointing, although effective palliation can be seen in some patients. A general strategy would be to use one or more drugs that the patient has not previously received from the following classes: (1) alkylating agents; (2) antimetabolites; (3) antitumor antibiotics; and (4) vinca alkaloids. For example, melphalan, mitomycin C, and vinblastine have all been associated with response rates of 20 to 30 percent when used as single agents in pre-

TABLE 1 Combination Chemotherapy Regimens

	Agents	*Dose*
CAF	Cyclophosphamide	100 mg/m² PO d 1–14
	Adriamycin	30 mg/m² IV d 1 + 8
	5-Fluorouracil	500 mg/m² IV d 1 + 8
	Repeat q 4 weeks	
AV	Adriamycin	60 mg/m² IV d 1
	Vincristine	1.2 mg/m² IV d 1 (maximum dose 2 mg per injection)
	Repeat q 3 weeks	
CMF(P)	Cyclophosphamide	100 mg/m² PO d 1–14
	Methotrexate	40 mg/m² IV d 1 + 8
	5-Fluorouracil	600 mg/m² IV d 1 + 8
	Prednisone	40 mg/m² PO d 1–14
	Repeat q 4 weeks	
CMFVP "Cooper" continous	Cyclophosphamide	80 mg/m² PO q d
	Methotrexate	40 mg/m² IV q wk
	5-Fluorouracil	500 mg/m² IV q wk
	Vincristine	1.0 mg/m² IV q wk (maximum dose 2.0 mg/injection)
	Prednisone	30 mg/m² PO q d × 21 days then taper to 0 over 7 days
	Continue for 12 wks; after a 2 wk break, maintenance therapy begins at week 15 with:	
	Cyclophosphamide	80 mg/m² PO q d
	Methotrexate	40 mg/m² IV q 3 wks
	5-Fluorouracil	500 mg/m² IV q 3 wks
	Vincristine (starting week 18)	1 mg/m² IV q 6 wks (maximum dose 2.0 mg/injection)
	Prednisone (starting week 18)	30 mg/m² PO q d × 7 days every 6 weeks.
CMFVP continous "SWOG"	Cyclophosphamide	60 mg/m² PO
	Methotrexate	15 mg/m² IV weekly
	5-Fluorouracil	300 mg/m² IV weekly
	Vincristine	0.625 mg/m² IV weekly × 10 weeks then discontinue
	Prednisone	30 mg/m² PO q d 1–14, 20 mg/m² PO q d 15–28, 10 mg/m² daily for d 29–42 then discontinue

viously untreated patients. The response rates of single agents in heavily pretreated patients are generally poor, and combination regimens in the salvage setting are more effective.

Patients who have received two or more combination regimens, have a poor performance status, have extensive visceral metastases, or have pre-existing cytopenias can be expected to respond poorly to chemotherapy.

DOSE MODIFICATIONS

Short-term toxicity from chemotherapy includes myelosuppression, alopecia, nausea and vomiting, mucositis, diarrhea, hemorrhagic cystitis (cyclophosphamide), and dermatitis (5-FU). General dose modification guidelines for myelosuppression are summarized in Table 2. If the nadir WBC is <2000 or platelet count <50,000, the doses should be reduced by 25 percent in the subsequent cycle. Therapy with most regimens can be delayed as long as 2 weeks to permit hematologic recovery.

The patient should be instructed to maintain adequate hydration while on cyclophosphamide therapy. The occurrence of microscopic hematuria should lead to dose reduction in the subsequent cycle. The occurrence of gross hematuria should prompt discontinuation of cyclophosphamide, with either substitution of another alkylating agent or a slight increase in the doses of the other agents in the regimen.

The occurrence of frank mucosal ulceration should mandate withholding fluorouracil, methotrexate, and Adriamycin until the ulcerations have resolved. The doses of these agents should be reduced by half in the subsequent cycle. Adriamycin and vincristine must be used cautiously in patients with hepatic dysfunction. Suggested dose modifications for hepatic dysfunction are outlined in Table 3. Methotrexate should be used cautiously in the presence of renal dysfunction. The dose should be reduced for those over age 65 and in those with creatinine >1 but >2, and the drug should generally be avoided in those with a serum creatinine >2.0.

The dose of vincristine should be reduced if mild neuropathy occurs. If more serious manifestations of neuropathy develop, such as muscle weakness or ileus, vincristine should be discontinued.

TABLE 2 Dose Modifications

WBC		*Platelets*	*Doses to give CYT, ADR, FU, MTX*
≥ 4000	and	≥ 1000,000	100%
2500–3999	or	75,000–99,999	50%
< 2500*	or	< 75,000*	0%

* If patient begins therapy with pre-existing cytopenia, initiate therapy at 25% doses.

TABLE 3 Dose Modifications for Hepatic Dysfunction

			Doses to Give	
Bilirubin (mg%)	*or*	*SGOT (I.U.)*	*ADR VCR*	*MTX FU CYT*
< 1.5		< 50	100%	100%
1.5–3.0		50–150	50%	100%
3.1–5.0		151–300	25%	100%
3.1–5.0		> 300	25%	25%
> 5.0		> 300	10%	25%

The dosage of prednisone may need to be reduced or omitted if untoward side effects such as psychiatric complaints, marked hyperglycemia, modest weight gain or edema, or serious gastrointestinal irritation develop.

Cardiomyopathy is a potential hazard with doses of adriamycin greater than 400 mg/m^2. Depending on the individual patient, the drug could be continued beyond 400 mg/m^2 if there are no electrocardiographic, radiographic, radionuclide, or clinical signs of cardiac dysfunction. Alternatively, another agent such as methotrexate could be substituted for Adriamycin. Other potential long-term toxicities include hepatic fibrosis from methotrexate, and the development of acute leukemia after therapy with alkylating agents.

Therapy frequently needs to be modified for individual patient toxicities. The guidelines noted above serve only in a general sense, and may need to be modified from patient to patient.

DIAGNOSTIC STUDIES AND FOLLOW-UP

Upon diagnosis of metastatic breast carcinoma, a metastatic work-up should include a complete blood count, chemistry survey, carcinoembryonic antigen (CEA), chest roentgenogram, and bone scan with plain radiographs of suspicious areas. Measurements of palpable disease should be performed. Hepatic involvement can be documented by a liver radionuclide scan or CT scan. New effusions should be sampled for cytologic analysis. Clinical symptoms may indicate the need for further diagnostic studies. The goal of follow-up examinations and studies is to evaluate the presence and extent of metastatic tumors, to evaluate the response to treatment, and to detect specific complications that can best be palliated by early intervention. The frequency of repeat diagnostic studies must be tailored to the individual patient's symptoms and involvement of vital organs.

GASTRIC CANCER

DANIEL G. HALLER, M.D.

In spite of an unexplainable decline in the death rate from gastric cancer during this century, this tumor remains the sixth most common cause of death from cancer in the United States. Numerous epidemiologic observations have documented wide variations in the relative risk for the development of gastric cancer among various countries, occupations, and socioeconomic groups. However, these observations have neither satisfactorily explained the decreasing incidence of this disease nor provided conclusive evidence for specific causative factors for the majority of patients. In countries with high-risk populations, such as Japan, screening for early gastric cancer may be a valuable method of decreasing the high mortality associated with this disease. In the United States, however, the relative risk of developing cancer of the stomach is too low to make widespread screening procedures cost-effective. Therefore, the practicing physician involved in the care of cancer patients must be aware of the therapeutic alternatives for the overwhelming majority of patients who present with symptomatic cancer of the stomach. Virtually all patients with gastric cancer present with symptoms; abnormal physical findings associated with the disease are hallmarks of surgical incurability.

The choice of these therapeutic alternatives rests firmly on an understanding of the natural history of gastric cancer. As with other malignant tumors, the relative patterns of spread are based on lymphatic and hematogenous drainage, as well as on the anatomic relationships of the stomach to other intra-abdominal viscera. Early hematogenous spread to the liver and lungs is common, and the majority of patients demonstrate distant metastases at autopsy. However, the extensive lymphatic network of the stomach also allows for early and widespread local extension of the tumor. Recent studies have documented the frequency of localized lymph node recurrences and peritoneal seeding in the absence of—or preliminary to—re-exploration after initial curative surgery. Although such loco-regional failures in the absence of distant metastases occurred in only one-quarter of patients, these data suggest that some form of effective local therapy may be beneficial in the postoperative period.

The prognosis for patients with gastric cancer relates directly to the extent of disease at the time of diagnosis. Even in patients who are operated on for cure, the 5-year survival is less than 25 percent. If any lymph nodes are found to be involved at the time of surgery, the chance of surviving more than 5 years is less than 10 percent.

SURGERY

Surgery should be considered for all patients with gastric cancer who do not present with obvious signs of metastatic or widespread intra-abdominal disease. When considering an initial surgical approach, it must be recognized that although the intent may be curative, the ultimate outcome is most often palliative. In the latter instance, appropriate gastric resection decreases the risk of obstruction or bleeding.

In general, the preferred surgical procedure for patients with gastric cancer is the radical subtotal gastrectomy. In this operation, approximately 80 percent of the stomach is removed with the omentum and the first portion of the duodenum. The local lymph nodes are sampled, and the spleen may also be removed if there is direct extension of the tumor to this organ. In general, lesser surgical procedures predispose to an increased risk of local and anastomotic recurrences. More extensive surgical procedures are rarely indicated since they are associated with increased morbidity and are often performed in the presence of extensive, essentially unresectable disease.

Immediate postoperative complications after gastric resection may be substantial and include typical nonspecific pulmonary and infectious complications after abdominal operations. Leaks at anastomotic sites may occur, leading to prolonged postoperative courses. In addition to these immediate complications, patients who have had gastric resections often develop specific long-term digestive and metabolic problems. Vitamin B_{12} deficiency occurs in virtually all patients who have had such surgery. Patients who have had total and near-total gastric resections may also develop dumping syndrome secondary to the rapid delivery of undigested, hypertonic foods directly into the small intestine. This syndrome typically manifests itself after large carbohydrate meals with symptoms related to hyperperistalsis and fluid shifts from the intravascular space into the small bowel lumen. Patients may obtain symptomatic relief from this postsurgical complication by taking frequent, small low-carbohydrate meals.

RADIATION THERAPY

Because of the relatively high risk of some element of loco-regional recurrence after surgery, regional nonsurgical therapeutic modalities, such as radiation therapy, should be considered in patients with gastric cancer. There is evidence that gastric cancer is a relatively radiosensitive malignant tumor, but the potential benefits of radiation therapy utilized alone or with surgery are limited by a number of factors. Although gastric cancer recurs locally to some degree in most patients, distant metastases—outside of a conventional radiotherapy port—are also common. In addition, the dose of radiation therapy which can safely be delivered to the gastric region is limited by the tolerance of surrounding organs such as small intestine, kidneys, and spinal cord. Precision radiation therapy techniques can partly, but not completely, overcome this limitation.

In general, radiation therapy alone has rarely been successful when utilized for long-term palliation of patients with gastric cancer. In some instances, radiation therapy may be administered to medically inoperable patients to relieve specific symptoms, e.g., bleeding. However, radiation therapy alone as an initial approach to patients with gastric cancer is not recommended. A more rational use of this modality is to utilize it in combination with surgery, when the extent of disease has been fully defined and the gross tumor maximally debulked. Such adjuvant radiotherapy has not been fully evaluated in a systematic prospective fashion. More complete data are currently available concerning the potential benefits of combined chemotherapy and radiotherapy in the postoperative patient. These will be discussed under combined modality therapies.

CHEMOTHERAPY

Adenocarcinoma of the stomach is relatively sensitive to chemotherapy. As with other tumors, there are a number of factors to be considered when evaluating the utility of chemotherapeutic agents in gastric cancer. Unlike other adenocarcinomas that are considered to be chemotherapy-sensitive, e.g., breast cancer, gastric cancer usually has been tested for activity in patients with bulky abdominal masses and extensive hepatic involvement. These features are commonly associated with modest response rates, at best, in even the most sensitive solid tumors. For the individual patient, a number of management considerations must also be taken into account before recommending chemotherapy treatments. In addition to the known response rate(s) of the drug(s) to be considered, these factors include:

1. *Anticipated goals of therapy*. The treating physician must have a realistic notion of the potential benefits of the treatments. In patients with advanced gastric cancer, the most likely benefits to be obtained involve palliation of symptoms. Less likely outcomes are significant prolongation of survival or complete eradication of disease.
2. *Natural history of the disease*. One must consider the tempo of disease progression in the individual patient and balance the potential risks and benefits of immediate vs. delayed chemotherapy. Since intent of therapy is palliative, rather than curative, the physician must judge the immediacy of the problems to be resolved by therapy.
3. *Threat of serious problems*. In addition to the speed of the disease process, judgments must be made concerning the gravity of the problems which the therapy is designed to improve.
4. *Consideration of other forms of supportive care*. In each patient, the physician should consider therapies other than chemotherapy for particular problems. These measures, such as pain management and nutritional support, can also be utilized in conjunction with anticipated drug therapy.
5. *Ancillary prognostic factors*. Above all, the physician should consider characteristics of the individual patient which will affect the anticipated benefits from therapy. Associated medical problems and age must be considered in all patients. In addition, the performance status, a powerful prognostic indicator, must be evaluated. Patients who are ambulatory, with a normal performance status, have a much higher likelihood of a beneficial response to therapy than the patient who is bedridden or severely symptomatic.

When the treating physician has considered all these factors, decisions must also be made concerning the type of chemotherapy to be utilized. Both single-agent and combination chemotherapy have been extensively evaluated in advanced, measurable gastric cancer.

Single-Agent Chemotherapy

A number of drugs have shown activity in gastric cancer, as defined by standard measures of response. Partial responses and short durations of response are the rule; complete responses are anecdotal, at best. Currently available agents which have shown reproducible activity in gastric cancer include: 5-fluorouracil, Adriamycin, mitomycin-C, and BCNU. The response rates for these drugs range from 15 to 20 percent and, as previously mentioned, are virtually all partial responses.

Combination Chemotherapy

Combination chemotherapy of gastric cancer has recently been the focus of research for two reasons. First, it is apparent that the responses to single-agent therapy are incomplete and transient; combinations of drugs may potentially increase both the completeness and duration of response. Related to this latter effect, the second goal of developing combination regimens is to develop more effective adjuvant therapies for patients who have been operated on with curative intent.

The combinations of drugs which have received the most attention include various combinations of 5-fluorouracil (5-FU), either with a nitrosourea (BCNU or methyl-CCNU) or with Adriamycin and mitomycin-C. Initial reports of 5-FU/nitrosourea combinations suggested response rates as high as 40 percent, but more recent evaluations have failed to confirm any benefit for the addition of a nitrosourea to 5-FU alone. Most recently, a number of investigators have studied combinations of 5-FU, Adriamycin and mitomycin-C. One of these programs, known as the FAM regimen, is administered in 8-week cycles:

	Week							
	1	2	3	4	5	6	7	8
5-FU 600 mg/m^2 IV	X	X			X	X		
Adriamycin 30 mg/m^2 IV	X				X			
Mitomycin-C 10 mg/m^2 IV	X							

Initial response rates of more than 40 percent have been reported with this regimen, including some clinical complete remissions. A number of clinical trials have since confirmed the apparent superiority of this regimen over single-agent therapies and various other Adriamycin- and nitrosourea-containing combinations.

It is unclear from these chemotherapy studies whether all patients with advanced gastric cancer require combination chemotherapy, or whether survival advantages are ultimately conveyed by the use of such treatment.

Given the caveats that introduce this chemotherapy section, combination chemotherapy with the FAM regimen appears to be a reasonable initial treatment for patients not entered into experimental protocols. As demonstrated in the trials that have evaluated this regimen, the toxicity—chiefly myelosuppression—is easily manageable by physicians trained in the use of chemotherapeutic agents. Approximately one-third of patients treated with this regimen are expected to achieve a clinically useful partial remission. Although patients who respond to this and other chemotherapies tend to survive longer than patients who do not respond, it is not clear whether this prolongation is due to unknown variables of natural history or to the treatment itself. In general, useful responses are seen early in the course of therapy. Patients who do not appear to have improvement of measurable disease by 10 to 12 weeks should not have their therapy continued, as they are unlikely to demonstrate late, meaningful responses. Response to combination chemotherapy are generally less than 9 to 12 months in duration, although investigators who treat many patients with this disease have observed occasional patients who have prolonged and apparent complete disappearance of metastatic disease. Second-time chemotherapies rarely provide meaningful responses, although investigations of drugs, such as cis-platinum and VP-16, continue in this population.

COMBINED MODALITY THERAPY

Combinations of chemotherapy and radiation therapy have been tested in patients with both unresectable and resectable gastric cancer. The intent of such combinations is to increase the effectiveness of radiation therapy on local control, with the administration of systemic chemotherapy to modify the growth of metastatic disease. Early reports from the Mayo Clinic have suggested that survival of patients treated with radiation and 5-FU appeared to be superior to patients treated with radiation or 5-FU alone. Radiation and combinations of 5-FU and nitrosoureas have also been tested, but the data from these studies have suggested significant additional toxicity without substantial or reproducible benefit. Such therapy of patients with locally unresectable disease should be considered experimental at this time. Simpler combinations of 5-FU and radiation therapy, such as those employed in the Mayo Clinic series, may be considered for selected patients with local residual disease. Future directions for combined modality therapy include (1) the use of more active, Adriamycin-containing combinations, (2) the sequencing of chemotherapy and radiotherapy to maximize tumoricidal effect and minimize toxicity, and (3) the use of combined modality therapy in earlier-stage disease to improve both local and distant control of disease.

Adjuvant Therapy of Gastric Cancer

Investigations of adjuvant therapy for patients who have had surgical resection are mandated by the 70 to 80 percent risk of recurrence documented in operable patients. Numerous single-agent (thiotepa, FUDR, 5-FU) and combination chemotherapy (5-FU + methyl-CCNU) trials have been reported; all but one have failed to show benefit from therapy in terms of disease-free or overall survival. One study, in which 5-FU + MeCCNU was compared to a no-treatment control, purports some benefit to such therapy. Similar studies have failed to confirm these findings, and analyses of these data are under way. Studies are actively in progress which are evaluating the role of the FAM combination as a postoperative adjuvant regimen. It is hoped that the high response rate seen with this combination will translate into a prolonged survival for treated patients. In addition, because of the high local recurrence rate, combined modality adjuvant protocols have also been activated for patients who have been operated on with curative intent. Adjuvant therapy of any type for gastric cancer should not be considered standard at this time.

PANCREATIC CANCER

RALPH R. DOBELBOWER Jr., M.D., Ph.D.
JOHN M. HOWARD, M.D.

Cancer of the pancreas is easily one of the most lethal of the neoplastic diseases, the overall 5-year survival being less than 1 percent. Approximately 25,000 new cases occur annually in the United States. It is the fifth most common cause of cancer death in this country. The disease is steadily increasing in incidence in males and females and in blacks and whites. The increase in the black population has recently been more dramatic than in the Caucasian population. The etiology of the disease still remains unclear, although specific factors such as consumption of alcohol, tobacco, and coffee have been postulated. Cancer of the pancreas is rarely diagnosed at an early stage; hence fewer than 20 percent of patients are candidates for surgical resection at the time of diagnosis. Resection with an operative mortality rate below 10 percent is being achieved by experienced pancreatic surgeons. Response rates to single-agent chemotherapy are generally less than 15 percent for this disease in cooperative group trials, and aggressive combination chemotherapy regimens produce response rates that are little better. Responses in this disease are characteristically short-lived. For years, pancreatic adenocarcinoma was regarded as radioresistant. Only recently has this notion been challenged.

PREFERRED APPROACH—RESECTABLE DISEASE

For patients with resectable adenocarcinoma of the pancreas, the treatment of choice is radical surgical excision. The operation should be preceded by

CT scan of the liver to delineate hepatic metastases and duodenoscopy to identify and obtain a biopsy of ampullary and duodenal cancers. Percutaneous transhepatic cholangiography with drainage may permit preoperative decompression of the bile ducts. Distant abdominal disease is a contraindication to extensive pancreatic resection.

After the peritoneal cavity is entered, the peritoneum and liver are carefully palpated and inspected. Dimpling or retraction at the base of the mesocolon may represent local extension of cancer. Dilated venous structures may imply obstruction by tumor. Entering the lesser sac permits inspection of the pancreas while a complete Kocher maneuver permits assessment of the distal common duct, the superior mesenteric artery, and the posterior aspect of the pancreatic head. These maneuvers permit detection of most contraindications to resection. Careful examination of the branches of the celiac axis, superior mesenteric vessels, portal vein, and porta hepatis often identifies suspicious lymph nodes, from which a biopsy should be obtained and sent to the laboratory for frozen section analysis.

If no tumor is encountered to this point, the common bile duct, hepatic artery, and portal vein are dissected and isolated with vascular tapes. The superior mesenteric vessels are identified, and the overlying peritoneum is incised over the caudal margin of the pancreas. The anterior aspect of the mesenteric vein is usually free of tributaries, so that the surgeon can develop a plane between this structure and the overlying portion of the pancreas and tunnel underneath the gland if invasion of the vein has not occurred. A Penrose drain may be used to elevate the tumor and the gland and facilitate further retropancreatic dissection. If no distant metastases or vascular involvement is found, the lesion can be considered resectable. To this point, the procedure may be terminated without resection, but further steps are generally irreversible.

The traditional definitive surgical approach is pancreaticoduodenectomy (Whipple resection) or total pancreatectomy. The pros and cons of these two operations are compared in Table 1. Surgical resection of the pancreas often lies at the limits of a surgeon's skill and the patient's endurance. For these reasons, surgical resection of cancer of the pancreas should only be undertaken by individuals who frequently perform this type of surgery. Patients with suspected resectable pancreatic adenocarcinoma diagnosed by most general surgeons in community hospitals should be decompressed by tube cholecystostomy and referred to major centers for definitive management. Palliative gastrointestinal and biliary bypass procedures may be indicated at the time of the first operation, but these should be done with cognizance of subsequent surgical procedures so that definitive treatment is not compromised. In general, the patient is better off if he is subjected only to a one-stage, definitive resection.

Following resection of the cancer, placement of radiopaque clips outlining the tumor bed will greatly facilitate delivery of postoperative external beam radiation therapy. Intraoperative consultation with the radiation oncologist is also of value, allowing him or her to better appreciate the original position of the tumor, to determine more precisely the volume to be irradiated, and to visualize the anatomic locations of surgical anastomoses and of loops of bowel used to construct biliary and gastrointestinal diversions. Intravenous hyperalimentation, adequate ventilatory support, and good intensive nursing care after operation are essential elements of pancreatic surgery.

TABLE 1 Surgical Treatment of Pancreatic Cancer

	Whipple Procedure	*Total Pancreatectomy*
Spleen removed	No	Yes
Biopsy diagnosis of cancer required before resection	When feasible	Yes
Pancreatic duct transection (possible spillage of tumor cells)	Yes	Seldom
Pancreaticojejunostomy (possible leakage)	Yes	No
Pancreatic remnant (possibly harboring residual disease)	Yes	No
Average number lymph nodes removed	33	41
Operative mortality	++	++
Long-term metabolic defects	±	+++

Recent data from Gastrointestinal Tumor Study Group Adjuvant Study for Cancer of the Pancreas suggest that post-resection radiation therapy in combination with 5-fluorouracil (5-FU) will enhance survival. Optimal radiation dosages and field arrangements have yet to be defined, as have the optimal chemotherapy agents and dosages. Available data suggest that a split-course radiation dose as low as 40 Gy in 6 weeks may be of benefit when combined with 5-FU therapy. The radiation therapy fields should be closely tailored to the target volume (tumor bed), and loops of bowel used in construction of biliary or gastrointestinal bypasses should be excluded from the fields, if feasible. Likewise, the anastomoses, except for the pancreaticojejunal anastomosis, should be excluded from the radiation field. Any pancreatic remnant should be included in the postoperative radiation fields.

When planning the target volume, the radiation oncologist must consider the location of the adjacent normal structures, particularly the spinal cord, kidneys, liver, and gut. A postoperative CT scan, with and without oral and intravenous contrast agent, usually suffices to define locations of most of these structures.

Radiation therapy should not be started until the patient has recovered from the surgical insult and any complications therefrom have been adequately managed. Development of pancreaticocutaneous fistula is a relative, but not absolute, contraindication to postoperative irradiation. A dose of 50 Gy in 1.8- to 2.0-Gy daily increments, five fractions weekly, is generally well tolerated after recovery from major upper abdominal surgery. Treatment should be interrupted or terminated if reaction to therapy is severe. Adjuvant 5-FU can be combined with these radiation doses on the first and last 3 days of radiation therapy in a dose of 500 mg/m^2. Weekly 5-FU should follow completion of external beam radiation therapy. The 5-FU should be delayed one week if the WBC is less than 3000 or platelet count less than 75,000. Nutritional support may be necessary during radiation or drug treatment. Patients should be followed closely by the radiation oncologist and medical oncologist (monthly intervals) to assess late radiation toxicity. Resultant gastritis should be managed by the usual medical means.

PREFERRED APPROACH—UNRESECTABLE DISEASE

The majority of patients with pancreatic cancer will present with unresectable disease. Approximately half of these will have no evidence of metastatic disease, but will be unresectable by virtue of local extension of disease into adjacent structures (e.g., portal vein, superior mesenteric vein or artery, stomach, colon, mesentery). Extensive surgical procedures in such patients may do more harm than good, but many can be treated with combined radiation therapy and chemotherapy. A few patients with such unfavorable disease may actually be salvaged with radiotherapeutic or combined modality approaches.

In light of this information, it is important to clearly establish the diagnosis histologically at the time of first laparotomy and it is important to outline the gross tumor margins with radiopaque clips for purposes of subsequent radiation therapy. Intraoperative consultation with a radiation oncologist is often helpful.

Many surgeons are reluctant to perform a biopsy of the pancreas because of the possibility of serious complication (pancreatic fistula). This surgical notion was conceived in the pre-antibiotic era, but persists even today. Recent reviews of experience with pancreatic cancer suggest that with current surgical and anesthetic techniques, and appropriate postoperative care, pancreatic biopsy is relatively accurate and safe. Neoplasms that obstruct the pancreatic duct can produce proximal dilatation of the pancreatic duct system via increased intraductal pressure. For this reason, pancreatic biopsy should be limited to the neoplasm itself or be performed from the duodenal side of the pancreatic neoplasm. Percutaneous or intraoperative needle biopsies may be safer (albeit less reliable) than open biopsy. A transduodenal needle biopsy can conceivably avoid the possibility of pancreaticoperitoneal fistula. Obstruction of the pancreatic duct by tumor often produces peripheral pancreatitis, which may be difficult to clinically distinguish from neoplasm; however, careful palpation can sometimes make this determination easier, as can the "feel" of the tissues during biopsy. The radiation oncologist is often quite accomplished in palpation of neoplastic tissues; hence his opinion regarding site of biopsy at the time of surgery may be as helpful as arranging clips to outline the gross limits of the neoplasm for subsequent external beam irradiation.

Radioisotope implanted directly into a pancreatic neoplasm is a mechanism for increasing the local radiation dose to the tumor, yet sparing the surrounding tissues (Fig. 1). The isotope most commonly employed for this purpose today is ^{125}I. Such isotope implants directly into the pancreas should only be performed by an experienced team under carefully controlled conditions because perioperative mortality rates as high as 25 percent have been reported from major centers. Thorough exploration of the abdominopelvic cavity, especially the liver, peritoneum, and mesentery, must be accomplished before a decision is made to implant a pancreatic neoplasm. Adequate surgical exposure of the anterior surface of the tumor and excellent hemostasis are mandatory for pancreatic implants. The radiation oncologist, who has the final word regarding adequacy of exposure, placement of radiopaque clips, and type of radioisotope implant to be performed, must be thoroughly familiar with the local anatomy in each case (e.g., location of major vessels, biliary system, pancreatic duct). The tumor is measured and the radioisotope implant is mapped intraoperatively by the radiation oncologist with the assistance of a radiation physicist. An external beam (or intraoperative) radiation dose of 5 Gy is administered preoperatively to minimize dissemination of tumor cells by the implant procedure.

It is important to implant only the neoplasm and to avoid the surrounding uninvolved (or inflamed) pancreas. This will minimize complications from high-dose irradiation of normal pancreatic parenchyma and from violation of inflamed parenchyma by needles. The thickness of the neoplasm is judged by the operator placing the needles as there is usually a difference in consistency between tumor tissue and the surrounding normal structures. Occasionally a needle penetrates a major blood vessel or a dilated pancreatic duct. Sustained local pressure with a "peanut" usually achieves hemostasis. The operator should not use his finger for such purposes if radioisotope has already been implanted. A record of placement of radioactive sources through the needles at the time of withdrawal is made intraoperatively, but radiographs of the implant generally are not taken in the operating room. Postoperatively, stereoshift or (preferably) orthogonal radiographs can be obtained for dosimetric purposes.

Biliary and gastrointestinal bypass procedures are best accomplished after the radioisotope implant has been performed. Because of the low energy of ^{125}I-emitted gamma rays, the dose to the operator in constructing gastrointestinal and biliary bypasses, even in the face of a large pancreatic implant, is rather low.

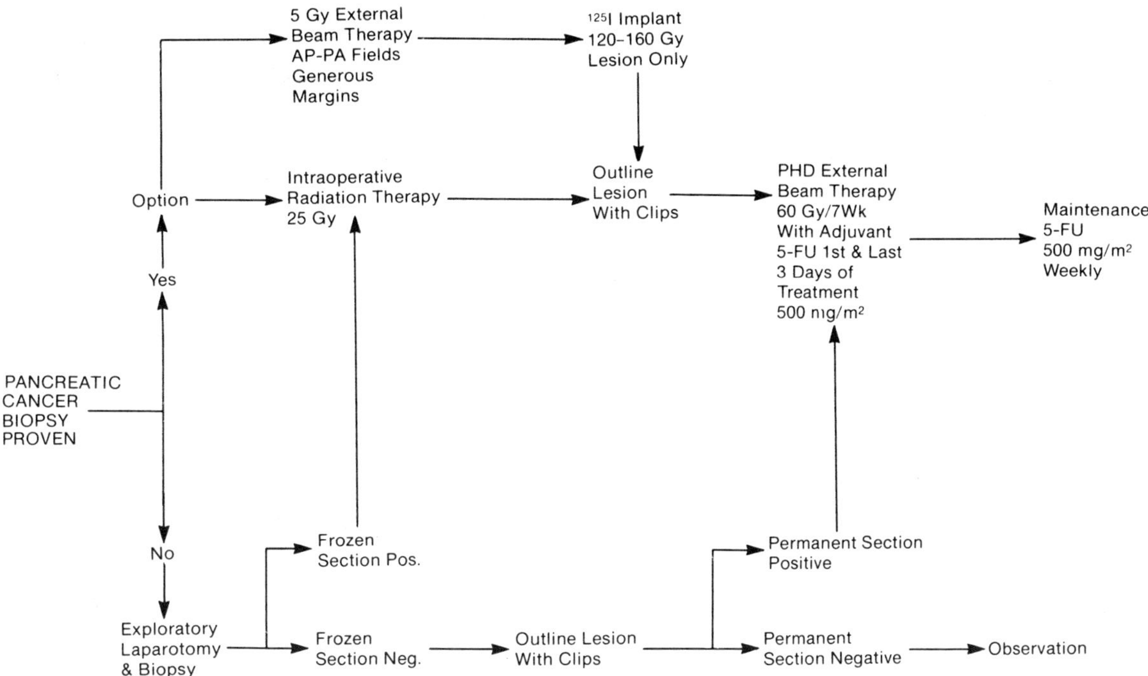

Figure 1 Management scheme of unresectable adenocarcinoma of the pancreas.

Both gastrointestinal and biliary diversions should be accomplished, even if "prophylactically", at the time of ^{125}I implant so as to minimize the necessity for subsequent surgical intervention. Choledochojejunostomy is preferred to choledochoduodenostomy because of the possibility of subsequent obstruction by tumor growth or radiation complication. If the anticipated life span is short, cholecystojejunal anastomosis is simpler. If the duodenum is not obstructed, a "circus movement" of food may follow a gastrojejunostomy and result in vomiting. Thus a jejunojejunostomy, anastomosing the proximal and distal limbs of the gastrojejunostomy, may prevent this by preventing the re-entry of food into the stomach.

Optimal radioisotope implant dosages have not been thoroughly worked out, but available evidence suggests that doses of 120 to 160 Gy over the period of complete isotope decay are well tolerated with ^{125}I. With other isotopes, the dosagees must be modified.

Because of occult local extension of disease, radioisotope implant for pancreatic tumors should be combined with precision high-dose external beam therapy and probably with chemotherapy as well (Fig. 1).

Pancreatic neoplasms require high local radiation doses to achieve control. These doses are in excess of the radiotolerance of surrounding normal tissues. High doses to the pancreas can be achieved with the use of *p*recision *h*igh *d*ose (PHD) *external beam* radiation therapy techniques. This implies accurate three-dimensional localization of the tumor and adjacent normal structures. This is best accomplished with CT scanning in conjunction with radiopaque clips placed at the margins of the neoplasm at the time of surgery. The renal parenchyma may be further localized by anteroposterior and cross-table lateral views of the kidneys during the nephrogram phase of an intravenous pyelogram. The location of the spinal cord is established with the radiation therapy simulator. The location of the stomach and liver is best established by CT scan. PHD irradiation techniques imply good patient immobilization, accurate reproduction of daily treatment set-up, careful simulation with attention to detail, the use of line lasers for reproducing patient set-up daily, and translation of information from simulation to treatment machine set-up with especially high technologic standards and much attention to detail. Beams are angled, blocked, and often extensively shaped to conform the three-dimensional dose profile to the disease profile.

External beam radiation therapy should not commence until the patient is well recovered from the surgical procedure. Field sizes should measure no more than 17 cm in greatest dimension. Doses of 1.8 Gy per fraction are well tolerated if the target volume is closely confined to the pancreatic mass. Only high-energy (over 4 meV) photons should be used for PHD external beam therapy. At the time of simulation for external beam radiation therapy, the excursion with respiration of the clipped pancreatic mass should be noted and the cephalic and caudal radiation field borders adjusted accordingly. If the excursion is minimal, a margin of 2 cm should suffice. The right and left lateral field margins should be more generous, especially in the region of the bile duct and the tail of the pancreas, as pancreatic tumors are known to spread along these planes in occult fashion. The anterior field margin can be less generous because this is the border best defined by surgical clips as the approach is generally from the anterior. The posterior margin is often the most difficult to establish, but in no case should it be less than 1 cm. It is important to ascertain that at least 50 percent of the functioning renal parenchyma is outside the high-dose treatment volume. The dose to the remaining kidney tissue should be kept below 25 Gy, and the dose to the spinal cord should be kept below 45 Gy. After a dose of 45 to 55 Gy, the field may be reduced to irradiate just the neoplasm with "tight" margins, continuing to doses as high as 75 Gy. If external beam therapy is used alone without ^{125}I seed implant boost, we have carried the dose to 67 Gy in most instances.

Five-fluorouracil can be administered in conjunction with PHD external beam radiation therapy in a dose of 500 mg/m^2 daily for 3 days at the beginning and at the end of external beam radiation therapy. Maintenance therapy can then continue with 5-FU in weekly doses of 500 mg/m^2. Drug administration should be delayed one week if the white count is less than 3000 or platelet count is less than 75,000.

If PHD external beam techniques are meticulously used for irradiation of pancreatic neoplasms, complications can be expected to be few. Acute reactions generally consist of mild nausea, vomiting, or anorexia. Nausea and vomiting can be treated with antiemetics or interruption of therapy. Anorexia is more difficult to manage. Delayed reactions may be seen in as many as 20 percent of patients (gastric bleeding, gastritis) 6 to 12 months post-treatment. These should be treated medically, if possible, but without undue pessimism, as there have been sporadic reports of pancreas cancer patients treated definitively with radiation therapy who have died because of neglect of complications (hemorrhage) or unrelated conditions (fecal impaction, appendicitis) and at autopsy have been found to be free of malignant disease.

With aggressive PHD external beam radiation therapy, with or without local boost dose by implantation of radioisotope, a median survival of 12 months for patients with locally unresectable cancer of the pancreas may be expected. The occasional patient (5%) will survive 5 years with radiation alone.

Occasionally the oncologist is presented with a patient with a *clinical* or *surgical* diagnosis of unresectable pancreatic cancer. Under no circumstances should such patients be treated with PHD external beam radiation therapy, with radioisotope implant, or with chemotherapy in the absence of histologic confirmation of disease (or the appearance of metastases) because myriad disease processes, most notably pancreatitis, mimic pancreatic cancer. The risks of chemotherapy and/or high-dose irradiation are not warranted in such situations. Lower doses of radiation therapy may preclude subsequnt definitive treatment. In such instances, attempts at histologic confirmation of the disease should be made.

PREFERRED APPROACH—METASTATIC DISEASE

For patients presenting with metastatic pancreatic cancer, cure is currently impossible. The goal for such patients should be palliation of symptoms. This may require a combined surgical/radiotherapeutic/chemotherapeutic approach. Radiation therapy is extremely effective for palliation of local symptoms of pancreatic cancer except for gastrointestinal or biliary obstruction. These should be treated surigically. Operation should include biopsy and, usually, cholecystojejunostomy, gastrojejunostomy, and, as already described, jejunojejunostomy to prevent reentry of food into the stomach. Careful attention to blood volume, serum albumin levels, and nutrition (IV hyperalimentation) is necessary to minimize operative mortality. Painful bone metastases regularly respond to a dose of 40 Gy administered in 15 equal increments over a period of 3 weeks. Likewise, upper abdominal pain and sometimes even nausea, vomiting, and anorexia are palliated by local upper abdominal irradiation, with or without adjuvant chemotherapy. Many studies have suggested that the palliative benefits of radiation in such instances are dose related, and it appears that one must achieve at least the radiobiologic equivalent of 45 Gy administered in equal 1.8 Gy increments over the course of 5 weeks in order to achieve a good response.

Obstruction of the gastrointestinal tract is best palliated surgically, whereas biliary obstruction can be treated by either surgical bypass or, perhaps in selected instances, with percutaneous transhepatic catheter drainage, with or without radioisotope placed per catheter. Palliative Whipple procedures and palliative total pancreatectomies are not recommended because the surgical morbidity and mortality outweigh the potential benefit in patients destined to die shortly of the disease.

Five-fluorouracil has been used extensively for pancreatic cancer, with response rates reported as high as 67 percent in retrospective reports. In prospective controlled cooperative group trials, response rates of less than 20 percent have generally been observed. The combination of Streptozotocin, mitomycin-C, and 5-FU is reported to have produced partial response in 43 percent of 23 evaluable patients so treated. Median duration of response was 5 months and duration of survival in responders was 9.5 months.

The patient who is asymptomatic after histologic proof of pancreatic cancer and appropriate palliative bypass surgery is best treated expectantly. Quality of

TABLE 2 Pancreatic Cancer: Particle Beam Therapy

Group	*Beam(s)*	*Dose (^{60}Co Equivalent) and Fractionation*	*Results*	*Complications*
M.D. Anderson (1981)	50 meV neutrons with or without 32 meVp photons	60 Gy, 10 weeks, Double split course	Survival enhancement with neutrons or "mixed beam" compared to photons alone	None observed
Fermilab (1981)	66 meV neutrons	58.5 Gy, 6–7 weeks	Alive NED, 4/31 Alive, with disease, 2/31 Local persistence, 25/31	GI hemorrhage, 2/31 Duodenal ulcer, 3/31 Pancreatic insufficiency, 4/31 Bowel obstruction, 1/31
Cleveland Clinic (1978)	25 meV neutrons plus 10 meVp photons	60 Gy 6–8 weeks	Alive, 4/30	GI hemorrhage, 4/30 Gangrene—small bowel, 1/30
Lawrence Berkeley Laboratory (1982)	934 meV Helium ions, Carbon ions or Neon ions	50–70 Gy 6-8 weeks	Local control, 11/55 Alive and well, 8/55	GI hemorrhage, 6/58 Bowel obstruction, 2/55
Mid-Atlantic Neutron Therapy Association (1981)	14 meV neutrons with or without 5-FU	52 Gy, 6 weeks	Partial response, 5/18 Alive NED, 1/14	GI hemorrhage, 6/58 Hepatopathy, 10/20 Colitis, 2/20 Radiation myelitis 1/25

Modified from Radiotherapeutic approaches to treatment of cancer of the pancreas. *Surgical Disease of the Pancreas,* Lea & Febiger

life is important. Liberal use of analgesic is the best treatment for selected patients with symptomatic refractory disease. Nutritional support and comfort measures may be the most important tools available to the clinician in such instances. When present, diabetes or exocrine insufficienty should be treated.

THERAPEUTIC ALTERNATIVES

Patients with unresectable (but nonmetastatic) cancer of the pancreas often are advised that there is nothing more to be done. Median survival of such abandoned patients is approximately 3 months in contrast to a median survival of approximately 12 months for patients treated aggressively with appropriate bypass surgery, radiation therapy, and chemotherapy. Simple observation may be appropriate for patients with rapidly advancing metastatic disease and rapid weight loss, but this is not appropriate for patients who are losing weight rapidly because of emotional depression. Depression is common with pancreatic cancer and can be successfully treated.

High linear energy transfer particulate radiation beams are being employed in clinical trials at several institutions for pancreatic cancer. Initial results of such therapy have been disappointing, with higher than anticipated complication rates and survival rates not demonstrably better than those of patients treated with PHD external beam therapy (Table 2).

For patients with curatively resected pancreatic cancer, a cooperative intergroup postopertive adjuvant study of PHD irradiation plus 5-FU vs PHD irradiation plus "sandwich" SMF combination chemotherapy is underway. For patients with locally unresectable pancreatic cancer, the Eastern Cooperative Oncology Group is currently testing PHD radiation therapy alone vs PHD radiation therapy plus radiation sensitizers (5-FU and mitomycin-C).

Complications of radiation therapy do not result from irradiation of tumors, but from irradiation of normal tissues. For external beam therapy, most of the radiation dose is deposited in transit tissues through which the beam must pass in order to reach the tumor. Intraoperative radiation therapy is a means by which normal tissues can be physically displaced from the radiation field surgically so that unresectable lesions or tumor beds may be exposed directly to radiation (Fig. 1). For pancreatic cancer, this necessitates having the abdomen open in the radiation therapy suite. In some centers, this is accomplished by transporting anesthetized patients from the surgical suite to the radiation therapy facility during laparotomy. It is our belief that such transportation presents additional risks and that intraoperative radiation therapy techniques should be explored in facilities that have appropriate radiation therapy equipment in an operating amphitheater. Early data from such treatment, either alone or in combination with chemotherapy and conventional irradiation, are encouraging.

CHEMOTHERAPY IN LUNG CANCER

DAVID S. ETTINGER, M.D.

Lung cancer is a major health problem in the United States with increasing incidence and mortality rates. Despite improvement in surgical and radiotherapy techniques, the overall 5-year survival rate of all lung cancer patients is less than 10 percent, reflecting the advanced stage of their disease at the time of diagnosis.

Based on differences in biological behavior and response to systemic therapy, lung cancers are classified as either non-small cell carcinomas (NSCC), with epidermoid carcinoma, adenocarcinoma, and large cell carcinoma being the most common histologic types (75 to 80%) or small cell carcinoma (SCC, 20 to 25%).

In addition there are several prognostic factors that affect survival rates. They include initial performance status, extent of disease, and weight loss. The effects of these prognostic variables on results of therapy can be considerable and must be kept in mind when evaluating therapeutic studies.

Different studies using the same drug(s), dosage(s), and schedule of administration report a wide range of response rates which can be accounted for by different criteria of objective response as well as different patient selection characteristics.

At present, extent of disease and histologic cell type are the major factors that determine whether a patient with lung cancer should receive chemotherapy. In NSCC, the decision to treat a patient with chemotherapy is made more difficult by its usual ineffectiveness. However, in SCC, chemotherapy is effective and indicated regardless of the extent of disease.

NON-SMALL CELL CARCINOMA

Staging of lung cancer according to the TNM classification provides a basis for selecting patients for a particular therapy. Radiation is the preferred treatment for patients with stage I or II disease who either refuse surgery or for whom surgery is contraindicated and in patients with stage III disease, limited to one hemithorax, but inoperable. Chemotherapy is usually reserved for patients with stage III disease, when there is known distant metastasis.

Chemotherapy has been utilized following surgical resection of primary NSCC, in theory to eradicate micrometastatic disease present at the time of surgery. Single agents, such as cyclophosphamide, nitrogen mustard, CCNU, and vinblastine, and combination chemotherapy, such as cyclophosphamide and methotrexate, CCNU and hydroxyurea, cyclophosphamide and methotrexate, and vinblastine and 5-FU, have been tried as adjuvant chemotherapy without success.

At present, there is no indication for the routine use of postoperative adjuvant chemotherapy. Its use should be restricted to patients entered on well-designed, randomized controlled clinical trials evaluating the use of adjuvant chemotherapy. Such trials, evaluating newer drug combinations (i.e., cyclophosphamide and Adriamycin and cisplatin) are in progress.

Since most patients with inoperable lung cancer, despite receiving definitive radiotherapy, die of metastatic disease, chemotherapy is sometimes given before, during, or after the radiation therapy. It is intended to destroy micrometastases and act as a radiation sensitizer, thereby improving local control of the disease.

Both single agents and combination chemotherapy following radiation therapy have been compared to radiation therapy alone with no significant benefit found. Single agents evaluated include cyclophosphamide, nitrogen mustard, 5-FU, vinblastine, hydroxyurea, and procarbazine. Drug combinations include cyclophosphamide and methotrexate, cyclophosphamide and methotrexate and CCNU, 5-FU and actinomycin D, and CCNU and hydroxyurea. In a nonrandomized trial, combination chemotherapy utilizing cyclophosphamide and Adriamycin and methotrexate and procarbazine (CAMP) after radiation therapy to the primary tumor gave a 51 percent objective response rate with a 15-month median survival rate for responders, which was better than historical controls who received radiation alone.

A number of studies are evaluating the use of chemotherapy before or during radiotherapy for inoperable NSCC. In the Eastern Cooperative Oncology Group (ECOG), three pilot studies have been initiated. In two of these, patients receive two cycles of either mitomycin C and vinblastine and cisplatin (MVP) or vinblastine and cisplatin (VP) prior to radiation therapy. In a third study, patients receive weekly escalating doses of cisplatin concomitantly with definitive radiation therapy.

At present, there is no evidence that the addition of chemotherapy in any sequence to radiation therapy significantly increases the survival of patients. These combined multimodality approaches should not be used routinely. When possible, patients should be entered on either pilot studies or randomized trials to determine the safety and efficacy of these combined approaches.

Since the majority of patients with NSCC have documented distant metastases at some point during their illness, there is a need for effective systemic chemotherapy.

The objective response rates for most single chemotherapeutic drugs are low (10 to 15%). Higher response rates have been reported with Adriamycin, mitomycin C, cisplatin, VP-16, and vindesine. Unfortunately, most objective responses achieved with single agents are partial; complete responses are rarely seen. The response duration is short (2 to 4 months), generally with no prolongation of survival.

Combination chemotherapy has been useful in controlling many other kinds of cancers; it is used in treating NSCC in the hope of producing similar benefits. The objective response rate, depending on the combination chemotherapeutic regimen, varies from 4 to 63 percent, with a complete response rate of 0 to 10 percent and a median survival rate of 4 to 13 months.

The most effective combination chemotherapeutic regimens in the treatment of NSCC appear to contain Adriamycin and/or cisplatin. Combinations in use today include:

CAMP

Cyclophosphamide	300 mg/m^2 IV day 1 and 8
Adriamycin	20 mg/m^2 IV day 1 and 8
Methotrexate	15 mg/m^2 IV day 1 and 8
Procarbazine	100 mg/m^2 PO day 2–11

Repeat cycle every 4 weeks.

CAP

Cyclophosphamide	400 mg/m^2 IV day 1
Adriamycin	40 mg/m^2 IV day 1
Cisplatin	40 mg/m^2 IV day 1

Repeat cycle every 4 weeks.

MVP

Mitomycin C	10 mg/m^2 IV day 1
Vinblastine	6 mg/m^2 IV day 1
Cisplatin	40 mg/m^2 IV day 1

Repeat cycle every 3 weeks.

The latter regimen has been the most active regimen in the ECOG randomized trials, with a 26 percent objective response rate. It is encouraging that 6 percent of the responses were complete responses.

Patients on combination chemotherapy should receive at least two cycles of the therapy. If no response is seen, treatment should be stopped. However, if the patient's disease has become stable while on chemotherapy and the associated toxicities are minimal, the chemotherapy should be continued. Patients who respond to chemotherapy should be maintained on it unless there is objective evidence of disease progression.

Most combination chemotherapeutic regimens used to treat NSCC can be administered in an outpatient setting because side effects are usually tolerable. Side effects common to most drugs used include: nausea, vomiting, alopecia, and myelosuppression. Drug-specific toxicities include: hemorrhagic cystitis (cyclophosphamide), cardiomyopathy (Adriamycin), and nephrotoxicity (cisplatin and methotrexate).

Patients with active cardiac disease, uncontrolled high blood pressure, unstable angina, congestive heart failure, or recent myocardial infarction should not receive Adriamycin. Patients receiving moderate doses of cisplatin require pre- and post-treatment IV hydration, usually on an outpatient basis. High-dose cisplatin (120 mg/m^2) requires inpatient administration, with extensive IV hydration plus furosemide and mannitol to maintain a brisk diuresis.

Despite the improvement in objective response rates with combination chemotherapy, there has been no improvement in the overall survival rate. It does appear, however, that responders to chemotherapy survive longer than nonresponders.

In general, patients with progressive disseminated NSCC who are ambulatory (ECOG performance status 0, 1, or 2), have no significant weight loss ($\leq$10% of body weight in the preceding 6 months), and have adequate bone marrow, liver, and renal function have the best chance of objectively responding to the therapy with the least amount of toxicity.

It is important to avoid waiting until the patient has symptoms before considering him a candidate for chemotherapy. Patients who are symptomatic because of their disease, are nonambulatory (ECOG performance status 3 or 4), have poor nutritional status, and are physiologically "old" not only do not respond to chemotherapy, but may also have significant side effects. Such patients should be given supportive care and not chemotherapy.

Progress, although slow, has been made in the use of chemotherapy in treating NSCC. Responders to chemotherapy live longer than nonresponders. Patients may derive some psychologic benefit from receiving chemotherapy. Since there is no standard chemotherapeutic regimen for NSCC, new regimens and new single agents are needed. Every effort should be made to enter eligible patients in investigative chemotherapeutic studies.

SMALL CELL CARCINOMA

SCC differs from NSCC in that it is a rapidly growing tumor, has a propensity for early metastatic dissemination, and is responsive to both chemotherapy and radiation therapy. Chemotherapy is the principal treatment modality because of early tumor dissemination.

During the past 15 years, a number of issues relating to the treatment of SCC have been addressed, but some remain unresolved. These issues include (1) choice of drugs, optimal drug number, intensity of the drug regimen, dose, and schedule of drug administration for induction therapy, (2) utilization of alternating non-cross-resistant combination chemotherapy, (3) value of late intensification chemotherapy and maintenance therapy, (4) role of radiation therapy, and (5) role of surgery.

Unlike the staging of NSCC, which uses the TNM classification, SCC uses a two-stage classification. This may soon change. With improvements in treatment and with definition of the role of surgery in SCC, a more precise tumor staging will be needed to plan therapy. Patients are now staged as having limited or extensive disease. Limited disease is defined as tumor confined to one hemithorax, including ipsilateral hilar and mediastinal lymph nodes. Some investigators include ipsilateral supraclavicular lymph node involvement and pleural effusion as limited disease; others do not. All patients with disease beyond the hemithorax have extensive disease (approximately two-thirds of patients at the time of diagnosis). The stage of disease has both prognostic and therapeutic implications. Complete response to therapy and increase in survival are much more likely to occur in patients with limited disease than with extensive disease.

Regardless of the stage of disease, systemic chemotherapy is the cornerstone of therapy of SCC. There are eight drugs that are active as single agents in the treatment of SCC: cyclophosphamide, Adriamycin, VP-16, vincristine, methotrexate, nitrogen mustard, hexamethylmelamine, and CCNU. Although objective response rates to these single agents are relatively good, complete response rates are under 5 percent, durations of response are brief (2 to 4 months), and there has been no significant improvement in survival rates.

With so many active chemotherapeutic agents, many different effective combination chemotherapeutic regimens have been employed in treating SCC. No regimen appears to be superior to another, although the more intensive chemotherapeutic regimens produce better overall response rates, median survival, and long-term survivors.

Three of the common induction chemotherapeutic regimens used are as follows:

CMC

Cyclophosphamide	1000 mg/m^2 IV day 1 and 22
MTX	15 mg/m^2 IV twice weekly
CCNU	100 mg/m^2 PO day 1

Repeat cycle every 6 weeks.

CAV

Cyclophosphamide	1000 mg/m^2 IV day 1
Adriamycin	50 mg/m^2 IV day 1
Vincristine	1.4 mg/m^2 IV day 1

Repeat cycle every 3 weeks.

CAVP-16

Cyclophosphamide	1000 mg/m^2
Adriamycin	45 mg/m^2 IV day 1
VP-16	50 mg/m^2 IV day 1–5

Repeat cycle every 3 weeks.

The concomitant use of radiotherapy with chemotherapy produces increased toxicity manifested by esophagitis and esophageal fibrosis, pneumonitis and pulmonary fibrosis, and pericarditis. Other potential late complications include acute leukemia and other malignant tumors.

In limited disease, over 50 percent of patients are expected to have a complete response; in extensive disease, over 25 percent are complete responders. In limited disease, the median survival is 12 to 18 months, with 10 to 20 percent of patients alive and free of disease at 2 years. In extensive disease, the median survival is 8 to 12 months, fewer than 5 percent of patients having relapse-free survival at 2 years.

Combination chemotherapy alone and combination chemotherapy plus radiation yield comparable complete response rates and median survival rates. In limited disease, chemotherapy plus radiation therapy may be more effective in increasing the percentage of long-term disease-free survivors. In addition, local control of the primary disease is improved in patients who have received radiation therapy.

Since SCC tends to involve the brain, prophylactic whole brain irradiation has been utilized to decrease the incidence of symptomatic CNS involvement. The use of prophylactic whole brain irradiation has reduced the CNS relapse rate from 20 percent to 6 percent; however, no survival benefit has been noted. Prophylactic whole brain irradiation is usually given to patients who achieve a complete response to chemotherapy.

In limited disease, there is renewed interest in surgical resection of the primary tumor following an initial response to chemotherapy. It is hypothesized that surgery removes tumor foci that may be resistant to chemotherapy and radiation therapy. Recent trials have demonstrated that in a small and highly select group of patients, surgical resection following response to chemotherapy is feasible and encouraging.

After the diagnosis of SCC is made, the first step is to determine whether the patient has limited or extensive disease. If the patient has limited disease, an outpatient induction regimen, preferably CAV or CAVP-16 should be given for at least 2 cycles after a complete response has been achieved (total, 6 to 8 cycles). Every attempt should be made to give full doses of chemotherapy despite low white blood cell and platelet counts. At the completion of the induction therapy, complete responders should receive radiation to the site of the primary tumor as well as prophylactic whole brain irradiation. At this point, consideration can be given to either stopping all therapy or utilizing maintenance chemotherapy.

Patients with limited disease who achieve only a partial response to the induction therapy, but still have a disease confined to the hemithorax, may benefit from chest irradiation. Prophylactic whole brain irradiation can be given at the same time despite the fact that the patient is only a partial responder. If the patient then achieves a complete response, maintenance chemotherapy with a non-cross-resistant regimen should be used. Patients with limited disease who fail to achieve a complete response following combined therapy usually have progression of their disease to distant sites and are candidates for investigational therapy.

Patients with extensive disease should be given induction therapy similar to that given to patients with limited disease. Patients who are considered "poor risk" because of poor performance status or have bone marrow involvement should have at least the first course of chemotherapy as inpatients. Complete responders should receive prophylactic whole brain irradiation and possibly radiation therapy to the primary tumor site when the induction therapy has been completed. Whether or not maintenance chemotherapy is needed in these patients is being evaluated by cooperative oncology group studies. Partial responders usually have rapid progression of their disease and, for the most part, have tumor that is resistant to further drug therapy.

Therapy of SCC has improved remarkably in the past 15 years; but only 5 to 10 percent of patients have long-term survival. Continued research is needed in both basic science and clinical areas in order to further advance our understanding and treatment of SCC.

CHEMOTHERAPY IN HEAD AND NECK CANCER

BARRY H. KAPLAN, M.D., Ph.D.
ROLAND T. SKEEL, M.D.

Cancers of the head and neck, excluding skin cancer, represent about 5 percent of all new cancer cases in the United States. In 1983, approximately 38,000 new cases were diagnosed and 12,850 patients died. This chapter will deal primarily with squamous cell cancer of the head and neck, by far the most common cancer in this region. Anaplastic carcinomas of the thyroid and carcinomas of the salivary glands will be mentioned briefly, but melanomas, lymphomas, and sarcomas are excluded from this discussion.

Squamous cancers may originate in the nasal sinuses (4%), nasopharynx (1%), oral cavity (55%), oropharynx (10%), larynx (25%), and hypopharynx (5%). The disease occurs predominantly in men (male:female > 3:1) over the age of forty with a history of smoking and alcohol use. The combination of the disfigurement and functional impairment associated with these cancers and the socioeconomic problems commonly found in this patient population have led to significant difficulties in evaluating therapy. It is only in the past few years that a systematic, multidisciplinary approach has been developed. It is hoped that this approach will yield new leads for managing these patients.

STAGING

Since treatment decisions and outcome are highly dependent on the extent of the primary tumor, local spread, and the presence of metastases, accurate staging is an essential part of the pretreatment assessment. Work-up includes at least panendoscopy with multiple biopsies, chest roentgenogram and CT scan. A bone scan is useful both to evaluate local invasion and to look for metastases. An esophogram can also be helpful in selected patients.

The American Joint Committee for Cancer Staging has devised a site-specific staging system for each of the primary regions and several subregions. As with other tumors, the T (tumor) stage is dependent on size and extension; the N (node) stage is based on the presence, number, size, and bilaterality of regional nodes; the M (metastases) stage indicates the presence or absence of distant metastases. Stage groupings for all sites are determined by the composite of tumor, node, and metastatic involvement shown in Table 1.

Unfortunately, the prognosis of a particular lesion depends on the site as well as the stage. An early lesion of the pyriform sinus or base of the tongue carries a much higher risk of relapse than a comparably staged lesion of the larynx. Similarly, even extensive nodal involvement in cancer of the nasopharynx can often be cleared with radiotherapy alone. There is no substitute for an experienced multidisciplinary team for evaluating these patients.

SELECTION OF TREATMENTS

In general, stage I and stage II cancers of the head and neck are treated with surgery and/or radiotherapy with cure rates in most sites greater than 50 percent. Even within these stages, however, there are patients who are good candidates for chemotherapy as part of their treatment. For example, patients with poor nutritional state at the time of diagnosis or who have other medical contraindications to immediate surgery may profit from 6 to 9 weeks of effective chemotherapy to allow for hyperalimentation and other supportive measures. Patients with stage I and II cancer of the pyriform sinus have such a high relapse rate that attempts to add chemotherapy to other modalities seem justified. In the future, it may well be that patients with early-stage cancer with significant relapse

TABLE 1 Stage Grouping for Carcinomas of the Head and Neck

Stage	*Groups*
I	T1 N0 M0
II	T2 N0 M0
III	T3 N0 M0
	Any T, N1 M0
IV	T4 Any N, Any M
	Any T, N2 or N3 Any M
	Any T, Any N, M1

rates benefit the most from adding chemotherapy to their management, but these patients are not commonly treated with chemotherapy at present.

Patients with stage III and IV disease without distant metastases are now usually treated with various combinations of surgery, radiotherapy, and chemotherapy. The value of chemotherapy in this group of patients will be discussed. Patients with metastases below the clavicle or recurrent disease following treatment with either radiation, surgery, or radiation and surgery are candidates for palliative chemotherapy.

CHEMOTHERAPY FOR RECURRENT OR METASTATIC DISEASE

Selection of Patients

Before recommending chemotherapy, the oncologist must be sure it is indicated. Two errors commonly occur. One mistake is to assume a mass or swelling represents recurrent cancer. Changes, especially edema, induced by radiotherapy, stitch granulomas, and intercurrent infections causing lymphadenopathy can mislead the treating physician. Biopsies or needle aspiration confirming the malignant nature of a suspicious mass should be carried out whenever possible. The other error is to assume a new mass is recurrent disease rather than a second, potentially curable primary. These patients, especially if they continue smoking, develop second primaries in the epithelium at risk (head and neck, lung, esophagus) at at the rate of 5 percent per year. A single coin lesion, for example, should be assumed to be a second, curable primary and should be resected.

Renal, cardiac, pulmonary, and bone marrow function are evaluated prior to therapy in order to guide the choice of drugs. Poor renal function with creatinine over 3.0 does not preclude the use of cis-platinum in moderate doses (e.g., 50 mg/m^2) as long as the patient can excrete a water load promptly. On the other hand, such a fluid load in a patient with congestive heart failure may be risky for that patient. By far the most dangerous drug used in these patients is methotrexate. Patients receiving this medication must be well hydrated, have creatinines less than 1.5, and have no third space fluid accumulations such as ascites, pleural effusions, or significant edema. Severe emphysema, common in this population of heavy smokers, should lead physicians to avoid bleomycin. Dosages must be reduced and patients carefully monitored for initial bone narrow suppression with a WBC less than 4000 or a platelet count less than 100,000. Even cis-platinum can cause significant myelosuppression.

Active Single Agents

Chemotherapeutic agents of established activity in squamous cancer of the head and neck include methotrexate, cis-platinum, bleomycin, 5-fluorouracil(5-FU), the vinca alkaloids, mitomycin, and mitoguazone. Weekly methotrexate at doses of 40 to 60 mg/m^2 has long been considered standard therapy, with response rates of 20 to 40 percent. There is no good evidence that higher doses of methotrexate with citrovorum rescue are better; in a controlled study by the Eastern Cooperative Oncology Group (ECOG), methotrexate at 260 mg/m^2 with rescue yielded a shorter response duration than standard methotrexate. High-dose methotrexate is also extremely dangerous in this debilitated patient population.

The response rate to treatment with cis-platinum as a single agent is comparable to the rate obtained with methotrexate. High-dose cis-platinum is no more effective than standard doses (50 mg/m^2). The vinca alkaloids and 5-FU appear to be more active when given as a continuous infusion over several days rather than as an intravenous bolus.

Combination Chemotherapy

The only combination of chemotherapeutic agents which has been shown in a prospective, randomized trial to have a higher overall and complete remission rate than methotrexate (M) alone is a regimen using methotrexate, bleomycin, and cis-platinum (MBD). In a study involving 163 patients, MBD produced responses in 48 percent compared to 35 percent for M alone, with 16 percent complete remissions versus 8 percent respectively. The difference is significant ($p = 0.04$) using a one-sided binary regression test. Ambulatory patients, those without fixed neck nodes, and those without distant metastases responded more often.

Unfortunately, median time to disease progression in this study among responders was only 5.8 months for MBD and 5 months for M, and median survival was identical at 5.6 months in each group. Poor performance status, distant metastases, history of heavy smoking, and adjacent organ invasion by the primary tumor were associated with shorter survival as were weight loss, the presence of tumor in the neck, and heavy alcohol consumption.

Either regimen can be given to patients safely in the office or clinic, although MBD requires a 2-hour intravenous hydration every 3 weeks. The toxicity is comparable except for the nausea and vomiting associated with cis-platinum administration. Lethal toxicity occurs in only about 3 percent of patients with either regimen and is usually associated with methotrexate-induced leukopenia and mucositis. Thus, since MBD more frequently provides effective palliative therapy, it is the treatment of choice except for those patients whose medical condition precludes the use of cis-platinum or who cannot tolerate the increased nausea and vomiting. For patients who do not wish to undergo any treatment toxicities when the duration of benefit is likely to be brief, symptomatic care may be most appropriate.

Another regimen, which has not been tested in a prospective, randomized trial, is now in common use in this country. The regimen was developed by Dr. Muhyi Al-Sarraf at Wayne State University and uses a combination of an IV bolus of 100 mg/m^2 cis-platinum and 4- or 5-day infusions of 5-FU at 1000 mg/m^2/day (DF). The initial report indicated a 27 percent complete remission rate and 70 percent overall response rate for DF, and an ECOG pilot study achieved about the same results. Median survival in these studies is 6 to 7 months. Toxicity with this treatment can be severe, especially in obese or cachectic patients or in patients over 65 years of age. The 5-FU dose should be reduced for these patients. The DF protocol requires extensive hospitalization, but is an option available for selected patients. The determination of whether DF or MBD provides the better palliative therapy remains for a clinical trial. The three regimens for the treatment of head and neck cancer (already discussed) are presented in Table 2.

CHEMOTHERAPY AS PART OF INITIAL MANAGEMENT

Resectable Cases

An enormous amount of excitement has been generated over the past several years because it has become apparent that patients who have not received prior radiotherapy have a very high response rate to chemotherapy. For example, two cycles of MBD given to previously untreated patients yielded a response rate of 80 percent. Even more interesting is a report of a response rate of 93 percent with 54 percent complete remissions, many documented at surgery, for patients treated with three cycles of DF using a 5-day infusion of 5-FU with cis-platinum.

There is no evidence that prior chemotherapy interferes with subsequent surgery and/or radiotherapy; indeed, many surgeons welcome the improved nutritional state and medical condition which several weeks of effective chemotherapy provide. The impression is that these patients become better surgical candidates with improved rates of healing. It is true, however, that about 25 percent of these patients refuse surgery following chemotherapy so that it is probably unwise to subject patients with a high surgical cure rate to preoperative chemotherapy except in highly selected cases.

The hypothesis that these high response rates to chemotherapy translate into improved survival for these patients remains to be proved. The one large controlled trial carried out thus far failed to show any benefit from the administration of one course of chemotherapy with bleomycin and cis-platinum prior to surgery and radiotherapy. Another randomized trial currently in progress uses three cycles of DF after surgery and before radiotherapy for half the patients; the control arm is surgery and radiotherapy alone.

Since the indications for combination chemotherapy in association with surgery or radiotherapy have not yet been clarified, selection of patients for multimodality therapy is made on a case-by-case basis. Most frequently, patients who require a period of hyperalimentation or other medical management receive several cycles of chemotherapy prior to definitive local therapy. Patients with a high probability of relapse and patients with bulky disease are also logical candidates for combined-modality approaches.

If preoperative chemotherapy is selected, it is critical that the lesions be mapped accurately endoscopically and tattooed or marked. Once the patient is given chemotherapy, it may be impossible to identify the original borders of the tumor. It is quite common to find small nests of viable tumor cells extending near to the original margin of the tumor even in patients who appear to have achieved a complete remission. Similarly, neither the surgical nor the radiotherapy treatment plan should be changed because the patient received chemotherapy.

Unresectable Cases

In general, these patients have been identified at the time of their initial staging as inoperable. Al-

TABLE 2 Regimens for Advanced Squamous Cell Carcinoma of the Head and Neck

Methotrexate (M)
  Methotrexate, 40 mg/m^2 IV bolus day 1. If no toxicity escalate to 60 mg/m^2 IV bolus day 8 and continue weekly.

MBD
  Methotrexate, 40 mg/m^2 IM days 1 and 15
  Bleomycin, 10 units IM days 1, 8, and 15
  Cis-platinum, 50 mg/m^2 IV day 4 with induced diuresis*
  Repeat cycle every 21 days
*Cis-platinum is given 30 minutes after starting a 2-hour intravenous infusion of 2 liters of 5% dextrose in half-normal saline with 10 mEq of KC1/liter. Furosemide, 40 mg, is given IV at the start of the infusion, and mannitol, 12.5 g, is given IV just before the administration of cis-platinum. The patient must void at least 200 cc or urine in the first 30 minutes of the infusion, or cis-platinum should be withheld and more intensive diuretic therapy administered until that rate of urine output is achieved.

DF
  Cis-platinum, 100 mg/m^2 IV day 1 with induced diuresis*
  5-FU, 1,000 mg/m^2 in 2000 ml 5% dextrose in half-normal saline to run over 24 hours daily × 4 or 5 days
  Repeat cycle every 21 days
*Forced diuresis using 2000 ml 5% dextrose in half-normal saline with 40 mEq KC1 24 hours prior to cis-platinum. Mannitol, 12.5 g IV bolus, immediately prior to cis-platinum and mannitol, 25 g in 1000 ml 5% dextrose in half-normal saline with 30 mEq KCl to run in over 4 hours after cis-platinum injection.

though preoperative treatment with chemotherapy can make these patients appear to become resectable, the results of surgery in controlling the disease is so poor that combined treatment with radiotherapy and chemotherapy is preferred to surgical intervention. Again, there are as yet no data that establish that combined modality therapy with chemotherapy improves survival in these patients.

There are two methods commonly used to combine chemotherapy and radiotherapy for this group of patients. One method is similar to the treatment for resectable patients; two or three cycles of MBD or DF are administered prior to starting radiotherapy. The disadvantages of this approach include potentially prolonged hospitalization prior to definitive therapy and patient refusal of definitive therapy. The other method for combining chemotherapy and radiotherapy is to give both treatments simultaneously, so that chemotherapy serves as a radiosensitizer for radiation therapy.

Experimental laboratory data have shown that cis-platinum enhances the effectiveness of radiotherapy. An ECOG pilot study in unresectable stage III and IV patients demonstrated that 20 mg/m^2 of cis-platinum can be given weekly concomitantly with intensive radiotherapy at 180 rads/day, 5 days/week, to 6800 to 7600 rads. At this dose, about 80 percent of these patients achieve a complete remission and 70 percent remain free of loco-regional disease for a median of 9 months. Only about 5 percent of patients suffer severe mucosal toxicity or myelotoxicity. Attempts to increase the dose of cis-platinum to 30 mg/m^2/week or to divide the dose of cis-platinum on a daily basis have met with unacceptable toxicity.

Cis-platinum is administered once a week on Tuesday, Wednesday, or Thursday immediately after radiotherapy during the entire radiotherapy course. Twenty-four hours before administration, a WBC, a platelet count, and a serum creatinine determination are obtained, and treatment is withheld for a WBC $<$ 2500, a platelet count $<$ 40,000, or a creatinine $>$ 1.5 mg/dl. A fluid intake of 2 to 3 liters is necessary for the 24-hour period prior to administration of cis-platinum. Patients receive cis-platinum within 2 hours following radiotherapy and should have urine output of at least 200 ml in the hour before cis-platinum administration. Thirty minutes prior to cis-platinum administration, an infusion of 5 percent dextrose in half-normal saline is started to run over a 2-hour period followed by a second liter also containing 10 mEq KCl to run over a 4-hour period. If the patient fails to void 200 cc in the hour prior to cis-platinum administration, mannitol, 12.5 g, is given IV push immediately before cis-platinum. The cis-platinum is given by slow IV push. Urine output is monitored for the next 3 hours, and Lasix, 20 mg by IV push, is given if the output falls below 200 ml/hour.

CANCER OF THE THYROID GLAND AND SALIVARY GLANDS

Only a modest number of reports deal with the chemotherapy of these tumors. One randomized study conducted by the ECOG compared Adriamycin alone to the combination of Adriamycin and cis-platinum in the treatment of patients with cancer of the thyroid. In order to be eligible, patients with differentiated carcinomas had to be refractory to radioiodine and to have progressed on suppressive hormone therapy. Eighty-four evaluable patients were entered in the study between 1976 and 1982. Although response rates on the two arms of this study, 17 percent for Adriamycin and 26 percent for Adriamycin and cis-platinum, were not significantly different, there were five complete remissions (four lasted over 2 years) for the combination treatment and none for Adriamycin alone. The addition of cis-platinum to Adriamycin appears to offer patients the only chance for long-term remission. Adriamycin was given at a dose of 60 mg/m^2 in this study, and cis-platinum at a dose of 40 mg/m^2, and both medications were repeated every 3 weeks. Anecdotal reports of responses of cancers of the salivary gland especially to Adriamycin and Adriamycin-containing regimens are in the literature, and the use of Adriamycin for palliative care can be recommended; much more information about the response of salivary gland tumors to chemotherapy will be needed before any firm conclusions can be developed.

THYROID CANCER

KATSUTARO SHIMAOKA, M.D.

Thyroid cancer is not a common malignant tumor. Based on data from the National Cancer Institute's surveillance, epidemiology, and end results program, the American Cancer Society predicted 10,300 new cases and 1100 cancer deaths from this malignant disease in 1984. The most important prognostic factor for thyroid cancer is histologic type. The international histologic classification of this tumor by WHO, published in 1974, is not too different from the previous American classification and has been adopted by the majority of pathologists and clinicians in most countries of the world (Table 1). Epithelial tumors, which are subclassified into five categories, are the most common malignant tumors of the thyroid and will be discussed in this chapter. The other tumors listed are rare, except for malignant lymphomas (these are mostly non-Hodgkin's lymphomas; Hodgkin's disease involving this gland is very rare), which

TABLE 1 Malignant Tumors of the Thyroid Gland

I. Epithelial tumors
   1. Follicular carcinoma
   2. Papillary carcinoma
   3. Squamous cell carcinoma
   4. Undifferentiated (anaplastic) carcinoma
      a. Spindle cell type
      b. Giant cell type
      c. Small cell type
   5. Medullary carcinoma

II. Nonepithelial tumors
   1. Fibrosarcoma
   2. Others

III. Miscellaneous tumors
   1. Carcinosarcoma
   2. Malignant hemangioendothelioma
   3. Malignant lymphoma
   4. Teratoma

IV. Secondary tumors

V. Unclassified tumors

should be evaluated and treated as malignant lymphomas.

In general, the disease tends to be more aggressive and more severe in patients over 45 years of age, even in the same histologic subclass. It is also rare for the younger age group to have undifferentiated and squamous cell carcinomas, which have a poor prognosis. Therefore, the therapeutic approach tends to be more aggressive in older patients.

The TNM system first included thyroid cancer in 1968 and was revised in 1977. However, neither the original nor the revision included the staging with consideration of histologic types and other variables because the system for thyroid cancer at that time was developed mainly for the purpose of data collection. In 1980, however, the American Joint Committee on Cancer revised the system and introduced staging. This is yet to be evaluated and examined on a larger scale. The new staging system appears to be somewhat complicated, partly because of the adoption of the original TNM system for thyroid cancer which conformed with that of the other head and neck tumors, the biologic behavior of which are vastly different from that of thyroid cancer.

PREFERRED APPROACH

The therapeutic approach to patients with thyroid cancer may differ considerably, depending on the histologic type of the tumor. Whenever feasible, the initial approach should be aimed at curative surgery.

Well-Differentiated Carcinoma

This category includes follicular carcinoma and papillary carcinoma. The latter may contain a varying degree of follicular component in its mixture. The biologic behavior of tumors with pure follicular component differs somewhat from that of papillary carcinoma with or without follicular component. The latter tends to spread via lymphatics, whereas the former spreads hematogenously. As a result, the initial presentation of the former may be a distant metastasis (e.g., pathologic fracture at the site of metastatic disease). The histologic features of the primary tumor may be difficult to distinguish from those of benign follicular adenoma; the microscopic evidence of capsular or vascular invasions may be the only diagnostic criterion for malignancy. Papillary carcinoma, on the other hand, spreads via regional lymphatics before producing distant metastases. The tumor is frequently associated with psammoma bodies, and the ground-glass appearance of the nuclei is diagnostic of this tumor.

Surgery. The surgical approach may differ from surgeon to surgeon. Conservative surgeons may choose to perform total lobectomy of the involved side and isthmusectomy for unilateral disease, whereas aggressive surgeons may choose to perform total or near-total thyroidectomy. The latter approach, if carried out by less experienced surgeons, may increase the rate of surgical complications. However, following this approach a thorough search could be made of the contralateral lobe for microscopic foci of multicentric disease and the patient can be adequately prepared for radioiodine therapy, if it is indicated.

If nodal disease is present at the time of initial surgery, some sort of modified neck dissection of the involved side is performed. A minority of surgeons may be satisfied with the removal of clinically evident nodal disease. The data from various institutions are in agreement that the presence of regional nodal disease, at least in younger patients, does not make the prognosis any worse. However, the data on older patients are not in complete agreement.

It has been well demonstrated that radiation therapy for benign conditions in the head and neck areas would result in an increased incidence in both benign and malignant thyroid diseases many years later. Thus, induced thyroid carcinomas are mostly differentiated carcinomas, except for the rare case of undifferentiated or squamous cell carcinoma. In approximately half the cases of differentiated carcinoma associated with previous radiation exposure, the condition was found to be minimal carcinoma (occult sclerosing carcinoma), which has an excellent prognosis with minimal treatment. Although there are some anecdotal episodes indicating that radiation-associated thyroid carcinoma may be more aggressive than non-radiation-associated thyroid carcinomas, treatment is the same for both.

Suppressive Therapy. Since the first observation by Dunhill of two young patients whose recurrent tumors completely regressed with thyroid therapy, suppressive therapy with thyroactive substances is widely utilized to treat thyroid cancer patients and to prevent recurrences. The basic principle is that the suppression of TSH secretion of the pituitary by saturating the nuclear receptors for thyroid hormones with the administration of exogenous thyroid hormones, will modify the biologic behavior of both benign and malignant thyroid lesions. This concept has been strengthened by the demonstration of cell membrane TSH receptors in the normal and diseased follicular cells of the thyroid. Two types of receptors—one low-affinity and the other high-affinity—have been demonstrated. The latter has been shown to be present in the follicular cells of the thyroid under normal and various disease conditions, as well as in the tumor cells of differentiated carcinoma. However, the high-affinity receptors are conspicuously lacking in the tumor cells of undifferentiated carcinoma. Any preparation containing thyroactive substances would be suitable for this purpose; liothyronine (T_3), levothyroxine (T_4), and desiccated thyroid are the most commonly utilized preparations. These drugs can be given by mouth; the only parenteral preparation available is T_4. We believe that the dosage of thyroactive substances should be individualized since there are wide differences in the individual requirement and tolerance. Once the diagnosis of thyroid carcinoma is confirmed, we gradually build up to the maximal tolerable dose. At this point we obtain a TRH stimulation test to confirm the refractoriness of TSH secretion by the pituitary to TRH. The most common side effects are the symptoms and signs of thyrotoxicosis, which occur if the dose should become excessive. The other side effects, such as skin rash, are very rare and can be handled by switching to other thyroactive preparations. Caution is advised in administering thyroactive substances to active cardiac patients; T_3 in particular appears to increase the frequency of angina attacks. Therefore, the administration of other preparations might be preferable in cardiac patients. The monitoring of suppressive therapy may be carried out by determinations of circulating thyroid hormones, but the normal laboratory values do not apply to patients receiving T_4 or T_3. Likewise, TSH determinations without TRH stimulation would be of little use, owing to limitation of the sensitivity of radioimmunoassay.

Prognostic Factors. As previously mentioned, minimal carcinoma, a single tumor less than 1 cm in diameter, has an excellent prognosis. Unlike the other malignant tumors, the presence or absence of regional lymph node involvement does not affect the prognosis, particularly in younger patients. The bad prognostic factors which have been recognized are primary tumor larger than 4 cm in diameter, multifocal carcinoma, gross findings of capsular or extraglandular invasion, and age over 45 years. Thyroid cancer is more common in females than in males, but the disease tends to be more aggressive in males than in females. Follicular carcinoma appeared to have a somewhat poorer prognosis than papillary carcinoma. Differentiated carcinoma in the pediatric group appears to present more aggressively, but the response to therapy is more favorable than in adults.

Radioiodine (^{131}I) Therapy. Many differentiated thyroid carcinomas retain the biologic characteristics of thyroid follicular cells; they are able to concentrate and organify radioiodine to synthesize and secrete thyroid hormones, although they are less efficient than the normal follicular cells. Therefore, in the lack of competition for radioiodine with normal thyroid tissue, thyroid cancer tissue can take up sufficient radioiodine to be irradiated internally. The obvious candidates for such treatment are differentiated carcinoma patients with known residual disease after surgery, with distant metastases, and with relapsed disease which may not be surgically resectable. In addition, some patients with multiple bad prognostic factors, as already mentioned, would be prepared for future radioiodine therapy at this institution. In many patients with differentiated carcinoma, the uptake of radioiodine by the tumor could not be demonstrated in the presence of residual normal thyroid tissue. The latter has to be removed surgically or has to be ablated by one or more thyroidectomy doses of radioiodine (50 to 100 mCi). It is not unusual to find a small amount of radioiodine concentration in normal thyroid tissue in the thyroid bed after total thyroidectomy was carried out by an experienced endocrine surgeon, and such remnants should be ablated before we can establish tumor uptake of radioiodine by the metastases. If surgery is contraindicated in the patients who initially had hemithyroidectomy, the ablation of the contralateral lobe could be achieved by radioiodine. However, the radioiodine administered in this kind of a situation would be incorporated into thyroid hormone, which would have a substantially longer biologic half-life in the body than inorganic radioiodine, thus increasing the radiation dose to the total body.

To prepare our patient for radioiodine ablation and/or therapy, we would withhold T_3 for 1 to 2 weeks prior to the date of radioiodine administration. If the patient is maintained on thyroactive substances other than T_3, suppressive therapy has to be withheld at least 4 weeks. In the event that radioiodine ablation is to follow total or near-total thyroidectomy, we would wait for 6 weeks without thyroid supplement. This measure is taken to ensure the development of hypothyroidism, which in turn provides the stimulation of the iodine-concentrating tissues by endogenous TSH. The patients receiving either ablative or therapeutic doses of radioiodine are isolated until the body burdens fall below 30 mCi (a federal requirement), at which time suppressive therapy with T_3 is resumed. Approximately 3 months after the ablation, a tracer study with 1 to 10 mCi of radioiodine is administered to the patient after withholding suppressive therapy for an adequate period. The whole body scan is done to establish the radioiodine uptake by the metastatic tumor and to localize clinically unrecognized tumor. When the presence of functioning tumor metastases is confirmed, a therapeutic dose of radioiodine, 150 to 200 mCi (sometimes higher), is given. If extrathyroidal tumor radioiodine uptake was not demonstrated, suppressive therapy is resumed and a tracer study is repeated at 3- to 6-month intervals. If the tumor uptake of radioiodine is established, the sequence of tracer study followed by therapeutic dose will be repeated, as long as the presence of persistent or new tumor uptake of radioiodine is demonstrated. The intervals for the therapeutic dose may vary from institution to institution; some may repeat the therapeutic dose at 3-month intervals whereas others may give only one therapeutic dose per year. Some tumors show evidence of tumor uptake of radioiodine even before the normal thyroid tissue is ablated, but in many instances the tumor uptake could only be shown after completion of the ablation. In some instances, it may take many months after the ablation to demonstrate tumor uptake of radioiodine. Therefore, not all patients with differentiated thyroid carcinoma can be treated with radioiodine; the reported series show that 50 to 80 percent of such patients would become treatable with radioiodine.

Various measures to enhance the radioiodine uptake by metastatic tumor, such as prolonged endogenous TSH stimulation, low iodine diet with or without diuretics, and the administration of exogenous bovine TSH, have not been shown to be effective. However, the administration of excess iodine should be avoided, since this may make the use of radioiodine completely ineffective. The often overlooked situations are CT scans with contrast and IVP. The contrast media involved in these studies can be excreted within a few weeks. On the other hand, the gallbladder dye usually persists as long as 6 months, and a single myelogram would make any radioiodine tracer study or treatment meaningless indefinitely. The therapeutic use of radioiodine may cause radiation sickness, radiation mumps, radiation reaction of the skin over the tissue where radioiodine was concentrated, cytopenia, and other acute effects. The development of leukemia was observed in 2 percent of the patients thus treated; we feel that this risk is reasonable. The chronic radiation changes may also appear in the organ where the metastatic tumor concentrated radioiodine (e.g., lungs).

External Radiation Therapy. The role of external radiation therapy in the management of differentiated thyroid cancer is considered to be of limited value. Limited residual disease or local recurrence with microscopic to small tumors are major indications. Treatment is delivered with megavoltage machines to cover the field, which includes all potential areas of tumor involvement. A dosage of 4000 to 5000 rads is delivered over a period of 4 to 5 weeks; then fields are reduced in size and area to cover the involved areas to deliver an additional 1000 to 1500 rads. Distant metastases also have been treated, with good palliative results.

Squamous Cell and Undifferentiated Carcinomas

The squamous metaplasia of a follicular epithelium in the thyroid has been observed in normal, nonneoplastic, and neoplastic pathologic conditions of the gland. Whether squamous carcinoma of the thyroid originates from such metaplasia or is transformed from differentiated carcinoma is still disputed. Squamous cell carcinoma of the thyroid can occur in a pure form or mixed with adenocarcinoma; the latter may be designated as adenoacanthoma. Approximately 50 such cases are reported in the world literature and probably constitute much less than 1 percent of all cases of thyroid malignant disease. On the other hand, undifferentiated carcinoma of the thyroid is seen in 15 to 20 percent of all cases of thyroid malignant disease in this country. Although the histologic findings are quite different, both conditions have similar clinical behavior and poor prognosis, the mean survival being less than 3 months from the time of diagnosis. Many pathologists and clinicians doubt whether there is a tumor with the subtype of small cell carcinoma, since many of the tumors with this diagnosis turn out to be non-Hodgkin's lymphoma on later pathologic and/or clinical review. The usual findings on light and electron microscopy make it extremely difficult to differentiate between these two conditions, but diagnosis is based on subsequent findings such as lymphoid cell markers, unusual radiosensitivity, or the disappearance of tumor after a single dose of chemotherapy such as vincristine.

By the time initial medical attention is sought, both squamous cell carcinoma and undifferentiated carcinomas of the thyroid are likely to be inoperable, and the surgical approach may be limited to obtaining a biopsy for histologic confirmation. However, if the tumor is found to be resectable, either partially or completely, the effort should be made. Because of the high probability of recurrence and relapse, surgical therapy should be followed by either external radiation and/or chemotherapy, even if complete resection of the tumor is confirmed surgically and pathologically.

Medullary Carcinoma of the Thyroid (MCT)

MCT originates from the parafollicular (C) cells of the thyroid, which belong to the APUD (Amine Precursor Uptake and Decarboxylase) system, and is characterized by the solid histologic pattern with amyloid in the stroma. The tumor has been shown to produce calcitonin and carcinoembryonic antigen (CEA) and other biologically active substances. MCT is also known to be associated with other endocrine tumors as multiple endocrine neoplasia (MEN), type II. This syndrome, may occur familially with autosomal dominance, and also sporadically. Clinically, the tumor is slow-growing, but regional lymph node and distant metastases are common and occur in early stages. The overall survival of patients with this tumor is between that of differentiated carcinoma and that of undifferentiated carcinoma. More recently, anaplastic variants of MCT, as well as MCT with papillary and/or follicular histologic variation, have been described. The significance of such pathologic findings should be investigated further by correlating histologic and clinical findings.

The surgical procedure of choice at our institution is total thyroidectomy and elective radical neck dissection. In some cases an exploration of the mediastinum with adequate node dissection may also be necessary.

We are not aware of any report demonstrating the presence of TSH receptors on the tumor cell membranes of MCT. Therefore, the use of thyroactive substances is aimed at the correction of thyroidal hypofunction, if present. There are, however, two case reports in the literature that indicate complete disappearance of metastases of MCT after suppressive therapy.

Since the parafollicular cells or the tumor cells of MCT have no ability to concentrate iodide and incorporate it into thyroid hormones, the therapeutic use of radioiodine in this tumor is not indicated. MCT is also only moderately radiosensitive; treatment with external radiation may prove to be beneficial in some cases.

CHEMOTHERAPY

Chemotherapy may be indicated in patients with inoperable differentiated carcinomas refractory to suppressive therapy and radioiodine therapy, differentiated carcinoma undergoing anaplastic transformation, and inoperable medullary and undifferentiated carcinomas. The number of patients requiring this modality of treatment is limited, and our experience at present is scanty in comparison to our experience with other more common malignant tumors. Some chemotherapeutic agents have been tried in sufficient numbers of patients as part of phase I trials or as case reports. We do not see much difference in response rate among various histologic types. Therefore, all histologic types are discussed as a group in this section. Doxorubicin is the only agent that has established its value as an antineoplastic agent for thyroid carcinoma. The results are summarized in Table 2, with the response rate varying from 31 percent to 45 percent. Bleomycin has also been tried in a sufficient number of patients with thyroid cancer and response rates in the earlier trials have been good (Table 3). However, subsequent experience has indicated that the responses are short-lived and that there is a high incidence of pulmonary and other toxicities. Several multiple-agent chemotherapy regimens have recently been evaluated in the treatment of this disease. Most combinations included doxorubicin as a constituent. No studies thus far have shown the superiority of combination chemotherapy over single agent chemotherapy with doxorubicin. Since most of these studies are single-arm studies run by single institutions, study design was such as to make comparison meaningless.

The Easter Cooperative Oncology Group has conducted a randomized trial to compare doxorubicin 60 mg/m^2 alone every 3 weeks and doxorubicin (60 mg/m^2) plus cisplatin (40 mg/m^2) every 3 weeks. This study was recently closed and analyzed: although there are no significant differences in the overall response rate, the difference in the quality of response was quite clear in favor of combination (Table 4). The combination arm also had significantly more severe GI and

TABLE 2 Doxorubican as Single Agent in Thyroid Cancer

Investigators	*No. Treated*	*CR*	*PR*	*Responders (%) (CR + PR)*
Bonadonna et al	11	2	3	45
Burgess Hill	53	0	17	32
O'Bryan et al	29	0	9	31
Shimaoka et al	19	1	6	38
Total	112	3	35	34

TABLE 3 Bleomycin as Single Agent in Thyroid Cancer

Investigators	*No. Treated*	*CR*	*PR*	*Responders (%) (CR + PR)*
Harada et al	29	2	7	31
Shimaoka et al	10	0	4	40
Total	39	2	11	33

TABLE 4 ECOG Study: Doxorubicin vs. Doxorubicin + Cisplatin (DDP)

	*Doxo.**			*Doxo. + DDP⁺*			*Combined*		
Cell Type	*No. Treated*	*CR/PR*	*%*	*No. Treated*	*CR/PR*	*%*	*No. Treated*	*CR/PR*	*%*
Differentiated	16	0/5	31	19	2/1	16	35	2/6	23
MCT	4	0/1	25	6	0/2	33	10	0/3	30
Undifferentiated	21	0/1	5	18	3/3	34	39	3/4	18
Total	41	0/7	17	43	5/6	26	84	5/13	21

* Doxorubicin, 60 mg/m^2

⁺ Doxorubicin, 60 mg/m^2; DDP 40 mg/m^2

TABLE 5 Combined Modalities

Investigator	*No. Treated*	*CR*	*PR*	*Responders % (CR + PR)*
Mimura at al* (all histologic types)	38	4	2	16%
Werner et al⁺ (undifferentiated)	19	3	Not stated	16%

* Doxorubicin 20 mg/m^2/d × 3, q 3 wks
RT to the neck, 200 rads/d to 4000–5000

⁺RT ≤3000 rads
5-FU, 500 mg IV twice per week
CTX, 200 mg/d IV for 3 wks
Bleo, 5 mg IM twice per week

Booster: the same for 1.5 wks, followed by 5 courses of 5-FU and CTX

hematologic toxicities. In this and other studies of thyroid cancer reported in the literature, side effects have been common to the agents studied, and no unusual or unique toxicities to thyroid cancer patients have been reported.

COMBINED MODALITY THERAPY

Earlier trials, called combined modality therapy, utilized chemotherapeutic agents as radiation sensitizers. As a result, it was not possible to obtain the full benefit of either radiation therapy or chemotherapy. More recently, such attempts are being made as shown in Table 5. Increased toxicities are likely to be anticipated, and more careful monitoring and observation of patients undergoing such therapy are obviously needed. Such an aggressive approach is probably necessary and desirable for some of the aggressive tumors.

CARCINOMA OF THE PROSTATE

DENNIS L. CITRIN, M.B., Ch.B., Ph.D.

Adenocarcinoma of the prostate gland is second only to lung cancer as the most common cancer affecting American males. Each year about 70,000 new cases are diagnosed, and approximately 24,000 patients die from the effects of the disease. Over half the patients with prostate cancer have established metastases at the time of initial presentation. A simplified staging system for the disease is shown in Table 1.

Prostate cancer spreads by direct extension and by lymphatic and hematogenous routes. Direct extension to seminal vesicles, bladder, and membranous urethra is common. Large pelvic masses are frequently encountered and are often associated with obstructive uropathy. Occasionally, tumor may obstruct the rectum by extrinsic compression, although direct invasion of the rectum is rare. The hypogastric and obturator lymph nodes are first involved by metastatic disease with late spread to external iliac, preaortic,

TABLE 1 Simplified Staging System for Prostate Cancer

Stage A	Clinically unsuspected; histologic diagnosis is made at time of surgery for benign prostate hyperplasia
Stage B	Cancer confined to prostate gland
Stage C	Extension of cancer through capsule into periprostatic tissues
Stage D1	Pelvic lymph node metastases
Stage D2	Metastatic disease beyond pelvic lymph nodes (e.g., bone or lung)

and ultimately para-aortic nodes. In about 5 to 8 percent of cases, massive retroperitoneal lymphadenopathy develops and may be associated with enlarged supraclavicular nodes. Approximately 90 percent of patients with advanced prostate cancer develop bony metastases, which characteristically involve the axial skeleton with predominantly osteoblastic lesions. As bone destruction (osteolysis) is less common than in other cancers that frequently metastasize to bone (e.g., breast, lung), pathologic fractures and hypercalcemia are rare.

In addition to the clinical stage of the disease, as determined by physical examination, several other factors of prognostic and therapeutic importance should be briefly mentioned.

The clinical stage of the disease is related to the histopathologic grade. Using the Gleason system of tumor differentiation, patients with well-differentiated tumors (Gleason scores 2 to 5) have a low incidence of positive pelvic lymph nodes, whereas those with high scores (Gleason 9 or 10) have an incidence of nodal metastases greater than 80 percent. The value of the Gleason count in terms of predicting pelvic node involvement is independent of serum acid phosphatase.

Mostofi has described a system for pathologic grading which emphasizes two factors, namely, the cellular architecture (degree of differentiation) of the tumor and the degree of anaplasia of individual tumor cells. Whichever system is used (Gleason or Mostofi), it seems clear that most well-differentiated (small or large glands) or moderately anaplastic tumors are associated with a good prognosis. In contrast, tumors that are undifferentiated (cells in solid sheets or columns and cords) or highly anaplastic have a high probability of early metastases and death.

Serum acid phosphatase elevation has been widely used as a marker for the presence of extra-prostatic disease. Although moderately useful, it lacks the high sensitivity of alpha fetoprotein (αFP) and βHCG in testicular tumors. Only 70 percent of patients with stage

D2 disease will have an elevated serum acid phosphatase. Measurement of bone marrow acid phosphatase is of little value.

Because of its low sensitivity and invasive nature, lymphangiography is not routinely recommended. CT scanning is preferred. Pelvic lymph node dissection is a low morbidity procedure that often demonstrates evidence of metastatic disease in lymph nodes that are not enlarged on CT scan. As a result, many surgeons advocate a limited pelvic lymph node dissection with frozen section examination of the nodes prior to performing a radical prostatectomy (to be discussed).

In a patient presenting with symptomatic prostate cancer, the diagnostic work-up should include a biopsy of the prostate gland, a routine serum chemistry to include serum acid phosphatase, a hematologic survey, a chest roentgenogram, an intravenous pyelogram, a pelvic ultrasound or CT scan to delineate enlarged pelvic lymph nodes, and a radioisotope bone scan. Following these studies, if there is no evidence of metastatic disease, consideration should be given to definitive treatment with curative intent. It should be stressed that, using the staging system suggested above, approximately 60 to 70 percent of all patients will be found to have metastatic disease and will not be candidates for curative therapy.

TREATMENT OF LOCO-REGIONAL DISEASE (STAGES A, B, AND C)

No treatment is recommended for patients with stage A disease when only a few chips of well-differentiated cancer are found. The prognosis for such patients is no different from that for age-matched patients without cancer. Many workers suggest that stage A disease with extensive microscopic involvement and/or poorly differentiated tumors should be given the same treatment as stage B disease.

The basic principle of treatment of patients with localized disease is to effectively extirpate all evidence of disease with minimal local morbidity. This can be achieved by using any one of a variety of techniques which include radical prostatectomy, interstitial irradiation combined with pelvic lymphadenectomy, or external irradiation to the prostate and pelvic lymph nodes. Each of these modalities will be briefly discussed. In all cases, surgical sampling of the pelvic lymph nodes is advised prior to definitive local therapy. Positive pelvic nodes (i.e., stage D1 disease) precludes radical prostatectomy (to be discussed).

Radical Prostatectomy

Radical prostatectomy is a technically demanding procedure. The principle is an *en bloc* removal of the prostate together with its capsule, the seminal vesicles, the vas deferens, and a cuff of bladder. Retropubic or perineal approaches can be utilized. (Surgical texts should be consulted for details.) Impotence occurs in almost all patients postoperatively. A significant number of patients (5%) develop urinary incontinence, which may require long-term use of a mechanical device (Texas catheter or penile clamp).

Radiation Therapy

Both external radiation and interstitial technique using ^{125}I and ^{198}Au have been employed in treatment. Interstitial irradiation is combined with surgical exploration and bilateral extraperitoneal lymph node dissection, whereas external radiation is generally delivered to the entire pelvic lymph node area in patients with stage C disease.

The optimal volume to be irradiated is not clearly defined. In stage B disease, interstitial radiation delivers very high doses (10,000 rads) to the prostate gland; for stage C disease, many recommend external radiation therapy delivering 5000 rads to the pelvic lymph nodes with a prostatic boost. Data from Stanford University would suggest, however, that radiation therapy following a negative lymph node dissection does not improve local control rate and increases the incidence of post-treatment lymphedema.

Complications of Radiation Treatment

During the course of radiation, most patients develop transient diarrhea, urinary frequency and dysuria, and tenesmus due to radiation effects on small bowel, bladder, and rectum. These symptoms can generally be controlled by Lomotil, high fluid intake, and antispasmodics for bladder spasms. More serious long-term problems include small bowel obstruction (5%), severe proctitis and stricture and lymphedema of the scrotum or lower extremities (20%), and erectile impotence which occurs in about 30 percent of patients and may be ischemic in origin. The incidence of small bowel obstruction can be reduced by employing an extraperitoneal approach to lymphadenectomy.

Choice of Local Therapy

Overall, the results of local therapy (surgical or radiation) for pathologically staged B and C disease are equivalent. Local control can be anticipated in about 90 percent of stage B and 80 percent of stage C patients. A 5-year disease-free survival rate of 80 percent (stage B) and 60 percent (stage C) can be anticipated. The addition of adjuvant hormonal therapy has not improved these figures. The choice of therapy depends to a great extent on local expertise and patterns of referral.

Treatment of Pelvic Lymph Node Metastases (Stage D1)

Despite effective local therapy, over 75 percent of patients with surgically documented pelvic lymph node involvement develop evidence of disseminated disease within 5 years. The median time to recurrence is about 30 months with an overall 5-year survival of about 50 percent. Neither radiation therapy (to full pelvic and paraortic nodes) nor hromonal therapy has yet made a significant impact on these figures. As a result, the treatment of stage D1 disease is not well defined. Many workers adopt an expectant policy, waiting until symptomatic metastases develop before initiating palliative hormonal therapy.

TREATMENT OF STAGE D2 (METASTATIC) DISEASE

At present the treatment of the patient with established metastatic disease (stage D2) is not curative. The major indication for treatment is the relief of symptoms, generally bone pain and such systemic symptoms as fatigue and weight loss.

The primary treatment modality employed in stage D2 disease is hormonal. The rationale for hormonal treatment is the observation that adult prostate epithelium (and prostate cancer) undergoes atrophy when the normal physiologic effect of androgens is reduced. This can be accomplished either by bilateral orchiectomy, exogenous hormones (generally estrogens), or antiandrogens.

Currently there are a large number of agents, some of which are still investigational, which can reduce the effect of androgens on prostate cancer (Table 2). The different mode of action of these compounds raises the possibility of combination therapy (e.g., orchiectomy and antiandrogen). Hypophysectomy and adrenalectomy are now rarely employed. Bilateral orchiectomy and diethylstilbestrol (DES) are most widely used. Orchiectomy reduces serum testosterone to castrate levels in approximately 90 percent of patients, although in rare instances significant serum levels of testosterone may be encountered even after technically adequate castration.

Approximately 75 percent of symptomatic patients respond following orchiectomy, with significant improvement in symptoms, return of acid phosphatase to normal, and at least partial response in bone scan. The median duration of response is approximately 18 to 24 months, although occasional excellent responses of many years' (5 to 10) duration are reported. Similar results can be obtained by the administration of DES in a dose of 3 mg per day. Studies of serial serum testosterone levels in patients receiving 1 mg per day have demonstrated that this dosage may not be effective in producing consistent suppression of testosterone secretion, whereas 5 mg per day produced a significant increase in deaths from cardiovascular causes.

TABLE 2 Hormone Treatment of Prostate Cancer

Inhibition of Gonadotropin Secretion	*Inhibition of Androgen Production*	*Inhibition of Androgen Action (Anti-androgens)*
LHRH Agonist	Orchiectomy	Cyproterone
Estrogens	Glucocorticoids	Flutamide
Progestins	Aminogluthethimide	

DES is currently considered the standard nonsurgical treatment for patients with symptomatic metastatic prostate cancer and is widely used in cases in which bilateral orchiectomy is unacceptable. The toxicity of DES in such patients is well documented, and includes nausea, vomiting, fluid retention, gynecomastia which can be reduced but not totally eliminated by prophylactic breast irradiation, and, most seriously, cardiovascular and thromboembolic disease, which may be fatal. An acceptable alternative to DES would be a drug that was equally effective but significantly less toxic.

There are two classes of compounds currently undergoing clinical trial which may satisfy these criteria. LHRH agonists are synthetic peptides which produce an initial rise in pituitary gonadatropin followed by a profound sustained decrease. This results in secondary testicular atrophy, with serum testosterone falling to castrate levels after 2 weeks. The major disadvantage of these compounds is the need for parenteral administration. Subcutaneous or intramuscular injection of a depot preparation may overcome this problem. Antiandrogens compete with endogenous androgen (5-dihydrotestosterone) and apparently prevent cellular uptake and binding to nuclear and cytosol receptors.

COMBINED MODALITY THERAPY

The combination of orchiectomy and DES is not widely advocated because of the experience of the Veterans Administration Cooperative Urology Research Group (VACURG), which observed increased mortality from cardiovascular disease in patients treated with DES in addition to orchiectomy. The VACURG studies did, however, show an apparent reduction in the number of deaths from prostate cancer in patients treated with both orchiectomy and estrogen (VACURG I) and in a group treated with high-dose estrogen (VACURG II). Critics of the VACURG studies have pointed out that the estrogen-treated patients had a 45 percent incidence of preexisting heart disease compared with only 21 percent in the placebo-treated group. A later VACURG report indicated that in patients with normal pretreatment electrocardiograms, there was no significant increase in cardiovascular complications associated with the administration of 5 mg DES, an observation confirmed by others.

As a result of these considerations, the combination of orchiectomy and additive hormones has been advocated by some workers. In general, however, concerns about unacceptable cardiovascular morbidity from estrogens have limited the use of combined modality therapy. Orchiectomy and estrogens are generally used sequentially, although responses to secondary estrogen therapy when the patient has relapsed following primary orchiectomy, and vice versa, are generally of short duration. As LHRH agonists and/or antiandrogens become more widely available, combined modality therapy producing total androgen blockade may prove to be more effective, although carefully randomized phase III studies will be required to prove that this approach is more effective than orchiectomy or DES alone.

TREATMENT OF PRIMARY HORMONE FAILURES

The prognosis for patients whose disease is no longer hormonally responsive is very poor; a majority of these patients die within 12 months. Reactivation of prostate cancer is not generally associated with secondary elevation of plasma testosterone levels. Response to secondary hormonal procedures (progestational agents, antiandrogens, adrenalectomy) are uncommon and rarely last more than a few months. Although experimental data to support this is sparse, it is thought that relapse or hormone resistance de novo is due to the presence of a clone of cells which lack steroid hormone receptors.

Systemic chemotherapy of hormone-resistant disease is currently investigational. A small number of drugs that have shown limited activity include cyclophosphamide, Adriamycin, and possibly 5-fluorouracil and cis-platinum. Combination chemotherapy has not yet shown any major advantage over single-agent therapy. Adriamycin is currently the most active cytotoxic agent against prostate cancer, producing responses in approximately 25 percent of patients. Because of cumulative cardiotoxicity, the drug can usually be employed for only 9 to 12 months.

Another promising new agent is estramustine phosphate, a conjugate of estradiol 17B and an alkylating agent (mechlorethamine). The precise mode of action of the drug is not clear. Toxicity is similar both quantitatively and qualitatively to that of low-dose DES. Estramustine has been reported to produce responses in 10 to 35 percent of patients with metastatic prostate cancer who no longer respond to conventional hormone treatment.

There are several preliminary reports of combination therapy with estramustine and cytotoxic drugs. The activity of both Adriamycin and estramustine as single agents in patients with hormone-resistant prostate cancer and the lack of overlapping major toxicity suggest that a combination of the two drugs may be valuable.

It should be emphasized that chemotherapy should be used with caution in patients with prostate cancer. Many patients are elderly and have cardiorespiratory disease. Additionally, there may be reduced renal function due to obstructive uropathy or bone marrow compromise secondary to bone metastases or prior radiation therapy. Despite these factors, when chemotherapy produces an objective response, survival is significantly prolonged. At present, many groups, including the National Prostate Cancer Project and Eastern Cooperative Oncology Group, are actively involved in phase II and III studies of chemotherapy.

MEDICAL COMPLICATIONS

Patients with prostate cancer may develop one or more medical complications and these must be properly recognized and actively treated (Table 3.)

Renal failure, generally of modest degree, but occasionally severe enough to require temporary dialysis, is common. The usual cause is obstructive uropathy often complicated by infection. A transurethral resection of prostate to reestablish proper drainage of the bladder is often all that is required, but on occasion, a ureteral stent or percutaneous nephrostomy may be life-saving in relieving obsruction while awaiting the anticipated response from orchiectomy or estrogen therapy. Rarely, acute renal failure may be precipitated by severe disseminated intravascular coagulation with microangiopathic hemolytic anemia. Hemodialysis and urgent hormonal treatment (orchiectomy or high-dose intravenous estrogen) are often effective in these seriously ill patients.

A number of hematologic abnormalities may be seen, the most common being anemia. A majority of patients with bone metastases (stage D2) are anemic, with a normochromic normocytic film and a hemoglobin level of about 10 g/dl. In patients with very extensive metastases (about 20% in our experience), a leukoerythroblastic picture with an occasional nucleated RBC and more primitive circulating WBCs is seen. On rare occasion, extensive bone marrow replacement by metastatic tumor may produce pancytopenia, but this is usually due to extensive radiation to bone and/or cytotoxic chemotherapy.

As bone metastases usually are not lytic in this disease, pathologic fractures (and hypercalcemia) are very uncommon in distinct contrast to their incidence in breast cancer. However, about 15 percent of patients develop evidence of spinal cord compression due to extradural tumor associated with extensive metastatic disease in vertebral bodies, without evidence of vertebral collapse. Radiation may be palliative.

Weight loss is a common problem in patients with metastatic prostate cancer, and hypoalbuminemia is

TABLE 3 Some Complications of Prostate Cancer

Renal failure
- Obstructive uropathy
- Disseminated intravascular coagulation

Hematologic complications
- Bone marrow failure
- Anemia
- Disseminated intravascular coagulation
- Venous thrombosis

Spinal cord compression

Cachexia

Lymphedema

Thromboembolic disease

Hypophosphatemic osteomalacia

common. Greater than 5 percent loss of body weight is a serious prognostic sign in this disease. Edema of the lower extremties is common and may be due to pelvic lymphatic obstruction from tumor or as a result of lymphatic damage from surgery, radiation, or a combination of both. Venous thrombosis is also common in this group of patients, many of whom are debilitated and bedridden, have pelvic vein obstruction by tumor, and/or preexisting cardiovascular disease. Estrogen therapy significantly increases the incidence of thromboembolic events in such patients, probably due to an effect on antithrombin III levels.

TESTICULAR CANCER

PATRICK J. LOEHRER Sr., M.D.
LAWRENCE H. EINHORN, M.D.

One of the most significant advances in medical oncology during the last decade has been the effectiveness of cisplatin-based combination chemotherapy for the treatment of metastatic germ cell neoplasms. Since current therapy can cure approximately 70 to 80 percent of patients with metastatic cancer, alternatives to the traditional surgical approach in early-stage disease have been proposed. This chapter will focus on the recent advances and current controversies in the treatment of early- and advanced-stage nonseminomatous germ cell tumors (NSGCT).

CLINICAL STAGE I TESTICULAR CANCER

When a patient presents with a testicular mass, exploration of the scrotal contents via an inguinal approach should be performed. Nearly half the patients with testicular cancer are initially misdiagnosed as epididymitis. In difficult cases, testicular ultrasound may be extremely useful and may even bring to light clinically nonpalpable testicular lesions in cases initially diagnosed as "primary extragonadal germ cell tumors".

Testicular biopsies or orchiectomy via a scrotal approach should never be performed as 90 percent of testicular tumors are malignant, and contamination of the tumor through the scrotum results in aberrant spread of tumor. In such cases, hemiscrotectomy is recommended, and when lymph nodes are palpable in this region, a superficial inguinal lymphadenectomy should be performed. In the absence of trauma or prior surgery, testicular cancer rarely spreads to the inguinal lymph node chains.

Histologically, testicular cancer may be separated into seminoma and NSGCT. The latter category includes the histologic subtypes of choriocarcinoma, embryonal carcinoma, immature and mature teratoma, and yolk sac carcinoma. Each cell type may occur alone or in combination with the other types. Serum markers such as the beta subunit human chorionic gonadotropin (beta HCG) and alpha fetoprotein (AFP) have been an important adjunct to the diagnosis and treatment of patients with testicular cancer. Any patient with a "pure seminoma" who demonstrates an elevated AFP or more than a minimal elevation of the beta HCG should be treated as a case of NSGCT.

Noninvasive staging should include serum markers (beta HCG, AFP), posterior-anterior and lateral chest roentgenograms, abdominal CT scan, and occasionally a lymphangiogram. If the chest roentgenogram is normal, whole lung tomograms or chest CT scans should be performed to rule out subclinical pulmonary metastases. Despite these noninvasive staging techniques, 20 to 35 percent of clinical stage I patients have metastatic involvement of the retroperitoneal lymph nodes discovered at retroperitoneal lymph node dissection (RPLND).

RPLND has remained an integral part of the diagnosis and treatment of early-stage testicular cancer. When performed, a RPLND should not be undertaken as a "staging" procedure, but rather as a curative operation. Indeed, 60 percent of patients with carcinoma found during a RPLND will be cured by surgery alone. In no other carcinoma with lymphatic involvement does surgery alone result in such high cure rates. The morbidity of a RPLND has been ejaculatory dysfunction. This has been ameliorated somewhat by the use of sympathomimetics (pseudoephedrine or desipramine) and unilateral lymph node dissections in patients without gross disease at time of RPLND. Following RPLND, abdominal recurrences are quite rare and early recurrences can be detected by physical examination, chest roentgenogram, and serum markers.

An alternative approach to clinical stage I testis cancer is careful observation alone, with more aggressive surgical or chemotherapeutic treatment reserved for patients with recurrent disease. One of the major arguments in favor of this approach is that approximately 70 to 80 percent of patients with clinical stage I testis cancer are truly pathologically negative and will not be benefited by a RPLND. Two institutions, Memorial Sloan Kettering Cancer Center and the Royal Marsden Hospital, are currently investigating the role of initial observation only in clinical stage I testis cancer. In the Memorial study, noninvasive staging includes history, physical examination, beta HCG and AFP, chest roentgenograms (posterior-anterior and lateral), ipsilateral pedal lymphangiogram, intravenous pyelogram, and CT scan of the abdomen and pelvis. Monthly follow-up for the first 2 years after orchiectomy consisted of physical examination, chest roentgenogram, serum markers, and abdominal plain films. A CT scan of the abdomen and pelvis was repeated every 3 months during the first 2 years and every 6 months during the third year of follow-up. When patients demonstrated a recurrence, treatment with cisplatin-based chemotherapy (VAB-VI) and/or surgery was undertaken. Of 45 patients followed in the foregoing fashion, 36 (80%) have remained continuously free of disease. Seven of the 9 patients who have relapsed developed recurrent disease within the abdomen (1 patient—IIA; 6 patients—IIB) and 2 patients had pulmonary metastases. One of the latter 2 patients subsequently died from progressive cancer. Royal Marsden has had a similar recurrence rate in over 50 patients, but a variety of treatment regimens were used for relapsing patients.

Prior to making broad recommendations regarding orchiectomy alone for clinical stage I testis cancer, caution must be exercised regarding this policy. In patients with stage I testicular cancer treated with a RPLND, relapses within the abdomen occur rarely (<1%). Thus physical examination, chest roentgenogram, and serum markers are sufficient to diagnose early recurrence. When patients are followed in this way, one should detect recurrent disease with either elevated markers or minimal pulmonary metastases. In this situation, a patient has virtually a 100 percent chance of being cured with cisplatin-based combination chemotherapy. In patients who relapse with a greater tumor burden (i.e., bulky abdominal disease and pulmonary metastases), chemotherapy cannot be expected to cure all patients. Although careful follow-up may be achieved in a protocol setting at institutions seeing large numbers of testis cancer patients, the practicing physician in the community who sees only an occasional patient with testicular cancer may not be as meticulous in follow-up. The lack of compulsive follow-up or inadequate support by radiologists who may infrequently read lymphangiograms and abdominal CT scans may also compromise results. Finally, although the morbidity of a RPLND can be avoided in a majority of patients by an observation-only arm, for the 20 to 30 percent of patients who are destined to have a recurrence, RPLND would have been a curative procedure in a majority of the cases with lymphatic involvement. For these relapsing patients, cisplatin-based combination chemotherapy cannot be considered a less morbid procedure than surgery.

Whether observation alone will ultimately replace the current recommendation of RPLND for clinical stage I testis cancer is uncertain. Physicians should be reminded of several important principles regarding this patient population. First, stage I testis cancer patients should be 100 percent curable when followed closely and subsequently treated appropriately when recurrence develops. Second, a RPLND should not be a "sampling" or a "staging" procedure. A limited procedure, however, can be performed in some (node-negative) cases and may decrease the morbidity. Finally, institutions investigating initial observation-only cases follow patients closely with chest roentgenograms, abdominal roentgenograms, serum markers, LAG, and abdominal CT scans. The proper frequency and sequencing of these noninvasive tests will ultimately need to be addressed, but casual follow-up is likely to result in delayed diagnoses. Patients who then present with more advanced disease are less likely to be cured.

STAGE II TESTICULAR CANCER

Stage II (or B) testis cancer is defined as cancer that has spread to the retroperitoneal lymph nodes. In patients with stage B_1 (microscopic involvement) or B_2 (disease noted on abdominal CT scan or ultrasound, but not palpable), RPLND alone can expect to cure approximately 40 to 60 percent of patients. Relapses generally occur within 1 to 2 years following RPLND and can be diagnosed by physical examination, chest roentgenogram, and/or serum markers, which should be obtained monthly during the first year and every other month during the second year. With this kind of follow-up, recurrences can be detected in the presence of minimal disease. When treated appropriately with cisplatin-based combination chemotherapy, in this setting virtually all patients will be cured.

Despite surgical cures in 90 percent of stage I patients and in 40 to 60 percent of stage II patients, the potential role for adjuvant chemotherapy has been questioned. Earlier adjuvant trials with non-platinum-containing regimens were not effective. Since platinum-based combination chemotherapy regimens have demonstrated marked effectiveness in metastatic disease, its extension to adjuvant therapy was logical. The intergroup testicular study is currently investigating the role of adjuvant therapy in stage II NSGCT. Preliminary data in 171 patients who were randomized to no further therapy versus two postoperative courses of cisplatin-based combination chemotherapy (PVB or VAB-VI) had demonstrated no recurrences in the adjuvant therapy group. In the patients who were randomized to close observation following RPLND in this study, an expected 40 percent of patients have developed recurrent disease. All of these patients who received cisplatin-based combination chemotherapy have attained complete remission and have remained free of disease. Until specific factors have been defined which will predict subgroups with a high risk for relapse, the implementation of adjuvant chemotherapy for all stage II disease would result in administration of combination chemotherapy in the majority of patients who were destined not to develop recurrence. Additionally, the long-term side effects of chemotherapy remain uncertain.

The decision whether or not to give adjuvant chemotherapy following RPLND may rest with patient compliance for continued follow-up, psychosocial reasons, or other undetermined risk factors which will be determined by the intergroup testicular study protocol. In patients in whom an incomplete resection is performed or who have elevated markers at the time of initiation of adjuvant chemotherapy, systemic treatment should be initiated (i.e., four courses of chemotherapy rather than two courses).

STAGE III DISEASE

One of the major achievements in medical oncology during the last decade has been the formulation of successful combination chemotherapy regimens for advanced-stage testicular cancer. Currently 70 to 80 percent of patients with stage III disease can expect to be cured with cisplatin-based combination chemotherapy. Prior to the utilization of cisplatin, various regimens frequently demonstrated responses, but only 10 to 25 percent of the patients maintained a durable complete remission. In 1974, cisplatin was added to one of the more successful two-drug combinations of the era, vinblastine and bleomycin (PVB). These three drugs demonstrated activity against testicular cancer, each having different mechanisms of action and different dose-limiting toxicities.

In the first 47 patients treated at Indiana University from August, 1974 to 1976 with PVB, 70 percent of patients achieved a complete remission with an additional 11 percent rendered free of disease with surgical excision of residual disease. With a minimal follow-up of 7 years, 57 percent of patients remained free of disease.

Granulocytopenia was a major toxicity with this initial PVB regimen, as 38 percent of the patients required hospitalization for granulocytopenic fever during therapy. Subsequent prospective randomized trials by Indiana University and the Southeastern Cancer Study Group have demonstrated that a lower dosage of vinblastine (0.3 mg/kg) afforded less myelosuppression without effect on survival. Additional data from the trial demonstrated that the addition of doxorubicin to the induction regimen or maintenance vinblastine therapy failed to improve results on the 12-week PVB regimen. This regimen included cisplatin, 20 mg/m^2, on days 1 through 5 and vinblastine, 0.3 mg/kg, on day 1, with both being repeated every 21 days for four courses. Additionally, bleomycin, 30 IU, was administered weekly for 12 weeks.

Although there is no role for "debulking surgery" as initial treatment in patients with advanced testicular cancer, excision of residual disease following chemotherapy is recommended. Approximately 10 to 15 percent of patients presenting with advanced disease can achieve a surgical complete remission following a partial remission induced by chemotherapy. In this setting histologic examination will reveal carcinoma (20%), fibrous or necrotic tumor (40%), or teratoma (40%). Although no further therapy is needed for the latter histologic findings, two postoperative courses of induction therapy are recommended for patients in whom residual carcinoma is resected.

Excision of teratoma is also believed to be an integral part of therapy as late relapses of testis cancer have been observed in patients with prior history of resected teratoma. This may suggest a possible dedifferentiation of benign tumor to a malignant neoplasm. Additionally, "benign" teratoma may grow locally and in some cases lead to death.

SALVAGE CHEMOTHERAPY

Unfortunately, for approximately 20 percent of patients who never achieve complete remission and for approximately 8 to 10 percent who relapse from complete remission, further PVB will not be curative. Etoposide (VP-16) has been demonstrated to have significant activity in testis cancer when used as a single agent. Nonetheless, single-agent etoposide is not curative. When etoposide (100 mg/m^2 on days 1 through 5) is combined with cisplatin (20 mg/m^2 on days 1 through 5), with or without bleomycin, in patients with refractory testicular cancer, approximately 30 to 35 percent will demonstrate durable complete remission which represents probable cure. Based on this high degree of activity in *refractory disease*, several cooperative groups are looking at etoposide as first-line therapy. As with vinblastine, the major dose-related toxicity of etoposide is myelosuppression. Unlike vinblastine, however, etoposide does not cause neuromuscular dysfunction, which can be debilitating in some patients receiving vinblastine. Other side effects associated with the etoposide include some mild nausea and vomiting, and rarely hypotension and anaphylactoid reactions.

IS THERE A DOSE RESPONSE RELATIONSHIP?

Although various institutions have recommended differing dosage schedules of cisplatin regimens, the optimal dosage of cisplatin has not been defined. Based on suspicion that attenuated dosages of cisplatin may adversely affect the response rate, the Southwest Oncology Group demonstrated a significantly superior response rate for high-dose cisplatin (120 mg/m^2) over lower-dose therapy (15 mg/m^2 on days 1 through 5) given concomitantly with vinblastine and bleomycin. A further extension of this concept has recently been reported by Ozols at the National Cancer Institute, where very high doses of cisplatin (40 mg/m^2 on days 1 through 5) were administered to patients with a poor prognosis along with hypertonic saline as well as vinblastine, etoposide, and bleomycin. This regimen was tolerated without significant nephrotoxicity. Whether this very high dosage of cisplatin will prove to be superior to conventional dosages (100 to 120 mg/m^2) remains to be determined by randomized trials.

TOXICITY OF CHEMOTHERAPY

Although nephrotoxicity is believed to be the dose-limiting toxicity for cisplatin, this is generally an uncommon clinical problem when strict adherence to pretreatment hydration is maintained. Current evidence suggests that hydration with normal saline, ensuring an adequate chloruresis, is important to minimize the nephrotoxicity. Unless clinically indicated, one should also avoid other nephrotoxic agents, such as aminoglycosides, during cisplatin therapy because apparent synergistic nephrotoxicity has been reported.

Gastrointestinal side effects (nausea and vomiting) have remained a significant problem, but have been ameliorated by the use of various antiemetic regimens including phenothiazines, cannabinoids, corticosteroids, and metoclopramide. Hypomagnesemia is common, but symptomatic neuromuscular toxicity is an infrequent finding. Supplemental treatment with parenteral magnesium can rapidly reduce the signs and symptoms of hypomagnesemia. Prophylactic administration of magnesium has not proved to be beneficial. When administered for prolonged periods, cisplatin therapy may be associated with neuropathies which may be dose-limiting.

Bleomycin is well known to cause pulmonary fibrosis as its dose-limiting toxicity. This toxicity is totally dose-related and occurs at an increased incidence in patients who have had prior radiation therapy. When careful attention is given to the physical findings of early toxicity (inspiratory rales or respiratory lag), symptomatic toxicity can usually be avoided. Pulmonary function tests and chest roentgenograms may be useful adjuncts, but should not replace careful physical examination. When any signs or symptoms of pulmonary toxicity develop, bleomycin should be discontinued. Other side effects of the drug include fevers and chills on the day of administration, and subacutely, stomatitis, weight loss, alopecia, and cutaneous striae may occur.

As mentioned previously, the major toxicity of vinblastine is myelosuppression. Additionally, myalgias, which at times may be quite severe, occur in approximately half of all treated patients. Bowel dysfunction leading to constipation and, rarely, ileus may also occur.

Raynaud's phenomenon, an interesting side effect, occurs in 30 or 40 percent of the patients treated with vinblastine and bleomycin. There are some suggestions that treatment with calcium channel blocking agents (e.g., nifedipine) may decrease these symptoms, which may be chronic in nature.

As testicular cancer generally occurs during reproductive years, the question of sterility is important to many patients. All patients who receive PVB become azospermic immediately following therapy. When followed for 3 or more years, however, approximately one-half of these patients have a return of normal spermatogenesis (normal concentrations and morphologic appearance of sperm). No obvious teratogenic effects have been noted in the offspring of treated patients.

SEMINOMAS

In contrast to nonseminomatous testicular cancer, early-stage seminoma can be treated with radiation therapy in lieu of a RPLND with an approximately 85 to 95 percent cure rate. Any seminoma having nonseminomatous elements or associated with an elevated AFP should be treated as a NSGCT. Although low levels of beta HCG may be observed in some patients with pure seminoma, levels above 100 mIU/ml generally represent the presence of undetected NSGCT, and patients should be treated accordingly.

In patients with bulky abdominal disease (stage IIB), some controversy exists regarding the most appropriate treatment regimen. Approximately 60 percent are cured by treatment with abdominal radiation therapy alone. Prophylactic mediastinal irradiation not only does not improve this cure rate, but significantly impairs the ability to give full dosage combination chemotherapy as salvage in cases of recurrence. In smaller numbers of patients, PVB appears to be equally as effective as radiation therapy in stage IIB disease, but a randomized trial comparing these treatments has not yet been performed. As long as prophylactic mediastinal irradiation is avoided, radiation therapy is probably still the preferred initial treatment as it has less morbidity than chemotherapy.

In patients with stage III (nodal disease above the diaphragm) or stage IV (distant disease including bone, lung, or liver), the 5-year survival rates with radiation therapy are 32 percent and 0 percent, respectively. Although chemotherapeutic trials in seminoma have been sparse, experience with PVB has demonstrated a similar if not better response rate than that seen with NSGCT. Although many patients with bulky abdominal disease do not have a normal abdominal CT scan following chemotherapy, resection of residual disease, in contrast to NSGCT, does not appear to be necessary because in nearly all cases necrosis or fibrotic tissue is found in resected specimens. As in NSGCT, follow-up should include monthly history and physical examination, chest roentgenogram *and serum markers* during the first year of follow-up and every other month during the second year. Particularly in patients who have received prior radiation therapy and are being treated with PVB, chemotherapy should be administered every 21 days despite the expected myelosuppression associated with therapy. In general, aggressive supportive care may be necessary in these patients receiving chemotherapy; however, less aggressive dosages and longer intervals between courses may lead to the development of resistant disease.

RENAL COMPLICATIONS OF CANCER

MARC B. GARNICK, M.D.
RICHARD E. RIESELBACH, M.D.

The renal complications of cancer cover a broad spectrum and may present as any of the ten basic syndromes in nephrology. Some of the clinical settings relating to cancer which result in each syndrome are noted in Table 1. Neoplastic processes may damage the kidney via immunologically mediated disease, tumor products, or tumor metabolites. Also, cancer may impair renal function by direct invasion of the kidney or by obstruction of urine flow. Finally, antineoplastic and associated therapy may produce substantial nephrotoxicity. Because acute renal failure (ARF) may represent a particularly catastrophic complication and occurs with alarming frequency in the cancer patient, in this chapter we will devote our attention to the prevention and management of this complication.

TABLE 1 Renal Complications of Cancer as Manifested by Ten Basic Syndromes in Nephrology

Syndrome	*Clinical Setting*
1. Acute nephritis	Glomerulopathies associated with carcinoma, lymphoma, leukemia, and dysproteinemic states
2. Nephrotic syndrome	Glomerulopathies (see #1); EN*
3. Asymptomatic urinary abnormalities	Glomerulopathies (see #1), tubular defects from tumor products and metabolites; primary renal and ureteral cancer; infiltrative and metastatic disease of kidney
4. Acute renal failure (ARF)	Prerenal AFR (volume or renal vascular disturbances); intrinsic ARF (glomerular, tubular, interstitial or vascular abnormalities); postrenal ARF (urethral, bladder neck or ureteral obstruction); (see Table 2)
5. Chronic renal failure	EN*; glomerulopathies (see #1); dysproteinemic states; hypercalcemia; cancer-related nephrolithiasis
6. Urinary tract infection	Cancer therapy-induced immune deficiency; obstruction; acute and chronic renal failure
7. Urinary tract obstruction	Primary renal and ureteral cancer; extrarenal cancer and lymphoma; cancer-related nephrolithiasis; intrarenal obstruction (uric acid, myeloma)
8. Renal tubular defects	Induced by tumor products (SIADH, ectopic hormones), acute leukemia (lysozymuria), hypercalcemia and amyloid
9. Hypertension	Renal artery compression by tumor; renal tumor infiltration; hypercalcemia
10. Nephrolithiasis	Cancer-related hypercalcemia and hyperuricemia

* EN = Exogenous nephrotoxicity due to cancer therapy.

In one large epidemiologic study, cancer was the underlying basic disease in 20 percent of all patients with ARF. ARF represents a major complication in the course of any patient, but especially in the presence of cancer. Approximately 60 percent of all patients with ARF require dialysis. If not properly controlled, uremia, with its infections and its hemorrhagic and metabolic complications, imposes a particularly difficult burden on the patient with cancer. Furthermore, the pharmacokinetics of cancer chemotherapeutic agents may be altered when the renal function is reduced. Because of the nature and number of potentially nephrotoxic agents employed both diagnostically and therapeutically for cancer, these patients are particularly susceptible to the development of ARF. Infiltrative, obstructive, and metabolic aspects of the primary cancer itself may lead to a reduction in renal function, thereby increasing vulnerability to further renal damage from potentially nephrotoxic agents. Also, cancer patients frequently undergo major surgery, with the attendant risk of intraoperative and postoperative hemodynamic instability which may lead to ischemic ARF. Finally, intrarenal hemodynamic disturbances may occur in association with severe hepatic parenchymal involvement or biliary tract obstruction due to cancer, thus leading to another type of ARF.

Although the onset of ARF is a particularly dreaded complication in the cancer patient, the potential for substantial recovery of renal function and our ability to replace renal function until such recovery occurs should allow morbidity and mortality to approximate that of the underlying disease, as is the case with patients who do not have cancer. Thus, in caring for the cancer patient, one is obligated to consider ARF as a manageable complication which should be addressed with vigor, if this approach is appropriate on the basis of the associated disease.

Table 2 lists some of the various etiologies of ARF which may be associated with cancer. First, we will discuss some general measures to prevent ARF, as well as to prevent or modify its course in the cancer patient. Then, we will discuss in some detail specific aspects of the prevention and management of ARF caused by cancer therapy.

GENERAL MEASURES TO PREVENT ACUTE RENAL FAILURE

An awareness of the precipitating factors of ARF in the cancer patiant is an important consideration in its prevention. The potential of increased immunoglobulin levels, hypercalcemia, or hyperuricemia for causing ARF should be remembered. Appropriate precautions must be instituted in employing cancer chemotherapy with potentially nephrotoxic agents or radiation therapy, as will be discussed subsequently in more detail. Early detection of the signs and symp-

Supported in part by PHS MO1 RROO-750-06 and Southeastern Cancer Study Group εCA19657.

TABLE 2 Etiology of Acute Renal Failure Associated with Cancer

I. Prerenal ARF	Hypovolemia Peripheral vasodilation Impaired cardiac function Bilateral extrarenal vascular occlusion Functional disorders of intrarenal circulation	
II. Intrinsic ARF	Glomerular abnormalities	Acute glomerulopathies
	Tubular abnormalities	Ischemic acute tubular necrosis Exogenous nephrotoxins Cancer chemotherapy Antimicrobials Radiocontrast media Anesthetic agents Endogenous nephrotoxins Myoglobin Hemoglobin Immunoglobulins Calcium and phosphorus Uric acid
	Interstitial abnormalities	Drug-induced acute tubulointerstitial nephritis (ATIN) Acute pyelonephritis Tumor infiltration Radiation nephropathy
	Abnormalities of intrarenal blood vessels	Acute bilateral renal cortical necrosis Malignant hypertension Vasculitis
III. Postrenal ARF	Urethral obstruction	
	Bladder neck obstruction	Prostatic or bladder cancer Functional; neuropathy or drugs
	Bilatral obstruction of ureters (or unilateral obstruction of single kidney)	Intraureteral Uric acid crystals Blood clots Stones Extraureteral Cancer: prostate/cervix Periureteral fibrosis Accidental ureteral ligation during pelvic surgery

toms of urinary tract obstruction may result in prompt resolution of postrenal ARF by appropriate measures, thus avoiding the complications of prolonged obstruction.

Cancer patients tend to have depleted extracellular fluid (ECF) volume as a result of (1) inadequate dietary intake, (2) gastrointestinal losses, (3) the diuretic effect of hypercalcemia or cholemia, (4) hypoalbuminemia, or (5) "third-spacing" due to malignant effusions. These contribute to the increased risk of ARF in the cancer patient. ECF volume depletion particularly increases the risk of ARF in cancer patients undergoing surgery or diagnostic procedures utilizing radiocontrast media, especially in the presence of pre-existing renal insufficiency, diabetic vascular disease, severe atherosclerotic disease, or old age.

When preparing a high-risk patient for surgery, preoperative expansion of ECF volume and maintenance of a solute diuresis with mannitol may be of value in preventing ARF. A suggested protocol is to initiate an infusion of 25 g mannitol in one liter of isotonic saline (or in 1 liter of 5 percent dextrose in water with supplemental bicarbonate if the patient is acidotic) one hour before surgery, to be administered continuously throughout the procedure at a rate of 150 ml/hour. In the case of a prolonged procedure, fluid and electrolyte losses in the urine should be replaced. Patients with substantial urinary excretion of uric acid or light chains require a vigorous regiment of saline hydration and alkalinization. ECF volume contraction is a particularly significant risk factor for aminoglycoside nephrotoxicity. Thus, ECF volume should be optimized prior to initiating therapy with these agents. Dosage of potentially nephrotoxic drugs must be modified according to renal function. Particular care must be exercised in the elderly or debilitated patients, in whom reductions in renal function are not accurately represented by the serum creatinine concentration because of their decreased muscle mass.

The course of ARF may be reversed effectively in many patients who have a prerenal or postrenal etiology, with resultant rapid return to normal renal function. In prerenal ARF, reversal may be accomplished by improving renal perfusion by expansion of ECF volume. Postrenal failure is resolved frequently through the correction of urinary obstruction once the diagnosis has been established.

ENDOGENOUS NEPHROTOXICITY ASSOCIATED WITH CANCER THERAPY

Treatment of cancer may result in the rapid generation of endogenous nephrotoxins such as uric acid, xanthine, and phosphorus. These possibilities are of particular concern in patients with rapdily growing tumors which are extremely sensitive to cytolytic therapy. As a consequence of massive cytolysis, intracellular products of malignant cells are released into the circulation and may produce hyperkalemia, hyperuricemia, hyperxanthinemia, and hyperphosphatemia with associated hypocalcemia. The magnitude of these biochemical alterations is related to tumor burden and is greatly magnified by prior renal dysfunction, since renal excretion is necessary for modulation of phosphate, potassium, uric acid, and xanthine concentrations. The foregoing metabolic aberrations have been described as part of the "acute tumor lysis syndrome", which has been observed in patients with acute leukemia and malignant lymphoma undergoing intensive cytoreductive therapy. Metabolic abnormalities are particularly severe in patients with Burkitt's lymphoma as a consequence of the rapid tumor cell proliferation and lysis following chemotherapy in this setting. Renal failure occurs owing to the intrarenal precipitation of uric acid, xanthine, or calcium phosphate, or a combination of these. Alkalinization of the urine in order to enhance uric acid and xanthine solubility may promote precipitation of calcium phosphate. Furthermore, therapy with allopurinol in order to decrease urinary acid excretion may increase the possibility of xanthine nephropathy owing to inhibition of xanthine oxidase, thereby increasing the formation of that purine metabolite.

When there is a potential for the acute tumor lysis syndrome, special precautions must be initiated in order to avert potentially fatal levels of hyperkalemia. The early management of these patients, particularly those with Burkitt's lymphoma, may constitute a medical emergency. Initial management is directed toward controlling pre-existing hyperuricemia with hydration, allopurinol, and alkalinization and thus maintaining a reasonable level of renal function to facilitate renal excretion of tumor breakdown products. For those patients without severe metabolic aberrations, chemotherapy usually can be initiated within 24 to 48 hours following initiation of the foregoing regimen. Thereafter, hydration is continued, whereas alkalinization is discontinued to avoid potential calcium phosphate precipitation within the kidneys. In patients with severe metabolic aberrations, diuresis, alkalinization, and allopurinol administration are pursued vigorously. Blood chemistries are monitored frequently, and therapy is not instituted until the urinary uric acid-to-creatinine ratio is less than 1.0.

When the foregoing management is not successful in preventing acute renal failure, hemodialysis is necessary. These metabolic abnormalities are rapidly responsive to hemodialysis, particularly if dialysis is carried out on a daily basis, thereby allowing cytolytic therapy to proceed without delay. The duration of metabolic aberration in patients with the acute tumor lysis syndrome is usually limited to 5 to 7 days because of the finite period of cytolysis.

EXOGENOUS NEPHROTOXINS

The kidney is highly susceptible to toxic injury from a number of currently utilized cancer chemotherapeutic agents, as well as from radiation therapy. Also, toxicity from cancer chemotherapy may be additive or synergistic with radiation therapy. Pretreatment renal insufficiency on the basis of the many renal complications of cancer (see Tables 1 and 2) may increase vulnerability to nephrotoxicity of these agents.

Cisplatin

Cis-diamminedichloroplatinum(II) (cisplatin) is a recently introduced agent with a broad spectrum of antineoplastic activity. Its role in the treatment of genitourinary cancer has been well established; it has also become an important component of many treatment programs in the management of other cancers. When cisplatin was initially introduced, nephrotoxicity seemed to be the dose-limiting side effect, although hematologic, gastrointestinal, and otic toxicity are significant problems with this agent. The incidence of renal damage in patients receiving the drug was 50 to 100 percent, regardless of the dose or schedule of administration. Renal biopsies revealed acute tubular necrosis, tubular degeneration, and interstitial edema; fatal acute renal failure occurred in some patients. From these early studies, it was concluded that renal toxicity was cumulative and appeared to be most profound 3 weeks after drug administration. Recently introduced measures to diminish cisplatin nephrotoxicity have allowed increased utilization of this effective agent. The incidence and severity of nephrotoxicity have been substantially reduced by utilizing hydration and diuretics with large amounts of parenteral fluid in conjunction with administration of the drug. Also, administering the drug as a continuous infusion has been helpful. Although the foregoing measures have all contributed to a lower incidence of nephrotoxicity, the optimal drug schedule and method of administration remain to be defined. Extensive studies have indicated that the same cumulative dosage of cisplatin can be given either as a bolus in one day, daily for 5 days, or continuously for 24 to 120 hours. One schedule is not superior to another in preventing nephrotoxicity, provided hydration status is closely monitored and urinary output is maintained. Recent studies indicate that high doses of cisplatin can be given with hypertonic saline solution with an acceptable risk of renal damage.

Hypomagnesemia is a prominent nephrotoxic effect of cisplatin therapy. We have found that hypomagnesemia develops in approximately 50 percent of patients receiving cisplatin; it occurs one to two weeks following drug administration. This complication is readily managed with administration of oral magnesium chloride solution (1 mEq/ml of magnesium) and usually does not rquire parenteral $MgSO_4$ administration. This tubular effect usually spontaneously remits over a period of weeks if cisplatin therapy is not instituted, although on occasion it may be longer-lasting.

Methotrexate

Although there is some controversy regarding the ultimate role of high-dose methotrexate followed by citrovorum factor "rescue" in the management of cancer, it has been used (1) as an adjuvant treatment for patients with osteosarcoma, (2) in the treatment of patients with penile cancer, non-Hodgkin's lymphoma of unfavorable histologies, head and neck cancer, and bladder cancer, and (3) in the management of selected patients with breast cancer. The cytotoxic activity of this analog of folic acid occurs as a consequence of tight binding to dihydrofolate reductase with subsequent inhibition and depletion of intracellular reduced folate pools.

MTX is excreted primarily by the kidneys. Any reduction in renal function, therefore, serves to increase plasma MTX level via a decrease in renal MTX clearance. MTX renal toxicity occurs with increasing frequency as its dose is increased from low levels (5 to 15 mg/m^2) to "high-dose" protocols (1 to 15 g/m^2); the latter require leucovorin rescue. Renal failure has been implicated in 10 percent of the deaths associated with high-dose MTX administration. Although the exact pathogenesis of MTX-induced renal failure has not been clearly defined, at least three hypotheses have been suggested as the basis for this lesion. The first and most widely accepted is that MTX or an MTX metabolite precipitates within the distal nephron, causing an obstructive nephropathy. The second is that MTX has a direct toxic effect on renal tubular cells. A third is that MTX directly affects the afferent arteriole, resulting in a decrease in GFR via glomerular hypoperfusion. The Dana-Farber Cancer Institute has extensive experience in utilizing high-dose methotrexate therapy. Moderate or severe nephrotoxicity has developed in only 7 percent of patients. The regimen currently employed is as follows:

1. After a baseline GFR and serum creatinine are obtained, patients are vigorously hydrated with 5 percent dextrose and water containing supplemental sodium bicarbonate in order to obtain a urinary pH greater than 7.0. Diamox may be added if necessary. Hydration generally begins 12 to 14 hours before MTX administration and continues for at least 2 to 3 days thereafter.
2. Twenty-four hours after MTX infusion, a repeat serum creatinine is obtained. A value of 50 percent or more above the baseline level is usually indicative of nephrotoxicity. If this occurs, leucovorin administration is continued until the methotrexate level falls below 7.5×10^{-8}M. Hydration and alkalinization should be maintained during this period.
3. If a greater degree of renal insufficiency supervenes, and the patient is not oliguric (as is usually the case), the foregoing hydration regimen is maintained and the dosage of leucovorin is increased tenfold from 15 to 150 mg IV every 3 hours. These supportive measures are continued until the serum methotrexate level is less than 10^{-7}M and the serum creatinine concentration has returned to the normal range. Recovery may require as long as 30 to 60 days.

Streptozotocin

Streptozotocin (streptozocin) is a nitrosourea antibiotic derived from the fermentation broth of *Streptomyces acromogenes*. The drug also has been chemically synthesized. It has a well-established role in the management of patients with metastatic islet cell carcinoma of the pancreas and carcinoid tumors. Additionally, clinical activity has been reported in Hodgkin's and non-Hodgkin's lymphoma, and it is being increasingly used in combination with other drugs for treatment of advanced colorectal cancer. Nephrotoxicity is the principal side effect which limits the usefulness of this drug. Acute renal failure, with a fatality rate of 5 percent, has been observed with this drug. This may be heralded by the development of proteinuria or multiple tubular defects. Renal damage is often manifest following a cumulative dose of 4 g/m^2. In order to minimize nephrotoxicity, the optimal dosage schedule may be either 1.5 g/m^2/wk or 0.5 g/m^2 daily for 5 days, with repeat courses every 3 to 4 weeks. The onset of proteinuria or any of the tubular defects compromising the Fanconi syndrome is an indication for discontinuance of the drug until these findings remit. Various hydration/diuretic regimens and/or a continuous infusion schedule may be of value in minimizing nephrotoxicity; firm data in this regard are not available as yet. It would appear that pre-existing renal dysfunction leads to an increased incidence of nephrotoxicity, thus streptozotocin is not recommended for patients with a reduced GFR.

Other Agents

Various other chemotherapeutic/immunologic agents have been associated with renal dysfunction. They include mitomycin-C, which is capable of causing glomerular sclerosis and the hemolytic uremic syndrome. Mithramycin has been known to cause acute tubular necrosis when used in tumoricidal doses. Renal function should be monitored closely when mithramycin is used in the management of hypercalcemia, as deterioration of renal function has been noted following lower doses. A variety of tubular defects have been found with 5-azacytidine, an antimetabolite used in the treatment of acute myelogenous leukemia. Recombinant leukocyte interferon may cause interstitial nephritis or the nephrotic syndrome.

RADIATION NEPHRITIS

The acute changes of radiation nephritis occur within 6 to 12 months of treatment and do not develop unless 2300 to 2500 rads have been delivered to both kidneys. Unfortunately, there is no good clinical dose-response curve for radiation renal damge. The threshold appears to be in excess of 2000 rads. Although the initial manifestations of renal damage are often managed successfully, the pathologic process is usually irreversible. Of 20 patients with acute radiation nephritis in one series, 6 of 8 patients who had associated malignant hypertension died within 3 to 12 months; a total of 10 patients in the series eventually died of renal failure. The fatal cases manifest a combination of hypertensive encephalopathy, congestive heart failure, and uremia. The early deaths were due to hypertensive disease; the later deaths were due to uremia.

In order to prevent acute renal failure from radiation nephritis, adequate renal localization at the time of radiation treatment planning must be accomplished as well as limitation of dose and volume. A dose of 2000 rads in 10 fractions over 2 weeks is generally regarded as a safe treatment plan. Nevertheless, it is not uncommon to exceed this dose to one kidney in the treatment of abdominal cancers. Provided the dose to one kidney does not exceed 2000 rads in 10 fractions, the dose to the other kidney is limited only by gastrointestinal tolerance. Since the kidney that received 2000 rads will continue to function, the injury to the contralateral kidney usually does not result in acute renal failure. Hypertension may ensure, however, and is managed with antihypertensive therapy.

The risk of radiation nephritis may be substantially increased for any dose fractionation scheme if the patient is receiving therapy with any of a number of radiation-potentiating or additively toxic drugs. These include actinomycin D, Adriamycin, cyclophosphamide, vinblastine, bleomycin, and nitrogen mustard. In several studies, radiation nephritis has occurred at lower radiation doses when the foregoing agents were utilized concurrently.

DIALYSIS THERAPY IN THE CANCER PATIENT WITH ACUTE RENAL FAILURE

When ARF cannot be prevented or reversed, dialysis may be necessary. In view of the multiple etiologies of ARF and the variability of its severity, as well as the broad spectrum of coexisting or underlying illness, it has been difficult to develop clear indications for dialysis based on data derived from well-designed clinical studies. Some key questions remaining to be answered in addressing this issue are: (1) What are the critical criteria in assessing the need for dialysis? (2) When does dialysis intervention truly affect patient outcome? Because of the lack of convincing data in this regard, indications for dialysis in patients with ARF may vary considerably from one center to another. Nevertheless, the current approach in many centers is to initiate dialysis early in the course of ARF so as to prevent uremic complications. This prophylactic approach appears to be of particular merit in the cancer patient.

Table 3 outlines indications for dialysis in the cancer patient with ARF, as applied by the Acute Dialysis Unit of the Mount Sinai Medical Center in Milwaukee. Many of these indications represent physiologic perturbations that require immediate intervention, such as pericarditis, the bleeding diathesis secondary to a defect in platelet function, marked overexpansion of the ECF volume, uremic encephalopathy, or uremic colitis. Other indications of somewhat less urgency, but rapidly reversible with dialysis, include (1) early and subtle signs of encephalopathy such as confusion, lethargy, or slowing of mentation; (2) anorexia and nausea preventing adequate nutrition (if due to uremia); and (3) marked electrolyte imbalance. In addition, dialysis should be considered when dialyzable endogenous nephrotox-

TABLE 3 Indications for Dialysis in the Cancer Patient with ARF

Indications	*Comments*
Pericarditis	If due to uremia rather than cancer; may not be rapidly reversible
Bleeding due to platelet dysfunction	Reversible with dialysis
ECF volume expansion causing CHF	Alternatively, may treat with ultrafiltration
Uremic encephalopathy	Reversible with dialysis
Uremic colitis	Reversible with dialysis
Anorexia, nausea, vomiting	If due to azotemia
Hyperkalemia	Relative; may be managed medically
Acidosis	Relative; may be managed medically
Hyponatremia	If <120 mEq/L and not amenable to treatment with hypertonic saline solution
Severe hyperphosphatemia	May be seen in rapid tumor lysis syndrome
Hypermagnesemia	Toxic levels >5.0 mEq/L
Hypercalcemia	If contributing to ARF or symptomatic
Hyperuricemia	If contributing to ARF
Presence of nephrotoxin	May not be dialyzable; consider removal by hemoperfusion
Prophylactic	Attempt to keep BUN <70 mg/dl

ins, such as calcium and uric acid, are present in high concentration in association with ARF. In view of the compounded risk faced by cancer patients with ARF, it would appear desirable to employ prophylactic dialysis in this group of patients in order to maintain the BUN concentration below 70 mg/dl, while simultaneously administering nutritional support. In order to achieve this goal, daily dialysis may be necessary, particularly in patients who have recently undergone surgery, are undergoing rapid tumor lysis, or are receiving high doses of corticosteroids which result in excessive catabolism.

HYPERCALCEMIA OF MALIGNANT DISEASE

I. CRAIG HENDERSON, M.D.

The type of therapy selected in the management of hypercalcemia in the cancer patient depends on the severity of the patient's symptoms, the underlying etiology of the hypercalcemia, and the availability of effective therapies for the patient's tumor. Although more than 10 percent of all cancer patients are likely to have some degree of hypercalcemia during their course, a smaller percentage have symptoms that are life-threatening, i.e., a hypercalcemic "crisis." Patients with nausea and vomiting, anorexia, abdominal pain, somnolence, obtundation, psychosis, seizures, severe muscle weakness, or coma should be hospitalized emergently. In addition, patients with a rapid rise in serum calcium to levels above 13 over a period of a few days to several weeks are also considered to be in hypercalcemic crisis. On the other hand, less severe degrees of hypercalcemia, in the range of 10.5 to 12 with a normal serum albumin, may be tolerated for long periods of time with minimal treatment as long as the calcium levels are stable.

INITIAL MANAGEMENT

The administration of fluids followed by diuresis should be the first step in the management of all patients with symptomatic or life-threatening hypercalcemia. Patients with hypercalcemia usually experience some degree of polyuria/polydipsia and have a volume contraction prior to diagnosis. The anorexia and obtundation associated with hypercalcemia often result in decreased fluid intake, and vomiting may further augment the loss of fluids. Thus the first goal of therapy is to replace these fluid losses, to increase plasma volume, to increase GFR, and thus to increase calcium excretion. This should be done with normal saline, since calcium clearance is linked to sodium clearance; increased sodium intake results in increased sodium *and* calcium clearance independent of the increase in GFR.

During the first 2 to 3 days it is recommended that the patient be given 4 or more liters of normal saline during each 24-hour period. Ideally a urine output of about 4 liters per day should be achieved. As soon as volume replacement has begun, furosemide may be given to augment the diuresis. Although furosemide doses of 80 to 100 mg every 1 to 2 hours have been recommended, it is not clear that such high doses are necessary in most patients, and a dose of 40 to 80 mg every 6 hours usually suffices. Some patients may be hypokalemic at the time of admission, and potassium should be routinely added to the IV fluids once a good urinary flow has begun. Patients should have their fluid balance carefully monitored since the major complication of such large fluid volume is congestive heart failure in patients with cardiac disease. Hypernatremia and hypomagnesemia are other complications that may occur in the absence of careful and frequent biochemical determinations. The use of fluids alone results in a significant reduction in the serum calcium in about 80 percent of patients, and up to one third of patients may have a return of serum calcium to normal levels following 2 to 3 days of adequate fluid replacement. However, the addition of diuretics hastens this process and decreases the total fluid volume needed to achieve a maximal result.

EVALUATION AND TREATMENT OF UNDERLYING CAUSES

In the majority of patients, no therapy other than fluids and diuretics is necessary during the first 24 hours, and a work-up to determine the underlying cause of the hypercalcemia should be initiated immediately following admission. Primary hyperparathyroidism, the use of thiazide diuretics, exogenous vitamin D, the use of calcium supplements, prolonged immobilization, and secondary hyperparathyroidism after renal failure are all causes of hypercalcemia which may coexist with cancer. Most of these etiologies can be ruled out by a careful history if the patient is alert. An immunoreactive parathormone (iPTH) level should be drawn, but it is not clear that a nephrogenous cyclic AMP level, a prostaglandin E_2 level, a 1,25-dihydroxyvitamin D level, or other markers are likely to be helpful in distinguishing the etiology of hypercalcemia in an individual patient. The history of acute onset hypercalcemia in a patient with a normal iPTH level and bone metastases is unlikely to be due to primary or secondary hyperparathyroidism. Hypercalcemia without bone metastasis is most frequently seen in patients with squamous cell carinoma of the lung, ovarian cancer, head and neck cancer, esophageal cancer, transitional cell carcinoma of the bladder, and clear cell carcinoma of the kidney. Hypercalcemia as the first manifestation of a previously undiagnosed cancer is extremely rare, but otherwise asymptomatic bone metastases from multiple myeloma may first be diagnosed during a hypercalcemic crisis.

Some episodes of hypercalcemia result from the use of a variety of endocrine treatments, especially estrogens, androgens, and tamoxifen in patients with breast cancer who have bone metastases. This phenomenon, sometimes called "flare," may begin within hours to a few days after the initiation of a new form of hormone therapy, and it has been observed in patients who have had prior hormone therapy without flare. In most cases the hypercalcemia is self-limiting even if the hormone therapy is continued, but at times the hypercalcemia from the endocrine therapy of breast cancer may be fatal. Fluids and diuretics should be administered as with any other form of hypercalcemia. If the hypercalcemia responds promptly to fluids, if the serum calcium is below 15, and if the patient's symptoms are mild and easily controlled, the endocrine therapy may be continued in spite of the hypercalcemia. Patients with a flare following endocrine therapy are as likely as, but not necessarily more likely than, patients without flare to eventually achieve an objective remission of their underlying cancer.

The various treatments of hypercalcemia lower serum calcium through one of five mechanisms, using one of four medications:

1. Increased urinary excretion of calcium (saline diuresis, gluocorticoids, calcitonin).
2. Inhibition of osteoclast activity (mithramycin, calcitonin, prostaglandin inhibitors, and possibly glucocorticoids).
3. Decreased bone resorption without an effect on osteoclast activity (diphosphonates, phosphates).
4. Decreased calcium absorption from the GI tract (oral phosphates).
5. Increased deposition in bone and soft tissues (intravenous or oral phosphates).

In some cases the primary effect of the antihypercalcemic agent may be to reduce the levels of a mediator, such as osteoclast activating factor or prostaglandins, which in turn results in decreased bone resorption.

The choice of therapy after the initial 24 hours of fluid replacement depends on the magnitude of the initial response to fluids, the persistence of symptoms, the underlying cause of the hypercalcemia, and the ability to treat the underlying cause of the hypercalcemia. For example, if the patient has a tumor that is likely to respond to chemotherapy or hormonal therapy, this therapy should be started as soon as possible, and the agents used to treat the hypercalcemia should not limit the selection of drugs or the dose of drugs used to treat the tumor. In patients with persistent symptoms in spite of anticancer therapy, the quickest but least durable response is likely to be achieved with calcitonin. A somewhat slower but more durable response may be achieved with mithramycin or diphosphonates, and both of these therapies should be considered in patients who have persistent hypercalcemia and tumors that are unlikely to respond to therapy. In circumstances in which mithramycin is unavailable, actinomycin D may serve with comparable efficacy. Finally, phosphates, glucocorticoids, diphosphonates, prostaglandin inhibitors, or combinations of these may be used with relatively few side effects to achieve long-term control in selected patients.

GLUCOCORTICOIDS

Although glucocorticoids have been shown to reduce hypercalcemia in a large number of different cancers, including lung and prostate, these agents are most often used in the treatment of multiple myeloma, lymphoma, and breast cancer. There are several potential mechanisms of glucocorticoid action. These include an antitumor effect on breast cancer and lymphomas, inhibition of osteoclast bone resorption, possibly inhibition of osteoclast-activating factor in patients with multiple myeloma, and increased renal excretion of calcium. Initially, 250 mg of hydrocortisone may be given intravenously every 8 hours; later a dose of 60 mg of prednisone should be administered daily in divided doses. Responses are usually seen in 72 hours, and the maximum effect may be seen between 5 days and 2 weeks after the initiation of the daily steroids. More recently glucocorticoids have been used in conjunction with calcitonin (to be discussed).

MITHRAMYCIN

This is one of the most effective of the various treatment options. It should be considered after an unsuccessful trial of saline diuresis and in patients with symptomatic hypercalcemia for whom no treatment of the underlying tumor is available. Mithramycin blocks RNA synthesis and is cytotoxic to osteoclasts. The usual dose is 25 μg/kg administered IV as a single dose over at least 10 minutes. This dose may be repeated every 2 to 4 days. Antihypercalcemic effects have been reported with smaller doses in the range of 10 μg/kg (and even as low as 2 μg/kg), but no large trials have been conducted to compare the efficacy of smaller doses with the standard recommended dose of 25 μg/kg/day. Relatively slow intravenous administration is recommended because hypotension may occur with a rapid IV push. Infusions of 4 to 6 hours result in less nausea and vomiting.

The major disadvantage of mithramycin is myelosuppression, which may result in a decreased ability to utilize other cytotoxic agents for the treatment of the underlying tumor. This is most often manifest as thrombocytopenia. Most patients experience nausea, and a few patients have intermittent vomiting with this dose of mithramycin. Larger doses of mithramycin administered daily for 10 days as antitumor therapy have been reported to cause hepatocellular necrosis and renal damage, but this is almost never seen with the single doses recommended for the treatment of hypercalcemia.

The response to mithramycin begins within 6 hours of treatment, but the effect usually is not measurable until 24 to 48 hours after therapy. The duration of the effect is variable and depends in part on the response of the underlying tumor to therapy. The average duration of response is 4 days and ranges between 3 and 16 days. Hypercalcemia may recur rather dramatically at the end of this period and may result in a second hypercalcemic crisis more life-threatening than the first.

CALCITONIN

Calcitonin is the most rapidly acting of all the antihypercalcemic agents and may temporarily control hypercalcemia in the majority of patients with a hypercalcemic crisis. It is also the least useful for chronic therapy over a period of months and years. Calcitonin may prove especially useful in the acute management of patients unable to handle a large saline diuresis. Since calcitonin is a physiologic regulator of osteoclast activity, its primary action is probably due to the inhibition of bone resorption by osteoclasts.

Calcitonin may be given intravenously, intramuscularly, or subcutaneously. Although a number of dose schedules have been recommended, initial therapy with 4 MRC units/kg of salmon calcitonin every 12 hours may be given subcutaneously or intramuscularly. If the response to this is unsatisfactory, the dose may be increased to 8 units/kg every 12 hours; and if the response is still inadequate, further escalation to 8 units/kg every 6 hours is warranted. Prior to the initiation of calcitonin therapy, skin testing with 1 MRC unit intradermally should be used to identify allergic individuals. Calcitonin should be administered in plastic syringes since it adheres to glass.

The effects of calcitonin can be seen within a few hours and are maximal between 12 and 24 hours after administration. The major drawback to the use of calcitonin is early onset of tachyphalaxis, usually within 48 hours. This "escape phenomenon" is thought to be due to a down-regulation of calcitonin receptors. It has been reported that the effects of calcitonin can be maintained for as long as 4 days and even as long as 3 months by the concomitant administration of daily oral predisone with the calcitonin.

Although the side effects from calcitonin are minimal, patients may experience flushing of the face 1 to 2 hours after administration, mild nausea, rare anorexia or vomiting, and severe hypocalcemia if calcitonin is used together with mithramycin.

INORGANIC PHOSPHATES

Inorganic phosphates have been used intravenously to acutely lower the calcium level and as an oral agent for chronic control of hypercalcemia. Phosphates remove calcium from the serum by the formation of complexes which deposit in bone and soft tissue. It may also decrease bone resorption and inhibit calcium absorption from the GI tract. Extraskeletal calcification, especially in the kidney, can be a serious side effect of phosphate therapy, but this has usually been seen following intravenous administration. Severe hypocalcemia and hypotension may also occur with IV phosphate administration. The toxicity of intravenous phosphates precludes its general use, and adequate saline diuresis usually results in rapid enough control of symptoms to make this hazardous approach unnecessary.

Chronic oral administration of 0.5 mg *bid* to 1.0 mg *tid* may be quite effective for long-term control of hypercalcemia in some patients. The major, and sometimas dose-limiting, side effect of oral phosphates is diarrhea. In addition, hyperphosphatemia may be seen, and oral phosphates are not recommended in patients with renal failure. Responses to phosphates may be transient in spite of continued administration. It is also possible that phosphates may potentiate the effects of calcitonin.

PROSTAGLANDIN INHIBITORS

There are abundant data suggesting that some tumor types induce hypercalcemia through a humoral mediator. Prostaglandins have been shown, in vitro and in vivo, to stimulate osteoclast activity and bone resorption, and this effect can be blocked in vitro with prostaglandin inhibitors such as indomethacin or aspirin. A small number of case reports of long-term control of hypercalcemia with the administration of indomethacin, 25 to 50 mg *tid*, have been published. These reports include patients with lung cancer, colon cancer, renal cell cancer, and pancreatic cancer. The drug must be continued indefinitely because withdrawal may result in return of symptoms. The correlation between measured prostaglandin levels and the response to prostaglandin inhibitors is not consistent, and the selection of patients for this approach is still poorly defined. At present, patients refractory to other antihypercalcemic therapies who need chronic therapy should be considered for this approach, and especially if their urinary PGE-M excretion is also elevated. Gastric distress, gastrointestinal bleeding, and thrombocytopenia are the most important side effects.

DIPHOSPHONATES

There are three drugs in this class of compounds: EHDP (ethane-1-hydroxy-1-diphosphonate), Cl_2MDP (dichloromethylene diphosphonate), and APD (3-

amino-1-hydroxypropylidine-1-diphosphonate). Only one of these compounds, EHDP (etidronate disodium, Didronel) has been approved by the FDA for general use, and none has been approved for the treatment of hypercalcemia. However, these agents may prove to be among the most effective of all antihypercalcemic agents for both acute and chronic control of hypercalcemia.

Diphosphonates are analogs of pyrophosphates, and these agents are absorbed onto the bone lattice where they inhibit resorption. However, high doses of EHDP may also inhibit remineralization. It is not clear whether the precise mechanism of action of these three different diphosphonates is the same. For example, Cl_2MDP may be cytotoxic to osteoclasts, in contrast to APD, which is not.

EHDP is available only in an oral form, and the response to EHDP is slower than that seen after the administration of the other diphosphonates. Both Cl_2MDP and APD can be given either intravenously or orally. The greatest experience is with Cl_2MDP given as an intravenous dose of 2.5 to 5.0 mg/kg daily for 6 days followed by an oral dose of 3200 mg per day for long-term control. The onset of the hypocalcemic effect may be seen as early as 12 to 48 hours after the start of therapy and may persist up to 72 hours. Normal calcium levels may be reached in some patients 2 to 6 days after an infusion of Cl_2MDP, but the calcium nadir may be seen as late as the fifteenth day.

In general, the diphosphonates are well tolerated. Asymptomatic hypocalcemia and transient diarrhea have been observed in patients treated with Cl_2MDP. EPHD has been given without side effects for periods of 7 to 30 days. APD appears to be the most toxic of these compounds, and gastric distress, transient fever, and a transient fall in WBC have all been reported to occur in some patients. Renal insufficiency has also been seen, but does not appear to be a common complication of therapy with diphosponates.

PAIN CONTROL IN THE CANCER PATIENT

ALLAN B. LEVIN, M.D.

The achievement of adequate pain control in the cancer patient, as indicated by personal experience, appears to work best if a team approach is used. The team approach allows for a multi-modality input into the therapeutic regimen. At a minimum, the team should consist of an oncologist, a radiotherapist, an anesthesiologist, and a neurosurgeon. It is also beneficial to have an additional person to coordinate the activities of these specialties.

There are three major modes of treatment of pain. The initial mode is to treat the underlying pathologic process causing the pain, i.e., treatment of a neoplasm with either radiotherapy or chemotherapy. The second mode is the use of *appropriate* analgesic agents, and the third mode consists of destructive procedures that interrupt pain pathways or augment endogenous analgesic systems. The use of one modality does not necessarily preclude the use of a second or even all three modalities simultaneously. The use of analgesic agents, and occasionally even destructive procedures, may be indicated while the underlying pathologic process is being treated.

ANALGESIC AGENTS

Analgesic agents are prescribed according to three basic principles: (1) combinations of drugs should be synergistic and not antagonistic, (2) begin with the simplest medication and progress as necessary to a medication that is most effective in the treatment of the pain with the least side effects, and (3) prescribe around-the-clock scheduled dosage. The simplest analgesics, aspirin and acetaminophen, can be surprisingly effective, even in relieving severe pain, when used on a regularly scheduled basis. The effect of either agent can be enhanced appreciably by the addition of codeine. Most of the newer drugs that are lavishly advertised for the treatment of pain are no more effective, although they are considerably more expensive, than the combinations just described. It is sometimes necessary to prescribe drugs that augment the effect of analgesic agents, such as (1) nonsteroidal anti-inflammatory agents, if the pain is caused in part by inflammation or irritation of nerve roots, or (2) the tricyclic antidepressants, to improve the sleeping patterns of the patient and, when adequate levels are reached, add significantly to overall pain relief. If control is not effected by the combinations just described, it may be necessary to prescribe stronger, narcotic analgesics. We prefer drugs that are absorbed well and achieve effective blood levels when taken orally. We avoid narcotic drug combinations, especially liquid combinations that offer mainly alcohol and very little in the way of true analgesic properties. Two specific drugs that are used frequently are methadone and levorphanol. Although adequate pain control with methadone can eventually be achieved with *q8h* dosing, it is advantageous to begin with 5 mg *q6h* and rapidly progress up to 15 or even 20 mg *q6* to *8h*. One must remember that because of the long half-life of methadone, patients become drowsy, and it takes a long time for the methadone to wear off. Levorphanol, with its shorter half-life is also well-absorbed orally and highly effective in doses of 1 to 4 mg *q4* to *6h* on a scheduled basis. These two drugs, along with the tricyclic antidepressants, give satisfactory pain relief to the majority of patients with cancer, especially during earlier phases of treatment.

The primary consideration in the neurosurgical treatment of cancer pain is always the question of *when* treatment should be instituted. The surgical control of pain should be considered whenever the patient cannot obtain adequate pain relief with oral analgesic agents or when the intake of analgesics interferes with normal activities of daily living. Basically, all accepted neurosurgical procedures for the control of cancer pain are destructive. These must effectively interrupt either the pain pathways or, by some other mechanism, interfere with pain transmission. In order to be considered a reasonable procedure for use in controlling pain, the following criteria should be met: (1) The procedure itself should be as simple as possible with a minimum of postoperative care and convalescence. (2) The procedure should have at least a 90 percent chance of giving a good to excellent result, which means that the patient's pain is controlled with small amounts of oral medication or no medication at all. (3) The pain relief should be anticipated to continue throughout the remainder of the patient's life. (4) The side effects of the procedure should be acceptable and should not interfere significantly with the patient's life. To provide a better understanding of the procedures available for the control of pain, a discussion of the basic techniques involved in neural-pathway interruption follows.

TECHNIQUES OF PAIN CONTROL

Surgical Methods

The most direct approach to the target, and theoretically the most complete method of interruption of the pain pathways, is surgical. The disadvantage of the surgical method is the need for an open operation to expose either the nerves within the cranial vault or spinal canal or to expose the spinal cord. In the already debilitated patient, a major surgical procedure is accompanied by an increased risk, and the recovery period is prolonged in most cases. Most patients and physicians tend to resist major surgical procedures.

Chemical Methods

The use of a chemical agent to denature the neural tissue and thereby interrupt the neural pathway is usually fairly simple. The procedures do not require a surgical incision, and the patient does not have to be put to sleep in the majority of cases. The disadvantages of chemicals lie in the lack of control of the amount and extent of destruction, and the adverse effect on surrounding tissue. Also, on occasion there may be return of neural function in an incomplete lesion. Absolute ethyl alcohol is the most commonly used neurolytic agent; however, it can cause tissue sloughing when used in the subcutaneous tissue for nerve blocks. In peripheral nerve blocks ammonium chloride or ammonium sulfate is the agent of choice. In the subarachnoid space, phenol can be used in place of ethanol.

Thermal Methods

Destruction of neural tissue by thermal degradation, either by heat or cold, is usually a procedure as simple as the chemical destruction, but with a greater degree of control and more permanent results. The use of cautery for thermal destruction can be painful, but the use of radiofrequency (RF) energy to induce heat is relatively painless. The radiofrequency current employed is approximately 500 kilocycles per second (KHz), which provides a well-circumscribed and uniform lesion with relative permanence. The lesion is produced as the current flows through the tissue, which represents a resistance to the flow of current. The resistance causes heat to be generated in the tissue and not in the electrical tip, which accounts for the relative painlessness of the procedure. The size of the lesion is dependent on the amount of current, hence the temperature, as well as the duration of the temperature and the electrode size.

Cryosurgical probes can be used for creating lesions in neural tissue, but the probes are very large in relation to the desired size of the lesion. Cold lesions also tend to be less permanent than radiofrequency lesions.

PROCEDURES

Rhizotomy

A rhizotomy usually involves the destruction of a single nerve or a component of that nerve. The severance of the nerve usually means the destruction of both motor and sensory functions mediated by that nerve, unless a more central lesion is made adjacent to the spinal canal, where just the posterior roots can be severed. Destruction of nerves or roots can be done by any of the previously mentioned techniques. Because of the difficulty in getting only sensory loss without affecting motor function short of doing a large laminectomy and open cutting of the posterior roots, it is best to restrict rhizotomies to areas where motor loss will not impair function. Even in areas where only sensory fibers are cut, function may still be lost because of the lack of proprioceptive feedback. Thus, one area of choice for rhizotomy is the sacral area. This is an effective mode of treatment in patients with deep midline perineal pain secondary to carcinoma of the rectum, vulva, or vagina, and occasionally even cervical carcinoma. In sacral rhizotomies a small incision is made and the bone over the superior aspect of the sacrum is removed. The S1 root is identified and all roots below this can be cut. Most of these patients already have colostomies, and therefore no anal sphincter abnormalities will be noted. Furthermore, most of these patients also have impaired bladder function and additional loss of bladder function will also be unnoticed. In our experience, approximately 50 percent of the patients who had preoperative bladder function will continue to have postoperative bladder function with only the S2 root intact. Sacral rhizotomies give rise to good relief of midline pain, and this relief is permanent.

This procedure can be done somewhat less effectively with phenol or alcohol injected at the L5–S1 level with care so as not to get the S1 roots. Thermal rhizotomies can also be performed if the patient does not want to lose bladder or sexual function. The radiofrequency lesions can be made following nerve root stimulation and more selective rhizotomies done. The more selective the rhizotomies the more chance of residual pain. In the thoracic region, surgical rhizotomies are again feasible over several levels. Individual thermal lesions can also be done if only a small area is involved. The use of hypobaric alcohol in the subarachnoid space by an experience anesthesiologist has proved to be extremely valuable in our institution. Some patients, however, will have weakness secondary to spinal cord involvement by the alcohol.

In the head and neck region, the trigeminal nerve carries sensation from the face, tongue, and alveolar ridge of the jaw and maxilla. Further, the trigeminal nerve is divided into three branches which are nicely layered in the retrogasserian space. Lesions can be made in this area by passage of a radiofrequency needle, under fluoroscopic control, through the foramen ovale into the retrogasserian space. With the use of the radiofrequency current, a lesion can be made in this space among the nerve fibers. The procedure is performed with the patient awake so that only the desired division is destroyed and sensation is preserved, especially in the V_1 division, where loss of sensation can lead to loss of corneal sensation with resultant corneal irritation and abrasion.

Cranial nerves IX and X exit through the jugular foramen and carry sensation to the tonsillar fossa, posterior aspect of the tongue, the nasal and oral pharynx, and the larynx. These areas are frequently involved in head and neck cancers. Under fluoroscopic control, a radiofrequency needle can be passed through the jugular foramen and a lesion made to destroy these nerves. The side effect can be difficulty in swallowing, but this effect is usually of short duration.

Cordotomy

From the nerve itself, the pain fibers travel in the posterior root entering the spinal cord and substantia gelatinosa. At this point it may travel up a segment or two, cross to the contralateral side, and travel in the lateral spinothalamic tract to the thalamus. The lateral spinothalamic tract contains the fibers for pain and temperature sensation. Interruption of this tract, therefore, causes loss of pain and temperature sensation at a level or two below the area of the lesion. Open surgical cordotomies have been done as far back as 70 years ago. Percutaneous techniques were introduced almost 20 years ago. At present there is no indication for an open cordotomy because more accurate, long-term results can be obtained with a closed percutaneous technique. In the hands of an experienced technician, the unilateral percutaneous cordotomy permits the interruption of the spinothalamic tract without fear of significant complications. It is simple to perform, requiring only some premedication and no general anesthesia. There should be no more discomfort than that of a myelogram and no significant convalescent period.

The procedure itself is performed under either fluoroscopic or x-ray control, with a spinal needle being placed in the area overlying the C1–C2 interspace on the side contralateral to the pain. Spinal cord and dentate ligament are outlined with a Pantopaque mixture. A radiofrequency electrode is directed to lie just above the dentate ligament and advanced into the spinothalamic tract. The electrode used is approximately 0.012 inches in diameter with a 2–mm active tip. Electrical stimulation localizes the area in which the tip lies, and minor readjustments can place the tip within a representation of the area of pain. With temperature monitoring of the electrode tip, a lesion in the range of 75 to 80° for 20 to 40 seconds can destroy portions of the spinothalamic tract. The size of the electrode allows for small discrete lesions, and in approximately 75 to 80 percent of the patients the lesion can be made to restrict analgesia to a quadrant of the body, depending on the area involved, with pain. To make a larger lesion, an elevated temperature of longer duration is used; it can affect the entire side of the body from approximately C3 to the sacral area. It is sometimes difficult to create a lesion in the lower sacral region because the sacral fibers may actually be tucked in the corticospinal tract. As the corticospinal tract lies just below the spinothalamic tract, any involvement of this tract could cause the patient to develop weakness in the ipsilateral side. As the procedure is carried out, motor function testing is performed to see that the corticospinal tract does not become involved.

The patient may experience some hypotonia from involvement of the extrapyramidal tracts. The unilateral lesion is attended with minimal risk, but bilateral lesions can involve the respiratory center in the spinal cord and give rise to sleep-induced-apnea. When this problem arises, the patient may note no difficulty in breathing when awake and there is little or no respiratory distress. However, when the patient goes to sleep, breathing becomes inadequate with resulting progressive hypercarbia and hypoxia, which can eventually lead to complete apnea. To prevent this in patients who undergo bilateral cordotomy, it is best to keep the sensory level low on one side, preferably on both sides. However, this is not always possible. In any event patients with bilateral cordotomies should be monitored for several days with a respiratory monitor and carefully observed for any evidence of confusion, especially in the morning, which may indicate some degree of hypoxia. They should also be observed for any evidence of generalized hypotonia, which may indicate involvement of extrapyramidal tracts, associated in many cases with involvement of the respiratory area. Sleep-induced apnea is treated with assisted ventilation while the patient is sleeping. This problem is self-limited, usually disappearing within a week.

Patients undergoing bilateral cordotomy may also have urinary problems. Facilitory pathways for initiation of micturition, which are located near the lateral spinothalamic tract, also become involved in percutaneous cordotomy. When they are involved bilaterally, the patient loses the ability to initiate micturition and may have to be placed on a catheter program. The incidence of this loss in our particular patient series has been approximately 90 percent. Our patients are routinely taught intermittent self-catheterization by a clean, unsterile technique. Women accept this readily; men do so with occasional hesitancy.

Approximately 2 percent of the patients undergoing cordotomy will also complain of some dysesthesias. Most of the dysesthesias are very mild, especially compared to the preoperative pain. Although some groups report dysesthesias that are quite severe, we have not seen this. Excellent results have been obtained in treating the dysesthesias with amitriptyline.

CENTRAL PROCEDURES

For patients with bilateral diffuse pain secondary to multiple areas of involvement, cordotomies sometimes have to be carried into the high cervical region bilaterally, with the attendant risk of respiratory difficulties, and this requires two separate procedures. It is preferable to do a single procedure more centrally to control pain. Pain is transmitted by the spinothalamic tract to the thalamic area and from there pain projects to cortical areas of the brain. In the past, cingulotomies done stereotaxically have been able to control the perception of pain in approximately 60 percent of the patients. This procedure involves the destruction of cortical projections that travel in the cingulate gyrus bilaterally. However, cingulotomies have some risk of undesirable personality changes. More recently, deep brain stimulators, stereotaxically placed in the midbrain in the periaqueductal area, have been used with varying degrees of success.

One central procedure that has been used in patients with hormonal tumors, specifically breast tumors, has been that of surgical hypophysectomy. Certain groups have reported good success in more than 75 percent of their patients. However, this does require a major surgical procedure and has been used only in hormonally responsive tumors. In 1975 we introduced the procedure of stereotaxic chemical hypophysectomy by injection of alcohol into the pituitary gland for the treatment of nonhormonal as well as hormonal tumors. The procedure is performed under a light plane of general endotracheal anesthesia, and under stereotaxic targeting and fluoroscopic control, a 20–gauge needle can be placed into the pituitary gland and a total of 3 to 6 cc of absolute ethyl alcohol can be instilled in the sella turcica. This causes complete pituitary destruction. Our experience now exceeds 100 patients with both hormonal and nonhormonal tumors. Overall, the percentage of good to excellent pain relief is the same in both the nonhormonal and hormonally responsive tumors and initially exceeds 90 percent. Six percent of the patients experiencing initial pain relief developed recurrent pain after one month and required another pain relieving procedure. The remaining 84 percent of the patients developed relief, which appears to last throughout the remainder of the patient's life. Approximately 20 percent of the patients had brief periods in which there was some exacerbation of pain, but it subsided spontaneously. This procedure appears to be most effective in relieving pain arising from bony metastases and, to a lesser degree, pain arising in the soft tissue. The patients for whom this procedure fails are those who had direct involvement of the nerve plexus. The question of mechanism of action of chemical hypophysectomy in pain relief has stimulated a fair amount of controversy and remains essentially unknown. The complications related to chemical hypophysectomy arise from the spread of alcohol around the pituitary gland or by expansion of the pituitary gland itself as the alcohol is injected. Major complications have been extraocular nerve palsies secondary to compression of either the third or the sixth cranial nerve. There have been no procedure-related deaths.

COMMUNICATING WITH THE PATIENT RECEIVING CHEMOTHERAPY

HOWARD LEVENTHAL, Ph.D.

As skilled clinicians, oncologists are accustomed to diagnosing and treating patients who present with a variety of physical, behavioral, and emotional symptoms and signs. Their emotions vary from the anger of the young patient, the shocked and distressed expression of the newly diagnosed patient, or the dejected and depressed visage of the terminal patient who cannot readily resign himself to an approaching death, to the optimistic, determined visage of the patient committed to battle against his cancer. Their tactics vary for coping with the disease, the treatment, and the staff. Some appear gluts for information, asking questions, seeking clarification, even coming with lists of concerns, whereas others seem indifferent, if not resistant, to being informed.

What can the oncologist do in the face of this ''splendid'' variety of human emotion and human problem-solving behavior? What does he or she have to offer? Oncologists are not psychotherapists and should not try to function as such. They should not attempt to alter personalities. Oncologists are not social workers or family therapists and should not try to function as such. Their job is not to alter long-term patterns of family interaction. Oncologists are at the center of that part of the patient's and family's world that is focused on cancer, and they must be prepared to do something about that. Within this focus, there are two things that an oncologist can offer in addition to technical or treatment competence: (1) information, and (2) an attentive ear! To do so skillfully, oncologists must view their relationship to the patient from two important perspectives: (1) the bio-psychologic and (2) the social psychologic.

THE BIO-PSYCHOLOGY OF RELATIONSHIPS

Animals of many types seek to be together: this is the common-sense and reasonable definition of social behavior. People are social animals. Our complex systems of social behavior have arisen over a long biologic and social evolutionary history. Our need to be together appears stronger when we are threatened. The biologic basis of our social action is seen in our neuromuscular make-up, our capacity for speech, and the complexity of our expressive behavior. In short, our biology is designed for verbal and expressive communication. Moreover, the evidence is now overwhelming that our autonomic and neuroendocrine systems respond as vigorously, if not more vigorously, to interpersonal or social stimuli than to physical assaults. In summary, our biologic system is designed to initiate and maintain social relationships, and the quality of our social relationships reverberates through our entire biologic system.

THE SOCIAL PSYCHOLOGY OF ROLES

The concept of *role* is central in social psychology. It is a concept at the social psychologic level which reflects our essential social nature. A role is a mutual set of expectations and obligations, i.e., what you expect to do, what you expect the other to do, and similar expectations on the part of the other. Roles are organized within the context of formal or informal social organizations. The medical care system is an institutional structure within which people fill and enact the roles of doctor and patient. These roles vary in content from, on the one hand, extreme passivity on the part of the patient and expert manipulation on the part of the physician (e.g., the patient in the operating room) to the often talked about, but rare, mutual exchange between the patient and the ''friendly'' family doctor. These roles or types of interaction vary for different practitioners, and they also vary by task and time: different types of treatment at different times in the history of the disease demand different modes of exchange. The doctor-patient roles depend, to a substantial degree, on the setting.

Practitioners and patients fulfill many roles in addition to those dictated by their participation in medical encounters. Each lives in a complex network of roles. The roles that comprise our everyday existence (for example, our roles as a spouse, parent, and family member) are sources of support and sources of stress. They are sources of support, as the family is the place within which we are given information about our self worth, given emotional support, and given direct help in managing the complexities of everyday life. The family is also the place where we can work through the stress produced by illness and other life problems. But these role relationships are also sources of strain as reciprocal demands come with support. Thus, we are expected to perform specific actions as spouses and parents. Our capacity to perform these duties, to provide our understanding presence, our concern and our economic support, are threatened by illness, which may absorb our energies and focus our attention on ourselves, disrupt our work, and terminate our lives. A cancer patient may be more concerned about his or her ability to continue at work or to function as a husband or wife than he or she is concerned about cancer. In short, one cannot ignore the social context of the patient and still be successful in patient management.

COMMUNICATION FROM A BIO-SOCIAL-PSYCHOLOGIC FRAMEWORK

Roles structure two-way communication, and communication requires that we listen as well as give information. How do roles structure what we are told?

What information are we supposed to give? Do the roles we occupy prevent us from sending or getting information critical for patient management? How we, both practitioner and patient, define our roles affects what we are willing to say and what we are willing and able to hear.

There is no end of articles on the psychosocial aspects of the cancer patient which recommend open communication. Few, however, provide any data relevant to the following critical questions. What do patients need to know? What are the effects of giving specific types of information? There are studies showing that patients may lack information about their diagnosis and about their treatment, both its expected outcome and course. But there are few investigations on whether the patients will be more or less well off when given information. This question should always be kept in mind. If we divide the various types of information into two classes, information about treatment and information about disease, we will find a number of studies on the effects of communication about treatment. Unfortunately, there are relatively few studies on communication about disease.

COMMUNICATION ABOUT TREATMENT

Communication about treatment is relatively easy to discuss as the studies in this area have distinguished between different types of information and evaluated their effects. Three types of information have been studied: (1) information about treatment procedures, e.g., telling the patient he will have surgery, radiation treatment, chemotherapy, and where, when, and how it will be given; (2) information about the sensory feel of treatment and how to cope with these effects, e.g., telling the patient about the various side effects of chemotherapy, how they feel, and how long they may last for different people; and (3) information about potential treatment outcomes. We will discuss each briefly.

Procedural Information

Information about procedures can provide the patient with a map of what will happen in the immediate future and reduce uncertainty. It can reduce distress and stabilize various autonomic and endocrine functions because events will happen according to expectations.

Giving procedural information is not necessarily easy; we tend to give it from the practitioners point of view. The patients may not understand the terminology, or they may be frightened by specific terms, such as surgery or radiation. It clearly pays to deliver such information in a simple organized fashion by providing booklets or appointment cards with maps and descriptions of the sequence of events in order to anchor the person and avoid arousing anxiety about forgetting. It also pays to systematically question the patient to locate specific areas of concern, e.g., does he or she have questions about radiation treatment, chemotherapy, the doctors, and so on. A review can bring out misinformation and misconceptions that can be corrected with simple explanations. It takes but a word or two to state that radiation is focussed to strike only the cancer to reduce the fears and threatening fantasies of someone who imagines that radiation will burn and destroy well parts of their body.

Care must also be taken to prepare the patient for variations in the procedure, if variation is likely. Unexpected events disturb one's sense that one knows what is happening and that things are going according to plan and can stimulate strong autonomic and endocrine response and alter the patients emotional and mental status.

Sensory and Coping Information

There is a substantial body of data showing the value of information about the sensory feel of treatment and how to cope in response to those specific sensations. A patient may know that he or she will receive chemotherapy, but may not know that nausea, vomiting, mouth sores, tiredness, and weakness are common experiences in treatment. If they are unprepared, they may place frightening interpretations on these symptoms. They may also have few ideas as to what to do if they have such experiences. Sensory information and coping tactics have been found effective in reducing gagging and lowering heart rate during endoscopic examinations, to facilitate patient cooperation during pelvic examinations, and to reduce postoperative hospital stays by 1 to 2 days following hysterectomy and cholecystectomy. In short, sensory and coping information are consistently superior to procedural information in reducing anxiety and distress.

The data on the effects of sensory information were gathered in randomized clinical trials. Information can be tested in the same way that one tests drugs. As with drugs, the information has the desired effect for most but not all patients. Thus, one must maintain a surveillance system to deal with the patient who is not helped by the information or the unusual patient who may become more distressed by it. Since information of this type is now given as a standard part of practice by oncology nurses, it might seem that the physician can ignore these issues. I think not. As a central figure in the treatment system it is worth the oncologist's while to distinguish between procedural, sensory and coping information to ensure that patients attend to and use this information.

Information on Treatment Benefits

Information about treatment outcomes are far more difficult to discuss. How does one communicate that treatment X has a 1 in 3 chance of working for 5 years of life whereas treatment Y has a 1 in 2 chance of working for 3 years? Will the patient understand the notion of probability? How do we turn a group probability into an individual figure? How do we describe and contrast two treatments which differ in immediate mortality and longer-term success yet have the same overall success rate?

Although it is clear that patients have difficulty understanding such information, it is less clear how to overcome their misunderstanding. It may help to use simple pictorial aids. It certainly would be advisable to ask questions and present information slowly. What needs to be remembered is that the meaning of a message depends on the emotional status and knowledge base of the recipient.

COMMUNICATION ABOUT DISEASE

Communication about treatment is designed to provide clear information to reduce uncertainty and ameliorate the distress produced by various treatment procedures. The intent is clear: to make it easier for the patient to handle treatment and to keep psychologic and physiologic distress to a minimum. The goal is consistent with the basic goal of chemotherapy, which is to increase the period of time for life and to increase the quality of life during that time. The goals for communication about illness are more complex. First, it is clear that the patient needs an accurate picture both of the probabilities of survival and of what to expect from treatment if he or she is to participate in decisions about entering and continuing treatment. In addition, the patient must make a variety of decisions and perform the varied tasks needed to put one's life in order in light of a new time frame and potentially changed competencies. Giving the patient the information needed to make these varied decisions cannot necessarily be evaluated against the same criteria used for evaluating information about treatment! Thus, a reduction in emotional upset during a procedure may be a sign of effective preparation for treatment, but it is not necessarily a sign of effective communication about illness. We have found, somewhat to our surprise, that a large proportion of cancer patients think their disease is an acute illness, as something that goes away, presumably for good, with treatment. Fully 54.8 percent of our lymphoma cases (n=52), 32.4 percent of our metastatic breast cases (n=34), and 42.2 percent of our adjuvant breast treatment cases (n=67) believed their illness to be similar to measles (in terms of being acute versus chronic) when asked to make this judgment prior to their second chemotherapy cycle. By the sixth cycle these percentages had declined slightly for the lymphoma and adjuvant breast patients (less than 6% drop), but had declined markedly for the patients with metastatic disease (to 12.5%). Was the original judgment of the patients with mestastatic disease a misperception that became a source of distress and disillusion? Will it be a source of distress and suspicion for the lymphoma and adjuvant breast patients if their disease recurs? We do not yet have answers to these questions, but it is clear that patients do not have an accurate view of their cancer or of what treatment can accomplish.

The information a patient needs to know about his or her disease can be highly distressing. Efforts to minimize this distress by giving reassurance may be inappropriate and harmful as there is the risk the patient will perceive these efforts as signs of indifference to the seriousness and enormity of his condition. No practitioner wants to appear to trivialize the patients problem, but empty reassurances can give that impression.

Although data bearing on the issue are sparse, various studies on the communication process suggest that stressful information needs to be given slowly, and the recipient needs time to assimilate it. Assimilating distressing news also means having the opportunity to ask questions and to fill in the gaps raised by questions about the impact of the disease upon one's physical, social, and economic being. It is also clear that patients may be less receptive to a variety of detailed information (e.g., about medications, appointments) if they are absorbed in and working through the implications and the feelings associated with just learning a diagnosis. Patients in the latter state often fail to hear, code, or retain other information.

Although it is clear that patients need time to adjust to the changed meaning of life given a diagnosis of cancer, it is also clear that nearly all patients have the cognitive and emotional capacity to adapt and cope with the disease. The patient is motivated to stay in control of his or her life and to minimize the intrusion of cancer.

ROLES AS BARRIERS TO COMMUNICATION

Many of the things a patient needs to know to restrict the impact of cancer on his life can be learned from other patients. But that does not detract from the physician's role in this key area. The practitioner can, at the very least, create opportunities for contact between patients by helping to establish self help groups and/or by informing patients of their existence. Many patients do not seek such contacts. But all patients are likely to appreciate and benefit from the physician's recognition of the patient's need for information and assistance in adjusting to the disease. Recognizing problems, being available if needed, suggesting that the patient consider informing key family members and/or bringing them to clinic to hear and ask questions about the patient's condition may be critical in assisting the adjustment to the disease. Bringing in key family members to ensure that they have a common understanding of the illness, its likely impact, the necessary treatment, and treatment goals can avoid a good deal of conflict and stress in the patient's role relationships.

Roles define perspectives on illness and treatment, and these perspectives may interfere with and bias communication. The biomedical orientation of the practitioner places a premium on those aspects of illness and its treatment which are related to the cellular nature of cancer. This orientation does not include concerns about the impact of the disease on activities in daily living and ability to function in roles as spouse, parent, and wage earner. Indeed, the biomedical or cellular perspective can focus the practitioner's attention to just a limited range of the impact of treatment, such as tumor mass, white cell count, and nausea and vomiting. These are of importance for monitoring the effectiveness of treatment and anticipating adverse side effects which may risk serious complications compromising the patient's life and causing reductions in treatment.

Of the aforementioned "side effects", only nausea and vomiting are likely to be noticed by the patient; he is not likely to directly feel the drop in white cell count, and for many cancers he will not feel the reductions in tumor mass that the clinician detects radiographically. On the other hand, there are side effects which may be of relatively little concern to the practitioner that are of very great concern to the patient. For example, weakness, tiredness and bone pain may lead a patient to feel sick rather than well, to believe that his or her disease is becoming increasingly serious, and that treatment is not working. Even the sensitive clinician who takes care to tell his patients about nausea and vomiting may fail to communicate about weakness, tiredness, and bone pain. Unlike nausea and vomiting, which may lead to dehydration and serious complications, weakness, tiredness, and bone pain may have little implication for treatment. If patients believe these side effects are due to progressive illness, not to treatment, they may become depressed and discouraged, and want to terminate treatment. In three studies with interviews of over 300 patients, we found virtually no one who believed nausea and vomiting were signs of advancing disease and a deteriorating condition. This was not the case for the side effects of tiredness and weakness. These more symptomatic events were related to worry about cancer for patients receiving adjuvant therapy and they were predictors of distress for patients with metastatic disease. These side effects were the obverse of the major cues used by patients to tell whether treatment is working, i.e., whether they are feeling good and energetic! In short, the relative importance of the side effects may differ from the perspective of the oncologist and the patient.

We are now testing an information package that will allow us to evaluate whether information on tiredness and weakness is beneficial. Given that there is not a great deal to do to overcome these feelings, it is not clear that making them salient will in fact be helpful! But the lesson in the contrast between nausea and tiredness is clear: different side effects and, indeed, the same side effect, may have different meaning to patient and clinician. These differences can only be discovered if communication is open and the physician takes the time to ask the patient whether he or she has questions about the meaning of any of the treatment effects or any of the things he or she is experiencing. Explicit recognition of the difference in perception from the two perspectives (e.g., "Do you have any questions about the different side effects of the drugs? I know they may seem different from the patient's point of view than from mine.") could facilitate communication.

The degree to which communication can be attenuated was brought home to us in the analysis of our most recent study. We were analyzing the responses of some 188 patients whom we have interviewed five times over six chemotherapy cycles. To our surprise, 40 percent of these patients said they had thought about quitting treatment. These thoughts were expressed, however, only to our interviewers! Fewer than 2 percent of the patients had mentioned these thoughts to their oncologist. While we do not know that patients suffered because they did not share these thoughts with their oncologist, we strongly suspect they were motivated not to relate them because they did not want to seem unappreciative or risk any possibility of rejection, no matter how slight! It is not easy to talk to an authority, and it is especially difficult to say things that you know may meet with disapproval. The finding was especially surprising to us, given the very attentive care and extraordinarily positive view of the cancer center and its practitioners voiced by our patients.

The role concept, particularly the idea that each of us lives multiple, overlapping roles, is critical to keep in mind if communication is to be successful. The patient's family may or may not hold the same view of treatment as does the patient: the procedures, sensory experiences, and coping suggestion, and expectations of treatment outcome are often different. This means that the patient receives information that contrasts with that coming from the medical care system which could be a source of concern and distress and even lead to doubts about the treatment plan and thoughts of discontinuing treatment.

ENDOCRINE AND METABOLIC DISORDERS

DIABETES INSIPIDUS

NED M. WEISS, M.D.
GARY L. ROBERTSON, M.D.

Diabetes insipidus is a disorder characterized by the excretion of abnormally large volumes (>2.5 liters/day) of dilute urine. It is caused by a deficiency of the antidiuretic hormone, arginine vasopressin, and can result from any of several different kinds of pathology (trauma, tumors, granulomas, infection, autoimmunity, idiopathic) that invade and/or destroy the neurohypophysis. In most patients with diabetes insipidus, the thirst mechanism operates normally. Hence, if given unrestricted access to water, they will always drink enough to replenish losses (polydipsia) and maintain nearly normal hydration. However, they are extremely bothered by the frequent thirst and urination and may suffer from chronic sleep deprivation as a result of nocturia. Moreover, if present for many years, the polyuria may lead to chronic dilation of the urinary tract with hydronephrosis, infection, and renal dysfunction. Thus, the goal of therapy is to reduce urinary flow to an acceptable level (usually <2.5 liters/day) by improving urinary concentration.

THERAPEUTIC ALTERNATIVES

The agents available for the treatment of diabetes insipidus can be divided into two categories. The first consists of several preparations of vasopressin, or analogs thereof, that are given as a form of hormonal replacement. The second consists of a variety of unrelated oral agents, primarily used to treat other disorders, that have been serendipitously found to be effective in diabetes insipidus.

Hormonal Replacement

Hormonal replacement is the conventional way of treating diabetes insipidus. The available agents are either injected or absorbed from the nasal mucosa. Several different preparations have been approved for use in the United States.

Pitressin tannate in oil was the standard hormonal replacement for many years. It is a synthetic form of vasopressin suspended in peanut oil. When injected intramuscularly in doses of 5 to 10 units, it affords prompt relief of polyuria lasting from 1 to 4 days. However, the duration of the antidiuresis may vary because of inadequate mixture of the suspension prior to its use. Occasionally, patients develop antibodies to the hormone which can lead to resistance to its antidiuretic effects. Because of these limitations and the discomfort and possible complications associated with intramuscular injections, the use of Pitressin Tannate in Oil has been largely superseded by other preparations in recent years. An *aqueous solution of synthetic vasopressin* is also available for parenteral use. However, when given by injection (IM or subcutaneously), its duration of action (1 to 2 hours) is too short to be convenient for chronic treatment. When infused intravenously (5 to 10 μU/kg/min), it may be useful in the short-term management of postoperative diabetes insipidus or for several diagnostic tests of antidiuretic function. However, in this setting, great care must be exercised to avoid accidental overdoses, which can produce severe abdominal cramping, vomiting, cutaneous vasoconstriction, and possibly hypertension or coronary ischemia as a consequence of its constrictive effects on smooth muscle of the intestines and blood vessels. *Synthetic 8-lysine vasopressin* is available as a nasal spray (Diapid). Its antidiuretic effects begin rapidly, but last only 4 to 6 hours, making it impractical for routine use.

Desmopressin (DDAVP-USV) is a synthetic analog of vasopressin in which the L-arginine in position 8 has been replaced with the dextro-isomer and the N-terminal amino group has been removed. These structural modifications enhance antidiuretic potency, eliminate smooth muscle effects, and significantly delay degradation of the hormone. The last-mentioned effect is responsible for a longer duration of action (8 to 24 hours). Desmopressin is available in two forms, one for nasal insufflation and the other for parenteral injection. The duration of action is the same in both forms, but the parenteral form is absorbed more efficiently and requires smaller doses. In most cases, 10 to 25 μg intranasally *bid* or 2 to 4 μg subcutaneously *bid* of the injectable form of desmopressin affords complete relief of polyuria. In a few patients the condition can be controlled with only one dose per day. Since the analog is largely devoid of pressor or other smooth muscle effects, it has virtually no toxicity. To date, antibody-mediated resistance to its antidiuretic effect has not been demonstrated. The presence of rhinitis and/or sinusitis may interfere with the absorption of the intranasal form and thus diminish its effectiveness. The main drawback to desmopressin is its high cost. Currently, one year of treatment costs an average of $2000 compared to $250 for the other commonly used agents.

Nonhormonal Oral Agents

Several nonhormonal oral drugs are also effective in controlling the polyuria in diabetes insipidus. These drugs have several advantages over vasopressin and its analogs because they are easier to administer and provide smoother and more predictable control of the polyuria. They also permit greater modulation of urinary output in response to fluctuations in water intake. However, they have the disadvantage of producing a weaker antidiuresis in some patients and the potential for more serious side effects and toxicities. The following drugs have significant antidiuretic effect in patients with diabetes insipidus.

Chlorpropamide (Diabinese) is an oral sulfonylurea used primarily to treat patients with type II diabetes mellitus. When it is given in a single daily dose of 250 to 500 mg, urine volume in patients with diabetes insipidus is invariably reduced by 25 to 75 percent (average 50%). Coincident with this reduction in urine volume, there is a proportionate rise in urine osmolality and improved hydration, as evidenced by a return in plasma osmolality to normal and an increase in body weight. The antidiuretic response to chlorpropamide varies considerably from patient to patient, and this variability seems to be independent of the etiology and severity of the diabetes insipidus. Many patients with severe if not complete diabetes insipidus respond as well if not better than others with partial deficiencies of the hormone. The mechanism of its antidiuretic action is unclear, but is most likely due to a direct action on the kidney since the bulk of the evidence now indicates that it does not promote the secretion of vasopressin from the neurohypophysis. A single oral dose usually takes effect within 1 to 2 hours and last for 2 to 3 days. However, if the patient has recently been treated with vasopressin, the full antidiuretic effect of chlorpropamide may not be manifested for as long as 10 days. The magnitude of the antidiuretic response is proportional to the amount of chlorpropamide administered, but doses in excess of 750 mg are associated with an unacceptable incidence of side effects and toxicity. When urinary volume cannot be reduced to asymptomatic levels with chlorpropamide alone, addition of a thiazide diuretic often does so (to be discussed). Like vasopressin, chlorpropamide has no antidiuretic effect in patients with nephrogenic diabetes insipidus.

The most troublesome side effects of chlorpropamide are hypoglycemic symptoms. It should not be given to children or to patients with coexisting defects in anterior pituitary function because they are particularly likely to develop severe hypoglycemia. Calorie restriction or severe exercise also accentuates the hypoglycemic effects of the drug. It is contraindicated in pregnancy because of its possible teratogenic effects. A relatively infrequent side effect is flushing induced by ingestion of alcoholic beverages. It is usually of minor inconvenience and rarely requires discontinuing the chlorpropamide. The other oral hypoglycemic drugs of the sulfonylurea class cannot be substituted for chlorpropamide because they are devoid of significant antidiuretic activity.

Carbamazepine (Tegretol) is an anticonvulsant medication most commonly used to treat several types of seizure disorders. When given in divided doses higher than 700 to 800 mg/day, it also reduces urine output, increases urinary concentration, and improves bodily hydration in patients with neurogenic diabetes insipidus. At a dose of 1000 mg/day, its antidiuretic potency is equivalent to that of chlorpropamide, with which it probably shares a common mechanism of action. At this dose, however, carbamazepine is also more liable to produce a number of serious side effects including ataxia, diplopia, jaundice, aplastic anemia, and cardiovascular collapse. Therefore, because equally effective yet safer agents are available, carbamazepine is rarely used to treat diabetes insipidus in the United States. However, it might be an appropriate choice in a patient with diabetes insipidus and a coexisting seizure disorder. Like vasopressin and chlorpropamide, carbamazepine has no antidiuretic effect in patients with nephrogenic diabetes insipidus.

Clofibrate (Atromid-S) is an oral drug commonly used to treat certain hyperlipidemic conditions. When given to patients with diabetes insipidus in divided doses of 1 to 2 g/day, it also reduces urine output, increases urinary concentration, and improves bodily hydration. Its mechanism of action is probably similar to that of chlorpropamide, but its antidiuretic effect is less potent. Because of this latter fact and its potential for serious long-term side effects (cholelithiasis and increased frequency of cardiovascular complications in patients with coronary artery disease), this drug is used infrequently to treat diabetes insipidus. It, too, is totally ineffective in patients with nephrogenic diabetes insipidus.

Thiazide diuretics have a paradoxical effect to reduce urinary output in patients with diabetes insipidus. They have a similar effect in patients with nephrogenic and dipsogenic diabetes insipidus and are thought to act, in part, by impairing urinary dilution in the distal nephron. The mechanism by which this leads to a reduction in urine volume is unclear, but may involve a secondary increase in the reabsorption of filtrate in the proximal tubules. Several thiazide preparations are now available on the market and are equally effective in reducing polyuria when given in the usual recommended doses. Because their antidiuretic potency is usually insufficient to reduce urinary output to asymptomatic levels, the thiazides are almost always used in combination with chlorpropamide in neurogenic diabetes insipidus (to be discussed). Thiazides have few toxic side effects apart from hypokalemia, hyperuricemia, and impaired carbohydrate tolerance which occasionally occur. It is important to exclude dipsogenic diabetes insipidus before prescribing thiazides because life-threatening water intoxication may result when they are given to patients with this disorder. In patients with nephrogenic diabetes insipidus, thiazides and salt restriction constitute the only form of therapy, since none of the various hormonal preparations or oral agents are effective in this disorder.

PREFERRED APPROACH

Before instituting therapy, it is usually best to determine whether the patient has neurogenic, nephrogenic, or dipsogenic diabetes insipidus because drugs commonly used to treat the first-mentioned may be ineffective or dangerous if used in the latter two conditions (to be discussed). Accurate diagnosis may require direct assay of vasopressin because the conventional indirect methods are unreliable for differentiating between partial defects in vasopressin secretion or action and dipsogenic diabetes insipidus. Diagnostic evaluation should also include a careful search for the etiology of the diabetes insipidus because it often involves another disorder, such as a tumor or sarcoidosis, which requires additional therapy. Anterior pituitary function should also be thoroughly evaluated because deficiencies of one or more of these hormones often accompany diabetes insipidus. In addition to requiring treatment in its own right, anterior pituitary failure may mask the severity or complicate the treatment of the polyuria.

Once the diagnostic studies are complete, the choice of therapy depends on a number of factors including the patient's age and associated medical or surgical conditions. Generally speaking, children, pregnant women, and patients with ACTH or growth hormone deficiency are treated exclusively with desmopressin. Treatment is initiated with a single dose of 10 μg intranasally at bedtime and increased to a maximum of 10 to 25 μg once or twice daily as needed to control polyuria. During the early phases of treatment, close monitoring for signs of water intoxication (excessive weight gain, hyponatremia) is necessary because some patients with longstanding diabetes insipidus continue to ingest large amounts of water for several days after antidiuresis is restored. In the presence of rhinitis or other conditions that interfere with absorption of DDAVP from the nasal mucosa, the parenteral form of the drug can be given until the condition abates.

Injectable desmopressin is also the preferred treatment in patients who develop acute diabetes insipidus after surgery or trauma. At the first appearance of polyuria, 2 to 4 μg of the drug should be injected subcutaneously and repeated every 12 to 24 hours or as often as needed to keep urine flow below 100 ml/hour. Intake, output, and plasma sodium should be monitored with particular care in this setting because the concurrent administration of intravenous fluids greatly increases the chances of water intoxication. After 7 to 10 days of such treatment, DDAVP should be discontinued for 24 to 48 hours to determine whether the diabetes insipidus was transient, as it often is following transphenoidal or other pituitary surgery. If polyuria does not recur, anterior pituitary function should be evaluated to ascertain that concomitant deficiency of ACTH or TSH is not masking the effects of vasopressin deficiency. If the polyuria recurs, the patient should undergo the usual evaluation as soon as other medical and surgical conditions permit.

Apart from these special circumstances, the choice of treatment should be dictated largely by patient preference. If oral therapy is selected, we start with chlorpropamide, 250 mg once a day. If satisfactory control of the polyuria is not achieved within 3 to 10 days, the dose is increased to 500 mg daily. This regimen provides satisfactory control of the polyuria (<3 liters/day) in slightly more than 50 percent of all patients with diabetes insipidus. In the remainder, satisfactory control is almost always achieved by addition of hydrochlorthiazide, 25 mg once or twice daily. If not, or if unmanageable side effects occur, the patient may be switched to desmopressin. Whatever the drug, however, the initial stages of therapy should be closely monitored (in hospital, if necessary) to document the response and observe for the development of water intoxication or other side effects (already discussed). Long-term management should include follow-up outpatient visits at least once a year to adjust drug doses and check for chronic side effects. Once established, vasopressin deficiency does not improve. Therefore, a decrease in therapeutic requirements for antidiuretic therapy should always point to possible progression of disease to involvement of other systems, particularly the pituitary adrenal axis or the thirst mechanism.

Suggested Reading

Berndt WO, Miller M, Kettyle WM, Valtin H. Potentiation of the antidiuretic effect of vasopressin by chlorpropamide. Endocrinology 1970; 86:1028.

Cobb WE, Spare S, Reichlin S. Neurogenic diabetes insipidus: management with DDAVP (1-Desamino-8-D arginine vasopressin). Ann Intern Med 1978; 88:183–188.

Meinders AE, van Leeuwen AM, De Vries LA. Antidiuretic effect of chlorpropamide. Folia Med Neerl 1969; 12:58–68.

Pokracki FJ, Robinson AG, Seif SM. Chlorpropamide effect: measurement of neurophysin and vasopressin in humans and rats. Metabolism 1981; 30:72–78.

Robertson GL. Diseases of the Posterior Pituitary. In: Felig P, Baxter JD, Broadus AE, Frohman LA, eds. Endocrinology and Metabolism. New York: McGraw Hill, 1981.

Vavra I, Machova A, Holecek V, Cort JH, Zaoral M, Sorm F. Effect of synthetic analogue of vasopressin in animals and in patients with diabetes insipidus. Lancet 1968; 1:948–952.

Webster B, Bain J. Antidiuretic effect and complications of chlorpropamide therapy in diabetes insipidus. J Clin Endocrinol Metab 1970; 30:215–227.

HYPOPITUITARISM

JOHANNES D. VELDHUIS, M.D.

Hypopituitarism embraces a spectrum of hormonal deficits, which range from isolated or monotropic deficiencies to panhypopituitarism. These deficits may have an abrupt onset or develop gradually over a period of years. Although individual hormonal deficiencies may develop in any order, progressive hypopituitarism classically evolves from sequential insufficiency of growth hormone (deficiency of which is largely asymptomatic in the adult), gonadotropic hormones, thyroid stimulating hormone (TSH), and/or adrenocorticotropic hormone (ACTH). Diminished prolactin secretion is typically asymptomatic, and its exact prevalence has not been thoroughly characterized. Hyperprolactinemia may actually be present in some cases of hypopituitarism associated with pituitary tumors. Thus, there is a wide range of clinical presentations for hypopituitarism, reflecting both the rate and the multiplicity of endocrine deficits that evolve in any individual.

Before hypopituitarism can be treated, the underlying etiology must be understood. Endocrine treatment usually results in the adequate physiologic replacement of hormones, but the underlying disease process producing hypopituitarism may create other serious problems. For example, expanding mass lesions in the region of the hypothalamus or pituitary can result in visual field deficits, extraocular nerve palsies, and hypothalamic syndromes. Alternatively, an underlying generalized disease such as metastatic carcinoma, vasculitis, or sarcoidosis may be progressive, with consequent morbidity or mortality arising from nonendocrine aspects of the illness. Thus, I believe that a clear knowledge of the cause of hypopituitarism is necessary, so that underlying diseases can be evaluated and treated appropriately. Thereafter, suitable endocrine replacement therapy can be organized according to the endocrine deficits recognized. Even so, patients must be monitored periodically to ascertain whether additional hormonal replacement becomes necessary as further deterioration of pituitary function occurs.

Fractional hypopituitarism can coexist with pituitary tumors that secrete excess glycoprotein or polypeptide hormones. For example, prolactin-secreting macroadenomas of the pituitary gland, growth hormone-secreting pituitary tumors, or pituitary-dependent Cushing's disease can be associated with partial hypopituitarism. (Partial hypopituitarism may typically involve the secretion of gonadotropins, growth hormone, or TSH.) In addition, such functioning pituitary tumors occasionally undergo spontaneous hemorrhagic infarction (apoplexy), with consequent acute or delayed development of partial hypopituitarism or panhypopituitarism. Pituitary apoplexy—which is usually heralded by headache, visual disturbances associated with symptoms of subarachnoid hemorrhage, and rapid reappearance of endocrine deficits—calls for urgent endocrine evaluation and treatment. Thus, hypopituitarism may coexist chronically with hypersecretion of other anterior pituitary hormones or develop acutely in the setting of a nonfunctioning pituitary tumor, which may or may not have been recognized earlier.

GENERAL CONSIDERATIONS

In general, patients with hypopituitarism can be treated effectively by providing an injectable or oral form of the hormonal product of the respective endocrine target gland, e.g., testosterone in the case of LH deficiency. In other cases, it is possible to administer the pituitary tropic hormone that is deficient. At present, hypothalamic peptides are not approved for clinical replacement therapy, but exciting preliminary clinical experience with gonadotropin-releasing hormone and growth hormone-releasing factor suggests that administration of these peptides may permit selective replacement of the correspondingly deficient hypothalamic peptides. Further research is under way to assess whether long-term intranasal instillation of hypothalamic peptides might be practical and effective.

TREATMENT OF SPECIFIC HORMONE DEFICIENCIES

Adrenocorticotropic Hormone (ACTH) Deficiency

Instructions to the Patient. All patients with established ACTH/cortisol deficiency should receive an identification card, bracelet, or pendant (Medi-Alert of Life Guard, Maurer Metal Specialties, Box 2493, Springfield, IL 62705) as well as injectable glucocorticoid for emergency use. Preassembled syringes of dexamethasone, 4 mg per ml, or 100 mg hydrocortisone phosphate or hemisuccinate (Solu-Cortef; Mix-O-Vial) are available. Patients with hypoadrenalism should be instructed in self-injection technique, so that they can receive additional glucocorticoid promptly after major stress or trauma, or if vomiting prevents oral intake.

For minor febrile illnesses (e.g., bladder or upper respiratory infections), the daily maintenance dose of glucocorticoid can be doubled until fever and acute symptoms resolve and remain so for 48 hours. Patients should be advised to seek medical assistance promptly whenever more serious systemic, traumatic, prostrating, or debilitating illnesses occur. For example, sustained vomiting, bacteremia, stroke, myocardial infarction, or other major illnesses require prompt hospitalization with an increase in daily hydrocortisone equivalent to 100 to 200 mg per day.

Maintenance Replacement. Symptoms and signs of cortisol deficiency appear within 12 to 36 hours of acute hormone deprivation, although low basal levels may support life in the absence of superimposed infection, surgery, or trauma. Glucocorticoid (rather than ACTH) constitutes preferred replacement therapy, because ACTH can cause allergic reactions and must be given by injection. The daily maintenance dose of oral cortisone acetate in adult patients is approximately 25 mg each morning and 12.5 mg each evening, or of hydrocortisone, 7.5 to 10 mg every 8 hours. A hydrocortisone schedule of three doses per day is suggested because of the relatively short biologic half-life of this steroid, although for some patients 20 mg in the morning and 10 mg 12 hours later provide adequate replacement.

In children, hydrocortisone administration should approximate the secretion rate of 12 (±3) mg per square meter per day, which is given in distributed doses, recognizing that patients typically require twice this dosage to account for incomplete oral absorption. Excessive glucocorticoid replacement should be avoided to ensure normal height progression in growing children. Although synthetic steroids such as dexamethasone, prednisone, and prednisolone have been commonly used as maintenance therapy, the metabolism of these compounds (but not of cortisone acetate or hydrocortisone) may be altered several-fold by other drugs administered concurrently (e.g., phenytoins, phenobarbital). Consequently, the dosages of such synthetic steroids required may vary markedly among different patients or in the same patient. For this reason, I prefer using hydrocortisone or cortisone acetate in most patients.

Adrenal Crisis. Acute adrenal insufficiency requires immediate parenteral (preferably intravenous) soluble glucocorticoid injection, e.g., IV hydrocortisone hemisuccinate (Solu-Cortef), 100 mg bolus, with additional doses thereafter (to be discussed). Cortisol replacement should be accompanied by intravascular volume restoration with dextrose in isotonic saline (without potassium initially) to replace sodium deficits and to avert hypoglycemia, which can occur in addisonian crises. Vigorous attention should be directed toward defining and treating any precipitating event (e.g., lobar pneumonia, pyelonephritis, perforated duodenal ulcer, myocardial infarction). Intravenous hydrocortisone infusion is continued at doses of 50 to 100 mg every 6 hours until resolution of the underlying illness, and then reduced by approximately 50 percent every 24 to 48 hours to oral maintenance levels.

Intramuscular cortisone acetate is not recommended as sole therapy under acute or urgent circumstances because it is absorbed slowly. Mineralocorticoid replacement is often not required in patients with panhypopituitarism (in contrast to primary Addison's disease), since aldosterone synthesis and release mechanisms are relatively intact. Furthermore, when doses of 300 to 400 mg per day of hydrocortisone or cortisone acetate are used (as in addisonian crisis), these glucocorticoids provide significant mineralocorticoid activity. Accordingly, combined treatment with saline and large amounts of hydrocortisone acting as mineralocorticoid can result in hypokalemia through renal sodium-potassium exchange in the distal tubule. Thus, during acute treatment, I recommend that electrolytes be monitored frequently as volume repletion is achieved.

Elective Surgery. For general anesthesia or major surgery, I administer 100 mg cortisone acetate intramuscularly (a long-acting preparation) the evening before surgery and 100 mg of hydrocortisone hemisuccinate (Solu-Cortef) intravenously immediately preoperatively and another 100 mg intraoperatively. Postoperatively, 50-mg intravenous infusions (or bolus injections) of hydrocortisone hemisuccinate should be continued at 6-hour intervals. This dose may be reduced by 50 percent the next day and again every 24 to 48 hours by a similar amount. Maintenance therapy is resumed when the patient is eating and afebrile. Persistence of low-grade fever should prompt evaluation for infection or thrombophlebitis and continuation of approximately 40 to 80 mg of hydrocortisone per day. If major postoperative complications arise or reoperation is necessary, resumption of larger amounts of glucocorticoid are required with the dosage decided on an individual basis.

As summarized in Table 1, ACTH/cortisol deficiency can represent one of the most urgent problems in hypopituitarism. Replacement of other hormonal deficits (to be discussed) is typically *less* an emergency.

TABLE 1 Relative Urgency for Endocrine Therapy in Acute Hypopituitarism*

Hormone(s)	*Urgency*
ACTH cortisol	Replace immediately (within hours) or Addisonian crisis may ensue.
ADH (vasopressin)	Replace when diabetes insipidus is documented. Use aqueous or synthetic ADH if permanent ADH deficiency is not certain.
TSH thyroxine†	Replace within hours to days (thyroxine half-life is approximately 1 week).
LH and FSH, testerosterone	Not life-threatening. Replace when endocrine emergency is stabilized.
Growth hormone, prolactin, β-lipotropin	No replacement currently indicated and/ or available in adults.

* E.g. after pituitary surgery or acute pituitary apoplexy. See text for special precautions re perioperative management.

† Caution: Do not begin thyroxine replacement until/unless ACTH/ cortisol deficiency is excluded or treated. Otherwise, an Addisonian crisis can be precipitated by increased metabolic demands superimposed upon diminished adrenal glucocorticoid reserve.

Thyroid-Stimulating Hormone (TSH) Deficiency

In patients with thyrotropin deficiency, a careful evaluation for coexistent glucocorticoid (ACTH) deficiency is necessary before thyroid replacement is initiated. *Augmentation of metabolic demands by starting thyroxine treatment while adrenal insufficiency is untreated could otherwise precipitate adrenal crisis.* This is of particular practical significance since isolated TSH deficiency is rare (reported sporadically and in association with pseudohypoparathyroidism), and hence unlikely to occur without other pituitary deficit(s).

A single daily dose of levothyroxine provides sustained, uniform, and predictable thyroid-hormone replacement. Adults require approximately 1.5–2 μg/ kg/day or 0.075 to 0.15 mg (range: 0.075 to 0.20 mg) daily. The lower dose range is appropriate in elderly patients. In children, 3 to 5 μg/kg/day of L-thyroxine approximates requirements. Adequacy of treatment can be confirmed by measurements of serum thyroxine levels assessed by age-adjusted norms and clinical examination. Unlike the situation in primary hypothyroidism, suppression of TSH levels cannot be employed to ascertain adequacy of replacement. On the other hand, triiodothyronine (T_3) as well as thyroxine (T_4) levels by radioimmunoassay should remain within the normal range during replacement with L-thyroxine alone, since the preponderance of endogenous T_3 derives from extrathyroid conversion of T_4 to T_3 (by 5″ monodeiodination) rather than from direct glandular secretion. In rare cases, patients manifest a T_4-to-T_3 conversion defect (the T_3 level is inappropriately low with a normal T_4), which can be corrected with triiodothyronine to achieve euthyroidism.

Triiodothyronine (Cytomel) exhibits a shorter half-life than L-thyroxine and therefore requires daily administration in divided doses: e.g., 25 μg orally three times daily in adults (range: 50 to 100 μg per day or 1 μg/kg/day in children). Serum T_3, rather than T_4, must be determined by radioimmunoassay to assess adequacy of hormone replacement, since T_3 is not back-converted to T_4.

Dessicated thyroid preparations are less desirable because of variable bipotency (inconstant T_4-T_3 ratios). If employed, the dose is 1 to 2 grains (60 to 120 mg) per day.

I would emphasize that tests of circulating thyroid hormone levels must be correlated with clinical parameters. The physician should not rely solely on the laboratory as a final arbiter of appropriate dosage. In addition, therapy should be started slowly in older patients, particularly those with known or suspected ischemic or arrhythmic heart disease. In these instances, one-eighth the usual replacement dosage is initiated and gradual increments made over a 3-month period, e.g., start with 25 μg L-thyroxine per day and increase by 25 μg every 3 to 4 weeks if angina or arrhythmias are not exacerbated.

Although the tripeptide, TSH-releasing hormone, is available for diagnostic studies, at present it has no practical utility in selective replacement in hypothalamic hypothyroidism.

Gonadotropin Deficiency

Monotropic Deficiency. Isolated FSH deficiency is exceedingly rare, and purified human FSH for selective replacement is not generally available. Monotropic LH deficiency may occur within the spectrum of hypogonadotropic hypogonadism as the "fertile eunuch" syndrome. Because of ready availability, human chorionic gonadotropin (hCG), not human luteinizing hormone (LH), is used as replacement therapy. Both hormones stimulate Leydig cell production of testosterone with suitable efficacy in males. However, in view of the cost and frequency of administration, direct replacement of testosterone (to be discussed) can be accomplished more practically than hCG administration (see Table 2).

Bihormonal Gonadotropin Deficiency. Gonadotropin deficiency may arise in the setting of partial or panhypopituitarism from a variety of causes, or in Kallmann's syndrome. Kallmann's syndrome is diagnosed when isolated hypogonadotropic hypogonadism occurs in males (or, less often in females) with anosmia, hyposmia, sometimes with a family history of infertility, delayed puberty or hypogonadism, or midline facial defects. Treatment of both sex-steroid deficiency and infertility should be considered in these conditions. In the future, selective replacement therapy with pulses of hypothalamic gonadotropin-releasing factor (GnRH) may be the treatment of choice for Kallmann's syndrome, which is believed to be caused by isolated GnRH deficiency. This approach is not yet approved for general clinical use, but holds promise as a means of restoring a virtually normal pituitary-gonadal axis.

TABLE 2 Therapy in Clinical Hypogonadism in Men

Treatment	*Advantages*	*Disadvantages*
1. Pulsatile Administration of GnRH	Can promote full physiologic responses and maturation of the gonadal axis	Not effective if pituitary or gonad is unresponsive; inconvenient because circhoral pulses are needed; not yet approved for use
2. Combined human LH and FSH injections (Pergonal)	Can restore fertility and androgen deficiency	Very costly; LH and FSH not individually available
3. hCG injections (500–2000 IU TIW)	Effectively acts as LH on testis; increases intra-testicular testosterone levels (hence useful to preserve fertility in some patients)	Injections are required twice or thrice weekly; relatively costly
4. Testosterone enanthate injections (200–300 mg IM q 2–3 wks)	Relatively inexpensive; given every 2–3 weeks; fully replaces androgen deficiency	Does not restore fertility; injections required
5. *Fluoxymesterone* (5–10 mg PO *bid*)	Orally active	May not restore full androgen potential; given at least daily

Treatment of testosterone deficiency in the adult may be accomplished by using an injectable repository ester of this steroid, e.g., testosterone enanthate in doses of 200 mg intramuscularly every 2 weeks, or 300 mg intramuscularly every 3 weeks (for details see chapter on *Hypogonadism: Androgen Therapy*). At the outset of therapy, serum testosterone levels should be monitored just prior to the next dose to help adjust the frequency of administration and thus maintain "trough" levels of this hormone within the normal adult male range.

The hypopituitary pubertal boy should receive correspondingly lower doses than an adult initially, e.g., 50 to 75 mg intramuscularly each month, in order to promote pubertal progression and minimize premature epiphyseal closure. Alternately, in the absence of associated testicular disease, exogenous hCG in doses of 500 to 2000 USP units three times per week intramuscularly will induce testosterone production and progressive male secondary sexual development. Clinical indices of androgenization and testosterone levels should be monitored at 2- or 3-month intervals to assess endogenous steroid production. The decision when to treat boys with hypopituitarism is beyond the scope of this chapter.

Undesired effects may occur during testosterone replacement, including gynecomastia, extracellular fluid retention, acne, and rarely prostatic hypertrophy with lower urinary tract obstruction (particularly in elderly men). In men with existing prostatic enlargement, a short-acting oral androgen preparation such as fluoxymesterone (5 to 10 mg per day) is appropriate for the first months of replacement, since this androgen can be stopped rapidly. However, in other circumstances, available oral preparations may not provide the clinical effects of full androgenic replacement. No androgen should be given if prostatic cancer is present or suspected.

When fertility is the therapeutic goal, replacement with pituitary hormones or their equivalent is necessary. Treatment is usually initiated with 500 to 2000 USP units of hCG three times per week intramuscularly. In patients with only a mild or relative deficiency of FSH, seminiferous tubular maturation and fertility can ensue after hCG treatment alone. However, if FSH levels are extremely low, a preparation containing this hormone (Pergonal, menotropins) may be required to provide concordant Leydig cell and seminiferous tubular stimulation. A reasonable clinical approach is to treat with hCG alone (1500 IU twice weekly) for 6 to 12 months, and thereafter add an FSH-containing preparation (25 to 35 IU/day) if needed. (The details are discussed in the chapter on *Hypogonadotropic Hypogonadism: Gonadotropin Therapy*). Such therapy is usually administered by an experience endocrinologist. In some cases of fractional hypopituitarism associated with pituitary tumors, concurrent hyperprolactinemia is present, which should be treated first before androgen replacement because in certain patients the gonadal axis recovers as prolactin levels decline.

In females, cyclic administration of sex steroids will induce withdrawal menses. Fewer adverse effects occur with lower doses of estrogens given as 20 to 30 μg ethinyl estradiol per day. A combination oral contraceptive may be employed. Alternately, daily oral conjugated estrogens, 0.625 to 1.25 mg (e.g., Premarin), or ethinyl estradiol, 20- to 50-μg tablets, for day 1 through 25 of each cycle may be used with the addition of 5 mg (1/2 tablet) or 10 mg (1 tablet) of medroxyprogesterone acetate on days 16 through 25. This schedule should result in cyclical withdrawal bleeding and protect the endometrium from unopposed estrogen effects. In peripubertal girls with hypopituitarism, initial replacement should include estrogen alone for 6 to 12 months to stimulate uterine and secondary sexual maturation (e.g., 0.625 mg of conjugated estrogens or 20 μg ethinyl estradiol on a continuous daily regimen). Thereafter, cyclic hormonal replacement is appropriate.

During long-term replacement, periodic (i.e., annual) endometrial biopsies should be considered as a means of monitoring endometrial hyperplasia, which can arise as a result of excessive estrogen doses. This precaution is warranted in light of recent evidence linking estrogen replacement therapy to endometrial carcinoma.

Pregnancy may be accomplished in bihormonal hypogonadotropism or in panhypopituitarism. A combination of human FSH and LH purified from postmenopausal urine is available as menotropins (Pergonal) for intramuscular administration. This treatment is costly. One major possible side effect of this therapy is ovarian hyperstimulation, which is associated with painful ovarian enlargement, ascites, pleural effusion, or ruptured ovarian cysts. Multifetation (usually twinning) develops in approximately 20 percent of patients and has resulted occasionally in live births of quintuplets and sextuplets. During ovulation induction, current practice requires frequent measurements of estrogens, and ovarian ultrasonography. The specialized laboratory support necessary for such monitoring limits use of ovulation induction to centers experienced in the administration of gonadotropic hormones.

As typical therapy, 1 to 3 ampules of Pergonal (75 IU FSH, 75 IU LH per ampule) are injected intramuscularly daily until follicular maturation is indicated by serum estradiol levels exceeding 350 to 500 picograms per ml (or total urinary estrogens exceeding 10 μg daily) and single-follicle development is complete by ultrasonography, or until 12 doses have been administered. Pergonal is stopped if there is any clinical, ovarian, biochemical, or sonographic evidence of hyperstimulation. Five or ten thousand USP units of hCG are then injected intramuscularly to induce ovulation. The latter event should be assessed by ultrasonography and serum progesterone or urinary pregnanediol determinations, by basal body temperature measurements, and by clinical evaluation of vaginal cytology and cervical mucus. Coitus is recommended on alternate days in proximity to anticipated ovulation.

Human Growth Hormone Deficiency

Human growth hormone (hGH) obtained from cadaver sources is available through the National Pituitary Agency for authorized research protocols or commercially (e.g., Serono, Calbio, or Kaby Pharmaceuticals). Genentech Inc. will soon provide synthetic hGH for clinical use. Moreover, studies are in progress to evaluate the utility of recently isolated hGH-releasing factor in clinical practice.

Unambiguous human growth hormone deficiency must be documented before treatment is begun, using two or more provocative tests. Adults do not require hGH replacement, but in children the principal indications are hypoglycemia, which is related to diminished gluconeogenetic substrate mobilization, and statural deficits prior to epiphyseal closure (bone age 15 or 16 years). Human growth hormone (hGH) is usually administered as 1 to 2 units intramuscularly three times each week. Precise height measurements and serum somatomedin C levels at 3-month intervals permit assessment of skeletal and hepatic responses. Height velocity may initially exhibit a ''catch-up'' increment exceeding norms adjusted for corresponding bone age. Subsequent height velocity approximates that of normal patients of equivalent bone age. Resistance to currently available human growth hormone is rare. Although antibody development does occur commonly, neutralization of hGH bioactivity is infrequent. Thus, if response to therapy is poor, other causes should be sought including intercurrent hypothyroidism (which may develop during hGH therapy and resolve with cessation of treatment); excessive or deficient cortisol replacement; premature epiphyseal closure, such as that related to overzealous sex steroid replacement; or nonendocrinologic systemic disease (e.g., sprue, renal disease).

Optimal preservation of the pubertal growth spurt requires continuation of hGH treatment during sexual maturation, whether spontaneous or induced.

Prolactin Deficiency

Rare families with asymptomatic isolated prolactin deficiency have been reported (e.g., in pseudohypoparathyroidism), but in most other cases pluritropic hypopituitarism is present. Exogenous human prolactin is not available for administration, nor are specific physiologic indications defined for its replacement.

Beta-Lipotropin

Isolated deficiency of β-lipotropin has not been reported. No replacement therapy is available or suggested.

Antidiuretic Hormone (ADH) Deficiency

Deficiency of antidiuretic hormone (ADH) most often implies a lesion in the supraoptic and paraventricular nuclei or the medium eminence of the hypothalamus, respective sites of neuronal synthesis and transport of ADH. Disease confined to the posterior lobe frequently permits continued ADH secretion by residual axons of the neurohypophyseal tract.

ADH replacement is discussed in detail in the chapter on *Diabetes Insipidus*.

Suggested Reading

Carter JN, et al. Prolactin-secreting pituitary tumors and hypogonadism in 22 men. N Engl J Med 1978; 299:847.

Costin G. Endocrine disorders associated with tumors of the pituitary and hypothalamus. Pediatr Clin North Am 1979; 26:1.

Veldhuis JD, Hammond JM. Endocrine function after spontaneous infarction of the human pituitary: Report, review, and reappraisal. Endocr Rev 1980; 1:100–107.

NONFUNCTIONING PITUITARY ADENOMA

BERNARD KLIMAN, M.D.
RAYMOND N. KJELLBERG, M.D.

CLINICAL PROBLEM

The most insidious type of pituitary gland tumor is the nonfunctioning pituitary adenoma since it is not heralded at an early stage by excess hormonal secretion and usually presents as an advanced mass lesion. Endocrine disturbances may develop at a late stage when normal pituitary functions are grossly impaired having failed to attract attention earlier because of the subtle nature of initial defects in growth hormone and gonadotropin secretion. Unlike craniopharyngioma, this tumor is rare in childhood so that growth failure is not a clinical feature. In several adolescent cases we have seen, delayed puberty was the first clinical warning. Adults may experience gonadotropin deficiency, but often elude diagnosis at this stage since they are tested either for alterations in serum prolactin levels, with negative results, or for serum gonadotropin levels, which may not be diagnostic owing to the pulsatile nature of follide-stimulating hormone (FSH) and luteinizing hormone (LH) secretion. In the more advanced stages associated with thyroid and adrenal deficiency, a very slow progression of hypopituitarism may escape attention unless an acute stress or illness supervenes. The recent discovery of isolated alpha subunit secretion by some of these tumors has not enhanced discovery because of the limited availability of the test and interference from gonadotropin cross-reactivity in the radioimmunoassay. Consequently, the detection and treatment of nonfunctioning pituitary tumors presents a greater challenge than that afforded by the functioning tumors, which can be detected in the microadenoma stage, when they are 10 mm or less in diameter. The functioning tumors declare their presence when they reach macroadenoma stage, have enlarged the sella, and may have invaded adjacent bone and neural and vascular tissues. Even when a fortuitous discovery is achieved because of a skull roentgenogram taken for head trauma or sinus disease or when a CT scan is done because of headaches, the tumor mass has usually reached macroadenoma stage in order to be visualized by these screening tests. The onset of hyperprolactinemia related to pituitary stalk compression, which releases the pituitary from the control of a hypothalamic inhibiting factor, is a very late complication of suprasellar extension.

EMERGENCY PROBLEMS

A variety of neurologic and endocrine problems may bring the patient to an emergency room or to a physician's office. First and most compelling is the onset of progressive visual loss or actual blindness. If the loss of vision is rapid over several hours or days, it is often due to an acute expansion of the tumor by internal hemorrhage or necrosis. When this results in bleeding into the subarachnoid space, excruciating headache and neck stiffness are prominent clinical signs of apoplexy. In this situation, an acute loss of pituitary gland function can occur and should be monitored by immediate plasma cortisol assays and follow-up thyroid hormone tests to screen for major functional loss. The possibility of gonadotropin deficiency should also be evaluated. Serious visual impairment must be considered as a true emergency requiring monitoring of vision with frequent bedside visual acuity card tests, constant ophthalmologic supervision, and prompt neurosurgical consultation for decompression by a surgical approach. Temporary reduction in chiasmal compression can usually be achieved by high-dose corticosteroid therapy with either Solu-Medrol, 40 mg IM or IV *q6h*, or dexamethasone, 4 mg IM or IV *q6h*. Stabilization or improvement in vision usually lasts for 48 to 72 hours and serves only to defer intervention to a more convenient time when operating room facilities and an experienced neurosurgeon are available. If apoplexy is not accompanied by visual loss, emergency surgery can and should be avoided by using corticosteroid therapy for several days at these high dosages followed by close observation as the treatment is gradually tapered. Such patients may experience total infarction of the tumor with subsequent development of an empty sella without need for additional therapy other than indicated pituitary hormone replacement.

Another type of emergency problem is represented by the onset of diplopia. Whether it is caused by infiltration and compression of oculomotor nerves in the cavernous sinus or by encroachment on these nerves as they traverse Meckel's cave (a spinal fluid-filled cavity near the posterolateral angle of the sella), the ability to prevent permanent nerve injury is limited by the duration of this event. Early decompression by craniotomy or, when possible, by transsphenoidal surgery affords the best prospect for saving functional vision and avoiding lifetime disability.

The formation of a large suprasellar mass can result in obstruction of the spinal fluid flow through the chiasmatic cistern with onset of hydrocephalus (visible on CT scan) and associated confusion or drowsiness. The initial care of this condition may require ventricular shunt surgery to improve the neurologic status before attempting to remedy the underlying tumor problem. In a recent case of an elderly woman who appeared to have adequate mental function, transsphenoidal removal of a pituitary adenoma was followed by progressive confusion and memory loss, which was relieved by insertion of a ventriculo-atrial shunt. The clinical change was attributed to pre-existing hydrocephalus, which was evident on the first preoperative CT scan and became clinically apparent after she had received general anesthesia and intravenous fluids.

An emergency situation can develop when thyroid-stimulating hormone (TSH) or adrenocorticotropic hormone (ACTH) function is inadequate, particularly during acute respiratory or other infections and after severe trauma. The recognition of hypothyroidism in a comatose patient may come too late to save the patient's life since recovery rates are only 25 to 50 percent at best, despite aggressive thyroid hormone therapy. Acute adrenal insufficiency is potentially reversible in all cases provided no time is lost in starting intravenous therapy with a bolus of 100 mg of Solu-Cortef after reserving a blood sample for plasma cortisol. If hypotension is not severe, there is time to perform a rapid Cortrosyn stimulation test using 25 units of synthetic ACTH (1–24), Cortrosyn, given IV or IM, and a plasma cortisol sample is drawn at least 30 minutes and preferably 60 minutes after the Cortrosyn dose. Hyponatremia may complicate thyroid hormone deficiency when associated with the syndrome of inappropriate antidiuretic hormone (ADH) secretion (SIADH). Hyponatremia may also be caused by ACTH deficiency, which can lead to a delayed response of aldosterone secretion. Fluid restriction is essential in SIADH whereas sodium and fluid volume replenishment is needed in hyponatremia caused by secondary adrenal insufficiency. If combined adrenal and thyroid deficiencies are suspected or if hypotension is present, central venous pressure monitoring will help in the regulation of fluid volume therapy. Urine and serum osmolality measurements are useful both for SIADH diagnosis and to monitor effects of treatment. Demeclocycline hydrochloride, 250 mg PO *q6h*, can provide immediate improvement in SIADH while awaiting return to normal thyroid hormone levels. If hyponatremia occurs in association with impaired ACTH function, sodium replacement and use of cortisol and its derivatives instead of synthetic steroids is the preferred approach. Daily losses of sodium should be measured. In some cases it may be necessary to give Florinef, 0.1 mg once or twice daily by mouth, to retain administered sodium. Accurate daily weights are useful in either SIADH or salt-wasting states in order to confirm desired changes in fluid balance during corrective therapy.

THERAPEUTIC OBJECTIVES

The major considerations in treatment of the nonfunctioning pituitary tumors are to correct or improve the visual, neurologic, and endocrine-metabolic disorders caused by the tumor mass and to prevent recurrence of the primary disease.

Preservation of vision is the most important of this triad of objectives. Partial or complete visual loss can cause major problems in the ability to work, to drive an automobile, to be productive, and to be independent of the need for care by family members. For these reasons, advanced age is not a barrier to effective treatment provided the medical risks are not excessive. If considerable impairment of vision persists, referral to a "low vision clinic" can be beneficial in obtaining practical help to augment visual function.

Neurologic problems are uncommon, but are very serious with regard to the future productivity and care requirements of these patients. Cerebrospinal shunt surgery usually provides dramatic relief of dementia related to the presence of hydrocephalus. Encroachment on the brain stem is uncommon but can be treated successfully by decompression of the tumor mass usually via a transsphenoidal approach. Since craniotomy can be followed by seizures, it is avoided when possible. Seizure disorders are responsive to anticonvulsive medications and to treatment of the lesion.

The consequences of pituitary function impairment deserve careful consideration in patients with pituitary tumors. In a few fortunate cases, such functions can be restored by relief of pressure on the normal gland. For the majority of cases, there is a prospect for retaining only existing function and a variable risk of further loss of function.

Preservation of fertility in both sexes and of potency in men is of major importance. Although replacement hormone therapy is corrective for libido and potency, restoration of fertility in patients with gonadotropin deficiency is time-consuming and expensive. It is possible to save semen in a sperm bank if the male patient is fertile prior to treatment. Pergonal (FSH and LH) and human chorionic gonadotropin (LH-like) are available for gonadal stimulation. LH-releasing hormone analogs are currently being tested for induction of ovulation. In cases in which fertility is not a primary consideration replacement of steroid hormones alone is needed. A "low-dose" oral contraceptive pill is sufficient for premenopausal women. Most men can be adequately maintained with oral fluoxymesterone, 10 mg daily, or depot testosterone preparations such as testosterone enanthate or cypionate, 200 mg IM every 3 weeks. Aside from the preservation of sexual function, such treatment has merit in terms of sustaining skeletal bone mass and promotion of general vigor and endurance.

Thyroid hormone replacement is uncomplicated and effective with suitable doses of L-thyroxine. The need for this treatment does expose the patient to hazards of under- or over-treatment or to complications of hypothyroidism if the medication is inadvertently discontinued. The use of a Medic Alert identification tag helps to reinforce the importance of taking lifelong uninterrupted therapy. Since thyroid hormone usage is common, and thyroid function tests are readily available, the regulation of treatment has become routine and not a hindrance to choice of therapy for the pituitary tumor patient. We advise at least annual hormone level measurements after more frequent testing in the first year in order to regulate thyroxine dosage.

The loss of ACTH function does present a significant hazard to the patient since it requires attention to constant corticosteroid replacement and prompt adjustments for trauma, illness, or other physical stress. Even when adrenocortical function is known to be adequate, it is prudent to give preparative steroid doses prior to use of a general anesthetic. Complications of steroid therapy can be avoided by following standard dosage schedules. If unexpected gastric ulceration develops, the possibility of a gastrin-producing pancreatic tumor should be investigated. It is desirable to provide each patient with written instructions describing a schedule for increases of steroid dosage during acute illness.

It is fortunate that craniotomy is now rarely required to treat pituitary tumors since it is likely to cause prolonged or permanent diabetes insipidus which presents a hazard for medical management and a great inconvenience to the patient. When possible, chlorpropamide, 250 mg PO daily, should be used provided hypoglycemia does not develop as a complication of this form of therapy. Otherwise, DD-AVP intranasal solution, 0.05 to 0.1 cc either once at bedtime or twice daily, is highly effective. There is often a gradual improvement in antidiuretic hormone function even after complete section of the pituitary stalk, so that the need for treatment should be assessed regularly. A low serum sodium or low osmolality is a sign of overtreatment. Long-term replacement of antidiuretic hormone is rarely needed after transsphenoidal surgery and is generally not observed after radiation therapy.

A discussion of these pituitary functions and how they are managed is an integral part of the care of patients prior to treatment of the tumor in order to educate the patient and to obtain proper informed consent. The physician in charge also has the obligation to provide follow-up of replacement therapy, either directly or by immediate transfer of responsibility to a physician available to the patient.

In some cases, the patient presents with one or more pituitary hormone deficiencies which must be recognized and treated as soon as possible, particularly if there is a prospect of surgery under general anesthesia. A panel of screening tests is obtained for all new patients. Reserve tests of pituitary function are indicated when screening tests are inconclusive or after treatment intervention.

CHOICES OF THERAPY

To a great extent the choices of various types of therapy may be limited by the stage at which the tumor is detected. Each treatment option also has its characteristic risk, complications, and success rate, which must be evaluated. No single form of therapy fits all stages of disease or all patient requirements, and more than one form of therapy may be necessary to provide relief of the initial problems and to prevent tumor recurrence. When excisional therapy is applied, the tumor has already developed to the macroadenoma stage and tends to regrow unless radiation therapy is given. Since no effective medical therapy is available for the nonfunctioning pituitary adenoma, the typical choices are limited to surgery and radiation, either alone or in combination. With respect to radiation, there is a further choice between conventional x-ray and proton-beam therapy.

As already mentioned, craniotomy is no longer the preferred surgical treatment and is restricted to those large tumors that cannot adequately be decompressed by the transsphenoidal route. Massive suprasellar extension does not preclude the use of transsphenoidal surgery since the tumor is often soft, and a supine, extended position of the head facilitates extrusion of the tumor into the operative field by virtue of the pressure of the cerebrospinal fluid on its suprasellar component. It is often worthwhile to attempt transsphenoidal decompression for relief of visual loss even if the prospects for tumor removal are limited. If the visual system is adequately decompressed by the surgery, radiation therapy can be directed at the remaining tumor with expectation of long-term gradual shrinkage of the mass. This may avoid preventable complications such as further tumor growth or pituitary apoplexy.

Current applications of radiation therapy are based on the wide availability of conventional x-ray therapy and the special option of proton-beam therapy. The dosage of x-ray is customarily based on daily fractions of 200 rads and a total delivered tumor dosage of 4500 rads. Dosage rates in excess of these limits carry an increased risk of neural and visual damage. Temporary epilation in the temporal regions is usual. An apparent risk of sarcoma development has been reported. The risk of resultant pituitary hormone deficiencies is not well defined for nonsecretory tumors; however, the identical x-ray dosage schedule given to patients with acromegaly who tend to have small tumors at the time of diagnosis results in a need for replacement thyroid hormone in 16.0 percent, adrenal hormone in 29.6 percent, and gonadal hormones in 47.4 percent within the first 10 years.

Heavy-particle therapy has been used extensively in the treatment of acromegaly and Cushing's disease, either with several fractions of alpha particles (Donner Laboratory, Berkeley, CA) or at a single sitting with the Bragg peak of the proton beam (Harvard Cyclotron, Cambridge, MA). The latter technique has been used for the past 20 years in selected patients with nonfunctioning pituitary tumors. Although a slight degree of suprasellar extension can be treated with a single portal technique and larger tumors can be treated with two portals in which the outer portal is limited to 600 rads in order to protect the optic nerves, most cases treated have had tumors confined to the sella. Invasion through the cavernous sinus into the parasellar area is considered a contraindication to proton-beam therapy. The primary advantages of this technique are its rapid application, avoidance of scalp epilation, and reduction of extrasellar radiation effects to less than 10 percent of the tumor dose. At the usual dosage of 6000 rads or less and a dose below 500 rads to the hypothalamus, loss of pituitary function has been relatively rare, about 3 percent after 5 to 20 years of follow-up.

Recurrence is a common problem after surgical treatment of nonsecretory pituitary tumors, but is considered to be less than 15 percent after x-ray therapy and under 5 percent after proton-beam therapy. If a postsurgical patient is followed without additional therapy, periodic CT scans are a necessity, at first annually and then triannually if no apparent recurrence is seen in the first 4 years.

INDICATIONS FOR SPECIFIC TYPES OF THERAPY

Unless acute loss of vision is a threat to the patient, it is worthwhile to obtain a prolactin assay on a stat basis since bromocriptine therapy is often effective in reducing tumor mass of prolactinomas, and prolactin hypersecretion may not be clinically detectable. Although compression of the pituitary stalk can elevate prolactin concentrations to a modest degree (up to 50 to 80 ng/ml), a tumor large enough to compress the stalk, if it is composed of prolactin-secreting cells, should be associated with much higher prolactin levels, hundreds or thousands of ng/ml. A rapid prolactin assay sufficient to make this discrimination can be performed in 24 hours. It is also possible for a nonsecretory tumor to release alpha subunit, identical to the common subunit of the glycoprotein hormones. This finding does not help in the choice of therapy since bromocriptine is not an effective treatment for alpha-secreting tumors, but it does indicate the presence of a relatively invasive tumor and provides a marker for future measurements.

The clinician is faced with a choice of the therapies just described. If the visual system is affected, either optic nerves or oculomotor nerves, surgical decompression is mandatory. The only exceptions are cases in which coexisting mental or physical disabilities would prevent achievement of a useful result or the procedure would present an extreme risk to health or life. If the tumor has been found at an earlier stage without visual impairment it does not require removal since it is either noninvasive and susceptible to radiation or invasive and not curable by surgery alone. The concept of "debulking" the tumor to render radiation therapy more successful is not relevant since the response rate of these tumors is excellent, regardless of size. There may be justification for surgical biopsy if the nature of the lesion is in doubt since the demonstration of a cystic lesion or calcium deposit suggests a craniopharyngioma. CT scans are so capable of confirming a diagnosis of pituitary adenoma that a diagnostic biopsy is rarely indicated. If contrast uptake is very dense, carotid aneurysm should be ruled out by digital subtraction angiography.

A microadenoma found by chance on skull films or CT scans taken for unrelated reasons can be followed expectantly for signs of active growth unless there is evidence of pituitary functional loss or an apparent association with headaches. For example, we have treated a patient of this type with impaired ACTH function. Proton-beam therapy was followed by recovery of responsiveness to metyrapone and development of a partially empty sella by CT scan. Another young woman, with amenorrhea, had restoration of menses and became pregnant after proton-beam therapy of a small nonsecretory tumor. A third example is that of a man who had tumor apoplexy with hypopituitarism, suffered from persistent headaches for more than a year, was then treated with the proton beam, and experienced a remission of headaches over the next 6 months. If no treatment is elected, long-term follow-up is essential since tumor growth can be extremely slow.

The intermediate-size tumors which have expanded the sella and may have extended into the sphenoid sinus can be followed or treated at that stage provided the risks are recognized. If the tumor is allowed to progress, there may be irreversible damage to the pituitary stalk or other structures. A low-risk treatment is a reasonable option and is afforded by surgery, conventional x-ray therapy, or proton-beam therapy. The long-term effectiveness of surgery is in doubt since recurrence is frequent unless radiation is used. As already mentioned, the lesser side effects of proton-beam therapy on pituitary function render it a more favorable choice than x-ray for these patients. Surgery and general anesthesia pose a minimal risk in terms of mortality whereas no fatalities occur with proton-beam therapy, and an uncertain number of cases may develop central nervous system sarcoma after x-ray therapy. We would therefore suggest proton-beam therapy as a reasonable first choice under these circumstances. It should be noted, however, that proton-beam therapy is not locally available.

Large tumors which have reached the optic chiasm or caused diplopia are most likely to be candidates for open surgical excision by the transsphenoidal route. In exceptional cases, vision may be normal due to a pre-fixed chiasm or long optic nerves. Surgical removal of tumor at this stage would avoid the risk of apoplexy with the rapid visual loss which could otherwise occur. The same argument applies to the use of x-ray therapy; however, the risk of side effects appears to be greater. Proton-beam therapy has been used in selected patients who had refused other treatment and has arrested tumor growth in these cases.

There is little or no controversy about the management of patients with signs of tumor expansion causing visual changes. Early decompression by surgery affords the best prospect of achieving a satisfactory reversal of visual loss. Diplopia is less likely to respond since it ordinarily signifies tumor invasion. If substantial tumor remnants are seen by a postoperative CT scan taken without 3 to 6 months after surgery, proton-beam therapy or conventional x-ray therapy is indicated. When CT scan findings are equivocal, follow-up scans serve as a guide to detection of recurrence in an early stage.

Whatever the initial choice of therapy, recurrence requires a new evaluation. A treatment that has failed should be avoided in a second attempt unless tumor progression allows no other option. In the event that x-ray therapy of 4500 rads has been given in 30 days, no additional radiation is allowed; however, a proton-beam supplement can be directed to the intrasellar zone if at least 3 years have elapsed after a lesser amount of x-ray therapy. Although it is possible to repeat transsphenoidal surgery, there is an undefined risk of hypopituitarism associated with additional curettage of the sella contents.

The choices of therapy in relation to tumor stage are summarized in Table 1.

FOLLOW-UP PROGRAMS

Throughout this discussion and analysis, follow-up has deserved frequent mention. The natural history of nonsecretory pituitary tumors is obscure because of the absence of a tumor marker substance that could be quantitated and the lack of specific clinical changes in its earliest stages. Although visual field examination remains important, it fails to detect recurrence except at an advanced stage. However, it may suggest continued disease when healing does not occur after treatment. The use of serial skull roentgenograms and hypocycloidal polytomes of the sella has declined as CT scan techniques have developed. At present, a CT scan with contrast enhancement directed at the sella is the mainstay of follow-up. Coronal plane scans are favored because of the sensitivity of detection for tumor tissue. Direct coronal scans may be difficult to obtain if neck flexion is a limiting factor or may be obscured by reflection artifacts from the teeth. For these reasons, we obtain axial scans with multiplanar reconstructions in the coronal and sagittal planes at close "section" intervals of 1 mm apart. There is further promise of the eventual routine application of Nuclear Magnetic Resonance scans, provided more rapid scanning time and thinner sections can be achieved. The lack of x-ray exposure and elimination of contrast infusion are desirable clinical features of this new instrumentation. Although it is important to monitor endocrine functions during follow-up, results of these studies do not usually serve as an early warning for tumor recurrence unless the tumor is invasive and causes pituitary damage.

An unusual complication of nonfunctioning pituitary tumors is the late development of a functional cell line. We have observed four cases in which classic Cushing's disease appeared several years after initial treatment for nonfunctioning tumors despite the early use of x-ray therapy in three cases and a low dosage of proton beam in the fourth case.

Varying degrees of pituitary functional loss may take place up to 10 or more years after conventional x-ray therapy. Patients who have received this treatment require close observation for possible hypopituitarism.

Regardless of the form of treatment applied and the nature of the initial results, all cases of nonfunctioning pituitary adenoma deserve lifetime follow-up. Likewise, the treatments chosen should have a goal of lifetime effectiveness in order to achieve the most beneficial results with the least risks and complications.

TABLE 1 Choices of Treatment for Non-Functioning Pituitary Adenomas

Clinical Problem	*Associated Complications*	*Therapy Choices*
Intrasellar microadenoma (less than 10 mm diameter)	Sella erosion, hypogonadism, headaches	Observe if asymptomatic; transsphenoidal surgery or proton-beam therapy if indicated
Intrasellar macroadenoma	Enlarged sella, possible hypopituitarism	Proton-beam therapy or transsphenoidal surgery
Suprasellar extension of macroadenoma	Visual loss due to chiasmal compression, possible hypopituitarism	Transsphenoidal surgery followed by proton-beam or x-ray therapy
Parasellar extension of macroadenoma	Cavernous sinus syndrome, possible temporal lobe seizures	Transsphenoidal surgery followed by x-ray therapy
Recurrent or invasive tumor after previous surgery, proton-beam therapy, or x-ray therapy	Visual loss, hypopituitarism, cavernous sinus syndrome	Consider for craniotomy or repeat transsphenoidal surgery followed by proton-beam or x-ray therapy if not used previously
Pituitary apoplexy	Headache, acute visual field loss, possible acute hypopituitarism	High-dose corticosteroids and close observation; transsphenoidal decompression if visual loss persists; replace pituitary hormone deficiencies

Suggested Reading

Feek CM, McLelland J, Seth J, Toft AD, Irvine WJ, Padfield PL, Edwards CRW. How effective is external pituitary irradiation for growth hormone-secreting pituitary tumors? Clin Endocrinol 1984; 20:401.

Hardy J. Transsphenoidal microsurgical removal of pituitary microadenoma. In: Morley JP (ed). Progress in Neurological Surgery. Philadelphia: WB Saunders, 1976, p 377.

Jenkins JS, Ash S, Bloom HJG. Endocrine function after external pituitary irradiation in patients with secreting and non-secreting pituitary tumors. Q J Med 1972; 41:57.

Kjellberg RN, Kliman B. Lifetime effectiveness—a system of therapy for pituitary adenomas, emphasizing Bragg peak proton hypophysectomy. In: Linfoot JA (ed). Recent Advances in the Diagnosis and Treatment of Pituitary Tumors. New York: Raven Press, 1979, pp 269-288.

Kliman B, Kjellberg RN. Pituitary tumors. In: Givens JR (ed). Endocrine Causes of Menstrual Disorders. Chicago: Year Book Medical Publishers, 1978, pp 165-180.
Pistenma DA, Goffinet DR, Bagshaw MA, Hanberg J, Eltringham JR. Treatment of chromophobe adenomas with megavoltage irradiation. Cancer 1975; 35:1974.
Sheline GE. Untreated and recurrent chromophobe adenomas of the pituitary. A J Roentgenol 1971; 112:768.
Sheline GE. Treatment of nonfunctioning chromophobe adenomas of the pituitary. Am J Roentgenol 1974; 120:553.
Wilson CB, Dempsey LC. Transsphenoidal removal of 250 pituitary adenomas. J Neurosurg 1978; 28:13.
Waltz TA, Brownell B. Sarcoma: A possible late result of effective radiation therapy for pituitary adenoma. J Neurosurg 1966; 24:901.

PROLACTINOMA

MICHAEL O. THORNER, M.B., F.R.C.P.

The therapy for prolactin-secreting pituitary tumors has changed considerably over the past 5 years. Initially it was thought that all pituitary tumors, including those secreting prolactin, should undergo active therapy directed primarily at the tumor itself, that is, surgery or radiotherapy or both. In this chapter I will consider the various therapeutic options that are open to the clinician in treating a patient with a prolactinoma and then specify why I believe that the primary mode of therapy for the vast majority of these tumors should be medical.

BACKGROUND

Prolactin-secreting pituitary tumors may present in a variety of ways. The female patient may complain to the gynecologist of menstrual disorders or infertility, and the male patient may go to the urologist because of impotence. Patients of either sex may consult a neurologist or ophthalmologist with complaints of headaches and visual field disturbances. In the past the mode of presentation has dictated the choice of therapy for the patient. For example, a patient presenting with visual field defects would automatically be immediately referred to a neurosurgeon for evaluation of a suprasellar mass compressing the optic chiasm, and almost certainly the patient would ultimately undergo surgery. Today, however, rather than approaching the management of pituitary tumors in a reflex manner, it may be beneficial to reconsider the objectives of the treatment of such tumors, especially in view of the advances in medical management. I consider the objectives to be (1) reduction or removal of the tumor mass, (2) preservation of anterior pituitary function, (3) correction of the hyperprolactinemic state, and (4) prevention of recurrence of the disease.

Prior to any treatment, it is imperative that the anterior pituitary function be properly assessed. I therefore always obtain, at the very least, measurements of basal (0800 hours) plasma cortisol, serum thyroxine and T_3 resin uptake, serum TSH, serum LH and FSH and, in addition, serum estradiol in women and serum testosterone in men. If all these are normal, and causes for the hyperprolactinemia, such as ingestion of drugs (which may elevate serum prolactin levels), have been excluded, no further endocrine studies need be performed. If there is any doubt about the interpretation of the basal hormone values we proceed to dynamic function tests; we perform a thyrotropin-releasing hormone test (TRH) for measurement of TSH and prolactin reserve and an insulin tolerance test (ITT) for growth hormone and ACTH reserve measurements. Evaluation of the anatomy of the pituitary is essential, and methods of doing this have changed in the last few years. In the past, plain skull x-rays, including a Caldwell (occipitomental) view and lateral view, were performed, and if these were equivocal, tomography of the sella was also performed. These evaluations have now been virtually completely replaced in major centers in the United States by CT scanning with fourth or later generation scanners. Using these scanners it is possible not only to discern the bony contour of the pituitary fossa but also to (1) see the soft tissues of the pituitary, (2) diagnose empty sella, and (3) diagnose both microadenomas and macroadenomas in the pituitary. It is also essential to get a neuro-ophthalmologic examination, including measurement of the visual fields on the Goldman apparatus.

THERAPEUTIC APPROACHES

When the diagnosis of prolactinoma has been established, the options for therapy are (1) to observe the patient and not treat; (2) to treat with external pituitary irradiation; (3) to treat with pituitary surgery (using a transsphenoidal approach); and (4) to treat with dopamine agonist drugs. One of the dilemmas in the evaluation of the optimal mode of therapy for this condition is that its natural history is not established and is clearly variable; however, the majority of microadenomas remain small and do not progress to macroadenomas. Unfortunately we cannot predict which will progress. Nevertheless, in my view any patient who is diagnosed as having significant hyperprolactinemia, particularly if he has gonadal dysfunction, deserves active intervention to restore gonadal function. An occasional patient will spontaneously develop return of gonadal function and lowering of prolactin levels, but this is highly unusual, and active treatment should be considered for the typical patient. Radiotherapy, either with conventional external pituitary irradiation, with proton beam therapy, or with implantation of radioactive yttrium, has been utilized to prevent further growth of the tumor and to reduce tumor size. Its effects on prolactin secretion are poorly described in the literature; however, the consensus is that serum prolactin levels fall in a similar way to serum growth hormone levels in acromegaly. Following external pituitary irradiation prolactin levels fall slowly; the nadir may not be achieved until up to ten years later and levels rarely reach the normal range. Therefore radiotherapy is not a satisfactory treatment for the prolactinoma. In the United States the most popular method for treatment of prolactinomas has been transsphenoidal surgery, an approach pioneered by Hardy and Guiot.

Results from several groups in the United States which have specialized in transsphenoidal surgery suggest that when prolactinomas are small, surgical therapy produces very good results; that is, if the prolactin level is less than 200 ng/ml, the chances of restoration of prolactin levels to normal and return of gonadal function are greater than 75 percent. However, these results are limited to centers that have the greatest experience. In centers where neurosurgeons do not operate on the pituitary every day, the results of surgery are less satisfactory and only a minority of patients are cured by surgery. Also, as the length of follow-up of patients after surgery increases, the number of patients with recurrence of hyperprolactinemia also increases and may be as high as 50 percent. Results of surgery are quite different when one is considering large prolactinomas with high prolactin levels (that is, those with prolactin levels greater than 250 ng/ml). In these cases, even in centers with the greatest experience, the chances of normalizing the prolactin levels and restoring gonadal function fall exponentially with the increase in the size of the prolactin-secreting tumor and the pretreatment basal level of prolactin. As an example, in Hardy's experience women with pretreatment prolactin levels of >250 ng/ml have only a 29 percent chance of achieving normal prolactin levels postoperatively. Furthermore, if there is any evidence of invasion of the dura by the prolactinoma, the results of surgery are extremely poor (<20% with normal prolactin levels).

MEDICAL THERAPY FOR PROLACTINOMAS

In 1971 the first prototype dopamine agonist drug was introduced for clinical trials. The drug, bromocriptine, is a semisynthetic peptide ergot. It was developed specifically as an inhibitor of prolactin secretion before it was known that dopamine could inhibit prolactin secretion directly at the anterior pituitary or that dopamine was itself one, if not the only, prolactin-inhibiting factor. Initial studies with bromocriptine showed that, regardless of whether a pituitary tumor was present, prolactin levels were suppressed by the administration of this compound and that when therapy was withdrawn, prolactin levels rose once more. Not only were prolactin levels lowered (usually into the normal range) by bromocriptine therapy, but gonadal function was also restored. This occurred in both men and women. Bromocriptine was in use in clinical research for the treatment of hyperprolactinemia for 5 years before it was realized that it also had profound effects on the volume of prolactin-secreting tumors. Most investigators initially treated patients with large prolactin-secreting tumors either with surgery or with irradiation, and when the patient was left with hyperprolactinemia, bromocriptine therapy was started.

Studies in several centers, including our own, have clearly demonstrated that the majority of large prolactin-secreting tumors respond to bromocriptine therapy with lowering of prolactin levels by over 80 percent (often into the normal range), restoration of gonadal and anterior pituitary functions, and a reduction in pituitary tumor volume. The size reduction of the tumors may occur very rapidly (within days of the initiation of therapy) and lead to decompression of the optic chiasm and to resolution of headaches and other symptoms and signs of raised intracranial pressure. These results may be expected in over 80 percent of patients (based on our own 18 cases). However, there does appear to be a spectrum of sensitivity of the tumors in terms of size reduction. Some tumors appear to be exquisitely sensitive and will shrink over 80 percent within 6 weeks of initiation of therapy.

Mechanism of Size Reduction by Bromocriptine

Based on animal data, it was considered that size reduction of these tumors possibly resulted from an antimitotic effect of bromocriptine. It has been clearly shown that bromocriptine can reverse the estrogen-induced increased rate of mitosis of the in situ pituitary in the rat. However, the mitotic activity in human prolactinomas is, in general, rather low. We have recently had the opportunity of studying pituitary tissue from untreated patients with prolactinomas, patients treated with bromocriptine, and patients withdrawn from treatment. Bromocriptine causes marked changes in the volumes of the prolactin-secreting cells. These marked reductions in cell volume are accounted for by reduction in both cytoplasmic and nuclear volumes. In the cytoplasm the amount of rough endoplasmic reticulum and size of the Golgi apparatus are markedly reduced, and the cell changes from appearing highly active to being quiescent. There is a similar reduction in both the nuclear and nucleolar areas. The changes are reversed after bromocriptine withdrawal.

An Approach to the Patient with Hyperprolactinemia

The correct approach to a patient with a prolactinoma depends on a variety of factors. These include the sex of the patient (and, in women, whether pregnancy is desired); the expertise in a given medical center where the patient is being seen; and the "prejudice" of the physician who is looking after the patient. My own personal view is that this disease process, which presumably reflects a spectrum from hyperplasia to isolated adenoma, is best treated by medical means. However, there are a number of problems with medical management, including (1) the risk of swelling of the tumor during pregnancy, (2) the cost of long-term treatment, and (3) the unknown effects of lifelong medical therapy.

If a patient has a small microadenoma and a prolactin level of less than 200, there is a good chance that transsphenoidal surgery performed by a skilled surgeon will be successful; under such circumstances, the patient will have an 80 to 90 percent chance of being euprolactinemic postoperatively and of needing no other form of treatment. However, in the patient who does not have a clear microadenoma, that is, one who has a prolactin level of less than 100 and an absolutely normal CT scan of the pituitary , or in a patient who may have a microadenoma but has a prolactin level of over 200, the chance of surgery being successful is probably less than 50 percent, even in the best hands. Similarly, in patients with very large prolactinomas and very high prolactin levels (above 250 ng/ml), the chances of restoring prolactin levels to normal by surgery are less than 30 percent. Thus surgery may be successful in decompressing the tumor, but will usually not be successful in curing the disease. With these large tumors the chance of surgically inducing hypopituitarism is considerable. It is interesting that these patients rarely have ACTH or TSH deficiency preoperatively. In my view all patients with hyperprolactinemia who do not have a clear microadenoma, or who have a prolactin level of over 200 ng/ml should be treated primarily with medical therapy. I would also treat such patients with microadenomas with medical therapy, provided they understand that the therapy probably has to continue throughout their lives; it is very unusual for a patient to remain euprolactinemic following the withdrawal of bromocriptine therapy, even after one or more years of such therapy.

At the present time only one drug has been approved by the FDA for the treatment of hyperprolactinemia in patients *without* tumors for up to 6 months only, and for treatment of infertility. Bromocriptine may be given starting with 1.25 mg taken with food on retiring. The dosage is gradually increased every 2 to 3 days to 1.25 mg *bid*, then *tid*, and then increased to 2.5 mg *tid*. Sometimes when patients have very large tumors, and 7.5 mg/day is not sufficient either to reduce the size of the tumor or to lower the prolactin levels by greater than 80 percent, it may be necessary to increase the dosage up to 15 mg per day. At the present time the drug has not been approved for treatment of prolactinomas, only for patients without obvious pituitary tumors.

I believe that patients with large prolactinomas should undergo primary therapy with bromocriptine rather than undergoing surgery. If there is good documentation of reduction in tumor size, the therapy should be continued indefinitely. If reduction in tumor size has not occurred within 3 months, it is unlikely that it will occur and medical therapy should be abandoned. However, if it does occur, size reduction may continue progressively up to one year or longer. We have seen no serious complications of this form of therapy other than return of the tumor to its pretreatment size following withdrawal of therapy as outlined above. One patient, after approximately 18 months of therapy, developed a hemorrhage into the pituitary which led to an increase in the volume of the pituitary. However, with conservative management this expansion spontaneously resolved, and the patient has remained on bromocriptine throughout. The rest of his anterior pituitary function was not compromised by this event. It is theoretically possible that bromocriptine may prevent the progress of prolactin-secreting pituitary tumors, although this had not yet been proved.

Pregnancy and Bromocriptine

Many women with hyperprolactinemia are infertile and desire pregnancy. The administration of bromocriptine lowers the prolactin levels and restores gonadal function. Thus there is little problem about the ability of the patient to conceive. There are, however, several considerations that must be stressed and recognized both by the physician and by the patient. First, the question of exposure of the fetus to bromocriptine and possible teratogenic sequelae merits consideration. There is no evidence for teratogenicity in animal studies. Furthermore, in over 1400 pregnancies in women who were taking bromocriptine when they conceived (and documented by Sandoz), there is no evidence of increased incidence of abortion, multiple pregnancy, or fetal abnormalities. However, until these babies have lived their own complete life cycles, the possibility of unexpected late effects cannot be excluded. So that the fetus is not exposed to bromocriptine for any longer than necessary, it is suggested that when the mother is initially treated with bromocriptine she takes mechanical contraceptive precautions. Once she has had three regular menstrual cycles she may discontinue contraceptive precautions and in that way pregnancy can be suspected as soon as her period is 48 hours overdue. At that time a serum beta HCG assay should be performed to confirm pregnancy and the patient should discontinue bromocriptine. Thus the fetus is exposed theoretically to bromocriptine for a maximum of 16 days.

The second problem relates to the risk of expansion of the tumor during pregnancy. There is little doubt that patients with pituitary tumors run a small but significant risk of expansion of the tumor during pregnancy. It is very difficult to assess the absolute risk. With microadenomas the incidence appears to be less than 1 percent and probably less than 0.5 percent. In patients with macroadenomas the incidence is probably higher; it may be between 5 and 20 percent. This risk is unrelated to bromocriptine therapy prior to the pregnancy; rather, it may occur when pregnancy is induced with other drugs, including exogenous gonadotropins and clomiphene, and even when no drug therapy is employed in patients with pre-existing pituitary adenomas.

In practice the problem of pregnancy is not great, since the vast majority of women who present with hyperprolactinemia only have microadenomas. To avoid major problems, it is extremely important that the patient undergo careful endocrine, neuoradiologic, and neuro-ophthalmologic evaluation prior to treatment. If there is no suprasellar extension and the patient harbors only a microadenoma, then the risk of swelling of the pituitary is extremely small and it is suggested that the patient be clinically evaluated at 2 month intervals throughout the pregnancy. If the patient has a macroadenoma and suprasellar extension, a strong case can be made for decompression of the tumor prior to pregnancy. However, it is possible for even these patients to go through pregnancy without developing visual disturbances. It is vital for patients to understand their condition and to take part in the choice of therapy. Outside the United States trials are under way evaluating the effects of continuing bromocriptine therapy throughout pregnancy in patients with macroadenomas in the hope of preventing swelling. I believe it is better to treat those patients who develop problems than to treat all patients throughout pregnancy in the hope of avoiding this problem.

If visual field defects or headaches from tumor expansion occur during pregnancy, a number of options are open. It should be stressed that thus far no patient has become permanently blind following expansion of the tumor during pregnancy. Following termination of the pregnancy, either by abortion or delivery, the tumor has become smaller with resolution of visual symptoms and headaches in all cases. Thus the approach will depend on at what stage of pregnancy the symptoms occur. If they occur early in the pregnancy, abortion may be indicated. If they occur in the eighth month of pregnancy, premature delivery of the baby may be decided upon, although if the field defects and symptoms are minor, careful observation may be all that is required. The most difficult time is when the field defects and symptoms occur in the middle trimester of the pregnancy. At that time I would suggest starting the patient on bromocriptine again in the hope of reducing the tumor size and at least preventing further swelling. If this is unsuccessful, high-dose dexamethasone can be used to achieve the same ends. This also has the advantage that, if the baby needs to be prematurely delivered, the chances of fetal respiratory distress syndrome are reduced. As a last resort, transsphenoidal surgery during the pregnancy can and has been used to decompress the tumor. In all events this complication is fortunately extremely rare, and for this reason no one has accumulated a large experience in dealing with it.

ACROMEGALY

LAWRENCE A. FROHMAN, M.D.

Acromegaly is a disease caused by excessive secretion of growth hormone (GH). It is characterized by excessive growth of soft tissues, bone, and visceral organs. If the disorder begins prior to the closure of long bone epiphyseal growth centers, i.e., during childhood and adolescence, increased long bone growth resulting in gigantism will occur. Tissue overgrowth and the metabolic consequences of GH hypersecretion result in specific features and complications of the disease, many of which require special therapeutic consideration. They include diabetes mellitus, hypertrophic osteoarthropathy, perineurial hypertrophy leading to nerve entrapment (i.e., carpal tunnel syndrome), and eustachian tube obstruction leading to recurrent serous otitis media.

PATHOGENESIS

In almost all patients the excessive GH secretion is caused by a somatotroph adenoma of the pituitary. In rare cases it may be caused by pituitary somatotroph hyperplasia or by ectopic GH production by an extrapituitary tumor.

Pituitary tumors are generally of two types: (1) those that exhibit relatively rapid growth and contain less stored hormone (macroadenomas) and (2) those that exhibit a slow growth rate and contain a large amount of stored hormone (microadenomas). The clinical features of acromegaly reflect the product of the plasma GH level and the duration of hypersecretion. Thus, the severity of clinical manifestations does not necessarily predict the type of tumor present. The GH-secreting macroadenoma, in addition to its hormonal effects, causes problems associated with an expanding intrasellar tumor: varying degrees of hypopituitarism caused by destruction of adjacent anterior and posterior pituitary tissue, headache caused by pressure on the diaphragma sella, and neurologic defects (visual field impairment, loss of cranial nerves III, IV and VI, and hypothalamic symptoms) due to extrasellar extension of the tumor. Therapy of the GH-secreting macroadenoma must therefore also take into consideration those facets of the disease. One-third of patients with GH-secreting adenomas also exhibit hyperprolactinemia, which can occur as a result of a mixed somatotroph-lactotroph tumor, a combination of separate somatotroph and lactotroph tumors, or production of both hormones from a single neoplastic cell type. No correlation has yet been found between tumor type and the response to therapy, with the possible exception of pharmacotherapy (to be discussed). Very rarely, a GH-secreting tumor may exhibit malignant potential with metastases both within and without the CNS.

On rare occasions, pituitary hyperplasia has been observed in patients with acromegaly due to ectopic production of GH-releasing factor (GRF). Although this histologic pattern was initially believed to be diagnostic of ectopic GRF production, it is now recognized to represent only an intermediary state of hyperfunction, which eventually leads to adenoma formation. No clinical features distinguish patients with somatotroph hyperplasia from those with adenomas.

A more significant classification of the etiology of acromegaly is provided in Table 1. Acromegaly may be considered a primary or secondary pituitary disease. Although the vast majority (perhaps up to 99%) of patients with acromegaly have a primary pituitary disorder, ectopic GRF production is responsible in a small number of patients. The prevalence of ectopic GRF-producing tumors from systemic sources is less than one percent, though that of intrapituitary and/or hypothalamic sources may be greater. Identification of the former group is of great importance since appropriate therapy should be directed at the extrapituitary tumor rather than at the pituitary. Therapy of ectopic GH production must also be directed at the extrapituitary tumor.

ESTABLISHING THE DIAGNOSIS

The diagnosis of acromegaly is established on a biochemical basis. Persistently elevated GH levels, a further rise after thyrotropin-releasing hormone (TRH), and a lack of suppression by glucose confirm the diagnosis. A computed tomographic (CT) scan of the pituitary provides anatomic identification of the tumor in 80 to 90 percent of patients. If evidence of suprasellar extension is present, visual field examination (Goldmann perimetry), visually evoked response, and digital subtraction angiography provide precise delineation of the anatomic and functional consequences of the extrasellar portion of the tumor. Elevated plasma levels of IgF-I (somatomedin C), a GH-dependent growth factor responsible for many of the effects of GH, are also present, but are less useful in diagnosis and therapy. Assessment of other pituitary function is indicated prior to therapy to serve as a baseline for future changes, to determine the extent of tumor to be removed if surgery is chosen, and to provide appropriate hormonal therapy in the perioperative period.

CT examination of the chest and abdomen to search for a remote source of ectopic GRF is not recommended because it is cost-ineffective, given the infrequency of the disease. However, measurement of plasma GRF levels provides a simple and effective means of excluding or confirming a disease that necessitates entirely different therapy. Elevated plasma GRF levels are present in patients with GRF-secreting tumors except in those with tumors of hypothalamic or pituitary origin, which do not secrete into the systemic circulation.

TABLE 1 Etiologic Classification of Acromegaly

Primary pituitary disease
Pituitary microadenoma
Pituitary macroadenoma
Pituitary carcinoma
Secondary pituitary disease
Ectopic GRF production
Pancreatic adenoma, carcinoid, small cell lung tumors
Intrapituitary gangliocytoma
Hypothalamic hamartoma
Eutopic GRF production (?) by hypothalamus
Eutopic GH production—pancreatic, carcinoid, or lung tumors

THERAPEUTIC POSSIBILITIES

The goals of treatment of acromegaly consist of (1) restoring GH secretion to normal, (2) ablation of the pituitary tumor mass with preservation of surrounding neurologic and pituitary tissue and function, and (3) prevention of recurrence. These goals are achievable in some but not all subjects. There are three options of therapy: surgery, irradiation, and pharmacotherapy—used alone or in combination.

Surgery

The most frequently used therapy for acromegaly is surgical removal of the tumor. The considerations and technical aspects are similar to those that pertain to nonfunctioning tumors. Most tumors can be removed by the transsphenoidal approach, and the older subfrontal approach is reserved only for tumors that exhibit extensive suprasellar extension and either encase surrounding blood vessels or nerves or are pedunculated. Knowledge of pituitary function preoperatively is an important determinant in the extent of tumor removed. In patients with intact pituitary function, a more conservative approach should be used and every effort made to preserve the remaining pituitary function (less than 10 percent of the pituitary is required) even if some tumor may be left. In these patients, postoperative radiation therapy is indicated to destroy the remaining tumor (to be discussed). In patients with preoperative loss of pituitary function, complete tumor removal should be attempted, since postoperative hormone replacement therapy will be required in any case.

Factors that predict therapeutic success relate to the size of the tumor and the plasma GH level. Likelihood of a true "cure", i.e., elimination of the tumor and restoration of normal GH levels (<5 ng/ml), approaches 90 percent in tumors totally confined within sella turcica and when GH levels are <40 ng/ml. With larger and more active tumors, the results are not as good. The age and sex of the patient, duration of disease, and association of hyperprolactinemia do not have predictive value on the therapeutic outcome. Overall operative mortality is about one percent and occurs primarily in patients with extensive suprasellar extension or those undergoing repeat surgical procedures. Complications of surgery include CSF rhinorrhea, bacterial or chemical meningitis, optic nerve damage, and loss of anterior and posterior pituitary function. The size of the tumor and the capabilities of the neurosurgeon are the major determining factors in both morbidity and mortality rates. Preoperative hormone therapy consists of hydrocortisone hemisuccinate (Solu-Cortef), 50 mg IM *q6h*, for 24 to 48 hrs with a gradual taper over the next few days, as permitted. If the patient is found to be hypothyroid preoperatively, the euthyroid state should be reestablished prior to surgery. The responses to surgery are dramatic. The decrease in GH levels occur immediately, and the effectiveness of the procedure can thus be rapidly evaluated.

In patients with ectopic GRF-secreting tumors in whom the diagnosis is made prior to pituitary surgery, successful removal of the extrapituitary tumor has been followed by a return of GH levels to normal and a disappearance of the pituitary tumor mass.

Radiation Therapy

Irradiation of pituitary tumors is also an effective method of destroying the tumor and reducing GH levels. The technique most commonly used is that of supervoltage irradiation. Any type of megavoltage beam is suitable for treating pituitary tumors, although the higher energy available from a linear accelerator is considered to be advantageous over that from a ^{60}Co source in limiting the radiation to surrounding tissues. A total dose of 4500 to 5000 rads is used and is administered over a 4- to 5-week period in order to minimize side effects and damage to surrounding tissues. Comparable effects can be obtained from proton beam and heavy particle therapy, which are available in only a few centers in the country. The main advantage of this type of irradiation is the ability to deliver the total dose in 1 or 2 days.

The effectiveness of radiation therapy, judged by the same criteria as that used for surgery, is somewhat different. First, the effects are slower in onset, i.e., decreases in GH are not seen for a few months, at least 2 years are required for a 50 percent reduction in GH levels, and even at 10 years, normalization of GH levels is achieved in only 70 percent of patients. Second, although many of the complications of surgery do not occur, an occasional patient experiences optic nerve damage, particularly when moderate suprasellar tumor extension is present, and the likelihood of anterior pituitary hormone loss is 30 to 50 percent at 10 years. However, the arrest of tumor growth is excellent and tumor shrinkage is observed in most patients.

Evaluation of Therapy

Short-term evaluation of therapy is based on relief of symptoms due to tumor mass effects, return of GH levels to normal, and regression of the clinical and laboratory features of GH hypersecretion. Although bony changes are permanent, dramatic decreases in soft tissue usually occur and carbohydrate tolerance is often restored to normal, as is androgen production and reproductive function. Although many of the changes occur even with incomplete reduction of GH levels, normalization is desired for optimal results.

Long-term assessment of therapy focuses on maintenance of normal GH levels and prevention of tumor regrowth. If tumor removal is incomplete at surgery or if GH levels do not decrease to 5 ng/ml or less, the likelihood of tumor regrowth and an increase in GH levels ranges from 25 percent to nearly 100 percent of patients in different series. For this reason, the use of radiation therapy postoperatively is recommended for all patients whose tumor is acknowledged to be incompletely removed at surgery or whose GH levels are not normalized postoperatively. There is some feeling that postoperative GH responses to TRH stimulation, even in the presence of normal basal GH levels, is an indication of persistent neoplastic tissue and an indication for radiation therapy. This has not yet been universally accepted. The radiation dose and method are the same as those used for primary therapy. The likelihood of recurrence after combined surgery and radiation therapy is less than 5 percent.

Pharmacotherapy

Although a number of agents, including estrogens and progestins, have been advocated in the past as being of value in the medical therapy of acromegaly, their efficacy was never firmly established and they are no longer used. One drug, bromocriptine, is effective in some patients in suppressing GH secretion and reducing tumor size. Bromocriptine is a lysergic acid derivative of ergoline which is approved for treatment of hyperprolactinemia. The drug binds with affinity to dopamine receptors and acts as a dopamine agonist. Its effectiveness in acromegaly depends on the presence of dopamine receptors on the neoplastic somatotrophs, which generally occur in tumors associated with hyperprolactinemia. In contrast to its effectiveness in hyperprolactinemia, however, bromocriptine suppresses GH levels in only about 20 to 25 percent of patients with acromegaly, and in many, the response is only partial. In addition, the doses required are higher than those for treatment of hyperprolactinemia and frequently may reach 30 to 60 mg/day. Even when the dose is increased gradually, side effects (primarily nausea, vomiting, and postural hypotension) are common and not tolerated in all patients.

Bromocriptine reduces tumor size in the majority of patients with prolactinomas, but in only about 5 or 10 percent of patients with acromegaly. When tumor reduction occurs, it is dependent on continued drug administration, and rapid tumor regrowth occurs when drug therapy is discontinued.

CHOICE OF THERAPY

The choice of a primary therapy rests between surgery and irradiation. In most patients with no contraindication to surgery, excision of the tumor is the preferred therapy in order to provide the optimal opportunity for regression of the clinical features. The availability of a neurosurgeon, well trained and experienced in transsphenoidal microsurgery, is critical, and close cooperation with an endocrinologist and neuroradiologist cannot be overemphasized. In the older patient, particularly in the presence of other medical problems, radiation therapy may be of advantage because of its lower short-term morbidity.

Bromocriptine cannot be recommended as primary therapy in acromegaly. However, it does have potential benefits in certain situations: (1) as initial therapy in an attempt to reduce tumor size preoperatively, (2) as interim therapy for the patient treated by irradiation in whom a more rapid decrease in GH is desired, and (3) in the patient already treated by surgery and irradiation in whom GH levels remain elevated.

THERAPY FOR SPECIFIC COMPLICATIONS

In addition to therapy directed at the source of GH overproduction, several of the consequences of GH hypersecretion may require treatment. Hypertrophic osteoarthropathy, particularly of the hip joint, may be very disabling and require total hip replacement. Nerve entrapment may require a nerve sheath release procedure to restore normal function. Eustachian tube mucosal hypertrophy and serous otitis media can be treated by a tympanic membrane fenestration procedure, and mandibular overgrowth may require surgical therapy to the temporomandibular joint or the mandible to re-establish normal dental occlusion. These procedures should be delayed whenever possible until primary therapy for acromegaly has stabilized the soft tissue changes. Hyperprolactinemia, if present, can generally be controlled with bromocriptine, and diabetes mellitus with insulin, bearing in mind that profound insulin resistance is frequently present. Adequate treatment of acromegaly usually allows discontinuance of insulin therapy.

Suggested Reading

Arosio M, Giovanelli MA, Riva E, Nava C, Ambosi B, Faglia G. Clinical uses of pre- and postsurgical evaluation of abnormal GH responses in acromegaly. J Neurosurg 1983; 59:402.

Baskin DS, Boggan JE, Wilson CB. Transsphenoidal microsurgical removal of growth hormone-secreting pituitary adenomas. A review of 137 cases. J Neurosurg 1982; 56:634.

Dons RF, Rieth KG, Gorden P, Roth J. Size and erosive features of the sella turcica in acromegaly as predictors of therapeutic response to supervoltage irradiation. Am J Med 1983; 74:69.

Frohman LA. Diseases of the anterior pituitary. In: Felig P, Baxter JD, Broadus AE, Frohman LA, eds. Endocrinology and Metabolism. New York: McGraw-Hill, 1981:151–231.

Melmed S, Braunstein GD, Horvath E, Ezrin C, Kovacs K. Pathophysiology of acromegaly. Endocrinol Rev 1982; 4:271.

Moses AC, Molitch ME, Sawin CT, Jackson IM, Biller BJ, Furlanetto R, Reichlin S. Bromocriptine therapy in acromegaly: use in patients resistant to conventional therapy and effect on serum levels of somatomedin C. J Clin Endocrinol Metab 1981; 53:772.

Schuster LD, Bantle JP, Oppenheimer JH, Seljeskog EL. Acromegaly: reassessment of the long-term therapeutic effectiveness of transsphenoidal pituitary surgery. Ann Intern Med 1981; 95:172.

SHORT STATURE

SELNA L. KAPLAN, M.D., Ph.D.

GROWTH HORMONE DEFICIENCY

At present, human pituitary-derived growth hormone is the appropriate treatment for GH deficient patients. The minimal effective dose is 0.3 U/kg/week administered in three divided doses weekly, either by the subcutaneous or the intramuscular route. The optimal range may be 0.6 U/kg/week, but supply limitations and financial constraints limit consideration of the use of higher doses at present. Preliminary studies suggest that doses of 0.3 U/kg/week, administered in divided doses daily, may induce greater increments in height than a thrice weekly administration schedule.

In neonates with hypothalamic hypopituitarism and associated hypoglycemia, growth hormone is administered every other day or daily to sustain a euglycemic state.

Treatment Period and Response

Accurate measurements of height and weight should be determined every 12 to 16 weeks. Either a wall-mounted metal tape or a stadiometer must be used; the measuring rod on the weight scales is inaccurate. Skeletal age is determined from a radiograph of the left hand obtained prior to therapy and at yearly intervals thereafter.

Therapy with growth hormone should be given continuously until epiphyseal fusion; the length of treatment may vary from 4 to 10 years. Interrupted treatment periods of more than 4 weeks will alter the optimal yearly growth rate. During the first few years of treatment, growth rates of 9 to 16 cm are attained. There is an inverse ratio of initial growth rate to skeletal age. The yearly growth rate decreases to 5 to 6 cm in subsequent years of therapy.

Sustainment of optimal rates of growth in later years of therapy may require higher doses of growth hormone. However, the current limited supplies necessitate conservative therapeutic regimens. The final height of treated GH-deficient patients has been 12 to 15 cm less than appropriate for parental height. Initiation of treatment at an earlier age with adequate doses may provide improved prognosis for final height.

TSH-thyroid and ACTH-adrenal function must be evaluated prior to initiation of growth hormone therapy. Thyroid function should be normalized before growth hormone therapy is initiated. L-thyroxine replacement doses are 0.05 to 0.1 mg daily. Hydrocortisone dosage should not exceed 5 mg twice daily during growth hormone therapy.

Inadequate increments in height during growth hormone therapy (<4 cm/year) may be the consequence of (1) development of tertiary hypothyroidism (replacement therapy with L-thyroxine restores normal growth); (2) induction of antibodies to hGH as determined by in vitro tests (increase dose of growth hormone or change preparation of growth hormone); (3) adolescent age of patient (addition of low-dose testosterone enanthate, 50 mg IM monthly, or Premarin, 0.3 mg, day 1 to 21 of each month may be necessary); (4) skeletal age more than 14 years in females and more than 15 years in males (discontinue growth hormone therapy), or (5) noncompliance (counseling and/or substitution of reliable individual to administer injections).

Alternative Sources of Growth-Stimulating Hormones

Recombinant DNA-derived human growth hormone has comparable biologic activity in growth hormone-deficient children. Its availability in the future will improve supplies of growth hormone.

Most patients with developmental defects (idiopathic) of growth hormone secretion have hypothalamic abnormalities associated with deficient release of hypothalamic growth hormone-releasing factor (GRF). This recently synthesized GRF peptide has been shown to stimulate growth in growth hormone-deficient children in short-term studies. Since frequent pulses of GRF are required to induce this effect, its use for chronic treatment is experimental at present. Synthesis of long-acting analog of GRF may provide an alternative effective mode of therapy for these patients.

NON-GROWTH-DEFICIENT SEVERE SHORT STATURE

This heterogeneous group includes children previously described in categories that include normal variant short stature, biologically inactive GH syndrome, and neuroendocrine GH dysfunction. They show the following characteristics: normal GH response to provocative stimuli; height at or below -2.5 SD (third percentile) for age; a 2-year or longer delay in skeletal age; growth rate at or less than 4 cm yearly. The somatomedin C may be low or normal for skeletal age. An improved rate of growth (an increment of 2 to 4 cm per year) is induced in 40 to 60 percent of these children in response to a 6-month course of pituitary growth hormone (0.1 to 0.2 units/kg/three times weekly).

The complete trial treatment course should include a 6-month to 1-year pretreatment observation period for baseline measurements of height and GH function, two 6-month interrupted treatment periods, and a 6-month interval nontreatment period. If the increment in height is more than 2 cm greater during growth hormone treatment than during periods off growth hormone, continued treatment should be considered. The potential beneficial effect, if any, of growth hormone therapy on the final height in these patients remains unknown at present.

INTRAUTERINE GROWTH RETARDATION

The deficits in height and weight which are inappropriate for gestational age at birth are sustained in many of these children throughout their lifetime. The range of final height is 137.2 to 152.4 cm (54 to 60 inches). Several reports suggest that 40 percent of these children exhibit an improved growth rate following daily administration of pituitary human growth hormone.

Preliminary data suggest that final height may not be altered significantly. The appropriateness of growth hormone therapy in this group of patients remains controversial.

GONADAL DYSGENESIS (TURNER SYNDROME)

Replacement therapy with low-dose estrogens can be initiated at age 12 to 13 years without jeopardizing final height. Ethinyl estradiol powder (5 to 10 μg) or conjugated estrogens (Premarin), 0.3 mg on days 1 to 21 of the calendar month, stimulates breast development and growth spurt during the first 6 months to one year of administration.

Induction of cyclic uterine withdrawal bleeding requires ethinyl estradiol in doses of 10 to 20 μg or Premarin, 0.6 mg on days 1 to 21 with 5 mg medroxyprogesterone acetate on days 12 to 21.

Improved growth following administration of human growth hormone either alone (0.2 U/kg three times weekly) or in conjunction with oxandrolone (0.1 mg/kg daily) has been reported. Beneficial effects on ultimate height cannot be determined in these short-term studies.

The use of androgen (fluoxymesterone) is not advisable owing to limited beneficial effects and associated undesirable side effects.

GROWTH RETARDATION ASSOCIATED WITH CHRONIC DISEASE

Growth failure with poor gain in height and weight is a major clinical manifestation of chronic illness. Undernutrition and poor utilization of nutrients are primary contributing factors. Treatment of the primary disorder and high caloric nutritional supplements can improve the associated growth failure.

Delayed growth and adolescent development is a concomitant abnormality seen in many patients with cystic fibrosis, sickle cell anemia, galactosemia, and thalassemia major. Replacement therapy with gonadal hormones is required.

PSYCHOSOCIAL DWARFISM (EMOTIONAL DEPRIVATION SYNDROME)

This pyschologic disorder is more easily diagnosed than treated. Transient diminished growth hormone secretion, retardation in growth rate, behavior disorder, and depressive mental state exist in children with this disorder. Most parents reject the need for family therapy and/or psychotherapy as treatment for the delayed growth in the child until the child becomes unmanageable at home. Rapid acceleration in growth rate and improved eating habits occur following hospitalization or transfer to a foster home. Deceleration of growth and emotional regression may occur if the child returns to the natural socially and emotionally deprived home environment.

Whether emotional deprivation and/or social upheaval in the home and at school of lesser severity can induce significant deceleration in growth rate in some children has not been adequately investigated.

GENETIC SHORT STATURE

Children with genetic short stature have yearly growth rates that are appropriate for age, a height between the first and the fifth percentile (-2 to -3 SD for age), and skeletal age that is normal or no more than 1 year less than chronologic age. Deviations from these criteria warrant further evaluation since growth hormone-deficient children may have short parents.

Human growth hormone treatment has not been beneficial in short children who have a normal rate of growth. It is not indicated in children with genetic short stature.

Suggested Reading

Kaplan SL, Fenno J, Stebbin N, Hintz R, Swift R. The biological effectiveness of pituitary-derived and biosynthetic methionyl-hGH in animals and man. In: Ahmad F, Schultz J, Smith EE, Whelan WJ (eds). From Gene to Protein: Translation into Biotechnology. New York: Academic Press, 1982, pp 419–428.

Kowarski Aa, Schneider J, Ben-Galim E, Weldom VV, Daughaday WH. Growth failure with normal serum RIA-GH and low somatomedin activity: somatomedin restoration and growth acceleration after exogenous GH. J Clin Endocrinol Metab 1978; 47:461–464.

Rudman D, Kutner MH, Blackston RD, Cushman RA, Bain RP, Patterson JH. Children with normal-variant short stature: treatment with human growth hormone for six months. N Engl J Med 1981; 035:123–131.

Schriock EA, Lustig RH, Rosenthal SM, Kaplan SL, Grumbach MM. Effect of growth hormone (GH)-releasing hormone (GRH) on plasma GH in relation to magnitude and duration of GH deficiency in 26 children and adults with isolated GH deficiency or multiple pituitary hormone deficiencies: Evidence for hypothalamic GRF deficiency. J Clin Endocrinol Metab 1984; 58:1043–1049.

Tanner JM, Whitehouse RH, Hughes PCR, Vince FP. Effect of human growth hormone treatment for 1 to 7 years on growth of 100 children with growth hormone deficiency, low birth weight, inherited smallness, Turner's syndrome, and other complaints. Arch Dis Child 1971; 46:745–782.

Van Vliet G, Styne DM, Kaplan SL, Grumbach MM. Growth hormone treatment for short stature. N Engl J Med 1983; 309:1016–1022.

HYPERTHYROIDISM IN GRAVES' DISEASE

SIDNEY H. INGBAR, M.D.

It is important to note that not all hyperthyroidism is due to Graves' disease, and not all thyrotoxicosis is a reflection of hyperthyroidism. To understand why this is the case requires a definition of terms. Thyrotoxicosis is the clinical and biochemical complex that results from the sustained delivery to the peripheral tissues of excessive quantities of thyroid hormones, wherever their source and whatever the cause. Hyperthyroidism is the term denoting that such hormone excess results specifically from sustained thyroid hyperfunction leading to increases in both hormone formation and hormone secretion. As can be seen in Table 1, which lists the major causes of thyrotoxicosis and their principal means of treatment, differentiation between the hyperthyroid and nonhyperthyroid varieties of thyrotoxicosis is of major importance because their treatment differs so radically. In the hyperthyroid variety, treatment is principally directed at bringing to an end the excess secretion of hormone. This is mainly accomplished with antithyroid agents or the use of radioactive iodine or surgery; iodine and glucocorticoids can be used, in addition, when hyperthyroidism is severe and life-threatening. Additional measures, such as the use of adrenergic blocking agents, sedation, and bed rest, are useful, often very much so, but are merely adjunctive. In the nonhyperthyroid varieties, thyrotoxicosis results from ingestion of excess quantities of hormone, from synthesis of hormone at some ectopic site, or, more commonly, from inflammatory disease that leads to the unregulated leakage of hormone from the gland. In all nonhyperthyroid varieties of thyrotoxicosis (which can be documented by very low values of the thyroid radioactive iodine uptake), new hormone synthesis is suppressed. Hence, measures intended to decrease hormone synthesis are to no avail. Instead, treatment comprises withdrawal of the exogenous hormone in the case of factitious thyrotoxicosis, destruction of the ectopic site when that is the source of hormone, or, in the case of inflammatory disorders, watchful waiting while the disease runs its course, often together with the palliative measures already mentioned when the patient is significantly symptomatic.

GENERAL CONSIDERATIONS REGARDING GRAVES' DISEASE

Several aspects of the pathogenesis and natural course of hyperthyroidism in Graves' disease bear importantly on its treatment. Graves' disease is one of several closely related autoimmune thyroid diseases, the others being Hashimoto's thyroiditis and primary myxedema. It is generally agreed that thyroid hyperfunction in Graves' disease results from the action of a class of IgG immunoglobulins that are probably antibodies to the thyrotropin (TSH) receptor. Antibody binding to the receptor activates adenylate cyclase within the plasma membrane of the follicular cell and initiates a chain of biochemical sequelae that result in thyroid growth and hyperfunction. Pathogenic IgG can be detected in vitro through their ability to inhibit the binding of TSH to thyroid membranes or through their thyroid-stimulating activity, as judged from activation of adenylate cyclase, increased radioiodine accumu-

TABLE 1 Disorders Associated With Thyrotoxicosis

Nature of Disorder	*Primary Mode of Therapy*	*Secondary Therapy*
Thyrotoxicosis with hyperthyroidism		
Syndromes of TSH excess		
TSH-producing tumor	Pituitary adenectomy	
Inappropriate TSH secretion	Uncertain*	
Graves' disease	Antithyroid agents	Adrenergic blocking agents
	Radioiodine	Iodine
	Subtotal thyroidectomy	Glucocorticoids
Toxic adenoma	Radioiodine	Adrenergic blocking agents
	Subtotal thyroidectomy	
Toxic multinodular goiter	Radioiodine	Adrenergic blocking agents
Thyrotoxicosis without hyperthyroidism		
Thyrotoxicosis factitia	Withdraw hormone	
Ectopic thyroid	Destroy ectopic tissue	
Hormone leakage (thyroiditis)		
Subacute thyroiditis	Analgesics	
	Glucocorticoids	
	Adrenergic blocking agents	
Chronic thyroiditis with transient thyrotoxicosis	Adrenergic blocking agents	

* Optimum treatment is uncertain. Hyperthyroidism can be controlled by the same measures as in Graves' disease, but tends to recur, and the concern is that a pituitary tumor might develop if the thyroid is ablated. Isolated reports suggest that treatment with bromocriptine, T_3, or 3, 5, 3′ — triiodothyroacetic acid (Triac) may be effective.

lation, or hormone release. Hence, they are designated TSH-binding inhibitory IgG (TBII) or thyroid-stimulating IgG (TSI), respectively.

As in other autoimmune disorders, hyperthyroidism in Graves' disease tends to be cyclic, undergoing periods of apparently spontaneous remission and exacerbation of varying duration. Because of associated chronic thyroiditis, there is a tendency over many years for such patients to develop evidence of progressive thyroid failure. These aspects of the natural history of the disease have an important bearing on the outcome, and therefore the choice, of therapy.

Unfortunately, there is as yet no mode of therapy directed at the underlying cause of the disease. The commonly used antithyroid agents, propylthiouracil (PTU) and methimazole (MMI), or carbimazole in the United Kingdom, act to inhibit both the organic binding of thyroid iodine and the coupling to yield iodothyronines. There is also some evidence that they may influence immune processes in vitro and may decrease the synthesis of thyroid-directed antibodies in vivo, but it is very unlikely that they have any effect that persists after their use is discontinued or that they influence the long-term course of the disorder. If this is indeed the case, then whether the patient experiences an immediate exacerbation of thyrotoxicosis when treatment is withdrawn or remains well for months, for years, or forever depends on the natural history of the disease in that particular patient. This undoubtedly accounts for the relatively low frequency of long-term or permanent remission that follows a course of antithyroid therapy.

Subtotal thyroidectomy and radioactive iodine destroy thyroid tissue, and if sufficient tissue is destroyed, the disease cannot manifest itself in hyperthyroidism. Their effect is long-lasting, therefore, and once a euthyroid state is achieved, recurrences of hyperthyroidism are quite rare. On the other hand, both surgery and radioactive iodine are prone to be associated with subsequent hypothyroidism with disturbing frequency. The cumulative frequency with which hypothyroidism follows ablative therapy increases progressively over the years as continuing chronic thyroiditis erodes the function of a gland that has been partly destroyed by these treatments.

Thus the relative long-term ineffectiveness of antithyroid therapy and the propensity of surgery and radioactive iodine to induce hypothyroidism pose a therapeutic dilemma in the management of the patients with hyperthyroidism in Graves' disease. As a result, and as a recent survey of thyroidologists discloses, there is no general agreement concerning the optimum mode of therapy in the patient who presents with an initial episode of hyperthyroidism. In general, the therapeutic decision depends on a number of factors. Mild disease, the absence of marked thyromegaly, and the fact that the patient is young weight the decision toward antithyroid therapy, especially if the patient is a woman. Patients with more severe disease and a large, highly vascularized goiter are less likely to experience a long-term remission after a course of antithyroid therapy; in such patients ablative therapy is more seriously considered—surgery for young women in the childbearing age and radioactive iodine in others. In patients in the fifth decade and older, I lean strongly toward the use of radioactive iodine. Superimposed on these considerations is a judgment concerning the likelihood of adequate patient compliance.

When an initial therapeutic recommendation has been formulated, I discuss with the patient in simple terms the nature of his or her disease, its natural course, and the therapeutic options available, including their advantages and limitations. In such discussions, the patient has the opportunity to express particular concerns, such as the fear of surgery or radioactive iodine, or the desire to "get it over with as quickly as possible". Ultimately, I make a strong therapeutic recommendation, which is almost always accepted, and a therapeutic plan is adopted to which both the physician and the patient are amenable. I find that this approach enhances patient confidence and compliance, minimizes later surprises, and in general fosters a favorable physician-patient relationship in respect to a disease whose care should extend over many years.

ANTITHYROID THERAPY

Owing in part to the age and sex distribution of patients with Graves' disease that I see, as well as to my personal inclination, I most often initiate treatment with antithyroid agents, usually 100 mg PTU given thrice daily, at 8-hour intervals. The approximately equivalent dose of MMI is 30 mg daily, but I usually employ PTU because of its additional effect of inhibiting the peripheral conversion of T_4 to T_3, hastening the therapeutic benefit that it brings. Patients with more severe disease, or those in whom a more rapid response is desired, are given higher doses, up to 600 mg PTU daily. Improvement is not immediate since PTU and MMI act by inhibiting hormone synthesis rather than its release. As a result, a decrease in hormone secretion and clinical improvement do not occur until significant depletion of intrathyroid stores of hormone has taken place. The duration of this apparent latent period varies with several factors, including the severity of the hyperthyroidism, the hormonal iodine content of the gland, and the dose of antithyroid agent administered. Generally, however, some improvement can be expected in about 2 weeks, with return to a normal metabolic state in 6 weeks to 2 months. Some patients, especially those with large vascular glands, are resistant to the usual doses of antithyroid agents; in them, larger doses, for example 1200 mg daily, may be required.

Clinical improvement is accompanied by a decrease in serum T_4 and T_3 concentrations, but such values do not always correlate well with the clinical state. Thus, some patients remain clinically thyrotoxic despite a normal serum T_4 concentration, probably because the serum T_3 concentration remains high. In others, a euthyroid clinical state is apparently sustained by a normal serum T_3 concentration, although the serum T_4 concentration is subnormal. Early evidence suggests that patients in whom serum T_3 concentrations remain relatively high during antithyroid therapy are less likely to experience a long-term remission after such therapy is withdrawn.

Once achieved, a euthyroid clinical state can usually be maintained by doses of PTU in the order of 150 to 200 mg daily, and once a maintenance dose is established, the patient is seen at monthly intervals and then every 2 months. An important element in following the patient is to observe the size of the thyroid gland. In about one-third of patients, the thyroid decreases in size. This is probably a reflection of a decreasing level of TSI and is a favorable sign that a long-term remission will follow withdrawal of antithyroid therapy. In some patients, the thyroid gland enlarges instead, often with the associated appearance of a thrill or bruit. This may signal overtreatment with resulting hypothyroidism, which may be symptomatic. Both symptoms and thyromegaly respond readily to a decreased dose of antithyroid agent or to the provision of supplemental thyroid hormone. On the other hand, in a smaller proportion of patients, enlargement of the thyroid gland during antithyroid therapy is a reflection of intensification of the disease that may require an increase in the dose of antithyroid agent.

Adverse reactions to antithyroid agents occur in a small percentage of patients. The most feared is agranulocytosis, an immunologic response that most often occurs after a few weeks of initial exposure to the antithyroid agent, but may occur after a much longer interval. During a second or third course of the agent, it may appear within a very few days. Agranulocytosis may be preceded by a period of drug-induced granulopenia; this may be hard to recognize since lymphocytosis and granulopenia occur in some patients with hyperthyroidism before therapy is initiated or may reflect the presence of an intercurrent viral infection. Dealing with this problem is difficult, but several measures are of assistance. I always obtain baseline total and differential leukocyte counts before therapy is begun, when the patient is seen again several weeks later, and when a euthyroid state has been achieved. Little benefit is to be derived from obtaining serial leukocyte counts thereafter, since granulopenia and agranulocytosis can appear precipitously within a few days after granulocyte counts have been shown to be normal. However, the patient is warned to call if a sore throat or fever (or rash) develops and to discontinue taking the antithyroid agent until he or she has been examined. This admonition should be repeated from time to time, and for medicolegal purposes, a note to the effect that this has been done should be placed in the patient's record. If granulopenia is found, frequent serial granulocyte counts are obtained, and if a downward trend is detected, the drug is discontinued. More often, granulopenia does remit, and therapy can be continued.

The other major toxic reaction to the antithyroid agents is a skin rash, which may be maculopapular or urticarial. Administration of antihistamines may alleviate the rash and allow treatment with the same antithyroid agent to continue. As an alternative, another antithyroid agent may be substituted. My own practice under these conditions is to discontinue antithyroid therapy altogether in view of the possibility that occult hypersensitivity reactions may take place, polyarteritis nodosa and lupus-like syndromes as a consequence of antithyroid therapy having been reported. Similarly, I never substitute one antithyroid agent for another in patients who have developed severe granulopenia or agranulocytosis, since studies have shown that lymphocytes of patients who have developed agranulocytosis while taking PTU undergo blast transformation when exposed in vitro to MMI.

The most common and difficult decision confronting the physician with respect to patients being treated with PTU or MMI is when to discontinue treatment, the hope being that a euthyroid state will persist. Unfortunately, there are no truly effective guidelines. As already noted, a decrease in goiter size during treatment is a reasonable indication that activity of the disease has abated and that a remission of reasonable duration may follow withdrawal of treatment. Efforts have been made to employ various laboratory tests as predictors of prognosis. Although statistically related to outcome, thyroid suppression and TRH tests are poor indicators of prognosis in the individual patient. There is some hope at present, however, that levels of TBII or TSI may be superior in this respect, their absence suggesting that the disease is in remission. In view of this uncertainty, the usual duration of a course of antithyroid therapy becomes somewhat arbitrary. The best data available indicate, not surprisingly, that the longer the course of treatment, the more likely a long-term remission after treatment is withdrawn. Generally, I employ a treatment period of 12 to 18 months. Treatment is then withdrawn and the patient is seen initially at 2- or 3-week intervals, and then at intervals progressively lengthening to one year. Serum T_4 and T_3 concentrations are measured at follow-up visits, since an elevation of the serum T_3 may presage the emergence of thyrotoxicosis while the patient still appears euthyroid.

Approximately 50 percent of patients treated in this manner experience a long-term remission; in the remainder, hyperthyroidism re-emerges within several weeks or recurs at some interval, sometimes many years, thereafter. When this occurs, I most often recommend a turn toward surgery or radioactive iodine therapy, but many patients prefer to undertake another course of antithyroid treatment, and there is no reason to discourage this approach if the patient is aware that the likelihood of a long-term remission after a second course of treatment is smaller than after the first.

SUBTOTAL THYROIDECTOMY

Subtotal thyroidectomy is an effective means of treating hyperthyroidism in Graves' disease, as many years of experience have demonstrated. It is infrequently followed by recurrence, but more often is followed by hypothyroidism, which sometimes occurs soon after operation, but also appears in succeeding years. The frequency of postoperative hypothyroidism varies inversely with that of recurrence, depending on the quantity of thyroid tissue removed and probably with the degree of associated thyroiditis. In the hands of experienced neck surgeons, subtotal thyroidectomy is quite a safe procedure, since both immediate and delayed postoperative complications occur in only a small percentage of patients. However, this is not always the case when the operation is performed by someone who lacks continued operative experience in this area.

Because of the tendency of subtotal thyroidectomy to lead to hypothyroidism, though less often than radioiodine does, and because the frequency of operative complications is greater than that of antithyroid therapy, I rarely recommend subtotal thyroidectomy as initial therapy in the patient experiencing a first episode of hyperthyroidism in Graves' disease, preferring to rely in general upon antithyroid agents in children and young adults and radioiodine in those whose who are older. Exceptions include patients with severe hyperthyroidism, usually with very large, hypervascular goiters, especially if they are young women or adolescents, in whom I prefer not to use radioactive iodine. In my experience, patients with severe thyrotoxicosis and very large goiters are often difficult to bring under control with antithyroid agents and, more importantly, are unlikely to experience a long-term remission after a course of antithyroid therapy. Another category of patients in whom I may recommend surgery as the initial mode of therapy comprises those young patients who for personal reasons strongly desire to deal with the disease quickly and definitively, and who do not wish to face possible recurrences after one or more courses of antithyroid agents.

Unlike other clinics, in which radioiodine is routinely recommended for the recurrences that follow one or more courses of antithyroid therapy, I often recommend surgery if the patient is a child or young adult, and especially if the patient is female. I also recommend surgery in young patients who are non-compliant with a medical regimen.

Unless there are compelling reasons to the contrary, I strongly believe in the importance of rendering the patient euthyroid with medical therapy before subtotal thyroidectomy is performed. Generally, I initiate therapy with antithyroid drugs, though I may use larger doses than usual in order to obtain control more rapidly. After a euthyroid state has been restored, and not before, iodides are added to the regimen, usually in the form of saturated solution of potassium iodide (SSKI), several drops two or three times daily. Although the value of iodides in bringing about involution of the gland and reducing its vascularity has been questioned, recent direct measurements have shown that the latter effect does take place. Some advocate discontinuing antithyroid therapy and replacing it with iodides once a euthyroid state has been achieved. I believe this to be an error, since it permits thyroid iodine stores to reaccumulate during the preoperative period. Some physicians, as a matter of convenience, set a target date for surgery on the presumption that a euthyroid state can necessarily be achieved within a defined period, a presumption that is infrequently justified.

Although it would certainly be both convenient and cost-effective if one could safely carry out thyroidectomy in a patient whose pre- and intraoperative regimen consisted only of a few days of treatment with adrenergic blocking agents, and although several reports suggest that this may be the case, I conservatively resist this approach, recognizing that thyroid storm can develop in patients receiving propranolol and believing that a prompt return of the patient to a normal routine after operation is more likely to occur if, before operation, the patient has undergone the return toward a normal state that the full preoperative regimen permits.

RADIOACTIVE IODINE

Early concerns about the use of radioactive iodine in the treatment of hyperthyroidism (i.e., the risk of leukemogenesis, carcinogenesis, and the induction of genetic damage) have proved to be unfounded, at least in adults, whereas indications of a low frequency of other late complications have given way to the realization that in a great many patients hypothyroidism either develops soon after ^{131}I therapy or continues to do so for years thereafter. I believe this to be due to the destructive effect of the radioiodine, and its possible inhibition of thyroid cell replication, combined with that of the chronic thyroiditis that is almost always associated with hyperthyroidism in Graves' disease. Nonetheless, because radioactive iodine is capable of curing hyperthyroidism in a way that antithyroid agents do not, and because it is essentially devoid of known complications apart from hypothyroidism, it plays a major role in the management of patients with Graves' disease. Opinions vary widely as to the type of patient in whom ^{131}I therapy can properly be used. Some use it to treat almost all patients, including children. However, children are prone to develop thyroid tumors and other nodular lesions after exposure to thyroid radiation, and the effects of hypothyroidism can be particularly damaging during childhood. Therefore, I and most others never use ^{131}I to treat children with hyperthyroidism. On the other hand, some who never use radioiodine to treat children use it routinely in almost any adult. Others, believing that long-term genetic effects have not been fully excluded, abjure its use in women who plan to have children. I lean toward the latter approach and resort to surgery in this group when ablative therapy is indicated. An additional consideration that also moves one toward this stance is the recognition that the younger the patient the more time there is for hypothyroidism to develop within the patient's life span. Hypothyroidism is also a complication of surgery, of course, but to a lesser degree. In patients who are middle-aged or older, or those whose family is complete, genetic damage is not a consideration, and delayed hypothyroidism is less a problem. As a consequence, I usually treat patients of this type with ^{131}I.

Research with respect to radioiodine therapy has concentrated on means of reducing subsequent hypothyroidism. Smaller than usual doses are less likely to do so in the short term, but more often fail to control hyperthyroidism, and there is no convincing evidence that they decrease the frequency of hypothyroidism in the long term. The latter is true whether or not antithyroid agents or iodides are employed to control hyperthyroidism in the early months after treatment. Similarly, the practice of administering larger doses per unit of thyroid weight in patients with larger glands and smaller doses for smaller glands has failed to achieve the objective of obtaining both early control of hyperthyroidism and a decreased frequency of delayed hypothyroidism. As a consequence, when I use radioactive iodine, I and the patient accept the fact that the patient has an approximately 20 percent likelihood of becoming hypothyroid in the first year and about a 50 percent likelihood of doing so by 10 years after treatment.

In patients who are to receive ^{131}I therapy, I first determine the 24-hour thyroid ^{131}I uptake and then administer a total therapeutic dose calculated to deliver about 80 μCi/g of estimated thyroid weight. Clinical improvement is usually delayed and progressive. Usually some improvement is evident in a few weeks, but the full early effect of treatment may not be realized for 3, 4, or even 6 months. During this period, propranolol is useful in controlling troubling manifestations of thyrotoxicosis.

Approximately 15 to 20 percent of patients, most commonly those with larger goiters, fail to achieve a euthyroid state within the first 6 months after radioiodine therapy. This is usually signaled by a lack of improvement in serum T_4 and T_3 concentrations by several months after treatment. In such patients, a second dose approximately two-thirds the magnitude of the first is administered. In a small proportion of patients, perhaps 5 percent, a third dose is required.

Though the likelihood of hypothyroidism is increased, I generally give somewhat larger doses of ^{131}I to elderly patients, particularly those with associated cardiovascular disease, in whom rapid and definitive control of thyrotoxicosis seems especially important. Furthermore, such patients are almost always brought to a euthyroid state with antithyroid agents before radioiodine is given so as to prevent the release of damaging quantities of hormone if radiation thyroiditis were to occur, as it commonly does approximately 2 weeks after radioiodine is administered. When this regimen is employed, antithyroid therapy is discontinued for 3 days, radioiodine is administered, and the antithyroid agent resumed 2 or 3 days later. Several months later, antithyroid therapy is gradually withdrawn so that the efficacy of the administered ^{131}I can be assessed.

A small proportion of patients become *transiently* hypothyroid several months after the dose of ^{131}I, as is also the case in patients treated surgically. This is difficult to distinguish from permanent hypothyroidism. If symptoms are mild, patients can merely be observed over the next several months to see whether symptoms and chemical evidence of hypothyroidism abate. When hypothyroidism is more pronounced, treatment with synthetic thyroxine in full replacement doses is initiated. Approximately one year later, measures are undertaken to determine whether the patient is permanently hypothyroid, and several options are available for doing so. One approach is to discontinue levothyroxine and to observe the patient for 6 weeks. At that time, serum T_4, T_3, and TSH concentrations will reflect the true functional capability of the thyroid. Prior to that time, evaluation may be misleading, since the TSH secretory mechanism that has been suppressed may require several weeks to resume its function. During this period, serum T_4 and T_3 concentrations fall to subnormal values and the patient may experience symptoms of hypothyroidism, whereas serum TSH concentrations and their response to TRH are inordinately low. An alternate approach can shorten the period of evaluation. Here, levothyroxine is discontinued and a replacement dose of liothyronine (approximately 75 μg daily) is substituted for a period of 4 weeks. At that time, the serum T_4 concentration is measured. Values less than 1.0 μg/dl indicate that the patient is truly hypothyroid; values greater than 1.0 μg/dl suggest that thyroid function is normal and that liothyronine can be discontinued. Intrinsic euthyroidism can then be verified by demonstrating a normal serum TSH concentration several weeks later. (This same procedure can be employed when one sees a patient already receiving replacement therapy for presumed hypothyroidism in whom one wishes to establish a definitive diagnosis.)

IODINE

Iodine is an extremely valuable agent in the treatment of hyperthyroidism under the special circumstances in which it is indicated. The action of iodine to decrease serum thyroid hormone concentrations and alleviate thyrotoxicosis is much more rapid than that of the antithyroid agents. This follows from the fact that iodine acts principally to inhibit the intrathyroid mechanisms that lead to hormone release, rather than synthesis. A secondary, and undesirable, effect of iodine is to increase glandular stores of hormone and iodine, creating a potential reservoir for subsequent excessive hormone release. For this reason, I do not undertake the use of iodine lightly and, except in patients being prepared for surgery, reserve its use for patients in whom rapid amelioration of thyrotoxicosis is critical. In this circumstance, concomitant use of antithyroid agents in large doses is strongly indicated for two reasons. First, patients in whom thyrotoxicosis is sufficiently critical to require treatment with iodine also require a major effort to inhibit ongoing hormone synthesis. Second, when used with iodine, large doses of antithyroid agents substantially decrease the degree of enrichment of thyroid iodine stores that would otherwise ensue. Patients sufficiently ill to receive iodine generally merit both hospitalization and adjunctive agents, such as adrenergic blocking agents and occasionally corticosteroids (to be discussed).

In patients who are not in actual or impending thyroid storm, but who are sufficiently ill to receive iodine, I initiate treatment with PTU in large doses, 600 mg daily or more, several hours before treatment with iodine is begun. SSKI is then begun in doses of several drops two or three times daily. The precise quantity of iodine required is admittedly uncertain and may vary from patient to patient, but in my experience, this quantity has been effective in almost all. Iodine therapy should not be discontinued too soon or too abruptly, since this may make possible accelerated release of hormonal stores that may have become somewhat enriched. For this reason, I continue administering iodine together with large doses of antithyroid agents for several weeks, until the effect of the latter to decrease hormone stores is strongly expressed and clinical improvement achieved. Doses of iodine are then tapered over the next several weeks.

ADJUNCTIVE THERAPY

Adrenergic Blocking Agents

The beta-adrenergic blocking agent propranolol plays an important role in managing patients with hyperthyroidism, owing to its ability to decrease many of the sympathomemetic manifestations of thyrotoxicosis. In patients with actual or impending thyroid storm, its use may be critical. In less severely ill patients, in the absence of contraindications, such as myocardial failure or bronchial asthma, I often use propranolol to decrease palpitations and lower heart rate, and to decrease perspiration and tremor. I use it in particular while awaiting the results of laboratory tests to confirm a diagnosis of hyperthyroidism and while awaiting the therapeutic response to antithyroid agents or radioactive iodine. Doses of 10 to 20 mg *qid* generally suffice; these are reduced and withdrawn altogether as the patient achieves a euthyroid state. As already indicated, I do not favor use of propranolol as the sole pre- and intraoperative therapy in patients undergoing subtotal thyroidectomy. Neither do I recommend chronic use of propranolol in the pregnant woman with hyperthyroidism. Although opinions concerning its safety in pregnancy vary, some indicate that growth retardation, low Apgar scores, and fetal hypoglycemia and bradycardia may attend its use.

Glucocorticoids

High doses of adrenal glucocorticoids play a poorly understood but useful role in the treatment of patients with Graves' disease and severe hyperthyroidism, in whom rapid relief of thyrotoxicosis is critical. One component of the beneficial effect of glucocorticoids stems from their ability to inhibit the peripheral deiodination of T_4 to yield T_3; this effect is not confined to patients with hyperthyroidism, being seen in euthyroid subjects as well. The second effect is more obscure in its origin, has been demonstrated only in patients with Graves' disease, and comprises a reduction in serum T_4 concentration that is evident within 1 or 2 days and is apparently due to inhibition of hormone release. In view of the slow turnover of IgG, this prompt effect is unlikely to reflect an inhibition of TSI synthesis, but it results from an effect of the glucocorticoids on some component of the immune system, possibly lymphocytes that are producing TSI within the thyroid itself. I have employed glucocorticoids only rarely, using doses of prednisone or dexamethasone equivalent to approximately 300 mg of hydrocortisone daily. My use of these agents has been confined to patients sufficiently ill to warrant concomitant treatment with iodides and propranolol.

Sodium Ipodate

This iodinated radiographic contrast agent is one of several that both inhibit the peripheral conversion of T_4 to T_3 and provide large quantities of iodine that act directly on the thyroid to inhibit hormone release. Doses of 1.0 g daily have been shown to produce a prompt decrease in serum T_4 and T_3 concentrations, together with alleviation of thyrotoxicosis. I have no direct experience with use of this agent, but would caution that large doses of antithyroid agents be administered concomitantly and ipodate withdrawn slowly, as in the use of iodine alone.

FOLLOW-UP

From their very first visit, patients with Graves' disease should be informed that they will require lifetime, if ultimately infrequent, follow-up. There are many reasons why this is the case. Approximately 50 percent of patients who remain euthyroid after one or more courses of antithyroid therapy develop thyroid failure 20 or more years later. Others, in contrast, develop recurrent hyperthyroidism; the longest interval between remission and later relapse that I have seen has been 28 years. On the other hand, among patients treated with radioiodine or surgery, continuing surveillance has revealed the development of hypothyroidism in several percent each year. Finally, the passage of years may permit the emergence of other autoimmune diseases with which Graves' disease is associated, such as pernicious anemia, idiopathic adrenal atrophy, or diabetes mellitus. These considerations make re-examination of the patient with Graves' disease at regular intervals mandatory, even though hyperthyroidism no longer appears to be a problem.

PRIMARY HYPOTHYROIDISM

DAVID H. SARNE, M.D.
SAMUEL REFETOFF, M.D.

In primary hypothyroidism, the thyroid gland fails to achieve tissue levels of thyroid hormone adequate to maintain euthyroidism. Patients with hypothyroidism form a clinical and biochemical spectrum. In its severest form, hypothyroidism or myxedema is characterized by gross cardiorespiratory, neuromuscular, and gastrointestinal dysfunction. In subclinical hypothyroidism, a lack of symptoms is accompanied by normal serum thyroid hormone levels. All patients have an elevated basal level of serum TSH (thyroid stimulating hormone, thyrotropin) and an exaggerated TSH response to TRH (thyrotropin releasing hormone). The goal of therapy is to restore thyroid hormone in tissues to a level sufficient to relieve all symptoms and reverse all the biochemical abnormalities of hypothyroidism.

Primary glandular dysfunction iis the most common cause of hypothyroidism. In the United States, chronic (autoimmune) thyroiditis and iatrogenic hypothyroidism are the most common etiologies in adults, whereas congenital athyreosis and inborn errors of hormonogenesis are more common in infants. Irrespective of the etiology, the treatment remains the same—exogenous hormone replacement. Exceptions are rare and include the administration of iodine to patients with an iodide-trapping defect or deiodinase deficiency and the withdrawal of iodine from patients with iodine-induced myxedema.

The normal thyroid gland synthesizes L-tetraiodothyronine (L-T_4) and L-triiodothyronine (L-T_3) within a large protein molecule, thyroglobulin. In this form, they are stored in the colloid of the thyroid follicles. As needed, the colloid is resorbed and hydrolyzed, and the hormones are released into the circulation. The normal intrathyroidal T_4 to T_3 molar ratio is 10 to 1. Whereas T_4 is only synthesized in the thyroid gland, 80 percent of the extrathyroidal T_3 is derived from peripheral monodeiodination of T_4.

PREPARATIONS AVAILABLE FOR CLINICAL USE

Thyroid hormone is available as synthetic hormone or as a crude extract from animal thyroid glands. Synthetic hormone is available as L-T_4, L-T_3, or a mixture of both. Natural preparations include hydrolyzed extracts and intact thyroglobulin (Table 1).

Sodium Salt of L-T_4 (Sodium Levothyroxine)

This is the most commonly used synthetic preparation. The use of a pure chemical ensures uniform potency. Absorption after an oral dose varies from 30 to 90 percent and is dependent on the binders in the tablet. Absorption is slightly higher in the fasting state. The half-life of the absorbed T_4 is 6 to 9 days. Most of it is reversibly bound to plasma proteins, and only the free fraction is immediately available to tissues. These properties are usually advantageous. Therapy may be taken once daily or, although less desirable, if necessary can be administered on a once weekly basis (1.5 to 2 mg per week). Once a steady state is achieved, ingestion of the daily dose and even an occasional missed dose produce only small, clinically insignificant alterations in the serum concentrations of T_4, T_3, or TSH.

Available strengths for oral administration range from 25 to 300 μg. Colors of the various dosages were formerly standardized by the manufacturers*. Tartrazine (yellow dye No. 5), used in the 100-μg (yellow) and 300-μg (green) tablets, may produce adverse reactions in patients sensitive to the dye. Sodium levothyroxine is also available in solution (100 μg/cc) or lyophilized in mannitol (100, 200, or 500 μg to be reconstituted in NaCl) for intravenous or intramuscular use.

Sodium Salt of L-T_3 (Sodium Liothyronine)

As with levothyroxine, the use of a pure chemical ensures uniform potency. After an oral dose, about 90 percent of the drug is absorbed. The half-life of the absorbed T_3 is one day. The drug is best administered in two or three daily doses. Even after a steady state is achieved, each dose produces a marked postabsorptive rise in the serum T_3 level. This variation in the hormone level should not produce symptoms. T_3 has a more rapid onset of action following the institution of therapy and a more rapid dissipation of its effects after its discontinuation. T_4 and T_3 both have distinct advantages. T_3 is the drug of choice when a rapid onset of action is needed, as in the treatment of myxedema, or when rapid dissipation of the hormonal effects is useful, as in the temporary withdrawal of therapy from thyrid cancer patients prior to scanning.

Liothyronine for oral administration is available in strengths of 5 to 50 μg. There is no commercially available preparation for parenteral administration unless obtained by special arrangement from Smith Kline & French laboratories. However, it can be prepared by dissolving crystalline L-T_3 in a slightly alkaline solution which is sterilized by passage through a Millipore filter.

Mixture of Synthetic L-T_4 and L-T_3 (Liotrix)

This preparation contains a 4 to 1 molar ratio of T_4 and T_3 for oral use. The product was developed to

---

*25 μg = orange; 50 μg = white; 100 μg = yellow; 125 μg = purple; 150 μg = blue; 175 μg = turquoise; 200 μg = pink; and 300 μg = green. Exception: Synthroid—75 μg = purple; 125 μg = brown.

supply T_4 as well as T_3 in order to more closely provide a normal hormone milieu. Only later was it recognized that most extrathyroidal T_3 is generated from T_4 in peripheral tissues. The absorption and half-life of each component remains the same as when they are administered separately. These preparations should be administered on a once-daily basis. Their hormonal potency is identified by approximate equivalence to desiccated thyroid. Despite the similar ratio of T_4 and T_3, the two available synthetic mixtures differ in their hormone content. One grain equivalent of Euthroid contains 60 μg L-T_4 and 15 μg L-T_3, whereas one grain equivalent of Thyrolar contains 50 μg L-T_4 and 12.5 μg L-T_3.

Dose equivalents in terms of approximate biologic activity of the synthetic products are 100 μg L-T_4, 40 μg L-T_3, and 1 grain equivalent of the L-T_4/L-T/$_3$ mixtures. The usual adult replacement dose is 100 to 200 μg L-T_4 per day (25 μg L-T_3 *bid* or *tid* or 1 to 2 grain equivalents L-T_4/L-T_3 per day).

Crude Hormone Preparations

These have been successfully used to treat hypothyroidism for over 75 years. Thyroid hormone extracts are prepared from the glands of slaughterhouse animals, usually cattle and pigs. The molar ratio of T_4 to T_3 in these products is usually 3 or 4 to 1, but pure pork products have even more T_3, with a ratio of 2.5 to 1. The US Pharmacopoeia sets a standard based only on the organic iodine content (0.17 to 0.23%). Determination of the actual content in T_4 and T_3 is not required, and thus inactive preparations containing other iodinated compounds have been marketed in the past. There is no legal safeguard to prevent variability in potency. However, reputable manufacturers currently standardize their own products by bioassay or chemical analysis, and any serious variation in potency is unlikely. Nevertheless, with the increasing use of generic prescriptions, the use of preparations from different manufacturers may lead to an inadvertent change in dosage. There are no side effects specifically associated with the crude hormone preparations.

These preparations can only be used orally. Available strengths range from 0.25 to 5 grains. Tablets of more than 3 grains desiccated thyroid contain hormone in excess of normal replacement therapy, and they should be avoided. Among the various preparations, the biologic potency per grain is roughly equivalent, except for Thyroid Strong Tablet (Marion Laboratories), which is 1.5 times more potent than most desiccated thyroid products. The approximate equivalent of 100 μg L-T_4 is 1 grain of desiccated thyroid. Thus, the usual adult replacement dosage is 1 to 2 grains daily.

Crude hormone in the form of pork thyroglobulin is also available. This compound is especially rich in T_3 content, but offers no advantages over other biologically active extracts and is more expensive.

As the price difference between the synthetic products and crude extracts has decreased, the former have become the drugs of choice. Except for special circumstances requiring rapid alterations in hormone effect, L-T_4 is preferable to L-T_3 as its longer half-life allows replacement with a single daily dose and provides a more stable hormonal blood level. As most tissue T_3 is normally derived from T_4, we do not ordinarily use the combination products.

TABLE 1 Thyroid Hormone Preparations Available for Oral Administration

Preparation	*Generic Name*	*Common Brand Name**	*Available Strengths*
Synthetic			
Sodium L-tetraiodothyronine (L-T_4)	Levothyroxine	Levothroid	0.025, 0.05, 0.1, 0.125, 0.15, 0.175, 0.2, and 0.3 mg.
		Synthroid	0.025, 0.05, 0.1, 0.15, 0.2, and 0.3 mg.
Sodium L-triiodothyronine (L-T_3)	Liothyronine	Cytomel	5, 25, and 50 μg
Mixture of L-T_4 and L-T_3	Liotrix	Euthroid	½, 1, 2, and 3 grain equivalents (1 gr eq = 60 μg T_4 plus 15 μg T_3)
		Thyrolar	¼, ½, 1, 2, and 3 grain equivalents (1 gr eq = 50 μg T_4 plus 12.5 μg T_3)
Crude hormone			
Powdered thyroid glands	Desiccated thyroid	Desiccated thyroid	¼, ½, 1, 1½, 2, 3, 4, and 5 grains
		Thyroid Strong Tablets†	½, 1, 2, and 3 grains
		S-P-T‡	1, 2, 3, and 5 grains
	Thyroglobulin	Proloid	½, 1, 1½, 2, and 3 grains

* Listed in Physicians' Desk Reference. Oradell, NJ: Medical Economics, 1984.
† 1 grain is equivalent to 1½ grains of other desiccated thyroid products.
‡ An encapsulated suspension in soybean oil.

APPROACH TO THERAPY

Institution of Therapy

The rapidity with which normal thyroid hormone levels should be restored depends on a number of factors including age, duration and severity of hypothyroidism, and the presence of other disorders (Table 2). In a young, otherwise healthy individual with a recent onset of hypothyroidism, therapy may be instituted with 100 μg L-T_4 daily. Further adjustment, usually an increase, is made at monthly or bimonthly intervals until the patient is euthyroid. In patients with recent onset of hypothyroidism after radioiodide treatment, hormone replacement should not be instituted until serum TSH levels have been elevated for 7 to 10 days without a documented increase in the serum T_4 level. In younger patients with longstanding hypothyroidism and in patients over the age of 45 without known heart disease, we begin therapy with 50 μg L-T_4 daily and after 4 weeks increase the dose to 100 μg per day. The dosage is further adjusted as described above. In adults, the usual replacement dose is 100 to 200 μg L-T_4 daily; only 20 percent of adults require the higher dose and very few require more than 200 μg daily.

In older patients with severe hypothyroidism and in patients with known ischemic heart disease, the initial dose should be only 25 μg L-T_4 daily. An EKG should be obtained before beginning therapy. The patient must be closely followed as the daily dose is increased by 25 μg increments at monthly intervals. Some patients may only tolerate increments of 12.5 μg L-T_4. In a few patients, angina may actually improve, but in most, the frequency and severity of the attacks could increase with higher doses of thyroid hormone. Even with the addition of β-blockers, nitrates, and calcium channel blockers, some patients cannot achieve euthyroidism without an unacceptable exacerbation of angina. Such patients should be evaluated for coronary artery bypass, and if they are otherwise appropriate candidates, they can undergo surgery despite only partial hormone replacement.

Rarely, the onset of visual field defects or pseudotumor cerebri has been reported during the initiation of replacement therapy in patients with longstanding hypothyroidism. Visual field defects, presumably related to transient pituitary enlargement, resolve over time as replacement is continued. Pseudotumor, which has occurred in children with longstanding hypothyroidism in whom thyroid hormone was rapidly replaced, responds to a reduction in dosage and more gradual replacement.

In hypothyroid neonates and infants, full maintenance therapy should be instituted rapidly in order to prevent or minimize the deleterious effects of thyroid hormone deprivation on the still developing nervous system. We recommend beginning therapy with 25 μg L-T_4 daily and increasing the dose to 37.5 μg by age 6 months and to 50 μg daily by age 1 year. It should be noted that the usual maintenance dose in children is on average 3.5 μg/kg body weight/day (or 100 μg T_4/m^2 body surface area) rather than the 2.1 μg/kg body weight/day recommended for adults.

Myxedema coma is the end stage of severe long-neglected or undiagnosed hypothyroidism. It represents a medical emergency with a high mortality rate even with proper treatment. If the diagnosis is apparent on clinical

TABLE 2 Administration of L-T_4

Patient	*Initial Dose*	*Next Increase*	*Added Doses*	*Maintenance*
Adult				
Under 45 years old, mild hypothyroidism	100 μg T_4 daily	25–50 μg T_4 at 4–8 weeks	25–50 μg T_4 at 4–8 weeks	100–200 μg T_4
Under 45 years old, marked hypothyroidism or Over 45 years old, mild hypothyroidism and without known cardiac disease	50 μg T_4 daily	25–50 μg T_4 at 4 weeks	25–50 μg T_4 at 4–8 weeks	100–200 μg T_4
Over 45 years old, marked hypothyroidism or Known cardiac disease*	25–50 μg T_4 daily	12.5 to 25 μg T_4 at 4 weeks	12.5 to 25 μg T_4 at 4–8 weeks	100–200 μg T_4
Myxedema coma	500 μg T_4 IV	12.5 μg T_3 q6h‡		100–200 μg T_4
Child				
Infants, neonates	25 μg T_4 daily	12.5 μg T_4 at age 6 months	12.5 μg T_4 at age 1 year	
2–10 years†	50 μg T_4 daily	12.5–25 μg T_4 at 4–8 weeks	12.5 to 25 μg T_4 at 4–8 weeks	150–200 μg T_4

* Recommended doses may produce unacceptable exacerbation of angina.
† Maintenance dose is usually about 3.5 μg/kg body weight.
‡ Until condition improves; T_3 should then be discontinued and the patient should be treated with 100 μg T_4 daily.

grounds, treatment should be instituted without awaiting laboratory confirmation. However, a blood sample for serum thyroid hormone determination should be obtained prior to the initiation of therapy. The proper method for hormone replacement in this condition remains controversial. Our goal is to rapidly restore serum levels of free T_4 and T_3, and this requires a loading dose to saturate the hormone-binding serum proteins. We recommend an intravenous bolus of 500 μg L-T_4 followed by 12.5 μg L-T_3 every 6 hours via nasogastric tube (except in patients with marked intestinal or gastric atony, who may require intravenous administration of T_3) until improvement is noted. The dosage is then reduced to a normal maintenance level. Adjunctive therapy—including cautious administration of intravenous fluids, ventilatory assistance, and treatment of hypothermia, infection, and other complications—should be administered in an intensive care unit setting.

Patients with subclinical hypothyroidism have no signs or symptoms of hypothyroidism. Serum levels of T_4 and T_3 may be within the normal range. The condition is detected by an elevated basal serum TSH level and an exaggerated TSH response to TRH. The need for treatment in this entity remains controversial. We supplement these patients with thyroid hormone when such treatment does not pose any significant risk since therapy may reverse subtle abnormalities and because most of these patients ultimately develop clinical hypothyroidism.

In patients with suspected adrenal dysfunction, evaluation of the hypothalamic-pituitary-adrenal axis should be performed and full-replacement glucocorticoid therapy began prior to initiating thyroid hormone therapy. In patients with inadequate adrenal reserve, thyroid hormone may precipitate adrenal crisis. If rapid treatment is required, cortisol levels before and one hour after the administration of cosyntropin should be obtained and hydrocortisone administered before thyroid hormone is given. Any patient with secondary (pituitary) or tertiary (hypothalamic) hypothyroidism must also be evaluated for adrenal insufficiency (see chapters on *Hypopituitarism* and *Hypothalamic Hypopituitarism*).

If a patient requiring elective surgery is found to be hypothyroid, the operation should be postponed until the patient is made euthyroid. If the operative procedure is urgent, it may be carried out with relative safety in a patient with partially treated hypothyroidism.

Maintenance Therapy

Once euthyroidism is achieved, patients can be maintained on the same single daily dose of L-T_4. Adjustments are rarely needed unless other disorders intervene. No dosage change is usually required during pregnancy because, although total T_4 levels rise secondary to increased levels of thyroxine-binding globulin (TBG), the absolute amount of thyroid hormone degraded each day remains unchanged. With aging, the daily requirement for thyroid hormone may be reduced. Reassessment of the replacement dose may be appropriate in elderly patients. It has been suggested that there may be a seasonal variation in thyroid hormone requirement, but we do not alter thyroid hormone replacement therapy on that basis.

With concomitant severe illness, the peripheral conversion of T_4 to T_3 is reduced. Since the appropriate serum level of T_3 in this setting is not known, we do not alter thyroid hormone therapy.

Monitoring Therapy

No available test can clearly document the achievement of physiologic tissue levels of thyroid hormone. Basal metabolic rate, cholesterol, CPK, and other parameters which indirectly quantitate the effect of thyroid hormone on peripheral tissues vary for other reasons and are not reliable indicators of euthyroidism. In the past, measurement of protein-bound iodine (PBI) and later total T_4 and T_3 in serum were used to monitor therapy. Interpretation of results requires particular attention to the hormone preparations used and the timing of blood sampling in relation to the treatment schedule. The ability to measure serum TSH levels has greatly improved the accuracy with which thyroid hormone replacement can be monitored in patients with primary hypothyroidism. The response of TSH to TRH is the most sensitive indicator of the adequacy of thyroid hormone replacement. Once a normal TSH response is achieved, an increment of only 10 μg of T_3 is sufficient to abolish it. In most cases, though, the basal serum TSH level is an adequate indicator of the proper replacement dose. We increase the dosage of thyroid hormone in the manner already described until the basal TSH level is within the normal range.

Although an elevated TSH level indicates inadequate replacement, the inability of most current routine assays to discriminate between low and normal TSH values limits the ability of this measurement to detect overdosage. The failure of TSH to respond to TRH does suggest overdosage in patients with primary hypothyroidism. The daily dose of T_4 should be decreased by 25 μg and by further monthly decrements according to the resulting TSH level. The appropriate dose is then the lowest that maintains the TSH within the normal range. Alternatively, a TRH test can be performed with each decrement, the appropriate replacement dose being that which no longer suppresses the response to TRH. It should be noted that in infants with neonatal hypothyroidism or in adults with longstanding hypothyroidism, TSH levels may remain elevated for months despite adequate thyroid hormone replacement therapy.

In patients with secondary hypothyroidism (pituitary dysfunction), serum free hormone levels interpreted in light of the hormone preparation and a knowledge of usual maintenance dose for different hormonal preparations must be used to judge the adequacy of therapy. In patients with tertiary hypothyroidism (hypothalamic dysfunction), although the basal TSH is not a reliable indicator, the TSH response to TRH can be used for monitoring therapy.

While receiving L-T_4 therapy, at a dosage sufficient to restore the TSH level to normal, most patients with primary hypothyroidism have normal values for total T_4 (TT_4), free thyroxine index (FT_4I), and total T_3 by radioimmunoassay (TT_3). TT_4 and FT_4I values tend to be high normal and TT_3 values low normal. In 10 to 25 percent of patients, TT_4 and FT_4I values are above the upper limit of normal. However, since the TSH remains elevated with a lower dose, we presume that this reflects the somewhat lower levels of TT_3. Following the recent introduction of high-pressure liquid chromatography to assay L-T_4 content, several manufacturers have increased the T_4 content of the tablets they produce. Patients who have been treated for several years may now require a slight reduction (25 to 50 μg) in their daily dosage to provide serum T_4 levels comparable to those on their previous regimen.

Patients treated solely with L-T_3 characteristically have low TT_4 and FT_4I values and elevated levels of T_3. Pituitary conversion of T_4 to T_3 appears to play a major role in the normal regulation of thyroid hormone; thus in the face of a low serum T_4, the serum T_3 level necessary to achieve TSH suppression is higher. Patients treated with L-T_4/L-T_3 mixtures or desiccated thyroid products often have TT_4, FT_4I values in the low range of normal.

If clinical or biochemical evidence of hypothyroidism persists despite suppression of serum TSH to normal, the response to TRH should be evaluated. If it remains exaggerated, the dosage of thyroid hormone should be increased. If the response to TRH is normal or suppressed, either the abnormalities are not related to thyroid hormone lack or the patient may have peripheral but not pituitary resistance to the action of thyroid hormone.

Some patients who became hypothyroid after the definitive treatment of hyperthyroidism require very small doses of thyroid hormone to achieve euthyroidism. It is likely that their glands retain autonomous function, but lack sufficient capacity to maintain euthyroidism.

PROBLEMS DURING THERAPY

Treatment Failures

Most adults achieve euthyroidism with a daily dose of 200 μg L-T_4 or less. If, after a 2- to 6-month trial on 200 μg L-T_4 daily, the patient still has symptoms of hypothyroidism, the following should be considered. The most common reason is failure to take the medication as prescribed. This can be documented by administration of the hormone under supervision. Other explanations include incorrect diagnosis, malabsorption, rapid degradation or excretion of the hormone, use of an inactive preparation, and tissue resistance to thyroid hormone (Table 3). The last two conditions are rare; incorrect diagnosis is much more common. Re-evaluation of the clinical and laboratory data should ensure the accuracy of diagnosis. Proper re-evaluation may require withdrawal of replacement therapy.

As thyroid hormone is recycled via the enterohepatic circulation, the failure of biliary reabsorption as well as decreased intestinal absorption may lead to increased fecal loss. Steatorrhea, the use of binding resins such as cholestyramine, and, in rare instances, a high soy bean diet may lead to excessive fecal loss of the ingested hormone. We have also observed a patient with inadequate absorption secondary to severe achalasia. Malabsorption may be documented by the measurement of protein-bound radioiodine following the simultaneous administration of oral and intravenous thyroid hormone, each labeled with a different radioactive iodine isotope. Rapid metabolism can be demonstrated by kinetic studies using radiolabeled hormone. An estimate of metabolic clearance can be made using the levels of bound and free hormone on the usual replacement dose, provided regular ingestion can be documented. Other than treatment of the underlying cause, increasing the daily dosage of hormone should provide adequate replacement in the aforementioned conditions.

Direct chemical analysis or bioassay can confirm the presence of an inactive preparation, but in practice, simply changing the preparation is sufficient. Resistance of the pituitary and peripheral tissues to thyroid hormone is a rare condition. With current techniques, the proof is time-consuming and requires a sophisticated investigation. It should be suspected when the other causes of treatment failure have been excluded.

Side Effects

Although a very rare patient may have a reaction to the dyes or other additives, true allergic or idiosyncratic reactions to the hormone are unheard of. Most common toxic effects relate to overdosage and are those of thyrotoxicosis. Headaches, palpitations, and anxiety are the most common complaints. Treatment consists of temporary cessation of therapy and resumption at a lower dose. Prolonged use of excessive amounts of thyroid hormone may contribute to the loss of bone mineral and the development of osteoporosis. Deleterious effects in the setting of adrenal insufficiency or cardiac disease have already been discussed. Nonspecific complaints which appear to be psychologic in origin and gastrointestinal symptoms can sometimes be relieved by changing the time of drug ingestion or by administering the hormone with meals or in divided doses.

TABLE 3 Evaluation of Patients Requiring Unusual Doses of L-T_4 for Subjective Improvement

Dose	Basal TSH	FTI	*Etiologies*	*Recommendation*
Subphysiologic Dose (< 100 μg/day)	Basal TSH Normal	FTI Low	1. T_3 Toxicosis	Check T_3
			2. Recent decrease in replacement dose	Repeat TSH, FT_4I in 2 weeks
			3. Taking preparation rich in T_3	Check T_3
			4. 2° or 3° hypothyroidism	TRH test
			5. Taking drugs which alter T_4 binding and metabolism (e.g., Dilantin) or suppress TSH (e.g., Bromocriptine)	Check drug history, increase T_4 if TSH is affected
		FTI Normal	1. Proper replacement	Verify with TRH test, continue with same dose
		FTI High	1. Nonsuppressible endogenous T_4	Reduce dose
			2. Patient taking more than prescribed dose	Check history, reduce dose
	Basal TSH High	FTI Low or Normal	1. Inadequate replacement	Increase dose
		FTI High	1. Inappropriate TSH secretion (pituitary adenoma or resistance to thyroid hormone)	Evaluation for adenoma vs. resistance
Supraphysiologic Dose (> 200 μg/day)	Basal TSH Normal	FTI Low or Normal	1. Incorrect diagnosis	Re-evaluate
			2. Poor absorption	Check absorption
			3. Rapid metabolism	Check metabolism
			4. Inactive preparation	Change preparation, recheck
			5. Patient taking less than prescribed dose	Check history
		FTI High	1. Incorrect diagnosis	Re-evaluate
			2. Overtreatment	Reduce dose 25 μg, repeat TSH, FT_4I in 4 weeks
			3. Peripheral resistance to thyroid hormone	Evaluate for resistance
	Basal TSH High	FTI Low or Normal	1. Poor absorption	Increase dose 25μg, repeat TSH, FT_4I in 4 weeks
			2. Rapid metabolism	Check metabolism
			3. Patient taking less than prescribed dose	Check history
			4. Inactive preparation	Change preparation
			5. Unusually high requirement	Increase dose 25 μg, recheck TSH, FT_4I in 4 weeks
		FTI High	1. Pituitary and peripheral resistance to thyroid hormone	Evaluate for resistance

Drug Interactions

Since alterations in metabolic status can affect the handling of a variety of drugs, patients should be carefully observed during the institution of therapy as the dose of other drugs may need adjustment. Requirements for insulin or oral hypoglycemic agents often increase with thyroid hormone therapy. The effects of anticoagulants are increased whereas those of digitalis and propranolol may be substantially decreased. Particular attention should also be paid to the dose of diuretics, sedatives, and opiates. As mentioned previously, cholestyramine and other binding resins may decrease the absorption of thyroid hormone; thyroid hormone should be administered several hours before the resin is ingested. Dilantin therapy may increase the metabolism of thyroid hormone and require an increase in the replacement dose.

WITHDRAWAL OF THERAPY

Re-evaluation of the diagnosis of hypothyroidism and the treatment of thyroid carcinoma with ^{131}I require the cessation of thyroid hormone therapy. Even with replacement doses of L-T_4, suppression of TSH may persist for 4 to 6 weeks after this hormone is discontinued. During this period, there is a progressive fall in the level of thyroid hormone, and transient signs and symptoms of hypothyroidism may develop even in patients who ultimately prove not to be hypothyroid. Only if serum T_4 levels fail to increase over a period of 7 to 10 days, during which TSH has been elevated, is the presence of primary hypothyroidism confirmed.

To shorten the period during which patients are subjectd to the symptoms of hypothyroidism, we switch patients from L-T_4 to an equivalent dose of T_3 administered *bid* or *tid* 4 weeks before hormone therapy is discontinued altogether. With this regimen, serum TSH should start rising within 10 to 14 days; however, on occasion, at least 21 days need to elapse. Patients with thyroid carcinoma resume therapy immediately after the scan is completed, unless they will be receiving a treatment dose of radioactive iodine, in which case the replacement is delayed until 24 hours after ^{131}I therapy.

Supported in part by US Public Health Grants AM 15070, AM 06169, and RR 305.

DIFFUSE NONTOXIC AND MULTINODULAR GOITER

LEONARD WARTOFSKY, M.S., M.D., F.A.C.P.

"Nontoxic" or "simple" goiter refers to a benign enlargement of the thyroid gland secondary to an impairment in the ability of the thyroid to produce amounts of thyroid hormone which are adequate to meet the hormonal needs of the patient. The impaired thyroid hormone production may be due to intrinsic defects in the gland, or to extrinsic factors such as iodine deficiency or exposure to various goitrogens. This group of disorders is generally "sporadic" in nature, whereas goiter due to iodine deficiency is often "endemic," a term that obtains when at least 10 percent of a population has the condition. (The treatment of endemic goiter is covered in the chapter by Dr. Fisher.) Whatever the cause, the basic underlying mechanism of this type of goiter relates to low circulating concentrations of thyroid hormone leading to a compensatory stimulation of the thyroid gland by thyrotropin (TSH). In most cases, there is true compensation with the re-establishment of euthyroidism, but at the cost of thyroid enlargement (goiter) due to the inherent inefficiency of the gland. Although serum TSH levels also may be within the normal range in these patients, the goiter probably is maintained by the chronic secretion of minimally supraphysiologic amounts of TSH.

Nontoxic goiter may be either diffuse or nodular. Diffuse goiter is commonly seen in patients exposed to pharmacologic levels of iodine or antithyroid agents such as prophylthiouracil or lithium carbonate. Nodular goiter is probably the result of chronic exposure of the thyroid to TSH stimulation with cycles of sequential hyperplasia and involution. The reponse of nontoxic goiter to medical treatment may be related to the stage of development present when the therapy is begun. The earliest lesion observed in nontoxic goiter is a diffuse hyperplasia, which will markedly or completely regress with thyroid hormone treatment. After more prolonged stimulation, areas of involution and hemorrhage are seen intermixed with hyperplasia, leading ultimately to nodule formation. Less predictable diminution in size with thyroid hormone therapy is to be expected with nodular goiter, and in fact it may be only the hyperplastic elements of the goiter that shrink and not the nodules per se. This phenomenon may result in a greater clinical appreciation by palpation of either the presence or the true size of nodules than was possible prior to treatment. In general, a significant diminution in size of diffuse goiter may be expected with thyroid hormone therapy in 75 to 85 percent of patients, whereas only approximately one-third of nodular glands will demonstrate shrinkage.

CLINICAL ASSESSMENT

Certain aspects of the history and physical examination determine the choice of treatment, and others may serve as parameters by which to judge response to therapy. A history is obtained to determine the presence of symptoms of hypothyroidism or hyperthyroidism, or of any exposure to goitrogens including iodine, lithium, or antithyroid drugs. Habitation in an iodine-deficient area should be ascertained, along with a family history of goiter or any thyroid disease. It is useful to assess the presence, initially and again after treatment, of such symptoms as cough, dysphagia, pressure sensation, pain, or hoarseness. The physical examination is concerned with a description of the size and consistency of the thyroid and the location and size of any nodules or lymph nodes. The metabolic status of the patient is assessed by the determination of serum levels of thyroxine (T_4), triiodothyronine (T_3), and TSH, and a 24-hour radioiodine uptake may be indicated.

We routinely perform a thyroid scan in patients whose thyroid gland is abnormal to palpation. Typically, the scan demonstrates heterogeneous distribution of radionuclide without major "hot" or "cold" areas. Scan visualization of several cold or hypofunctioning areas would not be unusual, but the multinodular goiter with a single, predominant (>1 to 1.5 cm) cold nodule warrants management comparable to that afforded the thyroid with a single cold nodule, as discussed elsewhere in this volume by Dr. Walfish. Suffice it to say that surgical excision of such a predominant nodule (subtotal thyroidectomy) may be preferable to medical therapy in such patients, and in other patients with increased risk of malignant tumor such as children or those with a history of irradiation therapy to the head and neck area in childhood. A scan suggesting multiple hyperfunctioning areas requires repetition when and if the patient is placed on thyroid hormone medication, in order to discern whether these areas are autonomous (nonsuppressible). When the initial scan result suggesting hyperfunctioning areas is obtained, our preferred management would include a thyrotropin-releasing hormone (TRH) test to determine whether supraphysiologic amounts of thyroid hormone are being produced. If the TSH response to TRH is flat, the aforementioned trial of thyroid hormone suppression with repeat scan is both unnecessary and contraindicated, but could be done to confirm autonomy on a test basis. In the absence of any symptoms, such patients should be followed without specific therapy, while recognizing that they may become hyperthyroid at some time in the future, especially after exposure to increases in stable iodine, as with radiocontrast dyes (Jod-Basedow phenomenon).

MULTINODULAR GOITER WITH AUTONOMY

Patients who have multinodular goiter with autonomous areas on scan, flat TRH responses, and symptoms should be treated for hyperthyroidism. The thiourea compounds (PTU, methimazole) constitute the mainstay of medical therapy of Graves' disease because of their antithyroid and possible anti-immune effects, which permit remission of active disease in a significant number of patients. The hyperthyroidism of multinodular goiter will not spontaneously remit as will Graves' disease (except in the rare event of infarction of toxic nodules). Hence, the choice for treatment in these patients is either radioactive iodine ablation or subtotal thyroidectomy. By and large, patients with toxic multinodular goiter tend to be over 35 years of age, making them more highly eligible candidates for ^{131}I treatment than for surgery. In either case, I do not think it wise to treat extremely toxic patients with radioiodine or by surgical thyroidectomy without first rendering them euthyroid, and therein lies the role for the antithyroid agents in toxic nodular disease, i.e., to prepare patients for ablative therapy. The rationale for such preparation is based on the potential danger (albeit small), that radioiodine may cause a radiation thyroiditis with resultant release of hormonal stores and aggravation of an already marginal clinical state; similarly, a thyroid crisis or "storm" may occur in the intra- or postoperative period of the operated patient who had not been properly prepared. By first treating these patients with antithyroid drugs for 4 to 8 weeks, one can render them euthyroid prior to either of these definitive therapies, as well as deplete the store of hormone in their thyroid glands and thus obviate the possibility of thyroid crisis.

When radioiodine is the choice of therapy, it is given according to the approximate formula:

$$\frac{160\ \mu c/g \text{ estimated thyroid weight} \times \text{No. of g estimated thyroid weight}}{\text{24-hr radioiodine uptake}}$$

This calculation results in a total dose which ranges between 12 and 30 mCi, representing a dose of 4 to 15 mCi to the thyroid. These doses are higher than those used in patients with comparably sized goiters due to Graves' disease, because of the relatively greater radioresistance of the multinodular goiter.

It is a matter of clinical judgment whether or not to treat the patient with one or more small autonomous areas in a multinodular gland, who is clincially euthyroid with an intact (normal) TSH response to TRH. Since the patient's thyroid is not fully suppressible by exogenous thyroid hormone, treatment carries the risk of complementing T_4/T_3 production from the gland and thereby converting a euthyroid goitrous individual into a hyperthyroid one. We treat such patients with thyroid hormone when there is a significant mass of goiter which is not hyperfunctioning, and do so especially when there are multiple hypofunctioning areas. The conversion of a normal TRH response to a flat one may be taken as the end point in adjusting thyroid hormone dosage, recognizing that a lesser dosage than usual will be required because of continuing hormonal output from the autonomous areas.

A rare patient with multinodular goiter will present with marginal to frank signs and symptoms of hypothyroidism with the expected low serum T_4 and high TSH, but a scan indicating hyperfunctioning areas which can be shown to be autonomous; the autonomous areas, albeit hyperfunctioning, are inadequate to maintain euthyroidism. Such patients may be treated with thyroid hormone with the recognition that smaller than usual replacement doses will be necessary to avoid iatrogenic thyrotoxicosis.

NONTOXIC GOITERS DUE TO GOITROGEN EXPOSURE OR IODINE DEFICIENCY

Goiters due to goitrogen exposure may be managed by discontinuation or removal of the responsible substance. When this is not possible, e.g., in a patient requiring lithium carbonate for severe manic depressive illness, or in a patient with iodine-induced goiter due to radiographic contrast dyes with a long half-life, thyroid hormone treatment may be given just as it is for intrinsic thyroid disease, in which case the continued presence of the offending goitrogen is moot. For large populations at risk, goiter due to iodine deficiency should be treated with iodine (daily requirement 100 to 200 μg/day), and dietary iodine supplements for goiter prophylaxis are most simply given in the form of iodized salt. Alternatively, iodized oil may be given by intramuscular injection at intervals of 3 to 4 years and has been successful in decreasing the prevalence of endemic goiter and cretinism. In individual patients, it may be simpler and more reliable to treat with thyroid hormone if practically and economically feasible.

EVALUATION OF THYROID HORMONE TREATMENT

Thyroid hormone treatment is categorized broadly as either "replacement" or "suppression" therapy. The best example of an indication for suppressive therapy is in patients with a history of thyroid cancer in whom it is desirable to suppress any TSH secretion which might stimulate residual tumor. Replacement therapy with thyroid hormone is required in frank hypothyroidism, of course, but also in those marginally euthyroid patients with significant intrinsic thyroid disease, such as children with congenital enzymatic defects in hormonogenesis, or the more common acquired thyroidal dysfunction with positive antithyroid antibodies representing Hashimoto's disease or chronic thyroiditis. In my opinion, when goiter is also present and fails to shrink significantly after 3 to 4 months of treatment, some compromise between replacement dosage and the higher doses used for suppression is warranted.

When replacement therapy is initiated in hypothyroid patients, the normalization of elevated serum TSH levels is an appropriate guideline to follow adequacy of treatment. In euthyroid patients with goiter receiving thyroid hormone, however, a basal TSH value will not tell us whether a given dosage is at a replacement or suppressive level owing to the limited sensitivity of routinely employed TSH assays. The best criterion on which to establish the desired dose level is obtained by assessing the TSH response to an injection of TRH. Thus, the most sensitive guide to supraphysiologic (suppressive) treatment would be the demonstration that TSH levels fail to increase after administration of TRH. Should the administration of TRH result in a measurable increase in serum TSH, the dose of thyroid hormone should be augmented gradually with results of TRH testing reassessed 3 to 6 weeks later. Whether such a slightly increased daily intake of thyroid hormone may have any long-term deleterious effects in the absence of clinical signs or symptoms is yet to be proved.

On the contrary, the optimal dosage range for replacement therapy in patients with nontoxic goiter is that dose which is consonant with a serum T_4 value within the normal range and with the persistence of a measurable ("normal") TSH response to TRH.

CHOICE OF THYROID HORMONE PREPARATION

A variety of thyroid hormone preparations are available at present for clinical use, but recent developments in our understanding of the physiology of thyroid hormone secretion and metabolism clearly help to narrow the choice to the singlemost physiologic preparation. Drawbacks to the use of desiccated thyroid include its variable potency, its relative instability, its variable absorption, and its standardization on the basis of iodine rather than T_4 content. Moreover, its T_3 content may cause acute relative increases in serum T_3, which can produce undesirable side effects, particularly in elderly patients. Use of triiodothyronine for treatment is expensive, causes difficulty in the monitoring and interpretation of routine thyroid function tests for most nonendocrinologists, and is associated with the same greater potential for the induction of signs and symptoms of thyroid excess. In my view, the best preparation is L-thyroxine. With their current standardization on the basis of T_4 measurement by high-pressure liquid chromatography, all thyroxine products on the market today should provide reliable potency, absorption, and bioavailability at a most reasonable cost. Because of endogenous conversion of ingested thyroxine to T_3, physiologic levels of both T_4 and T_3 are maintained by replacement therapy with thyroxine alone. In view of this, no indication is apparent to me for the use of the more expensive combination T_4/T_3 preparations, and L-thyroxine is the drug of choice for either replacement or suppressive therapy of nontoxic goiter.

In most patients, the ideal replacement dosage correlates directly with their weight, with only very large subjects requiring as much as 200 to 300 μg/day. My guideline for therapy is a dose of approximately one microgram per pound body weight. Since the majority of patients with goitrous thyroid disease are women, and the majority of women range in weight from 105 to 150 lbs, the usual recommended dosage falls between 100 and 150 μg/day (and a 125-μg tablet is available). After treatment is started, the patient is seen monthly for several visits to ascertain the absence of undesirable side effects and the effect of treatment on goiter size, and to establish the presence of acceptable levels of serum T_4, TSH, or the TSH response to TRH, as described above. Once we are satisfied that the dose is appropriate, the patient need return no more often than annually for routine reassessment on clinical grounds and by laboratory parameters. The evaluation of goiter response to treatment includes an estimate of any overall decrease in thyroid size or a change in the size of specific nodular areas of the gland. This assessment can be done by palpation and estimation with a small ruler, or by measurement with a tape measure of the change in neck circumference, with fixed reference points such as the spinous process of T7 posteriorly and a horizontal line across the approximate middle of the thyroid gland anteriorly. Some workers have been employing ultrasonographic estimates of thyroid volume for this purpose. The intent of follow-up evaluations is to ensure also that no existing nodules enlarge or that no new nodules appear while the patient is on thyroid hormone therapy, either of which would constitute grounds for immediate consideration for subtotal thyroidectomy.

In the very elderly patient, some clinical judgment is warranted regarding the necessity to consider any treatment at all. If the baseline studies indicate that the patient is euthyroid, and it is likely that the goiter may have been present for several decades, I would question the wisdom of advocating a therapy that may aggravate angina or provoke an arrhythmia or myocardial infarction. In the absence of a worrisome or enlarging solitary thyroid nodule, I am usually content to follow such patients at quarterly intervals without thyroid hormone therapy. If some element of hypothyroidism is present, replacement therapy is indicated even in the elderly patient with cardiac disease, but the physician should settle for less than optimal replacement since the patient may not tolerate full replacement to the euthyroid state.

INDICATIONS FOR SURGERY

Surgery should be necessary only rarely in euthyroid patients with simple diffuse goiter except in unusual cases associated with obstructive symptoms that are incompletely responsive to medical treatment. Patients with nodular goiters are sent to surgery with greater frequency, usually because of patient or physician fears of possible malignancy. In these patients, persistent or progressive symptoms of pressure, pain, or dysphagia while on thyroid hormone therapy are indications for thyroidectomy, as is a history of radiation treatments to the head and neck. Growth of a nodule while on thyroid hormone therapy represents an indication for more immediate surgery, although these nodules occasionally turn out to be merely benign hyperfunctioning adenomas, and a preoperative thyroid scan (with the patient still taking thyroid medication) could be revealing in this regard. Should the surgery reveal the presence of thyroid cancer, the patient will need to be managed according to its histologic type, extent of disease, and other criteria as discussed by Dr. DeGroot elsewhere in this volume. If the surgical specimen is benign, we believe that lifelong thyroid hormone therapy is warranted even when only a partial thyroidectomy or lobectomy is performed. We believe that such management should prevent the evolution of future thyroid nodules and obviate subsequent consideration of a second thyroid surgery with its attendant greater risks of injury to the recurrent laryngeal nerves or parathyroid glands.

SINGLE THYROID NODULE

PAUL G. WALFISH, M.D., F.R.C.P.(C), F.A.C.P.

In the assessment and management of the single thyroid nodule, the primary goal has been to select for surgery patients whose thyroid nodules are at risk for malignant change and to avoid unnecessary operations on those whose nodules are likely to be benign. Thyroid nodules are relatively common in North America, occurring in approximately 4 to 7 percent of the population. Since the majority of nodules are benign, there has been an increasing demand for improvement in the previous surgical selection criteria: clinical assessment, thyroid scintiscanning, and the response to thyroid hormone feeding. Over the past decade, several new noninvasive and invasive techniques have become available for the preoperative evaluation of nodular goiter disease that have assisted in more accurately distinguishing between benign and malignant thyroid lesions. Such techniques have resulted in a several-fold increase in the surgical incidence of thyroid cancer (i.e., from 5–10% to 30–40%) and neoplasia (i.e., from 40% to over 80%).

In my approach to the single thyroid nodule, routine radioisotope scintiscanning is the first important laboratory test for assessing the risk of thyroid malignant disease and the need for surgery. Once a hypofunctioning thyroid nodule has been identified, further testing is done with ultrasonography (US) or, preferably, immediate routine fine-needle aspiration biopsy (FNB). Owing to the known limitations of FNB, some hypofunctioning nodules without evidence of overt thyroidal cancer may be selected for surgery on the basis of suggestive clinical features. More recently the routine use of fine-needle aspiration biopsy in the assessment of all solitary nodules has been advocated for reasons of cost-effectiveness and reduction in radioisotope exposure. However, if such an approach is to be utilized, the limitations and appropriate principles of management to be followed should be recognized (to be discussed).

INITIAL CLINICAL ASSESSMENT

Information obtained by history and physical examination may suggest a high risk for malignant thyroid tumor, i.e., a past history of head and neck irradiation, recent growth and change in size of the nodule, local compressive symptomatology, and lymphadenopathy. Moreover, when thyroid nodules are greater than 2 cm in diameter, firm and fixed on deglutition, or associated with signs of local anatomic compression of trachea, esophagus, vocal cord and cervical sympathetic nerves and/or superior vena cava, the probability of malignancy is increased. Although such features may also occur in the presence of benign nodular goiter and thereby lack specificity, they do favor an indication for surgery to relieve compression on important mediastinal structures as well as to exclude malignancy. Whenever there has been an acute onset of swelling and pain, differentiation of hemorrhage into a nodule from other acute or subacute inflammatory lesions is required, and evidence of fever, leukocytosis, increased ESR, antithyroid antibodies, and thyroid functional laboratory information may be of assistance. Hypofunctioning thyroid nodules are usually asymptomatic, and additional special laboratory aids are required to determine their risk for cancer.

Patients with hyperfunctioning thyroid nodules are assessed for possible thyrotoxic symptoms such as weight loss, nervousness, sweating, palpitations, and/or cardiac arrhythmias. Most autonomous hyperfunctioning single nodules must attain a size greater than 3 cm in diameter in order to produce sufficient thyroid hormone to cause toxic symptoms.

Radioisotope Scintiscanning

Once a single thyroid nodule has been identified by palpation, a radioisotope scintiscan is routinely performed using pinhole columnation to obtain anterior and oblique views. Results of the scan must be directly correlated with the palpable nodule to ensure its correct functional assessment. In order to minimize the diagnostic radiation dose to the thyroid, technetium-99m (^{99m}Tc) or iodine-123 (^{123}I)—the latter is preferable when available—is the scanning agent of choice; ^{131}I is no longer recommended for routine scintiscanning. Nodules that take up relatively little isotope (cold and cool nodules) as well as those whose uptake is similar to that of adjacent normal tissue (warm or isofunctional) are considered to be hypofunctioning nodules and merit further study to exclude possible underlying thyroid cancer or neoplasm.

Nodules that take up more isotope relative to adjacent normal or contralateral thyroid gland tissue are diagnosed as being hyperfunctioning, i.e., hot nodules. However, nodules determined to be hyperfunctioning by ^{99m}Tc scintiscanning require further assessment by a radioactive iodine scan since 6 to 8 percent of nodules found to be hyperfunctioning by technetium scan may be hypofunctioning by iodine scans and represent underlying adenoma or carcinoma lesions. Such disparate imaging results occur in some hot nodules because of established differences in thyroidal handling between radioiodine and technetium, with the latter reflecting primarily blood flow and trapping. However, nodules which are hypofunctioning by technetium scintiscanning will have similar findings by radioactive iodine and do not require further isotopic studies.

The hypofunctioning thyroid nodule (representing approximately 75 to 80 percent of all single nodules) must be further assessed for the risk of underlying thyroidal malignancy, whereas the hyperfunctioning thyroid nodule (representing approximately 15 to 20 percent of nodules) is rarely of concern for underlying malignancy, but instead requires evaluation for possible toxicity and/or autonomy.

Hypofunctioning thyroid nodules may result from a variety of causes, both benign and malignant (Table 1). Hence, surgical treatment based solely on the presence of a hypofunctioning thyroid nodule yields only a 5 to 10 percent histologic incidence of thyroid cancer. Accordingly, our center has been systematically evaluating the routine application of ultrasonography (US) and fine-needle aspiration biopsy (FNB) in the further assessment of hypofunctioning thyroid nodules.

Ultrasonography

Ultrasonography (US) as a noninvasive test has no diagnostic features that can differentiate solid benign from malignant lesions. Even the most sophisticated real-time high-resolution US or nuclear magnetic resonance diagnostic methods cannot reliably distinguish benign from malignant thyroid nodules. The chief value of US is in recognizing single cystic lesions which have a lower risk for malignancy and may be initially treated conservatively by repeated fine-needle aspirations. Furthermore, since over 80 percent of hypofunctioning nodules are solid or mixed (solid and cystic), the incidence of surgical referral based on a combination of scintiscan and US selection criteria is high, i.e., 60 to 80 percent of the single hypofunctioning nodules referred to surgery, but does result in a 20 percent incidence in thyroid cancer (representing a two- to four-fold increment in incidence over our previous experience). Because only more direct invasive techniques can determine the underlying pathology of the hypofunctioning lesion, US is no longer routinely employed, but has been replaced by FNB.

Fine-Needle Aspiration Biopsy (FNB)

After scintiscanning, the next most important routine laboratory aid in determining underlying pathology in hypofunctioning thyroid nodules is an FNB procedure. This simple office procedure is well tolerated by the majority of patients, usually without local anesthesia, when 22- to 27-gauge needles are used. FNB of hypofunctioning nodules provides direct diagnostic information regarding the physical and cytologic characteristics of the nodule (Table 2).

FNB has a diagnostic accuracy of over 80 percent in single hypofunctioning thyroid nodules. Unsatisfactory or acellular cytologic results occur initially in approximately 25 percent of all single

TABLE 1 Heterogeneous Causes of Hypofunctioning Thyroid Nodule and Estimates of Their Frequency

Cause of Nodule	*Frequency*
Solid	
Carcinoma	10%
Adenoma	30%
Colloid nodules and miscellaneous degenerative calcified, acellular, nodular goiter, localized subacute or chronic thyroiditis	40%
Cystic and mixed (solid and cystic)	
Carcinoma	1–2%
Degenerative adenomas and colloid nodule, thyroid, parathyroid and thyroglossal duct benign cysts	18%
Total	100%

From Walfish PG. New approaches to thyroid nodules. Drug Therapy 1983;13:104–118. With permission.

TABLE 2 Classification of Fine-Needle Aspiration Biopsy (FNB); Results on Hypofunctioning Nodules Based Upon the Physical and Cytologic Features Observed*

Category (No.)	*FNB Physical Diag.*	*FNB Cytol. Diag.*	*Additional Features*
I	Solid	Malignant	Primary/secondary undiff. diff. carcinoma
II	Solid	Suspicious	Cellular and atypical adenomas
III	Solid	Benign/inadequate	High risk/low clinical risk for carcinoma
IV	Cystic†	Malignant	Sediment cytology: carcinoma/atypia
V	Cystic†	Suspicious	>4 cm hemorrhagic and recurrent
VI	Cystic†	Benign	<3 cm nonhemorrhagic and nonrecurrent

* Categories I, II, and some III (with high clinical risk) solid FNB results as well as categories IV and V for cystic or mixed FNB results are referred to surgery if patient consents and there are no medical contraindications.

† Also applicable to mixed (solid and cystic thyroid nodules).

From Walfish PG: New approaches to thyroid nodule. Drug Therapy 1983;13:104–118. With permission

hypofunctioning thyroid nodules that are subjected to biopsy, and FNB tests should be repeated to exclude a sampling error. Since patients tolerate the repeated use of FNB, it may also be used routinely in the long-term follow-up of apparently benign lesions selected for conservative, nonsurgical intervention (Fig. 1).

APPROACH TO MANAGEMENT OF THE HYPOFUNCTIONING SINGLE NODULE

Based on follow-up US and/or FNB assessment of single hypofunctioning thyroid nodules, our center has observed that their physical characteristics can be further subdivided into approximately 80 to 85 percent that are solid and 15 to 20 percent which are cystic or mixed. Solid lesions have the greatest risk for malignancy. However, contrary to previous dogma, we have documented that thyroid cancer may also occur in cystic or mixed lesions, but with a 10- to 20-fold lesser frequency than in solid nodules (see Table 1). Hence, in every hypofunctioning thyroid nodule, FNB results (see Table 2) have been used to assist in further management (see Fig. 1).

Solid Hypofunctioning Nodules

Hypofunctioning solid nodules assigned to category I (i.e., overt cytologic evidence of either differentiated or undifferentiated thyroid cancer) have a 90 to 95 percent surgical incidence of thyroidal malignancy with less than a 5 percent chance of a false-positive result. Hence, the selection of category I nodules for surgery results in high diagnostic specificity (95%) for the laboratory detection of thyroid cancer, but low diagnostic sensitivity (i.e., only a 50% detection of all the surgical cancers observed in hypofunctioning nodules).

It is difficult to differentiate follicular and Hürthle cell adenomas from their well-differentiated adenocarcinomas by any needle biopsy technique without careful histologic examination of a surgical specimen for vascular, capsular, or lymphatic invasion. For this reason, I classify the solid hypofunctioning nodules of category II (i.e., evidence of increased cellularity with or without atypia) as "suspicious" and recommend surgery for the majority of such nodules. Cases in category II (see Table 2) represent approximately 25 to 30 percent of all solid hypofunctioning thyroid nodules, have a 30 percent incidence of thyroid cancer, and have been confirmed to contribute an approximately equal number of surgically proven thyroid cancers as obtained in category I solid nodules, which have FNB cytology of overt malignancy. Hence, according to our current state of knowledge, category II patients require surgery to maximize the detection of thyroid cancer and enhance the diagnostic sensitivity of FNB to > 90 percent. Although some centers have attempted to further refine surgical selection of category II lesions by performing a cutting needle biopsy, particularly for nodules greater than 2 cm in diameter to obtain a core of tissue as well as some capsule, we prefer repeated and multiple FNB sampling because of the increased morbidity and the risk of needle tract implantation of thyroid cancer that might occur with large-needle biopsy procedures. Since microfollicular adenomas are three times more frequent than macrofollicular adenomas, and have a 25 percent risk of thyroidal malignant tumor, the cutting needle biopsy technique does not appear to offer sufficient improvement in surgical selectivity (i.e., avoiding surgery on macrofollicular lesions) to recommend its routine application and the concomitant increased morbidity risk associated with its use.

As shown in Figure 1, some patients from category III (solid hypofunctioning nodules with benign or inadequate cytology but with high clinical risk) may still require selection for surgery because of infrequent occurrence (less than 5%) of false negatives owing to sampling or diagnostic limitations associated with FNB. Increasing growth of a solid hypofunctioning and apparently benign thyroid nodule while the patient is receiving thyroid hormone suppression therapy, retrosternal or posteriorly located lesions that cannot be easily sampled or may be subject to geo-

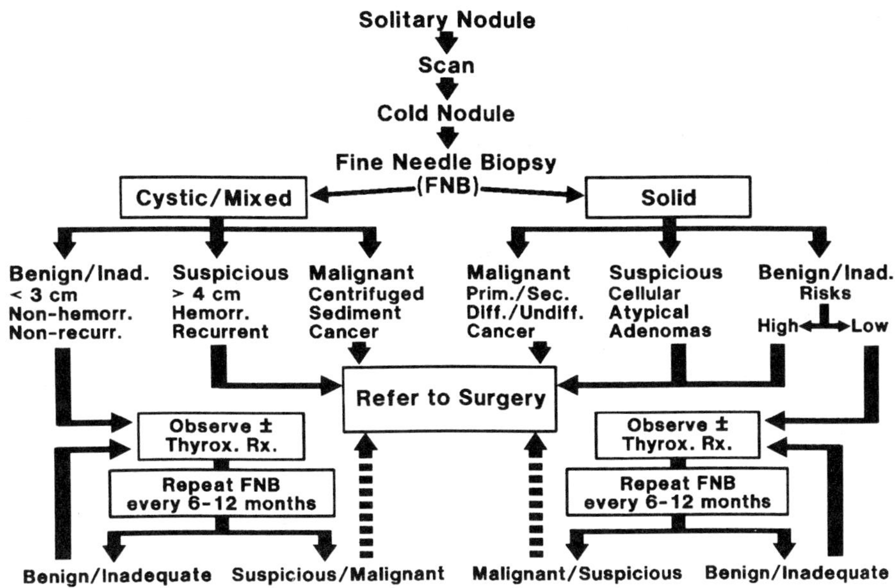

Figure 1 Schematic flow diagram of assessment and management of the hypofunctioning (i.e., cool, cold, warm [isofunction or nondelineated]) thyroid nodule, which utilizes routine initial thyroid scintiscan followed by fine-needle aspiration biopsy (FNB) on all hypofunctioning thyroid nodules to determine physical and cytologic characteristics as categorized in Table 2.

graphic errors, and a past history of increasing growth and exposure to head and neck irradiation could justify surgery in the absence of overt or suspicious cytologic information (i.e., category III with high clinical risk [see Table 2 and Fig. 1]).

In order to achieve adequate sensitivity from the FNB technique on solid hypofunctioning nodules, all category I and II lesions, as well as a few with high clinical risk in category III must be referred to surgery (see Table 2 and Fig. 1). Using such selection criteria, we have observed that approximately 30 to 40 percent of the hypofunctioning thyroid nodules (which represent 80% of all single nodules) have been referred to surgery (i.e., 24 to 32% referral rate among all single nodules and a 30 to 40% operative incidence of thyroid cancer). With this approach, the surgical incidence of thyroid cancer has increased three- to sixfold, i.e., 30 percent compared to the 5 to 10 percent incidence from unselected hypofunctioning thyroid nodules. The overall incidence of neoplasia has increased to over 80 percent, while simultaneously reducing the referral rate to surgery from previous approaches by 33 to 50 percent.

Occasionally, lesions due to medullary thyroid cancer can be diagnosed preoperatively by the presence of spindle or anaplastic-appearing FNB cytology. Such cytologic material may be positive for amyloid by Congo Red stains on polarizing light studies which demonstrate its characteristic apple-green birefringence. Concomitant basal and provocative responses of serum calcitonin to pentagastrin and calcium stimuli may be useful in confirming the diagnosis in such subjects and in following their clinical course after surgery. However, routine measurement of serum calcitonin in all hypofunctioning thyroid nodules is not cost-effective owing to the nonspecificity of serum calcitonin as a tumor marker of medullary cancer within the general population, as well as the much lower prevalence of medullary compared to papillary-follicular thyroid cancer.

More recently it has been proposed that FNB be performed as the first routine diagnostic test on all thyroid nodules even before a scintiscan. Since routine FNB of all thyroid nodules is less expensive than a scintiscan, and a scintiscan procedure may be averted when acellular or degenerative lesions are present, a favorable cost-benefit and an overall reduction in radiation exposure to the general population has been postulated.

When using routine initial FNB before scintiscan, physicians should be aware of the limitations of such an approach and follow certain principles of management. As the FNB of benign hyperfunctioning thyroid nodules could yield cellular and/or atypical cytology (i.e., Category I or II results) which can be misdiagnosed as malignancy, there is a greater risk for false-positive FNB results when hyperfunctioning thyroid nodules are subjected routinely to biopsy. Hence, when such cytology has been observed, it is important to perform a scintiscan routinely in order to exclude the presence of a hot nodule. Since almost all primary hyperfunctioning nodules by radioiodine scintiscans are invariably benign and may even be hyperfunctioning (toxic), routine scintiscanning of all category I or II lesions is required to avoid unnecessary surgery on benign hot nodules. Furthermore, it is my custom never to refer a patient to surgery without obtaining a thyroid synthoscan preoperatively, in order to accurately document preexisting pathology. Moreover, when utilizing a routine initial needle biopsy approach, a large (i.e., 14- to 18-gauge) cutting needle biopsy should not be used, since the inadvertent biopsy of hyperfunctioning nodules can risk bleeding and hematoma complications. When inadequate or absent cellularity results are obtained, FNB tests should be repeated routinely to check for a possible sampling error before concluding that neoplasm or cancer pathology has been excluded.

Although further systematic prospective studies are required to determine the relative merits of initial routine FNB followed by selective scintiscan on all single thyroid nodules in comparison to initial routine scintiscanning followed by FNB only on hypofunctioning thyroid nodules, it is likely that either approach will result in similar detection rates for thyroid cancer, provided the aforementioned diagnostic and management guidlines are followed.

Cystic or Mixed Hypofunctioning Thyroid Nodules

When FNB yields cyst fluid, underlying disease may be diagnosed from the fluid color, protein, hormonal and crystal content, and cytologic study of its sediment after nucleopore filtration or centrifugation. Cyst fluid that is amber to yellow in color usually represents a benign thyroidal cyst, which has only a small risk for neoplasia and malignancy. However, lesions that are frankly hemorrhagic or have chocolate-colored fluid and recur in spite of several aspirations, either immediately or within several days, have a greater risk for underlying neoplasia or carcinoma. In particular, large hemorrhagic lesions, i.e., >3 to 4 cm, which reaccumulate chocolate-colored or hemorrhagic frank blood on repeated aspirations and have an underlying residual solid component (mixed lesions), have been observed in our center to have a surgically proved 33 percent incidence of carcinoma and overall neoplasia of 66 percent. All cyst fluid is sent for routine nucleopore filtration and/or centrifugation to rule out a concomitant cytologic abnormality. Cystic or mixed lesions with overt evidence of malignancy in the sediment, i.e., category IV, and those with hemorrhagic lesions, >3 to 4 cm in diameter, which recur after several aspiration attempts over a 3- to 6-month interval (i.e., category V) and are "suspicious" for malignancy or neoplasia, even in the absence of exfoliative cytology in the sediment of cyst fluid, require careful consideration for surgical referral to exclude thyroid cancer.

Although parathyroid cysts may vary in color, fluid that is crystal-clear and colorless is virtually diagnostic. Such a diagnosis can be confirmed by comparing measurements of parathyroid hormone and protein content in the plasma with those in cyst fluid. A >3- to 4-fold increase in cyst fluid parathyroid hormone concentrations above serum levels in association with a lower protein (ultrafiltrate) and thyroid hormone content is confirmatory of a parathyroid cyst. While the majority of parathyroid cysts are secondary to an embryonic parathyroid retention cyst, routine measurement of serum calcium should also be performed to exclude the lesser possibility of coexisting underlying parathyroid neoplasia, which is reported to be more common in males. Simple FNB aspiration of such parathyroid cysts on one or two occasions in an office setting has usually resulted in a complete resolution of any palpable simple (non-neoplastic) parathyroid cyst lesion.

Amber to yellow cyst fluid usually occurs in association with a benign, simple non-neoplastic thyroid or thyroglossal duct cyst, which contains similar or higher thyroid hormone and protein concentrations than the patient's own serum values. A branchial cleft cyst lesion usually occurs anterolaterally and more superiorly in the neck, frequently yielding a gelatinous butterscotch-colored cyst fluid. This fluid has little cellularity and often contains many cholesterol crystals, which characteristically have a plate-like rhomboidal shape with an irregular edge and are birefringent on polarizing light microscopy.

Occasionally, acute asymmetric enlargment of the thyroid gland may occur in association with fever and pain, as well as laboratory evidence of leukocytosis and increase in sedimentation rate, as manifestations of acute suppurative thyroiditis. Such a diagnosis can be confirmed rapidly by fine-needle (22-gauge) aspiration of the dominant swelling, which often yields frankly purulent material. This material should be kept in the syringe and the needle tract capped with a cork to be sent immediately for aerobic and anaerobic bacteriologic studies. More rarely, asymmetric dominant nodules apparently caused by acute, subacute, or chronic thyroiditis of benign inflammatory etiology have been discovered to have underlying malignant thyroid disease when assessed by routine FNB, representing the so-called syndrome of "malignant pseudothyroiditis".

Patients with apparently benign cystic or mixed lesions (category VI) are placed on exogenous thyroid hormone suppression therapy and followed at regular intervals for repeat FNB of cyst fluid on at least two more occasions. The cyst fluid is assessed on each occasion by nucleopore filtration or centrifugation, and attempts are made to obtain by FNB material from the remaining solid portion of a mixed nodule. Cystic or mixed nodules which disappear or decrease to <1 cm in diameter are treated conservatively by long-term thyroid hormone suppression therapy and observation, particularly when cyst fluid is nonhemorrhagic. However, lesions that are recurrent, particularly when hemorrhagic, and >3 to 4 cm in diameter, are considered to be suspect for malignancy and/or neoplasia (category V) and are then referred for surgery (see Fig. 1).

For patients who appear to be in a benign category or are poor candidates for surgery, prevention of the reaccumulation of cyst fluid has been attempted by the routine administration of such sclerosing agents as sodium tetradecyl sulfate and tetracycline. However, in my experience, such treatment rarely prevents recurrences and is frequently associated with acute local pain at the injection site. Also, there is the concomitant risk of anaphylactic reactions when sodium tetradecyl sulfate is used. Accordingly, I no longer recommend, and will seldom use, such sclerosing agent therapy.

SURGERY ON THE HYPOFUNCTIONING THYROID NODULE

Simple nodulectomy is considered to be inadequate, and the minimum standard procedure should be a hemithyroidectomy. However, in some centers such as our own, who have an experienced endocrine head and neck surgeon, the extent of surgery routinely performed for a single thyroid nodule may increase to a total lobectomy on the side of the lesion, as well as removal of the isthmus and a portion of the contralateral lobe. In fact, over the past several years, most of our patients with category I and IV nodules underwent near-total thyroidectomy (i.e., leaving a fringe of thyroid tissue in the contralateral lobe to ensure the preservation of at least one parathyroid gland), and nearly all our patients in categories II and V undergo near-total thyroidectomy. When the quick-section diagnosis is positive for malignancy and central nodes do not appear to be affected, routine sampling of jugular chain lymph nodes has yielded a surprising 30 percent unsuspected microscopic positivity, thereby facilitating the possibility of an immediate concomitant modified radical neck dissection in a one-stage procedure.

Our rationale for a near-total thyroidectomy in the management of thyroid nodular disease is based on the following experience: (1) a 40 percent incidence of false-negative quick-section diagnoses of malignancy in type II lesions, which would require reoperation, (2) the frequent finding of benign or malignant lesions in the contralateral lobe, which may require reoperation in the future for recurrences of thyroid problems, and (3) a history of head and neck irradiation in at least 30 percent of our center's recent series of thyroid nodules taken to surgery. Nevertheless, the extent of surgery remains controversial, and the availability of appropriate surgical expertise capable of performing the more extensive surgery in a one-stage procedure without significantly enhancing the morbidity, i.e., risk of vocal cord paralysis or parathyroid insufficiency, should determine the type of surgery undertaken.

Regardless of whether a complete lobectomy or near-total thyroidectomy is performed and whether benign or malignant pathology is encountered, I usually recommend long-term L-thyroxine replacement therapy for almost all patients to ensure normal thyroid function and to avert the recurrence of nodular goiter disease in unresected thyroid tissue.

APPROACH TO MANAGEMENT OF THE HYPERFUNCTIONING (HOT) SINGLE NODULE

Whenever a primary hyperfunctioning (hot) thyroid nodule has been demonstrated, not only by technetium-99m, but also by a radioiodine scintiscan (preferably ^{123}I), thyroidal malignancy is assumed to have been virtually excluded. Furthermore, routine US or FNB studies of such lesions are no longer indicated, since all such lesions are solid and would have cytologic evidence of increased cellularity and atypia that could lead to a false-positive result.

Additional management of hot nodules depends on the results of thyroid function tests which determine the presence or absence of thyrotoxicosis. Routine serum total L-thyroxine (T^4) and total L-triiodothyronine (T^3) and T^3 uptake studies are obtained; elevated values indicate the presence of an autonomous toxic nodule. If such studies are not abnormal, further investigations are undertaken to determine whether the thyroid nodule is an autonomous or nonautonomous hot nodule (Fig. 2).

Autonomous hyperfunctioning thyroid nodules that are 3 cm or larger have the greatest risk for toxicity and merit careful assessment. Nodules that are not overtly toxic, as determined by routine measurement of circulating serum thyroid hormone levels and clinical assessment, are further assessed by a TRH test (thyrotropin-releasing hormone, thyrotropinone [Relefact]) using a 400 μg dose intravenously. An absent or impaired TSH response to TRH is compatible with an autonomous hot nodule and may be associated with either overt or subclinical hyperthyroidsm with an increase in serum total and free T^3, i.e., the "T^3 toxicosis" syndrome. Although a normal TSH response to TRH excludes the presence of hyperthyroidism, it does not rule out a nontoxic autonomous hot nodule. However, an enhanced TSH response to TRH suggests the presence of overt or subclinical hypothyroidism and favors the diagnosis of a nonautonomous hot nodule. This nodule probably represents residual normal or compensatorily hypertrophied thyroid tissue, which would be responsive to exogenous thyroid hormone therapy (i.e., suppressible) and should regress in size in response to such treatment.

Further assessment for the presence or absence of an autonomous hot nodule can be achieved using a trial of treatment of exogenous thyroid hormone with either L-triiodothyronine or L-thyroxine to assess the 50 percent suppressibility of the thyroidal radioiodine uptake (Werner's test); when using L-T^3, the 50 percent suppressibility of serum T^4 may also be determined. In addition, radioiodine scintiscans may be performed before and after intramuscularly administered bovine TSH to determine the presence of sup-

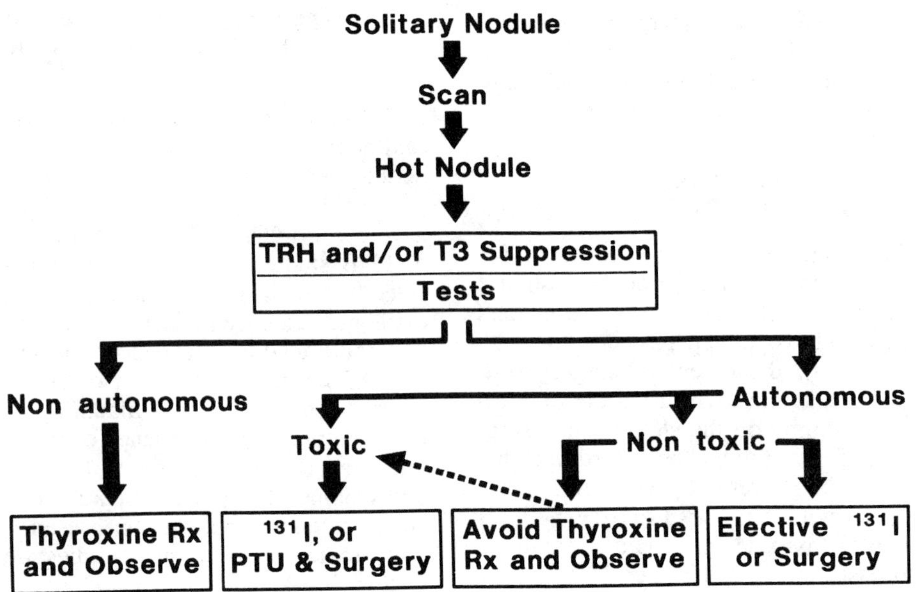

Figure 2 Schematic flow diagram of approach used in the assessment and management of the hyperfunctioning (hot) thyroid nodule using special laboratory tests to determine evidence of nonautonomous (suppressible with exogenous thyroid hormone) vs. autonomous toxic or nontoxic hyperfunctioning thyroid nodules.

pressed normal adjacent or contralateral thyroidal tissues. However, such approaches may be hazardous, particularly in the elderly, owing to the risk of provoking hyperthyroidism secondary to either the exogenous thyroid hormone feeding (suppression test) or the release of thyroid hormone from the suppressed normal tissue after bovine TSH administration (stimulation tests) which are additive to the hormonal secretion from autonomous nontoxic hot nodules. However, the absence on scintiscan of functioning thyroid tissue on the contralateral side after exogenous TSH stimulation in a patient with a thyroid scintiscan, which had the so-called "hockey stick" appearance of a congenital hemiagenesis (absence of contralateral functioning tissue), assists in its differentiation from a hyperfunctioning thyroid nodule with impending toxicity. In the latter there is usually complete suppression of functioning paranodular and contralateral tissue, which can be demonstrated after exogenous TSH stimulation.

For thyroid nodules that are demonstrated to be autonomous, further management is based on whether they are toxic or nontoxic (see Fig. 2). There are a variety of therapeutic choices for toxic hot nodules, depending upon the patient's age (whether in the childbearing years), coexisting cardiovascular disease, and the degree of radioactive iodine uptake in the nodule. In general, radioiodine therapy is avoided for single hot nodules in subjects under 40 years of age, particularly for females in the childbearing years, owing to the risks of ionizing irradiation to the patient and future offspring. In such situations, the patient is prepared for elective hemithyroidectomy with propylthiouracil or methimazole therapy to render the patient euthyroid over a 2- to 3-month interval, followed by exogenous iodine therapy before surgery, i.e., Lugol's iodine, 3 drops *tid* for 5 to 7 days preoperatively. After subtotal thyroidectomy in young subjects with single hot nodules, it is my custom to recommend long-term exogenous thyroid hormone substitutional therapy to avoid compensated hypertrophy and recurrent nodular disease in the remaining unresected thyroid gland tissue.

In patients who have autonomous nontoxic nodules, the risk of toxicity is small in nodules <2 cm in diameter, and these subjects may be followed without any specific therapy and observed at yearly follow-up intervals. However, the administration of thyroxine therapy to such patients is to be avoided as it could precipitate hyperthyroidism owing to the nonsuppressibility of an autonomous hot nodule. Patients over 40 years of age who have 3-cm or larger hot nodules, borderline toxicity, and coexisting problems such as cardiovascular disease may be selected for treatment with radioiodine therapy, usually after pretreatment with antithyroid drugs for 4 to 6 months to ensure a return to euthyroid status before administering radioiodine therapy. Patients with toxic single or multiple nodules receive much larger doses than those usually administered to patients with a diffuse toxic goiter of Graves' disease (e.g., 50 to 150 mCi ^{131}I, depending on their active tissue size and radioiodine uptake to deliver an estimated retained dose of 10 to 15 mCi of ^{131}I to the adenoma) to facilitate the ablation of hyperfunctioning tissue that characteristically has a lesser avidity for radioiodine than in Graves' disease. Also, the long-term risk for post-radioiodine-induced hypothyroidism is lower, particularly among toxic hot nodules which are accompanied by complete suppression of extranodular tissue. Owing to the poor uptake of the radioiodine therapy dose into the suppressed normal tissue, such thyroid tissue usually recovers its function after radioiodine therapy, whereas the risk for hypothyroidism after radioiodine therapy is higher in nontoxic nodule with incompletely suppressed extranodular tissue function.

Nontoxic autonomous nodules may be managed without any therapy by serial observations of nodule size and function at 12-month intervals (see Fig. 2). Studies of the long-term natural history of such lesions indicate that about 25 percent may have an increase in the size of the nodule to over 3 cm in diameter within a few years, as well as clinical and laboratory evidence of toxicity, i.e., elevated serum T^3, absent TSH response to TRH, and a complete suppression of extranodular tissue on thyroid imaging. The remainder may have little change in size or function for many years or may revert spontaneously to become hypofunctioning nodules secondary to degeneration and hemorrhage. Acute involution due to hemorrhage may rarely be associated with spontaneously resolving hyperthyroidism. Also, there is a risk for acute thyrotoxicosis in patients with nontoxic autonomous hot nodules who receive iodine x-ray contrast dyes or medications, which may be protected by thionamide therapy (e.g., propylthiourasil or methimazole) 24 to 48 hours before exposure and/or a beta-blocker (e.g., propranolol) for 10 days afterward. Nontoxic nodules that evolve to toxicity are treated in accordance with various therapeutic choices which will be determined by the activity of the thyroid nodule, clinical factors, and patient preference for choices of therapy (see Fig. 2).

As outlined in Figure 2, lesions that are not autonomous, e.g., characterized by a hyperreactive TSH response to TRH or >50 percent suppression of the previous radioiodine uptake value after exogenous thyroid hormone suppression, can be treated with thyroid hormone and may be anticipated to have a reduction in the size of the nodule when appropriate dosage has been administered. Patients receiving L-thyroxine are followed initially at 6-month intervals to determine the correct maintenance dose and ensure that iatrogenic hyperthyroidism has not been induced inadvertently from either excessive dosage or the presence of an unsuspected autonomous hot nodule.

Suggested Reading

Clark OH, Okerhurst MD, Cavalieri RR, et al. Diagnosis and treatment of thyroid, parathyroid, and thyroglossal duct cysts. J Clin Endocrinol Metab 1979; 48:943.

Ginsberg J, Young JEM, Walfish PG. Parathyroid cysts: Medical diagnosis and management. JAMA 1978; 240:1506.

Hamburger JI. The autonomously functioning thyroid adenoma: Clinical considerations. N Eng J Med 1983; 309:1512.

Klonoff DC, Greenspan FS. The thyroid nodule. In: Stollerman GH, ed. Advances in Internal Medicine. Chicago, Illinois: Yearbook Medical Publishers, 1982; 27:101.

Mazaferri EL, Young RL, Oertel JE, et al. Papillary carcinoma: The impact of therapy in 576 patients. Medicine 1977; 56:171.

Miller JM, Hamburger JI, Keene S. Diagnosis of thyroid nodules. Use of fine-needle aspiration and needle biopsy. JAMA 1979; 21:481.

Rosen IB, Wallace C, Strawbridge HTG, Walfish PG. Re-evaluation of needle aspiration cytology in the detection of thyroid cancer. Surgery 1981: 90:747.

Rosen IB, Palmer JA, Bain J, Strawbridge HTG, Walfish PG. Efficacy of needle biopsy in postradiation thyroid disease. Surgery 1983; 94(6):1002.

Walfish PG, Miskin M, Rosen IB et al. Application of special diagnostic techniques in the management of nodular goiter. Can Med Assoc J 1975; 15:35.

Walfish PG, Hazani E, Strawbridge HTG et al. Combined ultrasound and needle aspiration biopsy in the assessment and management of the hypofunctioning thyroid nodule. Ann Intern Med 1977; 87:270.

Walfish PG. New approaches to thyroid nodules. Drug Therapy 1983; 13:104.

THYROIDITIS

TERRY F. DAVIES, M.D., M.R.C.P.

Inflammation of the thyroid may be acute and associated with rampant bacterial infection or subacute with a less dramatic presentation and thought to be viral in etiology. Pain in the thyroid appears to depend on the speed with which the inflammation causes increased pressure within the thyroid capsule. Hence the rarer painless variety of subacute thyroiditis is a lower grade of inflammation. Similarly, the most common form of thyroiditis, the chronic autoimmune variety (Hashimoto's disease), usually causes a slowly progressive thyroid gland enlargement and is, therefore, rarely painful (Table 1).

AUTOIMMUNE THYROIDITIS

The Problem

All varieties of autoimmune thyroid disease are associated with a mononuclear cell infiltrate, but the term autoimmune thyroiditis is generally restricted to Hashimoto's disease. Up to 20 percent of the general population have easily detectable titers of antibodies to thyroglobulin and to a cell surface component present in microsomal fractions of thyroid homogenate. However, only about 1 percent of the population develop autoimmune thyroid failure, indicating that other, perhaps more important, risk factors need also be present (for example, T-cell abnormalities and appropriate HLA antigens). Patients with thyroid autoantibodies and a mildly raised TSH concentration progress to clinical thyroid failure at a rate of approximately 3 to 5 percent per year; hence the term

TABLE 1 Classification of Thyroiditis

Type	*Etiology*	*Treatment*
Acute	Bacterial	High-dose broad-spectrum antibiotics
Subacute	Viral (?)	For pain—aspirin/prednisone Hyperthyroid phase—propranolol Hypothyroid phase—low-dose T_4
Chronic	Autoimmune	T_4 replacement
Postpartum	Transient Autoimmune	Hyperthyroid phase—propranolol Hypothyroid phase—low-dose T_4

subclinical thyroid failure has been applied to such a disease state.

Patients with autoimmune thyroiditis may present with, or without, an obvious goiter (the goitrous and atrophic varieties), and it has been suggested that they represent two distinct varieties of the disease on the basis of HLA typing and natural history (for example, the early goitrus variety may show periods of remission). Whether or not goitrous and atrophic autoimmune thyroiditis are distinct entities is academic since their treatment remains the same. It is also important to remember that the term "primary myxedema" almost always depicts a patient with atrophic autoimmune thyroiditis.

Medical Treatment of Autoimmune Thyroiditis

Patients who have symptoms consistent with thyroid failure and whose thyroid function studies indicate reduced free thyroxine hormone concentrations combined with increased TSH levels should be given thyroid hormone replacement therapy (100 to 150 μg T_4 daily). It is inappropriate to prescribe thyroid hormones on the basis of suspicion alone; there must always be clearly documented evidence of thyroid failure. *Caution* should be exercised in the treatment of elderly patients and those with coronary artery disease. These patients should be given small initial doses of T_4 (25 to 50 μg daily) and monitored carefully for dysrhythmias and an influence on concurrent drug therapy. It may not be necessary to reduce their TSH levels to within the normal range, allowing them to remain in the 8 to 12 μU/ml range. Most patients, however, should be replaced with sufficient T_4 to normalize their TSH levels, preferably without removing the TSH response to TRH. An absent response to TRH suggests excess thyroid hormone and the possible long-term effects of such therapy on bone structure.

Occasionally, patients with autoimmune thyroiditis may present with hyperthyroidism, a condition sometimes referred to as "Hashitoxicosis." Acute autoimmune-mediated lysis of thyroid tissue appears to lead to an outpouring of thyroid hormone from the gland as colloid is released from within and without the cells. Serum T_3 and T_4 are increased, as is thyroglobulin, and there is no TSH response to TRH. This hyperthyroidism may be caused by local thyroid stimulators, such as prostaglandins from damaged cells, which act upon the remaining functional follicular cells. The treatment is beta-adrenergic blockade (for example, propranolol, 20 to 40 mg *qid*). The condition may be difficult to distinguish from hyperthyroid Graves' disease. A low 24-hour radioiodine uptake may be helpful, although local conditions may not have progressed sufficiently to reflect this. High titers of thyroid antibodies may also suggest thyroiditis, but treatment will need to be initiated before such data are available. These patients may rapidly become hypothyroid if antithyroid drugs are used, and their underlying autoimmune thyroiditis will be revealed after drug withdrawal.

Surgery and Autoimmune Thyroiditis

Surgery is rarely indicated in autoimmune thyroiditis, although particularly firm areas of the gland are often mistaken for an indication for surgery since such localized lesions are indistinguishable from a firm carcinoma (Table 2). In such patients, thyroid biopsy may not be helpful since many of the cells may appear atypical. Hence, there is little alternative to a hemithyroidectomy.

A large Hashimoto gland occasionally may cause pressure effects on the trachea, or even on a recurrent laryngeal nerve, which is best relieved by a careful surgeon. Postoperative precautions must be taken to prevent tracheal collapse when there has been pressure atrophy of the supporting cartilage.

POSTPARTUM THYROIDITIS

The Problem

Thyroid antibody titers consistently fall as a pregnancy progresses toward parturition, and autoimmune thyroid disease characteristically improves during pregnancy. This phenomenon is thought to be secondary to the presence of a variety of factors which favor immunosuppression during gestation. After delivery, antibody levels rebound (3 to 6 months postpartum) to titers often greater than before pregnancy and then gradually return to normal. This rebound may be associated with a variety of postpartum thyroid syndromes which are usually transient and may occur in up to 8 percent of women.

Lethargy associated with hypothyroid function tests and increasing titers of thyroid autoantibodies in

TABLE 2 Indications for Surgery in Thyroiditis

Localized cold nodule with negative serum thyroid antibodies
Tracheal compression and airway obstruction
Recurrent laryngeal nerve palsy
Localized suppuration following bacterial infection
Continued pain after repeated therapy with glucocorticoids

the postpartum period may be diagnostic or postpartum thyroiditis. The condition is usually painless and transient. In the mother who is not breast-feeding the diagnosis can be confirmed by low or absent radioiodine uptake. Thyroid biopsies in such cases show profuse mononuclear cell infiltration with follicular destruction.

Treatment of Postpartum Thyroiditis

Treatment depends on severity of the disease. Most episodes are tansient, and rapid recovery can be expected over a 2- to 4-month period. Symptoms of thyroid failure and a hypothyroid response to thyroid function tests should be treated with T_4 replacement therapy (50 to 150 μ daily), and the T_4 and TSH should be monitored. Since only replacement therapy is prescribed, the problem of drugs in breast-feeding mothers does not arise. As thyroid autoantibody levels fall, thyroid cell regeneration becomes possible, and thyroxine replacement should be reduced and withdrawn. It is uncertain what percentage of such patients obtain full recovery. Many patients no longer require thyroxine supplementation, but have evidence of continuing thyroiditis on the basis of high titers of thyroid antoantibodies and have a relapse following their next pregnancy. In other patients, full functional recovery clearly does not ensue and classic autoimmune (Hashimoto's) thyroiditis develops. Such patients require long-term thyroxine replacement.

Early Hyperthyroid Phase of Postpartum Thyroiditis

The early period in this form of thyroiditis may be associated with thyrotoxic symptoms and hyperthyroid response to function tests as a consequence of widespread thyroid cell destruction, as seen in autoimmune thyroiditis (see above). It may be even more common in the postpartum period than in the early phase of autoimmune thyroiditis. Antithyroid drugs are not helpful because of the long delay before they are effective and the transient nature of the condition. Appropriate treatment is beta-adrenergic blockade (e.g., propranolol, 20 to 40 mg *qid*) during the usually brief hyperthyroid phase prior to the onset of thyroid failure. Caution should be exercised in breast-feeding mothers. The thyroid status has to be distinguished from the onset of true Graves' disease. This may be on the basis of a low radioiodine uptake (if it is possible to perform the test) or by the natural evolution of the condition.

SUBACUTE THYROIDITIS

The Problem

Subacute (de Quervain's) thyroiditis presents most often with general malaise, fever, and a localized *thyroid tenderness*, usually bilateral. The prevalence varies widely between different countries and has been associated with evidence for a variety of viral infections. Such thyroiditis may even be a common presentation for multiple varieties of viral insults, and a single type may not be responsible. It is likely that many individuals experience a mild form of the disease, but only with the onset of pain do they present to their physician. Painless thyroiditis is a well-recognized, although must less common, form of de Quervain's thyroiditis, presumably associated with a lower grade of inflammation. The sedimentation rate is increased, and thyroid autoantibody levels may be transiently present during subacute thyroiditis.

Treatment of Subacute Thyroiditis

Most patients require no more than aspirin therapy to relieve the neck tenderness. However, severe tenderness may be devastating, and in this situation, prednisone, 30 to 40 mg daily over a 5- to 10-day period with dosage gradually reduced over the subsequent 2 weeks, is highly effective.

Massive destruction of thyroid tissue leads to an outpouring of thyroid hormone which may require beta-adrenergic blockade in the form of propranolol (20 to 40 mg *qid*). This transient hyperthyroidism is then followed by a period of marked hypothyroidism while the gland is undergoing regeneration. T_4 supplementation may be required at this stage, depending on both the symptoms and the serum T_4/TSH results, and may be continued for 6 to 8 weeks. However, thyroid cell regeneration may be enhanced by increased serum TSH levels in this and all other forms of thyroid destruction, and thyroxine supplementation should not be excessive (recommended dosage 50 to 100 μg daily) unless the symptoms become gross. Gradual withdrawal should lead to the return of normal thyroid function. It has been suggested that serum thyroglobulin may be a useful marker to assess the degree of thyroiditis during thyroid hormone supplementation.

Patients who have the painless variety of subacute thyroiditis may present during the initial hyperthyroid phase or, more commonly, during the onset of clinical hypothyroidism. The diagnosis may be made by the increased sedimentation rate and a low radioiodine uptake at 24 hours. Thyroid antibodies may be transiently present in lower titers than are seen in autoimmune thyroiditis. Treatment should be as described above, with beta-adrenergic blockade during the hyperthyroid phase and thyroxine supplementation as required, with emphasis on keeping serum TSH somewhat above normal (e.g., 8 to 12 μU/ml).

SUPPURATIVE THYROIDITIS

Both septicemia and local infection may spread to the thyroid gland itself and cause acute suppurative thyroiditis. The gland may be enlarged and acutely tender, with systemic symptoms of fever, tachycardia, and malaise. Thrombophlebitis of the external jugular veins may complicate the presentation. Treatment involves appropriate high-dose antibiotics combined with incision and drainage when indicated. Thyroxine replacement may be necessary if there is much destruction of the gland, but full recovery usually ensues.

PERINEOPLASTIC THYROIDITIS

Examination of thyroid tissue around a thyroid tumor or metastatic infiltration within the gland often reveals a variable degree of reactive thyroiditis. In almost every case, this occurs in patients who have detectable circulating thyroid autoantibodies. It appears that thyroid antibodies may have an increased prevalence in thyroid cancer, although the significance of this observation is uncertain and it is not known whether the presence of thyroiditis influences the natural history of a thyroid tumor. Autoimmune thyroiditis itself may show variable degrees of infiltration within the same gland, and a localized area of heavy infiltration may present as a suspiciously hard nodule. Often, if serum thyroid autoantibodies are negative, the nodule may need to be removed, particularly in a young patient. Thyroid aspiration may help, although many cytopathologists admit to having difficulty distinguishing atypical cells from the damaged cells resulting from thyroiditis. When facilities are available, autoantibody culture from the aspirate may be attempted.

REIDEL'S THYROIDITIS

This previously well-recognized chronic form of fibrous replacement of the thyroid is no longer seen clinically, and its etiology is uncertain. There may be fibrosis of associated tissues including the retroperitoneum. The only effective treatment is surgical correction of any resulting obstruction.

Suggested Reading

Davies TF ed. Autoimmune Endocrine Disease, New York: John Wiley, 1983.

Volpe R. Sub-acute thyroiditis. Prog Clin Biol Res 1981; 74:115.

ADRENOCORTICAL INSUFFICIENCY

J. LESTER GABRILOVE, M.D.

Adrenocortical insufficiency results from primary destruction of the adrenal cortex by idiopathic (autoimmune) atrophy, tuberculosis, amyloid, hemorrhage, fungal disease (such as histoplasmosis), metastatic carcinomatosis, or adrenalectomy. In addition, it can occur secondary to pituitary insufficiency due to pituitary or hypothalamic disease. The adrenal cortex elaborates cortisol, aldosterone, and androgens and estrogens as the termini of 3 biosynthetic pathways. Adrenocortical insufficiency thus reflects the loss of physiologic effects of these hormones. However, in clinical practice, only the loss of cortisol and of aldosterone are significant in primary insufficiency, and only cortisol in secondary insufficiency. Aldosterone production is regulated by the juxtaglomerular apparatus in the kidney via the renin-angiotensin system, which is independent of hypophyseal control. Loss of hypothalamic (CRH)-pituitary function (ACTH) results in secondary adrenocortical insufficiency manifested chiefly by cortisol lack, except under conditions of severe sodium restriction. By contrast, in primary destruction of the adrenal cortex, the picture reflects the loss of both cortisol and aldosterone.

INTERCRITICAL PHASE

In patients in whom the diagnosis of primary adrenal cortical insufficiency is made in the absence of crisis, treatment is effected by the oral administration of cortisone acetate, 12.5 to 37.5 mg a day, and fludrocortisone acetate (Florinef), 0.05 to 0.2 mg a day or every other day. The latter is given for its mineralocorticoid effect and the former as a glucocorticoid. I prefer cortisone to prednisone and dexamethasone for its added effectiveness in sodium conservation. Cortisone may be given on a schedule that reflects the normal diurnal variation of cortisol, with twice as much being given in the morning (25 mg) as in the evening (12.5 mg), although there is very little to indicate a difference in effectiveness clinically between such administration and that afforded by the use of equal divided doses. The equivalent doses of cortisol are 20 mg and 10 mg in in the morning and evening respectively. A liberal salt diet is recommended. Indications of adequate control are afforded by the sense of well-being, the maintenance of weight and blood pressure, the absence of edema, and normal serum levels of sodium. Measurement of serum ACTH is not necessary to monitor the patient's progress. Overtreatment, particularly with a mineralocorticoid, may result in hypokalemic alkalosis and/or hypervolemia or even in the precipitation of heart failure. This is probably of more concern in the overvigorous treatment of the patient in adrenocortical crisis who receives large amounts of intravenous fluids.

In the physiologic glucocorticoid dosage employed, dissemination of tuberculosis is extremely uncommon. However, if tuberculosis is the cause of the Addison's disease, antituberculous therapy should be instituted.

ADRENAL CRISIS

Prevention of Adrenal Crisis

Adrenocortical crisis is ordinarily precipitated by infection or "stress" such as an operative procedure. In the patient who is known to have adrenocortical insufficiency and has been receiving a salt-retaining compound, a modest or severe stress (such as surgery) can increase the need for glucocorticoids, which should be given immediately. Hydrocortisone (cortisol) sodium succinate (Solu-Cortef) or cortisol sodium phosphate is given intravenously in a dosage of 300 mg a day in divided doses *q6h*. Alternatively, cortisone acetate may be given in one daily intramuscular dose of 300 mg a day after one or more intravenous doses of 100 mg of hydrocortisone. The use of intravenous glucocorticoid is preferable when there is any doubt as to the presence of circulatory insufficiency, since the intramuscular depot may not be adequately absorbed and utilized under such circumstances. However, after the restoration of circulatory sufficiency, the intramuscular administration may be considered. When given in a dosage of 100 mg or more a day, cortisol and cortisone exert sufficient mineralocorticoid effect to obviate administration of additional mineralocorticoid. When the dosage is reduced below 100 mg/day, a mineralocorticoid (i.e., Fludrocortisone) may be needed. If an oral route for the mineralocorticoid is not feasible, deoxycorticosterone acetate (1 to 5 mg) may be given daily intramuscularly. In the presence of infection, antibiotics are concomitantly administered as indicated by the site of infection and the type of organism. For mild bacterial respiratory infections, the administration of penicillin parenterally or penicillin or erythromycin orally, depending on the condition of the patient, is usually sufficient. In more serious situations, ampicillin or other synthetic penicillins, or a cephalosporin, or antibiotics particularly effective against gram-negative organisms, such as the aminoglycosides, or some combination may be necessary. The antibiotics used are determined by the type of precipitating infection and the results of cultures and sensitivity tests. However, antibiotic treatment should be started promptly together or with the adrenocortical replacement therapy while results of the cultures are awaited.

Treatment of Adrenal Crisis

If the diagnosis of adrenocortical insufficiency is first made in the face of crisis, vigorous replacement of electrolyte (i.e., sodium) is indicated as well as antibiotics and glucocorticoid. This is carried out by the administration of 5 percent dextrose in normal saline at a rate of 100 to 150 ml/hour, or more rapidly at first in order to correct the calculated sodium deficit and rehydrate the patient, if necessary, as rapidly as it is clincally feasible. Large doses of IV cortisol (300 mg/day) are given as described above. In the treatment of crisis a psychosis may be precipitated in the rare case. This would ordinarily improve as the adrenocortical crisis is brought under control and the patient's clinical status improves.

In the patient who was adequately treated prior to crisis, electrolyte depletion is unlikely. Therefore, intravenous fluids in the form of 5 percent dextrose in $^{1}/_{2}$ strength saline may be given at the rate of 100 to 150 ml/hour or more, depending on the electrolyte, hydration, and circulatory status of the patient.

As the patient improves, the dosage of glucocorticoids is slowly decreased over a period of 10 to 12 days until an oral maintenance dose is reached. The switch from intravenous to oral medication is dictated by the degree of hydration and the clinical state of the patient. When the dosage of cortisone or cortisol is less than 100 mg a day, a supplement of mineralocorticoid (fludrocortisone) may become necessary. Antibiotic administration is stopped as clinically warranted.

In the face of an emergency or nonemergent operative procedure, a similar regimen is followed to prevent crisis: the equivalent of 300 mg of cortisone or cortisol a day, gradually decreasing the dosage by 25 mg a day over the course of 10 to 12 days if no surgical complications supervene. Electrolytes are replaced according to the general principles for replacement following surgical procedures plus those detailed under the treatment of crisis.

In minor episodes of infection, such as a cold, the dosage of oral cortisone is increased from the maintenance dosage to 50 to 100 mg a day or more, depending on the severity of infection. No adjustment of the mineralocorticoid is necessary.

SECONDARY ADRENOCORTICAL INSUFFICIENCY

Patients with secondary adrenocortical insufficiency due to pituitary disease, craniopharyngioma, or Sheehan's syndrome are treated in the intercritical phase with glucocorticoids alone, as described previously. Under ordinary circumstances, save in the face of severe sodium restriction, sodium balance is maintained, and no mineralocorticoid need be added to the regimen. However, the sodium-retaining effect of cortisone does afford a potential safeguard.

In the presence of crisis, treatment is carried out for glucocorticoid insufficiency, as described for primary adrenocortical insufficiency.

SPECIAL FORMS OF ADRENOCORTICAL INSUFFICIENCY

Removal of an Adrenocortical Tumor in Cushing's Syndrome

Following the removal of an adrenocortical tumor for Cushing's syndrome, since the contralateral adrenal is ordinarily suppressed, the untreated patient manifests glucocorticoid insufficiency. Prevention of adrenocortical insufficiency under these circumstances is afforded by the administration of 300 mg of cortisol sodium succinate intravenously in divided doses on the day of operation or 300 mg of cortisone acetate intramuscularly. The route of administration is dictated by circumstances described under the *Treatment of Adrenal Crisis*. The dosage of glucocorticoid (cortisone or cortisol) is slowly decreased and changed from a parenteral to an oral route over the postoperative course of 10 to 14 days to a level of 50 to 75 mg of cortisone by mouth. No mineralocorticoid is necessary. Then the glucocorticoid is gradually decreased over a period of 6 to 9 months in order to prevent symptoms of adrenocortical insufficiency, which may be characterized by weakness, aches and pains in the joints, fever and dermatitis to the point of exfoliation. It ordinarily takes 6 to 9 months for the contralateral adrenal to recover sufficiently to permit complete withdrawal of exogenously administered glucocorticoid.

Since the contralateral adrenal suppression noted in Cushing's syndrome due to an adrenocortical tumor results solely in glucocorticoid insufficiency, the use of prednisone or dexamethasone in equivalent doses can be substituted for cortisone or cortisol. This is of particular importance in the treatment of patients in whom excessive sodium retention is to be avoided, as in the presence of heart failure.

Congenital Adrenocortical Hyperfunction

In the 21-hydroxylase form, this disorder is characterized by a paradox of hyperfunction in regard to androgen and hypofunction in respect to glucocorticoid, and in the severest form, hypofunction in regard to glucocorticoid and mineralocorticoid production. In the intercritical phase the principles are similar to those described above. Glucocorticoids, such as cortisone or, in the absence of any mineralocorticoid defect, prednisone or dexamethasone, are given to minimize any virilization. In these circumstances dexamethasone is preferable. The effectiveness of therapy may be monitored by measuring the serum levels of 17α-hydroxyprogesterone or androstenedione or the urinary content of neutral 17-ketosteroids. In the presence of salt wasting, fludrocortisone is added to the regimen.

If the patient is first seen in crisis, parenteral treatment is indicated. In the salt-wasting form this may include, in addition to glucocorticoid, the intramuscular administration of deoxycorticosterone acetate (1 to 5 mg) for its mineralocorticoid effect. When the patient can take oral medication, fludrocortisone is given in addition to the glucocorticoid.

Pregnancy

The pregnant woman with Addison's disease may be given maintenance therapy until delivery, at which time the dosage of glucocorticoids should be increased as dictated by the added strain of delivery, particularly if she is to undergo cesarean section.

Patients on Long-Term Steroid Therapy

A patient treated with long-term steroid therapy is still considered to have glucocorticoid adrenocortical insufficiency in the face of an impending operative procedure or in the presence of a serious infection or fracture. The principles of treatment are those for a major or minor glucocorticoid adrenocortical crisis.

Patients who travel should carry both an antibiotic and a parenteral form of cortisone, cortisol, or dexamethasone. It is advisable for the patient to have in his possession, on a card or "dog tag" (Medic-Alert), the fact that he has Addison's disease and a statement as to his daily medication needs.

CUSHING'S SYNDROME

LAWRENCE M. FISHMAN, M.D.

Although corticosteroids are life-maintaining substances that in appropriate concentrations act to facilitate a variety of biologic functions, prolonged exposure to excess glucocorticoid is deleterious. Cushing's syndrome is the constellation of clinical and laboratory abnormalities that results from a chronic surfeit of glucocorticoid action. Increased morbidity and mortality in this condition relate predominantly to cardiovascular and infectious complications and to the profound antianabolic effects of high levels of glucocorticoids; in children, growth retardation is an additional sensitive and clinically important phenomenon that lends further urgency to the need to correct the metabolic abnormality. Since systemic corticosteroid therapy is a widely used tool in the management of a variety of disease states, in practice Cushing's syndrome is most commonly encouuntered as a complication of the pharmacologic use of glucocorticoids.

The goal of minimizing or avoiding the consequences of glucocorticoid excess in the setting of exogenous steroid administration is an important clinical problem that is dealt with in detail elsewhere in this volume.

Endogenous hypercortisolemia can result from (1) a primary adrenal abnormality, involving a cortical neoplasm (benign or malignant) autonomously oversecreting steroid hormones; (2) secondary adrenal overactivity produced by ACTH excess of pituitary origin, the pathogenesis of which is a primary hypothalamic-pituitary abnormality in the regulation of trophic hormone secretion (Cushing's disease); (3) adrenal hyperplasia caused by a primary abnormality relating to ectopic and autonomous secretion of ACTH (and often other peptides) by a nonpituitary tumor not usually associated with production of trophic hormone. The need to distinguish among these widely differing pathogenetic mechanisms if specific therapy is to be applied is obvious. Available techniques make it possible to do this with accuracy today in virtually every patient with Cushing's syndrome, though diagnostic error as a basis for therapeutic misadventure will always remain a possibility.

Orth and Liddle have formulated the objectives of ideal therapy for Cushing's syndrome as normalization of cortisol secretion, eradication of potentially harmful space-occupying lesions, prevention of permanent endocrine deficiency, and avoidance of the necessity for continuing dependence on medications; to these should be added, of course, the absence of any untoward effects of the therapeutic modality itself. As with many other disorders, in practice the results of therapy for Cushing's syndrome are only occasionally ideal, but quite often satisfactory and almost always adequate at least to relieve the burden of glucocorticoid excess. As will be seen, the lack of a universally applicable theraputic approach to any of the forms of hyperadrenocorticism, especially Cushing's disease, requires that management decisions take into account the severity of the disorder, the age and general condition of the patient and the relative availability of highly specialized therapeutic resources.

CUSHING'S DISEASE (PITUITARY ACTH-DEPENDENT ADRENOCORTICAL HYPERPLASIA)

Cushing's disease (pituitary ACTH-dependent hyperadrenocorticism) is the most common form of endogenous cortisol excess, accounting for approximately 65 percent of such patients. Treatment choices for this disorder have broadened over the past decade with the widespread availability of transsphenoidal pituitary microsurgery. Much of the appeal of this approach is that it may represent relatively low-risk therapy specifically directed toward correction of the primary abnormality in ACTH oversecretion. Other treatment modalities aimed toward this goal and with which experience is more extensive are, of course, various types of pituitary irradiation. Ablative surgical therapy directed at the adrenal has a long tradition and demonstrated effectiveness in relieving the burden of hyperadrenocorticism; pharmacologic approaches to the same end are less reliable and fraught with ongoing difficulties in application. Continuing uncertainties regarding the seemingly theoretic question of the specific locus of the central abnormality in Cushing's disease and the more pragmatic but possibly related clinical issue of the role of transsphenoidal surgery in this disorder make it necessary to continue to individualize treatment. Although transsphenoidal surgery is the preferred approach in most patients with Cushing's disease, other modalities may be more appropriate as primary treatment in certain circumstances and as important secondary management alternatives.

Transsphenoidal Surgery

Careful preoperative radiologic examination of the pituitary area is indicated as an important overall guide to the neurosurgeon, but false-positive (~30%) and false-negative (~30%) results abound, and there is generally poor correlation between the results of such studies and the surgical findings. The decision to carry out transsphenoidal exploration in a patient with Cushing's disease should not depend solely on the radiologic findings.

The sellar contents are exposed by careful dissection beginning with a gingival incision and carried through the nasal septum and sphenoid sinus, using intraoperative magnifying fluoroscopy. Meticulous hemostasis and careful exploration of the pituitary fossa are necessary to identify a focal abnormality in the substance of the gland, which may not be evident on its surface and only becomes apparent after cruciate incisions through the capsule. Adenomatous tissue is completely removed, leaving intact as much of the normal gland as possible. The identification of a discrete abnormality in the gland is the most prognostically favorable operative finding. The neurosurgeon and attending endocrinologist must be prepared by prior discussion, however, to confront the dilemma of an apparently normal gland, as occurs in 15 to 30 percent of cases. In this circumstance, I favor limited surgical intervention, restricted to thorough exploration and biopsy only of suspicious areas, thereby accepting an increased likelihood of operative failure. Exceptions to this policy, when more aggressive evacuation of the pituitary fossa and a higher risk of hypopituitarism are warranted in pursuit of a cure, include the following: (1) older patients in whom reproductive capacity is not at issue and for whom persistent hyperadrenocorticism and a second surgical procedure are highly undesirable because of intercurrent illness or debility; (2) repeat procedures, especially if adenomatous tissue was previously incompletely resected; (3) patients with findings suggesting biologically aggressive disease, such as very high nonsuppressible ACTH levels, extrasellar extension or other evidence of invasiveness, or Nelson's syndrome. The clinical problem in (2) and (3) is not usually a normal sella, but rather the low likelihood of total extirpation of tumor tissue.

In contrast to the prolonged disability of transfrontal neurosurgery, patients are usually alert and fully responsive within hours of undergoing transsphenoidal exploration, complaining only of headache and the annoyance of the nasal packing; hospital stay is typically only a few days. Aside from anesthetic risks, significant complications (<2%) are limited to the rare occurrence of perioperative hemorrhage or meningitis and occasional cerebrospinal fluid leak requiring repair. Transient diabetes insipidus is frequent, but permanent posterior pituitary insufficiency or loss of existing normal anterior pituitary function is exceptional. On the other hand, an almost universal finding in patients undergoing successful transsphenoidal resection of pituitary adenomas with subsequent remission of their Cushing's disease has been postoperative ACTH deficiency and secondary hypoadrenalism, resembling in all particulars pituitary-adrenal suppression occurring after prolonged exposure to high levels of glucocorticoids. Recovery takes weeks to months and is typically complete within a year. The rare patient does not recover.

Those responsible for attending patients subjected to transsphenoidal surgery for Cushing's disease must thus be aware of the anticipated course of pituitary-adrenal function in such patients if they are to manage steroid administration appropriately so as to avoid adrenal insufficiency, be able to assess outcome correctly, and work toward ultimate complete steroid withdrawal. In relation to the stress of surgery, adrenal insufficiency should be prevented by the administration of hydrocortisone, 100 mg or equivalent intravenously every 8 hours beginning with the operative procedure. In the immediate postoperative period, this dose should be tapered by 50 percent each day, if no significant complications occur, to a single morning oral replacement dose of hydrocortisone by about day 5 to 7, with the understanding that manifestations of the steroid withdrawal syndrome are common during the first days or weeks after any rapid cure of Cushing's syndrome. Hormone measurements just prior to the single morning replacement dose of short-acting steroid 2 to 3 weeks after surgery will usually clearly elucidate the postoperative status of the patient, since low values of both plasma cortisol and ACTH will accompany a successful outcome. Recovery from secondary adrenal insufficiency in cured patients should be monitored and managed as for those undergoing steroid withdrawal after hypothalamic-pituitary-adrenal suppression.

The advent of transsphenoidal surgery for Cushing's disease was heralded by reports from several large centers of cure rates for microadenomas of 85 to 95 percent and infrequent (<5%) recurrences. Other advantages of this approach included prompt response, low morbidity, and rare hypopituitarism. While the latter benefits apparently continue to characterize this procedure in other hands, initial enthusiasm for its success has been tempered by the recognition that remission rates of 50 to 60 percent are more realistically to be expected, as are more frequent recurrences than reported early on. The possibility must be considered that Cushing's disease represents a pathogenetically heterogeneous disorder, with varying outcomes resulting in different patient subsets. The most important basis for these variations, however, is almost certainly that expertise in identifying the very small lesions typically causing this disorder, frequently <6 mm in diameter and located deep within the substance of the gland, depends entirely on a specialized neurosurgical experience that cannot be assumed to be generally available. Furthermore, the follow-up period for patients undergoing transsphenoidal surgery for Cushing's disease has been brief in comparison with other treatments. More realistic assessments of recurrences and complications and a more balanced perspective on the role of this procedure in the management of Cushing's disease will require careful long-term studies.

Pituitary Irradiation

Two principal forms of pituitary irradiation are currently in use for the treatment of Cushing's disease: conventional supervoltage irradiation employing cobalt-60 sources or linear accelerators and proton-beam irradiation utilizing a specialized high-energy particle generator available for clinical application only in Boston. There would appear to be no significant role for the stereotactic implantation of radiation sources occasionally advocated in the past as a means of pituitary irradiation, since this technique requires highly specialized skills, is associated with other significant disadvantages and risks, and confers no special benefits as compared with other available treatments, especially transsphenoidal surgery.

Conventional irradiation is administered through multiple ports in a total of 4500 rads given in divided doses over 4 to 6 weeks in a radiotherapy regimen that has been well standardized over the years; the complication rate increases as the total dose exceeds 4800 rads with fractional daily doses above 200 rads. The advantages of this approach are: wide availability; minimal risk (neurologic complications or hypopituitarism are extremely unusual); and significant likelihood of prevention of subsequent Nelson's syndrome (enlarging pituitary tumor, often with neurologic manifestations, and hyperpigmentation accompanied by very high levels of ACTH), even if cure of hyperadrenocorticism is not achieved. Accordingly, when successful results occur, the outcome approximates closely the ideal objectives of treatment. Disadvantages of conventional irradiation are its relatively low remission rate (15 to 25% in adults, but as high as 80% in patients treated before age 18), the variable and occasionally prolonged lag period before cure occurs (3 to 18 months) or the outcome is known, and the likelihood that any subsequent neurosurgical approach to the pituitary will be made more difficult by scarring. Delayed development of cranial neoplasms is a feared but rarely documented complication of all forms of pituitary irradiation. (*Editor's note*:

In some series the remission rate reported for radiation in adults has ranged as high as 46 to 83 percent, of which two-thirds represent cures.)

Conventional irradiation may be preferrable as primary therapy for patients with mild Cushing's disease or in whom surgery is contraindicated, and it should be considered as alternative treatment in patients who are not cured by transsphenoidal surgery. The particularly favorable long-term results documented with conventional pituitary irradiation in children with Cushing's disease and the much more limited experience with transsphenoidal surgery in such patients suggest that radiation should still be strongly considered as a primary approach in children if there is any reason to doubt that the neurosurgical procedure would be carried out under optimal circumstances. In my judgment, conventional irradiation should be administered to all patients undergoing bilateral adrenalectomy for Cushing's disease, since there is suggestive if not incontrovertible evidence that the development of Nelson's syndrome in this circumstance (5 to 20% of adults; as many as 45% of children) is prevented or delayed. Another potentially promising role for conventional pituitary irradiation with which there is only limited experience is its combination with lower-dose, less toxic regimens of the adrenolytic agent o,p'-DDD (mitotane, Lysodren; see below), with apparently synergistic effect.

Heavy-particle irradiation requires detailed radiographic study of sellar anatomy and utilizes the localizing properties of the Bragg-peak phenomenon to deliver approximately 10,000 rads to the pituitary at a single sitting, with little radiation of surrounding structures. Patients with significant extrasellar extension or who have undergone previous conventional irradiation are usually not considered suitable candidates for this treatment. Advantages include higher remission rates (60 to 90%) than with conventional irradiation and short treatment periods. Disadvantages include limited accessibility and significantly greater likelihood of neurologic impairment or hypopituitarism than with either conventional radiation or selective transsphenoidal microsurgery; subsequent pituitary surgery is again likely to be relatively contraindicated. Heavy-particle irradiation should be reserved for special circumstances involving refractory or recurrent disease in adults, for which cure by nonsurgical hypophysectomy is acceptable.

Adrenalectomy

The introduction of reliable steroid replacement therapy more than three decades ago made possible bilateral adrenalectomy the first effective treatment for the hyperadrenocorticism of Cushing's disease. As indicated previously, in the vast majority of cases the pituitary lesions in this disorder are small, and morbidity relates almost entirely to hypercortisolism rather than to an expanding pituitary mass. Accordingly, adrenalectomy has remained an important therapeutic alternative when rapid, reliable correction of the metabolic derangement is urgent, despite subsequent recognition that the primary pathogenetic abnormality in Cushing's disease is central rather than adrenal.

The preferred surgical approach, because of more rapid postoperative convalescence and decreased morbidity, is through bilateral flank incisions rather than through the abdomen and peritoneal cavity. Pneumothorax is common with this procedure, but is usually small and easily managed. Care must be taken at surgery insofar as possible to resect the glands in toto and inspect the operative sites thoroughly so as to minimize the likelihood of persisting cortical function from an adrenal remnant. Here again, there is no substitute for a surgeon experienced with the specific procedure, and interactions with such individuals should be cultivated to the ultimate benefit of patients requiring this treatment. Complications may include postoperative infection, poor wound healing, and thromboembolic phenomena. Even in the most experienced hands, perioperative mortality may be as high as 5 percent; it should be recognized that this relates in large part to the circumstance that severely ill, debilitated patients are being subjected to major surgical intervention.

Steroid administration in relation to surgery follows the general pattern prescribed for the transsphenoidal procedure, except that after tapering to near-physiologic doses of cortisol, both glucocorticoid and mineralocorticoid replacement will be needed. The results of surgery can be ascertained in a patient maintained on a short-acting steroid preparation by predose morning determinations of plasma cortisol and by other hormone measurements, such as urinary free cortisol, if indicated. In fact, of course, the desired outcome is complete and permanent primary adrenal insufficiency. Steroid replacement therapy and the requirements for appropriate patient education, for carrying relevant identifying medical information, and for emergency availability of steroids parenterally are identical thereafter with policies mandated for the management of addisonian patients.

Remissions are virtually universal following bilateral adrenalectomy for Cushing's disease, though persisting adrenal function and eventual recurrence of hyperadrenocorticism as a result of continued stimulation of remnant or aberrant cortical tissue have been reported in as many as 10 percent of patients. The temptation to subject patients with recurrent hypercortisolemia after adrenalectomy to repeat surgery in an endeavor to extirpate remaining adrenal tissue should be resisted; a pituitary approach usually is far more fruitful. The major long-term complications of adrenalectomy for Cushing's disease relate to the alarming incidence of Nelson's syndrome and the substitution for the presenting problem of another permanent, potentially life-threatening disorder, adrenal insufficiency. As indicated previously, the risks of the former can probably be minimized by pituitary irradiation;

the hazards of the latter require life-long vigilance and are by no means inconsequential, since a small but irreducible increase in mortality from adrenal insufficiency remains an unsolved problem. Reimplantation in an accessible site of a fragment of resected adrenal tissue in order to obviate permanent adrenal insufficiency incurs little risk but in practice has rarely been successful in achieving the desired normalcy of adrenal function. Except perhaps as part of a research protocol involving combined therapies, planned partial adrenalectomy is a long-discredited form of therapeutic "fence-sitting" that, in my opinion, has no role in the treatment of patients with Cushing's disease.

Bilateral adrenalectomy seldom is indicated today as primary treatment for Cushing's disease, but may have a role in selected patients with relatively severe disease in whom a neurosurgical approach is unavailable or contraindicated, the results of pituitary irradiation judged to be too delayed or unreliable, and medical therapy found to be unacceptable. Obviously, such cases represent unusual circumstances occurring in relation to a relatively rare disorder. The role of adrenalectomy in bilateral nodular hyperplasia and the ectopic ACTH syndrome, both of which are sometimes confused with Cushing's disease, is discussed subsequently.

Pharmacologic Therapy

Three categories of drugs working through different mechanisms have been utilized in attempts to interfere with the pathophysiologic process resulting in the hyperadrenocorticism of Cushing's disease: centrally-acting agents that modify hypothalamic-pituitary activity so as to ameliorate the ACTH hypersecretion; drugs interfering relatively specifically with one or more biosynthetic reactions in the adrenal cortex, thereby inhibiting steroid secretion; and, more generally, adrenolytic agents that probably have a variety of effects but ultimately decrease the mass of functioning adrenal tissue. None of these drugs has been found suitable as primary therapy for Cushing's disease, but some may serve important adjunctive roles in this disorder and have even more important applications in states of hyperadrenocorticism involving relatively autonomous cortisol and ACTH overproduction.

Of the centrally active agents, the best documented successes have been with cyproheptadine (Periactin). In normal subjects, this drug interferes with the hypothalamic-pituitary responses to metyrapone and to insulin-induced hypoglycemia. Various lines of evidence suggest that the ACTH-suppressing effects of cyproheptadine are mediated predominantly by its serotonin-blocking action, though it has antihistaminic and anticholinergic properties as well. Clinical and biochemical improvement have been reported in a number of patients with Cushing's disease and in a few with Nelson's syndrome. The overall experience with cyproheptadine has been disappointing, however, with clinically useful responses occurring only infrequently and unpredictably. Even in successfully treated patients, relapse ensues almost universally upon withdrawal of the drug, so that its administration must be continued indefinitely. Somnolence is a prominent side effect, but can usually be minimized by beginning therapy with smaller total doses (6 to 8 mg per day) than are eventually needed in most cases (24 mg per day) and using a divided treatment schedule with increases prescribed initially at bedtime. The development of a marked increase in appetite and resulting weight gain is a distressing complication that may occur even if hypercortisolism is lessening and frequently renders treatment with this agent unacceptable to the patient. The results of cyproheptadine administration in Cushing's disease must be considered of interest at present primarily because of the insights they may provide into the underlying defects in this disorder, rather than as the basis for a clinically applicable approach. Such treatment should be considered in an individual patient only under the very unusual circumstances in which other more accepted therapies are not appropriate.

The dopaminergic agent bromocriptine (Parlodel) and a variety of other drugs affecting neurotransmitter function have been reported to decrease ACTH levels in occasional patients with Cushing's disease and Nelson's syndrome, but the responses achieved are rarely adequate for clinical purposes. The potential for enhancing our understanding and management of such patients in the future through the study of these agents is considerable, but at present they must be considered solely investigational tools.

Several drugs that act as adrenal enzyme inhibitors have the potential for decreasing cortisol biosynthesis in states of hyperadrenocorticism. The best-characterized of these are metyrapone, an agent that works predominantly on the final step in glucocorticoid formation, the hydroxylation of 11-deoxycortisol to cortisol; and aminoglutethimide, which blocks a very early enzymatic reaction in steroidogenesis, the conversion of cholesterol to pregnenolone. Inhibition of steroid biosynthesis is incomplete at concentrations of these agents that can be attained clinically, and significant problems often complicate their use. Metyrapone (Metopirone) is regularly associated with gastrointestinal side effects and occasionally with skin rash, is relatively short-acting and usually must be given in frequent divided doses (at least every 6 hours), and is very expensive for prolonged administration. Aminoglutethimide (Cytadren) has significant central nervous system toxicity, with lethargy, ataxia, and dizziness occurring frequently, and regularly causes distressing if often transient skin rash.

The effectiveness of these adrenal enzyme inhibitors alone in diminishing cortisol production in Cushing's disease might be expected on theoretic grounds to be limited, and such in fact is the case: ACTH secretion in this disorder is regulated around a higher set-point than normal, but is not in fact autonomous;

the increase in ACTH release elicited in otherwise untreated patients with Cushing's disease by any fall in circulating glucocorticoid thus overcomes the partial block in steroidogenesis that can be achieved with any of the currently available agents, and cortisol production is thereby restored to pretreatment levels. Accordingly, these drugs are not suitable as primary therapeutic agents in the long-term management of Cushing's disease. When no compensatory increase in the concentration of ACTH reaching the adrenal can occur, however, as in most patients with Cushing's syndrome related to autonomous hypersecretion of ACTH in the ectopic ACTH syndrome or of cortisol with adrenal neoplasms, these agents may be very useful clinically in reducing cortisol secretion (as is subsequently discussed).

Adrenal enzyme inhibitors can be effective in Cushing's disease, however, under circumstances in which pituitary ACTH reserve is compromised. These agents may thus be used as adjunctive therapy in reducing hypercortisolism in patients awaiting the delayed outcome of pituitary irradiation or in those experiencing incomplete remission after such treatment. They may occasionally also be helpful while awaiting the beneficial effects of o,p'-DDD, but the toxicity of such combined drug therapy is usually prohibitive. Attempts to prepare patients with severe Cushing's disease to withstand planned surgery better by a period of medical therapy with enzyme inhibitors is generally ill-advised in my experience, with little clinically significant overall improvement resulting from the delay in definitive treatment. Promising results have been reported in limited trials involving combined administration of metyrapone and aminoglutethimide, making use of the enhanced effectiveness of the two agents acting at different sites in the steroid biosynthetic sequence, while toxicity is lessened by reduced doses of each. This approach, which requires very careful clinical titration, probably deserves further exploration, but at best merely represents an improved temporizing measure, since the effects of these inhibitors quickly dissipate after their discontinuation.

Persistent pharmacologic interference with adrenocortical function has been achieved clinically only with the adrenolytic agent o,p'-DDD (mitotane, Lysodren). The actions of this drug are still not fully understood despite its use for more than two decades, but it apparently acts initially for the most part as an adrenal enzyme inhibitor, with a cytotoxic effect superimposed after a variable interval. A curious but as yet unexplained observation is that in some patients with Cushing's disease DDD seems to have a partial suppressive effect on ACTH as well.

The use of DDD is fraught with difficulties, for reasons that include the following: (1) Onset, duration and dissipation of its effects, both toxic and clinically desirable, are often delayed and prolonged, at least in part because of the tendency of the drug to be sequestered in adipose tissue depots. (2) Drug toxicity is appreciable and often limiting and includes frequent gastrointestinal symptoms and neurologic manifestations, as well as skin rash, gynecomastia, and hyperlipidemia. (3) Effects of the agent on the peripheral metabolism of steroids may confound the interpretation of hormone determinations, especially those involving urinary metabolites, making it necessary to rely on direct measurements of cortisol and aldosterone. (4) It is often difficult to distinguish permanent from reversible interference of the drug with adrenal function. (5) The development of transient or permanent adrenocortical (especially glucocorticoid) insufficiency is a significant possibility, thus incurring the need for steroid replacement therapy. If this litany of problems does not suffice to interdict the use of DDD as primary therapy for Cushing's disease, one must further consider that, with the primary pituitary abnormality left untreated, the possibility of Nelson's syndrome becomes an additional significant long-term risk even if hypercortisolism is successfully corrected in such patients.

Nevertheless, several studies have attempted to define a role for DDD in the management of patients with Cushing's disease. This would seem most appropriately limited to adjunctive therapy in patients treated with pituitary irradiation. Such patients might include those in whom pituitary irradiation has failed and pituitary and adrenal surgery are contraindicated or patients undergoing pituitary irradiation in whom an attempt to correct the hypercortisolism more promptly than might otherwise occur following such treatment is considered necessary. Under such selected circumstances, the following regimen has been reported to be associated with significant likelihood of remission and with reversible toxicity of an acceptable degree: DDD is administered in a daily total of 4.0 g, divided so that the largest dose is given at bedtime to minimize disability from side effects. An attempt is made to taper this dose after 3 to 4 months to maintenance levels of 1.5 to 2.0 g daily. A decrease in various indices of cortisol secretion to normal within this period heralds likely cure; if DDD cannot be withdrawn, a decision concerning continued long-term administration depends on patient tolerance of the agent and specific clinical circumstances. Vigilance must be maintained concerning the possible need for cortisol replacement therapy, especially in relation to intercurrent illness; mineralocorticoid deficiency is less likely except with higher doses or chronic administration. Treatment of adrenocortical carcinoma with DDD, of course, requires a more aggressive approach (as is subsequently discussed).

ADRENOCORTICAL TUMORS

The preferred and only curative treatment for functioning adrenal tumors, including those causing Cushing's syndrome, is complete surgical removal. If the clinical manifestations of glucocorticoid excess are particularly debilitating, the possibility should be considered of improving the patient's overall status and likely tolerance of surgery by correcting the hypercortisolism for a period of time prior to operation. In contrast to the circumstance in Cushing's disease, the hyperadrenocorticism resulting from adrenal tumors is usually readily responsive to treatment with adrenal enzyme inhibitors, though administration for several weeks is usually necessary for clinically significant improvement. Either metyrapone or aminoglutethimide may be used, but I prefer the former agent for such relatively short-term therapy because of its less troublesome side effects, particularly in the relatively low doses (250 to 500 mg every 6 hours, given with food or milk) that are usually adequate to normalize cortisol secretion here. Enhanced effectiveness of metyrapone apparently comes about because a secondary site of its inhibitory action on steroidogenesis, the conversion of cholesterol to pregnenolone, is made available in the absence of countervailing ACTH stimulation to augment its potency. The choice between prompt definitive therapy and delayed surgical resection in a somewhat better prepared patient requires the considered judgment of those familiar with the relevant clinical particulars, but is only rarely a difficult decision.

The great majority of functioning adrenocortical neoplasms are unilateral, but mention should be made of the unusual variant of Cushing's syndrome resulting from bilateral nodular adrenal hyperplasia, a heterogeneous condition that can easily be confused with hyperadrenocorticism of the primary pituitary variety. In nodular hyperplasia, adrenal hyperfunction is not predominantly dependent on ACTH stimulation at the time of diagnosis, though there is reason to believe that the condition may evolve from an earlier state in which such was the case. Therapy is probably best directed at the adrenal, with total adrenalectomy the less than ideal but nonetheless preferred treatment. Long-term follow-up for evidence of possible development of pituitary changes is indicated.

With the availability of greatly improved radiographic techniques, the anatomic relationships of adrenal masses can usually be defined with considerable accuracy preoperatively and this information used to plan appropriate surgical strategy. With small unilateral lesions clearly confined to the suprarenal area, a posterior extraperitoneal flank approach results in adequate exposure and lessened morbidity. If bilateral nodular hyperplasia is suspected or radiographic studies leave any doubt as to the discreteness or localization of the adrenal lesion, or with obviously bulky masses, an anterior approach allows for more extensive exploration and the possibility of en bloc dissection of tumor and adjacent involved organs. When transabdominal surgery is contemplated, angiography, careful assessment of renal function, and sterilization of the bowel may be indicated preoperatively in view of the increased likelihood of nephrectomy and colonic resection. Although surgical morbidity is certainly increased in patients with hyperadrenocorticism, this risk must be balanced against the desirability of complete removal of all neoplastic tissue, often requiring an aggressive surgical approach, if there is to be any prospect of cure when adrenocortical carcinoma is present; the dilemma may be heightened by the difficulty sometimes encountered in making this diagnosis with confidence even on the operating table.

The same regimen of steroid administration should be adhered to with surgery for resection of an adrenal tumor causing Cushing's syndrome as with transsphenoidal surgery for Cushing's disease. The possibility of prolonged hypothalamic-pituitary-adrenal suppression, whose management is described elsewhere, should be anticipated. Indeed, except for surgical complications, this potentially vexing sequela is the only obstacle in achieving an ideal result in the vast majority of patients with benign adrenocortical tumors, since recurrences are virtually unknown.

Adrenocortical carcinoma, on the other hand, is a highly malignant neoplasm with a generally dismal prognosis. Metastasis to the lungs, lymph nodes, liver, or, not infrequently, the contralateral adrenal, or locally invasive disease is present at diagnosis in more than two-thirds of patients. The overall 5-year survival rate is less than 25 percent, and even when potentially curative resection is undertaken, fewer than half the patients live this long. In addition to being rare, this malignant growth can manifest unusual variability in biologic behavior, with changes in functional status occurring not infrequently during its evolution and occasional well-documented instances of indolent course and prolonged survival despite metastatic spread. Accordingly, controversy exists concerning the efficacy of any therapeutic approach.

Guidelines that may be useful in managing patients with adrenal carcinoma include the following:

1. Surgical resection should be as extensive as practical, even if a curative procedure is out of the question, since there is reason to believe that the course of the disease and the likelihood of response to chemotherapy are favorably affected by minimizing tumor burden in a given patient. In selected patients with prolonged survival, repeat surgery to remove recurrent or even metastatic disease in order to accomplish this should be considered.
2. Despite some doubt concerning the effectiveness of o,p'-DDD in prolonging survival, this agent represents the only relatively specific chemotherapy available. DDD was first introduced clinically for its cytotoxic actions in adrenocortical carcinoma, its previously alluded to application in benign adrenal hyperplasia constituting a derivative application. A therapeutic trial with this drug is indicated whether or not the malignant adrenal tumor is hormonally active. Objectively measurable disease responses result in about one-third of patients, but these are usually partial and almost always temporary. Occasionally, dramatic and long-lasting regression occurs and it is highly likely that significant benefit accrues from the use of this drug and from aggressive management in selected pa-

tients. The caveats previously set forth concerning the time-course of action of DDD, its toxicity, the potentially misleading effects seen on certain hormone assays, and the risk of adrenal insufficiency apply with greater relevancy to its use in treating adrenal carcinoma, since the usual approach involves administering the maximally acceptable dose, at least initially. Therapy may be started with 3.0 g per day, increased over a period of weeks to a total of as much as 8 to 20 g per day, if tolerated; an attempt should be made to minimize side effects by using a divided-dose regimen (higher dose at bedtime), but toxicity is inevitably appreciable. It is noteworthy that clinically significant improvement, if it is to occur, almost always becomes evident within 4 to 6 weeks of initiating therapy, and thus there is little point in continuing DDD beyond that time in the face of significant toxicity and lack of any indication of response. If regression does occur, lower doses of DDD should be used for maintenance indefinitely, since the impaired quality of life of patients treated with large doses over an extended period renders such therapy unacceptable.

3. The efficacy of radiation therapy is highly doubtful, but radiation is worth considering as attempted palliation for symptomatic local disease in view of the limited toxicity of such treatment.
4. Adrenal enzyme inhibitors may be useful in ameliorating the effects of steroid excess (Cushing's syndrome, virilization) if these are not adequately controlled by DDD. There is no reason to believe that metyrapone or aminoglutethimide has any effect on tumor growth, however, and the use of these agents should be restricted solely to improving hormonal status, if this is felt necessary.

A favorable effect on prognosis in adrenal carcinoma of earlier diagnosis as a result of new technology is a prospect whose realization remains to be demonstrated.

ECTOPIC ACTH SYNDROME

The primary clinical problem in patients with ectopic ACTH production is almost always the presence of a rapidly progressive malignant tumor, and therapy should be directed toward this process if at all possible. In most cases, at diagnosis the tumor is obvious, unresectable, and poorly differentiated, and the prognosis defined by its behavior is usually limited to weeks or months. Although the florid clinical picture of Cushing's syndrome associated with primary pituitary or adrenal disease frequently is not present, hypertension, hypokalemia, edema, glucose intolerance, profound weakness, and muscle wasting are common manifestations of cortisol and mineralocorticoid excess in patients with ectopic ACTH production and may contribute significantly to morbidity.

If a decrease in tumor mass can be achieved by whatever means, ACTH and steroid levels will fall and metabolic improvement ensue. In rare instances, permanent cure of the underlying neoplasm has been accomplished, but most often response is transient. In the absence of successful primary tumor therapy or while awaiting its outcome, an attempt may be made to reduce excess steroid production by utilizing the adrenal enzyme inhibitors previously described.

Either metyrapone or aminoglutethimide may be useful in this circumstance, and the combination of the two agents (metyrapone, 250 to 500 mg, and aminoglutethimide, 125 to 250 mg, both three or four times daily) especially recommends itself because of reduced toxicity and enhanced efficacy. Here again, as with adrenal tumors causing hyperadrenocorticism, enzyme inhibitors are likely to be more effective in reducing steroid production than in Cushing's disease because the malignant tumor does not compensate for the fall in cortisol caused by these agents by increasing its ACTH output. In certain patients, rapid and profound decreases in steroid secretion may occur, and steroid replacement therapy may be required. Not infrequently, however, the level of autonomous ACTH production by the tumor is so high that the incomplete block in steroidogenesis wrought by these inhibitors is only partially effective in normalizing steroid levels. Ancillary supportive measures, such as potassium supplementation, insulin administration, and the use of mineralocorticoid antagonists, may also be helpful in managing patients with ectopic ACTH syndrome.

Isolated cases have been documented in which prolonged survival occurs despite the persistence of a metastatic ACTH-producing malignant tumor, obviously of indolent behavior. We have helped care for one such patient who has survived 12 years; bilateral adrenalectomy was successfully carried out after 7 years of medical management in order to simplify her care, and consideration of such extreme measures may be appropriate in rare circumstances.

Suggested Reading

Aron DC, Findling JW, Fitzgerald PA, Forsham PH, Wilson CB, Tyrrell JB. Cushing's syndrome: Problems in management. Endocrine Rev 1982; 3:229–244.

Bertagna C, Orth DN. Clinical and laboratory findings and results of therapy in 58 patients with adrenocortical tumors admitted to a single medical center (1951 to 1978). Am J Med 1981; 71:855–875.

Boggan JE, Tyrrell JB, Wilson CB. Transsphenoidal microsurgical management: Report of 100 cases of Cushing's disease. J Neurosurg 1983; 59:195–200.

Cohen KL, Noth RH, Pechinski T. Incidence of pituitary tumors following adrenalectomy. Arch Intern Med 1978; 138:575–579.

Didolkar MS, Bescher RA, Elias EG, Moore RH. Natural history of adrenal cortical carcinoma. Cancer 1981; 47:2153–2161.

Fitzgerald PA, Aron DC, Findling JW, Brooks RM, Wilson CB, Forsham PH, Tyrrell JB. Cushing's disease: Transient secondary adrenal insufficiency after selective removal of pituitary microadenomas; evidence for a pituitary origin. J Clin Endocrinol Metab 1982; 54:413–422.

Gold EM. The Cushing syndromes: Changing views of diagnosis and treatment. Ann Intern Med 1979; 90:829–844.

Hardy J. Cushing's disease: 50 years later. Can J Neurol Sci 1982; 9:375–380.

Jennings AS, Liddle GW, Orth DN. Results of treating childhood Cushing's disease with pituitary irradiation. N Engl J Med 1977; 297:957–962.

Kelly WF, MacFarlane IA, Longson D, Davies D, Sutcliffe H. Cushing's disease treated by total adrenalectomy: Long-term observations of 43 patients. Quart J Med 1983; 206:244–231.

Krieger DT. Cushing's syndrome. New York: Springer-Verlag, 1982.

Lubitz JA, Freeman L, Okun R. Mitotane use in inoperable adrenal cortical carcinoma. JAMA 1973; 223:1109–1112.

McArthur RG, Hayles AB, Salassa RM. Childhood Cushing's disease: Results of bilateral adrenalectomy. J Pediat 1979; 95:214–219.

Moore TJ, Dluhy RG, Williams GH, Cain JP. Nelson's syndrome: Frequency, prognosis and effect of prior irradiation. Ann Intern Med 1976; 85:731–734.

Salassa RM, Laws ER Jr, Carpenter PC, Northcutt RC. Transsphenoidal removal of pituitary microadenoma in Cushing's disease. Mayo Clinic Proc 1978; 53:24–28.

Styne DM, Grumbach MM, Kaplan SL, Wilson CB, Conte FA. Treatment of Cushing's disease in childhood and adolescence by transsphenoidal microadenomectomy. N Engl J Med 1984; 310:889–893.

PRIMARY ALDOSTERONISM

GAIL K. ADLER, M.D., Ph.D.
GORDON H. WILLIAMS, M.D.

Primary aldosteronism, hypersecretion of aldosterone in the absence of definable stimulus, is most commonly associated with a unilateral adrenal adenoma. However, a significant minority of patients have bilateral adrenal hyperplasia. In rare cases, an adrenal carcinoma, an ectopic source of aldosterone, or glucocorticoid-suppressible cortical nodular hyperplasia can cause primary aldosteronism. Primary aldosteronism usually is detected in individuals between the ages of 30 and 50 and has an incidence of approximately 1 percent in populations of unselected hypertensive patients. Since aldosterone causes sodium reabsorption and hydrogen and potassium ion excretion, signs and symptoms of primary aldosteronism are attributable to the hypertension (headache and infrequently visual disturbances) or, more commonly, to potassium depletion (fatigue, polyuria, muscle weakness, and cramps). Unfortunately, on the basis of the symptoms alone, patients with primary aldosteronism cannot be readily distinguished from patients with other forms of hypertension.

SCREENING FOR PRIMARY ALDOSTERONISM

Even though primary aldosteronism occurs relatively infrequently, because it is a potentially curable disease it is important to have a simple, inexpensive screening test. In our opinion, no clinical characteristics distinguish the patient with primary aldosteronism. Studies conducted a number of years ago suggested that a low plasma renin activity may be an effective screen for primary aldosteronism. This was based on the observation that patients with primary aldosteronism are volume expanded and therefore would have suppressed renin levels. Unfortunately, we as well as others have not been particularly enchanted with plasma renin activity as a screening test since it is relatively expensive ($30 to $50) and not very specific (roughly 20 percent of patients with essential hypertension also have low renin levels). We believe that if certain precautions are taken, a more reliable, and certainly cheaper, screening test is a serum potassium level. In our experience, *spontaneous* hypokalemia in a hypertensive patient is almost invariably a sign of aldosterone excess. Whether it is primary or secondary, aldosteronism can readily be distinguished by measuring plasma renin activity (Fig. 1).

Unfortunately, spontaneous hypokalemia is unusual in hypertensive patients. In most instances a low serum potassium is a result of treatment with potassium-wasting diuretics. Thus, if a patient is hypokalemic and taking potassium-wasting diuretics, the diuretics need to be discontinued for 10 to 14 days and serum potassium remeasured. If it is still low, this would suggest that the patient has mineralocorticoid excess.

What is the sensitiivity of this procedure? Theoretically, all patients with primary aldosteronism should have hypokalemia unless they are on a low sodium diet (thereby preventing the reabsorption of sodium, a necessary prerequisite for the potassium wastage with aldosterone), are ingesting potassium-sparing diuretics, or have renal failure. Thus, in interpreting a serum potassium level, we take the following precautions to prevent a false-negative result. If patients are on potassium-sparing diuretics, these drugs are discontinued for 10 to 14 days and serum potassium is remeasured. During this period the patient should be maintained on a normal sodium (100 to 200 mEq) and potassium (60 to 100 mEq) intake. If the serum potassium is normal while the patient is on a liberal sodium intake, off potassium-sparing diuretics, and free of evidence of renal failure (by BUN and/or creatinine), we believe that primary aldosteronism is effectively excluded.

In our experience several concerns need to be addressed in performing what appears to be a relatively simple procedure. First, discontinuing diuretic therapy for 14 days may produce a rise in blood pressure which could be intolerable for the patient. Under these circumstances, if other antihypertensive agents are not effective and one is concerned about whether a low serum potassium level is secondary to potassium-losing diuretic or excess aldosterone, one could simply measure a 24-hour urine potassium after discontinuing the drug. Under most circumstances, if the hy-

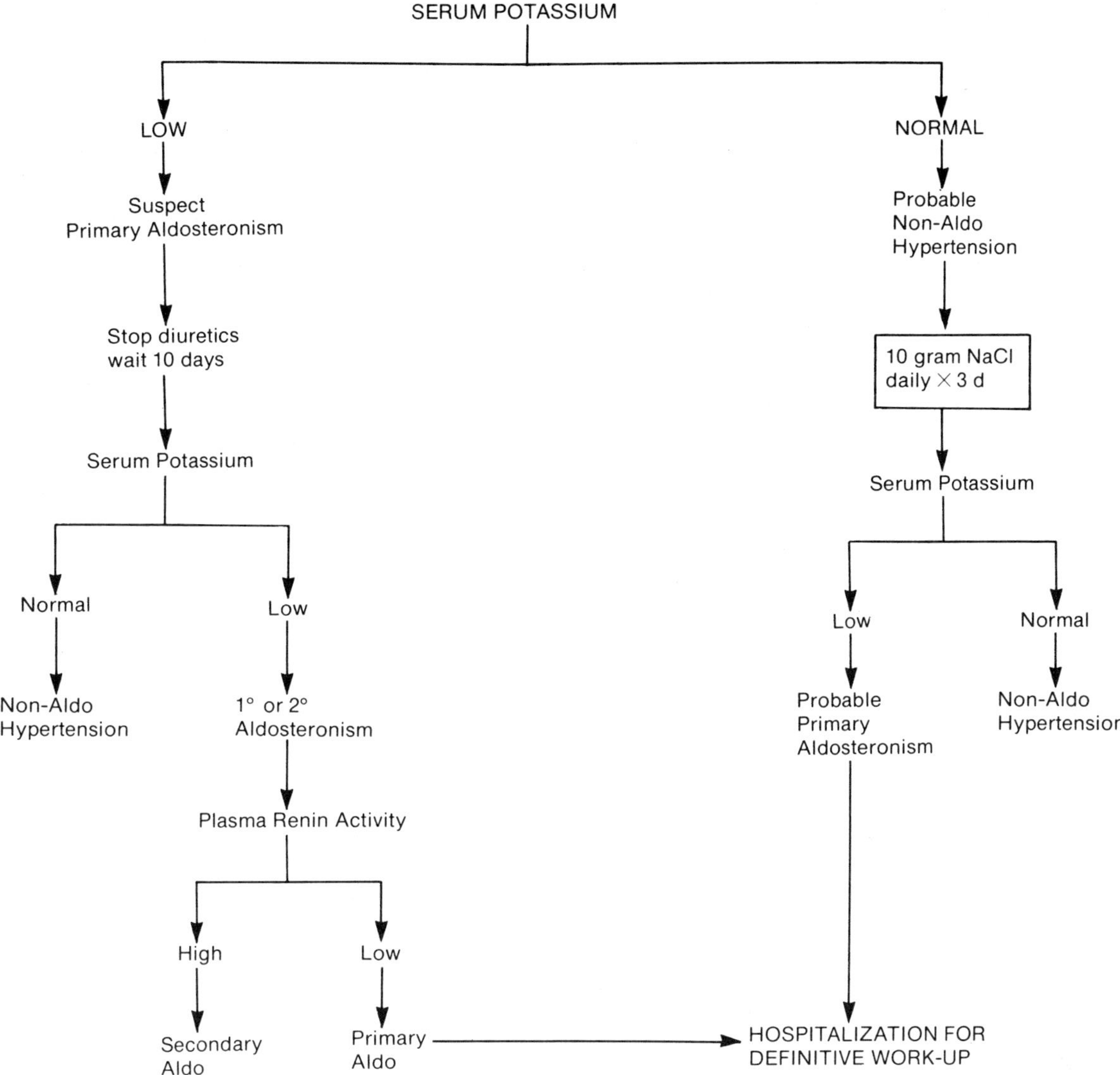

Figure 1 Flow sheet for office screening of hypertensive patients for hyperaldosteronism. (Reprinted with permission from Williams GH, Dluhy RG. How to evaluate and manage hypokalemic high blood pressure. In: Wolf GL. Eliot RS (ed). Contemporary problems in cardiology. Vol 2 Practical management of hypertension. Mt. Kisco, NY: Futura Publishing Company, Inc 1975).

pokalemia is drug-induced, urinary potassium excretion declines markedly (less than 30 to 40 mEq per 24 hours). On the other hand, if the hypokalemia is secondary to aldosterone excess, the urinary potassium excretion rate remains elevated (greater than 50 to 60 mEq/24 hrs). Second, care should be taken when increasing a patient's dietary sodium intake, particularly in those who may have severe hypertension or incipient congestive heart failure. Finally, in our opinion, sodium should never be administered to a hypokalemic patient in whom you suspect primary aldosteronism. If the suspicion is correct, salt losing will promote further potassium loss, more hypokalemia, and potentially severe adverse cardiac manifestations of the hypokalemia.

Recently, a screening test for primary aldosteronism has been suggested whereby patients are given 25 mg of captopril by mouth and their plasma aldosterone and renin levels measured 2 hours later. A nomogram is used to determine whether the patient's response is normal. It is suggested that in patients with primary aldosteronism no change in renin or aldosterone levels will occur, whereas other patients show a rise in renin and a fall in aldosterone. We have had limited experience with this test, but are concerned about two potential shortcomings: (1) the cost is probably greater than $100, and (2) the results are highly dependent on the reliability of blood sample collection and the processing of the laboratory samples. Both reasons in all probability exclude this test as a standard screening procedure.

DEFINITIVE DIAGNOSIS OF PRIMARY ALDOSTERONISM

If the techniques outlined above reveal a hypertensive patient with spontaneous hypokalemia and a suppressed plasma renin activity, admission to a metabolic unit for a definitive work-up of primary aldosteronism should be arranged. In our experience, the definitive diagnosis of primary aldosteronism should be made on the basis of the following four criteria: (1) plasma or urinary aldosterone levels that do not suppress when salt loaded, (2) plasma renin activity that cannot be stimulated with salt restriction and upright posture, (3) potassium wasting and/or hypokalemia when salt loaded, and (4) normalization of serum potassium with sodium restriction. We believe the easiest way to definitively evaluate a patient suspected of having primary aldosteronism is as follows. The patient is admitted to a metabolic unit and placed on low (10 mEq) sodium and relatively high (100 to 150 mEq) potassium intake. After approximately 5 days when balance is achieved on this diet, supine and upright plasma renin activities are obtained. The individuals then are given a saline load—3 liters of normal saline intravenously over a 6-hour period. Plasma aldosterone and cortisol levels are obtained before starting the saline infusion and at 6 hours. In our laboratory the normal 6-hour aldosterone value should be less than 5 ng/dl. The cortisol level is obtained to rule out a false-positive elevation of aldosterone secondary to stress and ACTH stimulation.

The advantages of this approach are as follows:

1. The low sodium diet prepares the patient for the appropriate renin stimulation test. In our laboratory the upright plasma renin activity has been less than 2 ng AI/ml/hr in every patient with primary aldosteronism whom we have studied on a sodium-restricted diet.
2. Often, by first restricting the patient's salt, both blood pressure and potassium are normalized. The saline load now can be given with less potential danger to the patient (hypokalemia and/or hypertension).
3. Since approximately 40 percent of patients with essential hypertension have difficulty handling the sodium load and may take longer than 4 hours to suppress their plasma aldosterone levels, we prefer a 6-hour saline infusion and do not recommend a shorter 4-hour infusion. Because the renin levels also fail to suppress normally in these patients, the false-positive elevation of aldosterone usually becomes apparent if one obtains a simultaneous plasma renin activity.

Two other parameters are assessed during the course of the saline infusion: (1) urine potassium excretion (in primary aldosteronism the increment in 24-hour potassium excretion is at least 30% over basal); and (2) serum potassium levels. Although serum potassium levels can fall precipitously, we often do not observe a significant change in serum potassium at the conclusion of the 6-hour saline infusion, but do observe it the following morning—24 hours after initiating the saline infusion. The reason we fail to see the rapid development of hypokalemia may be in part our preparation of the patients—high potassium, low sodium intake.

We have had an occasional patient in whom we were unable to carry out the foregoing procedures. These individuals had concomitant mild-to-moderate renal failure; thus, the sodium restricted intake produced a deterioration in renal function and the development of hyperkalemia. In these individuals, we elected to perform a 4-hour saline infusion under very closely monitored conditions both for blood pressure and potassium shifts. In each case, we observed no change in the plasma aldosterone levels over the 4-hour infusion. Each had an aldosterone-secreting adenoma removed at surgery, with lowering of blood pressure and normalization of the hypokalemia. However, each has required continued medication to normalize the blood pressure. The saline infusion should not be performed in patients with severe hypertension or in patients who have a stroke, myocardial infarction, or congestive heart failure within the past 6 months (Fig. 2).

BILATERAL ADRENAL HYPERPLASIA VERSUS AN ALDOSTERONE-PRODUCING ADENOMA

Once the diagnosis of primary aldosteronism is established, its etiology should be determined since the treatments for an adenoma and bilateral adrenal hyperplasia differ. Initially, a high-resolution computed tomography scan should be obtained. The CT scan will detect approximately 90 percent of all adenomas with a less than 1 percent false-positive rate. In our experience, if both adrenal glands are visualized and a unilateral adrenal mass is found, further work-up is unnecessary, and the patient can be assumed to have an aldosterone-producing adenoma. Adenomas that are less than 1 cm in diameter are most difficult to detect by CT scan, especially if they are isodense with surrounding tissues and have not changed the contour of the gland. These small adenomas account for most of the 10 percent false-negative rate associated with CT scans.

If by CT scan both adrenals are of equal size, or if one adrenal is not seen, we believe that the patient should undergo adrenal vein sampling. This study should be performed by an experienced radiologist because technical problems can lead to inadequate adrenal vein sampling and significant complications including adrenal vein thrombosis, adrenal infarction, rupture of the adrenal vein, and extravasation of contrast. The sensitivity of adrenal venous sampling is greater than 90 to 95 percent. Bilateral adrenal vein sampling for determination of aldosterone and cortisol concentrations should be obtained to look for lateralization of aldosterone secretion. Lateralization indicates an adenoma, and equal aldosterone levels indicate bilateral hyperplasia. The cortisol levels indicate whether the samples are adequate and should show no lateralization although differences in levels be-

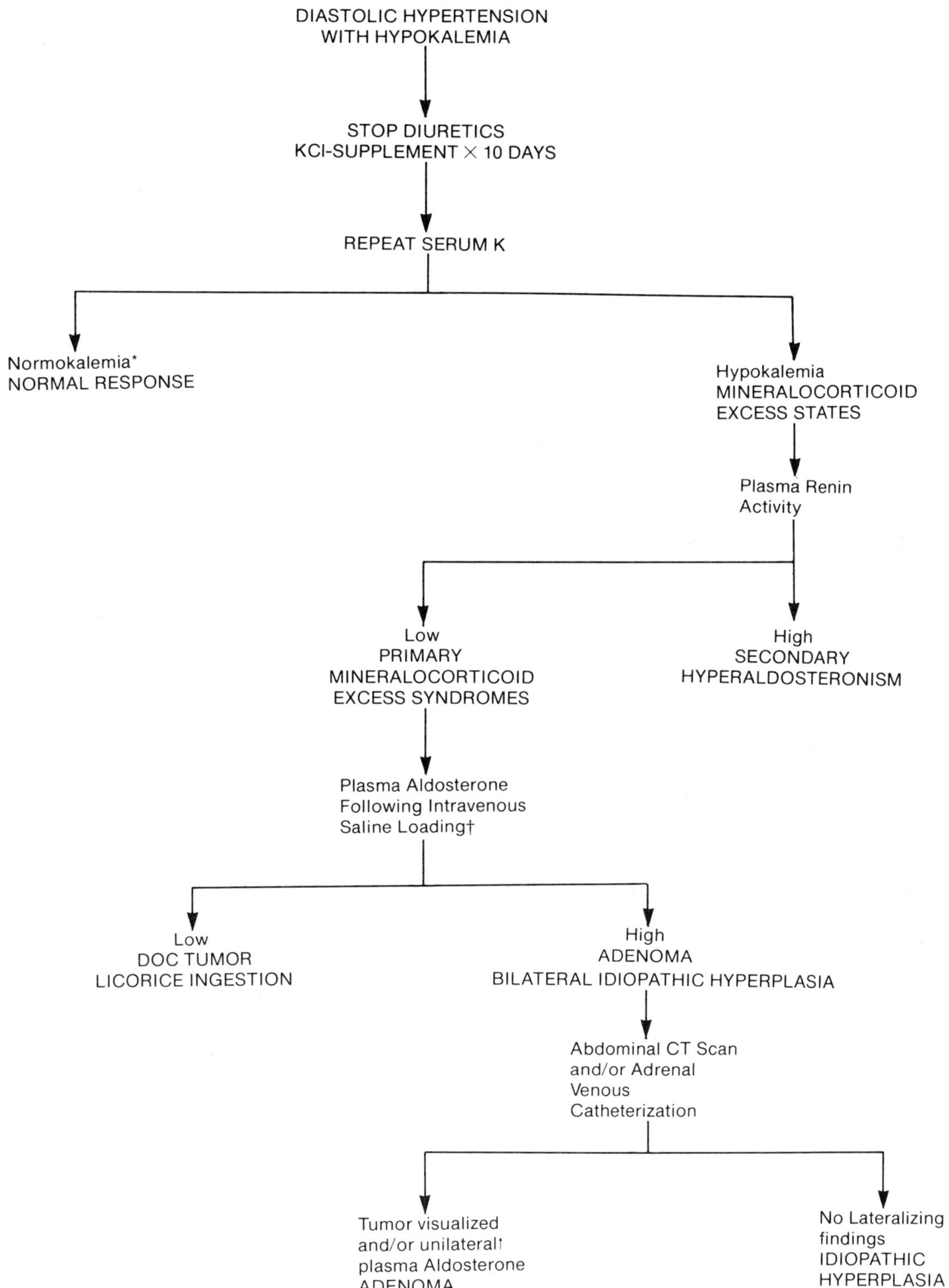

Figure 2 Diagnostic flowchart for evaluating patients with suspected primary aldosteronism.

* Serum K may be normal in some patients with hyperaldosteronism who are taking potassium-sparing diuretics (spironolactone, triamterene) or ingesting low sodium-high potassium intakes.

† This step should not be taken if hypertension is severe (diastolic> 115 mm Hg) or if cardiac failure is present. Also, serum potassium levels should be corrected before the infusion of saline. (Reprinted with modifications from Williams GH, Dluhy, RG. Diseases of the adrenal cortex. In: Harrison's principles of internal medicine. 10th Ed. New York: McGraw Hill Book Company, Inc. 1983.)

tween the two sides if samples are not obtained concomitantly, may result from the normal episodic secretion of this steroid. Adrenal venography has a lower sensitivity of 75 to 90 percent with up to 30 percent false-positives and a slightly higher complication rate than just adrenal venous sampling. However, once the catheter is in place for adrenal venous sampling, the added risk of adrenal venography is minimal in experienced hands, and useful information can be obtained. Unfortunately, adrenal venography may be prohibitively expensive in some institutions.

The adrenal iodocholesterol scan is less sensitive (70 to 90% sensitivity) and more expensive, and it results in 5 to 10 times more adrenal radiation than a CT scan. In addition, the radioisotopes used are not yet FDA approved except for research purposes. For these reasons, we do not perform adrenal iodocholesterol scintigraphy routinely. We have found that other procedures which have been advocated to distinguish an adenoma from hyperplasia are less reliable. They include plasma aldosterone response to upright posture. About 80 percent of patients with an aldosterone-producing adenoma have a decrease in their aldosterone level after 2 hours of upright posture. However, up to 25 percent of patients with bilateral hyperplasia also show this decrease in aldosterone. A second discriminant is an elevated 18-OH corticosterone level in a supine patient on an ad lib sodium intake. In our experience, there are both false-negatives and false-positives with this test.

Consideration should also be given to the rare causes of primary aldosteronism. An adrenal carcinoma probably would be detected by CT scan since these tumors tend to be inefficient producers of aldosterone and would be large by the time the patient developed symptoms of primary aldosteronism. Overproduction of additional adrenal hormones would also suggest carcinoma. Since our initial treatment for both adrenal adenomas and carcinomas is surgical removal of the affected adrenal, further preoperative testing to distinguish between these possibilities is seldom warranted. Finally, patients with a family history of primary aldosteronism should be evaluated for glucocorticoid-suppressible hyperaldosteronism. Prednisone, 5 mg twice a day for 4 to 6 weeks, will normalize blood pressure, potassium, plasma renin activity, and plasma aldosterone in patients with glucocorticoid-suppressible hyperaldosteronism. A *transient* decrease in aldosterone production during the first few days of prednisone suppression will occur in some patients with primary aldosteronism.

THE APPROACH TO TREATMENT

While waiting for study results, patients with suspected primary aldosteronism should be given a trial of medical therapy. Patients should be placed on less than an 80-mEq sodium diet. With less sodium available for exchange with potassium in the distal renal tubule, patients tend to conserve potassium. In addition, the mild volume depletion that accompanies a low sodium diet may lead to a decrease in the patient's blood pressure. Compliance with the low sodium diet can be monitored by obtaining a 12-hour urine for sodium and creatinine. At the same time, treatment with a potassium-sparing diuretic should be initiated (Table 1).

We usually use spironolactone, a competitive antagonist for the mineralocorticoid receptor. We start at 50 mg twice a day. The dose can be increased in increments of 100 mg at 1- or 2-week intervals up to 300 to 400 mg a day. The patient's blood pressure and serum potassium should be followed weekly. With spironolactone there is an average increase in serum potassium levels of 1.5 mEq/L. In addition, the majority of patients with primary aldosteronism become normotensive with spironolactone therapy. Unfortunately, up to 20 percent of patients develop side effects with spironolactone. In males these include decreased libido, impotence, gynecomastia, lassitude, and gastrointestinal disturbances. The gastrointestinal complaints can be minimized, however, if spironolactone is taken with meals.

An alternate potassium-sparing diuretic, amiloride, acts on the distal renal tubules to block sodium channels. Thus, sodium and chloride excretion is increased and potassium excretion decreased. Amiloride does not directly inhibit aldosterone's action. The initial oral dose is 10 mg a day, which may be increased at 10 mg intervals up to 40 mg a day. As with spironolactone therapy, average serum potassium levels rise by roughly 1.5 mEq/L. Again the majority of patients with an aldosterone-producing adenoma become normotensive. A somewhat smaller decrease in

TABLE 1 Drug Therapy for Patients with Primary Aldosteronism

Medication	*Initial dose*	*Maximum dose*	*Cost/Tablet**	*Side effects*
Spironolactone	50 mg *bid*	200 mg *bid*	10¢–13¢ for 25 mg (generic) 16¢ for 25 mg (Aldactone) 75¢ for 100 mg (Aldactone)	Impotence, decreased libido, gynecomastia, lassitude, gastrointestinal complaints
Amiloride	10 mg qd	40 mg qd	20¢–26¢ for 5 mg	Headaches, lassitude, muscle cramps, impotence, gastrointestinal complaints, increased BUN and uric acid

* Cost/Tablet was obtained from a sampling of pharmacies in the Boston area.

blood pressure is seen in patients with bilateral adrenal hyperplasia. The side effects of amiloride are mild. They include headaches, lassitude, muscle cramps, gastrointestinal complaints, and occasionally impotency. A mild increase in blood urea nitrogen and uric acid can occur.

A combination of triamterene and thiazide has been tried, but in our opinion is less effective than spironolactone or amiloride in reversing potassium depletion. The dose of triamterene/thiazide (50 mg/25 mg) tablets is up to 2 tablets twice a day. Side effects include blood dyscrasias, liver damage, gastrointestinal disturbances, weakness, headaches, and anaphylaxis.

Rarely, a low sodium diet and maximum therapy with either spironolactone or amiloride does not control a patient's hypokalemia. In these cases, we have begun potassium supplementation. Potassium supplementation and a potassium-sparing diuretic should not be started simultaneously because of the danger of hyperkalemia. Rather than initiating potassium supplementation, there is theoretic support for considering a combination of amiloride and spironolactone to control resistant hypokalemia. Spironolactone and amiloride exert their effects by different mechanisms and could have a synergistic effect on serum potassium. However, we have no practical experience with this approach.

If the patient's blood pressure is not controlled with a low-salt diet and a potassium-sparing diuretic, an aldosteronoma alone is unlikely. The patient has bilateral hyperplasia and/or renal damage secondary to the elevated blood pressure. In these patients, we have found a β-blocker or a converting enzyme inhibitor (captopril) good first choices. Calcium channel blockers decrease aldosterone levels in isolated glomerulosa cells and also may prove to be effective in treating primary aldosteronism. Cyproheptadine, an antiserotoninergic agent, and bromocriptine, a dopamine agonist, have both proved to be ineffective in treating primary aldosteronism. These medications were tested because of the hypotheses that aldosterone production is under tonic dopaminergic inhibition and that there exists a pituitary-aldosterone-stimulating hormone under serotoninergic stimulation.

If test results indicate bilateral adrenal hyperplasia, patients should be continued on medical therapy. For unknown reasons, bilateral adrenalectomy, despite correcting the biochemical abnormalities in patients with bilateral adrenal hyperplasia, is generally ineffective in reversing hypertension, with only 15 percent of patients becoming normotensive after surgery. In addition, these patients face the problem of adrenal insufficiency. Because of the complications associated with long-term steroid administration, patients with glucocorticoid-suppressible hyperaldosteronism may need to be treated in the same way as patients with bilateral adrenal hyperplasia if a large glucocorticoid dose is required.

The treatment for a patient with an aldosterone-producing adenoma is surgical removal of the adenoma and the affected adrenal gland. Patients who refuse therapy or who are poor surgical candidates because of other medical problems may be treated medically. Our surgeons usually use a posterior rather than a transabdominal surgical approach. With the posterior approach, patients tend to recover more rapidly and have fewer complications. In our experience, roughly 95 percent of patients who undergo adrenalectomy for an aldosterone-producing adenoma become normotensive and normokalemic in the first 3 to 6 months after surgery. Over the next 2 to 3 years, however, 20 to 25 percent again develop hypertension. When hypertension recurs, it is usually easier to control and is not associated with hypokalemia.

Preoperatively, patients should be treated with a low sodium diet, potassium-sparing diuretics, and antihypertensive agents as needed to control serum potassium and blood pressure. Intraoperatively, a patient's potassium level should be monitored, and because the remaining adrenal may not produce cortisol adequately, a patient should receive high-dose steroids. The intraoperative steroid dose is 10 mg hydrocortisone per hour by constant intravenous infusion. This dose also prevents rebound mineralocorticoid deficiency. Postoperatively, the patient can be switched to oral steroid supplementation and the dose gradually tapered to zero over a 2- to 6-week period. In the postoperative period, a patient may develop hypoaldosteronism with elevated serum potassium levels due to inadequate functioning of the remaining adrenal cortex. It may take 3 to 6 months before the adrenal cortex fully recovers from the long-term suppressive effects of high aldosterone levels produced by the tumor. During this time a patient should follow a liberal sodium diet, follow daily weights, and be alert for signs of hypovolemia. Fluorohydrocortisone should be avoided since this can further suppress the adrenal cortex.

Finally, how does one treat a patient with an aldosteronoma who refuses surgery? We have had several such patients. All have been treated with spironolactone with normalization of blood pressure. The longest treatment has been 14 years. We have been successful with this approach only in women. No complications have occurred in them. We have not had any men who have tolerated the side effects, i.e., impotency, associated with long-term spironolactone therapy.

Suggested Reading

Bravo EL, Tarazi RC, Dustan HP, Fouad FM, Textor SC, Gifford RW, Vidt DG. The changing clinical spectrum of primary aldosteronism. Am J Med 1983; 74:641–651.

Ferriss JB, Beevers DG, Boddy K, Brown JJ, Davies, DL, Fraser R, Kremer D, Lever AF, Robertson JIS. The treatment of low-renin ("primary") hyperaldosteronism. Am Heart J 1978; 96:97–109.

Geisinger MA, Zelch MG, Bravo EL, Risius BF, O'Donovan PB, Borkowiski GP. Primary hyperaldosteronism: comparison of CT, adrenal venography, and venous sampling. AJR 1983; 141:299–302.

Lyons DF, Kem DC, Brown RD, Hanson CS, Carollo ML. Single-dose captopril as a diagnostic test for primary aldosteronism. J Clin Endocrinol Metab 1983; 57:892–896.

Williams GH, Dluhy RG. Diseases of the adrenal cortex. In: Harrison's Principles of Internal Medicine. 10th ed. New York: McGraw-Hill Book Company, 1983.

HIRSUTISM

ROGER LOBO, M.D.,
RICHARD HORTON, M.D.

The skin and its appendages are the largest target tissues for the sex hormones. The hair follicle and the sebaceous glands, in particular, are very sensitive to levels of androgens or changes in androgen production that occur at puberty. Perhaps because of this tissue sensitivity, and evidence that the control factors for adrenals (ACTH and other proopiomelanocortin-derived products) and ovaries (gonadotropins) are related primarily to glucocorticoid and estrogen respectively, the regulation of androgens and androgen prehormones are imprecise. Hirsutism is said to be the most common endocrine disorder in women. Although it is almost always a benign process, the social and psychologic implications and potential reduction in fertility make it an important problem that should be handled by the physician with concern and sensitivity.

Testosterone in both men and women has a dual function. Acting directly, it is anabolic, inducing protein synthesis and growth in muscle, liver, and probably bone. However, the second action, that of a sex hormone, is primarily expressed through dihydrotestosterone (DHT), which represents a quantitative and qualitative alteration in hormone action. DHT is required for prostate development in the male and appears to be the active hormone in sexual hair development, acne, and frontal balding. This was best demonstrated in studies of peripheral enzyme 5α-reductase deficiency. Individuals with this disorder are genetic males with pseudohermaphroditism at birth who at puberty develop male genitalia and spermatogenesis, but no prostate appears, and these individuals have little or no facial and sexual hair, frontal balding, or acne formation at the time of purberty.

CAUSES OF HIRSUTISM

Virilizing Tumors

Endocrine-related hirsutism can be divided into two types. First, hirsutism results from increased levels of testosterone reaching the hair follicle. The most dramatic example is that resulting from an ovarian virilizing tumor or, less often, a tumor of the adrenal cortex. These are very rare tumors, associated with a marked increase in testosterone production (plasma testosterone >150 ng/dl, normal 20 to 60) and evidenced clinically by virilization (e.g., menstrual irregularity, amenorrhea, and clitoral hypertrophy). The ovarian tumors synthesize and secrete testosterone directly. Adrenal tumors usually secrete DHEA and DHEA sulfate and androstenedione. Levels of DHEA-S above 3 μg/ml implicate a role of the adrenal gland; levels above 8 μg/ml suggest the presence of an adrenal tumor.

Polycystic Ovary Syndrome

Another example is the polycystic ovary (Stein-Leventhal) syndrome, which is a much more common cause of hirsutism than virilizing tumors. Unfortunately, it remains a syndrome difficult to precisely define. Current understanding suggests an abnormality in neuroendocrine regulation of luteinizing hormone (LH), with inappropriate release of LH and induction of a hyperstimulation state of the ovary. This leads to secretion of increased testosterone and androstenedione. The result, starting at puberty, is menstrual irregularities of all degrees, hirsutism, and failure to ovulate. Associated problems often include obesity and increased insulin levels. The characteristic laboratory findings are LH/FSH ratios >3, and the reduction in FSH is probably the result of increased formation of estrogen from androgen. Subcapsular cysts of the ovary develop and often the ovaries are enlarged. However, the ovaries need not be enlarged. Ultrasonography may be helpful to confirm these anatomic changes. In blood, androstenedione, DHEA sulfate, and testosterone are increased, but levels of androgens capable of producing virilization rarely occur. A variant of PCO is the rare, often familial entity, hyperthecosis, which tends to be associated with increased secretion of androgen from ovarian elements.

Idiopathic Hirsutism

The second category is that of disorders in which circulating testosterone is normal or only slightly increased. This is idiopathic hirsutism (IH), which makes up the overwhelming group (>90%) of patients with increased sexual hair. Some patients with completely normal steroid tests, but positive family history, can also be considered in this category. Slight or subtle increases in unbound testosterone concentrations are present in many, perhaps a majority, of these patients. However, a considerable number appear to have either testosterone in the normal range or only increased DHEA and androstenedione. This was previously confusing, since these ketosteroids are not potent androgens. Our understanding has been clarified by evidence that these androgen prehormones can be further processed by skin to testosterone and DHT. Indeed, hair follicles from patients with idiopathic hirsutism form increased DHT from these precursors in vitro. These observations suggest that peripheral formation of androgens may be poorly reflected by circulating levels of androgens. Importantly, these studies support the concept that IH is primarily a peripheral disorder of skin. A recent further support of this theory is the fact that the metabolite androstanediol glucuronide (3α-diol G) which appears to represent peripheral 5α-reductase activity and DHT formation, is increased not only when circulating testosterone and DHT are increased, but also in IH.

Hirsutism Associated with Adrenal Disease

Hirsutism associated with adrenal tumors, Cushing's syndrome and congenital adrenal hyperplasia are covered in other chapters of this book.

OUR APPROACH TO TREATMENT

The treatment of hirsutism should be directed at normalizing abnormal androgen production and action. For this reason we recommend the measurements of serum testosterone (T) and dehydroepinandrosterone sulfate (DHEA-S), and androstenediol glucuronide (3α-diol G).

Among the methods used to treat hirsutism, only oral contraceptives, corticosteroids, and antiandrogens should be considered. Ovarian wedge resections should never be done because of the limited success and short- and long-term morbidity of that procedure. Parenteral administration of long-acting progestins, such as depo-medroxyprogesterone acetate, should not be used in women in the reproductive age group because of its long-lasting effects.

Our general approach would be to suppress androgen production in disorders such as PCO where testosterone and DHEA-S are increased with oral contraceptives. Antiandrogens appear to be rational agents in idiopathic hirsutism.

Hair Removal

Only after suppressive therapy has been instituted, and the increased androgen production normalized, should existing hair be removed. The rate of growth of existing hair will be slowed by treatment, but it will not disappear until it has been mechanically removed. On the other hand, once treatment has started, new hair growth should be suppressed. Various depilatory agents have been used for the removal of unwanted hair; however, electrolysis is the only method that offers a permanent effect. Some caution should be exercised in selecting an experienced electrologist because improper treatment may result in permanent scarring.

Oral Contraceptives

Oral contraceptives (OCs) have been effective in the treatment of hirsutism. The progestin-dominant OC is responsible for lowering LH-mediated ovarian androgen production primarily from the ovarian stroma, as there is little follicular development while the patient is taking OCs. At the same time, the synthetic estrogen (mestranol or ethinylestradiol) suppresses gonadotropins, but also increases SHBG. Therefore, the lowering of T with treatment is accompanied by greater SHBG binding of T, which results in lower levels of biologically active free T. Ovarian androgen production is decreased with OCs, as is adrenal androgen production (approximately 30%). The latter findings are only true for OCs containing certain progestins. Although norethindrone-containing OCs (e.g., Ortho Novum) are effective, norgestrel-containing OCs are ineffective (e.g., Ovral, Lo-Ovral). Norgestrel pills should also be avoided because of the inherent property of this 19-nor-gestogen to be androgenic and to inhibit the binding of T to SHBG. Therefore, we have used norethindrone-containing OCs almost exclusively, although others have also had success with ethynodioldiacetate (e.g., Demulen). The dose of estrogen is less important, as 30 μg of estrogen is extremely effective in raising SHBG. We advocate the use of OCs containing less than 50 μg of estrogen. It has recently been demonstrated that OCs may also decrease peripheral androgen formation by decreasing tissue 5α-reductase activity. Although this finding is an important adjunctive mechanism for the success of treatment with OCs, OCs may not be as effective as receptor blocking agents for treating patients who exhibit only increased peripheral androgen production.

Glucocorticoids

Corticosteroids are only indicated for the treatment of hirsutism if there is evidence of significant adrenal androgen production. Levels of serum DHEA-S up to 4 μg/ml may be normalized by treatment with OC. If a patient has high levels of DHEA-S and no evidence of an adrenal neoplasm, low-dose corticosteroids may be administered. We prescribe 0.5 mg of dexamethasone or less until DHEA-S is lowered and clinical improvement occurs. We then decrease the dose of dexamethasone to the minimum dose required to keep DHEA-S levels suppressed (<1 μg/ml). Cortisol levels at 8AM are usually 2 to 5 μg/dl or more on 0.25 mg. This regimen is safe for even relatively long periods of time. The dose of corticoid is best administered at night. Prednisone has also been used effectively in equivalent doses and may be safer for prolonged use.

In a few patients in whom T is elevated and DHEA-S is >5–6 μg/ml, a combination of OCs and corticoids may be prescribed. This combination of 2 agents has an additive effect on suppressing androgen production and has been safely administered with good clinical results.

Corticoid therapy is also most appropriate for the hirsute women with adult manifestation of congenital adrenal hyperplasia (covered in another chapter). These present as patients resembling those with polycystic ovary syndrome (PCO), but usually have elevated levels of serum 17OH progesterone (17OHP) (>3 ng/ml) and exaggerated responses of 17OHP after ACTH (>20 ng/ml). Although we do not advocate screening all hirsute patients for this disorder, serum 17OHP should be measured in patients who are shorter, have significant hirsutism and/or virilism at a young age, resemble patients with PCO, and have high levels of T and/or DHEA-S. Doses of dexamethasone that normalize 17OHP and androgen levels result in normal ovulatory menses and improvement in hirsutism.

Antiandrogens

These agents have a key role in the treatment of hirsutism when there is increased peripheral androgen production. Indeed, most patients with hirsutism have evidence of increased peripheral androgen production regardless of their primary disorders. However, we have chosen these agents only when T and DHEA-S levels have been near normal and if other treatments (OCs or corticoids) have not been clinically effective.

In this category of peripheral blocking agents, cyproterone acetate and spironolactone are most effective, but cimetidine and cyproheptadine have also had limited success. In our hands, cimetidine has not been as effective as spironolactone, and has been associated with hyperprolactinemia. Cyproterone acetate, a progestin, has been used in Europe, either alone or in combination with ethinylestradiol, the so-called "reverse sequential" oral contraceptive (Diane). However, despite its reported success, concern about toxic effects has prevented its use in the United States. Spironolactone is therefore the drug of choice in the USA for inhibiting increased androgen production and action.

Spironolactone

Spironolactone, an aldosterone antagonist, increases the clearance of T and decreases its production via inhibition of cytochrome P450 oxidation. In addition, it blocks the androgen receptor, and we have recently shown that it is a 5α-reductase inhibitor. In doses of 100 to 200 mg daily, spironolactone has been effective in about 70 percent of patients without producing major side effects. Apart from a mild transient diuresis, no electrolyte imbalance, blood pressure changes, or other problems have been encountered in patients with normal renal function. A minority of patients may occasionally complain of mild dizziness, headaches, and nausea. These symptoms appear to be dose-related and are completely reversible. Menstrual function is unpredictable. Although women with normal menses before treatment often become irregular, some anovulatory, oligomenorrheic women may start having normal menstrual cycles. In the former group, menstrual function usually improves with the addition of an OC.

Improvement in the clinical score of hirsutism or in hair shaft diameters appears to be dose-related with the use of sprionolactone. We start treatment with 100 mg of spironolactone daily, and if no improvement occurs in 2 to 3 months, we increase the dose to 100 mg *bid*. The first objective change in hair growth can be appreciated by the second or third month, with continued improvement occurring for another 6 months. Serum T is consistently decreased with either dose, reflecting the changes in secretion and kinetics. However, DHEA-S is not affected by treatment. Indeed, the major mechanisms for the effectiveness of spironolactone treatment (receptor blockade and decrease in 5α-reductase activity) cannot be measured by parameters in blood. Preliminary data suggest that measurements of 3α-diol G will not be helpful or predictive of the clinical response to spironolactone.

A major problem in the treatment of hirsutism is the assessment of the effectiveness of therapy. Clinical scoring is helpful, as is the frequency with which hair is removed. However, measurements of anagen hair shaft diameters before and after treatment have been useful. Most patients will notice a change in their appearance, or that the need for using depilatory agents has decreased, some patients will not be able to notice differences when in fact change may be occurring. For this reason, photographs before and during treatment are advised. The physician should be patient and reassuring that oral contraceptives and/or antiandrogen therapy will improve and control the hirsute process.

GOUT

TSAI-FAN YU, B.A., M.D.

Management of gout should be directed to prevention and treatment of acute gouty arthritis, tophaceous gout, uric acid nephropathy, and recurrent nephrolithiasis. With marked progress in the development of various therapeutic agents nowadays, it is most important to know how to use these drugs intelligently.

TREATMENT OF ACUTE GOUTY ARTHRITIS

An attack of acute gouty arthritis must be treated with an appropriate anti-inflammatory drug without delay, and in the correct dosage. An experienced sufferer of gout usually knows enough to begin taking medication even during the prodromal stage of an acute attack, and he also knows his exact degree of tolerance toward an anti-inflammatory drug. Nonetheless, the physician should guide him carefully so as to help ameliorate suffering as soon as possible, and to prevent adverse reactions.

Colchicine

Colchicine used to be the sole agent for acute gouty arthritis. Owing to the introduction of new anti-inflammatory drugs and the toxic symptoms following a therapeutic course of colchicine, colchicine has somewhat lost its pre-eminent position.

Colchicine is an alkaloid, derived from the corm and seeds of the autumn crocus (Colchicum autumnale). It is so named because it originally grew in Colchis, an ancient country in Asia Minor bordering on the Black Sea. After oral administration, colchicine is absorbed from the gastrointestinal tract, metabolized in the liver, and excreted mostly into the intestinal tract by the bile, with some 20 percent excreted by the kidney. Colchicine is cleared from plasma rapidly, but it stays much longer in the leukocytes. The anti-inflammatory action of colchicine is through the inhibition of the crystal-induced chemotactic factor produced by polymorphonuclear leukocytes and a decrease in the release of lysozyme enzymes.

My personal experience in using colchicine for acute gouty arthritis has been favorable. In order to avoid toxic effects of colchicine on the gastrointestinal tract, I have been using colchicine orally, 0.6 mg *q2h*, after an initial dose of 1.2 mg. By taking colchicine, 0.6 mg *q2h*, not to exceed 5 doses on day 1, most patients improve considerably. The dosage may thereafter be reduced to 3 times a day for 1 or 2 days, and finally once or twice daily. The therapeutic program may be modified according to the progress in symptomatic relief. If the patient discontinues colchicine as soon as some suggestion of nausea or gastrointestinal discomfort appears, few patients develop alarming symptoms.

A colchicine preparation for intravenous use is available. It may be employed in severe attacks, particularly if the patient is not able to tolerate it by mouth because of a coexisting gastrointestinal disorder. If given early in the course, a single injection of 0.6 or 1.2 mg is usually sufficient to terminate an attack. In some instances, a second injection of 0.6 mg or 1.2 mg may be necessary 4 to 5 hours after the first one. Although intravenously administered colchicine does not as a rule give rise to intestinal upset, occasionally nausea has been observed after repeated injections. Extravasation of colchicine could cause much pain and adjacent tissue necrosis.

Most physicians prescribe oral colchicine, 0.6 mg every hour, after an initial dose of 1.2 mg. If the drug is ordered to be given every hour until diarrhea, nausea, or vomiting develops, it may provoke a lot of unpleasant side effects. Many patients recall such experiences and develop abdominal cramps as soon as the word colchicine is mentioned.

Phenylbutazone (Butazolidin)

This pyrazolone derivative is a potent anti-inflammatory agent. Following its ingestion, it is well absorbed from the gastrointestinal tract. The biologic half-life is relatively long, 72 hours in man. Two metabolites are formed in the liver. One metabolite, oxyphenbutazone (Tandearil), formed with the introduction of a phenolic group to the para-position in one of the benzene rings, has pharmacologic properties similar to those of phenylbutazone. Both drugs have been used effectively for acute gouty arthritis. With a dosage schedule of 200 mg 3 to 4 times a day for 1 or 2 days, the agony usually disappears promptly. Phenylbutazone and oxyphenbutazone may sometimes cause bone marrow depression, but this is extremely rare following a brief period of use. Since phenylbutazone (or oxyphenbutazone) tends to cause retention of sodium and water, it is contraindicated in cases of cardiac insufficiency. It is also sometimes ulcerogenic. Because of such potential hazards, many physicians tend to use phenylbutazone (or oxphenbutazone), 100 mg instead of 200 mg, three or four times a day. Because of the reduced efficacy with small dosages, an acute attack may develop into a subacute stage and the drug may have to be used for a longer period of time, thus increasing the risk of undesirable side effects.

Indomethacin

This indole-acetic acid derivative inhibits prostaglandin synthetase and also interferes with the migration of leukocytes into sites of inflammation. Like phenylbutazone, it is rapidly nd completely absorbed from the gastrointestinal tract, and it is strongly protein-bound. But the metabolites formed in the liver, unlike those from phenylbutazone, are inactive. Like phenylbutazone, it may cause peptic ulceration or gastrointestinal bleeding, but hemopoietic toxicity is rare. The most common annoying side effects are dizziness and headache. In view of the undesirable side effects, I prefer to use a lower dosage than the conventional dosage. By giving 25 mg instead of 50 mg, 3 or 4 times a day after meals for 2 to 4 days, an acute attack is terminated effectively without side effects.

Probenecid

This agent inhibits the renal tubular secretion of indomethacin. When both drugs are used together, indomethacin dosage should be reduced in order to avoid side effects, although its anti-gout effect is enhanced. Combined use of salicylate and indomethacin, on the other hand, decreases the urinary excretion of indomethacin, which is diverted to bile, and thus increases excretion in the stool.

Naproxen

This propionic acid derivative is another inhibitor of prostaglandin synthetase. Like the other anti-inflammatory drugs, naproxen is well absorbed from the gastrointestinal tract and is likewise strongly protein-bound and metabolized in the liver. Its metabolite is a glucuronide, which is inactive. Its prolonged anti-inflammatory action is due to a long biologic half-life, exceeding 12 hours, and high drug concentration in synovial fluid. Naproxen, 250 mg *bid* for 2 to 3 days, is effective treatment for mild to moderate attacks of acute gouty arthritis. In patients with low-grade chronic pains, naproxen, 250 mg a day, may be continued for a week or two without apparent side effects. Some patients may develop gastrointestinal symptoms, but gastrointestinal bleeding has been rare.

Corticotropin (ACTH)

When there is failure to respond, or when treatment is long delayed in patients who have very severe acute attacks involving several joints, ACTH is the drug of choice. The initial dose should be 40 to 100 units intramuscularly on the first day, gradually lowering the dosage as the clinical picture dictates. Before discontinuing corticotropin, colchicine, 0.6 mg *bid*, should be added to the regimens.

PREVENTION OF ACUTE GOUTY ARTHRITIS

An attack of acute gouty arthritis may be incited by physical stress, emotional disturbance, excessive ingestion of rich food, or overindulgence in alcoholic drinks. Most of the time, however, no inciting cause may be recognized. Generally speaking, the daily use of colchicine to prevent recurrent attacks of acute gouty arthritis is well accepted by physicians and by gouty sufferers as well. However, the efficacy of prophylactic colchicine is not necessarily uniform. Factors contributing to failure of the prophylaxis are mostly related to associated uncontrolled medical complications, intemperate habits in eating and drinking, and irregular life style, such as on and off starvation diet for weight reduction.

In most patients, colchicine, 0.6 mg once or twice a day, is sufficient to achieve satisfactory prophylaxis. Two tablets of colchicine taken at one time are usually more potent than one tablet taken twice a day. With one or two 0.6-mg tablets of colchicine a day, its concentrations in the body are extremely low. The possibility exists that such minute doses may affect the initiation of some immune responses, resulting in a gradual but steady suppression of chemotactic activity.

Long-term evaluation of the efficacy of colchicine prophylaxis revealed excellent results in 83 percent of 540 patients, satisfactory results in 12 percent, and unsatisfactory results in 5 percent only. Very few patients were colchicine intolerant. No hematologic or renal toxic effects and no chromosomal aberration or infertility were observed.

Discontinuance of the prophylactic program may be attempted in any patient who has been free from recurrent attacks for a reasonable period of time. It may be discontinued sooner in early uncomplicated gout with infrequent attacks and controlled uricemia. It should be continued longer in those with frequent and severe acute attacks prior to prophylaxis. As one gets older, the patient as a rule becomes less sensitive to provocative factors in precipitating acute gouty arthritis. Thus the dosage may be gradually reduced, and eventually discontinued altogether, in elderly patients who have no medical complications. Colchicine does not prevent the appearance of tophi, since it does not modify the serum uric acid or the amount of uric acid in urine.

TREATMENT OF TOPHACEOUS GOUT

Although acute gouty arthritis is usually brief and episodic, tophaceous gout is indeed a storage disease, in that the body is unable to excrete uric acid at a rate sufficient to balance the rate of formation. Human plasma is saturated with monosodium urate at a concentration of about 7 mg/dl. Precipitation of sodium urate sufficient to form tophi that are visible grossly or on roentgenogram seems to require a plasma concentration well above 7 mg/dl; even then the process of precipitation is remarkably slow. The rate of overt tophaceous depositis in the joints is, in general, a function of both the degree and the duration of hyperuricemia. A retrospective study of a large number of gouty patients before appropriate drug therapy revealed 70 percent of patients remained free of tophi 1 to 5 years after the first attack of acute gouty arthritis. The proportion of nontophaceous cases slowly declined to 28 percent after 20 years. With a serum urate of 7 or 8 mg/dl, >90 percent of the patients were free of tophi. When serum urate was maintained between 9 and 11 mg/dl, about 50 percent of them became tophaceous; with >11 mg/dl, <30 percent remained free of tophi. Tophi are usually located at the periarticular areas of the peripheral joints where they appear as soft tissue swellings. Most frequently involved areas include first metatarsophalangeal joints, olecranon bursae, Achilles tendons, and finger joints. Minute juxta-articular punched-out erosions may be found on x-ray examination. Increasing destruction of articular ends of the bones may lead to narrowing of the joint space and eventually chronic pains, joint deformity, and disability.

The principle of management for chronic tophaceous gout is to promote a negative balance between the production and excretion of uric acid. With prolonged negative uric acid balance, joint mobility may be promoted. Tophus already present in the periarticular spaces may become smaller and eventually disappear. Further precipitation of sodium urate may be prevented.

Probenecid

Probenecid (benemid; [p-di-n-propylsufamyl] benzoid acid) was originally developed to sustain high blood levels of penicillin by interfering with its renal tubular secretion at a time when penicillin was in short supply. Utilizing its similar capacity to inhibit the renal tubular reabsorption of uric acid, probenecid has been used as a uricosuric agent since 1949, thus ushering the era of modern therapy of gout.

After its ingestion, probenecid is rapidly and completely absorbed from the gastrointestinal tract. It is about 90 percent protein-bound. It has a pKa of 3.4 and a high lipid solubility; hence its excretion is pH-dependent. In acid urine, it is mainly reabsorbed from tubular lumen by non-ionic diffusion in relatively distal segments of the nephron. In alkaline urine, its excretion exceeds the amount filtered, and this is indicative of tubular secretion.

When probenecid is given to a gouty man, a profound uricosuric effect may be observed for a long time. Thus the expanded miscible uric acid pool is gradually reduced, and in turn, urate deposits in the tissues are mobilized. On the other hand, when probenecid is given to a normouricemic man, the uricosuric effect is short-lived because of rapid exhaustion of the miscible uric acid pool. Probenecid is not an anti-inflammatory agent. Unfortunately this is often misunderstood by many. Probenecid is not indicated in patients who excrete an excessive amount of uric acid or who have a history of renal calculus. When probenecid is being used, it is always important to maintain an adequate urine volume, at least 2 L daily, so as to prevent renal complications such as calculus formation.

Sulfinpyrazone

Sulfinpyrazone (anturane; 1,2 diphenyl-4- [2-phenylsulfinethyl], 3,5-pyrazolidinedione) was discovered to be a potent uricosuric agent in a systematic evaluation of more than 80 phenylbutazone analogs. This sulfoxide derivative does not have anti-inflammatory or sodium- and water-retaining properties. After oral ingestion, gastrointestinal absorption is rapid and virtually complete. Sulfinpyrazone, pKa 2.8, is a more acidic compound than phenylbutazone, is almost totally bound to plasma proteins, and is largely confined to the extracellular compartment. Very little is filtered by the glomerulus; renal excretion is mainly by tubular secretion. Its rate of renal excretion is not affected by change in urine pH. The biologic half-life is short, averaging 3 hours. Its metabolite, p-hydroxy-sulfinpyrazone, is also uricosuric. Sulfinpyrazone is a much more potent uricosuric agent than probenecid, a daily dosage of 200 to 400 mg of sulfinpyrazone being equivalent to 0.5 to 1.0 g of probenecid daily. Sulfinpyrazone may be used in patients who do not tolerate probenecid or do not respond satisfactorily to probenecid. Combined use of sulfinpyrazone and probenecid may exert additive uricosuric effects, in part because probenecid inhibits the tubular excretion of sulfinpyrazone, thus prolonging its uricosuric action.

Careful administration of appropriate dosages of probenecid or sulfinpyrazone in more recent years has not been associated with untoward side effects except for occasional complaints of gastrointestinal discomfort or drug allergy. Complete blood counts periodically are advisable.

Allopurinol

Allopurinol (Zyloprim; [4-hydroxypryrazolo-3.4-] pyrimidine) was originally selected as a prospective antitumor agent, but proved to be ineffective. However, it proved to be effective in blocking the formation of uric acid from hypoxanthine and xanthine by inhibiting the enzyme xanthine oxidase. After its administration, a striking reduction in serum and urinary uric acid is found, and yet hypoxanthine and xanthine do not accumulate in the blood, because they are rapidly cleared by the kidneys. Allopurinol has a relatively short biologic half-life of 1 to 3 hours, being rapidly excreted by the kidneys and oxidized by xanthine oxidase to form oxipurinol. Oxipurinol noncompetitively inhibits xanthine oxidase, and it has a more prolonged half-life, 17 to 40 hours. It is extensively reabsorbed in the kidney, and its renal clearance is about three times greater than the uric acid clearance. Because of the relatively longer half-life of oxipurinol, the effectiveness of allopurinol in reducing the rate of uric acid production is sustained for a long time. The reduction in uric acid excretion in most gouty subjects does not correlate stoichiometrically with an increase in urinary excretion of hypoxanthine and xanthine. However, in Lesch-Nyhan syndrome and in gout with partial deficiency of hypoxanthine-guanine-phosphoribosyl transferase (HGPRT), the decreased excretion of uric acid is in balance with the increase in hypoxanthine and xanthine. This is apparently related to the loss of the feedback inhibition mechanism in purine biosynthesis.

Allopurinol offers an alternative to uricosuric drugs in preventing and mobilizing tophaceous deposits, especially in patients who are intolerant or refractory to uricosuric agents. The interaction between allopurinol and probenecid is rather complex. The biologic half-life of probenecid is usually prolonged with concurrent allopurinol administration. On the other hand, probenecid facilitates the renal excretion of oxipurinol as well as of uric acid, thus lowering the plasma oxipurinol level, and hence diminishing the xanthine oxidase suppression. Because allopurinol is both a substrate and an inhibitor of xanthine oxidase, it can inhibit its own metabolism. Nevertheless, combined use of probenecid and allopurinol often facilitates the more rapid mobilization of urate deposits.

Concurrent use of allopurinol and dicumarol slows the metabolism of the latter by reducing the activity of hepatic microsomal drug-metabolizing enzyme systems. In a gouty patient with associated coronary heart disease requiring both drugs, the dosage of allopurinol and dicumarol should be reduced, and prothrombin time regularly determined.

Although allopurinol is well tolerated, with a low order of toxicity, serious reactions such as drug rash, epidermal necrolysis, exfoliative dermatitis, hepatitis, vasculitis, and bone marrow suppression have been reported. It is therefore advisable to use allopurinol, 100 mg daily, only for 1 to 2 weeks before the dosage is increased to 200 mg daily. Most patients require only 200 mg daily, but secondary gout due to blood dyscrasia, deficiency of HGPRT, or neoplastic disease with unusually excessive production of uric acid may require 300 mg of allopurinol daily. With 200 to 300 mg per day, untoward reactions are rare except for an occasional patient who manifests drug allergy. It is not advisable to place all patients with gout on 300 mg daily, regardless of the degree of hyperuricemia or the amount of urinary uric acid. With chronic use of allopurinol, periodic examination to check liver enzymes, blood counts, and blood and urine uric acid are indicated.

Indiscriminate use of probenecid, sulfinpurazone, or allopurinol for just anyone with joint pains is to be discouraged. After prolonged use of either drug for a few years, normouricemia may last for weeks or months after its discontinuance. Drug dosage may have to be adjusted periodically. There is no justification for prescribing a particular drug indefinitely since the patient's biochemical state may change with time. Also, life-long commitment discourages patients' compliance.

Aspirin

Acetylsalicylic acid was used widely for gout prior to the development of various antigout drugs. In more recent years, it has been used for prevention of coronary heart disease morbidity among elderly patients by virtue of its inhibition of platelet aggregation. Since many patients with gout belong to this age group, many are taking a small amount of aspirin daily.

Aspirin is rapidly hydrolyzed to salicylic acid after its administration, with a biologic half-life of 4 to 5 hours. Salicylic acid has a pKa of 3.0, and approximately 30 percent of plasma salicylate is not bound to plasma proteins in man and is thus filtrable at the glomeruli. In acid urine, the filtered salicylate is reabsorbed by the proximal tubule. Of the salicylate appearing in acid urine, only a small part, about 20 percent or less, is excreted as free salicylate. The major portion is conjugated, 55 to 65 percent with glycine to form salicyluric acid and 20 to 30 percent with glucuronide; the remaining 20 percent or so is converted to gentisic acid and other degradation products. In alkaline urine, there is great enhancement of urinary excretion of free salicylate, which suppresses the tubular reabsorption of uric acid, resulting in a uricosuric effect. Hence, the competitive action between free salicylate and uric acid at the renal tubular level depends on the urinary free salicylate concentration, as determined by the salicylate dosage, and on the pH of the urine.

Probenecid uricosuria, which is produced by inhibition of the tubular reabsorption of urate, is counteracted by small doses of salicylate, in part because of concurrent suppression of tubular secretion of urate. Probenecid likewise exerts a moderate inhibitory effect on the tubular secretion of free salicylate which in turn affects the uric acid excretion. The interaction of salicylate with probenecid is complex.

In patients whose serum uric acid has been satisfactorily maintained for a long time, it is not necessary to discourage the use of small doses of aspirin for a worthwhile purpose, such as inhibition of platelet aggregation. Small doses of aspirin, 0.3 to 0.6 g per day, have only a minimal effect in elevating serum uric acid.

Aches and pains in chronic gouty arthritis associated with degenerative joint changes frequently require small doses of aspirin. When deformities are corrected with disappearance of tophi, the use of aspirin for analgesia can be discontinued. Physical therapy also helps.

Acetohexamide

About 8 to 10 percent of patients with gout also have diabetes mellitus. Acetohexamide (Dymelor), a cyclohexyl derivative of sulfonylurea, is used in the treatment of diabetes. It has a uricosuric property in addition to its hypoglycemic action. Acetohexamide is readily metabolized with a short half-life, a little over an hour. The major metabolite is hydroxyhexamide, which is metabolically active, exerting a uricosuric action. Although the hypoglycemic action is due mainly to a metabolic effect on the β cells of the islets of Langherhans, the uricosuric property depends on an inhibition of renal tubular reabsorption of uric acid. In patients with renal insufficiency, acetohexamide does not exert any uricosuric action. Thus, a disassociation of the hypoglycemic and uricosuric action may be observed in such patients. Acetohexamide is recommended for patients with gout and diabetes mellituus.

Surgical Intervention

With timely diagnosis and the availability of effective drugs to prevent and treat the tophaceous stage of the disorder, the deformities and disabilities of advanced chronic gouty arthritis have become much less common. However, surgical intervention may be indicated in a few patients. Debridement is useful in accelerating the disappearance of ulcerating and discharging superficial tophi. Impairment of joint mobility or joint deformity with structural erosion and destruction may require corrective surgery.

ASYMPTOMATIC HYPERURICEMIA

The most common problem that confronts the physician nowadays is what to do about the patient who is discovered to have hyperuricemia, but who has never had symptoms referable to gout. Approximately 5 to 10 percent of men past the age of 30 years have some degree of asymptomatic hyperuricemia. Development of gout may be correlated with the degree of hyeruricemia, as observed in population and family studies.

A study of hyperuricemia among asymptomatic relatives of patients with primary gout reveals wide fluctuation of serum uric acid throughout the years of follow-up. Thus a single determination of serum uric acid can be misleading. Although the hyperuricemia trait may be inborn, it certainly can be modified by environmental changes. Appropriate dietary restriction and gradual weight reduction often lead to a decline in serum uric acid levels.

Alcohol consumption has traditionally been associated with hyperuricemia. Studies have indicated that it is related to elevation of blood lactate level, which leads to inhibition of urinary uric acid excretion. Other studies indicate that alcohol-induced hyperuricemia may be associated with hyperuricosuria due to enhancement of uric acid synthesis related to adenine nucleotide turnover. Normouricemia resumes when alcohol is entirely oxidized and eliminated from the body.

Hyperuricemia, sometimes of marked degree, may appear during starvation or after a high fat diet. The induced ketosis apparently suppresses urinary uric acid excretion. A high protein diet usually increases uric acid excretion, with a relatively modest increase in serum uric acid. The hyperuricemia may be greater when there is also some renal function impairment. With appropriate adjustment in diet, hyperuricemia should improve.

Hyperuricemia may be drug-induced, such as after chlorothiazide or furosemide used for hypertension, or after pyrazinamide or ethambutol used in treating tuberculosis. Drug-induced hyperuricemia is apparently due to inhibition of renal uric acid excretion.

Hyperuricemia associated with blood dyscrasia, as in polycythemia and leukemia, is usually accompanied by excessive urinary uric acid excretion. Dietary regulation is frequently unable to control the hyperuricemia and hyperuricosuria. The use of allopurinol is rational, particularly when chemotherapy is contemplated.

In asymptomatic hyperuricemia and excessive hyperuricosuria among members of families with deficient (HGPRT), an increased phosphoribosyl pyrophosphate synthetase (pp-ribose-p-synthetase), or other purine metabolizing enzyme abnormalities, use of allopurinol again is indicated.

Generally speaking, in persistent hyperuricemia of more than 9 or 10 mg/dl, despite careful dietry restriction and modification of medications, or in hyperuricosuria in the order of 1.0 g or more per day, with the uric acid nitrogen to total nitrogen ratio of the 24-hour urine being more than 2.0 percent, drug therapy using allopurinol is justified. If the ratio of urinary uric acid nitrogen to total nitrogen is within the normal range of 1.5 ± 0.3 percent, small doses of uricosuric agent, either probenecid or sulfinpyrazone, may be used. When asymptomatic hyperuricemia is associated with reduced urinary uric acid and evidence of significant renal damage, it is more advisable to seek possible causes of intrinsic kidney disease first.

GOUT AND NEPHROPATHY

The number of gout patients with severe renal damage is relatively small. Renal disease secondary to gout is not causally related to the severity of hyperuricemia and duration of gout, although a correlation does exist. In an analysis of a large number of patients with gout in the past 3 decades, the incidence of nephropathy has decreased over time due to rational therapy. In general, the incidence of nephropathy is greater in those with tophi. Nephropathy in gout in most cases is due to associated independent conditions, or to nephrolithiasis and infection.

The most frequent underlying disease causing nephropathy in gout is cardiovascular in nature, particularly essential hypertension. Although the incidence of hypertension in gout has been on the rise in recent years, nephropathy in gout is on the decline, reflecting the benefits of therapy.

A substantial number of gout patients have had chronic renal disease antedating gout for many years. As renal damage progresses, hyperuricemia may become more extreme, but not accompanied by increased uric acid excretion or higher incidence of renal calculi. Not many of those develop tophi, because of their relatively short life expectancy. Treatment is mainly supportive.

In saturnine gout, with a history of lead intoxication for many years, the damage to interstitium and renal tubules frequently overshadows the hemopoietic changes. Hyperuricemia is striking, but there is no high excretion of uric acid in urine. Allopurinol is preferred since uricosuric therapy is not efficient in such cases with renal insufficiency. Deleading with EDTA may help in some patients.

Gout may contribute more directly to nephropathy in those with fulminating gout, gout in HGPRT deficiency, or gout secondary to blood dyscrasias and certain neoplastic diseases. Microtophi in the renal interstitium do not necessarily cause damage of renal function. However, in the situations just cited, nephropathy may result from obstructive uropathy due to recurrent uric acid nephrolithiasis, either spontaneous due to overproduction or iatrogenic due to the use of uricosuric agents.

By using allopurinol, 200 to 400 mg per day, uric acid production becomes less and urinary uric acid excretion and concentration may decrease. Urine volume should not be less than 2 L per day, so as to keep the uric acid concentration adequately low; optimal urine pH should be maintained between 6.0 and 6.6.

IDIOPATHIC EDEMA

DAVID H.P. STREETEN, M.B., D.Phil., F.R.C.P.

Despite the profusion of diuretics available for the treatment of most types of fluid accumulation, many patients with idiopathic edema tend to become resistant to conventional diuretic therapy. A short summary of what is known about the pathogenesis of this group of disorders is essential to an understanding of their most effective treatment.

PATHOGENESIS

When one has excluded the many known causes of noninflammatory edema, ranging from such common conditions as congestive heart failure, intrinsic renal diseases, and cirrhosis to more unusual causes such as hypothyroidism, hyperthyroidism, Cushing's syndrome, protein-losing enteropathy, other types of hypoproteinemia, and many others, there remain a group of patients whose edema is of unknown origin. In most of these patients, perhaps 80 percent of them in the United States, a strong orthostatic component can easily be demonstrated. When these patients remain on their feet or in the seated position for several hours, their excretion of sodium and water or of water alone falls to a greater extent than it does in healthy, nonedematous subjects. The excessive fall in excretion appears to result from a disorder of the vasculature causing undue transudation of fluid from the capillaries in the dependent limbs, since the entire pathogenetic sequence that follows can be largely prevented by application of external pressure to the legs and pelvis. In the absence of such external pressure, continuing transudation leads to a greater orthostatic fall in plasma volume than occurs in normal subjects under the same conditions. Presumably in consequence of this hypovolemia, there follows (1) an excessive stimulation of vasopressin release resulting in orthostatic water retention, or (2) an excessive production of aldosterone, perhaps via renin release, and an abnormally profound fall in glomerular filtration rate, together leading to orthostatic sodium (and water) retention. The fluid retained by these mechanisms replenishes the depleted plasma volume and permits continuing transudation and measurably excessive swelling of the legs while the upright posture is maintained. When recumbency is resumed, the described chain of events is broken by the fall in hydrostatic pressure in the legs. Thus, the accumulated fluid is redistributed to the upper parts of the body, often causing edema of the eyelids, the face, and the hands the following morning and allowing at least some of the retained fluid to diffuse back into the vascular compartment, where it is excreted as the orthostatic hyperaldosteronism and/or hypervasopressinism subside.

It is not known why patients with these types of orthostatic edema transude excessively from the capillaries in their dependent limbs in the upright posture. Whether it results from a thickening of the capillary basement membrane or from the action of a local dilator of the precapillary sphincter (bradykinin? prostaglandin?) or from deficiency of a specific vasoconstrictor, such as dopamine, or from some other cause remains to be determined.

It should be added that, since there is no understanding of the pathogenic mechanism(s) of fluid retention in the minority of patients whose idiopathic edema is of the nonorthostatic type, no special therapeutic measures can be recommended for these patients.

TREATMENT

Since idiopathic edema is a chronic disorder that seldom remits, it is important for both the physician and the patient to appreciate that all medications are capable of doing harm as well as good and that the smallest amount of medication compatible with reasonable comfort should be used. A few patients with idiopathic edema have a tendency to escalate the dosage of their drugs in a compulsive desire to get rid of any vestige of excessive fluid. This tendency should be resisted.

A good general principle is to prescribe medications one at a time, monitoring the effects of each addition to the therapeutic program on body weight. This should be measured and recorded each morning on arising and each evening before retiring, always after emptying the bladder, for at least 2 weeks, preferably 4 weeks, before any new medication is begun. These records serve to determine whether mean weight gain from the beginning to the end of orthostasis (usually from morning to evening), over at least a 2-week period, is excessive—more than 1.5 lbs (0.7 kg)—since such excessive weight gain is the hallmark of orthostatic fluid retention. They also serve to document the presence of any premenstrual increment in body weight. Continued measurements during successive changes or additions to therapy indicate whether the treatment is or is not effective in producing a gradual downward trend in morning weight and/or a consistent reduction in mean weight gain *intra diem* to less than 0.7 kg and preferably less than 0.5 kg. Therapy that fails to produce improvement in at least one of these respects during a trial lasting 4 weeks or more should clearly be abandoned.

Posture

Since, by definition, orthostatic edema accumulates exclusively when the patient is in the upright posture, the patient should be made aware of this fact and encouraged to reduce the length of time spent sitting and standing each day as much as is compatible with a reasonable life-style. Whenever the opportunity is available, the patient should sit or lie down with the legs elevated. This often requires minor adjustments of social habits. It may be advisable for some severely affected patients to lie down on a couch for 2 or 3 hours after lunch each day and/or after dinner each evening in order to reduce the total duration of orthostatic fluid retention and to promote its excretion in recumbency.

Food and Fluid Intake

When obesity is present in these patients, caloric restriction is required. In the majority of instances in which there is orthostatic sodium retention, reduction of sodium intake is helpful and should be prescribed to an extent compatible with individual needs. Some patients are able, by purchasing low-salt foods, to restrict sodium intake to 10 to 30 mEq daily, with benefit. In others, it may be possible only to exclude obviously salty foods such as ham, pickles, salted potatoes or peanuts, either because low-salt foods are too expensive or unavailable or because of noncompliance with recommendations. Requirements for diuretic drugs are obviously reduced or obviated if sodium intake can be sufficiently restricted, and in this way, diuretic-induced potassium losses can be minimized.

Some patients consume unusually large volumes of fluids either because of habit or because of an excessive thirst. It is worthwhile to estimate average daily fluid intake and, when this exceeds a reasonable amount (about 1000 to 1200 ml daily), to recommend a reduction in the volume of liquids imbibed. Reduction of excessive thirst by drug therapy is not practicable at present, but might be a useful therapeutic adjuvant in the future.

Conventional Diuretic Drugs

In patients whose fluid retention is mild or intermittent, a thiazide diuretic (e.g., hydrochlorothiazide, 50 mg) may be all that is required. Frequently, however, such therapy loses its initial effectiveness when administered at the beginning of the active part of the day (the morning in most people, or the evening in workers on night shifts). When this happens, it is almost invariably helpful to recommend that the patient try to elevate the legs and to take the diuretic after the daily chores have been completed. In this way, a brisk diuresis will almost always ensue, facilitating rapid excretion of fluid retained during the preceding hours of orthostasis, so that diuretic action is complete before the patient goes to bed, and nocturia (often a troublesome complaint even before treatment of orthostatic edema) can be reduced or prevented. Chlorthalidone has been particularly useful in my experience, but there is no objective evidence of its superiority to other diuretics in these patients. The rapidity and effectiveness of furosemide might commend its use during the few recumbent hours before sleep. Occasional or more frequent measurement of serum potassium concentration is advisable. If and when hypokalemia occurs, it should be treated either with potassium supplements or by changing to a potassium-sparing diuretic. Spironolactone has been widely employed for this purpose, and its use is appropriate, a priori, as a direct means of preventing the effects of the secondary hyperaldosteronism which so many of these patients manifest. Since spironolactone has prolonged action, it may be given at any time of the day. Dosages less than 100 mg daily are preferred, since higher doses may cause breast tenderness, menstrual irregularities, amenorrhea, or occasionally mild hirsutism. Triamterene may also be used in doses of 100 mg daily. Amiloride has lived up to its promise of being another effective potassium-sparing diuretic. The use of such proprietary combinations as Aldactazide, Dyazide, and Moduretic is not generally recommended since they often have insufficient potassium-sparing activity to prevent the occurrence of hypokalemia. However, their use in a dose of 2 tablets each evening does simplify therapy in individuals in whom hypokalemia does not supervene during a trial of their use.

Drugs to Reduce Orthostatic Weight Gain

Diuretics often become ineffective in reducing the accumulation of fluid during the time of the day spent in the upright posture. This can be shown by measuring mean weight gain from the beginning to the end of orthostasis on successive days. The only medications that are known to be effective in reducing orthostatic weight-gain are sympathomimetic amines. Of these ephedrine is the simplest to administer and should be prescribed if the treatment described above fails to reduce the discomfort resulting from edema formation. A dose of 25 mg three times daily is often beneficial, as evidenced by a reduction of weight gain *intra diem* toward normal limits. When ephedrine causes palpitations or fails to reduce weight gain from morning to evening, its use should be abandoned. In such circumstances, dextroamphetamine is frequently effective and often restores weight gain *intra diem* to about 0.5 kg without other therapy. It should be prescribed in a dose of 10 mg as a sustained-release capsule or Spansule each morning. If there is slight but inadequate reduction in weight gain from morning to evening, a dose of 15 mg in the morning or 10 mg upon awakening and again at noon may be more effective. Occasionally 25 mg daily may be needed. If there is no improvement in weight gain *intra diem*, the amphetamine should be discontinued. Some patients become unduly tense, nervous, or excitable for the first few days of amphetamine therapy. If these symptoms persist, the treatment should be combined with a barbiturate or stopped. Usually any initial excitement or garrulousness subsides in a few days, and the dextroamphetamine appears almost to have a tranquilizing action after several weeks. As long as the drug is taken for its action on fluid accumulation and not for its psychic, mood-elevating effects, which are relatively transient unless dosage is progressively escalated, addiction, dependence, and any other serious side effects have not been observed by us to result from the use of dextroamphetamine in more than 150 patients with idiopathic edema over the past 27 years. In many patients I have stopped the administration of dextroamphetamine abruptly without withdrawal effects except for some sleepiness for a day or two. The most valuable aspects of its use are its safety in the doses prescribed and its continued effectiveness in reducing weight gain from morning to evening as long as it is administered—as long as 20 years in some patients whom I have studied repeatedly. Newer sympathomimetic drugs, such as Midodrine (still unapproved in the United States), have shown promise in early studies conducted in Syracuse.

Other Drugs

Kuchel et al showed that dopamine excretion in the urine was subnormal in a group of patients with idiopathic edema in the recumbent, albeit not in the upright, posture. The finding suggested that deficiency of this natriuretic catecholamine might actually be the cause of orthostatic edema in some patients. For this reason, the dopamine agonist bromocriptine (Parlodel) has been used for the treatment of idiopathic edema. Unfortunately, my own observations and those of others have cast doubt on the usefulness of this form of therapy in more than a small minority of patients. A similar rationale has led to a trial of L-dopa in a few patients with idiopathic edema. This, too, has been transiently effective in a few but not in most patients. Unlike dopamine, bromocriptine has relatively slight natriuretic action. It is possible that the efficacy of dextroamphetamine may depend on endogenous dopamine release, which the amphetamine probably induces. For these reasons, the usefulness of dopamine agonists that might be developed in the future will be worthy of full investigation.

Propranolol has been prescribed by some clinicians, but its effectiveness in idiopathic edema has not been convincingly documented. Since captopril blocks the conversion of angiotensin I to angiotensin II, its use would be expected to reduce hyperaldosteronism and perhaps even excessive vasopressin release in patients with orthostatic edema. The usefulness of captopril in orthostatic edema is currently under investigation. It is important to appreciate that hypotensive responses to this drug might constitute serious "side effects" when captopril is administered for the treatment of orthostatic edema.

Special Stockings

Since elastic bandages and pressure garments (e.g., MAST suits) have been shown to reduce edema, and to promote normal excretion of sodium and water in the upright posture, it seemed obvious that elastic stockings or individually fitted Jobst garments might be therapeutically useful. On some patients they can be used with advantage and will reduce or eliminate the need for medication. Unfortunately, most patients stop using stockings or garments after a disappointingly short period because they are uncomfortable, or difficult to put on, or tend to aggravate swelling by raising the temperature of the legs, particularly on hot days when orthostatic edema tends to be most severe.

RESULTS OF TREATMENT

It is usually possible to reduce morning weight by at least 2–4 kg and to decrease the mean weight gain during the orthostatic portion of each day to or toward the normal range of 0.7 kg or less, in consequence of the therapeutic program described above. Patients almost always experience symptomatic improvement, including reduction of discomfort in the legs and abdomen, loss of numbness and tingling in the hands and fingers (thus occasionally obviating surgical treatment of the carpal tunnel syndrome), and disappearance of headaches, periorbital edema, and the impaired cerebration of which they frequently complain. Irritability and depression are diminished and should not be treated with tranquilizers, some of which aggravate fluid retention. Weight records serve to document the improvement in fluid retention objectively, and pitting edema of the legs or ankles, which is demonstrable at the end of the day, before therapy, should be reduced or completely overcome. The extent to which these desirable results are accomplished should dictate the vigor with which the suggested therapeutic measures are applied.

Suggested Reading

Edwards OM, Bayliss RIS. Idiopathic oedema of women. A clinical and investigative study. Quart J Med 1976; 45:125–144.

Kuchel O, Cuche JL, Buu NT, Guthrie GP Jr, Unger T, Nowaczynski W, Boucher R, Genest J. Catecholamine excretion in "idiopathic" edema: decreased dopamine excretion, a pathogenic factor? J Clin Endocrinol Metab 1977; 44:639–646.

Streeten DHP. Idiopathic edema: pathogenesis, clinical features and treatment. Metabolism 1978; 27:353–383.

Streeten DHP, Dalakos TG, Souma M, Fellerman H, Clift GV, Schletter FE, Stevenson CT, Speller PJ. Studies of the pathogenesis of idiopathic oedema: the roles of postural changes in plasma volume, plasma renin activity, aldosterone secretion rate and GFR in the retention of sodium and water. Clin Sci 1973; 45:347–373.

HYPOGONADISM: ANDROGEN THERAPY

ALVIN M. MATSUMOTO, M.D.,
WILLIAM J. BREMNER, M.D., Ph.D.

Testosterone was identified nearly fifty years ago as the main virilizing principle synthesized and secreted by the testes. Soon after its identification, more potent ester analogs of testosterone were prepared and used to treat male hypogonadism, often with dramatic clinical responses. Androgen administration has been used to promote protein anabolism and to stimulate erythropoiesis in various clinical conditions. However, the primary use of androgens remains replacement therapy in androgen-deficient men, and it is this indication that is the focus of this chapter.

PHYSIOLOGY

Testosterone is the major steroid product of the testis. It is synthesized by the Leydig cells of the interstitial compartment of the testis and is under the control of the pituitary gonadotropin, luteinizing hormone (LH). The daily production rate of testosterone is approximately 7 mg per day. Plasma levels of testosterone are maintained between 3 and 10 ng/ml and fluctuate in a circadian rhythm, with maximal levels early in the morning. Circulating testosterone is largely (98%) bound to protein, primarily to sex hormone-binding globulin (60%) and albumin (38%). The unbound or free fraction is thought to be the major biologically active fraction. Free testosterone is rapidly metabolized by the liver (with a serum half-life of approximately 20 minutes) and its metabolites are excreted in urine.

In some target tissues (e.g., prostate, seminal vesicles, epididymides, and skin), the action of testosterone depends on intracellular conversion to 5 alpha-dihydrotestosterone (DHT). In other tissues (e.g., skeletal muscle), testosterone itself may be the active intracellular hormone. In the central nervous system, a part of testosterone action may require intracellular aromatization to estradiol. For the remainder of this chapter, "testosterone" will be used to include testosterone itself and the intracellular metabolites (e.g., DHT and estradiol) important in its biologic effects.

PATHOPHYSIOLOGY

The manifestations of androgen deficiency depend on the stage of development of an individual. Testosterone is required for normal fetal and pubertal development, as well as for the maintenance of adult sexual characteristics. During embryogenesis, testosterone is required for the differentiation of the wolffian ductal system and the indifferent anlage of the external genitalia into normal male internal and external genitalia, respectively. Androgen deficiency during this period of development results in varying degrees of ambiguous genitalia. During puberty, testosterone is responsible for the development of male secondary sex characteristics (such as the male pattern of hair growth, growth of penis and scrotum, enlargement of larynx and consequent deepening of voice, development of skeletal musculature, and redistribution of body fat). Testosterone also stimulates the pubertal spurt of long bone growth and eventually the closure of long bone epiphyses. Finally, androgens stimulate libido and potency and participate in the initiation of spermatogensis, eventuating in fertility. Androgen deficiency prior to the onset of puberty results in failure to develop normal male secondary sex characteristics, a eunuchoidal body habitus (with excessive long bone growth, as a result of delayed closure of the epiphyses), and failure to develop normal sexual functioning. In the adult, androgens act primarily to maintain libido and potency and participate in the maintenance of spermatogenesis. Normal levels of testosterone are also required to maintain some secondary male sex characteristics (such as skeletal muscle development, body fat distribution, and the male pattern of hair growth). Therefore, adult-onset androgen deficiency is usually manifested primarily by abnormalities of sexual performance and infertility and, to a lesser degree, by loss of secondary sex characteristics.

Androgen deficiency may result from a primary testicular defect in testosterone production (primary hypogonadism, as in Klinefelter's syndrome, congenital anorchia, traumatic or surgical castration, mumps) or from lack of adequate gonadotropin stimulation of Leydig cells (secondary hypogonadism, as in pituitary or hypothalamic insufficiency). In general, the therapeutic goal of androgen therapy in any of these states of hypogonadism is the same: induction of the normal physiologic effects of testosterone. The specific goals of treatment depend on the age and wishes of the patient. In hypogonadism causing delayed puberty, the aim of androgen replacement is to stimulate and maintain male secondary sex characteristics, libido, and potency and to induce the pubertal growth spurt without compromising adult height by premature closure of the epiphyses. In hypogonadism developing after puberty, the main objective of testosterone treatment is to maintain libido, potency, and secondary sex characteristics. Testosterone therapy cannot correct the ambiguous genitalia resulting from androgen deficiency during fetal life, although it has been used as an adjunctive treatment to surgery in selected cases of microphallus and hypospadius. Initiation and maintenance of human spermatogenesis is thought to require a very high concentration of testosterone within the testes. Exogenous testosterone cannot be practically administered in sufficiently high dosages to stimulate spermatogenesis.

GOALS OF ANDROGEN REPLACEMENT THERAPY

In general, the indications for androgen replacement therapy in any individual patient, regardless of age, are the clinical symptoms and signs of androgen deficiency. Often, particularly in adults with gradual onset of hypogonadism (as in slow-growing pituitary tumors) or partial, long-standing gonadal failure, clinical manifestations are subtle and may go unnoticed by patients and their physicians. In other instances, patients may have the clinical syndrome of androgen deficiency, but may have serum testosterone levels in the low normal range. This situation occurs in some men with Klinefelter's syndrome. In addition to having serum testosterone levels in the low normal range, these men have elevated serum gonadotropin levels, suggesting that their hypothalamic-pituitary axis senses inadequate negative feedback. Testosterone therapy is generally accompanied by an improvement in their symptoms and signs of androgen insufficiency. When a patient has subtle clinical manifestations and low-normal testosterone levels, a therapeutic trial of testosterone therapy (6 months) may help to identify patients with very mild androgen deficiency.

Androgen therapy is contraindicated in men with cancer of the prostate. These cancers are known to be androgen-sensitive, and rapid tumor growth has been documented to occur during androgen treatment, often with catastrophic results. Therefore, careful examination of the prostate gland should be performed prior to and during institution of androgen therapy. Fully androgenic dosages of testosterone may be inappropriate for men with severe psychopathology or mental retardation and for older men with severe bladder neck obstruction secondary to benign prostatic hyperplasia, particularly if they are not good surgical candidates. Low-dosage testosterone or an oral preparation may be administered to preserve bone mineral mass. Androgen therapy may be particularly indicated in patients with risk factors for the development of osteoporosis, such as pharmacologic glucocorticoid usage.

THERAPEUTIC ALTERNATIVES

Gonadotropin and LHRH

In men with primary testicular failure, there is no therapeutic alternative to androgen therapy to accomplish the goals outlined above. Infertility in these men is untreatable, and if children are desired, the patient and spouse should be counseled to pursue adoption or artificial insemination using donor semen. On the other hand, secondary hypogonadal men may achieve normal testosterone levels with gonadotropin therapy or, in some cases, treatment with luteinizing hormone releasing hormone (LHRH). Both gonadotropin and LHRH therapy require much more frequent administration and expense compared to testosterone therapy and therefore are not practical alternatives to androgen treatment if virilization is the therapeutic goal. However, because they stimulate endogenous testicular function, both gonadotropin and LHRH treatment offer the potential of stimulating spermatogenesis and therefore are the treatment of choice if fertility is desired. Prior androgen therapy does not adversely affect subsequent testicular responses to gonadotropins. The uses of gonadotropins and LHRH for hypogonadism are considered in other chapters of this book.

Testosterone

Soon after the identification of testosterone as the major androgenic product of the testis, it was realized that the native form of the hormone had minimal androgenic effects when administered orally or parenterally. Unmodified testosterone is rapidly absorbed from the gastrointestinal tract or injection vehicle and promptly metabolized by the liver. Currently, there are no oral forms of unmodified testosterone available in the United States. A microparticulate form of testosterone has been used in small numbers of patients in Europe and shown to be therapeutically effective orally. However, since very large dosages are required (200 to 400 mg/d) and only short-term toxicity data are available, this preparation cannot be viewed too optimistically as a viable alternative to currently available preparations. Although aqueous testosterone is still available for intramuscular injection, the rapidity of absorption and hepatic degradation make it impractical to sustain physiologic testosterone levels and androgenic effects. Subcutaneous surgical implants of unmodified testosterone have been used by some as a means of achieving sustained release and prolonged effect of testosterone for several months. This is not practical and is unacceptable for the majority of hypogonadal men. With the recent development of injectable matrices for drug administration, there is hope for the development of a slowly released form of unmodified testosterone to sustain physiologic levels of testosterone for prolonged periods.

Synthetic Androgens

To achieve the higher and more sustained blood levels of androgen necessary for the chronic replacement in hypogonadal men, chemical modifications of the testosterone molecule were undertaken to diminish the rate of absorption from the injection vehicle and/or reduce the rate of hepatic metabolism. There are two major forms of androgen preparations that are available for replacement therapy in the United States: the parenteral forms, which are all 17 beta-hydroxy ester derivatives of testosterone, and the oral androgen preparations, which are all 17 alpha-alkyl derivatives.

Esterification at the 17 beta-hydroxyl group prolongs the duration of action by decreasing the polarity of the molecule, resulting in increased solubility of the preparation in the injection vehicle and slowed release into the circulation. These testosterone esters all require hydrolysis to native testosterone prior to biological action and degradation. Because testosterone esters cross-react poorly in testosterone radioimmunoassays, serum testosterone levels may be used to monitor therapy. Three testosterone esters are available for parenteral androgen replacement therapy: testosterone propionate, a relatively short-acting preparation and testosterone enanthate and testosterone cypionate, both longer-acting preparations. Testosterone enanthate and cypionate are equivalent for clinical purposes (Table 1). Compared to unmodified testosterone, which has to be given in very large doses several times a day, testosterone propionate need only be given in a single dose daily or every other day. The duration of action is prolonged further in testosterone enanthate and testosterone cypionate, which are typically administered every 2 to 3 weeks. Recently, an orally effective testosterone ester preparation, testosterone undecanoate, became available for clinical use in Europe. Because of its long aliphatic side chain, it is very nonpolar and is absorbed from the gastrointestinal tract via the lymphatics into the systemic circulation. Although apparently effective in the treatment of hypogonadism and free of hepatotoxity, the requirement that large doses be administered several times daily may limit its practical use in long-term androgen replacement therapy.

TABLE 1 Commonly Used Androgen Preparations

Medication	*Dose**	*Route*	*Schedule**	*Liver Toxicity*	*Cost/ Month†*
Testosterone enanthate‡ cypionate‡	150–200 mg	IM	every 10–14 days	No	$5
Testerone propionate	25–50 mg	IM	3 times/ week	No	$7
Methyltestosterone	25–50 mg 10–25 mg	PO Buccally	daily daily	Yes §	$16
Fluoxymesterone	10–20 mg	PO	daily	Yes §	$25

* Dosage schedule for adult hypogonadal men

† Based on retail pharmacy costs in Seattle, WA, April, 1984, for testosterone enanthate, 200 mg IM every 2 weeks; testosterone propionate, 50 mg IM 3 times/week; methyltestosterone, 25 mg buccally daily; and fluoxymesterone, 10 mg PO daily.

‡ Preferred preparations for chronic androgen replacement therapy in male hypogonadism.

§ Hepatic cholestasis. Rarely, peliosis hepatis (blood-filled cysts in liver) and hepatoma.

Alkylation at the 17 alpha-position impedes hepatic inactivation and allows oral or buccal administration of androgen preparations. In contrast to testosterone esters, 17-alpha alkylated androgens do not have to be metabolized prior to their action at the target organs or their excretion. These preparations exhibit variable cross-reactivities with testosterone radioimmunoassays, and therefore serum testosterone levels cannot be used to monitor therapy. In addition to 17 alpha-alkylation, many of the orally active androgen preparations have incorporated other structural modifications (such as 5 alpha reduction, removal of the methyl group at the 19 position, and substitutions at the 2, 9, or 11 position) to modify their androgenic potency. Two preparations, methyltestosterone and fluoxymesterone, have been advocated for androgen replacement treatment of hypogonadal men (see Table 1).

The cost of androgen replacement with oral androgens is usually much greater than that with parenteral preparations. More importantly, all orally active androgen preparations available in the United States (including methyltestosterone and fluoxymesterone) are 17 alpha-alkylated and share the potential for serious hepatotoxicity. In contrast, liver toxicity has not been reported with replacement dosages of parenteral testosterone esters. Finally, oral androgens are less potent than parenteral preparations, and full androgenic effects are difficult to achieve with these preparations. Therefore, because oral androgens have potentially greater risk and less benefit than parenteral preparations, long-acting esters of testosterone (testosterone enanthate and cypionate) are the preferred preparations for the androgen replacement therapy in male hypogonadism.

PREFERRED APPROACH

Adult Replacement

Testosterone enanthate and testosterone cypionate are the most effective, safe, and practical preparations currently available for androgen replacement therapy. Intramuscular injection of either preparation results in peak serum testosterone levels in 24 to 48 hours, at the upper limits of, or slightly above, the normal adult male range. Testosterone levels remain in the eugonadal range for a variable length of time, usually for 10 to 14 days. We institute testosterone enanthate or cypionate treatment at an initial dosage of 200 mg IM every 2 weeks. Although some patients have adequate therapeutic responses to this dose every 3 weeks, it is clear that, in most patients, administration of these preparations every 4 weeks is inadequate to maintain eugonadal testosterone levels, induce full virilization, and maintain libido and potency. In general, patients are taught to give their own deep intramuscular injections (usually in the thigh). In the unusual circumstance that patients cannot or will not inject themselves, family members are instructed to administer testosterone or injections are given by nurse assistants.

Assessment of therapeutic efficacy is accomplished by careful monitoring of the clinical response. Initially, patients are seen in clinic one month after institution of testosterone, and then at 3- to 4-month intervals. Within a few weeks after the institution of testosterone replacement, most hypogonadal men experience stimulation of libido and potency and notable improvement in energy level and general feeling of well-being. Such responses are even noted by patients with long-standing or mild androgen deficiency, who previously considered themselves asymptomatic. Within a few months, patients experience an increase in physical and social drive and aggressiveness. Some men note a decrease in libido and sense of well-being a few days prior to their next testosterone injection. If these symptoms persist for several months, adjustment of the dosage interval from every 2 weeks to every 10 days may be indicated.

The changes in sexual behavior and aggressiveness experienced by hypogonadal men beginning testosterone treatment may be quite distressing to the patients as well as their spouses, both of whom may have grown accustomed to the patient's behavior prior to androgen replacement. Often, problems can be avoided if patients and their spouses are counseled prior to the institution of testosterone. The initial frequent clinic visits with patients (and spouses) often help to detect problems in sexual adjustment that may require further counseling. In addition to monitoring clinical response and potential side effects of testosterone treatment, these visits also help in the assessment of medication compliance.

In the young eunuchoidal patient, testosterone therapy also results in marked stimulation of male secondary sex characteristics and somatic growth. In these patients, initiation of testosterone replacement stimulates growth of the penis, scrotum, pubic and axillary hair, prostate and seminal vesicles (with increase in ejaculatory volume), and later the growth of beard and body hair in a male pattern of distribution (chest, perianal area, inner thighs, external auditory canal). Within the first year, the larynx grows and the voice deepens, skeletal muscle development and strength increase (especially in shoulder and pectoral muscles), body fat is lost from the lower abdomen and thighs, and long bone growth is stimulated. In older eunuchoidal and adult hypogonadal men, the response of secondary sex characteristics and somatic growth may be much less dramatic. In most hypogonadal men, hematocrit and hemoglobin increase under the influence of testosterone therapy. The stimulation of erythropoiesis by testosterone is responsible for the normal difference in hematocrit and hemoglobin between males and females.

In older hypogonadal patients with symptoms of bladder neck obstruction and/or a large prostate gland on physical examination, it is prudent to begin testosterone replacement gradually with a short-acting testosterone preparation, such as testosterone propionate. The rapid onset and offset of action of this preparation permit rapid withdrawal of androgen stimulation of prostatic growth if urinary obstruction and/or a prostatic nodule develops. In these men, testosterone propionate, 25 to 50 mg IM three times weekly, is employed for androgen replacement with frequent examinations of prostate size.

Pubertal Replacement

Androgen replacement therapy for the patient with delayed puberty, in whom full adult height has not yet been achieved, is more complicated. One of the difficulties is that the physician may not be able to differentiate patients with constitutional delayed puberty, who require only transient androgen therapy, from truly hypogonadal patients, who require permanent testosterone treatment. In addition, overzealous premature androgen replacement, while leading to rapid virilization and increase in long bone growth, can lead to premature closure of epiphyses, resulting in compromised potential adult height.

Therefore, in the patient with delayed puberty, androgen replacement therapy is intermittent and the dosage of testosterone is generally reduced. Testosterone treatment should be instituted for periods of 4 to 6 months, and then stopped for 4 to 6 months to determine whether there are signs of progression of spontaneous pubertal development. Testis size is the most important clinical parameter to monitor as an indicator of spontaneous onset of puberty. If no increase in testis size is measured during the 4 to 6 months off testosterone therapy, another course of androgen treatment is instituted. In patients whose changes in testis size are equivocal, measurement of serum testosterone and gonadotropins may aid in the detection of spontaneous puberty. It is generally recommended that patients not be treated until age 15 to 16 years. However, delay in sexual maturation often results in profound emotional stress and trauma to patients and their families, and treatment should be undertaken earlier if this is the case. Depending on the age of the patient, testosterone enanthate or cypionate is started at a dosage of 100 to 200 mg IM every 2 weeks. The dosages of testosterone enanthate or cypionate are gradually increased over several years to adult dosages with increasing age and height of the patient.

In our experience, it is uncommon for patients to refuse parenteral androgen therapy. In these rare patients, the use of oral androgen preparations can be considered. In undertaking oral androgen therapy, both the physician and the patient should understand that treatment carries with it potentially greater risk (i.e., hepatotoxicity) and cost as well as reduced benefit. Fluoxymesterone, 5 to 10 mg PO daily, or methyltestosterone, 25 to 50 mg PO or 10 to 25 mg buccally daily, are usually used for replacement therapy in hypogonadism.

Adjunctive Therapy

Hypogonadism is often associated with significant gynecomastia; in fact, gynecomastia may be the patient's chief complaint. Large breasts are a source of embarrassment and psychologic trauma, particularly in the adolescent patient. Significant gynecomastia often does not reverse with androgen replacement therapy; occasionally it worsens. In these cases, surgical reduction mammoplasty is indicated. As discussed above, androgen therapy does not stimulate growth of testicular size. In many hypogonadal patients, especially those with Klinefelter's syndrome, testes are extremely small. In some hypogonadal men, small testes are a source of severe emotional stress. Surgical implantation of testicular prostheses may be indicated in some of these men.

Side Effects

Local Side Effects. Occasionally local pain, hemorrhage, or irritation is experienced at the site of intramuscular injection of testosterone esters. In our experience, with the proper instruction in the techniques of deep intramuscular injection, these local side effects can be avoided. Subcutaneous injection of testosterone esters can cause irritation that is related to the injection vehicle.

Androgenic Side Effects. Symptoms of excessive androgenic stimulation of libido and erections are uncommon. This complication usually occurs in young boys and men with long-standing, severe androgen deficiency. Often these symptoms resolve with continued androgen therapy. If excessive libido and frequent erections occur to a point of disturbance, they can be overcome by reduction in the dosage of testosterone replacement. Patients receiving androgen therapy for induction of puberty often develop acne, which can usually be treated satisfactorily with local skin measures and antibiotics. Acne almost always spontaneously improves with continued testosterone treatment. Testosterone therapy should be used with caution in elderly men, especially those with large prostate glands and/or symptoms of bladder outlet obstruction. Although urinary obstruction has been reported to occur as a result of testosterone-induced growth of benign prostatic hyperplasia, in our experience it is extremely uncommon in the absence of prostatic carcinoma. Androgen therapy generally results in mild-to-moderate weight gain as a result of sodium retention and the protein anabolic effects of testosterone. Patients with underlying congestive heart failure, nephrotic syndrome, or hepatic cirrhosis may develop gross edema during testosterone treatment.

Estrogenic Side Effects. Testosterone is aromatized to estradiol in peripheral tissues. Patients who are receiving testosterone esters demonstrate increased serum levels of estradiol as well as testosterone. Gynecomastia occasionally develops in patients receiving testosterone therapy, especially in children receiving testosterone for the induction of puberty and in adult men receiving high dosages of testosterone and/or who have a predisposing condition such as cirrhosis of the liver.

Hepatotoxicity. All 17 alpha-alkylated androgens have been reported to cause hepatic cholestasis with elevation of serum alkaline phosphatase and bilirubin and occasionally clinical jaundice. Hepatic function is frequently disordered during oral androgen therapy, as manifested by the increase in certain plasma proteins (haptoglobin, plasminogen, inhibitor of the first component of complement), decreased conjugation of adrenal steroids, and decreased serum clotting factors (I, V, VII, and X). Although very rare, a more serious and potentially life-threatening complication of oral androgen treatment is the development of peliosis hepatis (hemorrhagic cysts in the liver) and hepatocellular carcinoma. It should be emphasized that most patients reported to have these complications have also had severe underlying illnesses (such as Fanconi's anemia). Regression of peliosis hepatis has been reported in some patients after discontinuation of oral androgens. If oral androgens are used in the treatment of hypogonadism, the liver should be examined frequently and liver function tests should be routinely monitored. Hepatotoxicity has not been reported to occur with replacement dosages of parenteral testosterone ester preparations.

Erythrocytosis. Occasionally, erythrocytosis above the normal male range occurs during androgen replacement therapy, often requiring therapeutic phlebotomy. Some of these men may have other reasons for developing erythrocytosis, such as hypoxia due to chronic obstructive lung disease. In other men who develop severe erythrocytosis, no predisposing factor is apparent. We have recently found that replacement dosages of testosterone in hypogonadal men can induce or worsen obstructive sleep apnea. These men had erythrocytosis on replacement dosages of testosterone, with normal oxygen saturation, pulmonary function testing, and respiratory drives while awake. However, during sleep, they exhibited significant oxygen desaturation associated with frequent apneic episodes. The frequency of apneic episodes was decreased markedly by discontinuation of testosterone therapy.

Allergic Side Effect. Rarely, individuals demonstrate an allergy to either the sesame oil vehicle of testosterone enanthate or the cottonseed oil vehicle of testosterone cypionate. Certain preparations of methyltestosterone or fluoxymesterone that contain tartrazine (FD&C Yellow No. 5) may cause allergic-type reactions (including bronchial asthma) in certain susceptible (usually aspirin-sensitive) individuals.

Suggested Reading

Dorfman RI, Shipley RA, eds. Androgen, Biochemistry, Physiology, and Clinical Significance. New York: John Wiley and Sons, 1956; 330:388.

Snyder PJ. Clinical use of androgens. Ann Rev Med 1984; 35:207–217.

Wilson JD, Griffin JE. The use and abuse of androgens. Metabolism 1980; 29:1278–1295.

HYPOGONADOTROPIC HYPOGONADISM: GONADOTROPIN THERAPY

STEPHEN J. WINTERS, M.D.
PHILIP TROEN, M.D.

Hypogonadotropic hypogonadism refers to congenital and acquired disorders in which gonadotropin secretion is insufficient to sustain normal adult testicular function. Neither the production of testosterone nor spermatogenesis is entirely normal in these men. However, the extent of Leydig cell and seminiferous tubular dysfunction is highly variable. The clinical presentation of affected individuals relates to the underlying disease and the chronologic age and extent of sexual development at the onset of the disease process. Congenital gonadotropin deficiency does not adversely affect male sexual differentiation in utero because of the predominant role of placental human chorionic gonadotropin (HCG) in the control of fetal Leydig cell function. Instead, patients with congenital (idiopathic) gonadotropin deficiency present in the teenage years with a lack of expected sexual development. Pubertal failure is also a common consequence of tumors of the hypothalamic-pituitary unit in children. Acquired hypogonadotropic hypogonadism in adult men is generally a subtle illness manifested by a decline in libido and potency as well as infertility. Often it is other aspects of the basic disease process, e.g., headaches and visual disturbances in subjects with pituitary adenomas, which lead to the diagnosis.

TREATMENT OF ANDROGEN DEFICIENCY

Androgen deficiency in either teenagers or sexually mature men is probably best treated with parenteral testosterone. Considerations of cost and frequency of administration favor the use of long-acting esters of testosterone, such as the cypionate or the enanthate. Human chorionic gonadotropin can also be used to stimulate Leydig cell function in hypogonadotropic men. HCG resembles human luteinizing hormone (LH) both structurally and biologically. Both gonadotropins bind to membrane receptors on Leydig cells and stimulate testicular steroidogenesis through a cyclic AMP-mediated process. Because it is purified from pregnancy urine, HCG, unlike pituitary LH, is readily available.

Several seemingly equivalent commercial preparations of HCG are available in vials containing 1000, 5000, 10,000 or 20,000 IU of powder to be reconstituted in an appropriate volume of diluent. The product names include: APL, Chorex, Follutein, Pregnyl, Profasi HP, and various generic preparations. Among these, we often choose Pregnyl (Organon), 10,000 IU/vial, because of considerable financial savings for the patients. Generally, doses of 1500 to 2000 IU intramuscularly will sustain normal serum testosterone levels for 4 to 7 days. Although the acute steroidogenic response to HCG is impaired in previously untreated patients with hypogonadotropic hypogonadism, long-term HCG therapy usually produces normal adult serum levels of testosterone. As with testosterone therapy, several years of HCG treatment are needed for complete virilization to occur. Recent observations in experimental animals and men, including gonadoptropin-deficient men, indicate that the frequent administration of HCG produces a state of refractoriness of Leydig cells to gonadotropin stimulation. Thus, circulating testosterone levels and the acute response during long-term HCG treatment should be monitored for optimum results.

A major advantage of HCG treatment in patients with prepubertal gonadotropin deficiency is the resultant growth of the testis. Although normal adult testicular size is not achieved with HCG therapy alone, some patients see demonstrable testis enlargement as an important goal of therapy. It has also been suggested that HCG produces greater virilization and enhanced sexual behavior than does testosterone in patients with panhypopituitarism. However, convincing support for this opinion is lacking. As will be discussed, HCG is needed to stimulate Leydig cells in the treatment of hypospermatogenesis.

Gonadotropin therapy often produces incomplete masculinization in hypogonadotropic subjects with coexistent bilateral cryptorchidism. In spite of orchidopexy, Leydig cells as well as seminiferous tubules appear to sustain damage when the testis is ectopic. It is unknown at present what effect early surgery (before age 5 years) will have on this process.

Several reports of the development of anti-HCG antibodies in subjects treated with HCG have appeared in the recent literature. Generally, these antibodies are of relatively low affinity and are not clinically significant. However, one patient with Kallmann's syndrome who became resistant to HCG has been described. Presumably, the extraction and purification for HCG may render it antigenic.

Gynecomastia may occur during treatment with HCG. Estradiol levels may exceed those of normal men, even when serum testosterone levels are within the range of normal. Although the mechanism for this unbalanced production of estradiol is uncertain, it may relate to the frequency of HCG administration. If breast development is recognized clinically, the frequency of administration or the dosage of HCG should be reduced. Occasionally, reduction mammoplasty is required.

Because of potential adverse effects of testosterone on the testis, it has often been suggested that HCG rather than testosterone be used to virilize hypogonadotropic men in whom future fertility is important. Several recent reports indicate, however, that men treated with parenteral testosterone for many years may become fertile when gonadotropin therapy is initiated. Slight weight gain and fluid retention, similar to that observed with testosterone treatment, may occur during HCG therapy.

INDUCTION OF SPERMATOGENESIS

Both LH and follicle stimulating hormone (FSH) are needed to initiate spermatogenesis. Presumably, the effect of LH is to stimulate Leydig cells to produce testosterone, thereby increasing intratesticular testosterone levels and, specifically, the androgen environment within the seminiferous tubule and seminal plasma. Testosterone almost certainly influences germ cell development through binding to two high-affinity androphilic proteins found within the seminiferous tubule, intracellular androgen receptors, and testicular androgen-binding protein. However, the details of these effects are not known. FSH binds to receptors on Sertoli cells, activates cyclic AMP-dependent protein kinase, and increases steroid, RNA, and protein synthesis within these cells. Whether gonadotropins also influence germ cells directly is not known.

Treatment With HCG

Selected patients with hypogonadotropic hypogonadism may produce sperm and successfully impregnate their spouses when treated with HCG alone in doses of 1500 to 2000 IU one to three times weekly. The optimum dosage and frequency of administration have not been clarified. It is likely that these subjects have some endogenous FSH secretion, since sperm output does not increase in most subjects with complete hypogonadotropic hypogonadism treated with HCG alone. Patients with pituitary adenomas, including prolactinomas, are included in this HCG-responsive subgroup, since destruction of the pituitary gland by a pituitary adenoma is rarely complete. In contrast, hypogonadotropic patients with diffuse infiltrative diseases of the hypothalamic-pituitary unit, such as hemochromatosis, are less likely to produce sperm during therapy with HCG.

A subgroup of men with congenital hypogonadotropic hypogonadism present with eunuchoidal body habitus, deficient secondary sexual characteristics, and testes that are larger than those of prepubertal children (greater than or equivalent to 5 ml), but considerably smaller than those of normal adult males (20 to 25 ml). Morning serum testosterone concentrations in these subjects range from prepubertal levels to those of boys in midpuberty. Circulating FSH concentrations and LH and FSH responses to LRH administration are usually similar to those of sexually mature men. Testicular biopsy reveals germ cell development beyond spermatogonia and absence of mature Leydig cells. The evidence suggests that these patients, known in the literature as "fertile eunuchs", have a partial deficiency in gonadotropin production. Anosmia and other midline defects are less common in this subgroup than in patients with complete hypogonadotropic hypogonadism, but have been reported. Generally, treatment with HCG alone will be sufficient to initiate spermatogenesis in these men.

Twelve to 18 months of HCG therapy may be required before sperm appear in the ejaculates of men with congenital partial gonadotropin deficiency. The response of men with hypogonadism acquired in adulthood is generally more rapid. Finally, treatment with HCG alone may also sustain sperm output in men who require HCG together with FSH to initiate spermatogenesis.

Treatment With HCG and HMG

There is considerable clinical experience with the use of HCG together with preparations containing FSH to induce spermatogenesis in hypogonadotropic men. Patients with pituitary adenomas and other forms of acquired gonadotropin deficiency, as well as patients with Kallmann's syndrome and its variants, are candidates for this form of treatment when pregnancy is desired. Because of the expense and the apparent need for frequent FSH injections, we initiate treatment with HCG and add FSH after a minimum of one year of HCG if the patient remains azoospermic. With this approach, adult Leydig cell function is restored, and the patient who may produce sperm with HCG alone can be recognized. It is important to bear in mind that the spouse should also be carefully evaluated for subtle reproductive disturbance.

Commercial preparations of FSH are derived from the urine of postmenopausal women, hence the designation human menopausal gonadotropins (HMG). This preparation, HMG, is available as Pergonal (Serono Laboratories), which contains 75 IU of FSH and 75 IU LH per vial. The amount of LH is small compared to the dosage of HCG administered. Human pituitary glands have not been used as a starting product to prepare FSH because of their limited availability. Because of potential antigenicity, nonhuman pituitaries have also not been used. The inexpensive production of human pituitary hormones using recombinant DNA methodology will undoubtedly be realized within the next decade.

The available literature in this field consists, for the most part, of case reports and the results of small series of patients. Further, the details of dosage and frequency of administration of HMG as well as HCG vary among different centers. Therefore, a precise estimate of the likelihood of achieving a pregnancy in the spouse is not possible. Yet it appears that the majority of hypogonadotropic men do produce sperm and impregnate their wives when treated with HCG/HMG since the testes in such patients are only lacking in gonadotropin exposure, but are not intrinsically abnormal. Subjects with coexistent bilateral cryptorchidism are an exception to this generalization since, in spite of orchidopexy, they respond poorly to gonadotropin treatment. Careful measurement of testis size with a ruler or orchidometer is important because lack of testis growth during treatment indicates a poor clinical response.

Most workers have used FSH intramuscularly in doses of 75 IU three times per week. However, there is evidence from one study in progress that one-half this dose may also be effective. As the maturation of spermatogonia to mature sperm requires 70 to 80 days, sperm do not generally appear in the ejaculate for at least 3 months. In fact, it may take as long as 12 to 18 months after initiating combination therapy for sperm production and pregnancy to occur. Thus, treatment should not be considered a failure before at least 12 months with this regimen. The dose of HMG can be increased to 150 IU if 75 IU is ineffective.

Patients with prepubertal gonadotropin deficiency achieve a testis size of 10 to 15 ml with HCG/HMG therapy; much of this growth is evident in the first 3 months. The sperm output is usually 2 to 10 million per ejaculate in these men. When compared to sperm outputs of 100 to 300 million per ejaculate observed among normal men, the fact that such relatively few sperm are compatible with fertility is intriguing. The motility of these sperm is generally normal, suggesting that the sperm produced are qualitatively normal. Whether lack of fetal, prepubertal, or postpubertal exposure to gonadotropins is responsible for the patients' inability to produce normal numbers of sperm is unknown. Since treatment with HCG/HMG is not entirely physiologic, refinements in product, as well as dosage and frequency of administration, may also result in greater numbers of sperm being produced.

Following conception we generally discontinue HMG and maintain therapy with HCG alone until it is determined that no further pregnancies are desired; at this point treatment is changed to testosterone enanthate. We have found that sperm production will be sustained in many subjects treated with HCG alone following the induction of spermatogenesis with HCG/HMG. If not, HMG can be reinstituted.

Use of HCG together with HMG to stimulate spermatogenesis appears to be without significant side effects. We are unaware of any reports of the development of neutralizing antibodies or allergic reactions to HMG in men. Compliance among these highly motivated patients is generally excellent, and most patients can be taught to self-administer the medications.

MALE INFERTILITY OF UNDETERMINED ETIOLOGY

H.W.GORDON BAKER, M.D., Ph.D., F.R.A.C.P.

Initial assessment of the male partner of an infertile union is directed at separating the small number of men who can be treated successfully and the larger number who are irreversibly sterile from the bulk who are subfertile and have conditions for which there are currently no clearly defined effective treatments.

CONDITIONS CAUSING INFERTILITY

Treatable Conditions

Gonadotropin deficiency and coital disorders are covered in other chapters. Obstruction of the ejaculatory ducts by cysts or inflammatory scarring is rare, but can be corrected by surgery. Suggestive findings are normal testicular size, palpable vasa, normal serum follicle stimulating hormone (FSH), and azoospermia with low semen volume and fructose concentration. Epididymal disorders causing obstructive azoospermia or partial obstruction with oligospermia are also potentially treatable by bypass surgery. Patients with epididymal obstructions have normal testicular size and serum FSH levels, but may have slightly enlarged and tender epididymal heads and histories of epididymitis, scrotal surgery, or bronchiectasis. In the future, patients with vasal agenesis may be treated by implantation of artificial spermatoceles or direct collection of sperm from the head of the epididymis and subsequent in vitro fertilization.

Irreversible Sterility

Untreatable conditions causing sterility are azoospermia due to primary seminiferous tubule failure, zero sperm motility, and total teratospermia. Primary tubular failure is suggested by reduced testicular size and elevated serum FSH levels. Zero sperm motility often results from structural defects in the sperm tails, such as absent dynein arms, and this may be associated with other evidence of the immotile cilia syndrome, such as bronchiectasis. Total teratospermia, in which all sperm show the same abnormality, such as pinheads or absent acrosomes, is rare but must be recognized to avoid fruitless attempts at treatment.

Oligospermia and Asthenospermia

Many infertile men have none of the aforementioned disorders. They have abnormalities in their semen—oligospermia (mean sperm concentration less than 20 million/ml, usually with poor sperm motility and increased abnormal morphology of mixed type) or asthenospermia (mean sperm concentration above 20 million/ml but motility less than 60 percent with poor forward progression). Results of semen analyses in these men are often highly variable, and at least three tests should be performed over a 6- to 8-week period. Causes for the poor semen quality, such as mumps orchitis or undescended testes, are found in some patients, but these conditions do not have any specific prognostic significance. Prognosis depends more on average sperm concentration. Reversible impairment of spermatogenesis from drugs such as androgens and sulfasalazine or exposure to heat from frequent saunas is rare. Associated disorders such as varicoceles, genital tract infections, sperm autoimmunity, and chronic ill health may be relevant in some patients. Treatments for varicocele and genital tract infections are discussed in other chapters. Sperm antibodies causing agglutination and immobilization of sperm are found in the sera of many men who have undergone vasectomy reversal, in some following orchitis or trauma to the scrotal contents, and in a few for unknown reasons. Overall, we find that 6 percent of infertile men have sperm-immobilizing activity in serum or antibodies on sperm detected by screening tests involving the attachment to motile sperm of polyacrylamide beads coated with rabbit antibodies to human immunoglobulins. In patients with severe oligospermia, the sperm antibodies in serum may indicate the presence of autoimmne orchitis or sperm agglutination in the genital tract, producing partial obstruction. With higher sperm outputs, the antibodies may or may not contribute to the infertility: additional evidence of the presence of antibodies in semen is required. Lack of sperm penetration of normal midcycle cervical mucus indicates a severe degree of infertility. On the other hand, men with sperm antibodies and sperm that will pentrate cervical mucus do not appear to be particularly more infertile than those with similar semen quality and duration of infertility but no sperm antibodies. Chronic illnesses or their treatments, for example, hepatic cirrhosis, renal failure, and cytotoxic therapy for malignant disease, are well known to impair testicular function. Provided the illness is controlled, the infertility can be dealt with in the same way as for other patients.

About three-quarters of men seen for infertility have oligospermia or asthenospermia. We will review various treatments used in the past and outline our current approach to management of this group.

THERAPEUTIC ALTERNATIVES

Many treatments have been recommended for oligospermia and asthenospermia on the basis of anecdotal experience or uncontrolled trials in which improvement in semen quality or pregnancies occurred. The natural variability of semen analysis results and the tendency to improve with time have been neglected, as has the fact that men with such disorders are subfertile rather than sterile and have some chance of producing pregnancies without treatment. Furthermore, there is usually no sound basis for the treatments. Some of these treatments were used in Melbourne, and results are summarized in Table 1. Pregnancy rates were calculated by life table analysis, which takes into account the time factor—when the pregnancies occurred and the duration of follow-up of unsuccessful couples. Although there were some individuals who might have responded to treatment with improved semen quality and pregnancy, when all subjects are considered, none of the treatments is significantly better than no treatment.

Drug Treatments

Androgens and Human Chorionic Gonadotropin (hCG). Androgens in low dose (methyltestosterone, 10 to 50 mg per day; mesterolone, 50 to 75 mg per day; fluoxymesterone, 5 to 20 mg per day) or hCG (1500 to 3000 IU twice or thrice weekly) has been given for 3 or more months in the hope that spermatogenesis might be stimulated or sperm maturation and motility improved by direct actions of androgens on the seminiferous epithelium and epididymis. Androgens are also used in high doses (testosterone enanthate, 250 mg every 2 weeks for 3 months) to sup-

TABLE 1 Treatments of Uncertain Value for Oligospermia and Asthenospermia

	Melbourne Experience (Logrank test)			
Treatment	*Number of Courses*	*Number of Pregnancies*	*Expected Pregnancies*	*Relative Pregnancy Rate*
Testosterone "rebound"	33	6	7.92	0.76
Mesterolone	49	7	12.93	0.54
hCG	10	2	2.15	0.93
Clomiphene	50	5	10.66	0.47
Antibacterial agents	95	25	18.83	1.33
Bromocriptine	13	3	3.15	0.95
Varicocelectomy	201	70	57.37	1.22
AIH	61	10	11.76	0.85
None	583	102	105.22	0.97

Note: Logrank $\chi^2 = 11.37$ p NS. Side effects or complications of the treatments were uncommon, although there were some instances of acne with testosterone rebound; dyspepsia, diarrhea, or rashes with antibacterial agents; nausea with bromocriptine; hydroceles following varicocelectomy; and anxiety and inability to produce semen during AIH (artificial insemination with husband's semen).

press gonadotropin secretion and spermatogenesis temporarily. Following treatment, a rebound rise in sperm output above pretreatment values is supposed to occur. In Melbourne, 92 patients receiving androgen or hCG therapy produced pregnancy rates no greater than those achieved by untreated men with similar degrees of subfertility. Sperm concentrations were significantly suppressed during treatment with high-dose testosterone and hCG, but there was no significant "rebound", and sperm motility was unchanged.

Gonadotropins. Extracts of human urinary or pituitary gonadotropins containing FSH and variable amounts of luteinizing hormones (LH) or pregnant mare serum gonadotropin have been injected alone (FSH, 75 to 600 IU) or with hCG twice or thrice weekly for several months in attempts to stimulate the seminiferous epithelium of men with idiopathic oligospermia. Gonadotropin-releasing hormone has also been used in small uncontrolled trials. In my opinion the results were unremarkable, and such expensive treatments should be reserved for patients with gonadotropin deficiency.

Antiestrogens. Clomiphene citrate (25 to 50 mg per day) and tamoxifen (20 mg per day) also increase circulating levels of FSH and LH. Treatment for 3 to 6 months is claimed to increase sperm output in men with idiopathic oligospermia. However, the trials were inadequately controlled. Fifty patients treated with clomiphene in Melbourne showed no significant change in semen quality, and the pregnancy rate was not significantly different from that for untreated infertile men.

Antibacterial Agents. Erythromycin (0.75 to 1.5 g per day), doxycycline (100 mg per day), trimethoprim with sulfamethoxazole (160 mg and 800 mg per day), or other antibacterial agents that enter prostatic fluid are often prescribed in prolonged courses (28 days or more) for infertile men with asthenospermia, leukocytes in the semen, or symptoms of inflammation of the prostate or genital tract. Courses of therapy with these agents in 95 patients, most of whom had asthenospermia, produced a slightly but not significantly better pregnancy rate than that for untreated patients. More recently a double-blind cross-over placebo-controlled trial of erythromycin for asthenospermia demonstrated no significant effect of the antibiotic on semen quality. However, there were twice as many pregnancies with erythromycin as with placebo, although there were too few to reach statistical significance. This trial will need to be repeated on a larger number of subjects to determine whether erythromycin improves infertility.

Glucocorticoids. Men with sperm antibodies have been treated with immunosuppressive doses of glucocorticoids, for example, prednisolone, 0.75 mg/kg per day for 4 months, or methylprednisolone, 96 mg per day for 5 days repeated at 2- to 3-month intervals. Antibody titers were often reduced, sperm motility and penetration of cervical mucus improved, and some pregnancies occurred. Marked improvement in sperm output has been noted in rare patients with severe oligospermia and sperm antibodies. However, no controlled trials have been reported. Also, such treatment has unpleasant and potentially serious side effects.

Other Drugs. Thyroxine, glucocorticoids in low doses, vitamins, minerals, and amino acids have been recommended for men with oligospermia or asthenospermia, but there is no reason to believe that they might help in the absence of a specific deficiency state. Bromocriptine has not proved useful for infertile men with normal or slightly elevated prolactin levels. Pathologic hyperprolactinemia appears to be uncommon in men with oligospermia or asthenospermia.

Surgical Treatment

Varicocelectomy. Spermatic vein ligation or embolization is commonly advised for infertile men with varicoceles. However, it is not certain that this procedure improves semen quality and fertility. From a follow-up of subfertile couples in Melbourne, it would appear that the presence of a varicocele is associated with a better chance of fertility whether or not it is surgically corrected.

Vasoepididymostomy. Because results of conventional vasoepididymostomy are so poor, the possibility that oligospermia might be due to partial epididymal obstruction usually is not investigated. However, new microsurgical procedures in which the epididymal tubule is anastomosed end-to-end to the vas appear to have much higher success rates. Thus the detection of men with partial obstructions may become more important in the future.

Other Methods

Coital Techniques. Some infertile couples are told to abstain from intercourse until the midcycle period of the wife's menstrual cycle because sperm concentrations usually rise with abstinence and fall with frequent ejaculation. However, the influence of ejaculatory frequency on sperm concentration is much less in oligospermic than in normospermic men, and many couples attempting this technique miss midcycle. Another method is the split ejaculate withdrawal procedure whereby only the first part of the ejaculate is deposited in the vagina. Although the first part of the ejaculate often contains a higher concentration of sperm with better morphology and motility than later parts, this is not invariably so and should be checked by a split ejaculate semen analysis. Although they have not been studied adequately, it is my opinion that these coital techniques are unlikely to improve fertility. In addition, they often distress the couple.

Artificial Insemination with Husband's Semen (AIH). AIH is a logical method of treatment when natural insemination is impossible, for instance, in cases of impotence or anejaculation and in cases in which the husband's semen was collected and stored before vasectomy or other treatment causing sterility. Pregnancies may occur following intravaginal or intracervical AIH with oligospermic or asthenospermic semen, but it is not clear that AIH provides a better pregnancy rate than natural insemination (see Table 1). Recently, a small controlled trial of intrauterine AIH produced a high conception rate of approximately 20 percent per cycle. Motile sperm suspensions were obtained from the poor quality semen by a method developed for in vitro fertilization, and insemination was carefully timed to coincide with ovulation. If confirmed in larger trials, this procedure will constitute a major breakthrough in the management of oligospermia and asthenospermia.

In Vitro Fertilization. Human ova can be fertilized in the laboratory with as few as 50,000 sperm, and in vitro fertilization and embryo transfer has produced some pregnancies when the only obvious cause for the couple's infertility was oligospermia. However, the fertilization rates are less than half those for couples in whom there is good semen quality, and therefore the overall pregnancy rates are likely to be low. New methods of separating the better sperm from poor specimens and for micromanipulating sperm and oocytes are being investigated.

General Advice

Many infertile men are told to avoid smoking, alcohol and unnecessary drugs, sauna and spa baths, stress at work, and unbalanced diets. While such exhortations are reasonable for general health purposes, compliance is not reliably associated with improved semen quality and fertility.

PREFERRED APPROACH

Our present strategy for managing subfertile men with oligospermia and asthenospermia has developed through disillusionment with empiric therapies and is mainly advisory. The lack of proof that such treatments improve fertility is explained to the couple. Their chances of achieving a pregnancy are estimated, and alternative methods for starting a family are discussed. We restrict drug treatments, varicocelectomy, and AIH to patients who volunteer to be included in controlled trials.

Prognosis for Fertility

A method for estimating the chances of conception occurring in a given time has been developed from a life table analysis of 250 pregnancies in 788 subfertile couples followed in Melbourne over the last 10 years. Overall, 25 percent achieved a pregnancy within one year and 30 percent within 2 years, but certain factors were associated with higher or lower pregnancy rates. The major prognostic factors were mean sperm concentration, duration of infertility, and age of the wife. The lower the sperm concentration, the longer the duration of infertility, and the older the wife, the worse the outlook. Also, the presence of a varicocele and previous pregnancies in the union were associated with better chances. We use these factors to predict the likelihood of a pregnancy occurring with each couple, and we emphasize the lack of treatments proved to increase pregnancy rates.

Alternatives and Planning

Following discussion of prognosis, the alternatives of adoption, artificial insemination with donor semen (AID), or childlessness are mentioned. In Melbourne there are few children for adoption, waiting lists are long, and guidelines for acceptance of adopting parents stringent. Thus, couples are advised to consider entering a waiting list early unless they are sure they would never want to adopt. At present, AID has an overall success rate of 70 percent in one year, which is clearly superior to the chances with the average subfertile men (25 percent in one year). For many couples the major decision is whether or not to have AID, and when. They must balance the desire to have their own children against the uncertainty of success while bearing in mind the declining fertility with increasing age of the women. We suggest that plans for the future be made at an early stage. For example, the average couple with 3 years primary infertility, a healthy wife aged 30, and a husband with mild oligospermia have a 25 percent chance of pregnancy in one year and 30 percent in 2 years. A reasonable plan is for them to continue trying for one or 2 years, during which time the husband might enter a therapeutic trial, and if no pregnancy occurs the wife will have

AID. Similar couples might decide this chance of success is too low and use AID sooner. Others are not interested in AID; they may wish to continue trying for a much longer period and are prepared to accept childlessness.

Female Factors

Unless the couple do not wish to pursue treatment, investigations of the wife are reviewed, and further consultations with gynecologists expert in the management of infertility are arranged as necessary. In our clinic, approximately 15 percent of female partners have ovulatory disorders, 13 percent tubal disorders, and 42 percent some problem prejudicial to fertility. Furthermore, the frequency of these female factors is inversely related to the severity of the semen disorder in the male partner, being more common with better semen quality. Easily correctable problems in the wife, such as anovulation, should be treated vigorously; pregnancies will occur on occasion even with very poor semen quality.

Timing of Intercourse

We believe it to be important that the couple have some understanding of the physiology of fertilization, particularly indications of ovulation and the requirement that coitus occur near the time of ovulation. We suggest they have intercourse at least every 48 hours over 8 to 10 days spanning ovulation. This should ensure the presence of the maximum possible number of sperm in the cervical mucus and female genital tract at the time of ovulation. Intercourse need not be restricted to this time, however, and may occur more frequently during the midcycle and at other times as desired.

Reduction of Anxiety and Acceptance of Infertility

Infertility presents a severe psychologic trauma to most couples. Denial, grief, and hostility reactions are common, and many patients take months or years before they come to terms with their infertility. The fact that no clear explanation of the cause and no effective treatment can be offered to the majority of infertile men causes further frustration. Stress and anxiety increase with each unsuccessful treatment. Furthermore, a significant proportion of couples end up with no children despite trying everything, including AID. We try to be frank yet empathetic when dealing with these difficult aspects of infertility. We request that both partners be present when results of investigations, prognosis, and alternatives such as AID are discussed, and we also mention the possibility of their seeking another option about their case and the availability of self-help groups for infertile couples.

PROS AND CONS OF TREATMENT

The aim of treatment of subfertile men is to improve fertility. The Melbourne results suggest that methods commonly used in men with poor semen quality—drugs, varicocele operations, and intracervical AIH—do not produce higher pregnancy rates than occur with no treatment. However, retrospective analysis may be subject to serious bias. Therefore, adequately controlled prospective trials are required. Multicenter trials of clomiphene for idiopathic oligospermia with normal gonadotrophin levels, AIH for oligospermia and asthenospermia, and prednisolone for sperm autoimmunity have been initiated.

In the future, clinical research may indicate that certain treatments do improve fertility. Alternatively, logical approaches to therapy may arise from basic research on the pathophysiology of disorders of spermatogenesis or sperm maturation. In the meantime, we believe drug and surgical treatments should not be used indiscriminately in men with oligospermia and asthenospermia.

Suggested Reading

Kerin JFP, Peek J, Warnes GM, Kirby C, Jeffrey R, Matthews CD, Cox LW. Improved conception rate after intrauterine insemination of washed spermatozoa from men with poor semen quality. Lancet 1984; 1:533–535.

Mahadervan MM, Trounson AO, Leeton JR. The relationship of tubal blockage, infertility of unknown cause, suspected male infertility, and endometriosis to success of in vitro fertilization and embryo transfer. Fertil Steril 1983; 40:755–762.

Pepperell RJ, Hudson B, Wood C. eds. The Infertile Couple. Edinburgh: Churchill-Livingstone, 1980.

Wang C, Chan C-W, Wong K-K, Yeung K-K. Comparison of the effectiveness of placebo, clomiphene citrate, mesterolone, pentoxifylline and testosterone rebound therapy for the treatment of idiopathic oligospermia. Fertil Steril 1983; 40:358–365.

Wood C, Trounson A. eds. Clinical In Vitro Fertilization. Berlin: Springer-Verlag, 1984.

ORAL STEROID CONTRACEPTIVES

DANIEL R. MISHELL Jr., M.D.

Oral steroid contraceptives (OCs) first became available for use by women in 1960. Shortly thereafter, they became the most widely used method of contraception in developed countries among both married and unmarried women. The main reasons for the popularity of this method of contraception were ease of administration combined with an extremely high rate of effectiveness. OCs are the most effective method of reversible contraception currently available. OC use steadily increased in the United States from 1960 to 1970. Between 1970 and 1975 about 35 percent of women practicing contraception in the United States used OCs. However, as a result of the risks of OCs being exaggerated to the consumer, retail sales of OCs have steadily declined in the United States after 1975.

MAJOR CONCERNS

Women have three major concerns about OCs. They are concerned about (1) an increased risk of developing cancer, (2) problems with future childbearing, and (3) an increased chance of developing heart attacks and stroke. These concerns are mostly unwarranted as the following discussion indicates.

Cancer

There is no valid evidence in the 22 years of study since OCs were introduced that their use increases the risk of any type of cancer including breast cancer, cancer of the uterus, cancer of the cervix, and cancer of the liver. Three large prospective studies initiated in 1968 compared large groups of women using OCs with a similar number of control women using other methods of contraception. To date, the majority of these studies have not been able to demonstrate an increased risk of any type of cancer. In our study an increased risk of cervical cancer was noted that may have been due to confounding factors such as earlier age of first intercourse and more sexual partners. Although data from a United States study suggest that women using OCs and exposed to large amounts of sunlight may have an increased risk of melanoma, this association has not been found in other studies.

Pregnancy After Discontinuing Use of Oral Contraceptives

Although OCs produce a period of temporary infertility in some women after their discontinuation, this infertility usually is not permanent. After a 2- to 3-year interval, fertility rates are the same among groups of former OC users and former users of other methods of contraception. Furthermore, the spontaneous abortion rate in women who conceive in the first or subsequent months of stopping OCs is the same as the spontaneous abortion rate in the general population or that in women who stop using other contraceptive methods.

Several studies of large numbers of babies born to women who stopped using OCs show that these infants have no greater chance of being born with any type of birth defect. The incidence of congenital anomalies was the same in babies born to women who had previously used OCs as in babies born to women who had previously used other methods of contraception or women who had not used any method of contraception.

Cardiovascular Disease

Analysis of the latest results from the three prospective OC studies indicates that a significantly increased risk of developing cardiovascular disease occurs only in current OC users over 35 years of age who smoke or those of any age who use OCs and also have some type of pre-existing vascular disease, such as hypertension, diabetes, or hypercholesterolemia. There is no reliable evidence that nonsmokers under age 45 and smokers under 35 who use OCs have an increased chance of dying from a heart attack provided they have no other vascular diseases. Thus, if a woman is under 35 and is a cigarette smoker, she can still use OCs. Likewise, a woman between 35 and 45 can continue to use OCs provided she does not smoke cigarettes or have any other type of vascular disease such as hypertension, diabetes, or hypercholesterolemia.

The incidence of deaths from cardiovascular disease does not increase with increased duration of OC use. This information, together with data from many other epidemiologic studies which show no increase in deaths from myocardial infarction in former users of OCs, indicates that the cause of myocardial infraction or stroke in OC users is due to arterial thrombosis, not atherosclerosis. These arterial thromboses occur mainly in women who have arterial narrowing produced by cigarette smoking or other arterial disease such as that caused by hypertension, diabetes, or hypercholesterolemia. Thus, despite data indicating that certain OC formulations lower HDL-cholesterol and raise LDL-cholesterol (changes which theoretically could be atherogenic), there is no evidence that long-term use of OCs produces a permanent harmful effect on the blood vessels such as development of atherosclerosis. Furthermore, the adverse lipid alterations produced by some formulations, especially those with high progestin potency, are small and within the normal range. There are no data to suggest that these small alterations in lipids increase the incidence of atherosclerosis in humans. Thus, women can take OCs for an unlimited time period no matter how old they are when they start taking them. In addition, there is no evidence that there is need for a rest period after a few years of OC use.

Other Concerns

Other concerns about taking OCs that have proved to be untrue are the belief that women need to take vitamin supplements because the OCs produce vitamin deficiency. Although OCs do lower the blood levels of the B-complex vitamins and vitamin C, these low vitamin levels are not accompanied by any clinical evidence of vitamin deficiency and vitamin supplementation is not necessary. There has also been concern that OCs should not be prescribed to young teenagers as their use might cause permanent changes in their hypothalamic-pituitary-ovarian axis as well as produce premature epiphyseal closure and cause them to stop growing. Both these concerns have proved to be unfounded, and OCs can be used by women of any age who have started to have regular menstrual cycles. Finally, OCs have been considered to be contraindicated in women who developed morphologic alterations in their vagina and uterus due to exposure to diethylstilbestrol during fetal life. However, in women with adenosis or other genital tract changes due to antenatal DES exposure, ingestion of OCs has not been associated with an increase in cancer or other harmful alterations. Therefore, OCs can be used safely by these women.

ADVERSE EFFECTS

It is important to realize that the OCs do produce adverse effects, although the incidence of these effects has been exaggerated. Fortunately, in most instances the more common adverse effects are relatively mild. The majority are produced by the estrogenic component of the formulation, while the rest are produced by the progestin component alone or by a combination of the two. The most frequent symptoms produced by the estrogenic component include nausea, breast tenderness, and fluid retention, which usually does not exceed 3 to 4 pounds of body weight.

The synthetic estrogen, ethinyl estradiol, used in OCs causes an increase in hepatic production of several globulins, and the amount of increase is related to the dosage of estrogen in the formulation. Increased levels of one of the globulins, angiotensinogen, may cause an increase in angiotensin II, which may result in the development of hypertension in certain individuals. Other globulins are involved in the blood clotting process, and their increase may cause a hypercoagulable state and cause the development of thrombosis in certain OC users. Although a small percentage of women taking OCs develop an increase in blood pressure, this elevation is temporary and disappears when the medication is stopped. Likewise, alterations in glucose metabolism, which are also produced by the estrogen component, are also only temporary and disappear when OC use is discontinued. There is no evidence that OC use produces diabetes mellitus or permanent hypertension.

Other adverse effects produced by the estrogen are changes in mood and depression produced by diversion of tryptophan metabolism from its minor pathway in the brain to its major pathway to the liver. The end product of tryptophan metabolism, serotonin, is thus decreased in the central nervous system. The resultant lowering of serotonin can produce depression in some women and sleepiness and mood changes in others. This is a reversible symptom that fortunately is not too common and disappears when the OCs are stopped. The incidence of all these estrogenic side effects occurs much less frequently now than a decade ago because the formulations in use today contain only one-fifth as much estrogen as the formulations that were used in the 1960s.

The progestogens, because they are structurally related to testosterone, produce certain androgenic adverse effects. These include weight gain and acne and a symptom perceived by some women as nervousness. Some women gain a considerable amount of weight when they take OCs, and this weight gain is produced by the anabolic effect of the progestin component. Although estrogens decrease sebum production, progestins increase sebum production and can cause acne to develop and/or worsen. Thus, patients who have acne should be given a formulation with a low progestin-estrogen ratio. The final symptom produced by the gestogenic component is failure of withdrawal bleeding or amenorrhea. Because the progestins decrease the estrogen receptors in the endometrium, endometrial growth is decreased, and some women have failure of withdrawal bleeding. Although this symptom is not important medically, since bleeding serves as a signal that the patient is not pregnant, it is desirable to have some amount of periodic withdrawal bleeding during the days the woman is not taking these steroids. Finally, both the estrogen and progestin portions of the formulation can act together to produce irregular bleeding and/or chloasma. Breakthrough bleeding which is usually produced by not enough estrogen or too much progestin or a combination of both, as well as failure of withdrawal bleeding, can be alleviated by increasing the amount of estrogen in the formulation or by switching to a more estrogenic formulation. The symptom of chloasma, pigmentation of the malar eminences, is accentuated by sunlight and usually takes a long time to disappear after OCs are stopped.

In addition to these more common adverse effects, there is an increased risk of developing more serious problems which can lead to death or severe morbidity. Although the incidence of cholelithiasis is increased about two-fold compared to its incidence in controls in the first few years of OC use, recent data indicate that after 4 years of OC use the incidence of cholelithiasis in OC users is decreased compared with controls. Thus OCs appear to accelerate the process of cholelithiasis, but do not increase its overall incidence. The risk of developing deep vein thrombophlebitis is also increased about three to four times, as is the risk of developing thromboembolism. However, the absolute incidence of these disorders, which are not necessarily related (i.e., patients with thromboembolism do not have to have clinical symptoms of thrombophlebitis), is on the order of about 1/10,000 users annually for thrombophlebitis and about 1/30,0000 users annually for thromboembolism. OCs probably increase the incidence of thrombotic and possibly hemorrhagic stroke, although the epidemiologic data relating OC use to stroke are conflicting and indicate that the increased risk of stroke in OC users, like MI, is mainly limited to women with underlying vascular disorders like hypertension or older women who smoke and use OCs. Although the relative risk of developing stroke in OC users is possibly increased about 3 times, the actual incidence remains quite low, about 1/20,000 to 1/30,000 users/year. Benign liver adenomas occur very rarely in OC users, with an estimated frequency of about 1/30,000 to 1/50,000 users/year. The incidence is increased in women who have used the formulations for more than 5 years. Also, as already mentioned, although there is epidemiologic evidence that women over 35 who smoke or have other associated risk factors, such as hypertension or hypercholesterolemia, have an increased risk of developing myocardial infarction with OC use, the actual incidence of myocardial infarction in this group is also low, about 1/5000 users/year.

CONTRAINDICATIONS TO ORAL CONTRACEPTIVE USE

OCs can be prescribed for the majority of women in the reproductive age group because they are young and healthy; however, there are certain absolute contraindications for their use. These include a present or past history of vascular disease, including thromboembolism, thrombophlebitis, atherosclerosis, stroke, or systemic vascular disease, such as lupus erythematosus or hemoglobin SS disease. In addition, hypertension, diabetes mellitus with vascular disease, and hyperlipidemia are contraindications to OCs, as use of these agents in women with these disorders can increase the risk of the patient's developing a stroke or myocardial infarction. One of the contraindications for OC use listed by the United States Food and Drug Administration is cancer of the breast or endometrium, although there are no data indicating OCs are harmful in women with these diseases. In addition, patients who are pregnant should not ingest OCs because of the masculinizing effect of the progestogens on the external genitalia of the female fetus. Concerns that ingestion of OCs while pregnant produce other deleterious effects on the fetus, such as limb reproduction defects and heart defects, have not proven to be valid. Patients with heart disease should not use OCs since the fluid retention produced by these agents could produce congestive heart failure. Finally, patients with active liver disease should not receive OCs, since the steroids are metabolized in this organ. However, patients who have had liver disease in the past, such as viral hepatitis, but whose liver function tests have returned to normal can receive these agents. Relative contraindications to OC use include heavy cigarette smoking, migraine headaches, amenorrhea, and depression. Migraine headaches can be made worse by OC use, and patients who develop a stroke while taking OCs frequently have an increased incidence of headaches of the migraine type, fainting, loss of vision or speech, or paresthesias prior to development of the CVA. If any of these symptoms develops in OC users, the patient should stop ingesting these agents. Patients who are amenorrheic for a cause other than polycystic ovarian syndrome should probably not receive OCs, as they may have a pituitary microadenoma. OC use masks the symptoms of both amenorrhea and galactorrhea, which are the symptoms produced by enlargement of the adenoma. Thus patients with amenorrhea should not receive OCs until the diagnosis for this symptom is established. Anyone who develops galactorrhea while taking OCs should stop these agents, and after 2 weeks, a serum prolactin level should be measured. If the prolactin is elevated, further diagnostic evaluation, such as x-ray studies of the sella turcica, are indicated. A recent NIH study confirmed findings of other studies which showed that OCs do not produce prolactin secretory pituitary adenomas, as the incidence of these tumors was the same in OC users and controls.

BEGINNING ORAL CONTRACEPTIVES

Adolescents

In deciding whether the pubertal, sexually active girl should use OCs for contraception, the clinician should be more concerned about compliance in this age-group than possible physiologic harm. Provided the postmenarcheal girl has demonstrated maturity of the hypothalamic-pituitary-ovarian axis by having at least three regular, presumably ovulatory, cycles, it is safe to prescribe OCs without being concerned about causing permanent damage to the reproductive process. It is probably best not to prescribe OCs to women of any age with oligomenorrhea, except those with polycystic ovarian syndrome, because of the increased likelihood of their developing postpill amenorrhea, and oligomenorrhea is more frequent in adolescence than later in life. One need not be concerned about accelerating epiphyseal closure in the postmenarcheal female. Their endogenous estrogens have already initiated the process a few years prior to menarche and the contraceptive steroids do not hasten the process.

Following Pregnancy

There is a difference in the relationship of the return of ovulation and bleeding in the postabortal woman and in the woman who has had a term delivery. The first episode of menstrual bleeding in the postabortal woman is usually preceded by ovulation. Following a term delivery, the first episode of bleeding is usually, but not always, anovulatory. Ovulation occurs sooner after an abortion, usually between 2 and 4 weeks, than after a term delivery, when ovulation is usually delayed beyond 6 weeks, but may occur as early as 4 weeks after delivery in a woman who is not breast-feeding.

Thus after spontaneous or induced abortion of a fetus of less than 12 weeks' gestation, OCs should be started immediately to prevent conception following the first ovulation. For patients who have a delivery after 28 weeks of gestation and are not nursing, the combination pills should be initiated 2 weeks after delivery. If the termination of pregnancy occurs between 21 and 28 weeks, contraceptive steroids should be started 1 week later. The reason for delay in the latter instances is that the normally increased risk of thromboembolism occurring postpartum may be further enhanced by the hypercoagulable state associated with contraceptive steroid ingestion. As the first ovulation is delayed for a period of at least 4 weeks after a term delivery, there is no need to expose the patient to this increased risk.

It is probably best for women who are nursing not to use combination OCs as their use may diminish the amount of milk produced since estrogen inhibits prolactin's action on the breast. Women who are breast-feeding every 4 hours, including the nighttime, will not ovulate until at least 10 weeks after delivery and thus do not need contraception before that time. Since only a small percentage of breast-feeding women will ovulate as long as they continue full nursing, either a barrier method or the progestin only OC can be used. The latter does not diminish the amount of breast milk and is effective in this group of women.

All Patients

At the initial visit, after a history and physical examination have determined that there are no medical contraindications for oral contraceptives, the patient should be informed about the benefits and risks. It is best to use a written informed consent signed by the patient and to note on the patient's medical record that the benefits and risks have been explained to her.

APPROACH TO TREATMENT

Type of Formulation

In determining which formulation to use, it is probably best to initially prescribe a formulation with 30 μg or 35 μg ethinyl estradiol. A study from Great Britain reported that the incidence of total deaths as well as death due to arterial causes alone was significantly decreased in patients using formulations with 30 μg ethinyl estradiol compared with those using formulations of 50 μg ethinyl estradiol. Furthermore, the incidence of ischemic heart disease and stroke was also significantly decreased in women using the lower-dose estrogen formulations. In addition, the increase in amounts of serum globulins, including angiotensinogen as well as those involved with coagulation, is related to the dose of estrogen administered. Thus, it would appear reasonable that lower doses of estrogen formulations should not cause as great or frequent an increase in blood pressure. As few randomized studies have been performed comparing the different marketed formulations, until large-scale comparative studies are performed, the clinician has to decide which formulation to use based on which formulations have the least adverse effects among patients in his or her practice. Unless acne is present, there is no evidence that some patients do better with formulations that are more estrogenic while other patients do better with formulations that are more gestagenic.

Evidence that some highly progestogenic formulations might lower HDL-cholesterol levels more than others has caused concern that these agents may increase the risk of myocardial infarction more than formulations producing less change in HDL-cholesterol. However, there is no evidence that artificially lowering or raising HDL-cholesterol levels in humans alters the increase of myocardial infarction. The alterations produced by oral contraceptives are minimal. Furthermore, as already noted, the cause of OC-related MI appears to be thrombotic, not atherosclerotic, as the risk is not increased in ex-users and is not related to duration of use of the compounds.

Follow-Up

If the patient has no contraindication to OC use, the only routine laboratory tests indicated are a complete blood count, urinalysis, and Pap smear. At the end of 3 months, the patient should be seen again; at this time a nondirected history should be obtained and the blood pressure measured. After this visit the patient should be seen annually, at which time a nondirected history should again be taken, blood pressure and body weight measured, and a physical examination, including a breast, abdominal, and pelvic examination (including a Pap smear), performed. It is important to perform annual Pap smears on oral contraceptive users as they are a relatively high-risk group for the development of cervical neoplasia. The routine use of other laboratory tests is not indicated unless the patient is over 35 or has a family history of diabetes or vascular disease. For patients over 35 who wish to continue taking OCs, it is advisable to obtain a lipid panel, including HDL and LDL cholesterol, total cholesterol, and triglycerides. If the lipid levels are abnormal, another method of contraception may be safer. In addition, because of the increased incidence of diabetes after age 35, a 2-hour postprandial blood glucose should be obtained; if this is elevated, a full glucose tolerance test should be performed. If results of this test are abnormal, the OCs should probably be stopped. Routine use of these tests in women under 35 is not indicated because the incidence of positive results is extremely low. However, if the patient has a family history of vascular disease, such as myocardial infarction occurring in family members under the age of 50, it would be advisable to obtain a lipid panel before and after starting OC use, and if the patient has a family history of diabetes or evidence of diabetes during pregnancy, a 2-hour postprandial blood glucose should be obtained before and after starting OCs. If patients have a past history of liver disease, a liver panel should be obtained to make certain that the liver function is normal before starting OCs.

Drug Interactions

Although synthetic sex steroids can retard the biotransformation of certain drugs, such as phenazone and meperidine, due to substrate competition, such interference is not important clinically. OC use has not been shown to inhibit the action of other drugs. However, some drugs can clinically interfere with the action of OCs by inducing liver enzymes that convert the steroids to more polar and less biologically active metabolites. Certain drugs have been shown to accelerate the biotransformation of steroids in the human. These include barbiturates, sulfonamides, cyclophosphamide, and rifampicin. Several investigators have reported a relatively high incidence of OC failure in women ingesting rifampicin, and these two agents should not be given concurrently. The clinical data concerning OC failure in users of other antibiotics, such as penicillin, ampicillin, and sulfonamides, and analgesics, such as phenytoin, as well as barbiturates, are less clear. A few anecdotal studies have appeared in the literature, but reliable evidence for a clinical inhibitory effect of these drugs, such as occurs with rifampicin, is not available. Until such time as controlled studies are performed, it would appear prudent when both agents are given simultaneously to suggest use of a barrier method in addition to the OCs because of possible interference with OC action by the action of the antibiotic on the gut flora. In addition, women with epilepsy requiring medication are best treated with 50 μg estrogen formulations because a higher incidence of accidental pregnancies has been reported in these women with the use of lower-dose estrogen formulations.

HEALTH BENEFITS

Finally the consumer should be made aware of the many noncontraceptive health benefits of OCs. As a result of the antiestrogen effect of the progestin compound, there is less endometrial growth in OC users. As a result there is less blood loss and less iron deficiency anemia in OC users. There are less menstrual irregularities, including dysfunctional uterine bleeding, and less endometrial hyperplasia and endometrial cancer in OC users. Other noncontraceptive medical benefits of OCs result from their main action, inhibition of ovulation. A major beneficial effect is a 2- to 3-fold reduction in the incidence of benign cystic breast disease in OC users. As a result of ovulation inhibition, there is significantly less premenstrual tension and dysmenorrhea in OC users as well as almost a complete absence of functional ovarian cysts. In addition, cancer of the ovary is reduced 2- to 3-fold in current and former OC users. A 50 percent reduction in rheumatoid arthritis and salpingitis has been found in several studies of OC users. Finally, use of OCs greatly reduces the chance of developing an ectopic pregnancy, a possibly lethal disorder.

To summarize these benefits, Ory recently estimated that in 100,000 women in the United States using OCs each year, their use will prevent 320 from developing iron deficiency anemia, 32 from developing rheumatoid arthritis, and 450 from developing PID which does not require hospitalization. In addition, there will be 150 less women hospitalized for PID, 235 less hospitalized for breast disease, 35 less hospitalized for ovarian tumors, and 117 less hospitalized for tubal pregnancies. Ory estimated that each year about 1 of every 750 women taking OCs will not develop a serious disease which she would have developed if she did not take this drug. He estimated that use of OCs prevents 50,000 women from being hospitalized in the United States each year. It is unfortunate that the infrequent adverse effects of OCs have received widespread publicity, while information about the more common noncontraceptive health benefits has attracted little attention.

Suggested Reading

Brinton LA, Vessey MP, Flavel R, et al. Risk factors for benign breast disease. Am J Epidemiol 1981; 113:203.

Centers for Disease Control Cancer and Steroid Hormone Study: Long-term oral contraceptive use and the risk of breast cancer. JAMA 1983; 249:1591.

Centers for Disease Control Cancer and Steroid Hormone Study: Oral contraceptive use and the risk of endometrial cancer. JAMA 1983; 249:1600.

Meade TW, Greenberg G, Thompson SG. Progestogens and cardiovascular reactions associated with oral contraceptives and a comparison of the safety of 50- and 30-μg estrogen preparations. Brit Med J 1960; 1:1157.

Mishell DR Jr. Noncontraceptive health benefits of oral steroidal contraceptives. Am J Obstet Gynecol 1982; 142:809.

Oral Contraceptives and Health: An Interim Report from the Oral Contraceptive Study of the Royal College of General Practitioners. New York: Pitman Publishing, 1974.

Ory HW: The noncontraceptive health benefits from oral contraceptive use. Fam Plann Perspect 1982; 14(4):182.

Ramcharan S, Pellegrin FA, Ray RM, Hsu JP. The Walnut Creek Contraceptive Drug Study: a prospective study of the side effects of oral contraceptives, v. III. NIH Publ. 81-564. Washington DC, US Gov't. Printing Office, 1981.

Royal College of General Practitioners' Oral Contraception Study: Further analysis of mortality in oral contraceptive users. Lancet 1981; 1:541.

Vessey MP, Wright NH, McPherson K, et al. Fertility after stopping different methods of contraception. Br Med J 1978; 1:265.

Vessey M, et al. A long-term follow-up study of women using different methods of contraception—An interim report. J Biosoc Sci 1976; 8:373.

MENOPAUSE

LUIGI MASTROIANNI Jr., M.D.

Management of the menopause is an increasingly important issue in practice today. Data from the 1980 census indicate that there were 32 million women over the age of 50 in the United States. Symptoms vary substantially from woman to woman; in fact, some women have no symptoms at all. Decisions as to when and how to treat are based largely on good clinical judgment. Laboratory evaluation has limited usefulness.

Technically, menopause occurs with cessation of menstrual flow. The symptom complex associated with the menopause often begins much earlier, however, as the ovaries begin to show signs of ovulatory failure and transition from estrogen-producing to androgen-producing organs. In general, there are fewer ovulations as the time of the menopause approaches. In the United States, the mean age of menopause is 49.5 years, with tremendous variation around that number.

The menopause may or may not be predicted by changes in menstrual pattern. When a change does occur, it is related to variations in ovulation. Cycles may be irregular, with periods which are very heavy or very light. When flow is not preceded by ovulation, it is often heavy from an endometrium that has been stimulated with unopposed estrogen without benefit of progesterone effect.

In the early perimenopausal years, levels of circulating estradiol in the proliferative phase are actually somewhat increased. This may be related to the increase in gonadotropins, both follicle stimulating hormone (FSH) and luteinizing hormone (LH), which occurs at about that time. The rise in FSH levels in the perimenopause is the most sensitive indicator of imminent ovarian failure. In practice, however, gonadotropin determinations are rarely useful to corroborate a clinical impression that menopause is impending. Gonadotropin determinations are somewhat helpful in the management of the amenorrheic patient in her forties who wishes to know whether it is safe to discard contraception. If FSH and LH levels are elevated, we can give her reasonable assurance that she is postmenopausal. Sporadic ovulations occasionally occur after several months of amenorrhea associated with menopausal symptoms, and gonadotropins are most useful in the evaluation of amenorrhea to corroborate a diagnosis of premature ovarian failure.

Symptoms of the menopause do not present any really typical pattern. Hot flashes are an early symptom and among the most annoying. Another important symptom, one that may not surface except through direct questioning, is dyspareunia. This is the result of the atrophic vaginitis that results from estrogen deficiency. A common symptom is fatigue. This is a rather nondescript symptom and there are many factors which could contribute to it. The usual explanation for menopause-related fatigue is the occurrence of nocturnal hot flashes and diaphoresis which interfere with sleep. Recent studies have shown a direct relationship between estrogen levels and sleep. As estrogen levels decline, there is an associated decrease in rapid eye movement (REM) sleep. Estrogen treatment promotes REM sleep.

Increasing awareness of the relationship between estrogen deficiency and osteoporosis has influenced attitudes toward estrogen treatment. Unfortunately, the patient is unaware that there is a problem until she experiences a fracture. Osteoporosis can begin during the perimenopausal interval and continue unabated as estrogen levels decline. Bone changes occur gradually, principally affecting the long bones and vertebrae. In some cases, spontaneous compression fractures of the vertebrae occur, producing the so-called "dowager hump". Women who have been surgically castrated are at greater risk, and with rare exceptions, should receive replacement therapy. Some women, in fact, never experience hot flashes. They may be efficient converters of androgen to estrogen and may more effectively utilize the steroids produced by the adrenals. Thin women have less peripheral conversion of androstenedione to estrogen and generally experience earlier, more pronounced symptoms.

TREATMENT

Treatment of the menopause requires considerable clinical skill. The most logical approach is to substitute for that estrogen which had previously been produced by the ovary. A strong case can be made for the use of replacement therapy unless there are contraindications. Since the troublesome symptoms are related directly to lack of estrogen, response is rapid. However, I have not made it a practice to treat patients who are completely asymptomatic. It is not unreasonable to assume that if a patient has no symptoms, i.e., no hot flashes, no atrophic vaginitis, she is probably producing sufficient circulating estrogen to protect her bones, although there are no data to support this position. When using estrogen, I like to start with a low dose. The dosage is increased if the symptoms do not respond. The aim is to provide sufficient estrogen to eliminate the symptoms without causing bleeding. In practical terms, this means an initial dose of 0.3 mg of conjugated estrogen or its equivalent, 5 micrograms of ethinyl estradiol. It is usually necessary to increase the dose of conjugated estrogen to 0.625 mg or more.

A good case can be made for adding a progestational agent to the regimen. The most common estrogen-associated long-term complication is carcinoma of the endometrium. Progesterone down-regulates the estrogen receptors in the endometrial cells and therefore controls the growth-producing effect of estrogen on endometrial tissue. Recent evidence suggests that progesterone may be effective in fairly low dosage, i.e., as little as 2.5 mg of medroxyprogesterone acetate daily. The estrogen is given cyclicly, 25 days on and 5 days off, and the medroxyprogesterone acetate added to the regimen in the last 10 days of each cycle. When the medication is given cyclicly, continuous stimulation of the breast is avoided. The combination of progesterone with estrogen may also have a protective effect on the breast. One of the difficulties associated with the use of combination of estrogen and progesterone is the occurrence of withdrawal bleeding. Some women respond with cyclic menstrual periods and find these undesirable. One should try to regulate the dosage, making it high enough to prevent symptoms, but low enough so that the endometrium is not stimulated sufficiently to bleed.

In addition to estrogen, diet is important in the prevention of osteoporosis. A daily intake of 1500 mg of calcium is recommended. We have found it useful to provide the patient with a rundown on the calcium content of various foods and their caloric value. She can then review this in relation to her standard daily diet. If she is ingesting less than 1500 mg of calcium daily, the diet should be modified or supplementary calcium prescribed. Yogurt is an excellent source of calcium and is low in calories. Calcium without estrogen is not very effective in preventing osteoporosis. Vitamin D and fluorides have been suggested, but there are few places in the United States where both vitamin D and fluoride intake is not adequate. Large doses of fluoride would have to be taken to have any impact at all, and these could be associated with unacceptable side effects, including peptic ulcer and arthralgias. Furthermore, bone that is formed under the influence of fluoride alone tends to fracture easily. There is no evidence that the addition of fluoride offers any advantage.

Since endometrial carcinoma is a critical issue, endometrial sampling should be seriously considered in selected cases. A sample should certainly be taken from any postmenopausal patient who bleeds, unless bleeding is consistently associated temporarily with withdrawal flow. Certainly, any perimenopausal woman who is having irregular menses with variable menstrual flow should have her endometrium sampled before estrogen therapy is instituted. There is generally no need for a full-dress dilatation and curettage, and some type of office aspiration generally suffices. If it is not possible to obtain an endometrial sample in the office, a dilatation and curettage should be carried out.

Unfortunately, there is no practical way to evaluate patients for osteoporosis and its progression. The most precise method is to measure bone mass by photon-absorption densitometry over a period of several months. The forearm, from the wrist to the elbow, is usually measured. The metacrapals also provide an excellent reference point. The equipment for these studies is expensive, and at this point the cost is unacceptably high to justify its routine use.

The risks of prolonged estrogen treatment are a matter of some concern and should be thoroughly reviewed with the patient prior to treatment. She should be made aware of the possibility of future osteoporosis. She should know that a relationship between carcinoma of the endometrium and estrogen therapy has been established, but its incidence appears to be decreased when progesterone is added to the regimen. She should be made aware that in the event of bleeding, endometrial sampling should be carried out. The relationship between estrogen treatment and breast carcinoma should also be discussed. The combination of estrogen with a progestational agent has not been shown to be associated with an increased incidence of carcinoma of the breast, but periodic breast evaluation is important. The use of substitution therapy has relieved many women from the debilitating and discouraging symptoms of the menopause. It is hoped that this therapy, in combination with appropriate calcium intake, will also decrease the incidence of osteoporosis with its debilitating sequelae.

THE ADULT DIABETIC PATIENT

STEFAN S. FAJANS, M.D.

It is the purpose of this chapter to discuss the management of the adult Type I, insulin-dependent diabetic patient as well as that of the Type II, noninsulin-dependent patient, whether noninsulin-requiring or insulin-requiring.

AIMS OF MANAGEMENT

The aims of ideal management and control for all types of diabetes mellitus are directed at several goals. First, we strive for the achievement of metabolic or biochemical control. This includes the normalization, or near-normalization, of fasting and postprandial plasma glucose concentration in the absence of insulin- or drug-induced hypoglycemia, the normalization of hemoglobin A1 concentration, and the normalization of plasma lipid levels. The second aim of ideal management is to prevent the development of the long-term complications of diabetes mellitus and to avoid or decrease cardiovascular risk factors. Third, attention must be paid to various sociopsychologic factors playing a role in any given patient's health. The whole patient must be considered, not only his disease.

ACHIEVEMENT OF AIMS

To achieve or approach these goals of management and control of diabetes the following therapeutic modalities are considered. Education of the patient and his/her family concerning the nature of diabetes, its control, and the possible development of acute and chronic complications is vital to achieve the aims of therapy and to institute specific therapy. Education includes instruction in the means to achieve metabolic control and to monitor the patient's progress. The importance of meal planning therapy and increased physical activity must be stressed and appropriate modifications instituted. Therapy with insulin is essential in the Type I diabetic patient. If an adequate trial of dietary modification and exercise fail to achieve the desired goals in a Type II diabetic patient, the use of diet plus pharmacologic intervention with either oral agents or insulin must be initiated to achieve or approach biochemical control. Although final proof for the thesis has not been established in man, present evidence strongly suggests that achievement of euglycemia has the potential to prevent the neurologic and microvascular complications of diabetes. The treatment of obesity and hypertension and the elimination of the use of cigarettes are important also for the aim of avoiding or decreasing cardiovascular risk factors.

Criteria for Biochemical Control

Realistic and achievable criteria for biochemical control must be individualized according to the type of diabetes (Type I, IDDM vs. Type II, NIDDM), the ease of correction of the metabolic abnormality, the stability vs. lability of plasma glucose levels on implementation of a constant therapeutic program, age of patient, activity, presence and severity of complications, other illness or stress. In addition, the patient's understanding, education, and level of motivation may influence the level of biochemical control achievable. If normalization of plasma glucose levels in a nongeriatric patient is the criterion of control, glucose concentration below 115 mg/dl in the fasting state and below 140 mg/dl two hours postprandially would be sought. Acceptable control, signifying realistic if not ideal control, would be a fasting plasma glucose concentration below 140 mg/dl and a two-hour postprandial plasma glucose concentration below 200 mg/dl. From epidemiologic evidence it appears that the specific microvascular complications of diabetes occur rarely when plasma glucose is below these levels. Control may be judged to be "fair", when fasting plasma glucose levels are between 140 and 200mg/dl, and control would be judged to be poor with fasting plasma glucose levels above 200 mg/dl. Postprandial plasma glucose levels can be judged to be fair between 200 and 230 mg/dl and poor above 230 mg/dl. Concentration of glycosylated hemoglobin to be achieved depends on the laboratory method, but usually below 8 percent. Plasma cholesterol is normal below 200 mg/dl, acceptable below 230 mg/dl, fair below 250 mg/dl, and poor above 250 mg/dl. Corresponding levels for fasting plasma triglycerides would be <150, 180, 200, and >200 ml/dl, respectively. These various concentrations given should be increased for elderly patients.

Education

Education of the patient and his family is the key to successful treatment of all types of diabetes mellitus. Education programs should be considered a management tool of high priority. Unless the patient understands his disease and its treatment, the recommended treatment plan, whatever its components, is bound to fail.

A team approach to education and treatment of diabetes is usually most effective. The patient and the patient's family profit from interaction with the physician, nurse, dietician, educator, psychologist, social worker, and community support groups. In the prevention and treatment of complications, various physician specialists and a podiatrist are helpful. All these health professionals provide instruction, advice, encouragement, motivation, and psychologic support. National standards for the implementation of diabetes education programs have been endorsed by the National Diabetes Advisory Board and published (National Standards for Diabetes Patient Education Programs, 7550 Wisconsin Avenue, Room 616, Bethesda, Maryland 20205). They should be followed in establishing or maintaining such a facility. Support groups organized by clinics, hospitals, physicians, and affiliates of the American Diabetes Association are most valuable.

Educational programs should include information on the nature and manifestations of diabetes and its control, self monitoring of blood glucose and urine glucose and ketone testing, causes, recognition and treatment of hypoglycemia, treatment of hyperglycemia, and prevention and treatment of ketosis. They should also include nutrition and dietary management, types of insulin and insulin injection techniques, medications, personal hygiene and foot care, exercise, causes, prevention and treatment of chronic complications, care during intermittent illness, and psychologic and family adjustment.

Specific techniques for helping the patient adjust to and comply and cope with the diagnosis, various aspects of the management plan, and the prognosis of diabetes are beyond the subject of this chapter.

Assessment of Metabolic Control

Accurate assessment of metabolic control is necessary to achieve the aims of normalization of fasting and postprandial concentrations of plasma glucose, to normalize hemoglobin A1 and to avoid insulin-induced hypoglycemia. Two means are available to the patient and physician for accurate assessment of metabolic control. One is self-monitoring of blood glucose (SMBG) and the other one is determination of concentration of hemoglobin A1 in blood.

Provided the patient is willing to self-monitor blood glucose levels several times daily so that appropriate changes in treatment can be made, SMBG provides the means to achieve near-normoglycemia for the majority of diabetic patients and is far more reliable than urine testing. It supplements and, if done accurately and reliably, may replace fasting and postprandial plasma glucose determinations during the periodic office or clinic visit, which may give limited information pertaining only to one day, particularly in a patient with fluctuating blood glucose levels. Before venous glucose determinations are abandoned in favor of SMBG, the patient should be asked to ascertain blood glucose concentrations by SMBG technique on the same blood that venous determinations are performed. This gives a measure of the accuracy of SMBG in any given patient. SMBG has proved to be feasible and acceptable as part of the treatment program for the majority of patients and presents few technical difficulties for the moderately well-motivated patient. The results of SMBG facilitates the patient's understanding of the major metabolic abnormality of diabetes, permits his assessment of glycemic control, and improves and reinforces his motivation to adhere to or adjust to the prescribed program. SMBG is a helpful component of the diabetes education program; it is most helpful in the management of patients with unstable diabetes and more valuable than urine-glucose monitoring. It improves glycemic control by allowing the physician and patient to adjust specifically any aspect of the therapeutic program, be it diet, exercise or insulin at specific times of the day. It is particularly important to the diabetic patient who takes multiple injections of insulin, including intermediate-acting or long-acting and short-acting insulin. Periodic SMBG during the day and occasionally at night allows patients with labile diabetes to avoid hypoglycemic reactions and is obligatory with intensified conventional insulin therapy or for continuous subcutaneous insulin infusion programs. SMBG is mandatory in pregnant women with diabetes to achieve optimum control and prevent the increased morbidity and mortality of the neonate of the diabetic mother. The frequency of SMBG during a 24-hour period (fasting, 1- to 2-hour postprandial and/or before the next meal or feeding), and/or frequency of testing during a week depend on the goals to be reached, stability vs. lability of blood glucose excursions, and previous findings with this technique. Most patients prefer SMBG to urine-glucose monitoring.

Self-monitoring of blood glucose can be done successfully with test strips with or without the use of reflectometers. Although many patients do not like pricking their finger, the use of an automated lance has facilitated obtaining the necessary drop of blood. The drop of blood is placed on a chemically treated pad on a test strip, the color developed during a prescribed period of time, and the color compared visually to a color chart. Some patients are able to interpolate the color on the test strip to within 10 to 20 mg/dl of that obtained by the reflectance meter whereas others interpret the strip as indicating a narrow range, such as within 40 mg/dl. At the very least, it will tell the patient whether blood glucose is low, normal, or high. Alternatively, the color strip can be read by a reflectometer that provides a numerical readout of the blood glucose value. Patients with visual problems or patients who feel insecure in interpreting colors may feel more secure with the use of reflectometers. Self-monitoring of blood glucose increases the cost of management of diabetes.

The patient should be instructed and encouraged to keep a daily record of insulin (or oral agent) dosage, fasting, post- and preprandial blood glucose determinations, urine glucose and ketones if indicated, occurrence and timing of hypoglycemic reactions, other symptoms, exercise, and deviations from the prescribed diet as well as weekly weight. This information is necessary for allowing judgment in regard to changes to be made in any aspect of the therapeutic plan and reinforces the importance of therapy for the patient.

Determination of the concentration of hemoglobin A1 during follow-up visits is the best tool in the assessment of long-term integrated glycemia. In one value it reflects the time-averaged blood glucose concentration over the preceding weeks to 2 months and gives an excellent assessment of overall control over that period of time. This measurement is not greatly influenced by day to day fluctuations in blood glucose levels and does not depend on patient cooperation. If elevated it indicates that control must be improved, but unlike SMBG, does not indicate how improved control can be achieved.

Urine glucose determinations are useful in patients who are unwilling or unable to utilize SMBG. It is an indirect measure of glucose control which depends on the level of the renal threshold. Urine ketone determinations are mandatory when the patient is symptomatic, or has severe hyperglycemia and glycosuria, particularly in the Type I diabetic patient.

Planning of Diet

General Principles. Establishment of an appropriate diet or modification of the patient's diet is an important element in the therapeutic planning for all patients with diabetes mellitus. Patients with Type I diabetes usually require a weight-maintaining diet, but must eat regularly and time meals and feedings to the time-activity course of their insulin and to their daily activity and exercise schedules. In the great majority of obese patients with Type II diabetes, the prescription of an appropriate reduction diet for correction of obesity is the most important and frequently the only therapeutic intervention needed for the effective control of metabolic abnormalities associated with the disease. In general, the principles to be kept in mind in the control of diabetes and the maintenance of proper nutrition are: (1) attention to the total number of calories being ingested for maintenance of proper nutrition, with foods that provide a well-balanced diet; (2) attention to the composition of the diet in terms of amount and type of protein, carbohydrate, and fat; and (3) attention to the distribution of calories and carbohydrates during the day, including frequency and timing of food ingestion. The physician needs to understand these principles to be able to determine and prescribe the appropriate diet. However, it is the unusual physician who can design and prescribe a detailed dietary plan, or has the time to do so, without the help of a trained dietician or nutritionist. In most instances the physician will define the objectives of dietary modification and leave the specifics of the plan and its implementation to the trained nutritionist. In almost all hospitals and diabetes clinics a nutritionist is available. In most communities, the physician in private practice is able to find a nutritionist who is qualified to help with the provision of diet therapy. Nevertheless, it is important for the physician to emphasize the importance of diet in overall management, to give encouragement for its implementation and to insist on frequent follow-up for evaluation and correction of misunderstandings. Without the patient's cooperation, a prescription for dietary modification is of little use. Patients are more likely to adhere to a dietary plan if they understand the importance and reasons for dietary modification. Diets must be individualized; the patient must be consulted in the planning stage to ensure that the dietary plan is one that he can adhere to. Patients' likes and dislikes and ethnic preferences should be considered in planning a diet. The use of standard hand-out sheets can never substitute for individualized planned dietary modification. In many obese patients, adherence to a weight reduction diet will not succeed without behavior modification therapy. Support groups such as Weight Watchers, Tops, and Weight Loss Clinics may be useful for many obese patients.

Total Caloric Intake. Adjustment of caloric intake is the most essential objective in the dietary management of diabetes. Nutritional requirements and daily caloric needs of patients with diabetes are essentially the same as those of individuals without diabetes. For nonobese patients, one estimates the daily caloric requirement to maintain body weight: 25 kcal/kg body weight per day is required for maintenance of basal metabolic weight, with additional calories depending on the level of activity of the patient. Sedentary individuals need approximately 30 kcal/kg body weight per day for maintenance of basal metabolic rate plus a modest activity level. Moderately active individuals need a total of approximately 35 kcal/kg body weight per day, while in those who engage in brisk physical exertion for prolonged intervals throughout the day, caloric expenditure may be 40 kcal/kg body weight per day or more. For patients with Type II diabetes who are overweight, significant caloric restriction leading to weight loss over time is most important. Significant caloric restriction is usually successful in lowering plasma glucose even before weight loss is achieved. Depending on the degree of initial hyperglycemia, the degree of obesity, and the amount of weight loss achieved, euglycemia can be maintained in many patients after the decided weight loss has been attained and a eucaloric diet has been initiated. The more recent the diagnosis of Type II diabetes, the more effective diet therapy will be in achieving euglycemia. There are various approaches to achieve weight reduction. A gradual reduction in daily intake of calories is more likely to succeed. Nutritionally sound, modestly restricted hypocaloric diets, such as a 1000- to 1600-calorie diet, depending on age, sex, and physical activity of the subject, achieve slow gradual weight loss over several months and may induce rapid or slow decreases in fasting hyperglycemia. A total caloric deficit of 3500 kcal will lead to a tissue weight loss of 1 lb. For patients with pronounced fasting hyperglycemia, a very low caloric diet such as 300 to 600 kcal/day containing some carbohydrates for 4 to 10 days in hospital may be useful either in achieving rapid control of fasting hyperglycemia or in deciding whether diet therapy alone will be effective as initial therapy. In addition, a very low caloric intake may induce initial rapid weight loss and may be of benefit from the psychologic and motivational point of view.

Protein. A generally accepted protein requirement is 0.8 to 1.0 g/kg a day for adults. The protein content of the diet usually comprises 12 percent to 20 percent of total caloric intake. For restriction of total fat calories of saturated fat (primarily animal fat) and of cholesterol intake, meat exchanges of low fat content should be used. The use of low fat fowl and fish in exchange for red meats should be encouraged several times a week, with limitation of butter, cheese, and eggs. When reduction diets are used, the daily protein intake should not be below 50 to 60 grams per day.

Carbohydrate. In the last 15 years previous recommendations to restrict total carbohydrate to approximately 40 percent of caloric intake have changed to a recommended liberalized carbohydrate intake of 50 to 60 percent of total calories. In the make-up of the carbohydrate portion of the diet, the physician and nutritionist should consider the proportion of complex versus refined carbohydrate, the inclusion of fiber in the diet, and new information about the glycemic responses to different carbohydrates. The major portion of carbohydrate intake should come from complex carbohydrates or starches. It has been conventional to think of complex carbohydrates in terms of bread exchanges, each bread exchange providing 15 g of carbohydrate and giving similar glycemic responses. Recently Jenkins has classified foods on the basis of the glycemic index which is the area under the blood glucose response curve for each food expressed as percentage of the same amount of glucose. The glycemic index for a variety of foods has been given as follows: glucose, 100 percent; sucrose, 59 percent; fructose, 20 percent; corn flakes, 80 percent; All-Bran, 51 percent; porridge oats, 49 percent; white bread, 69 percent; whole meal bread, 72 percent; buckwheat, 51 percent; spaghetti, 42 percent; apples, 39 percent; oranges, 40 percent; orange juice, 46 percent; bananas, 62 percent; milk, 33 percent; ice cream, 36 percent; yogurt, 36 percent; carrots, 92 percent; instant potato, 80 percent, new potatoes, 70 percent; sweet potatoes, 48 percent; butter beans, 36 percent; harricot beans, 31 percent; kidney beans, 29 percent; soya beans, 15 percent; and lentils, 29 percent. Thus, it is apparent that the glycemic response for bread and potatoes is considerably higher than for lentils and pasta. More work needs to be done before precise recommendations can be made in regard to the effects of various carbohydrate-containing foods, taken singly or in combination, on blood sugar excursion in diabetic patients. Sucrose is no longer forbidden as part of the diabetic diet. If taken as part of a mixed meal and divided over several feedings, up to 5 percent of total carbohydrate may be consumed as sucrose. Sucrose in concentrated form when taken by itself, such as the sole nutrient in soft drinks or candy, is still inadvisable. Fructose is a simple carbohydrate which is somewhat sweeter than sucrose and has a substantially lower glycemic index.

Dietary Fiber. An increased fiber content in diets used in the treatment of diabetes can effectively reduce plasma glucose and lipid concentrations and promote satiety. Digestible and undigestible dietary fiber slow gastric emptying and reduce the rate at which the small intestine absorbs nutrients. Useful high-fiber containing foods include brans, unrefined grains, cereals, breads, raw vegetables, and fruits rather than juices. At least 10 to 15 g of high-fiber foods are needed per meal to achieve the desired effects.

Fat. Patients with diabetes mellitus have a greater than normal prevalence of atherosclerosis and hyperlipidemia, indicating a need to reduce fat intake. Since protein and carbohydrate make up approximately 70 percent of the caloric intake, the total fat intake should not exceed 30 percent. The fat intake should be high in polyunsaturated fats and low in saturated fats (not to exceed 10 percent of total daily caloric intake) in an attempt to prevent accelerated macrovascular disease. Ideally, cholesterol intake should not exceed 450 mg/day and should be reduced to 300 mg/day in patients with hypercholesterolemia.

Sweeteners. Fructose may be used as a nutritive sweetener. Saccharin and aspartame are popular non-nutritive sweeteners.

Alcohol. If the patient expresses a wish to use alcoholic beverages in moderation, they may be included in the diabetic diet. It is customary to reduce the patient's fat intake for the calories consumed by alcohol. The caloric value of alcohol is 7 calories per gram. Two ounces of an 80 proof alcoholic beverage will provide approximately 160 calories. Before including alcohol in the diet plan, other potential problems associated with alcohol consumption should be considered.

Distribution, Frequency, and Timing of Meals. In the Type II diabetic patient who is on a weight reduction diet but is not taking oral agents or insulin, the frequency of meals, timing of meals, and distribution of carbohydrate are simple. Calories and carbohydrates may be distributed evenly over three meals or, as shown on line 1 of Table 1, as one-fifth for breakfast, two-fifths for lunch, and two-fifths for dinner. Patients who take insulin should almost always have a bedtime meal. Other insulin-requiring patients may need a midafternoon feeding to prevent hypoglycemia (line 3, Table 1). Patients with unstable diabetes or pregnancy may need feedings as indicated on line 4 of Table 1. Preceding or during periods of exercise, additional carbohydrate-containing snacks or drinks may have to be ingested to avoid hypoglycemia.

Physical Activity and Exercise

Regularity of activity and exercise facilitates blood sugar control in the Type I diabetic patient. Exercise ameliorates glucose intolerance and hyperglycemia in the Type II diabetic patient and may contribute to the weight loss achieved by a hypocaloric diet by increasing energy expenditure. An exercise program must be individualized and adjusted to the ability and physical status of the patient. Daily walking is usually the initial exercise program suggested. Other exercises are added as appropriate. In general, an exercise program is the least quantitative of the therapeutic modalities suggested. Physical acitivity increases sensitivity to insulin, increases caloric expenditure (and thus may contribute to weight loss), improves cardiovascular fitness and decreases cardiovascular risk factors and hypertension, decreases plasma lipids, enhances work capacity, and increases the well-being of the patient. However, there are few published data that document the beneficial effect of exercise in the treatment of diabetes. Increased physical activity is an adjunct and not a substitute for proper nutrition and hypocaloric diets.

TABLE 1 Distribution, Frequency, and Timing of Meals (Calories and Carbohydrates)

Breakfast	*Interval*	*Lunch*	*Interval*	*Dinner*	*Interval*	*H.S.*
1/5		2/5		2/5		
1/6		2/6		2/6		1/6
1/7		2/7	1/7	2/7		1/7
2/18*	1/18	5/18	2/18	5/18	2/18	1/18

* Applicable to patients with unstable diabetes or diabetes and pregnancy

In Type I diabetic patients who are poorly controlled, exercise may exacerbate hyperglycemia and lead to ketonemia. On the other hand, in well-controlled Type I diabetic patients and in some Type II diabetic patients, exercise may lead to hypoglycemia unless the patient prevents this by taking additional carbohydrate or decreases the intake of insulin. On a day of exercise the patient ingests extra carbohydrate feedings prior to and during exercise, depending on the severity of exercise, to counteract increased energy expenditure and more rapid absorption of injected insulin. If extremely strenuous exercise is anticipated, a decrease in the daily insulin dose of 10 to 25 percent would be advised. Self-monitoring of blood glucose has become most useful in helping patients adjust to meal planning and insulin dosage. In both types of patients, exercise may constitute an increased risk of complications of arteriosclerotic cardiovascular disease, angina, myocardial infarction, arrhythmias, and death. Exercise may aggravate certain complications, such as diabetic proliferative retinopathy.

INSULIN THERAPY IN TYPE I DIABETES

In the Type I diabetic patient with absolute insulin insufficiency, partial or total, administration of insulin is essential to prevent hyperglycemia, glycosuria, and ketonemia. The aim of insulin therapy is to mimic as closely as possible physiologic insulin delivery. In the fasting state appropriate insulinization of the liver is essential to prevent excessive hepatic glucose release due to accelerated gluconeogenesis and glycogenolysis. During the day, appropriate delivery of insulin should prevent postprandial hyperglycemia and glycosuria. Thus, insulin should be administered in such a way as to prevent fasting as well as postprandial hyperglycemia. Intermediate-acting insulin or long-acting insulin, particularly if given late in the day, is used to prevent excessive hepatic glucose output in the fasting state. Short-acting insulin given before breakfast and other meals is used to prevent postprandial hyperglycemia. Table 2 provides idealized representations of the time course of action of short-

TABLE 2 Time Course of Action of Insulin Preparations Available in the United States

Insulin Preparation	*Maker*	*Species*	*Approximate Onset of Action*	*Approximate Peak Action*	*Approximate Duration of Action*
Short-Acting Standard					
Regular Iletin I	Lilly	Beef and pork			
Regular Insulin	Squibb-Novo	Pork			
Short-Acting Purified					
Regular Iletin II	Lilly	Pork or beef	15–30 minutes	2–4 hours	5–7 hours
Purified Regular	Squibb-Novo	Pork			
Actrapid	Novo	Pork			
Velosulin	Nordisk	Pork			
Humulin R	Lilly	Human	Slightly shorter than beef and pork		
Actrapid Human	Squibb-Novo	Human			
Intermediate-Acting Standard					
NPH Iletin I	Lilly	Beef and pork			
Lente Iletin I	Lilly	Beef and pork			
Isophane NPH	Squibb-Novo	Beef			
Lente	Squibb-Novo	Beef			
Intermediate-Acting Purified					
NPH Iletin II	Lilly	Pork or beef			
Lente Iletin II	Lilly	Pork or beef			
Purified Isophane NPH	Squibb-Novo	Beef			
Purified Lente	Squibb-Novo	Beef			
Protophane NPH	Novo	Pork			
Lentard—Lente	Novo	Pork and beef	1–2 hours	6–12 hours	16–24 hours
Monotard—Lente	Novo	Pork			
Insulatard — NPH	Nordisk	Pork			
Mixtard—NPH 70%, Regular 30%	Nordisk	Pork			
Humulin N—NPH	Lilly	Human			
Monotard Human—Lente	Squibb-Novo	Human			
Long-Acting Standard					
Ultralente Iletin I	Lilly	Beef and pork			
PZI Iletin I	Lilly	Beef and pork			
Ultralente	Squibb-Novo	Beef			
PZI Insulin	Squibb-Novo	Beef	4–6 hours	12–24 hours	32–36 hours
Long-Acting Purified					
PZI Iletin II	Lilly	Pork or beef			
Ultratard	Novo	Beef			

acting, intermediate-acting and long-acting insulin preparations. Timing of peak action and duration of action pertain to subjects not previously treated with insulin, but may differ in patients with insulin-binding antibodies.

The method of insulin administration can be classified in three ways. In conventional insulin therapy the patient receives one or two doses per day. Intensified conventional insulin therapy consists of multiple daily injections such as three to four injections per day. Continuous subcutaneous insulin infusion with an insulin pump delivers short-acting insulin at a near constant rate during 24 hours with superimposed bolus injections of insulin before meals. A high level of motivation and understanding of diabetes is necessary on the part of both the patient and the physician to institute intensified conventional insulin therapy or continuous subcutaneous insulin infusion. Either of these two programs, and particularly the latter, can normalize 24-hour plasma glucose profiles in selected insulin-dependent patients.

There is tremendous variability in the total dose of insulin required by any patient, depending on whether one is dealing with a newly diagnosed Type I patient or with an established Type I diabetes; the presence of insulin-binding antibodies; the patient's activity level, diet, and environmental stress; and other factors. One can give general directions for total doses that may be used for initiation of therapy to achieve optimal diabetic control, with variations to be instituted depending on need. Newly diagnosed IDDM will need approximately 0.5 units per kg/day, whereas established IDDM patients usually use from 0.6 to 0.7 units per kg/day. Increments and decrements of 2 to 4 units in various timed doses of insulin must be made depending on blood glucose values in the fasting state and following meals. Total insulin dose during pregnancy may be 0.7 units kg/day during the first trimester, 0.8 units kg/day during the second trimester, and 0.9 to 1.0 units kg/day during the third trimester.

Table 3 gives several possible types of insulin regimens employed in increasing order of complexity depending on the need of the patient. Some newly diagnosed Type I diabetic patients, and often for a few years after their diagnosis, can be controlled on a single dose of intermediate-acting insulin a day to control fasting and postprandial hyperglycemia. Most frequently, rapid-acting insulin will have to be added, in the same syringe, to intermediate-acting insulin to prevent postbreakfast hyperglycemia. The true requirement for short-acting insulin does not become apparent until fasting hyperglycemia has been controlled. In most Type I diabetic patients, after one to four years of diabetes, two doses of mixed insulins, one before breakfast and one before dinner, become necessary to prevent fasting hyperglycemia and to prevent postprandial hyperglycemia after breakfast and dinner. The action of a single dose of intermediate-acting insulin is not long enough to prevent fasting hyperglycemia 24 hours after its injection. If increased to sufficient doses to do so, it may cause hypoglycemia in the afternoon, approximately 8 to 9 hours after its injection. Patients who require two or three injections of insulin a day of both intermediate-acting and short-acting insulin usually take approximately two-thirds of their total insulin dose before breakfast and approximately one-third of their insulin dose before supper, or before supper and at bedtime. The example given in Table 4 is a patient requiring 42 units of insulin. In the morning he takes two-thirds of the total or 28 units of insulin. The morning dose is split further into approximately two-thirds as intermediate-acting insulin and one-third as regular-acting insulin. Intermediate-acting and short-acting insulin are given as a mixture in one syringe, 20 to 30 minutes before breakfast. One-third of the total daily dose, or 14 units, is given before supper or dinner. Half of this is given as intermediate-acting insulin and half as regular insulin. In some patients in whom fasting euglycemia is difficult to achieve because intermediate-acting insulin does not have sufficient activity to last from its injection before dinner until the following morning, the evening insulin is split into 7 units of regular insulin before supper to prevent postprandial hyperglycemia and 7 units intermediate-acting insulin given at bedtime to achieve better inhibition of excessive hepatic glucose output. In some extremely labile diabetic patients, four injections of insulin may be necessary to obtain the best control. Ultra Lente or Lente insulin is given at bedtime (and before breakfast) to

TABLE 3 Types of Insulin Regimens

1. Intermediate-acting—once daily	a.c. breakfast
2. Intermediate-acting—twice daily	a.c. breakfast and supper
3. Intermediate-acting mixed with Short-acting	(a) a.c. breakfast (b) a.c. breakfast and supper
4. Intermediate-acting Short-acting	a.c. breakfast and h.s. a.c. breakfast (mixed) and supper
5. Intermediate-acting Short-acting	a.c. h.s. a.c. breakfast, lunch, supper
6. Long-acting—once or twice daily Short-acting	a.c. breakfast and/or supper a.c. breakfast, lunch, supper
7. Continuous subcutaneous insulin infusion	Basal, pre-meal boluses 2 basal modes

TABLE 4 Example of Split and Mixed Insulin Distribution—Insulin Dosage: 42 Units (total)

	Breakfast	*Supper*	*H.S.*
Total:	4/6	2/6	
Total:	28 units 2/3 19 NPH (Lente) 1/3 9 R (Regular)	14 units 1/2 7 NPH 1/2 7 R	
	or		
	19 NPH 9 R	7 R	7 NPH

control the fasting blood sugar level by preventing excessive hepatic glucose output. Regular insulin is given before breakfast, lunch, and dinner to prevent postprandial hyperglycemia. The patient taking the same 42 units of total insulin might receive 12 units of regular before breakfast, 10 units of regular before lunch, 10 units of regular before dinner, and 10 units of lente or ultra lente at bedtime. Usually somewhat more regular insulin is necessary to prevent postbreakfast than the postdinner hyperglycemia.

Rotation of insulin injection sites should be practiced. Absorption is faster from the abdominal region than from the femoral or gluteal region or the arm. Exercise will speed up absorption from the injected limb. Injection into sites of insulin tissue hypertrophy should be avoided.

The physician can ascertain the degree of glycemic control for the preceding 2 months by the determination of the concentration of the glycosylated hemoglobin. This will indicate whether control has been adequate or whether it must be improved. At the time of the follow-up visit, the physician can also as-ascertain fasting and postprandial blood glucose concentrations.

A record of the patient's determination of blood glucose concentrations in the fasting state, 1 to 2 hours postprandially, and/or before meals by self-monitoring of blood glucose will give the best indication of how glycemic control can be improved. If the fasting plasma glucose is elevated, intermediate-acting insulin in the morning, or particularly in the evening or at night, should be increased by 2 to 4 units at a time. If there are large increases in plasma glucose following meals, short-acting insulin before meals should be introduced or increased. If hypoglycemia occurs at night or in the fasting state, intermediate-acting insulin is decreased. If postprandial hypoglycemia occurs, short-acting insulin before meals is decreased. The introduction of interval feedings or snacks may also be used to prevent hypoglycemia between meals.

In general, three types of insulin preparations are available for use (see Table 2). Standard insulins contain impurities and usually are composed of mixtures of beef and pork insulin. They continue to be used for many patients who do not have specific problems, indicating the use of highly purified pork or synthetic human insulins. Beef insulin is more antigenic than pork insulin. Highly purified pork insulin contains concentrations of proinsulins of less than 10 parts per million and frequently less than 1 part per million. Synthetic or semi-synthetic human insulins, Lilly Humulin NPH and Regular, and Squibb-Novo Monotard Lente and Actrapid Regular have the exact amino acid composition of human insulin and are free of proinsulin and other contaminations. The highly purified and human insulins are more expensive than standard insulins. The complications with the use of impure insulin and indications for highly purified pork or synthetic human insulin are insulin lipodystrophy, severe insulin resistance due to insulin antibodies causing large insulin requirements, and insulin allergy. The intermittent use of insulin as during surgery, pregnancy, infection, and stress is an indication for the use of highly purified insulins to avoid enhanced antigenicity. Some patients prefer to use highly purified or human insulin without specific indications for them. In general, to avoid insulin lipodystrophy, purified insulins are used preferentially in new insulin-requiring diabetic patients under the age of 40 years.

TREATMENT OF TYPE II DIABETES

There is general agreement that the most important steps in the treatment of Type I diabetes are the correction of obesity and inactivity. If an adequate trial of dietary modification and increased physical activity fails to achieve normoglycemia, pharmacologic intervention with either oral hypoglycemic agents or insulin should be added to the therapeutic plan. The choice between an oral antidiabetic agent and insulin must be made depending on the particular patient under consideration, including such factors as age, body weight, severity of fasting hyperglycemia, the patient's acceptance of the two pharmacologic modalities, and the patient's motivation and education about diabetes.

Therapy With Oral Agents

Sulfonylurea drugs are the only oral agents available in the United States. Sulfonylureas exert their effect by stimulation of insulin release as well as by potentiation of the action of insulin. This may occur by an increase of activity at athe postreceptor level as well as by an increase in the number of insulin receptors. They may be effective and useful in NIDDM patients whose hyperglycemia is not controlled adequately on diet. However, sulfonylurea drugs are not substitutes for diet in obese or nonobese diabetic patients. Patients are most likely to respond to sulfonylurea drugs if they have had onset of diabetes after 40 years of age, have had known diabetes for fewer than 5 years, have fasting plasma glucose levels below 250 to 300 mg/dl, and have not received insulin or have been well controlled on less than 20 to 40 units of insulin per day. Patients with maturity-onset type diabetes of the young (MODY), a subtype of NIDDM inherited in an autosomal dominant fashion, may have fasting hyperglycemia under the age of 40 and even under the age of 20 years. Such patients do respond to sulfonylureas for decades. In patients who are likely to respond well to sulfonylureas, these drugs may be useful when patients are emotionally or physically incapacitated to take insulin, when they afford greater convenience than insulin injections, and in a few patients with large insulin requirements due to antibodies or allergies to insulin.

Before using an oral antidiabetic agent, contraindications to their use ought to be considered. They are contraindicated in Type I diabetic patients, in Type

II diabetic patients during pregnancy or lactation, in the presence of hepatic and renal disease, and with intercurrent stressful situations such as infection, trauma, or acute myocardial infarction. They are contraindicated in patients with known allergies to sulfonylurea compounds. Although in the 1970s there were major concerns about the safety of oral agents in regard to their being associated with an increased cardiovascular mortality (University Group Diabetes Program [UGDP] Study), sulfonylureas are being used freely in the 1980s since the interpretation of the UGDP data has been questioned by the majority of experts. Nevertheless, the FDA guidelines for the patient package insert carries a required warning that "The patient should be informed of the potential risks and advantages of (name of drug) and of alternate modes of therapy."

The major complication of sulfonylurea therapy is drug-induced hypoglycemia. This occurs most frequently in elderly patients who are not obese, who have a tendency to skip meals, who have impaired hepatic and renal function, and who are treated with long-acting sulfonylurea compounds such as chlorpropamide. Gastrointestinal, hematologic, hepatic, and skin reactions or laboratory changes are infrequent complications.

Table 5 gives the older sulfonylurea preparations as well as two second-generation sulfonylureas which have become available in the United States.

In older patients, and particularly in those with underlying heart disease, chlorpropamide can cause significant water retention and hyponatremia due to potentiation of antidiuretic hormone action at the renal tubular level. An Antabuse-like reaction, i.e., chlorpropamide-alcohol flushing, is seen most commonly with this agent. Tolbutamide may also cause water retention, while Tolazamide, Acetohexamide, Glipizide, and Glyburide have diuretic activity.

In selecting a sulfonylurea agent for therapy, the physician should consider the compound's duration of action, metabolism, side effects, and dosage range; the age and nutrition of the patient; his likelihood of skipping meals; and his cardiovascular status, renal status, and other pertinent history.

The interaction of sulfonylurea drugs with other drugs must be considered in their use. Drugs that may potentiate the action of sulfonylurea drugs are: alcohol, beta-adrenergic blockers, monoamine oxidase inhibitors, phenylbutazone, oxyphenbutazone, clofibrate, bishydroxycoumarin, sulfonamides, salicylates, diphenylhydantoin. Drugs that may antagonize the action of sulfonylureas are: thiazide and loop diuretics, phenytoin, estrogens, glucocorticoids.

The initial dose to be prescribed should not exceed one-half the maximal dose unless the patient is thought to be a marginal candidate for effective therapy with sulfonylureas. The dose should be increased every week or two until satisfactory glycemic control or the maximum dose is reached. A patient who does not respond to sulfonylureas initially is called a primary failure. When glycemic control is achieved initially with an oral agent and then this control is not maintained, the patient is considered a secondary drug failure. The percentage of patients who do not respond to sulfonylurea therapy depends on the selection of patients and their degree of adherence to a prescribed therapeutic program. Occasionally a patient responds to a second agent when the first one tried has not resulted in satisfactory glycemic control.

At present there are no well-established indications for the combination of sulfonylurea therapy and insulin.

Insulin Therapy in Type II Diabetes

When dietary modification and increased physical activity fail to achieve satisfactory control, and pharmacologic therapy with an oral agent is either contraindicated (as already discussed) or fails to achieve the desired results, the use of insulin is demanded. The principles for insulin therapy in Type II diabetes are similar to those in Type I diabetes. However, since in Type II diabetic patients, residual insulin secretory capacity is present, and labile or unstable diabetes is

TABLE 5 Characteristics of Sulfonylurea Agents

Generic Name	*Trade Name*	*Daily Dosage Range (g)*	*Duration of Action (hr)*	*Dose/Day*	*Metabolism*
Tolbutamide	Orinase	0.5–3.0	6–12	2–3	By liver to inactive product
Tolazamide	Tolinase	0.1–1.0	10–14	1–2	By liver to active and inactive products
Acetohexamide	Dymelor	0.25–1.5	12–18	1–2	By liver to active metabolites
Chlorpropamide	Diabinese	0.10–0.5	60	1	By liver to less active metabolites and excreted by kidney intact. Also see text.
		(mg)			
Glipizide	Glucatrol	5.0–40	12–24	1–2	
Glyburide-Glybenclamide	Diabeta Micronase	2.5–20	12–24	1–2	By liver to inert products

not present, most Type II diabetic patients can be controlled on one, or at most two, doses of insulin. Patients with mild or moderate fasting hyperglycemia may be adequately controlled with one injection of intermediate-acting insulin before breakfast. In patients with more pronounced fasting hyperglycemia, signifying greater insulin secretory defect, mixtures of intermediate-acting and short-acting insulin may be necessary. Although some obese patients with Type II diabetes who require relatively large doses of insulin (60 to 100 units) may be well or adequately controlled with a single dose of insulin, the majority of patients who require 60 units or more of insulin can be better controlled with two doses of insulin. Particularly in obese patients with insulin resistance, large doses of insulin, i.e., well in excess of 100 units per day, may be required for adequate control. If insulin is given in appropriate doses, whatever the requirement of insulin, almost all patients with Type II diabetes can be controlled. Nonadherence to diet, however, may make this difficult. After initiation of insulin therapy the patient may experience an increase in appetite, gain weight, and become more insulin-resistant, which may lead to further fasting hyperglycemia and increasing insulin requirement.

Insulin therapy is essential in Type II diabetic patients during pregnancy or during acute metabolic stress such as injury, infection, or surgery, when sulfonylurea compounds in addition to diet fail to achieve metabolic control or if there is allergy to sulfonylurea compounds.

MANAGEMENT OF DIABETES DURING SURGERY

The objectives of the management of diabetes before, during, and immediately after an operation are to prevent excessive hyperglycemia and glycosuria, to prevent ketosis, and to prevent hypoglycemia. Fluid and electrolyte balance and adequate intake of carbohydrate calories in the form of intravenous glucose solutions on the day of surgery and postoperatively are given to avoid starvation ketosis. Insulin therapy should be continued in the insulin-dependent or insulin-requiring diabetic, or initiated in the diet-treated or diet-plus-sulfonylurea-treated patient in the presence of significant hyperglycemia.

There are many possible ways in which to administer insulin to the surgical patient. One way is to give, on the morning of surgery, approximately one-half of the usual total dose of insulin as a long-acting insulin preparation and to cover each liter of glucose solution with 10 to 15 units of short-acting insulin in the infusion fluid, depending on total insulin requirements and severity of stress. Supplemental doses of short-acting insulin can be given as necessary. Intravenous insulin infusion ensures systemic delivery during circumstances of possible decreased absorption of subcutaneously given insulin (hypotension, shock) and allows control over the speed of its administration.

Suggested Reading

Schiffrin A. Treatment of insulin-dependent diabetes with multiple subcutaneous insulin injections. Med Clin North Am 1982; 66:1251–1267.

Skyler JS. Self-monitoring of blood glucose. Med Clin North Am 1982; 66:1227–1250.

The Physician's Guide to Type II Diabetes (NIDDM): Diagnosis and Treatment. American Diabetes Association, 1984.

DIABETIC KETOACIDOSIS

DANIEL W. FOSTER, M.D.

Diabetic ketoacidosis is the end stage of acute decompensation in patients with insulin-dependent diabetes mellitus. It is induced by a rise in the glucagon:insulin ratio, which can be produced either by omission of insulin or by the presence of physical or emotional stress. The latter mechanism operates primarily through release of glucagon and the other catabolic hormones: catecholamines, cortisol, and growth hormone. These hormonal changes cause the two major pathophysiologic events: hyperglycemia, which leads to osmotic diuresis and volume depletion, and metabolic acidosis due to the overproduction of acetoacetic and beta-hydroxybutyric acids from long-chain fatty acids passing to the liver from adipose tissue stores. Large deficits of potassium and phosphate accompany the acidosis and osmotic diuresis, although initial plasma levels of both may be high. Other metabolic abnormalities, such as elevated triglycerides, are not of major clinical import and reverse with treatment of the primary condition.

Ketoacidosis can also be seen in the absence of diabetes in certain alcoholics, with prolonged fasting in pregnancy, and in the postpartum state when nursing mothers are calorically deprived. These conditions represent exaggerated starvation ketosis and usually are easily reversed by intravenous glucose with or without a small amount of insulin. Diabetic ketoacidosis, on the other hand, is a serious complication which can be fatal.

Diagnosis of ketoacidosis usually is not difficult. Since many intercurrent illnesses are accompanied by inability to eat, the presence of ketones in the urine is not sufficient to distinguish starvation ketosis from true ketoacidosis. If the plasma ketones (measured semiquantitatively by serial dilution using reagent sticks) are strongly positive at a dilution of 1:1 or higher, it is likely that total ketone concentrations are in the ketoacidotic range. The differential diagnosis includes the following anion gap acidoses: renal failure, lactic acidosis, and poisons such as ethylene glycol or methyl alcohol (most often seen in alcoholics).

PREFERRED TREATMENT

The treatment of diabetic ketoacidosis requires administration of fluids, insulin, glucose, and potassium. Phosphate and bicarbonate are optional (Table 1).

Fluids

Sodium chloride, 0.9 percent, or lactated Ringer's solution is given intravenously immediately on admission. If cardiac function is not impaired, I administer the first liter very rapidly (30 to 60 minutes), with subsequent rates determined by response. Three to 5 liters of saline usually are required in the first 24 hours, the first 3 over the initial 6 to 8 hours. Restoration of the extracellular fluid volume and stimulation of urine flow lowers plasma glucose by dilution, by urinary excretion, and by decreasing counterregulatory hormone release even in the absence of insulin. Dextrose (5%) is usually added when the plasma glucose reaches the 250 to 300 mg/dl range in an attempt to forestall osmotic disequilibrium in the central nervous system and the appearance of cerebral edema. It also provides free water as glucose is metabolized. The dextrose should be given by separate infusion as dextrose in water and not added to the saline solution (to avoid hypertonicity). Occasionally, severe hyperosmolality accompanies ketoacidosis; in such circumstances 0.45 percent saline may be given after the initial 1 to 2 liters of 0.9 percent saline is administered.

Insulin

I prefer to give insulin intravenously in larger doses than are popular throughout the country. I use an initial bolus of 50 units of regular insulin followed by 20 units per hour by constant infusion. (NPH and Lente insulin should never be used in diabetic emergencies.) As the pH rises, infusion rates may be slowed to 10 units per hour. In my opinion this approach is safer than low-dose insulin schedules since significant insulin resistance is present in a small, but not unimportant, fraction of patients suffering from diabetic ketoacidosis. Under no circumstances should less than 10 units per hour be given. Insulin should be continued until the urine (not plasma) is free of ketones. If ketones remain in the urine it is a sign that the liver is still activated for ketogenesis. The reappearance of any stress (e.g., fever or chills, hypoglycemia) may then reinitiate ketoacidosis by mobilization of free fatty acids. It is a common mistake to stop or slow insulin when the plasma glucose falls without considering the state of ketosis.

Extreme insulin resistance is a rare phenomenon. It may occur in patients previously treated with insulin because of the appearance of insulin antibodies in high titer. Occasionally, profound resistance occurs in women with androgen excess (e.g., polycystic ovary syndrome) or in the context of collagen vascular disease. In the former case, insulin receptors are markedly diminished; in the latter, autoantibodies against the insulin receptor block access of insulin to the binding site. The possibility of insulin resistance should be entertained if acidosis remains unchanged after 4 to 6 hours of routine treatment. Insulin dosage should be briskly increased at this point to a hundred or more units per hour. If there is no response over the next 2 to 3 hours, the hourly dose should be jumped again. On rare occasions, more than 50,000 units of insulin have been required. Commercial solutions of U-500 insulin should be used under these circumstances. Life-threatening insulin resistance should also be treated with high-dose glucocorticoids (e.g., 60 to 100 mg prednisone) against the possibility that anti-insulin or antireceptor antibodies are present. Short-term steroids are not a significant risk in the diabetic subject.

TABLE 1 Typical Treatment Sequence in Diabetic Ketoacidosis

1. Draw complete blood chemistries on admission; repeat full chemistries q2h.; monitor capillary glucose and urine at bedside every 30 minutes.
2. Regular insulin 50 units by IV bolus, 20 units per hour IV until urine is free of ketones.
3. Rapid infusion of 1 liter of 0.9% saline or Ringer's lactate over 30 to 60 minutes; 3 to 5 liters of saline over first 24 hours.
4. Start glucose infusion when plasma glucose falls to 250 to 300 mg/dl
5. Infuse potassium salts when plasma potassium is 4.0 mEq/liter (care required if urine output is low).
6. Give bicarbonate only if pH is less than 7.0.

Potassium and Phosphate

Potassium is always needed in the treatment of ketoacidosis. Although initial plasma levels are usually high, total stores in the body are depleted. Once glucose metabolism is re-established and the plasma pH begins to rise, potassium shifts rapidly into cells. Failure to give potassium at this time can result in fatal cardiac arrhythmias. Potassium levels should be checked on admission and repeated every 2 hours during the acute phase of treatment. I start potassium intravenously at a rate of 40 mEq/hour when the plasma K^+ concentration is 4.0 mEq/L. (Slower infusion rates are used if urine flow is not adequate.) Although recovery is not influenced by provision of phosphate, I usually give potassium initially as the phosphate salt (40 to 100 mM). Potassium is usually required about the third or fourth hour into treatment, but if the initial value is 4.0 mM or below, potassium needs to be given within the first hour.

Bicarbonate

The use of bicarbonate is controversial. I given sodium bicarbonate if the initial pH is less than 7.0 and stop when the pH is 7.2. Usually 50 to 100 mM is all that is required, provided other treatment is optimal. Severe acidosis should be treated because it can cause vascular collapse in and of itself, especially when accompanied by volume depletion.

Nonroutine Measures

Although leukocytosis is common in ketoacidosis, fever is not and strongly suggests the presence of infection. If fever is present and the patient is very ill, antibiotics should be given until cultures are returned, even if a site of infection is not identified. Septicemia and gram-negative infections are not rare in ketoacidosis. If pain resembling sinusitis and bloody nasal discharge is present, the ketoacidosis-associated infection, mucormycosis, should be considered. Treatment requires amphotericin B. Acute gastric dilatation can occur and requires nasogastric suction if present. Because of this possibility, patients with ketoacidosis should not be fed. Erosive gastritis may occur and cause significant bleeding. Treatment is no different from that required in nondiabetic subjects. Intravascular thrombosis is not uncommon. The most important prophylaxis is the administration of fluids, but it may be useful to give 325 mg acetylsalicylic acid on arrival to blunt platelet aggregation. Late cerebral edema is a rare problem usually seen in children. It is often fatal. Appearance is heralded by worsening stupor or coma after initial improvement with or without neurologic, cardiovascular, or respiratory signs. Diagnosis is confirmed by CT scan. Treatment involves administration of mannitol 1 g/kg body weight as an intravenous bolus (20% solution). Although of questionable benefit, dexamethasone can be given simultaneously—12 mg initially, then 4 mg *q6h*. If there is no response, hyperventilation to a P_{CO_2} of 28 should be carried out by an anesthetist in an attempt to reduce cerebral blood flow.

Monitoring Therapy

It is important to keep careful written records during therapy. The flow sheet should have columns for insulin, fluids, potassium, phosphate, blood chemistries, urine volume, urine ketones and glucose, and vital signs. Capillary blood glucose and urine glucose and ketones should be measured at the bedside every 30 minutes initially. Plasma glucose, sodium, potassium, bicarbonate, chloride, and BUN or creatinine should be measured at 2-hour intervals until it is clear that the patient is responding to therapy, after which the frequency can be decreased. The best early sign of response is narrowing of the anion gap since bicarbonate usually stays low for a number of hours. The anion gap is calculated as follows: anion gap = $[Na^+ + K^+] - [Cl^- + HCO_3^-]$. The usual course is a rise in bicarbonate to only 12 to 14 mM while the gap progressively narrows to normal due to a replacement of ketone anions by chloride. The pH also rises with effective therapy and may be normal in the face of a low bicarbonate. As noted above, insulin should be continued (covered by glucose infusion) until the urine is ketone-free. Clues to complications are shown in Table 2.

TABLE 2 Clues of Complications of Diabetic Ketoacidosis

Complication	*Clues*
Acute gastric dilatation or erosive gastritis	Vomiting of blood or coffee-ground material
Cerebral edema	Obtundation or coma with or without neurologic signs, especially if occurring after initial improvement
Hyperkalemia	Cardiac arrest
Hypoglycemia	Adrenergic or neurologic signs; rebound ketosis
Hypokalemia	Cardiac arrhythmias
Infection	Fever
Insulin resistance	Unremitting acidosis after 4–6 hours of adequate therapy
Myocardial infarction	Chest pain, appearance of heart failure; appearance of hypotension despite adequate fluids
Mucormycosis	Facial pain, bloody nasal discharge, blackened nasal turbinates, blurred vision, proptosis
Vascular thrombosis	Stroke-like picture or signs of ischemia in non-nervous tissue

Suggested Reading

Alberti KGMM, Hockaday TDR. Diabetic coma: a reappraisal after five years. Clin Endocrinol Metab 1977; 6:421–455.

Clements RS Jr, Vourganti B. Fatal diabetic ketoacidosis: major causes and approaches to their prevention. Diabetes Care 1978; 1:314–325.

Foster DW, McGarry JD. The metabolic derangements and treatment of diabetic ketoacidosis. N Engl J Med 1983; 309:159–169.

Kreisberg RA. Diabetic ketoacidosis: new concepts and trends in pathogenesis and treatment. Ann Intern Med 1978; 88:681–695.

HYPEROSMOLAR, NONKETOTIC COMA

GEORGE F. CAHILL Jr., M.D.

The treatment of the typical patient with hyperosmolar coma requires knowledge of its pathogenic origin. The classic patient is elderly, has documented or undiagnosed diabetes, and has some recent additional process such as bronchopneumonia, urinary tract infection, cholecystitis, or a myocardial infarction. This intercurrent process diminishes his or her already limited insulin secretion and inhibits insulin's peripheral effects, the result being progressive hyperglycemia leading to the hyperosmolar state. Early there may be some polyuria, which also leads to hyperosmolarity by dehydration. Also required for the process to occur is an underlying diminished renal function, most frequently senile nephrosclerosis, which occurs in all elderly individuals to a greater or lesser degree. Should renal failure be so severe that glycosuria is minimized, severe hyperglycemia can appear without any other gross clinical symptoms or signs, and the patient may gradually lapse into coma for no apparent reason.

Hyperosmolar coma can also appear in otherwise previously healthy individuals in association with severe infection or trauma, in which case the renal failure component is essentially prerenal due to blood or other fluid loss, and with sufficient adrenergic suppression of endogenous insulin release. This often occurs with severe major trauma, particularly large burns, especially if the subject is given glucose and water intravenously without proper monitoring and is then literally pushed into hyperosmolar coma by the attending physicians or surgeons.

PREFERRED TREATMENT

The First Hour

In the treatment of all acute emergencies and all unconscious patients, rapid precise diagnosis is required. The unconscious or semiconscious patient suspected of being in hyperosmolar coma should rapidly be cannulated with a large-bore needle, well-positioned and capable of conducting appropriate volumes of fluid. If no adequate vein can be found, a cutdown is indicated. The blood is then sampled at bedside for glucose, using one of the currently available test tapes or sticks, and also for the presence or absence of ketoacids. A value on the top of the color chart for glucose and negative for ketoacid or perhaps trace-positive corroborates the diagnosis; however, blood samples should be sent off to the laboratory for definitive diagnosis as well as determination of other parameters.

The large-bore needle is then connected to a liter of isotonic saline solution, which is rapidly administered (10 to 20 ml/minute), since the highest priority is to maintain effective vascular volume, meaning extracellular volume. Assuming that the initial physical examination and history had been completed rapidly, a more definitive investigation is now in order. Careful physical and neurologic examinations, hematologic studies, and emergency radiologic examination are done at this time to unmask the triggering factor or factors. During this period, the laboratory will be processing the various tests initially requested, and of these, probably the most important are the repeat blood glucose determination to check the bedside value and the bicarbonate level to rule out a severe acidosis such as lactic acidosis or ketoacidosis.

Of next importance is the serum potassium, particularly when insulin therapy is being considered. Performance of an arterial puncture for blood gases and placement of a central venous line to monitor venous pressure might be of help. The typical patient has a blood glucose of 600 to 1000 mg/dl, an increase of approximately 30 to 50 milliosmolar; a slightly reduced bicarbonate value of about 18 to 22 due to the mild renal failure; and perhaps minimal lactic acid and ketoacid increases. The blood urea nitrogen is usually about 40 to 60 mg/dl. The syndrome can occur in children with glucose levels as low as 400 mg/dl, and conversely, values over 2000 mg/dl have been reported in some cases in adults; thus the levels of glycemia are variable.

Again, it should be emphasized that small amounts of ketoacids can be found and, in fact, there is a complete spectrum. On one end is the diabetic in ketoacidosis in its pure form, as seen in the youngster acutely insulin-deficient and with normal renal function who might have glucose levels in the 200 to 300 mg/dl range in the presence of severe ketonemia. On the other end of the spectrum is the elderly dehydrated patient with classic hyperosmolar coma in its pure form with no detectable ketoacids and only extreme hyperglycemia. At both ends of the spectrum there may be variable degrees of lactic acidosis. Thus, some patients may have a mixture of hyperosmolar coma and lactic acidosis, others a mixture of diabetic ketoacidosis and lactic acidosis, as occasionally seen in diabetic alcoholics, and still others may have components of all three, namely, severe hyperglycemia, modest ketoacidosis, and modest lactic acidosis. Fortunately, however, the initial therapy for all three is identical: intravenous isotonic saline administered rapidly into an easily accessible vein or cutdown.

Hours 2 Through 12

Assuming one is dealing with the classic patient with hyperosmolar, hyperglycemic, nonlactic acidotic, nonketotic coma, saline itself may be sufficient to reverse the process without any other therapy. Replenishment of fluid volume may simply permit the endogenous insulin to again capture glucose homeostasis, and blood sugar may gradually fall back toward normal levels. Some physicians urge that this initial mode of therapy be used alone and insulin be avoided in order to prevent too rapid a fall in blood glucose, which would result in major and dangerous fluid shifts (to be described), leading to other more severe problems such as vascular collapse or cerebral edema. Ideally, then, with the second liter of saline now running at the end of an hour, if the initial blood glucose had been 800 mg/dl and now after 1 to $1^1/_2$ hours of therapy a value of 700 mg/dl were obtained, saline might be the only therapy necessary, at least for the present. By the second or third hour, another 100 mg/dl fall might be considered to be right on schedule, and the hope is that over the next 8 to 12 hours, the glucose value might gradually fall to 200 mg/dl after 3 or perhaps even 4 liters of saline. However, in the elderly patient one has to be alert to overloading the individual and producing congestive failure.

One might ask why saline alone in the initial therapy when common sense would state that the loss of water had been greater than the loss of electrolyte and therefore hypotonic solutions should be the fluids of choice. As mentioned above, vascular collapse due to the loss of the osmotic effect of the high glucose value leading to diminished extracellular fluid volume is one complication to be avoided, as is a too rapid a shift of fluid from the extracellular to the intracellular space, particularly into the brain. Thus, isotonic saline, at least for the first 2 liters, is the fluid of choice, and can be followed by more hypotonic solutions. Should the patient be alert, simply drinking free water is the safest and most physiologic fluid therapy. Some have suggested that a nasogastric tube could be inserted in many for this purpose at or near the start of therapy once a diagnosis has been made.

If elevated glucose levels persist at the end of 2 hours and after as many liters of saline have been infused, insulin can be administered. Experts differ in how this should be given, some prescribing 10 units infused over 1 hour, others recommending a simple bolus of 5 or 10 units of insulin, and some suggest both. However, the patient should be closely monitored since the response to the insulin may be extremely variable from case to case. In some it may be ineffective and therefore a second bolus or infusion of 10 to 20 units may be necessary for the succeeding hour; in most, the insulin produces a rapid fall in blood glucose. Too rapid a fall should be detected and corrected by administering solutions made up of equal volumes of isotonic saline and isotonic glucose. Such a solution would still be isotonic, but would effectively administer free water as the glucose is metabolized and prevent the blood glucose level from falling too rapidly. Once the blood glucose level approaches 200 to 300 mg/dl, glucose-containing solutions must be administered again to prevent the fluid shifts described above, and to prevent hypoglycemia. Oral fluids such as juices may be safely administered if the patient is alert.

Use of Insulin

If insulin is administered, no matter how small the dose, the potassium level should be watched closely, both by hourly determinations of its level in the serum and by repetitive precordial electrocardiograms to monitor T-waves. If the initial potassium (on admission) was in the normal or low range, a situation in which one would expect mild hyperkalemia, small amounts of potassium can be administered in the intravenous infusion, but with caution in case of renal failure. Forty milliequivalents of potassium per liter of saline or 40 milliequivalents of potassium given per hour, for the first 2 hours, is a reasonable dose; if the initial phosphate level had been normal or depressed, potassium could be given as the phosphate salt in solution. If there had been a more moderate degree of renal failure and phosphate levels were elevated, then potassium can be given as the chloride.

Other Treatment and Supportive Therapy

Usually, some other process has triggered the event, and the hyperosmolar coma is really a secondary process. Thus the white count, blood cultures, cardiograms, roentgenograms, and other diagnostic measurements should be carefully evaluated to be sure one is not overlooking a major process. Other supportive therapy, such as oxygen, antibiotics, and cardiac drugs, may be in order. Not mentioned so far has been catheterization of the urinary bladder, and it is my opinion that this should never be done as a routine procedure unless there is evidence of a distended bladder, in which case the catheterization is indicated urologically and not medically. My reason is that any finding in the urine would not alter the initial therapy to any great degree, and if urine can be obtaied without catheterization the patient might be spared subsequent urinary tract infection. Obviously, if there has been a history of incontinence, frequency, or pyuria, this anti-catheter stance could be reversed.

Finally, another word of caution: elderly diabetics who are taking sulfonylureas can occasionally lapse into protracted hypoglycemia and present in the emergency ward unconscious with a history not unlike that of the patient with hyperosmolar coma. Although they lack the dehydrated ill-appearing look of the latter, this entity should not be forgotten and, of course, the bedside glucose and corroborating laboratory glucose values can simplify the differential diagnosis.

Suggested Reading

Arieff AE, Carroll HJ. Nonketotic hyperosmolar coma with hyperglycemia: clinical features, pathophysiology, renal function, acid-base balance, plasma-cerebrospinal fluid equilibria and the effects of therapy in 37 cases. Medicine 1972; 51:73–94.

Feig PU, McCurdy DK. The hypertonic state. N Engl J Med 1977; 297:1444–1454.

Feig PU. Hypernatremia and hypertonic syndromes. Med Clin N Amer 1981; 65:271–290.

Gennari FJ. Serum osmolality. N Engl J Med 1984; 310:102–105.

Podolsky S. Hyperosmolar nonketotic coma: death can be prevented. Geriatrics 1979; 34:29–42.

DIABETIC NEUROPATHY

EDWARD C. LaCAVA, M.D.
JEFFREY B. HALTER, M.D.
EUGEN HALAR, M.D.
DANIEL PORTE Jr., M.D.

Diabetic neuropathy has been a clinically recognized syndrome for well over a hundred years, yet even today our understanding of its pathophysiology, progression, and therapy is incomplete. Rather than being one disease process, diabetic neuropathy represents several processes with distinct syndromes, some due to defects in neural carbohydrate metabolism and others due to vascular impairment.

Onset of signs and symptoms of any one of these syndromes, with the notable exception of acute mononeuropathies (which correlate with vascular disease), is rarely correlated with any one characteristic (e.g., polyol pathway abnormalities, degree of glycemic control, myoinositol levels, duration or type of diabetes, or degree of vascular impairment). In fact, neuropathy may be the only presenting sign at first diagnosis of diabetes mellitus.

Diabetic neuropathy is perhaps best divided into three separate categories: first, diffuse symmetric peripheral polyneuropathy; second, diffuse diabetic autonomic nervous system (ANS) involvement; and third, other diabetic neuropathies, which include the acute mononeuropathies, radiculopathy, amyotrophy, and diabetic neuropathic cachexia.

DIFFUSE SYMMETRIC PERIPHERAL POLYNEUROPATHY

This disorder is a generalized, sensorimotor polyneuropathy most commonly of insidious onset. The initial symptoms are in the distal extremities, with legs and feet affected more often than arms and hands. Subsequent proximal progression, over months to years, is the rule. With time, some patients develop symmetric muscle atrophy and weakness in the distal extremities. The loss of sensory symptoms may lead to other complications such as painless arthopathy (Charcot joints), plantar foot ulcerations, and predisposition to secondary infection. Patients typically describe varying degrees of associated pain (both sharp and dull) and a tingling and burning sensation, sometimes greatest at night. A clinical neurologic exam usually demonstrates symmetrically decreased perception of pinprick, temperature, light touch, and vibration in the distal extremities and diminished or absent reflexes (usually ankle first). However, the correlation between symptoms and objective measures of nerve function in diffuse symmetric peripheral polyneuropathy can be very poor.

Clinical symptoms of neuropathy are very common both in patients with insulin-dependent diabetes mellitus (IDDM) and in those with noninsulin-dependent diabetes mellitus (NIDDM). The onset of symptoms and their severity are generally related to the duration of diabetes, although this relationship may be quite variable. Objective measures of nerve function, such as nerve conduction velocity, are abnormal in most, if not all, diabetics regardless of whether clinical symptoms are present. This objective evidence of nerve dysfunction can be demonstrated early in the course of diabetes.

The progression of diabetic peripheral polyneuropathies is considered at present to be irreversible, although intermittent apparent improvement of some of the symptoms is often seen. Diabetic autonomic neuropathy is also believed to be characterized by this same progression. It is also becoming clear that other types of diabetic neuropathies (i.e., radiculopathy, amyotrophy) may coexist. The lancing asymmetric pains that many patients describe may be due to other diabetic neuropathies superimposed on previous symmetric peripheral disease.

Although the pathogenetic mechanisms of diabetic peripheral polyneuropathy are not clearly known, it is likely that the principal mechanism is metabolic rather than vascular in nature. It remains uncertain at present which combination of biochemical abnormalities—sorbitol accumulation from increased polyol pathway activity, loss of intracellular myoinositol, neuronal membrane defects, or axonal protein transport problems—results in the presentation of clinically demonstrable peripheral neuropathy.

Of importance prior to beginning a treatment program in these diabetics is a careful historical review to exclude additional causes of peripheral symmetric polyneuropathy, such as exposure to toxins including heavy metals (i.e., arsenic, lead, gold, mercury), drugs (vincristine, diphenylhydantoin, isoniazide, hydralazine), solvents, or organophosphate compounds. Metabolic disorders which must be ruled out include B-vitamin deficiences, uremia, hypothyroidism, amyloidosis, and chronic alcoholism. Inflammatory diseases (such as polyneuritis, sarcoidosis, syphilis, or leprosy) and familial peripheral neuropathy syndromes (rare) must also be considered as additional causes of peripheral neuropathy.

Although there have been several new avenues of study over the past few years, there is no specific treatment currently available to arrest or reverse diabetic neuropathy, and most of our efforts as practitioners have been directed at daily patient foot care, neuropathic pain management, and blood glucose control. Foot care is extremely important as neuropathy, vascular disease, and infection are interrelated.

Since approximately 50 percent of all nontraumatic amputations in this country are in diabetics and probably half of these could have been prevented, it is important to recognize that impaired sensory perception may lead to unrecognized trauma either from extremes of temperature or poorly fitting shoes. Poor attention to injury may lead to serious infections and occasionally loss of limb. All diabetics should be strongly urged to examine their feet and hands daily, and the clinician should reinforce this instruction by including an examination of both the hands and feet at every office visit.

The approach to pain management in diabetic neuropathy remains an area of therapy meeting variable success, with many drugs used on a trial and error basis. The approach to the management of symptomatic pain involves several medications. The most frequently employed are phenytoin (Dilantin), 100 to 300 mg daily, and carbamazepine (Tegretol), 200 mg initially, gradually increasing to 800 mg daily in two divided oral doses. Logic for usage relates to their known benefit in suppressing abnormal epileptiform neuronal discharge and to a presumed additional effect on peripheral nerves, as is seen in pain management of trigeminal neuralgia with carbamazepine. Other drugs frequently employed include amitriptyline (Elavil), 25 to 100 mg orally at bedtime; fluphenazine (Prolixin) 1 to 3 mg orally, sometimes in combination with amitriptyline, at bedtime; and diazepam (Valium), 2 to 5 mg orally one to three times daily. As with all medications, effort should be made to keep the dose to the minimally effective level and to carefully monitor for side effects by periodic laboratory tests. In their usual therapeutic dose range, all of these drugs have met with variable success. If there is no response within 10 to 14 days, the test drug is unlikely to be of benefit and should be discontinued. Often the associated pain is so severe that use of narcotic analgesics may be necessary as a treatment of last resort. We recommend beginning with acetaminophen (Tylenol) with codeine prior to other, stronger analgesics.

In addition to attempting strict glycemic control, there are a few new medications in investigative trials directed at specific metabolic causes of diabetic neuropathy. These are the aldose reductase inhibitors (e.g., Sorbinil), which block the intracellular production of sorbitol, and dietary myoinositol supplementation. Neither of these approaches can be recommended at this time until further positive results of controlled clinical trials are reported. Since improvement of motor nerve conduction velocity has been documented with improved glycemic control, it seems reasonable to recommend, when possible, tight glycemic control for patients instructed in home glucose monitoring. However, it should be emphasized that the relationship between degree of hyperglycemia and the development and/or severity of neuropathy has not been defined. Thus, it is not yet clear whether tight glycemic control is more effective than standard management as an approach to this complication of diabetes. Symptomatic improvement has been reported by many diabetics following periods of good glycemic control.

DIABETIC AUTONOMIC NEUROPATHY

Neuropathy affecting the autonomic nervous system (ANS) is often an insidious process which does not lead to clinical signs until the impairment of ANS function is severe. Subclinical ANS dysfunction is probably very common.

Orthostatic Hypotension

Impaired function of the parasympathetic (vagal) innervation of the heart may be one of the earliest signs of autonomic neuropathy and may often be asymptomatic. However, this abnormality may become clinically significant, eventually resulting in a fixed resting tachycardia and abnormal cardiac response to postural changes or exercise. Patients with moderate-to advanced cardiovascular diabetic autonomic neuropathy often complain of sudden dizziness, weakness, nausea, and/or lightheadedness with occasional syncopal episodes.

The definition of orthostatic hypotension is arbitrary, but can be said to be present when there is a drop of 20 mmHg or more of the diastolic arterial pressure from supine to sitting upright (or standing), when measured every 2 minutes up to a maximum of 10 minutes' duration. Before ascribing this syndrome to diabetic autonomic neuropathy, we rigorously eliminate other important etiologies. The most common potentially reversible causes are volume depletion and drug-induced states of orthostatic hypotension. Any factor that leads to intravascular volume depletion will worsen the underlying tendency to postural hypotension.

Treatment may be difficult and usually involves three different approaches. Symptomatic relief is often obtained by:

1. Mechanical support measures such as fitted support hose (Jobst stockings) and commercially available antigravity suits.
2. Plasma volume expansion, by use of high sodium diet (>6 g/day) and/or medications with sodium-retaining effects such as 9 α-fluorocortisone (Florinef). The dose required for clinical response to Florinef (0.1 to 0.4 mg per day) is often quite high. Slow titration usually provides clinically symptomatic improvement and minimizes the potentially severe complications of *supine hypertension*, hypokalemia, and/or congestive heart failure. Occasionally, indomethacin (Indocin), up to 150 mg per day in divided doses, has been used.
3. Other medications, such as phenylephrine (intranasal), have been tried with limited success. In addition, pindolol (Visken), a beta-adrenergic antagonist with partial intrinsic sympathomimetic (agonist) activity, in divided doses from 10 to 15 mg orally per day, has been of reported benefit in

several empiric trials. Clonidine (Catapres) has also been found to be of some paradoxic benefit, with the dose titrated (0.1 to 0.4 mg per day) for therapeutic effect. The last three medications are experimental and should be undertaken in a controlled setting in which the patients blood pressure can be closely followed for judgment of response to a clinical trial.

Gastroesophageal Dysfunction

Gastric reflux (heartburn), nausea, vomiting, anorexia, and/or a bloated sensation are common clinical presentations. Combined abnormal esophageal motility and gastroparesis diabeticorum are believed to be principally secondary to parasympathetic (vagal) denervation. Diagnostic work-up is necessary to exclude other problems, either intrinsic to the gastrointestinal tract (GI) or systemic in nature. Prolonged gastric-emptying time can pose problems for glycemic control in insulin-treated diabetics because the delayed and irregular emptying of the stomach makes glycemic effects of meals unpredictable. Changing the dietary plan to multiple small meals per day may be of some help. Metoclopramide (Reglan) appears to be useful on the basis of enhancing tissue responsiveness to acteylcholine and/or dopaminergic inhibition. If symptoms are severe, initial parenteral or intramuscular administration may be helpful to insure drug availability. Otherwise, 10 mg orally approximately 30 minutes before meals and at bedtime may be effective. Bethanecol (Urecholine), 25 mg orally three to four times daily, can be tried if metoclopramide fails.

Diabetic Diarrhea

Lower intestine diabetic ANS involvement is characterized by diarrhea, often nocturnal or postprandial, and usually without warning. Other etiologies of diarrhea should first be eliminated by standard work-up. In fact, a proportion of diabetics with diarrhea are thought to have bacterial overgrowth due to small bowel stasis from abnormal motility. Such cases generally respond to broad-spectrum antibiotic therapy (e.g., tetracycline, 250 mg orally four times daily for approximately 7 to 10 days). Symptomatic relief for diabetic diarrhea, usually a transient syndrome, is probably best achieved by the opiate-like antidiarrheals, Lomotil and loperamide (Imodium).

Loperamide, probably the more effective of the two, is given as 4 mg (two capsules) initially, followed by 2 mg (not to exceed a daily total of 16 mg) after each loose stool, usually resulting in clinical improvement within 48 hours.

Genitourinary Diabetic Autonomic Dysfunction—Diabetic Neurogenic Bladder

The diabetic neurogenic bladder is a late finding clinically, heralded by the onset of symptoms of urgency, overflow incontinence, and difficulty voiding which develops as progressive failure of detrussor and sphincter function occurs, causing urinary retention. Complications, such as urinary tract infections, ureteral reflux with possible hydroureter and hydronephrosis, as well as pyelonephritis and decreasing renal function, may result from neuropathic bladder dysfunction.

In addition, examination should be performed to exclude prostatic disease or phimosis in men and descensus of the bladder (cystocele) in women. Once a diabetic neurogenic bladder has been diagnosed, immediate short-term (1 to 2 weeks) catheterization may be necessary if there is significant urinary retention. This often helps to restore bladder tone. All urinary tract infections, after appropriate laboratory culture and sensitivity testing, should be treated. Subsequently, bladder training (using intermittent catheterization, by patient and nurse) every 3 to 4 hours is performed and gradually replaced by Credë and Valsalva. The addition of bethenechol (Urecholine), a parasympathomimetic agent, can be given in a dose of 20 to 50 mg orally four times daily as a helpful adjunct. If medical therapy fails, surgical bladder neck resection (which simply eliminates resistance of the vesical outlet internal sphincter) is necessary. Retrograde ejaculation is a complication of this surgery.

Impotence

Impotence is a common problem in diabetic men. Those affected commonly complain of slowly progressive inability to achieve satisfactory erection despite intact libido and ejaculatory capacity. A careful history, physical examination, and appropriate laboratory screen for other endocrine causes are important to the assessment of this problem, since it may involve both psychic and organic components. Open communication with the patient and spouse regarding all aspects of work-up and therapy remain particularly important, as well as the routine review of sexual history with all diabetic men, with special emphasis on potentially aggravating drugs (usually antihypertensives).

Insertion of a penile prosthesis in the appropriately selected patient is often successful and has been met by wide acceptance. There are three basic types, each consisting of a pair of silicon rods implanted within the two corpora cavernosa: (1) chronically semierect (Small-Carrion), flexible (least expensive); (2) malleable (containing a silver wire within the rods which retains the shape in which last positioned); and (3) inflatable/deflatable rods with subcutaneous storage well (most expensive).

OTHER DIABETIC NEUROPATHIES

Acute Mononeuropathies/Radiculopathy

Of all the forms of diabetic neuropathy, the acute mononeuropathies appear to have the most clear-cut mechanism: localized thrombosis or ischemia of a nerve. The most common presentations are the acute extraocular muscle palsies, involving principally cranial nerves III, IV, and VI, alone or in combination with each other. These lesions are characteristically abrupt in onset, sometimes occurring with localized sharp pains along the nerve pathway, and are followed by a self-limited course of paralysis of approximately 5 to 12 weeks' duration, usually with spontaneous resolution.

Truncal mononeuropathies, although readily defined by a *careful* neurologic examination (revealing their dermatome-like distribution), have been commonly mistaken for a variety of medical and surgical emergencies (e.g., angina pectoris and acute myocardial infarctions, renal colic, appendicitis, acute cholecystitis). The electromyogram may be of limited help, only on a retrospective basis, in the diagnosis. Two additional and important causes of severe, sharp pain, similar to that of acute mononeuropathies, are the early dermatomal distribution of pain preceding the lesions of herpes zoster and the unilateral or bilateral pain which may be the only early sign of an epidural abscess.

Generally, a conservative approach serves best, with adequate explanation to the patient and reassurance that the overwhelming majority of acute mononeuropathies resolve spontaneously.

Amyotrophy

Amyotrophy is a syndrome of *asymmetric* pain and proximal muscle weakness, typically involving the muscles of the pelvic girdle and proximal thigh. It is most often seen in older men with mild diabetes and is reversible after a few months' duration. Reasons for this progressive atrophy and weakness remain unclear. In the presence of diabetes, this syndrome generally has few other causes and it is generally quite rare.

Diabetic Neuropathic Cachexia

Unexplained profound weight loss, peripheral sensory neuropathy, pain, and associated depression describe this syndrome in elderly noninsulin-dependent diabetic (NIDDM) men. Because of the striking presentation, many patients are at first thought to harbor occult malignant disease. Typically, in accordance with the original description, there is spontaneous recovery within 12 to 18 months. The relationship of this condition to a possible associated major endogenous depression needs further study. This syndrome may coexist with acute painful neuropathy with either lower limb or truncal involvement or may occur with diabetic amyotrophy.

DIABETIC RETINOPATHY

LAWRENCE I. RAND, M.D.

Diabetic retinopathy, a major complication of diabetes, is treated primarily by someone other than the endocriology and metabolism specialist. Future proof of a definitive role of metabolic control in preventing or delaying retinopathy may change all that, but at present all known effective means of therapy are in the hands of the ophthalmologist. Since this volume does not address ophthalmologists, it would be of limited value to discuss here the ophthalmologist's role in the treatment of diabetic retinopathy. Perhaps of more value, and certainly more unique, would be a discussion, from this ophthalmologist's perspective, of what the role of the internist, endocrinologist, and metabolism specialist is in the treatment of this common complication of a very common disease, for which they provide care in most other aspects.

RETINOPATHY DETECTION MECHANISMS

The job of the metabolic specialist is to ensure that no diabetic patient develops severe retinopathy or loses sight from retinopathy without having the opportunity of receiving timely therapy from a qualified ophthalmologist. The patient must be informed about the importance of regular eye evaluations, examined on a regular basis, and referred at the appropriate time to a single or several ophthalmologists known to be interested in diabetic eye disease. Close attention must be paid to the ophthalmic follow-up given to each patient.

Diabetic retinopathy is the leading cause of new blindness in adults aged 20 to 74. A significant proportion of these patients have become blind unnecessarily—because they did not receive sightsaving laser photocoagulation in time. All too frequently, a patient first visits the ophthalmologist after hemorrhage into the vitreous has already caused loss of vision. Although many of these eyes can still be saved, the optimal time for treatment is before any sight is lost, when the patient may be asymptomatic but warning signals are detectable on ophthalmoscopy. It is the responsibility of the person caring for the patient's diabetes to know what is going on in his patient's eyes because early assessment and timely intervention should markedly reduce blindness from diabetes.

A most important foundation for establishing a follow-up and referral pattern is a thorough knowledge of the natural history of the disease. Diabetic retinopathy eventually affects just about all persons with diabetes. Over time, retinal blood vessels—in particular the capillaries—become incompetent. They swell, forming microaneurysms; they leak blood, lipids, and proteins; and they may close down completely, depriving the retina of needed oxygen and nutrients. The process usually begins focally, but may become diffuse and involve a large portion of the retina. No one knows what aspect of diabetes initiates this process. It could be hyperglycemia; it could be hypoinsulinemia; it could be something entirely different. It is quite clear, though, that at a certain stage, the course of the disease represents a retinal reaction to damage and probably proceeds independent of the diabetes itself.

Diabetic retinopathy is usually divided into two stages: nonproliferative diabetic retinopathy (NPDR), a less severe form, and proliferative diabetic retinopathy (PDR), the chief cause of blindness in patients with diabetes. Lesions in a third grouping, preproliferative diabetic retinopathy (PPDR), while usually considered part of NPDR, will be discussed separately because of their clinical importance.

The retinal changes described here vary in degree of visibility. They are easiest to detect when fundi are examined through a dilated pupil. A physician who knows what abnormalities to look for, however, will be able to find many of them even when looking through an undilated pupil. Fortunately, some of the most ominous signs (e.g., optic disc neovascularization) are often observable in time for referral and treatment.

STAGES OF DIABETIC RETINOPATHY

Nonproliferative Diabetic Retinopathy (NPDR)

Almost all people with diabetes develop some retinopathy. Its earliest manifestations are usually microaneurysms, which are small outpouchings in the vessel walls visible as red dots on fundus examination. Small, roundish, deep intraretinal "dot-and-blot" hemorrhages are also characteristic.

Microaneurysms and dot-and-blot hemorrhages are present in some patients after 5 to 7 years of diabetes and after 20 years, almost all diabetic patients have these lesions. Some lesions are remarkably stable; while others may come and go over periods of months and years. The rare patient with no evidence of retinopathy after 35 to 50 years of diabetes may well have experienced some minimal degree of it previously.

I like to refer to this very early stage of NPDR as "background diabetic retinopathy" (BDR) to highlight its ubiquitous occurrence and lack of prognostic significance. The term BDR has previously been used synonymously with NPDR, but over the past few years I have found the term increasingly less useful and now prefer to use a more restrictive definition. This usage is not uniformly accepted, however.

Hard exudates near the macula and macular edema, which often occur together, are the most common cause of visual impairment from diabetes, particularly in older patients. Macular edema is a thickening of the retina with some loss of macular transparency, although this is difficult to see. The hard exudates are readily visible as waxy yellow deposits that tend to form rings or partial rings.

Vision in eyes with macular involvement is distorted, but usually not reduced below 20/200, and can fluctuate in the 20/40 to 20/100 range for long periods. Macular edema without hard exudate is fairly typical of younger patients and may be a sign that significant retinal damage is taking place. Any macular involvement warrants referral of the patient to an ophthalmologist, preferably an expert in diabetic retinal disease. (Nonmacular hard exudates are usually asymptomatic and need cause no concern unless extensive, in which case they may represent a different problem that warrants referral.)

At present, there is no commonly accepted treatment for macular exudates and edema. Lipid-lowering agents, such as Atromid-S, to treat exudates were once popular, but are not recommended because of equivocal benefits and reported adverse side effects. Laser treatment of macular edema is currently being evaluated in the Early Treatment Diabetic Retinopathy Study (ETDRS), a multicentered clinical trial sponsored by the National Eye Institute. After two years of follow-up, that study has not yet reported its results.

Transitional and Preproliferative Diabetic Retinopathy (PPDR)

Some lesions, while usually classified as BDR, in its broader sense, probably represent a more advanced degree of retinopathy. This group includes soft exudates ("cotton-wool spots"), venous caliber abnormalities ("beading" or a "link-sausage" appearance), arteriolar abnormalities (white threads, as those seen in hypertension), and intraretinal microvascular abnormalities (IRMA), which appear as irregular and tortuous retinal vessels. The first occurrence of these lesions (usually soft exudates or IRMA) places an eye into a new category of retinopathy. These eyes, which correspond to P1 retinopathy classification used in multicentered studies such as the ETDRS, are now in a transitional stage of retinopathy. Some eyes remain rather stable for many years and only then gradually develop further changes. Other eyes, however, can rapidly progress. Only regular follow-up can distinguish between these two groups. Certain combinations of these lesions, along with more extensive degrees of intraretinal hemorrhages, are frequently referred to as preproliferative diabetic retinopathy (PPDR).

Although not all eyes with PPDR develop PDR, these eyes are at significant risk for proliferative disease. In fact, when lesions characteristic of PPDR are seen, PDR may already be present. The appearance of transitional or particularly preproliferative retinopathy is indication for referral to an ophthalmologist.

Another lesion of diabetic retinopathy, more common than previously thought, is optic disc edema. It is often asymptomatic and detected on routine examination; its course is usually benign—most cases resolve spontaneously over a period of months with no apparent residual. A few, however, seem to occur with, or just preceding, neovascularization of the optic disc (a form of PDR), so that ophthalmologic referral is recommended as a precaution. (Neurologic evaluation may also be advisable if edema is bilateral, as it is not easily distinguishable from papilledema.)

Eyes with transitional and PPDR are being treated by photocoagulation as part of an ETDRS experimental protocol, but photocoagulation is not yet standard therapy.

Proliferative Diabetic Retinopathy (PDR)

The latest to appear and most dangerous stage of retinopathy is marked by proliferation of new blood vessels outside the retina. This phase may occur in as many as 60 percent of diabetics by the time they have diabetes for 40 or more years. It usually develops following extensive capillary closure and may represent an abortive attempt by the eye to revascularize an ischemic retina. Whereas in NPDR, pathology is generally within the retina, in PDR, a network of convoluted new vessels grows over the retinal surface and onto the posterior vitreous. In additon, the walls of these vessels are thin and "leaky," likely to rupture and bleed. Should the vitreous contract, as it frequently does in diabetics, these fragile vessels are pulled forward, causing bleeding into the preretinal space or vitreous gel. Patients may experience small hemorrhages as "cobwebs" or "floaters" in the field of vision. Large hemorrhages cause a sudden, painless loss of vision.

Vitreous or preretinal hemorrhage in the presence of neovascularization, particularly on the optic disc (NVD), places an eye at great risk of severe visual loss, even if vision is good at the time. If new vessels cover more than one-third of the disc, even in the absence of hemorrhage, that eye is also at high risk. These high-risk characteristics carry a 25 to 40 percent risk of severe visual loss over 2 years, and in most cases, demand prompt photocoagulation, which reduces the risk by about 60 percent. Lesser degrees of PDR may be treated, but because of risks associated with photocoagulation it may be prudent to treat one eye and postpone treatment of the other until high-risk characteristics develop.

Photocoagulation halts retinal neovascularization before repeated hemorrhages into the vitreous cause their devastating damage. Most eyes go through an active phase of disease, characterized by new vessel growth and possible recurrent vitreous hemorrhages, and, after a period of several years, may go into remission. Photocoagulation may accelerate this cycle, bringing about an early remission while vision is still preserved.

Remission

PDR is usually followed, after a time, by the proliferation of fibrous tissue, signalling remission. Unfortunately, this process is not without hazards. The fibrous tissue usually develops along abnormal vessels, but may also spread between retina and vitreous and over the posterior vitreous surface. When fibers contract, they may wrinkle the retina; anterior-posterior traction can drag it forward, causing retinal detachment.

Until the development of closed vitrectomy by Machemer about 10 years ago, eyes with diabetic retinal detachment or massive vitreous hemorrhages could not be treated effectively. In the vitrectomy procedure, a small instrument inserted into the eye nibbles and sucks away the blood-filled vitreous and membranes while simultaneously infusing clear fluids. The bloody gel is thus removed and traction on the retina released, restoring sight to a significant proportion of eyes.

The major risk of vitrectomy is neovascular glaucoma, which occurs in as many as 25 percent of cases. It is characterized by new blood vessel growth on the iris (rubeosis iridis) extending into the filtration angle and blocking drainage of fluid from the eye. Neovascular glaucoma may occur in eyes that have not had vitrectomy, especially those with extensive new vessel growth or a long-standing retinal detachment. Once full-blown glaucoma develops, little can be done to save the eye, but laser treatment for neovascularization may abort its development. Vitrectomy may also lead to iatrogenic retinal tears, which require immediate treatment.

Following the period of fibrous proliferation, most eyes eventually enter a full remission phase, known as involutional or quiescent diabetic retinopathy. It is characterized by thinned retinal arterioles, a pale optic nerve head, and wispy, fibrous proliferation frequently extending into the vitreous. If central vision has not been destroyed during the active phase, it may be quite good for many years, though electrophysiologic activity may gradually deteriorate. Eyes in remission following photocoagulation behave similarly, and though they may require periodic retreatments, many have retained 20/20 vision for more than 15 years with no further problems. In addition to knowledge of retinopathy itself, a good background in how retinopathy may relate to other demographic and medical factors is of great value.

RISK FACTORS

Our knowledge of the causes and determinants of retinopathy is fairly rudimentary, but certain associations have been documented and may be helpful in clinical practice. Duration of diabetes is the most well-established factor. Juvenile-onset (insulin-dependent) patients rarely develop serious problems before 15 years of diabetes and almost never before 10 years. Those who develop diabetes at an older age may develop significant retinopathy after 5 to 10 years. We usually recommend yearly evaluation by an ophthalmologist after 5 years in juveniles and shortly after onset in adult-onset patients. This recommendation is rather ambitious, and a delay of several years would not miss a large number of serious but asymptomatic patients.

Other factors that may identify patients at risk of developing PDR are joint contractures in young patients and pregnancy in patients who already have some retinopathy. Both these patient groups should be quickly referred to an ophthalmologist. The presence of hypertension or diabetic complications such as neuropathy or renal disease should also alert the physician to possible PDR. Approximately 50 percent of PDR patients have accompanying renal disease. If renal disease (proteinuria) is not present at the time PDR is diagnosed or within the next year or two, it is unlikely to develop.

A knowledge of how ophthalmologists experienced in diabetes examine and treat patients should be helpful in selecting an ophthalmologist for your diabetic patient.

OPHTHALMIC EXAMINATION AND TREATMENT

Examination

A complete ophthalmic examination for diabetic retinopathy by an ophthalmologist should include a best corrected visual acuity, slit-lamp examination, intraocular pressure measurement, and direct and indirect ophthalmoscopy. At least the last two should be done at each subsequent visit. Contact lens biomicroscopy of the vitreous and macular region of the retina is frequently included, and is necessary for detection of subtle macular edema. Important adjuncts to the clinical examination are fundus photography and fluorescein angiography. Stereo photography of seven standard areas of the retina and, recently, wide-angle photography significantly improve on the diagnostic capabilities of the clinical examination and provide an invaluable permanent reference. Fluorescein angiography can also add significantly to the clinical examination, but except in certain special circumstances, it does not add enough to warrant its routine use, considering its invasiveness and the possibility of serious allergic reactions. We currently reserve fluorescein for research purposes and for identification of leakage points prior to treatment for macular edema. Many capable ophthalmologists, however, use angiography considerably more frequently.

For the nonophthalmic specialist, examination should include a history, covering areas such as blurred vision lasting more than a day or so and not associated with changes in blood sugar, floaters, or flashing lights, or sudden loss of vision in one or both eyes. Examination should be direct ophthalmoscopy, if possible through a dilated pupil. Once a patient has been examined and dilated by an ophthalmologist, there is little chance that future dilation would precipitate an acute angle closure attack, unless a narrow angle configuration has been found. In the nonretinopathic or BDR patient, a yearly examination by an ophthalmologist with interim examinations by the physician treating the diabetes should provide optimum follow-up. The examination should focus on two principle areas: the optic disc and the macula. If the presence of new vessels on the optic disc (NVD) is ruled out, this eliminates the most frequent cause of severe visual loss, while the absence of edema or exudates threatening the macula eliminates the most common cause of less severe visual loss. Scanning the vascular arcades and the area between them superiorly, inferiorly, temporally, and nasally should identify areas of new vessels elsewhere (NVE). Early microaneurysms may first appear in the area temporal to the macula or nasal to the disc. Soft exudates and venous abnormalities frequently occur nasal to the disc. A good examination with the direct ophthalmoscope through a dilated pupil should provide a large proportion of the information available on the status of the diabetic retina, and should be able to rule out all but peripheral neovascularization. It should become part of the armamentarium of anyone providing overall care for diabetic patients. Physicians who would prefer not to dilate pupils or even examine eyes, could opt for more frequent ophthalmologic evaluations, or might look into nonmydriatic fundus cameras.

Photocoagulation

This term refers to the use of light to destroy tissue. In diabetes, the tissue being destroyed is retina, and the modalities used are xenon arc white light, and argon or krypton laser. Both xenon-arc and argon laser were proved effective in treating PDR by the DRS. Argon laser is used in the vast majority of treatments, primarily because of ease of application. Krypton laser, a new red laser which penetrates blood, has been used recently to treat eyes when adequate argon photocoagulation is not possible due to vitreous hemorrhage or other opacities. While most people assume that krypton will be as effective as other photocoagulation modalities, and our clinical impressions are that it is effective, since it has not been tested for effectiveness against argon, the proven therapy, it should not be substituted for argon in clear media cases routinely.

At this time, photocoagulation is routinely applied to eyes with high-risk characteristics. Treatment consists of 1200 or more burns placed one-half burn diameter apart, avoiding the macula, papillomacular bundle, optic disc, and major vessels, and extending out to the equator. Application of only 100 to 200 burns at a time several weeks apart may not be effective and should not be considered acceptable therapy unless there are extenuating circumstances. Treatment is usually applied in two to four sessions, and may require retrobulbar anesthesia. Unfortunately, not all photocoagulation is the same. If you look into the eye of a patient who has received panretinal photocoagulation, the entire retina except the area around the macula should be covered by burns. Focal treatment of macular edema, a treatment whose efficacy is being tested at present, can involve considerably less treatment, confined to the macular region. Treatment to macular ring exudates should be aimed at the center of the rings. To be sure your patients are receiving the accepted forms of therapy, know the background and capability of your local ophthalmologists and select those most interested and best trained in diabetes to treat your patients. Any ophthalmologist may be capable of applying expert photocoagulation treatment, but the most expert have usually received subspecialty training in retinal surgery or retinovascular disease.

Vitrectomy

When photocoagulation fails to stem the course of retinopathy and recurrent vitreous hemorrhage or a traction detachment of the macula develops, vitrectomy surgery may become necessary. Surgery is usually not performed unless hemorrhage has been present for several months, or detachment actually involves or imminently threatens the fovea. The Diabetic Retinopathy Vitrectomy Study (DRVS) is currently investigating vitrectomy in eyes before hemorrhage or detachment occurs, as well as the timing of vitrectomy once hemorrhage does occur. Numerous instruments are available to perform surgery, each with its own advantage. It is difficult surgery, and results are not uniformly good. With increasing timely photocoagulation, fewer diabetic eyes are undergoing vitrectomy than 5 years ago. Decreasing volume results in less total experience for vitrectomy surgeons in a community. It would probably be of value to send patients to those with the greatest diabetic vitrectomy experience, who are open and straightforward about their results. If they do not know their results, perhaps it would be a useful, if not humbling, experience for them to have them tabulated.

Counseling and Support

Although the most important task from a medical standpoint is probably assuring timely referral and treatment, possibly almost as important for the patient's overall well-being is the ability of the endocrinology and metabolism specialist to integrate the patient's ocular status with all the other components that make up this complicated disease. The way in which patients are told they have retinopathy and what meaning they should place on it in the overall spectrum of things can be very important.

For the specialist to find minimal diabetic retinopathy (BDR) in a patient after 10 years of diabetes is important, but certainly much more so for the patient than the physician. Since no treatment is indicated, the patient may have to be watched more closely. From the patient's point of view, this is something he has been dreading for the past 10 years. This disease, which to this point has been a major nuisance, may just be getting the best of him. What did he do wrong? What did his physician do wrong? Does he need laser treatment? How long before he needs one of those white canes? All these questions and many more are going through his mind, and no matter how hard an ophthalmologist may try to play down the seriousness of the problem, he is likely to be less successful than the patient's own physician in allaying these fears. He should be told that after 10 years of diabetes, most people with the disease may have some evidence of retinopathy, and that no one is at fault. What's more, at this level his risk of ever developing vision-threatening retinopathy probably has not been increased. However, closer follow-up is indicated, as is referral to an ophthalmologist. The reassurance that there are no significant changes in his kidney or nerves and that his current regimen for managing his diabetes is reasonable, should provide the patient with the support he needs at this time.

In addition to the first development of retinopathy, other major landmarks appear to be the development of PDR or a need for laser treatment, and the development of vitreous hemorrhage or other vision-affecting event. Each of these can have a devastating effect on the patient. In fact, we have recently uncovered a significant association between metabolic control and negative life events in patients with PDR and/or laser, but not in patients without PDR. How the patient reacts to these events can influence the ability of the ophthalmologist to treat and can directly affect how the patient responds to that treatment.

Suggested Reading

The Diabetic Retinopathy Study Research Group: Preliminary report on effects of photocoagulation therapy. Am J Ophthalmol 1976; 81:383–396.

The Diabetic Retinopathy Study Research Group: Photocoagulation of prolifertive diabetic retinopathy. The second report of Diabetic Retinopathy Study findings: Ophthalmology 1978; 85:82.

Klein R, Klein BE, Moss SE, Davis MD, DeMets DL. The Wisconsin epidemiologic study of diabetic retinopathy. II. Prevalence and risk of diabetic retinopathy when age at diagnosis is less than 30 years. Arch Ophthalmol 1984; 102:520–526.

Rand LI. Recent advances in diabetic retinopathy. Am J Med 1981; 70:595.

INSULIN ALLERGY AND INSULIN RESISTANCE

C. RONALD KAHN, M.D.

INSULIN ALLERGY

Clinical Syndromes

Although insulin provides lifesaving therapy for patients with type I diabetes mellitus and is a useful adjunct to the therapy of many patients with type II diabetes, almost all individuals exhibit some immune response to injection of the protein antigen. With the introduction of more purified preparations of porcine insulin in the United States in 1980 and the addition of human insulin in 1983, these complications of diabetes therapy have become relatively rare. However, allergic reactions have still been observed in patients receiving human or purified pork insulins, and in patients in whom these reactions occur, the clinical features can be dramatic and the management difficult.

The most common clinical manifestations of the immune response to insulin are local and generalized urticaria. Local cutaneous reactions to insulin usually occur within 6 months after the initiation of insulin treatment, but occasionally do not appear until several years after institution of therapy. The reaction may consist simply of a stinging, burning, or itching sensation at the site of injection or may be accompanied by local swelling, erythema, induration, and wheal formation. Local reactions usually occur immediately after injection and subside rapidly, but in some patients their appearance is delayed. These delayed reactions may progress to painful local induration that persists for 2 or 3 days. Up to 50 percent of patients with insulin allergy give a history of allergy to other drugs, particularly penicillin.

Systemic allergic reactions are rare, but generalized responses—such as serum sickness, purpura, angioedema (with or without respiratory compromise and shock), or an Arthus phenomenon with LE cells, eosinophilia, and hypergammaglobulinemia—have been observed in some patients. About 50 percent of patients with systemic insulin allergy have a history of insulin treatment that was interrupted and then reinstituted.

Certain patients develop changes at the site of insulin injections consisting of either an increase or a decrease in subcutaneous fat. Although the exact pathogenesis of these lipodystrophies is unclear, they are probably unusual manifestations of immune reactions to insulin or pharmacologic reactions to impurities in the insulin preparation, since both occur much less frequently in patients receiving purified insulins, and patients who have already developed these reactions often improve when therapy is changed to purified insulins. In general, lipoatrophy is observed more commonly in children and young women within the first few months of insulin therapy. Lipohypertrophy is said to occur more frequently in males.

Diagnosis and Treatment

The diagnosis of insulin allergy is basically a clinical diagnosis. Skin tests with insulin are positive in up to 80 percent of patients with histories of insulin allergy and are useful in identifying the most and least antigenic insulin. In most cases, the skin test shows an immediate reaction, but about 10 to 15 percent of patients also show a delayed reaction. The presence of insulin allergy can be confirmed by analysis of IgE antibodies against insulin, but this test is usually available only at research centers.

To approach the therapy of insulin allergy rationally, it is necessary to understand some of the antigenic features of the insulin molecule as well as the methods used to evaluate the immune response. Insulin is a polypeptide hormone composed of two chains joined by two disulfide bonds. The A-chain has 21 amino acids, the B-chain has 30. The major variations in structure occur in the region between the intrachain disulfide bridge of the A-chain (A8, 9, 10) and in the carboxy-terminal region of the B-chain, particularly the B-30 residue (Table 1). Human and porcine insulin are identical except for substitution of alanine for threonine at position 30 of the B-chain, whereas beef insulin differs from human insulin in positions 8 and 10 of the A-chain, as well as position 30 of the B-chain. It is not surprising, therefore, that beef insulin is more antigenic than pork insulin, which is slightly more antigenic than human insulin. Most of the standard commercial insulin used in the United States is still a mixture of beef and pork insulins and thus provides a significant antigenic stimulus in susceptible individuals.

In addition, insulin preparations obtained by pancreatic extraction may be contaminated with small amounts of other peptides. These include proinsulin, the single-chain precursor of insulin, as well as other peptide hormones, such as glucagon, pancreatic polypeptide, vasoactive intestinal peptide, and somato-

TABLE 1 Approach to Therapy of Insulin Allergy or Insulin Resistance

Change to a less antigenic form of insulin
Human insulin
Monocomponent pork insulin
Sulfated insulin
Fish insulin
Desalanine pork insulin
Desensitization
Immunosuppressive therapy
Prednisone
Other

statin. Antibodies to these noninsulin contaminants, especially proinsulin and pancreatic polypeptide, which differ greatly in sequence from species to species, have been identified in significant numbers of insulin-treated patients. Over the past several years, the concentration of these impurities has been substantially reduced by means of chromatographic and ion-exchange processes. Human insulin made by recombinant DNA techniques obviously is not contaminated with such peptides, but probably contains other very minor contaminants from the bacterial fermentation process or denatured molecules which inevitably occur in the processing protein samples.

Other factors may also play a role in the immunogenicity of insulin. These include the pH of the mixture, the zinc content, and the nature of the insulin preparation (long-acting forms of insulin are more immunogenic than rapid-acting forms). Finally, individuals with certain HLA types appear to be more likely to develop an exaggerated immune response to insulin, particularly those with HLA types A2, BW44, DR4, and DR7.

Management of patients with abnormal immune response to insulin depends on the degree and nature of the immune response and the necessity for insulin treatment. In a few patients with insulin allergy, a careful history reveals that the skin irritation results from faulty, i.e., intradermal, injection of insulin or improper cleansing or use of syringes. In others the reaction is mild, consisting of only local swelling or soreness. Such reactions frequently subside spontaneously, and no treatment is necessary. In many obese, type II diabetic patients, insulin may be discontinued, and the patients may be managed by dietary restriction with or without concomitant oral hypoglycemia agents. This should not be done, however, if the patient is likely to need insulin at some later time since intermittent insulin therapy predisposes to more severe allergic reactions.

In patients in whom insulin must be given, the simplest approach to therapy is to switch to a more purified, single-species insulin. A skin test containing beef, pork, and human insulins is available from Eli Lilly and Company, and skin testing may help in the selection of the least antigenic insulin. In almost all cases, this is either human insulin or single-component pork insulin. Changing from beef-pork to purified pork or human insulin results in an improvement in insulin allergy in up to 70 percent of patients. Other less antigenic insulins are listed in Table 2. Of these, sulfated insulin is also effective since it has a low degree of immunogenicity, but it is currently commercially available only in Canada.

TABLE 2 Differences in Amino Acids of Mammalian Insulins

Insulin	*A-Chain (α-loop)*			*B Chain*
	Position 8	Position 9	Position 10	Position 30
Human	Threonine	Serine	Isoleucine	Threonine
Pork	Threonine	Serine	Isoleucine	Alanine
Beef	Alanine	Serine	Valine	Alanine

Simultaneous injection of an antihistamine, such as diphenhydramine (Benadryl or equivalent), has been used successfully in some patients; the antihistamine can even be mixed in the same syringe with the insulin. Some antihistamines, however, such as methapyrilene hydrochloride (Histadyl), are not compatible with insulin.

When these methods fail, desensitization should be undertaken. If possible, the patient should be taken off insulin for a short while and the allergic reaction allowed to subside before desensitization is begun. Skin testing using serial ten-fold dilutions allows one to determine the least antigenic insulin and the highest concentration of insulin that does not cause an immediate wheal and flare response. Desensitization is begun with this amount of insulin administered subcutaneously (occasionally the first few doses are given intradermally). The dose of insulin is then progressively doubled and administered at 30-minute intervals until therapeutic doses are achieved. If allergic symptoms appear during desensitization, a more gradual increase in dosage can be used. Antihistamines may be added to suppress allergic symptoms, but should be avoided if at all possible. Conventional insulin therapy is instituted after desensitization using the species of insulin selected for desensitization.

INSULIN RESISTANCE

Clinical Syndromes

Insulin resistance may be said to exist any time a given concentration of insulin produces a less-than-normal biologic response. Insulin resistance is a common feature of non-insulin-dependent forms of diabetes. In these patients, the resistance is usually manifested by normal or impaired glucose tolerance accompanied by increased levels of endogenous insulin. Insulin resistance is also a relatively rare complication of insulin therapy. Excluding patients with known causes of tissue resistance to insulin action, such as obesity, infection, and steroid excess, insulin resistance occurs in about 0.01 percent of insulin-treated patients. In most of these patients, insulin resistance represents the development of anti-insulin antibodies. Since the average rate of secretion of endogenous insulin in the adult is between 20 and 60 U per day, any patient who requires more than 60 U per day has at least some degree of insulin resistance. For practical reasons, however, most patients are not considered significantly insulin-resistant unless their daily dose of insulin exceeds 150 U or, for a child, 2 U/kg body weight.

In addition to the accompanying clinical features, major clues to the underlying cause of the resistance are the duration of insulin therapy and the insulin dose required. Patients with tissue resistance to insulin action, owing to defects in the insulin receptor or insulin action at the cellular level, are resistant from the initiation of therapy. In these patients, the degree of insulin resistance is quite variable, but in the extreme examples, insulin requirements exceed 2000 and even 100,000 units of insulin per day. In patients with anti-insulin antibody, the duration of insulin treatment before the onset of insulin resistance ranges from one month to 15 years. Commonly, there is a history of intermittent or interrupted insulin treatment. The amount of insulin required for treatment may be high, but seldom exceeds 2000 units per day. In about 25 to 35 percent of patients with insulin antibodies, there is also a history of insulin allergy.

Diagnosis and Treatment

The differential diagnosis of the cause of the insulin resistance ultimately depends on reliable measurements of anti-insulin antibodies, and, when available, assays of insulin receptors and antireceptor antibodies. Virtually every patient treated with commercial mixtures of beef-pork insulin develops some insulin-binding antibodies within a few months, and thus quantitative estimates of antibody are required. The concentration of such antibodies in noninsulin-resistant patients, as measured by binding capacity, rarely exceeds 5 U of insulin per liter of plasma. Most patients who require insulin in excess of 100 U per day due to anti-insulin antibodies have significantly higher binding capacities. Since there are many causes of insulin reistance, laboratory confirmation of high-titer insulin antibodies is useful in patients with suspected immunologic resistance. Abnormalities in the cellular response to insulin should be suspected in all patients with insulin resistance and low titers of insulin antibodies. In the absence of assays for insulin receptors or receptor antibodies, these patients can often be identified by the clinical syndrome they present.

Treatment of the insulin resistance must be directed at the underlying cause. In patients with cellular causes, treatment includes weight reduction in obese patients, ablation of the pituitary gland or adrenal glands in patients with acromegaly or Cushing's disease, and immunosuppression in patients with antireceptor antibody.

Insulin resistance due to anti-insulin antibodies tends to be a self-limited disorder that spontaneously remits in about 60 percent of patients within 6 months. Treatment of these patients, therefore, should be directed primarily at prevention of metabolic complications associated with insulin resistance. Three general approaches in therapy have been used. As with insulin allergy, the first is a change to a less antigenic form of insulin. Since most insulin antibodies have a lower affinity for pork or human insulins than beef insulin, switching to porcine monocomponent insulin or human insulin should be the first therapeutic maneuver attempted. The latter results in a decrease in insulin requirement in about 50 percent of the patients with high-titer insulin antibodies. This has little or no immediate effect in the other 50 percent of these patients, who have antibodies that cross-react among all insulins, and no effect in patients with cellular resistance to insulin action. Sulfated insulin (when available) is even more effective in patients with immunologic insulin resistance. On average, when switched to sulfated insulin, patients with insulin resistance require only 15 percent of their former insulin dose, and this will fall even further as the antigenic stimulus is removed and the antibody titer falls. In some patients with insulin resistance, changing from U-100 to U-500 insulin has also resulted in decreased insulin requirements. The mechanism of this effect is unknown.

In the patient who does not respond to a change in insulin, but has high-titer anti-insulin antibodies, treatment with glucocorticoids may be useful. The patient should be started on high doses (60 to 80 mg prednisone per day). This will result in a decreased insulin requirement in up to 75 percent of patients, usually within a few days. The individual response is erratic and unpredictable, however, and side-effects from steroid treatment are prominent. Thus, the dosage should be tapered as rapidly as possible (usually in 2 to 3 weeks) and discontinued when the patient is no longer resistant to insulin. Cytotoxic drugs, such as cyclophosphamide and 6-mercaptopurine, have also been used; however, since the disease is self-limited and alternative methods of treatment are available, such aggressive therapy is rarely warranted.

FUNCTIONAL AND REACTIVE HYPOGLYCEMIA

RONALD A. ARKY, M.D.

Few medical topics evoke more feelings and controversies than that of reactive hypoglycemia. Although lay literature on the subject of reactive hypoglycemia abounds, the number of reports based on the pathophysiologic understanding of glucose homeostasis is relatively small. That reactive hypoglycemia exists is not questioned; what is questioned is its frequency as a cause of symptoms. Clinical investigators with knowledge of glucose homeostasis and the counterregulatory mechanisms that ensure homeostasis consider spontaneous, symptomatic reactive hypoglycemia an uncommon event, whereas the authors of popular books on the subject contend that reactive hypoglycemia is extremely common and the basis for many major and minor clinical disorders. The American Medical Association, Endocrine Society, and the American Diabetes Association warn the public against the overdiagnosis of the entity and the potential consequences of misdiagnosis.

In healthy individuals, there is a normal fall in the level of the blood glucose to below the fasting value as a response to the hyperglycemia induced by a meal. Reactive hypoglycemia refers to a set of nonspecific symptoms that occur in the postprandial period and accompany this fall in blood glucose. Since these symptoms may simulate those experienced after an injection of epinephrine or overactivity of the sympathetic nervous system, they may appear in anyone unrelated to the level of glucose. These symptoms invariably include palpitations, anxiety, tremor, sweating, pallor, and hunger. For the diagnostic criteria of reactive hypoglycemia to be fulfilled, all or a combination of these symptoms must be related to the postprandial fall in blood glucose and must subside when the blood glucose is normalized. Reactive hypoglycemia may occur under a variety of clinical circumstances, and as early as 1 hour and as late as 5 hours after eating.

Although the entity of reactive hypoglycemia was first described by Seale Harris in 1924, there are still many clinical questions about the entity and its definition. These controversies do not usually center about the symptomatic rebound hypoglycemia that may occur in some patients after extensive gastric surgery or in the rare individual whose symptoms are the first indications of diabetes mellitus and glucose intolerance, but about those individuals who are otherwise healthy and have normal glucose tolerance. At present, these controversial questions can be summarized under the following headings:

1. *Criteria for diagnosis*. Must the symptoms coincide with the nadir glucose value? Can the diagnosis of reactive hypoglycemia be made at glucose levels above 50 mg/dl (2.77 mM)?
2. *Diagnostic tests*. Is the oral glucose tolerance test (5 to 6 hours) appropriate as a diagnostic tool? Since the standard oral glucose tolerance tests employ "unphysiologic" concentrations of carbohydrate, should a standard mixed meal be employed? Are measurements that consider the rate of the glycemic fall reliable diagnostic devices?
3. *Blood sampling*. Is constant glucose monitoring necessary to confirm a diagnosis of reactive hypoglycemia and to detect the absolute nadir of blood glucose? Is intermittent sampling (i.e., half-hourly) adequate?
4. *Hormonal changes*. Is reactive hypoglycemia characterized by an abnormal or excessive response in one of the counterregulatory hormones? Is epinephrine overresponsiveness characteristic of symptomatic reactive hypoglycemia?
5. *Psychologic concomitants*. Why do so many individuals with reactive hypoglycemia exhibit evidence of a hyperactive autonomic nervous system? What is the relationship between reactive hypoglycemia and the abnormal responses to several psychologic testing screens?

The specific levels of blood glucose cited in texts and papers as being crucial for the diagnosis of reactive hypoglycemia vary from 60 mg/dl (3.9 mM) to 40 mg/dl (2.2 mM). This variation reflects the fact that some individuals experience symptoms at glucose levels routinely encountered after meals whereas others are symptomatic only at unphysiologic levels. Absolute levels of glucose are not relevant without symptoms, whereas symptoms are essential for the diagnosis. Approximately 25 percent of normal subjects have blood glucose levels of 50 mg/dl (2.77 mM) within the 6-hour postprandial period after a 75-g load of glucose, yet are asymptomatic.

Controversy persists as to the ideal challenge test to document reactive hypoglycemia. In the past, the 6-hour oral glucose tolerance test with appropriate preparation was regarded as the "gold standard" for the diagnosis. However, in recent years, a number of authorities have belittled the value of this test and discourage its use. The obtainment of a low level of glucose during the occurrence of symptoms is not considered tantamount to a diagnosis. Plasma levels of glucose of 45 mg/dl (2.5 mM) or less during a symptomatic period establishes the diagnosis. For those who persist in the use of the standard 6-hour glucose tolerance test, several caveats are offered. Inappropriate intake of carbohydrate (150 to 300 g) prior to such testing exaggerates the initial phase of hyperglycemia and the consequent hypoglycemia rebound. Intermittent sampling may obscure the absolute nadir level; frequent or even constant monitoring is often necessary to detect the lowest glucose fall. Most importantly, the glucose challenge presented in the standard test is unphysiologic, and the correlation between the glucose responses after such challenges and standard meals is poor, so that the relevance of the tolerance test to the glucose fluxes of routine life is highly questionable.

Rarely are the symptoms of reactive hypoglycemia so severe as to induce unconsciousness or syncope. However, in patients with preexisting central nervous system disease or cardiovascular disease, syncopal episodes are reported after a rapid fall in blood glucose. Although the hypoglycemic rebound to the initial postprandial hyperglycemia is physiologic, there are several factors that may exaggerate the glucose decline. Among these are (1) the magnitude of the carbohydrate challenge and the subsequent level of hyperglycemia, (2) the quantity of the insulin response and the co-ingestion of insulin secretogogues as alcohol, and (3) the uptake of glucose by peripheral tissues and factors such as activity and exercise that exaggerate that uptake.

This summary describes the several clinical settings in which reactive hypoglycemia may be encountered (Table 1).

ALIMENTARY HYPOGLYCEMIA

After extensive gastric surgery, a small percentage of individuals (approximately 5%) experience symptomatic hypoglycemia between $1^1/_2$ and 3 hours after a meal. Actually, up to 80 percent of individuals who have had a partial or total gastrectomy, gastrojejunostomy, or pyloroplasty may demonstrate chemical hypoglycemia when challenged with a concentrated solution of glucose, yet do not experience classic symptoms. When present, the symptomatic hypoglycemia of postgastroenterostomy is distinct from the classic "dumping syndrome", which may appear 15 to 45 minutes after eating. The magnitude of the hypoglycemia correlates directly with the hyperglycemia that occurs immediately after the ingestion of a meal. Glucose levels may exceed 200 mg/dl (11.1 mM) and stimulate the release of excessive amounts of insulin from pancreatic beta cells. Such hyperinsulinemia causes an abrupt fall in glucose and the resulting hypoglycemia. In the absence of a stomach and/or the surgical bypass of the pyloric valve, the load of glucose delivered rapidly into the jejunum probably releases insulin-stimulating enteric hormones (gastric inhibitory polypeptide and possibly others), which augment the insulin secretagogue action of the hyperglycemia.

Case reports of reactive hypoglycemia in patients with peptic ulcer disease who have not had surgery and in other patients with alleged rapid gastric emptying appear intermittently in the literature. Such patients are said to secrete excessive quantities of insulin following a standard challenge, although the precise mechanism for their symptoms is vague. As with individuals who have undergone gastric surgery, it is unclear what differentiates the symptomatic patient with an ulcer or rapid gastric emptying from others with the same disorder who are asymptomatic.

Diets low in simple carbohydrate content help to alleviate symptoms in these patients. To offset the reduction in calories provided by carbohydrate, the protein intake should be increased to the level of 100 to 130 g per meal. The amino acids supplied by such protein feedings serve as a source for endogenous production of glucose by the liver. Instead of the standard three meals per day, such patients should consume six small feedings, none of which contains an excess of 25 g of carbohydrate. If these dietary manipulations are unsuccessful, some investigators suggest propantheline, 7.5 mg, three times per day before meals. Others have prescribed the oral hypoglycemic, chlorpropamide, but I am skeptical of the value of this sulfonylurea in postgastrectomy patients with reactive hypoglycemia. Although beta-adrenergic blockers, such as propranolol, may inhibit the secretion of insulin and thus theoretically diminish the occurrence of rebound hypoglycemia in postgastrectomy patients, these agents may in fact exaggerate the hypoglycemia and its symptoms and so should not be prescribed.

TABLE 1 The Reactive Hypoglycemias

Type	*Clinical Characteristics*	*Therapies*
Alimentary	Gastric surgery in past Symptoms 1–2 hours after meals Very high blood glucose immediately after meal Hypersecretion of insulin	Reduce dietary carbohydrate Frequent small feedings Propantheline before meals Modify surgical bypass
Early diabetes mellitus or Impaired glucose tolerance	Often obese; family history Glucose intolerance or type II diabetes Symptoms 3–5 hours after meals Insulin secretion delayed, but excessive	Reduce weight, if obese Reduce simple carbohydrates Oral hypoglycemics if other methods unsuccessful
Idiopathic postprandial hypoglycemic syndrome	Anxious, tense, thin Hyperkinetic personality Symptoms 3–5 hours after meals Glucose tolerance normal Insulin kinetics variable, usually normal	Restrict simple carbohydrates Frequent feedings Reduce or eliminate alcohol Propantheline or tranquilizer

DIABETES MELLITUS AND IMPAIRED GLUCOSE TOLERANCE

In rare instances, reactive hypoglycemia may serve as a harbinger of diabetes mellitus (type II, or non-insulin-dependent) or impaired glucose tolerance. Such patients have a normal fasting level of glucose, yet exhibit an early excessive increase in the levels of postprandial glucose, allegedly because the beta cells of the islets of Langerhans are sluggish and release insulin in a delayed fashion. This excessive degree of glycemia provides a continuing stimulus for insulin release, and consequently, the delayed but excessive quantity of insulin results in a severe rebound hypoglycemia. The latter occurs $3^1/_2$ to 5 hours after eating, and is accompanied by the classic signs of adrenergic overactivity. The number of individuals with mild, recent-onset diabetes who manifest this form of reactive hypoglycemia is unknown, but in my experience, only a very small percentage of those individuals who present with type II diabetes or impaired glucose tolerance complain of symptoms that might coincide with rebound hypoglycemia. Those few people who have symptomatic reactive hypoglycemia demonstrate insulin kinetics that do not differ from those of asymptomatic subjects with a like degree of glucose intolerance. Whether differences in c unterregulatory responses account for the symptoms is uncertain at this time.

Those few patients in whom reactive hypoglycemia accompanies diabetes mellitus are often obese and have a strong family history of diabetes mellitus. The symptoms are usually mild and may disappear with deterioration of the diabetes. Weight reduction induced with hypocaloric intake is often the best therapeutic measure for both the diabetes and the reactive hypoglycemia. Tolbutamide (500 mg, 30 minutes before meals) may prevent the postprandial hyperglycemia and, consequently, the hypoglycemic rebound.

IDIOPATHIC POSTPRANDIAL HYPOGLYCEMIC SYNDROME

Each year, many thousands of individuals seek medical attention because of the onset of adrenergic-like symptoms that occur after eating. The overwhelming majority of these individuals fail to fulfill the diagnostic criteria for reactive hypoglycemia. Most of these individuals are either self-diagnosed or are referred for testing by physicians who are unfamiliar with the specific diagnostic criteria for symptomatic reactive hypoglycemia. The best estimate is that less than 5 percent of the individuals referred for the possible presence of reactive hypoglycemia fulfill the diagnostic criteria and are considered to demonstrate "idiopathic postprandial hypoglycemia". The remainder of the patients are "nonhypoglycemics".

Individuals with IPHS are most often hard-driving, anxiety-prone personalities with a dimension of the compulsive-perfectionist type. Although women are said to predominate among the IPHS group, I believe that males are equally affected. Most of these individuals range between 30 and 40 years of age, are gainfully employed, and often occupy a "tension-filled" position. Most of these individuals complain of symptoms such as an irritable bowel, gastric hypermotility, or other problems that might relate to a hyperactive autonomic nervous system. To confirm the diagnosis, a low blood glucose must be recorded at the time of symptoms.

When individuals with IPHS are challenged with unphysiologic glucose loads, their tolerance curves are within normal range and the insulin responses are variable. Some display early hyperinsulinism, possibly related to an abnormal stimulus from one of the gastrointestinal secretogogues of insulin, but most show normal insulin kinetics, with regard to both the temporal release of insulin and the quantity of insulin secreted. A number of recent reports reveal that some individuals with IPHS secrete excessive quantities of epinephrine after nadir glucose values are reached, and that this defect is the cause of the symptoms. In summation, the pathogenesis of IPHS has not been definitely elucidated, but evidence indicates a multifactorial etiology.

Individuals with IPHS are more symptomatic during periods of extreme emotion stress and less so when relaxed, so that their complaints may wax and wane. Many insist that their symptoms are dramatically reduced when they lower their carbohydrate intake. However, recent studies concerned with the glycemic indices of foods emphasize that equal quantities of carbohydrate do not necessarily induce similar glycemic responses. At present, patients with IPHS should avoid foods and beverages with high concentrations of simple sugars such as sucrose. They should be encouraged to consume legumes, pasta, and even rice—foods known not to induce marked degrees of hyperglycemia. Foods with a high content of fiber may also be appropriate for patients with IPHS, since crude fiber may decrease gastric emptying time and absorption, and thus induce a lesser glycemic response. Fats delay gastric emptying, and should not be unduly restricted. Just as with the symptomatic gastrectomy patient, patients with IPHS should avoid the standard heavy meal and instead consume six or more small feedings during the day. Alcohol and caffeine-containing foods should also be restricted.

When dietary manipulations are unsuccessful, propantheline (7.5 to 15.0 mg, 30 minutes before each meal) is recommended. The dose may be increased up to 30 mg before each meal. Sedatives or tranquilizers, such as phenobarbital (30 mg, 2 to 3 times daily) or diazepam (2.5 mg, twice daily) may be tried.

HYPERLIPIDEMIA

SCOTT M. GRUNDY, M.D., Ph.D.

The recognition of hyperlipidemia is of clinical significance for three reasons: (1) some forms of hyperlipidemia are risk factors for coronary heart disease (CHD); (2) other forms increase the risk for acute pancreatitis; and (3) hyperlipidemia may be a sign of an underlying disease, such as diabetes mellitus, renal disease, or endocrine disturbance. The aims of therapy thus differ depending on the cause and form of hyperlipidemia. To recognize the various categories of hyperlipidemia, the basic mechanisms of transport of lipids in plasma must be understood. Therefore, before discussing treatment of hyperlipidemia, I will review the pathways of lipid transport in plasma.

PLASMA LIPID TRANSPORT

The major lipids of plasma are cholesterol and triglycerides. Both are insoluble in aqueous solutions, and special mechanisms are required foor solubilizing them in plasma. The major mechanism is the formation of lipid-protein complexes called lipoproteins. Lipoproteins enter plasma from either the gut or the liver. Most lipoproteins secreted by either organ are rich in triglycerides. The triglycerides ingested in the diet are hydrolyzed in gut lumen to fatty acids and monoglycerides; these are resynthesized to triglycerides in the intestinal mucosa and are incorporated into chylomicrons.

Chylomicrons are composed of a hydrophobic core, containing triglycerides and cholesterol esters, and a hydrophilic coat composed of unesterified cholesterol, phospholipids, and apolipoproteins. The major apoprotein of chylomicrons is a form of apoprotein B called apo B-48. Other apoproteins are apo AI, apo CI, CII, and CIII, and apo E. Chylomicrons are secreted into chyle and pass into the systemic circulation through the thoracic duct. As they pass into capillaries, they come into contact with lipoprotein lipase, an enzyme located on the surface of capillary endothelial cells. This enzyme is activated by apo CII, and it hydrolyzes chylomicron triglycerides. In this process, the apo Cs and apo AI are released and become associated with high-density lipoproteins (HDL), and chylomicrons become chylomicron remnants. The latter contain about equal amounts of triglycerides and cholesterol esters in the lipid core. The liver quickly removes chylomicron remnants from the circulation. This organ seemingly has chylomicron-remnant receptors that bind to the apo E or possibly to apo B-48 remaining on the remnant.

The liver secretes very low-density lipoproteins (VLDL) that also are rich in triglycerides. Figure 1 outlines the basic steps of VLDL metabolism. These lipoproteins contain the same apoproteins as chylomicrons except that their apoprotein B, called apo B-100, is a larger molecule than apo B-48. VLDL triglycerides also undergo lipolysis by lipoprotein lipase, and VLDL remnants are formed. The latter can have either of two fates. Normally about one-third to one-half of VLDL remnants go directly to the liver. They bind to another receptor called the B-100/E receptor. Apo B-100 specifically directs VLDL remnants to this receptor, but apo E apparently enhances their binding to receptors. The remainder of remnants undergo degradation to another particle, low-density lipoprotein (LDL). In this degradation process, most triglycerides disappear from the particle. The mechanism for loss of remnant triglycerides is unknown, but another enzyme, hepatic triglyceride lipase, may catalyze their hydrolysis.

LDL contains apo B-100 as essentially its only apoprotein. Its core consists almost exclusively of cholesterol esters. LDL particles leave the circulation in two ways: (1) they bind to B-100/E receptors at the surface of cells, and the resulting LDL-receptor complexes are internalized and degraded; (2) LDL can exit the circulation by nonreceptor-mediated pathways, presumably by nonspecific pinocytosis. The liver seemingly accounts for about two-thirds of LDL removal, and extrahepatic tissues dispose of the rest.

The HDL constitute another class of lipoproteins. They arise in plasma as the end product of several processes. Their major apoproteins are apo AI and apo AII, but they also contain small quantities of apo Cs and apo Es. HDL act as a reservoir for these latter apoproteins and can transfer them to newly secreted chylomicrons and VLDL. HDL also serve as a shuttle for cholesterol by accepting it from tissues and transferring it to VLDL. Thus, most of the components of HDL are exchangeable with other lipoproteins. Whole HDL particles nonetheless can exit from the circula-

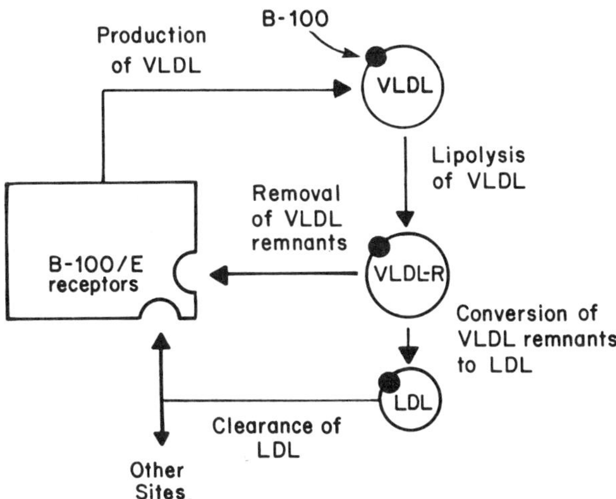

Figure 1 Metabolism of lipoproteins containing apolipoprotein B-100. The major steps in this metabolism are shown.

tion intact, but how this occurs remains to be determined.

Lipoproteins have their greatest clinical impact by accelerating atherosclerosis. However, different lipoproteins differ in their atherogenic potential. Chylomicrons probably are not atherogenic; they contain little cholesterol, and their large size seemingly prohibits their filtration through the intact endothelium. For similar reasons, VLDL probably are only mildly atherogenic. In contrast, VLDL remnants seem moderately atherogenic, and the small, cholesterol-rich LDL are markedly so. On the other hand, HDL are not atherogenic, and when they are present in high concentrations, they may actually retard the development of atherosclerosis. Several dyslipoproteinemias are associated with premature atherosclerotic disease, and these will receive primary attention in this article.

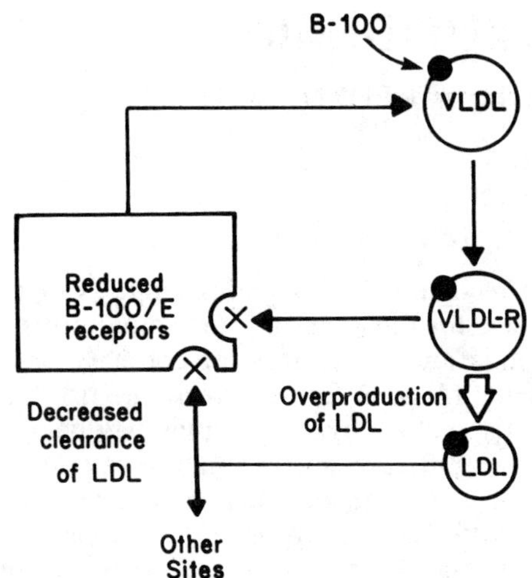

Figure 2 Metabolic consequences of a decreased activity of B110/E receptors. Reduction in receptor activity decreases hepatic uptake of VLDL remnants (VLDL-R) and causes increased transformation of VLDL-R to LDL. Clearance of LDL also is retarded.

HYPERCHOLESTEROLEMIA

For present purposes, hypercholesterolemia is defined as a plasma total cholesterol (or LDL cholesterol) associated with accelerated atherosclerosis. Whether there is in fact a cholesterol level above which atherogenesis is accelerated is a matter of dispute. However, several epidemiologic studies suggest such a threshold. When all epidemiologic studies are considered together, the level for plasma total cholesterol at which risk for CHD seems to rise strikingly is about 200 mg/dl. This corresponds to an LDL cholesterol of approximately 125 mg/dl. Values below these levels thus can be considered in the desirable range. Higher levels constitute hypercholesterolemia, but this term will be modified according to the degree of cholesterol elevation.

The most common cause of hypercholesterolemia seemingly is a decrease in activity of B-100/E receptors. The consequences of reduced receptors are twofold (Fig. 2): (1) clearance of LDL is delayed; and (2) VLDL remnants are removed less efficiently by the liver. The second defect causes more VLDL to be converted to LDL, i.e., overproduction of LDL.

Mild Hypercholesterolemia

This condition is defined as a plasma cholesterol of 225 to 275 mg/dl, assuming a normal plasma triglyceride and HDL cholesterol. LDL cholesterol should be in the range of 150 to 200 mg/dl. The risk for CHD imparted by mild hypercholesterolemia is about $1^1/_2$ to 2 times that of cholesterol levels in the desirable range. The risk is greater in men than in women, and it is accentuated further by smoking, hypertension, obesity, and diabetes mellitus.

The causes of mild hypercholesterolemia are largely dietary, i.e., high intakes of cholesterol, saturated fatty acids, and total calories (obesity). Both dietary cholesterol and saturated fatty acids appear to reduce the activity of LDL receptors (see Fig. 2). Excess caloric intake stimulates the synthesis of VLDL which in turn leads to a high input of LDL. Genetic factors also can contribute to development of mild elevations of LDL, although the nature of these factors has not been defined.

The aim of treatment of mild hypercholesterolemia is to bring total cholesterol and LDL cholesterol into the desirable range. This objective usually can be achieved by diet. The American Heart Association has recently published a dietary approach for treatment of hypercholesterolemia. The approach uses a stepwise reduction in intakes of fat and cholesterol. Phase I is a reduction of total fat to 30 percent of calories and saturated fatty acids to 10 percent; intake of cholesterol is restricted to 300 mg/day. Weight reduction to achieve the desirable range of weight also is recommended. These changes should bring LDL and total cholesterol to near 200 mg/dl in most patients with mild hypercholesterolemia. Modification of other risk factors should further reduce risk for CHD.

Moderate Hypercholesterolemia

Moderate elevations of plasma cholesterol are defined as total cholesterol of 275 to 350 mg/dl, or LDL cholesterol of 200 to 250 mg/dl. In patients with cholesterol levels in this range, risk for CHD is increased two- to fourfold above that found with cholesterol levels in the desirable range. Most patients of this type have a decreased activity of LDL receptors (see Fig. 2). Dietary factors undoubtedly contribute to moderate hypercholesterolemia in many patients. However, genetic factors are increasingly important, although the precise mechanism by which they reduce the activity of LDL receptors is unknown.

Since patients with moderate hypercholesterolemia are at a distinctly increased risk for CHD, an attempt should be made to lower their LDL levels. Dietary therapy should be tried first. Again, the American Heart Association's regimen can be used. Intakes of total fat should be reduced stepwise to about 20 percent of total calories, and saturated fatty acids should be reduced as much as possible. Cholesterol intakes should be lowered to 150 mg/day, and body weight should be decreased to desirable levels.

If diet does not induce a satisfactory lowering of cholesterol, drug therapy can be considered. The first drug to use is a bile acid sequestrant. Either cholestyramine (8 g *bid*) or colestipol (10 g *bid*) can be employed. Recently, the efficacy of sequestrant therapy in preventing CHD was demonstrated in the Lipid Research Clinic's Coronary Primary Prevention Trial. This trial provides a strong justification for treatment of patients with moderate hypercholesterolemia with bile acid sequestrants. However, drug therapy should not be started until a distinct elevation of cholesterol levels is proved by multiple measurements (at least three). Lipoprotein fractionation also should be carried out to confirm that the cholesterol elevation resides in the LDL fraction.

Bile acid sequestrants are inconvenient to take, and they also can cause constipation. Some patients cannot tolerate them, and it may be necessary to resort to other drugs. All drugs unfortunately have their drawbacks. Nicotinic acid (1 g *qid*) is an excellent lipid-lowering drug, but it causes flushing and itching of the skin, gastrointestinal upsets, hepatic dysfunction, a rise in uric acid, and a worsening of glucose tolerance. Neomycin (1 g *bid*) blocks the absorption of cholesterol and is an effective hypocholesterolemic agent; however, it has not be approved by the FDA for this purpose. Its major side effect is diarrhea. Probucol (1 g *bid*) causes a moderate reduction in LDL levels, but unfortunately, it also lowers HDL concentrations; therefore, the full benefit of LDL lowering may be lessened. Gemfibrozil (1.5 g *bid*) in hypercholesterolemic patients both lowers LDL and raises HDL. Although in most patients the LDL reduction is moderate, the drug has potential side effects, e.g., development of cholesterol gallstones and myalgias. Therefore, the responses and possible side effects of drugs other than the bile acid sequestrants must be monitored carefully.

Severe Hypercholesterolemia

Total cholesterol levels persistently over 350 mg/dl frequently are due to familial hypercholesterolemia. In this condition, tendon xanthomas commonly are present, and patients are prone to premature CHD. Men often develop CHD in their 20s and 30s and women in their 40s and 50s. The underlying defect is a structural abnormality in LDL receptors. Most patients are heterozygotes for the disease, i.e., they have inherited it from only one parent and thus have half the normal number of LDL receptors.

Dietary therapy should be employed in severe hypercholesterolemia, but it rarely produces sufficient lowering of LDL levels when used alone. Therefore drugs must be employed in addition. The bile acid sequestrants should be used first. Higher doses than those recommended for moderate hypercholesterolemia can be tried. The sequestrants remove bile acids from the enterohepatic circulation. Consequently, more cholesterol is converted into bile acids, and hepatic levels of cholesterol fall. This fall triggers an increase in the synthesis of LDL receptors that in turn lowers LDL levels. Even in familial hypercholesterolemia the synthesis of receptors can be increased above the usual half-normal level. Still, most patients with severe hypercholesterolemia fail to have an adequate lowering of LDL levels with bile acid sequestrants alone, and a second drug must be used in combination.

One such drug is nicotinic acid. This drug blocks the formation of lipoproteins by the liver. Doses should be started low (100 mg *tid*), but increased gradually to 3 to 6 g per day. With high intakes of both sequestrants and nicotinic acid, plasma LDL levels decline to an acceptable level in most patients. Unfortunately, tolerance of nicotinic acid is not good in many patients for the reasons already cited.

An alternate second drug is neomycin. This drug blocks cholesterol absorption, decreases return of cholesterol to the liver, reduces hepatic cholesterol concentrations, and thereby increases the synthesis of LDL receptors. The dose of neomycin is 1 g *bid*. Neomycin can be used successfully in many patients, although it has not been approved for cholesterol lowering by the FDA. Diarrhea occurs commonly when the drug is used alone, but this symptom usually is avoided when neomycin is used in combination with bile acid sequestrants.

Probucol is still another drug that can be tried with sequestrants. This drug enhances the clearance of LDL by unknown means. Its action to lower LDL levels is additive to that of sequestrants, and thus an adequate lowering of LDL can be achieved in many patients with severe hypercholesterolemia.

Finally, a new class of drugs should be mentioned. These agents inhibit the synthesis of cholesterol by competitive inhibition of the rate-limiting enzyme in cholesterol synthesis, namely, 3-hydroxy-3-methylglutaryl coenzyme A (HMG CoA) reductase. The agents currently under trial are compactin and mevinolin. They are effective at low doses, e.g., 10 to 20 mg *bid*. At present these drugs appear to have great promise for treatment of severe hypercholesterolemia.

HYPERTRIGLYCERIDEMIA

An elevation of plasma triglyceride (TG) is clinically significant for three reasons: (1) hypertriglyceridemia is frequently associated with CHD; (2) severe elevations of TG levels can produce acute pancreatitis; and (3) high TG concentrations often occur secondarily to other diseases. Although hypertriglyceridemia is commonly found in patients with CHD, the relation between plasma TG levels and atherosclerosis has been a subject of dispute. Most epidemiologic studies show a positive correlation between plasma TG levels and rates of CHD when data are examined by univariant analysis; however, when a multiple variant analysis is carried out, the correlation between TG levels and CHD loses its significance. The latter analysis gives primacy to other known risk factors, i.e., total cholesterol and HDL cholesterol, and when these are factored out, the residual risk remaining for TGs is small or nonexistent. Unfortunately, this analysis can be confusing to the clinician. The fact remains that many and perhaps most patients with hypertriglyceridemia are at increased risk for CHD. So far, the mechanisms leading to the increase risk in hypertriglyceridemic patients are unknown. For the physician, however, it is prudent to assume that the patient with hypertriglyceridemia is at higher than normal risk.

As in the case of hypercholesterolemia, the severity of hypertriglyceridemia can be used in part to make clinical decisions and judgments. In contrast to cholesterol levels, however, there is not a continuous relation between TG concentrations and risk of CHD. For this reason, it is difficult to define the limit between desirable TG levels and those associated with enhanced risk. Current practice therefore is to define hypertriglyceridemia as a plasma TG level over the 90th or 95th percentile for the general population. For adult men in the United States, an abnormal TG level by these criteria would be above 250 mg/dl.

Mild Hypertriglyceridemia

This condition can be defined as a TG level between 250 to 500 mg/dl. When TGs are in this range, the increase in plasma TG is limited almost entirely to the VLDL fraction. This is the pattern of type 4 hyperlipoproteinemia (HLP). There can be two causes of high VLDL levels. One is overproduction of VLDL, the other a decrease in VLDL catabolism. Our studies suggest that mild hypertriglyceridemia in most patients is due to overproduction of VLDL. An excess production of VLDL can occur on a primary or secondary basis. The most common causes of the latter are obesity with a high caloric intake, adult onset diabetes mellitus, and the nephrotic syndrome. The causes of primary lipoprotein overproduction are unknown; whether the basic defect lies in the overproduction of hepatic TG or hepatic apo B-100 remains to be determined.

The lipoprotein patterns resulting from overproduction of VLDL are shown in Figure 3. One pattern is depicted in Figure 3A. Some patients have excess synthesis of VLDL, but because of rapid clearance rate of VLDL, IDL, and LDL, hyperlipidemia does not develop. These patients have an increased flux of lipoproteins without elevated levels. Other patients show hyperlipidemia, by mechanisms depicted in Figure 3B. For example, if hepatic synthesis of TG is increased concomitantly, the VLDL will be enriched with TG; the high influx of VLDL consequently leads to a high VLDL-TG level (type 4 HLP). Type 4 HLP

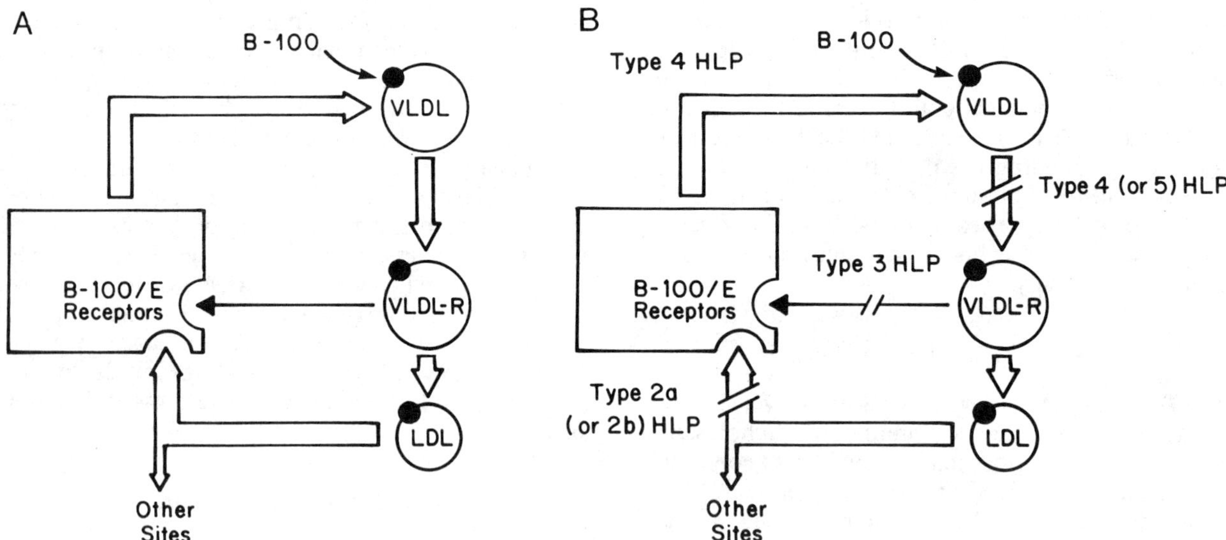

Figure 3 Consequences of overproduction of VLDL. *A* (left), Hypersecretion of VLDL leads to increased formation of VLDL remnants (VLDL-R) and LDL. The turnover of all lipoproteins is increased, but if clearance rates also are rapid, hyperlipidemia does not develop. *B* (right), Mechanisms of hyperlipidemia associated with overproduction of VLDL. Increased outputs of triglycerides with VLDL can cause type 4 HLP. If catabolism of VLDL is defective, the result is either type 4 HLP or type 5 HLP. If clearance of VLDL remnants is retarded, owing to a defect in apo E, these lipoproteins accumulate, producing type 3 HLP. Finally, defective clearance of LDL causes a rise in LDL, with either type 2a or type 2b HLP.

also is produced if the patient simultaneously has overproduction of VLDL and a mild defect in lipolysis of TG. Also, in the rare patient who has an abnormality in the structure of apo E, remnant removal by the B-100/E receptor is delayed, and small VLDL (beta VLDL) accumulate. This is type 3 HLP. Finally, if clearance of LDL is defective, overproduction of VLDL causes an increase in LDL levels (type 2 HLP). Elevated LDL alone is called type 2a HLP, whereas a combined increase in LDL and VLDL is named type 2b HLP. Thus, multiple lipoprotein phenotypes are possible in single families. When multiple phenotypes occur in families with primary lipoprotein overproduction, the term "familial combined hyperlipidemia" is used. However, the same clinical picture can occur in secondary lipoprotein overproduction due to excessive caloric intake (associated with obesity), adult-onset diabetes mellitus, and the nephrotic syndrome.

Patients with overproduction of VLDL appear to be at increased risk for CHD regardless of their lipoprotein phenotype, whether types 4, 3, 2a, 2b, or normolipidemic, and whether the cause is primary or secondary. For clinical purposes it can be assumed that the patient with mild hypertriglyceridemia has overproduction of VLDL and thus is at increased risk for CHD. Therefore, it is reasonable to treat patients with TG levels in the range of 250 to 500 mg/dl. Many such patients have secondary lipoprotein overproduction, and depending on the cause (obesity, diabetes mellitus, or nephrotic syndrome) they should be treated appropriately. The remaining patients can be assumed to have primary lipoprotein overproduction. A decision to treat these patients with drugs depends on clinical judgment of the patient's degree of risk. Men are more prone to CHD than women, and the former should be treated first. Other risk factors (e.g., smoking, hypertension, hypercholesterolemia) apparently accentuate the danger of hypertriglyceridemia. If smoking cannot be stopped or hypertension corrected, drug therapy of hypertriglyceridemia should be seriously considered. If hypercholesterolemia and/or premature CHD is present in other family members, the hypertriglyceridemic patient under investigation can be assumed to be at elevated risk. Finally, if the patient has clinical evidence of atherosclerotic disease, it is reasonable to attempt to retard the progression of atherosclerosis. On the other hand, if the patient with mild hypertriglyceridemia is devoid of other risk factors, has a low cholesterol level, and has no family history of atherosclerotic disease, one might take a calculated risk and withhold drug treatment. Still, the advice to keep weight in the desirable range and to increase exercise is fully justified because both reduce TG levels.

One of the problems in using drugs for mild hypertriglyceridemia associated with primary lipoprotein overproduction is that the ideal drug has not been developed. Theoretically, the ideal agent would be one that blocks the synthesis of VLDL. One drug that has this effect is nicotinic acid. Its primary action is to retard the production of VLDL, and this change decreases both VLDL and LDL levels. Therefore, nicotinic acid can be recommended for patients with mild hypertriglyceridemia who are judged to be at increase risk for CHD. Unfortunately, this drug is associated with a variety of side effects, as already discussed, and many patients cannot tolerate nicotinic acid or adhere to it for a long time. Alternate drugs therefore must be considered for those who cannot take nicotinic acid.

One possible alternative is clofibrate. This drug can be highly effective in lowering TG levels in many hypertriglyceridemic patients. Several studies indicate that the primary action of clofibrate is to increase the activity of lipoprotein lipase and thus to promote clearance of TG-rich lipoproteins. Our studies have shown that clofibrate has little or no effect on the production of VLDL. Therefore, it does not significantly modify the underlying defect in primary lipoprotein overproduction. Consequently, clofibrate may not be beneficial in most patients with mild hypertriglyceridemia, even though it may lower TG levels.

On the other hand, newer analogs of clofibrate appear to be more powerful lipid-lowering agents. For example, we have shown that one such analog, gemfibrozil, not only promotes lipolysis of VLDL, but also inhibits production of VLDL. Therefore, gemfibrozil may be useful in the treatment of primary lipoprotein overproduction. Although gemfibrozil may not be quite so effective in inhibiting the production of VLDL as nicotinic acid, it is better tolerated. With either drug, lowering of plasma TG usually causes a rise in HDL cholesterol levels, another apparently beneficial change.

If a patient with mild hypertriglyceridemia is treated with either nicotinic acid or gemfibrozil, a rise in LDL cholesterol frequently accompanies the fall in TG levels. In many patients this rise is relatively small, and LDL remains in the low-normal to mid-normal range. In a few patients, however, the increment is greater, and the LDL level may become distinctly elevated. For such patients the use of a second drug may be necessary; the best choice probably is a bile acid sequestrant. Although the LDL-lowering response to sequestrants rarely is dramatic in such patients, it is usually satisfactory.

The potential of dietary therapy for primary lipoprotein overproduction has not been adequately tested. The American Heart Association advocates a low fat-high carbohydrate diet on the assumption that the major risk associated with this disorder derives from abnormalities in the metabolism of cholesterol and LDL. This assumption unfortunately has not been validated. Some investigators advocate a diet rich in polyunsaturated fatty acids, but again, adequate investigation has not proved the usefulness of these fats. Recently, several reports indicate that fish oils, which are rich in omega-3 fatty acids, are highly effective in the lowering of TG levels. Fish oil fatty acids have long carbon chains and are highly unsaturated; they appear to interfere with the synthesis of VLDL. Intakes of 20 to 30 g of fish oil per day seem to be required. Future studies may prove them useful in therapy of mild hypertriglyceridemia.

Moderate-to-Severe Hypertriglyceridemia

Most patients with triglyceride levels over 500 mg/dl have a lipolytic defect for TG-rich lipoproteins. They thus are prone to accumulation of both VLDL and chylomicrons. Three types of lipolytic defects have been identified: (1) a congenital absence of lipoprotein lipase; (2) a congenital defect of apo CII, the apoprotein responsible for activation of lipoprotein lipase; and (3) a partial defect in the activity of lipoprotein lipase.

A *congenital absence of lipoprotein lipase* produces marked hypertriglyceridemia. In patients with this disorder, chylomicrons of dietary origin are the major lipoprotein to accumulate in plasma. An excess of chylomicrons in fasting plasma without a marked increase in VLDL levels is called type 1 HLP. When the diet contains moderate amounts of fat, TG levels can be as high as 2000 to 10,000 mg/dl. Patients frequently have eruptive skin xanthomata, and they are prone to acute pancreatitis. Withdrawal of fat from the diet is urgent to prevent development of pancreatitis. Patients with type 1 HLP do not respond to lipid-lowering drugs. The only therapy is removal of long-chain fatty acids from the diet. Fat should constitute less than 10 percent of calories. Most of the decrease in fat intake should be replaced by carbohydrate, but partial replacement by medium-chain triglycerides (MCT) can be tried. MCTs are not incorporated into chylomicrons. Type 1 HLP apparently does not enhance the risk of development of atherosclerosis. A similar clinical picture is produced by a *congenital absence of apo CII*, the apoprotein required for activation of lipoprotein lipase, and the clinical approach to the patient also is the same.

A *partial deficiency of lipoprotein lipase* appears to be the most common cause of a lipolytic defect in moderate-to-severe hypertriglyceridemia. Most patients with TG levels above 500 mg/dl seem to have this abnormality. In many cases, the reduction in lipoprotein lipase activity presumably is a genetic defect. Other causes are insulin-deficient diabetes mellitus and hypothyroidism. A partial deficiency of lipoprotein lipase alone usually is not sufficient to produce severe hypertriglyceridemia; an overproduction of VLDL also is required. The combination of overproduction of VLDL and defective lipolysis causes an increase in concentrations of both VLDL and chylomicrons, a pattern called type 5 HLP. The hypersecretion of VLDL can be on either a primary or secondary basis. A significant portion of type 5 patients have adult onset diabetes mellitus or obesity or both.

The most pressing need in type 5 HLP is to prevent the development of acute pancreatitis. Pancreatitis can occur when TG levels exceed 2000 mg/dl. Since TG levels can abruptly rise in patients with levels over 500 mg/dl, any such patients must be considered candidates for pancreatitis. There has been a dispute whether patients with type 5 HLP are at increased risk for CHD. In view of the fact that most type 5 patients have overproduction of VLDL, and since this abnormality is commonly associated with premature CHD, it is reasonable to assume that patients with it are at enhanced high risk.

Because of the danger of acute pancreatitis, patients with TG levels over 500 mg/dl should be treated. If the patient's elevated TG concentrations have a secondary component, this should be treated first. Obese patients should undergo weight reduction. Diabetic patients should be treated appropriately, with insulin if necessary. If hypertriglyceridemia persists despite correction of these conditions, drug therapy can be employed. The desirable drug for treating the overproduction component is nicotinic acid. Some patients with type 5 HLP show a remarkable response to this drug. The lipolytic defect can be treated with a fibric acid which will increase the activity of lipoprotein lipase. Since gemfibrozil both increases lipolysis and inhibits the synthesis of VLDL, it would seem to be the preferred fibric acid for type 5 HLP. In addition to drug therapy, the fat intake of type 5 patients should be curtailed to decrese the influx of chylomicrons. If possible the dietary fat should be reduced to 10 to 15 percent of total calories.

Type 3 Hyperlipoproteinemia

A rare form of hypertriglyceridemia is type 3 HLP. This is proved by direct actions of androgens on the seminiferous epithelium and epididymis. Androgens are also used in high doses (testosterone enanthate, 250 mg every 2 weeks for 3 months) to suppress gonadotropin secretion and spermatogenesis temporarily. Following treatment, a rebound rise in sperm output above pretreatment values is supposed to occur. In Melbourne, 92 patients receiving androgen or hCG therapy produced pregnancy rates no greater than those achieved by untreatd men with similar degrees of son remnants. The latter defect is due to an abnormality in the structure of apo E so that this apoprotein binds poorly with hepatic receptors. The poor binding leads to accumulation of lipoproteins. In the absence of overproduction of VLDL, the apo E defect alone usually does not cause hyperlipoproteinemia. The treatment of type 3 HLP is twofold. Curtailment of VLDL overproduction can be achieved by appropriate treatment of secondary disorders (e.g., obesity or diabetes mellitus) or by treatment with nicotinic acid in those with primary lipoprotein overproduction. The clearance defect for remnants can be largely corrected with a fibric acid (clofibrate or gemfibrozil).

HYPOALPHALIPOPROTEINEMIA

A low level of HDL cholesterol is another risk factor for CHD. For men, HDL cholesterol levels in the range of 35 to 50 mg/dl can be considered normal. Higher levels (i.e., over 50 mg/dl) may be protective against CHD. Such high levels are common in Caucasian women and may be one reason why they are not as prone to CHD. HDL cholesterol concentrations in the range of 25 to 35 mg/dl appear to be associated with a mild-to-moderate increase in risk for CHD, and levels below 25 mg/dl signify high risk.

The causes of low HDL cholesterol include some factors that cannot be modified and others that can be. Those of the former category include sex (male versus female) and genetic factors. On the other hand, most factors that reduce HDL cholesterol—obesity, hypertriglyceridemia, smoking, lack of exercise, and certain drugs (diuretics, beta-adrenergic blocking agents, and anabolic steroids)—can be modified. Although the mechanisms by which a low HDL concentration contributes to acceleration of atherosclerosis are unknown, it is reasonable to attempt to raise HDL levels when possible. Thus, in patients with a low HDL, one can recommend weight loss in obese patients, stopping smoking, increasing exercise, and treatment of hypertriglyceridemia. Also, it is worthwhile to review the patient's drug regimen to determine whether modifications are needed.

Suggested Reading

American Heart Association Ad Hoc Committee to Design a Dietary Treatment of Hyperlipoproteinemia (Gotto AM Jr, Bierman EL, Connor WE, Ford CH, Frantz ID, Glueck CJ, Grundy SM, Little JA). Recommendations for treatment of hyperlipidemia in adults. Edited by SM Grundy. Circulation 1984; 69:1067A-1090A.

Grundy SM (Chairman), Barrett-Connor E, Bierman EL, et al. The Consensus Development Conference on Treatment of Hypertriglyceridemia. National Institutes of Health. JAMA 1984; 251:1196-1200.

Grundy SM, Bilheimer D, Blackburn H, Brown WV, Kwiterovich PO Jr, Mattson F, Schoenfield G, Weidman WH. Rationale of the diet-heart statement of the American Heart Association. Circulation 1982; 65:839A-854A.

The Lipid Research Clinics Coronary Primary Prevention Trial Results. I. Reduction in the incidence of coronary heart disease. Lipid Research Clinics Program. Lipid Metabolism—Atherogenesis Branch. National Heart, Lung, and Blood Institute. JAMA 1984; 251:351.

The Lipid Research Clinics Coronary Primary Prevention Trial Results. II. The relationship in incidence of coronary heart disease to cholesterol lowering. Lipid Research Clinics Program. Lipid Metabolism—Atherogenesis Branch. National Heart, Lung, and Blood Institute. JAMA 1984; 251:365.

OSTEOPOROSIS

ROBERT LINDSAY, M.B., Ch.B., Ph.D., M.R.C.P.

In general, therapy for osteoporosis should be clearly divided into prevention and treatment of the established disease, although many of the current therapeutic approaches overlap and the end point, prevention of fracture, is obviously the same. In practice, however, prevention and treatment should be thought of separately. If they are not, it is easy to lose sight of the fact that the pathophysiologic status of the skeleton may differ between younger asymptomatic individuals and patients who have either vertebral or hip fracture. Future developments in treatment are likely to require more objective measures of skeletal turnover and provision of therapy tailored to the status of the skeleton in each individual.

PREVENTION OF BONE LOSS

With increasing frequency, asymptomatic young individuals are requesting an assessment of their potential for development of osteoporosis. Although there are many associated risk factors for bone loss (Table 1), we currently consider three to be of likely major importance, among those that are correctable: (1) dietary deficiency of calcium, (2) sedentary life style, and (3) early menopause or oophorectomy. In giving preventive advice, however, it is useful for general good health reasons to eliminate or at least reduce alcohol and cigarette consumption, however poor compliance with such measures is liable to be. In our experience, when osteoporosis occurs in premenopausal females or in males, a history of chronic alcohol abuse can often be obtained.

TABLE 1 Factors thought to place Women at Increased Risk from Osteoporosis

Race: white or oriental
Reduced weight for height
Early menopause or oophorectomy
Positive family history for osteoporosis
Poor diet
Low calcium intake
Low vitamin D intake
High caffeine intake
High alcohol intake
High protein intake
Cigarette smoking
Sedentary lifestyle

Calcium

The evidence that the human species is generally deficient in calcium intake is much stronger than the evidence that increasing calcium intake can reduce bone loss. However, provision of extra calcium is simple, and as far as can be determined, it is a safe procedure in normocalcemic individuals with no active history of renal calcium stones or without significant hypercalciuria on a normal diet. Since the average diet contains only about 500 mg calcium per day (in comparison to an RDA of 800 mg), we generally recommend an increment in total intake to obtain 1500 to 2000 mg per day for most women, especially if postmenopausal. Although this can be obtained by increasing the intake of milk products, in general patient compliance with this type of regimen is not good. (One quart of milk yields approximately 1200 mg calcium.) Usually, therefore, calcium supplementation is required, generally in the form of calcium carbonate, since 40 percent of the tablet weight is calcium and a higher intake of calcium is achieved with a lesser number of tablets. In this recommendation, no consideration is given to any possible effect of the anion, since there are insufficient data to indicate whether this should be of concern. Since there is no comparability data (as for bioavailability, etc.), the least expensive form of calcium carbonate should be provided. In most instances, despite the lower quantity of calcium per tablet, this form is, in effect, generic calcium carbonate. However, with tablets containing 500 mg elemental calcium, compliance is usually better, simply because fewer tablets are required for adequate supplementation; therefore, often we recommend the more expensive commercial preparations.

Exercise

Repetitive, gravity-resistive exercises, such as walking, jogging, and the various forms of aerobic exercise, are believed to benefit bone mass in the axial skeleton, where the beneficial effects are required. Exercise prescription should take into account the general state of health of the individual. Therefore, the recommendations of the American Heart Association can also form the basis of exercise suggestions for prevention of osteoporosis. To obtain maximum benefit from exercise, some recent evidence suggests that an adequate supply of dietary calcium must be provided, and therefore calcium supplementation is given routinely in combination with exercise programs. Competitive sporting activities are also helpful, since patient compliance is liable to be better. Tennis, racquet ball, and squash are ideal in that they can be year-round activities. There is no evidence that swimming is beneficial to the skeleton.

Sex Steroids

Calcium and exercise by themselves may not be sufficient to prevent bone loss, particularly in postmenopausal women. Therefore, for patients who may be particularly at risk, we routinely offer estrogen therapy. The following can be used as a rough guide for prescription of estrogens:

1. Small, thin, white or oriental women
2. Early menopause or surgical oophorectomy
3. Evidence of continued bone loss after calcium and exercise
4. Nulliparity
5. Strong family history of osteoporosis
6. Prolonged amenorrhea or oligomenorrhea during the normally fertile period of life (e.g., exercise induced)

For women with more than one of these risk factors, after menopause, we provide conjugated equine estrogens 0.625 mg/day (or equivalent) unless greater amounts are required to treat menopausal symptoms. The patient is carefully informed of the reasons for the prescription and the fact that therapy will probably be required for a minimum of 5 years. Thus, patient and physician are undertaking a long-term commitment. We stress the importance of careful follow-up. At present, we do not cycle estrogen therapy, but we do induce a progestogen withdrawal bleed for all women who have a uterus. Many various regimens of such therapy are possible, but usually we most commonly provide medroxyprogesterone, 2.5 or 5 mg for 2 weeks, either monthly or three-monthly. Prior to therapy we request a gynecologic consult and usually obtain a mammogram, and we invite the gynecologist to assist in patient follow-up. The most likely future development in this area will be introduction of combination continuous estrogen-progesterone preparations.

Use of Bone Mass Measurements

Noninvasive techniques of bone mass measurement using a variety of methods are becoming increasingly available. At present, however, such estimates offer no more than a supplement to clinical assessment, and perhaps a method for determining the efficacy of therapy. Decisions to provide preventive therapy should not be based solely on a single bone mass determination, especially of peripheral bone. Nor should the unavailability of such measurements deter the clinician from providing therapy if it is clinically indicated.

TREATMENT OF ESTABLISHED DISEASE

Patients with fracture present a different set of problems when the physician is considering treatment of the underlying problem of reduced bone mass. Therapy for patients with an acute fracture must be directed toward both the reduction of those symptoms associated with the fracture itself and the prevention of further fracture.

Back Pain

Following vertebral fracture, there is often a period of acute back pain, which may be of sufficient severity to require the use of narcotic analgesics. Generally, we combine analgesics with alternative pain relief modalities including hot packs and transcutaneous nerve stimulation (TENS). The aim is to minimize the period of bed rest. In most instances, mobilization can begin within one week of the fracture, if possible within 48 to 72 hours. If pain is of sufficient severity to prohibit mobilization, a lumbodorsal support may be used temporarily to increase mobility. The painful spasms of the paraspinal muscles that occasionally follow fracture can be alleviated by the use of diazepam or another muscle relaxant. Whirlpool therapy also is often beneficial during this period. For those patients who are maximally affected by pain, 4 to 6 weeks may elapse before maximum mobility is achieved. Generally, however, we expect most patients to be fully mobile within a 2 to 3 week period, and we stress earliest possible mobilization for all patients. Fractures of the femoral neck are treated by orthopedic surgical intervention.

Treatment of Osteoporosis

Once fracture has begun, it is now generally appreciated that treatment of the underlying problem, low bone mass, is problematic. Several reasons can be suggested for this:

1. Few therapeutic maneuvers are available to increase bone mass.
2. There is insufficient understanding of the underlying causes of the disease.
3. There is a widespread failure to understand the physiologic status of the skeleton in affected individuals.
4. Fracture occurrence predisposes to further fractures (low bone mass, increased likelihood of falls, fear, and anxiety).

Currently, therapy should be directed toward prevention of falls and prevention of further bone loss.

Attacking the problem of reduced bone mass requires a knowledge of the status of the skeleton. Seventy-five to 90 percent of all patients with osteoporosis exhibit low bone turnover on biopsy, presumably equating to a low rate of bone loss. In such circumstances, it can be argued that pharmacologic therapy aimed at further reducing bone turnover is illogical. Therapeutic modalities that reduce bone turnover include calcium, calcitonin, estrogens, and diphosphonates. However, such agents are still commonly used.

Calcium

Because of the growing evidence suggesting generalized calcium deficiency, the use of calcium as therapy appears simplistically to be logical. Declining calcium absorption efficiency in the gastrointestinal tract would be countered. The likelihood of further reducing bone turnover is probably a small price to pay for an adequate calcium supply, and some patients do relatively well with calcium intakes of 1.5 to 2.5 g/day (elemental calcium).

Estrogens

Estrogen usage also reduces bone turnover, but may improve intestinal calcium absorption and increase the efficiency with which the patient utilizes available calcium. Prescription of estrogen should be done on the same basis as for preventive therapy. In patients in this age group, endometrial stimulation often fails to occur at 0.625 mg conjugated equine estrogens per day, and we do not cycle therapy, nor do we add progestogens. Gynecologic follow-up should be recommended, however.

Other Drugs

Although calcitonin has been shown in two studies to increase total body calcium, patient compliance is poor. The available preparations must be given by subcutaneous or intramuscular injection on a schedule ranging from daily to twice-weekly, often with uncomfortable side effects of nausea, flushing, and headache. Diphosphonates have not been used yet to any extent in the treatment of osteoporosis.

Stimulation of Bone Mass

Although the most sensible approach to therapy for the patient with fracture is to stimulate the production of new bone, currently there is no established method by which this can be achieved with consistency. Fluoride in high doses does induce new bone formation, but doubts remain about the quality of bone. Additionally, there is a close relationship between response rate and dose, and an equally close relation ship between side effects (gastric irritation and bleeding, arthopathy) and dose. Currently, fluoride is not approved by the FDA for use in osteoporosis and should be reserved for use only in a clinical investigational setting until the results of two major studies are completed. Clearly, however, this drug will have some role to play in the future.

Exercise

Potentially, exercise should stimulate new bone formation as well as prevent loss of bone mass. Unfortunately, it is difficult for most patients with osteoporosis to participate in programs providing significant gravity-resistive exercise. In the rehabilitation period following fracture, we use water exercises and swimming to provide a program of gradually increasing activity. As indicated, there is no evidence that such exercise benefits the skeleton; however, the well-being of the patient is dramatically improved. As early as is feasible, we introduce walking, encouraging all patients to attain a level of activity of at least one mile per day.

Anabolic Agents

Although most sex steroids prescribed reduce bone turnover, there is some circumstantial evidence that anabolic agents may directly stimulate the osteoblast. However, we do not routinely use such compounds except in osteoporosis in males, since our general experience is that they are less well tolerated among females than other agents.

HYPOCALCEMIA

NORMAN H. BELL, M.D.

Hypocalcemia almost always results from an abnormality in the metabolism of parathyroid hormone or vitamin D. Since about half of the calcium in the circulation is bound to albumin, hypoalbuminemia can cause a low serum total calcium which is associated with a normal serum ionized calcium. It is important to be certain that a finding of hypocalcemia does not result from hypoalbuminemia, since this does not itself require further evaluation or treatment.

Hypocalcemia can cause tetany, cataracts, diarrhea, laryngeal stridor, grand mal seizures, and increased intracranial pressure with papilledema. In children, chronic hypocalcemia may produce mental retardation, behavioral abnormalities, and psychoses. Early detection and treatment therefore are essential. The causes of hypocalcemia are listed in Table 1.

TABLE 1 Pathogenesis of Hypocalcemia

Absence of or impaired secretion of parathyroid hormone
Hypoparathyroidism
Magnesium deficiency
Abnormal response to parathyroid hormone
Pseudohypoparathyroidism
Abnormal metabolism of vitamin D
Deficiency
Inadequate intake
Poor exposure to sunlight
Malabsorption syndromes
Impaired vitamin D-25-hydroxylation
Liver disease
Impaired 25-hydroxyvitamin D-1a-hydroxylase
Chronic renal failure
Hypoparathyroidism
Hypophosphatemic rickets
Pseudohypoparathyroidism
Tumor-induced osteomalacia
Vitamin D resistant rickets type I
Impaired response to 1,25-dihydroxyvitamin D
Anticonvulsant therapy
Vitamin D-dependent rickets type II
Miscellaneous
Acute pancreatitis
Osteoblastic metastases
Phosphate therapy
Chemotherapy

METABOLISM OF VITAMIN D

Vitamin D_2 (ergocalciferol) from the diet is absorbed via the intestinal lymphatic system. Absorption requires bile acids and takes place in the proximal small intestine. Vitamin D_3 (cholecalciferol) is produced in the skin by photochemical synthesis from 7-dehydrocholesterol. Upon exposure to ultraviolet light, 7-dehydrocholesterol absorbs one photon of light energy and is converted to previtamin D_3, which is thermally labile. Previtamin D_3 then undergoes a temperature-dependent rearrangement of double bonds to form vitamin D_3, which is thermally stable. Vitamin D_3 is removed from the skin by way of the dermal capillaries by vitamin D-binding protein, which has a high affinity for the vitamin and a low affinity for previtamin D_3. The remaining previtamin D_3 is slowly converted to vitamin D_3 by the temperature-dependent process.

Vitamin D_2 and vitamin D_3 themselves have little in the way of biologic activity. Both undergo hydroxylation in the liver to form 25-hydroxyvitamin D by action of the enzyme vitamin D-25-hydroxylase. 25-hydroxyvitamin D is the major storage form of the vitamin. The normal range in the circulation is from 8 to 60 ng/ml. 25-Hydroxyvitamin D undergoes further hydroxylation to form 1,25-dihydroxyvitamin D by action of the enzyme 25-hydroxyvitamin D-la-hydroxylase. This hydroxylation takes place primarily, but not exclusively, in the kidney and is tightly regulated by circulating parathyroid hormone. Production is not as well regulated in children. The normal range of serum 1,25-dihydroxyvitamin D in adults is from 20 to 50 pg/ml. Values in infants and children are somewhat higher. In man, the metabolites of vitamin D_3 are present in higher amounts than those of vitamin D_2. The biologic activities of the metabolites of vitamin D_2 and D_3, however, are thought to be the same. 1,25-Dihydroxyvitamin D inhibits the hepatic production of 25-hydroxyvitamin D. Thus, there is feedback regulation by 1,25-dihydroxyvitamin D of synthesis of its precursor 25-hydroxyvitamin D, a mechanism which protects against abnormal increases in circulating 1,25-dihydroxyvitamin D.

25-Hydroxyvitamin D is converted to 24,25-dihydroxyvitamin D by action of the enzyme 25-hydroxyvitamin D-24-hydroxylase. The enzyme is induced by 1,25-dihydroxyvitamin D. This reaction also takes place primarily, but not exclusively, in the kidney. There is considerable controversy as to whether this metabolite has a physiologic role with regard to bone and mineral metabolism. Evidence on the one hand indicates that 24,25-dihydroxyvitamin D may be important in healing osteomalacia and rickets, and on the other hand that 24-hydroxylation may be of importance only as a pathway for degradation. Both 24,25-dihydroxyvitamin D and 1,25-dihydroxyvitamin D undergo further hydroxylation to form 1,24,25-trihydroxyvitamin D before cleavage of the side chain and excretion.

Vitamin D, 25-hydroxyvitamin D, 24,25-dihydroxyvitamin D, and 1,25-dihydroxyvitamin D are all transported in the circulation by the vitamin D-binding protein, an a_2 globulin which is also the group specific component protein or Gc protein. Patients with heavy proteinuria sometimes lose significant amounts of the metabolites in the urine and thus are at risk for developing vitamin D deficiency. Vitamin D and the metabolites listed above undergo an enterohepatic circulation and are conjugated in the liver to form sulfates and glucuronides. Vitamin D deficiency can result from disruption of the enterohepatic circulation.

Clinical and basic studies show that hydroxylations of vitamin D in both the 25 and la positions are necessary for optimal biologic activity. Dihydrotachysterol (DHT) resembles la-hydroxyvitamin D_3 in structure: the A ring is rotated 180° so that the hydroxyl group in the 3 position acts as a "pseudo" la-hydroxyl group. Both la:hydroxyvitamin D_3 (which is not clinically available in the United States) and dihydrotachysterol must undergo 25-hydroxylation by the liver for full biologic activity. Indeed, dihydrotachysterol is inactive. The rank order of biologic activity as determined experimentally is: $1,25(OH)_2D_3 > 1a,25\text{-}OHD_3 > 25\text{-}DHT > 25\text{-}OHD_3 > D_3 > DHT$.

MECHANISM OF ACTION OF VITAMIN D

1,25-Dihydroxyvitamin D_3 binds to a cytosol receptor in target organs, predominantly the intestine and skeleton, and is transported to the nucleus where it initiates events that are related to translation and transcription. The major actions are to augment the intestinal transport of calcium and phosphorus and to stimulate release of these ions from the skeleton. Inhibition of secretion of parathyroid hormone is mediated indirectly through increases in the intestinal absorption of calcium. In vitamin D intoxication, serum 25-hydroxyvitamin D is markedly increased and serum 1,25-dihydroxyvitamin D_3 is normal or only slightly increased because 25-hydroxyvitamin D-la-hydroxylase is tightly regulated. At high concentrations, 25-hydroxyvitamin D is thought to occupy and activate the receptors in target organs.

DRUGS USED IN TREATMENT OF HYPOCALCEMIA

The preparations of vitamin D and its metabolites which are available for clinical use in the United States are listed in Tables 2 and 3. The onset of optimal biologic activity, duration of effect after cessation of treatment, dosage forms available, and trade names are listed in Table 2. The pharmacologic advantages and disadvantages of the drugs are listed in Table 3.

Vitamin D_2 and 25-hydroxyvitamin D_3 have the theoretical advantage of being the precursors of the other vitamin D metabolites including 24,25-dihydroxyvitamin D, which may prove to be of value in treating rickets. Also, 25-hydroxyvitamin D_3 should be used in patients with liver disease who have decreased activity of the enzyme vitamin D-25-hydroxylase. The major practical advantage of vitamin D_2 is that it is inexpensive and can be used in selected patients. In contrast to 25-hydroxyvitamin D_3, however, vitamin D_2 tends to be chemically unstable and to lose its activity with storage. It also tends to accumulate in fat and muscle during long-term administration, so that its effects may become cumulative. With both compounds, the therapeutic dose approaches the toxic dose, a long period is required for optimal biologic effect, and activity may persist after cessation of administration, a disadvantage in the event of intoxication. Also, the two sterols are not consistently effective, especially when the metabolism of vitamin D is abnormal.

The advantages of dihydrotachysterol and 1,25-dihydroxyvitamin D_3 are that they require only a short

TABLE 2 Preparations of Vitamin D and its Derivatives

Drug	*Dose Required (µg/day)*	*Period for Optimal Activity (weeks)*	*Duration of Action (weeks)*	*Available Preparations (µg)*	*Trade Name*
Vitamin D_2 (ergocalciferol)	250–2500	4–8	6–18	250 solution* 1250 capsules	Drisdol Drisdol
25-Hydroxyvitamin D_3 (calcifediol)	50–200	2–4	4–12	20 capsules 50 capsules	Calderol
Dihydrotachysterol	125–1000	1–2	1–3	125 capsules 200 capsules 400 capsules	Hytakerol, Dihydrotachysterol
1,25-Dihydroxyvitamin D_3 (calcitriol)	0.5–3	0.5–1	0.5–1	0.25 capsules 0.50 capsules	Rocaltrol

50,000 IU of vitamin D is 1,250 µg.
* 250 µg per ml.

TABLE 3 Advantages and Disadvantages of Vitamin D and Its Derivatives

Drug	*Advantages*	*Disadvantages*
Vitamin D_2	Inexpensive Precursor of vitamin D metabolites	Therapeutic dose approaches toxic dose Long period for onset of biologic effect Prolonged period of effect after cessation May not be effective, particularly when vitamin D metabolism is defective Unstable, undergoes oxidation, photochemical decomposition, and loss of activity with storage
25-Hydroxyvitamin D_3	Chemically stable Precursor of vitamin D metabolites Should be useful in liver disease when 25-hydroxylation is impaired	Moderately expensive Except for stability, disadvantages are same as for vitamin D_2
Dihydrotachysterol	Does not require la-hydroxylation; can be used when this is impaired Short period for onset of biologic effect Period of effect after cessation usually short but may be prolonged	Therapeutic dose approaches toxic dose Moderately expensive 25-hydroxylation required for biologic effectiveness; may be ineffective in liver disease May be less effective in osteomalacia than in osteitis fibrosa cystica
1,25-Dihydroxyvitamin D_3	Short period of onset for biologic effect Short period of effect after cessation Can be highly effective when la-hydroxylation is impaired and may provide normal or near normal growth	Expensive May be less effective in osteomalacia than in osteitis fibrosa cystica Toxicity may occur spontaneously

period of administration for optimal biologic activity and have a short period of effect after cessation of treatment. The biologic activity of dihydrotachysterol, however, may be prolonged on occasion. Also, both drugs are effective when la-hydroxylation of 25-hydroxyvitamin D is defective. On the other hand, both drugs are relatively expensive, neither may be completely effective in curing rickets in patients who are deficient in some of the other metabolites, and toxicity can occur spontaneously in patients who are on long-term treatment with them. The hypercalcemia, however, is easily managed by stopping the drug and is prevented by reducing the dose. 1,25-dihydroxyvitamin D_3 may be highly effective in promoting normal or near-normal growth and development in some children with deficiency of the metabolite. This may also be the case with optimal treatment when the other preparations of vitamin D are utilized.

SIDE EFFECTS AND COMPLICATIONS OF TREATMENT

Intoxication can occur with vitamin D or any of its metabolites and can be a major problem. Patients with intoxication are often asymptomatic, but may have anorexia, nausea, vomiting, constipation, lethargy, weakness, weight loss, polyuria, polydipsia,, a dry mouth, and alterations in mental status. Children and infants often show listlessness and are hypotonic. Hypercalcemia and hypercalciuria result from increased intestinal absorption of calcium and mobilization of calcium from the skeleton, and this may lead to impairment in renal function, nephrocalcinosis, nephrolithiasis, urinary tract infections, renal failure, and death. In patients who are on long-term treatment, the development of hypercalcemia and hypercalciuria are not uncommon. Unfortunately, there is no way of predicting when or in whom intoxication will occur.

Intoxication with vitamin D, 25-hydroxyvitamin D_3, and dihydrotachysterol are related to the fact that there is very little difference between toxic and therapeutic doses. On the other hand, toxicity occurring with 1,25-dihydroxyvitamin D_3 appears to be related to an alteration in the metabolism of the drug. There are suggestions that this may be the case with regard to vitamin D since lower doses are sometimes required after a hypercalcemic episode. Factors that may contribute to the development of vitamin D intoxication include selection of an inappropriately high dose, increases in dose over too short an interval, change in dietary calcium intake, lack of follow-up evaluation of serum and urinary calcium, administration of thiazides, and improvement in underlying disease.

The treatment of intoxication is to stop the drug and to force fluids. If intoxication is profound, a short course of steroids or salmon calcitonin may be required, usually only when hypercalcemia is produced by the longer-acting sterols. Use of lower doses of the drugs after episodes of hypercalcemia usually prevent recurrences. Patients who are difficult to treat with vitamin D may be more easily managed with 1,25-dihydroxyvitamin D_3.

The best treatment for intoxication is prevention. Patients should be closely followed at regular intervals of 4 to 6 weeks with measurement of serum calcium and creatinine. When placed on treatment, they should be informed of the possibility of intoxication, the symptoms of intoxication, and the potential harmful effects.

PREFERRED TREATMENT OF HYPOCALCEMIA

The goals are (1) to correct hypocalcemia, alleviate related symptoms, and prevent grand mal seizures and cataracts, (2) to prevent or alleviate the skeletal deformities of rickets or osteomalacia and excess parathyroid hormone when present, (3) to prevent hypercalcemia, hypercalciuria, and their sequellae, and (4) to promote normal growth and development in children and infants. Treatment must be individualized according to pathogenesis and severity of the hypocalcemia.

Administration of elemental calcium is useful. Calcium content varies with oral preparations: calcium carbonate (40%), calcium chloride (36%), calcium lactate (13%) and calcium gluconate (9%). Thus, 2.5 g, 2.8 g, 7.7 g, and 11.0 g are required, respectively, to provide 1.0 g of elemental calcium daily. Calcium chloride is irritating and should be given only with milk or meals. One preparation, calcium lactate powder, can be obtained from health food stores; one level teaspoonful provides about 1.0 g of elemental calcium. It can be administered in a glass of water and is well tolerated.

Hypocalcemia, usually presenting with tetany and grand mal seizures, is sometimes a medical emergency, especially when it is acute and severe. Treatment is needed to prevent laryngeal stridor, which may produce asphyxia and death. For this, calcium gluconate should be given slowly intravenously, 20 to 40 ml of a 10 percent solution over a period of 1 to 2 hours. It should be noted that each milliliter of this solution contains 9 mg of elemental calcium. Calcium can then be given by mouth together with vitamin D as outlined below.

Vitamin D Deficiency

Regardless of age, the patient with vitamin D-deficient rickets is treated by the daily administration of 125 μg (5000 IU) of vitamin D_2 and 1.0 g of elemental calcium for 4 to 6 weeks or until the rickets is healed. thereafter, the dose is 10 μg (400 IU) per day. Additional calcium is required only if the dietary intake is not adequate.

Malabsorption Diseases

Hypocalcemia frequently occurs in diseases associated with intestinal malabsorption and may result from impaired absorption of calcium or magnesium (e.g., due to rapid transit, formation of soaps) or vitamin D deficiency (e.g., due to rapid transit, interruption of the enterohepatic circulation). Hypomagnesemia, if present, should be treated since administration of calcium alone, even in large amounts, will be ineffective in correcting hypocalcemia. Treatment must be adapted for the individual patient. Initially, 1.0 to 3.0 g of calcium can be given orally in divided daily doses together with 0.62 mg (25,000 IU) of vitamin D_2 per day. Serum calcium and creatinine should be measured at intervals of 4 to 6 weeks. The dose of vitamin D can be increased as necessary, depending on the response of the serum calcium. Treatment with 25-hydroxyvitamin D_3, beginning with a dose of 50 μg per day, may be required in patients with associated hepatic disease.

Magnesium Deficiency

Magnesium deficiency may result from diminished intake or from excessive loss of the ion from the gastrointestinal tract or kidneys. Hypocalcemia commonly occurs and results from impaired secretion of parathyroid hormone, from diminished response of target organs to parathyroid hormone, or both. Initially, 2.0 g magnesium sulfate (16.3 mEq of magnesium) should be given intramuscularly every 4 hours for a total of five doses the first day. In instances where more rapid treatment is deemed necessary, 2 g of magnesium sulfate can be given intravenously over a period of several minutes, and a constant infusion can be administered at a rate of 1 mEq/kg body weight for the first day. Thereafter, 0.5 mEq/kg body weight per day may be given either intramuscularly or intravenously for several days or until the serum magnesium returns to normal. Correction of hypomagnesemia almost always corrects the hypocalcemia.

Anticonvulsant Therapy

Phenobarbital and Dilantin impair the target-organ response (intestine and skeleton) to 1,25-dihydroxyvitamin D_3 and may cause rickets. Anticonvulsant drugs also cause the production of more polar, biologically inactive metabolites of vitamin D by the liver. Rickets can be treated and prevented by small but pharmacologic doses of vitamin D, 125 μg (5000 IU) per day.

Hypoparathyroidism and Pseudohypoparathyroidism

Serum 1,25-dihydroxyvitamin D values are diminished in hypoparathyroidism and pseudohypoparathyroidism because of lack of parathyroid hormone and abnormal response to parathyroid hormone, respectively. Patients with rickets may respond to vitamin D_2. The dose is from 1.25 to 2.5 mg (50,000 to 100,000 IU) per day. Elemental calcium should be given in an initial dose of 1.0 g per day in divided doses. The dose can be increased to as much as 3.0 g per day to bring the serum calcium to the lower range of normal. The serum phosphate will often then decrease to within the normal range. If hypocalcemia persists, the dose of vitamin D can then be increased, but this should be done very slowly at intervals of 1 to 2 months.

If rickets and hypocalcemia persist, vitamin D should be stopped, and treatment with 1,25-dihydroxyvitamin D_3, 0.5 μg per day, should be started.

The dose can be increased at about 2-week intervals if required to correct hypocalcemia. Healing of the rickets may require 2 months or longer.

Vitamin D-dependent Rickets Type I

Rickets in this disease is caused by impaired renal production of 1,25-dihydroxyvitamin D_3, 0.5 to 2.0 μg per day (or 0.04 μg/kg/day). This results in correction of the hypocalcemia, hypophosphatemia and increased alkaline phosphatase and in healing of the rickets within 1 to 2 months.

Vitamin D-dependent Rickets Type II

Rickets in this disease is caused by defective target-organ response to 1,25-dihydroxyvitamin D_3. The disease is particularly severe in patients with associated alopecia who may be refractory to as much as 20 μg a day of 1,25-dihydroxyvitamin D_3. Some patients respond to large doses of vitamin D. Therefore, vitamin D_2 in doses of 1.25 to 2.5 mg (50,000 to 100,000 IU) or more and 3.0 g a day of elemental calcium should be tried initially. If the response is poor, treatment with 1,25-dihydroxyvitamin D_3 may be tried with an initial dose of 1.0 to 2.0 μg per day.

Hypophosphatasia

This disease of unknown cause is characterized by rickets and low serum alkaline phosphatase. There is no known treatment.

Hypophosphatemic Rickets

Hypophosphatemic rickets is caused by a defect in renal tubular transport of phosphate, which results in renal phosphate wasting and hypophosphatemia. Serum 1,25-dihydroxyvitamin D is inappropriately low for the serum phosphorus, does not respond normally to exogenous parathyroid extract, and may represent a secondary impairment resulting from the abnormal renal transport of phosphate.

Treatment is with elemental phosphate, 2.0 to 4.0 g per day by mouth, and 1,25-dihydroxyvitamin D_3, 1.0 to 2.0 μg per day (or 0.04 μg/kg/day). With this regimen, the serum phosphorus may be brought into the normal range, and there is a decline in the serum alkaline phosphatase toward normal and healing of the rickets. Treatment is lifelong.

Corrective osteotomies should be carried out after cessation of growth. Reduction of the dose of 1,25-dihydroxyvitamin D_3 may be required during prolonged bed rest because of immobilization and the potential development of hypercalcemia.

Suggested Reading

Avioli LV. The therapeutic approach to hypoparathyroidism. Am J Med 1974; 57:34–42.

Bell NH, Stern PH. Hypercalcemia and increases in serum hormone value during prolonged administration of 1a,25-dihydroxyvitamin D. N Engl J Med 1978; 298:1241–1243.

Davie M, Adams PH. The continuing risk of vitamin D intoxication. Lancet 1978; 2:621–623.

Harrison HE, Lifshitz F, Blizzard RM. Comparison between crystalline dihydrotachysterol and calciferol in patients requiring pharmacologic vitamin D therapy. N Engl J Med 1967; 276:894–900.

Kumar R, Riggs BL. Vitamin D in the therapy of disorders of calcium and phosphorus metabolism. Mayo Clin Proc 1981; 56:327–333.

Pierides AM. Pharmacology and therapeutic use of vitamin D and its analogues. Drugs 1981; 21:241–256.

HYPERCALCEMIA

BAYARD D. CATHERWOOD, M.D.
LEONARD J. DEFTOS, M.D.

In this chapter we shall review our approach to the therapy of hypercalcemia. The clinical objectives of therapy should be: alleviation of symptoms related to the elevated serum calcium, reversal or prevention of the complications of hypercalcemia, and control of hypercalcemia while diagnosis and management of the underlying cause are accomplished.

The symptoms of hypercalcemia are shown in Table 1 and are related to the effects of extracellular calcium on function of many tissues, including brain, peripheral nerve, visceral smooth muscle, cardiac muscle, and kidney. Symptoms specific to the etiology of the hypercalcemia, such as the bone pain of hyperparathyroidism or metastatic bone disease and the pulmonary and ocular symptoms of sarcoidosis, will not be alleviated by lowering the serum calcium. The symptoms in Table 1 correlate in a general way with the degree of severity of the hypercalcemia and, while they may have other causes, they should respond to effective treatment if due to the hypercalcemia in a given case. Rapid worsening of hypercalcemia may be precipitated by tumor progression in malignancy, acute immobilization in Paget's disease, sunlight exposure in sarcoidosis, or dehydration with any etiology of hypercalcemia. These clinical events may produce more severe symptoms for a given degree of hypercalcemia, but this is by no means invariably the case. Poorly defined complaints of abdominal discomfort may be seen in hypercalcemia

TABLE 1 Symptoms of Hypercalcemia

Lethargy
Impaired mentation
Confusion
Anorexia
Nausea
Vomiting
Constipation
Polyuria
Polydipsia

without specific abdominal pathology; however, it should be noted that abdominal pain, nausea, and vomiting may also represent the complications of peptic ulceration or pancreatitis, which cannot be expected to resolve optimally with subsequent treatment of the hypercalcemia alone.

A number of complications may result from the hypercalcemic state (Table 2). The most common consequence of hypercalcemia is dehydration. It is essential to proper therapy to understand that this is a direct consequence of inhibition of the renal medullary concentrating mechanism by the hypercalcemia. Dehydration is commonly present in moderate to severe hypercalcemia of any cause unless the hypercalcemia is of very short duration or renal salt wasting cannot occur because of intrinsic renal disease. In addition, other effects of hypercalcemia, such as vomiting or gastrointestinal bleeding, may contribute to dehydration. Decreased glomerular filtration and, in turn, decreased renal calcium clearance exacerbate hypercalcemia, thus creating a vicious cycle. Potentially life-threatening complications of profound dehydration include stroke, myocardial infarction, and acute renal tubular necrosis. Other life-threatening complications of hypercalcemia on the brain, cardiovascular system, and kidneys include coma with the potential for aspiration of oral and gastric secretions, cardiac arrhythmias and metastatic calcification in the heart with conduction blocks, and nephrocalcinosis, which may be reversible if of short duration, but otherwise progresses untreated to permanent renal failure.

We shall not discuss in detail the etiologies of hypercalcemia, their mechanisms, and their diagnosis, which are described in detail in general endocrinology textbooks. The basic mechanisms of hypercalcemia are (1) increased bone resorption, (2) increased calcium absorption, and (3) decreased renal calcium excretion; the first is by far the most common. Thus, treatment can theoretically be directed to (1) inhibit bone resorption, (2) decrease calcium absorption, and (3) increase urinary calcium excretion. In practice, however, the treatment is not necessarily aimed at the abnormal mechanism. Decreased renal calcium excretion is seldom a cause of hypercalcemia, but promoting the renal excretion of calcium is commonly used for treatment. Although increased calcium absorption may contribute to some cases of hypercalcemia, attempts to decrease dietary calcium intake and absorption are seldom useful. Drugs to inhibit bone resorption are commonly used for treatment of hypercalcemia because increased bone resorption is a common mechanism of hypercalcemia. Specific causes of hypercalcemia are summarized in Table 3. Although some therapies for hypercalcemia are generally applicable regardless of etiology, the utility of other treatment modalities, especially glucocorticosteroids and prostaglandin synthesis inhibitors, is limited, and these should be used only when the mechanism of the hypercalcemia indicates a possibility of success. It should be noted that primary hyperparathyroidism or malignancy is the cause of hypercalcemia in the overwhelming majority of cases. Although most cases of severe hypercalcemia persisting after correction of dehydration result from progression of a previously known malignant tumor, hypercalcemia can be the presenting manifestation of a

TABLE 2 Complications of Hypercalcemia

Dehydration
Renal
Nephrolithiasis
Nephrocalcinosis
Renal failure
Cardiac
Hypertension
Arrhythmias
Gastrointestinal
Peptic ulceration
Pancreatitis
Neurologic
Coma

TABLE 3 Etiologies of Hypercalcemia

Hyperparathyroidism
Primary (common)
Multiple endocrine neoplasia
Parathroid carcinoma
Hypercalcemic secondary
Familial hypocalciuric hypercalcemia
Malignant tumor (common)
With skeletal involvement
Without detectable skeletal involvement (humoral hypercalcemia of malignant disease)
Drugs
Vitamin D/Vitamin A
Calcium (massive)
Thiazide diuretics
Lithium
Granulomatous disease
Sarcoidosis
Other
Endocrinopathies
Thyrotoxicosis
Pheochromocytoma
Addison's disease
Other
Miscellaneous
Immobilization
Acute renal failure recovery
Infantile (e.g., William's syndrome)

tumor. When no alternative diagnosis is apparent after admission to the hospital and initial evaluation, hyperparathyroidism or malignant tumor should be considered most likely. The possibilities for direct treatment of the underlying cause represent an important consideration in the symptomatic management, especially in hypercalcemia of malignant disease.

The severity of hypercalcemia and urgency of its treatment are assessed by consideration of the patient's symptoms, the presence of established complications, and the degree of elevation of the serum calcium. Calcium blood levels can be measured as total calcium by autoanalyzer methods or atomic absorption spectrophotometry or as ionized calcium by calcium selective electrode. Usually only small differences, if any, are seen between the two methods for total serum calcium. However, since approximately half of the circulating calcium is protein-bound, mostly to albumin, determination of total serum calcium may underestimate or occasionally overestimate the degree of elevation of unbound calcium ion concentration, which is most directly related to symptoms and complications. The most common circumstance resulting in underestimation of the severity of hypercalcemia is a decrease in the protein-bound fraction due to hypoalbuminemia from malnutrition, intrinsic hepatocellular disease, metastatic liver disease, or excessive albumin losses. Conversely, hemoconcentration may be partly responsible for mild increases in total serum calcium seen in conditions of volume depletion such as diuretic therapy, adrenal insufficiency, and pancreatic cholera. Exaggerated levels of total serum calcium have also been seen in a few cases of plasma cell dyscrasia with very high levels of a monoclonal immunoglobulin of high calcium-binding capacity. In cases of hypoalbuminemia, it is usually sufficient to mathematically correct the observed total serum calcium by the addition of 0.8 mg Ca/dl for every g/dl of albumin deficit, but this is only an approximation, and if necessary, unbound ionic calcium should be measured directly. In addition to these abnormalities of protein binding, the severity of the hypercalcemic diathesis can be masked by countervailing disorders that usually cause hypocalcemia, the most well known of which is acute pancreatitis. The presence of even mild hypercalcemia in this disorder should alert the physician to the possibility that the hypercalcemia was much more severe prior to this complication and may rebound.

The upper limit of normal total serum calcium is usually 10.5 mg/dl; slight decreases in serum calcium with age due to altered protein binding are usually unimportant in the immediate management of hypercalcemia since levels up to 12 mg/dl represent mild hypercalcemia. In this range symptoms are subtle, frequently representing dehydration in the older patients, and may be discernible only in retrospect following rehydration and other treatment. Calcium concentrations between 12 and 14 mg/dl represent moderate hypercalcemia. The severity of symptoms may be variable, depending on the degree of dehydration and the chronicity of the hypercalcemia. The activity of the underlying bone resorption which is responsible for the hypercalcemia may be variable since some patients with previously mild disease may be made much worse by administration of diuretics or laxatives, and by vomiting or diarrhea. Thus the severity of the problem should be reassessed after clinical evidence of adequate volume repletion. Serum calcium levels greater than 14 mg/dl represent severe hypercalcemia with significant risk of complications and should be treated as a medical emergency. Many patients with rapid osteolysis in hypercalcemia of malignant disease continue to be severely hypercalcemic in spite of vigorous attempts at therapy and represent the most challenging problems.

CALCIURETIC THERAPY

The cornerstone of the emergency management of hypercalcemia is the promotion of urinary calcium excretion by the administration of saline followed by diuretics. We divide calciuretic therapy into three stages (Table 4). The rationale for this sequence is the action of hypercalcemia to impair renal concentrating ability and cause dehydration. In stage I, the degree of dehydration should be assessed by physical examination and laboratory evidence of prerenal azotemia. An orthostatic drop in blood pressure usually indicates at least 5 to 10 percent volume deficit. Saline should be infused at 200 to 250 ml per hour or more, depending on the severity of hypercalcemia, the presence of target organ damage, the age of the patient, and cardiovascular and renal function. During the rehydration stage of treatment, most patients with good cardiac function can be managed by careful clinical observation, although invasive monitoring of right atrial or pulmonary capillary wedge pressure should be considered in patients with heart failure and severe hypercalcemia. As extracellular volume repletion and urinary calcium excretion are both directly related to the amount of sodium infused, it is not generally rational to use hypotonic saline because the delivery of sodium at any chosen rate requires the infusion of twice as much water. Failure to achieve adequate rehydration may impair the clinical response to other therapies directed at inhibition of bone resorption.

TABLE 4 Calciuretic Therapy

Stage	*Action*	*Rationale*
I	Volume repletion with normal saline	Hypercalcemia causes renal sodium wasting and dehydration
II	Volume expansion with normal saline	Increasing renal sodium clearance increases calcium clearance
III	Assist sodium excretion with furosemide as necessary	Do not start diuretic until after stage II to avoid recurrent dehydration

In patients with mild to moderate hypercalcemia whose condition has recently been worsened by dehydration, intravenous rehydration may be the only intervention necessary to bring the calcium into a safe range until more definitive therapy can be instituted. In that case intravenous lines may be discontinued if proper care is taken to prevent recurrent dehydration. If previous diuretic therapy contributed to the dehydration, alternative drugs should be used if possible; consideration should also be given to liberalization of dietary sodium allowances to prevent recurrence of dehydration pending the institution of direct treatment of the underlying cause. Some textbooks have suggested that oral salt supplements can be used for chronic treatment of hypercalcemia. In our experience, this treatment is limited by palatability to about 9 g NaC1 per day (equivalent to only 1 liter of saline solution) and is useful only for mild hypercalcemia.

For moderate to severe hypercalcemia, the second stage of calciuretic therapy is extracellular volume expansion. The therapeutic rationale is the direct relationship between calcium clearance and sodium clearance due to linkage of renal tubular reabsorption of the two cations. If hypercalcemia has not responded to volume repletion, urinary clearance of 5 to 6 liters per day of saline is usually necessary for the adequate treatment of hypercalcemia until bone resorption can be controlled by one or more of the agents to be discussed below. At these rates of saline infusion, most patients develop some sodium retention, and older patients, even without known heart disease, develop pulmonary venous hypertension or edema. Careful recording of intakes and urinary volume and sodium, as well as repeated clinical evaluation, is thus essential to maintain sodium balance; monitoring pulmonary capillary wedge pressure should seriously be considered in patients with significant heart failure. When other therapeutic options are limited and hypercalcemia is not responding, saline infusion may be increased to as much as 500 ml per hour if renal function is good, but this probably should not be attempted except in an intensive care unit.

The third stage of calciuretic therapy is a loop diuretic such as furosemide (Lasix) or ethacrynic acid (Edecrin) to assist the renal excretion of the infused saline and with it the filtered load of calcium. To avoid recurrent dehydration, it is important not to institute the diuretic until mild extracellular volume expansion has been achieved. The dose of furosemide should be determined to just prevent further sodium retention and may be 10 to 40 mg intravenously every 2 to 6 hours. Significant decreases in serum potassium and magnesium may result and should be replaced appropriately. At the highest rates of saline infusion, profound abnormalities of these other electrolytes may result, and repeated measurement of actual urinary losses is required for effective replacement. (See below for discussion of serum phosphorus.)

In patients with mild intrinsic renal disease, therapy with saline and furosemide can be used as long as an effective response to the diuretic can be achieved. In patients with significant renal failure, this mode of therapy is not possible, and if the serum calcium must be rapidly lowered because of life-threatening cardiac or central nervous system effects, emergency dialysis is the only sure means to rapidly and safely lower their serum calcium. In patients who are not already receiving maintenance hemodialysis, establishing vascular access may be the rate-limiting step in obtaining this treatment.

INHIBITION OF BONE RESORPTION

Calcitonin

Treatment of hypercalcemia associated with malignancy is an approved use of salmon calcitonin in the United States. This hormone has many clinical advantages. It is a potent inhibitor of osteoclastic bone resorption, can act rapidly against hypercalcemia, and has few serious complications. Accordingly, it can be considered for almost every patient with hypercalcemia. However, calcitonin treatment does have several drawbacks. Although it can rapidly lower blood calcium, normal levels are seldom achieved. Furthermore, resistance to the hypocalcemic effect of calcitonin is commonly seen after several days of treatment. Concomitant treatment with glucocorticosteroids has been reported to imporve the initial effectiveness of calcitonin treatment in the first 4 days and may be worth trying in patients whose long-term prognosis is poor, but controlled studies of its long-term efficacy are not available. We thus use calcitonin in patients with contraindications to the use of plicamycin (Mithracin), not uncommon in malignant disease, or for patients who have initially received plicamycin and in whom we anticipate recurrent hypercalcemia because the underlying disease has not been controlled. We administer 100 to 200 units of salmon calcitonin subcutaneously every 12 hours if the patient can tolerate treatment without nausea and flushing. We believe allergic reactions with current formulations of salmon calcitonin are very uncommon. Salmon calcitonin in our experience is more effective in the treatment of hypercalcemia due to immobilization either in patients with Paget's disease or in adolescents. In such patients, treatment can be started at 100 units every 12 hours and tapered with control of the hypercalcemia.

Plicamycin (Formerly Called Mithramycin)

Plicamycin is a highly reliable treatment currently available in the United States for the treatment of severe hypercalcemia that is unresponsive to volume repletion and saline diuresis. We use a single dose of 25 $\mu g/kg$ intravenously. This is infused over 4 hours to minimize associated nausea, and unless contraindicated, we premedicate the patient with an antiemetic. Some response is usually seen by 24 hours; however, the time course of plicamycin action is variable, and the nadir of serum calcium frequently occurs after 2 days and sometimes later. It should be noted that this is less intensive treatment than the dosage schedule contained in the package insert, which recommends daily infusions until the hypercalcemia has responded or four consecutive doses have been given. If the serum calcium has not begun to fall 48 hours after the first infusion of plicamycin, the patient should be reassessed to ensure that dehydration has been corrected.

Plicamycin is a cytotoxic agent, and although a single infusion at the recommended dose is relatively specific for the osteoclast, the drug can cause thrombocytopenia, qualitative platelet function disorders, and hepatic and renal damage. These adverse effects should almost never occur from a single infusion of plicamycin in patients with normal platelet, liver, and renal function. In patients with preexisting disorders of these systems or who are receiving cancer chemotherapy regimens with similar toxicities, we do consider the possibility of using other means of treatment first, even though other therapies are not so uniformly effective as plicamycin. In such patients, the benefits should be very carefully weighed against the risks. Reduction of the dose to 15 μg/kg may lessen the toxicity of plicamycin, but also fail to control the hypercalcemia. The mechanisms of inactivation and clearance of plicamycin are not well characterized. However, we have successfully used plicamycin without toxicity in a patient with end stage renal failure on maintenance hemodialysis in whom nephrotoxicity was not a concern. Although we usually use plicamycin in patients with malignant tumors, a few patients with primary hyperparathyroidism have severe hypercalcemia in the face of saline infusion. We believe one course of the drug is indicated in such patients, with parathyroidectomy planned during the ensuing normocalcemic period.

The duration of initial response to plicamycin is unpredictable and may range from 3 days to 2 weeks. The return of hypercalcemia can be extremely rapid, and serum calcium should be determined daily. After the initial treatment of severe hypercalcemia, if no toxicity has developed; we give another infusion as soon as the serum calcium exceeds 11 mg/dl. Repeated doses of plicamycin carry increased risk of toxicity, especially if treatment must be given at frequent intervals.

Diphosphonates

Several newer agents of this class of drug appear very promising for the treatment of hypercalcemia. Etidronate disodium (Didronel), the first diphosphonate developed, is not effective against hypercalcemia in the oral form available for general use in the United States. However, several investigational drugs are under study which are very effective. Intravenous infusion of dichloromethylene diphosphonate (Cl_2MDP), 300 to 500 mg/day or 5 mg/kg/day, or aminohydroxypropylidine diphosphonate (APD), 30 mg/day, markedly lowers the serum calcium within 6 to 7 days and, in most patients, restores the serum calcium to normal. Initial therapy with the oral form of either of these agents—Cl_2MDP, 800 to 3200 mg/day, or APD, 4 to 17 mg/kg/day—is less uniformly effective, but may be useful as maintenance therapy once normocalcemia has been achieved by intravenous infusions of the drug. Neither of these agents is approved for general use in the United States, and dichloromethylene diphosphonate has been reported to cause acute leukemia in a small number of cases.

Oral Phosphorus

Hypophosphatemia can be seen due to the phosphaturic action of parathyroid hormone, phosphaturic humoral factors produced by tumors, and direct effects of hypercalcemia on the kidney. Since bone resorption is in part controlled by the extracellular calcium-phosphate product, correction of hypophosphatemia can inhibit bone resorption. However, calcification of vital organs is one of the complications of hypercalcemia dependent on the calcium-phosphate ion product, and thus hypophosphatemia may be protective with respect to these complications. For this reason we avoid its use, unless serum phosphorus has fallen to a level where complications of hypophosphatemia per se are of concern (i.e., <2 mg/dl). If administered, it should be given only by mouth in doses of up to 1.5 g of phosphorus per day, usually a neutral phosphate solution, and renal function must be observed very closely. Intravenous phosphate infusions are extremely hazardous and seldom if ever indicated. Intravenous infusion of EDTA is also dangerous because of nephrotoxicity and renal failure.

OTHER GENERAL MEASURES

The accretion of extracellular calcium by bone is stimulated by weight-bearing, possibly through the generation of electromagnetic forces in bone mineral crystal. The effect of physical mobility is most easily seen when patients with high bone turnover rates, such as adolescents or patients with Paget's disease, are forced by trauma or another severe illness to observe complete bed rest. In such cases hypercalcemia results from an abrupt decrease in the rate of calcium accretion in the face of continued bone resorption, with an increased net flux of calcium from bone to blood. Such patients should be ambulated as soon and as much as possible, although other measures usually are needed to treat the hypercalcemia. Decreased weight-bearing may have a contributory role in any cause of hypercalcemia, and bed rest should not be ordered unnecessarily. Dairy products and other foods high in calcium may be restricted in hypercalcemic disorders with increased intestinal calcium absorption such as hyperparathyroidism, vitamin D intoxication, and sarcoidosis, but strict low calcium diets are not more effective.

Hypercalcemia may especially cause ventricular arrhythmias in patients receiving digitalis glycosides. In this setting, meticulous care should be given to replacement of urinary potassium and magnesium losses and treatment of deficiencies. If ventricular arrhythmias do not respond to the standard drugs, magnesium infusion may antagonize the cardiac effects of hypercalcemia, but the clinical efficacy of this treatment has not been well documented. Severe hypercalcemia can also cause heart block, and then a temporary pacemaker may be needed before treatment of ventricular ectopy.

SPECIFIC TREATMENTS

Glucocorticoids

Glucocorticoids are not generally effective inhibitors of bone resorption and should be reserved for cases in which a specific glucocorticoid-responsive etiology for the hypercalcemia is suspected. These include vitamin D intoxication per se and sarcoidosis and other granulomatous diseases in which unregulated synthesis of 1,25-dihydroxyvitamin D is believed to mediate the hypercalcemia. In such cases of severe hypercalcemia, treatment should be initiated with 300 mg/day of hydrocortisone in divided doses intravenously. Sarcoidosis with less severe hypercalcemia may respond to lower doses (e.g., prednisone, 20 mg daily). The dose should subsequently be reduced even further if not needed for the treatment of other sarcoid complications.

A second group of patients in whom glucocorticoids are indicated are those with glucocorticoid-responsive malignant disease, including myelomas, lymphomas, lymphocytic leukemias, and possibly breast cancer. In these situations, initiation of glucocorticoid therapy may be helpful prior to, or even in the absence of, other chemotherapy. Hypercalcemia due to other solid tumors does not respond to this treatment.

Prostaglandin Synthesis Inhibitors

Indomethacin and aspirin, which inhibit the synthesis of prostaglandins, enjoyed an initial wave of enthusiasm following a report that some cases of malignant hypercalcemia responded to this treatment. percalcemia recurs or progresses, the drug should be promptly discontinued.

Treatment of Underlying Disease

The generally effective measures to inhibit bone resorption only provide days to weeks of control of the hypercalcemia, and more definitive treatment of the underlying etiology must be promptly undertaken when possible and appropriate. A few patients with solid tumors with apparent humorally mediated hypercalcemia may have resectable primary lesions, and a history of hypercalcemia per se is not necessarily a contraindication to surgical treatment. However, most patients with cancer have more or less advanced disease and receive radiation therapy or chemotherapy; the chance of a long-term disease-free period depends on the responsiveness of the tumor. When the primary tumor fails to respond to direct treatment, control of the hypercalcemia becomes progressively more difficult, and the decision to continue antihypercalcemic Subsequent experience has been very disappointing, and these agents are considered to be rarely effective. We believe that it is most dangerous to attempt to use these agents in place of known and generally effective treatments for moderate to severe hypercalcemia. We would attempt a therapeutic trial of these drugs only in patients with malignant tumors of the genitourinary tract who either present with mild hypercalcemia or have undergone initial treatment with plicamycin or other agents. Precautions against, and careful observation for, GI ulceration should be taken, and if hytherapy is frequently made on the basis of other considerations such as need for pain control. In contrast, the treatment of hyperparathyroidism and sarcoidosis is usually very effective.

Suggested Reading

Broadus AE. Mineral metabolism. In: Felig P, et al. eds. Endocrinology and Metabolism. New York: McGraw Hill, 1981: 963–1080.

Deftos LJ, Neer RM. Medical management of the hypercalcemia of malignancy. In: Creger WP, Cloggins DH, Hancock EW, eds. Annual Review of Medicine, Palo Alto, California: Annual Reviews, Inc., 1974; 25:323–331.

First BP, Deftos LJ. Hypercalcemia in malignancy. In: Klastersky J and Staquet M, eds. Medical Complications in Cancer Patients. New York: Raven Press, 1981; 155–169.

Stewart AF, Horst R, Deftos LJ, Cadman EC, Lang R, Rasmussen H, Broadus AE. Biochemical evaluation of patients with malignancy-associated hypercalcemia: evidence for humoral and non-humoral groups. New Engl J Med 1980; 303:1377–1383.

PAGET'S DISEASE OF BONE

MELVIN HORWITH, M.D.

Paget's disease (osteitis deformans) is a fairly common disease of bone characterized by a localized disturbance of bone architecture secondary to abnormally increased osteoclastic activity. The lesions may be monostotic or polyostotic. Clinical manifestations depend on location. Fractures, proximity to neural tissue, and involvement of large joints are the most common causes of clinical problems. Since this disease affects chiefly the elderly, our increasingly aging population will undoubtedly present more frequently with the sequelae of Paget's disease. Europeans (with the exception of Scandanavians) are more likely to have this disease as are Australians, New Zealanders, and North Americans. Although relatively infrequent in Africa, native-born blacks in North America may also have Paget's disease. A genetic predisposition may make certain ethnic groups more susceptible to this chronic disturbance of orderly bone remodeling. Recent histologic and immunologic evidence have suggested the possibility of a slow-virus infection of the osteoclasts as an etiologic agent. Infection may also be dependent on a genetic predisposition of certain population groups.

PATHOPHYSIOLOGY

Paget's disease of bone represents a disturbance in the normally coupled resorption and formation of bone. The markedly accelerated resorptive process leads to abnormal architecture with lamellar bone replaced by "woven" or amorphous bone. The basic defect appears to be abnormal osteoclastic cell hyperfunction as well as an increase in the numbers of these cells. The osteoclast, which has its origin from hematopoietic cell lines (macrophage) becomes "deregulated" so that each cell (of which there are increased numbers in local areas) becomes hyperfunctional, as indicated by the ruffled borders and increased numbers of nuclei. This resorptive process in turn stimulates osteoblastic activity. Increased osteolysis with the appearance of localized osteoporosis often precedes the deposition of sclerotic bone. This abnormal bone is structurally weaker and thus more susceptible to fracture. There is increased vascularity of the bones and of overlying soft tissue, leading to increased cardiac output. However, high output failure, even with generalized Paget's disease, is uncommon. The pagetic lesion is in reality a benign neoplasm of the osteoclast. However, malignant degeneration to osteosarcoma, chondrosarcoma, or fibrosarcoma may occur rarely. Giant cell tumors have also been reported in pagetic bone.

Clinical Aspects

Although we do not have adequate information regarding the natural history of Paget's disease, it is apparent that it is a chronic disease of the skeleton, possibly present for 20 to 30 years before becoming clinically apparent. It is also evident that most patients with monostotic Paget's disease are not clinically handicapped and, as a matter of fact, may have no pain or other disability. Many patients are detected solely by automated chemical screening and the detection of increased alkaline phosphatase or via routine films often taken for nonskeletal complaints. The areas of the skeleton most frequently involved are the skull, spine, thoracolumbar and sacral areas, pelvis, and lower extremities (femur and tibia). Any other bones, however, may be involved. Complications of involvement of the skull include cranial nerve entrapment and also basilar invagination with brain stem syndromes. Deafness is common. Involvement of the vertebrae may lead to syndromes of myelopathy and radiculopathy. Pagetic involvement of bone around large joints (hip, knee) may be admixed with concurrent osteoarthritis, and the primary cause of arthropathy may be impossible to define. Hip involvement is especially common and is often progressively disabling. Fractures are a common occurrence in pagetic areas of the long bones. It is important to recognize that pain in Paget's disease is more often related to joint involvement, fractures, and neural entrapment than to bone involvement per se.

Laboratory Evaluation of Patients with Paget's Disease

Increased Serum Alkaline Phosphatase. This enzyme is a reflection of bone formation. Elevated alkaline phosphatase in the presence of normal gamma glutamyl transpeptidase excludes causation by liver disease. If both enzyme levels are elevated, determination of alkaline phosphatase isoenzymes is necessary to quantify bone alkaline phosphatase. Very high alkaline phosphatase levels are often seen in Paget's disease and may be particularly associated with skull involvement.

Increased Urinary Hydroxyproline. This is a reflection of bone resorption.

Serum Calcium. This parameter is usually normal except in the immobilized patient or in a patient with concurrent disease such as primary hyperparathyroidism, metastatic disease to bone, or malignant disease leading to hypercalcemia. Primary hyperparathyroidism is not uncommonly associated with Paget's disease.

Examination of Bones. Blastic skeletal metastases from cancer of the prostate or other tumors may be differentiated from Paget's disease by the x-ray finding of bone enlargement in Paget's disease. Radiologic examination of the skeleton is generally the primary visualization technique used to study Paget's disease. However, the radioisotope bone scan is a far more sensitive detector. The x-ray examination can then be used to focus on particular sites indicated by positive bone scan. The bone scan often identifies pagetic sites, such as the base of the skull and vertebral bodies, which may not be radiologically apparent. CT scanning may be particularly helpful with regard to basilar invagination and also in evaluating possible malignant degeneration of a pagetic lesion. Nuclear magnetic resonance imaging may be particularly useful in lesions of the base of the skull and spinal column. Bone biopsy is employed only when the diagnosis is not certain or when there is a question of sarcoma or metastatic bone disease, for example, in dealing with patients who may have carcinoma of the prostate.

AN APPROACH TO THERAPY

Many patients with localized and/or asymptomatic disease do not require treatment and can be followed with periodic re-evaluations. In general, the indications for treatment of Paget's disease are: (1) pain and/or limited mobility, and/or progressive deformity, and/or fracture, due to strategic lesions involving joints, long bones, or neural tissue; and (2) generalized extensive bone disease, with high elevations of chemical parameters. Unfortunately, we are unable to cure Paget's disease; we are, however, able to control the progression of the pathology. The aim of therapy is to decrease discomfort and to prevent further deformity and disability by suppressing the metabolic activity of the pagetic bone, that is, by inhibiting "turnover". Inhibition of bone resorption (osteoclasts) leading to an overall decrease in bone "turnover" is reflected by a decrease in urinary hydroxyproline and in serum alkaline phosphatase. On the average, these parameters decrease to approximately 50 percent of pretreatment values. In a few patients the parameters may almost normalize. In others, the response may be very limited. Response may not plateau for up to 6 months or longer after initiation of treatment. The customary fluctuations of laboratory indices in untreated Paget's disease may make it difficult to ascertain that the changes are caused by treatment.

My initial approach to therapy is to discuss the nature of the problem with the patient and the concerned family. Understandably, the diagnosis of Paget's disease produces anxiety, often needlessly or inappropriately exaggerated. I review the films and bone scans with the patient and also discuss the results of the laboratory studies. It is important for the patient to understand the nature of the disease and the fact that, generally, the impairment produced is minimal and not life-threatening. The indications for therapy (or lack of indications) are reviewed, and the therapeutic regimens currently available are discussed. The informed patient appreciates more fully that we are trying to control rather than cure the bone disease. I also emphasize that not all patients respond to a given regimen and that response may take weeks to become evident.

THERAPEUTIC AGENTS

Calcitonin

I favor calcitonin as the initial treatment for Paget's disease. This hormone acts specifically to inhibit the osteoclasts and thus decrease bone resorption. The lowering of increased osteoblastic activity is not a direct calcitonin effect, but the result of coupling to decreased osteoclastic activity. *Calcimar* is a synthetic preparation of salmon calcitonin. This hormone may be self-administered subcutaneously in a manner similar to the administration of insulin. Calcitonin is generally well tolerated. However, many patients complain of gastrointestinal manifestations, especially nausea, and some complain of a disturbing facial flush shortly after the injection. Synthetic "human" calcitonin and porcine calcitonin are available in some countries (not in the United States) and produce the same side effects.

Beneficial effects should be apparent by 3 to 4 weeks of administration. There is generally a good correlation of benefit with a decrease of serum alkaline phosphatase and urinary hydroxyproline. The patient should be aware that these values may not return to normal. Maximum benefits occur in 3 to 6 months. Some start therapy with 100 units of salmon calcitonin per day, but I generally utilize 50 units/day (to minimize side effects I suggest administration before retiring) and gradually decrease the dose to 50 to 100 units every other day. After protracted administration of salmon or porcine calcitonin, antibodies are likely to develop. The antibodies may inhibit both the hypocalcemic and the clinical response—or the clinical response alone. Development of antibodies to human calcitonin is most infrequent.

Therapy is continued for at least 6 months as long as the patient tolerates the medication and treatment appears to be of benefit. Serum alkaline phosphatase is determined every 4 to 6 weeks and urinary hydroxyproline obtained somewhat less frequently. A good stopping point may be after chemistries are at a plateau for 2 months. Occasionally, there may be a slight increase in alkaline phosphatase, but this is not an indication that therapy is failing. Chemical and clinical improvement may persist for variable periods of time after discontinuance of calcitonin, occasionally up to one year, permitting intermittent therapy.

Calcitonin is preferable to diphosphonates in (1) immobilized patients, (2) hypercalcemic patients (at least until the etiology of the hypercalcemia is determined), (3) patients undergoing bone surgery for fractures, neural entrapment, and the like, and (4) patients with an osteolytic wedge on radiologic examination, which suggests impending fracture.

The disadvantages of calcitonin are (1) route of administration (subcutaneous injection), (2) side effects (facial flush, nausea, diarrhea, abdominal pain), and (3) antibody formation and resistance of biochemical and clinical effects (true for salmon and porcine). The thrice-weekly calcitonin injections of 50 units are slightly more costly than diphosphonate, 400 mg daily.

Diphosphonates

These agents represent an interesting group of compounds that bear similarities to the pyrophosphates and are known to inhibit mineralization. The diphosphonates are "bone seekers", and their bone localization favors areas of high turnover, making them useful as bone-scanning agents. These agents are also inhibitory to osteoclasts, exerting a calcitonin-like action, which makes them useful in the treatment of Paget's disease. Unfortunately, diphosphonates, to varying degrees and in dose-dependent fashion, interfere with osteoblastic function and mineralization of bone. These effects appear to be direct actions of the chemical agent, separate from the indirect osteoblast-inhibiting effect resulting from "coupling" between resorption and formation. Some of the newer diphosphonates apparently selectively inhibit resorption (osteoclasts), with only minimal direct effects upon formation (osteoblasts). It is hoped that these newer agents will be available in the near future. At this time, the only diphosphonate available in this country is the disodium salt of etidronate or EHDP (Didronel). This agent should not be used in doses greater than 5 mg/kg body weight per day, and generally for no more than a 6-month period of continuous therapy. At this dose level, and for this duration, the inhibitory effect on the osteoblasts is not considered to be clinically significant. For an individual of average body weight, the dose is usually 400 mg per day (two 200-mg tablets). Following a successful course of therapy for 6 months, one should wait until there is evidence (clinical and/or chemical) of relapse, before a repeat course of therapy is administered. Remissions are sometimes protracted, occasionally lasting up to 3 years. Results of diphosphonate therapy are quite similar to those of calcitonin, but perhaps with a somewhat greater quantitative chemical response and with longer remissions in many patients. There are many patients in whom I am constrained to begin treatment with diphosphonate because of dislike for injections or because of intolerance of such reactions as flushing and nausea.

Whether one begins treatment with disodium etidronate or with calcitonin, one may eventually consider adding the other drug if response is incomplete. In certain patients with severe disease, one may elect to use combined therapy from the start. It is important to anticipate that a small number of patients will report increase in arthralgia or in bone pain during therapy with disodium etidronate. This may be severe enough to warrant discontinuance. I have, on occasion, added a nonsteroidal anti-inflammatory agent to the regimen when pain develops during diphosphonate therapy. I have also halved the dose of diphosphonate to minimize the discomfort. It is difficult to be certain of the cause and effect relationship of therapy to the discomfort in Paget's disease since there is often fluctuation of clinical status in the untreated patient.

The disadvantages of diphosphonate therapy are (1) they cause increased arthralgia or bone pain in some patients; (2) they cause diarrhea (somewhat unusual); (3) they cause hyperphosphatemia, seen generally only with doses higher than 5 mg/kg body weight; and (4) they should not be taken with food containing calcium, but must be taken on an empty stomach 2 hours before eating.

Combined calcitonin and diphosphonate therapy may be employed in (1) patients totally or partially refractory to either agent alone, (2) severe generalized bone disease, or particularly threatening local lesions, (3) neurologic complications, and (4) impending surgery for basilar invagination.

Mithramycin

Mithramycin is an antibiotic that inhibits RNA synthesis and is known to be cytotoxic to osteoclasts. This agent is used to treat hypercalcemia of malignant disease since most hypercalcemia syndromes associated with malignant disease are secondary to increased bone resorption. I use this therapy infrequently for Paget's disease since it is fairly toxic and must be administered by IV infusion. The dose is 10 to 15 μg/kg body weight every other day (8–12 hr infusions) for up to 10 treatments. There are the usual hepatotoxic and nephrotoxic effects associated with the use of this agent, but more frequently gastrointestinal manifestations, such as nausea and vomiting are encountered. Platelet number and function may also be impaired. The side effects appear to be dose-related. Mithramycin therapy should be reserved for patients with severe neurologic manifestations resulting from compression by pagetic bone. If sufficient preoperative time is available, I would prefer to use combined calcitonin and diphosphonate therapy prior to surgical decompression.

Other Therapies

Numerous other treatment regimens have been used in Paget's disease. Most of these have not been proved effective or are less effective than calcitonin, diphosphonates, or mithramycin. Oral calcium supplementation plus a thiazide diuretic have been claimed to be of clinical value, but chemical parameters improve in very few patients. The mild hypercalcemia induced by this regimen is supposed to increase calcitonin secretion. However, there is no evidence that calcitonin secretion is increased or that any improvement occurs on radiologic examination. Certainly this regimen is relatively easy and less costly for the patient; however, if the patient is having significant clinical manifestations of Paget's disease, I use either the diphosphonates or calcitonin.

PRINCIPLES OF ESTROGEN THERAPY

JUDITH L. VAITUKAITIS, M.D.

For more than 50 years estrogen replacement therapy has been used to alleviate symptoms associated with the menopause. In most cases clinicians prescribe estrogens to alleviate hot flushes and symptoms of genital tract atrophy, which include urinary frequency and dysuria, dyspareunia, vaginal burning, itching, and even genital bleeding. In 1941, Albright and his colleagues suggested an association between osteoporosis and menopause. Since that time considerable evidence has accumulated to support a relationship between decreased estrogen production and development of osteoporosis, a setting in which the total skeletal mass is decreased but its composition remains normal. It is not clear whether estrogen replacement therapy significantly affects emotional lability, insomnia, depression, anxiety, and other related symptoms attributed to menopause, even though some double-blind studies suggest a significant therapeutic benefit in the alleviation of these symptoms.

The concentrations and analogs of estrogens suggested for replacement therapy vary considerably. Since the complications attributed to estrogen therapy appear to be dose related, it behooves clinicians to use the lowest effective dose to correct or minimize the patient's symptoms. In most cases estrogen therapy is given in pill form for convenience although parenteral formulations are available. There is a general consensus that unopposed estrogen replacement therapy should not be used in women with primary gonadal failure or in any other setting in which a uterus is present because of the increased risk of endometrial cancer. Even in those women who have undergone hysterectomy, some clinicians advocate using combined estrogen and progestin to counteract the effects of estrogen on breast tissue and the presumptive increased risk of breast cancer in that ssetting. There is some doubt about the adverse effect of estrogens on breast tissue, especially since results of some studies are consistent with a relative decreased risk of breast cancer among those postmenopausal women treated with estrogen alone.

Unfortunately, there are no good longitudinal studies which carefully assess the role of dietary calcium intake along with ascertaining the concentration of estrogen needed to minimize or stop bone loss and the development of osteoporosis. Moreover, there is essentially no information as to whether estrogen therapy need be given indefinitely in low concentrations combined with a progestin to induce those beneficial effects. Studies are sorely needed to dissect out the relative contributions of calcium versus estrogen deficiencies on the rate of bone loss or osteoporosis in women. Studies assessing dietary calcium intake strongly support insufficient intake of that element as a contributing factor in the development of osteopenia and its attendant risks. Finally, study designs and the techniques used to monitor bone loss leave much to be desired in most published studies. Although a wide array of different estrogen analogs and doses have been used to treat the consequences of gonadal failure, it is difficult to compare those studies because there is no good way to normalize the biochemical effects induced by different forms of estrogen administered alone or combined with progestins. Moreover, dietary calcium is frequently ignored in those studies. Perhaps the most widely used form of estrogen for ovarian failure is estrone sulfate, usually marketed in the form of Premarin in the United States. Unfortunately, it is one of the most expensive forms of estrogen replacement and probably offers no therapeutic advantage over other estrogen analogs. Further confounding those clinical studies is the fact that a wide variety of progestins are incorporated in combined estrogen-progestin therapy. Some may minimize bone loss in postmenopausal women. In addition, progestin analogs exert differential effects on lipid metabolism and have different intrinsic androgenic effects.

The other major group of women receiving estrogens are those who use combinations of estrogen and progestins for contraceptive purposes. Although birth control pills initially contained significantly higher concentrations of estrogen analogs, more recent formulations contain significantly lower concentrations of estrogen in view of accumulating information strongly supporting a dose-related effect between the concentration of estrogen and many of the side effects of the ''pill''. Additionally, some of the progestins may increase the risk for vascular disease as a result of altering glucose and lipid metabolism. All oral contraceptives currently marketed in the United States contain both an estrogen and a progestin.

Use of oral contraceptives containing an estrogen and a progestin may be beneficial since their use results in protection against development of pelvic inflammatory disease, ovarian cancer, benign breast disease, ectopic pregnancy, and endometrial cancer. Some of these benefits reflect the fact that current formulations contain lower concentrations of sex steroid. Most oral contraceptives contain one of two estrogens—ethinyl estradiol or mestranol. The form of progestin present varies considerably. The progestins present within those formulations contain differential androgenic and progestational activities. Of the two estrogen preparations commonly present within those formulations, mestranol exerts approximately two-thirds the estrogenic effect that ethinyl estradiol induces. Mestranol must be metabolized to ethinyl estradiol in the liver prior to inducing its effects. Some progestins may exert weak estrogenic activity.

HOT FLUSHES AND ENDOMETRIAL CANCER

Approximately three of four women who undergo spontaneous physiologic menopause or undergo surgical removal of the ovaries experience hot flushes. Approximately 20 percent of affected women continue to experience their symptoms for at least 5 years, and approximately half of these (or 10% of all postmenopausal women) require therapy. Hot flushes per se are not an indication for therapy since most women tolerate those symptoms, which decrease over several months to a few years. Moreover, many postmenopausal women are not enamored with the periodic menstrual bleeding that accompanies combined estrogen and progestin therapy. Interestingly, the symptoms of hot flushes correlate positively with decreasing estrogen levels. Women receiving parenteral forms of estrogen may experience hot flushes when the circulating estrogen levels decrease but are at supraphysiologic levels. Estrogens have proved to be more effective than placebo in alleviating hot flushes and other signs and symptoms associated with the perimenopausal or postmenopausal state. It is interesting that the subjective symptoms of the hot flush precede measurable changes in skin conductance and an increase in skin temperature by approximately one minute. The intensity and frequency of hot flushes may be alleviated with estrogen therapy. Nonsteroidal medications may also alleviate those symptoms.

I recommend starting treatment with a low-dose estrogen-progestin combination (20 μg ethinyl estradiol and a progestin) when treating women with hot flushes and consider increasing the dose of estrogen only if symptoms are not markedly alleviated. Starting with formulations with higher estrogen content and then attempting to decrease the dose usually is not well tolerated. It has been suggested that the circulatory changes associated with hot flushes result from a transient increase in sympathetic activity. Symptoms may be alleviated with estrogens (10 to 20 μg ethinyl estradiol), progestins (e.g., Provera, 10 mg *bid*), propranolol (20 mg *bid*), or clonidine (0.1 to 0.2 mg *bid*). Alleviation of the hot flushes experienced by some women receiving antiestrogen therapy (Tamoxifen, for example) for breast cancer can be attained with clonidine. A dose of clonidine 0.1 mg *bid* usually suffices.

Based on several case control studies, the risk of developing endometrial cancer among women receiving unopposed estrogen therapy (no progestin) was significantly greater than that of controls; the risk increased with the dose and duration of estrogen therapy. That relationship is not surprising in view of the apparent relationship between endometrial hyperplasia, induced by unopposed estrogen, and the risk of neoplasia. Interestingly, although the incidence of endometrial cancer was increased significantly, the mortality associated with that cancer was unchanged. The addition of a progestin to cyclic estrogen therapy is associated with a significantly lower incidence of endometrial cancer than that observed among women receiving estrogens alone. Ideally one would wish to combine low-dose estrogen with a progestin that does not significantly affect HDL cholesterol levels.

OSTEOPOROSIS

Osteoporosis and its attendant symptoms and complications is a significant public health problem among women. Beginning in the fourth or fifth decade, men and women begin to lose total bone mass. If a woman undergoes a complete hysterectomy or develops primary ovarian failure prior to that time, the foregoing process begins earlier. It has been estimated that 20 percent of all women will have suffered a hip fracture by the time they attain the age of 90. At least 80 percent of those women will have had pre-existing osteoporosis. The mortality associated with hip fractures is also high in that approximately 1 in 8 dies within 3 months. In addition to that type of fracture, approximately 25 percent of all Caucasian women over the age of 60 develop compression fractures of vertebrae as a complication of osteoporosis. Other bony fractures occur at a greater rate among women over the age of 60. The annual cost of medical care is astronomic within this group because of complications of osteoporosis. Although osteoporosis is frequently attributed to decreased estrogen, as already noted, several studies have documented that a deficiency of dietary calcium intake is undoubtedly a contributing factor to the development of this disorder. The decreased dietary intake is further complicated by the fact that efficiency of gut calcium absorption decreases with age. The recommended daily allowance of elemental calcium has been established at 800 mg/day. That requirement may even be higher among the elderly. If a woman consumes significantly lower levels of calcium per day, that effect is magnified over time and results in significant bone loss. One must remember that there is currently no form of therapy that stimulates bone formation. Therapy is directed to decreasing bone resorption by administering estrogen or by adding dietary calcium to prevent bone loss. Several studies support a relationship between insufficient dietary calcium ingestion and the risk of bone fractures among older women. Although adequate studies have not been completed, estrogen treatment appears to be superior to calcium treatment alone when postmenopausal bone loss is monitored. However, whether high dietary calcium supplements are sufficient to significantly retard bone loss is unknown. Although essentially all studies support a therapeutic effect for estrogen in terms of significantly retarding bone loss, as monitored by x-ray techniques or by single- or double-beam photon absorptiometry, the optimal dose of estrogen and duration of therapy needed, in the setting of adequate dietary calcium, has not been determined. Moreover, whether estrogen alone can significantly retard the dire consequences of already established osteoporosis in the absence of adequate dietary calcium would seem unlikely. A minimum dose of 0.625 mg of estrone sulfate or its equivalent is apparently required to significantly retard bone loss. That dose level is higher than that usually needed to minimize hot flush. An appropriate progestin should also be incorporated in the therapeutic regimen and may include 5 mg of Norlutate or 10 mg of medroxyprogesterone acetate (Provera). Comparable doses of other estrogen-progestin combinations undoubtedly would be effective as well. For more details see the chapter on Osteoporosis.

BREAST CANCER AND ESTROGENS

In the early 1980s, several case control studies examined the relative risk of breast cancer and estrogen replacement therapy. Several suggested a slightly increased risk of development of breast cancer, but more recent studies do not support that contention. In fact, recent studies support a decreased risk of breast cancer among patients using combined estrogens and progestins, implying that progestin incorporation within the regimen decreases the risk of breast cancer. However, other studies observed that beneficial effect with estrogens alone. Undoubtedly, part of that confusion results from the time of collection of data in terms of the dose of estrogens to which the women were exposed. If there is a strong family history of breast cancer or if the patient has had breast cancer, estrogen replacement therapy is not recommended.

ADVERSE EFFECTS OF SEX STEROID REPLACEMENT

Up to this point therapeutic considerations of estrogen therapy have been addressed. However, clinicians and patients alike have many concerns regarding adverse effects of estrogens. Interestingly, if one compares coronary arteriosclerotic disease among women undergoing castration prior to the age of 50 with women of normal reproductive status, the former have a higher incidence of coronary artery disease. That disparity is more evident among women undergoing castration prior to age 40. However, younger women who take estrogens and are cigarette smokers are at higher risk of having a myocardial infarction than women who take estrogens and do not smoke. Administration of estrogen increases HDL cholesterol concentrations. As a result of the foregoing studies as well as other similar studies, a beneficial effect of estrogen replacement therapy on arteriosclerotic heart disease has been suggested. However, when a cohort of men given graded doses of estrogen after having had a myocardial infarction were studied, no benefit of the estrogen therapy was observed. Since most therapeutic regimens for estrogen replacement includes progestins and estrogens of different concentrations and ratios, a discernible protective effect is tenuous at this point. Just as for other adverse effects of estrogen, the potential for adverse effects on the cardiovascular system appears to be related to the dose and duration of estrogen therapy in terms of the risk of myocardial infarction. One of the difficulties in assessing the relative risk of myocardial infarction and combined estrogen and progestin therapy is the fact that after it became realized that the side effects associated with those medications was related to the concentration of estrogen, current formulations of combined estrogen and progestin have lower estrogen content. Consequently, although older epidemiologic data may be valid, it may not relate to current forms of estrogen-progestins prescribed. As already noted, estrogen tends to increase HDL cholesterol whereas progestins related to 19-nor testosterone tend to have the opposite effect. Moreover, pills containing combined estrogen and progestins have varying concentrations of both forms of sex steroid. In general, epidemiologic studies tend to support the hypothesis that oral contraceptives may magnify the effects of other risk factors for increasing the risk of myocardial infarction and stroke. Autopsy studies of women who died while taking oral contraceptives are consistent, with myocardial infarction resulting from a thrombotic rather than an atheromatous cause. Estrogens alter platelet aggregation and decrease antithrombin III activity as well as the plasminogen-activator content of endothelium. Those effects are not correlated with duration of use, but reflect biochemical effects of estrogens.

Because of the effects of oral contraceptives (containing both estrogens and progestins) on intravascular coagulation, an increased risk of venous thromboembolic disease and subclinical thrombosis has been reported. The risk of subclinical thrombosis appears to be three times that of nonpregnant women of the reproductive age group who are not taking sex steroids. Again, most of these data are derived from studies in which women took oral contraceptives containing higher concentrations of estrogens. Recent observations based on oral contraceptives containing lower concentrations of estrogen suggested lower risk of development of, and risk of death from, pulmonary embolism. No correlation with progestin content has been observed to date.

Estrogens affect hepatic lipid metabolism, resulting in an increase in the cholesterol fraction of bile. That increased concentration of cholesterol in bile may result in stone formation. Such effects are dose-dependent.

Suggested Reading

Avioli LA. Postmenopausal osteoporosis: prevention versus cure. Fed Proc 1981; 40:2418–2422.

Gambrell RD, Maier RC, Sanders BI. Decreased incidence of breast cancer in postmenopausal estrogen-progestin users. Obstet Gynecol 1983; 62:435–443.

Judd HL, Meldrum DR, Deftos LJ, Henderson BE. Estrogen replacement therapy: indications and complications. Ann Intern Med 1983; 98:195–205.

Lindsay R, Hart DM, Clark DM. The minimum effective dose of estrogens for prevention of postmenopausal bone loss. Obstet Gynecol 1984; 63:759–763.

Oral contraceptive. Population Reports. Series A, Number 6, 1982.

Schiff I, Ryan KJ. Benefits of estrogen replacement. Obstet Gynecol Surv 1980; 35:400–411.

Weinstein MC. Estrogen use in postmenopausal women—costs, risks, and benefits. N Engl J Med 1980; 303:308–316.

Wynn V, Adams PW, Godsland I, et al. Comparison of effects of different oral contraceptive formulations on carbohydrate and lipid metabolism. Lancet 1979; 1:1045–1049.

PRINCIPLES OF SYSTEMIC CORTICOSTEROID THERAPY IN NONENDOCRINE DISEASE

NICHOLAS P. CHRISTY, M.D.

Over the past thirty years corticosteroids have found a place in the treatment of more kinds of disease than any other class of pharmaceutical agents. The strictly endocrine uses of corticoids in the replacement therapy of adrenocortical insufficiency and suppression of the hypothalamic-pituitary-adrenal (HPA) system in adrenal virilism account for only a small portion of the steroids dispensed annually. Most are given for a broad range of disorders which appear to have no common denominator. The main pathologic disorders ameliorated by these compounds are allergic, inflammatory, and neoplastic diseases in which pharmacologists and cellular biologists now understand, at least superficially, why glucocorticoids are beneficial. But for several other conditions as different as cerebral edema, myxedema coma, and septic shock, the mechanism of therapeutic efficacy remains mysterious.

ACTIONS OF GLUCOCORTICOIDS

Cellular research of the past fifteen years has yielded much information about the nature of glucocorticoid action. Nevertheless, the accumulated data do not provide complete biochemical explanations for all of the biologic and clinical effects of these hormones.

On a superficial level, investigators have made some clear observations which, upon classification, form a fairly coherent picture of general corticosteroid effects. In the basal state, *normal* levels of circulating glucocorticoids exert a *permissive* effect on physiologic processes, allowing the maintenance of blood pressure and euglycemia and, to a limited extent, retention of sodium by the renal tubule.

Glucocorticoids, secreted in *supranormal* quantities during physiologic and pathologic stress (muscular exercise, trauma) are *protective* in, for example, sustaining circulatory processes. This protective property is that applied when the investigator or physician administers large amounts of exogenous cortisol to the stressed adrenalectomized animal or to the patient in addisonian crisis.

Most of the corticoid effects which are regarded by physiologists as *deleterious* are catabolic, or, more specifically, antianabolic; these follow the administration of large *supraphysiologic* doses of the hormones over long periods of time, as in the treatment of serious human disease. In patients so treated, those antianabolic characteristics of glucocorticoids account for many of the familiar untoward signs, e.g., muscle weakness and atrophy, impaired collagen synthesis with delayed or inadequate wound healing, and osteoporosis. Paradoxically, the antianabolic actions are probably those most closely linked with the therapeutically useful properties of the glucocorticoids, i.e., their anti-inflammatory, antineoplastic, and antiallergic actions.

Something is known about the mechanism of corticoid action on anabolism, that is, on protein synthesis. The corticoisteroid molecule passes across the cell membrane and binds to a specific cytoplasmic receptor protein. The steroid-receptor complex then enters the nucleus where it stimulates, depresses, or otherwise influences the process of RNA transcription from the DNA template. The rate of synthesis of certain proteins is thereby changed, but it should be noted that the production rate of some cellular proteins is augmented by corticoids in the absence of steroid-induced stimulation of specific mRNA.

As to the generality of glucocorticoid effects on virtually all cells of the body, it is now clear that glucocorticoid receptors are present ubiquitously. Further, with respect to the general mode of action of these hormones, it is clear that corticosteroids modify the lipid composition of cellular membranes, causing an increase in their sphingomyelin content. This effect may be only transient, however.

Such observations, taken together, explain some of the actions of corticoids. For instance, the antianabolic property accounts for muscle wasting, for osteopenia with consequent calcium loss, for hormonal inhibition of every phase of the immune response, and for lysis of lymphocytes and eosinophils. The protein synthesis-stimulating property accounts for the augmentation of hepatic gluconeogenetic (and other) enzymes and hence the promotion of hyperglycemia. But the known activities of the hormones fail to provide clear or intimate understanding of many of their effects, e.g., the inhibition of catecholamine-mediated lipogenesis in the fat cells of the extremities with a directly opposite effect on adipose cells of the abdomen and dorsal fat pad. Similarly, many of the therapeutically beneficial effects remain unexplained, e.g., prevention of capillary leakage, stabilization of traumatized lysosomal and plasma membranes, a general protective effect against cellular damage regardless of the nature of the noxious stimulus, the inotropic effect of corticoids on the heart, their multiple actions on the microcirculation, and the protective action against the shock associated with endotoxin or anaphylaxis.

Thus the observed cellular activities of glucocorticoids provide an incomplete theoretic basis for the diverse and often divergent effects of corticoids in different organs and tissues. As set out in the section immediately following (Toxicity), it will be seen that the antianabolic action of glucocorticoids—their most obvious property—explains some but not all of their untoward clinical effects.

Toxicity of Glucocorticoids

Since glucocorticoids exert a basic action upon cells and affect an early stage of protein synthesis, it follows that their somatic actions would be many, various, and inseparable from the *toxic* or untoward effects: myopathy, osteoporosis, peptic ulceration, impaired wound healing, hypertension, hypokalemic alkalosis, precipitation of diabetes mellitus, and suppression of the immune response with consequent increase in susceptibility to every kind of infection—viral, bacterial, fungal, and parasitic. Further untoward effects not easily predictable from the known actions of glucocorticoids are steroid-induced psychosis, pseudotumor cerebri (especially when there is an abrupt change in the dosage or specific type of steroid), glaucoma, and posterior subcapsular cataracts. It is noteworthy that pseudotumor, glaucoma, cataracts, pancreatitis, aseptic necrosis of bone, panniculitis, and vasculitis are almost unique to the iatrogenic form of Cushing's syndrome, a restriction perhaps related to the exclusive use of semisynthetic steroids, not the naturally occurring hormone cortisol, in pharmacotherapeutics.

Actions of Glucocorticoids on the Endocrine System

Glucocorticoids exert a permissive effect on the capacity of catecholamines to stimulate vasoconstriction; this is one mechanism whereby corticoids regulate the circulation and is not a property of mineralocorticoids. The corticoids stimulate hyperinsulinemia, probably secondary to hypergluconeogenesis and hyperglycemia, and hyperglucagonemia, perhaps as a result of the demonstrated hyperaminoacidemia. Because 10 percent of administered C_{21} corticosteroid is metabolized to C_{19} androgens, amenorrhea, hirsutism, and virilism occur in some women receiving corticoids. The C_{19} metabolites are 11-oxygenated (the mammalian organism has no enzyme for removal of =O or —OH from the C-11 position, probably because of steric hindrance); such compounds are weak androgens. Therefore, very large doses of corticoid are required to produce virilism, which appears far less frequently in iatrogenic than in natural Cushing's syndrome, wherein the host's adrenal cortex sometimes secretes large amounts of the more potent 11-deoxy C_{19} androgenic hormones (for example, dehydroepiandrosterone). Administered glucocorticoid inhibits pituitary growth hormone response to insulin hypoglycemia (probably not an important element in steroid-induced growth failure) and transiently blunts the adenohypophyseal release of thyrotropin; the consequent "corticogenic hypothyroidism" is chemically demonstrable but not of clinical importance. The steroids promote water diuresis; the mechanisms are not completely understood but may entail both a blunting of neurohypophyseal ADH release and a renal tubular action that is partly dependent on and partly independent of corticoid-ADH interactions at the level of the renal collecting ducts. Corticoids do not affect aldosterone secretion; the hypokalemic alkalosis induced by glucocorticoids is due to their own intrarenal kaliuric actions and to the potassium loss accompanying the general cellular breakdown associated with the antianabolic property of these agents (potassium loss is roughly proportional to negative nitrogen balance).

Suppression of the Hypothalamic-Pituitary-Adrenal (HPA) System by Glucocorticoids

HPA suppression with adrenocortical failure is the most discussed, most thoroughly studied, and most feared endocrine consequence of long-term corticosteroid administration.* This fear has been greatly exaggerated in the clinical literature for two reasons. First, three cases were reported in 1952 and 1953 of fatal postoperative shock with apparent addisonian crises and adrenal atrophy following year-long cortisone treatment; these caused great alarm, which still persists. Second, the function of the HPA system can be assessed by fairly simple provocative tests which have been widely used. The voluminous data obtained provide ample biochemical evidence of HPA suppression, but two major uncertainties remain: the relevance of this biochemical lesion to the patient's competence in mounting an appropriate HPA response to a clinical stress, and the length of time clinically important HPA suppression may last after corticosteroids are withdrawn. The available information does not permit definite answers to these two questions, but thirty years' experience validates the following statements.

First, anatomic evidence of a steroid effect upon the adrenal cortex, anterior pituitary, and hypothalamus appears within 5 days after starting the administration of corticoids. The clinical significance is minor within that short period.

Second, steroids induce a fall in pituitary ACTH release within minutes to hours; this acute decrease is not clinically dangerous.

Third, the "short" synthetic ACTH test with plasma cortisol response provides an adequate assessment of total HPA function and turns out to yield results that correlate more closely with clinical HPA

---

*It is assumed that the reader is familiar with the negative feedback inhibition exerted by cortisol upon the adenohypophyseal secretion of corticotropin: the higher the plasma level of cortisol, the less ACTH released, and vice versa. Corticoid administration induces adrenal atrophy and failure of adrenocortical response to stress in animals, but it does not prevent the adrenocorticotropic effect of administered ACTH. The cortisol feedback action takes place at at least three levels: the anterior pituitary corticotroph cells, the CRF (corticotropin releasing factor) secreting neurohumoral cells of the medial basal hypothalamus, and the limbic system of the CNS. In human beings, tests of HPA function usually show blunted responses after long-term administration of natural or semisynthetic corticosteroids; urinary and plasma corticosteroid values tend to be low and rise subnormally during provocative tests with ACTH, metyrapone, insulin hypoglycemia, vasopressin, bacterial pyrogen, and in a very few cases, during the clinical stress of trauma, surgery, or explosive, acute disease.

response to stress than do tests specifically designed to give theoretically more complete information about all the elements of HPA activity. These procedures (metyrapone, insulin hypoglycemia, vasopressin, bacterial pyrogen) are more cumbersome, more time-consuming, and, in some instances (the last three), more traumatic (see next chapter for ACTH test).

Fourth, careful analysis of such test results has not permitted precise definition of the smallest dosage of steroid or the shortest time of its administration that causes HPA suppression. Nevertheless, the evidence suggests that any patient who has received a glucocorticoid dosage equivalent to 20 to 30 mg of prednisone/prednisolone daily for 3 to 4 weeks or more should be considered to ave *biochemically evident* HPA suppression that may or may not be clinically significant. HPA function remains biochemically intact in patients who have been treated with 4 to 5 mg of prednisone equivalent daily for 8 years or longer.

Fifth, after prolonged treatment with large doses of glucocorticoid (>30 mg prednisone equivalent per day), biochemically demonstrable HPA suppression persists for 12 months or more after cessation of steroid therapy. By biochemical criteria, hypothalamic-pituitary recovery occurs first, within 5 to 9 months; adrenocortical response lags, recovering in 9 to 12 months; and the total capacity of the HPA system to react appropriately to clinical stress may not be restored until as late as 12 to 16 months following steroid withdrawal.

Sixth, this biochemically detectable HPA suppression can be muted by administering the glucocorticoid as a single daily morning dose; the HPA axis is more susceptible to steroid-induced inhibition in the evening. The alternate-day schedule of corticoid administration often ameliorates or prevents biochemically evident HPA suppression (see chapter on *Corticosteroid Withdrawal*).

Seventh, the use of ACTH as a therapeutic agent instead of glucocorticoids is not accompanied by biochemical or clinical evidence of HPA suppression, but ACTH has many disadvantages (see section on *Therapeutic Alternatives* and chapter on *Corticosteroid Withdrawal).*

Eighth, it follows from statements four and five above that the high probability of biochemically detectable HPA suppression in patients receiving prolonged, high-dose glucocorticoid therapy compels the use of steroid cover for intercurrent stresses (trauma, surgery, acute illness) to avoid collapse due to acute adrenocortical insufficiency. The physician is theoretically constrained to take this precaution during the treatment period and for a year or more after steroid withdrawal (see section on *Preferred Approach).*

Ninth, a sufficiently powerful neurogenic stress can break through the negative feedback inhibition imposed by corticosteroids, that is, such a stress can provoke a strong HPA response with a measurable rise of plasma cortisol level in patients whose HPA systems are biochemically suppressed by long-term administration of glucocorticoids.

Tenth, *biochemically proved acute adrenocorticoid failure due to HPA suppression in steroid-treated patients has been conclusively demonstrated only a few times in the entire world literature*. There are several reasons for this. Detailed studies of HPA function are rarely performed during acute medical emergencies. Few investigations have been published relating biochemical behavior of the HPA system to the patient's endocrine response to stress. Such reports as there are indicate that blood pressure and plasma cortisol concentrations show irregular and inconstant correlations: Blood pressure may be low in the face of normal or raised plasma cortisol level, or the converse may be true. Other clinical signs of adrenocortical insufficiency correlate poorly with plasma cortisol values. Finally, the "breakthrough" capacity of the HPA system under stress (already discussed) may in many instances preclude adrenocortical failure.

Eleventh, it appears to follow, from the preceding paragraph, that clinically important HPA failure due to suppression in patients undergoing prolonged high-dose glucocorticoid therapy occurs infrequently, and that plasma cortisol concentration and its response in provocative tests are not the only or necessarily the prime determinants or indices of the patient's overall reaction to clinical stress.

Twelfth, the steroid cover given to such patients for intercurrent clinical crises should therefore be recognized for what it is: a precautionary measure taken in *all* cases to ward off theoretically possible adrenocortical failure with collapse in a *small minority* (see section on *Preferred Approach*).

Finally, flare-ups of the basic disease, corticosteroid dependence (bordering on addiction in some patients), and other manifestations of iatrogenic Cushing's syndrome are more troublesome complications of prolonged steroid therapy than is suppression of the HPA system (see chapter on *Corticosteroid Withdrawal*).

PHARMACOLOGIC CONSIDERATIONS

The foregoing review of glucocorticoid action and toxicity applies equally to the naturally occurring hormone cortisol and to its semisynthetic derivatives and congeners. The organic chemists have synthetically introduced many changes into the steroid nucleus and its side chains and have succeeded in producing pharmacologically useful alterations in the ratio of anti-inflammatory (carbohydrate regulating) to sodium retaining effects. Nevertheless, no steroid analog has been synthesized in which the therapeutically desirable and seriously toxic effects are completely divorced. This is perhaps not surprising in view of the basic and therefore general action of glucocorticoids upon early phases of cellular synthesis of protein. Stated briefly, five specific chemical configurations must be present in the steroid molecule for the fullest expression of glucocorticoid and anti-inflammatory action: the 4,5 double bond and the 3-ketone in ring A, the 11β-hydroxyl of ring C, and the 17α-hydroxyl and 21-hydroxyl groups in the 2-carbon side chain at carbon 17 of ring D. Leaving these configurations intact while introducing a double bond at 1,2 of cortisol's ring A (prednisone/prednisolone) augments fourfold the anit-inflammatory potency and reduces by 20 percent the mineralocorticoid activity; 6α-substitution in ring B of prednisolone (methylprednisolone) produces the same two changes, but quantitatively somewhat greater, in the same directions. 9α-Fluorination in ring B (9α-fluorocortisol, Florinef) greatly increases all corticosteroid activities, but the enhancement of mineralocorticoid (125-fold) is so much greater than of anti-inflammatory potency (tenfold) that sharp reduction in dosage fractions of milligrams (0.05 to 0.1 mg daily or less often) virtually eliminates the latter effect, so that a "pure" salt-active action can be clinically achieved, as in the maintenance therapy of Addison's disease. Even in the presence of the 9α grouping, 16α-hydroxylation (triamcinolone), 16α-methylation (dexamethasone), or 16β-methylation (betamethasone) in ring D completely does away with the mineralocorticoid effect, but further augments glucocorticoid and anti-inflammatory potency only slightly.

The practical result of this chemical manipulation has been the creation of corticosteroid drugs which possess diminished salt-retaining activity—usually not a life-threatening untoward effect and in any case manageable with modern diuretics—but which also have augmented anti-inflammatory potency along with a roughly proportionate* increase in the characteristic and apparently inseparable capacity of all therapeutically effective glucocorticoids to impair growth and wound healing, promote osteoporosis and diabetes mellitus, and suppress the HPA system. Thus the most troublesome untoward effects of corticosteroid therapy have not been eliminated. To achieve palliation of disease ranging from acute lymphocytic leukemia to chronic bronchial asthma, the physician and the patient must still accept the risk of the major complications of steroids conferred by their fundamental actions upon the nuclear synthesis of cellular protein.

The foregoing considerations will determine the use or avoidance of corticosteroids, the dosage, timing, route of administration, and choice of specific compound. In HPA-suppressive therapy of adrenal virilism, the aim is simple: to inhibit pituitary ACTH secretion, which can be achieved with a small dose of glucocorticoid. Replacement therapy for Addison's disease and other forms of adrenocortical insufficiency requires, by definition, only physiologic doses of steroid, enough to sustain the *permissive* actions of the missing adrenocortical secretion upon the rates of cellular biochemical processes. Successful palliation of inflammatory, immunologic, and neoplastic disease requires larger doses whose toxicity is inescapable, but the fundamental actions of the corticosteroid are the same whether the dose is physiologic or pharmacologic. In the latter instance, the untoward effects only appear to be qualitatively different; most of them are mere exaggerations deducible from the physiologic effects of these potent hormones.

The therapist now has several methods whereby he or she can mitigate but not prevent the complications of glucocorticoid therapy (see *Preferred Approach*).

Interactions of Glucocorticoids with Other Drugs. Drug interactions rarely preclude administration of corticosteroids, but may necessitate adjustments in dosage. Patients receiving corticoids along with one or more other drugs simultaneously or in close time sequence usually react to them simply as if each were being given independently. With other agents, either the corticosteroid or the other drug shows diminished pharmacologic activity; with still others, such activity is enhanced. Unexpected or unintended effects may also occur.

Fifteen to twenty drug interactions have been reported. Some of these are clinically important. *Two kinds of central nervous system-active drugs* reduce

---

*It is important to emphasize the fact that the proportionality is only approximate. In general, structural alterations in the steroid molecule enhance anti-inflammatory activity of glucocorticoids in parallel with their carbohydrate activity and other effects on organic metabolism. In the literature of the past two decades it has been fashionable to convey the impression that the anti-inflammatory and HPA suppressive potencies of a given steroid are equal. This is not true. For example, prednisone/prednosolone has an anti-inflammatory action three to five times that of cortisol; the enhancement of HPA suppressive potency is about seven times that of the parent compound. Sources of error in making such comparisons are several. The dose of steroid is critical. Different results emerge from in vitro versus in vivo bioassays. The time at which the assay end point is determined influences the result; different reactions reach the point of maximal stimulation at different times after application of the steroid.

The chemical changes introduced into the steroid molecule have also given rise to differences in the transport, plasma and biologic half-life, and metabolism of the synthetic analogs as compared with cortisol. They are all less firmly bound to plasma corticosteroid-binding globulin (transcortin), yet all are metabolized less rapidly than is cortisol. The influences of these differences on steroid availability at the cellular level and on duration of action are not in harmony with one another nor with observed biologic effectiveness in the treatment of disease. Different indices of potency are affected differently; for instance, the HPA-suppressive action of a single dose of an analog lasts several hours longer than does the hyperglycemic effect. Doses of prednisone or dexamethasone too small to inhibit HPA function are sufficiently anti-inflammatory to suppress the clinical manifestations of rheumatoid arthritis. *It appears that the enhanced therapeutic effectiveness of the steroid analog cannot be satisfactorily explained by differences in their metabolism.* Those differences, as set out above, fail to account for the quantitative advantages one sees in the clinic. The more likely explanation is to be found in the cellular receptor. Only at that level does it seem likely that, for example, the *unique* toxicities of the corticosteroid analogs will be elucidated (already discussed). It is noteworthy that the pharmaceutical manufacturers have abandoned the search for a nontoxic corticosteroid. No novel steroids are being introduced nowadays—they have been replaced by a spate of new nonsteroidal anti-inflammatory and bronchodilating agents.

the effectiveness of corticoids: barbiturates as a class and diphenylhydantoin. The presumed mechanism is induction by these agents of hepatic microsomal enzymes that inactivate corticoids. Increasing the dose of steroid may be necessary. A number of *hormones and hormonelike substances* affect corticosteroid action. Estrogens and estrogen-containing oral contraceptives are said to enhance the anti-inflammatory and glucogenic actions of glucocorticoids, perhaps by increasing transcortin binding of the latter and thus delaying their inactivation. This is probably a minor clinical effect and not therapeutically useful or harmful; it has no visible bearing on the steroid treatment of the pregnant woman. Ephedrine diminishes dexamethasone activity; the mechanism is not understood. Corticoid interactions with thyroid hormone are discussed below under *Pathologic Considerations*. *Antidiabetic agents* oppose the glucogenic effect of corticoids; put another way, corticosteroids blunt the hypoglycemic actions of these drugs. This interaction is of clinical importance and necessitates titrations of dosage. Corticosteroids considerably augment the potassium loss promoted by most *diuretics* (except spironolactone and triamterene) through additive kaliuretic actions on the renal tubule. This also is a significant interaction; doses of both drugs must be monitored and potassium supplements added with more than ordinary care. Among the *antibiotics*, amphotericin B and corticoids work additively, presumably on the renal tubule, to provoke a high degree of potassium loss. The precautions necessary with steroid-diuretic combinations apply. Rifampin reduces corticoid efficacy by inducing steroid-inactivating enzymes in hepatic microsomes. Glucocorticoids have been reported to promote the growth of antibiotic-resistant strains of bacteria in patients treated with tetracycline. This is almost certainly not an interaction unique to tetracycline. Corticosteroids appear to operate additively, perhaps synergistically, with the *anti-inflammatory agents* indomethacin and aspirin in causing peptic (especially gastric) ulceration. Doses may have to be reduced or one or the other agent discontinued. The important action of corticosteroids in regulating blood levels of salicylate is dealt with in the next chapter. Glucocorticoids have no significant effect in evoking hypercoagulability of the blood as was formerly thought; the contrary, when given together with oral *anticoagulants*, corticosteroids may act additively to promote superficial bleeding because of their subcutaneous tissue wasting action and their adverse effects on the integrity of dermal blood vessels. *Vitamin A* has been reported to inhibit locally the steroid-mediated impairment of wound healing; there is no systemic counterpart. Finally, reduction in dose of a simultaneously administered corticoid may permit excessive activity of the *cytotoxic agent* cyclophosphamide. The mechanism is not certain and further studies are needed to determine the generality of this interaction. If the observation is confirmed, one may have to lower the dose of Cytoxan if the corticoid is reduced or discontinued.

PATHOLOGIC CONSIDERATIONS

Extreme Physiologic States that Modify Corticoid Action. In *childhood*, the metabolism of corticosteroids is not substantially different from that of adult life, but corticoids markedly inhibit linear growth through their antianabolic properties. The alternate-day schedule of hormone administration mitigates this effect (see *Preferred Approach*). In extreme *old age*, corticoid metabolism is slowed down; smaller than usual doses are probably indicated. *Postmenopausal women* are exceedingly susceptible to the protein-wasting actions of administered corticosteroids, probably because the opposing anabolic activity of ovarian estrogen and androgen is lacking. Easy bruising and a worsening of osteopenia are the familiar consequences. Steroid dosage should be moderated or alternative therapies used when possible. The marked hyperestrogenemia of *pregnancy* greatly increases the binding of cortisol to plasma transcortin. Despite the observed enhancing effect of administered estrogen on the glucogenic and anti-inflammatory properties of cortisol, pregnant women apparently do not require less corticosteroid to achieve a given clinical effect. Large doses of glucocorticoids have not been convincingly shown to harm the fetus.

Pathologic States that Modify Corticoid Action. Diseases of the liver provide the most vivid demonstrations of pathologic states affecting the therapeutic actions of glucocorticoids. The liver is the principal site of corticosteroid metabolism; through a series of microsomal enzymatic and other reactions, the liver reduces the steroid nucleus and its side chains and substituent groups and brings about the formation of sulfate and glucuronide conjugates, polar metabolites readily excreted in the urine. Any hepatic disease—such as the acute or chronic viral hepatitides, alcoholic hepatitis, poisoning with any hepatotoxic agent, hepatic metastases, or the many forms of cirrhosis—impairs the metabolism and slows the rate of disposition of glucocorticoids. The result is that the slow rate of steroid inactivation permits the same clinical effect to be achieved with about half the expected or premorbid dose of hormone. An interesting detail is that prednisolone is probably preferable to prednisone in patients with major hepatic disease; such people show defective reduction of the 11-keto group to a hydroxyl, a step essential to the biologic effectiveness of a glucocorticoid.

Terminally ill patients show a marked slowing in the rate of corticosteroid metabolism; an administered dose remains in the blood stream for hours. The detailed implications are not clear.

Hypothyroidism also slows the inactivation of administered corticoids. The effect may be exerted through the liver. As in cirrhosis, a half or less of the expected or previously established dose of corticoid may suffice. There are many reports of iatrogenic Cushing's syndrome occurring in people treated with standard or even with modest amounts of steroid hormone in the face of unrecognized myxedema. Restoration of the patient to a euthyroid state is corrective and the signs of hypercortisolism then disappear. Although corticosteroid metabolism is much accelerated in *hyperthyroidism*, no cogent clinical evidence suggests that unusually large dosages of steroid hormone are needed. It should be noted that corticoids transiently suppress pituitary release of thyrotropin, with a consequent lowering of most indices of thyroidal function. This lesion is biochemically detectable but not of much clinical moment.

Pre-Existing Disease Made Worse by Corticoids. There are many of these, as stated above. Whether an established disease will be a relative or absolute contraindication to corticosteroid therapy or no contraindication at all is determined by how much is at stake, how long steroid treatment will have to be given, what dosage will be required, and the probable effectiveness of the steroid as a therapeutic agent for the specific disease to be treated in the particular patient. Even the pre-existence of the six major hazards associated with glucocorticoid therapy need not preclude the use of corticosteroids. Hypertension is usually not exacerbated in the absence of renal involvement as signaled by proteinuria. If blood pressure rises significantly, one can usually control it by increasing or changing the antihypertensive agents without stopping the steroids. Patients who have congestive heart failure from any cause may be safely treated with corticosteroids as long as there is concomitant administration of digitalis and diuretics and employment of the 16-substituted steroids, which are virtually without salt-retaining effect. Diabetes mellitus may be precipitated or worsened; this is usually controllable with modifications in the insulin and dietary regimen. The urgency of the clinical need for steroid therapy is a determinant. If an existing peptic ulcer cannot be managed effectively with antacids and cimetidine, the steroid dosage may have to be reduced or stopped. Major complications of ulcer, such as bleeding or perforation, usually mandate reduction of steroid dosage for the sake of the ulcer, but in an emergent clinical situation that dosage may have to be greatly increased for the sake of the "whole" patient because of his need for greater adrenocortical support during stress and in the face of HPA suppression (already discussed). Osteoporosis should not preclude careful administration of steroids. The special predilection of the postmenopausal woman has been discussed. Anabolic steroids have not proved useful in combating the corticoid effects on bone; use of a combined calcium, fluoride and vitamin D regimen for steroid induced osteopenia may be valuable, but supporting data are not yet at hand. As for major psychologic disorders, the available information indicates that the presteroid personality does not provide a basis for predicting the patient's psychic reaction to corticosteroid therapy. It is known that the emotional disturbances of psychotic patients are unaffected by large doses of corticoids. If the clinical indication is strong, the steroid should be given, regardless of the patient's emotional state. The exception is the addicted subject: persons addicted to other drugs tend to become corticosteroid dependent. Corticosteroids may perhaps be life-saving in some existing infections as in gram-negative sepsis. Disseminated tuberculosis is probably not an absolute contraindication; again, if the clinical need for steroid is compelling enough, it may be cautiously given together with appropriate antituberculous chemotherapy. When specific antibiotics for any infection are available, corticoid treatment may be started or continued along with such agents, but only if the indication for steroids is powerful. Intercurrent infections may require adrenocortical support, as is the case with any clinical stress; the rule is to hold corticosteroid doses to the minimum that will protect against adrenal insufficiency or clinical collapse.

Two disorders of the eye deserve mention. Glaucoma is worsened by corticosteroids. If the clinical need for steroids is great, they may be cautiously continued at the minimum possible dose and with frequent measurement of intraocular pressure and appropriate use of miotic agents. Herpes simplex of the cornea constitutes an absolute contraindication to the use of corticoids, which may augment the virus-induced opacification of the cornea with consequent blindness.

THERAPEUTIC ALTERNATIVES

Alternatives to systemic corticosteroid therapy are the use of ACTH, corticosteroid therapy administered locally or topically, and the employment of other anti-inflammatory, antiallergic, or antineoplastic agents. Modifications of oral or parenteral dosage schedules as alternative methods are discussed below in the section on *Preferred Approach*.

ACTH therapy is not a satisfactory substitute for glucocorticoid therapy. The arguments are given in the next chapter.

The complications of systemic glucocorticoid treatment can be attenuated and sometimes avoided entirely by judicious employment of local, topical, and some forms of parenteral routes of steroid administration. Whenever possible, diseases of the anterior segment of the eye, skin disorders, affections of the bronchi and colon, and many musculoskeletal ailments can be treated effectively by direct application of the corticosteroid (for specific and most appropriate steroid preparations, consult textbooks of pharmacology). The therapist can often circumvent major systemic effects of corticosteroids by prescribing steroid-containing ophthalmic solutions for some cases of iritis; corticoid-containing dermal lotions, ointments, and creams for innumerable skin diseases; steroid aerosols, such as beclomethasone dipropionate, for bronchial asthma and some cases of pulmonary emphysema; corticosteroid enemas for exacerbations of chronic, nonspecific ulcerative colitis; and intrasynovial injection of suitable corticosteroid esters in patients having rheumatoid or osteoarthritis with involvement of only one or two joints. Direct injections of steroid into bursae or musculoskeletal lesions are also feasible.

The physician and patient must be prepared to pay some price for these evasive tactics. If dermal ointments are applied under film, absorption will be considerable and systemic effects may follow. Steroid aerosols and steroid enemas are associated with ample absorption, sooner or later, of glucocorticoid, so that the desired avoidance of untoward effects may be thwarted. The tactic in all these instances should be to space the steroid applications as widely as is consistent with controlling the disease to a reasonable degree. In patients with generalized arthritides, intra-articular injection of corticoids indeed obviates systemic therapy and its complications, but the usefulness is limited by the possibility that such intense local treatment may lead to more rapid breakdown of the joint; therefore, applications of this sort are usually not performed at intervals of less than 4 to 6 weeks.

Physicians have begun to adopt the use of other agents to replace corticosteroid therapy. The process has to be one of trial and error, starting and stopping, and frequently having to change direction. In some disorders, the decision to abandon steroids and use something else is easy; in others, difficult or impossible. Rheumatologists now agree that systemic treatment of rheumatoid arthritis with glucocorticoids in no way alters the natural history of the disease; the number of disabled joints is the same in patients treated or not so treated. Therefore, a decision to carry out therapeutic trials with such "intermediate" anti-inflammatory drugs as indomethacin, Motrin (ibuprofen) or Clinoril is straightforward. In contrast, treatment of Hodgkin's disease or acute lymphocytic leukemia consists of complex regimens which combine cytotoxic agents, vinca alkaloids, immunosuppressive agents and corticosteroids in elaborate predetermined dosage schedules; these rigid protocols forbid easy cessation of their glucocorticoid moiety. The general approach would be something like this: In disorders that are not life-threatening, for example, chronic bronchial asthma and rheumatoid arthritis, alternative nonsteroidal therapies, such as various bronchodilating inhalants or indomethacin, should be given a thorough trial, either alone or in combination with other agents. For the serious, sometimes catastrophic diseases in which corticosteroids are used, e.g., disseminated lupus, the combination of steroids with other drugs (for example, immunosuppressants) may permit use of lower steroid doses. In these situations, nevertheless, steroid toxicity may not loom large as a disadvantage to the patient when compared with the complications of immunosuppressive therapy or with the consequences of the potentially lethal disease under treatment.

PREFERRED APPROACH

The mechanisms of action of corticosteroids, their untoward actions, and the complications of steroid therapy have been discussed. It remains to deal with dosage regimens that blunt the severity of those untoward actions and assessment of therapeutic response.

To dispose of the last point first, a thorough analysis of the methods whereby the physician estimates the quantitative and qualitative aspects of disease response to corticosteroid therapy would entail an encyclopedic exploration of the subject appropriate to a multivolume treatise on medicine. The indices of therapeutic response are, Does the patient survive? Do the objective manifestations of his disease remain in abeyance? For the purposes of this chapter, it is enough to say that there are five major categories of disease in which glucocorticoid therapy is useful in those terms: (1) replacement therapy for the various kinds of adrenocortical insufficiency—here physiologic dosages (the equivalent of 20 mg of cortisol daily) are sufficient; (2) suppressive therapy to inhibit pituitary ACTH secretion in the various forms of adrenal virilism (0.5 to 0.75 mg of dexamethasone, betamethasone or equivalent nightly, because the adenohypophysis is more prone to steroid suppression of ACTH at night); (3) intensive short-term therapy for catastrophic illness; (4) prolonged high-dose therapy to contain a potentially lethal disease; and (5) chronic low-dose palliative therapy. The following paragraphs will deal with items (3) through (5), which are also analyzed elsewhere (see next chapter).

Corticoid treatment of catastrophic illness is usually desperate and for the most part empiric, having no solid basis in pathophysiology. Such illnesses include thyrotoxic crisis ("storm"), acute cerebral edema of any cause, septic shock, and myxedema coma. Disorders for which glucocorticoids ought to be effective in terms of their known mode of action include hypoglycemic coma, water intoxication, acute hypercalcemia due to vitamin D intoxication or androgen therapy for osseous metastases from mammary carcinoma, and allergic emergencies (for example, anaphylaxis due to bee sting or penicillin hypersensitivity). In all these conditions, whether or not the mode of therapeutic action of corticoids is understood, the hormones must be intravenously administered in large doses as fast as possible. A conventional series of doses would be 100 to 500 mg of cortisol hemisuccinate given as a single bolus, followed by infusion of the steroid ester at a rate of 100 to 300 mg in 250 to 1000 ml of dextrose and water or saline every 4 to 6 hours. Still larger doses of steroid, the equivalent of 2 to 4 g prednisone/prednisolone per day, are said to be required for a favorable effect on blood pressure in septic shock. The point remains controversial. There are no special toxicities associated with these huge doses. Dexamethasone phosphate, available in a concentration of 4 mg/ml is equally effective. Equivalent doses are 1/25 those just described for cortisol. The therapist must remember that, where available, the primary therapeutic agent (e.g., an antibiotic in overwhelming infection) is more important than the corticosteroid as a life-saving measure. A prime example is allergic anaphylaxis; parenteral epinephrine administration is of more immediate value than steroid injection, which should be viewed as supplementary. As discussed in the following chapter, steroids, no matter how high the daily dose, can be withdrawn with impunity as abruptly as they were started. In such patients, treated for no more than a few days, the only complications are the occurrence of itching at mucocutaneous junctions, punctate ulcerations of the gastric mucosa (rare), or premature ventricular contractions (very rare).

Therapeutic response in patients with serious disease treated with prolonged high-dose steroids (15 to 120 mg of prednisone per day) is assessed in the following chapter. The problems are to keep the manifestations of the disease suppressed on one hand, and to minimize the devastating signs of iatrogenic Cushing's syndrome on the other. The best method yet devised for walking this narrow path is the use of the *alternate day schedule of glucocorticoid dosage*. The rationale is twofold: (1) it is taken for granted that the disease can be sufficiently suppressed with inconstant or waxing and waning quantities of administered steroid; and (2) it is assumed that this intermittency of exposure to supraphysiologic amounts of glucocorticoid spares the patient serious HPA suppression, physical signs of hypercortisolism, osteopenia, diabetes, psychosis, and so on. Whatever the intellectual merits of the hypothesis, the method is often empirically successful. Most diseases—the notable exception being temporal (giant cell) arteritis with the threat of blindness—respond as well to the alternate-day treatment schedule as to daily administration of glucocorticoids in divided doses. Further, patients maintained on this schedule for years show fewer signs of Cushing's syndrome than patients who have received daily steroid, and the indices of function of the immune system and of phagocytic capacity are better preserved.* Children managed by the alternate-day scheme have less impairment of growth than do their coevals treated with steroid every day. HPA suppression is absent or less pronounced, and steroid withdrawal is said to be easier. It is important to use a relatively short-acting corticoid in the alternate-day schedule, for example, prednisone/prednisolone or methylprednisolone. If the longer-acting compounds (dexamethasone, betamethasone) are given, their biologic half-life is long enough so that intermittency of exposure to glucocorticoid is not achieved and the organism is not, so to speak, put to rest at intervals; biologically, the regimen is not alternate-day. For those patients whose basic disease is not adequately controlled by the alternate-day administration of corticoid, the therapist may give a single daily dose in the morning. This modified schedule partially spares the HPA system and controls temporal arteritis in most instances, but does not mitigate the outward signs of Cushing's syndrome.

Simply stated, the alternate-day schedule entails giving twice the daily amount of steroid in a single matutinal dose every other day; for example, a patient with lupus nephritis who would ordinarily be given 60 mg of prednisone equivalent daily, receives 120 mg every other morning. For patients already on daily divided doses of steroid, conversion to the alternate-day dosage may be accomplished by gradually increasing the steroid dose on odd days, and commensurately reducing it on even days, until double the original daily dose is attained on the odd day, zero on the even. This can usually be completed within 2 weeks; control of manifestations of the basic disease governs the rate of conversion. The role of the alternate-day dosage schedule in the process of discontinuing corticoid therapy is dealt with in the next chapter. Why this technique is efficacious, controlling the disease while causing fewer and less toxic complications of the administered steroids, is a challenging question that has not yet been answered.

Acute intercurrent medical or surgical emergencies, including sudden exacerbations of the basic disease, prompt the use of the so-called steroid cover during and for a short time after the emergency. The strengths and weaknesses of the arguments for and against this procedure are listed above in the section on *Suppression of the HPA System by Glucocorticoids*. The suggested protocol, which is modified to suit the needs of individual patients, was originally designed for people receiving prolonged high-dose continuous steroid therapy. For the reasons detailed in previous sections, it is difficult to determine which patients receiving the alternate-day or any other intermittent dosage schedule have significant HPA suppression and which do not. Therefore, patients being treated with the interrupted steroid courses should also be given steroid cover.

All patients receiving prolonged high-dose therapy for a serious disease should wear an identification bracelet or carry a card describing the steroid treatment and the need for added hormone during stress—acute medical illness, surgery, or trauma. For minor (office) surgical procedures, no extra steroid should be needed. The same is true for illnesses the patient and his family can treat at home, such as viral gas-

---

*With continuous prolonged high-dose glucocorticoid therapy, the physician must keep in mind the danger that the anti-inflammatory, antipyretic, and generally supportive properties of corticosteroids may mask infection and, because of the inhibitory effect on wound healing, may permit the spread of an infection that would be walled off in a patient not treated with corticoids. I have seen a woman, treated with high-dose prednisone for nephrotic syndrome and ascites due to disseminated lupus whose hitherto unsuspected peptic ulcer perforated without clinical signs. There was no fever and the white blood cell count was not elevated. Abdominal signs were minimal. An upright abdominal film done for some other reason showed air under the diaghragm. Bacteriologic study of the ascitic fluid showed generalized peritonitis.

This kind of untoward event is less likely to occur in persons treated by the alternate-day method, but the possibility is always present. The doctor must still be vigilant, particularly with patients known to harbor a chronic infection that might become active, either because of the steroid therapy or for any other reason.

troenteritis, influenzalike respiratory ailments, or bacterial pharyngitis; for these, the patient must be instructed to continue, not stop, his steroid (as a diabetic person takes more, not less, insulin in similar circumstances). Specific antimicrobial treatment is added as necessary. If the patient is vomiting, the physician may have to administer a parenteral, rapidly acting water-soluble steroid preparation, for example, cortisol hemisuccinate, either intravenously or (since blood pressure will usually be well maintained) intramuscularly. One hundred milligrams per day for 2 to 3 days should suffice, with immediate return to the maintenance dosage for the underlying disorder. For major intercurrent stresses—a threatening flare-up of the disease being treated with steroids, a major surgical procedure, large-scale trauma—the treatment is entirely intravenous with a daily dose of up to 300 mg of cortisol hemisuccinate (or equivalent) given by infusion aroung the clock. Higher doses of parenteral corticoid may be needed to maintain blood pressure; there is no contraindication to such doses in the range of several hundred milligrams daily. Gradual reduction of the dose in these patients is not necessary, since their maintenance doses are so high. As the emergency subsides, the patient can be switched to an oral dose of his usual steroid analog in a range of 30 to 60 mg of prednisone equivalent. This can then be adjusted as the status of the basic disease dictates. Special and attentive care of surgical wounds usually overcomes the steroid-induced impairment of wound healing. For acute infections, it is axiomatic that antibiotics are the central therapeutic agents; steroids are merely supportive.

Patients in this group who have been withdrawn from prolonged high-dose glucocorticoid regimens are conventionally assumed to be at risk for a year or so after withdrawal (see above and the following chapter). During that time, minor illnesses, minor trauma, and office surgical procedures can be treated with oral doses of cortisone or hydrocortisone, 50 to 100 mg daily two or three doses for 1 to 3 days, tapering carefully to zero within 5 to 10 days. The reduction can almost always be done within that time. For major medical emergencies, daily intravenous infusions containing 100 to 300 mg of a cortisol ester usually are sufficient; the number of days of treatment at that dosage level is governed by the status of the emergent condition. Transient falls in blood pressure can sometimes be corrected by rapid intravenous injection of boluses of cortisol hemisuccinate, 50 to 100 mg at a time. The steroid dosage must then be reduced gradually when the patient can be switched to oral cortisone or cortisol. Complete withdrawal of the steroid cover can usually be accomplished successfully within 2 weeks. If the acute intercurrent illness happens during the period of corticosteroid withdrawal, the emergency dosage plan is the same, except that the corticosteroid tapering is cautiously resumed, when the acute event has run its course, at a level 10 to 25 percent above the dose the patient had been taking just before the emergency.

The treatment plans described above are similar to those for acute adrenocortical insufficiency associated with Addison's disease, except that mineralocorticoid is unnecessary. Since the adrenal cortex may be unresponsive ACTH as a therapy is contraindicated.

The difficulties in managing patients with rheumatoid arthritis, bronchial asthma, and regional enteritis who are treated with long-term (often life-time) low-dose palliative corticoid are spelled out in the following chapter. In this category the dosage is generally below 10 mg of prednisone equivalent daily. The alternate-day schedule usually does not work; the patients will not tolerate the recurrent symptoms on the day off steroids. These patients require careful titration of the steroid dosage, which should be set at the level of reasonable palliation, not total relief, to avoid the large doses that would evoke the signs of iatrogenic hypercortisolism. In most instances, the patients also need adjunctive therapy: other anti-inflammatory agents, bronchodilators, anticholinergic drugs. Keeping the corticoid dosage as low as possible is overridingly important in these people, who have a curious propensity to develop corticosteroid dependence, which often makes weaning the patient from the hormone impossible.

The elaborate steroid cover described for prolonged high-dose glucocorticoid regimens is usually not required in patients receiving low-dose palliative steroid treatment. Close observation during acute intercurrent illnesses will show whether modified steroid cover is indicated.

Suggested Reading

Axelrod L. Glucocorticoid Therapy. Medicine 1976; 55:29–65.

Christy NP. Iatrogenic Cushing's syndrome. In: Christy NP, ed. The Human Adrenal Cortex. New York: Harper & Row, 1971:395–425.

Christy NP, Wallace EZ, Jailer JW. Comparative effects of prednisone and of cortisone in suppressing the response of the adrenal cortex to exogenous adrenocorticotropin. J Clin Endocrinol Metab 1956; 16:1059–1074.

David DS, Grieco MH, Cushman P Jr. Adrenal glucocorticoids after twenty years. A review of their clinically relevant consequences. J Chron Dis 1970; 22:637–711.

Jasani MK, Freeman PA, Boyle JA et al. Studies of the rise in plasma 11-hydroxycorticosteroids (11-OH-CS) in corticosteroid-treated patients with rheumatoid arthritis during surgery: correlations with the functional integrity of the HPA axis. Quart J Med 1968; 37:407–421.

Kehlet H, Binder C. Adrenocortical function and clinical course during and after surgery in unsupplemented glucocorticoid-treated patients. Brit J Anaesth 1973; 45:1043–1048.

Keller-Wood ME, Dallman MF. Corticosteroid inhibition of ACTH secretion. Endocr Rev 1984; 5:1–24.

Melby JC. Systemic corticosteroid therapy: Pharmacology and endocrinologic considerations. Ann Intern Med 1974; 81:505–512.

CORTICOSTEROID WITHDRAWAL

NICHOLAS P. CHRISTY, M.D.

Successful withdrawal of a patient from corticosteroid therapy requires the physician to have a firm grasp of essential background information and to formulate clear answers to several questions. One must define "successful withdrawal". One needs to be fully acquainted with the disease the steroids have been used to suppress. One must be certain why corticoids were chosen in the first place and why they are now being stopped. The physician has to know in detail the duration of steroid treatment, the exact dosage schedule, and the pharmacologic characteristics of the specific corticosteroid the patient has been receiving. One must be prepared to identify and then deal with any of the various forms of the "corticosteroid withdrawal syndrome". Finally, it need hardly be said that the physician ought to possess intimate knowledge of all pertinent aspects of the patient's personality and the features of the underlying disease which are peculiar to that patient.

PRINCIPLES

Definition of Successful Steroid Withdrawal

An ideal course of steroid withdrawal would be a smooth and rapid transition from the induced state of "tissue" hyperadrenocorticism to total deprivation of exogenous corticosteroid without recrudescence of the basic disorder and without the emergence of either adrenocortical insufficiency due to adrenal suppression or of corticosteroid dependence (to be discussed). This untroubled state of affairs can often be achieved. For example, self-limited, short-lived disorders, such as severe penicillin reactions for which steroid treatment is highly effective, do not recur when corticosteroids are withdrawn. Neither adrenal suppression nor steroid dependence is likely to develop in patients given very small doses—the equivalent of prednisone, 5 mg or less per day even over periods as long as several years, a dosage schedule often used by gynecologists in treating mild forms of adrenal virilism. Nor does clinically significant suppression or dependence occur with large doses—the equivalent of 60 mg or more of prednisone daily—administered over periods as short as 7 to 10 days, a scheme frequently employed in treating, for example, severe acute *Rhus* dermatitides (poison ivy, poison oak, poison sumac).

These rules are generally applicable, but it must be recognized that, as with other drugs, patients show wide individual variations in their responses to a given quantity of a given corticoid.

When the ideal smooth withdrawal from steroids cannot be achieved, successful management is then defined as gradual stepwise reduction of the corticosteroid dosage, with intermittent increases when and if necessary to control flare-ups of the basic disorder or to palliate the symptoms and signs of adrenal insufficiency or corticoid dependence. This kind of interrupted downward titration demands vigilance on the part of the physician; in practical terms, frequent follow-up visits by the patient are required.

The Underlying Disease

As suggested above, some acquaintance with the disease being suppressed or controlled by the corticoids will enable the physician to predict the likely course of steroid withdrawal and to gauge the probability that signs and symptoms of the disorder in being treated will ensue. Such acquaintance will alert the physician as to how vigilant he or she must be and will provide the basic information necessary to design appropriate history taking, physical examination, and laboratory tests to detect evidence of recrudescence early, before symptomatically unpleasant or clinically threatening events occur or get out of control.

In inflammatory or noninflammatory disorders which are immediately life-threatening, steroid withdrawal and the rate of steroid dosage reduction are dictated to a degree by the subsidence of the clinical condition. These disorders include, among other medical emergencies, acute adrenocortical insufficiency, allergic crises, shock associated with infection, hypoglycemic coma, water intoxication, central hyperthermia, thyroid storm, and myxedema coma. These conditions, with the exception of adrenal insufficiency, for which steroid therapy is crucial, *may* be improved by high-dose, short-term corticoid therapy, but steroids are not the central mode of therapy. One must of course treat the underlying disease with the appropriate primary modalities as well. Steroid withdrawal can usually be abrupt, without tapering, for the presence or absence of pharmacologic hypercortisolism is not the essential determinant of the patient's recovery.

Most of the patients the physician will encounter who present major difficulties in steroid withdrawal suffer from serious hematologic, inflammatory, and immunologic diseases. This is because the diseases themselves are systemic and more or less catastrophic and because large doses of corticosteroid are administered over long periods of time, usually as the principal means of palliating or suppressing the disease. These diseases include acute lymphocytic leukemia, idiopathic thrombocytopenic purpura, and Hodgkin's disease; ulcerative colitis, chronic active and acute alcoholic hepatitis, subacute hepatic necrosis, temporal (giant cell) arteritis, polymyositis, classic dermatomyositis; disseminated lupus erythematosus; autoimmune hemolytic anemia and severe asthma.

A detailed discussion of all the possible signs, symptoms, and abnormalities of laboratory tests which might mark the resurgence of these disorders during corticoid withdrawal would constitute a virtual textbook of internal medicine. The few essential points to be made are these. In many of the conditions listed above, early signs of recurrence may be straightforward, if rather general. Fever, for example, may characterize, and be the first evidence of, flare-up of leukemia, Hodgkin's disease, lupus, ulcerative colitis, the hepatitides, and the mesenchymal disorders. The physician, knowing this, will regulate the rate of steroid withdrawal in part by the presence or absence of fever. Petechiae of skin and mucous membranes and dermal ecchymoses may mark a recurrence of idiopathic thrombocytopenic purpura; abdominal pain, diarrhea, and blood in the stool herald the return of colitis. Appearance of such signs dictates slowing the rate of steroid withdrawal and, in most instances, a temporary increase in steroid dosage. For other diseases, one resorts to a combination of clinical and laboratory findings. An example is the nephrotic syndrome of lupus. If ascites appears, the clinical need is obvious, but recurrent peripheral edema may be subtle. If it is, one is forced to measure the daily loss of urinary protein, which is a more sensitive and earlier marker for escape of the renal lesion from the suppressive effects of the diminishing quantity of circulating corticosteroid. In the hepatitides that can be treated with steroids, the most prudent course is to monitor hepatic function tests frequently. These are more likely to give early warning of recurrence than are clinical signs, such as fever or jaundice. Resorting to such subtleties is clearly not necessary in asthma; the obvious clinical sign, bronchial wheezing, inform patients and doctor that the disorder is no longer controlled and the steroid dosage is regulated accordingly.

Some patients with rheumatoid arthritis, many with regional enteritis (Crohn's disease), some with asthma, and the subset of people with disseminated lupus who have arthritis as the principal manifestation, comprise another special group of steroid-responsive entities. These are treated with chronic low-dose palliative doses of corticosteroids. They are troublesome to treat during withdrawal of corticoids, not because of adrenal suppression, but because of apparent flare-ups of the disease upon the slightest reduction in dosage. I have had one patient with regional enteritis whose gastrointestinal symptoms were well controlled with a prednisone dose of 7.5 mg daily; reducing the amount to 5 mg was followed by recurrence of bloody diarrhea. Almost all rheumatologists have treated patients with rheumatoid arthritis who are satisfactorily free of articular pain and stiffness on daily prednisone doses as small as 2.0 to 2.5 mg of prednisone equivalent, but whose arthritic symptoms become insupportable when the dosage of steroid is cut, not necessarily abruptly, to 1.0 mg or to zero.

Faced with the problem of withdrawing patients with these four conditions from corticosteroids, the physician is well advised to prepare the patient for a long and tedious period, usually measured in terms of many months to a year, during which the dose of corticoid is diminished very slowly and by minuscule degrees. One must also keep in mind the peculiar tendency of some rheumatoid patients to develop a panmesenchymal reaction, the so-called steroid pseudorheumatism, during steroid withdrawal. Such an occurrence may require the reinstitution of corticosteroids at far higher dosages than the palliative levels that had been used to suppress the basic rheumatoid disease.

Another category of patients, those receiving relatively low-dose chronic corticoid treatment to suppress the secretion of ACTH by the adenohypophysis, includes persons with idiopathic hirsutism, presumably due to acquired adrenal hyperplasia (acquired adrenal virilism), and those with the several forms of congenital adrenocortical hyperplasia with virilism. The first type, found in adolescent or adult women, requires only modest dosages of prednisone equivalent, on the order of 7.5 mg per day or less. These women generally need treatment only during reproductive life, except those few who have associated hypertension. Further, the small doses do not produce untoward effects, and their withdrawal can be accomplished abruptly without eliciting any of the manifestations of corticosteroid withdrawal syndrome, adrenal suppression or corticoid dependence.

As for congenital adrenal hyperplasia, most patients can be treated with relatively small daily doses, so that difficulties with steroid withdrawal are generally not severe. This statement must be qualified, however. One must know precisely what type of adrenal enzymatic lesion is present. For the majority of subjects, the disorder is 21-hydroxylase deficiency, with "relative", that is, usually incomplete, lack of cortisol biosynthesis and secretion. Once pituitary-adrenal suppressive therapy with corticoids has brought them successfully through the periods of growth, sexual development, and reproductive function, these individuals do not require further corticosteroid treatment into late adult life and old age. Withdrawal can be carried out abruptly and with impunity. One may wish to add extra steroid cover for intercurrent, severe, acute illnesses in patients still on suppressive therapy. For the other forms of congenital adrenal hyperplasia, characterized by more nearly complete cortisol deficiency and by blocked aldosterone biosynthesis or hypertension, corticosteroid therapy is both ACTH-suppressive and a form of adrenal steroid replacement. These patients—those with deficits in 3β-hydroxysteroid dehydrogenase, 17α-hydroxylase, 11β-hydroxylase, and 18-hydroxysteroid dehydrogenase—are committed to a lifelong regimen of steroid medication. Like persons with Addison's disease, these people should never be subjected to steroid withdrawal.

A word should be said about patients, other than those just discussed, who are receiving lifelong adrenal replacement therapy. These are people with Addison's disease (primary adrenocortical insufficiency), those who have had total bilateral adrenalectomy (as for neoplastic disease), patients with secondary adrenocortical insufficiency due to hypopituitarism, and those few who are permanently adrenal deficient because of hypothalamic-pituitary-adrenocortical (HPA) suppression caused by prolonged high-dose corticosteroid administration (see below). The main point to be made about these chronically adrenal deficient patients is that the *replacement* doses of steroid, which are small and not associated with untoward effects, *should never be withdrawn*. The absolute contraindications to *pharmacologic* doses of corticoids—steroid induced psychosis, herpes simplex, tuberculosis and other infectious diseases—are not applicable to the small amounts needed for replacement, namely the equivalent of cortisol, 25 mg per day (the normal daily secretion rate of cortisol normally not exceeding 20 mg). On the contrary, it is worth reemphasizing the need for *larger* doses of steroid during most acute intercurrent infectious illnesses in these patients, not smaller ones. One other point concerning the secondary adrenal insufficiency states should be made: Unlike Addison's disease and the salt-losing forms of congenital adrenal hyperplasia, significant aldosterone deficiency does not occur. Measurements of plasma electrolytes will therefore be normal in acute emergencies, but these findings do not signify that there is no cortisol deficiency.

The Reasons for Starting and Stopping Corticosteroid Therapy

These are plain enough when the managing physician has personally made all the decisions, less so when he or she has inherited a patient from another doctor or another locale. It is essential to familiarize oneself thoroughly with the rationale for the patient's receiving corticoids in the first place. We have seen that the basic indications for corticosteroid therapy may be summarized in this way: supportive-"curative", keeping a serious disease at bay, palliative, ACTH-suppressive, and as replacement. The last two categories are dealt with in other chapters. Knowing which of the other three categories a given patient occupies provides clear signals as to what has been expected of the steroid therapeutically, how long it has been given, and what dosage has been used, large or small. This information in turn permits accurate and detailed predictions concerning the likelihood and specific nature of possible recurrences and the probability of HPA suppression. Whether or not corticoid dependence will supervene appears to be an individual and unpredictable matter.

The rationale for withdrawal of pharmacologic—that is, supraphysiologic—dosages of corticosteroids should be clear and definite. If the corticosteroid is no longer deemed to be therapeutically effective, it should be discontinued. In cases of herpes simplex, corticosteroids are thought by most clinicians to be *absolutely* contraindicated and should be stopped as rapidly as possible. The appearance of most other viral, bacterial, fungal, protozoan and metazoan infections during steroid therapy, which increases host susceptibility to all those infectious diseases, is regarded by most authorities as a *relative* contraindication. The procedure is to weigh the seriousness of the disease for which the steroid is being given against the threat posed by the intercurrent infectious insult. One cannot make a general rule.

As for the untoward effects of steroids themselves (iatrogenic Cushing's syndrome, for example), only a few dictate discontinuance of the drugs. The most definite of these is steroid induced psychosis. Less commonly, the induction of uncontrollable diabetes in a patient with genetic diabetes will force one to stop corticoid treatment. The same is rarely true of steroid related severe hypertension which can usually be controlled by antihypertensive agents even if the steroid is continued at an undiminished dosage. Incapacitating osteoporosis with pathologic fractures is an uncommon indication for withdrawing corticoids, as is pseudotumor cerebri (benign intracranial hypertension). Other untoward effects that may indicate withdrawal are peptic ulceration of the stomach, severe inhibition of growth in children, and crippling impairment of wound healing. The decision to withdraw steroids in each instance is again made by balancing the risks of the untoward effect against the benefit with respect to the underlying disease. As before, there is no simple rule applicable to all cases.

Duration of Therapy, Dosage Schedule, Specific Steroid Used

This information enables the doctor to assess the likelihood of clinically significant steroid-induced HPA suppression with concomitant inability of the patient's HPA system to respond to clinical stress. It should be apparent that the longer the course of steroid therapy and the higher the dosage the more likely is HPA suppression to occur. The relation between duration of dosage and magnitude of dose is complex and information is incomplete. A few definite statements can be made. Patients' susceptibility to HPA suppression by steroids is extraordinarily variable. Some patients may receive corticoids for years without impairment in their response to provocative tests of HPA function. Others, treated with prednisone, 15 mg daily for a week, show flattening of the adrenocortical response to ACTH. In general, patients treated with chronic low-dose palliation (as for rheumatoid arthritis), that is, with prednisone equivalent of 10 mg daily or less, show little or no impairment of HPA activity. Most patients with serious diseases treated with prolonged high-dose therapy (leukemia, lupus) have biochemical evidence of HPA suppression. Most people undergoing intensive short-term therapy (as for infectious shock) are not suppressed. People treated with large doses over long periods with the alternate-day schedule of corticoid administration have relative or partial preservation of HPA function, but given the present state of knowledge, they must still be considered at risk.

In numeric terms, any patient who has received the corticoid equivalent of 20 to 30 mg prednisone per day for more than 3 to 4 weeks should be suspected of having biochemical (if not clinically significant) HPA suppression. Since there are so few data relating duration and magnitude of corticoid therapy to rate of recovery of a putatively suppressed HPA axis, a suppressed patient should be considered to have possible HPA suppression, at least biochemically, for a year after cessation of the corticoid. This view is probably too conservative from the scientific point of view, but clinically it is prudent and thoroughly safe.

Further numeric data from stress tests (bacterial pyrogen) indicate that patients given 12.5 mg or more of prednisone equivalent daily for 1 month to 8 years uniformly show HPA suppression, while those receiving 4 mg or less for the same period do not. Suppressed patients are still suppressed one month after withdrawal from steroid therapy, but have recovered by 5 months; alternate-day treatment usually does not suppress the HPA axis. It should be noted that the range of dosage between 4 and 12.5 mg of prednisone equivalent constitutes an area of ambiguity. The prudent therapist will probably consider such patients as having received the 12.5 mg or greater dose.

In the light of such information, we see that detailed knowledge of duration and dosage schedule permits a fairly accurate calculation of probability that the of HPA system will be suppresed.

The only point to be made about the specific corticosteroid used relates to the duration of drug action. Cortisone and cortisol (the ''native'' hormone), rarely used in pharmacotherapy because of their salt-retaining property in susceptible individuals, have short half-lives in plasma. The semisynthetic corticoid analogs are all less firmly bound to specific plasma corticosteroid binding globulin (transcortin) and albumin than is cortisol, but all have longer plasma half-lives than cortisol; in the cases of prednisone, prednisolone and methylprednisolone, slightly longer; triamcinolone, somewhat longer; dexamethasone and betamethasone, much longer. Although the relationship between duration of action and plasma half-life is irregular, these properties mean in general that the longer lasting steroids tend to induce a more constant state of ''tissue'' hyperadrenocorticism, a constancy conducive to a greater likelihood of HPA suppression for an equivalent dose.

The Various Forms of Corticosteroid Withdrawal Syndrome

The specific biologic type of steroid withdrawal syndrome determines its management. This section defines the types and sets out the methods for identifying them.

No Withdrawal Syndrome. Many, perhaps most, patients of the millions receiving steroids undergo withdrawal without clinical difficulty. An unknown number may have subtle recrudescences of underlying disease or minor degrees of HPA suppression, but these are not clinically visible to patient or physician. No treatment is indicated.

Hypothalamic-Pituitary-Adrenocortical (HPA) Suppression. The incidence and prevalence of true adrenocortical insufficiency due to HPA suppression are not known because the symptoms are often vague and difficult to distinguish from those of corticosteroid dependence, because systemic tests of HPA function are not routinely made, and because not enough data are available to allow firm correlation between tests of HPA function and effective response of the HPA system to clinical stress. Normal biochemical behavior in a provocative test of the HPA system does not necessarily mean a normal adrenocortical capacity to withstand an acute episode of illness, and biochemical evidence of HPA suppression does not always predict inability to make an adequate and appropriate hormonal response to acute illness or trauma or surgery. Nevertheless, tests of HPA response are the only objective guides available, so such tests should be done where possible and the results cautiously interpreted as if they were predictive (to be discussed).

The symptoms and signs of corticoid-induced adrenal insufficiency are much like those of Addison's disease. The most common manifestations are weakness, lassitude, easy fatigability, mental depression, hypotension, postural hypotension, and undue prostration in the face of minor illnesses, such as coryza and mild viral gastroenteritis. Addisonian pigmentation is not seen because pituitary ACTH secretion is suppressed, and hyponatremia and hyperkalemia do not occur because corticosteroid suppression of ACTH has no lasting or quantitatively major effect upon aldosterone production. The nonobjective elements of this clinical picture cannot easily be separated from those of psychologic or physiologic dependence on corticosteroids except by provocative tests of HPA function.

The clinician has a choice of many procedures that test the whole HPA system: insulin hypoglycemia, vasopressin, and bacterial pyrogen, for example. These are cumbersome, stressful, and require hospitalization. The adrenocortical response to ACTH is simpler, less traumatic, correlates well with the other tests of HPA function, and parallels most closely the response of the adrenal cortex to clinical stress. The preferred method is to withhold the corticosteroid for 12 to 24 hours, determine baseline plasma cortisol level, at 8 AM, administer 250 μg of synthetic (proportional to amino acids 1–24) ACTH extra- or intramuscularly, and repeat the plasma cortisol measurement 60 and 120 minutes later. This procedure is safe and virtually devoid of side effects; the unexplained hypotension and prostration during administration of conventional ACTH to some patients with Addison's disease do not occur. Normal baseline values for plasma cortisol are 7 to 23 μg/dl, post-stimulation values are 19 to 43 μg/dl, and the normal increment is greater than 6 to about 30. A deficient rise in plasma cortisol level after synthetic ACTH should be interpreted as evidence of HPA suppression; a subnormal cortisol response renders untenable the exclusive diagnosis of psychologic dependence on corticoids.

Establishing the presence of HPA suppression rests on four elements: a plausible clinical syndrome, absence of recurrent disease whose symptoms mimic those of HPA suppression, rigorous laboratory demonstration of HPA insufficiency, and relief of the clinical syndrome by *replacement* doses of corticoid, not pharmacologic doses.

Psychologic or Physical Dependence Upon Corticosteroids. The diagnosis is made by elimination: recrudescent disease is absent and HPA suppression is biochemically excluded. In those circumstances, a patient who cannot tolerate steroid withdrawal or who demands increased doses, and who evinces weakness, lethargy, mood changes, or delirium when the amount of hormone is being reduced can be considered as corticoid-dependent or, in a sense, habituated. In the presence of anorexia, nausea, weight loss, fine desquamation of the skin of the face, hands, and feet, musculoskeletal aches, arthralgias, and fever the clinician can reasonably suspect physical dependence on corticosteroids. The symptoms and signs are alleviated by *pharmacologic* doses of steroid, not by replacement or physiologic doses.

The phychologic and subjective features of this type of withdrawal syndrome were originally ascribed to underlying and preexisting (that is presteroid) psychologic disturbances. Longer experience has shown that the presteroid personality has no detectable bearing on the likelihood of corticoid habituation, with the single exception that persons known to be or to have been addicted to narcotics tend to become dependent upon steroids as well.

Symptomatic Flare-Up of the Underlying Disease. Detection of this kind of withdrawal syndrome depends upon the reappearance of the subjective and objective manifestations of the disease being treated with steroids. The principles and methods are outlined above. If HPA function tests are normal, a given clinical picture cannot be attributed to adrenal insufficiency. Corticoid dependence is not always so easy to differentiate. For example, many of the symptoms and signs listed in the section above on corticoid dependence would be indistinguishable from those of a recurrence of rheumatoid arthritis. But the distinction between disease flare-up and steroid dependence is usually clear and straightforward in patients with asthma and the severe illnesses for which long-term high-dose corticoid treatment is given.

Combination. Finally, perhaps the most common form of steroid withdrawal syndrome is a combination of the three syndromes just discussed. The best way to deal with this set of problems is to inject as much objectivity as possible into the clinical setting. This is done by routinely performing the simple ACTH-plasma cortisol test of HPA function and by undertaking careful physical and laboratory investigations for objective criteria of recrudescent disease.

Peculiarities of Patient and Disease

For optimal management of the patient undergoing steroid withdrawal, the physician must be aware of relevant aspects of that patient's personality; his or her tolerance for pain and willingness or unwillingness to undergo a long and tedious process of dosage reduction; the interplay of the patient's illness with his or her family, occupation, and social life; and whether or not there is a history of prior addiction to other pharmacologic agents. The physician must know about absolute and relative contraindications, for example, the status of tuberculin reactivity, which should be monitored every 6 months, and about the details of possible drug interactions between the corticosteroid and other medications the patient is receiving. With respect to the disease being treated with steroids, the therapist must know precisely what symptoms and signs predominate in the particular patient and which manifestations tend to appear earliest during recurrences. For most asthmatics, cough, dyspnea, or wheezing, or combinations of these are the straightforward harbingers of recurrence. As suggested above, there is more variety in other diseases. One patient with leukemia may evince easy bruising, and another, fever as the first sign that steroid treatment is failing. Some patients with rheumatoid arthritis may complain of myalgias and stiffness during corticoid withdrawal, others of objective arthritis in two or three joints. Knowledge of the natural history of the disease in the specific patient and of his or her specific reactions to treatment is thus essential to permit early detection of the need for slowing the rate of steroid reduction and for temporarily increasing the dosage of corticosteroid.

THERAPEUTIC ALTERNATIVES

These consist of using other nonhormonal drugs in place of corticosteroids, small or homeopathic doses of steroids, the alternate-day schedule of glucocorticoid therapy, or ACTH.

In the severe diseases often treated with long-term high-dose steroids, other immunosuppressive agents may enable the physician to avoid corticoids if there is good reason to do so, that is, if absolute or relative contraindications exist. Immunosuppressives may sometimes suffice in lupus, leukemia, and the hepatitides. In asthma, inhaled steroids may induce less HPA suppression than steroids given systemically; other nonsteroidal inhalants, cromolyn, or other bronchodilators, singly or in combination, may palliate the disease without steroids. As for rheumatoid arthritis, corticosteroids are being used less and less, and other anti-inflammatory agents, for example, indomethacin, are given instead.

Very small doses of corticosteroids may control the manifestations of inflammatory and immunologic disease, but this is usually not possible. The physician may then resort to larger doses but on the alternate-day schedule, which is discussed in another chapter. It should be noted here that patients may be converted from the daily to the alternate day schedule in mid course of their treatment or of steroid withdrawal; this change permits HPA recovery to occur but does not accelerate that process.

Corticotropin (ACTH) has been used in intermittent dosage schedules *during steroid therapy* in attempts to prevent adrenocortical insufficiency due to HPA suppression. Although biochemical HPA response to both insulin and ACTH response tests is usually preserved, the subjective and objective signs of steroid withdrawal syndrome are as severe as with steroid therapy alone. The method has no value.

ACTH given *after a course of steroids* accelerates the return of adrenocortical function, but this return is transitory; the post-steroid hyporesponsiveness can be detected again within a week after the ACTH treatment. One would not expect to improve hypothalamic or pituitary function in these circumstances. In fact, ACTH may sometimes exert a negative feedback inhibitory influence upon endogenous ACTH secretion, and anti-ACTH antibodies against the native hormone may be formed. This method is without value.

ACTH given *instead of steroids* has a few advantages. Allegedly there are fewer serious undesirable effects. Growth curves in children are more nearly normal. Some clinicians believe it is easier to withdraw patients from ACTH than from steroids. The HPA system is more likely to remain biochemically intact. But these benefits are outweighed by the disadvantages. ACTH has to be given by injection. No disease responds better clinically to ACTH than to steroid therapy. A moderate number of patients have sustained severe hypersensitivity reactions to ACTH and a few have suffered intra-adrenal hemorrhage. Rarely, acute and catastrophic collapse, presumably due to adrenal failure, has occurred after a prolonged course of ACTH therapy, especially in the face of simultaneous anticoagulant therapy. The maximum amount of endogenous cortisol secretion that can be stimulated by exogenous ACTH is not more than 250 mg per day (or the equivalent of 60 mg of prednisone); many diseases (acute leukemia, lupus nephritis) require more than that. Finally, there is some evidence that exogenous ACTH may interfere with biosynthesis and release of pituitary ACTH. These seem sufficient reasons to discard this method.

PREFERRED APPROACH

Textbooks and treatises on therapeutics provide recommendations and recipes for corticosteroid withdrawal as if the only hazard were HPA suppression, but there are others as well (see above). The foregoing analysis indicates that the disease that has been treated, its recurrence or failure to recur, the therapeutic indications for steroid therapy, the details of the corticosteroid regimen and its duration, the exact type of corticosteroid withdrawal syndrome, and the idiosyncrasies of the particular patient and the particular disease all influence the choice of method for withdrawing a patient from corticosteroids. No single, simple approach will do for all.

General Considerations

The category of disease dictates the intensity and duration of steroid treatment, and that regimen indicates in general the method of withdrawal.

For acute, catastrophic conditions (such as septic shock) treated for no more than 2 to 6 days with high-dose steroids (hundreds of milligrams to grams of prednisone equivalent daily), the physician can stop the steroid therapy as abruptly as it was started. The activity of the precipitating condition dictates the need for tapering the steroid dose, not HPA suppression.

For the serious inflammatory, immunologic, and hematologic disorders (such as disseminated lupus) treated with prolonged high-dose steroid therapy (more than 15 mg of prednisone daily), withdrawal must be gradual because of HPA suppression and the danger of recurrent disease. Further, in those patients acute secondary adrenal insufficiency may be precipitated or exacerbated if the disease flares up during steroid withdrawal. If the patient has not been maintained throughout the course of steroid treatment on the alternate day schedule it does no good to switch to it as a prelude to steroid withdrawal since the process of HPA recovery is not accelerated thereby. The integrity of the HPA system is more or less maintained by the alternate day schedule only when it is maintained throughout most of the course.

In the inflammatory disorders (e.g., rheumatoid arthritis) managed with prolonged low-dose palliative steroid therapy (2 to 10 mg of prednisone per day), corticoid withdrawal must be gradual because of recurrence of the disease and because of corticosteroid dependence. HPA suppression is probably not much of a factor. The doses have to be decreased by very small steps and very slowly, usually with intermittent plateaus or slight increases in dosage. Withdrawal may take a year or more and a small portion of patients will not tolerate the total elimination of steroid therapy.

As suggested above, the small doses used in deliberate long-term inhibition of pituitary ACTH secretion (0.75 mg dexamethasone or equivalent daily as in congenital adrenal hyperplasia) do not seriously impair the cortisol-secreting facet of HPA function. Gradual lowering of steroid doses is therefore not necessary.

Specific Methods of Corticosteroid Withdrawal

For HPA Suppressed Patients. Patients in this category are chiefly those with a serious disease that has been treated with prolonged high-dose daily steroid therapy. A good rule of thumb is that any patient who looks cushingoid probably has significant HPA suppression. The critical dose of corticosteroid above which cushingoid appearance almost universally occurs is 15 mg of prednisone daily or the equivalent. Since the dosage range for this category of patients is approximately 15 to 120 mg of prednisone per day and the duration of treatment more than 3 to 4 weeks, one assumes that all patients in this group are biochemically HPA suppressed, whether the clinical degree of HPA suppression (generally difficult to detect) is significant or not.

A second rule depends on the reasons for stopping steroid treatment. The rate of withdrawal should be as rapid as possible in the face of major untoward effects of steroids or absolute contraindications to them, such as herpes simplex, varicella infections, or the abrupt appearance of psychosis. If the aim of withdrawal is to take advantage of a strong likelihood that the disease is in remission (when, for example, it has been possible to lower the steroid dosage considerably without recurrence), then the rate of dosage reduction should be gradual. This is the procedure in many instances of disseminated lupus, ulcerative colitis, and acute lymphocytic leukemia.

A third precept is that the physician should subdue his or her own excessive anxiety about corticoid withdrawal. With minimal vigilance, no patient dies from this process. Adrenal insufficiency does not happen suddenly and HPA suppression as a cause of death has been proved only rarely. Disease recurrences, with the rare exception of such entities as grand mal seizures due to cerebral microvascular disease in lupus, are not fatal. The aim is to spare the patient avoidable sudden, intense flare-ups of disease. Since corticosteroids seldom eradicate the chronic disorders for which they are used, steroid removal merely allows a condition, hitherto apparently held in check, to show itself. During withdrawal, one wishes to blunt these manifestations as much as possible.

The fourth rule concerning this group of patients is that steroid dependence in a few, HPA suppression in very few, and flare-up of disease in most will govern the rate of withdrawal from steroids. This gradual lowering of dosage is directed toward reducing the probability both of clinically significant adrenocortical insufficiency and of recrudescent illness.

In this category of persons given long-term high-dose steroid therapy, the clinical problem is that the disease (to the extent that one can separate disease from host) tolerates steroid withdrawal poorly; the host (with the same reservation) tolerates withdrawal relatively well.

Method. No prescription can be given which will suit all patients and all diseases. What follows is a practical outline that is generally applicable but must be modified to fit individual needs.

For the patients whose steroid therapy is interrupted because of an acute emergency which contraindicates corticoid administration (generalized viral infection, psychotic break), the principle is to cut the dose rapidly to an amount just enough above the physiologic level (prednisone, 5 mg, or cortisone, 20 to 25 mg) to sustain a presumably HPA suppressed, that is, adrenal-deficient patient through the stress of the intercurrent illness. Specifically, for the infectious complications, one reduces the daily steroid dosage from the maintenance level of 30 to 120 mg prednisone to 10 to 15 mg within 1 to 2 days, carefully observing vital signs and the activity of the basic disease. Since disseminated herpetic infection, for example, can be immediately fatal, whereas the steroid-treated systemic diseases are not, one errs on the low side of corticoid administration to minimize the immunosuppressive effect, that is, one lowers the dose still further to 5 to 10 mg of prednisone daily or 5 mg and 10 mg on alternate days, or less if possible. In managing steroid psychosis, the dosage can be at that level or lower—that is, physiologic—depending on the hyperactivity of the disturbed patient. In the event of severe trauma or a surgical emergency, patients receiving high-dose steroid therapy should be treated with larger doses of parenterally administered corticosteroids, as for the steroid cover described in the preceding chapter.

For the majority of patients in this high-dose category whose steroids are being eliminated in anticipation of a partial or complete remission, withdrawal can usually be accomplished quite smoothly within four weeks. Before starting withdrawal, the physician carefully notes and records all objective physical signs of the basic disease and obtains the essential laboratory data that will be used as indices of its activity. If one is starting from a dosage range of 15 to 40 mg of prednisone or equivalent daily, one can reduce the amount of steroid by decrements of 2.5 to 5 mg every second or third day until a physiologic level, 5 mg daily, is reached within 1 to 2 weeks. This can usually be done with impunity. Beginning at the higher dosage ranges, above 40 to 120 mg of prednisone per day, the dosage is lowered by decrements of 2.5 to 5 mg every 3 to 7 days. The reduction can be continued through minor recurrences of the basic disease, but if the flare-up is serious or incapacitating, the dosage is raised again to an amount just sufficient to suppress the clinical or laboratory manifestations and a more gradual reduction is attempted. It may be necessary to add other therapeutic agents, for example, immunosuppressants or cytotoxic drugs, if these are not already being given. Switching the patient to the alternate day steroid schedule during attempted steroid withdrawal is probably not useful and may only interpose another time-consuming step in an already lengthy procedure. By the third to fourth week, after a steady decrement of steroid dosage or after a series of decrements, brief increments, further decrements or periods of plateau, the amount of steroid ought to have arrived at a physiologic level, 5 mg of prednisone daily or 0.75 mg of dexamethasone. At this point, after the patient has been shown to tolerate this dosage for 3 to 7 days, the steroid is changed to 20 to 25 mg of hydrocortisone or cortisone, a physiologic dose of the physiologic hormone, the steroid with the shortest biologic action, given as a single morning dose to allow the maximum opportunity for resurgence of the HPA system.

During the fourth week, an 8 AM, plasma cortisol determination is made and that day's cortisone dose is withheld. Most patients will then have a cortisol level <10 μg/dl, a value likely to persist for 6 to 9 months after the initiation of corticoid withdrawal. At about the fourth to sixth week, the cortisone dosage is again reduced to 10 mg of cortisone, given as a single morning dose; this is not enough steroid to foster the continuance of iatrogenic Cushing's syndrome nor to suppress the HPA system, but it is sufficient to provide a cushion against adrenocortical insufficiency under basal conditions. In medical emergencies, such as acute infections, trauma, or surgery, and in minor illnesses or small-scale interventive procedures (endoscopy, dental work), steroid cover is necessary. By the sixth to ninth month, the 8 AM plasma cortisol level, which may be measured about every 2 months, should have returned to >10 μg/dl. Then the physician can assume that basal HPA function has recovered and the morning dose of cortisone can be stopped, but steroid cover for emergencies will still be required.

Nine or more months after the start of withdrawal, the integrity of the entire HPA system should have been restored. There is not much point in performing an ACTH stimulation test until this time, because full HPA capacity to respond to provocative tests may take 9 to 12 months or more. During this period, a synthetic ACTH (Synacthen, Cosyntropin) test is done; when the increment of plasma cortisol is in the range of >6–30 μg/dl HPA recovery is judged to be complete, and steroid cover for medical emergencies should theoretically not be required. Nevertheless, the correlation between biochemical tests of HPA function and HPA capacity to react to clinical stress is uncertain, so that for the first 12 to 16 months after the beginning of corticoid withdrawal steroid cover should be instituted for acute stresses or in the event that manifestations which suggest adrenocortical insufficiency appear.

As stated above, ACTH has no place in the treatment of the corticosteroid withdrawal syndrome or in the management of steroid withdrawal. Since the HPA suppressed patient has an inadequate adrenocortical capacity to respond to endogenous or exogenous corticotropin, ACTH administration will not stimulate enough cortisol secretion to protect the patient from adrenal insufficiency during stress.

For Corticosteroid-Dependent Patients. This category includes patients with rheumatoid arthritis and some asthmatics maintained on long-term low-dose palliative therapy. Despite the low dosages (<15 mg of prednisone daily), these people are more difficult to withdraw than those on prolonged high-dose corticosteroid regimens. For unknown reasons, this group evinces a greater tendency to become dependent upon corticosteroids. It is not known whether the dependence is psychologic or physiologic or both. The dangers of corticosteroid withdrawal are less than in high-dose patients, but the likelihood of failure to achieve withdrawal is greater. The clinical problem is that the disease tolerates withdrawal relatively well; the host tolerates it poorly or not at all.

For practical purposes, HPA suppression does not present difficulties during withdrawal, except that the cautious physician will provide steroid cover if medical emergencies supervene during the process. Plasma cortisol measurement and ACTH tests are unnecessary. Particularly in rheumatoid arthritis, reduction of the steroid dosage must be regular and deliberate. The physician has to make every effort to enlist the full cooperation and tolerance of the patient. Decrements in dosage should not exceed 1 mg of prednisone equivalent every 1 to 2 months; at that rate withdrawal may require a year or more. The physician should not try to hasten the withdrawal or attempt alternate-day schedules; such maneuvers may precipitate "steroid pseudorheumatism"—more likely a manifestation of corticoid withdrawal than of recurrent arthritis—which requires raising the steroid dosage again, sometimes to levels above the dosage from which one started. For mild to moderate exacerbations, increased amounts of salicylate may be given and indomethacin added. The physician must be careful about salicylates; corticosteroids enhance renal clearance of aspirin, and when the steroid dosage is reduced blood values of salicylate may rise to the toxic range in some patients. Monitoring of plasma salicylate levels permits appropriate titration of aspirin dosage.

Patients with asthma are almost as difficult to withdraw as are those with rheumatoid arthritis. Reduction of the steroid dose must be gradual, but the decrements need not be as exquisitely small as for rheumatoid patients, and the variety of other effective medications (e.g., systemic or inhaled bronchodilators) offers a broader choice in mitigating flare-ups during steroid withdrawal. As in the arthritic subjects, these patients must be persuaded to cooperate fully with the withdrawal procedure.

In this category, the physician must be prepared to fail. An unknown proportion of people with these two diseases cannot or will not tolerate life without corticosteroids. In my opinion, this is because of corticosteroid dependence or habituation, not uncontrollable disease; but a clinical impression of steroid dependence does not give the physician license to adopt a high moral tone toward his dependent—some might say "addicted"—patient. The corticosteroid dependency syndrome, comprising objective and subjective signs, might as well be viewed as an organic illness. The only effective treatment is the lowest possible dosage of steroid, as little as 1 to 2.5 mg of prednisone daily. Such small amounts lie below the physiologic secretion rate of cortisol in equivalence. Why these few milligrams should effectively relieve symptoms is not known, but since there is no danger of HPA suppression or iatrogenic Cushing's syndrome with minute dosages of corticosteroid, the physician has no good reason to withhold what the patient will demand in any case.

For Flare-Ups of the Steroid-Treated Disease. Consideration of *recurrent disease* during steroid withdrawal is necessarily woven into the foregoing discussions concerning *HPA suppression* and *corticoid dependence*. This interweaving emphasizes the difficulty in separating, on clinical grounds, the manifestations of the three elements. This is not difficult in flagrant systemic disease like ulcerative colitis and disseminated lupus or disorders like asthma, which are marked by some clear and unmistakable sign. But in rheumatoid arthritis, for example, a syndrome—occurring during steroid withdrawal—of weakness, lassitude, muscle aches, joint stiffness with only minimal swelling or redness, and low-grade fever can reasonably be interpreted as HPA insufficiency, corticoid dependence, or a mild recrudescence of the rheumatoid process. Serologic tests for mesenchymal disease may be somewhat informative but only rarely provide a definite diagnosis of recurrence. Provocative tests of HPA function may show normal or subnormal biochemical response, but the relation between test and clinical adequacy or deficiency of the HPA system is irregular and obscure. The physician must therefore be prepared to deal with some patients in whom the three threads—status of the HPA system, corticoid dependence, mild flare-up of disease—are almost impossible to disentangle. In such people, the clinical syndrome is relieved by administration of low-dose corticosteroids. This is not intellectually rewarding for the doctor but leads to a satisfactory clinical result for the patient.

Suggested Reading

Amatruda TT, Hurst MM, D'Esopo ND. Certain endocrine and metabolic facets of the steroid withdrawal syndrome. J Clin Endocr Metab 1965; 25:1207–1217.

Byyny RL. Withdrawal from glucocorticoid therapy. N Engl J Med 1976; 295:30–32.

Collins TR, Byyny RL. The clinical use of glucocorticoids. Comprehensive Ther 1980; 6:63–72.

Dixon RB, Christy NP. On the various forms of corticosteroid withdrawal syndrome. Am J Med 1980; 68:224–230.

CARCINOID TUMORS

RICHARD R. P. WARNER, M.D.

Carcinoid tumors are generally so slow growing that they may be considered "malignancies in slow motion". Appendiceal carcinoids comprise two-thirds of these neoplasms. The appendiceal carcinoids rarely spread or cause the carcinoid syndrome and almost never produce clinically significant amounts of vasoactive humoral substances. They are usually found at the time of surgery for appendicitis, and most of the time simple appendectomy is sufficient treatment for them. Of greater importance and often presenting problems in treatment are the extra-appendiceal carcinoids, of which approximately 25 percent arise from the small intestine, one-tenth from the lung (bronchial adenomas of carcinoid type), and the remainder from assorted sites such as colon, esophagus, stomach, rectum, biliary tract, pancreas, testes, ovary, and, very rarely, other unusual extraintestinal sites. In 10 percent of patients presenting with the carcinoid syndrome, the primary tumor is not found during life. Though a reasonable effort to find the primary tumor should be exerted, location of the primary site is usually not critical to therapy of the carcinoid syndrome.

The major manifestations of the carcinoid syndrome which require therapy are flushing and diarrhea, which occur in almost all cases; cardiac disease in 25 percent of cases (congestive failure, carcinoid fibrotic valvular lesions, metastatic carcinoid tumor involvement of myocardium and/or pericardium), bronchospasm in 10 percent of cases, and sometimes painful hepatic enlargement due to neoplasm. Minor features are peptic ulcer, severe hypoalbuminemia, pellagra, muscle wasting, myopathy, arthropathy, retroperitoneal fibrosis and fibrosing reaction in other sites, brawny edema, and hyperglycemia. Except for low serum albumin and peptic ulcer, clinically significant minor features occur in only a small percentage of cases.

Most patients with carcinoid metastases do not manifest the functioning carcinoid syndrome. Since these tumors vary in their degree of production of chemical substances (serotonin, bradykinin, prostaglandin-PGE_2, neurotensin, and sometimes histamine) that cause the pharmacologic effects resulting in most of the manifestations of the syndrome, there is great variation in the signs and symptoms of the syndrome and its severity. Unless the tumor arises in an organ that drains its venous blood into the caval system, fairly large deposits of carcinoid metastases are needed in the liver before the carcinoid syndrome will occur. Carcinoid tumors usually spread in a predictable and fairly orderly fashion, with local extension and then regional node involvement before liver metastases occur. Only one-fifth to one-quarter of patients with metastases in the liver actually manifest carcinoid syndrome. Even in the absence of the syndrome, almost all patients with distant carcinoid metastases show modest increases in levels of urinary indole metabolites and blood serotonin, and decreases in blood tryptophan. Although there is not close correlation between the severity of the syndrome and levels of these substances, patients with a more florid syndrome have more abnormal values, and in any individual case these chemical parameters serve as helpful markers in assessing the efficacy of various forms of treatment.

The development of carcinoid syndrome is usually gradual and insidious, and once it is present, cure by surgical excision of tumor is not possible except in very rare instances in which a highly functioning primary tumor drains into the caval system and has no metastases. This sometimes occurs in carcinoid of the ovary and testis. Hence, the therapeutic approach to carcinoid syndrome is usually to relieve symptoms and prolong life rather than to cure.

Carcinoid tumors without metastases can be cured by surgical extirpation. When metastases have occurred, but are relatively nonfunctioning and not causing the carcinoid syndrome, their slow growth is often compatible with many years or even decades of life. However, when the carcinoid syndrome is present, the timetable is faster, and the majority of these patients succumb to the pharmacologic effects of the humoral substances produced by their tumors. About one-half die from cardiac complications, and the rest die from infection and nutritional, electrolyte, bleeding, and renal disorders indirectly resulting from the effects of the products of their tumors. As occurs in patients who do not have the functioning syndrome, some patients with the carcinoid syndrome also die from mechanical and invasive effects of their neoplasm. For optimum results in carcinoid disease, treatment must be highly individualized in each case, i.e., with the aggressiveness and vigor of therapy being determined in large part by the size of the carcinoid tumor, the extent of its spread, and the degree of its chemical function. Because of the usually slow rate of growth of carcinoid tumors, even when producing the carcinoid syndrome, more aggressive treatment is justified in such patients than one would consider in patients with equally extensive spread of a more rapidly growing adenocarcinoma. Often in carcinoid syndrome vigorous treatment can effectively palliate the disease and prolong life for several years or longer.

TREATMENT OF NONFUNCTIONING TUMORS

Carcinoid tumors of the intestine, lung, or other organs, whenever found, and even in the absence of symptoms, should be removed. Limited en bloc resection is sufficient for small tumors, but those over 2 cm in diameter require wider resection since invasiveness correlates with tumor size. The small intestinal carcinoid tends to be multiple, and a search for additional primary growths should be made when one is found. Even though an adequate cuff (10 cm) of uninvolved bowel should be included in the resection of larger carcinoids of the small intestine, as much intestine as possible should be conserved in order to avoid problems of a shortened intestine superimposed on the carcinoid syndrome which might later develop. Sometimes simply bypassing a kinked or obstructed loop of bowel, when the primary is inoperable and extensive metastases are present, may prove palliative for years. Because of the slowness of regrowth, occasional debulking of an unresectable tumor may palliate the disease and extend life for a worthwhile period. A portion of a resected carcinoid should be preserved, frozen and unfixed, for serotonin assay. If the tumor has any chemical production of serotonin, the blood level should be monitored every 6 months along with the urinary excretion of indole metabolites. Such measurements can sometimes provide early evidence of tumor spread or beginning carcinoid syndrome.

In patients with intestinal carcinoid there is an increased frequency of metachronous or subsequent development of adenocarcinoma of the colon. Hence, new abdominal complaints in a patient who previously underwent surgery for GI tract carcinoid must be thoroughly investigated.

Most carcinoids do not respond to radiotherapy. Experience with chemotherapy in nonfunctioning carcinoids has been limited, but the response appears to be less promising than that of the functioning tumors. About one-half of the carcinoid syndrome patients respond favorably to one of the combination chemotherapy regimens now available.

TREATMENT OF THE CARCINOID SYNDROME

Since most symptoms and the patient's eventual deterioration are mainly due to the effects of the substances that the carcinoid tumor produces, stores, and releases, treatment is directed to preventing or reducing the tumor's chemical production, inhibiting release of these substances, or blocking their effects on target organs. In addition, a number of general supportive measures are very important.

General Supportive Measures

Niacin synthesis is deficient in carcinoid syndrome since utilization of its precursor, tryptophan, is abnormally increased and diverted by the functioning tumor to form serotonin. In some untreated patients, this can even lead to the development of pellagra. Hence, all carcinoid syndrome patients should be given niacin, at least 50 mg, three times a day by mouth as well as multiple vitamins. Also, because of the diversion of tryptophan metabolism, protein synthesis in these patients is subnormal. Therefore, a high protein diet should be given. Intestinal motility is tremendously altered in the carcinoid syndrome, and small intestinal transit time is exceedingly rapid. Malabsorption may be present. The rapid passage of intestinal contents can result in relative pancreatic insufficiency, as well as inadequate reabsorption of bile salts in the terminal ileum. If there has been resection of a portion of the small intestine previously, these mechanisms of diarrhea are further enhanced. For these reasons many patients benefit from medium-chain triglyceride oil supplements (2 to 4 tablespoons, three times a day) and cholestyramine (Questran, 1 packet with each meal). Between-meal high protein elemental diet supplements are desirable, but usually provoke diarrhea.

Symptomatic treatment of the diarrhea sometimes is successful with diphenoxalate hydrochloride with atropine sulfate (Lomotil, 1 to 2 tablets with meals and at bedtime) or Loperamide (Imodium, 2 to 4 mg before meals and at bedtime), and with antiserotonin and antihistamine agents such as cyproheptadine (Periactin) and methysergide (Sansert) (to be discussed).

Since adrenergic agonists provoke acute vasomotor symptoms of the carcinoid syndrome (carcinoid crisis), these patients must avoid adrenergic drugs and must be shielded from abrupt release of endogenous catechols. Physical and emotional stress must be minimized. Hypotension or even shock may occur in a severe carcinoid crisis and must not be treated with sympathomimetic vasopressors, except for the direct-acting vasoconstrictor, methoxamine (Vasoxyl). Epinephrine must not be used in the treatment of carcinoid asthma since it may induce worse or even intractible bronchospasm, hypotension, and even shock. The use of sympathomimetic nasal decongestants must also be strictly limited. Alcohol often produces attacks and should be forbidden. MAO inhibitors (many antidepressant drugs) block the degradation of serotonin and can potentiate some of the symptoms of the carcinoid syndrome; they should not be used in these patients. Individuals with carcinoid syndrome tolerate surgery and anesthesia poorly. Even minor procedures can induce severe respiratory and cardiac complications if the patient has not been specifically pretreated in preparation for the procedure with antiserotonin and antikinin agents. The safest anesthesia we have found utilizes thiopentone, pancuronium and nitrous oxide.

Although others have noted good results in treating carcinoid diarrhea with cimetidine (Tagemet, 300 mg four times a day), I have not. Anticholinergic preparations (Pro-Banthine, 15 to 30 mg three times a day) are sometimes helpful. Often large amounts of potassium and magnesium are needed to replace diarrheal losses. Parachlorophenylalanine (PCP), an experimental inhibitor of serotonin synthesis, has been effective in controlling the diarrhea, but it has a high incidence of serious allergic side effects and is not generally available. The new experimental antiserotonin, ketanserin, shows considerable promise of being helpful, according to preliminary reports, but it is still limited to investigative use.

Surgery

When technically feasible it is sometimes palliative to debulk large functioning tumor masses, to destroy or resect large discrete functioning metastases in the liver, or even to perform partial hepatectomy. Unless intestinal obstruction, infarction, or bleeding requires intervention, there is no proven benefit in simply resecting a small primary intestinal carcinoid which has already produced extensive metastases. Sometimes surgery may be required to catheterize and/or ligate the hepatic artery when this is not technically possible by a percutaneous approach. In rare cases of severe progressive and intractible congestive heart failure due to carcinoid valvular disease, prosthetic valve replacement can produce dramatic and prolonged improvement.

Chemotherapy

Cytotoxic drugs in combination with other modalities are used in the treatment of almost all carcinoid syndrome patients. The more potent the drug and the more sensitive the tumor, and the more severe the carcinoid syndrome being treated, the worse the paradoxical exacerbation of the symptoms will be in response to the treatment. This is the result of release of their vasoactive products from the injured carcinoid cells.

The severity of this paradoxical reaction is somewhat related to the dosage of the cytotoxic agent administered. Conventional dosages of these drugs must not be utilized in the active carcinoid syndrome patient because of the risk of precipitating a severe or, on rare occasions, even fatal attack. The schedule and dosage for treatment must be highly individualized and should not be started until the lability of the patient's carcinoid syndrome has been evaluated. This can be done by carrying out an epinephrine provocative test, as described later in this chapter. If a strongly positive response is obtained, chemotherapy should not be started until a protective drug regimen has been initiated in the patient and its effectiveness confirmed by a weak or negative response to a repeat epinephrine provocative test. The agents available for this protective treatment regimen (antiserotonins, bradykinin antagonists, and alpha adrenergic blockers) are discussed below in the pharmacologic therapy section.

Since lower than usual dosages of chemotherapeutic drugs are used in most active carcinoid syndrome patients, their conventional side effects (e.g., mucositis, bone marrow suppression, nephrotoxicity) are usually only mild; therefore, after initial in-hospital treatment, the repeated treatment, which these patients require for years, can usually be done on an outpatient basis.

The currently preferred chemotherapy programs involve combinations of 5-fluorouracil and streptozotocin, 5-fluorouracil and CCNU or BCNU, 5-fluorouracil and Adriamycin, and DTIC. Earlier experience with methotrexate, cyclophosphamide, and melphalan showed them to produce some, but more limited, benefits. It is my opinion that whatever chemotherapy is used should be administered by an oncologist and the dosage adjusted to the tolerance of each patient.

Hepatic Artery Treatment—Occlusion and Injection

Current experience points to hepatic dearterialization as the most effective way to palliate the carcinoid syndrome and, when combined with chemotherapy, to also prolong life. This procedure usually can be done by percutaneous catheterization with injection of Gelfoam emboli, Ivalon, or other material. When percutaneous catheterization of the hepatic artery is not technically possible, ligation of the artery by a surgical approach can be utilized. Once correct placement of the catheter has been confirmed angiographically, I usually precede the injection of embolizing material with a bolus injection of 5-fluorouracil and streptozotocin. Subsequently, the patient is continued on a prolonged regimen of systemic chemotherapy. In order to prevent provocation of a severe carcinoid crisis during or after the procedure and to protect against liver abscess, peritoneal and systemic reaction from tumor necrosis, hepatic failure, and hypoglycemia, extensive treatment is required before, during, and after the procedure. The following contraindications would exclude a carcinoid syndrome patient from undergoing hepatic dearterialization: portal vein occlusion, replacement of more than 75 percent of the liver by metastases, signs of a significant degree of liver failure (e.g., jaundice, encephalopathy) hyperurecemia, uncorrectable bleeding diathesis, extensive extrahepatic carcinoid metastases, and persisting, very severe and uncontrollable manifestations of carcinoid syndrome in spite of the use of various antagonists and blocking drugs available for dampening the syndrome.

Preparation of a patient for hepatic dearterialization should include confirmation of an effective and well-tolerated drug regimen for blocking carcinoid syndrome attacks. As already noted, the repeated use of the epinephrine provocative test before and after drug treatment is helpful in severe cases to establish objective evidence of effective treatment. The most used drugs are: cyproheptadine (Periactin) or phenoxybenzamine (Dibenzyline). Beta adrenergic blockers are of no apparent benefit. The carcinoid crisis blocking effects of IV bolus injection of glucagon and methotrimeprazine (Levaprome) should also be tested. The usual dose of cyproheptadine is 2 to 4 mg orally one to four times daily. The usual dose of phenoxybenzamine is 10 mg orally once a day, gradually increasing to no more than 40 mg twice a day. Patients undergoing hepatic dearterialization should receive 3 days of pretreatment with prednisone, 30 mg a day, for kinin and prostaglandin inhibition, and 3 liters of 5 percent dextrose in water per day, with 10 units of regular insulin per liter, to build up glycogen stores and hydration. Twelve hours and 6 hours before the procedure, IV cefazolin (Kefzole), 0.5 g, is given. The percutaneous hepatic artery catheterization, angiography, chemotherapy, and embolus injection are performed under either local anesthesia following preoperative Demerol and Valium, and with the anesthetist standing by, or, in the more labile cases, under general anesthesia with airway intubation and the anesthetic agents recommended earlier in this chapter. Additional corticosteroids are given intraoperatively. In Europe, preoperative and intraoperative intravenous administration of large doses of the protease inhibitor, aprotinin (Trasylol), has been found to be exceedingly helpful in preventing and treating provoked carcinoid attacks. Unfortunately, this agent is not available for human use in the United States.

Bronchospasm and hypotension during a procedure are treated with IV injection of methotrimeprazine (Levoprome), 2.5 to 5 mg; glucagon, 0.5 to 1 mg IV; and IV hydrocortisone (Solucortef), 100 mg. When hypotension persists, IV methoxamine (Vasoxyl), 3 to 5 mg, may be used.

Following the procedure, most patients are treated in the intensive care unit for several days. Nausea, vomiting, and right upper quadrant pain are common sequelae to the procedure. They are controlled with perchlorperazine (Compazine), methotrimeprazine (Levaprome), and Demerol injection. IV infusion of glucagon, 0.1 mg per hour, is continued for 48 hours to enhance portal blood flow to the liver and to suppress functioning carcinoid symptoms. Blood sugar levels must be monitored and insulin given when indicated. IV antibiotics must be continued for at least 3 days. Corticosteroids are continued, but tapered to lower dosage by the end of the first week if marked hepatic tenderness has subsided and functioning carcinoid symptoms have waned. Oral medications and feeding are resumed 2 or 3 days after the procedure, or as soon as nausea, vomiting, and peritoneal reaction permit. Liver function tests are monitored daily for the first week. Approximately 1 month after the procedure, the patient is started on long-term systemic chemotherapy. Usually the first combination I use is 5-fluorouracil and streptozotocin, on a schedule of treatment varying from weekly to monthly, depending on the patient's response. Urinary excretion of 5-HIAA and, when the assays are available, excretion of the other indole metabolites, as well as blood serotonin and tryptophan, are measured at 2-month intervals for 8 months and thereafter at more prolonged intervals.

Pharmacologic Therapy

Alpha adrenergic blockers, phentolamine (Regitine), 25 to 50 mg PO one to three times a day, and phenoxybenzamine (Dibenzyline), 10 mg PO, slowly increased to 30 mg once a day, are given for the control of flushing. Perchlorperazine (Compazine), 5 to

10 mg PO or IM *q4h*, and chlorpromazine (Thorazine), 10 to 25 mg PO or IM *q6h*, have both antiserotonin and antinausea properties and may help flushing. More potent antiserotonins are methysergide (Sansert), 2 mg PO *tid*, and cyproheptadine (Periactin), 2 to 8 mg *tid*. Prolonged use of Sansert can cause retroperitoneal, pleural, and peritoneal fibrosis. Periactin also has strong antihistamine properties. Both these drugs are often helpful in controlling diarrhea. Flushing is sometimes responsive to combined use of H_1 and H_2 antagonists, particularly when due to foregut carcinoids producing histamine. Useful for this purpose are diphenhydramine (Benadryl), 50 mg PO *qid*, and cimetidine (Tagamet), 300 mg PO *qid*. The gastric carcinoid variant syndrome with its patchy cherry red flush, excessive histamine production, and absence of diarrhea and heart lesions also sometimes responds well to methyldopa (Aldomet), 250 mg PO *tid*.

Corticosteroids and chlorpromazine are helpful, and even occasionally lifesaving, in those bronchial carcinoids with the variant syndrome, characterized by severe prolonged flushing preceded by disorientation, anxiety, and tremor, and accompanied by facial edema, lacrimation, hypotension, tachycardia, bronchospasm, diarrhea, nausea, vomiting, and sometimes pulmonary edema.

I have not observed any good response of flushing or diarrhea to indomethacin (Indocin). For this reason, and because of the known tendency of carcinoid syndrome patients to develop peptic ulcer, I consider it prudent not to use this drug in this disease.

Methotrimeprazine (Levoprome), 5 to 20 mg IM or IV every 4 to 6 hours, has antiserotonin, analgesic, and sedating properties which make it particularly useful. Demerol in conventional dosage seems well tolerated in carcinoid syndrome patients, but morphine, a serotonin liberator, should be avoided.

Somatostatin and some of its experimental analogs, acting through unknown mechanisms, have been found to be extremely effective in preventing spontaneous and provoked carcinoid flushes and diarrhea. These drugs are still experimental, and their beneficial effects last only for the brief period during which the parenteral treatment is given. However, if safe and longer-acting analogs are developed in the future, I would expect them to provide the most effective means of treating the carcinoid syndrome crisis.

The Epinephrine Provocative Test as a Guide to Therapy

At the patient's bedside, with an IV of 5 percent D/W running slowly, the blood pressure and heart rate are measured and recorded every 30 seconds until a stable baseline is obtained. Thereafter, at 5-minute intervals, starting with 1 μg, a bolus of epinephrine is rapidly injected intravenously in progressively larger doses until a positive response occurs or a dose of 10 μg is reached. Heart rate and blood pressure are measured every 60 seconds after the injection. The patient is observed for flushing, hypotension, tachycardia, and other symptoms of carcinoid attacks. The appearance of a flush alone and/or a fall in blood pressure of at least 20 mmHg systolic and 10 Hg diastolic, between 45 and 120 seconds after the injection and lasting 1 minute or more, is a positive response. In some active carcinoids even the smallest dose of epinephrine can precipitate a serious hypotensive episode. This can usually be reversed by the immediate (within 2 to 4 minutes) IV injection of 5 mg of phentolamine (Regitine). This test should not be done casually, and phentolamine should be ready for injection before epinephrine is injected. In addition, methoxamine (Vasoxyl), 3 mg, should also be available to reverse hypotension in the rare event that phentolamine fails to do so.

Suggested Reading

Harris Al. Chemotherapy for the carcinoid syndrome. Cancer Chemother Pharmacol 1981; 5:133-38.

Jager RM, Polk HJ Jr. Carcinoid apudomas. In: Hickey RC ed. Current Problems in Cancer. Chicago: Year Book Medical Publishers 1977; 1:1–53.

Levine RJ, Sjoerdsma A. Pressor amines and the carcinoid flush. Intern Med 1963; 58:818–28.

Maton PN, Camilleri M, Griffin G, Allison DJ, Hodgson HJF, Chadwick VS. Role of hepatic arterial embolization in the carcinoid syndrome. Br Med J 1983; 287:932–35.

Miller R, Patel AU, Warner RRP, Parnes I. Anesthesia for the carcinoid syndrome: A report of nine cases. Can Anaesth Soc J 1978; 25:240–44.

GASTROINTESTINAL AND ACCESSORY ORGAN DISEASES

GASTROESOPHAGEAL REFLUX: MEDICAL TREATMENT

THOMAS R. HENDRIX, M.D.

Gastroesophageal reflux occurs daily in everyone. In most individuals these episodes are asymptomatic, and if symptoms are produced, they usually are not considered as abnormalities requiring medical attention. In a study of hospital staff and employees considered in good health, 7 percent experienced heartburn, the characteristic symptom of gastroesophageal reflux, daily, and more than one-third had the symptom at least once a month. Despite these symptoms, none sought medical advice nor considered they had any dysfunction or disease.

If our discussion is limited to those patients demonstrated to have gastroesophageal reflux in the course of evaluation of their presenting complaints, we find a wide spectrum of symptoms ranging from troublesome heartburn at one extreme to serious damage to the esophageal mucosa at the other. The serious end of the spectrum comprises erosive esophagitis and its sequelae, such as peptic stricture and Barrett's esophagus, a complication of reflux in which the ulcerated squamous mucosa is replaced with columnar mucosa having a considerable potential for malignant transformation. It seems likely that our convention of lumping all of these consequences of gastroesophageal reflux into a single entity, gastroesophageal reflux disease (GERD), obscures important pathophysiologic features which, if better understood, could lead to more rational therapy.

The recognition that there are two, not mutually exclusive, patterns of reflux *postprandial* and *nocturnal*, is an important first step towards making sense of the heterogeneity of GERD. While everyone has some postprandial reflux, nocturnal reflux is not seen in "normal" individuals. Symptomatic postprandial reflux may be merely an exaggeration of a "normal phenomenon," whereas nocturnal reflux is clearly pathologic. Nocturnal reflux is frequently associated with the complications of reflux, i.e., esophagitis, stricture, Barrett's esophagus, and pulmonary aspiration. It is particularly treacherous because: (1) it is less likely to produce symptoms that warn the individual that something is wrong; (2) swallowing is only one-tenth as frequent during sleep as when awake; (3) rate of production of alkaline saliva is reduced during sleep; and (4) gravity does not aid in the clearing of the esophagus. Until we have a better understanding of the factors underlying symptomatic and pathologic reflux, our treatment of necessity must be empiric.

A second important concept in understanding reflux and planning for its treatment is that gastroesophageal reflux causes a vicious cycle which, if not interrupted, leads to progression of symptoms and esophageal damage. Reflux of irritant material into the esophagus interferes with effective peristalsis and leads to delayed clearing of the esophagus. The latter is associated with decreased sphincter tone, thus setting the stage for further reflux, which, if not interrupted, may progress to esophagitis and its complications.

TREATMENT MODALITIES

Treatment is aimed at improving the function of the elements that protect the esophagus from the irritant nature of refluxed gastric contents. These elements are (1) the gastroesophageal reflux barrier, which is primarily the function of the lower esophageal sphincter (ES); (2) the combined effects of peristalsis and gravity to produce rapid clearing of refluxed material from the esophagus; (3) the acid neutralizing capacity of saliva; and (4) the squamous epithelial barrier, which prevents the penetration of noxious material, primarily H^+ ions, into the mucosa. Successful treatment must reduce reflux sufficiently to permit the restoration of the normal squamous epithelial barrier. It is analogous to treating sunburn (damage to another epithelial barrier). If the damaged epithelium is not well protected from the damaging factor, ultraviolet light in the case of sunburn and gastric contents in reflux, healing will not occur.

In practical terms treatment aims at (1) decreasing the frequency and duration of reflux episodes, (2) increasing the rate of clearing of refluxed material from the esophagus, and (3) decreasing the noxious nature of refluxed gastric contents.

Decreasing Frequency and Duration of Reflux Episodes

The frequency and duration of reflux episodes may be decreased by improving LES tone and function, elevating the head of the bed, and weight reduction.

Improving Lower Esophageal Sphincter Function

Sphincter function may be improved by *dietary* and *drug* therapy. Protein meals have been shown to increase sphincter tone, whereas fatty meals decrease it. In addition, chocolate, caffeine, peppermint, and alcohol decrease sphincter tone. Sphincter tone is increased by antacids, cholinergic agents (bethanechol), and metoclopramide. A variety of drugs decrease sphincter tone, including theophylline, anticholinergic agents, calcium channel blocking agents, beta-adrenergic agonists (isoproterenol), alpha-adrenergic antagonists (phentolamine), diazepam, and progesterone containing contraceptives. Smoking also is associated with increased reflux. Gastric distention is associated with decreased sphincter pressure; thus small meals, low in fat, empty promptly, thereby avoiding impairment of the sphincter's barrier function. In addition, since dyspepsia is often associated with delayed gastric emptying, those foods that the patient associates with dyspepsia should be avoided. Finally, bethanechol and metoclopramide increase both the rate of gastric emptying and sphincter tone. Aerophagia and inspiring air into the esophagus lead to gastric distention and eructation, thus interfering with sphincter function.

Elevation of Head and Chest When Reclining

Elevation of the head of the bed on 6-inch blocks has been shown, by continuous intraesophageal pH recording, to decrease the frequency and duration of nocturnal reflux episodes.

Weight Loss

Overweight patients with reflux should be urged to lose weight. Although the reflux symptoms are often increased with increases of 10 or more pounds, and unmanageable reflux symptoms become tractable with weight loss, the mechanisms responsible are poorly understood. Realistically, however, if we had to rely on the patient's ability to lose weight to control reflux symptoms, only a few patients would improve.

Increasing Esophageal Clearing

Effective esophageal clearing of refluxed acid from the stomach depends upon the combined action of effective peristalsis and bicarbonate secretion in saliva. Maneuvers that improve esophageal peristalsis and increase salivary flow improve esophageal clearing. Those factors outlined above which decrease the frequency and duration of reflux episodes are probably the most important in improving esophageal clearing because they interrupt the vicious cycle which perpetuates reflux of irritant gastric contents.

Bethanechol has been shown to improve esophageal clearing. This action is widely attributed to increased amplitude of esophageal peristaltic contractions, but more likely the reason is its cholinergic stimulation of salivary flow. Other means of stimulating salivary flow, such as sucking hard candy or chewing gum, although not formally tested are reported by some patients to be helpful in controlling heartburn. Nocturnal esophageal clearing is facilitated by enlisting the aid of gravity by raising the head of the bed.

Decreasing Irritant Quality and Volume of Gastric Juice

Antacids

Antacids have been the mainstay of dyspepsia and reflux treatment for as long as any of us can remember. Aluminum-magnesium hydroxide antacids taken 1 and 3 hours after meals and at bedtime have been shown to control gastric acidity sufficiently to heal peptic ulcers of the stomach and duodenum. Patients report that antacids of all types give prompt but usually only transient relief of heartburn; hence the large volume of sales of over-the-counter antacid preparations. Calcium carbonate antacids, e.g., Tums, enjoy considerable popularity because of their quick effect. Because they may be sucked, neutralization of the esophageal surface is prolonged and sucking stimulates endogenous "antacid" production by stimulating increased salivary flow.

To prolong the effect of antacid and to decrease the irritant nature of refluxed material, antacids have been mixed with *alginic acid* (Gaviscon), which is supposed to form a viscous antacid foam that floats on top of the gastric contents so that when sphincter failure allows reflux, the material entering the esophagus is not pure gastric juice but rather alginic acid with its associated antacid. In spite of the attractiveness of this approach, Gaviscon's control of reflux symptoms was significantly superior to placebo in only two of four placebo-controlled studies of 244 patients.

Recent preliminary reports of sucralfate "slurry" being helpful in experimental and human esophagitis may lead to an important additional treatment in some patients with resistant esophagitis.

Histamine$_2$ Receptor Antagonists

The introduction of histamine$_2$ receptor antagonists *cimetidine* and *ranitidine* has provided a convenient, acceptable, and effective means of decreasing the volume and acid content of gastric juice. It seems likely that the major contribution of these agents to the treatment of reflux is more effective and longer lasting control of nocturnal acid secretion, which thus provides increased protection of the esophagus in its most vulnerable period which is unattainable with antacids. Doubling the traditional doses of cimetidine to 600 mg, or of ranitidine to 300 mg at bedtime provides even greater suppression of nocturnal acid secretion.

TREATMENT STRATEGIES

Most practitioners advocate a gradual approach in treatment of gastroesophageal reflux. The first step is "lifestyle" modifications, such as elevation of the head of the bed, weight loss, cessation of smoking, eating small meals, avoiding dyspeptic foods, and use of antacids. If these measures fail to produce improvement, then drugs with specific effects on motility, e.g., bethanechol or metoclopramide, and on gastric secretion, e.g., cimetidine or ranitidine, should be added.

There is an old military axiom that you will get on target sooner with less expenditure of ammunition if the first salvo is over the target. This philosophy is also applicable to therapeutics, especially in disorders in which dysfunction is perpetuated by a cycle of events. In addition, if therapy is promptly successful in controlling symptoms, the patient is much more likely to take the physician's advice regarding changes in lifestyle than if control is achieved only after passage through several treatment phases over 1 or 2 months.

My approach to the treatment of gastroesophageal reflux is to institute therapy with an intensive 2-week treatment schedule. The aim is to interrupt the cycle so that a simpler, less demanding schedule may then be followed to maintain control of reflux symptoms. The patient is told that it is a 2-week trial.

The intensive 2-week trial consists of the following:

1. Elevation of head of bed on 6-inch blocks.
2. Small meals with decreased fat intake and avoidance of chocolate, coffee, alcohol, and foods the patient associates with dyspepsia. No food intake after evening meal.
3. Decrease or stop smoking.
4. Histamine$_2$ receptor antagonist—cimetidine, 300 mg 3 times daily before meals and 600 mg at bedtime or ranitidine, 150 mg in the morning and 300 mg at bedtime.
5. Aluminum-magnesium antacid, 30 ml after meals and at bedtime.
6. Bethanechol, 25 mg at bedtime. Metoclopramide is associated with troublesome side effects too frequently to be used in this initial treatment trial.
7. It is possible that a slurry of sucralfate may prove to be useful therapy in some patients.

The sequence of simplifying the regimen in patients who have responded is empiric. Usually the treatment that the patient has found the least tolerable, e.g., elevation of the head of the bed, omission of coffee, or antacids, is the first to be discontinued. The evening dose of histamine$_2$ receptor antagonist is usually maintained for a prolonged period of time.

If treatment fails to improve the patient's symptoms one of the following must be considered: first and most likely, the diagnosis is wrong and symptoms that have been attributed to reflux actually have a different origin; or second, the patient has such severe reflux disease that medical means are inadequate to interrupt the destructive cycle. Failure of medical therapy is often manifested by return of symptoms as the intensive treatment is relaxed to a level compatible with long-term maintenance therapy or by failure of the regimen to heal erosive esophagitis. Regardless of the cause of failure of therapy, diagnostic tests should be performed to establish whether or not the patient has pathologic reflux and whether the reflux episodes are associated with the pain that brought the patient to the physician in the first place. In my experience continuous ambulatory intraesophageal pH recording for 18 to 24 hours is the most direct method of getting the needed information. The patient who has symptoms attributed to reflux but no erosive esophagitis should never be referred for surgical therapy until it is clearly demonstrated that pathologic reflux exists and that reflux is the cause of the patient's pain. Finally, only about 5 percent of reflux patients are candidates for antireflux surgery. The most frequent indication is failure to heal erosive esophagitis or the presence of late complications of esophagitis, e.g., progressive Barrett's esophagus, stricture, or both.

DIFFUSE ESOPHAGEAL SPASM AND RELATED DISORDERS

ALAN G. SUNSHINE, M.D.
SIDNEY COHEN, M.D.

The precise cause of angina-like chest pain is sometimes difficult to determine. Approximately 10 to 30 percent of patients with anginal syndromes have normal coronary arteries or minimal atherosclerosis at cardiac catheterization. Patients without significant coronary disease are being referred for esophageal manometric studies in hopes of determining a cause for their symptoms. It is well established that the esophagus can cause serious chest pain, and it is suggested in the literature that patients with chest pain of esophageal origin will have either diffuse esophageal spasm or gastroesophageal reflux. In recent years, esophageal manometric laboratories have notably improved with the development of catheters and precise low compliant infusion systems. These systems have resulted in an increased incidence of the diagnosis of esophageal motility disorders but have also generated confusion as to the specific manometric patterns responsible for a patient's symptoms. The sensitivity of esophageal manometry in determining the cause of chest pain is unknown. More patients are found to have a nonspecific motor disorder of the esophagus instead of classic diffuse esophageal spasm, and only a minority of patients will have definitive manometric changes associated with their typical symptoms at the time of manometry. Because of the wide variability in the results of esophageal manometry, controlled trials designed to characterize the precise manometric abnormality and their specific therapies have been difficult. Therefore, most of the discussion in this chapter will outline the *empiric* treatments that are available to the clinician in the hope of conveying an organized approach to a difficult problem.

CLINICAL MANIFESTATIONS

The symptoms most frequently encountered in patients with esophageal motor disorders are those of dysphagia and chest pain. *Dysphagia* is seen in about 70 percent of patients, is provoked by eating either solids or liquids, and is nonprogressive. Occasionally, in the case of liquids, the patient is conscious of the fluid being forcefully ejected from the esophagus back into the nasopharynx, but frank regurgitation is uncommon.

Chest pain is one of the most characteristic manifestations, especially in younger patients. Chest pain is usually described as squeezing, is substernal in location, and radiates in the back, neck, jaw, or arms, making it sometimes indistinguishable from angina-like pain. The pain is usually associated with deglutition, especially foods that are of extreme temperatures. The pain, however, may also awaken a patient from sleep, be unrelated to meals, and be unprovoked in many cases. Weight loss is uncommon but occasionally a patient will avoid eating to prevent the occurrence of symptoms.

The incidence of esophageal dysfunction as a cause of chest pain is difficult to ascertain. In one prospective trial evaluating 200 patients, only 23 percent had abnormalities of the gastrointestinal tract, primarily of the esophagus. The classification of esophageal manometric abnormalities has evolved over the years in an arbitrary fashion. A wide range of manometric findings has been used to characterize patients with the diagnosis of *diffuse esophageal spasm* (DES). As can be seen in Table 1, there is overlap between the diagnosis of DES, the nutcracker esophagus, and other nonspecific motor disorders. This is in contrast to achalasia, in which total aperistalsis and a hypertensive nonrelaxing lower esophageal sphincter are definitive diagnostic criteria. The difficulty in diagnosis in patients with chest pain arises from the lack of specific presenting symptoms, manometric criteria, and the intermittent nature of the manometric changes at the time of patient evaluation. To overcome this ambiguity we have routinely utilized *provocative agents*, such as edrophonium chloride, to enhance the value of esophageal manometry. All patients with chest pain undergoing esophageal manometry who have had a negative cardiac evaluation are given 10 mg of intravenous edrophonium. In 120 patients evaluated with normal baseline manometry, provocative testing demonstrated significant manometric abnormalities and the development of typical symptoms in 34 percent. Seventeen percent of patients with negative baseline manometric results either developed typical chest pain or had manometric change but not both. As reported by others, approximately 50 percent of patients will have no significant change from baseline manometry despite the use of provocative agents. Ergonovine,

TABLE 1 Manometric Criteria for Esophageal Motor Disorders

Diffuse Esophageal Spasm
Simultaneous, nonperistaltic contractions (> 30% of swallows)
Prolonged, repetitive contractions
Spontaneous contractions
High-amplitude contractions
Periods of normal peristalsis
Normal LES function in 70%, elevated LES pressure with or without impaired relaxation in 30% of patients
High Amplitude Esophageal Contractions (Nutcracker)
High-amplitude contractions (mean > 120 mm Hg)
Prolonged contractions
Normal peristalsis
Nonspecific Motor Disorders
Hypertensive (LES pressure > 35 mm Hg with normal relaxation)
Combination of abnormal peristaltic sequences (< 30% of swallows)
Simultaneous contractions
Spontaneous contractions
Low-amplitude contractions
Repetitive contractions
Prolonged contractions

another provocative agent, has been used to induce coronary spasm. We have evaluated those patients with negative coronary arteriograms and chest pain after ergonovine administration and found their symptoms to be esophageal in origin. The potential side effects and the lack of proven efficacy over edrophonium, however, has limited the use of ergonovine in our laboratory. Effective and accurate evaluation of patients with esophageal chest pain will occur if proper patient selection, provocative agents, and characterization of the esophageal motility disorders are utilized (Fig. 1).

TREATMENT

The treatment of esophageal motility disorders is quite variable, with no single agent being totally effective for any group of patients (Table 2). Because the symptoms are intermittent, it has been very difficult to define the correct agent for a specific symptom or even for any unique manometric abnormality. Secondary causes of esophageal spasm, such as gastroesophageal reflux, should be suspected in any patient with vague chest pain and a hypotensive lower esophageal sphincter (LES) pressure. Because the treatment for reflux disease is very effective, a Bernstein acid perfusion test should be administered in the hope of reproducing the patient's symptoms. This test, at the time of esophageal manometry, allows for the simultaneous documentation of any specific motor abnormality believed to be contributing to the patient's symptoms.

Anticholinergic Agents

Once secondary causes have been excluded, initial treatment involves the use of anticholinergics, such as *dicyclomine hydrochloride* (Bentyl) in doses up to 20 mg 4 times a day. The use of anticholinergics is based on the assumption that there may be supersensitivity to endogenous substances and neural transmitters, such as acetylcholine, leading to the development of esophageal spasm and symptoms. Because the symptoms are usually associated with eating, it is recommended that the patient take the medication 30 minutes before each meal.

TABLE 2 Therapy for Esophageal Causes of Chest Pain

Treatment	*Dose*	*Side Effects*
Gastroesophageal Reflux		
Antacids		
Gaviscon	30 cc PO 1 hr p.c. and h.s.	Avoid with tetracyclines
H_2 Antagonists		
Cimetidine	300 mg PO q.i.d.	Diarrhea, somnolence, dizziness, rash
Ranitidine	150 mg PO b.i.d.	Somnolence, headache, rash
Dopamine Antagonists		
Metaclopramide	5–20 mg PO ½ hr a.c. and h.s.	Dystonic reactions, depression
Motility Disorders		
Anticholinergics		
Dicyclomine	10–20 mg PO q.i.d.	Dry mouth, blurred vision, dizziness
Nitrates		
Isosorbide dinitrate	10–30 mg PO q.i.d.	Headache, flushing, dizziness
Calcium-channel blockers		
Nifedipine	10–20 mg PO q.i.d.	Dizziness, headache
Verapramil	80 mg PO t.i.d.	
Diltiazem	30–60 mg PO q.i.d.	
Smooth muscle relaxant		
Hydralazine	25–50 mg PO t.i.d.	Lupus-like reaction, dizziness, edema
Bouginage	50–54F as needed	
Pneumatic dilatation	8–10 PSI for 20 sec	Perforation
Esophageal myotomy		Gastroesophageal reflux

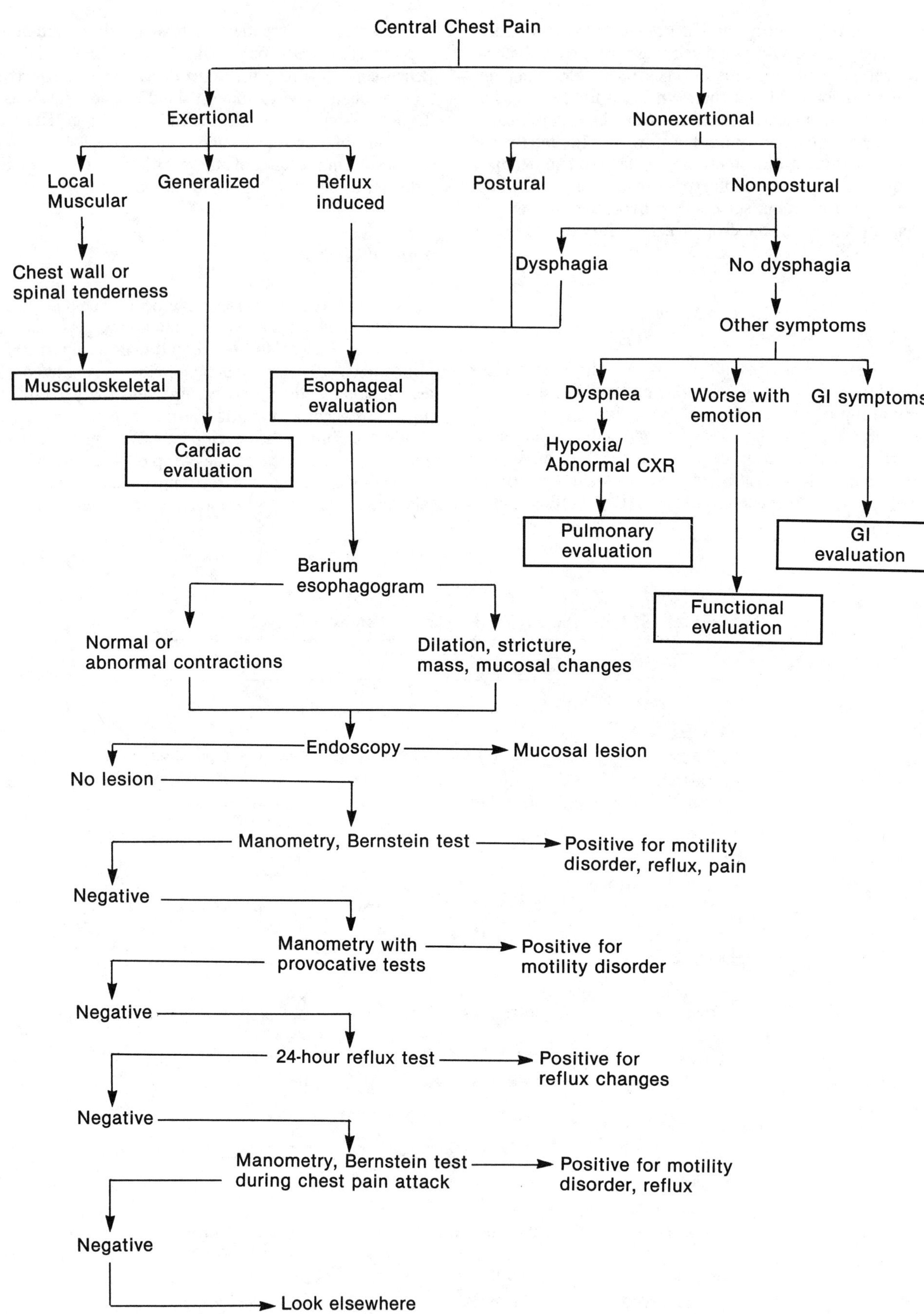

Figure 1 Evaluation of chest pain.

Nitrates

If anticholinergic treatment is unsuccessful, oral or sublingual nitrates can be used. Because the basic pharmacologic action of nitrates is to relax smooth muscle, one would anticipate that nitrates would be beneficial in relieving esophageal spasm. Although some reports have noted no objective response, others have found that acute as well as chronic administration of nitrates relieves and prevents the recurrence of chest pain and associated symptoms. Either *isosorbide dinitrate* (Isordil), 10 to 30 mg 4 times a day, or *erythrityl tetranitrate* (Cardilate), 10 to 15 mg 4 times a day, has been shown to reduce the frequency of symptoms and lower the high-amplitude contractions in the esophageal body. The frequency of side effects, most notably headache, usually precludes increasing the dosage of these drugs.

Calcium-channel Blockers

Calcium ions play an essential role in muscle contraction. The calcium-channel blockers inhibit calcium ionic flux and relax coronary artery smooth muscle. Various reports have described the effects of *nifedipine* on some parameters of esophageal smooth muscle. Nifedipine has been shown in a dose response relationship to lower LES pressure preferentially to decrease amplitude of esophageal high-amplitude contractions. In contrast, *verapamil* is noted to decrease contraction amplitude and wave duration in the baboon. Finally, another preliminary report notes the beneficial effects of *diltiazem* 30 to 60 mg 4 times a day, on esophageal spasm. Because nifedipine has preferential effects at the LES it is more beneficial in patients who have a hypertensive LES and whose primary symptom is dysphagia. In my experience, side effects prevent the beneficial effects at higher dosages. If the patient's symptoms are *primarily chest pain*, then *verapamil* is instituted at 80 mg 3 times a day. As reported by others, despite the initial enthusiasm for calcium-channel blockers to alleviate chest pain thought to be of esophageal origin, we have encountered only a 40 to 50 percent response rate. Elucidation of the potential benefit of calcium-channel blockers for esophageal motor disorders requires well-controlled protocols to investigate specific motor disorders and continued research into the development of new calcium-channel antagonists specifically for the smooth muscle of the gastrointestinal tract.

Smooth Muscle Relaxants

There is marked varibility in smooth muscle response to other pharamacologic agents. *Hydralazine* acts by direct relaxation of arteriolar smooth muscle, with minimal effect on other vessels. Because of its specific actions on smooth muscle, a single report of long-term administration of 25 mg 4 times a day suggested efficacy in preventing recurrent chest pain due to esophageal spasm upon bethanechol provocation. My experience with this drug has been of limited success because of fluid retention and postural hypotension-associated side effects.

Esophageal Dilatation

If the medical regimen described above fails to alleviate most of the patient's symptoms, repeated esophageal dilatation may be necessary. Again several studies have demonstrated conflicting results with bouginage. Most notably, there was no significant change in LES pressure or amplitude of contractions or significant reduction in major symptoms. There was, however, a sense of improvement once the study interval had ended, suggesting that a benefit may result due to the close physician-patient relationship. In general, patients who are refractory to medical therapy and who have normal LES pressures will be treated with *bouginage*. Patients who have failed to improve with medical therapy and are also found to have *hypertensive LES* pressure are candidates for *pneumatic dilatation*. I have seen dramatic results in relief of symptoms, most notably dysphagia, with dilatations.

Surgery

Only rarely will a patient be refractory to the regimen described above such that a *surgical* approach must be taken. When necessary, a long *myotomy* of the esophagus can be performed. A left thoracotomy provides excellent exposure for involvement of the distal two-thirds of the esophagus and the lower esophageal sphincter. When there is more extensive esophageal involvement, a right-sided approach to include the entire esophagus may be necessary. The length of the myotomy is determined by *preoperative manometric assessment*, and the incision should spare the normal lower esophageal sphincter. Lateral dissection of the muscle wall from the mucosa is essential to discourage subsequent healing of the myotomy.

Although symptomatic improvement is reported in 70 to 80 percent of patients, there is a definite risk of reflux esophagitis following extended myotomy. The lower esophageal sphincter should be involved in the myotomy if sphincter pressure is elevated or relaxation is impaired. If the myotomy includes the sphincter, a loose fundoplication is indicated.

Experience with long myotomy has not been good for several reasons: (1) persistent pain from spasm of the upper third of the nonmyotomized esophagus, (2) dysphagia secondary to myotomy or impaired sphincter function, and (3) post-thoracotomy chest wall pain. The best results have been achieved with a full myotomy of the entire esophagus, including the sphincter, together with a loose fundoplication.

PHARYNGEAL DYSPHAGIA

WILLIAM J. RAVICH, M.D.

Pharyngeal dysphagia is not a disease but a symptom. In order to direct therapy, an accurate understanding of the nature and severity of swallowing impairment is essential. Neither the interest nor the skills of any single subspecialty, however, is comprehensive enough to analyze or treat the various causes of pharyngeal symptoms. It is difficult in many cases even to determine which subspecialty should be involved.

The Johns Hopkins Swallowing Center is a multidisciplinary center formed in recognition of the diverse skills required for the care of the dysphagic patient. Subspecialties involved include dentistry, gastroenterology, neurology, otolaryngology, radiology, and rehabilitation medicine.

Many patients referred to the center have symptoms suggesting a pharyngeal disorder. In this chapter I will describe some observations derived from the Swallowing Center experience with patients presenting with pharyngeal dysphagia, concentrating on the techniques available for the treatment of these patients.

BASIC PRINCIPLES

A number of basic principles govern the evaluation and treatment of patients with pharyngeal dysphagia, and attention to these principles is critical in directing therapeutic efforts.

First, the events of a pharyngeal swallow are too fast for either the eye to see (with fluoroscopy) or the hand to catch (on spot films). Significant structural, as well as motor, abnormalities can be missed when a routine barium swallow is used to assess the pharynx. A dynamic study (cine- or videoradiography) of swallowing by a radiologist experienced in the technique is essential in the evaluation of any patient suspected of having a pharyngeal disorder.

Second, patients who localize their dysphagia to the neck often have disorders of the oral cavity or the esophagus. Clinical and radiographic assessment should routinely include evaluation of the entire swallowing mechanism and not be limited to pharyngeal structure and function. The esophagus is a particularly frequent cause of pharyngeal symptoms.

Third, cough is an unreliable symptom of airway penetration. Many physicians and patients assume that if a patient does not cough, the airway is not in jeopardy. Unfortunately, a substantial proportion of patients with neurologic impairment of pharyngeal function also appear to have a deficient cough reflex. We frequently see patients who fail to cough even as barium is pouring down the trachea. Objective evaluation based on a dynamic contrast study is essential in assessing airway competence.

Fourth, a vigorous search for a structural obstruction should be part of the evaluation of every patient with dysphagia in whom the radiographic evaluation does not adequately explain symptoms. In practice, the onus is on the physician who withholds endoscopy as part of the evaluation.

Fifth, in patients with evidence of a neurogenic or myogenic cause of pharyngeal symptoms, treatable causes such as polymyositis, myasthenia gravis, hypothyroidism, hyperthyroidism, and Parkinson's disease must be excluded.

Sixth, an empiric approach is the best guide to therapy. For a variety of reasons, the precise influence of detected derangements in function and structure on the patient's symptoms is often unclear. In addition, the effect of specific interventions on swallowing cannot always be predicted. A step-by-step approach, relying on a combination of past experience and observation of effect based on a careful analysis of baseline and follow-up dynamic radiographic studies, is generally preferable.

Finally, the nutritional status of the patient is a critical, but often neglected, aspect of management. Whether the swallowing impairment is temporary or permanent, assurance of adequate caloric intake may require alternative means of feeding.

ANALYSIS OF DYSFUNCTION

The initial approach to management relies heavily on a careful analysis of clinical, radiographic, and endoscopic (pharyngoscopy and/or esophagoscopy) findings. Because the knowledge and skills required to evaluate all patients are not available within any one subspecialty, multiple consultations may be required to provide a complete assessment of the factors underlying symptoms and of the therapeutic options available. A joint discussion with all personnel who are or might become involved is often the best means of overcoming the intellectual distance between the subspecialties traditionally involved in the care of patients with pharyngeal dysphagia.

Clinical Examination

A clear description of symptoms is critical, as any physical, radiographic, or endoscopic findings must be put into context. Coughing or choking during swallowing strongly suggests the presence of an oral or pharyngeal disorder, while coughing after the meal or at night suggests esophageal disease.

Particular attention should be paid to the specific types of food which cause symptoms. Contrary to popular opinion, patients with neurogenic dysphagia often have the most trouble with liquids. These patients frequently do best with foods that have a gelatinous consistency and have enough intrinsic cohesiveness to pass an incompetent larynx without dripping into the airway.

Dysphagia with solids alone should be assumed due to a structural obstruction until proven otherwise. Because of its luminal diameter, the esophagus is likely to be responsible for solid food dysphagia. Patients often have modified their own diets prior to seeking medical attention. Such modifications should be specifically elicited. Occasionally patients presenting with pulmonary symptoms due to swallowing impairment deny difficulty swallowing because they have long before excluded solids from their diets.

Clinical examination should include an assessment of *oral cavity* structure and function. The condition of the teeth, including the adequacy of occlusion, is obviously important in the preparation of food for swallowing. A dry oral cavity should suggest xerostomia or the use of drugs with anticholinergic properties. Congenital or acquired (usually surgical) defects in maxilla, mandible, tongue, or hard and soft palate should be looked for.

The *tongue* should be evaluated for bulk and movement. Tongue enlargement can result from hypothyroidism, amyloidosis, or tumor. A serrated appearance on the margin of the tongue, representing the impression by the teeth, may be a subtle sign of enlargement. Wasting of the tongue or fasciculations suggests a neurologic disorder, though mild fasciculations present on extension only may be a normal, effort-related finding.

Additional signs of neurologic disease include buccal and tongue weakness, poor lip closure, an asymmetric palatine arch, or deviation of the uvula. The gag reflex should be assessed bilaterally. An absent gag reflex suggests the presence of a bulbar lesion which could involve the swallowing center, the neurologic area controlling swallowing which extends through much of the pons and medulla. The neurologic examination should include particular attention to cranial nerves V through XII, the nuclei of which are stretched out along the course of the swallowing center.

When abnormalities are noted, the appropriate subspecialty should be consulted for a more thorough assessment.

Radiographic Examination

A careful review of the findings on *cine-* or *videoradiography* is an essential part of the evaluation of any patient presenting with known or suspected pharyngeal dysfunction. This review is best done jointly by the clinicians and radiologist involved, and should assess not only the findings but also the adequacy of the study in answering pertinent clinical questions. Some patients have modified head position or bolus size to minimize symptoms. These self-imposed maneuvers should be noted. A conscious attempt by the radiologist to reproduce the situation that elicits symptoms may be required, including the use of a variety of barium-coated or barium-impregnated material.

The analysis of the dynamic study can be divided into oral, pharyngeal, and esophageal phases.

Oral Phase. The control of the bolus before, during, and after the initiation of swallowing should be assessed. Some patients have difficulty keeping material in the mouth during the oral preparation of food owing to impaired separation of oral cavity and pharynx. This can result in premature leakage into the pharynx. Others have an inadequate propulsion due to weak or uncoordinated movement of the tongue, causing oral retention often followed by post-swallow leakage into an unprotected larynx.

Pharyngeal Phase. The strength, symmetry, and completeness of the pharyngeal stripping wave; the adequacy of laryngeal closure, which involves both elevation of the larynx and tilt of the epiglottis; and the timing and extent of opening of the pharyngoesophageal segment should be assessed.

In addition to the presence of abnormal masses, pharyngeal pouches and webs involving the pharynx or pharyngoesophageal segment should be looked for. Though most gastroenterologists think of a Zenker's diverticulum whenever a pouch is mentioned, the majority of pharyngeal pouches are lateral and located in the valleculae. Most often these pouches represent an incidental finding and are not responsible for symptoms. If the pouch cannot be shown to retain material after the pharyngeal peristaltic wave has passed, its significance in the genesis of symptoms is dubious.

A worthwhile distinction can be made between direct penetration into the larynx during swallowing (*penetration*) and the inhalation of barium retained in the hypopharynx after pharyngeal swallowing is completed (*aspiration*). Direct penetration is most often due to neurologic or myogenic dysfunction. Though also frequently due to a neurologic or myogenic process, aspiration may result from a pouch, web, or an isolated disorder of upper esophageal function. In addition, review of radiographic studies done at the Swallowing Center indicates that pharyngeal dysfunction resulting in pharyngeal retention commonly occurs in association with esophageal dysmotility or structural disease. The possibility that esophageal disease may produce secondary dysfunction in the pharynx must be considered.

Esophageal Phase. Of patients presenting to the Swallowing Center with previously unexplained pharyngeal dysphagia, one-fourth have an isolated abnormality of esophageal function or structure on radiographic evaluation, while about one-third have combined disorders of the pharynx and esophagus in which either is capable of causing symptoms. Among the esophageal abnormalities demonstrated are esophageal stricture, Schatzki's ring, achalasia, and esophageal spasm. The treatment of these esophageal disorders usually results in symptomatic improvement of pharyngeal symptoms.

THERAPEUTIC APPROACHES

It is important for those caring for the dysphagic patient to have some understanding of how different subspecialties approach treatment. The following is intended as a brief overview of some of the therapeutic options and their indications.

Prosthodontics

The capacity to chew is obviously helpful in the ingestion of solid foods. In addition, the teeth are important in maintaining the proper alignment of the oral cavity. Though only occasionally implicated as the sole cause of swallowing difficulties in patients at the Swallowing Center, poor dentition or ill-fitting dentures may exaggerate the symptoms produced by disordered function or structure downstream.

In patients with congenital or acquired structural defects of the mandible, maxilla, tongue, or palates, a combination of oral reconstruction and prosthetic devices can produce dramatic improvement in swallowing. Obdurators are used to fill in the defects, preventing food from extruding into empty spaces where oral control and bolus preparation cannot occur. In patients with severe malocclusion, plates with specially designed ramps may be used to guide teeth into proper position for mastication. It is easier to secure these devices in an oral cavity in which at least some of the patient's own teeth remain.

Although not as successful for the neurologically impaired, similar devices can be tried in patients in whom loss of tongue mass or problems with alignment result from muscle wasting rather than structural abnormaliies.

Treatable Neurogenic and Myogenic Disease

The detection of pharyngeal paresis or inadequate elevation of the larynx suggests the presence of a neurologic or myogenic cause of dysphagia. Determining a specific diagnosis depends heavily on the detection of other physical findings and the judicious use of specific laboratory tests.

Disorders that require particular consideration are those susceptible to pharmacologic intervention. Polymyositis, myasthenia gravis, myopathies associated with hypo- and hyperthyroidism, and Parkinson's disease will respond to appropriate medical therapy.

Dysphagia associated with Huntington's disease can be ameliorated by phenothiazine compounds and haloperidol, drugs often used to decrease the severity of the choreiform movements that are the hallmark of this disease.

Chorea makes introduction of an appropriate-sized bolus into the mouth difficult. In addition, chorea of the tongue is often present, making control of the oral bolus difficult. Premature or delayed leakage into the pharynx is a common problem. Prolixin or haloperidol is useful in improving dysphagia.

What is remarkable in the few patients in whom the effects of this therapy on swallowing has been evaluated is the small, even subtherapeutic, doses of the medication to which they respond. In addition, as the dose is increased or as serum levels equilibrate, improvement can be followed by deterioration, possibly resulting from a sensitivity to the dyskinetic effects of the drugs which is not noted in normal individuals until much higher doses are used. Careful titration to obtain an optimal result in terms of swallowing is mandatory.

The Role of Pharyngeal Surgery

The frequency with which surgery is performed in patients with pharyngeal dysphagia varies considerably from institution to institution. Aside from the management of tumors, the otolaryngologist is most often asked to consider cricopharyngeal myotomy or resection of pharyngeal pouches.

Cricopharyngeal myotomy involves the incision of the cricopharyngeus—the main component of the upper esophageal sphincter—through a lateral neck incision. Its major indication is the presence of an isolated abnormality of upper esophageal sphincter function. This diagnosis is usually entertained on the basis of an incompletely opening pharyngoesophageal segment seen on barium swallow. Careful analysis of cineradiographic studies in patients referred to the Swallowing Center with a diagnosis of "cricopharyngeal achalasia" or "cricopharyngeal spasm" however, usually demonstrates profound abnormalities of pharyngeal function as well. Manometric confirmation that the upper esophageal sphincter is functioning improperly can only rarely be obtained. Cricopharyngeal myotomy in patients with diffuse impairment of pharyngeal function—as opposed to isolated upper esophageal sphincter dysfunction—is of questionable value, especially as additional damage to the peripheral nervous system and scarring at the pharyngoesophageal segment may actually make matters worse in an already impaired pharynx.

The role of *resection*, usually combined with *myotomy*, in Zenker's diverticulum is well established in otolaryngology. The myotomy is included because of manometric evidence of upper esophageal sphincter dysfunction and the clinical impression that diverticula are more likely to recur if myotomy is not performed. It is postulated that the pouch occurs through an area of relative weakness in the presence of increased pharyngeal pressure during swallowing resulting from sphincter dysfunction. Unfortunately, it is often impossible to intubate patients with large Zenker's diverticuli because the manometric catheter tends to preferentially pass directly into the pouch.

The surgical resection of lateral pharyngeal pouches is only rarely indicated. Most lateral pouches are incidental findings. Only pouches that remain filled after passage of the pharyngeal peristaltic wave should be considered potentially responsible for symptoms. In the Swallowing Center experience, these pouches are often associated with dysfunction elsewhere in the swallowing mechanism. In most cases, symptoms seem to correlate with these other abnormalities. A *double swallow rehabilitation* technique (see section on rehabilitation) is usually effective in diminishing symptoms from a pouch sufficiently to avoid surgery.

Gastroenterologic Considerations

As previously mentioned, patients often are inaccurate in localizing the level of obstruction. About one-third of individuals with obstructive lesions in the distal esophagus localize their symptoms to the neck. Conversely, about one-fourth of patients presenting to the Swallowing Center with pharyngeal dysphagia have a purely esophageal cause for their symptoms. This finding has two implications: first, that a careful examination of the esophagus is essential in patients presenting with pharyngeal dysphagia, and second, that esophageal disorders should be treated vigorously when they are found. The most common esophageal disorders causing pharyngeal dysphagia are esophageal stenosis (either due to Schatzki's ring or peptic stricture), gastroesophageal reflux without evidence of stricture formation, and idiopathic esophageal spasm. The treatment of these and other esophageal disorders is covered elsewhere in this book.

Rehabilitation Approach

The rehabilitation approach is aimed at the most efficient use of available resources. In terms of swallowing it concentrates on strengthening weak muscles where possible and consciously altering the way in which the patient swallows to *maximize pharyngeal clearance* and *minimize airway soiling*. The ultimate goals, as with other methods of treatment, include improved comfort, adequate nutrition, and airway safety. The rehabilitation approach, however, accepts that these goals often require substantial adjustments in the way the patient obtains his nutrition, adjustments that may be less than ideal from the patient's viewpoint.

The most obvious intervention is avoidance of foods that cause the greatest difficulty. Patients with problems in the oral preparation of foods or with a structural lesion obstructing the esophagus clearly recognize that foods that are chewy or stringy cause the greatest difficulty. Often patients have modified their diets to minimize symptoms. Depending on the alternatives available and the type of restriction required, modification of diet may be more or less acceptable.

For patients with impaired control of the oral phase of swallowing or incomplete laryngeal closure, thin liquids often cause particular difficulty, as they easily drip over the back of the tongue or into the incompletely protected larynx. Foods with a thicker consistency, such as thick liquids, puddings, jellos, and mashed potatoes, often are handled best. It appears that some degree of intrinsic cohesiveness prevents separation and diversion of a portion of the swallowed bolus. Some individuals who are unable to swallow either liquids or solids can be sustained entirely by means of a gelatinized diet.

As opposed to patients with masticatory or obstructive problems, neurologically impaired patients are less likely to have modified their diets appropriately. This failure may be due to the natural, but often inaccurate, impression that liquids are easiest to swallow, the relatively circumscribed role of foods with the necessary quality of cohesiveness in the average diet, and the influence of associated sensory and cognitive defects which limit the patient's ability to discriminate degrees of difficulty.

Beyond modification of diet, attempts to rehabilitate the neurologically impaired swallow involve the conscious alteration of a process that usually occurs without thought. Patients who leak before or after swallowing must learn to limit the quantity of material in the mouth at any one time and ensure that the mouth is cleared of material before the introduction of additional food. Chewing with the chin down may prevent leakage. Patients with a weak tongue may find that a coordinated extension of the head at the time of swallowing improves the efficiency with which food is introduced from mouth to pharynx.

In patients with *direct laryngeal penetration*, neck flexion decreases the distance that the larynx needs to elevate in order to protect the airway. This maneuver, in combination with the modification of the diet toward more cohesive foods, can often provide the margin of benefit required for adequate and safe hydration and nutrition.

In those with *pharyngeal retention*, the use of a *double swallow technique* is usually helpful. Because aspiration occurs during inspiration when substantial amounts of material remain in the pharynx at the end of a swallow, the goal is to minimize residual pharyngeal contents at the time of inspiration. Normally, swallowing occurs at any time during respiration and is associated with a temporary cessation of respiration. With the double swallow technique, the patient is instructed to consciously inhale just prior to swallowing. Post-swallow resumption of respiratory activity will begin with expiration, during which airway soiling is unlikely to occur. The patient is then instructed to swallow a second time before the next inspiration to clear the pharynx of as much residual material as possible.

SPECIAL PROBLEMS

Combined Dysfunction

Combined dysfunction of pharynx and esophagus is quite common in the Swallowing Center experience. In a series of 40 patients presenting with previously unexplained pharyngeal dysphagia, more than a third had combined disorders of pharynx and esophagus, either one of which could account for their symptoms (defined as the presence of a 50 percent decrease in luminal diameter or evidence of retention on barium study). In this situation, a decision must be made as to the most likely cause of the patient's symptoms. In many cases intensive treatment of the most treatable of the problems detected represents the best course, the response to therapy being used to confirm or deny its importance to the patient's clinical presentation.

Presumed Psychogenic Dysphagia

Many patients referred to the Swallowing Center have been previously diagnosed as having dysphagia of psychogenic origin. A careful investigation of these individuals reveals a cause for dysphagia in approximately three-fourths. In a series of 23 such patients, we were able to establish a cause in 16. Even in those in whom a cause is not found, it is not always clear that the problem is only emotional in origin. Only two patients were strongly suspected of having a purely psychogenic dysphagia on the basis of diffuse anxiety and unexplainable multisystem complaints. For the others, it is equally plausible that current technology does not permit proper assessment of the cause.

This is not to say that anxiety plays no role in dysphagia. Fear of cardiac disease, cancer, or sudden death from choking all represent legitimate reasons for anxiety. Often the anxiety produced by the symptoms has an important role in exaggerating the severity of symptoms beyond that expected from the degree of impairment detected. When the problem cannot be directly treated, and when reassurance fails to alleviate anxiety, *behavior modification* therapy may be useful.

Sedatives must be used with extreme caution in patients with impaired swallowing. These drugs are unlikely to help, except in doses at which mental acuity is severely impaired. In the presence of swallowing difficulties, the decreased attention to the act of oral preparation of food and the initiation of swallowing caused by sedatives may exacerbate the degree of disability. This is particularly dangerous in patients with symptoms suggesting airway soiling, such as coughing or choking during eating. Patients with both neurogenic and structural causes of dysphagia almost uniformly have more trouble when treated with tranquilizers than when these agents are withdrawn.

Alternative Means of Feeding

All too often patients are referred to the Swallowing Center in a severely malnourished condition. Consideration of tube feeding should not await severe weight loss. A starving patient is unlikely to be able to cooperate in a rehabilitation program. Often the patient compensates by taking an excessively long time to eat. For many, a major portion of the day is taken up in an often vain attempt to ingest an adequate number of calories. Such efforts are quite disruptive to normal activity. In addition, eating may be exhausting to those with swallowing difficulties, resulting in increasing difficulty as the meal goes on.

The reluctance of patients and physicians to implement tube feeding is unfortunate. Tube feeding is an excellent means of ensuring adequate caloric intake in patients in whom treatment is unlikely to bring rapid results. Because an already neurologically impaired pharynx may have increased trouble swallowing around a tube, an endoscopically or surgically placed feeding gastrostomy is generally preferable in anyone in whom tube feeding is likely to be required for an extended period of time. If oral feeding can be subsequently resumed, removal of the gastrostomy tube is followed by rapid closure of the surgical fistula. In patients who are able to eat food safely, but only in decreased amounts, tube feeding may be used to supplement oral feeding, taking pressure off the patient to eat unreasonable amounts of food.

The approaches to evaluation and management discussed here have evolved from the work of The Johns Hopkins Swallowing Center. They therefore represent the combined efforts of my colleagues in the Center, including Martin Donner, Bronwyn Jones, James Bosma, Susan Kramer, and Steven Rubesin (Radiology); Thomas Hendrix (Gastroenterology); Bernard Marsh and Haskins Kashima (Otolaryngology); David Buchholz (Neurology); Arthur Siebens, Patricia Linden, and Jeffrey Palmer (Rehabilitation Medicine); and Lowell Wiener (Dentistry).

DUODENAL ULCER

BASIL I. HIRSCHOWITZ, B.Sc., M.B., B.Ch., M.D., F.A.C.P., F.R.C.P.E., F.R.C.P.

Duodenal ulcer (DU), which at some time affects one person in ten in our society, is in most cases a disease of long duration with multiple recurrences of a single ulcer crater in the duodenal bulb. Duodenal ulcers tend to heal spontaneously. About 20 percent of patients have only one or two attacks, and another 20 percent have, at some time, a major complication such as bleeding, pyloric obstruction, or perforation. Duodenal ulcer is not associated with later development of cancer. Several factors (e.g., smoking, anti-inflammatory drugs, and excessive acid secretion) may promote ulcer recurrence or delay healing.

DIAGNOSIS AND EVALUATION

Since the symptoms of duodenal ulcer may not always be typical or may be mimicked by other conditions (e.g., irritable bowel syndrome, biliary tract or pancreatic disease, hiatal hernia, or gastric ulcer), the first step in treatment requires that the diagnosis of DU be firmly established. In many cases barium contrast studies may be diagnostic, but radiologic diagnosis (positive or negative) should be further supported by upper gastrointestinal endoscopy, which is the more definitive means of diagnosing a DU crater. Endoscopy provides additional information on the esophagus (e.g., esophagitis or hernia) and stomach (e.g., gastritis or gastric ulcer) which may further define the individual case. Every DU patient should have a fasting serum gastrin measured to rule out an underlying gastrinoma; if elevated, a gastric analysis should be performed to confirm gastric hypersecretion and to rule out the false hypergastrinemia of gastric atrophy. The diagnosis and treatment of gastrinoma (Zollinger-Ellison syndrome) is dealt with in a separate chapter in this volume.

Once the diagnosis of DU is established, the next step is to define the individual patient's disease profile and response to therapy over a period of time and to educate the patient in the symptoms, natural history, and complications of his or her disease, so that later relapses can be treated without full reinvestigation. It is perhaps self-evident that the best treatment of a chronic relapsing disease involves the physician and the patient in a mutually understood enterprise.

BASIS FOR TREATMENT

The factors predisposing to DU (DU disease) and the immediate or proximate causes of DU recurrence or complication are not well understood. What we know at present forms the basis for much of current therapy. In many, but not all, patients with DU there is a higher rate of basal and stimulated acid and pepsin secretion, moreso in males, so that the amount and concentration of both these digestive compounds entering the duodenal bulb per unit time in patients with DU is greater than in those without DU. Whether the pathophysiology can be equated with etiology is not clear, but reduction of secretion by a variety of medical or surgical means to levels in the normal range alleviates symptoms, promotes healing, and reduces the rate of relapse. The principal modes of therapy thus are directed toward reduction in acid (and pepsin) secretion. Conventional or traditional methods (e.g. diet, phenobarbital, and other psychotropic drugs) are not considered to be of value in current ulcer therapy. Coffee in any form may produce symptoms and should be proscribed. The patient should know that smoking, anti-inflammatory drugs, and strong family predisposition may make therapy less effective or may contribute to relapses. Women tend to have milder disease and fewer relapses than men.

TREATMENT STRATEGIES

Reduction of Acid. There are several ways in which we can reduce the acid/peptic load on the duodenal bulb: (1) postsecretory and surface coating agents, (2) alteration of neurohormonal controls, and (3) alterations of cellular mechanisms.

Postsecretory Therapy

Once acid is secreted, it can be neutralized in the stomach by food and by antacids. The average basal acid secretion in DU is about 6 mEq per hour compared to about 2 mEq per hour for normals, and with the stimulation by meals, the rate for perhaps half the day may be three or four times that amount. Thus, about 250 to 300 mEq per 24 hours require neutralization. Since food probably provides about one-fourth of this neutralization, at least 200 mEq of antacids are required per day for effective partial neutralization. Anatacids vary in potency from 0.3 to 4.2 mEq per milliliter (for potency and cost, see Table 1). If antacids are chosen, my preference is for a higher-potency (40 mEq/dose) liquid antacid, 1 and 3 hours after meals, continued for 4 to 6 weeks after the onset of a relapse. Antacids are also of value for occasional use for sporadic symptoms that may occur without an ulcer recurrence. Most patients learn to keep antacids handy for such use. Nowadays, however, the ease of use and effectiveness of other treatments, especially H_2 antagonists, have greatly reduced the role of anatacids as primary ulcer treatment.

Surface Coating Agents

As an alternative to antacid therapy, these agents act by combining with the slough in the ulcer base to form a protective coating, presumably allowing the ulcer to heal more readily. They include bismuth preparations, such as PeptoBismol or DeNol (DeNol is not available in the

TABLE 1 Antacid Grouping According to Neutralizing Capacity and Cost

Approximate Dose for 40 mEq Antacid	*Names of Antacids*	*Approximate Monthly Cost of 200–300 mEq/day ($)*
10 ml	Titralac, Maalox TC, Delcid, Mylanta II	13–22
15 ml	Camalox, Gelusil II, Maalox Plus, Basaljel ES	17–35
20 ml	Gelusil, Riopan Plus	28
30 ml	Amphojel*	40
130 ml	Phosphajel*	175

* Contain only aluminum salts

United States) and sucralfate (1 g four times a day for 6 weeks). Efficacy in promoting healing is similar to that of other drugs (Fig. 1). One possible advantage is a lack of systemic effects. Bismuth preparations cause black stools. Pepto Bismol contains salicylates and some authors caution against its use in peptic disease (see chapter on *Gastric Ulcer*).

Neurohormonal Alteration

The cause of basal hypersecretion in DU is believed to be due to the vagus, acting directly via acetylcholine as well as through the release of gastrin. This activity can be altered by medical (cholinergic muscarinic antagonists such as atropine and the synthetic anticholinergics or pirenzepine [not available in the United States]) or surgical means (vagotomy, preferably confined to the fundus). The vagus is highly sensitive to anticholinergics, and a dose of atropine, 0.4 to 0.6 mg sublingually 15 minutes before meals and at bedtime or its equivalent, is adequate for modest control of acid. However, these medications tend to have side effects (e.g., dry mouth, urinary retention, delayed gastric emptying), which make them less desirable as first-line drugs for the treatment of DU. They

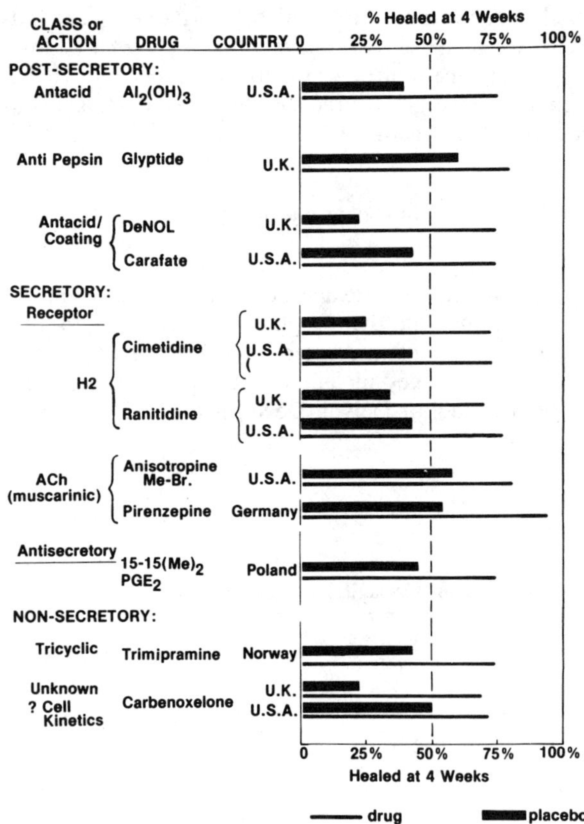

Figure 1 Duodenal ulcer healing with different classes of drugs. Relative percentage of patients healed with each class of drug (thin line), each compared to placebo treatment (thick line). *Note*: Most patients in the placebo group used antacids for relief of symptoms.

may be useful as supplemental therapy, especially for hypersecretors, who are not fully responsive to H_2 antagonists.

For patients with ulcers that are difficult to treat or for patients with complications who qualify for surgical treatment (to be discussed), vagal denervation of the fundus has the advantage of permanently reducing acid secretion with virtually no mortality or morbidity.

Cellular Mechanisms

The parietal cell may be suppressed by different kinds of treatment. The most widely used are the H_2 histamine receptor antagonists. Two are currently on the market: cimetidine, 300 mg four times a day, and ranitidine, 150 mg twice a day are equally effective, and several others are in various stages of clinical testing. These drugs, which inhibit acid in the basal state as well as acid stimulated by all stimuli, have few side effects. At present they may be considered the first line of drugs for treating active DU. Healing rates without treatment, except antacids taken for symptoms only may reach 40 to 50 percent at 4 to 6 weeks. With H_2 antagonist treatment, 60 to 70 percent are healed at 4 weeks, 70 to 80 percent at 6 weeks, and 85 to 92 percent at 8 weeks, leaving some 10 percent of patients unhealed. Relapse rates after treatment is discontinued are high; as many as 80 percent of ulcers recur within a year of stopping medication regardless of the length of active treatment.

One group of drugs, now in the test stage, inhibits acid secretion by blocking the H^+-K^+-ATPase enzyme responsible for secreting acid into the lumen (the proton pump). These drugs are the class of substituted benzimidazoles. One of these, *Omeprazole*, has been tested clinically, and at a single daily dose of 40 to 60 mg, it completely inhibited acid secretion and produced 100 percent healing of DU in 2 weeks, thereby proving the underlying dictum of ulcer treatment: "No acid, no ulcer." However, the development of histologic gastric mucosal abnormalities resembling carcinoid tumors in female rats led to the temporary suspension of clinical testing for the present. Testing in the United States and abroad resumed in late 1985. The question raised is whether "no acid, no ulcer" carries some sort of price such as the problems of gastric tumors and possible susceptibility to orally ingested bacteria, as seen in patients with total anacidity due to pernicious anemia.

Another class of drugs being tested is the *prostaglandin E_2* series; several synthetic orally effective analogues have been tested with beneficial reduction in acid secretion (presumably acting on [adenosine 3′:5′ cyclic phosphate] cAMP-dependent pathways of acid stimulation) and on ulcer healing. Because these agents have widespread effects, the full range of side effects have not yet been evaluated. An additional benefit may accrue from an effect that has been described as "cytoprotective;" the exact nature of this phenomenon and particularly its specific effect, if any, on duodenal mucosa, including alkaline secretion, are not yet well enough understood for a thorough theoretic underpinning of the therapeutic potential of prostaglandins in DU.

Non-acid Active Drugs

Carbenoxelone (not available in the United States) and *trimipramine* (a tricyclic antidepressant) are at least two drugs that have been shown to lead to the healing of DU better than placebo (see Fig. 1). Mechanisms of action are unknown. With the availability of drugs of known action and effectiveness, they probably do not offer useful alternative treatment.

Overall, many treatments are equally effective in healing ulcers in the short term (see Fig. 1), but relapse is common after all of these. Medicines may heal duodenal ulcers, but do not cure the underlying disease.

SIDE EFFECTS OF TREATMENTS

Antacids. Diarrhea may be caused by Mg^{++}-containing antacids, constipation and phosphate depletion by aluminum hydroxide, and renal damage by sodium bicarbonate or calcium carbonate in excess.

Anticholinergics. These may cause dry mouth and urinary and gastric retention.

H_2 Antagonists. Cimetidine may produce mental changes, especially in sick or elderly patients, and antiandrogenic effects may cause gynecomastia and impotence in cases of prolonged maintenance therapy for hypersecretors. Ranitidine is much less likely to cause these effects and may be used safely in the place of cimetidine in such cases.

Carbenoxelone. Side effects are sodium retention and potassium depletion.

Trimipramine. This drug causes constipation and, at times, drowsiness. It may also cause excessive weight gain.

SPECIAL CASES

Renal failure. Doses of H_2 antagonists should be reduced by one-third for creatinine levels of 2.5 to 4 mg per deciliter and by one-half for creatinine levels over 4 mg per deciliter. Redosing after dialysis is needed. Antacids should be free of magnesium; aluminum toxicity may be a factor in both antacid and Carafate use.

Acutely Ill Patients. The evidence for prevention of DU activation due to physical stress is not very strong, and the routine use of H_2 antagonists intravenously in intensive care units and postoperatively is not justified by the evidence.

Patients with Rheumatoid Arthritis Receiving Continuous Steroid or Non-Steroidal Anti-inflammatory Therapy. If some of these patients develop DU, the dose of anti-inflammatory drug should be reduced or another drug should be substituted. H_2 antagonists should be given and, if effective, continued as long as other medications are needed. However, H_2 antagonists or antacids may not be effective in such cases.

Bleeding DU. There is no evidence that immediate intravenous administration of H_2 antagonists or other ulcer therapy is of benefit in controlling bleeding from a DU. Longer-term treatment to heal the ulcer should be considered on its own merits.

DU Relapses. Treating acute ulcer attacks with any one of a number of classes of drugs (see Fig. 1) leads to an improvement of 10 to 40 percent over placebo at 6 weeks, but relapse occurs after discontinuation of therapy. Since relapse is somewhat unpredictable in the individual case, Table 2 and the following schema provide a framework for management of DU.

TABLE 2 Objectives of Treatment of Uncomplicated Active DU

Relief of symptoms
Healing the active crater
Prevention of relapse and of complications
Minimizing the socioeconomic consequences, preferably by keeping the patient ambulatory

SUGGESTED METHOD OF TREATMENT

The following steps are suggested for the treatment of duodenal ulcer:

1. For the acute attack (first encounter with patient), after confirming the presence of DU and measuring fasting gastrin, treat for 6 to 8 weeks with (a) H_2 antagonists or (b) antacids or (c) Carafate (a, b, c is my order of preference), expecting 75 to 90 percent healing rate. Watch compliance; symptoms usually disappear after 2 to 5 days and patients tend to stop taking medication when they feel better.
2. Stop treatment and await relapse. Retreat relapse as above and await relapse again. The type of therapy does not affect relapse. If relapse occurs rapidly when the patient is off treatment or if complications occur, place patient on partial or full long-term therapeutic maintenance with H_2 antagonists.
3. If the patient relapses on *maintenance* therapy or has complications, review compliance and possible deleterious habits or medication and re-evaluate the ulcer, including study of gastric secretion to rule out nongastrinemic hypersecretion. Increase dosage, change or add medication, and observe effects on gastric secretion and on the ulcer. Include follow-up endoscopy in the evaluation.
4. If, after obtaining the best possible medical result, the patient still has a nonhealing ulcer or has complications, fundic vagotomy should be recommended.

GASTRINOMA

ROBERT T. JENSEN, M.D.
JERRY D. GARDNER, M.D.

Zollinger-Ellison syndrome (ZES) is characterized by hypersecretion of gastric acid due to hypergastrinemia secondary to a nonbeta islet cell tumor. Because these tumors contain and release large amounts of gastrin into the circulation, they are referred to as gastrinomas. A gastrinoma is found at surgery in 65 percent of patients, occurring in the pancreas in 42 percent, in the duodenum in 14 percent, and in other sites in 9 percent of cases—such as regional lymph nodes near the pancreas, or rarely, within the liver, ovary, or hilum of the spleen. Gastrinomas are malignant in 60 to 90 percent of cases, but they tend to grow slowly and are slow to metastasize. Currently 77 percent of patients with gastrinomas present with pain, usually due to a typical peptic ulcer. Up to 13 percent have esophageal symptoms, 50 percent have diarrhea, and in 18 percent diarrhea is the only symptom. Except for patients with far advanced metastatic disease, all symptoms in patients with gastrinomas are caused by excessive gastric acid secretion.

Approximately 25 percent of patients with gastronomas have evidence of multiple endocrine neoplasia type 1(MEN-1). MEN-1 is an autosomal dominant trait characterized by tumors or hyperplasia of multiple endocrine organs with hyperparathyroidism occurring in 98 percent, functional islet cell adenomas in 80 percent of patients and pituitary adenomas less commonly. Almost all patients with MEN-1 and ZES have multiple gastrinomas, and thus have a very low probability of surgical cure.

TREATMENT PHILOSOPHY

In patients with gastrinoma two therapeutic aims need to be considered. First, therapeutic decisions must be made to control gastric acid hypersecretion both short and long term. Second, because of the malignant potential of the gastrinoma, therapeutic decisions need to be made about the treatment of the gastrinoma itself. With the recent availability of potent antisecretory agents, hypersecretion of gastric acid can now be controlled medically in almost every patient, making routine total gastrectomy unnecessary. With the ability to control gastric hypersecretion, the natural history of the gastrinoma is becoming a more important determinant of long term prognosis.

CONTROL OF HYPERSECRETION OF GASTRIC ACID

Medical Treatment of Gastric Hypersecretion

The single most important determinant of successful medical management of hypersecretion of gastric acid is an adequate dosage of the antisecretory agent. Most studies show that relief of symptoms is not a good guide to ulcer healing or adequacy of therapy, although persistence of symptoms, especially diarrhea or epigastric pain, usually indicates the drug dosage is inadequate. *If gastric acid secretion is reduced to less than 10 mEq per hour for the last hour prior to the next dose of medication, peptic ulcers will heal and further peptic disease will be prevented.* In the small group of patients who have previously had a vagotomy and partial gastrectomy with a Billroth II gastroenterostomy, gastric acid secretion should be reduced to less than 5 mEq per hour. To assess the adequacy of antisecretory control a nasogastric tube should be passed into the antrum of the stomach, gastric secretion collected for 1 hour prior to the next dose of medication, a sample of the gastric secretion titrated to pH 7.0, and the acid secretory rate determined and expressed in milliequivalents per hour. The nasogastric tube can be properly placed without flouroscopy by passing the tube 50 to 55 cm and checking the recovery of instilled fluid by adding 50 cc of saline or water, of which 90 percent should be recovered. It cannot be overemphasized that *only by determining adequacy of suppression of gastric acid secretion can the adequacy of medical management be assessed.* In addition, long term medical management will be successful only in a compliant patient. The small number of patients who cannot or will not take medication regularly should not be considered for medical therapy with the antisecretory medications currently available, and should undergo total gastrectomy.

Intravenous Therapy

Most patients with ZES present with a long history of peptic ulcer disease, diarrhea, or esophageal symptoms, and treatment can be started with oral antisecretory medications. A few patients present with severe electrolyte or metabolic abnormalities and acute complications of their ulcer disease and cannot take oral medication. These patients should be treated with appropriate fluid and electrolyte replacement, nasogastric suction, and intravenous cimetidine or ranitidine. Ranitidine has been shown to be three to four times more potent than cimetidine, but either drug can be used and should be administered by continuous intravenous infusion after an intravenous bolus injection. Continuous intravenous infusion can be accomplished by adding intravenous cimetidine (or ranitidine) to 5 percent dextrose/water such that if the intravenous infusion rate is 75 ml per hour the patient will receive 3 mg per kilogram of body weight per hour of cimetidine (or 1 mg per kilogram per hour of ranitidine). If cimetidine is used, first administer a bolus injection of 150 mg, begin the intravenous cimetidine infusion at 1 mg per kilogram per hour (25 ml per hour), and after a few hours determine the gastric secretory rate for 1 hour. If gastric secretion is greater than 10 mEq per hour, give 2 mg per kilogram per hour of cimetidine (50 ml per hour), recheck the acid secretion, and continue increasing the cimetidine up to 6 mg per kilogram per hour until gastric secretion is controlled. If gastric acid secretion is still not less than 10 mEq per hour when giving 6 mg per kilogram per hour, an anticholinergic agent, such as Pro-Banthine, 15 mg IM every 6 hour, should be added.

Oral Therapy

For long term oral treatment, either cimetidine or ranitidine alone or with an anticholinergic agent should be used. Antacids are ineffective even in large amounts, probably because of the high acid secretion and rapid gastric emptying that occur in patients with gastrinoma. Ranitidine is preferable to cimetidine in men because high doses of cimetidine cause antiandrogen side effects (breast tenderness, gynecomastia, impotence). Ranitidine is also preferable in patients taking other medications that are metabolized by the hepatic mixed function oxidase system (Dilantin, Coumadin, theophylline, etc.) because cimetidine but not ranitidine, affects metabolism of drugs by the hepatic mixed function oxidase system. In women who are not taking medication that is metabolized by the hepatic mixed function oxidase system either cimetidine or ranitidine can be used, because equipotent doses of both drugs have the same duration of action. Even though ranitidine is three times more potent than cimetidine, ranitidine is three times more expensive.

If sufficient doses of cimetidine or ranitidine are used, gastric hypersecretion can be controlled in almost every patient with ZES. Patients should first be treated with cimetidine, 300 mg every 6 hours, or ranitidine, 150 mg. every 8 hours, and the gastric acid secretory rate determined the next day, 1 hour before the next dose of medication. If gastric acid secretion is greater than 10 mEq per hour in this hour, cimetidine should be increased to 600 mg every 6 hours or ranitidine to 150 mg every 6 hours and the secretory rate determined again. If the gastric acid secretory rate continues to be greater than 10 mEq per hour, cimetidine should be increased to 900 mg every 6 hours or ranitidine to 300 mg every 6 hours. If gastric hypersecretion is still not controlled, an oral *anticholinergic* agent such as isopropamide 5 mg every 6 hours can be added. Anticholinergic agents alone only inhibit gastric hypersecretion by 15 to 25 percent, but when combined with cimetidine or ranitidine can greatly increase the effectiveness of the histamine H_2 receptor antagonists. Anticholinergic agents should be continued for at least 3 days before the gastric secretory rate is redetermined. Side effects with anticholinergic agents, such as dry mouth, constipation, and visual changes, are usually dose related so that if the side effects become significant, the dose can be reduced. Anticholinergic agents should generally not be used in patients with prostatism, glaucoma, partial gastric outlet obstruction, or significant esophageal disease.

Dosage Requirements. To control gastric hypersecretion, most patients with gastrinoma require more than 1.2 g per day of cimetidine or 0.3 g per day of ranitidine, the doses used in treating routine duodenal ulcer. In recent large studies the median doses required were 3 to 5 g per day of cimetidine or 1 to 1.5 g per day of ranitidine. Patients with gastrinoma have been treated for more than one year with doses as high as 12 g per day of cimetidine or 6 g per day of ranitidine. High doses of either drug have been well tolerated without evidence of dose-related hepatic, renal, or central nervous system toxicity. The continued effectiveness of antisecretory control should be checked every 6 to 12 months even if the patient is asymptomatic or if at any time diarrhea, esophageal, or peptic symptoms develop and persist for more than one week.

Newer Drugs

Recently, several new drugs have been described which promise to facilitate medical management of patients with ZES but have not been approved for use by the Food and Drug Administration. More potent histamine receptor antagonists, such as famotidine, which is 40 times more potent than cimetidine, will probably soon be available. Other classes of drugs, such as omeprazole, a substituted benzimidazole which inhibits H^+-K^+-ATPase on the gastric parietal cell, also may soon by available. Famotidine has only a slightly longer duration of action than cimetidine or ranitidine, whereas omeprazole has a duration of action of at least 3 days. Recent studies suggest that hypersecretion of gastric acid will be controlled in most patients with omeprazole taken once a day.

Surgical Treatment of Gastric Hypersecretion

Parietal Cell Vagotomy

Most studies have shown that long-term medical management with cimetidine or ranitidine is effective, but many patients require more than 4.8 g per day of cimetidine or 1.5 g per day of ranitidine to control gastric acid hypersecretion. Furthermore, medication dose requirements slowly increase with time; thus, medication expense will become an increasingly important determinant of the feasibility of long-term medical management. Therefore, until more potent antisecretory agents such as omeprazole become available, in many patients with high antisecretory drug requirements, a parietal cell vagotomy should be considered. A recent study demonstrates that a parietal cell vagotomy will decrease basal acid secretion by 56 percent, decrease antisecretory drug requirement in more than 90 percent of patients, and allow control of acid secretion with less than 3.0 g per day of cimetidine. Although it is likely that drug requirements will increase with time as the gastrinoma progresses, in the patients followed for up to 24 months after a parietal cell vagotomy only one patient required an increased cimetidine dose to control gastric hypersecretion. If parietal cell vagotomy is considered, a surgeon who routinely performs this operation should be selected. The patient should realize that this operation reduces the drug requirement, but in no case will a patient be able to stop all antisecretory medication.

Parathyroidectomy

In patients with gastrinoma with the MEN-1 syndrome, medical control of gastric hypersecretion can be facilitated by correction of the hyperparathyroidism, which is almost invariably present by the time Zollinger-Ellison syndrome develops. Correction of the hyperparathyroidism may reduce the fasting gastrin concentration, increase responsiveness to a given dose of antisecretory medication, and decrease the basal acid output, all of which facilitate medical control of gastric hypersecretion. Correction of the hyperparathyroidism is recommended in those gastrinoma patients with MEN-1 in whom the hyperparathyroidism is symptomatic (for example, renal stones, and so on) or in those who have a high antisecretory drug requirement.

Total Gastrectomy

Total gastrectomy should now be reserved for patients who cannot or will not take antisecretory medication. In a recent review of all series published since 1978 involving 248 patients with gastrinoma undergoing total gastrectomy, the operative mortality was 5.6 percent overall and 2.4 percent for elective procedures. The true morbidity rate associated with total gastrectomy, however, is not apparent from most series. When total gastrectomy is performed, gastrinoma patients should be treated with oral calcium, vitamin D, iron, and monthly injections of vitamin B_{12}.

TREATMENT OF THE GASTRINOMA

All physicians agree that the ideal treatment of gastrinoma is total surgical excision. In long-term studies of patients with gastrinoma who survived total gastrectomy and subsequently died, at least 50 percent of the deaths were due to tumor progression. Aggressive surgery, however, is not warranted in most patients because the overall prognosis for most patients is good. In recent studies the 5-year survival for patients with metastatic or unresectable locally invasive gastrinoma was 14 to 70 percent, and for all patients with gastrinoma it was 42 to 80 percent. Recent studies provide a number of results that help identify which patients should be considered for exploratory surgery. Present studies report that preoperative imaging studies, such as CT scan, angiogram, and ultrasound, can identify more that 90 percent of patients with gastrinoma metastatic to the liver and 38 percent of primary gastrinomas. Almost every study demonstrates that the possibility of surgical cure is very low (<2%) in patients with MEN-1 and gastrinoma, probably because of the multiplicity of gastrinomas. In early studies up to 1981 involving 157 patients with gastrinoma, the surgical cure was only 5 percent, whereas in recent studies in patients with sporadic gastrinoma (i.e., without MEN-1) the cure rate was 20 percent overall and up to 50 percent in patients with an extrapancreatic gastrinoma. In most studies, in at least one-third of patients, no gastrinoma is found and, after long-term follow-up, none of these patients have died from tumor progression. Some studies suggest that excision of all gastrinoma visible at surgery will improve long-term prognosis. No studies have demonstrated that aggressive surgery in patients with advanced metastatic disease improves long-term survival.

Approach to Patients With Nonmetastatic Gastrinoma

The results outlined above suggest that, among patients in whom the gastrinoma has not metastasized to the liver, the gastrinoma is potentially resectable, and who do not have MEN-1, approximately 60 percent will have a tumor found at surgery. In 40 percent the resection will not be curative and in 20 percent the resection will be curative (in 40% no tumor will be found). If no tumor is found, present evidence suggests that it is very likely that tumor progression leading to death will not occur in the 10 years following surgery.

Therefore, at present it is recommended that all patients with sporadic gastrinoma, i.e., gastrinoma not associated with MEN-1, undergo preoperative imaging studies. First, a CT scan with intravenous contrast should be performed, which will identify more than 80 percent of patients with gastrinoma metastatic to the liver. If hepatic metastatic disease is not present and even if the CT scan demonstrates a probable primary gastrinoma, ultrasound and selective pancreatic and hepatic angiography should be performed. All patients without gastrinoma in the liver or gastrinoma that is judged unresectable should undergo surgical exploration. Even the 60 percent of patients with negative localization studies should undergo exploratory laparotomy, because recent studies suggest that small gastrinomas (≤1 cm) are frequently not identified preoperatively but may be found by an experienced surgeon. Preoperative transhepatic selective venous sampling for gastrin from portal venous tributaries has been claimed to be helpful by some workers but not by others, and until its value is proven further, it should not be performed routinely.

The single most important factor in achieving good surgical results is the expertise of the surgeon. Even many experienced pancreatic surgeons have little experience with islet cell tumors, with the difficulty in identifying extrahepatic gastrinomas, and with the technique of enucleating lesions within the pancreas. At surgery the entire pancreas shoud be examined, with a Kocher maneuver performed to examine the pancreatic head; and the duodenum, stomach, mesentery, liver, and splenic hilum should be examined carefully. Any suspicious lymph node or mass should be biopsied. Gastrinomas are occasionally multiple; therefore, even if one tumor is found, examination for others should be continued. If at laparotomy a gastrinoma is found in the pancreatic head and cannot be enucleated, a Whipple procedure is not recommended because at present no studies have demonstrated that this will enhance survival. In fact, given the morbidity and mortality associated with this procedure coupled with the slow growth of the tumor, a Whipple procedure may possibly decrease long-term survival. Gastrinoma in the pancreatic body and tail, as well as involved lymph nodes, should be resected when safe and possible. Solitary gastrinomas or a few isolated areas of gastrinoma in the liver should also be resected if safe and possible because some such tumors may represent multifocal primaries. If no tumor is found, a blind pancreatic resection should not be performed because this does not increase the cure rate. If cure is unlikely either because no tumor is found or because tumor is found but is not completely resectable, and if the preoperative antisecretory drug requirement is high, a parietal cell vagotomy should be performed.

Prior to surgery the dosage of intravenous cimetidine or ranitidine that reduces gastric acid secretion to less than 10 mEq per hour should be determined for each patient. This dose of antisecretory agent should be given by continuous intravenous administration throughout surgery and the postoperative period until the patient can resume oral medication. The antisecretory medication should not be stopped postoperatively until it is clear the patient has been cured. Because results of gastrin assays may take a number of days, a reasonable course is to treat the patient with the same antisecretory medication that was taken preoperatively and perform a fasting gastrin and secretin provocative test. If either of these two tests suggests incomplete resection, the patient should be maintained on oral medication and the minimum antisecretory dose to reduce gastric acid secretion to less than 10 mEq per hour should be determined. Patients with a normal fasting gastrin concentration and a normal secretin test postoperatively should be maintained on antisecretory medication for 3 months and then reassessed yearly with measurement of fasting gastrin concentration and a secretin provocative test.

Approach To Patients With Metastatic Gastrinoma

When gastric acid hypersecretion is adequately controlled almost all patients with metastatic gastrinoma remain asymptomatic until the gastrinoma becomes quite extensive. At what point chemotherapy should begin has still not been established. The response to chemotherapy is usually slow (months); and therefore, it should not be used as an attempt to control gastric acid hypersecretion. Streptozotocin and 5-fluorouracil, either alone or with Adriamycin, have been reported to reduce tumor mass. No cases of cure or even of complete disappearance of the gastrinoma have been reported with these chemotherapeutic agents. Approximately 60 percent of patients will show a decrease in tumor size, but the gastrinoma usually starts to grow again within 24 months of beginning chemotherapy even with continued treatment. Streptozotocin causes significant nausea and vomiting and can cause renal toxicity, requiring frequent monitoring of renal function. Of the two groups with considerable experience treating metastatic gastrinoma, one group recommends chemotherapy be used when there is objective evidence of metastatic tumor growth in the liver by CT scan or angiogram over a three to six month period. The other group does not use chemotherapy until the tumor becomes symptomatic (with local pain, anorexia, and so on).

LONG-TERM FOLLOW-UP

All patients with gastrinoma should be assessed for the adequacy of antisecretory therapy by determining the gastric acid secretion rate every 6 to 12 months or at any time that symptoms such as diarrhea, epigastric pain, or heartburn recur and persist. Possible tumor progression should be assessed at least every 2 years with a CT scan and ultrasound. All patients with gastrinoma with MEN-1 should be assessed at least every 2 years for hyperactivity of other endocrine glands. Hyperparathyroidism should be excluded by serial determinations of serum calcium and phosphate and a parathyroid hormone determination. Pituitary status should be assessed with serum prolactin determinations and pituitary sella size evaluated by CT scan. Adrenal status should be assessed by abdominal CT scan and an overnight dexamethasone suppression test.

ACUTE UPPER GASTROINTESTINAL BLEEDING

J. LOREN PITCHER, M.D., F.A.C.P.

There are few medical emergencies that provoke more urgency and anxiety for both the physician and the patient than acute upper gastrointestinal (UGI) bleeding. This common clinical problem accounts for an estimated 100 to 150 hospital admissions per year per 100,000 population in the United States and continues to be a therapeutic and economic challenge.

Despite major diagnostic and management advances, overall mortality from acute UGI hemorrhage has not decreased in the past 30 years. During this period, however, there has been a significant increase in the percentage of patients with UGI bleeding who are elderly, who often have serious underlying medical conditions, and in whom mortality may often be due to conditions other than the UGI bleeding. Thus, real improvements in reduced mortality, complications, transfusion requirements, and need for surgery in patients with certain bleeding lesions and in younger patients may be obscured by overall outcome data for all patients.

The cardinal rule that any amount of UGI bleeding is life-threatening until proven otherwise should prevail. A trickle of blood must always be considered as a harbinger of exsanguination even though 80 to 90 percent of patients will spontaneously cease bleeding.

In the past decade, seven prospective trials provided

no evidence that a correct endoscopic diagnosis of the cause(s) of bleeding had any significant effect on either morbidity or mortality. Within these studies, however, were serious flaws in protocol design, inadequate stratification of patients, and often a lack of application of effective therapies for specific bleeding lesions, all of which make these studies of questionable value. Regardless, no one questions that endoscopy is the most safe, effective, and accurate method of diagnosing the cause(s) or site(s) of UGI bleeding in most patients. Recent advances in endoscopic techniques that (1) can effectively treat actively or recently bleeding lesions, (2) can identify lesions with a high probability of rebleeding or the need for surgical intervention, and (3) may preclude the use of unnecessary, ineffective, or potentially harmful therapies have opened a new era of optimism and realistic enthusiasm in the treatment of patients with UGI bleeding.

INITIAL PATIENT EVALUATION AND MANAGEMENT

Acute UGI bleeding may be massive, moderate, or mild and may be a single episode, intermittent episodes, or continuous. Fresh blood or "coffee grounds" in the emesis or in the gastric lavage return proves UGI bleeding if one can exclude paradoxic bleeding from the mouth, nasopharynx, or tracheobronchial tree and factitious bleeding (the swallowing of either human or animal blood). True melena is rarely found from a small bowel or proximal colonic source and hence its presence serves as a reasonable clue to UGI bleeding. Hematochezia, however, can occur in both UGI and lower GI bleeding. When bleeding is from the former rather than the latter source, the patient more often has signs and symptoms of significant blood volume loss.

A gastric lavage that is negative for gross or occult blood but is bile stained usually implies bleeding distal to the ligament of Treitz; however, a lack of duodenal-pyloric reflux of luminal contents, cessation of previous bleeding, or poor technique may yield a false-negative gastric lavage result.

The most common judgmental errors made in the initial evaluation and care of bleeding patients are to underestimate both the degree of blood loss (often due to a false reliance upon initial hematocrit values) and the potential gravity of the situation.

The patient's hemodynamic status must be rapidly and accurately assessed and monitored while resuscitative efforts are simultaneously initiated. Recumbent hypotension with or without clinical findings or hypovolemia and/or shock indicates a blood volume loss of 25 to 40 percent or more. For patients with recumbent normal blood pressures, a positive "tilt test" manifested by a rise in pulse rate of greater than 20 to 25 beats per minute and a diastolic pressure drop of greater than 10 to 15 mm Hg predicts a 10 to 20 percent loss of blood volume.

A relevant and expeditious history, physical examination, and review of available medical records should be accomplished while blood samples are drawn, large intravenous lines are established, and fluids, colloid, and blood replacement are initiated. In selected patients, a Swanz-Ganz catheter with thermodilution cardiac output capabilities and/or arterial monitoring lines may be indicated. Numerous studies have shown that the prediction of the actual bleeding site based upon history, physical examination, and prior known diagnoses is fraught with considerable error and cannot be relied upon.

Initial resuscitation always takes precedence over specific diagnostic and/or therapeutic measures; these can, however, usually be performed simultaneously.

Specific laboratory tests, always tailored to the patient's age, clinical history, symptoms, physical findings, and suspected or known underlying diseases should include complete blood count, urinalysis, prothrombin time, partial thromboplastin time, and careful review of the peripheral blood smear, with particular note taken of evidence of chronic anemia, hemolysis, vitamin B_{12} or folate deficiency, and platelet estimation. Blood chemistries should include, at minimum, blood glucose, creatinine, blood urea nitrogen, and liver function tests. Samples of blood may be obtained and stored and other tests run at a more expeditious time. In selected patients, serum and/or urinary amylase, electrolyte, and arterial blood gas measurements may be indicated. An electrocardiogram should be obtained in selected patients at admission and repeated in 24 to 48 hours or the patient monitored to uncover silent myocardial ischemia or infarction.

A portable chest roentgenogram, physical examination, and arterial blood gases provide reasonable assessment of pulmonary function status.

More detailed coagulation studies may be required when consumptive coagulopathy, liver disease, blood dyscrasias, drug ingestions, purpura, uremia, or other bleeding tendencies are suspected or apparent. Although it is often difficult to be certain when or if identified coagulation disorders are contributing to or causing the UGI bleeding, judicious replacement of appropriate clotting factors is usually indicated. Unless fresh whole blood less than one day old is available, this is usually best accomplished with fresh frozen plasma, platelets, or both. Specific clotting factor concentrates are rarely needed. Care must be exercised in using prothrombin complex concentrates, especially in patients with serious liver disease, because of the potential for inducing disseminated intravascular coagulation.

Critical vital signs and physiologic variables should be monitored and a flow sheet initiated to serially record all data and therapy. Patients with moderate and severe bleeding should have hourly measurement of urinary outputs obtained via an indwelling urinary catheter.

Deaths associated with UGI bleeding are often related to delayed resuscitation and/or insufficient volumes and rates of replacement therapy. Whole blood or packed red blood cells with isotonic fluids, colloid, or both are preferred when active bleeding and hypovolemia are present.

While one awaits blood products, Ringer's lactate (preferred if metabolic acidosis is present) or isotonic fluids should be infused at a rapid rate until the blood volume is minimally restored as indicated by improvement in blood pressure, pulse, clinical signs of hypovolemia, and other monitored, indicators of the patient's hemodynamic status.

Preference is given to maintaining a stable hematocrit above 30 to 34 percent with due precautions to avoid overexpansion of blood volume in patients at risk for congestive heart failure, variceal bleeding, or those with renal failure.

A team effort, to include *early surgical consultation* and intensive care provided by highly skilled nursing personnel, is important to optimal care and outcome.

Gastric lavage through a large-bore or a gastric tube is indicated when there is blood in the stomach. Although controlled studies are lacking to prove that iced or room temperature saline or water for gastric lavage either slows, halts, increases, or has no effect on active bleeding, clinical experience indicates that gastric lavage does slow or halt bleeding and is safe. Most importantly, lavage clears the stomach of blood to allow adequate endoscopic examination and/or therapy while precluding regurgitation and aspiration of blood during such procedures.

Gastric lavage should be accomplished using vigorous and forceful flushing and infusions of 100 to 250 ml of lavage solution with a 50-ml syringe, not a gravity flow system, so that organized clots can be broken up and blood flushed off the gastric mucosa. Return flow should be by either gravity or very gentle suction aspiration to avoid suction artifacts and damage to the gastric mucosa. Typically, the vigorous lavage will yield clear to pink return within 30 minutes. The lavage should not be discontinued until just before any diagnostic and/or therapeutic endoscopic procedures are performed.

Lavage solutions containing various vasoconstrictor agents are not commonly used or proven effective. One controlled, double-blind study comparing normal saline with an Aramine solution (300 mg per liter of normal saline) showed a benefit from the latter in reducing bleeding in a small number of patients.

SPECIFIC THERAPEUTIC ALTERNATIVES

Acid Neutralization or Secretory Inhibition

The use of antacids or histamine$_2$ (H_2) receptor antagonists has not been proved effective in stopping active bleeding from any lesion but may prevent rebleeding from ulcers; may be effective prophylaxis against bleeding in stress gastric erosions, as seen in patients on medical, surgical, trauma, and burn intensive care units; and may promote uncomplicated ulcer healing.

It is possible that the unproven or equivocal efficacy of these agents in some trials may be related to inadequate attention to proper doses to achieve near intragastric neutrality and to obviate the adverse effects on intragastric coagulation that may result from an intragastric pH of less than 6 to 7.

I prefer a combination of *cimetidine*, 300 to 400 mg IV every 4 to 6 hours by bolus injection or 50 to 65 mg per hour by constant infusion, plus a *potent antacid* (e.g., Mylanta II or Maalox T.C.) in doses of 15 to 45 ml every hour titrated to identify those amounts of both medications needed to maintain an intragastric pH of 6 to 7 for patients with peptic ulcer, reflux esophagitis with or without ulcer, and acute erosive gastritis/duodenitis secondary to drug, alcohol or gastric irritant ingestion.

I initially withhold H_2 receptor blockers in patients with gastric "stress" erosions or ulcers except those with central nervous system injuries or heptic coma. Reasonable but theoretical evidence suggests that, in other forms of gastric fundal "stress" bleeding, a secreting mucosa may be less vulnerable to erosions and ulceration than one blocked by an H_2 receptor antagonist.

Except in reflux esophagitis, with or without esophageal ulcer, and in patients with esophageal varices, antacids should be initiated via a nasogastric tube. After 48 to 72 hours of no significant bleeding and the necessary titration-calibration of the antacid/cimetidine therapy, comparable and then reduced oral doses may be utilized with due attention paid to the known side effects, contraindications, and drug interactions of these agents.

Angiotherapy

Selective and subselective catheterization of the mesenteric vasculature is now possible and allows the delivery of vasoconstrictor drugs and embolization therapy. I reserve this technique for very high-risk patients who fail to improve with more conventional and/or less hazardous and invasive procedures to control bleeding. No well-controlled studies are available, but control of bleeding has been reported in ulcer disease, diffuse mucosal erosions, Mallory-Weiss tears, and variceal bleeding when intravenous vasopressin fails.

Endoscopic Therapy

Thermal and Photocoagulation Methods. Of the endoscopic, hemostatic techniques evaluated to date, the most promising results, short of controlled studies, favor the application of techniques of coaptive electrocoagulation with either the available multipolar (BICAP) probe or the experimental heater probe. The combination of pressure and "slow" tissue heating from these instruments is felt to be more effective in controlling arterial bleeding. Neodymum: yttrium, aluminum, garnet (Nd:Yag) and argon lasers have proved effective in treating ulcer lesions to control bleeding and oozing and to prevent rebleeding. These have a greater erosive and perforation/penetration potential and are extremely costly, less portable, and less generally available than mono bipolar or multipolar electrocoagulation.

Injection Therapy. Injection sclerotherapy of esophageal varices has been shown to be relatively safe and effective in the control of acute, actively bleeding varices, rebleeding from recently bleeding varices, and long-term control of variceal bleeding once obliteration of the varices is achieved. Control of bleeding has unfortunately not always and unequivocally been equated with increased short-, mid-, or long-term survival after an acute bleed but cost effectiveness has been demonstrated in one study. There is an excellent, well-referenced review of sclerotherapy by Conn and Grace.[1]

Of the sclerosing agents available in the United States, I prefer tetradecyl (Sotradecol) over sodium morrhuate or 95 percent ethanol. I specifically favor a mixed solution of equal volumes of 3 percent tetradecyl, 95 percent ethanol, and normal saline with methylene blue added as a marker (so-called TES solution). Such a mixture yields a solution of 1 percent tetradecyl, 32 percent ethanol, and 0.3 percent saline. This is an effective solution with a reasonable balance between efficacy and mucosal injury potential; it causes less fever, pleural effusions, chest pain, and other complications than fatty acid sclerosants such as sodium morrhuate. The use of single agents in full strengths yields too high an incidence of mucosal injury, ulcers, and other side effects. Perivariceal injections of these agents should be avoided when possible.

The technique is to inject 0.5 to 2.0 ml of TES solution at each site, with total volume not to exceed 26 ml per session. Varices should be injected in a circumferential fashion beginning at the esophageal gastric junction after the injection of the bleeding point of a recently bleeding or actively bleeding varix. I repeat injections in 48 hours in recently bleeding patients and then at 4- to 7-day intervals for three or four more sessions, followed by monthly injections until total obliteration of the varices has been achieved.

I consider reasonable indications for sclerotherapy to include active bleeding from esophageal varix at the time of diagnostic endoscopy; proven recent or recurrent variceal bleeding in Child's category B or C patients (especially those with severe clotting disorders); the absence of definitive therapy which would lead to a cure (i.e., splenic vein thrombosis); and proven, relatively recent variceal bleeding in a patient with large varices and a demonstrable cherry red spot, clot on a varix, submucosal hematoma around a varix, varix on a varix, black spot, red wale, or the so-called Mt. St. Helen's sign.

Limited reports on the effectiveness of 95 percent ethanol injections to control ulcer and other arterial bleeding points and the use of endoscopic clipping and suturing techniques are too preliminary to recommend use of these techniques. Likewise, topical agents applied through the endoscope have no role in endoscopic therapy at this time.

Transhepatic Obliteration of Varices

Transhepatic obliteration of varices is of limited value because of the lack of controlled studies, the technical expertise required, the ease and accessibility of endoscopic sclerotherapy, and the theoretical disadvantage that this therapy may obliterate the paraesophageal veins which may act as a desirable portasystemic shunt.

Vasopressin

By its effect on splanchnic vasoconstriction and perhaps its reduction in intramural esophageal venous flow through its effect on smooth muscle action in the esophageal wall, both peripheral intravenous and mesenteric intra-arterial infusions of vasopressin may be equally effective in variceal bleeding. Because of its easy administration, the intravenous route is preferred at a rate of 0.2 to 0.9 units of vasopressin per minute. Close attention must be paid to the many adverse side effects of vasopressin, especially the unpredictable decrease in cardiac output, which may respond to appropriate doses of isoproterenol. A few patients who fail to respond to intravenous vasopressin may respond to mesenteric arterial infusions at doses of 0.1 to 0.4 units per minute. I prefer hemodynamic and cardiac output monitoring capabilities to be available during vasopressin infusion.

Vasopressin for the treatment of other sources of nonvariceal bleeding usually requires mesenteric intra-arterial infusion and often selective or subselective infusion into the vessel(s) directly supplying the bleeding site. Alcohol- or drug-induced gastritis may rapidly respond to vasopressin.

The use of sodium nitroprusside and propranolol for the control of acute bleeding, particularly variceal bleeding, cannot be recommended at this time.

Balloon Tamponade

Either the Sengstaken-Blakemore (S-B) tube with the Boyce modification or the Linton tube (the latter is preferred for gastric variceal bleeding only or Mallory-Weiss tear tamponade) can be safe and effective in the hands of experienced physicians. Permanent hemostasis utilizing this technique, however, occurs in only 40 to 50 percent of patients, and therefore it is generally relegated to the role of a procedure to halt acute variceal bleeding temporarily when vasopressin therapy and/or sclerotherapy fails. Details of a recommended safe and effective technique for the use of the S-B tube are available[2]. These instructions differ from those usually offered by the manufacturers of the various tamponade tubes.

Miscellaneous Medical Treatment

A number of therapeutic agents, including glucagon, anticholinergic drugs, somatostatin, prostaglandins, and sucralfate, are under investigation but none can be recommended at this time for routine use in the United States in actively bleeding patients. Seemingly, patients with diffuse erosive gastritis, may be the beneficiaries of some of these medications that have "cytoprotective" effects in the stomach.

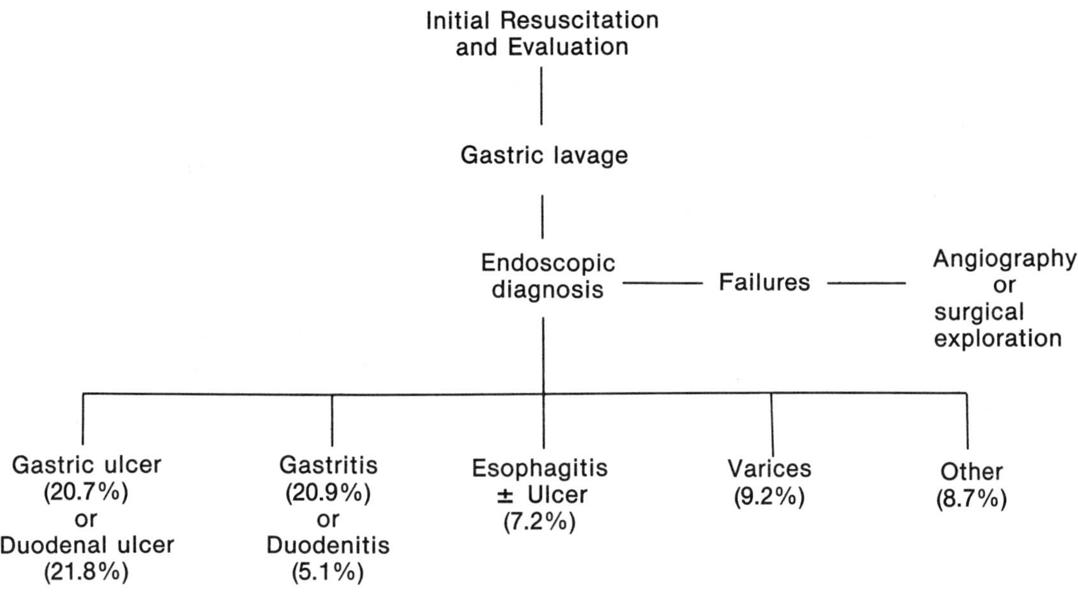

Figure 1 Initial management of acute upper gastrointestinal hemorrhage and approximate frequency of bleeding lesions.

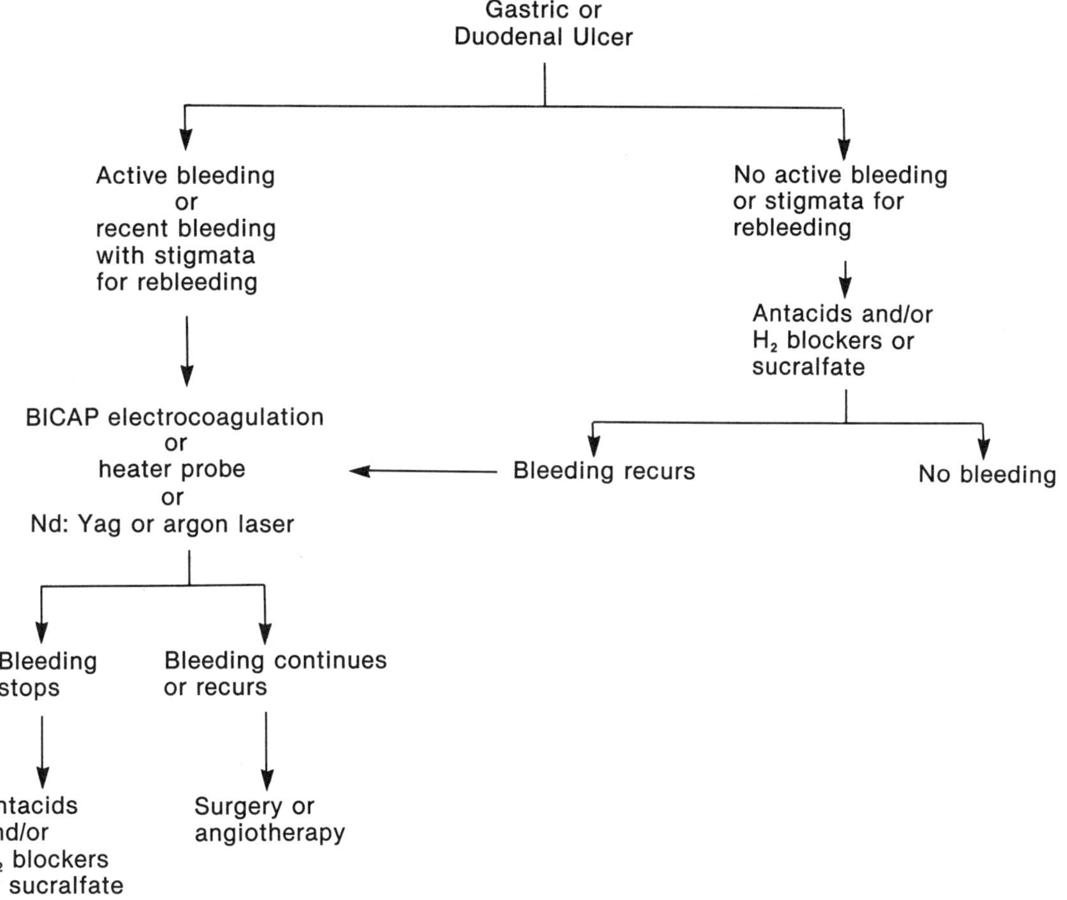

Figure 2 Management of acute hemorrhage from gastric or duodenal ulcer.

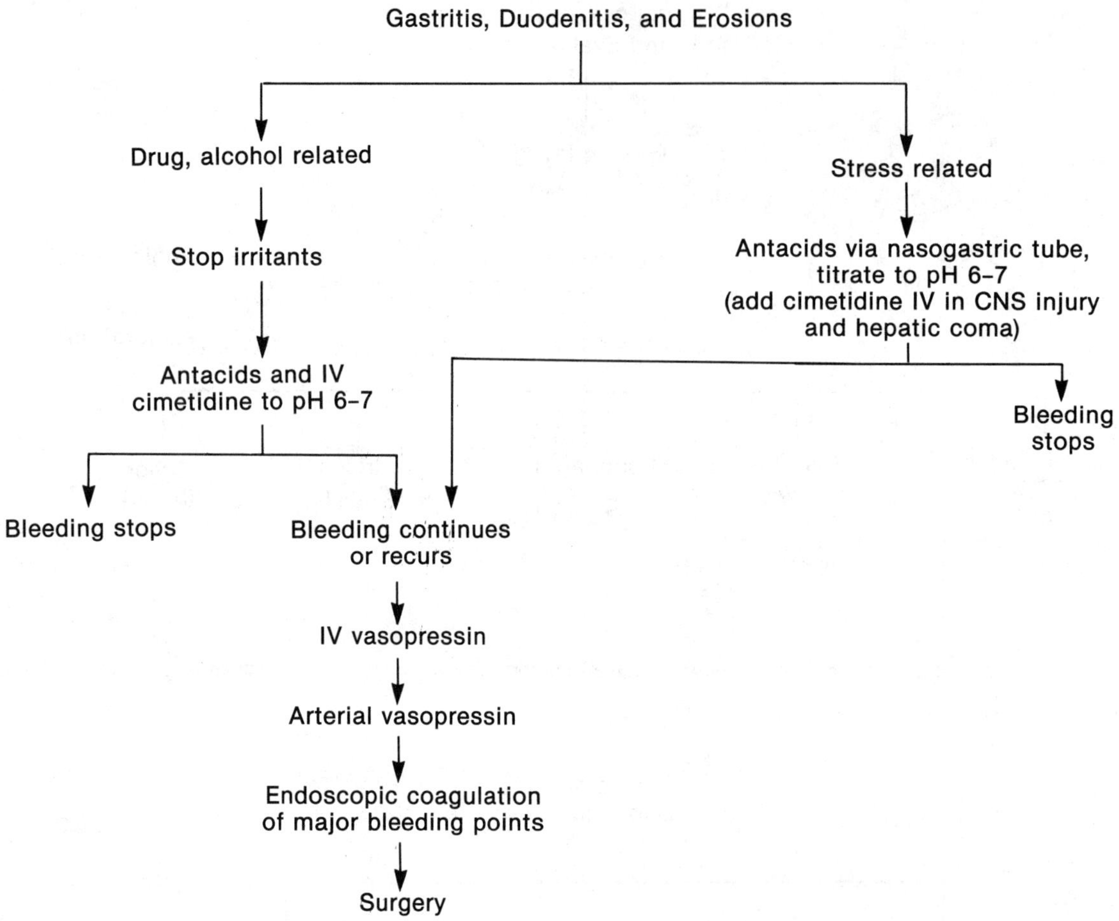

Gastritis, Duodenitis, and Erosions
Drug, alcohol related
Stress related
Stop irritants
Antacids via nasogastric tube, titrate to pH 6–7 (add cimetidine IV in CNS injury and hepatic coma)
Antacids and IV cimetidine to pH 6–7
Bleeding stops
Bleeding stops
Bleeding continues or recurs
IV vasopressin
Arterial vasopressin
Endoscopic coagulation of major bleeding points
Surgery

Figure 3 Management of acute hemorrhage from gastritis, duodenitis and erosions.

Esophagitis with or without Ulcer
Antacids and
H₂ blockers orally
Antireflux measures
Bleeding continues or recurs
Bleeding stops
? Sucralfate liquid
IV vasopressin
Surgery

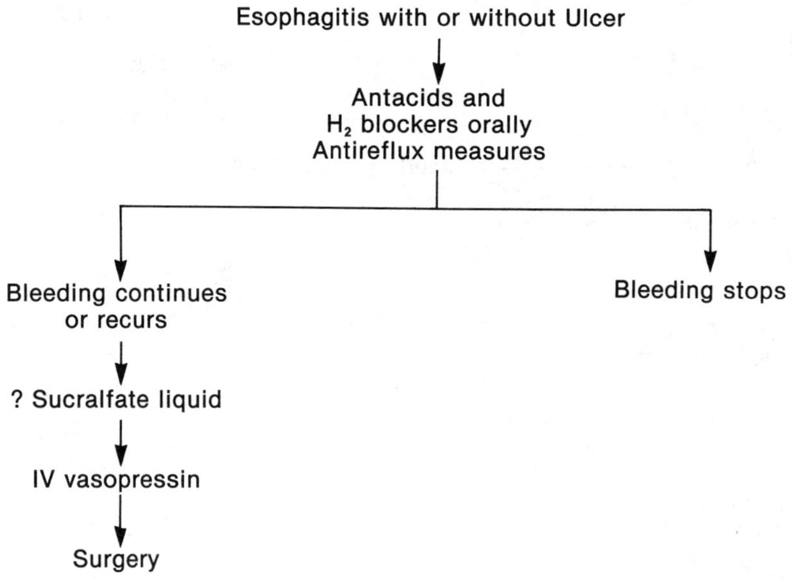

Figure 4 Management of acute hemorrhage from esophagitis, with or without ulcer.

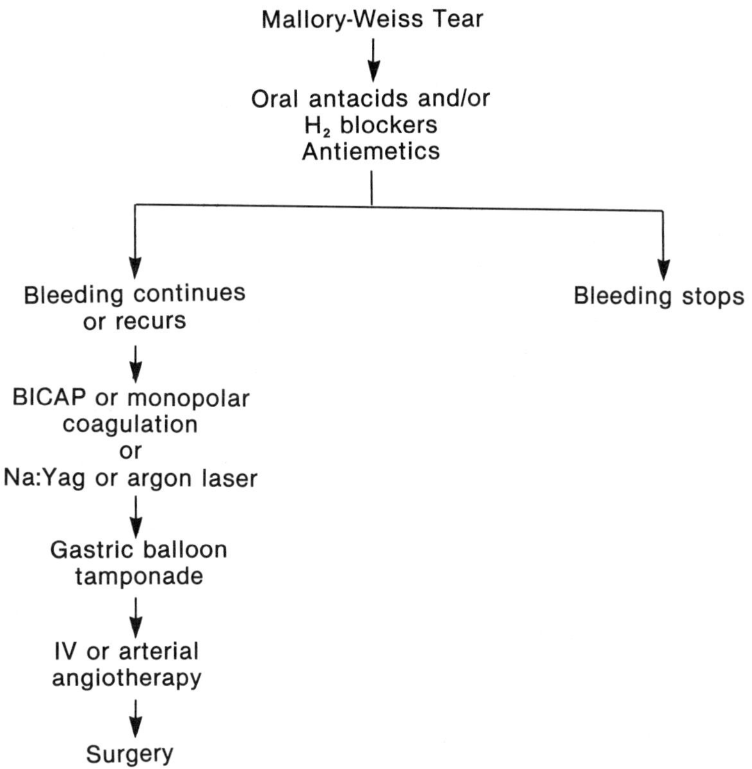

Figure 5 Management of acute hemorrhage from a Mallory-Weiss tear.

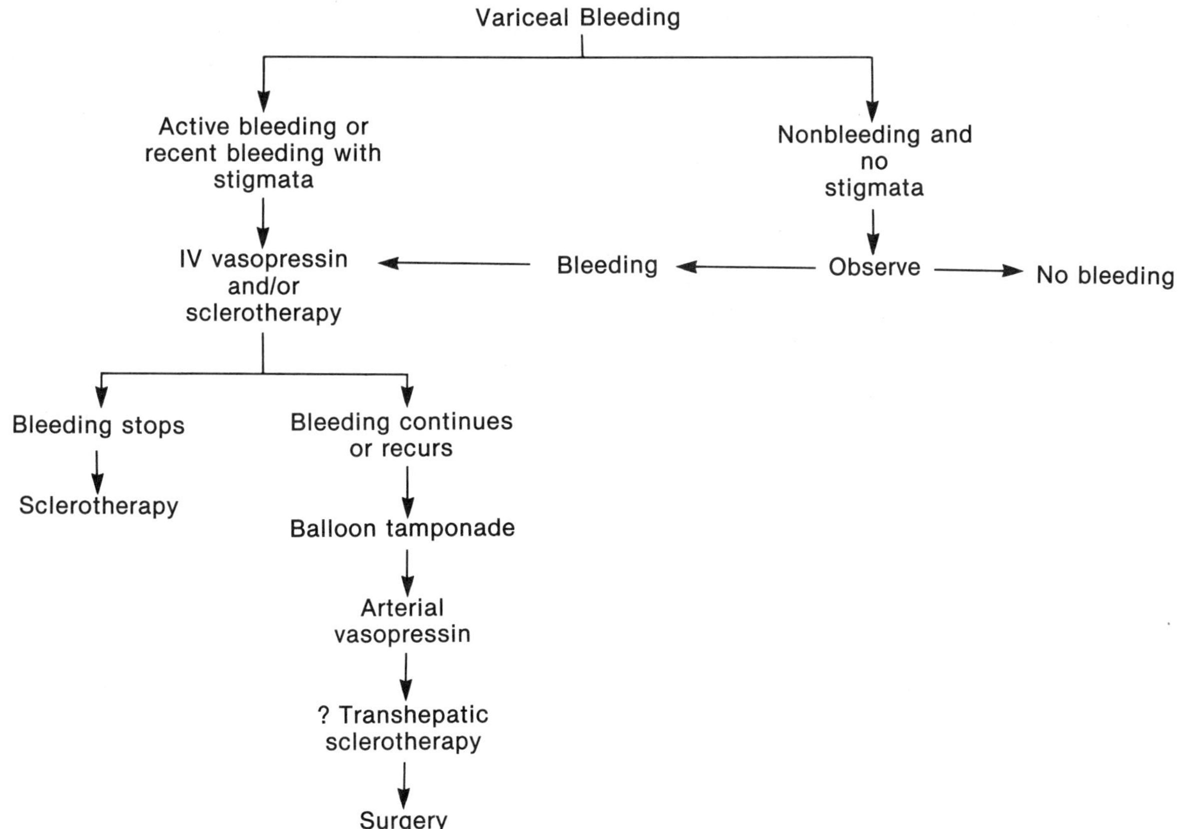

Figure 6 Management of acute hemorrhage from gastroesophageal varices.

Surgery

Surgical intervention to control bleeding is reserved for those who fail to stop bleeding spontaneously, have recurrent or continuous bleeding despite other modes of therapy, or who have specific lesions that are best treated and/or cured by surgery. Many factors, such as patient age, underlying medical conditions, the specific nature of the bleeding site, the amount, frequency, and rapidity of bleeding, the surgical expertise available, transfusion difficulties, patient's physiologic response and tolerance of the bleeding, and the availability of nonsurgical effective therapies, enter into the decision of when and on which patients surgery should be performed. No hard or fixed formulas can replace sound judgment and clinical experience in this arena. In some patients, surgical intervention may be the primary and most conservative approach to therapy.

TREATMENT OF SPECIFIC CAUSES OF ACUTE UPPER GASTROINTESTINAL BLEEDING

A national, multicenter study involving 2,225 patients with 2,486 causes of UGI bleeding diagnosed by endoscopy identified eight common conditions which accounted for 93.9 percent of all final diagnoses. In order of frequency these causes were (1) duodenal ulcer (21.8%), (2) gastric erosions—gastritis (20.9%), (3) gastric and stomal ulcer (20.7%), (4) varices (9.2%), (5) esophagitis—esophageal ulcer (7.2%), (6) Mallory-Weiss tears (6.4%), (7) erosive duodenitis (5.1%), and (8) neoplasms (2.6%). It should be noted that several patients (11.7% of all patients) bled from or had more than one potential bleeding source identified in this study.

Figure 1 outlines the general and initial approach to most patients with acute UGI bleeding and displays the common specific causes and their approximate frequencies from a large multicenter study.

Figures 2 through 6 depict my current general preference for a stepwise approach to treating the major specific bleeding lesions. For specific details on each therapeutic alternative in the schematic diagrams, reference should be made to that section on specific therapeutic alternatives in this chapter. Fixed rules must be avoided, however, and each patient's care must be individualized based upon a multitude of clinical factors present. There can be no substitute for sound clinical judgment and extensive clinical experience in treating these patients with acute upper GI bleeding.

In selected patients with torrential bleeding, endoscopy and/or other forms of medical therapy are impossible or futile and surgical intervention is mandated.

Regardless of the immediate therapy being rendered or the status of the patient's bleeding, physicians should always be contemplating the next logical therapeutic step to be taken should the current therapy fail or complications of therapy develop.

Some recommended treatments in Figures 2 through 6 may not have been proved to be safe and effective in well-controlled studies. A combination of factors, however, such as relative safety of a treatment, the cumulative weight of uncontrolled clinical trials, current concepts of pathophysiologic mechanisms, and experimental/theoretical considerations have been incorporated in the recommendations. Occasionally, when the stakes are high, when the remaining therapeutic options are limited or carry a known high mortality rate for a specific patient's overall condition; and when a relatively simple, safe, clinically effective albeit unproven therapy is available, one may elect to "have a shot at it" after obtaining informed consent.

Other Bleeding Lesions

Bleeding arteriovenous malformations and angiodysplasia may be treated by BICAP electrocoagulation, Nd:Yag or argon laser, or monopolar electrocoagulation in that order of preference. Bleeding neoplasia may be treated by the same modalities above plus surgical resection or snare coagulation (when the lesion is polypoid). Bleeding aortoenteric fistula requires surgical intervention.

REFERENCES

1. Conn HD, Grace ND. Portal hypertension and sclerotherapy of esophageal varices; a point of view. Endoscopy Review 1985; May/June:39–53.
2. Pitcher JL. Safety and effectiveness of the modified Sengstaken-Blakemore tube: a prospective study. Gastroenterology 1971; 61:291.

FUNCTIONAL DISORDERS OF THE UPPER GASTROINTESTINAL TRACT

GARY A. NEWMAN, M.D.
RICHARD W. McCALLUM, M.D., F.A.C.P., F.R.A.C.P.(Austral), F.A.C.G.

NONULCER DYSPEPSIA

Dyspepsia, or more appropriately nonulcer dyspepsia, refers to a symptom complex which includes heartburn, indigestion, abdominal/epigastric pain or burning, postprandial bloating and early satiety sensations, and even nausea and vomiting. The syndrome, which can account for up to 40 to 60 percent of all patients referred to gastroenterologists, includes various functional problems such as nervous dyspepsia, abdominal pains for which no organic cause can be found, and the visceral or somatic manifestations of psychiatric disease.

In dealing with nonulcer dyspepsia, a brief understanding of its presumed pathogenesis is necessary. First of all, the existence of gstroesophageal reflux, complicated esophageal disease (i.e., strictures, achalasia), peptic ulcer disease, pancreatic disease, small bowel mucosal disease, or biliary tract disease must be ruled out. Once this is accomplished endoscopically or otherwise, the treatment of nonulcer dyspepsia can be directed toward the suppression or neutralization of gastric acid, the enhancement of gastrointestinal motility, or the psychologic and emotional aspects of the disease.

Recent reports have suggested that patients with nonulcer dyspepsia have histologic increases in the gastroduodenal mucosal neutrophil count, possibly indicative of ongoing low-grade inflammation that is not yet endoscopically visible. This patient group, however, has never been shown to be hypersecretors and significant bile reflux has never been documented. Further, while patients have reported significant improvement of their symptoms with antacid ingestion, acid neutralizing compounds have not been consistently shown to be significantly more effective than placebo. Along these lines, H_2 antagonists, most notably cimetidine, have not been shown to be significantly better than placebo in controlling the long-term or recurrent symptoms of nonulcer dyspepsia.

Anticholinergic agents have also been used, but again there is little controlled evidence of a significant advantage over placebo. Nonetheless, *pirenzepine*, a new anticholinergic, acid-suppressing drug with selective antimuscarinic (MI) activity (thus avoiding antimotility side effects), has shown promise. Preliminary reports in peptic ulcer disease indicate that, used alone, its acid-suppressing properties are not impressive. Its most useful role may be to augment the acid inhibition induced by other agents. It may also be of some use if nocturnally administered.

Another new component in the increasing spectrum of nonulcer dyspepsia and gastroduodenal inflammation is the entity of "infectious" gastritis. Investigators from Australia have described the presence of a specific organism, *Campylobacter pyloridis*, in 95 percent of the patients they studied with chronic active gastritis of the antrum with or without ulceration. This finding raises the question of in situ antibacterial treatment for the symptoms of nonulcer dyspepsia patients. Whether or not the surface-acting agents such as sucralfate and prostaglandins offer any bactericidal action, rather than a specific ability to bind acid/bile or to cytoprotect, will obviously need investigation.

Turning to the role of gastrointestinal motility in the approach to nonulcer dyspepsia, the typical symptoms of abdominal distention/bloating, indigestion, and feelings of fullness after meals strongly suggest a disturbance in gastric emptying. Expanding on this aspect of abnormal gastrointestinal motility, one can interconnect the functional diseases of irritable bowel syndrome and nonulcer dyspepsia. The irritable bowel syndrome can be viewed as a diffuse disturbance of gastrointestinal motility, not just a colonic disorder. When patients have this diffuse "unhappiness" of the gastrointestinal tract smooth muscle, it seems reasonable that symptoms can certainly extend to the upper tract.

In investigating the role of a motility disturbance in patients with nonulcer dyspepsia, we and other investigators have identified the role of *duodenogastric dyssynchrony*. Normally there is a coordination of aborally conducted contractions that begin in the proximal stomach, extend into the antrum, and then progress through the duodenum and small bowel. Observations in patients with duodenogastric dysfunction show that multiple and often high-amplitude contractions of the duodenum can be observed without any indication that they initiated in the antrum. Moreover, these contractions seemed to be conducted toward the antrum rather than aborally toward the small intestine. This creates a relative duodenal block and presumably contributes to abdominal pain, duodenogastric reflux, bile reflux gastritis, nausea, and even vomiting.

In accordance with the above, manometric abnormalities have been recently documented in patients with functional upper gut symptoms. Measurements in the stomach revealed decreased antral phasic pressure activity after a solid meal, while probes in the small intestine showed unpropagated bursts of phasic and tonic activity.[1]

Another interesting aspect of gastric motility and its relationship to nonulcer dyspepsia is the concept of *electrical dysrhythmias* of the stomach and small bowel. At this point, longer and better studies in normal subjects are a prerequisite before one goes beyond the stage of postulating that some groups of patients with symptoms consistent with nonulcer dyspepsia may have dysrhythmias of the wavelike electrical rhythms of the stomach and small intestine. These abnormalities could vary from tachy- to bradyarrhythmias using the cardiology blueprint. The accompanying impairments in motility and/or gastric emptying could explain the patient's symptoms.

With the lack of specific gastrointestinal antiarrhythmic agents, treatment of these profound postprandial symptoms is currently aimed at reorchestrating a normal aboral propagation of motility. This is best accomplished by the prokinetic agents metoclopramide (note its similarity to procainamide, Fig. 1) and domperidone (still experimental in the United States, Fig. 2), which are the most promising drugs at this time.

Metoclopramide is a dopamine antagonist and partial cholinergic agonist that stimultes motility of the upper gastrointestinal tract without stimulating gastric, biliary, or pancreatic secretions. It increases the resting tone of the lower esophageal sphincter and increases and coordinates the tone and amplitude of gastric (primarily antral) contractions while relaxing the pyloric sphincter and duodenal bulb. It also increases aboral peristalsis in the duodenum and jejunum. *Domperidone* is similar to metoclopramide in that it is a dopamine antagonist and prolactin releasing agent, but it does not cross the blood-brain barrier and does not enter the central nervous system, resulting in no extrapyramidal side effects. In addition, domperidone neither augments acetylcholine release nor sensitizes muscarinic receptors as metoclopramide does. Therefore, it is not antagonized by either atropine or other anticholinergic agents.

Both domperidone and metoclopramide have been evaluated in patients with postprandial upper gastrointestinal distress or chronic postprandial dyspepsia. In placebo controlled trials, both metoclopramide (Reglan in the United States and Maxalon in England), given in a dose ranging from 5 to 15 mg orally one-half hour before meals, and domperidone (to be marketed as Motilium), given in a dose ranging from 10 to 30 mg orally prior to eating, have shown significant benefit over placebo.

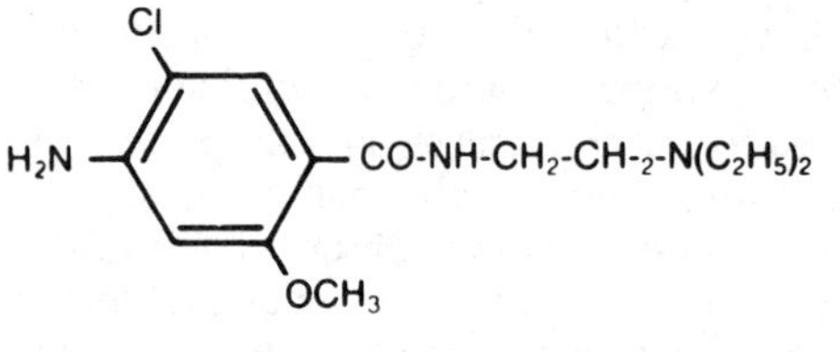

Cl

H_2N — CO-NH-CH_2-CH-$_2$-N$(C_2H_5)_2$

OCH_3

Metoclopramide

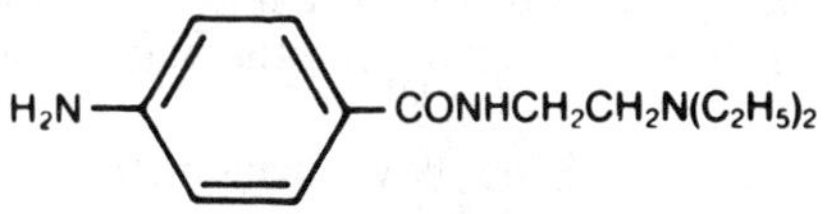

H_2N — $CONHCH_2CH_2N(C_2H_5)_2$

Procainamide

Figure 1 Structural formula of metoclopramide and procainamide.

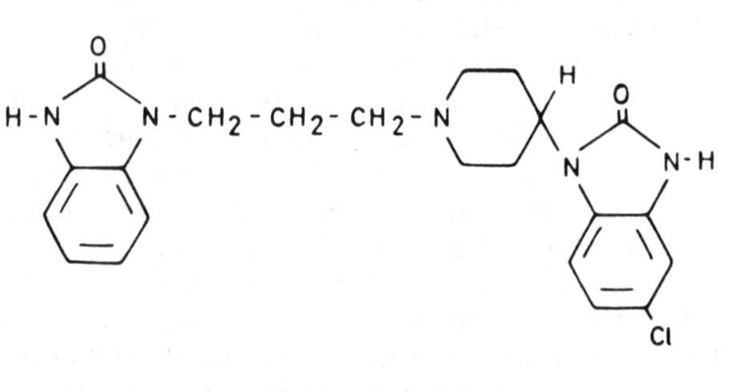

O H O

H-N N-CH_2-CH_2-CH_2-N N N-H

Cl

Figure 2 Chemical structure of domperidone.

Finally, the psychologic stresses and emotional tensions that are known to affect bowel function may be playing a role in some patients with classic nonulcer dyspepsia. In reviews of the Scandinavian experience with nonulcer dyspepsia, a majority of the patients showed signs and symptoms of inner tension, autonomic disturbances, and complaints of fatigability, irritability, and hostile feelings. The patients were also found to have an increased incidence of phobias, sleep disturbances, and obsessive-compulsive symptoms. Further, recent reports in the United States indicated that many patients with functional upper tract symptoms and normal manometry of the stomach and proximal small bowel had some level of psychiatric problems.

The experience with the treatment of irritable bowel syndrome (IBS) is clearly an appropriate area for comparison. Patients with classic IBS are often sensitive, anxious, depressed, and may have abnormalities in learned illness behavior. Medical therapy in association with intensive psychotherapy has been shown to be more efficacious in IBS than medical therapy alone. This ''holistic'' approach in the absence of response to the standard medical therapies noted above may be necessary in selected patients with refractory, chronic, and relapsing dyspeptic symptoms. The chapter *Functional Illness* provides additional suggestions. Further information on nonulcer dyspepsia can be found in articles by Lagarde and Spiro[2] and Petersen[3].

NAUSEA AND VOMITING

The characterization and treatment of nausea along with unexplained vomiting is a difficult diagnostic challenge. While a precise description of the sensation of nausea is elusive, vomiting is a more physical and objective complaint and involves a complex interaction between the gut and central nervous system (Fig. 3).

The differential diagnosis of nausea and vomiting is wide-ranging (Table 1). Because of the multiple etiologic factors involved, extensive investigations are often necessary to pinpoint the cause and direct therapy at the appropriate source.

First of all, the usual history and physical examination, standard laboratory tests, and plain abdominal films are obtained. The determination of acute versus chronic/recurrent symptoms, the temporal relationship of vomiting to meals, and the association of other systemic complaints are the most significant points. In this initial part of the investigation, it is important to keep in mind that vomiting can occur in healthy people as part of a strong emotional response, or in neurotic patients as a manifestation of underlying pathologic factors. Psycho-

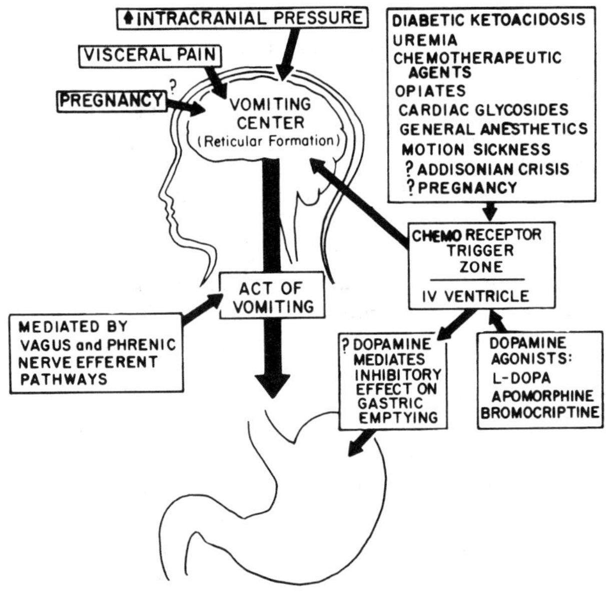

Figure 3 The central control of vomiting.

TABLE 1 Differential Diagnosis of Nausea and Vomiting

Acute onset of symptoms
- Viral gastroenteritis
- Bacterial enterotoxins
- Drugs, including chemotherapeutic agents
- Visceral pain
- Viral hepatitis
- Vestibular disorders
- Metabolic disturbances
- Acute mechanical obstruction
- Postoperative

Chronic symptoms
- Esophageal
  - Achalasia
  - Zenker's diverticulum
- Mechanical gastric outlet obstruction
  - Peptic ulcer disease
  - Gastric ulcer
  - Gastric carcinoma
  - Pancreatic disease
- Motility disorders
  - Gastroparesis
  - Drug-induced gastric stasis
  - Chronic intestinal pseudo-obstruction
  - Postviral gastroenteritis
  - Irritable bowel syndrome
  - Postgastric surgery
  - Idiopathic gastric stasis (? role of electrical dysrhythmias)
  - Anorexia nervosa—spectrum of bulimia and psychogenic vomiting
- Miscellaneous
  - Pregnancy
  - Increased intracranial pressure
- Psychogenic vomiting
  - Self-induced
  - Rumination

genic vomiting can be recognized early by its classic pattern. The patient often has a long personal or family history of vomiting. Although the vomiting can often be suppressed, delayed vomiting is less common than vomiting directly after a meal. Stressful situations are often a precipitating factor in the reflex. Concealed vomiting and cyclic vomiting usually also fall into this psychogenic category.

In the further investigation of unexplained vomiting, a standard saline load test may be useful in ruling out gastric outlet obstruction or gastric atony, but the key to revealing true mechanical obstruction or mucosal disease involves the use of upper endoscopy and/or barium studies. Peptic ulcer disease, pancreatic disease, or an upper tract malignancy can usually be defined and appropriately treated.

If mechanical obstruction is not present, more general disease states must be considered, and endocrine, neurologic (both central and peripheral), and more intensive psychiatric assessments are reasonable. At this point, therapeutic trials can be attempted, but if the patient's symptoms remain refractory, a thorough search for motility disorders is necessary.

Gastroparesis can be idiopathic or can occur secondary to drugs (anticholinergics, beta-adrenergic agents, opiates, tricyclic antidepressants). It is also seen after gastric surgery (e.g., after gastrectomy or vagotomy), in the diabetic patient, in metabolic disorders (e.g., acidosis, hypothyroidism), in connective tissue disease (primarily scleroderma), and in achlorhydric states, such as pernicious anemia. Disorders of gastric electrophysiology (dysrhythmias) have been reported in patients with unexplained nausea and vomiting, and upper tract symptoms can be seen in patients with classic irritable bowel syndrome.

While gastric manometry and electrophysiology studies can be obtained in some centers, radioisotope scanning is currently the most useful and available method for measuring both solid and liquid gastric emptying and is the test primarily relied upon to document emptying dysfunction.

Drug therapy for nausea and vomiting should always be aimed at the cause, if it can be delineated. Patients with symptomatic gastrointestinal upset from a labyrinthine source, i.e., motion sickness, can best be treated with *meclizine hydrochloride, diphenhydramine* preparations, *promethazine hydrochloride*, or *scopolamine* patches. Patients with immediate postoperative gastrointestinal distress often respond to *benzquinamide hydrochloride, prochlorperazine, trimethobenzamide hydrochloride, haloperidol* preparations, or to *phenothiazines*.

Patients receiving cancer chemotherapy develop severe nausea and vomiting both as a learned response prior to the actual administration of the drugs and, of course, secondary to the actual instillation of the noxious agents. The control of emesis in this case depends on the suppression of the peripheral and central pathways of emetogenesis and the chemoreceptor trigger zone. While prochlorperazine has been of little consistent use, particularly when the intensely emetogenic agent cisplatin is used, high-dose intravenous *metoclopramide* is useful in increasing the number of patients without vomiting at all. Further, intravenous *dexamethasone* has been found useful in controlling nausea and vomiting in these chemotherapy patients, and *tetrahydrocannabinol*, acting centrally, has been used with varying success.

In the postgastrectomy, postvagotomy patient with nausea and vomiting, the symptom complex may be due to either the disruption of motility or to bile reflux gastritis causing delayed emptying. Therapy with either prokinetic agents (discussed below) or with drugs such as cholestyramine, aluminum containing antacids, or sucralfate is reasonable. Bile reflux gastritis is discussed in a separate chapter.

The treatment of delayed gastric emptying without true mechanical obstruction deserves an additional note as the newer prokinetic agents are becoming more widely used. Metoclopramide, whose pharmacology has already been described, acts centrally as an antiemetic agent and peripherally to accelerate gastric emptying by increasing gastric tone and amplitude of the antral contractions. The drug also decreases relaxation of the proximal stomach, relaxes the pylorus and duodenal bulb, increases peristalsis in the duodenum and jejunum, and accelerates intestinal transit time from the duodenum to the ileocecal valve.

Domperidone is a benzimidazole derivative that is a specific dopamine antagonist. It stimulates the gastrointestinal tract and has antiemetic properties but does not readily cross the blood-brain barrier and rarely, if ever, causes extrapyramidal side effects. The usual dose of domperidone in various studies has ranged from 40 to 120 mg orally every day usually in four divided doses. While the oral form may be available soon in the United States, an intravenous preparation will not be pursued. The drug does have a potent effect on prolactin secretion, with other reported side effects including dry mouth, headache, and nervousness. While domperidone appears to be no better than metoclopramide as a prokinetic agent, its minimal side effects make it an attractive agent for long-term use, which can often be necessry in patients with diabetic gastroparesis or idiopathic gastric stasis. The drug may also be particularly useful in the treatment of the nausea and vomiting accompanying levodopa therapy for patients with Parkinson's disease, as it will not deplete central dopamine stores.

A mention of *naloxone* in the treatment of delayed gastric emptying should be made. The opiate peptides have been identified in the entire gastrointestinal tract, and it is well known that morphine has an inhibitory effect on gastric emptying which can be demonstrated by the systemic or intracerebroventricular administration of the gent. Naloxone is a potent opiate (mu) receptor antagonist and may be able to accelerate gastric emptying by antagonizing endogenous inhibitory peptides or by a direct effect on smooth muscle. While small isolated doses (2 mg via intravenous bolus) of naloxone may inhibit gastric emptying, sustained doses (1.6 mg subcutaneously daily) have been shown to markedly accelerate both solid emptying and small intestinal transit in a group of patients with intestinal pseudo-obstruction. Further studies on naloxone and its oral equivalent *naltrexene* are necessary.

A summary of the effective antinauseants/antiemetics currently available in the United States is presented in Table 2.

It is also important to note that there are multiple *behavioral strategies* for reducing nausea and vomiting. Hypnosis with guided imagery for relaxation, progressive muscle-relaxant training, multiple muscle-site electromyographic biofeedback, and system desensitization have all been used with some success. While these techniques have been primarily used in the anticipatory nausea seen in chemotherapy patients, their application, along with psychotherapy and counseling, may be extended to patients with functional nausea and vomiting.

If all attempts at symptomatic control fail, a trial of therapy with parenteral feeding may become necessary. Finally, the consideration of surgery involving a gastric bypass or drainage procedure is a difficult decision and lies beyond the scope of this chapter. There is a review of nausea and vomiting by Hanson and McCallum[4] and a discussion of unexplained vomiting by Malagelada and Canillieri[5].

HICCUPS

Hiccups, defined as the brief involuntary inspirations cut short by glottic closure, can be precipitated by many stimuli. While peripheral causes of persistent hiccups include gastric distention, intra-abdominal/diaphragmatic inflammation, and even tympanic membrane irritation, central causes encompass any central nervous system insult from infection to tumor. To complete the list, one should remember that intractable hiccups also occur in the setting of uremia and hyponatremia and also secondary to various drugs (e.g., Aldomet, diazepam, and sodium pentothal).

The management of hiccups is usually aimed at inhibiting or interrupting the irritated reflex arc. The traditional home remedies of gagging, breathing into a paper bag, ingesting granulated sugar, or drinking a glass of water while bending over head down are all worth a try. More complicated approaches include nasogastric intubation with gastric decompression, pharyngeal intubation, or high pressure O_2 inhalation.

Drug treatment with chlorpromazine (25 to 50 mg PO or IV) and metoclopramide (10 mg PO or IV) may be effective. Quinidine, atropine, amphetamines, and ephedrine have also been used. Hiccups are reviewed by Kaufman[6].

Eructation/Bloating

Excess upper gastrointestinal tract gas can result in repetitive and excessive eructation or complaints of upper abdominal bloating and pain. The gases involved in-

TABLE 2 Effective Antinauseant and Antiemetic Agents Available in United States

Phenothiazines (Prochlorperazine, Trifluoperazine)	
Mechanism:	Acts primarily through the chemoreceptor trigger zone and on the vomiting center itself
Adverse Effects:	Extrapyramidal reactions, drowsiness, dizziness, hypotension, hypersensitivity reactions, blood dyscrasias, gynecomastia, cholestatic jaundice
Dosage:	Trifluoperazine (Stelazine) 1–2 mg PO b.i.d./t.i.d. 1–2 mg IM b.i.d./t.i.d. Prochlorperazine (Compazine) 5–10 mg PO t.i.d./q.i.d. 1–2 mg IM t.i.d./q.i.d. 25 mg PO t.i.d./q.i.d. (as a suppository)
Butyrophenone (Haloperidol)	
Mechanism:	Acts as a dopamine antagonist and antagonizes the chemoreceptor trigger zone
Adverse Effects:	Marked extrapyramidal effects, insomnia, confusion, lethargy, decreased seizure threshold
Dosage:	Haloperidol (Haldol) 1–5 mg PO b.i.d./t.i.d. 2.5–5.0 mg IM with dose titrated for symptoms
Metoclopramide Hydrochloride	
Mechanism:	Dopaminergic antagonist and partial anticholinergic agent with both peripheral and central effects; increases antral contractions, increases jejunal and duodenal peristalsis, increases lower esophageal sphincter pressure
Adverse Effects:	Extrapyramidal reactions, sedation, restlessness, prolactin elevation, galactorrhea
Dosage:	Metoclopramide hydrochloride (Reglan) 10–20 mg PO ½ hr p.c. and q.h.s. 1–2 mg/kg IV ½ hr prior to treatment and then 22 hr × 3 (for cancer chemotherapy-induced emesis)
Trimethobenzamide Hydrochloride	
Mechanism:	Acts on chemoreceptor trigger zone; useful for postanaesthetic and postsurgical nausea/vomiting
Adverse Effects:	Extrapyramidal symptoms, hypersensitivity reactions
Dosage:	Trimethobenzamide hydrochloride (Tigan) 250 mg PO t.i.d./q.i.d. 200 mg IM t.i.d./q.i.d. 200 mg PO t.i.d./q.i.d. (as a suppository)
Benzquinamide Hydrochloride	
Mechanism:	Nonphenothiazine with antiemetic, antihistamine, and mild anticholinergic actions; primarily used for postsurgical nausea/vomiting
Adverse Effects:	Drowsiness, dry mouth, tremors, fatigue, blurred vision, sedation
Dosage:	Benzquinamide hydrochloride (Emete-Con) 50 mg IM × 1, then q1h × 1, then q3–4h p.r.n.
Promethazine Hydrochloride	
Mechanism:	Phenothiazine derivative with additional antihistamine activity
Adverse Effects:	Dry mouth, blurring of vision, dizziness
Dosage:	Promethazine hydrochloride (Phenergan) 12.5–25.0 mg PO/IM presurgery
Dimenhydrinate	
Mechanism:	Depresses hyperstimulated labyrinthine function; useful in motion sickness
Adverse Effects:	Drowsiness, dizziness, dry mouth
Dosage:	Dimenhydrinate (Dramamine) 50–100 mg PO q4h
Scopolamine	
Mechanism:	Belladonna alkaloid with anticholinergic effects; probably acts to prevent motion sickness nausea by inhibiting the vestibular input of the chemoreceptor trigger zone
Adverse Effects:	Dry mouth, difficulty urinating, acute narrow-angle glaucoma, disorientation, memory disturbances
Dosage:	Scopolamine (Transderm Scop) One disk applied cutaneously (4 hr prior to expected insult) then q3 days p.r.n.

clude O_2, N_2, H_2, CO_2, and CH_4, with their primary sources being swallowed air, gut production via chemical reactions or bacterial metabolism, or diffusion from the blood into the gut lumen.

Swallowed gas, primarily O_2 and N_2, can arise from gases trapped in foods, during ingestion of liquids or solids (particularly in the supine position), and via the nervous habit of swallowing or aspirating air (aerophagia). The latter can occur at any time but may be worse during times of stress. It may result from the actual gulping of air, but much of the problem in patients who complain of "belching" rests with the unconscious inhalation of air. It is thought to be an unconscious "sucking in" or actual "aspiration" of air at points during the day associated with an automatic and unconscious relaxation of the upper esophageal sphincter. This then causes esophageal distention and the resultant rejection of the air based on an esophageal burping mechanism; the net result is eructation. Studies have shown that such air does not actually end up in the stomach, but is expelled efficiently by the esophagus after it reaches different levels, probably quite proximal within the esophagus. This cycle falls into the realm of an unconscious nervous tendency and may be very difficult to treat.

Gas can be produced in the gut when gastric acids or fatty acids produced from lipid metabolism react with endogenously produced bicarbonate to produce CO_2. Further, intestinal bacteria can produce large amounts of H_2 from nonabsorbable carbohydrates, and gut anaerobes can produce significant quantities of CH_4. Gases can be removed from the gut via eructation, passage of flatus, metabolism by intestinal bacteria, or via diffusion back into the blood. Eructation, the primary focus of this discussion, may occur when the basal pressure of the lower esophageal sphincter (LES) is low, when a transient increase in intragastric pressure occurs, or during transient but complete LES relaxation associated with swallowing. Further, some transient relaxations may be nonswallow-related and can be precipitated by esophageal or gastric distention.

Most of the patients who complain of repetitive belching are simply expelling swallowed air that has lodged in the esophagus. Cycles of purposeful air swallowing to precipitate belching may occur in an effort to relieve any discomfort but only exacerbate the problem. The patient rarely recognizes this and instead views his problem as increased gas production from some digestive abnormality.

Nonetheless, ruling out true organic abdominal or thoracic disease is necessary in many cases. Gastric outlet obstruction of any origin can result in trapped air and belching. Foul-smelling belching may be seen in patients with gastric bezoars. Milk/carbohydrate intolerance will usually not result in excessive upper tract gas but may be useful to investigate. Finally, we have seen severe eructation in diabetics with gastric stasis and have also seen complaints of abdominal bloating and belching in patients with small bowel overgrowth and in achlorhydric patients. Beyond the use of prokinetic agents, the use of ingested acids to minimize bacterial colonization has proved useful.

If true disease is not found, treatment is often difficult. For the patient with excessive eructation, the ingestion of hot water is a home remedy with variable results. The beneficial effect of simethicone, 40 to 80 mg orally four times a day, is also poorly documented. Acting as a surfactant, this agent may break up air bubbles but probably does little to the resulting gas released. Charcoal has been widely presented as an absorber of gas, but again, controlled studies on proven gastric gas diminution or a significant clinical effect on eructation are lacking. Metoclopramide and the newer prokinetic agents may be of some use in patients with complaints of bloating where there is really no evidence that they actually have excessive intestinal gas, but there is evidence that they tolerate the gas present poorly and/or could have slow gastric emptying. The patient should also be alerted to the fact that his complaints may be related to excessive air swallowing and, although bothersome, are benign. The patient should avoid reclining after meals and may benefit from a low-fat, low-nonabsorbable carbohydrate, low-lactose diet. Behavioral training is evidently of some help in patients with minimal symptoms but rarely helps those with severe complaints.

RUMINATION

Rumination is a process whereby food is transferred from the stomach to the mouth, usually within 15 to 20 minutes after ingestion. Some of the food is chewed and reswallowed while some is ejected from the mouth. The act itself can either be involuntary, or voluntary with some patients actually putting their fingers down their throats or contracting their abdominal muscles to bring the food into their mouths.

Ruminators tend to be young patients, some younger than 17, with the onset of symptoms often becoming apparent by age 10 or younger. The patients usually seek medical evaluation on the advice of concerned family members who are either repelled by the habit or fear a more severe, more widespread problem. While the young ruminators tend to downplay the disorder and appear quite cheerful, the adult ruminators can often be depressed and anxious.

The possible association of significant regurgitation and vomiting in infants and rumination later on in the young adult is an interesting but totally unproven one. It is felt that gastroesophageal reflux in infancy is transient between the ages of 6 months and 2 to 3 years and that a resolution usually occurs over time. Infants with severe problems can present with either failure to thrive or pulmonary complications, and we have reported a delay in gastric emptying of liquid formula in this group which apparently improves with time.

We have been intrigued by the possibility of anatomic defects being present in the population of young adult and adult patients with rumination. While LES pressure measurements have been normal in this group, it is possible that some impairment of the angle of His or in the gastric sling fibers could lead to a failed valve mechanism and free reflux. These patients often present to the gstroenterologist for the evaluation of reflux disease, but true complaints of heartburn are rare. Further, despite the long duration of presumed rumination, complicating problems of weight loss, aspiration, coughing, or nocturnal regurgitation are usually absent. While pH studies of the esophagus can show an acid milieu during the events of reflux, motility studies and endoscopy are usually normal and gastric emptying studies have shown normal or even rapid emptying rather than delayed rates. We have actually recommended fundoplication of the gastroesophageal junction in one patient in whom the volume and social embarrassment of the problem were not acceptable. The outcome was successful, and this should be kept in mind as a last resort.

Other approaches include psychotherapy and mechanical restraints, including a device known as a "ruminator cap" which keeps the patient's jaws shut when placed postprandially, plugging the nostrils, or restraining the arms so that self-gagging cannot be carried out. The passage of time and reassurance of patient and family that a disease process is not being missed and that severe complications do not occur play an important role.

ABDOMINAL EPILEPSY

Abdominal epilepsy is a rare cause of abdominal pain in children and young adults. The criteria for diagnosis include intermittent abdominal pain of unknown cause associated with occasional alterations of mental status during the attacks, an abnormal EEG, and a response to anticonvulsant therapy.

The pains are often periumbilical, are described as sudden in onset, and can last from minutes to hours. The patients can complain of nausea and vomiting during the attacks and there are reports of altered consciousness and postattack fatigue.

While the EEG abnormalities seen in these patients are somewhat nonspecific, generalized slow wave dysrhythmia and paroxysmal 6 and 14 per second positive spikes seem the most prominent findings. Sleep studies may be necessary for case detection.

Whether anticonvulsants such as phenytoin (Dilantin, 300 mg orally daily) or phenobarbitol (90 mg orally daily) control the reported pain centrally or peripherally is unknown. there have been no studies evaluating the effect of Dilantin on either gastrointestinal motility or disorders in which an abnormal gastrointestinal electrical rhythm is suspected. The one study of Dilantin in irritable bowel syndrome showed it to be more effective than placebo. Occasionally a teenager with unrecognized lactose intolerance may present with recurrent abdominal pain. Zarling has published a review of abdominal epilepsy[7].

REFERENCES

1. Malagelada J–R, Stanghellini V. Manometric evaluation of functional upper gut symptoms. Gastroenterology 1985; 88:1223.
2. Lagarde SP, Spiro HM. Non-ulcer dyspepsia. Clin Gastro 1984; 13:347.
3. Petersen H. Further investigations and treatment of non-ulcer dyspepsia. Scand J Gastro 1982; 17 (Suppl 72):130.
4. Hanson JS, McCallum RW. The diagnosis and management of nausea and vomiting: a review. Am J Gastro 1985; 80:210.
5. Malagelada J–R, Canillieri M. Unexplained vomiting: a diagnostic challenge. Ann Int Med 1984; 101:211.
6. Kaufman HJ. Hiccups: causes, mechanisms, and treatment. Pract Gastro 1985; 9:12.
7. Zarling EJ. Abdominal epilepsy: an unusual cause of recurrent abdominal pain. Am J Gastro 1984; 79:681.

OBESITY

THOMAS POZEFSKY, M.D.

The physician is justifiably concerned with the overweight patient when the degree of obesity is sufficient of itself to constitute a physical health hazard, or when a coexisting medical condition, such as diabetes or hypertension, is exacerbated by the increased weight. While such physical health considerations should and frequently do motivate the obese patient to attempt weight reduction, this is not always the case. Very commonly patients are motivated simply by unhappiness with their appearance. To them their weight constitutes a "mental health" hazard; and, of course, the patient's psychological well-being is also the physician's legitimate concern. Achieving and maintaining weight loss is a difficult and lifelong undertaking. To facilitate this process it is important for the physician to provide or reinforce motivation by clearly defining the physical health benefits to be derived from weight reduction, by understanding the patient's objectives (even when cosmetic), by helping to define realistic weight goals, by providing a specific diet plan, and by empathizing with the patient's ongoing struggle to deny himself food.

INITIAL EVALUATION

The primary purposes of the initial history, physical examination, and laboratory evaluation are self-evident. Onset and progression of the weight problem are characterized, the degree of obesity is quantified, the presence of underlying genetic or endocrine-metabolic disease of etiologic significance is sought, and symptoms or disease processes complicating the obesity and potentially ameliorated by weight reduction are identified (Table 1). Details of the initial physical examination should not be compromised. Obese patients frequently view themselves as metabolically abnormal, capable of gaining weight while consuming no more, and often fewer, calories than those around them. Consequently, confidence in the physician and the therapeutic program can be jeopardized if the clinical evaluation is viewed as too superficial to detect underlying metabolic disease. In this context it is useful to ask the question: "Why do you think you are overweight?" Some will frankly assume responsibility by acknowledging overeating (even binging), or lack of exercise. Others will respond in metabolic terms, and it is these patients who must come away from the initial examination feeling that their "metabolism" has been adequately evaluated. It is likely that patients with the "metabolic mentality" are more inclined to seek therapy from an internist, endocrinologist, or related subspecialist, while those who frankly acknowledge overeating gravitate toward more psychiatrically oriented programs.

Just as obesity can be caused by and/or lead to abnormalities in the patient's physical health, so it can be caused by and result in psychiatric disturbance. In such patients overeating is often stimulated by anxiety, depression, boredom, fatigue, and cravings rather than by hunger. It is estimated that binging (complete loss of control over food intake) occurs in one-half to two-thirds of overweight patients. Desperate attempts to prevent weight gain include the induction of vomiting and the abuse of diuretics and laxatives. Not only depressed by their weight, such patients are mortified by their inability to control such a fundamental biologic activity as food intake. The whole problem takes on the character of a substance abuse, and as such, it is obvious that there must be a psychologically oriented component to the evaluation and management of these patients. The evaluation outlined in Table 1 does not adequately define the psychological dimension. Most internists (and gastroenterologists) are not comfortable doing a detailed psychologic assessment. Yet sensitivity to this aspect of the problem is important in establishing rapport with the patient. As outlined later in this discussion, it may be wise at some point in the therapeutic program to collaborate with a behavioral psychologist in undertaking a formal analysis of eating behavior. One explanation for the poor overall results of nutrition-metabolism oriented programs on one hand and behavior oriented pro-

TABLE 1 Initial Evaluation of the Obese Patient

Onset and Progression	*Etiology*	*Complications*
History:		
Age at onset and first diet Weight at high school graduation, college graduation, marriage, discharge from service, after deliveries, menopause, one year ago Success of previous efforts (diet clubs, physician supervised diets, personal diets, use of diet pills): amount of weight lost, how long sustained Lowest, highest adult weight and "typical" weight last 5–10 years	Symptoms of: Hypothyroidism Hypogonadism Polycystic ovary Hypoglycemia Intracranial mass Depression Anxiety Family history of obesity Use of antidepressants Exercise level	Symptoms of: Diabetes Hypertension Congestive heart failure Pickwickian syndrome Sleep-apnea Degenerative joint disease Gout Gallstones Esophageal reflux Menstrual irregularity
Physical Examination:		
Height Weight Wrist circumference*	Slow reflexes, goiter Striae, buffalo hump, central fat distribution Hirsutism Small testes Papilledema Retinitis pigmentosa, polydactyly (Bardet-Biedl syndrome) Hypotonia, mental retardation (Prader-Willi syndrome)	Hypertension Right upper quadrant tenderness Varicose veins, phlebitis Asterixis, facial rubor, somnolence Intertrigo Joint tenderness or deformity
Laboratory Tests†:		
	Thyroxine, TSH 24-hr urine free cortisol Testosterone, FSH and LH Androstenedione CT scan of head	HDL and LDL cholesterol Triglyceride Blood sugar, GTT Blood gases, spirogram Roentgenograms of back, knees, hips Uric acid Gallbladder sonogram

* Used to calculate body frame size (see text and Table 2).

† A minimum laboratory evaluation includes a CBC, urinalysis, spirogram, EKG, chest film, serum thyroxine, multichannel blood analysis (glucose, creatinine, electrolytes, uric acid, liver function studies), triglycerides, and HDL and total cholesterol.

grams on the other is that both disciplines are required for the proper management of practically all patients.

FIRST RETURN VISIT

Discussion of Results

The purpose of the first return visit is to review the findings of the initial evaluation and present the specifics of the diet program to the patient. In most instances the obesity is found not to be secondary to an identifiable underlying disease process. Consequently, it should be made clear that the principal component of the weight control program will be restriction of food intake. One need not directly contradict those patients who perceive themselves to be metabolically abnormal. It is fair to tell them that medical researchers have identified several metabolic and hormonal differences between obese and thin people. However, as these differences disappear when the obese patient loses weight, they are the result rather than the cause of obesity. The patient's perception of a primary metabolic error may be correct, but since the error has thus far escaped detection, control of food intake must be the basic therapeutic approach. An increase in fat cell number is associated with early onset obesity and persists despite weight reduction. The significance of this finding in terms of ability to lose weight and maintain weight loss is speculative, although long-term success is poorest in those with obesity of adolescent or preadolescent onset.

Coexistent risk factors identified in the patient and known to be responsive to weight reduction (hyperglycemia, hypertriglyceridemia, increased low-density lipoprotein, cholesterol, decreased high-density lipoprotein cholesterol, and hypertension) should be discussed. Physical conditions complicating obesity and their potential response to weight reduction require elaboration. All this serves to reinforce whatever motivation the patient brings to the process.

Set Weight Goals

At this point weight goals should be discussed. Body frame size is estimated from the ratio of height to wrist circumference (Table 2). Ideal body weight is determined from the Metropolitan Life Insurance Company table (Table 3) as the midpoint of the ideal weight range for a given height and frame size. Percent overweight is the ratio of the patient's actual weight to his ideal weight. A weight greater than 120 percent of ideal shortens life expectancy even in the absence of coexistent risk factors. Such patients are considered obese. Patients 110 to 120 percent of ideal are considered overweight.

The initial objective should be to decrease weight to 120 percent of ideal. When this is achieved, risk factors and residual physical symptoms can be reassessed as a guide to further weight reduction. In the patient without risk factors or physical symptoms who is within 120 percent of ideal, the need for weight reduction lies in the psychological sphere. Cosmetic considerations are usually paramount, and the patient must suggest the weight goal. The role of the physician is to be sure the desired weight is not inappropriately low as gauged both by the patient's weight history and the ideal weight range indicated in Table 3.

TABLE 3 Ideal Body Weight According to Sex and Height*

Height Feet	Height Inches	Small Frame	Medium Frame	Large Frame
		Men		
5	2	128–134	131–141	138–150
5	3	130–136	133–143	140–153
5	4	132–138	135–145	142–156
5	5	134–140	137–148	144–160
5	6	136–142	139–151	146–164
5	7	138–145	142–154	149–168
5	8	140–148	145–157	152–172
5	9	142–151	148–160	155–176
5	10	144–154	151–163	158–180
5	11	146–157	154–166	161–184
6	0	149–160	157–170	164–188
6	1	152–164	160–174	168–192
6	2	155–168	164–178	172–197
6	3	158–172	167–182	176–202
6	4	162–176	171–187	181–207
		Women		
4	10	102–111	109–121	118–131
4	11	103–113	111–123	120–134
5	0	104–115	113–126	122–137
5	1	106–118	115–129	125–140
5	2	108–121	118–132	128–143
5	3	111–124	121–135	131–147
5	4	114–127	124–138	134–151
5	5	117–130	127–141	137–155
5	6	120–133	130–144	140–159
5	7	123–136	133–147	143–163
5	8	126–139	136–150	146–167
5	9	129–142	139–153	149–170
5	10	132–145	142–156	152–173
5	11	135–148	145–158	155–176
6	0	138–151	148–162	158–179

* Weights at ages 25 to 59 based on lowest mortality. Weights are in pounds, in indoor clothing weighing 5 pounds in men and 3 pounds in women, and shoes with 1 inch heels. Metropolitan Life Insurance Company, 1983. (Source of basic data, 1979 Build Study Society of Actuaries and Association of Life Insurance Medical Directors of America, 1980.)

General Principles of the Diet

The patient must now be told what to eat. The only imperative in the design of a diet is that it be hypocaloric. The balanced low calorie diet recommended by most nutritionists and diet clubs, and typified by the American Diabetes Association exchange list diet, is widely used. Its attractiveness follows from its nutritional adequacy (except for calories), and from the flexibility it gives patients in food selection. Theoretically, it can be followed indefinitely, with minor upward adjustments in calorie intake when the patient achieves his weight goal. Unfortunately, fewer than 30 percent of patients following a balanced low calorie diet lose more than 20 pounds; fewer than 5 percent lose more than 40 pounds. Hence, this diet rarely has a significant impact on the more obese patient who is of greatest medical concern. It is precisely the diet's variety that appears to be at fault. The overweight patient needs rigidity rather than flexibility—the fewer choices the better. He has already demonstrated an inability to make appropriate food selections, and prefers explicit guidance by the physician. Beyond this, poor control over the intake of certain specific foods appears to be characteristic of many very obese patients. These foods are generally rich in carbohydrate and sweet (chocolate, ice cream, Coca-Cola, cookies, cake), "starchy" but not sweet (bread, pasta, crackers, pizza), or salty and crunchy (chips, pretzels). The small amounts of such foods permitted on the balanced low calorie diet stimulate overeating just as small quantities of alcohol in the diet of the

TABLE 2 Estimation of Frame Size from the Ratio of Height to Wrist Circumference*

Frame Size	Male	Female
Small	> 10.4	> 11.0
Medium	9.6–10.4	10.1–11.0
Large	< 9.6	< 10.1

* Height (inches); wrist circumference (inches)

alcoholic lead to its overindulgence. Consequently, although the low calorie diet makes sense nutritionally, it may not behaviorally.

One reason for surprisingly good initial adherence to the protein-supplemented modified fast by very obese patients and accompanying large weight losses is the removal of all food choices, including binge stimulators. The central problem with the protein-supplemented modified fast is that patients living exclusively on this synthetic diet do not learn how to control the intake of real food during the period of weight loss. When appetizing foods are finally reintroduced (as eventually they must), control is lost and weight regained. On theoretical grounds a diet that is very restrictive intially, giving the patient few choices and eliminating potential binge stimulators (particularly carbohydrate), would seem best. As weight is lost and the patient gains confidence in his control over food intake, flexibility in the form of food choices can be introduced, variety increased, and the diet balanced nutritionally. Aggressive dieting is particularly well suited to the very overweight patient who, while losing some weight with previous dieting efforts, may never have reached an acceptable weight goal. Rapid weight loss strongly reinforces the patient's dieting effort. He can, perhaps for the first time, anticipate success in realizing goal weight in months rather than years.

In behaviorally oriented weight control programs rigid diet is usually scrupulously avoided. A limit on total caloric intake may be the only nutritional recommendation (e.g., 1,200 kcal for women, 1,500 kcal for men). The emphasis instead is on eating behavior. The therapist's presumption is that the more rigid the diet, the more likely is deviation to occur along with the attendant risk that the first "cheat" will beget a second, and ultimately a binge ("I've already blown it so what's the difference what I eat?"). This concern is real, but has to be balanced against the fact that the dieter initially is well motivated and often can follow a rigid diet for relatively long periods of time as experience with large resultant weight losses as experienced with the protein-supplemented modified fast has shown. Failure to capitalize on this opportunity may jeopardize the obese patient's chance to lose enough weight to make a difference physically and psychologically, and thereby to provide the motivation necessary to maintain weight loss. Weight reduction has amounted to only 10 to 15 pounds on average in programs that are exclusively behaviorally oriented. Obviously, when a rigid diet of the type described below is prescribed, the physician must be alert to the potential for binges induced by excessive rigidity, and be prepared to respond to transgressions by increasing flexibility.

Semistarvation

Diets are outlined in Tables 4 through 6 that meet the needs of virtually all adult patients. (The nutritional composition of each diet is given in Table 7). The highly motivated individual who is grossly overweight (for example, a man with more than 65 pounds to lose or a woman with more than 45 pounds to lose) can be started on a semistarvation regimen of calorie-free fluids and vegetable salads for a week (see Table 4). Since carbohydrate intake is substantially below 100 g per day, ketosis develops; ketosis suppresses the appetite in many patients. Urine ketones are monitored by the physician as a check on compliance. The patient can also monitor urinary ketones and, having been told that this is an index of massive fat breakdown and utilization, is reinforced in the dieting effort. After initiation of the diet, brief office visits are set up weekly. Foods of low carbohydrate content are added on a weekly or biweekly basis as indicated in Table 4 and discussed below in the section Follow-Up Visits. Carbohydrate-containing foods are cautiously added as goal weight is approached. Within a few pounds of weight goal greater flexibility is introduced by the addition of a fixed number of calories daily (e.g., 150 kcal for women, 200 kcal for men). The specific food choices are left to the dieter with instructions to avoid foods traditionally poorly controlled. The anticipated rate of weight loss is greater the higher the initial weight , and is greater in men than women of the same weight. Males over 250 pounds can expect to lose 45 pounds or more in the first ten weeks. For females over 200 pounds the anticipated weight loss in the same time frame is 25 pounds or more.

Despite the aggressiveness of this approach, side effects are few and easily managed. Postural lightheadedness due to salt and water loss is the most common complaint and can be controlled by salt supplementation. Insomnia responds to a mild hypnotic, headache to over-the-counter analgesics. Hyperuricemia routinely occurs because of competition between uric acid and ketones for excretion by the renal tubules. Gouty arthritis is infrequent, mild, and responds to Indocin or colchicine. If there is a prior history of uric acid elevation, gout, or uric acid stones, a 24-hour urine collection to measure uric acid excretion should be obtained before and after the first week of dieting. Hyperuricosuria which increases as a result of the diet mandates a different dietary approach. Ketogenic diets are contraindicated during pregnancy because of potential harm to the developing fetal central nervous system.

Low Calorie Ketogenic Diet

When lesser amounts of weight are to be lost (25 to 65 pounds for men, 20 to 45 pounds for women), or for the larger patient who rejects the semistarvation approach as "too radical," a ketogenic diet as outlined in Table 5 may be used. Food intake initially is equivalent to that reached after about 8 weeks of dieting by the semistarvation method described above. Because carbohydrate intake is very limited ketosis will develop, but ketonemia and ketonuria are less intense, as is the attendant dehydration. Patients are seen every 10 to 14 days, and noncarbohyrate-containing foods are added as shown in Table 5 (and further elaborated in the section Follow-Up Visits). Ultimately, as goal weight is approached, specific carbohydrate-containing foods are cautiously added, followed by the introduction of greater flexibility in food

TABLE 4 Semistarvation Diet*

Week 1: Unlimited fluids include coffee, tea, club soda (or Perrier), and water. Minimum of 48 oz water required. Six oz skim milk to "lighten" coffee or tea. Unlimited unsweetened lime or lemon juice (to make lime- or lemonade). Artificial sweetener (saccharin, aspartame). Three 8-oz cups of salad (four cups for men) using lettuce, tomato, celery, cucumber, radish, green pepper, mushroom, onion, and carrot. Unlimited diet dressing (up to 25 kcal/tbsp) or vinegar and lemon. Seasonings (including salt), herbs, and spices. Supplemental multivitamin (Theragran-M), potassium (50 mEq as Kaylite), calcium (400 mg as two Tums), and if postural lightheadedness develops, 3–5 g salt (Thermogram).

Week 2: Boiled or steamed vegetables, such as string beans, asparagus, broccoli, cauliflower, brussels sprouts, zucchini, spinach, eggplant, cabbage, may be substituted for salads.† Add unlimited diet sodas.

Week 3: Add 3½ oz can of water packed tuna fish (7 oz can for men). Add 2 cups bouillon (Lipton Trim).

Week 4: May substitute 3½ oz cooked weight (7 oz for men) of poultry, fish, or shellfish for tuna fish if desired.

Week 5: Add an egg (2 eggs for men). If scrambled or fried use Pam or Teflon pan.

Week 6: Add 1 tbsp diet mayonnaise or margarine.

Week 7: Add 6 oz 1% fat cottage cheese (8 oz for men). The carbohydrate in cottage cheese will reduce the degree of ketosis.

Week 8: Increase chicken, fish, or shellfish allotment to 6 oz (9 oz for men). Veal or liver may also be included.

Week 9: Add 1 oz hard cheese (cheddar, Swiss, American, etc.) or 2 oz low-fat hard cheese (Lite-Line).

Week 10: May substitute beef, lamb, or pork for poultry, fish, shellfish, veal, or liver, but only twice a week (3 times a week for men).

Weeks 11 and thereafter: No additions until the patient is 20 pounds from goal weight (25 pounds for men), or until weight begins to plateau. Then add 1 fruit selection (2 for men) from fruit list below.‡ This probably will terminate ketosis.

10 Pounds from Goal Weight (15 pounds for men): Add either a small baked potato, ½ cup (boiled and drained) rice, beans, or corn, or 2 thin slices bread (e.g., Hollywood bread).

5 Pounds from Goal Weight (8 pounds for men): Add a fixed number of calories of the patient's choice, avoiding binge triggering foods. The number of calories added depends on the concurrent rate of weight loss but might be 150 kcal per day (200 kcal per day for men). If weight loss is rapid, a greater number of calories may be added.

* The schedule of food additions, in terms of amount and timing, can be viewed as flexible. Physician initiated alterations in the precise amount of food added and the timing of additions should conform to the overall strategy of adding as little as possible consistent with the patient's capacity to comply, and avoiding carbohydrate containing foods (particularly potential binge stimulators) until goal weight is approached. Daily rations are shown unless otherwise stated.

† Other vegetables (cooked or raw) that may be included are bean sprouts, beet greens, chard, chicory, collard greens, dill pickles, dandelion greens, escarole, kale, mustard greens, okra, sauerkraut, summer squash, watercress, and wax beans.

‡ Fruit list (unsweetened if canned, or fresh):

Apple (2-in diameter)	1	Figs (dried)	1 small	Papaya	⅓ medium
Applesauce	½ cup	Fruit cocktail	½ cup	Peach	1 medium
Apricots (fresh)	2 medium	Grapefruit	½ small	Pear	1 small
Apricots (dried)	4 halves	Grapefruit juice	½ cup	Pineapple	½ cup
Blackberries, raspberries, strawberries	1 cup	Grapes	12	Pineapple juice	⅓ cup
Blueberries	⅔ cup	Grape juice	¼ cup	Plums	2 medium
Cantaloupe (6-in diameter)	½	Guava	1 small	Prunes	2
Cherries	10 large	Honeydew (7-in diameter)	¼	Raisins	2 tbsp
Cider	⅓ cup	Mango	½ small	Relish	2 tbsp
Dates	2	Nectarine	1 medium	Tangerine	1 large
Figs (fresh)	2 large	Orange	1 small	Watermelon	3×1×½-in slice
		Orange juice	½ cup		

selection by the addition of a fixed number of calories daily. The specific food choices to be left to the dieter. Weight loss in the first 10 weeks is about 30 pounds for men, 15 to 20 pounds for women. Side effects are insignificant, although hyperuricemia and hyperuricosuria are potential problems.

Balanced Low Calorie Diet

A balanced diet of 1,200 kcal and 150 g of carbohydrate daily is shown in Table 6. It can be used for women with less than 20 pounds of weight to lose and, in slightly liberalized form, (1,500 kcal and 170 g of carbohydrate daily) for men with less than 25 pounds to lose. While carbohydrate is present in the form of fruit, some starchy vegetables, and bread, the patient's choices are still limited and most of the binge provoking foods mentioned previously are excluded. Because carbohydrate intake exceeds 100 g per day, ketosis does not develop. Patients are seen every 10 to 14 days initially for the addition of specific foods, then for the introduction of greater flexibility in food selection by the addition of a fixed number of calories daily.

Body Measurements

Although the patient's total caloric intake may vary only slightly from week to week, the rate of weight loss will not be constant. This is explained largely by variations in the state of hydration. For example, fluid retention may follow for a day after a meal of high sodium content; and in women it may occur simply on a cyclic basis. Concomitant fat loss can thereby be obscured. Nothing is more frustrating to the dieter than a week of no weight loss or even weight gain despite diligent dieting. In this setting patients often comment on an apparent loosening of their clothes despite the absence of weight loss. This is because fat loss leads to a reduction in certain body dimensions which are unaffected by the retention of fluid. Reductions in body dimensions can be quantified and knowledge of them will help sustain moti-

TABLE 5 Low Calorie Ketogenic Diet

Initial Diet:*

Breakfast: Cup of bouillon (Lipton Trim).
One egg (two for men). If scrambled or fried use Pam or Teflon pan.

Lunch: One 8-oz cup of vegetable salad (two for men). Use lettuce, tomato, celery, cucumber, radish, green pepper, mushroom, onion, and carrot. Unlimited diet dressing (up to 25 kcal/tbsp) or vinegar and lemon.
6 oz 1% fat cottage cheese (8 oz for men).

Supper: One Lipton Cup of Soup.
5 oz cooked weight (8 oz for men) poultry, fish, or shellfish (boiled, baked, broiled, or steamed).
One 8-oz cup of vegetable salad with dressing (two for men), see lunch above; or one 8-oz cup (two for men) of boiled or steamed vegetables such as string beans, asparagus, broccoli, cauliflower, brussel sprouts, eggplant, zucchini, spinach, and cabbage.†

Bedtime: One 8-oz cup of vegetable salad with dressing or cooked vegetables (two for men) as described above.

Fluids: Unlimited fluids include water, black coffee, tea (with or without lemon), club soda, diet sodas, and unsweetened lime and lemon juice (to make lime- or lemonade). Six oz skim milk to "lighten" coffee or tea.

Other: Seasonings, spices, herbs, and artificial sweetener.
1 tbsp diet mayonnaise or margarine. Supplemental multivitamin (Theragran-M), potassium (50 mEq as Kaylite), calcium (400 mg as 2 Tums), and if postural lightheadedness develops, 3–5 g salt (Thermogram).

Changes at 10 to 14 Day Intervals:

Increase poultry, fish, and shellfish allotment to 7 oz (10 oz for men).
Substitute beef, lamb, pork, veal, or liver for poultry, fish, or shellfish twice a week (3 times a week for men).
Add 1 light beer, 6 oz dry wine, or 1½ oz liquor.
Add 1 oz hard cheese (cheddar, Swiss, American, etc.) or 2 oz low-fat hard cheese (Lite-Line). For men, 2 oz of any hard cheese may be added.

10 Pounds from Goal (15 for Men):

Add 1 fruit from the fruit list (see Table 4, third footnote). For men add 2 fruits.

5 Pounds from Goal (8 for Men):

Add either a small baked potato, ½ cup (boiled and drained) rice, beans, or corn, or 2 thin slices bread (e.g., Hollywood bread).

Within a Few Pounds of Goal:

Add a fixed number of calories of the patient's choice, avoiding binge triggering foods. The number of calories added depends on the concurrent rate of weight loss but might be 150 kcal per day (200 kcal per day for men). If weight loss is rapid, more calories may be added.

* Although the specific foods are divided into three meals and a bedtime snack, this is for convenience only. The patient may change the timing and sequence of foods to accommodate his life style.

† Other vegetables (cooked or raw) that may be included are listed in Table 4, second footnote.

vation. The following body dimensions should be measured by the patient (undressed) at the start of the diet, and before each subsequent visit: bust (or chest), waist, hips, thigh (at the level of the pubic symphysis), and upper arm (largest circumference). From the behavioral viewpoint, the initial prediet data may so mortify the patient as to underscore the need to lose weight. As time goes on, careful measurements keep the patient in better touch with bodily change than weight which is, after all, only an abstraction. Other factors which contribute to variations in weekly weight loss include the drop in basal metabolic rate which occurs within the first two weeks of dieting, variations in exercise, and differences in the weight of clothing and of bladder, bowel, and stomach contents at the time of weigh-ins.

FOLLOW-UP VISITS

Brief follow-up visits should be scheduled weekly for patients dieting most aggressively (semistarvation), and at intervals of 10 to 14 days for the remainder. These continue until goal weight is achieved. The interval between visits is then lengthened to 3 weeks or longer if weight is well maintained. The ultimate objective is to have the patient managing independently. The entire process often extends beyond a year. The purposes of these follow-up visits are to measure weight change, to determine urine ketones semiquantitatively (when a ketogenic diet has been recommended), to record changes in body dimensions, to make food additions as shown in Tables 4 through 6, to treat physical complaints to introduce other important behavioral components such as diet diary keeping and exercise, and to respond sympathetically to the emotional stresses incident to giving up food and losing weight. The physician is viewed as an authority figure and his or her personal approval is important to the dieter. Success should be commended. The patient who is doing poorly will be depressed and guilt-ridden and sees the physician as impatient, critical, and disapproving. Inevitably these projections are partly true. Nevertheless, encouragement is the appropriate response to the dieter who slips! An unkind word from a frustrated physician can make follow-up visits more painful for the patient and lead to his dropping out of the weight control program.

The Diet Diary

The diet diary is a powerful behavioral tool for helping patients regain control over food intake. At the second or third follow-up visit the dieter is asked to record the foods eaten and their estimated caloric content immediately after each meal. He then calculates total daily calorie intake. At subsequent follow-up visits the calorie total for each day is reported to the physician, who notes high values indicating loss of control. The foods eaten and the specific reasons for overeating on these days should be discussed briefly. In this way the physician can develop a feeling for the circumstances surrounding overeating. The average daily calorie intake for the 1- to 2-week period between visits is then calculated and recorded. Diary keeping may be further refined by having the patient record carbohydrate intake as well to scrutinize the in-

TABLE 6 Balanced Low Calorie Diet

Initial Diet*:

Breakfast (select 1 or 2)

Breakfast 1

One fruit (see Table 4, third footnote).
One cup cereal (bran or corn flakes, puffed rice or wheat, oatmeal or farina).
8 oz skim milk

Breakfast 2

One fruit.
One egg (two for men). If scrambled or fried use Pam or Teflon pan.
One thin slice bread (two for men), e.g., Hollywood bread.
One tsp butter or margarine or 1 tbsp cream cheese or Neufchatel cheese.

Lunch: One fruit
One 8-oz cup of vegetable salad (two for men). Use lettuce, tomato, celery, cucumber, radish, green pepper, mushroom, onion, and carrot. Unlimited diet dressing (up to 25 kcal/tbsp) or vinegar and lemon.
Select either A,B, or C
A. 6 oz 1% fat cottage cheese (8 oz for men) *or* 3 oz farmer cheese (4 oz for men) *or* 1½ oz mozzarella, ricotta, feta, parmesan, or Lite-Line cheese (2 oz for men)
B. 2 eggs, if scrambled or fried use Pam or a Teflon pan
C. 3½ oz shellfish, or water packed tuna fish.

Supper: One fruit.
One Lipton Cup of Soup
5 oz cooked weight of poultry, fish, veal, or liver (8 oz for men), or 7 oz shellfish (9 oz for men).
A starchy vegetable or bread (select 1): Either a small baked potato, a small ear of corn, ½ cup of rice or beans, 2 thin slices bread, 4 melba toast, or 6 saltines.
One 8-oz cup of salad (two for men) as described for lunch, or an equivalent amount of boiled or steamed vegetables. Use string beans, broccoli, asparagus, cauliflower, brussel sprouts, eggplant, zucchini, spinach, or cabbage.†
2 tbsp of sour cream, or 1 tsp of butter, margarine, or mayonnaise.

Fluids: Unlimited fluids include water, black coffee, tea (with or without lemon), club soda, diet sodas, bouillon (Lipton Trim), and unsweetened lime and lemon juice (to make lime- or lemonade). Six oz skim milk to "lighten" coffee or tea. 6 oz of tomato or V8 juice.

Other: Seasonings, spices, herbs, and artificial sweetener. Supplemental mulivitamin (Theragran-M).

Changes at 10 to 14 Day Intervals:

Substitute 5 oz beef, lamb, or pork (8 oz for men) for poultry, fish, shellfish, veal, or liver twice a week (3 times a week for men).
Add 1 light beer, 6 oz dry wine, or 1½ oz liquor.
Add a second starchy vegetable selection from the supper list.
Add a fixed number of calories of the patient's choice when the dieter is within 5 pounds of goal weight. Avoid binge triggering foods. The number of calories added depends on the rate of weight loss but might be 150 kcal per day (200 kcal per day for men). If weight loss is rapid more calories may be added.

* Although the specific foods are divided into three meals and a bedtime snack, this is for convenience only. The patient may change the timing and sequence of foods to accommodate his life style.
† Other vegetables (cooked or raw) that may be included are listed in Table 4, second footnote.

take of foods over which control may be poor. Behavioral psychologists ask for a detailed description of the setting in which food is consumed and the feeling states surrounding food ingestion. Discussions of this material are time consuming and generally beyond the scope of the internist or gastroenterologist and are best left to those specifically trained in this area.

Beyond helping the patient and physician to understand the causes of overeating, the diet diary is of value in other important respects. First, the recording of food intake is a "consciousness raising" experience that serves to discourage deviations from the diet. The principle that the act of observation itself alters behavior appears to apply in the behavioral sphere as it does in the physical sciences. The patient is embarrassed to present a diary replete with "cheats" to the physician. Far more important, the dieter is uncomfortable confronting his own lack of control. While some will fabricate information, most see this as pointless, particularly if the physician takes the information seriously and uses it as a basis for discussion at follow-up visits. Rather, resistance takes the form of not having the data, along with attendant excuses (e.g., "It was too time-consuming." "I simply forgot." "It was lost." "I ate out frequently and didn't know how the foods were prepared."). Second, the patient acquires valuble nutritional information. Many are surprised at the high caloric content of the foods they had not considered "fattening." A patient's frustrating and self-defeating perception of an intrinsic metabolic defect as the explanation for his obesity may thus be altered. Third, an estimate of the patient's actual caloric requirement can be made from the weekly averages of caloric intake and the rate of weight loss. The central assumptions are that a pound of fat is lost for every 3,500 kcal of negative caloric balance, and that all of the patient's weight loss is fat. These assumptions are approximately true if the degree of ketosis is about the same on the starting and termination dates used for the calculation (to minimize errors due to changes in state of hydration incident to varying degrees of ketosis). The period of observation should be long enough (perhaps 8 to 12 weeks) and the amount of weight lost large enough to minimize the impact of small errors in estimates of caloric intake and in the actual measurement of weight change. In the final analysis, for the dieter to maintain weight loss he must have some concept of the caloric content of the foods he eats and of his daily caloric requirement. This information is best derived from diary keeping.

TABLE 7 Daily Caloric and Nutrient Intake

	Women				Men			
	Kcal	Protein (g per day)	Fat (g per day)	Carbohydrate (g per day)	Kcal	Protein (g per day)	Fat (g per day)	Carbohydrate (g per day)
Semistarvation Diet								
Week 1	301	16	7	52	369	19	9	65
2	307	21	7	51	377	25	10	63
3	445	47	10	53	634	75	16	65
4	456	46	11	54	656	72	16	66
5	545	52	18	54	832	86	30	67
6	595	52	23	55	882	86	35	68
7	715	73	25	61	1,042	114	37	76
8	841	92	29	63	1,167	130	42	79
9	943	102	36	64	1,375	143	59	80
10	1,063	102	50	64	1,645	142	90	78
11+[1]	1,103	102	50	73	1,725	144	91	98
12+[2]	1,193	105	50	92	1,815	146	91	117
Low Calorie Ketogenic Diet								
Basic Diet	863	84	29	76	1,316	125	47	112
Change 1	937	96	31	76	1,390	138	49	112
2	1,116	98	50	78	1,747	141	88	113
3	1,234	98	62[3]	81	1,865	141	100[3]	116
4	1,336	109	68	82	2,073	154	116	117
5[4]	1,376	109	68	92	2,153	155	117	136
6[5]	1,466	112	69	111	2,243	158	118	155
Balanced Low Calorie Diet								
Breakfast 1								
Basic Diet	1,221	94	27	158	1,508	120	38	183
Change 1	1,318	93	39	157	1,749	119	66	182
2	1,436	93	51[3]	160	1,867	119	78[3]	185
3	1,526	96	51	179	1,957	122	78	204
Breakfast 2								
Basic Diet	1,171	88	39	127	1,585	122	56	160
Change 1	1,268	87	50	126	1,826	122	84	159
2	1,386	87	62[3]	129	1,944	122	96[3]	162
3	1,478	90	63	148	2,034	124	96	181

[1] 20 pounds from goal weight in women, 25 pounds in men.
[2] 10 pounds from goal weight in women, 15 pounds in men.
[3] Alcohol is considered a fat for purposes of this table.
[4] 10 pounds from goal weight in women, 15 pounds in men.
[5] 5 pounds from goal weight in women, 8 pounds in men.

Exercise

Exercise is the only practical and effective way to enhance the disposal of ingested calories. Dieters frequently abuse diuretics and laxatives for this purpose with resultant dehydration rather than calorie loss. Some attempt to induce vomiting; this is both dangerous and abhorrent to the patient. Effecting a life-style change that includes regular exercise is difficult. Lack of time is a commonly cited and often real obstacle. Important, too, but less often verbalized, is self-consciousness about appearance while exercising. Sometimes the problem is simply ignorance of how to go about exercising and what kind of exercise to do. Exercise diary keeping helps to establish a regular pattern of exercise. Once the patient has begun to keep his diet diary consistently, he is asked to begin monitoring exercise. The number of calories burned for each planned exercise period is calculated and recorded by the patient using Table 8. Although the dieter need not exercise every day, a reasonable initial goal would be to average 700 kcal per week (equivalent to about 1 mile of walking daily at a comfortable pace). This combusts about 10 pounds of fat yearly, a value that may seem trivial from the point of view of weight loss, but is significant for weight maintenance. The patient is often surprised by the relatively small caloric dividends of exercise, but it is important that he recognize the substantial amount of physical effort required to burn "harmless" snacks. This reinforces adherence to the diet. Beyond increased caloric expenditure, an anticipated improvement in cardiovascular conditioning should be stressed. Patients will find that, with time, they can do more with less effort. It should be pointed out that exercise can help compensate for the drop in basal metabolic rate incident to diet-

TABLE 8 Calories Used for Each Minute of Continuous Exercise*

Activity	*120*	*150*	*170*	*200*	*220*	*250*
	Weight in pounds					
	kcal/min					
Volleyball, moderate	2.7	3.4	3.9	4.6	5.0	5.7
Walking, 3 mph	3.2	4.0	4.6	5.4	5.9	6.8
Table tennis	3.2	4.0	4.6	5.4	5.9	6.8
Bicycling, 5.5 mph	3.8	4.7	5.3	6.3	6.9	7.9
Calisthenics	3.9	4.9	5.6	6.6	7.2	8.2
Golf	4.3	5.4	6.1	7.2	7.9	9.0
Skating, moderate	4.3	5.4	6.1	7.2	7.9	9.0
Walking, 4 mph	4.6	5.8	6.6	7.8	8.5	9.7
Aerobics	4.6	5.8	6.6	7.8	8.5	9.7
Tennis, doubles	4.8	6.0	6.9	8.1	8.9	10.1
Badminton	5.2	6.5	7.4	8.7	9.6	10.9
Canoeing, 4 mph	5.6	7.0	7.9	9.3	10.2	11.6
Swimming, breaststroke	5.7	7.2	8.1	9.6	10.5	12.0
Tennis, singles	6.0	7.5	8.5	10.0	10.9	12.5
Bicycling, 10 mph	6.5	8.1	9.2	10.8	11.9	13.6
Swimming, crawl	6.9	8.7	9.8	11.6	12.7	14.5
Jogging, 11 min mile	7.3	9.1	10.4	12.2	13.4	15.3
Skiing, downhill	7.6	9.5	10.7	12.7	13.9	15.8
Racquetball	7.6	9.4	10.7	12.7	13.9	15.8
Handball	7.6	9.5	10.7	12.7	13.9	15.8
Mountain climbing	8.0	10.0	11.3	13.3	14.6	16.6
Squash	8.1	10.2	11.5	13.6	14.9	17.0
Skiing, cross-country	8.7	10.8	12.3	14.5	15.9	18.0
Running, 8 min mile	11.3	14.1	16.0	18.8	20.7	23.5
Running, 5 min mile	15.7	19.7	22.3	26.3	28.9	32.8

* The figures were developed under standardized conditions at the Human Performance Research Center at Brigham Young University, Provo, Utah. Factors such as ambient temperature and clothing can affect values.

ing. Exercise is often associated with an improvement in mood. It influences the changes in body composition occurring with dieting in a salutary way by reducing loss of lean muscle mass. Its effect on appetite is debated; studies show both stimulation and inhibition. In either event the effect is small. Excessive exercise is time consuming, painful, and hazardous, and should be discouraged.

ADDITIONAL SUPPORTIVE MEASURES

Most dieters starting the program described above do well initially. Rigid adherence to the diet and rapid weight loss may continue for 6 months or more in the very obese. For all patients weight loss eventually decelerates and ultimately stops. Some will reach goal weight, but the majority will not. One strategy for the patient whose weight loss has stopped near goal weight and in whom risk factors have been normalized is simply to revise the goal upward. In this instance the reason for additional weight loss is aesthetic, and the selected goal not an absolute. In patients far from goal weight additional supportive measures are necessary.

Formal Psychologically Oriented Therapy

Reasons for the deceleration of weight loss include the decline in basal metabolic rate with dieting, the lowered caloric requirement incident to the patient's becoming smaller, and the gradually increasing caloric intake called for by the diet. Unquestionably most important, however, is deviation from the diet. The reasons for deviation are multiple; almost invariably they are fundamental to the cause of obesity in the first place. The patient may now know them, or knowing them feel powerless to affect them. Frustration over the slowing rate of weight loss is frequently mentioned, as is boredom with the limited food selections. These can be dealt with respectively by removing some of the foods previously added or by adding new ones, perhaps some suggested by the patient. This occasionally is effective, but in most instances the problem lies not with the diet. The most important reasons are the most difficult to reverse, and sometimes even to identify. This is not surprising in view of the well-known refractoriness of obesity to all forms of therapy.

Common underlying reasons for deviations from the diet include eating to satisfy emotional needs rather than hunger (depression, anxiety, boredom, fatigue), specific food cravings, and premenstrual (and possibly hormonally mediated) food cravings. Dieting, rapid weight loss, and thinness attract attention to the dieter who is often shy, unaccustomed to such attention, and uncomfortable with it. There is an abiding fear about what others who have been so supportive during the dieting process will think but not say if and when weight is regained. Also, there may be disappointment when long held fantasies about life as a thinner person prove unrealistic. Surprisingly, hunger is rarely offered as an explanation. Dieters sometimes refer to "poor eating habits" as the cause of deviation, implying a somewhat more benign underlying psychologic process. Even if a significant emotional disturbance does not appear to motivate eating in such patients, it may follow dieting simply because of interference with familiar and comfortable patterns of food intake.

It is thus obvious that in some patients, and probably in most, a psychologically oriented component to the weight reduction program should be introduced. This may take the form of counseling by a therapist interested in the problem of substance abuse as it applies to overeating. The patient's spouse and other family members can be included. Lay support groups such as Overeaters Anonymous are helpful, particularly when they include role models who have dieted successfully. For many, a formal behavior modification program is best. The patient should be an important guide as to which form of psychologically oriented therapy might be best. Some will reject a group format, others will already have had negative experiences with individual counseling.

It is beyond the scope of this chapter to describe behavior modification techniques in detail. Patients must be referred to an existing program which may be found in a university setting, at a local psychiatric hospital (or the psychiatry department of a general hospital), or perhaps in the private sphere. Generally, it is done in a group setting, on a weekly basis, and with an experienced therapist. Diet diary keeping is central and the information recorded includes the foods eaten, their caloric content, the reasons for eating, the location of and activities surrounding eating, and associated feeling states. An attempt is then made to identify internal cues (e.g., anxiety) and external cues (e.g., passing a bakery, seeing food advertisements on television) for eating. Alternative outlets for internal cues, such as calling a friend or exercising, are sought. External cues are either removed or minimized. The location and circumstances of eating are restricted. A system is developed to reward the attainment of short-term goals either through group recognition or by self-administered rewards, e.g., the purchase of new clothes in a smaller size. Flexibility is important at this point in the dieting process. Minor deviations should not be viewed as tantamount to failure, a perception that justifies further discouragement, deviation, and even binging. A group setting is particularly useful because it helps the patient realize that he is not alone in the difficult struggle to control food intake. The transition from a metabolically oriented program supervised by the internist or gastroenterologist to one that has a behavioral focus primarily is difficult to orchestrate in the private practice of medicine. This accounts in significant measure for poor long-term results.

Appetite Suppressants

A wide variety of drugs (digitalis, thyroid hormone, chorionic gonadotropin, "starch blockers") have been used to facilitate weight reduction, but only appetite suppressants have established efficacy. Appetite suppressants are structurally related to the naturally occurring sympathomimetic amines. They are presumed to act by releasing norepinephrine or dopamine from adrenergic nuclei in the central nervous system. In addition to appetite suppression they produce psychomotor stimulation. With respect to enhancement of weight reduction they all seem to be equally effective. The established duration of efficacy is limited to 20 weeks because high dropout rates in longer term studies preclude firm conclusions. Tachyphylaxis is common and side effects can be significant, particularly insomnia and blood pressure elevation.

Although not to be recommended for all dieters, appetite suppressants can be a useful adjunct when compliance falters with episodic loss of control. Schedule II drugs like dextroamphetamine (Dexedrine), methamphetamine (Desoxyn), and phenmetrazine (Preludin) should be avoided because of their high potential for abuse. Phendimetrazine, a Schedule III drug, can be administered either one hour before meals (17½ to 70 mg in short-acting form, supplied generically as 35-mg tablets) or as a single dose before 3 PM (long-acting form, supplied in 105-mg capsules as Prelu-2). Fenfluramine (Pondimin) produces drowsiness rather than central nervous system stimulation, and can be useful before the evening meal in patients who snack throughout the evening (20 to 40 mg one hour before supper, supplied as short-acting 20-mg tablets). The nonprescription sympathomimetic agent phenylpropanolamine is promoted directly to the public for weight reduction. Studies lasting 2 to 4 weeks show it to have significant, though minimal, appetite suppressing effect. No more than a 2-week supply of an appetite suppressant should be prescribed at one time. Effectiveness, either as continued weight loss or weight maintenance, should be closely monitored. It may be well to recommend that regular daily use be avoided; rather, the medication can be used "as a crutch" only when an impending loss of control is anticipated. Intermittent use may minimize the development of tachyphylaxis and the potential for dependence.

WEIGHT MAINTENANCE

Obese patients who have lost weight previously recognize that weight maintenance is at least as difficult as weight reduction, having already succeeded at losing weight and failed at maintaining the loss. It is clear to them that a long-term perspective is necessary. Those who are dieting for the first time must be educated early to the fact that dieting, i.e., the conscious exercise of restraint over food intake, does not end with the attainment of goal weight. Failure to accept this harsh reality will inevitably lead to weight gain. Theoretically, the process ends only when the patient is able to maintain optimal weight comfortably and independently through control of food intake and regular exercise. This ideal is rarely, if ever, totally accomplished.

Operationally, the process of weight reduction should blend imperceptibly into that of weight maintenance. This will follow from the previously outlined strategy of gradually increasing caloric intake so that the patient approaches goal weight asymptomatically rather than abruptly. At goal weight the diet must come close to meeting the patient's need for nutritional balance and variety, with subsequent minor adjustments being made early in the period of weight maintenance. Office visits are spaced farther apart but the self-monitoring of calorie (and carbohydrate) intake and of exercise continues. If the patient falters, the time interval between office visits can be shortened. Patients have a need to "internalize" control of food intake, i.e., to function independent of the physician. They may wish to discontinue visits prematurely, and great care must be taken to endorse the cessation of visits only when control seems good. The patient who has lost substantial weight but nevertheless has stabilized above goal may suggest discontinuation of visits, stating: "I don't see that progress is being made." Either he has failed to learn that stabilization at a lower weight is a significant accomplishment; or, he perceives that the physician is disappointed with his failure to lose more weight. These misconceptions must be clarified. Particularly at risk for weight gain is the dieter whose weight, after a period of stabilization, begins to fluctuate wildly from week to week, with the general trend being slowly upward. Clearly, such patients are losing control, alternating fasting with feasting, and need more rather than less reinforcement. Long-term follow-up studies show that continued contact with the therapeutic program and regular exercise characterize successful patients.

Patients who discontinue treatment and return to diet again after regaining weight merit comment. For them very rigid dieting seems to work poorly. Excessive dietery restriction must lead first to minor deviations, then binges followed by fasts. In such patients it is probably best to prescribe a flexible regimen consisting of a fixed total daily calorie and carbohydrate intake (e.g., 1,000 kcal and 100 g of carbohydrate for women, and 1,500 kcal and 150 g of carbohydrate for men) without reference to specific foods, along with regular follow-up visits and the other self-monitoring techniques described above.

SURGERY

Surgical intervention to alter nutrient ingestion or absorption may be considered for the morbidly obese patient (more than 100 pounds or 100 percent above ideal weight) who cannot control his weight by dieting. The risk:benefit ratio has proved most favorable in patients aged 20 to 50 years. Jejunoileal bypass was introduced for this purpose first, and results in dramatic weight loss through a combination of malabsorption and decreased appetite. Though it is generally effective, initial enthusiasm has waned because of side effects. Diarrhea may be intractable, leading to very uncomfortable proctitis and hemorrhoids. Patients are afraid to eat because of the almost immediate need to defecate. Fatal cirrhosis has been reported, along with serious nutritional deficiencies resulting from malabsorption and the blind loop syndrome. Polyarthralgias and renal stones also occur. For these reasons gastric bypass, and more recently gastroplasty, have become more popular. The latter procedure involves partitioning the stomach, creating a small (35 to 50 ml) upper reservoir emptying into the larger distal portion of the stomach through a narrow channel (9 to 12 mm in diameter). Early satiety is then experienced. Overeating leads to nausea and vomiting. The incidence of long-term complications of gastroplasty is not known as yet, but the problems reported thus far appear to be less serious than with jejunoileal bypass. Gallstones frequently develop. Deficiencies in water-soluble vitamins, loss of bone mineral, and hepatic damage resembling alcoholic hepatitis have also been reported. Although patients lose only 50 percent of excess weight on average, they usually are gratified by the results. Unfortunately, some weight gain after the first year is common owing to dilatation of the upper gastric reservoir and/or the channel between the upper and lower segments of the stomach. A conscious effort by the patient to curtail binging is necessary to prevent dilatation of the upper reservoir. External banding of the channel has recently been introduced to prevent its dilatation. Surgical revision may prove necessary in a significant number of patients as weight is regained. Gastroplasty can also be defeated by the continuous sipping of calorie-dense liquids.

For patients who lose large amounts of weight either by dieting or surgical intervention, cosmetic surgery may be desirable to remove unsightly skin folds about the abdomen, thighs, and upper arms. This surgery should be delayed until weight loss has been successfully maintained for at least 6 months. Suction lipectomy is an effective procedure to remove localized accumulations of fat no more than 8 inches in diameter.

FUNCTIONAL ILLNESS

PHILIP A. TUMULTY, M.D.

A very large proportion of the patients seen by a clinician have illnesses that are entirely or in part due to emotional factors. One of our most brilliant internists, Dr. Louis Hamman, once reported that one-third of the patients he saw in consultation had illnesses that were entirely functional, and in another one-third, psychophysiologic factors played an important role. Experiences in my own practice echo his.

Physician Attitude

I smile when I hear young clinicians say, "I wish I were a consultant like you—you must get only interesting organic problems referred to you." They don't realize that the more one becomes recognized as a consultant, the more functional illness one must deal with because very often referring physicians are not sure whether a patient has a functional disorder or some obscure organic disease; they may be anxious, for a variety of reasons, to pass on to a consultant a difficult functional problem they do not want to handle themselves. Make no mistake: The proper management of a major functional illness requires the very best efforts of a skilled clinician, certainly no less than does a complicated organic problem.

It has been my impression through the years that many patients with functional illnesses are not well managed, for a variety of reasons. In many instances, the functional aspects of a patient's health problem are quickly passed over or even completely ignored, and the patient is treated for some inconsequential or even nonexistent organic disorder, such as a hiatus hernia, hypoglycemia and so forth. The result is that the patient's symptoms become more and more deeply embedded, and finally immutable, as each new physician whom the patient sees fails to make clear the real nature of the illness, and what must be done to manage it effectively. The physician's failure may be compounded, because in a sense, functional illness is an "infectious" disease which is often contracted by other members of the family; children and spouse eventually may be affected by it.

Why are many patients who have functional disorders so frequently managed so poorly? There are a variety of reasons.

Many physicians are "turned off" by functional illness. One hears it said by young physicians that "I got into this specialty to get away from those kinds of patients. They are a nuisance, they take up a lot of your time, and they keep coming back with the same old complaints, or new ones that are even worse. You simply cannot get them well. They just don't want to become well. They enjoy being sick!"

During their clinical education, many young physicians feel an intense pressure to learn about a welter of technical matters concerning organic disorders, and they may regard the functional aspects of their patient's health problems as secondary matters for which they have neither the time nor the interest. Alas, their instructors or clinical models may likewise have little of either. Current clinical education of our young physicians stresses the disease state and its recognition and treatment through the employment of a variety of special techniques and not the management of the *total* factors—functional as well as organic—which actually comprise the patient's illness. It is only through meaningful dialogue with the patient that all of these factors can be disclosed and effectively altered. While the modern clinician is, indeed, a doer, he or she is often unfortunately not a conversationalist, and the ability to carry on meaningful dialogue with patients may not be a technique that has been taught or acquired. To have a meaningful dialogue with sick persons means that one must understand something about human nature and its reactions to various stimuli and circumstances, which differ from patient to patient, depending upon such factors as intellectual capacity, ethnic, social, and economic background; experience; and so forth.

Clearly, these matters are not taught in medical school, and probably they cannot be. Perhaps only through working closely with many people can they be learned, and this to a large degree depends upon the individual physician's interest and sensitivity. Unfortunately, both these requisites are sometimes lacking, and the ability to have a positive impact upon a patient through conversation is never acquired. The result is that the physician becomes a technician—one who does things to the patient, some of them scientifically quite remarkable, but who cannot sensitively discern the human issues and reactions and who cannot positively affect these through the strength of his or her own spirit expressed through conversation.

A practical and most important corollary to the failure of some physicians to conduct effective dialogue with their patients is the fact that to accomplish this takes time, a very great deal of time, which is very costly for both the physician and the patient. In the time required for a follow-up visit with one of my patients who has an emotional problem, for example, a colleague in some specialty area can perform some type of technical procedure upon a patient and realize a much larger fee. Most unfortunately, insurance companies and other agencies fail to adequately reimburse a clinician merely for *talking* with patients—one must *do* something to them to really earn one's keep! And yet, truthfully, isn't effective conversation with a patient the most valuable diagnostic and therapeutic "technique" of all?

Inappropriate Psychiatric Referral

Poor management of functional illness also results when the physician tells the patient that all of the diagnostic studies are normal, the patient's symptoms are emotional in origin, and that therefore the patient should see a psychiatrist in consultation.

I realize that I am broaching delicate issues at this point in my discussion, but frankly, I am of the opinion that most patients with functional illness do not need formal psychotherapy, and furthermore it is much wiser *not* to urge them to seek psychiatric help, at least not initially, although it may become appropriate later.

I believe this for two main reasons, first, despite the sophistication of this era, to many patients, being advised that they need to see a psychiatrist is a serious indication that they are losing control of themselves emotionally; that they are no longer able to call their own shots; and that there is something lacking or unsound or weak or different about them. Therefore, at a time when the patient needs so badly to maintain and, if possible, increase his self-esteem, the advice that he must see a psychiatrist may undermine what little self-confidence remains and even cause panic.

I believe that the key concept that must be presented to the patient at the outset of the management of a functional illness is that, while it is evident that here and now the patient is going through a very stormy period, and the storm is a severe and distressing and frightening one, the patient is still very much in control of the situation. He has a strong arm at the helm and can ride out the storm. The premature insistence that the patient must see a psychiatrist will, in some instances, destroy this feeling of still being in control of self.

Secondly, I am convinced that many patients with functional illness do not get sufficient practical help from the type of therapy they are given by some psychiatrists. Specifically, I refer to the type of psychotherapeutic approach which seeks to explain and to reveal to the patient through detailed analysis of self and past *why* he reacts as he does. The patient is not primarily concerned with the question, "*Why* do I react as I do?" nearly so much as with the question, "Reacting as I do, what in a practical way can I do about it? I am what I am—I am not seeking a theoretical explanation of why I am this way, but being what I am, in practical terms, what can I do to control and to modify and to manage myself in these particular situations more effectively, so that I am no longer made sick by them?"

Common Sense Support

Patients want positive direct, uncomplicated, straightforward, sensible, realistic help with the problems of everyday living as they exist within themselves, and not a detailed unearthing and analysis of how the problems got there in the first place. They want practical help and not explanations, in useful terms, not theoretical ones, not magical in scope, but realistically forward-moving and positive.

Another reason some physicians are highly reluctant to become involved in their patient's emotional problems, is that they simply do not fully understand what their role should be, and they are fearful of their inability to play it adequately. Thus, they are concerned that the patient will expect them to have quick, smart, satisfying answers and solutions to their sometimes very involved problems. The physician is afraid that he or she will be expected to create something for the patient that cannot possibly be produced and to achieve results that simply cannot be had. Actually, all such patients really want is understanding, a chance to tell their story fully and reassuring common sense support and sound direction which has practical meaning.

Since most of the problems patients have usually involve matters that are common to so many of us, a clinician of any experience and sophistication should be able to give needed support, understanding, and practical advice.

PATIENT MANAGMENT STEPS

What should be the general approach of a clinician to the management of the patient with functional illness? For the sake of conciseness, let us consider this question in a series of steps.

Diagnostic Evaluation

In the first step, the clinician must reasonably exclude the possibility of latent organic disease by carrying out appropriate studies and consultations. Without such a survey, it is impossible to exclude organic factors. It is the experience of all of us that some exceedingly important organic disorders may exactly duplicate the manifestations of classic functional illness and, the experienced clinician has learned the hard way that the early stages of serious organic disease may masquerade as a functional illness. Furthermore, in this day of "scientific medicine," many patients will simply not accept the fact that they have a functional disorder until organic possibilities have been reasonably excluded by appropriate investigation. This does not mean that the clinician "shoots the works" diagnostically just to please the whim of a patient. What it does mean is that at the conclusion of the initial conference with the patient, following completion of the history and physical examination, the physician explains in terms the patient understands that his particular symptoms could be due either to an organic disorder or to the stresses of circumstances and interpersonal relationships, and that the role of the physician is to evaluate meticulously all of the clinical evidence until the true cause of the illness is fully understood. In coming to a final diagnosis, the physician will, of course, look carefully at both sides of the street. If the physician has carried out a very thorough history and physical examination, he or she will at this point already have won the patient's confidence and set the stage for a satisfying relationship.

Review of Study Results

When the diagnostic evaluation has been completed, the clinician takes the second step at the next meeting by reviewing with the patient the results of the studies, explaining the scope and significance of each test in meaningful terms so that the patient appreciates that the cause of his symptoms has been pursued in a very careful and organized way. The physician concludes this step by stating that a careful and logical synthesis of the total evidence gathered indicates that the symptoms are not due to any significant organic disorder, but rather to psychophysiologic or functional factors.

Explanation of Functional Illness

The third step is to explain to the patient, in easily understood terms, what is meant by functional illness, and then, just as important, what is *not* meant by functional illness. Often, at this stage of the interchange, the patient will be resentful and conclude that the doctor is telling him that his symptoms are imaginary or put on, or that he is "crazy" or losing control of himself, or that he is peculiar or different or odd.

Therefore, it is critically important at this point to make it crystal clear to the patient that his symptoms are exceedingly real and very valid, but that they are not the product of structural abnormalities but rather the result of the physiologic response to stress. Several examples of this interrelationship between stress and body function should be presented to the patient in keeping with the patient's intellectual capacities. For example, when we are embarassed, we flush, when we are frightened, we sweat and our hearts beat faster, when we are under pressure our bowels may stop functioning or overfunction; and so forth. We are all familiar with the expression, "What a headache he is!"

Patient's Reactions. The patient's reaction at this juncture is often one of disbelief, anger, resentment, or insincere acceptance at a very superficial level. The physician must be prepared to accept this unhappy and negative response and not be perturbed or discouraged and above all, the physician must not be forced into backing off and suggesting that possibly some minor organic factors might be playing some role. Unequivocal recognition and understanding by the patient of what is truly causing the illness, and the significance of what the physician is saying, are of the greatest importance at this juncture if the patient is to be cured.

It is at this stage, unfortunately, that many physicians fumble the ball, and the patient grabs it and runs away with it. When the patient demurs, the physician must be understanding but persistent in firmly restating his or her conclusions. Unfortunately, the fear of legal suits which haunts many physicians and sometimes directs their philosophy of patient care, holds them back from dealing with patients who have these sorts of problems in this straightforward, positive, definite approach that is so essential. So they hedge, and they back and fill, as they become self-protective. The patient limps on with his chronic functional illness, no better and probably worse because his convictions of hidden organic disease have become deeper and deeper as a result of his encounter with a physician who practices what might be called "self-defensive medicine."

Discussion of Interpersonal Factors

The fourth step is to discuss with the patient the kind of factors in his life which are most commonly responsible for the development of a functional illness. I have given much thought to this issue, and while the specific causes of functional illness are as varied as the human personality, I think one can make certain basic generalizations. First, the factors are always interpersonal. Second, they are always items that affect us in our most sensitive areas. They are most often little items, but ones that have very special and major significance for us, sometimes for reasons that are quite unclear to us.

At this stage of our conversation, I find it helpful to tell my patient that if he and I were playing a game in which I would list on a piece of paper all the various things that affect me in my areas of deepest reactivity and sensitivity, and he would do likewise, and if we then exchanged our lists and compared them, he would say, after looking over my list, "Doctor, you don't mean to tell me that this or that item could possibly be important and significant to you!" And I'm certain I would say the same thing about his list. Some of these items I am sure are the products of our genes, and still others the result of little things and big things that have happened to us since our very earliest days. Like a computer, little circuits have been turned on within us, through the years, to which we continue to react.

As I perceive it, there are two major mechanisms most often responsible for functional illness in the area of interpersonal relationships: First, *frustration*—something is keeping me from achieving some need which means a great deal to me; secondly, *ambivalence*,—for one set of reasons which mean a great deal to me, I want to walk sharply to the right, and for another set of reasons, meaning an equal amount to me, I want to walk sharply to the left, and so I find myself pulled apart and torn in the middle.

Self-Treatment Measures

Lastly, the patient is advised that there are a series of steps which he must take to recover from this functional illness, which he can do completely, though it may take considerable time, much self-discipline, and a great deal of patience. There will be periods of success, followed by some perids of discouragement, but ultimately the regaining of peace and well-being will be the reward.

The first of these curative steps the patient has already accomplished, namely, the completion of a very meticulous *evaluation* of his symptoms to determine the role and proper management of any organic factors.

The second step is to develop an *understanding* of the real nature of functional illness, and how it differs from organic illness, and especially how it differs from imaginary illness, or wanting to be sick, or putting on, or hysteria, or losing control of one's self, or being emotionally unstable, and so forth.

The third step to *comprehend* fully that functional illness is as natural as human nature itself, and just as common, and that there is no one who goes through life who does not sooner or later suffer the consequences of functional illness to a greater or a lesser degree, and frequently over and over again.

Finally, the patient must *appreciate* that functional illness is particularly likely to occur in individuals who are perceptive and sensitive and thoughtful and imaginative and reactive, and those who are somewhat perfectionistic and obsessive, for these are the kind of persons who feel deeply and who respond keenly to people and to life's encounters. So, having a functional illness is nothing to be ashamed of or to fear. It is simply something that must be overcome, and this the patient can do with your help.

In attempting to understand the nature of functional illness—what it is and also what it isn't—the patient should ask himself the difficult question, "What are the factors in my life which might be responsible for this illness? What items might be causing frustration? What items might be causing ambivalence?" All of these various factors must be ferreted out and examined, recognized and accepted as real, and be understood for what they are and for the negative effects they are producing.

Having recognized the factors, the patient must then ask the hardest question of all: "What can I do about them?"

In attempting to answer this question, it is well to think in terms of *modification* rather than in terms of *change*. Once in adult life, how many of us can realistically think in terms of producing major changes either within ourselves or without? How many of us can completely rid our lives of the factors that are causing frustration and ambivalence? No, modification is surely the word, and not change, and many times, although we surely wish it could be otherwise, it is modification not of the situation, but of our reaction to it.

Practical Measures

Another key word to add to the concept of modification is the word practical, for our decisions and our resolutions and our actions must have practical meaning and be within the reach of attainment. Thus, recovering from a functional illness usually has to be thought of in terms of achieving practical modifications in those features of one's life which self-questioning has indicated are causing illness.

What are the courses of action a wise man adopts when he cannot rid himself of something that is noxious to him? They are few, they are practical, and they are simple: (1) he attempts to avoid it as best he can; (2) he tries to substitute something for it; (3) he endeavors to alter it or to modify his own reaction to it; and (4) he learns to adapt to it, and to put up with it. A wise man does not continue to chew on the same old bone.

These are the alternatives open to the patient in meeting his problems. There is no mystic formula, there is no magic wand, there are no easy solutions. Complete bliss and happiness and self-satisfaction are not the goals, for who on earth has them? The goal is simply not to be made chronically sick by factors from which we cannot escape, and this can be brought about only through persistent effort based on self-discipline and maturity.

Some practical aids are the development of interests and hobbies, and the practical organization of one's work and responsibilities so that they create less unremitting stress. Most important of all is the advice that the patient learn to heal himself in the wounds of others by devoting a significant portion of time and energies to activities that deal with the problems and miseries of persons even more ill and unfortunate than himself.

What must be done is clear. The goal is a middle ground of a reasonable degree of satisfaction and peace, which comes only to those who, with wisdom and maturity and self-discipline, walk through the steps I have outlined. It should be made clear to the patient that either he can make these necessary adjustments, or his sick way of living will undoubtedly continue. There is no alternative route. The choice is his, but the physician will be helping and advising the patient during the long journey.

Finally, which patients with functional illness should be referred to psychiatrists? Certainly patients who have major emotional and personality disturbances should seek psychiatric help, but also those patients who simply cannot accept the fact that their illness is a functional one, or who despite your best efforts, cannot comprehend the nature of functional illness or cannot discern for themselves the factors in their lives which are responsible for their illness. Finally, patients who are thoroughly incapable of altering or affecting in any significant way the things in their lives that are making them sick should be referred to a psychiatrist.

This then, is one physician's approach to the management of functional illness. Does it work? My impression is that it is reasonably successful, for it is based upon telling the patient the truth about himself and his problems in a kind and gentle way. It is based upon interest and understanding. The nature of man is such that his intellect cannot reject the truth when it is presented clearly, and his spirit will always respond to genuine interest and caring.

CARBOHYDRATE MALABSORPTION

JAY A. PERMAN, M.D.

Malabsorption of carbohydrate results in a predictable set of symptoms, including diarrhea, gas, bloating, cramping, and borborygmi. These symptoms can be understood in light of the pathophysiology of sugar malabsorption. Passage of significant quantities of carbohydrate to the colon causes an osmotic diarrhea. In addition, fermentation of carbohydrate by colonic bacteria results in gas production and release of short-chain fatty acids, which contribute to the osmotic load and stimulate peristalsis.

Malabsorption of sugar may be secondary to a variety of conditions which have specific treatments. Therapy for the underlying condition is thus essential. For example, lactose malabsorption associated with gluten-sensitive enteropathy usually resolves within several months following institution of a gluten-free diet. Restriction of lactose alleviates symptoms during the recovery process, but is no longer necessary following regeneration of mucosa. In contrast, intolerance to lactose caused by primary or adult-onset lactase deficiency requires persistent restriction of lactose in the diet. Rapid alleviation of symptoms attributable to malabsorption of sugar depends on restriction of the offending sugar in both secondary and primary forms of carbohydrate malabsorption.

LACTOSE INTOLERANCE

When lactose malabsorption is suspected as a basis for the patient's symptoms, I generally perform a lactose hydrogen breath test before instituting dietary therapy. In my experience, history sometimes, but not always, identifies the patient with lactose malabsorption. Confirmation of lactose malabsorption by breath hydrogen determination provides objective evidence to both the physician and the patient of inability to digest and absorb lactose, and allows both physician and patient to proceed confidently with dietary restriction.

The patient should understand that primary lactase deficiency is not a disease. I find it helpful to tell patients that this disorder occurs in the majority of the world's population, and those with normal lactase activity throughout life are in fact "abnormal." A distinction should be made between lactose malabsorption and milk allergy. This distinction has therapeutic implications because the individual allergic to cow's milk protein will require strict elimination of dairy products from the diet. In contrast, the individual with lactose malabsorption need not strictly eliminate dairy products from the diet except for an initial diagnostic period.

Dietary modification should begin with strict avoidance of lactose for a short time. This interval is determined by the frequency with which the patient's symptoms occur. If the patient has symptoms daily, strict restriction of lactose for the purpose of determining whether lactose malabsorption is the basis for the symptoms can be limited to 1 or 2 weeks. On the other hand, strict elimination of lactose-containing products for a month's time is reasonable when symptoms attributable to lactose malabsorption occur only once or twice a week.

It is particularly important to reassure patients, especially children, that adherence to a strict diet will not be necessary once it is confirmed that elimination of all lactose from the diet ends the symptoms. The prospect of a life devoid of lactose-containing foods is dismal to most individuals, and it should be pointed out that the strict restriction is being undertaken for confirmation of diagnosis only. In my experience, most patients will accept a strict restriction on this basis.

I provide patients with a lactose-free diet including not only foods avoided but foods *allowed* (Table 1). This assists patients in accepting what might otherwise appear to be a very restrictive diet, and also helps to ensure that the resulting diet will be reasonably well balanced.

Upon confirmation of the symptomatic response to elimination of lactose from the diet, reintroduction of lactose-containing foods to the degree consistent with control of symptoms can be undertaken. The patient should be given information on the lactose content of various foods (Table 2).

A variety of strategies are available to the patient who is a lactose malabsorber, but who prefers dairy products in his diet. Microbial sources of lactase are available which may be added to milk or taken at the time that lactose-containing foods are ingested. LactAid (LactAid, Inc, Pleasantville, NJ) may be added to milk which is then refrigerated for 24 hours. This procedure results in hydrolysis of the bulk of lactose present, reducing the symptoms associated with lactose malabsorption. Some patients, however, will find the resulting milk too sweet for their taste. Capsules containing lactase (Lactrase, Kremers-Urban Co, Milwaukee, WI) or LactAid can be taken orally just before and during ingestion of dairy products or foods containing added milk solids. The dose is titrated upward until symptoms are controlled. Recent evidence indicates that yogurt containing active culture, i.e., not pasteurized, is an autodigesting source of lactose. Bacterial lactase present in the yogurt apparently survives passage through the stomach and is activated in the duodenum, thus substituting for the lack of endogenous lactase in individuals with low lactase activity.

Consideration should be given to supplementation of calcium and riboflavin in the diet of those patients who severely curtail their intake of dairy products. Calcium gluconate or other calcium-containing products can be used. For example, the individual can take calcium-containing antacids or wafers rich in calcium. Riboflavin can be economically given using a riboflavin-containing multivitamin.

SUCROSE MALABSORPTION

Isolated sucrase-alpha-dextrinase deficiency causes symptoms of carbohydrate malabsorption in early childhood. Occasionally, however, an adult previously thought to have an irritable bowel syndrome may be diagnosed as having the disorder. Despite the deficiency of alpha-dextrinase (isomaltase), starch is generally well tolerated by these individuals because of hydrolysis by other pathways. Restriction of sucrose is required to control symptoms. The patient is instructed on how to follow a sucrose-restricted diet which again emphasizes both foods allowed and foods avoided (Table 3). Some affected patients may demonstrate increasing tolerance to sucrose as they grow older.

Sucrose malabsorption may occur as a result of sucrase deficiency secondary to mucosal injury, short gut, or intestinal bypass. Since disaccharidase deficiency in these situations is not limited to sucrase activity alone, concomitant restriction of lactose-containing foods is also necessary.

MONOSACCHARIDE AND SORBITOL MALABSORPTION

Congenital glucose-galactose malabsorption is a well-established but fortunately rare inability to digest and absorb all sugars other than fructose. This disorder presents in very early infancy. A mono- and disaccharide-free formula to which fructose can be added is utilized to manage these infants. In other infants, severe mucosal injury may result in transient inability to transport glucose. Continuous feedings of modular formulas permitting titration of the quantity of sugar, or parenteral alimentation is necessary for a variable period of time.

Recent evidence indicates that healthy adults may have symptoms associated with malabsorption of fructose. A dietary history indicating intake of large amounts of fructose-containing food or drink may suggest this diagnosis (Table 4). Since both the degree of malabsorption and associated symptoms are dose related, dietary counseling designed to decrease fructose intake will be useful to these individuals.

Similarly, healthy individuals malabsorb sorbitol. When diet history suggests considerable intake of sorbitol (Table 5) in individuals with symptoms suggesting carbohydrate malabsorption, a trial of a sorbitol-free diet is appropriate.

TABLE 1 Lactose-Free Diet

This diet is for the patient who must eliminate *all* sources of lactose from the diet. Lactose is the sugar found in milk, so all foods containing milk are to be excluded from the diet.

Read the label carefully. Avoid any food containing *milk, nonfat milk solids, skim milk, butter, cream,* and *lactose.*

FOODS ALLOWED		*FOODS AVOIDED*
MILK:	None	All milk, milk drinks—including whole, skim, low fat, dried, evaporated, and condensed milk—human breast milk Yogurt—any type Cream—sweet or sour Infant formulas other than those permitted Frappes, ice cream sodas
BEVERAGES:	Powdered, fruit-flavored drinks, ginger ale, carbonated beverages, cocoa without added milk solids, coffee, tea	Any made with milk, such as frappes, eggnog, hot chocolate
MEATS:	Any baked, broiled, roasted, and boiled, except those to be avoided	Creamed or breaded meat, fish, or poultry, and prepared meats that may contain dried milk solids, including bologna and cold cuts, frankfurters, salami, commercially prepared fish sticks, and some sausage
EGGS:	As desired	Any made with milk—use specific formula; do not prepare with butter
CHEESE:	None	
BREADS:	Breads made without milk only, such as French bread, Italian bread, water bagels, or "pareve" breads; saltines, graham, oyster, and soda crackers, Triscuits	Made with any form of milk Any baked product made with milk (muffins, biscuits, waffles, pancakes, donuts, sweet rolls) Commercial mixes
CEREAL:	Any made without milk, cooked or ready to eat (read labels). Macaroni, spaghetti, pasta, rice, all prepared without milk or cheese	Any prepared cereal that contains dry milk solids
VEGETABLES AND POTATOES:	All—cooked, canned, frozen, or fresh	Any vegetable prepared with milk, butter, milk solids, bread or bread crumbs; no cheese or cream sauces
FRUIT:	All	
DESSERTS:	Any made without milk or milk products, such as gelatin desserts, fruit crisp, snow puddings, fruit and water sherberts, pie with fruit filling, angel cake, milk-free cookies (fig bars, ginger snaps, lemon snaps), tofu ice cream	All commercial cake and cookie mixes, ice cream, custard puddings, junket, ice milk, or sherberts that contain milk; frostings made with milk or butter, dessert sauces, cheese cakes
SOUP:	All prepared without milk or milk products; homemade or canned, e.g., chicken rice	All creamed soups, chowders; no cheese
FATS:	Milk-free margarine or "pareve" margarine; oils, nuts, peanut butter	Butter, margarine, some commercial salad dressings (check labels)
SUGAR AND SEASONINGS:	Sugar, honey, molasses, maple syrup, corn syrup, jelly and jam, hard candy, gum drops, marshmallows, hard peppermints, fondant Salt, pepper, spices, herbs, condiments, vinegar, catsup, relish, pickles, olives, tomato sauce, coconut, wheat germ Artificial flavoring and extracts	Any product made from milk, butter, cream, chocolate, toffee, cream mints, caramel candy, candy with cream centers, butterscotch
MISCELLANEOUS:	Coffee Rich, Coffee Mate	Medications that may contain lactose as filler or bulk agents; party dips; nonprescription vitamins, spice blends, Easter egg dyes; dietetic foods and foods advertised as "high protein" sometimes contain lactose or dry milk solids *Check all labels carefully*

TABLE 2 Lactose Content of Selected Milk, Milk Products, and Substitutes

Product	*Unit*	*Lactose (Approx. g/unit)*
Milk	1 cup–244 g	11
Low-fat milk, 2% fat	1 cup–244 g	9–13
Skim milk	1 cup–244 g	12–14
Chocolate milk	1 cup–244 g	10–12
Sweet Acidophilus	1 cup–244 g	9–10
Sweetened condensed whole milk	1 cup–244 g	35
Dried whole milk	1 cup–128 g	48
Nonfat dry milk, instant	1½ cup–91 g	46
Buttermilk fluid	1 cup–245 g	9–11
Whipped cream topping	1 tbs–3 g	0.4
Light cream	1 tbs–15 g	0.6
Low-fat yogurts	8 oz	8–15
Cheese		
Blue	1 oz–28 g	0.7
Camembert	1 oz–28 g	0.1
Cheddar	1 oz–28 g	0.4–0.6
Colby	1 oz–28 g	0.7
Cream	1 oz–28 g	0.8
Gouda	1 oz–28 g	0.6
Limberger	1 oz–28 g	0.1
Parmesan, grated	1 oz–28 g	0.8
Cheese, pasteurized, processed		
American	1 oz–28 g	0.5
Pimento	1 oz–28 g	0.5–1.7
Swiss	1 oz–28 g	0.4–0.6
Cottage cheese	1 cup–210 g	5–6
Cottage cheese, low-fat (2% fat)	1 cup–226 g	7–8
Butter	2 pats–10 g	0.1
Oleomargarine	2 pats–10 g	0
Ice cream		
Vanilla, regular	1 cup–133 g	9
French, soft	1 cup–173 g	9
Ice milk, vanilla	1 cup–131 g	10
Sherbert, orange	1 cup–193 g	4
Ice, orange	100 g	0

From Welsh JD. Carbohydrate Malabsorption. In: Bayless T, ed. Current therapy in gastroenterology and liver disease. Toronto: BC Decker, 1984, p 136.

TABLE 3 Sucrose-Restricted Diet

FOODS ALLOWED	*FOODS AVOIDED*
Milk, unsweetened evaporated milk, and cream	Sweetened condensed milk and formulas containing sucrose
Asparagus, broccoli, Brussels sprouts, cabbage, cauliflower, celery, chard, chicory, cucumber, lettuce, mushrooms, spinach, tomatoes bamboo shoots, radishes, and potatoes (0.3 g/100 g)	Peas, dried beans, lentils, turnips, parsnips, and other vegetables not listed in foods allowed or those not tolerated
Grapes, fresh cherries, dried Kadota figs, blackberries, cranberries, currants (red and white), lemons, loganberries, and medium ripe strawberries (0.3 g/100 g)	Those not on the list of fruits allowed or those not tolerated
Fried, hard-cooked, soft-cooked, and poached eggs	
Fresh meat, fish, and ham	Check all commercially prepared meats and fish
All cheeses	
Bread (homemade), spaghetti, and macaroni (without sugar)	Breakfast cereals, wheat germ, rice, and bran
Butter, margarine, cooking oil, lard, and salad dressing (oil and vinegar)	Mayonnaise, salad dressing (French, Roquefort, Thousand Island, Russian)
Cocoa, coffee, tea (all unsweetened), and vegetable juice	Malted milk, milk shake, Kool-Aid, and pop
Salt, pepper, gravy, spices, herbs, and vinegar	Olives, pimento, and pickles (sweet and sour)
Chicken and beef broth, bouillon, and consommé	
Glucose (dextrose) and artificial sweeteners	Sugar (cane, beet, granulated, powdered, brown), jam, honey, jelly, candy, molasses, maple syrup, and frosting
Homemade cake, cookies, ice cream using glucose, gelatin, tapioca, and diabetic chocolate	Commercially prepared pies, cookies, cakes, diabetic products (unless mentioned elsewhere), ice cream, sherbert, and any food prepared with sugar
	Salad dressing, pickles, chutney, and medicines made up in syrup

From Perman JA, Watkins JB. Malabsorptive syndromes and intestinal disaccharidase deficiencies. In: Gellis SS, Kagan BM, eds. Current pediatric therapy 10. Philadelphia: WB Saunders, 1982, p 222.

TABLE 4 Fructose Content of Foods

Figs*	30.9 g†
Dates*	23.9 g†
Prunes*	15.0 g†
Grapes*	8.0 g†
Soft drinks containing high fructose-syrup	37.5 g‡

* Dried
† Per 100 g edible portion
‡ Per 18–19 oz of soda
From Ravich WJ, et al. Fructose: incomplete intestinal absorption in humans. Gastroenterology 1983; 84:26.

TABLE 5 Sorbitol Content of "Sugar-free" Products and Various Foods

"Sugar-free" gum	1.3–2.2 g/piece
"Sugar-free" mints	1.7–2.0 g/piece
Pears	4.6*
Prunes	2.4*
Peaches	1.0*
Apple juice	0.3–0.9 g*

* Expressed as grams of sorbitol per 100 g dry matter or per 100 g juice. Dry weight equals approximately 15% of fresh weight.
From Hyams JS. Sorbitol intolerance: an unappreciated cause of functional gastrointestinal complaints. Gastroenterology 1983; 84:30.

OTHER FORMS OF CARBOHYDRATE MALABSORPTION

Limited evidence indicates that some individuals with functional intestinal complaints will respond to a gluten-free diet despite the absence of gluten-sensitive enteropathy. Starch malabsorption may occur in healthy individuals ingesting foods containing both starch and gluten, e.g., breads made from wheat. Further study is required, but it appears that gluten restriction may reduce functional complaints attributable to sugar malabsorption in some otherwise normal individuals. Similarly, further study is required of carbohydrate malabsorption in the elderly. For the present, reduction of the total amount of carbohydrate ingested in a meal may be useful in some elderly individuals should the degree of symptomatology warrant intervention.

FOOD FADS AND ALTERNATIVES

SIMEON MARGOLIS, M.D., Ph.D.

One dictionary defines a fad as "a practice or interest followed for a time with exaggerated zeal." Food fads are also characterized by their divergence from the dietary practices of the general population, and often, by the belief of the faddist that the diet provides health benefits despite the lack of scientific evidence to support this viewpoint. Among the more common fad diets are vegetarian and macrobiotic diets and those employed for weight reduction. Alternative dietary practices include an emphasis on the use of organic or natural foods, as well as supplementation of the diet with specific nutrients, such as vitamins, minerals, protein, lecithin, or fiber.

Many factors contribute to the popularity of food fads and alternative dietary patterns. Some individuals follow vegetarian diets because of philosophical or religious convictions opposing the ingestion of animal foods. Others have adopted fad diets in an attempt to control problems, such as obesity, which have not been successfully managed by more conventional dietary or medical approaches. Common motivations for the use of alternative dietary practices are the widespread beliefs that the usual American diet is nutritionally inadequate and that the American public is slowly being poisoned by food additives and by the agricultural use of fertilizers and pesticides. These misconceptions foster the intake of nutritional supplements and the purchase of organic or natural foods.

Abetting these factors is the enormous proliferation of books, newspaper and magazine articles, radio and television shows, and advertisements concerning nutritional issues. Although some of this outpouring disseminates worthwhile nutritional information, the majority contains misinformation, at times because the author is well meaning but poorly informed. All too often, however, the promotion of nutritional fallacies is motivated by the profit from sales of books or nutritional products.

I am convinced that the usual American diet is nutritionally adequate and that organic or natural foods add no health benefits. In fact, a healthy adult in the United States who can afford to buy enough food and is not an alcoholic would have to follow a most unusual diet to become significantly deficient in any nutritional requirement, with just a few exceptions in women. Nutritional needs are increased during pregnancy and lactation; moreover, many women need iron supplementation prior to menopause and additional calcium intake following, and for at least a decade before, menopause. Although the contamination of our food with pesticides and other environmental pollutants is deplorable, organic foods do not contain smaller amounts of these undesirable substances. Food additives have been carefully tested for safety and most are essential to prevent food spoilage.

Some disadvantages and health risks are associated with fad diets and alternative food habits. Nutritional supplementation and the purchase of specially grown or prepared products add unnecessary expense to the food budget. Some patients may rely upon ineffective nutritional measures rather than seek or follow medical advice for treatable illnesses. Finally, toxic side effects may result from excessive amounts of some nutritional supplements and from the use of some exotic foods. The dangers of a fad diet depend upon the magnitude of its nutritional imbalance and how long the diet is followed. Fortunately, most fad diets are monotonous or unpalatable enough to limit their use to a relatively short time.

FAD DIETS

Vegetarian Diets

The health risks of vegetarian diets vary with the degree of avoidance of animal foods. Partial vegetarian diets, which eliminate only specific animal foods such as red meats, pose no risks and may indeed provide some health benefits. The most common vegetarian diets limit the intake of animal foods to dairy products (*lacto-vegetarian*) or dairy products and eggs (*lacto-ovo-vegetarian*). Such diets are usually adequate in nutrients other than iron. Bioavailability is greater for heme iron, which is present only in animal foods, than for the nonheme sources of iron found in other foods. Strict vegetarians, or *vegans*, consume no foods of animal origin. Vegan diets require careful planning to avoid nutritional deficiencies of calories, protein, minerals and vitamins.

Caloric needs may not be met, particularly in children, because vegan diets are high in bulk. Although vegans can easily ingest enough protein to meet the recommended daily allowance (RDA), many plant proteins are deficient in one or more of the essential amino acids. Therefore, meals must include an appropriate combination of foods that contain proteins which together provide all of the essential amino acids. For example, an adequate intake of essential amino acids can be achieved by the combination of cereal proteins, which are high in methionine and relatively deficient in lysine, with legumes, which contain ample lysine but are low in methionine. It is possible to avoid shortfalls in calcium and iron by careful selection of foods, but the inclusion of fortified soybean milk or an iron supplement may be necessary to ensure adequate intakes. Most vegan diets contain enough vitamins except for vitamin B_{12}. Fortified meat substitutes or a vitamin supplement should be used.

The potential risks of vegan diets are considerably increased in infancy, pregnancy, lactation, and when individuals are ill. It is also important to recognize that some vegetarians ingest large amounts of unconventional nutrient supplements and employ unorthodox sources of health care and advice. Vegans who also have the irritable bowel syndrome may be quite uncomfortable with the gas-producing legumes that are a major part of that diet.

Macrobiotic Diets

Adherents of macrobiotic diets move through a series of rice-rich diets that are progressively more limiting in nutritional content. The ultimate macrobiotic diet consists almost exclusively of unpolished rice. The obvious nutritional dangers of such diets are compounded by their being advocated to treat diseases in lieu of standard medical care. Complications of strict macrobiotic diets include scurvy, anemia, hypoproteinemia, renal dysfunction, severe emaciation, and death.

Reducing Diets

Nutritionists recommend low-calorie diets that are well balanced with respect to their content of carbohydrate, fat, and protein. The effectiveness of such diets depends upon controlling the quantity of food intake rather than restricting its variety. The popularity and frequent short-term success of fad diets for weight reduction are due to the common inability of obese individuals to limit food quantity without a concomitant restriction in food variety.

A bewildering array of fad diets has been tried for weight loss, and new formulas for weight reduction grace the best-seller lists almost every year. The central features of these fad diets involve a wide assortment of ways to limit food variety. Most are low in carbohydrate, but some high carbohydrate diets have been recommended. Some low carbohydrate diets emphasize the use of certain foods, such as grapefruit and even wine; others are high in fat or protein content. Although the risks and benefits of these diets have not been studied carefully, it is *not* evident that they have caused serious ill effects, because most are only moderately unbalanced and the "single food" diets are followed for a short time. Of greater concern are a widely used group of diets that employ a form of protein-sparing modified fasting. Such diets, limited to 200 to 800 calories daily, can be dangerous because of their severely restricted nutrient intake. The underlying principle of these diets is to avoid the protein breakdown and negative nitrogen balance that accompany total starvation by using hydrolyzed protein as the exclusive source of calories. In addition to moderate complications of orthostatic hypotension and attacks of gout, more than 50 deaths, due to myocardial degeneration and arrhythmias, have been reported in patients utilizing protein-sparing modified starvation. These deaths were generally attributed to the use of protein hydrolysates deficient in essential amino acids. Even with a nutritionally adequate source of protein, however, such diets should be undertaken only with close medical supervision and for periods no longer than 2 months. The diet must provide supplemental vitamins, minerals, and fluid.

ALTERNATIVE DIETARY PATTERNS

Organic and Natural Foods

Although neither term is formally defined, organic foods are those grown without the use of chemical fertilizers, herbicides, or pesticides, while natural foods undergo no processing and contain no synthetic ingredients or additives. The purveyors and users of these special foods claim that they are more nutritious, better tasting, and safer than regular foods. Food analyses and blind taste tests have shown no differences from regular foods in either the composition or the taste qualities of organic and natural foods. Two studies in New York, a decade apart, demonstrated that organic and regular foods had similar contents of pesticides. This finding, attributed to the widespread contamination of American soil with environmental pollutants, suggests that it is now difficult to avoid their presence in food products by organic farming. The use of organic or natural foods poses no health hazard, but these products are significantly more expensive than ordinary foods.

Most food additives are used to prevent spoilage from the growth of bacteria or molds and to slow the development of rancidity due to the oxidation of unsaturated fats. The geographic separation between the producers and consumers of food products in this country fully justifies the employment of preservative substances. Some additives, such as artificial sweeteners and synthetic dyes used as food colorings, are not essential to protect the food supply. The safety of such additives has been thoroughly tested, however, and the Food and Drug Administration has banned cyclamates and food dyes when animal studies suggested health risks for humans.

The ultimate example of the avoidance of food additives is the diet recommended initially by Feingold for the management of children with the hyperactivity syndrome. This diet restricts not only all foods with artificial coloring or flavoring but also a number of fruits and vegetables that contain natural salicylates. The severe limitations of the diet have created difficult problems for parents trying to follow this recommendation, and there is no valid evidence for the effectiveness of the diet.

Nutritional Supplementation

Supplementation of the diet with vitamins and other nutrients is widespread in this country. Some estimates indicate that almost half the elderly population regularly uses some form of nutritional supplement. With the exception of calcium and iron in women, healthy individuals do not need such supplements. At best, such practices are an added expense, but not harmful. The costs of vitamin supplements are compounded by claims that "natural," more costly forms are more effective than synthetic vitamins. Dangers arise when the diet is supplemented with megadoses (10 to 100 times the required daily allowances) of certain vitamins. Excessive intake of the fat-soluble vitamins, *A* and *D*, has long been recognized as a cause of toxic manifestations that may persist for many months because of the tissue storage of these vitamins. More recently, toxic manifestations have been identified from the consumption of more than a gram daily of *pyridoxine* (RDA = 2 mg per day) for a period exceeding 2 months. Side effects of megadoses of *niacin* were recognized from its use in the treatment of patients with hyperlipidemia. The untoward effects of each of these

TABLE 1 Side Effects of Megavitamin Use

Vitamin	*Side Effects*
A	Headaches due to increased intracranial pressure; nausea, vomiting and anorexia; fatigue and somnolence; petechiae and epistaxis; skin desquamation and hair loss; hypercalcemia; bony tenderness. Chronic toxicity may also cause papilledema and fibrotic changes in the liver.
C	Hemolysis in individuals with glucose-6-phosphate dehydrogenase deficiency; diarrhea; possibly kidney stones.
D	Hypercalcemia; polyuria and polydipsia; anorexia, nausea, vomiting, constipation; headaches, fatigue, weakness, confusion; nephrocalcinosis and renal failure.
Niacin	Cutaneous flushing, pruritus, urticaria; peptic ulcer; impaired glucose tolerance; hyperuricemia and gouty arthritis.
Pyridoxine	Progressive sensory ataxia; impaired position and vibratory sensation.

vitamins, as well as *vitamin C*, are listed in Table 1. Physicians must be aware of the toxic manifestations of these vitamins and routinely determine the vitamin intake of their patients. It is ironic that individuals risk the side effects of these vitamins either unwittingly, because of the high content of vitamin A in some multivitamin preparations, or in the unproven expectation that large doses of vitamin C prevent colds and cancer or that megadoses of pyridoxine ameliorate the premenstrual syndrome or hyperactivity or are useful in body-building regimens.

Other nutritional supplements are equally ineffective but relatively harmless. For example, lecithin and vitamin E have no proven efficacy in preventing the complications of atherosclerosis even though the former is widely used for that goal and the latter is probably the most common nutritional supplement. Many *fiber-containing* pills and other products are available, but any benefits of a high fiber diet should be obtained through the appropriate selection of food products rather than by adding supplements to the diet.

RECOGNITION, ASSESSMENT, AND THERAPEUTIC INTERVENTION

Physicians frequently obtain inadequate nutritional data from the history and physical examination. The usual questions about dietary practices are perfunctory and superficial. Instead, physicians should always obtain certain salient information about a patient's nutritional status, including weight changes, appetite, alcohol history, and problems that may interfere with the ingestion or absorption of food, such as difficulty in chewing, loss of taste, dysphagia, vomiting, diarrhea, or prior abdominal surgery. Anthropometic measurements and detection of specific signs of malnutrition are important parts of the physical examination. Physicians should also take the time to discover whether the patient follows a fad diet or alternative dietary habits. In many instances patients are reticent about mentioning unusual dietary habits and do not recognize the relevance of their diet unless the physician asks about it directly. The presence of most unusual dietary practices will be uncovered by asking the questions presented in Table 2. Identification of unusual dietary habits is worthwhile because they may have significant diagnostic and therapeutic implications. Moreover, most patients on fad diets have an intense interest in nutrition and great faith in the health benefits of their particular diet, and therefore they may doubt the interest and skills of a physician who does not even ask about their diet.

Once unusual dietary habits are discovered, the physician must decide what to do about them. This decision depends on the extent of variance of the diet from sound nutritional practices and the likelihood that the patient's diet has, or will have, serious adverse health effects. It is especially important to consider the health consequences

TABLE 2 Questions to Ask Patients to Determine Whether They Are At Risk from Unusual Diets

Question	*Rationale*
Has your doctor prescribed any special diet?	The special diet may need modification or more detailed explanation by a nutritionist.
Are you on any other special diet, such as a vegetarian or weight loss diet?	Such diets are apt to be nutritionally inadequate unless well planned.
Do you take any vitamins, minerals, or other supplements such as fiber?	Very large doses of vitamins may be toxic.
Do you exclude any types of foods (animal foods, processed foods, convenience foods) or food groups from your diet?	Restrictions on types of foods, especially entire food groups, raise the possibility of nutritional shortfalls and imbalances.
How long have you adhered to this diet?	In general, the longer the patient has been on the regimen, the greater are the health risks.
Do you indulge in fasting, self-induced vomiting, or extreme use of enemas?	These practices suggest anorexia nervosa or bulimia.
Why have you adopted special dietary practices?	Exploring the rationale for the use of the diet often permits insight into other health beliefs and provides clues to acceptable dietary advice.

of unusual diets during adolescence, pregnancy or lactation, and when the presence of disease, such as diabetes, dictates specific dietary measures.

In many instances the physician can easily assess the nature and extent of the unusual practices by asking a few more questions about the diet. Time spent in discussion may help to establish patient rapport and later compliance with nutritional and other therapeutic measures. A more detailed dietary history, with the assistance of a trained nutritionist, is recommended to ensure the adequacy of the diet when patients have followed, or plan to follow, a fad diet for a considerable period. Depending on the type and duration of the diet, the physician may choose to perform laboratory tests to assess current nutritional status. Thus, measurements of serum albumin or transferrin levels may be indicated to determine adequacy of protein intake in patients on a strict vegetarian diet.

Physician intervention to alter unusual dietary habits may be difficult. Patients are quite confident of the health benefits of their diets and of their own knowledge of nutrition, though much of it may be faulty. Even physicians well versed in nutrition may be unable to convince patients that their dietary practices are not beneficial and may be harmful. When the dietary habits are unnecessary, but safe, such as modest supplements with vitamins, minerals, lecithin or fiber, I point out the economic disadvantages and make no serious effort to alter the diet. I do not intervene when patients are on most fad diets for weight reduction, but rather insist on close follow-up with the anticipation that the diet will be discontinued before the occurrence of serious consequences. Although I may not agree with these dietary choices, prolonged battles with the patient are not worth the risk that he will abandon medical follow-up.

In contrast, more firm measures must be taken to interrupt or control dietary practices with serious health implications. Patients taking megadoses of vitamins or minerals are informed of the toxic effects of vitamins A and D and pyridoxine and are strongly urged to discontinue their use. Those on reducing diets containing fewer than 800 calories per day are warned of their nutritional inadequacies and told to stop the diet. If they refuse, this group of patients, along with those committed to strict vegetarian diets, are referred to a nutritionist for more complete evaluation of the diet and for detailed advice on measures to minimize the dangers of their diet.

PARENTERAL NUTRITION

C. RICHARD FLEMING, M.D.

Parenteral and enteral nutrition are not mutually exclusive techniques with which to feed our patients. There are many patients with patent intestinal tracts who simply cannot or will not eat enough; therefore, parenteral nutrition as supplemental rather than the sole nutrition is appropriate.

The terminology available to describe various forms of parenteral nutrition is confusing, and there is no uniformly accepted nomenclature. Hyperalimentation, parenteral alimentation, total parenteral nutrition, central parenteral nutrition, peripheral hyperalimentation, and protein-sparing therapy are terms which do not convey the same meaning to all readers. We will use central parenteral nutrition (CPN) to mean the use of a large-diameter central vein through which to administer hypertonic formulas. Peripheral parenteral nutrition (PPN) will refer to the use of small-diameter peripheral veins to infuse isotonic or hypotonic solutions.

QUALITY CONTROL

The assignment of one person, rather than a committee, to oversee the day-to-day supervision of parenteral nutrition is ideal. That individual is usually a nurse, dietitian, or pharmacist who works very closely with physicians and other health care professionals who comprise a nutritional support group. Specifics that require close supervision include the following:

Flow monitors for all patients on CPN. The use of either a pump or drip regulator reduces metabolic complications and optimizes nutrient utilization.

Catheter care should be carefully controlled either by continuing education of floor nurses or, if the hospital size permits, one nurse managing all catheters placed in large-diameter central veins.

Flow sheets with which to record serial chemistries that allow early detection of nutrient excesses or deficiencies.

A *monograph* for hospital staff which details the basic information needed for day-to-day patient care.

Incompatibilities between specific nutrients or between drugs and nutrients.

A nutritional support team is active in most large medical centers. Most are run on a consultative basis, but a few hospitals make a consultation mandatory for any patient started on enteral or parenteral nutrition.

NUTRIENTS

The basic nutrients delivered in parenteral nutrition are fat, carbohydrates, amino acids, electrolytes, macroelements, trace elements, and vitamins. Table 1 lists the usual composition of 1 L of CPN.

TABLE 1 Central Parenteral Nutrition with Standard Electrolytes*

	Final Concentration			
Dextrose	☐ 10%	☐ 15%	☐ 20%	☐ 25%
Amino acids		4.25%		
Sodium		36.5 mEq		
Potassium		30.0 mEq		
Calcium		4.8 mEq		
Magnesium		5.0 mEq		
Chloride		35.0 mEq		
Phosphorus		15.0 mmol		
Acetate		67.5 mEq		
Grams nitrogen		7.15 g/L		
Total kilocalories	510	680	850	1,020
Approx. osmolarity	1,090	1,340	1,595	1,845
Approx. volume		1,000 ml		

* One liter of standard central parenteral nutrition. The standard adult multivitamin injection is added to one bottle daily. Generally, a standard adult trace element injection is added to one bottle daily (4 mg of zinc, 1 mg of copper, 500 μg of manganese, and 10 μg of chromium/ml).

Fat

Intravenous fat emulsions are available as emulsions of soybean or safflower oils, egg phospholipid, and glycerol. Ten and 20 percent concentrations of isotonic fat emulsions can be administered with PPN or CPN. All patients on parenteral nutrition more than a week should receive at least enough fat each week (e.g., 1 to 1.5 L of 10% fat emulsion for the average adult) to prevent biochemical evidence of essential fatty acid deficiency.

Carbohydrate

Dextrose is a safe and efficiently used caloric source. Solutions of alcohol, sorbitol, xylitol, and fructose have all been tested and proved to be less safe or more expensive (or both) than dextrose.

The use of dextrose as the only nonprotein energy source in CPN solutions is associated with several problems. Infusion of dextrose in excess of that which is readily oxidized results in net synthesis of body fat and water accumulation. Complications observed in patients receiving excess glucose are fatty liver and mild elevations in serum amino transferase and alkaline phosphatase values, and, in patients on respirators, an increase in carbon dioxide production with only minimal increase in oxygen consumption. The dual energy system (dextrose and fat) appears more efficient than glucose alone in replenishing protein and avoiding water retention. The apparent advantage of using the dual energy system in all patients must be weighed against the disadvantage of the added expense of the fat emulsions.

Protein

Synthetic crystalline amino acids are available in concentrations of 3 to 10 percent, with and without electrolytes. Most amino acid preparations consist of approximately two-thirds nonessential and one-third essential amino acids. These preparations are very efficiently used; the mean nitrogen retention when 1 g per kilogram of body weight per day of a 10 percent amino acid mixture was given was equivalent to high biologic value protein given orally to healthy adults.

Electrolytes

Single package electrolyte solutions added to parenteral nutrition will meet most patients' needs. There are exceptions when alterations are needed, such as in patients with cardiac, renal, or hepatic disease or when there are large gut losses of electrolytes as can occur in patients with short bowel syndrome or high output, proximal enterocutaneous fistulas.

Trace Elements

Commercial solutions with multiple trace elements (e.g., copper, zinc, chromium, and manganese) are available; however, some of these trace elements, such as chromium and manganese, are often not needed. Also, patients with large stool losses may lose zinc in excess of what the multitrace element formula will contain (4 mg zinc). Vials containing single trace elements allow for adequate flexibility in nutrient mixing and for maintaining normal blood levels.

Iron is not routinely added to parenteral nutrition solutions. Iron dextran can be added in small amounts to daily CPN, or it can be given by a bolus infusion designed to replace body stores. Parenteral iron has been associated with anaphylaxis or a constellation of symptoms including myalgias, fever, and headache. A small test dose of parenteral iron should be given prior to initiating the replacement of larger amounts of iron. Preliminary reports that parenteral ferrous gluconate was safer than iron dextran have not yet been followed by its commercial availability.

Vitamins

There are vitamin preparations with both water-soluble and fat-soluble vitamins. Vitamin K is not routinely added, but it can be supplemented either orally or parenterally. The multivitamin preparation MVI-12 (Armour Pharmaceutical, Kankakee, IL) results in normal blood levels of almost all vitamins when added to 1 L of CPN each day.

Most hospital pharmacies provide dextrose, amino acids, vitamins, electrolytes, and macroelements (calcium, phosphorus, and magnesium) in a "standard" CPN formula. This formula is not "total" as implied in the label *total* parenteral nutrition because several nutrients are not routinely added, including vitamin K, essential fatty acids, iron, and trace elements. The likelihood of deficiencies of each of these nutrients increases with the duration of nutritional support.

TYPES OF PARENTERAL NUTRITION

Peripheral Vein Parenteral Nutrition

The advent of safe, isotonic fat emulsions in 10 and 20 percent concentrations created great hope that one could meet the needs of most patients requiring parenteral nutrition by PPN. These hopes, however, have been tarnished by frequent episodes of phlebitis and soft tissue infiltrations, with the end result being the inability to feed the patients adequately. The addition of small amounts of heparin and corticosteroids to PPN solutions decreases the incidence of phlebitis and thrombosis. A double-blind, prospective study showed that the use of a 0.22-μ filter decreased the incidence of phlebitis by approximately two-thirds compared to that in patients receiving PPN without filters. This latter study suggested that the phlebitis is caused by microparticulate components present in the infusion fluids which are removed by in-line filtration.

Peripheral vein nutrition should be reserved for patients whose nutritional status is near normal and in whom the treatment goal is to maintain and not to replace lean body mass. Such patients may be undergoing elective surgery, in which case one can anticipate a 3- to 7-day period of nothing by mouth. Several alternatives exist:

First, dextrose-in-water, 100 to 150 g daily, with multivitamins and 20 to 30 mEq potassium chloride per liter. This is usually given as 2 or 3 L of 5 percent dextrose in water. The administration of dextrose and the stimulation of insulin, the premier anabolic hormone, will decrease urinary nitrogen losses by 50 percent compared with the administration of saline without calories. This mainstay has served patients well and remains the usual short-term postoperative nutrition for patients undergoing elective surgery.

Second, crystalline synthetic amino acids can be given as isocaloric replacements for dextrose. This "protein-sparing therapy" was initially promoted as a better alternative than dextrose-in-water because amino acids decrease urinary nitrogen losses by 50 percent when compared with isocaloric amounts of 5 percent dextrose. This response is independent of insulin and glucagon secretion, and the critical ingredient for "protein sparing" appears to be the administered protein itself—in this case, amino acids. The response is dose dependent—1 g per kilogram ideal body weight per day results in a cumulative nitrogen loss in patients undergoing elective surgery whereas 2 g per kilogram ideal body weight per day promotes a cumulative nitrogen retention. Although it provides a good lesson in nutritional metabolism, the use of intravenous amino acids alone has little clinical use. There are no data to show that there is clinical benefit (such as reductions in hospital stay, postoperative complications, and rehabilitation time) to justify the extra expense of amino acids instead of hypotonic dextrose for the uncomplicated patient undergoing elective surgery.

Third, combinations of hypotonic dextrose, amino acids, and fat emulsions plus vitamins, minerals, and trace elements can meet the average patient's basal energy and protein needs provided that 50 percent of the calories are given as fat calories. The dextrose and amino acids have traditionally been mixed together along with the micronutrients and given through the main line while the fat emulsions are given through a Y-connector placed downstream from the filter. Table 2 itemizes the usual components in 1 L of peripheral parenteral nutrition solution used in our hospitals. Most adult patients will receive 2 or 3 L of PPN and 500 ml of a 10 percent fat emulsion each day.

More recently, three-in-one mixtures have been marketed. These allow the mixture of dextrose, amino acids, and fat emulsions in the same bag. At least one control study has shown a significantly higher rate of catheter occlusion when the three-in-one system was used compared with the conventional system of dextrose and amino acids in one bottle and the fat emulsion in another.

Central Vein Parenteral Nutrition

Catheter Placement and Care

Generally, the infraclavicular approach to the right subclavian vein is used in adults. In small children, the jugular vein is often catheterized and the proximal end

TABLE 2 Peripheral Parenteral Nutrition with Standard Electrolytes*

	Final Concentration
Dextrose	5%
Amino acids	4.25%
Sodium	36.5 mEq/L
Potassium	30.0 mEq/L
Calcium	4.8 mEq/L
Magnesium	5.0 mEq/L
Chloride	35.0 mEq/L
Phosphorus	15.0 mEq/L
Acetate	67.5 mEq/L
Grams nitrogen	7.15 g/L
Total kilocalories	340 kcal/L
Approx. osmolarity	835 mOsm/L
Approx. volume	1,000 ml

* The standard adult multivitamin injection is added to one litre of standard peripheral parenteral nutrition daily. Generally, a standard adult trace element injection is added to one bottle daily (4 mg of zinc, 1 mg of copper, 500 μg of manganese, and 10 μg of chromium/ml).

of the catheter is tunneled subcutaneously to exit through an incision behind the ear. Dressings should be changed 3 times a week, using the same aseptic techniques that were followed when the catheter was inserted. A filter, either 0.22 or 0.45-μ pore size, is inserted between the intravenous tubing and catheter; the tubing and filter are changed daily. Careful taping at tubing connections and/or Luer locks are used to prevent accidental disconnections and the potential for air embolism. Intravenous drugs, colloid, and blood should not be given through the central line except under unusual circumstances when no other venous access is available.

Indications

Rigid guidelines as to when and in whom to use CPN often disintegrate on hospital wards, but most patients for whom enteral nutrition is impossible or inadequate for more than 10 days and who have lost 10 percent or more of their usual weight are candidates. Most such patients have gastrointestinal diseases or conditions (Table 3). Although the usual CPN formulas are applicable to most, specialized solutions have been marketed for patients with renal or hepatic failure and "stress formulas" for those experiencing marked catabolism. Of these special formulas, the high branched chain preparations for trauma patients appear to have the soundest and most reproducible results.

Fistulas. The combination of CPN and bowel rest for traumatic or surgically induced fistulas will result in nonoperative, permanent closure in 70 to 80 percent of cases. The same treatment for fistulas arising in cases of Crohn's disease, radiation enteritis, or malignancies may result in temporary closure, but the fistulas will usually reopen soon after resumption of oral food. Although CPN and bowel rest rarely result in a "cure" in the latter circumstances, they are important adjuncts to optimize nutrition prior to surgery.

Unresolving Pancreatitis. These patients should probably not be fed with tube enteral infusions placed downstream from the pancreas. Instead, CPN and bowel rest interrupt the predictable sequence of oral food → postprandial pain → ↓ oral intake → malnutrition. One must monitor plasma glucose levels at least once each day, because marked hyperglycemia may occur. If hypertriglyceridemia is present at presentation, I do not use intravenous fat emulsions. In the absence of elevated serum triglycerides, fat emulsions are used to give 20 to 30 percent of nonprotein calories and minimize the risk of severe hyperglycemia. Intravenous fat emulsions have not been shown to increase pancreatic enzyme outputs through pancreatocutaneous fistulas or alter the course of experimental pancreatitis in animals.

TABLE 3 Common Indications for Central Parenteral Nutrition

Gastrointestinal Diseases

- Fistulas
- Unresolving pancreatitis
- Intestinal pseudo-obstruction
- Radiation enteritis
- Inflammatory bowel disease
- Prolonged postoperative ileus
- Severe diarrhea in infants

Specially Designed Formulas

- Hepatic failure
- Renal failure
- "Stress" high branched chain amino acid formulas for catabolic patients

Diffuse Motility Disorders. Patients with pseudo-obstruction from scleroderma or amyloidosis are extremely difficult to manage over long periods with CPN because of their multisystem involvement. The chronic idiopathic intestinal pseudo-obstruction syndromes, however, are relatively easy to manage and patients usually fare well with normal body weights and periods of less severe symptoms when some enteral nutrition is possible.

Radiation Enteritis. Most patients who experience pain, diarrhea, and rectal bleeding following abdominal radiation have self-limiting symptoms and minimal long-term morbidity. Another group who undergo total abdominal radiation develop diffuse submucosal edema and subsequent fibrosis, which results in chronic small bowel obstruction at multiple sites, often requiring long-term home parenteral nutrition. Yet a third group are those who develop a picture of subacute intestinal pseudo-obstruction following total abdominal radiation for which CPN for several months is necessary.

Inflammatory Bowel Disease. Central parenteral nutrition with or without "bowel rest" is often used in patients with inflammatory bowel disease as an adjunct to conventional medical or surgical treatment, to prepare the debilitated patient for surgery, or as primary therapy for patients with extensive Crohn's disease and gut failure.

Dickinson and colleagues conducted the only randomized trial of CPN and bowel rest in patients with acute colitis, most of whom had chronic ulcerative colitis. Control patients were fed an ad lib oral diet and the treatment group received CPN and bowel rest. Controls and CPN treated patients were taking comparable amounts of prednisone. Half of each group required surgery during the same hospitalization. Among those not requiring surgery, the duration of medical treatment required to induce clinical remissions was comparable in the two groups. Thus, there was no difference in the outcome in the controlled and CPN groups with regard to frequency of surgery or duration of medical therapy. These data should not discourage the use of CPN in malnourished patients with chronic ulcerative colitis for whom enteral nutrition is inadequate.

Uncontrolled data suggest that 60 to 70 percent of patients with *Crohn's disease* who are refractory to medical treatment and are treated with CPN and bowel rest undergo an initial in-hospital remission, but only 50 percent of those followed for 3 months remain in clinical remission. These observations need to be tested in a randomized trial comparing CPN and bowel rest with other means of nutritional support, such as tube enteral and peripheral parenteral nutrition. Lochs and associates conducted a randomized trial comparing CPN with bowel rest to CPN without bowel rest in 20 patients with Crohn's disease. There was no apparent advantage by clinical scores or nutritional indices in the patients with complicated Crohn's disease with 12 weeks of CPN and bowel rest. No medications were given. Although surgery was initially avoided in 25 to 30 patients, the cumulative relapse rate was 60 percent after 2 years and 85 percent after 4 years. This was compared with the results of resection, obtained from a 10-year period before CPN was begun at the same hospital, showing the cumulative recurrence rates after CPN to be four times higher than after resection. The available data on CPN in adults with Crohn's disease punctuates its importance as an adjunctive tool to reverse the frequent protein-calorie malnutrition; however, it is not a substitute for corticosteroids and surgery, which are the mainstays of treatment.

Thirty percent of children or adolescents with Crohn's experience growth retardation. Adequate nutritional supplementation alone, regardless of the form, stimulates growth. The calorie and protein requirements revert to those of the newborn infant—75 to 100 Kcal per kilogram and 2 g of protein per kilogram per day. Although most of these patients can be managed with aggressive enteral nutrition, CPN is necessary in some of the most severe cases.

Complications

Discussion of the major metabolic complications in patients receiving TPN, shown in Table 4, is beyond the scope of this chapter. Sequential measurements of blood and/or urine concentrations of most of these nutrients will alert one to evolving deficiencies or excesses.

One of the most common mistakes made is *overfeeding* the cachectic patient—too much nutrition in too short a period of time. Sudden deaths have been reported in this setting. Although the exact cause of such deaths is unknown, the most likely possibilities include cardiac arrhythmias and/or severe hypophosphatemia. When refeeding the severely protein-calorie malnourished patient, one should start at approximately one-third the estimated maintenance calories and slowly (every third day) increase the caloric load to the maintenance level.

Patients with hypoalbuminemia who are started on parenteral nutrition will frequently reduce their serum albumin levels even lower during the first 1 to 2 weeks. This reduction usually reflects only rehydration and should not be managed by increasing the amino acids infused. The half-life of albumin is approximately 19 days; therefore, serum albumin levels are not good indicators of protein synthesis over a shorter period of time.

The malnourished patient who is hypoproteinemic and edematous will frequently lose weight shortly after starting CPN. This initial weight loss is accompanied by a diuresis and mobilization of edema fluid. This may be interpreted as inadequate parenteral nutrition and the volume or concentration of CPN (or both) will inappropriately be increased. Weight gain in hospitalized paients on TPN is often erratic. For instance, patients who are adequately fed may not gain for several days and then the weight may suddenly increase by 1 pound per day. Only after a stable course of 2 weeks do we see a desirable, steady weight gain of ¼ to ½ pound per day.

TABLE 4 Major Metabolic Complications in Patients Receiving Total Parenteral Nutrition

Nutrients	*Presentations*
Excess of:	
Glucose	Hyperglycemia, polyuria, polydipsia
Amino acids	Hyperammonemia in patients with liver disease Azotemia in renal failure
Calcium	Hypercalcemia, pancreatitis, renal stones
Vitamin D	Hypercalcemia, negative calcium balance, osteopenia, long bone pain (reported in long-term home parenteral nutrition patients)
Deficiency of:	
Copper	Neutropenia, anemia, scorbutic bone lesions, ↓ ceruloplasmin
Zinc	Nasolabial and perineal acrodermatitis, alopecia, ↓ T cell function, ↓ alkaline phosphatase
Chromium	Glucose intolerance
Selenium	Myalgias, cardiomyopathy, ↓ glutathione peroxidase
Molybdenum	Amino acid intolerance, tachycardia, tachypnea, central scotomas, irritability, ↓ uric acid
Essential fatty acids	Eczymoid dermatitis, ↑ 20:3/20:4
Vitamin A	Night blindness, ↓ dark field adaptation
Vitamin K	Easy bruising, hypoprothrombinemia
Vitamin E	In vitro platelet hyperaggregation and H_2O_2-induced red blood cell hemolysis
Vitamin D	Osteomalacia, long-bone pain, low serum 25-OH vitamin D
Biotin	Dermatitis, alopecia, hypotonia
Thiamine	Wernicke's encephalopathy
Taurine	Impaired vision, abnormal retinogram
L-carnitine	Inadequate data

HOME PARENTERAL NUTRITION

Patients with gut failure from any cause are candidates for home parenteral nutrition (HPN). Most such patients suffer from severe short bowel syndrome, extensive Crohn's disease of the small bowel, extensive radiation enteritis, chronic adhesive small bowel obstruction, or intestinal pseudo-obstruction. Because of the complexity of our HPN cases, we organize our efforts by means of a multispecialty team consisting of physicians, nurses, a pharmacist, dietitians, and a social worker. Venous access is achieved with a subcutaneously tunneled catheter that is inserted in the operating room. The training of patients in the hospital takes approximately 2 weeks and is done by HPN nurses and a pharmacist who rely heavily on our HPN training manual. A home health care company delivers supplies to patients' homes at monthly intervals according to our prescription. After discharge, patients return to see us at 3-month intervals initially; the frequency of visits lessens as stabilization occurs. Almost all of our HPN patients eat, but their intakes are often limited by fear of diarrhea or increased abdominal pain.

HPN has significantly improved the quality of life for gut failure patients. Nutritional repletion is dramatic and approximately 70 percent return to active routines as students or homemakers, or to gainful employment. Only 4 percent of the total HPN days (656/15,035) of our 41 active patients in 1983 were spent in the hospital.

One-third of patients will experience a catheter-related septicemia at some time during their course of HPN. Considering that our patients have been on HPN for an average of 30 months, the frequency of these infections is one for every 3.5 patient years of HPN. A small cluster of patients have repeated infections, perhaps due to faulty aseptic technique. The most common problem is damage to the external segment of the catheter, which is easily repaired with a repair kit. Catheter occlusions are surprisingly rare and can usually be managed by instillation of streptokinase into the catheter.

The estimated average daily price for HPN in 1984 was $200 (or $73,000 per year for a patient who infuses nightly), compared with $25 per day ($9,125 per year) 10 years ago. Our patients' HPN bills range from $35,000 to $70,000 per year and depend on the number of nights they infuse, their formulas, and the vendor. Most third-party carriers will pay 80 percent of the HPN expenses, but most patients cannot realistically pay the remaining 20 percent.

ENTERAL FEEDING: LIQUID FORMULA DIETS

ROLANDO H. ROLANDELLI, M.D.
JOHN L. ROMBEAU, M.D., F.A.C.S

Enteral feedings by tube have been used for many centuries. Until the advent of safe techniques for parenteral nutrition in the late 1960s, enteral feeding was the only means to nourish patients who were unable to eat. As parenteral nutrition became popular, the use of enteral nutrition declined. A major factor in this decline was that enteral feeding was commonly associated with complications and was poorly tolerated by the patient.

Parenteral nutrition was advocated as a better method of alimentation for the critically ill because it eliminated the "lag time" produced by intestinal and hepatic processing of nutrients. Furthermore, because of the theoretical advantage of bowel rest, parenteral feeding was recommended as the primary treatment for some gastrointestinal diseases. Recent reports, however, have shown that bypassing the digestive system via parenteral nutrition is not entirely innocuous. Complications, such as fatty liver, occur frequently in parenterally fed patients. Moreover, several controlled clinical studies have failed to show an improvement in clinical outcome with the use of parenteral nutrition for patients in need of bowel rest for inflammatory bowel disease.

While the hypothesis of parenteral feeding was being clinically tested, remarkable advances were made in the development of feeding techniques and dietary formulas for enteral nutrition. Thin, soft, radiopaque feeding tubes were developed that allowed longer periods of nasoenteric intubations with less discomfort. New enteral diets were formulated for specific nutrient needs, and they were delivered efficiently via the soft tubes. New feeding methods, such as continuous, pump-assisted feeding into the jejunum, were developed for the patient at high risk of aspiration. Finally, and perhaps most importantly, a significant reduction in dietary costs due to the use of enteral feeding was documented. Although the costs of parenteral nutrition have undergone a marked reduction in the last few years, they are still significantly greater than those for enteral feedings.

These new enteral feeding techniques are currently available in almost every hospital, and they are being used more frequently as better life-sustaining methods and treatment become available. The availability of these improved techniques makes the use of the gastrointestinal tract more efficient and less risky. "Starving" the hospitalized patient is considered today to be malpractice. For all of the aforementioned reasons a new trend in clinical nutrition has evolved which reemphasizes an old concept: "If the gut works, and can be used safely, use it." This chapter will discuss the rationale, indications, routes of access, formula composition, delivery methods, monitoring techniques, and complications of the delivery of liquid formula diets by tube.

RATIONALE

A major rationale for the use of enteral feeding is the physiologic benefit that accrues from the influence of food on the gastrointestinal tract. This benefit results from increased hormonal secretions and direct trophic effects on the intestinal mucosa. Enteral diets stimulate the secretion of diverse enterohormones, such as gastrin, gastric inhibitory polypeptide (GIP), and enteroglucagon. Some of these enterohormones, e.g., gastrin, are essential to maintain the structure and function of the intestinal epithelium. Other enterohormones, e.g., GIP, participate in the metabolism of absorbed nutrients. GIP, also called "glucose insulinotropic polypeptide," because of its effect on insulin secretion, may mediate the greater insulin response when carbohydrates are delivered enterally as compared to parenterally.

The intestinal mucosa itself is an active cellular mass that requires continuous nutrition. Mucosal cells have selective needs for fuels, such as glutamine for the small bowel and short-chain fatty acids for the colon. These fuels are utilized preferentially when present in the lumen of the gut rather than in the bloodstream. When the intestine lacks enterohormonal stimuli and luminal nutrients, villous atrophy occurs; digestive enzyme secretion is reduced and absorption is impaired.

As noted previously, the role of the gastrointestinal tract in nutrition is more than a mode of passive transference of metabolic substrates to the bloodstream. Nutrients delivered enterally are processed in the intestinal wall and the liver before reaching the systemic circulation. The induced hormonal secretion that results from enteral feeding provides a more efficient utilization of metabolic substrates.

INDICATIONS

Our selection of enteral feeding methods is based on an algorithm, as shown in Figure 1. Before initiating nutritional therapy, one must first obtain baseline nutritional data via a thorough medical history, dietary review, complete physical examination, and laboratory evaluation. To establish the need for enteral feeding, it must be demonstrated that the patient's volitional intake is insufficient to meet his nutrient needs.

The objectives of enteral feeding must be clearly identified. Enteral feedings by tube can be used as primary treatment for various gastrointestinal disorders, or secondarily for conditions causing impaired oral intake, surgery, chemotherapy, and radiotherapy (Table 1).

TABLE 1 Indications for Enteral Feedings

*Primary Treatment**
Malabsorption syndromes
Inflammatory bowel disease
Short bowel syndrome
Fistulas
Oropharyngeal disorders
Esophagogastric obstructions
Secondary Treatment
Anorexia nervosa
Neurologic disorders
Burns
Renal failure
Hepatic failure
Cardiac disease
Respiratory insufficiency
Perioperative
Cancer

* It is acknowledged that enteral feeding may also be used as a secondary modality for some of these indications.

ROUTES OF ACCESS

Enteral feedings are delivered through nasoenteric tubes or tube enterostomies. For one to decide on the appropriate route, the duration of feeding and the risk of aspiration need to be considered. If enteral feedings are to be given for less than 6 weeks, a nasoenteric tube should be used. If the patient is at potential risk of aspiration, a nasojejunal tube should be placed.

Several small-bore tubes are available for transnasal passage into the stomach, duodenum, or jejunum. These tubes are placed in the stomach with the aid of a stylet. Passage into the duodenum and jejunum is accomplished by gastrointestinal propulsion of the weighted tip. Positioning of the patient in the right lateral decubitus position and the intravenous administration of metoclopamide help promote passage across the pylorus. The tube can be manipulated into the duodenum with the aid of fluoroscopy or endoscopy if the weighted tip does not advance in 48 hours. If gastric contents cannot be aspirated with a syringe after initial placement of the tube, radiographic confirmation of the position of the tube in the stomach is mandatory before infusion of the diet. This will identify inadvertent intubation of the tracheobronchial tree. Once the correct position is confirmed, the tube is secured to the malar skin. In instances of repeated accidental removal of the feeding tube, a special bridle can be constructed to secure the tube to the nasal pharynx.

Feeding tube enterostomies can be placed by surgical procedures in several locations in the gastrointestinal tract. The most common types are pharyngostomies, gastrostomies, and jejunostomies. Pharyngostomy is a useful adjunct to head and neck surgery and has also been recommended as an easy technique for any patient requiring long-term tube feedings.

Gastrostomies are the most common type of tube enterostomies. They are performed via different surgical techniques, such as those described by Stamm and Janeway. The Stamm technique is used for temporary needs and the Janeway is a permanent gastrostomy. Recently the *percutaneous placement of a feeding gastrostomy* by endoscopic technique has gained in popularity.

Pulmonary aspiration of gastrostomy feedings is a potential complication in high-risk patients. For these patients a new tube has been devised which combines a decompression gastrostomy with a feeding jejunostomy (Fig. 2). When the risk of aspiration is overcome, the gastric port of the tube can be used for feedings or medications. As with the other temporary gastrostomies, the tube is easily replaceable.

There are two basic types of feeding jejunostomies: the Witzel and the Delany techniques. A sutured tunnel is created in the Witzel technique, and a 14-gauge needle of the type used for subclavian vein catheterization is used in the Delany method. The Delany method is an easier

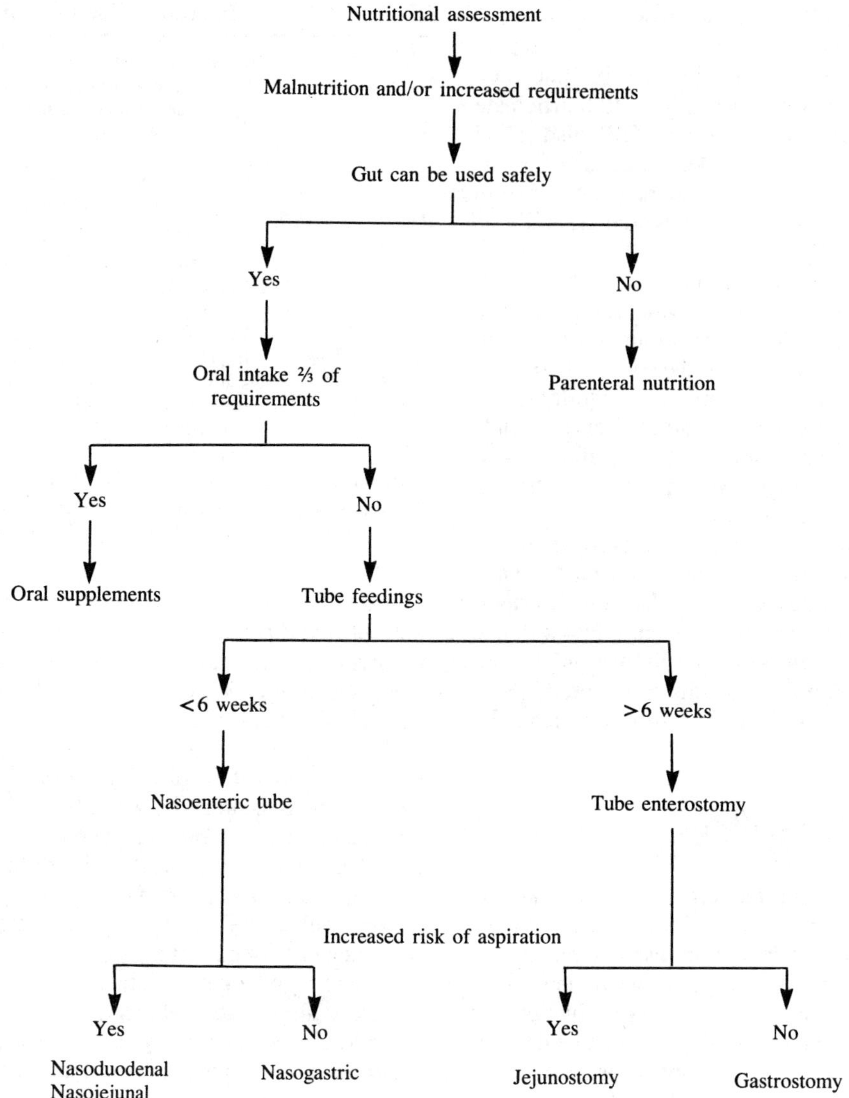

Figure 1 Decisions for enteral feeding route access.

technique with fewer surgical complications, but its limitation is that a No. 15 French catheter is used, while a No. 16 French tube is used for the Witzel jejunostomy. The resultant diameter, 1.5 mm versus 5 mm, mandates the use of low-viscosity (expensive) elemental diets for needle catheter jejunostomy feedings.

FORMULAS

Many liquid diets for enteral feeding are currently available in the United States. Several classifications of these diets have been proposed, but unfortunately, none is completely satisfactory. The problem with existing classifications is that the dietary categories are often intermingled as to both composition and clinical use. We have chosen the following classification which is based on nutrient composition: (1) polymeric, (2) elemental, and (3) modular.

Polymeric Diets

In polymeric diets the three basic nutrients—proteins, carbohydrates, and fats—are in complex forms, i.e., polymers. Carbohydrates are present in the form of oligosaccharides, maltodextrins, or polysaccharides; fats consist of medium- or long-chain triglycerides. The protein source is a natural protein which may be intact or partially hydrolyzed. In general, these diets are isotonic, lactose-free, "ready to use," and available in liquid form. Many polymeric diets can be used either for tube feedings or for oral supplementation. Selection of these diets is made on the basis of calorie, protein, and fluid requirements. Polymeric diets can be further divided according to their caloric density (Table 2). The caloric density of polymeric formulas is 0.6, 1.0, 1.5, or 2.0 Kcal per milliliter. The group with 1 Kcal per milliliter includes the largest number of commercially available diets. The nonprotein caloric content in these diets is derived from either

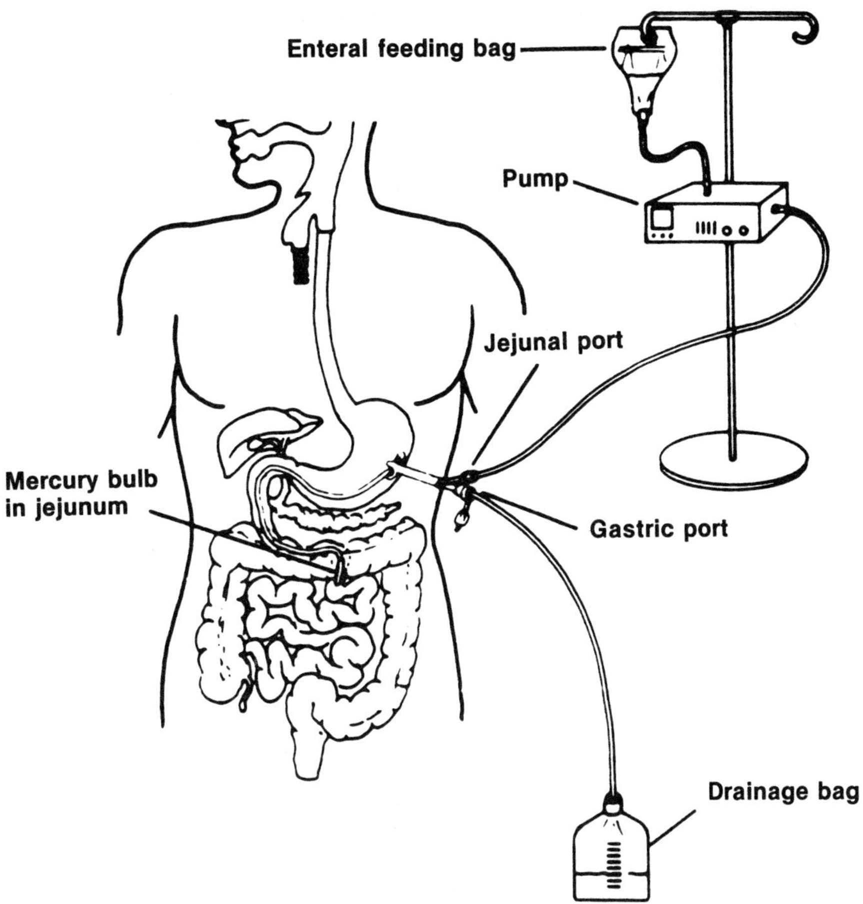

Figure 2 Enteral feeding with combined decompression gastrostomy and feeding jejunostomy. With permission from Delrio et al. Enteral Nutrition. California: Medical Specifics Publishing; p. 133.

carbohydrates or lipids. Polymeric diets formulated with carbohydrates as the main caloric source have higher osmolality than isocaloric diets containing lipids. Hypertonic diets, which are carbohydrate based, are well tolerated when infused intragastrically and reasonably well tolerated when administered directly into the small bowel. Carbohydrate based diets are advantageous for patients with steatorrhea and hyperlipidemias. Polymeric diets, which are fat based, may be more appropriate for patients who have diarrhea associated with tube feedings, especially when the feedings are infused directly into the small bowel. High-fat diets are useful for patients on mechanical ventilatory assistance, since they reduce the carbon dioxide production and thereby facilitate ventilator weaning. Most polymeric diets are formulated to provide approximately 6.25 g of protein (1 g of nitrogen) for every 150 Kcal. The concomitant provision of sufficient calories at this ratio promotes the utilization of nitrogen for synthesis of structural compounds, i.e., visceral and muscle protein. If the caloric content of the diet does not meet the patient's requirements, the protein content is utilized as an energy source and the nitrogen intake results in increased ureagenesis. Diets with high calorie:nitrogen ratios are recommended for patients with renal and hepatic insufficiency. Diets with higher caloric density, 1.5 and 2.0 Kcal per milliliter, are used for patients with increased energy requirements, e.g., hypercatabolism, or fluid restrictions, e.g., respiratory distress syndrome, renal failure, and so on.

Elemental Diets

Elemental diets, also called "chemically defined" or "synthetic" diets, include basic nutrients in monomeric forms. All elemental diets contain crystalline amino acids as the protein source, but the composition of these amino acids is variable. The source of carbohydrates varies from dextrose to oligosaccharides, while fats are usually in the form of medium-chain triglycerides. Elemental diets are hypertonic, usually in powder form, and are not palatable. Because of this lack of palatability, they are rarely used for oral supplements. Elemental diets were initially formulated with a ratio of essential:nonessential amino acids of 35 percent:65 percent, as recommended by Rose. These ratios were chosen because they resembled the high biologic value of proteins such as egg albumin and human milk.

In addition to this standard formulation of amino acids, new elemental diets have been developed with

TABLE 2 Polymeric Defined Formula Diets*

Kcal/ml	Protein (g/L)	Carbohydrate (g/L)	Fat (g/L)	Product
0.66	40	121	1.7	Citrotein
	26–45	217–249	1.3–13.5	Criticare, Precision LR & HN, Vital HN, Travasorb HN & STD
1	25–49	115–176	25–40	Isocal, Ensure, Enrich,† Precision Isotonic, Osmolite, Travasorb MCT, Renu, Vipep
	60	130	23	Sustacal
1.5	55–61	190–200	53–57	Ensure Plus, Sustacal HC
	62	105	92	Pulmocare
	83	143	68	Traumacal
2.0	70–75	225–250	80–91	Magnacal, Isocal HCN

* Caloric density and nutrient contents are based on the information provided in the product's literature.
† Enrich includes 21 g of soy polysaccharide per liter of diet as a fiber source.

different compositions of amino acids (Table 3): (1) "*stress*" formulas enriched in the branched-chain amino acids (leucine, isoleucine, and valine); (2) *hepatic* formulas containing increased branched-chain amino acids and decreased aromatic amino acids (phenylalanine, tryptophan, and tyrosine) and the sulfur amino acid methionine, and (3) *renal* formulas containing all essential amino acids and histidine and lacking the other nonessential amino acids. These three types of elemental diets consist of crystalline amino acids, monosaccharides, and low amounts of fats in the form of medium-chain triglycerides. "Stress" formulas have been developed from metabolic studies on hypercatabolism which demonstrate that branched chain amino acids may improve nitrogen balance by serving as the precursors of muscle protein. Renal formulas have been used to nourish non-dialysis patients with renal failure to promote the re-utilization of urea nitrogen for synthesis of nonessential amino acids by transamination in the liver. The hepatic formulas were initially formulated to reduce the availability of precursors of neurotransmitters (aromatic amino acids) synthesized in excess in the development of hepatic encephalopathy. The purported benefits of these three "disease-specific" elemental diets need to be documented in controlled clinical trials.

Modular Formulas

Despite the availability of numerous formulated enteral diets, there are some patients in whom standard, "fixed ratio" formulas may not be optimal. In these patients the use of modular formulas may obviate the need for parenteral nutrition. Modular diets are those formulated as separately packaged nutrient sources for each substrate. The modules consist of single or multiple nutrients that can either be combined to produce a nutritionally complete feeding or used individually to enhance an existing "fixed ratio" formula, i.e., polymeric or elemental diets. The modular system allows the physician to alter the ratio of a constituent nutrient without affecting the concentration of other constituents. One can select not only the

TABLE 3 Elemental Diets*

	Amino Acids (g/package)									
		Essential								
Formula	Total	Total	B–C	A	Nonessential	CHO (g/L)	Fat (g/L)	Kcal/g N	Kcal/ml	Product Name
Standard (stress)	38	20.1	12.6 (33%)	3.8	18.2	206	3	164	1.0	Vivonex T.E.N.
Stress	37	23.2	16.4 (44%)	3.4	14.0	140	23	90	1.2	Stresstein
	28	18.4	13.9 (50%)	2.7	9.6	166	12	87	1.0	Traum-Aid HBC
Renal	19	18.3	6.4 (33%)	6.0	0.6	366	19	380	1.9	Amin-Aid
	23	14.5	5.9 (25%)	3.9	8.4	274	18	362	1.3	Travasorb Renal
Hepatic	43	24.4	13.8 (32%)	1.3	18.5	289	36	215	1.7	Hepatic-Aid
	29	20.7	12.5 (43%)	0.8	7.8	210	15	218	1.1	Travasorb Hepatic

* Nutrient contents and caloric density are based on the information provided by the product's literature.
B–C = branched amino acids. The numbers in parentheses refer to the percentage of essential amino acids provided as B–C. The amount given for nonessential amino acids includes histidine, which may be regarded as essential amino acid for renal patients.
A = aromatic amino acids and includes methionine.

amount of each nutrient, substrate, mineral, vitamin, etc, but also the type of nutrients most appropriate for the patient, e.g., whole protein versus partially hydrolyzed versus crystalline amino acids.

It is often difficult to select the appropriate enteral formula, although choices may be limited because of an incomplete selection at any one institution. Our decision process is summarized in Figure 3. Polymeric diets are the first choice for patients with normal intestinal function and without dietary restrictions and in whom standard-sized feeding tubes have been placed. Elemental diets usually have specific disease-related indications, such as impaired enzymatic digestion, reduced absorptive surface, renal or hepatic failure, and hypercatabolic states. Modular diets are reserved for the rare patient who cannot be fed with the two previously mentioned formulas.

DELIVERY METHODS

Once the optimal diet and access site are selected, it must be decided whether to infuse the diet intermittently or continuously. Advantages of *intermittent feedings* are that a pump is not required for their administration and they may be more physiologic, since they resemble the periodicity of normal alimentation. Experimental evidence suggests that nutrients delivered intermittently are more efficiently converted into storage forms of energy than when delivered continuously. This improved utilization of nutrients appears to be mediated by the increased activity of hepatic enzymes that are involved in the conversion of carbohydrates into lipids. Intermittent feeding is also associated with improved nitrogen balance and protein synthesis. In patients with normal gastric emptying and intestinal transit, we prefer to feed intermittently into the stomach. This is particularly advantageous if the patient has a large-bore feeding tube and needs to continue enteral feedings at home. In these patients, viscous formulas or blenderized foods can be infused intermittently. Disadvantages of intermittent feeding include an increased risk of gastroesophageal reflux and aspiration. Furthermore, it is difficult to feed intermittently via a jejunostomy, especially when using hyperosmolar diets.

Advantages of *continuous feedings* include a reduction in side effects such as diarrhea and abdominal cramps. Continuous feedings are preferable for patients with delayed gastric emptying, accelerated intestinal transit, or need for hyperosmolar diets. The disadvantages of continuous feedings include the physical and psychological ''attachment'' of the patient to the pump and the expenses involved with the use of the pump.

MONITORING TECHNIQUES

Patients who receive enteral feedings require the same careful monitoring as those who receive parenteral nutrition. A protocol should be established and followed to ensure that the specified nutritional goals are met. This is especially relevant in institutions where individuals with varying experience are responsible for writing orders.

Most patients who require enteral feedings are malnourished. Malnutrition per se or other underlying conditions may be the cause of gastrointestinal intolerance to enteral diets. Therefore, it is essential to start infusing small volumes of the diet with a gradual increase in the

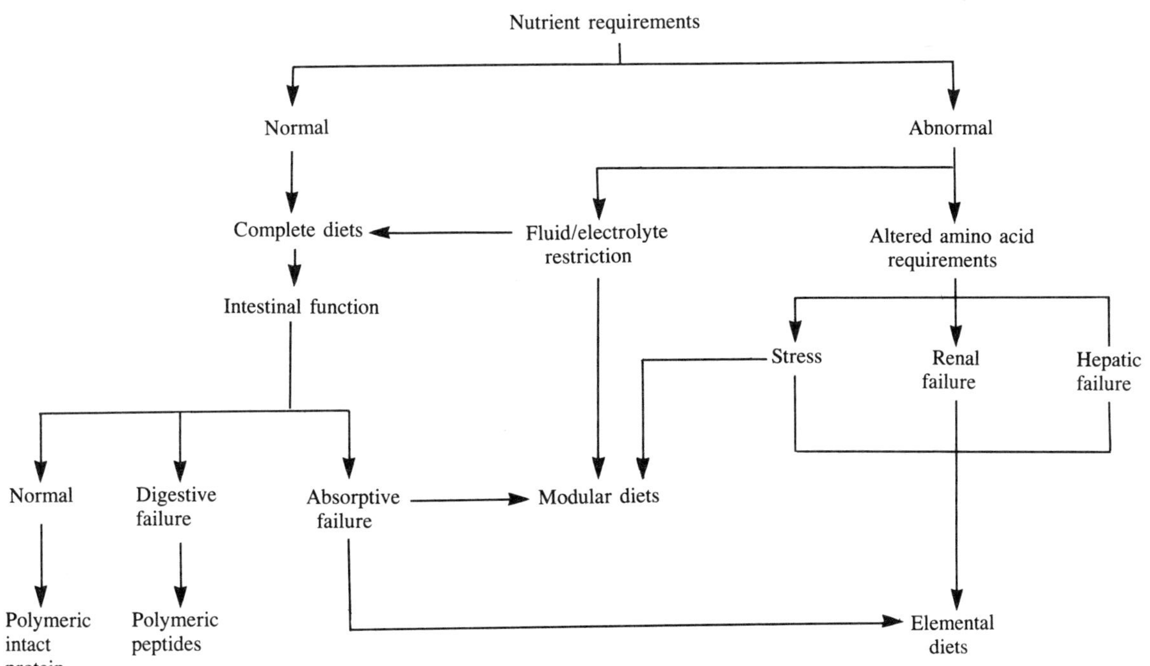

Figure 3 Selection of enteral feeding formula.

rate of delivery according to the tolerance of the patient. When increasing the rate of continuous feedings into the jejunum, we prefer to increase the volume prior to increasing the concentration of the diet. Continuous feedings can be started at a rate of 50 ml per hour and increased by 25 ml per hour daily in the absence of gastrointestinal side effects. When feeding intermittently into the stomach, volumes of 200 ml can be administered every 4 hours over a period of 15 minutes and increased by 50 ml per feeding. If the caliber of the feeding tube is sufficient, gastric residuals are checked before each feeding or every 6 to 8 hours with continuous feedings. If the residual is greater than 150 ml the patient must be evaluated for delayed gastric emptying and the feeding withheld temporarily.

COMPLICATIONS

There are two major types of complications of enteral feeding: tube-related—improper placement, dislodgment, or occlusion of the feeding tube—and gastrointestinal—delayed gastric emptying, diarrhea, and constipation. The improper placement or dislodgment of the feeding tube may lead to aspiration. The gastrointestinal complications are important. Diarrhea is the most common gastrointestinal complication and its cause is often multifactorial. Hypertonic liquid diets may cause diarrhea by an osmotic mechanism that is aggravated if the patient is hypoalbuminemic. After long periods of malnutrition and/or diminished oral intake the activity of digestive enzymes may decline. Acquired disaccharidase deficiencies may cause malabsorptive diarrhea. Perhaps the most important cause of diarrhea is the administration of antibiotics concomitantly with enteral feedings. Broad-spectrum antibiotics cause perturbation of the colonic flora, which in turn reduces the production of short-chain fatty acids. Bacterially produced short-chain fatty acids are required for sodium absorption, and when the colon is deprived of them the luminal concentration of sodium increases, thereby leading to watery diarrhea. Contamination of enteral diets has also been implicated as a cause of the diarrhea in tube feedings.

Several measures may help in the treatment of diarrhea. If the patient is receiving hyperosmolar diets the concentration should be reduced. If diarrhea is reduced the solute deficit may be compensated for by increasing the volume of the diluted diet or by switching to an isoosmolar diet. If malabsorption is suspected in a patient receiving a diet containing polymeric nutrients, the formula should be changed to an elemental diet. The deleterious effect of antibiotics on the colonic flora may be partially overcome by adding a noncellulosic fiber such as pectin to the enteral diet. Maintenance of the colonic flora depends on the availability of energy substrates in the form of fiber polysaccharides. One percent pectin can be added to enteral diets without impairment of formula delivery. Antidiarrheal agents such as paregoric (1 ml per 100 ml formula) can be used if diarrhea becomes severe. Enteral feedings should be discontinued in patients with diarrhea who are resistant to all of these therapeutic measures.

Constipation may be a serious problem in patients receiving elemental diets. The addition of bulk agents such as soy polysaccharide or mucilage (Metamucil) may improve colonic emptying.

SUGGESTED READING

Greene HL (ed). Enteral nutrition. Mead Johnson Symposium Series No. 2. Princeton NJ, Excerpta Medica, 1984.

Heimburger DC, Weinsier RL. Guidelines for evaluating and categorizing enteral feeding formulas according to therapeutic equivalence. JPEN 1985; 9:61.

Rombeau JL, Barot LR. Enteral nutritional therapy. Surg Clin North Am 1981, 61:605.

Rombeau JL, Caldwell MD (eds). Clinical nutrition, vol I. Enteral and tube feeding. Philadelphia: WB Saunders Co, 1984.

Torosian MH, Rombeau JL. Feeding by tube enterostomy. Surg Gynecol Obstet 1980; 150:918.

HYPEROXALURIA AND NEPHROLITHIASIS

JOHN W. DOBBINS, M.D.

Since the 1960s, patients with idiopathic inflammatory bowel disease have been noted to have an increased incidence of nephrolithiasis. The incidence of this condition has also increased since the advent of the jejuno-ileal bypass for obesity. The overall incidence of nephrolithiasis in inflammatory bowel disease is not great, probably only in the 2 to 3 percent range; however, prior surgical treatment increases the risk of nephrolithiasis. The incidence of nephrolithiasis in patients with Crohn's disease, who have undergone an ileal resection, is approximately 10 percent; the majority of stones, when analyzed, are composed of calcium oxalate. The incidence of nephrolithiasis in patients with ulcerative colitis who have undergone an ileostomy is also approximately 10 percent; however, in these patients uric-acid stones make up a significant proportion of the calculi. The incidence of nephrolithiasis in patients who have undergone jejuno-ileal bypass for obesity is the highest, the incidence being in the 20 percent or greater range.

URINARY CONSTITUENTS IN INTESTINAL DISEASE

Examination of the urine in patients with stone formation reveals a number of abnormalities (Table 1). The urine volume is low as is the sodium and chloride content. This indicates dehydration and extracellular volume deficit. The urine citrate, the pH, and the carbon dioxide content is low and the ammonia concentration is high. This is indicative of a metabolic acidosis, although, as will be discussed later, other factors control urinary citrate levels. Magnesium and pyrophosphate levels are also low. Magnesium, pyrophosphate, and citrate are considered inhibitors of calcium-oxalate stone formation because they either chelate the calcium or form stable complexes with the calcium or the oxalate. Urinary oxalate excretion is normal in patients who have undergone a total colectomy or who have had an ileostomy, whereas excretion is elevated in patients who have undergone an ileal resection, have either all or part of the colon in the alimentary stream, or have undergone a jejuno-ileal bypass for obesity. As a general rule, all of these urinary abnormalities, except for oxalate levels, are attributable to the malabsorption of water, electrolytes, and alkali thereby accounting for the acidosis and hypocitraturia. The increased absorption of oxalate is the sole exception and, as will be discussed, is primarily attributable to the increased absorption of dietary oxalate. In the following sections I will discuss how intestinal disease, resection, or bypass can result in the urinary abnormalities listed in Table 1.

TABLE 1 Urinary Constituents Important in Stone Formation

Urinary Constituents	*Small Bowel Resection or Bypass*	*Ileostomy*
Volume	Normal or ↓	↓
pH	Normal or ↓	↓
NH_4	↑	↑
CO_2	↓	↓
Na,C1	Normal or ↓	↓
K	↓	↓
Calcium	Normal or ↓	Normal
Mg	↓	↓
Pyrophosphate	↓	↓
Citrate	↓	↓
SO_4	↓	Normal
PO_4	↓	↓
Oxalate	↑	Normal
Urate	Normal	Normal

↓ value lower than normal
↑ value higher than normal

ENTERIC HYPEROXALURIA

Oxalic acid is an organic acid composed of two molecules of carboxylic acid; it is a strong acid that is ionized at the physiologic pH. The calcium salt of oxalic acid is only slightly soluble in water. Oxalate is a metabolic end-product in man and serves no known purpose. Oxalate is excreted almost exclusively by the kidney.

In normal individuals, approximately one-half of urinary oxalate is derived from the endogenous catabolism and one-half from the absorption of oxalate in the diet. In a normal diet oxalate is present in many foods; however, less than 10 percent is absorbed. In hyperoxaluria resulting from intestinal disease, there is increased absorption of dietary oxalate; this is designated enteric hyperoxaluria. Hyperoxaluria can also result from increased endogenous production of oxalate (primary hyperoxaluria), or present as secondary to a number of conditions such as ethylene-glycol poisoning (where ethylene glycol is converted to oxalate), pyridoxine deficiency, or excessive intake of oxalate-containing foods (rhubarb "poisoning"). Primary hyperoxaluria and secondary or acquired hyperoxalurias, other than enteric hyperoxaluria, are rare.

The mechanism of enteric hyperoxaluria is twofold. First, when intestinal disease results in steatorrhea, there is an increased *solubility* of oxalate. Normally, dietary calcium binds to dietary oxalate, forming an insoluble precipitate which prevents oxalate from being absorbed—better to form the stone in the intestine than in the kidney. When intestinal disease, resection, or bypass surgery results in malabsorption of fat calcium will bind to fatty acids more avidly than to oxalate, thereby leaving oxalate in solution and allowing more to be absorbed. Second, when bile acids and fatty acids are not absorbed in the small intestine because of disease, resection, or bypass, and spill into the colon, the *permeability* of the colon to oxalate is increased. This increased permeability is probably the result of bile acids and fatty acids chelating calcium in the tight junctions, thus making them loose or more permeable to small molecules like oxalate.

Of interest is that patients who have had a total colectomy or an ileostomy do not exhibit increased absorption of dietary oxalate or hyperoxaluria (Table 1). This suggests that increased colonic permeability to oxalate is important in the genesis of enteric hyperoxaluria. Bile acids and fatty acids do *not* appear to increase the permeability of the small intestine to oxalate. Recent evidence suggests that oxalate can be actively transported by the colon. However, the clinical significance of these observations remains to be determined. It is known that dietary protein contributes to hyperoxaluria in patients who have had a jejuno-ileal bypass for obesity; however, this contribution is small at best. In these patients, dietary protein may be converted to oxalate by bacteria in the colon.

HYPOCITRATURIA

Profound hypocitraturia has been noted in patients who have had an intestinal resection and bypass. Hypocitraturia is multifactorial in origin. Acidosis is known to decrease urinary-citrate excretion, and patients with hypocitraturia develop a metabolic acidosis secondary to bicarbonate loss in diarrheal stool. Urinary magnesium excretion has a profound effect on urinary-citrate excretion, and since hypomagnesuria is common in these patients, hypocitraturia is undoubtedly related to this problem. It was once thought that malabsorption of dietary citrate may play a role in hypocitraturia; however, removal of citrate from the diet has no effect on urinary citrate excretion in normal subjects; thus it appears that dietary citrate is unnecessary for the maintenance of a normal citrate excretion.

HYPOMAGNESURIA

The mechanism of normal magnesium absorption is not well understood; therefore, our understanding of the role of the intestine in hypomagnesuria associated with intestinal resection and bypass is limited. However, it is known that fatty acids and bile acids can precipitate magnesium and that some magnesium malabsorbtion probably occurs on this basis. It appears likely that when there is extensive resection or bypass that some magnesium is malabsorbed because of the loss of intestinal surface area. Some magnesium malabsorption may be obligatory simply because of the volume of diarrheal stool.

TREATMENT

Calcium Oxalate Nephrolithiasis

Increase Urine Volume. In general, the goal of therapy in nephrolithiasis should be to reverse all the urinary abnormalities that increase the likelihood of stone formation (Table 1). This can be difficult in a patient with an extensive ileal resection that results in the short bowel syndrome. Urine volume should be increased by increasing fluid intake and by decreasing diarrhea. Since most of the urinary abnormalities in Table 1 are attributable to diarrhea, considerable attention should be directed toward decreasing it. In general, diarrhea is treated by reducing the malabsorption of fat and carbohydrates as much as possible and by using antidiarrheal agents (codeine, loperamide, etc).

Low Oxalate Diet. If hyperoxaluria is present, a low oxalate diet should be instituted (Table 2). This will significantly reduce urinary oxalate excretion in most patients. Foods with a high oxalate (>40 mg per serving) should be avoided and even foods with a moderate oxalate content (>10 mg per serving) should be limited.

Decrease Steatorrhea. If there is significant steatorrhea (>20 g per day), then a low fat diet should be instituted. A low fat diet decreases fatty-acid concentration in the colon resulting in a decrease in fatty-acid-mediated alteration in colonic permeability. There is also less calcium-fatty-acid soap formation, and more calcium will be available to precipitate oxalate, thus preventing the absorption of oxalate. Unfortunately dietary fat cannot be decreased below approximately 50 g per day without making the diet unpalatable. This problem can be overcome somewhat by using medium-chain triglycerides. Medium-chain fatty acids neither increase the permeability of the colon to oxalate nor do they chelate calcium; thus, they do not affect the permeability or the solubility of oxalate.

Anion Binding Agents. "Anion binding agents" work by binding to bile acids and fatty acids, thereby decreasing bile acid and fatty-acid induced diarrhea. Thus they prevent the increase in colonic permeability induced by these acids, which bind to oxalate, and prevent its absorption. Anion-binding agents that can be used include cholestyramine, calcium, aluminum, magnesium, and bismuth. Cholestyramine however, can make the steatorrhea worse and should not be used if fecal-fat excretion is greater than 20 g per day. Also cholestyramine should be used with caution if the fecal fat excretion is greater than 10 g per day. The usual dose is 4 g (one packet) up to 4 times a day; however, this varies from patient to patient. Cholestyramine is also expensive. To avoid making the aluminum phosphate depletion significantly worse, aluminum hydroxide must be used with care (Table 1). Likewise, one must keep an eye on urinary-calcium excretion when administering this agent. Patients with significant small-bowel resection or bypass, however, usually have hypocalciuria. Of the alkali-metal preparations, I prefer Camalox, which is a combination of calcium carbonate, aluminum hydroxide, and magnesium hydroxide. The calcium, magnesium, and aluminum bind to oxalate, bile acids, and fatty acids. Magnesium is provided to help correct hypomagnesuria and alkali is provided to help increase urinary pH and to correct any hypocitraturia. Camalox usually does not worsen the diarrhea. I begin with 1 tablespoon (3 tablets) 3 times a day with meals, and I adjust the dose until urinary oxalate excretion is less than 50 mg per 24 hours.

Increase Urinary Magnesium Excretion. Urinary magnesium is important because it increases the solubility of oxalate and helps prevent hypocitraturia. Hypomagnesium can be difficult to correct because magnesium-salt ingestion can make the diarrhea worse. Diarrhea may be less of a problem when magnesium is administered along with calcium (i.e., Camalox). Some investigators have claimed success with magnesium oxide and magnesium gluconate. Various preparations can be tried. The amount of magnesium administered should be increased until urinary magnesium excretion is normal or a significant increase in diarrhea occurs. When using Camalox, administer it as already described. If using magnesium oxide, begin wtih 150 mg 4 times a day and increase until urinary magnesium excretion is normal or diarrhea is significantly worse.

Increase Urinary Citrate Excretion. To correct hypocitraturia it is necessary to restore urinary magnesium excretion to a level as close to normal as possible and to give alkali, such as calcium carbonate or sodium bicarbonate. Citrate can be given, but this is expensive. One advantage of citrate is that it comes in fairly concentrated forms. One ounce of Polycitra is equivalent to a 60 milliequivalent of bicarbonate, and it takes eight 650-mg

TABLE 2 Oxalate Content of Common Foods*

Oxalate Content	*Foods*	*Serving Size*	*Serving Weight (g)*	*Oxalate Content*	*Foods*	*Serving Size*	*Serving Weight (g)*
>100 mg/serving:	Beets	½ cup	83	10–20 mg/serving (continued):	Rutabagas	½ cup	100
	Chard	½ cup	90		Turnip greens	½ cup	90
	Rhubarb	½ cup	100		Blueberries	½ cup	120
	Spinach	½ cup	90		Blackberries	½ cup	70
	Cocoa	Tbsp.	7		Currants	½ cup	100
70–100 mg/serving:	Collard	½ cup	90		Strawberries	10 large	100
	Leeks	½ cup	90		Oranges	½ small	120
	Okra	8–9 pods	100		Fruit cake	1 slice	60
	Gooseberries, raw	⅔ cup	100		(WW) Allison's bread	1 slice	30
	Peanuts	½ cup	75	5–10 mg/serving:	Corn on the cob	1 small ear	100
40–70 mg/serving:	Raspberries	¾ cup	100		Mustard greens	½ cup	90
20–40 mg/serving:	Beans, green and wax	½ cup	62–100		Potato	1 small	100
					Parsnips	⅔ cup	100
	Carrots	⅔ cup	100		Parsley	1 Tbsp.	3.7
	Onion, fresh	½ cup	100		Tomato	½ cup	100
	Grapes	½ cup	100		Grapefruit	½ cup	100
	Squash, summer	½ cup	90		Prunes	5 large	50
	Chocolate	1 oz	28		Biscuits	1 small	30
10–20 mg/serving:	Beans, pinto	½ cup	100		Kidney	3 oz	90
	Eggplant	½ cup	100		Liver	3 oz	90
	Celery	½ cup	100		Sponge cake	1 slice	60
	Dandelion greens	½ cup	100		Orange peel	1 Tbsp.	4
	Fruit cocktail	½ cup	100		Lemon peel	1 Tbsp.	4
	Pepper, green	2 cups	100				

Beverages

Oxalate Content	*Beverage*	*Serving Size (oz)*	*Oxalate Content*	*Beverage*	*Serving Size (oz)*
10–20+ mg/serving:	Tea	8	0–5 mg/serving:	Apple juice	6
	Cola (Coke)	12		Grape juice	6
5–10+ mg/serving:	Coffee (ground)	8		Orange juice	6
	Coffee (instant)	8		Pineapple juice	6
	Ovaltine	8		Tomato juice	6
	Red Wine	6		White wine	6
				Milk	8

Foods With Little If Any Oxalate

Apple	Cucumbers	Mango	Plums	Sugar, salt
Avocado	Grapefruit	Melons	Radishes	Turnip
Cauliflower	Grapes	Nectarines	Squash	Flavoring extracts
Cherries	Lime, lemon	Olives, pickles	Starches (except potato)	

* The following table presents dietary constituents according to oxalate content per average serving. Oxalate content was obtained from standard reference sources. Foods not listed have either less than 5 mg oxalate/serving *or* the oxalate content is uncertain. The standard serving is presented as both volume and weight. Foods containing more than 10 mg oxalate/serving should be avoided, and those containing 5 to 10 mg/serving used only sparingly. (From: Earnest DL. In: Bayless TM ed. Current therapy in gastroenterology and liver disease. Toronto: BC Decker 1984:176.)

TABLE 3 Treatment of Nephrolithiasis Associated with Intestinal Disease

Modality		Amount
Calcium Oxalate Nephrolithiasis		
Increase urine volume		
Increase fluid intake		
Decrease diarrhea		
Low oxalate diet		<75 mg/day
Low fat diet		50 g/day
Anion binding agents		
Cholestyramine		Up to 4 g q.i.d.
Calcium	Camalox	Variable, must monitor urinary oxalate excretion
Magnesium	Camalox	
Aluminum	Camalox	
Bismuth		
Pepto Bismol		
Magnesium		
Camalox		Enough to normalize urinary citrate excretion
Mg oxide		
Mg gluconate		
Citrate		
$NaHCO_3$		Enough to normalize urinary citrate excretion
Polycitra		
Urate Nephrolithiasis		
Increase urine volume		
Increase urine pH		
$NaHCO_3$		Increase until urine pH is in the 6.5 range
Polycitra		

sodium bicarbonate tablets to give the same amount of bicarbonate. I start with a half ounce of Polycitra twice a day or 2 tablets of sodium bicarbonate 4 times a day and increase the dose until urinary citrate levels are in the normal range. Alternatively, one can monitor serum bicarbonate and urinary pH. Keep in mind that dehydration can result in a contraction alkalosis, thereby making serum bicarbonate levels difficult to evaluate.

Urate Nephrolithiasis

Uric acid stones are seen primarily in patients with an ileostomy, and generally speaking, these patients do not have increased excretion of uric acid in the urine (Table 1). Uric acid stone formation in these patients is attributable to decreased urine volume and low-urine pH; low-urine pH is the most important factor. Urinary volume can be increased as described previously. Urinary pH should be increased by administration of bicarbonate or citrate in amounts sufficient to keep the urinary pH consistently in the 6.5 range; patients should be given nitrazine paper so they can monitor their own urinary pH. Allopurinol should be used only if urinary urate excretion increases or if the patient continues to form uric acid stones after correcting volume and pH changes as much as possible.

Approaches to the treatment of nephrolithiasis associated with intestinal disease are summarized in Table 3.

CROHN'S DISEASE OF THE SMALL BOWEL

STEPHEN B. HANAUER, M.D.

Crohn's disease is a chronic variant of inflammatory bowel disease for which neither the cause nor the cure has been identified. Hence, when making therapeutic decisions, the physician must consider the short- and long-term consequences of the actual illness as well as the potential benefit and "cost" of medical therapy. Furthermore, since surgery is almost never curative for Crohn's disease, one must constantly balance the less immediate rewards of continuing medical therapy against the short-term benefits of surgery followed by almost certain recurrence.

In initially managing the patient with Crohn's disease, it is important to confirm the diagnosis and to exclude complications such as intercurrent enteric infections, lactose intolerance, or bile-acid-induced diarrhea. A review of the original diagnosis and, if necessary, an update of studies to assess the current location and extent of the inflammatory process are essential.

The diagnosis of active Crohn's disease can be confirmed by the presence of inflammatory symptoms and signs (fever, night sweats, abdominal tenderness and so on) supported by laboratory findings of an increased white blood cell count, elevated sedimentation rate, fecal leukocytes, an increase in fecal $alpha_1$-antitrypsin and radiographic or endoscopic evidence of mucosal edema or ulceration. Any patient presenting with a sudden exacerbation of symptoms should have stool cultures for enteric pathogens, a fecal smear for ova and parasites, and an assay for *Clostridium difficile* toxin. More chronic or progressive symptoms require a review of the current therapy for possible adverse consequences, or postsurgical or noninflammatory complications. The latter may range from partial obstruction in areas of scarred bowel with poor motility and bacterial overgrowth to the short bowel syndrome with profuse diarrhea and malnutrition.

A thorough evaluation (or reevaluation) of each patient is essential to determine the site of activity of the Crohn's inflammation, and to exclude superinfection or additional complications. A review of the dietary history and an updated nutritional profile are important whenever new or changing symptoms arise. The extent of the evaluation will depend upon the complaints and the previous history of the individual patient.

MEDICAL APPROACH TO TREATMENT

The potential medical therapy for small intestinal Crohn's disease ranges from changes in diet to immunosuppressant medication. Many of the therapeutic alternatives, including steroids, are nonspecific and are directed at symptoms rather than the actual disease process. The ultimate goal of treatment often is supportive, aiming to control symptoms and to maintain an active lifestyle until the disease activity is brought under control.

Each patient will require an individualized program of therapy incorporating dietary modifications, medications, and recommendations regarding necessary changes in lifestyle. A complete nutritional assessment and dietary plan must ensure replacement and/or maintenance of essential nutrients which are administered in a manner to minimize adverse symptoms. Antidiarrheal agents and additional adjunctive medications should be prescribed to reduce symptoms. Antibacterial agents are indicated for such complications as bacterial overgrowth or abscess or, in a more general role, to supplement or spare steroid therapy. Sulfasalazine presumably has specific gut-related anti-inflammatory activity and is often used as a first-line therapy or combined with steroids to treat mild to moderate intestinal Crohn's disease. Steroids remain the mainstay of medical therapy for more moderate to severe small bowel Crohn's disease, but they require judicious monitoring of the cost-benefit ratio. *Specific objectives of therapy* should be identified prior to administering steroids, immunosuppressant agents or hyperalimentation.

Nutritional Therapy

Diet and nutritional factors are of the utmost importance in the management of patients with intestinal ailments. In small intestinal Crohn's disease in which the normal absorptive mechanisms have been disrupted, nutritional evaluation and planning are indispensable. Whether the patient complains of weight loss, abdominal pain, diarrhea, or nonintestinal symptoms, a review of the dietary history is an important first step. Lactose intolerance should be ruled out by breath hydrogen or blood sampling. A nutritional profile including the assessment of iron stores, folate, vitamin B_{12}, and fat-soluble vitamins is important, as are the more routine measurements of electrolytes, calcium, magnesium, phosphate, and serum albumin. Trace mineral deficiencies should be considered in patients with protracted, severe diarrhea or malnutrition.

While no dietary factors are known to cause or activate intestinal inflammation, modifications in the diet can provide relief from a variety of symptoms, and a dietary plan for the individual patient is an important practical measure.

Most patients can be managed with an oral dietary program. Sufficient calories and protein to maintain body weight and replenish intestinal losses are essential. Milk products should be withheld or modified by one of the available lactase products (e.g., LactAid or Lactrase) for patients with lactose intolerance. In either case, sufficient calcium (1 g daily) should be provided. Replacement of diminished vitamin stores by either the enteral or parenteral route will depend on the deficient factors and the patient's tolerance of these compounds. The amount of fat allowed in the diet will depend on the individual's tendency to develop steatorrhea.

In most patients with small bowel Crohn's disease I institute a modified low-residue diet that avoids large amounts of "hard roughage" such as raw fruits and vegetables, nuts, and seeds in favor of cooked, canned, or peeled fruits and vegetables. Highly seasoned foods also are proscribed in patients prone to diarrhea.

More refined or elemental diets have been useful as an adjunct in patients with more severe disease. While controversy still exists regarding the ultimate role of highly modified diets, there is no question that a change to elemental feedings can markedly reduce the symptoms of patients with active disease or luminal narrowing. Unfortunately, the lack of palatability of the available preparations over prolonged periods limits the length of time that most patients will tolerate this modification. In some situations, such as children with growth retardation, nocturnal enteral elemental feedings via a nasoenteric feeding tube may be a useful supplement to the daily oral intake.

Parenteral nutritional support may be useful to (1) provide supplemental feedings in patients unable to tolerate sufficient oral calories, (2) improve the nutritional status in malnourished patients scheduled for elective surgery, (3) reduce symptoms in patients with active disease, (4) reverse growth retardation in children, and (5) provide maintenance therapy for the short bowel. The role of total parenteral nutrition and bowel rest is the subject of continued controversy. A regimen of complete bowel rest often is of symptomatic benefit in situations in which the added caloric intake cannot be tolerated without aggravating symptoms. Fistulas and perianal suppuration often improve with the reduction in intestinal output, although permanent closure of fistula tracts unfortunately is rare. It also has been speculated that the reduction in orally derived antigens may beneficially alter the local gut immune response and allow healing. I have observed marked reductions in inflammatory masses and have avoided surgery in patients with complicated courses by the prolonged (3 to 6 months) use of hyperalimentation. tation.

Adjunctive Medications

Medications often are administered to reduce symptoms. Antispasmodics may be effective in alleviating abdominal cramps and pain. Anticholinergic agents can be administered safely in patients with luminal narrowing, although they should be closely monitored and warned to discontinue antimotility agents in the presence of progressive or severe pain or abdominal distention. I tend to prescribe such drugs on a continual rather than "as needed" basis to maintain control of the symptoms. Antidiarrheal drugs also are of benefit in patients with small (and large) bowel Crohn's disease. Again, these agents should be discontinued in the presence of toxic symptoms, severe abdominal pain, or suspicion of obstruction.

Histamine$_2$ receptor antagonists may help relieve symptoms in patients with Crohn's disease of the upper gastrointestinal tract. Sucralfate may be similarly helpful, although neither has been studied in a controlled clinical trial.

Cholestyramine is useful in patients who have undergone surgery with bile-salt-induced diarrhea. In this setting, the dose is titrated to the point of maximal symptomatic benefit. One may begin with one-half packet or one-half scoopful (2 g of resin) administered twice daily and adjusted upward to three to four packets daily. I often note benefit at lower doses, and higher doses may actually worsen symptoms if the bile salt pool becomes depleted. Care should be taken to avoid administering this resin with other medications, levels of fat-soluble vitamins need to be monitored, and the drug should be discontinued in the presence of partial obstruction, as formed contents may worsen or complete the blockage.

Sedatives or anxiolytics have a role in individual patients but should be carefully regulated because of the hazard of possible drug dependency. Accordingly, I *almost never* prescribe narcotic analgesics. Pain severe enough to require narcotics should be evaluated for more sharply focused therapy. Cramps may be treated with antispasmodics, partial obstruction with a more refined diet , abscess by drainage, and so on. Partial obstruction may be aggravated by narcotics (increased intraluminal pressure) and, conversely, can be eased by dietary adjustments and antispasmodics. Other causes of chronic pain are never resolved by narcotics. Many patients are referred who are already addicted to narcotics and thus require inpatient admissions for detoxification. In these situations, I emphasize the alternative approaches to the treatment of pain (biofeedback, transcutaneous electrical nerve stimulation, physiotherapy, and so on) and withhold potent analgesia for the perioperative setting.

Patient support measures include literature from the National Foundation for Ileitis and Colitis (NFIC), 444 Park Ave. South, New York, 10016 as well as local NFIC chapter support groups.

"Specific" Medications

Sulfasalazine. Many experienced clinicians have found sulfasalazine therapy useful to reduce enteric inflammation and to maintain patients once the active phase has subsided. Although sulfasalazine had only limited but significant benefit in small intestinal Crohn's disease in the National Cooperative Crohn's Disease Study (NCCDS), I have found the drug helpful in some patients with mild to moderate small bowel disease even in the absence of active colonic inflammation. For mild symptoms, the drug may be administered as the solitary "specific" medication in quantities of 2 to 4 g daily in divided doses. If symptoms improve, a maintenance dose of 2 g daily may be continued almost indefinitely. Here again, little benefit in preventing relapses was observed in the NCCDS; however, I frequently observe flare-ups in patients when sulfasalazine therapy is suddenly withdrawn. In the presence of more severe inflammatory symptoms, sulfasalazine may be administered in conjunction with corticosteroids and maintained as the steroids are gradually withdrawn. Sulfasalazine (or other antibiotics, see below) may behave as a "steroid-sparing" agent, and can maintain quiescent symptoms as the steroids are tapered.

The mode of action of sulfasalazine in inflammatory bowel disease has not been elucidated (see the chapter *Ulcerative Colitis).* Although once regarded mainly as an antibacterial drug, the 5-aminosalicylic acid moiety is the more active component, at least for colonic disease. Both the parent compound and 5-aminosalicylic acid interact at various levels within the arachidonic cascade of inflammatory mediators.

Sulfasalazine is best tolerated when taken with meals to avoid the side effects of headache and nausea. A gradual dose increment is useful to initiate therapy, at which time patients can be observed for intolerance. Allergic side effects, such as skin rashes or drug fever, are not uncommon and can be overcome by a desensitization program beginning with very low doses of sulfasalazine suspension (1 to 50 mg initially), with doubling of the dose every 3 days. More severe allergic reactions, such as hepatitis, agranulocytosis, or hemolytic anemias, are less common and require discontinuation of the drug. Sulfasalazine is known to inhibit the absorption of folic acid from the diet; hence, 1 mg daily of folic acid is added to the regimen of patients receiving chronic therapy.

Antibacterial Agents. Antibiotics also have been found to be useful either alone or in conjunction with steroids. *Metronidazole* has been used extensively lately, following reports of its value in the treatment of perianal Crohn's Disease. Subsequently, the European Cooperative Crohn's Disease Study found metronidazole to be as effective as sulfasalazine for colonic Crohn's disease and somewhat better than sulfasalazine for the treatment of ileal Crohn's disease. The optimal dose of metronidazole has not been determined, although a cooperative study of metronidazole as the sole treatment of Crohn's disease in the United States in evaluating both 10 and 20 mg per kilogram per day, while 20 mg per kilogram per day has been recommended for perianal disease.

Most patients will tolerate between 500 and 1,500 mg daily. The common side effects include a metallic taste in the mouth, a coated tongue, and occasional nausea. Peripheral neuropathy has been the most troublesome complication of metronidazole. In my experience this occurs more commonly in malnourished patients. Therefore, I prescribe supplemental vitamins for all patients taking metronidazole with a warning to discontinue the drug should they develop any signs of tingling or numbness in the extremities. The neuropathy seems reversible in most instances, although there have been a few reports of persistent changes. Patients also should be warned of the interaction between metronidazole and ethanol producing an Antabuse-like effect. Potential tumorigenicity and mutagenicity in laboratory animals have been observed, causing concern over the long-term use of this drug in humans. The potential benefit (response) in this chronic illness needs to be weighed against reports of animal toxicity, although no such effects have been described in humans. I maintain patients on the lowest possible dose of metronidazole (assuming an initial response) and warn women against becoming pregnant while on the drug.

Alternative antibiotics have not been extensively studied in clinical trials, although most gastroenterologists who treat Crohn's disease utilize antibacterials in a nonspecific manner. Individual practitioners have favored regimens which employ either a single drug or alternating antibiotics in a serial fashion (as one might treat bacterial overgrowth). The *tetracyclines, sulfonamides, ampicillin, erythromycin,* and *sulfamethoxazole-trimethoprim* each have proponents. Again, I tend to prescribe a single antibiotic as primary therapy either alone or in combination with steroids for patients who have failed to improve with or are tolerant of sulfasalazine. These drugs also are indicted for treatment of suspected bacterial overgrowth or evidence of an abscess or septic focus and may be of benefit for patients with enteric arthropathies or cutaneous manifestations of Crohn's disease.

Corticosteroids. Steroids have been the most consistently effective agents for the treatment of active small bowel Crohn's disease in all clinical trials. Unfortunately, the efficacy has been at the expense of a wide spectrum of adverse consequences. Furthermore, as with all drugs studied to date in Crohn's disease, corticosteroids have a palliative rather than curative action. Steroids appear to be of no benefit in maintaining remissions of quiescent disease or in preventing recurrences after surgical resection.

Nevertheless, steroids are the most commonly used (and often abused) medications for small bowel Crohn's disease. Steroids are indicated if sulfasalazine or antibiotic therapy has not been adequate to control symptoms of mild ileitis or ileocolitis and should be prescribed alone, or in combination with sulfasalazine or an antibiotic, as initial treatment for moderate or severe disease. One can expect a prompt reduction of symptoms and a return to a feeling of well-being with an improved appetite and associated weight gain. Corticosteroids are potent antidiarrheal agents in small intestinal Crohn's disease, can reduce inflammatory masses, will reduce luminal narrowings due to active disease (in the presence of mucosal edema and ulceration, but not fibrotic strictures, manifest by pseudodiverticula and the absence of inflammation), may improve perianal disease (partially by decreasing diarrhea), but have not been effective in closing enteric fistula. These drugs may be hazardous in the presence of sepsis (abscess or peritonitis) unless they are administered in "stress doses" to patients with adrenal suppression from prior steroid therapy.

Adrenocorticotropic hormone injections or intravenous drip infusions may be of similar benefit for patients with flare-ups of Crohn's disease, and appear to be best suited for patients who have not been receiving other forms of steroids.

A variety of preparations are available for oral or parenteral use, and change from one form to another may be associated with clinical improvement in patients who seem to be no longer responsive to steroid therapy. The most widely used preparation is *prednisone,* usually prescribed as 40 to 60 mg daily in a single morning dose. The once a day schedule mimics the diurnal variation of endogenous cortisone, allows convenient tapering, and appears appropriate for alternate day dosing and an eventual return of adrenal function with gradual weaning. Alternatively, split doses may be necessary for patients with persistent nocturnal symptoms. *Prednisolone* and *methylprednisolone* are alternatives which can be used in a similar manner. *Hydrocortisone* may also be prescribed in divided doses (initially 50 mg 4 times daily) and may be of use in patients who fail to improve with prednisone, although at the expense of enhanced salt retention (as may be seen also with *triamcinolone*).

Once a clinical remission has been achieved, tapering should begin, but the exact schedule will depend upon the individual patient's response to the initial decrease in dosage. I find that the most frequent cause of referrals for active disease is an exacerbation of the disease due to too rapid tapering of steroids. In general, the weaning process correlates with the length and severity of symptoms and prior therapy. Patients with the acute onset of ileitis may have their dose decreased from 40 mg by 5 mg per week, whereas patients who have been under therapy for many months or years require a more gradual approach. In these patients a reduction by 5 mg per month down to a 20-mg dose and a 2.5 mg per month reduction thereafter, may be necessary to wean a chronically ill patient from steroids. Some patients may remain at a dose of 20 mg daily and have trouble with further tapering. In this situation, the addition or change to a different antibiotic and/or steroid preparation can be useful in renewing the tapering process.

Alternate day therapy may be useful in selected patients and has the benefit of lessened adrenal suppression. In children with small bowel Crohn's disease, alternate-day therapy can be effective in avoiding the problem of growth retardation. In adults it is presumed, though not tested in clinical trials, that alternate day therapy will reduce the adverse consequences of long-term steroid therapy. Unfortunately, this worthy goal is difficult to achieve in most adults, although some patients with chronic, low-grade symptoms can be maintained on alternate-day prednisone.

The adverse effects of steroid therapy are well known and need not be detailed in this review. There are, however, a few complications more characteristic of small intestinal Crohn's disease which should be emphasized. First, the physician should be cautious about initiating steroid therapy in a patient with a potential suppurative complication for which antibiotics and/or surgical drainage are likely to be more helpful. In children steroids can aggravate growth retardation, and we have found that in both children and adults steroid therapy is most beneficial in terms of a more rapid response if the nutritional status has been restored toward normal. Metabolic bone disease is seen without steroids in Crohn's disease, and the addition of steroids to regimens for patients with insufficient calcium, magnesium, and vitamin D intake may accelerate bone demineralization and osteoporosis. It is essential that vitamin D stores be maintained and adequate calcium supplemented as part of the nutritional program.

Immunosuppressant Agents. Immunosuppressive agents have been used sporadically for 20 years despite a number of clinical trials that have not as yet provided clear evidence of their efficacy in Crohn's disease of the small bowel. The acute and chronic course of Crohn's disease, the wide spectrum of clinical situations, and the length of time necessary to evaluate objectively a response to these drugs probably have made it difficult to document proof of benefit in randomized controlled trials. Hence, it is not surprising that the NCCDS was unable to identify improvement in the patients treated with azathioprine (2.5 mg per kilogram) as a single therapeutic modality over 17 weeks when steroid withdrawal was mandatory. Other investigators have recognized that azathioprine may have a role as an adjunct to steroid therapy or in the prevention of relapse of medically or surgically treated patients. Most recently, Present and Korelitz have utilized 6-mercaptopurine in a 2-year placebo-controlled, crossover protocol.[1] These two investigators were able to identify a favorable response in two-thirds of their patients manifested as significant improvements in symptoms, improvement in fistulas, and a reduction in the steroid dose. In this study and in subsequent reports, many patients required up to 6 months to respond, so that the short-term efficacy probably cannot be evaluated. Furthermore, many patients were receiving concurrent steroid treatment which was gradually tapered, compared with the NCCDS which demanded regular reduction of steroids and termination of azathioprine at 17 weeks.

The immunosuppressive drugs probably are effective in a subgroup of patients with Crohn's disease. The fears of long-term consequences, most notably susceptibility to malignancy, as yet have not been borne out in the large series of patients from New York. Nevertheless, patients must be followed closely for the development of neutropenia. Pancreatitis was observed in 5 percent of patients receiving azathioprine in the NCCDS and probably occurs with a similar frequency with 6-mercaptopurine. Possible hepatotoxicity and malignancy have yet to be confirmed in patients with Crohn's disease.

I reserve the use of immunosuppressants in small bowel Crohn's disease (1) for patients with refractory disease activity which persists despite steroids or recurs with tapering; (2) as adjunctive therapy for patients with postoperative recurrences in an attempt to avoid additional surgery; (3) in patients with diffuse small bowel Crohn's disease (jejunoileitis) in whom surgery would be impractical; (4) in patients with intractable perianal disease; (5) in patients with fistulas for whom surgery is not desirable; and (6) in patients with extra-intestinal manifestations of inflammatory bowel disease (arthritis, erythema nodosum, iritis and so on) out of proportion to the bowel disease. I begin with 50 mg daily of either azathioprine or 6-mercaptopurine and follow the complete blood count weeky for the first month. After 2 weeks the dose is increased to 100 mg daily and eventually to a total dose of 2 to 2.5 mg per kilogram per day. Blood counts are followed monthly after a stable dose has been achieved. Many patients respond to lower doses (e.g, 50 to 100 mg per day), which diminish the risk of neutropenia. Abdominal pain or nausea should be evaluated by measuring serum amylase or lipase, and liver function tests should be followed every 3 to 4 months. I generally begin to taper steroids after a stable clinical course has been achieved. Although up to 6 months may be required to determine efficacy, most patients tolerate these drugs well. Unfortunately, experience indicates that disease activity typically recurs after withdrawal of these medications, so that long-term therapy, albeit at reduced dosages, may be necessary.

ACUTE DISEASE

Patients presenting with new or recurrent disease should be assessed as described above for the location and activity of the Crohn's disease as well as for possible complications. Those with milder symptoms of diarrhea, abdominal cramping, limited weight loss and no abdominal mass or fistula may begin to receive sulfasalazine (2 to 4 g per day) alone or an alternate antibiotic and instructed as to a diet (usually low-residue with or without milk products according to their lactase status). Adequate protein, calcium, and vitamin supplements should be provided. If symptoms persist, a trial of mild antispasmodics, antidiarrheal agents, or both should be instituted prior to advancing to steroid therapy. Therapy is then continued until a complete response is achieved. Even though symptoms remit, I will maintain the initial dose of sulfasalazine for up to 5 to 6 months before beginning to taper down to a maintenance dose of 2 g per day.

Patients with moderate disease manifested by fever, significant weight loss, more severe diarrhea and abdominal pain and tenderness usually will require steroids. While the benefit of combination therapy remains controversial, I commonly prescribe both prednisone and an antibiotic (or sulfasalazine) beginning with 40 mg of prednisone until a complete response is achieved. At that point, the prednisone can be decreased rapidly by 5 mg every week or 2 (as tolerated) down to 20 mg, and by about 5 mg per month thereafter. While this schedule probably is slower than many physicians prescribe, I have been impressed by the frequency of incomplete responses or exacerbations with the rapid tapering schedules frequently employed. I maintain the antibiotic therapy while the steroids are tapered and often will change drugs if there is a worsening of symptoms prior to complete withdrawal. Dietary and nonspecific, symptomatic therapy are, of course, continued.

Patients with more severe disease manifested by malnutrition or a tender inflammatory mass or abscess, or those appearing septic require hospitalization. They should be stabilized with intravenous hydration and broad-spectrum antibiotics (after appropriate cultures of blood, urine, and so on), such as metronidazole and an aminoglycoside; clindamycin and an aminoglycoside; or cefoxitin. Steroids should be withheld (unless the patient has been taking adrenal suppressive doses) until a suppurative process has been excluded. Once an abscess or perforation has been ruled out, parenteral steroids should be administered in divided doses equal to 40 to 60 mg per day of prednisone. This can be changed to an oral regimen as the patient improves.

The decision whether or not medical therapy should be continued in acute disease will depend upon associated complications. I consider evidence of an abscess, persistent obstruction, continuing hemorrhage, or complicated fistula (enterosigmoid, enterovesical, and so on) as indications for surgical intervention. Surgery usually is recommended as soon as the patient has been stabilized, rehydrated, and prepared with preoperative antibiotics.

Patients who respond to initial medical intervention may be considered for further medical and nutritional therapy. For severely malnourished individuals with significant abdominal pain, an inflammatory mass, or partial obstruction, a period of hyperalimentation and bowel rest will allow the steroids (and time) to determine whether surgery will be necessary. For those who respond the diet can be gradually advanced. Less ill patients who can tolerate oral feedings may be placed on elemental feedings or a low-residue diet as discussed previously. With clinical improvement, the diet then may be advanced as tolerated, with constant monitoring of weight, nutritional stores, and calorie counts. The patients then are gradually weaned off steroids as described for less severely ill individuals.

CHRONIC DISEASE

Chronically ill patients require a separate decision analysis because of their failure to respond completely to medical therapy, inability to eliminate steroids, a persistent mass, or recurrent obstruction. These patients are caught in a dilemma because medical treatment has been less than optimal, prior surgery has provided only temporary improvement, or the patient is a poor surgical candidate owing to diffuse or multifocal disease. The objectives of medical therapy in this setting are to create a less toxic, but effective long-term treatment regimen or to modify the intestinal inflammation to the point that a well-planned, elective operation will successfully eliminate a specific problematic segment of bowel.

Depending upon the individual situation, a modification of medical therapy will often shift the course in a more favorable direction. Often, a change in steroids (e.g., prednisone to methylprednisolone or hydrocortisone) as well as the use of an alternate antibiotic may be beneficial. Some small bowel symptoms may be related to bacterial overgrowth or malabsorption, which justifies the change in antibiotic and allows further dietary modifications. Elemental feedings or a period of total parenteral nutrition may provide a respite from symptoms, induce a more prolonged symptomatic remission, reduce the size of an inflammatory mass, or resolve the bowel narrowing resulting from active inflammation. This approach may require up to 3 to 6 months to produce a lengthy clinical response. Total parenteral nutrition is of little benefit (aside from nutritional repletion prior to elective surgery) in permanently closing enteric fistulas or in opening tight fibrotic strictures. While I have found TPN to be most useful in patients with chronic or unrelenting Crohn's disease, some patients will not improve sufficiently to resume total enteral diets. In many of these individuals the course of TPN will have further confined and delineated the small bowel inflammation sufficiently to limit the extent of a necessary surgical resection, or, rarely, patients may require long-term home TPN.

Another option for these patients is the introduction of an immunosuppressant drug to assist in steriod tapering or possibly to be used in conjunction with dietary modifications (elemental feedings or TPN). A few patients will be unable to eliminate steroids and they then should be transferred to an alternate day schedule to reduce the potential for long-term steroid toxicity.

The decision to recommend surgery in chronic Crohn's disease needs to be weighed against the likelihood of recurrence. Chronicity itself is a favorable feature, as extended intervals between operations appears to be a good prognostic indicator for prolonged remissions. By this time, the active disease has "burned out" and physicians and surgeons are dealing with problems related to scarring and fibrosis. Indications for surgery include stricture formation, suspicion of malignancy in a newly narrowed segment or excluded loop of bowel, and failure to wean patients of TPN or down to acceptable levels of steroids or immunosuppressants or both. The latter indication is, of course, the most subjective and often creates one of the most difficult decisions for experienced clinicians and their well-informed patients.

RECURRENT DISEASE

When patients present with symptoms after a surgical resection in Crohn's disease, it is necessary to determine whether the symptoms are related to active Crohn's disease or represent a complication of the surgery. Inflammatory symptoms, fever, extraintestinal symptoms, and an abdominal mass or new fistula indicate disease activity. Diarrhea, abdominal pain, and weight loss are less specific and warrant a reevaluation because of the possibility that the new symptoms are related to intercurrent infection of *Clostridium difficile,* malabsorption (lactose, and so on), a short-bowel syndrome, bacterial overgrowth, or bile salt induced enteropathy.

An examination of the stool for fecal leukocytes is a simple initial test that should be followed by a 72-hour collection for stool volume and fecal fat. Steatorrhea, with the daily excretion of more than 10 to 20 g of fat, usually responds to a low-fat diet (which can be supplemented with medium-chain triglycerides if necessary). Patients excreting less than 10 g of fecal fat often will respond to the introduction of cholestyramine to reduce the conversion of colonic bile salts to bile acids.

Loss of the ileocecal valve alone can lead to more frequent bowel movements. Additionally, many patients without inflammatory symptoms or signs will have symptoms of an irritable bowel which can be treated with dietary modifications, antispasmodics, and antidiarrheals. The chapter on small bowel resection provides additional details of management.

Patients who present with recurrent Crohn's disease require a great deal of patience, understanding, and supportive therapy to deal with their disappointment over the need for reinstitution of medical therapy. Once again, all of the nonspecific supportive measures, including dietary adjustments and symptomatic medications, sulfasalazine or antibiotics, should be used prior to reinstituting steroids. If immunosuppressants have not previously been employed, then these agents may be useful to control extending or refractory inflammatory disease.

COMPLICATIONS

Many of the local complications of small bowel Crohn's disease have been discussed previously (inflammatory mass, fistula, strictures). Crohn's disease of the upper digestive tract rarely occurs independently of intestinal Crohn's disease, but aphthous ulcerations in the mouth, esophagitis, and Crohn's ulcerations of the stomach and duodenum will occasionally produce symptoms requiring therapy in addition to that for small bowel disease. Usually, these manifestations improve as the intestinal disease is treated, especailly with systemic steroids. *Oral ulcerations* can be treated topically with Kenalog in Orabase. *Esophageal involvement* tends to mimic peptic disease of the distal esophagus and may symptomatically respond to acid reduction therapy. Theoretically, liquid sulfasalzine therapy might be helpful because of the anti-inflammatory action of the parent compound. *Gastroduodenal* Crohn's disease also is difficult to separate from peptic ulcer disease except for the increased tendency toward gastric outlet obstruction from either impaired motility and pyloric or duodenal narrowing. A low-residue or liquid diet may be beneficial and many patients will respond to H_2 receptor antagonists. Steroids are occasionally effective in improving the obstruction, which may require palliative (bypass) surgery. Crohn's disease *fistulas* involving the duodenum present some of the most complicated problems because of their intractability and the potentially serious surgical complications.

Exraintestinal Complications

Growth retardation and *hyperoxaluria* are topics of other chapters. *Ocular manifestations,* including iritis, iridocyclitis, and uveitis rarely occur with small bowel involvement and usually improve with topical steroids or with systemic steroids administered for the intestinal inflammation. Peripheral *arthritis* is more common with colonic disease and also responds to treatment of the bowel disease. In a few patients the arthropathy is more severe and troublesome than the intestinal inflammation but may improve with the *cautious* use of nonsteroidal anti-inflammatory agents. Intra-articular injections of steroids or a brief course of systemic steroid therapy may improve the arthropathy. I have found immunosuppressives useful in a group of patients who would otherwise require maintenance steroids to control the joint manifestations. While symptoms of peripheral joint involvement frequently improve coincident with improving bowel disease, the HLA B27-related arthropathies of ankylosing spondylitis and sacroiliitis tend to run a course independent of the bowel disease. Occasionally, a course of antibiotics will improve these "enteric arthropathies."

The cutaneous manifestations of Crohn's disease, *erythema nodosum* and *pyoderma gangrenosum,* occur more often with colonic than small bowel Crohn's disease and usually improve with treatment of the intestinal disease, although pyoderma gangrenosum may require intensive local therapy with a combination of topical steroids and antibiotics and may occasionally benefit from oral high-dose antibiotics (tetracycline, erythromycin, or dapsone).

Pericholangitis requires no specific treatment. *Sclerosing cholangitis* has a rather unpredictable course which typically is unassociated with the intestinal manifestations. *Cholelithiasis* most often is related to bile salt malabsorption associated with ileal disease or resection. A number of patients have developed acute *cholecystitis* after a course of TPN and subsequent refeeding due to the formation of sludge in an atonic, unstimulated gallbladder. Protocols under investigation to avoid this complication include small, intermittent feedings interspersed with TPN, or daily injections of cholecystokinin.

Pregnancy and inflammatory bowel disease has been the topic of several recent reviews.[2,3] Despite the expected influence of a chronic illness and potent medications upon the menstrual cycle, it appears that women with Crohn's disease are as fertile as the general population, although in the presence of active disease there is an increased risk of a spontaneous abortion. Pregnancy does not seem to activate quiescent Crohn's disease and has little impact upon the overall course of Crohn's disease, although a number of women may have flare-ups subsequent to delivery. There is no increased risk to the fetus as a result of the inflammatory bowel disease, and most obstetricians are more concerned that the expectant mother be maintained under good control. Despite the theoretical effects of steroids and sulfasalazine upon the fetus, there have not been reports of significant effect upon the fetal outcome or significant birth defects. Because of the mutagenic and teratogenic potentials of metronidazole and the immunosuppressants, I continue to warn women taking these drugs against becoming pregnant and will attempt to taper off or change the medical regimen prior to conception. Some women may require TPN for nutritional support, which has been used successfully during pregnancy.[4] Sulfasalazine can affect sperm count and motility and can be a factor in male infertility.

Crohn's disease of the small bowel is a most challenging clinical problem for the physician, who must contend with a chronic, remitting, and as yet, incurable illness. Potent and effective, but potentially toxic medications can be used or, alternatively, surgery, but this can never be considered curative and has potential adverse consequences. The physician must approach each patient and consider the underlying pathophysiologic processes, in order to define an optimal diet, to prescribe supportive and specific medications, and to control problems unique to each individual. Throughout the course of treatment, the physician must maintain an optimistic attitude with the patient and his family; this will help preserve a positive outlook. For certainly, the underlying cause and the eventual cure of Crohn's disease will be discovered.

REFERENCES

1. Present, Korelitz. Treatment of Crohn's disease with 6-mercaptopurine. N Engl J Med 1980; 302:981–987.
2. Management of medicine problems in pregnancy—inflammatory bowel disease. N Engl J Med 1985; 312:1616–1619.
3. Crohn's disease in pregnancy. Gut 1984; 25:52–56.
4. Successfully completed pregnancy in patient maintained on home parenteral nutrition. Br Med J 1983; 286:602–603.

ULCERATIVE COLITIS AND PROCTITIS

MARK A. PEPPERCORN, M.D.

Ulcerative colitis is a recurrent inflammatory process of unknown etiology involving predominantly the mucosa and submucosa of the colon. The disease may be limited to the rectum or rectosigmoid, involve the left colon to the splenic flexure, or in a continuous fashion extend to the cecum with associated mild superficial changes in the terminal ileum (backwash ileitis). Although worldwide in distribution, ulcerative colitis tends to be a disorder of developed countries, with about 10,000 new cases diagnosed yearly in the United States. Its peak incidence is between ages 20 and 40 years, although it can occur at any age. Approximately 20 percent of patients afflicted have a close relative with either ulcerative colitis or Crohn's disease. More common in whites than nonwhites, it also has a greater incidence in Jewish than in non-Jewish populations. The disease is characterized by its chronicity, with repeated attacks of bloody diarrhea, tenesmus, and abdominal pain with a potential for complications (perforation, massive bleeding, intractability) leading to colectomy. Patients with extensive longstanding colon involvement are at increased risk for the development of carcinoma of the colon. Ulcerative colitis can usually be distinguished from acute forms of colitis (bacterial, amebic, ischemic) by appropriate investigations, and from the other major cause of chronic colitis—Crohn's disease—which often spares the rectum, is predominantly right-sided, involves the colon transmurally, and may show granulomas microscopically on colonic biopsy.

THERAPEUTIC ALTERNATIVES

Drugs form the mainstay of any therapeutic program for patients with ulcerative colitis and proctitis. Topical therapy with corticosteroids and systemic therapy with oral sulfasalazine, prednisone, or parenteral corticosteroids are the major alternatives. Immunosuppressive agents, metronidazole, antibiotics, and nonspecific antidiarrheal drugs also may be part of the therapeutic program at a given time for such patients. New studies based on sulfasalazine's metabolism suggest that we are on the threshold of discovering new topical and systemic agents containing 5-aminosalicylate. In addition, new, rapidly metabolized forms of topical steroid therapy should soon be available. Other aspects of medical therapy may include dietary manipulations, psychiatric intervention, and behavior modification. When medical therapy fails to provide a satisfactory result or when the disease becomes rampant, surgery can be life-saving and curative. Before any therapeutic program can be satisfactorily devised, however, a number of factors must be assessed, including extent of disease, severity of symptoms, nutritional status, and the emotional make-up of the patient.

Extent of Disease

Ulcerative colitis always involves the rectum, although on occasion the severity of the rectal disease may be less prominent than that of more proximal areas. Ulcerative proctitis refers to disease limited to the distal 12 cm of colon, while distal colitis or proctosigmoiditis does not extend more proximally than the sigmoid colon. A high percentage of patients whose initial presentation is proctitis or proctosigmoiditis will progress with subsequent flares to more extensive disease. Most patients whose disease involves only the rectum or rectosigmoid have limited symptoms, are not at increased risk for carcinoma, and are candidates for topical forms of therapy.

Although many patients eventually have evidence of disease beyond the sigmoid, it is not unusual for the disease process to stop at the splenic flexure (left-sided colitis). These patients can have a range of symptoms from mild to severe, are at some increased risk for colon cancer, and usually require some form of systemic drug, although they may also be helped by topical agents.

The remainder of patients with ulcerative colitis have

disease involving the transverse colon often extending to the cecum (universal colitis). Such patients tend to have more severe symptoms, are at a high risk for colon cancer when the disease is present for more than 8 years, and almost always will require one of the systemic treatment alternatives.

Since the most important initial determination with regard to extent of disease is whether the process is limited to distal involvement or extends proximal to the sigmoid colon, flexible sigmoidoscopy should be considered as part of the early evaluation of all patients with ulcerative colitis. Total colonoscopy, on the other hand, need not be done initially, since information gathered from the procedure rarely contributes to the initial therapeutic approach, and in the setting of active disease may increase the risk of megacolon or perforation. Once the disease quiets down, colonoscopy should be considered, since documentation of universal colitis will likely influence subsequent cancer surveillance. The barium enema can also contribute to morbidity in the acutely ill patient and often does not provide as much information as a flexible sigmoidoscopy.

Severity of Symptoms

In choosing from a variety of therapeutic alternatives, it is convenient to classify patients' symptoms as mild, moderate, or severe. Patients with mild symptoms may have only occasional rectal bleeding and/or mild diarrhea with fewer than four bowel movements per day. Tenesmus and mild cramping are common in such patients but severe pain, fever, and poor nutrition are not part of the spectrum of mild disease. These patients usually have more limited disease, although on some occasions active universal colitis can be associated with minimal symptomatology. When the symptoms are mild and the disease limited in extent, topical forms of therapy are usually desirable as an initial approach. If the disease is more extensive systemic therapy may be necessary, but the risks of side effects of the available systemic agents have to be weighted against the degree of morbidity from the mild symptoms.

Patients with moderate symptoms may have up to ten loose stools a day with frequent bleeding and mild anemia, but they usually do not need transfusion. Abdominal pain though often present, is not severe. Fever, if any, is low grade (less than 100 °F), and although weight loss is common, the overall nutritional status is adequate. Most such patients will require some form of systemic drug therapy, although on occasion patients with distal colitis may present with moderate symptoms and a trial of topical therapy can be initiated. Moreover, topical therapy may be added to the regimen of systemic drugs for such patients. Although patients with moderate symptoms can usually be managed as outpatients the symptoms are such that some form of treatment is usually indicated, and when the disease is refractory hospitalization has to be considered.

Patients with severe symptoms who have more than ten bowel movements per day, bleeding often requiring transfusion, severe pain, fever at times as high as 103 °F, and poor nutritional status almost always require hospitalization and therapy with parenteral agents. Patients who are toxic with or without magacolon will require early surgery if they fail to improve on medical therapy.

Nutrition

Perhaps in recognition of its being one aspect of their disease that they themselves might control, patients usually want dietary instructions. It is often discouraging for them to be told that there is no evidence that specific diets (e.g, low roughage, bland) are of significant help in ulcerative colitis. Although I usually suggest eliminating products that might contribute to diarrhea, gas, and cramps when symptoms are active (e.g. fresh fruits and vegetables, nuts, seeds, caffeine, monosodium glutamate, diet gum). I try to emphasise normalization of diet and adequate caloric intake to guard against excessive weight loss and nutritional depletion. Lactose intolerance, on the other hand, is worth considering in such patients, and it should be documented or excluded if there is any question. In lactose-intolerant patients supplemental calcium should be prescribed. Multivitamins are often part of a general therapeutic program, although their efficacy is dubious except in specifically documented deficiencies. Since chronic blood loss is a feature in many patients with ulcerative colitis and proctitis, iron replacement is often indicated.

Patients with unrelenting chronic disease activity may gradually become seriously nutritionally depleted (20 percent below optimal body weight). Such malnutrition alters the immune system and puts the patients at greater risk should surgery be needed. Although the nutrition of most such patients cannot be significantly improved until their disease is controlled, on occasion they will benefit from dietary supplements with an elemental diet.

For severely ill patients who require hospitalization, appropriate replacement of fluid and electrolytes is essential. If I suspect the hospitalization may be short I will try to temporize by placing such patients on peripheral hyperalimentation, usually with total bowel rest or clear liquids. This form of therapy does not provide adequate caloric repletion and is not tolerated for long periods because of discomfort due to phlebitis. For most seriously ill patients total parenteral nutrition (TPN) is indicated. In all such patients TPN will maintain and improve the nutritional status. The benefits of such therapy are reflected in reduced postopertive morbidity and mortality. This form of therapy, however, has no role as a primary treatment modality in ulcerative colitis and does not seem to influence the course of active disease.

Emotional Make-up

There is little evidence to support the concept that psychic disorders are etiologic factors in ulcerative colitis or that intervention with psychotherapy benefits the patient's course. On the other hand, some patients will manifest overt evidence of severe psychoneurosis, depression, or even psychosis and will require psychiatric consultation and psychotropic drug therapy. I have recently found behavior modification, usually with relaxation techniques, helpful for certain patients who themselves feel that stress and tension exacerbate disease activity. Some patients have a coexistent irritable bowel syndrome that had developed previously. All patients with ulcerative colitis seem to need, and benefit from, a caring physician who is willing to answer questions, be available at all times, and show a sincere interest in all aspects of their care.

PREFERRED APPROACH TO THE USE OF SPECIFIC DRUGS

Sulfasalazine

Sulfasalazine, which consists of sulfapyridine linked to 5-aminosalicylate via an azo bond, was first used for patients with ulcerative colitis in the late 1930s. Subsequent studies have shown that it will benefit 80 percent of patients with active mild or moderate disease whether the disease is limited to the rectum or rectosigmoid or involves the entire colon. It is not known whether the drug is of any benefit in severe colitis, but it is almost never used alone in such situations. Patients should begin therapy with 500 mg twice a day with gradual advancement of the dose to 3 or 4 g per day over a 1-week period. Most patients will respond within 2 to 3 weeks. Some will show a striking early response while others may take up to 2 to 3 months to show the full benefit of the drug. On occasion patients not responding to 4 g per day will respond to 5 or 6 g per day; such high doses, however, are not well tolerated by most patients.

Although sulfasalazine is often used adjunctively with both topical and oral steroid preparations, there are no data to support or refute such a role in ulcertive colitis and proctitis. In my own practice, although I often use sulfasalazine in combination with other agents, I try to stop the drug if it seems clear that it is having no therapeutic benefit on the course of the patient's illness.

A major role for sulfasalazine is in preventing relapses of ulcerative proctitis and colitis in patients who have gone into remission on some form of medical therapy. About 75 percent of patients maintained on 2 g of sulfasalazine per day will stay in remission for an idefinite period, compared with 35 percent of patients treated with placebo therapy. Four grams per day is actually a more effective prophylactic dose than 2 g per day but less well tolerated and therefore not usually used as a maintenance level.

Once patients have a clinical and sigmoidoscopic remission on standard therapeutic doses of sulfasalazine the drug can be tapered and maintained at the 2 g per day maintenance level. In those instances when the remission has been induced by corticosteroids, sulfasalazine is usually introduced at a maintenance level once the prednisone has been tapered to a range of 20 to 30 mg per day.

Does every patient in remission after an initial episode of ulcerative proctitis or colitis need to receive prophylactic sulfasalazine? If the episode has been moderate or severe with an extent of disease beyond the rectosigmoid, my own answer is yes. For such patients I tend to continue the drug at maintenance levels indefinitely, although there are no available data showing prophylactic benefit beyond 3 years. For patients with mild distal disease it is often worth a period of observation, and for those with early or frequent recurrences institution of prophylactic sulfasalazine once remission again is achieved may be helpful.

Because sulfasalazine and its metabolites cross the placenta and are secreted into breast milk, there has been valid concern over the use of the drug during pregnancy and nursing. Several large clinical studies suggest that the drug has no adverse effects on the fetus or on the pregnancy. Moreover, since its sulfa metabolite is a weak competitor for biliribin binding to albumin, jaundice does not seem to be a problem. Sulfasalazine, therefore, can be initiated and/or maintained in pregnancy as in the nonpregnant patient with ulcerative colitis, and can be continued during the nursing period.

One of the drawbacks of sulfasalazine is a high rate of intolerance and untoward reactions. Almost 20 percent of patients will experience nausea, headache, anorexia, or dyspepsia. A smaller percentage will have evidence of hemolysis and neutropenia. Mild allergic reactions characterized by fever and rash are seen as with other sulfa-containing drugs, but serious idiosyncratic reactions such as hepatitis, pancreatitis, alveolitis, and a serum-sickness-like illness are fortunately very uncommon. Two recently recognized adverse effects include an *exacerbation of the underlying ulcerative colitis* and reversible *infertility* in males. Although sulfasalazine may interfere with dietary folate absorption, routine folate replacement usually is not necessary.

The common untoward effects as well as hemolysis correlate with serum levels of the sulfapyridine moiety. These effects, as well as mild degrees of neutropenia, can be reversed simply by lowering the dose of the drug. Dyspepsia can be averted at times by the use of an enteric-coated prepartion. In patients with infertility, exacerbation of colitis, or the more serious systemic reactions the drug shoud be discontinued. It has been shown, however, that many patients who experience mild allergic reactions, such as fever and rash, can be desensitized to the drug. Although several desensitization schema have been proposed, two are particularly convenient for patients. One involves stopping the drug for a period of 1 to 2 weeks with reinstitution at a dose of 250 mg to 500 mg per day for 7 to 10 days and a gradual increase by 250 mg a week until maintenance or therapeutic levels of the drug are reached. However, the use of a new liquid oral suspension of sulfasalazine should make desensitization even easier than it has been. Another regimen begins with one-eighth of a 500-mg tablet daily with doubling of the dose every 3 to 7 days until therapeutic levels are reached. Clearly patients have to be monitored closely during this period for recurrence of their prior symptoms and laboratory abnormalities.

Despite its clinical availability for more than 45 years little was known about sulfasalazine's pharmacology until the past decade. Now studies of the drug's metabolism and distribution along with information about its toxicity have led to the development of a new generation of related drugs. The parent drug is partially absorbed from the proximal small intestine and then partly excreted unchanged in the urine, importing to the urine a strong yellow or light orange color. The remaining absorbed portion is excreted unchanged in the bile, and together with the unabsorbed drug reaches the distal ileum and colon where intestinal bacteria split sulfasalazine into its two components, sulfapyridine and 5-aminosalicylate. The sulfapyridine moiety is absorbed, metabolized by the liver, and excreted in the urine. The 5-aminosalicylate portion is largely unabsorbed and excreted in the stool.

The observation that 5-aminosalicylate is largely unabsorbed after sulfasalazine degradation and stays in contact with distal colonic mucosa led to the suggestion that it might actually be the active moiety of the parent drug, with sulfasalazine serving merely as the vehicle for delivery of the 5-aminosalicylate to distal disease sites. This speculation, coupled with the known findings about sulfapyridine's role in the drug's toxicity, led to the development of agents that deliver 5-aminosalicylate by itself to diseased areas of bowel. There are now several controlled trials which show convincingly that 5-aminosalicylate enemas and suppositories are efficacious in the treatment of mild and moderate distal ulcerative colitis and proctitis. Moreover, many such patients whose disease is refractory to conventional therapy with both sulfasalazine and topicl corticosteroids will respond to 5-aminosalicylate. An analogue of 5-aminosalicylate, 4-aminosalicylate, appears to be equally effective in these clinical settings. The hoped for safety of these agents has been realized, since patients previously allergic or intolerant to sulfasalazine can usually take topical aminosalicylate preparations without adverse effect.

In addition, there are currently four oral forms of 5-aminosalicylate under study in patients with inflammatory bowel disease. Disodium azo-disalicylate links two 5-aminosalicylate molecules via an azo bond. Balsalazide, on the other hand, links 5-aminosalicylate to an inert carrier molecule, aminobenzoylalanine, again via an azo bond. Asacol is a delayed release preparation wich coats 5-aminosalicylate with an acrylic-based resin which breaks down at pH 7. Finally, Pentasa is another slow-release preparation in which 5-aminosalicylate in microgranules is coated with a semipermeable membrane of ethylcellulose. Bioavailability, toxicity, and early efficacy studies suggests that one or more of these agents will be clinically effective and useful in patients with more proximal ulcerative colitis in whom topical agents are less likely to be effective. They may also be useful in patients with Crohn's disease of the ileum. Although there are no currently available commercial preparations of 5-aminosalicylate or 4-aminosalicylate in the United States, it seems clear that in the near future enema and oral forms of the drug will become available and emerge as front-line therapy for patients with inflammatory bowel disease.

It is hoped that an understanding of sulfasalazines and 5-aminosalicylate's modes of action might shed light on the pathogenesis of ulcerative colitis itself. Both sulfasalazine and 5-aminosalicylate are weak inhibitors of the cyclo-oxygenase pathway of arachidonic acid metabolism leading to prostaglandin synthesis inhibition. Although levels of prostaglandins are increased in active ulcerative colitis and diminished after successful therapy with sulfasalazine, other more potent inhibitors of prostaglandin synthesis are not efficacious in treating the disorder. In fact, indomethacin therapy actually may be associated with worsening of active colitis. An alternative explanation for sulfasalazine action suggests that sulfasalazine and 5-aminosalicylate, by inhibiting the lipoxygenase pathway of arachidonic acid metabolism, decrease the formation of leukotrienes and certain fatty acids which are potent chemotactic agents in recruiting polymorphonuclear leukocytes to sites of inflammation. At present, however, the actual mechanism of action of these agents remains unclear.

Corticosteroids

Topical Agents. For patients with ulcerative proctitis and proctosigmoiditis the therapeutic choice is usually between sulfasalazine and a topical steroid enema preparation. The latter becomes a clear choice if the patient has a known sulfa or salicylate allergy, wants to avoid the potential adverse effects of sulfasalazine, and can't tolerate pills. Steroid enemas in the form of hydrocortisone or methylprednisolone in 60 ml of water are efficacious in such patients; more than 80 percent achieve a remission or significant improvement with the use of one enema nightly over a 2- or 3-week period. Systemic steroid side effects are usually not seen over such short periods of therapy. Occasionally a partial response will be obtained and the enema may be continued for a longer period on a nightly or every-other-night basis. Some positive response is usually noted within the first 2 weeks of treatment. If not, a twice daily steroid enema regimen is worth trying, but therapy for longer than 1 month with no clear improvement is not warranted. Occasionally, in the most limited forms of proctitis, steroid foams or even suppositories may be helpful in the same manner as the enema preparations.

The issue of whether steroid enemas work locally or through limited systemic absorption has been subjected to some study over the years. It is clear that the absorbed portion of an administered dose can lead, in some patients, to the usual adverse effect associated with chronic steroid administration. There are two new forms of topical steroid, however, which do appear to act locally with avoidance of chronic adverse reactions. One agent, *beclomethasone dipropionate*, is as clinically effective as hydrocortisone in enema form, but because of gut wall and first pass liver metabolism avoids suppression of the pituitary-adrenal axis. Similarly, a non-glucocorticoid, nonmineralocorticoid steriod, *Tixocortal pivolate*, also has rapid first pass metabolism, avoids suppression of the adrenal glands, is not salt retaining, and appears to be as effective in ulcerative proctitis and proctosigmoiditis as standard steroid enema preparations. Although neither of these preparations is currently available commercially in the United States each should emerge as an important form of therapy for distal ulcerative colitis and proctitis.

Systemic Agents. Oral corticosteroids were introduced into clinical medicine in the mid 1940s and quickly established themselves as useful in the therapy of ulcerative colitis. Prednisone, the oral agent most often used, is most helpful clinically in patients with moderate symptoms and disease proximal to the rectosigmoid who either cannot take or do not improve with sulfasalazine. More than 75 percent of such patients will achieve a remission or significant improvement. The drug is started at 30 to 60 mg per day, depending on the level of symptoms, and continued at the initial dose for about 2 weeks. Should the hoped for response be noted as assessed by disappearance of diarrhea and bleeding and improvement in the sigmoidoscopic appearance then a progressive reduction in dosage can be attempted at a rate of 5 mg per week. Somewhat paradoxically, patients with more limited distal colitis and proctitis not responding to topical steroids or sulfasalazine usually do not respond to prednisone, and its use in such patients should be discouraged or minimized.

A small proportion of patients with ulcerative colitis will present with severe or even fulminant symptoms and require hospitalization. The major therapy for such patients is some form of parenteral corticosteroid. For patients already receiving oral steroids the treatment of choice is either hydrocortisone, given as a continuous infusion at a dose of 300 mg per day, prednisolone, 60 to 80 mg per day, or methylprednisolone, 48 to 60 mg per day. I favor the latter drugs because salt retention is less of a problem. On occasion a refractory patient seems to respond to a brief trial of extremely high doses of these agents (e.g., 200 mg per day of prednisolone). Although most investigators have found corticotropin (ACTH) to be similar in efficacy to corticosteroids, recent experience suggests that ACTH may be more effective for patients with severe colitis who have not recently received oral steroid therapy. Corticotropin can be given as a continuous infusion at a dosage of 120 units per day.

Most patients with moderate symptoms and many with severe disease will obtain remission with systemic corticosteroid therapy. Such patients should be gradually weaned off steroids while continuing to receive sulfasalazine when possible. Unfortunately, low daily doses of corticosteroid (e.g., 7.5 to 10.0 mg of prednisone) do not appear to be effective in maintaining a remission in patients with ulcerative colitis. A recent trial, however, found that prednisolone, 40 mg every other day, was more effective than placebo in preventing relapses. Although chronic adverse effects may still occur on an alternate-day regimen, this type of therapy may be effective for patients with frequent flares of disease who are either unable to tolerate sulfasalazine as a maintenance drug or who have flare-ups despite its use.

Immunosuppressive Agents

Although increasingly used in Crohn's disease, azathioprine and 6-mercaptopurine thus far have played a more limited role in ulcerative colitis. Indeed, it has been difficult to show that these agents are of any benefit when used as single drugs in patients with ulcerative colitis and proctitis. In my own experience their major use is in the patient who is only partially responsive to prednisone and repeatedly flares when the dose is tapered below 20 to 40 mg per day. For many such patients the addition of azathioprine or 6-mercaptopurine at a dose of 1.5 mg per kilogram per day will permit a lowering of the steroid dose or withdrawal of the drug while the patient's disease continues at a quiescent level. Some preliminary information suggests that, as in Crohn's disease, these agents may be helpful in maintaining a remission in ulcerative colitis. Because of concern over the potential for neutropenia and infection and the unknown long-term risk of malignancy, I tend not to use these agents in patients with ulcerative colitis beyond 1 year.

Antibiotics

Broad-spectrum parenteral antibiotics such as ampicillin and an aminoglycoside have to be considered in toxic patients with ulcerative colitis with and without magacolon. In the face of impending perforation an agent active against the anaerobic colonic flora is usually added. Standard oral agents (e.g., ampicillin, tetracycline, cephalexin) are not helpful in less severe forms of ulcerative colitis and at times seem to trigger flares of the disease even in the absence of positive *Clostridia difficile* toxin titers. Metronidazole, however, may be one such agent that will find a role in the outpatient management of ulcerative colitis as it has in treatment of Crohn's disease involving the colon and perineum. There are as yet no available controlled studies of metronidazole in ulcerative colitis, but I have used the drug with apparent success in a small number of patients who are not responding to other measures. Its routine use in ulcerative colitis cannot at this point, however, be recommended.

Nonspecific Antidiarrheal Agents

Drugs such as loperamide, diphenoxylate with atropine, codeine, deodorized tincture of opium, and belladonna are useful in the treatment of diarrhea in patients with ulcerative colitis with mild, well-established chronic symptoms. Although the addictive potential of such drugs is a concern, their limited judicious use can make the difference between multiple trips to the bathroom at night and a good night's rest. These agents should be avoided, however, in patients with acute symptoms and more severe forms of the disease because of the risk of precipitating ileus and even megacolon.

SURGICAL CONSIDERATIONS

Surgery can be life-saving for patients with unresponsive fulminant colitis, some of whom may have already suffered a perforation or be having an exsanguinating bleed. A subtotal colectomy in such instances may be preferable to a total colectomy, since it is a lesser procedure in the severely ill patient and preserves the options for an alternative to a permanent ileostomy. With severe bleeding or fulminant disease clearly involving the rectum, a total colectomy may be necessary.

Another group of patients in whom colectomy has to be considered includes those with severe dysplasia on mucosal biopsy. It is hoped that the regular use of surveillance colonoscopy in patients at high risk (extensive disease for more than 8 years) will have an impact on the cancer problem in ulcerative colitis. This is also the topic of a separate chapter.

The majority of patients requiring an operation are not those with fulminant disease or in whom cancer is an immediate threat, but rather those with chronic symptoms who are often steroid-dependent and have suffered the physical and emotional ravages of the disorder over a number of years. Although once in place the standard permanent ileostomy is well tolerated by most patients, the specter of an ileostomy bag keeps many patients from surgery long after it may have been medically advisable. Now the surgical alterntives to a permanent conventional ileostomy may make decision-making easier for such patients.

POLYPS OF THE COLON

JEROME D. WAYE, M.D.

A colon polyp is any tissue protuberance above the surface mucosa. Polyps may be neoplastic or non-neoplastic (Fig. 1); the majority of neoplastic polyps are adenomas, which are premalignant lesions. Most polyps larger than 1 cm in diameter are adenomas, but it is usually impossible for the radiologist, internist, endoscopist, or surgeon to predict the histologic type of adenoma, i.e., tubular, villous, or mixed, from the gross appearance of the polyp. Small polyps, less than 6 mm in diameter, are more often adenomas than not, but the differentiation can only be made histologically. Five to 10 percent of adenomas will become malignant, but it is not possible to predict accurately which adenomas will develop cancer. The incidence of cancer in adenomas correlates directly with their size and with the proportion of villous architecture present. Prior to the advent of colonoscopy, polyps at risk of malignancy or those that contained cancer were pooorly identified because, although polyp size could be estimated by a barium enema x-ray examintion, it was not possible to assess polyp histology. In the precolonoscopy era, polyps within reach of the sigmoidoscope were removed and those more proximal were evaluated by interval colon roentgenograms. The polyp with smooth contours and no growth tendency from one x-ray film to the next was followed periodically by repeat colon roentgenograms; removal of a proximal colon polyp required surgical laparotomy for the indications of surface irregularity, size, or a change in the polyp's shape or diameter on successive roentgenograms.

The ease and safety with which polyps can be removed colonoscopically has markedly altered the treatment of colon polyps. Since a nonsurgical approach is feasible and generally available, it is inappropriate to follow outmoded practice and observe polyps with serial roentgenograms. If a barium enema x-ray film demonstrates a polyp of 1 cm in diameter, it should be removed because of the 1 percent incidence of carcinoma in adenomas of this size. Malignancy in small polyps is extremely difficult to diagnose by gross visual inspection, a factor that mandates their resection for microscopic examination. Removal of the early carcinoma confined to a polyp is curative. The resection of polyps at high risk for cancer will undoubtedly interrupt the adenoma-carcinoma sequence. The small polyp with a high malignant potential can only be identified when the amount of villous component is seen histologically.

DIMINUTIVE POLYPS DISCOVERED ON BARIUM ENEMA X-RAY FILM

The occurrence of carcinoma in a polyp less than 0.5 cm in diameter is so rare that such a finding on a barium enema x-ray film may not, in itself, be sufficient indication for the performance of colonoscopic polypectomy. The clinician must be alert, however, to the probability that the symptoms that prompted the x-ray examination are not explained by a diminutive polyp and that occult or overt bleeding requires investigation by total colonoscopic examination, since blood loss is uncommon with these small polyps. The management of patients with polyps 0.5 to 1.0 cm in diameter is controversial; decisions should be based on the patient's symptoms, age, past history, family history, presence of other illnesses, and the physician's judgment. If a small polyp is detected on barium enema, and there are no symptoms or signs that require urgent colonoscopy, the patient may properly be scheduled for an interval follow-up surveillance examination by colonoscopy rather than by barium enema with the purpose of reevaluating the entire colon and removing the previously identified polyp.

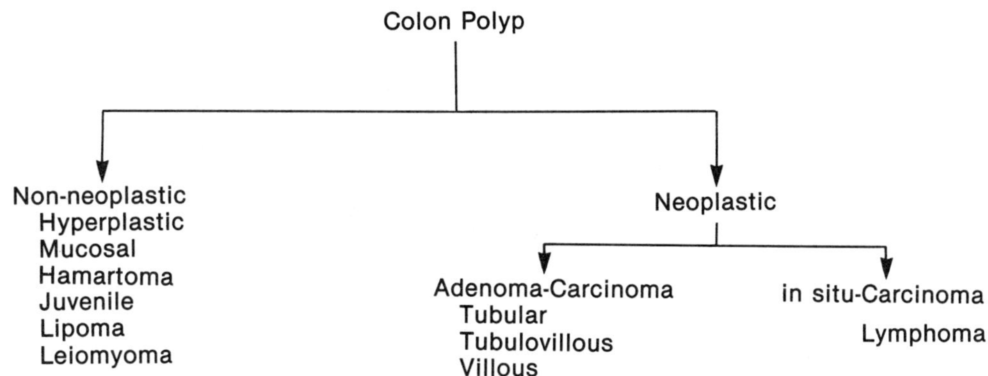

Figure 1 Nomenclature of colon polyps.

SYNCHRONOUS ADENOMA

Whenever one polyp is discovered in the colon, total colonoscopy is mandated, since there is a 50 percent probability of discovering a synchronous adenoma. Whenever polyps are encountered during colonoscopy, they should be removed and biopsied. Even small polyps are now known to often contain adenomatous tissue, and if discovered during colonoscopy they should be sampled and ablated with the hot biopsy forceps. The majority of polyps are less than 2 cm in diameter, and experience has shown that most polyps seen during colonoscopy can be completely removed by simultaneous biopsy and fulguration or by cautery snare. In view of the current expertise in the field of colonoscopy, there are few occasions when a patient should be requested to return at some future time for removal of a polyp discovered during the endoscopic examination.

POLYPECTOMY

Complications

Serious complications, such as hemorrhage or perforation, occur in 1.8 percent of all colonoscopic polypectomies, with bleeding being the most frequent. Thermal injury to the bowel wall can occur during polypectomy and may result in a syndrome of peritoneal irritation characterized by abdominal pain, fever, and leukocytosis in the absence of free air on plain x-ray films of the abdomen. Symptoms of this "colon coagulation syndrome" usually subside with symptomatic therapy in 24 to 48 hours.

Surgical Polypectomy

The morbidity, mortality, and cost of colonoscopic polypectomy are significantly less than when polypectomy is performed surgically. The decision to remove a polyp surgically should be made by an experienced endoscopist who can directly assess the feasibility of endoscopic polypectomy by observing size of the polyp base, its position in the colon, and its accessibility for snare placement. The obviously malignant polyp with a waxy, irregular, ulcerated surface should properly be resected surgically. Some adenomas with a wide base or those that straddle an interhaustral fold may require several separate polypectomy sessions with only a small chance of total endoscopic removal; the endoscopist must weigh the risks and benefits of the endoscopic versus surgical approach for each patient before reaching a decision as to which route should be recommended.

Preparation for Colonoscopic Polypectomy

Preparation for a polypectomy should be a routine part of any diagnostic colonoscopic examination in order to avoid repetitive procedures and to control endoscopic costs. These preparations should encompass many areas, the most important of which is the preparation of the endoscopist.

Preparation of the Physician. The physician who performs colonoscopy must be trained in (not just familiar with) the techniques of colonoscopic polypectomy. This cannot be undertaken lightly, and adequate polypectomy experience will ensure the lowest possible rate of complications. The technique of polypectomy should be learned in a preceptor-type of relationship, during a specified training program only after the physician is completely capable of handling the colonoscope well. Initially, small pedunculated polyps can be removed, and with further experience, the physician can resect sessile polyps endoscopically, either with single snare application or in piecemeal fashion. Every endoscopist must be thoroughly knowledgeable with principles of electrosurgery and be familiar with the specific cautery unit available in the endoscopy suite.

Preparation of the Patient. Prior to any colonoscopic examination, the patient should be informed that polyps identified during the procedure will be removed at that time. Informed consent to include the polypectomy should be obtained from the patient before embarking upon any colonoscopic examination. The patient should be made aware of the risks involved in polypectomy, namely, perforation and bleeding. When colonoscopy is being performed specifically to remove a colon polyp, the patient should know that surgery is an alternative method of polyp removal. It is the responsibility of the physicians or an interested staff member to give instructions on the importance of bowel cleansing and to explain the possibility of not performing the procedure if the large bowel is poorly prepared.

Preparation of the Colon. Gases within the lumen of the unprepared bowel may be present in explosive proportions. Placing patients on a liquid diet for 48 hours has been shown to be effective in markedly decreasing the concentration of combustible gases. When this diet is coupled with a purgative, the level of explosive gas further decreases to where it is safe for electrocautery to be performed without the need for carbon dioxide insufflation. A colonic explosion related to the use of mannitol as an osmotic cathartic has been reported, and the use of this cathartic cannot be condoned for bowel preparation if electrocautery current is to be used. Adequate cleansing of the colon may be accomplished by giving the patient a low-residue diet, cathartic, and enemas. Castor oil (2 oz) or citrate of magnesia (10 oz) may be taken in the evening prior to the procedure. A full liquid diet for 24 or 48 hours prior to endoscopy is recommended, as are cleansing enemas on the day of the examination to be completed 2 hours prior to colonoscopy, allowing evacuation of excess water. Balanced electrolyte preparations are excellent cathartics but may leave a considerable amount of fluid within the bowel. Approximately one out of every 20 patients using the electrolyte preparation has a poorly prepared colon that may interfere with the ability to complete the examination. Two major factors account for this problem; a distaste for the solution and a reluctance to ingest the large volume of fluid required.

The patient should receive two instructions approximately 1 week prior to any colonoscopic examination, especially if polypectomy might possibly be performed. These are: (1) discontinue iron-containing medications (because they cause a dark residue in the colon); and (2) discontinue the use of aspirin-containing drugs (to decrease the risk of bleeding in the postpolypectomy period). The patient's coagulation status should be ascertained historically, by specifically inquiring as to previous bleeding episodes, especially with prior operations or tooth extractions. There is no need to obtain a "coagulation work-up" before polypectomy, unless a particular reason exists. In general, the use of carbon dioxide is not necessary for the performance of polypectomy. Adequate preparation of the colon is sufficient to prevent an explosive mixture of gases.

Preparation of the Equipment. For the performance of polypectomy, the following equipment must be available: hot biopsy forceps, two snares, and an electrosurgical unit. Each piece of apparatus should be individually inspected daily to ensure proper function. Since a number of incompatible items are commonly purchased from individual manufacturers, all connections should be checked and appropriate adapters employed.

Preparation of the Gastrointestinal Assistant. A trained gastrointestinal assistant should be available for the performance of colonoscopy and polypectomy. The assistant must be familiar with the principles of polypectomy and with the electrosurgical unit, its dial settings, the need for a ground-plate return, and so on. It is the assistant's role to identify the polypectomy site on the resected specimen with a pin or thread and to label each specimen in the order of its removal, permitting precise site location when the pathologist's report is received. It is customary for the assistant to close the snare around the polyp pedicle or base upon the physician's request. However, the force with which the wire loop guillotines the polyp while electric current is applied mandates training, practice, and experience to prevent complications. The use of an untrained assistant may be detrimental to the patient's safety.

The Site of Polypectomy

There is no contraindication to removal of colon polyps in whatever setting colonoscopy is performed. Most polyps may be removed in an ambulatory facility, either in a hospital endoscopy suite or in a physician's specially equipped office.

The *indications for hospitalizing* patients for polypectomy are as follows: (1) Age or infirmity may make it difficult for patients to ambulate, and they may not tolerate an in-home preparation requiring enemas and frequent trips to the bathroom; (2) the presence of known coagulopathy; (3) the need for prophylactic antibiotics; and (4) multiple polyps, large polyps, or suspected complications may justify hospitalization for observation following the polypectomy procedure.

The low frequency of complications that require hospitalization after polypectomy means that polyps may be removed in a physician's office as well as in the hospital outpatient department. Whenever polypectomy is to be performed on an ambulatory basis, emergency resuscitation equipment must be available for the treatment of the rare but potentially disastrous complications of medication administration. An endotracheal tube should be available with an Ambu-bag, along with various drugs for resuscitation. Narcan should be available to reverse the effect of narcotics. Many physicians administer Narcan routinely to ambulatory patients who have received meperidine for the procedure. Whenever endoscopy is to be performed on an ambulatory basis, it is imperative that the patient bring a companion to assist the partially sedated patient in traveling home.

THE MALIGNANT POLYP

Lymphatic channels are not present superficial to the muscularis mucosa in the polyp head. Because of the lymphatic distribution, malignant cells that do not penetrate the muscularis mucosa have no potential for metastatic spread. The adenoma with carcinoma-in-situ or noninvasive carcinoma may, once resected, be subsequently followed as any other benign adenoma. The three absolute criteria for surgically operating on the malignant polyp are: (1) invasion of lymphatic or vascular channels, (2) the presence of poorly differentiated carcinoma, and (3) malignancy at the resection margin of a sessile adenoma. Any sessile adenoma with malignancy invading beyond the muscularis mucosa is at risk for metastasis, and the patient may properly be advised to have a surgical resection of the colon to remove this site and adjoining lymph nodes. There is controversy concerning the need for such surgery, and the decision may be altered by the condition of the patient (elderly or infirm), the location of the malignant polyp (whether it requires an abdominoperineal resection), and the histopathologic findings in the polyp (only a small amount of malignancy at a distance from the resection margin).

Pedunculated adenomas with cancer invading the polyp head need not be surgically resected unless the malignancy satisfies the above-mentioned absolute criteria for surgery. When the pedicle contains carcinoma, even though the resection margin is not involved, surgery (with the above caveats) should be recommended. The pedicles of some polyps are broad-based and represent a portion of the colon wall pulled upon by peristalsis; these are pseudo-pedicles and should be treated as sessile polyps.

FOLLOW-UP AFTER ENDOSCOPIC POLYPECTOMY

Polyps recur in 30 to 50 percent of patients in whom adenomas are resected. Patients who have multiple adenomas are at greater risk of recurrence than those with a single adenoma resected. If no polyps were missed during the index polypectomy, then the follow-up interval to seek and remove metachronous adenomas should properly be at a time just prior to the development of cancer; more frequent examinations will permit the removal of adenomas but the risk of cancer in small adenomas is extremely slight. Since adenomas may, however,be missed at the time of the index examination, the first surveillance colonoscopy should be scheduled one year following the index polypectomy, and residual polyps removed. Because the growth rate of adenomas is unknown, as is the duration of time required for the development of carcinoma in an adenoma, no exact time period can be suggested for follow-up examinations. It does, however, take a few years for an adenoma to grow to 1 cm in size, when the realistic risk of cancer begins. A suggested surveillance plan would be to perform total colonoscopy every 2 or 3 years after the initial follow-up examination when patients have had multiple polyps removed, and every 3 years when one adenoma was originally resected.

LOWER GASTROINTESTINAL BLEEDING

JAMES H. JOHNSTON, M.D.

Lower gastrointestinal (GI) bleeding is a challenging problem in terms of both diagnosis and treatment, often requiring the coordinated efforts of the gastroenterologist, radiologist, surgeon, and nursing staff. In contrast to upper GI bleeding, in which endoscopy has assumed an important role with rapid accurate diagnosis as well as definitive hemostatic therapy, there is often no single approach to lower GI hemorrhage.

The management of major acute lower GI hemorrhage is quite different from minor hematochezia or occult bleeding. These topics will be discussed separately, while the primary focus of the chapter will be on management of the patient with acute bleeding.

MAJOR ACUTE HEMORRHAGE

Massive bleeding is a true medical emergency that must be handled in an expedient manner. After initial passage of a formed stool with blood, further bowel movements typically consist of frank blood and clots. In contrast to the common delay in recognition of the significance of melena, the patient with hematochezia usually seeks medical attention urgently. Resuscitative measures should begin immediately with correction of hypovolemia by rapid infusion of intravenous fluid via large-bore catheter. Blood is typed and crossmatched for transfusion as needed. Relatively minor changes in blood pressure and pulse may reflect significant deficits in blood volume. Coagulopathies should be corrected if present.

Diagnostic Approach

History and Physical Examination

Initial evaluation includes general medical assessment with a concise but thorough history and physical examination. With major hemorrhage of suspected lower GI origin, it is important to search for clues suggesting a possible upper GI source of bleeding (history of peptic ulcer or dyspepsia, liver disease, alcoholism, anti-inflammatory drugs, and so on). Abdominal pain precedes rectal bleeding in ischemic bowel disease, whereas a history of diarrhea and anal fistulas suggests inflammatory bowel disease. Prior radiation therapy is an important clue. Acute major lower GI bleeding is most often due to either a colonic diverticulum or a vascular ectasia in patients over 45 years of age, but other lesions, such as a Meckel's diverticulum, inflammatory bowel disease, and colonic polyps, are more important causes in young patients. Causes of lower GI bleeding are listed in Table 1.

TABLE 1 Causes of Lower Gastrointestinal Bleeding

Disorder	Major Acute Hemorrhage	Minor Chronic Hemorrhage
Hemorrhoids		*
Anal fissure		*
Colonic diverticulum	*	
Vascular ectasia	*	*
Polyp		*
Cancer		*
Solitary colonic ulcer	*	
Colonic varices	*	
Post-polypectomy	*	
Ischemic colitis		*
Inflammatory bowel disease		*
Radiation colitis		*
Small bowel lesion		
Meckel's diverticulum	*	
Tumor		*
Upper gastrointestinal lesion	*	

After the patient is stabilized in an intensive care unit, the search for a specific diagnosis continues (Fig. 1).

Anorectal Examination

Careful digital, anoscopic, and proctosigmoidoscopic examination is the next step. This usually reveals copious blood and clots coming from above the proctoscopic level. It is important, however, not to overlook a hemorrhoidal source of massive bleeding, especially in a cirrhotic patient with portal hypertension. Similarly, a minute rectal ulcer with arterial bleeding should be carefully excluded, as well as signs of inflammatory bowel disease. The rigid proctoscope permits much better suctioning, but the flexible fiberoptic instrument provides a superior image if large rectal clots are removed manually or rendered dependent by changing the patient's position and examining the exposed mucosa. Retroflexion of the flexible instrument may aid in inspection of the anorectal junction. Careful exclusion of the uncommon anorectal source of major hemorrhage is an important but often underemphasized task. Its significance can be stressed by considering the implications of a subtotal colectomy done for uncontrolled hemorrhage, only to discover postoperatively an anorectal cause for the persistent bleeding.

Exclude Upper Gastrointestinal Source of Bleeding

Traditionally, the next diagnostic step is passage of a nasogastric tube in search of gross blood. If there was syncope or orthostatic hypotension, however, or if dark stools preceded passage of red blood, then a negative nasogastric aspirate is not sufficient to rule out a bleeding duodenal ulcer with competent pyloric sphincter, and upper endoscopy should be performed.

After exclusion of anorectal and upper GI sources of hemorrhage, the evaluation becomes considerably more difficult. Further diagnostic studies include radionuclide scanning, arteriography, and/or colonoscopy. There is no longer a place for barium x-ray studies in the setting of acute GI hemorrhage.

Bleeding Scan

The radionuclide scan frequently receives mixed reviews regarding its usefulness in the evaluation of a patient with GI bleeding. Many clinicians have been disappointed with its low sensitivity and specificity. It is true that the yield is low, but this is primarily because active bleeding has stopped by the time the test is performed. When positive, the bleeding scan provides valuable localization of the source of hemorrhage with little discomfort, risk, or expense to the patient (especially as compared with the alternatives of arteriography, colonoscopy, and surgery).

I order the bleeding scan only if I believe the patient is continuing to bleed actively at that moment. A nuclear medicine technician is on call 24 hours a day for emergency scanning. Nocturnal participation by the radiologist is required only when there is immediate diagnostic confusion; most scans can be fully interpreted later and do not have urgent therapeutic implications. An unequivocal hot spot on scan that appears in the first few minutes after injection is considered to be useful; overinterpretation of subtle findings is fraught with error. The diagnostic accuracy of the technetium sulfur colloid scan is claimed to exceed that of the technetium-labeled red blood scan, although the latter technique allows delayed scanning to detect intermittent hemorrhage. In my experience, however, delayed scans are of limited benefit for specific localization because the isotope migrates substantially by the time the scan is done. If the bleeding scan is negative, this implies that active bleeding has stopped at least temporarily and the urgency for specific diagnosis and therapy may be reduced.

Arteriography

If major lower GI bleeding persists or recurs, requiring therapeutic intervention, then emergency arteriography may offer specific localization of the bleeding site as well as definitive therapy by selective vasoconstrictor infusion. This procedure requires an interested, readily available and experienced radiography team, and, in practical terms, this service is not universally available. It is important to maintain the intensive care unit environment while in the radiography suite, including attentive nursing care and monitoring. Many angiographers require a positive bleeding scan (proving active bleeding) before proceeding with full arteriography. The active bleeding point is seen as a localized zone of extravasated contrast. Most bleeding lesions lie within the distribution of the superior mesenteric artery, which includes the small bowel

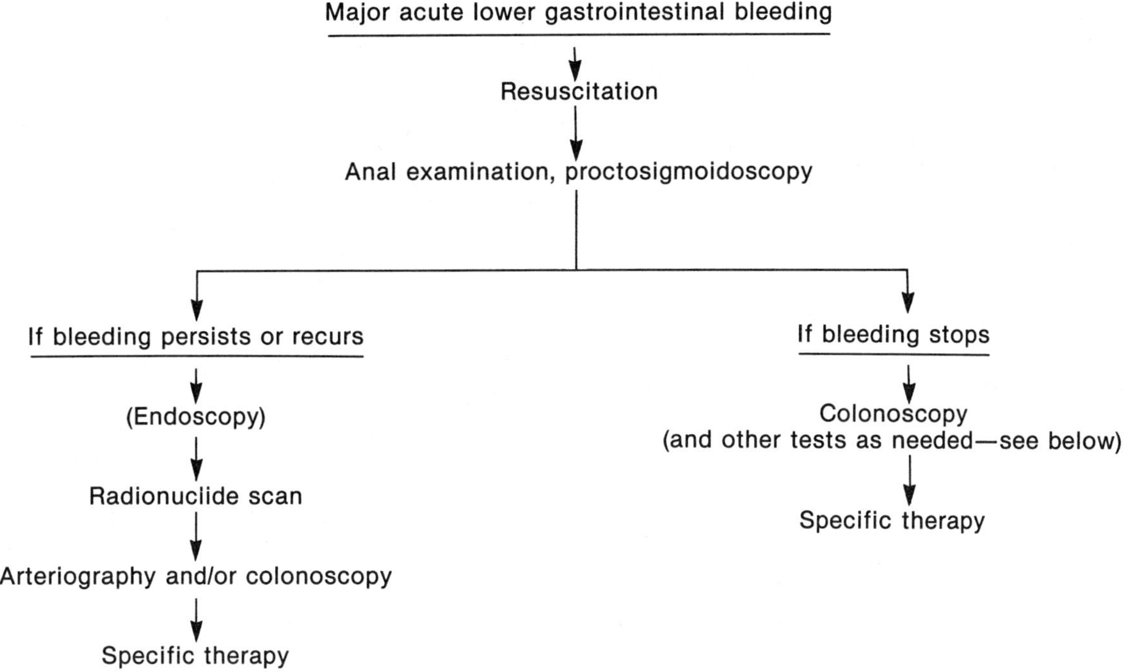

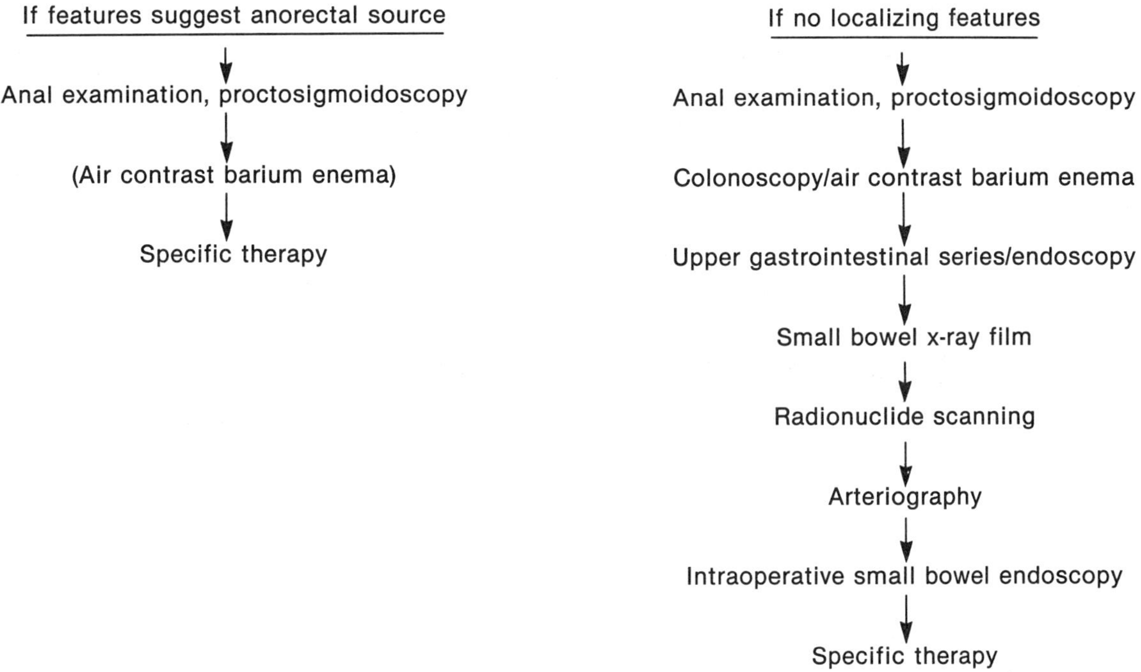

Figure 1 Algorithms for management of lower gastrointestinal bleeding.

and proximal two-thirds of the colon. Although angiography may not define the precise nature of the bleeding lesion, there often are helpful diagnostic signs with particular lesions (to be discussed below). Following a positive angiogram and successful selective catheter placement, vasopressin infusion may be employed with a high success rate. Complications of arteriography include serious allergic and nephrotoxic reactions to the contrast media, as well as local catheter problems.

Emergency Colonoscopy

Once considered to be impractical in the setting of massive lower GI hemorrhage, Golytely preparation now permits successful total colonoscopy in the majority of cases. Within several hours of Golytely administration by mouth or by nasogastric tube, colonoscopy can usually be performed.

Although the technical feat of colonoscopy is usually possible during active major hemorrhage, I have mixed feelings about its usefulness as an emergency procedure. On one hand, valuable information is gained when the site and nature of the bleeding lesion are accurately determined. Additionally, there are certain bleeding lesions which can be effectively and safely treated endoscopically, thereby avoiding surgical intervention. On the other hand, the Golytely preparation may be arduous and stressful when coupled with major hemorrhage and adds a risk of aspiration. There is no current information that assures us that this purge does not aggravate or prolong active bleeding. Moreover, the lesions that can be treated colonoscopically will still be present after active bleeding has stopped spontaneously, and endoscopic diagnosis and therapy is considerably easier, safer, and more precise under elective, blood-free conditions.

To summarize, in the setting of active lower GI bleeding, invasive tests such as arteriography or emergency colonoscopy are best reserved for those few patients with continued or recurrent major hemorrhage that requires urgent therapeutic intervention. If the bleeding stops on its own, then elective colonoscopy is preferable to its emergency counterpart. In general, the ability to localize the bleeding site has greatly enhanced our therapeutic efforts. The bleeding source can now be accurately determined preoperatively in most patients who require emergency surgery for major lower GI hemorrhage, and this key information directs the surgical approach.

Ninety percent of patients with acute lower GI hemorrhage are bleeding from a colonic diverticulum or a vascular ectasia. Common as well as uncommon causes of acute lower GI bleeding will now be discussed.

SPECIFIC BLEEDING LESIONS AND THERAPY

Diverticular Hemorrhage

Colonic diverticular bleeding emanates from a small (0.25-mm range) artery characteristically located in the base or perimeter of the diverticulum (recall that a diverticulum forms at the relatively weak point where serosal vessels pierce the muscularis). Despite a preponderance of diverticulae in the left colon, diverticular bleeding occurs from the right colon in 60 percent of cases. This arterial source explains the acute and abrupt nature of diverticular hemorrhage. As with arterial bleeding from a peptic ulcer, active bleeding is often intermittent in nature. Most episodes are self-limited and cease spontaneously. Chance of recurrent hemorrhage after the initial hospitalization is less than 50 percent (I suspect that the older data regarding rebleeding tendency inadvertently included some patients with unrecognized vascular ectasias).

The mainstay of treatment of diverticular bleeding is good supportive care and transfusion as needed. There is little evidence that any medication administered systemically (e.g., intravenous vasopressin) is effective in halting diverticular hemorrhage; this therapy cannot be recommended because of dangerous problems with myocardial and mesenteric ischemia in this elderly population.

If *specific* therapy is needed because of persistent hemorrhage, then it depends upon accurate localization of the bleeding point. Localization may occasionally be accomplished by bleeding scan. If good emergency arteriography is available, this generally is the best way to obtain accurate localization of the site of persistent bleeding. With intraluminal pooling of extravasated contrast material, the outline of the bleeding diverticulum may be seen, otherwise the precise nature of the bleeding lesion may not be defined by arteriography. In the best of hands, successful localization of the bleeding diverticulum is possible in 60 to 70 percent of cases.

Regarding emergency colonoscopy, only occasionally have I been able to find the bleeding diverticulum (either as active bleeding from a single diverticulum, an adherent sentinel clot in the base of a diverticulum, or localization of active bleeding to a specific zone of the colon). I advise caution in interpreting the location of "freshest" blood, since there is frequent proximal backwash, and, additionally, retention of bowel contents by the sigmoid colon is a physiologic function.

Any attempt to localize the colonic bleeding point at the time of surgery, including intraoperative colonoscopy, is notoriously inaccurate.

If profuse diverticular bleeding persists or recurs requiring specific invasive therapeutic intervention, the main options currently include angiographic vasoconstrictor therapy or surgical resection. If the bleeding artery is selectively catheterized, *intra-arterial vasopressin* can be infused locally. If successful in halting bleeding, vasopressin infusion is usually continued for 24 hours, then gradually tapered. If rebleeding occurs, repeat vasopressin infusion can be performed, but surgical treatment is usually recommended. Most angiographers are reluctant to consider embolic therapy in the superior mesenteric artery circulation.

Surgical resection is required as definitive therapy if profuse bleeding persists or recurs repeatedly and if nonoperative measures are not successful or available. In general, surgery is required sooner in an elderly patient with other serious medical problems than in a younger healthy patient. There may be less enthusiasm for early operation if subtotal colectomy will be required as opposed to segmental resection. Surgical resection is not generally recommended following a single self-limited hemorrhage from a colonic diverticulum. I agree with most authorities who currently recommend segmental resection if the bleeding point has been accurately localized preoperatively. Although there apparently have been rare instances of simultaneous hemorrhage from two different diverticulae, it is generally considered that diverticular hemorrhage is solitary and can be treated effectively by segmental resection if preoperative localization is truly accurate. Attempts to find the bleeding diverticulum at surgery are typically frustrating, often misleading, and generally have been abandoned by most surgeons. If accurate preoperative localization has not been possible, then subtotal colectomy is the procedure of choice. Before this operation is performed, it is important to take a second careful look at the anorectal zone to exclude a distal bleeding source.

In passing, I note a couple of instances in which high-risk patients have been found at colonoscopy to have active arterial bleeding from a single diverticulum, and I employed the heater probe to halt bleeding effectively. In each case, the probe was gently inserted into the diverticulum with just enough pressure to tamponade active bleeding, at which point heat was delivered and coaptive coagulation was achieved. This new and unorthodox therapy was considered reasonable in view of the absence of any acute erosive potential with the heater probe, our large experience with this device, and the high-risk status of each of these patients. Further experimental study of this technique is in progress.

Bleeding Vascular Ectasia

Vascular abnormalities of the colon have been increasingly recognized as a frequent cause of gastrointestinal hemorrhage. Although a variety of terms have been used to describe these lesions (angiodysplasia, vascular ectasia, arteriovenous malformation, telangiectasia, and so on), for the purpose of this chapter our attention will be directed to the vascular ectasia[1]. The vascular ectasia, occurring predominantly in the right colon, may be viewed endoscopically as a discrete mucosal red spot, often intensely red in color and sharply demarcated with a fern-like perimeter. Lesions may be single or multiple, and size may vary from less than 1 mm to larger than 1 cm. Three-dimensional morphologic study has revealed these lesions to be similar to an oak tree, with a mucosal canopy of dilated venules and capillaries that converge into a large draining submucosal vein. The vascular ectasia is confined to the submucosa and mucosa, in contrast to a hemangioma, which may be transmural in location. Angiographically, the vascular ectasia may be seen as a vascular tuft on the tip of the feeding artery. There may be early filling of a draining vein, indicating a significant arteriovenous connection. Histologically, the elderly patient with a vascular ectasia in the right colon typically has a preponderance of dilated submucosal veins. Vascular ectasias are occasionally found incidentally at colonoscopy, without history of overt bleeding or anemia, and these lesions do not require treatment.

The patient with a vascular ectasia may present with chronic anemia from intermittent low-pressure oozing. The same lesion may also mimic diverticular arterial bleeding when a direct arteriovenous communication is present. Endoscopically, a white spot or erosion in the center of a vascular ectasia may represent a stigma of recent hemorrhage and is helpful in deciding which of several lesions may have been the true bleeding culprit. Histologically, there may be only a thin layer of epithelial cells overlying the vascular channels, and it is common for endoscopic trauma to induce transient bleeding. Induced hemorrhage is usually an ooze, although in rare instances we have observed pulsatile arterial bleeding from these lesions.

Treatment options include angiographic, endoscopic or surgical therapy. At *angiography* selective vasopressin infusion might be used to halt active bleeding, but this would not represent definitive therapy because of the high rebleeding rate with these lesions. Embolic therapy is considered unwise in the right colon by most angiographers.

There has been increasing interest and experience with *endoscopic* methods for coagulation and destruction of vascular ectasias. Thermal modalities include monopolar electrocoagulation (e.g., "hot biopsy" forceps), bipolar electrocoagulation (BICAP unit, American ACMI, Stamford, CT), thermal cautery (Heat Probe, Olympus Corp., Lake Success, NY), and laser photocoagulation (Neodymium: YAG and argon lasers). The most promising nonthermal method is injection sclerotherapy. These hemostatic modalities were recently comprehensively reviewed.[2]

In general, the vascular ectasia is an easy lesion to treat with any of these endoscopic hemostatic methods. I currently prefer the nonerosive contact probes (Heat Probe or BICAP) because of low cost, portability, precise control of tissue heating, no potential for tissue erosion, adjustable depth of coagulation, and potential for coaptive coagulation.

Regarding treatment technique, I recommend applying thermal treatment directly at the vascular lesion to produce tissue coagulation or whitening. Suggested initial instrumental settings include the following: heat probe, 10 joule pulses, light touch; BICAP (25 watt unit), 1- to 2-second pulses of power 5, light touch; "hot biopsy" forceps, grasp and "tent" the lesion, then apply short pulses with a low power coagulation setting; YAG laser, 40 to 60 watts, 2-cm treatment distance, 0.5-second pulses; argon laser, 5 watts, 2-cm treatment distance, 1- to 2-second pulses. Induced bleeding is common in treatment of the vascular ectasia regardless of which modality is used. It is important to deliver only enough thermal energy to ultimately destroy the lesion, but it is unwise to overtreat just to control "cosmetic" induced bleeding.

Unfortunately, precise guidelines for "safe and effective" energy limits cannot be defined, but in general, it is better to undertreat initially than to overtreat.

"Ideal" therapy for the vascular ectasia involves coagulation down to the submucosa but avoids a full-thickness burn. It is not necessary to treat the normal mucosa surrounding a vascular ectasia. The peripheral parts of a large lesion may be treated quite superficially, whereas the deeper central vessels may require deeper coagulation (increased energy setting and appositional force with the contact probes). Because of endoscopic problems with accurate lesion identification and traumatic artifacts, I recommend searching for and treating vascular lesions as the colonoscope is introduced, rather than on withdrawal. I see no reason to take the risk of biopsying a typical appearing vascular ectasia.

The main risks of endoscopic treatment of the vascular ectasia include perforation of the thin-walled cecum and delayed hemorrhage. Acute perforation can be prevented by using a nonerosive contact probe or by avoiding high power density with the lasers or electrical sparking with the monopolar probe. Delayed perforation one to seven days after treatment is possible after any full-thickness bowel injury but is prevented by keeping intraluminal pressure low (liquid diet and avoiding repeat endoscopy) and by the body's effective response in sealing the injured bowel with adjacent bowel loops and omentum. Delayed hemorrhage, an uncommon but potentially serious complication, may be caused by thermal-induced ulceration of a normal underlying submucosal artery. It is unwise to assume that rebleeding during the week following thermal treatment is due to inadequate coagulation of the vascular ectasia and attempt repeat endoscopic treatment. If the patient is supported and hemorrhage ceases spontaneously, then repeat colonoscopy 1 month later will usually reveal complete tissue healing with no residual vascular ectasia.

Although *surgical* resection has traditionally played a major role in definitive treatment of colonic vascular ectasia, I now reserve surgery (usually right hemicolectomy) for patients with widespread or particularly large vascular lesions, or when poor endoscopic orientation prevents effective endoscopic therapy. Typically, vascular ectasias are difficult or impossible to see at surgery or in the resected specimen, and special techniques with silicone rubber injection followed by tissue clearing are required.

Upper Gastrointestinal Bleeding

In the setting of major hemorrhage manifest as hematochezia and hypotension, endoscopy is indicated to exclude a bleeding lesion in the upper gastrointestinal tract, most of which are now amenable to endoscopic therapy. In the absence of hypotension or significant transfusion requirement, it is unlikely that an upper GI source explains passage of red blood from the rectum.

Colonic Ulcer

A solitary ulcer of the colon with arterial bleeding is an uncommon but important cause of major lower GI hemorrhage (cecum and rectum are the most frequent sites in our experience). Size of the bleeding artery is typically small, and direct endoscopic coagulation can usually be easily accomplished. Surgical oversewing of the ulcer or limited resection may be employed if effective endoscopic therapy is not possible.

Colonic Varices

In the setting of portal hypertension, colonic varices are an uncommon but potentially treatable cause of lower GI bleeding. As with their esophageal counterpart, injection sclerotherapy can be tried if the specific point of bleeding can be found, although portocaval shunt surgery is usually required.

Meckel's Diverticulum

An ulcerated Meckel's diverticulum should be considered as a cause of major hemorrhage in a young patient. Technetium sulfur colloid or technetium-labeled red blood cell scan may be helpful during active bleeding, whereas a technetium pertechnetate scan or small bowel x-ray film may show the diverticulum after bleeding has ceased. Lateral films or delayed films after barium enema or small bowel series may help demonstrate a Meckel's diverticulum. Surgical resection is required.

Postpolypectomy Bleeding

Delayed major hemorrhage during the week following colonic polypectomy occurs infrequently and usually subsides spontaneously with observation. Whereas the acutely bleeding stalk can be resnared and tamponaded by pressure, with delayed hemorrhage the polypectomy site is ulcerated and the bleeding artery may be retracted deeply into the submucosa. Spontaneous hemostasis is most desirable, but if therapeutic intervention is required, either injection sclerotherapy or coaptive coagulation with a nonerosive contact probe is optimal for this deep arterial bleeding site; caution must be exercised regarding the weakened wall.

Hemorrhoids

Hemorrhoids are a rare cause of major lower GI bleeding, most often associated with obstructed venous return from the superior hemorrhoidal veins (cirrhosis, cancer, and so on). Injection sclerotherapy with a variety of agents is typically effective in the control of acute bleeding. Other definitive therapy, such as rubber band ligation or possibly operative hemorrhoidectomy, may subsequently be required for third-degree hemorrhoids.

Radiation Colitis

Major hemorrhage from radiation colitis is distinctly uncommon. Whereas minor bleeding may be due to diffuse proctitis with granular, friable mucosa and characteristic telangiectasias, major bleeding usually implies an arterial source within the base of a radiation-induced ulcer. Although minor bleeding may respond to steroid enemas, persistent major hemorrhage requires definitive endoscopic or surgical therapy. If the bleeding point is found endoscopically, my treatment technique is similar treatment of a bleeding peptic ulcer (namely tamponade of bleeding with a nonerosive contact probe, followed by coaptive coagulation). If massive bleeding cannot be controlled endoscopically, surgery is needed to oversew or resect the bleeding ulcer. Unfortunately, diverting colostomy alone is not usually sufficient to control major hemorrhage.

Inflammatory Bowel Disease

Crohn's disease will rarely cause major bleeding from a deep ulcer which has eroded into an artery. This may require surgical intervention if the hemorrhage does not cease spontaneously. In contrast, the superficial ulceration of chronic ulcerative colitis characteristically produces only minor intermittent bleeding.

MINOR CHRONIC OR OCCULT BLEEDING

Small volume intermittent hematochezia typically implies a bleeding source in the left colon, rectum or anus, with benign anal causes predominating (see Table 1). Clues obtained from a careful history may be helpful. Passage of fresh blood after normal stool suggests an anal lesion, especially if there is dripping of bright red blood into the toilet. Hematochezia associated with painful defecation suggests an anal fissure. Streaks of blood on the stool or blood mixed in the stool suggests a lesion higher in the rectum or colon.

When historical features strongly suggest an anorectal cause of bleeding, and if careful digital, anoscopic and proctosigmoidoscopic examinations confirm a likely source of bleeding, then full colonic examination may not be required. There is additional support for this approach if a stool specimen, obtained from the sigmoid colon at the time of endoscopy, is negative for occult blood. However, if the patient is over age 40, or if a convincing distal source of bleeding is not found, or if features of bleeding suggest a higher bleeding site, then full colonic examination by good quality air contrast barium enema and colonoscopy or both should be performed.

Occult GI bleeding does not have any inherent localizing features and therefore requires examination of the entire GI tract. The main worry with occult bleeding is neoplasia, especially of the colon. Evaluation includes anorectal examination, proctosigmoidoscopy, and air contrast barium enema or colonoscopy. If the barium enema is negative except for diverticulae, colonoscopy is indicated and will reveal a missed colonic lesion in approximately 40 percent of cases. Conversely, if the colonoscopy is technically suboptimal or if the entire colon is not carefully examined, then air contrast barium enema is needed. Examination of the upper GI tract is accomplished either by air contrast x-ray film or endoscopy, depending upon clinical suspicions. With occult or recurrent overt GI bleeding and negative examination of the colon and upper GI tract, further possible diagnostic tests include small bowel x-ray films (enteroclysis is preferred), radionuclide scans, arteriography and use of a bleeder tube. A peroral attempt to endoscope the small bowel beyond the ligament of Treitz is usually not very rewarding, and the length of ileum that can be inspected at the time of colonoscopy is limited. As a last resort, if the clinical situation warrants, laparotomy with intraoperative small bowel endoscopy can be performed. Although a variety of techniques have been suggested, I have found that it is best to make a single small enterotomy in the mid small bowel, then pass the gas-sterilized colonoscope proximally and distally to inspect the entire small bowel. This is accomplished by a patient surgeon gently passing the endoscope as the endoscopist carefully observes the mucosa. Telescoping over the endoscope can be very traumatic to mucosal as well as serosal surfaces of the bowel, and it is therefore important to inspect adequately on insertion, since artifacts may preclude a satisfactory examination as the endoscope is withdrawn.

Evaluation of intermittent melena is similar to the approach outlined for occult bleeding except that suspicion of an upper GI source is greater and upper endoscopy should be considered earlier.

Once a precise diagnosis has been established, specific treatment options depend upon the particular lesion (see other chapters for full discussion). For example, medical therapy may include steroids for inflammatory bowel disease or stool softeners for anal fissure. Endoscopic therapy may be effective for removal of a bleeding polyp, for coagulation of bleeding telangiectatic vessels with localized radiation colitis, or for palliative treatment of a bleeding rectal malignancy. Surgery may offer definitive treatment of colon cancer, an intractable anal fissure, third-degree hemorrhoids, a Meckel's diverticulum, or ischemic colitis with peritoneal signs.

REFERENCES

1. Boley SJ. On the nature and etiology of vascular ectasias of the colon: degenerative of aging. Gastroenterology 1977; 72:650.
2. Johnston J. Endoscopic thermal treatment of upper gastrointestinal bleeding: overview and guidelines. Endoscopy Rev 1982; 2:12–33.

IRRITABLE BOWEL SYNDROME

MARVIN M. SCHUSTER, M.D.

Although irritable bowel syndrome is the most common gastrointestinal condition, little is known concerning its etiology. Recently acquired knowledge concerning pathophysiology and precipitating factors permits a rational approach to treatment based on these factors as well as empiric observation. Irritable bowel syndrome is characterized by abdominal pain and altered bowel habits, usually alternating constipation and diarrhea with one of the two symptoms predominating. The syndrome is recognized as a motor disorder which is strongly influenced by emotional stress and by food intake, and occasionally by specific food intolerances.

GENERAL PRINCIPLES OF TREATMENT

Since the etiologic determinants of irritable bowel syndrome are unknown, treatment focuses on correcting the underlying motor disorder and modifying those factors which are known to precipitate or aggravate the motor disorder and associated symptoms (Table 1). Treatment is therefore multidimensional and predominantly symptomatic. A consistent approach with persistent attention to details and a sensitive understanding of the individual patient can lead to significant improvement with time.

TABLE 1 Treatment of Irritable Bowel Syndrome

General Principles of Treatment
- Establish confidence
- Educate and reassure
- Dispel fears and misconceptions
- Schedule return visits

Dietary Management
- Investigate and treat lactose intolerance
- Eliminate offending foods
- High-fiber diet
- Hydrophilic colloids

Medications (as appropriate)
- Antispasmodics
- Antidiarrheals
- Intestinal stimulants
- Analgesics
- Antiflatulents

Psychological Management
- Anxiety
  - Manage situational stressors
  - Improve coping techniques
  - Relaxation training
  - Mild tranquilizers as needed
- Depression
  - Manage situation stressors
  - Support
  - Tricyclic antidepressants
- Illness Behavior
  - Avoid reinforcement of illness behavior
  - Reward healthy behavior
  - Push toward maximal performance

Adapted from Schuster MM. Irritable bowel syndrome. a coordinated approach to therapy. Drug Therapy 1962; August.

Establishing Confidence

The initial visit sets the stage and begins the ongoing process of the developing doctor-patient relationship. The interest and compassion shown by the physician at this time serves not only to inspire confidence but also to assist in the diagnostic pursuit of relevant information concerning the patient and the factors affecting his illness. A dogged pursuit of details can produce helpful and rewarding results.

Education and Reassurance

It is important that the patient understand that irritable bowel syndrome is an intestinal motor disorder, that it is chronic and recurrent, and that it is influenced by a number of factors, including emotional stress, food intake, and drugs. The patient will then be more likely to accept recurrence as part of the disease process rather than as an indication of inappropriate diagnosis or inadequate treatment. This will alleviate one of the stresses that every person with irritable bowel syndrome undergoes, namely, concern about the significance of persistent, recurrent, or intensified symptoms. It is often helpful to utilize as an analogy chronic disorders, such as hypertension or diabetes, which, like irritable bowel syndrome, are not cured but can be controlled.

Managing Fears and Misconceptions

A frank and open invitation to discuss concepts and concerns is perhaps the best way to elicit information which may be highly specific to the individual. This invitation may have to be repeated in subsequent sessions as the patient develops confidence and as the physician develops knowledge of the patient. Relatives may also be quite helpful in providing useful information in this regard. Patients also should understand that, although bothersome, irritable bowel syndrome does not lead to any serious disorder such as ulcerative colitis or cancer, nor does it in any way influence life expectancy.

Scheduling Return Appointments

A scheduled return visit will provide reassurance of continued interest, will avoid a sense of abandonment, will provide support, and will permit the continued gathering of information that can help to fine-tune the treatment program. During subsequent visits the patient's response to the therapeutic regimen can be ascertained and modifications can be made in the program as indicated. The support provided by this expression of ongoing interest, while not tangible, may be extremely meaningful and useful. Subsequent visits may be more brief and less frequent as improvement occurs and the patient is encouraged to assume a more active and independent role in the management of his disorder.

DIETARY MANAGEMENT

Investigate and Treat Lactose Intolerance

Symptoms of lactose intolerance can mimic in every way the symptoms of irritable bowel syndrome. In addition, lactose intolerance can aggravate the symptoms of irritable bowel syndrome. For these reasons lactose intolerance should be ruled out in every patient presenting with symptoms of irritable bowel syndrome. This can be achieved by performing a lactose tolerance test, or more simply by placing the patient on a lactose-free diet for a trial period of 2 weeks. Initially this diet should be quite strict, eliminating all milk and milk products. At a later stage, if lactose intolerance is demonstrated, the level of intolerance can be tested by gradually adding small quantities of the milk-containing products which the patient misses most until a threshold is reached at which symptoms recur. Only about 2 percent of patients who present with symptoms of irritable bowel syndrome will have lactose intolerance as the sole basis for their symptoms. Though small in number, this will be a very grateful group of patients who are cured by control of the quantity of lactose in their diets. In a larger number, about 40 percent, lactose intolerance is superimposed upon irritable bowel syndrome. Elimination of lactose in this group will improve but not alleviate symptoms completely. I generally reserve lactose tolerance tests for patients who appear to have lactose intolerance but refuse to accept the concept that small quantities of milk can be deleterious. Intolerance of other foodstuffs is a highly individual phenomenon and best demonstrated by the keeping of a careful dietary diary.

High-Fiber Diet

Diets high in bran (and perhaps other fibrous foods) may be helpful especially when constipation is a dominant feature of irritable bowel syndrome. One may begin by prescribing bran cereals, whole wheat or rye bread, and progress as needed to unprocessed bran which can be sprinkled on foods. It is perhaps best to start with small doses, increasing as needed and as tolerated to 16 g per day (2 tablespoons 3 times daily). More palatable forms of brans such as crackers (Fibermed) are also available. A transient increase in gas and bloating occurs not infrequently for the first several weeks but often disappears. Patients should therefore be encouraged to continue with the diet for about 3 weeks unless symptoms are extremely disturbing. Only about 15 to 20 percent cannot tolerate bran because of the intensity of the symptoms or because they persist for longer than 3 weeks.

Hydrophilic Colloids

Bulk agents containing psyllium seeds are particularly helpful when alternating constipation and diarrhea exist, since these agents are hydrophilic and tend to solidify diarrheal stools and also soften hard stools. They are therefore safer than antidiarrheal agents to treat the diarrheal phase and safer than laxative agents to treat the constipated phase. Dosage requirements are highly individual; one should begin at small doses, increasing as required until an effective dose is reached. The preference for one hydrophilic colloid over another is based predominantly on palatability, and in some specific instances on salt and sugar content for patients who require restriction of these ingredients. Some of the more popular agents are Metamucil, Perdiem plain, LA formula, Hydrocil, Konsyl, and Mitrolan. These agents may be more effective when administered with meals rather than at bedtime, because then they mix with the stool as it is being formed. Because of taste factors and because some swelling of the psyllium seeds takes place in the stomach, there may be some appetite suppression if administered before meals. Therefore these agents should be taken by obese people before meals and by thin people after meals.

DRUG THERAPY

Antispasmodic Agents

Although they are the most physiologically reasonable drugs for treatment of the intestinal motor disorder of irritable bowel syndrome, antispasmodics have been less than dramatic in their success. Still, they do play a role and provide varying degrees of relief for many sufferers of irritable bowel syndrome. Antispasmodics may be particularly useful in patients who have postprandial symptoms induced by increased intestinal motor activity. Anticholinergic drugs that have more spasmolytic than antisecretory activity are the logical choice for the treatment of the majority of patients with irritable bowel syndrome who do not have dyspepsia. In the United States, dicyclomine hydrochloride (Bentyl) is used; it has a high ratio of spasmolytic to antisecretory action. Therefore, side effects of dry mouth and decreased gastric secretion are less prominent. While it is generally prescribed in dosages of 20 mg 4 times daily, a recent study indicates that as much as 40 mg 4 times daily may be required. It is probably wise to start with doses of 10 mg 4 times daily for elderly patients, who are often not able to tolerate higher doses. At least 3 weeks should be allowed to judge clinical efficacy. Spasmolytic agents are generally best administered half an hour to an hour before meals and at bedtime (particularly in those patients with meal-aggravated symptoms). This allows time for peak blood levels to be reached during the postprandial period.

Blurred vision, urinary retenion, and aggravation of glaucoma are possible side effects with any anticholinergics.

When dyspeptic symptoms suggest hyperacidity, anticholinergics with more antisecretory activity may be preferred. Tincture of belladonna has the advantage of permitting graded dosage, starting with 10 drops and increasing until side effects of dry mouth or blurred vision appear, then dropping back to the dosage immediately preceding the one that caused the side effects. The liquid form may, however, be inconvenient outside the home. Other anticholinergics, such as propantheline, Levsin, and Cantil, are often used.

Antidiarrheal Drugs

Although mild diarrhea usually responds to hydrophilic colloids or dietary manipulations, severe diarrhea may require drugs such as diphenoxylate and atropine (Lomotil), one or two 2.5-mg tablets every 4 to 6 hours as long as diarrhea persists, or loperamide (Imodium), which has a rapid but longer duration of action and generally need be given as 2 or 4 mg only every 8 hours. When diarrhea is unremitting or accompanied by severe disabling pain, codeine, 30 to 60 mg every 4 to 6 hours, may be helpful but carries the danger of addiction. Since the effective antidiarrheal dose of codeine remains constant over time, increased dose requirements should suggest problems with addiction and possible need for withdrawal from the medication. Another problem associated with antidiarrheal agents of this type is induction of constipation, especially in patients with alternating diarrhea and constipation.

Stimulant Laxatives

As with antidiarrheal agents, stimulant laxatives should be used only when absolutely necessary, because they may induce diarrhea in patients with alternating constipation and diarrhea. They are also habit forming and should be prescribed only in the smallest possible effective doses and for the briefest period of time. Stimulants such as milk of magnesia, cascara, Senokot, and Dulcolax may aggravate a painful condition by stimulating intestinal spasm.

Analgesic Medication

The pain of irritable bowel syndrome can often be relieved by antispasmodic medications. When pain is severe and unresponsive to anticholinergics, analgesics may be required, but they should be reserved only for acute stages of severe pain. A heating pad applied to the abdomen or warm baths may also be helpful. When a chronic pain syndrome is present, referral to a pain treatment center may be appropriate. Non-steroidal anti-inflammatory agents, including aspirin, 2 tablets every 6 hours, may alleviate acute exacerbations of pain. Pentazocine (Talwin), 50 to 100 mg every 6 hours, should be used in preference to opiates for severe, acute, limited situations. Morphine particularly is to be avoided because of its addiction potential as well as the fact that it aggravates spasm even though its central action may diminish perceived pain.

Antiflatulents

The effective antiflatulent is yet to be discovered. Trial and error seems to be the most useful way of finding drugs that provide some relief. Simethicone (Mylicon), two to four tablets, or activated charcoal (4 tablets), may be prescribed with meals and at bedtime. Pancreatic supplements, Phazyme 95, Ilozyme, Pancrease, Viokase, Cotazyme, and so on, 1 to 2 tablets before meals and at bedtime, are helpful for some.

MANAGEMENT OF PSYCHOLOGIC FACTORS

Since emotional stress is one of the most commonly recognized factors aggravating irritable bowel syndrome, and since 70 to 80 percent of patients with irritable bowel syndrome demonstrate psychopathologic factors on psychological tests, psychological management is an important aspect of treatment. In the vast majority of instances this can be effectively handled by the primary physician or consulting gastroenterologist. Psychiatric referral is appropriate only for those conditions that would require psychiatric referral whether or not irritable bowel syndrome were present. A life history chart compiled by the patient can be quite helpful in detecting stressful factors that are associated with exacerbation of symptoms. This information is best obtained simply by probing into life events that surround periods of exacerbation and remission.

Anxiety

Although anxiety is easily recognized by patients, somatization (which represents an internalization of anxiety) is less readily detected. Correlation of life events with anxious periods provides useful clues. In some instances direct environmental manipulation may successfully remove the stressful stimulus. For example, with the physician's questions acting as a catalyst, a patient may arrive at the conclusion that his interest would be better served by changing jobs or locations. This type of milieu therapy can produce dramatic improvement. Often, however, these changes are either impossible or inadvisable, and the patient must be helped to learn appropriate coping techniques for dealing with stresses that cannot be removed. A number of audiotapes are available for relaxation training e.g., Budzynski narration MV 3–B (BMA Audiocassettes Department C1, 200 Park Avenue South, New York, NY 10003). Infrequently tranquilizers may be required for brief periods of intensive anxiety, but long-term use should be avoided if possible.

Depression

Depression is less readily recognized than anxiety, since it is often masked and expressed as somatic symptoms. As with anxiety, precipitating factors can sometimes be altered but more commonly they cannot. Supportive therapy is often helpful. Tricyclic antidepressants may be useful when given in a single night-time dose, e.g., 25 to 50 mg of amitriptyline (Elavil), or 50 to 100 mg of maprotiline (Ludiomil).

There is some evidence that symptoms of irritable bowel syndrome represent illness behavior learned in early childhood and perpetuated by social reinforcement (secondary gain). A behavioral approach to this aspect is the most direct, and often the most successful. Patients and relatives are instructed to avoid disscussion of illness and by all means to avoid rewarding illness by attention, while focusing on and rewarding healthy behavior. Patients are asked to distract themselves from thinking about their symptoms whenever they become more aware that they are doing so. They are told to avoid discussion of symptoms except during their routine visits with their physicians. Patients are instructed to view their irritable bowel syndrome as they would view a physical disability which they would try to overcome. Rather than give in to the illness, they are encouraged to push themselves to maximal performances as they would if they had visual impairment, hearing deficit, or other physical disability.

While no single drug or therapeutic maneuver may be curative, gratifying relief can result for a coordinated program based on sound physiological principles and empiric observations.

CONSTIPATION

ALASTAIR M. CONNELL, M.D.
ALVIN M. ZFASS, M.D.

To be normal is to be "regular." While gastroenterologists have traditionally minimized the need for "a stool a day," epidemologic studies have suggested reasonably convincing benefit associated with a large daily stool! But what is a "normal" stool, and precisely what is the definition of "normal bowel habits?" What is meant by constipation?

Constipation can be defined according to frequency of the stool and/or consistency of the stool. Most surveys show that "a stool a day" is most commonly experienced in healthy populations, but the frequency varies. For example, in the United States, approximately 5 percent of healthy subjects report two or fewer stools per week; others consider three stools per day as "regular" or healthy.[1]

As noted, constipation is also a term used to describe the consistency of stool. A hard or desiccated stool contains little water, usually 50 percent. Normal stools contain 70 percent water, and "liquid" stools contain more than 95 percent water.

In summary, terminology is confusing. Hard, infrequent stools that are associated with straining represent a consensus example of constipation. However, there are unusual examples where definitions fail. Consider the soft effortless stool that happens every 4 days or the pellet-like stool that is passed only with considerable straining! A working definition of constipation is often best provided by the patient: any change in defecation, due to a decrease in frequency and/or an increase in the consistency, may be considered "constipation."

PHYSIOLOGY

Constipation usually represents a disordered function of the colon or of the anorectal region. For example, transit through the upper gut in patients with constipation has been shown to be only slightly prolonged, and this is of no clinical significance.[2]

The precise abnormalities in colonic function that result in constipation have not been satisfactorily identified. Three major normal functions of the colon have been identified: (1) the extraction (conservation) of water, which is a function of the colonic epithelial cell, (2) the maintenance of an abundant intraluminal bacterial population, and (3) the capacity to control the delivery of feces (colonic motility and the act of defecation). The constipated patient has been poorly studied, and it is not possible in any given case to assess which of the aforementioned functions is abnormal.

Careful observation of colonic contraction and flow of intraluminal colonic contents suggests that the colon is broken into three distinct functional segments. In the proximal part of the colon, there is little regular propulsive movement, and the colonic content tends to remain in the cecum for long periods. This type of motility results in a longer contact time of intraluminal contents and increased water absorption.

In the transverse and descending colon, the major muscular activity is segmenting contracting caused by contraction of the circular muscle. This results in a to-and-fro movement of the content with a gradual forward progression toward the sigmoid and rectum.

Occasional strong contractions occurring in the colon move the fecal mass caudad. These movements occur infrequently, but the fecal mass, when moved, is transported over long segments. One such contraction occurring approximately once daily results in defecation.[3]

Although the process of defecation is incompletely understood, it is generally accepted that distention of the sigmoid or rectum by stool entering it stimulates pressure receptors. This stimulus causes forward movement of a bolus of stool and a reflex relaxation of the internal anal sphincter accompanied by the "urge" to defecate. Continence is ensured by a variety of mechanisms, including a reverse gradient of contraction in the sigmoid and the existence of the internal anal sphincter. The external anal sphincter also maintains continence. This striated muscle sphincter is under voluntary control and provides the appropriate "emergency" squeeze when necessary. When the rectum is suddenly distended, the internal anal sphincter relaxes involuntarily and defecation is imminent. The area of mucosa proximal to the anal margin acts on a sensory zone and can discriminate between water or solid. It is response to the sensory discrimination that provides input for voluntary consent to defecation.

The rectal vault is also important in maintaining continence since it may act as a reservoir. Its ability to do so is related to rectal compliance and the ability of the rectum to allow an increase in volume without a concomitant increase in pressure. Although not adequately studied, this "receptive relaxation" may be similar to that observed in the gastric fundus.

CONTROL MECHANISMS

Control of the movement of colonic contents is poorly understood. A brief overview of the important factors follows.

Myogenic Factors

Myogenic factors include electrical activity of smooth muscle cells (periodic depolarization and repolarization) of the colon. This activity is irregular, but conforms to the basic "slow waves" and "spike bursts" described in the stomach and small intestine. A relationship between slow waves, contractions, and movement of intraluminal contents has been suggested in man. Slow wave frequencies occur over a range of 2 to 12 cycles per minute and frequently occur irregularly. Slower frequencies have been described in constipation, but the data are not convincing. It is probable that myogenic control mechanisms play a more important role in the proximal colon than in the distal colon. Exercise has an important role in preventing constipation and has an effect on colon motility, but the exact mechanism is not clear.

Neuro-endocrine Factors

The motor nerves to colonic muscle can be broadly classifed as (1) excitatory nerves, which are both cholinergic and noncholinergic, and (2) inhibitory nerves, which are adrenergic and nonadrenergic. Lesions of the spinal cord, especially destruction of the lumbosacral cord, cause severe and sometimes intractable constipation. Recently, the classic model of the autonomic nervous system with only cholinergic or adrenergic neurotransmitters has been greatly expanded, and noncholinergic and nonadrenergic regulatory peptides have been identified not only in the gut, but in the brain and other tissues. These peptides are released from specialized endocrine cells in the gut or from autonomic nerves. In the human colon, enteroglucagon, gastric inhibitory polypeptide, and neurotensin are confined to the specialized endocrine epithelial cells. Vasoactive intestinal polypeptide (VIP), substance-P, and bombesin-like peptides have been demonstrated exclusively in nerves. VIP is likely to be the most important "relaxant" or inhibiting neurotransmitter in the gut.

The gastrocolic responses, which result in increased motor activity during or following eating certain foods and may contribute toward bowel regularity, are mediated in part by gastrointestinal hormones. It is important, but may prove difficult, to identify the specific roles of these peptides in constipation. In Hirschprung's disease (aganglionosis), however, there is a depletion of VIP- and substance-P-containing nerves in the myenteric plexus. The absence of the inhibitory neurotransmitters is related to the segment of contracted bowel, and this area of contraction, which does not relax, leads to the development of megacolon.[4] Recent studies have demonstrated abnormalities in the myenteric plexus in idiopathic pseudo-obstruction.[5] In another study, women with severe intractable constipation were also found to have abnormalities of the myenteric plexus.[6]

Water Absorption

Mucosal absorption of water by the colon determines the consistency of stool at the time of defecation. Mucosal surface area, mixing, contact time, and intraluminal pressure are important factors. An increased "avidity" for water absorption has not been demonstrated in constipation, although carefully designed studies have not been reported.

Transit-Pressure Alterations

In constipated subjects, transit (radiopaque markers, barium, telemetering devices) through the colon is delayed. The usual pattern of prolonged transit is a uniform delay in passage throughout the entire colon so that intraluminal contents remain in each segment of the colon for longer than normal periods of time. In some patients, especially the young and elderly, delay occurs in the rectal segment. Persistent fullness of the rectum is abnormal and used to be known as dyschezia. Addition of fiber to the diet decreases transit time by as much as 50 percent, but the precise factors that promote this acceleration have not been elucidated. Gastrointestinal hormones may be implicated.

Pressure studies using small balloons as sensors or open-tipped catheters have demonstrated higher than normal resting pressure in the left colon (10 to 30 cm from the anal verge) in some constipated patients. Although exaggerated colonic response (increased pressure) after food or other stimuli has been reported, it has not been noted consistently. In general, the overall motility responses of groups of constipated subjects are not significantly different from those of subjects with normal elimination.

CLINICAL CONSIDERATIONS

Constipation with No Structural Abnormalities Identifed

Deficient bulk. This deficiency is probably the most common cause of constipation in western countries. Dietary changes designed to increase fecal bulk and fecal water are helpful. Wheat bran, oatmeal, certain fruits, and root vegetables such as carrots are beneficial.

Poor Defecation Habits. During the rush of daily life, the suppressed urge to defecate or disagreeable toilet facilities result in continued filling of the rectal ampulla or vault. The need to defecate is suppressed and normal anorectal sensation diminishes. The stool becomes desiccated while remaining in the rectum. This hardened stool makes subsequent defecation difficult and uncomfortable. Management consists of behavioral modification by the patient. Use of simple glycerin suppositories help to restore rectal sensation, lubricate the stool, and facilitate emptying of the rectum. Rarely, operant conditioning (biofeedback) with rectal training programs are needed to restore normal rectal reflexes.

Irritable Colon Syndrome with Constipation. Treatment in this disorder is for the underlying irritable bowel syndrome. An adequate explanation of the pathophysiology of constipation in conjunction with a high fiber diet is usually effective. Stool bulking agents such as psyllium seed can help. Occasionally, antispasmodics such as mebeverine or dicyclomine are useful.

Idiopathic (Slow Transit) Constipation of Women. In this interesting group of patients, transit time is strikingly prolonged, and as noted, the constipation is most common in women. Abdominal distention, pain, and laxative abuse are also commonly noted. Treatment is unsatisfactory and, specifically, dietary fiber supplementation may increase or aggravate the symptoms. Frustration with all forms of medical management may lead to consideration of colonic resection.

Constipation with Structural Disease of the Colon

Laxatives are rarely necessary for treatment of constipation and should always be used under supervision. Laxative abuse, especially with phenolphthalein, has become a major problem, particularly with elderly persons or young females.

Anal Pain. Any disease of the anus associated with pain may interfere with defecation. Common disorders include anal fissures or hemorrhoids. Medical management is effective and includes stool softeners, sitz baths, and application of local anesthetic ointments or suppositories. Anal dilation under general anesthesia may be required in some cases.

Aganglionosis. This disease is usually diagnosed in childhood, but may be recognized for the first time in adult life. Anal manometry and rectal biopsy establish the diagnosis with certainty. Surgery is indicated.

REFERENCES

1. Connell AM, Hilton C, Irvine G, Lennard-Jones JE, Misiewicz JJ. Variation of bowel habit in two population samples. Brit Med J 1965; 2:1095–1099.
2. Eastwood HDH. Bowel transit studies in the elderly:radio-opaque markers in the investigation of constipation. Gerontol Clin 1972; 14:154–159.
3. Christensen J. Motility of the colon. In: Johnson LR, ed. Physiology of the gastrointestinal tract. New York: Raven Press, 1981, Chapter 14, pp 445–471.
4. Tsuto T, Okamura H, Fukui K, Obata HL, Terubayashi H, Iwai N, Majima F, Yanaihara N, Ibata Y. Immunohistochemical investigation of vaso active intestinal polypeptide in the colon of patients with Hirschsprung's disease. Neurosc Letter 1982; 34:57–62.
5. Schuffler MD, Jonak Z. Chronic idiopathic pseudo-obstruction caused by a degenerative disorder of the myenteric plexus: the use of Smith's method to define the neuropathology. Gastroenterology, 1982; 82:476–486.
6. Krishnamurthy S, Schuffler MD. Severe idiopathic constipation is caused by a distinctive abnormality of the colonic myenteric plexus. Gastroenterology 1983; 84:1218.

HEPATORENAL SYNDROME AND ASCITES

H. FRANKLIN HERLONG, M.D.

ASCITES

Ascites, the accumulation of fluid within the abdominal cavity, may develop because of hepatic, cardiogenic, neoplastic, or inflammatory disorders. Modest amounts of ascites are not reliably detectable on physical examination. In one study the overall accuracy of detection was only 58 percent when the presence of ascites was questionable, with many false-positive assessments. If there is any doubt as to the presence of ascites, a blind paracentesis should not be performed. Since ultrasonographic examination of the abdomen can reliably detect even small amounts (100 ml) of ascites, this procedure should be used to confirm its presence. The sonogram can not only locate a site at which a paracentesis can safely be performed but also can detect abdominal or pelvic masses or organomegaly.

When a patient develops ascites for the first time, or when a patient with chronic ascites develops unexplained fever, encephalopathy, or other significant changes, he should be hospitalized and should undergo a diagnostic paracentesis. A Z-track technique is employed to avoid a post-paracentesis leak. Under asceptic conditions, 100 ml of ascitic fluid is removed and the syringe is immediately capped. A portion of the fluid is sent for routine studies, including protein and glucose determinations, cell counts with differential, and bacteriologic cultures. The rest of the specimen should be transported to the laboratory anaerobically and on ice for a pH determination. If cancer is suspected an additional 100 ml of fluid should be obtained for cytopathologic examination. Appropriate analysis of these tests should allow a correct diagnosis to be made and institution of appropriate therapy.

The most common cause of ascites is cirrhosis, which accounts for approximately 70 percent of all cases. Extrahepatic disorders also produce ascites. Table 1 summarizes the laboratory and clinical features of some diseases associated with ascites. When possible, therapy is directed toward underlying conditions; this often leads to resolution of the ascites. There is no effective treatment for some of the conditions, however, and the ascites can only be palliated.

Treatment of Ascites in Patients with Underlying Liver Disease

In most patients with underlying liver disease, ascites develops as a complication of the cirrhosis itself; however, patients with cirrhosis may have coexistent disorders that contribute to the production of ascites. For instance, alcoholic cirrhotics are predisposed to tuberculous peritonitis, and patients with chronic hepatitis B infection may develop hepatocellular carcinoma with peritoneal metastases.

Spontaneous Bacterial Peritonitis

Patients with cirrhosis are also predisposed to developing spontaneous bacterial peritonitis. Early recognition and prompt institution of therapy for this disorder dramatically reduce mortality. If the condition is diagnosed before patients become febrile or develop peritoneal signs, the mortality can be reduced by 50 percent.

The presence of more than 500 polymorphonuclear (PMN) leukocytes per cubic millimeter in ascitic fluid is evidence of bacterial peritonitis even if the patient is asymptomatic. Immediate antibiotic therapy should be instituted in such cases or for patients who have evidence of systemic infection, even if the fluid PMN cell count is less than 500 per cubic millimeter.

Antibiotic therapy should be appropriate for gram-positive organisms, including streptococci and staphylococci, and gram-negative bacilli until culture results are available. Anaerobic infections are uncommon except in patients who have recently undergone abdominal surgery. I recommend either *cefamandole* or a combination of *ampicillin* and *gentamicin*. When possible I avoid aminoglycosides, since patients with cirrhosis are at increased risk of aminoglycoside-induced nephrotoxicity. The choice of antibiotics should be adjusted once the results of the ascitic fluid culture are known.

Potential Aggravating Factors

Some medications may precipitate ascites formation in patients with cirrhosis. Nonsteroidal anti-inflammatory agents which inhibit prostaglandin synthetase cause retention of sodium by the kidneys. This increased renal sodium retention may expand the plasma volume sufficiently to cause ascites. Discontinuation of these medications results in mobilization of the ascitic fluid.

Perhaps one of the most important management steps is to look for reversible components of the underlying liver disease. Treating these components may make it unnecessary to prescribe specific therapy for the ascites. For instance, when patients with severe alcoholic hepatitis are forced to abstain from drinking alcohol over several weeks, they may have enough improvement in their liver function that they may not need diuretic therapy. Restoration of blood volume after a gastrointestinal hemorrhage may also promote ascites reabsorption (Table 2).

Primary Treatment of Ascites

Once complicating extrahepatic conditions have been excluded or treated, therapy may be directed specifically toward mobilization of ascites. Patients with only mild ascites do not need therapy. Use of diuretics should be restricted to those patients in whom ascites has become uncomfortable or causes specific complications, since injudicious use of diuretics may lead to serious complications.

While a mild to moderate amount of ascites may be cosmetically unattractive, it rarely harms the patient. Specific therapy is indicated when the ascites becomes extensive enough potentially to cause complications. For example, respiratory compromise due to decreased diaphragmatic excursion may predispose to pneumonia. Associated pleural effusions can exacerbate the respiratory compromise. In addition, ascites may increase risk of variceal bleeding by increasing portal pressure. Other important complications are anorexia and development of inguinal and umbilical hernias.

The mainstays of therapy for ascites caused by cirrhosis are *sodium restriction* and/or *diuretics*. The rationale for this approach is based on the three factors that produce ascites in patients with cirrhosis. Ascites develops in patients with cirrhosis because of increased renal retention of sodium in combination with portal hypertension and decreased plasma colloid oncotic pressure. All three factors favor the transudation of fluid from the liver into the abdominal cavity. When the production of fluid overcomes the removal of fluid by the lymphatic system, ascites accumulates.

TABLE 1 Causes of Ascites

Associated Diseases	*Fluid Analysis* WBC (/mm³)	RBC	Protein (g/dl)	*Other Laboratory Features*	*Clinical Features*
COMMON					
Cirrhosis	< 250 (mono)	Few	< 2.5	pH > 7.4	Signs of portal hypertension frequently present
Infection					
Bacterial	> 500 (poly)	Few	> 2.5	pH < 7.35	Fever, rebound tenderness; some patients are asymptomatic
Tuberculous	> 500 (mono)	Few	> 2.5	pH < 7.35	Low-grade fever, cachexia, alcoholic liver disease
Tumor	Few	Many	> 2.5	pH < 7.35 (tumor cells present)	Cachexia, abdominal pain, primary site may be occult
Pancreatitis	> 500 (poly)	Many	> 2.5	Fluid amylase > 1,000 IU/L	Severe abdominal pain, leukocytosis
Congestive heart failure	Few	Few	< 2.5		
RARE					
Nephrotic syndrome	Few	Few	< 2.5		Urinary protein > 2 g/24 hr
Pseudomyxoma peritonei	Few	Few	< 2.5	Gelatinous fluid, occasionally with tumor cells	Marked abdominal distention, pain, cachexia
Chylous ascites	Few	Few	Variable	Fluid triglycerides elevated > 400 mg/dl	Results from lymphatic obstruction; may be due to tumor, trauma, tuberculosis

TABLE 2 Treatment for Ascites in Patients with Cirrhosis

1. Hospitalize patients with new onset of ascites.
2. Perform diagnostic paracentesis
   If > 500 PMNs/mm³ in ascitic fluid, treat empirically for bacterial peritonitis with either cefamandole or ampicillin/gentamicin. Adjust antibiotics depending on culture results.
3. Discontinue drugs that increase sodium retention.
4. If ascites is uncomplicated, collect 24-hour urine to measure sodium excretion.
5. Base diuretic therapy on urinary sodium excretion.

Urinary Na+ Excretion (mEq/24 hr)	*Dietary Sodium (g/day)*	*Therapy*
> 50 (= 1 g Na+)	2.0	None
25–50 (0.5–1.0 g)	1.5	Spironolactone (100–300 mg/day)
10–25 (250–5 mg)	1.0	Spironolactone (100–300 mg/day) and furosemide (40–160 mg/day) or bumetanide (2–8 mg/day)
< 10(<250 mg)	0.5	Maximal diuretic dose Therapeutic paracentesis (?) Peritoneovenous shunt (?)

The limited capacity to reabsorb ascites must be taken into consideration in designing therapy. When patients have peripheral edema in addition to ascites, a maximum of 3 L of fluid can be mobilized within a 24-hour period. In the absence of edema, a maximum of only 900 ml of ascitic fluid can be removed in 24 hours.

If diuresis exceeds these amounts, the extra fluid is removed at the expense of the intravascular space and hypoperfusion may ensue. Therefore, in treating ascites the goal is to use the simplest regimen that will produce a diuresis of about 900 ml (1 to 1½ lb) a day in patients without peripheral edema, and 2 L (3 to 4 lb) a day in patients with edema. Once edema has resolved, the diuretic regimen may have to be adjusted to ensure continued safety.

Since renal retention of sodium is one of the most important factors responsible for the development of ascites, assessing quantitative renal sodium excretion is of value in planning a quantitative therapeutic regimen. Before beginning diuretic therapy, 24-hour urinary sodium excretion should be measured while the patient is on a 1-g sodium diet. This allows accurate prediction of diuretic effectiveness at the start of therapy, rather than using the trial-and-error method of adding various agents depending on patient response. Table 2 outlines various dietary and diuretic regimens based on renal excretion of sodium. Fluid restriction is not necessary unless the patient develops hyponatremia.

In most patients, ascites will resolve with a combination of salt restriction and diuretics. If patients fail to lose weight on an appropriate diuretic regimen, however, it is useful to remeasure their urinary sodium excretion. Excretion of an adequate amount of sodium without the mobilization of ascites suggests surreptitious ingestion of extra salt. Refractory ascites is defined as excretion of less than 10 mEq of sodium in 24 hours while taking less than 500 mg of sodium in the diet and maximum doses of diuretics. In these patients the tendency to form ascites is so severe that ascites accumulates at a rate exceeding reabsorption despite intravascular volume depletion sufficient to cause prerenal azotemia. Patients with intractable ascites may, if they are suitable candidates, require surgical therapy to mobilize their ascites.

Alternative Treatment

Alternatives for removing ascites include *portosystemic shunting, therapeutic paracentesis,* and *ascites reinfusion* via *peritoneovenous shunt*. Portosystemic shunts will reduce portal hypertension and mobilize ascites, but surgical morbidity and/or subsequent encephalopathy makes shunting unacceptable therapy for ascites.

Therapeutic Paracenteses

Several recent studies have demonstrated the efficacy and safety of therapeutic paracenteses for patients with resistant ascites. In these patients, paracenteses of up to 6 L per day led to effective ascites control, with no more complications than diuretic therapy. These large-volume paracenteses did not cause a higher incidence of renal insufficiency, systemic hypotension, or plasma protein depletion compared with diuretic therapy. I have used this technique successfully in a number of patients whose ascites was refractory to a potent diuretic regimen.

An 18-gauge plastic catheter is placed in the linea alba inferior to the umbilicus and attached via plastic tubing to evacuated bottles to facilitate large-volume fluid removal. Continuous removal of ascites at a fixed rate may be accomplished by attaching the plastic tubing to a continuous infusion pump (I-Med).

Ascites Reinfusion

Ascites may be reinfused into the intravascular space through *peritoneovenous shunts*. These shunts allow ascitic fluid to flow unidirectionally from the peritoneal cavity into the superior vena cava. Several pressure-sensitive valves have been developed which allow fluid to flow up the shunt when the intraperitoneal pressure exceeds the intrathoracic pressure. The LeVeen shunt is the most popular. It consists of a silicone valve that remains open and permits ascites flow when a pressure gradient between the intraperitoneal limb and intrathoracic limb exceeds 5 cm H_2O. Two modifications of the LeVeen shunt have been developed and are commercially available: the Cordis-Hadin shunt and the Denver shunt. These newer shunts include pumping mechanisms which create turbulence within the valves and reduce the chances of mechanical shunt failure because of valve occlusion.

Soon after the peritoneovenous shunt is implanted, diuresis and natriuresis produce significant decreases in abdominal girth and body weight. Some patients have an increase in creatinine clearance accompanied by a fall in renin and aldosterone secretion.

Unfortunately, a number of potential complications limit the usefulness of peritoneovenous shunts. In about 30 percent of patients, the shunt fails for mechanical reasons. In some of these patients, repositioning the distal end of the shunt may restore function. In others the valve becomes clogged and needs to be replaced. Some patients with underlying heart disease fail to increase their cardiac outputs in response to the increased delivery of fluid into the right heart. Unless left ventricular function improves, the shunt will fail.

The most serious complication of peritoneovenous shunts is associated *coagulopathy*. Patients with acute liver disease such as alcoholic hepatitis seem particularly predisposed. Although the etiologic agent of this coagulopathy has not been clearly established, the problem seems to result from introduction of thromboplastic substances from the peritoneal fluid into the intravascular space. Complete removal of ascites with partial replacement by normal saline at the time of surgery has been reported to reduce the risk of severe coagulopathy.

When disseminated intravascular coagulation is accompanied by significant bleeding, heparin and/or epsilon-aminocaproic acid may be necessary to control the hemorrhage. Some patients require shunt removal. Low-grade fever is common during the first week after the peritoneovenous shunt is placed. Most patients have negative cultures and the fever resolves without therapy.

Expansion of intravascular volume in some patients may increase portal pressure and flow, precipitating variceal hemorrhage. Therefore, peritoneovenous shunts should not be used in patients who have recently bled from esophageal varices. Another absolute contraindication to peritoneovenous shunting is intrinsic renal disease, such as acute tubular necrosis, which prevents the kidneys from excreting the additional salt load. Since patients with active hepatocellular injury are predisposed to severe bleeding, the shunt is also contraindicated in patients with active hepatocellular disease such as alcoholic hepatitis.

HEPATORENAL SYNDROME

Progressive oliguria and renal insufficiency may complicate both acute and chronic liver disease. Patients with liver disease may develop renal insufficiency from hypoperfusion caused by intravascular volume depletion or a reduced cardiac output, from acute tubular necrosis because of ischemia or nephrotoxic agents, and from obstructive uropathy.

The initial approach to oliguria in patients with liver disease should include a vigorous search for reversible precipitating factors. Insertion of a urinary catheter will promptly relieve prostatic obstruction in men. An ultrasonogram may reveal ureteral dilatation in patients who have obstruction at the level of the urinary bladder.

Patients should be examined carefully to assess intravascular volume status. When doubt exists as to whether they are volume depleted, measurement of central venous pressure is necessary. In addition, all potentially nephrotoxic drugs should be discontinued.

In some patients with advanced liver disease, no specific cause is found for the renal insufficiency and the disorder is termed the "hepatorenal syndrome." The hepatorenal syndrome is a disorder of unknown origin that develops in patients with severe acute or chronic liver disease and is characterized by progressive oliguria and azotemia. It may develop insidiously, with a gradual decrease in urine volume over days to weeks, or it may develop suddenly, with profound oliguria or even anuria developing within a few days. Most patients have cirrhosis and portal hypertension with ascites; however, there are reports of the hepatorenal syndrome developing in the absence of ascites. The hepatorenal syndrome may also complicate acute liver failure.

In patients with the hepatorenal syndrome, the kidneys are anatomically and morphologically normal. There is, however, a profound shift in intrarenal blood flow, from the cortical nephrons to the medullary nephrons. This shift may be produced by afferent vasomotor constriction of vessels supplying the cortical nephrons, perhaps mediated by prostaglandins. This shift in blood flow results in avid reabsorption of sodium, with preservation of the kidneys' capacity to concentrate the urine.

Using urinary electrolyte measurements and urinalysis, one can often differentiate between the hepatorenal syndrome and oliguria produced by acute tubular necrosis. The urine osmolarity in the hepatorenal syndrome is normal but contains virtually no sodium (<3 mEq per 24 hours). The urinary/plasma creatinine ratio is often greater than 30. In contrast, in acute tubular necrosis the urinary/plasma creatinine concentration is approximately 1, and significant quantities of sodium are found in the urine (Table 3).

Many patients with the hepatorenal syndrome are hyponatremic and have a compensated respiratory alkalosis. Most patients have modest systemic hypotension. Despite prolonged oliguria the serum creatinine and urea concentration may remain minimally elevated because of reduced muscle mass and impaired hepatic urea synthesis. The urine sediment is unremarkable in patients with the hepatorenal syndrome, but in patients with acute tubular necrosis it contains cellular debris and casts.

Urinary biochemical tests and urinalysis results in patients with the hepatorenal syndrome are indistinguishable from those seen in patients with prerenal azotemia in the absence of acute tubular necrosis. Careful assessment of intravascular volume is essential in all patients with liver disease and renal insufficiency. This may be difficult from the physical examination alone. Frequently it is necessary to measure the central venous pressure. If the central venous pressure is less than 6 cm H_2O, patients should receive a trial of volume expansion, preferably with 50 g of albumin, or with blood if patients are anemic. Overexpansion of the intravascular volume should be avoided (central venous pressure >12 cm H_2O), as the excess volume may increase portal flow and/or pressure, precipitating variceal hemorrhage. If initial volume expansion does not increase urine output and sodium excretion, volume expansion with intravenous fluid should be discontinued.

TABLE 3 Treatment for Acute Renal Insufficiency in Patients with Liver Disease

1. Rule out obstruction, urinary tract infection.
2. Obtain 24-hour urine collection to measure sodium and creatinine for differential diagnosis.

	Urinary Sodium (mEq/L)	*Urinary/Plasma Creatinine Ratio*
Prerenal azotemia	< 10	> 30
Acute tubular necrosis	> 30	< 20
Hepatorenal syndrome	< 10	> 30

3. If urine Na^+ < 10 mEq/L, carefully assess intravascular volume.
4. If central venous pressure < 6 cm H_2O, try volume expansion with albumin or blood.
5. Therapy for hepatorenal syndrome
   - Diet: 3,000 calories, 40 g protein, 40 mg potassium, 1 g sodium.
   - Avoid *indwelling* catheter to prevent infection.
   - Avoid drugs that adversely affect renal function: nonsteroidal anti-inflammatory agents, demeclocycline

   No specific therapy (i.e., vasodilator drugs, diuretics, ascites reinfusion) is of proven efficacy.

   Dialysis depends on reversibility of underlying liver disease.

   Liver transplantation (?)

Management of patients with the hepatorenal syndrome is similar to that of patients with other forms of acute renal failure (see Table 3). Dietary protein should be restricted and electrolyte disturbances corrected. If oliguria persists, complications of renal insufficiency and azotemia will develop.

Dialysis

Although peritoneal or hemodialysis may improve metabolic acidosis and associated complications of azotemia (platelet dysfunction with bleeding, altered mental status, and pericarditis), these benefits are usually transient without improvement in survival. I make the decision to dialyze patients with renal insufficiency and advanced liver disease based primarily on the potential reversibility of their underlying liver disease. I dialyze patients with advanced cirrhosis and portal hypertension only if they have treatable complicating factors and/or reversible components of their liver disease.

Vasodilating drugs and peritoneovenous shunting have been used in attempts to reverse the hepatorenal syndrome. Unfortunately, none of these has been consistently effective. Orthotopic liver transplantation cures the hepatorenal syndrome but can be considered only if the patients are appropriate candidates for this procedure.

PORTOSYSTEMIC ENCEPHALOPATHY

LAURENCE M. BLENDIS, M.D., F.R.C.P., F.R.C.P.(C)

Portosystemic encephalopathy (PSE) is a potentially reversible neuropsychiatric syndrome occurring in patients with chronic liver disease. It can occur at any age but is more common in older patients. Its pathogenesis is unknown but there are several theories. Portosystemic encephalopathy may be due to a number of factors including; toxic nitrogenous substances, false neurotransmitters, and decreased physiologic neural excitation (Table 1).

Toxic nitrogenous substances, e.g., ammonia, are produced by and absorbed from the right side of the colon and normally detoxified by the liver. In cases of severely decompensated liver disease, with or without shunting, these substances pass to the brain with toxic effects. This is an old theory and has stood the test of time despite many imperfections.

The theory of *false neurotransmitters* as a cause of PSE is based on the observation of increased circulating levels of aromatic amino acids, e.g., phenylalanine, and decreased levels of branched chain amino acids competing for the same amino acid transport system across the blood-brain barrier. The possible result is increased phenylalanine concentrations in the brain, with saturation of the normal neurotransmitter metabolic pathway to form dopamine and norepinephrine. This results, via alternate pathways, in the production of weak or false neurotransmiters such as octopamine, which block normal neurotransmission. The problem with this theory is that the altered amino acid ratios in patients with PSE compared to those with uncomplicated cirrhosis are not different and are probably a manifestation of liver dysfunction rather than encephalopathy. Thus the development of PSE by this theory remains controversial.

Another theory is that involving *decreased physiologic neural excitation*, e.g., due to glutamate or increased physiologic neural inhibition due to gamma-aminobutyric acid (GABA), in which GABA synthesized from glutamate in presynaptic neurons interacts with specific receptors or postsynaptic neurons to exert its inhibitory effect. This appears to result from increased chloride ion conductance across the postsynaptic neural membrane with generation of an inhibitory postsynaptic potential. Support for this hypothesis includes evidence that GABA is generated by gut bacteria and that serum levels of GABA-like activity are increased in patients with PSE and in cirrhotic patients following gastrointestinal hemorrhage. Other precipitating factors, however, do not closely relate to nitrogen metabolism (see Table 1), thus supporting the concept that PSE is multifactorial.

Whatever the pathogenesis of PSE, it is clear that it can be induced by a number of clearly defined precipitating factors, most of which are treatable or reversible (see Table 1).

ACUTE PORTOSYSTEMIC ENCEPHALOPATHY

Diagnosis

Diagnosis of acute PSE requires a clinical suspicion of chronic liver disease aroused by clues in the history, if available, or by signs of hepatic dysfunction on physical examination. In addition, there may be neuropsychiatric signs of a metabolic encephalopathy, e.g., fetor,

TABLE 1 The Precipitating Causes of Portosystemic Encephalopathy

Precipitating Cause	*Diagnosis*
Increased Colonic Nitrogen Load	
Excessive protein intake	History
Upper gastrointestinal hemorrhage	Rectal examination—melena, occult blood
Constipation	Abdominal examination Rectal examination Abdominal x-ray films
Metabolic Disturbance	
Excess sedation	History
Infection	White blood cell—total and differential
Pneumonia	Chest x-ray films
Urinary tract infection	Urinalysis—microscopy, culture, and sensitivity
Peritonitis (ascites)	Peritoneal tap—polymorph count
Acid-Base disturbance	Blood gases
Electrolyte abnormality	Serum electrolytes
Intravascular Volume Depletion	Clinical—postural drop in blood pressure, absent jugular vein, elevated BUN, creatinine

asterixis, cogwheel rigidity, hyperreflexia, ankle clonus, and so on. Frequently the patient will come to the emergency department at a time of day when confirmatory diagnostic tests such as arterial ammonia measurement or electroencephalogram may be difficult to obtain. Therefore the diagnosis may have to be entirely clinical.

Once the diagnosis is made, the next problem, management of the disease, requires the detection and treatment of the precipitating cause(s) (see Table 1) as well as specific treatment of PSE. Once again a history of recent excessive protein load to the gastrointestinal tract, either exogenous, such as a large steak, or endogenous; melena or constipation; or diuretic or sedative therapy may provide a clue to the precipitating cause. A full clinical examination is essential and may reveal melena or severe constipation. Intravascular volume depletion is diagnosed by a postural drop in blood pressure and absent jugular veins. The presence of a fever may indicate infection. Pneumonia can be diagnosed clinically, whereas spontaneous peritonitis in the presence of ascites may produce little in the way of physical signs and can be very difficult to diagnose.

Tests at the bedside, such as that for fecal occult blood, are important. In addition, routine laboratory investigations, e.g., blood count, serum electrolytes, BUN and creatinine, and urine for microscopy, culture, and sensitivity, may reveal the precipitating cause. Other tests, such as blood gas measurements, indicate the consequence, and not the cause of the disorder. In the presence of ascites with negative preliminary results, a diagnostic peritoneal tap is indicated to exclude peritonitis. A chest roentgenogram for evidence of pneumonia is essential, and an abdominal roentgenogram to assess colonic fecal content is useful.

General Therapeutic Measures

Management initially requires securing the patient's airway if necessary and maintaining the vital signs. In patients who have had a gastrointestinal bleed, glucose and colloid infusions prior to blood replacement are preferable to saline, which is likely to be "third spaced." In patients with nonhemorrhagic intravascular depletion, colloid is preferred if possible. Electrolyte disturbances, such as hyponatremia due to excessive diuretic therapy, are best managed by complete cessation of diuretic therapy and strict fluid restriction to about 1,200 ml per day in patients who can drink, or 50 ml per hour of intravenous fluid in the comatose patient. When infection is diagnosed, a broad-spectrum antibiotic regimen is begun until culture results are available. For pneumonia, ampicillin is used; for peritonitis a cephalosporin and an aminoglycoside are chosen.

Specific Therapeutic Measures

In patients with acute PSE, with or without coma, oral protein intake can be withheld completely for two to three days with the patient receiving intravenous fluids only. Colonic washout with tap water enemas until the returns are clear should be started immediately and continued every 6 to 12 hours. At the same time lactulose, the specific treatment of choice (Table 2), in a dosage of 30 ml (20 g lactulose) by mouth every 2 to 4 hours should be instituted to produce at least two or three loose watery stools. If the patient cannot cooperate, a thin nasogastric feeding tube should be passed and, after one is certain that it is indeed in the stomach, lactulose can be administered via this route. In the comatose patient it is preferable to give lactulose per rectum as an enema, e.g., 300 ml lactulose made up to 1 L with water, but only after the tap water enema has been completed. When lactulose enemas are given from the first, the importance of colonic cleansing is forgotten by both nursing and medical staff. The result is that the lactulose remains in the sigmoid or descending colon while the right side of the colon remains full of feces.

Most patients will respond within 3 to 5 days to this combined treatment of the precipitating cause and the encephalopathy. In any event, by the third day, as the patient recovers, oral protein intake should be reinstituted at 20 g per day, often in the form of enteral feedings. At the same time the dose of lactulose should be reduced to not more than 30 ml 4 times per day. With further improvement the lactulose dose should be reduced again, provided the patient continues to have one to two loose bowel movements daily. It is most important to reduce the dose of lactulose as soon as possible, otherwise the patient may become severely dehydrated and in addition develop an anion gap metabolic acidosis.

Resistant Comatose Patients

Differential Diagnosis

In some cases the patient does not appear to respond to standard medical therapy, i.e., resistant coma. First it is essential to exclude the possibility of a missed precipitating cause perpetuating the hepatic coma, such as a masked spontaneous peritonitis, other cerebral disease, and so on. We would, however, repeat or perform for the first time an electroencephalogram to confirm the diagnosis and to assess the severity of PSE. A decrease rather than an increase in wave amplitude or an absence of recognizable wave forms would indicate a poor prognosis and the necessity of additional measures.

Management

In my experience, the majority of these patients will eventually respond to continued standard therapy (5 to 7 days) without altering the management. Theoretically, the addition of neomycin to lactulose does not make sense, since the therapeutic effect of lactulose is thought to result from the alteration of the colonic flora by creating an acidic pH with the suppression of urease-containing bacteria (see Table 2). Thus, at that stage the antibacteri-

TABLE 2 Specific Therapy for Portosystemic Encephalopathy

Medication	Mode of Action
Proven	
Lactulose	Laxative Acidification of colon: Converts ammonia to ammonium, decreases faster nonionic diffusion across colonic mucosa Suppresses bacterial reproduction or metabolism Increases fecal bacterial ammonia excretion
Neomycin Metronidazole	Antibacterial action in colon
Unproven	
L-dopa	Increased cerebral dopamine production
Bromocriptine	Dopamine agonist
Branched chain amino acid	Promotes cerebral neurotransmission production

al effect of neomycin should not be beneficial. Nonetheless, there is some evidence that the combination of neomycin and lactulose may result in an additional therapeutic effect.

Nonproven Treatment of Acute Portosystemic Encephalopathy

L-Dopa

The suggestion that PSE might be due to a relative deficiency of the neurotransmitters led to the use of L-dopa. Although initial anecdotal reports indicated that it might be beneficial, carefully controlled trials failed to show any significant improvement in patients so treated.

Bromocriptine

Similarly, it was suggested that the dopamine agonist bromocriptine might be helpful. Again, although initial studies were optimistic, a controlled trial showed no beneficial effects.

Branched Chain Amino Acids

The controversy still rages as to whether branched chain amino acids (BCAAs) are beneficial either intravenously or orally in PSE. In comatose patients there are few controlled data in favor of their use and a considerable number of controlled trials showing no obvious improvement in the level of PSE with amino acid infusions rich in BCAAs. The longer the patients remain in coma, however, the more they are at risk of developing serious effects of protein malnutrition. Thus an argument can be made that in this regard there is an indication to use amino acid solutions that do not use hepatic metabolic pathways, such as BCAAs. The benefits may be marginal, however, and insufficient to compensate for the high costs even if the solutions are available. Therefore I do not use them in this situation.

Finally, it is important to emphasize that cirrhotic patients who are in coma with resistant PSE often have severely decompensated or end-stage liver disease and may have entered the final, irreversible stage of their disease. Thus it is important to resist heroic measures, particularly if the electroencephalogram shows marked flattening of the wave forms.

CHRONIC PORTOSYSTEMIC ENCEPHALOPATHY

Cirrhotic patients with chronic PSE present a different group of problems. First there is the question of diagnosis. It is well recognized that stage I PSE may be difficult to diagnose. The patients can present with myriad symptoms, e.g., changes in personality, such as becoming more irritable or being depressed, possibly associated with a failure to recognize a deterioration in mental function or absent-mindedness. Deterioration of mental function is an important symptom because, if the cause goes unrecognized, it can lead to loss of employment. These presentations are much more common than the classic reversal of sleep pattern with a tendency to sleep during the day and for which sedatives at night can have disastrous consequences.

Diagnosis

In the treatment of chronic PSE the first prerequisite is to make the diagnosis and then treat. In the absence of clear-cut history or neurologic signs, such as asterixis, hypertonicity with cogwheel rigidity, and hyperreflexia, the diagnosis may be difficult. In such patients the use of a simple psychometric test, such as the number connection test, is invaluable. It can be performed immediately in the office and, particularly if there is a previously normal test (i.e., less than 40 seconds), an increase in the time taken to complete the test to more than 90 seconds is highly suggestive of PSE. Other tests, such as a fasting arterial ammonia level or an electroencephalogram, are much more difficult to obtain.

Treatment

There are several proven therapeutic regimens for the treatment of chronic PSE.

Lactulose to Prevent Constipation. This in itself may be sufficient to treat very mild cases of PSE. Lactulose is still the drug of choice but is expensive. I usually start treatment with a dose of 30 ml four times a day to produce two loose bowel movements daily before decreasing to a maintenance dose of 30 ml twice a day. Similar laxative effects may be achieved by other cheaper combinations, including a fiber substitute (Metamucil), or stool softener (Colace), as well as an osmotic laxative (sorbitol). Alternatively, a high-fiber diet is a more natural way of preventing constipation. As previously stated, however, the benefit of lactulose is not simply due to its laxative effect but is multifactorial (see Table 2).

Reduction in Animal Protein. There is no doubt that a reduction in protein intake is an effective treatment of PSE. Yet many of these patients are already suffering from protein malnutrition. It is therefore often necessary to decrease the protein from the normal amount of about 70 g per day to 40 g, which is usually the reduction required to achieve a therapeutic effect. Vegetarian diets, which are higher in fiber, appear to be less encephalopathogenic than animal protein diets. It is extremely difficult, however, to convert a life-long meat eater to vegetarianism but relatively easy to encourage someone to increase the fiber content of his diet.

Antibiotics. A small group of patients either cannot tolerate lactulose or are resistant to it, the alternative medication for many years has been neomycin. Because of its side effects of ototoxicity and nephrotoxicity which occur in about 5 percent of the patients, alternatives have been sought. Recently metronidazole, in a dosage of 250 mg 3 times daily, has been shown to be as effective as neomycin and therefore it is now the alternative drug of choice.

Subclinical Portosystemic Encephalopathy

It has become clear in the past few years that many cirrhotic patients who appear totally asymptomatic may have a subclinical form of PSE. More sophisticated techniques, such as a battery of psychometric tests, can show a classic pattern of abnormalities in patients with clinical PSE. Similar abnormalities have also been found in asymptomatic patients, even with apparently normal electroencephalograms.

In the future we will be faced with the necessity of developing even more sensitive diagnostic tools, such as visually evoked potentials, and better therapeutic regimens that will not necessitate the reduction in dietary protein with its possible drastic nutritional and metabolic consequences.

ACUTE VIRAL HEPATITIS

LEONARD B. SEEFF, M.D.

The remarkable advances of the past two decades in diagnostic serology and molecular virology of viral hepatitis have, unfortunately, not been paralleled by improved techniques for treatment of the disease. On the contrary, current management of the acute illness is characterized by the omission of certain approaches that were common a decade ago, items such as mandatory hospitalization, mandatory bed rest, the use of special diets, and treatment with glucocorticoids in certain circumstances. Prevention of the disease, however, or at least some of its forms, has made dramatic progress, testimony to the persistent and innovative research of the clinical epidemiologist, virologist, and molecular biologist.

DIAGNOSTIC CONSIDERATIONS

A prerequisite for specific and effective treatment of any disease is the ability to establish a definitive diagnosis. In the case of acute hepatitis that has no pathognomonic features, diagnosis depends on the accumulation of historical facts, clinical findings, and biochemical alterations that, taken together, suggest the presence of acute hepatocellular necrosis. Attention must then be directed toward finding a specific etiology, since the liver responds in only a limited number of ways to numerous, diverse noxious stimuli. For example, it is now recognized that viruses other than those of hepatitis A and B can induce identical acute liver disease, namely, those causing delta hepatitis, non-A, non-B hepatitis (of which there are almost certainly two), and epidemic non-A, non-B hepatitis. The illness can be mimicked also by adverse reactions to certain drugs, by congestive cardiac failure, and by severe hypotension. Finally, a similar although generally distinguishable liver disease can result from other infectious agents (e.g., cytomegalovirus, Epstein-Barr virus, herpes simplex virus, coxsackievirus, rubella, and so on), in association with acute choledocholithiasis, from alcohol excess (alcoholic hepatitis), and occasionally in connection with certain metabolic disorders (Wilson's disease, alpha$_1$-antitrypsin deficiency). Thus, etiologic identification is imperative not only as a guide to specific therapy but also as an aid in the institution of appropriate preventive measures.

PRELIMINARY EVALUATION

In persons with apparent acute liver disease, a presumptive etiologic diagnosis can generally be achieved through the combination of a detailed historical interview (with special emphasis on the circumstances that favor exposure to viral hepatitis), extensive questioning regarding the use of all drugs (prescription and over-the-counter), a carefully administered physical examination, and the use of appropriate biochemical and serologic tests. If the diagnosis remains unclear, additional evaluation is necessary, as dictated by clinical circumstances. This may include ultrasound and computed tomographic scanning of the abdomen, immunologic tests, screening procedures for Wilson's disease, and so on. A liver biopsy is no longer considered a routine procedure when acute viral hepatitis is strongly suspected. The biopsy is now reserved for instances in which there is a diagnostic dilemma that is likely to be resolved by the finding of characteristic morphologic changes, or for the further evaluation of a bout of acute viral hepatitis that follows a disturbing course or persists for an unusual period of time (more than 4 to 6 months).

Once a diagnosis of acute viral hepatitis is established, the next step is definition of the severity of the disease and of the responsible virus. The basis for the latter exercise is to permit the adoption of the appropriate preventive and prophylactic measures for contacts of the patients.

Biochemical Tests

Routine biochemical tests should include measuring the activities of the aminotransferases (SGOT or AST; SGPT or ALT) and alkaline phosphatase, the levels of serum bilirubin and the serum proteins, and the prothrombin time. Of these, the tests that best define severity and prognosis are the prothrombin time and the serum bilirubin value. A prothrombin time in a patient which exceeds that of the control by 3 to 4 seconds is a disturbing finding, as is deep jaundice (> 25 mg/dl, unless superimposed hemolysis is the basis for the increased value). There is little correlation between the height of the aminotransferase values and the severity of the disease.

Serologic Tests

The most useful panel of serologic tests are HBsAg, IgM anti-HBc, and IgM anti-HAV, with the addition of HBeAg and IgM anti-delta (anti-HD) as needed. Thus, acute liver disease associated with a positive test for IgM anti-HAV establishes a diagnosis of acute hepatitis A. It must be noted, however, that in about 15 percent of instances, this antibody persists for 200 days or longer. Hepatitis B is diagnosed by the presence of HBsAg and/or IgM anti-HBc. If, instead, IgG anti-HBc is present together with HBsAg, the diagnostic consideration is a superimposed bout of acute hepatitis A, non-A, non-B hepatitis, or delta hepatitis, or a flare of hepatitis B (which sometimes occurs when HBeAg spontaneously seroconverts to anti-HBe) in an HBsAg carrier. Acute non-A, non-B hepatitis requires the exclusion of all known causes of acute hepatitis and the absence of IgM anti-HAV and of IgM anti-HBc.

MANAGEMENT OF ESTABLISHED ACUTE VIRAL HEPATITIS

There are two aspects to management when the precise diagnosis is finally made, namely, active treatment and prevention and prophylaxis.

Active Treatment

Site

The site of treatment is dictated by the severity of the disease and the adequacy of home support. If the disease is not classified as severe (bilirubin <25 mg per deciliter, prothrombin time <4 seconds prolonged), and there is an acceptable level of home care available, hospitalization is not needed. Adequate care implies that there is a household member willing to observe the patient daily for any signs of unusual physical or mental change, and to supply the necessary nursing and subsistence support. Such patients need not be seen by the physician any more frequently than is necessary for appropriate blood testing (see below).

Hospitalization will, however, need to be considered at the outset of the illness or during its course if the patient has persistent vomiting with the threat of dehydration, has a serum bilirubin value that is greater than 25 mg per deciliter or a prothrombin time that is greater than 4 seconds prolonged, has clinical evidence of encephalopathy, shows rapidly declining aminotransferase activity in the face of a rising bilirubin level, or develops other evidence of hepatic failure (falling albumin level, ascites, and so on).

Evaluation

Ideally, biochemical evaluation should be performed twice weekly while values continue to rise, once a week after they have reached a plateau and begin to decline, and at 1- to 2-week intervals when a slow but inexorable reduction toward normal becomes apparent. It is worth recording normalization of all values even though this may require a prolonged period of observation. It is also important in persons with proven hepatitis B to establish the loss of HBsAg and, if possible, the appearance of anti-HBs (although this may take many months).

Bed Rest

There is now general agreement that complete bed rest is not essential. Indeed, physical activity within the bounds of fatiguability can be permitted without fear of permanent damage. The exception to this rule is evidence of persistent biochemical or neurologic worsening, particularly in an older person (>40 years of age), even though there are no scientific data that demonstrate a beneficial effect of bed rest.

Diet

Contrary to earlier practice, it is no longer believed necessary to restrict fats. A nutritious diet should be encouraged which need not include vitamin supplementation unless there is evidence of a specific deficiency. If there is persistent nausea and vomiting, repeated small feedings of caloric liquid formulas may be helpful. Occasionally nausea and vomiting may be severe enough to culminate in dehydration, which would require appropriate intravenous fluid and electrolyte replacement. Protein restriction is required only if overt encephalopathy develops.

Drugs

There are no drugs available for the treatment of acute hepatitis. Because corticosteroids accelerate the reduction in bilirubin levels and aminotransferase activity, they have been used in the past therapeutically in different stages of the disease, (e.g., during the early acute phase, for fulminant hepatitis, in suspected subacute hepatic necrosis, for chronic viral hepatitis). Available data suggest that they are not only unhelpful, but they may well be harmful by increasing viral replication. Certain experimental drugs (e.g., cyanidanol, isoprinosine, ribavirin, levamisole, high-titer anti-HBs) have also been evaluated in patients with acute viral hepatitis but without demonstrable benefit.

Because the liver is the major site of metabolism of many drugs, all medications, particularly narcotics, analgesics, and tranquilizers, should be strictly avoided during the acute illness. The reduction in drug clearance when there is widespread necrosis may promote hepatic encephalopathy or even respiratory depression. If sedation is essential, reduced doses of benzodiazepines can be employed, or preferably oxazepam, a drug whose metabolism is not impaired in the presence of acute liver damage. Protracted nausea and vomiting may require the judicious use of phenothiazines or antihistamines. Rarely, pruritus may be sufficiently severe and persistent as to warrant the use of medication, such as the exchange resin cholestyramine. Vitamin K_1 is often administered in the hope of preventing or improving coagulation abnormalities; however, no benefit derives from its use in acute hepatocellular disease, although it may be effective in cholestatic liver disease.

A question that sometimes arises is whether or not alcohol can be used. Generally this is in reference to the period after recovery but occasionally it relates to the taking of alcohol during the acute illness as symptoms begin to wane. It has been traditional to proscribe its use during the acute illness and for a period of 6 to 12 months after recovery based on early data which suggested that fulminant hepatitis could be provoked or that relapse of acute hepatitis could result. Despite the lack of firm data to support these observations, it seems prudent to continue this approach, if for no other reason than to reduce confusion regarding the meaning of subsequent enzyme abnormalities (alcohol effect versus disease exacerbation). If, on the other hand, enzyme abnormalities persist for more than 12 months, suggesting transition to chronic hepatitis, it is wise to recommend to the person who strongly desires alcohol to use it in moderation and infrequently.

Finally, while the use of oral contraceptives can be continued during acute hepatitis without fear of harm, sexual activity during the early acute phases of hepatitis should be discouraged so as to avoid transmission of the virus to the partner.

Preventive Measures and Prophylaxis

Prevention

The institution of appropriate preventive public health measures is predicated on a thorough knowledge of the modes of spread of hepatitis. The *hepatitis A virus* is excreted in stool from the latter half of the incubation period to approximately the time of peak illness, generally within a week of onset of overt disease. Transmission from person to person is via fecal-oral contact; accordingly, those at risk are susceptible household or institutional contacts. Because of this pattern of viral excretion, many of these contacts are likely to have been exposed by the time the index case is brought to medical attention. Nevertheless, to curtail further spread, the modes of disease transmission should be discussed with the patient, and strict standards of personal hygiene should be imposed. This includes regular hand washing, particularly after using the toilet (separate facilities are not required), a warning against intimate contact, and a prohibition of the sharing of food and drink. With regard to eating utensils, either disposable or regular crockery can be used as long as a hot-water dishwasher is available, which provides adequate sterilization. If hospitalization is required, there is no need to impose reverse isolation procedures or require the use of separate bathroom facilities. Needle precautions continue to be advised even though there is no carrier state for hepatitis A and percutaneous transmission of hepatitis A is uncommon (but by no means unheard of).

The *hepatitis B virus* is present in blood and in all physiologic and pathologic body fluids, with the exception of stool; presumably the same holds true for the viruses of *non-A, non-B hepatitis* and the *delta agent*. Thus, blood and body secretions are the source of transmission, and high-risk individuals are those who are likely to come into contact with blood or its products or who have close intimate contact with the index case. Nonpercutaneous transmission other than through sexual contact also occurs but the precise mechanism often cannot be established. Consequently, preventive measures that can be adopted include efforts to reduce the number of blood transfusions; the development and maintenance of hospital surveillance to identify HBsAg carriers; the requirement that gloves be worn by personnel who are in regular contact with blood, followed by careful hand washing; the requirement that needles be appropriately disposed of and that instruments in contact with blood and secretions be adequately cleaned (with soap and water), disinfected (sodium hypochlorite, formalin, glutaraldehyde), and sterilized (autoclaving, ethylene oxide); and the recommendation that sexual abstinence be followed during the acute disease and that sexual contact be limited by the carrier. Finally, as will be discussed, if immune prophylaxis is provided for all susceptible high-risk individuals, many of these problems would be avoided.

Prophylaxis

Prophylaxis is the area of most impressive gains. For *hepatitis A*, passive protection with immune globulin (IG, formerly ISG) remains the backbone of prophylaxis, and, provided IG is administered to susceptible contacts within 2 to 4 weeks of exposure, complete inhibition or modification of the disease can be anticipated. A practical dose formulation is the administration intramuscularly of 0.5 ml of IG to children weighing less than 50 lb, 1.0 ml to persons weighing 50 to 100 lb, and 2.0 ml to those who weigh more than 100 lb (based on a dose of 0.02 ml per kilogram of body weight). Now that the hepatitis A virus has been cultured, an attenuated, live hepatitis A vaccine has been developed. Recombinant vaccine, made possible by the cloning of hepatitis A, is also in the process of development. Early studies with the live vaccine indicate that it is immunogenic, and human studies are now in progress to determine its efficacy.

Hepatitis B prophylaxis is more complex because of the carrier state of this virus, often in totally asymptomatic individuals. Therefore, prevention has to be considered in two contexts, namely, postexposure prophylaxis that follows an episode of known contact (e.g., percutaneous exposure to a contaminated needle, sexual contact with a partner incubating the disease or carrying the virus, the birth of an infant to a mother with acute disease or who is a carrier), or preexposure prophylaxis (e.g., high-risk individuals in whom contact can be anticipated in the future). In the former situation, hepatitis B immune globulin should be administered intramuscularly to contacts as soon as possible after exposure (5 ml on two occasions to an adult, 0.5 ml once to a newborn). Adults who already have adequate titers of anti-HB^s (10 sample ratio units or more by radioimmunoassay or positive by enzyme immunoassay) do not require prophylaxis; pre-screening of exposed neonates is unnecessary. The "needlestick" and neonatal contacts should also receive hepatitis B vaccine (20 μg for adults, injected into the deltoid; 10 μg for neonates, injected into the thigh immediately and 1 and 6 months after exposure). Postexposure prophylaxis for sexual contact is controversial; the current official recommendation is that either IG or HBIG be administered once only, with the addition of the vaccine reserved for contacts of a carrier but not of a person with acute hepatitis B. Preexposure prophylaxis with hepatitis B vaccine is strongly recommended for all susceptible high-risk contacts. There is overwhelming evidence that it provides a high rate of immunogenicity, protection, and safety. Deltoid injection may induce a more consistent response than buttocks injection. The current plasma-derived vaccine may be replaced in the future by vaccines that are genetically engineered or synthesized from defined immunogenic HBsAg peptide sequences. In a population with a high prevalence of hepatitis B, such as homosexually-active men or nurses in a dialysis unit, screening for hepatitis B antibody is cost-effective.

No specific prophylactic measures are available for the delta agent or non-A, non-B hepatitis. None is needed for delta hepatitis; this agent is entirely dependent for its expression on the coexistence in the human host of hepatitis B, and hence prevention and prophylaxis of the latter affords equal protection for the former. The development of passive or active immunizing products against non-A, non-B hepatitis obviously awaits the identification of the responsible viral agents. In the interim, since this disease has many epidemiologic similarities to hepatitis B, the same general preventive measures should be instituted as those described for hepatitis B. Indeed, the use of IG as postexposure prophylaxis for the same circumstances as it is used in hepatitis B has become common practice. This should probably continue even though it is impossible to determine whether a specific lot of IG contains any or sufficient concentrations of specific antibody. Research in this area continues.

CHRONIC HEPATITIS

RAYMOND S. KOFF, M.D.

Chronic hepatitis refers to a set of necro-inflammatory liver disorders in which clinical, biochemical, and histologic abnormalities persist for more than six months. Chronic hepatitis can be caused by viral hepatitis (persistent hepatitis B virus (HBV) infection, delta agent infection of HBV-positive individuals, persistent non-A, non-B hepatitis virus infections, but not hepatitis A virus infection), adverse hepatic drug reactions, and metabolic disorders such as Wilson's disease, $alpha_1$-antitrypsin deficiency, and iron overload disorders. In a large proportion of patients no etiologic agent can be defined and the term *idiopathic chronic hepatitis* seems appropriate. Some of these may be examples of autoimmune-initiated disease (autoimmune chronic hepatitis), but it is likely that primary defects in immunoregulation are responsible for only a minority of cases. Patients with primary biliary cirrhosis may have features resembling those seen in chronic hepatitis. Similarly, patients with alcoholic liver disease occasionally may present with features typical of chronic hepatitis (this disorder is also discussed elsewhere in this volume). In this chapter, the treatment of viral and idiopathic chronic hepatitis will be discussed.

Liver biopsy is essential for confirmation of the diagnosis of chronic hepatitis, histological classification of the form of chronic hepatitis present, and identification of severity of the lesion. The presence of sequelae and some clues to etiology may also be provided.

Three major forms of chronic hepatitis have been recognized: chronic persistent hepatitis, chronic lobular hepatitis, and chronic active hepatitis.

CHRONIC PERSISTENT HEPATITIS

Chronic persistent hepatitis is a benign form of chronic hepatitis characterized histologically by the presence of a dense infiltrate of mononuclear cells in the portal tracts, with minimal stromal collapse, slight or no periportal hepatocyte necrosis, and little if any fibrosis. While some authorities have suggested that liver biopsy may be unnecessary because management of this form of hepatitis is not altered by confirmation of the diagnosis, biopsy confirmation provides reassurance that a more serious disorder is not present and seems an appropriate measure. Hepatitis B virus (the hepatitis B surface antigen [HBsAg] is detected in the sera of 10 to 40% of patients) and non-A, non-B viral hepatitis are responsible for most cases. Chronic persistent hepatitis is a nonprogressive disorder which rarely, if ever, evolves into cirrhosis. An identical lesion may be seen, however, following spontaneous or treatment-induced remission in some patients with chronic active hepatitis. In this case, the natural history of the disease is that of chronic active hepatitis, and relapses may occur with clinical, biochemical, and histologic progression. One additional exception to the general benign course of chronic persistent hepatitis is the occurrence of delta agent superinfection of patients with HBsAg-positive chronic persistent hepatitis. In this event, the disease may be progressive and can lead to the development of chronic active hepatitis and cirrhosis.

Most, but not all, patients with chronic persistent hepatitis are asymptomatic and appear healthy. Such patients come to medical attention because of the detection of persistently elevated levels of serum aminotransferases or during the evaluation of the HBsAg carrier state. Nonspecific complaints of mild fatigue, anorexia, and abdominal discomfort or pain may be seen in a few patients, but physical findings are usually absent except for minimal hepatomegaly. Serum bilirubin levels are mildly elevated in about 10 percent of patients, but with the exception of the serum aminotransferases other liver tests are usually within normal limits.

No specific therapy has been shown to alter the natural history of this disorder irrespective of its etiologic agent. Neither immunosuppressive therapy nor antiviral therapy has established a role in the management of affected patients. Treatment of chronic persistent hepatitis is limited to reassurance, simple supportive measures, the avoidance of known hepatotoxins (small amounts of alcohol may be permitted if well tolerated), avoidance of parenteral exposures that might result in delta agent superinfection of HBsAg-positive patients, and annual follow-up to ascertain that the disease remains nonprogressive as determined by physical examination and serial liver chemical tests. Liver biopsy is not repeated unless clinical or biochemical deterioration suggests that the original diagnosis of chronic persistent hepatitis may have been erroneous. This is a rare event. The disease may persist for many years before resolution, which is signaled by normalization of the serum aminotransferase levels and, in some instances of HBV-induced disease, seroconversion from HBeAg-positive to anti-HBe-positive and loss of HBsAg.

CHRONIC LOBULAR HEPATITIS

This uncommon form of chronic hepatitis appears to be a sequel of hepatitis B and non-A, non-B viral hepatitis in which the features of acute hepatitis may persist for a prolonged period, with moderately increased levels of serum aminotransferases typical of those found in acute hepatitis. The course is characterized by multiple biochemical remissions and relapses over many years. During the relapses the hepatic histopathologic lesion is that of acute hepatitis. During remissions the lesion resembles chronic persistent hepatitis. Physical findings are minimal; about one-third of patients have hepatomegaly. Signs of portal hypertension are absent. Neither cirrhosis nor hepatic failure is a sequela of chronic lobular hepatitis. No specific therapy is available. Biochemical and histologic resolution may occur after years of follow-up, as in chronic persistent hepatitis.

CHRONIC ACTIVE HEPATITIS

Chronic active hepatitis is the most serious form of chronic hepatitis because, in its most severe and aggressive form, the disorder may progress to fatal hepatic failure and/or the development of cirrhosis with associated complications of portal hypertension. Liver biopsy reveals enlarged portal tracts which are infiltrated with mononuclear and plasma cells, spilling out into the hepatic parenchyma and eroding and obscuring the limiting plate. Periportal (piecemeal) necrosis is a characteristic feature. In some patients a more aggressive form of confluent, bridging hepatic necrosis is prominent and fibrous septa appear to isolate clusters of hepatocytes into precirrhotic nodules. Cirrhosis may be present upon initial examination in as many as one-third of patients with the severe form of chronic active hepatitis and may develop in a similar proportion during follow-up, whether or not such patients are treated with currently available regimens. In contrast, patients with the less severe forms of chronic active hepatitis (without bridging necrosis) infrequently develop cirrhosis and, in general, have a more favorable prognosis.

Identification of orcein-positive, ground-glass hepatocytes in the biopsy specimen strongly suggests that the patient has persistent HBV infection; similarly, recognition of intracytoplasmic, acidophilic PAS-positive, diastase-resistant alpha$_1$-antitrypsin globules suggests the presence of alpha$_1$-antitrypsin deficiency rather than idiopathic or viral-induced chronic active hepatitis. Identification, by immunohistologic techniques, of delta antigen in the hepatocytes of patients with HBsAg-positive chronic active hepatitis or the presence of IgG anti-delta antibody in such patients indicates that superinfection by this defective, pathogenic RNA virus may have occurred. Because the delta agent requires HBV for its expression and replication, delta infections are limited to HBsAg-positive patients. Although the severity of delta-induced liver disease appears to be variable, a rapidly progressive and fatal form of HBsAg-positive chronic active hepatitis has been described in association with delta infection, and cirrhosis may be a consequence of persistent delta infection.

Because ideal treatment for chronic active hepatitis is predicated on the etiologic agent of the disease, discussion of management will focus on the etiologic factors. All patients with chronic active hepatitis, with or without cirrhosis, should be immunized with the polyvalent pneumococcal vaccine. This may be particularly important for those patients who will receive immunosuppressive therapy.

Chronic Active Hepatitis-HBV

Between 5 and 10 percent of adults with clinically apparent acute hepatitis B will become persistent carriers of HBV and are identified by the prolonged presence (more than 6 months) of HBsAg in sera. Of this group about half are asymptomatic carriers without aminotransferase abnormalities and without histologic evidence of chronic hepatitis. In many of these individuals, markers of viral replication are absent or low, or decrease on follow-up over many years. Available longitudinal studies suggest that these individuals will not develop signs or symptoms of chronic hepatitis in the future unless superinfection with the delta agent occurs. In those in whom HBV-DNA has become integrated into the genome of the host hepatocyte, however, malignant transformation into primary hepatocellular carcinoma may occur after a variable, but generally long, latent period (several decades).

In most of these asymptomatic infections inhibitors of viral replication would appear to have little therapeutic value. Elimination of clones of hepatocytes containing HBV-DNA or which have undergone malignant transformation is the major goal. Monoclonal antibody-toxin conjugates have been studied in experimental models but therapeutic studies in man are not available. Management of HBsAG carriers is currently limited to prevention of contact transmission by vaccination of susceptible household members, prevention of delta agent superinfection by avoidance of parenteral exposure, and periodic screening for early hepatocellular carcinoma by polyclonal or monoclonal assays for alpha-fetoprotein.

In addition to the 50 percent of carriers without evidence of liver disease, about one-third of adults identified as HBsAg carriers after recognized HBV infection will have histologic evidence of chronic active hepatitis (the remaining 20% of carriers have chronic persistent hepatitis or nonspecific minor histologic lesions). Two phases of HBsAg-positive chronic active hepatitis have been identified. The initial phase is characterized by the presence in serum of markers of viral replication, i.e., HBeAg, HBV-DNA polymerase, and HBV-DNA. In the subsequent phase viral replication is dramatically reduced and HBV-DNA may be integrated into the DNA of the infected hepatocyte. Therapeutic trials have focused primarily upon HBsAg-positive patients with active viral replication. As in the case of chronic persistent and chronic lobular hepatitis, therapy of HBsAg-positive chronic active hepatitis is largely supportive.

Recent studies using monoclonal assays for HBsAg and hybridization techniques for the detection of HBV-DNA in serum and liver suggest that some HBsAg-negative patients with chronic active hepatitis also may have persistent HBV infection. Few therapeutic trials have been directed toward the use of immunosuppressive drugs, antiviral chemotherapy, immunostimulant drugs, or other agents in HBV-infected patients without HBsAg.

Immunosuppressive Therapy

Immunosuppressive treatment with prednisone (or prednisolone) with or without azathioprine appears to have little therapeutic value in HBsAg-positive chronic active hepatitis. In HBeAg-positive patients, markers of HBV replication increase in titer and seroconversion to anti-HBe positivity appears to be delayed. In patients with negative tests for both HBeAg and anti-HBe, immunosuppressive therapy may result in the reappearance of HBeAg. Abrupt discontinuation of short-term corticosteroids, resulting in "rebound immune stimulation," also has failed to have a clearly beneficial influence on the course of the disease. Despite the nearly overwhelming evidence that corticosteroid therapy has no value in the treatment of these patients, anecdotal data suggest that a few patients with severe, progressive HBsAg-positive chronic active hepatitis may receive short-term benefit from high-dose steroid therapy. Such therapy should be restricted to those patients in whom the clinical course has been inexorably downhill. Setting a time limit for the trial seems reasonable. At present there are no unequivocal means of identifying HBsAg-positive patients likely to respond. Delta agent superinfection is clearly not such a marker. In fact, because the liver injury associated with persistent delta agent infection is believed to be a consequence of a direct cytopathic effect, it is not surprising that immunosuppressive therapy with corticosteroids and azathioprine appears to have no beneficial influence on the course of the disease.

Antiviral Therapy

The use of antiviral drugs in the management of HBsAg-positive chronic active hepatitis remains experimental. Trials of human leukocyte or fibroblast interferon have revealed that such therapy may transiently reduce HBV replication and aminotransferase elevations in some patients, but that following drug withdrawal no consistent beneficial effect can be recognized. Whether interferons produced by recombinant DNA technology will have greater efficacy when used alone or in combination with other antiviral drugs remains to be determined. Combination therapy with interferon and the aqueous salt of adenine arabinoside (ARA-A), adenine arabinoside 5″ monophosphate (ARA-AMP), is currently in progress in controlled clinical trials. Despite in vitro activity as inhibitors of DNA polymerase, ARA-A and ARA-AMP appear to have a minimal or inconstant favorable influence on markers of HBV replication when used individually. Furthermore, severe neuromuscular toxicity has been reported in several patients treated with these agents. Therapy combining immune stimulation and inhibition of viral replication resulting from discontinuation of a short-course of corticosteroids followed by ARA-AMP may be more effective than either therapy alone and may reduce the frequency and severity of neuromuscular side effects.

Acyclovir appears to reduce markers of HBV replication, but a consistently beneficial effect on disease activity has yet to be described. Other antiviral agents, such as ribavirin, isoprinosine, intercalating agents such as quinacrine, and phosphonoformate analogues also have yet to be shown to have any beneficial effects. Until the results of large-scale controlled trials are available, all treatment with antiviral chemotherapy must be considered experimental.

Other Drugs

Levamisole and other agents with potential immunostimulant activity have been studied but none appears promising. Active immunization with the hepatitis B vaccine and passive immunization by infusion of anti-HBs have no beneficial effect on established HBV infection. The efficacy of transfer infection remains uncertain.

Non-A, Non-B Chronic Active Hepatitis

Chronic active hepatitis is believed to be a common sequela of non-A, non-B viral hepatitis. As many as 33 to 85 percent of patients with transfusion-associated non-A, non-B hepatitis will have persistent aminotransferase abnormalities 6 months after the recognition of hepatitis, and the majority of these have histologic evidence of chronic active hepatitis. The frequency of progression to chronic active hepatitis appears to be lower in sporadic non-A, non-B hepatitis, and chronic persistent hepatitis may be at least as common as chronic active hepatitis in this setting. Most patients with chronic active hepatitis associated with persistent non-A, non-B viral hepatitis have a generally mild disease and many are entirely asymptomatic. Despite this benign picture as many as 10 to 15 percent may develop cirrhosis after a relatively short follow-up period of 2 to 5 years.

Treatment is supportive. Corticosteroids appear to have little, if any, efficacy, and a limited study of the antiviral agent acyclovir has failed to provide convincing evidence of clinical value.

Idiopathic Chronic Active Hepatitis

The origin of idiopathic chronic active hepatitis is multifactorial. Some patients may have previously unrecognized persistent non-A, non-B hepatitis infection and some may have HBV infection despite the absence of circulating HBsAg. Although an autoimmune-initiated form (autoimmune or lupoid hepatitis) has long been recognized as a serious, progressive disease of young women associated with HLA type B8, DRw3, fewer than 20 percent of patients with severe HBsAg-negative chronic active hepatitis have other associated autoimmune disorders. Furthermore, serologic markers of autoimmunity, such as the LE factor, antinuclear antibody, and smooth muscle antibody, are found in more than 50 percent of patients with idiopathic chronic active hepatitis. Despite the belief that autoimmune hepatitis is a form of chronic active hepatitis that is highly responsive to immunosuppressive therapy with corticosteroids, the rates of remission, treatment failure, progression to cirrhosis, death from hepatic failure, and 5-year survival are similar in HBsAG-negative patients with or without LE cells or antinuclear antibodies and in patients with or without associated autoimmune disorders. These data suggest that a corticosteroid-responsive subset of patients with autoimmune chronic active hepatitis cannot be readily identified with current markers of autoimmunity.

Immunosuppressive Therapy

Although the mortality of severe idiopathic chronic active hepatitis (severity defined by prolonged and progressive symptoms of liver disease associated with jaundice, signs of portal hypertension, and the presence of bridging necrosis or cirrhosis on liver biopsy) is high in the absence of corticosteroid therapy, cirrhosis and complications of portal hypertension may develop despite prolonged treatment with corticosteroids. The course of asymptomatic or mild forms of idiopathic chronic active hepatitis has not been shown to be influenced by such therapy.

In light of this information *corticosteroid* therapy should be reserved for patients with symptomatic disease. Therapy is initiated with a maintenance dose of 20 mg of prednisone. (There are no data supporting increased efficacy resulting from the use of a higher dose tapered to this maintenance dose.) If 20 mg is not sufficient to reduce symptoms and return the serum aminotransferases to near-normal levels within several weeks, 50 mg of *azathioprine* may be added. Azathioprine also may be useful if corticosteroid-induced side effects are prominent, since its addition may permit reduction of the prednisone dose. Whether supplemental oral calcium and vitamin D reduce the frequency of prednisone-induced bone thinning is uncertain.

Most patients require treatment for one or more years before histologic remission is likely. Alternate-day therapy has no value in achieving histologic remission. Cessation of therapy is associated with relapse in about 50 percent of patients. While a number of tests, such as serum bile acid concentration, ^{14}C-aminopyrine breath test, molar ratio of branched chain to aromatic amino acids, and antibodies to liver-specific protein, have been used to assess the probable outcome of corticosteroid withdrawal, all are imperfect prognostic indicators. For those patients who relapse on corticosteroid withdrawal a second course of therapy may reinduce remission. Overall, remission is achieved in 60 percent of patients within 3 years of beginning therapy. The 5-year survival rate of treated patients is about 90 percent. About 30 percent will develop cirrhosis during the treatment period and another 10 percent will develop cirrhosis after cessation of therapy. Despite histologic evidence of cirrhosis, clinically important complications of portal hypertension are infrequent in treated patients.

Treatment failure may be most common in patients with non-A, non-B hepatitis associated disease or in those with HBsAg-negative HBV infection. However, data to support this hypothesis are not yet available. No treatment of patients who have failed to respond to corticosteroid therapy is known to influence the course of the disease.

DRUG-INDUCED LIVER DAMAGE

MACK C. MITCHELL, M.D.

Drug-induced liver damage is becoming an increasingly common cause of both acute and chronic liver diseases. Injury may result from an idiosyncratic reaction to medication or from exposure to known hepatotoxic chemicals. Management of drug-induced liver damage requires prompt recognition of hepatic injury and elimination of exposure to the offending agent. In some instances, administration of specific agents may be useful in preventing injury or reducing its severity. One example, which will be discussed in detail later in this chapter, is acetaminophen overdose. With the majority of drugs, however, therapy for hepatotoxicity is limited to supportive treatment for the complications of resulting hepatic dysfunction.

CLASSIFICATION

Drug-induced liver damage may be classified according to the histologic features of liver injury (Table 1) or the mechanism of injury (Table 2). Both classifications are useful and are by no means mutually exclusive. Classification based on histopathology is valuable in recognition of the offending agent, since the features of injury are often characteristic for a particular hepatotoxin. For example, chlorpromazine typically causes cholestasis and periportal inflammation, whereas isoniazid most often causes centrilobular necrosis and patchy lobular inflammation. Classification by mechanism of injury is likewise helpful because it provides a rational basis for prevention and treatment of the injury.

As shown in Table 1, both acute and chronic liver diseases may result from drug hepatotoxicity. Furthermore, the length of time between exposure to the drug and development of clinical manifestations of liver disease may vary. Acute injury from exposure to intrinsic hepatotoxins, such as carbon tetrachloride, results in rapid elevation of aminotransferases and clinical signs of injury when severe. These abnormalities are usually apparent within several days of exposure.

By contrast, idiosyncratic drug hepatotoxicity almost always requires a longer period of exposure before development of damage. Adverse hepatic reactions to medications and other pharmaceuticals is more often idiosyncratic than due to intrinsic hepatotoxicity, since most drugs known to be hepatotoxic are eliminated during preclinical testing. With few exceptions, intrinsic hepatotoxins cause liver injury in animals similar to that which might occur in man, thereby preventing widespread exposure of patients to these agents. However, idiosyncratic injury may be equally severe and can result from immunologic hypersensitivity or because of metabolic abnormalities that might alter normal drug detoxification within an individual (see Table 2). Hypersensitivity reactions may involve organs other than the liver and frequently produce systemic manifestations such as fever, arthralgias, and rash. Peripheral eosinophilia and granulomatous inflammation in the liver are common. These reactions usually develop within 2 weeks to 2 months after initiation of therapy but recur promptly upon rechallenge after discontinuation. Reactions due to host metabolic idiosyncrasy may require a longer exposure before clinical signs become manifest. In many instances a minor but potentially toxic metabolite of the drug is responsible for the injury. The dose of drug given, and the rate of formation and elimination of the metabolite(s) will determine the concentration of the metabolite to which the patient is ultimately exposed. For this reason, it is difficult to predict a time for onset of symptoms.

TABLE 1 Classification of Drug-Induced Liver Disease by Histopathology

Type of Injury	Biochemical Abnormalities (× normal)		Examples
	Aminotransferase	*Alkaline Phosphatase*	
Hepatocellular			
Acute necrosis	10–500	1–2	Acetaminophen, carbon tetrachloride
Acute hepatitis	10–200	1–2	Isoniazid, alpha-methyldopa, aspirin, phenytoin
Chronic hepatitis	5–50	1–2	Isoniazid
Steatosis			
"Steatohepatitis"	5–10	1–3	Tetracycline, valproate, corticosteroids
Cholestasis	5–10	1–3	Ethanol, amiodarone, perhexiline maleate
Inflammatory	1–10	3–10	Chlorpromazine, erythromycin
Noninflammatory	1–5	1–5	Oral contraceptives, rifampicin
Granulomatous inflammation	5–25	2–10	Numerous
Vascular			
Peliosis hepatis	1–2	1–2	Anabolic steroids, oral contraceptives
Hepatic vein thrombosis	2–5	1–2	Oral contraceptives
Veno-occlusive disease	2–5	2–5	Several antineoplastic agents
Tumors			
Hepatic adenomas	Variables	1–3	Oral contraceptives
Hepatocellular carcinoma	Variables	1–3	Anabolic steroids, oral contraceptives
Angiosarcoma	Variables	1–3	Vinyl chloride

TABLE 2 Classification of Drug-Induced Liver Damage by Mechanism of Injury

Mechanism	*Example*
Intrinsic Toxins	
Direct	Carbon tetrachloride, arsenic
Metabolite-mediated	Acetaminophen, carbon tetrachloride, chlorpromazine
Idiosyncratic Toxins	
Hypersensitivity	Phenytoin, sulfonamides, para-aminosalicylic acid, halothane
Host idiosyncrasy metabolic	Phenytoin?, valproate, isoniazid?, halothane?

MONITORING

Since most adverse hepatic drug reactions are idiosyncratic, it is often difficult to identify which patients are at risk. However, the incidence of hepatic drug reactions appears to be higher in women, in elderly patients, and in those individuals who have a previous history of drug reactions, including nonhepatic reactions. The incidence of reactions to some agents, although idiosyncratic, may be high enough to justify periodic monitoring of liver enzymes. The anticonvulsants *phenytoin* and *sodium valproate* both may cause hepatitis in susceptible individuals. Although the occurrence of hepatitis is rare, it is serious and potentially fatal. Monitoring serum aminotransferase levels may be helpful in predicting which patients will develop serious liver injury. Not all patients with elevated aminotransferase levels develop serious hepatic necrosis, but these patients are at highest risk and thus require close supervision. A similar situation exists with *isoniazid*, which is associated with a 10 percent incidence of abnormal aminotransferase levels, but only a 1 percent incidence of serious toxicity. *Nonsteroidal anti-inflammatory drugs, antidepressants*, and *antiarrhythmics* are other categories of drugs for which periodic monitoring of aminotransferases may be indicated. Patients given medications known to cause hepatotoxicity should be alerted to report any symptoms of hepatitis, such as anorexia, nausea, abdominal pain, jaundice, or dark urine, to their physician immediately.

When confronted with an asymptomatic patient in whom liver enzymes have become abnormal, the physician must decide whether the suspected drug is necessary and whether another compound might be equally effective. If the medication is the only effective therapy for a patient's illness, such as life-threatening arrhythmia, the drug could be continued with careful monitoring of enzymes. In these instances liver biopsy may help to determine the severity of liver damage. If the patient develops symptoms of hepatitis, hypersensitivity, or jaundice, the drug should be stopped. Continuing therapy in a symptomatic patient with hepatitis is hazardous.

A more difficult problem is determining whether abnormal liver enzymes are drug-related or are related to another condition, such as non-A, non-B viral hepatitis.

Assuming that no other cause for liver disease is found in a patient with hepatitis, discontinuation of the presumed offending agent usually results in improvement, although not necessarily complete resolution, in symptoms and liver enzymes within 2 weeks. There are exceptions to this general rule, but failure to improve in this time suggests an alternative cause for liver disease. Rechallenge is often carried out in an attempt to determine whether the presumed agent was responsible for the liver disease. There is always a risk involved in rechallenge, and it is probably greatest for those drugs that cause allergic hypersensitivity. For example, fatal hepatic necrosis may occur after only the second administration or "rechallenge" with halothane. Rechallenge does not always produce prompt increases in aminotransferases or recurrence of symptoms. For some drugs that are hepatotoxic because of metabolic idiosyncracy, several weeks or months may be required before recurrence becomes apparent. Whenever rechallenge is carried out, the physician should be prepared for an exaggerated response to readministration of the drug. Hospitalization is advisable in most instances. For these reasons, I do not believe that rechallenge is necessary in the majority of patients with suspected drug-induced liver damage.

TREATMENT

In cases of suspected drug hepatotoxicity, *discontinuation* of the presumed offending agent is the first step in treatment. Asymptomatic patients do not usually require hospitalization, but careful follow-up must be ensured. Occasionally patients will continue to self-administer medications which they believe to be beneficial for a medical problem other than liver disease. If the patient does not have symptoms of liver disease, he may not recognize the potential danger in continuing therapy. The physician must be alert to such a possibility and instruct the patient carefully. Patients with jaundice or other symptoms of liver injury require more thorough evaluation. Prolongation of the prothrombin time and/or development of hepatic encephalopathy are poor prognostic signs. Liver biopsy, when possible, is helpful in determining the severity of injury as well as the histologic pattern of damage.

In patients with fulminant hepatic failure, supportive care and close monitoring in an intensive care unit is indicated. These patients may require vasopressor therapy for hypotension, administration of intravenous dextrose solutions to prevent hypoglycemia, fresh frozen plasma for active bleeding, and judicious management of fluids and electrolyte balance. The routine use of cimetidine as prophylaxis against gastrointestinal bleeding should be avoided, since cimetidine may interfere with metabolism and elimination of some drugs. Lactulose may be indicated for encephalopathy and mannitol may be helpful in patients with cerebral edema.

Corticosteroid therapy does not directly alter the cause of fulminant hepatic failure and should not be used routinely. In patients with fever, skin rash, or other signs of allergic hypersensitivity, however, steroids may attenuate the exaggerated immune response and further reduce hepatic injury that is immunologic rather than due to direct toxic effects of the drug. For example, steroids may be beneficial in patients with phenytoin or halothane hepatitis, both of which involve allergic hypersensitivity.

Charcoal or *resin hemoperfusion* has been used successfully in some patients to increase the rate of elimination of highly lipid-soluble drugs with a long half-life. Experience with these techniques is limited and both may cause complications, such as thrombocytopenia. Hemodialysis is seldom necessary, except for associated renal failure, since most drugs that can be easily eliminated with this technique have short half-lives.

These recommendations are general measures that apply primarily to management of patients with idiosyncratic drug-induced liver damage. A few drugs and unusual lesions associated with drug injury merit special attention.

Acetaminophen Poisoning

Acetaminophen is becoming the most widely used analgesic in Western countries. In general, the drug has a wide therapeutic index with toxicity occurring at doses more than ten times the usual therapeutic dose of 1 g every 4 hours. In some individuals, particularly alcoholics, this therapeutic index may be narrower for reasons discussed below. Fulminant hepatic failure and death may occur in individuals after massive overdoses of this drug. Acetaminophen hepatotoxicity develops because of excessive formation of a highly reactive electrophilic metabolite which is formed by a minor metabolic pathway of elimination, cytochrome P-450 mediated oxidation. Usually this reactive metabolite is further detoxified by hepatic glutathione; however, after massive overdose, glutathione is depleted, allowing the reactive metabolite to damage cellular macromolecules. Long-term heavy alcohol consumption or use of phenobarbital causes induction of cytochrome P-450 and enhances the formation of the toxic metabolite of acetaminophen.

Symptoms of acetaminophen hepatotoxicity usually appear after 24 hours, often resulting in delay in the patient seeking medical attention. The clinical course of hepatotoxicity is outlined in Table 3. Symptoms of liver failure usually begin after 48 to 72 hours. Patients with bilirubin levels over 4 mg per deciliter and prolongation of prothrombin time more than two and a half times that of controls are at highest risk for serious liver damage.

The key to management of acetaminophen overdose is prompt recognition and initiation of treatment. If the patient is seen 24 or more hours after ingestion, therapy is supportive only. Less than 12 to 18 hours after ingestion, specific treatment with N-acetylcysteine (Mucomyst) can prevent or reduce the severity of liver damage. Treatment may be initiated up to 24 hours after poisoning but is most effective when given early. For oral administration, the recommended dose is 140 mg per kilogram mixed in juice or soft drinks to disguise the unpleasant taste and odor. Repeat doses of 70 mg per kilogram should be given at 4-hour intervals for a total of 72 hours. N-acetylcysteine can also be given by gavage. If the patient vomits within

TABLE 3 Clinical Course of Acetaminophen Hepatotoxicity

Time After Ingestion	*Signs and Symptoms*	*Laboratory Studies*
1–8 hr	Nausea, vomiting, anorexia	Normal
24–48 hr	Nausea, vomiting, anorexia, right upper quadrant pain	Aspartate aminotransferase and prothrombin time
48 hr	Jaundice	Aspartate aminotransferase and prothrombin time, bilirubin
72 hr		Peak of all tests
4–6 days	Encephalopathy, coma, death	

1 hour the dose should be repeated. In Europe intravenous therapy has been used: 150 mg per kilogram in 200 ml of 5 percent dextrose over 15 minutes, followed by 50 mg per kilogram over the next 4 hours, and 100 mg per kilogram over the following 16 hours. Both routes of administration are effective, although at present an intravenous formulation is not available in the United States. If signs of liver failure develop, additional doses should be withheld to prevent worsening of hepatic encephalopathy.

Liver Disease Associated with Oral Contraceptives

A variety of liver diseases, including intrahepatic cholestasis, hepatic tumors, Budd-Chiari syndrome, and peliosis hepatis (blood-filled ''lakes''), have occurred in patients taking oral contraceptives. Intrahepatic cholestasis is usually mild and always responds to discontinuation of the pill. There may be a higher frequency of this lesion in women with a history of jaundice during the third trimester of pregnancy. Hepatic adenomas and hepatocellular carcinoma also occur, although the incidence is low. Hepatocellular carcinoma should be resected, if possible, as medical and radiation therapy are mostly palliative. Although hepatic adenomas may regress after withdrawal of the drug, the propensity of this tumor to bleed massively into the peritoneal cavity suggests that surgical resection is advisable.

Budd-Chiari syndrome and peliosis hepatis are both vascular lesions associated with oral contraceptive use. Peliosis may rupture and bleed into the peritoneum. Surgical treatment is recommended only if there is hemoperitoneum. Otherwise, the drug should be withdrawn and the patient followed conservatively. *Budd-Chiari syndrome* is a dramatic illness characterized by abdominal pain, hepatomegaly, and ascites. Although the outlook for these patients is usually poor with only medical management, one recent report suggests the prognosis may be better in those women who develop Budd-Chiari syndrome while taking oral contraceptives. In patients in whom there is complete occlusion of both hepatic veins, either side-to-side portocaval or mesocaval shunting is indicated to relieve the severe outflow obstruction and prevent further loss of hepatocytes. With associated thrombosis of the vena cava, mesoatrial shunting is the preferred operation. In cases in which only one vein is obstructed, a trial of medical therapy is permissible although surgery may ultimately be needed.

Liver Disease Associated with Anabolic Steroids

Anabolic steroids, particularly methyltestosterone, are widely used by weight lifters and some other athletes. Although the incidence of liver disease in these individuals is low, peliosis hepatis, hepatocellular carcinoma, and angiosarcoma have been reported. Treatment for peliosis is withdrawal of the drug. Hepatocellular carcinoma should be resected, if possible. Angiosarcoma has a dismal prognosis and is not amenable to any therapy.

Occupational Liver Disease

Since discontinuation of the widespread open use of carbon tetrachloride in dry cleaning and other industries, the incidence of documented hepatotoxicity through occupational exposure has diminished. Nonetheless, there are still many potentially hepatotoxic organic compounds to which workers are exposed which may cause liver damage. Haloalkanes (tetrachlorethane, trichloroethane, and TNT), arsenic, beryllium, and vinyl chloride all cause liver damage or hepatic tumors or both. Pesticides, particularly chlordecone (Kepone), may cause damage to liver and other organs. The herbicides paraquat and diquat have been reported to cause hepatic necrosis, although pulmonary damage is more commonly seen. Prevention of exposure to these potentially hazardous compounds is vital, since there is no specific treatment for hepatotoxicity once it has occurred.

CHOLELITHIASIS

HANS FROMM, M.D.
MAURO MALAVOLTI, M.D.

New data regarding the epidemiology and natural history of gallstones have removed much of the controversy which surrounded the indications for medical versus surgical treatment of gallstones. Although there was little disagreement as to the need for surgical intervention in acute biliary tract disease, considerable differences of opinion existed concerning the management of gallstone carriers with either no symptoms or nonspecific ones. In this chapter, the role of surgical vis-a-vis that of medical treatment will be delineated in the different clinical settings of cholelithiasis.

DIFFERENTIAL DIAGNOSTIC CONSIDERATIONS AND MANAGEMENT OF ACUTE GALLBLADDER DISEASE

Although this chapter is primarily aimed at discussing the key elements of the medical and surgical treatment of gallstone disease, a few comments regarding the differential diagnosis of acute biliary tract disease and the indications for gallbladder surgery are in order. On one hand, the diagnosis is not always easy to establish because of the variability of the clinical manifestations of gallbladder disease. On the other hand, nonspecific symptoms are frequently used as indications for a cholecystectomy, in spite of the fact that they are neither caused by, nor significantly associated with, the presence of gallstones. In most cases the clinical picture of an acute gallbladder attack is marked by a so-called biliary colic. The term "colic" is not entirely appropriate, since biliary pain is usually steady rather than "colicky." It is typically located in the epigastrium and/or right upper quadrant of the abdomen, lasting several hours with a crescendo-plateau-decrescendo sequence. A biliary colic can also begin suddenly and end abruptly; however, since gallstones are very common, they frequently coexist with other conditions such as irritable colon, peptic ulcer, reflux esophagitis, and ischemic heart disease, any of which may stimulate symptoms of a gallbladder attack. Therefore, if the presence of gallstones is documented by ultrasonography or other imaging techniques in a patient with acute abdominal pain, acute gallbladder disease represents only one of several differential diagnostic possibilities. It is thus necessary to corroborate the clinical impression of acute biliary tract disease by laboratory tests, such as the measurement of serum alanine aminotransferase, asparate aminotransferase, alkaline phosphatase, and/or amylase, which are frequently abnormal within a 24-hour period after an attack. Even if the biliary origin of the pain has been established, the decision to operate should not be an automatic one. Although an elective cholecystectomy is, in the hands of an experienced surgeon, very safe, the operation carries a significant mortality rate in elderly debilitated patients, especially if they present with cardiovascular and/or pulmonary disease in addition to biliary complications. The frequency of biliary colic attacks varies considerably, with some patients experiencing them weekly and others only once in a lifetime. It is therefore advisable to treat high-risk patients medically to determine both their chances of improving with medical treatment and the likelihood of their remaining free of symptoms and complications after improvement has taken place. If a cholecystectomy is indicated, the operation should be performed by an experienced surgeon, regardless of whether a "difficult case" or only a "routine" elective cholecystectomy is involved. It is not unusual that anatomic variations of the biliary tree and other unexpected intraoperative findings change a "routine" case into a difficult one.

MANAGEMENT OF GALLSTONE PATIENTS WITH EITHER NO SYMPTOMS OR NONSPECIFIC SYMPTOMS

Expectant Management

Several carefully conducted prospective studies in both the United States and Italy have shown that the risk of subjects with silent stones developing biliary pain is very low, i.e., approximately 1 to 2 percent per year. The risk of development of complications from gallstones is even lower. Only about 10 percent of the patients with biliary pain develop complications. Furthermore, biliary complications, such as gallbladder perforation, bile duct obstruction, and ascending cholangitis, are virtually always preceded by attacks of biliary pain. A risk-benefit analysis based on these data convincingly shows that prophylactic cholecystectomy does not increase life expectancy. Patients with silent stones who are managed expectantly and undergo cholecystectomy only if they develop biliary pain or complications live as long as those who choose prophylactic cholecystectomy. The latter mode of treatment, however, has been estimated to be almost four times as expensive as expectant management. A prophylactic cholecystectomy should therefore not be considered in patients with silent stones. The same recommendation applies to patients with gallstones who have nonspecific symptoms, such as "dyspepsia," heartburn, fat intolerance, and irritable bowel-induced pain. These symptoms bear no significant relation to the presence of gallstones and thus do not represent an indication for cholecystectomy.

Bile Acid Dissolution Treatment

General Criteria For and Features of Gallstone Dissolution Therapy. A select group of patients with gallstones, namely those with cholesterol stones, may benefit from treatment with either chenodeoxycholic acid (cheno) or its 7β-epimer, ursodeoxycholic acid (urso), or a combination of the two. Cheno and urso are bile acids that naturally occur in both man and several animal species. Ingestion of either 14 to 15 mg per kilogram of body weight per day of cheno or 10 to 13 mg per kilogram per day of urso results in the dissolution of gallbladder stones in 50 to 90 percent of the patients. The gallbladder has to be functioning, as evidenced by its adequate filling with contrast medium during an oral cholecystogram, and the gallstones have to be radiolucent. Nonvisualization of the gallbladder and calcification of the stones make it unlikely that the dissolution treatment will succeed. Small and floating stones respond best and fastest to the bile acid treatment. In contrast, stones larger than 1.5 cm in diameter dissolve poorly. The success rate of cholelitholytic therapy is thus mainly determined by the composition and size of the stones as well as by gallbladder function. The length of treatment varies from 6 to 24 months, depending upon the individual stone and gallbladder characteristics. The treatment can be considered a failure if there is no change in stone size after 1 year. The progress of gallstone dissolution is documented by follow-up oral cholecystograms after 1 and 2 years. The advantage of oral cholecystography over ultrasonography of the gallbladder lies in the ability of the radiographic technique to provide information on gallbladder function. Ultrasonography, however, is more sensitive for the detection of small stone remnants that may remain in the gallbladder as a result of incomplete dissolution. These residues may act as a nidus for the formation of new concrements, probably explaining, at least in part, the stone recurrence that is observed in approximately 10 percent of the cases per year. It is therefore our practice to follow patients after successful dissolution therapy with twice yearly ultrasonograms. If stones recur, they usually respond to a relatively short course of cholelitholytic therapy with either bile acid.

Differential Therapeutic Features of Cheno and Urso. Cheno and urso are equally efficacious. Although they both are safe for medical use, urso is safer. Cheno treatment is associated with minor to moderate elevations of serum transminases in about 20 percent of cases. These occur during the first 3 to 6 months of treatment and are almost always transient, in spite of continued cheno administration. There is no evidence that chemo causes any permanent functional or histologic abnormalities of the liver. The changes, if any, always disappear after discontinuation of cheno, although this is, as noted above, not usually necessary.

The second side effect of cheno relates to its cathartic action, which results in the development of diarrhea in a significant number of patients. The occurrence of diarrhea is dose-dependent and therefore more common in the patients who adhere to the optimal dose of 15 mg per kilogram per day than in those who take lower doses. The diarrheal effect of cheno is less pronounced and can often be avoided if the optimal therapeutic dose is built up slowly over several weeks, allowing for an adjustment of the intestine to the secretory action of this bile acid.

The third side effect of cheno is a minor one. In the National Cooperative Gallstone Study it was observed that, during the 2-year treatment period, cheno caused an approximately 10 mg percent increase of serum cholesterol in the low-density lipoprotein fraction. There is little reason to believe that this rise poses any significant cardiovascular risk, especially since the duration of cheno treatment does not exceed 2 years.

In contrast to cheno, urso has no known side effects. Neither liver test abnormalities nor diarrhea have been observed as a result of urso treatment. There is also no evidence that urso affects serum cholesterol levels. For these reasons, urso has become the drug of choice as far as gallstone dissolution therapy is concerned. There are, however, several reasons for keeping cheno available for cholelitholytic treatment. First, the concern regarding the described side effects of cheno is most certainly exaggerated in view of the considerable experience which now exists with this compound. Cheno is safe if the patient is properly monitored with measurements of serum transaminases during the first 6 months of treatment. Second, cheno is, in contrast to urso, approved by the Food and Drug Administration (urso is currently under review for approval). Third, cheno is less expensive than urso. A fourth and important reason for continuing the use of cheno lies in the potential this compound has in combination with urso. Our preliminary experience and that of other investigators suggest that a combination of half of the optimal doses of cheno (about 7.5 mg per kilogram per day) and urso (about 6.5 mg per kilogram per day) causes no side effects and is as effective as the optimal doses of either compound alone. The reason for the apparent safety of the cheno–urso combination probably relates to both the relatively low dose of cheno and a possible hepatoprotective effect of urso.

A 1-year course of treatment with cheno at a dose of 15 mg per kilogram per day costs about $1,200. The cost for urso would be somewhat higher. A 2-year treatment with either bile acid, however, would still be significantly less expensive than a cholecystectomy.

Common Duct Stones. The presence of common duct stones in patients after cholecystectomy usually is an indication for endoscopic papillotomy (the exceptions are patients immediately after a cholecystectomy who have a biliary tube in place and are found to have retained common duct stones. In selected cases, in which the stone causes no significant obstruction of the common duct, however, bile acid treatment can be considered. It is probably safer to use urso than cheno, especially since the common duct stones can be associated with intermittent liver test abnormalities. Experience gained in studies of patients with chronic active hepatitis treated with urso indicates that this bile acid can also be safely used in the presence of abnormal liver tests.

Other Clinically Applicable Methods of Gallstone Dissolution. Current research efforts are directed at devising treatment methods which not only allow a speedier dissolution of cholesterol gallstones, but also are effective against pigmented and calcified stones. Although tangible progress has been made in regards to the first goal, no agent has yet been found which is both effective and safe for the dissolution of pigmented and calcified stones. The first progress concerning accelerated gallstone dissolution was recently reported by investigators from the Mayo Clinic. Cholesterol gallstones were dissolved in the gallbladder using *methyl tert-butyl ether*, which is instilled via a catheter placed transhepatically through the gallbladder bed. Following exposure of the stones to the ether, the gallbladder content is aspirated through the catheter. By repeating the instillation and aspiration several times, cholelitholysis can be accomplished within a few hours. The procedure has so far been tested only at the Mayo Clinic. Further experience is necessary before its utility for medical practice can be assessed. The relatively invasive nature of the procedure, however, will probably limit its application to patients with biliary pain and/or complications who either present a high surgical risk or refuse a cholecystectomy.

MANAGEMENT OF CHOLELITHIASIS IN DIABETES MELLITUS

There is only limited information regarding the natural history of gallstones in diabetic patients. Contrary to common belief, there are no solid data supporting the need for prophylactic cholecystectomy in patients with diabetes mellitus and gallstones. In the absence of convincing proof that patients with diabetic gallstones are at increased risk of developing biliary pain and/or complications, either expectant management, or cholelitholysis appears to be advisable in this condition, as long as the stones cause no symptoms.

MANAGEMENT OF PATIENTS WITH NONVISUALIZING GALLSTONES

The term "nonvisualization of the gallbladder" refers to the failure of this organ to fill with contrast medium during oral double-dose cholecystography. This may be due to either inadequate hepatic extraction of the dye (hepatic dysfunction, intrahepatic cholestasis), gallbladder dysfunction (insufficient intestinal release of cholecystokinin or inadequate contractile response of the gallbladder to this hormone), cholecystitis, or cystic duct obstruction. A cholecystectomy should certainly be considered if nonvisualization occurs because of the latter two conditions. In contrast, expectant management is probably reasonable if the patient has neither evidence of active gallstone disease nor a history of previous gallbladder attacks. Long-term studies are needed to further define the prognosis of asymptomatic gallstone patients with nonvisualizing gallbladders.

ACALCULOUS CHOLECYSTITIS

Cholecystitis seldom occurs in the absence of gallstones. Acalculous cholecystitis usually represents a complication of serious systemic illnesses, such as severe burns and sepsis. In addition, so-called cholesterolosis of the gallbladder can, although rarely, cause abdominal pain suggestive of gallbladder disease. With these rare exceptions, however, the diagnosis of acute gallbladder disease becomes most unlikely if neither gallstones nor gallbladder sludge can be found by ultrasonography.

CONCLUSION

Careful prospective studies and surveys of relatively large population groups in the United States and Western Europe have shown that the majority of gallstones are silent and never lead to complications. Expectant management is therefore advisable in both patients with silent stones and those in whom they are associated with nonspecific symptoms. A cholecystectomy should be considered only after the development of biliary pain and/or complications.

ACUTE CHOLECYSTITIS

JOEL J. ROSLYN, M.D.
HENRY A. PITT, M.D.

Acute cholecystitis has traditionally been associated with cystic duct obstruction, which usually results from impaction of a gallstone either in the cystic duct or in Hartmann's pouch. In addition, cholecystitis can develop in the absence of gallstones (acalculous cholecystitis) as a result of cystic duct obstruction secondary to edema, fibrosis, or the congenital presence of a long, tortuous cystic duct of small diameter. Although numerous theories have been proposed and countless experiments performed, the mechanisms by which cholecystitis develops in patients, with or without gallstones, remain unclear. It would seem, however, that both disease entities are in fact related and that their causes are multifactorial. Cystic duct occlusion, either mechanical or functional, in combination with alterations in gallbladder biliary lipid composition, would seem to initiate a series of events that culminate in the local release of inflammatory agents resulting in acute cholecystitis.

The clinical hallmark of acute cholecystitis is persistent right upper quadrant pain. The onset and character of this pain are similar to those occurring in patients with biliary colic; however, in contrast to the case with biliary colic, the pain of acute cholecystitis persists and is generally unremitting for several days. With time and progression of the inflammatory process, the gallbladder becomes more distended, inflammation develops in the contiguous parietal peritoneum, and the patient complains of more localized right upper quadrant pain. This sometimes subtle change in pain patterns reflects the shift from visceral to parietal pain. Many of these patients will have anorexia, nausea, and vomiting associated with a low-grade temperature.

During physical examination, the patient is usually reluctant to move, reflecting the peritoneal component of the discomfort. Palpation will elicit localized tenderness in the right upper quadrant associated with guarding and rebound. The classic finding of acute cholecystitis is a positive Murphy's sign, which refers to inspiratory arrest during deep palpation in the right upper quadrant. The complaints and physical findings of patients with acute cholecystitis, however, vary considerably, and therefore the persistence of right upper quadrant discomfort for a prolonged period may be an important clue to the diagnosis of acute cholecystitis. Most patients with uncomplicated acute cholecystitis have a mild leukocytosis in the range of 12,000 to 15,000 per cubic millimeter. Mild jaundice may be present in up to 30 percent of patients and is often due to contiguous inflammation rather than acute obstruction by common duct stones. Elevated alkaline phosphatase and transaminase levels may also be found.

DIFFERENTIAL DIAGNOSIS

The differential diagnosis of acute cholecystitis includes other common causes of an acute abdomen, such as appendicitis or perforated ulcer. In addition, pancreatitis, pyelonephritis, right lower lobe pneumonitis, and myocardial infarction must all be considered. One of the most difficult problems in differential diagnosis is distinguishing acute cholecystitis from acute cholangitis. The latter problem results from obstruction of the extrahepatic or intrahepatic bile ducts, whereas acute cholecystitis is generally associated with cystic duct obstruction.

The median age of patients with acute cholecystitis is in the 50s, compared with the 60s for patients with acute cholangitis. Acute cholecystitis is seen slightly more often in women (female:male ratio of 3:2), whereas acute cholangitis is seen with equal frequency in men and women. Patients with acute cholecystitis are more likely to have right upper quadrant pain and tenderness, and patients with acute cholangitis are more likely to have chills and jaundice. While leukocytosis is common to both entities, a white blood cell count above 20,000 per cubic millimeter occurs more frequently with cholangitis. Similarly, a bilirubin concentration greater than 5.0 mg per deciliter and other liver function test abnormalities occur more often in patients with cholangitis.

DIAGNOSIS

During the past fifteen years, new diagnostic modalities, such as ultrasound and cholescintigraphy, have been introduced and have revolutionized our approach to the patient with suspected cholecystitis. Before discussing these tests, however, the value of plain roentgenograms and of oral and intravenous cholangiography will be discussed. Supine and upright radiographs of the abdomen may be useful in the overall evaluation of patients with abdominal pain but are rarely diagnostic in patients with cholecystitis. Visualization of gallstones on a plain abdominal radiograph is possible in the 15 to 20 percent of patients whose stones are partially calcified. Plain radiographs of the abdomen may also demonstrate air in the wall or lumen of the gallbladder or in the biliary tree of those rare patients with emphysematous cholecystitis or cholecystoenteric fistula.

While oral cholecystography (OCG) has been the gold standard for the diagnostic evaluation of patients with chronic cholecystitis since its introduction more than 50 years ago, its value is severely limited in the patient with suspected acute cholecystitis. Similarly, intravenous cholangiography, which had once been the test of choice for acute cholecystitis, is now rarely used because of poor imaging associated with jaundice, severe allergic reactions, and less accuracy than newer tests.

During the past several years, abdominal ultrasonography has become a mainstay in the evaluation of patients with suspected cholelithiasis or cholecystitis. Numerous studies have confirmed that ultrasonography is more than 90 percent accurate for diagnosing cholelithiasis, and it is being used with increasing frequency to diagnose cholecystitis. Specific criteria for identifying acute inflammation of the gallbladder based on ultrasonography include the size and shape of the gallbladder, gallbladder wall thickness, and the presence of pericholecystic fluid collections. The overall accuracy of ultrasonography in diagnosing acute cholecystitis is probably somewhere between 80 and 85 percent, because some patients are "gassed out" and others have a single small stone obstructing the cystic duct which is missed by ultrasound.

Currently, the most accurate means of diagnosing acute cholecystitis, and our test of choice, is hepatobiliary scintigraphy. Cholescintigraphy had a rather limited role in the evaluation of patients with cholecystitis until 1975, when Harvey introduced the technetium 99 labeled and substituted iminodiacetic acid derivatives as new and improved agents to facilitate hepatobiliary scanning. A group of related analogues of technetium 99 iminodiacetic acid are now being used. These radionuclide substances are administered intravenously, taken up by the liver, and then excreted unconjugated and unchanged by the hepatocytes. While this imaging technique is not a suitable diagnostic test for cholelithiasis, cholescintigraphy is a very accurate means of diagnosing cystic duct obstruction, which is the sine qua non of acute cholecystitis.

Failure to opacify the gallbladder by cholescintigraphy after 60 minutes is diagnostic of cystic duct obstruction and, in the right clinical setting, is highly suggestive of acute cholecystitis. Delayed visualization of the cystic duct and gallbladder after 4 hours, even in patients with altered hepatocellular function, is diagnostic of cholecystitis except in those patients receiving total parenteral nutrition or in those who are on a prolonged fast. Extreme caution must be exercised in the interpretation of a scan in which imaging of the liver is obtained without any evidence of radionuclide in any portion of the extrahepatic biliary system. While this situation occasionally may be due to complete extrahepatic obstruction, more frequently it indicates diffuse parenchymal disease.

TREATMENT

Supportive Measures

Almost without exception, patients with suspected cholecystitis should be admitted to the hospital for diagnostic evaluation and management. The diagnosis of acute cholecystitis is based largely on clinical criteria as outlined above. Confirmation of the diagnosis can generally be made with either biliary scintigraphy or ultrasonography. In view of the fact that most cases of cholecystitis are self-limited, the early management of this disease focuses on patient comfort, restoration of homeostasis, and prevention of disease progression. In recent years, we have become less rigid in employing nasogastric tubes for gastric decompression, and generally reserve this intervention for the patient who is extremely nauseated or who has been vomiting.

Nevertheless, oral intake should be restricted in all patients to avoid further gallbladder contraction and increased intragallbladder pressure. Intravenous fluid therapy will therefore be necessary to restore fluid and electrolyte balance in patients who have been vomiting and to maintain normal intravascular volume. Traditionally, relief of pain by the parenteral administration of *meperidine* has been a priority. We generally attempt to avoid the use of morphine in patients with acute cholecystitis because of its deleterious effects on sphincter of Oddi motor activity. Meperidine also has this problem but to a lesser degree. Thus, the recent report suggesting that *indomethacin* is excellent for pain relief in acute cholecystitis may have some merit, but this study needs confirmation.

Antimicrobial Therapy

Septic complications continue to be a source of significant morbidity following cholecystectomy in patients with acute cholecystitis. Several studies have demonstrated a direct correlation between the presence of bacteria in bile at the time of surgery and postoperative infective complications. In most cases the organisms leading to wound infection and other septic complications are similar to those found in the patient's bile. In normal healthy subjects without gallstones, the incidence of positive bile cultures is essentially zero. In contrast, the incidence of positive bile cultures in patients with acute cholecystitis ranges between 30 and 70 percent. Several studies have demonstrated that the incidence of positive bile cultures increases significantly with age. Moreover, a recent study suggests that the incidence of positive cultures also correlates with the duration of the patient's illness. This observation supports the concept that bacterial infection is not a primary pathogenic mechanism in acute cholecystitis but is a secondary complication.

The most common organism cultured from the gallbladder bile in patients with acute cholecystitis is *Escherichia coli*. Other common bacteria include *Klebsiella pneumoniae* and *Streptococcus faecalis* (enterococcus), which are also of enteric origin. Although anaerobes, including *Bacteroides fragilis*, have been reported to occur in as many as 20 to 40 percent of patients undergoing biliary surgery, anaerobes are most likely to be recovered from elderly patients, those with complex biliary problems, and those presenting with cholangitis. The incidence of anaerobic infection in patients with "routine" acute cholecystitis is less than 10 percent. Those subgroups of patients with acute cholecystitis most likely to harbor anaerobes include patients with emphysematous cholecystitis and those with empyema of the gallbladder.

Although some authors have questioned the routine use of antibiotics in patients with acute cholecystitis, we feel that appropriate antimicrobial therapy is advisable in the management of most of these patients. A common argument against routine use of antibiotics in this situation is that therapeutic levels of antibiotics in the biliary system are not achieved if there is obstruction of the cystic or common duct. The goal of antimicrobial therapy in this clinical situation, however, is not to sterilize an infected biliary tree but rather to obtain adequate tissue levels so as to reduce the incidence of wound and intra-abdominal infections.

Antibiotics are begun immediately in patients who present with fever, leukocytosis, leukopenia, or septic shock. If the patient has no fever and minimal or no leukocytosis, however, antibiotics are withheld until the diagnosis is established and the patient is about to undergo surgery. In this subset of patients with "mild" cholecystitis, the incidence of positive bile cultures is low, and antibiotic administration may be limited to a short perioperative course. In patients with more severe cholecystitis, antibiotics are continued postoperatively until the patient has become afebrile and his leukocytosis has resolved for at least 24 hours. In most patients these criteria are met by the fifth postoperative day.

With the recent proliferation of newer antibiotics the choice of specific agents has become a matter of considerable debate. For many years, most experts recommended the combination of a *penicillin* and an *aminoglycoside* for patients with biliary infections. This combination provides excellent coverage for the gram-negative aerobes and synergistic action against enterococci. The one problem with this choice is the toxicity of the aminoglycosides, especially in elderly patients, in those with preexisting renal disease, and in those who present with jaundice or septic shock. Thus, newer, potentially less toxic antibiotics, such as *piperacillin, mezlocillin,* and *cefoperazone*, which have broad spectra against biliary organisms and high biliary excretion, are now being suggested. Whether these agents truly are less toxic and equally efficacious, however, must await the results of ongoing randomized trials. In patients with empyema or emphysematous cholecystitis coverage for *Clostridium perfringins* and *B. fragilis* should be part of the antibiotic regimen.

Timing of Cholecystectomy

In most cases, cholecystectomy, either early or delayed, is mandated in patients with acute cholecystitis. The optimal timing for cholecystectomy in such patients has been another area of controversy. For many years, the standard of practice was to admit patients with acute cholecystitis to the hospital for a period of intense medical management. These patients would be allowed to "cool down" and then would be discharged home. They would return in approximately 6 to 10 weeks for an elective cholecystectomy. The rationale for this mode of therapy was to allow resolution of the acute inflammatory process and to facilitate the operative procedure.

A series of studies, however, has questioned this rationale and demonstrated that the morbidity and mortality rates are similar for patients undergoing either early or delayed cholecystectomy. In addition, these prospective trials have identifed a recurrence rate of 15 to 20 percent for patients undergoing delayed cholecystectomy and have documented increased cost for the delayed procedure. Moreover, it was the impression of these authors that the operation, when performed early in the course of the clinical disease, is technically easier than when performed electively 6 to 10 weeks later. Further support for early cholecystectomy for patients with acute cholecystitis is provided by the finding of significantly increased morbidity and mortality for those patients who fail to improve after a trial of conservative medical management and require emergency cholecystectomy 5 to 10 days following the onset of their symptoms.

Currently, we perform *urgent cholecystectomy* on most patients with acute cholecystitis within 2 to 4 days after the onset of their symptoms. Following a diagnosis of acute cholecystitis, which is usually a rapid process, these patients are managed with intravenous hydration, nasogastric decompression, and broad-spectrum antibiotics as outlined above. If they demonstrate signs of clinical improvement, we perform an urgent cholecystectomy during the next operating day. If there is no initial improvement, however, or if there are signs of clinical deterioration, we will proceed with *emergency cholecystectomy*. Occasionally, cholecystectomy may be ill advised in extremely high-risk patients. In this clinical setting we will not hesitate to perform a *cholecystostomy*, under local anesthesia if necessary. In our opinion, percutaneous cholecystostomy is almost never indicated because it does not allow observation of a gangrenous gallbladder that must be resected.

Another consideration for the surgeon performing cholecystectomy in patients with acute cholecystitis is whether to perform operative cholangiography or common duct exploration. Because of acute inflammation, cystic duct cholangiography may be more difficult to perform than in patients undergoing cholecystectomy for chronic cholecystitis. Nevertheless, we recommend that every attempt be made to perform *cholangiography* either via the cystic duct or by direct, fine-needle puncture of the common bile duct.

Approximately 15 to 20 percent of patients with acute cholecystitis will also have common duct stones. Moreover, the incidence of choledocholithiasis is higher in patients with a preoperative bilirubin concentration above 5.0 mg per deciliter. Thus, *common duct exploration* in patients with acute cholecystitis is indicated when operative cholangiography is positive and when patients have severe jaundice. In this latter group, we usually perform either percutaneous or endoscopic cholangiography preoperatively.

COMPLICATIONS OF CHOLECYSTITIS

Gallbladder Perforation

Gallbladder perforation, either acute free perforation with bile-stained peritoneal fluid, subacute perforation with pericholecystic right upper quadrant abscess, or chronic perforation with formation of either cholecystoenteric or cholecystocutaneous fistula occurs in less than 5 percent of patients with acute cholecystitis. The preoperative diagnosis of gallbladder perforation is difficult in that the symptoms are frequently comparable to those of patients with uncomplicated cholecystitis. The successful management of gallbladder perforation is based on early recognition. A recent study from UCLA has suggested that acute free perforations tend to occur in patients who are immunocompromised without any antecedent history of gallstone disease. In contrast, a chronic perforation with fistula formation tends to develop in elderly patients who have a longstanding history of chronic gallstone disease. The clinical suspicion of gallbladder perforation should prompt early evaluation with cholescintigraphy or ultrasonography. Aggressive treatment with fluid resuscitation, nasogastric decompression, and intravenous broad-spectrum antibiotic therapy should be instituted, followed by an expeditious laparotomy, especially for patients with free perforations. The management of cholecystoenteric fistulas is beyond the scope of this chapter.

Emphysematous Cholecystitis

Emphysematous cholecystitis, defined by the radiographic demonstration of gas within either the gallbladder wall or lumen, is associated with a significant morbidity and mortality rate. Emphysematous cholecystitis is more common in elderly men and is associated with gangrene and perforation of the gallbladder. Clostridial organisms are present in almost 50 percent of these patients and frequently account for the remarkable radiographic features of this disorder. Despite the severity of this problem and the magnitude of the associated complications, many patients with emphysematous cholecystitis do not appear overtly septic. In any event, the potential for serious morbidity and mortality is so great that prompt cholecystectomy is indicated.

Empyema of the Gallbladder

Another complication of untreated cholecystitis is empyema of the gallbladder. Empyema also occurs more commonly in the elderly population and in the compromised host. Empyema is usually found unexpectedly at laparotomy for acute cholecystitis. Antibiotic coverage for anaerobes should be added when empyema is encountered. Even though many of these patients are elderly and extremely ill, every effort should be made to perform a cholecystectomy as opposed to cholecystostomy. To leave the infected gallbladder wall by performing cholecystostomy may delay or prevent recovery. This principle also applies to emphysematous and gangrenous cholecystitis.

CONCLUSIONS

Acute cholecystitis is the most common complication of gallstone disease. The diagnosis of this entity is based largely on clinical criteria, and confirmatory evidence is generally available either by biliary scintigraphy or abdominal ultrasonography. In most instances, early cholecystectomy performed within the first 3 to 4 days after the onset of symptoms is our preferred choice for definitive treatment. Survival for patients with acute cholecystitis is related to age, extent of disease, and the host's immune status. Nearly all patients who expire are either over 60 years of age or are immunocompromised.

ACUTE PANCREATITIS: MEDICAL CONSIDERATIONS

PETER A. BANKS, M.D.

Acute pancreatitis is an inflammatory process triggered by activated pancreatic enzymes. The factors that mediate this activation are poorly understood. The factors that govern its intensity once inflammation occurs are also poorly understood. In mild pancreatitis, the inflammatory response is characterized mainly by edema and is confined predominantly to the pancreas. In severe pancreatitis, the response is more injurious and includes pancreatic necrosis and hemorrhage. In addition, pancreatic exudate containing activated pancreatic enzymes, toxins, and vasoactive material spills out of the pancreas into retroperitoneal spaces, into the lesser sac, and at times into the peritoneal cavity. This exudate produces an extensive chemical burn that permits the loss of protein-rich fluid into these third spaces. If activated enzymes and materials are then reabsorbed into the systemic circulation, they may produce additional harmful effects: first, they increase capillary permeability and induce systemic vasodilation, thereby intensifying hypovolemia and hypotension; second, they may damage end organs directly, causing respiratory failure, renal failure, congestive heart failure, and coma.

There is no treatment at present either to inhibit the activation of enzymes or to modify the intensity of the inflammatory response. Treatment is therefore supportive: during the first few days of severe pancreatitis, when events are dominated by harmful effects of enzymes and toxins both locally and systemically, the goals of therapy are correction of hypovolemia and prevention (or treatment) of organ failure; later, after 5 to 7 days, additional treatment may be required for complications of pancreatic necrosis, including pancreatic abscess and pancreatic pseudocyst.

This chapter will outline first the criteria for determining the severity of pancreatitis and then fundamentals of medical treatment of mild and severe pancreatitis.

DETERMINATION OF SEVERITY OF PANCREATITIS

In mild pancreatitis, mortality is usually less than 5 percent; in severe pancreatitis, it is approximately 30 percent. Approximately one-half of all deaths occur during the first several days as a result of cardiovascular instability, respiratory failure, and renal failure; the remaining deaths occur after the first week as a consequence of pancreatic abscess and other complications.

During the first several days, the distinction between mild and severe pancreatitis is at times difficult. Clinical clues suggestive of severe pancreatitis include tachycardia, hypotension, dyspnea, and oliguria. Additional help is provided by etiology and circumstances. For example, idiopathic and postoperative pancreatitis have a far higher mortality (approximately 15% to 50%) than alcohol-related or gallstone-related pancreatitis (each approximately 5%). Also, the likelihood of a fatal outcome is greatest during the first or second episode, far less during a subsequent one.

More objective criteria of severity of pancreatitis are provided by Ranson's 11 prognostic signs (Table 1). If fewer than three of these 11 signs are positive, pancreatitis is usually mild and rarely fatal; if three or four are positive, pancreatitis is usually more severe and fatal in

TABLE 1 Prognostic Signs in Acute Pancreatitis

At Admission or Diagnosis
Age over 55 years
White blood cell count over 16,000/mm^3
Blood glucose over 200 mg/100 ml
Serum lactic dehydrogenase over 350 IU/100 ml
Serum glutamic oxaloacetic transaminase over 250 IU/100 ml
During Initial 48 Hours
Hematocrit fall greater than 10 percentage points
Blood urea nitrogen rise more than 5 mg/100 ml
Serum calcium level below 8 mg/100 ml
Arterial PO_2 below 60 mm Hg
Base deficit greater than 4 mEq/L
Estimated fluid sequestration more than 6 L

approximately 15 to 20 percent of patients; as the number of positive signs increases, mortality also increases. Since all 11 prognostic signs are measured within 48 hours of admission (5 at the time of admission and 6 during the next 2 days), the clinician can rapidly assess the severity of disease and prognosis. This assessment need not consume a full 48 hours. Of the six signs that are documented within 48 hours, only the criterion of fluid sequestration requires this entire time interval; the remaining five criteria are valid at any time during the 48-hour interval. For example, whenever the serum calcium level falls below 8 mg per 100 ml during the initial 48 hours (even if this occurs at the time of admission), this prognostic sign is recorded as positive.

Other criteria have been proposed to gauge severity of pancreatitis. One method utilizes three characteristics of peritoneal fluid recovered by diagnostic aspiration: the ability to aspirate more than 10 ml of free peritoneal fluid of any color, the aspiration of any quantity of free fluid that is brown in color, or the recovery following saline lavage of any amount of mid-straw-colored or darker fluid have all been considered valid markers of severe pancreatitis. Finally, a poor prognosis may be indicated by a computed tomographic (CT) scan that shows an intense and severe pancreatic and peripancreatic inflammatory response.

Once the clinician has determined whether pancreatitis is mild or severe, appropriate therapeutic strategy can be structured as outlined below.

TREATMENT OF MILD PANCREATITIS

Intravenous Rehydration

Although third space losses of fluid are not severe in mild pancreatitis, significant hypovolemia may occur because of inadequate fluid intake, severe vomiting, and diaphoresis. Unless hypovolemia is treated vigorously, splanchnic vasoconstriction may ensue, and the arterial circulation of the pancreas may be compromised. If pancreatic ischemia is thereby allowed to occur, the inflammatory response intensifies, and an episode of mild pancreatitis is converted into severe pancreatitis.

For these reasons, the most important requirement of therapy in patients with mild pancreatitis is vigorous intravenous rehydration. A reasonable mixture is 5 percent dextrose in half-strength saline containing appropriate amounts of potassium. A *metabolic flow sheet* is strongly advised during the first several days to plan the rate of fluid replacement. Measurements that help in this assessment include postural vital signs, accurate charting of intake and output every 8 hours, urine specific gravity, daily weight, and daily measurement of hematocrit, blood urea nitrogen, and electrolytes. It is strongly recommended that instructions pertaining to intravenous hydration be reevaluated by a physician at least every 8 hours to ensure adequacy of fluid replacement and thereby avoid hypovolemia. This advice is particularly applicable during weekends, where there may be a tendency to anticipate fluid needs for a 24-hour interval (or longer).

Nasogastric Suction

A nasogastric tube is not required in all cases of mild pancreatitis. The need to "put the pancreas to rest" by preventing gastric acid from reaching the duodenum and stimulating basal pancreatic secretion (by liberation of the hormone secretin) has been overstated. Available evidence now indicates that basal acid is not harmful in acute pancreatitis. Therefore it is not necessary either to aspirate gastric acid or to reduce secretion of acid (by the use of a histamine$_2$ (H_2) receptor blocker, anticholinergic agent, or glucagon). A nasogastric tube should be inserted if there is gastric or intestinal ileus or if nausea and vomiting are intractable.

Pain Control and Antibiotics

Control of abdominal pain can usually be achieved by *meperidine* in conventional dosages. Morphine is generally not recommended because it may cause spasm of the sphincter of Oddi and thereby impair the outflow of biliary and pancreatic secretions into the duodenum. Available evidence indicates that antibiotic therapy is not helpful in mild pancreatitis. Accordingly, I prescribe an antibiotic only if a source of infection is documented, such as in the urinary tract or biliary system.

Reintroduction of Oral Feedings

Once abdominal pain and tenderness have subsided, serum amylase has returned to normal, and the patient is once again hungry, it is reasonable to initiate nourishment by mouth (usually by the fourth to seventh day). During the first several days of oral intake, it would appear prudent to reduce the delivery of acid stimulated by food into the duodenum and also to reduce the stimulation of pancreatic enzyme secretion. These goals are sensible in view of the experience that excessive food intake on occasion leads to a significant exacerbation of pancreatitis. The delivery of acid into the duodenum following oral intake can be reduced by a *liquid antacid* prescribed 1 hour after meals and at bedtime and at times by an H_2 receptor blocker as well. Pancreatic enzyme secretion can be reduced first by providing food in *six small feedings*, next by emphasizing foods that are rich in *carbohydrate* rather than fat and protein, and finally by providing calories as *liquids* (which stimulate less pancreatic secretion than solid food).

TREATMENT OF SEVERE PANCREATITIS

Strategy During the First Few Days

Transfer to Intensive Care Unit

Severe pancreatitis requires very close supervision which is best provided in an intensive care unit. A variety of measurements and requirements during the first several days are listed in Table 2. Measurement of central venous pressure is required in almost all patients to gauge adequacy of fluid replacement. A low central venous pressure (e.g., 0 to 2 mm Hg) clearly demonstrates a need for additional vigorous rehydration. Even if the central venous pressure is in a normal range, vigorous rehydration may still be required. In this circumstance, measurements provided by a Swan-Ganz catheter inserted into the pulmonary artery help enormously in the assessment of fluid needs and the capacity of the heart to tolerate additional rehydration. A Swan-Ganz catheter is of particular help when fluid requirements are massive, respiratory function is deteriorating, and cardiovascular status is unstable. This type of catheter provides a wide variety of important measurements, including pulmonary artery pressure, central venous pressure, and cardiac output. Whenever necessary, pulmonary artery wedge pressure (indicative of left atrial pressure) can also be measured and compared with pulmonary artery diastolic pressure: if wedge pressure is normal, an increased pulmonary artery diastolic pressure is caused by pulmonary complications of pancreatitis; if elevated, it is caused by congestive heart failure.

TABLE 2 Appropriate Measurements and Bedside Care in Severe Pancreatitis

Vital signs, at least hourly
Central venous pressure, at least hourly
Pulmonary artery pressures (from Swan-Ganz catheter), if indicated
Arterial blood gas analysis, at least every 12 hours and at times every 1 to 3 hours
Measurement of intake and output, at least every 8 hours
Foley catheter to gravity drainage, measure urine output every hour
Nasogastric tube to low intermittent suction, maintain intragastric pH at 7 by instilling liquid antacid every 2 hours
Humidified oxygen at 2 L/min via nasal prongs or mask
For pain, Demerol 100 mg and Vistaril 25 mg every 3 to 6 hours IM
Daily weight
Daily electrocardiogram
Blood tests, one or more times daily, CBC, blood sugar, electrolytes, BUN, creatinine, calcium, magnesium, prothrombin time, platelet count, total protein with albumin, and lipase (or amylase)
Blood tests, every 2 to 4 days, liver function tests

In most intensive care units, a bedside console provides a visual recording of the electrocardiogram, the pulmonary artery wave form of systolic and diastolic pressure, and a radial artery pressure wave form (if a transducer is placed in the patient's radial artery). In additon, there is a continuous digital print-out of pulse, pulmonary artery systolic and diastolic pressure, and radial artery systolic and diastolic pressure. Only in an intensive care unit setting can sophisticated equipment such as this be utilized to best advantage and appropriate measurements made often enough for optimal patient care.

Fluid Resuscitation

The important word is *resuscitation*. The amount of fluid required each 24 hours to compensate for excessive third space losses and to prevent hypovolemia is at times enormous. Measurements provided by a central venous pressure catheter or a Swan-Ganz catheter are required to gauge adequacy of fluid resuscitation. During the first several days, daily replacement is often in excess of 5 to 6 L. When there is substantial loss of albumin and significant hypotension, fluid replacement should include colloid. If there is retroperitoneal hemorrhage, whole blood or packed red blood cells is required.

Nasogastric Tube

A nasogastric tube is a definite help in cases of severe pancreatitis. Aspiration of gastric contents counteracts intractable nausea and vomiting, thereby reducing the threat of aspiration, and helps in the treatment of gastric and intestinal ileus. In addition, a nasogastric tube serves as a conduit to instill liquid antacids to maintain the intragastric pH as close to 7 as possible and thereby prevent stress ulcerations. The parenteral use of an H_2 receptor blocker may also be helpful in maintaining intragastric pH at 7.

A variety of measures that reduce pancreatic flow of fluid, including glucagon, anticholinergic agents, calcitonin, and somatostatin do not improve mortality and morbidity in severe pancreatitis. The concept of "resting the pancreas" in patients with acute pancreatitis really means the avoidance of oral alimentation until pancreatic inflammation has subsided.

Respiratory Care

Hypoxemia may occur for many reasons, including atelectasis, pneumonia, pleural effusions, fatigue, congestive heart failure, and—after the first 2 or 3 days—adult respiratory distress syndrome. Humidified oxygen should be provided by mask or nasal prongs. If hypoxemia persists, endotracheal intubation and assisted ventilation may become necessary. It is essential to determine whether hypoxemia is caused by congestive heart failure (characterized by an increased pulmonary artery wedge pressure) or by adult respiratory distress syndrome (characterized by a normal pulmonary artery wedge pressure). If there is evidence of adult respiratory distress syndrome, positive end expiratory pressure is also required.

Cardiovascular Care

Congestive heart failure should be treated by parenteral digitalization and diuretic therapy. Cardiac arrhythmias, myocardial infarction, and cardiogenic shock are treated by conventional pharmacologic strategy.

Renal function may deteriorate despite adequate fluid resuscitation. If there is evidence of acute tubular necrosis, an intravenous diuretic at a high dosage (or intravenous mannitol) and at times peritoneal dialysis are required. Since furosemide increases pancreatic volume flow, an alternate diuretic should be utilized.

Pain Relief

Severe pain should be treated with an effective medication such as meperidine, 75 to 100 mg IM or IV as required every 3 to 4 hours. At times, meperidine is needed every 2 to 3 hours to relieve agonizing pain. The effects of meperidine can be enhanced with medications such as Vistaril. Instructions for narcotic medications should be reevaluated several times each day to titrate this requirement. The source of pain should also be reevaluated to exclude a complication such as myocardial infarction, infarction of small or large bowel, or acute gastric dilation caused by a poorly functioning nasogastric tube.

Treatment of Infection

There is no evidence that the prophylactic use of antibiotics improves morbidity or prevents the development of a pancreatic abscess. Accordingly, I refrain from using antibiotic therapy until a specific infection is documented, such as biliary tract sepsis, urinary sepsis, or pneumonia. Some clinicians advise antibiotic use if a large phlegmon is seen on CT, hoping to prevent abscess formation.

If a pancreatic abscess is documented, appropriate antibiotic therapy should be instituted and surgical debridement of infected retroperitoneal tissue should be performed. A reasonable combination of antibiotics includes gentamicin, ampicillin, and either Flagyl or clindamycin. Antibiotic therapy by itself cannot cure a pancreatic abscess, and mortality is virtually 100 percent without surgical debridement.

The distinction between a pancreatic abscess and an infected pancreatic pseudocyst should be clearly understood. An abscess is a spreading infection involving necrotic tissue in the retroperitoneum that requires extensive surgical debridement. An infected pseudocyst is an infection of fluid contained within this structure. The latter also requires antibiotic therapy as well as either surgical drainage or percutaneous drainage using a pigtail catheter (if a safe route of entry can be confirmed by CT scan). Serial CT determinations may prove helpful during this critical phase of management.

Treatment of Metabolic Complications

Hyperglycemia may occur early in the course of severe pancreatitis, but blood sugar levels then normalize as the inflammatory process subsides. Because an elevated blood sugar level may spontaneously return to normal, insulin should be administered with great caution and usually at intervals of at least 6 to 8 hours. A determination of blood sugar level should be obtained just prior to each dose to avoid hypoglycemia. In general, a blood sugar less than 250 mg per 100 ml does not require insulin therapy. Blood sugar levels that continue to be higher than 250 mg per 100 ml (and particularly 300 mg per 100 ml) should be treated cautiously with subcutaneous or intravenous regular insulin.

Hypocalcemia may occur either because of a decrease in unionized or ionized calcium. Reduction in serum unionized calcium is usually caused by the loss of calcium bound to albumin into third spaces. This decrease has no physiologic importance and does not require intravenous calcium administration. Infusion of fluids that contain albumin usually restores unionized serum calcium to normal levels.

Signs of neuromuscular irritability may occur when serum ionized calcium levels are decreased. A reduction in ionized calcium could occur through several potential mechanisms, including deposition of ionized calcium within areas of fat necrosis and the development of hypomagnesemia. A reduction in ionized calcium not associated with a reduction in magnesium levels can be treated with calcium gluconate. A 10-ml ampule of 10 percent calcium gluconate can be administered intravenously in 1,000 ml of replacement fluid over 4 to 6 hours. Additional calcium can be infused over a similar interval until there is clinical improvement. The clinician should bear in mind that a 10-ml ampule contains 1 g of calcium gluconate but only 93 mg of calcium. Since 400 mg of dietary calcium are absorbed daily, calcium replacement provided by this protocol is not excessive. In an emergency, two 10-ml ampules of 10 percent calcium gluconate can be safely administered intravenously over a 10- to 15-minute period. Before initiating calcium replacement at a rapid rate, the clinician must be sure that the patient is not hypokalemic and is not receiving treatment with digitalis. In either situation, a rapid infusion of calcium may induce a fatal arrhythmia because infused calcium binds to myocardial receptors and may intensify harmful effects of hypokalemia on the heart.

If a reduction in ionized calcium is caused by coexisting hypomagnesemia, a 2-ml ampule of 50 percent magnesium sulfate can be diluted in 1,000 ml of replacement fluid and infused over 4 to 6 hours. One ampule contains only 8 mEq of magnesium, which is slightly less than the amount of dietary magnesium absorbed daily by the small intestine. Accordingly, if magnesium deficiency is more severe, 2 ampules can be safely administered as above. If magnesium deficiency is extreme and renal function is normal, it is safe to dilute 5 ampules (40 mEq) of 50 percent magnesium sulfate in 500 ml of replacement fluid and infuse it slowly over a 6-hour period. The adequacy of magnesium replacement can be gauged by increases in serum calcium and magnesium. In addition, when serum magnesium levels are restored, urinary magnesium levels increase.

Removal of Activated Pancreatic Enzymes

Currently available protease inhibitors are ineffective when administered intravenously. Hemodialysis is also ineffective in improving survival. In recent years, there has been increased interest in the efficacy of *peritoneal lavage* to remove activated pancreatic enzymes and toxins contained in ascitic fluid before they can be reabsorbed into the circulation. While there have been anecdotal reports of improvement following peritoneal lavage and one earlier prospective study that suggested an improved survival, a recent multicenter prospective randomized study did not demonstrate any improvement in survival among patients who underwent peritoneal lavage compared with those who did not. Nonetheless, it is possible that additional studies will demonstrate that a subset of patients benefits from peritoneal lavage. For example, variables that were not considered in this recent study were the volume of ascites and the quantity of toxic materials in the ascitic fluid. Until further studies are performed, I am willing to attempt peritoneal lavage as a potentially life-saving strategy if there is *considerable ascitic fluid* and if a patient with severe pancreatitis is *deteriorating rapidly* because of refractory *hypotension*, progressive *respiratory or renal failure*, or deepening *coma*.

If there is little or no ascitic fluid, peritoneal lavage cannot be expected to be beneficial, since this technique does not dialyze enzymes or toxins from the systemic circulation. Faced with a severely ill and failing patient, the clinician now has only two options. One is an emergency laparotomy in the hope of preventing a fatal outcome. Before considering this option, I would suggest an emergency CT scan in an effort to find a treatable condition. For example, if an early pancreatic abscess is confirmed by the presence of retroperitoneal air bubbles, a surgical approach has a reasonable expectation of being beneficial. If a large pancreatic fluid collection is discovered within the lesser sac, the anterior pararenal space, or the posterior pararenal space, an experienced radiologist can aspirate this fluid via a safe percutaneous route guided by CT scan. The purpose of this aspiration—much like the theory of peritoneal lavage—is to remove as much fluid containing enzymes and toxins as possible before they gain access to the circulation. Although this strategy has not as yet been subjected to a prospective trial, it is a reasonable effort in my view to stabilize blood pressure and improve organ function in a patient who is failing rapidly. If CT scan does not show an abscess or a significant fluid collection, an emergency laparotomy can still be considered.

Nutritional Support

Patients seriously ill with pancreatitis cannot be fed orally for several weeks. Some patients require nutritional support for several months. Nutrition is best achieved by instituting total parenteral nutrition within a few days of hospitalization. Intravenous fat emulsions have not caused an exacerbation of pancreatitis among patients with normal triglyceride levels. If serum triglyceride levels are markedly increased, fat emulsions should not be utilized.

Once pancreatitis has improved clinically, a final CT scan should be performed. If a large phlegmon is still demonstrated, and especially if there is residual abdominal tenderness or hyperamylasemia, total parenteral nutrition should be continued until there is complete clinical improvement and additional radiologic improvement. Oral feedings can then be initiated very cautiously. This strategy is outlined in the section on mild pancreatitis.

Miscellaneous

Disseminated intravascular coagulation is an infrequent but serious complication of acute pancreatitis. The use of intravenous heparin is controversial. Initial strategy should be directed toward intravenous replacement of coagulation factors (fresh frozen plasma and platelets as needed).

Gastrointestinal bleeding may occur for a variety of reasons including stress ulcerations and esophageal varices. Maintenance of intragastric pH in an alkaline range helps prevent stress ulcerations. *Intestinal obstruction* caused by an extension of inflammatory exudate into the mesentery of the small intestine may require surgical treatment if either a nasogastric tube or long tube is not helpful. *Bowel infarction* may occur because of thrombosis of blood vessels or encroachment by inflammatory exudate, and requires surgical treatment. Occasionally ischemic colitis of the splenic flexure or proximal descending colon may cause rectal bleeding.

Metabolic acidosis occurs for a variety of reasons, including renal insufficiency, lactic acidosis, ketoacidosis (either diabetic or alcoholic), and drug intoxification (such as with salicylates, methanol, or ethylene glycol). All are characterized by an increased serum anion gap. Lactic acidosis occurs in acute pancreatitis on the basis of severe hypotension and occasionally on the basis of metabolism of alcohol. Treatment includes copious intravenous fluid replacement, colloid therapy, and the administration of sufficient amounts of bicarbonate intravenously to maintain an arterial pH greater than 7.1. The treatment of alcoholic ketoacidosis includes the administration of intravenous fluids that contain glucose and sodium chloride and the infusion of sodium bicarbonate to maintain the arterial pH greater than 7.1.

Pancreatic encephalopathy may be manifested by a wide variety of neurologic and psychiatric signs and symptoms. Various mechanisms include high fever, hypotension, respiratory failure, electrolyte derangement, hypocalcemia, alcohol withdrawal, metabolic acidosis, and coagulopathy. Pancreatic enzymes may also be responsible by either inducing brain damage directly or causing a toxic state. There are anecdotal reports of improvement in pancreatic encephalopathy following initiation of peritoneal lavage.

Obstructive jaundice has several explanations, including edema of the head of the pancreas compressing the distal common bile duct and the presence of retained stones. Pancreatic edema usually recedes following several days of medical treatment of pancreatitis. Retained common bile duct stones pose a more serious problem. If there is ascending cholangitis, surgical decompression of the common bile duct is usually required. In the absence of sepsis, a cautious interval of medical management of pancreatitis is warranted until a more elective operation can be performed during the same admission after severe pancreatitis has subsided. The role of endoscopic papillotomy for retained stones in acute pancreatitis has not as yet been defined. The risks and benefits of endoscopic papillotomy compared with conventional surgical treatment have not been studied in a prospective, randomized, controlled trial. A firm recommendation can therefore not be made. If an extremely poor risk patient requires emergency surgical decompression of the common bile duct, it is reasonable to consider endoscopic papillotomy as an alternative if an endoscopist is available with skill and experience in this procedure.

Strategy After the First Week

A pancreatic abscess usually does not occur until after the first week. Even if appropriate antibiotics are utilized, mortality is virtually 100 percent unless aggressive surgical debridement is performed.

A sterile pancreatic pseudocyst requires urgent treatment if it is expanding rapidly, becomes secondarily infected, or causes significant bleeding. The role of pigtail catheter drainage of a sterile pancreatic pseudocyst has not yet been defined. A rapidly expanding pseudocyst can be decompressed at least temporarily by percutaneous aspiration. An infected pancreatic pseudocyst can be treated by surgical drainage or by an indwelling pigtail catheter if a safe portal of entry can be found to insert the catheter. A pseudocyst associated with bleeding is best treated by surgical ligation of bleeding vessels and at times by a limited pancreatic resection once the site of bleeding has been localized by arteriography.

An uncomplicated pancreatic pseudocyst is usually treated medically for 4 to 6 weeks. It would seem reasonable to curtail or avoid oral intake in an effort to reduce pancreatic secretion and thereby prevent further accumulation of pancreatic fluid within the pseudocyst. If total parenteral nutrition is required during this interval because of the severity of pancreatitis, the advisability of oral intake is not an issue. If pancreatitis has subsided, however, and the patient would otherwise be receiving oral intake, it is not known whether the institution of total parenteral nutrition is more helpful than oral nutritional strategy, such as an elemental diet, in promoting shrinkage of a pseudocyst. If a pancreatic pseudocyst has not resolved spontaneously after 4 to 6 weeks, surgical decompression is usually required if it is causing symptoms or is more than 6 cm in diameter. The chapter *Pancreatitis: Surgical Considerations* also discusses this issue.

TREATMENT OF RECURRENT PANCREATITIS

Recurrent pancreatitis caused by biliary calculi is best treated by a cholecystectomy. It is much more difficult to prevent recurrent episodes of pancreatitis caused by alcohol, and the patient should be strongly urged to discontinue the use of alcohol. Recurrent pain severe enough to cause narcotic addiction requires serious consideration of surgery, especially if the main pancreatic duct is dilated. Recurrent pancreatitis caused by metabolic abnormalities such as hypertriglyceridemia or hypercalcemia is treated by conventional methods to lower the serum values.

Recurrent pancreatitis secondary to sphincter of Oddi stenosis or dysfunction is best diagnosed by endoscopic manometry and treated by either endoscopic papillotomy or surgical sphincteroplasty.

The discovery of pancreas divisum on endoscopic retrograde cholangiopancreatography raises the possibility that this anatomic variant is the cause of recurrent pancreatitis. It is important to exclude other causes of pancreatitis. Endoscopic manometric evaluation of the sphincter of Oddi and cholecystectomy are important steps in this evaluation. Therapeutic approaches directed toward the accessory papilla in an effort to improve drainage of the dorsal duct include endoscopic dilation, endoscopic stinting, and surgical sphincteroplasty. These various procedures have not yet been subjected to a prospective clinical trial, and no firm recommendation can be made among them at present. In addition, criteria that would enable the clinician to determine which patients with pancreas divisum are likely to benefit from one of these approaches have not yet been rigorously defined.

CHRONIC PANCREATITIS: EXOCRINE AND ENDOCRINE INSUFFICIENCIES

PHILLIP P. TOSKES, M.D.

Patients with chronic impairment of pancreatic exocrine function usually present with abdominal pain or diarrhea, steatorrhea, and weight loss. Those patients who have abdominal pain as their chief complaint may develop diarrhea, steatorrhea, and weight loss or always have abdominal pain as their major symptom and never evolve into frank exocrine insufficiency. Approximately 15 percent of patients with chronic pancreatitis will never manifest abdominal pain and will present initially with diarrhea, steatorrhea, and weight loss.

In adults the usual causes of pancreatic exocrine impairment are alcohol-induced chronic pancreatitis, pancreatic resection, pancreatic cancer, and idiopathic chronic pancreatitis. In children the usual cause is cystic fibrosis.

The diagnosis of chronic pancreatitis in general is difficult to make and is often done by exclusion. This is especially true of those patients whose main manifestation is pain, since they often have just mild to moderate impairment of exocrine function, while those with steatorrhea have severe impairment of exocrine function. Often the diagnosis of chronic pancreatitis has necessitated the use of invasive tests that are uncomfortable for the patient, time-consuming for both patient and physician, and expensive; consequently, the diagnosis is often not made. Now, however, a group of pancreatic function tests (bentiromide, trypsin-like immunoreactivity) are emerging that are simple to perform and that provide the clinician with very good sensitivity and specificity, especially in those patients with pancreatic steatorrhea. Such tests may also be valuable in assessing the response to therapy, e.g., an improvement in the bentiromide test after administration of pancreatic extract. These tests of pancreatic function are characterized by their ease of performance and excellent acceptance by patients. They are noninvasive, inexpensive, and can be performed in an office or clinic setting. For those patients with mild to moderate impairment of exocrine function, i.e., the patients with chronic abdominal pain and no steatorrhea, direct tube tests, such as the secretin test or endoscopic retrograde cholangiopancreatography (ERCP), remain the most consistent way to make the diagnosis of chronic pancreatitis.

PANCREATIC EXTRACT THERAPY

The cornerstone of the therapeutic approach to patients with chronic pancreatitis is the use of pancreatic extracts. This is true whether one is treating steatorrhea or pain, since the principles of therapy are similar. A potent pancreatic enzyme formulation must be employed to ensure that the relevant enzymes (lipase for steatorrhea, proteases for pain) escape destruction by gastric acid and reach the duodenum.

Treatment of Steatorrhea

Since pancreatic extract traditionally has been used to decrease steatorrhea in patients with pancreatic insufficiency, the treatment of pancreatic steatorrhea will be discussed first. Steatorrhea does not occur until lipase output is less than 10 percent of normal. I direct therapeutic efforts toward administering exogenously to the patient a source of lipase that will replace the endogenous lipase that the damaged pancreas cannot secrete. The goals of therapy are to decrease diarrhea and steatorrhea, enable the patient to gain weight, and increase the patient's sense of well-being. These goals are quite readily achieved, despite the fact that steatorrhea can rarely be completely corrected.

Selection of the Best Pancreatic Extract

The ideal pancreatic extract preparation does not yet exist. A preparation is needed with ten times the amount of lipase that is currently available. This would allow the patient to take fewer tablets or capsules—an important practical point, since therapy is lifelong. Thus the lipase content of the preparation is a critical factor. Of the many preparations available, only the following, listed in order of decreasing lipase content, have enough lipase to consider their use: Ilozyme, Ku-Zyme HP, Festal, Cotazym, Pancrease, Cotazym-S, and Viokase. Therapy should be initiated with an appropriate dose of pancreatic extract, as detailed in Table 1. If the patient does not respond adequately, the following should be considered: (1) Is the diagnosis correct? (2) Is there concomitant disease, such as bacterial overgrowth or sprue? (3) Is there a need for adjuvant therapy? My experience indicates that as many as 25 percent of patients with chronic pancreatitis may have concomitant small intestine bacterial overgrowth due to previous gastrointestinal surgery or perhaps hypomotility of the intestine from chronic abdominal pain or frequent usage of narcotics. These patients may need both pancreatic extract and antimicrobial therapy before diarrhea and steatorrhea can be effectively treated.

Adjuvant Therapy

Probably the most important factor leading to less than satisfactory treatment of steatorrhea following the administration of a potent pancreatic extract preparation is the destruction of lipase within the acid environment of the stomach. Pancreatic lipase is irreversibly inactivated below a pH of 4. Thus, the goal is to maintain the intragastric pH above 4 for as long as possible after the ingestion of the pancreatic extract preparation. In my opinion this is best achieved with the use of sodium bicarbonate. This is an effective, inexpensive therapy which, in the doses detailed in Table 1, has not led to any significant complications. My extensive experience has demonstrated that histamine$_2$ receptor antagonists (cimetidine, ranitidine) and other antacids (calcium carbonate, magnesium-aluminum hydroxide) are not very effective. The latter antacids may actually make steatorrhea worse by the formation of calcium or magnesium soaps.

Theoretically the use of enteric-coated microspheres (Pancrease or Cotazym-S) should obviate the need for adjuvant therapy, since these preparations will not release their contents until a pH of approximately 5.5 exists. Although these preparations are effective in some patients, other patients respond best to conventional preparations with sodium bicarbonate. Some of the problems with the microsphere preparations are that they do not contain enough lipase, they are large, and may empty slowly from the stomach. It is important to consider adjuvant therapy if the approach suggested in Table 1 fails, because increasing the dose above that listed in the table does not achieve much more reduction in steatorrhea, yet leads to a marked increase in bloating and cramps.

Treatment of Pain

The treatment of the pain associated with chronic pancreatitis follows the same approach with respect to pancreatic extract preparations and adjuvant therapy as the treatment of steatorrhea outlined in Table 1. The pathogenesis of the pain associated with chronic pancreatitis is not understood, with the exception of the pain related to a pseudocyst. Drainage of a pseudocyst often will bring dramatic relief of pain. If no pseudocyst is found, two patterns emerge: (1) some patients have minimal or no abnormalities on ERCP and an abnormal secretin test, and (2) others will have dilated ducts or strictures or both detected by ERCP. Traditionally, the abnormalities of the latter group have been thought to be amenable to surgery.

TABLE 1 Approach to Treatment of Pancreatic Maldigestion

Pancreatic Extract

Schedule: Before meals (and at bedtime if the patient experiences pain)

Dose: Viokase, 8 tablets each time *or*
Cotazym, 6 capsules each time *or*
Ilozyme, 4 capsules each time *or*
Pancrease, 3 capsules each time (enteric coated)

If no significant improvement occurs with extract alone add:

Sodium Bicarbonate*†

Schedule: Before and after each meal (and at bedtime if the patient experiences pain)

Dose: Sodium bicarbonate, 650 mg before and after meals
(and 1,300 mg at bedtime if needed)

* I have not noted hypercalcemia or milk-alkali syndrome with this dose of sodium bicarbonate.

† I do not recommend concomitant treatment with sodium bicarbonate and enteric-coated enzyme preparations, since increased gastric pH may cause premature release and inactivation of enzymes.

The findings at ERCP largely dictate the surgical approach, but the surgical procedure of choice has been pancreatic duct drainage.

Rationale

Treatment of the former group, i.e., those with normal ducts at ERCP, has been completely unsatisfactory, but recent data suggest that large doses of pancreatic extract may relieve the pain in these patients. It appears that pharmacologic doses of proteases may inhibit pancreatic exocrine secretion, thus putting the pancreas at rest and affording relief of pain. These clinical observations fit with a large amount of data in experimental animals which indicates that the amount of trypsin and chymotrypsin within the lumen of the proximal duodenum exerts a controlling influence on pancreatic exocrine secretion.

It would thus seem reasonable to approach the patient with chronic pancreatitis and pain in the following manner (Fig. 1). After other causes of abdominal pain have been appropriately excluded, an ultrasound or computed tomographic scan of the pancreas should be performed. If no abnormality is found, a secretin test should be done. Invariably, if the pain is related to chronic pancreatitis, the secretin test will be abnormal. If the secretin test confirms the clinical impression of chronic pancreatitis, a trial of pancreatic extract therapy is indicated (e.g., Viokase, 8 tablets with meals and at bedtime) for 30 days. If relief from pain is achieved, no further steps need to be taken. If the result is unsatisfactory, the pancreatic extract should be enhanced with sodium bicarbonate (650 mg before and after each meal and 1300 mg at bedtime). If the results still are unsatisfactory, ERCP should be performed, looking for an inflammatory stricture or other lesion that might be corrected with surgery. It is noteworthy that few patients progress all the way to ERCP. The clinical course of patients receiving pancreatic extract for pain has not been fully defined as yet. I have had some patients receiving this therapy for 4 years who suffer a relapse when the therapy is stopped. Others have had the pancreatic extract stopped after shorter periods of treatment with no relapse.

Pharmacologic suppression of pancreatic exocrine secretion with proteases has been demonstrated in patients with chronic pancreatitis and in healthy subjects. Pancreatic proteases in the proximal small intestine apparently modulate pancreatic exocrine secretion in humans. The clinical implications of pharmacologic suppression of pancreatic output are exciting. By increasing the intraluminal concentration of pancreatic enzymes with orally administered exogenous enzymes, endogenous production of pancreatic enzymes is either directly or indirectly decreased. In patients with chronic pancreatitis, pancreatic extract reduces secretion and alleviates pain. Pancreatic extract should be considered the treatment of choice for most patients with chronic pancreatitis and recurrent abdominal pain.

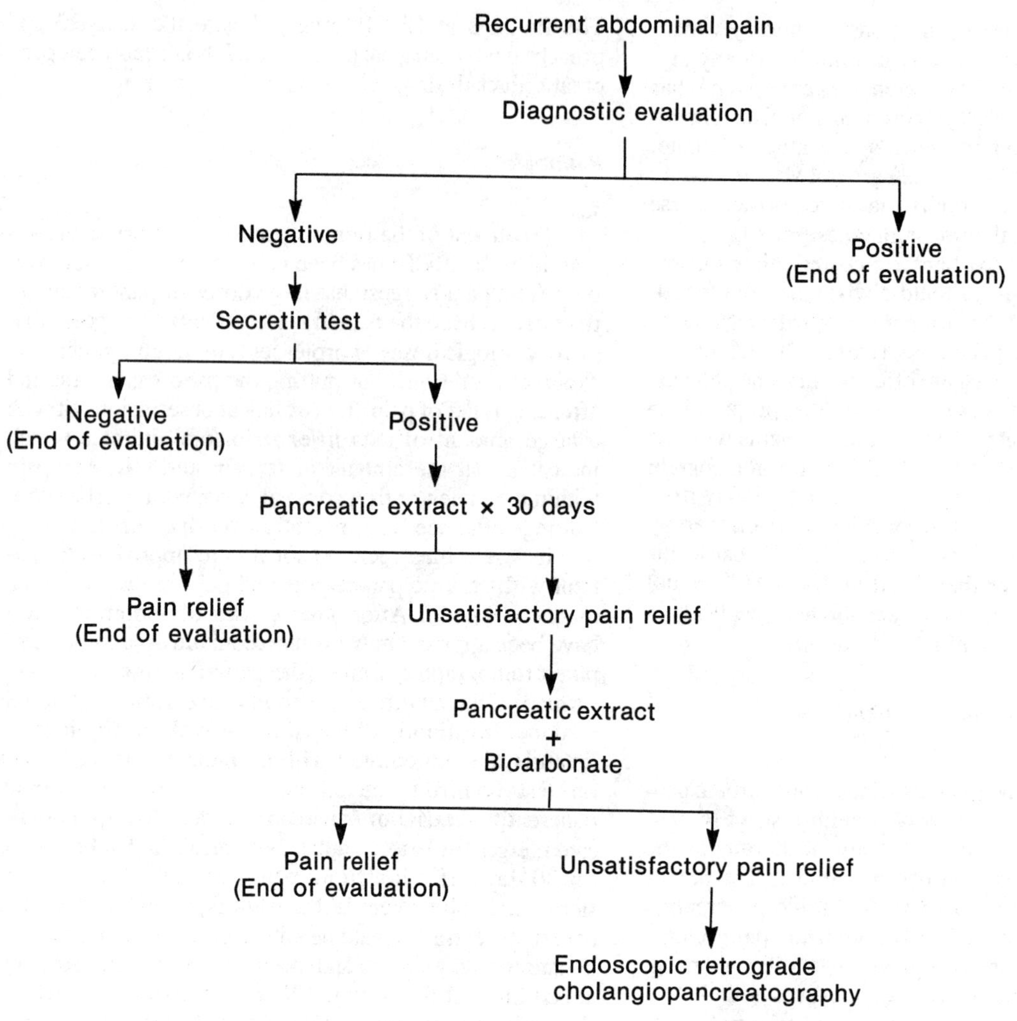

Figure 1 Algorithm for evaluating patients with recurrent abdominal pain.

DIET

I individualize the diet for each patient depending on the severity of the disease, etiology, and so on; however, there is no specific diet for pancreatic insufficiency per se. I recommend that alcohol in any form or quantity be avoided, since it can exacerbate pancreatitis, thereby worsening pancreatic insufficiency. Also, in some patients, meals with high fat content may increase the frequency and intensity of pain. In these patients fats should be restricted to 25 percent of the caloric intake. The diet in patients with pancreatic insufficiency should also be rich in protein to avoid protein deficiency, and low in fiber, since fiber may inhibit pancreatic enzymes. In the rare patient who has documented pancreatic steatorrhea but who does not respond to the program suggested in Table 1, reduction of long chain triglyceride fat in the diet to 40 percent of fat and substitution of 60 percent of fat by medium chain triglycerides may increase weight gain and decrease steatorrhea.

ENDOCRINE INSUFFICIENCY SECONDARY TO EXOCRINE INSUFFICIENCY

Glucose intolerance may be demonstrated in up to 90 percent of patients with diffuse calcification of the pancreas, and overt diabetes in up to 70 percent of patients. Thus, abnormalities in pancreatic endocrine function are common in patients with severe pancreatic exocrine insufficiency. It is almost impossible to take meaningful therapeutic steps in controlling the glucose intolerance until optimal control of steatorrhea has been achieved. In these patients, who are very sensitive to insulin, significant changes in absorption will greatly affect the insulin response. Although such patients may not require large doses of insulin, their situation is often precarious because they may have a decreased reserve of pancreatic glucagon and may not be able to respond appropriately to hypoglycemia.

RESPIRATORY DISEASES

UPPER AIRWAY OBSTRUCTION

ROGELIO J. PEREZ-PADILLA, M.D.
MEIR H. KRYGER, M.D., F.R.C.P.(C)

Acute upper airway obstruction (UAO) can lead rapidly to death. Chronic upper airway obstruction, which may be due to anatomic obstruction or related to the sleep state, may mimic other disorders such as asthma, or it may give rise to the sleep apnea syndrome.

Acute UAO is one of the most dramatic emergencies in which proper management is essential for survival of the patient. Acute obstruction is generally caused by diseases that rapidly diminish the caliber of the airway by causing enlargement of its structure, as by infection or inflammation (Table 1). Acute UAO can progress rapidly, increasing the work of breathing until ventilation cannot be sustained and death ensues.

CLINICAL FEATURES

The clinical presentation of UAO depends on its severity, location, cause, acuteness of onset, and the pre-existing size of the airway. Disorders that cause little physiologic impairment in the adult can cause life-threatening obstruction in the small upper airway of the child. With upper airway obstruction, symptoms may not occur until obstruction is severe. Initially the patient may complain of dyspnea, especially during exercise and sometimes in certain positions (neck flexion, extension, or rotation). The voice may be hoarse, the sleep might be poor, and the patient might have a cough with an unusual sound. Stridor is the hallmark of extrathoracic UAO, presenting initially on inspiration during exercise or hyperventilation, then on inspiration during rest, and finally during the whole respiratory cycle. With acute extrathoracic obstruction (e.g., epiglottitis), patients often have a slow breathing rate with supraclavicular and intercostal indrawing and may also have severe sore thorat and drooling. Intrathoracic lesions can produce localized, unilateral, or bilateral wheezes mainly in expiration. Some patients are diagnosed as having asthma and are treated with bronchodilators with no response.

DIAGNOSIS

Pulmonary function tests are useful in the diagnosis of UAO and assessment of its severity. Typically there is limitation of airflow at high lung volumes, producing a plateau in the flow volume loop. The pressures acting on the extrathoracic airway are the tracheal pressure (inside) and atmospheric pressure (outside). In the intrathoracic airway the pressures are tracheal pressure (inside) and pleural pressure (outside). Because of the differences in the outside pressures, the extrathoracic airway tends to collapse with inspiration (tracheal pressure is less than atmospheric), but the intrathoracic airway tends to collapse with expiration(tracheal pressure is less than pleural pressure). That is why stridor and flow limitation are mainly inspiratory in extrathoracic UAO, and expiratory (with wheezes) in intrathoracic UAO. In these conditions, the airway resistance is increased with a normal distribution of ventilation and the diffusing lung capacity of carbon monoxide (D_LCO). Flows improve when the patients breathe helium-oxygen mixtures. In pure UAO, arterial blood gases may remain normal until death is imminent.

Radiologic studies (including neck upright soft tissue views, conventional and computerized tomograms, and contrast tracheograms), laryngoscopy, and bronchoscopy usually define the nature, diameter, length, and location of the obstruction. If visual examination of the pharynx or epiglottis is attempted in a child with suspect epiglottitis, extreme care should taken. The examination should be done in an operating room. The child should be sitting during the examination since the supine position may result in acute occlusion.

There may develop in some patients repetitive occlusion of the upper airway during sleep. The main features are excessive daytime sleepiness, heavy snoring, restless sleep, and, in some patients, the development of awake respiratory failure (see chapter on *Obesity Hypoventilation Syndrome*).

Many patients with obstructive sleep apnea have a pre-existing upper airway obstruction. The combination of this pre-existing obstruction and the loss of upper airway muscle tone associated with the sleep state result in periodic upper airway occlusions in sleep. In some patients, a pathologic loss of tone of the upper airway musculature can also result in sleep apnea.

TABLE 1 Some Causes of Upper Airway Obstruction

Nasopharynx and Oropharynx	
Enlarged tonsils and adenoids	Can cause sleep apnea syndrome and cor pulmonale
Ludwig's angina	Indurated cellulitis of the floor of the mouth after mucosal laceration or dental infection
Epiglottitis	Swollen red epiglottis, dysphagia, high fever, sore throat, drooling, leukocytosis
Pharyngeal abscess	Fever, dysphagia, trismus, drooling, cervical adenopathy, hoarseness, stridor; mixed flora infection
Sleep apnea syndrome	Hypersomnia, snoring, disturbed sleep, obesity with or without awake hypoventilation
Larynx	
Bilateral vocal cord paralysis	Stridor, dyspnea, usually after thyroid surgery; voice may be surprisingly good
Edema	
Angioedema	Frequently associated with urticaria or anaphylaxis; atopic or familial history may be present
Infection (diphtheria)	Pseudomembranous pharyngitis, myocarditis, palatal paresis
Postintubation	Stridor and distress usually beginning within one hour after extubation
Tumors	Progressive hoarseness, smoking history, UAO is late
Trachea	
Tumors of trachea	Paroxysmal dyspnea (''asthma''), hoarseness, hemoptysis
Tumors of mediastinum	Chest pain, retrosternal pressure, cough, myasthenia gravis, superior vena caval syndrome, hoarseness, clubbing, tracheal deviation, mediastinal mass
Thyroid enlargement	Dyspnea, goiter, previous thyroid surgery, positive thyroid scan
Tracheomalacia	
Postintubation	Stridor, ineffective cough, recurrent infections
Relapsing polychondritis	Progressive inflammation and destruction of cartilage (most commonly of ears and nose), autoimmune features, episcleritis, iritis, anemia, abnormal liver function, aortic insufficiency, cataracts, hearing loss
Tracheal strictures	UAO occurring several weeks after tracheostomy or prolonged endotracheal intubation; localized wheezes, lung collapse

Foreign bodies, acute trauma, and upper airway burns can produce obstruction at different levels of the upper airway.

The sleep apnea syndrome is suspected on clinical grounds and confirmed by recording of oxygen saturation and observation of the sleeping patient. For more precise diagnosis, a polygraphic recording during sleep in a fully equipped sleep laboratory is required to define sleep stages, to differentiate central from obstructive apneas, to detect cardiac arrhythmias and to quantitate oxygen desaturation.

MANAGEMENT

Intubation

Patients with acute UAO require a stable, reliable patent airway. Awake endotracheal intubation with the tube inserted blindly, or under direct laryngoscopy, or through a fiberoptic laryngoscope or bronchoscope can often bypass the obstruction. In UAO, especially in acute cases with severe edema (e.g., epiglottitis), there is always the risk of worsening the obstruction by attempting endotracheal intubation. In such cases, or when endotracheal intubation is likely to fail, a tracheostomy should be performed. Children with epiglottitis can be treated with nasotracheal intubation.

In an emergency, an adequate PaO_2 can temporarily be maintained by administering oxygen through a bronchoscope bypassing the obstruction, or through a large-bore needle inserted through the cricothyroid membrane. Ventilation can be sustained by means of a pediatric endotracheal tube inserted through a cricothyroidotomy. Such measures are temporary and used only until a definitive procedure establishes a stable adequate airway.

Avoidance of Respiratory Depressants

This cannot be emphasized enough. Agents such as sedatives, hypnotics, and opiate analgesics can have disastrous consequences in patients with upper airway obstruction. These agents depress chemical drives to breathe and may also blunt the compensating reflexes that increase the drive to breathe in the presence of obstruction.

Oxygen

Although a low PaO_2 is not usually a problem, inspired O_2 concentration should be increased to maintain a normal PaO_2. A proper humidification system should be used. If the hypoxemia is due to hypoventilation, inspiratory arrest may soon occur.

Inhaled Epinephrine

Because of the alpha-adrenergic stimulant effect of epinephrine, one would expect mucosal vasoconstriction with reduction in edema and airway obstruction. Epinephrine has been shown to be useful in children with laryngotracheitis, but there have been no convincing controlled studies in other causes of UAO. However, as edema is commonly present in several diseases causing acute UAO, it is possible that epinephrine could help.

A 2.25 percent solution of racemic epinephrine is available for nebulization through a face mask, hand nebulizer, or IPPV machine; L-epinephrine is probably as useful as the racemic mixture and more potent. For adults, 1.5 to 2.5 ml of either the racemic mixture (Vaponephrine) or 1 percent epinephrine is nebulized in 10 to 15 minutes. The effect lasts for 1 to 2 hours, and a rebound increase in UAO can occur if the basic cause of obstruction has not been corrected or bypassed. It should be used carefully in patients with hypertension, cardiac arrhythmias, or angina and in the elderly. In a desperate situation, the epinephrine may be injected through the cricothyroid membrane.

Corticosteroids

Corticosteroids have been shown to be useful in viral laryngotracheitis, but there have been no controlled trials in other types of UAO. Corticosteroids are used in high doses, usually as soon as the diagnosis is made. Dexamethasone, 0.3 to 0.5 mg per kilogram, or methylprednisolone, 30 mg per kilogram is usually recommended for viral croup and for prevention of the laryngeal edema occurring after removal of endotracheal tubes. The medication is administered 2 to 6 hours prior to removal of the endotracheal tube in patients most likely to develop obstruction—those with prolonged intubation or those in whom movement of the tube has traumatized the airway. In viral croup the dose of corticosteroid is repeated after 2 hours.

Helium-Oxygen Mixtures

Helium is a gas with a density one-seventh that of nitrogen. Flow in upper airways in turbulent and resistance is dependent on gas density. Resistance is reduced in the presence of UAO when the patient is breathing a He-O_2 mixture.

Patients with UAO achieve higher flows and have less respiratory distress and stridor while breathing He-O_2. Some patients who would otherwise need endotracheal intubation or tracheostomy can sometimes be managed with He-O_2. Even if intubation or tracheostomy is eventually performed, He-O_2 can give precious time for assessment and preparation.

SPECIFIC THERAPY

The first principle in treating upper airway obstruction is to ensure an adequate airway. Some diseases causing UAO require additional specific therapy, as indicated in Table 2. Because of the increasing frequency of beta-lactamase-positive *H. influenzae*, ampicillin alone is not recommended as primary treatment for epiglottitis. One must either add chloramphenicol or use the agents listed in Table 2. Note that young household contacts require chemoprophylaxis. Foreign bodies are discussed elsewhere.

SLEEP APNEA SYNDROME (SAS)

All factors predisposing to sleep apnea should be corrected (Fig. 1). Obese patients can have substantial improvement after weight loss. Alcohol *must* be avoided in the 6 hours prior to bedtime. When enlarged tonsils and adenoids are present, they should be removed. With deformity of the jaw (e.g., micrognathia or retrognathia), reconstructive surgery may be helpful. Surgically correctable forms of nasal obstruction should be referred for surgery. Patients with allergic or chronic rhinitis may be treated with the recently introduced nonsedating H_1 receptor blockers, terfenadine (60 mg twice a day) or astemizole (10 mg daily), or with a trial of topical corticosteroids, or with topical cromoglycate.

Patients with severe obstructive sleep apnea require a more aggressive therapeutic approach. Severity is defined by clinical findings (severe hypersomnia, bizzare behavior, heart disease), socioeconomic factors (altered social, family, or job relationships), and polygraphic data (many apneas, severe oxygen desaturation associated with cardiac arrhythmias). Such patients usually have 20 to 60 apneic episodes each hour of sleep.

Protriptyline

Protriptyline is a nonsedating tricyclic antidepressant that can improve patients with SAS. The usual dose is 10 to 30 mg (taken before retiring), which is well tolerated on a long-term basis in about half the patients treated. A trial of protriptyline is recommended for patients with mild obstructive sleep apnea or those who refuse more invasive forms of treatment. Although patients on protriptyline are less somnolent, they still have quite abnormal sleep with many apneas and arousals. Protriptyline reduces REM sleep, which is associated with the longest apneas and the most severe oxygen desaturation, and so improves oxygenation. Some patients lose weight on protriptyline; this can also improve the SAS. The side effects are mainly due to the anticholinergic effects of the medication (dry mouth, urinary retention, constipation, impotence) and can force some patients to discontinue the drug. Tricyclic antidepressants can induce cardiac arrhythmias, but in our experience patients with SAS have fewer cardiac arrhythmias while receiving protriptyline, probably because of the improved oxygenation.

TABLE 2 Specific Treatment for Upper Airway Obstruction

Condition	*Treatment*
Ludwig's angina	Penicillin or clindamycin
Epiglottitis	First choice: cefuroxime, cefotaxime, or moxalactam; second choice: chloramphenicol; household contacts <4 years of age: rifampin (20 mg/kg/day to maximum 600 mg/day × 4 days).
Peripharyngeal abscess	Surgical drainage, antibiotics (clindamycin, cefoxitin or penicillin)
Diphtheria	Antitoxin, erythromycin, or penicillin
Angioneurotic edema	Epinephrine SC or IM, antihistamines
Hereditary angioneurotic edema	Androgens, antifibrinolytics (prophylactic)
Tracheal stenosis	Bronchoscopic dilatation, surgical repair, laser resection
Vocal cord paralysis	Surgery, tracheostomy
Tumors	Endoscopic resection, surgery, radiation, laser resection
Relapsing polychondritis	Steroids, dapsone, immunosuppressants
Papillomatosis	Endoscopic resection, transfer factor?

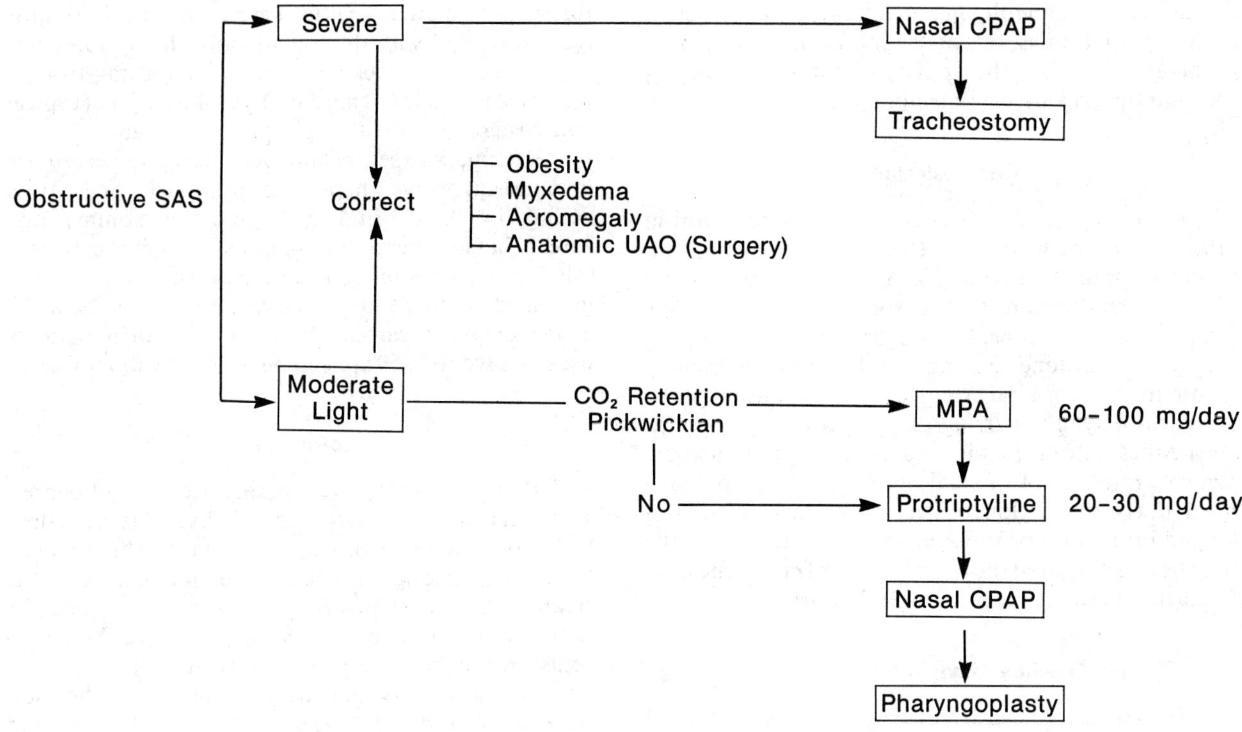

Figure 1 Treatment of obstructive sleep apnea syndrome.

Medroxyprogesterone

Medroxyprogesterone acetate (MPA) treatment is discussed in detail elsewhere. This agent can be useful for some patients, especially those with the obesity-hypoventilation syndrome. The recommended starting dose of medroxyprogesterone is 60 mg orally once a day.

Continuous Positive Airway Pressure

Continuous positive airway pressure (5 to 15 cm of water), applied through the nose (nasal CPAP), may prevent obstructive apneas and can be tolerated chronically in many patients. It is especially well suited to hospital treatment of very sick SAS patients. Nasal CPAP units that are convenient to use are now available for home use.

Uvulopalatopharyngoplasty

Evaluations should be performed to determine the structural cause of the upper airway obstruction. Cephalometrics, endoscopic evaluation, and CT scans may be used. Patients found to have mandibular insufficiency may require maxillo-mandibular surgery.

Surgical enlargement of the pharyngeal airway by resecting the excessive mucosa, uvulopalatopharyngoplasty (UPPP) can improve SAS significantly and make tracheostomy unnecessary. In many centers, when uvulopalatopharyngoplasty is performed, a tracheostomy is also performed. This is because the apnea may temporarily worsen after the surgery of the pharynx. After several weeks, the patient is evaluated with the tube plugged. If results are satisfactory, the tracheostomy tube may be removed. Initially it appeared that about 50 percent of patients responded to this operation. With more detailed evaluations and selection of the upper airway, the success rate is much higher.

Tracheostomy

Permanent tracheostomy is the gold standard of therapy of obstructive sleep apnea. It is recommended when the sleep apnea is severe (hypersomnia, severe oxygen desaturation, serious cardiac arrhythmias) and when the aforementioned therapeutic measures are ineffective or cannot be tolerated. It is beyond the scope of this text to review surgical techniques, but a few points will be emphasized. Tracheostomy in obese patients is more difficult to perform than in thin people, and occasionally the tracheostomy is done too low in the neck, particularly if the jowls are large. Some surgeons prefer to perform the tracheostomy using topical anesthesia, since these patients are difficult to intubate when anesthetized conventionally. Because of the potential danger of anesthetic agents, some anesthetists intubate the patient without a preanesthetic agent or with only a small amount. After tracheostomy we usually monitor the patient for 1 or 2 nights to ensure proper tube function. We monitor the endotracheal CO_2 by means of an infrared analyzer, SaO_2, using an ear oximeter and the electrocardiogram.

We usually use a silver fenestrated tracheostomy tube or one of the newer Silastic tracheostomy tubes. In some centers the Silastic tubes are custom-fenestrated. The optimal location for the fenestration is found by placing a metal marker on the tube and then determining roentgenographically whether it is an appropriate position.

Patients and their families must take part in an intensive education program to ensure that they take proper care of the airway.

Patients with central SAS or patients with treated obstructive SAS who have abundant central apneas might require further treatment. In most cases, these residual central apneas regress within several months.

SUGGESTED READING

Burns JE, Hendley JO. Epiglottitis. In: Mandell GL, Douglas RG, Bennett JE (eds). Principles and Practice of Infectious Diseases. New York: Wiley 1985.

Chow AW. Infections of the Oral Cavity, Neck and Head. In: Mandell GL, Douglas RG, Bennett JE (eds). Principles and Practice of Infectious Diseases. New York: Wiley,

Kryger M (ed). Symposium on Respiration During Sleep. Chest Clin North Am December, 1985.

Riley RW. Guilleminault C, Powell N, et al. Palatopharyngoplasty failure, cephalometric roentgenograms, and obstructive sleep apnea. Otolaryngol Head Neck Surg 1985; 93:240–244.

ACUTE UPPER AIRWAY INFECTION

HANS PASTERKAMP, M.D.
VICTOR CHERNICK, M.D.

Acute upper airway infection with severe increase in *inspiratory* airflow obstruction is a common occurrence in young infants and children, but may occur in the adult. In the United States, approximately 45,000 children per year are hospitalized with viral croup for an average length of stay of about 3 days. About 3,000 children per year are hospitalized with epiglottitis for an average length of stay of 6 days. The susceptibility to upper airway obstruction with infection in infants and children is related to the small size of the triangular glottic inlet (7 × 4 mm in an infant) and the narrow diameter of the subglottic area (5 to 6 mm in an infant). Reduction of these diameters results in increased turbulent flow and production of a harsh whistling sound (stridor) during inspiration (negative intraluminal pressure). Obstruction is less severe during expiration because of the positive intraluminal pressure (dilating effect) and is not associated with sound production in these conditions. Therapy is aimed at relieving obstruction and reducing the inspiratory work of breathing.

The major cause of croup used to be diphtheria, but several distinct clinical entities are currently recognized: laryngotracheobronchitis (viral croup), spasmodic croup, epiglottitis, and bacterial tracheitis. Management of each is different, and precise diagnosis is important to avoid such complications as severe hypoxia and death.

VIRAL CROUP (LARYNGOTRACHEOBRONCHITIS)

The major cause of this condition is the parainfluenza virus (usually type 1), but it may be caused by influenza, respiratory syncitial virus, adenovirus, and, rarely, *Mycoplasma pneumoniae*. Infection results in inflammation, swelling, and edema of the subglottic area of the trachea. The condition usually occurs in children under 3 years of age, during the fall or winter. It is characterized by signs and symptoms of an upper respiratory tract infection including coryza, followed after several days by onset of inspiratory stridor, a barking cough, and mild tachypnea.

The diagnosis is confirmed by the typical clinical course and absence of epiglottitis noted on *gentle* direct examination of the pharynx. If this is not possible, a lateral roentgenographic study of the neck may demonstrate subglottic swelling and a normal-sized epiglottis. The disease is usually self-limited (3 to 5 days), and treatment is largely symptomatic.

Management

Mist Therapy

The mainstay of therapy for patients with croup is the provision of high humidity (running the shower in the bathroom) or mist (home mist generator or mist or croup tent in the hospital). Rigid scientific documentation on the efficacy of this therapy has not been done, but most clinicians and nurses attest to its effectiveness. Precisely how mist or high humidity works is unclear. It is thought that increased airflow through a narrowed trachea may have a local drying effect, stimulate irritant receptors, and cause local smooth muscle constriction. Alternatively, large-particle mist that rains out in the upper airway may reflexly slow respiration, resulting in a decrease in inspiratory flow rate, less decrease in intraluminal pressure during inspiration, and a decrease in inspiratory work.

Oxygen

Since most patients with croup severe enough to require hospitalization have some degree of hypoxemia, the mist tent is a convenient way of providing a low concentration of O_2 (30% to 35%), which is sufficient to relieve the hypoxemia.

Racemic Epinephrine

Administration of aerosolized 2.25 percent racemic epinephrine (0.25 ml in 1.5 ml saline for patients 5 kg body weight or less; 0.5 ml in 1.5 ml saline for patients of more than 5 kg body weight) by simple face mask is effective in relieving obstruction in patients with viral croup within a few minutes. We do not believe that there is a "rebound" phenomenon with this therapy, but some patients may require this treatment as often as every hour. Usually the therapy is effective for 2 to 4 hours. If a child has obstruction severe enough to warrant this therapy, hospitalization and close observation are mandatory.

Sedation

Although many clinicians prescribe sedation with phenobarbital or chloral hydrate in the treatment of this condition, we believe that this practice is dangerous to a patient with severe obstruction. We do not recommend the use of sedatives since anxiety is a sign of severe obstruction and hypoxemia, and sedation may hasten sudden respiratory arrest.

Steroids

The use of steroids in the treatment of children with viral croup is controversial. There are no convincing data to support their routine use in this condition. However, the occasional child with a prolonged course of croup does respond to dexamethasone (0.5 mg per kilogram). In such cases, one should suspect another cause for the prolonged obstruction such as tracheomalacia, subglottic tumor, or a foreign body.

Helium and Oxygen Breathing

Theoretically, breathing a mixture of 80 percent helium and 20 percent oxygen—a mixture that is one-third as dense as air—should greatly reduce the resistance to turbulent airflow that characterizes upper airway obstruction. This therapy has not been extensively studied in children with croup, but theoretical considerations and a few case reports indicate that it is effective in relieving inspiratory work of breathing. The lowest effective concentration of helium is contained in a mixture of 60 percent helium and 40 percent oxygen (about one-half the density of air). This therapy is expensive and unlikely to be widely adopted.

Intubation

Intubation for relief of obstruction from viral croup is only required in a small percentage of patients. Prior to the use of racemic epinephrine, about 6 percent of children with viral croup were intubated or had a tracheotomy. In more recent years, and in association with the use of aerosolized epinephrine, this rate has dropped to less than 1 percent. We do not recommend tracheotomy. Nasotracheal intubation under anesthesia by a skilled anesthesiologist or surgeon is our preferred method of therapy in the vast majority of patients since the artificial airway is rarely required for more than 4 or 5 days. This subject is considered in greater detail in the subsequent section on Epiglottitis.

Follow-up Studies

Long-term follow-up studies of patients with viral croup indicate that 35 percent have increased bronchial reactivity to inhaled methacholine and 50 percent have exercise-induced bronchospasm. Baseline pulmonary function may be normal, and enhanced bronchial reactivity is not related to allergies. The reason for this long-term effect is not known, but some of these patients may require inhaled bronchodilator.

SPASMODIC CROUP

Spasmodic or recurrent croup is a poorly understood clinical entity that usually occurs in children, but may occur in adults. It presents as recurrent attacks of croup with a sudden onset, usually at night without signs of upper respiratory tract infection or fever. Acute adductor spasm of the vocal cords has been considered the major cause of the obstruction, but a pale edema of the subglottic area has been noted at laryngoscopy. These children have a distinct response to histamine challenge, which affects both the inspiratory and the expiratory portion of the flow-volume loop, suggesting the presence of both extrathoracic and intrathoracic airway hyperactivity.

Management

One study reports that although dexamethasone (0.6 mg per kilogram IM in a single dose) was ineffective in viral croup, it was effective in relieving spasmodic croup. Adults have been successfully treated with intermittent positive pressure breathing (IPPB) or continuous positive airway pressure (CPAP). Aerosolized racemic epinephrine may also be effective.

EPIGLOTTITIS

In contrast to viral croup, epiglottitis is an acute fulminating infection of the epiglottitis, aryepiglottic folds, and surrounding tissues. It has a sudden onset with fever, sore throat, inspiratory stridor, and progressive toxicity. The patients are usually between 2 and 6 years of age, but the condition may occur at any age and even in adults. As the obstruction worsens, stridor may disappear, and the patient has slow, deep breathing, a muffled voice, and drooling. The condition is diagnosed by the typical clinical course and visualization of a cherry-red, swollen epiglottis. Examination of the pharynx *must* be done *gently*. Vigorous attempts that make the child cry may cause sudden, complete airway obstruction. In no case should the pharynx be examined unless the physician is in a facility that is prepared for an emergency intubation. If the pharynx cannot be visualized, a lateral x-ray study of the neck demonstrates the swollen epiglottis ("thumb-print" sign) and aryepiglottic folds. The causative organism in the majority of cases is *Haemophilus influenzae* type B, but in rare instances, it may be *Streptococcus* or *Staphylococcus*. This condition constitutes a medical emergency and must be treated promptly in order to avoid the significant morbidity and mortality associated with severe hypoxemia.

Management

Intubation

The mainstay of therapy in patients of any age is provision of an adequate airway for 36 to 48 hours. In our institution, we have abandoned tracheotomy, and all children with epiglottitis are intubated immediately on admission without waiting for signs of worsening obstruction. Nasotracheal intubation should be done in the operating room under anesthesia administered by a skilled anesthesiologist or surgeon. A rigid bronchoscope should be available if intubation is difficult. We have used nasotracheal intubation for this condition for a decade, have not had any failed intubations, have zero mortality, and have no significant complications. In the majority of cases, it is possible to remove the endotracheal tube after 48 hours of antibiotic therapy. Extubation should be done in the operating room where a staff is prepared to re-intubate if necessary.

Antibiotics

Since the emergence of resistant strains of *H. influenzae*, it is prudent to use both ampicillin, 200 mg per kilogram per day in four to six divided doses, and chloramphenicol, 50 to 100 mg per kilogram per day every 6 hours; the total adult dose of chloramphenicol is 2 to 4 g per day). Once culture and sensitivity results are known, the antibiotic may be discontinued. Antibiotics are given intravenously for the first 3 or 4 days and then continued orally for a total of 10 days.

BACTERIAL TRACHEITIS

This condition, also known as pseudomembranous croup, membranous laryngotracheobronchitis, or bacterial tracheobronchitis, was well recognized in the early third of this century. It has recently re-emerged with a number of reports from various centers across North America. Bacterial tracheitis is an infection of the trachea and bronchi by either *Staphylococcus aureus* or *H. influenzae* and is associated with the formation of thick purulent secretions in the large airways. Symptoms resemble those of viral croup: croupy cough and inspiratory stridor. The patients affected may be 1 month to 7 or 8 years of age, and the illness is more progressive than with viral croup, but less acute than epiglottitis. It is associated with fever and leukocytosis. The hallmark is the presence of thick purulent secretions. In practice, the condition may be difficult to distinguish from viral croup or epiglottitis. The latter is ruled out when the normal epiglottis is seen on direct examination or on the lateral x-ray study of the neck. Subglottic swelling is usually absent, but secretions may be seen as a vague density or as a "dripping candle" effect on the tracheal mucosa. The diagnosis is confirmed by smear and subsequent culture of tracheal secretions.

Management

Intubation and Pulmonary Toilet

These patients cannot handle the copious purulent secretions and are in danger of sudden complete obstruction with large plugs of material. The hallmark of therapy is nasotracheal intubation (as described for epiglottitis). Patients must be managed in an intensive care unit, where frequent and vigorous pulmonary toilet is mandatory. Saline should be instilled into the endotracheal tube prior to suctioning. In only one instance of 14 cases that we have seen, that of a 3-year-old child, was intubation unnecessary since he was able to cough out the secretions. Extubation may be accomplished 5 to 6 days after beginning antibiotic therapy, but we have seen cases in which prolonged (7 to 10 days) intubation was required.

Antibiotics

Appropriate antibiotics (antistaphylococcal or anti-*H. influenzae* as for epiglottitis) are required for 10 to 14 days. They are given intravenously for the first 4 to 6 days and then orally.

SUGGESTED READING

Cramblett HG. Croup. In: Kendig EE, Cernick V, eds. Disorders of the respiratory tract in children. 4th ed. Philadelphia: WB Saunders 1983, 268–274.

Loughlin GM, Taussig LM. Upper airway obstruction. Semin Resp Med 1979; 1:131–146.

Newth JJL, Levison H, Bryan AC. The respiratory status of children with croup. J Pediat 1972; 81:1068–1073.

Sofer S, Duncan PD, Chernick V. Bacterial tracheitis, an old disease rediscovered. Clin Pediatr 1983; 22:407–411.

PULMONARY INFECTION INVOLVING AEROBIC GRAM-POSITIVE COCCI

JOHN G. BARTLETT, M.D.

Gram-positive cocci, which are important pulmonary pathogens, include the *Pneumococcus, S. aureus*, and *S. pyogenes* (group A beta-hemolytic streptococci). Occasional reports suggest that the enterococcus, *Streptococcus viridans*, and *S. epidermidis* may cause lower airway infections, but either these cases are rare or the occasional anecdotal reports do not provide compelling evidence regarding their pathogenic role. Anaerobic and microaerophilic streptococci are relatively common organisms in aspiration pneumonia or lung abscess (see chapter on *Anaerobic Bacterial Pulmonary Infection*).

The pneumococcus is the most frequently recognized bacterial pathogen of the lower airways, account for 40 to 60 percent of infections in adults over the age of 35 years who acquire their disease in the community. *S. aureus* accounts for about 2 percent of community-acquired infections and 10 to 20 percent of nosocomial pneumonias. *S. pyogenes* is a relatively rare pulmonary pathogen, but has been implicated in some epidemics of pneumonia, particularly in military recruits.

Management strategies include certain general principles, which apply to any patient with an infection of the lower airways, and selection of an antibiotic regimen that is optimally based on reliable microbiologic data. With regard to the latter, the etiologic diagnosis is considered secure when a likely pulmonary pathogen is recovered from a reliable specimen source that is not subject to contamination from the upper airways (cultures of blood, pleural fluid, transtracheal aspirate, or transthoracic aspirate) or from a site of distant dissemination (cerebrospinal fluid or joint fluid). The diagnosis is considered tentative on the basis of expectorated sputum studies showing a dominance of an appropriate morphotype accompanied by a large number of neutrophils on a direct Gram stain and/or the recovery of this organism on culture in large concentrations with a specimen showing evidence of lower airway secretions according to cytologic screening.

DIAGNOSIS

The time-honored method for detecting an etiologic agent in lower respiratory tract infections consists of a Gram stain and culture of the expectorated sputum specimen. The utility of this diagnostic exercise is often questioned owing to numerous errors that result from contamination of the specimen by the normal flora of the oral cavity during passage through the upper airways. Both the Gram stain and the culture of expectorated secretions are recommended, provided their limitations are recognized and cytologic screening is performed as a condition for culture. With the Gram stain, the greatest source of error is a false-positive reading for pneumococci. These organisms may be difficult to distinguish from the streptococci that comprise the dominant flora in the upper airways. The Quelling reaction provides this distinction. Pneumococci are also relatively fastidious, and so false-negative cultures are common. By contrast, *S. aureus* is rather easily cultivated, and failure to recover this organism is rather strong evidence against their role in a lower respiratory tract infection.

Alternative specimen sources include blood cultures, which should be obtained from virtually all patients with suspected bacteremia, and pleural fluid cultures, which should be obtained from all patients with a pleural effusion. Other specimen sources include transtracheal aspirations and transthoracic aspirations, which are generally reserved for cases that satisfy the following criteria: (1) technical expertise is available; (2) the severity of the disease justifies the risk incurred; (3) an etiologic diagnosis cannot be established with alternative, noninvasive specimen sources; and (4) patients do not have contraindications to the procedure. It should be noted that prior antibiotic treatment rapidly alters the cultivable flora of the lower airways, and any specimen other than blood cultures or pleural fluid cultures obtained after treatment must be interpreted with considerable caution.

Pleural Effusions

These should be aspirated for culture, cell count, and pH determination. When the effusion is large, the thoracentesis is done for both diagnosis and therapy. The decision for chest tube drainage depends on multiple interrelated factors, but the usual criteria are positive pleural fluid cultures, a pH less than 7.0, purulent collections that do not flow readily with needle aspiration, large effusions that reaccumulate rapidly, or loculated collections.

MANAGEMENT

General Principles

Hospitalization

Surveys of office practice indicate that most patients, perhaps 60 to 75 percent, with infections of the lower airway may be managed as outpatients. Thus, in many instances the initial decision concerns the advisability of inpatient versus outpatient management. This decision is largely based on the severity of the infection according to the history and physical examination.

Initial laboratory tests advocated for all patients when a lower respiratory tract infection is suspected include a chest roentgenogram and a complete blood count. The chest roentgenogram is considered the definitive test to distinguish pneumonia with involvement of the pulmonary parenchyma from infections limited to the major airways (bronchitis) or infection restricted to the upper airways (e.g., sinusitis, URI, allergic rhinitis). There are occasional patients with pulmonary infections who do not demonstrate an infiltrate during the first day of the infection, but this is uncommon. It is worth emphasizing that most adult patients with a pulmonary infiltrate and systemic findings compatible with a lower respiratory tract infection have an infection involving a treatable agent, whereas those with a negative chest roentgenogram and otherwise typical findings usually have bronchitis, which is most commonly caused by viruses. In the latter case, the major pathologic changes may be in the upper airways and must be approached differently. The purpose of the complete blood count is to determine the presence of anemia, which would indicate a systemic disease necessitating investigation; an abnormal peripheral leukocyte count, either very high or very low; or a prevalence of eosinophils, which would introduce many additional considerations in the differential diagnosis of the patient with a pulmonary infiltrate.

There are three general indications for hospitalization: (1) a patient who is seriously ill and requires either supportive care or intravenous antibiotics; (2) a patient who by history or by screening laboratory tests has evidence of an underlying disease that requires diagnostic evaluation; and (3) a patient whose social circumstances merit hospitalization simply because the resources for supervised care as an outpatient are limited. Critical factors in outpatient treatment include observation for evidence of response, compliance with the treatment regimen, and adequate long-term follow-up.

Supportive Care

Tracheobronchial Toilet. The clearance of pulmonary secretions should be stimulated by adequate hydration, encouraging the patient to cough, and, if necessary, a steam vaporizer or water nebulizer. Expectorants are of questionable benefit. It has not been proved that recovery is promoted by pulmonary physiotherapy, including intermittent positive pressure breathing. A possible exception is the patient with large volumes of secretions, particularly one with large abscesses or severe bronchiectasis, for whom postural drainage may prove useful when supervised by a pulmonary physiotherapist. Additional methods to facilitate drainage in this setting include nasotracheal suction and bronchoscopy. A debilitating cough may be suppressed with codeine in doses of 45 to 60 mg, as necessary. This drug or similar agents may also be used to relieve severe pleuritic pain. The use of sedatives or large amounts of nacrotics for pain relief may cause suppression of respiration and should be avoided.

Oxygenation. Patients who have hypoxia may benefit from oxygen therapy. This may be delivered with a nasal cannula at a flow rate of 6 L per minute, although great caution is necessary in patients with chronic lung disease. Patients with a history of respiratory insufficiency who require supplemental oxygen should receive this with considerable caution to avoid suppression of the hypoxic drive, using 24 to 28 percent oxygen by Ventimask or a nasal cannula with a flow rate of 1 to 2 L per minute.

Small bowel ileus or gastric dilatation may cause elevation of the diaphragm and further compromise pulmonary function. Patients with this complication may benefit from nasogastric suction or a rectal tube.

Antipyretics. The decision to use antipyretics is often difficult, particularly in patients managed at home, since these drugs are widely available in virtually all drug store remedies for respiratory infections. There are several disadvantages to eliminating fever: (1) elevated temperatures appear to enhance the immune response to a microbial infection, (2) fever is a major parameter for judging response to treatment, and (3) the intermittent use of these agents may result in wide fluctuations in the temperature profile, which may contribute to the patient's misery. Antipyretics are advised for patients with high fever who do not tolerate temperature elevations well or have medical contraindications to high fever (e.g., myocardial ischemia). In these settings, the usual regimen is Tylenol or aspirin in doses of 0.6 g every 4 to 6 hours.

Corticosteroids. Corticosteroids are not advocated for the patient with severe pneumonia, but patients who have previously received these agents chronically should have an increased dosage to prevent addisonian crisis. Doses as high as the equivalent of 300 mg of hydrocortisone may be required during the period of acute illness.

Other Measures. Other supportive measures for the seriously ill patient include intravenous fluids for dehydration, correction of electrolyte imbalance, intravenous sodium bicarbonate for lactic acidosis, and digitalis or diuretics for patients with congestive failure and fluid retention, preferably confirmed by the measurement of pulmonary wedge pressure or the monitoring of central venous pressure.

Epidemiologic Considerations

The source of infection in patients with bacterial pneumonia is often difficult to establish, although the possibility of transmission within the hospital setting is the subject of considerable concern and sparse data. Our policy is adherence to the CDC guidelines, which provide a medical-legal document with at least some rationale. No particular precautions are necessary in patients with pneumococcal pneumonia except for those with penicillin-resistant strains. Patients with pneumonia caused by penicillin-resistant pneumococci or by *S. pyogenes* are placed in a single room, where secretion precautions are observed for 24 hours after the initiation of appropriate antibiotic therapy. Patients with staphylococcal pneumonia are kept in strict isolation for the duration of the illness.

Antibiotic Selection

The major problem with pulmonary infections is detection of an etiologic agent, since antibiotic selection is markedly simplified if the culprit is known. Guidelines are provided in Table 1 for the agent of choice, alternative regimens if there is a contraindication to the primary agent, and drugs that are considered acceptable subsitutes if there is a polymicrobial infection or if there are additional etiologic possibilities.

Streptococcus pneumoniae

Penicillin is the drug of choice, the only matters of controversy being the route of administration, dosage, and duration of treatment. The only possible exception is the patient with an isolate that is resistant to penicillin. These strains are unusual, except in children who have received multiple or extensive courses of penicillin. Sensitivity testing using an oxacillin disc is recommended for blood and spinal fluid isolates, and possibly even sputum isolates for patients in the high-risk categories. Most of these strains are only "moderately" resistant (MIC values of 0.1 to 1.0 μg per milliliter) and presumably should respond to penicillin given parenterally at somewhat higher dosages. The alternative agent with assured activity for strains that are highly resistant to penicillin and multiply resistant to other agents is vancomycin.

The dosage and route of administration for the usual patient with pneumoccocal pneumonia depends on the severity of illness, the decision for inpatient versus outpatient management, and the presence or absence of extrapulmonary, suppurative complications. Most patients with pneumococcal pneumonia may be treated at home using penicillin V in doses of 250 to 500 mg four times daily until the patient has been afebrile for 2 to 5 days. Patients who are hospitalized are treated with either procaine penicillin G, 600,000 units every 8 to 12 hours, or aqueous penicillin G in doses of about 2,000,000 units per day. Treatment is continued until the patient has been afebrile for 2 to 5 days, although this course may be completed with oral penicillin V on an outpatient basis. High doses of penicillin (10 to 20 million units of aqueous penicillin G per day) are reserved for patients who have cases complicated by pneumococcal meningitis, septic arthritis, or endocarditis.

The alternative agent used for outpatient management in patients with a contraindication to penicillin is erythromycin in a dosage of 250 to 500 mg four times daily. This drug has been particularly attractive in patients without an established etiologic diagnosis, since it is active against *Mycoplasma* and *Legionella* as well as *Pneumococcus*. In many patients, erythromycin causes gastrointestinal complications that are dose-related. Most will tolerate the lower dosage recommended if there is appropriate emphasis on the importance of compliance. The preferred alternative agents for parenteral use are cephalothin or cefazolin. Patients with a contraindication to beta-lactam antibiotics may be treated with clindamycin or several other agents listed in the table.

TABLE 1 Initial Treatment of Staphylococcal and Streptococcal Pulmonary Infections

Agent	*Preferred Regimen*	*Alternatives*	*Comments*
S. pneumoniae			
Outpatient therapy	Penicillin V 250–500 mg PO q.i.d.	Erythromycin 250–500 mg PO q.i.d.	Acceptable alternatives: Ampicillin, penicillin G, tetracycline, clindamycin, sulfa-trimethoprim
Hospitalized patients	Moderately ill: Procaine penicillin G, 600,000 units q8–12h	Cephalothin, 0.5–1 g IV q6h Cefazolin 0.5 g IM or IV q8h	Acceptable alternatives: Other cephalosporins, clindamycin, nafcillin, chloramphenicol, vancomycin
	Severely ill: Aqueous penicillin G, 500,000 units IV q6h		
	Complicated: Aqueous penicillin G, 3–5 million units q4–6h		"Complicated" refers to patients with meningitis, septic arthritis, or endocarditis
S. aureus			
Methicillin-sensitive	Nafcillin 1–3 g IV q4–6h	Cephalothin, 1–2 g q4–6h	Strains sensitive to penicillin at 0.1 μg/ml may be treated with penicillin G, 1–2 million units q4–6h
		Clindamycin (erythromycin + clindamycin-sensitive strains) 600 mg IV q8h	Oxacillin and methicillin are considered equivalent to nafcillin
		Vancomycin, 500 mg IV q6h	Cefamandole and cefazolin are considered equivalent to cephalothin
Methicillin-resistant	Vancomycin 500 mg IV q6h	(None)	For overwhelming or refractory cases: vancomycin plus rifampin (300 mg PO b.i.d.) *or* an aminoglycoside
S. pyogenes	Aqueous penicillin G, 500,000 units IV q4–6h	Cephalothin, 0.5–1 g IV q6h Clindamycin, 600 mg IV q8h	Acceptable alternatives: Ampicillin, other cephalosporins, (preferably cefazolin, cefotaxime, or cefamandole), erythromycin, vancomycin, chloramphenicol

Staphylococcus aureus

Penicillinase-resistant penicillins are regarded as the drugs of choice for methicillin-sensitive strains. Nafcillin, oxacillin, and methicillin are considered therapeutically equivalent, and all are given intravenously in relatively high doses (8 to 12 g per day) for rather extended periods. The total duration of therapy cannot be specified, since so much depends on the nature of the initial infection and response in individual cases. As a general rule, patients with staphylococcal bronchopneumonia are treated parenterally until they have been afebrile for at least 7 days, and this may be followed by an oral agent, such as dicloxacillin (2 g per day), cephalexin (2 g per day), or clindamycin (1.2 g per day) following discharge. Parenteral antibiotics are usually given for 4 to 6 weeks for patients with lung abscess, empyema, and suspected or established endocarditis. This includes patients with right-sided staphylococcal endocarditis and septic emboli to the lung, which are commonly seen in association with intravenous drug abuse. Rifampin (600 mg per day) or an aminoglycoside (usually gentamicin) may be added to the penicillinase-resistant penicillin or cephalosporin for patients who do not respond or are critically ill.

Cephalosporins are considered therapeutically equivalent to penicillins in the treatment of serious staphylococcal infections, particularly cephalothin, cefazolin, or cefamandole. These drugs may be preferred for the patient with a possible hypersensitivity reaction to penicillins or poor tolerance to intravenous administration of penicillins, which is particularly common with nafcillin. Cefazolin is the preferred agent when intramuscular treatment is necessary. For patients who have a history of an IgE-mediated response to penicillin, as indicated by anaphylaxis or giant urticaria, or a positive skin test to penicillin major or minor determinants, an agent other than beta-lactam agents should be given. Clindamycin has established efficacy, but should be reserved for strains that are sensitive to both erythromycin and clindamycin. The reason is the phenomenon of disassociated cross-resistance between these two drugs, indicating the probability of rapid emergence of clindamycin resistance in erythromycin-resistant strains. Vancomycin, another alternative to the beta-lactam drugs, is active against virtually all strains.

In recent years there has been an alarming increase in the incidence of methicillin-resistant strains of *S. aureus*. These strains are also resistant to virtually all cephalosporins, although they may appear sensitive with the routine in vitro sensitivity tests. Some of the strains are susceptible to aminoglycosides, sulfa-trimethoprim or tetracycline, although there is limited clinical experience with these drugs. The only agent that can be advocated is vancomycin, given in doses of 2 g per day to adults with normal renal function. This drug is advocated for all patients with pneumonia involving methicillin-resistant strains, and it is often the preferred drug for empiric treatment for nosocomial infections in which *S. aureus* is an established or suspected pathogen in hospitals where these strains are highly prevalent. In this situation, the antibiotic may be changed when in vitro sensitivity data are available.

Streptococcus pyogenes

The preferred regimen is aqueous penicillin G given intravenously in doses of 2 to 4 million units daily for initial treatment. This is continued until the patient has been afebrile for 2 to 5 days, and it may be followed by oral penicillin G or penicillin V (2 g per day) following discharge. There are multiple agents that may be given as alternatives, including cephalosporins and clindamycin. Many of these patients have pleural effusions or empyema, requiring drainage.

FOLLOW-UP

One of the most important facets in the treatment of pneumonia is to know what to expect in terms of response. The published experience with pneumococcal pneumonia shows that penicillin therapy has not altered the natural mortality rate of this disease during the first 3 to 5 days following treatment, and about 20 percent of patients with pneumococcal bacteremia expire despite appropriate use of antibiotics. For those who do respond, about one-third become afebrile in 24 hours, one-third become afebrile in 1 to 2 days, and one-third require longer. Patients should appear clinically improved with decreased temperatures within 24 to 48 hours. There is less information about pneumonia due to *S. aureus* or *S. pyogenes*, except that these patients tend to respond more slowly. The best parameters to follow are the temperature profile, leukocye count, and clinical appearance. Serial chest roentgenograms are not very helpful since there may be progressive infiltrates or new cavities in patients who are otherwise doing well. I recommend follow-up roentgenograms early in the treatment course only in patients who are doing poorly by clinical criteria, and to evaluate pleural effusions. Nevertheless, long-term follow-up roentgenogram examinations are important to document clearance of roentgenographic changes and detect any underlying lesions. This applies to patients over 35 years of age; routine follow-up chest films are not advocated for younger patients who respond well clinically.

The following should be considered for patients who fail to respond to the initial antibiotic regimen:

1. Inappropriate antimicrobial agent: This depends largely on the security of the etiologic diagnosis as defined above. The sensitivity of *S. aureus* to methicillin should be confirmed. Sensitivity of pneumococci to penicillin should also be confirmed in the appropriate setting.
2. Inadequate dosage or route of administration: This is seldom a problem when using the regimens enumerated in Table 1.
3. Compliance: This is a major concern in outpatients.
4. Inadequate host: Some patients simply do not

respond despite optimal management. This is most common in patients with overwhelming infections, those who are treated relatively late in their course, and patients with inadequate host defenses, as in chronic granulomatous disease, neutropenia, and severe chronic lung disease.

5. Associated lesions or complications: Major concerns are empyema requiring drainage, an underlying obstructing lesion, or a distant metastatic site of suppuration. Pleural effusions should be aspirated and bronchoscopy should be performed whenever bronchial obstruction is suspected.
6. Superinfection: Patients with this compliance usually respond and then deteriorate. Cultures of sequentially collected sputum specimens are of limited value except to provide guidelines for treatment when clinical observations clearly support the impression of superinfection.
7. Infection at another anatomic site: These include urinary tract infections, phlebitis at IV infusion sites, and tracheitis in patients with tracheostomies or endotracheal intubation.
8. Alternative diagnoses: Included are infections due to alternative agents (e.g, mycobacteria, chlamydia, fungi, rickettsia, viruses, mycoplasma, legionella, aerobic gram-negative bacilli, anaerobes) and non-infectious diseases (e.g, hypersensitivity pneumonitis, tumor infiltrates).
9. Adverse drug reaction, especially drug fever: These patients often appear deceptively well compared to their temperature profile. The most likely antibiotics are sulfonamides and beta-lactam antibiotics, although almost any drug may be responsible. Eosinophilia may or may not be present.

SUGGESTED READING

Bartlett JG. Diagnostic accuracy of transtracheal aspiration bacteriologic studies. Am Rev Resp Dis 1977; 115:777–782.

Dans PE, Charache P, Fahey M. Management of pneumonia in the prospective payment era. Arch Intern Med 1984; 144:1392–1398.

LaForce MF. Community-acquired lower respiratory tract infections. Am J Med 1985; 78:52–57.

Murray PR, Washington JA III. Microscopic and bacteriologic analysis of sputum. Mayo Clin Proc 1975; 50:339–344.

AEROBIC GRAM-NEGATIVE PNEUMONIA

HERBERT Y. REYNOLDS, M.D.

The aerobic gram-negative bacilli that commonly cause pneumonia are in the families of Enterobacteriaceae (*Klebsiella pneumoniae, Escherichia coli, Serratia maracescens*) and Pseudomonadeaceae (*Pseudomonas aeruginosa*). Normally these bacteria are part of the bowel flora or can reside on moist, intertriginous skin areas, but are found infrequently on the pharyngeal and nasal mucosa (occurrence is about 15% in area swabs taken from the mouth of healthy people). Normal flora of the naso-oropharynx is dominated by anaerobic bacteria and common commensals such as *Neisseria* species, *Streptococcus, Branhamella catarrhalis* and, perhaps, *Haemophilus* species and *Streptococcus pneumoniae* in people with chronic bronchitis. Almost any form of stress (hospitalization, intensive care stay, or a surgical procedure), metabolic derangement (uncontrolled diabetes mellitus, renal or hepatic failure), chronic illness, or immunosuppressive therapy with antineoplastic chemotherapy or anti-inflammatory agents is associated with a striking increase in colonization of bowel, skin, and upper respiratory tract mucosa with the gram-negative rods mentioned. This has been well documented in medical and surgical intensive care units where acquisition of these organisms in the oropharynx is rapid, occurring within 1 to 3 days of admission, and frequent, as over half of patients can become colonized. Thus, the stage is set for a hospital-acquired or so-called nosocomial pneumonia to develop, and approximately 1 to 5 percent of all hospital infections are considered to be a nosocomial pneumonia. Moreover, the impact on health care of these respiratory infections is appreciable for mortality can be high (30% to 50%) and morbidity plus an added hospital stay are usual. The most direct relationship between upper airway colonization and the etiology of acquired pneumonia was documented among patients in intensive care units. They had a high probability of developing pneumonia with the same gram-negative rod bacterium that had been found to colonize their oropharynx, probably by aspirating oropharyngeal secretions. This has led to thoughts about the value of monitoring flora to predict susceptibility to pneumonia and about ways to intervene prophylactically with topical antibiotics or immunization. However, no consensus for overall management has seemed to evolve, although the problem remains as large and dangerous as ever. Finally, the aftermath of a gram-negative rod pneumonia may be more severe than that of pneumonia caused by gram-positive bacteria. The lung usually repairs itself and restores much of its architecture after pneumococcal or some similar infection, but following *Pseudomonas* or *Klebsiella* infections, fibrosis and persistent scarring may remain. Telltale chest roentgenographic shadows persist, and lung function can be diminished as well. The more complex cell surface and wall structure containing lipopolysaccharides, plus the secretion of various exotoxins and proteases by these bacteria, probably cause more direct injury to tissue and elicit more inflammation, all contributing to the severe infection produced. As shown in some animal models of aerosol bacterial infection, when gram-negative bacteria are deposited on the air-space surface, the host defense response is a combined one of alveolar macrophages and an intensive influx of polymorphonuclear granulocytes. Certainly, one of the most obvious defects in overall host defense that predisposes to gram-negative rod infections is bone marrow failure due to primary tumor or to cytotoxic chemotherapy. This results in an inability to mount a sufficient polymorphonuclear granulocyte (PMN) inflammatory response. Thus, a lack of PMNs enhances susceptibility to gram-negative bacteria and to certain fungi (*Aspergillus* species). Ironically, the host who can mount an appropriate inflammatory response to combat these bacteria may suffer the consequence of the heavy PMN fire power and excessive tissue damage that may ensue. The point is that gram-negative rods, which usually are docile commensals that have become opportunistic microbes, quickly become aggressive in the susceptible host and are able to wreak havoc. Therefore, a good defense plan to compensate for the host who may be deficient in natural mechanisms is to anticipate respiratory infection, diagnose it precisely, and move quickly to treat it decisively. We will focus on these three topics.

ANTICIPATING THE SUSCEPTIBLE PATIENT

As mentioned, almost any unusual stress, serious illness, and hospitalization, especially in an intensive care facility, promotes acquisition of, and oropharyngeal colonization with, common but potentially pathogenic gram-negative rods. These bacteria probably originate with the patient who autoinoculates his upper respiratory tract with his hands or bodily secretions; health care personnel and such innocuous things as uncooked food, salad, or even flowers and plants in the room also can be a vehicle. Colonization develops quickly and may not be preventable. Its ultimate consequence depends somewhat on the integrity of host defenses and individual resistance of the patient. However, cachexia and immunosuppression are so frequent in hospital patients that most might be considered vulnerable. Therefore, it is important to know what the patient's baseline microbial flora is, to monitor its change so that when the potential culprits appear one knows where they are residing, and to obtain preliminary antibiotic sensitivity tests. As part of the admission laboratory evaluation, nasal, oropharyngeal, perirectal, and axillary skin swabs should be obtained for routine bacterial cultures. Any potential pathogens isolated can be tested for antibiotic sensitivities, especially if the hospital is having any problems with resistant species. The cotton-tipped applicators should first be dipped in transport medium such as Stuart's bacterial transport medium containing glycerophosphate, thioglycolate, calcium chloride, and water (Culturette, Marion Scientific, Kansas City, MO) to moisten them before they are rubbed over the skin sites or in the nares. A swab of the perianal area and around the anal opening seems to give as good a yield of bowel flora as a stool specimen. In the mouth, liberal swabbing of the buccal and soft palate areas should be done. All of the individually labeled specimens must be taken promptly to the microbiology laboratory for culture. The cost for routine culture and enumeration of the flora in each sample is about \$15 to \$20; for antibiotic sensitivity analysis of the principal pathogens, the laboratory fee is about \$20. Thus, four baseline surveillance cultures and possible sensitivity testing have added about \$100 to the patient's initial hospital bill. A daily naso-oropharyngeal culture should be obtained for the first 3 days of hospitalization since the majority of patients acquire the potential pathogen and colonize the nose and throat quickly. Also, as it requires a day or so to process the initial admission cultures, it might take several days to assess the baseline colonization pattern. If the potential pathogen is recovered in the original naso-pharyngeal or sputum culture, subsequent daily cultures just planned can be cancelled. However, if several days of unrevealing cultures from the nose and mouth are received, clinical judgment must be used to decide whether continued surveillance with cultures is required. The patient's clinical course influences this decision.

An alternative approach is to judge the patient's potential for colonization with a gram-negative bacterium by assessing in vitro the adherence of a test bacterial species (usually a *Pseudomonas aeruginosa* isolate) to squamous buccal epithelial cells collected by scraping the inner cheek. Good correlations between the quantitative binding of bacteria to the cells and subsequent colonization following surgery, for example, make the use of such an assay attractive. My colleagues and I have examined the feasibility of using ciliated epithelial cells obtained by brushing the nasal mucosa and tracheal surface for the same purpose. Obviously, this is a laboratory research procedure whose validity must be substantiated better before it is used as a screening test; however, these tests underscore a major problem for many patients in the clinical setting I am describing—adequate nutrition. The overall nutritional status of the patient, who is perhaps cachectic to begin with or catabolic because of recent surgery or is now showing nutritional improvement from skillful hyperalimentation and/or parenteral feeding, seems to influence the degree of bacterial adherence and binding to these buccal or airway cells. My colleagues and I noted in a group of patients with chronic tracheostomies that the better their prognostic nutritional index (lower score), the fewer bacteria bound to their tracheal epithelial cells. This direct relationship could be modulated in patients by improving nutritional status and general health. Two points merit emphasis: (1) it may become feasible soon to use a laboratory test to help judge susceptibility to colonization, but bacterial cultures for surveillance also will be needed; and (2) nutrition is an important ingredient in the patient's medical therapy and may relate directly to the integrity of local airway defenses and to a mucosal surface that is more resistant to colonization and potential infection. This topic is too broad for more discussion here, but should be given further thought because physicians are now much more enlightened about the treatment of poor nutrition.

Colonization with a potentially pathogenic gram-negative rod found in the oropharynx of an at-risk patient presents a therapeutic dilemma. Is this an indication for a prophylactic antibiotic or for enhanced surveillance? As already mentioned, prior immunization with a basic core lipopolysaccharide antigen that would raise potentially cross-reacting, protective antibodies to many gram-negative bacteria has not become a feasible option yet. However, use of a topical antibiotic sprayed into the nose and mouth has been tried to prevent colonization with *Pseudomonas* and reduce the risk of nosocomial pneumonia. It is worthwhile recalling the following experience.

Clinical Study. In the Respiratory-Surgical Intensive Care Unit of Boston's Beth Israel Hospital, there was, over a 2-year period, a 21 percent incidence of acquired pneumonia, often with *Pseudomonas*, which caused a 70 percent mortality rate. In an attempt to prevent *Pseudomonas* colonization, polymyxin B was aerosolized into the oropharynx or down a tracheostomy tube. In the first report on a feasibility study, 33 randomly selected patients entering the unit received polymyxin B and 25 controls did not (9-day stay for treated versus 6-day stay for controls). This treatment significantly reduced gram-negative bacterial colonization to 21 percent in the treated patients, in contrast to 68 percent in the controls. Infection with *Pseudomonas aeruginosa* was completely prevented in the polymyxin B-treated group. Indications were good that this preventive approach might be successful.

These results led to a study of all patients entering the unit, divided into 2-month cycles. Of 744 patients admitted over 22 months, 374 were given polymyxin B and 370 were not: only six of the 374 treated patients (1.6%) developed *Pseudomonas* colonization, in contrast to 36 of the 370 controls (9.7%). Colonizattion with *E. coli, Klebsiella,* and *Enterobacter* species was three times higher in the control group (62 of 370) than in the treated group (22 of 374). Colonization with *Staphylococcus aureus* occurred in about 2 percent of both groups (9 treated patients, 8 controls). *Serratia* and *Proteus* infections were ominously high in both groups (8 treated patients and 6 controls).

Because the treatment's aim, preventing *Pseudomonas aeruginosa* pneumonia, was well achieved, the study then went on to treat all patients entering the unit with aerosol polymyxin B. Over 7 months, 69 of 292 patients (24%) became colonized with bacteria, but only three with *Pseudomonas*, and only one of these developed *Pseudomonas* pneumonia (0.3%). However, 11 patients did develop pneumonia. When colonization occurred, 74 percent of the gram-negative isolates were polymyxin-resistant and included *Proteus, Pseudomonas cepacia, Ps. maltophilia, Flavobacterium,* and *Serratia* species. Of the 11 patients who acquired pneumonia, 10 had pneumonia caused by organisms resistant to polymyxin. Seven of the 11 patients (64%) died. In this study, as in one conducted by Johanson et al, colonization preceded the development of pneumonia. In 10 of the 11 patients, pneumonia was caused by the same organism that had colonized. Although continuous prophylactic use of aerosol polymyxin B lowered the incidence of *Pseudomonas aeruginosa* pneumonia, it helped to create antibiotic-resistant strains that caused other, perhaps even worse, pneumonias.

This unfortunate clinical outcome greatly deterred further attempts to manipulate bacterial flora with aerosol antibiotics. Instead, the occurrence of pneumonia in ICU patients has been reduced appreciably by such hygienic measures as assiduously cleaning ventilatory equipment. Increasing awareness among members of the staff of their role in transmitting microorganisms to patients is another important factor in controlling infection.

In summary, anticipating respiratory infection may be the best approach to diagnosing it quickly and treating it promptly, specifically, and vigorously. Unfortunately, nothing can completely prevent colonization. But severe respiratory infection often follows the acquisition of certain bacteria in the oropharynx that are later aspirated into the lungs. Therefore, monitoring patients closely after specific bacteria appear alerts the health care team that respiratory infection may occur and helps the team to select the initial antibiotics. Thus an appropriate strategy for coping with nosocomial respiratory infection should include (1) assessing which patients are likely to develop colonies of potentially pathogenic organisms in the oropharynx, (2) monitoring the patient when colonization occurs, (3) concentrating special attention on the highly susceptible patient (which might include using an aerosol antibiotic), giving special care to control of secretions and increasing general surveillance, and (4) knowing which organisms are sensitive to which antibiotics. Underlying all of this interest in microbial colonization are fundamental questions about the dynamic interaction between bacteria and host cells.

DIAGNOSIS AND ETIOLOGY

In elderly, severely ill, or immunocompromised patients in whom nosocomial pneumonia is most likely to occur, early detection of respiratory infection may not be easy, nor is its onset always obvious. The usual clinical parameters, including fever and leukocytosis, can be trivial, and respiratory symptoms may be subtle. Patients may have an unimpressive amount of cough and scant expectoration, if any. In many cases, they are intubated and on assisted ventilation so that they cannot speak and readily report their chest complaints. Fever can be deceptively absent, especially if renal or liver failure exists, or if bone marrow insufficiency precludes the anticipated whole blood cell count rise and blunts the inflammatory response so that an infiltrate on a chest roentgenogram may be hard to discern or slow to blossom. Agitation or altered mentation frequently ushers in the infection; an elevated pulse rate and more difficulty with fluid balance, especially diminished urine output, are clues. The point is that the presentation can be atypical and a high index of suspicion plus subtle clues often suggest the diagnosis. When respiratory signs are minimal, only after excluding infection systematically in other organ systems (urinary tract, wound/catheter sites, decubitus areas, occult meningitis) does the respiratory tract receive more consideration. In some intensive care units where daily portable chest films are almost routine, one may depend on the development of, or changing appearance of, parenchymal shadows for the clue that pneumonia is present. The roentgenographic pattern may lag behind the actual onset of infection, and valuable time is lost in initiating treatment. However, it is difficult to make (or accept) a diagnosis of nosocomial pneumonia without definite roentgenographic changes as some objective evidence is required. Unfortunately, auscultation of the chest may not reveal early pneumonitis if secretions are scant or if the patient is attached to a ventilator. The ventilator and endotracheal tube apparatus generate too much confusing background noise for precise auscultation and, importantly, the patient cannot be positioned optimally or cooperate well for a careful physical examination. For the intubated patient, the question inevitably arises whether occult aspiration has caused the pneumonia, but this can never be decided with certainty. Just as a healthy person can aspirate oropharyngeal secretions during sleep, so can patients with a disoriented sensorium from many causes, including prescribed sedation. Aspiration around the inflated endotracheal cuff also occurs. Suctioning hyperalimentation liquid or small food particles from the endotracheal tube may heighten the diagnosis. Measuring pH of respiratory fluid or the glucose content to identify tube feeding material is touted as being helpful in picking up small, recurrent aspiration. Rarely has this proved decisive in my experience.

Realizing that pneumonitis exists, the most expeditious means for making a microbial diagnosis must be decided. This may precipitate the most controversial step in patient management—one that can become the weakest link in the treatment process. The issue focuses on how invasive one should be in obtaining an adequate specimen for bacteriologic diagnosis, for these patients, invariably it seems, never make much sputum or cannot cough well. The initial choice of antibiotics to cover the spectrum of infectious agents responsible will be somewhat empiric because the coverage should be broad to include an unsuspected microbe. However, the crucial step of narrowing the antibiotic coverage, based on recovery of a specific infectious agent, for the duration of therapy may be difficult unless adequate specimens were cultured originally. Several blood cultures are an indispensable part of the work-up, but their yield will not be known for a few days. In such cases, the baseline surveillance cultures can be expected to reveal some of the flora of the patient and, importantly, to identify which of the potentially pathogenic gram-negative rods have already colonized the naso-oropharynx or are present in expectorated secretions. Such bacteria are likely to be causative, at least partially. Initial antibiotic coverage certainly should include such probable pathogens. The problem of obtaining actual lung secretions or tissue persists. For the intubated patient, a deep tracheal suction with a firm curved catheter that can be advanced into a major bronchus may suffice. Attempts to aerosol nebulized water particles into the airways to stimulate secretions are usually worthless and, at best, provide a stimulus for coughing that might produce some sputum. In many cases this dilemma arises: should transtracheal aspiration (if a skilled person is available) or fiberoptic bronchoscopy be performed or should one go straight to an open lung biopsy, if the diagnosis is not going to be obtained with one of the first procedures and if the patient can tolerate a minithoractomy? Each patient requires a thoughtful assessment of these options based on the patient's condition and prognosis.

Transtracheal aspiration is a direct approach and it avoids most of the oropharyngeal flora that can confuse culture results; this specimen usually contains the offending pathogen. These aspirates should be cultured for anaerobic bacteria as well as for aerobic flora. According to the literature, the procedure is reliable, yet its utilization varies from not at all to frequently in different medical centers. Fear of acute cricothyroid artery bleeding and reluctance of the patient are inhibiting factors. However, transtracheal aspirates should be obtained more frequently because they provide reliable cultures. The procedure could be performed by a surgical colleague, who is capable of gaining control of the airway and stemming acute bleeding should it develop. A small amount of subcutaneous air in the neck and some blood-tinged sputum with coughing may occur after the procedure, but these are self-limited complications. It is important that this procedure be performed by competent doctors otherwise many complications may occur.

Fiberoptic bronchoscopy can be done readily, even if the patient is on a ventilator through a side-port attachment to the endotracheal tube (minimal size, 8 mm). If the patient is thrombocytopenic, platelet transfusions given just before bronchoscopy largely prevent endobronchial bleeding. The brush catheter seems to cause the most trouble with bleeding. Transbronchial biopsies can be done in this setting, with care obviously. Oxygen should be given through the bronchoscope. With a combination of cultures from a telescoping protected-tip catheter, brushings, and transbronchial biopsies, the yield of a probable pathogen is approximately 50 percent in the immunocompromised host. Upper airway flora are included in the culture reports because some pharyngeal secretions are picked up during passage of the bronchoscope and the various specimen catheters. In many cases the bronchoscopic examination permits a view of the bronchial orifices to rule out endobronchial obstruction. Serious complications from bronchoscopy are not frequent. With transbronchial biopsy, a pneumothorax occurs in about 5 percent of cases and may require placement of a chest tube. Transthoracic needle aspiration of a lung area involved with an infiltrate can be used to diagnose infection, but this requires fluoroscopic or CT scan guidance and is not a bedside procedure. This procedure does not seem too popular for adults, but is used more by pediatricians confronted with undiagnosed pneumonia in infants.

The need to do a small open thoracotomy to obtain lung tissue often becomes apparent. This approach gives the best piece of tissue and is tolerated surprisingly well by the sickest patient. Generally, thoracic surgeons are extremely skillful in managing this situation. Open lung biopsy is often necessary in the immunocompromised patient with an advancing, undiagnosed pulmonary infiltrate and pneumonia. However, two failings often are observed with the procedure. Medical personnel procrastinate and wait too long to get the biopsy, thus delaying appropriate antimicrobial therapy, or they do not coordinate the handling of the tissue with the microbiologist and pathologist to ensure optimal analysis. A brief presurgical consultation with all the principals is most helpful. The pathologist can often suggest the best area of lung to biopsy, and having the microbiology laboratory prepared can ensure that the most appropriate cultures are quickly planted.

MANAGEMENT

The initial therapy must be chosen on the basis of the skillful interpretation of essentially clinical phenomena and must be heavily weighted toward protecting the patient against the most dangerous of the conceivable diagnoses in the particular set of circumstances. Appropriate support with parenteral fluids, antipyretic drugs, supplemental oxygen, airway suction or postural drainage, bronchodilator therapy for some patients, and the other modalities employed to treat serious lung infection must be instituted as needed. These will not be discussed. Antimicrobial therapy remains the cornerstone of medical management, but intelligent use of antimicrobial drugs is not easy, and frequent reappraisal of their choice and the patient's response must be made.

For the bacteria under consideration—aerobic gram-negative bacilli—a broad selection of antibiotics exists: aminoglycosides (gentamicin, tobramycin, and amikacin), semisynthetic penicillins that are active against pseudomonas principally (carboxypenicillins such as carbenicillin and ticarcillin) or have an extended spectrum (ureido penicillins including piperacillin and mezlocillin), and cephalosporins, which are divided into three generations based on general features of antimicrobial activity. Representative cephalosporins most active against the bacteria under discussion are first-generation agents such as cephalothin or an oral form cephalexin, second-generation choices such as cefamandole or cefoxitin, and third-generation agents represented by cefotaxime and moxalactam. Several third-generation cephalosporins have especially good antipseudomonas activity (ceftazidime, cefoperazone, and cefsulodin). A newer group of beta-lactam antibiotics called thienamycins will not be included; however, these agents do have activity against certain *Enterobacteriaceae* and *Pseudomonas* species that are resistant to cephalosporins, but laboratory susceptibility testing is required for their selection. As aspiration pneumonia is a frequent consideration in patients with nosocomial pneumonia, antibiotics to cover anaerobic flora are often given in addition to the gram-negative rod coverage outlined; suitable antibiotics for anaerobics in the lung include penicillin G, clindamycin, and perhaps metronidazole. Finally, standby antibiotics, ampicillin, or amoxicillin, are often used to treat respiratory infection of unknown cause because of their gram-positive and gram-negative antibacterial activity and general efficacy as respiratory tract antibiotics. If urosepsis is contributing to the infective process and *E. coli* is a possible lung pathogen, ampicillin may be used.

The list of antibiotics is not inclusive, only representative, and each physician has favorites and is more comfortable using certain agents. There is continuing proliferation of new cephalosporins seemingly more potent and active against certain bacteria such as *Pseudomonas*, but still broad in overall coverage and more expensive to prescribe. Some of these agents need more clinical experience before they are given a special place in the armentarium of antibiotics for serious gram-negative infections. It should be remembered that as the higher generations of cephalosporins have been developed with greater activity against gram-negative bacteria, some of the activity against gram-positive ones has been lost, and so these drugs may not offer suitable therapy for species of staphylococci, enterococci, and *Streptococcus pneumoniae*. On the other hand, much of the commerical literature about these newer cephalosporins suggests that a single agent will give broad coverage and alone may suffice for treatment of serious infection. However, a single antibiotic has not generally proved to be adequate in eradicating or curing pneumonia caused by a *Pseudomonas* or *Klebsiella* species, especially if the host is in any way immunocompromised. Dual or multiple antibiotics are still recommended for predictable coverage. Cephalosporins, as do other antibiotics, have special side effects that must be recognized and anticipated for each agent employed. Finally, as bacterial resistance to antibiotics increases, appropriate selection must be based on probable sensitivities of the bacterium in question, which must be confirmed in the laboratory for the particular isolate.

Patterns of bacterial resistance may be unique for individual hospitals, and one must keep abreast of the current susceptibility tests monitored by the hospital epidemiology service. These changes directly affect one's initial selection of antibiotics. For example, at the Yale New Haven Hospital, our most recent communication about antibiotic susceptibility of bacteria indicated that gentamicin-sensitive isolates of *Pseudomonas aeruginosa* had decreased from about 93 to 84 percent in the past 2-year interval; *Serratia marcescens* dropped from 96 to 59 percent against this aminoglycoside. However, other major gram-negative pathogens generally remained susceptible to gentamicin, i.e., *E. coli* (97%), *Klebsiella* species (about 90%), *Enterobacter* species (about 90%), and *Proteus mirabilis* (98%). In surveying gram-negative bacteremia, 21 of 172 isolates were resistant to gentamicin and most of these were *Serratia marcescens* and *Pseudomonas aeruginosa*. However, many of these isolates came from patients with nosocomial pneumonia or sepsis in the medical and surgical intensive care units and from the oncology service, as might be anticipated.

With this background of antibiotics choices and a somewhat unique pattern of microbial resistance to these antibiotics in our hospital setting, let us plan treatment for a patient with pneumonia, possibly nosocomial in origin and likely to be caused by a pathogenic gram-negative rod. The patient is colonized in the oropharynx with a probable pathogen, and so there is a reasonably certain bacterial etiology for which a rational selection of antibiotic's) is possible. However, it was necessary to obtain better samples of respiratory secretions, and so fiberoptic bronchoscopy was done and specimens obtained have been cultured appropriately. Blood cultures are incubating as well. Keep in mind that we want to treat the most probable infectious agent, based on our surveillance cultures and current analysis of a carefully gram-stained smear of the respiratory secretions, but one must also cover the patient for the unsuspected bacterium that could be the most devastating in this clinical setting. I am always concerned about covering for *Pseudomonas* infection because it is the most frequent cause of nosocomial pneumonia. It becomes a virulent infection in the elderly or immunocompromised host and can progress rapidly. Aided by the many endo- and exotoxins possessed by the microbe and its propensity to cause vasculitis as well as pneumonitis, *Pseudomonas* can be destructive to tissue. If *Pseudomonas* is judged to be a reasonable infectious cause, initial antibiotic coverage must be adequate for *Pseudomonas* until culture results rule out this etiology. Concomitant septicemia with pneumonia have to be considered. If gram-negative sepsis exists, a nonpulmonary nidus of infection is likely (urinary tract or bowel), and the resulting pulmonary infection is from metastatic seeding and a secondary problem. Attention has to be directed to treating the primary source. Urosepsis and *E. coli* pneumonia often are coupled in this way.

For therapy of a newly diagnosed nosocomial pneumonia, the initial antibiotic combination should include an aminoglycoside and a semisynthetic broad-spectrum penicillin to cover the aerobic gram-negative rods. If a component of aspiration is evident, pencillin G or clindamycin should be given, too. The need for antistaphylococcal coverage also must be weighed. Gentamicin is preferable because of its broad activity and good general efficacy, plus the desire to save other aminoglycosides for later use, should resistance to gentamicin develop. However, this initial choice of gentamicin is contingent upon the likelihood that *Pseudomonas aeruginosa* infection exists and upon the status of the medical unit where the patient is located (potential of microbial resistance). A loading dose of 1 mg per kilogram IV is given, followed by doses of about 1.7 mg per kilogram every 8 hours. Intermittent (given over 30 minutes, diluted in saline or 5 percent dextrose solution), not continuous, intravenous administration is preferred. The aim is a daily total of about 5 mg per kilogram per day, assuming that the patient has normal renal function. After 2 or 3 days at this high dose, it is scaled down to 3 mg per kilogram per day total dose for the duration of therapy, which is usually 7 to 10 days. However, if *Pseudomonas* is a likely possibility from the start, tobramycin is the better choice because it is more potent on a weight basis against this bacterial species. After a loading dose of 1 mg per kilogram IV, subsequent doses of 1.7 mg per kilogram are given every 8 hours for a total daily dose of 5 mg per kilogram. This total dose should be reduced to 3 mg per kilogram daily in several days for the duration of treatment, which is also 7 to 10 days. As all aminoglycosides are excreted by the kidneys, nephrotoxicity can occur. With renal insufficiency, the daily dose in terms of amount and frequency of administration must be adjusted according to the degree of renal impairment. Nomograms and formulas based on serum creatinine and/or urine creatinine clearance must be consulted to determine the appropriate dose. After gentamicin or tobramycin therapy is underway for about 48 hours, the peak level (serum sample obtained at completion of dose) and a trough level (before next dose) should be measured. It is desirable not to exceed 12 μg per milliliter at the peak. It is important to know the trough value for it gives a clue to how well antibiotic levels are maintained between doses. The lower value should be at least 4 μg per milliliter to ensure continuous bactericidal activity against the gram-negative rods. Generally, these organisms are sensitive to a mean inhibitory concentration of 2 to 4 μg per milliliter or less.

Amikacin should not be used in the initial antibiotic combination unless specific microbial resistance is known and dictates its use because this is the back-up, last-resort aminoglycoside. This antibiotic does not perform better than the others discussed, but it is likely to be active if resistance to gentamicin and tobramycin has developed. If possible, it should be reserved for use in the immunocompromised patient or the patient with cystic fibrosis who may have repeated respiratory infections with *Pseudomonas*. When used, amikacin is given in three divided doses for a total daily dose of 15 mg per kilogram. The same caution about renal toxicity and side effects applies for amikacin as for the other aminglycosides.

As the choice for a broad-spectrum semisynethetic penicillin, mezlocillin is now preferred to the others listed in this category. It is a bactericidal antibiotic with a potent and impressive range of activity against important gram-positive and gram-negative bacteria. With an aminoglycoside it gives a synergistic effect against *Pseudomonas aeruginosa, Klebsiella pneumoniae*, and perhaps *Serratia*. One of these broad-spectrum penicillins is a necessity in patients with granulocytopenia, if they are to have a reasonable chance of survival. In a lethal granulocytopenic canine model of *Pseudomonas aeruginosa* pneumonia, we found that the combination of carbenicillin and gentamicin gave a survival rate of about 70 percent, almost comparable to that attained with daily granulocyte transfusions (90%); use of gentamicin alone resulted in mortality of all infected dogs. This continues to be my clinical impression of this excellent antibiotic group. Whereas the original antibiotics in this category, carbenicillin and ticarcillin provide good activity, mezlocillin has several desirable qualities that make it preferable. Mezlocillin is more active against streptococci and *Haemophilus influenzae*; it inhibits more Klebsiella isolates at lower concentrations than the others; it is the least likely of the broad-spectrum penicillins to alter bleeding times; and it is relatively low in its sodium content. The intravenous dose is 200 to 300 mg per kilogram per day given in four divided doses (or about 4 g every 6 hours). In cases of renal failure, the dose intervals should be lengthened to 8- to 12-hour intervals.

Finally, the question arises whether a cephalosporin should be used as a single drug or in combination with an aminoglycoside in the treatment of one of the serious gram-negative pneumonias under consideration —*Pseudomonas, Klebsiella*, or *Serratia*. The combination of cephalothin and gentamicin has been an acceptable one for *Klebsiella pneumoniae* for some time and needs to be evaluated only because of microbial resistance to these two antibiotics or because better drug choices exist. As mentioned, the first-generation cephalosporins have some activity against gram-negative organisms that might be considered adequate (*E. coli, Klebsiella pneumoniae*, and *Proteus mirabilis*), and this activity is more potent in the second- and third-generation cephalosporins. Only a subset of third-generation agents are active against *Pseudomonas aeruginosa*, and the clinical experience with them is still limited. One advantage of these cephalosporins is their effectiveness as an alternative antibiotic for the patient with penicillin allergy in whom there is a reasonable possibility that cross-reactions are unlikely. In my judgment, they should be used in combination with an aminoglycoside and not relied on as a single agent. This is especially true for primary *Klebsiella pneumoniae* respiratory infection. For *Pseudomonas* pneumonia, sole use of cefoperazone would seem to be insufficient, and the drug should be combined with an aminoglycoside; whether the substitution of cefoperazone for mezlocillin in the combination already discussed is equally good will need further laboratory and clinical assessment.

Once the patient's therapy is under way, the physician cannot relax, but must remain alert for complications that can develop. A resurgence of fever after an initial period of defervescence is a frequent clue. One of a number of problems could be the cause. Poor coughing and an accumulation of secretions or a mucous plug can obstruct an airway, leading to partial collapse of a lung lobe or segment. Vigorous postural drainage and endotracheal suction may remove secretions and help to re-expand the lung portion and should be tried, if possible, for 24 hours before resorting to bronchoscopy. The development of loculated pleural fluid could be the cause and usually requires thoracentesis and possibly chest tube drainage. Secondary bacterial infection or superinfection occurring after broad-spectrum antimicrobial therapy may cause fever and worsening of the patient's condition; thus, reculturing sputum and blood is necessary. Drug allergy causing mild blood eosinophilia and lingering fever is a frequent and often unsuspected complication that requires discontinuation or substitution in the antibiotic regimen. Finally, complete resolution of the pneumonic process or closure of a lung abscess, for example, must be observed, for failure of this part of the healing phase may require additional attention. Cytologic examination of sputum and bronchoscopic examination might be indicated to rule out a partially obstructing airway lesion or endobronchial tumor.

SUGGESTED READING

Matthay RA, Moritz ED. Invasive procedures for diagnosing pulmonary infection. Clin Chest Med (Reynolds HY, Editor) 1981; 2:3–18.

Niederman MS, Raferty TD, Sasaki CT, Merrill WW, Mattay RA, Reynold HY. Comparison of bacterial adherence to ciliated and squamous epithelial cells obtained from the human respiratory tract. Am Rev Respir Dis 1983; 127:85–90.

Reynolds HY. Pneumonia due to *Klebsiella* (Chapter 263). In: Wyngaarden JB, Smith LH (eds). Cecil's Textbook of Medicine. 17th ed. Philadelphia: WB Saunders, 1985, pp. 1509–1510.

Reynolds HY. Pneumonia caused by aerobic gram-negative bacilli (*Pseudomonas, Escherichia coli, Serratia*) (Chapter 264.) In: Wyngaarden JB, Smith LH (eds). Cecil's Textbook of Medicine. 17th ed. Philadelphia: WB Saunders, 1985, pp. 1510–1513.

Reynolds HY. Aspiration pneumonia (Chapter 265). In: Wyngaarden JB, Smith LH (eds). Cecil's Textbook of Medicine. 17th ed. Philadelphia: WB Saunders, 1985, pp. 1513–1516.

Wolfson JS, Swartz MN. Drug therapy: serum bactericidal activity as a monitor of antibiotic therapy. N Engl J Med 1985, 312:968–975.

ANAEROBIC BACTERIAL PULMONARY INFECTION

GERARD J. SHEEHAN, M.B., M.R.C.P.I.
ALLAN R. RONALD, M.D., F.R.C.P.(C), F.A.C.P.

Anaerobic lung infections generally present as an aspiration pneumonia, a necrotizing pneumonia, a lung abscess, or an empyema. These syndromes blend into each other and one may evolve to another, depending on the stage of the illness at diagnosis and the interaction of therapy and host defenses. With the exception of *Fusobacterium necrophorum*, a rare pathogen now but common in the pre-antibiotic era, the virulence of the infecting organism is not an important determinant of the course of the illness. In about 90 percent of cases, a recognizable underlying predisposition is found, most important of which are gross aspiration (or predisposition to aspiration), peridontal disease, and pulmonary neoplasm or infarction. Thus, patients with community-acquired infections commonly have alcoholism, epilepsy, or drug overdoses. Patients with hospital-acquired infections often have aerobic gram-negative rods and *Staphylococcus aureus* as copathogens; they frequently present with a more virulent illness and require different concomitant therapy.

The usual community-acquired anaerobic pulmonary infection presents with a history of gradually worsening cough, purulent foul-smelling sputum, anorexia, weight loss, and sometimes hemoptysis and pleuritic chest pain. The illness has often been present for weeks or even months and may mimic cancer. Physical findings are those of pneumonia and pleural effusion, along with those of the underlying prediposition. Sometimes amphoric breath sounds associated with a large abscess cavity are heard. The chest film shows an infiltrate or an abscess cavity, most commonly in the dependent portions of the lung. Anemia and other laboratory evidence of chronic inflammatory disease are often present. Attempts to isolate the anaerobic pathogens by culture of sputum should not be made because of inevitable contamination from the oropharyngeal flora. However, sputum culture is useful at excluding other causes of necrotizing pneumonia such as aerobic gram-negative rods and *S. aureus*. Cultures of lower respiratory secretions obtained by transtracheal aspiration reliably identify the multiple anaerobic and facultative organisms involved, but are not generally advocated as a diagnosis can be made on clinical and radiologic grounds alone. Bacteremia occurs in less than 10 percent of cases, and the blood isolate may only be one of several pulmonary pathogens. In general, culture of empyema fluid yields reliable microbiologic data.

The anaerobes most commonly isolated are *Fusobacterium nucleatum, Bacteroides melaninogenicus, Bacteroides fragilis* group, *Bacteroides gracilis*, and anaerobic streptococci. *B. fragilis* is generally resistant to penicillin, and in recent years, *B. melaninogenicus* has also been resistant in 40 percent of patients. With few exceptions, the anaerobic flora of pulmonary abscesses is susceptible to clindamycin. *Bacteroides* species are uniformly susceptible to metronidazole, but this drug is ineffective against the facultative aerobic organisms such as streptococci and peptostreptococci. Cefoxitin is effective against 80 to 90 percent of *Bacteroides* species, as well as the facultative flora, but cannot be prescribed orally. Essentially all anaerobic pulmonary pathogens are sensitive to chloramphenicol, but its hematologic toxicity precludes its use except for very ill patients. Some third-generation cephalosporins such as moxalactam are active against most anaerobic flora, but its expense, requirement for intravenous administration and lack of in vivo proof of clinical efficacy preclude its routine use. Similarly, the antipseudomonas penicillins (carbenicillin, ticarcillin, piperacillin, azlocillin, and mezlocillin) are all active against anaerobes when used in high doses, but are not ordinarily prescribed for this indication. Thus, the antibiotic regimens that are generally used for anaerobic pulmonary infections are penicillin alone, clindamycin alone, or a combination of penicillin and metronidazole.

MANAGEMENT

The patient should be admitted to the hospital and a clinical and radiologic evaluation obtained along with aerobic culture of sputum. Features suggestive of other etiologies of lung necrosis should be sought (such as aerobic gram-negative rods, *S. aureus, Mycobacterium tuberculosos*), especially in patients without predisposition to anaerobic lung abscess. Underlying carcinoma of the lung should be suspected in smokers, in patients with hemoptysis, and in those who are edentulous. In typical patients with putrid sputum, invasive techniques to obtain lower respiratory tract secretions are not indicated. These should be considered for those who are critically ill with atypical clinical features or who fail to respond to appropriate therapy.

Antibiotics

Clindamycin is the preferred antibiotic regimen; it is initially given intravenously, 450 mg every 6 hours, until defervescence, abolition of putrid sputum, and return of the patient's sense of well-being. This generally takes 1 week or less, at which time therapy can be altered to clindamycin, 150 mg PO four times a day, and continued until 6 weeks of therapy have been completed. Clindamycin is well tolerated intravenously without causing thrombophlebitis and is well absorbed orally (90%), with only rare instances of upper gastrointestinal upset. In the 1970s it was implicated as the major cause of pseudomembranous colitis. These initial cases had a significant morbidity and some mortality. The syndrome is now known to be associated with the penicillins, particularly ampicillin, and many other antibiotics, and its cause has been defined as superinfection due to *Clostridium difficile*. It occurs in 0.01 to 10 percent of clindamycin-treated patients. It is not directly related to dose and may occur after oral or parenteral therapy. It may begin during, or as long as several weeks following, a course of clindamycin. The toxin of *C. difficile* can be detected in the stool in nearly all patients with pseudomembranous colitis and in about 20 percent of those with antibiotic-associated diarrhea. Clindamycin-associated diarrhea readily responds to withdrawal of the drug. In such patients, we generally switch therapy to a combination of penicillin, 1 million units every 4 hours, and metronidazole, 500 mg every 8 hours IV. Diarrhea should be investigated with *C. difficile* cultures and toxin, and sigmoidoscopy is indicated if it persists for 48 hours or more after clindamycin is discontinued. Because of heightened awareness of diarrhea and alteration of antibiotics early in its course, pseudomembranous colitis is no longer a serious impediment to the use of clindamycin. Minor elevations of transaminases are commonly reported with clindamycin, especially with parenteral administration, but some of these are false-positive reactions due to use of a colorimetric method. However, rare cases of frank hepatotoxicity with jaundice have been reported. Similarly, allergic reactions such as skin rash, fever, anaphylaxis, or erythema multiforme have rarely been reported.

Immediately following an intravenous infusion of 450 mg of clindamycin, serum levels of 8 μg per milliliter are achieved. After single oral doses of 150 mg, peak levels are 2.5 μg per milliliter, and at 6 hours, 0.7 μg per milliliter. Most relevant anaerobic species are inhibited by concentrations less than 2 μg per milliliter. The half-life is 2.4 hours. Significant dose modifications are indicated only for patients with combined severe renal and hepatic impairment as the drug is inactivated in the liver. Clindamycin has been shown to concentrate in polymorphonuclear leukocytes and macrophages, and is present in relatively high concentrations in relation to peak serum values in experimental abscess.

In a recent prospective randomized trial of therapy for lung abscess, clindamycin was shown to be superior to penicillin (Table 1). There were two major problems with this study: (1) The low numbers recruited (39 patients from 8 centers), suggesting a possible bias in selection, and (2) the definition of failure, which was based on an absence of improvement after 10 days of therapy. In the older trials that proved the efficacy of penicillin, fever persisting beyond 10 days was not uncommon, and did not predict ultimate failure. However, statistically significant differences between the two antibiotics were demonstrated in (1) response of fever (4.4 vs 7.6 days), (2) disappearance of foul sputum (4.2 vs 8 days), and (3) overall failure rate (7 of 20 patients treated with penicillin and 0 of 19 patients treated with clindamycin). It is possible that some of the seven patients who failed with penicillin treatment could have been cured by penicillin if radiologic deterioration occurring in the first few days were ignored, if a longer course were given, or if persistent fever beyond 10 days were ignored. The older data showed response occurring beyond 10 days in five of 35 patients receiving penicillin. Thus, clindamycin is superior to penicillin in terms of failure rate, morbidity, and length of hospital stay. A combination of penicillin and metronidazole, given intravenously, may be as efficacious as, or perhaps superior to, clindamycin alone. However, owing to the potential adverse effects, we believe that selection of two drugs is not justified. The combination should only be used for patients who have overwhelming sepsis due to anaerobes or in the rare case in which a virulent *Fusobacterium necrophorum* is thought to be involved. This organism should be considered when pulmonary abscesses are occurring in association with widespread head and neck anaerobic infection and septic thrombophlebitis with emboli.

TABLE 1 Comparison of Treatment Response Between Treatment Groups

Treatment Response	*Penicillin*	*Clindamycin*
Duration of fever (>38.3 °C rectal)	7.6±1.4 days	4.4±0.8 days
Duration of fetid sputum	8.0±1.2 days	4.2±0.6 days
Patients with failed treatment after 10 days	4/20	0/19
Persistent fever	1	
Pulmonary lesions	1	
Empyema	2	
Patients with failed treatment after 10 to 21 days	2/11	0/13
Patients with relapse less than 1 month after therapy		
3-week course	1/4	0/7
6-week course	0/5	0/6

From Levison et al. Ann Intern Med 1983; 98:466–471.

Physiotherapy

Physiotherapy is an important adjunct in maintaining adequate drainage through the bronchial tree. Using auscultatory and radiologic findings, the therapist can determine the optimal position for drainage from the infected area and augment such drainage by percussion and vibration.

LUNG ABSCESS

Necrotizing anaerobic pneumonia, a variant of lung abscess, is characterized by a more rapid course, greater systemic toxicity, and multi-lobe involvement, sometimes bilateral, with cavities smaller than 2 cm (radiologically). There is usually an accompanying empyema. The course is such that an organized fibrotic abscess capsule does not form. Most of these cases are adequately managed with clindamycin alone, provided aerobic pathogens are excluded by sputum culture. In the occasional patient with a particularly virulent course, we may elect to use penicillin and metronidazole intravenously.

Surgical therapy for lung abscesses is generally contraindicated, as a cure can be obtained by antibiotics alone, and drainage occurs spontaneously through the tracheobronchial tree. Furthermore, there is a hazard of intrabronchial spread of infection or even drowning during surgery due to spillage of pus from large abscess cavities. Surgical management is indicated only for those with underlying carcinoma, massive or chronically recurring hemoptysis, and empyema (to be discussed). Surgery rarely is justified in the patient who remains critically ill after 2 to 3 weeks of appropriate antibiotics, and whose drainage through the tracheobronchial tree is impaired by diminished cough reflex. Late roentgenographical resolution was a common indication for surgery in the treatment of lung abscess in the 1950s, but can no longer be justified. Bronchoscopic evaluation is indicated in patients suspected of carcinoma or other forms of obstruction such as aspiration of a foreign body, and in those with hemoptysis. Massive hemoptysis of more than 200 ml per day can be life-threatening, and in such patients urgent bronchoscopic evaluation is indicated, along with pulmonary or bronchial angiography in selected patients. Clotting defects should be sought and corrected. Emergency lobectomy should be considered when bleeding is sufficient to require transfusion.

EMPYEMA

Empyema may occur in association with necrotizing pneumonia or abscess. Its presence is indicated by gross pus, organisms seen on the Gram stain, a pH of less than 7.2, a low glucose concentration, or an LDH greater than 1,000. Our practice is to insert a thoracostomy tube as soon as such a diagnosis is established. This is invariably effective in the early exudative phase, and at this stage, open drainage should be avoided as it leads to collapse of the lung. We generally continue drainage for 10 to 14 days, and when the effusion is less than 50 milliliters, we slowly withdraw the tube. As the fibropurulent phase develops, closed-tube drainage may not suffice. In about one-quarter of cases, either open drainage with rib resection or surgical resection of the pleural space (empyemectomy) is indicated. Since the former requires 3 to 4 months to heal, the latter is preferred in selected younger patients who are good surgical risks and have large thick-walled cavities. A bronchopleural fistula may close spontaneously if it is small, but a large fistula requires appropriate surgical management such as the use of a muscle flap.

Studies of the natural history of anaerobic lung abscess in the preantibiotic era showed that about one-third died, one-third developed chronic debilitating disease, and one-third recovered. With modern therapy and evaluation, the vast majority of patients achieve a cure without complications. Failure of therapy is often related to poor compliance, to underlying disease, or to complications that had begun before antimicrobials were initiated. Scars or thin-walled cavities may persist for years on roentgenographs but have no consequence. Rarely, mycetomas may form and require surgical excision for resultant hemoptysis.

SUGGESTED READING

Bartlett JG, Gorbach SL. Penicillin or clindamycin for primary lung abscess? Ann Intern Med 1983; 98:546.

Finegold SM. Respiratory tract and other thoracic infections. In: Anaerobic bacteria in human disease. Chapter 9. New York: Academic Press, 1977, pp 223.

Levison ME, Mangura CT, Lorber B, Abrutyn E, Pesanti EL, Levy RS, Macgregor RR, Schwartz AR. Clindamycin compared with penicillin for the treatment of anaerobic lung abscess. Ann Intern Med 1983; 98:466–471.

Mandell GL, Douglas RG, Bennett JE. Principles and practice of infectious diseases. 2nd ed. New York: Wiley, 1985.

NOSOCOMIAL PULMONARY INFECTION

JAY P. SANFORD, M.D.

Pneumonia is considered to be nosocomial if the clinical and radiographic onset is 48 or more hours after the patient's admission to the hospital.

ETIOLOGIES

The nature of the patient's underlying disease and treatment are major factors in determining the etiology of such pneumonias. Unique environmental conditions may impose additional important etiologic considerations; for example, legionnaires' disease is far more prevalent in some hospitals than in others, and aspergillosis is a more common cause of opportunistic pulmonary infections on oncology units than on others. These differences are illustrated in Table 1.

DIAGNOSIS

Gram stain and culture of expectorated sputum are still the most widely used techniques. However, contamination with oropharyngeal microorganisms significantly limits the value of the sputum culture. These limitations can be minimized if both the patient and the person collecting the specimen understand that a deep cough specimen is desired, if the patient brushes his teeth to include the surface of the tongue before the collection, and if the specimen is transported promptly to the laboratory. The laboratory should examine the specimen microscopically. If the number of squamous epithelial cells exceeds 25 per low power microscopic field, the specimen is too contaminated to allow interpretation of a smear or culture. Transtracheal aspiration (TTA) has been used as a means of avoiding pharyngeal contamination; however, even with TTA, more than one bacterial species is usually isolated and complications, although infrequent, do occur. Yet in the critically ill patient, other than the immunocompromised one who is unable to produce an expectorated sputum, TTA is the procedure of choice. In the immunocompromised patient including individuals with the acquired immunodeficiency syndrome (AIDS) more invasive techniques are required. Such techniques include fiberoptic bronchoscopy with collection of specimens using a protected specimen brush, bronchial washings, or transbronchial biopsy, direct lung aspiration, or open lung biopsy.

Blood cultures should be obtained from all patients with nosocomial pneumonia. Bacteremia occurs in one-fourth to one-half of the patients. Procedures such as counter-immunoelectrophoresis (CIEP) and coagglutination to detect antigens in sputum or urine are being developed and appear very promising.

TABLE 1 Etiology of Nosocomial Pneumonias by Clinical Epidemiologic Group

	Clinical-Epidemiologic Group (percentage)			
Microbial Etiology	*Community Hospital**	*VA Hospital†*	*Immunosuppressed Leukemia/Lymphoma Patients‡*	*Renal Transplant Patients§*
Viral	NR	NR	4	46
Bacterial	83	82	16	13
Gram-negative aerobes	27	22	12	2
Legionelliaceae	13	47	NR	0
Strep. pneumoniae	6	3	0	0
H. influenzae	17	0	0	2
Aspiration	6	9	0	6
Other	12	0	4	6
Fungal	NR	NR	12	10
Pneumocystis carinii	NR	NR	12	NR
Polymicrobial	—	—	—	31
Unknown—no specific Dx	17	18	56	NR

* 30 episodes in 28 patients. Muder et al. JAMA 1983; 249:3184.
† 32 patients. Muder et al. JAMA 1983; 249:3184.
‡ 25 patients. Singer et al. Am J Med 1979; 66:110.
§ 52 episodes. Peterson et al. Medicine 1982; 61:360.
NR = not recorded.

MANAGEMENT

Antimicrobial Therapy

Empiric treatment is usually initiated while results of sputum cultures and antibiotic sensitivity studies are awaited. Such treatment must take into consideration any microbiologic feature that is unique to the area or hospital and must be based on a knowledge of the susceptibility patterns of organisms within the specific hospital or area of the hospital. The choice of aminoglycoside (gentamicin vs. tobramycin vs. amikacin) varies, depending on the specific organisms that make up the bacterial flora of an individual hospital or specialized care unit and their resistance-susceptibility patterns. When the results of cultures and subsequent sensitivity studies are available, empiric regimens should be modified by discontinuing unneeded drugs and using the least toxic effective drugs. In the treatment of pneumonias caused by Enterobacteriaceae and Pseudomonadaceae in the critically ill patient, especially the immunocompromised, combination drug therapy is indicated.

The use of aerosolized antibiotics has been recommended by some. The evidence that they have therapeutic benefit is controversial; I do not recommend them.

Adjunct Therapy

Among nosocomial infections, nosocomial pneumonia has the highest case:fatality ratio; hence prompt diagnosis and initiation of appropriate antimicrobial and pulmonary supportive care are critical. Attention to hydration and ventilation are essential. Intermittent positive pressure breathing and chest physiotherapy have not been shown to hasten the rate of resolution.

Preventive Measures

Since most of these patients receive some type of inhalation therapy, equipment for this purpose must be protected from contamination, so that its use will not contribute to suprainfection. Most of these patients also have residual pulmonary damage, which places them at increased risk of significant morbidity and mortality from influenza and pneumococcal pneumonia. They should receive polyvalent pneumococcal vaccine at the time of discharge and annual influenza vaccine.

The following recommendations for empiric treatment are based on the radiographic pattern and various clinical-epidemiologic circumstances (Table 2). The specific antimicrobial agents that belong to the classes, dosage, and route of administration are presented in Table 3. Duration of therapy should be based on clinical response and should be continued until the patient has been afebrile approximately 7 days. Radiographic resolution usually takes much longer.

SUGGESTED READING

Gross PA, Neu HC, Aswapokee P, et al. Deaths from nosocomial infections: experience in a university hospital and a community hospital.

TABLE 2 Empirical Treatment of Nosocomial Pneumonia

Radiographic Pattern/Clinical Epidemiologic Circumstances	*Microbial Etiologies (likely)*	*Initial Empiric Antibiotic Therapy*	*Comments*
Broncho- or diffuse pneumonia "Noncompromised" (ex. COPD without tracheostomy)	*H. influenzae* *Klebsiellae pneumonia* + other enterobacteriaceae Legionelliaceae	Antipseudomonal aminoglycoside plus First generation cephalosporin plus Erythromycin	If type A influenza is epidemic, add amantadine, 100 mg orally b.i.d. If patient with legionnaires' disease is not responding in 96 hours, increase erythromycin to 1.0 g IV every 6 hours, then add rifampin 600 mg PO daily. If enterobacter, Citrobacter, Serratia, Proteus, Acinetobacter are common in your hospital setting, use second-generation cephalosporin.
Postinfluenza A virus	*Strep. pneumoniae* *Staph. aureus*	Penicillinase-resistant penicillin	If *H. influenzae* is found on sputum smear, add cefuroxime or third-generation cephalosporin (ceftazidime) or imipenem-cilastin or aztreonam or amoxicillin-clavulanic acid.
Compromised—not neutropenic (ex. COPD with tracheostomy, azotemia, adult respiratory distress syndrome)	Pseudomonadaceae Enterobacteriaceae; Enterobacter, Serratia, Proteus, Providencia, Klebsiella, Acinetobacter *Staph. aureus* (rare)	Antipseudomonal aminoglycoside plus Antipseudomonal penicillin or Third-generation cephalosporin	If pseudomonas, give antipseudomonal penicillin plus tobramycin or amikacin. If *E. coli,* Klebsiella, or Serratia: give cefotaxime plus amikacin. If enterobacter, give trimethoprim-sulfamethoxazole IV If *Staph. aureus*, give penicillinase-resistant penicillin or vancomycin. If patient is penicillin-allergic, use third-generation cephalosporin.
Compromised—neutropenic (neutropenic $<500/mm^3$) (ex. acute leukemia—induction chemotherapy)	As with non-neutropenic plus: *Pneumocystis carinii* Cytomegalovirus *Candida* sp. *Aspergillus* sp. Legionellaceae Nocardia	Antipseudomonal aminoglycoside plus Antipseudomonal penicillin plus Trimethoprim-sulfamethoxazole plus Erythromycin	If candida or fungal elements on smear or if patient does not respond in 96 hours, add amphotericin B. (Ketoconazole not as effective.) Even with isolation of a single organism, combination therapy is more effective than single drug therapy.
"Aspiration"—Mendelson's syndrome (ex. acute aspiration of gastric contents during anesthesia)	None initially, Late: compromised—not neutropenic	None or low-dose penicillin G	Bronchoscopy. Value of steroids controversial.
Abscess			
Nonputrid	Enterobacteriaceae: *E. coli*, Klebsiella, Enterobacter *Staph. aureus*	First-generation cephalosporin plus Antipseudomonal aminoglycoside	If staph. predominate on smear, substitute vancomycin, clindamycin, or penicillinase-resistant penicillin for the cephalosporin. Bronchoscopy to rule out obstruction.
Putrid	*Bacteroides* spp. (about 15% *B. fragilis*) Peptostreptococci *Fusobacterium* sp.	Clindamycin or Penicillin G (high dose) or Cefoxitin	Bronchoscopy to rule out obstruction.

TABLE 3 Classes of Antimicrobial Agents, Dosage, and Route of Administration

Class of Agent	*Specific Agents (Trade Name)*	*Usual Dosage**	*Route of Administration*
Penicillins			
—	Penicillin G	low dose: 600,000 units q12h	IM
		high dose: 5 million units q6h	IV
Penicillinase-resistant	Methicillin	2.0 g q4h	IV
	Nafcillin	1.0 g q4h	IV
	Oxacillin	1.0 g q4h	IV
Antipseudomonal	Carbenicillin	5.0 g q4h	IV
	Ticarcillin (Ticar)	3.0 g q4h	IV
	Piperacillin (Pipracil)	3.0 g q4h	IV
	Azlocillin (Azlin)	3.0 g q4h	IV
	Mezlocillin (Mezlin)	3.0 g q4h	IV
Combination with beta lactamase inhibitor	Amoxicillin-clavulamic acid (Augmentin)	0.5 g q8h	PO
Cephalosporins			
First generation	Cephalothin (Keflin)	3.0 g q6h	IV
	Cefazolin (Ancef, Kefzol)	2.0 g q6h	IV or IM
	Cephapirin (Cefadyl)	2.0 g q6h	IV
	Cephradine (Anspor, Velosef)	2.0 g q6h	IV
Second generation	Cefamandole (Mandol)	2.0 g q4h	IV
	Cefoxitin (Mefoxin)	2.0 g q4h	IV
	Cefuroxime (Zinacef)	1.5 g q6h	IV
Third generation	Cefotaxime (Claforan)	2.0 g q4h	IV
	Cefoperazone (Cefobid)	2.0 g q12h	IV
	Moxalactam (Moxam)	4.0 g q8h	IV
	Ceftazidime (Fortaz)	2.0 g q8h	IV
	Ceftizoxime (Cefizox)	4.0 g q8h	IV
Aminoglycosides	Gentamicin (Garamycin, Apogen, Bristagen)	5.0 mg/kg/day	IV
	Tobramycin (Nebcin)	4.5 mg/kg/day	IV
	Amikacin (Amikin)	15 mg/kg/day	IV
	Netimicin (Netromycin)	6.0 mg/kg/day	IV
Newer beta lactams	Aztreonam (Azactam)	2.0 g q8h	IV
	Imipenem-cilastatin (Primaxin)	1.0 g q6h	IV
Miscellaneous			
Chloramphenicol	Chloromycetin	0.5 g q6h	PO
Erythromycin	Erythromycin glucoheptonate (Ilotycin glucoheptonate)	0.5 g q6h	IV
	Erythromycin lactobionate (Erythroxin)	0.5 g q6h	IV
Trimethoprim-sulfamethoxazole	(Bactrim, Septra)	5.0 mg/kg q6h	IV
Clindamycin	(Cleocin)	600 mg q6h	IV
Amantadine	(Symmetral)	100 mg b.i.d.	PO

* The dosages presented are for adults of average size (60 to 70 kg) with normal renal and hepatic function. In elderly patients renal clearances may decrease without elevation in BUN or creatinine. Dosages are also given for nosocomial pneumonia of "life-threatening" severity.

Am J Med 1980; 68:219.

Karnad A, Alvarez S, Berk SL. Pneumonia caused by gram-negative bacilli. Am J Med (Suppl 1A) 1985; 79:61.

Parry MF, Stampleman L, Hutchinson JH et al. Waterborne Legionella bozemanii and nosocomial pneumonia in immunosuppressed patients. Ann Int Med 1985; 103:205.

Rodriguez JR, Ramirez-Ronda CH. Efficacy and safety of aztreonam versus tobramycin for aerobic gram-negative bacilli lower respiratory infections. Am J Med (Suppl 2A) 1985; 78:42.

Salata RA, Gebhart RL, Palmer DL et al. Pneumonia treated with imipenem/cilastatin. Am J Med (Suppl 6A) 1985; 78:104.

Simmons BP, Wong ES. CDC guidelines for the prevention and control of nosocomial infections. Guidelines for the prevention of nosocomial pneumonia. Am J Inf Cont 1983; 11:230.

VIRAL RESPIRATORY DISEASE

GEORGE G. JACKSON, M.D.
MARY E. RUBENIS, B.S.
ROLAND A. LEVANDOWSKI, M.D.

Viral respiratory infections are caused by many different viruses, each of which can produce a variety of clinical syndromes that overlap in clinical manifestations from one viral cause to another. Each infection is further modified by the age, constitution, and prior experience of the host. With so many variables affecting the resultant clinical illness, the diagnosis, evaluation, and treatment of viral respiratory infections are resolved by different means for different purposes depending on the epidemiology, the anatomic site of the major symptoms, and detection of the specific viral etiology. Each of these approaches provides understanding of a part of the clinical problems, the likely cause, possible treatment, and expected course of the disease. Only identification of the virus permits an accurate etiologic diagnosis and offers the possibility of specific antiviral therapy. Other treatments, including most of those in common practice, are nonspecific and consist mostly of symptomatic and supportive care.

SEASONAL EPIDEMIOLOGY OF RESPIRATORY VIRUSES

The epidemiologic patterns of occurrence of the different taxonomic groups of viruses that cause most of the acute clinical illnesses have contributed to the factual biology of the viruses. The seasonality of occurrence tends to be consistent, and the prevalence of infection may be endemic (parainfluenza 3) or epidemic with twice yearly (rhinoviruses), annual (respiratory syncytial virus, influenza A), biannual (parainfluenza 1, 2), or sporadic (influenza B, pandemic influenza A) episodes of occurrence. In the northern temperate climates, the season in which most of the viral respiratory disease occurs is from September to May. The biology of the viruses regulate this pattern to some degree, but it is augmented to a large extent by climatologic and sociologic modalities. The respiratory disease season starts with an epidemic of acute rhinovirus infections from September through November. In the beginning, the etiology of the outbreak may be pure, but in October and November, the epidemic spread of parainfluenza viruses type 1 or 2 occurs with an increase in the baseline occurrence of parainfluenza type 3. Annually a sharp outbreak of respiratory syncytial virus (RSV) infections occurs alternately in the Fall and Spring. This mixed group of respiratory viruses continues to cause infections through the early winter months. Rhinovirus infections almost disappear after the occurrence of severe cold weather, and influenza viruses make a sharply inserted midwinter appearance with some displacement of the paramyxoviruses. The peak of epidemic influenza may occur any time between early December and late February and affects school children, parents, working adults, and shut-ins, sometimes in discernible successive waves. About 80 percent of the time, the epidemic strain is influenza A, and on average, once in 5 years the cause is influenza B. A continual drift in the surface antigens, hemagglutinin (HA) and neuraminidase (NA), characterizes influenza viruses. Pandemics tend to occur in 10- to 15-year cycles, based on the emergence of a strain with a major antigenic shift; the last major antigenic shift in influenza A virus was H_3N_2 in 1968. In the years when respiratory syncytial virus (RSV) does not appear in November, the epidemic occurs in the following February. These myxoviruses (influenza A and B) and paramyxoviruses (parainfluenza and RSV) continue to cause sporadic infections into the Spring. By March or April, influenza has disappeared, and in April or May, a second wave of rhinovirus infections occurs. Infectious summer colds are usually caused by a rhinovirus or parainfluenza 3. Adenoviruses types 3, 4, 7, 14, and 21 cause up to 5 percent of acute respiratory infections in civilian populations which, during the summer, may be asymptomatic. Occasional outbreaks of adenoviral disease occur in school dormitories. In military recruit camps, adenovirus infections become endemic, infect almost all recruits, and account for a large amount of acute respiratory disease. Some types of Coxsackie A and B and ECHO viruses cause respiratory infections, usually in the summer months. Coronaviruses and influenza C can be related to outbreaks of common colds in the winter. Reoviruses and perhaps several other viruses cause asymptomatic infections of the respiratory tract. Herpesviruses are commonly recovered from respiratory secretions during an acute infection, but they are not considered to be primary in the cause of disease other than ulcerative stomatitis. Viral respiratory infections with systemic manifestations such as EBV, measles, varicella, and others replicate in the mucosal cells of the respiratory tract and cause local as well as systemic symptoms. They can be clinically differentiated from the common causes of acute respiratory infections. Mycoplasmal pneumonia must be differentiated from pneumonia of viral origin, and *Chlamydia* can cause bronchiolitis of newborns resembling viral infections.

SYNDROMES BY ANATOMIC SITES

The anatomic site of the main symptoms of infection has a correlation with the viral etiology, but the site of infection does not permit a reliable etiologic diagnosis. The exception is that during an epidemic in which the viral cause has been demonstrated, the clinical diagnosis can be specific with about 70 percent accuracy. The clinical description of common infections is divided into categoric anatomic diagnoses as upper respiratory infection (URI) including the common cold with coryza and nasopharyngitis, acute laryngitis (croup), bronchitis/bronchiolitis, pneumonia, and febrile respiratory disease with respiratory and systemic symptoms (flu).

The relation of these syndromes to the most common respiratory viruses is illustrated in Figure 1. Each syndrome represents an acute infection with a short incubation period of 1 to 3 days. During this time and preceding the onset of symptoms, infectious virus can be found in the respiratory tract secretions. With influenza, viremia may occur, but it is of short duration and usually disappears before the abrupt onset of clinical disease occurs.

The virus replicates in permissive cells of the respiratory tract, involving an increasing area of the airway. The difference in temperature between the anterior nares, 33^{-}C, and the distal bronchioles, 37^{+}C, and perhaps also the density and histologic arrangement of virus-susceptible cells influence the locality in which viral replication occurs most rapidly and achieves the highest titers. The amount of virus collected in washings of respiratory secretions usually is between 10^2 and 10^5 tissue culture infectious doses. In the normal respiratory tract, the secretions contain no plasma proteins except albumen and no cellular or humoral products of inflammation. In the initial asymptomatic phase of infection, serum globulins begin to appear in the secretions followed transiently by polymorphonuclear leukocytes, and then with increasing symptoms, all components of the serum, lymphocytes, interferon, secretory mucus, antibody, and other immunoreactive products appear along with exfoliated cells of the respiratory mucosa. Sometimes, especially with influenza, there is hemorrhagic denudation at the site of infection. The time relation of some of these events, as observed in influenza in volunteers, is shown in Figure 2.

In the peripheral blood there is transient lymphopenia with specific reduction of T-helper cells. In influenza and perhaps other respiratory viral infections, a reversal of cell-mediated delayed dermal hypersensitivity occurs. The cause and effect relation between the symptoms and the sequence of virologic and immunologic manifestation is not entirely clear. The replication of virus that initiates the process is initially asymptomatic, and the virus titer, although usually related to the severity of disease, does not uniformly parallel the symptomatology. Interferon is delayed in appearance following the onset of symptoms and declines following the decrease of symptoms. From these temporal relations, its production could cause, reflect, or ameliorate the symptoms. Clinical improvement has almost always occurred before a demonstrable rise of antibody in the secretions or serum. The antibody in the secretions may be secretory IgA, IgM, or IgG. The appearance of antibody is correlated with the termination of virus shedding.

Laryngeal stridor (croup) and bronchiolitis are dangerous pathophysiologic consequences of infection with parainfluenza viruses 1 and 2 and RSV respectively. Respiratory insufficiency and pneumonia of viral

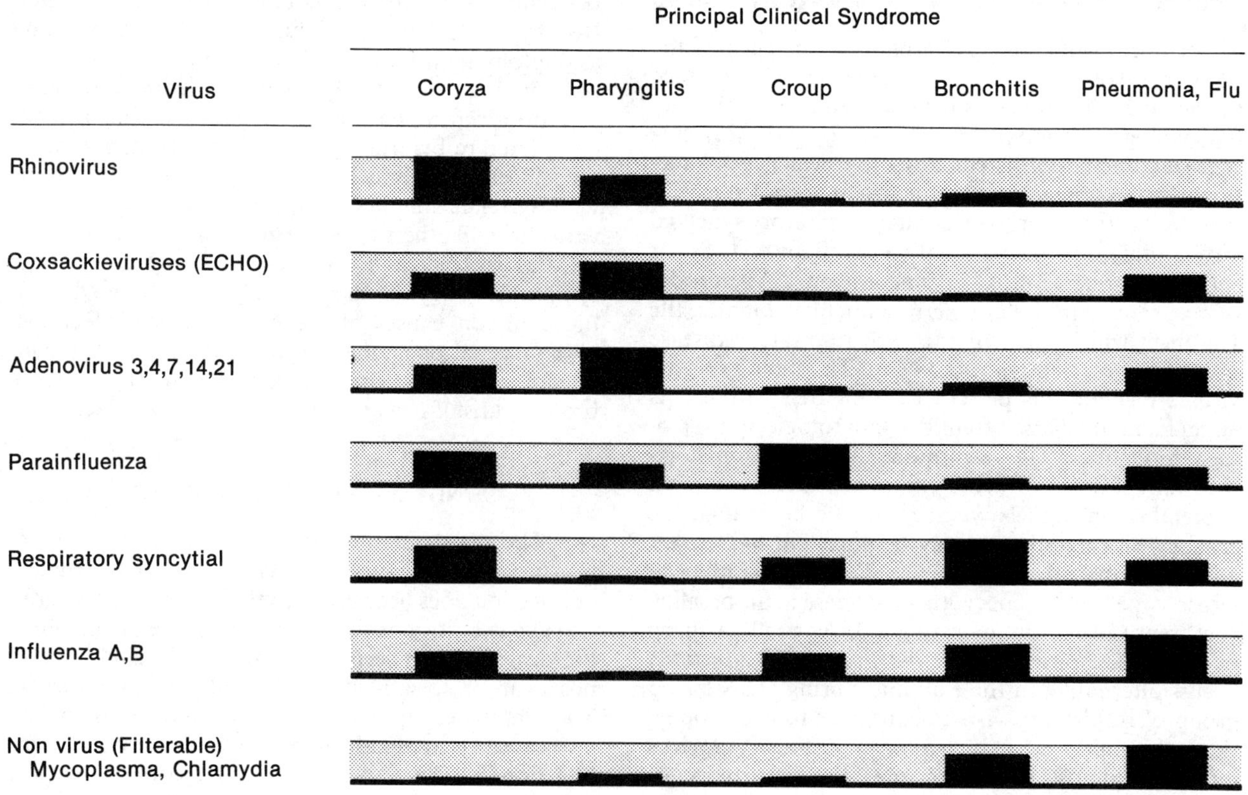

Principal Clinical Syndrome

Virus — Coryza — Pharyngitis — Croup — Bronchitis — Pneumonia, Flu

Rhinovirus

Coxsackieviruses (ECHO)

Adenovirus 3,4,7,14,21

Parainfluenza

Respiratory syncytial

Influenza A,B

Non virus (Filterable)
Mycoplasma, Chlamydia

Figure 1 Schematic representation of the relative frequency of different clinical manifestations of respiratory infection with particular viruses.

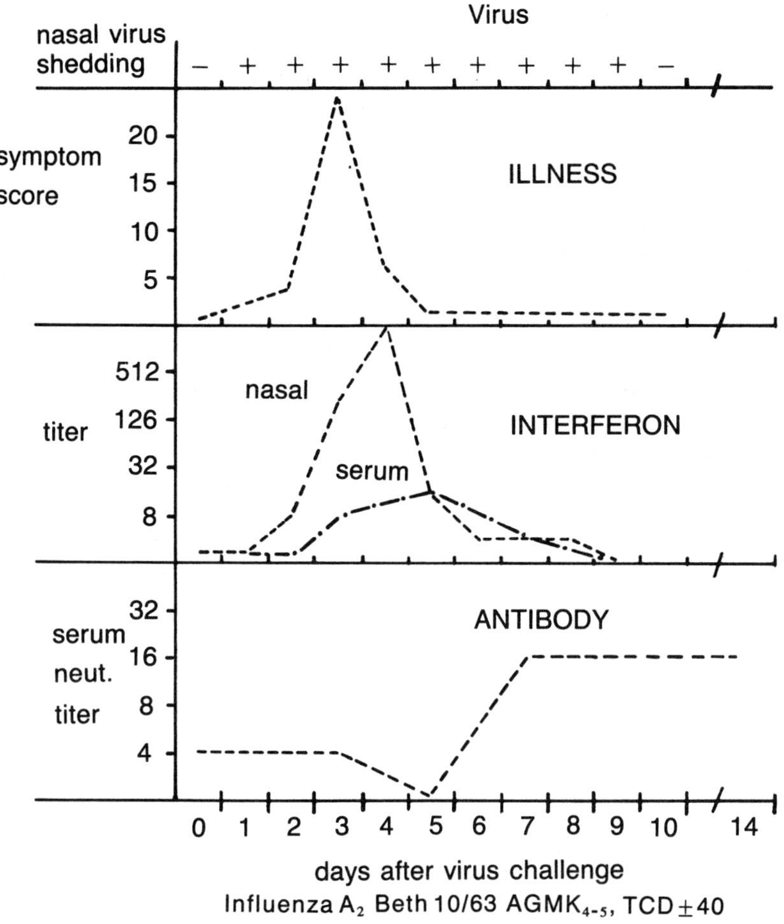

Figure 2 Characteristics of viral respiratory infection in volunteers.

and/or bacterial cause complicate influenza. Infection with parainfluenza 3 is a common cause of "walking pneumonia." Although rhinoviruses infrequently cause systemic manifestations, they can provoke asthma and produce altered ciliary function of the lower respiratory tree. The latter is most disturbed in influenza. The nature and effect of the disruption in the numbers and functions of immunoreactive cells that occurs during the acute viral infection is still mostly in the descriptive phase of investigation. The early changes may be pathogenic in producing symptoms, and the later changes components of the curative immune response. What relation, if any, the immune responses have to the apparent increased susceptibility to bacterial infections in the convalescent phase is unknown. If the transient acquired immune insufficiency persists into the convalescent period, reactivation of latent infections (e.g., herpes and tuberculosis) can be observed in some persons.

DIAGNOSIS

Most of the viral respiratory infections cause only a brief period of acute morbidity with a benign outcome. Thus, the justification for more than a categoric diagnosis and nonspecific symptomatic treatment, except for influenza and RSV, has not been compelling or cost-effective. Specific viral diagnosis heretofore has been done mostly for research and epidemiologic purposes. Surveillance of influenza is done by the U.S. Public Health Service and WHO. Different research groups have provided data about the prevalence and specific etiology of some of the other types of respiratory infections. Now the increasing availability of virology laboratories, the accomplishment of rather complete classification of the respiratory viruses, the standardization and simplification of viral diagnostic methods, and the development of useful virus-specific antiviral drugs all promise increasing need and application of rapid specific viral diagnosis of patients with acute viral respiratory infections.

Classically, specific diagnosis is made by recovery of the virus from respiratory secretions in tissue cultures or embryonated eggs and demonstration of a fourfold or greater rise in the titer of specific antibody in the convalescent phase serum. Virus isolation permits characterization of the strain, including recognition of antigenic drift and drug resistance. Therefore, it remains the fundamental standard for an etiologic diagnosis. However, classic virologic and serologic methods do not satisfy the clinical need for rapid diagnosis with a high level of sensitivity as well as selectivity. To satisfy the need for rapid specific diagnosis, methods using the technology of fluorescent antibody, biotin-avidin conjugation of specific antisera, and enzyme-linked immunoabsorbent antigen-antibody reactions are being developed and are available for RSV and influenza. In addition to early detection, these methods approach the sensitivity of virus isolation with high specificity. Methods that further increase the sensitivity of antigen detection are desirable and necessary for early diagnosis in one-third of the patients. Hybridization blots using labeled specific probes and kinetic assays for enzyme-specific products have the promise of meeting this need. Whether or not we will see wide application of molecular diagnostic technology for the rapid specific viral diagnosis of respiratory viruses will depend on the cost and utility of the information gained and the capability for specific treatment.

MANAGEMENT

Nonspecific Treatment

Most of the experience with the treatment of viral respiratory infections is nonspecific, testimonial, uncontrolled, and, in a scientific sense, unevaluable—partly because of the nature of the problem. The variability in the number and virulence of the viruses, the sites and pathologic manifestations of different syndromes, and the effects of specific host modification make trials of therapeutic measures difficult and rife with artifacts as the basis for conclusion. The only animal model for controlled therapeutic studies that has been useful is for influenza. Proper, moral, ethical, and economic considerations prevent many controlled observations in humans. It is also difficult to disprove treatment regimens that are ineffective. In this milieu there is much room for opinion and individual experience that is meaningful in limited application, but much effort has gone into the proclamation of ideas or products with inconclusive data and of doubtful value with the hope for fame or profit. Topical inactivators of viruses (e.g., treated tissues, sprays), products for increased host resistance (e.g., vitamins, including ascorbic acid), various host remedial measures (e.g., antihistamines and minerals), and symptomatic remedies (e.g., aspirin, decongestants, mucolytics, secretion inhibitors, antitussive agents, expectorants) have been developed or recommended and may be applicable at particular times for special persons and specific symptoms, but they are without any general value in the prevention and management of viral respiratory infections. Zinc gluconate, specic amino acids, and other substances are sometimes claimed by faddists to have an antiviral effect. Even if this is true, they have no clinical value. The short benign course of most of these illnesses requires absolute assurance that the treatment will "do no harm." In spite of the difficult constraints on the treatment of viral respiratory infections and the unavailability or deficient use of immunoprophylaxis (for influenza), the prevalence of the infections in all ages and classes of people and their severity with life-threatening or fatal effects in some demand a continued effort for improved specific management. The increasing availability of selective, safe, and effective prophylactic and treatment measures marks progress in this direction with a promise of increasing success.

Supportive Treatment

Recognizing the need for, and maintaining, an adequate patent airway and minimizing anoxia are the paramount objectives of nonspecific treatment of acute viral respiratory infections. In infants and children, the problem is far greater than in adults. The physician must be alert to the potential need and prepare for intubation or tracheotomy to bypass laryngeal obstruction and decrease dead space in the airway. Specific measures for other pathophysiologic manifestations such as excessive fever and dehydration may be necessary, and attention to supportive measures to provide rest and promote the comfort of the patient is desirable. High humidity created by a cold water vaporizer has generally been considered useful in decreasing laryngeal spasm and liquefying secretions in croup.

Specific Treatment

The control and management of specific viral respiratory infections should be considered in terms of immunoprophylaxis, chemoprophylaxis, and therapy.

Immunoprophylaxis for Influenza

Inactivated influenza virus vaccine is effective in preventing the currently circulating strains of influenza A, H_1N_1, H_3N_2, and influenza B. After 17 years without a major antigenic shift in the H_3 hemagglutinin and 28 years for the N_2 neuraminidase of influenza A viruses, most persons have been exposed to these antigens. Influenza A, H_1N_1 was prevalent prior to 1957 and then reappeared in 1977. People over 25 years of age had a prior primary exposure, but in younger persons who have not been vaccinated or have not had natural infection since 1977, successive primary and booster doses of vaccine are indicated. Annual immunization is recommended to produce a booster response and heighten protection. The vaccines can be used with a high degree of confidence that they will be at least 70 percent effective in preventing influenza of the present types.

The formulation of the vaccine is reviewed annually and changes made to match the antigenic character of the prevalent strains. Inactivated trivalent vaccines contain 15 μg of each of three hemagglutinin antigens H_1, H_3 and B per 0.5-ml dose. A single subcutaneous or intradermal dose elicits an adequate antibody response in 90 percent of vaccine recipients. Intradermal injection of 0.1 ml has sometimes been used as a booster, but it has no advantages and some drawbacks. The present inactivated vaccines have limitations imposed by (1) the number and amount of antigens that can be included without eliciting an unacceptable reaction and (2) the short duration of a strain-specific response. The character of the antibody elicited is affected by the prior immunologic experience of the person vaccinated. These conditions require annual or nearly annual reimmunization. Attenuated live virus vaccines have been developed and are expected to bring about a broader longer-lasting response, easy modification of the antigens, and acceptable reimmunization, but they are not approved for widespread use. The purity of the present vaccines has greatly diminished the occurrence of adverse local and systemic reactions. With the recommended dose, only 10 to 15 percent of recipients have a noticeable local reaction and about 1 percent of adults have fever and systemic symptoms. For children who are more prone to significant febrile reactions, split-hemagglutinin vaccine is recommended. The Guillian-Barré syndrome, which may have been associated with the swine flu antigen, has not been associated with the vaccine preparations used since 1976 and not considered to be a risk with currently recommended vaccines. The vaccines are prepared from viruses grown in embryonated eggs, and a high degree of hypersensitivity to eggs is a contraindication to vaccination.

The use of influenza vaccine is specifically directed toward protection of the individual recipient and not as a general public health measure to decrease transmission of influenza. People who are recognized to be at high risk of acquiring severe influenza are categorized in Table 1. In the high-risk groups, immunization with influenza vaccine not only decreases the rate of influenza infection, but also appears to reduce the number of hospitalizations for any cause, including decompensation of the underlying disease during the influenza season. Although there are occasional paradoxical failures in the protective effect of influenza vaccines, the principal problem in the application of immunoprophylaxis for influenza lies in the attitudes and practices of physicians. Most physicians accept the effectiveness of influenza vaccine, but they fail to make specific recommendations to their patients and do not prepare for and accomplish their immunization. Surveys show that most patients who are hospitalized for influenza have been seen by a physician in the preceding 3 months. Adult patients dislike having "shots," and only about 15 percent of selected populations who are eligible for free vaccination seek and take it. In America, implementation of the vaccine policy rests with individual physicians, with only education as a prod to performance and personal awareness as a basis for evaluation of the practice adopted.

TABLE 1 Conditions Placing Patients at High Risk from Influenza

Acquired or congenital heart disease with altered hemodynamic flow including valvular heart disease, congestive failure, and pulmonary edema or excessive vascular load.
Chronic pulmonary disease of any type accompanied by compromised ventilation or respiration, or by bronchial secretions, or a history of lung infection. Pregnancy in the third trimester may place women in this category.
Chronic metabolic disease associated with renal failure, diabetes, or severe anemia.
Immunodeficiency resulting from disease, certain malignant tumors, or immunosuppressive therapy.
Advanced age, especially over 65 years; the risk of excessive mortality begins after 45 years and is significant after age 65.
Exposure while providing essential community services.

Chemoprophylaxis

Amantadine. The most effective use of amantadine is for prophylaxis against influenza A. The recommended dose is 100 mg twice daily for 3 days, then once or twice daily for the duration of prophylaxis. Under defined conditions, amantadine or rimantadine can prevent influenza A infection in 70 percent or more of exposed persons and has been highly successful in preventing the occurrence of illness. Results from some prospective double-blind controlled studies of this effect in representative groups are given in Table 2.

Fear of drug intoxication has diminished as experience and further definition of its occurrence have been developed. Mild central nervous system side effects occur in about 7 percent of persons taking the recommended dose of 100 mg twice a day. They may disappear with subsequent doses and do so quickly after discontinuation of the drug with no sequelae. It is recommended that vaccine be given simultaneously with chemoprophylaxis, which is continued as protective cover for 10 days thereafter. Otherwise, chemoprophylaxis must be continued for the entire period of risk as there is no post-treatment protection.

Interferon. Inducers of interferon in situ, interferon derived from leukocytes, and alpha-interferon produced by a cloned gene in bacteria have all been shown to be capable of reducing the frequency and severity of rhinovirus infections. The last product has been available for field trials in which rhinovirus, but not other viral respiratory infections, were decreased. Although the original description of interferon showed the protection of mice against influenza, controlled trials against influenza in man have given equivocal results, partly because of problems of dosage. When given topically in the repeated mega-unit doses that are necessary for prophylaxis, cloned alpha-interferon commonly produces congestion and bleeding of the nasal turbinates. Some preparations of $alpha_2$-interferon produce myalgia and other systemic symptoms that are similar to the "flu syndrome." At this time the biology of interferon and its potential prophylactic and therapeutic role in viral respiratory infections remain questions of investigative interest, but temporarily cannot be beneficially applied.

Chemotherapy

Amantadine. This drug has a therapeutic effect on influenza A when given early in the course of illness. It has no effect on influenza B. The effect is more subtle than with prophylaxis and can be shown best when the

TABLE 2 Studies of Amantadine Prophylaxis of Influenza A

		Clinical and Serologic Influenza		Serologic Antibody Rise Only		Not Infected	
	No.	No.	(%)	No.	(%)	No.	(%)
Families (H_2N_2)*							
Amantadine	48	0	(0)	7	(15)	41	(85)
Placebo	69	10	(15)	27	(39)	32	(46)
Hospital ward (H_2N_2)†							
Amantadine	50	0	(0)	2	(4)	48	(96)
Placebo	61	7	(12)	5	(8)	49	(80)
Students							
Amantadine (H_1N_1)‡	136	8	(6)	18	(13)	110	(81)
Placebo	139	28	(20)	14	(10)	97	(70)
Amantadine (H_3N_2)§	113	2	(2)	5	(4)	106	(94)
Placebo	132	27	(20)	5	(4)	100	(76)

* Galbraith, 1969.
† O'Donahue, 1973.
‡ Monto, 1979.
§ Dolin, 1984.

illness (as determined from untreated control patients) is destined to be severe with fever and symptoms lasting for several days. This is most likely to occur with certain strains of virus and in people in the designated high-risk groups. In young, healthy, ambulatory patient, the disease can be of too short duration to demonstrate a significant difference between treated and untreated patients. Whenever objective measures are available for evaluation, such as fever or increased terminal airway resistance, the effect of amantadine has been beneficial. In other cases, the benefit may be reflected by a more rapid return to usual duties, but the difference has not been documented to have statistical significance.

The approved dose of amantadine or rimantadine is 100 mg twice a day. However, much remains unknown about the optimal therapeutic dose. Amantadine and its congener, rimantadine, have different pharmacokinetics. Oral administration of rimantadine gives a lower plasma level and, on this basis, causes somewhat fewer side effects at equivalent doses than amantadine, presumably because of a larger volume of distribution. If confirmed to have equal absorption, these characteristics of rimantadine would appear to be favorable for therapy. Both compounds have a long half-life (±16 hours), are not biodegraded, and are excreted almost completely in the urine. There is progressive accumulation of drug even in people with normal kidney function, but the dose does not need to be adjusted for short courses of therapy or in the absence of severe renal insufficiency. The therapeutic activity should be enhanced by initial loading and a sequential decrease in the amount and frequency of drug given. The use of this strategy is handicapped by the direct relation between the amount of the individual dose and the symptoms of acute intoxication. A personal recommendation for therapy is that 100 to 200 mg be given initially, and a dose of 100 mg given at 6 and 12 hours, then twice daily for 3 days, then once daily for 3 days. Prophylactic administration of amantadine should be considered for the household or ward contacts of the case and for nonimmunized health care personnel with close exposure (Table 3).

Ribavirin. The administration of ribavirin in mono-dispersed, small-particle aerosol has had a significant beneficial effect on severe influenza A or B in adults and on infants hospitalized with bronchiolitis from RSV infection. In both instances, the benefit was demonstrated by objective physiologic measurements, rapidity of defervescence, and a faster rate of improvement of impaired oxygenation respectively, and by more rapid disappearance of virus from respiratory secretions. Various dosage regimens have been used. The initial equilibration of the tissues with the drug concentration in the aerosol is rapid, and the dose delivered to the patient depends on the duration of aerosol administration. In prior studies, the concentration of ribavirin in the liquid reservoir was 20 mg per milliliter. The aerosol generated with compressed air at 50 p.s.i. had particles with a

TABLE 3 Indications for Amantadine

Prophylaxis

- Household contacts of an index case of influenza A.
- Hospital patients at risk for nosocomial spread when patients with influenza A are admitted.
- Elderly patients in semiclosed institutions when influenza A is causing disease.
- Unvaccinated adults with a serious underlying disease during epidemic influenza A.
- Vaccinated adults who are at high risk of serious consequences from influenza A.
- Well university and boarding school students during periods of epidemic influenza A.
- Specialized health care workers during periods of pandemic influenza A.

Therapy

- Patients with acute influenza A within 48 hours of onset and/or manifestations of severe influenza A.

median diameter of 1.6 μm, of which 95 percent were less than 5.0 μm and contained an average of 190 μg of ribavirin per liter. The dose deposited in the lungs was calculated to be 55 mg per hour. The small-particle aerosol has been administered for several hours or continuously each day, usually for 2 to 5 days, but to infants for as long as 22 days. The average dose given the patients treated for influenza was 3.0 g, but the optimal dose and regimen must still be determined. No adverse local responses have been observed, nor any apparent systemic toxicity. Although small-particle aerosol has been used to show the applicability and effectiveness of ribavirin treatment against severe influenza A or B and RSV, only the treatment of RSV bronchiolitis is currently approved. The need for aerosol rather than oral administration of the drug in the treatment of aduls has yet to be established.

Investigational Drugs. Several new drugs with activity against rhinoviruses, paramyxoviruses, or myxoviruses are under investigation and some of them have had preliminary clinical trials. Inhibition of viral replication usually is not the limiting factor; rather, the difficulties pertain to the pharmacokinetics of in vivo drug delivery to the target tissue, adverse reations which —although mild—disqualify the compound from general applicability, or drug activity that is virustatic without a lasting effect. The full investigation and development of new drugs with specific antiviral action against the respiratory viruses is a difficult, laborious, and expensive process, but it is proceeding with experience and skill that will yield products for more effective and specific treament of viral respiratory infections.

SUGGESTED READING

ACIP. Prevention and control of influenza. MMWR 1985, 34; 19:261–275.

Dolin R, Reichman RC, Madore HP, Maynard R, Linton PN, Webber-Jones J. A controlled trial of amantadine and rimantadine in the prophylaxis of influenza A infection. N Engl J Med 1982; 307:580–585.

Hall CB, McBride JT, Walsh EE, Bell DM, Gala CL, Hildreth S, Ten Eyck LG, Hall WJ. Aerosolized ribavirin treatment of infants with respiratory syncytial viral infection. N Engl J Med 1983; 308:1443–1447.

Jackson GG. The development and clinical evaluation of amantadine for the prophylaxis and treatment of influenza A. J Mol Biol (in press). 1985.

McClung HW, Knight V, Gilbert BE, Wilson SZ, Quarles JM, Devine GU. Ribavirin aerosol treatment of Influenza B virus infection. JAMA 1983; 249:2671–2674.

MYCOPLASMAL PULMONARY INFECTIONS

THEODORE C. EICKHOFF, M.D.

Pulmonary infection due to *Mycoplasma pneumoniae* is the single largest component of that entity known as "primary atypical pneumonia" or, more recently, the atypical pneumonia syndrome. The term "primary atypical pneumonia" was first used in 1938 by Reimann, to denote a form of pneumonia with generally milder symptoms and less toxicity, and nonproductive of the obviously purulent sputum that characterized most bacterial pneumonias. Furthermore, it became apparent that patients with "primary atypical pneumonia" did not respond to sulfonamides or penicillin in the dramatic way that most patients with bacterial pneumonia responded.

The major contribution of *Mycoplasma pneumoniae* infection to the atypical pneumonia syndrome was not fully defined until the early 1960s. Although it is now possible to identify most, but not all, of the organisms that cause the atypical pneumonia syndrome, the concept remains a clinically useful one in patients who are less severely toxic, whose sputum is not typically purulent, and in whom the Gram stain of expectorated sputum fails to reveal bacterial pathogens. The atypical pneumonia syndrome includes, in addition to *Mycoplasma pneumoniae* infection, pulmonary infection caused by a rickettsial organism, Q fever; a chlamydial organism, psitticosis; viral infection such as adenovirus or influenza virus pneumonia; and, in more recent years, *Pneumocystis carinii* pneumonia and legionnaires' disease.

None of the specific entities that comprise the atypical pneumonia syndrome are readily diagnosable by the usual techniques of examination of sputum. Consequently, the epidemiologic setting must be relied upon to suggest possible etiologies and often reveals useful clues. Thus, an atypical pneumonia in a patient whose occupation provides exposure to cattle, sheep, or goats should suggest the possibility of Q fever. Patients with pet birds at home may be at risk of psitticosis. During a major outbreak of influenza, patients with atypical pneumonia may have influenza virus pneumonia. In the hospital setting, and increasingly in some communities in the United States, legionnaires' disease occurs as a community-acquired atypical pneumonia, frequently accompanied by gastrointestinal distress and/or diarrhea. In the immunocompromised host, as in patients with acquired immune deficiency syndrome (AIDS), *Pneumocystis carinii* is the major cause of the atypical pneumonia syndrome. In mycoplasmal pulmonary infection, the epidemiologic setting is much less specific, and it is really the absence of other risk factors that suggests the clinical diagnosis.

Infection rates with *Mycoplasma pneumoniae* are highest in school-age children, and although rates decrease thereafter substantially, they remain elevated through young adulthood and in adults through the age of 50 to 60 years. Although infection rates subside in adults of increasing age, it is important to recognize that *Mycoplasma pneumoniae* infections do occur in the elderly, albeit infrequently.

The principal recognized infection caused by *Mycoplasma pneumoniae* is, of course, pneumonia. In some patients, however, its clinical expression is varied and includes bronchitis and bronchiolitis (especially in infants and older children), tracheobronchitis, pharyngitis, rhinitis, and myringitis. However, pneumonia is the principal clinical expression of *Mycoplasma pneumoniae*, and this organism is the most common cause of pneumonia in adolescence and through adulthood into the fiftieth year.

Specific etiologic diagnosis is possible, but in most patients with relatively mild disease (walking pneumonia), the benefit is probably not worth the cost. However, it is possible to isolate the organism from expectorated sputum, but most clinical microbiology laboratories are not equipped to do so. Furthermore, definitive identification of the organism may take several weeks. Serologic diagnosis is established by the complement fixation test, demonstrating a fourfold or greater rise in specific antibodies to *M. pneumoniae* between acute and convalescent sera. This test is positive in the majority of patients with *Mycoplasma pneumoniae* pneumonia, but the diagnosis is again retrospective in nature, since most patients have either fully recovered or are recovering from their disease by the time the diagnosis is confirmed. Contemporary techniques of genetic analysis using DNA probes are expected to provide much more rapid etiologic diagnosis in future years.

Cold agglutinin titers may be helpful, but the test is neither highly specific nor sensitive. Cold agglutinin titers of 1:128 or higher correlate well with infections caused by *M. pneumoniae*, but at least half the patients with mycoplasma pulmonary infection may not demonstrate elevated cold agglutinins.

Thus, if a patient with the atypical pneumonia syndrome is suspected of having mycoplasma pulmonary infection, the physician must rely on the clinical and epidemiologic setting to exclude or to minimize the other possible causes and manage the patient on the basis of a working clinical diagnosis.

SPECTRUM AND COMPLICATIONS

Many patients wih mycoplasmal pulmonary infection never consult a physician, and only a minority become ill enough to require hospitalization. The onset of the disease is typically gradual, with headache, malaise, and fever. Headache is generally more pronounced in adults than in children. After several days, cough begins and usually becomes such a predominant complaint that its absence should make the diagnosis of *Mycoplasma pneumoniae* infection highly unlikely. Typically, the cough is nonproductive, although occasional flecks of purulent materia or blood may be seen. A general soreness in the substernal area is common, but frank pleuritic pain is rare. Typically, fever varies between 100° and 103°F. Chilly sensations are common, but frank shaking chills are rare. Marked dyspnea and cyanosis are similarly rare. The disease is generally benign, and death is rare. In untreated patients the disease usually runs a course of 2 to 4 weeks, with slow, gradual improvement. Cough and roentgenographic abnormalities may persist for as long as 6 weeks. Small pleural effusions may be seen in as many as 25 percent of patients, but large pleural effusions are infrequent.

Occasional patients develop extensive and severe disease, accompanied by marked tachypnea, dyspnea, and hypoxemia. A few such patients develop respiratory failure, requiring intubation, ventilatory assistance, and even positive end-expiratory pressure. Infants, in particular, should they acquire *Mycoplasma pneumoniae* infection, are at increased risk of developing severe respiratory distress, requiring intubation and ventilatory support. In addition, patients with sickle cell disease appear to have an increased risk of developing large multilobar pneumonias and major pleural effusions with mycoplasmal pulmonary infection.

Complications of mycoplasmal pulmonary infection are relatively infrequent and include respiratory insufficiency (as previously noted), clinical relapse in as many as 10 percent of patients, maculopapular skin rashes, urticaria, and erythema multiforme. *Mycoplasma pneumoniae* infection appears to be one of the major antecedent infections causing erythema multiforme major, or the Stevens-Johnson syndrome. Other complications include intravascular hemolysis in association with high titers of circulating cold hemagglutinins, Raynaud's phenomenon, and, in rare instances, disseminated intravascular coagulation. Myocardial and pericardial involvement have been reported, and although arthralgia is a common complaint, frank arthritis is rare.

A variety of neurologic complications have been associated with mycoplasmal pulmonary infection, including meningoencephalitis, mono- or polyneuritis, and transverse myelitis. It has not been established whether such neurologic complications are immunologically mediated or result from direct spread of the organism to the central nervous system or possibly both.

MANAGEMENT

Antibiotics

Only two classes of drugs are known to be clinically effective in the treatment of mycoplasmal pulmonary infection: the tetracyclines and erythromycin. Clindamycin has been reported to be active against *Mycoplasma pneumoniae* in vitro, but has not been found to be clinically effective. Both the tetracyclines and erythromycin act by inhibiting protein synthesis in *Mycoplasma pneumoniae* and thus are primarily mycoplasmastatic in nature, rather than mycoplasmacidal. This is supported by the observation that *Mycoplasma pneumoniae* can continue to be recovered from the sputum of many patients being treated with either tetracycline or erythromycin, and may indeed by recoverable for several weeks after chemotherapy has been discontinued. Since mycoplasmas lack a rigid cell wall, none of the cell-wall-active antibiotics such as the beta-lactam drugs are effective against them.

The decision whether to treat with erythromycin or tetracycline must be made purely on clinical grounds and based on severity of illness and similar risk-benefit considerations. Since the costs and adverse reaction risks with either drug are so relatively modest, I would suggest treating any patient with significant symptomatic pneumonia in whom mycoplasmal infection was suspected.

Several clinical considerations should influence the choice of antibiotic. The tetracyclines have been proved effective in the treatment of psittacosis and Q fever, in addition to mycoplasmal infections; thus, if either psittacosis or Q fever is significant in the differential diagnosis, tetracycline would obviously be the preferred drug. Because of its particular binding and staining qualities, however, it is not generally used in children under the age of 10 years.

Erythromycin, on the other hand, is known to be effective in legionnaires' disease, as well as in pneumococcal pneumonia. Thus, particularly in adults in whom legionnaires' disease cannot be confidently ruled out, or in communities in which legionnaires' disease is known to be a relatively frequent community-acquired infection, or in settings in which pneumococcal pneumonia cannot confidently be ruled out, erythromycin would logically be the drug of choice. All of the aforementioned considerations relative to the choice between tetracycline or erythromycin point to erythromycin as the preferred drug in most clinical settings.

The dosage of erythromycin for adults is 20 to 25 mg per kilogram per day, given in three equal doses every 8 hours; for children, the dosage is 35 to 50 mg per kilogram per day, also in three equal doses, given every 8 hours. The adult dosage should be used in children who weigh more than 25 kg. For tetracycline, the adult dosage is 15 to 30 mg per kilogram per day in four equal doses given every 6 hours. For children, the dosage is 25 mg per kilogram per day, also in four equally divided doses given every 6 hours.

At the clinical level, the tetracyclines and erythromycin appear to be equally effective. Among the various erythromycin preparations available, none is documented to be superior to any other. Erythromycin estolate has been associated with infrequent hepatotoxicity, estimated to be on the order of 1 per 1,000 treatment courses, consisting of reversible cholestatic jaundice; this complication has been only rarely observed with other erythromycin preparations. Consequently, lacking any evidence of superiority of erythromycin estolate over other erythromycin preparations, it would be prudent to avoid erythromycin estolate. Similarly, no tetracycline congener has been found to be superior to tetracycline hydrochloride in treating patients with mycoplasmal pulmonary infection; if drugs other than tetracycline HCl or oxytetracycline are used (e.g., doxycycline), the dosage should be adjusted as appropriate.

Patients who are too severely ill to take medication by mouth may be safely treated with either of the intravenous preparations of erythromycin or with intravenous tetracycline.

Adverse reactions commonly encountered with erythromycin include gastrointestinal intolerance, occasional skin rashes, and rare hepatotoxicity. Similarly, adverse reactions encountered with tetracycline therapy include gastrointestinal intolerance, occasional skin rashes, mottling of tooth enamel, and photosensitivity. Vertigo, ataxia, nausea, and vomiting have been uniquely associated with minocycline therapy, and it would therefore be prudent to avoid the use of that drug.

Most patients begin to show some symptomatic improvement after 72 hours of therapy with either erythromycin or tetracycline. However, the clinical response is not dramatic, and the patient should not be expected to become afebrile and generally improved after 48 hours of therapy, as may often happen in treated cases of pneumococcal pneumonia. The effect of antibiotic therapy in mycoplasmal pulmonary infections consists simply of a decrease in the duration of fever, other clinical manifestations, and infiltrates on chest film, as compared to patients who are not treated or are treated with ineffective drugs.

In most patients, however, some degree of clinical improvement is apparent after 72 hours of therapy. The patient might not yet be afebrile, however, and it is not at all unusual for the x-ray findings to worsen somewhat, even during the first several days of antibiotic therapy.

Treatment for 7 to 10 days usually results in significant improvement. However, there is a significant relapse rate, and therapy should probably continue for 2 weeks or, in patients with extensive disease, as long as 3 weeks. As a working rule of thumb, 2 weeks of therapy appears appropriate.

Other Therapeutic Measures

The mild-to-moderate degree of hypoxemia that almost invariably is seen in patients ill enough to require hospitalization usually can be managed satisfactorily with oxygen delivered by nasal cannulae, at flow rates of 1 to 3 liters per minute. As previously indicated, however, only rarely do patients with extensive disease develop frank respiratory failure, requiring intubation, ventilatory support, and occasionally positive end-expiratory pressure as well. Fortunately, such severe illness is rarely caused by *Mycoplasma pneumoniae.*

Cough or headache is sometimes so severe and incapacitating as to merit therapy with judicious amounts of codeine, 16 to 32 mg PO every 4 to 6 hours. There is little reason to use antipyretic drugs. In particular, external cooling should be avoided in severely ill patients who have high titers of circulating cold hemagglutinins since a hemolytic crisis may be precipitated.

SUGGESTED READING

Cassell GH, Cole BC. Mycoplasmas as agents of human disease. N Engl J Med 1981; 304:80.

Levine DP, Lerner AM. The clinical spectrum of *Mycoplasma pneumoniae* infections. Med Clin North Am 1978; 62:961.

Murray HW, Masur H, Senterfit LB, et al. The protean manifestations of *Mycoplasma pneumoniae* infection in adults. Am J Med 1975; 58:229.

Reimann HA. An acute infection of the respiratory tract with atypical pneumonia. A disease entity probably caused by a filterable virus. JAMA 1938; 111:2377.

LEGIONELLOSIS

VICTOR L. YU, M.D., F.A.C.P.

The members of the family Legionellaceae are newly recognized agents in the causation of pneumonia. Legionnaires' disease is pneumonia caused by *Legionella pneumophila*. The natural reservoir for these organisms appears to be water. The method of transmission of these organisms to the human host is unclear, but there is evidence for airborne transmission, direct inoculation of organisms into the respiratory tract via invasive respiratory tract devices, and possibly aspiration.

CLINICAL FEATURES

The primary manifestation of disease caused by these organisms is pneumonia, although wound infections, perirectal abscess, pericarditis, and endocarditis have been reported in the absence of pneumonia. Bacteremia has been documented. *L. pneumophila* has also been isolated from kidney, lymph nodes, spleen, liver, bone marrow, and myocardium.

In the original description of legionnaires' disease, severe indicators of clinical illness were emphasized including high fever, diarrhea, abdominal pain, encephalopathy, and signs of multi-system failure, including renal and hepatic failure. Newer information shows that the clinical presentation is nonspecific and that specialized laboratory tests are necessary for accurate diagnosis. Clinical clues that should alert the physician to consideration of legionnaires' disease in a patient with pneumonia include the presence of hyponatremia, a Gram stain of respiratory secretions with large numbers of neutrophils but without a corresponding number of organisms visualized, and failure of the pneumonia to respond to beta-lactam (penicillins and cephalosporins) and aminoglycoside antimicrobial agents. A major epidemiologic context for legionnaires' disease is that of an outbreak of undiagnosed pneumonias in the community or acquisition of pneumonia during hospitalization.

Pontiac fever, a non-pneumonia syndrome caused by *L. pneumophila*, is characterized by fever, headache, myalgia, and malaise. It has an incubation period of 2 to 4 days, a high attack rate, and a completely benign prognosis. All reported cases have recovered, usually within 2 days, without specific antibiotic therapy. Diagnosis is established by demonstration of seroconversion in the context of the characteristic clinical syndrome.

DIAGNOSIS

The most reliable method for diagnosis of legionnaires' disease is isolation of *L. pneumophila* from respiratory secretions. Isolation, by culture of transtracheal aspirate specimens is currently the most sensitive method for making the diagnosis. However, with the use of selective dye-containing media, sputum culture is now feasible. Visualization of the organism by direct immunofluorescence (DFA) stains is the most rapid method of making the diagnosis, but not a particularly sensitive one. The DFA test may be negative if there are only few organisms in culture or if the pneumonic process has just begun.

Serologic detection of *Legionella* antibodies is both sensitive and specific. However, a convalescent sera is usually required 4 to 6 weeks after the onset of pneumonia so as to detect a possible fourfold rise in antibody titer. Thus, serology may be useful only in retrospect. On the other hand, if the seroprevalence rate of elevated *Legionella* titers is known to be low in the community, a level equal to or greater than 1:128 (indirect fluorescent antibody method) obtained during or following the pneumonia constitutes presumptive evidence of *Legionella* infection.

MANAGEMENT

Antimicrobial Agents

Antimicrobial therapy must often be administered empirically because specialized diagnostic tests are not readily available. I use erythromycin, 1 g every 6 hours intravenously. In most patients, defervescence occurs within 72 hours. When a clinical response has been noted, I usually switch to oral erythromycin, 500 mg every 6 hours. Thus, the majority of my patients with legionnaires' disease require less than a 1-week course of intravenous antibiotic therapy and conclude their therapy with oral erythromycin.

The most common side effects are phlebitis induced by the intravenous preparation and nausea and vomiting with both intravenous and oral preparations. The relatively large volume of fluid in which the intravenous preparation is administered can pose problems for patients with underlying cardiac or renal dysfunction. Hepatotoxicity is a rare complication of some forms of erythromycin. Ototoxicity is a rare complication of erythromycin therapy and tends to occur in patients with renal dysfunction.

The patient with community-acquired pneumonia without serious underlying disease usually responds readily to erythromycin therapy and can be treated comfortably with a 10- to 14-day course. For patients who are diagnosed late in the course of pneumonia, respond poorly to initial therapy, or are immunosuppressed, therapy of longer duration should be considered. Twenty-one days of therapy has been recommended for treatment of legionnaires' disease in the immunosuppressed host (organ transplant recipients, neutropenic hosts) to prevent relapse.

Monitoring Therapy

Defervescence and feeling of well-being usually occur within 72 hours. The chest roentgenogram lags behind clinical recovery and thus is not a useful guide for therapy. If the patient fails to respond within 72 hours, culture and repeat DFA should be performed; if these tests remain positive, I add rifampin. I use rifampin orally at a dosage of 600 mg every 12 hours. However, only a minority of patients would require the addition of a second antibiotic. Tetracycline and trimethoprim-sulfamethoxazole have also been efficacious in selected cases.

Infection Control Measures

Hospital personnel and patient contacts can be reassured that the disease is not contagious. Identification of the disease requires notification of the county health department. Since legionnaires' disease has been reported in outbreak and nosocomial situations, epidemiologic investigation may be fruitful. Since the reservoir in nosocomial legionellosis has been shown to be the water distribution system, environmental culturing and further case finding is indicated.

PITTSBURGH PNEUMONIA AGENT

Pittsburgh pneumonia agent (*Tatlockia micdadei, Legionella micdadei*) is also a newly recognized cause of pneumonia. The clinical presentation is similar to that of legionnaires' disease, although the organism has greater predilection for the immunosuppressed host. Erythromycin is also the treatment of choice for this organism, and addition of rifampin should be considered in patients who fail to respond to erythromycin.

OTHER LEGIONELLA SPECIES

Other Legionellaceae species have also been implicated in cases of pneumonia, including *Legionella longbeachae, Legionella wadsworthii, Legionella (Fluoribacter) bozemanii, Legionella (Fluoribacter) dumoffi*, and *Legionella feelii*. The treatment of choice for these organisms is also erythromycin, although clinical experience is limited.

SUGGESTED READING

Muder RR, Yu VL, Zuravleff JJ. Pneumonia due to the Pittsburgh pneumonia agent: new clinical perspective with a review of the literature. Medicine 1983; 62:120–128.

Parry MF, Stampleman L, Hutchinson J, et al. Waterborne *Legionella bozemanii* and nosocomial pneumonia in immunosuppressed patients. Ann Internal Med 1985; 103:205–210.

Thornsberry C, et al (eds). Legionella. Proceedings of the 2nd International Symposium, Washington, DC: Amer Soc Microbiol, 1984.

Winn WC. *Legionella* and legionnaires' disease: a review with emphasis on laboratory diagnosis. CRC Crit Rev Clin Lab Sci 1984; 21:323–381.

Yu VL. Nosocomial legionellosis: current epidemiologic issues. In: Swartz M, Remington J (eds). Current clinical topics in infectious diseases. New York: McGraw-Hill, 1986.

Zuravleff JJ, Yu VL, Shonnard J, Davis B, Rihs JD. Diagnosis of legionnaires' disease: an update of laboratory methods with new emphasis on isolation by culture. JAMA 1983; 250:1981–1985.

THORACIC ACTINOMYCOSIS

MANUEL RIVERA, M.D., F.A.C.P., F.C.C.P.
M. BROOKE NICOTRA, M.D., F.A.C.P., F.C.C.P.
RICHARD J. WALLACE Jr., M.D., F.A.C.P., F.C.C.P.

Human actinomycosis represents an uncommon and frequently misdiagnosed bacterial infection. Although several species of *Actinomyces* and *Arachnia propionica* can produce disease, *Actinomyces israelii* is responsible for over 80 percent of human infections. The fungus-like morphology of these bacteria, their fastidious growth characteristics, and the insidious onset and slow development of disease are largely responsible for the difficulty in diagnosing this condition. Although the term *Actinomyces* means "ray fungus," these organisms actually represent true bacteria; although *A. israelii* grow best anaerobically, some strains are microaerophilic. The normal habitat of this organism is the oropharyngeal cavity; from here the organism can gain access to the surrounding cervicofacial area, the gastrointestinal tract, and the chest cavity, giving rise to the three main forms of the disease.

Thoracic disease accounts for 15 to 50 percent of all cases of actinomycosis. In the thoracic form, *Actinomyces* gain entrance to the chest by aspiration of mouth contents. In the presence of an adequate inoculum, they may initially produce a pulmonary parenchymal infection. Systemic or local depression of the host defense mechanisms may allow the organism to thrive and expand and eventually cause a necrotizing pneumonia. If the infection is locally contained, it may adopt a well-circumscribed form resembling a neoplasm. On the other hand, the process may progress with dissection through anatomic boundaries to cause bronchopleural fistulas and empyema. On occasion the process may create an early pneumonic focus and, without overt pleural involvement, extend directly to the chest wall, leading to bony destruction and draining cutaneous sinuses. The varying behavior in the chest cavity of this infectious process gives rise to its protean clinical and roentgenographic presentations.

Pathologically, the infection with *Actinomyces* initially causes an acute pneumonic phase. This subsequently evolves into a chronic granulomatous and suppurating abscess with hard fibrous walls and soft central loculations containing pus. The abscess wall consists of cellular fibrous tissue containing acute and chronic inflammatory cells. Lymphocytes are present in moderate numbers and, on occasion, present as dense collections at the periphery of the lesion. Plasma cells are more numerous than lymphocytes and are often present as sheets and clusters. A few multinucleated giant cells may be seen. Frequently, large macrophages with foamy cytoplasm accumulate around the purulent centers.

Typically the abscesses contain within them the characteristic sulfur granules. These granules are round or oval, basophilic or amphophilic masses with a radiating fringe of eosinophilic clubs. All granules contain numerous branching gram-positive bacilli. The organisms are slender and beaded and average 0.5 micron in width and 13 microns in length. Branching is present in all granules and consists of at least one short branch for every 10 to 20 organisms.

CLINICAL FEATURES

Thoracic actinomycosis most often affects male patients in their third to sixth decade of life. The initial presentation is that of a chronic illness. Examination of the patient and the chest roentgenogram usually reveals one of the following findings: (1) well-circumscribed parenchymatous infiltrate resembling a tumor and, if cavitary, a lung abscess, (2) necrotizing pneumonia frequently accompanied by pleural extension with or without fluid, or (3) a chest wall mass with draining sinuses.

Symptomatically, cough, chest pain, weight loss, and fever are the most common complaints, having generally persisted for weeks or months. Physical examination frequently confirms a low-grade fever and reveals a chronically ill and wasted subject. Poor dental hygiene is a common although not universal finding. Examination of the chest varies from being normal to demonstrating an obvious chest wall mass, sometimes with draining sinuses.

DIAGNOSIS

Thoracic actinomycosis is a difficult disease to diagnose. Therefore a high index of suspicion is necessary so that appropriate specimens can be obtained. In addition, special care in the handling of these specimens for microbiologic studies and the choice of proper culture media is necessary.

In general, the disease should be suspected in the presence of complaints of cough, chest pain, weight loss, and fever when accompanied by clinical or roentgenographic evidence of a pneumonic infiltrate suggesting a tumor, an undiagnosed pleuropulmonary infiltrate, or a chest wall mass. Establishment of a definitive diagnosis requires a positive anaerobic culture, the finding of granules with clubs in tissue sections, or the presence of gram-positive branching bacilli on a Gram stain of exudate in the setting of anaerobic disease.

Commonly used diagnostic tools include a sputum Gram stain and culture, sputum cytology, fiberoptic bronchoscopy with anaerobic cultures of "sterile" brushings, anaerobic cultures of empyema fluid or sinus drainage, percutaneous needle aspirate of pulmonary lesions with cytologic and bacteriologic analysis (including anaerobic cultures), and resectional surgery.

The findings on Gram's stain of sputum are usually nonspecific, but they are helpful. They suggest an inflammatory process by the invariable presence of large numbers of polymorphonuclear leukocytes (PMNs). Additionally, because actinomycosis usually represents mixed anaerobic infection, mixed flora with intracellular organisms with morphologic features suggestive of other anaerobes are present. We have seldom made a diagnosis of actinomycosis on the basis of finding the gram-positive organisms in Gram's stain of sputum. As previously mentioned, the normal habitat of this organism is the oropharyngeal cavity, and the identification of this microbe in coughed-up bronchial secretions contaminated in their passage through the mouth always raises the question whether such an identified organism came from the mouth or had a bronchopulmonary origin.

Sputum cytology in our experience is useful, suggesting that inflammation rather than tumor is the cause of the problem. The cytologic study reveals many PMNs and, on occasion, reveals branching filamentous organisms that suggest the diagnosis.

Fiberoptic bronchoscopy usually discloses bronchitis, as evidenced by mucosal erythema, thickening, and edema, on occasion causing narrowing of the bronchial lumen. Frequently the bronchial lumen exhibits large amounts of thick purulent secretions. Gram's stain of bronchial brushings obtained through a sterile, sheathed catheter may reveal gram-positive beaded and branching bacilli. Anaerobic cultures of material so obtained usually grow a mixed group of anaerobic organisms, including *Actinomyces*. The bacteriologic evaluation of pleural fluid, drainage from chest wall sinuses, or material obtained from needle aspiration of lung masses may reveal similar results. Analysis of lung material obtained via percutaneous needle aspirate may demonstrate colonies of organisms morphologically consistent with *Actinomyces*.

Despite utilization of some of these diagnostic tools and frequently owing to a failure to suspect the diagnosis, tissue specimens obtained at thoracotomy or soft-tissue biopsy may be required to establish a definitive diagnosis. As a result, among all types of proven actinomycosis, more than 50 percent are diagnosed on the basis of histopathologic findings rather than culture results.

Two caveats are worth mentioning: a major and relatively frequent diagnostic pitfall is that of ordering fungal cultures when attempting to diagnose actinomycosis under the erroneous assumption that this organism is a fungus; another potential mistake is that of confusing the aerobic *Actinomyces, Nocardia*, with the anaerobic *Actinomyces, A. israelii*. By Gram's stain, these two organisms are morphologically indistinguishable and this should be borne in mind. To distinguish them, we resort to various measures: clinically, *Nocardia* usually produces pulmonary infection only in an immune-compromised host (malignancy, immunosuppressive therapy), whereas *Actinomyces* usually affects an otherwise immune-competent host. As previously mentioned, *Actinomyces* infection may occur in a mixed form with other anaerobes, whereas *Nocardia* usually produces infection alone. Using microbiologic techniques, *Nocardia* is weakly acid-fast, and this feature may separate them. To make this separation a modification of the Ziehl-Nielsen stain, a weaker acid is used as a decolorizer (Kenyon's stain). Additionally, although *Nocardia* grows under aerobic conditions on blood agar plates provided sufficient time is allowed, *Actinomyces* requires an anaerobic or microaerophilic environment for its growth.

MANAGEMENT

A review of the literature, as well as our own experience, indicates that while the drug of choice for therapy is well known, optimal duration of therapy for thoracic actinomycosis has not been well defined. This failure stems from several factors: the protean manifestations of the disease and the consequent need for therapy tailored for the individual needs, the difficulty in establishing a definitive diagnosis prior to resectional surgery (which in and by itself might be therapeutic by major "debulking" of the infected tissue), and the fact that the majority of papers on this subject concern either a small number of cases or lack a significant number of patients treated by any one method.

The following recommendations are largely based on our own limited experience. For this purpose, we find it convenient to categorize thoracic actinomycosis as follows:

1. Lung abscess (well circumscribed necrotizing parenchymatous process)
   a. Diagnosed by resectional surgery (debulking)
   b. Diagnosed without surgical removal or drainage
2. Necrotizing pneumonia (extensive poorly demarcated process with multiple abscesses)
3. Pleural empyema with and without overt parenchymatous involvement
4. Chest wall (bone, cutaneous, subcutaneous tissue) involvement with and without sinus drainage

For practical purposes, all these categories require antibiotic therapy; in addition, surgical resection or drainage may be necessary. Surgical drainage alone is not recommended, even though on occasion it has proved successful in the treatment of a chest wall abscess without underlying pleuropulmonary infection or a tumor-like pulmonary lesion. Removal of the source of infection by improving the dental hygiene is also essential.

Antibiotic therapy in general should be given until all clinical and roentgenographic evidence of active disease has resolved. The goal is that of resolution of the disease and prevention of recurrences (late relapse), which may occur months after what was thought to be initial adequate therapy.

1. *Specific treatment of lung abscess.* Intravenous (IV) aqueous penicillin, 10 to 20 million units per day for 30 days; follow with oral penicillin, 2.0 to 3.0 g per day for 6 months.
2. Treatment of lung abscess after surgical excision (no significant roentgenographic evidence of residual disease). IV penicillin, 10 to 20 million units for 15 to 30 days; follow with oral penicillin, 2.0 to 3.0 g per day for 3 months.
3. Treatment of necrotizing pneumonia. IV aqueous penicillin, 10 to 20 million units for 30 days; followed with oral penicillin, 2.0 to 3.0 g per day for 6 to 12 months.
4. *Treatment of pleural empyema.* Surgical drainage (to be tailored to suit individual needs and taking into consideration the "operability" of the individual patient); optimally, the patient should undergo open thoracotomy with removal of empyema/decortication under large-dose parenteral antibiotic (penicillin) coverage. Alternative, and on occasion necessary, approaches include multiple needle thoracentesis, closed (usually multiple) chest tube drainage, open chest tube thoracotomy with rib resection, and, rarely, additional thoracoplasty to obliterate a residual pleural space. Adequate surgical drainage needs to be followed by prolonged antibiotic therapy, i.e., IV penicillin, 10 to 20 million units per day for 30 days, and subsequently, oral penicillin, 2.0 to 3.0 g per day for a minimum of 6 months.
5. Treatment of chest wall actinomycosis. Surgical drainage and debridement followed by IV penicillin, 10 to 20 million units daily for 30 days, and subsequent oral administration of penicillin, 2.0 to 3.0 g per day for 3 months. It should be mentioned that penicillin is the antibiotic of choice and it should always be used. On occasion, serious allergy to this antibiotic precludes its use. Under this circumstance, other effective antibiotics can be beneficial.

In the presence of serious penicillin allergy, alternative antibiotic therapy is recommended. Although there are few data in this regard, we favor the use of tetracycline, 2.0 to 3.0 g per day, doxycycline, 200 mg per day, or clindamycin, 1.2 to 2.4 g per day. The length of therapy with any of these drugs probably should not be less than 6 months.

SUGGESTED READING

Bates M, Cruickshank G. Thoracic actinomycosis. Thorax 1957; 12:99.

Bennhoff DF. Actinomycosis: diagnostic and therapeutic considerations and a review of 32 cases. Laryngoscope 1984; 94:1198.

Flynn MW, Felson B. The roentgen manifestations of thoracic actinomycosis. Am J Roentgenol 1970; 110:707.

Jara FM, Toledo-Pereyra LH, Magilligan DJ. Surgical implications of pulmonary actinomycosis. J Thorac Cardiovasc Surg 1979; 78:600.

PULMONARY NOCARDIOSIS

EVERETT R. RHOADES, M.D., F.A.C.P.

Pulmonary nocardiosis is an acute or chronic infection of the lungs associated with one or more members of the genus *Nocardia*. Most infections are caused by *Nocardia asteroides, N. brasiliensis,* or *N. caviae*, with the great majority being associated with *N. asteroides*. Mycetoma, the other prominent syndrome, is more often associated with *N. brasiliensis*.

Nocardia species are aerobic saprophytic bacteria distributed in soil throughout the world. A variety of animals are susceptible to the organisms, which presumably enter the body through inhalation, causing pulmonary disease, or by cutaneous inoculation, causing mycetoma. In either instance, disease may progress by contiguous spread or by hematogenous seeding to many organs. Draining sinuses are one of the hallmarks of the disease. The disease is basically noncontagious, but the possibility of human-to-human spread, at least under hospital conditions, has been suggested.

MICROBIOLOGY

Nocardia species share the family Actinomycetaceae with the anaerobe *Actinomyces*. The family name implies that these organisms are fungi; they are not. They are gram-positive filamentous rods that fragment readily into coccoid and bacillary forms. The order name, Mycobacteriales, is more appropriate, implying organisms that appear both mycotic and bacterial. The cell wall, like that of mycobacteria, contains waxes that render the organism acid-fast positive when stained by the Ziehl-Neelson technique. *Nocardia* species are sometimes described as weakly acid-fast, so that less vigorous decolorizing, using acid-water instead of acid-alcohol, is necessary to demonstrate the property. However, this is not usually an important distinction and should not confuse the diligent microscopist. In virtually every instance, true acid-fastness can be demonstrated in *Nocardia* by careful search. It is true that acid-fastness is modified by growth conditions; it is enhanced by growth in glycerol-containing media. Part of the confusion regarding acid-fastness arises because authors often do not state whether the variation in acid-fastness applies to single organisms that stain poorly or to groups of organisms, some of which stain and some of which do not. At any rate, in my experience, the use of a modified Ziehl-Neelson stain using acid-water for decolorization is only rarely necessary.

In the laboratory, *Nocardia* grows readily on a variety of media at both room temperature and 37°C. It is important to note that, in contrast to most bacterial pathogens, growth may not be apparent for 72 hours or longer, so that the organisms are not inadvertently discarded when routine incubation ends at 48 hours. When *Nocardia* is suspected as a causative agent, the laboratory should be alerted to incubate specimens for as long as 3 weeks. *Nocardia* species are pleomorphic organisms that should be differentiated from diphtheroids, streptomyces, and the rhodochrous complex. This is not always as easy as one would wish. Speciation requires certain techniques often beyond the means of the routine laboratory and does not appear to be required as far as management of the patient is concerned.

CLINICAL FINDINGS IN PULMONARY INFECTIONS

There are no characteristic clinical findings in nocardiosis. The diagnosis should be suspected in any person with an unexplained pulmonary infiltrate. Certain underlying diseases such as malignant disease of the hemopoietic and lymphopoietic systems, pulmonary alveolar proteinosis, and other immunosuppressed states are frequent, reported to be present in 30 to 80 percent of cases.

The symptoms of pulmonary nocardiosis, as in most pulmonary infections, vary widely and are not helpful in establishing an etiologic diagnosis. Cough is the most common symptom and is usually accompanied by a modest-to-moderate amount of sputum of variable purulence. In hematogenous pulmonary involvement, sometimes still referred to as "miliary," there is less exudation, and consequently sputum production may be nearly absent. Various other complaints may be present such as fever, malaise, and pain or discomfort in the chest.

Physical findings depend on the location, extent, and severity of involvement. There may be a few localized rales or evidence of consolidation with dullness, egophony, and tubular breath sounds. As in many subacute pulmonary conditions, the physical examination may produce nonspecific findings and often does not correspond to the roentgenographic appearance.

The blood count may show leukocytosis with a slight increase in young neutrophils. Microscopic examination of sputum or other purulent material should be carefully examined by Gram's stain for the presence of gram-positive pleomorphic, thread-like rods sometimes containing granules; and by the Ziehl-Neelson technique. All the difficulties associated with microscopy of sputum apply to the search for *Nocardia*. The significance of organisms found in pus or drainage not contaminated with pharyngeal flora is much greater than that of organisms found in the presence of obvious pharyngeal organisms or epithelial cells.

The radiographic appearance of pulmonary nocardiosis is not characteristic and may vary from small patch pneumonitis to consolidated areas with lobular or lobar distribution. Cavitation is frequent, as are pleural effusion and empyema. Dense consolidation in apical and subapical areas with volume loss and cavitation should alert one to the possibility of nocardiosis. Involvement of surrounding tissue, including the bony structures of the thorax, may suggest malignant disease.

The histologic response to *Nocardia* infections may be virtually absent or may be an intense polymorphonuclear leukocyte infiltration with microabscess formation. Granulomas are rare, as are "sulfur granules." Skin and serologic testing are not helpful in clinical diagnosis or management.

MANAGEMENT

The optimal treament of pulmonary nocardiosis has not been finally established largely because the disease is relatively uncommon, and no controlled comparisons of therapy have been made. This applies to choice of antimicrobial, route of administration, dosage, and duration of therapy.

It must be emphasized that successful treatment depends as much, if not more, on duration of therapy as on selection of the appropriate drug. It is not unusual to encounter difficult cases in which the patient has received multiple short courses of antibiotics, including those appropriate for *Nocardia*, which have unfortunately been stopped too soon. The response to therapy is seldom dramatic, but is usually heralded within several days by diminution in fever, decreased toxicity, and decreased drainage. Roentgenographic clearing usually is not seen until after several days, sometimes weeks. The clinical response is a more important indicator of appropriate therapy than are in vitro drug susceptibility studies.

The optimal duration of therapy has not been clearly established and depends on the nature of the lesion, especially the presence of underlying fibrocavitary change, involvement of other tissue, dissemination, and the immunologic status of the patient. In acute pneumonitis, therapy for 3 to 6 months is not unreasonable. However, when there is involvement of other thoracic or chest wall tissue, such as mediastinitis or osteomyelitis, the burden rests with the physician who discontinues therapy before 6 to 12 months have been completed. In spread beyond the lung, as long as 3 years or more may be required to prevent relapses.

Although a number of antimicrobials exhibit anti-*Nocardia* effects in vitro, there is general agreement that the most appropriate therapy at present is the trimethoprim-sulfonamide combination containing 80 mg of trimethoprim and 400 mg sulfamethoxazole, although this ratio may not be optimum for *Nocardia*. Oral administration produces satisfactory blood levels under ordinary conditions, and the usual adult dose is two tablets twice daily. A suspension is available for children who should receive the following dosages: from age 6 weeks to 5 months, 20 mg trimethoprim and 100 mg sulfamethoxazole (2.5 ml) twice daily; from age 6 months to 5 years, 40 mg trimethoprim and 200 mg of sulfamethoxazole (5.0 ml) twice daily; from age 5 to 12 years, 80 mg trimethoprim and 400 mg sulfamethoxazole (10 ml) twice daily.

A difficult problem arises in the person who cannot take trimethoprim-sulfa because of hypersensitivity or in whom this drug has failed. A number of cases have been reported in which various regimens, often combined, have been used. Examples are minocycline, ampicillin combined with erythromycin, or antibiotics combined with sulfonamides. In hypersensitivity reactions to a trimethoprimm-sulfonamide combination, care should be given to avoid inadvertent administration of other sulfonamides.

Cycloserine has been reported to be effective in treating patients who do not tolerate sulfonamides, but its use is limited by frequent association with central nervous system (CNS) toxicity, which may be severe. The CNS toxicity is dose-related and is most often seen with peak blood levels of 30 μg per milliliter or more. However, I have found that careful attention to dose permits most patients to successfully complete a course of therapy. An attempt should be made to use no more than 250 mg three times daily in adults, in which case CNS toxicity has not been prominent and clinical response has been satisfactory. There is insufficient experience to guide possible combinations of cycloserine and other drugs.

In summary, therapy should begin with trimethoprim-sulfonamide. If this cannot be given, cycloserine is an effective second choice. Should this also fail, a combination of erythromycin and ampicillin should be tried, reserving minocycline as a last choice.

It is unwise to feel secure about prognosis at the beginning of therapy. However, depending on the severity of the infection, the underlying status of the patient, promptness in therapy, and the regimen chosen, arrest or cure of the disease should be achieved in two-thirds to three-quarters of cases.

SUGGESTED READING

Frazier AR, Rosenow EC III, Roberts GD. Nocardiosis: A review of 25 cases occurring during 24 months. Mayo Clinic Proc. 1975; 50:657-663.

Geiseler PJ. Results of therapy in systemic nocardiosis. Am J Med Sci 1979; 278:188-194.

Kucers A, Bennett NMcK. The use of antibiotics. 3rd ed. London: Heinemann, 1979.

Maderazo EG, Quintiliani R. Treatment of nocardial infection with trimethoprim and sulfamethoxazole. Am J Med 1974; 57:671-675.

Palmer DL, Harvey RL, Wheeler JK. Diagnostic and therapeutic considerations in *Nocardia asteroides* infection. Medicine 1974; 53:391-401.

Stevens DA. Clinical and clinical laboratory aspects of nocardial infection. J Hygiene 1983; 91:377-384.

HISTOPLASMOSIS

HANS EINSTEIN, M.D.

Histoplasmosis is the most common of the pulmonary mycoses and one of the most frequently occurring infectious diseases. It has been estimated that there are 40 million individuals with past infections in this country and about 500,000 new cases annually. A recent epidemic in Indianapolis involved approximately 100,000 victims with 495 clinically recognized cases. Widely disseminated fatal histoplasmosis is found increasingly among the microbial complications in the acquired immune deficiency syndrome (AIDS).

The disease is caused by a dimorphic fungus, *Histoplasma capsulatum*, a soil mycelium of world-wide distribution. The airborne spores (microconidia) lodge in distal airways where they rapidly transform into yeasts, and a granulomatous reaction results.

Investigation of point-source epidemics has established a definite connection between the occurrence of these outbreaks and the presence of chicken coops; starling, pidgeon, or blackbird roosts; decaying hollow trees; lofts; attics; barns; or caves inhabited by bats. With the exception of the bats, the animals themselves do not become ill, but their feces promote fungal growth in the soil.

PATHOGENESIS

Following inhalation of spores by a nonimmune person, a primary complex consisting of a granulomatous parenchymal focus with usually regional lymphadenopathy results. The infection may remain localized or spread by lympho-hematogenous dissemination. The rapidly developing cell-mediated immunity usually succeeds in limiting further spread, and healing occurs by fibrosis and ultimately calcification.

CLINICAL FEATURES

The outcome of any *H. capsulatum* infection depends on the size of the inoculum and the immune status of the host. An astonishing and at times confusing array of syndromes can be produced. Roughly 90 percent of cases are mild and subclinical, and their previous occurrences are discovered only when a histoplasmin skin test is performed or characteristic calcifications are detected. These are frequently multifocal, producing numerous so-called buckshot calcifications, varying from innumerable small to several large conglomerate histoplasmomas. The former can be a source of broncholiths; the latter can enlarge and resemble neoplasms.

Extensive primary pneumonia can be symptomatic (cough, fever, chest pain); cavities or pleural or pericardial effusions are seen occasionally.

Reinfection after reexposure may well be a mechanism for maintaining immunity. Clinical disease can be produced under these circumstances if the inoculum is large enough or the host's immunity has waned owing to intercurrent disease, therapeutic manipulations, or age. Whereas the initial infection has an incubation period of 10 to 16 days, endogenous reinfection occurs after a shorter incubation period of 3 to 7 days. The disease is usually less severe and there is no lymphadenopathy. Endogenous reinfection is the result of severe breakdown of systemic immunity; widespread dissemination is the usual result. The latter, therefore, can occur far removed in time and place from the endemic area, which is the humid south central region of the United States, particularly along the areas of the great rivers and their tributary basins. Microfoci also have been found in states as divergent as Florida, New York, Minnesota, and New Mexico. Histoplasmosis does not occur west of the Rockies.

Unusually heavy exposures result in a syndrome of acute or epidemic histoplasmosis. After an incubation period of 10 to 23 days, there is extensive bilateral involvement, patients are acutely and severely ill with respiratory distress, chest pain, and fever. X-ray shows patchy, frequently bilateral areas of pneumonitis with hilar lymphadenopathy. Recovery is usually spontaneous and calcification results.

Disseminated disease ranges from a fulminating, generalized, rapidly fatal disease in infants to a subacute or chronic lingering illness in adults who are in most cases male and immunosuppressed. This is characterized by weight loss, fever, bone marrow depression with anemia and leukopenia, hepatosplenomegaly, and oral-pharyngeal ulcerations, particularly on the tongue. Other sites of the gastrointestinal tract can be involved. Adrenal insufficiency, endocarditis, meningitis, cerebritis, and renal and prostatic involvement can occur.

Another complication of disseminated disease is excessive fibrosis of the pericardium and other mediastinal structures; this fibrosis produces a syndrome of superior vena caval obstruction resembling that caused by malignant neoplasia. Ocular involvement remains a subject of some controversy as to its existence and significance.

Chronic pulmonary histoplasmosis is an important cause of progressive respiratory insufficiency. Usually seen in white males with preexisting emphysema, it resembles chronic pulmonary tuberculosis clinically and roentgenographically. It is estimated that 20 percent go on to develop progressive respiratory failure and die from respiratory insufficiency and cor pulmonale. Others heal with extensive fibrosis and frequent relapses.

DIAGNOSIS

The definitive diagnosis of histoplasmosis requires demonstration of the organism in culture or tissue. Recently, cytologic staining of sputum, pus, and serous fluid has been found to be a useful screening procedure.

Immunologic tests are available and basically reliable. The skin test using the standard histoplasmin (mycelial extract) or the newer yeast phase skin test is of use only for epidemiologic purposes or to assess cell-mediated immunity. Their diagnostic value is limited to the examination of small children or known recent converters. The mycelial skin test antigen can elicit a false-positive complement fixation result.

Immunodiffusion testing is a readily available, sensitive, and specific screening test and is followed by the standard quantitative complement fixation test using both mycelial and yeast-phase antigens. This test has both diagnostic and prognostic value in that it is performed serially during the management of a case.

MANAGEMENT

The majority of histoplasma-related syndromes are self-limited and do not require active therapy. Respiratory support and occasionally corticosteroids may be needed in cases of acute respiratory insufficiency due to acute epidemic disease. Progressive cavitary disease, metapulmonary dissemination including meningitis, and disease in immunoincompetent individuals require antifungal chemotherapy. Amphotericin B remains the drug of first choice. The initial course of treatment for an adult generally consists of 2 g, total following which the response and toxicity are reevaluated and further plans are made. There have been some recent reports that shorter courses, some consisting of as little as 500 mg, have been effective, but controlled studies have not been done. Generally, histoplasmosis requires 2 to 6 g for control.

I give amphotericin as follows: a freshly mixed colloidal suspension of a 10 percent solution of amphotericin B in 5 percent glucose and distilled water is infused over 1 hour. It has been well shown that more rapid installation than the customary 4 to 6 hours is better tolerated by the patient, equally effective, and facilitates outpatient administration. I do not use the frequently troublesome 1-mg test dose, but give an initial dose of 5 to 10 mg, which is followed by daily increments of 10 mg. The usual maintenance dose is 1 mg per kilogram per day, but I do not give more than 50 mg daily. Once the dose is established, the medication is given daily to hospitalized patients and three times weekly to outpatients; the alternate-day administration takes advantage of the long (36-hour) half-life of amphotericin B. The dose-response curve of serum levels flattens at the 50 mg per day point, and thus larger daily amounts are not necessary. Rapid infusion through small needles in the peripheral veins has made phlebitis a minor problem, and therefore heparin no longer needs to be added.

Premedication with a phenothiazine antiemetic and aspirin is usually adequate to control nausea, vomiting, and chilling. Should the latter be severe, meperidine can be given before or at the end of the infusion to control chilling. Azotemia is the most serious side effect and is invariably present. I do not modify administration of amphotericin B until the serum creatinine level exceeds 3.0 mg. Salt replenishment has recently been shown to ameliorate azotemia. The drug is kaliopenic, and potassium monitoring and oral supplementation are mandatory. Magnesium also should be monitored, but its loss is rarely a clinical problem. In rare instances, corticosteroids are required if side effects are severe.

TABLE 1 Treatment Choices in Histoplasmosis

Syndromes	*Treatment*
Self-limited histoplasmosis	
Asymptomatic primary infection	No treatment
Symptomatic primary infection	No treatment
Asymptomatic reinfection	No treatment
Symptomatic reinfection	No treatment
Acute epidemic histoplasmosis	Occasional respiratory support, steroids
Progressive Histoplasmosis	
Chronic pulmonary histoplasmosis	(1) Ketoconazole* (2) Amphotericin B†
Disseminated histoplasmosis	(1) Amphotericin B† (2) Ketoconazole*
Late sequelae	
Mediastinal fibrosis	Surgery rarely effective
Solitary cavity	Consider surgery
Histoplasmoma	Observe
Broncholithiasis	Rarely bronchoscopy
Adrenal insufficiency	Amphotericin B,† steroids
CNS involvement	Amphotericin B†

* Ketoconazole: 400 to 600 mg per day for 6 months to 2 years.

† Amphotericin B dose: usually at least 2 g total (50 mg three times weekly).

Local administration of amphotericin B should be used in the treatment of arthritis, osteomyelitis, peritonitis, pleuritis, empyema, meningitis, and other localized and accessible lesions. Other self-limited side effects of amphotericin include a normocytic normochromic anemia, which is probably due to bone marrow suppression. Transfusions are rarely necessary, and blood counts return to normal at the end of therapy.

It should be emphasized again that although the amphotericin B toxicity is formidable, it is reversible in most cases and should not become a reason for withholding amphotericin in situations in which it is needed clinically. Attempts have been made for years to develop rational approaches to amphotericin dosing. None has worked well, and as a result dosage schedules remain empiric based on experience. The chronic indolent nature of histoplasmosis and other fungal infections makes critical evaluation difficult, particularly when the natural history of the disease and the condition of the host are frequently as important as the chemotherapy.

The recent introduction of the imidazoles has broadened the therapeutic armamentarium significantly. Ketoconazole, a dioxalane imidazole, has been under evaluation since 1981. It blocks the oxidative demethylization of lanosterol to ergosterol; the latter is a vital constituent of yeast membranes and thus cytoplasmic leakage results. The drug is useful in the management of chronic progressive cavitary disease, frequently arresting the progressive component. Like amphotericin B, ketoconazole is fungistatic rather than fungicidal, and thus relapses are frequent. The recent use of larger amounts (400 to 600 mg) each morning for longer periods than the initial 3 to 6 month courses may improve results further. At present it is recommended that the patient be given 400 mg of ketoconazole before breakfast with orange juice for a period of at least 6 months, extending this to a year if there has been clinical, roentgenographic, and serologic improvement. Relapses occur in approximately 20 percent of cases following cessation of therapy. This may improve with larger amounts for longer periods of time. The drug is somewhat more toxic than originally anticipated; hepatitis is seen in approximately 1 of every 10,000 courses. Androgen and cortisol synthesis is definitely suppressed, thereby causing gynecomastia and impotence, but the suppression appears to be reversible. Gastritis and occasional dermatitis are seen. Ketoconazole is surprisingly effective against chronic fibrocavitary histoplasmosis, but treatment has to continue for a full year. It will probably emerge as the drug of choice for this syndrome. Ketoconazole is a secondary agent to amphotericin in the treatment of disseminated histoplasmosis or in the treatment of children. Neither drug plays a major role in the treatment of late sequelae, except in cases of histoplasma meningitis, for which amphotericin B is the drug of choice. A summary of treatment choices is given in Table 1.

SUGGESTED READING

Schwartz J. Histoplasmosis. New York: Prager Publishers, 1981.

Slama TG. Treatment of disseminated and progressive cavitary histoplasmosis with ketoconazole. Am J Med 1983; 74:70–73.

Wheat LJ, French ML, Kohler RB, et al. Diagnostic laboratory tests for histoplasmosis: analysis of experience in a large urban outbreak. Ann Intern Med 1982; 97:680–685.

COCCIDIOIDOMYCOSIS

ROBERT A. BARBEE, M.D.

For many years, therapeutic decisions in this disease were limited to the question: Who should be treated? Once a decision to treat was made, only one nonsurgical therapy was available: amphotericin B. Currently, the availability of two additional drugs, miconazole and ketoconazole, has added a new dimension to coccidioidomycosis management. Which therapeutic approach is best in which specific clinical circumstance? Although it is doubtful that any single answer to this question would be uniformly accepted, the discussion that follows provides guidelines in making the decision to treat, and the choice of therapy once the decision has been made. Each drug, with its advantages and disadvantages, will be presented separately, followed by a discussion of the clinical stages of disease in which treatment decisions must be made.

GENERAL CONCEPTS OF THERAPY

The clinical outcome of an infection with *Coccidioides immitis* is predicated not only on the number of inhaled organisms, but also on the development of an appropriate cell-mediated immune response. For practical purposes, this repsonse is measured by the development of a positive delayed skin reaction to either coccidioidin or spherulin antigens. Under normal circumstances, this response occurs 2 to 4 weeks following infection. As a general rule, when active cocci exists in the absence of the skin test positivity, because of either prior immunosuppression or overwhelming infection, therapeutic intervention is indicated. In this setting, the goal of therapy, irrespective of the medication employed, is to control the disease until an appropriate immune response is mounted. None of the three drugs currently available is fungicidal in vivo; all are fungistatic. Although "cure" can and does occur, it is difficult to achieve in the absence of a return of cell-mediated immunity, documented by the return of a positive skin test. Therefore, from a practical standpoint it is unrealistic, when starting therapy, to predetermine the duration of treatment or total dose required. Similarly, one can expect a relatively high relapse rate when therapy is discontinued, even after several months, when the immune status of the patient is as inadequate at the end of a course of therapy as it was initially.

Amphotericin B

For over 20 years, the only effective nonsurgical therapy available for the treatment of the deep mycoses was amphotericin B. Because of its toxicity and inconvenient intravenous delivery, the decision to treat or not to treat a cocci infection was often determined by whether the disease or the drug was the worse of the two evils. Despite the current availability of miconazole and ketoconazole, it continues to be the standard against which the others are measured.

Pharmacologically, amphotericin is a polyene, insoluble in water, dispersed with a bile salt as a colloidal dispersion. In this form it is stable in light for at least 8 hours. Thus, covering the infusion bottle with a brown bag during administration is not required. Its mode of action is to bind to steroids in the fungal membrane, producing cell leakage. With a serum half-life of 24 hours, therapeutic levels persist for many hours, and excretion is not complete for 6 to 8 weeks. Less than 5 percent of the administered dose is excreted in the urine, so that it is not necessary to alter the dose in patients with renal failure.

Traditionally, therapy has been started with a 1 or 2 mg test dose to minimize major immediate side effects. It is uncertain that such a test dose is really necessary. Such side effects as chills, fever, nausea, and vomiting are common at the beginning of therapy, and do not appear to be dose-related. Thus, an initial dose of 5 to 10 mg is appropriate, doubling the dose daily until a maintenance dose of 40 to 50 mg (0.7 to 0.9 mg per kilogram) is reached. The concentration of the administered drug should never exceed 10 percent, and is best delivered in 5 percent dextrose in water, over a period of 45 to 90 minutes. Use of this more rapid delivery rate in recent years appears to have decreased the incidence of side effects and has facilitated more convenient outpatient management.

In addition to the obvious therapeutic objective of controlling the disease, two more immediate goals relate to the administration of the drug itself: (1) to minimize the untoward side effects, and (2) to settle on a schedule that will accomplish the therapeutic goal with minimal interruption of the patient's life style. The former involves premedication with 50 mg of diphenhydramine hydrochloride (Benadryl) and analgesics 30 minutes before treatment. Hydrocortisone (25 to 50 mg) mixed in the intravenous solution further reduces chills and fever and is helpful early in the treatment course. Rarely, antiemetics may be necessary. Heparin (500 to 1,000 U) has traditionally been added to the infusion to prevent thrombophlebitis, but with the more rapid infusion schedule, it probably is not necessary. As a general rule, reactions are more severe at the beginning of a treatment course, and the drug becomes much more tolerable after the first week or two of therapy.

To accomplish the objective of minimizing the effect of therapy on the patient's life style, a maintenance treatment schedule must be adopted which allows patients an opportunity not only to recover from the specific toxic effects of the drug between doses, but also to "feel good" on a relatively regular basis. There is no convincing evidence that a three-times- or even twice-a-week maintenance schedule is any less effective than one in which the drug is administered more frequently. Also, patient tolerance is enhanced and renal toxicity minimized by the less aggressive schedule.

Side Effects

Three major toxic reactions are experienced by patients receiving amphotericin:

1. Because of renal artery vasoconstriction, the glomerular filtration rate is decreased, with a concomitant rise in both creatinine and BUN and a lowering of the creatinine clearance. Values for all three should be measured prior to beginning therapy with repeat creatinine measurements on a weekly basis. It is my usual practice to omit a dose if and/or when the creatinine level reaches 2½ times the pretreatment level or exceeds a level of 3.0 mg per deciliter. With careful monitoring, all toxic renal effects are reversible, returning to or near their pretreatment levels 2 to 4 months following the discontinuation of therapy.
2. Hypokalemia, secondary to decreased renal tubular reabsorption of K^+, occurs almost universally in patients undergoing amphotericin therapy. Serum potassium levels should be monitored weekly, and supplements provided when indicated.
3. Mild-to-moderate anemia is common. The mechanism for this is uncertain. Some have ascribed it to bone marrow suppression, others to hemolysis. Because of this, Hgb and Hct levels must be followed weekly. Blood replacement is not usually necessary, as counts generally stabilize at a hematocrit of 22 to 25 mm and a hemoglobin of 7 to 8 g per deciliter.

Miconazole

This imidizole became available in the mid 1970s as an alternative to amphotericin and has fewer serious side-effects. Therapeutically, it has no advantage, and its three-times-per-day intravenous administration requirement limits its use to the hospital setting. A full course over a 3-week period or longer provides for a total dose of approximately 0.9 gram per kilogram body weight.

Side Effects

Although this drug is less toxic to the kidneys, significant side effects do occur. The most common include phlebitis, hyponatremia, anemia, thrombocytosis, nausea, and a bothersome pruritus, which may persist for varying periods following the completion of therapy. Relapses are common. At present, the use of miconazole is limited to those circumstances in which a previous failure or intolerance to amphotericin exists and a more rapid therapeutic response than can be achieved with ketoconazole is required.

Ketoconazole

Following extensive clinical trials, ketoconazole became available in 1981 as a broad-spectrum antifungal agent. Like amphotericin and miconazole, it is fungistatic in vivo. Its major advantage is that it is rapidly absorbed from the stomach following oral administration, with relatively mild side effects. Therefore, because it is administered orally, it offers a significant alternative to amphotericin in terms of both convenience and toxicity. As originally proposed, the drug is taken as a single morning dose, before or with breakfast. Peak blood levels occur after 1 or 2 hours, and primary excretion takes place through the gastrointestinal route.

At present, the optimal dose for control of cocci infections is uncertain. Initial reports of its use were based on data collected during clinical efficacy trials in which a starting dose of 200 mg per day was standard. This dose was subsequently increased to 400 mg. It would appear that 600 mg or 800 mg per day are required for maximal therapeutic benefit.

Side Effects

In addition to the obvious advantage of once-per-day oral administration, early studies with ketoconazole produced only minor side effects. The most common is gastrointestinal irritation with nausea, diarrhea, and/or anorexia. This appears to be dose-related, and can be minimized somewhat by taking the drug with the morning meal. Mild headache and dizziness have also been observed. The capacity of ketoconazole to interfere with steroid synthesis by the adrenal has been reported. Rare instances of gynecomastia have been observed. Perhaps the most serious potential toxicity is hepatocellular dysfunction, apparently on an idiosyncratic basis. In most instances the hepatitis is transient, disappearing following the cessation of therapy. Current recommendations include an assessment of liver function prior to therapy, with monthly follow-up throughout the course.

Despite its obvious advantages of convenience and relatively rare major side-effects, ketoconazole has not replaced amphotericin as the drug of choice for all patients who require therapy. Clinical responses following the initiation of therapy often are relatively slow, requiring several weeks. Therefore, in life-threatening situations, amphotericin is still recommended. Finally, relapses following even 6 or 9 months of therapy are common (probably more than 25%). Despite these drawbacks, ketoconazole has become a valuable therapeutic tool in the treatment of this disease.

THERAPEUTIC DECISIONS IN VARIOUS CLINICAL SETTINGS (TABLE 1)

Inapparent Infection

Approximately 60 percent of exposures to *C. immitis* are followed by skin test conversion in the absence of a recognizable clinical illness. Radiologic and

TABLE 1 Clinical Stages of Cocci—Therapeutic Recommendations

Disease Form	*Therapy*
Inapparent infection/acute infection without pneumonia (skin test conversion to positive)	None
Acute cocci pneumonia (skin test positive)	None
Residual pulmonary lesions	
Solitary nodule (young or nonsmoker)	None; radiographic follow-up
Solitary nodule (smoker)	Bronchoscopy; needle biopsy, followed by excision if cocci dx uncertain
Cavity (no systemic activity—negative complement fixation titer)	Radiographic follow-up; excision if unstable after 6 months
Cavity (systemic activity present—positive complement fixation titer)	Ketoconazole 400–600 mg, 3–6 months, followed by excision if unresolved
Chronic progressive pulmonary disease	Ketoconazole 400–600 mg/d indefinitely or Amphotericin 2–3 ×/wk, minimum 2 g total dose
Disseminated disease	
Miliary—life-threatening	Amphotericin 10 mg → daily doubling to 50–60 mg, daily for 7–10 days, then 2–3 ×/wk, minimum 2–3 g
Skin, soft tissue, bone and/or joint—not life-threatening	Ketoconazole 400–600 mg/d, minimum 6–9 months Amphotericin 2–3 ×/wk, minimum 2–3 g
Central nervous system	Amphotericin IV (as above) plus cisternally 0.1 mg doubled daily to 0.5 mg daily, then 3 ×/wk until CSF response. Continue 1–2/month, indefinitely.
Pregnancy	
1st trimester	Ketoconazole 400–600 mg
2nd or 3rd trimester	Amphotericin (as above)

Note: 1. Miconazole may be substituted for amphotericin when patient intolerance prevents amphotericin therapy or prior therapy was unsuccessful or was followed by relapse.
2. See text for details and discussion.

serologic assessment of possible clinical activity is reasonable when it can be documented that skin test conversion is recent, but therapy is not indicated.

Acute Coccidioidal Pneumonia

In the vast majority of instances, cocci pneumonia in the immunocompetent patient resolves uneventfully, without a residual lesion. Also, there is no convincing evidence that ketoconazole either shortens the acute course or prevents nodular or cavitary residuals. Thus, specific antifungal therapy is not recommended in this setting. A possible exception may be made in the diabetic or in the patient with significant prior pulmonary disease, for whom ketoconazole (400 to 600 mg per day) may be helpful. However, no conclusive evidence currently exists to support this. Rarely, pleural effusion may occur alone or in conjunction with the pneumonic infiltrate. Although complement fixation titers are frequently high in this setting (1:16 or greater), therapy is not generally required.

Residual Pulmonary Lesions

Solitary Nodules

By far the most common residual lesion, the nodule is generally peripheral, less than 3 cm in diameter, does not calcify, and, in the middle-aged smoker, is easily confused with primary carcinoma of the lung. Serologic tests are usually negative, and the skin test is of little help diagnostically, especially in endemic areas. When findings from bronchoscopy and/or needle biopsy are nonspecific, and no prior cocci history is evident, surgical excision is recommended. In the young patient or nonsmoker, roentgenographic follow-up is appropriate. Such nodules seldom cavitate and are generally stable. Ketoconazole has no role in these lesions.

Cavities

Residual cocci cavities share all the potential problems of cavities resulting from other infections. Some close spontaneously, others are stable and produce few symptoms, and a significant number are mechanically unstable—enlarging and/or shrinking almost monthly. Predicting their course is both difficult and unreliable. When the cocci serology is negative (as it often is), it is my usual practice to follow such cavities for approximately 6 months. An increase in size, hemoptysis, pleuritic pain—any or all of these are indications for surgical excision. Pre- or postoperative therapy with either amphotericin or ketoconazole is not routinely required. Recurrent cavities occur with increased frequency in diabetics, often with continued serologic evidence of active disease. Pretreatment with 400 to 600 mg of ketoconazole per day for 3 to 6 months, or amphotericin (usually 500 μg) is recommended, followed by surgical resection. Ketoconazole may be continued for several months following excision.

Chronic Progressive Pulmonary Disease

For as yet unexplained reasons, a small percentage of otherwise healthy individuals fail to control the local spread of apparently routine cocci pneumonia. The result is a progressive destructive process, usually involving the upper lobes. Surgical excision in the absence of antifungal therapy generally is not curative, and local recurrence is the rule. Long-term ketoconazole (400 to 600 mg) is preferable, with control a more realistic goal than cure.

Disseminated Disease

Life-Threatening Disseminated Disease

The vast majority of patients in this category are either very young, very old, or immunocompromised. The latter include those with lymphomas, cancer undergoing chemotherapy, organ transplants, or conditions that require high-dose corticosteroids. Rapid diagnosis and therapy are imperative. A miliary pattern on chest roentgenogram, extrathoracic lymph node enlargement, and/or diffuse hematogenous spread with hepatosplenomegaly are commonly present. An initial dose of amphotericin (10 or even 20 mg) is followed by doubled daily doses until the 50- or 60-mg maintenance level is reached. Daily administration is continued for 7 to 10 days, when, almost invariably, renal impairment requires shifting to an every-other-day regimen. When disease stability or control is achieved, dosage intervals may be extended to three times or even twice per week. As long as the reason for the immunocompromised state exists, no treatment end point can be determined. With careful monitoring of renal function, amphotericin doses of 5 g, or even 7 g, may be successfully given. No conclusive data exist concerning the efficacy of amphotericin and ketoconazole given simultaneously. However, in a limited number of patients, I have used the two drugs concurrently for 2 to 3 weeks following the achievement of disease control, prior to switching to ketoconazole alone (400 to 600 mg) for chronic maintenance.

Chronic Disseminated Disease

In racially susceptible individuals (blacks and Filipinos) and, rarely, in otherwise apparently immunocompetent caucasians, dissemination may occur on a more chronic basis, either following an acute cocci pneumonia or without clinically evident acute disease. Areas of involvement generally include the skin, soft tissues, bones, and/or joints. Frequently these patients feel quite well, and invariably, the skin test is negative. Ketoconazole (400 to 600 mg) is appropriate first-line therapy. Clinical responses may not be evident for several weeks, with skin and soft tissue lesions the earliest to show resolution. Bone and joint lesions respond more slowly. Therapy must be continued for a minimum of 6 to 9 months, and relapses are not uncommon, especially when skin test conversion to positive has not occurred during the course of therapy. Some investigators have advocated increasing the daily dose to 800 mg or more in difficult or poorly responsive disease. Because results with high-dose ketoconazole have not been reported, it is impossible to compare the efficacy of ketoconazole with that of amphotericin in this setting.

Central Nervous System Involvement

Management of CNS cocci is properly the province of the neurologist, and will not be discussed in detail. Because all available systemic antifungal agents penetrate the blood-brain barrier either poorly or unpredictably, disease involving the CNS requires intrathecal therapy. Several approaches to intrathecal amphotericin have been employed, all associated with a relatively high complication rate. Arachnoiditis is common, especially when administration is by the lumbar route. Currently, the cisternal or lateral cervical routes are usually preferred. Intracisternal hemorrhage is a complication of the former. The Omaya ventricular shunt has been used extensively, but the complication rate is high. The usual starting dose for intrathecal administration is 0.1 mg, increasing by 0.1 daily or every other day until a maintenance dose of 0.5 mg is reached. Therapy is continued on a two- or three-times-per-week basis until abnormalities of the CSF have cleared. The frequency of therapy may then be decreased, but usually must be continued for many months or even years, until CSF findings have remained normal for at least 6 months. Occasional patients have been reported to benefit from high-dose (800 to 1,200 mg) ketoconazole.

Pregnancy

Routine cocci infections during pregnancy, especially when they occur in the third trimester, are associated with a high rate of dissemination, leading to maternal and fetal death in many cases. Thus, clinically evident disease at any time during pregnancy requires treatment. The choice between amphotericin and ketoconazole is not clear-cut. I would recommend ketoconazole when the disease occurs during the first trimester, with careful observation and substitution with amphotericin if control is not achieved. For disease in the third trimester, amphotericin would be my drug of choice.

From the foregoing discussion, it is apparent that the vast majority of patients with cocci require no treatment. However, when the ability of the patient to develop an appropriate cell-mediated immune response is compromised, therapy not only is necessary, but becomes a long and often frustrating experience for both patient and physician.

SUGGESTED READING

Bayer AS. Fungal pneumonias; pulmonary coccidioidal syndromes. Part I. Primary and progressive primary coccidioidal pneumonias—diagnostic, therapeutic, and prognostic considerations. Chest 1981; 79:575–583.

Bloom JW, Camilli AE, Barbee RA. Disseminated coccidioidomycosis: a ten year experience. In: Coccidioidomycosis. Proceedings of Fourth International Conference on Coccidioidomycosis, San Diego, CA, March 14–17 1984:369–378.

Dismukes WE, Stamm AM, Graybill JR, et al. Treatment of systemic mycoses with ketoconazole: emphasis on toxicity and clinical response in 52 patients. Ann Int Med 1983; 98:13–20.

Drutz DJ, Catanzaro A. Coccidioidomycosis. Part I. Am Rev Respir Dis 1978; 117:559–584.

Drutz DJ, Catanzaro A. Coccidioidomycosis. Part II. Am Rev Respir Dis 1978; 117:727–771.

Graybill JR. Current recommendations for treatment of coccidioidal meningitis. In: Coccidioidomycosis. Proceedings of Fourth International Conference on Coccidioidomycosis, San Diego, CA, March 14–17 1984:466–473.

BLASTOMYCOSIS

JOHN P. UTZ, M.D.

Blastomycosis is a chronic disease that is caused by the dimorphic fungus, *Blastomyces dermatitidis*. The tissue reaction to this fungus is both suppurative and granulomatous. The disease is acquired by the respiratory route from a still unidentified source in nature. The primary focus of infection is the lung, but there is hematogenous dissemination, in declining order of frequency, to the following organs or tissues: cutaneous, subcutaneous, genitourinary (usually male), osseous, mucous membrane, and reticuloendothelial (and others in about 10% of patients).

In assessing need for treatment, there are two major considerations: diagnosis and activity.

The diagnosis is established unequivocally by the culture and identification of *B. dermatitidis* from a specimen appropriate to the disease present. The diagnosis is more quickly arrrived at—and only slightly less certainly—by the finding of approriate-sized budding yeast forms on microscopy by an experienced mycologist examining direct preparations (especially KOH) of fresh specimens of sputum, pus, skin lesions, and prostatic massage secretions. Histopathologic studies of specially stained tissue (e.g., periodic-acid–Schiff stain) that show microscopic forms that are consistent in size and form in the eyes of an experienced mycologist or pathologist also establish the diagnosis.

However, the last-mentioned method does not establish activity of disease, the second consideration. Such activity is established by culture of the fungus (or seeing it on direct examination of specimens as just described). Laboratory values that support the presence of inflammation (e.g., leukocyte count, erythrocyte sedimentation rate, lactic dehyrogenase and other enzymes, hemoglobin, changes in roentgenographic findings, and ventilatory measurements) assess activity and also document response to therapy. Adherence to an updated protocol for work-up helps to avoid embarrassing oversights in doing such tests.

Serologic studies are not generally available primarily because they have not been helpful to physicians: a negative test does not rule out disease, and a positive test is inadequate proof of diagnosis or activity. No skin test material is available.

Determination of status of immune competence (cell-, serum-, or phagocyte-mediated) seems important, but less relevant than in other opportunistic infections (e.g., cryptococcosis, candidosis, aspergillosis, or zygomycosis [mucormycosis]).

An undetermined pulmonary lesion may be diagnosed tangentially by culture of *B. dermatitidis* from another site, notably a skin lesion. However, such a lesion at another site has no protective effect against bronchogenic carcinoma, which may coexist, especially in older white men, who are most prone to blastomycosis.

Furthermore, there are no symptoms, signs, or laboratory or chest film findings that are specific for blastomycosis. Cough, chest pain, sputum production, and hemoptysis may occur with nuances of frequency only slightly more suggestive of one etiology than of another. For example, generalized findings of inflammation (e.g., fever, chills, night sweats, anorexia, weight loss, depression, and malaise) may be more frequent than in bronchogenic carcinoma, but are usually less frequent than in bacterial pneumonia. Series of cases of pulmonary blastomycosis have emphasized the protean rather than distinctive patterns on chest film.

MANAGEMENT

Chemotherapy

Amphotericin B

Although not the first chemotherapeutic agent, *amphotericin B* remains the gold standard to which all older and more recent agents must be measured. Moreover, experience with it covers almost 30 years. Although new aspects (e.g., immunostimulatory and immunosuppressive) continue to come to light, knowledge of its effects and side effects on disease and patient seems stable and well established. One does not expect surprises, early or deferred down the years, and it is therefore the preferable agent.

The mode of action of the drug is its binding to steroids, chiefly ergosterol, in the fungal cell membrane. That binding is irreversible and renders the cell permeable, so that small molecules, notably potassium, leak out. Conversely, such defects in the membrane permit entry of other antifungals (e.g., flucytosine, which in other fungal infections thereby enters the cell and further impedes growth by interfering with nucleic acid synthesis, specifically blocking the enzyme thymidylate synthetase). Ketoconazole, which interferes with ergosterol *synthesis* and thus reduces binding sites on the membrane, interferes with and reduces amphotericin B activity in vitro and in experimental infections in animals.

Amphotericin B is administered intravenously. To the vial containing 50 mg, 10 ml of sterile water is added. (I routinely put the vial in my pocket thereafter for an hour or so during walking rounds to allow maximal suspension.) The dose to be given is then added to 5 percent glucose in water, at a concentration not to exceed 10 mg amphotericin B per 100 ml of infusion. A Y-tube assembly and infusion pump are necessary. I prefer an initial dose of only 1 mg. Subsequent doses can be increased daily by increments of 5 or 10 mg, depending on the reaction to the previous day's dose. Since the work of Bindschadler and Bennett, I have not given a daily dose greater than 50 mg (approximately 0.7 mg per kilogram of the patient's body weight). Although various authors give various total dosages (up to 2.5 g) and duration of therapy (up to 10 weeks), I favor 2.0 g given in approximately 6 weeks. Despite impressive experience of a few others, the predictable and quantifiable cardiotoxicity in our dog experiments has kept me from giving the infusion over a period shorter than 2 to 4 hours, again depending on the patient's tolerance and preference. As an additional precaution, the patient's pulse, temperature, blood pressure, and state of well-being are measured every half hour during the infusion, and thereafter as indicated by the values during the infusion. Never add potassium or sodium salt solutions or attempt to dilute the vial in them, as they precipitate the already precarious colloid suspension. I do not use a membrane filter with a pore size less than 0.45 μm, and studies in our lab showed that the infusion need not be protected from light. As a prudent step, I have never given the drug except in a hospital setting, although not necessarily on an inpatient basis. When reactions are severe (q.v.), 50 mg of hyrocortisone sodium succinate may reduce or lessen severity of reactons when given into the tubing or bag at the beginning. Aspirin (1,200 to 1,500 mg) or diphenhydramine (25 to 50 mg) or prochlorperazine (5 to 10 mg) may be given orally 15 to 30 minutes before the infusion, but these premedications are slightly less effective. I do not use heparin (final concentration 5 U per liter) routinely, although it has been recommended by a few others.

Complications. I know of no antimicrobic drug that has such severe side effects. Chills, fever, nausea, vomiting, anorexia, headache, and shortness of breath are clearly perceptible and unpleasant for the patient. Paradoxically, these usually occur more often and to a greater degree with the earlier infusions and lower doses (which phenomenon has led me to a more conservative initial dose than in the package insert). These side effects are not predictable (a few patients escape almost completely), but have prompted the use of the aforementioned premedications. Hypotension is less symtomatic and, if severe or symptomatic, is relieved by elevation of the foot of the bed, by 15 to 50 mg ephedrine subcutaneously, or by infusion of normal saline by the alternate Y (after clamping off the amphotericin B) arm.

With daily infusions of any drug, but especially one

suspended in glucose solution (pH 3.5 to 5.0), phlebitis is a problem. This is reduced by using a pediatric, 23-gauge, butterfly needle. Poor veins should never be an excuse for discontinuing a course of therapy: a Broviac or Hickman catheter solves the problem of access immediately.

With the larger (i.e., 50 mg) daily dose, impaired glomerular filtration, as measured by blood urea nitrogen or, better, serum creatinine levels, occurs in approximately 85 percent of patients. Temporary interruption of therapy is the only response. The indications are arbitrary, but values of 50 and 3.0 mg per deciliter respectively are useful cut-off points. Salt depletion, either intentional or asymptomatic and accidental, increases azotemia.

Anemia occurs in approximately 75 percent of patients and complicates a subtle hemolytic process usually present from the infection. The anemia from treatment seems a function of suppression of erythropoietin. The hemoglobin or hematocrit stabilizes as the infection is controlled. Transfusions are not necessary, and iron administered orally is useless. Thrombocytopenia rarely occurs and is not severe.

Hypokalemia is a threat to virtually all patients, and serum values should be monitored at least twice weekly. Unrecognized hypokalemia has led to frightening muscle weakness and electrocardiographic changes. Foods rich in potassium help, but 20 to 40 mEq of potassium intravenously (again not in the infusion bottle) are more immediately helpful. The mechanism of loss is from cells, although amphotericin B levels in blood are never high enough to produce the hemolysis and loss of potassium into serum that occurs in vitro, and by excretion in the urine. Anorexia, diarrhea, and vomiting may also contribute.

There have been reports of deterioration in respiratory function when amphotericin B is given shortly after leukocyte transfusions; this has been denied by others. Such reactions have support of experimmental studies, and prudent caution is recommended. Fortunately, pulmonary blastomycosis is rarely an opportunistic infection, and agranulocytopenia or even leukopenia is rarely encountered.

Monitoring Response. Painstaking initial study and work-up, best done by an updated protocol, facilitate assessment of therapeutic response. Regular monitoring during treatment of abnormalities present before treatment, in addition to tests necessary by virtue of the drug itself, document response. Patients usually report symptomatic improvement within a week, provided they can distinguish this from counterbalancing ill effects from the drug itself. Repeat chest films, ventilatory studies, culture of sputum or other specimens, blood tests, and occasionally radionuclide studies are appropriate and sensible. For reasons cited earlier, I do not monitor the serology, and determinations of either peak or trough levels of amphotericin B are not routine.

Relapse after treatment has occurred in increasing numbers. In contrast to cryptococcosis, in which relapse almost invariably occurs within 12 months, that in blastomycosis may occur many years later. The record is not yet in the Guiness *Book of Records*, although a recurrence after 9 years has been reported.

Hydroxystilbamidine

The older drug, hydroxystilbamidine, was almost abandoned when amphotericin B appeared because relapse seemed to occur so frequently. When the side effects of amphotericin were appreciated, interest in the older drug revived, and a randomized, prospective study was organized. Early failures in an unexpected form of disease (central nervous system) led to refinements in indications. At present hydroxystilbamidine is reserved for amphotericin B treatment failures (rarely encountered) and for nonprogressive, noncavitary pulmonary disease or cutaneous disease.

Miconazole

Miconazole, like ketoconazole, has demonstrated in vitro and in vivo activity and has been used successfully in a few patients. Comparative studies have not been done; the intravenous route of administration vis-a-vis ketoconazole (but not amphotericin B or hydroxystilbamidine) is a disadvantage. Pruritus has been a sufficiently severe side effect to lessen interest, and thus there is no defined role of this drug.

Ketoconazole

Ketoconazole has a better (oral) route of administration than the three preceding agents and it has proven efficacy: in one cooperative study, it was effective in seven (44%) of 16 patients. However, its side effects, hepatotoxicity and suppression of adrenocortical and testicular function, are at least as serious as those of amphotericin B. Moreover, dramatic failures have been reported. A summary of drug therapy for blastomycosis is given in Table 1.

Surgery

Surgery is often of initial importance, but it is never definitive treatment. Open lung biopsy is only occasionally needed for diagnostic purposes. Drainage of abscesses is most helpful for both diagnostic and therapeutic reasons. Excision of a sequestrum in a bone lesion or repair of bronchopleural fistula is rarely necessary. As in the case of tuberculosis, thoracic surgery for cavitary or other pulmonary disease is also rarely necessary now.

PROS AND CONS OF TREATMENT

Once the diagnosis and evidence of disease activity have been established, there is no reason to delay onset of therapy.

Should every patient with acute, primary, pulmonary blastomycosis receive treatment? It is clear that some patients, especially those recognized after a single site infection, have recovered without treatment. Initial recovery in other series has been tarnished by subse-

TABLE 1 Chemotherapy of Blastomycosis

Drug	Indications	Route	Dosage: Initial	Dosage: Optimal (mg)	Dosage: Total	Duration (weeks)	Side Effects	Remarks
Amphotericin B	All forms	IV	1.0	1.0/kg (not to exceed 50)	c.2,000	c.6	Azotemia, hypokalemia, anemia, fever, chills, nausea, vomiting	Gold standard
Ketoconazole	Except for central nervous system	Oral	400–600	same	c.100,000	26	Hepatoxicity, depression of testosterone and adrenal corticoids, diarrhea	Role being defined
Hydroxystilbamidine	Nonprogressive, noncavitary pulmonary and cutaneous	IV	25	225	8,000	c.6	Dizziness, flushing, dyspnea	After other drug failures (rare); hepatic disease a relative contra-indication
Miconazole	Pulmonary	IV	600	3,000–3,600	120,000	c.6	Nausea, vomiting, pruritus	Role will probably never be defined

c. = approximately (circa)

quent relapses. Even so, the relapses seem to be in a minority. But how does one distinguish the patient with active disease who does not need treatment or the one who will relapse later? These questions have not been answered to date.

What is the ultimate role of ketoconazole? Clearly its value at present, vis-a-vis amphotericin B, must be considered inferior. Will the larger dose (800 mg per day) for 6 months in the cooperative, prospective, blinded study currently under way, show it to be better than the lower dose (400 mg per day)? The study seems on shaky grounds already, owing to the list of side effects that seem to be increasing and to the number of fatalities from hepatotoxicity. The drug already has been proscribed for meningeal disease and for pulmonary disease more menacing than the slowly progressive form.

Should every patient in whom blastomycosis is encountered unexpectedly at thoracotomy be treated? A well-organized, complete protocol to establish (or rule out) activity is helpful for the individual patient. Even so, activation of dormant disease has occurred frequently enough to prompt thoughtful physicians to recommend chemotherapy "routinely" in such patients.

SUGGESTED READING

Bindschadler DD, Bennett JE. A pharmacologic guide to the clinical use of amphotericin B. J Infect Dis 1969; 120:427–436.

Cockerill FR, Roberts GD, Rosenblatt JE et al. Epidemic of pulmonary blastomycosis (Namekagon Fever) in Wisconsin canoeists. Chest 1984; 86:688–692.

Evans ME, Haynes JB, Atkinson JB et al. *Blastomyces dermatitidis* and the adult respiratory distress syndrome. Am Rev Resp Dis 1982; 126:1099–1102.

Parker JD, Doto IL, Tosh FE. A decade of experience with blastomycosis and its treatment with amphotericin B. Am Rev Resp Dis 1969; 99:895–902.

Thiele JS, Buechner HA, Cook EW Jr. Failure of ketoconazole in two patients with blastomycosis. Am Rev Resp Dis 1983; 128:763–765.

PNEUMOCYSTOSIS

PETER D. WALZER, M.D.

Pneumocystis carinii was discovered in 1909 by Chagas during his studies of American trypanosomiasis. The organism's status as a human pathogen was first demonstrated when it was found to be the cause of "interstitial plasma cell pneumonia," a disease of institutionalized premature and malnourished infants in Europe following World War II. In the 1960s, *P. carinii* became recognized as a leading cause of pneumonia in the compromised host; major targets included children with primary immune deficiency diseases and patients of all ages who received corticosteroids and other immunosuppressive agents for the treatment of cancer, organ transplantation, and collagen vascular diseases. *P. carinii* declined somewhat in prominence in the 1970s with the development of trimethoprim-sulfamethoxazole (TMP/SMZ) as an effective therapeutic and prophylactic agent. However, in the 1980s, the organism returned to haunt clinicians with the discovery of the acquired immune deficiency syndrome (AIDS). Not only is AIDS the most common underlying disease in pneumocystosis, but *P. carinii* is the principal opportunistic infection and leading cause of death in AIDS.

The clinical manifestations of pneumocystosis are similar regardless of the underlying disease. Typically these include dyspnea, tachypnea, nonproductive cough, and fever with minimal findings on lung ascultation. Pulmonary function studies reveal hypoxemia, increased alveolar-arterial oxygen gradient, respiratory alkalosis, and impaired vital capacity and diffusing capacity. There are bilateral diffuse infiltrates on the chest roentgenogram and increased uptake on gallium scan. Pneumocystosis presents as an acute illness in most immunocompromised hosts, whereas in AIDS the infection follows a more chronic indolent course lasting many weeks or even months.

The clinical features of pneumocystosis can be mimicked by many other organisms as well as noninfectious agents, and so proper management necessitates establishing a specific etiologic diagnosis. This can only be done by histopathologic demonstration of the organism. The most popular stains are those that selectively stain the cell wall of *P. carinii* cysts; examples include methenamine silver, toluidine blue, cresyl echt violet, and Gram Weigert. Stains such as Giemsa, Diff Quik, Wright's, or Gram's stains are rapid and provide data on the internal structures of *P. carinii*; since these stains also stain host cells, they require some experience for proper interpretation.

An invasive procedure must be performed to obtain adequate tissue specimens for the hisologic diagnosis of *P. carinii*. Transtracheal aspiration has a low yield, but has not been widely studied in this disease. Needle aspiration or biopsy is performed mainly in pediatric patients. Fiberoptic bronchoscopy is the most common diagnostic procedure in adults. Bronchial brushings and washings were formerly used, but have now been largely replaced by transbronchial biopsy (TBB) bronchoalveolar lavage (BAL). The higher diagnostic yield of bronchoscopy with TBB or BAL in patients with AIDS (90%) than in other immunocompromised hosts (40%) probably reflects the greater organism burden in AIDS. Open lung biopsy is performed in cases of nondiagnostic bronchoscopy, failure to respond to anti-*P. carinii* therapy, or suspected infection with another organism. Open lung biopsy is also much more reliable than bronchoscopy in diagnosing pulmonary involvement with Kaposi's sarcoma in patients with AIDS.

The natural history of untreated pneumocystosis in the immunocompromised host is one of progressive respiratory insufficiency leading to death. Prognosis in response to specific therapy is related to such factors as the status of the patient's nutrition and underlying disease, degree of respiratory functional impairment and prior lung damage, total leukocyte and lymphocyte counts, and the presence of concomitant infection with other opportunistic pathogens.

MANAGEMENT

General supportive measures, including adequate oxygenation and careful fluid and electrolyte balance, are important adjuncts in management. Since *P. carinii* is communicable, patients should be placed in respiratory isolation or at least separated from direct contact with other susceptible hosts.

The drug of choice in the treatment of pneumocystosis in non-AIDS patients is TMP/SMZ, which is effective in 50 to 80 percent of cases in different series. TMP/SMZ inhibits folic acid synthesis, but its mode of action against *P. carinii* is unknown. The drug is administered orally or intravenously in a dose of 20 mg per kilogram per day TMP and 100 mg per kilogram per day SMZ in four divided doses for 14 days. Dosage of TMP/SMZ should be adjusted according to serum concentration; optimal levels for TMP are 3 to 5 μg per milliliter in children and at least 5 μg per milliliter in adults, and those for SMZ are 100 to 150 μg per milliliter. TMP/SMZ is usually well tolerated. Adverse reactions occur in 10 to 15 percent of patients and consist mainly of a skin rash and gastrointestinal disturbances; more serious effects (e.g., bone marrow depression) are uncommon. Folinic acid has been suggested as a possible aid in preventing the bone marrow effects of TMP/SMZ, but has not been widely used.

The other major drug in the therapy of pneumocystosis is pentamidine isethionate. Formerly available to physicians in this country only on an investigational basis through the Centers for Disease Control, pentamidine has recently been licensed. Pentamidine is an old drug and has been used to treat other parasites, but its mechanism of action against *P. carinii* is unclear. Pentamidine is administered intramuscularly or intravenously in a single dose of 4 mg per kilogram per day for 14 days.

Several studies have shown that pentamidine is as effective as TMP/SMZ in the treatment of pneumocystosis, but is considerably more toxic. About 50 percent of patients experience adverse reactions to pentamidine, some of which can be quite serious. These reactions have been broadly categorized as follows: local (induration, abscess formation), systemic (hypotension, cardiac arrhythmias), renal (azotemia), hepatic (abnormal function tests), hematologic (leukopenia, thrombocytopenia), and metabolic (hypo- and hyperglycemia).

The increased incidence of pneumocytosis in the last few years has renewed investigative interest in pentamidine. Simple assays are being developed to measure serum concentrations of pentamidine, which should lead to better knowledge of the drug's pharmacology and more precise dosing schedules. For example, it is unknown whether pentamidine is dialyzable or what dosage reduction is needed in the presence of renal insufficiency. There has also been an increasing tendency to administer pentamidine by the intravenous route. The data so far suggest that diluting pentamidine in 50 to 250 ml of a 5 percent dextrose solution (the drug is poorly soluble in saline) and infusing over a period of at least 60 minutes is no more hazardous than intramuscular injection of the drug. It is prudent to monitor the patient, even after completing a course of pentamidine, for changes in blood glucose.

The average time to begin to observe a response to TMP/SMZ or pentamidine is after 4 days of therapy, although there is considerable variation among individual patients. The response is characterized initially by improvements in dyspnea, fever, and hypoxemia; changes in the chest roentgenogram may be delayed. A question that arises frequently is what to do if no response to TMP/SMZ or pentamidine is observed. In general, it is reasonable to continue with the initial drug as long as the patient's condition has stabilized. However, if there is no improvement by about day 5 or 6, it is prudent to consider switching to the other drug. There is no clinical or experimental evidence to suggest that the use of TMP/SMZ and pentamidine together is any more efficient than the use of either agent alone; in fact, this combination probably increases the risks of adverse reactions. Repeat bronchoscopy or open lung biopsy should also be considered to determine whether *P. carinii* is still present and to look for other treatable entities not covered by anti-*P. carinii* agents.

Another question that frequently arises in the treatment of non-AIDS patients is what to do with the corticosteroid dose if the patient is receiving this class of drugs. Since the symptoms of pneumocystosis often begin after the corticosteroid dose has been tapered, it has been suggested that the host inflammatory response plays a role in this process. In a few individual cases, successful treatment of pneumocystosis has only occurred after the corticosteroid dose was increased; however, these are uncontrolled observations. All available data indicate that corticosteroids are the most important factor predisposing to *P. carinii* pneumonia. Since corticosteroids have broad deleterious effects on host defenses, they may facilitate the propagation of other opportunistic pathogens. Thus, it seems best to taper the corticosteroid dose to as low a level as permitted by the patient's underlying disease.

Pneumocystosis in AIDS presents new therapeutic problems. As a group, these patients have a longer duration but milder form of the illness than do other immunocompromised hosts. The overall survival rate for treatment of the initial episode of pneumocystosis among AIDS patients is similar to that for non-AIDS patients; however, AIDS patients generally take longer to show a clinical response.

TMP/SMZ and pentamidine appear to be equally efficacious in the treatment of pneumocystosis in AIDS. The major difference is the high frequency (60% to 80%) of adverse reactions to TMP/SMZ in these patients. The principal side effects include fever, rash, and leukopenia; hepatic abnormalities and thrombocytopenia have also been reported. These reactions usually appear during the second week of therapy and are frequently severe enough to necessitate discontinuation of TMP/SMZ. Whether these effects represent some form of hypersensitivity reaction or whether other mechanisms are involved is unclear at present. The bone marrow effects of TMP/SMZ are not prevented by the administration of folinic acid. The few patients rechallenged with TMP/SMZ have exhibited a variety of responses ranging from no ill effects to very severe toxic reactions.

The frequency and severity of adverse reactions to pentamidine in patients with AIDS are generally similar to those experienced by other compromised hosts. However, some studies have found a higher incidence of leukopenia in AIDS patients administered the drug.

The decision whether to use TMP/SMZ or pentamidine as primary therapy of pneumocystosis in AIDS is largely a matter of personal preference. TMP/SMZ still seems to be favored by most authorities because of familiarity with its pharmacokinetics and because it covers some other infectious causes of pulmonary infiltrates in this patient population. Because AIDS patients tend to respond more slowly to therapy than do other compromised hosts, it seems reasonable to wait for a longer period of time before declaring treatment failure with a particular drug.

Pneumocystosis recurs at a considerably higher frequency in AIDS patients (20% to 30%) than in other immunosuppressed hosts (1% to 2%), except in certain pediatric oncology institutions, where the recurrence rate is 10 to 15 percent. It is unclear whether these recurrences represent episodes of relapse or reinfection. *P. carinii* persists in the lungs for weeks to months following a conventional course of TMP/SMZ or pentamidine, and even may be found if drug treatment has been continued for up to 4 to 6 weeks. The viability of these persisting organisms and their clinical significance remain to be determined.

Therapy of pneumocystosis in AIDS patients should be continued for at least 21 days, although the optimal duration has not yet been established. Repeated bronchoscopy following completion of therapy is controversial. Since the presence or absence of organisms in BALF or TBB may not correlate with the clinical status of the patient, some authorities believe that bronchoscopy is unnecessary. Others believe that the presence of *P. carinii* on repeated bronchoscopic examination suggests a higher chance of recurrence, and hence the need for more prolonged treatment. I favor the latter approach. Recurrent episodes of pneumocystosis in AIDS patients are frequently refractory to all forms of therapy and carry a high mortality rate.

The problems associated with treatment of pneumocystosis in patients with AIDS emphasize the need to develop alternative drugs. Pyrimethamine and sulfadiazine have been successful in a small number of patients, but have never undergone controlled clinical trials. Moreover, these drugs have the same potential problems in AIDS patients as does TMP/SMZ. Dapsone has been effective in an animal model of *P. carinii* pneumonia and is currently undergoing clinical evaluation. It is unclear whether dapsone will have the toxicity problems of TMP/SMZ. Difluoromethylornithine (DFMO), which inhibits the synthesis of polyamines, is effective against African trypanosomiasis and other related protozoa and has shown promising activity in a few cases of human pneumocystosis. It is currently undergoing further testing.

Another goal in the development of new anti-*P. carinii* drugs is an effective prophylactic agent. TMP/SMZ in a dose of 5 mg per kilogram per day TMP and 25 mg per kilogram per day SMZ has been shown to prevent pneumocystosis in selected high-risk patient populations, such as children with acute lymphatic leukemia, patients with severe combined immunodeficiency disease, and bone marrow transplant recipients. The long-term administration of TMP/SMZ in these patients is associated with few side effects, but the indiscriminate use of the drug has been discouraged. TMP/SMZ does not kill *P. carinii*, and thus is only effective as long as it is being given. TMP/SMZ has not found much use as a prophylactic agent in AIDS patients because of the high risk of adverse reactions.

SUGGESTED READING

Gordin FM, Simon GL, Wofsy CB, et al. Adverse reactions to trimethoprim-sulfamethoxazole in patients with the acquired immunodeficiency syndrome. Ann Intern Med 1984; 100:495–499.

Kovacs JA, Hiemenz JW, Macher AM, et al. Pneumocystis carinii pneumonia: a comparison between patients with the acquired immunodeficiency syndrome and patients with other immunodeficiencies. Ann Intern Med 1984; 100:663–671.

Murray JF, Felton CP, Gray SM, et al. Pulmonary complications of the acquired immunodeficiency syndrome. N Engl J Med 1984; 310:1682–1688.

Shelhamer JH, Ognibene FP, Macher AM, et al. Persistence of *Pneumocystis carinii* in lung tissue of acquired immunodeficiency syndrome patients treated for pneumocystis pneumonia. Am Rev Respir Dis 1984; 130:1161–1165.

Walzer PD, Perl DP, Krogstad DJ, et al. Pneumocystis carinii pneumonia in the United States: epidemiologic, diagnostic, and clinical features. Ann Intern Med 1974; 80:83–93.

Young LS, ed. Pneumocystis carinii Pneumonia: Pathogenesis., ed. Diagnosis, Treatment. New York:Marcell Dekker Inc., 1984.

LUNG ABSCESS

BEN V. BRANSCOMB, M.D., F.A.C.P., F.C.C.P.

DIAGNOSIS

Sixty percent of lung abscesses (purulent cavitary parenchymal lesions) are of the primary or nonspecific type, usually considered secondary to aspiration of mixed oropharyngeal organisms. There usually is a history of a circumstance predisposing to aspiration, often in a person with poor oral hygiene and impaired resistance to infection. Consequently the clinical circumstances, initial findings, and bacterial flora are usually those of the aspiration pneumonia from which the abscess evolves. In occasional patients, the acute onset will have passed unnoticed. Such persons may complain of malaise, fever, weight loss, night sweats, anorexia, pleuritic pain, cough, and hemoptysis. Clubbing of the fingers is an uncommon finding. If the abscess does not communicate well with the bronchi, the sputum volume may be small and the systemic manifestations pronounced. Conversely, with a communicating abscess, there may be less fever and malaise, but a large volume of frankly purulent foul-smelling sputum, often deeply colored or bloody. Occasionally, intermittent drainage of the cavity is reflected in an alternation between these two symptom patterns.

Most aspirational abscesses are located peripherally in the posterior segments of the upper lobes or superior segments of the lower lobes, more often on the right than on the left, the areas most dependent during recumbency. Initially the roentgenogram demonstrates the inhomogeneous opacities of the bronchopneumonia with a central dense zone indistinguishable from consolidation or tumor. The process frequently extends to the pleura, and free, loculated, or interlobar effusions are common. As the process becomes less acute, the pneumonia subsides, although some reaction in the lung around the cavity typically remains until treatment is initiated. The cavity becomes visible, usually with a fluid level, when communication with a patent bronchus permits the entry of air. However, air in the cavity does not mean that effective drainage exists; better criteria are abrupt reduction in cavity size, fall in the fluid level within the cavity, reduction in fever and other systemic manifestations, and increased production of the characteristic purulent sputum.

Primary lung abscess must be differentiated from a large number of other cavitary lung diseases by appropriate methods. The factors that predispose to the development of purulent pulmonary cavitation are summarized in Table 1. Table 2 is a partial listing of organisms that can cause lung abscess. The most important diagnosis to exclude is carcinoma, which occurs in about 20 percent of persons suspected of having a primary lung abscess and half of those above the age of 50 who are smokers. Fungal and mycobacterial infections should also be considered initially because of the length of time required for culturing these organisms. The predisposing circumstances and organisms most frequently associated with primary lung abscess are indicated in the tables by an asterisk.

Bacteriology

Of the mixed anaerobic organisms which, in combination with normal oral aerobic flora, are responsible for most primary lung abscesses, the predominant ones are *Bacteroides melaninogenicus*, other *Bacteroides* species, *Fusobacterium nucleatum* and other species, anaerobic or microaerophilic streptococci, and *Peptostreptococcus. Bacteroides fragilis* is present in 15 percent of cases. In hospitalized patients, persons who have been receiving antibiotics, or immunosuppressed patients, gram-negative bacilli and staphylococci are common. Gram staining and routine aerobic culture of

TABLE 1 Lung Abscess: Predisposing Factors

Massive inoculum
- Aspiration*
  - Stupor, coma, seizure, intoxication
  - Anesthesia
  - Laryngeal dysfunction
- Dental and gingival infection*
- Hematogenous dissemination
  - Intravenous drug abuse
  - Right-sided endocarditis
  - Septic phlebitis
  - Osteomyelitis or other septic focus

Local pathology
- Obstructing neoplasm
- Foreign body
- Distortion by fibrosis
- Bronchostenosis
- Cysts, bullae
- Sequestration
- Contusion or trauma
- Gastric acid

Necrotizing vascular disorders
- Embolic infarction
- Vasculitis
  - Wegener's, RA, polyarteritis
- Necrosis within neoplasm
- Necrotizing conglomerate pneumoconiosis
- Chronic eosinophilic pneumonia

Impaired host resistance
- Alcoholism*
- Diabetes
- Chronic debilitating disease
- Malnutrition*
- Impaired humoral resistance
  - Leukopenia
  - Hypoglobulinemia
- Impaired tissue-mediated immunity
  - Acquired immunodeficiency
  - Radiation exposure
  - Chemotherapy
  - Steroid therapy
  - Neoplasia; Hodgkin's disease, lymphomas

* Circumstances commonly associated with primary lung abscess

the sputum should be carried out initially to exclude specific necrotizing aerobic organisms. Subsequent cultures are required only if a significant change in bacterial flora is suggested by failure to improve after 2 or 3 weeks of treatment, by an exacerbation of an abscess that has been responding, or by the development of new pulmonary opacities.

The first indication that the abscess is not of the simple aspirational type may consist of a failure to respond after several weeks of treatment. Therefore, tuberculosis skin testing with controls and smears and culture of the sputum for mycobacteria and fungi should be performed initially if there is any possibility that these organisms are present. The bacteriologic findings in the sputum are helpful in identifying specific aerobic organisms responsible for acute pneumonia with cavitation and, of course, if a specific pathogen such as *Klebsiella, M. tuberculosis*, or fungi (other than *Candida* or *Aspergillus*) are found. Otherwise the sputum findings are generally misleading: gram-negative and other saprophytes nearly always are found after the

TABLE 2 Lung Abscess: Partial List of Etiologic Organisms

Pyogenic aerobic bacteria
- *Staphylococcus aureus*
- Gram-negative bacilli (*Klebsiella, Proteus,* and others)
- *Streptococcus pneumoniae*
- Group A streptococci
- *Legionella*

Pyogenic anaerobes*
- *Fusobacterium nucleatum* and other species
- *Bacteroides melaninogenicus, B. fragilis,* and other species
- Peptostreptococci
- *Treponema macrodentium*

Nocardia

Mycobacteria
- *M. tuberculosis, M. kansaii, M. intracellularis* and other species

Fungi
- *Histoplasm, Coccidioides, Blastomyces, Actinomyces, Sporothrix, Aspergillus, Cryptococcus, Phycomycetes*

Parasites
- *Entamoeba histolytica*
- *Paragonimus*
- *Echinococcus*

* Primary lung abscess is caused by combinations of these anaerobes with *S. viridans, Neisseria sp.*, and other normal oral flora.

onset of hospitalization or antibiotic therapy. Furthermore contamination of the cavitary exudate by the upper airway and pharynx is inevitable. In addition, the cavity must communicate openly with the bronchi for valid sputum to be obtained.

Bronchoscopy

Bronchoscopy is used to rule out malignant tumor and other local pathologic processes, to evaluate hemorrhage, and to obtain material for bacteriologic examination. It is performed at some time during the management of almost all patients. Bronchoscopy should be postponed until the acute illness subsides, if possible, particularly in persons with reduced pulmonary function. Even a few days of antibiotic treatment reduces toxicity, improves oxygenation, and enhances visibility during the procedure. Since postobstructive pneumonias may respond to antibiotics, improvement during treatment does not eliminate the possibility of endobronchial neoplasm, foreign body, or other local disease. Bronchoscopy is unnecessary in nonsmoking patients with straightforward primary abscess who respond well to treatment. Sosenko and Glassroth compared patients with primary lung abscess with those who had malignant tumors and noted that the former had more roentgenographic evidence of pneumonitis around the cavity, more systemic symptoms, frequent history of circumstances predisposing to aspiration, temperatures above 37.5°C, and white counts greater than 11,000. If three of the last four of these criteria were present, there was a 91 percent probability that there was no underlying malignant tumor. In such persons, bronchoscopy is indicated only if the clinical response is unsatisfactory.

Bronchoscopy is usually ineffective in establishing drainage of an abscess that does not communicate freely with the bronchi. However, sometimes irrigation and aspiration are followed by improved drainage of the cavity. Antibiotics, postural drainage, and attention to concomitant disease problems are generally effective in establishing drainage. As already noted, culture from the cavity is needed only when the clinical circumstances, the routine sputum culture findings, or the failure to respond to treatment raises the question of specific infectious causes other than the usual mixed anaerobic flora. Bronchoscopic culture is helpful in these special circumstances, especially to recover mycobacteria or fungi. The shielded brush technique should be used when the suspected pathogen, particularly gram-negative rods and staphylococci, may also occur as a saprophyte in the upper airway. Bronchoscopy is also occasionally used to verify the site of pulmonary hemorrhage if resection for control of bleeding is contemplated. Occasionally, bronchoscopy causes massive eruption of purulent material that results in widespread airways obstruction, aspiration pneumonia, or death. Tracheal intubation with bronchoscopy through the tube allows better control of ventilation and secretions in high-risk patients. Rigid bronchoscopy is used in rare cases to aspirate life-threatening massive secretions.

MANAGEMENT

Antibiotics

Because of difficulties in obtaining and evaluating anaerobic cultures, the diagnosis of primary abscess is usually established on clinical grounds. When the clinical circumstances and bacteriologic findings indicate that specific pathogens such as *Klebsiella* are causative, antibiotic therapy is selected on the basis of cultures and sensitivity studies. If the differentiation between gram-negative and anaerobic etiology is unclear, semisynthetic penicillin or other drugs to which both groups of organisms are sensitive should be used initially. In primary lung abscess, penicillin, by virtue of long experience and low incidence of side effects, is the drug of choice. Clindamycin, 600 mg every 8 hours intravenously, is equally effective and should be used when the response to penicillin is unsatisfactory or in persons who are allergic to it. The initial penicillin dose should be 6 to 10 million units intravenously daily, although doses as small as 1.2 million units have been used successfully. Although 15 percent of patients harbor penicillin-resistant *B. fragilis*, these patients respond to penicillin just as well as those in whom all of the anaerobic organisms are penicillin-sensitive. After toxicity subsides, cavitary drainage becomes established, and a favorable response is evident, treatment is changed to 750 mg of oral penicillin V four times daily. Occasionally, a good response, one that permits the patient to be discharged from the hospital, may occur quickly, but it generally requires 2 to 4 weeks. Subsequent antibiotic therapy is based on the principle that resolution of lung abscess is usually extremely slow, commonly requiring 4 weeks to 4 months. As long as the cavity remains unchanged or becomes smaller, or the cavity wall becomes thinner, penicillin is continued. Progress is evaluated clinically and roentgenographically every 2 to 4 weeks. If the disease is stable or improving, sputum cultures are misleading and unnecessary. Treatment is discontinued when the abscess disappears or only a thin-walled asymptomatic lesion remains. Currently, the mortality in primary lung abscess is reported to be 3 to 11 percent.

Bronchial Clearance

Postural drainage, deliberate expulsive coughing maneuvers, early ambulation, and avoidance of sedation are required to remove pulmonary secretions. Chest percussion is not often helpful, and its use should be evaluated by the immediate response to these treatments. Repeated bronchoscopic examinations for aspiration of secretions are not used. Concomitant diseases, including malnutrition, alcoholism, circumstances leading to aspiration, and chronic obstructive pulmonary disease, must be treated.

COMPLICATIONS

Delayed resolution is not a cause for alarm unless a thick-walled cavity is unchanged for 2 or 3 weeks. Cessation of drainage with a persistent fluid level, increase in cavity diameter, increased surrounding pneumonitis, or resumption of fever and malaise suggests, first, noncompliance with the prescribed medications. Failure to control concomitant disease problems such as diabetes, malnutrition, or other factors affecting host resistance should be considered. If bronchoscopy was not performed earlier, it should be done to rule out neoplasm or a radiolucent foreign body. Bronchoscopic irrigation and aspiration of an impacted mucous plug may also restore cavity drainage.

Failure to respond may also indicate that the abscess is not secondary to the usual anaerobic flora. Bronchoscopically obtained cultures using the protected brush technique can resolve this problem. Occasionally, *B. fragillis* is the principal organism, particularly if the abscess is secondary to gastrointestinal or gynecologic infection. Clindamycin, chloramphenicol, or cefoxitin is then indicated.

Hemoptysis occurs in one-third of primary lung abscesses and is not usually massive. Brisk hemoptysis is treated by placing the cavity in the dependent position. Massive hemoptysis may be sudden and require emergency lobectomy. Intubation with a divided tube allows ventilation of the opposite lung until the hemorrhage is controlled or the abscess resected.

Septicemia with hemodynamic consequences, dissemination of infection including brain abscess, adult respiratory distress syndrome, and pneumonia from bronchial spread of infected secretions may occur before treatment has become effective. A severely ill person, particularly if the patient has been on antibiotic therapy, immunosuppressed, or hospitalized, should receive broad-spectrum antibiotics against gram-negative and staphylococcal organisms, and sometimes treatment for legionella and tuberculosis, until the diagnosis is established.

Sterile parapneumonic effusions are common and empyema occurs occasionally. Thoracentesis is therefore necessary when significant pleural fluid is present, but need not be done for small effusions in patients who are responding well. Many abscesses and the surrounding pneumonia are pleural-based. Bronchopleural fistulas sometimes occur, and it can be difficult to determine whether the fluid level is in the pleura or located within an abscess cavity. The CT scan is effective in determining whether the disease process is located entirely within the lung.

SURGERY

In contrast to the pre-antibiotic era, surgery is rarely used in the management of primary lung abscess. A stable abscess with minimal symptoms or one that is becoming smaller intermittently or slowly over many weeks requires only continuation of antibiotics and supportive measures. Resection is sometimes required for massive hemorrhage. If delay is possible, even a few days of antibiotic treatment of the acutely infected patient can reduce the risks involved in operating in the presence of acute pneumonia, and the hemorrhage may cease. In a small number of patients, in spite of adequate antibiotics, supportive measures, and bronchoscopy, severe systemic toxicity and failure to obtain drainage of the cavity may persist. Resection is sometimes required in these cases, particularly if septic complications are occurring.

Cavernostomy is rarely needed, but can be used in patients with uncontrolled hemorrhage or uncontrollable progressive disease in whom resection cannot be carried out because of the severity of concomitant diseases, including diminished pulmonary function. The two-stage Monaldi procedure is used to prevent empyema when pleural symphysis has not occurred.

SUGGESTED READING

Bartlett JG, Gorbach SL, Tally FP, Friegold SM. Bacteriology and treatment of primary lung abscess. Am Rev Respir Dis 1974; 109:510–518.

Sosenko A, Glassroth J. Fiberoptic bronchoscopy in the evaluation of lung abscesses. Chest 1985; 87:489–494.

Snow N, Lucas A, Horrigan T. Utility of pneumonotomy in the treatment of cavitary lung disease. Chest 1985; 87:731–734.

TUBERCULOSIS

PHILIP C. HOPEWELL, M.D.

Although commonly regarded as a disease of the past, tuberculosis remains an important problem in many parts of the developed world and is of even greater concern in developing countries. For tuberculosis, as opposed to most communicable diseases, treatment serves as the major public health measure for reducing spread of the infection; thus, the incidence of tuberculosis is determined in large part by the effectiveness and availability of chemotherapy. Of course effective treatment is equally important for the health of the individual patient. To achieve coequal benefits to the patient and to society it is essential that chemotherapy be properly administered. The physician who undertakes treatment of tuberculosis is assuming a responsibility not only to the patient but to the community as well. Fulfilling this responsibility requires both a thorough understanding of the principles and practice of treatment for tuberculosis on the part of physicians prescribing treatment and an organization capable of ensuring that the regimen is adhered to by the patient. A treatment program that is poorly designed and conducted carries a high likelihood not only of failure to cure the illness, but of induction of drug resistance and perpetuation of the patient's infectiousness.

BASIC PRINCIPLES OF ANTITUBERCULOSIS CHEMOTHERAPY

Truly effective chemotherapy for tuberculosis became a reality in 1952 with the introduction of isoniazid. Although streptomycin was introduced six years earlier, lack of a suitable companion agent to inhibit the emergence of resistant organisms prevented it from becoming a striking therapeutic success. Shortly after streptomycin was introduced it became apparent that patients whose condition initially improved with the drug subsequently worsened. Investigators quickly determined that the organisms isolated from patients who had relapsed were no longer susceptible to streptomycin and thereby defined an important bacteriologic principle that underlies successful chemotherapy for tuberculosis: populations of *Mycobacterium tuberculosis* are not uniform in their susceptibility to antimycobacterial agents. For this reason it is always necessary to use more than one drug to which the organisms are susceptible. The concept of multiple-drug chemotherapy was first validated in a British Medical Research Council study in which streptomycin was supplemented by para-aminosalicylic acid. Since that time, treatment with at least two agents has been standard in the management of patients with tuberculosis.

Subsequent to the clinical observations already described, the frequency of drug resistant mutants among wild-strain *M. tuberculosis* was determined to be

1×10^{-5} for isoniazid and 1×10^{-6} for streptomycin. Based on these frequencies, a bacillary population of more than 10^{11} organisms would be required to contain a mutant resistant to both agents.

Having established the need for, and the basis of, multiple-drug therapy using isoniazid, plus streptomycin and/or para-aminosalicylic acid, there remained a need to determine the optimum duration of therapy. In 1962, the Medical Research Council reported that in patients with cavitary pulmonary tuberculosis the relapse rate was significantly less with 24 months of therapy than with 12 months (4% versus 22% relapses).

In the ensuing 10 to 15 years there were a number of important modifications in treatment regimens for tuberculosis. Hospitalization, which had been regarded as an essential component of care for all or part of the treatment period, was shown to confer no benefit compared to treatment at home. In addition, it was shown that chemotherapy was very effective in reducing or eliminating the infectiousness of patients, thereby greatly decreasing the need for their isolation. Diet and rest were shown not to be important factors in determining outcome. Surgical procedures became of less and less importance in patient management. Finally it was recognized that antituberculosis drugs could be given in single daily doses or, in some instances, even twice weekly without decreasing their effectiveness.

In 1967 the effectiveness of ethambutol as a substitute for para-aminosalicylic acid was documented. Ethambutol was readily accepted as a much more tolerable and less toxic companion drug for isoniazid.

The next advance in chemotherapy for tuberculosis resulted from the discovery of the antimycobacterial effect of rifampin, and the demonstration that using the combination of isoniazid and rifampin, generally with ethambutol, streptomycin, or pyrazinamide, the necessary duration of treatment could be shortened dramatically. A series of studies from East Africa demonstrated that, under controlled circumstances, a regimen consisting of 6 months of isoniazid, streptomycin, and rifampin was as effective as 18 months of isoniazid and thioacetazone with streptomycin given in the first 2 months. Although these studies clearly indicated that shorter durations of treatment using regimens that included rifampin and isoniazid were of great potential usefulness, the applicability of such treatment under working program conditions remained to be defined. The British Thoracic and Tuberculosis Association conducted an operational evaluation of regimens that consisted of isoniazid and rifampin given for 6, 9, 12, or 18 months plus either streptomycin or ethambutol for the initial 2 months. The rate of treatment failure and relapse in the 6-month regimen was 5.6 percent whereas in the 9-month regimen there were no failures or relapses.

The success of a 9-month regimen was substantiated by a report from Arkansas showing that a regimen consisting of isoniazid and rifampin given daily for 1 month and twice a week for 8 months was highly successful as administered by the Tuberculosis Control Program throughout the State. In the initial report there were 5.4 percent failures and 0.5 percent relapses. Longer term follow-up has shown an overall success rate of 96.1 percent.

Preliminary information from recent studies suggests that the combination of isoniazid and rifampin, given for 6 months, supplemented by pyrazinamide in the initial 2 months has a very high rate of success.

Concomitantly, with information on short durations of chemotherapy, there has been an increasing understanding of the effects of antituberculosis drugs on various subpopulations of mycobacteria. These principles complement the earlier observations on the nonuniform susceptibility of populations of mycobacteria to antituberculosis drugs. Streptomycin, rifampin and isoniazid are bactericidal for rapidly growing *M. tuberculosis* in vitro. The in vitro conditions could be likened to the conditions under which the large pool of extracellular organisms in tuberculous lesions are living.

Although both rifampin and isoniazid are bactericidal, rifampin appears to be more effective in killing organisms that grow in spurts rather than in those that grow continuously. If there is a subpopulation of organisms that grow intermittently, this suggests an additional beneficial effect of rifampin.

Finally, it has long been known that pyrazinamide is active in an acid environment such as exists within macrophages. It seems logical to assume that the beneficial effects of pyrazinamide noted in clinical trials may be due to its ability to kill intracellular organisms.

These basic principles described in this section are summarized as follows, and will be enlarged upon in the following sections:

1. Treatment should always include two drugs to which the organisms are presumed or documented to be susceptible. In the presence of treatment failure or relapse at least two new agents should be given. Definitions of treatment failure are as given previously. Relapse after treatment with an isoniazid regimen should be subsequently treated with the same agents.
2. The necessary duration of treatment is much longer than for "usual" bacterial infections. At present 6 months is the minimum duration.
3. Antituberculosis drugs act on different subpopulations of bacilli in tuberculous lesions.

FIRST-LINE ANTITUBERCULOSIS DRUGS

The antituberculosis drugs that are available currently in the United States and Canada are listed in Table 1 together with their doses and adverse effects.

These agents are in general potent, easily administered, and possess relatively low toxicity. Of these isoniazid and rifampin have the highest ratio of peak-serum-concentration to minimal-inhibitory-concentration. Ethambutol, although not particularly potent, is an effective companion agent for isoniazid and rifampin and has a very low rate of adverse reactions. Pyrazinamide may be useful because of its effect on intracellular organisms. Streptomycin has the disadvantage of requiring parenteral administration and is the most toxic of the first line drugs.

Isoniazid

Isoniazid in many respects is an ideal drug: it is very effective, relatively non-toxic, easily administered, and inexpensive. It is highly active against *M. tuberculosis*, most strains being inhibited by concentrations of 0.05 to 0.20 μg per milliliter. Peak blood concentrations of approximately 5 μg per milliliter occur 1 to 2 hours after oral administration of 3 to 5 μg per kilogram of body weight. The serum half-life varies from 2 to 4 hours in slow acetylators and 0.5 to 1.5 hours in rapid acetylators. The drug penetrates well into all body fluids and cavities producing concentrations similar to those found in serum.

Isoniazid is bactericidal for *M. tuberculosis* and probably acts by inhibiting mycolate synthetase.

Side Effects. Hepatitis is the major toxic effect of izoniazid. In a study of 13,838 patients who were given isoniazid alone as preventive therapy, the rate of "probable" isoniazid-related hepatitis was 10.4 cases per 1,000 patients with an additional 10.2 "possible" cases per 1,000 patients treated. The rate increased directly with increasing age being 0 percent for those less than 20; 0.3 percent in those aged 20 to 34; 1.2 percent in those aged 35 to 49; and 2.3 percent in those aged 50 to 64. Alcohol consumption was identified as another risk factor.

Peripheral neuropathy associated with isoniazid administration may occur especially in persons with other diseases that may cause neuropathy (diabetes, uremia, alcoholism). The neuropathy can be prevented or reversed by administration of pyridoxine in doses of 10 to 25 mg per day.

Rifampin

Rifampin rapidly halts the growth of *M. tuberculosis* and subsequently is bactericidal. The drug is easily administered and is relatively nontoxic. It is quickly absorbed from the gastrointestinal tract with serum concentrations of 6 to 7 μg per milliliter occurring 1.5 to 2 hours after ingestion. The half-time in blood is 3 to 3.5 hours, although this may be accelerated in persons who have been taking the drug for several weeks. The half-time increases with increasing doses of the drug. For sensitive strains of *M. tuberculosis* the minimum inhibitory concentration of rifampin is approximately 0.5 μg per milliliter. Although approximately 75 percent of the drug is protein-bound, it penetrates well into tissues and cells. Penetration through noninflamed meninges is poor, but therapeutic concentrations are achieved in cerebrospinal fluid when the meninges are inflamed.

TABLE 1 Drugs Used in the Treatment of Mycobacterial Disease

Antituberculosis Drugs	*Adult Dosage*		*Most Common Adverse Effects*	*Tests for Adverse Effects*
	Daily	*Twice Weekly*		
Isoniazid	5–10 mg/kg, up to 300 mg PO or IM	15 mg/kg PO or IM	Peripheral neuropathy, hepatitis, hypersensitivity	SGOT (not as routine)
Ethambutol	15–25 mg/kg PO	50 mg/kg PO	Optic neuritis (reversible with discontinuation of drug; very rare at 15 mg/kg), skin rash	Red-green color discrimination and visual acuity*
Rifampin	10–15 mg/kg up to 600 mg PO	600 mg PO	Hepatitis, febrile reaction, purpura (rare), drug interactions	SGOT (not as routine)
Streptomycin	15 mg/kg, up to 1 g IM	25–30 mg/kg IM	Eighth nerve damage, (vestibular) nephrotoxicity	Vestibular function, audiograms, BUN, and creatinine
Pyrazinamide	25 mg/kg, up to 2 g PO	50 mg/kg up to 3.5 g PO	Hyperuricemia, hepatotoxicity	Uric acid, SGOT
Capreomycin	12–15 mg/kg, up to 1 g IM		Eighth nerve damage, (auditory), nephrotoxicity, vestibular toxicity (rare)	Vestibular function, audiograms, BUN, and creatinine
Kanamycin	12–15 mg/kg, up to 1 g IM		Eighth nerve damage, (auditory), nephrotoxicity, vestibular toxicity (rare)	Vestibular function, audiograms, BUN, and creatinine
Ethionamide	15 mg/kg, up to 1 g PO		GI disturbance, hepatotoxicity, hypersensitivity	SGOT
p-Aminosalicylic acid (aminosalicylic acid)	150 mg/kg, up to 12 g PO		GI disturbance hypersensitivity, hepatotoxicity, sodium load	SGOT
Cycloserine	15 mg/kg, up to 1 g PO		Psychosis, personality changes, convulsions, rash	

* Determine at the start of treatment and subsequently as clinically indicated. BUN, blood urea nitrogen; GI, gastrointestinal; IM, intramuscularly; PO, by mouth; SGOT, serum glutamic-oxaloacetic transaminase.

Rifampin has activity against many bacteria including mycobacteria. The major effect of the drug is an inhibition of DNA-dependent RNA polymerase.

Side Effects. When it is given daily, adverse reactions to rifampin include skin eruptions, hepatitis, gastrointestinal upset, and rarely, thrombocytopenia. The rate of these reactions is variable, but in general is quite low. Hepatitis occurred in 3.1 percent of the patients in the United States Public Health Service (USPHS) study of 6-month isoniazid-rifampin treatment. Twice weekly administration of higher doses of rifampin is associated with several immunologically mediated reactions. These include thrombocytopenia, an influenza-like syndrome, hemolytic anemia, and acute renal failure. Rifampin turns body secretions orange. Although this is not a side effect per se, it may discolor soft contact lenses. The drug is also a potent inducer of hepatic microsomal enzymes and as such may accelerate the metabolism of many drugs. Documented interactions have occurred with methadone, oral contraceptive agents, Coumadin, oral hypoglycemic agents, cortisone-like drugs, and others as well.

Ethambutol

Ethambutol in usual doses is generally considered to have a bacteriostatic effect on *M. tuberculosis.* The drug is easily administered and has a low frequency of adverse reactions. Peak-plasma concentrations occur 2 to 4 hours after ingestion. With doses of 15 mg per kilogram the peak concentration is approximately 4 μg per milliter. The concentration increases proportionately with increasing doses. In persons with normal renal function the half-time in blood is approximately 4 hours. Minimum inhibitory concentrations of the drug for *M. tuberculosis* range from 1 to 5 μg per milliliter. Cerebrospinal fluid concentrations of ethambutol, even in the presence of meningeal inflammation, are low, averaging 1 to 2 μg per milliliter after a dose of 25 mg per kilogram. The mechanism of action of the drug is not known.

Side Effects. Retrobulbar neuritis is the main adverse effect of ethambutol. Symptoms include blurred vision, central scotomata, and red-green color blindness. This complication is dose related, occurring in 15 percent of patients given 50 mg per kilogram, approximately 5 percent with 25 mg per kilogram and less than 1 percent with 15 mg per kilogram. The frequency of ocular effects is increased in patients with renal failure presumably related to increased serum concentrations of the drug.

Pyrazinamide

Pyrazinamide is very active against *M. tuberculosis* but only at an acid pH; this suggests that the drug is activated under this condition. The drug is particularly active against organisms in macrophages presumably because of the acid environment within the cell. It is rapidly bacteriostatic but only slowly bactericidal. Absorption from the gastrointestinal tract is nearly complete with peak serum concentrations occurring approximately 2 hours after ingestion. Concentrations generally range from 30 to 50 μg per milliliter with doses of 20 to 25 mg per kilogram. The serum half life is 9 to 10 hours. At a pH of 5.5 the minimal inhibitory concentration of pyrazinamide for *M. tuberculosis* is 20 μg per milliliter. Penetration of the drug into cells and tissues seems to be fairly good, although data with regard to tissue concentrations are limited. The mechanism of action of pyrazinamide is not known.

Side Effects. The most important adverse reaction to pyrazinamide is liver injury. This appears to be a dose-related occurrence. In a large USPHS study in which pyrazinamide was given in a dose of 25 mg per kilogram daily for 6 months, hepatotoxicity occurred in 2 to 3 percent of patients. At a dose of 40 mg per kilogram per day, also given for 6 months, 6 percent of patients developed hepatitis. It should be noted, however, that all patients were receiving isoniazid and para-aminosalicylic acid in addition to pyrazinamide.

Administration of pyrazinamide impairs renal urate clearance. Because of this, hyperuricemia is very common in patients taking the drug. Clinical gout is not common; however, diffuse arthralgias, apparently not related to the hyperuricemia, occur frequently.

Streptomycin

Streptomycin is rapidly bactericidal although its effectiveness is inhibited to a great degree by an acid pH. Because the drug is not absorbed from the gut it must be given parenterally. Peak serum concentrations of approximately 40 μg per milliliter occur 1 hour after an intramuscular dose of 15 mg per kilogram. The usual half-time in blood is 5 hours. Sensitive strains of *M. tuberculosis* are inhibited by streptomycin in a concentration of 8 μg per milliliter. The drug has good tissue penetration; however, it enters the cerebrospinal fluid only in the presence of meningeal inflammation.

Streptomycin exerts its effect by interfering with ribosomal protein synthesis. Some protein synthesis is necessary for the action of the drug to be irreversible. Resistance rapidly emerges when the drug is used alone.

Side Effects. Of the first-line drugs, streptomycin contributes the most to toxicity when used in combination chemotherapy. The most serious adverse effect of streptomycin is ototoxicity. This usually results in vertigo, but hearing loss may also occur. The risk of ototoxicity is related to cumulative dosage and to peak serum concentrations. In general, peak concentrations of greater than 40 to 50 μg per milliliter should be avoided and a total dose of more than 100 to 120 grams should not be given.

SECOND-LINE ANTITUBERCULOSIS DRUGS

The second-line agents in general are less effective and more toxic and therefore more difficult to use.

Currently, in the United States there are 5 second-line antituberculosis agents, para-aminosalicylic acid, ethionamide, cycloserine, kanamycin and capreomycin.

Amakacin, although not commonly used in treating tuberculosis, is active against *M. tuberculosis* and may be helpful in some situations. Each of these drugs has important limitations that interfere with their general usefulness in treating tuberculosis.

Para-aminosalicylic Acid

Para-aminosalicylic acid is associated with a very high frequency of gastrointestinal upset. Hypersensitivity reactions occur in 5 to 10 percent of patients taking the drug. In addition, the usual dose of 10 to 12 g per day requires ingestion of 20 to 24 tablets.

Ethionamide

Ethionamide likewise causes a very high frequency of gastrointestinal side effects often necessitating discontinuation of the drug.

Cycloserine

Cycloserine causes behavioral disturbances in a large number of patients to whom the drug is given. These behavioral disturbances range from irritability and depression to frank psychosis. In addition, seizures and peripheral neuropathy occur, especially with higher doses, and when cycloserine and isoniazid are given together. These neurologic effects may be prevented by high doses of pyradoxine.

Kanamycin and Capreomycin

Kanamycin and capreomycin are not absorbed from the gastrointestinal tract and thus they require parenteral administration. Both drugs may cause hearing loss related both to peak concentrations and cumulative doses. In addition, they may cause impairment of renal function.

MANAGEMENT

It is clear that at least in the initial phase of treatment for tuberculosis, isoniazid and rifampin are essential components of the drug regimen. Using isoniazid and rifampin as the core, a variety of potential treatment options are available (Table 2), the basic goal being to provide the most effective therapy in the shortest period of time. Recent clinical trials allow a number of important generalizations to be made that can provide guidance in constructing drug regimens:

1. Isoniazid should be used throughout the course of treatment unless there is a well substantiated reason for its exclusion (intolerance or bacterial resistance).
2. Rifampin given at least for 2 months is an essential component in regimens of less than 9 months and probably with any regimen less than 12 months. Regimens of less than 8 months are probably more effective if rifampin is used throughout.
3. Although there are scattered reports of good results with regimens of less than 6 months, in general, relapse rates with regimens of this duration are unacceptably high.
4. Pyrazinamide given in the initial phase improves the efficacy of regimens of less than 9 months duration. It does not appear, however, that continuing pyrazinamide beyond the initial 2 months improves the outcome of a "good" regimen.
5. At least in the doses usually given, ethambutol is not an adequate substitute for pyrazinamide. However, it appears that ethambutol may be substituted for streptomycin without decreasing the potency of a regimen.
6. Continuation of streptomycin beyond the initial 2 months does not improve outcome.

TABLE 2 Chemotherapy for Tuberculosis

Regimen	*Disadvantages*	*Advantages*
Standard Situations		
2IRZ/41R*	Less experience, Z toxicity	Shorter allowing better supervision
2IRE/7IR or 2IRE/$7I_2R_2$**	Longer	More experience, "Safe" in presence of I resistance
9I R or 2IR/$7I_2R_2$	Longer May fail in presence of I resistance	Simpler, cheaper
Special Situations		
12–18IE	Very long	Can be used if R cannot be included
12–18RE	Very long Less experience	Can be used if I cannot be included
IS (variable duration)	S Toxicity	Can be given parenterally
18–24/any combination not including I or R	Very long Less likely to be successful and more toxic	Only options when I and R cannot be used or are ineffective

I-Isoniazid; R-Rifampin; Z-Pyrazinamide; E-Ethambutol; S-Streptomycin.
* Numbers preceding drugs indicate months of administration
** I_2R_2 - administration 2 times per week

7. There is good evidence that intermittent administration of appropriate doses of the drugs after an initial daily phase of treatment produces results equal to those of daily administration.

These generalizations apply only to patients who have drug-susceptible organisms. Resistance to isoniazid and/or streptomycin as well as to other agents is associated with much lower rates of success and is of major concern. Although in the United States, Canada, and Western Europe overall rates of initial drug resistance are low (3% to 5% for isoniazid), there are geographic areas and ethnic groups where rates are much higher. Moreover, in much of the developing world, reported rates of resistance to isoniazid, streptomycin, or both, among previously untreated patients are commonly in excess of 20 percent and occasionally above 50 percent.

Patients with organisms that are resistant to isoniazid and who are given isoniazid and rifampin alone are likely to develop resistance to rifampin. The occurrence of resistance to rifampin in those with isoniazid resistance is in sharp contrast to the nearly 100 percent maintenance of susceptibility to rifampin in patients who have fully sensitive organisms at the time treatment is begun and who relapse.

The findings concerning the effects of resistance strongly suggest that in segments of the population of developed countries or in developing countries, where the prevalence of initial resistance to isoniazid is likely to be great, treatment regimens should contain an initial three- or four-drug phase, depending on the planned duration, and rifampin should be given for a minimum of 4 to 6 months. The risk of not taking this approach is the development of rifampin resistance.

PATIENT-RELATED CONSIDERATIONS IN CHOOSING A DRUG REGIMEN

History of Previous Treatment for Tuberculosis. Persons who have been treated previously with regimens that did not contain both isoniazid and rifampin and who have a recurrence are much more likely to have drug-resistant organisms than untreated patients. In one survey, 23 percent of patients who had been treated previously with isoniazid in combination with other agents for 1 to 6 months and who subsequently relapsed had isoniazid-resistant organisms. The prevalence of isoniazid resistance increased to 53 percent in patients treated 12 to 24 months and 72 percent in those treated for more than 24 months. Because of the likelihood of bacillary resistance, patients who have been treated in the past cannot be managed using the guidelines described in the preceding section but must be assumed to have organisms that are resistant to the drugs that had been used. Regimens then must be tailored to include at least two agents that the patient has not received previously. The management of these patients will be discussed subsequently. Patients who relapse after apparently successful treatment with an isoniazid-rifampin regimen generally have susceptible organisms and can be treated with the same regimen.

Probability of Primary Isoniazid Resistance. Tuberculous infection acquired in a developing country is much more likely to be caused by isoniazid-resistant organisms than infection acquired in the United States or Canada. Thus, in general, persons from developing countries should be treated at the outset with a regimen that would likely be effective even if the organisms were resistant to isoniazid. This can be accomplished by the addition of ethambutol to the initial phase of treatment until the results of drug suceptibility tests are available. If the organism is fully susceptible, ethambutol can be discontinued and if not, the regimen can be modified as necessary.

Assessment of Patient Compliance. The major reason for failure of antituberculosis chemotherapy is failure of the patient to adhere to the regimen as prescribed. Predicting who will and who will not comply with therapy is difficult at best; however, patients who have a history of antisocial behavior or substance abuse can be anticipated to present problems; younger age and unmarried status are also predictive of poor compliance. Perhaps the best assessment is the patient's behavior early in the course of treatment. In patients who are predicted to be noncompliant, several approaches can be used. First, in this group, the shortest duration of effective treatment is the most likely to be completed, hence, a 6-month isoniazid, rifampin, pyrazinamide regimen should be employed. Strong consideration should be given to providing directly observed therapy – daily in the initial phase and twice weekly in the continuation phase. In patients not given directly-observed therapy, techniques to monitor compliance (pill counts or urine checks) should be used.

Presence of Coexisting Diseases. Whenever possible, drugs having toxicities that may add to the effects of coexisting diseases should be avoided. In patients with impaired renal function, streptomycin, kanamycin and capreomycin should be avoided. In addition, these agents should not be given to patients with hearing loss or disturbances of balance. Similarly, ethambutol should not be used in patients with significant loss of vision.

The use of isoniazid and rifampin in patients with preexisting liver disease represents an exception to this general rule. Although both isoniazid and rifampin may have adverse effects on liver function they are of such crucial importance that they should not be withheld. However, patients should be carefully monitored with both clinical and laboratory evaluations and it should be recognized that changes in clinical status or in liver function tests may be caused by the underlying disease rather than the drugs.

Necessary Routes of Administration. The necessary route of administration of antituberculosis drugs may also influence the choice or formulation of agents used. Patients who cannot take drugs by mouth, but whose gut function is intact, can be given any but the injectable agents via nasogastric tube. Only isoniazid, streptomycin, kanamycin and capreomycin are available in injectable form for use in patients who cannot absorb drugs from the gut. In such patients, a regimen of isoniazid and streptomycin given intramuscularly should be used.

Results of Drug Susceptibility Tests. Generally, the results of drug susceptibility tests are not available at the time treatment is initiated. Thus, initial therapy should be based on the considerations discussed previously and the regimen modified, if necessary, when the sensitivity of the organism is known. At a minimum, susceptibility testing should be performed on the isolates from patients who have been treated previously and from those in whom there is a suspicion of initial drug resistance. Generally it is prudent to perform susceptibility testing as a matter of routine on all initial isolates. However, it should be kept in mind that susceptibility studies for mycobacteria are somewhat difficult to perform. The physician supervising treatment should be familiar with the capability and experience of the laboratory performing the tests and should be very cautious in interpreting results from laboratories that do not process many specimens.

History of Adverse Reaction. If there is a clear history of either a toxic or hypersensitivity reaction to an agent administered previously, the drug should be avoided. However, if the nature and cause of the reaction is not certain, especially with isoniazid or rifampin, a careful challenge with the suspected drug may be necessary.

EVALUATION OF RESPONSE TO THERAPY

In patients whose pretreatment sputum contains *M. tuberculosis*, elimination of the organisms is the most important indicator of a favorable response. For this reason sputum examinations should be performed at least at monthly intervals and perhaps more frequently early in the course of treatment. After 2 months of treatment with an isoniazid-rifampin regimen, 80 to 90 percent of patients should have negative smears and cultures and after 3 months the proportion should be over 90 percent. Patients whose sputum is not negative after 2 to 3 months of treatment should be carefully reevaluated. Susceptibility testing should be performed on the organism isolated from the 2- to 3-month specimen. Prior to obtaining the results, strong consideration should be given to directly observing therapy. When the results of susceptibility tests are available the regimen can be modified if necessary. Unless resistance is demonstrated the initial regimen should be continued under close supervision.

Once bacteriologic conversion has been achieved further routine examinations are not necessary until therapy is completed. However, it is desirable to obtain a sputum specimen at the time treatment is completed to document that the patient is truly cured.

Clinical evaluations are also of importance early in the course of treatment. Attention should be paid to resolution of fever, weight gain, and decrease in cough frequency. Patients should also be questioned for symptoms that may be indicative of adverse reactions to any of the drugs.

Unless there is concern about the possibility of a pulmonary process other than tuberculosis, routine radiographic examinations are of less importance than either clinical or bacteriologic follow-up in patients who had positive sputum at the outset. In patients having abnormalities on chest film, consistent with tuberculosis, but whose sputum is negative, radiographic evaluations are of greater importance. The intervals at which chest films are obtained should be determined by the clinical status of the patient and the differential diagnosis being considered. In general, lack of radiographic response or any worsening after 3 months of treatment should be taken to indicate that either the abnormality is not of tuberculous origin or that it is the residual of an old, not a current, tuberculosis. In either instance, the drugs should be discontinued. However, if the person has a positive tuberculin skin test and no other cause for the radiographic abnormality is determined, isoniazid should be continued for a full course of preventive therapy (usually 12 months).

In general patients who responded promptly to treatment and who successfully completed one of the described "standard" chemotherapeutic regimens require no further routine follow-up. Those patients who are slow to convert their sputum, who have significant residual radiographic abnormalities, or who have associated illnesses will need further follow-up. The intervals and kinds of evaluations must be determined on an individual basis. All patients should be instructed to be aware of symptoms that may indicate a recurrence of tuberculosis and to report these symptoms promptly.

MANAGEMENT OF PATIENTS WHO HAVE FAILED TREATMENT OR HAVE RELAPSED

Treatment failure is defined as persistence or recurrence of positive sputum during the course of drug therapy. If the sputum is positive after 4 to 6 months of treatment, the regimen should be considered to have failed. This may be due either to drug resistance or to noncompliance with the drug regimen. If good compliance has been documented, the patient should be assumed to have organisms that are resistant to the drugs that had been used, and treatment should be modified. The patient should be given at least two and generally three new agents. This new regimen can then be adjusted based on the results of susceptibility tests. Relapse is considered to have occurred when a patient, who has apparently successfully completed treatment, develops a recurrence of tuberculosis. If such patients have been treated with regimens containing *both* isoniazid and rifampin, it is likely that their organisms are still sensitive to these agents and the same treatment regimen can be reinstituted. Drug susceptibility testing should be performed and the regimen changed if necessary.

Patients who relapse after treatment with a regimen that did not contain *both* isoniazid and rifampin should be assumed to have organisms that are resistant to all the agents that they had received previously. As in the case of treatment failures, these patients should be given a minimum of two and generally three new agents. In general, patients with organisms that are resistant to isoniazid alone can be treated with rifampin and ethambutol, perhaps supplemented initially by pyrazinamide, for a total of 12 months. Patients whose organisms are resistant to isoniazid and rifampin should be treated for a minimum of 18 months. Evaluations during treatment and follow-up after completion of treatment should be determined on a case-by-case basis.

SPECIAL PROBLEMS IN TREATMENT

Children

The basic principles that apply in the management of adults with tuberculosis are equally applicable in children. Although children have been excluded from nearly all clinical trials of shorter durations of chemotherapy there are several reports documenting the usefulness of 6 and 9 month regimens in children. However, there are some important differences in managing tuberculosis in children. Children in general have fewer adverse reactions to antituberculosis drugs and tolerate higher doses. At least in younger children, sputum specimens for bacteriologic evaluations cannot usually be obtained; consequently, the response to treatment is assessed by clinical and radiographic criteria. For this same reason drug susceptibility or resistance must often be inferred from epidemiologic information rather than being determined in the laboratory.

Pregnancy and Lactation

Active untreated tuberculosis represents a much greater hazard to a pregnant woman and her fetus than does treatment for the disease. In a pregnant woman or a mother of a young infant, it is important that the most effective therapy for tuberculosis be given. Only streptomycin has been documented to have harmful effects on the fetus. Streptomycin interferes with development of the ear and may cause congenital deafness. This potential is presumably shared by kanamycin and capreomycin; however, there is little or no specific information on the fetal effects of these two drugs nor is there information on cycloserine, ethionamide and pyrazinamide.

Although several of the antituberculosis drugs are present in breast milk, their concentrations and the total amounts that could possibly be ingested by a nursing infant are such that adverse effects would be very unlikely.

Extrapulmonary Tuberculosis

The same basic principles that underlie the treatment of pulmonary tuberculosis apply to extrapulmonary forms of the disease as well. Although there have not been the same kinds of carefully conducted clinical trials of treatment of extrapulmonary tuberculosis as for pulmonary disease, increasing experience is indicating that shorter durations of treatment are effective. As with children, bacteriologic evaluation may be limited by the relative inaccessibility of the sites of disease. Thus, response to treatment is often judged on the basis of clinical and radiographic findings.

SURGICAL TREATMENT OF TUBERCULOSIS

Surgical therapy, once an important component of the management of tuberculosis, currently has only limited indications. In pulmonary tuberculosis resection of an involved portion of the lung may be necessary because of massive hemoptysis or localized post-tuberculous bronchiectasis with persisting or recurring bacterial infections. Resection may also be considered in patients who have localized tuberculosis caused by multiple drug resistant organisms.

The need for surgery is more common in extrapulmonary tuberculosis, particularly in establishing diagnoses. In lymphatic tuberculosis, incision and drainage may be necessary to prevent spontaneous drainage and formation of fistulas. Open drainage may also be necessary for tuberculous empyema and cold abscesses. Occasionally bone and/or joint lesions may require debridement, and decompression procedures may be required for vertebral tuberculosis with spinal cord compression. Tuberculous pericarditis may cause cardiac tamponade early in its course or cause constrictive pericarditis later. Either of these occurrences requires pericardiectomy. Finally, surgery may be necessary for removal of a kidney destroyed by tuberculosis that has persistent or recurring bacterial infections or is the source of bleeding.

CORTICOSTEROIDS IN TUBERCULOSIS

Corticosteroid treatment may be beneficial in patients with severe pulmonary tuberculosis and marked hypoxemia. It may also be of benefit in patients with extensive lung involvement who have marked systemic effects of the disease such as fever, weight loss, and hypoalbuminemia.

In extrapulmonary tuberculosis the use of corticosteroid treatment may hasten the resolution of tuberculous pericardical effusion and decrease the risk of subsequent constrictive pericarditis. Steroids may also reduce cerebral edema associated with tuberculous meningitis and in addition, decrease the likelihood of cerebrospinal fluid block associated with severe inflammation.

SUGGESTED READING

Glassroth J, Robins AG, Snider DE Jr. Tuberculosis in the 1980s. N Engl J Med 1980; 302:1441–1450.

Grzybowski S, Enarson DA. The fate of cases of pulmonary tuberculosis under various treatment programmes. Bull Internat Union Tuberc 1978; 53:70–75.

Hopewell PC, Ganter B, Baron RB, Sanchez-Hernandez M. Operational evaluation of treatment for tuberculosis: results of 8 and 12-month regimens in Peru. Am Rev Resp Dis 1985; 132:737–741.

Iseman MD. Tailoring a time bomb: inadvertent genetic engineering. Am Rev Resp Dis 1985; 132:735–736.

Snider DE Jr, Graczyk J, Bek E, Rowgowski J. Supervised six-months treatment of newly diagnosed pulmonary tuberculosis using isoniazid, rifampin and pyrazinamide with and without streptomycin. Am Rev Resp Dis 1984; 130:1091–1094.

MYCOBACTERIUM KANSASII INFECTION

CURTIS F. VEAL Jr., M.D.
WILLIAM C. BAILEY, M.D.

The nontuberculous mycobacteria are well-known causes of pulmonary and extrapulmonary disease in man. Of these, the M. avium-intracellulare/scrofulaceum (MAIS) complex and *M. kansasii* are second only to *M. tuberculosis* as agents of human pulmonary mycobacterial disease. The prevalence of disease caused by *M. kansasii* is increasing, not only in this country but around the world; indeed, in some areas of the world it is the most common nontuberculous mycobacterium. Although *M. kansasii* may cause lymphadenitis, cutaneous disease, synovial infection, pericarditis, and even disseminated infection, by far the most common disease manifestation in the United States is pulmonary infecion. The treatment of such infections will be the subject of this brief review.

Disease due to *M. kansasii* was first described as "yellow bacillus" disease in 1953 by Buhler and Pollak. The gross appearance of the organism on culture media is distinctive owing to the induction of beta-carotene crystal formation on prolonged exposure to light, a phenomenon known as photochromogenicity. *M. kansasii* also presents a characteristic appearance on acid-fast smears, which reveal unique large cross-barred bacilli; detection of this feature by an astute microbiologic technician may suggest *M. kansasii* even before culture results are available.

Although most other nontuberculous mycobacteria are found in a wide variety of environmental sources, *M. kansasii* is exceptional in that the natural reservoir is unknown. A number of reports have described isolation of *M. kansasii* from tap water, shower heads, and other water systems, suggesting a potential role for aerosolization in colonization or infection of the respiratory tract. Unlike tuberculosis, person-to-person spread of nontuberculous mycobacteria, including *M. kansasii*, has never been demonstrated. *M. kansasii* is more prevalent in the central and southwestern parts of this country than in other areas. Unlike the MAIS complex, it is more common in urban than in rural areas.

CLINICAL FEATURES

The clinical presentation of the patient with *M. kansasii* pulmonary infection is similar to that of patients infected with the MAIS complex. The majority of patients present with cough or are incidentally noted to hae an abnormal chest roentgenogram. Approximately half of these patients are middle-aged or older males who have some underlying lung disease, most commonly chronic obstructive pulmonary disease. It should be noted, however, that the disease affects a significant number of younger men and women without apparent lung disease or immune deficiency; this is in contrast to those infected with the MAIS complex, few of whom are free of predisposing conditions, and may be related to the relatively greater virulence of *M. kansasii.*

DIAGNOSIS

Diagnosis of disease due to the nontuberculous mycobacteria relies on a number of conventional criteria: (1) repeated isolation of the organism from the same site (e.g., expectorated sputum, preferably over several weeks time); (2) clinical evidence of a compatible disease process (e.g., parenchymal opacities or cavitary lesions on chest roentgenogram); and (3) no other demonstrable etiology for the disease process.

M. kansasii rarely occurs as a casual isolate, so that the recovery of this organism even once may reflect disease. Hurst and Ahn have recommended distinguishing infection from colonization in patients with sputum cultures positive for *M. kansasii*, based on the presence or absence of cavities on chest roentgenogram or tomogram; those with cavitary lesions are considered to be infected and clearly should begin a course of chemotherapy, whereas those with parenchymal opacities alone are considered potentially colonized and may undergo a period of "bronchial hygiene" with roentgenographic and microbiologic re-evaluation after a 6-week period. If a patient in this latter group has persistently positive sputum cultures or progression of the density on chest films, that patient is considered infected and chemotherapy is begun. Otherwise, patients are followed for evidence of active disease every 4 to 6 months. Although we use bronchial hygiene as a part of our overall therapy for *M. kansasii* and other nontuberculous mycobacterial infections, we use this method of distinguishing infection from colonization more often in patients at our institution who have a positive sputum culture for the MAIS complex.

Before addressing the specifics of therapy, it is useful to review the natural history of untreated disease. One short-term follow-up study (7.5 months to 3 years) of 19 patients with untreated *M. kansasii* pulmonary disease revealed evidence of active or progressive disease in nine (47%). A more recent review of four patients with *M. kansasii* pulmonary infection, followed without treatment for 10 to 14 years after diagnosis, found spontaneous resolution of active disease occurring 5 years after diagnosis in one patient, but slowly progressive disease in the absence of significant symptoms in the other three over a 12- to 14-year period. These cases illustrate the potentially indolent nature of this disorder, especially in patients with relatively minimal underlying pulmonary disease. Furthermore, should the physician choose to withhold chemotherapy in a patient who is believed to be colonized rather than infected, meticulous and protracted follow-up care is imperative.

MANAGEMENT

In all of our patients with nontuberculous mycobacterial infections and underlying obstructive lung disease, we use a program consisting of both antituberculous chemotherapeutic agents and bronchodilator drugs.

The chemotherapy of pulmonary infection due to *M. kansasii* is generally safe and effective. Indeed, *M. kansasii* is the prototype of the "easy to treat" nontuberculous mycobacteria. This is largely due to the nearly universal effectiveness of rifampin in the treatment of these infections. In agreement with the recent ATS position paper, we do not use in vitro sensitivity data in choosing initial therapy in this disorder. At our institution, we use a combination of isoniazid, 300 mg per day, rifampin, 600 mg per day, and ethambutol, 15 mg per kilogram per day. All of these are given as a single oral dose. Streptomycin is used if the foregoing three drugs cannot be tolerated or if bacteriologic conversion has not been achieved within 4 months. When used, streptomycin is usually given in doses of one gram intramuscularly three times weekly. The aforementioned drugs are the only chemotherapeutic agents required in the vast majority of cases. When other drugs are necessary owing to lack of response or drug intolerance, pyrazinamide, ethionamide, and cycloserine may be effective oral drugs; of these, pyrazinamide has the advantage of being administered as a single daily dose. Para-aminosalicylic acid is notoriously ineffective in this disorder and has no role in the therapy of infections due to *M. kansasii*. We have rarely found it necessary to substitute any other injectable antituberculous agent for streptomycin, but if necessary, one might use capreomycin, amikacin, viomycin, or kanamycin.

Treatment regimens used before 1976 did not include rifampin; the recommended duration of therapy in that era was to continue the three most effective drugs for at least 2 years after the sputum cultures became negative. Today, we would continue the chosen regimen for a total of 18 months. Therapy is usually well tolerated, and the relapse rate for such a regimen is extremely low.

The efficacy of shorter courses of therapy is receiving increasing attention. Ahn et al studied 40 patients treated with isoniazid, rifampin, and ethambutol daily for 12 months and with streptomycin twice weekly for the first 3 months; this regimen resulted in rapid conversion to negative sputum cultures (mean 5.5 weeks) and only one relapse (2.5%) after an average follow-up of 31 months. Banks et al reviewed 35 patients treated with regimens containing rifampin and ethambutol (and nine of these treated with those two drugs alone) for an average of 15 months, and found 100 percent sputum conversion and no relapses after an average follow-up of 5-½ years. Dutt and Stead recently treated 23 patients with isoniazid and rifampin alone for only 9 months; the results of this regimen were less promising, with only an 82 percent rate of sputum conversion, and bacteriologic relapse in three patients. As more data are accumulated on these various regimens, it is likely that the recommended duration of therapy will decrease.

Relapse

As already noted, relapses are extremely uncommon when rifampin is a part of the drug regimen. A relapse may reflect inadequate compliance, and a full course of isoniazid, rifampin, and ethambutol may be all that is required. In cases of relapse that do not respond to this approach, in vitro sensitivity data may be useful in guiding the selection of drugs to be used in the retreatment regimen; in general, we would use three drugs to which the organism is sensitive and would probably use rifampin again as well. Since there are only anecdotal data on duration of such therapy, we would arbitrarily continue treatment for 2 years after sputum conversion in these unusual cases.

Surgery

Surgery, which played a significant role in the therapy of pulmonary disease due to *M. kansasii* in the pre-rifampin era, has become largely unnecessary with the use of rifampin-containing regimens. The patient with massive hemoptysis due to this disease may still be considered for surgical resection, but the combination of therapeutic embolization and aggressive chemotherapy may eliminate the need for surgery even in this unusual circumstance.

Side Effects and Drug Toxicity

The major toxic effect of both isoniazid and rifampin is on the liver, with an incidence of hepatotoxicity from this combination ranging from 1 to 4 percent. Elderly women, or those with a history of previous liver disease or heavy alcohol use, may be at increased risk of this complication. Those in the latter category are urged to limit alcohol use during the course of therapy.

We obtain baseline liver function tests on all patients prior to the institution of therapy. In those with a history of previous liver disease or alcohol abuse, we repeat these tests at monthly intervals throughout the first 6 months of treatment. If a rise in SGOT greater than three to five times baseline is noted, we withhold both INH and rifampin until the SGOT reverts to normal, at which time we resume treatment with these drugs, beginning with rifampin, at lower doses. We spend considerable effort to resume therapy with rifampin, but if more than a minor amount of intolerance is demonstrated to isoniazid, we replace it with another agent.

Streptomycin causes dose-related renal and eighth nerve toxicity; thus, the dose of this and other injectable aminoglycosides should be reduced in the elderly and in others with impaired renal function.

Other side effects of the antituberculous drugs are less common and generally less severe. In addition to its potential hepatotoxicity, isoniazid may cause peripheral neuritis in nutritionally depleted individuals (e.g., the alcoholic or pregnant patient). We routinely administer pyridoxine in daily doses of 50 to 100 mg to such patients. Rifampin may cause malaise, nausea, and vomiting as well as hepatitis. Other problems seen with intermittent high-dose rifampin therapy (such as acute renal failure, flu-like syndrome, and thrombocytopenia) are rarely encountered with the daily therapy necessary in this infection. Ethambutol may cause retrobulbar neuritis when doses exceed 20 mg per kilogram for prolonged periods, but this is rarely seen when the dose is 15 mg per kilogram. Pyrazinamide may cause hepatotoxicity and hyperuricemia; up to 7 percent of patients on daily therapy with Pyrazinamide may complain of arthralgias, which are usually easily managed with an analgesic. The main side effects of ethionomide are gastrointestinal, whereas cycloserine may cause CNS toxicity ranging from personality changes to convulsions.

SUGGESTED READING

Ahn CH, Lowell JR, Ahn SS, Ahn SI, Hurst GA. Short-course chemotherapy for pulmonary disease caused by *Mycobacterium kansasii*. Am Rev Respir Dis 1983; 128:1048–1050.

Banks J, Hunter AM, Campbell IA, Jenkins PA, Smith AP. Pulmonary infection with *Mycobacterium kansasii* in Wales, 1970-1979: review of treatment and response. Thorax 1983; 8:271–274.

Pezzia W, Raleigh JW, Bailey MC, Toth EA, Silverblatt J. Treatment of pulmonary disease due to *Mycobacterium kansasii*: recent experience with rifampin. Rev Infect Dis 1981; 3:1035–1039.

Wolinsky E. Nontuberculous mycobacteria and associated diseases. Am Rev Respir Dis 1979; 119:107–159.

CHRONIC ASTHMA

TIMOTHY J.H. CLARK, B.Sc., M.D., F.R.C.P.

Asthma is, by definition, a variable condition, and in many patients it only causes intermittent symptoms. In a substantial minority, however, these symptoms become more persistent and may be present almost every day and persist throughout the seasons and the years. Under these circumstances, asthma can be regarded as chronic, with problems of management that differ from those of intermittent asthma.

The underlying pathogenesis of chronic asthma is probably similar to that of the intermittent variety. Airway hyperreactivity is a cardinal feature of asthma, and the consequent airway irritability leads to bronchoconstriction and its associated symptoms of chest tightness, wheeze, and dyspnea. Airway reactivity is in part hereditary, but may also be amplified by environmental factors such as allergens or occupational agents. Patients with atopy and airway reactivity are particularly at risk of developing asthma, and mediator release from mast cells and alveolar macrophages are now thought to play a role in both allergen-induced asthma and the nonimmune variety, as well as under such circumstances as cold air challenge or exercise.

Mediator release is also likely to be important in the production of inflammation, which is now regarded as an important component of asthma. Not only do mediators excite inflammation, but some recruit, via chemotaxis, other inflammatory cells such as neutrophils and eosinophils, which further promote inflammation, particularly on a chronic basis. These events may themselves also increase airway reactivity so that there is a complicated interaction between reactivity, mediator release, and inflammation (Table 1). All these events lead to bronchoconstriction either on a chronic basis or when stimulated by trigger factors.

CLINICAL FEATURES

The basic mechanism of asthma includes airway reactivity and inflammation, and these provide the basis for the most important symptomatic features of wheeze, dyspnea, and cough. In some patients wheeze and dyspnea associated with chest tighteness are predominant, but in others a more exudative and presumably inflammatory presentation occurs, with a productive cough

TABLE 1 Mechanisms of Asthma Pathogenesis

Asthma triggers (e.g., allergens, exercise)
Mediator release
Inflammation
Bronchial hyperreactivity
Bronchoconstriction

dominating the clinical features. The latter, bronchitic, variety is more common in older patients and young children. It is commonly mistaken for infective bronchitis, and antibiotics are prescribed needlessly and without effect. The proper diagnosis of asthma can be established on the basis of diagnostic features of asthma as well as a therapeutic trial; many children are condemned to symptoms and loss of schooling because recurrent episodes of cough are not recognized to be asthmatic in origin. Similarly, in the older patient, the condition is often diagnosed as chronic bronchitis or emphysema, and the treatable condition of asthma is missed.

Circadian Rhythm. The symptoms of asthma, be they bronchitic or bronchospastic, often display a circadian rhythm, with the patient being reasonably well by day, but symptomatic at night. This is a reflection of the underlying circadian variation in lung function observed in asthma. This diurnal rhythm describes the fall in lung function, which reaches its lowest at about 3:00 AM before gradually recovering to reach peak values during the afternoon some 12 hours later.

This diurnal rhythm of asthma is probably an exaggeration of a healthy circadian variation and is produced by increased reactivity of airways. A number of other factors may be important, such as sleep and cyclic variations in plasma epinephrine, but the important thing to remember is that the cycle has a 24-hour basis, and therefore there is no specific nocturnal event that needs to be treated. Asthma needs to be managed on a 24-hour basis and not largely at night.

Trigger Factors. In a substantial minority of patients with asthma, a specific cause can be identified. This is usually of an allergic nature but occupational agents are being found with increasing frequency. Allergic causes can often be confirmed by specific tests, but usually bronchial challenge is required to demonstrate the authenticity of an apparent association noted by the patient. This assumes importance when treatment is directed toward removing the cause and controlling immunopathologic mechanism (to be discussed).

ASSESSMENT

In the management of chronic asthma, it is important to monitor response to therapy, and this requires a critical approach to assessment. Traditionally, clinicians have relied on a symptomatic response, and this continues to be the case, even with modern techniques at our disposal. Careful clinicial inquiry can reveal changes in exercise tolerance and the frequency of asthmatic episodes. It is also important to inquire about sleep disturbance and how often a bronchodilator aerosol is used for treating breakthrough symptoms. Signs of deterioration in chronic asthma are (1) increasing exertional dyspnea, (2) increasing sleep disturbance with increased use of bronchodilator aerosol at night, and (3) early morning chest tightness that is relieved for shorter and shorter periods of time by the early morning bronchodilator aerosol. Cough frequency and severity are also important indicators, as are other features suggesting an increased allergic state such as nasal hypersecretion and early morning sneezing.

In addition to this basic clinical information, it is important to measure lung function, and repeated estimation of a simple test such as peak expiratory flow rate is more valuable than the occasional comprehensive measurement of rather more recondite lung function. Peak flow, measured last thing at night and first thing in the morning before medication, provides useful information about absolute levels of lung function as well as the diurnal rhythm and, in particular, the extent of the morning dip (Table 2).

It is seldom necessary to carry out further assessments, although there is increasing use of tests of bronchial reactivity to indicate the need for therapy and to monitor response of this important pathogenetic mechanism of asthma.

MANAGEMENT

The most effective treatment is usually provided by medication; only occasionally can environmental control or immunotherapy be of value to these patients. I remain to be convinced that immunotherapy plays an important role in the treatment of chronic asthma and indeed would relegate it to the margin. Only a minority of patients have a clearly defined allergic cause for their asthma which is amenable to immunotherapy. Whereas desensitization regimens may be of help to patients with hay fever, their value in asthma is less well established, and it is seldom possible to find patients who have a single allergic cause that can be treated in isolation. The technique itself is not without danger when compared with pharmacologic measures that are usually effective.

Having clearly stated my view on this subject, I recognize that immunotherapy offers a real prospect for effective treatment by altering host factors, and therefore the position may change and we must keep an open mind as to future benefits. I also recognize the need to consider immunotherapy when drug treatment has proved ineffective or can only be effective at the cost of side effects. Under these circumstances, immunotherapy may play a useful role, but not as a first-line treatment for allergic asthma.

Before discussing individual therapies, it is worthwhile briefly to invoke some general principles.

TABLE 2 Assessment of Asthma

Symptoms
Exercise tolerance
Sleep disturbance
Cough frequency
Use of bronchodilator aerosol
Length of relief from aerosol
Lung function
Peak flow rate
Amplitude of diurnal rhythm
Bronchial reactivity

Twenty-Four Hour Control. In view of the diurnal nature of asthma, the aim of therapy should be to both raise the mean level of lung function and reduce the amplitude of the circadian rhythm. Such an approach ensures that treatment given during the day can improve symptoms at night by raising daytime values and preventing the nocturnal decline in lung function.

Specific nocturnal events are unlikely to play an important role in causing nocturnal asthma, and treatment need not be timed to coincide with sleep. The full 24 hours needs to be encompassed by therapy and the effect monitored by changes in the diurnal rhythm as well as absolute measure of lung function.

Intermittent or Regular Treatment. Although chronic asthma, by definition, implies regular symptoms, some patients have symptoms that are present throughout the year but not every day. In some of these patients the symptoms may be recurrent and treatment is therefore intermittent. If symptoms last more than 2 or 3 weeks and there is less than 1 month of freedom from symptoms between episodes, treatment should continue throughout the year both to control the episodes and to prevent them. Less frequent episodes of chronic asthma may require intermittent therapy as it becomes less profitable to use treatment for 365 days of the year to prevent a limited number of weeks of symptoms. Where a balance is struck depends largely on the patient and the severity and frequency of the episodes.

Route of Administration. Another important guiding principle to treatment of chronic asthma is choice of route of administration. I favor the inhaled route as this delivers a small but effective dose directly to the airway, thus enhancing prospects for success and minimizing the risks of adverse systemic side effects.

There is growing evidence that the bronchial epithelium may play an important role both in pathogenesis and in propagation of asthma, and this may explain the potency and success of inhaled therapy. Small doses delivered to the airway can achieve results as good as those from oral or parenteral administration. This occurs despite severe airflow obstruction, as in patients with status asthmaticus, although for these patients nebulized therapy usually is required to replace a hand-held aerosol. Aerosol delivery can therefore be used at all levels of asthma severity, and the benefits are the same, with fewer side effects, as the benefits of the drug (e.g., albuterol) administered by the oral route. Two inhalations equivalent to 180 μg albuterol can achieve the same therapeutic effect as 4,000 μg (4 mg) taken by mouth. Thus therapeutic potency is achieved by the inhaled route with much less likelihood of systemic side effects. The reduction of risks of systemic activity is of particular importance when considering corticosteroid therapy, and inhaled steroids have now largely replaced systemic steroids in the treatment of chronic asthma.

The major disadvantage of inhaled therapy lies in drug delivery systems, but these are rapidly being improved, and today the majority of patients should be able to use the inhaled route without much difficulty. Pressurized aerosols remain the most common hand-held delivery system, and spacer devices may improve prospects of patient compliance and better drug delivery. These new spacer devices are still being examined, but I suspect that they will only prove of real benefit in reducing local side effects from inhaled steroids.

I personally prefer powdered aerosol systems rather than spacer devices as a substitute for the pressurized aerosol because these devices are easy to load and are patient-actuated, enhancing patient compliance considerably. The use of powdered beclomethasone dipropionate has clearly been shown to improve prospects of asthma control in children, and these devices are highly satisfactory. However, they do not improve particle penetration into the lung, but this may not be an important problem. In practice, powdered aerosols have proved valuable, with increases in dose compensating for any minor inefficiency of the system as compared to the pressurized aerosols.

The increasing use of nebulization for delivery of drugs by inhalation has caused some concern because of the difficulties in supervising the much larger doses given via nebulizers. The great merit of the inhaled route is its ability to deliver effectively a small dose of drug, and this advantage is being lost by use of nebulizers, which are often employed to deliver substantially greater doses of bronchodilators. The role of nebulizers remains to be evaluated. I reserve them for the few patients who critically depend on high-dose inhaled therapy to treat incipient status asthmaticus or to decrease dependence on hospital care.

Bronchodilators

As with intermittent asthma, bronchodilators play a key role in managing chronic symptoms. Bronchodilators used on a continuous basis are able to suppress attacks of asthma and may achieve this by mechanisms other than bronchodilatation. Beta-adrenergic agonists, which have been shown to prevent the release of mediators from sensitized mast cells, may have beneficial effects in mucociliary transport. Whatever the mechanism, regular bronchodilator therapy can be used to protect patients from chronic asthma and is often successful.

Despite current evidence regarding the relative merits of various bronchodilators in the treatment of *acute* asthma, there is still speculation about the best bronchodilator for *chronic* asthma. In many countries, oral theophylline therapy provides the main treatment, and in the United States, this therapy has been shown to provide protection comparable to that provided by sodium cromoglycate, although at a slightly greater risk of side effects. In other countries, beta-adrenergic agonists are widely used on a regular basis to suppress asthma and are usually given by inhalation as this route of administration minimizes adverse systemic side effects. Both theophylline and beta-adrenergic agonists can protect against exercise-induced asthma. However, there has been less experience with regular administration of anticholinergic bronchodilators, and this treatment is usually reserved for acute episodes. In the elderly patient, however, they may have a useful role when taken regularly.

Bronchodilator Dosage. Regular administration of bronchodilators often controls symptoms, but not always. Under these circumstances, the clinician must decide what to do next. In the majority of these patients, the dose of bronchodilator, whether oral theophylline or inhaled beta-adrenergic agonist, is frequently suboptimal, and at this stage, it seems worthwhile to increase the dose in the hope of obtaining greater benefit without increasing the risks of side effects. Because adverse effects are a much greater problem with theophylline therapy, blood level monitoring is necessary. It is for this reson that I prefer to use regularly inhaled beta-adrenergic agonists as my first-line regular bronchodilator therapy. The usual dose of a beta-adrenergic agonist such as albuterol, 2 puffs four times a day, can be used as basic therapy, but the dose should be increased to 4 or even 6 puffs four times a day if required. This apparently large dose of inhaled albuterol, given over 24 hours (2.4 mg), is still less than that delivered by an oral dose from a 4-mg tablet, and thus the safety margin is larger than that offered by oral theophylline therapy.

Although clinical experience suggests that some patients are more sensitive and responsive to one type of bronchodilator than to another, in general there is little merit in adding in a second or third bronchodilator when the first is not proving effective. If inhaled beta-adrenergic agonist therapy is employed, a similar effect can be achieved by increasing the dose rather than adding another bronchodilator. The main problem associated with multiple bronchodilator therapy, using different types by different routes, is that this might obscure deteriorating asthma and delay the introduction of more effective therapy. In general, if the patient is responding poorly to 4 or 6 puffs of albuterol or equivalent four times a day, the addition of other bronchodilators is unlikely to be helpful and even may be harmful in that it delays the effective treatment of asthma, perhaps putting the patient at risk.

Other Suppressive Therapy

If bronchodilators are proving ineffective in controlling chronic asthma, particularly if the patient is still waking at night with symptoms, other suppressive treatment is required. Of these, the most effective agents are sodium cromoglycate and corticosteroids. There is interest in the role of calcium-channel blocking drugs as well as newer antihistamines such as ketotifen, but these drugs seem unlikely to replace sodium cromoglycate or inhaled steroids.

Sodium Cromoglycate. Sodium cromoglycate is an effective treatment for asthma when taken regularly to suppress its symptoms. Its mode of action is unknown, but its role is likely to be particularly valuable in childhood asthma. It is difficult to predict when it will be successful, and as its success rate does not appear to be as high as with inhaled corticosteroids in adults, I tend to reserve its use for childhood asthma, against which it is effective. In the treatment of adults, it may take 1 or 2 months before a trial of cromoglycate is shown to be unsuccessful, further delaying effective therapy.

Sodium cromoglycate has a good safety record and can be taken either by powdered or pressurized aerosol as well as by nebulizer. This means that children have a variety of delivery systems to chose from, and provided they take it regularly, effective control of asthma can be achieved. If cromoglycate is unsuccessful and corticosteroids are added, there is little need for both treatments, and treatment with sodium cromoglycate can be discontinued.

As with bronchodilators, sodium cromoglycate can block asthma produced by exercise or allergen challenge, although in practice, inhaled beta-adrenergic agonist therapy is usually found to be the most convenient and effective.

Corticosteroids. After some initial hesitation, corticosteroids were found to be effective in the treatment of chronic asthma, and only the development of side effects has limited their use. With the introduction of inhaled steroids, the situation has changed substantially, as chronic steroid treatment can now be given by inhalation to provide effective and safe treatment.

Inhaled steroids can therefore be used as a substitute for chronic oral therapy and can provide an equipotent dose of about 15 mg per day of prednisolone if higher-dose regimens are employed. Oral steroids are reserved for the few patients whose asthma is still uncontrolled by inhaled steroid therapy as well as for short courses to treat an acute attack of asthma.

Since their introduction in the early 1970s, inhaled steroids have proved to be free from adverse systemic side effects, and millions of patient-years of experience have been gained with their use. This safety record, plus the fact that inhaled steroids can provide effective topical anti-inflammatory therapy, has lead to their increasing use in chronic asthma, so that in some countries, they now compete with sodium cromoglycate and bronchodilators as the drugs of choice following failure of inhaled beta-adrenergic agonist therapy to control symptoms. Thus, rather than add sodium cromoglycate or oral theophylline, many clinicians sometimes choose inhaled steroids, and I support this strategy (Table 3). Recent evidence also shows that inhaled steroids can be effective when given twice daily, a regimen that is more

TABLE 3 Choice of Drug for Chronic Asthma

Condition	*Drug*
Episodic asthma	Inhaled beta-adrenergic agonist as required
Chronic asthma	Regular inhaled beta-adrenergic agonist up to equivalent 2.5–3.0 mg albuterol per day in divided doses
If still symptomatic and especially if sleep is being disturbed by asthma, one of the following:	Sodium cromoglycate Inhaled steroid Oral sustained-release theophylline

convenient and is likely to improve patient compliance.

In contrast to the other options, inhaled steroids have many advantages. They provide anti-inflammatory therapy and are clinically effective in treating chronic asthma. They are more potent than sodium cromoglycate and bronchodilators, and the safety record of inhaled steroids compares favorably with that of oral theophylline with respect to both morbidity and mortality.

SUGGESTED READING

Brompton Hospital/Medical Research Council Collaborative Trial. Long-term study of disodium cromoglycate in treatment of severe extrinsic or intrinsic bronchial asthma in adults. Br Med J 1972; 4:383–388.

Brompton Hospital MRC Collaborative Trial. Double-blind trial comparing the dosage schedules of beclomethasone dipropionate aerosol in the treatment of chronic bronchial asthma. Lancet 1974; ii:303–307.

BTTA Controlled Trial. Inhaled corticosteroids compared with oral prednisolone in patients starting long-term corticosteroid therapy for asthma. Lancet 1975; ii:469–473.

Klein JJ, Leftowitz MS, Spector SL, Cherniack RM. Relationship between serum theophylline levels and pulmonary function before and after inhaled beta-agonists in "stable" asthma. Am Rev Resp Dis 1983; 127:413.

Tattersfield AE. Bronchodilators in the prevention of asthma. In: Clark TJH, ed. Bronchodilator therapy. Auckland: Adis Press, 1984.

CHRONIC BRONCHITIS

THOMAS L. PETTY, M.D.

Chronic bronchitis is a common condition encountered by primary care physicians. Acute exacerbations of chronic bronchitis with symptoms of cough, expectoration, fever, and malaise are seen throughout the year, but periods of sudden worsening are most prevalent during the winter season in cold climates. Both acute and chronic symptoms can be improved with a variety of medications. Whether or not chronic airflow limitation, which occurs in only a small proportion of those suffering from chronic bronchitis, can be prevented or altered in its natural course is often debated. But it is clear that most patients with chronic bronchitis can be improved both symptomatically and objectively, and it is likely that the natural course of emerging chronic airflow limitation can be altered by systematic management in the primary care physician's office. The purpose of this chapter is to present the rationale and details of therapy for patients with acute or chronic cough and sputum.

EPIDEMIOLOGY

The epidemiology of chronic obstructive pulmonary disease, in which chronic bronchitis is commonly present, is well documented. Data from the National Health Interview Survey estimate that at least 7.5 million Americans have chronic bronchitis and more than 2 million have emphysema, and at least 6½ million more have some form of asthma. Data from the Tecumseh Community Health Survey of over 9,000 men and women in all age groups revealed approximately 14 percent of adult males and 8 percent of adult females with chronic bronchitis, obstructive airway disease, or both. In addition, days of disability as defined by restricted activity are considerable and averaged 12 days per year for patients with chronic bronchitis, 68 days per year for patients with emphysema, and roughly 17 days for asthmatics. In 1981 there were at least 60,000 deaths from chronic obstructive pulmonary disease and related conditions, making this the fifth leading cause of death. All estimates point to the fact that deaths are increasing from chronic obstructive pulmonary disease (COPD). The estimated economic cost for COPD in 1979 was 6.5 billion dollars, and health care costs are rising for this spectrum of disease. Therefore, there is no question of the importance of this disease spectrum as a major health problem in our country, representing a major challenge to physicians who care for patients in their clinics and offices.

COURSE AND PROGNOSIS OF CHRONIC OBSTRUCTIVE PULMONARY DISEASE

The accepted definition of chronic bronchitis is chronic cough and expectoration for at least 3 months for a minimum of 2 years. Many patients fulfilling this definition have no abnormality of airflow, and the prognosis for these patients is good. By contrast, patients with airflow limitation suffer premature morbidity and mortality. Recent evidence clearly indicates that the course and prognosis in patients with chronic cough and expectoration, labeled chronic bronchitis, are not related to the symptom complex at all, but rather to the degree of airflow obstruction as judged by forced expiratory volume obtainable by simple spirometry and the age at which spirometric abnormalities are first identified. The rate of change of ventilatory function is also a powerful prognostic indicator. Patients who lose ventilatory function rapidly die sooner than those with slower rates of lung function deterioration. Most patients become symptomatic in their 40s or 50s, with disability occurring in the late 50s or early 60s. Living to the late 60s or early 70s with severe chronic airflow obstruction is not unusual.

ASSESSMENT

It is now clear that the development of chronic airflow obstruction in chronic bronchitis is a problem that clusters in families. The presence or absence of a family history of chronic airflow obstruction is an important indicator of the likelihood of airflow obstruction in the patient. Airflow obstruction is also related more closely to smoking than to any other factor. Thus a recording of age of onset of smoking, years of smoking, and amount consumed daily is important. It is now known that ventilatory function in children who smoke is lower than in nonsmoking children of the same age, suggesting an adverse effect of tobacco smoke on lung growth. An assessment of ventilatory function is of paramount importance in judging prognosis of patients with chronic cough and expectoration as an indicator of the degree of severity of airflow obstruction. The availability of simple, accurate, dry, direct recording office spirometers makes simple measurements of forced vital capacity (FVC) and forced expiratory volume in one second (FEV_1) practical and highly useful. These measurements are the key indicators of volume and flow respectively and are the only tests tht are needed to estimate prognosis and to evaluate response to therapy.

MANAGEMENT

Smoking Cessation. Smoking cessation is the single most important therapeutic maneuver that can alter the course of chronic bronchitis with airflow obstruction. Thus, an effort toward behavioral modification leading to smoking cessation should be made. The newly available nicotine-containing gum (Nicorette) may help to counteract the addictive features of nicotine as part of an overall smoking cessation program. The value of smoking cessation on the course and prognosis of disease has been well established. Susceptible smokers demonstrating premature loss of ventilatory function who stopped smoking before the age of 50 and had relatively good remaining ventilatory function showed a rate of loss of ventilatory function equivalent to the age-related rate after they stopped compared to the continued accelerated loss of ventilatory function in those who continued to smoke. Even patients who stopped smoking at age 65 with severe ventilatory function impairment averaging only 30 percent of predicted FEV_1 at age 25 had a better survival than those who continued to smoke. Thus there can be no doubt that discontinuance of smoking is the fundamental therapy for chronic bronchitis.

Vaccines. The use of influenza virus vaccine is recommended by the Centers for Disease Control; it is believed to provide a substantial degree of protection against common A type strains of influenza in COPD. Little doubt remains as to the cost-effectiveness of influenza virus vaccine. When there is insufficient time to offer vaccine during epidemics, the use of oral amantadine or rimantidine also offers substantial protection. These drugs are likely to shorten the course of an exacerbation of chronic bronchitis caused by influenza if given when symptoms first appear. Whether or not pneumococcal vaccine offers significant benefit to patients with COPD is also debatable. Newer vaccine preparations have introduced an increased number of antigenetic strains (from 14 to 23). It is my belief that both influenza virus vaccine and pneumococcal vaccine are valuable in the treatment of COPD, and can be given simultaneously. Influenza virus vaccine should be given each fall if epidemics are predicted, and because of the antigenic shift of the organism, repeated yearly vaccination is recommended. According to current opinion, polyvalent pneumococcal vaccine need be given only once in a lifetime.

Bronchodilators. Bronchodilators are widely used in patients who demonstrate at least a small degree of reversibility of airflow obstruction as judged by simple office spirometry. At least a 15 percent improvement over baseline probably should be considered significant improvement. The systematic treatment of the nonspecific bronchial hyperreactivity that may accompany COPD could possibly prevent accelerated losses in lung function over time. The first step in bronchodilator management is the use of an inhaled beta-adrenergic agonist aerosol delivered by a metered-dose device. Increasing numbers of more selective, longer-acting preparations are now available. These preparations are listed in Table 1 along with older agents. The proper use of a metered-dose aerosol is probably as effective as any bronchodilation. Nonetheless, some physicians still prefer to use beta-adrenergic agonist aerosols and pump-driven nebulizers. Table 2 lists selected solutions for use in powered nebulizers.

Theophyllines also are widely used for bronchodilation (Table 3). Theophyllines are also known to improve respiratory muscle function and to prevent or

TABLE 1 Selected Bronchodilator Aerosols (Metered-Dose Device)

Nonprescription
Epinephrine (Bronkaid, Primatene)
Prescription
Albuterol (Proventil, Ventolin)
Bitolterol (Tornalate)
Fenoterol (Berotec)*
Isoetharine (Bronkometer)
Isoproterenol (Isuprel)
Metaproterenol (Alupent, Metaprel)
Terbutaline (Brethaire)

* Soon to be released

TABLE 2 Selected Solutions for Nebulizers

Isoetharine (Bronkosol or generic)
Isoproterenol (Isuprel or generic)
Metaproterenol (Metaprel)
Metaproterenol (Alupent)
Racepinephrine (Vaponefrin or generic)

TABLE 3 Common Oral Products That Are Time-Release Theophylline

Short-acting products* (usually taken 3 or 4 times a day)
- Aminophylline (generic)
- Bronkodyl
- Choledyl
- Theophylline USP

Long-acting products (usually taken twice a day)
- Bronkodyl S-R
- Choledyl SA
- Constant T
- Resbid
- Theo-Dur
- Theo-24†
- Theovent
- Uniphyl†

* Among others.
† Usually prescribed once a day.

reduce respiratory muscle fatigue in states of severe chronic airflow obstruction. Both beta-adrenergic agonists and theophyllines can improve mucociliary clearance, but it is not known whether this fact is clinically significant.

Corticosteroids. It is well established that corticosteroids are useful in the treatment of exacerbations of chronic bronchitis resulting in acute respiratory failure. One controlled clinical trial has demonstrated objective improvement in airflow from corticosteroids as compared to results of placebo. Even patients believed to have irreversible airflow obstruction may respond to oral corticosteroids. Thus it is believed by most, including myself, that a short-term trial of corticosteroids should be offered nearly every patient with chronic airflow obstruction on a trial basis for approximately 2 weeks. A single morning dose of 40 mg of prednisone, guided by symptoms and spirometric measurements, will be able to determine those patients with responsive features resulting in reversible airflow obstruction. Inhaled corticosteroids are not usually so effective as oral agents in steroid-responsive patients. For patients who have no improvement, steroids can simply be stopped. Tapering is not necessary. For those with improvement, strategies to capitalize on benefits and minimize long-term side effects, such as osteopenia and eye complications are required.

Antibiotics. Antibiotics are probably the most widely used pharmacologic agents in the treatment of exacerbations of chronic bronchitis. Whereas the initial insult resulting in increased cough and expectoration is likely to be viral, the fact of bacterial invasion in many patients is also well established. However, an infective organism is not found in all patients. *Streptococcus pneumoniae and Haemophilus influenzae* species are the most commonly cultured organisms. In addition, *Mycoplasma* is occasionally present, and the possibility of anaerobes must be considered. It is now well established that culture of expectorated sputum is not necessary in most cases because purulent sputum is an indication for antimicrobial therapy. Oral antimicrobials can be selected on epidemiologic grounds, based on a knowledge of the organisms that are usually present. Table 4 lists the antibiotics in roughly their order of incidence. These antimicrobials are empirically effective in reducing the symptom complex of chronic bronchitis exacerbations. Special mention of chloramphenicol is in order because of the fears of devastating hematologic complications (i.e., aplastic anemia). In fact, these complications are exceedingly rare, occurring in roughly one in 10,000 to 40,000 individuals. Since chloramphenicol remains the drug of choice for *Haemophilus* and since chloramphenicol is often effective against *Pneumococcus* and highly effective against anaerobes, its use, when other antimicrobials are ineffective, is entirely appropriate. Chloramphenicol has been found to be superior to ampicillin in patients with severe exacerbation of chronic bronchitis. Trimethoprim with sulfamethoxazole (Bactrim or Septra) is also effective in the treatment and prevention of purulent exacerbations of chronic bronchitis and is generally a first or early choice in antimicrobial management. The effectiveness of tetracycline in acute exacerbations of bronchitis in hospitalized patients with chronic bronchitis has been seriously questioned in a recent double-blind controlled clinical trial.

Controversy still surrounds the role of infection in the pathogenesis of chronic obstructive pulmonary disease. It would appear that repeated viral and bacterial invasion with infection of the conducting airways could participate in airway narrowing and perhaps damage to the surrounding parenchyma via release of proteases and/or free radicles from polymorphonuclear leukocytes that respond to invading organisms.

A growing body of evidence relates childhood respiratory infections to the later development of chronic bronchitis with airflow obstruction (COPD). Repeated childhood infections could be a marker of the patient with inadequate natural antimicrobial defense mechanisms. An alternate hypothesis is that early and subtle injury of the lungs makes later infection more likely. Bronchial reactivity may follow viral illnesses in chil-

TABLE 4 Common Antimicrobial (Antibiotic) Drugs Used for Exacerbations of Chronic Bronchitis

Name	*Usual Dose*	*Side Effects*
Ampicillin	250 or 500 mg	Rash, diarrhea
Trimethoprim-sulfa (Bactrim and Septra)	1 capsule twice a day	Rare gastrointestinal upset
Tetracycline	250 mg 4 times a day—some other preparations once a day	Stomach upset, diarrhea, vaginal yeast infections
Erythromycin	250 or 500 mg	Stomach upset
Chloramphenicol	500 mg 4 times a day	Rare GI upset, mild anemia (common), aplastic anemia (rare)

dren. This bronchial hyperreactivity may persist into adult life and perhaps become a factor in progressive airflow obstruction.

The effect of repeated infections on the course and prognosis of adults with COPD is not well known. Some patients suffer step losses in ventilatory function following bronchopulmonary infections, suggesting a major impact of infection on the progress of disease. The use of antimicrobials can shorten the symptomatic period of exacerbations of chronic bronchitis. Some evidence exists that the prophylactic use of antimicrobials reduces the frequency of winter exacerbations in patients who often suffer from acute attacks of purulent bronchitis. However, no controlled clinical trial has shown a favorable influence in the long-term course and prognosis with antimicrobial agents. Nonetheless, the weight of clinical experience and the high likelihood of improving the symptom complex of acute attacks have helped to establish the widespread use of antimicrobial agents for episodes of acute purulent bronchitis. It has become established practice to institute a 7- to 10-day course of antimicrobials for each episode on empiric grounds. Sputum culture and sensitivity tests are not useful in this context.

A Systematic Approach to Therapy

No chapter can define all of the strategies of therapy that apply to all patients. A combination of smoking cessation, influenza virus vaccine, and pneumococcal vaccine once in a lifetime is the most effective preventive approach available. The systematic use of inhaled and oral bronchodilators, corticosteroids when indicated, and antimicrobials constitutes effective therapy for most patients.

Other Therapies

Pulmonary rehabilitation techniques are useful in patients with severe airflow obstruction. Breathing retraining, physical reconditioning, and oxygen all play their roles. That oxygen can alter and improve survival and quality of life is no longer in doubt based on two multicenter trials in both the United Kingdom and North America.

FUTURE TRENDS

More needs to be learned about the role of childhood chest infections and exposure to tobacco, both actively and passively, as a prelude to the development of chronic bronchitis with airflow obstruction. The early identification of patients with airflow abnormalities also predicts those who will become the respiratory cripples of the future. Although no controlled trials have proved this, it is likely that the early identification and management of patients via smoking cessation and use of bronchodilating aerosol to combat nonspecific bronchial hyperreactivity, known to be present probably in 15 to 20 percent of patients with early stages of disease, might well forestall or curtail the premature loss of ventilatory function that results in premature morbidity and mortality. At this writing, controlled clinical trials to test this hypothesis are underway sponsored by the National Heart, Lung, and Blood Institute. In any case, it seems appropriate to offer not only symptomatic management, but specific pharmacologically oriented therapy, designed to improve airflow obstruction and to deal with bacterial invasion on a regular basis as maintenance management for patients with all stages of chronic bronchitis.

BRONCHIECTASIS

JOHN G. KIRBY, M.B., M.R.C.P.I., F.R.C.P.(C)
MICHAEL T. NEWHOUSE, M.D., M.Sc., F.R.C.P.(C), F.A.C.P.

Bronchiectasis is a dilatation of the bronchial tree, usually with severe injury or destruction of the mucosal elements and cartilage within its wall. It may be congenital or acquired. In acquired bronchiectasis, the ectasia is thought to be caused by extramural traction phenomena due to adjacent pneumonitis and atelectasis, acting on severely damaged airway walls. Bronchiectasis is almost always due to a failure of normal lung defenses with infection (pneumonia) and a failure to clear bronchial secretions. This may be due to primary or secondary ciliary dysfunction, gastric acid or foreign body aspiration, bronchial obstruction by tumor, or the abnormal mucus clearance of cystic fibrosis or allergic aspergillosis. Failure of the immune system, cell-mediated or humoral or both, may also predispose to infection leading to bronchiectasis. These various factors often coexist and are more likely to cause severe, chronic airway and pulmonary injury in the developing bronchial tree of the child. We have displayed the most important interrelationships in Figure 1.

DIAGNOSIS

The diagnosis of bronchiectasis is primarily clinical, and the features of the history and physical examination are well known. Pulmonary function abnormalities are nonspecific, frequently being a combination of obstructive and nonobstructive abnormalities.

We usually perform spirometry, assess lung volumes and diffusing capacity, and, in many cases, perform a standard maximum exercise study to determine if desaturation develops. The purpose of these tests is to document existing pulmonary function as a baseline for

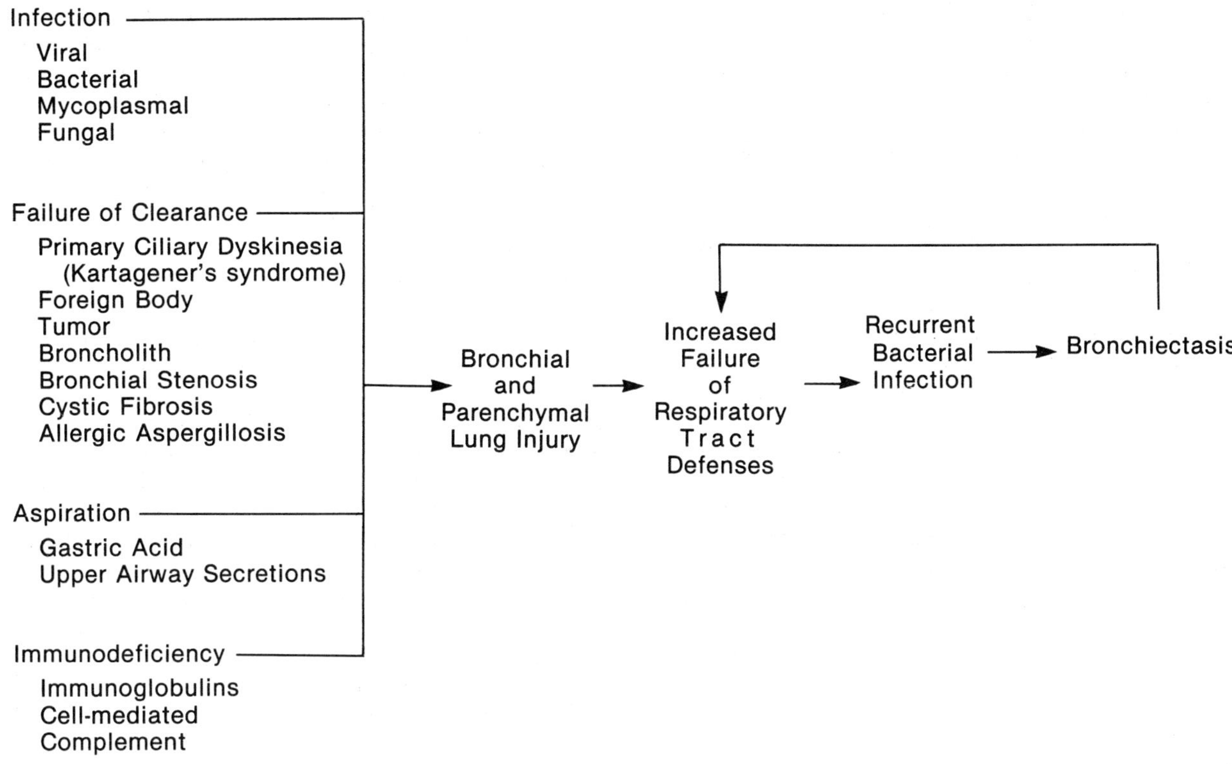

Figure 1 Pathogenesis of bronchiectasis.

future comparison, detect patterns of pulmonary function abnormality (obstructive, restrictive, or mixed ventilatory defect), and assess whether there is reversible airflow obstruction by the response to an inhaled adrenoceptor agonist or anticholinergic bronchodilator.

The chest film may show signs that are typical of (ring shadows or "tram lines") or consistent with bronchiectasis. However, roentgenographic changes may also be nonspecific or absent. This, once again, points to the importance of the clinical diagnosis of bronchiectasis. Sinus films are obtained to evaluate the presence of fluid. Rubbery brown mucous plugs, blood eosinophilia, and proximal upper zone fingerlike shadows on the chest film may suggest allergic aspergillosis. The diagnosis can be confirmed with skin prick tests and serum precipitins as well as fungus cultures.

There have been suggestions that computed tomography (CT) of the lung may be useful in assessing the presence and extent of bronchiectasis, although another view is that the bronchiectasis that is detected by CT is also obvious on a plain chest film. We are only just beginning to employ CT in the diagnosis of bronchiectasis at present, and its use in this condition will require further validation.

Bronchography is the gold standard at present for confirming the clinical diagnosis and assessing the extent of disease. It is our usual practice to defer this procedure until patients are considered for surgical resection of diseased lung on clinical grounds. We then obtain bilateral bronchograms by means of a transcricothyroid instillation of contrast medium, although some bronchoscopists are now instilling contrast medium through the bronchoscope, which is manipulated under fluoroscopic control.

MANAGEMENT

Prevention

Bronchiectasis is often a sequel of severe bacterial, mycoplasmal, or viral pulmonary infection, particularly in childhood. The decline of bronchiectasis in developed countries is probably due to better nutrition and living conditions, use of antibiotics early in the treatment of pulmonary infection, and immunization against childhood infections, particularly pertussis and measles. It is a matter for concern that the decline of full immunization due to fear of adverse reactions appears to have resulted in resurgence of pertussis, especially in some developed countries. We would strongly recommend full immunization of all children except the relative few with definite contraindications due to a severe systemic reaction to previous injection with the same vaccine, ongoing neurologic disorders, and immunodeficiency states.

General Measures

Causes of continuing lung damage or failure of lung defense should be treated, if possible. We refer patients with recurrent sinusitis and persistent purulent drainage to an otolaryngologist for evaluation and a possible drainage procedure, if chronic aspiration of purulent sinus secretions seems to be a significant factor. We treat patients with gastroesophageal reflux and aspiration vigorously with ranitidine, 150 mg twice a day; metoclopramide, 10 mg 30 minutes before the evening meal; and Gaviscon, 400 mg 2 hours after meals and 800 mg at bedtime. We also advise that the head of the bed be elevated 6 to 8 inches on blocks: we recommend a light evening meal before 7 PM and no coffee, tea, cola, alcohol, or bedtime snack afterward. The minority who fail to respond to this regimen are referred for surgical correction unless other contraindications are present. We perform a bronchoscopic examination initially on patients who have hemoptysis, recurrent infection, or persistent atelectasis in one lobe or segment to detect the presence of a foreign body, tumor, broncholith, or bronchial stenosis. We advise vaccination against influenza annually, pneumococcal vaccine once, and the cessation of smoking.

Patients whose bronchiectasis is a result of recurrent bacterial infection due to IgG deficiency may be treated with intramuscular injections of 0.6 ml per kg of a 16.5 percent solution of gamma globulin, up to a maximum of 20 ml per dose, every 2 to 4 weeks (maximum 5 ml per IM site). Treatment usually starts in childhood and continues indefinitely. Occasionally, patients who get reactions to this treatment or who respond poorly may benefit from regular infusions of plasma, preferably from a single, infection-free donor. However, treatment of specific mucosal IgA deficiency is not possible in this way.

Antibiotics

The most important feature of antibiotic use is individualization of treatment, which still remains an art, rather than a science, in the treatment of bronchiectasis (Table 1). Most patients with bronchiectasis have large amounts of chronically infected sputum, usually due to mixed aerobic and anaerobic "normal" respiratory flora or to *Haemophilus influenzae, Pseudomonas aeruginosa*, or, much less frequently, *Staphylococcus aureus*. Complete eradication of the airway infection is rarely possible for more than a short period even with large doses of intravenous antibiotic and optimal physical therapy. We use antibiotics for alteration of the sputum character (purulence, increased volume, or tenacity) together with change in symptoms, especially increase in dyspnea or hemoptysis. We treat episodes of deterioration individually unless they follow one another at short intervals. Continuous antibiotic therapy may then be tried and this frequently results in improved well-being, decreased exacerbations, and fewer hospitalizations.

Some recent work has suggested that even patients who appear clinically stable may have an increased amount of neutrophil-derived elastase in their sputum, which damages epithelium, inhibits normal ciliary function, and can be cleared by antibiotics. If confirmed, this would be a useful marker for continuous antibiotic therapy, although it is our practice, at present, to start treatment based on clinicial deterioration.

We use ampicillin, 500 to 1,000 mg four times a day; tetracycline, 500 mg four times a day; or cotrimoxazole (trimethoprim, 160 mg, and sulfamethoxazole, 800 mg), twice a day orally for 14 to 21 days. However, the response of the frequently present *Pseudomonas* organisms is negligible. Some studies suggest that these doses may not produce adequate tissue levels of antibiotic and have suggested that high doses (e.g., amoxicillin, 3 g twice a day PO) result in a higher response rate and longer period before clinical relapse. Others have cautioned against these high doses because of their effect on gut flora and the possibility of selecting out resistant organisms. This controversy must await further work on the benefits and hazards of such treatment.

Patients with cystic fibrosis, or those who fail to respond to a couple of antibiotic courses, or those who have a more severe initial infection with systemic features usually have a *Pseudomonas* infection. For many years we treated this with a combination of ticarcillin, 3 g IV every 4 hours, and tobramycin, 1 mg per kilogram IV every 8 hours (normal renal function), for 10 to 14 days but more recently we have started using ceftazidine 150 mg per kilogram intravenously daily in three divided doses, which has been shown to be more efficacious. Infection with *S. aureus* is usually treated with

TABLE 1 Antibiotic Therapy

Infection Severity	*Initial Treatment*	*Continuing Treatment*
Mild	Tetracycline, 500 mg q.i.d., *or* ampicillin, 500 mg q.i.d., *or* cotrimoxazole, 2 tablets b.i.d. - PO for 14–21 days	Continued for recurrent infection
Severe	Ampicillin 1 g IV q.i.d.	Continued for recurrent infection
Pseudomonas	Ticarcillin 3 g IV q.i.d. + Tobramycin 1 mg/kg IV q8h	Nebulized tobramycin, 160 mg t.i.d.
S. aureus	Cloxacillin 1 g IV q.i.d.	
Anaerobes	Penicillin G 2–3 million units IV q4h *or* metronidazole 500 mg IV/PO t.i.d.	

cloxacillin, 1 g IV four times a day for 10 to 14 days, unless the organism is resistant to this antibiotic, in which case we use vancomycin 500 mg intravenously four times a day (normal renal function). Sometimes a patient with mixed respiratory flora continues to produce large amounts of purulent sputum with troublesome symptoms. In this situation, anaerobic infection may be responsible, and we use penicillin G, 2 to 3 million units IV every 4 hours, or metronidazole, 500 mg PO three times a day for 14 days.

Previously, the need to use intravenous antibiotics required hospitalization, but patients can be taught to administer all or part of an antibiotic course themselves through an intravenous cannula. Recently, another approach in the maintenance therapy of cystic fibrosis has been to use antibiotics inhaled as an aerosol from a nebulizer to reduce the total lung burden of *Pseudomonas* infection. We nebulize tobramycin, 160 mg three times a day, with a Devilbiss D646 nebulizer, but carbenicillin, 1 g, and gentamicin, 80 mg, both nebulized twice a day, have been used by others for prolonged periods of 6 weeks to several months. The poor systemic absorption of aminoglycosides has been confirmed by measuring blood levels, and this approach is likely to be free of the renal complications of the systemically administered drug.

Bronchodilators

There is some evidence that many patients with bronchiectasis may have increased airway hyperreactivity, although the mechanism by which this might occur is unclear, and in the presence of a component of fixed airflow obstruction, measurements of airway responsiveness such as methacholine inhalation may be unreliable. We rely on the demonstration of an increase in FEV_1 of more than 15 percent after an inhaled bronchodilator. We have found salbutamol, 200 μg every 4 to 6 hours, and/or ipratropium bromide (Atrovent), 40 to 80 μg every 6 hours, to be useful. We use long-acting theophylline preparations for maintenance in rare instances, and then only if we have been able to demonstrate additional bronchodilatation after the maximum effect has been achieved with inhaled bronchodilators. The additional small benefit to airflow, if any, is often outweighed by frequent side-effects especially gastrointestinal symptoms of nausea and gastric acid reflux, which would obviously be undesirable because of the risk of further aspirational pulmonary injury. The starting dose of long-acting theophylline is 200 mg every 12 hours, increasing after a few days to 300 mg every 12 hours or more. We check the serum theophylline level to confirm a therapeutic serum level and to help minimize possible side effects.

We often find that a patient who gives a good history of variable airflow obstruction demonstrates a response to bronchodilator therapy both subjectively and by spirometric criteria. However, if we cannot demonstrate some objective evidence of reversibility after a reasonable clinical trial over 3 to 4 weeks, when the patient's condition is relatively stable, bronchodilator therapy would be discontinued or used only intermittently. Nevertheless, there may be an indication for bronchodilator therapy along with antibiotics and occasionally steroids in such patients during infective exacerbations.

Physical Therapy

For raising moderate amounts of secretions, vigorous frequent self-directed coughing has been shown to be as effective in most patients as formal physiotherapy programs, which include percussion and postural drainage. There is still some controversy regarding the best type of cough maneuver, and vigorous end-expiratory cough (huffing) is thought by some investigators to be more effective than cough initiated at high lung volumes.

However, there may be situations in which a patient becomes ill with an infection and cannot cough effectively. In this setting, we would suggest that, in association with rehydration, postural drainage supplemented by percussion and vigorous cough may help to clear secretions, particularly if these are copious. The relative merits of manual percussion versus mechanical vibration has recently been reviewed by Wanner.

We are not convinced that there is any evidence to justify the use of oral or inhaled mucolytic agents and do not use them.

Allergic Aspergillosis

Bronchiectasis due to allergic bronchopulmonary aspergillosis occurs almost invariably in asthmatics of long standing whose clinical features of airflow obstruction, mucus plugging, and mainly upper lobe patchy atelectasis respond to therapy with systemic steroids, while antifungal agents are of no value. We usually start such patients on prednisone, 0.5 mg per kilogram, and continue this until symptoms, spirometry, lung volumes, and the roentgenogram approach normal or plateau. Prednisone is then gradually decreased by 5 mg a week until a minimum maintenance dose is achieved. To minimize adrenal suppression, alternate-day therapy is used for maintenance whenever possible.

Surgery and Other Measures

The clinical criteria for removing the bronchiectatic area of lung have changed somewhat in the last 20 years. We recommend surgery if bronchiectasis is confined to one lobe and the patient experiences recurrent infection, frequent severe cough and sputum that impairs the quality of life, or frequent major hemoptysis of 100 ml or more not readily controlled by antibiotic therapy. We would advise lobectomy for profound or life-threatening hemorrhage, even if disease is not confined to one lobe, provided the patient has sufficient reserve of pulmonary function to avoid becoming a respiratory invalid, assuming that one lung might have to be removed. If pulmonary function is thought to be marginal, an isotope ventilation-perfusion scan might be helpful preoperatively to predict adequate residual function after the planned resection. It should be remembered that the area being removed is usually nonfunctioning, and its removal probably will not further decrease functional reserve. As a general guide, an FEV_1 less than 50 percent of predicted and a PaO_2 less than 60 mm Hg at sea level while breathing room air are relative contraindications to pulmonary resection.

When hemorrhage is profuse or life-threatening, this problem is best managed by a thoracic surgeon with measures such as rigid bronchoscopy to identify and isolate the uninvolved lung and achieve tamponade of a bleeding segmental or subsegmental bronchus with a Fogarty catheter. In the face of massive hemorrhage threatening to cause asphyxiation (>200 ml per 24 h), selective intubation and ventilation of the unaffected lung is often a prelude to emergency lobectomy or pneumonectomy due to persistent bleeding.

For patients with severe or life-threatening hemorrhage, who are not surgical candidates because of severely impaired pulmonary function, the technique of therapeutic embolization by selective bronchial arterial catheterization usually arrests bleeding with relatively little risk, unless the arteries feeding the spinal cord are inadvertently embolized, resulting in neurologic damage from spinal cord ischemia or infarction. It is essential that this risk is explained to the patient beforehand and written consent obtained. The risk of cord injury can be minimized by injecting a small bolus of contrast material to visualize the vessels before gelfoam is injected.

On occasion, we have had some success using irradiation to an area of lung from which recurrent severe hemorrhage originated, but where bronchial artery catheterization could not be achieved. The dose of irradiation we used was 2,000 rads in two divided doses one week apart, but we would suggest discussion with a radiotherapist to assess the needs of an individual case.

Frequently, foreign bodies can be removed transbronchoscopically unless they have gone undetected for long periods and are completely encased in granulation tissue. An open surgical procedure may then be needed to resect the involved area of bronchus or the entire lobe if, as is often the case, there is marked destruction of the parenchyma distal to the obstruction.

SUGGESTED READING

Hodson ME, Penketh ARL, Batten JC. Aerosol carbenicillin and gentamicin treatment of *Pseudomonas aeruginosa* infection in patients with cystic fibrosis. Lancet 1981; 2:1137–1139.

Rossman C, Waldes R, Sampson D, Newhouse MT. Effect of chest physiotherapy on the removal of mucus in patients with cystic fibrosis. Am Rev Respir Dis 1982; 126:131–135.

Stockley RA, Hill SL, Morrison HM. Effect of antibiotic treatment on sputum elastase in bronchiectatic outpatients in a stable clinical state. Thorax 1984; 39:416–419.

Wanner A. Does chest physical therapy move airway secretions? Am Rev Respir Dis 1984; 130:701–702.

CYSTIC FIBROSIS

IAN MacLUSKY, M.B., B.S., F.R.C.P.(C)
HENRY LEVISON, M.B., F.R.C.P.(C)

Cystic fibrosis (CF) is the most common inherited lethal disease in Caucasians, with an incidence of approximately one in 2,300. Based on family studies, it is believed to be inherited on an autosomal recessive basis, although there is no method yet available of reliably detecting heterozygotes. It is rare among blacks (approximately 1 in 19,000) and orientals (1 in 90,000).

Cystic fibrosis is characterized by a heterogeneous group of abnormalities involving the mucus-secreting glands of the respiratory, gastrointestinal, and hepatobiliary systems, as well as the sweat glands and reproductive system. Although the underlying biochemical defect is not known, the primary defect appears to be an abnormality in the control of the water content of exocrine secretions. Thus secretions from serous glands, such as sweat and saliva, are characterized by increased levels of inorganic ions. Secretions from mucus-secreting glands appear to be hyperviscid, resulting in obstruction of the glands and leading to the major pathologic sequelae of the disease.

DIAGNOSIS

Cystic fibrosis may present at any age, from infancy to adulthood. Diagnosis is based on clinical presentation (Table 1), and confirmed by an elevated sweat chloride level. Sweat chloride analysis, using the pilocarpine iontophoresis technique, is the most consistent diagnostic test available, but even this test has a 2 percent false-positive and false-negative rate. A sweat chloride concentration greater than 60 mEq per liter is considered diagnostic. If borderline, or if there is some question about the clinical presentation, repeated testing may be necessary.

Although other diagnostic techniques have been suggested, none have shown enough sensitivity or specificity to be used for the diagnosis of CF, although they may be useful as screening techniques.

There is no known cure for cystic fibrosis. Without knowledge of the underlying biochemical defect in CF, treatment remains aimed primarily at the disease sequelae. Despite marked improvement in prognosis since CF was first described, the disease remains uniformly fatal, the median age of death being approximately 22 for women, 28 for men.

TABLE 1 Clinical Presentation of Cystic Fibrosis

Age	*Clinical Features*
Infancy	Meconium ileus, protracted neonatal jaundice, hyponatremic dehydration
Childhood	Recurrent/chronic chest infection, malnutrition, intussusception, volvulus, rectal prolapse, portal hypertension, meconium ileus equivalent, fat-soluble vitamin deficiency, pancreatitis, recurrent nasal polyps, chronic sinusitis
Adolescence	Recurrent/chronic chest infection, cor pulmonale, diabetes mellitus, male infertility

RESPIRATORY DISEASE

Outside the neonatal period, respiratory disease is the major cause of both morbidity and mortality in patients with CF.

Patients with CF have normal lungs at birth. The earliest pathologic changes seen, occurring in the first few months of life, are dilatation and hypertrophy of the bronchial glands, initially in the smaller bronchioles. Coincident with these changes, the patients develop chronic colonization of the airways with a specific group of organisms (Table 2). This leads to irritation of the airways, goblet cell hyperplasia, loss of ciliated epithelium, and progressive peribronchial inflammation, with plugging of the airways by mucopurulent exudate. This results in progressive air trapping and patchy atelectasis, with ventilation/perfusion mismatching and progressive hypoxemia. Thus patients with CF usually die from a combination of progressive cor pulmonale and respiratory failure.

MANAGEMENT

Treatment is aimed at (1) minimizing the bronchial plugging, and (2) attempting to inhibit the bacterial colonization.

Mucous Plugging

Physiotherapy

Physiotherapy is a time-honored part of the treatment of cystic fibrosis. Using standard techniques of chest percussion and postural drainage, the aim is to aid the patients in expectorating mucus from the various pulmonary segments. We recommend that the parents perform physiotherapy for 20 minutes either twice or three times daily, depending on the amount of sputum produced by the children. When the children are old enough, usually about 8 to 10 years old, we encourage the children to perform their own physiotherapy, using a variety of mechanical percussors available, which appears to be as effective as manual percussion.

Although physiotherapy is an integral part of treatment for CF, some questions remain. It is probably the most time-consuming part of the treatment and, as the child grows, can form a major area of both contention and noncompliance. Improvements in pulmonary function have been shown following physiotherapy, but these have been mainly in short-term trials on patients who have significant sputum production. However, there are no long-term trials of the effect of physiotherapy, particularly as to whether it has any "prophylactic" value in patients who are non-sputum-producing. In the clinic population at The Hospital for Sick Children, approximately 20 percent of the patients admit to performing no physiotherapy, yet do not appear to fare any worse than the more compliant patients. This is a self-selected group, with presumably mild chest disease, but obviously further studies are necessary to identify the exact role of physiotherapy in patients with CF. Until this information is available, we recommend routine physiotherapy for patients with evidence of significant pulmonary disease.

Inhalation Therapy

Mist tents, using humidified air, were originally used in an attempt to hydrate the retained secretions. However, this was associated with a significant risk of inducing both bacterial colonization and bronchospasm, as well as causing marked family disruption, yet with little evidence of therapeutic benefit; this treatment has been generally discontinued. Mucolytics, such as N-acetylcysteine (Mucomyst), can be given by inhalation (Table 3). Whether it is clinically effective remains unproven, although it may induce both bronchospasm and hemorrhagic tracheitis with long-term use. Its use should therefore be tailored to individual patients.

Bacterial Colonization

Cystic fibrosis is characterized by chronic bacterial colonization of the airways associated with progressive inflammatory changes and by steady deterioration in pulmonary function. With decreasing pulmonary status, there are increasing episodes of acute deterioration, associated with anorexia, weight loss, increased production of purulent sputum, decreased exercise tolerance, and increasing shortness of breath. Elevated white cell count and fever may occur, but are not necessarily present. Up to 40 percent of these episodes of deterioration may be precipitated by viral upper respiratory tract

TABLE 2 Approximate Incidence of Sputum Colonization by Specific Organisms*

Organism	*Incidence (%)*
Staphylococcus aureus	18
Pseudomonas cepacia	20
Haemophilus influenzae	20
Klebsiella	8
Pseudomonas aeruginosa	70

* Colonization by multiple organisms is common.

infections. However, since bacterial colonization appears to be the primary process, antibiotic therapy is a logical part of treatment.

Acute Disease

For patients with evidence of significant deterioration in pulmonary status, hospitalization is usually required because therapy administered at home is frequently ineffective. Unlike patients with other pulmonary diseases, the sputum culture in patients with CF is usually representative of the colonizing organisms. Therapy can therefore be appropriately instituted on the basis of sputum cultures. In children younger than 2 years, *Staphylococcus aureus* is the principal organism isolated. We therefore initiate treatment with intravenous cloxacillin until sputum cultures are available. In the older child, *Pseudomonas aeruginosa* is the most frequently isolated organism. To date, the most effective treatment is a combination of an aminoglycoside and a ureidopenicillin. However, bacterial resistance is a common problem, and substitution with either a third-generation cephalosporin, co-trimoxazole, or chloramphenicol may be necessary. Owing to the risk of inducing bacterial resistance, combination therapy is usually required. The duration of therapy is empiric. In most cases, 10 days is optimum, less than this being associated with reexacerbation on discontinuing the antibiotics; a longer duration, except in specific cases, has not been shown to have any apparent increased benefit.

There is no convincing evidence of transmission of *Pseudomonas aeruginosa* between patients with cystic fibrosis. We therefore do not isolate the patients.

Pseudomonas cepacia is seen increasingly in older patients and usually shows multiple antibiotic resistance. Most patients with *Pseudomonas cepacia* colonization show a rate of decline in pulmonary status similar to that seen in patients with *Pseudomonas aeruginosa.* However, in a small group of patients, *Pseudomonas cepacia* has been associated with a frank pneumonic picture, with elevated temperature, white count, and sedimentation rate, resulting in rapid deterioration, usually ending in death.

Long-Term Antibiotic Therapy

Oral Antibiotics. In an attempt to inhibit bacterial colonization, long-term oral antibiotics are prescribed in many centers (Table 3). Treatment is usually initiated with oral cloxacillin in an attempt to prevent staphylococcal colonization; this drug is replaced with ampicillin, cephalosporin, or co-trimoxasole when *Pseudomonas* superinfection occurs.

Although long-term oral antibiotic therapy in patients with CF is a common practice, there is little scientific basis for their use. When CF was first described, *Staphylococcus aureus* was the major pathogen identified and has subsequently, coincident with the use of oral cloxacillin "prophylaxis," become far less a problem. However, over the same period there appears to have been a decrease in staphylococcal infections in people without CF. Moreover, the long-term use of cloxacillin might merely lead to colonization of the sputum with resistant *Pseudomonas* rather than *Staphylococcus aureus.* Thus, long-term placebo-controlled trials are warranted to determine the true effectiveness of long-term oral antibiotics.

Inhaled Antibiotics. Inhaled antistaphylococcal antibiotics have been tried without apparent therapeutic effectiveness. Long-term inhaled aminoglycoside has been recommended in an attempt to suppress colonization by *Pseudomonas aeruginosa.* However, this is an inefficient method of administering a medication, since less than 10 percent of any inhaled drug is absorbed, and penetration of the antibiotic is least to the areas of atelectasis, where the infection is probably greatest. Although initial reports have suggested some improvement, this is an expensive form of therapy and requires further study before it can be routinely advocated.

"Tune-Ups"

Some patients may show steady, progressive deterioration in pulmonary status desite maximal at-home therapy. Admission to the hospital for intravenous therapy may effect some improvement. However, the use of "routine" intravenous antibiotics for patients who show no evidence of acute exacerbation is debatable. Repeated hospitalization causes significant home and school disruption, and there is little evidence that repeated courses of intravenous antibiotics significantly alter the long-term prognosis. We therefore reserve intravenous antibiotic therapy for those with evidence of acute or persisting decline in clinical status.

Cough

With progression in the pulmonary disease, persistent productive cough becomes a major feature of the illness. This is frequently worse at night and on rising. Antitussives are contraindicated, since suppression of cough may lead to further mucous plugging and deterioration in respiratory status. Physiotherapy immediately before the patient goes to sleep and on his or her rising in the morning may help to alleviate the cough. In the rare patient with persistent nonproductive cough due to apparent hyperreactive airway disease (to be discussed), an inhaled bronchodilator such as ipatropium bromide (Atrovent, not yet approved for general use in the United States) may be effective (Table 3).

Airway Hyperreactivity

Up to 25 percent of patients with cystic fibrosis have evidence of airway hyperreactivity, presumably secondary to chronic airway irritation. This may be exacerbated by physiotherapy. Thus, in patients with evidence of airway hyperreactivity, inhaled bronchodilators such as salbutamol should be taken immediately prior to physiotherapy. Sodium chromoglycate and oral theophyllines may be required by patients with frank asthma.

Respiratory Complications

Pulmonary Osteoarthropathy

Clubbing is a frequent finding in patients with significant lung disease from CF and is usually proportional to the severity of the disease.

Pulmonary osteoarthropathy causes swelling and tenderness of the long bones, with roentgenographic evidence of periosteal elevation. Treatment is primarily aimed at the underlying lung disease, if at all possible, and nonsteroidal anti-inflammatory agents may be effective for analgesia.

Occasional patients may present with a nonspecific form of polyarthralgia, unassociated with the severity of the lung disease, possibly arising as a form of immune complex disease. Again, treatment is primarily with anti-inflammatory agents.

Atelectasis

Patchy atelectasis is a common finding in CF and in some patients, it is associated with collapse of a whole lobe. Repeated bronchoscopy and bronchial lavage has been tried in various centers for all patients with CF. This was associated with significant morbidity and a questionable effect on the long-term outlook. The procedure has been generally abandoned. However, in patients with evidence of persisting lobar atelectasis, despite vigorous physiotherapy, bronchoscopy is probably warranted in an attempt to reinflate the lobe.

Bronchiectasis

Diffuse, progressive bronchiectasis is a major feature of CF. Occasionally, a localized area of bronchiectasis may cause marked bronchorrhea, leading to severe intractable coughing productive of large volumes of

TABLE 3 Drugs Used in the Treatment of Cystic Fibrosis

Drug	*Route*	*Dosage*	*Schedule*
ANTIBIOTICS			
Penicillins			
Amoxicillin	PO	50–100 mg/kg/day	q6h
Cloxacillin	PO/IV	50–200 mg/kg/day	q6h
Ticarcillin	IV	200–300 mg/kg/day	q4–6h
Piperacillin	IV	100–300 mg/kg/day (max 24 g/day)	q4–6h
Cephalosporins			
Cephalexin	PO	100–200 mg/kg/day	q6h
Cefamandole	IV	50–150 mg/kg/day	q4–6h
Ceftazidime	IV	200 mg/kg/day	q6h
Aminoglycosides			
Gentamicin*	IV	5–10 mg/kg/day	q8h
Tobramycin*	IV	5–10 mg/kg/day	q8h
Others			
Co-trimoxazole: trimethoprim-sulfamethoxazole	PO	8 mg/kg/day 40 mg/kg/day	q12h
	IV	5–10 mg/kg/day 25–50 mg/kg/day (max adult dose 640 mg trimethoprim/day)	q6–12h
Chloramphenicol	PO/IV	50–100 mg/kg/day	q6h
BRONCHODILATORS			
Salbutamol (2-mg or 4-mg tabs)	PO	0.05–0.1 mg/kg/day	q6h
Metered aerosol (100 μg/puff)	Inhalation	1–2 puffs	q4–6h
Inhalation solution (5 mg/ml)	Inhalation	0.01–0.03 ml/kg/dose	q4–6h
Fenoterol			
Metered aerosol (200 μg/puff)	Inhalation	1–2 puffs	q4–6h
Orciprenaline (tabs/syrup)	PO	0.3–0.5 mg/kg/dose	q6–8h
Metered aerosol (650 μg/puff)	Inhalation	1–2 puffs	q6–8h
Inhalation solution 2%	Inhalation	0.01–0.02 ml/kg/dose	q6–8h
Ipratropium bromide (Atrovent)			
Metered aerosol (20 μg/puff)	Inhalation	2–5 puffs	q4h
Theophylline* (anhydrous)	PO or IV	18–24 mg/kg/day	
Short-acting PO preps			q6h
Long-acting PO preps			q8–12h
MUCOLYTICS			
N-acetylcysteine Inhalation (20% solution)		1–2 ml	q8h
SCLEROSING AGENTS			
Quinacrine Intrapleural		100 mg in 50 cc	1/day × 3

* Increased drug clearance in CF: therefore requiring close monitoring of serum levels.

purulent sputum, out of proportion to the general severity of the lung disease. Initial treatment consists of intensive physiotherapy and intravenous antibiotics. If this is unsuccessful, resection of the bronchiectatic lobe may be effective. However, there are no clear guidelines as to the timing of surgery, which has to be individualized for each patient. Diffuse bronchiectasis is a usual feature of the disease, the severity of which may not be readily apparent on plain chest film. Thus, bronchoscopy and/or bronchography, particularly of the neighboring, apparently noninvolved segments, is usually necessary to delineate the exact extent of the disease. As long as the patient is adequately evaluated and receives intensive pre- and postoperative physiotherapy, intravenous antibiotics as necessary, and early postoperative mobilization, operative morbidity and mortality should be minimal.

Reflux

Esophageal reflux is known to occur with increased frequency in patients with chronic lung disease, presumably owing to a combination of (1) increased intra-abdominal pressure with coughing and (2) hyperinflation of the chest with distortion of the diaphragm. Not surprisingly, reflux is frequently seen in patients with CF, although the exact incidence is unknown. Clinically, reflux presents with symptoms of esophagitis and increase in cough, particularly at night. However, the esophagitis may be relatively asymptomatic and the nocturnal cough interpreted as due to deterioration in pulmonary disease alone. Evidence of reflux should be actively searched for, both by appropriate questioning and by barium swallow or esophagoscopy if necessary, in patients with a history of nocturnal exacerbations. Treatment is usually medical, with antacids, metoclopramide, and elevation of the head of the bed. Surgical correction is frequently prohibited by the severity of the lung disease.

Hemoptysis

There is a proliferation of bronchial vessels around the areas of bronchiectasis, forming a rich vascular anastomosis around the bronchiole. With progression of the disease, hemorrhage through the overlying areas of granulation tissue is common. Usually the hemorrhage is transient, presenting as painless blood-streaked sputum or, occasionally, as episodes of coughing up frank blood clots. Treatment is aimed primarily at the underlying infection. We usually hospitalize all but the mildest cases and treat with intravenous antibiotics as appropriate. Physiotherapy is discontinued for the first 24 hours, until bleeding has resolved, and any associated coagulopathy is treated as necessary.

In the occasional patient, bleeding may be either persistent or profuse (more than 300 ml in 24 hours) and may even be life-threatening. In these cases, more aggressive therapy is warranted. Bronchoscopy with endobronchial tamponade has been successful in some hands as long as active bleeding is minimal. However, rebleeding is common, and with active bleeding, isolation of the bleeding point is frequently difficult.

Surgical excision of the bronchiectatic lobe arrests the bleeding. However, in most patients, the pulmonary disease is too extensive to permit safe surgery. Alternatively, identification of the bleeding point by angiography, with arrest of hemorrhage by the instillation of Gelfoam particles into the supplying bronchial arteries, can usually be safely performed, even in patients with advanced pulmonary disease.

Pneumothorax

Chronic air trapping due to mucous plugging frequently leads to the development of apical cysts, which may eventually rupture. Thus pneumothorax is common; its incidence, which increases with age, approaches 20 percent among patients over the age of 13. Recurrence may occur in as many as 50 percent of cases.

Symptomatic pneumothoraces should be treated by intercostal drainage. Because of the morbidity associated with prolonged or recurrent drainage, if the air leak stops, pleural sclerosis should be performed with quinacrine or tetracycline. If the air leak continues or sclerosis fails, a parietal pleurectomy should be performed.

Bronchopulmonary Aspergillosis

Patients with CF have an increased incidence of positive *Aspergillus* precipitins, and aspergillus can be isolated from the sputum of 10 to 15 percent of patients. However, in the majority it is a commensal, having no discernible effect on the pulmonary disease. In approximately 10 percent of patients, proliferation of *Aspergillus* within the airways leads to overt hyperreactive pulmonary disease, manifested as deteriorating pulmonary status, scattered areas of consolidation on chest film, eosinophilia, elevated IgE, and increased serum *Aspergillus* precipitins. Treatment consists of high-dose steroids. This treatment is usually successful, but recurrence is not uncommon and may require repeated or even long-term steroids for suppression.

Cor Pulmonale

Progressive plugging of the airways leads to atelectasis and air trapping, as well as shunting through the bronchopulmonary anastomoses around areas of bronchiectasis. These events lead to progressive ventilation/perfusion mismatching and result in progressive hypoxemia. This condition is frequently exacerbated during sleep owing to the fall in residual volume, which increases the ventilation/perfusion imbalance. The resultant hypoxemia causes pulmonary vasoconstriction, which is initially reversible but eventually becomes fixed, leading to progressive cor pulmonale and eventual right heart failure.

Diagnosis may be difficult; clinical signs are frequently masked by the underlying lung disease. Routine electrocardiogram may show evidence of right ventricular hypertrophy or strain, although this may be obscured by the thoracic cage distortion seen in patients with advanced pulmonary disease. Similarly, pulmonary hyperexpansion may obscure right ventricular enlargement on the chest film. M-mode echocardiography, by demonstrating delayed opening of the pulmonic valve, correlates well with pulmonary hypertension. However, protrusion of the hyperexpanded left lung anterior to the heart restricts the "echographic window" available and limits the usefulness of this test. Vectorcardiography is usually successful in demonstrating abnormalities in right ventricular function. However, practically speaking, cor pulmonale can be expected in patients with advanced lung disease; it is usually present in patients with resting arterial Po_2 less than 50 mm Hg, particularly with a Pco_2 greater than 45 mm Hg. Similarly, clinical signs of right heart failure may be obscured by the overlying pulmonary disease and may simply be manifested by deteriorating pulmonary status and unexplained weight gain.

Treatment

Since there is usually little that can be remedied in the lung disease, treatment is aimed at the sequelae.

Oxygen. Supplemental oxygen helps to reverse the pulmonary vasoconstriction due to hypoxemia and improves myocardial performance. We therefore prescribe nocturnal oxygen, via nasal cannula, to all patients in whom daytime resting arterial oxygen is less than 60 mm Hg, and continuous oxygen to those in whom it is less than 50 mm Hg.

Patients with CF are usually able to maintain a normal Pco_2 until late in the disease process. However, with severe lung disease, there is frequently blunting of the CO_2-dependent respiratory drive. Oxygen should therefore be used cautiously in patients with advanced lung disease because it can cause suppression of the hypoxemic respiratory drive and resultant hypercapnia and carbon dioxide narcosis.

Pulmonary Vasodilators. These have no place in the treatment of cor pulmonale due to cystic fibrosis, since they also increase perfusion to areas of consolidation or atelectasis, causing further hypoxemia.

Diuretics. Biventricular failure is a common finding in patients with advanced cystic fibrosis. Fluid restriction and long-term diuretic administration is an obvious effective supplemental therapy. Inappropriate antidiuretic hormone production also occurs in these patients, and diuretics should be used cautiously owing to the risk of electrolyte imbalance. Digoxin is of questionable benefit in patients with right ventricular failure alone. However, since many of these patients have biventricular failure, digoxin may have therapeutic value, but it should be used cautiously in view of the hypoxemia and hypokalemia frequently seen in these patients.

Respiratory Failure

Patients with cystic fibrosis eventually succumb to progressive respiratory and cardiac failure. They are usually able to maintain a normal arterial Pco_2 until late in the disease process. An elevated Pco_2, which carries a poor prognosis, may occasionally be treated effectively with intravenous aminophylline owing to its bronchodilator, cardiac and respiratory stimulant, and diuretic effects. However, mechanical ventilation is not usually warranted, since we are rarely able to produce sufficient improvement to subsequently wean them off the ventilator. Thus, for progressive respiratory failure, palliative care, such as effective analgesics to treat the respiratory muscle strain commonly seen with respiratory failure, should be considered.

NUTRITION

Eighty-five percent of patients with CF have steatorrhea. Even in those treated with supplemental pancreatic enzymes, fat malabsorption remains around 10 percent of intake (compared to less than 2% in normals). Provided these patients receive a high calorie diet, normal growth should be achieved. A retardation in growth, particularly weight for height, is a poor prognostic sign, presumably since deterioration in pulmonary status causes both increased work of breathing and anorexia.

We therefore emphasize adequate nutrition, with supplemental fat-soluble vitamins and high calorie formulas as necessary. If adequate intake cannot be maintained orally, supplemental feeding—either intravenously or via a gastrostomy—may be necessary. However, these treatments probably have no significant effect on the long-term prognosis of the lung disease.

SUGGESTED READING

Lloyd-Still JD. Textbook of Cystic Fibrosis. Boston: John Wright Publishing Inc, 1983.

Marks MI. The pathogenesis and treatment of pulmonary infections in patients with cystic fibrosis. J Pediatr 1981; 98:173–179.

Moss AJ. The cardiovascular system in cystic fibrosis. Pediatrics 1982; 70:728–741.

Scanlin TF. Cystic fibrosis: current trends in research. Clin Chest Med 1980; 1:423–427.

Wood RE, Boat TF, Doershuk CF. Cystic fibrosis: state of the art. Am Rev Resp Dis 1976; 113:833–877.

ALPHA$_1$-PROTEINASE INHIBITOR DEFICIENCY

ROBERT A. SANDHAUS, M.D., Ph.D.

Life-threatening genetic diseases that strike the young are rare. The hereditary deficiency of alpha$_1$-proteinase inhibitor (α_1PI), which was previously known as alpha$_1$-antitrypsin, is such a disease. It can lead to cirrhosis in the perinatal period and precocious emphysema in young adults. The molecular biology of this disease has been revealed by recent investigations, and rudimentary treatment protocols are being devised. In addition, our understanding of the events leading to the development of precocious emphysema in individuals with α_1PI deficiency has provided us with important clues about the etiology of all forms of pulmonary emphysema.

Our understanding of the cellular and molecular basis of this disease began in the mid-1960s with two unrelated investigations. In the United States, Paul Gross and his co-workers found that instillation of a proteinase capable of degrading elastin produced an animal model of pulmonary emphysema. In Sweden, Eriksson and Laurell were looking at the serum proteins of individuals with familial emphysema and found that all individuals with this disease have a deficiency in the proteins that migrated in the alpha$_1$ region of a serum protein electrophoretogram. They further identified the deficient protein as alpha$_1$-antitrypsin (now referred to as alpha$_1$-proteinase inhibitor because of its broad range of activity).

Janoff and co-workers found that the human polymorphonuclear leukocyte (the neutrophil) contains a potent elastase within its azuraphil granules. Moreover, this elastase is extremely sensitive to inhibition by α_1PI. Thus a link was found between the Swedish population studies and the animal models of emphysema. This information has led to a better understanding of the processes leading to the production of emphysema in individuals who are not deficient in α_1PI. Most current research suggests that oxidation of α_1PI by environmental agents, primarily products of tobacco combustion, leads to inactivation of the lung's α_1PI screen and subsequent elastin degradation by neutrophil elastase. It may be, therefore, that all emphysema is the result of α_1PI deficiency: Rarely, this is due to a genetic deficiency of this protein; more commonly, there is a functional deficiency induced by the action of cigarette smoke on the lung's α_1PI screen.

The diagnosis of α_1PI deficiency is dependent on the clinical picture of precocious emphysema, a family history of emphysema or neonatal cirrhosis, and/or the laboratory evaluation of the serum protein of interest, α_1PI. This laboratory evaluation usually includes obtaining a quantitative analysis of α_1PI in the serum and, if that is abnormal, an evaluation of the α_1PI phenotype (Pi-typing). Thus far, although there are well over 25 different phenotypes of α_1PI identified the most important factor leading to development of precocious emphysema is the amount of protein in the serum.

MANAGEMENT

Currently, the lung disease associated with α_1PI deficiency is usually relentlessly progressive, although individuals with the genetic abnormality have been identified who live without lung disease throughout their lives. The reasons for this are not clear, but there is some evidence that these individuals may have a compensatory lack of elastase in their neutrophils.

Treatment should first concentrate on factors that accelerate the lung destruction of pulmonary emphysema. Thus, smoking cessation is of utmost importance. Bacterial infections of the lungs should be treated promptly to reduce the neutrophil influx. The use of steroids to achieve this same goal is extremely controversial and currently without clear support.

Genetic Counseling

An important aspect of therapy is genetic counseling. Evaluation of living family members is often indicated, and education regarding the inheritance of this abnormality should be provided. The homozygote deficiency state (typically in individuals with the Z or S phenotypes; the normal phenotype is M) is the only abnormality clearly associated with an increased incidence of precocious emphysema. There is some evidence that certain heterozygous combinations (MZ, MS) may be associated with an increased risk of lung disease, perhaps when they are present in association with risk factors such as smoking.

It is important to note that, like those afflicted with the more typical tobacco-related emphysema, individuals with emphysema due to α_1 PI deficiency often have an element of reversible obstructive airway disease, and this "asthmatic" component should be fully evaluated and treated.

Treatment of Airflow Limitation

The individual with precocious emphysema due to α_1PI deficiency should be approached in exactly the same way as the individual with emphysema of any etiology. The degree of reversible disease should be assessed and treated with theophylline, beta-agonists, and the entire array of asthma medication. A steroid trial may be indicated. (See chapter on *Chronic Asthma*.)

Oxygen

If evaluation reveals cor pulmonale, or if there is demonstrable decrease in oxygen saturation of the blood, especially with exercise, supplemental oxygen therapy is indicated. Treatment of cor pulmonale requires the continuous use of supplemental oxygen for at least 8 to 12 hours out of every 24. This is usually administered during sleep. When exercise desaturation is demonstrated, oxygen administration during exercise can often greatly improve exercise tolerance. In many cases, continuous oxygen therapy is eventually required.

Rehabilitation

Physical rehabilitation may do more than any other form of therapy to affect the lives of individuals with α_1PI deficiency and emphysema. Muscle training can improve exercise tolerance without any improvement in lung function per se. Instruction in the most effective use of space in the home can allow an individual to live a much more independent life.

Surgery

There is little surgical therapy available for emphysema due to α_1PI deficiency. Bullectomy of large lower-zone blebs is sometimes considered. However, in spite of the disease's predilection for lower lung zone destruction, virtually all lobes are affected, and the remaining upper zone parenchyma may not be capable of sustaining adequate respiratory function. Lung transplantation usually is not a consideration because most centers do not offer transplantation to an individual with a genetic cause for continued lung damage.

Experimental Approaches

Experimental therapies exist and should be considered in the context of current research in this area. Individuals with α_1PI deficiency are currently receiving chronic replacement therapy using pooled human serum-derived α_1PI. Bacterially synthesized, cloned human gene product will soon be available for study. Whether these therapies will prove safe and effective is not yet known. It is important to realize that even if these therapies are completely effective, they are entirely prophylactic: they will not reverse lung destruction that has already occurred, but will prevent further lung destruction from taking place.

The use of hormonal therapy to increase the production of α_1PI by the liver was proposed earlier in this decade after studies showed a slight, but significant, increase in serum levels of α_1PI with this therapy. However, long-term follow-up has failed to show any clinical effect of this therapy. In view of the side effects associated with this therapeutic approach, this method of therapy is no longer recommended.

Because the α_1PI of the lung is exquisitely sensitive to oxidative inactivation by both endogenous oxidants and environmental oxidants, the use of antioxidants to protect the existing α_1PI in the lungs of α_1PI-deficient individuals has been proposed. Currently there is no evidence as to the effectiveness of this approach.

Finally, the development of synthetic elastase inhibitors that can be given orally, parenterally, or by inhalation is on the therapeutic horizon. This prophylactic therapy, if proved safe and effective, could be given to individuals at risk on a continuous basis and would provide a great impetus to promote early detection of α_1PI deficiency and emphysema in general.

SUGGESTED READING

Kueppers F, Black LF. Alpha$_1$-antitrypsin and its deficiency. Am Rev Respir Dis 1974; 110:176–194.

Morse JO. Alpha$_1$-antitrypsin deficiency. N Engl J Med 1978; 299:1045–1048 and 299:1099–1105.

EXTRINSIC ALLERGIC ALVEOLITIS

JAMES E. FISH, M.D.

Extrinsic allergic alveolitis, also referred to as *hypersensitivity pneumonitis*, is an immunologic disorder characterized by alveolar filling and diffuse parenchymal interstitial infiltration following exposure to airborne antigens. The immunopathogenesis of this group of disorders has not been clearly established, but it is thought to involve immune-complex and cell-mediated hypersensitivity mechanisms leading to inflammation of alveolar and peripheral airway structures. The causative agents in extrinsic allergic alveolitis are usually contained in finely dispersed organic dust. In particular, antigens derived from microorganisms, animal proteins, and plant proteins are common causes, although reactive chemical substances have recently been found responsible for some cases (Table 1). The disease manifestations are largely determined by level of exposure, immunologic reactivity of the host, and duration of disease activity. Recurrent or chronic parenchymal inflammation can lead to pulmonary fibrosis and ultimately to death from respiratory failure. Since extrinsic allergic alveolitis can be prevented by avoidance of exposure, early recognition of disease as well as the responsible antigen are the key elements of succesful management.

CLINICAL FEATURES

The disease may present in *acute* or *chronic* form, depending largely on the type of inhalation exposure. In general, the acute form of disease occurs with short-term, intermittent exposure and manifests as a flu-like illness. Chills, fever, headache, and myalgias, as well as

TABLE 1 Extrinsic Allergic Alveolitis

Disease	*Offending Agent*	*Agent*
Farmer's lung	Thermophilic actinomycetes	Moldy hay
Bagassosis	Thermophilic actinomycetes	Moldy bagasse
Mushroom worker's lung	Thermophilic actinomycetes	Mushroom compost
Humidifier lung	Thermophilic actinomycetes	Contaminated water in forced-air systems
Malt worker's lung	*Aspergillus* species	Moldy barley
Maple bark disease	*Cryptostroma corticale*	Maple bark
Woodworker's lung	*Alternaria*	Wood dust
Cheese worker's lung	*Penicillium casei*	Moldy cheese
Suberosis	Cork dust mold	Cork dust
Bird fancier's lung	Avian proteins	Avian dust
Enzyme worker's lung	*Bacillus subtilis*	Enzyme detergents
Epoxy resin lung	Reactive chemical-protein conjugate	Trimellitic anhydride Phthalic anhydride
Isocyanate hypersensitivity pneumonitis	Isocyanates	Toluene diisocyanate Diphenylmethane diisocyanate

cough and dypsnea, are usual complaints. Physical findings include fever, bilateral inspiratory rales, tachypnea, and tachycardia. A polymorphonuclear leukocytosis is usually present, but eosinophilia is uncommon. The chest roentgenogram may be normal in the acute form of disease, but more frequently it reveals poorly defined, diffuse, small nodular interstitial infiltrates. At the height of an episode, pulmonary function studies tend to reveal a pattern of restrictive ventilatory impairment; the forced vital capacity (FVC) and the 1-second forced expiratory volume (FEV_1) are both decreased without a reduction in the FEV_1/FVC ratio. Gas exchange abnormalities include resting hypoxemia as well as a reduction in the pulmonary diffusing capacity. As a rule, clinical recovery from the acute form of the disease is spontaneous and occurs within 12 to 24 hours, attendant with partial or complete resolution of corresponding laboratory abnormalities. Because acute symptoms mimic those found with viral or bacterial pneumonia, the illness is often mistaken for an acute respiratory infection.

The chronic form of extrinsic allergic alveolitis occurs more commonly with long-term, regular antigen exposure. In this form, symptoms tend to be more insidious and progressive. The most prominent symptom is dyspnea with exertion, although weight loss, easy fatiguability, and cough with or without sputum production are also frequently noted. The chest roentgenogram is indistinguishable from that seen in idiopathic diffuse fibrosing alveolitis, showing diffuse reticular and nodular infiltrates or fibrotic changes with honeycombing. Evidence of pleural disease and hilar adenopathy, on the other hand, are not among the roentgenographic manifestations of extrinsic allergic alveolitis. Typical pulmonary function findings include a restrictive ventilatory impairment with reductions in vital capacity, total lung capacity, and residual volume; an abnormal diffusing capacity; and hypoxemia at rest or with exercise. Because an obliterative bronchiolitis can also occur with the chronic form of disease, some patients may demonstrate evidence of airflow obstruction. Hence, a combined restrictive and obstructive pattern of ventilatory impairment may be found. In the advanced stages of disease, chronic respiratory failure with hypercapnea may also be present.

DIAGNOSIS

The most critical element in the diagnosis of extrinsic allergic alveolitis is suspicion that an environmental agent is responsible for respiratory symptoms. Once this is suspected, a thorough clinical history is needed to establish a relation between symptoms and exposure. In general, suspicion is easily aroused by a history of classic delayed-onset symptoms typical of the acute form of disease in a patient with known exposure to established offending agents. The more insidious nature of symptoms in the chronic form of the disease makes the history somewhat less conspicuous, however. In my view, the best approach is to consider extrinsic allergic alveolitis as a diagnostic possibility in all patients with clinical, physiologic, and roentgenographic findings compatible with a diffuse interstitial infiltrative process of unknown etiology.

Since successful management depends largely on limiting further exposure, a complete diagnosis requires not only recognition of the presence of disease, but also specific identification of the causative agent. Examination of serum for precipitating antibodies to the suspected antigen is most helpful in this regard. It is emphasized, however, that the presence of precipitins does not distinguish between individuals with true disease and those who have been exposed and, despite sensitization, remain in good health. The demonstration of antibody thus merely confirms exposure and sensitization, and it should be regarded only as presumptive evidence of disease. By contrast, a negative test is generally useful as a screening procedure to exclude a particular antigen as a causative factor. The major limitations of antibody screening include an unknown rate of false-negative reactions due to deficiencies in purity and potency of commercially available antigens, as well as the current availability of only a small number of standardized antigens despite a growing list of incriminated agents. Nevertheless, if suspicion of disease is high, any crude organic material obtained from the source of exposure can be used for antibody screening. If a positive reaction is obtained, this crude material may be further extracted and purified to gain more specific identification of the agent. Lung biopsies as a rule are nonspecific, although they may be used to rule out other causes of diffuse lung disease such as pulmonary infection, lymphangitic spread of malignant disease, or other interstitial processes with characteristic histologic features such as sarcoidosis.

Recent evidence indicates that patients with extrinsic allergic alveolitis have increased numbers of T-lymphocytes in bronchoalveolar lavage fluid as compared to lavage fluid obtained from patients with many other forms of interstitial pneumonias. Although increased numbers of T-lymphocytes in lavage fluid are also found in sarcoidosis, extrinsic allergic alveolitis may be distinguished by a relative increase in the T8+ (T-suppressor/cytotoxic) lymphocyte subset as compared to an increase in the T4+ (T-helper/inducer) subset in sarcoidosis. However, because of limited application and because the sophistication required for cell identification and lymphocyte subset classification is not widely available, the diagnostic usefulness of bronchoalveolar lavage procedures remains promising but uncertain.

The diagnosis is most often confirmed when avoidance of the suspected antigen results in demonstrable improvement in symptoms, the chest roentgenogram, and pulmonary function tests. Confirmation of diagnosis can also be obtained by monitoring the patient's response after exposure to the suspected antigen. This can be accomplished in the setting of natural environmental exposure or under controlled laboratory conditions. Documentation of lung function changes and/or leukocytosis and fever in association with respiratory symptoms 4 to 8 hours after exposure furnishes confirmatory evidence that a particular antigen is responsible. If the patient is exposed in his own natural environment or undergoes laboratory inhalation challenge using antigen levels that are equal to or less than those likely to be encountered in the natural environment, these procedures are generally safe and involve only minimal discomfort. For a number of antigens, however, it is difficult to accurately estimate the level of exposure that causes symptoms. For this reason, and also because minute concentrations of an agent may provoke severe life-threatening reactions in patients with extreme sensitivity, I recommend that controlled laboratory challenges be performed by individuals experienced in such procedures in a setting where severe reactions can be anticipated and properly managed.

MANAGEMENT

Prevention

Avoidance of the causative agent remains the most effective means of preventing extrinsic allergic alveolitis as well as the treatment of choice for established disease. Absolute avoidance, though ideal, often requires either complete elimination of the antigen or complete removal of the patient from the environmental source of exposure. Because these disorders most commonly occur in association with a specific occupation (e.g., farmers, mushroom workers, sugar cane workers) or avocation (bird fanciers), the impact of such drastic alterations in life style and livelihood as imposed by absolute avoidance may be unacceptable or impractical for personal, social, and economic reasons.

If strict avoidance cannot be achieved, alternative environmental control measures should be instituted to effectively reduce exposure. For example, the redesign of barns to improve ventilation patterns as well as the treatment of vegetable material with chemicals, or by wetting, or by exposing them to high temperatures may inhibit growth and dissemination of thermophilic actinomycetes spores. Rigorous efforts to decontaminate and clean air conditioner and humidifier systems can similarly reduce exposure to antigenic spores in the home or work environment. Changing the patient's personal environment can also be accomplished by the use of mask respirators. Most masks designed to filter 1-μm spores may impose too much airflow resistance to be useful in the occupational setting. However, I have had good experience with mask respirators that incorporate an airflow line to provide a constant source of fresh air from an external source such as an air compressor.

The prophylactic value of drugs, particularly corticosteroids in either oral or inhaled form, has not been evaluated in controlled clinical trials. Lacking scientific support for their use and owing to the potential risks of such therapy, I cannot recommend preventive therapy with corticosteroids as standard practice.

Therapy of Established Disease

Recommendations concerning the treatment of established disease are largely empiric, as controlled studies to establish optimal principles of management have not been carried out. With regard to the acute form of disease, symptoms and physiologic impairment generally tend to resolve spontaneously within a 12- to 24-hour period. Accordingly, I recommend only supportive care with bed rest and nonsteroid anti-inflammatory agents to control fever and discomfort from myalgias. Proper management includes arterial blood gas analysis to assess the presence and severity of hypoxemia. If present, hypoxemia should be treated with supplemental oxygen at an inspired concentration sufficient to keep arterial tension greater than 60 mm Hg. Although there are no controlled studies to support the use of corticosteroids in the acute form of disease, it is my contention that such therapy is warranted under extraordinary circumstances. Specifically, I believe that steroids are indicated for severe episodes in which hypoxemia responds poorly to oxygen therapy despite high fractional concentrations of inspired oxygen (>40% O_2) and for episodes in which spontaneous resolution is prolonged. In these circumstances, it is my practice to administer prednisone, 60 mg per day, until there are objective signs of improvement of symptoms and physiologic abnormalities. Tapering of prednisone is then carried out according to the needs and response of the patient. I prefer to continue prednisone at a lower alternate-day dose until the vital capacity and pulmonary diffusing capacity show no further signs of improvement.

In the chronic, more progressive form of disease, I recommend the use of corticosteroids in conjunction with avoidance procedures to hasten resolution of symptoms and physiologic impairment. In the chronic form of disease, however, resolution is apt to occur more slowly or not at all. As a rule, I administer prednisone (60 mg per day) for a period of approxiately 3 weeks as a means of documenting the reversibility of pulmonary function alterations as well as a means of hastening improvement. The patient is then placed on alternate-day therapy with a gradually tapering dose as pulmonary function continues to improve. Objective measurements should always be used to monitor the response to treatment, and for this I use measurements of the lung volume compartments and the diffusing capacity. Steroid therapy should be discontinued when pulmonary function returns to normal or when there is no evidence of further improvement. It is emphasized, however, that many patients may present with irreversible fibrotic changes at the time of diagnosis. Therefore, it should be assumed that physiologic impairment is more likely due to irreversible fibrosis than to reversible inflammation if no objective improvement in lung function can be demonstrated after 3 weeks of steroid therapy. Treatment at this point should be discontinued, as the risks of therapy tend to outweigh any anticipated benefits.

SUGGESTED READING

Allen DH, Williams GV, Woolcock AJ. Bird breeder's hypersensitivity pneumonitis: Progress studies of lung function after cessation of exposure to the provoking antigen. Am Rev Resp Dis 1976; 114:555–566.

Braun SR, Dopico GA, Tsiatis A, et al. Farmer's lung disease: Long-term clinical and physiologic outcome. Am Rev Resp Dis 1979; 119:185–191.

Salvaggio JE, Karr RM. Hypersensitivity pneumonitis: State of the art. Chest 1979; 75(suppl):270–274.

LOEFFLER'S SYNDROME

E. LESLIE CHUSID, M.D., F.C.C.P., F.A.C.P.

In 1932, Loeffler described a syndrome characterized by the following features: (1) variable chest film shadows that were "fleeting" and recurring, (2) peripheral (blood) eosinophilia, and (3) mild respiratory symptoms. The disease or syndrome is now described as respiratory illness characterized by "mild" clinical and roentgenologic pneumonitis, blood eosinophilia, concomitant findings of an allergic disorder in the patient, transience of pulmonary disease, and excellent response to corticosteroid medication.

Since the symptoms vary, and the chest film infiltrates vary in size and location from patient to patient, and the blood eosinophilia may not be present initially, the illness may masquerade as infectious pneumonitis and cause considerable confusion in management. There are no classic hallmarks except possibly the following signs: (1) nontoxic appearance of the patient despite pneumonia and leukocytosis, denoting what has been called the "benign" nature of the illness, (2) previous history of a similar pneumonitis and illness, (3) a transient change in the chest film pattern on serial films with variable locations of infiltrates, and (4) a significant blood eosinophilia and/or elevation of serum IgE levels.

In 1969, a similar entity, chronic eosinophilic pneumonia (CEP), was described. Since then Loeffler's syndrome has been viewed by some as a variant of CEP and has been called "eosinophilic pneumonia of brief duration" or acute eosinophilic pneumonia (AEP). Differentially, CEP has a more clearly defined chest film pattern, described as parietal or laterally placed edema, and a more prolonged clinical course. Furthermore, AEP has been associated, since 1932, with various etiologies, making its management dependent on the inclusive or exclusive diagnostic results obtained in ferreting out the cause. These etiologies must be considered carefully in decisions regarding therapy, since the therapy can be definitive in the resolution of the disease. The currently recognized causes of AEP include:

- Parasite infection
- Drug hypersensitivity
- Aspergillus infection (allergic aspergillosis)
- Allergic disorder with or without asthma
- Blood transfusion reaction
- Smoke inhalation
- Carcinomatosis
- Nickel hypersenstivity
- Investigative intravenous dye reaction
- Acute vasculitis/angitis

The parasites associated with Loeffler's syndrome and the drugs for their treatment are listed in Table 1. Medications that produce the syndrome are nitrofurantoin,

TABLE 1 Parasitic Infestation Associated with Loeffler's Syndrome

Parasite or Disease	*Drugs*
Ascariasis	Pyrantel pamoate, piperazine citrate, mebendazole, bephenium hydroxynaphthoate
Strongyloidosis	Thiabendazole
Larva migrans	Thiabendazole, diethylcarbamazine
Schistosomiasis	Niridazole, stibophen, antimony
Ancylostomiasis	Thiabendazole, diethylcarbamazine, diethylamine acetarsol
Dirofilariasis	Diethylcarbamazine
Necator americanus	Thiabendazole, mebendazole
Trichinosis	Thiabendazole
Fasciola hepatica	Emetine, metronidazole
Wuchereria malayi	Diethylcarbamazine, diethylamine acetarsol
Toxocara canis	Diethylcarbamazine

para-amino salicylic acid, penicillin, sulfonamides, mephenesin, thiopramine, chlorpropamide, gold salts, isoniazid, streptomycin, tolbutamide, methotrexate, aspirin, mecamylamine, imipramine, hydrochlorothiazide, cromolyn sodium, azathioprine, and carbamazepine.

Thus, if a specific etiology is found, specific therapy must be directed toward that etiology in conjunction with antiallergic therapy. This "specific" therapy would include antiparasitic treatment (see Table 1), discontinuance of a drug suspected of being the cause, treatment of a fungal infection, treatment of a specific carcinoma when found, and treatment of a diagnosed vasculitis.

MANAGEMENT

After having excluded infectious lung disease as the cause of pneumonitis, or having excluded all of the eosinophilic/allergic lung diseases of *specific etiology* (see Table 1), one is left with the management of idiopathic eosinophilic lung disease, which would be either CEP or AEP. If the chest film pattern and severity of illness that characterize CEP are absent, the presumptive diagnosis is AEP. The diagnosis may be established by fiberoptic lung biopsy, open lung biopsy, transcutaneous needle lung biopsy, or a therapeutic trial of corticosteroids to elict an immediate response.

The route of administration of corticosteroids may be oral, intramuscular, or intravenous. Dexamethasone phosphate, 8 mg IM twice a day for 1 or 2 days, or prednisone, 60 mg PO daily for 1 or 2 days may be given. In AEP there is usually a dramatic subsidence of fever, clinical symptoms, and chest film infiltrates following the therapeutic trial. With this type of response, a regimen of oral prednisone is then begun, starting with 60 mg daily given as one dose in the morning or two divided doses (30 mg twice a day), morning and evening. If lung biopsy is performed and confirms the diagnosis, in association with the clinical, laboratory, and chest film pattern, the 60-mg oral dose of prednisone is begun immediately on a daily basis. In rare instances, the initial dose of prednisone is 80 mg daily, but in general the response to corticosteroids is similar at 60 mg daily. The dose of prednisone is reduced by either 5 mg or 10 mg every 4 to 7 days, each dose not having to be as prolonged as in the management of CEP. However, the patient should be evaluated every 2 weeks to ensure proper resolution of the disease. Evaluation includes temperature, chest films, serum IgE determination, peripheral blood count, sedimentation rate, and especially eosinophil count and spirometry. Serial nasal smears, whereby nasal secretions are stained by Wright's stain on a slide, are a means of observing the subsidence of eosinophils. Serum IgE levels fall gradually over months, not as precipitously as the peripheral eosinophilia.

When the dose of daily prednisone has been reduced to 20 mg, further reduction must proceed more slowly and cautiously. Some patients suffer an exacerbation of the disease at daily doses below 20 mg if too rapid a reduction of dosage is pursued. At this stage, the dose should be reduced by either 2.5 mg or 5 mg daily, about every 2 weeks, until a dose of 5 to 7.5 mg daily is reached. Then, after 1 to 2 weeks, the dose (5 to 7.5 mg) may be given on alternate days and finally stopped after one month. The whole course of therapy with reduction in corticosteroids takes about 3 to 6 months to complete if the final diagnosis is *idiopathic* AEP. If there is a specific etiology to be treated (the so-called eosinophilic lung disease of specific etiology), the reduction of corticosteroids may proceed every 2 to 3 days and is completed in 1 to 3 weeks.

Approximately 20 percent of patients with idiopathic AEP have a recrudescence of the illness 1 to 4 weeks after the corticosteroids are discontinued, or when the corticosteroid dosage drops below 20 mg per day. When this occurs, one must boost the corticosteroid dosage back to at least 40 mg daily or even 60 mg daily, and again go through the gradual reduction over 3 to 6 months. However, at the level of 20 mg, in such a patient, a concomitant medication should then be given to allow further reduction in the corticosteroids with recrudescence. The medication could be an aerosol corticosteroid such as triamcinolone or beclomethasone (three inhalations three times daily) or an anticellular anti-immune medication such as Imuran (one 50-mg tablet daily). Treatment with the aerosol corticosteroid or Imuran is maintained while the oral steroids are gradually reduced to the alternate-day dose or discontinued. In the patient who experiences recrudescence, the combination regimen of prednisone, 5 mg daily or 5 mg every other day, plus Imuran or aerosol steroid may have to be continued for 6 to 12 months, similar to the CEP management. Table 2 summarizes the treatment of Loeffler's syndrome.

Since the therapy of Loeffler's syndrome (AEP) consists mainly of corticosteroids, management must include protection of the patient from steroid complications. These hazards include osteopenia, weight gain with edema, hyperglycemia, hypertension, and hyper-

TABLE 2 Treatment of Loeffler's Syndrome

Etiology	*Medical/Drug Approach*	*Concomitant Medication*
Specific AEP	Antiparasitic agents	Oral corticosteroids, 60 mg daily with rapid tapering[*]
	Discontinue causative drug	"
	Antifungal agent	"
	Discontinue transfusion	"
	Chemotherapy for carcinoma	"
	Cytotoxic agent for angitis	"
Idiopathic AEP	Oral prednisone, 60 mg daily with slow tapering[†]	
Recrudescent AEP	Oral prednisone, 40–60 mg daily with slow tapering	Aerosol corticosteroid[‡] Imuran[‡] Cromolyn sodium[‡] Ketotifen[‡]

* Rapid tapering = 1 to 3 weeks
† Slow tapering = 3 to 6 months
§ To be used when prednisone level = 20 mg prednisone daily and below 20 mg

acidity with dyspepsia. Concomitant medications should include, when necessary, calcium compound (1 g daily), vitamin D (50,000 units weekly), sodium fluoride (30 to 90 mg daily), hydrochlorthiazide (25 to 50 mg daily), cimetidine (300 to 400 mg four times a day) or ranitidine (150 mg twice daily), and anatacids. Generally, alternate-day corticosteroid therapy, when the level of 30 mg daily (60 mg on alternate days) is reached, eliminates some of the hazards of corticosteroid therapy.

Recently, antiallergic or antimediator agents such as cromoglycate (cromolyn sodium) and ketotifen ([Zaditen]) not yet available in the United States) have been suggested as prophylactic agents in idiopathic AEP. Cromoglycate may be used as the powder (20-mg capsule three times a day) for inhalation or the solution for inhalation (20 mg per 2-cc ampule three times daily). Ketotifen, in a 1-mg tablet, is given twice daily. When either agent is used, corticosteroid therapy is continued, starting at the prednisone level of 20 mg daily; the antiallergy agents are used concomitantly while the prednisone is reduced to low levels and then later discontinued.

SUGGESTED READING

Carrington CB, Addington WW, Goff AM, et al. Chronic eosinophilic pneumonia. N Engl J Med 1969; 280:787–798.

Fraser RG, Pare JAP. Diagnosis of Diseases of the Chest. Philadelphia: WB Saunders, 1978:900–906.

Mayock RL, Saldana MJ. In: Fishman AP (ed). Pulmonary Diseases and Disorders. New York:McGraw-Hill, 1980:926–932.

Shaba JK. In: Fishman AP (ed). Pulmonary Diseases and Disorders. New York:McGraw-Hill, 1980:1184–1186.

IDIOPATHIC PULMONARY FIBROSIS

GERALD S. DAVIS, M.D.

Idiopathic pulmonary fibrosis (IPF) usually leads to severe respiratory impairment and often death over several years if left without treatment. Most patients are above age 45, the peak incidence being about age 65. It is a disease of unknown cause and produces diffuse interstitial inflammation and fibrosis, resulting in progressive disorganization of pulmonary architecture, stiff lungs with a high work of breathing, and impaired gas exchange. IPF is characterized by dyspnea with exertion, dry cough, basilar crackles, digital clubbing, diffuse small irregular shadows on chest roentgenogram, and restrictive lung function tests with hypoxemia that worsens with exercise. Surgical open lung biopsy is usually required to accurately establish the diagnosis and to indicate the choice of therapy.

It is believed that IPF develops through the mechanism of a chronic immune-inflammatory reaction mediated by activated macrophages with the participation of lymphocytes, neutrophils, and fibroblasts. The inciting cause for initiating and perpetuating this response is unknown. Initial inflammation, secondary tissue injury, and finally fibrosis are believed to occur in sequence, but these processes may all take place simultaneously in nearby alveolar units. Anti-inflammatory and immunosuppressive drug therapy is aimed at controlling inflammation before tissue injury and fibrosis take place.

Treatment is only partially effective in most cases, but disease progression may be arrested sometimes even if lung function does not return to normal. Many patients deteriorate despite the best available therapy. The median survival is about 9 years for patients who respond to therapy, and 2 years for those who do not respond. Overall, approximately half the patients with IPF remain alive 5 years after initial diagnosis. The drugs used to treat IPF are toxic, and most patients experience at least minor side effects during therapy. There are many similarities between cancer and IPF in both course and management. These features all highlight IPF as a serious illness that requires definitive and detailed diagnosis, aggressive therapy, and skilled management.

CLINICAL PRESENTATION

Patients with IPF complain of gradually progressive shortness of breath on exertion. About three-quarters are bothered by dry cough. These symptoms have usually been present for several months, and sometimes for several years, before medical attention is sought. Climbing stairs or hills, carrying packages, or moderate exercise usually brings on dyspnea. Constitutional symptoms are common, and most patients report general fatigue, malaise, lack of energy, and reduced endurance which are out of proportion to their measured impairment in pulmonary function. Sputum production, chest pains, episodes of paroxysmal coughing, and wheezing are usually absent. Symptom levels remain stable from day to day. Table 1 summarizes the clinical features of IPF.

The most striking physical finding in IPF is the presence of high-pitched end-inspiratory crackles (dry or "Velcro" rales) over the lower one-third or two-thirds of both lung fields. Breath sounds may be enhanced, and tactile fremitus is often increased. In late disease, findings of cor pulmonale may appear. Digital clubbing is common, occurring in two-thirds of patients, but without the other features of symptomatic hypertrophic pulmonary osteoarthropathy.

The chest roentgenogram typically shows a diffuse symmetrical pattern of small irregular shadows predominantly in the lower lung zones. The fine vascular markings and the adjacent heart borders and pleural surfaces become blurred. A definite fraction of patients, perhaps 5 to 10 percent, appear with symptoms and physiologic abnormalities before the chest roentgenogram becomes abnormal. Both the extent (profusion) and coarseness of the infiltrate noted on roentgenogram increase as the disease progresses. A destructive "honeycomb" pattern, with small airspaces surrounded by dense linear shadows, may be seen in advanced disease. Pleural effusion generally is not part of IPF, and hilar lymph node enlargement is not seen.

Pulmonary function testing in IPF documents the nature and extent of abnormality, and provides important benchmarks for measuring the effect of treatment. A pattern typical of "restrictive" disease is seen. The vital capacity and total lung capacity are reduced. Pulmonary compliance is decreased, with the pressure-volume curve shifted down and to the right, evidencing stiff lungs which are hard to inflate. Air flow rates are normal or even super-normal, and thus the FEV_1/FVC ratio is preserved or increased. Abnormalities of oxygenation and gas transfer are present in most patients at rest, and in virtually

TABLE 1 Clinical Features of Idiopathic Pulmonary Fibrosis

Symptoms
Dyspnea with exertion
Dry cough
Malaise, reduced energy and endurance
Lack of occupational exposure
Physical findings
Bibasilar dry end-inspiratory rales
Digital clubbing
Laboratory tests
Elevated erythrocyte sedimentation rate
Positive antinuclear antibodies
Chest roentgenogram
Small irregular shadows
Diffuse symmetrical pattern
Lower lung zone predominance
High diaphragms
Pulmonary function
Reduced vital capacity
Normal airflow rates
Small lung volumes
Reduced diffusing capacity
Hypoxemia without hypercarbia
Hypoxemia worse with exercise
Reduced lung compliance
Lung biopsy tissue
Interstitial lymphocytes and macrophages
Alveolar inflammatory cells
Alveolar exudates
Interstitial collagen deposition
Hyperplasia of fibroblasts
Hyperplasia of interstitial contractile cells
Obliteration of small blood vessels
Distortion of alveolar architecture

all patients during exercise. The single-breath diffusing capacity for carbon monoxide (D_LCO) is usually decreased to 50 percent of predicted or less. Hypoxemia with normal or slightly reduced arterial blood carbon dioxide tension is usually found. Hypercarbia is almost never present until late disease with end-stage respiratory failure. The arterial blood oxygen tension (Po_2) is often normal or nearly normal at rest, but falls dramatically with moderate treadmill or bicycle exercise. Arterial Po_2 levels of 45 to 55 torr during exercise are common in patients who may have normal or nearly normal lung volumes and resting arterial blood gases. Exercise testing is usually essential to bring out the degree of abnormality and to follow the impact of treatment.

Laboratory tests are not helpful in IPF. The erythrocyte sedimentation rate is often moderately elevated; antinuclear antibodies are frequently present in low titer. Neither of these findings seems to be of particular diagnostic or prognostic value. Obviously, laboratory tests may be useful in excluding other diseases and before administering drugs whose side effects might change test results.

ESTABLISHING THE DIAGNOSIS

It is essential to establish the diagnosis of IPF with certainty, to estimate the likelihood of response to treatment, and to document the severity of impairment before beginning therapy. The clinical picture already described makes IPF likely if features of other diseases are absent. Unfortunately, these features alone do not make the diagnosis certain, and lung tissue biopsy is required in almost all cases. We have found that as many as 20 percent of patients with suspected IPF proved to have other diseases upon open lung biopsy. Sarcoidosis, hypersensitivity pneumonitis, eosinophilic granuloma, lymphangitic carcinomatosis, environmental dust diseases, and other causes can all be mistaken for IPF without tissue proof.

I obtain an open lung biopsy on almost all patients with suspected IPF. A limited thoracotomy is performed under general anesthesia, with a small anterior submammary intercostal incision. Small portions from the margins of two lobes are obtained; the tip of the lingula is avoided since it may be scarred in normal individuals. A thoracostomy tube is left to suction drainage for about 24 hours. Most patients leave the hospital 4 to 6 days after surgery. Some centers perform outpatient lung biopsy in this manner. The safety record for open biopsy is good, with little morbidity and less than 1 percent mortality in the reported series. Patients are excluded from open biopsy if they are elderly or have serious cardiovascular disease, severe pulmonary impairment, or other major operative risk factors. Patients who are poor candidates for open lung biopsy may still undergo bronchoscopic transbronchial biopsy in an attempt to confirm the diagnosis, and particularly to exclude other diseases.

MANAGEMENT

The therapy of IPF is aimed at suppression and elimination of this chronic immune-inflammatory response. The agents that have been proved useful in the treatment of IPF are believed to work by "quieting down" the proinflammatory actions of activated macrophages and lymphocytes, by reducing neutrophil chemotaxis and adherence, and by selectively reducing the number of these cells in the lung and the circulation.

Diagnosis should be established as early as possible and treatment should be instituted in order to intervene before tissue destruction and fibrosis become extensive. Treatment should be aimed at suppressing the immune-inflammatory response and ideally should be monitored by observing the activity of this response. Future treatments should modulate and normalize fibroblast replication and collagen production (Table 2).

TABLE 2 Current Therapy of Idiopathic Pulmonary Fibrosis

Drug therapy
- Corticosteroids
- Cyclophosphamide
- Azathioprine

Supportive treatment
- Home exercise program
- Diet counseling
- Stationary home oxygen therapy
- Portable oxygen for exertion
- Cough suppressants
- Lung transplantation
- Compassionate health professionals

Corticosteroids

Corticosteroids are the major drugs used for the treatment of IPF. Oral prednisone or methylprednisolone, taken in moderate to high doses on a daily or alternate-day basis, is the most common regimen. The glucocorticoids are believed to work in IPF by suppressing inflammation, by impairing activated lymphocyte function, and by their lympholytic effects. Although steroids have been used in almost every case series of IPF that has been reported, the dosage, schedule, and end-points for success have varied widely within most series as well as between them. A few patients achieved impressive improvement, while most had slight or no objective improvement and only partial relief of symptoms. Unfortunately, most authors do not distinguish the patients who stopped getting worse (arrested disease) from those who continued to deteriorate (progressive disease). Higher doses appear to have somewhat greater effectiveness than lower doses. The incidence of complications usually is not described, but anecdotal experience suggests that minor side-effects are usual and significant ones are not rare. As a crude estimate, 20 to 30 percent of patients with IPF achieve stabilization of disease or improvement with steroid therapy alone.

Cyclophosphamide

Cyclophosphamide (Cytoxan) has been used to treat IPF in several published trials and has demonstrated apparent effectiveness in preliminary results from an ongoing randomized study in Great Britain. Anecdotal clinical experience supports its effectiveness in some patients. Curiously, cyclophosphamide can also cause pulmonary fibrosis in patients treated for cancer with this agent. Cyclophosphamide is an alkylating agent of the nitrogen mustard group. It is well absorbed orally and activated in the liver to several cytotoxic compounds. The drug is believed to work by depleting lymphocyte numbers and by suppressing the function of those that remain. Cyclophosphamide is usually administered in daily oral maintenance dosage (to be discussed). Cyclophosphamide is usually reserved for use in patients in whom steroid therapy has proved unsuccessful. An additional 20 to 30 percent of patients may achieve stabilization or improvement with this drug. Preliminary results of cyclophosphamide used as initial primary therapy for IPF look encouraging. It must be emphasized that cyclophosphamide has not been approved by the Food and Drug Administration for use in the treatment of this particular disease.

Azathioprine

Azathioprine (Imuran) has been reported to have some effectiveness in the treatment of IPF in several small trials. Azathioprine is a purine analogue that is slowly converted to mercaptopurine in body tissues. It appears to act both by substitution for purines in DNA synthesis and, perhaps more importantly, as an inhibitor of adenine deaminase. Lymphocytes are particularly susceptible to adenine deaminase deficiency, resulting in impairment of both cellular and humoral immunity. This action might explain the particular sensitivity of T-lymphocytes to azathioprine and its utility as an immunosuppressive drug. It is usually given daily by mouth. Azathioprine, like cyclophosphamide, has been used mainly for patients who have already failed to respond to steroid therapy. Several small studies suggest that an additional 20 to 30 percent of patients respond to this agent. These may be the same patients who respond to cyclophosphamide, and there is no direct evidence that patients who fail to respond to one cytotoxic drug will respond to another. Azathiaprine was no more effective than steroids in the preliminary results of one recent randomized study. It has not been approved by the Food and Drug Administration for use in the treatment of IPF.

D-Penicillamine

Because of its effectiveness in the treatment of several of the rheumatologic diseases, D-penicillamine has been considered for use in IPF. Although the trials have been small and generally not randomized or controlled, the results are not encouraging. The use of D-penicillamine for treatment of IPF is not warranted until further evidence supports its effectiveness.

The drug treatment programs available for IPF do not work in all patients, and most only achieve a partial response at best. Although most clinicians use steroids as the first line of treatment, in many cases the patient's condition does not improve but continues to worsen during therapy. Since the disease progresses to disability and death, attempts to achieve remission through the use of drugs that are not yet fully approved seems justified and appropriate. Cyclophosphamide and azathioprine are used for this reason. Available therapies may effect improvement or stabilization in 50 to 60 percent of patients. Large-scale multicenter treatment trials with proper randomization are needed; multiple-drug schedules as well as single-drug treatments should be considered. The models developed for the conduct of multicenter treatment programs in oncology should be applicable to the treatment of IPF. The treatment schedules that follow are clearly not an ideal drug therapy program for IPF, but they are believed to be the best available therapy at present.

Selection of Patients for Therapy

The course of IPF is highly variable among patients. Whether to treat at all, and if so what program to use, must be individualized for each patient. Factors that predict advancement of the disease are listed in Table 3; these factors also seem to predict a more likely response to therapy. Patients who exhibit these features deserve aggressive therapy. Acceptance of a higher rate of side effects and complications seems justified by the greater likelihood of a favorable result.

Some patients appear to have disease that is not likely to respond to therapy (see Table 3). These patients deserve a more conservative approach. Treatment is probably still indicated, since our ability to precisely anticipate response and outcome is limited. Treatment should be closely monitored, secondary drugs may not be justified, and therapy should probably be reduced or discontinued if significant or uncomfortable side effects develop. We do not wish to make the cure worse than the disease.

Patients with severe complicating diseases may not be candidates for aggressive therapy. Mild IPF that appears to be progressing slowly may not warrant treatment if the patient is aged or infirm.

Occasional patients may not require therapy at the time of presentation. These individuals usually have few or no symptoms and normal or nearly normal pulmonary function. Most importantly, they fail to show evidence of disease progression over time. These patients may be young, in contrast to the middle-aged predominance for IPF. Typically, these patients are referred for evaluation because of an abnormal chest roentgenogram that demonstrates a diffuse pattern of small irregular shadows in low profusion. When they are available, old films often show that the same pattern has been present for years. Lung biopsy shows minimal fibrosis, with no cellularity or inflammation. Perhaps these individuals carry an inactive scar that is the evidence of some previous infection, inhaled insult, or self-limited inflammatory process.

Drug Treatment Program

Patients who present with suspected IPF undergo a defined initial evaluation and follow a specific treatment algorithm. This treatment plan, which is shown schematically in Figure 1, is similar to that used for a multicenter study of bronchoalveolar lavage, which is currently in progress. The initial evaluation is designed to establish the diagnosis, to assess the prognosis and likelihood of

TABLE 3 Prognostic Factors in Idiopathic Pulmonary Fibrosis

Favorable predictors
Cellular lung biopsy
Immune complexes in lung and serum
Lymphocytes in bronchoalveolar lavage (?)
Early disease
Mild lung function abnormalities
Younger age at presentation
Female sex
Unfavorable predictors
Fibrotic biopsy without inflammation
Neutrophils and eosinophils in lavage (?)
Late disease
Honeycomb pattern on chest roentgenogram
Severe function impairment
Older age at presentation
Male sex

response to therapy, and to provide baselines against which future progress can be measured. It must be emphasized that this treatment program is empiric and somewhat arbitrary in dose and schedule. These choices need to be validated by proper randomized and controlled trials.

Patients are interviewed for a careful medical and occupational history, with emphasis on precise description of their current level of dyspnea, any complicating medical conditions, and any occupational or environmental exposures that might provide an explanation for their respiratory disease. Current body weight and blood pressure are recorded. Physical examination documents current findings and focuses on detecting complicating illnesses. The eyes are carefully examined for cataracts and glaucoma. Excellent quality 72-inch posteroanterior and lateral chest films, made with a small focal spot and high kilovoltage technique, are essential for proper definition of small irregular shadows. Laboratory tests include a complete blood count, a sedimentation rate, an antinuclear antibody determination, measurement of electrolytes, renal function tests, fasting glucose test, and a urinalysis. These measurements are important primarily to establish normality before possible drug toxicities appear. Pulmonary function testing must be meticulous, including measurement of lung volumes, flow rates, single breath diffusing capacity for carbon monoxide, and measurement of arterial blood gases and oxygen consumption at rest and during exercise. As already discussed, an open surgical lung biopsy is obtained in almost all patients.

Patients who have progressive disease, as evidenced by a cellular biopsy and other features shown in Table 3, should receive full therapy. They are treated with high daily doses of corticosteroids for 3 months. The high initial dose is prescribed so that failure of the patient to respond can be attributed to lack of sensitivity to the drug, rather than too low a dose of the drug. Patients are allowed 2 or 3 weeks to recover from their biopsy surgery before treatment is begun. Treatment is started with prednisone, 1.5 mg per kilogram body weight, taken as a single oral dose each morning. Total dose is not to exceed 100 mg per day, even if body weight exceeds 70 kg. Methylprednisolone would be used in equipotent doses (1.2 mg per kilogram) for patients in whom sodium retention, preexisting congestive heart failure, or hypertension is a problem.

The many side effects of steroid therapy must be discussed with each patient before treatment is started. I warn all patients beginning this high-dose steroid program that they can expect a change in their body habitus and self-image; cushingoid changes are universal. They have to fight hard against increased appetite and weight gain. Their face becomes rounded, often red and flushed. Body hair may become coarser. They bruise easily as their skin becomes more delicate, and acne may develop. Many patients feel emotionally labile or irritable. I assure them that all of these changes are fully reversible and are related to the dose of the drug. These side effects will disappear as dosage is reduced or stopped. Somewhat more serious side effects are common as well: mild glucose intolerance, mild hypertension, obesity, frequent urinary tract infections, vaginitis, or bronchitis are often seen. The risk of peptic ulcer disease and gastrointestinal bleeding may be increased, but this remains controversial. Loss of bone density, osteoporosis of the spine, and vertebral compression fractures are a particular problem in older women. Some physicians recommend supplemental calcium and vitamin D for women who are receiving steroid therapy.

The most serious side effects of steroid treatment are fortunately rare. Although host defenses against infection are theoretically (and measurably) impaired, serious infections are uncommon and opportunistic pathogens are almost never involved in IPF patients. The clinician must remain alert for early signs of infection, since symptoms are suppressed by the anti-inflammatory drug effects. Myopathy may occur. Posterior subcapsular cataracts develop rarely, and then only in patients who have been treated for a long time.

Patients receiving high-dose steroid therapy must be cautioned not to stop treatment abruptly under any circumstances. The risk of adrenal insufficiency is real, particularly under stress. Steroids must be tapered gradually once dosage is below the level of estimated normal endogenous production. These patients require supplemental steroids at times of physical stress, surgery, or trauma for as long as one year after this treatment course. It may be helpful for patients to enroll in the Medicalert program, and carry a warning bracelet or other identification that states that they are receiving steroid therapy.

The patient returns for brief follow-up 7 to 14 days after steroid therapy has been started. The purpose of this visit is solely to monitor drug side effects; no impact on IPF is expected. Blood pressure, urine glucose, and possibly blood glucose and potassium are checked. Most patients have many questions, and this visit is a good time for teaching and reassurance.

Prednisone dosage is reduced to 1.0 mg per kilogram per day after 6 weeks of therapy. Limited re-evaluation is carried out at this time, including measurement of vital capacity and of arterial blood gases at rest, and a chest roentgenogram. Some early treatment response or deterioration may be seen. These interval tests help to indicate the extent of day-to-day variability in these measurements. Evidence of adverse steroid side effects should be sought at each visit; the patient is checked for diabetes, hypertension, excessive potassium loss, infections, and other common complications.

A detailed re-evaluation is performed after 3 months of steroid therapy to determine whether treatment is succeeding. A symptom history is obtained in an attempt to quantitate the level of dyspnea as precisely as possible. Complete lung function testing is performed, including studies of gas exchange at rest and during exercise. Chest roentgenograms and laboratory blood tests are repeated.

The next step in therapy depends on whether the patient's condition can be classified as better, worse, or unchanged. For some patients, the changes over 3 months are so obvious that classification is easy, but for many it may be difficult. Each test variable should be assessed independently and as objectively as possible. Vague symptoms related to energy, endurance, and general well-being

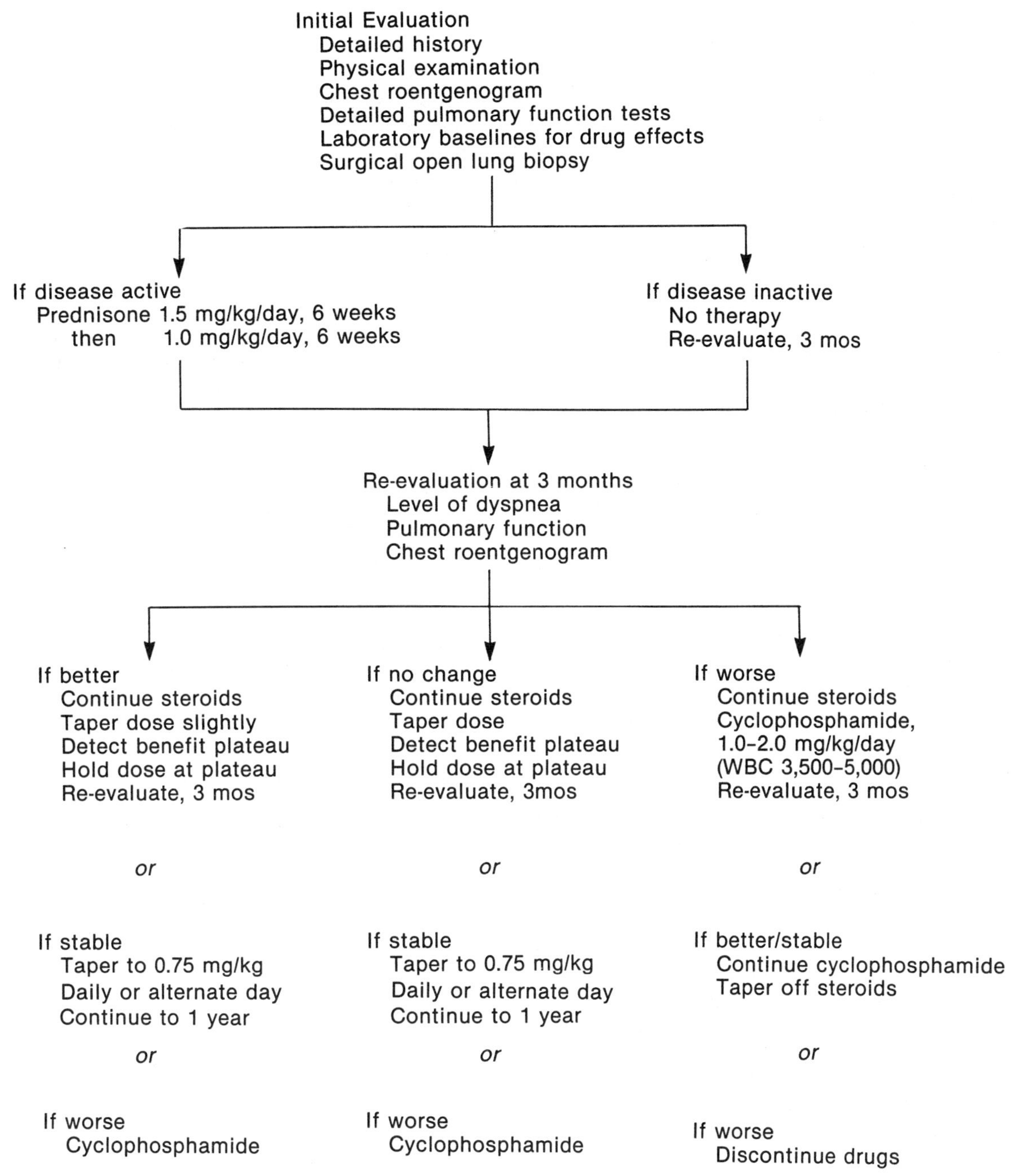

Figure 1 Drug treatment algorithm for idiopathic pulmonary fibrosis

are important as regards the quality of life of the patient; however, they are nearly impossible to quantitate and are susceptible to placebo effects and the euphoria of steroids. Semi-quantitative assessment of dyspnea is useful, as measured by the ability to perform routine activities that are repeated frequently. Roentgenographic changes are important, but these are often minimal or evolve more slowly than other variables. Pulmonary function tests should receive the most weight; changes for better or worse that are greater than 5 to 10 percent are probably significant. I have found that exercise arterial blood oxygen tensions are often the most sensitive reflection of improvement or deterioration, and may change significantly when lung volumes do not. The clinician should attempt to develop a composite assessment based on a synthesis of all of these factors.

Patients whose condition is improved on steroid therapy should continue on this treatment with re-evaluations at frequent intervals until a plateau is reached. The dose may be reduced slightly, and gradual transition toward alternate-day treatment should keep side effects to a minimum. Doses in the range of 0.75 to 1.0 mg per kilogram every other day might be reached in another 2 or 3 months, and then maintained until repeat evaluations no longer show interval improvement. Evaluation, as just described, should be repeated every 2 or 3 months. When maximal beneficial effect is achieved, steroids may be tapered further and re-evaluations stretched to 4- or 6-month intervals. Maintenance prednisone dosage at 20 to 30 mg every other day may be reached about 6 to 8 months after treatment is begun and should be continued empirically for a total course of about one year. Patients should be re-evaluated frequently as therapy is withdrawn so that recrudescence can be detected. In many cases, after a year of treatment, drug therapy can be tapered without a reappearance of active disease.

Patients whose condition deteriorates despite high-dose steroid therapy are candidates for cytotoxic drug treatment. The decision to use agents whose side effects can be serious or life-threatening and whose effectiveness is not yet fully proved must be based on firm evidence that the patient is experiencing a progressive downhill course expected to result in respiratory insufficiency and death. Both a secure tissue-proven diagnosis and clear objective evidence of active disease are required. Cyclophosphamide appears somewhat more effective than azathioprine in the limited studies available to date. Initially the cytotoxic drug is added to a moderate dose of steroids.

I begin with cyclophosphamide in a dose of about 1.5 mg per kilogram body weight per day, and increase to 2.0 mg per kilogram per day if tolerated and needed. Doses greater than 150 mg per day are rarely required. The target for proper dosage is a total peripheral white blood cell count (WBC) between 3,500 and 5,000 per cubic millimeter. The dose should be increased up to 2.0 mg per kilogram per day until this slight-to-moderate WBC depression is achieved. Dosage should be reduced if the WBC dips below 3,500. Patients should be cautioned to drink liquids aggressively and to void frequently in order to minimize the concentration and residence time of the drug in the bladder, and thus reduce the risk of hemorrhagic cystitis. Some patients experience nausea and anorexia. Most patients experience hair thinning, and women may wish to purchase a wig before alopecia becomes apparent. Once again, patients should be assured that this bothersome cosmetic change can be reversed in almost every case when treatment is completed. The WBC and a urinalysis should be monitored every several weeks as treatment is begun and dosage is adjusted. The frequency of these tests can be decreased somewhat once a stable dosage is obtained, but frequent re-evaluation is still necessary. With these moderate doses of cyclophosphamide, and with close observation for toxicity, severe side effects are uncommon. Dosage often has to be reduced as treatment progresses in order to avoid excessive WBC depression.

Clinical progress and detailed pulmonary function testing should be reassessed after 3 months of combined prednisone-cyclophosphamide treatment. The techniques and criteria already described are used to determine whether patients are better, worse, or unchanged. Patients who show definite improvement on cyclophosphamide, and probably those whose condition worsened during steroid therapy but stabilized with cyclophosphamide treatment, should continue on this drug for one year of therapy. The concomitant steroid treatment can be discontinued by tapering over the next 2 or 3 months, and cyclophosphamide continued as a single drug for the last 6 months. It can be stopped without tapering when treatment is completed or if intolerable side effects appear. If pulmonary function continues to deteriorate despite the combination of cyclophosphamide and prednisone, the former drug should be stopped and the latter drug tapered off as quickly as possible. No alternative drug treatments have been shown to be effective for these unfortunate patients.

Azathioprine is an alternative cytoxic drug that could be used in place of cyclophosphamide. Preliminary results suggest it may be less effective than cyclophosphamide, but its side effects are probably more manageable as well. Hair loss is not a problem; WBC depression is less pronounced. A dose of 1 to 3 mg per kilogram body weight as a single dose each day is standard. This drug may be useful for patients who are unable to tolerate cyclophosphamide, but are shown to be good candidates for aggressive therapy. If patients fail to respond to full doses of prednisone and cyclophosphamide, I would not expect azathioprine to be useful.

The cytotoxic agents, cyclophosphamide and azathioprine, theoretically increase the risk of neoplasia in patients who receive them. Data supporting this risk come from relatively young patients whose malignant disease developed a number of years after drug treatment. This risk may be of less concern in the older age group of patients with IPF. These drugs are also teratogenic, but most IPF patients are beyond the childbearing years. The cytotoxic agents are generally much better tolerated than are high-dose steroids, and patients seem much less aware of their day-to-day side effects.

The patient whose symptoms, pulmonary function, and chest roentgenogram remain unchanged during treatment presents a difficult problem. On the one hand, such a patient may have had inactive and nonprogressive disease all along. Drug therapy would have no effect in that case, and the side effects would be incurred with no benefit to counterbalance them. Alternatively, an active and progressive inflammatory process may have been arrested successfully, and a downhill course may have been stopped. The residual, but now stable, pulmonary dysfunction may represent irreversible lung scarring. This frequent therapeutic dilemma emphasizes the need for careful documentation of the degree of disease activity before treatment is begun. If definite activity and progressive disease have been documented previously, treatment should be considered a success and should be continued. We may not have been able to make this patient better, but we have stopped him from getting worse. I would manage this patient in the same way as a patient who shows clear improvement.

Supportive Care

Patients with IPF require considerable supportive care in addition to specific drug therapy. Of greatest importance is their need and their family's need for supportive and compassionate physicians and other health care providers. These patients have a serious and often progressively disabling disease, which may impair their quality of life and constrain their activities as it progresses. The drugs used to treat this disease produce unsightly and sometimes uncomfortable side effects. These patients need encouragment and understanding, advice regarding ways to accomplish their activities of daily living, and clear explanations about their illness. Hospice care or home nursing is recommended to help family members if dyspnea becomes severe and patients are bedridden.

Exercise programs for IPF patients can help to maintain muscle strength and ambulation. Daily walks are excellent. A stationary bicycle used with supplemental oxygen can help most patients to get daily exercise. Diet counseling should help patients to avoid excessive weight gain while on steroids and to maximize nutrition when dyspnea makes eating difficult.

Oxygen therapy is needed by many IPF patients, particularly with exertion. Exercise tolerance in IPF is often limited by hypoxia as well as by the high work of breathing; the hypoxia can be effectively relieved by portable supplemental oxygen. A number of my IPF patients have been able to resume shopping, light housework, socializing, and full-time sedentary jobs after portable oxygen therapy was begun. Portable oxygen for use while walking or otherwise exercising is probably helpful if the Po_2 during exercise measures less than 55 torr, or the saturation measures less than 88 to 90 percent. I believe that both the need for portable oxygen and the efficacy of supplemental oxygen during exercise should be documented by testing with a treadmill or bicycle. A transcutaneous ear or digital oximeter is particularly useful for this type of testing. Oxygen dosage can be adjusted during moderate steady-state exercise until a saturation greater than 90 percent is achieved. Oxygen during exercise usually provides a higher saturation, greater exercise endurance, greater comfort, a lower pulse rate, and a shorter recovery time after exercise stops. Many patients with severe IPF require high oxygen flow rates by nasal cannulae to reach these goals. Oxygen therapy should be continued for 5 to 10 minutes after exertion.

Small portable aluminum or stainless steel oxygen tanks weigh about 6 pounds, carry enough oxygen for about one hour of use, and can be refilled by patients from a large reservoir cylinder at home. Liquid oxygen systems also provide convenient portable units; they can be refilled by patients from reservoirs at home, and each provides several hours of oxygen. They may be more suitable for patients who require very high flow rates. The liquid units weighs 8 to 11 pounds, and thus are somewhat more difficult for frail or elderly patients to carry while walking.

With more advanced disease, supplemental oxygen may also be required to relieve hypoxia at rest. Arterial blood gases that show a Po_2 less than 55 torr (or less than 60 torr with evidence of heart failure) at rest indicate likely benefit from continuous home oxygen therapy at flow rates adequate to raise the Po_2 to about 65 to 70 torr or the saturation to about 92 to 94 percent. Oxygen concentrators, which operate on home electric power and concentrate oxygen from room air, are useful for patients who require continuous oxygen therapy. They are reliable, relatively quiet, unobtrusive, and cost-effective. They can be transported from room to room as activities change during the normal day. Liquid oxygen systems for continuous stationary use may be a good choice for IPF patients who are active and also require oxygen with exercise.

Cough is a troublesome manifestation of IPF, interrupting sleep and meals, and often making conversation difficult and embarrassing. Codeine cough suppressants work for a few days at a time, but tolerance soon appears. They are best reserved for occasional use at night and for patients with terminal disease and intractable cough.

Ventilatory support usually is not appropriate for IPF patients who slide gradually into progressive respiratory failure. These patients typically have run a course of several years of progressive disease and already have been treated aggressively with the drugs that are available. Unfortunately, there is little hope of reversing the disease in these patients, and they are dependent on a ventilator for the remainder of their lives. Conversely, ventilatory support usually is indicated for the patient with IPF who experiences acute respiratory failure due to a potentially reversible intercurrent illness. Support is also indicated for the patient with rapidly progressive probable IPF who has not yet received definitive diagnosis or therapy. The mortality rate is high, but some of these patients can achieve a remarkable reversal of their disease.

Lung transplantation remains an experimental procedure, but it holds great promise for some patients with IPF. Only a few centers throughout the world have undertaken lung transplantation, but IPF patients have enjoyed some of the most successful outcomes in several of these programs. Patients should be considered for referral who are relatively young, who do not have any other complicating medical illnesses, and who have severe progressive IPF that has been resistant to other forms of therapy.

This work was supported in part by grant HL-14212 (SCOR) from the National Heart, Lung and Blood Institute and by grant RR-109 from the General Clinical Research Centers Program of the National Institutes of Health.

SUGGESTED READING

Crystal RG, Bitterman PB, Rennard SI, Hance AJ, Keogh BA. Interstitial lung diseases of unknown cause: disorders characterized by chronic inflammation of the lower respiratory tract. N Engl J Med 1984; 310:154–166 and 235–244.

Dreisin RB, Schwarz MI, Theofilopoulos AN, Stanford RE. Circulating immune complexes in the idiopathic interstitial pneumonias. N Engl J Med 1978; 298:353–357.

Turner-Warwick M, Burrows B, Johnson A. Cryptogenic fibrosing alveolitis: clinical features and their influence on survival. Thorax 1980; 35:171–180.

Turner-Warwick M, Burrows B, Johnson A. Cryptogenic fibrosing alveolitis: corticosteroid treatment and its effect on survival. Thorax 1980; 35:593–599.

Winterbauer RH et al. Diffuse interstitial pneumonitis: clinicopathological correlations in 20 patients treated with prednisone/azathioprine. Am J Med 1978; 65:661–672.

COLLAGEN VASCULAR LUNG DISORDERS

JOHN I. KENNEDY, M.D.
JACK D. FULMER, M.D.

The collagen vascular disorders are a diverse collection of diseases that are grouped together because of common clinical and pathologic features. All are systemic diseases and may involve multiple organs including the musculoskeletal, cardiovascular, respiratory, and digestive systems. The major pathology of these diseases is inflammation of blood vessels and connective tissue.

Thoracic involvement by specific connective tissue diseases is varied and ranges from chest wall diseases to parenchymal disease. Although the thoracic pathology of some of these diseases is unique (i.e., the rheumatoid nodule), most exhibit a nonspecific acute or chronic inflammatory pattern, and the diagnosis of each can be made only by the clinical features in concert with serologic studies.

In the discussion to follow, an overview of the thoracic complications of each of the collagen vascular diseases and specific treatment regimens will be presented. Finally, an overview of the general principles of management of the thoracic complications of these diseases will be presented.

RHEUMATOID ARTHRITIS

Rheumatoid arthritis (RA) is a chronic inflammatory disease of unknown etiology that mainly affects synovial joints, but has a variety of extra-articular manifestations. Six types of thoracic diseases have been associated with RA and include (1) pleural disease, (2) necrobiotic nodules, (3) diffuse interstitial fibrosis, (4) Caplan's syndrome, (5) pulmonary arteritis, and (6) chronic airways disease. In general, the thoracic manifestations of RA follow the development of classic or definite RA. In many cases, however, the thoracic manifestations precede the development of clinical joint disease.

Pleural Disease

Pleural disease, with or without effusions, is the most common thoracic manifestation of RA. Necropsy studies indicate that half of these patients have pleural disease, but in practice, it is noted in 7 to 9 percent of men and 2.0 percent of women. Effusions may be unilateral or bilateral and are generally small and recurrent, although they may be persistent. The pleural fluid is almost always exudative with a high protein and low pH, and typically it has a low glucose (<30 mg per deciliter).

Management

Most patients with pleural disease may require no therapy. Pain can almost always be managed with nonsteroidal anti-inflammatory agents. If salicylates fail, indomethacin, 25 to 50 mg three times a day, is usually effective. Ibuprofen and sulindac, given in standard doses, do not appear to be as effective as indomethacin. Large symptomatic pleural effusions should be drained by needle aspiration. If the effusion recurs, a course of prednisone, 35 mg daily for 3 days followed by rapid taper over 10 days to 2 weeks, is generally effective. Failure to respond or rapid recurrence of the effusion should alert one to the possibility of another underlying disease such as an infection, neoplasia, or heart failure.

For the rare refractory rheumatoid effusion, tube thoracostomy and obliteration of the pleural space by a sclerosing agent is indicated. Chemical sclerosis can be accomplished by instilling 500 mg tetracycline with 100 to 150 mg of lidocaine by tube thoracostomy. We recommend premedication with 0.6 to 0.8 mg of atropine. Once the sclerosing agent is instilled, the tube is clamped and the patient is turned every 20 to 30 minutes for approximately 3 hours. The chest tube is then attached to water-seal drainage and removed after 24 hours, if the drainage stops.

Necrobiotic Nodules

Usually appearing as multiple well-circumscribed lesions, necrobiotic nodules range from a few millimeters to several centimeters in diameter. Necrobiotic nodules are usually pleura-based, but can be deep in lung parenchyma. Generally, necrobiotic nodules are asymptomatic, but they can pose a diagnostic dilemma in a middle-aged smoker in whom carcinoma must be excluded. Excisional biopsy may be required in these patients.

Management

Once a diagnosis of necrobiotic nodules is established, treatment is rarely required; they generally wax and wane with the activity of the underlying RA. Excision may be required if they cavitate, become infected, or rupture into the pleural space to form a bronchopleural fistula. Large nodules that compromise ventilation or obstruct airways generally respond to moderate-dose prednisone (35 mg daily) for 1 to 2 months, followed by a rapid taper over 3 to 4 weeks.

Diffuse Interstitial Lung Disease

Often termed "rheumatoid lung," diffuse interstitial disease is a well-described feature of RA. Clinically, diffuse interstitial disease associated with RA is similar to idiopathic pulmonary fibrosis (IPF), but it may not be as aggressive. The decision to treat patients with interstitial disease can be made on the basis of objective evidence of progression. Physiologic and radiologic data are preferable. We generally recommend open lung biopsy to exclude more treatable causes of interstitial disease, or to exclude more aggressive types of interstitial disease (e.g., pulmonary vasculitis), and to accurately stage the disease. Bronchoalveolar lavage and gallium lung scans have been recommended for initial staging and follow-up, but their effectiveness has not been proved and they remain research procedures.

Management

Once the decision is made to treat the patient, the initial treatment of choice is prednisone, 1 mg per kilogram ideal body weight per day, or up to 80 mg daily. Treatment is continued for 6 to 8 weeks at that dosage; then the dose of prednisone is slowly tapered (5 to 10 mg per wk) to a maintenance dose of 15 to 20 mg daily. Repeat physiologic testing is performed at 6-month intervals, and if the patient's data indicate continued progression of the disease, high-dose corticosteroids are reinstituted along with cyclophosphamide, 1.0 to 1.5 mg per kilogram ideal weight per day. The dosage of cyclophosphamide is adjusted to maintain the white cell count at about 3,000 cells per cubic millimeter. Corticosteroid dosage is tapered, as already described, and then maintained at 15 to 20 mg daily. Azathioprine, 2.0 to 2.5 mg per kilogram ideal body weight per day, is a useful alternate drug. Treatment is generally maintained until pulmonary function has been stable for a year, and then both drugs are slowly tapered.

Caplan's Syndrome

Pneumoconiosis associated with RA and pulmonary nodules is termed Caplan's syndrome. Initially described in soft coal workers in South Wales, this syndrome has been observed in silicosis and in other pneumoconioses. Multiple peripheral well-defined nodules that range from 0.5 to 5 cm in diameter are most typical. The nodules develop rapidly and are often associated with subcutaneous nodules. Their appearance often signals excerbation of the RA.

Management

Treatment generally is not indicated, although compromise of ventilatory function or cavitation and rupture of the nodules may necessitate surgical excision.

Pulmonary Arteritis

A rare complication of RA, pulmonary arteritis can occur with or without pulmonary hypertension. In general, pulmonary arteritis occurs as part of a disseminated vasculitis in RA. Several clinical presentations of rheumatoid vasculitis have been described. The clinical and laboratory manifestations of pulmonary arteritis can be identical to those of idiopathic pulmonary hypertension. In these patients, arteritis should be considered because of the underlying connective tissue disease. In rare cases, acute pulmonary arteritis can result in localized infiltrates that mimic pneumonia or pulmonary infarction. Lung biopsy is necessary to confirm the diagnosis, however.

Management

In patients with necrotizing vasculitis, we recommend a combination of corticosteroids and cyclophosphamide in dosages as already described.

Airway Disease

Patients with RA can have chronic obstructive disease of small airways. Pathologic studies have described both bronchiolitis and peribronchiolar fibrosis with narrowing of small airways. Some studies have shown bronchiolitis obliterans with intraluminal polyps of granulation tissue in respiratory bronchioles. In some patients, presumably those with bronchiolitis, airflow may improve with corticosteroid therapy when the drug is prescribed as for rheumatoid lung.

Management

We generally treat these patients with standard dosages of a long-acting oral theophylline preparation, but rarely can document physiologic improvement. However, improved mucociliary clearance with therapeutic theophylline could be an added benefit.

There also appears to be a small subgroup of patients with RA who develop progressive small airway obliteration in the absence of chronic bronchitis or emphysema. The etiology of the bronchiolitis obliterans in this disease is unclear, but may be part of the autoimmune process affecting pulmonary interstitium. However, limited pathologic studies have not shown parenchymal lung disease or mucous gland hypertrophy. Treatment with bronchodilators and corticosteroids is recommended, but often is not effective. We add cyclophosphamide in dosages as described for progressive disease. A severe obstructive defect with ventilatory insufficiency may result.

Drug-Induced Lung Disease

Patients with RA are treated with a wide variety of drugs, many of which have been associated with lung disease. Gold salt therapy has been associated with acute pneumonitis characterized by dyspnea, fever, and malaise. Rechallenge with parenteral gold salts can precipitate life-threatening respiratory insufficiency. High-dose, short-term corticosteroids generally reverse the acute disease. Uncommonly, gold salts can cause progressive interstitial disease. Lung biopsy in most patients with gold-salt-induced chronic interstitial disease is of little value, and a trial without gold and corticosteroids is indicated. We generally use a dose similar to that prescribed for rheumatoid lung. Chest roentgenograms and pulmonary function studies should be used to monitor the response to treatment. If the patient is to improve on corticosteroids and without the gold salts, a 6-week trial generally suffices.

Pulmonary infiltrates, with or without eosinophilia, have resulted from treatment with several nonsteroidal anti-inflammatory drugs (e.g., naproxen, sulindac) and with penicillamine. Corticosteroids may be useful if discontinuance of the agent fails to improve the roentgenograms or pulmonary function. There is at least one report of association between penicillamine and bronchiolitis obliterans in RA; however, the relationship has not been established.

SYSTEMIC LUPUS ERYTHEMATOSUS

Systemic lupus erythematosus (SLE) is a chronic inflammatory disease of unknown etiology that mainly affects skin, joints, and kidneys, although thoracic disease is relatively common. Six thoracic manifestations of SLE are described: (1) pleural disease, (2) atelectasis, (3) acute pneumonitis, (4) pulmonary hemorrhage, (5) diffuse interstitial disease, and (6) respiratory muscle dysfunction.

Pleural Disease

Pleural disease is the most frequent thoracic abnormality associated with SLE. Generally the pleuritis is symptomatic and coincides with a clinical exacerbation of the disease. Effusions are usually small and bilateral and rarely need therapeutic drainage or sclerosis. Diagnostic tap is indicated because of the high incidence of infection in these patients. Persistent effusions and pain should be managed like those associated with RA.

Atelectasis

Usually basilar and peripheral, atelectasis is a common roentgenographic finding in SLE. Respiratory muscle dysfunction probably contributes to recurrent atelectasis, although multiple etiologies such as pneumonitis and impaired perfusion of parenchyma also exist. The treatment consists of managing the infections or the respiratory muscle dysfunction (to be discussed).

Acute Lupus Pneumonitis

Generally presenting with high fever, tachypnea, hypoxemia, and diffuse or patchy infiltrates on the chest roentgenogram, acute lupus pneumonitis is a well-described entity. Careful evaluation to exclude an infectious etiology must be undertaken in these patients.

Management

Until an infectious agent is excluded, we frequently treat with a first-generation cephalosporin in concert with erythromycin and an aminoglycoside. High-dose corticosteroids (methylprednisolone succinate, 80 mg every 6 hours) are given simultaneously. Patients typically improve in 48 to 72 hours, but for the rare patient who does not, we add cyclophosphamide, 1.5 to 2.0 mg per kilogram ideal body weight per day. Alternatively, azathioprine, 2.5 to 3.0 mg per kilogram ideal body weight per day, may be used. For the rare patient with aggressive lupus pneumonitis that progresses to an ARDS-like picture, we recommend 3 days of intravenous high-dose cyclophosphamide (5 mg per kilogram ideal body weight per day) followed by oral (enteric) cyclophosphamide at previously stated dosages.

Pulmonary Hemorrhage

Pulmonary hemorrhage with glomerulonephritis is a recognized manifestation of lung involvement in SLE. Patients generally present with dyspnea, cough, hemoptysis, and bilateral lower lobe alveolar infiltrates. However, hemoptysis may be absent even with massive intra-alveolar hemorrhage. In patients with nephritis, renal biopsy with immunofluorescent and ultrastructural studies is the initial procedure of choice to exclude Goodpasture's syndrome. Once the diagnosis of SLE pulmonary hemorrhage is made, the objectives are to control the alveolar hemorrhage and prevent irreversible damage to the kidneys.

Management

We use high-dose pulse corticosteroid therapy in dosages of 1 to 2 g per day of methylprednisolone succinate for 3 days, followed by a maintenance dose of prednisone at 1 to 2 mg per kilogram ideal body weight per day. Plasmapheresis is recommended for Goodpasture's syndrome, but generally is not used in other forms of alveolar hemorrhage. High-dose pulse methylprednisolone appears to be effective in pulmonary hemorrhage associated with SLE, but cyclophosphamide may be used to treat the refractory patient.

Diffuse Interstitial Lung Disease

Interstitial lung disease in SLE is much less common than diffuse interstitial disease in RA; most patients with diffuse disease have had SLE for years. Clinically, these patients mimic those with rheumatoid lung or IPF. Whether therapy can alter the natural history of this disease is unclear. However, we manage patients with progressive disease just as we do patients who have rheumatoid lung.

Respiratory Muscle Dysfunction

A recently recognized complication of SLE, respiratory muscle dysfunction may present as lower lobe atelectasis, a restrictive ventilatory defect without parenchymal disease, or as hypoxic-hypercarbic respiratory failure. Either diaphragmatic dysfunction alone or in combination with chest wall dysfunction, may occur. Efforts should be made to document an active myositis with biochemical, electromyographic, or histologic studies.

Management

Myositis can be responsive to large or medium dosages of corticosteroids (prednisone at a dosage of 0.5 to 1.0 mg per kilogram per day). Patients may initially present with dyspnea in the supine position. A permanent tracheostomy with nocturnal ventilation may suffice in these cases, but ultimately continuous home ventilatory support may be needed. In rare cases, we have seen phrenic nerve neuritis in association with small vessel vasculitis produce diaphragmatic dysfunction. Corticosteroids in dosages similar to those used in diffuse interstitial lung disease may be helpful.

ADULT STILL'S DISEASE

Patients with adult Still's disease may develop pleuritis and an effusion. In rare cases, mild interstitial disease may co-exist.

Management

Most patients can easily be managed with aspirin or nonsteroidal anti-inflammatory drugs, as described for lupus pleuritis. If there is progressive interstitial disease, its management is the same as for rheumatoid lung.

PROGRESSIVE SYSTEMIC SCLEROSIS

Physiologic or roentgenographic evidence of diffuse interstitial disease is present in most patients with progressive systemic sclerosis (PSS). Additional thoracic diseases include pulmonary vascular disease, aspiration pneumonia due to esophageal dysfunction, and chest wall restriction due to sclerosis of thoracic skin.

Management

Usually, the interstitial disease of PSS is not responsive to steroids. However, there are some reported cases of steroid-responsive disease, and a trial of prednisone at dosages used in rheumatoid lung may be indicated.

Most patients have pulmonary hypertension by catheter study; approximately one-third have clinical pulmonary hypertension with cor pulmonale. There have been reports of response of the pulmonary hypertension to vasodilator agents such as hydralazine and nifedipine. Such treatment must be viewed as experimental, but if attempted should be performed with pulmonary artery pressure and cardiac output monitoring in an ICU setting.

Aspiration pneumonitis is a potential problem in all patients with esophageal disease. We routinely recommend elevation of the head of the bed and delaying bedtime until 3 or 4 hours after the ingestion of food.

POLYMYOSITIS-DERMATOMYOSITIS

Thoracic diseases in polymyositis-dermatomyositis (PM-DM) include interstitial lung disease, aspiration pneumonia, and ventilatory failure secondary to respiratory muscle weakness. The development of interstitial disease appears to be unrelated to the severity or duration of the myopathy, and may precede the muscle disease. Clinically and roentgenographically, the interstitial disease mimics IPF.

Management

Generally, corticosteroid therapy is effective in reversing or delaying progression of the disease. When corticosteroid therapy fails, we recommend cyclophosphamide in doses similar to those prescribed for rheumatoid lung.

Pharyngeal muscle disease with aspiration pneumonia constitutes a major problem in patients with PM-DM. Aggressive treatment of the myositis is indicated; therapy with cyclophosphamide may be indicated, but alternate agents such as methotrexate do not appear to be more effective than corticosteroids alone.

In the uncommon case, respiratory muscle myositis can result in respiratory insufficiency with hypoxemia and hypercarbia. Corticosteroid therapy with prednisone, 1.0 mg per kilogram per day, is generally effective.

SJÖGREN'S SYNDROME

Sjogren's syndrome consists of a triad of keratoconjunctivitis sicca, xerostomia, and recurrent parotid gland swelling. Glandular dysfunction appears to result from infiltration with lymphocytes.

Pleuropulmonary involvement occurs in as many as 50 percent of patients and includes tracheobronchitis, chronic nonspecific pneumonitis-fibrosis, lymphocytic interstitial pneumonitis (LIP), recurrent pneumonitis, pleural effusions, pseudolymphoma, and malignant lymphoma. Only the lymphoid diseases and xerotracheobronchitis are specific for Sjogren's syndrome.

Lymphoid infiltration of tracheal and bronchial mucous glands results in drying of airways with tracheobronchitis and recurrent pulmonary infections.

Management

Management of this problem involves treatment of infections, bronchodilator therapy, artificial humidification of airways, and corticosteroids. Expectorants are not helpful, but ingestion of spicy foods is said to increase production of mucus.

Lymphoid lung disease can range from LIP to malignant lymphoma or lymphocytic infiltration of pleura with pleural effusion. Benign lesions have been known to progress to malignant tumors. Early benign lymphoid disease is generally steroid-responsive and can be managed with prednisone in the same dosage prescribed for rheumatoid lung. Untreated LIP has been known to progress to end-stage "honeycomb" lung. Nonspecific pneumonitis and fibrosis are managed the same as rheumatoid lung. Malignant lung disease should be treated according to cell type and the biologic behavior of the disease with the aid of a medical oncologist.

MIXED CONNECTIVE TISSUE DISEASE

Mixed connective tissue disease (MCTD) is a syndrome characterized by an admixture of clinical features found in SLE, PSS, and PM-DM. However, pleural effusions, interstitial disease, and pulmonary vascular disease are dominant.

Management

In general, the interstitial disease is responsive to corticosteroids when treated in the same way as the interstitial disease of RA and SLE. However, there is a small group of patients with severe, rapidly progressive interstitial disease who respond poorly to corticosteroids; for these patients, a combination of corticosteroids and cyclophosphamide or chlorambucil (8 to 10 mg per day) has been recommended.

RELAPSING POLYCHRONDITIS

Relapsing polychronditis (RP) is an uncommon disease characterized by (1) destruction of articular and nonarticular cartilage, and (2) inflammation of eyes and ears. The pulmonary manifestations of RP occur as a result of involvement of laryngeal, tracheal, or bronchial cartilage. Laryngeal or tracheal flaccidity can result in severe airflow obstruction with suffocation. Bronchial involvement can result in recurrent bronchitis and pneumonitis with bronchiectasis.

Management

Treatment consists of permanent tracheostomy, if indicated, and bronchodilators with broad-spectrum antimicrobials for bronchitis or pneumonitis. Corticosteroids improve acute episodes and reduce the frequency and severity of recurrences, but may not stop the progression of the disease. Acute episodes may require as much as 200 mg of prednisone daily, but most patients can be maintained on 15 to 20 mg per day of prednisone. Resistant disease may respond to immunosuppressive drugs. Dapsone has been used in doses of 25 to 200 mg per day and compares favorably to prednisone.

ANKYLOSING SPONDYLITIS

Ankylosing spondylitis is characterized by progressive inflammation and sclerosis with ankylosis of sacroiliac joints, spine, costovertebral joints, and occasionally hips and shoulders. Fixation of costovertebral joints can occur, but rarely causes disability. Pulmonary function testing reveals an increase in FRC and RV, with a reduction in vital capacity. One of the most common pulmonary findings is upper lobe fibrobullous disease of indeterminate etiology. These bullae are susceptible to the development of aspergillomas.

Management

There is no therapy for the fibrobullous disease. Although amphotericin and, more recently, ketoconazole have been prescribed, their efficacy in treating

TABLE 1 Complications of Corticosteroid Therapy

Side Effects	*Monitoring*	*Precautionary Measures*
Sodium retention (edema, hypertension, CHF)	Weekly weights, physical examination	2–4 g sodium restriction
Hyperglycemia	History (e.g., polydipsia), serum glucose	Weight reduction, Vanderbilt diet
Gastric ulceration	History of GI upset, stool for occult blood	Antacids in patients with history of peptic ulcer
Adrenal suppression	Blood pressure, electrolytes	Slow withdrawal of steroids
Osteoporosis	—	Shortest possible duration of therapy
Posterior subcapsular cataracts	Slit lamp examination for visual symptoms	—
Mood alteration/psychosis	—	Use lowest effective dosage
Increased appetite/weight gain	Weekly weights	Caloric restriction (Vanderbilt diet)

TABLE 2 Complications of Cytotoxic Agents

Side Effect	*Monitoring*	*Precautionary Measures*
Cyclophosphamide		
Bone marrow suppression	Weekly WBC and differential	Adjust dose to maintain WBC $\geq$3,000
Hemorrhagic cystitis	History of hematuria, monthly urinalysis	Force fluids (10–12 glasses H_2O daily)
Nausea and vomiting	—	Antiemetics (e.g., metoclopramide)
Alopecia	—	—
Gonadal suppression	—	—
Potential carcinogenesis	—	—
Azathioprine		
Bone marrow suppression	Weekly WBC and differential	Adjust dose to maintain WBC $\geq$3,000
Nausea and vomiting	—	Antiemetics
Oral ulcers	—	—

aspergillomas has not been established. In rare instances, invasive aspergillosis can result and is responsive to amphotericin. Resection or embolization may be necessary for control of massive hemoptysis.

GENERAL MANAGEMENT

Certain general principles of management apply to all the pulmonary manifestations of the collagen vascular disorders. Current concepts of the pathogenesis of the interstitial diseases are that there is some type of injury to alveoli which results in alveolitis. Unchecked, the alveolitis progresses to destruction of alveoli and fibrosis. The overall objectives of treatment are to suppress the alveolitis to prevent progression of the disease, to treat the complications of the disease (i.e., infection, hypoxemia), and to try to restore activity. Corticosteroids are the mainstay of therapy, but immunosuppressive or cytotoxic therapy is indicated in the more aggressive diseases. Therapy may not restore ventilatory function, but may prevent progression of the disease. The side effects of corticosteroids and cytotoxic agents are formidable, but can be easily controlled if drugs are given under close supervision (Tables 1 and 2).

Preventive and supportive measures are also important in the management of thoracic manifestations of the collagen vascular diseases. Airway disease and interstitial disease constitute an important host defense problem. Influenza and pneumococcal vaccines are recommended, and acute bronchitis should be treated aggressively with antimicrobials, using sputum cultures as a guide. Supplemental oxygen is appropriate in acute conditions when there is documentation of a PaO_2 below 60 mm Hg or arterial saturation below 90 percent. Long-term oxygen therapy is indicated for patients who have a PaO_2 below 55 mm Hg after being on an optimal medical regimen for at least 30 days. Long-term oxygen therapy should be considered if there is evidence of hypoxic organ dysfunction such as secondary pulmonary hypertension, cor pulmonale, secondary erythrocytosis, or central nervous system dysfunction. Patients who demonstrate PaO_2 values of 55 mm Hg or less during exercise, and in whom O_2 administration improves exercise duration, performance, or capacity should be considered for long-term O_2 therapy. Oxygen should be given at lowest dosage to alleviate hypoxemia (e.g., increase the PaO_2 to 60 to 80 mm Hg) or the hypoxic organ dysfunction.

Depending on the type of lung disease, patients are generally tapered off corticosteroids after the disease has been stable for at least one year. There are recorded cases in which exacerbations occurred during tapering of corticosteroids, and for this reason, close clinical and physiologic monitoring must be maintained. In our experience, ventilatory function lost during the tapering of corticosteroids is often not regained once a high dose is reinstituted.

Supported in part by a grant from the Veterans Administration Research Service and the American Lung Association.

SUGGESTED READING

Eisenberg H, Dubois EL, Sherwin RP, Balchum OJ. Diffuse interstitial lung disease in systemic lupus erythematosus. Ann Intern Med 1973; 79:37–45.

Hunninghake GW, Fauci AS. State of the art: Pulmonary involvement in the collagen vascular diseases. Am Rev Respir Dis 1979; 119:471–503.

Matthay RA, Schwarz MI, Petty TL, et al. Pulmonary manifestations of systemic lupus erythematosus: Review of twelve cases of acute lupus pneumonitis. Medicine 1974; 54:397–409.

Peters-Golden M, Wise RA, Schneider P, et al. Clinical and demographic predictors of loss of pulmonary function in systemic sclerosis. Medicine 1984; 63:221–231.

Schwarz MI, Matthay RA, Sahn SA, et al. Interstitial lung disease in polymyositis and dermatomyositis: Analysis of six cases and review of the literature. Medicine 1976; 55:89–104.

Sullivan WD, Hurst DJ, Harmon CE, et al. A prospective evaluation emphasizing pulmonary involvement in patients with mixed connective tissue disease. Medicine 1984; 63:92–107.

DRUG-INDUCED LUNG DISEASE

VINCENT A. TARASKA, M.D., F.R.C.P.(C), F.A.C.P., F.C.C.P.

Physicians have a growing number of drugs with which to prevent, diagnose, and treat disease. These agents can themselves cause reactions and produce serious illness and death in a variety of ways. Although it is difficult to estimate the number of drug reactions in the general population, some data are available from hospital and outpatient studies. Hospitalized adults receive an average of 10 drugs during their hospital stay, and outpatients receive an average of two drugs daily. Five to 10 percent of hospitalized medical patients have drug reactions; a lower incidence prevails among surgical and other patients. Adverse reactions may account for 3 percent of acute medical admissions. Drug reactions are considered to be of one or more of the following types: intolerance, toxicity (overdosage), indirect effects (e.g., hypercoagulation from birth control medication), drug interaction, idiosyncratic reactions, and allergic or pseudoallergic reactions. In general, toxic reactions are more common than allergic reactions, drug allergy being estimated to account for 10 to 20 percent of reactions. These data stress the magnitude and importance of drug reactions. Precise figures of the incidence of drug-induced pulmonary reactions are not available.

The large number of drugs that can cause drug-induced lung disease (DILD) precludes my discussing each of them in detail. The more commonly used drugs will be discussed to illustrate principles of treatment. The diagnosis and management of drug-induced lung disease involves a knowledge of the specific mechanism of injury as well as a recognition of the various clinical syndromes in which drug reactions may be involved (Tables 1 and 2).

The principles of management of drug reaction are seen in Table 3. The specific combination of measures chosen depends on the drug involved and the nature and severity of the reaction.

TABLE 1 Classes of Drugs Causing Drug-Induced Lung Disease

Antibiotics	Analgesics/Narcotics
Nitrofurantoin	Heroin
Sulfonamides	Morphine
Antituberculous drugs	Methadone
Aminoglycoside	Propoxyphene
Chemotherapeutics	Antiarrhythmics
Chlorambucil	Procainamide
Methotrexate	Amrinone
Cyclophosphamide	Anticonvulsants
Procarbazine	Dilantin
Bleomycin	Tegretol
Adriamycin	Antihypertensives
Nitrosourea	Beta-blocker
Anti-inflammatory/ immunosuppressives	Methyldopa
Salicylate	Antipsychotics
Indomethacin	Imipramine
Ibuprofen	Antituberculous Drugs
Fenoprofen	Isoniazid
	Miscellaneous Drugs
	Methysergide
	Dantrolene

ANTIBIOTICS

Antibiotics may affect the respiratory system by causing one or more of the following: (1) acute pulmonary infiltrates with or without eosinophilia, (2) chronic progressive pulmonary fibrosis, and (3) acute muscle paralysis (curare-like effect). A short review of a few classic examples follows.

Nitrofurantoin

Nitrofurantoin may cause either acute or chronic pulmonary infiltration. The acute syndrome presents as fever (98%), dyspnea and unproductive cough (65%), chest pain, gastrointestinal symptoms, and/or myalgia and rash (17% to 22%). Although symptoms may present as early as 1 to 2 hours after exposure, symptoms usually appear in 6 to 12 days. Physical examination, chest roentgenogram, and pulmonary function tests confirm an acute pneumonitis with a restrictive defect showing bilateral crackles, alveolar and interstitial infiltrate, reduced lung volumes, and low diffusing capacity.

TABLE 2 Clinical Syndromes of Drug-Induced Lung Disease

Clinical Syndrome	*Causes*
Asthma—bronchospasm	Aspirin, ibuprofen, fenoprofen, indomethacin, propranolol and other beta-blockers, penicillin and other drugs associated with immediate-type hypersensitivity, drug additives
Drug-induced pulmonary infiltrate with eosinophilia	Nitrofurantoin, sulfonamides, penicillin, methotrexate, procarbazine, carbamazepine, cromolyn, salicylates, isoniazid, and para-aminosalicylic acid
Acute and chronic fibrosing alveolitis	Chemotherapeutic drugs (bleomycin, busulfan), antibiotics (nitrofurantoin), gold, cromolyn sodium
Pulmonary edema (capillary leak syndrome)	Morphine Demerol Propoxyphene Aspirin
Pleural effusion	Nitrofurantoin, methysergide, drug-induced SLE
Mediastinal widening	Dilantin, steroids
Respiratory muscle paralysis	Aminoglycosides

TABLE 3 Management of Drug Reaction

Prevent further drug administration
Discontinue intravenous and oral administration
Induce emesis or gastric lavage
Administer oral charcoal
Promote drug elimination
Cathartic
Diuresis
Dialysis
Antagonize drug effect
Treat immunologic reaction
Epinephrine
Antihistamines
Steroids
General supportive measures
Oxygen
Assisted ventilation
Maintain blood pressure and cardiac output
Treat organ disfunction

Lung biopsy, which demonstrates fibrosing alveolitis, is not useful except to rule out other diseases with a more specific histologic picture. In distinguishing drug-induced pneumonitis from other causes of bilateral pulmonary infiltrates, eosinophilia is a valuable clue. Immunologic tests demonstrating lymphocyte transformation and/or macrophage migration inhibition are also valuable evidence confirming an immunologically mediated reaction.

Reoccurrence of the reaction with rechallenge establishes the diagnosis, but the clinical situation and ancillary tests usually do not require this potentially dangerous step.

Management

Treatment consists of stopping the drug. Its short half-life and rapid complete elimination results in prompt resolution of pulmonary infiltrates. Steroids should be reserved only for severe reactions associated with respiratory failure.

Nitrofurantoin may also cause progressive pulmonary fibrosis in patients on long-term nitrofurantoin therapy. This form of the disease differs from the acute form by virtue of its tempo, the absence of eosinophilia, and the possibility of incomplete resolution with residual fibrosis. Treatment recommendations, apart from stopping the drug, are largely anecdotal, and the place of steroids is uncertain.

Many other antibiotics listed in Table 1 may cause a similar acute picture of infiltrates, and these reactions are managed similarly.

AMINOGLYCOSIDES, POLYMIXINS, AND MUSCLE PARALYSIS

Severe neuromuscular paralysis can occur in patients given aminoglycosides and/or polymixin. This reaction is dose-dependent and may be seen in accidental overdose or in patients with renal disease. The simultaneous use of muscle relaxants or the presence of neuromuscular disease may combine with subtoxic doses to produce marked muscle weakness.

Management

Treatment usually includes assisted ventilation, supplemented with neostigmine, until muscle strength returns. Repeated intravenous doses of neostigmine, 0.125 mg every 5 minutes until maximum benefit is noted, or incremental doses of oral neostigmine, 7.5 mg every 2 hours, may be used to diagnose and treat this rare complication. In cases of severe renal failure, dialysis may be required to reduce toxic levels.

CHEMOTHERAPEUTIC DRUGS

These agents are used in the treatment of a variety of neoplastic and nonneoplastic diseases. Since they all may cause progressive bilateral pulmonary infiltrates (acute fibrosing alveolitis), they present a major diagnostic problem; differential diagnosis often includes infection (in the immunocompromised host), carcinomatosis, leukemia or lymphomatous pulmonary infiltration, radiation pneumonitis, and drug reaction. Although the detailed investigation of infection in the immuncompromised host is beyond the scope of this chapter, a few pertinent comments are in order.

First, the probability that certain infectious agents will cause disease varies with the nature of the immunosuppression. For example, the development of acute bacterial pneumonia would be highly likely in patients with acute leukemia who were neutropenic (WBC < 500 per cubic millimeter) and had no previous respiratory disease. The spectrum of possible etiologies would be quite different if a patient with recent bone marrow transplant developed bilateral pulmonary infiltrates.

Second, the management plan, including investigation and initial therapy, depends on the disease for which immunosuppressive therapy was given, which agents were used, and the immediate state of health of the patient. For example, the rapidity with which you would proceed to open lung biopsy would depend on the extent of pulmonary disease, the degree of respiratory failure, and the likelihood of an unusual infection that could be rapidly fatal if not identified and treated within the first few days.

The diagnosis of drug-induced lung disease is difficult in this situation since there is no reliable test that establishes the diagnosis without the need for provocative testing. Lung biopsy is nonspecific, although some authors believe that chemotherapeutic agents produce bizarre diagnostic changes in the alveolar type II cell. Double-blind studies or single-blind studies evaluating the predictive accuracy of this observation have not been published to my knowledge. Therefore, the diagnosis of DILD remains one of exclusion.

Bleomycin

This potent cytotoxic agent forms a part of many multidrug chemotherapeutic regimens and could be used as a prototype of drug-induced lung disease caused by chemotherapeutic agents. Its mechanism of cytotoxic injury includes inhibition of DNA synthesis, the generation of oxidants, and direct damage by granulocytes. The vascular endothelium shows the first sign of injury, followed rapidly by the alveolar type II cell. The neutrophil may be the effector cell in bleomycin-induced pneumonitis. Bronchoalveolar lavage reveals large numbers of neutrophils, and animals made neutropenic show decreased lung injury. However, the precise mechanism of injury is not known. Bleomycin injury is dose-related, but with a wide range of susceptibility and an increasing incidence from a cumulative dose of 50 to 400 mg.

Bleomycin produces the symptoms and signs of progressive alveolitis and fibrosis. Since this toxicity is predictable, considerable effort should be expended in its prevention. Early signs of toxicity include the appearance of basal crackles, spirometric evidence of a reduced vital capacity, and an abnormal chest roentgenogram showing bilateral basal interstitial shadows. Since none of these signs is more sensitive than any other, all three should be used as a screen for early disease.

Management

If bleomycin-induced pneumonitis occurs, it may progress for several weeks before undergoing spontaneous resolution even if the drug is discontinued. The value of steroids remains unproven for most cases, but the tendency of some patients to relapse after steroid withdrawal provides evidence for a continuing immune injury.

Other chemotherapeutic agents (see Table 1) can cause a subacute or chronic pulmonary fibrosis similar to that caused by bleomycin. In rare instances, they cause acute pulmonary infiltrates with peripheral blood eosinophilia. These acute reactions resolve quickly after the drug has been discontinued and are identical to reactions caused by antibiotics and other therapeutic agents.

ANTI-INFLAMMATORY/IMMUNOSUPPRESSIVE AGENTS

Salicylates

Salicylates may cause a number of reactions affecting the respiratory system, including acute asthma, pulmonary infiltrates and eosinophilia, and pulmonary edema. Aspirin sensitivity occurs in about 5 percent of asthmatics, often appearing in a syndrome of nasal polyps and asthma. The pronounced bronchospasm that may occur is not IgE-mediated, but reflects the ability of acetylsalicylic acid to interfere with prostaglandin synthetase. The diagnosis of aspirin-induced asthma is based on the clear temporal relationship of aspirin ingestion and acute bronchospasm. Since these reactions can be life-threatening, confirmation by challenge test is not recommended except in special circumstances.

Management

Therapy consists of the usual treatment of acute asthma with inhaled $beta_2$ agonist such as Ventolin liquid, 2.5 mg every 2 to 4 hours, intravenous aminophylline, and corticosteroids in severe unresponsive cases.

Pulmonary infiltrates with eosinophilia respond to prompt withdrawl of aspirin and only occasionally require a short course of steroids. Pulmonary edema usually appears only after toxic blood levels are attained. It is treated by alkaline diuresis, supplemental oxygen, mechanical ventilation, and occasionally dialysis. Toxic blood levels can cause a pulmonary capillary leak syndrome.

NONSTEROIDAL ANTI-INFLAMMATORY DRUGS

For the most part, these drugs, because of their ability to interfere with the cyclo-oxygenase pathway, produce severe bronchospasm in susceptible subjects (to be discussed).

Gold

When gold was first being used therapeutically, it was prescribed in large doses once per week. These large doses (> 50 mg per week) caused a high incidence of toxic reactions and responded to a reduction to the common present regimen of 25 mg per week. Occasional reactions still occur, and although skin rash is the most common, pulmonary reactions are significant.

Pulmonary toxicity, which consists of an acute or chronic fibrosing alveolitis, may be seen in patients who have received as little as 175 mg of gold or may present late in the course of treatment after as much as 1 g of gold. Symptoms, signs, chest roentgenogram, and pulmonary function tests are typical of fibrosing alveolitis and not specific for gold toxicity. Lung biopsy is not helpful except to exclude diagnosis with a more characteristic histology. Gold can be demonstrated within the lung, but occurs as a natural consequence of gold therapy and is not predictive of toxicity.

Eosinophilia does occur in approximately 40 percent of patients with gold-induced pneumonitis and is helpful in suggesting that diagnosis.

Management

Gold reactions usually respond promptly to the cessation of further gold administration. Rarely, the reaction may proceed and result in respiratory failure and death. Treatment of respiratory failure with oxygen and ventilator support and high-dose steroid therapy has been effective in most cases. One group attempted, without success, to remove gold by administering British anti-lewisite. However, the interrelationship of dose-dependent toxicity and immunologic factors suggests that this therapy deserves further evaluation.

ANALGESICS

Morphine, Heroin, and Methadone

These drugs gain rapid access to the central nervous system because of their high lipid solubility. In mild doses, they depress respiratory drive and decrease ventilatory responses to hypoxia and hypercarbia. In large doses, they produce complex effects that may result in profound respiratory depression, hypoxia, and death. In addition to these central effects, they can produce profound pulmonary edema in association with a normal pulmonary arterial wedge pressure. This capillary leak syndrome is caused by a variable loosening of endothelial junctions without structural damage. The mechanism of this reaction is not clear, but may involve histamine since histamine increases capillary permeability, and plasma histamine levels are elevated after heroin injection.

It seems that immunologic mechanisms are not important, since acute pulmonary edema can occur on first exposure to narcotic analgesics despite the occasional demonstration of low complement levels, decreased IgM, and immune complexes in pulmonary tissues.

Propoxyphene

This medication is administered orally as propoxyphene hydrochloride or propoxyphene napsylate. The hydrochloride is more rapidly absorbed (peak concentration in 1 to 2 hours) than the napsylate (peak serum concentration in 3 to 4 hours). Proxyphene undergoes metabolic conversion to an active metabolite norproxyphene with a half-life of 36 hours. The drug is associated with profound toxicity and significant mortality from ingestion of even 15 to 20 tablets. It is rapidly taken up and bound by tissues, resulting in low serum levels but important toxicity (serum level 0.8 to 1.1 mg). Overdose produces rapid respiratory depression and coma which, with oral administration, occurs within one-half to 1 hour, and with intravenous administration, may occur within minutes. As with other narcotics, there is danger in combining the medication with alcohol or other sedatives. Pulmonary edema may occur, but is not a common occurrence.

Management

Treatment of these narcotic toxic effects includes induction of emesis and administration of oral charcoal, although this is of limited value since propoxyphene is so rapidly absorbed. Naloxone antagonizes the respiratory depression of narcotics and propoxyphene and should be administered in a dose of 0.4 to 0.8· mg intravenously. The management of pulmonary edema may require assisted ventilation, PEEP, or CPAP with oxygen supplementation. Reduction of pulmonary capillary pressure reduces the transudation of fluid and assists in the clearance of pulmonary edema.

MISCELLANEOUS DRUGS

Penicillamine

Penicillamine is used primarily in the treatment of Wilson's disease because of its chelating properties and, in experimental protocols, in the treatment of rheumatoid arthritis. It has been associated with four different reactions: drug-induced systemic lupus erythematosus, diffuse fibrosing alveolitis, Goodpasture's syndrome, and bronchiolitis obliterans. If reactions occur, the drug is discontinued and complete resolution usually occurs.

Methysergide

This is the only drug known to produce chronic pleural effusion. It can also cause pulmonary fibrosis, which resolves completely after the drug is discontinued. If resolution is incomplete, a short course of steroids is in order.

DRUG-INDUCED SYTEMIC LUPUS ERYTHEMATOSUS

Some drugs, such as hydralazine, procainamide, diphenylhydantoin, isoniazid, and chlorpromazine, cause systemic lupus erythematosus (SLE) commonly; some others cause it only rarely. Pulmonary physicians must recognize both the possibility of drug-induced SLE and features that may help distinguish the reaction from SLE.

Systemic lupus erythematosus is a systemic multisystem inflammatory disease of unknown etiology. It causes arthralgia, polyarthritis, malaise, and fever with frequent involvement of the respiratory system including pleuritis, pericarditis, and diffuse pneumonitis.

Drug-induced SLE is indistinguishable from non-drug-induced SLE in the individual patient. Although drug-induced SLE has a low incidence of renal disease, central nervous system disease, myalgia, lymphadenopathy, and skin disease, when this group of patients is compared to age-matched patients with SLE, the pattern of disease is not significantly different.

Management

After the drug has been discontinued, treatment with aspirin or other nonsteroidal anti-inflammatory agents usually controls symptoms until remission is complete, but in 10 to 15 percent of cases, steroid therapy may be required. The absence of serious organ dysfunction in drug-induced SLE, such as cerebritis and nephritis, reduces the necessity for steroid administration. Occasionally continuation of the drug is essential to treatment, in which case aspirin or low-dose steroids may be required to control symptoms.

DRUG-INDUCED ASTHMA

Drugs may cause acute bronchospasm by three mechanisms: inhibition of cyclo-oxygenase, antagonism of beta agonists, and interaction with specific IgE-mediated antibody.

Cyclo-oxygenase Inhibitors

Salicylates, nonsteroidal anti-inflammatory drugs (NSAID), tartrazine, and azo dyes can cause allergic-like responses in approximately 1 percent of the population. Nonasthmatics develop rhinitis, urticaria, and angioedema, but asthmatics may also develop life-threatening asthma. Approximately 10 to 20 percent of all adult patients with asthma experience a respiratory reaction to ASA and NSAID, and these reactions occur almost exclusively in patients with rhinosinusitis and asthma. The weight of evidence suggests that these drugs cause acute symptoms because of their ability to inhibit cyclo-oxygenase. All NSAIDs that inhibit cyclo-oxygenase cross-react with ASA, and the degree of cross-reactivity parallels the degree of inhibition. NSAIDs that act by inhibiting lipo-oxygenase pathways do not cross-react with ASA. Therefore, should anti-inflammatory drugs be required, acetaminophen, propoxyphene, sodium salicylate, or benoxaprofen may be used.

Beta-Blockers

The common and widespread use of beta-blockers in the treatment of hypertension has caused increased symptoms in known asthmatics and produced symptoms in subjects with minimal bronchial reactivity. These symptoms are seldom severe and respond quickly to discontinuance of the beta-blocker.

Drug Additives

The pharmaceutical industry uses many additives in the preparation and preservation of drugs. Most have not been found to produce symptoms, but benzoates, sulfites, and azo dyes have been shown to cause severe hypersensitivity reactions. Both parabens (aliphatic esters of parahydroxy-benzoic acid) and sulfites have been shown to cause IgE-mediated reactions including urticaria, angioedema, and asthma. Of particular importance to pulmonologists is the recognition that sulfites are contained in bronchodilator solutions (e.g., Bronoksol, Isuprel, Alupent, Micronefrin, Vaponefrin), adrenalin, local anesthetics, corticosteroids, and certain antibiotics (e.g., gentamicin, amikacin, tobramycin). Since it has been estimated that 5 to 10 percent of asthmatics may be sensitive to sulfites, all medications should be carefully examined for the presence of sulfite before administration.

Management

Treatment of drug-induced asthma is similar to the treatment of severe asthma, whatever the cause, once administration of the sensitizing drug is stopped.

SUGGESTED READING

Goldstein RA. Drug allergy: prevention, diagnosis and treatment. J Allergy Clin Immunol 1984; 74(4) Part 2, Suppl.

Klassen CD. Toxicology. In: Gilman AG, Goodman LS, Gilman A, eds. The pharmacologic basis of therapeutics. 6th edition, New York: Macmillan, 1980:1602.

Melman KL, Morrelli HF. Drug reactions. In: Melman KL, Morrelli HF, eds. 2nd ed. New York: Macmillan, 1978:951.

Rosenow EC III. Drug-induced lung disease. In:Petty T, Cherniack R, eds. Seminars in Respiratory Medicine. New York: Thieme-Stratton 1980:2(2).

SARCOIDOSIS

D. GERAINT JAMES, M.A., M.D.(Cantab), F.R.C.P.(Lond), L.L.D.(Hon)

Sarcoidosis, a multisystem disorder of unknown etiology, most commonly affects young adults and presents most frequently with bilateral hilar lymphadenopathy, pulmonary infiltration, and ocular and skin lesions.

The course and prognosis of the disorder correlates with the mode of onset; an acute onset usually heralds a self-limiting course with spontaneous resolution, whereas an insidious onset may be followed by relentless progressive fibrosis.

Corticosteroids relieve symptoms, suppress granuloma formation including the Kveim-Siltzbach skin test, and normalize serum angiotensin-converting enzyme (ACE) levels.

PATHOGENESIS

T4 helper cells are mobilized to all points of activity where they cooperate with macrophages leading to B-cell overactivity (Fig. 1). Activated T4 helper cells secrete a 20,000-dalton glycoprotein, interleukin 2, which leads to a tenfold clonal proliferation of the same T4 cells to augment their presence at sites of activity (Fig. 2). This phenomenon does not include blood T-lymphocytes and hence the relative anergy away from sites of activity.

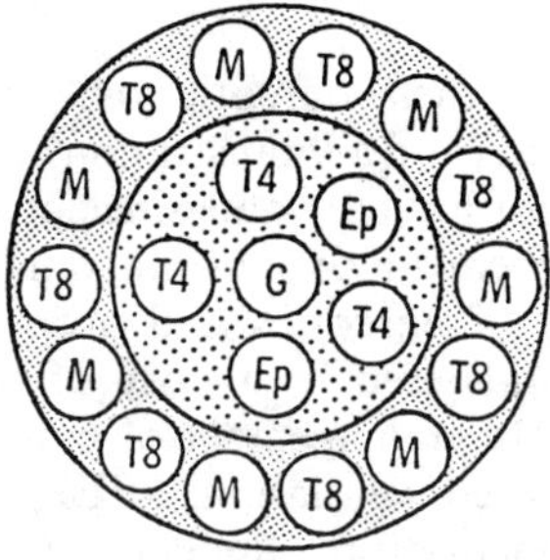

Figure 1 The sarcoid granuloma. M = Macrophage; Ep = Epithelioid; G = Giant; T4 = Helper; T8 = Suppressor.

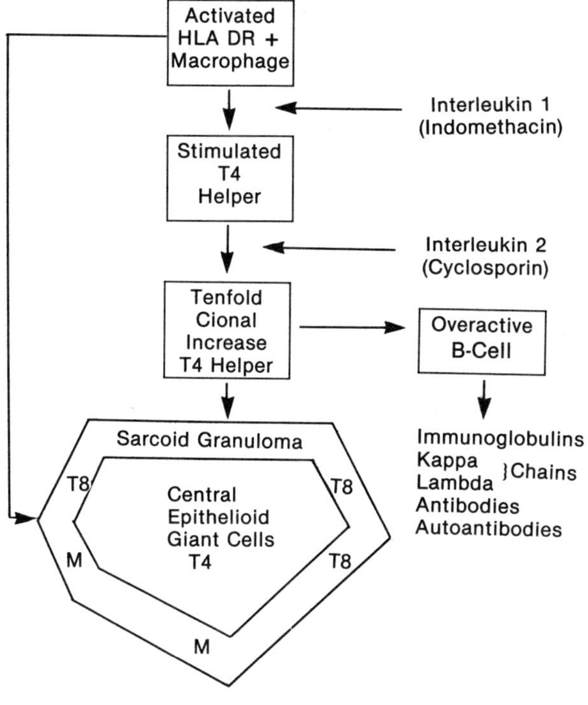

Figure 2 Influence of interleukins on granuloma formation.

DIAGNOSIS

Patients with sarcoidosis are usually in the 20- to 40-year age group and are usually seen first by the chest physician, ophthalmologist, or dermatologist. In our Royal Northern Hospital series, the chest roentgenogram was abnormal in 90 percent of patients, and ocular or skin sarcoidosis was evident in about 25 percent (Table 1). The diagnosis is established most securely when well-recognized clinical and roentgenographic findings are supported by histologic evidence of widespread epithelioid cell granulomas in more than one system. Markers of activity of the disease include a positive Kveim-Siltzbach skin test, elevated serum angiotensin-converting enzyme (ACE) levels, hypercalciuria and hypercalcemia, and intrathoracic uptake of radioactive gallium.

When sarcoidosis is suspected, the following investigative routine is recommended:

1. Full general medical examination, including ophthalmoscopy.
2. Slit-lamp examination of the eyes for otherwise silent lesions that may be overlooked.
3. Chest film.
4. Serum calcium level, which is elevated in up to 20 percent of cases. It is also preferable to do routine

TABLE 1 A Comparison of Sarcoidosis in London with the Worldwide Survey

	Royal Northern Hospital, London		*Worldwide Survey*	
Sarcoidosis	*Number*	*%*	*Number*	*%*
TOTAL	818	100	3,676	100
Female	500	61	2,082	57
Presentation under 40 years	604	74	2,504	68
White	728	89		
West Indian	81	10		
Intrathoracic	700	88	3,224	87
Erythema nodosum	251	34	640	17
Other skin lesions	147	21	324	9
Ocular lesions	224	27	539	15
Parotid enlargement	52	6	160	4
Nervous system	77	9	134	4
Bone	31	3	109	3
Lymph nodes and spleen	326	39	1,031	28
Lymphadenopathy	225	27		
Splenomegaly	101	12		
Hepatomegaly	82	10		
Heart	27	3		
Lacrimal gland	22	3		
Kidney	10	1		
Upper respiratory tract	53	6		
Systemic corticosteroid therapy	344	42	1,738	47
Skin tests				
Positive Kveim-Siltzbach	550/657	84	1,714/2,189	78
Negative tuberculin test	488/702	70	2,093/3,268	64
Hyperglobulinemia	161/526	31	808/1,832	44
Hypercalcemia	99/547	18	200/1,760	11
Mortality due to				
Sarcoidosis	25	3	84	2.2
Other causes	23	3	54	1.4

24-hour urine calcium levels, for hypercalciuria may occur despite normal serum calcium levels.
5. Histologic confirmation by fiberoptic bronchoscopy or biopsy of lymph node, skin, liver, minor salivary gland, gum or muscle, or Kveim-Siltzbach skin test.
6. Serum angiotensin-converting enzyme determination, which offers a monitor of progress of the disease.
7. Tuberculin skin test, which is negative in two-thirds of patients.
8. Special situations may include fluorescein angiography for suspected posterior uveitis, radioactive thallium for evidence of myocardial involvement, and CT scanning for neurosarcoidosis.

MANAGEMENT

Corticosteroids

Corticosteroids are the mainstay of treatment and are indicated if the following manifestations are present.

The Eyes

The inflamed iris is rested by local atropine eye drops to maintain a dilated pupil. Topical corticosteroids should always be administered for iridocyclitis in the form of eye drops applied frequently during the day, reinforced with a corticosteroid eye ointment at night. If there is no substantial and continuing improvement after one week, the concentration of corticosteroids in the anterior segment of the eye may be increased by a local subconjunctival depot of cortisone. Oral prednisolone is indicated if local treatment does not lead to a rapid response or if ophthalmoscopy reveals posterior uveitis. The latter is best visualized by fluorescein angiography, which demonstrates leakage of dye due to retinal vasculitis. This responds well to oral prednisolone, 40 mg daily. Treatment is continued for about 3 months, depending on the degree of involvement of other systems.

A raised intraocular pressure during treatment with steroid eye drops is a signal to switch to fluormethalone eye drops, which are least likely to cause a rise in pressure, and also to consider Timoptic eye drops, which return the intraocular pressure to normal.

Hilar Adenopathy

Bilateral hilar lymphadenopathy is likely to subside without treatment, and this is particularly so if there is associated erythema nodosum. It has therefore been traditional, worldwide, not to treat stage 1 hilar adenopathy. However, we now know, from lung biopsy experience, that there are active sarcoid granulomas in the lungs even when they are not evident in the chest film. Raised serum angiotensin-converting enzyme levels and radioactive gallium scans disclose their activity. The fire must surely be extinguished in these widespread granulomas, for otherwise they may lead eventually to pulmonary fibrosis. Therefore, I do treat hilar adenopathy if there is a significantly elevated serum ACE level.

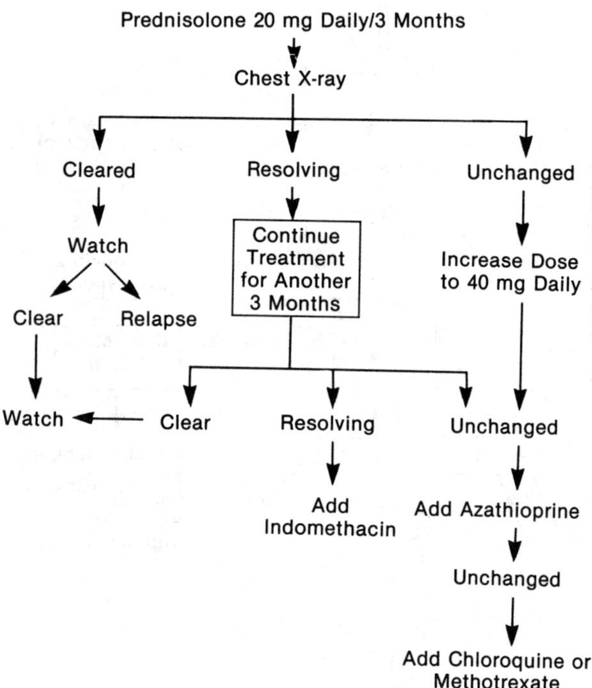

Figure 3 Treatment schedule for pulmonary sarcoidosis.

Pulmonary Infiltration

Pulmonary infiltration that remains static or worsens during the course of 3 months is an indication for oral prednisolone, again in an effort to prevent eventual irreversible pulmonary fibrosis. Several factors influence the likelihood of resolution of the chest film. The younger the patient, the more likely it is to clear. The presence of chronic skin lesions and/or bone cysts would confer an unfavorable prognosis, for these are the hallmarks of chronicity. Their presence would suggest that the pulmonary lesions are unlikely to subside. Substantial improvement in the chest film is also related to the length of time before treatment is given. Results are considerably better in those treated within 2 years of onset of the disease (Fig. 3).

Breathlessness

If this symptom is present, the patient has already reached a stage of irreversible pulmonary fibrosis or disturbed gas transfer. Oral steroids provide symptomatic relief, but do not influence the natural history of the disease or its grave prognosis at the irreversible stage of breathlessness.

The impact of steroids in our series of 700 patients in London with a chest roentgenographic abnormality is shown in Table 2. Complete radiologic resolution was eventually achieved in 363 (52%); one-third achieved radiologic resolution with steroids, and two-thirds without steroids. Although there was no evidence that steroid therapy influenced the resolution of roentgenographic changes in pulmonary sarcoidosis, it is possible that without such treatment, the number of patients

TABLE 2 Resolution of Intrathoracic Sarcoidosis in Relation to Steroid Therapy

		With Steroids			*Without Steroids*				
			Resolution			*Resolution*		*Total Resolution*	
Chest X-ray Stage	*No. of Patients*	*Total No.*	*No.*	*%*	*Total No.*	*No.*	*%*	*No.*	*%*
1	458	208	93	45	250	175	70	268	59
2	150	82	28	34	68	31	46	59	39
3	92	56	10	18	36	25	69	35	38
Total	700	346	131	38	354	231	65	362	52

Chest X-ray Stage 1 = Hilar lymphadenopathy only
2 = Hilar adenopathy + pulmonary infiltration
3 = Pulmonary infiltration without hilar adenopathy, ± fibrosis, scarring, cavitation.

with chronic persistent disease and its attendant morbidity might have been greater. Moreover, steroid therapy certainly provided symptomatic relief and overcame many manifestations of extrathoracic sarcoidosis.

Upper Respiratory Tract

Involvement of the pharynx and larynx may cause edema, hoarseness, and stridor due to laryngeal obstruction. Intravenous steroids may be a matter of urgency, relieving life-threatening stridor. If intravenous therapy is given early enough it may obviate tracheostomy.

Skin

Steroid therapy is indicated for unsightly skin lesions such as lupus pernio, involving nose, lips, eyelids, cheek, and/or ears. Steroids shrink the disfiguring lesions, but these lesions recur when treatment is discontinued. Methotrexate, in a small dose of 5 mg once weekly, is also most effective in overcoming unsightly lupus pernio. When given with steroids, it allows the dose of prednisolone to be reduced to a minimum (Table 3).

Abnormal Calcium Metabolism

Disordered calcium metabolism is due to overactivity of calcitriol. The natural form, cholecalciferol (vitamin D_3), is metabolized first in the liver to 25-hydroxycholecalciferol and then a second hydroxy group is added in the kidney to produce the potent highly active 1,25-dihydroxycholecalciferol (calcitriol).

TABLE 3 Response of Lupus Pernio to Various Drugs

Treatment	*Dose*	*Months*	*Result*
Prednisolone	Smallest possible	Shortest possible	Good
Chloroquine	250 mg alternate	9	Moderate
Methotrexate	5 mg weekly	3	Very effective
Potassium paraminobenzoate	12 g daily	12	Slight
Levamisole	150 mg daily	1	Unchanged
Antituberculous	Full	6	Unchanged

Calcitriol causes increased intestinal calcium absorption leading to hypercalcemia and hypercalciuria. This can also be induced by sunlight. It is overcome swiftly by steroid therapy.

Nervous System

The more acute the disease, the more likely it is to respond to systemic corticosteroids, which should be administered as soon as the diagnosis has been established. Resolution of neurosarcoidosis is more likely to occur in younger patients whose sarcoidosis has an explosive sudden onset. The response to treatment is better in those with accompanying erythema nodosum rather than chronic skin lesions, or with acute rather than chronic uveitis; and with hilar adenopathy rather than old diffuse pulmonary infiltration.

Glandular Involvement

Corticosteroids are used particularly if there is disordered function—e.g., dry eyes due to lacrimal gland involvement, dry mouth due to salivary gland enlargement, and hypersplenism due to sarcoidosis of the spleen. The indication for treatment is disordered function rather than anatomic enlargement of the gland in question.

The Heart

It is easy to include involvement of the heart in a theoretic list of indications for corticosteroid therapy, but much more difficult, in practice, to recognize myocardial sarcoidosis. It is suspected and treated when a patient with multisystem sarcoidosis develops cardiac arrhythmia or bundle branch block.

Treatment demands steroids for resolution of the granulomas, chloroquine as an antifibrotic agent, betablockade, nifedipine as a calcium antagonist, and amiodarone or equivalent as an antiarrhythmic agent.

Bone

Bone cysts cause pain, swelling, and deformity of the hands and feet. Steroids provide relief of symptoms, but bone cysts persist despite treatment and symptoms recur when steroids are discontinued. Methotrexate or indomethacin may be a helpful alternative treatment.

Other Drugs

Treatment with other drugs may be necessary when there are contraindications to steroid therapy.

Indomethacin

The activated macrophage produces interleukin 1, which in turn influences T4 helper lymphocytes. The macrophage-T-lymphocyte feedback axis is prostaglandin-mediated. Indomethacin is a potent inhibitor of prostaglandin synthetase, and this may be its site and mode of action (see Fig. 2). It should be considered in acute exudative sarcoidosis. It is particularly valuable in patients with acute uveitis, phlyctenular conjunctivitis, sarcoid polyarthritis, and erythema nodosum.

Chloroquine

The way in which chloroquine acts is unknown, but it controls some instances of chronic fibrotic sarcoidosis involving lungs and skin. It is particularly helpful in the management of lupus pernio and pulmonary fibrosis. In view of its ocular toxicity, it should only be given in a dose of 250 mg on alternate days for as long as 9 months.

Methotrexate

This drug is helpful in the treatment of chronic skin lesions, particularly lupus pernio. Since it is known to cause hepatic fibrosis when taken daily for prolonged periods, I restrict it to a small dose of 5 mg taken just once weekly for courses of 3 months. Patients are soon aware of its value, for it shrinks the cosmetically unacceptable lupus pernio effectively. However, when the course of treatment is discontinued, lupus pernio slowly recurs during the following 3 months. Repeated courses every 6 months, possibly in conjunction with oral steroids or chloroquine and cosmetic camouflage, constitute the best treatment regimen at present.

Potassium Para-Aminobenzoate (Potaba)

This drug is known to have an antifibrotic effect in Peyronie's disease, scleroderma, and rheumatoid arthritis. It is worth considering in pulmonary fibrosis and lupus pernio due to sarcoidosis. Three-gram capsules should be taken by mouth four times daily for several months. This form of treatment is an alternative to corticosteroids, methotrexate, and chloroquine, and giving all four in rotation helps to overcome the undesirable long-term complications of any one drug.

Azathioprine (Imuran)

I have observed clinical improvement in four, chest clearing in two, and improved respiratory function in one, out of a group of ten patients given azathioprine. These ten patients had already failed to respond to corticosteroids, oxyphenbutazone, and chloroquine, and so they can be regarded as cases of hard-core chronic fibrotic sarcoidosis which has resisted all other therapy. Azathioprine may be helpful in sharing the burden of steroid therapy when the patient is developing complications to steroids.

Sodium Cellulose Phosphate (Calcisorb, Riker Laboratories)

This drug is indicated for the treatment of absorptive hypercalciuria associated with recurrent formation of renal calculi. It is an ion-exchange compound with a particular affinity for divalent cations. It binds calcium ions in the lumen of the stomach and intestine, and the calcium-complex is excreted harmlessly in the feces. It is a white-to-beige fibrous powder. Each 5-g sachet binds 250 mg of calcium. The usual adult dose is 5 g three times daily.

Effervescent Phosphate (Sandoz)

Each effervescent phosphate tablet provides 500 mg elemental phosphorus to bind calcium. The daily adult dose is 1 to 2 g.

Radiotherapy

Before steroids were available, hilar adenopathy was treated by radiotherapy with good results. Corticosteroids swept aside this vogue, which is once again returning to favor. Henry Williams and colleagues report a patient with sarcoid meningitis associated with grand mal seizures. The patient failed to respond to corticosteroid therapy, but demonstrated improvement of symptoms, CT scan, and cerebrospinal fluid after receiving low-dose whole brain irradiation.

Still Untried

Cyclosporin A

Cyclosporin A is a fungal metabolite with interesting immunosuppressant properties. It seems to act selectively on T-lymphocytes and has virtually no effect on other white blood cells. It acts at an early stage of T-cell stimulation, interfering with interleukin 2 production (see Fig. 2) and preventing organ rejection; hence its current popularity in the field of organ transplantation. Cyclosporin A exerts profound effects on experimental epithelioid cell granulomas, produced in rats by subcutaneous injections of various opportunistic mycobacteria, and then treated with oral cyclosporin A in a daily dose of 20 mg per kilogram. In the course of one month it prevented the formation of epithelioid cell granulomas or the development of caseous necrosis. Macrophages, containing well-preserved mycobacteria, accumulated at the local site and in the regional lymph node, but there was no generalization of infection. Inhibition of T-lymphocyte activation by cyclosporin A presented harmful mycobacterial infection in this experimental model. The mycobacterial infection remained circumscribed and even showed signs of regression. Thus far it has not been evaluated in sarcoidosis.

Ineffective and Harmful Regimens

Calciferol

This substance is positively harmful for it gives rise to hypercalcemia and hypercalciuria. Multivitamin preparations containing vitamin D are best avoided during pregnancy. Likewise, ultraviolet light should not be administered to patients with active sarcoidosis.

Antituberculous Chemotherapy

This is of no benefit in sarcoidosis. The only possible indication is that the physician is undecided whether the patient has sarcoidosis or tuberculosis.

Invalidism

Patients with sarcoidosis should not become invalids in sanatoriums. They should be encouraged to return to work and to lead normal lives. Women can be encouraged to become pregnant.

Levamisole

This anthelmintic has been extensively investigated for its immunotherapeutic potential in restoring impaired cellular immunity in cancer and autoimmune disorders. A short-term trial of 150 mg daily for 4 weeks in 22 patients with chronic sarcoidosis had no effect on the clinical course or on the skin reactivity of patients with active chronic sarcoidosis.

SUGGESTED READING

Fleming HA. Sarcoid heart disease. Sarcoidosis 1985; 2:20–24.
James DG, Jones Williams W. Sarcoidosis and other granulomatous disorders. Philadelphia: WB Saunders, 1985.
Johns C, ed. Transactions of Tenth World Congress on Sarcoidosis. Ann NY Acad Sci 1986 (In press)
Scadding JG, Mitchell DN. Sarcoidosis. London: Chapman and Hall, 1985.

PULMONARY ALVEOLAR PROTEINOSIS

RICHARD J. MARTIN, M.D.

Pulmonary alveolar proteinosis (PAS) is a disease of uncertain origin in which the alveoli are filled with proteinaceous material and the interstitium remains intact. Symptoms are a nonproductive cough (unless the patient is also a smoker), progressive dyspnea, a "heavy" sensation in the chest, and weight loss. Physical examination of the lungs usually reveals fine inspiratory rales, but lung sounds may be normal even with extensive disease involvement. The other common physical finding is clubbing of the nail beds. The chest roentgenogram can reveal many different patterns from alveolar to a combined alveolar and interstitial pattern. The clinical picture is nondiagnostic. The differential diagnosis includes pulmonary fibrosis, pneumonconiosis, carcinoma, sarcoidosis, pulmonary edema, immunologic processes, and pulmonary infections with fungi, viruses, and *Pneumocystis carinii*. The infectious processes and pulmonary edema can usually be differentiated on clinical grounds, but for the other, more chronic diseases, some form of tissue analysis has been required.

Since the pathologic process involves filling of the alveolar spaces, the basic physiologic abnormality is shunting. Thus, with a simple, noninvasive shunt measurement in the appropriate clinical setting, one could determine whether the physiologic event causing the hypoxemia is a shunt. Putting this together with another simple laboratory test, the lactic acid dehydrogenase (LDH) level, helps to guide the physician toward the diagnosis of pulmonary alveolar proteinosis. The reason for the elevation of LDH in pulmonary alveolar proteinosis is unknown.

For any diffuse lung disease, an open-lung biopsy would certainly give the diagnosis; however, there is a significant amount of morbidity and a slight mortality rate (that of general anesthesia) associated with it. The transbronchial biopsy has less morbidity and mortality associated with it. However, for pulmonary alveolar proteinosis, the diagnosis can easily be missed by this technique because, although it is a diffuse lung disease on chest roentgenogram, the histologic picture is more that of a patchy diffuse process, and thus, with the 2-mm transbronchial biopsy forceps, the appropriate tissue may not be obtained. But with the fiberoptic bronchoscope, bronchoalveolar lavage using 20 to 50 ml of saline can provide the diagnosis. The effluent is a milky appearing substance which, when spun down and processed, shows the PAS-positive material as it is seen on open lung biopsy.

Complications of pulmonary alveolar proteinosis are related to the hypoxemia at rest or with exercise and associated infectious diseases. The hypoxemia over time leads to pulmonary hypertension and cor pulmonale. In the rare patient who is unresponsive to therapy, biventricular failure develops. Since the basic underlying physiologic problem is a shunt, supplemental oxygen does not correct the problem of hypoxemia. This statement, in general terms, is true, but depends on the percent of the shunt. Furthermore, some patients may have significant disease on chest roentgenogram, but their oxygen tension improves on supplemental oxygen, probably because the proteinacious material filling the alveolar sacs is so arranged as to act more as a diminished ventilation-to-perfusion abnormality than as a zero ventilation-to-perfusion process, i.e., a shunt.

The infectious diseases associated with pulmonary alveolar proteinosis are gram-negative pneumonia, Nocardia infection, and fungal infections. The gram-negative pneumonias are generally associated with the inappropriate use of corticosteroids in the treatment process. Steroids are not of benefit in this disease. *Nocardia* and fungal infections are primarily located in the lung, but brain abscesses have been reported. The apropriate therapeutic intervention for *Nocardia* is sulfadiazine, 4 to 6 g per day. The optimal duration of therapy is uncertain. It is usually continued for many months after apparent cure because of the pronounced tendency for relapse or the appearance of metastatic abscesses. At times, surgical drainage of abscesses and empyemas is needed. The treatment of individual fungal infections is discusssed in their respective chapters in this book.

MANAGEMENT

At present, the most reliable and successful means of treating these patients is total lung lavage. A double-lumen endotracheal tube is used to ventilate one side while the other is being totally "washed out." Many other types of therapy, including inhalation of trypsin, acetylcysteine, bronchodilators, and the use of intermittent positive pressure breathing machines have all had occasional positive reports in the literature. These treatment modalities are not used at the present time. There have also been reports of successful treatment of alveolar proteinosis with multiple segmental lavages via the fiberoptic bronchoscope. This is probably an inferior means of totally "washing out" the patient's lung. Several such patients referred to me were initially treated with mutiple segmental lavages without success.

The initial decision must be the timing of the total lung lavage (Fig. 1). This depends both on the patient's subjective limitations in his daily activities and objective laboratory data. If the patient is limited by this disorder so as to interfere with work and social activities, this plays a major role in the decision process. Uncommonly, symptoms exceed the objective data, but the patient still responds to lung lavage. The laboratory tests that are most useful in helping to determine whether therapeutic intervention is indicated are the resting arterial oxygen tension, the oxygen saturation (or tension) during exercise, and the diffusing capacity. Resting hypoexemia, to various degrees, exists at presentation. Virtually all the patients that need lavage have further oxygen desaturation with exercise. The reduction of the diffusing capacity reflects to a degree the amount of alveolar filling that is present.

Mild Disease

If the patient is only mildly limited by the disease process and has minimal physiologic abnormalities, the choice is to clinically follow the patient or try segmental lavages via the fiberoptic bronchoscope. There are reports of spontaneous remissions with pulmonary alveolar proteinosis; thus immediate intervention at this stage is not mandatory. The segmental lavages may improve the clinical status enough at this stage to give symptomatic improvement.

Moderate-to-Severe Disease

For moderate-to-severe symptoms and abnormal test results, total lung lavage is the treatment of choice. This is performed under general anesthesia through a double-lumen endotracheal tube. In this manner, one lung can be lavaged with warm saline while the other lung is being ventilated; 15 to 50 liters of saline may be used per lung. The use of chest percussion and vibration

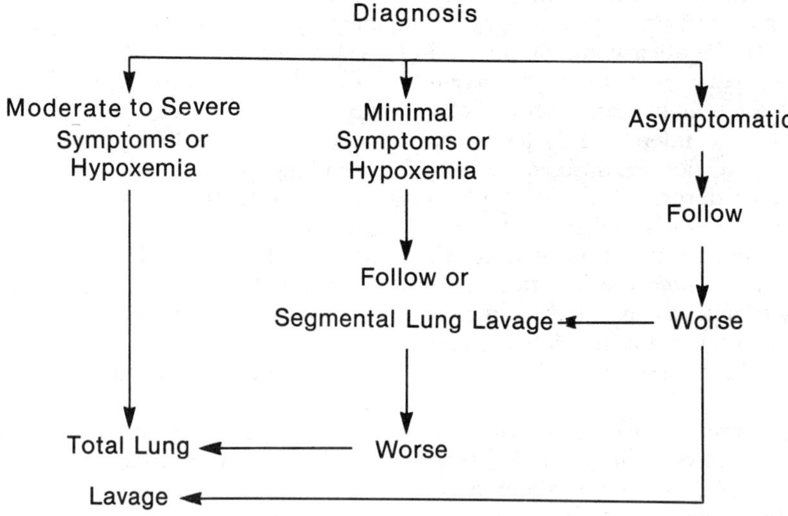

Figure 1 Algorithm for management of pulmonary alveolar proteinosis

(manual is more efficacious than mechanical) increases the proteinaceous material in the effluent. An interval of 3 to 6 days is usually allowed before lavage of the other lung is performed.

COMPLICATIONS

Most complications of this procedure result from poor placement of the endotracheal tube. Time and effort need to be given to the appropriate placement of the tube even if it necessitates extubation and reintubation with a different double-lumen catheter. Isolation of both lungs is mandatory to prevent leakage. Proper positioning of the tube is also important to allow free inward and outward flow of the saline. Since breath sounds can be transmitted with this system, auscultation alone to determine whether the lungs are isolated can be misleading. Ventilating one side and having the proximal part of the other catheter under water can determine whether all leaks are sealed, i.e., no bubbling of the water is seen after 5 to 10 breaths.

Another complication of this procedure is wide fluctuations in temperature. Hypothermia or hyperthermia can occur if the lavage fluid is under- or overheated. The PaO_2 and $PaCO_2$ need to be checked throughout the procedure as these variables can change greatly.

In following 25 patients over a 12-year period, the response to total lung lavage has been varied. Some patients need only one lavage and appear to remain in remission. Other patients need repeated lavages at 4- to 5-year intervals, while a few patients need lavages every 8 months to 1 year. The reason for the varied response is not known. However, with segmental lavage via the fiberoptic bronchoscope for diagnostic purposes, the patients in remission can also be detected. Their histologic appearance is different from the true active pulmonary alveolar proteinosis case. Thus, if a patient's pulmonary function studies or oxygen level have a slow, downward trend, the question is whether this is due to pulmonary alveolar proteinosis or some other factor. By performing a segmental lavage, determination of reactivation of the pulmonary alveolar proteinosis can be made and appropriate treatment reinstituted.

SUGGESTED READING

Martin RJ, Coalson JJ, Rogers RM, Horton FO, Manows LE. Pulmonary alveolar proteinosis: the diagnosis by segmental lavage. Am Rev Respir Dis 1980; 121:819–825.

Martin RJ, Rogers RM, Myers NM. Pulmonary alveolar proteinosis: shunt fraction and lactic acid dehydrogenase concentration as aids to diagnosis. Am Rev Respir Dis 1978; 117:1059–1062.

Rogers RM, Levin DC, Gray BA, Mosely LW. Physiologic effects of bronchopulmonary lavage in alveolar proteinosis. Am Rev Respir Dis 1978; 118:255–264.

Rogers RM, Tantum KR. Bronchopulmonary lavage: a "new approach" to old problems. Med Clin North Am 1970; 54:754–771.

WEGENER'S GRANULOMATOSIS

NANCY BATES ALLEN, M.D.
HERBERT A. SALTZMAN, M.D.

Wegener's granulomatosis is a distinct clinicopathologic entity characterized by upper and lower airway involvement, glomerulonephritis, arthritis, palpable purpura, ocular inflammation, neurologic involvement, and constitutional symptoms. The hallmark pathologic finding is that of necrotizing granulomatous inflammation involving small arteries and veins. Typically, a definite diagnosis is based on the multisystem nature of the disease and specific pathologic findings on an open lung biopsy. Occasionally, biopsy of other tissue sites yields a specific diagnosis.

The disease was originally described in the 1930s and remains rare, but reports are increasing in the literature. The largest series reported to date is that of Fauci et al from the National Institutes of Health in 1983, a study involving 85 patients over 21 years. Age at onset ranges from 8 to 80 years, with a mean of 40 to 45 years. The male-to-female ratio in reported series is approximately 3 to 2, and the disease appears to affect Caucasians predominantly.

The etiology of Wegener's granulomatosis remains unclear, with hypersensitivity to an unknown agent or inhaled antigen strongly suspected. Important in the pathogenesis are such immunologic factors as immune complex disease in the kidney, elevated IgE or IgA levels in the serum of some patients, granuloma formation, and possible defects in cellular immunity.

The clinical features of Wegener's granulomatosis are shown in Table 1. Upper airway symptoms are the most frequent, occurring in 90 to 95 percent of cases. Pulmonary symptoms include cough, dyspnea, hemoptysis, and, less commonly, pleuritic chest pain and symptoms of tracheal obstruction. Chest roentgenograms show pulmonary infiltrates that are often fleeting, cavitary lesions, and occasionally pleural effusions. Obstructive airway disease is noted on pulmonary function testing in more than half the patients. Subglottic stenosis and endobronchial lesions have been described in some patients.

The concept of "limited" Wegener's granulomatosis, meaning pulmonary involvement without renal involvement, has been debated in the literature. Many of the patients believed to be free of renal involvement

TABLE 1 Clinical Manifestations of Wegener's Granulomatosis

Organ System	*Clinical Manifestations*	*% Patients*
Lungs	Cough, dyspnea, hemoptysis; pulmonary infiltrates, nodules, cavities	90
Upper Airways	Sore throat, epistaxis, hearing loss, sinusitis, serous otitis media, "saddle nose deformity"	90–95
Kidney	Active urinary sediment (proteinuria, red cell casts), biopsy with focal and segmental glomerulonephritis	85
Musculoskeletal	Polyarthralgias, arthritis, myalgias	80
Ocular	Conjunctivitis, episcleritis, scleritis, orbital mass lesions	60
Skin	Palpable purpura, cutaneous nodules, leukocytoclastic vasculitis	45
Neurologic	Mononeuritis multiplex, cranial nerve palsies, diabetes insipidus	20–30
Cardiac	Pericarditis, carditis	10
Constitutional symptoms	Fever, weight loss, malaise, fatigue	70

because of normal renal function and normal urinary sediment findings have actually had abnormalities on renal biopsy, making this concept more tenuous.

Laboratory abnormalities include a normochromic, normocytic anemia, leukocytosis, elevated Westergren erythrocyte sedimentation rate, thrombocytosis, hypergammaglobulinemia, and positive rheumatoid factor (50% of cases). Antinuclear antibodies, serum cryoglobulins, and anti-DNA antibodies are usually absent. Circulating immune complexes by a variety of methods have been found during active disease in up to 50 percent of cases.

MANAGEMENT

In early reports of Wegener's granulomatosis, the disease was uniformly fatal within 2 years. Corticosteroids alone lengthened survival by a few months, but did not otherwise beneficially affect patients with this disease, except perhaps those patients with truly "limited" disease. The current preferred approach to therapy of all patients with a confirmed diagnosis includes a combination of corticosteroids and cyclophosphamide, with greatly improved survival. Complete remissions occur in approximately 90 percent of patients treated with this combination of drugs, and relatively few victims relapse after therapy is discontinued.

Prior to initiation of therapy, the diagnosis should be established on the basis of clinical organ system involvement and appropriate tissue biopsies. Infectious, malignant, and other inflammatory conditions should be ruled out. Although therapy is effective for Wegener's granulomatosis, toxic responses do occur and should not be taken lightly. Each patient should be approached individually and educated regarding the disease, the proposed therapy, and the benefits and risks of therapy.

Preferred Therapeutic Approach

Corticosteroids, cyclophosphamide, azathioprine, methotrexate, chlorambucil, and nitrogen mustard have all been used in the treatment of patients with Wegener's granulomatosis.

Cyclophosphamide

Cyclophosphamide is currently the drug of choice because of its proven ability to induce remission, its acceptable side effect rate, and the collective experience gained in its use for treating this disease. Corticosteroids are generally administered in combination with the cyclophosphamide initially.

Cyclophosphamide is administered orally in doses of 2 mg per kilogram per day in nonfulminant cases, and in doses of 3 to 4 mg per kilogram per day intravenously or orally in fulminant cases. After 3 to 4 days, this higher dose is reduced to 2 mg per kilogram per day. The medication is taken in the morning with a liquid intake of at least 2 liters per day to prevent hemorrhagic cystitis. Careful monitoring of blood counts must be done on patients treated with cyclophosphamide. The maximal leukopenic effect is seen approximately 7 to 10 days after the initiation of the drug or after a change in dosage. Thus, the adage "this week's lab reflects last week's dose" applies. Initially, white blood cell counts should be obtained every other day until stable, then twice weekly, then weekly. The white blood cell count should be kept above 3,000 to 3,500 per cubic millimeter, with the polymorphonuclear leukocyte count above 1,000 to 1,500 per cubic millimeter, in order to prevent infectious complications from therapy. One important point to remember is that a patient receiving tapering doses of corticosteroids often shows a gradual reduction of the white blood cell count while receiving a stable cyclophosphamide dose. This phenomenon probably reflects a mild bone marrow protective effect of corticosteroids against the toxic effects of cyclophosphamide. Often, a patient begins with a cyclophosphamide dose of 100 to 150 mg per day while receiving corticosteroids and, 6 to 12 months into therapy, require only 50 to 75 mg per day of cyclophosphamide while off corticosteroids.

Cyclophosphamide should be continued for at least 12 months following clinical remission, as noted by resolution of symptoms ascribed to Wegener's granulomatosis and by return of the erythrocyte sedimentation rate to normal. If cyclophosphamide is discontinued prior to this time, recurrence is more likely. In our experience, late recurrences may be seen even when optimal therapy has been given. After cyclophosphamide is discontinued, the patient should be observed carefully with frequent history, physical examination, chest roentgenograms, urinalysis, erythrocyte sedimentation rate, and complete blood counts. We see our patients every 3 months for the first year off therapy, every 6 months for the second and third years, and then annually.

We generally discontinue cyclophosphamide without a final tapering schedule, often because our patients are on only 50 mg per day as maintenance dosage. However, an alternative approach is to gradually taper the dosage by 25-mg decrements every 4 to 8 weeks until the drug is discontinued. With this method, milder disease flares may be controlled by increasing that dosage of cyclphosphamide by 25 mg per day.

Corticosteroids

Corticosteroids are initiated at the time of diagnosis in one of several ways. In nonfulminant cases, prednisone 1 mg per kilogram per day, is administered in two to four divided daily doses for one week, and then consolidated to a single, morning dose of approximately 60 mg per day. This provides maximal anti-inflammatory and milder immunosuppressive effects until the cyclophosphamide has a chance to become effective. In fulminant cases, methylprednisolone, 1 to 2 mg per kilogram per day, is administered intravenously in four divided doses until the patient is stable and then converted to oral prednisone in equivalent doses. The regimen of prednisone 60 mg per day is continued until the end of the first month of therapy, followed by a tapering schedule leading to alternate-day therapy over the next month. By the beginning of the third month of treatment, the patient should be receiving 60 mg prednisone on alternate days and continue this dose for the next 1 to 2 months. Then, the dose is further tapered so that the patient will be off corticosteroids at the end of the first 6 months of therapy. Some patients require longer treatment periods of corticosteroids, but this regimen usually suffices. Occasionally, alternate-day prednisone is not sufficient to control symptoms, but this is the exception rather than the rule. If daily prednisone must be used, the lowest dose possible should be given. Patients receiving corticosteroids should be monitored closely for the development of hypertension and diabetes. Therefore, they should be educated about the symptoms of these conditions and participate in the monitoring process. Older patients in particular should be checked frequently while on the higher doses of prednisone.

Upper Respiratory Tract Involvement

Patients with Wegener's granulomatosis often develop intercurrent sinus and upper airway infections and should be treated with appropriate antibiotics. The most common organism cultured from the upper airways is *Staphylococcus aureus*. Nasal saline douches two to four times daily and topical steroid spray preparations are often advised in patients with ongoing upper airway symptoms. Caldwell-Luc or other drainage procedures are often necessary in patients with severe sinus involvement. Myringotomy tubes are of some benefit to patients with chronic serous otitis media. Correction of saddle nose deformities and other functional abnormalities in the nose may be performed after the disease is in remission.

Renal Involvement

If chronic renal failure develops in patients with Wegener's granulomatosis, appropriate dietary and medical care are given. The disease appears to remit in some patients receiving hemodialysis, so that the immunosuppressive therapy can then be tapered and discontinued. Successful renal transplants have been performed in these patients, and we prefer to use cyclophosphamide rather than azathioprine as their immunosuppressive agent. Disease recurrence in the transplanted kidney has been reported.

Other Immunosuppressive Agents

Other immunosuppressive agents may be used once the disease is in remission and if a side effect of therapy occurs. For example, if hemorrhagic cystitis develops in a patient receiving cyclophophamide, azathioprine may be substituted. A purine analogue rather than an alkylating agent, this drug often sustains a remission with fewer potential side effects. The dose of azathioprine initially is 2 mg per kilogram per day, and the white blood cell count must be monitored weekly until stable, then every 2 to 4 weeks. Chlorambucil, another alkylating agent, is rarely used in this condition. Studies using methotrexate in Wegener's granulomatosis are not available.

TOXIC SIDE EFFECTS AND COMPLICATIONS OF THERAPY

The potential side effects of corticosteroids are numerous and include diabetes, hypertension, adrenal suppression, salt retention, cataracts, osteoporosis and compression fractures, cushingoid effects, increased susceptibility to infection, aseptic necrosis of bone, decreased wound healing, peptic ulceration, and central nervous system effects. Daily corticosteroids are much more hazardous than alternate-day administration, particularly with respect to the occurrence of infections and adrenal suppression via the hypothalamic-pituitary axis.

Cyclophosphamide is an aklylating agent and a potent immunosuppressive agent. The side effects include bone marrow suppression, alopecia, hemorrhagic cystitis, mucosal ulcerations, nausea and vomiting, gonadal dysfunction, and oncogenesis. Careful laboratory monitoring should be done as noted in the previous section. If nausea and vomiting remain a problem, prochlorperazine, 5 to 10 mg can be administered orally 30 to 60 minutes before the morning dose of cyclophosphamide. Adequate hydration and administration of cyclophosphamide in the morning are important for the prevention of hemorrhagic cystitis. The oncogenic potential is real, but appears to be small: leukemia and lymphoma have been reported in a few cases of Wegener's granulomatosis treated with cyclophosphamide. Gonadal dysfunction and sterility are major problems in younger patients with Wegener's granulomatosis treated with cyclophosphamide. Consideration should be given to sperm-banking for young men who are starting treatment with this drug. Women with childbearing potential should be treated with oral contraceptives for two reasons: (1) pregnancy is contraindicated because of risk of birth defects, and (2) suppression of normal cyclic ovarian function may actually protect against infertility following completion of therapy. The efficacy of this latter statement is not yet fully known.

A special complication of cyclophosphamide therapy, which may produce significant morbidity or even mortality, is massive pulmonary hemorrhage into a resolving cavity. We have observed the occurrence of this event within 1 to 4 weeks following open lung biopsy and initiation of therapy. Presumably, a large vessel becomes eroded in the early healing process, since this event usually follows rapid roentgenographic and clinical improvement in pulmonary findings. This vascular erosion leads to hemopneumothorax and, if not treated promptly, may progress rapidly to cause hypoxemia, acute respiratory distress syndrome, and death.

SUGGESTED READING

Carrington CB, Liebow AA. Limited forms of angiitis and granulomatosis of Wegener's type. Am J Med 1966; 41:497.

Fauci AS, Haynes BF, Katz P, Wolff SM. Wegener's granulomatosis: prospective clinical and therapeutic experience with 85 patients for 21 years. Ann Intern Med 1983; 98:76.

Godman GC, Churg J. Wegener's granulomatosis. Pathology and review of the literature. Arch Pathol 1954; 58:533.

Wegener F. Uber generalisierte, septische Gefasserkrankungen. Verh Dtsch Ges Pathol 1936; 29:202.

SPONTANEOUS PNEUMOTHORAX

ROBERT M. TATE, M.D.

Pneumothoraces can be categorized as spontaneous or traumatic. Spontaneous pneumothoraces obviously occur without any recognizable antecedent trauma, direct or indirect, to the chest. It is useful to further subdivide spontaneous pneumothoraces into primary versus secondary spontaneous pneumothorax. The primary form occurs in otherwise healthy individuals. Secondary spontaneous pneumothorax occurs as a consequence of a variety of underlying lung diseases (Table 1).

Primary spontaneous pneumothorax is more common in males. The approximate incidence is 8 per 100,000 per year for males and 1 per 100,000 per year for females. The usual etiology is the rupture of subpleural blebs that are frequently located in the lung apices. The origin of these blebs is unclear, but they are most likely the result of congenital abnormalities of the lung or of inflammation or degeneration of lung tissue. An additional pathophysiologic mechanism is suggested by the observation that primary spontaneous pneumothorax seems to occur more frequently in tall, thin individuals. The increased height of the lung in these people results in a larger range of alveolar-pleural pressure gradients in the thorax, with higher distending pressures at the lung apex. (Alveolar pressure is similar from lung apex to base, whereas pleural pressure is more negative at the apices.) Long-term exposure to these higher distending forces could lead to apical subpleural bleb formation. In a minority of cases at surgery, no pulmonary bleb formation can be demonstrated. In these cases, the cause is shown to be tears of the visceral pleura at the site of pleural adhesions or near an area of subpleural fibrosis.

TABLE 1 Underlying Lung Disorders in Secondary Spontaneous Pneumothorax

Emphysema
Chronic bronchitis
Tuberculosis
Interstitial pneumonitis
Eosinophilic granuloma
Sarcoidosis
Cystic fibrosis
Pneumonia
Lung abscess
Asthma
Bronchogenic carcinoma
Metastatic neoplasms
Pulmonary infarction
Pneumoconioses

Secondary spontaneous pneumothorax occurs with a variety of lung disorders, most commonly chronic obstructive pulmonary disease. However, virtually all lung disorders have been complicated by spontaneous pneumothorax. A classic example of a disease that predisposes to pneumothorax is eosinophilic granuloma. Other common associated disorders are listed in Table 1.

DIAGNOSIS

The clinical presentation of a pneumothorax is usually straightforward, and the condition is easily diagnosed. Chest pain, often pleuritic in nature, and dyspnea are nearly always present. Characteristically in secondary spontaneous pneumothorax, the shortness of breath is often out of proportion to the degree of pneumothorax owing to the already limited pulmonary reserve. Nonproductive cough is occasionally present. The onset of symptoms is usually sudden, but may be insidious or transient in as many as one-third of patients.

Diagnosis is confirmed by visualizing the visceral pleural line on chest roentgenogram. Occasionally, it is difficult to be certain about a small pneumothorax. In these circumstances, a chest roentgenogram taken during full expiration may be helpful. During maximal expiration, the volume of the lung is reduced. The pneumothorax now occupies a proportionately greater volume of the hemithorax and becomes more obvious. The increased density of the lung during expiration may also accentuate the pneumothorax. Another technique is to obtain a lateral decubitus view in which the air in the pleural space may be seen more clearly against the lateral chest wall. Approximately 20 percent of these patients have a small pleural effusion.

MANAGEMENT

Therapeutic alternatives in the management of spontaneous pneumothorax include observation, needle aspiration, and tube thoracostomy. The initial choice between procedures depends on the size of the pneumothorax, the severity of symptoms, the status of the underlying lung, and whether the pneumothorax is progressing. Each of the treatment options will be considered separately here.

Observation

In a minority of cases, the patient is simply observed. Clinical characteristics leading to this decision include a small pneumothorax (< 15%), which is not progressing in a patient who is minimally symptomatic and reliable. Appropriate inpatient or outpatient facilities and personnel must be available to observe the patient. Although symptoms usually subside in a few days, complete resolution of the pneumothorax requires 3 to 4 weeks in most patients. It has been calculated that pleural air is resorbed at a rate of 1.25 percent of the hemithorax volume per day. Therefore, even a small pneumothorax (e.g., 10%) requires several days to resorb. The rate of pleural air absorption may be enhanced by inhalation of high FIO_2. A lowering of the partial pressure of nitrogen in the blood increases the gradient for reabsorption of pleural space nitrogen.

The major disadvantage of observation is the potential that the lung leak will re-open and perhaps allow a large or even tension pneumothorax to develop. However, the frequency of this complication is low.

Needle Aspiration

Another conservative approach to spontaneous pneumothorax is needle aspiration of the pleural space. This technique is appropriate only when the pneumothorax is relatively small and not progressing. The goal is not necessarily to remove all pleural gas, but rather to substantially reduce the size of the pneumothorax so that it can then be observed.

The technique is to use a small-gauge (16- to 20-gauge) needle or plastic cathether inserted into the second or third anterior interspace in the midclavicular line. The patient should be in the upright or semi-upright position. Careful use of a three-way stopcock prevents accidental introduction of additional air into the pleural space.

Needle aspiration has been reported to have a 40 percent failure rate. This high figure suggests that the technique was being tried in inappropriately large pneumothoraces or that data collection was not complete.

Complications of needle aspiration include puncturing the lung, re-opening the leak by expanding the lung, and possibly empyema. These complications should be managed by proceeding to tube thoracostomy.

Tube Thoracostomy

Certainly the majority of pneumothoraces require drainage by chest tube. Owing to the more severe symptoms and occasional mortality (15%) of secondary spontaneous pneumothoraces, essentially all of these should be treated initially with tube thoracostomy. A properly placed chest tube allows complete re-expansion of the lung, even if a lung leak persists. Tube thoracostomies may be performed in a variety of locations, depending on the preference of the surgeon and the location of the pneumothorax on the chest roentgenogram. The anterior second interspace and the high midaxillary line are two popular sites. For cosmetic reasons, I prefer the midaxillary approach. The tube should be placed fairly high in the hemithorax, where escaped air generally collects. A dependently placed tube often does not completely evacuate the air.

Tubes of a moderate size (20 to 28 F) should be used. Smaller tubes develop problems with kinking, collapse, and obstruction with secretions. With small pneumothoraces, it is usually sufficient to connect the tube to underwater seal without suction. Larger pneumothoraces are best initially managed by applying suction to the tube (-20 cm H_2O). In general, I prefer placement of the tube by surgical dissection and clamp puncture of the parietal pleura as opposed to trocar insertion. The major disadvantage of the trocar technique is that the operator may not detect adhesions at the insertion site and the trocar may puncture the lung. This becomes less an issue with large pneumothoraces.

The tube should be checked frequently for patency and communication with the pleural space. This is indicated by respiratory fluctuation of the fluid column in the chest tube. If the fluid level does not fluctuate with tidal breathing, the patient should be asked to perform a maximal inspiration. Failure of the fluid level to fluctuate indicates kinking of the tube, obstruction of the lumen by blood or fibrinous material, that the tip of the tube has been sealed off in a pleural space pocket, or that the tube has slipped out of the pleural space.

It may be more difficult to assess tube status if the tube is attached to suction, since the negative pressure in the suction-control chamber is constant and transmitted continuously to the pleural space. Pleural space pressure is constant, and little if any respiratory fluctuation is observed. The suction can be temporarily discontinued, and then fluctuation in the water-seal fluid level should be observable if the tube is patent.

If the fluid level in the chest tube fails to fluctuate, either patency should be re-established or the tube should be removed. Clots or fibrinous material can be stripped from the extrathoracic portion of the tube manually or with a special chest tube roller device. If patency cannot be re-established, the tube should be removed before it becomes colonized with bacteria and acts as a source of contamination of the pleural space. Flushing the tube with air or liquid is discouraged owing to the risk of contaminating the pleural space with bacteria-laden material.

In addition to a frequent assessment of chest tube patency, the amount and type of drainage and the presence or absence of an air leak should be noted daily. In spontaneous pneumothorax, pleural fluid drainage should be minimal ($<$ 150 cc per 24 hours) and serous. Cloudy or thick drainage should raise the question of an infected pleural space. The presence of an air leak is suggested by bubbles escaping through the water seal. If no bubbles are seen initially, the patient should be asked to cough. The positive intrathoracic pressure that is created drives air out of the chest and through the water seal. If bubbling is noted and the tube is attached to suction, the clinician must discriminate between a true lung leak and a leak in the tubing-collection system. For instance, a loose connection may allow air to be pulled into the tube and thus mimic a lung leak. Connections should be checked, and if doubt remains, a clamp can be placed on the tube as it exits from the chest. If the bubbling persists, it indicates a leak in the collection system.

One other misleading situation can be created by allowing one or more holes in the chest tube to remain outside the chest. In this circumstance, air enters the pleural space through the chest tube and is then evacuated. To rule out this possibility, the chest tube is inspected and the chest roentgenogram evaluated.

A chest tube placed for spontaneous pneumothorax alone should be removed 24 to 48 hours after indications of an air leak disappear. Chest tube removal is a fairly simple procedure. The patient is asked to perform a Valsalva maneuver while the tube is removed, and the wound is quickly covered with petrolatum gauze and an occlusive bandage. Tube thoracostomy is expected to be successful in more than 90 percent of cases.

It is unusual to require more than one chest tube to treat spontaneous pneumothorax. Occasionally, failures with a single tube result from loculation of a pneumothorax or occlusion of the tube. In secondary spontaneous pneumothorax, and rarely in primary spontaneous pneumothorax, higher levels of negative suction are necessary to re-expand the lung. This is apparently due to the increased stiffness and higher elastic recoil of the underlying diseased lung. Pressures of -30 to -40 cm H_2O usually are effective in these circumstances.

Tube thoracostomies are occasionally complicated by excessive subcutaneous emphysema, empyema, dissection or migration of the tube into the lung, and re-expansion pulmonary edema. The latter is uncommon, but seems to correlate with the size and duration of the pneumothorax.

Thoracotomy

The indications for thoracotomy are persistent pneumothorax and air leak or recurrent pneumothorax. Spontaneous pneumothorax recurs in one-third to one-half of patients. After the second pneumothorax, the recurrence rate increases to 60 to 80 percent. Therefore, with the second episode, it is usually appropriate to proceed with a pleural symphysis procedure. At thoracotomy, the surgeon can either excise the bleb or, preferably, oversew or staple the involved area. He can then encourage pleural symphysis by pleural abrasion or parietal pleurectomy. Parietal pleurectomy is essentially 100 percent effective. In this procedure, the parietal pleura is mobilized as completely as possible and resected. However, it is not necessary to include the mediastinal or diaphragmatic pleura. The most critical area is the superior aspect of the chest where subpleural blebs are most common. The major disadvantages of parietal pleurectomy are (1) it is a long procedure and (2) it may be complicated by hemorrhage.

Pleural abrasion, whereby the parietal pleura is abraded with dry surgical gauze, appears to be almost as effective as parietal pleurectomy and is the treatment of choice for recurrent pneumothoraces.

Sclerosing Procedures

Intrapleural sclerosing agents are accepted therapy for malignant effusions and can be used similarly for pneumothorax. Certain patients with recurrent pneumothoraces are not desirable candidates for thoracotomy. This is frequently the situation in patients with significant underlying lung disease. Moreoever, it is in this fragile group of patients that the physician most wants to avoid a recurrence. I recommend an attempt at chemical sclerosis to treat the second episode in a patient with underlying lung disease and to treat selected patients with primary spontaneous pneumothorax. I avoid this technique in patients with a persistent significant air leak since there would be some risk of the agent flooding lung parenchyma and causing severe pneumonitis. I also avoid chemical sclerosis in young patients with a long life expectancy since there is the theoretic risk of a fibrothorax developing in later years. At this time, there are no studies that describe the long-term results of chemical sclerosis.

In patients at high risk for surgery and with a limited life expectancy, I proceed with tetracycline sclerosis. I use tetracycline, 20 mg per kilogram, according to the technique of Good and Sahn. This can be a painful procedure. Effective pain control requires parenteral analgesics and sedatives. In addition, I instill 15 ml 1 percent lidocaine into the pleural space 15 minutes before the tetracycline instillation.

SUGGESTED READING

Good JT, Sahn SA. Intrapleural therapy with tetracycline in malignant pleural effusions. Chest 1978; 74:602.

Killen DA, Gobbel WG. Spontaneous Pneumothorax. London: J. and A. Churchill Ltd., 1968.

Light RW. Pneumothorax. In: Light RW, ed. Pleural Disease. Philadelphia: Lea & Febiger, 1983.

Sahn SA. Pneumothorax. In:Sahn SA ed. Pulmonary Emergiencies. New York: Churchill Livingstone, 1982.

PLEURAL EFFUSION

GERALD R. KERBY, M.D.

Therapy of pleural effusion is based on accurate diagnosis of the etiology. In some instances, the etiology is obvious, based on the associated disease in the patient. In most instances, thoracentesis with analysis of pleural fluid establishes or aids in the diagnosis. Specific microorganisms or malignant cells found in pleural fluid point to the diagnosis. Other studies on pleural fluid—specific gravity, total protein, lactic dehydrogenase, glucose, pH, amylase—help to narrow the diagnostic possibilities, but do not establish a specific diagnosis.

Other diagnostic techniques of value in the assessment of pleural effusion include (1) lateral decubitus chest roentgenograms and sonography to establish the presence and/or location of the effusion; (2) computed tomography to better define the extent and location of effusion, and the presence of associated parenchymal lung or mediastinal disease; (3) closed needle or, rarely, open surgical biopsy to provide a histologic diagnosis. Bronchoscopy has a low diagnostic yield in pleural effusion unless associated with parenchymal lung disease.

Details of the diagnostic approach are well outlined in the monographs recommended at the end of this chapter. The remainder of this section will address therapy of pleural effusions seen most frequently by the clinician.

MANAGEMENT

Transudative Pleural Effusions

These effusions are characterized by a specific gravity less than 1.015, pleural fluid/serum ratio of total protein less than 0.5, and pleural fluid/serum ratio of LDH less than 0.6.

Congestive Heart Failure

This is the most common cause of transudative pleural effusion. It may be seen with either left or right heart failure, usually in patients with typical symptoms and signs of heart failure. It is usually bilateral; the presence of unilateral effusion or of normal cardiac size on the chest roentgenogram should lead to a search for another cause.

The effusion generally responds to treatment of heart failure. Thoracentesis is indicated to verify the presence of a transudate and to remove large effusions that compromise lung function. The effusion often resolves more slowly than other manifestations of heart failure. On rare occasions, repeated thoracentesis or tetracycline sclerosis may be required to prevent recurrence of effusion when medical therapy fails to compensate the heart failure. Pulmonary embolism and infarction commonly complicate heart failure. When the effusion or the response to therapy is atypical, pulmonary embolism should be suspected.

Liver Cirrhosis with Ascites

Unilateral or bilateral pleural effusions may be present in patients with massive ascites whether due to liver disease or malignant peritoneal implants. In the latter instance, the effusion usually is an exudate. The peritoneal fluid enters the pleural space through diaphragmatic lymphatics or anatomic defects in the diaphragm. Control of pleural effusion requires control of ascites. Thoracentesis may be required because of compromised lung function, but the effusion usually reaccumulates rapidly. Attempts at drainage via chest tube usually result in massive loss of fluid, electrolytes, and protein. If the ascites cannot be controlled, there is usually no good solution to the pleural effusion.

Miscellaneous Transudative Effusions

Myxedema, renal disease, peritoneal dialysis, and misdirected central venous lines with infusion of parenteral fluid into the pleural space may result in transudative effusion. Thoracentesis may be necessary for respiratory compromise; otherwise treatment of the underlying cause solves the problem.

Exudative Pleural Effusions

These effusions are characterized by a specific gravity greater than 1.015, pleural fluid/serum total protein ratio greater than 0.5, and pleural fluid/serum ratio of LDH greater than 0.6.

Malignant Pleural Effusion

Malignant effusions occur because of pleural implants and/or lymphatic obstruction due to mediastinal node involvement. The diagnosis is usually established by pleural fluid cytology or closed needle biopsy. Less frequently, thoracoscopy, thoracotomy, or mediastinoscopy (in the presence of enlarged mediastinal nodes on CT scan) may be required to prove a malignant etiology.

Small effusions require no specific therapy. Symptomatic effusions should be drained as completely as possible with an Intracath or similar catheter. About one-fourth do not recur.

Sclerosis of the Pleural Space. With recurrence that produces symtoms, sclerosis of the pleural space should be attempted. Many agents have been used, but tetracycline is the most popular since it produces an adequate chemical burn and avoids the marrow suppression sometimes associated with alkylating or antimetabolic agents. Attention to detail and an adequate dose of tetracycline are important in achieving sclerosis.

A chest tube should be inserted and the effusion maximally drained. The patient should be premedicated with morphine or a similar agent. Lidocaine, 150 to 200 mg, may be instilled (in 50 ml saline) prior to the tetracycline or incorporated with the tetracycline. The tetracycline, 20 to 25 mg per kilogram in 100 to 200 ml saline, is instilled, the tube clamped, and the patient rapidly rotated to assume the following positions—prone, supine, both decubitus, sitting, and Trendelenburg—over 15 to 20 minutes to distribute the solution over the entire pleural surface. The chest tube is connected to suction and maximal expansion of the lung maintained for 48 to 72 hours. If drainage is greater than 200 to 250 ml per day, prolongation of chest tube suction may enhance successful sclerosis.

Recurrence of effusion after sclerosis is usually related to failure of the lung to expand to fill the pleural space. The usual mechanisms are a visceral pleural peel, parenchymal lung disease (metastases or radiation fibrosis), and bronchial obstruction. Definition of the mechanism may allow correction. In difficult cases in which there is rapid reaccumulation of fluid after attempt at sclerosis, mediastinal radiation (when malignant nodes are present) or surgical pleurectomy may be useful. The latter consideration must balance the potential length of survival against the morbidity of the procedure.

Parapneumonic Effusion and Empyema

Pleural effusion is present in 25 to 40 percent of pneumonias. Many are small and require no therapy beyond appropriate antibiotic treatment of the pneumonia. Formerly, pneumonias due to gram-positive aerobic organisms were the most common cause of parapneumonic effusion or empyema. In recent years, anaerobic organisms appear to be the most common cause of effusions progressing to loculation and empyema. It is imperative to include an antibiotic with activity against anaerobes in the treatment of pneumonia associated with significant pleural effusion unless an alternative specific etiology can be established by blood or sputum culture.

Thoracentesis should be performed early in the treatment of pneumonia with effusion of more than minimal volume (extending above the dome of the diaphragm on upright roentgenogram) or greater than 1 cm in thickness on lateral decubitus films). This is the most accurate way of differentiating benign parapneumonic effusion from early or frank empyema. Benign parapneumonic effusions are usually characterized by a pH greater than 7.2, glucose greater than 40 mg per deciliter, LDH less than 1,000 IU per liter, and white blood cell count less than 15,000 per cubic millimeter. Early empyema usually has a pH below 7.0, glucose less than 40, and white blood cell count greater than 20,000 to 25,000. Frank empyemas contain gross pus and organisms on Gram stain.

Benign parapneumonic effusions generally require no therapy beyond antibiotics and supportive therapy for pneumonia. Early or frank empyemas require immediate chest tube drainage via one or more large-bore catheters. Effusions intermediate between benign parapneumonic effusion and early empyemas require close observation. Some resolve with antibiotic therapy alone; some require one or more thoracenteses; those that progress require tube drainage.

Failure of the patient to improve clinically after treatment with antibiotics and tube drainage indicates the presence of additional loculations of pus that are not being adequately drained. Sonography may be useful in localizing loculations, but on occasion cannot differentiate between fluid filled with cells and debris and consolidated lung. Computed tomography is the best imaging technique for evaluating the extent and location of pleural disease.

Decortication. Multiple loculations that cannot be drained by tubes require surgical decortication if the patient can tolerate it. Timing of decortication is important. Toxicity should be reduced by means of tube drainage and antibiotic therapy prior to surgery. The peel is easier to remove when it is inflammatory and fibrinous, but becomes increasingly adherent as fibrosis progresses. Generally, the second or third week is optimal for decortication. Patients who are too ill to undergo decortication may require localized surgical drainage procedures with lysis of adhesions. Fibrinolytic agents such as streptokinase may be of value to promote drainage in difficult situations.

Decortication may also be needed to remove thick pleural peels that are likely to significantly compromise lung function. The decision can be difficult since it needs to be made in the first few weeks when the operation is easier while recognizing that impressive inflammatory pleural thickening may eventually scar down to minimal pleural fibrosis. The age and activity level of the patient as well as extent and thickness of the inflammatory peel are major factors to be weighed in the decision.

Tuberculous and Fungal Pleural Effusions

Granulomatous pleuritis occurs less frequently than in prior years, but remains a significant cause of pleural effusion. The effusion is usually a lymphocytic exudate. The diagnosis is established by the presence of granulomas on closed pleural biopsy as well as results of skin tests, serologic titers, and recovery of specific organisms from pleural fluid, pleural biopsy, or sputum. Culture of the pleural biopsy specimens enhances recovery of organisms.

The effusions generally are not large and usually resolve with chemotherapy for the causative agent. Rarely, frank empyema deelops and bronchopleural fistula may occur. The principles discussed under bacterial empyema apply to that situation .

Collagen Vascular Diseases

This group of diseases, especially rheumatoid arthritis and systemic lupus erythematosus, may be associated with pleural effusion. Rhematoid effusions are characterized by low glucose levels. Lupus erythematosus cells may be present in the effusion of SLE. These effusions rarely require specific therapy unless they are large, but occasionally they produce significant pleural fibrosis.

Asbestos Pleural Effusion

In addition to effusion associated with mesothelioma, some asbestos-exposed individuals develop exudative pleural effusions. These effusions, although usually small and self-limited, on rare occasions may be large and/or produce sufficient restriction to require thoracentesis or decortication.

Pulmonary Infarction

Pulmonary infarction may be associated with pleural effusion, usually exudative, and rarely transudative or bloody. They are usually small and resolve with treatment of thromboembolism.

SUGGESTED READING

Light RW. Pleural diseases. Philadelphia: Lea & Febiger, 1983.

Light RW, ed. Symposium on pleural disease. Clin Chest Med 1985; 6:1–2.

EMPYEMA

STEVEN A. SAHN, M.D.

The Greek word "empyema" is defined as the accumulation of pus in a cavity of the body, especially in the chest, where it is actually termed a pyothorax. Today, empyema most commonly occurs in the setting of bacterial pneumonia, but also can occur following thoracic surgery, following chest trauma, as a result of esophageal or subdiaphragmatic disorders, and from iatrogenic insults (thoracentesis). In adults, anaerobes are the most common cause of empyema today, gram-negative aerobes being second in incidence. Infection occurs in the pleural space following penetration of a large inoculum of microorganisms that cannot be killed by phagocytes or removed adequately by the parietal pleural lymphatics. The normal pleural cavity is relatively resistant to the development of established infection and, therefore, empyema generally occurs only in the setting of a damaged pleura and/or a good culture medium for bacteria such as exudative pleural fluid or blood. Direct extension of the pneumonic process into the pleural space, seepage of anaerobic organisms through an esophageal fistula, spread of infection through the diaphragm from below, a leaky bronchial stump, penetrating chest trauma, and thoracentesis with poor aseptic technique are all possible portals of entry for bacteria into the pleural cavity.

Since empyema (and complicated parapneumonic effusions—effusions that behave clinically like empyema, but are not purulent and are negative bacteriologically) most commonly occurs following pneumonia, the discussion will be directed toward that disease. It is important in considering therapy of empyema to understand the pathogenesis of pleural fluid formation in pneumonia and the time course of development of empyema or a complicated parapneumonic effusion. Since pneumonias tend to have a nidus in a peripheral subpleural location and spread centrifugally toward the hilum, the pleura is vulnerable to the inflammatory response induced by the bacterial infection. Probably during the first 72 hours of a bacterial pneumonia, owing to the accumulation of polymorphonuclear leukocytes in a subpleural location and the release of a number of mediators of the inflammatory response, capillary dilatation occurs with the leakage of protein-rich fluid into the subpleural interstitium. Owing to direct pleural inflammation and/or "loosening" of the visceral mesothelial junctions, sterile interstitial fluid leaks into the pleural cavity. This fluid generally is slightly turbid and high in protein concentration with a moderate number of polymorphonuclear leukocytes; the biochemical characteristics are a normal glucose (pleural fluid to serum ratio more than 0.5), a pH of 7.30 or higher, and an LDH less than 500 U per liter. If the pneumonia at this stage is treated with an appropriate antibiotic, the pleural fluid is resorbed over several days and adhesions and fibrosis do not occur in the pleural space. From day 4 to day 10, the natural history of pneumonia with pleural effusion progresses to an infected pleural space that does not resolve without pleural space sequelae with antibiotic therapy alone. During this interval, the pleural fluid forms a gelatinous "clot" owing to the relatively high concentrations of intravascular clotting factors that have accumulated in the pleural space and impaired fibrinolysis due to the damaged pleural membrane and inhibitors in the pleural fluid. This coagulum serves as a lattice-work to which fibroblasts adhere as they migrate into the pleural space. At this stage, loculations are evident on chest roentgenogram, and pleural drainage with a chest tube becomes more difficult. By 2 weeks, collagen begins to be laid down and eventually an isolated empyema cavity forms, increasing both morbidity and therapeutic difficulties.

DIAGNOSIS

It would be advantageous if it could be determined at the time of admission whether or not a free-flowing parapneumonic effusion will resolve with antibiotic therapy only or will require chest tube drainage. Unfortunately, the clinical presentation usually is not helpful in this regard since both patients with empyemas and those with uncomplicated parapneumonic effusions usually have similar peripheral leukocyte counts, peak temperatures, incidences of pleurisy, and extent of pneumonia. However, patients with anaerobic infections usually have a predisposing factor (alcoholism, impaired consciousness) and an indolent course and are more likely to have empyema.

If the chest roentgenogram shows loculation, the clinician can assume that the parapneumonic effusion is complicated, and drainage of the pleural space should be strongly considered depending on the clinical situation; if the presentation suggests anaerobic pleuropulmonary infection, chest tube drainage is almost always indicated. However, in pneumococcal pneumonia with a few small loculations, a nonacute history, and absence of sepsis, observation is warranted. The aspiration of pus from the pleural space establishes the diagnosis of empyema and necessitates adequate pleural space drainage beginning with the tube thoracostomy.

The biochemical characteristics of the pleural fluid help the clinician to decide on the proper course of management if the fluid is not loculated, not purulent, and has a negative Gram stain. The details pertaining to this decision will be discussed below.

Both ultrasonography and computed tomography (CT) are effective in diagnosing and locating infected, loculated pleural fluid. If the fluid is free-flowing on lateral decubitus roentgenogram, thoracentesis should be attempted directly. If loculation is present, clinical judgment dictates whether thoracentesis should be attempted on the basis of physical examination or under ultrasound guidance. A clearly defined echo-free or septated abnormality located by real-time ultrasonography to be situated under the chest wall and seen to change in shape with respiration usually represents aspirable fluid. Thoracentesis can be done simultaneously with the ultrasound study or following localization and mapping of the chest wall. In the latter situation, the thoracentesis must be accomplished with the patient positioned the same as for his ultrasound examination. Ultrasound usually allows sampling of the fluid portion of a suspected empyema and avoids fruitless aspiration of fibrinous pleural adhesions.

When infection is suspected in the region of the diaphragm, ultrasound study demonstrates the location of the fluid—in the pleural space or in the subdiaphragmatic space—and the relationship of the fluid to the diaphragm. Ultrasonography can also guide the placement of chest tubes into individual locules. Advantages of ultrasound study are the rapidity and ease of the procedure, portability for ill patients, lack of ionizing radiation, and relatively low cost.

The anatomic delineation of the abnormal pleural space by CT scan is superior to that of conventional chest roentgenogram of ultrasound and does not depend on the expertise of the examiner for quality as does ultrasonography. The differentiation of empyema from lung abscess is often difficult as the exact location of the air-fluid levels (lung vs pleural space) may be impossible to predict based on the chest roentgenogram. Unfortunately, characteristics such as thin and smooth wall, vertically oriented cavity, difference in air-fluid levels on different projections, and extension of the air-fluid level across the entire hemithorax may not convince the clinician that he should proceed with tube drainage. CT scanning is useful in making this differentiation; findings of empyema on CT scan are uniform internal and external cavity walls, compression of adjacent lung parenchyma, tendency toward lenticular as opposed to round shape, and an obtuse angle with the pleural margin. The CT scan may reveal other unsuspected pleural loculations, and positional scanning may demonstrate communications of these locules with the primary focus, especially following a drainage procedure.

The basic decision facing the clinician regarding the treatment of a parapneumonic effusion is straightforward: (Table 1). Does the patient need pleural space drainage or not? As already suggested, the decision usually cannot be made on clinical grounds alone but requires laboratory tests, including pleural fluid analysis and chest roentgenogram. If the chest roentgenogram demonstrates free-flowing pleural fluid and pleural fluid analysis shows a nonpurulent fluid with a negative Gram stain, a pH of 7.30 or greater, a pleural fluid to serum glucose ratio greater than 0.5, and an LDH less than 1,000 U per liter, then the only therapy required is an antimicrobial agent or agents directed at the pneumonia. In general, the dose of antibiotic does not need to be increased over that recommended for the pneumonia as pleural fluid antibiotic concentrations approach that of serum. In almost all instances, antibiotic therapy at this stage effects relatively rapid absorption (several days) of fluid from the pleural space, resulting in an essentially normal pleural space on roentgenogram and no impairment in pulmonary function. If the pleural fluid is purulent, immediate chest tube drainage should be established. These two extremes provide simple decision

TABLE 1 Treatment of Parapneumonic Effusions

Classification	*Clinical Presentation*	*Treatment*	*Comments*
Uncomplicated parapneumonic effusion	Short time between initial symptom and presentation; small-to-moderate free-flowing effusion; turbid fluid, pH≥7.30, glucose PF/S>0.5, LDH<500 U/L, negative bateriology	Antibiotics directed at pneumonia	Antibiotic dose does not have to be increased; effusion resolves over days; no pleural space sequelae
Complicated parapneumonic effusion (empyema)	Longer time between initial symptom and presentation; moderate-to-large loculated effusion; turbid fluid or pus, pH<7.00, glucose <40 mg/dl, LDH>1,000 U/L, positive bacteriology	Antibiotics; closed chest tube drainage; open drainage if closed not effective; empyemectomy if sepsis continues	Antibiotic dose same as for pneumonia alone with exception of ↑ penicillin for anaerobes; effusion resolves over days to weeks; usually a restrictive defect on PFTs
Indeterminate parapneumonic effusion	Variable time between initial symptom and presentation; moderate free-flowing fluid; turbid fluid, pH 7.10–7.29, glucose 40–60 mg/dl, LDH 500–1,000 U/L, negative bacteriology	Antibiotics; repeat thoracentesis at 6–12 hrs; if pH stable or ↑, observe; if pH ↓, chest tube	Frequently received antibiotics before hospitalization; may act like an empyema despite lack of criteria; follow closely

making for the clinician. However, like many decisions in medicine, this one is not always straightforward. In any patient who has received previous antibiotic therapy outside the hospital and who has turbid, nonloculated pleural fluid, the biochemical characteristics of the fluid are particularly helpful in guiding decision making. Experience has shown that the pleural fluid markers of severe inflammation, the development of acidosis, and the utilization of glucose in the pleural space tend to predict an unfavorable pathologic resolution of the pleural space inflammation. Therefore, in low-pH, low-glucose effusions, the prudent course is early chest tube drainage. There is good evidence that when the pleural fluid pH is less than 7.00, the glucose is less than 40 mg per deciliter, and the LDH is greater than 1,000 U per liter, those parapneumonic effusions do not resolve without adequate drainage. There are some parapneumonic effusions, albeit a small number, with a pH in the range of 7.10 to 7.29 and a glucose level in the range of 40 to 60 mg per deciliter that loculate in the pleural space and cause morbidity for the patient if chest tube drainage is not established early. In borderline situations in which the pH is in the range of 7.10 to 7.29, a repeat thoracentesis in 6 to 12 hours is advisable. If the patient is improving clinically, the fluid is still free-flowing, and the PH is stable or rising, antibiotic therapy alone should be sufficient. However, if the fluid has loculated or the pH is falling, immediate tube drainage should be instituted.

Since the pleural fluid pH may alter clinical decision making, the clinician must be confident about laboratory measurement and ensure accuracy by meticulous collection and handling. Three to 5 ml of pleural fluid should be aspirated anaerobically in a syringe rinsed with 0.2 ml of 1:1000 heparin and kept on ice until subjected to measurement with a blood gas analyzer. Since arterial pH influences pleural fluid pH, a difference of at least 0.15 pH units is necessary to define pleural fluid acidosis. The pH of pus aspirated from the pleural space does not need to be measured as it does not provide information that affects therapy and may damage the blood gas analyzer.

Occasionally, the patient who presented with an uncomplicated parapneumonic effusion is seen to be improving clinically except for persistence of fever. If no other cause of the fever can be found, thoracentesis with removal of a collection of pyrogens from the pleural space may be therapeutic.

MANAGEMENT

Chest Tube Drainage

Once the decision has been made to proceed with chest tube drainage, the tube should be inserted as quickly as possible, since the transition from free-flowing to loculated fluid can occur over several hours. Large-diameter chest tubes should be used for purulent fluid and placed in the most dependent part of the pleural effusion. Water-seal or negative-pressure drainage may be used. If several large loculations exist, the thoracic surgeon may prefer to place more than one chest tube in the operating room setting where he can "break-up" fibrinous adhesions with finger dissection and facilitate drainage.

Following proper chest tube placement with drainage, there is often dramatic defervescence and an improved feeling of well-being. By 48 hours, clinical improvement should be substantial. In the setting of an acute complicated parapneumonic effusion or empyema, the chest tube can be removed when no large loculations exist on chest roentgenogram, the patient is no longer febrile, and pleural space drainage is serous and less than 75 ml per day. There is no need for open drainage (to be discussed); in fact, it may be deleterious to the patient because in the acute or subacute disease, there is no well-formed empyema cavity.

Reasons for lack of improvement include a severely debilitated host, inadequate pleural space drainage (either an occluded chest tube or additional undrained locules), severe necrotizing pneumonia, and incorrect antibiotic therapy. The microbiologic data should be re-evaluated, and either an ultrasound study or a CT scan done to search for additional loculations or unsuspected disease.

Intrapleural Fibrinolytic Agents

If inadequate pleural space drainage is the problem, the alternatives include insertion of another chest tube, intrapleural instillation of streptokinase, or thoracotomy. Intrapleural fibrinolytic agents have not received widespread use in the United States. If these agents are effective, it would appear that the timing of use is critical. They are more likely to be effective when fibrinous adhesions are present early in the course of a complicated effusion than later when collagen is laid down in the pleural space. Prior to inserting another chest tube for failed drainage early in the course of the empyema, a trial of streptokinase, 250,000 units intrapleurally, may be attempted. If it appears to increase drainage, the drug should be continued at the same dose for 7 to 10 days. The regimen requires clamping of the chest tube for 1 to 3 hours following streptokinase instillation and having the patient change positions. Adverse effects are virtually nil.

Open Pleural Drainage

If closed drainage is unsuccessful (pleural loculations remain associated with fever and leukocytosis), a surgical procedure is necessary. Open drainage provides more complete evacuation of pleural space contents, but is done only if a well-defined empyema cavity exists. Development of this cavity usually takes at least 2 weeks from the initial involvement of the pleural space. Opening the chest tube to the atmosphere or instillation of a small amount of contrast into the pleural space through the chest tube can define the pleural pathology; the development of pneumothorax or contrast dispersement in the pleural space contraindicates an open drainage procedure.

Open drainage of a well-established empyema cavity can be accomplished with rib resection and either tube insertion or open-flap (Eloesser) technique. Portions of as many as three ribs are resected at the caudad part of the emyema space and a cut-off large-diameter chest tube is inserted into the cavity. The cavity should be irrigated daily with an antiseptic solution and the drainage collected in a colostomy bag. The tube is gradually advanced from the cavity as it closes. Cavity closure is a prolonged process, frequently taking 4 to 6 months. The Eloesser flap technique entails lining the tract between pleural space and chest wall with skin and muscle, creating a skin-lined fistula and eliminating the need for chest tubes.

Decortication

When pleural sepsis cannot be controlled with closed tube drainage, empyemectomy with or without decortication should be done in patients who can tolerate a thoracotomy. This procedure involves complete debridement of the pleural space and evacuation of pus. Chest tubes are then placed under direct vision. Necrotic lung is sometimes found at thoracotomy, necessitating lobectomy. Sepsis usually is well controlled by empyemectomy and decortication, which has a high morbidity and substantial mortality in debilitated patients, and generally requires 2 additional weeks of hospitalization.

A thoracotomy may be necessary to control sepsis in empyema, but decortication alone is rarely indicated for the restrictive ventilatory defect that occurs following pleural space infection. Data indicate that pulmonary function (FVC and TLC) improve progressively over the 6 to 9 months following empyema, with return to baseline function if the underlying lung parenchyma was not severely affected. Late decortication should be considered in individuals who have a persistent restrictive defect that interferes with their life style. Prior to decortication, a CT scan of the thorax should be done to assess the extent of pleural and pulmonary disease. Decortication can only be successful if the pleural disease has made the largest contribution to restriction. Lung function returns to baseline approximately 6 to 12 weeks following decortication in the properly selected individual.

BRONCHOPLEURAL FISTULA

Bronchopleural fistula deserves special attention since it is a dreaded complication of pulmonary resection and necrotizing pneumonia. Postoperative bronchopleural fistulas can result from technical error, postoperative radiotherapy, failure of the remaining lung to fill the pleural space, and positive pressure ventilation. Following pneumonectomy, the diagnosis is suspected when the patient develops fever, sudden dyspnea, subcutaneous emphysema, expectoration of pleural fluid, a contralateral shift of the mediastinum, and a change in the air-fluid level. Following lobectomy, a persistent air leak with purulent drainage and expectoration of purulent secretions are clinically diagnostic. When the fistula develops following chest tube removal, it is signaled by fever, purulent sputum, and a new air-fluid level. The diagnosis can be established by thoracentesis, and the anatomy of the fistula defined by bronchography, bronchoscopy, or sinogram. Fistulas that develop in the first few days postoperatively usually can be closed by resture of the stump with pleura or muscle pedicle. Small fistulas that develop later usually respond to antibiotics and tube drainage but occasionally require surgery.

A postpneumonia bronchopleural fistula usually is heralded by fever, leukocytosis, and a new air-fluid level on chest roentgenogram. Chest tube drainage with apposition of the visceral and parietal pleura may result in closure of the fistula. The amount of chest tube suction leading to the minimum gas flow through the fistula varies from individual to individual on mechanical ventilation and may require precise gas flow measurements through the chest tube to promote the most rapid closure. Clinical judgment dictates the timing of surgical closure of chronic fistulous tracts.

SUGGESTED READING

Bartlett JG, Finegold SM. Anaerobic pleuropulmonary infections. Medicine 1972; 51:413–450.

Bartlett JG Gorbach SL, Thadepalli H, Finegold SM. Bacteriology of empyema. Lancet 1974; 1:388–340.

Light RW, Girard WM, Jenkinson SG, George RB. Parapneumonic effusions. Am J Med 1980; 69:507–511.

Morin JE, Munro DD, Maclean LD. Early thoracotomy for empyema. J Thorac Cardiovasc Surg 1972; 64:530–536.

Potts DE, Levin DC, and Sahn SA. Pleural fluid pH in parapneumonic effusions. Chest 1976; 70:328–331.

Samson PC. Empyema thoracis: essentials of present-day management. Ann Thorac Surg 1971; 11:210–220.

ADULT RESPIRATORY DISTRESS SYNDROME

JOHN M. LUCE, M.D.

The adult respiratory distress syndrome (ARDS) is a form of acute respiratory failure characterized by severe dyspnea, hypoxemia refractory to normal amounts of supplemental oxygen, diminished lung compliance, diffuse chest roentgenographic infiltrates, and a normal left atrial filling pressure. ARDS is also known by such terms as capillary leak syndrome, congestive atelectasis, post-traumatic pulmonary insufficiency, and shock lung.

ETIOLOGY AND PATHOGENESIS

The exact cause of ARDS is uncertain. Nevertheless the syndrome occurs in such well-known clinical settings as the following: (1) sepsis, (2) trauma, (3) multiple emergency transfusions, (4) prolonged hypotension, (5) fat embolism, (6) pancreatitis, (7) oxygen toxicity, (8) lung contusion, (9) drug overdosage, (10) pulmonary irradiation, (11) aspiration, (12) infectious pneumonia, and (13) pulmonary thromboembolism. Of the conditions associated with ARDS, the most common is bacterial sepsis. ARDS occurred in 18 percent and 23 percent of septic patients, most of whom were hypotensive, in two retrospective series. The incidence of ARDS among intubated patients with sepsis was 38 percent in a recent prospective series by Pepe and associates. This incidence increased to 47 percent if sepsis was accompanied by any two of the other conditions associated with a high incidence of ARDS in this series, including lung contusion, aspiration of gastric contents, and multiple emergency transfusions.

Damage of the alveolar-capillary membrane is the common denominator of the conditions associated with ARDS. This damage involves both the capillary endothelium and the alveolar epithelium. As capillary permeability increases, water and protein leak into the pulmonary interstitium. Lymphatic drainage is overwhelmed as the leakage progresses, and the alveoli are flooded with protein-rich fluid. Hyaline membranes form around the air spaces as the proteinaceous exudate is deposited. Although this deposition occurs in other injuries, it once was considered so specific for ARDS that the syndrome was called adult hyaline membrane disease.

To a greater or lesser degree, the formation of pulmonary edema is accompanied by interstitial inflammation involving activated complement and neutrophils that give off toxic oxygen radicals. These substances in turn cause destruction of the type 1 cells that line the alveoli. Type 2 cells also are affected, disturbing their production of the surfactant that normally limits alveolar collapse at low lung volumes. Reactive pulmonary vasospasm, in situ thrombosis, and vascular remodeling increase pulmonary vascular resistance in many patients with ARDS. Lung collagen also is increased, and extensive pulmonary fibrosis may be seen during the resolution of injury. This scarring also may be associated with emphysematous changes that relate either to the initial insult or to the high concentrations of oxygen and positive pressure ventilation used in its therapy.

CLINICAL PRESENTATION AND CHEST ROENTGENOGRAPHIC PATTERN

It should be emphasized that ARDS may manifest abruptly in patients with previously normal lungs. Similarly, although focal roentgenographic infiltrates attributed to lung contusion or pneumonia may precede the development of diffuse infiltrates, the chest roentgenogram often is normal to begin with and remains so for hours after certain insults such as shock. This underscores the fact that ARDS represents a delayed reaction to injury in many individuals.

PULMONARY FUNCTION ABNORMALITIES

ARDS is a restrictive disease characterized by a reduced lung compliance. This reduction is due to interstitial fluid, inflammation, and ultimately fibrosis that impairs lung expansion and requires that a higher transplumonary pressure be generated to achieve a given volume change. The reduced compliance in turn causes a decrease in total lung capacity and in functional residual capacity (FRC), the resting volume of the lungs. This means that the airways and alveoli are abnormally small at the end of a quiet exhalation.

In normal persons, the FRC remains greater than the volume at which airway and alveolar closure occurs during exhalation. Airway and alveolar closure takes place first in the dependent lung regions, where blood flow is greatest, because the transpulmonary pressure is less there than at the top of the lung. FRC is so reduced in patients with ARDS that it may be exceeded by their closing volume, which may increase because interstitial disease impinges on airways and alveoli. As a result, many air spaces are collapsed at the end of exhalation and cannot participate in gas exchange. Other alveoli are flooded with edema fluid. The combination of alveolar flooding and collapse causes such a profound mismatching of ventilation and perfusion that mixed venous blood cannot be oxygenated in the lungs. This condition, which is called intrapulmonary shunt, is responsible for the refractory hypoxemia that is a hallmark of ARDS.

Carbon dioxide exchange is not severely reduced early in ARDS. Most patients even are hypocapnic at this point because mechanical reflexes in the lungs or the hypoxemia stimulates them to overbreathe. However, carbon dioxide production increases as the work of breathing does in these patients. Their dead space ventilation also rises owing to a functional or anatomic loss of the pulmonary capillary bed that may be reflected in a low diffusing capacity for carbon monoxide. Unless minute ventilation can keep pace, which is unlikely in sick patients with decreased lung compliance, carbon dioxide excretion is impaired and hypercapnia may ensue.

DIAGNOSIS

ARDS is a clinical diagnosis that requires the presence of dyspnea, hypoxemia, diminished lung compliance, and diffuse roentgenographic infiltrates in the appropriate setting. It is also essential that the pulmonary edema of ARDS be due to increased capillary permeability rather than increased hydrostatic pressure, that is, left atrial filling pressures must be shown to be normal or low. Although direct measurement of left atrial pressure rarely is convenient, an estimate may be made through determination of the pulmonary arterial wedge pressure by means of a Swan-Ganz catheter. Measurement of the protein content of edema fluid may help to distinguish ARDS from elevated hydrostatic pressure, but this technique cannot be substituted for Swan-Ganz catheterization at the present time.

MANAGEMENT

The three aims in treating ARDS are (1) to anticipate the syndrome in associated clinical settings, (2) to apply specific therapy for underlying causes, and (3) to use supportive therapy to keep patients alive while waiting for their lungs to heal (Table 1). In regard to the first objective, conditions such as shock should be treated as quickly as possible to prevent pulmonary injury. Similarly, aspiration can be avoided by positioning patients upright while eating, withholding food and oral fluids in patients without a gag reflex, and intubating patients who need airway protection. Ongoing infections should be treated with antibiotics or surgical drainage as indicated. If sepsis develops, broad-spectrum antimicrobial coverage should be provided until the causative organisms can be identified. A reasonable combination in most patients would be ampicillin, 1 g; clindamycin, 0.5 g; and tobramycin, 1.5 g—all given intravenously every 6 hours.

TABLE 1 Prevention and Treatment of the Acute Respiratory Distress Syndrome

Limit aspiration
Reverse shock
Treat sepsis
Administer oxygen
Use positive end-expiratory pressure
Maintain normal to low wedge pressure
Give fluids judiciously
Support cardiac output with vasoactive drugs

Some clinicians routinely provide coverage for gram-positive and gram-negative bacteria in all patients with ARDS regardless of whether pneumonia or sepsis is demonstrated. However, giving prophylactic antibiotics is of unproven benefit and may lead to superinfection with resistant microorganisms. Corticosteroids also are given in high doses (as much as 30 mg per kilogram 4 times daily) to ameliorate shock, sepsis, and other disorders associated with ARDS. This approach is supported by recent studies demonstrating that corticosteroids inhibit complement-induced leukocyte aggregation and prevent increased capillary permeability in sheep following the injection of endotoxin. Nevertheless, despite these studies, clinical and experimental evidence does not support the prophylactic use of corticosteroids in ARDS, save perhaps for that associated with fat embolism and pulmonary irradiation.

Given the possibility that platelets and intravascular coagulation play a role in ARDS, some clinicians give heparin to patients with the syndrome. Yet heparin has never been shown to prevent or resolve ARDS, and because of potential complications, its use should be limited to individuals with pulmonary thromboembolism. Whether drugs that affect platelet aggregation (e.g., sulfinpyrazone) can alter the course of ARDS is uncertain. Also of unclear benefit in ARDS are agents such as cyclosphamide, which are used to prevent pulmonary fibrosis in other individuals.

Oxygen is the one essential drug for patients with ARDS. It should be given as soon as possible and in concentrations sufficient to reverse hypoxemia regardless of its potential toxicity. After hypoxemia has been corrected, oxygenation can be supported and the risk of oxygen toxicity reduced in most patients by the application of positive end-expiratory pressure (PEEP). PEEP can be administered to mechanically ventilated patients and to those breathing spontaneously, in which case the form of PEEP usually employed is called continuous positive airway pressure (CPAP). Intubation is not required for spontaneously breathing patients wearing a tightly fitting CPAP face mask. Most investigators assume that PEEP improves arterial oxygenation primarily by increasing FRC to pre-injury levels and thereby preventing airway and alveolar collapse during exhalation. Although PEEP does not diminish extravascular lung water, it may redistribute fluid within the lungs and normalize the surface area available for gas exchange.

In addition to using PEEP therapeutically, some clinicans apply it prophylactically to abort or reverse the pathologic process responsible for ARDS. One rationale for prophylactic PEEP is that surfactant function is improved and the effects of complement activation are limited in airspaces that are not allowed to collapse in the early stages of lung injury. Several studies have demonstrated the possible benefits of prophylactic PEEP. Nevertheless, PEEP did not influence the resolution of experimental lung injury in a recent animal study. Nor did it prove useful in a prospective study of intubated patients with risk factors for ARDS. As a result, prophylactic PEEP is not generally recommended at the present time.

Deciding how much PEEP to use in patients with ARDS often is difficult. One group defined optimal PEEP as that level at which respiratory system compliance was highest; this appeared to correlate with oxygen transport, the product of arterial oxygen content and cardiac output. By contrast, other investigators consider the best PEEP to be that level which reduces intrapulmonary shunt to the greatest extent. Neither of these two approaches has proved to be universally applicable, and it is just as likely that the optimal PEEP is that level which allows the least amount of supplemental oxygen to be used while not compromising oxygen transport.

Since oxygen transport reflects cardiac output as well as the arterial oxygen content, it is essential that cardiac output be monitored in patients receiving high levels of PEEP. This can be accomplished with the Swan-Ganz catheter, which also can be used to guide fluid administration. In most patients with ARDS, left atrial filling pressure should be high enough to ensure an adequate cardiac output, but not so high that pulmonary edema due to elevated hydrostatic pressure occurs. A pulmonary artery wedge pressure of 5 to 10 mm Hg is reasonable in most individuals.

Nitroprusside, which has a relatively balanced effect in dilating both arterial and venous vessels, has been shown to reduce pulmonary vascular resistance and to be as effective as fluid restriction or depletion in lowering the wedge pressure in an animal model of ARDS. This model differs from human ARDS due to sepsis, in that systemic vascular resistance is high in the animals and low or normal in humans. Unfortunately, nitroprusside drops the blood pressure to unacceptable levels in many patients. It also may reduce arterial oxygenation by inhibiting hypoxic pulmonary vasoconstriction. Thus, nitroprusside and hydralazine, another agent with more specific arteriolar vasodilating properties, should only be given to patients whose blood pressure and arterial oxygen tension are continuously monitored.

When they are administered to lower wedge pressure or reduce pulmonary vascular resistance, nitroprusside and hydralazine often must be combined with inotropic and vasoconstricting agents. Dopamine is the drug most commonly used for circulatory support in patients with ARDS, especially when the syndrome is associated with sepsis. Low doses of dopamine (0.05 to 2.0 μg per kilogram per minute) stimulate dopaminergic receptors in the kidneys and cause selective dilation of renal arterioles. At doses between 2 and 10 μg per kilogram per minute, dopamine acts primarily on beta-adrenergic receptors and improves myocardial contractility and cardiac output. At doses of 10 to 20 μg per kilogram per minute, the drug has mixed beta- and alpha-agonist properties. At doses above 20 μg per kilogram per minute, dopamine stimulates alpha-agonist receptors and causes vasoconstriction in most vascular beds. In this range, the drug may increase pulmonary vascular resistance and wedge pressure.

Dobutamine is a newer synthetic catecholamine with predominantely beta-1 agonist properties. Myocardial contractility is enhanced with doses ranging between 2 and 20 μg per kilogram per minute; systemic vascular resistance and wedge pressure usually fall in this range. Dobutamine rarely is effective in improving cardiac output when hypotension is present, as it often is in patients with ARDS. However, when given in combination with dopamine, dobutamine may support the cardiac output sufficiently to allow a low wedge pressure to be used. This in turn limits the formation of pulmonary edema in patients with ARDS.

The proper use of supplemental oxygen, PEEP, judicious fluid therapy, and vasoactive drugs should support tissue oxygenation by improving the arterial oxygen content and the cardiac output in most patients. Clinicians should remember that the treatment of ARDS is purely supportive and that their challenge is to prevent infections and other complications inherent in the intensive care unit. Such support remains the major therapy for ARDS until we better understand the syndrome and can apply more selective treatment modalities.

PROGNOSIS

ARDS is associated with an overall mortality of about 50 percent in most centers. The mortality of mechanically ventilated patients with post-traumatic pulmonary insufficiency who were between 20 and 49 years of age was 23 percent in the series from San Francisco General Hospital in the early and mid 1970s; mortality rose to 53 percent in this series among mechanically ventilated patients older than 60 years of age. Mortality exceed 90 percent in the 90 patients enrolled in a study of extracorporeal membrane oxygenation who had extensive inflammation, fibrosis, and necrosis on lung biopsy. The mortality in 741 patients considered for enrollment in this study, who were mechanically ventilated for longer than 24 hours and received greater than 50 percent oxygen, was 66 percent. In most instances, death was due to multiorgan failure.

Although these figures underscore the severity of ARDS, pulmonary function is surprisingly good in those individuals who survive the syndrome. Most survivors have residual dyspnea, but they are able to live productively. This is particularly true of young persons with otherwise normal lungs who sustain a limited insult such as trauma. That such individuals can function after ARDS should inspire clinicians to approach the syndrome hopefully and aggressively.

SUGGESTED READING

Luce JM. The cardiovascular effects of mechanical ventilation and positive end-expiratory pressure. JAMA 1984; 252:807–811.

Pepe PE, Potkin RT, Reus DH, et al. Clinical predictors of the adult respiratory distress syndrome. Am J Surg 1982; 144:124.

Pontoppidan H, Geffin B, Lowenstein E. Acute respiratory failure in the adult. N Engl J Med 1972; 287:9690.

Rinaldo JE, Rogers R. Changing concepts of lung injury and repair. N Engl J Med 1982; 306:900.

ACUTE RESPIRATORY FAILURE IN ASTHMA

ALAN L. PLUMMER, M.D.

Asthma is a common disorder affecting more than 7 million people in the United States. Patients with asthma have underlying bronchial hyperreactivity ("twitchy airways") and react to a multitude of allergic, chemical, irritative, emotional, and other factors. Acute severe asthma, leading to respiratory failure, is less common, but in 1982 more than 3,100 deaths occurred from asthma (1.4 per 100,000 population). The asthmatic may develop a sudden severe attack leading to death in less than an hour, but more commonly the patient has had increasing symptomatology over a period of days or weeks. Perhaps as many as one-half of these deaths are preventable if the patient seeks timely assistance and the proper therapy is instituted.

PATHOLOGY AND PATHOPHYSIOLOGY

Patients with stable asthma of varying severity have airway inflammation manifested by shedding or loss of the airway epithelium. In patients who develop acute severe asthma and die, the airway inflammation is marked with widespread mucous plugging of the airways, loss of epithelium and replacement with goblet cells, thickened basement membrane, vascular congestion, submucosal edema, eosinophilic infiltration, and smooth muscle hyperplasia. Mast cells are abundant and are free in the bronchial lumen, in the bronchial mucosa, and subpleural areas. The mast cells contain a large number of chemicals that, when released, have been shown to cause bronchospasm and mucosal edema (particularly histamine, leukotrienes, prostaglandins, and platelet-activating factor); to release chemotactic factors for neutrophils and eosinophils setting the stage for inflammation; to cause mucous secretion; and to cause desquamation and basement membrane thickening (particularly oxygen radicals, peroxide, and proteolytic enzymes). Allergens and other agents that stimulate mast cell degranulation can reach the luminal mast cells as well as those mast cells exposed by the diffuse airway inflammation that occurs in the asthmatic. If the stimulus is strong enough, sudden bronchospasm, in addition to marked intensification of the airway inflammation, can result in an acute attack, leading to respiratory failure. Physiologically this is manifested by a marked increase in residual volume and functional residual capacity, a normal or increased total lung capacity, and a marked decline in pulmonary flows (peak expiratory flow [PEF], forced expiratory volume in one second [FEV_1]). As the severity of the attack progresses, hypoxemia intensifies and the $PaCO_2$ rises from a low level to the normal range and finally to a level above normal. The presence of respiratory failure is heralded by a PaO_2 less than 55 mm Hg or a $PaCO_2$ greater than 45 mm Hg, an FEV_1 less than 1 liter or a PEF less than 80 liters per minute. Patients with these values are at great risk of dying and require immediate and intense therapy.

CLINICAL EVALUATION

The patient with acute severe asthma, particularly if he has acute respiratory failure, is severely dyspneic and fatigued and may have impairment of mental faculties. Rapid institution of therapy is essential; thus the historical review and physical examination must be efficient and brief. Once the patient has improved with therapy, a more detailed history and physical examination must be performed. It is important to ascertain the nature of the precipitating event, the duration of symptoms, and the medications and doses taken by the patient prior to his recent episode. The presence of other organ system disease, particularly cardiovascular disease, should be determined. A brief physical examination should be performed in search of signs of severe airway obstruction such as (1) respiratory rate greater than 25 per minute, (2) depressed diaphragms, (3) decreased diaphragmatic excursion, (4) distant breath sounds, (5) faint wheezing or rhonchi, (6) pulsus paradoxus, (7) hypertension, (8) sinus tachycardia, (9) cardiac arrhythmias, (10) fatigue, and (11) decreased mental clarity. The use of two or three sets of accessory muscles, a high level of pulsus paradoxus, a heart rate greater than 120 per minute, signs of fatigue, and decreased mentation all indicate existing or impending acute respiratory failure. Measurements of peak flow and/or FEV_1 should be obtained quickly to document the level of airway obstruction. Arterial blood gases should be measured rapidly to ascertain the degree of hypoxemia, the level of $PaCO_2$, and the acid-base status. Patients with acute respiratory failure (as already defined) should be placed in the intensive care unit for monitoring and treatment. A chest film should be obtained to determine whether a pneumothorax, pneumomediastinum, mucoid impaction, or pneumonia is present.

MANAGEMENT

There are two basic pathologic events that must be overcome with treatment: bronchospasm and airway inflammation, including mucous plugging. Bronchodilating agents are most effective against bronchospasm, whereas steroids and, if an acute infection is present, antibiotics are effective against airway inflammation.

Reversal of Bronchospasm

Beta$_2$ Agonists

The initial treatment should be instituted with the beta$_2$ agonists. Beta$_2$ agonists bind to beta-receptors on bronchial smooth muscle and mast cells. Adenylate cyclase becomes activated, leading to the production of intracellular cyclic AMP (cAMP). The cAMP then activates specific protein kinases, which in turn modulate the intracellular effects of the beta-agonists, including bronchodilation from smooth muscle relaxation and inhibition of the release of mast cell products.

Treatment should be initiated quickly with subcutaneous terbutaline, 0.25 mg, repeated at 30 and 60 minutes. Subcutaneous epinephrine could be substituted as the side effects are similar, but the duration of action is shorter (Table 1). As soon as it can be arranged, an aerosol of a beta-agonist, terbutaline, 1 mg diluted to 2 cc total volume by sterile water, should be administered via a hand-held nebulizer. A respiratory therapist should supervise the aerosol administration and monitor the patient properly. An aerosolized beta$_2$ agonist delivered by an IPPB device is contraindicated. Aerosolized terbutaline should be repeated in one hour and then at 2- to 4-hour intervals, depending on the clinical response. Other aerosolized beta$_2$ agonists are available (see Table 1), but these are associated with a higher incidence of side effects. Albuterol and fenoterol currently are not available in solution for nebulization; however, they can be substituted for terbutaline when they become available. The principal side effects of the beta$_2$ agonists are tachycardia, cardiac arrhythmias, shakiness, tremor, and muscle cramps. Potassium loss also may occur. If side effects occur with aerosol therapy, the dose can be reduced and/or the interval can be lengthened.

TABLE 1 Beta-Agonists Used in the Treatment of Acute Respiratory Failure in Asthma

	Mechanism of Action				*Drug Dosages and Route of Administration*		*Duration of Action*
Drug	*α*	B_1	B_2	*Subcutaneous*	*Aerosol**	*Intravenous*	*(hrs)*
Epinephrine	+	+	+	0.3–0.5 cc of 1:1,000 aqueous solution	2.5–12.5 mg per treatment	—	1–2
Isoproterenol	−	+	+	—	0.63–3.8 mg per treatment	0.04–0.225 μg/kg/min	1–2
Isoetharine	−	+	++	—	1.25–7.5 mg per treatment	—	2–3
Metaproterenol	−	+	++	—	10–15 mg per treatment	—	3–4
Terbutaline	−	±	++	0.25 mg	0.5–1.5 mg per treatment†	up to 0.5 μg/kg/min†	4–6
Fenoterol	−	±	++	—	0.5–1.5 mg per treatment†	up to 0.5 μg/kg/min†	4–6
Albuterol	−	±	++	—	0.5–1.5 mg per treatment†	up to 0.5 μg/kg/min†	4–6

* Optimal dose not established. Side effects limit doses used.
† Not FDA-approved.
Adapted from Plummer AL. Bronchodilator drugs in the cardiac patient. In: Kaplan JA (ed). Cardiac anesthesia. Vol II, Cardiovascular Pharmacology. New York: Grune and Stratton, 1983:586.

Theophylline

Another class of effective bronchodilators consists of the methylxanthines, of which theophylline is the major agent. Aminophylline is the ethylenediamine salt of theophylline. Theophylline increases the cellular level of cAMP by the inhibition of phosphodiesterase in bronchial smooth muscle cells and mast cells, but its major influence on bronchodilation may be its effect on the entry and intracellular distribution of calcium.

If the patient has not taken a theophylline product, an aminophylline loading dose of 6 mg per kilogram (ideal body weight) should be given intravenously over 20 to 30 minutes (Table 2). After that, a maintenance drip should be continued, the amount depending on the age and clinical status of the patient (see Table 2). If the patient has been taking theophylline products, an educated guess will have to be made as to whether the patient needs a partial loading dose before initiating maintenance therapy. If serum theophylline levels can be determined rapidly, it is preferable to draw blood for this test, start a maintenance drip, and adjust the dose after the serum theophylline level is reported. Once the adjustments have been made, a serum theophylline level should be drawn within 1 to 2 hours so that the serum level can be kept within the therapeutic range, 10 to 20 μg per milliliter. Therapeutically, a level of 15 to 20 μg per milliliter is preferable. If the serum theophylline level is not in the therapeutic range or needs to be increased (or decreased), an increase (or decrease) in aminophylline of 1 mg per kilogram ideal body weight will increase (or decrease) the serum theophylline level by approximately 2 μg per milliliter. To effect an increase, this dose should be given as a loading dose over 20 to 30 minutes, after which the intravenous maintenance dose for 24 hours should be increased by a similar amount. The serum theophylline level should be rechecked within 1 to 2 hours to ensure that a proper therapeutic level has been achieved. To effect a decrease, the 24-hour maintenance dose should be decreased by the amount calculated and the level rechecked in 18 to 24 hours. Theophylline is metabolized in the liver. Certain drugs and diseases affect theophylline clearance (Table 3); if any of these conditions is present, the maintenance dose of aminophylline must be adjusted accordingly (see Table 2). Theophylline metabolism is particularly slowed by congestive heart failure and liver failure, necessitating a markedly reduced maintenance dosage (see Table 2). Many of the side effects of theophylline are similar to those of the $beta_2$ agonists: tachycardia, cardiac arrhythmia, shakiness, in addition to nausea, vomiting, diarrhea, and seizure activity.

TABLE 2 Intravenous Aminophylline Dosage

Group	*Loading Dose* (Over 20–30 min)*	*Maintenance Dose**
Children: 6 mo–9 yr	6 mg/kg	1.2 mg/kg/h
Children: 9–16 yr Young adult smokers	6 mg/kg	1.0 mg/kg/h
Otherwise healthy non-smoking adults ≤50 yrs	6 mg/kg	0.8 mg/kg/h
Patients >50 yrs	6 mg/kg	0.6 mg/kg/h
Patients with cor pulmonale	6 mg/kg	0.3 mg/kg/h
Patients with CHF, liver disease	6 mg/kg	0.1–0.2 mg/kg/h

* Based on ideal body weight:
105 + 5 lbs per inch, above 5 feet (female)
106 + 6 lbs per inch, above 5 feet (male)

TABLE 3 Conditions and Drugs that Affect Theophylline Metabolism

	Decreased	*Increased*
Age	Prematurity Neonates	1–16 years
Smoking		Cigarettes Marijuana
Disease states	Hepatic diseases Moderate-severe CHF Acute pulmonary edema Cor pulmonale Pneumonia Acute viral illnesses	
Drugs	Oral contraceptives (smokers only) Cimetidine Erythromycin Lincomycin Troleandomycin (TAO)	Phenobarbital Benzodiazepines Alcohol

Both $beta_2$ agonists and theophylline have nonbronchodilator actions, including the inhibition of mast cell mediator release, an increase in mucociliary clearance, an improvement in diaphragmatic contractility, and a delay in diaphragmatic fatigue. All of these actions should be beneficial to the asthmatic who is in respiratory failure.

Reversal of Inflammation

Corticosteroids

The underlying inflammatory changes and mucous plugging probably are responsible for the initial irreversible component in patients with acute asthma. This component must be reversed in order to effect improved airflow in the patient. Corticosteroids probably have their greatest application in this reversal since they have anti-inflammatory properties. There is evidence that corticosteroids have other beneficial actions: a direct relaxation of bronchial smooth muscle; inhibition of the synthesis and release of chemical mediators such as histamines, leukotrienes, and prostaglandins; an improvement in mucociliary clearance and a decrease in mucous production; and a reversal in drug tolerance (tachyphylaxis) of $beta_2$ agonists. Intravenous steroids should be begun immediately in all patients in acute respiratory failure from asthma, since the beneficial effects of the steroids do not appear for 4 to 6 hours.

Initially, a loading dose of hydrocortisone, 4 mg per kilogram IV, should be given (Table 4). A continuous drip of hydrocortisone can be given, but because of the simultaneous administration of intravenous amino-

TABLE 4 Intravenous Corticosteroid Dosage

Drug	*Loading Dose**	*Maintenance IV Drip*	*Bolus Dose**
Hydrocortisone	4 mg/kg	0.5 mg/kg/h	4 mg/kg/q4h
Methylprednisolone	0.8 mg/kg	0.1 mg/kg/h	0.8 mg/kg/q4h

* Based on ideal body weight (see Table 2).

phylline, it is easier to administer boluses of hydrocortisone intravenously (see Table 4). These doses ensure a serum cortisol level greater than 150 μg per 100 ml, which appears to be necessary for optimum treatment. Intravenous methylprednisolone can be substituted for hydrocortisone (see Table 4). There usually are no side effects from high-dose intravenous corticosteroids over a period of a few days, nor is a state of steroid dependency induced. Well-known side effects, which occur with chronic therapy, are not evident. However, if corticosteroids are not instituted immediately or if an inadequate (low) dosage is given, the patient's condition could deteriorate or his hospital course could be unnecessarily prolonged.

Anticholinergic Agents

There have been no adequate studies on the efficacy of anticholinergic drugs used in the treatment of patients with acute asthma or acute respiratory failure from asthma. In acute asthma, the cholinergic system is stimulated by mast cell mediators and airway inflammation, leading to bronchoconstriction. Theoretically, the administration of an anticholinergic agent might be beneficial. If the patient has not responded satisfactorily to the bronchodilator agents, steroids, and other measures, atropine should be administered via a hand-held nebulizer in doses of 0.025 mg per kilogram every 4 to 6 hours. In order to achieve this dose, the pharmacy must have a concentrated solution available, since the stock solution comes in 1 mg dissolved in 2.5 cc, which is near the largest volume (around 3 cc) that one would want to nebulize. Side effects are dry mouth, headache, difficulties with vision and micturation, and tachycardia. A cogener of atropine, ipratroprium bromide, has yet to be released in the United States, but appears to be an effective bronchodilator agent that has few reported side effects, i.e., a bitter taste and dryness of the mouth or trachea. Atropine has been shown to decrease mucociliary clearance, but ipratropium bromide appears to have no effect on mucociliary clearance.

Relief of Hypoxemia

Oxygen

Oxygen therapy should be instituted in all patients who have a PaO_2 less than 60 mm Hg or have an A-a gradient greater than 35 mm Hg. Nasal O_2, 2 to 4 liters per minute, should be instituted immediately after the blood gas results are drawn and continued until the patient has shown significant improvement in gas exchange. A PaO_2 equal to or greater than 65 mm Hg should be maintained.

Other Measures

If the patient's condition was precipitated by acute bronchitis, a broad-spectrum antibiotic should be administered orally. Ampicillin or tetracycline, 500 mg every 6 hours, or trimethoprim 160 mg/sulfamethoxazole 800 mg every 12 hours should started. If bacterial pneumonia is present, the offending agent should be identified and the proper antibiotic(s) administered intravenously. The patient should receive intravenous hydration in order to thin the mucous. As much as 4 liters may be required during the first 24 hours, depending on the degree of dehydration. Thereafter, maintenance fluids can be administered.

Tranquilizers and sedatives are contraindicated because of their adverse effects on the CNS respiratory centers. Many deaths from asthma are directly related to the use of these agents. Other drugs are also contraindicated during acute asthma, including cromolyn sodium, atomized steroids, acetylcysteine, and beta-blocking agents. The former three inhaled agents may precipitate bronchospasm by irritation of the airways. Beta-blocking agents may promote bronchospasm by reducing the effect of $beta_2$ agonists.

MONITORING AND ASSESSMENT OF THERAPY

The patient should be carefully monitored by the nursing staff, the respiratory therapists, and the physician for changes in the symptoms and the signs of severe airway obstruction (already discussed). Timely monitoring of PEF and/or FEV_1 is essential. They should be monitored within the first 2 hours after the bronchodilator agents have been given and intravenous steroid therapy begun. A 20 to 25 percent improvement in pulmonary flows is desirable, but not always achievable. Pulmonary flows should be monitored every 4 to 6 hours until the patient shows significant improvement, after which time they can be monitored once or twice per day. Arterial blood gases should be repeated within 1 hour after oxygen therapy has begun to determine whether sufficient oxygen is being administered, the acid-base status, and the effect of therapy on $PaCO_2$. Usually progressive CO_2 retention is not a problem unless the patient has been sedated or fails to respond to therapy. The frequency of arterial blood gas determinations thereafter is dictated by the patient's clinical condition.

MECHANICAL VENTILATION

Prompt institution of therapeutic doses of $beta_2$ agonists, aminophylline, corticosteroids, and the other measures listed previously (Table 5) usually results in significant improvement of the patient's symptoms, physical signs, airflow, and gas exchange. Rarely, however, a patient may deteriorate in spite of intense therapy. If this occurs in a child, intravenous isoproterenol should be started using a dose of 0.1 μg per kilogram per minute (see Table 1), which should be increased by increments of 0.1 μg per kilogram per minute every 15 minutes until the PaO_2 begins to fall or a heart rate of 200 beats per minute is reached. Once improvement occurs, the dose can be decreased by 0.05 μg per kilogram per minute every 1 to 2 hours, depending on the continuing improvement in arterial blood gases and the patient's symptoms and signs. Intravenous isoproterenol has been used sparingly in adults because of cardiovascular side effects. A reasonable adult starting dose of isoproterenol is 0.04 to 0.05 μg per kilogram per minute (see Table 1). This dose can be increased by increments of 0.02 μg per kilogram per minute until clinical improvement occurs as well as a decrease in $PaCO_2$ and an improvement in pulmonary flows. Once improvement occurs, the dose can be decreased by 0.02 to 0.05 μg per kilogram per minute every 1 to 2 hours, depending on the continued improvements in arterial blood gases, pulmonary flows, and the patient's symptoms and signs. Intravenous albuterol, once it is approved by the FDA, would be a worthy substitute for isoproterenol (as would intravenous terbutaline or fenoterol) since side effects are decreased and cardiac function is improved (see Table 1). Every effort should be made to avoid intubation and mechanical ventilation because of the associated high morbidity and mortality.

If the patient deteriorates (demonstrates declining pulmonary flows, increasing $PaCO_2$, fatigue, and mental deterioration), if the patient develops superimposed sudden bronchospasm leading to cardiopulmonary arrest, or if the patient arrives at the hospital in a terminal state, he or she should be intubated with an endotracheal tube possessing a large-volume, low-pressure cuff and be ventilated with a volume mechanical ventilator. The use of a pressure-cycled ventilator is contraindicated.

Because of the high pressures required to overcome the airway obstruction, an intermittent manditory ventilation (IMV) set-up with a rate of 4 to 6 per minute should be used to improve ventilation. The ventilator tidal volume should be set at a volume that allows for 9 cc per kilogram ideal body weight plus the peak pressure times the compliance factor of the ventilator tubing. (The tidal volume usually is between 11 and 13 cc per kilogram ideal body weight.) Once the patient is receiving mechanical ventilation, sedation is required. Diazepam, 2.5 to 5 mg IV, or morphine sulfate, 1 to 2 mg IV, at appropriate intervals to maintain adequate sedation is helpful. If, in spite of these measures, the patient fights the ventilator or if the ventilator peak pressure rises above 60 cm H_2O, the patient should be paralyzed immediate-

TABLE 5 Flow Chart for Therapy of Acute Respiratory Failure in Asthma

*Time**	*Drug and Dosage*	*Monitor*
0–2 hours	Start the following rapidly and in sequence: 1. Subcutaneous terbutaline, 0.25 mg; repeat at 30 and 60 minutes 2. Aerosolized terbutaline, 1.0 mg in 1 cc H_2O; repeat in 1 hour 3. IV aminophylline, 6 mg/kg IBW† load over 20–30 minutes (*no* prior theophylline), then maintenance dose (Table 2) OR maintenance alone (if theophylline taken) 4. IV hydrocortisone, 4 mg/kg IBW† load, then 4 mg/kg IBW† bolus q4h 5. Nasal oxygen, 2–4 L/minute	1. FEV_1 and/or PEF before medication and after 2 hours 2. Stat serum theophylline 1–2 hours after load and maintenance began, if patient *not* on theophylline; measure theophylline before maintenance drip begun if patient on theophylline products 3. ABGs before O_2 therapy and again 1 hour after therapy begun
2 hours until chest wheeze-free or nearly so	Maintain the following medications: 1. Subcutaneous terbutaline *only* prn 2. Aerosolized terbutaline q2–4h initially, then q4h when improved 3. IV aminophylline maintenance drip 4. IV hydrocortisone, 4 mg/kg IBW,† q4h 5. Nasal O_2	1. FEV_1 and/or PEF q4–6h decreasing to once/day as patient improves 2. Maintain serum theophylline 15–20 μg/ml 3. Maintain PaO_2 ≥65 mm Hg 4. Measure ABCs only as needed to monitor $PaCO_2$ or PaO_2 changes
Switch to oral medications when chest wheeze-free or nearly so	Maintain the following: 1. Aerosolized terbutaline q4h during day and prn at night 2. Calculate 80% of the 24-hour aminophylline dose and give ½ of it q12h as long-acting theophylline tablets 3. Give prednisone, 30–40 mg q12h for several days, then 60–80 mg as a daily *am* dose 4. Stop oxygen when PaO_2 >60 mm Hg and A-a gradient <35 mm Hg 5. Begin education on home program	1. Measure peak serum theophylline level and maintain theophylline dose in 10–20 μg/ml range 2. Measure pulmonary function tests before discharge

* Time after first seeing patient
† Ideal body weight

ly with pancuronium bromide (0.06 to 0.1 mg per kilogram by IV bolus) to reduce the hazard of barotrauma. Sedation must be continued while the patient is paralyzed, and pancuronium bromide boluses, 0.02 to 0.04 mg per kilogram at varying time intervals, are needed to maintain paralysis. Once the patient is paralyzed, someone must be in the patient's room at all times. The ventilator rate must be increased to deliver to the patient a minute ventilation (rate × tidal volume) equal to 4 × the body surface area (BSA) for males and 3.5 × BSA for females, and a normal $PaCO_2$.

An FIO_2 should be provided to keep the PaO_2 at or above 65 mm Hg. During this period, aerosolized and intravenous bronchodilators, steroids, and other therapy should be continued. If ventilation sufficient to normalize pH cannot be accomplished or if the ventilator peak pressure cannot be kept below 60 cm H_2O, the ventilator tidal volume should be reduced and the pH normalized by administration of a bolus (44 to 88 mEq) of sodium bicarbonate followed by an intravenous drip (22 to 44 mEq per hour) of sodium bicarbonate. Once the peak pressure falls below 45 cm H_2O, the tidal volume can be increased and the sodium bicarbonate drip can be slowed and stopped. Once the patient's wheezing has nearly subsided and the peak pressure on the mechanical ventilator drops below 40 to 45 cm H_2O, the pancuronium bromide can be stopped, sedation lightened, and weaning begun. During the weaning period, respiratory therapists should monitor the vital capacity, tidal volume, inspiratory and expiratory forces as the IMV rate is decreased. The patient can be safely extubated if he or she is able to maintain a normal $PaCO_2$ with a PaO_2 at or above 65 mm Hg, a vital capacity greater than 15 cc per kilogram ideal body weight, an inspiratory force greater than −25 cm H_2O, and an expiratory force greater than +40 cm H_2O on an IMV rate of zero for 4 to 6 hours.

PREPARATION FOR HOME TREATMENT

Once the patient's symptoms have subsided, the signs of severe airflow obstruction (already discussed) have been reversed, and the patient has become wheeze-free or nearly so, the intravenous theophylline can be replaced by oral theophylline and corticosteroids while aerosolized bronchodilators are continued every 4 hours (see Table 5). The oral theophylline dose is calculated by taking 80 percent of the 24-hour dose of aminophylline and half the amount every 12 hours given with a sustained-released theophylline product. Intravenous steroids can be stopped, and a regimen of prednisone, 30 to 40 mg orally every 12 hours, can be started. Decisions on whether to reinstitute or start aerosolized steroids and/or cromolyn sodium should be made at this time (see chapter on *Chronic Asthma*). Oxygen therapy can be stopped if the PaO_2 is greater than 60 mm Hg and the A-a gradient is less than 35 mm Hg on room air.

The patient should be educated regarding the pathophysiology of asthma, the rationale behind the treatment program outlined for home care, and the use of MDIs or any other devices. The patient and responsible family members should be instructed in the technique of administering subcutaneous terbutaline (or epinephrine), which may be life-saving if a sudden, severe attack of bronchospasm occurs. Before going home, the patient should have a good grasp of the pathophysiology of asthma and understand the rationale behind the drug treatment program and the nature of side effects. He must know how to use a metered-dose inhaler and other equipment. He must receive written instructions for his home care program sufficiently in advance of discharge to allow time for discussion and clarification. The patient should return for follow-up 1 to 2 weeks after discharge.

SUGGESTED READING

Fanta CH, Rossing TH, McFadden ER, Jr. Glucocorticoids in acute asthma. A critical controlled trial. Am J Med 1983; 74:845–851.

Plummer AL. Bronchodilator drugs in the cardiac patient. In: Kaplan JA, ed. Cardiac anesthesia. Volume II, Cardiovascular Pharmacology. New York: Grune and Stratton, 1983, 581–605.

Scoggin CH, Sahn SA, Petty TL. Status asthmaticus. A nine-year experience. JAMA 1977; 238:1158–1162.

Westerman DE, Benatar SR, Potgieter PD, Ferguson AD. Identification of the high-risk asthmatic patient. Am J Med 1979; 66:565–572.

ACUTE RESPIRATORY FAILURE IN CHRONIC OBSTRUCTIVE PULMONARY DISEASE

ANTHONY S. REBUCK, M.D., F.C.C.P., F.A.C.P.
ARTHUR S. SLUTSKY, M.D.

Although the development of hypercapnia is regarded as the hallmark of respiratory failure, the life-threatening aspect of inadequate alveolar ventilation is usually its accompanying and inevitable hypoxemia. The objectives of therapy should be to improve oxygenation and, by treating the precipitating cause, reduce the work of breathing. Patients with chronic bronchitis suffer acute deterioration from a variety of causes: bronchoconstriction, cardiac failure, pulmonary embolus, pneumonia, or the excessive use of oxygen or sedation. By far the most common cause is an acute exacerbation of their chronic bronchitis, either as a result of infection or from heavy atmospheric pollution. So common is respiratory infection as the precipitating factor that an increase in sputum volume or a change in its color from whitish-gray to yellow or green should be interpreted as an indication for antibiotic therapy.

The objective of this chapter is to present a personal view of the therapeutic approach to patients with chronic airway obstruction who present with an acute exacerbation of their disease.

MANAGEMENT

The therapeutic modalities available to the physician all involve decisions to be made in the face of controversies, changing fashion, and the need for repeated evaluation of physiologic response. The questions that are most puzzling are:

1. What are the indications for antibiotics?
2. What is the ideal oxygen dose?
3. When is mechanical ventilation required?
4. What is the role of respiratory stimulants?
5. How can the patient be helped to clear his retained secretions?

In addition to the foregoing controversial issues, our views on bronchodilators, Digoxin, ventilator settings, and weaning protocols will be summarized in this chapter.

Dealing with Retained Secretions

Clearly the first priority is to secure a clear airway, thereby promoting appropriate ventilation and adequate oxygenation. Measures as simple as supervised coughing and changing the patient's position from side to side may be sufficient. The compassionate and constant care of a physiotherapist is ideal for this purpose; if a physiotherapist is not available, this care must be administered by the attending medical or nursing staff. Coughing of secretions is facilitated by inhaled bronchodilator treatment, our current approach being a combination of sympathomimetic and anticholinergic therapy. The regimen that we have found to best tolerated has been 1.25 mg fenoterol or salbutamol respirator solution plus 0.5 mg ipratropium in saline, nebulized and administered by mouthpiece over 10 to 15 minutes. We are, in general, cautious in our use of intravenous aminophylline, as the majority of presenting patients have been taking maintenance doses of slow-release theophylline preparations. Accordingly, bolus doses of aminophylline are not given unless it is definitely known that the patient has not been taking oral theophylline or until blood theophylline levels are available. Patients with a history of bronchial hyperreactivity or those who have previously required corticosteroids are given methylprednisolone, 50 mg intravenously, followed by prednisone, 30 mg per day in divided doses. Therapeutic aspiration of bronchial secretions by bronchoscopy or angle-tipped catheter is undertaken only when endotracheal intubation is required for assisted mechanical ventilation.

Treating Hypoxemia

In this group of patients, characterized by hypercapnia, oxygen enrichment of inspired air is mandatory, the goal being to achieve an arterial oxygen saturation of around 90 percent. Ideally, ear oximetry is used to register this end point, the alternative being an arterial oxygen tension of 55 mm Hg. Our preferred oxygen delivery system is one of high flow and low concentration, preferably 24 or 28 percent oxygen via masks based on the Venturi (or more correctly Bernoulli) principle. This approach ensures a known, constant inspired oxygen concentration, uninfluenced by the patient's pattern of breathing, and permitting calculation of the A-a O_2 difference. Alternatively, but less satisfactorily, oxygen can be administered at flow rates of 1 to 2 liters per minute by nasal cannula, adequate humidification being essential. Low-flow oxygen delivery by nasal cannula does not permit even an estimate of inspired oxygen concentration as entertainment of room air and altered ventilatory pattern influence the oxygen dose received. An oxygen-induced increase in $PaCO_2$ reflects a combination of (1) the reduced ability of oxyhemoglobin to carry CO_2 (Haldane effect), (2) removal of the hypoxic stimulus to breathe, and (3) worsening of ventilation/perfusion ratio ($\dot{V}/\dot{Q}$) inhomogeneities due to removal of compensatory hypoxic vasoconstriction. In any event, oxygen therapy should never be discontinued abruptly; the danger of inadequate oxygenation far exceeds that of hypercapnia. A rise in P_{CO_2} following oxygen administration indicates a need for more intense concomitant therapy, not for removal of the oxygen.

Ventilatory Support

Endotracheal intubation and mechanical ventilation is used if adequate respiratory effort cannot be maintained by assisted coughing, physiotherapy, bronchodilators, and supplemental oxygen. The situation is characterized either by deterioration in the level of consciousness or by a persistently high or rising Pco_2, causing significant respiratory acidosis (pH < 7.25) despite the best efforts of the health care delivery team to ensure a clear airway and adequate oxygenation. Intubation is conducted in the conscious patient after explanation and reassurance, the procedure being accompanied by careful use of sedatives. Owing to the altered pulmonary compliances in patients with COPD, positive-pressure ventilation can be associated with a relatively large increase in pleural pressure, leading to decreased venous return, increased pulmonary vascular resistance, and decreased left ventricular compliance, all tending to cause a decrease in cardiac output and arterial blood pressure. These cardiovascular complications can usually be treated adequately with intravenous fluids.

Volume-cycled machines are used, the settings arranged to deliver 6 to 8 liters per minute at a rate of less than 20 breaths per minute. As patients frequently experience difficulty synchronizing their ventilatory effort with the selected ventilator rate, a single dose of morphine is administered, and the machine is set in its "control" rather than "assist" mode. Inspired gas is subjected to a temperature-controlled heated humidifier. The timing of tracheostomy is a topic of considerable controversy, but it is our practice to perform this procedure electively in the operating room if weaning clearly cannot be achieved within 5 days. The cuffs of endotracheal tubes are deflated for a brief period every 2 hours, and strict asepsis is observed during tube manipulation or suctioning.

A number of maneuvers can be used to increase Po_2. If the patient has unilateral lung disease, oxygenation may improve greatly if he is placed in a position that causes the "good" lung to be dependent. Pulmonary blood flow is then preferentially distributed by gravity to the "good" lung, thus improving $\dot{V}/\dot{Q}$ inhomogeneity and blood gases. Another method to increase Po_2 at a given respiratory frequency and tidal volume is to increase inspiratory flow rate to 70 or 100 liters per minute, thus lengthening the time for exhalation. By allowing a longer time for exhalation in these patients with severe airflow obstruction, we probably improve ventilation to poorly ventilated regions.

Weaning

Weaning protocols are tailored to the individual patient, the length of the weaning period generally being related to the duration of mechanical ventilation. Weaning protocols are always initiated during the daytime; generally the patient is ventilated throughout the night during the first 24 to 72 hours of weaning.

We do not use respiratory stimulants, viewing them at best as short-term measures that stimulate nonrespiratory as well as respiratory muscles and thus increase CO_2 production. We concede that in acute situations respiratory stimulants may "buy time" and assist clearing of secretions, but confine their use to aminophylline, which may have a role in the treatment of diaphragmatic fatigue.

A common cause of failure-to-wean is respiratory muscle fatigue, and should it occur during an attempt to wean, mechanical ventilation should be resumed. The diaphragm is the only muscle that can cause the abdomen to protrude, thus indrawing of the abdomen during inspiration (paradoxical abdominal motion) is a sign of diaphragmatic fatigue. Similarly, indrawing of the rib cage during inspiration (rib cage paradox) can indicate accessory muscle fatigue. A common sign of respiratory muscle fatigue is alternating abdominal and rib cage paradoxical motion. This is usually associated with an increased respiratory rate.

If weaning proves to be difficult, a number of treatable conditions should be ruled out. An endotracheal tube that is too narrow can greatly increase the resistive work of breathing and make it difficult for a patient to wean. Adequate nutrition must be ensured, especially in patients who have not had sufficient calories for prolonged periods of time. However, care must be taken to avoid giving too many calories, because the increased CO_2 production (which usually only occurs during parenteral alimentation) may present an excessive load. Other metabolic causes should also be ruled out, such as hypophosphatemia, hypomagnesemia, hyperthyroidism, and muscle weakness, which can be caused by aminoglycosides.

Respiratory Infections

If an ambulatory patient with chronic bronchitis has a change in sputum color with an increase in sputum volume, with or without fever, a high white cell count, or infiltrate on chest roentgenogram, an oral broad-spectrum antibiotic is given. If the chest film shows a pneumonic infiltrate, every effort is made to isolate a specific pathogen. If the infiltrate has developed during the patient's hospital stay, a gram-negative pneumonia is suspected and treated appropriately.

Cardiac Failure

Digitalis is used only when biventricular failure develops; it is not prescribed for cor pulmonale. Diuretics are used if edema is present, but because of their tendency to cause metabolic alkalosis, our choice of agent is the carbonic anhydrase inhibitor Diamox, 0.5 g given intravenously on alternate days, with careful attention to fluid balance and hypokalemia.

SUGGESTED READING

Cherniack RM, Cherniack L. Management of acute respiratory failure. In:Cherniack RM, Cherniack L, eds. Respiration in health and disease. 3rd ed. Philadelphia: WB Saunders, 1983, 389–410.

McCaffree DR, Gray BA, Rogers RM. Respiratory failure. In: Simmons DH, ed. Current pulmonology. Vol. 2. Boston: Houghton Mifflin Professional Publishers, 1980, 135–160.

Roussos C, Macklem PT. The respiratory muscles. N Engl J Med 1982; 307:786–797.

Sykes MK, McNicol MW, Campbell EJM. Respiratory failure. 2nd ed. Oxford: Blackwell Scientific Publications, 1976.

OBESITY HYPOVENTILATION SYNDROME

RICHARD W. ROBINSON, M.D.
CLIFFORD W. ZWILLICH, M.D.

Without coexisting lung disease, obesity itself rarely causes significant respiratory dysfunction. However, a small minority of obese individuals develop a syndrome of alveolar hypoventilation and hypersomnolence. This entity, formerly called the Pickwickian syndrome, is more appropriately termed the obesity hypoventilation syndrome (OHS). This chapter will briefly review the clinical features and pathophysiology of this disorder and discuss in detail our approach to its diagnosis and management.

CLINICAL FEATURES

The triad of obesity, alveolar hypoventilation, and hypersomnolence is seen in all patients with the OHS. Obesity is frequently severe, and often a history of recent weight gain precedes clinical presentation. Occasionally, however, patients are only moderately obese. Alveolar hypoventilation results in arterial hypercapnia and hypoxemia, and these gas exchange abnormalities account for many of the clinical features, including pulmonary hypertension, right-sided heart failure, cyanosis, erythrocytosis, and headache. Left-sided heart failure is frequently seen also, and probably results from coexisting heart disease, systemic hypertension which may be particularly severe during sleep, and the expanded blood volume of obesity. Hypersomnolence is usually profound and often associated with serious adverse personal and vocational sequelae. The hypersomnolence is a direct consequence of severe obstructive sleep apnea seen with the OHS.

PATHOPHYSIOLOGY

Obesity imposes a variety of respiratory burdens that predispose to the development of hypercapnia. These include increased carbon dioxide production, decreased chest wall and lung compliance, increased work of breathing, abnormal breathing pattern, ventilation-perfusion mismatching, and respiratory muscle dysfunction. Despite these many disadvantages, the majority of obese people do not hypoventilate, and the correlation between body weight and arterial carbon dioxide tension is poor. Furthermore, OHS patients can normalize their arterial CO_2 tension with voluntary hyperventilation, implying that there is a basic defect in ventilatory control responsible for the hypoventilation. Markedly depressed ventilatory responses to laboratory-induced hypoxia and hypercapnia have been demonstrated in OHS patients. It is likely that a combination of this depressed chemosensitivity and the respiratory burden of obesity is required for the OHS to develop.

DIAGNOSIS

The diagnosis of OHS is easily made in the grossly obese patient with profound hypersomnolence. However, the clinical presentation is occasionally more subtle. For example, a moderately obese person may present with unexplained congestive heart failure, erythrocytosis, or a psychiatric disturbance. Correct diagnosis in such patients requires the determination of arterial blood gas tensions to demonstrate the presence of alveolar hypoventilation (hypercapnia).

In evaluating any patient with alveolar hypoventilation, it is essential to determine whether the hypoventilation is due to a mechanical impediment to breathing or to disordered control of breathing. Spirometry in OHS usually reveals a mild-to-moderate restrictive deficit that is not sufficient to cause alveolar hypoventilation. We find that measurement of arterial blood gases following a 2-minute period of voluntary hyperventilation is helpful. In OHS patients, CO_2 tension falls to or below the normal range and O_2 tension rises, indicating the basic defect in ventilatory control crucial to the pathogenesis of this syndrome.

Careful questioning of the patient or spouse usually reveals classic symptoms of obstructive sleep apnea. Overnight polysomnography should be performed in all obese, hypercapnic patients to document the presence and define the severity of sleep apnea. Many clinicians refer to obesity with obstructive sleep apnea as the OHS (Pickwickian syndrome). This is improper since the diagnosis of OHS requires the presence of awake hypercapnia, which is not seen in most sleep apnea patients. Moreover, obstructive sleep apnea clearly may occur in nonobese individuals.

Myxedema may present with a clinical picture of obesity and alveolar hypoventilation. In addition, hypothyroidism, particularly with obesity, is commonly associated with sleep apnea. Appropriate replacement therapy in these patients reverses all clinical manifestations, eliminating the need for high risk and more expensive therapeutic interventions. Therefore, we recommend excluding this diagnosis in all patients presenting with OHS.

MANAGEMENT

Appropriate treatment for the OHS is crucial; without proper therapy the mortality is high. Treatment should be individualized, depending on the severity of clinical manifestations. In less symptomatic patients, proper initial therapy may consist only of low-flow oxygen and a weight reduction program, whereas in patients presenting with severe gas exchange abnormalities and neurologic dysfunction, immediate intubation and mechanical ventilation may be necessary. The relative rarity of the OHS, together with the lack of controlled studies dealing with its management, requires us to warn the reader that our therapeutic recommendations are largely based on personal experience in treating this disorder.

Weight Reduction

A modest amount of weight loss (5 to 10 kg) is frequently associated with dramatic clinical improvement accompanied by improvement in arterial blood gases. Consequently, elevated pulmonary artery pressure falls with a lessening of symptoms of right heart failure. The effect of weight loss on nocturnal apnea is less consistent, but some patients have strikingly fewer episodes of apnea with reduced hypersomnolence.

It is likely that most OHS patients have a critical weight above which clinical manifestations are likely to occur. Patients themselves frequently recognize this fact. Accordingly, weight loss should be a primary therapeutic aim in OHS patients, particularly those with only moderate obesity and less severe manifestations. The help of hospital dieticians or nurses interested in nutrition may be invaluable in this regard. Unfortunately, sustained weight loss is usually difficult to maintain with diet alone. Surgical approaches to the treatment of obesity may be useful in carefully selected OHS patients. Gastric partitioning procedures are currently the most popular, but their long-term efficacy is still unproven. In addition, OHS patients, by virtue of their disordered ventilatory control and right heart failure, are probably more susceptible to postoperative respiratory failure, atelectasis, and thromboembolic complications. Until more data become available demonstrating the efficacy and safety of these procedures in patients with OHS or sleep apnea, we would only recommend their use in special circumstances (e.g., patient refuses tracheostomy and all other therapies have been unsuccessful).

Oxygen Therapy

Oxygen therapy for the OHS is rational since many of the clinical manifestations are direct consequences of hypoxia, and time may elapse before other therapeutic modalities (weight loss, progestational agents) exert their effects. Oxygen should be given by nasal cannula at low flow rates (2 to 4 liters per minute) to maintain an O_2 saturation of approximately 90 percent. Moderate amounts of worsening hypercapnia and acidosis may occur, but this does not contraindicate the continued use of supplemental O_2. In fact, these risks seem minor compared to the benefits of improved arterial O_2 saturation. Oxygen therapy is particularly warranted in patients with clinical signs of right heart failure, overt pulmonary hypertension, or erythrocytosis. A vigorous diuresis often ensues after institution of therapy, eliminating the need for diuretics. The effects of oxygen on obstructive sleep apnea are less clear. Episodes of apnea decrease in some patients. In others, although apnea duration is prolonged, the degree of O_2 desaturation is less with less dramatic increases in pulmonary and systemic arterial pressures during the apnea.

We recommend the use of 24-hour low-flow oxygen in virtually all OHS patients at the time of diagnosis. Therapy should be continued until other treatment interventions maintain an awake O_2 saturation greater than 90 percent. Nocturnal apnea and O_2 desaturation may persist even with improvement in daytime symptoms and blood gases. The role of nocturnal oxygen therapy in these instances is unclear. If used, its efficacy should be demonstrated by either overnight polysomnography or ear oximetry monitoring during sleep.

Progestational Agents

When progesterone is physiologically increased (pregnancy; luteal phase of menstrual cycle), hyperventilation and hypocapnia occur. The synthetic progestin, medroxyprogesterone acetate (MPA), if given to normal men, causes hyperventilation and increases both hypoxic and hypercapnic ventilatory responses. When given to OHS patients, MPA stimulates ventilation, thus normalizing arterial CO_2 tension and improving oxygenation, with resultant decreases in pulmonary artery pressure, right heart failure, and hematocrit. These effects are seen within a few days of drug administration and occur without weight loss. The effect of MPA on sleep disordered breathing in OHS is not known. Symptoms of hypersomnolence frequently improve, but the available evidence from nonhypercapnic sleep apnea patients suggests that MPA does not decrease apnea frequency or duration. We recommend the use of MPA in most OHS patients, particularly those with more severe hypoventilation and those in whom appreciable weight loss seems unlikely. Therapy with MPA may eliminate the need for more expensive and cumbersome daytime supplemental oxygen. Patients maintained on MPA should have a sleep study performed to determine whether more aggressive therapy directed toward obstructive sleep apnea is required. The recommended dose of MPA is 20 mg, either orally or sublingually, three times daily. Side effects are minimal except for impotence in some of these men.

Sleep Apnea Therapy

Severe obstructive sleep apnea is invariably seen in the OHS. The need for overnight sleep studies in all OHS patients has already been mentioned. These studies may been done prior to the institution of therapy in less severe cases, but may be done after beginning any of the aforementioned treatments in more symptomatic patients.

Tracheostomy is the most effective and time-honored treatment for obstructive sleep apnea. Newer modalities, including the use of nasal CPAP and uvulopalatopharyngoplasty, have recently become available. The former seems promising, but requires that the patient use cumbersome equipment each night. The latter is a major surgical procedure and is effective in only some patients. Many OHS patients respond dramatically to tracheostomy with improved sleep quality, diminished hypersomnolence, massive diuresis, and even improved daytime blood gases. Despite this, we do not routinely recommend immediate tracheostomy in OHS patients for several reasons. Tracheostomy is cosmetically unappealing and poorly accepted by many patients. In addition, the procedure is often technically difficult in these patients owing to their obese, short necks. Therefore it should only be performed by surgeons experienced in performing this procedure on such patients. Some OHS patients develop significant central apnea following tracheostomy. Thus, sleep disordered breathing may occasionally remain a clinical problem despite tracheostomy. Finally, in some patients a combined regimen of weight loss, low-flow oxygen, and progestational agents may sufficiently reduce apnea frequency and the severity of associated O_2 desaturation so that tracheostomy is not required. It should be mentioned, however, that the effects of these less aggressive treatment modalities on sleep disordered breathing in the OHS is not known. Therefore, we strongly suggest that overnight sleep studies be performed in all patients on these therapeutic regimens to document that severe nocturnal apneic desaturation is not occurring.

Despite attempts at more conservative management, many OHS patients eventually require a tracheostomy. The most common indications are failure of conservative management or the presence of such severe sleep apnea that the procedure is mandatory. Many patients have severe hypersomnolence with hundreds of episodes of apnea causing profound oxygen desaturation (less than 60%) and bradyarrhythmias each night. If a therapeutic response to oxygen or progesterone is to occur in such patients, it should be seen within several days. Therefore, a sleep study should be repeated within 5 to 7 days of instituting combined oxygen-progesterone therapy in these severely affected patients. If no improvement is seen, tracheostomy or other definitive therapy for obstructive sleep apnea is indicated. We treat persistent central sleep apnea following tracheostomy with nocturnal low-flow oxygen and progestational drugs.

Mechanical Ventilation

Some OHS patients present with such severe symptomatology and gas exchange abnormalities that immediate endotracheal intubation and mechanical ventilation are necessary. The abnormal upper airway anatomy of these patients may make intubation extremely difficult and potentially hazardous if attempted by inexperienced individuals. Several days of intubation and mechanical ventilation may benefit these patients greatly, and fear of ventilator dependence should not prevent this approach. Such therapy rests respiratory muscles, corrects hypoxemia, lowers CO_2 tension, and restores normal, apnea-free sleep. A vigorous diuresis may occur, and the patient may be in better condition to breathe independently after several days. Overventilation must be avoided to prevent severe alkalosis. Arterial CO_2 tension should only be lowered enough to maintain a normal arterial pH. Low concentrations of inspired oxygen (less than 35%) usually suffice to maintain adequate O_2 saturation (greater than 90%). If higher concentrations are required, an additional process (atelectasis, pneumonia, or thromboembolism) should be suspected. Therapy with medroxyprogesterone should be started after intubation in these patients.

Extubation may be attempted after at least 48 hours of mechanical ventilation provided the patient is reasonably alert, can maintain adequate oxygenation, and does not develop more than a few torr rise in arterial CO_2 tension after breathing low concentrations of inspired oxygen through a T-piece for at least 2 hours. The narrow pharyngeal aperture of OHS patients makes them vulnerable to severe upper airway obstruction following extubation from endotracheal tube-induced edema. Nebulized racemic epinephrine should be available for administration if this occurs, and personnel skilled at intubation and emergency tracheostomy should always be nearby. If extubation is successful, the usual therapies for OHS should be continued. If a patient cannot be weaned from the ventilator after several days, we recommend tracheostomy followed by a more gradual schedule of weaning, which incorporates a weight reduction program. These more difficult patients should be mechanically ventilated throughout the night during the weaning program. This not only rests respiratory muscles for the following day, but also insures against disordered breathing during sleep.

Other Considerations

The clinical course of many OHS patients is characterized by remissions and exacerbations. Common reasons for exacerbation include recent weight gain, obstructive lung disease, congestive heart failure, and use of central nervous system depressants. The difficulties in maintaining weight loss have already been mentioned. Obstructive lung disease should be vigorously treated with bronchodilators. Diuretics and digoxin should only be used for manifest left-sided heart failure. These agents are ineffective in treating right-sided heart failure and may produce dangerous side effects, including hypokalemia, metabolic alkalosis, arrhythmias, volume depletion, and azotemia. For predominantly right-sided heart failure, oxygen and progesterone are the appropriate treatment modalities. Central nervous system depressants such as alcohol, sedative-hypnotics, and narcotics are contraindicated in the OHS. They depress respiratory drive, resulting in greater hypoventilation, and worsen obstructive sleep apnea. These drugs should never be given as premedication for tracheostomy or other surgical procedures, as fatalities from complete upper airway occlusion have been reported following their administration to sleep apnea patients.

Prophylactic heparin therapy should be given to all hospitalized and immobile patients to reduce the high risk of thromboembolic complications. Erythrocytosis is commonly seen as a result of hypoxemia. Excessive amounts of erythrocytosis raise blood viscosity, increasing pulmonary and systemic vascular resistance. This results in impaired systemic oxygen delivery. Therefore, phlebotomy should be considered in all patients whose hematocrit exceeds 55 to 60 percent.

Finally, the mechanical burdens and ventilation-perfusion mismatching seen with obesity are worse when patients are in the supine position. Accordingly, OHS patients should be kept out of bed in a chair as much as possible, and when they are lying in bed the head of the bed should always be elevated.

SUGGESTED READING

Luce JM. Respiratory complications of obesity. Chest 1980; 78:626–631.

Morgan EJ, Zwillich CW. The obesity-hypoventilation syndrome. West J Med 1978; 129:387–393.

Rochester DF, Enson Y. Current concepts in the pathogenesis of the obesity-hypoventilation syndrome. Am J Med 1974; 57:402–420.

Sutton FD, Zwillich CW, Creagh CE, Pierson DJ, Weil JV. Progesterone for outpatient treatment of pickwickian syndrome. Ann Intern Med 1975; 83:476–479.

SLEEP DISORDERED BREATHING

DAVID C. FLENLEY, Ph.D., F.R.C.P., F.R.C.P.(Edin)
NEIL J. DOUGLAS, M.B., Ch.B., M.D., F.R.C.P.(Edin)

In recent years, disordered breathing and hypoxemia during sleep have become recognized in chronic obstructive lung disease (COLD: chronic bronchitis and emphysema), in bronchial asthma, and in the sleep apnea syndromes. However, it is also now apparent that irregular breathing in sleep, with some hypoxemia, is more common as age advances, as in apparently healthy normal subjects of both sexes aged over 55 years. This must dictate caution in prescribing therapy (which may be both expensive and carry side effects) for older patients with minor abnormalities of breathing patterns during sleep, if their ear oxygen saturation (SaO_2) does not fall below 80 percent for we do not yet know whether this carries adverse implications.

SLEEP DISORDERED BREATHING IN CHRONIC OBSTRUCTIVE LUNG DISEASE

"Blue Bloaters" and "Pink Puffers"

Patients with chronic airflow limitation, as indicated by persistently low peak expiratory flow rate (PEFR or FEV_1/FVC), tend to be either "pink and puffing," or "blue and bloated." "Pink puffers" are usually breathless, with marked chest hyperinflation, yet with relatively mild hypoxemia and low or normal arterial Pco_2. They have no cor pulmonale, normal pulmonary arterial pressure when at rest, and no secondary polycythemia. In contrast, "blue bloaters" are centrally cyanosed, usually have cor pulmonale, ankle edema (unless on diuretic therapy), pulmonary hypertension even when at rest, and secondary polycythemia. Their arterial hypoxemia is combined with a high Pco_2 even when in a stable state. The old idea that "pink puffers" have mainly emphysema and "blue bloaters" only bronchitis is not supported by detailed pathologic studies, and it is possible that the "blue bloaters" have a low hypoxic drive to breathing even before developing COLD, whereas "pink puffers" have a high drive at this time, but this still needs to be proved.

REM Hypoxemia in "Blue Bloaters"

"Blue bloaters" usually develop profound arterial hypoxemia during rapid eye movement (REM) sleep with irregular breathing (Fig. 1). Recent studies suggest that the degree of desaturation in REM sleep is predictable from the arterial oxygen saturation when awake. Thus a patient with COLD who is hypoxemic when awake is likely to become much more profoundly hypoxemic during REM sleep. Does this matter? In "blue bloaters" this profound transient hypoxemia can

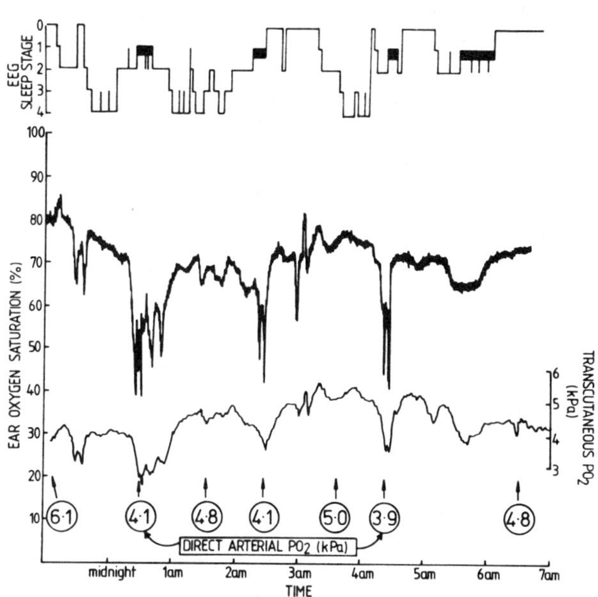

Figure 1 EEG sleep stage (1 = wakefulness, 4 = deep sleep, rapid eye movement (REM) sleep, ear oxygen saturation, and transcutaneous oxygen tension throughout the night in a patient with the "blue and bloated" pattern of chronic bronchitis and emphysema, showing severe transient hypoxemia during REM sleep.

increase pre-existing pulmonary hypertension and increase cardiac output, and is associated with irregular breathing and probably worsening of ventilation-perfusion relationships. Some of the depression and intellectual deterioration that are common in "blue bloaters" may be related to their sleep hypoxemia. In British trials of long-term oxygen therapy, those who died who were not receiving oxygen did so at night, whereas those who died despite long-term oxygen (always given during sleep) did so in the day. Thus, REM-associated hypoxemia in "blue bloaters" is probably dangerous and contributes to shortening of life, development of cor pulmonale, disturbed sleep, cardiac irregularities, and possibly intellectual deterioration.

MANAGEMENT

Oxygen Treatment

Two controlled trials have now shown that long-term domiciliary oxygen therapy, given for at least 19 hours in the 24 hours, can prolong life in hypoxic "blue bloaters." Some of this no doubt is due to relief of REM hypoxemia in sleep. I therefore use long-term domiciliary oxygen for such patients, provided they, when in a stable state (as shown by constant FEV_1 body weight, Po_2 and Pco_2 while receiving maximal therapy with diuretics, oral slow-release theophylline, inhaled $beta_2$ agonist, and ipratropium to give the best FEV_1), still show an arterial Po_2 below 55 mm Hg when awake. Most patients also have CO_2 retention, and strictly speaking, the trial results apply only to such patients. Formal polysomnography, with recording of EEG, SaO_2, and breathing movements throughout the second of two nights of sleep, is not necessary before long-term oxygen therapy is started in such "blue bloaters," nor is routine measurement of pulmonary arterial pressure (PAP). Nonetheless, it may be that long-term oxygen therapy has the most to offer if PAP falls by at least 5 mm Hg when oxygen, 2 liters per minute, is administered by nasal prongs, but this needs to be confirmed.

In Britain, long-term oxygen is most economically provided by an oxygen concentrator, but other systems, such as liquid oxygen (the only method of giving oxygen during exercise when away from home) or even oxygen in tanks, may need to be considered. Costs of this therapy are being reduced by oxygen-conserving devices, most of which are still experimental, but this is clearly a rapidly growing field. Modern concentrators are small and quiet, and many find that they are now acceptable in the bedroom, providing a flow of 1 to 3 liters of oxygen per minute delivered by nasal prongs. Oxygen masks are not used during sleep, but nasal prongs do stay in place and are well accepted. I do not give oxygen to patients who continue to smoke, as shown by carboxyhemoglobin levels (COHb) over 3 percent at two visits 3 weeks apart, because (1) long-term oxygen therapy does not reduce red cell mass in patients who continue to smoke, (2) death from burning can occur in people who smoke while receiving long-term oxygen therapy, and (3) I am disinclined to provide an expensive resource from the public purse to patients who will not help themselves by giving up smoking.

Almitrine

Drugs may also improve nocturnal hypoxemia in "blue bloaters." Almitrine, a new and still investigational French drug, stimulates the carotid chemoreceptors and improves ventilation/perfusion ($\dot{V}/\dot{Q}$) relationships. Almitrine, in a dosage of 50 mg twice daily by mouth, improves arterial Po_2 and reduces Pco_2 even in awake "blue bloaters," and can largely prevent REM-associated hypoxemia during sleep (Fig. 2), probably by improving arterial oxygenation when awake, this effect persisting into sleep. Almitrine does not impair EEG quality of sleep, but we do not yet know whether it is an alternative to long-term oxygen therapy, or whether Almitrine combined with oxygen therapy is

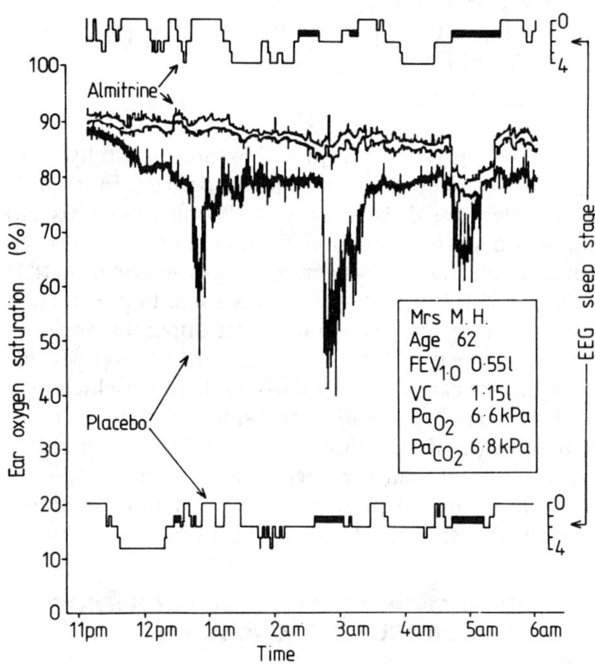

Figure 2 Ear oxygen saturation and EEG sleep stage recorded throughout the night in a "blue bloated" breathing air, on one night when he was receiving 50 mg of Almitrine by mouth twice daily for 14 days previous, and on another night when he had received a placebo tablet twice daily for 14 days before the sleep study. Note that Almitrine improves ear oxygen saturation and greatly improves hypoxemia in REM sleep, as compared to placebo effects. This result was entirely due to improvement in waking oxygen saturation as the arterial Po_2 probably fell by 10 to 15 mm Hg during sleep on both nights. However, as this fall was from a higher oxygen saturation, the curvilinear shape of the oxygen dissociation curve prevented this Po_2 fall being reflected in such a profound fall in oxygen saturation on the Almitrine night. (From Connaughton JJ, Douglas NJ, Morgan AD, Shapiro CM, Critchely JAJH, Pauly N, Flenley DC. Almitrine improves nocturnal oxygenation in patients with chronic bronchitis and emphysema. Am Rev Respir Dis 1985; 132:206–210.

even better. If the patient does not suffer from the "overlap syndrome" (to be discussed), any rise in arterial Pco_2 during sleep with oxygen is trivial, provided the patient is not in an acute exacerbation. Almitrine may have side effects such as peripheral neuropathy (which seems to resolve when the drug is discontinued) and a minor increase in pulmonary arterial pressure (PAP), which is of no importance at rest but can become more pronounced on exercise. However, the importance of these potential adverse effects, as compared to the undoubted improvement in Po_2 and PcL_2 with Almitrine remains to be determined by long-term trials.

Medroxyprogesterone Acetate

Medroxyprogesterone acetate (MPA) can stimulate ventilation in some patients with COPD. Although MPA can improve blood gases in a few patients, both awake and asleep, this action seems to be unpredictable, and most "blue bloaters" do not respond to MPA, whereas so far nearly all patients have responded to Almitrine. However, the only treatment so far *shown* to prolong life in "blue bloaters" has been long-term domiciliary oxygen therapy. I therefore use oxygen, but consider Almitrine for patients who will not quit smoking. Again, oxygen usually slightly lowers PAP during sleep in these patients, but although no measurements of PAP with Almitrine in sleep are yet available, measurements taken when the patient is awake and exercising suggest that such a fall in PAP is unlikely to occur with Almitrine.

THE "OVERLAP SYNDROME"

The confusing earlier literature on the effects of oxygen in the sleeping patient with COPD has led me to suggest the existence of the "overlap syndrome," a combination of obstructive sleep apnea with COPD. Few such patients have so far been described, but it seems probable that such common syndromes sometimes occur simultaneously in the same patient. The picture is emerging of an obese, smoking snorer with chronic airflow limitation, who has severe hypoxemia during sleep with widening of the baseline of the SaO_2 trace throughout the night owing to recurrent episodes of obstructive apnea with superimposed REM-associated hypoxemia (Fig. 3). These patients seem to be particularly prone to develop a potentially dangerous rise in Pco_2, with prolongation of sleep apnea, if given oxygen during sleep. I therefore now request a full polysomnographic study in a "blue bloater" who is somnolent or obese, particularly if he is a snorer. Oxygen at night could be dangerous in these patients, and they probably need nasal CPAP (to be discussed) or even permanent tracheostomy to correct the obstructive sleep apnea, as well as oxygen to correct the REM-associated hypoxemia.

All hypnotics are dangerous in patients with hypoxemia and CO_2 retention; these include barbiturates, nitrazepam, benzodiazapines, and alcohol. Weight reduction is good for any of these patients, but is particularly important in cases of the "overlap syndrome."

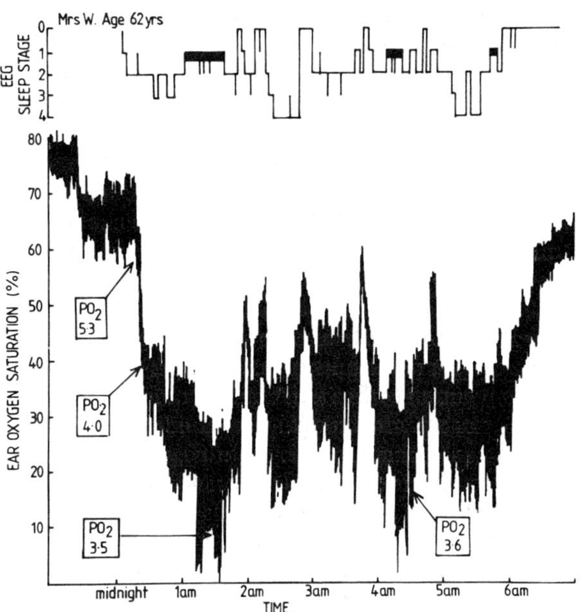

Figure 3 EEG sleep stage, and ear oxygen saturation throughout the night in a "blue and bloated" bronchitic who probably also suffered from obstructive sleep apnea, constituting therefore the "overlap syndrome." Note the thick baseline, presumably due to recurrent apneic episodes, compounded with more severe hypoxemia to profound degrees during rapid eye movement sleep.

BRONCHIAL ASTHMA

Most asthmatics, particularly young ones, say "yes" to the question, "Do you ever wake at night wheezy and short of breath?" Monitoring of PEFR at home (particularly recording it first thing in the morning and on awakening at night) clearly shows the problem. It seems probable that a child who is often awakened at night by his asthma will not perform well at school, or in examination, and increasing frequency of these wheezy awakenings suggests that a potentially life-threatening acute severe attack of asthma may be impending. These nocturnal awakenings are often associated with hypoxemia, SaO_2 falling to 80 to 85 percent, but this is not so profound as in "blue bloaters." Hypoxemic episodes probably also occur with nocturnal bronchoconstriction that does not awaken the patient, but this is difficult to prove. Exact mechanisms of nocturnal bronchoconstriction are still debatable, but a REM-associated bronchoconstriction is superimposed on a circadian pattern, with the lowest PEFR at 4 AM, when circulating catecholamines are also low in the asthmatic. The morning dip in PEFR and wheeziness are as common in atopic as in nonatopic asthmatics, disproving the earlier data that inhalation of the potent allergen of house-mite fecal pellets in sleep causes the bronchoconstriction.

What can be done about the nocturnal wheeze and hypoxemia? The mainstay of asthma treatment, inhaled $beta_2$ agonists, are rarely totally effective, as they last only 4 to 6 hours. Nonetheless, allergen avoidance studies suggest that maintaining the airways fully dilated does reduce bronchial hyper-reactivity in the asthmatic. Thus, good treatment of the asthma by day appears sensible, but in addition, specific therapy is required to control nocturnal awakenings. This is the particular role of slow-release theophyllines, the desired therapeutic plasma level of which is 10 to 20 μg per milliliter. I usually start with 225 mg Phyllocontin twice daily for a 70-kg adult, doubling the dose on retrial after 3 or 4 days if there is no anorexia, nausea, or undue tremor, unless the lower dose has already controlled the symptoms. I prefer to have the patient measure his own PEFR at home for the first week or so, to ensure that the morning dip has been adequately controlled. I also prescribe an inhaled beta$_2$ agonist, to be taken at bedtime to improve the amount of drug delivered to the lungs. High-dose inhaled topical steroids (250 μg beclomethasone, 200 μg Budesonide/puff) are also useful for such brittle asthmatics, and are administered by nebulizer in divided doses for a daily dose of 1,000 to 1,500 μg. However, such large doses can inhibit the pituitary-adrenal axis, causing aphonia and oral thrush both of which improve when the drug is discontinued. If this combination of inhaled topical steroid, slow release theophylline, and inhaled beta$_2$ agonist does not control noctural wheeze, oral steroids should be added, but if possible, never exceeding a dose of 10 mg per day in the adult, otherwise side effects almost certainly develop.

SUGGESTED READING

Barnes PJ, Greening AP, Neville L, Timmers J, Poole GW. Single-dose slow-release aminophylline at night prevents nocturnal asthma. Lancet 1982; 1:299–301.

Connaughton JJ, Douglas NJ, Morgan AD, et al. Almitrine improves oxygenation both awake and asleep in patiens with hypoxia and CO_2 retention due to chronic bronchitis and emphysema. Am Rev Respir Dis 1985; 132:206–210.

Douglas NJ, Calverley PMA, Leggett RJ, Brash HM, Flenley DC, Brezinova V. Transient hypoxemia during sleep in chronic bronchitis and emphysema. Lancet 1979; 1:1–4.

Flenley DC. Long-term home oxygen therapy. Chest 1985; 87:99–103.

Fletcher EC, Levin DC. Cardiopulmonary hemodynamics during sleep in subjects with chronic obstructive pulmonary disease. The effect of short- and long-term oxygen. Chest 1984; 85:6–14.

Goldstein RS, Ramcharan V, Bowes G, McNichols WT, Bradley D, Philipson EA. Effect of supplemental nocturnal oxygen on gas exchange in patients with severe obstructive lung disease. N Engl J Med 1984; 310:425–429.

PULMONARY EMBOLISM

THOMAS M. HYERS, M.D.

Standard treatment for pulmonary embolism and its antecedent, deep venous thrombosis, consists of heparin followed by warfarin. In patients with massive embolism who are hemodynamically compromised, thrombolytic agents can be given acutely followed by heparin and warfarin. In the most severely compromised patients, surgical removal of the embolus is attempted. In individuals with venous thromboembolic disease who are at high risk of bleeding or who have recurrence on adequate doses of heparin, placement of a vena caval filter can be lifesaving. In the past few years a great deal of progress has been made in prevention of venous thromboembolism. Each of these areas will be discussed in this article, and my approach to treatment and prevention of venous thromboembolism will be outlined.

MANAGEMENT

Heparin

Heparin is an acidic glycosaminoglycan and is a highly effective antithrombotic agent. Clinical preparations vary in molecular weight from 5,000 to 25,000 daltons, but the native molecule may be larger. Currently, smaller fragments of active heparin molecules are being tested clinically. The drug combines with a naturally occurring plasma inhibitor, antithrombin III, to make the inhibitor more effectively inactivate clotting factors, notably thrombin (factor IIa) and factor Xa. Heparin only works intravascularly in combination with antithrombin III. The unit of heparin is measured in animals using a biologic assay. Unitage may vary by as much as 50 percent on a weight basis, and consequently heparin is properly prescribed by units not by weight.

Intensity of Administration. Blood levels of heparin are not easily predictable, and specific plasma assays for the drug have not been widely applied. It is clear, however, that patients maintained on a constant blood heparin level via continuous intravenous infusion have fewer bleeding episodes than patients who receive intermittent intravenous bolus heparin treatment. In any heparin regimen, a minimum level of heparin anticoagulation must be maintained to achieve an antithrombotic state. In clinical terms this seems to mean that the activated partial thromboplastin time must be consistently prolonged beyond 1½ times the control value. Lesser degress of anticoagulation result in unacceptably higher rates of recurrent thromboembolism. Heparin requirements are usually greatest in the first few days after the acute thromboembolic event, and consequently therapy should be monitored most closely then. After the first few days, the monitoring tests usually can be obtained daily. It is wise to check a platelet count every 3 or 4 days when administering heparin since the drug can induce thrombocytopenia. Fortunately, this problem is rare. Use of heparin for periods longer than 3 months at doses over 15,000 units a day can lead to severe osteopenia.

If full-dose heparin is contraindicated for a patient with acute venous thromboembolism, as it would be for someone with an actively bleeding central nervous system lesion, the only acceptable alternative is vena caval interruption or filtering. Substitution of low-dose prophylatic heparin for full-dose heparin in this setting is inappropriate.

Duration of Anticoagulation. Heparin can be conveniently administered intravenously for 7 to 10 days to recovering patients. Unfortunately, such short periods of treatment do not seem to be sufficient in many patients with acute venous thromboembolic disease. Consequently, many clinicians use coumarin derivatives for long-term oral coagulation. The alternative is to give heparin to outpatients in a larger subcutaneous dose, which maintains the anticoagulated state.

TABLE 1 Antithrombotic Therapy with Heparin and Warfarin in Venous Thromboembolism

Disease suspected
Obtain baseline APPT,* PT,† and platelet count and give heparin bolus (7,500–10,000 units) intravenously. Order diagnostic test, e.g., ventilation-perfusion lung scan, pulmonary angiogram, contrast venogram.
Disease confirmed
Give loading dose of heparin (7,500 units) and start constant intravenous infusion at approximately 1,000 units/hr.
Monitor APTT at 4–6 hours and thereafter until the APTT is stabilized at beyond 1½ times control value.
Monitor platelet count while administering heparin.
Start warfarin early by instituting the estimated daily maintenance dose (usually 4–5 mg).
After at least 4 to 5 days of joint therapy, stop heparin and check PT 4 hours later.
Maintain PT off heparin at 1.25 to 1.5 times control value.
Full-dose anticoagulation for at least 3 months in patients without continuing risk factors, longer in other patients.

*APTT = activated partial thromboplastin time
†PT = one stage prothrombin time performed with rabbit brain thromboplastin (equivalent to a prothrombin time of 2 times control performed with human brain thromboplastin)

Coumarin Derivatives

These drugs are chemical derivatives of 4-hydroxycoumarin. They are well absorbed in the gut and transported in plasma bound to albumin. The drugs are metabolized by the liver and excreted in hydroxylated form in the urine. Coumarins act in the liver by inhibiting the synthesis of 4 vitamin K-dependent coagulation proteins, factors II, VII, IX, and X. The synthesis of a number of other vitamin K-dependent proteins is also impaired, although the significance of this inhibition is uncertain. The major mechanism of action seems to be the inhibition of a specific post-translational event in protein synthesis: the gamma carboxylation of multiple glutamic acid residues near the amino terminus of the polypeptide chains of the clotting factors. This failure of gamma carboxylation of glutamic acid interferes with the function of the proteins as clotting factors.

Coumarins do not act immediately since time is required for normal coagulation factors already present in the plasma to be cleared. This lag period varies according to the plasma survival times of the K-dependent factors, being shortest for factor VII and longest for factor II. Accordingly, the one-stage prothrombin time might appear therapeutically prolonged 24 hours after a large loading dose of warfarin because of the relatively short half-life of factor VII, but plasma levels of the other three factors would still be high. For this reason, it is more reasonable to initiate warfarin therapy early with an estimated daily maintenance dose and allow 4 to 5 days of overlap of heparin and warfarin before discontinuing heparin (Table 1).

Monitoring Coumarin Therapy. Therapy is most commonly monitored with the one-stage prothrombin time. The clotting time is measured after mixing citrated plasma with calcium and a well-characterized tissue thromboplastin. The major source of this lipoprotein is rabbit brain. Commercially available tissue thromboplastins vary in potency, and consequently prothrombin times with different thromboplastins are not always directly comparable; this has resulted in much confusion over the years as to the intensity of the anticoagulant effect required.

A major difficulty with coumarin therapy is the number of factors that influence coumarin metabolism and action. A complete review of these factors is beyond the scope of this article, but they can generally be divided into those that interfere with albumin binding of warfarin and those that increase or decrease the clearance of warfarin (Table 2). Other interactions can occur with changes in clotting fraction or concentration, with vitamin K absorption, and the introduction of separate hemostatic defects. The ideal patient for treatment with warfarin would be on no other drugs, would not use alcohol, and would be consuming a diet that contained a decreased but constant amount of vitamin K. Consequently, it is important that individuals receiving warfarin be instructed in a low vitamin K diet and that they adhere to this diet.

TABLE 2 Some Coumarin Interactions*

Enhancers (prolonged prothrombin time)	Suppressors (decreased prothrombin time)
Allopurinol	Adrenal corticosteroids
Anabolic steroids	Barbiturates
Clofibrate	Cholestyramine
Disulfiram	Diuretics
Hepatic disease	Griseofulvin
Hypermetabolic states	Hereditary resistance
Low vitamin K diet	High vitamin K diet
Metronidazole	Oral contraceptives
Phenylbutazone	Rifampin
Quinidine	Uremia
Trimethoprim-sulfamethoxazole	

* The use of any other drug with warfarin requires careful monitoring until stability of the prothrombin time is ensured.

Intensity of Coumarin Therapy. As with heparin, a minimum level of anticoagulation seems necessary to achieve the antithrombotic state. Recently, it has been recognized that because of the current potency of commercial rabbit brain thromboplastins in North America, the minimum effective level seems to be reflected by prothrombin time prolongation of 1.25 to 1.5 the control value. This level of anticoagulation is equivalent to two times prolongation of the prothrombin time when human brain thromboplastin is used. It should be noted that the less intensive anticoagulation recommendations for warfarin currently only apply to the treatment of venous thromboembolic disease. These results should not be extrapolated to other indications for warfarin anticoagulation until controlled studies are performed.

Duration of Anticoagulant Therapy. The duration of anticoagulation must be tailored to the individual patient. Patients with slowly resolving risk factors, e.g., prolonged immobilization, should be treated for at least 3 months; patients with tumors should be treated indefinitely. In many patients whose risk factors can be interrupted, the optimum length of treatment may be as short as 4 to 6 weeks. However, 2 weeks of anticoagulation does not seem to be sufficient. In the absence of well-controlled clinical trials on the duration of anticoagulation, the current recommendation would be a minimum of 3 months for the patient whose risk factors can be interrupted and longer for patients with continuing risk factors.

Complications of Anticoagulant Therapy

The major complication associated with coumarin use is hemorrhage. The incidence of bleeding is crudely related to prolongation of the prothrombin time, but bleeding also occurs in patients with prothrombin times prolonged only 1.5 to 2 times control value using rabbit brain thromboplastin. Any vascular site in the body can bleed with warfarin therapy, but many observers have been impressed with the frequency with which organic lesions (tumors, ulcers, cerebral aneurysms) bleed following induction of anticoagulant therapy. If bleeding is serious, warfarin effects can be reversed within 24 hours by large doses of parenteral vitamin K. More severe bleeding can be treated acutely with fresh frozen plasma infusions.

Much is made of the bleeding complications associated with warfarin and heparin, and for this reason it is instructive to remember the high mortality and morbidity rates associated with untreated and undertreated venous thromboembolic disease.

Another complication associated with the coumarins is a vascular purpura that causes skin necrosis and occurs occasionally in the first weeks of therapy. Coumarins cross the placenta and cause spontaneous abortion and specific embryopathies if given in the first trimester of pregnancy. There is also concern that warfarin may cause fetopathic effects during the second trimester of pregnancy and fetal bleeding during and after delivery. Consequantly, warfarin should be avoided during pregnancy, and heparin, given subcutaneously in adjusted dose, is the therapy of choice.

Cost-effectiveness of Anticoagulant Therapy

The most cost-effective anticoagulant therapy must prevent recurrent venous thromboembolism, have a low incidence of bleeding complications, and be easy and inexpensive to administer. A recently published cost-effectiveness analysis has ranked the different anticoagulation regimens. These regimens all begin with a 7- to 10-day course of intravenous heparin followed by long-term therapy for at least 3 months. Low-dose subcutaneous heparin as long-term therapy is ineffective and is associated with the highest cost due to recurrent venous thromboembolism. Less intensive oral anticoagulant therapy with warfarin is the most cost-effective and is associated with a low incidence of bleeding. More intensive warfarin anticoagulation effectively prevents recurrent venous thromboembolism, but is associated with a high frequency of bleeding. Adjusted-dose subcutaneous heparin is effective and is associated with a low incidence of bleeding, but it is slightly more expensive than the low-intensity warfarin regimen. Less intensive warfarin therapy should be chosen for long-term anticoagulation of most patients, and adjusted-dose subcutaneous heparin would be the treatment of choice for pregnant patients or those with hypersensitivity to warfarin.

Thrombolytic Therapy

Fear of bleeding and uncertainty about laboratory monitoring of thrombolytic agents have discouraged the use of thrombolytic agents for pulmonary embolism and deep venous thrombosis. Heparin, though an effective anticoagulant and antithrombotic agent, is not the ideal therapy for either condition. Chronic deep venous insufficiency develops in the affected leg of some patients with deep venous thrombosis, and chronic pulmonary hypertension develops in a few patients with pulmonary embolism despite heparin therapy. Thrombolytic agents offer the possibility of nearly complete thrombolysis in both of these settings. However, it is not clear yet whether these agents reduce the incidence of the postphlebitic syndrome or of chronic pulmonary hypertension following pulmonary thromboembolic disease.

The two purified thrombolytic agents currently available in the United States for clinical use are streptokinase (Kabikinase, Streptase) and urokinase (Abbokinase, Breokinase). Both agents work by activating circulating plasminogen to form the active enzyme plasmin that degrades fibrin clots, fibrinogen, and some clotting factors. Compared with heparin, both agents show similarly enhanced thrombolytic effects. Thrombolytic agents seem to be most useful clinically in acute massive pulmonary embolism in hemodynamically compromised patients and in acute deep venous thrombosis of the popliteal and proximal veins. Patients whose thrombi have occurred in the previous 5 days are more likely to respond than are patients with more prolonged symptoms. Both agents are given with an intravenous loading dose followed by a constant infusion. Based on clinical trials, streptokinase is recommended for 24 hours in pulmonary embolism and 48 to 72 hours in deep venous thrombosis. Urokinase is given for 12 hours in pulmonary embolism. (Urokinase is currently not approved for treatment of deep venous thrombosis.)

Close bedside observation of a patient receiving thrombolytic agents can be helpful in judging response. In the hemodynamically compromised patient with pulmonary embolism, blood pressure requires less support and oxygenation improves as therapy progresses. In the affected lower extremity, decreased swelling and improved color can be seen. Although clinical improvement does not always indicate complete thrombolysis, it is a useful noninvasive way to follow therapy, and some studies indicate reasonable correlation between clinical improvement and thrombolysis.

Minimizing bleeding. The contraindications to thrombolytic therapy are similar to those for anticoagulant therapy. Specifically, patients with any active bleeding process should be excluded. Also, patients who have undergone major surgery, childbirth, or major trauma within the previous 10 days should not be treated. Individuals who have had a stroke or undergone central nervous system surgery within the previous 2 months should not be treated. Relative contraindications include severe hypertension, coagulation factor deficiency, or any other propensity to bleed. If these exclusions are observed and patients with recent thrombosis are selected, thrombolysis can be expected, and an acceptable incidence of bleeding should result. A major caveat in regard to bleeding is that patients undergoing thrombolytic therapy should not be subjected to unnecessary invasive procedures. Arterial blood gas determinations should be strictly limited, and central placement of intravenous lines should be avoided if possible. No intramuscular injections should be performed.

In case of severe bleeding, thrombolytic therapy should be stopped and blood loss controlled and corrected. After 2 to 4 hours, the coagulation system usually returns to normal. If no further bleeding occurs, anticoagulation with heparin may be cautiously attempted to achieve a partial thromboplastin time greater than 1.5 times the control value.

Monitoring Thrombolytic Therapy. Any number of in vitro anticoagulant tests can be used to monitor thrombolytic therapy. One is seeking to determine that a "lytic" state has been achieved, at least as manifested by in vitro testing. In this way, prolongation of the partial thromboplastin time or thrombin time, elevation of fibrinogen degradation products, and lowered plasma fibrinogen levels all reflect the action of the thrombolytic agent. However, none of these tests correlates well with in vivo thrombolysis, and excessive reliance on laboratory testing complicates thrombolytic therapy unnecessarily.

The doses of thrombolytic agents have been chosen on the basis of clinical evidence that these doses activate the system in more than 90 percent of patients. Consequently, the need for any laboratory monitoring or dosage adjustment is minimal. I use a 10-second prolongation of the thrombin time or the activated partial thromboplastin time to indicate activation of the lytic state (Table 3).

Rarely, with streptokinase, the coagulation test remains unchanged after several hours of therapy. When this occurs, one can double the loading dose. If no effect is seen after infusion of the larger loading dose, streptokinase therapy should be stopped and either urokinase or heparin infused.

Restarting Anticoagulant Therapy. Since thrombolytic agents are rapidly cleared from the blood, one can simply turn off the infusion and wait 2 to 4 hours. If at this time the clotting test has returned to near baseline, heparin therapy can be restarted with a loading dose followed by a continuous intravenous infusion. The estimated daily maintenance dose of warfarin can also be instituted at this time. In this way, after 4 to 5 days, the heparin can usually be discontinued and warfarin continued for the necessary period of time for long-term anticoagulation.

Vena Caval Filtering

Current experience indicates that Greenfield vena caval filter is superior to other methods of vena caval interruption. However, no controlled studies have been performed comparing this method to other methods of vena caval interruption. The filter is usually inserted when a patient cannot be anticoagulated, either because of excessive bleeding or because of some absolute contraindication to anticoagulation. Other indications include recurrent embolism in the presence of adequate

TABLE 3 Using Thrombolytic Therapy in Venous Thromboembolism

Initial evaluation
- Suspect acute venous thromboembolism.
- Give heparin 7,500 to 10,000 u IV; order diagnostic test.

Diagnosis
- Positive pulmonary angiogram or contrast venogram.

Starting therapy
- Check contraindications to thrombolytic therapy.
- Show dissipation of anticoagulant: thrombin time or APTT within 10 sec of control value.

Thrombolytic infusion (12–72 hr)
- Deep venous thrombosis: streptokinase (48–72 hr)—250,000 IU/load; 100,000 IU/h
- Pulmonary embolism: urokinase (12 hr)—2,000 IU/lb/load; 2,000 IU/lb/h ; streptokinase (24 hr)—250,000 IU/load; 100,000 IU/h
- (Optional) 2–4 hr into therapy, show lytic state: thrombin time or APTT more than 10 sec beyond control.

Restarting anticoagulation (1–4 hr)
- Stop thrombolytic agent and show dissipation of thrombolytic effect: thrombin time or APTT within 10 sec of control.
- Start heparin and warfarin therapy as outlined in Table 1.

anticoagulation and as an adjunct to pulmonary embolectomy. The filter can be inserted from either the jugular or femoral route, and either route of insertion seems to result in an acceptably high long-term patency rate. Since recurrent venous thromboembolism does occur after insertion of the filter, anticoagulants should be reinstituted once the danger of severe bleeding is passed.

Surgical Pulmonary Embolectomy

In patients with greater than 70 percent occlusion of the pulmonary vasculature by pulmonary embolism, surgical embolectomy is probably the only method that will salvage a patient. The technique is performed either by cardiopulmonary bypass or, more recently, by transvenous suction catheter developed by Greenfield. Controlled studies have not been done to compare the two techniques of embolectomy to each other or to medical therapy. With proper use of anticoagulant therapy, preventive therapy, and thrombolytic therapy, pulmonary embolectomy should only rarely be necessary.

PREVENTION

Pulmonary embolism can now be prevented in nearly every high-risk patient with the large number of preventive regimens available. Low-dose subcutaneous heparin is effective and safe in most medical patients and surgical patients undergoing elective abdominal and gynecologic surgery. Patients at higher risk, including patients undergoing orthopaedic procedures of the lower extremity and urologic procedures, can be given effective prophylaxis with higher doses of heparin adjusted to achieve slight prolongation of the activated partial thromboplastin time, with less intensive warfarin therapy, with Dextran, and with intermittent pneumatic compression of the leg. In addition, a new combination of heparin and dihydroergotamine appears promising as a prophylactic agent in high-risk patients. Consequently, one cannot argue that prophylaxis is not available for high-risk patients. With more widespread application of prophylactic measures, the incidence of massive pulmonary embolism and unexpected postoperative fatalities from this event should decrease.

SUGGESTED READING

Greenfield LJ. Vena caval interruption and pulmonary embolectomy. Clin Chest Med 1984; 5:495–505.

Hull RD, Raskob G, Hirsh J, Sackett DL. A cost-effectiveness analysis of alternative approaches for long-term treatment of proximal venous thrombosis. JAMA 1984; 252:235–239.

Hyers TM, Hull RD, Weg JG. Antithrombotic therapy for venous thromboembolic disease. Chest, Suppl. Feb. 1986.

Sharma GVRK, Cella G, Parisi A, Sasahara AA. Thrombolytic therapy. N Engl J Med 1982; 306:1268–1276.

PRIMARY PULMONARY HYPERTENSION

LEWIS J. RUBIN, M.D.

Primary pulmonary hypertension (PPH) is a rare disease that is characterized by pronounced elevations in pulmonary artery pressure and pulmonary vascular resistance. It attacks primarily young women, although both sexes can be affected at any age. The symptoms associated with this disorder are nonspecific and are largerly manifestations of an impaired cardiac output, such as exertional dyspnea, chest pain, syncope, and lower extremity edema. The cause of PPH is unknown, and the prognosis is poor; most patients die from right ventricular failure within 3 to 5 years of the time of diagnosis.

DIAGNOSIS

A diagnosis of PPH can be established only by excluding conditions that secondarily raise pulmonary artery pressure. Accordingly, clinical evaluation should begin with a detailed history, particularly as regards prior use of illicit drugs, oral contraceptives, or appetite-suppressants since the use of these compounds has been associated with the development of pulmonary hypertension. Since a familial association with PPH has been reported, a detailed family history may provide clues to the diagnosis. Physical examination may disclose signs of systemic diseases that can cause secondary pulmonary hypertension, particularly the connective tissue diseases.

Laboratory evaluation should include (1) perfusion lung scanning or pulmonary angiography to exclude unresolved major vessel thromboembolism, (2) pulmonary function studies including a diffusing capacity for carbon monoxide and a chest roentgenogram to exclude significant parenchymal lung disease, and (3) a complete cardiac catheterization to exclude valvular or congenital heart disease.

Controversy exists whether an open lung biopsy should be performed routinely in patients suspected of having PPH. Proponents argue that diseases other than PPH that have not been suspected clinically are frequently diagnosed only by lung biopsy, while opponents feel that the risks of a surgical procedure in these hemodynamically fragile patients often outweigh the theoretic benefits. Our policy is to recommend an open lung biopsy only when a confident diagnosis of PPH cannot be made on clinical grounds because of conflicting or confusing clinical information. For example, a patient with evidence of pulmonary hypertension who has normal-appearing lung fields on roentgenogram and a mild-to-moderate restrictive defect and impaired diffusing capacity for carbon monoxide as demonstrated by pulmonary function testing poses a difficult challenge. Differentiating between PPH, which can be associated with a mild restrictive defect, and interstitial lung disease secondarily producing pulmonary hypertension has both therapeutic and prognostic significance and warrants further investigation.

MANAGEMENT

Vasodilators

There is neither a cure nor a definitive form of treatment available for patients with PPH. However, the pathologic findings of medial hypertrophy and muscular hyperplasia of the arteries and arterioles in the lungs of PPH patients suggests that active vasoconstriction may play a role in the pathogenesis of primary pulmonary hypertension, and has served as the rationale for approaching therapy with vasodilating agents. There is, at present, no selective pulmonary vasodilator, but several systemic vasodilators have been shown to exert pulmonary vasodilator effects in experimentally induced pulmonary hypertension. Although a variety of systemic vasodilators have been used to treat PPH with conflicting results, several important lessons can be learned from these disparate observations.

The major hazard entailed in administering a vasodilator to a patient with PPH is the risk of inducing life-threatening systemic hypotension if systemic vasodilation is unaccompanied by any pulmonary vascular effects. The possibility of encountering adverse hemodynamic effects is greatest when long-acting medications are administered intravenously. It is therefore advisable to evaluate an individual's "pulmonary vasoreactivity," using a potent, titratable intravenous agent that possesses a rapid onset of action but a brief half-life once the infusion is discontinued. I use prostaglandin I_2 (PGI_2, prostacyclin) in the routine evaluation of patients with PPH prior to instituting therapy with long-acting vasodilators. Although prostacyclin is not currently available for general use, intravenous nitroglycerin has been used in a similar role in some centers.

Patients who manifest a reduction in pulmonary vascular resistance of at least 20 percent in response to prostacyclin, resulting from either a decrease in pulmonary artery pressure or an increase in cardiac output, or both, are considered candidates for a trial of oral vasodilator therapy. Although there is controversy whether a fall in calculated pulmonary vascular resistance resulting primarily from an increased cardiac output without reducing pulmonary artery pressure may be considered a beneficial hemodynamic response, many patients who respond hemodynamically in this manner experience improvement in their symptoms. It is not known at this point whether vasodilator therapy prolongs survival in PPH.

The selection of an oral vasodilator is often difficult since there are few studies comparing the effects of these agents in the same patients. I have noted that individual patients may respond to one drug but not to others. Accordingly, it is best to approach the treatment of PPH with a carefully outlined protocol, employing the drugs that have been most extensively studied as the first line of therapy. At our institution we have had more experience with nifedipine and hydralazine than with other agents, and we therefore prefer to use these agents initially. Long-acting nitrate preparations have also been used successfully, particularly in patients who have developed side effects with the other drugs.

Although cardiac catheterization is associated with an increased risk of complications in PPH patients, I feel that it is important to evaluate the hemodynamic responses to vasodilators prior to embarking on continuous therapy. Empiric therapy should be avoided, since adverse hemodynamic effects do not always manifest themselves symptomatically. Noninvasive techniques of evaluating cardiac function to monitor the long-term effects of therapy such as radionuclide angiocardiography or echocardiography may become useful in the future, but there has been limited experience with these tools in this setting to date. For reasons of both patient comfort and safety, I prefer to repeat right heart catheterization several days after instituting oral vasodilator therapy rather than monitor hemodynamic parameters continuously for several days in an intensive care unit.

Anticoagulation

Patients with PPH are at risk for developing pulmonary thromboembolism by virtue of their low-flow circulatory state and sedentary life style, and sudden death occurs frequently. Additionally, the clinical differentiation between PPH and recurrent microthromboembolism is often difficult. Accordingly, I treat PPH patients with oral anticoagulants (coumarin) unless contraindications exist. Subcutaneous heparin (usually 10,000 to 15,000 units subcutaneously twice daily) adjusted to keep the partial thromboplastin time (PTT) 1½ times control may be a reasonable alternative in patients who have experienced bleeding complications with oral anticoagulants. A recently published retrospective study from the Mayo Clinic found that patients who were treated with anticoagulants lived longer than those who were not, supporting the potential importance of thromboembolism as a serious complication of this disease.

Cardiac Glycosides and Diuretics

Cardiac glycosides have no utility in the management of PPH unless supraventricular tachyarrhythmias are present. Diuretics are useful in controling edema once right heart failure develops, but with precautions against over-diuresis since the failing right ventricle is highly susceptible to changes in preload. I have seen good results with metolazone (Zaroxolyn) in low doses when an effective diuresis cannot be accomplished with increasing doses of furosemide (Lasix).

TABLE 1 Recommended Outline for the Diagnosis and Therapy of Primary Pulmonary Hypertension

I. History, physical examination, perfusion lung scanning and pulmonary function testing to exclude other conditions

II. Cardiac catheterization to confirm the presence of pulmonary hypertension and to exclude valvular, ischemic, or congenital heart disease

III. Incremental infusion of a short-acting vasodilator to evaluate pulmonary vascular responsiveness:

A. Prostacyclin (PGI_2), 1–12 ng/kg/min in incremental doses of 1–2 ng/kg/min every 15 minutes

or

B. Nitroglycerin, 0.5–4.0 μg/kg/min in incremental doses of 0.5 μg/kg/min every 15 minutes

IV. If pulmonary vascular resistance falls by >20% without an increase in pulmonary artery pressure, a decrease in cardiac output, or a symptomatic decrease in systemic artery pressure, begin therapy with an orally active agent:

A. Nifedipine, 10 mg PO t.i.d.–q.i.d., increasing to a maximal dose of 20–30 mg PO q.i.d.

or

B. Hydralazine, 10 mg PO q.i.d., increasing to a maximal dose of 50–75 mg PO q.i.d.

or

C. Isosorbide dinitrate, 5 mg PO q4–6h, increasing to a maximal dose of 25–30 mg PO q4–6h

or

D. Nitroglycerin patch, 5 mg daily, increasing to a maximal dose of 25 mg daily

V. If no contraindication to anticoagulation exists, begin oral coumarin and adjust dose to maintain prothrombin time at 1½ to 2½ times control.

VI. Trial of supplemental oxygen, 2–4 liters per minute by nasal cannula, for symptomatic relief of dyspnea.

VII. If unresponsive to vasodilators, consider referral for combined heart-lung transplantation.

Oxygen

The pulmonary vasodilator effects of supplemental oxygen in the setting of chronic hypoxemic lung disease have been well established, but oxygen usually has little hemodynamic effect in PPH since hypoxic vasoconstriction does not play a role in the pathogenesis of this disease. Nevertheless, low-flow oxygen occasionally provides partial relief from dyspnea, and a trial of oxygen therapy for symptomatic patients may be warranted.

Combined Heart-Lung Transplantation

Patients who are unresponsive to vasodilator therapy are candidates for combined heart-lung transplantation. Although the experience to date with this procedure is limited and the expertise is available at only a few centers, the results have been encouraging, particularly in light of the poor prognosis of this disease.

A suggested outline for the evaluation of patients suspected of having PPH and the institution of therapy is presented in Table 1.

SUGGESTED READING

Fuster V, Steele PM, Edwards WD, Gersh BJ, McGood MD, Frye RL. Primary pulmonary hypertension: Natural history and the importance of thrombosis. Circulation 1984; 70:580–587.

Peter RH, Rubin LJ. The pharmacologic control of the pulmonary circulation in pulmonary hypertension. In: Stollerman GH, ed. Advances in Internal Medicine. Chicago: Year Book Medical Publishers, 1983; 29:495–520.

Rubin LJ. Cardiovascular effects of vasodilator therapy for pulmonary arterial hypertension. Clin Chest Med 1983; 4:309–319.

Voelkel N, Reeves JT. Primary pulmonary hypertension. In: Moser KM, ed. Pulmonary vascular diseases. New York: Marcel Dekker 1979; 573–628.

PULMONARY REHABILITATION

JOHN E. HODGKIN, M.D.

Rehabilitation was defined by the Council on Rehabilitation in 1942 as the restoration of the individual to the fullest, medical, mental, emotional, social and vocational potential of which he or she is capable. Rehabilitation has found widespread use, particularly for patients with musculoskeletal and neuromuscular disorders, and rehabilitation programs for patients with cardiac disease have become popular. However, the application of the process of rehabilitation to patients with pulmonary disorders is relatively recent.

In an effort to clarify the meaning of pulmonary rehabilitation, an Ad Hoc Committee of the American College of Chest Physicians developed the following definition:

> Pulmonary rehabilitation may be defined as an art of medical practice wherein an individually tailored multidisciplinary program is formulated which through accurate diagnosis, therapy, emotional support, and education stabilizes or reverses both the physio- and psychopathology of pulmonary diseases and attempts to return the patient to the highest possible functional capacity allowed by his pulmonary handicap and overall life situation.

This statement was published in the American Thoracic Society's *Basics of Rd* series in 1975.

In the late 1970s, more and more pulmonary rehabilitation programs came into existence around the United States. Because of (1) the concern that some of these programs seemed to be more intent on making money by selling and servicing respiratory therapy equipment than on providing good care for patients, as well as (2) a recognition that the term "pulmonary rehabilitation" had different meanings to pulmonary specialists, an Ad Hoc Committee of the Scientific

Assembly on Clinical Problems of the American Thoracic Society developed a statement that not only defined pulmonary rehabilitation, but also listed the essential components of such a program. A pulmonary rehabilitation program should be able to provide all the services described in this official position statement of the American Thoracic Society, published in the November 1981 issue of the *American Review of Respiratory Disease.* This comprehensive statement includes a definition, recommended sequence, required services, expected benefits, and limitations of pulmonary rehabilitation. In defining pulmonary rehabilitation, this ATS statement concludes that "in the broadest sense, pulmonary rehabilitation means providing good, comprehensive respiratory care for patients with pulmonary disease."

The process of rehabilitation is most beneficial for individuals with chronic obstructive pulmonary disease (COPD), e.g., patients with emphysema, chronic bronchitis, bronchial asthma, bronchiectasis, or some combination of these disorders. However, certain aspects of care would also be appropriate for patients with other pulmonary disorders, e.g., restrictive disorders related to neuromuscular dysfunction and kyphoscoliosis. The two principal objectives of pulmonary rehabilitation are (1) to control and alleviate as much as possible the symptoms and pathophysiologic complications of respiratory impairment, and (2) to teach the patient how to achieve optimal capability for carrying out his or her activities of daily living.

Impairment and disability from pulmonary disorders constitute a significant economic concern. A Task Force from the National Institutes of Health (NIH) reported that the economic cost for patients with emphysema and chronic bronchitis in 1977 totaled $5.7 billion and for asthma patients in 1972 exceeded $1.5 billion. In addition, these figures do not take into account the cost in terms of human suffering. Rehabilitation for patients with respiratory disease can result in direct health benefits to patients and significant economic benefits to the country.

SEQUENCE OF PULMONARY REHABILITATION MEASURES

In order to develop an individualized comprehensive care program, it is helpful to follow a certain sequence, as was recommended in the ATS statement on pulmonary rehabilitation:

1. Select patient.
2. Evaluate patient.
3. Develop goals.
4. Outline components of care.
5. Assess patient's progress.
6. Arrange long-term follow-up.

Numerous factors can affect the success of rehabilitation including the presence of other coexisting disabling diseases, age, intelligence quotient, occupation, family support, and personal motivation. In general, however, any patient with symptomatic COPD is an appropriate candidate for pulmonary rehabilitation.

The initial evaluation of the patient should include spirometry, chest roentgenography, electrocardiography, and, in appropriate patients, arterial blood gas analysis, sputum analysis, blood theophylline measurement, and an assessment of behavioral considerations. An exercise evaluation as a preliminary to outlining an exercise training program is essential. Team members participate in this initial assessment to help determine the individual's needs. An evaluation of personal and environmental assets available to the patient, including potential employment skills and opportunities, family and social support, and community resources, is important in outlining an appropriate treatment program and long-term care.

It is essential that short and long-term goals be developed in conjunction with the individual and his or her family. One of the reasons patients and families become displeased with their physicians is that they have unrealistic expectations because physicians fail to develop and discuss goals with them.

A comprehensive treatment plan designed to meet the patient's needs is developed by the pulmonary rehabilitation team. Once the treatment plan has been implemented, the patient's progress needs to be monitored closely. Any necessary changes can then be initiated prior to the completion of the program. Crucial to successful rehabilitation of the patient is arrangement for long-term care. Generally, the responsibility for continuing care will be assumed by the patient's primary care physician. The pulmonary rehabilitation team should be willing to reassess the patient in the future if desired by the patient and/or referring physician. This allows for objective evaluation of the patient's progress as well as educational reinforcement.

COMPONENTS OF CARE

Pulmonary rehabilitation requires the use of individually tailored treatment modalities designed to help the patient achieve and maintain the highest functional capacity possible. The components of a comprehensive respiratory care program are listed in Table 1. Although all pulmonary rehabilitation programs have reported multiple benefits achieved by patients participating in their programs, there is not uniform agreement concerning the benefits derived from each individual component listed in Table 1.

General Care

Attempting to educate patients and their families about respiratory disease, its adverse effects, and the various treatment modalities utilized is a core part of most pulmonary rehabilitation programs. Helping a patient and his or her family to understand the underlying pulmonary disease process and the components of the treatment plan should improve the patient's motivation and compliance. There is a better chance of achieving the goals outlined by the team if the patient complies

TABLE 1 Components of Pulmonary Rehabilitation

- General measures
  - Patient and family education
  - Proper nutrition including weight control
  - Avoidance of smoking and other inhaled irritants
  - Avoidance of infection (e.g., immunization)
  - Proper environment
  - Adequate hydration
- Medications
  - Bronchodilators
  - Expectorants
  - Antimicrobials
  - Corticosteroids
  - Cromolyn sodium
  - Digitalis
  - Diuretics
  - Psychopharmacologic agents
- Respiratory therapy techniques
  - Aerosol therapy
  - Oxygen therapy
  - Home use of ventilators
- Physical therapy modalities
  - Relaxation training
  - Breathing retraining
  - Chest percussion and postural drainage
  - Deliberate coughing and expectoration
- Exercise conditioning
- Occupational therapy
  - Evaluate activities of daily living
  - Outline energy conserving maneuvers
- Psychosocial rehabilitation
- Vocational rehabilitation

with the team's recommendations.

Cessation of the smoking habit is critical to achieving optimal improvement. Reported benefits of discontinuance include improved appetite, reduced dyspnea, decreased cough and sputum, and improved pulmonary function. Nonsmoking has also been reported to reduce the risk of influenza. Multiple techniques have been advocated for curing the smoking habit. Most of these have similar success rates, i.e., 20 to 30 percent of those who quit smoking remain off cigarettes for one year after participating in the program. A strong recommendation from a nonsmoking physician is probably the most successful technique in getting patients to abstain from cigarettes. Nicotine chewing gum has been shown to be a helpful adjunct for some patients who are addicted to nicotine.

An initial nutritional assessment is important. A weight-reduction program for obese patients can lessen the work of breathing, resulting in reduced dyspnea. For patients who are losing weight inappropriately, a diet with adequate protein is essential to improve muscle strength. For patients who get full quickly in spite of consuming small amounts of food, multiple feedings, e.g., six feedings per day, can improve the caloric intake. For debilitated and anorexic patients, enteral alimentation may help to reverse the malnutrition. Proper nutrition should help the patient resist respiratory infections and may restore the ventilatory response to hypoxemia in severely malnourished individuals.

Adequate hydration, i.e, 10 to 12 glasses of fluid per day, is generally recommended to prevent the adverse consequences of dehydration. Yearly flu shots and a single dose of the pneumococcal vaccine are recommended to reduce the prevalence of these infections in patients with respiratory disease. The avoidance of large crowds when respiratory infections are prevalent may also reduce the risk. The use of a cold-weather mask or scarf over the nose and mouth may help to prevent cold-air-induced bronchospasm in patients with reactive airway disease. Air conditioners should be considered for patients living in hot climates. Moving from an area of high altitude to a lower altitude may be useful for patients with hypoxemia.

It is crucial to control rhinitis and sinusitis in COPD patients since aspiration of postnasal drainage into the airway can provoke significant airway irritation and inflammation. One must also be alert to the possibility of aspiration of refluxed gastric contents as a reason for exacerbations of chronic bronchitis or asthma. If either of these problems remains untreated, it becomes more difficult to achieve satisfactory improvement in the patient's respiratory status.

Medications

Although various medications are useful for patients with COPD, most of them have adverse effects. A judicious use of these agents is crucial to achieving optimal improvement for patients in a pulmonary rehabilitation program. In addition to relieving bronchospasm, bronchodilators have been reported to enhance mucociliary clearance and improve diaphragmatic contractility. Many COPD patients report a reduction of dyspnea after starting bronchodilator therapy, even though spirometric studies do not demonstrate a significant improvement following bronchodilator inhalation. Sympathomimetics are best utilized by inhalation since they work faster by this route and provoke fewer side effects than when the same medication is taken orally or parenterally. Oral, long-acting anhydrous theophylline preparations allow for administration only one to three times per day and complement the effect of sympathomimetics in patients with airway obstruction. Inhalation of atropine-type medications may be a helpful adjunct to sympathomimetic and theophylline-type bronchodilators in some patients.

Antimicrobials limit the airway inflammation that results from bacteria and should be used at the first sign of respiratory infection. Corticosteroids are clearly beneficial for patients with reactive airway disease. Inhaled corticosteroids, i.e., beclomethasone, flunisolide, and triamcinolone, provide benefit to the airways while avoiding the adverse consequences of systemic corticosteroids. Cromolyn sodium inhalation has been particularly helpful in young asthmatics, reducing the need for hospitalization and systemic corticosteroids. Digitalis is useful in patients with left ventricular failure and may be tried in patients with cor pulmonale. The dose of digitalis has to be monitored carefully in patients with COPD since hypoxemic patients are particularly sensitive to digitalis. Diuretics are indicated in both right and left heart failure. Potassium-sparing diuretics such as amiloride and triamterene should be considered in those who develop hypokalemia on thiazide diuretics or furosemide, thus eliminating the need for potassium chloride supplements. Psychopharmacologic agents should be considered for patients with anxiety or depression. Doxepin, which provides both tranquilizer and antidepressant effects, is generally free of significant adverse effects such as arrhythmias and respiratory center depression; when taken once daily, at bedtime, it can improve the quality of sleep.

Respiratory Therapy Techniques

Aerosol Therapy

Various solutions have been aerosolized, including bronchodilators, corticosteroids, mucolytic agents, bland mist, antimicrobials, and, most recently, cromolyn sodium. Inhaled bronchodilators and corticosteroids clearly benefit the airway while reducing systemic effects. There is little evidence, on the other hand, that inhalation of mucolytic agents or bland mist helps to liquefy lower airway secretions. If inhalation of a mucolytic agent, e.g., acetylcysteine, is tried, it should be combined with a bronchodilator to help prevent bronchospasm induced by the mucolytic medication. Inhalation of bland mist by an ultrasonic nebulizer may be of benefit in some patients with cystic fibrosis or severe bronchiectasis, but is not indicated for the usual patient with COPD. Aerosolization of an antibiotic such as gentamicin should only be considered in the patient who gets recurrent *Pseudomonas* pneumonias in spite of optimal care and adequate systemic antimicrobial therapy. Inhalation of gentamicin may reduce colonization of the airway with *Pseudomonas* and lessen the frequency of *Pseudomonas* pneumonias. However, this mode of therapy should be considered only rarely. Inhalation of corticosteroid or cromolyn sodium powder 10 minutes or so after bronchodilator inhalation may facilitate deeper inhalation and better deposition of the medication.

Various devices have been used to aerosolize medications including metered-dose cartridge inhalers, hand-bulb nebulizers, compressor pumps, and intermittent positive pressure breathing (IPPB) devices. The first choice for most patients is the metered-dose cartridge inhaler because it provides for immediate inhalation of bronchodilator from a compact portable device. Because of its ease of administration, there is a risk that patients will abuse the device by inhaling the medication too frequently. Spacer devices have been used with cartridge inhalers to (1) reduce side effects from inhalation of large particles and (2) facilitate administration in patients who have difficulty in coordinating inhalation with activation of the inhaler. By reducing large-particle deposition in the mouth, soreness of the oral pharynx from corticosteroids and systemic side effects from rapid absorption of bronchodilators through the oral mucosa may be minimized. However, most COPD patients are maintained satisfactorily without the use of these spacer devices. Rinsing the mouth with water after inhalation of corticosteroids may also lessen the prevalence of sore mouth and monilial infection of the oropharynx.

Hand-bulb nebulizers are difficult for older patients since they require repetitive squeezing of the hand-bulb for aerosolization of the medication. Although IPPB therapy has been used for many years in patients with pulmonary disorders, there is no evidence that continuous use of IPPB in outpatients has any advantage over less expensive and simpler methods of aerosol therapy. The recently completed National Heart, Lung and Blood Institute sponsored cooperative study comparing IPPB with compressor nebulizer therapy in outpatients with COPD showed no difference in morbidity or mortality between subjects in the two groups (Fig. 1). A compressor nebulizer does provide the opportunity to vary the concentration of the medication being administered and allows for administration of such things as liquid cromolyn sodium, atropine, and acetylcysteine.

Oxygen Therapy

In hypoxemic COPD patients, supplemental oxygen has been shown to help reverse pulmonary hypertension, cor pulmonale, polycythemia, and neuropsychologic dysfunction. The National Heart, Lung and Blood Institute study comparing continuous oxygen therapy with nocturnal oxygen only in COPD patients showed a definite advantage to continuous oxygen in patients with significant hypoxemia (Fig. 2). Specifically, patients with an arterial Po_2 of 55 mm Hg or less on room air or a Po_2 less than 60 mm Hg and evidence of right heart dysfunction, when stable, survived significantly longer with continuous oxygen than with nocturnal oxygen only. Patients who develop significant hypoxemia during exercise testing can improve their exercise tolerance by using supplemental oxygen during exercise training periods, and nocturnal oxygen is helpful for patients with sleep apnea or arrhythmias resulting from nocturnal hypoxemia.

Oxyen is usually administered to outpatients by means of a nasal cannula (nasal prongs). The goal is to achieve a PaO_2 of approximately 60 mm Hg in COPD patients. In patients with chronic CO_2 retention, achieving a PaO_2 greater than 60 mm Hg can result in worsening CO_2 retention and respiratory acidosis. Other devices or techniques for administering oxygen are currently being considered, including the use of reservoirs in close proximity to the nasal prongs, the use of only one nasal prong, and a transtracheal catheter to help reduce the amount of oxygen consumed. Administering oxygen through a transtracheal catheter has been reported to not only reduce the amount of oxygen required to maintain a satisfactory PaO_2, but to eliminate the undesirable consequences of nasal oxygen administration, i.e., nasal irritation and the adverse aesthetic effects of a visible oxygen cannula.

Several oxygen systems are available for providing

this gas. Cylinders or tanks of oxygen have been the usual source for oxygen. However, liquid oxygen devices are a popular means for providing portable oxygen to ambulatory patients. Oxygen concentrators (which concentrate O_2 by extracting nitrogen from the air) are advantageous for patients using higher flows of continuous oxygen since they eliminate the inconvenience and cost of having oxygen tanks delivered to the home on a regular basis. See Table 2 for a comparison of advantages and disadvantages of the various home oxygen systems.

Home Use of Ventilators

The transfer of ventilator-dependent patients from hospitals to extended care facilities and homes is becoming more common. It is far less expensive to care for these patients out of hospitals than to utilize intensive care unit beds or even acute care hospital beds. Home ventilator care has been used most commonly for patients with chronic respiratory failure from neuromuscular causes. However, since Medicare switched from a system of reimbursement that pays for care delivered to hospitalized patients to prospective reimbursement based on the patient's diagnosis, it is no longer profitable for hospitals to maintain ventilator-dependent patients in an acute care facility on a long-term basis. In addition, many patients would prefer to be on long-term ventilator support in their home rather than in a hospital. Careful planning and education of the patient's family, prior to transfer of these individuals out of an acute care facility, and the support of a home care agency are crucial for satisfactory care for these patients.

Physical Therapy Modalities

Relaxation Training

Listening to soothing music and biofeedback can reduce fear and tension in anxious patients. Techniques such as contracting and then relaxing skeletal muscle groups can help patients to cope with the stress and tension of COPD. Although these techniques are particularly useful for patients with asthma, they may also help some individuals with emphysema and chronic bronchitis.

Breathing Retraining

One of the most important elements of dyspnea or panic control is for the patient to slow the respiratory rate, with a prolonged exhalation, during acute episodes of shortness of breath. Slowing of the respiratory rate in this manner, with or without the use of pursed lips, results in improved ventilation and a reduced alveolar-arterial oxygen difference. Such a breathing pattern can also improve the patient's ability to exercise and carry out daily living.

Multiple studies have been published in the last several years evaluating respiratory muscle training. Inspiratory muscle training through voluntary hyperpnea can improve the patient's exercise capacity and increase respiratory muscle strength and endurance. Benefits are rapidly lost, however, if the training is not continued on a regular basis. I prefer to have patients achieve improved exercise capacity through an aerobic-type exercise training program whenever patients are capable of such training and reserve respiratory muscle training for patients who are incapable of participating in such a program, i.e., patients with paraplegia or degenerative arthritis of the lower extremities.

Cough, Chest Percussion, and Postural Drainage

Teaching patients how to cough properly can result in more effective expectoration. Postural drainage, accompanied by chest clapping, percussion, or vibration, has been recommended to help clear secretions from obstructed airways. In the outpatient setting, this technique should be reserved for individuals with large amounts of spu-

TABLE 2 Advantages and Disadvantages of the Three Home Oxygen Systems

	Advantages	*Disadvantages*
Cylinders	Most economical Can be stored for long periods without loss of oxygen Two or more cylinders can be joined together, resulting in fewer monthly deliveries	Heavy—cannot be carried or moved easily High pressure—potential explosive hazard Requires an expensive pressure regulator Frequent deliveries may damage carpets in patients' homes
Liquid	Reservoirs more attractive than cylinders Portable unit is lightweight Portable unit permits more time away from home Nationwide network of dealers makes traveling easy	Most expensive of the three systems Oxygen lost by venting when not used continuously Reservoir requires frequent refilling
Concentrators	Provides constant, inexhaustible home oxygen supply Attractive equipment Most economical for long-term oxygen use Negligible fire hazard Casters permit easy movement within the home	Increases monthly electrical expense Is relatively noisy Requires periodic maintenance by vendor Patients on continuous oxygen require portable cylinder when away from home Requires backup cylinder and regulator in event of electrical failure

From McLean DL. et al. Respiratory therapy techniques. In: Hodgkin JE, Zorn EG, Connors GL, eds. Pulmonary rehabilitation: guidelines to success. Boston: Butterworth, 1984.

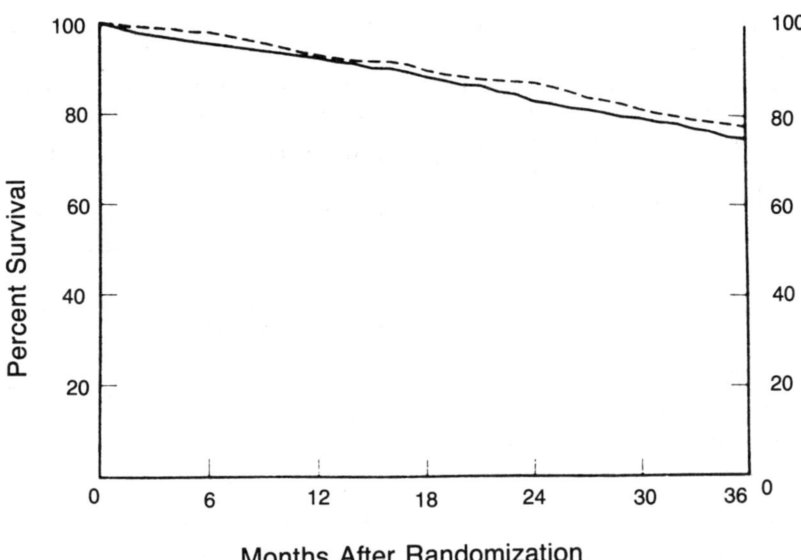

Figure 1 Survival of randomized patients. Dotted line = intermittent positive pressure breathing patients; solid line = compressor nebulizer patients. (From The IPPB Trial Group. Intermittent positive pressure breathing therapy of chronic obstructive pulmonary disease. Ann Intern Med 1983; 99:612–620.)

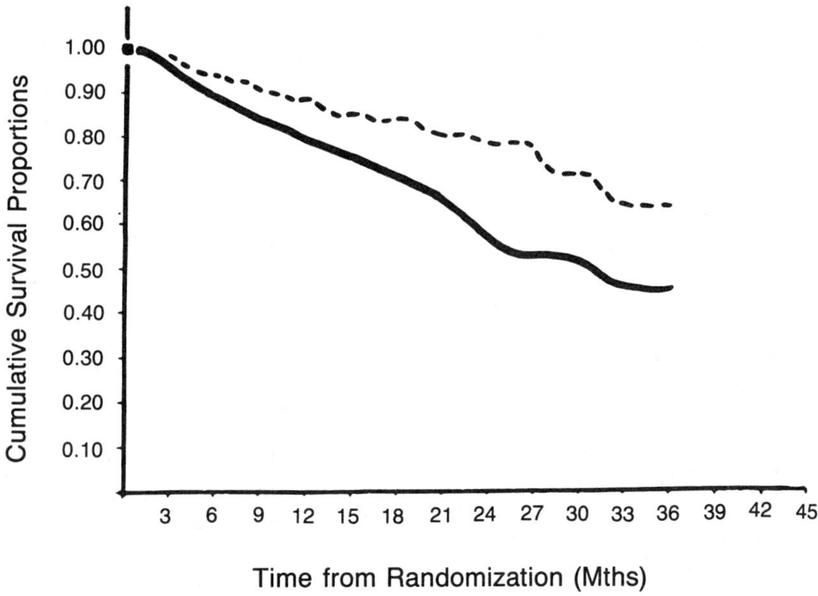

Figure 2 Overall mortality. Ordinate is fraction of patients surviving; abscissa is time from randomization of duration of treatment. Dashed line represents continuous O_2 therapy group; solid line represents nocturnal O_2 therapy group. Of the total group, 80 nocturnal O_2 and 87 continuous O_2 therapy patients were followed for 12 months, and 29 nocturnal O_2 and 37 continuous O_2 therapy patients were followed for 24 months. (From Nocturnal Oxygen Therapy Trial Group. Continuous or nocturnal oxygen therapy in hypoxemic chronic obstructive lung disease. Ann Intern Med 1980; 93:391–398.)

tum, i.e., greater than 30 ml per day, who are having difficulty expectorating the secretions spontaneously. There is no evidence that postural drainage is helpful in COPD patients with lesser amounts of sputum or with uncomplicated pneumonia. In addition, clapping and postural drainage have been shown to result in bronchospasm and temporary worsening of hypoxemia in patients with obstructive airway disease.

Exercise Conditioning

Many patients with COPD reduce their physical activity because of dyspnea and fatigue, resulting in a worsening cycle of deconditioning. Reported benefits of exercise training include an enhanced exercise capacity, improved ability to perform daily activities, increased tolerance of dyspnea, and improved appetite and sleep.

Some type of exercise evaluation should be performed to determine the ability and safety of exercise. A continuous incremental exercise test to maximum exercise capacity can be used for three basic purposes: (1) to determine the etiology of dyspnea, (2) to evalaute the level of impairment as part of a disability evaluation, i.e., to help determine the individual's ability to continue to work in his or her present occupation, and (3) to help in the outlining of an exercise training program that is appropriate and safe. If the only reason for the exercise test is to evaluate the feasibility and safety of an exercise training program, monitoring of heart rate and rhythm, blood pressure, and O_2 saturation at the level of work to be performed during the exercise conditioning program is acceptable.

There are four components to an exercise prescription: (1) mode, (2) intensity, (3) duration, and (4) frequency. To improve exercise tolerance significantly, one should train at 60 to 80 percent of his or her maximal oxygen consumption (about 70% to 85% of the achievable maximal heart rate), with sessions lasting 20 to 30 minutes, at least three times per week. In patients with COPD, the mode of exercise usually selected is walking, although some prefer swimming, bicycling out of doors, or using a stationary bicycle or treadmill indoors. Most pulmonologists recommend exercise sessions lasting 20 to 30 minutes, 3 or 4 times per week; however, the approach to determining the intensity of exercise to be used for COPD patients remains controversial. Target heart rates are commonly used in "normals" and in patients participating in cardiac rehabilitation programs; however, in patients with severe COPD, the heart rate may not be an accurate reflection of the level of oxygen consumption. Target heart rates generally can be used in patients with mild-to-moderate COPD.

Since patients with significant COPD generally cannot exercise to a high enough intensity to reach the predicted maximal heart rate, it would be more sensible to start exercising at approximately 70 percent of the peak heart rate on a maximal exercise stress test. An approach to selecting a target heart rate which takes both the patient's resting heart rate and maximal achievable heart rate into account was advocated by Karvonen. If a target heart rate is to be selected that would approximate 60 percent of the patient's maximal oxygen consumption, Karvonen's formula would be:

$$THR = 0.6\ (PHR\text{-}RHR) + RHR$$

where 0.6 = the factor for 60 percent of the patient's achieved maximal oxygen consumption

PHR = the peak heart rate achieved during a maximal exercise stress test

RHR = the patient's true resting heart rate, e.g., at home, first thing in the morning

If sophisticated exercise equipment is available, one can select, as the target heart rate, the heart rate at which the patient's oxygen consumption is approximately 60 percent of the achieved maximal oxygen consumption. When a target heart rate is selected, the patient should exercise at that heart rate with cardiac and O_2 saturation monitoring to determine the safety and appropriateness of that level of exercise. For some patients, particularly those with severe impairment of function, patients should simply be encouraged to exercise to tolerance, and a 12-minute walk test can be used to determine whether the patient is making progress with his or her exercise training program.

Supplemental oxygen can allow severely hypoxemic patients to achieve improved exercise conditioning. Supplemental oxygen at 2 to 4 liters per minute is recommended for patients in whom the PaO_2 is less than approximately 55 mm Hg or the oxygen saturation is less than approximately 87 percent before, during, or immediately after exercise. Oxygen should also be considered even when the PaO_2 or O_2 saturation is higher than these levels for patients with exercise-induced arrhythmia or myocardial ischemia.

Enhanced exercise tolerance generally results in greater independence and an improved sense of well-being. However, the increased exercise capacity is dependent on a sustained regular exercise training program at home.

Occupational Therapy

An occupational therapy evaluation can disclose tasks important to the patient that are precluded by functional limitations. The individual can then be taught alternative ways of performing these activities so that energy can be conserved and oxygen utilization minimized. The home assessment may disclose architectural barriers that can be altered, allowing the patient to function much more satisfactorily in his or her world.

Psychosocial Rehabilitation

Patients with severe COPD commonly exhibit emotional reactions such as depression, fear, anxiety, hostility, and denial, all of which impair functional capacity.

Psychotherapy, sometimes requiring a psychologist or psychiatrist, and the appropriate use of psychopharmacologic agents can help such patients to better cope with their disease process. Special attention should be paid to the common problem of sexual dysfunction since avoidance in this area can result in a failure to achieve optimal improvement in the patient.

Vocational Rehabilitation

Some patients are able to continue to work in their current occupations; however, many others need to either quit their jobs or modify the type of work performed. Proper evaluation and categorization of the patient's capacities are important.

The ability of a maximal exercise stress test to determine a patient's ability to work in his or her current occupation was described in an official position statement of the American Thoracic Society, published in the November 1982 issue of the *American Review of Respiratory Disease*. This statement concluded that if the oxygen consumption required by the patient's job exceeded 40 percent of the patient's maximal achievable oxygen consumption, the individual would not be able to sustain this work for an 8-hour period. Thus, determining the patient's maximal oxygen consumption with an exercise stress test and then comparing it with the oxygen requirement of the individual's job can be useful as part of the vocational rehabilitation process. If an individual is employed in an unhealthy environment, or progression of disease is anticipated and continued employment therefore unlikely, it may be beneficial to train the patient for a sedentary occupation in anticipation of the future course of the disease.

STRUCTURE OF THE PULMONARY REHABILITATION TEAM

A physician who is knowledgeable about respiratory disease is a key part of any pulmonary rehabilitation team. The physician should perform the initial history and physical examination and assist in developing the components of care appropriate for the individual patient. The specific provider of essential services may vary from program to program. A multidisciplinary team that includes a respiratory nurse, respiratory therapist, occupational therapist, physical therapist, dietician, social worker, chaplain, and psychologist or psychiatrist is particularly useful for programs to which large numbers of patients are referred and for teaching or research purposes. However, it is possible to perform a thorough assessment and deliver similar services with fewer individuals if they are appropriately trained in the evaluation and management of COPD patients. Pulmonary rehabilitation is generally accomplished in an outpatient setting. However, it is often useful to perform the initial evaluation and outline the treatment program while the patient is still hospitalized for an acute exacerbation.

Benefits of Pulmonary Rehabilitation

Most patients participating in pulmonary rehabilitation programs can expect to achieve the benefits listed in Table 3. In addition, some patients are able to continue or return to gainful employment.

The decrement in FEV_1 for the normal population is approximately 20 to 30 ml per year. The reported decrement in FEV_1 for patients with COPD is in the range of 40 to 80 ml per year. No study of patients participating in a pulmonary rehabilitation program has yet reported a significant alteration in the mean rate of decline in the FEV_1 in COPD patients with significant respiratory impairment. However, implementing therapy early in the course of a patient's disease may result in an alteration of the natural course of COPD, since it has been shown that a mild reduction in FEV_1 may be reversed in individuals who quit smoking. A cooperative study supported by the National Heart, Lung and Blood Institute to evaluate the results of early intervention in mild COPD, i.e., smoking cessation and bronchodilator therapy, is currently in progress.

Most pulmonary rehabilitation programs have reported that survival curves for patients with COPD are similar whether or not pulmonary rehabilitation is utilized; however, once again, this may be related to the fact that most of the patients in these reported studies had severe impairment of respiratory function at the time they entered the pulmonary rehabilitation programs. The possibility that a comprehensive pulmonary rehabilitation program, including close follow-up, may improve survival was suggested by the survival curve for patients in the NIH IPPB study (see Fig. 1), in which mortality was less for the 3 years of follow-up than in most previously published studies.

It seems reasonable that in order to achieve a significant reduction in the rate of deterioration of respiratory function and definite prolongation of life, good comprehensive care must be applied earlier in the course of the disease rather than waiting until severe, irreversible impairment of function is present. Prolongation of life has been reported in selected patients, such as those COPD patients with severe hypoxemia who use supplemental oxygen continuously.

TABLE 3 Demonstrated Benefits of Pulmonary Rehabilitation

Reduction in respiratory symptoms
Reversal of anxiety and depression, and improved ego strength
Enhanced ability to carry out activities of daily living
Increased exercise ability
Better quality of life
Reduction in hospital days required
Prolongation of life in selected patients, i.e., use of continuous oxygen in patients with severe hypoxemia

SUGGESTED READING

Hodgkin JE, ed. Chronic obstructive pulmonary disease: current concepts in diagnosis and comprehensive care. Park Ridge, IL: American College of Chest Physicians, 1979.

Hodgkin JE, Gray LS, Connors GA, eds. Pulmonary rehabilitation and continuing care (special issue). Resp Care 1983; 28:1419–1528.

Hodgkin JE, Zorn EG, Connors GL, eds. Pulmonary rehabilitation: guidelines to success. Boston: Butterworth, 1984.

Lertzman MM, Cherniack RM. Rehabilitation of patients with chronic obstructive pulmonary disease. Am Rev Respir Dis 1976; 114:1145–1165.

Petty TL, ed. Chronic obstructive pulmonary disease. 2nd ed. New York: Marcel Dekker, Inc., 1985.

Pulmonary rehabilitation: official ATS statement. Am Rev Respir Dis 1981; 124:663–666.

CARDIOVASCULAR DISEASES

UNCOMPLICATED MYOCARDIAL INFARCTION

AUBREY PITT, M.D., F.R.A.C.P, F.A.C.C.

The routine management of a patient presenting with an acute mycardial infarction (MI) includes measures to prevent complications. To this extent the concept of the uncomplicated case is contrived, but it has merit in facilitating discussion of the general and specific principles of management.

In this chapter, "uncomplicated" is defined as the absence of severe cardiac failure, cardiogenic shock, major arrhythmias, and conduction disturbances. Other chapters in this book address each of these problems.

PREHOSPITAL, DOMICILIARY, AND EMERGENCY ROOM CARE

The availability in many centers of specially equipped ambulances staffed by highly trained paramedical personnel has improved the mortality rate from acute MI, particularly mortality from ventricular arrhythmias. If such ambulance services are available, they should be used to transport patients with suspected infarction to hospital. Treatment that should be started in the prehospital phase includes relieving pain, inserting an IV line, monitoring cardiac rhythm, and correcting significant arrhythmias.

Domiciliary care has little or no role to play in the modern management of patients presenting in the early stage of acute MI. Occasionally, a patient is first seen 24 hours or later after an MI, a time when complications are unlikely. Management may be continued at home if the patient's condition and home circumstances are satisfactory.

Measures should be taken to expedite the patient's passage through the emergency room. Patients should not be detained in this area to wait for a diagnosis; this is the responsibility of the coronary care unit. If not already in place, an intravenous line should be inserted and rhythm monitoring started. Pain relief is mandatory; serum biochemistry studies should be performed, an electrocardiographic examination done, and chest films taken.

CORONARY CARE UNIT

All hospitals treating acute medical problems should have a coronary care unit (CCU) for patients with coronary artery disease syndromes, including acute MI. The unit's layout is important, with the best design having the nurses' station centrally placed surrounded by the patients in cubicles. This permits the nursing staff to maintain visual contact with each patient.

Although some institutions have nursing or technical staff who constantly observe the central monitors, this is an unnecessary expense. Appropriate ward design, with careful placement of the central and bedside monitors, can make this approach unnecessary.

Monitoring units with well-designed alarm facilities and suitable electronic storage and retrieval systems for cardiac arrhythmias are useful but not essential aids to patient management.

Although each patient's management should be individualized, there are advantages in having predetermined protocols that have been developed in consultation with all members of the unit, including nursing staff, physiotherapists, occupational therapists, and physicians. Such protocols should be widely distributed and displayed.

INVESTIGATION

Certain routine investigations are typically performed daily for 2 or 3 days. They include a full electrocardiographic examination and serum biochemistry studies, including blood urea nitrogen, electrolytes, and cardiac enzymes. It is usual to continue the last-mentioned until peak levels are established. Preferably, the enzyme profile should include a cardiac isoenzyme, such as creatinine phosphorinase (CK) MB. This is of particular importance if total CK elevation may have resulted from skeletal muscle release such as after an intramuscular injection.

A daily chest film is also recommended. At times, the film may show pulmonary venous congestion or even frank interstitial pulmonary edema, although cardiac failure is not apparent clinically.

Other typical investigations include those for serum glucose, full blood count, urinalysis, and serum lipids.

DIET

In the early phase of acute MI, there is no merit in a restrictive dietary program. A light but palatable diet is appropriate. Excess salt and fatty foods should be avoided. Specific diets previously prescribed for patients with diabetes mellitus or established hyperlipidemia should be continued.

NURSING CARE

No advantage accrues to confining patients with acute MI to prolonged bed rest. I allow patients to sit out of bed the day after admission. A written mobilization plan is helpful to patients and attending staff, and patients should use the bedside commode from the first day.

Appropriate physiotherapy should be administered early and should include breathing exercises, shoulder exercises to lessen the chance of peritendinitis, and leg exercises to lessen the risk of deep venous thrombosis.

REHABILITATION

Appropriate programs should begin the day of admission and be tailored to the patient's needs. An adequate explanation of the illness and the patient's future prospects is a vital part of proper care; the patient's immediate family should be included in these discussions. Written material, such as explanatory brochures, are invaluable in developing the patient's confidence.

Most patients leave the CCU after 48 hours and are discharged from hospital after 7 or 8 days. There is some advantage in having the patient enter an intermediate care or "step-down" ward after the CCU.

Formal rehabilitation programs should be implemented after hospital discharge. They facilitate rehabilitation and return to normal activities. Most patients recommence work 6 to 12 weeks after infarction, depending upon the severity of the infarct and the occupation.

SPECIFIC TREATMENT

Pain Relief

Apart from maintenance of the patient's comfort, evidence shows that early pain relief helps to ease the hemodynamic complications of infarction. The drug of choice is morphine, preferably given intravenously in a dose of 5 to 15 mg. If there is evidence of increased vagal tone, atropine (0.5 to 1.0 mg) should be given simultaneously. Other analgesics, such as meperidine, have only a limited role in suppressing pain from MI.

For patients with early postinfarction angina, the usual treatment is nitrates, often given as an intravenous infusion of nitroglycerin, 25 to 200 μg per minute.

Pericardial pain is common in the first 72 hours after transmural infarction and must not be confused with infarct extension. The pain of pericarditis is typically central, worsened by inspiration and coughing, and improved by sitting up and leaning forward. A rub is seldom useful. Pericardial pain usually responds to aspirin.

Control of Anxiety

The sudden precipitation of a patient into CCU can naturally cause severe anxiety. Explanation and reassurance are important. Occasionally, medication such as diazepam (5 to 10 mg) is appropriate. Rarely are the services of a psychiatrist required.

Lidocaine and Ventricular Arrhythmias

Although some units administer lidocaine routinely, there is no evidence that this lessens morbidity or mortality and it is therefore not recommended. As well, the use of lidocaine to suppress the "warning" arrhythmias is still controversial. Hence, current practice varies, but we continue to treat frequent ventricular premature beats (VPBs), multiform VPBs, R-on-T VPBs, couplets, and longer runs with lidocaine. A typical intravenous infusion rate of lidocaine is 2 to 3 mg per minute. In patients with cardiac failure in whom liver metabolism of lidocaine is impaired, the dose is decreased by one-third to one-half.

Electrolyte Control

Hypokalemia is common in patients with acute MI, particularly if they have previously received diuretic therapy. As hypokalemia promotes ventricular irritability, intravenous potassium chloride is often required. Serum potassium should be maintained at levels greater than 4.0 mEq per liter.

Less well documented is the importance of hypomagnesemia. In some patients, it appears to relate to ventricular arrhythmias, and treatment is indicated.

Diabetes Mellitus

This is a major risk factor in the development of coronary disease and is commonly seen in patients with acute infarction, either being known previously or first diagnosed in the CCU. Insulin supplements are often needed, at least in the first few days, and the dose should be individualized, depending upon blood glucose levels.

Incipient Cardiac Failure

Although cardiac failure is an important complication of acute infarction, its recognition and management are beyond the scope of this chapter. The initial features of cardiac failure can be subtle, and they may not be clinically apparent. An unexplained sinus tachycardia, particularly one that is present when the patient is asleep, may be the first sign. As stated previously, radiologic features may precede clinical signs. Early treatment with conventional medication is important.

Anticoagulant Therapy

No benefit has been established for the routine use of full anticoagulation in the acute or long-term management of patients with MI. Anticoagulation with heparin and warfarin is therefore reserved for specific indications, such as systemic embolism or an established deep venous thrombosis. A difficult judgment decision occurs when left ventricular mural thrombosis is seen on echocardiographic study, a common situation particularly with acute anterior wall infarction. We reserve anticoagulants for patients in whom the thrombus is observed to bulge into the cavity or to be mobile and not firmly attached to the ventricular wall. Full-dose anticoagulation is also routinely given to patients who have received thrombolytic therapy.

Pulmonary embolism is a rare complication of acute MI. However, deep vein thrombosis of the leg is common, occuring in as many as 30 percent of patients confined to bed because of a recent MI. Low-dose heparin is a useful prophylactic; the recommended dose is 5,000 units given every 12 hours while the patient has limited mobility.

Thrombolytic Therapy

The role of intravenous or intracoronary streptokinase (SK) or newer agents, such as tissue plasminogen activator, is not established. The role of such therapies in limiting infarct size and lessening morbidity and mortality is suggested by some but not all clinical studies. Pending more conclusive evidence, we do not recommend the routine use of intracoronary SK. Intravenous SK is more easily given and can begin earlier in the course of the infarction than can the intracoronary drug. In patients presenting within 4 hours of infarction with no contraindications, we administer 1 million units of SK intravenously over 30 minutes. Recent evidence, however, indicates that the intravenous route is not as efficacious as the intracoronary one.

Percutaneous Coronary Transluminal Angioplasty

Several reports confirm that angioplasty can be successfully performed in the acute stage of infarction alone or combined with the administration of a thrombolytic agent. Such treatment is not yet established and must still be regarded as experimental. Less controversial is the established role of coronary angioplasty in the management of postinfarction angina.

Beta-Adrenergic Blockage

Several studies from Europe and the United States have established that mortality is lowered in patients receiving metoprolol, timolol, or propranolol after acute MI. Such benefit has been demonstrated to continue for more than 2 years. Evidence shows that patients with certain high-risk features, such as previous infarction, poor ventricular function, diabetes mellitus, arrhythmias, and hypertension benefit most from long-term treatment. However, it is not always easy to predict which patients are most likely to benefit from beta-blockade. We therefore recommend treatment in all patients in the absence of contraindications such as hypotension, bradycardia, or obstructive airway disease. We begin treatment before hospital discharge, a typical regimen is metoprolol, 50 to 100 mg twice daily. Beta-blocking drugs with intrinsic sympathomimetic activity may not confer the same advantage as those drugs without such activity.

Recently, two studies specifically addressed the role of intravenous beta-blockade that was started within 24 hours of infarction in lowering early mortality and morbidity. Only marginal improvement has been demonstrated, and we do not routinely use early beta-blockade in the absence of a specific indication, such as hypertension or arrhythmias.

Because of widespread use of beta-blocking therapy, as many as 30 percent of patients who present with acute infarction are already receiving therapy. Beta-blockade should then be continued unless there are specific contraindications.

Calcium-Channel Blocking Therapy

There is no evidence that such treatment alters either short- or long-term morbidity or mortality. Specific indications for calcium antagonists are few, most typically when coronary artery spasm is likely to be present. In patients receiving calcium-channel blockers at the time of presentation, the medications are usually continued.

Treating Hypertension

An aggressive approach to controlling hypertension is important during both the acute and later stages of MI. The first step is to relieve pain. If hypertension persists, several options are available. For rapid control, nitroprusside, started at 0.5 μg per kilogram per minute, is given intravenously, and the dose is adjusted upward as required. Intravenous administration of nitroglycerin is less efficacious, but it is occasionally used. Ongoing treatment consists of conventional therapy with emphasis on beta-adrenergic blockade.

Hemodynamic Monitoring

It is fashionable in some units to use a Swan-Ganz catheter for tenuous indications. We recommend measurement of intracardiac pressures or cardiac ouput only when specific indications exist, such as hypotension or cardiac failure.

Limiting Infarct Size

Various strategies have been tried to limit infarct size, including beta-blockade, calcium antagonists, nitrates, steroids, thrombolytic agents, angioplasty, intra-aortic balloon pumping, and acute coronary artery surgery. No method is of proven efficacy.

FOLLOW-UP INVESTIGATIONS

Exercise Stress Testing

There is evidence to show that an exercise stress test is a useful noninvasive way to determine which patients may require coronary angiography and interventional therapy with angioplasty or surgery. Some clinicians perform a modified test before hospital discharge. I prefer to delay the test a few weeks and then perform a full-symptom limited test. If it causes ECG ischemia and chest pains at a low work load, coronary angiography is usually recommended.

If the ECG stress test is equivocal or cannot be done (for instance, in the presence of a left bundle branch block) nuclear stress testing with thallium myocardial perfusion imaging or gated blood-pool scanning is used.

Coronary Angiography

I routinely recommend angiography in younger patients—arbitrarily defined as younger than age 50 years. I also perform it if stress testing is positive at a low work load, indicating reversible ischemia. The development of early postinfarction angina is a further indication for coronary angiography.

Testing for Ventricular Arrhythmias

There is accumulating evidence that ventricular arrhythmias are important predictors of death, particularly sudden death, in the first year after an MI. Evidence of electrical instability may be observed clinically and specifically pursued, using stress testing as well as electrophysiologic laboratory testing and Holter monitoring. The appropriate role for these latter has not yet been established, and they cannot be recommended as routine investigations. A new approach, not yet established, is the analysis of after-potentials as evidence of fragmented ventricular electrical activity.

In conclusion, the mortality from uncomplicated MI is low. Many of the management decisions are aimed at anticipating complications and preventing further progression of the disease. As yet, no clear role has emerged for techniques designed to limit infarct size or for routine prophylaxis against major rhythm disturbances. However, there is accumulating evidence that functional testing and anatomic assessment with coronary angiography can identify patients in whom active interventions with medication, angioplasty, or surgical revascularization are appropriate.

ARRHYTHMIAS AND CONDUCTION DISTURBANCES COMPLICATING MYOCARDIAL INFARCTION

ARTHUR J. MOSS, M.D., F.A.C.C.

Cardiac dysrhythmia—including atrial and ventricular ectopic beats, as well as various types of atrioventricular and intraventricular conduction disturbances—are frequently observed during both the coronary care unit and the in-hospital convalescent phases of acute myocardial infarction. The clinical significance of these arrhythmias, their requirements for treatment, and the type of therapy that is indicated are determined in part by the potential risk posed by the arrhythmia, the patient's comorbidity, degree of hepatic and renal dysfunction, and the age of the patient. Each patient is different, and there is no simple therapeutic algorithm or formula that is universally applicable for all patients with a given arrhythmia. Rather, therapy needs to be tailored to each patient, and in many clinical situations the wisest course of action is to observe and monitor the arrhythmia without specific therapeutic intervention. In this chapter, general as well as specific therapeutic guidelines are provided for major cardiac dysrhythmias which frequently complicate the hospital phase of acute myocardial infarction. However, the treating physician must appreciate the fact that the protocols which follow are guidelines only and that they require updating and modification in terms of newly introduced drugs and the unique aspects of each clinical situation.

VENTRICULAR FIBRILLATION

Ventricular fibrillation may appear with or without premonitory ventricular arrhythmias, and defibrillation with 400 joules should be carried out immediately if less than 2 minutes have elapsed after the onset of the observed fibrillation. With longer elapsed times, full cardiopulmonary resuscitation should be provided with establishment of a clear airway and adequate ventilation before initiating external cardiac massage and the defibrillating shock. When the elapsed time is longer than 4 minutes, or the initial countershock is ineffective in defibrillating the heart, or both, cardiopulmonary support with oxygenated ventilation and external massage should be used as a temporizing measure. During this time, the rapidly evolving metabolic acidosis should be corrected with sodium bicarbonate, 80 mEq IV bolus, and defibrillation reattempted. If a fibrillation rhythm persists, more aggressive cardiopulmonary, metabolic, and antiarrhythmic support should be provided, including additional sodium bicarbonate and bretylium tosylate, 300 mg IV. Once an intrinsic cardiac rhythm is established—either supraventricular or ventricular in origin—effective oxygenated ventilation should be continued; blood pressure maintained with dopamine, 1 to 10 μg per kilogram per minute, if the systolic blood pressure is less than 100 mm Hg; and antiarrhythmic therapy initiated with lidocaine, 100 mg IV bolus, followed by a constant IV drip at 3 mg per minute. An additional 75 mg IV bolus of lidocaine should be given 10 minutes later if the patient was not receiving antiarrhythmic therapy before onset of the ventricular fibrillation. In a patient with large infarction complicated by hypotension, recurrent ventricular fibrillation may occur, necessitating intra-aortic balloon counterpulsation to achieve hemodynamic stabilization in addition to the aforementioned pharmacologic measures.

VENTRICULAR ECTOPIC BEATS: EARLY CORONARY CARE UNIT PHASE

During the first 48 hours of an acute myocardial infarction, ventricular ectopic beats with varying frequency and complexity are almost always present. Although ventricular fibrillation may occur without preceding ventricular ectopy, patients with increasingly frequent ventricular ectopy—particularly those manifesting early-cycle and repetitive patterns—are at an increased risk of primary ventricular fibrillation. Generally, intravenous antiarrhythmic medication should be administered prophylactically when contact is first made with the patient, regardless of whether or not ventricular ectopy is evident. If during coronary-care unit monitoring, ventricular irritability is evident despite "routine" antiarrhythmic prophylaxis and correction of metabolic factors, such as hypoxia and hypokalemia, then upward dose adjustment of the initial agent or change to a second drug is indicated. In patients younger than age 75 years without evidence of heart block, I start with a loading dose of lidocaine, 100 mg IV bolus, followed in 10 minutes with a 75-mg IV bolus; concomitantly, I initiate maintenance intravenous lidocaine therapy at a dose rate of 40 μg per kilogram per minute which in the average 70-kg adult approximates 3 mg per minute. I maintain the lidocaine for 48 hours. This therapy usually suffices to control ventricular irritability, has been associated with a marked reduction in the incidence of primary ventricular fibrillation, and is generally well tolerated. If ventricular irritability is not adequately suppressed, an additional 50- to 75-mg IV bolus of lidocaine should be given and the dose rate increased to 60 μg per minute (4 mg per minute). At this dose rate, adverse and toxic side effects—such as slurred speech, confusion, hypotension, or seizures—may develop with sustained lidocaine administration, and the patient must be monitored closely.

If lidocaine is not effective in controlling frequent, early-cycle, or repetitive ventricular ectopic beats and rhythms despite a full-dose regimen, I usually switch to procainamide, another class-I antiarrhythmic agent that is pharmacodynamically similar to lidocaine. For reasons that are not clear, some patients respond more favorably to procainamide than to lidocaine, and vice versa. Thus, if the initially chosen agent is not effective, it is worth trying a sister drug. The dosage schedule for procainamide is roughly the same as that for lidocaine. The major adverse effect of short-term intravenous procainamide therapy is hypotension, but it occurs in only a small percentage of patients.

If recurrent, complex, and potentially life-threatening ventricular irritability persists during the early phase of myocardial infarction despite full-dose lidocaine or procainamide therapy, the addition of beta-blocker therapy should be tried. The combination of a class I antiarrhythmic agent (lidocaine or procainamide) with a class II beta-blocker, such as propranolol, frequently results in effective control of the more troublesome ventricular irritability. Propranolol has potent antiadrenergic effects, and it results in a reduction in the heart rate and the myocardial oxygen consumption—two results that favorably influence myocardial oxygen balance and reduce the ischemic contribution to ventricular irritability. If blood pressure permits and overt pulmonary congestion is absent, propranolol should be initiated at a dose of 20 mg PO every 6 hours with a progressive increase in the dose to 60 mg PO every 6 hours if the drug is well tolerated. If complex ventricular rhythms persist, especially runs of ventricular tachycardia, despite the administration of combined class I and class II antiarrhythmic agents, special therapy with investigational agents may be required, and appropriate consultation or referral is indicated.

In patients older than age 75 years, the risks of therapy with potent antiarrhythmic agents are considerable. Hence, I do not routinely administer prophylactic antiarrhythmic agents to patients in this older age group. Rather, I simply observe nonlife-threatening ventricular irritability and initiate therapy only when repetitive ventricular rhythms are manifest. Older patients require approximately one-half the loading and maintenance dosage of lidocaine or procainamide as compared to younger patients, since in the former the hepatic and renal function is generally reduced, the clearance of the antiarrhythmic drugs is diminished, and tissue sensitivity to the drugs may be increased. The net result is that older patients frequently develop major complications from antiarrhythmic agents that are administered in the dose usually given to younger patients.

VENTRICULAR ECTOPIC BEATS: PREDISCHARGE PHASE

Several recent studies have substantiated the increased posthospital risk to patients of frequent and repetitive ventricular ectopic beats recorded by Holter monitoring prior to their hospital discharge. To date, no satisfactorily conducted studies have demonstrated a reduction in posthospital mortality with "routine" prophylactic administration of any of the available antiarrhythmic agents. These findings indicate that if any benefit is to be achieved with antiarrhythmic therapy in the posthospital period, the drugs should be administered only to patients at high arrhythmic risk, i.e., those with potentially life-threatening ventricular rhythms.

I obtain 24-hour Holter recordings prior to their hospital discharge on all postinfarction patients. Most patients are on beta-blocker therapy at the time of the recording. Only patients who manifest one or more runs of sustained ventricular tachycardia (10 beats or longer) at a rate of 150 beats per minute or faster or a "torsades de pointes" rhythm are candidates for discharge antiarrhythmic therapy. I initiate therapy with either quinidine sulfate (or one of the sustained-release preparations), 400 mg PO every 6 hours; procainamide 500 mg PO every 6 hours; or tocainide hydrochloride, 400 mg PO every 8 hours. The choice of the agent is determined in part by both my clinical experience with these drugs and the patient's prior exposure and tolerance to these agents. After 48 hours or more of therapy, I check a trough drug blood level and repeat the Holter recording. Dose adjustment is made on the basis of the persistence of the life-threatening arrhythmia, the adequacy of the blood level, and the patient's tolerance of the drug. When arrhythmia control is achieved, I maintain therapy for 2 to 3 months, taper the patient off the drug, and then obtain a follow-up, 24-hour Holter recording and a treadmill exercise test. Antiarrhythmic therapy is reinitiated only if potentially life-threatening ventricular tachyarrhythmias (sustained ventricular tachycardia or torsades de pointes rhythms) are found.

SUPRAVENTRICULAR ARRHYTHMIAS

New-onset supraventricular tachyarrhythmias (atrial flutter-fibrillation or paroxysmal supraventricular tachycardia) infrequently complicate acute myocardial infarction. When they occur, they are often a consequence of left ventricular dysfunction or pericarditis; these atrial tachyarrhythmias may compound an already embarrassed circulatory state. The aims of therapy are three-fold: (1) to control the ventricular rate, (2) to reconvert the arrhythmia to sinus rhythm, and (3) to prevent recurrence. If the supraventricular tachyarrhythmias are at a rapid rate (>160 beats per minute), and there is acute hemodynamic compromise or increased ischemia, or both, synchronized electrical cardioversion should be utilized for rapid restoration of sinus rhythm. After administration of diazepam, 5 to 10 mg IV, for sedation and amnesia, cardioversion should be initiated at 50 joules, with sequential increases to 100, 200, and 400 joules being made as required if the initial or lower energy levels are not successful. In less time-demanding situations, pharmacologic conversion and rate control should be used. Digoxin, 0.75 mg IV administered immediately then followed in 2 hours with 0.5 mg IV, is effective, but it may take a few hours to achieve the desired result. If blood pressure permits, I use verapamil, 5 mg IV over 2 minutes followed by another 5 mg IV 5 minutes later, for both prompt slowing of the ventricular response to atrial fibrillation and conversion of paroxysmal supraventricular tachycardia to sinus rhythm. The sequential administration of digoxin and verapamil is particularly effective, and maintenance thereafter with digoxin, 0.25 mg IV or PO every day, and verapamil, 40 to 80 mg PO every 8 hours, usually prevents recurrence.

In patients with low-output states, or hypotension, or both, verapamil is contraindicated. In such situations, quinidine sulfate, 200 to 400 mg PO every 6 hours, can be given for conversion once the ventricular response rate of atrial flutter and/or fibrillation is controlled with digoxin. Quinidine should also be continued thereafter to prevent recurrence of the arrhythmia. In patients who do not tolerate quinidine, procainamide should be used as alternative therapy. Disopyramide is also effective, but its cardiopressant effects preclude its use in patients with hemodynamic dysfunction. As a general rule, I have not used heparin anticoagulation prior to attempting the initial, urgent electrical or pharmacologic cardioversion. However, since patients with these atrial tachyarrhythmias are likely to have recurrences and are also at increased risk of thromboembolic complications, I routinely start warfarin anticoagulation and continue it throughout the hospitalization.

Sinus bradycardia, with rates in the 40 to 50 beats per minute range, is frequently seen with inferior-wall infarctions as a result of increased vagal tone. Therapy is usually not required, but if the bradycardia is dysfunctional, atropine, 1 mg IV, is usually effective in augmenting the rate. In the elderly, more profound sinus bradycardia, and occasionally transient 2- to 3-second episodes of sinus arrest, may occur. If these bradyarrhythmias persist despite withdrawal of beta-blockers or other offending agents and the administration of atropine, a temporary transvenous atrial or ventricular demand pacemaker should be placed. In most medical centers this can be rapidly and safely done, using a percutaneous subclavian or internal jugular approach.

CONDUCTION DISTURBANCES

Prolongation of the PR-interval and the Wenckebach conduction block (Mobitz I) are frequently seen in patients with inferior-wall infarctions, and intervention therapy is rarely required. Atropine, or a temporary pacemaker, or both, are indicated only if the conduction block progresses to a higher degree and bradycardia is significant. The arrhythmia is almost always transient, and normal conduction usually returns within a few days.

In patients with anterior infarctions, compromise of blood supply to the septum may affect conduction in the right and left bundle branches. The development of a new right or left bundle branch block pattern has potentially serious implications, and patients with this complication should be monitored closely for indications or warning signs of incomplete trifascicular block, a prelude to life-threatening complete heart block. In the setting of an acute anterior infarction, I place a prophylactic temporary ventricular demand pacemaker for any newly evolving conduction disturbance which indicates trifascicular block including, (1) right bundle branch block with left or right axis deviation and PR interval greater than 0.24 seconds; (2) left bundle branch block and PR interval greater than 0.24 seconds; or (3) Mobitz type II block (isolated blocked sinus beat without preceding PR-interval prolongation) with or without right or left bundle branch block. Patients with anterior infarction who develop transient complete heart block are at increased risk for recurrent heart block if they survive the acute coronary episode. I have implanted permanent pacemakers in such patients, but agreement on this point is not universal.

Therapy for arrhythmias and conduction disturbances complicating acute myocardial infarction should be tailored to the risk posed by the dysrhythmia. Overtreatment carries more risk than undertreatment. When there is a serious question about the need for aggressive antiarrhythmic intervention, a conservative therapeutic approach is recommended.

HYPOTENSION AND SHOCK FOLLOWING MYOCARDIAL INFARCTION

KANU CHATTERJEE, M.B., F.R.C.P.

Cardiogenic shock is defined as a clinical syndrome in which shock is precipitated by abnormalities in cardiac function. The clinical manifestations of shock are characterized by hypotension and decreased organ perfusion, such as oliguria, cold, clammy skin, and mental obtundation. However, hypotension may exist as a complication of acute myocardial infarction (MI) without other manifestations of shock. A number of complications of acute MI may induce hypotension, low cardiac output, and clinical shock syndrome (Table 1).

Bradyarrhythmia may be associated with hypotension and low cardiac output. Cardiac output is the product of heart rate and stroke volume. When heart rate is markedly reduced, cardiac output tends to decline, particularly when there is lack of compensatory increase in stroke volume, such as occurs in patients with acute MI. Treatment of choice is temporary transvenous pacing to increase the ventricular rate to an adequate range. Ventricular pacing alone may not increase cardiac output adequately, particularly in patients with right ventricular infarct. The increase in stroke volume during atrioventricular sequential pacing with timed atrial contribution is significantly greater and, therefore, preferable to ventricular pacing, if increase in cardiac output is inadequate. Both sustained supraventricular and ventricular tachycardia can precipitate hypotension and low cardiac output. Tachycardia precipitates low cardiac output due to decreased ventricular filling and impaired relaxation. Systolic function is also impaired during ventricular tachycardia.

TABLE 1 Complications of Acute Myocardial Infarction that can Precipitate Hypotension and Shock

- Bradyarrhythmia
- Tachyarrhythmia
- Hypovolemic shock
- Right ventricular infarct
- Left ventricular failure:
  - With mechanical defects
  - Without mechanical defects
- Cardiac tamponade due to cardiac rupture
- Pulmonary embolism

Myocardial perfusion is compromised because of reduced diastolic filling time, and myocardial oxygen requirements are also concomitantly increased. There is, thus, the potential for myocardial ischemia and further compromise of left ventricular function. The immediate therapy for both supraventricular and ventricular tachyarrhythmia is direct-current cardioversion. Subsequent therapy aims to maintain sinus rhythm with antiarrhythmic drugs. Although tachyarrhythmias, bradyarrhythmias, and conduction abnormalities are important complications of acute MI, the low-output state that frequently accompanies these complications may not always improve when the dysrhythmias are controlled. In addition to the management of dysrhythmias, attention should be directed to the diagnosis and appropriate management of the other associated complications of MI.

HEMODYNAMIC MONITORING

In patients with acute MI, hemodynamic monitoring permits both the diagnosis of the mechanism of low-output state and the prompt assessment of therapeutic results. The hemodynamic abnormalities of the various complications of acute MI, which can be associated with low-output state, hypotension, and shock, are summarized in Table 2. In hypovolemic shock, both right atrial and pulmonary capillary wedge pressures are lower than normal in addition to relative hypotension and low cardiac output. Minor differences in opinion exist about the optimal level of left ventricular filling pressure in patients with acute MI. In some studies, the maximum increase in stroke volume in-

TABLE 2 Low-Output State in Acute Myocardial Infarction: Hemodynamic Diagnosis

Abnormality	*Diagnostic Finding*
Hypovolemic shock	↓RAP, ↓PCWP
RV infarction	RAP/PCWP > .65, RAP = PCWP, PADP = PCWP
LV failure	PCWP > RAP, RAP/PCWP < .65, PADP = PCWP
Mitral regurgitation	Giant early "V" wave, no step up in PaO_2 saturation
Ventricular septal rupture	Step up in PaO_2
Pulmonary embolism	RAP > PCWP, RAP/PCWP > .65, PADP > PCWP
Cardiac tamponade	RAP = PCWP, PADP = PCWP

Abbreviations: ↓ = decreased; RAP = right atrial pressure; PCWP = pulmonary capillary wedge pressure; PADP = pulmonary artery end-diastolic pressure; Pa = pulmonary artery.

dex was obtained with pulmonary capillary wedge pressures between 14 and 18 mm Hg. In other investigations, the maximum cardiac index or stroke volume index was obtained when the left ventricular end-diastolic pressure range was between 20 and 24 mm Hg. Since the left ventricular end-diastolic pressure is usually higher than the simultaneously measured mean pulmonary capillary wedge pressure, these differences are not clinically significant.

Clinical evaluation, electrocardiography, echocardiography, and myocardial scintigraphy can provide diagnosis of predominant right ventricular infarction in the large majority of patients. However, hemodynamic monitoring is required to determine the severity of right ventricular failure and to assess therapeutic results when low cardiac output is present. Disproportionate elevation of right atrial pressure compared to pulmonary capillary wedge pressure is the most common hemodynamic abnormality. The ratio of right atrial pressure to pulmonary capillary wedge pressure usually exceeds 0.65. In patients with severe right ventricular failure, right atrial pressure may be equal to pulmonary capillary wedge pressure, simulating effusive constrictive pericarditis. In these patients, no significant difference betwen pulmonary artery end-diastolic pressure and pulmonary capillary wedge pressure is observed.

Studies in experimental animal models have demonstrated that the equalization of the diastolic pressures following isolated right ventricular infarction results from increased intrapericardial pressure from acute right ventricular dilatation. In patients with predominant left ventricular failure, pulmonary capillary wedge pressure is significantly higher than the right atrial pressure. However, right atrial pressure may also be elevated when right ventricular failure is present. In these patients, pulmonary artery pressure is frequently increased. However, the pulmonary vascular resistance may remain normal, and no significant gradient between pulmonary artery end-diastolic pressure and pulmonary capillary wedge pressure is observed.

Papillary muscle infarct or rupture can produce severe acute mitral regurgitation and can be diagnosed at bedside with hemodynamic monitoring. Severe acute mitral regurgitation is recognized by either a giant, peaked "V" wave in the pulmonary capillary wedge pressure tracings or the reflected "V" wave in the pulmonary artery pressure tracings. However, a giant "V" wave in the pulmonary capillary wedge pressure tracings can be observed in the *absence* of mitral regurgitation. In patients with large left-to-right shunt, in coronary artery disease, and in aortic valve disease, the normal "V" wave in the wedge pressure tracing may be markedly accentuated and simulate the regurgitant wave of severe acute mitral regurgitation. The onset of the regurgitant wave, however, is earlier and coincides with the QRS complex of the electrocardiogram (ECG). The reflected "V" wave in the pulmonary artery pressure tracing, however, is almost always associated with acute or subacute severe mitral regurgitation. Left-to-right shunt due to ventricular septal rupture complicating acute MI is also diagnosed at bedside by significantly higher (more than 5 volume %) oxygen saturation in pulmonary arterial blood compared to that in right atrial blood samples. Pulmonary capillary wedge pressure and right atrial pressure are elevated, and pulmonary hypertension is frequently observed. No difference between pulmonary artery diastolic end-pressure and mean pulmonary capillary wedge pressure is seen in the absence of increased pulmonary vascular resistance.

The hemodynamic abnormalities in cardiac tamponade are very similar to those in patients with severe right ventricular infarct. For differential diagnosis, it is necessary to perform noninvasive—preferably echocardiographic—investigations. An echocardiogram in cardiac tamponade demonstrates pericardial effusion and decreased right and left ventricular volumes, as well as right ventricular compression. In acute right ventricular infarction, the right ventricle is dilated and the systolic function of the right ventricle is markedly depressed.

Massive pulmonary embolism is an infrequent complication of acute MI. In pulmonary embolism associated with right ventricular failure, right atrial pressure is disproportionately higher than the pulmonary artery wedge pressure. Pulmonary artery pressure is markedly elevated, and a significant gradient between pulmonary artery end-diastolic pressure and mean pulmonary capillary wedge pressure is seen.

THERAPY OF LOW OUTPUT STATE AND CARDIOGENIC SHOCK

Hypovolemic Shock

Hypovolemic shock is a relatively uncommon complication of acute MI. Repeated administration of diuretics or nitrates and severe diaphoresis and vomiting may precipitate hypovolemic shock. Patients with hypovolemia are treated with intravenous fluid to increase right atrial and pulmonary capillary wedge pressure to an optimal range. The choice of intravenous fluid is not critical. In most patients with acute MI in whom the size of the left ventricle is relatively normal, there usually is no further increase in cardiac output when pulmonary capillary wedge pressure exceeds 18 to 20 mm Hg during volume expansion. In some patients with the hemodynamic features of hypovolemia, cardiac output and stroke volume may not increase adequately despite pulmonary capillary wedge pressure being maintained in the optimal range. Significant left ventricular dysfunction coexists in these patients, and therefore therapy should be similar to that for treatment of pump failure, while optimal filling pressure is maintained with intravenous fluid therapy.

Right Ventricular Infarct

Predominant right ventricular infarction occurs almost exclusively in patients with inferior or inferoposterior MI. The incidence of right ventricular infarction in patients with inferior wall infarction is between 30 and 40 percent. However, only a small percentage of patients develops severe low-output syndrome. Right ventricular infarction should be suspected when physical findings of right ventricular failure are present in the absence of significant left ventricular failure. An elevated jugular venous pressure with positive Kussmaul's sign, a right ventricular gallop, and tricuspid regurgitation in the absence of physical findings of pulmonary venous and arterial hypertension all suggest predominant right ventricular infarction. An ST elevation in the right precordial leads (V_1–V_4) without loss of "r" waves in the presence of electrocardiographic evidence of inferior or inferoposterior wall MI also indicates involvement of the free wall of the right ventricle. Leads V_3R and V_4R may demonstrate ST elevation and loss of "r" waves. An echocardiogram and gated blood-pool scintigraphy reveal a dilated and poorly contracting right ventricle, whereas the left ventricular ejection fraction is near normal. A technetium pyrophosphate scan demonstrates uptake of pyrophosphate by the free wall of the right ventricle. In the absence of low-output state or hypotension, no specific therapy is required. However, one should avoid diuretics or venodilators, such as nitroglycerin, which may both precipitate hypotension and decrease cardiac output due to decreased intravascular volume or venous return. When low-output state complicates right ventricular infarction, aggressive therapy is required, and hemodynamic monitoring is necessary both to determine the severity of hemodynamic abnormalities and to assess therapeutic results.

The mechanism for the decreased systemic output in predominant right ventricular infarction appears to be due to reduced left ventricular preload. In experimental isolated right ventricular infarction, decreases in left ventricular transmural pressure and diastolic volume have been observed in association with increases in right ventricular transmural pressure and diastolic volume. The reduction of left ventricular preload results from both decreased right ventricular stroke output and restricted filling of the left ventricle due to an increase in intrapericardial pressure. The objective of therapeutic intervention is to increase left ventricular preload so that systemic output can be increased.

Intravenous fluid administration, despite elevated right atrial pressures, increases systemic output. The precise mechanism for this improvement is unclear. In experimental right ventricular infarction, volume loading improves right ventricular stroke output and increases left ventricular transmural pressure and diastolic volume. Thus, increased left ventricular preload results from the improvement in right ventricular systolic function. Passive filling of the left ventricle with volume loading is also a potential mechanism for increasing left ventricular preload. Excessive fluid administration may cause marked dilatation of the right ventricle and a greater increase in intrapericardial pressure, which may compromise left ventricular filling. Furthermore, excessive right atrial dilatation may cause right-to-left intracardiac shunt through a patent foramen ovale and precipitate significant arterial desaturation. Therefore, excessive fluid administration should be avoided, and changes in right atrial and pulmonary capillary wedge pressure should be monitored during intravenous fluid therapy. Clinical experience suggests that when right atrial pressure exceeds 20 mm Hg during volume loading, there is no further increase in systemic output. It is preferable to keep right atrial pressure at 20 mm Hg or less during intravenous fluid administration.

Right ventricular stroke volume can also increase from the concomitant use of vasodilators, such as nitroglycerin or nitroprusside, that have the potential to decrease right ventricular afterload (pulmonary artery pressure and pulmonary vascular resistance). Vasodilators should not, however, be used without concomitant administration of intravenous fluids because left and right ventricular preload may decline due to decreased venous return. Also, vasodilators can significantly aggravate hypotension. As a result, vasodilators are contraindicated as initial therapeutic agents in significant hypotension. If cardiac output does not increase adequately and hypotension persists despite intravenous fluid therapy, inotropic agents are frequently effective in improving cardiac output. Dobutamine, a $beta_1$- receptor agonist, can cause a reduction in pulmonary arterial pressure and pulmonary vascular resistance, besides enhancing the inotropic state. Dobutamine is useful in increasing systemic output when used in conjunction with volume loading. Dopamine is also useful in improving systemic output; however, it has the potential to increase pulmonary arterial pressure and pulmonary vascular resistance (right ventricular afterload). It is likely to be less effective than dobutamine in improving systemic output in patients with predominant right ventricular infarction. Thus, dopamine is restricted to patients with severe hypotension.

The right ventricular pneumatic pump and pulmonary artery balloon counterpulsation have been used in some patients with acute right ventricular failure, and hemodynamic and clinical improvements have been noted. However, such measures are rarely needed to manage predominant right ventricular infarction.

Hypotension with low cardiac output can occur when bradyarrhythmias complicate right ventricular infarction. The incidence of complete atrioventricular block in patients with right ventricular infarction is considerably higher than the reported overall incidence in patients with acute MI. Loss of timed atrial contraction appears to be particularly detrimental to patients with predominant right ventricular infarction. During ventricular pacing, stroke volume is significantly lower than it is during atrioventricular sequential pacing at an identical pacing rate. Thus, atrioventricular sequential pacing is preferable to ventricular pacing in patients with right ventricular infarction complicated by atrioventricular block. The therapeutic management of right ventricular infarction is outlined in Table 3.

Left Ventricular Failure

Left ventricular failure is the most common cause of low-output state, hypotension, and cardiogenic shock in

TABLE 3 Therapeutic Management of Predominant Right Ventricular Infarction

In the absence of low cardiac output and hypotension:
- Avoid diuretics and vasodilators, particularly nitroglycerin.

In the presence of low systemic output:
- Administer intravenous fluids to maintain right atrial pressure around 20 mm Hg;
- Add vasodilators (nitroglycerin or nitroprusside) with concomitant administration of intravenous fluids;
- Add dobutamine if the increase in cardiac output is inadequate; or,
- In the presence of significant hypotension, add dopamine.

In the presence of bradyarrhythmia and low systemic output:
- Check for sinus bradycardia—atrial pacing
- Check for A–V block—A–V sequential pacing

patients with acute MI. The diagnosis and management of the mechanical defects, such as severe mitral regurgitation and ventricular septal rupture, have been discussed earlier. The hemodynamic abnormalities of left ventricular failure consist of elevated pulmonary capillary wedge pressure and reduced cardiac output. Cardiogenic shock is the clinical expression of severe left ventricular failure.

In patients with adequate cardiac output but elevated pulmonary capillary wedge pressure, diuretics decrease pulmonary venous pressure and relieve symptoms of pulmonary venous congestion. Changes in pulmonary capillary wedge pressure should be monitored during diuretic therapy to avoid lowering the filling pressure to hypovolemic levels.

If the pulmonary capillary wedge pressure remains elevated despite diuretic therapy, nitroglycerin and other organic nitrates can be used to reduce pulmonary venous pressure. In patients with more severe pump failure, left ventricular stroke volume and cardiac output are significantly decreased, and pulmonary capillary wedge pressure and systemic vascular resistance elevated. In the absence of significant hypotension, vasodilator therapy appears to improve left ventricular performance. For the treatment of pump failure, the most common vasodilators are sodium nitroprusside and nitroglycerin. Although they produce qualitatively similar hemodynamic effects, there are significant quantitative differences in their hemodynamic response. The major hemodynamic effects of sodium nitroprusside are a significant decrease in systemic vascular resistance, an increase in cardiac output, and a significant reduction in right atrial and pulmonary capillary wedge pressures. In most patients, there is a modest reduction in arterial pressure as well.

Nitroglycerin is predominantly a venodilator. But when it is given intravenously, particularly in larger doses, an arterial dilatating effect is also observed. The hemodynamic effects of nitroglycerin or nitrates are a significant reduction in right atrial and pulmonary capillary wedge pressures, with only a modest—or even no—increase in cardiac output. Thus, the choice between nitroprusside and nitroglycerin in the management of pump failure complicating acute MI should depend on the associated hemodynamic abnormalities. In patients with elevated systemic vascular resistance, low cardiac output, and elevated pulmonary capillary wedge pressure, nitroprusside is the drug of choice, provided that severe hypotension is absent. However, if the cardiac output is adequate or only slightly decreased and pulmonary capillary wedge pressure is markedly elevated, nitroglycerin may be the more appropriate vasodilator. In certain patients, nitroprusside and nitroglycerin can be combined to optimize the increase in cardiac output and the decrease in pulmonary capillary wedge pressure.

Hemodynamic monitoring is essential during vasodilator therapy in patients with acute MI. But one of the potential hazards of such therapy is hypotension. If marked hypotension occurs during vasodilator therapy, the potential exists for enhancement of myocardial ischemia irrespective of the vasodilating agent used. The major objective of vasodilator therapy in patients with pump failure is to decrease left ventricular resistance to ejection and to increase cardiac output. If the increase in cardiac output is proportional to the decrease in systemic vascular resistance, mean arterial pressure remains unchanged. Thus, during vasodilator therapy, it is necessary to monitor not only the changes in pulmonary capillary wedge pressure and cardiac output but also the changes in arterial pressure and systemic vascular resistance.

The initial infusion rate of the vasodilators (nitroprusside: 10 μg per minute; nitroglycerin: 10 μg per minute) should be small, and the dose increased gradually. If cardiac output increases, along with a reduction in pulmonary capillary wedge pressure, the vasodilator therapy should be continued. If hypotension occurs before any significant change in cardiac output or pulmonary capillary wedge pressure, vasodilator therapy should be discontinued. In these latter patients, therapy can be initiated with an inotropic agent, such as dobutamine. Later, vasodilators can be added.

If significant hypotension complicates left ventricular failure, vasodilators cannot be used as initial therapy because of the potential risk of further hypotension. Vasopressive agents, such as dopamine or norepinephrine can be used to increase and maintain arterial pressure until hemodynamic abnormalities are determined. The common vasopressor and inotropic agents are dopamine, dobutamine, and norepinephrine. Norepinephrine, in a dose of 5 to 15 μg per minute, increases systemic vascular resistance and arterial pressure. However, cardiac output may not be significantly raised. Dopamine, on the other hand, increases cardiac output as well as arterial pressure. Pulmonary capillary wedge pressure and pulmonary arterial pressure may not change or may even increase.

Dobutamine also increases cardiac output, but there is also a reduction in pulmonary capillary wedge and pulmonary arterial pressure; arterial pressure may not change or it may even decrease. Thus, the choice between dopamine and dobutamine should depend on associated hemodynamic abnormalities, besides reduced cardiac output. In the absence of significant hypotension and elevated pulmonary capillary wedge pressure, dobutamine is preferable to dopamine. On the other hand, in the presence of significant hypotension, dopamine is more effective in maintaining arterial pressure. A new inotropic agent, amrinone, is also available in combination with other catecholamines, such as dopamine or dobutamine, to optimize the increase in cardiac output. Amrinone is a phosphodiesterase inhibitor and reduces systemic vascular resistance while increasing contractility. With larger doses of amrinone, there is the potential risk of inducing hypotension and tachycardia.

In patients with severe hypotension or in whom hypotension is not easily corrected with vasopressors and inotropic agents, intra-aortic balloon counterpulsation should be considered. With the advent of percutaneous techniques, intra-aortic balloon counterpulsation can be instituted rapidly.

With this device, several hemodynamic benefits can be achieved. The balloon is inflated during diastole, which increases arterial diastolic pressure (diastolic augmentation); this helps to maintain coronary arterial perfusion pressure. The balloon is rapidly deflated at end-diastole, which is associated with decreased peak systolic arterial pressure. Thus, the resistance to left ventricular ejection declines, associated with an increase in cardiac output. The other hemodynamic benefits include reductions in left ventricular diastolic volume and pressure. Pulmonary venous pressure is also concomitantly reduced. Lower arterial pressure and decreased left ventricular diastolic volume reduce myocardial oxygen requirements; increased arterial diastolic pressure maintains coronary artery perfusion pressure. Furthermore, an increase in transmyocardial pressure gradient (aortic diastolic pressure–left ventricular diastolic pressure) has the potential to enhance myocardial perfusion. The global coronary blood flow, however, tends to decrease despite diastolic augmentation; this is probably due to a significant reduction in myocardial oxygen requirements.

One major advantage of intra-aortic balloon counterpulsation is that vasodilators can be added to improve hemodynamics without compromising perfusion pressure. However, intra-aortic balloon counterpulsation without corrective surgery does *not* improve the immediate prognosis of patients with cardiogenic shock. With intra-aortic balloon counterpulsation alone, hospital mortality remains extremely high, nearly 90 percent. However, if surgery can be performed (e.g., mitral valve replacement; ventricular septal rupture; or infarctectomy with or without coronary artery bypass surgery), about a 50 percent survival rate can be expected. Thus, once intra-aortic balloon counterpulsation therapy is instituted and the patient stabilized, the feasibility of surgical intervention should be determined by cardiac catheterization. Hemodynamic monitoring is essential to the appropriate management of severe left ventricular failure with hypotension, with or without clinical features of cardiogenic shock. The stepwise therapeutic approach based on hemodynamics is outlined in Figure 1.

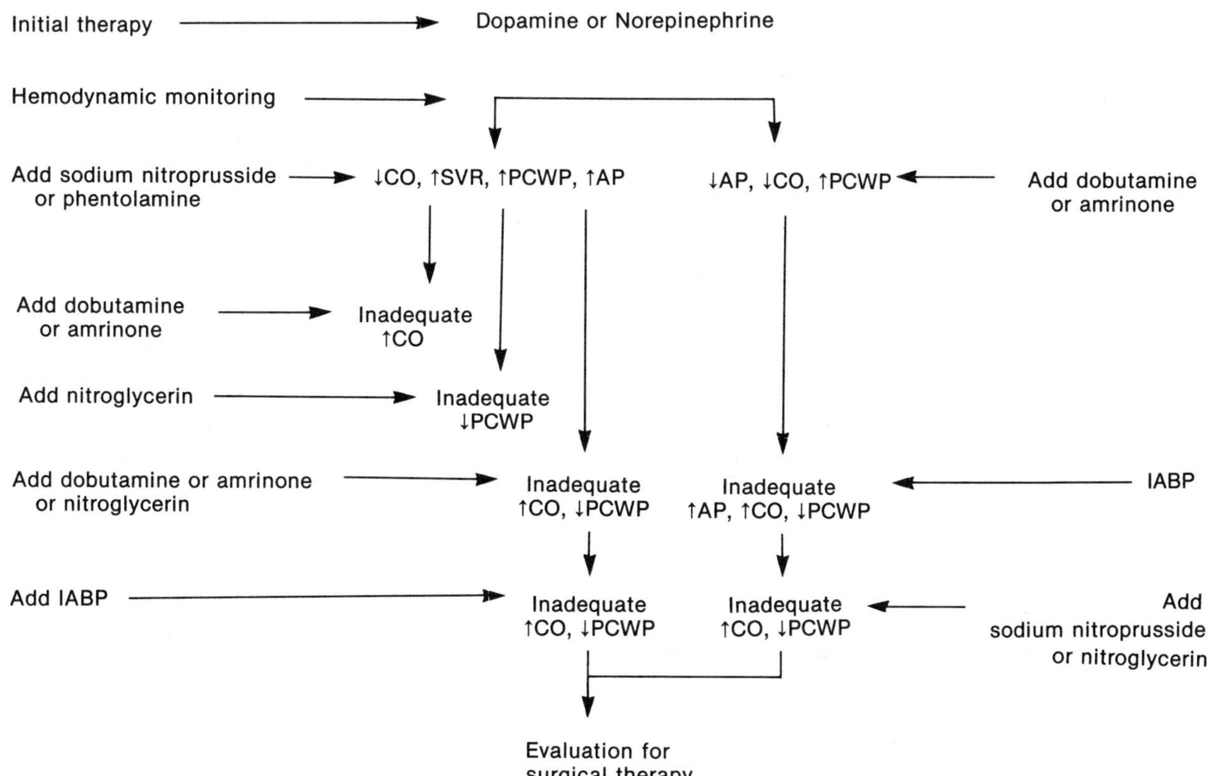

Figure 1 The therapeutic approach to hemodynamic monitoring.

Vasopressor therapy with dopamine or norepinephrine should be immediately instituted to maintain arterial pressure. Hemodynamics should then be determined and, based on the hemodynamic abnormalities, subsequent therapy decided on. If cardiac output remains low after the use of a vasopressor, and systemic vascular resistance is elevated and arterial and pulmonary capillary wedge pressures are increased, sodium nitroprusside or phentolamine should be added. If there is still an inadequate increase in cardiac output after the addition of nitroprusside, inotropic agents, such as dobutamine or amrinone, may help to increase cardiac output significantly.

If, however, pulmonary capillary wedge pressure remains elevated, then nitroglycerin can be added along with diuretics to decrease pulmonary capillary wedge pressure. If arterial pressure remains low despite vasopressor therapy, consider intra-aortic balloon counterpulsation therapy, the addition of vasodilators, such as nitroprusside, and inotropic agents, such as dobutamine or amrinone. If arterial pressure and cardiac output remain low, and if pulmonary capillary wedge pressure remains elevated despite initial vasopressor therapy with dopamine or norepinephrine, add dobutamine or amrinone to increase cardiac output and initiate intra-aortic balloon counterpulsation therapy. Once the patient's hemodynamics and clinical status are stabilized with the latter therapy and the addition of the vasodilator and inotropic agents, he or she should undergo cardiac catheterization with a view to surgical correction.

STABLE ANGINA PECTORIS

NICHOLAS J. FORTUIN, M.D.

Managing the patient with stable angina pectoris begins with establishing the diagnosis of coronary artery disease properly. This is not difficult in the majority of patients and can be done most readily by careful history-taking. Other cardiac disorders that cause angina, such as aortic stenosis or hypertrophic cardiomyopathy, usually can be excluded by physical examination. When the setting is unusual, for example, in a younger woman, or the discomfort is not typical, further studies may be needed to provide objective evidence of the presence or absence of myocardial ischemia. A discussion of the role of exercise stress testing, radionuclide studies, or coronary angiography in the diagnostic process is beyond the scope of this chapter. It is sufficient to note that such studies usually are not required for diagnostic purposes, but are employed more profitably in establishing prognosis once the diagnosis has been made.

After establishing the diagnosis of angina due to coronary artery disease and before beginning specific treatment, the physician must determine, insofar as is possible, the patient's prognosis. He must decide whether the patient is in a high-risk group for future coronary events or in a low-risk group. This distinction is the deciding factor in whether to proceed to a coronary angiographic study as part of the initial work-up in anticipation of surgical therapy. I do not recommend angiography for all patients with the newly established diagnosis of angina pectoris, but only for those who, on clinical grounds, appear to be at high risk. Table 1 describes the clinical factors that aid in assessing prognosis. All can be analyzed by simple clinical tools. The function of the left ventricle and the age of the patient are the two most powerful prognostic indicators, followed by the severity of myocardial ischemia. I find the resting ECG (evidence of old infarction), chest film (evidence of cardiomegaly), and duration and blood pressure response to treadmill exercise adequate to assess ventricular function for prognostic purposes and have not relied routinely on radionuclide ventriculography or echocardiography to further evaluate the left ventricle. If the patient's ventricular function is so poor that clinical congestive heart failure has occurred, angina is not the presenting complaint since physical activities are severely curtailed by the left ventricular disease. The severity of ischemia may be assessed by careful history-taking. Increased frequency of angina, the precipitation of discomfort by minor effort, and the occurrence of rest or prolonged pain, excessive fatigue, or reduced activity level may signify severe disease. When symptoms indicate severe ischemia, there is little to be learned by treadmill testing, and it is best to proceed directly to catheterization. In a minority of patients with angina, symptoms are not a good guide to severity of ischemia, and treadmill testing may be of value. I do not find yearly or twice-yearly treadmill testing to be helpful in managing the patient with stable symptoms. Generally, I recommend catheterization for patients with angina who show evidence of severe ischemia or left ventricular dysfunction in order to more accurately determine prognosis. Table 2 describes angiographically determined variables that have a bearing on prognosis. Again left ventricular function has primacy, but involvement of the main left coronary artery, multiple vessel obstructions, and proximal obstruction of a large coronary artery supplying a large area of myocardium (''risk area'') are important indicators of adverse prognosis. The angiographic variables bear stronger relation to prognosis when considered with the clinical variables. For example, three-vessel occlusive disease is more ominous when there is clinical evidence of severe ischemia than when ischemia is mild. Clinical and angiographic indicators of prognosis are important in deciding on the proper timing of surgical revascularization (to be discussed). For many patients with stable angina pectoris, the prognosis for long life is excellent. Patients with mild symptoms who have a normal resting ECG and blood pressure have a prognosis only slightly worse than that of age-matched controls. Most studies in

TABLE 1 Clinical Factors Influencing Prognosis in Stable Angina Pectoris

Severity of left ventricular dysfunction
Previous myocardial infarction
Cardiomegaly
Poor treadmill performance
Severity of ischemia
Easily provoked symptoms
Dyspnea with discomfort
Unstable presentation
Resting ECG change
Severe ECG changes during ischemia
Early symptoms on treadmill
Poor response to medical therapy
Age of patient
Hypertension
Other medical problems, e.g., diabetes

TABLE 2 Angiographic Prognostic Variables in Stable Angina Pectoris

Left ventricular function
Left main coronary involvement
Number of vessels obstructed
Location of obstruction—risk area
Status of distal vessels

the literature describing prognosis are based on patients with severe symptoms referred for surgical management to tertiary care facilities. Data from these studies may not be relevant to patients seen in primary care settings. One of the major benefits of the several randomized trials comparing medical and surgical treatment of patients with stable angina pectoris has been the recognition that these patients, even with advanced three-vessel disease, have a better prognosis than had been thought previously.

GENERAL MEASURES

General measures aim to retard progression of atherosclerosis and help the patient to live with his condition. Patients with angina invariably improve when they are placed in the hands of an understanding, calm physician who ministers to their personal and medical needs and reassures the patient that he understands the disease thoroughly. Overzealous laboratory testing or other manifestations of anxiety by the physician inevitably engender fear and may cause more severe symptoms in the patient. Since the disease process is a long one, it is important for the physician to get to know his patient as a person. Many environmental influences on the emotional life of the patient may manifest themselves as worsening symptoms, which may be best dealt with by personal rather than pharmacologic or surgical action. Patients should be told as much about the nature of the underlying disease process as they can be expected to understand. They should be made aware of precipitating events such as eating, emotion, or cold weather and advised to curtail physical activities when these are present. They should be advised to avoid activities that produce excessive fatigue from mental or physical stress. In some cases, a change of job or even retirement may have beneficial results. Dietary measures aimed at reducing weight and serum cholesterol should be employed. I generally employ lipid-lowering agents if the serum cholesterol cannot be brought below 250 mg per deciliter by diet in patients under the age of 60. Blood pressure control is usually abetted by antianginal agents. The most important risk factor modification is complete cessation of smoking, which must be emphasized repeatedly. Exercise enhances self-esteem and reassures the patient that his disease is not severely disabling. I encourage patients to continue recreational sports such as golf or doubles in tennis, but I discourage active competitive sports such as squash or singles in tennis. Brisk walking or stationary cycling are effective dynamic exercises and are easy to perform. Some patients like the communal and structured atmosphere of a rehabilitation center, but I do not recommend this routinely. Patients readily learn to exercise until they have a premonition of angina and stop at that point. Exercise is often easier to perform after taking sublingual nitroglycerin or isosorbide dinitrate. The same can be said for sexual intercourse, which the patient may be afraid to pursue vigorously because of the precipitation of angina. Normal sexual functioning should be encouraged; sometimes this may require counseling by the physician and alteration of drug regimens. Other medical problems such as anemia, thyroid disease, or poorly controlled diabetes may adversely affect anginal frequency as may many bronchodilators used in patients with chronic pulmonary disease.

PHARMACOLOGIC THERAPY

Not all patients with angina pectoris require drug therapy. Patients with mild symptoms may prefer not to take medication. These patients have learned to live with their disorder and instinctively avoid activities that might bring on discomfort. All patients should be instructed in the use of nitroglycerin (to be discussed), although many reject the use of the drug because of headache or because the chest discomfort is too short-lived. The aim of long-term prophylactic drug therapy is to allow the patient to function in normal activities free of anginal pain or intolerable drug side effects. I usually begin with a single drug, adjust the dose to maximal efficacy, and add additional agents if symptoms are not alleviated. I discourage the shotgun approach of multiple drugs as initial treatment. I sometimes obtain a treadmill test after drug therapy has been maximized to assess objectively the clinical prognosis.

Beta-Adrenergic Blocking Agents

I prefer to start treatment of most patients with beta-blocking drugs because they are generally effective and well tolerated and can be given once daily. Cardioselective agents (atenolol and metoprolol) may be better tolerated at low doses, but these drugs lose their cardioselectivity at higher doses and act on both $beta_1$- and $beta_2$- receptors. I usually begin with atenolol, 50 mg daily (25 mg daily for older patients), and use resting and light exercise heart rate as well as clinical response to assess therapeutic efficacy. A resting heart rate of 50 to 60 per minute usually indicates adequate beta-blockade. It is useful to become familiar with all of the beta-blocking drugs because some patients have adverse reactions from one, but not another of the class. There is no evidence that one beta-blocker is more effective than another in managing patients with angina. They all reduce myocardial oxygen demands during exercise by reducing heart rate, systolic pressure, and ventricular contractility. Many are effective if given in one daily dose. Table 3 describes the characteristics of currently available beta-blockers.

There are several matters to consider in the selection of beta-blocking drugs for the individual patient. Physician familiarity is one. A second is whether to employ a cardioselective or nonselective agent. Cardioselective beta-blockers block $beta_1$- receptors in lower dosage. These receptors are responsible for cardiac stimulation (contractility and heart rate), renin release by the kidney, and lipolysis. $Beta_2$- receptors, which are not affected, produce bronchodilation, vasodilation, and glycogenolysis when stimulated. $Beta_2$- stimulation by epinephrine may also produce mild and transient hypokalemia as a result of movement of potassium ions into cells. Thus, cardioselective agents may be preferable for patients with lung disease, diabetes mellitus, or peripheral vascular disease. A theoretic drawback of cardioselective agents may be transient hypokalemia and resultant potentiation of arrhythmias during stressful periods. This latter action has not been definitely proved to be a problem in man. Another characteristic of certain beta-blocking agents (pindolol, acebutolol, and labetalol) is intrinsic sympathomimetic activity (ISA), which refers to the ability of those drugs to provide partial beta-agonist activity. This usually occurs when basal sympathetic tone is low, as in the resting state. Such drugs may be useful in patients with sinus bradycardia or in those with reduced ventricular function when partial agonist activity may cause less depression of ventricular performance.

Contraindications to the use of beta-blockers include moderate or severe ventricular dysfunction, asthma, or marked sinus bradycardia. I use cardioselective agents with caution and in low doses in patients with chronic obstructive pulmonary disease, diabetes mellitus, or peripheral vascular disease, and use all agents cautiously in patients with SA or AV node dysfunction. Although most patients tolerate these drugs well, side effects limit their use in some patients. These include a sense of fatigue and muscle weakness (the ''beta-blocker blahs''), cool extremities, Raynaud's phenomenon, depression, and impotence. Switching from one agent to another may eliminate side effects. Beta-blockers have been employed in the treatment of angina for nearly 20 years. There have been no reports of long-term ill effects. A 20 to 40 percent increase in exercise capacity has been documented in many studies. Many patients with angina can be rendered pain-free for normal activities with the use of a single daily dose. An additional benefit may be improved longevity, if one can extrapolate the results from trials employing beta-blockers in patients after myocardial infarction to results in patients with stable angina pectoris.

Calcium-Channel Blocking Drugs

These drugs can be used as sole agents for managing patients with angina or in combination with beta-blocking drugs. They provide roughly the same improvement in exercise capacity as beta-blockers, and the effects of the two types of drugs are additive. They are effective in stable effort angina as well as in vasospastic angina. The three agents currently available—diltiazem, nifedipine, and verapamil—are a heterogeneous group of drugs that

TABLE 3 Pharmacology of Beta-Adrenergic Blocking Drugs

Drug	*Dosage (mg)*	*No. of Doses*	*ISA**	*Cardioselectivity*	*Excretion*
Atenolol (Tenormin)	25–200	1	No	Yes	Renal
Propranolol (Inderal)	80–360	1–4	No	No	Hepatic
Nadolol (Corgard)	20–320	1	No	No	Renal
Metoprolol (Lopressor)	50–200	1–2	No	Yes	Hepatic
Pindolol (Visken)	7.5–22.5	3	Yes	No	Hepatic and renal
Timolol (Blocatren)	10–40	2	Minor	No	Hepatic and renal
Acebutolol (Sectral)	400–1200	2–4	Yes	Yes	Hepatic and renal
Labetalol† (Normodyne or Trandate)	300–1200	3	Yes	No	Hepatic

* ISA = intrinsic sympathomimetic activity
† Labetalol has mild alpha-receptor blocking activity

act predominantly as potent arterial and weak venous vasodilators by interfering with calcium transport in smooth muscle cells. They reduce ventricular afterload, lower blood pressure, reduce coronary arterial vasomotor tone, and relieve coronary artery spasm. I generally prefer to add one of these drugs to a beta-blocker, but also employ these agents as single drugs in patients who are intolerant of beta-blockers. Calcium blockers are preferred therapy when the clinical history suggests that variability in coronary vascular tone is responsible for symptoms. Such patients often describe a "variable threshold" of activity to their anginal spells or a major emotional component. Table 4 describes the clinical pharmacology of calcium-channel blockers. They all must be administered three or four times daily. Because the drugs are so different, each may have a role in some therapeutic situation, so that it behooves the physician to become familiar with all agents available. I prefer diltiazem as initial therapy in combination with a beta-blocker because, of the three, it has the lowest incidence of side effects. I usually begin with 30 mg four times daily and advise the patient to double the dose after 3 days if there have been no side effects. Where sinus or AV node disease is present, nifedipine would be preferable. I find verapamil the best agent as single therapy because of its effect on heart rate and contractility. Verapamil can be used with beta-blockers, but some patients may not tolerate the combination because of summated effects on sinus or AV node and on the left ventricle. Nifedipine is probably the most efficacious drug of the three in reducing arterial pressure and thus is useful in hypertensives. All calcium-channel blockers depress ventricular function and can precipitate pulmonary congestion when compensation is marginal. Nifedipine has the least depressant action and should be used when ventricular performance is reduced, but even this drug may cause heart failure in the barely compensated patient.

Nitrates

All patients with angina should be familiar with the actions and use of sublingual nitroglycerin. They should be taught to use the drug for relief of chest discomfort and to use it before activities which predictably bring on discomfort such as sexual intercourse. They should recognize the side effects of headache, light-headedness, flushing, palpitation, and occasionally syncope. Many patients do not realize that the drug is rapidly metabolized so that it can be taken repeatedly without ill effect or the development of tolerance. It is important that patients realize that nitroglycerin tablets deteriorate on exposure to air or sunlight, and that potency of tablets is lost after 3 to 6 months.

TABLE 4 Pharmacology of Calcium-Channel Blocking Drugs

	Verapamil	*Nifedipine*	*Diltiazem*
Dosage (mg)	240–480	30–120	120–360
Vasodilation			
Venous	+	+	+
Arterial	+	+ +	+
A–V node conduction	↓↓	O	↓
Contractility	↓↓	O/↓	↓
Heart rate	↓	↑(Reflex)	O/↓
Hypotension	+ +	+ + +	+
Edema	+	+ + +	+
Headache	+	+ +	+/O
Constipation	+ +	O	O/+

With the advent of calcium-channel blocking drugs, I have used long-acting nitrates less frequently for prophylactic management. For many years, nitrates were the only effective drugs for treating angina, so that many physicians are reluctant to abandon their use because of long-term familiarity and historic sentimentality. Several factors make them less appealing than beta- or calcium blockers for long-term therapy. These include (1) side effects, particularly intolerable headache, in a significant proportion of users, (2) poor absorption and rapid metabolism by oral route, (3) short half-life requiring frequent dosing (they are not really long-acting), (4) absence of clinical or blood level guide to adequacy of dose, (5) development of tolerance and reduced efficacy with round-the-clock dosing.

Nitrates work by reducing myocardial oxygen demand by virtue of their action as potent systemic venodilators and weak arteriolar dilators; they may improve myocardial blood flow to ischemic areas and reduce coronary spasm by action on coronary arteries and the coronary microvasculature. They are absorbed well through the buccal mucosa when administered by sublingual or chewable preparations and rapidly reach active sites. Oral absorption is less reliable, and first-pass liver metabolism renders some of the orally administered drug inactive. Adequate levels in the blood can be achieved after oral administration by giving large doses, i.e., 20 to 40 mg of isosorbide dinitrate. Because of rapid metabolism and elimination, nitrates should be administered every 3 to 4 hours. Nitroglycerin can be absorbed through the skin by means of an ointment, applied thinly in a dose of 1 to 3 inches every 6 hours, or as a transdermal delivery system. The latter approach has achieved widespread popularity with patients and physicians. Unfortunately, blood levels, when measured, are too low for therapeutic efficacy unless several "patches" or the newer larger patches are applied. These systems do not provide for 24-hour absorption. There has been conflicting evidence concerning clinical effectiveness, and the cost of transdermal patches is high. I do not recommend the use of current, single-dose transdermal delivery systems.

I do not use long-acting nitrates as sole treatment for patients with angina. In patients who cannot tolerate calcium blockers, I use nitrates as adjunctive therapy to beta-blockers, usually isosorbide dinitrate orally. I have not seen convincing evidence that nitrates add significant antianginal effect in the patient who is taking maximal doses of calcium blockers as a vasodilator. I find the best use of nitrates as periodic prophylactic therapy before activities. I usually advise patients to take sublingual or chewable isosorbide dinitrate, 2.5 to 5.0 mg, before activities that are known to produce angina, such as a long walk or jog, a game of tennis, or 9 holes of golf. The patient can expect 2 hours of protection. This kind of "pulse" nitrate therapy may be effective and prevents the development of tolerance. I use nitroglycerin ointment (2%) applied at bedtime (0.5 to 2.0 inches) for patients with nocturnal angina. The ointment is generally too messy to be used regularly during the day in ambulatory patients.

SURGICAL THERAPY

Rational planning for surgical treatment of the patient with chronic ischemic heart disease requires proper understanding of what coronary bypass surgery can be expected to accomplish. The operation can be done safely with an expected operative mortality of less than 1 percent in patients with stable angina. Symptomatic improvement, which is dramatic, occurs in 90 percent of patients, and most of these are completely free of symptoms without taking antianginal medications. There are salutary emotional responses since the patient may feel more confident about the future, even returning to demanding physical employment. Patients are often motivated to modify risk factors more rigorously after surgery. There is little controversy about any of this—the major question revolves around who can be expected to live longer as a result of operation. Several randomized studies have attempted to answer this question. In spite of the fact that all have been rigorously attacked and vigorously defended, the studies show a remarkable similarity of results. To date, relatively few subgroups of patients have shown improved survival as a result of surgery. Longer-term follow-up may even swing some of these results back toward no benefit of surgery as atherosclerosis affects grafts in later years of follow-up. Symptomatic patients with left main coronary obstruction show major improvement in survival, particularly if there is left ventricular dysfunction. Symptomatic patients with three-vessel disease and normal ventricular function show small increases in survival at 5 to 7 years, as do minimally symptomatic patients with three-vessel disease, but only with significant ventricular dysfunction, not with normal function. Final answers are not in, but at this time it seems clear that most patients with angina will not show prolonged survival as a result of coronary bypass, but some important subgroups will. As noted earlier, clinical evaluation combined with judicious use of catheterization permits recognition of most of the subgroups in whom enhanced survival can be expected.

Physicians should not frighten patients into having surgery by invoking dire predictions of the outcome without operation. I like to tell patients the facts about bypass surgery as a part of the recommendation for surgery. I tell them that the operation is not curative, but palliative, and that the basic disease process, atherosclerosis, affects the grafts even more aggressively than the native arteries, and this process seems to accelerate in later years. In the Montreal Heart Institute studies, the graft closure rate was 2.1 percent per year from years 1 to 7 following surgery, but increased to 5.2 percent per year from years 7 to 12. By the tenth postoperative year, 30 percent of previously open grafts were occluded, and an additional 33 percent had significant atherosclerotic narrowings in them. These data apply to saphenous veins used for bypass. By contrast, internal mammary arteries show a 90 percent or greater patency rate at 10 years, strong reason to insist that surgeons utilize the internal mammary artery whenever feasible. Paralleling the change in grafts is a return of mild angina in one-third of patients at 10-year follow-up and more severe and limiting angina in another one-third of patients. Thus, the beneficial effects of bypass are not permanent. To date, no randomized study has shown that bypass surgery prevents myocardial infarction, even in high-risk subgroups. Second operations are possible and may be beneficial, but carry increased risk of failure, morbidity, and mortality. For these reasons, it seems prudent to delay bypass surgery as long as possible so that the patient will obtain maximal symptomatic and prognostic benefit.

I recommend surgery for patients who are significantly limited in spite of an adequate trial of medical therapy. For patients who have progressive and severe symptoms and angiographic evidence of severe disease, I recommend surgery without medical therapy. I tend to be more aggressive with patients who develop angina after myocardial infarction, either acutely or chronically, because these patients most often have three-vessel disease with ventricular dysfunction, and prognosis may be improved by surgery. For patients who cannot tolerate medication or do not wish to be dependent on medication, surgery is a logical alternative. Younger patients who wish to remain active often feel better with surgical treatment, but early operation makes it more likely that second operations will be needed. I often refer patients for surgery when there is evidence of severe ischemia, or poor treadmill performance, even when symptoms are mild or appear easy to control. I tend to be more conservative with older patients because getting through an operation may be difficult with a prolonged convalescence, and associated disease in cerebral circulation may lead to perioperative stroke. However, surgery should not be denied because of age if the patient has unmanageable symptoms, no other severe medical problems, and a satisfactory anatomic situation for bypass. Some diabetics show severe distal coronary disease, which makes grafting more difficult, but many do not show these changes, and in those that do, effective bypasses can be created, so that diabetes is not a reason to reject surgical management. I do not use severe ventricular dysfunction as a reason to exclude patients, since the best improvement in survival occurs in this group of patients, and surgical mortality is not high. Generally, if patients have enough ventricular function to allow them to have angina, they can get through surgery with beneficial results. Some patients with angina and concomitant pulmonary disease require bypass surgery to allow proper use of bronchodilator medication.

The decision to recommend surgery to a patient with angina is a major one and requires that the physician understand well the emotional state and social milieu of the patient as well as his cardiovascular status, general medical condition, and coronary arteriogram. The decision cannot be made with knowledge of only the latter.

ANGIOPLASTY

Indications for the use of angioplasty (PTCA) expand almost monthly. To date there are no long-term studies on patency or the effects of the procedure on prognosis, so that current indications are guided largely by the patient's symptoms and the intuitive reaction of the cardiologist. In general, I recommend angioplasty when feasible. In part this posture is predicated on the idea that patients found to be candidates for angioplasty have undergone catheterization for a clinically defined problem related to myocardial ischemia. Single-vessel disease is optimal, but double-vessel disease, particularly after infarction, and selected three-vessel disease may be amenable to improvement by this technique.

UNSTABLE ANGINA PECTORIS

STEPHEN C. ACHUFF, M.D.

Unstable angina is a common clinical syndrome of acutely deteriorating ischemic heart disease that carries substantial risk of myocardial infarction or cardiac death. Although new-onset effort angina or a worsening pattern of chronic angina can be considered "unstable," the term is generally reserved for more dramatic situations in which patients experience angina at rest and transient electrocardiographic signs of ischemia are demonstrable. Upon initial presentation, it may even be difficult to distinguish between unstable angina and acute myocardial infarction, and recent studies indicate that the two syndromes have much the same underlying pathophysiologic mechanisms. Our increasing awareness and understanding of these mechanisms has led to a more rational and, it is hoped, a more effective approach to the management of these dynamic conditions.

PATHOPHYSIOLOGY

Exercise-induced, chronic stable angina can be viewed as a problem of inadequate myocardial oxygen delivery in circumstances of increased demand. The anatomic substrate is one of fixed atherosclerotic coronary artery narrowings. Medical treatment is designed to reduce cardiac work load and thus decrease the demand side of the supply: demand equation. By contrast, unstable angina usually involves the additional problem of reduction in oxygen delivery in the face of relatively unchanged demands. In well over 90 percent of such patients, the same advanced coronary atherosclerotic narrowings seen with stable angina are present, but something new precipitates the unstable syndrome. Exactly what is new may not be discernible in many cases, but among factors to consider are progressive atherosclerotic narrowing, plaque rupture and hemorrhage, spasm in the area of a fixed lesion, and thrombosis causing acute occlusion. Platelet aggregation with release of vasoactive substances may be operative in both coronary vasospasm and thrombosis. It is important to mention these dynamic factors early in this discussion because (1) they raise therapeutic possibilities that might not be relevant in the management of stable angina, and (2) they highlight the need for aggressive and expeditious evaluation and therapy in this group of patients.

GENERAL PRINCIPLES OF MANAGEMENT

These critically ill patients have the potential for sudden decompensation and therefore warrant admission to an intensive care area. The only important diagnostic information to be established is whether or not a myocardial infarction is evolving or has already occurred. Serial ECGs and serum enzymes should be obtained for the first 24 hours after admission. In particular, when patients are having recurrent bouts of pain, ECG localization of reversible ischemic changes should be sought as this may aid in the overall analysis of which coronary artery needs particular attention, for example, with reperfusion by balloon angioplasty.

In the initial assessment of patients with unstable angina, it is important not to overlook readily treatable precipitating factors such as new anemia due to an occult ulcer or colon cancer, uncontrolled hypertension, infection with associated fever and tachycardia, new-onset atrial fibrillation with a rapid ventricular response, and hyperthyroidism. Correction of these aggravating conditions may be all that is required to restore complete stability, and such patients need not undergo rigorous diagnostic and therapeutic maneuvers.

Once a patient is admitted to a monitored unit, the goal of therapy is to achieve an angina-free state as promptly as possible, beginning with simple forms of treatment and working through to the more complex. This approach allows for flexibility and maintenance of as many options as possible, depending on individual circumstances and unforeseen developments. Lack of predictability is one of the features inherent in the unstable angina syndrome, and the physician must guard against inadvertently closing an important diagnostic or therapeutic "door." With regard to drug therapy, for example, it is preferable to begin with short-acting parenteral regimens so that effects (both beneficial and adverse) can be assessed quickly and the drug can be stopped or the dosage changed readily as needed. Critical time may be lost waiting for the effect of an orally administered, long-acting drug to dissipate. Specific examples include: using propranolol rather than atenolol when the adequacy of left ventricular function is not known, intravenous heparin instead of warfarin (or even aspirin) in case the patient requires an intra-aortic balloon pump or coronary bypass surgery, and intravenous nitroglycerin as opposed to oral isosorbide dinitrate if hypotension becomes a problem, as it often does with multiple drug regimens. Once it is clear that a patient's condition is stabilized and a long range plan of management can be devised, it is appropriate to begin changing to forms of therapy that are suitable and convenient for outpatient use.

DRUG THERAPY

Nitrates

The cornerstone of pharmacologic therapy for unstable angina is nitroglycerin. Although seldom wholly effective alone in controlling symptoms and signs of ischemia, it should be the first drug used once patients are admitted to the hospital. Intravenous nitroglycerin, in my opinion, is clearly the preparation of choice as opposed to cutaneous or oral forms. It can be titrated precisely to achieve maximal benefit with minimal adverse effects. Dosages usually begin at 2 to 5 μg per minute and can be increased frequently up to 200 to 300 μg per minute, depending on systemic arterial pressure. Intolerance because of headaches is uncommon if the dosage is low initially and increased gradually, although some patients may experience this side effect and require additional analgesics. If hypotension develops, one must be certain that the patient has an adequate intravascular volume and left ventricular filling pressure. This can usually be assessed clinically, but occasional patients require pulmonary artery catheterization for accurate hemodynamic monitoring.

Cutaneous nitrates, specifically nitroglycerin ointment, can be useful for the hospitalized patient once the acute phase of his illness has passed. This form of administration is best viewed as transitional between the intensive care unit, where precise dosage is critical, and the outpatient setting, where more standardized dosages of an oral preparation can be employed. Nitroglycerin ointment should be applied every 4 to 6 hours and in doses between 1 and 4 inches spread thinly and evenly over a hairless area of skin. If hypotension occurs, the drug can be wiped off quickly and the amount of the next dose reduced. Because of its relative inconvenience, it is not practical for outpatient use so that prior to a patient's discharge I generally convert to an oral preparation, for example, isosorbide dinitrate, 20 to 40 mg every 6 hours. At the time of this writing there is no once-daily patch preparation of cutaneous nitroglycerin that is effective for more than 8 to 12 hours. Because of this as well as the greater expense as compared with oral nitrates, I cannot recommend their use at present.

Beta-Blockers

The vast majority of patients with unstable angina benefit from beta-blockade despite opinions to the contrary. Concern about using a beta-blocker stems from the largely theoretic rationale that alpha-adrenergic-mediated coronary vasoconstrictive influences are unopposed if beta-blockade is instituted, and the net effect is an exacerbation of myocardial ischemia. In clinical practice, this has been observed only in occasional patients with purely vasospastic angina, but these represent a small minority of the overall population of unstable angina. Most patients are treated concurrently with a calcium-channel blocking agent to prevent spasm, and it has now been shown conclusively that a regimen of beta-blockers in conjunction with nitrates and a calcium-channel blocker is superior to therapy with the latter two alone.

The primary practical concerns regarding the use of beta-blockers are their potential for causing undue bradycardia and congestive heart failure. They are ideal for patients who present with tachycardia or develop tachycardia after being started on intravenous nitroglycerin, and for hypertensive patients with hypertrophic, hyperkinetic left ventricles. But great caution must be exercised in patients whose admission heart rate is only in the 60s or 70s or those whose left ventricular function may be compromised by previous infarction or valvular disease. One should always make a careful bedside assessment of ventricular function prior to initiating beta-blocker therapy, and if questions remain, an objective test such as echocardiography or radionuclide ventriculography should be obtained. In some situations, it may be impossible to accurately predict the patient who will respond adversely to a beta-blocker, and for this reason I prefer to use propranolol because of its short duration of action. This preparation also has the advantage of being available for parenteral use when lowering of the pulse and/or blood pressure quickly is deemed important. The only other parenteral beta-blocker now available is metoprolol, and this might be preferable in the occasional patient with significant bronchospastic lung disease, although its duration of action is much longer than that of propranolol. As with chronic, stable angina, one uses doses that maintain a resting heart rate of 50 to 60 beats per minute. With oral propranolol, most patients can be started safely on a dose of 40 mg every 6 hours, and subsequent doses are adjusted accordingly.

Longer-acting beta-blockers such as atenolol, nadolol, metoprolol, and timolol are reserved for patients who have stabilized and are out of the critical phase of their illness, perhaps anticipating hospital discharge. At that point, one tries to simplify the medical regimen as much as possible, and cutting down the number of pills a patient has to take is one component of this approach.

Calcium-Channel Blockers

Three agents in this class of drugs are currently available: nifedipine, diltiazem, and verapamil. Although each has been shown to be effective in patients with unstable angina, I prefer to use nifedipine unless there is some specific contraindication, such as previous intolerance to the drug. I think it is probably the best coronary vasodilator of the three, it has the least negative inotropic effect and the least tendency to alter cardiac conduction (important considerations in patients who are also taking a beta-blocker), and it can be squeezed from the capsule and administered sublingually for prompt onset of action. The usual starting dose is 10 mg every 6 hours, and this may be increased to as much as 40 mg every 6 hours or even every 4 hours.

Diltiazem may be prescribed for patients who do not tolerate nifedipine, but I regard it as a second-line calcium blocker whose main advantage is that it is least likely to cause side effects. An occasional refractory patient is seen whose angina can be better controlled by adding diltiazem to nifedipine, although one has to be cautious about producing excessive hypotension from multiple vasodilator drug regimens.

Verapamil's role in the management of unstable angina is hardest to define, but its advantages include its ability to suppress supraventricular arrhythmias and its negative inotropic properties. The patient with documented hypertrophic cardiomyopathy or similar left ventricular pathophysiology, or the patient with persistent tachycardia (or paroxysmal supraventricular tachycardia) that is refractory to beta-blockade might be started on verapamil as the initial calcium-channel blocker in preference to nifedipine or diltiazem. Verapamil is the only one in this class of drugs that is currently available for parenteral use, and there may be unusual situations in which this mode of administration can be helpful.

Antiplatelet and Anticoagulant Drugs

With our present understanding of the pathophysiology operative in some cases of unstable angina implicating transient thrombosis of a narrowed coronary artery, it seems rational to use anticoagulants as part of the treatment regimen. In fact, two randomized trials have shown a striking benefit from aspirin, in one study, and heparin, in the other, in patients with well-documented unstable angina. Use of these drugs is not intended to replace the other agents discussed earlier, but as supplemental therapy. The difficulty with giving them routinely, especially early in the course of treating unstable angina, is that they may create logistic problems with respect to procedures. Cardiac surgeons do not like to operate on patients who have been treated recently with aspirin for fear of excessive surgical bleeding. Likewise, a patient who is receiving heparin therapy cannot undergo urgent percutaneous cardiac catheterization or intra-aortic balloon pump insertion. One has to either reverse the effects of heparin by giving protamine, which has its own risks, or wait 4 to 6 hours for the anticoagulated state to resolve.

Despite the aforementioned problems, I believe that there are circumstances where antiplatelet or anticoagulant therapy can be helpful. Patients who have been treated with maximum conventional therapy but continue to experience angina at rest sometimes can be controlled with full anticoagulating doses of heparin intravenously. Infusions are given for 48 to 72 hours, and then aspirin, 324 mg once daily, is begun (the dose used in the Veterans Administration Cooperative Study) as the heparin is stopped. This assumes that the patient will not be undergoing coronary artery bypass grafting or balloon angioplasty, in which case heparin is stopped 6 hours prior to the procedure. In patients having surgery, dipyridamole, 100 mg 4 times a day, is begun 24 to 48 hours preoperatively according to the protocol used by the Mayo Clinic in patients undergoing surgery for stable angina. With balloon angioplasty, assuming the feasibility of the procedure has already been demonstrated by prior angiography, both aspirin and dipyridamole are begun 24 to 48 hours beforehand. Patients who are inoperable and cannot undergo PTCA are kept on aspirin, 324 mg daily, indefinitely. I know of no studies that involve patients treated with warfarin for unstable angina syndrome and generally do not use this drug after the period of intravenous heparinization is completed.

INTRA-AORTIC BALLOON COUNTERPULSATION

There is no question that the majority of even the most refractory patients with unstable angina can be controlled at least temporarily by intra-aortic balloon counterpulsation. However, this is not a step to be taken lightly, for at least two important reasons. First, having inserted the balloon pump, one is obligated to proceed with definitive evaluation and treatment promptly. Catheterization must be done soon (usually within 24 hours) and revascularization by some means shortly thereafter. If for any reason one is concerned that the patient might not be a candidate for surgery or angioplasty, the balloon pump probably should not be used in the first place. There are few more difficult management problems than having to deal with a patient who is balloon-dependent and who has no additional options available. Second, the intra-aortic balloon pump has its own complications, some of which can lead to significant morbidity. These are mainly related to vascular injury or compromise of the circulation to the limb where the device is inserted. Despite these important reservations, intra-aortic balloon pumping can be life-saving in patients with recurrent rest angina on maximal pharmacologic therapy. It is an extremely valuable component of the cardiologist's armamentarium in the treatment of unstable angina. Skill in the techniques of percutaneous insertion and subsequent maintenance of optimal counterpulsation hemodynamics should be readily accessible in any hospital with a cardiac catheterization laboratory.

CARDIAC CATHETERIZATION

As a general rule of management, allowing for exceptions as with all guidelines in medicine, patients admitted with unstable angina should undergo cardiac catheterization to define the coronary anatomy before they are discharged from hospital. Preferably, the patient should be stabilized to the point where the procedure is considered virtually elective. However, if good control of the angina is not feasible, there should be no delay in proceeding with catheterization because of unfounded fears regarding safety of the procedure. In all likelihood the risks of not knowing the anatomy exceed the risks of catheterization in these refractory patients.

I think it is important to obtain coronary angiography in patients with unstable angina because a certain proportion (5 to 10%) have normal or near-normal arteries, and for this group nitrates, calcium-channel blockers, and/or antiplatelet therapy is by far the most appropriate. An additional 10 to 15 percent of patients have significant left main coronary artery obstruction, and for this group coronary artery bypass grafting is indicated. Decisions regarding optimal management in the remaining 75 to 85 percent of patients can be made on an individual basis, but I find these decisions easier if I know the details of the coronary anatomy. Furthermore, several years ago we made decisions *not* to perform catheterization on some patients based on a judgment that they could not be surgical candidates because of advanced age, poor left ventricular function, significant noncardiac disease, and the like. However, with current expanded criteria for what constitutes surgical candidacy and, perhaps more importantly, the availability of nonsurgical means of revascularization (thrombolysis, PTCA), most of the barriers to performing a diagnostic catheterization have been removed.

Immediately on completion of the coronary angiography, while the patient is still in the laboratory and before the arterial catheter is removed, a decision should be made regarding thrombolytic therapy and/or balloon angioplasty, assuming these techniques are available. These topics are addressed in more detail in other chapters, but both forms of therapy, alone or in combination, have been applied successfully to patients with unstable angina in many centers. At present, intracoronary streptokinase is the agent used for thrombolysis, but in the future one can expect this to be supplanted by tissue plasminogen activator made by recombinant DNA techniques (rTPA).

SUBSEQUENT THERAPY

Assuming that the patient does not undergo thrombolytic therapy or PTCA after diagnostic coronary angiography, how does one proceed with a rational treatment plan? Patients who continue to experience angina at rest or with minimal exertion should have coronary artery bypass grafting done as soon as feasible if they have operable vessels. Those whose angina can be more completely controlled become like patients with chronic stable angina. They need not undergo urgent surgery, but this can remain an option, depending on several factors: symptomatic status, the particular coronary anatomy demonstrated at catheterization, and physiologic testing. For the patient whose angina has become quiescent on medical therapy, I try to devise the simplest regimen that can be followed as an outpatient. I then obtain a treadmill exercise ECG and 24-hour Holter monitor reading prior to hospital discharge, seeking signs of ischemia at low levels of activity. If these are found, I generally recommend elective surgery, but if not, I simply follow the patient indefinitely in the usual fashion. As with all patients coming to medical attention because of ischemic heart disease, a vigorous attempt to modify risk factors for atherosclerosis is an important aspect of long-term therapy.

REHABILITATION AFTER MYOCARDIAL INFARCTION

GARY J. BALADY, M.D.
DONALD A. WEINER, M.D.

Major efforts and millions of dollars are expended each year to establish and implement new methods of caring for the patient with acute myocardial infarction (MI). Once the patient has survived a MI, continued efforts must be made both to promote maximum recovery and to prevent its recurrence. Well-designed cardiac rehabilitation exercise programs have thus become part of the standard treatment for patients with coronary artery disease. The goals of a cardiac rehabilitation program include (1) restoration of optimal physiologic, psychological, and vocational status to program participants; (2) attainment of a physiologic "training effect," which would increase the efficiency of the heart and peripheral muscles so that myocardial oxygen consumption is reduced at any given level of work; and (3) reduction of risk factors for the development or progression of coronary artery disease.

CARDIAC REHABILITATION PROGRAM

Inhospital Phase

Once the patient has been admitted to the coronary care unit (CCU) with the diagnosis of a MI, an individualized cardiac rehabilitation program should be implemented. If the patient has stable blood pressure and heart rate and does not require invasive hemodynamic monitoring, initial activity orders should call for him to be at bedrest with commode privileges. Use of the bedpan is associated with a greater increase in myocardial work than use of the commode. The second day after admission, he should begin to sit on the side of the bed and dangle his feet or sit in the chair. This early progression of activity in an otherwise stable patient has been shown (1) to reduce the incidence of orthostatic hypotension, which develops after prolonged bedrest, and (2) to lead to a greater exercise capacity at the time of discharge. Continued increases in activity should be monitored by the physician, nurses, and inpatient cardiac rehabilitation team (if available). Early ambulation, as well as stretching and range-of-motion exercises, can begin after the patient has been transferred from the CCU to the ward (Table 1). The patient should be able to climb a flight of stairs without developing angina or marked shortness of breath prior to discharge.

Certainly, early post-MI patients are a "captive" audience and are usually amenable to making changes in their lifestyle that might reduce the chances of reinfarction. An educational program, whether formal or informal, is an integral part of post-MI therapy. Topics to be addressed are (1) definition of coronary artery disease—angina versus infarct; (2) medications—schedule, uses, and side effects; (3) risk factors for the development of coronary artery disease; (4) functional status postdischarge—e.g., work, sexual activity, exercise, and driving; (5) diet; and (6) name and telephone number of person to be contacted with a problem or question.

The inhospital phase of cardiac rehabilitation should include recommendations for diet. Unquestionably, example is the best teacher. Thus, prudent diet orders while the patient is in the hospital should feature foods low in fat and cholesterol and containing no added salt. Diet orders should then be tailored to meet individual needs for obese, diabetic, hypertensive, or hypercholesterolemic patients. Fasting cholesterol and HDL levels drawn during hospitalization are useful in both risk-factor assessment and diet therapy.

A predischarge modified exercise stress test should be performed about 9 to 10 days post-MI in the stable patient (Table 2). The test is modified in two ways—it starts at a lower work load and increases with smaller increments. The test is most safely performed by patients who have completed an inhospital rehabilitation program without complications. Patients with rest pain, angina at low activity levels, congestive heart failure (CHF), a changing ECG profile, complex ventricular arrhythmias, and rest or postural hypotension should be excluded. Endpoints of exercise should include the occurrence of mild angina, complex ventricular arrhythmias, 1 to 2 mm of ischemic ST-segment depression, or the attainment of a target heart rate (usually 60 to 70% of the age-predicted maximal heart rate) or workload (usually 4 to 5 multiples of resting energy expenditure [METS]). The test can provide useful information in assessing prognosis, adequacy of current medication, and functional capacity and in guiding posthospital rehabilitation.

Walking remains the most available method of exer-

TABLE 1 Boston University Medical Center Cardiac Rehabilitation: Phase 1

*Stage**	*Activities*	*METS†*	*Education and Exercise*
I	Complete bed rest	1.0	*Active assistive* ROM to all extremities in a semi-Fowler position twice per day
	Complete bath by nurse	1.0	Breathing exercises twice per day
	Brush teeth	1.5	Emotional support: patient/family orientation to CCU
	Feed self (tray prepared by nurse)	1.0	
	Bedside commode	1.5	
II	Bedside commode	1.5	Active ROM to all 4 extremities in semi-Fowler position twice per day
	Bathe and shave in bed	1.5	Breathing exercises twice per day
	Sit in armchair:		Orientation to cardiac rehabilitation program
	1st day (1 × 30 min)	1.0	
	2nd day (2 × 1 hour)	1.0	
III	*Patient out of CCU*		
	Bathroom privileges	2.0	Active exercises in sitting position
	Bathe seated:		Breathing exercises
	at sink	1.7	Job and home assessment
	at bedside	1.7	Risk factors
	Shower seated	1.8	
	Sit in armchair as tolerated	1.5	
	Walk in room at will	2.0	
IV	Shower standing	3.5	As above: exercise
	Walk in hall with assistance	2.0	Review risk factors
			Discussions of healing and limitations
			Medications and diet
V	Walk in hall at will	2.5–3.0	Discharge plans
	Climb stairs with therapist	3.0	Active exercise standing
	Home program		Home care and activities
			Medications and diet teaching

**Criteria for advancement through stages:*

1. Free from angina
2. Controlled congestive heart failure
3. No adverse ECG changes
4. No new elevation in enzymes
5. No significant arrhythmias
6. Patient tolerates present activity level

† METS = Multiples of resting energy expenditure

TABLE 2 Representative Predischarge Modified Treadmill Exercise Stress-Test Protocols

Stage	*Speed (mph)*	*Grade (%)*	*METS*
Modified Bruce			
0	1.7	0	1.7
½	1.7	5	2.9
1	1.7	10	4.0
Modified Naughton			
1	2.0	0	2
2	2.0	3.5	3
3	2.0	7	4
4	2.0	10.5	5

cise in the first 3 weeks after hospital discharge. Patients should be encouraged to begin a walking program as early as possible. Guidelines for this program should include:

1. Location—no inclines initially; shopping malls or indoor running tracks are optimal, especially during inclement weather;
2. Dress—loose-fitting clothes appropriate for ambient temperature; and
3. Program—the patient should walk at least three times per week on alternate days; he should start walking for about 10 minutes per day, increasing to 20 minutes by the third week of exercise; walking pace should be about 80 steps per minute for the first week, gradually increasing to 120 steps per minute as tolerated; he should keep nitroglycerin at hand if needed and report any symptoms of angina to the physician.

Recommendations about return to work should be individualized for each patient, depending on his or her occupational requirements and functional capacity 6 to 8 weeks postdischarge, which may be assessed by exercise stress testing. Driving an automobile is a task that in general adds little to overall myocardial work. A patient should be allowed to drive within a few weeks of discharge, providing that his condition is stable, and at least initially he should avoid stressful driving conditions. Similarly, resumption of sexual activity can begin early postdischarge. Sexual activity increases myocardial oxygen demand to an extent similar to climbing a flight of stairs or completing stage I of a Bruce Protocol Treadmill Test. Therefore, ease of performance in these activities may be used as a guide. Reassurance by the physician to *both* patient and spouse regarding sexual activity is strongly recommended.

Out-of-Hospital Phase

Once the patient has been discharged from the hospital, he must continue his efforts to accomplish the goals of cardiac rehabilitation. He should be evaluated within 3 to 4 weeks and entered into an outpatient cardiac rehabilitation program. Patients will benefit most from such a program if it is begun early in the posthospital course.

The outpatient program staff consists of a medical director (usually a cardiologist), registered nurse-coordinator, exercise physiologist, dietician, and psychologist. This multidisciplinary team, in conjunction with the referring physician, works to design and implement an individualized exercise, diet, and stress-reduction program for each patient. Patients are initially evaluated by a history, physical examination, and exercise stress test. The exercise stress test assesses functional capacity and determines an individualized target heart rate for training.

Patients should be excluded from participation in the cardiac rehabilitation program if they (1) have unstable angina, (2) suffer from class III or greater CHF, (3) have uncontrolled arrhythmias, (4) have uncontrolled hypertension, or (5) do not have the permission of their personal physician. Exercise sessions are held three times per week on alternate days. Each session includes the following:

1. Stretching exercises and calisthenics, used to reduce muscle strains during continued exercise.
2. Warm-up—5 minutes of dynamic exercise to allow redistribution of circulating blood to the exercising muscles. Dynamic exercise, which involves high repetition movements against a low resistance, is performed on a bicycle ergometer, rowing machine, or treadmill.
3. Training—20 to 30 minutes of dynamic exercise at target heart rate. That is, the pulse rate is maintained at 75 to 85 percent of the maximum heart rate achieved during the exercise test at which the patient was free from angina or ischemic ST changes. Target heart rate is similarly determined for patients taking beta-adrenergic blocking agents. For patients unable to determine their heart rate, instruction about the *rate of perceived exertion* has been useful. This method correlates the patient's exertion levels with the desired heart-rate training levels.
4. Cool-down—5 minutes of low-resistance exercise. This prevents postexercise orthostatic hypotension.

This regimen should lead to a training effect within 8 to 12 weeks. Dynamic upper extremity exercise training should be part of any cardiac rehabilitation program, especially in patients whose occupation requires work with their arms, e.g., carpenters and painters. Lower extremity training alone will not serve to blunt the heart-rate response to exercise when performing upper extremity work. Therefore, arm ergometry, light weights, or pulleys should be employed to increase the strength and efficiency of the upper extremities and lead to decreased myocardial oxygen demand during upper extremity work. The cardiac rehabilitation program also should be designed to implement methods for risk-factor reduction. Diet therapy, along with exercise, can promote weight loss and decrease total cholesterol levels. Individual and group diet counseling should be available. The basic principles of nutrition need to be stressed in a practical, useful manner. Advice about how to prepare foods and what foods to choose or avoid when dining out is an important adjunct to any diet plan. What is kept simple will be easy to remember and more likely to be employed.

Psychosocial counseling is integral to the succesful rehabilitation of any patient. Methods of stress reduction, elimination of smoking, and other behavior modification activities should be employed. A psychologist experienced in dealing with cardiac patients can serve to guide the efforts of the personnel who work directly with the patients. Much support and lifestyle modification can take place through the nurse and exercise physiologist during each session. The psychologist can give periodic group lectures, as well as be available for individual referrals.

DISCHARGE PLANNING

One of the most important goals of cardiac rehabilitation is that patients continue to practice what they have learned about exercise, nutrition, stress, and risk-factor reduction, long after leaving the close supervision of a formal program. Therefore, participants must be slowly tapered from supervised sessions to home or outside exercise, rather than being abruptly discharged or ''graduated'' from a given program. The scheduling of visits should initially be three times per week and then taper, depending on individual progress. Patients should not be completely weaned from the supervised sessions unless they have achieved certain goals. That is, patients must demonstrate that they have attained a functional capacity adequate to their occupation and appropriate to their lifestyle. They should have a fundamental understanding of their cardiovascular disease process and should demonstrate knowledge of the signs and symptoms of their disease. They should also have a clear understanding of the benefits of physical activity in improving functional capacity, the importance of a safe heart range and limiting symptoms of physical activity, the benefits of optimal nutrition in weight and blood-lipid control, and the importance of modifying personal stress.

The medical director and cardiac rehabilitation team should meet weekly to discuss new patients and review the progress of current program participants. Changes in the exercise prescription should be made if needed, and problems such as weight, stress, noncompliance, or change in cardiac status should be identified and appropriate plans made. Forwarding periodic progress reports to the referring physician ensures a continued working relationship among patient, cardiac rehabilitation team, and personal physician.

RECORD KEEPING

Maintenance of adequate and complete records is invaluable to optimal patient care. All patients records should contain (1) dictated history, physical, and medication list based on initial visit data collected; (2) reports of exercise tests; (3) exercise prescription; (4) daily exercise session data, including rest, peak and postexercise heart rate achieved, and peak work load achieved; (5) attendance records; (6) referring physician's name, address, telephone number, and written permission; (7) laboratory data; (8) patient consent form; and (9) care plan evaluation and update.

TABLE 3 Emergency Equipment and Drugs

Emergency Equipment:

Defibrillator
ECG cable, electrodes, parts, and paper
Oxygen tank: not to read less than 500 cc
Crash cart: fully stocked with emergency drugs, intravenous bags and tubing, endotracheal tubes, and laryngoscope

Emergency Drugs:

Atropine
Bretylium tosylate
Sodium bicarbonate
Calcium
Epinephrine
Dopamine
Lidocaine
Procainamide

PROGRAM BENEFITS

A well-planned inpatient and outpatient cardiac rehabilitation program can be beneficial to an individual in many ways. Attainment of a training effect should lead to an increased tolerance for activities, while concomitantly reducing cardiac risk factors. Increased HDL levels, decreased blood pressure, decreased weight, and elimination of smoking all can be achieved. Patients acquire a sense of confidence and well-being and are therefore more likely to return to a productive life. Whether subsequent cardiovascular morbidity and mortality are actually reduced remains inconclusive.

RISKS

Organized cardiac rehabilitation programs pose little risk to its participants. The incidence of cardiac death or ventricular fibrillation during exercise in a supervised program remains low. Program safety should be maintained by both experienced staff and clearly outlined emergency procedures and policies. Resuscitation equipment must be readily available and in proper working order at all exercise sessions (Table 3).

ALTERNATIVES TO SUPERVISED EXERCISE

Well-motivated, low-risk patients may be able to exercise safely at home using the same principles as previously outlined for a supervised exercise program. Careful heart-rate monitoring with occasional transtelephonic transmission of the ECG can minimize the risk. Drawbacks of this approach include the loss of the camaraderie of a group and a subsequently increased dropout rate.

MITRAL STENOSIS

ARTHUR SELZER, M.D.

Mitral stenosis is the only valve lesion that is always related to rheumatic fever. Almost always acquired in childhood, the clinical course of mitral stenosis extends over many decades. Management of a patient thus becomes of lifelong duration and involves several problems, including prophylactic therapy, guidance and management of the asymptomatic stage, management of the symptomatic stage, treatment of complications, timing of valve surgery, and management of prosthetic-valve problems.

PROPHYLACTIC THERAPY

Prophylactic therapy involves the use of drugs aimed at the prevention of recurrences of rheumatic fever and the prevention of infective endocarditis.

Rheumatic fever prophylaxis is aimed at prevention of streptococcal infections, which are capable of triggering the autoimmune reaction, manifesting itself as acute rheumatic fever. This, in turn, may produce or increase valve damage. Standard therapy involves the use of penicillin, either as an oral dose of 500,000 units daily or, preferably, as monthly injections of 1.2 million units of penicillin benzathine. The superiority of parenteral penicillin is presumably related to the elimination of the problem of patient compliance. In patients with penicillin sensitivity, sulfadiazine or tetracycline may be used.

All patients with known valvular lesions have high susceptibility to bacterial infection. Proneness to infective endocarditis is low in mitral stenosis (unassociated with mitral regurgitation); nevertheless, the usual prophylactic therapy is indicated in every patient. Standard prophylaxis consists of drug therapy at the time of dental manipulations and operations on the respiratory or urinary tract, as well as manipulations in the lower gastrointestinal tract. The standard drug is penicillin, with erythromycin as the second choice. Many dose schedules are available. The most widely used one is the administration of oral penicillin V: 2 g before the dental procedure followed by 500 mg every 6 hours for 4 to 8 doses.

MANAGEMENT OF PRESURGICAL STAGE

Management of patients with early stages of mitral stenosis involves (in addition to prophylaxis) counseling about vocational and recreational activities, as well as recommendations about pregnancy. Mitral stenosis differs from other valve lesions in that the principal cause of disability—high pulmonary capillary pressure—is inherent in the lesion rather than appearing late as a result of myocardial failure. Consequently, some limitation of activities due to dyspnea is often a lifelong feature of patients with mitral stenosis. While it is not unusual to see patients with severe aortic regurgitation indulging without difficulty in athletic activities, patients with mitral stenosis tend to lead inactive lives. Although many patients are guided by symptoms, those who are able to perform normally should be discouraged from strenuous activities. Furthermore, asymptomatic patients may respond to unusual exercise or to water and salt overload with acute pulmonary edema. Appropriate warnings are in order. Women in the childbearing age with mild or moderate mitral stenosis may deliver children without major problems, but they need careful medical supervision; however, it is prudent to discuss with such patients the higher-than-average risk of pregnancy.

Treatment of the symptomatic stage requires a great deal of thought. Surgical treatment of mitral stenosis is a palliative procedure, aimed at relief of symptoms. The clinician has to decide at which point the patient is sufficiently symptomatic to warrant mitral valve surgery. Yet symptoms in mitral stenosis are, as already explained, often variable, related to variation in lifestyle, and may be manageable medically for long intervals without difficulty. Thus, unless mitral stenosis is shown to be severe, management initially should be nonsurgical. The most effective drug controlling effort dyspnea and protecting patients from the risk of pulmonary edema is one of the diuretic agents, either one of the thiazide series or a loop diuretic (furosemide). Mild restriction of dietary sodium is also advisable. Some patients develop an early tendency to retain fluid, in which case monitoring of body weight is used as a guide in diuretic therapy.

Medical treatment of mitral stenosis includes management of complications, which play a very important role in the natural history of this lesion. Aggressive management of the serious direct manifestation of mitral stenosis may become necessary in patients in whom surgical treatment is contraindicated or who refuse surgical treatment. Patients with advanced mitral stenosis are frequently in atrial fibrillation, in which case control of rate by digitalis, or beta-blocking agents, or both is essential. Aggressive diuretic therapy with appropriate control of water and electrolyte balance is often needed. The treatment is similar to that of "intractable cardiac failure," even though the cause of congestive phenomena is mechanical and not myocardial "pump" failure.

Complications play a major role in the course of mitral stenosis. The most common and most important group of complications are *atrial arrhythmias*. Atrial fibrillation develops so frequently in older patients that it almost becomes the expected sequel to mitral stenosis. As a rule, atrial fibrillation appears first in paroxysmal form. Attacks of paroxysmal atrial fibrillation represent the most common cause of the first appearance of cardiac symptoms. Rapid ventricular rate may produce frightening onset of severe dyspnea or even pulmonary edema. Prompt control of ventricular rate by intravenous digoxin or verapamil may not only slow ventricular rate to relief dyspnea, but may also terminate the paroxysm. Patients who have repeated attacks of atrial fibrillation may be given quinidine (not more than 1.2 g per 24 hours) as a means of prevention of attacks or — if attacks occur only occasionally — a daily maintenance dose of digoxin.

When atrial fibrillation is present in its persistent

form, the choice of management rests between restoration of sinus rhythm and control of ventricular rate while leaving the patient in atrial fibrillation (Fig. 1). The decision as to which of these two choices to accept rests with the clinician's appraisal of the probability that sinus rhythm can be maintained. Three factors contribute to persistence of chronic atrial fibrillation: the patient's age, the size of the left atrium, and the duration of the arrhythmia. Thus, an older patient with a large left atrium, who is first seen months after the onset of arrhythmia, has a low enough probability of staying in sinus rhythm that no attempt of conversion to sinus rhythm is indicated. Patients with new onset of atrial fibrillation are worthy of an attempt to restore sinus rhythm even if the other conditions are unfavorable. Patients are pretreated by quinidine (0.2 g every 6 hours) for 1 or 2 days—some patients may return to sinus rhythm on quinidine alone. Thereafter, direct-current shock is administered under anesthesia or heavy sedation. After sinus rhythm is restored, a maintenance dose of quinidine is administered indefinitely.

Patients who remain in atrial fibrillation can usually be managed without difficulty with digitalis. The dose of the drug should be individually adjusted using ventricular rate similar to that of sinus rhythm as a target. Some patients develop inordinate acceleration of the ventricular rate during activity-producing disability. Often an increase in digitalis dose which slows the resting rate to about 50 contractions per minute may alleviate this problem. A minority of patients cannot be adequately controlled by digitalis. The addition of a beta-blocking agent or verapamil, may help to attain the desired responses of the ventricular rate.

Other atrial arrhythmias occurring in mitral stenosis include atrial flutter and supraventricular tachycardia. They are as a rule paroxysmal. Effective control can usually be accomplished by quinidine, verapamil, or a beta-blocking agent. As in paroxysmal atrial fibrillation, rare attacks are best treated when they develop; frequent attacks may require maintenance therapy of one of these drugs or of digitalis.

Systemic embolization represents another common and often devastating complication of mitral stenosis. Emboli originate in the left atrium and occur preferentially, although not exclusively, in the presence of atrial fibrillation. Cerebral embolism leading to hemiplegia occurs frequently in mitral stenosis and represents a common cause of clinical disability. Management of hemiplegia involves conventional rehabilitation. The principal therapeutic intervention related to thromboembolism is the controversial use of anticoagulants as a preventive treat-

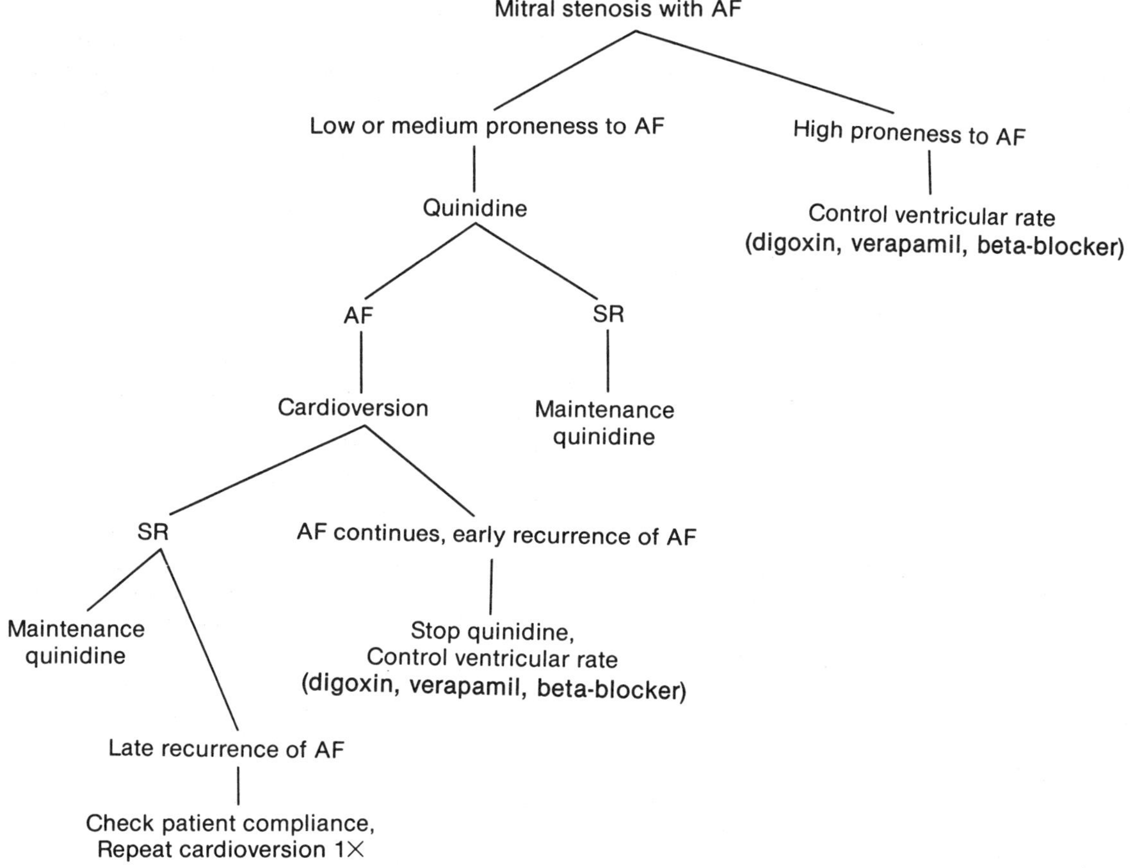

Figure 1 Management choices when atrial fibrillation is present.

ment. The controversy centers around the question of when anticoagulants should be used. It is generally agreed that patients with mitral stenosis who suffered cerebral embolism need continuous and permanent anticoagulant therapy with drugs of the coumarin series (warfarin is the standard drug). Considering that oral anticoagulant therapy is a high-risk intervention (it is estimated that this treatment carries a 1 percent annual mortality), some experts question whether the development of atrial fibrillation per se represents an indication of anticoagulant therapy. A reasonable approach to this dilemma is to use anticoagulants in those patients who show the presence or the suspicion of mural thrombi in the left atrium by echocardiography and in those who have grossly enlarged left atria.

Other complications of mitral stenosis include *hemoptysis*. In the great majority of patients, this is a self-limiting complication that requires no treatment. Rarely, massive pulmonary hemorrhage may occur (“pulmonary apoplexy”), which may require blood transfusion.

Other complications include infective endocarditis, which is, as stated, rare in pure mitral stenosis. Patients with mitral stenosis have a high susceptibility to upper respiratory infections, which are occasionally a starting point of clinical disability.

SURGICAL THERAPY

Timing of surgical intervention represents the most important decision-making process in the management of this lesion. The decision relates to two points: when to operate and what type of operation to recommend.

One of the common misconceptions regarding mitral stenosis is the opinion that this lesion is a “surgical disease,” with the implication that every patient should undergo surgical treatment. Two points need to be reemphasized: (1) mitral valve surgery is not curative, but palliative, i.e., a residual narrowing of the mitral orifice is the rule, and (2) results of surgery are not permanent; in most instances further operations are needed.

Optimal management of a patient with mitral stenosis thus requires a thoughtful analysis of all the factors before surgical treatment is recommended. The following factors need to be considered when surgical treatment is being contemplated.

1. Clinical disability, as already explained, varies considerably and is frequently nonpermanent. Thus, effort dyspnea or paroxysmal dyspnea may respond to medical management. Consistent (not episodic) progression of symptoms or failure of medical therapy are the most important indications that surgical relief may be required.
2. Complications of mitral stenosis—which account for many clinical manifestations—are not necessarily related to the severity of the lesion and may not be relieved by the operation, if stenosis is mild. They include atrial fibrillation, systemic embolization, and hemoptysis.
3. On the other hand, some patients, particularly middle-aged women with severe mitral stenosis, may have intuitively restricted themselves to a point that they deny symptoms, even though they may have severe pulmonary hypertension with right ventricular failure. Symptoms may be a poor guide for surgical selection.

In terms of risk– benefit relationships, each patient should be individually considered for surgery with specific objectives in mind. The two major objectives are (1) relief of critical mitral stenosis, particularly when pulmonary hypertension is present, regardless of disability, and (2) the relief of symptoms related to the mechanical aspects of mitral stenosis (not to complications). As a corollary of this approach, one should consider that symptoms present in patients who have mild or moderate degrees of mitral stenosis often persist after successful operations. One frequently encounters middle-aged women with mitral stenosis within the range of 1.0 to 1.5 cm^2 with dyspnea, excessive fatigability, or fluid retention, who are in atrial fibrillation and whose heart rate cannot be adequately controlled, remaining unchanged after mitral valve replacement.

The choice of operation presents a point worthy of serious consideration. The successful development of mitral valve replacement led to an eclipse of mitral valvotomy. Yet, experience with mitral valvotomy, the origin of which dates back to 1948, has been satisfactory, even spectacular, in suitable patients. This operation is successful when stenosis is predominantly related to fusion of commissures; it fails when mitral leaflets are heavily calcified and immobile. This operation is mostly used in younger patients: it is eminently successful in developing countries in which severe rheumatic heart disease often produces critical mitral stenosis at an early age. That we frequently encounter patients ready for mitral valve replacement who had mitral valvotomy performed as long as 20 to 25 years earlier demonstrates the success of mitral valvotomy performed in younger patients. The advantages of mitral valvotomy are obvious: the risk of the operation is lower and the many potential complications of prosthetic valves are absent.

Indications for valve surgery for mitral stenosis include (1) patients with moderately severe or severe mitral stenosis who show progressively increasing disability directly related to the stenosis; (2) patients with severe mitral stenosis and pulmonary hypertension whose symptoms are uncertain; and (3) patients with significant mitral stenosis and stable or episodic disability, not adequately controlled by optimal medical regimen. In western countries, surgical treatment of mitral stenosis is at present performed predominantly in patients in their 50s or 60s, hence mitral valve replacement is usually mandatory. However, in younger patients an evaluation of valve mobility should be performed in order to consider the possibility that the lesser operation—mitral valvotomy—has a prospect of attaining good results.

POSTSURGICAL TREATMENT

Management of Prosthetic Cardiac Valves

Routine care of patients with prosthetic mitral valves includes the decision as to whether anticoagulant therapy is indicated. The incidence of thromboembolism originating upon valve prostheses is related to the type of the valve. Ball valves and disc valves are known to have a high enough incidence of thromboembolic complications that routine use of anticoagulants is generally recommended, unless specific contraindications exist. Bioprostheses are associated with a lower, although not negligible, incidence of embolic complications. In those, long-term anticoagulant therapy may be omitted, although in many centers such therapy is used, particularly in patients who are in atrial fibrillation. The alternative approach is to use anticoagulants during the initial 6 to 8 weeks after the operation and then to stop them.

Atrial fibrillation, as a rule, persists after valve replacement. The success of restoration of sinus rhythm after valve replacement in patients in chronic atrial fibrillation is only slightly higher than that prior to the operation, so that it is questionable whether cardioversion is worthwhile after surgery, if it failed prior to it. However, this arrhythmia develops commonly in the immediate postoperative period in patients who were in sinus rhythm prior to the operation. If this is the case, restoration or sinus rhythm is indicated and is usually successful either within the first 2 weeks after the operation or if this cannot be accomplished, 6 to 8 weeks later.

Infective endocarditis develops in about 1 to 3 percent of patients with prosthetic valves. "Early" endocarditis, defined as that occurring within 60 days, is considered to be more serious and less responsive to therapy. In part, this is because it is often caused by organisms resistant to antibiotics. Reoperations with re-replacement of prosthetic valves may be necessary in treatment-resistant cases, but even so, the mortality is considerable. "Late" endocarditis is considered to be less ominous, being within the range of infection in unoperated patients with a comparable response in terms of therapy and prognosis.

Cardiac failure develops occasionally in patients following valve replacement, even if prior to the operation none was present. Before medical therapy of cardiac failure is instituted, it is necessary to evaluate the cause of failure, since different forms of management may be needed. Failure may develop as a result of intraoperative myocardial damage, or as a result of prosthetic valve malfunction, or because of a mismatch between the valve opening and flow demands (valve too small for the orifice, producing continuation of mitral stenosis). This last cause is apt to occur preferentially in patients who were in cardiac failure prior to the operation. The last two causes usually require repeat surgical intervention. Another possible cause of cardiac failure, usually benign and self limiting, is an autoimmune reaction, "postcardiotomy syndrome," in which case a course of anti-inflammatory drugs, including, if necessary, steroids, usually brings relief.

In summary, management of mitral stenosis, which extends throughout the lifetime of a patient, presents many difficulities. The most critical decision relates to the choice between medical and surgical treatment. Optimal therapy requires that this decision be based on careful clinical considerations in each patient.

MITRAL REGURGITATION

ROBERT C. SCHLANT, M.D.

Mitral regurgitation is the most frequent type of valve disease. And the most common type of mitral regurgitation is "functional" and secondary to left ventricular enlargement from many causes, including systemic hypertension, dilated cardiomyopathy, chronic high-output state (anemia and A-V fistula, among others), and aortic valve disease. In such patients, the amount of regurgitation can vary from mild to severe. Basic treatment is to the underlying disease; if mitral regurgitation is more than mild, treatment should usually include arterial vasodilators, such as hydralazine, captopril, or prazosin, which decrease peripheral resistance, help to decrease the amount of mitral regurgitation and lower the load on the left ventricle.

Primary mitral regurgitation may be divided into two types, acute and chronic. The distinction, which may depend upon how rapidly mitral regurgitation develops, can often be made clinically. In addition, a patient with chronic mitral regurgitation can also develop acute mitral regurgitation.

ACUTE PHASE

The most common causes of acute mitral regurgitation are (1) myocardial ischemia from coronary atherosclerosis with ischemia of the ventricular wall at the base of a papillary muscle, or ischemia of a papillary muscle, or both, at times with actual rupture of the papillary muscle at any point from its base to its tip; (2) infective endocarditis with perforation of a mitral valve leaflet or rupture of chordae tendineae; and (3) other causes of rupture of chordae tendineae, including idiopathic rupture, trauma to patients with chronic mitral valve prolapse, or chronic rheumatic mitral valve disease.

Ischemic heart disease, including acute myocardial infarction (MI) and chronic coronary artery disease, is one of the more frequent causes of acute (and chronic) mitral regurgitation in middle-aged and older patients. Transient, acute mitral regurgitation develops in some patients during episodes of angina pectoris and may contribute to the frequent association of dyspnea. In patients with acute MI, acute mitral regurgitation may be related to a variety of mechanisms, including diffuse ventricular ischemia; left ventricular dilatation; ischemia of the ventricular wall at the base of a papillary muscle; ischemia, or rupture of a papillary muscle, or both; and rupture of chordae tendineae. Acute mitral regurgitation can be extremely severe, producing acute pulmonary edema and cardiogenic shock. In some instances, the onset of mitral regurgitation occurs suddenly with the development of a loud holosystolic murmur and pulmonary congestion a few days after the MI and is due to rupture of either the body or the tip of a papillary muscle. If the regurgitation is due to actual rupture of the body of a papillary muscle, the mitral regurgitation is severe and virtually always fatal within 24 hours unless the mitral valve is replaced. In other patients with only rupture of chordae tendineae or part of the tip of the papillary muscle, the mitral regurgitation is less severe and the patient may survive with only medical therapy.

In patients who have sustained acute MI and who develop acute mitral regurgitation, therapy should consist of intravenous administration of dopamine and sodium nitroprusside in addition to general measures, such as digoxin and intravenous furosemide. Most of these patients should receive careful hemodynamic monitoring, utilizing a Swan-Ganz catheter. Other useful procedures in assessing the patient include chest roentgenography, echocardiography, and, in selected patients, cardiac catheterization, including coronary arteriography and left ventriculography. Patients who respond well to medical therapy should be reevaluated regularly to determine whether or not replacement of the mitral valve is necessary. In general, surgical treatment is better tolerated after 1 to 3 weeks; however, in patients who have mitral regurgitation that either persists despite optimal medical therapy or is due to rupture of the body or tip of a papillary muscle, it may be necessary to proceed with emergency valve replacement. At times, such patients are helped by an intra-aortic counterpulsation balloon, which supports the circulation prior to valve replacement.

Patients with infective endocarditis may also develop acute severe mitral regurgitation. Many patients who develop pulmonary edema in this setting will ultimately require mitral valve replacement. In some patients in whom pulmonary edema responds well to therapy with digoxin, furosemide, and arterial vasodilators, such as sodium nitroprusside or hydralazine, it may be possible to postpone surgical treatment until antibiotic therapy has eradicated the infection. Occasionally, surgical treatment can be postponed for several years. But in patients who do not respond promptly to medical therapy, valve surgery is appropriate.

Rupture of chordae tendineae may occur in apparently healthy individuals as well as in those with myxomatous degeneration of the mitral valve and mitral-valve prolapse syndrome. Patients who develop acute mitral regurgitation and pulmonary edema require therapy with furosemide, digoxin, and arterial vasodilators, such as sodium nitroprusside. Hydralazine and captopril are also useful in some patients. If medical therapy produces effective relief of pulmonary congestion, it may be possible to postpone mitral valve surgery. Valve replacement is appropriate, however, if the patient's response to medical therapy is not satisfactory.

CHRONIC PHASE

Chronic mitral regurgitation is often secondary to left ventricular dilatation from a variety of causes, including systemic hypertension; dilated cardiomyopathy; aortic valve disease; and high-cardiac output states, such as chronic anemia or arteriovenous fistula. In such patients, therapy is directed at the underlying disease and often includes agents to decrease afterload and the volume of mitral regurgitation.

Primary chronic mitral regurgitation is often due to mitral valve prolapse or rheumatic heart disease. Less frequent causes include healed infective endocarditis, ischemic heart disease, calcified mitral annulus, lupus erythematosus, Marfan's syndrome, methysergide therapy, congenital anomalies, and traumatic heart disease.

All patients with mitral regurgitation should have appropriate antibiotic prophylaxis before any dental surgical procedure or cleaning as well as before procedures that may produce bacteremia. It is well to obtain a baseline electrocardiogram, echocardiogram, and chest film. If the patient's symptoms or signs indicate more than mild or trivial mitral regurgitation, consider obtaining a radionuclide ventriculogram with the patient both at rest and doing exercise as an additional measure of ventricular performance. In many patients, mitral valve surgery will not be necessary. In others, however, it will be ultimately necessary. In the latter group it is important to recommend surgical treatment promptly; do not wait until the development of relatively irreversible changes in the left ventricle when operative mortality increases and the benefits of surgery may decrease. However, valve surgery should not be recommended too early, namely, before evidence of a significant decrease in left ventricular systolic function or when the cardiac symptoms are primarily due to permanent, irreversible myocardial dysfunction or scarring rather than to severe mitral regurgitation.

Patients with chronic mitral regurgitation are particularly susceptible to both infective endocarditis and atrial arrhythmias, especially atrial fibrillation. The clinical course and overall cardiac function are often significantly impaired by atrial fibrillation. When a patient with mitral regurgitation develops atrial fibrillation, consider whether or not to attempt cardioversion. Factors associated with failure of cardioversion or recurrence of the atrial fibrillation include a long duration of the atrial fibrillation, a large left atrium, and patient age over 50 years. Patients with rheumatic mitral regurgitation who are to undergo electrical cardioversion are given oral doses of the anticoagulant sodium warfarin for 3 to 6 weeks before cardioversion. A regimen of quinidine sulfate, 1,200 to 2,400 mg per day in 3 or 4 divided doses, is started 36 to 48 hours before cardioversion. After cardioversion, quinidine is administered to achieve a plasma concentration of 2 to 5 μg per milliliter to help maintain normal sinus rhythm.

SPECIFIC DRUG THERAPIES

Prophylaxis for Recurrent Rheumatic Fever

Patients with rheumatic mitral regurgitation should be maintained indefinitely on a drug regimen to prevent recurrent rheumatic fever, even after prosthetic valve replacement. For adults, penicillin V, 125 or 250 mg twice a day, or sulfadiazine, 1 g once a day, is satisfactory. Alternatively, one may use intramuscular benzathine penicillin G, 1.2 million units every 4 weeks.

Prophylaxis for Infective Endocarditis

Patients with either mitral regurgitation from any cause or a prosthetic heart valve should receive antibiotic prophylaxis to prevent bacterial endocarditis under a variety of circumstances, including:

1. All dental procedures likely to induce gingival bleeding, including routine cleaning
2. Tonsillectomy or adenoidectomy, or both
3. Surgical procedures or biopsy involving respiratory mucosa
4. Bronchoscopy, especially with a rigid bronchoscope
5. Incision and drainage of infected tissue
6. Genitourinary and gastrointestinal procedures likely to be associated with bacteremia, including vaginal hysterectomy and urethral catheterization in the presence of infection
7. Open-heart surgery

The recommended antibiotic regimen for dental or respiratory-tract procedures is penicillin V, 2.0 g orally 1 hour before the procedure, then 1.0 g 6 hours later. For patients unable to take medications orally, 2 million units of aqueous penicillin G, IV or IM, 30 to 60 minutes before a procedure, and 1 million units 6 hours later may be given instead. Patients allergic to penicillin may be given either erythromycin 1.0 g orally before the procedure, then 500 mg 6 hours later, or vancomycin, 1.0 g IV slowly over 1 hour, starting 1 hour before the procedure with no repeat dose. Patients with prosthetic valves, in whom maximal protection is desired, should receive ampicillin, 1.0 to 2.0 g IM or IV, plus gentamicin, 1.5 mg per kilogram IM or IV, one-half hour before the procedure followed by either 1.0 g oral penicillin V 6 hours later or the same doses of ampicillin and gentamicin 8 hours later.

The standard recommended systemic antibiotic regimens for genitourinary and gastrointestinal tract surgery and instrumentation are ampicillin, 2.0 g (50 mg per kilogram for children) IM or IV, plus gentamicin, 1.5 mg per kilogram IM or IV (children, 2.0 mg per kilogram). The initial doses are given one-half to one hour before the procedure and repeated 8 hours later. For patients allergic to penicillin, administer vancomycin, 1.0 g for adults (20 mg per kilogram up to 1 g for children) IV slowly over 1 hour plus gentamicin, 1.5 mg per kilogram IM or IV (2.0 mg per kilogram for children) 1 hour before the procedure. These doses are repeated once 8 to 12 hours later. A regimen for minor or repetitive procedures in low-risk patients is amoxicillin, 3.0 g (50 mg per kilogram for children) orally 1 hour before the procedure, and 1.5 g (25 mg per kilogram or up to 1.5 g for children) 6 hours later unless renal function is compromised.

Patients requiring valve replacement who also need dental treatment should have the latter performed under full antibiotic coverage before valve replacement whenever possible to decrease the risk of late postoperative endocarditis. Patients undergoing open-heart surgery, particularly placement of prosthetic heart valves, should have short-term antibiotic prophylaxis at the time of cardiac surgery, especially against *Staphylococcus aureus*. The choice of agents depends upon the hospital's recent antibiotic susceptibility data but will usually include penicillinase-resistant penicillins or "first-generation" cephalosporins. In general, prophylaxis is started immediately before surgical treatment and continued for 2 days postoperatively.

Digitalis

Most patients with moderate or severe mitral regurgitation should be treated with digoxin, whether they have normal sinus rhythm or atrial fibrillation. The average dose is 0.25 mg (range, 0.12 to 0.5 mg) daily. Absorption of digoxin is interfered with by kaolin pectate, cholestyramine, neomycin, salicylazosulfapyridine, and possibly antacids. Plasma concentrations of digoxin are sometimes significantly increased by quinidine and verapamil. Older patients and those with renal insufficiency require smaller doses of digoxin. In patients with atrial fibrillation, the proper dose is best determined by measuring the patient's ventricular response rate at rest and especially after moderate exertion, which should not increase the ventricular response rate more than 110 to 120 beats per minute. In some patients in whom it is not possible satisfactorily to control the ventricular rate with only digoxin because of toxic effects, it is often helpful to increase the A-V block and slow the ventricular response with verapamil, 40 to 80 mg every 6 to 8 hours. Since verapamil can depress left ventricular contractility, it must be used very cautiously. Small doses of propranolol, 10 to 20 mg every 6 to 8 hours may also be cautiously tried if the drug is needed to control the ventricular response, although it also depresses left ventricular contractility.

Diuretics

In patients with moderate or severe mitral regurgitation who do not have acute pulmonary edema or chronic renal insufficiency, a thiazide diuretic once or twice a day helps to relieve pulmonary and systemic congestion. The dietary limitation of sodium intake to 2 g (5 g sodium chloride) per day lessens the severity of hypokalemia and helps to control pulmonary and peripheral congestion. In general, the lowest effective dosage should be used. Many patients are able to weigh themselves each morning on the same scale and to keep a weight diary to learn when they need an extra "water pill."

Patients with acute pulmonary edema require IV furosemide, which produces venodilatation in addition to a brisk diuresis. Chronic oral therapy with furosemide may be necessary in patients with renal insufficiency, although otherwise thiazide therapy is preferred. The beginning daily dose of furosemide is 20 to 40 mg, increased to 200 mg daily. Patients with very severe renal failure may require 500 to 1,000 mg daily.

Afterload-Reducing Agents

Intravenous sodium nitroprusside, which is most safely administered by an infusion pump, is a potent arterial and venous vasodilator. The usual dose is 0.25 to 8.0 μg per kilogram per minute or about 10 to 200 μg per minute. Patients should be carefully monitored to prevent excess hypotension. At times, the drug can be given simultaneously with an inotropic agent, such as dopamine or dobutamine.

Prazosin is an orally effective arterial and venous vasodilator. The first dose of 1 mg should be given in the evening when the patient is supine. The dose in most patients is 2 to 5 mg every 6 hours. Tolerance develops in some patients after a few weeks or months and may require high doses or increased use of diuretics for several weeks.

Hydralazine causes direct vasodilatation of the arteriolar resistance vessels and also has a slight direct inotropic effect. When used in patients with chronic heart failure, usually little or no reflex tachycardia develops. The usual dose is about 50 to 75 mg every 6 hours, but total daily dosages up to 2,400 mg have been reported. A drug-induced "lupus-like" syndrome may occur after several months, particularly in those patients receiving more than 300 mg daily.

Captopril is an angiotensin-converting enzyme (ACE) inhibitor that produces both arterial and venous vasodilatation. After an initial dose of 6.25 mg and measurements of supine and upright blood pressures, the dose is gradually increased over several days to 25 to 50 mg every 8 hours. It should be used with caution in the presence of azotemia or potassium-sparing diuretics.

Intravenous Inotropic Agents

Dopamine in low-to-moderate doses (1 to 5 μg per kilogram per minute) produces a strong inotropic effect in association with peripheral and renal vasodilatation. At doses above 5 μg per kilogram per minute, some alpha-receptor vasoconstriction develops; at doses above 30 μg per kilogram per minute, its peripheral effects resemble norepinephrine except for some persistent renal vasodilatation. Occasionally, dopamine causes pulmonary capillary pressure to rise, although it can be reduced by sodium nitroprusside.

Dobutamine, a strong patent inotropic agent with relatively less effect upon heart rate or the peripheral circulation, in low doses (below 7.5 μg per kilogram per minute), produces mild peripheral vasoconstriction. In higher doses (above 10 μg per kilogram per minute), it produces predominately peripheral vasodilatation. The usual initial rate of infusion is 3.5 μg per kilogram per minute. Dobutamine alone is more likely to reduce an elevated pulmonary capillary pressure than is dopamine alone. In some patients with very severe heart failure due to severe mitral regurgitation, it may be necessary to use dopamine together with dobutamine and sodium nitroprusside.

AORTIC REGURGITATION

DEREK G. GIBSON, M.B., F.R.C.P.

The hemodynamic problem posed by aortic regurgitation, namely, left ventricular disease secondary to volume overload, would seem a simple one, and its prevention in all moderate and severe cases by aortic valve replacement straightforward. Yet, the treatment of this apparently simple lesion has given rise to much controversy and uncertainty, casting doubt on the comfortable view that unambiguous hemodynamic criteria can be developed for the management of all patients with valve disease. The problem is that moderately severe aortic regurgitation is well tolerated by many patients for many years without intervention. On the one hand, premature operation exposes the patient to the risks of embolism and anticoagulant therapy with a mechanical prosthesis or of reoperation with a xenograft. On the other, the penalty for delayed intervention is the development of severe left ventricular disease, with cavity enlargement developing to an extent rarely seen in other types of heart disease. The slow and variable rate of progression of the disease means that rigorous assessment of selection criteria for operation or of treatment designed to delay the appearance of ventricular disease will require trials involving thousands of patients extending over many years. Not surprisingly, therefore, little definite information is available on many of these important questions.

MEDICAL TREATMENT

Many patients with aortic regurgitation do not require operation. This is self-evident in those who are asymptomatic, with physical signs suggesting trivial or moderate regurgitation, in whom heart size and lung fields are normal on chest film, and in whom there are no T-wave changes on electrocardiogram (ECG). Further confirmation comes from demonstrating a normal or only slightly increased left ventricular cavity size by M-mode echocardiography. Such patients require only annual review and antibiotic prophylaxis. Pregnancy presents no additional problem. In young patients, excessive athletic activity may be associated with enlargement of the left ventricular cavity out of proportion to the degree of regurgitation, so that more frequent review is necessary. The benefits of long-term drug treatment in such patients remain undetermined. The weak inotropic effect of digitalis does not seem to have any particular advantage, whereas its effect on the ECG prevents changes in the T waves being used to follow the disease's progression. Administration of thiazide diuretics may delay left ventricular dilatation, but the incidence of side effects with these drugs is surprisingly high. There is a case for chronic administration of a beta-blocking drug if the underlying cause of the aortic regurgitation is Marfan's syndrome, particularly if the ascending aorta is significantly dilated. Rare cases with syphilitic aortitis should receive a full course of penicillin.

EMERGENCY SURGICAL MANAGEMENT

At the other end of the scale of severity, patients with severe aortic regurgitation, particularly when its onset is acute, require emergency operation. The commonest underlying cause is acute infective endocarditis. The patient presents with pulmonary edema, often with evidence of low forward output. The physical signs may be atypical with no early diastolic murmur but a low-pitched early diastolic sound instead. The diagnosis is readily made echocardiographically by demonstrating an active left ventricle, vegetations on the aortic valve, and disruption of the usual pattern of cusp movement. Aortic root abscess may be detected. Premature closure of the mitral valve on the M-mode indicates severe elevation of ventricular diastolic pressure while premature aortic opening denotes actual equalization of aortic and ventricular diastolic pressures with its implication for coronary flow. Demonstration of either of these manifestations is a strong indication for immediate surgical treatment. It may be preceded by intubation and artificial ventilation if warranted by the severity of the pulmonary edema. Our experience with vasodilators in these circumstances is disappointing. Cardiac catheterization has little to contribute to the management of such patients; operation is delayed, plasma volume expanded, and catheter manipulation in the aortic root may cause emboli. At operation, the vegetations can be cultured, the valve bed disinfected, and abscess cavities drained and obliterated. Other indications for early operation in infective endocarditis include the persistence of pulmonary congestion; prolongation of the PR interval of the ECG, which may reflect involvement of the septum and deteriorate to complete heart block with disastrous hemodynamic consequences; and progressive renal disease with elevation of the blood urea level and persistent hematuria. Large vegetations on the aortic valve and fungal etiology are also relative indications for early replacement. Another condition requiring early operation is aortic regurgitation secondary to acute dissection. In this case, surgery is preemptive: it is performed with the aim of preventing further deterioration, rather than on hemodynamic grounds, so that the exact severity of the regurgitation is not of great significance.

AORTIC REGURGITATION

Chronic severe aortic regurgitation is another clear indication for aortic valve replacement. Such patients are frequently but not always symptomatic. A collapsing pulse and left ventricular hypertrophy are present. Chest films show that heart size is increased, and pulmonary congestion is evident. An ECG is likely to show ST-T wave changes and, in more advanced cases, interventricular conduction delay. The extent of the volume overload can be semiquantitatively assessed from the M-mode echocardiogram, which is likely to show an end-diastolic dimension of 6.5 cm or more, which falls to normal at end-systole. Two-dimensional echocardiography demonstrates a uniform contraction pattern of the left ventricle; it also allows the size of the aortic root to be gauged, and the dilatation of the ascending aorta detected. Some indication of the severity of the regurgitation can also be gained from Doppler ultrasonography or from the difference between right and left ventricular outputs on blood-pool scanning. If necessary, the diagnosis can be confirmed by cardiac catheterization and coronary artery anatomy determined in patients older than age 40 years. Such patients do well with aortic valve replacement, which can be performed with low mortality and morbidity. Symptoms regress, and left ventricular cavity rapidly returns to normal, often within a few days of operation.

MODERATELY SEVERE AORTIC REGURGITATION

Considerable uncertainty exists over the management of this group of patients, who are usually asymptomatic and may present because either a murmur has been heard on routine examination or a chest film has demonstrated cardiac enlargement. Evidence of significant pulmonary congestion is absent; enlargement of the left ventricular cavity is moderate, within the range of 6 to 6.5 cm on M-mode echo, and left ventricular function is well preserved. The ECG either is normal or shows voltage criteria of left ventricular hypertrophy only. Such patients may do well for many years with conservative treatment so that premature operation should be avoided. The most significant factor in determining the optimum timing for surgical intervention is not to demonstrate values of one or more parameters outside some arbitrary range on a single occasion, but rather to document the onset of changing hemodynamic state, with evidence of increasing severity of left ventricular disease. This may manifest itself as the development of ST-T wave changes on the ECG and increasing heart size on chest films, or left ventricular cavity size on echocardiography.

Symptoms of pulmonary congestion may occur only when ventricular disease is far advanced, but should they do so, it is a significant development. Regular exercise testing may be useful in monitoring these patients, although a normal exercise capacity does not preclude severe left ventricular disease. A number of more sophisticated measurements of systolic function have been proposed in such patients. "Contractility" can be assessed from end-systolic pressure-volume or pressure-dimension relations. The extent to which wall stress is normalized by hypertrophy can also be measured; lack of appropriate hypertrophy causes systolic wall stresses to increase and may herald the onset of cavity dilatation and "heart failure." Although such approaches are of theoretical interest, their use in patients in whom simpler methods give equivocal results has not been validated. In addition, the first evidence of ventricular disease may appear as impaired diastolic rather than systolic function. Even when all these measurements are taken into account, the timing of surgery may not be clear.

In the literature, it is implicitly assumed that information is potentially available in every case that allows unequivocal determination of the optimum timing of operation. This approach has led to the development of a plethora of parameters of increasing complexity. However, there are confidence limits of measurement in individual patients of any physiologic variable, whereas the mechanism of progression of ventricular disease is unclear and almost certainly not deterministic. It is possible, therefore, that such information will never be available so that for many patients there is effectively a period, which may last for many years, in which there is no practical difference between the results of operating and of conservative treatment. This conclusion can be reflected in management, so that it seems reasonable to allow the timing of surgery to be determined by nonmedical factors when they are clear cut.

LEFT VENTRICULAR DISEASE

An appreciable number of patients with aortic regurgitation do not present until left ventricular disease is far advanced. They typically remain asymptomatic until a late stage of the disease, often presenting with pulmonary edema after some unusual exertion. Volume overload is still considerable, but the left ventricle is greatly dilated with a reduced ejection fraction and elevated end-diastolic pressure. Such patients do significantly less well with operation than those with aortic stenosis and corresponding cavity enlargement. The risks of operation are increased, not usually at the operation itself, but over the first few postoperative days. Cavity size does not shrink as in uncomplicated cases, so with loss of the volume load, ejection fraction is further reduced, often with striking asynchrony of wall motion. Postoperative treatment with diuretics and vasodilators may be required.

As with a dilated left ventricle from any other cause, ventricular arrhythmias occur, so that Holter monitoring should be undertaken. Although rigorous proof is lacking, it seems reasonable to give appropriate treatment if advanced ectopy is present and if repeated monitoring confirms a therapeutic response. Postoperative atrial fibrillation is also a major problem in such patients and may be associated with striking clinical deterioration. Hence, a patient who was asymptomatic until just before operation now has, as the result of one's treatment, severe limitation of exercise tolerance. If control of the ventricular rate with digoxin does not correct this defect, we perform DC shock, repeatedly if necessary, and give quinidine in an attempt to maintain sinus rhythm. In view of the poor results of surgery, it is a moot question whether it is worth operating at all on this group of patients. I believe that it is since the results of conservative treatment are uniformly bad, even in the short term, whereas those of surgery are unpredictable. Significant improvement occurs early after operation in a minority of patients; in some of the remainder, a modest response to medical treatment over months is seen.

The role of surgery is much more questionable in those in whom the left ventricular disease is not the result of aortic regurgitation but of some associated condition, so that it is out of proportion to the magnitude of the volume load. This may be seen when the main clinical problem is hypertension associated with mild aortic regurgitation. In such cases, the aortic diastolic pressure is elevated, in contrast to the systolic hypertension that accompanies uncomplicated aortic regurgitation. Treatment should be directed toward the hypertension, since the results of valve surgery are unsatisfactory. The same applies to the combination of moderately severe aortic regurgitation and impaired left ventricular function from coronary artery disease, which is not improved by concomitant vein grafting. A major indication for valve replacement, however, is the combination of moderately severe regurgitation and a small, stiff left ventricular cavity. This combination may be seen when a patient with aortic stenosis develops reflux, due possibly to infective endocarditis or a postoperative paraprosthetic leak. A relatively minor increase in stroke volume causes a striking increase in end-diastolic pressure—and hence of pulmonary congestion—although systolic function of the ventricle remains intact. If the condition is left untreated, the patient may develop atrial fibrillation and even pulmonary hypertension, the clinical picture resembling that of mitral valve disease.

ASSOCIATED MITRAL VALVE DISEASE

If aortic regurgitation is rheumatic in origin, it is virtually always accompanied by mitral involvement. When mitral stenosis dominates the clinical picture, the resulting low stroke volume may mask the physical signs of aortic regurgitation, so that the potential importance of a significant leak is not recognized. Successful mitral valve surgery unmasks the aortic regurgitation, which may cause an enlarged heart and pulmonary congestion. Hence, it is essential that both lesions be dealt with at the same time, or a second operation may be necessary. If the aortic regurgitation dominates the clinical picture, the mitral valve disease may not be apparent clinically, although it can readily be diagnosed echocardiographically. The commonest manifestation is mild-to-moderate mitral stenosis, which requires an additional open valvotomy rather than replacement. Such patients do well, since symptoms develop early due to mitral obstruction rather than left ventricular disease. The combination of organic mitral and aortic regurgitation occurs in connective tissue diseases, such as Marfan's syndrome, or may result from aortic infective endocarditis. The resulting volume overload on the left ventricle is severe, and the natural history of the combined lesion seems appreciably more rapid than that of either condition alone, so that earlier operation is justified. In general, replacement of both valves is required, the nature of the mitral valve involvement making a conservative procedure at this site frequently unsatisfactory.

CHOICE OF OPERATION

Surgical treatment of aortic regurgitation almost invariably requires aortic valve replacement. Conservative operations rarely give satisfactory long-term follow-up, and we would restrict them to aortic regurgitation associated with subaortic ventricular septal defect (VSD). My own preference for valve replacement in a young or middle-aged patient in whom durability is a major requirement is for a mechanical prosthesis. I have been particularly impressed with the performance of the Starr-Edwards prosthesis on long-term follow-up of more than 20 years with an acceptably low incidence of emboli and anticoagulant-induced complications. A mechanical prosthesis is also particularly suitable on technical grounds, when there is associated disease of the aortic root and ascending aorta from infective endocarditis or aneurysm. In view of their relatively limited life, we restrict biologic valves to the elderly, to young women who wish to become pregnant, and to those in whom anticoagulant therapy is contraindicated, knowing that a second operation may be necessary.

PARAPROSTHETIC AORTIC REGURGITATION

Aortic regurgitation may follow aortic valve replacement with either a biological or a mechanical prosthesis. Although paraprosthetic aortic regurgitation obviously has much in common with the naturally occurring condition, often its main clinical significance arises from its being a manifestation of a more serious prosthesis-related complication rather than simply in its causing a volume load on the left ventricle. If aortic regurgitation appears early after operation, the possibility of infective endocarditis must be actively excluded. Infection associated with a prosthesis responds poorly to medical treatment, and operation is often required to eradicate it. Dehiscence of the prosthesis by endocarditis can be diagnosed radiologically and is an indication for emergency operation. Moderately severe regurgitation around a mechanical prosthesis may cause hemolysis severe enough to lead to anemia and even to require transfusion. In such cases, reoperation is usually required. If the valve bed was heavily calcified at the first operation, mild aortic regurgitation may persist postoperatively. Much can be said for managing this condition conservatively if it is well tolerated hemodynamically and if anemia can be prevented, if necessary by ferrous sulfate and folic acid administration, since a second operation is unlikely to be any more successful than the first. The commonest failure of a biologic aortic valve substitute, whether a xenograft or a homograft, is the development of regurgitation. In the absence of infection, the process is slow and predictable, initially manifesting itself only as a short early diastolic murmur, which can be treated conservatively, often for several years. Reoperation can thus be elective and should be undertaken only with increasing heart size or pulmonary congestion.

CALCIFIC AORTIC STENOSIS

MARY E. FONTANA, M.D.
RICHARD P. LEWIS, M.D.

The three major causes of calcific aortic stenosis in adults are congenital, inflammatory, and degenerative. Despite different original anatomy, all three types of valves become stenotic because of calcification. Significant aortic stenosis unassociated with valve calcification is distinctly uncommon after age 30 years. Recent studies have shown that the calcification can occur rapidly (in as little as 1 or 2 years), particularly in the degenerative type. The mechanism of calcification is unclear, but blood turbulence in the ascending aorta—with resultant trapped flows and platelet deposition on the leaflets—probably plays a major role in initiating the process. As the obstruction worsens, a vicious cycle develops. A therapeutic hope for the future is to interrupt this process.

PATHOLOGIC FACTORS

Approximately one-third of congenital bicuspid (but not inherently stenotic) aortic valves develop calcification leading to stenosis. This process begins in the fourth decade of life, and new cases continue to appear up to the eighth decade. Such patients may have a long history of a murmur and often have some aortic regurgitation.

The inflammatory form of calcific aortic stenosis has its peak incidence in the sixth and seventh decades of life. Whether these cases represent milder forms of rheumatic disease (the mitral valve is often thickened) or some other inflammatory process is unclear. The valve is tricuspid and shows commissural fusion as well as extensive calcification within the valve leaflet. Mild aortic regurgitation is often present.

The degenerative (Mönckeberg) type of calcific aortic stenosis is becoming the most common etiology as the population ages. Such valves are thought to be normal valves on which calcification occurs, predominantly at the base of the leaflets. There is no commissural fusion. The anatomy of these valves is such that there may not be a prominent jet lesion. As a result, the murmur is often less coarse (frequently musical) and softer and has less extensive radiation. There is usually no aortic regurgitation. The peak incidence occurs after age 65 and increases each decade thereafter. Mitral annular calcification and atrioventricular conduction defects are frequently associated with the degenerative type of valve.

PATHOPHYSIOLOGIC FACTORS

In contrast to other valvular lesions, aortic stenosis has a symptomatic course lasting only a few years—most patients are dead within 3 to 5 years after the onset of syncope, angina, or exertional dyspnea. Ten percent die suddenly, often during exertion. Once the patient progresses to frank congestive heart failure (CHF), death within 2 years is usual.

Traditionally, it has been thought that patients have a long "asymptomatic" period wherein significant aortic stenosis is present, but well compensated for, by concentric left ventricular hypertrophy. When compensation becomes inadequate, symptoms develop. It now appears far more likely that calcific stenosis develops within a very few years and that symptoms quickly follow. Indeed, most patients who present with symptoms other than CHF have well-preserved resting left ventricular function.

Syncope in aortic stenosis most likely is of the vasodepressor type, involving baroreceptors in the left ventricle. In more advanced cases, ischemic arrhythmias may develop after the vasodepressor reaction. Syncope in aortic stenosis is a harbinger of sudden death.

Patients with aortic stenosis may have angina pectoris with normal coronary arteries. Studies have shown that subendocardial ischemia develops as a result of excessive myocardial oxygen demand and inadequate diastolic coronary perfusion; these defects are largely due to low systemic diastolic pressure and high left ventricular end-diastolic pressure. On the other hand, significant coronary disease is present in 25 to 50 percent of patients, and the basis for angina pectoris cannot be clarified short of coronary arteriography. Recurrent ischemic episodes likely play a major role in the diffuse subendocardial fibrosis and subsequent left ventricular failure that develops in the unoperated patient.

CLINICAL DIAGNOSIS

Because of both the unique problems of aortic stenosis in the elderly and the increasing incidence of this disorder, much of the following discussion will focus on this group of patients. However, the principles are applicable to younger patients as well.

Therapeutic decisions regarding aortic stenosis in the elderly are often not as difficult to reach as establishing the diagnosis and determining the severity of the obstruction. Systolic ejection murmurs heard in the aortic area are extremely common in the elderly. Many are due to sclerosis of the valve without enough reduction in leaflet mobility to cause significant obstruction. The classic findings of significant aortic stenosis in younger age groups, i.e., slowly rising carotid upstroke, small pulse pressure, and paradoxic splitting of the second heart sound, are generally absent in the people older than age 65 years. Sclerosis of the peripheral vessels lead to increased pulse-wave transmission velocity, resulting in a "normal" carotid upstroke and normal or increased pulse pressures despite severe stenosis. Hypertension is a frequent finding (systolic, or diastolic, or both) in the older population; its presence does not preclude significant aortic stenosis—the left ventricle can generate up to 300 mm HG of pressure. Calcification of the leaflets leads to reduced mobility and results in an inaudible aortic component of the second heart sound—a useful clinical sign in this group. The intensity of the murmur, as noted earlier, may be unimpressive, especially when the cardiac output is low.

The electrocardiogram is less useful for diagnosis of aortic stenosis in elderly patients, since left ventricular hypertrophy is frequently encountered in patients without significant aortic valve disease. As in younger individuals, the absence of left ventricular hypertrophy does not exclude significant aortic stenosis. The chest film can be normal despite severe obstruction. Consequently, more specific tests are required to assess severity.

Systolic time intervals may show a prolongation of the left ventricular ejection time, but a slow carotid upstroke is often not present in the elderly. Echocardiography can establish the presence or absence of stenosis but is not useful to assess severity. The addition of Doppler techniques to echocardiography improves the accuracy, especially in patients with severe obstruction, but misses some significant disease. However, as technology improves, Doppler studies may become extremely useful in this category of patient. Image-intensification fluoroscopy can be very useful—the absence of aortic valve calcification excludes significant valvular obstruction. In summary, the major value of noninvasive laboratory tests in this setting is to exclude significant aortic valve disease. If there is evidence of aortic valve disease, diagnostic catheterization is required.

Cardiac catheterization definitively assesses the severity of aortic stenosis and is necessary to establish the presence or absence of associated diseases. Recording the pressure gradient across the valve, with cardiac output determinations under identical conditions and as closely as possible in time, is mandatory since a modest gradient can mean significant obstruction if the output is depressed. Elderly people, even with relatively normal left ventricular function, often have a low cardiac output. This can be aggravated by left ventricular dysfunction or aggressive diuresis. Calculation of the valve area is essential in this group of patients for reasons already noted. Even the valve area calculated from the Gorlin formula may underestimate the severity of the obstruction in older patients. This may be related to the dense calcification of these valves as well as to higher systemic arterial pressures. A calculated aortic valve area of less than 0.75 cm^2 indicates severe obstruction; a valve area of 0.75 to 1.0 cm^2 indicates moderate obstruction.

Selective coronary arteriography should also be done because coronary artery disease affects the surgical approach. Quantitative evaluation of left ventricular function should also be performed, although poor left ventricular function is not a contraindication for surgical management as it is for other valvular lesions.

MEDICOSURGICAL THERAPY

Aortic stenosis is a surgical disease. The major contraindication to surgical treatment is the presence of noncardiac illness (central nervous system disease or cancer, among others). In patients older than age 80 years, the decision for surgery must be highly individualized. Aortic stenosis is the only valvular lesion for which there is evidence that valve replacement prolongs life as well as improves (in most cases abolishes) symptoms. Currently, operative mortality in patients with intact left ventricular function should be less than 5 percent, even if coronary bypass is also required.

Angina pectoris is often relieved by aortic valve replacement, even if coronary artery bypass is not done. This relates to two facts. First, many patients with angina pectoris have normal coronary arteries. Second, the coronary arteries enlarge as concentric hypertrophy develops to accommodate the increase in resting coronary flow required, which can be up to three times normal. Thus, a 70 percent lesion in an enlarged vessel may not be hemodynamically important after valve replacement surgery, when left ventricular hypertrophy regresses. Nonetheless, it is now common to bypass significant lesions because this practice does not increase, and may in fact decrease, operative risk.

In elderly patients, we often place permanent pacemaker wires at the time of surgical management, despite the absence of proved conduction-system disease, since postoperative bradycardias and heart block commonly occur in this group. This is likely related to the surgical removal of calcium deposits close to the atrioventricular junction. In addition, elderly people are more likely to have fibrotic degeneration of the conduction system.

As noted earlier, left ventricular dysfunction is seldom a contraindication to surgery, although the operative risk is higher (20 percent). Relief of the aortic obstruction usually results in dramatic improvement in left ventricular function. It is manifested as soon as the patient is removed from cardiopulmonary bypass. Studies performed 3 to 6 months after surgery show improvement in left ventricular function with regression of both hypertrophy and dilatation. Nonetheless, it is desirable to perform surgery before left ventricular dysfunction develops and before severe symptoms occur because long-term follow-up (greater than 10 years) shows a striking difference between those whose preoperative New York Heart Association functional class was I to II (90 percent 10-year survival) and those in class III to IV (less than 40 percent 10-year survival).

In older patients, a thorough evaluation of other organ systems is necessary prior to surgical intervention, as postoperative morbidity is often related to other coexisting medical problems. Renal function tests, pulmonary function tests, and gastrointestinal evaluation for sources of bleeding or malignancy are all indicated in the elderly patient with stable symptomatic aortic stenosis who is to undergo surgery. The patient with severe heart failure or unstable angina may not tolerate a thorough evaluation and must undergo surgical treatment urgently. Delaying surgical treatment in an effort to stabilize angina or aggressively to treat heart failure may produce more problems and increase mortality, since aggressive use of diuretics, vasodilators (arterial or venous), or negative inotropic agents, such as beta- blockers or calcium-channel antagonists, is often ineffective and potentially deleterious. The obstructed valve mitigates the beneficial effects of decreasing afterload on the cardiac output, since the left ventricle cannot "see" the reduced resistance. Hence, an arterial vasodilator may produce hypotension with syncope or myocardial ischemia.

Venodilators, such as nitrates are helpful if the left ventricular end diastolic pressure is high, and significant pulmonary congestion is present; however, lowering filling pressure excessively may sharply lower cardiac output, resulting in syncope, shock, or myocardial ischemia. Similarly, negative inotropic agents may produce intractable heart failure if used to treat angina in this group. Excessive use of diuretics may lower filling pressure by contracting intravascular volume. The noncompliant, hypertrophied ventricle of aortic stenosis may not have adequate preload at "normal" filling pressures.

APPROACH TO ASYMPTOMATIC PATIENTS

Asymptomatic aortic stenosis is a difficult management problem. In many cases, it is simply a matter of an early diagnosis having been made in patients with mild-to-moderate disease. Such patients invariably develop surgical disease and require both close follow-up and activity restriction. Occasionally, an asymptomatic patient with severe aortic stenosis is seen. Careful questioning may reveal that symptoms are indeed present. Cautious use of a nuclear angiographic exercise study to document the asymptomatic state may be indicated. It does appear that the incidence of sudden death is low (less than 1%) in asymptomatic patients, and this must be balanced against an operative mortality of 5 percent. Scrupulously close follow-up, as well as activity limitation, is clearly required in this group of patients if surgery is not performed.

SELECTION OF A PROSTHESIS

Once the surgical decision is made, the choice of a prosthesis becomes the primary consideration. In patients younger than age 65 years, the more durable mechanical prostheses are the best choice, provided there is no contraindication to long-term anticoagulant therapy. The Starr-Edwards ball valve has the longest proved durability of the mechanical prostheses.

The valve of choice in those individuals older than age 65 years is a tissue valve, the current choice being the porcine heterograft. The tissue valve is preferred over mechanical prostheses because of its more effective orifice area and lack of need for long-term anticoagulant therapy. The significant failure rate of porcine valves at 10 years is less of a problem in the elderly. In patients with a small aortic root, the porcine prosthesis may be too obstructive, so that a low-profile tilting disc prosthesis is used in these patients. The Björk-Shiley, or St. Jude prosthesis is preferred. The St. Jude prosthesis has the most effective orifice area of the prosthetic valves, but its durability past 5 years is yet to be determined. Any mechanical prosthesis requires long-term anticoagulant (warfarin) therapy, with all of the risks of bleeding complications, which are more common in older than in younger patients.

Some surgical groups are attempting debridement procedures in selected valves where the valve tissue seems relatively intact. Long-term results of such procedures are not yet established. Laser technology is in its infancy but may prove useful in the future management of calcific aortic valve disease.

MITRAL VALVE PROLAPSE

W. PROCTOR HARVEY, M.D.

Before treatment of mitral valve prolapse is discussed, it is appropriate that a description of the general clinical features of this interesting and prevalent condition should be outlined. The basic lesion is the result of myxomatous degeneration of the mitral valve. The mitral valve normally is made up of two basic components, a fibrosa element and a spongiosa element. Normally, the fibrosa element predominates, but with mitral valve prolapse, the spongiosa proliferates. There is, therefore, an increased amount of mitral valve tissue, which results in a scalloping or hooding effect of the valve. In other words, there is more tissue in the mitral valve than is needed. This condition is a common one, affecting approximately 15 million Americans. It is the commonest familial cardiac condition, followed next by the congenital bicuspid aortic valve. Most of the patients with mitral valve prolapse are undiagnosed although, increasingly, diagnosis is being accomplished. This change is explained by an increased awareness by the members of the medical profession, so the physicians are more likely to search for this abnormality. Also, with the frequent use of the echocardiogram today, the condition is being detected by this useful procedure. Mitral valve prolapse remains a major topic of discussion and presentation at annual meetings and symposia, such as those of the American Heart Association and American College of Cardiology; it has been a major topic of interest, presentation, and discussion for the past 15 years. It can also be demonstrated on cardiac angiograms. However, what is often not appreciated, but is a fact, is that the stethoscope is still the most valuable and accurate instrument in the diagnosis of this condition.

Various terms are synonymous with mitral valve prolapse. They include the systolic click-murmur syndrome, billowing mitral valve leaflet syndrome, floppy valve syndrome, Barlow's syndrome, and others. Probably 90 percent of patients have no symptoms referable to this common condition, and the 10 percent who are symptomatic may have chest discomfort, palpitations, dizziness, nervousness, and other complaints that might be labelled as "neurotic." As a rule, the chest discomfort can be easily differentiated from that of coronary artery disease by careful history, although at times it may simulate angina pectoris or coronary insufficiency. Various symptoms are often described by the patient as "palpitation" of the heart. They may result from varying causes, such as premature beats, both ventricular and atrial; paroxysmal atrial tachycardia or fibrillation; and nodal, and even ventricular, tachycardia. The diagnosis is frequently overlooked—mainly because it is not specifically searched for by the physician.

AUSCULTATORY DIAGNOSIS

There are a number of detectable variants of mitral valve prolapse, which represent a spectrum of auscultatory findings, that must be actively looked for when examining a patient. Most commonly, the patient has a systolic click (or clicks) that generally occurs in mid or late systole or a systolic murmur most commonly occurring in mid to late systole. Both a click and a murmur may be present (hence, the term "systolic click-murmur syndrome"). A large number of varying findings can be present to identify this syndrome. It is necessary that the examining physician be aware of these variants so as not to overlook their presence. It is also important that he be aware of the fact that these findings may be transient in a patient and at one time be easily heard, whereas at another time they may be poorly heard or even absent. For example, only a single mid-systolic click may be detected on one evaluation, and at other times both a click and a murmur are present; on another occasion several clicks may be present, or a musical systolic murmur may be heard, referred to as a "whoop" or "honk." Even in the same patient, these findings may "come and go" or be "brought out" by various positions, such as by having the patient turn to the left lateral position, sit, stand, or squat. The patient should be examined using the simple bedside maneuver of squatting. In some patients, this can result in the auscultatory notation of movement of findings to another part of systole, such as the systolic clicks occurrring more at the latter part of systole than in the mid part; or a systolic murmur, not heard before, may now be elicited by listening in the various positions. Care also must be taken to listen specifically during the various phases of respiration. At times, the typical auscultatory findings are heard only on inspiration, at other times only on expiration. It is worthy of emphasis that mitral valve prolapse is not a new condition. For example, in 1935 Drs. Samuel A. Levine and William B. Thompson described the sound now known as systolic click heard in 35 patients examined over 16 years. The following features were described at that time: the extra sound had a variable intensity in different patients as well as in the same patient. The sound might appear or disappear without apparent cause. Most patients were nervous and presented with bizarre complaints. A murmur and a degree of chest discomfort and palpitations were noted. The age range was 11 to 71 years. Younger than age 40 years, there was no evidence of heart disease.

None of the patients was dead at the time of the report, whereas 40 percent of a group with a diastolic gallop observed over the same period had already died. It was concluded that the auscultatory finding was more frequent than previously supposed. Heart disease was more often absent than present, although serious heart disease might also be present. The syndrome has no unfavorable influence on prognosis. The findings described by these authors 50 years ago are, of course, characteristic of what we find in our patients today; in fact, they referred to a paper by Cuffer and Barbillion approximately 100 years ago, that also described the systolic click; these authors also stated that it would "come and go without apparent cause over a period of hours or days at a time."

There is no epidemic of mitral valve prolapse today. It is merely being detected with increasing frequency. It is true in medicine as in other aspects of life that we find what we look for. However, there is a counterpart to this statement: to find what we look for we must know what we are looking for. The most serious complication is rupture of a chorda tendineae, which may occur spontaneously or, because of infective endocarditis on the valve, damage the valve itself or rupture a larger chorda tendineae, thereby resulting in acute mitral regurgitation. Among the complications associated with mitral valve prolapse may be increasing severe mitral regurgitation with or without rupture of chordae tendineae. Rupture of the valve leaflet itself can result from either infective endocarditis or unknown cause. There may be calcification of the mitral annulus. The patient may have transient ischemic attacks (TIAs) with cerebral emboli. Various arrhythmias, (atrial, ventricular, or both) can occur. Chest discomfort of varying degrees and of nonspecific nature are present in some patients. Symptoms compatible with neurocirculatory asthenia (Da Costa's syndrome or effort syndrome) have been described; patients with these symptoms may be anxious or nervous or have a cardiac neurosis. Sudden death has been described, but it is worthy of emphasis that it is a rare occurrence; it has been overemphasized in the past as being a significant feature of this problem.

To be remembered is that the majority of patients with mitral valve prolapse are asymptomatic.

TREATMENT

Since the majority of patients are asymptomatic, no treatment is necessary. When the diagnosis is first made, the main treatment is reassurance. Only a minority of patients needs any form of medication. Education of the patient and explanation of what mitral valve prolapse represents are part of the treatment. The use of a heart model in which the various chambers can be shown to a patient is an excellent way to enlighten the patient, the physician pointing out where the mitral valve is located, and its normal anatomy and function. This can be followed by the description of the movement of the prolapsed mitral valve with systolic contraction of the left ventricle. It is useful to use one's hands to illustrate the mitral valve to show that with diastole the valve opens (the two hands opening to allow blood to flow into the left ventricle from the left atrium). With systole the hands swing back together, illustrating how the mitral valve closes and seals. Placing one's necktie or piece of cloth or handkerchief on one hand can simulate the extra mitral valve tissue. With systole, this extra material can be shown to bulge or prolapse into the left atrium. It can be analogous to the billowing that takes place with the opening of a parachute, which is checked by its strings or guy ropes.

It is recommended that the patient be given the educational pamphlet supplied by the American Heart Association entitled "Mitral Valve Prolapse." This assists in educating the patient and helps him to understand the condition.

The only necessary treatment in the majority of patients is reassurance. Only a minority (perhaps less than 10%) needs any form of medication. Time should be taken by the physician and other involved medical personnel to carefully explain mitral valve prolapse to the patient as well as to family members, particularly the spouse or parents. This can be accomplished by the use of actual photographs or a drawing of the normal mitral valve as well as one showing prolapse. In fact, the pamphlet "Mitral Valve Prolapse" has excellent diagrams illustrating this. Most patients have never been aware of this condition in themselves or in others; neither have they been aware of any complications associated with it. I make it a practice in explaining mitral valve prolapse to the patient to tell him that the prognosis is excellent. I use anecdotes to personalize the fact that longevity is similar to that of the normal population. Examples of the following people may be cited: a physician who died at age 88 years, one whose medical course I had the opportunity to follow over a couple of decades: his symptoms could be traced back to when he was a teenager. He had systolic clicks, a systolic murmur, and premature beats every time I examined his heart. He had no symptoms referable to these findings. His death at age 88 years was from cancer. This was more than a 70-year follow-up of his condition.

Another patient, my mother-in-law, has mitral valve prolapse. She is now age 77 years, and her symptoms date back to when she was in her early teens. Auscultation of her heart sometimes reveals a systolic click (or clicks), and, at other times, an associated systolic murmur at the latter part of systole. This represents more than a 60-year follow-up of her condition. She does, however, represent one of a small number of patients (probably less than 10%) who have had symptoms. Hers are those of palpitations, dizziness, chest discomfort, weakness, and nervousness. I had the opportunity to observe her carefully during the time that she was symptomatic. Her palpitations were related to multiple ventricular premature beats, which caused her chest discomfort (not typical of coronary insufficiency pain, however). She is basically a stoic lady, even though education and understanding of her problem did not eliminate her symptoms. She was given propranolol, one 40-mg tablet 4 times a day, which controlled her symptoms.

Complications

I ask the following question when first evaluating my patient: "What have you been told concerning this condition?" I ask it to see if the patient has heard of any serious complications of this condition, such as sudden death. (Unfortunately, this rare complication has been mentioned in the literature that goes to the laity as well as to members of the medical profession). If the patient is unaware of any dire event such as this, it is unwise to mention it. Instead, emphasize the positive aspect of the patient's condition, giving reassurance that there is no reason for him or her not to continue to lead a normal life. If the patient is aware of sudden death as a complication of mitral valve prolapse, enough time should be spent explaining the fact that it is indeed a rare condition, greatly overemphasized; I make sure that the patient goes out of the office not fearing this complication.

It should be explained to the patient that the main complication could be damage to the mitral valve, such as ruptured chordae tendineae, which can occur with infective endocarditis or spontaneously; acute mitral regurgitation can result. However, it should be stressed that this too is an unusual, although serious, complication that may take place. Prevention of the condition by antibiotic prophylaxis prior to dental work, operations, and certain diagnostic procedures of the gastrointestinal and genitourinary tracts should be stressed. Patients can develop infective endocarditis from the simpler dental procedures, such as cleaning and filling of teeth, as well as from extractions. At our institution some years ago, we had five patients in approximately 22 months with infective endocarditis from cleaning and filling of teeth. *Streptococcus viridans* was the infecting organism. Three of these patients died of complications of their endocarditis. These five patients had rheumatic or congential heart disease, and we emphasized the fact that endocarditis could occur from these dental procedures as well as from tooth extractions. Patients should be given the AHA-sponsored pamphlet that has instructions on the specific doses of antibiotics for gastrointestinal and genitourinary-tract surgical procedures (Fig. 1).

Antibiotic prophylaxis as outlined in this pamphlet is recommended for our patients with mitral valve prolapse. They may develop infective endocarditis, resulting in severe mitral regurgitation.

Some physicians state that they give antibiotic prophylaxis only when a systolic murmur is present and not if only a systolic click (or clicks) is heard with the stethoscope. However, I believe that those patients with a click, as well as those with a systolic murmur, should also receive antibiotic prophylaxis. I have seen patients with infective endocarditis occurring on the mitral valve when only a systolic click (no murmur) was heard. Also, I have observed many patients who at first have only a click and no murmur; subsequently, listening to the patient in various positions—left lateral, sitting, standing, and after various bedside maneuvers (such as squatting or Valsalva)—a murmur is also heard. If one listens for longer periods, or sometimes after the patient performs exercise, a murmur can be heard. Also, on continuous recordings of the phonocardiogram, we have documented clinical findings varying from no murmur or click to clicks, murmurs, "whoops," and "honks," which were transient and intermittent.

Arrhythmias causing palpitations as a bothering symptom to the patient can occur. More commonly, the symptom reflects ventricular premature beats occurring frequently. When premature ventricular beats are infrequent and cause the patient no concern or if the patient is unaware of them, there is no need for specific medical treatment. Reassurance as to the benign nature of these premature beats is generally all that is necessary for treatment. On the other hand, if these beats are frequent and cause genuine symptoms, antiarrhythmic drugs may be prescribed similar to what is prescribed for these rhythms in other patients who do not have mitral valve prolapse. Some patients have episodes of supraventricular tachycardia, i.e., paroxysmal atrial tachycardia or atrial fibrillation. If this is an isolated event, no treatment is necessary. At times, one detects frequent multiform ventricular premature beats; for these patients, Holter monitoring is indicated. If this represents a persistent finding, treatment may then be indicated. Propranolol or other beta-blocker drugs may be helpful in such patients. It is also possible that some of the newer antiarrhythmic drugs may have a place in treatment of this symptomatic group in the future. The symptomatic group of patients with mitral valve prolapse probably represent only about 10 percent or less with the condition.

For Gastrointestinal and Genitourinary Tract Surgery and Instrumentation

1. For most patients: **Ampicillin** plus **Gentamicin**	**Adults:** 2.0 g ampicillin IM or IV plus gentamicin 1.5 mg/kg IM or IV given 30 minutes before procedure. May repeat once eight hours later. **Children:** Same timing of medications as adult schedule. Dosages are ampicillin 50 mg/kg and gentamicin 2.0 mg/kg.
2. For patients allergic to penicillin: **Vancomycin** plus **Gentamicin**	**Adults:** 1.0 g vancomycin IV given over 60 minutes plus 1.5 mg/kg gentamicin IM or IV, each given 60 minutes before procedure. Doses may be repeated once 8-12 hours later. **Children:** Timing as above. Doses are vancomycin 20 mg/kg and gentamicin 2.0 mg/kg.
3. Oral regimen for minor or repetitive procedures in low-risk patients: **Amoxicillin**	**Adults:** 3.0 g amoxicillin one hour before procedure and 1.5 g six hours after initial dose. **Children:** Same timing of doses: 50 mg/kg initial dose and 25 mg/kg follow-up dose.

Note: In patients with compromised renal function, it may be necessary to modify or omit the second dose of antibiotics. Intramuscular injections may be contraindicated in patients receiving anticoagulants. Children's doses should not exceed adult doses.

Adapted from A Statement for Health Professionals by the Committee on Rheumatic Fever and Infective Endocarditis: Prevention of Bacterial Endocarditis. *Circulation* 1984; 70:1123A-1127A (also excerpted in *J Am Dent Assoc* 1985;110:98-100).

Please refer to these joint American Heart Association–American Dental Association recommendations for more complete information as to which patients and which procedures require prophylaxis.

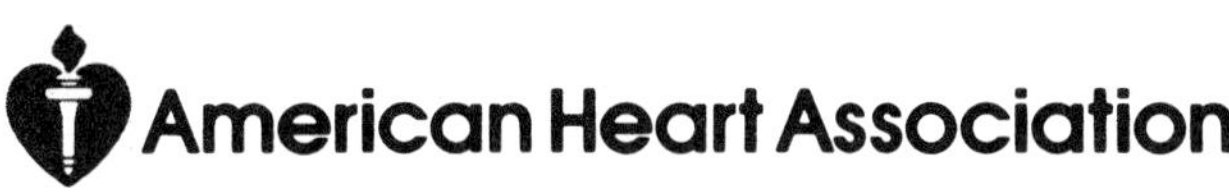

National Center
7320 Greenville Avenue
Dallas, Texas 75231

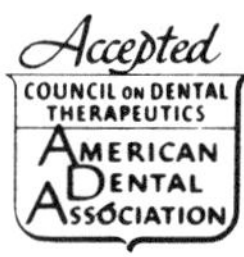

The Council on Dental Therapeutics of the American Dental Association has approved this statement as it relates to dentistry.

Name: ____________________
needs protection from
BACTERIAL ENDOCARDITIS
because of an existing
HEART CONDITION
Diagnosis: ____________________
Prescribed by: ____________________
Date: ____________________

For Dental Procedures and Surgery of the Upper Respiratory Tract

1. For most patients: **Oral Penicillin**	**Adults:** 2.0 g of penicillin V one hour prior to procedure and then 1.0 g six hours after initial dose. **Children less than 60 pounds:** 1.0 g of penicillin V one hour prior to procedure and then 500 mg six hours after initial dose.
2. For those allergic to penicillin (may also be selected for those receiving oral penicillin as continuous rheumatic fever prophylaxis): **Erythromycin**	**Adults:** 1.0 g orally one hour prior to procedure and then 500 mg six hours after initial dose. **Children:** 20 mg/kg orally one hour prior to procedure and then 10 mg/kg six hours after initial dose.
3. For those patients at higher risk of infective endocarditis (especially those with prosthetic heart valves) who are not allergic to penicillin: **Ampicillin** plus **Gentamicin**	**Adults:** Ampicillin 1.0-2.0 g plus gentamicin 1.5 mg/kg IM or IV, both given 30 minutes before procedure; then penicillin V 1.0 g orally six hours after initial dose. **Children:** Timing of doses is same as for adults. Dosages are ampicillin 50 mg/kg and gentamicin 2.0 mg/kg.
4. For higher risk patients (especially those with prosthetic heart valves) who are allergic to penicillin: **Vancomycin**	**Adults:** Vancomycin 1 g IV over 60 minutes, begun 60 minutes before procedure; no repeat dose is necessary. **Children:** Vancomycin 20 mg/kg IV over 60 minutes, begun 60 minutes before procedure; no repeat dose is necessary.

Figure 1 Antibiotic prophylactic instructions recommended by the Amercian Heart Association.

The question of participation in sports, particularly for young patients may arise. Of course, each case must be individualized; in general, my policy is to suggest that the patient avoid sports of the highly competitive, vigorous contact type, such as football. Instead, he should focus on sports such as tennis, swimming, or volley ball, if he is so inclined. Again, Holter monitoring may be indicated to see if any serious rhythms develop with increasing degrees of exercise. It is, of course, wise for us to remember that a young person who is prevented from participation in all sports may develop an even more difficult medical problem, that of psychoneurosis. As far as a young person is concerned, time itself usually solves the problem. As a person grows older, the desire to continue in an active sports program, as in high school or college, has an abrupt decrease after graduation from college.

It is true that many patients with mitral valve prolapse are of a more nervous temperament, so occasionally some form of sedation may be prescribed that can be helpful in treating the related symptoms.

The main serious complication of mitral valve prolapse is development of significant mitral valve regurgitation. This can occur from rupture of a chorda tendineae, either spontaneously or from infective endocarditis. If mitral regurgitation is of a severe degree, surgery may be necessary for repair of the mitral valve by annuloplasty or valve replacement. Valve repair without replacement may be possible; it has been successful in a number of patients when mitral annuloplasty was performed. Any of the patients with findings of the broad spectrum of mitral valve prolapse (even a single click or clicks) can develop mitral regurgitation of a severe degree. As already mentioned, it may result from a ruptured chorda tendineae or be due to increasing degrees of mitral regurgitation in a patient with a flail leaflet. As Dr. Jesse Edwards and Howard Burchell taught us some years ago, "Mitral regurgitation begets mitral regurgitation." When the condition progresses to severe regurgitation, surgery (usually valve replacement) is indicated. It should be remembered however that this complication occurs in only a small number of patients.

It is wise to follow patients with mitral valve prolapse at intervals of every 1 or 2 years even though they are asymptomatic. One example of a benefit of this follow-up is the fact that during the past year the American Heart Association has come out with new, revised recommendations for antibiotic prophylaxis against infective endocarditis; these measures are much easier and simpler to follow than those previously recommended. In addition, any change in the patient's condition can be detected by an office evaluation. Frequent repeat echocardiograms are usually an unnecessary expense and should be discouraged. The echocardiogram, however, can be helpful if there is a change in the baseline that has previously been observed in the physician's office.

There have been instances of transient ischemic attacks (TIAs). It is now well documented that small emboli from the mitral valve can break off and can land in the arteries supplying the brain, ophthalmic arteries, or elsewhere.

Concerning infective endocarditis, some physicians state that, in the first place, since it is a rare condition, and therefore statistically uncommon, why give prophylaxis to the large number of people with mitral valve prolapse? The answer to that is that, even though statistically this is not a common complication, as far as an individual patient is concerned, when it does occur, it represents a 100 percent chance of involvement in his or her case.

I have never recommended surgical replacement of the mitral valve for a patient in whom the valve is prolapsed, but who does not have a ruptured chorda tendineae or flail leaflet that causes significant mitral regurgitation. Occasionally, these patients have been treated and helped medically by psychiatric care. This medical management includes specifically the element of having patients understand their condition, to a large extent through plenty of reassurance and education. Close follow-up may be necessary to demonstrate that they can manage their problems.

I would like to relate an anecdote concerning a patient I saw about 20 years ago. She was seen on an outpatient basis recently; when talking to her, I remembered that I had first seen her 20 years previously. She was from a small town in Pennsylvania. She had mitral valve prolapse. A single mid-systolic click was heard. She had had some symptoms at the time that consisted of palpitations, chest pains, slight dizziness, and nervousness. Through reassurance, the patient's symptoms disappeared, and she was able to return to a normal life. She had gotten along well for 20 years until she read a medical news bulletin on her condition of mitral valve prolapse. In it, she noted that sudden death could occur. After reading this report, she began to have symptoms similar to, and even more aggravated than the ones she had had originally. She became so disturbed and fearful of sudden death that she called for an appointment. Her examination revealed no change from the previous one. She had the typical mid-systolic click, and her baseline findings were essentially unchanged from her previous evaluation. In discussing this with her, I reasurred her again that her mitral valve prolapse was compatible with her leading a perfectly normal life and that she was no different now than she was before. No specific cardiac medication was necessary. There was no indication that anything like sudden death was likely. Once again, as was done 20 years earlier, a careful detailed explanation concerning her condition was given, and plenty of time was afforded to answer her questions. She had taken prophylaxis against infective endocarditis as previously outlined, which she was advised to continue. She seemed reassured when her evaluation was completed. As she was leaving (to further emphasize the benign nature of her condition and to give her even more reassurance), I said "Why don't you make an appointment to come back to see me again, 20 years from now?"

DILATED CARDIOMYOPATHY

KENNETH L. BAUGHMAN, M.D.
ARTHUR M. FELDMAN, M.D., Ph.D.

INCIDENCE AND PROGNOSIS

Although epidemiologic studies differ as to the incidence of heart failure, all investigators recognize the magnitude of the problem. Over 4 million Americans suffer from congestive heart failure (CHF). Earlier studies, such as the Framingham prospective evaluation, demonstrated that an average of 3.7 per 1,000 men and 2.5 per 1,000 women were diagnosed yearly with myocardial failure. The incidence of CHF may be increasing. The number of hospitalizations partially or wholly for the treatment of CHF has nearly doubled from 1970 to 1979, and over 250,000 new cases of heart failure now occur yearly, according to figures compiled by a recent NIH study group.

Of patients suffering from heart failure, approximately 40 percent have a primary heart muscle disorder (cardiomyopathy). The remaining patients have myocardial dysfunction due to other primary disorders, such as hypertension, coronary artery disease with infarction-associated segmental wall motion abnormalities, or valvular disease. Many of the principles of treatment of heart failure are the same regardless of the etiology of the myocardial dysfunction.

Primary heart muscle disorders are classified by their gross pathologic appearance and their hemodynamic abnormalities into dilated, hypertrophic, and restrictive varieties (Table 1).

All the primary cardiomyopathies may develop high end-diastolic pressures and resultant symptoms of pulmonary or systemic venous congestion. Incomplete diastolic relaxation occurs with hypertrophic and restrictive cardiomyopathies due to muscular hypertrophy or muscle infiltration, respectively. This incomplete relaxation and/or small cavity size may limit the forward cardiac output. Dilated cardiomyopathy is characterized by a thin-walled heart muscle with hypodynamic systolic contraction and diastolic relaxation. The damaged heart muscle mandates an increased diastolic pressure. Although the heart cavity is large and the heart rate often elevated, the decreased contractility of the heart muscle results in a depressed cardiac output.

The prognosis, once heart failure is present, is poor regardless of the etiology and whether or not the disorder is primary or secondary. In the Framingham study, the 5-year mortality after the diagnosis of CHF was approximately 50 percent. Dilated cardiomyopathy is a particularly devastating disease; it affects young patients, has an obscure etiology and is poorly responsive to medical therapy. In dilated cardiomyopathy, the 1-year mortality varies from 15 to 25 percent, and the 5-year mortality is approximately 80 percent.

It is only with this background that the treatment of patients with dilated cardiomyopathy can be appreciated. The incidence of the disease is increasing, the etiology unclear, the prognosis poor, and the disease usually affects otherwise healthy young to middle-aged persons. In the remainder of this article we will outline the medical therapy available to treat this disorder.

REVERSIBLE CAUSES

In over 90 percent of patients with dilated cardiomyopathies, the etiology of the muscle dysfunction remains unknown. Several systemic disorders have been identified that can cause cardiac dysfunction resulting in a dilated cardiomyopathy. These disorders should be sought since treatment of these systemic disorders may result in an improvement in cardiac function.

Before addressing reversible causes of cardiomyopathy, one must ensure that the patient with cardiomegaly and CHF has a cardiomyopathy and not "reversible" primary valvular disease, pericardial disease, or focal coronary artery disease with left ventricular aneurysm. Cardiomyopathy "look-alikes" include: focal coronary artery disease (left ventricular aneurysm); primary valvular disease (aortic stenosis, aortic regurgitation, and mitral regurgitation); and pericardial disease (pericardial effusion).

Left Ventricular Aneurysm

Patients with a single myocardial infarction, particularly in the left anterior descending (anterior wall) distribution, may form massive left ventricular aneurysms. Our increasing awareness of silent ischemia and infarction makes the possibility of an undiagnosed infarction greater than was previously considered. These massive transmural infarctions may be difficult to diagnose because of associated electrocardiographic changes, such as interventricular conduction delay, and atypical symptoms, such as acute pericardial irritation simulating acute pericarditis. Aneurysms may be large enough to obscure the remaining functional myocardium, and certain noninvasive studies, such as gated blood pool scan, may report virtually no cardiac contractility. Patients suspected of having left ventricular aneurysm should undergo definitive diagnostic studies. If the remaining myocardium shows reasonably well-maintained function, the patient should be referred for aneurysmectomy, regardless of the size of the focally abnormal area.

Valvular Heart Disease

Rarely, patients with chronic primary valvular heart disease present with severe secondary ventricular dysfunction resulting in massive cardiomegaly and CHF. The advanced state of ventricular dysfunction that these patients display alters the usual physical examination hallmarks of the presence of valvular disease. Significant aortic stenosis with severe left ventricular dysfunction may be in-

TABLE 1 Primary Cardiomyopathies

Form	Incidence (%)	*Pathology*		*Hemodynamics*	
		Wall	*Cavity*	*Systole*	*Diastole*
Dilated	95	Thin	Large	Hypodynamic	Slow
Hypertrophic	5	Thick	Small	Hyperdynamic	Slow, incomplete relaxation
Restrictive	<1	Normal	Normal	Normal (until advanced)	Rapid, restricted relaxation

apparent due to the low cardiac output crossing the valve orifice, rendering the heart nearly silent and preventing recognition of delayed carotid upstroke. Similarly, significant valvular aortic regurgitation with a low cardiac output and severe left ventricular dysfunction may be less apparent due to the associated high left ventricular end-diastolic pressure (LVEDP). The high LVEDP decreases the diastolic pressure gradient across the aortic valve, which coupled with low blood pressure may decrease the murmur of aortic regurgitation. This same high LVEDP, decreased diastolic gradient, and low cardiac output blunt the usual hyperdynamic pulses of significant aortic reflux. Mitral regurgitation is a particular problem because many patients with cardiomyopathy display mitral annular dilatation and secondary mitral reflux. In this instance, a history of preceding murmur or evidence of mitral valve disease by echocardiogram is paramount in determining if definitive studies should be done. The advanced state of left ventricular dysfunction with which these patients usually present makes them poor candidates for surgical intervention, particularly those displaying valvular regurgitation as opposed to stenosis. The degree of left ventricular dysfunction often makes one suspicious of a mixed primary muscular and primary valvular disorder. Regardless, if a primary valvular lesion is suspected, definitive catheterization studies should be performed and surgical management undertaken if the patient is otherwise an appropriate candidate.

Pericardial Disease

A large chronic pericardial effusion may be reflected by an enlargement of the cardiothoracic ratio on chest films, pulmonary and venous congestion, and low cardiac output. Again, physical examination criteria may be blunted. A paradoxical pulse may be difficult to discern, particularly with any irregularity of cardiac rhythm, and jugular venous distention is common to both myopathy and pericardial effusion. The echocardiogram is diagnostic of this disorder. Patients should have the etiology of the effusion sought and diagnostic and therapeutic pericardiocentesis performed as soon as possible.

REVERSIBLE CAUSES

As the disorders just mentioned are all easily diagnosed by echocardiographic examination, every patient with a suspected cardiomyopathy should have an echocardiogram to rule out coronary, valvular, or pericardial disease. An echocardiogram will also confirm the diagnosis of dilated cardiomyopathy. If a dilated cardiomyopathy is confirmed, reversible causes of cardiomyopathy should be sought. Reversible causes of cardiomyopathy include: inflammatory (infective myocarditis, noninfective myocarditis, and autoimmune myocarditis); metabolic, both nutritional (thiamine or carnitine deficiency) and endocrine (thyroid disease and pheochromocytoma); toxic (alcohol or drug abuse); infiltrative (sarcoidosis or hemochromatosis); fibroplastic (Löffler's syndrome); and postpartum.

Inflammatory Conditions

The most frequently suspected etiology of dilated cardiomyopathy is "viral" myocarditis. An animal model exists, which confirms that this mechanism is possible. Viral myocarditis results in antibodies being directed against the heart, and there is some evidence that patients with dilated cardiomyopathy may have a defective immune system with a diminished capacity to "turn off" the antibody response stimulated by the viral invasion. There is also evidence that some selected patients with myocardial inflammation and dilated cardiomyopathy can improve their ventricular function with immunosuppressive therapy. However, the incidence of acute myocarditis in patients with dilated cardiomyopathy is less then 5 percent; treatment entails considerable risk and is effective in only 50 percent of those treated. Whereas some patients with cardiomyopathy improve spontaneously, it is naive to consider all such cases of spontaneous improvement as being due to myocarditis. Furthermore, the efficacy of immunosuppressive treatment has not been proved in a prospective placebo-controlled trial. The disorder is only "diagnosed" by endomyocardial biopsy. We perform biopsy studies on patients who are most likely to have ongoing myocarditis, including those younger than age 50 years, with heart failure symptoms of a duration of less than 1 year, with or without an appropriate "myocarditis" history. Myocarditis may also be part of a systemic autoimmune disorder, such as lupus erythematosus, and appropriate serologic testing should be done. It is important to have the results of the heart biopsy interpreted by an experienced cardiac pathologist because the pathologic diagnosis is fraught with hazard and often incorrectly made. Patients with biopsy-proven myocarditis should be treated with prednisone, 50 mg per square meter, and azathioprine, 75 mg per square meter. Weekly clinical, metabolic, and hematologic examinations are necessary once treatment is initiated. Treatment should be continued for 6 weeks at which time complete assessment should be repeated, including noninvasive determination of ventricular function and endomyocardial biopsy. If the patient has not improved, it is unlikely that further treatment with immunosuppressives will be of benefit. If severe myocarditis continues, however, higher dose therapy or cyclosporine should be considered. If the patient is improving, treatment taper should be attempted. Most patients require 6 months of treatment; a too-rapid taper has resulted in a recurrence of symptoms and deterioration of ventricular performance in some patients.

The possibility of myocarditis, however remote, exists in every patient. In addition, endomyocardial biopsy may demonstrate pathologic features that are diagnostic of other disorders (to be discussed), or it may provide some indication of the severity of the heart muscle disorder. Therefore, an endomyocardial biopsy may be justified in every patient with a dilated form of cardiomyopathy. We prefer to exercise some clinical judgment in the performance of biopsies of the heart and do not do a biopsy examination on every patient with a dilated cardiomyopathy.

Metabolic Abnormalities

Thiamine deficiency exists even today and can result in a hypodynamic heart syndrome (beriberi). Thiamine deficiency should be suspected in alcoholics, persons on "fad" diets (particularly exclusive carbohydrate diets), and patients subjected to long-term diuretics with parenteral forms of nutrition. Thiamine levels can be measured or estimated by red cell transketolase levels. Thiamine deficiency tends to allow peripheral vasodilation and heart muscle dysfunction, resulting in the characteristic "high output" heart failure. Repletion with thiamine may reverse the vasodilation before improving heart contractility, and a transient worsening of heart failure symptoms may occur soon after treatment is initiated. We give thiamine, 100 mg intravenously or orally each day for repletion, and hemodynamic improvement can be expected within 1 week.

Carnitine is a quaternary ammonium compound, which transports long-chain fatty acids into the mitochondria for cardiac metabolism. Several forms of deficiency are evident, and carnitine deficiency should be suspected both in patients with a family history of cardiomyopathy and in patients with cardiomyopathy and electrocardiographic spiked "T" waves across the precordium, with or without a peripheral neuritis or peripheral myopathy. Patients who show improvement on oral administration of carnitine have all had low levels when subjected to direct measurement. The deficiency will likely require lifelong replacement.

THYROID DISEASE

Hypothyroidism can cause a hypodynamic heart with bradycardia, cardiomegaly, and slightly elevated filling pressures. Replacement should be undertaken cautiously, particularly in the elderly, as indolent coronary atherosclerosis may suddenly become manifest. We begin with 0.05 mg per day, increasing the dose every 3 to 4 weeks as judged by symptoms and thyroid-stimulating hormone levels.

Pheochromocytoma

Pheochromocytoma has caused three unexpected deaths from dilated cardiomyopathy in the Baltimore area in the last 2 years. Removal of a pheochromocytoma resulted in normalization of left ventricular function in a patient with a dilated form of cardiomyopathy in this same interval. We find nothing to differentiate these patients from others with dilated cardiomyopathy, although excessive sweating, tachycardia, and diaphoresis may provide a clue. We measure metanephrines in all patients with dilated cardiomyopathy and proceed with other more definitive tests if indicated.

Alcohol

Although alcohol is demonstrated to cause acute diminution of left ventricular function and to alter myocardial metabolism, definitive proof that it can cause a dilated form of cardiomyopathy is lacking. Few clinicians, however, believe that alcoholic cardiomyopathy does not exist. Men appear to be more susceptible than women, and a certain level of alcohol consumption is probably necessary over at least a 5-year interval to initiate significant cardiac damage. Approximately 60 percent of patients with alcoholism and dilated cardiomyopathy who abstain from alcohol improve, and those who stop alcohol consumption as soon as symptoms of CHF appear have the greatest chance of significant improvement. Every patient with dilated cardiomyopathy should be suspected of having alcoholic cardiomyopathy; an appropriate history of alcohol consumption should be obtained from family or friends. We recommend that all patients with dilated cardiomyopathy abstain from alcohol, regardless of the etiology of their disorder.

Drug Toxicity

Doxorubicin is well recognized for its ability to cause cardiac dysfunction. A dose-response deterioration in ventricular function may appear with as little as 350 mg per square meter and becomes apparent in most patients at a level higher than 500 mg per square meter. Greater toxicity can be expected in those of advanced age, those who have had prior chest radiation or cyclophosphamide treatment, or those with known cardiac dysfunction before therapy. In those patients at risk, serial endomyocardial biopsies and noninvasive assessment of left ventricular function are necessary. Once the diagnosis of myopathy is established, little can be done to improve left ventricular performance. In addition to doxorubicin, a number of other drugs can cause cardiac dysfunction, including phenothiazines, methyldopa, and penicillin, among others. Therefore, every patient with a dilated form of cardiomyopathy should have his current and previous drug history reviewed, and potentially offending agents should be removed.

Infiltrative Disease

Sarcoidosis may cause left ventricular dysfunction as well as valvular and pericardial disease. Whereas 25 percent of patients dying with sarcoidosis have cardiac involvement, it is suspected clinically in only about 5 percent. The clinical significance of cardiac sarcoidosis is dependent on the amount and location of granulomatous involvement. Steroids may allow stabilization or regression of myocardial dysfunction. Cardiac biopsy can provide a definitive diagnosis, but endomyocardial sarcoidosis may be missed because of the spotty character of the involvement. Hemochromatosis should be suspected in the cardiomyopathic patient with excessive skin pigmentation, diabetes, and hepatic abnormalities. Involvement in other organs may be inapparent or cardiac dysfunction may precede other organs with regard to systemic manifestations. Iron and iron-binding capacity should be evaluated in all patients with dilated cardiomyopathy, and a heart biopsy may prove definitive if the tissue is appropriately stained. Phlebotomy or chelation may improve ventricular performance.

Fibroplastic

Löffler's syndrome associates eosinophilia with endomyocardial inflammation and eventual fibrosis. Patients suspected of having Löffler's syndrome because of an elevated eosinophil count and dilated cardiomyopathy should have an endomyocardial biopsy examination to confirm the diagnosis. Treatment with steroids to control the eosinophil count may prevent progression of the disease.

Postpartum Cardiomyopathy

Acute cardiomyopathy affecting women in the final trimester of their pregnancy or in the 6 months following delivery defines postpartum cardiomyopathy. Some investigators suggest that this form of cardiomyopathy is due to myocarditis and should be treated with immunosuppressive therapy. We perform biopsy examinations on all patients with postpartum cardiomyopathy to evaluate for possible myocarditis. In our experience, myocarditis is infrequently present; when present, it may either resolve without immunosuppressive therapy or continue despite therapy and improvement in heart function. Well over one-half of those patients affected improve "spontaneously," whether or not myocarditis is present. We treat patients with postpartum cardiomyopathy as we do patients with dilated cardiomyopathy and gradually withdraw therapy over a 6-month period after their condition has stabilized.

INOTROPIC THERAPY

Digitalis

Despite a number of recent advances, digitalis remains the only clinically acceptable inotrope. Although digitalis effects a dose-response improvement in ventricular function, it has considerable toxicity in the cardiomyopathy population. We usually give patients with dilated cardiomyopathy a loading dose of 1 to 1.5 mg over 24 hours and then give no more than 0.125 mg per day. This schedule normally establishes a low "therapeutic range" serum level, but avoids the potential for increased myocardial oxygen consumption and ventricular ectopy. Although one may wish to control the ventricular response to atrial fibrillation with digoxin in patients with dilated cardiomyopathy, this mode of treatment often becomes impractical, and higher-than-normal heart rates must be accepted to avoid toxicity.

Other Inotropes

Amrinone and milrinone both vasodilate and provide inotropic support. Amrinone is limited to short-term intravenous use. We utilize a bolus of 0.75 mg per kilogram over 2 to 3 minutes followed by a dose of 5 to 10 μg per kilogram per minute or as adjusted to effect as estimated by invasive hemodynamic assessment. Milrinone is not yet clinically available. A number of other oral-form inotropes are being investigated at this time. All true inotropes share the potential risk of increasing the myocardial oxygen consumption and causing myocardial cellular ischemia and/or ventricular ectopy. Most inotropes tested so far appear to improve the patient's quality of life but may decrease longevity.

Patients with advanced CHF occasionally require intravenous inotropic support with dopamine or dobutamine. Dopamine exerts an inotropic effect by stimulation of the beta $_1$- adrenergic receptor and release of myocardial norepinephrine. At low doses, dopamine vasodilates selected arterial beds, including the coronary and renal arteries, probably by stimulation of specific dopamine receptors. Dobutamine stimulates cardiac beta $_1$- receptors as well as providing mild stimulation of beta $_2$- and alpha-1 receptors. Dobutamine is a less potent vasopressor than dopamine. Both these pressor agents mandate invasive hemodynamic monitoring with careful dose-response assessment. Neither of them should be used unless the situation demands prompt and immediate action. This therapy should not be primary at the time of presentation unless shock or severe deterioration is present. Often these agents are initiated prematurely before standard therapy for heart failure has been tried; this results in excessive initial therapy and a difficult weaning process as oral therapy is initiated. In some patients, the hemodynamic benefit of even short-term pressor infusion may persist for several weeks, further delaying establishment of an appropriate chronic oral regimen.

A limited number of patients have been treated with long-term dopamine infusion through Hickman catheters from external portable infusion pumps or through implanted devices. This form of therapy should be undertaken only in patients who fail to respond to conventional therapy and who demonstrate a beneficial response to dopamine or dobutamine infusion. Therapy with continuous or long-term intermittent infusion remains experimental, while investigators attempt to find the appropriate dose and duration of therapy to balance beta-receptor stimulation and protection. Oral levodopa is decarboxylated to dopamine and has been demonstrated to cause a modest inotropic and vasodilating response. As large doses of the agent are necessary (4 g per day) and as patients selected for this therapy have poor gastrointestinal tolerance, it is of limited practical benefit.

DIURETICS

In the 25 years since diuretics were introduced, no form of therapy has proved to be safer or more effective for the management of acute and chronic heart failure. Diuretics can be divided into four groups by their site of action and into three groups by their ability to excrete sodium (Table 2).

Proximal Tubular Agents

While two-thirds of the filtered sodium is resorbed in the proximal tubule, no diuretic effectively influences this area of the nephron. In addition, renal adaptation compensates for diminished proximal sodium absorption by increased distal sodium resorption with a resultant decreased diuretic effect.

Acetazolamide (Diamox) inhibits carbonic anhydrase and decreases sodium and bicarbonate absorption. The drug is supplied as 125-mg tablets or ampules of 500 mg for IV use. The usually effective heart failure dose is 250 to 375 mg per day. The drug's effect is limited by the small quantities of carbonic anhydrase available in the nephron. Diminished diuretic efficacy is usually due to excessive carbonic anhydrase suppression or excessive bicarbonate loss with resultant systemic acidosis. The diuretic effect is mild and the drug cannot be recommended routinely.

Mannitol is a small molecular weight agent that serves as an osmotic diuretic in the proximal tubule. The drug is of limited efficacy in heart failure because of its obligate volume load and intravascular expansion.

Henle's Loop Diuretics

Diuretics affecting this portion of the nephron are the most effective agents currently available and include furosemide, ethacrynic acid, bumetanide, and piretanide. Mercurial diuretics, the predecessors of this group, are infrequently utilized.

Furosemide (Lasix) has a potent saluretic effect because of its inhibition of chloride transport. Furosemide also results in acute dilatation of the venous bed after intravenous administration. The diuretic effect is apparent in 5 minutes, peaks in 20 to 30 minutes, and is completed in 3 to 4 hours. The dose of furosemide should be individualized. Patients not previously exposed to intravenous furosemide may demonstrate a profound diuretic effect to 20 mg. Most patients require 40 mg intravenously; rarely are doses of up to 200 to 500 mg necessary. Patients with severe CHF not responding to an intravenous dose after 1 hour should have twice that dose given until a diuretic effect appears or until unacceptable levels of the drug are given. Furosemide is 50 to 60 percent bioavailable after oral administration. Oral therapy is usually initiated with 20 to 40 mg and increased daily as needed.

Bumetanide (Bumex) is similar to furosemide yet is fortyfold more potent by weight with possible diminished ototoxicity, decreased potassium loss, and increased efficacy in patients with renal insufficiency. These advantages may become less apparent as increased clinical experience is obtained with this drug. The usual initial oral dose is 0.5 mg and may be increased to 2 mg as needed every 4 to 6 hours. Up to 15 mg per day may be necessary in patients with edema and renal insufficiency. Intravenously, 0.5 mg is usually effective and rarely is a dose of more than 1 mg every 2 to 3 hours needed.

Ethacrynic acid (Edecrin) shares the pharmacokinetics of furosemide as well as the dose recommendations. Oral tablets of 25 or 50 mg are available, and a dose range of 50 to 200 mg per day is usually required for heart failure therapy. Intravenously, 0.5 to 1 mg per kilogram is usually necessary for an effective diuresis. Ethacrynic acid is more ototoxic than furosemide and should not be used with other ototoxic agents. Ethacrynic acid, however, is not a sulfa derivative and is the only "loop" diuretic available for patients with a history of sulfa allergy or furosemide sensitivity.

Early Distal Tubule Agents

Thiazide diuretics (thiazide, hydrochlorothiazide, and dichlorothalidone) all have minimal carbonic anhydrase inhibition and mild saluresis due to a yet undefined mechanism. These agents differ in their duration of action and frequency of administration. Chlorthalidone has a half-life of 40 to 50 hours, thiazide 24 hours, allowing these drugs to be given every day or every other day as needed. Hydrochlorothiazide has a half-life of 6 to 8 hours and may be given once or twice per day. This group of agents is used for patients with mild fluid retention. These early distal tubule agents are ineffective in patients with renal insufficiency and should not be used when the glomerular filtration rate falls below 20 ml per minute. Metolazone is similar to other benzothiadiazines with a naturetic effect, which may persist for 11 to 24 hours. This drug is the only agent in this group with maintained efficacy in patients with depressed renal function. The usually effective dose of metolazone is from 2.5 to 10 mg per day in edematous patients.

Late Distal Tubule Agents

The saluretic effect of this group of agents is limited, but their usefulness is balanced by the potassium-sparing effect of these drugs. Spironolactone is an aldosterone-competitive antagonist and therefore prevents the normal sodium retention, potassium-losing effects of this mineralocorticoid. Aldosterone levels are elevated in patients with CHF, particularly those with right-sided failure and hepatic congestion. Spironolactone is available as 25-, 50-, or 100-mg capsules, and the normal dose varies from 50 mg to 200 mg per day. The diuretic and potassium-sparing effect of spironolactone may not be apparent for 3 or 4 days. Therefore, the dose should not be altered until the efficacy of the last change in therapy is apparent, and potassium supplements should be carefully reassessed 3 to 5 days after the drug is initiated. Aldosterone antagonists will have limited efficacy in patients whose aldosterone levels are already suppressed by angiotensin-converting enzyme inhibitors. Triamterene and amiloride inhibit sodium resorption and promote potassium and hydrogen retention independent of aldosterone. Triamterene has a diuretic effect for up to 8 to 10 hours with a dose range from 50 to 150 mg twice per day. Capsules of 50 and 100 mg are available for oral administration. Amiloride has a longer duration of action of up to 24 hours. The usual dose is 5 mg per day with a maximum of 20 mg per day. The potassium-sparing drugs should never be used in combination with one another.

Diuretics and Congestive Heart Failure

Even the limited listing of diuretics (Table 2) demonstrates the tremendous variability of treatment alternatives available to manage states of salt and water excess. It is important to match the "power" of the therapy utilized to the clinical need. Patients with very mild heart failure may be managed with dietary salt restriction alone. Many patients with mild heart failure may be managed with dietary salt restriction and mild-to-moderate saluretics, such as the early distal tubule (thiazide) and late distal tubule (potassium-sparing) agents. Patients requiring hospitalization because of CHF usually should be treated with loop diuretics, at least until the acute excess of salt and water is resolved. Only those patients with signs and symptoms of refractory CHF or those with pulmonary edema should be subjected to intravenous diuretic therapy. Excessive initial diuretic therapy or excessive persistent diuretic therapy can lead to acute intravenous volume depletion, hyponatremia, hypotension, renal hypoperfusion, and renal insufficiency.

Acute intravenous loop diuretic therapy should be monitored hourly. Failure to promote an effective diuresis in the face of persistent pulmonary edema requires repeated bolus injections of higher dose diuretic therapy until a response is apparent. Most loop diuretics display a "threshold" phenomenon. The diuretic response is inapparent until this threshold is reached. The diuretic response above this threshold appears to be dose responsive. Once the threshold is established, at least this quantity of drug should be administered as necessary to maintain an adequate and effective diuresis. One must be aware of the increased potential toxicity from higher-dose drug therapy. Patients requiring hospitalization due to CHF without pulmonary edema should be treated with oral loop diuretics. Again, the threshold dose of diuretics should be sought and then given twice per day. The best means of determining response to therapy is by accurate daily weights with intake and output measurement confirmation when possible and appropriate. Once an intravenous or oral regimen is initiated, it is often difficult to prevent excessive diuresis, and the drug should be adjusted to allow a steady weight loss of one to two pounds per day. Regardless of the initial agent used and frequency of utilization, the patient should be adjusted to a once daily, or at most twice daily, diuretic regimen before discharge. The onset of action of the diuretic chosen should be noted to insure that the diuretic effect occurs during the patient's waking hours.

Patients with renal insufficiency requiring diuretics should be treated with loop diuretics or metolazone. Metolazone is the only early distal tubular agent with retained efficacy in renal insufficiency. The distal tubular agents may cause significant hyperkalemia if used in patients with renal insufficiency.

Hypokalemia is a virtual certainty when patients require loop diuretics. To prevent hypokalemia and its potentially toxic manifestations, we initiate potassium supplementation with the loop diuretics. The vigor of potassium replacement should match the degree of diuretic response, since a greater saluresis virtually always implies a greater kaluresis. This vigorous replacement response is blunted if the patient is taking an angiotensin-converting enzyme inhibitor or a potassium-sparing agent. Patients requiring long-term diuretic therapy, particularly without adequate food intake, may become depleted in magnesium or thiamine, and repletion may occasionally become necessary.

TABLE 2 Diuretics in Treatment of Congestive Heart Failure

Site	*Location*	*Agents*	*Maximal Fraction of Excretion (%)*
I	Proximal tubule	Osmotic: Mannitol and isosorbide Carbonic anhydrase inhibitor: Acetazolamide	<5
II	Henle's ascending limb	Phenoxyacetic acids: Ethacrynic acid Sulfamoyl benzoates: Furosemide, bumetanide, and piretanide	>15
III	Early distal tubule	Benzothiadiazines: Thiazide and hydrochlorothiazides Related compounds: Chlorthalidone and metolazone	5–10
IV	Late distal tubule	Aldosterone antagonist: Spironolactone Pteridines: Triamterene and amiloride	<5

Combination Diuretic Therapy

Patients with refractory CHF may require combination diuretic therapy. As effective diuretic agents (the proximal tubule) in site I remain impractical, this implies a combination of agents from sites II, III, or IV (the loop of Henle or distal tubule). As agents in each group share the renal site and mechanism of action, only one agent at a time—active in each site—should be chosen. Therefore, a single site II agent might be combined with a single site III and/or site IV agent. Combination therapy should not include combination of agents active within the same area of the nephron. No patients should receive more than one site II, III or IV agent at a time. The most frequent combinations are the potassium-sparing agents with the more powerful loop diuretics or, not infrequently, with the benzothiadiazines and other agents active in the early distal tubule. The combination of loop diuretics with early distal tubular active diuretics results in an effective but almost assuredly marked hypokalemia. Rarely, in refractory patients, the thiazide agents must be added on an intermittent basis (every other day or every third day) to patients receiving loop diuretics and potassium-sparing agents.

Diuretics in Combination with Other Drugs

Diuretics may affect or be affected by other drugs. The ototoxicity of the loop diuretics may be enhanced by aminoglycoside antibiotics. Similarly, the nephrotoxicity of certain cephalosporins may be enhanced by Henle's loop diuretics. The efficacy of diuretics may be diminished by the nonsteroidal anti-inflammatory agents or display decreased absorption if given with meals.

Theophylline, or other active xanthines, may enhance renal blood flow and provide a proximal tubular saluresis, both of which may provide diuretic action.

VASODILATOR AGENTS

Patients with decreased cardiac output must increase systemic resistance to stabilize organ perfusion pressure. The patient with dilated cardiomyopathy often has an elevation of systemic resistance out of proportion to the depression of cardiac output. Vasodilator drugs decrease this resistance and may improve forward cardiac output and organ perfusion. Despite the attractiveness of this pathophysiologic proposition, vasodilators have demonstrated only mild-to-moderate benefit for patients with heart failure. These agents can be divided into three major categories (Table 3).

TABLE 3 Vasodilator Agents

Direct-acting	*Neurohumoral*	*Calcium-channel Antagonist*
Nitrates	Prazosin	Nifedipine
Hydralazine	Captopril/Enalapril	Verapamil
Minoxidil	Trimazocin	Diltiazem

Direct-Acting Agents

Nitrates produce vasodilatation in the venous circulation to a much greater extent than in the arterial circulation by activation of vascular nitrate receptors. Whereas cutaneous nitrates have the advantage of once per day convenience, there is increasing evidence that persistent stimulation of the nitrate receptor results in "down regulation" of its vasodilatation site and diminished efficacy. Patients with a dilated form of cardiomyopathy, therefore, are increasingly being treated with oral nitrate preparations. Isosorbide dinitrate in doses of 20 to 40 mg every 4 to 6 hours has been utilized in a number of clinical trials, which have shown improvement in acute and chronic (3 months) rest and exercise hemodynamics. The oral nitrates have a peak effect within 1 hour, and their duration of action is from 4 to 6 hours. The hemodynamic improvement is modest at best and, as already noted, most prevalent in the venous circulation.

Hydralazine is an arterial smooth muscle vasodilator. Acutely, hydralazine has demonstrated hemodynamic benefit with as much as a 40 to 50 percent increase in cardiac output. The long-term results are variable, and some prospective double-blind trials report unfavorable results. The peak hemodynamic effect develops within 1 to 2 hours after oral administration and the duration of action is approximately 6 hours. Patients require between 50 and 100 mg every 6 hours to provide systemic vasodilation. We usually initiate patients at 10 mg every 6 hours and increase the dose every other dosing interval (every 12 hours) until 50 mg every 12 hours is achieved. Increases in drug dose beyond this level are done more gradually, and we allow 3 to 4 days for maximum drug effect. Angina may be provoked in patients with dilated cardiomyopathy with or without coronary artery disease due to vasodilatation, decreased myocardial perfusion, and primary myocardial stimulation. While large doses of hydralazine are utilized, patients with dilated cardiomyopathy infrequently develop drug-induced lupus erythematosus.

Hydralazine is a primary arterial vasodilator, whereas nitrates affect the venous circuit. These two drugs used in combination are effective for acute and long-term vasodilatation in patients with dilated cardiomyopathy.

Neurohumoral Agents

Prazosin is a vascular smooth muscle dilator that blunts the alpha–receptor of the sympathetic nervous system, thereby diminishing sympathetic tone. Prazosin has the advantage of arterial and venous dilatation from a single agent. It improves hemodynamics in acute rest and exercise studies. The long-term hemodynamic improvement noted in prospective double-blind trials is varied, depending on the severity of the patient's hemodynamic deterioration and duration of follow-up. After oral administration, the drug has a peak effect in 1 to 2 hours and a persistent dilating effect for approximately 6 hours. Prazosin demonstrates a "first-dose" phenomenon characterized by dramatic hypotension following the initial but not subsequent doses. Treatment is initiated at 0.5 to 1 mg administered at bedtime. If patients develop hypotension, they will be in a supine position and are unlikely to suffer symptomatic consequences. The dose is then increased on a weekly basis by 1 mg 4 times per day until an appropriate dose is reached. Patients are judged clinically by symptomatic improvement, and their tolerance is estimated by blood pressure response. The maximum dose is approximately 5 mg every 6 hours.

Captopril is an angiotensin-converting enzyme inhibitor. This drug prevents the conversion of angiotensin I to angiotensin II and similarly diminishes bradykinin degradation. Angiotensin II is a potent vasoconstrictor and bradykinins are mild vasodilators. The effect of captopril is to produce arterial and venous dilatation. The medication is most effective in those patients who have stimulation of the renin-axis system. Measurement of renin levels is impractical and expensive, and renin-angiotensin stimulation can usually be assumed if hyponatremia is present. Captopril is capable of producing a first-dose phenomenon similar to prazosin. Patients are started on a dose of 6.25 mg, and the first dose is administered while the patient is supine. Those patients most likely to develop this first-dose phenomenon are those with marked hyponatremia and/or a recent dramatic diuresis. The dose is gradually increased as tolerated. Approximately 10 to 20 mg of captopril per day blocks the available angiotensin, and larger doses tend to prolong its effect as opposed to increasing its hemodynamic benefit. Most patients utilize between 12.5 and 25 mg 3 times per day. The peak effect of the drug develops within 1 to 2 hours, and its duration of action is 4 to 6 hours. The efficacy of captopril has been demonstrated in a prospective, acute and chronic double-blind multicenter trial. Patients with renal insufficiency or proteinuria may be liable to the adverse renal effects of this drug, so renal function must be monitored closely. As captopril also diminishes aldosterone levels, patients on diuretic therapy may be less likely to develop hypokalemia. Potassium replacement should be monitored closely after initiation of captopril. Similarly, diuretics that are aldosterone-competitive inhibitors (spironolactone) should be discontinued if captopril is initiated.

Calcium-Channel Antagonists

Nifedipine results in an alteration in calcium flux in the vascular smooth muscle and ventricular myocardium. This results in systemic vasodilation, but a negative inotropic effect in the myocardium. In our experience with nifedipine, the vasodilatory effects are predominant over the negative inotropic effects if doses under 20 mg every 6 hours are utilized. Nifedipine has arterial and venous dilating properties and is of proven hemodynamic benefit in acute rest and exercise studies. A limited number of chronic studies has been performed, which appear to show persistent efficacy. The drug has a peak effect approximately 1 hour after oral administration and a duration of effect for approximately 6 hours. The limitations of nifedipine are hypotension, edema, gastrointestinal side effects, and in higher doses a negative inotropic effect. Nifedipine may have the advantage of dilating the coronary artery circulation and improving myocardial cellular perfusion.

A limited number of studies has been performed in patients with dilated cardiomyopathy and heart failure with diltiazem and verapamil. Both agents have some efficacy with regard to short-term improvement in ventricular function; however, the negative inotropic effect of verapamil is likely to limit its long-term utilization. Insufficient studies have been performed on the efficacy of long-term administration of diltiazem, and at this time neither verapamil nor diltiazem can be recommended.

There is no "perfect" vasodilating agent. The most efficacious drug available is captopril. In an assessment of the efficacy of vasodilators, clinical judgment of symptomatic improvement and exercise testing are likely to be more beneficial then repeated hemodynamic measurements. Lack of drug efficacy must raise the question of (1) an ineffective vasodilator, (2) an inadequate dose of medication, (3) failure to adjust other medications, or (4) tachyphylaxis. Every vasodilator as a result of blockade at its primary site of action may result in stimulation of a compensatory vasoconstricting site. For instance, alpha-receptor blockade may result in stimulation of the renin-angiotensin system and secondary fluid retention. Therefore, the continuation of vasodilator drugs often requires repeated assessment of the patient and adjustment of the vasodilator itself or alterations in diuretic therapy. Vasodilators tend to be more effective in patients with larger hearts, higher jugular venous pressure, and severe hemodynamic deterioration. There is, as yet, no definitive evidence that vasodilators prolong life in patients with dilated cardiomyopathy. Vasodilators, however, do appear to improve the quality of life.

BETA-BLOCKING AGENTS

Some investigators have demonstrated that the activity of the sympathetic nervous system (as measured by plasma norepinephrine levels) is directly related to the risk of death in patients with dilated cardiomyopathy. Therefore the activity of the sympathetic nervous system is a sensitive measure of the severity of cardiovascular decompensation.

Persistently high sympathetic tone results in a selective down regulation of beta-receptors. The number of beta-receptors is decreased in failing human hearts. This adrenergic fatigue results in a diminished inotropic and chronotropic response to sympathetic stimulation. More recently, it has been demonstrated that beta$_2$- receptors do not appear to be down regulated in failing myocardium.

Because of the negative inotropic effect of beta-blockers, physicians are reluctant to give adrenergic antagonists to patients with myocardial failure. There are several potential benefits of beta-blocker therapy in this patient group. They include: (1) decreased heart rate, (2) decreased myocardial oxygen consumption, (3) protection from the probable toxic effects of elevated circulating catecholamines, (4) decreased incidence of arrhythmia, (5) membrane stabilization and (6) upregulation of the beta-adrenergic receptor. "Upregulation" implies an increase in the density and responsiveness of beta-receptors as a result of their protection from sympathetic stimulation by beta-blockade. Several small studies have demonstrated the efficacy of beta-blockers in selected patients with dilated cardiomyopathy. While these studies are pathophysiologically attractive, larger number of patients must be examined and prospective randomized trials performed before this form of therapy can be recommended to the population with cardiomyopathy at large. It is likely, however, that a subset of the cardiomyopathy population will benefit from these drugs in the future.

ANTIARRHYTHMIC AGENTS

Patients with dilated cardiomyopathy are subject to supraventricular and ventricular arrhythmias. Atrial premature contractions, atrial tachycardia, and most frequently, atrial fibrillation may occur. Ventricular arrhythmias are frequently due to myocardial damage and myocardial cellular dysfunction.

Supraventricular Arrhythmias

Atrial tachycardia and atrial fibrillation both result in a dramatic deterioration in cardiac output due to the rapid ventricular response, diminished ventricular filling, and heightened end-diastolic pressure associated with these arrhythmias. Digoxin remains the most efficacious agent for supraventricular arrhythmias. Beta-blockade and verapamil may similarly control the ventricular response, but their negative inotropic effect makes them unsatisfactory for this group of patients.

Ventricular Arrhythmias

All patients with dilated cardiomyopathy have ventricular arrhythmias. These arrhythmias virtually always include ventricular tachycardia when patients with dilated cardiomyopathy are in a decompensated state. Therefore, unless the patients have symptoms of syncope or near-syncope, we do not assess their need for chronic antiarrhythmic suppression until their myocardial failure has stabilized. Once patients' conditions are reasonably stable, they receive at least 24 hours of Holter monitoring. If patients demonstrate ventricular tachycardia on Holter monitoring, we treat them with chronic suppressive therapy. Patients with symptomatic ventricular arrhythmias must be treated with chronic antiarrhythmic therapy as soon as the diagnosis is made. While most antiarrhythmic drugs have some negative inotropic effect, it usually is not clinically apparent during treatment. There is no indication that suppression of ventricular arrhythmias improves the long-term prognosis of patients with dilated cardiomyopathy. Nonetheless, as approximately 50 percent of these patients suffer a sudden and unexpected death, we feel obligated to attempt antiarrhythmic treatment. We characteristically utilize quinidine or procainamide. Disopyramide can initiate a dramatic deterioration in left ventricular function and is therefore not used in the group. Amiodarone is used only for demonstrated failure by symptoms or Holter monitoring, demonstrated prorhythmic effect, or drug toxicity of standard agents. Quinidine should always be initiated with a 100-mg oral test dose while the patient is under hospital observation as an idiosyncratic hypotensive reaction has been demonstrated with the first dose in some patients. As virtually all antiarrhythmic agents increase the effective level of digoxin, digoxin toxicity must be assessed after initiation of these drugs.

ANTICOAGULANT AGENTS

Patients with dilated cardiomyopathy are prone to systemic and pulmonary embolization. Pulmonary emboli occur because of venous stasis, low cardiac output, and diminished activity displayed by most cardiomyopathy patients. Systemic embolization may occur because of increased ventricular cavity size and blood stasis. The risk of symptomatic systemic embolization is approximately 10 to 15 percent per year in this population and is likely twice this figure with atrial fibrillation. We treat all patients with dilated cardiomyopathy and an ejection fraction below 30 percent with warfarin unless there is a contraindication to anticoagulation. As this group of patients requires close observation for their primary disorder, the frequent evaluation of prothrombin time is often beneficial to help adjust the patients' other medical therapy. Patients with right sided CHF must be followed closely because alterations in the degree of hepatic congestion may significantly affect warfarin metabolism. Because of this alteration in hepatic congestion, patients with dilated cardiomyopathy treated with warfarin are more susceptible to systemic bleeding complications than the routine patient population, and this fact must be considered when determining if therapy should be initiated.

Our understanding of the pathophysiology, pathology, and etiology of dilated cardiomyopathy is likely to be dramatically improved in the next several years. At the present time, dilated cardiomyopathy must be considered to be one of the last remaining frontiers of ignorance in the field of cardiology. The lack of understanding of the pathology and pathophysiology involved in patients with presumed "idiopathic" dilated cardiomyopathy leads to undirected therapy. The results of current therapy have not significantly improved the prognosis for this group of patients. Not infrequently all forms of medical therapy fail and patients require transplantation. This is not a procedure for all patients with cardiomyopathy even assuming an endless supply of donor heart availability. We look forward to the intellectual explosion that will occur in the area of dilated cardiomyopathy over the next decade.

HYPERTROPHIC CARDIOMYOPATHY

E. DOUGLAS WIGLE, M.D., F.R.C.P.(C), F.A.C.P., F.A.C.C.
SUSAN WILANKSY, M.D., F.R.C.P.(C)

Hypertrophic cardiomyopathy (HCM) may be defined as an idiopathic form of ventricular hypertrophy that principally involves the left and, to a lesser extent, the right ventricle. In our experience, the left ventricular (LV) hypertrophy is concentric in about 5 percent of cases and asymmetric in 95 percent of cases. The asymmetric hypertrophy most commonly involves the ventricular septum, but in a small percentage of cases the involvement is primarily apical or midventricular. In this discussion, we will deal with HCM due to ventricular septal hypertrophy, which may be localized to the subaortic area or may extend down to the papillary muscles or to the LV apex, in which case anterolateral wall involvement is almost invariably present. This tremendous variation in the extent of hypertrophy in HCM is an important determinant of the clinical manifestations and prognosis in patients with this abnormality. Thus, patients with extensive septal and anterolateral wall hypertrophy are more likely to demonstrate obstruction to left ventricular outflow in systole (muscular subaortic stenosis [MSS]) and impaired LV relaxation during diastole, as well as atrial and ventricular arrhythmias. Treatment of HCM is principally directed at the amelioration or abolition of these three manifestations of the disease. A detailed account of our views on the pathophysiology and management of HCM has recently been published (Wigle ED, Sasson Z, Henderson MA, et al. Hypertrophic cardiomyopathy. The importance of the site and the extent of hypertrophy. Prog Cardiovasc Dis 1985; 28:1–83).

MECHANISM OF OBSTRUCTION TO LEFT VENTRICULAR OUTFLOW IN HCM

Therapeutic Implications

Since one of the principal aims of therapy in HCM is the amelioration or abolition of the obstruction to left ventricular outflow, it is desirable (and indeed necessary) to review current concepts with regard to the pathophysiology of the obstruction in order to understand the rationale for the various forms of therapy. Figure 1 depicts our concept of the mechanism of systolic anterior motion of the anterior (or posterior) mitral leaflet(s), and how mitral leaflet-ventricular septal apposition results in obstruction to left ventricular outflow and the invariable and concomitant mitral regurgitation. Crucial to these considerations is the fact that there is a high velocity, nonobstructed flow of blood through the narrowed outflow tract at the onset of systole, which draws the anterior mitral leaflet toward the septum by a Venturi effect or similar mechanism. Any pharmacologic intervention that decreases the velocity of ejection (decreased contractility by negative inotropic agents and increased afterload by vasopressor agents) will lessen or abolish the Venturi forces—and hence mitral leaflet systolic anterior motion—with resultant amelioration or abolition of the obstruction to outflow and mitral regurgitation. Surgical widening of the outflow tract (ventriculomyectomy) will lessen or abolish the obstruction to outflow by reducing the velocity of ejection and displacing the path of ejection away from the mitral leaflets, thus lessening the Venturi forces on these leaflets. Mitral valve replacement can also abolish the outflow tract obstruction by the removal of the offending mitral leaflet(s).

HEMODYNAMIC SUBGROUPS

Not only is it important to understand the mechanism of obstruction and the therapeutic implications thereof but also to appreciate the principal hemodynamic subgroups of HCM based on whether there is resting, latent, or no obstruction to LV outflow (Table 1). Patients with resting obstruction (MSS) consistently have obstruction to LV outflow due to mitral leaflet-ventricular septal contact under control conditions. In latent (provocable) obstruction, there is no obstruction to outflow at rest, but one may be provoked by amyl nitrite inhalation, isoproterenol infusion, or in the postextrasystolic beat. In nonobstructive HCM, there is no obstruction to outflow at rest or on provocation. Aside from these three major hemodynamic subgroups of HCM, there are two relatively

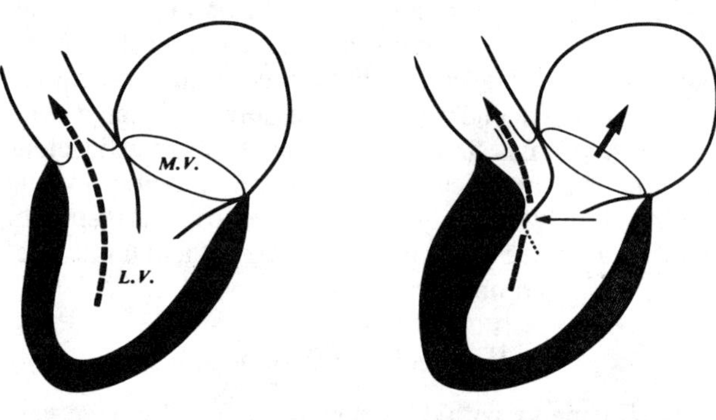

Figure 1 Proposed mechanism of systolic anterior motion of the anterior mitral leaflet and obstruction to left ventricular outflow in hypertrophic cardiomyopathy (MSS). In normal subjects, blood is ejected from the left ventricle in a relatively direct path into the aorta through a wide open outflow tract. In MSS, the ventricular septum is thickened (left horizontal arrow), resulting in a narrow outflow tract. Because of this narrowing, ejection of blood from the ventricle occurs at high velocity, and the ejection path is closer to the anterior mitral leaflet than normal. As a result, the anterior leaflet is drawn into outflow tract toward the septum by a Venturi effect (right horizontal arrow). Mitral leaflet-septal contact results in obstruction to left ventricular outflow. Mitral regurgitation (upper right oblique arrow) results from the anterior mitral leaflet being out of its normal systolic position. LV = left ventricle, MV = mitral valve.

TABLE 1 Major Hemodynamic Subgroups of Hypertrophic Cardiomyopathy

Hemodynamic Subgroup	*Hemodynamics*	*Echocardiography*	*Doppler Echocardiography*	*Nuclear Angiography*	*Clinical Signs*
Resting obstruction	Pressure gradient at rest	Severe SAM, LAE, and AVN; thickest septum; and extensive hypertrophy	Subaortic gradient: mitral regurgitation	Increased EF*;impaired relaxation	3-4/6 M; reversed split S_2; ML–SC sound; triple apex; spike and dome arterial pulse
Latent obstruction	Provocable pressure gradient	Mild-to-moderate SAM; LAE and AVN rare; septal hypertrophy usually restricted to subaortic area	Provocable subaortic gradient; provocable mitral regurgitation	Increased EF*; relaxation usually normal	1-2/6 M; S_2 normal; no signs of obstruction
Nonobstructive HCM	No pressure gradient	Mild or No SAM; LAE rare; no AVN; moderately extensive hypertrophy	No gradient; no significant mitral regurgitation	Increased EF*; impaired relaxation	0–1/6 M; S_2 normal; no signs of obstructin

SAM = Systolic anterior motion of anterior (or posterior) mitral leaflet(s)
LAE = Left atrial enlargement
AVN = Aortic valve notch
EF = Ejection fraction
* = Ejection fraction may occasionally be reduced
M = Murmur
S_2 = Second heart sound
ML–SC = Mitral leaflet-septal contact

rare minor subgroups, i.e., patients with labile or midventricular obstruction. Patients with labile obstruction, in which the MSS appears to come and go for no apparent reason, are managed in the same manner as those with resting obstruction. Midventricular obstruction (at the level of the papillary muscles) is rare and will not be discussed further.

PATIENT INVESTIGATION

All patients with HCM should undergo a careful history and physical examination. Laboratory investigations should include an electrocardiogram (ECG), chest film, and one- and two-dimensional echocardiographic examinations.

Patients with resting obstruction have a significantly greater incidence of angina, dyspnea, and presyncope-syncope, than do patients with latent or no obstruction, as well as a significantly louder apical systolic murmur (due to the outflow obstruction and mitral regurgitation) and reversed splitting of the second heart sound. These patients may have other characteristic findings that reflect resting outflow tract obstruction, e.g., a mitral leaflet-septal contact sound, a double systolic or triple apical impulse, and a spike and dome arterial pulse (Table 1).

Echocardiographic examination of patients with resting obstruction reveals severe systolic anterior motion (SAM) of the mitral leaflet(s) with prolonged mitral leaflet-septal contact, aortic valve notching, left atrial enlargement due to mitral regurgitation and impaired relaxation, a significant degree of septal thickening, and usually an extensive degree of hypertrophy (Table 1). Doppler echocardiography can estimate the magnitude of the subaortic pressure gradient and the degree of mitral regurgitation, whereas nuclear angiography is best for evaluating LV systolic function and impairment of LV relaxation (Table 1). Patients with latent or no obstruction to outflow are usually, but not always, less symptomatic and have less loud apical systolic murmurs and none of the other signs of resting outflow obstruction. In these patients echocardiography does not reveal severe SAM or aortic valve notching, rarely shows left atrial enlargement, and usually reveals the least extensive hypertrophy in latent cases, in which septal thickening is frequently restricted to the subaortic area (Table 1). The limited degree of hypertrophy in these patients explains why they usually do not have problems with diastolic filling.

Ambulatory rhythm monitoring should be carried out in all HCM patients with a history of palpitations and/or presyncope-syncope, in those with resting obstruction, and in all patients with extensive hypertrophy as detected by echocardiography or as reflected by the presence of left ventricular hypertrophy and/or strain on the ECG. We have found that the incidence of atrial and ventricular arrhythmias is greatest in those patients with resting obstruction and extensive hypertrophy.

Hemodynamic and angiographic investigation of patients with HCM should be undertaken: (1) to establish definitively the hemodynamic subgroup when this is in doubt after noninvasive investigation; (2) to test acutely the effect of various pharmacologic agents on the degree of outflow tract obstruction and impairment of relaxation; and (3) for preoperative assessment.

PATIENT MANAGEMENT

Having discussed the mechanism of outflow obstruction, the different hemodynamic subgroups, and the importance of the extent of hypertrophy in determining the presence of arrhythmias and impaired relaxation, the therapeutic principles for the management of patients with HCM can be readily understood (Table 2).

TABLE 2 Treatment of Hypertropic Cardiomyopathy by Hemodynamic Subgroup

Hemodynamic Subgroup	Aim of Therapy	Medical Therapy: Preferred	Medical Therapy: Alternative	Surgery: Preferred	Surgery: Alternative
Resting obstruction	Relief of obstruction to IV outflow (which will also improve relaxation)	Disopyramide*	Calcium antagonists† Beta-adrenergic blocking drugs	Ventriculomyectomy	Mitral valve replacement (only under special circumstances; see text)
Latent obstruction	Prevent provocation of obstruction	Beta-adrenergic blocking drugs	? Calcium antagonists† ? Disopyramide*	Ventriculomyectomy (rarely)	Mitral valve replacement (only under special circumstances; see text)
Nonobstructive HCM	Improve IV relaxation	Calcium antagonists	Beta-adrenergic blocking agents	N/A	N/A

* Disopyramide lessens or abolishes resting obstruction and thereby improves relaxation; in latent obstruction, negative inotropic action of disopyramide could impair relaxation.

† Calcium antagonists (particularly nifedipine but also verapamil) by their vasodilator action can provoke or worsen obstruction to outflow.

Resting Obstruction

Medical treatment of HCM patients with resting obstruction involves the administration of a negative inotropic agent to lessen the velocity of early LV ejection, which reduces the Venturi forces on the mitral leaflets and thus diminishes or abolishes the systolic anterior motion of these leaflets and the accompanying obstruction to outflow and mitral regurgitation (Table 2). In the 1960s and 1970s, we and others used beta-adrenergic blocking agents in the medical therapy of MSS. Employing a dose of propranolol (160 to 240 mg per day) that was sufficient to reduce the resting heart rate to 60 per minute, together with a blunted heart rate response to exercise, as a dosage guide, we found that symptomatic benefit was limited and temporary in patients with moderate-to-severe obstruction to outflow, in whom beta-blockade prevented provocation of obstruction but did not significantly affect the degree of resting obstruction. Patients with mild obstruction and mild symptoms seemed to benefit most from this form of therapy. Propranolol did not reduce the incidence of arrhythmias or sudden death or the need for surgical intervention in those patients with hemodynamically significant obstruction to outflow. As the result of this experience, we no longer use beta-adrenergic blocking agents as primary drug therapy for these patients. Some authors, however, have reported benefit from huge doses of propranolol (500 mg per day or more). Our patient population was unable to tolerate larger doses of propranolol than those administered, without suffering from increased presyncope and/or fatigue.

A number of groups of investigators have reported on the use of calcium antagonists in the therapy of patients with resting obstruction. The negative inotropic effect of these drugs tends to lessen the outflow obstruction, whereas their vasodilator action has the opposite effect. A lowering of myoplasmic calcium tends to improve LV relaxation. It is our belief that nifedipine should not be used in patients with resting obstruction because of its potent vasodilator properties, which would worsen the outflow obstruction. Verapamil has been widely used and generally lessens the degree of outflow obstruction, but occasionally it intensifies it. In as many as 10 percent of patients with resting obstruction, verapamil will unpredictably result in pulmonary edema and in some, this is associated with cardiogenic shock and death. Considerable caution must therefore be used in administering verapamil to patients with resting obstruction and elevated ventricular filling pressures. Verapamil may also result in significant impairment of sinus and AV nodal function.

As a result of the foregoing considerations, we currently favor the use of the negative inotropic and antiarrhythmic agent, disopyramide in the medical management of HCM patients with resting obstruction. Its effectiveness can be tested acutely in the heart catheterization laboratory by administering it intravenously at the rate of 10 mg per minute to a total dose of 100 to 150 mg, while studying its effect on the pressure gradient. Acute administration of disopyramide usually results in marked amelioration or abolition of the subaortic stenosis and mitral regurgitation, together with a lessening of left ventricular end-diastolic pressure and ejection time and an increase in cardiac output.

Subsequently or alternatively, disopyramide may be administered orally, beginning with a dose of 100 mg 4 times daily while observing the loudness of the apical systolic murmur, the degree of systolic anterior motion on echocardiography, and/or the Doppler estimated gradient as evidence of pharmacologic effect. Each dose is increased by 50 mg every 24 hours until the patient is receiving 200 mg 4 times daily. At each dose level, the ECG QT interval is checked, and inquiry made regarding the drug's atropine-like side effects (blurred vision, dry mouth, and difficulty in micturition). Long-term dosage is usually 200 mg 4 times daily but may be less, depending on the side effects. Long-term patient response can be determined by repeated exercise testing, assessment of symptoms and the loudness of the apical systolic murmur, or by echocardiographic and/or Doppler assessment of the degree of obstruction to outflow. After treating about 40 patients in this manner, we have the impression that it is most effective in those with a mild-to-moderate degree of subaortic stenosis. Patients with severe obstruction to outflow may temporarily benefit, but usually they require surgical management within 2 to 3 years or less. Disopyramide has the advantage over other negative inotropic agents because of its antiarrhythmic action and has proved to be effective in suppressing both atrial and ventricular arrhythmias in patients with resting obstruction. A potential adverse effect of disopyramide is that it may impair LV relaxation directly by its negative inotropic action. However, an improvement in relaxation results from the relief of the obstruction to outflow, and this effect appears to be dominant.

There is the potential of using a combination of negative inotropic agents in HCM patients with resting obstruction. We have utilized a combination of disopyramide and beta-adrenergic blocking agents in treating a few patients, whereas others have used a combination of beta- and calcium-channel blocking agents. Such combinations, particularly if used in addition to antiarrhythmic agents, have the potential of further impairing LV relaxation and causing heart failure. We would use double or triple negative inotropic therapy only in extenuating circumstances and only if the patient was not a surgical candidate.

Patients who do not respond favorably to acute and/or chronic administration of medical therapy and/or who are intolerant of their physical limitations are advised to undergo the ventriculomyectomy operation. The mechanisms by which this form of surgery has such dramatic effects in patients with MSS is outlined in Figure 2. By decreasing septal thickness, the ventriculomyectomy increases the size of the left ventricular outflow tract (LVOT) and results in the early systolic ejection path being displaced away from the mitral leaflets, thus reducing or abolishing the Venturi forces on these leaflets. This action results in the abolition of the mitral leaflet systolic anterior motion (SAM) as a result of which the obstruction to outflow and mitral regurgitation is abolished. The abolition of the obstruction normalizes aortic flow, the result of which is that the spike and dome aortic flow and

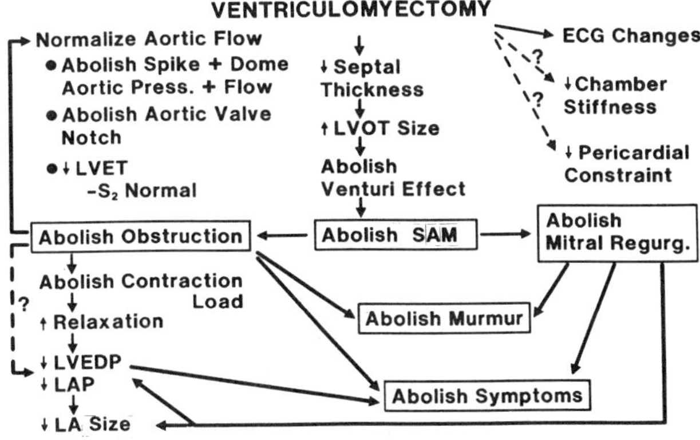

Figure 2 Proposed mechanism(s) by which the ventriculomyectomy operation affects the hemodynamic and clinical findings in HCM patients with resting obstruction (muscular subaortic stenosis) (see text).

pressure profiles and aortic valve notch are abolished. Left ventricular ejection time (LVET) is no longer prolonged, and splitting of the second heart sound (S2) becomes normal. The abolition of the obstruction abolishes the early systolic contraction load on the left ventricle, which results in improved LV relaxation and a reduction in LV end-diastolic (LVEDP) and left atrial pressures (LAP). The abolition of the obstruction, together with the lowering of LVEDP, should also improve relaxation by increasing the hemodynamic coronary filling load that is applied to the relaxing myocardium. Abolition of the mitral regurgitation would also decrease LVEDP and LAP as well as LA size, thus rendering the patient less liable to atrial arrhythmias. The abolition of the apical systolic murmur results from the abolition of obstruction and mitral regurgitation, while these latter two factors plus the lowering of LVEDP and LAP result in a lessening or abolition of the patient's symptoms. It is not known whether a decrease in chamber stiffness or in the degree of pericardial constraint might also favor symptomatic benefit following ventriculomyectomy. There is evidence that surgically induced ventricular conduction defects do not explain the beneficial effects of this surgical procedure.

In our experience, a successful ventriculomyectomy is far more effective in abolishing the pathophysiologic features as well as the symptoms and signs of resting obstruction than is any form of medical therapy. Approximately 120 of our patients have undergone this operation with a mortality rate of less than 4 percent, and there were no deaths in the last 40 operations. Completely successful surgery brings about a truly dramatic change in a patient's lifestyle. Even partially successful surgical treatment results in significant benefit, in that pharmacologic therapy is then more effective. We clearly indicate to these patients, however, that the operation is for the relief of the obstruction to outflow and does not affect the underlying heart muscle abnormality. It is preferable that this form of surgery be carried out in centers that are experienced in doing it. Patients who have structural mitral valve abnormalities and significant mitral regurgitation or who have outflow obstruction in the absence of a greatly thickened septum are candidates for mitral valve replacement.

Latent Obstruction

The great majority of patients with latent obstruction to outflow have only limited hypertrophy and therefore are not troubled with problems of impaired relaxation or significant arrhythmias. However, the limited degree of septal hypertrophy is located in the subaortic area, and therefore they have the potential of developing obstruction to outflow with suitable provocation. For 20 years we have managed these patients with beta-adrenergic blocking agents to prevent provocation of the obstruction by adrenergic stimuli. This form of therapy in about 70 patients has resulted in significant symptomatic benefit so that we rarely have advised surgery for these patients, nor have we felt the need to try disopyramide or calcium-channel blocking agents in this hemodynamic subgroup. Disopyramide has the disadvantage of impairing relaxation in these patients, whereas the vasodilator action of the calcium antagonists (particularly nifedipine) has the unwanted potential of provoking obstruction to outflow.

Nonobstructive Hypertrophic Cardiomyopathy

The calcium antagonists (verapamil, nifedipine, and diltiazem) represent the preferred line of therapy for HCM patients without obstruction to outflow. Lowering of myoplasmic calcium should improve LV relaxation, while vasodilatation should improve LV systolic function (when it is impaired) by means of afterload reduction. The negative inotropic effect of these drugs can depress LV systolic function, and this action can trigger heart failure in these patients if systolic function is impaired to begin with. The latter has been reported with both nifedipine and verapamil. In spite of this potential danger, the use of these agents is clearly the therapy of choice in symptomatic patients with nonobstructive HCM. All three agents improve the indices of LV relaxation and result in symptomatic improvement in these patients. Verapamil has been used most extensively for this purpose in doses varying from 240 to 480 mg per day in 3 divided doses. We have used nifedipine in doses of 40 to 80 mg a day and found significant symptomatic improvement in 50 percent of cases, but a significant percentage of these patients complained of flushing, dizziness, headache, and postural hypotension, which limited the usefulness of the drug. Long-acting forms of nifedipine may circumvent these problems. We have not used diltiazem chronically in these patients, but others have. At present, we use verapamil in preference to nifedipine but only because of the frequency of the side effects to the latter in this patient population.

MANAGEMENT OF ARRHYTHMIAS

Both atrial and ventricular arrhythmias are a significantly greater problem in HCM patients with resting obstruction than in those with latent or no obstruction. Atrial fibrillation in HCM patients is almost invariably associated with left atrial enlargement, which is the rule with resting obstruction (due to the concomitant mitral regurgitation) and is rare in the other hemodynamic subgroups.

Atrial arrhythmias in HCM result in dramatic hemodynamic and clinical deterioration as the result of loss of atrial transport function; everything possible must be done to restore sinus rhythm. Recurrent or established atrial fibrillation in patients with resting obstruction is an indication for surgical intervention, which will result in a decrease in left atrial size and restoration of normal sinus rhythm in patients younger than age 40 to 45 years. Successful surgery does not usually decrease atrial size or restore sinus rhythm in older patients with large left atria, but postoperatively they are better able to tolerate the lack of atrial transport function. Patients with chronic or recurrent atrial fibrillation require long-term anticoagulant therapy because of the risk of systemic emboli.

First-line drug therapy for atrial arrhythmias in HCM consists of the use of quinidine, procainamide and disopyramide, preferably in their long-acting formulations. Although some authors favor amiodarone, we reserve its use for both older patients and those who do not respond to either type 1 antiarrhythmics or surgical intervention.

The increased incidence of ventricular arrhythmias in patients with obstruction at rest is believed to be due to the more extensive hypertrophy as well as to the obstruction itself. In our experience, type 1 antiarrhythmics usually control the malignant ventricular arrhythmias in HCM but if they do not, we utilize amiodarone. It is of interest that some investigators have reported that patients with HCM showed symptomatic improvement while taking amiodarone. The mechanism of this clinical improvement, unrelated to the antiarrhythmic action of the drug, is unknown in that it has been reported with and without alleviation of the obstruction to outflow.

Medical or surgical therapy in HCM is based on the presence or absence of (1) obstruction to left ventricular outflow, (2) impairment of left ventricular relaxation, and (3) atrial and/or ventricular arrhythmias. A rational approach to management based on these principles has been presented. Surgery (ventriculomyectomy) is considerably more effective than currently available medical therapy in alleviating the obstruction to left ventricular outflow and the accompanying mitral regurgitation. Successful surgery can also improve left ventricular relaxation and abolish atrial arrhythmias.

ACUTE AND RECURRENT PERICARDITIS

DAVID H. SPODICK, M.D., D.Sc.

Acute pericarditis presents problems of local disease (mainly symptomatic) when it is part of an acute or chronic generalized syndrome. The latter includes infection, immune processes, systemic diseases, singly or in combination. *Recurrent pericarditis* usually indicates flares of a preexisting condition and only rarely represents reinfection by an organism. Most recurrences of local, originally infective pericardial disease are probably immunopathic.

Treatment aims to (1) conrol symptoms, (2) destroy etiologic agents, (3) suppress inflammation, and (4) manage any systemic disorder.

THERAPEUTIC ALTERNATIVES

The main symptom is pain, usually pleuritic, and very often—especially in recurrent pericarditis—disabling. Anti-inflammatory agents usually control pain as well as inflammation and, if there is an inflammatory systemic disorder, will attack that simultaneously. For the mildest attacks, aspirin (650 mg every 6 hours for 3 or 4 days) will probably suffice. However, there are frequent therapeutic failures with aspirin, and a different nonsteroidal anti-inflammatory agent will be needed. If the patient is not too uncomfortable, increased doses of aspirin may first be used, (e.g., 650 to 975 mg every 4 hours). Nonsteroidal anti-inflammatory agents include ibuprofen, a propionic acid derivative, 400 to 1,000 mg every 6 hours (usually 600 mg per dose); indomethacin, 25 to 50 mg every 8 hours; naproxen, 375 to 500 mg every 12 hours; piroxicam, 20 mg every day; or sulindac, 200 mg every 12 hours. In stubbornly resistant (usually recurrent) cases, phenylbutazone (100 mg every 6 hours) may be tried for 3 or 4 days. All of these agents, particularly phenylbutazone, must be used with a vigilant eye to their gastrointestinal and hematologic effects. Corticosteroid agents, usually prednisone, may be prescribed, usually with success, but *should always be the last resort*, because there is anecdotal evidence that both therapeutic success and failure with corticosteroid agents predispose to recurrent pericarditis as well as to all the side effects of steroid administration.

PREFERRED APPROACH

Therapy should begin immediately, on presentation of the patient, with a nonsteroidal anti-inflammatory medication. Oral therapy is usually quite effective, and in most cases pain is relieved before serum levels peak (usually 2 to 4 hours in this group of agents). (Corticosteroids may be used intravenously or orally.) Side effects are uncommon except in some patients with gastrointestinal intolerance for whom cimetidine or antacids can be prescribed. Usually a 3- to 6-day course of a nonsteroidal anti-inflammatory agent is sufficient. Therapeutic response means absence of symptoms with subsequent return of acute phase reactants (sedimentation rate and white blood cell count) to normal and disappearance of electrocardiographic changes (although inverted T waves may take weeks to disappear and in rare cases may remain indefinitely).

In systemic disorders involving the pericardium (e.g., uremic pericarditis, or lupus pericarditis), there may be an inadequate response. It may be necessary to use corticosteroid therapy for lupus and for uremic patients. For those patients already on dialysis, aggressive maximal dialysis is needed to try to prevent significant pericardial effusion and tamponade. For infectious pericarditis of any kind, specific antimicrobial agents should be added. Most antibiotics appear in excellent concentration in the pericardial fluid despite the inflammation.

RECURRENT ACUTE PERICARDITIS

If, on the one hand, acute pericarditis returns as a flare of an underlying systemic disorder, increased therapy for that disorder is indicated. On the other hand, the most vexing therapeutic problems are in a group of patients almost all of whom have had corticosteroid therapy, either as an initial treatment or as a last resort when other therapy has not been effective (although usually only one agent has been tried). There are two forms: (1) recurrent pericarditis in a patient who can never completely be weaned from a corticosteroid (or, rarely, another agent), or (2) discrete recurrences requiring corticosteroid therapy each time. The latter is considerably less common and less difficult to manage. The approach here is to taper the corticosteroid very slowly. For example, prednisone, if at 60 mg per day, can be tapered to 2.5 mg per day. If this is unsuccessful and there is a threshold below which the patient has recurrence, tapering can be attempted every third or fourth day. This is a trial-and-error method, which occasionally is reduced to 1 mg reductions as infrequently as every week or every 2 weeks. Simultaneously, a nonsteroidal anti-inflammatory agent should be introduced. I favor ibuprofen, 600 mg every 6 hours (begun just before, or concomitantly with, tapering).

Occasionally, while waiting for therapy to take effect in a patient with either new pericarditis or recurrent pericarditis, you can give him Sir William Osler's treatment—an icebag on the precordium (not for coronary patients)—or, alternatively, a hot-water bottle.

SURGICAL CONSIDERATIONS

Surgery of the pericardium is usually reserved for resistent cardiac tamponade, wounds, or constrictive pericarditis. However, pericardiectomy has been resorted to in desperation for patients who were resistant to nonsurgical management or who had unacceptable side effects of, usually corticosteroid, therapy. In my experience, surgery is likely to be ineffective in that the recurrences will begin either immediately after or weeks to months after the operation, and many patients must resume some form of medical therapy. Occasionally, however, individuals seem to respond. The reason for the ineffectiveness of surgery is probably that most of the pericardium cannot be resected: posteriorly, it is closely applied to the left atrium; pericardial prolongations go over the aortic arch; and the phrenic nerves lie on the pericardium so that after any pericardiectomy, two "tapes" of pericardium are left to support them.

CARDIAC TAMPONADE

RALPH SHABETAI, M.D.

In the final analysis, the treatment of cardiac tamponade hinges on removing the offending fluid from the pericardial sac. However, as for all therapeutic decisions, this central truth must be modified according to clinical circumstances. Except in the direst of emergencies, pericardiocentesis mut not be attempted without first determining the amount and location of pericardial fluid. In some cases, tamponade is mild, caused by a readily reversible condition, such as acute pericarditis; it may resolve with anti-inflammatory treatment and not require pericardiocentesis. At the other extreme, the wise and compassionate physician, who has a patient with widespread neoplasm in whom tamponade is a terminal event, may elect not to treat it.

ACUTE SEVERE (SURGICAL) FORM

This is the classic cardiac tamponade characterized by raised venous pressure, hypotension, pulsus paradoxus, and a small quiet heart. Commonly, the patients are victims of blunt or sharp chest trauma. In extreme cases, consciousness may be lost or impaired and hypotension may be so severe that blood pressure and the pulsus paradoxus cannot be ascertained. These are the circumstances under which it is fully justified, indeed mandatory, to explore the pericardial sac with a needle without waiting for confirmatory evidence of cardiac tamponade. The pericardium is highly resistant to rapid stretching; this is why severe cardiac tamponade can occur rapidly and be produced by a relatively small volume of fluid under these circumstances. Furthermore, when the pericardium is rapidly expanded, its pressure-volume relation is steep, and removal of a small quantity of the tamponading fluid causes both a sharp drop in a pericardial pressure and dramatic relief of symptoms and signs. Although it is true that hemorrhagic pericardial fluid does not clot, blood rapidly accumulating in the pericardium clots rapidly; furthermore, its hematocrit is close to that of simultaneously obtained venous blood samples.

The emergency treatment of cardiac tamponade by pericardiocentesis is not definitive. As soon as the patient's condition sufficiently improves, full cardiovascular evaluation, including echocardiography and at least the determination of central venous pressure, must be carried out. This examination is followed by definitive drainage, usually by surgical exploration, at which time the source of intrapericardial bleeding when found is repaired. In a small but significant proportion of cases, there is accompanying cardiovascular trauma, such as rupture of the chordae tendineae of the mitral or tricuspid valve; or rupture of the aortic valve, the aorta, or a cardiac chamber. Persistently elevated central venous pressure after complete drainage of the pericardium is a strong clue to complicating cardiac trauma. When such trauma is found, surgical treatment often is indicated. Some patients with traumatic hemopericardium also suffer myocardial contusion; this abnormality must be treated essentially as an acute myocardial infarction (MI).

CARDIAC TAMPONADE AS A MEDICAL EMERGENCY

Hyperacute hemopericardium with severe cardiac tamponade may occur in medical patients as when myocardial infarction, dissecting hematoma of the aorta, or aortic aneurysm ruptures into the pericardium. This development produces a clinical picture comparable to that of acute surgical cardiac tamponade, except that the physical findings of cardiac tamponade are usually obscured by those of preexisting heart disease, including cardiogenic shock or congestive heart failure. Those abnormalities complicate the interpretation of hypotension, the absence of pulsus paradoxus, and the analysis of the jugular venous pressure. In this setting, pericardiocentesis, performed when necessary without first documenting pericardial fluid, seldom produces satisfactory results because most of the patients die from underlying cardiac condition.

CARDIAC TAMPONADE IN MEDICAL PATIENTS

Cardiac tamponade may occur under various nonsurgical conditions. Pericardial effusion complicates several common medical conditions. When one of them is present and the patient exhibits cardiovascular deterioration, cardiac tamponade should be considered. The conditions include not only neoplasm particularly of the breast and lung, but also lymphoma, chronic dialysis, mediastinal radiation, and some instances of acute, idiopathic, or viral pericarditis. Tuberculosis and histoplasmosis are now much less common. Cardiac tamponade can complicate many other illnesses, but the ones just cited represent most of the conditions encountered in medical patients. When cardiac tamponade is severe, the venous pressure is elevated. Careful inspection of the neck veins shows that the venous pressure declines slightly during inspiration; the predominant pulsation is the *x* descent, whereas the *y* descent is greatly attenuated or absent. Pulsus paradoxus is usually present, although blood pressure most often is normal. In contrast to surgical tamponade, the heart is not necessarily small, and the cardiac impulse is often palpable.

The physical findings of pericardial effusion are so insensitive and so nonspecific as hardly to be worth describing. On the other hand, there may be clincial evidence of pericarditis, such as pericardial pain and friction rub; the electrocardiogram may show the characteristic diffuse ST–segment elevation and, sometimes, PR-segment depression. If an earlier x-ray film of the chest is available, another taken at the time of the illness usually shows considerable increase in the cardiac silhouette, which may have a globular configuration, characteristically with unexpectedly clear lung fields.

Before embarking on pericardiocentesis to relieve

cardiac tamponade under these circumstances, the clinician must establish the diagnosis of pericardial effusion, preferably by echocardiography. The M-mode study should show at least a moderate pericardial effusion. One can be reasonably confident of success at pericardiocentesis if the echo-free space between the pericardium and heart is 1 cm or more by M-mode study, particularly if fluid is also visible anterior to the right ventricle.

In addition to proving the presence of intrapericardial fluid, the echocardiogram may show specific findings related to cardiac tamponade. The most important of them are right atrial compression and diastolic collapse of the right ventricle. In the severest cases, a rocking motion of the heart can be identified and is often associated with electrical alternans.

The next step is relief of cardiac tamponade by removal of intrapericardial fluid. The decision must be made whether to do this by pericardiocentesis or by open surgical drainage. To a great extent, the choice is a matter of local preference and circumstances. Pericardiocentesis is cheaper, quicker, and less traumatic and allows accurate determination of hemodynamics in the cardiac catheterization laboratory. Open surgical drainage has the advantages that adequate biopsy can be obtained; and the procedure is peformed under direct vision and to that extent is safer. Often a subxiphoid drainage suffices; when necessary, the procedure can be carried out under local anesthesia.

Pericardiocentesis

Except in emergencies, pericardiocentesis should be performed in the cardiac catheterization laboratory, or at any rate in a facility equipped with electrocardiographic, pressure, and radiographic monitoring devices. The safety of pericardiocentesis has been enhanced by the introduction of two-dimensional echocardiography. It enables the operator to locate where the effusion is closest to the skin and thus to select the easiest and most profitable entry site. Before starting pericardiocentesis, the operator should place a catheter in the right atrium for continuous pressure monitoring. An intra-arterial needle or catheter should also be placed; arterial pressure is then monitored throughout the procedure. The pericardium is penetrated by a sharp, short-beveled needle attached to an electrocardiograph; to detect ST–segment elevation if the needle touches the epicardium, an event usually accompanied by ventricular extrasystole. When the needle lies freely in the pericardium, the operator replaces it with a soft catheter, using the Seldinger technique and fluoroscopy. Correct positioning of the needle or catheter is ascertained by the location, pressure wave form, and nature of the aspirate; it can be confirmed by injecting a small amount of contrast agent, which pools in the pericardial space and does not circulate. Pericardial pressure should then be measured and compared with right atrial pressure.

If the diagnosis of tamponade is correct, the right atrial and intrapericardial pressures should be equal, the latter should show absence of *x* descent, and both should decline during inspiration. Pericardial fluid is then aspirated, samples being taken for analysis. As this is done, the patient should be observed for progressive increase in blood pressure and cardiac output, together with disappearance of pulsus paradoxus and decline of atrial and intrapericardial pressures. When complications are absent, right atrial pressure returns to normal and intrapericardial pressure falls considerably below right atrial pressure. If the right atrial pressure remains abnormal in magnitude or wave-form, consider complicating cardiac disease or effusive-constrictive pericarditis.

LOW-PRESSURE CARDIAC TAMPONADE

Severe cardiac tamponade is associated with increases in intrapericardial pressure from the normal subatmospheric level to values in the range of 15 to 25 mm Hg or more. Circulation can be maintained only by equal elevation of the central venous pressure. If intrapericardial pressure rises to a level that the venous pressure cannot attain, circulation ceases. Consequently, severe cardiac tamponade is associated with high central venous pressure. However, cardiac tamponade is not an all-or-nothing phenomenon; it may develop when the central venous pressure is only slightly elevated, for example from 7 to 10 mm Hg. This phenomenon may either represent mild cardiac tamponade, or develop in the early stages of a more slowly developing severe cardiac tamponade, or be attributable to heavy diuresis or major blood loss from another site. Critical to detecting low-pressure cardiac tamponade is recognizing a slightly increased venous pressure with a prominent *x* descent, although in these low-pressure cases, the *y* descent may partially persist. Often, intrapericardial pressure is not high enough to generate pulsus paradoxus; certainly, the blood pressure is usually normal. The diagnosis is suspected when modest elevation of central venous pressure appears in a patient with an underlying condition that may affect the pericardium. This development should signal the need for an echocardiogram to confirm pericardial effusion. Right atrial compression and right ventricular diastolic collapse may be found, even though pulsus paradoxus is absent.

It is important to recognize low-pressure cardiac tamponade because it may deteriorate into more severe tamponade. However, it is not always necessary to drain pericardial fluid. For instance, when low-pressure cardiac tamponade develops in a patient undergoing hemodialysis, the patient should be carefully observed to see whether increased frequency of dialysis removes pericardial fluid and abolishes cardiac tamponade. Similarly, when this situation develops in acute pericarditis, the patient can be carefully followed while receiving anti-inflammatory treatment, which may resolve the pericarditis and obviate the need for pericardial drainage. Evidence of progression is usually an indication to drain even low-level cardiac tamponade. When pressure measurements are carried out, even in these low-pressure cases, pericardial and right atrial pressures are equal, although considerably lower than in classic cardiac tamponade; sometimes, they are less than pulmonary wedge pressure.

EFFUSIVE CONSTRICTIVE PERICARDITIS

One of the arguments for pericardiocentesis over open surgical drainage is that recognizing the hemodynamics of effusive constrictive pericarditis is easier in the cardiac catheterization laboratory than it is when pressure measurements are attempted in the operating room. Effusive constrictive pericarditis occurs when the pericardium is thickened; it can constrict the heart when pericardial fluid is still present. The condition is found in both neoplastic and postradiation pericardial disease and in the subacute state of tuberculous pericarditis. The presentation is usually that of cardiac tamponade. However, following pericardiocentesis, the right atrial pressure fails to normalize. Instead, it remains variably elevated and shows absence of respiratory variation and a prominent *y* descent. Many of the patients require subsequent pericardiectomy.

CHRONIC RENAL DISEASE

Disagreement is still considerable regarding the best approach to cardiac tamponade that occurs during chronic dialysis. Early low-pressure cardiac tamponade can be managed by increasing the frequency of dialysis. Satisfactory response is judged by a drop in the level of venous pressure with reestablishment of a *y* descent and disappearance of pericardial fluid as viewed on the echocardiogram. More severe cardiac tamponade requires fluid drainage. In many centers, this is done by pericardiocentesis, at least for an initial event. In other centers, even the first episode of significant cardiac tamponade is regarded as an indication for surgical drainage. Most authorities agree that recurrent cardiac tamponade in a patient undergoing dialysis should be managed by both open surgical drainage and the removal of a portion of pericardium, usually by the subxiphoid route. When pericardiocentesis is used, it can be followed by instilling nonabsorbable steroid, such as triamcinolone, into the pericadial space. Diagnosis can be particularly difficult because (1) pulsus paradoxus may be absent despite severe cardiac tamponade, (2) cardiac enlargement may be due to heart failure or fluid overload, and (3) raised venous pressure may be due to overhydration.

NEOPLASTIC DISEASE

The guiding principle in treating cardiac tamponade in most patients with malignant pericardial effusion is to manage it as conservatively as possible. This means that whenever possible pericardiocentesis rather than open surgical drainage should be used. But when the latter is required, it should be done, when feasible, from a subxiphoid approach. Recurrence of pericardial effusion with tamponade can be delayed or even prevented by instilling a sclerosing agent, such as tetracycline, into the pericardial space.

ENDOCARDITIS CAUSED BY GRAM-POSITIVE ORGANISMS

STEVEN G. ALSIP, M.D.
C. GLENN COBBS, M.D.

Gram-positive bacteria are a major cause of infective endocarditis (IE); overall, 75 percent of patients with this disorder have a gram-positive microorganism identified as the etiologic agent. However, compared to the preantibiotic era, the relative number of cases caused by different varieties of gram-positive bacteria has changed. Viridans streptococci, responsible for over one-half of the cases of IE in early series, are now responsible only 30 to 40 percent of the time, whereas other streptococci and staphylococci have assumed more importance, especially in patients with prosthetic heart valves and in intravenous (IV) drug abusers.

GENERAL THERAPEUTIC CONSIDERATIONS

The diagnosis of IE is suggested in several clinical situations. In patients with known valvular heart disease, the new onset of fever, emboli, and cutaneous manifestations of immune injury are highly suggestive of that diagnosis. In the addict who injects drugs by the intravenous route, fever and bacteremia, especially if caused by *Staphylococcus aureus*, are very likely to represent IE even in the absence of a heart murmur reflecting right-sided cardiac disease. In other patients, persistent bacteremia may reflect endocardial infection even if there is no evidence of prior valve disease.

In any case, following the initial evaluation of a patient with suspected IE, the diagnosis may be either very likely or only possible. In the first instance, it is reasonable to obtain three to four blood cultures drawn by separate venipunctures over several hours and then initiate antimicrobial therapy. Table 1 summarizes guidelines for choice of initial antibacterial agents. In general, one should choose therapy directed against the most resistant streptococcus (the enterococcus) and add antistaphylococcal therapy if there is a history of narcotic addiction, if the patient is postcardiovascular surgery, or if the patient's illness is following a fulminant clinical course. In other patients in whom the diagnosis of IE is possible and who are not critically ill, it is reasonable to obtain blood cultures as just described and observe. The demonstration of bacteremia in a patient with ''possible'' IE is obviously sufficient cause to justify initiation of antimicrobial therapy directed against the specific microorganism isolated

TABLE 1 Empiric Antimicrobial Therapy

Treat for enterococcal endocarditis:
penicillin G, 18–24 million units per day, plus gentamicin, 1 mg/kg q8h* (vancomycin, 500 mg q6h* if penicillin-allergic)

Except:

In narcotic addicts	Add antistaphylococcal therapy; nafcillin, 9–12 g per day
Following cardiac surgery	
Acute fulminant course	

*If renal function is normal.

TABLE 2 Indications for Valve Replacement in Gram-Positive Native Valve Endocarditis

Absolute:
- Moderate or severe heart failure
- Uncontrolled infection

Relative:
- Mild heart failure
- Emboli
- Myocardial abscess
- Organism other than sensitive *streptococcus*

from blood. In 95 percent of previously untreated patients, the initial blood cultures will be positive, allowing the clinician to switch to specific antimicrobial therapy guided by in vitro sensitivity data.

A number of laboratory tests for monitoring the response to therapy are available to supplement the physician's clinical assessment. Follow-up blood cultures, preferably utilizing technology to neutralize the effects of administered antibiotics, should be obtained every day or two until the bacteremia has cleared, and then weekly for four times after therapy to detect relapse. Persistently positive blood cultures during presumed adequate antimicrobial therapy signal both the failure of therapy and the need for a change in antibiotic regimen and/or surgical debridement and valve replacement. Determination of serum bactericidal activity (the Schlichter test) may be used to assess the effectiveness of antibacterial therapy. Killing the causative organism by serum diluted 1:8 or greater has generally been accepted as a suitable level of activity, although definitive data addressing the implications and applications of the test are scanty.

At present, the major cause of death in patients with IE is congestive heart failure (CHF). In patients who are hemodynamically unstable, close monitoring in an intensive care unit is necessary. Appropriate support with pressors, diuretics, and vasodilators, as well as careful attention to fluid balance, is crucial to the patient's survival. Cardiac complications, such as progressive valvular insufficiency, embolic myocardial infarction, myocardial abscess causing conduction defects, pericarditis, and, in the case of prosthetic valve endocarditis (PVE), valve dehiscence or obstruction should be searched for with careful daily physical examination as well as with cardiac monitoring and periodic electrocardiographic testing.

In certain patients, cardiac surgery will be necessary during active infection (Table 2). The most common indication for operative intervention is heart failure. The development of heart failure during IE is clearly associated with increased mortality. Cardiac surgery also carries a greater risk as a patient's heart failure worsens. However, in a study that compared medical and medical plus surgical therapy during IE, members of the group who did not receive indicated surgery had a mortality rate of 51 percent compared to 9 percent in those who underwent cardiac surgery. In a large group of patients undergoing valve replacement at this institution for all indications, the 6-month mortality for those patients in NYHA class I was 1.4 percent compared to 8.9 percent if in NYHA class IV heart failure. The risk of subsequent PVE following replacement of an infected native valve in the face of active infection is small, about 2 percent. Thus, valve replacement is life saving and should be undertaken as soon as moderate or severe heart failure develops.

The other absolute indication for urgent valve replacement is persistent valvular infection, manifested by bacteremia and other signs of toxicity in the absence of metastatic abscess. Relative indications for surgery include mild heart failure, one or more systemic emboli, valvular vegetation on echocardiographic examination, a relatively resistant causative organism, and a myocardial abscess. Although clear guidelines concerning the timing of surgery in the presence of one or more relative indications are not available, in general the development of any of these complications in a patient likely to require valve replacement or the presence of multiple relative indications for valve replacement should lead to early surgery.

Noncardiac complications of endocarditis include glomerulonephritis, mycotic aneurysms and other embolic phenomena, and metastatic abscesses. Glomerulonephritis associated with IE is secondary to immune injury and generally improves with appropriate antimicrobial therapy. Rarely is aggressive therapy, such as dialysis, required. Management of mycotic aneurysms depends on their location. Intracerebral aneurysms may cause severe morbidity or mortality, primarily by leaking or rupturing. Optimal therapy of a large, enlarging, or leaking mycotic aneurysm is surgical removal, if possible. There have been reports of resolution of stable or inaccessible mycotic aneurysms with medical therapy alone. Intra-abdominal mycotic aneurysms are often difficult to detect until they leak or rupture.

Larger emboli are commonly distributed to the extremities, the renal bed, and the brain. In the latter case, major morbidity can occur. Management is supportive except when a large embolus to a peripheral artery can be removed. Anticoagulation in native valve endocarditis (NVE) is not indicated due to a higher incidence of hemorrhagic sequelae associated with emboli. In PVE, therapeutic anticoagulation should be maintained. If emboli occur, most authorities withhold anticoagulation for 3 days and then resume it if there is no evidence of hemorrhage.

Virulent organisms, such as *Staphylococcus aureus*,

are more likely to cause metastatic abscesses. Persistent fever or leukocytosis or intermittently positive blood cultures, despite apparently appropriate therapy, should prompt a careful search for metastatic abscesses. Surgical drainage usually results in prompt improvement.

SPECIFIC ANTIMICROBIAL THERAPY

A summary of our recommendations for antimicrobic therapy of IE caused by gram-positive organisms is shown in Table 3. In general, due to the relative ineffectiveness of host defenses in IE, bactericidal agents are necessary. Oral antibiotic therapy rarely produces sufficiently high or sustained blood levels of antibiotics to effectively treat IE. Thus, parenteral administration is necessary except under unusual circumstances.

Streptococci that cause endocarditis can be divided into two groups according to their susceptibility to penicillin. Highly susceptible streptococci, defined by a minimum inhibitory concentration (MIC) to penicillin G of less than 0.2μg per milliliter, are usually members of the viridans group but may also include nonenterococcal group D streptococci as well as anaerobic and microaerophilic species. Native valve endocarditis caused by such bacteria is relatively easily treated by any one of three penicillin-containing regimens listed in the table, all of which produce cure rates of 95 to 98 percent. Four weeks of intravenous penicillin G has been the traditional therapy for such patients and is still the treatment of choice in patients who are prone to suffer from streptomycin tox-

TABLE 3 Antimicrobial Therapy for Gram-Positive Native Valve Endocarditis

Causative Organism	*Regimen of Choice*	*Alternative Regimens*
Streptococci:		
Penicillin-sensitive (MIC≤0.2 μg/ml to penicillin G)	Aqueous penicillin G, 10–20 million units IV (in 4–6 divided doses) daily for 4 weeks or Aqueous penicillin G, (as above) or procaine penicillin G, 1.2 million units IM q6h for 4 weeks plus Streptomycin, 0.5 g IM q12h for 2 weeks or Aqueous penicillin G or procaine penicillin G (as above) daily for 2 weeks plus Streptomycin (as above)	Cephalothin, 2 g IV q4h, or cefazolin, 1 g IV q6h, for 4 weeks or Cephalothin, 2 g IV q4h, or cefazolin, 1 g IV q6h, for 4 weeks plus Streptomycin, 0.5 g IM q12h for 2 weeks or Vancomycin, 0.5 g IV q6h for 4 weeks
Penicillin-resistant (MIC>0.2 μg/ml to penicillin G)	Aqueous penicillin G, 20 million units IV (in 6 divided doses) daily for 6 weeks plus Gentamicin, 1 mg/kg IM or IV q8h for 6 weeks	Vancomycin, 0.5 g IV q6h for 6 weeks or Vancomycin (as above) plus Gentamicin, 1 mg/kg IM or IV q8h for 6 weeks
Staphylococcus aureus:		
Methicillin-sensitive	Nafcillin, 1.5–2 g IV q4h for 6 weeks	Cephalothin, 2 g IV q4h or cefazolin, 1 g IV q6h, for 6 weeks or Vancomycin, 0.5 g IV q6h for 6 weeks
Methicillin-resistant	Vancomycin, 0.5 g IV q6h for 6 weeks	None
Staphylococcus epidermidis:		
Methicillin-sensitive	Nafcillin, 1.5–2 g IV q4h for 6 weeks	Vancomycin, 0.5 g IV q6h or cephalothin, 2 g IV q4h or cefazolin, 1 g IV q6h, for 6 weeks
Methicillin-resistant	Vancomycin, 0.5 g IV q6h for 6 weeks plus Rifampin 0.3 g PO q8h for 6 weeks plus Gentamicin, 1 mg/kg IM or IV q8h for 2 weeks	None
Corynebacterium sp:		
Gentamicin-sensitive (MIC≤4 μg/ml)	Aqueous penicillin G, 20 million units IV (in 6 divided doses) for 4–6 weeks plus Gentamicin, 1 mg/kg IM or IV q8h for 4–6 weeks	Vancomycin, 0.5 g IV q6h for 4–6 weeks
Gentamicin-resistant (MIC>4 μg/ml)	Vancomycin, 0.5 g IV q6h for 4–6 weeks	

icity, such as the elderly and the hearing-impaired, or who have had symptoms for more than 3 months. The 2-week regimen of penicillin and streptomycin is a cost-effective alternative in uncomplicated cases. In patients allergic to penicillin, cephalothin plus streptomycin, or vancomycin alone, can be used.

"Resistant" streptococci, those with an MIC to penicillin higher than 0.2μg per milliliter, are usually enterococci. Disc-susceptibility patterns are unreliable for these isolates and should not be relied upon to guide antimicrobial therapy. Penicillin or ampicillin in high doses plus gentamicin is the treatment of choice. Vancomycin alone or in combination with gentamicin should be used in penicillin-allergic patients. Currently, we favor 6 weeks of combination parenteral antimicrobial therapy for enterococcal endocarditis, although recent data suggest that certain patient subgoups may do well with shorter courses.

Staphylococcus aureus can, on the one hand, cause a fulminant illness with rapid valve destruction and metastatic abscess formation. Involvement of the aortic or mitral valve can lead to rapid hemodynamic deterioration. On the other hand, involvement of the right side of the heart, as is often seen in intravenous drug users, may be manifested primarily by multiple pulmonary abscesses, causing cough and pleuritic chest pain without much in the way of cardiac signs or symptoms. Therapy with a penicillinase-resistant penicillin, such as nafcillin, should be initiated as early as possible. Cephalothin or vancomycin are alternatives in the penicillin-allergic patient, while vancomycin should be used when the isolate is resistant to penicillinase-resistant penicillins (methicillin-resistant). Six weeks of parenteral therapy is the rule, although some drug abusers with right-sided involvement may be cured with shorter parenteral courses followed by oral therapy. Emergent or urgent cardiac surgery for mitral or aortic valve replacement associated with uncontrollable heart failure, for myocardial abscess drainage, or for tricuspid or pulmonic valvulectomy, when infection persists, is frequently necessary in staphylococcal disease.

Staphylococcus epidermidis is more commonly a cause of PVE, but has been observed occasionally in patients with NVE. When the organism is susceptible to penicillin G or to a penicillinase-resistant penicillin, such a drug is the treatment of choice. However, most isolates are methicillin-resistant and require treatment with vancomycin and rifampin for 6 weeks plus gentamicin for the initial 2 weeks of therapy.

Corynebacterium species, commonly known as diphtheroids, rarely if ever cause NVE but may be seen in patients with PVE. The bacteria is fastidious and difficult to grow, making susceptibility testing difficult. When sensitivity to gentamicin can be demonstrated, high-dose penicillin G plus gentamicin is the preferred therapy. When the isolate is gentamicin-resistant or cannnot be tested, vancomycin should be employed.

ENDOCARDITIS CAUSED BY GRAM-NEGATIVE ORGANISMS AND FUNGI

MILAGROS P. REYES, M.D.
A. MARTIN LERNER, M.D.

Aerobic gram-negative organisms are the etiologic agents in 1.3 to 4.8 percent of cases of infective endocarditis seen today. In the 1960s, only 1.7 percent of 452 valvular infections were caused by these gram-negative organisms. However, more recent series report an increased incidence of 7 percent. Fungi comprise 2 to 4 percent of all causative agents of infective endocarditis. The overall occurrence is increasing owing to the practice of intravenous drug abuse and the increasing use of prosthetic valve replacements in cardiac surgery. Gram-negative bacillary endocarditis and fungal endocarditis will be discussed separately.

GRAM-NEGATIVE ENDOCARDITIS

Etiologic Agents

Enterobacteriaceae. Although they are relatively common causes of bacteremia, these bacilli are uncommon causes of infective endocarditis. In early reports, *Salmonella* species were most common. The majority of cases were due to *S. choleraesuis, S. typhimurium, and S. enteritidis*. Salmonellae have an affinity for abnormal heart valves, usually on the left side of the heart. Valvular perforation and/or destruction, atrial thrombi, myocarditis, and pericarditis were common complications. The outlook for the affected patient is poor. In a review of forty-four cases of endocarditis due to enterobacteriaceae the following organisms were identified: *Escherichia coli*-17; *Citrobacter* sp.-1; *Klebsiella-Enterobacter* sp.-9; *Serratia marcescens*-13; *Proteus* sp.-2; and *Providencia* sp.-2. In narcotic addicts from San Francisco, *Serratia marcescens* has also caused endocarditis. All of these patients had previously normal valves and the majority of infections were on the aortic or mitral valves. Large vegetations were common, and occlusion of the valve orifice without underlying valvular destruction occurred. Medical therapy alone usually is not sufficient and the mortality rate is high.

Pseudomonas aeruginosa. Infective endocarditis due to *Pseudomonas aeruginosa* appeared in Detroit in 1969. Patients with *Pseudomonas* endocarditis are, characacteristically, young black men with a mean age of 29 years who are intravenous drug users. Underlying heart disease is infrequent. The source of this organism is the standing water that contaminates paraphernalia used for illicit injections. Infection of the tricuspid valve is subacute, but involvement of the mitral or aortic valve precipitates more acute disease. Fever is a presenting manifestation of *Pseudomonas* endocarditis; however, it may be absent in some patients with persisting bacteremia. Eighty-seven percent of 37 patients seen by us had a cardiac murmur on admission. Several weeks after admission, every patient had developed a murmur. The tricuspid valve is most commonly affected, but the pulmonic, mitral, or aortic valves, as well as the atrium, may be involved. In patients with tricuspid disease, repetitive septic pulmonary emboli produce cough, hemoptysis, sputum, pleuritic chest pain, pulmonary infiltrates (sometimes with abscesses), and pleural effusions.

In left-sided *Pseudomonas* endocarditis, intractable heart failure and large, systemic arterial emboli are seen. Cerebritis, brain abscess, and mycotic aneurysms occur. Splenomegaly with septic infarcts and frank abscesses may be present.

Most valvular infections are due to a single pseudomonad immunotype, but 20 percent of the cases are mixed, either with two types of pseudomonads or a single *Pseudomonas* immunotype with *Staphylococcus aureus* or viridans streptococci. Mortality remains high despite optimal use of available antibacterial agents. Delay in initiation of drug therapy, age over 30 years, the presence of left-sided disease, mural vegetations, and mixed infection involving *Pseudomonas aeruginosa* and *S. aureus* are deterrents to medical cure.

Other Gram-Negative Bacteria. *Haemophilus* species, predominantly *H. paraphrophilus, H. parainfluenzae*, and *H. aphrophilus*, account for 0.8 to 1.3 percent of all cases of infective endocarditis. This disease usually occurs in the presence of preexisting valvular disease and runs a subacute course. Major central nervous system complications and emboli to peripheral arteries are relatively frequent.

Actinobacillus actinomycetemcomitans, an organism closely related to *Haemophilus* sp., is a rare cause of subacute endocarditis. The mortality rate is 34 percent. Endocarditis due to *Cardiobacterium hominis* closely resembles the endocarditis due to *Haemophilus* sp.

Neisseria gonorrhoeae is now rarely implicated as a cause of infective endocarditis. Endocarditis due to *N. gonorrhoeae* is typically characterized by a double-quotidian fever pattern and involvement of the right side of the heart in half of cases. Nonpathogenic *Neisseria* sp. (*N. perflava, N. flava, N. pharyngis, N. mucosa,* and especially *Branhamella catarrhalis*) are now isolated more frequently than gonococci in cases of infective endocarditis. These newly recognized organisms usually produce infection on abnormal or prosthetic heart valves.

Diagnosis

Fever, heart murmur, embolic phenomena, and underlying heart disease are the classic signs of infective endocarditis (IE). Even in the absence of underlying heart disease, intravenous drug abuse predisposes to the development of gram-negative and fungal endocarditis. The tricuspid valve is commonly involved, and emboli occur to the pulmonary circulation.

The single most important laboratory test in the diagnostic work-up of IE is the blood culture. The bacteremia is low-grade and persistent. Blood cultures are positive in approximately two-thirds of cases. The first two blood cultures yield the etiologic agent more than 90 percent of the time when bacteremia is present. Prior administration of antibiotics significantly decreases the yield in blood culture isolations.

During the first 24 hours after admission, at least three sets of blood cultures should be obtained. Patients with subacute illnesses, or those who have received antibiotics during the previous 2 weeks and who are not acutely ill, may need two or three sets of blood cultures obtained daily for the next 48 to 72 hours. Five milliliters of blood should be inoculated into both trypticase soy (or brain-heart infusion) and thioglycollate broth. Daily inspection for macroscopic growth should be performed and routine subcultures done on days 1 and 3. Cultures should be held for at least 3 weeks. Positive blood cultures should be saved for special microbiologic studies. In patients with culture-negative endocarditis, routine subculturing onto supplemented chocolate agar or incubation in atmospheres of 5 to 10 percent CO_2 may be necessary for the isolation of fastidious gram-negative organisms such as *Haemophilus* sp., *Actinobacillus* sp. and *Cardiobacterium* sp.

Echocardiography is an adjunctive test in the diagnosis of infective endocarditis. The use of two-dimensional echocardiography has improved the diagnostic accuracy over M-mode methods. Owing to the variable sensitivity for detection of vegetations, a negative study does not exclude endocarditis. False-positives occur, but are rare. Echocardiography may also be useful in localizing vegetations in culture-negative endocarditis, in detecting large friable vegetations, and in assessing the severity of acute aortic insufficiency in cases of active IE. Unfotunately, echocardiography has not been of special value in prosthetic valve endocarditis because of poor resolution around the prosthetic device.

In patients who are candidates for surgery, cardiac catheterization and cineangiography provide valuable hemodynamic and anatomic information. Anemia, elevation of the sedimentation rate, positive rheumatoid factor, and the demonstration of circulating immune complexes also support the diagnosis of IE.

Definitive diagnosis is made only by histopathologic and microbiologic studies of valve tissue obtained either at surgery or at autopsy.

Antimicrobial Therapy

Management of IE due to gram-negative organisms should include careful consideration of the choice of the agent to be used, its dosing, and the duration of administration. Bactericidal agents must be used. Their choice is guided by the minimum inhibitory concentration(s) as well as the minimum bactericidal concentration(s) of the selected antibiotic(s) versus the organism isolated from the patient's blood. The use of at least two agents in combination is necessary for gram-negative endocarditis caused by *Pseudomonas aeruginosa* or members of the family Enterobacteriaceae. Regimens are based on in vitro synergy studies using standard techniques of Mueller-Hinton broth dilutions, microtiter "checkerboards," or time-kill curves. Aminoglycosides are often used, and with these agents, serum concentrations of the antibiotic are done to ensure adequate peak and trough therapeutic levels and to monitor toxicity. Serum bactericidal levels do not predict therapeutic cures in cases of gram-negative, particularly *Pseudomonas*, endocarditis.

For IE due to *E. coli* or *P. mirabilis*, we suggest a combination of ampicillin (2 g IV q4h) with an aminoglycoside, usually gentamicin (1.7 mg per kilogram q8h). For *Klebsiella* endocarditis, we recommend cephalothin and an aminoglycoside (either gentamicin or amikacin). Invariably, replacement of the affected valve is necessary for left-sided endocarditis due to *S. marcescens* since it is refractory to medical therapy alone. The duration of antimicrobial therapy in all cases is at least 6 weeks.

The prognosis in patients with *Pseudomonas* endocarditis has improved with aggressive antibacterial therapy. We recommend a combination of a beta-lactam (preferably ticarcillin) with an aminoglycoside (either gentamicin or tobramycin) at high doses of 8 mg per kilogram per day. We aim for maximum peak concentratins of 12 to 20 μg per milliliter for the aminoglycoside. Treatment should be continued for a minimum of 6 weeks. In this group of young patients, clinically significant ototoxicity is infrequent, and rises in levels of serum creatinine revert to normal after cessation of treatment.

Infective endocarditis due to beta-lactamase-negative *Haemophilus* sp. is usually responsive to ampicillin (2 g q4h) with an aminoglycoside, given for 4 to 6 weeks. For ampicillin-resistant *Haemophilus*, third-generation cephalosporins (e.g., cefotaxime) plus an aminoglycoside are recommended.

We use penicillin, 20 million units IV per day for 4 weeks for gonococcal endocarditis. Again, beta-lactamase-producing strains of *Neisseria gonorrhoeae* should be tested for susceptibility to third-generation cephalosporins such as cefotaxime (Claforan).

Surgical Therapy

The indications for surgical intervention during active gram-negative IE are (1) refractory congestive heart failure, (2) persistent bacteremia with appropriate medical therapy, (3) more than one serious systemic embolic episode suggesting a large vegetation, and (4) local suppurative complications including perivalvular or myocardial abscess with conduction system abnormalities or heart block. Some also consider the presence of a large vegetation by echocardiography a sufficient cause for surgical intervention.

For right-sided *Pseudomonas* endocarditis, if bacteremia persists 2 weeks after initiation of medical therapy, or if bacteremia recurs after cessation of a 6-week course of appropriate antibiotic therapy, we recommend tricuspid valvulectomy without valve replacement. A prosthetic valve is inserted at a second operation 6 to 8 months later if the patient is not an intravenous drug user. After confirmation of the diagnosis of left-sided *Pseudomonas* endocarditis, we recommend immediate valve replacement. In either case, surgery is accompanied by a 6-week course of the high-dose combined drug regimen. All four valves are inspected at surgery because an unsuspected valve(s) may also be affected. Prior to valve replacement we routinely search for splenic abscesses by abdominal computerized tomography. If an abscess is found prior to cardiac surgery, we remove the spleen.

FUNGAL ENDOCARDITIS

Numerous fungi may cause infective endocarditis including *Candida* sp., *Aspergillus, Histoplasma, Coccidioides immitis, Cryptococcus neoformans, Torulopsis glabrata, Phycomyces, Penicillium* sp., *Curvularia geniculata, Phialophora, Rhedotorula, Saccharomyces cerevisiae, Coprinius* sp., and *Paecilomyces varioti*.

Candida endocarditis is the most common type of infective endocarditis caused by fungi. Among 319 reported cases, species of *Candida* were found in 67 percent. *Aspergillus* and *Histoplasma* were the next most frequent. *Candida* endocarditis is common in herion addicts, in patients recovering from cardiovascular surgery, and in others who have been treated with intravenous fluids and broad-spectrum antibiotics for prolonged periods. The most common blood culture isolate among heroin users is *C. parapsilosis*, the next most common being *C. tropicalis*. *Aspergillus* infection often follows prosthetic valve replacement. *C. albicans* is usually isolated following long-term use of intravenous fluids and antibiotics.

Clinical Manifestations

Fever is the major presenting symptom. New or changing murmurs are usually present and indicate valvular insufficiency or stenosis. Myocarditis (characterized by chest pain), unexplained heart failure, conduction disturbances, and arrhythmias are seen. The skin should be inspected for such cutaneous abnormalities as erythematous, generalized maculopapular or macronodular eruptions. Petechiae, Osler's nodes, splinter hemorrhages, and Janeway lesions are frequent. Endophthalmitis may provide the clue that IE is present.

Embolization to a major blood vessel such as a cerebral, femoral, or brachial artery is characteristic of fungal endocarditis. Vegetations are large (2 cm or more); they may be as large as 8 cm. The aortic or mitral valves are commonly involved. At microscopic section, vegetations are masses of fibrin with large fungal colonies in yeast, or hyphal forms, or both. Fungi are seen easily at section with methenamine silver stain.

Diagnosis

Persistent fungemia without a known source establishes the diagnosis of fungal endocarditis. In 50 to 82 percent of cases, blood cultures are positive. Occasionally the diagnosis is difficult because blood cultures are sterile. In these cases, echocardiography may help to establish the diagnosis. Definitive diagnosis is sometimes possible after embolectomy from peripheral vessels and staining with methenamine silver. Cultures of the extracted clot are positive. Exploratory cardiac surgery is necessary at times. The possible value of serologic tests for *Candida* and *Aspergillus* antigens (e.g., mannan) or antibodies (e.g., precipitins) in the diagnosis of fungal endocarditis has not yet been defined.

Therapy

Neither antifungal therapy nor surgery alone is sufficient to cure fungal endocarditis. Prolonged intravenous administration of amphotericin B (minimum total dose of 1 g) plus surgical intervention as *soon* as the diagnosis is made constitute the best mode of treatment. For right-sided endocarditis, valvulectomy without valve replacement is the initial procedure of choice. Valve replacement is done as a second-stage procedure when infection is no longer present. For left-sided involvement, valve replacement with either a natural heterograft valve or prosthetic heart valve is necessary.

Prognosis of fungal endocarditis is bleak. The overall cure rate in cases treated since 1968 is only 14.5 percent. The large, bulky vegetations, the tendency for fungal invasion of the myocardium, poor penetration of antifungal agents into vegetations, and the low therapeutic-toxic ratio of amphotericin B account for the poor prognosis. Drug combinations, such as amphotericin B plus 5-fluorocytosine or amphotericin B plus rifampin, should be studied in vitro as well as in vivo in animal models.

PROSTHETIC VALVE ENDOCARDITIS

ADOLF W. KARCHMER, M.D.

Based upon its frequency and morbidity, prosthetic valve endocarditis (PVE) is an important disease of medical progress. Actuarial analysis of patients undergoing cardiac valve replacement surgery at two major university hospitals indicates that 4 to 5.5 percent of valve recipients are at risk for PVE during the 48 months after surgery. The risk of endocarditis is greatest during the initial year after surgery. Further, the severity of this infection is underscored by the 50 to 65 percent mortality experienced by patients with PVE reported from 1965 through 1975. Only since 1975 has the prognosis for this infection improved.

DIAGNOSIS

Bacteremia that persists for several days or more in the absence of an extracardiac source is the hallmark of PVE, as it is for native valve endocarditis (NVE). Persistent bacteremia occurring in association with clinical evidence of new prosthesis dysfunction, systemic emboli, or immunopathologic signs of endocarditis allows a clinical diagnosis of PVE and mandates therapy. However, not all bacteremias are indicative of PVE, and conversely, not all patients with endocarditis have demonstrable bacteremia; some are culture negative. Patients with an extracardiac infection or an indwelling intravenous line may have a transient bacteremia without infecting their prosthetic valve. Documented transient bacteremias eradicated by a brief course of antibiotics allow this conclusion. Prosthetic valve endocarditis should be suspected when recently developed prosthesis dysfunction or perivalvular disease is noted. Clinical clues to this process include murmurs of prosthesis incompetence or stenosis, cine-fluoroscopic or echocardiographic evidence of excessive prosthesis motion, evidence of prosthesis dysfunction by cardiac catheterization, systemic emboli, and new or progressive atrioventricular or bundle branch electrocardiographic conduction disturbances. When one or more of these clues is noted, four to six blood cultures should be obtained in 24 hours. To design an effective antimicrobial regimen for treating PVE, it is necessary to know the antimicrobial susceptibility of the causative organism. Therefore, it is essential to obtain adequate blood cultures before initiating antimicrobial therapy. Anemia, microscopic hematuria, an elevated sedimentation rate, and an increased concentration of circulating immune complexes support the diagnosis of PVE as they would NVE.

In diagnosing PVE, remember that the time elapsed since valve surgery determines, in part, the conditions that should be considered as alternative diagnoses. Immediately after surgery and for several months thereafter, nosocomial infections, particularly pneumonia, empyema, mediastinal abscess, cryptic sternal wound infection, and sternal osteomyelitis must be considered. In addition, the postpericardiotomy syndrome and cytomegalovirus infection cause fever during this period. Three or more months after surgery the differential diagnosis approaches that which would be considered in regard to NVE.

CLINICAL CONSIDERATIONS

The treatment of PVE is based upon understanding the bacteriology, pathology, and pathophysiology of this entity as well as the requirements for effective antimicrobial therapy of endocarditis in general. A wide range of organisms has caused isolated cases of PVE; nevertheless, the microbiology of this infection is relatively predictable (Table 1). Prior to 1975, *Staphylococcus epidermidis, S. aureus,* enteric and nonfermentative gram-negative bacilli, diphtheroids, and fungi were common causes of PVE occurring within 2 months of surgery. Since 1975, *S. epidermidis* and diphtheroids, particularly the former, have been the predominant pathogens in cases occuring within 2 months of surgery. Cases developing more than 2 months after surgery are frequently due to *S. epidermidis, S. aureus,* and streptococci (enterococci, *Streptococcus bovis,* and the viridans streptococci). The fastidious gram-negative coccobacilli, ie, *Haemophilus* species, *Actinobacillus actinomycetemcomitans,* and *Cardiobacterium hominis,* are also important pathogens during this later period.

In contrast to NVE wherein infection is usually confined to the valve leaflet, PVE is not restricted to the device itself. In fact, infection is primarily localized to the interface of the prosthesis and the valve annulus. Frequently, invasion beyond the annulus results in abscess formation in the adjacent cardiac tissue. In patients with infected mechanical prosthetic valves, annular invasion and myocardial abscesses are found in 60 and 40 percent of cases, respectively. In 15 percent of cases, bulky vegetations obstruct the valve orifice; this occurs more commonly at the mitral than at the aortic site. Destruction of paravalvular tissue by infection commonly causes dehiscence of the prosthesis from the annulus and hemodynamically significant valve incompetence. This is particularly common with infection of an aortic valve prosthesis. Initial reports of infection involving porcine bioprosthetic valves (a leaflet of tissue rather than a mechanical prosthesis) suggested that infection was frequently confined to the leaflet and was not invasive. However, invasion of paravalvular tissue occurs commonly in this setting. Invasive infection is present in more than 50 percent of patients with porcine bioprosthetic valve endocarditis that presents during the initial year following cardiac surgery. The pathology and hemodynamic consequences of infection in these patients resemble those seen with infected mechanical valves. Infection limited to the porcine leaflet tissue is more common when the valve becomes infected more than 1 year after implantation. Occasionally, infection will destroy the porcine leaflets and produce hemodynamically significant valvular incompetence.

Selected patients with PVE experience uniquely high mortality rates. These patients have one or more of the following: moderate-to-severe congestive heart failure (CHF); murmurs or noninvasive studies (echocardiography or cine-fluoroscopy) indicating valve dehiscence or dysfunction; new or progressive electrocardiographic conduction abnormality, and persistent unexplained fever despite appropriate antimicrobial therapy. These features are clinical correlates of invasive and destructive infection. They are clues to underlying pathology that is unlikely to be corrected by antimicrobial therapy in the absence of surgical intervention. Given the therapeutic implications, serial observations to detect these features should be included in the routine monitoring of patients who are being treated for PVE.

TREATMENT

Antibiotic Therapy

The general principles that guide therapy for NVE serve equally well to direct the antibiotic therapy of PVE. Bactericidal antibiotics or combinations of antibiotics that

TABLE 1 Bacteriology of Prosthetic Valve Endocarditis

	*Published before 1975**		*Cases 1975–1982†*	
	Onset following surgery		*Onset following surgery*	
Organism	*2 months*	*2 months*	*2 months*	*2 months*
S. epidermidis	41	36	22	29
S. aureus	30	22	2	8
Gram-negative bacilli	30	19‡	2	10‡
Streptococci (viridans and other nonenterococci)	9	41	0	13
Enterococci	6	14	0	6
Pneumococci	2	0	0	0
Diphtheroids	12	6	4	1
Fungi	18	9	2	3
Others	--	--	3	3
Culture-negative	3	7	3	5
Total	151	154	38	78

* From Karchmer AW, Swartz MN. Infective endocarditis in patients with prosthetic heart valves. In: Kaplan EL, Taranta AV, eds. Infective endocarditis: an American Heart Association Symposium Monograph No. 52. Dallas, American Heart Association, 1977; 58.

† From Calderwood SB, Swinski LA, Waternaux CM, Karchmer AW, Buckley MJ: Risk factors for the development of prosthetic valve endocarditis. Circulation 1985; 72:31–37.

‡ Numbers not specified but largely fastidious gram-negative coccobacilli.

are bactericidal are selected and administered parenterally in large doses for extended periods. An effort should be made to minimize drug toxicity when selecting antimicrobial agents and doses. For a given pathogen, generally, parenteral antibiotic treatment for PVE is longer than standard therapy for NVE.Most patients with PVE receive at least 6 weeks of antibiotic therapy. Those with endocarditis due to more virulent or resistant organisms are sometimes treated for 8 weeks. The decision to initiate antibiotic therapy prior to isolating the causative organism should be made after careful consideration. Given the importance of precise susceptibility data in the planning of optimal antibiotic therapy, it is essential that antibiotics not be administered prematurely and thus obscure the etiology of the infection. If the endocarditis has been indolent and the physical examination does not reveal deteriorating hemodynamics that require early surgical intervention, antibiotics should be withheld pending the isolation of an organism from blood cultures. This delay is particularly important if, prior to obtaining blood cultures, antibiotics have been given orally. These antibiotics may supress the infection and render initial cultures negative. In this setting, repeat cultures 3 to 5 days later may yield the causative organism. If, however, the endocarditis is acute or if hemodynamic deterioration due to valve dysfunction suggests that prompt valve replacement will be required, multiple blood cultures should be obtained over several hours and empiric antibiotics (as used for "culture-negative" prosthetic endocarditis) started immediately thereafter. Therapy can be revised when the etiology is known.

For a specific causative organism, the antibiotic regimen recommended for treating PVE would be the same as that used for NVE (see tables in chapter on *Endocarditis Caused by Gram-Positive Organisms).* Antimicrobial therapy for *S. epidermidis* and endocarditis-causing diphtheroids merits special mention, as these organisms are uniquely involved in PVE.

Although the susceptibility of diphtheroids to the penicillins and cephalosporins is unpredictable, these organisms are uniformly susceptible to the bactericidal effect of vancomycin. Furthermore, if the strain is susceptible to gentamicin, a synergistic bactericidal effect can be anticipated from the combination of gentamicin and penicillin, regardless of the penicillin susceptibility of the strain. The treatment of diphtheroid PVE is based upon these in vitro observations and clinical experience. In patients who can tolerate penicillin and who are infected by a diphtheroid strain that is susceptible to gentamicin, treat for 6 weeks intravenously with aqueous penicillin G, 4 million units every 4 hours, plus gentamicin, 1.5 mg per kilogram every 8 hours. If the patient is allergic to penicillin or if the strain is resistant to gentamicin, treat for 6 weeks with vancomycin, 7.5 mg per kilogram every 6 hours. As always, vancomycin and gentamicin doses must be adjusted for renal insufficiency.

The majority of *S. epidermidis* strains causing PVE are resistant to methicillin and other semisynthetic, penicillinase-resistant penicillins and cephalosporins. These strains may appear susceptible to beta-lactam antibiotics by routine testing, using the Bauer-Kirby disc diffusion method and on determination of the minimum inhibitory concentration, using a standard 10^5 inoculum. However, the resistance to methicillin and other beta-lactam antibiotics can be reliably detected by special studies (Table 2). Notably, more than 75 percent of *S. epidermidis* strains isolated from patients with PVE occurring within 12 months of valve implantation are methicillin-resistant; approximately 25 percent of those strains causing endocarditis with onset more than 12 months after surgery are also methicillin-resistant. These methicillin-resistant strains are uniformly susceptible to vancomycin and usually susceptible to rifampin and gentamicin. Patients with PVE caused by methicillin-resistant *S. epidermidis* (susceptible to rifampin and gentamicin) are more likely to be cured when treated with vancomycin in combination with rifampin or gentamicin, or both, than when treated with a beta-lactam antibiotic alone or a beta-lactam agent in combination with rifampin or an aminoglycoside, or both.

A 6-week regimen is recommended for the treatment of PVE due to methicillin-resistant rifampin and gentamicin-susceptible *S. epidermidis*. Vancomycin, 7.5 mg per kilogram intravenously every 6 hours, and rifampin, 300 mg orally every 8 hours, are given for 6 weeks. Gentamicin, 1 mg per kilogram intravenously every 8 hours is also administered during the inital 2 weeks of therapy. If infection is due to a *S. epidermidis* strain whose susceptibility to methicillin is definitively established, oxacillin, nafcillin, cephalothin, cephapirin, or cephradine (150 mg per kilogram per day IV in divided doses every 4 hours) is preferred for therapy. The need for combina-

TABLE 2 Staphylococcus Epidermidis: Tests for Methicillin Susceptibility*

1. Pick four or five colonies of strain and grow overnight in brain-heart infusion broth (organisms = 5×10^8 CFU†/ml)
2. Inoculate with 0.1 ml (5×10^7 CFU) by spreading on surface:
   Meuller-Hinton agar with 20 μg methicillin/ml
   Meuller-Hinton agar with 12.5 μg methicillin/ml
3. Incubate agar plates 72 hours at 37 °C
4. Read:
   Colonies on agar with 20 μg methicillin/ml = methicillin-resistant strain (also resistant to cephalosporins)
   No colonies on agar with 20 μg or 12.5 μg methicillin/ml = methicillin-susceptible strain

* Modified from Archer GL. Antimicrob Agents Chemother 1978; 14:353–359.
† CFU = Colony Forming Unit

tion antibiotic therapy in this later situation has not been established.

Given the spectrum of bacteria that cause PVE, putative "culture-negative" PVE should be treated with the combination of vancomycin, gentamicin, and ampicillin. Ampicillin is particularly important in view of the prominent role of fastidious gram-negative coccobaccilli as causes of endocarditis, beginning a year or more after surgery. Blood cultures are often negative in fungal endocarditis, especially forms due to fungi other than *Candida* species. The likelihood of fungal endocarditis must be carefully considered when embarking upon antibiotic therapy for culture-negative endocarditis. Bacteriologic and histologic study of surgically removed peripheral emboli may provide an etiologic diagnosis in some patients with negative blood cultures.

TABLE 3 Clinical Settings Warranting Possible Surgical Intervention in Prosthetic Valve Endocarditis

1. Moderate to severe heart failure and valve dysfunction
2. Clinical evidence of invasive and destructive disease:
   Partial valve dehiscence
   New or progressive conduction system disturbances
   Fever persisting 10 days despite antibiotic therapy
   Purulent pericarditis
3. Selected organisms associated with increased mortality:
   Fungi
   S. aureus
   *S. epidermidis**
4. Persistent bacteremia despite maximal antibiotic therapy
5. Relapse of infection after adequate antibiotic therapy
6. Recurrent emboli

* If associated with features noted in #2

SURGICAL INTERVENTION

Surgery to debride infected perivalvular tissue and to correct valvular dysfunction by placing a new prosthesis has become increasingly important in the management of PVE. Among patients recently treated for PVE, 50 percent have required surgery during the initial antibiotic therapy. It is desirable to suppress infection with antibiotic therapy for 10 to 14 days prior to surgery; however, surgery must be undertaken before hemodynamic deterioration becomes severe and irreversible. As with NVE, the likelihood of surviving valve replacement surgery is inversely related to the severity of heart failure at the time of surgery.

The clinical situations that warrant possible surgical intervention are noted in Table 3. Moderate-to-severe heart failure (New York Heart Association class III or IV) associated with valve dysfunction is one of the most commonly accepted and invoked indications for surgery. Survival is clearly increased in patients with moderate-to-severe heart failure when aggressive early surgery is undertaken to restore valve function. Patients with clinical evidence of invasive and destructive disease, e.g., murmurs of valve dysfunction, excessive valve motion indicating dehiscence, new or progressive conduction system disturbances, and unexplained fever persisting beyond 10 days despite appropriate antibiotic therapy, usually do poorly unless treated surgically. Some organisms causing PVE themselves serve as an indication for surgery. Fungal endocarditis is an absolute indication for early surgical intervention. The outcome of PVE caused by *S. aureus* may also be improved by early surgical therapy. Similarly, endocarditis due to *S. epidermidis* when associated with clinical signs of invasive pathology warrants surgical intervention. If blood cultures remain positive despite maximal antibiotic therapy or if endocarditis relapses after appropriate antibiotic therapy, surgery is indicated. Recurrent emboli have occasionally been cited as the sole indication for surgery. More commonly, a systemic embolus is used to support the argument for valve replacement based upon one of the previously stated indications. If the tissues removed at surgery harbor viable organisms or active inflammation is noted histologically, a full course of antibiotic therapy, dating from surgery, is recommended.

Selected patients with PVE can be cured with antibiotic therapy alone. Usually these patients have endocarditis that presents a year or more after surgery and is caused by organisms that are relatively avirulent and are highly susceptible to antibiotics. Antibiotic therapy alone is most likely to be effective when PVE is due to streptococci, fastidious gram-negative coccobacilli, or methicillin-susceptible *S. epidermidis*. In addition, these patients have uncomplicated disease; they have no evidence of invasive infection and are hemodynamically compensated.

ANTICOAGULANT THERAPY

Systemic emboli have been reported in 15 to 30 percent of patients with PVE. Hemorrhagic central nervous system events have complicated PVE, particularly when anticoagulation therapy has been excessive. In one retrospective study of mechanical valve endocarditis, the mortality rate among patients maintained on careful warfarin anticoagulation therapy was similar to the rate among those who were not given anticoagulants. However, morbidity due to central nervous system and systemic emboli was significantly greater among patients who were not given anticoagulant therapy. As a consequence of this study and our experience, careful anticoagulation (prothrombin time increased approximately 1.5 times the control value) is advocated during endocarditis if the infected prosthetic device is one that would usually merit maintenance anticoagulant therapy. If a hemorrhagic complication occurs, anticoagulation should be promptly reversed until the bleeding threat resolves. Anticoagulation is not recommended for patients with infection of a prosthetic valve that does not require anticoagulation under usual circumstances.

The prognosis of patients with PVE has been significantly improved by the treatment outlined in this chapter. Experience with this disease since 1975 indicates that an overall survival rate of 70 percent can be expected. Despite these favorable results with improved antimicrobial therapy and aggressive surgical intervention, morbidity and mortality due to this infection remain high. Vigorous efforts to prevent PVE are indicated. Patients with prosthetic valves should be carefully instructed about the risk of endocarditis and protected through the assiduous application of the prophylactic regimens recommended by the American Heart Association (Circulation 1984; 70:1123A). In the interim, through early recognition and continued refinements in both antibiotic therapy and the indications for surgical intervention, the morbidity and mortality of this disease may be further reduced.

CHRONIC CONGESTIVE HEART FAILURE

MILTON PACKER, M.D.

Congestive heart failure (CHF) is a clinical syndrome characterized by a functional limitation of exercise capacity of varying severity that results from an impairment of cardiac performance. Exertion may be limited by dyspnea or fatigue, or both; cardiac performance may be limited by disorders of ventricular or valvular function, or both. This article considers the management of patients whose heart failure is the result of irreversibly impaired left ventricular performance, i.e., left ventricular ejection fraction of less than 30 to 35 percent, resulting from ischemic or nonischemic causes, in the absence of primary valvular stenosis or regurgitation.

APPROACH TO THE PATIENT WITH HEART FAILURE

The primary goal in the management of the patient with CHF is to improve functional capacity by relieving dyspnea and fatigue. Consequently, we titrate therapy so that the patient is able to carry out activities of daily living commensurate with his needs and desires, and we judge the success of treatment by the relief of symptoms. Noninvasive measures of left ventricular performance correlate poorly with functional capacity and thus are *not* a therapeutic end point. Similarly, the severity of CHF is graded according to the degree of functional impairment and not by the degree of left ventricular dysfunction.

The treatment of the patient with CHF consists largely of a sequential approach, in which diuretics, digoxin, and vasodilator drugs are successively added to the therapeutic regimen in an attempt to control symptoms. The decision to utilize the next step in the sequence depends not on the severity of illness, but on the ability of previously utilized drugs to control symptoms. Hence, the approach to the patient with mild, moderate, or severe CHF is conceptually *identical*; all three classes of drugs just mentioned may be utilized at each stage in a patient's illness to minimize the degree of functional impairment.

DIURETICS AND LOW-SALT DIET

One of the earliest pathophysiologic abnormalities of the patient with CHF is the development of a sodium-avid state, such that sodium excretion is less than sodium intake; hence, the first goal in the treatment of the patient with heart failure is the restoration of sodium balance. This can be achieved by a combined approach in which dietary sodium is restricted and diuretic agents are administered to bring sodium excretion in line with a reduced salt load. Given the potency of currently available diuretic drugs, it is generally not necessary to impose severe dietary restriction of sodium; attempts to do so may result in poor patient compliance and an altered quality of life, which may diminish the benefits of treating the heart failure state. A 2-g sodium diet is sufficient in nearly all patients.

Clinical End Points for Diuretic Therapy

Although the purpose of diuretic therapy is the restoration of sodium balance, this goal is not precisely applicable to clinical practice, since such an approach conceptually requires the serial measurement of 24-hour urinary sodium excretion. Instead, diuretics are titrated to relieve the signs and symptoms of heart failure; the end point that we utilize most frequently is the relief of peripheral edema, since this finding is linked directly to changes in sodium balance. Diuretics also serve to relieve pulmonary congestion and exertional fatigue in patients with heart failure, but these symptoms may also be related to changes in cardiac contractility or in loading conditions and thus provide an imprecise end point for the titration of diuretic drugs. Although these agents may relieve dyspnea in the patient with heart failure who has no peripheral edema, such benefits are unpredictable and may be accompanied by signs and symptoms of intravascular volume depletion.

Choice of Diuretic Drug

The diuretic drug most frequently utilized in the management of CHF is furosemide. Its efficacy is largely determined by factors that affect the delivery of sodium and drug to the renal tubule; hence, patients with reduced renal blood flow (from a low cardiac output) or renal insufficiency (serum creatinine level greater than 2.5 mg/dl) generally require higher doses of furosemide to achieve a diuresis than do patients with normal renal perfusion and function. Its actions on the loop of Henle permit furosemide to be effective (albeit in high doses) in states of altered renal perfusion and function; in contrast, the efficacy of conventional thiazide diuretics is nearly abolished under these circumstances.

Clinical Use of Diuretics

The starting dose of furosemide is 20 to 40 mg daily. Should patients fail to respond, larger doses are prescribed until a diuresis is noted. We administer furosemide in a single daily administration, *not* in divided doses. Clinical experience has shown that subtherapeutic doses of furosemide remain ineffective even if given multiple times during the day. Once a diuresis is achieved, it can be reproduced daily as needed; twice- or thrice-daily dosing is not necessary and may lead to excessive depletion of intracellular cations (potassium and magnesium).

As the heart failure state progressively worsens and as cardiac output falls, furosemide becomes progressively less effective in restoring sodium balance, despite increments in the oral dose to 200 mg daily. Under these circumstances, the drug may be given intravenously for short periods of time; such parenteral administration ensures the direct and rapid delivery of the drug in states in which its oral absorption may be impaired by bowel edema. With the relief of such edema after several days of intravenous therapy, the efficacy of oral furosemide may be restored. Unfortunately, as cardiac function deteriorates, even this approach eventually fails. At this time, we resort to the simultaneous administration of multiple diuretics, which are added to (not substituted for) furosemide. Our diuretic of choice for this purpose is metolazone; its addition to furosemide frequently results in a profound diuresis, which is often complicated by profound hypokalemia. Hence, great care must be exercised when such multiple diuretic regimens are initiated. We have also found hydrochlorothiazide and spironolactone to be useful when added to furosemide. Should all of these approaches fail, sodium balance may be achieved only by the *direct* removal of fluid by techniques such as hemofiltration or ultrafiltration; fortunately, such approaches are generally needed only when renal failure complicates the clinical picture.

Complications of Diuretic Therapy

The principal complications of diuretic therapy are the depletion of intracellular cations (potassium and magnesium) and the activation of reactive neurohormonal vasoconstrictor systems (particularly the sympathetic nervous system and the renin-angiotensin system). These events, acting alone or in concert, may predispose patients to malignant ventricular arrhythmias that are so frequent in these patients and may be an underlying cause of sudden death. Hence, restoration of potassium and magnesium balance may exert more potent antiarrhythmic effects in patients with CHF than the use of conventional antiarrhythmic drugs. Although aggressive potassium supplementation may prevent hypokalemia, it does little to prevent magnesium depletion, which can be effectively treated only by potassium-sparing diuretics or converting-enzyme inhibitors. It is not known to what extent the activation of vasopressor systems by diuretic therapy contributes to the excessive loading conditions of the failing heart and, thereby, serves to accelerate progression of the underlying heart disease.

In patients whose cardiac output is extremely reduced, diuretic therapy may be complicated by increasing azotemia, as renal blood flow is decreased by natriuretic effects of treatment. Contrary to conventional wisdom, such circumstances are not usually the result of an excessive lowering of ventricular filling pressures; right heart catheterization in these patients usually reveals marked increases in both mean right atrial and pulmonary capillary wedge pressures, which may be lowered by continued diuresis. Hence, the development of azotemia during diuretic therapy should not generally be a cause for a reduction in the dose or the discontinuation of these agents, especially if the therapeutic end point (abolition of peripheral edema) has not been reached.

DIGITALIS

Although used in the treatment of CHF for over 200 years, the place of digitalis remains undefined. There is little doubt that, by its ability to impair atrioventricular conduction, the drug can produce hemodynamic and clinical improvement in patients whose heart failure is complicated by atrial fibrillation. Yet, although the drug also increases cardiac contractility, it is not clear that this action is helpful in patients with heart failure in normal sinus rhythm. Present evidence indicates that digitalis produces sustained hemodynamic and clinical benefits in *some* of these patients, but it is not clear how frequently this occurs, in which patients such improvement is seen, and how often it is accompanied by serious drug toxicity. Until such evidence is gathered, the use of digitalis remains a matter of tradition and personal preference.

Clinical Use

Because of these uncertainties, most physicians in the United States employ small doses of digitalis in patients with heart failure, in the hope that some therapeutic benefit may be achieved without major toxicity. Our drug of choice is digoxin, usually administered in a daily oral dose of 0.25 mg. In patients older than age 70 years and in those with a serum creatinine concentration greater than 1.5 mg per deciliter, the dose is commonly reduced to 0.125 mg daily or every other day, since the renal excretion of the drug is impaired in the elderly and in patients with reduced renal function. Doses greater than 0.25 mg daily are rarely utilized at the present time, unless atrial fibrillation with a rapid ventricular response is present.

Digitalis is commonly instituted in patients with CHF at the same time as diuretic therapy is begun. It is important to note, therefore, that the drug is usually administered in empirically determined doses and is *not* generally titrated to a therapeutic end point, since the clinical benefits of digitalis cannot be distinguished from the improvement that is expected following diuretic therapy. Digitalis should *not* be titrated to achieve "therapeutic" serum levels since there is no evidence that circulating levels of the drug correlate with therapeutic efficacy.

Complications

Although low doses of digitalis are generally prescribed in patients with CHF, digitalis toxicity is still frequent, although it usually occurs in the presence of defined risk factors, particularly hypokalemia and sinoatrial and atrioventricular conduction disease (sick sinus syndrome). Under these circumstances, the most frequent manifestations of digitalis toxicity are cardiac brady- or tachyarrhythmias; gastrointestinal distress, xanthopsia, and altered mentation are rarely seen at the present time except in cases of intentional poisoning. The detection of potentially toxic arrhythmias in the digitalized patient presents the physician with a therapeutic dilemma, since such arrhythmias may occur in patients with a severely diseased left ventricle in the absence of digitalis; indeed, most of the arrhythmias in patients with heart failure are *not* related to digitalis therapy. Although serum levels of the drug are frequently utilized to resolve this dilemma, the correlation between circulating levels of the drug and toxicity is not as close as is commonly believed; hence, measurement of serum digoxin levels usually serves to confirm a well-established clinical impression. To securely implicate digitalis toxicity as the cause of an arrhythmia, the rhythm disturbance must disappear upon discontinuation of the drug and recur when digitalis is readministered. This is rarely done, however, in clinical practice.

The most serious potential adverse effect of digitalis is that the drug may exert a direct deleterious effect on the prognosis of patients with heart failure, either by its arrhythmogenic actions or by its ability to accelerate progression of the underlying heart disease. Such fears derive from retrospective studies performed in patients recovering from an acute myocardial infarction, but similar concerns about the risks of inotropic therapy have been raised in patients with CHF treated with investigational nonglycosidic inotropic drugs. Future studies are needed to confirm or refute this potential adverse effect of digitalis on survival.

VASODILATOR DRUGS

Although it is well established that excessive systemic vasoconstriction plays a critical pathophysiologic role in patients with CHF, the use of vasodilator drugs to attenuate these peripheral mechanisms (and thereby favorably alter loading conditions in the failing heart) generally produced disappointing results until the introduction of the converting-enzyme inhibitors.

Experience with Direct-Acting Vasodilators

The first orally active class of drugs introduced for the treatment of CHF were the organic nitrates. Although effective hemodynamically and clinically in some patients, the usefulness of nitrates has been hampered by their short duration of action; hence, sustained delivery systems for nitroglycerin were developed, which result in continuous blood levels of the drug with once-daily application. Unfortunately, these nitroglycerin discs and patches have not been shown to be effective during long-term treatment, probably because pharmacologic tolerance develops to the actions of the drug when administered continuously. The only nitrate preparation that has been demonstrated to be effective in the treatment of CHF is oral isosorbide dinitrate, administered in a dose of 40 mg orally, 4 times a day. In our experience, however, the drug is only moderately effective in the relief of symptoms, and hence it is most frequently utilized as adjunctive therapy in association with other vasodilator drugs.

Hydralazine produces marked hemodynamic responses in patients with CHF, but large doses (usually 300 mg or more daily) are generally necessary to achieve these effects, and clinical benefits are largely restricted to patients whose heart failure is complicated by marked left ventricular dilatation, in whom the drug effectively reduces the magnitude of secondary mitral regurgitation. Unfortunately, long-term treatment with the drug is frequently (20 to 25%) accompanied by dose-limiting adverse effects (particularly nausea and vomiting) and by the development of drug-specific hemodynamic and clinical tolerance (25 to 30%). The overall response rate to hydralazine is only 30 to 40 percent; hence, it is not surprising that the drug has not been shown to be effective in double-blind, placebo-controlled trials.

Like hydralazine, prazosin also produces marked short-term hemodynamic effects in patients with CHF, but, unlike hydralazine, the drug is well tolerated and is rarely discontinued because of adverse reactions. Unfortunately, long-term treatment with prazosin is frequently (60 to 65%) accompanied by the development of hemodynamic and clinical tolerance that may be seen as early as 48 hours after institution of treatment with the drug. Such pharmacologic tolerance appears to be the result of changes in the interaction of prazosin and its receptor and is not due to fluid retention; thus, it cannot generally be overcome by alterations in the dose of concomitantly administered diuretics. Like hydralazine, the overall response rate to prazosin is also low (30 to 40% of consecutively evaluated patients), and hence the drug has also failed to produce consistent benefits in double-blind, placebo-controlled trials.

Experience with Converting-Enzyme Inhibitors

By inhibiting the angiotensin converting enzyme, captopril (and its analogue, enalapril) interferes with angiotensin II biosynthesis in patients with heart failure, and this action leads to short- and long-term hemodynamic and clinical improvement. Both drugs have been shown to be effective in double-blind, placebo-controlled trials; the incidence of hemodynamic tolerance with both agents is low (10 to 15%), and both drugs are well tolerated during long-term treatment. Approximately 60 to 65 percent of consecutively evaluated patients with CHF improve clinically during long-term converting-enzyme inhibition; these benefits are generally greater than can be achieved with hydralazine or prazosin.

There is no reliable means of selecting patients with heart failure who are likely to benefit from long-term converting-enzyme inhibition. Measurements of plasma renin activity or of hemodynamic variables do not reliably predict long-term response. Although many physicians evaluate the acute hemodynamic efficacy of first doses of captopril or enalapril (during right heart catheterization) in order to select those patients likely to improve clinically, recent evidence indicates that acute hemodynamic determinations are of little value in predicting long-term hemodynamic and clinical response. Such data raise serious questions about the need for invasive measurements during the initiation of vasodilator therapy in patients with severe heart failure. The only means of determining which patients with heart failure may improve during treatment with converting-enzyme inhibitors is by a therapeutic trial with these drugs.

Converting-enzyme inhibitors are generally initiated in patients with CHF who remain symptomatic on digitalis and diuretics; the initial doses should be 6.25–12.5 mg of captopril or 2.5–5.0 mg of enalapril. We generally keep concomitant therapy with digoxin and diuretics constant when starting treatment in patients at low risk of hypotension; in patients with severe hyponatremia (serum sodium concentration <130 mEq/L) or in those who have recently experienced a vigorous diuresis, we prefer to reduce the dose of diuretics before institution of therapy. It is important for the clinician to determine that the first dose of captopril or enalapril does not produce symptomatic hypotension before prescribing long-term treatment with the drug; such assurances are easier to gain with captopril, since its peak effects are seen within 90 minutes of drug administration. If test doses are well tolerated, long-term therapy may be instituted at a dose of 12.5–25 mg of captopril 3 times daily or 5–10 mg of enalapril twice daily; these doses may be increased to 150 mg daily of captopril or 40 mg daily of enalapril, but more data are needed to determine if higher doses are superior to low doses in producing long-term benefits. If the dose of concomitantly administered diuretic has been reduced, we generally attempt to restore its dosage to pretreatment levels during the first week of therapy. Decreases in the dose of diuretics are made only if symptomatic dizziness or worsening azotemia are seen during the course of treatment. Therapy is maintained for at least 3 to 4 weeks, at which time the patient's therapeutic response is assessed; if symptoms are improved, long-term treatment is maintained indefinitely and can be expected to be accompanied by progressive clinical benefits. As with diuretics, assessment of the success or failure of treatment is based on the relief of symptoms, not on changes in ventricular function.

The principal adverse effects of converting-enzyme inhibition are symptomatic hypotension and functional renal insufficiency, both of which are related to interference with the homeostatic functions of the renin-angiotensin system. These reactions may occur at any time during the course of treatment, are commonest in patients who have recently undergone a notable diuresis, and usually can be controlled by reducing the dose of concomitantly administered diuretic; neither reaction generally requires discontinuation of therapy. Hyperkalemia can occur during converting-enzyme inhibition (because of its ability to reduce aldosterone secretion), but almost invariably it is seen in patients who are taking oral potassium supplementation or potassium-sparing diuretics; hence, we generally discontinue these drugs when treatment with converting-enzyme inhibitors is begun. Other adverse reactions of concern include rash and dysgeusia; they occur in approximately 5 to 10 percent of patients with heart failure taking captopril and in less than 1 percent of patients taking enalapril.

INOTROPIC AGENTS

Many new inotropic drugs are being developed that directly stimulate cardiac contractility by mechanisms that differ from that of the digitalis glycosides. At the present time, however, these agents (dopamine, dobutamine, or amrinone) can be given only intravenously, although orally active analogues are at present under intense investigation. Unfortunately, in preliminary trials, the long-term administration of these drugs has not produced impressive clinical results and has been associated with an unexpectedly high mortality rate, possibly because inotropic agents may serve to increase myocardial oxygen consumption, exacerbate underlying ventricular arrhythmias, and accelerate progression of the underlying heart disease. Until further work is done, such therapeutic approaches must be considered strictly investigational.

ARTERIAL OCCLUSIVE DISEASE

JAMES F. BURDICK, M.D.

Most patients who present with chronic atherosclerotic peripheral vascular disease show one of several patterns, and there is general consensus about the preferred surgical approach to these situations. Differentiation between an acute embolus to an extremity and rapid progression of an underlying atherosclerotic lesion to total occlusion of the vessel occasionally may be in question in the patient with acute presentation. Generally, however, the distinction is easily made.

PATTERNS OF CHRONIC OCCLUSIVE DISEASE

Patients typically present with either predominately arterial occlusive disease or aneurysmal disease. Atherosclerotic disease is often found at many sites, but only one or two critical occlusions occur at one time to prompt medical intervention. It is important that the patient understand that the underlying atherosclerosis is not curable.

Involvement of the aortoiliac system generally is worse in the distal aorta and proximal iliac arteries. On the angiogram, the distal external iliac arteries may appear relatively uninvolved with disease, but generally they are much more diseased, with plaque deposited posteriorly when they are actually examined. Leriche's syndrome may occur in male patients. It consists of absence of femoral pulses, claudication, and impotence due to complete occlusion of the distal aorta and proximal iliac arteries. Involvement of the mesenteric arteries sufficient to produce symptoms is uncommon, although angiographic narrowing or even occlusion of either the superior mesenteric artery or the celiac axis is not at all rare. Intestinal angina may be produced if both of these vessels are severely narrowed or occluded. At present, the importance of occlusion of the internal iliac arteries in impotence is under study. Investigators at some centers feel that impotence may occasionally be helped by revascularization of the pelvic vasculature.

Disease in the superficial femoral artery typically occurs in the region of the adductor hiatus, often with proximal progression so that the patient presents with an occlusion from the origin of the superficial femoral artery to the popliteal artery, with only an open common femoral artery and a profunda femoris artery remaining. The distal popliteal region, including the origins of the three tibial vessels, may be free of atherosclerosis. The disease in the popliteal artery is typically severer proximally than distally. Occlusion of the profunda femoris artery as an isolated problem is not common and usually not symptomatic. However, the profunda femoris artery is a critical vessel for protecting the leg from severe ischemia should the superficial femoral artery become occluded. This fact should be taken into account in assessing patients and in planning revascularization.

Disease of the tibial vessels distally is particularly common in diabetic patients. Open vessels in the lower leg is key to revascularization because inability to provide inflow to them prevents successful revascularization. In either the presence or absence of diabetes, occasionally the distal tibial vessel disease may be severe enough to cause lesions in the foot. However, the neuropathic lesions, altered collagen biochemistry, and immune impairment in the diabetic patient typically represent more important reasons for the characteristic indolent chronic toe or distal plantar ulcers that develop. Hence, the diabetic patient with a foot lesion may have palpable pedal pulses and no indication for revascularization.

EVALUATION

History and Physical Examination

If the patient smokes, strongly encourage him to stop. Whether diabetes, hypertension, or other atherosclerotic manifestations are present should be determined. Intermittent claudication is reproducible with a certain degree of activity and resolves after 5 to 15 minutes of rest. Rarely, neurogenic claudication due to lumbar disk disease may be confused with intermittent claudication. Neuropathic features sometimes complicate the assessment of rest pain but are usually distinguishable because they do not improve with dependency. Typically, patients complain progressively of claudication; this is followed by rest pain. Eventually necrotic lesions develop and the loss of a limb is imminent. A more sudden presentation of severe ischemia should raise the suspicion of an embolus. Careful assessment for a distal pulse is important, since if present, it is a much better assessment of the status of the vasculature than other diagnostic means. However, the absence of a pulse is not necessarily serious since many patients may have minimal or no symptoms despite proximal occulsion of a major blood vessel from collateral circulation. Effectiveness of arterial perfusion is made by noting temperature, color, appropriate motion, and sensation. Chronicity of the change is signaled by loss of hair and thin, shiny skin. The most reliable determinant of the degree of acute ischemia of a limb is whether the patient is capable of pedal dorsiflexion. If he has severe rest pain, the relief afforded by keeping the extremity dependent most of the time may produce a paradoxical edema.

The typical transient ischemic attack with recurrent, focal, severe, neurologic deficits, alternating with entirely normal status, is a strong indication for carotid arterial evaluation. However, more global symptoms of brain ischemia, including dizziness or impaired mentation, are also occasional manifestations of hemodynamically significant carotid artery disease.

Vascular Laboratory

For the patient with no palpable distal pulses, assessing the vasculature through the Doppler signal and either pressures or wave forms of the extremity vessels is valuable. Sometimes, a patient with excellent vascular laboratory findings or even a palpable pulse in the extremity at rest complains of claudication. An exercise Doppler examination may document an abnormal post-exercise decrease in the pressure. Artifacts, particularly the degree of sclerosis in the wall of a diabetic femoral artery, may interfere with pressure and wave-form measurements. Therefore, the initial Doppler pressures obtained are particularly useful as a baseline for longitudinal study of the patient. For carotid disease, the oculoplethysmographic examination correlates well with the degree of hemodynamically significant carotid stenosis, but not with an ulcerated plaque. In some centers, plethysmography or pressure in the penis is used to determine the degree to which impotence is related to pelvic vascular compromise.

Angiography

In general, arteriograms should not be done for diagnosis. They should be reserved for situations in which surgical evaluation is contemplated. It is important to communicate with the radiologist so that the greatest benefit can be obtained from the study. It is often useful to do pressure measurements below an iliac or femoral lesion of questionable significance, before and after injection of a vasodilator, to determine the significance of the lesion. For all these reasons, and because surgical complications occasionally occur after angiography, it is important to have a vascular surgeon examine the patient before the study. The importance of intravenous fluid hydration in the hours before and immediately after the angiographic study to protect the kidneys from damage caused by the dye cannot be overemphasized. Noninvasive tests, such as a computed tomography (CT) scan are of particular value in aneurysmal, but not occlusive, peripheral vascular disease. Brain CT is a useful study before carotid endarterectomy.

OPERATIVE INDICATIONS AND CONSERVATIVE MANAGEMENT

Threatened Limb Loss

Revascularization is mandatory in most cases of threatened limb loss from severe ischemia or nonhealing lesions. If (1) the patient is severely demented, (2) the limb in question is paralyzed from a stroke, (3) the limb has been devascularized for longer than 1½ to 2 days, or (4) severe clostridial infection is present, primary amputation should be performed. Otherwise, regardless of risk, a reconstruction should be carried out. The risk of an amputation, if reconstruction is not performed, is close to the risk of the reconstructive procedure in general. Even in high risk patients, it is usually possible to provide some combination of operative approach and anesthetic management to allow the reconstruction to be done with reasonable safety. The value of two sound legs in a patient who is older and failing in other ways is incalculable and should be taken into account in making decisions about threatened limb loss.

Rest Pain

If the patient has pain at rest but is reasonably comfortable, if no lesions have developed, and if there is no evidence of neurologic damage, the urgency in revascularization is not as great. However, if reconstruction is deferred, ischemic neuropathic problems or ascending infection may complicate the outcome of an otherwise successful revascularization.

Claudication

Intermittent claudication in a patient who is asymptomatic at rest and has no lesions threatening the foot is never an absolute indication for operation, no matter how markedly abnormal the patient's physical and angiographic findings are. Occasionally, a patient has misunderstood this or received other information from the referring physician. When claudication first develops, the average patient's chances are about even that it will progress, recede, or remain the same in the ensuing 6 months. There are series that report remarkable improvement after initial onset of claudication if the patient undergoes a rigorous program of exercise, follows a diet, and stops smoking. After this 6-month waiting period, the patient with stable or increasing claudication may still wish to consider revascularization, which is often appropriate. In the younger patient, claudication may interfere with work. Compromise of the patient's self-image, unwillingness to accept a stigma of old age, or interference with appropriate exercise for cardiopulmonary health may all represent appropriate considerations in favor of revascularization, as long as he or she understands that this is not the only option. The degree of enthusiasm with which revascularization is recommended should be modified, depending on both the ease of the revascularization and the patient's age and general physical status.

Several pharmacologic approaches to mild peripheral vascular disease have been recommended, including administration of PGE_2, prostacyclin, calcium chelation, calcium-channel blockers, pentoxifylline, or other vasodilators. These approaches in general have not been shown to ease claudication.

Carotid Artery Disease

Two major categories of patients exist. If the patient is symptomatic and has an otherwise reasonable operative risk, carotid endarterectomy should be undertaken. In appropriate hands, the subsequent risk of stroke is greater than the risk of endarterectomy. If the patient is asymptomatic, there is a vaguer recommendation for revascularization before other major surgery, which may cause fluctuations in the patient's blood pressure intraoperatively or in the early postoperative period. Otherwise, it is not currently established that the truly asymptomatic patient, regardless of the angiographic picture, benefits from carotid endarterectomy. Many investigators surmise, however, that in the appropriate hands, a major asymptomatic lesion is best treated by endarterectomy.

Mesenteric Artery Disease

Atherosclerosis leading to intestinal ischemia is uncommon and variable. But, occasionally, a patient with postprandial pain or episodes of frank ischemia and severe disease of both the superior mesenteric artery and celiac axis may be a candidate for revascularization, usually of the superior mesenteric artery. Not performing this procedure increases the risk of an acute occlusion with bowel infarction.

SURGICAL OPTIONS

Aortic Graft Reconstruction

The graft is generally placed from the aorta to the femoral vessels because of the likelihood of progression of iliac disease. It is necessasry to obtain revascularization of one or the other internal iliac arteries, or of the inferior mesenteric arteries, or both, so that appropriate revascularization of the lower colon is ensured. Generally, unilateral revascularization from aorta to iliac artery is not indicated since the risk is not much greater if both vessels are replaced. Most commonly, patients with severe aortoiliac disease have reasonable femoral vessels for outflow anastomoses in the groin. This arrangement may consist only of an open profunda femoris artery, which usually provides excellent outflow. It should always be preserved, even if the superficial femoral artery is open at the time of the procedure, to prevent future problems if superficial femoral artery occlusion develops. Mortality is generally lower than 5 percent, with morbidity lower than 15 percent, even in the older patients with other atherosclerotic disease in whom it is typically performed. Complications include pulmonary dysfunction or pneumonia, wound infection, and nonfatal complications of atherosclerosis, such as myocardial infarction (MI), cerebrovascular accident, or renal failure.

Femorofemoral Grafts

The femorofemoral graft, since it is a more superficial procedure, has associated mortality of 1 percent and morbidiy of 10 percent. It is a prudent alternative for patients who are at poor risk for undergoing aortofemoral graft and who have a healthy contralateral aortoiliac segment. The donor limb need not be angiographically perfect, but should have normal pressure measurements after peripheral vasodilatation. If inflow is sufficient, a steal from the noninvolved limb is not a problem. The possibility of placing a femorofemoral graft should be included as an option for any patient with strikingly unilateral disease. The long-term patency of these grafts, however, is poorer, so that an aortofemoral graft is perferable in the good-risk patient.

Axillobifemoral Grafts

These procedures are definitely inferior to aortofemoral grafts in long-term patency. Hence, they are generally reserved for severely ill patients with limb-threatening ischemia. In most centers, the axillofemoral graft is used only for patients with a recent MI, prohibitive chronic obstructive pulmonary disease, or an infected aortic graft requiring removal. The success of the graft depends on inflow and although proximal brachial vessel disease is uncommon, it should be assessed. The mortality directly associated with placement of this graft should be less than 1 percent, but the patient population in which it is usually performed is such that the reported mortalities usually are 10 percent or greater within 1 month of operation. The morbidity is low, in the range of 5 percent.

Aortic and Femoral Endarterectomy

Aortoiliac endarterectomy is now rare. This is because of the great success of aortic bifurcation grafts, which can be placed safely with excellent long-term patency. Endarterectomy involves increased blood loss and much longer operating time. A profunda femoris endarterectomy may form an important adjunct to placement of a graft, however. A unilateral iliac endarterectomy for a specific diseased segment is generally unsafe without obtaining proximal control and arteriotomy on the contralateral iliac to allow flushing and clot prevention. Superficial femoral endarterectomies are not successful.

Femoropopliteal Grafts

Femoropopliteal grafts are more superficial than aortofemoral grafts. They typically carry about a 2 percent mortality. There may be a 15 percent or greater morbidity due to minor wound problems and reexplorations. Whether or not an intact saphenous vein of appropriate caliber can be employed determines the expected results. Saphenous vein bypass grafts to the popliteal artery have a greater than 90 percent expectancy of patency for many years. Prosthetic grafts, including the common polyexpanded tetrafluoroethylene ones, are much less successful. Often, however, with rethrombectomy upon occlusion, the graft may be kept open for years. The extent of distal disease in the outflow for the graft is an important factor, regardless of the graft material, so that patients with only an isolated popliteal segment or extensive disease in the distal tibial vessels are much less likely to show satisfactory long-term results than are those with an open distal system.

Femoral-Distal Grafts

These bypasses may be performed using vein or prosthetic material to any of the three distal vessels. They carry a mortality of lower than 2 percent and a morbidity of 15 percent. The key problem with these procedures is a marked early drop in patency rate so that 50 percent to 75 percent of the grafts have failed by 1 year. However, those that remain open during the first few months generally enjoy long-term success. Sequential anastomoses to more than one distal destination appears to improve the likelihood of success. Another approach is by means of the in situ graft. In this approach the saphenous vein valves are destroyed and the tributaries ligated; the vein is not removed from the subcutaneous tissue, instead it is anastomosed proximally to the femoral artery and distally to an outflow tibial vessel.

Carotid Endarterectomy

Carotid endarterectomy is aided by the natural tendency of the disease to occur in a localized area right at the bifurcation of the common carotid artery. Generally, operative mortality and risk of stroke are less than 5 percent; the risk of other complications is approximately 10 percent. The risk of the procedure is largely due to the possibility of air or a small particle migrating up the internal carotid artery at the time of reanastomosing flow to this vessel. In addition, cardiovascular stress appears to be great even for this superficial procedure, and perioperative MI is not uncommon. Occasionally, cranial nerve damage, particularly to nerves X or XII is a complication. Acute endarterectomy for a stroke is not generally beneficial. A recent nonresolving neurologic deficit should be regarded as a stroke, and revascularization deferred until at least 1 month after it has occurred.

ACUTE THROMBOPHLEBITIS

CRAIG M. KESSLER, M.D.

Thrombosis of the venous system is diagnosed clinically in at least 180,000 to 250,000 patients per year in the United States. The number is expected to rise as the use of sensitive diagnostic screening techniques for the detection of subclinical deep venous thrombosis (DVT) becomes more prevalent. The acute mortality associated with DVT is produced primarily by the propensity of the thrombi to embolize to the lung. Pulmonary emboli are the sole or major contributing cause of death in approximately 200,000 patients per year in the United States. Many of these deaths could have been prevented in high-risk individuals if increased clinical suspicion had been combined with improved diagnostic and prophylactic procedures. The long-term sequelae of acute DVT are related to the development of the postphlebitic syndrome (PPS), which is characterized by extremity pain with dependent edema, skin hyperpigmentation, chronic ulceration with recurrent infection, and local inflammation with subcutaneous fibrosis. The syndrome occurs as the direct physiologic consequence of destruction of the venous valvular system mediated by thrombus formation, organization, and slow recanalization. These developments in turn permit the retrograde transmission of increased venous pressure through the communicating veins to the subcutaneous veins and tissues. Hypoxia, extravasation of blood, cell death, and ulceration may follow. The syndrome is estimated to affect at least 60 percent of patients within 5 years of their DVT, despite adequate anticoagulation therapy, and is associated with considerable socioeconomic consequences for the patient and society. A 1977 study from the Tufts-New England medical center estimated that patients with PPS would have spent almost $40,000 in medical expenses alone for these sequelae of DVT over a 10-year period.

These data clearly indicate that more effective and efficient approaches to the treatment of DVT are required. Ideally, DVTs should be clinically suspected and diagnosed early enough so that pharmacologic intervention can be instituted to furnish complete removal of the offending thrombus and prevent recurrence. Complete or partial thrombolysis should decrease the risk of fatal pulmonary emboli and (theoretically) preserve venous valvular integrity and vascular patency to provide ultimate relief of long-term sequelae of PPS.

DIAGNOSIS

The signs and symptoms of DVT are nonspecific, and the diagnosis is often suspected only following an embolic event. On the one hand, less than 50 percent of patients with overt clinical features consistent with DVT may be expected to have confirmatory positive venograms; on the other hand, it is not unusual for high-risk patients, e.g., those following general surgical treatment and hip operations, to have documented evidence of DVT in the absence of clinical findings or subjective complaints.

Despite the search for noninvasive diagnostic techniques to establish DVT, venography remains the reference method against which all other procedures are compared. Venographic radiopaque contrast studies are useful in delineating the location and extent of DVT in any venous system of the body. Ascending venography, in which the contrast medium is injected into a dorsal foot vein, almost always provides adequate visualization of the deep veins of the calf, the popliteal vein, and the common and external iliac veins. Pulmonary emboli are thought to arise mainly from ileofemoral thrombi, although approximately 20 percent of clots that originate in the calf veins and which ordinarily do not pose a significant threat for embolization may propagate proximally and eventually break off. Some physicians are often reluctant to subject their patients to this definitive but invasive procedure, particularly if the clinical examination is strongly suggestive. Venography may be painful, may induce DVT formation in as high as 5 percent of patients, and may not be readily available in all hospitals; however, the frequency of these complications is much lower than the incidence and seriousness of side effects of empirical long-term anticoagulation.

None of the noninvasive techniques developed so far for the diagnosis of DVT is as reliable or as accurate as venography when used alone. Recent evidence indicates that the combined approach of impedance plethysmography (IPG) and leg scanning may be sensitive and specific enough to replace venography in patients with clinically suspected DVT. The accuracy and reproducibility of these procedures require specialized expertise and equipment not readily available in all institutions.

Impedance plethysmography is an indirect and noninvasive means to detect thrombosis in the popliteal, femoral, or iliac veins, but also may be used in the upper extremities. The technique measures changes in lower extremity venous volume following the rapid deflation of a midthigh pneumatic cuff previously inflated to a pressure of 45 mm H_2O to distend the venous system fully. Any compromise of proximal venous outflow, e.g., extrinsic venous obstruction, usually by tumor, or intrinsic obstruction due to thrombosis, will produce abnormal results. Normal findings do not exclude the diagnosis of calf-vein thrombosis or old proximal DVT with well-developed collateral circulation. False positive results on IPG may be associated with Baker's cysts compressing the popliteal vein, large calf and thigh hematomas, and technical difficulties in performing the procedure. Doppler ultrasonography essentially has the same limitations as, and appears to be less sensitive than, IPG in detecting partially occlusive proximal DVT. Doppler recordings may be more useful than IPG in clinical situations in which access to the extremities is limited by orthopaedic immobilization casts.

The diagnosis of DVT by scanning with radionuclide-labeled protein or platelets depends upon incorporation of the material into the thrombus with subsequent detection of localized radioactivity by a gamma camera. The most extensive clinical experience has been gained with ^{125}I-fibrinogen scanning, which in the leg appears to be most sensitive to DVTs in the calf and distal part of the thigh. The technique is limited by false positive results produced by isotopic accumulation in areas of inflammation and hematoma. The risk of hepatitis transmission by this plasma-derived protein is minimized by careful donor screening.

In our institution and several others, indium 111-labeled platelet scans are performed to diagnose DVT. This technique detects thrombi in any venous or arterial system, and the risk of hepatitis can be circumvented by employing autologous platelets. The use of indium 111-labeled platelet scans is limited currently by the time-consuming and labor-intensive necessity of radiolabeling freshly collected platelets and by decreased ability to detect DVTs once heparin anticoagulation has been initiated.

In summary, the diagnosis of DVT should be established by venography, the most definitive technique available. This need is especially crucial if fibrinolytic intervention is anticipated. If there is a medical contraindication for this radiographic procedure, e.g., iodine hypersensitivity, pregnancy, or limited venous access, among others, noninvasive procedures may be considered, and their results should be interpreted in light of their limitations. Impedance plethysmography combined with an isotope-scanning technique, e.g., ^{125}I-fibrinogen or indium 111-labeled platelet scan, approaches 90 percent specificity and sensitivity when performed by experienced and skilled personnel.

The diagnosis of DVT often may be facilitated by recognizing the clinical situations and risk factors associated with an increased incidence of venous thromboembolism (Table 1).

TREATMENT

Superficial Thrombophlebitis

Management of isolated superficial thrombophlebitis is directed toward symptomatic relief of the accompanying edema and pain. The affected extremity should be rested and elevated until discomfort and swelling subside. Nonsteroidal anti-inflammatory agents and local wet heat compresses may facilitate clinical improvement. Although scattered reports advocate administration of ana-

TABLE 1 Clinical Situations Predisposing to Increased Incidence of Deep Venous Thrombosis

History of previous DVT or varicose veins
Abdominothoracic, orthopaedic, and intracranial surgery
Cast immobilization of lower extremities or pelvic fractures
Situations and illnesses requiring prolonged physical immobilization, e.g., quadraplegia, myocardial infarction, and congestive heart failure
Obesity
Malignant neoplasms, e.g., adenocarcinomas or acute progranulocytic leukemia
Pregnancy
Oral contraceptives and other estrogen-containing medications
Transvenous catheters for diagnostic or therapeutic purposes, e.g., Hickman catheters, transfemoral pacemaker electrodes, hepatic vein catheters for localized chemotherapy delivery, or parenteral nutrition catheters
Significant muscular effort or stress-producing DVT of upper extremities, e.g., baseball pitchers, weight lifters, or air hammer operators
Anatomic compression of venous systems, e.g., thoracic outlet syndrome
Polycythemia rubra vera
Paroxysmal nocturnal hemoglobinuria
Behçet's syndrome and other vasculitides, e.g., systemic lupus erythematosis
Homocystinuria
Dysfibrinogenemia
Antithrombin III deficiency
Plasminogen abnormality
Heparin-induced thrombocytopenia
Infusions of concentrates of vitamin K-dependent clotting factors

bolic steroids to enhance secretion of tissue plasminogen activator from venous endothelial cells and thus hasten clot lysis, no adequately controlled studies support its use.

If the superficial phlebitis extends proximally above the knee, a brief treatment with heparin may be indicated until symptoms resolve and physical activity is resumed. If no improvement occurs, venous ligation should be considered. Migratory recurrent superficial phlebitis may occur as a manifestation of occult or obvious malignancies (Trousseau's phenomenon).

Septic Thrombophlebitis

The incidence of septic thrombophlebitis has been gradually increasing with the use of indwelling central venous catheters in chronically ill patients. The catheters should be removed and treatment initiated with full doses of appropriate antibiotics and heparin followed by oral preparations of anticoagulants. Lytic therapy may be considered only if the thrombus is of recent origin (less than 7 to 10 days old) and if antibiotics are administered concomitantly.

Septic thrombophlebitis may also originate in pelvic vessels, particularly following septic abortions, and should be treated similarly. If no improvement occurs despite adequate antibiotic and anticoagulant therapy, surgical removal of the thrombus is indicated.

Iliofemoral Deep Venous Thrombosis

The rationale for treating iliofemoral DVT is to prevent lethal pulmonary emboli and to preserve venous value integrity to avoid the postphlebitic syndrome. Several studies suggest that these aims can be achieved best by employing fibrinolytic agents initially as adjuncts to subsequent conventional anticoagulation. Heparinization alone may prevent propagation of the thrombus, but early substantial clot lysis and venographic improvement are unusual. The degree of therapeutic benefit of lytic therapy is related to the age of the clot and the extent of thrombosis.

Patients with extensive clot involvement and with DVT symptoms of less than 1 week's duration appear to respond best, and the existing risk factors associated with development of DVT do not influence the success of the lytic therapy. Hence, thrombolytic therapy should be considered the initial treatment of choice for proximal DVT in any individual in whom the diagnosis is firmly documented by venography and in whom there are no contraindications (Table 2).

Proximal DVT in pregnant females requires alternative approaches to diagnosis and treatment. Invasive venography potentially exposes the fetus to undesirable irradiation, particularly if the DVT occurs in the first trimester. The irradiation effects of noninvasive radionuclide-labeled proteins or platelets should also be avoided. In addition, the sensitivity and specificity of IPG may be compromised by vascular compression from the enlarging uterus. When a DVT is suspected, IPG combined with limited venography in which the fetus is shielded should provide adequate information upon which therapeutic decisions can be reached. Full-dose heparin anticoagulation treatment should be initiated only if there is confirmatory venographic evidence of a proximal DVT. Heparin should be administered in some form up to the time of delivery, but then discontinued during labor or 4 to 8 hours before caesarean section. It should be resumed in moderate doses postpartum and continued until the patient is ambulatory. Anticoagulation treatment should be continued for at least 3 months.

TABLE 2 Clinical States Contraindicating Thrombolytic Therapy

Absolute contraindications
Major active bleeding site(s)
History of cerebrovascular accident within previous 2 months
Intracranial neoplasm, primary or metastatic
Malignant hypertension
Major surgery within previous 10–14 days
Postpartum state within previous 10–14 days
Organ biopsy within previous 10–14 days
Cardiopulmonary resuscitation within previous 10–14 days
Hemorrhagic diabetic retinopathy
Relative contraindications
Hemorrhagic diatheses associated with coagulation factor deficiencies, qualitative/quantitative platelet defects, or severe renal or hepatic disease
Recent major trauma
Recent significant gastrointestinal bleeding
Pregnancy
Bacterial endocarditis
High likelihood of left-side heart thrombus formations, e.g., mitral stenosis with atrial fibrillation or mural thrombus

If the DVT occurs in the third trimester, oral anticoagulant preparations can replace heparin postpartum for the remainder of the 3-month treatment. In either case, breast feeding is not recommended. Although both heparin and sodium warfarin have been associated with teratogenicity when administered in pregnancy, the latter is absolutely contraindicated because of the frequency and severity of its complications to the fetus. Heparin-associated defects are rare, but because they may occur, it is incumbent on the clinician to establish the diagnosis definitively and to analyze the risk-benefit ratio before initiating therapy. If the pregnant female has a calf-vein thrombosis, one may elect to withhold anticoagulation therapy unless serial IPG examinations demonstrate the gradual extension of the thrombus into the popliteal or iliofemoral veins.

CALF-VEIN THROMBOSIS

A DVT limited to calf veins is associated with low incidence of clinically significant pulmonary emboli; left untreated, however, approximately 20 percent of these clots will propagate proximally and increase the risk of embolic complications. In addition, calf-vein thrombi, which do not lyse spontaneously, may damage venous valves and produce sequelae of PPS. Therefore, unless contraindicated, conventional heparinization and oral anticoagulation therapy for 6 weeks to 3 months is recommended. If patients are at high risk for hemorrhagic complications, anticoagulation therapy can be deferred until serial IPGs reflect proximal extension of the clot. Because of the relatively low mortality and morbidity associated with calf-vein DVT, thrombolytic therapy with its potential complications is not usually considered. Randomized controlled studies remain to be performed to determine if lytic therapy can reduce the PPS consequences that may occur in 5 to 30 percent of patients with calf-vein DVT.

UPPER EXTREMITY DEEP VENOUS THROMBOSIS

Upper extremity DVT makes up less than 2 percent of all DVTs and is not usually complicated by clinical pulmonary emboli. In the upper extremity, PPS and propagation and recurrence of DVT are critical problems and should prompt the clinician to employ therapy for complete thrombolytic resolution, if possible. Thromboses of the major veins of the upper extremities are associated with muscular activity and stress to the upper arms, indwelling catheters in the central venous system, or compression of the venous vessels by tumor or anatomic structures, such as cervical ribs. In the superior vena cava syndrome (SVC) central DVT from compression by tumor or metastatic lymph node is considered to be a medical emergency and should be treated with high-dose steroids, radiation, and occasionally chemotherapy. One recent study described more rapid symptomatic improvement in patients who also received thrombolytic and anticoagulation therapy. Because of the increased intracranial pressure and risk in intracranial bleeding that may accompany the SVC syndrome, these latter modalities should be used cautiously, if at all.

THROMBOLYTIC THERAPY

Streptokinase (SK) and urokinase (UK) are the two most frequently administered fibrinolytic agents; UK, however, has neither been thoroughly evaluated in the treatment of DVT nor approved specifically for that indication. Nevertheless, several controlled studies support its lytic effectiveness. Both drugs promote the generation of the active lytic enzyme plasmin through their proteolytic action on the zymogen plasminogen; UK directly proteolyzes plasminogen, whereas SK must first form a complex with circulating plasminogen. The SK-plasminogen complex then functions as a proteolytic activator of residual circulating plasminogen, or fibrin-bound plasminogen, or both. Thus, the lytic state produced by SK often is associated with plasminogen depletion and the production of a potential, paradoxical hypercoagulable state.

Thrombolysis occurs when fibrin is degraded by the plasmin generated within a thrombus. This central location protects the plasmin from its specific circulating inhibitors. Circulating plasmin is available to degrade fibrinogen and other clotting factors and is more readily inactivated by inhibitors. Therefore, the pharmacologic ability to induce and sustain a lytic state can be monitored in the laboratory by (1) detecting circulating fibrinogen-fibrin degradation products (FDP) and their effects on clotting assays, (2) measuring absolute decreases in plasma fibrinogen concentrations, and (3) demonstrating that plasminogen has been consumed. These changes are reflected in any one of the following coagulation assays: partial thromboplastin time (PTT), thrombin time (TT), euglobulin clot lysis time, and titer of fibrinogen-fibrin degradation products. The clinician should be aware that the accuracy of plasma fibrinogen assays in lytic states may be compromised by large quantities of FDP and that the euglobulin clot lysis time may be unreliable in hypofibrinogenemic states. Recently, rapid enzyme-linked immunosorbent assay (ELISA) techniques have become available to measure the $Beta_{B1-42-}$ and $Beta_{15-42-}$ peptides, which are specifically cleaved from fibrin I and fibrin II by plasmin.

The in vivo effectiveness of fibrinolysis can be evaluated superficially by assessing changes in the physical signs and symptoms and more objectively by carrying out serial IPG, venograms, or indium 111-labeled platelet scans.

The rationale for administrating SK as the initial treatment of proximal DVT of recent onset is provided by the results of numerous randomized, controlled studies. Specifically, the rapid resolution of the thrombus, with restoration of venous patency and preservation of venous value integrity, clearly reduces the incidence of future PPS sequelae. Nevertheless, this possible benefit must be weighed against the potential increased risks of hemorrhagic complications as compared to routine anticoagulation therapy. Much of the risk of bleeding can be minimized by both careful patient selection and judicious patient manipulation during fibrinolytic therapy (Table 2).

Once the decision is made to pursue thrombolytic therapy, the patient's baseline coagulation time and hematologic status should be assessed. Previous use of acetylsalicylic acid-containing medications may increase the risk of hemorrhage. If hepaιin was initiated prior to documentation of the DVT and consideration of thrombolytic therapy, it should be discontinued to allow the PTT to return to a relatively safe level (between 1 ½ to 2 times normal control). At that time, SK can be administered according to the protocol listed in Table 3. Pretreatment with intravenous hydrocortisone is useful to minimize or prevent the allergic reactions (urticaria, pruritus, flushing, bronchospasm, and musculoskeletal pain) and febrile reaction (temperature elevations to 0.5° C) that develop in a significant proportion of patients. They are not an absolute indication to discontinue SK, and they should be treated symptomatically with additional corticosteroids, acetaminophen, or diphenhydramine.

Thrombolytic therapy should be maintained for 48 to 72 hours with repeat IPG or indium 111-labeled platelet scans to evaluate the success of achieving venous vessel patency. Theoretically, there is a risk of fragmenting the DVT and predisposing the patient to subsequent pul-

TABLE 3 Guidelines for Streptokinase Administration in Treatment of Proximal Deep Venous Thrombosis

Optimal patient selection
- Absence of absolute contraindications
- Evidence that potential benefits will outweigh potential risks
- Venographic documentation of proximal major venous vessel thrombosis
- Symptoms of DVT for less than 7 days
- No recent infections with streptococcal organisms
- No recent (less than 1 year) SK administration for previous DVT or pulmonary emboli

Therapeutic approach
- Obtain baseline laboratory tests (PT, PTT, TT, fibrinogen, FDP, hematocrit, and platelet count)
- Pretreat with 100 mg hydrocortisone IV
- Administer loading dose of SK, 250,000 U IV, over 20–30 minutes followed by continuous infusion of SK, 100,000 U/hour for 48–72 hours
- At conclusion of SK infusion, begin full-dose continuous heparin infusion without bolus *after* allowing TT or PTT to return to about twice control value
- Maintain heparin infusions for 5–7 days and then begin patient on oral anticoagulation or subcutaneous heparin regimens; overlap heparin and sodium warfarin for at least 5 days
- Continue maintenance anticoagulation for at least 3 months to prevent recurrent DVT

Laboratory monitoring
- Measure TT or PTT 4 hours after initiating SK therapy and then every 12 hours for duration of lytic therapy
- Maintain TT or PTT 1.5 to 5 times control levels
- If TT or PTT exceeds 5 times control levels, decrease or discontinue SK until laboratory values return to desired range; titrate SK dose thereafter

Patient management
- Pressure dressings or sandbags over sites of previous venotomy or arterial punctures
- Avoid unnecessary venipunctures and intramuscular injections
- Use small-gauge needles for venipunctures
- Monitor urine and stool specimens for blood daily
- Avoid unnecessary patient manipulation and movement
- Apply manual pressure to minor accessible bleeding sites
- If there is excessive bleeding locally or in vital organs, discontinue SK and administer fresh frozen plasma—or in extreme situations epsilon-aminocaproic acid—to reverse the lytic state.
- Advance activity and ambulation of patient as tolerated without discomfort during heparin therapy

monary embolization. In practice, however, this occurs no more frequently than with conventional anticoagulation alone (lower than 10 percent incidence) and is probably of little consequence if an adequate lytic state exists. The PTT or TT should be maintained between 1.5 and 5 times their normal control levels. There is no correlation between the degree of circulating lytic activity and the effectiveness of fibrinolysis. A direct correlation does exist, however, between the degree of circulating lytic activity and the incidence of hemorrhagic complications when the PTT or TT exceeds 5 times normal. The hemorrhagic complications of lytic therapy are attributable to the non-specific action of generated plasmin on pathogenic thrombi, normal hemostatic fibrin clots, and circulating fibrinogen. The inability to achieve a lytic state with SK may indicate high levels of antistreptococcal antibodies, and use of UK should be considered with a loading dose of 4,400 units per kilogram IV over 30 minutes followed by a continuous infusion of 4,400 units per kilogram per hour. The guidelines for SK are appropriate also for UK therapy. In the future, tissue plasminogen activator will be available as another alternative treatment of DVT. This agent is more specific for fibrin and should be associated with fewer hemorrhagic complications than has been either SK or UK.

Heparinization and eventual oral anticoagulation therapy are crucial to prevent rethrombosis at the site of endothelial injury and clot lysis. If an underlying malignancy is associated with recurrent or migratory DVT, sodium warfarin may be ineffective in preventing rethrombosis.

When heparin anticoagulation is the treatment of choice for DVT in any location, a loading dose of 5,000 to 7,500 units IV should be administered followed by 1,000 units per hour IV, titrated upward or downward to maintain the PTT between 1.5 to 2.5 times normal control values. After 5 to 7 days, sodium warfarin should be started orally at a daily dose of 10 to 15 mg, depending on the patient's age, liver function, concomitant medications that would inhibit or potentiate warfarin's effects, and body weight. Heparin and warfarin should be continued simultaneously for about 5 days, with the PT being maintained between 1.5 and 2.5 times normal control. This approach of concomitant overlapping therapies theoretically assures the maintenance of an adequate antithrombotic state during the time when the warfarin initially interferes with carboxylation of protein C (a vitamin K-dependent protein, the deficiency of which is associated with hypercoagulable states) and eventually increases antithrombin III levels and functional activity. Although conventional warfarin therapy is effective in preventing recurrent DVT, it is associated with a 20 percent incidence of bleeding complications. Therefore, new therapeutic options are being studied, including low-intensity warfarin therapy to maintain the PT at 15 seconds and adjusted-dose subcutaneous heparin every 12 hours to maintain the PTT at 1.5 times normal at 6 hours. These strategies appear equally effective in preventing rethrombosis without excessive bleeding. If rethrombosis occurs after 3 months of adequate anticoagulation therapy, the patient should be examined for any of the conditions predisposing to hypercoagulability (see Table 1), and anticoagulation therapy should be reinstituted for at least another 3 to 6 months. Caval interruption may also need to be considered.

Besides the bleeding complications of heparin and warfarin, the clinician should be alert to the onset of heparin-induced thrombocytopenia and the rare occurrence of warfarin-associated necrosis, both of which abnormalities are observed relatively early in therapy. Platelet counts should be monitored every 3 days for the first 2 to 3 weeks of heparin administration.

SURGICAL VENOUS INTERRUPTION FOR RECURRENT DVT

In patients who cannot be adequately anticoagulated, cannot tolerate anticoagulant medications, or continue to rethrombose or embolize despite adequate treatment with anticoagulant drugs, venacaval interruption remains a useful alternative therapy.

Surgical vena caval ligation, or clipping, is associated with a high incidence of chronic venous insufficiency and recurrent pulmonary emboli, as well as with significant operative mortality and morbidity. Vena caval filters can be inserted easily under local anesthesia and can be maintained without anticoagulation therapy. The Greenfield filter is associated with the fewest complications and has a high long-term patency rate, thereby reducing subsequent venous stasis sequelae. Recurrent pulmonary emboli have occurred in 3 percent of patients.

Surgical thrombectomies are rarely indicated because of their technical difficulty and rethrombosis rate. However, thrombectomies may be required when septic thrombophlebitis does not respond to conventional therapies.

POSTPHLEBITIC SYNDROME

JOHN N. CLASSEN, M.D.

For many years, deep venous thrombosis has been a dreaded disease primarily because of the danger of pulmonary embolism. Only in the last few decades has one come to respect, recognize, and understand pathophysiology of another complication, namely, the postphlebitic syndrome.

This syndrome is characterized by aching pain in the legs on standing, dependent edema leading to brawny induration, recurrent cellulitis, stasis dermatitis, secondary varicosities, ulceration, liposclerosis, venous claudication, causalgia, and leg cramps. The postphlebitic syndrome is not lethal as is pulmonary embolism. Nevertheless, its prolonged morbidity, representing a great economic burden to sufferers as well as to the community, makes it mandatory that we (1) take the necessary prophylactic steps to limit the condition and (2) recognize its earliest manifestations so that an educational and therapeutic program can be instituted that adds comfortable years to the lives of patients with this syndrome.

In 1984, deep venous thrombosis of the lower limbs was diagnosed in hospitals in the United States roughly 500,000 times. Only one study suggests that the incidence may be decreasing. Careful follow-up data reveal that after 6 months, 3 to 5 percent of patients will have developed signs of the post-phlebitic syndrome; after 10 years, 35 percent of patients will have had ulcerations. Historical figures cite that 0.5 percent of the population of Great Britain and the United States suffer from the syndrome.

ANATOMIC CONSIDERATIONS

To treat the condition properly, both the physician and the patient must understand the anatomic and pathophysiologic features of the venous drainage of the leg. The three main circulatory systems are the superficial, the deep, and the communicating. The first has little support since it is embedded in loose areolar connective tissue and normally transports at low pressure a minute percentage of the blood to the heart. The greater saphenous vein, draining the medial aspect of the leg, and the lesser saphenous vein, draining the lateral side, with their tributaries make up the superficial system. The deep veins lying beneath the investing fascia are well supported by muscle. Below the knee each artery is paralleled by two small veins known as venae comitantes. These vessels converge in the inferior posterior aspect of the popliteal space to form the popliteal vein, which also normally receives the lesser saphenous vein. The popliteal vein passes through the adductor foramen to Hunter's canal, where it becomes the superficial femoral vein. The superficial femoral vein, despite its name, is a deep vein and should not be confused with the long saphenous vein. About 2 inches below the inguinal ligament, the superficial femoral vein joins the deep femoral vein, which receives blood from the muscles of the thigh, and forms the common femoral vein. This vessel accepts the greater saphenous vein and then passes beneath the inguinal ligament to become the external iliac vein. Communicating veins connect the superficial and deep venous systems.

Normally, physiologic flow is from superficial to deep system. Competent valves prevent both retrograde flow and flow from deep to superficial system.

PATHOPHYSIOLOGIC CONSIDERATIONS

For the last 40 years, the cause-and-effect relationship between extensive deep vein thrombosis and the postphlebitic syndrome has been universally accepted. The thrombosis may be limited to either small veins, the popliteal vein, or the entire iliofemoral tract. Usually, symptomatic severity of the postphlebitic syndrome is proportional to the extent of the initial thrombosis and the frequency of recurrent phlebitis. Recurrent thrombosis adds further insult to an already inefficient peripheral pump.

When thrombosis occurs in a peripheral deep vein, it creates mild venous hypertension, reflected as mild edema. Later, this vein may recanalize and malignant venous hypertension may ensue. The vein then becomes a rigid tube with ravaged incompetent valves. The peripheral tissues are subjected to pressure of gravity as well as the force developed by the contractions of the gastrocnemius muscle. As the muscle contracts, blood is propelled caudad as well as cephalad. Because there are no proximal valves (in the thigh) to hold this blood column, it recedes when the muscle relaxes. Since the valves are incompetent below the knee, blood rushes toward the foot and horizontally to the skin through the lowest communicating vein. Ambulatory venous pressures in the foot may rise to 150 cm of water. Further dilatation develops rendering deep and communicating valves incompetent.

Bidirectional flow occurs in all three systems, but with muscle contractions, the predominant flow through the perforators is from deep to superficial systems. The more distal the incompetent valve, the severer the ravages to the subcutaneous tissue. The lowest perforators are in the gaiter area, so it is natural that this area suffers the most from venous hypertension when all three systems are defective. This great pressure must be absorbed by minute venules and capillaries. These vessels dilate and become permeable, and plasma escapes into the subcutaneous tissue. Fibrinogen is converted to fibrin. This conversion leads to depressed fibrinolysis and pericapillary fibrin cuffing. Proliferation of abnormal capillaries occurs. And oxygen exchange suffers.

SYMPTOMS AND TREATMENT

Edema

Edema, which collects primarily in the subcutaneous tissue, is the most common symptom. It may be mild and soft or massive, tense, and brawny. It can usually be controlled by a conservative regimen of rest, elevation, and support of the limb. Sometimes a diuretic must be administered. Chlorthalidone, 50 to 100 mg every day, plus a potassium supplement is far more effective than furosemide. Mechanical compression with the Jobst therapeutic pump may be useful. For extreme indurated swelling, a Lymphpress apparatus is indicated.

Prolonged swelling may produce brawny edema, liposclerosis, and even ossification of the subcutaneous tissues. Fibrosis of the structures about the ankle joint leads to talipes equinus. Although limitation of motion in the ankle joint reduces the efficiency of the peripheral venous pump, physical therapy and exercise help to restore normal function.

Sometimes liposclerosis develops. This condition is painful and incapacitating. It is best treated with stanozolol, an anabolic steroid. A regimen of 5 mg by mouth twice a day for 3 months is prescribed. Weight gain and virilization are rare undesirable side effects. Occasionally, the area must be excised.

Ulcers

Ulcers are a frequent unpleasant complication of the postphlebitic syndrome. They occur after many years of venous hypertension in the gaiter area where ambulatory venous pressures are greatest due to the low incompetent communicating veins. An ulcer is initiated by minor trauma to the skin and edematous subcutaneous tissue. Once the skin is broken, secondary infection ensues. The ulcer is difficult to heal and likely to recur in the atrophic scar.

Each ulcer should be cultured and cleaned and proper support placed. If surrounding cellulitis and marked swelling develop, continuous warm compresses are applied from the knee to and including the foot, and strict bedrest with a 15 degree elevation of the foot is instituted. Appropriate systemic antibiotics are prescribed. When the cellulitis subsides, an Unna boot is applied. At first, it should be changed every 3 to 5 days, depending on the amount of secretion. Later, it should be replaced every 2 to 3 weeks until the ulcer heals, a process that may take 2 to 3 months. Prolonged indolence suggests malignancy (Marjolin's ulcer). Although rare, it indicates the need to have a biopsy of the tissue. Failure of the ulcer to heal in 4 months warrants hospitalization. Usually excision of the ulcer and its bed as well as the incompetent perforating vein must be performed. A split-thickness meshed graft may be used to cover the defect. Occasionally, pinch grafts on clean granulation also lead to healing. When the ulcer heals, the regimen of rest, elevation, and support is continued.

Topical agents to the ulcerated area must be used judiciously. Ointments tend to mascerate, steroid creams are contraindicated, and many preparations appear to precipitate or aggravate existing stasis dermatitis.

Stasis Dermatitis

With chronic edema, the skin of the legs—particularly around the ankles—may become eczematous. The dermatitis may arise independently or around an ulcer. It can be caused by either irritation from the ulcerous ooze or sensitivity to local applications. By absorption of the sensitizing substance, the eczema may become widespread and even generalized. Id reactions on the hand are seen. Treatment is aimed at eradicating ulcerous secretions. As infection subsides, secretions diminish. Warm saline compresses are beneficial. Steroid creams should be applied to the area of dermatitis but not to the ulcer. No other medications should be used locally. Severe generalized reactions may dictate systemic steroid therapy for 3 to 5 days.

Pain

Pain is a prominent symptom for many patients. It is described as a dull ache that develops on standing and increases as the day passes. The pain is more noticeable when the patient is stationary and eases with movement. Elevation of the feet for 5 to 10 minutes relieves the symptoms. Muscular cramps may occur. A quinine sulfate preparation (Quinamm) is curative. Infected ulcers and diffuse cellulitis are associated with severe pain, but eradication of the infection by proper antibiotic therapy brings prompt relief.

Occasionally, a causalgia-like pain (unremitting) develops in a leg exposed to severe and prolonged stasis. Lumbar sympathetic blocks can relieve the pain and break the cycle. Sympathectomy is rarely necessary. Neuritis of the long saphenous nerve has also been reported; entrapment of the nerve in a large fibrotic medial patellar fat pad is the cause. Resecting the fat pad with careful skeletization and isolation of the nerve can remedy the neuritis.

Cellulitis

Cellulitis may either be associated with an ulcer or develop independently. Some clinicians believe that the infection in an ulcer is only on the surface, and hence antibiotic therapy is contraindicated. Frequently, I see patients who are neglected because of this misconception. Some ulcers, which have been present for months or years, heal when they are cultured and appropriate drug therapy is instituted.

Cellulitis developing de novo is precipitated by a focal portal of entry or by a transient bacteremia. The capillary stasis in the leg allows bacteria to multiply and become entrenched. Each attack of cellulitis causes more scarring and stasis, thus making the tissues more susceptible to infection. The streptococcus microorganism is frequently the culprit and may produce the classic picture of erysipelas. Erythromycin or ampicillin and continuous warm compresses with elevation comprise the desired treatment. Sometimes several attacks occur yearly. In that case, a regimen of prophylactic chemotherapy must be programmed to prevent unacceptable long periods of absenteeism.

Venous Claudication

This term refers to a bursting pain in the thigh associated with occlusion of the iliac vein on that side. A contralateral saphenous vein bypass to the ipsilateral femoral vein is then in order.

Psychosis

Many physicians, attempting to alert patients who have had one bout of deep vein thrombosis to the dangers of recurrent deep venous thrombosis and possible pulmonary embolism, precipitate great mental anguish in the patient and his family. Every twinge of pain in the calf or chest may be regarded as potentially catastrophic. Many patients live a life of fear, entering the hospital often for repeated diagnostic studies or even heparin therapy. Continual reassurance rather than antiocoagulant therapy is the desired approach.

SURGICAL APPROACH

Once the acute symptoms have been eased, all patients must be investigated to define the exact anatomicophysiologic deficit.

In recent years, the value of noninvasive tests to reveal the degree of reflux and stasis has been documented. Photoplethysmography is a useful clincial screening test. Directional Doppler and foot volumetry studies, as well as plethysmography, may be used. Phlebography, however, should be performed to demonstrate the exact location of incompetent veins before surgical treatment is undertaken. Both descending and ascending phlebographic studies have a definite role. The former is particularly helpful when one is considering valvuoplasty or vein transplantation in the femoral region. Ascending phlebography with tourniquets at appropriate levels can demonstrate incompetent perforators. Many patients are not good candidates for surgery. Nevertheless, adequate studies reveal that a few patients benefit from ligation and stripping of the greater saphenous system. More patients have the incompetent posterior perforator syndrome of Crockett. Local extrafascial ligation of these three communicating veins can be curative if the major symptoms are related to this area. However, most patients have many incompetent perforators on the lateral and medial side of the leg. Subfascial ligation of these communicating veins through a long stocking-seam incision is proper.

Although not curative, these operations should lessen the pressure exerted on the soft tissues in the gaiter area. All patients must adhere to the basic regimen of rest, elevation, and support of the limb.

In recent years, attention has turned to direct venous reconstruction. Valvuloplasty and transposition of a vein with a competent valve from the femoral region into the iliofemoral tract have been performed. Even free vein grafts have been inserted. Initial enthusiasm for the first attack waned rapidly as follow-up studies revealed that venous pressures tended to return to high presurgical levels in 6 to 24 months. Husni, one of the early investigators in this work, no longer performs the procedures and questions their justification. Certainly, more clinical investigation is needed. At present, this work cannot be regarded as an acceptable modality for routine use.

Femorofemoral venous bypass for isolated iliac obstruction, using the contralateral saphenous vein, is beneficial, and the effects are long lasting.

Although helpful, these modalities are not curative. Although the postphlebitic syndrome cannot be cured, it can be controlled. Every patient, regardless of how symptoms present or are treated, must realize this fact and be prepared to stay on a rigid conservative regimen of rest, elevation, and support for life. Many patients are controlled by this way of life.

Foot hygiene must be meticulous. Fungal infection leads to recurrent phlebitis or cellulitis. Routine potassium permanganate soaks can control fungal infection. The foot of the bed should be elevated 6 inches on shock blocks or a 6-inch foam rubber wedge placed between the mattress and boxspring. Elevation of feet on pillows is not a satisfactory substitute. A gradient compression stocking or garment must be worn at all times. Knee-length hose suffice for most patients. Many of them prefer the leotard garment. Long leg stockings are not satisfactory and indeed are contraindicated since an abnormality other than swelling does not occur above the knee. Although custom-made gradient compression stocking is preferable, expense may dictate a ready-made one. Support products lose their effectiveness in 4 to 6 months, but infrequent washings can extend the life of the garment or stocking.

Furthermore, early diagnosis of deep venous thrombosis and prompt treatment to limit extension of the clot are twin imperatives. Patients with the postphlebitic syndrome are in the high-risk group to develop recurrent deep venous thrombosis when placed in stressful medical and surgical situations. Accordingly, prophylactic use of heparin or intermittent venous compression therapy should be instituted in these settings.

The postphlebitic syndrome is an incapacitating and incurable condition, best controlled by following a regimen of rest, elevation, and support and preventing recurrent bouts of deep venous thrombosis. Individual symptoms require specific conservative measures. Occasionally surgical treatment to reduce local venous hypertension is helpful, but it is not a panacea.

SINUS NODE DYSFUNCTION

M. IRENÉ FERRER, M.D.

Viewed in a clinical setting, disordered function of the sinoatrial node comprises a constellation of signs, symptoms, electrocardiographic abnormalities, cerebral dysfunctions, and the trilogy of sinus bradycardia, arrest, and exit block (these last three are often but not always simultaneously or sequentially present). Periodic rapid atrial arrhythmias and chronic atrial fibrillation can also be seen.

The incidence of the dysfunction is still as yet uncertain, although statistics on pacemakers suggest that patients with the sick sinus syndrome may even exceed in number those with atrioventricular or intraventricular block.

At present, the greatest difficulty in diagnosing disease of the primary pacemaker is to spot its earliest falterings. The disorder, which goes on slowly but relentlessly in most cases, can start with intermittent failures. When seen, the patient may present no clue, either spontaneously or during provocative interventions with drugs, exercise, or pacing. This sick sinus disorder is not rare, and the problem of documenting its incidence is real since no prospective survey is yet available. For example, if one seeks the end stage of the syndrome, when pacing is essential, recent statistics show that approximately 400,000 people throughout the world are now living with a pacemaker; nearly 156,000 of them live in the United States (1 out of every 1,300 Americans).

In the United States, the rate of implantation for pacemakers is 270 per million; that means that 60,000 people per year receive a pacing unit.It is now thought that at least one-half (perhaps more) of these patients need pacing for a failing sinoatrial node, and most of the rest for complete heart block. Thus, perhaps 30,000 individuals are being diagnosed as having late stages of sinoatrial nodal disease. The only prospective attempt to determine incidence comes to us from Devon, England, where Shaw and Kekwick surveyed the same community of 600,000 people for 8 consecutive years to determine the incidence of heart block and sinoatrial disorders. A total of 436 patients with the sick sinus sydrome were seen in 8 years (79 or 18 percent of them had pacemakers). The calculated incidence of the sick sinus syndrome is 108 per million.

ETIOLOGY

In a cellular aggregate such as the sinoatrial (SA) node, faltering of function might be explained by the pathologic etiology. Unfortunately, such is not the case. Early in our knowledge of the sick sinus and its effects, only one or two cases were studied pathologically. Coronary arterial disease was blamed; however, in a recent review (adding eight cases of their own), Evans and Shaw found no evidence that coronary arterial atherosclerosis was the cause of nodal disorder; rather, they found atrophy and fibrosis of the nodal tissue. Those investigators agree that the etiology of a disturbed node is multifactorial and include in their list not only infiltrative diseases (such as amyloidosis, tumor cells and leukemia), fibrosis of unknown post-infectious or autoimmune origin, and idiopathic degenerative processes, but also, when pathologic defects appear totally absent, enzyme disturbances of the P cells, such as abnormal metabolism of cholinesterase. Since the syndrome is most common in the elderly, it was assumed, incorrectly, that atherosclerosis of the SA nodal artery might play a role. However, any consistent association has been ruled out, especially since the artery supplying the SA node is not of a size usually affected by atherosclerosis, although it may be the site of emboli, arteritis, or necrotic lesions. Investigators agree that the etiology of SA node dysfunction is multifactorial (Table 1). The syndrome is seen in patients with myocarditis and other inflammatory conditions, various collagen diseases (e.g., rheumatoid arthritis), and infiltrative diseases affecting the atria (specifically, amyloidosis and hemochromatosis).

TABLE 1 Diseases Producing Sinus Node Dysfunction

Ischemic, sclerotic, rheumatic, and other inflammatory conditions
Pericarditis
Cardiomyopathies
Friedreich's ataxia
Muscular dystrophy
Collagen disease
Surgical injury to SA node
Metastatic disease
Amyloidosis
Hemochromatosis
Fibrotic infiltration of unknown cause
Familial SA node disease
Surdocardiac state

According to the limited pathologic data that we have, a nonspecific degenerative fibrosis is definitely involved in some cases. Further, the fibrosis, when present, is evidently not limited to disturbing the SA node. The atrioventricular (AV) node, as well as the bundle of His and bundle branch systems at times, is also "nibbled at," if not grossly damaged. This factor may become critical when the SA node fails completely and other pacemaker tissues must take over to rescue the heart. When anatomic lesions are absent, the cause of SA nodal disease may be an enzyme disturbance in pacemaker cells. Abnormal cholinesterase metabolism has been implicated.

It is relevant, of course, that this region of the heart is subject to biochemical influences through the cholinergic and adrenergic postganglionic fibers, which are so abundant in the vicinity of, but not within, the SA node. Parasympathetic and sympathetic effects are carried to the node by chemical neurotransmitters (acetylcholine and norepinephrine) liberated from these fibers. The neurotransmitters must reach and effectively bathe the pacemaker cells within the SA node by traversing the surrounding matrix of collagen. As a corollary, some cases of the sick sinus syndrome may represent a combination of a partial anatomic lesion and vagal stimulation, causing the release of acetylcholine from nerve terminals. When relieved of the effect of marked vagal discharge (e.g., by atropine), the SA node may become functional again. Conversely, a dysfunctional node may not be recognized as such because endogenous catecholamines, liberated by various stimuli, can speed up the rate of a failing SA node and fool us.

The association of sick sinus syndrome with acute myocardial infarction deserves special mention. The SA node is often damaged in patients who develop atrial arrhythmias after infarction. However, atrial damage seldom occurs in patients with isolated occlusion of the left anterior descending artery (anteroseptal infarcts), and atrial arrhythmias do not appear with disease of this vessel alone. Atrial damage is common, by contrast, after occlusion of the main right coronary artery (inferior infarcts) and left circumflex artery (anterolateral infarcts). This should not be too surprising, since one or the other of these vessels provides the SA node and surrounding atrium with its nutrient artery. Dysfunction of the SA node develops in about 15 percent of patients with inferior infarcts.

Postinfarction disruption of the SA node also deserves mention. We have noted that there are cholinergic terminals near the SA node, and ischemia at these sites may cause marked slowing of the sinus rate. Sinus bradycardia in this setting may result from cholinergic stimuli, therefore, and not from primary anatomic damage to the SA node. True nodal dysfunction, if it is to arise, usually does so in the first 4 days of the infarction. Patients who show signs of nodal dysfunction during this period, but appear to recover, should have careful follow-up indefinitely. The more chronic manifestations, probably due to a gradual fibrosis, may take several months or even years to become permanent. If this possibility is overlooked, a late syncopal episode could be fatal.

CLINICAL MANIFESTATIONS

The manifestations of the sick sinus syndrome are those of hypoperfusion of critical circulations due to sinus bradycardia, sinus arrest, or the trachyarrhythmias that arise as escape rhythms. Thus, syncopal attacks, dizziness, and lightheadedness are common symptoms when cerebral blood flow is reduced. But one must be alert also to more subtle changes, such as irritability, fleeting memory loss, or nocturnal wakefulness. The patient may be less aware of such symptoms than are his family or friends and, therefore, may give a negative history. If the patient is elderly, symptoms are often ascribed to senility, and that diagnosis is missed.

Transitory but repeated sinus bradycardia sets the stage for mild ventricular failure, especially if there is underlying coronary disease. Then, tachyarrhythmia follows—usually either atrial fibrillation with a rapid ventricular response or atrial tachycardia—and severe ventricular failure with pulmonary edema brings the patient to the emergency room. By this time, however, the tachyarrhythmia may have ceased, and one finds a patient in respiratory distress with an inappropriately slow sinus rate. This picture should immediately suggest the sick sinus syndrome.

Symptomatology thus varies considerably with the state of vital organs, e.g., the brain, heart, and kidneys, as well as with the type of rhythmic disturbance. Patients with cerebrovascular, cardiac, or renal disease may have dramatic symptoms, with episodes of bradycardia or tachycardia being triggered. Others, without associated disease, may have no significant symptoms. In the latter group, occasional palpitations, unexplained fatigue, muscle aches, or periodic oliguria may seem to be so vague a constellation of complaints that the underlying cardiac disorder is overlooked.

DIAGNOSIS

At present, the diagnostic criteria for full-blown failure of the SA node are still to be found in the clinical electrocardiogram (ECG); however, provocative testing by atrial pacing methods can uncover less definite dysfunction. In a study of 51 patients with sinus bradycardia, Reiffel and Bigger searched for the electrocardiographic criteria of spontaneously occurring SA nodal dysfunction, using continuous electrocardiographic monitoring (Holter) coupled to functional testing (by atrial pacing) of the SA node; these two methods together represent our best means of finding the patient with the sick sinus syndrome. Neither test alone was as effective in sorting out subjects with basically disturbed SA nodes from the physiologic (nonpathologic) variants. A new approach to testing the function of the SA node has been initiated by Cramer et al, whose recent physiologic information describes direct action potentials from the SA node now observed in man.

An unfortunate side effect of the great interest in the sick sinus syndrome is that some subjects with sinus bradycardia alone are incorrectly labeled as having disordered behavior of the SA node and even have been offered pacemakers. It is urgent to disseminate knowledge concerning the normal effects of the autonomic nervous system (ANS) on the SA node, effects that may be extreme and produce the slow rate, sinus arrest, and exit block. Vagotonia is common; its production springs from many areas, e.g., gastrointestinal causes, pain, and the mechanical effects of pregnancy and labor. Again, continuous electrocardiographic monitoring (for 24 hours) and (possibly) functional testing should precede any diagnosis of the sick sinus syndrome, especially if the diagnosis is based solely on the presence of sinus bradycardia. By the same token, primary dysfunction of the ANS, in contrast to physiologic (or normal) effects, can produce all the characteristics of the sick sinus syndromes. Hence, autonomic activity should be tested by mechanical or pharmacologic means. Finally, the SA node may become either unresponsive to appropriate autonomic activity or hypersensitive to vagal stimuli, both of which are forms of dysfunction of the SA node.

The human pacemaker is a highly complex structure whose numerous interacting components must be delicately tuned to ensure integrated, effective control of the heart's electrical behavior. Normal function of the SA node depends on a complex and delicately balanced interaction between intrinsic electrophysiologic properties of the SA node, SA conduction, and extrinsic factors outside the region. The ANS has probably the most important role of all the extrinsic influences. The multifaceted influences on nodal function are predictive of the statement that can be made today of the sick sinus syndrome, namely, that this syndrome is not a homogenous physiopathologic entity, as recently stressed by Jordan and associates, and that intrinsic failure of the node, as opposed to disorders of the extrinsic regulators (autonomic) of the pacemaker, must be differentiated to arrive at rational pacing or medical therapy.

ELECTROCARDIOGRAPHIC FINDINGS

The failing SA node expresses dysfunction by a slowing of its automaticity, so that the pacemaker discharges less frequently. This is somewhat paradoxical, since other automatic cardiac tissues, such as the His-Purkinje or specialized atrial fibers, respond to noxious stimuli with acceleration of their automaticity. Be that as it may, the sick sinus syndrome usually begins with episodes of sinus bradycardia, which may be sustained or intermittent. Despite the slowing of rate, the ECG shows a normal P wave followed by both a normal QRS and a normal P-R interval. By definition, sinus bradycardia is present when the heart rate slows to fewer than 60 beats per minute. In SA nodal dysfunction, one not only sees such bradycardia, but also may get inappropriate responses to normally tachycardic stimuli. For example, the rate may fail to rise in response to an exercise test or with severe pain, febrile episodes, or acute left ventricular failure. Such a patient has a relatively slow sinus rate, perhaps due to a dysfunctional SA node.

In fact, the sick sinus syndrome often escapes notice at an early stage because only sinus bradycardia is present in its inception. Sinus bradycardia has been presented as essentially harmless, if not advantageous, and indicative of athletic conditioning. Another pitfall is the slow heart rate of a patient receiving digitalis for congestive heart failure. The usual assumption is that the slow heart rate is drug-induced, especially in the elderly. The possibility of a failing SA node, most likely in this age group, therefore can be overlooked. Instead, digitalis dosage may be reduced or eliminated entirely, leaving the patient without life-preserving inotropic support.

Both sinus bradycardia and SA exit block in its various forms are evidence that function of the SA node is depressed. At a later stage, sinus function deteriorates further, and sinus arrest appears intermittently for one, two, or (rarely) three beats at a time. Cardioactive drugs (e.g., digitalis, quinidine, and procainamide) can elicit periodic sinus arrest or SA exit block, as can excess potassium. Therefore, other possibilities have to be excluded before diagnosing intrinsic SA nodal dysfunction.

All three of the arrhythmic states mentioned—sinus bradycardia, SA exit block, and sinus arrest—can be mimicked exactly by excess vagal discharge. Moderate or even severe vagotonia may have many causes, ranging from strong emotion to acute illness associated with retching or pain. Gastrointestinal disorders are likely to stimulate the vagus nerve.

ESCAPE RHYTHMS

With advancing SA node disease, there may be longer periods of pacemaker silence, leading to complete cessation of sinus rhythm. This may provoke a fatal arrhythmia or death from cardiac arrest itself, although neither event occurs often. Generally, at the stage when sinus rhythm ceases entirely, a nonsinus rhythm takes over for the silenced SA node, at least temporarily. The escape rhythm may be atrial or junctional in origin, occurring at relatively slow rates (55 to 75 beats per minute). When SA dysfunction is even more severe, the escape rhythm is usually atrial fibrillation. However, there is really no way to distinguish atrial fibrillation of this type from atrial fibrillation in patients without sick SA nodes, unless previous cardiac rhythms are known to be present in the patient.

One clue to differential diagnosis is a slow ventricular rate accompanying atrial fibrillation, without concurrent administration of drugs such as digitalis or propranolol. The slow rate is evidence that organic disease in the AV node is producing some degree of AV block. (At least 30 percent of patients with the sick sinus syndrome have binodal disease). This distinction is important, since treatment to eliminate atrial fibrillation can be disastrous if the SA node is inoperative or failing.

There is a reverse side to the coin, moreover, when episodes of atrial fibrillation occur in the absence of AV disease and block. In this situation, basic sinus bradycardia is present at most times; then paroxysms of atrial fibrillation appear and are repeated, causing rapid ventricular rhythms. The usual approach, given a patient with chronic atrial fibrillation and a rapid ventricular rate, is to administer digitalis to control the arrhythmia; if this does not work, cardioversion may be employed. Sinus rhythm does not resume, however, if the SA node is sluggish or silent.

The atrial or junctional escape rhythms that take over when sinus rhythm ceases tend to be unstable and often slow, and they may cease entirely. Such patients require artificial pacing at once, but the need for pacing may be only temporary if atrial fibrillation resumes. Unlike some other investigators, we have not found atrial fibrillation to be a permanent rescue rhythm, although it often persists for long periods. It, too, can be an unstable atrial rhythm. When it ceases, a slow heart rate (due to sinus bradycardia, slow junctional or atrial rhythm, or SA exit block) soon returns. The patient is whom pacing is not instituted may then be left without any safe rhythm at all.

Disease of the SA node of the type just described is referred to as the bradycardia-tachycardia syndrome. Sinus bradycardia is punctuated by episodes of atrial arrhythmia with fast ventricular rates (often atrial fibrillation, atrial flutter, and atrial tachycardia in the same patient). In flagrant forms of the bradycardia-tachycardia syndrome, the patient may switch from severe bradycardia to fast heart rates during atrial fibrillation and do this many times in the course of a few hours. Unless there is some degree of AV block, the ventricular response may produce rates as high as 200 beats per minute.

Extraordinary fluctuations of heart rate can occur. For example, during an ECG recording, an 89-year-old woman was found to have sinus bradycardia at a rate of 20 to 46 beats per minute, atrial fibrillation with a ventricular rate of 180 beats per minute, and post-tachycardia pauses (with no escape rhythm intervening) of 1.5 to 2.5 seconds; one pause lasted 11.4 seconds, the equivalent of a heart rate of five to six beats per minute. Continuous ambulatory ECG monitoring has revealed many more such sequences in patients than were suspected before the technique became available. Not surprisingly, the bradycardia-tachycardia syndrome may have serious hemodynamic consequences, producing heart failure and syncope.

Diagnosing the sick sinus syndrome may be a problem because the disorder often takes a slow and erratic course, with eventual progression to final and permanent failure of the SA node. In the interim, the patient may have intermittent sinus arrest or intermittent SA exit block, neither of which is ever evident on a routine ECG, which samples electrical activity only for brief periods. SA exit block with dropped beats may be missed if, instead of having a regular sinus rate, the patient has a marked sinus arrhythmia. Similarly, a routine ECG may be inadequate for showing the mechanism of a paroxysmal atrial fibrillation, that is, its appearance as an escape rhythm after a long sinus pause.

Continuous ECG monitoring often documents the presence of a failing SA node when it is otherwise inapparent. Certainly, any patient with sinus bradycardia and suggestive symptoms should be monitored in this fashion. All complexes are recorded for a 24-hour period and should include at least one complete sleep-awake activity cycle. Severe sinus bradycardia (<20 to 30 beats per minute) or periodic sinus arrest often appears only during sleep or becomes maximal at that time. An attempt to stimulate a flagging SA node by moderate exercise (e.g., rapid arm or leg flexion, hopping up and down) may also be useful. In these patients, the rise in heart rate during exercise is blunted.

NATURAL HISTORY

The deficiency of knowledge regarding the basic natural history of the sick sinus syndrome is gradually being diminished. The splendid report by Lien et al from the Republic of China on the longitudinal survey of 52 patients provides important data in this sector, showing duration of the disease as long as 29 years and stressing the intermittency of the dysfunction in many subjects. Boal and Kleinfeld also have noted long durations (up to 33 years) of the syndrome; however, adequate prediction of the stage of the dysfunction has eluded us to date. Especially weak in the young or middle-aged patient, the ability to tag the danger zone of malfunction in any one person is perhaps best now in the elderly patient, in whom the dysfunction usually progresses more rapidly. The correct timing of insertion of a pacemaker depends on the prediction of dangerous symptoms. This problem of timing remains difficult to solve until the natural history of the syndrome is better known.

DECISIONS IN THERAPY

The treatment of choice for the present is to substitute an electrical demand pacemaker for an ailing SA node. Ventricular pacing is preferred since associated disease of the AV conduction system is often present as well. When tachyarrhythmias are part of the syndrome and no organic AV block exists, it is best to provide pharmacologic AV block to control atrial fibrillation, flutter, or tachycardia to limit the ventricular rate. As a rule, long-term pacing does not prevent the reappearance of tachycardiac arrhythmias. However, they can be rendered almost imperceptible to the patient if the controlled ventricular rate approximates the pacing rate. It is rare for ectopic ventricular activity to appear in patients with sick sinus syndrome, so no treatment is needed in this respect.

One would like to be able to predict the crucial time for inserting an artificial pacemaker. But although it is agreed that around 20 or 30 percent of patients with the sick sinus syndrome need pacing, prognosis is uncertain with respect to any individual patient. Sinus bradycardia may progress to various forms of exit block or may simply become increasingly severe until no sinus beats occur. The escape rhythms, at first only periodic rescuers, eventually become the basic mechanism. In fact, atrial fibrillation is the only stable long-term replacement rhythm that arises, but it may not remain so for long.

Failure of the SA node may proceed slowly at first but then speed up, producing a disastrous asystole or cardiac failure if therapy is delayed or ignored.

A tragic example comes to mind of a child who had periods of sinus arrest and SA nodal dysfunction first documented when he was 3 months old. A conscientious pediatrician followed up with periodic functional testing until the child was 12 years old, at which time he was doing so well that the parents refused further care. The boy died suddenly at age 15 years.

Thus, the dilemma is real. It is difficult to inflict a permanent pacemaker on a patient (especially a young one) unless the indications are clear-cut. Yet once symptomatic disease is diagnosed, one probably should consider artificial pacing in the near future for safety's sake, since the exact progression and timing of complications are unknown. An asymptomatic disorder of the SA node can be watched, of course, unless rates are excessively slow or the rapid arrhythmias appear to be dangerous.

DIGITALIS AND THE SA NODE

Antiarrhythmic drugs directed at episodes of tachyarrythmia generally are not effective in the syndrome. Digitalis therapy is a controversial issue. Judging from animal studies, the risk to an already severely bradycardic subject would be a further slowing of the heart rate. In addition, by prolonging the pause following a bout of tachycardia or atrial premature depolarizations, digitalis could increase the likelihood of syncope or other complications. Ambulatory monitoring, maximal treadmill tests, and atrial stimulation techniques all have been utilized to define more clearly the effects of digitalis in the SA node. In fact, most such studies have shown insignificant changes in exercise or resting sinus rates, slight prolongation of SA conduction time, and a shortening of postoverdrive sinus node recovery time in response to digoxin or ouabain.

For example, Reiffel et al studied a group of 35 patients with SA nodal dysfunction, using atrial stimulation and pacing techniques. After digoxin (0.75 mg IV), sinus cycle length increased in some patients and decreased in others. For the group as a whole, the rate was unchanged, SA conduction time was increased, and maximal sinus node recovery time was shortened. Some of the patients had clinical indications for digitalis therapy and had not been receiving it previously; they were continued on digoxin therapy after the study. Of the nine patients available for follow-up, all but one tolerated long-term digitalization without difficulty. The remaining patient, who had developed SA block of the Wenckebach type during electrophysiologic study, was given a permanent pacemaker but continued to have SA block.

If carefully evaluated, probably most patients with sick sinus syndrome can be given digitalis for an accompanying cardiac arrhythmia or ventricular failure. If symptoms are amenable to pacemaker therapy, e.g., syncope from SA arrest or AV block, pacing should be instituted by all means. If symptoms are due to a condition that may be controlled with digitalis, e.g., ventricular failure or syncope from post-tachycardia pauses, digitalis should be given as necessary. It may be wise to evaluate the effects of digitalis by acute digitalization during an in-hospital electrophysiologic study; the same protocol probably should be used in selecting other antiarrhythmic drugs to control episodes of atrial fibrillation or rapid ventricular response. Each drug being tested is administered in increasing doses, carefully monitored, to arrive at the best drug or dosage for the purpose.

ATRIAL AND VENTRICULAR ECTOPIC BEATS

BERNARD TABATZNIK, M.D., F.R.C.P.

To find a proper accommodation between overkill and underplay in the treatment of the patient with extrasystoles requires a careful assessment of the importance of a particular ectopic rhythm in a particular individual, mature judgment, and a modicum of courage. The ventricular ectopic beat (VEB) has been described as a ''trick of the healthy heart'' (Evans) and a ''harbinger of sudden death'' (Lown). Factors that determine the prognostic role of the VEB in an individual patient are, first and foremost, 'the company it keeps,'' and second, certain qualitative features of the ectopic activity. These, together with a critical appreciation of the efficacy and dangers of antiarrhythmic drug therapy, form a clinical tripod that determines treatment in a given patient.

VENTRICULAR ECTOPIC ACTIVITY: CLINICAL CONTEXT

A simplistic view of sudden death is that it results from an interaction between the ''seed'' (ventricular ectopic activity), the ''soil'' (the state of the myocardium), and ''spring rains'' (a variety of factors, including acute ischemia; central and autonomic nervous system factors; and metabolic factors, such as hypokalemia, drug effects, anoxia, and extremes of heat and cold, which may render cardiac tissue abnormally excitable and act as the trigger mechanism for ventricular fibrillation). Thus, it is understandable that even highly complex ventricular ectopic activity, such as ventricular tachycardia, seldom progresses to ventricular fibrillation if the heart is structurally normal; that bizarre ventricular arrhythmias in patients with mitral valve prolapse may be observed for long periods of time without leading to sudden death; and that the risk of sudden death is seemingly lessened in the surgically revascularized patient even though ventricular ectopic activity has not been substantially reduced.

On the other hand, even minor ventricular ectopic activity may be compounded by ventricular tachycardia or fibrillation in the patient with an acutely injured heart as, for example, in acute myocardial infarction or acute myocarditis. Between these categories are patients with VEBs in association with chronic ischemic heart disease, hypertrophic cardiomyopathy, and the concentrically hypertrophied hearts of hypertension and aortic valve stenosis, the dilated hearts of chronic rheumatic valvular disease and congestive cardiomyopathy, the long QT syndromes, and survivors of ventricular fibrillation, all with varying degrees of susceptibility to sudden death. Within the category of chronic ischemic heart disease itself, the risk varies appreciably, from the very high risk in the first 6 months after infarction, particularly in patients with compromised left ventricular function, to a much lower risk in the long-term survivor with efficient myocardial function. In the high-risk groups, the most intensive measures needed to suppress ventricular ectopic activity are justified, whereas in low-risk groups, antiarrhythmic drug therapy should be undertaken only after due consideration of the total clinical picture.

CHARACTERISTICS OF VENTRICULAR ECTOPY

Numerous studies have confirmed a prognostic role for complex ventricular ectopy in patients with chronic ischemic heart disease. Although there have been different definitions of complexity and much argument about the value and limitations of various grading systems for Holter-identified arrhythmias, there has been an association in most studies between complex ventricular ectopic rhythms and both sudden and nonsudden cardiac death. Some studies (including my own) have shown a linear association between complexity and sudden death; others have indicated a prognostic role for only the severer grades of ectopy, such as ventricular tachycardia. And many studies have demonstrated a prognostic power for ventricular ectopy independent of other factors, such as myocardial dysfunction. Much of the confusion in this area has stemmed from the fact that left ventricular dysfunction is also an important predictor of mortality; it has been difficult to separate the respective prognostic roles of ventricular ectopy and ventricular dysfunction, particularly when the two conditions coexist. However, there is sufficient evidence to indicate a prognostic role for ventricular ectopic activity over and above that which is seen in patients with severe left ventricular dysfunction to warrant a positive approach to the treatment of patients with frequent (>20 per min) VEBs, multiformity, pairs, runs, and the R-on-T phenomenon.

There are other qualitative features of ventricular ectopic activity, less important than complexity, that may be helpful in deciding whether or not to treat a particular patient. Both elimination and enhancement of the VEBs occur on exercise in patients with both diseased and normal hearts; it is only in the patient with known ischemic heart disease that enhancement during or immediately after exercise can be regarded as a prognostic sign for subsequent cardiac events.

Ventricular parasystole may have a lower risk of ventricular fibrillation than have VEBs with a fixed coupling interval, since it is an automatic rather than a reentrant rhythm that is protected against a rapid discharge rate by the phenomenon of exit block. Parasystole can be recognized on the standard electrocardiogram (ECG) by the marked variation in coupling interval between the ectopic beat and the preceding sinus beat; paired beats and fusion beats are frequently seen. Ventricular escape beats, easily recognizable by their prolonged coupling intervals, are protective and should not be suppressed.

CONTEMPORARY DRUG THERAPY

Pharmacologic therapy in the patient with VEB must be considered within the following context:

(1) No randomized study has yet demonstrated a reduction in sudden death mortality in groups of patients on antiarrhythmic drug therapy.

(2) The adage that "the treatment may be worse than the disease" is applicable. Membrane-stabilizing or type 1A agents, such as quinidine, procainamide, and disopyramide, may prolong the Q-T interval and lead to the polymorphic type of ventricular tachycardia known as "torsade de pointes". Even in the absence of Q-T prolongation, these agents may exacerbate the arrhythmia under treatment. The frequency with which these drugs aggravate or induce major arrhythmias is estimated at approximately 10 percent, with a somewhat greater frequency for quinidine.

(3) There are no well-defined end points in the treatment of the asymptomatic patient, other than reduction in mortality. Whereas it is comforting to the physician to see a reduction of 70 percent to 90 percent in the frequency of VEBs or to eliminate the more complex forms, such as pairs or runs of ventricular ectopic activity, these may not necessarily result in a reduction in ventricular fibrillation and sudden death. Conversely, failure to reduce ventricular ectopic activity may not be synonymous with failure to prevent ventricular fibrillation. One recent study suggests that the end point of treatment should be a consistently maintained therapeutic drug level in the serum, regardless of the effect on the frequency or complexity of the ectopic activity. The management of ventricular arrhythmias would be revolutionized should this theory be confirmed.

Despite these considerations, there should not be undue pessimism in prescribing antiarrhythmic agents for the patient with ventricular ectopy. Treatment directed specifically at controlling VEBs in a patient with a drug of proven efficacy for that individual is different from treating a group of patients with an agent that may be effective for some and not for others. Individualized therapy of this type, selected on the strength of either acute drug testing or electrophysiologic studies, has been demonstrated to protect against fatal arrhythmias. It is essential that the physician set realistic objectives when treating the patient with ventricular ectopy; it is seldom possible to eliminate the arrhythmia entirely. For the symptomatic patient, the prime goal should be the control of symptoms. For the asymptomatic patient with potentially dangerous arrhythmias, the goal should be a reduction of the higher grade of ectopy. If it cannot be achieved, one should aim at maintaining an adequate blood level of the drug. For all patients with ventricular ectopic activity short of ventricular tachycardia and fibrillation, the principle of treatment should be to treat "cheaply," that is, to strive for a defined therapeutic goal without inducing significant side effects.

Based on these principles, the initial antiarrhythmic drug of choice should, whenever possible, be a beta-blocking agent, since they are far freer of side effects than the membrane-stabilizing drugs. Unfortunately, their efficacy in controlling ventricular ectopic activity is often less than that of quinidine, procainamide, and disopyramide. They are more likely to be effective when the resting heart rate is above 70 beats per minute, and they are particularly effective in exercise-induced ventricular ectopy. However, their use is limited in the presence of sinus bradycardia, and they are contraindicated in the patient with congestive heart failure (CHF). Differences between beta-blocking drugs in terms of their membrane-stabilizing activity are of little practical importance; all of the currently available agents have adequate antiarrhythmic activity in standard dosages. Their side effects and contraindications are well known.

The type IA antiarrhythmic agents are generally effective, either alone or in combination with a beta-blocking drug, in controlling VEBs. However, the high incidence of side effects with all three agents of this type is a major limiting factor. Quinidine is the prototype antiarrhythmic drug. It is available in sulfate, gluconate, and polygalacturonate forms; it is hoped that the latter two forms produce fewer gastrointestinal side effects. The slow-release forms seem to maintain adequate blood levels. The standard therapeutic dose is between 800 and 1,600 mg of quinidine per 24 hours. Immediate side effects are diarrhea and other gastrointestinal symptoms. These occur within 1 or 2 days of starting the drug and may affect as many as 25 percent of patients using quinidine. An additional 10 percent of patients develop a fever approximately 10 days after starting the drug. If a patient has previously been sensitized to quinidine, fever or other major side effects, such as thrombocytopenic purpura or agranulocytosis, may occur after a single dose. Symptoms of cinchonism may appear in sensitive persons. Quinidine augments serum digoxin levels and may induce toxicity in patients on a previously well-tolerated dose of digitalis. It prolongs appreciably the Q-T interval and may lead to torsade de pointes or "quinidine syncope." It is estimated that it may aggravate ventricular arrhythmias either through the mechanism of Q-T prolongation or through other mechanisms in 15 percent of patients. Hence, only about one-half the patients treated with quinidine are able to use the drug on a long-term basis.

The side effects of procainamide therapy are equally common. Although early gastrointestinal side effects and hypersensitivity are much less frequent than with quinidine, the late development of a positive antinuclear antibody (ANA) titer occurs in approximately 70 percent of patients and the clinical lupus erythematosus syndrome in over one-half of them. There are some patients in whom the drug may be cautiously continued even in the presence of a positive ANA test, provided they have no symptoms of the lupus syndrome. However, it should be appreciated that arthritic and pleuritic manifestations of lupus syndrome, when they occur, may persist for months after the drug has been discontinued. The relatively recent introduction of the slow-release forms of procainamide has made its long-term use practical in those patients who remain free of side effects. Long-term therapy must be monitored by repeated blood tests for ANA activity and for serum levels of both procainamide and its active metabolite, N-acetyl-p-aminophenol (NAPA). A daily dose between 1 and 4 g of the sustained release form, given at 6-hourly intervals, usually provides adequate blood levels; however, therapeutic success often depends on the rate at which acetylation occurs, and NAPA levels do exceed procainamide levels in rapid acetylators. It is likely that slow acetylators are more susceptible to the lupus syndrome. Prolongation of intraventricular conduction time (QRS duration) and Q-T interval occur with procainamide as well as with quinidine, and it is estimated that procainamide may be arrhythmogenic in approximately 10 percent of patients.

Disopyramide (Norpace) has an antiarrhythmic spectrum similar to that of quinidine and procainamide, but it is often effective when the latter has failed. Unfortunately, it has an even greater frequency of side effects than its counterparts. Anticholinergic side effects, including urinary hesitancy and retention, constipation, dryness of the mouth, and blurring of vision, limit its usefulness appreciably, particularly in older male populations with potential prostate problems. Furthermore, the unusually potent negative inotropic action of disopyramide contraindicates its use in the presence of impaired ventricular function. It prolongs the Q-T interval and has often been incriminated as a cause of torsades de pointes. Like quinidine, it can depress sinus node automaticity in patients with sinoatrial dysfunction. The effective daily dosage range is between 300 and 800 mg.

Phenytoin sodium (Dilantin) has electrophysiologic effects similar to those of lidocaine. It is probably the least effective of the currently available antiarrhythmic agents, except in the case of digitalis-induced atrial or ventricular arrhythmias. Its use in the management of patients with symptomatic or asymptomatic VEBs is generally confined to those who have either developed side effects or who have not responded to a combination of beta-blocker and a type 1A antiarrhythmic drug. It may be used in combination with other antiarrhythmics; however, it does reduce serum quinidine levels. The usual maintenance dose is between 300 and 400 mg a day; the most important side effects are neurologic (drowsiness, nystagmus, ataxia, and nausea) and generally correlate with elevated blood levels of the drug.

On the other hand, tocainide HCL (Tonocard), another type IB (lidocaine-like) antiarrhythmic agent recently approved for the suppression of VEBs, may prove to be as effective as the type IA agents, but with the advantages of not prolonging the Q-T interval; not affecting sinus node function, AV conduction, or His-Purkinje conduction; and not depressing myocardial contractility. A response to intravenous lidocaine predicts a response to tocainide in the majority of cases. The daily dose is 1,200 to 1,800 mg in divided doses of either 400 or 600 tablets 3 times a day. The important side effects are neurologic (lightheadedness, parasthesia, and tremor), nausea, and rash.

Although other drugs, such as digitalis, atropine and isoproterenol, have been used for the treatment of ventricular ectopy in certain specific clinical settings, they are more likely to induce ectopy than to control it. Imipramine (Tofranil) has recently been shown to have antiarrhythmic properities, but has not yet been approved for this indication. Lidocaine and bretylium are widely used parenterally, but do not have any role in long-term management of ventricular ectopy. None of the calcium-channel blocking agents in current use has any direct effect on ventricular ectopy; some of the slow channel blockers under investigation do seem to show promise in this regard. Numerous other antiarrhythmic agents are at present under intensive study.

MANAGING THE PATIENT WITH VENTRICULAR ECTOPIC BEATS

The patient presents to the physician either with symptoms directly attributable to ventricular ectopic activity or because ventricular ectopy has been detected by examination, ECG, or Holter monitor. Symptoms range from a sensation of palpitations in most patients to significant hemodynamic embarrassment in a few. At times, it may be difficult to correlate certain symptoms—such as shortness of breath, chest or epigastric distress, and dizziness or near syncope—with ventricular ectopic activity, even though the latter has been documented. It has now been established that, contrary to popular belief, patients with an awareness of extrasystoles actually feel the ectopic beat and not the forceful postextrasystolic beat. Why some patients are exquisitely sensitive to each heart beat, whereas others are totally oblivious is not understood. While neuroses and anxiety undoubtedly potentiate awareness in some patients, certain physical properties of the VEB, such as prematurity, may play a role in others.

The physician must make a detailed evaluation of possible etiologic precipitants of the ventricular ectopic activity and the impact of this activity on the patient's life. He then must judge its potential for adversely affecting longevity, considering the characteristics of the ventricular ectopy and the context in which it occurs. Historical information on potential precipitants requires an assessment of the effect of cigarette smoking, alcohol, caffeine intake, physical activity, rest, fatigue, and emotional stress on the frequency and severity of symptoms. An intimate inquiry regarding medications being used, particularly psychotropic drugs, agents containing ephedrine or epinephrine, appetite suppressants, thyroid replacement drugs, digitalis, and diuretics may yield a remediable cause for the arrhythmia. It is satisfying indeed to discover a diuretic-induced hypokalemia as the cause of significant ventricular ectopy and to treat it accordingly. Recently, hypomagnesemia has also been recognized as a potent cause of ventricular arrhythmia.

Physical examination is directed at determining clinical associations—such as a normal heart, mitral valve prolapse, and other forms of valvular disease, chronic ischemic heart disease with or without ventricular aneurysm, and hypertrophic or dilated cardiomyopathy—and at assessing the severity of the disease in view of the established correlation between ventricular ectopy, ventricular dysfunction, and mortality. Characterization of the ventricular ectopy requires careful analysis of the ECG, rhythm strips, and a 24-hour Holter recording. A treadmill stress test provides additional information on the response of the ectopic rhythm to exercise and may uncover rhythm disorders of prognostic importance, particularly in the patient with chronic ischemic heart disease but also in the patient with mitral valve prolapse. The treadmill test, together with the Holter recording, should be regarded as part of the routine work-up of the patient with ventricular ectopy. Cardiac catheterization is indicated in only a small subset of patients who present solely with ventricular ectopy and is based, not on the ectopy per se, but on other suspicions of possible critical coronary obstructive disease. Laboratory studies are directed specifically at renal and electrolyte function with emphasis on both serum potassium and magnesium levels.

Once the arrhythmia and its relation to the patient's symptoms, underlying heart disease and prognosis have been defined, the physician is obliged to explain the findings to the patient in as much detail as the patient is expected to understand. For the patient with symptomatic ventricular ectopy and a normal heart or mitral valve prolapse, this is perhaps the most important overall aspect of management. The patient should be reassured in unequivocal terms of the benign nature of the ectopic rhythm in his or her particular clinical context. In addition, the cyclic behavior of ectopic rhythms should be emphasized, since the patient may wonder whether the "skipped beats" rhythm will ever disappear. In contemporary clinical practice, the patient with mitral valve prolapse and ventricular ectopy is at greater risk of suffering intractable neuroticism than of dying of ventricular fibrillation. Only the patient who has massive prolapse as seen on the ECG, associated with documented ventricular tachycardia or exercise-induced ventricular ectopy and repolarization abnormalities on the resting ECGs, should be singled out for treatment if he or she is asymptomatic. In discussing the significance of ventricular ectopy with the patient with chronic ischemic heart disease or cardiomyopathy, emphasize the potential hemodynamic benefits of suppressing ventricular ectopic activity and not the risk of sudden death.

Although it is the exception rather than the rule for ectopic rhythms to respond to the withdrawal of cigarettes, alcohol, and caffeine, an attempt to eliminate these cardiac stimulants should always be made. Greater success might be anticipated from the discontinuation of a medication that has arrhythmogenic properties or from the correction of an electrolyte abnormality.

Before drug therapy is initiated, the patient must be fully informed that the treatment program is a matter of trial and error, since each patient responds differently to different medications. Patience and cooperation are more likely to be achieved if the patient is cognizant of his or her role in the clinical "experiment." The clinical goals, namely, control of symptoms in the symptomatic patient or suppression of the more complex forms of ectopy in the asymptomatic patient, are defined in the context of potential side effects.

The choice of the appropriate antiarrhythmic agent is often difficult and arbitrary. Beta-blocking drugs have relatively few side effects and are preferred for initial treatment, unless they are relatively contraindicated by sinus bradycardia or absolutely contraindicated by CHF. Propranolol is still the beta-blocker of choice, 40 to 80 mg a day, in divided doses. The dosage range is wide and can be adjusted according to the therapeutic response. Thereafter, longer-acting beta-blockers can be used as desired for patient convenience and compliance. The overall effectiveness of beta-blocking agents in suppressing ventricular ectopy is not particularly great and, in a majority of patients treated in clinical practice, a type I antiarrhythmic agent is required as well.

When introducing either quinidine, procainamide, or disopyramide, one prefers to use the "trendscription" technique described by Lown and his associates. The patient is requested to devote 3 hours to the initial study, which is performed on an outpatient basis. He is attached to the "trendscriber," which records the electrocardiographic signal on a slowly revolving drum so that 3 hours of electrocardiographic activity is recorded on six sheets of paper. The first hour is used as a control, after which a loading dose of the medication of given. This is generally one-half the anticipated daily maintenance dose (i.e., 600 mg of quinidine, 1,500 mg of procainamide, and 300 mg of disopyramide). The patient should not have received a type I antiarrhythmic agent for at least 24 hours before receiving an acute loading dose. The loading dose technique should be used for disopyramide only when ventricular function is normal. The immediate response to an acute loading dose is readily apparent on inspection of the trendscription sheets, the maximum effect generally occurring 1 to 2 hours after administration. A positive response to the loading dose is usually an accurate indication of a long-term response. Furthermore, side effects immediately become apparent, particularly the cholinergic side effects of disopyramide. The trendscription technique can be used to assess the long-term efficacy of therapy; it is less expensive and less cumbersome than repeated Holter recordings, although the latter provide better information on ectopic activity under nonbasal conditions.

I generally choose quinidine over procainamide as the initial type I agents, mainly because tolerance is established within 2 weeks, whereas the lupus syndrome may take months to develop. Disopyramide, by virtue of its common anticholinergic and negative inotropic side effects, is kept in reserve for those situations in which the combination of a beta-blocking drug and either quinidine or procainamide has failed. The quinidine-treated patient is apprised of two hurdles that have to be overcome in the initial 2 weeks of therapy—diarrhea and other gastrointestinal side effects, which become apparent within 24 to 48 hours, and a fever that may occur in the tenth day of treatment. Once the patient has successfully crossed these barriers, the dose and the type of preparation can be selected for efficacy and convenience. The usual maintenance dose is between 800 and 1,600 mg per day in divided doses; the slow-release form of quinidine sulfate (Quinidex) appears to maintain excellent blood levels and can be used in a dose of 600 mg every 12 hours; the gluconate (Quinaglute) and polygalacturonate (Cardioquin) forms are used 2 or 3 times a day and seem to induce diarrhea less frequently. Monitoring of therapy should include an analysis of the ECG for prolongation of the QRS duration (>50 percent prolongation over baseline is an indication to discontinue the drug) and Q-T interval, periodic measurements of serum quinidine levels, and periodic electrocardiographic recording of either long rhythm strips, trendscription patterns, or 24-hour Holter studies.

Procainamide is used when quinidine has failed. Early signs of intolerance, such as fever, gastrointestinal symptoms, skin rash, and hypotension, occur much less frequently than with quinidine. It is therefore possible to adjust the dosage level of the drug and to achieve a therapeutic effect more rapidly. Similar attention must be given to prolongation of the QRS duration and Q-T interval. The slow-release form of the drug (Procan-SR) is preferred since it is reasonable to prescribe this preparation on a 6-hourly basis. The initial dose of 250 mg every 6 hours can be steadily increased to a dose of 1 g every 6 hours, depending upon therapeutic response, side effects, and blood levels. Blood levels define the slow acetylators and give an indication of those patients most likely to develop the lupus syndrome. The development of a positive ANA titer without symptoms of arthritis or pleuritis presents a major therapeutic dilemma. I prefer not to use procainamide when the ANA titer has become positive, except when all other measures have failed and suppression of ventricular ectopy is mandatory. Although both procainamide and quinidine have negative inotropic effects, they may be used in the presence of CHF and cautiously in the patients with bundle branch block.

Disopyramide, on the other hand, is contraindicated in actual or impending heart failure. Although it was a highly effective antiarrhythmic drug that held much promise when first released in 1977, its role in the suppression of VEBs has now become severely limited as a result of its side effects. I avoid its use in elderly male patients and those with significant ventricular dysfunction. I now use it only in symptomatic patients who are willing to tolerate the anticholinergic side effects in preference to the palpitations and in those in whom other forms of treatment have failed. In such patients, it is still often possible to use the acute loading dose technique. I try to maintain the patient on the lowest effective maintenance dose, starting at 100 mg 3 or 4 times daily, and then converting to the slow-release capsule for patient convenience. The dosage level can be increased to 800 mg or even 1 g a day, but tolerance is poor at the larger dosage range.

I have used phenytoin sparingly in the management of ventricular ectopic activity. Its main usefulness has been in combination with a type IA antiarrhythmic drug; however, on some occasions, it has been successful on its own where the other drugs have failed. It has the advantage of low toxicity and the disadvantage of relative ineffectiveness except in the presence of digitalis toxicity.

To date, my personal experience with tocainide, while limited, has been encouraging. The drug seems to be effective in suppressing ventricular ectopy and if it proves to be as effective as lidocaine (as is claimed), it is likely to become the initial therapy for ventricular ectopy. The electrophysiologic and hemodynamic effects make it theoretically preferable to the type IA antiarrhythmic agents. However, side effects could be a significant problem, since initial reports are that 15 percent to 20 percent of patients are unable to tolerate the drug.

On rare occasions, "overdrive" electronic pacing has a role in the suppression of ventricular ectopic activity. These are generally situations in which both the ectopy has produced hemodynamic embarrassment and drug therapy has failed or is limited by factors such as sinus bradycardia or CHF. Whereas it is the treatment of choice for torsade de pointes at one end of the ventricular ectopy spectrum, it is seldom indicated in the management of the average ambulant patient with ventricular ectopic beats.

MANAGING THE PATIENT WITH ATRIAL ECTOPIC BEAT

Most of the principles of management of the patient with ventricular ectopic activity apply equally to the patient with atrial ectopic activity. There are, however, three major differences:

(1) Atrial ectopic beats are the precursors of atrial tachycardia, atrial flutter, and atrial fibrillation. None of these rhythm disorders pose a threat to life, except perhaps indirectly through embolic complications or occasionally through hemodynamic consequences. Hence, the only indications for suppression of atrial ectopic beats are for symptomatic relief or for prevention of atrial tachyarrhythmias, a topic beyond the scope of this chapter. Reassurance, general hygienic measures, and a willingness on the part of the patient to live with the condition should therefore be preferred to antiarrhythmic drug treatment; the asymptomatic patient who has not had a tachyarrhythmia requires no treatment at all.

(2) Although atrial and ventricular ectopic beats occur in a similar pathologic spectrum, certain states are more conducive to the emergence of atrial ectopy. Notable among them are sinoatrial dysfunction, which may result from intrinsic disease of the sinus node (sick sinus syndrome), either primary sclerodegenerative or secondary to coronary occlusive or myocardial disease; excessive vagal tone; potentially reversible conditions, such as hypothyroidism and hyperkalemia; and the administration of a variety of drugs. Included in the drug causes of sinoatrial dysfunction are the beta-blocking agents, quinidine, and disopyramide. Hence the importance of determining when atrial ectopic activity is a manifestation of sinoatrial dysfunction. Electronic pacemaker therapy plays a prominent role in the management of sick sinus syndrome. Pulmonary conditions, such as emphysema and even bronchial neoplasm, may also be clinical associates of atrial ectopic activity. Treatment is directed at the control of anoxia and bronchial infection in patients with chronic obstructive lung disease and atrial ectopy. Antiarrhythmic drug therapy for anoxic pulmonary disease is often associated with toxicity and should be avoided except to prevent multiform atrial tachycardia and other atrial tachyarrhythmias.

(3) The beta-adrenergic blocking agents and the type IA antiarrhythmic drugs are all effective against atrial ectopic beats. The choice of drug and technique of administration are essentially as outlined for management of the individual patient with venticular ectopic activity. There is in addition an occasional role for digitalis, verapamil, and atropine in the management of the patient with atrial ectopic activity. Although neither digitalis nor verapamil suppress atrial ectopic beats, they may prevent atrial tachycardia by slowing atrioventricular conduction, as well as slowing the ventricular response should atrial fibrillation or atrial flutter ensue. Atropine may be indicated on rare occasions in younger patients who have symptomatic atrial ectopic activity in association with sinoatrial dysfunction and vagotonia.

SUPRAVENTRICULAR TACHYCARDIA

ALBERT A. DEL NEGRO, M.D., F.A.C.C.
ROSS D. FLETCHER, M.D., F.A.C.C.

Supraventricular tachycardias are usually thought to be benign, but occasionally may be life-threatening. They usually produce symptoms, and the description provided by patients can sometimes give clear clues to the sorts of rhythmic disturbances that occur. Although the term "supraventricular tachycardia" implies that the rhythmic disturbance arises from and involves only the atria, certain of these rhythms may in fact be initiated by ventricular activity and utilize the ventricles in a tachycardia circuit. Often, aberrant ventricular conduction of supraventricular beats may give the mistaken impression of a ventricular arrhythmia.

ELECTROPHYSIOLOGIC FEATURES

Cardiac impulse formation originates in the sinoatrial (SA) node by the spontaneous depolarization of this tissue. A calcium current (slow channel) is responsible for SA node depolarization, and the excitation wave spreads to the atrium over the internodal tracts that connect the SA node with the atrioventricular (AV) node. Atrial tissue utilizes the sodium-fast channel to initiate depolarization as do the bundle of His, the right and left bundle branches, the Purkinje fibers, and the ventricular muscle itself. The AV node, on the other hand, is like the SA node in that is uses a calcium current to initiate depolarization.

The autonomic nervous system plays an important role in the regulation of cardiac rhythm and conduction. A predominance of sympathetic influences over parasympathetic influences speeds the rate of discharge of the SA node and speeds conduction through the AV node. This is effected by adding sympathetic influences (epinephrine or isoproterenol) or by subtracting parasympathetic influences (atropine). A predominance of parasympathetic influences can slow the sinus rate and prolong AV nodal conduction time. This effect is achieved by adding parasympathetic influences (neostigmine or carotid massage) or by diminishing sympathetic influences (beta-blockers).

These facts have important implications for the treatment of supraventricular tachycardias, since drugs should be used for the treatment of arrhythmias depending on the unique electrophysiologic features of the tissue through which the arrhythmia occurs. For example, arrhythmias utilizing the AV node are best treated by drugs that inhibit the calcium slow channel. Similarly, an arrhythmia utilizing only the atrium during a tachycardia is best treated pharmacologically by a drug that interferes with the sodium-fast channel.

MECHANISMS OF ARRHYTHMIA

Irrespective of the location in the heart, tachycardias may be triggered by one of two mechanisms. The first is the mechanism of increased automaticity. This occurs during exercise when the sinus rate speeds to greater than 100 beats per minute or during shock states when sinus tachycardia is the usual rhythm observed. Under pathologic conditions, automaticity may be increased, as in digitalis intoxication with atrial tachycardia and AV block. The second mechanism is the mechanism of reentry wherein the arrhythmia reenters through an estblished circuit, as seen during reentry through the AV node or through the atrium itself during atrial flutter.

Occasionally, neither reentry nor increased automaticity can be invoked as the arrhythmia mechanism although they may introduce it. This is the case during atrial fibrillation when there is chaotic, rapid, and unorganized depolarization throughout the atria, resulting in no organized mechanical contraction.

ARRHYTHMIAS AND INCREASED AUTOMATICITY

Sinus Tachycardia. This common tachycardia is due to increased automaticity of the sinus node. The mechanism of this arrhythmia is a catecholamine-induced increase in the firing rate of the sinus node so that the rate increases to over 100 beats per minute. Generally, the rate is no greater than 150 beats per minute in adults, although it may be faster than that in young children. This tachycardia is normally encountered during exercise, during which the rates may be in excess of 180 beats per minute in young adults, but it may also be secondary to a pathologic process, such as congestive heart failure (CHF), hypoxia, hypovolemic shock, fever, and thyrotoxicosis. When this tachycardia is secondary to a pathologic process, therapy should obviously be aimed at correction of the underlying problem. Sinus tachycardia is too frequently overlooked in the differential diagnosis of rapid heart action. Its accurate diagnosis avoids useless, occasionally harmful, therapy.

Paroxysmal Atrial Tachycardia with Block. The hallmarks of paroxysmal atrial tachycardia (PAT) with block are an atrial rate of 150 to 220 beats per minute and a degree of AV block. The P waves are usually upright in lead II, III, and aVF, and the AV block is usually 2:1, but there may be any ratio of AV conduction. This is an important arrhythmia to recognize because the most common cause is intoxication with digitalis. The arrhythmogenic effects of digitalis create the atrial tachycardia, and the vagomimetic effects create the AV block. Continued administration of digitalis results in dangerous ventricular arrhythmias, including ventricular tachycardia and ventricular fibrillation.

Therapy for this arrhythmia includes discontinuation of digitalis preparations and administration of potassium chloride calculated to raise the serum potassium level to the 4.5 to 5.0 mEq per liter range. This usually returns the tachycardia to normal. Of course, this arrhythmia should never be cardioverted if it is due to digitalis intoxication. Finally, when the ventricular response is rapid, with little or no AV block present, treatment with a low-dose beta-blocker or verapamil in the absence of CHF can enhance AV block and slow the tachycardia to clinically acceptable rates.

Frequently, since monitoring digitalis levels has led to a more conservative use of the drug, this tachycardia may occur in patients who have not been given digitalis. The most common setting for this is that of chronic pulmonary insufficiency, and therapy should be directed at improvement of pulmonary function. When the AV block is low grade, resulting in a relatively rapid rate, judicious use of verapamil slows the ventricular response.

Multifocal Atrial Tachycardia. Multifocal atrial tachycardia (MAT) is commonly noted in patients with chronic respiratory insufficiency. The diagnosis is made by the findings of a heart rate greater than 100 beats per minute, a chaotic rhythm, and the recongnition of P waves of at least three morphologies. As the name implies, MAT is due to multiple atrial pacemakers coming to threshold at irregular intervals. Diagnostically, this tachycardia is most often confused with atrial fibrillation because of its gross irregularity. This error occurs when the physician fails to note the presence of discrete atrial activity in the form of P waves; it can lead to inappropriate repeated attempts at cardioversion. This rhythm never responds to cardioversion.

Treatment is aimed at improving oxygenation, which decreases the hypoxic stimulus to the diverse atrial pacemakers. Quinidine-like antiarrhythmics are used, but are of little benefit if hypoxia cannot be relieved. Treatment with digitalis and/or verapamil may create greater degrees of AV block and slow the ventricular response without affecting the atrial ectopy and make the tachycardia better tolerated hemodynamically. The discontinuation of drugs that stimulate the release of endogenous catecholamines is often helpful.

Nonparoxysmal Atrioventricular Junctional Tachycardia. This tachycardia is also commonly seen in digitalis intoxication in which the agent is given in increasing doses to control the rapid ventricular response to atrial fibrillation. Often the clinician fails to note the extreme regularity of the ventricular response, which is the earliest clue to the presence of this tachycardia and digitalis intoxication. Continued administration of digitalis results in lethal ventricular arrhythmias. The usual rate is 130 to 150 beats per minute, and retrograde AV block is often present. Sinus beats may capture the ventricle. In sinus rhythm, the diagnosis is more easily made since the presence of an accelerated junctional rhythm is relatively obvious.

Nonparoxysmal AV junctional tachycardia may occur in the absence of digitalis administration and is seen in acute ischemic states, as well as in respiratory insufficiency. Occasionally, this tachycardia occurs immediately after open heart surgery.

As with PAT with block, cardioversion is not helpful, withdrawal of digitalis being the chief therapeutic step when digitalis overdose is the etiology of the tachycardia. When the etiology is respiratory insufficiency, improvement in pulmonary function is the chief therapeutic aim. Occasionally, when this tachycardia is persistent, it may be modified by treatment with beta-blockers or the quinidine-related antiarrhythmic agents or even digitalis itself.

ARRHYTHMIAS AND REENTRY

Sinus Node Reentry. As the name suggests, this tachycardia uses a reentry circuit within the sinus node. It is usually introduced by a premature atrial beat, and the P waves are identical to those seen in normal sinus rhythm. The usual rate of this tachycardia is 130 to 180 beats per minute, but the rate depends on the conduction time through the sinus node, which may be extremely slow, accounting for a rate as low as 90 to 110 beats per minute.

The sinus node is a vagally innervated structure and uses the calcium slow channel for depolarization. Consequently, vagomimetic drugs, such as digitalis, and calcium-channel blockers, such as verapamil, may be used for reversion to normal rhythm and or prophylaxis against recurrence. Beta-blockers withdraw sympathetic drive and thereby accentuate vagal effects, indirectly achieving the same result as direct vagomimetic drugs. Often quinidine-like drugs may be helpful because of their effect on adjacent atrial tissue and because they may diminish the frequency of premature atrial beats that introduce the tachycardia.

Carotid sinus massage can normalize this tachycardia in a large number of patients, and the "all-or-none" response can be diagnostic, either causing reversion of the rhythm to normal or having no impact on the tachycardia at all. As with virtually all reentrant tachycardias, pacing overdrive can return sinus node reentry tachycardia to normal rhythm. This form of therapy is little used, however, unless a significant bradyarrhythmia also complicates the clinical picture.

Paroxysmal Supraventricular Tachycardia. Paroxysmal supraventricular tachycardia(PSVT) is commonly noted in patients with no organic heart disease. Reentry within the AV node that has adjacent portions of differing refractoriness and conduction speed is the mechanism of this tachycardia and like sinus node reentry, it is often introduced by a premature atrial beat or, less commonly, by a premature ventricular beat. Rates during the tachycardia are in the 140 to 200 beats per minute range, and the diagnosis is made by the recognition of a (usually) narrow QRS tachycardia, with P waves being either concealed within the QRS or just barely seen at the end of the QRS. The P waves, when visible, are negative in the inferior leads, since atrial depolarization occurs in a retrograde fashion from the low atrium.

Reversion to normal rhythm depends on vagomimetic stimulation. Numerous therapies exist and include carotid sinus massage, eliciting the diving reflex (face in ice water), Valsalva maneuver, and drugs such as digitalis, beta-blockers, and calcium-channel blockers. All of the drug therapies can be used not only to return tachycardia to normal, but also to provide prophylaxis against recurrence of arrhythmia. In addition, quinidine-like drugs can reduce the frequency of premature atrial and ventricular beats, which may introduce the tachycardia.

Approximately 30 percent of patients with PSVT have concealed Kent bundles (AV bypass tracts) as the retrograde part of their reentrant circuit. This is the postulated reason why the quinidine-like drugs may be helpful, since the Kent bundle is atrial tissue and uses the sodium-fast channel for depolarization. Of course, quinidine is a drug that slows conduction and prolongs refractoriness in sodium-depolarizing structures.

Intracardiac electrophysiologic examination is a useful tool in the management of patients who are poorly controlled with medications. Such studies may confirm the contributory presence of a Kent bundle, against which therapy may be added, and more precisely define the mechanism of tachycardia, thereby aiding treatment. Finally, intracardiac electrophysiology may be used to treat patients who are medical treatment failures by creating an AV block or at least modifying AV conduction. This end is achieved by transcatheter electroshock ablation, with a shock being delivered directly to the AV node. Of course, only the tiny minority of patients with this tachycardia are so poorly controlled that this form of therapy is necessary.

Atrial Flutter. This tachycardia uses the atria for its reentry circuit. The initial wavefront pattern of its reentry is almost superior, and so superiorly directed P waves are the rule, accounting for the negative flutter waves in leads II, III, and AVF. The atrial rate is usually 280 to 320 beats per minute, but may be slowed with the use of quinidine-like drugs to the 200 beats per minute range. The ventricular response is usually one-half the atrial rate, but occasionally a patient may have such brisk AV nodal conduction that rates close to 300 beats per minute are possible.

The initial goal of therapy, if cardioversion is not immediately contemplated, is to slow the ventricular response. Removing contributory factors is indicated. Hypoxia should be corrected, CHF treated, and the possibility of thyrotoxicosis investigated. Correcting hypovolemia, fever, and anemia also aids in control of ventricular response. Pharmacologic control can be achieved with digitalis, which used to be the early drug of choice for this purpose, but atrial flutter is such an orderly attack on the AV node that it takes very high doses of digitalis to achieve greater degrees of AV block. The result is that by the time sufficient digitalis is given to slow the ventricular rate from 150 beats per minute (2:1 conduction) to 100 beats per minute (3:1 conduction), digitalis intoxication ensues. Consequently, increasing AV nodal block with beta-blockers or verapamil is the treatment of choice. This allows the use of cardioversion to normalize rhythm at any time without the fear of digitalis-related arrhythmias.

Cardioversion to normal rhythm is feasible by medical or electrical means. Medical therapy involves the administration of increasing doses of a quinidine-like drug, which increases refractory periods to the point that reentering wavefronts are unable to excite the atrium. In addition, while slowing conduction initially favors reentry, complete block of pathways in the reentrant circuit allows sinus rhythm to dominate. The hazard of this approach is that often patients require very large doses to convert to normal. Postreversion, extremely slow rates may also occur, especially in patients with the sick sinus syndrome already receiving verapamil or beta-blockers for the control of the ventricular response. For this reason, direct-current cardioversion is the favored means of reversion to normal, since bradyarrhythmias can accurately be identified and treated. Furthermore, the mean electrical dose for reversion of atrial flutter to normal is low, making the likelihood of digitalis-related arrhythmias in patients on that drug relatively small.

Chronic maintenance therapy includes a drug for the control of ventricular response should atrial flutter recur (digitalis, verapamil, or beta-blockers) and a drug to reduce the likelihood of premature atrial beats, which can introduce atrial flutter (quinidine or procainamide).

For patients with recurring and resistant atrial flutter who may be susceptible to pacing overdrive to normal rhythm, permanent pacing therapy is available. One pacemaker under clinical evaluation at present senses the atrial flutter and thereafter delivers a burst of atrial pacing at a rate in excess of the flutter rate known by empiric testing to be able to return the flutter to normal.

REENTRANT ARRHYTHMIAS IN THE WOLF-PARKINSON-WHITE SYNDROME

Wolf-Parkinson-White (WPW) is a syndrome of preexcitation of the ventricles from the atrium by an atrial muscle fiber that bypasses the AV node by bridging the AV sulcus. The conduction time in atrial tissue and hence in such bypass tracts, or Kent bundles, is vastly more rapid the conduction along the AV node. In such patients, the QRS is the offspring of two parents, the AV node and the Kent bundle. The QRS resembles conduction down the AV node or the Kent bundle, depending on which contributes more to ventricular excitation. The result in normal sinus rhythm is that most beats are a form of fusion. The morphologic criteria for the diagnosis of WPW are the classic findings of a short P–R interval, a wide QRS, and a delta wave, which presents the earliest ventricular activation by way of the Kent bundle.

Approximately half of all patients with WPW electrocardiograms have tachycardias, and the majority of these have a form of atrioventricular reentry. The mec hanism of this tachycardia is that a premature atrial beat may find one pathway to the ventricle unrecovered from the previous depolarization while the other path to the ventricle is at least partially recovered. Usually, the premature atrial beat encounters the Kent bundle in its refractory period, whereas the slower conducting AV node may be able to pass the impulse to the ventricle. The QRS is usually narrow in this circumstance. The Kent bundle being spared depolarization initially, it now has the chance to propagate the return to the atrium, creating a retrograde P wave, which then reciprocates antegrade down the AV node to reexcite the ventricle. In this way, a reentrant atrioventricular tachycardia is established, usually with a narrow QRS, at a rate of 160 to 220 per minute.

Because of the retrograde P waves, the narrow QRS, and the rate that overlaps precisely, there may be some diagnostic confusion with PSVT, which reenters within the AV node. That WPW is the diagnosis during the tachycardia is established by the presence of P waves clearly after the QRS, and occasionally by recognizing negative P waves in V6, which implies atrial activation from the lateral wall, a likely location for a left atrial'left ventricular Kent bundle. Of course, the finding of classic WPW morphologies on reversion to normal rhythm is also diagnostic.

As mentioned earlier, approximately 30 percent of patients with PSVT and no evidence during sinus rhythm of WPW may actually have Kent bundles with no property of antegrade conduction, but with intact retrograde conduction. In this manner, premature atrial beats always find the Kent bundle refractory to antegrade conduction, but often able to conduct from the ventricles to the atrium to establish a classic reentrant tachycardia. The discovery that such a concealed retrograde Kent bundle is operant in PSVT requires invasive electrophysiologic study, which may be done because of medically refractory arrhythmias.

The medical therapy of reentrant tachycardia in WPW syndrome is similar to that for PSVT because the tachycardia circuit uses the AV node as one limb of its circuit. The other limb of the circuit is the Kent bundle, which is atrial tissue, uses the sodium fast channel for depolarization, and is susceptible to quinidine-like drugs. For this reason, chronic therapy for reentrant tachycardia in WPW syndrome always includes a drug to prolong AV nodal conduction and refractoriness (digitalis, verapamil, beta'blockers) as well as a drug to slow conduction and prolong refractoriness in the Kent bundle (quinidine, procainamide, disopyramide).

SUPRAVENTRICULAR TACHYARRHTHMIA AND ATRIAL FIBRILLATION

This rhythm disturbance is common in mitral valve disease and CHF. The diagnosis is based on the absence of organized atrial activity and the finding of a random and irregular ventricular response. The ventricular rate in atrial fibrillation depends on the conduction properites of the AV node in the absence of the Wolff-Parkinson-White syndrome, and so the first step in treating atrial fibrillation is to control the ventricular response by increasing AV node refractoriness and slowing its conduction. The classic drug for this is digitalis, which has direct and indirect vagal effects on the AV node. Other drugs capable of this effect are verapamil and the beta-blockers.

Reversion to normal rhythm is usually desirable, especially if the atrial fibrillation is of short duration. As with atrial flutter, medical or electrical conversion is feasible. Medical conversion is achieved by the administration of increasing doses of quinidine. This drug has a moderate vagolytic effect and therefore is never the initial drug of choice before rate control has been established. Reversion in this fashion is spontaneous and often unsupervised. Significant bradyarrhythmias may attend this reversion, and for these reasons direct-current synchronized cardioversion is the method of choice for conversion to normal rhythm.

The role of anticoagulation prior to reversion to normal rhythm has long been debated. There is no question that anticoagulation is desirable in the presence of mitral valve disease, especially in patients with mitral stenosis and in those with a prosthetic mitral valve. In patients with no organic heart or valvular disease, the incidence of postreversion systemic emboli is small but real and justifies initial rate control with medication and a 2-week course of full-dose anticoagulation with sodium warfarin, which lessens the chance of postconversion emboli. Continued anticoagulation is recommended after conversion for a full 2 to 4 weeks based on the fact that the peak incidence of postconversion emboli is about 4 days after conversion.

Chronic maintenance therapy after conversion should consist of both a drug to promote AV nodal refractoriness in the event of recurrence of atrial fibrillation and a quinidine-like drug to reduce the incidence of premature atrial beats and make atrial fibrillation more difficult to establish. Attention to predisposing factors, such as CHF, also reduces the chances for recurrence.

There are numerous patients who are easily and comfortably maintained in atrial fibrillation chronically. They are individuals who have failed to remain in normal rhythm and who need only rate control achieved with digitalis or other AV nodal blocking drugs.

ATRIAL FIBRILLATION IN THE WOLF–PARKINSON–WHITE SYNDROME

About 20 percent of WPW patients with tachycardias have atrial flutter or atrial fibrillation. Of those patients, many have Kent bundles with extremely short refractory periods capable of rapid conduction to the vnetricles, achieving rates of close to 300 per minute. This occurs by way of antegrade conduction along the Kent bundle, and the prime goal of therapy in this critical situation is to slow the ventricular response. The classic drug for this in the absence of WPW is digitalis, but AV nodasl conduction is not one's conc ern in this situation. Digitalis is lethal for such patients because it shortens refractoriness in the atrium and also in the Kent bundle and thereby speeds the ventricular rate. Verapamil likewise may speed the already too-fast ventricular response, and hence these two drugs are absolutely contraindicated in this situation. Intravenous procainamide is the drug of choice. Lidocaine masy also cause slowing, and reversion of the atrial fibrillation with sinus rhythm by DC cardioversion immediately removes the patient from danger.

Patients with WPW and atrial fibrillation that achieve rates of 250 to 300 beats per minute are candidates for surgical therapy to divide the Kent bundle; because of the nearly 50 percent incidence of sudden death from ventricular fibrillation induced by the extremely rapid ventricular response during atrial fibrillation. Alternatively, for patients with this complication and suitably located Kent bundles, endocardial shock therapy delivered through an electrode catheter positioned in the region of the bypass tract may destroy, or at least modify, the properties of conduction of the bypass tract, and remove the patient from the risk of sudden death. This latter procedure is new and applies to a small percentage of patients with WPW.

Electrophysiologic study is recommended for WPW patients who demonstrate atrial fibrillation and a rapid ventricular response as has been outlined. This study is done to define the risk as well as to map the location of the bypass tract in preparation for surgery or catheter ablation.

Supraventricular tachycardias are noted in patients with heart disease as well as in persons with no demonstrable abnormality. In most circumstances, identification is simple, and treatment based on a knowledge of the type of arrhythmia and its anatomic and physiologic substrate is appropriate. As in the circumstance of atrial flutter with one-to-one ventricular conduction or the patient with Wolff-Parkinson-White syndrome with atrial fibrillation and an extremely rapid ventricular response, supraventricular tachycardia may be life threatening. Furthermore, the fact that inappropriate therapy may be lethal underscores the importance of accurate diagnosis and treatment.

VENTRICULAR TACHYCARDIA: DRUG THERAPY

DAN M. RODEN, M.D.

The majority of the 400,000 sudden cardiac deaths in the United States each year are due to ventricular tachycardia (VT) and ventricular fibrillation. Most patients who die suddenly have extensive coronary artery disease; however, those patients resuscitated from out-of-hospital ventricular fibrillation only rarely have evidence of an *acute* myocardial infaraction (MI). Patients who have been resuscitated from one episode of non-MI-related sudden death are at high risk for recurrence, presumably because the electrophysiologic instability that contributed to their initial cardiac arrest is unchanged. Long-term survival rates in these patients can be improved by drug therapy, as well as by surgical procedures and implantable devices discussed in other chapters.

The desirability of aggressive antiarrhythmic management in other patient populations is not as clear as in patients with aborted sudden death. Patients with electrophysiologic and clinical features most closely resembling those with aborted sudden death have advanced coronary disease and recurrent sustained VT, i.e., VT that is relatively well tolerated for variable periods of time, which usually requires some intervention—drugs, pacing, or cardioversion—for its termination, and which has not (yet) culminated in cardiac arrest. This entity is particularly important to recognize for two reasons. First, it is frequently misdiagnosed as supraventricular tachycardia with aberrant ventricular activation; intravenous administration of verapamil can then result in, at best, treatment delay and, at worst, cardiovascular collapse. And second, correct diagnosis is important since these patients have clinical electrophysiologic features resembling those with aborted sudden death and are themselves at high risk for sudden death, presumably from rapid VT. A patient with a wide-complex tachycardia and a history of advanced coronary disease should be regarded as having VT; unless there is a history of a supraventricular tachyarrhythmia (AV nodal reentrant tachycardia, a bypass tract, or atrial flutter or fibrillation), exceptions to this rule are rare. Methods to establish definitively the diagnosis include vagal maneuvers, electrocardiographic discriminators, esophageal electrocardiography, and intracardiac recordings, any or all of which can and should be used in the patient whose condition is stable. As much information as feasible should be gathered in patients with hypotension, angina, or pulmonary edema but without delaying definitive treatment, usually synchronized cardioversion.

Sustained VT occurring in the setting of an MI obviously requires prompt therapy. Nonsustained ventricular arrhythmias in acutely ischemic patients are usually treated, but it is no longer thought that these are specific or sensitive indicators of risk for sustained VT. Patients with stable coronary artery disease and salvos of nonsustained VT (three or more consecutive ventricular beats at a rate > 100 per min) are at increased risk for sudden death. However, studies of the effects of arrhythmia suppression have not been shown to alter that risk, primarily because of drug-related side effects. With the advent of newer, better tolerated agents, large scale studies to assess the impact of antiarrhythmic drug therapy on risk for sudden death in this patient population have been initiated. Rapid, sustained VT can occur in the absence of coronary disease; underlying etiologies include cardiomyopathies, mitral valve prolapse, or no identifiable structural disease. These patients generally require therapy for symptoms. Prognosis in patients with noncoronary heart disease and nonsustained ventricular arrhythmias depends on the underlying disease, and antiarrhythmic treatment has not been shown to reduce a (perceived) risk of sudden death. Rarely, patients with normal hearts will be highly symptomatic with premature beats; prognosis in this group is excellent and antiarrhythmic drugs are not requried except for symptoms.

PRINCIPLES OF MANAGEMENT

Antiarrhythmic drugs have narrow margins between the doses required to achieve a desired end point and the doses that produce toxicity. It is therefore mandatory that the physician who uses these agents has a clear idea of what is an acceptable clinical end point in a particular patient, what toxicity may be anticipated (and how it may be avoided), and how to administer the drugs so as to minimize the likelihood of toxicity and maximize the likelihood of a favorable outcome. It should also be self-evident that reversible precipitating factors (such as hypokalemia, digitalis toxicity, and unstable myocardial ischemia) should be sought and eliminated prior to contemplating treatment with antiarrhythmic drugs.

Clinical End Points

Before any therapy for VT is initiated, it is critical to know the patient's baseline rhythm status. Only when rhythm in a drug-free state is known can the physician make a rational judgment on whether a particular treatment is effective. The modality of treatment is irrelevant: every patient should be assessed initially—be it by ambulatory monitoring, treadmill exercise, or programmed ventricular stimulation—in the absence of antiarrhythmic drugs. Although physicians are frequently loath to withdraw what they perceive as potentially or partially effective therapy to establish a suitable baseline, there is really no other way in which to begin to assess drug efficacy. Moreover, occasional patients (10% to 20%) will have their rhythmic status markedly improved (even to the point of abolition of inducible, sustained VT) by withdrawal of antiarrhythmic therapy.

The modality used to assess drug efficacy depends on the arrhythmia being treated and its associated risk for sudden death as already discussed. Some patients have frequent episodes of well-tolerated (sustained or nonsustained) VT and can have their therapy guided by ambulatory monitoring. Total suppression of all ventricular arrhythmias is an unrealistic goal in this group (and in fact carries a risk of serious drug toxicity), so abolition of VT events, which is usually accompanied by 70 to 80 percent reduction in total ventricular arrhythmia frequency, should be the therapeutic end point. Rarely, patients have consistent exercise-related VT; management in this group can be guided by repetitive exercise testing; it must be kept in mind, however, that the reproducibility of this technique is unestablished. Patients with rare clinical events (including those with aborted sudden death in the absence of an MI) but inducible VT that resembles their spontaneous arrhythmia should have their therapy guided by programmed electrical stimulation. An inability to induce VT on drugs improves prognosis in this group. Unfortunately, this end point can be achieved only in a minority (50% or less) of these patients. Drug-related slowing on VT rate may improve hemodynamic stability, but is not shown to be associated with an improved outcome (either decreased incidence of sudden death or fewer hospitalizations). It is in this group which fails to respond to trials with multiple drugs, that surgical management, automatic defibrillators, and amiodarone have their place.

My own bias is to test at least two or three agents with different electrophysiologic characteristics as well as at least one drug combination before considering these other modalities. There are no firm guidelines in this area, and clinical judgment—tempered by such factors as the patient's age, left ventricular function, the patient's anticipated degree of physical activity, and availability and expertise in alternative modes of therapy—plays a critical role in this decision-making process. These patients frequently remain hospitalized for long periods of time, and the physician must provide intensive psychological support, emphasizing the high likelihood of an ultimate excellent outcome.

Drug Toxicity

Antiarrhythmic drug toxicity can be divided into two major categories: that which is related to excessive doses or plasma concentrations and that which is not. The former group is, by definition, predictable in a population, although not necessarily in a given patient. On the other hand, toxicity unrelated to dose or plasma concentration ("idiosyncratic reactions"—a term that serves merely to betray our ignorance of the underlying mechanisms) is a common feature of antiarrhythmic therapy. Examples of side effects of antiarrhythmic drugs that are predictable and dose related include tremor and nausea with lidocaine, mexiletine, and tocainide, and blurred vision and ataxia with flecainide and encainide. Other side effects are predictable and dose related, but also depend on an interaction between drug and host characteristics. Examples include rapid development of the lupus syndrome among slow acetylators of procainamide and urinary retention in elderly males receiving disopyramide. On the other hand, patients at risk for certain common and serious antiarrhythmic drug reactions cannot yet be identified with certainty. Examples include quinidine-induced diarrhea and amiodarone toxicity of all types (which appears to be related to cumulative dose as much as to anything).

Provocation of sustained VT by antiarrhythmic drugs is probably the most feared complication of therapy. This takes one or two forms, either "torsades de pointes" or monomorphic VT, both of which have distinctive clinical features. Torsades de pointes is a polymorphic VT (rate 160 to 240 beats/min) seen during treatment with QT-prolonging drugs (quinidine and disopyramide are the most frequently implicated antiarrhythmics). Amiodarone does not appear to be a frequent cause despite the marked QT prolongation that it can cause. Left ventricular dysfunction is not a prerequisite for the development of torsades de pointes, and in fact about one-half the affected patients are receiving these drugs for atrial arrhythmias. An episode of torsades de pointes most frequently starts after abrupt slowing in heart rate, and the first beat of the tachycardia usually arises on the downslope of the T wave of a markedly prolonged QT interval (>600 msec). Hypokalemia, either absolute (<3.5 mEq/L) or relative (3.5 to 4.0 mEq/L) in association with diuretics is common, being present in up to 60 percent of patients. Most patients develop torsades de pointes within 1 to 2 days of starting the drug, but in a small minority, it can develop during chronic treatment, usually in the setting of hypokalemia or bradycardia.

The most effective treatments are potassium replacement and measures to increase heart rate (isoproterenol or temporary pacing). At Vanderbilt University Hospital, we estimate that at least 1.5 percent of patients for whom quinidine is prescribed develop this complication. It is not clear that there are ever circumstances under which patients who develop torsades de pointes during therapy with one of the associated agents should receive another. Even if there were important associated precipitating causes that have been corrected, patients who have had one episode have demonstrated an "at risk" substrate and remain at risk.

A second form of induction of sustained VT by antiarrhythmic drugs is seen most commonly with the newer agents flecainide, encainide, and others, that markedly slow intracardiac conduction (although it can occur with any sodium-channel blocking agent). This form of arrhythmia exacerbation may occur in as high as 20 percent of patients, with a history of sustained VT and large left ventricular scars related to remote transmural infarctions, who receive these drugs. Such exacerbation may take several forms (marked increase in frequency of episodes, new hemodynamic instability, and/or difficulty in cardioverting a previously easily reverted rhythm), and fatalities have occurred in hospital despite prompt resuscitative measures. Patients at high risk either for this type of arrhythmia exacerbation or for torsades de pointes can be identified, but exceptions are frequent enough that antiarrhythmic drugs should only be started in inpatients whose rhythm is continuously monitored. If a rhythm disturbance is sufficiently serious to warrant treatment, it seems paradoxical to initiate that treatment in an outpatient setting.

Successful Drug Therapy

Drugs exert their effects by interacting with subcellular constituents, such as ionic channel receptors. The intensity of the pharmacologic response is dependent on both host factors and drug concentration. While we cannot measure concentrations at the effector sites, concentrations of drugs in plasma generally parallel effect well. Hence, monitoring plasma concentrations and trying to keep them within a prescribed "therapeutic range," comprise a common method of improving the chances of successful drug therapy. A plasma concentration value is no substitute for clinical judgment: some patients tolerate and require "toxic" concentrations for an effect; others display side effects at low concentrations. Nevertheless, monitoring plasma concentrations can establish that a reasonable amount of drug is present, and hence a reasonable drug effect should, in general, be anticipated. This is, for example, useful when serial programmed electrical stimulation is being used to guide therapy and it is undesirable to "waste" a test if plasma concentrations are for some reason particularly low. Monitoring concentrations may also help to avoid serious side effects; for example, induction of VT by flecainide is most common at concentrations above 1,000 ng per milliliter, and so one current recommendation is to keep flecainide concentrations below this value.

The major pharmacokinetic factors that determine drug disposition are clearance, volume of distribution, and elimination half-life. *Clearance* is a measure of the efficacy of the drug removal processes and determines (along with dose) the ultimate plasma concentrations achieved with any particular drug dosage regimen. *Volume of distribution* is a term derived from mathematical descriptions of drug disposition; its major clinical utility lies in guiding adjustments of loading regimens. *Elimination half-life*, which is actually a function of both a volume of distribution term and of clearance, determines the time required to achieve steady-state plasma concentrations. In one elimination half-life on a given drug regimen, one-half the ultimate steady state level is achieved; in two, 75 percent; in three, 87.5 percent, and so on. Therefore, for practical purposes, steady-state conditions can be assumed to prevail after four to five elimination half-lives have elapsed.

Loading doses are useful if an arrhythmia requires urgent treatment or if the effects of an acute dose of a drug are to be tested in patient over a short period of time (e.g., in the electrophysiology laboratory). Obviously, in these settings, waiting until steady-state conditions are present is not appropriate. Otherwise, the use of loading doses neither accelerates the time to steady state (a function of elimination half-life) nor alters the ultimate steady-state plasma concentration achieved (a function of clearance); it only exposes the patient to needless risk for no benefit. Hence, to test a particular chronic drug regimen, a loading dose not only is unnecessary, but can be misleading or even potentially dangerous.

The entire premise of monitoring plasma concentrations of drugs rests on a sound correlation between concentrations in plasma and those at effector sites. This correlation may break down for a number of reasons. For example, as long as drug concentrations at these two sites are not in equilibrium, plasma concentrations may be high while an antiarrhythmic action is small. This effect has been well documented for many drugs (quinidine, disopyramide, procainamide, and flecainide), but the lag time is usually short (under 20 minutes). It is nevertheless important to be aware of this phenomenon since, if a desired effect is not seen during intravenous loading, waiting 10 to 30 minutes (rather than administering more drug) may be the correct strategy. A long (days or weeks) time to equilibrium between plasma and effector sites may also explain the lag seen early during amiodarone administration. Another important reason for a noncorrelation between drug concentration and effect is the generation of active drug metabolites that may themselves actually have different pharmacologic properties from those of the parent drugs. An excellent example is procainamide; although it is common practice to add concentrations of procainamide to those of its active metabolite N-acetylprocainamide, this step is inappropriate since the two compounds have different electrophysiologic characteristics in vivo and in vitro, and each has been shown to suppress arrhythmias resistant to the other. Other drugs with major active metabolites that may disturb the relationship between parent drug concentration and effect include encainide, lidocaine, and (possibly) quinidine, propafenone, lorcainide, and amiodarone. For some drugs (encainide, propafenone, and procainamide), formation of these active metabolites, and hence net drug effect, appears to be under genetic control.

Interactions between antiarrhythmic drugs and other agents or concomitant disease can alter effect by altering pharmacokinetics. Such interactions can decrease drug effect by increasing the drug-metabolizing ability of the liver; for example, concentrations of quinidine, disopyramide, or mexiletine fall dramatically when phenytoin, phenobarbital, or rifampin is added. On the other hand, interactions may increase net drug effect by raising plasma concentrations: mechanisms include interference with drug metabolism (cimetidine increases quinidine concentrations; heart failure reduces lidocaine clearance), lowering liver blood flow, which is the major determinant of disposition of some agents (propranolol raises lidocaine concentrations through this mechanism), and delaying drug excretion (renal failure increases procainamide concentrations by this mechanism).

Effect can also be altered by nonpharmacokinetic-based drug interactions. For example, the anticholinergic side effects of disopyramide appear to be reversible by the addition of pyridostigmine, which leaves the antiarrhythmic activity intact. Also, improved drug efficacy and reduced side effects appear to be possible in some cases by combining low doses of two antiarrhythmic drugs with different electrophysiologic properties; this effect has been convincingly shown for the combination of quinidine and mexiletine, and further work is required before it can (or should) be more universally applied. Thus, not only can the interactions of concomitant drug therapy or disease alter pharmacokinetics thereby causing unexpected drug accumulation, but these interactions can occasionally be exploited to actually improve drug therapy.

MANAGEMENT OF ACUTE VENTRICULAR TACHYCARDIA

Synchronized DC-cardioversion is the treatement of choice for sustained, hemodynamically compromising VT. Drug therapy should be initiated or modified to prevent recurrence. Patients with frequently recurring episodes of hemodynamically stable sustained VT can occasionally be managed by ventricular pacing techniques (most often burst pacing), thereby avoiding frequent cardioversions while drug therapy is optimized. Patients with frequent episodes of nonsustained VT in whom urgent therapy is deemed necessary (e.g., in the setting of acute MI or for presyncope with each episode) should be managed with drugs alone.

The patient with reasonably preserved left ventricular function in whom active ischemia may be playing a role should receive a intravenous trial of propranolol; if this is successful, aggressive anti-ischemic therapy is indicated. With this exception, intravenous administration of lidocaine remains the treatment of choice for the acute management of VT. A loading dose of approximately 3 to 4 mg per kilogram should be administered to achieve a prompt antiarrhythmic effect. This should be given either as a series of slow boluses of 50 to 100 mg each over a total of 20 minutes or as a single 75 to 100 mg slow bolus followed by a rapid infusion of 8 to 10 mg per minute for 15 to 20 minutes (Tables 1 and 2). A physician should be in attendance during lidocaine loading for VT and if side effects—most commonly dysarthria or dysesthesias—occur, the loading process should be slowed. If arrhythmias persist after an adequate load, a plasma concentration should be measured to document adequate levels. If side effects are absent, continued cautious loading can be undertaken. If arrhythmias do not recur after lidocaine loading, a maintenance infusion (20

TABLE 1 Loading Doses of Antiarrhythmic Drugs in Ventricular Tachycardia

Agent	*Loading Dose*
Lidocaine	100 mg over 2–3 min followed by 50 mg over 2–3 min every 8 min to total of 3–4 mg/kg, *or* 75 mg over 3 min followed by 8 mg/min for 20 min, reduce by 50% in congestive heart failure
Procainamide	20/mg/min infusion to a maximum of 2 g
Bretylium	300–600 mg over 30 min; avoid in situations when markedly reduced afterload may be detrimental (aortic stenosis or pulmonary hypertension)
Amiodarone	300 mg over 30 min (IV); orally: many regimens; at Vanderbilt: 2,000 mg/day × 1 day 1,400 mg/day × 3 days 1,000 mg/day × 10 days 800 mg/day × 14 days 600 mg/day × 30 days If arrhythmia recurs on any given dose, that and subsequent dosages should be continued longer than scheduled.

TABLE 2 Maintenance Doses of Antiarrhythmic Drugs in Ventricular Tachycardia*

Agent	*Maintenance Dose*
Lidocaine	1–4 mg/min (IV); reduce in congestive heart failure, prolonged infusions, cimetidine, propranolol, or liver disease
Procainamide	2–6 mg/min (IV); 3–6 g/day (oral: q3h or, with sustained release, q6h); reduce in renal failure
Bretylium	1–4 mg/min (IV)
Amiodarone	200–600 mg/day
Quinidine sulfate	200–400 mg q6h
Disopyramide	300–900 mg/day (given q6h or, with controlled release, q12h); reduce in renal or hepatic disease
Tocainide	200–600 mg q8h; reduce in renal disease
Mexiletine	100–300 mg q8h
Flecainide	100–200 mg q12h; reduce in renal disease
Encainide	25–60 mg q8h; reduce in renal disease (accumulation of active metabolites)
Propafenone	300 mg q8–12h

* Doses are oral unless otherwise indicated.

to 60 μg/kg/min = 1 to 4 mg per min) should be started. This infusion achieves steady-state plasma concentrations in four to five elimination half-lives (8 to 10 hours), and the level achieved depends solely on clearance and rate of administration. Hence, arrhythmia recurrence several hours after successful lidocaine loading suggests that the maintenance infusion rate was too low; a small (50 to 75 mg) bolus followed by a higher maintenance infusion rate should be administered. On the other hand, late lidocaine toxicity and often subtle central nervous system symptoms (e.g., "CCU psychosis") suggest an excessive maintenance infusion rate.

Congestive heart failure reduces both volume of distribution and clearance of lidocaine; both loading and maintenance doses should be lowered. Severe liver disease, on the other hand, reduces only clearance; thus loading doses are unaltered, but maintenance infusions should be reduced. Cimetidine and propranolol both reduce lidocaine clearance, and lowered maintenance doses are required. For reasons that are not yet certain, lidocaine clearance falls during prolonged (>24 hours) infusions; plasma concentrations should therefore be monitored daily and infusion rates adjusted to maintain levels of 3 to 5 μg per milliliter.

If lidocaine fails to control VT (i.e., the arrhythmia recurs in the face of plasma concentrations above 5 μg per milliliter or in the presence of symptoms), intravenous procainamide or bretylium should be used. A loading dose of up to 2 g of procainamide can be administered as a 20 mg per minute infusion (again with a physician in attendance); hypotension is the most common effect that requires termination or slowing of the loading procedure. If the loading dose appears to be effective, a maintenance infusion of 2 to 6 mg per minute should be started. Plasma concentrations should be monitored, particularly when arrhythmia is suppressed and if arrhythmia recurs. Concentrations as high as 20 μg per milliliter can be used acutely, although levels above 8 to 10 μg per milliliter are rarely tolerated during chronic treatment. Bretylium is also highly effective, but its autonomic effects (orthostatic hypotension) complicate patient care. Also, once oral antiarrhythmics are started, bretylium effects may take several days to be eliminated, a distinct disadvantage compared to lidocaine (8 to 10 hours) or procainamide (12 to 18 hours). Rarely, patients whose VT persists after effective trials of lidocaine, procainamide, and bretylium require combination therapy (e.g., lidocaine and procainamide), intravenous administration of amiodarone, or urgent antitachycardia surgical intervention (with coronary artery bypass grafting and aneurysmectomy, if indicated).

MANAGEMENT OF CHRONIC RECURRENT VENTRICULAR TACHYCARDIA

In patients on parenteral therapy, oral agents should be started and permitted to come to steady-state (four to five elimination half-lives) levels before the drug is stopped. If side effects develop during this combined therapy, the dose of the intravenous agent can be cautiously lowered. Once chronic oral therapy is established, the common practice of "tapering" lidocaine is inappropriate. It is more reasonable simply to discontinue the drug, anticipating that plasma concentrations will approach zero in 8 to 10 hours. Thus, between 5 and 6 AM is the best time of day to stop lidocaine, since arrhythmias will then recur (if they do) during the midmorning hours. In all patients in whom chronic oral therapy is undertaken, an adequate baseline record of arrhythmia frequency and/or inducibility should be obtained, if at all possible, prior to the initiation of therapy. Each drug trial should begin

TABLE 3 Usual Range of Plasma Concentration Associated with Maximal Efficacy and Minimal Side Effects ("Therapeutic Range")

Agent	*Concentration*
Lidocaine	1–4 μg/ml
Procainamide	4–10 μg/ml (associated NAPA: 10–20 μg/ml; NAPA above 20 μg/ml frequently causes gastrointestinal intolerance)
Bretylium	....
Amiodarone	1–2 μg/ml
Quinidine	2–5 μg/ml
Disopyramide	2–5 μg/ml (associated free concentration dependent on protein binding, which is variable over this therapeutic range)
Tocainide	3–9 μg/ml
Mexiletine	0.5–2.0 μg/ml
Flecainide	0.2–1.0 μg/ml
Encainide	.... (major metabolite: ? 0.02–0.15 μg/ml)
Propafenone	? 0.2–1.0 μg/ml

TABLE 4 Relative Indications/Contraindications for Antiarrhythmic Drugs

Abnormality	*Used (with caution):*	*Avoid:*
Congestive heart failure	Quindine, procainamide, ?tocainide, ?mexiletine, ?encainide, or amiodarone	Disopyramide, flecainide, verapamil, beta-blockers, or propafenone
Conduction system disease	Quinidine, procainamide, disopyramide, tocainide, mexiletine, or amiodarone	Flecainide, encainide, or propafenone
Chronic pulmonary disease		Amiodarone
Prostatism		Disopyramide
Long QT	Mexiletine or tocainide	Quinidine, procainamide, or disopyramide
Atrial fibrillation	Quinidine, procainamide, disopyramide, amiodarone, ?flecainide, ?encainide, or ?propafenone	Not active; mexiletine, tocainide, or lidocaine

at low dosages. If with any agent, side effects develop and arrhythmia persists, that agent can be declared a failure. If, on the other hand, no side effects develop, each drug regimen should be evaluated only after steady-state conditions are assumed to be present (four to five elimination half-lives); loading doses do not decrease the time to achieve steady-state plasma concentrations. For patients undergoing evaluation of therapy by repetitive electrophysiologic testing, follow-up tests should only be performed at steady-state, in the absence of side effects, and when plasma concentrations are in the mid-to-high range of therapeutic concentrations (Table 3).

Although many drugs have been shown to be effective in the management of VT, there is no method of predicting response in an individual patient. For patients whose management is being guided by programmed electrical stimulation, failure of intravenous procainamide has been shown to be a predictor that other drugs will also fail. This may simply reflect the fact that effective drug therapy is found in only a minority of these patients. It is convenient to group antiarrhythmic drugs by subtype, depending on their major electrophysiologic actions in vitro and in vivo. Most available agents block cardiac sodium channels (and therefore slow conduction velocity) as their major mode of action. Failure of an arrhythmia to respond to one member of a subclass of drugs does not necessarily predict failure with other members of that class, particularly since drug "failure" is often a reflection of noncardiac side effects. Selection of drugs for testing then hinges on the likelihood of side effects and concurrent medical problems (Table 4). Quinidine is among the first drugs that should be tried. If the patient has a history of quinidine-related diarrhea or if diarrhea develops on quinidine, the drug should be stopped since it is unlikely to be tolerated for chronic therapy. Procainamide is effective but eventually causes the lupus syndrome in a high proportion of patients.

Disopyramide should be tested in patients who do not have severely depressed left ventricular function and no other contraindications (such as prostatism). Therapy with the lidocaine analogs, tocainide, and mexiletine frequently causes side effects (nausea or tremor). They can be avoided by giving the drug with food, which slows but does not decreases the extent of absorption. Combinations of low doses of quinidine and either of these lidocaine analogs are frequently well tolerated and produce additive (and possibly synergistic) antiarrhythmic effects. Phenytoin, which has some electrophysiologic properties in common with lidocaine, can be effectively combined with procainamide. The major problem with phenytoin therapy is induction of hepatic metabolism of several other agents, including quinidine, disopyramide, mexiletine, and digitoxin. Patients receiving these other agents therefore require high doses to achieve therapeutic effects; if phenytoin therapy is stopped, these patients run high risk of serious drug toxicity if dosages of the other drugs are not reduced as well.

A number of members of a novel subclass of sodium-channel blocking drugs have been (flecainide) or are close to being marketed (encainide, propafenone, indecainide, and lorcainide). These agents appear to share a number of unusual clinical features: they are more effective (and better tolerated) than standard therapies (such as quinidine) for patients with nonsustained VT and near-normal left ventricular function, but appear to confer a high risk (5% to 20%) of exacerbating sustained VT in patients with a history of this arrhythmia and depressed LV function. The high reported incidence of this adverse effect may be related in part to excessive dosages used early in drug development, and drugs of this type do not appear to be out of the question for patients with sustained VT. (In fact, in the rare case of a patient with recurrent sustained VT and an otherwise apparently normal heart, they may be the drugs of choice.) These drugs markedly slow cardiac conduction even at normal heart rates, and 20 to 40 percent increases in PR and QRS duration are routine during therapy; marked QRS widening (>40%) may be a warning of impending sustained VT, but some cases of exacerbation of sustained VT by drug have occurred in the absence of QRS widening. Bundle branch block and complete AV block are a real risk, especially in patients with conduction system disease. There are only a few points to consider in choosing among drugs of this subtype: flecainide and propafenone appear to exert negative inotropic effects, whereas encainide does not. On the other hand, there is a great degree of interindividual variability in metabolism of encainide and propafenone (and both have active metabolites), making plasma concentration monitoring difficult or impossible to interpret, whereas flecainide does not appear to have highly variable metabolism or active metabolites. Flecainide has a very long elimination half-life (up to 24 hours), allowing twice daily dosing, but mandating infrequent dosage regimen increases (no more often than every 4 days). Some studies with propafenone indicate that patients may have a satisfactory clinical outcome despite persistently inducible VT during programmed electrical stimulation. As with all new agents, the real place of these drugs becomes apparent only after they have been released for general use and their side-effect profile becomes better delineated.

A drug in a category of its own is amiodarone. Amiodarone was originally developed for the therapy of angina but has its greatest application in the treatment of supraventricular and ventricular arrhythmias. It has an extraordinarily long elimination half-life (at least several weeks). In order to achieve a prompt (within days) antiarrhythmic effect, a loading regimen of some sort is required. However, once an effect is seen, pills can be taken once a day, and missing a dose is unlikely to result in recurrence of arrhythmia. The major problem with amiodarone is side effects; in contrast to most other agents, side effects are *unusual* early in therapy but appear progressively during treatment. If side effects requiring discontinuation of amiodarone develop, the drug effect may persist for months, making the choice of alternative antiarrhythmic therapy particularly difficult. The most common side effects are corneal microdeposits (which are generally asymptomatic), pulmonary fibrosis (5%), abnormal liver function, hyper- or hypothyroidism, ataxia and weakness, photosensitivity, and bluish skin discoloration (which can be disfiguring).

Many reports suggest that arrhythmia recurrence is unlikely even in the face of continued inducibility of sustained VT during programmed electrical stimulation. Amiodarone is a very useful drug in the management of sustained VT. Patients who decline operation or antitachycardia devices are strong candidates, as are patients who are not candidates for repetitive electrophysiologic study (e.g., the elderly or mentally incompetent). Amiodarone was released on the United States market in early 1986. It is well tolerated, particularly during the first 6 to 12 months of therapy, but it is not a first-line drug because of the likelihood of serious late side effects and the difficulty in managing patients who develop them.

Ventricular tachycardia is one of the most difficult problems in clinical medicine. The first decision is whether a patient should be treated. Assuming treatment is undertaken, a method to assess its adequacy is required. Drugs are the first line of treatment, but other modalities should be available if drugs fail. Each drug trial should be well documented in terms of efficacy, side effects, and plasma concentrations. Psychological support is an integral part of the management of these patients during prolonged hospitalizations. With a multitude of drugs now available and in the late stages of preclinical investigation, it is becoming increasingly important for physicians caring for these patients to have a sound knowledge of general pharmacokinetic and electrophysiologic principles and of how they apply to each of the drugs that a patient receives.

ATRIOVENTRICULAR BLOCK AND IMPLANTATION OF PERMANENT CARDIAC PACEMAKERS

LEONARD SCHERLIS, M.D.

There is concern about the use and abuse of cardiac pacemaker insertion for the treatment of cardiac dysrhythmias. It is estimated that about 500,000 people in the United States have pacemakers implanted and that over 500 units are implanted per million population each year. In one 1981 survey, 5,700 physicians from 3,300 hospitals were implanting permanent pacemakers. As is to be expected, the criteria for the implantation of pacemakers may vary, as may the training and experience of the physicians and the adequacy of the facilities available in the hospitals.

Unlike earlier pacemakers, which were comparatively simple units and subject to unpredictable failures, the present implantable cardiac pacemaker is a far more reliable and complex device. It reflects many technical changes including hermetic sealing, complementary metal oxide semiconductor circuits, long-life batteries, multiprogrammability, and dual-chamber pacing. Pacemakers are now available that can restore normal atrial and ventricular sequence and selectively sense and pace either at the atrial or ventricular level or both. One recent development is the atrioventricular universal pacemaker, which combines atrial synchrony with atrioventricular sequential and ventricular inhibition. These models may be widely programmed for output and sensitivity, and the minimum and maximum rates are independently variable as are the atrioventricular delays.

The wide variety of available permanent pacemakers has required a 5-position coding system designating the chamber or chambers sensed, the chamber or chambers paced, the mode of response (triggered or inhibited), programmability (simple, multiple, communicating: telemetry), and special antiarrhythmic features. Recent changes have been made in the nomenclature code for implantable cardiac pacemakers. The 5-position code now recommended is contained in Tables 1 and 2 from the Inter-Society Commission for Heart Disease Resources Report on Permanent Pacemakers. Some of the dual chamber (A-V sequential) models are capable of being programmed to innumerable settings. Programmable features include rate (minimum and maximum), output (pulse duration and amplitude), sensitivity, refractory period, mode, A-V interval, hysteresis, and polarity (unipolar or bipolar). Telemetry, while not truly programming, permits interrogating the pacemaker for three categories of data: record keeping, pacemaker status, and physiologic information.

As the electrical stimulus arises normally in the sinus node and spreads through the atria, AV junction, bundle branches, and ventricles, there is a measurable period of time normally involved between atrial and ventricular activation. First-degree AV block is an increased delay (i.e., prolonged P-R interval [>0.20 sec]). This may be due to increased parasympathetic tone, drug effect, or-

TABLE 1 Nomenclature Code for Implantable Cardiac Pacemakers

Chamber Paced	*Chamber Sensed*	*Mode of Response*	*Generic Description*	*Previously Used Description*
V	O	O	Ventricular pacing; no sensing function	Asynchronous; fixed rate; set rate
A	O	O	Atrial pacing; no sensing function	Atrial fixed rate; atrial asynchronous
D	O	O	Atrioventricular pacing; no sensing function	AV sequential fixed rate (asynchronous)
V	V	I	Ventricular pacing and sensing, inhibited mode	Ventricular inhibited; R inhibited; R blocking; R suppressed, noncompetitive inhibited; demand; standby
V	V	T	Ventricular pacing and sensing, triggered mode	Ventricular triggered; R triggered; R wave stimulated, noncompetitive triggered; following; R synchronous; demand; standby
A	A	I	Atrial pacing and sensing, inhibited mode	Atrial inhibited; P inhibited; P blocking; P suppressed
A	A	T	Atrial pacing and sensing, triggered mode	Atrial triggered; P triggered; P stimulated; P synchronous
V	A	T	Ventricular pacing, atrial sensing, triggered mode	Atrial synchronous; atrial synchronized; AV synchronous
D	V	I	Atrioventricular pacing, ventricular sensing, inhibited mode	Bifocal sequential demand; AV sequential

TABLE 2 ICHD Five-Position Pacemaker Code

Position	*I*	*II*	*III*	*IV*	*V*
Category	*Chamber(s) Paced*	*Chamber(s) Sensed*	*Modes of Response(s)*	*Programmable Functions*	*Special Antitachyarrhythmia Functions*
Letters used	V-ventricle	V-ventricle	T-triggered	P-programmable (rate and or output)	B-bursts
	A-atrium	A-atrium	I-inhibited	M-multiprogrammable	N-normal rate competition
	D-double	D-double	D-double* O-none	C-communicating	S-scanning
		O-none	R-reverse	O-none	E-external
Manufacturer's designation only	S-single chamber	S-single chamber			

* Triggered and inhibited response.

ganic lesions, and so on. The site of the block is usually at the level of the AV node. The P-R interval is prolonged beyond 0.20 seconds and the QRS duration remains unchanged. No therapy is indicated, but the patient should be monitored for the possibility of developing second- or third-degree block.

In Mobitz type I second-degree AV block, (Wenckebach periods), delay in conduction between the atria and ventricles at the AV node becomes progressively longer until an impulse is blocked and the cycle is then resumed. The prognosis is usually favorable, and the disturbance in rhythm temporary. The causes are usually related to drug effect or increased parasympathetic tone. Second-degree AV block may occur during the course of an inferior myocardial infarction. The patient should be observed for the development of third-degree heart block. Therapy usually is not indicated unless the ventricular rate is very slow. In these instances, atropine may be necessary or a temporary pacemaker may be required.

In Mobitz type II second-degree AV block, there is a sudden nonconducted beat without the progressive prolongation of the P-R interval as seen in Wenckebach periods. This is usually due to an organic lesion in the infranodal conduction pathway at the bundle branch level or, less frequently, at the bundle of His level. It may indicate the development of complete heart block; the use of a permanent pacemaker is usually indicated.

In third-degree AV block, there is no conduction between the atria and ventricles. If the block is at the level of the AV node, the impulse for ventricular depolarization is present at the junctional level, and the rate varies between 40 and 60. This type of AV block is usually well tolerated even with an acute inferior myocardial infarction; a permanent pacemaker is seldom indicated. Atropine or a temporary pacemaker may be of help. The block is usually infranodal in location if in association with an acute anterior myocardial infarction. The rate is slower (i.e., less than 40 beats per minute), and a permanent pacemaker is indicated although the effect on prognosis may not be significant.

In general, pacing is appropriate for control of symptomatic bradyarrhythmias, particularly those unresponsive to medical management. Permanent pacemakers are indicated in instances of complete heart block (i.e., third-degree AV block with a slow subsidiary pacemaker site), particularly with accompanying symptoms such as syncope, seizures, confusion, or easy fatigue, or symptoms of congestive heart failure. Rates of 40 or more are usually well tolerated. Pacemakers are not generally indicated in instances of Mobitz type I second-degree AV block (Wenckebach periods) in the presence of a narrow QRS complex. These patients rarely have symptoms since there are only periodic absent ventricular contractions due to failure of AV conduction. Permanent pacemakers are not indicated in first-degree block (i.e., P-R interval prolongation with AV conduction delayed but not blocked).

In the presence of Mobitz type II block (sudden transient complete AV block for one or more beats), there is greater concern since it may be a warning of the development of complete heart block with severe symptoms.

With increasing pacemaker technology, indications for permanent pacing have expanded. Synchronized capability and atrioventricular sequential modes have extended treatment to complex brady- and tachyarrhythmias. Indications are not always clear and remain controversial in bundle branch block with acute ischemic heart disease in bifascicular and trifascicular blocks, and in intermittent or undocumented symptomatic low cardiac output syndromes attributable to bradycardia. Electrophysiologic testing, rapid pacing, or drug-induced stress assessment of the conducting system is of value in many, but not all, pacemaker candidates; often, physiologic assessment is impractical. Generally accepted indications are listed in Table 3.

There is difficulty in attempting to be dogmatic in the recommendations for permanent pacemaker implantation. Indications have been extended as electrophysiologic studies have increased and various conduction disorders have been documented at a basal state or provoked by various maneuvers. There is general agreement on the favorable impact of permanent pacemaker implantation in sinoatrial disease. However, the leading indication for permanent pacemaker implantation is now "sick sinus syndrome," that is, sinus node dysfunction. The relationship of appropriate symptoms to this disorder can be difficult to demonstrate in an individual patient, and relief of symptoms may not follow permanent pacemaker implantation. The clinical significance of such data as prolonged H-V intervals, sinoatrial conduction time, or sinus recovery time is controversial in the absence of an appropriate relationship of a dysrhythmia and symptoms. However, at times it may be difficult to document the occurrence of symptoms with the recordings of transient arrhythmias. The use of electrophysiologic studies, including the assessment of sinus node and AV function, may be of value in selected patients with unexplained syncope.

Permanent pacemakers have been utilized for bifascicular and trifascicular block in the absence of symptoms, since there is concern that these lesions will progress to complete heart block. Even in the presence of prolonged His-Purkinje conduction time, data are lacking on the prolongation of life by the prophylactic implantation of

TABLE 3 Indications for Permanent Pacemaker

- Bradyarrhythmia
  - Atrioventricular block, congenital or acquired
    - Third degree (complete)
    - Second degree, below the AV node (Mobitz II)
- Sick sinus syndrome, symptomatic
  - Sinus node dysfunction
    - Severe sinus bradycardia
    - SA block
  - Atrial dysrhythmia with profound bradycardia
    - Atrial fibrillation
  - Bradycardia—Tachycardia
- Tachyarrhythmia
  - Overdrive suppression of ventricular tachycardia
  - Conversion of supraventricular tachycardia
- Deficiency of myocardial function
  - AV dissociation (need for atrial augmentation)

a permanent pacemaker. The prognosis is usually related to the severity of the underlying heart disease.

In the presence of a dysrhythmia, usually a bradycardia, which is demonstrated to be related to symptoms, there is clear agreement regarding the implantation of a permanent pacemaker. Pacemakers may be inserted in the presence of less severe dysrhythmias when available data indicate the probable progression of the rhythm disturbance to one producing significant symptoms. Care must be given to avoid the use of a permanent pacemaker when the disturbance of rhythm is drug-related and the drug is not critical for the patient's therapy.

Attempts must be made to demonstrate the correlation of the dysrhythmia with the symptoms of the patient in order to justify the use of a pacemaker and to help select the appropriate device. A carefully kept diary in conjunction with 24-hour dynamic electrocardiographic monitoring, transtelephonic electrocardiographic transmission, or patient-activated electrocardiographic recordings are of value. Such monitoring provides documentation of the presence of the rhythm disturbance and its relationship to the patient's symptoms, as well as data on transient changes in specific activities. It should be noted that the presence of transient bradyarrhythmias without symptoms or occasionally during sleep is rarely in itself an adequate reason for permanent pacemaker implantation.

Patients who have been resuscitated from cardiac arrest and who have not had an acute myocardial infarction or other documented cause should be subjected to electrophysiologic studies, including programmed electrical stimulation, for the selection of appropriate drug therapy or for the implantation of antitachycardia pacing devices or defibrillators. The use of rapid atrial pacing for serious recurrent supraventricular tachyarrhythmias is promising and is an additional use for complex pacemakers. The automatic implanted defibrillator, while still under investigation, may be of significant value in patients who have experienced sudden death and who remain candidates for ventricular fibrillation or life-threatening ventricular tachycardia.

As yet not determined is the role for the more advanced pacemakers, which permit normal synchrony between atrial and ventricular activity as well as physiologic responses of heart rate. Most pacemakers inserted have been of the VVI or VVT type. The availability of more complex pacemakers, DDD, VDD, or DVI permits many additional options for patient management. However, the need for such pacemakers remains controversial except in certain specific clinical entities. AV sequential pacemakers, for example, are only indicated when the atrial contribution to cardiac output is significant and provides a necessary increment in cardiac performance. In selected patients, over 20 percent of the cardiac output may depend on effective atrial systole. However, in most patients, AV sequential pacing is not necessary. The additional benefits to selected patients must be weighed against the increased cost, complexity, and difficulty in programming of these units for specific patient needs. The question of how many patients will derive additional significant benefits from such units beyond the benefits derived from pacemakers that do not permit atrial and ventricular synchrony remains to be determined. Additional problems may also be presented by the effects of retrograde (ventricular-atrial) conduction after ventricular depolarization when VDD or DDD units are implanted.

Although the cost of the pacemaker is in the thousands of dollars, present-day pacemakers last longer, have enhanced reliability, are more complex, and can be programmed in numerous ways. They represent a class of devices that are all too infrequently available in medical practice. Their implantation can enable an individual to live a relatively normal life with a minimum of device maintenance and with minimal inconvenience. In many instances, there is both a significant prolongation of life and an enhanced quality of life. Individuals can be restored to a productive life, and the likelihood of syncope or of sudden death is significantly reduced. However, the indications for pacemaker insertion require careful definition, and the requirements for training and resources must be defined because of the complexity of the devices and the specific electrophysiologic criteria to be met for implantation.

The decision to insert a permanent pacemaker is critical and must be made only after careful consideration of all the factors involved for the individual patient. The experience, training, and skills of the implanting physician are critical, particularly given the large choice of pacemakers now available. Several groups have addressed the problem of what constitutes optimal training for implanting physicians; there has been emphasis on the need for specific documentation of such training. The pacemaker study group of the ICHD has recently addressed this issue, and I recommend review of its detailed report. In this report, it is emphasized that the cardiologist or surgeon who implants pacemakers should have the clinical and electrophysiologic skills and knowledge necessary to make informed decisions. Training requirement should include documentation that the necessary clinical and electrophysiologic skills have been acquired during formal training in cardiology. The individual performing the implantation should be skilled in right heart catheterization and should have experience in implantations, reoperations, insertions of temporary pacemakers, and electrophysiologic studies. Interpretation of electrocardiography by physicians requires that they have adequate training and verified skills in routine electrocardiography and a knowledge of the electrocardiograms related to cardiac pacing. The implanting physician should be knowledgeable in the basic mechanical and electrical aspects of pacemaker technology, electrocardiography, and the safe and appropriate use of radiologic equipment. He should be trained in the recognition and management of complications and emergencies that may arise during implantation, during the postoperative period, and during long-term follow-up. The presence of a manufacturer's representative during implantation can only be condoned under isolated and extremely unusual circumstances.

Although permanent pacemakers are implanted in

many hospitals, there is a significant difference in the number inserted in each hospital. The minimum normal hospital case load should be 50 implantations per year. The insertion of a permanent pacemaker requires the availability of both the necessary physical facilities and well trained and experienced personnel. In the absence of these resources, the implantation should be assigned to an institution where such resources are available.

CORONARY ARTERY SPASM

CHARLES R. LAMBERT, M.D., Ph.D.
CARL J. PEPINE, M.D.

Coronary artery spasm is an important pathophysiologic mechanism in the genesis of both acute and chronic myocardial ischemic syndromes. These syndromes may include silent myocardial ischemia, chronic stable-effort angina, unstable-rest angina, and acute myocardial infarction (MI). Coronary artery spasm may occur in angiographically normal arteries or, more commonly, be superimposed on atherosclerotic obstructive disease. The latter is probably the more important clinically and forms the basis for complex interactions between passive changes affecting vascular caliber, vasomotion, "fixed" obstruction, and mediators of thrombosis, all of which appear to modulate myocardial ischemia in vivo.

Whenever possible, making a definitive diagnosis of coronary artery spasm is very important so that appropriate treatment can be instituted. A definitive diagnosis also aids the primary-care physician in interpreting and managing the highly variable clinical course that many patients with coronary artery spasm follow. The diagnosis of coronary artery spasm is suggested by angina when the patient is often at rest or during ordinary activity without elevation of heart rate or blood pressure. At times, angina due to coronary spasm may be associated with serious dysrhythmias or syncope. Other findings associated with coronary artery spasm include a variable threshold for exercise-induced angina and an almost-universal responsiveness of spasm-related angina to nitroglycerin. Coronary spasm may be associated with ST-segment depression or T-wave changes. Although the finding of transient perfusion defects associated with angina and ST-segment elevation is highly suggestive of coronary artery spasm, definitive diagnosis requires coronary angiography. During angiographic examination, spasm that occurs spontaneously or is provoked by ergonovine can be visualized. Care must be taken to ensure that any change observed in the size of the coronary artery is neither catheter-related nor due to other problems, such as dissection, thrombus, or embolus.

Certain general considerations should be taken into account when treating patients with coronary artery spasm in any setting. Factors contributing to precipitation or exacerbation of coronary artery spasm include exposure to cold, smoking, and emotional stress. These factors should be removed whenever possible. Known vasoconstrictors should be avoided and patients cautioned against use of "over-the-counter" sympathomimetic drugs. Recent withdrawal of nitrates or calcium antagonists should be sought as a possible exacerbating factor. Recent therapeutic institution of beta-adrenergic blocking agents should also be considered in the coronary-spasm patient with worsening symptoms.

TREATMENT IN THE ACUTE CARE SETTING

Relieving the Acute Episode in the Hospitalized Patient

As already noted, coronary artery spasm can play an important role in the genesis of unstable anginal syndromes. Thus, spasm should be considered in the treatment strategies employed for all coronary-care unit patients with acute myocardial ischemia. In this setting, the agent of choice is intravenous nitroglycerin, although isosorbide nitrate and nitroprusside may also be used intravenously. The infusion rate of nitroglycerin should be started at 5 to 10 μg per minute and titrated to achieve resolution of signs (e.g., ST-segment shifts) and symptoms of myocardial ischemia and not to an arbitrary reduction in blood pressure. The latter strategy may provoke ischemia by reducing coronary perfusion pressure while causing a reflex increase in heart rate in patients with severe atherosclerotic obstructive disease. In many cases, a bolus of 100 to 200 μg, given just before the continuous infusion, is helpful in achieving more rapid resolution of spasm-related ischemia. Coronary artery spasm is usually very sensitive to nitrates, and it is not usually necessary to achieve high blood levels.

In the rare instance in which acute ischemia caused by coronary artery spasm appears refractory to parenteral nitrates, buccal administration of nifedipine or intravenous administration of verapamil or diltiazem should be added. When administered by the sublingual route, a single 10-mg nifedipine capsule should be punctured and its contents expelled by chewing. Alternatively, if the patient finds this difficult or is under anesthesia, the contents can be withdrawn by a large needle and syringe and then expressed to the buccal area from the syringe. For intravenous use, we recommend verapamil (0.15 mg per kilogram) or diltiazem (0.25 mg per kilogram) given over 2 minutes. Care must be taken to avoid triggering systemic hypotension when calcium blockers are added to the nitrate infusion. However, if hypotension occurs, restoration of systemic blood pressure is usually readily achieved by temporarily discontinuing the calcium blocker and nitroglycerin, or careful fluid administration, or both. Of the three calcium blockers available, diltiazem is usually the best tolerated and has highly desirable pharmacologic properties that act to relax coronary vascular smooth muscle, prevent spasm, and reduce myocardial oxygen requirements.

In the rare situation in which a patient does not respond to these measures, the intra-aortic balloon pump can relieve the acute episode of ischemia due to spasm. Coronary artery bypass surgery is of no proven value and probably harmful in patients with acute ischemia due to an acute episode of coronary artery spasm.

Preventing Recurrent Episodes

Shortly after parenteral nitrates are started, calcium antagonists should be orally administered to prevent recurrent episodes. Therapy with the combination of nitrates and calcium antagonists inhibits both primary activational mechanisms in vascular smooth muscle and thus has a firm pharmacologic basis. The choice of an oral calcium blocker, in general, is not critical; however, a few general guidelines must be followed. Verapamil should be avoided in patients with bradydysrhythmias, heart block, and severe impairment of left ventricular function. Nifedipine and other dihydropyridine compounds are potent peripheral vasodilators and should be used with caution in patients with tachycardia and fixed, obstructive disease unless another agent is used concomitantly to avoid further reflex sympathetic stimulation. Such an agent may be either a beta-adrenergic blocking agent or another antagonist of a different class with negative chronotropic activity, such as verapamil or diltiazem. The dose range we employ for diltiazem is 30 to 120 mg 4 times per day; for verapamil, 40 to 120 mg, 3-to-4 times per day; and for nifedipine, 10 to 30 mg, 3-to-4 times per day.

When patients are controlled in the acute setting, parenteral administration of nitrates should be changed to oral or topical preparations, or both. We usually follow a progression from parenteral administration of nitrates to nitroglycerin paste and then to an oral form of isosorbide dinitrate which may be administered on a 4- or 6-hour schedule or, in sustained release form, twice per day. Transdermal patches may also be utilized, but their sustained effectiveness in patients with coronary artery spasm has not been demonstrated. The choice of nitrate preparation, in our opinion, is not critical and should be tailored to patient response and physician familiarity.

In the rare patient with recurrent episodes of coronary spasm despite these drugs being given in maximum tolerated doses, the intra-aortic balloon pump can help in preventing recurrent episodes for several days, while more definitive studies are carried out. Coronary artery bypass surgery can be effective in the patient with recurrent spasm limited to the site of an important atherosclerotic-type narrowing. If, however, spasm involves multiple vessels, is diffuse in the same vessel, or is not associated with an important atherosclerotic obstruction, coronary artery bypass surgery is of no value. In any patient with suspected coronary spasm undergoing operation (coronary artery bypass or other), it is essential to provide effective prophylaxis against coronary spasm. Conventional coronary artery bypass surgery can be combined with denervation (e.g., plexectomy), but there is no objective evidence that this procedure improves results. Likewise, percutaneous transluminal angioplasty can be effective in managing selected patients with coronary spasm associated with important atherosclerotic narrowings. With either form of revascularization, the patient is likely to require continued drug therapy. The frequency of graft occlusion after coronary artery bypass surgery or restenosis after angioplasty is considerably higher than when these procedures are used in patients without coronary spasm.

TREATMENT IN THE AMBULATORY SETTING

The treatment principles for coronary artery spasm in ambulatory patients are similar to those for patients in the acute setting; they differ only in the routes by which medications are administered. Sublingual nitroglycerin is used for relief of the acute episode. Both nitrates and calcium antagonists remain the mainstays of chronic therapy. Many patients require an agent of both classes, although some patients may do well with monotherapy. The clinical course of patients with coronary artery spasm is highly variable and typically displays periods of exacerbation and remission even with seemingly optimal therapy. During flares of activity, after the measures already listed are instituted, our general approach is to increase doses of calcium antagonists and nitrates and to utilize topical nitroglycerin ointment as an adjunct to oral preparations of isosorbide dinitrate. Topical nitrate therapy allows the physician and patient to optimize nitrate levels at times of anticipated symptomatic exacerbation, which may be remarkably cyclic in some patients with coronary artery spasm. In some patients, symptoms tend to recur in the early morning.

MONITORING THERAPY

After institution of an effective ambulatory treatment regimen, several options are available to monitor patients with coronary artery spasm. Simply monitoring their symptoms is sufficient for many patients; however, there is evidence that as many as 90 percent of all ischemic episodes in coronary spasm patients may be silent. Thus, it may be beneficial to attempt more objective assessment of therapeutic efficacy, especially in patients with severe ischemia or sequelae, such as tachydysrhythmias, pump dysfunction, or conduction disturbances related to coronary artery spasm. Some investigators have advised repeat catheterization with ergonovine provocation during therapy to assess efficacy. We have not employed this method for documenting therapeutic success. It has obvious disadvantages in cost and risk, and results can be misleading. Ambulatory ECG monitoring is a useful objective method to monitor effectiveness of therapy in patients with coronary artery spasm. The indicator of greatest usefulness is ST-segment depression, and the frequency of this finding in a given period can be a guide to therapeutic efficacy. Elevation of the ST segment and changes in T wave are much less reliable because it is difficult to distinguish ischemic changes from positional changes and other artifacts during ambulatory ECG monitoring. If spasm-related dysrhythmias are present in a given patient, they can also be used to follow efficacy of therapy.

UNRESOLVED ISSUES

The basic pathophysiologic mechanisms underlying coronary artery spasm are unknown, but experimentation in this area has led to questions about the clinical relevance of various therapeutic modalities. There is no current clinical evidence that either aspirin or prostanoid compounds (e.g., prostacyclin) modify coronary spasm in the clinical setting. Although aspirin clearly seems effective in preventing untoward events in the larger group of patients with unstable angina and may be given for this reason, there is no proven role for aspirin in the subset of patients with coronary spasm. Likewise, there is no proven role for other antiplatelet drugs (e.g., dipyridamole, sulfinpyrazone, ticlopidine) in patients with coronary artery spasm. Clinical trials with ketanseran suggest no important role of the serotonergic system in clinical coronary artery spasm, and the contribution of the histaminergic system and histamine-blocking agents remains speculative. The issue of whether beta-adrenergic blocking agents should be used in patients with coronary spasm is unresolved. There are patients in whom removing endogenous $beta_2$- adrenergic receptor dilator tone seems to be detrimental, in that the frequency or duration of ischemic episodes increases. However, some other patients, particularly those with multiple-vessel disease, have improved effort tolerance when a beta-blocker is added to an effective antispasm treatment plan. Along similar lines, controlled trials have realized no benefits from alpha-adrenergic blockade in patients with coronary artery spasm. Whether patients with coronary artery spasm should be placed on antidysrhythmic agents is unresolved. We reserve this form of therapy for patients with specific rhythm disturbances for which specific therapy can be instituted.

Treatment of patients with coronary artery spasm relies upon nitrates and calcium antagonists. In most patients, an agent of both classes should be used; however, monotherapy may be effective. In the acute setting, a parenteral preparation of nitroglycerin is the agent of choice and should be supplemented with oral administration of calcium antagonists. In the ambulatory monitoring setting, both oral agents and topical nitrates are usually effective but must be tailored to the individual patient. An ambulatory ECG may be a useful adjunct in assessing the efficacy of a given therapeutic regimen. Infrequently, a revascularization approach designed to bypass or dilate important atherosclerotic stenoses associated with localized spasm can be helpful when combined with antispasm drug treatment.

DIGITALIS TOXICITY

THOMAS L. WENGER, M.D., F.A.C.C.

Digitalis toxicity has been a problem of clinical management for 200 years. It is estimated that as many as 500,000 patients per year become toxic (10%), of which perhaps 50,000 are considered to be severe (1%). The proper management of digitalis toxicity requires early recognition of the problem, which is no easy matter, as there are few highly selective criteria for establishing the diagnosis. Serum digitalis glycoside concentrations offer diagnostic insight, but cannot in themselves establish the diagnosis. A serum digoxin concentration above the "therapeutic range" suggests only a statistically increased likelihood of digitalis toxicity in such patients. The most common symptoms and signs are nonspecific and include the following: listlessness, anorexia, nausea, vomiting, and uniform or multiform ventricular extrasystoles and runs of ventricular bigeminy or trigeminy. These abnormalities alone or together cannot establish the diagnosis. An acute decrease in color discrimination or onset of blurred or yellow vision should be sought, since visual disturbances are not uncommon and are fairly specific for digitalis toxicity. Atrial tachycardia with block, although suggestive of digitalis toxicity, can occur in other situations, may be difficult to diagnose, and is a rare manifestation of the condition. Bidirectional ventricular tachycardia is also highly suggestive of digitalis toxicity, but is only rarely encountered.

Thus, physicians treating patients for digitalis toxicity often do so despite some uncertainty as to the correct diagnosis. On the other hand, massive digitalis intoxication, although rare, lacks subtlety. These patients often have severe bradyarrhythmias with heart block. A variety of supraventricular and ventricular arrhythmias can occur, with death ensuing from ventricular fibrillation or asystole.

THERAPEUTIC ALTERNATIVES

Withdrawal of Digitalis

Most patients suspected of digitalis toxicity can be handled simply by withdrawing the digitalis glycoside in question for several half-lives to see if the abnormalities dissipate (Table 1). A digoxin withdrawal trial may require 2 or 3 days observation in patients with normal renal function or more than 1 week in patients with severely impaired renal function to determine if resolution of the

TABLE 1 Alternative Treatments for Digitalis Toxicity

Treatment	*Setting*	*Time Course of Response*	*Comments*
Digitalis withdrawal	All cases	Days or longer	Response can aid in diagnosis
Potassium supplements	Patients with hypokalemia or severe toxicity and low or low-normal serum K^+	Hours	Administration must be done slowly and cautiously with frequent monitoring; massive digitalis toxicity can cause hyperkalemia
Lidocaine	Hemodynamically significant ventricular arrhythmias	Minutes	Seizures, other CNS toxicity, or asystole can occur
Phenytoin	Hemodynamically significant ventricular arrhythmias	Minutes	Hypotension and cardiac arrest can occur if agent is given too rapidly
Other antiarrhythmics	Back up to lidocaine and phenytoin	Minutes	CHF, hypotension, SA and AV block, or asystole can occur
Atropine	Severe bradycardia or heart block	Seconds	Effect is often too short lasting; belladonna toxicity must be avoided; CNS toxicity of atropine can be confused with CNS toxicity of digitalis
RV pacemaker	Rapidly progressive or severe bradycardia or heart block	Time to placement	Prophylactic placement is debatable in terms of risk:benefit ratio
Digoxin-immune Fab(ovine)	Life-threatening toxicity	Minutes to hours	Rapid reversal of digitalis effects can precipitate CHF, hypokalemia, rapid ventricular response in AFib
Cardioversion	VT/VF	Immediate	Recurrent episodes are likely; use lowest effective energy; Fab also indicated
Activated charcoal	Massive ingestion	Hours	Absorption is reduced; may enhance elimination of digitalis undergoing enteroenteric recycling
Glucose, insulin, or bicarbonate	Hyperkalemia	Minutes	Death from other effects of digitalis is likely
Potassium-binding resins	Hyperkalemia	Hours	Death from other effects of digitalis is likely; exacerbation of total body potassium deficit
Dialysis	Hyperkalemia	Hours	Death from other effects of digitalis; exacerbation of total body potassium deficit; rapid electrolyte shifts may worsen arrhythmias

AFib = Atrial fibrillation

abnormalities coincides with elimination of the drug. In the case of digitoxin, resolution of toxicity occurs over a longer time course. In general, the severer the toxicity, the longer the time to resolution following withdrawal of the drug. Although dissipation of abnormalities, such as arrhythmias, in coordination with drug withdrawal is considered to be the standard means to establish a relationship between an adverse event and a drug, the lengthy time course for digitalis elimination, coupled with the known variability in cardiac arrhythmias caused by heart disease, decreases the usefulness of withdrawal observation in establishing causality. I therefore recommend prolonged monitoring both to establish the diagnosis and at the same time to assure complete resolution of toxicity. A serum digoxin concentration obtained at the time of resolution offers a useful guide to future treatment of the individual patient.

Potassium Therapy

The availability of potent diuretics capable of depleting body stores of potassium probably caused a substantial increase in digitalis toxicity during the 1960s and 1970s. An effort to maintain normal body stores of potassium reduces this risk. The mechanism for this increased sensitivity has to do with the fact that extracellular potassium competes with binding of digoxin to the membrane Na^+, K^+ pump catalytic enzyme (Na^+, K^+)–ATPase and stimulates that pump, whereas the toxic effect of digitalis is thought to be through binding to (Na^+, K^+)–ATPase with inactivation of the Na^+, K^+ pump. Thus, hypokalemia increases the sensitivity of the heart to digitalis, whereas a high extracellular concentration of potassium decreases the heart's sensitivity to digitalis. Based on this relationship, it is suggested that toxic patients be administered judicious amounts of potassium supplements, aiming for a high normal serum potassium concentration in the range of 4.5 to 5 mEq per liter.

My own approach is to administer potassium to patients with mild digitalis toxicity only when hypokalemia is present. In patients with severer toxicity, one can give cautious potassium supplements even if the serum potassium concentration is in the normal range, depending on the baseline concentration and renal function. Potassium supplementation can worsen heart block caused by digitalis and should not generally be used in the setting unless severe hypokalemia is present or the block is related to digitalis-induced atrial tachycardia.

It is essential that recent massive digitalis intoxication be ruled out before potassium supplements are given, since severe inactivation of the Na^+,K^+ pump will cause loss of large quantities of intracellular potassium into the extracellular space. In this setting, severe *hyper*kalemia can ensue. The hyperkalemia in such massive overdose cases may not be apparent at the time of admission to the hospital but tends to develop 4 to 8 hours after ingestion of digoxin and over (perhaps) 8 to 16 hours after the ingestion of digitoxin.

The amount of potassium supplement to be administered depends on whether the patient is an adult or a child, the renal function of the patient, and the degree of hypokalemia. Obviously, potassium salt should be administered slowly. In adults, potassium chloride can be given in oral doses of 40 to 80 mEq of potassium every 4 hours, provided acidosis is not present and renal function is adequate. When correction of the arrhythmia is urgent and serum potassium concentration is low or normal, potassium can be administered intravenously in saline or 5 percent dextrose. For adults, a total of 40 to 80 mEq diluted in 500 to 1,000 ml may be given at a rate of 20 mEq per hour or slower if limited by pain from local irritation. The electrogram should be monitored to watch for both evidence of potassium toxicity and effects on the arrhythmia. Serum potassium concentrations must be carefully monitored.

Antiarrhythmic Drugs

Ventricular arrhythmias not responsive to withdrawal of the drug and potassium supplementation often respond to antiarrhythmic drug therapy.

Lidocaine and phenytoin are the antiarrhythmic drugs of choice for treating ventricular tachyarrhythmias caused by digitalis toxicity. Both are highly effective and less likely than other antiarrhythmic drugs to potentiate sinus node depression or sinoatrial or antrioventricular block. These drugs should be used according to standard guidelines for treatment of arrhythmias, with particular care being taken to administer them slowly by the intravenous route to avoid seizures or hypotension. The usual dose of lidocaine is 50 to 100 mg IV over 1 to 2 minutes repeated up to 200 mg and followed by an infusion of 1 to 4 mg per minute. Phenytoin can be given slowly intravenously and never faster than 50 mg per minute, at a dose of 250 to 1,000 mg over 1 hour. It should not be added to intravenous infusion solutions because it may precipitate.

The role of other antiarrhythmic drugs, should lidocaine or phenytoin fail, is no longer clear. Whereas experience shows that patients occasionally respond to intravenous procainamide or beta-receptor adrenergic blockers—even if ventricular arrhythmias did not respond to lidocaine or phenytoin—the possibility of complications from multiple antiarrhythmic drugs coupled with the lower likelihood of success if first-line therapy has failed favors use of antibody fragments that bind digoxin and digitoxin as a specific means of reversing the toxicity. Beta-adrenergic receptor blockers and verapamil can potentiate heart block and asystole in patients who are digitalis-toxic. The hypothetical use of a calcium-channel blocker to reduce intracellular calcium and thereby decrease triggered arrhythmias has little confirmation in the clinic. Bretylium has been used in patients with ventricular fibrillation to help restore hemodynamically viable rhythm. I believe bretylium to be contraindicated in patients with digitalis toxicity who are not in ventricular fibrillation because this drug is known to release catecholamines, which sensitize the heart to the effects of digitalis. Intravenous magnesium sulfate may be useful to treat refractory digitalis-toxic arrhythmias, especially in the setting of hypokalemia and hypomagnesemia induced by diuretics.

Treatment of Bradycardia and Heart Block

Severe sinus bradycardia and heart block can occur from digitalis toxicity and are particularly prominent in subjects with normal hearts who have taken a massive ingestion of digitalis by accident or with the intent to commit suicide. Bradycardia and heart block are also particularly prominent in the pediatric population. First-degree atrioventricular block that is not progressive requires only a reduction or temporary discontinuation of digoxin therapy. Rapidly progressing heart block or severe second-and third-degree block require more aggressive management. Atropine given as a 0.5-mg intravenous bolus, which can be repeated once or twice acutely to obtain the desired effect, is often useful in transiently reversing severe bradycardia or atrioventricular block. Since digitalis toxicity is often long lasting and atropine has a short duration of effect, further administration is often required; belladonna toxicity can easily result if atropine is used to treat persisting or recurrent bradycardia or block. Atropine excess is easily missed, since both digitalis toxicity and atropine toxicity can cause acute psychosis. Atropine is most useful as a short-term treatment for the vagal effects of digoxin or as a preliminary measure before inserting a temporary pacemaker.

Temporary right ventricular pacing is a highly effective means for maintaining heart rate during bradycardia or heart block induced by digitalis toxicity. Problems with pacemaker therapy include technical problems with insertion, increased vagal tone during insertion, and the potential for precipitating ventricular tachycardia or fibrillation if the pacemaker wire gives rise to ectopic beats by mechanical stimulation of the ventricle. In the case of massive digitalis intoxication, the threshold for ventricular stimulation may rise to the point that the pacemaker will not successfully capture. In a setting where the risks of these complications to pacemakers are high, reversal of the toxicity with digoxin-specific antibody fragments is a reasonable alternative to pacemaker implantation.

Although antiarrhythmic drugs and pacemakers are often effective measures for treating digitalis-toxic rhythm disturbances, digoxin-specific antibody fragments (digoxin-immune Fab[ovine]) offer physicians an opportunity specifically and completely to reverse digitalis toxicity. Since this new treatment should soon be available to practicing physicians, it is helpful to describe its benefits and risks.

Digoxin-Immune Fab(ovine) for Treating Digitalis Toxicity

Antibodies highly specific to digoxin were successfully developed in the late 1960s and formed the basis for the serum digoxin concentration immunoassay. Although the whole antibody was shown to reverse digitalis toxicity when given intravenously to experimental animals, the known side effects of whole nonhuman-derived antibodies, such as anaphylaxis and serum sickness, slowed development of these antibodies for use as an antitoxin. Modern techniques for fractionation and purification of immunoglobulins were applied by Drs. Smith, Butler, and Haber. They digested digoxin-specific IgG derived from sheep with papain to obtain Fab fragments that specifically bind digoxin. The digoxin-specific Fab fragments (digoxin-immune Fab[ovine]) were then separated and purified to eliminate the F_c fragments and other serum proteins through a process called immunoadsorption. Since the Fab fragment lacks both the immune determinants and the complement-binding portion of the F_c fragment and is much smaller than the intact immunoglobulin, it is much less immunogenic and is rapidly excreted by the kidney.

These highly purified digoxin-specific Fab fragments (digoxin-immune Fab[ovine]) have been shown both in experimental animal and in man to reverse rapidly and specifically massive intoxication with digoxin. Since digoxin-immune Fab(ovine) cross-reacts substantially with digitoxin, it has been used successfully for digitoxin toxicity as well. Little data are available on the cross-reactivity of these digoxin-specific antibody fragments with other digitalis drugs or other naturally occurring glycosides, such as oleander. Nevertheless, it would seem reasonable to attempt reversal of massive intoxication from any of these causes with digoxin-immune Fab(ovine) fragments, if clearly life-threatening intoxication exists that is not responsive to other modes of therapy.

In patients, digoxin-immune Fab(ovine) has an onset of effect within 30 minutes, with complete reversal of toxicity usually within 3 or 4 hours after administration of a neutralizing dose. In some instances, heart failure has occurred that may have been due to withdrawal of the digitalis effect. By reversing the inhibition of the Na^+,K^+ pump, caused by severe digitalis intoxication, administration of the digoxin-immune Fab(ovine) can cause rapid return of potassium inside the cell. If total body potassium depletion is present, hypokalemia may ensue within hours of Fab administration. This is most likely if digitalis toxicity is severe and longstanding, if potassium-binding resins are administered, or if potassium-depleting diuretics have been administered.

Another potential problem relating to the rapid reversal of digitalis effect is the precipitous return of a rapid ventricular response in patients with atrial fibrillation. Since redigitalization can be difficult for several days after giving digoxin-immune Fab(ovine), patients with atrial fibrillation may be difficult to treat. This is especially so if they have concomitant severe left ventricular dysfunction because such patients are not ideal candidates for control of the ventricular response with verapamil or beta-adrenergic receptor blockers.

Allergic reactions have been absent. In more than 150 patients treated so far, there have been no anaphylactic or delayed hypersensitivity reactions to these antibody fragments. Reexposure of previously treated patients has not been studied.

In patients whose manifestations of toxicity are severe enough to warrant aggressive therapeutic intervention, the nonspecific but established effectiveness and safety profile of antiarrhythmic drugs for tachyarrhythmias or pacemaker therapy for bradyarrhythmias need to be assessed in comparison to the high specificity and effectiveness use of digoxin-immune Fab(ovine). Depending on the severity of the intoxication and likelihood of a beneficial response with standard therapy, the physician may elect to use conventional measures until more experience with the antibody fragments is obtained. In patients who are likely to do poorly with conventional therapy, it is my inclination to move quickly to use the antibody fragments because they are highly effective, rapid in effect, and, in addition, offer confirmation of the diagnosis of digitalis intoxication if abnormalities improve within 30 minutes of an appropriate dose.

MASSIVE DIGITALIS INTOXICATION

Most physicians have had experience treating mild-to-severe digitalis intoxication resulting from difficulty in management of patients who require the drug for congestive heart failure or atrial fibrillation. On the other hand, few physicians have had experience treating massive digitalis ingestion. Whereas patients with underlying heart disease may develop life-threatening digitalis toxicity even with (usually) therapeutic levels of digoxin in the body, persons with normal hearts require much higher amounts of the drug to cause severe toxicity. Bradycardia and heart block are especially common in such cases. Experience suggests that cardiac arrest is likely to occur in otherwise healthy adults who ingest more than 10 mg of digoxin or in previously healthy children who ingest more than 4 mg of digoxin. These patients usually have steady-state serum digoxin concentrations above 10 ng per milliliter. Although some persons with healthy hearts will develop arrhythmic manifestations and even ventricular fibrillation at lower ingestions, such patients often can be managed using standard measures.

All patients with massive digitalis ingestion should receive large doses of activated charcoal. The usual dose is 50 to 100 mg in adults and 15 to 20 mg in children. Activated charcoal may not only prevent absorption of a massive ingestion but binds digoxin in the gut during enteroenteric recirculation. Activated charcoal should be administered as an aqueous or sorbitol slurry. Electrolyte imbalance caused by diarrhea should be carefully avoided. Emesis or gastric lavage may be indicated, especially if ingestion has occurred within 30 minutes of the patient's presentation at the hospital. Emesis should not be induced in patients who are obtunded. The usual dose of ipecac syrup is 30 ml in the adult and 15 ml in children aged 1 to 12 years. Ipecac is often not effective when given within 1 hour of activated charcoal. If the patient presents more than 2 hours after ingestion, I believe it unsafe to induce vomiting or attempt passage of a gastric tube, because such maneuvers may induce an acute vagal episode that can worsen digitalis-toxic arrhythmias. The benefit of gastric emptying declines with time after ingestion, whereas the likelihood of this adverse effect increases with time after ingestion.

If a patient with massive digitalis ingestion presents to the emergency room within 2 or 3 hours of ingestion, there may be little immediate evidence of toxicity. Deterioration is likely to begin about 2 or 3 hours after ingestion of digoxin and reach a peak effect by 6 to 12 hours. There appears to be a fairly long plateau of 12 to 24 hours before improvement occurs unless the toxicity is reversed with digoxin-immune Fab(ovine) fragments. This time course results from the known kinetics of digoxin once absorbed into the body, since there is slow distribution of the drug from the blood to its sites of action. Toxicity may not only persist but even worsen between 12 and 24 hours after ingestion. This phenomenon may be the result of delayed absorption from the gut. Accordingly, patients with large ingestions of digoxin should be observed carefully for 24 to 48 hours to establish that their toxic manifestations are truly on the decline before they are removed from an intensive care setting. The onset and duration of digitoxin toxicity are substantially longer than those observed with digoxin toxicity.

It is common for physicians to administer potassium supplements to patients who have digitalis toxicity. A patient who ingests a massive amount of digoxin and appears in the emergency room 2 hours later is likely to have a normal serum potassium concentration from his blood drawn at admission. Over the next 3 or 4 hours, the potassium concentration may well rise rapidly to levels as high as 8 or 9 mEq per liter. This hyperkalemia is caused by digitalis-induced inactivation of (Na^+, K^+)−ATPase, which catalyzes the pumping of sodium outside the cell in exchange for potassium to the inside of the cell. It is most important that patients such as these not be treated with potassium supplements at the time of admission to the hospital.

Hyperkalemia caused by digitalis toxicity often signals a fatal outcome. The standard treatment has been the same as treatment of hyperkalemia from other causes, namely, administration of potassium-binding resins to enhance excretion of potassium; administration of glucose, insulin, and bicarbonate to drive potassium back into the cell; and dialysis to remove potassium from the blood. Dialysis will not effectively remove digoxin from the body and may precipitate arrhythmias by causing a too-rapid fall in serum potassium concentration. Use of binding resins or dialysis to enhance elimination of potassium aggravates the depletion of total potassium. In my opinion, hyperkalemia that is directly related to digitalis toxicity constitutes a clear indication for early use of digoxin-immune Fab(ovine) fragments. These antibody fragments reverse hyperkalemia in 3 to 4 hours or less, while treating all other manifestations of digitalis toxicity as well.

In patients who have ingested large amounts of digitalis in a suicidal effort, one must be alert to the possibility that other drugs have been ingested concomitantly. This is a particular problem in patients with heart disease who are on other cardioactive drugs. Likely coadministered drugs include tricyclic antidepressants, beta-adrenergic blockers, and calcium-channel blockers. These drugs may be arrhythmogenic (tricyclics) and aggravate heart block, bradycardia, or hypotension. A patient with an elevated serum digoxin concentration and arrhythmias consistent with digitalis toxicity may show only partial reversal in this setting after treatment with antibody fragments because many of the presumed digitalis toxic manifestions may actually be related to the other drugs.

AORTIC DISSECTION

ROBERT M. DOROGHAZI, M.D.
EVE ELIZABETH SLATER, M.D.

The successful treatment of acute aortic dissection is based on early diagnosis and meticulous managment, since the events that most influence survival occur early in the course of the disease. This chapter reviews the classification, initial management, indications for definitive medical and surgical therapy, and follow-up in patients with aortic dissection. A knowledge of the classification of aortic dissection is essential for recognition and proper management of the disease. Classification is based upon duration and location of the dissecting hematoma.

Acute aortic dissection is defined as being less than 2 weeks in onset. In chronic dissection, more than 2 weeks will have elapsed from the onset of symptoms to the institution of therapy.

We prefer to classify aortic dissection according to the presence or absence of involvement of the ascending aorta. This decision derives from the findings that involvement of the ascending aorta is an important determinant of both choice of therapeutic modality and prognosis. In type A dissection, the dissecting hematoma involves the ascending aorta. The aortic arch or distal aorta may or may not be involved, and the intimal tear, while usually within several centimeters of the aortic valve, may be located anywhere in the aorta. All dissections that do not involve the ascending aorta are referred to as type B. Previous classifications were based upon location of the intimal tear in either proximal (DeBakey types I and II) or distal (DeBakey type III) aorta.

THERAPEUTIC MANAGEMENT

There are two phases in the therapy of a patient with suspected acute aortic dissection. Initial management involves institution of medical therapy, stabilization of vital signs, and definitive diagnosis by retrograde aortic angiography. This protocol is followed by definitive therapy, in which medical therapy is continued and surgical intervention may or may not be undertaken.

Initial therapy is begun in all patients whose clinical presentation is strongly suggestive of aortic dissection. Patients should be admitted to an intensive care unit (ICU) where vital signs, including blood pressure, heart rate, and heart rhythm can be continuously monitored. A Foley catheter should be placed to monitor urine output. An intra-arterial cannula and Swan-Ganz catheter are highly desirable to monitor blood pressure and cardiac filling pressures, respectively, during the administration of potent cardioactive and vasoactive drugs.

Drug administration during the first several days of treatment should be by the parenteral route, since in acutely ill patients gastrointestinal absorption is unreliable and the need for an immediate drug effect urgent. Moreover, surgical intervention may be imminent.

The goals of medical therapy of aortic dissection were originally outlined by Wheat and colleagues. One objective is to lower systolic blood pressure. Lowering arterial pressure reduces the shearing forces exerted against the diseased and damaged aortic wall. The other objective is to reduce the force and velocity of ventricular contraction, referred to as dp/dt. Although definitive data do not exist for man, laboratory investigation strongly suggests that reduction of dp/dt is the more important variable in medical therapy. This fact provides the rationale for medical therapy in normotensive and postoperative patients.

Thus, the objectives of initial therapy are to reduce blood pressure and control dp/dt, as well as to control pain. The pain of acute aortic dissection is often refractory to the administration of opiates, but usually subsides once the progression of the hematoma is halted. The objective of hypotensive therapy is to reduce systolic blood pressure to 90 to 120 mm Hg or to the lowest level commensurate with maintaining vital organ perfusion. Urinary output should be maintained above 20 ml per hour. Therapy to reduce dp/dt is begun in all patients, including those who are normotensive or free of pain on admission.

Drug Therapy In Initial Management

Sodium Nitroprusside

The most effective agent for the immediate reduction of blood pressure is sodium nitroprusside, given with concomitant beta-adrenergic blockade (Table 1). A solution of 50 or 100 mg in 500 ml of D5W is infused at an initial rate of 20 μg per minute, and the dosage is titrated against

TABLE 1 Initial Management of Acute Aortic Dissection

Drug	*Dosage*	*Effect on Blood Pressure*	*Effect on dp/dt*	*Side Effects and Complications*	*Comment*
Sodium nitroprusside	50–100 mg in 500 ml D5W, infused initially at 20 μg/min with maximum dosage; dosage not more than 200 μg/min; not more than 1 mg/kg should be given in first 3 hrs and 0.2–0.3 mg/kg/hr thereafter	↓↓↓	↑	Hypotension, cyanide and thiocyanate toxicity, methemoglobinemia, nausea, agitation, somnolence, and dp/dt	Light sensitive, requires intensive monitoring
Trimethaphan	500 mg–2 g in 500 ml D5W infused initially at 1 mg/min	↓↓↓	↓↓	Hypotension, respiratory arrest, somnolence, ganglionic blockade, rapid development of tachyphylaxis	Requires intensive monitoring
Propranolol	0.5 mg IV, followed by doses of 1 mg every 5 min, until total dose of 0.15 mg/kg or adequate effect is achieved	⟷	↓↓↓	Congestive heart failure, bradycardia, and bronchospasm	
Reserpine	0.5–2 mg IM q4–8h	↓ to ↓↓	↓	Depression, somnolence, and acute gastric ulceration	Antacids and cimetidine should be given concomitantly
Methyldopa	500–1,000 mg in D5W (100 mg/ml) infused over 30–60 min q6h	↓↓	↓↓	Hypotension, somnolence, orthostatic hypotension, delayed onset of action	Long duration of action
Labetalol	20–80 mg IV at 10-min intervals	↓↓	↓↓	Pressor response possible or failure to respond in patients already receiving beta-blockers, hypotension, bradycardia, bronchospasm, congestive heart failure, and urinary retention	Its use in aortic dissection has not been reported

↑ = increased, ↓ = decreased

blood pressure response to a maximum dose of approximately 3 μg per kilogram per minute (200 μg per min). Not more than 1 mg per kilogram should be given in the first 3 hours and a maximum of 0.2 to 0.3 mg per kilogram per hour (approximately 200 μg per min) thereafter. The solution must be prepared immediately prior to use and is light sensitive so that the bottle containing it should be covered with aluminum foil. Blood pressure reduction occurs within seconds and "overshoot" hypotension can occur. Intravenous nitroglycerin should not be substituted for sodium nitroprusside to reduce blood pressure, since intravenous nitroglycerin is principally a venodilator and not a hypotensive agent per se.

The most important complications of high-dose nitroprusside therapy are cyanide and thiocyanate toxicity, which may develop after more than 48 hours of use. The earliest indication of cyanide toxicity is metabolic acidosis. Thiocyanate toxicity may be indicated by neurologic signs, including confusion, hyperreflexia, and (later) convulsions. Blood thiocyanate levels can be monitored, and levels below 10 mg percent generally are well tolerated.

Sodium nitroprusside decreases platelet adhesiveness in vitro, but clinically apparent difficulties with hemostasis have not been reported. By inhibiting pulmonary vasoconstriction mediated by hypoxia, sodium nitroprusside may worsen ventilation-perfusion mismatching. However, the resulting hypoxia is usually of little consequence unless the patient is severely hypoxemic prior to therapy. Methemoglobinemia rarely occurs.

Restlessness, somnolence, and nausea occur frequently with sodium nitroprusside therapy. These side effects may be disconcerting to both patient and family members, but should not lead to an alteration of otherwise successful hypotensive therapy.

Sodium nitroprusside alone or in combination with inadequate doses of propranolol can cause reflex tachycardia and an increase in dp/dt, which can conceivably accelerate the dissection process. Therefore, adequate simultaneous beta-adrenergic blockade is mandatory when sodium nitroprusside is used.

Trimethaphan

If sodium nitroprusside is ineffective or poorly tolerated, the ganglionic blocker trimethaphan is the drug of second choice. Because trimethaphan can both lower blood pressure and reduce dp/dt, it is the hypotensive agent of choice when propranolol is contraindicated. A solution of 500 mg to 2 g of trimethaphan in 500 ml of D5W is mixed immediately prior to use and infused initially at 1 mg per minute with the dosage titrated against blood pressure response. The head of the bed should be elevated to 45 degrees to potentiate the orthostatic effect of this drug.

Side effects of trimethaphan are common and often include overshoot hypotension and ganglionic blockade manifested by urinary retention, paralytic ileus, constipation, and pupillary dilatation with blurred vision. Respiratory arrest by an unkown mechanism can occur. Tachyphylaxis to trimethaphan usually occurs within 48 hours. Trimethaphan has become the drug of second choice in therapy because of these numerous side effects and the tachyphylaxis just noted. In addition, physicians and ICU personnel often have more experience with sodium nitroprusside and thus are more comfortable with its use.

The hypotensive effects of both sodium nitroprusside and trimethaphan can be blunted by fluid retention, so concomitant administration of intravenous diuretics, such as furosemide or bumetanide, is often necessary.

Hypertension requiring massive dosages of hypotensive agents should raise the possibility that the dissection involves one or both renal arteries, resulting in renovascular hypertension. This should be confirmed by either aortography or renal scan. In such cases, surgical intervention is almost always required to decompress the dissecting hematoma.

Therapy to reduce dp/dt is mandatory in all patients, including those who are normotensive or pain-free on admission. Beta-adrenergic blockade is our therapy of choice to achieve this effect. In patients with acute dissection, the rapid effect of an intravenously administered beta-blocker is required. However, it should be noted that intravenous beta-blockade has only minimal hypotensive effect. Propranolol is the only beta-blocking agent currently approved for intravenous use. An initial dose of 0.5 mg is given intravenously, followed by incremental doses of 1 mg every 5 minutes until either there is evidence of adequate beta-adrenergic blockage or a total dose of 0.15 mg per kilogram has been given.

Although there are no set criteria for "adequate beta-adrenergic blockade," a heart rate of 50 to 60 beats per minute usually indicates sufficient beta-blocking effect. Higher heart rates may be acceptable temporarily in patients who are in pain or critically ill or after a maximal dose of propranolol has been given. Contraindications to the use of propranolol or other beta-adrenergic blocking agents, include preexisting sinus bradycardia of less than 45 beats per minute, congestive heart failure, severe bronchospastic pulmonary disease, or second- or third-degree AV block.

Reserpine

Reserpine can both lower blood pressure and reduce dp/dt and can be used when propranolol is contraindicated. Reserpine is given in doses of 0.5 to 2 mg intramuscularly every 4 to 8 hours and begins acting after 1 to 3 hours. Side effects include drowsiness, depression, and gastric ulceration secondary to stimulation of gastric acid secretion. The risk of peptic ulceration can be minimized by nasogastric suction and the concomitant administration of antacids, as well as the H_2-receptor antagonist cimetidine in 300-mg intravenous doses every 6 hours.

Other Agents

Of the other hypotensive agents available for intravenous use, diazoxide and hydralazine are contraindicated because they increase dp/dt. Methyldopa has a negative intropic effect and thus can be used to lower both blood pressure and dp/dt; however, it has a delayed onset (4 to 6 hours) and prolonged duration (10 to 16 hours) of action. The dosage is 250 to 500 mg (initial) to 1.0 g (maximum) in D5W (100 mg/ml) infused over 30 to 60 minutes every 6 hours.

Labetalol, the combined nonselective $beta_1$- and $alpha_1$- blocker, administered intravenously in doses of 20 to 80 mg at 10-minute intervals can rapidly lower blood pressure levels in patients with severe hypertension and, of course, reduce dp/dt. Thus, it should be ideal for use in both acute and chronic treatment of aortic dissection, although we are unaware of any clinical reports that address themselves specifically to this use. One potential contraindication to its use in acute aortic dissection, however, is that labetalol given intravenously may cause a pressor response in patients concurrently receiving beta-blocking therapy.

Whereas sublingual nifedipine has been shown to result in relatively rapid blood pressure lowering, its positive inotropic effect contraindicates a use in acute aortic dissection.

Adequate sedation and analgesia are of great importance in acute management. Blood pressure may be well controlled when the patient is quiet or asleep only to rise dramatically when he is awake or agitated. This is especially common in a patient with a prior history of hypertension. We prefer sedatives with minimal cardiovascular effect, such as haloperidol, given in 1- to 10-mg doses intravenously every 4 to 6 hours.

As soon as the patient's condition is adequately stable, retrograde aortic angiography should be performed. If the patient is in a community hosptial that lacks angiographic and experienced cardiovascular surgical capabilities, he should be transferred at this time to a center where these facilities are available.

Aortic angiography not only confirms the diagnosis of aortic dissection, but also provides essential information regarding subsequent medical or surgical management. This information includes the site and extent of the dissecting hematoma, the presence or absence of aortic valvular insufficiency, and the patency of aortic tributaries. Although other techniques, such as intravenous and intra-arterial digital subtraction angiography, computed tomography (CT) scanning, echocardiography, and nuclear magnetic imaging can diagnose aortic dissection, they have not replaced retrograde aortic angiography for rapid diagnosis in patients suspected of having acute disease.

Following initial stabilization and diagnosis by angiography, a decision is made whether to proceed with surgery. Although some authors recommend that all patients with acute aortic dissection be treated surgically, we recommend a more selective approach.

SURGICAL MANAGEMENT

Surgical therapy is the treatment of choice for all patients with acute type A (proximal) dissection (Table 2). Involvement of the proximal aorta is associated with a high incidence of immediately life-threatening complications, many of which are surgically remediable. They include acute aortic valvular insufficiency, loss of a major arterial pulse, and rupture into the pericardial sac with pericardial tamponade.

TABLE 2 Indications for Definitive Therapy of Aortic Dissection

Surgical:
1. All patients with type A dissection unless site of origin cannot be identified or dissection limited to the aortic arch
2. Patients with type B dissection complicated by rupture, circulatory compromise of a vital organ, inability to control pain or blood pressure, extension as manifested by recurrent pain, or appearance of a new complication or localized aortic expansion
3. All patients with Marfan's syndrome

Medical:
1. All patients with uncomplicated type B dissection
2. Patients with type A dissection complicated by prohibitive surgical risk, inability to identify the site of origin, or involvement confined to the aortic arch

Medical therapy can be undertaken rarely in patients with proximal dissection who are poor surgical candidates or in whom the site of origin cannot be identified. Although the Stanford surgical group advocates replacement of the proximal aorta in this latter circumstance, its view has not gained wide acceptance except for patients who are considered to have low surgical risks.

Medical therapy is also recommended for dissections originating in the aortic arch, since surgical correction is associated with high mortality and is technically difficult to perform.

Patients with uncomplicated acute distal dissection can be treated medically (see Table 2). In a recent series from the Massachusetts General Hospital, we showed that medically treated patients with uncomplicated distal dissection had a significantly better hospital survival than those treated surgically. Surgical intervention, however, is advised in distal dissection complicated by rupture, compromise of blood supply to a vital organ, inability to control pain or blood pressure medically, extension of the dissecting hematoma as manifested by recurrent pain or the appearance of a new complication, or localized expansion of the aorta.

Patients with Marfan's syndrome, with either proximal or distal dissection, should be treated surgically. In addition, concomitant aortic valve replacement should always be performed in the patient with Marfan's syndrome with proximal aortic dissection to preclude subsequent development of aortic regurgitation.

The principal complications of surgical intervention in aortic dissection include bleeding, renal failure, hypotension or myocardial dysfunction, respiratory failure, and CNS deficit.

MEDICAL MANAGEMENT

Whatever the mode of definitive therapy, all patients require long-term chronic medical therapy, including those who have undergone successful surgical intervention. As during the acute phase of therapy, beta-adrenergic blockade is a requisite of therapy and should be used regardless of whether or not hypertension is present. The most frequently used beta-blocking agent in initial management has been propanolol, given in divided doses of 40 to 480 mg total per day. Physicians now favor beta-blockers which can be given on a once or twice daily basis. Other nonselective beta-blockers include nadolol, administered as a single dose of 40 to 480 mg per day, and timolol, given twice daily in doses of 20 to 80 mg per day total. In patients with bronchospastic pulmonary disease, the more selective beta-receptor antagonists metroprolol, given in divided doses of 100 to 300 mg per day, or atenolol, given as 50 to 100 mg once a day, may be better tolerated. Other drugs with beta-blocking effect include pindolol, a nonselective beta-blocker with intrinsic sympathomimetic activity, given in twice-daily doses of 20 to 60 mg per day, and labetalol, an adrenergic-receptor blocking agent, which has both selective $alpha_1$- and nonselective beta-adrenergic receptor blocking activity, given in twice daily doses of 200 to 1,200 mg per day. Because the intrinsic sympathomimetic property of pindolol might aggravate dp/dt, we do not advise its use. Experience with labetalol in aortic dissection is not known. Patients who cannot tolerate beta-blocking agents should receive one of the negative inotropic agents described subsequently.

Systolic blood pressure should be maintained at 120 mm Hg or less if tolerated by the patient. If blood pressure cannot be controlled at this level by a beta-blocker and a diuretic or if the patient cannot tolerate beta-blockers, oral drugs that reduce both blood pressure and dp/dt are required. They include methyldopa, clonidine, guanabenz, reserpine, prazosin, guanethidine, or guanadrel. Vasodilators, because of the reflex tachycardia and increase in dp/dt, should be used only in conjunction with adequate beta-blockade. They include hydralazine, prazosin, and minoxidil. Captopril and enalapril could conceivably increase dp/dt if an element of myocardial dysfunction is extant, and thus we do not favor their cautious use unless other alternatives have failed. The calcium antagonists verapamil, nifedipine, and diltiazem have variable effects on peripheral dilatation and cardiac contractility and should also be used only in conjunction with adequate beta-blockade, if such a combination can be tolerated.

No definite guidelines exist regarding the rate of mobilization of medically treated patients with aortic dissection. We apply an empiric program of increasing activity paralleling that used after extensive myocardial infarction, namely, limb dangling on days 3 and 4, sitting on days 5 through 7, and gradually increasing ambulation, with discharge at about 2 weeks if the patient's condition is stable. Some degree of orthostatic hypotension is commonly observed when patients begin to ambulate, with methyldopa therapy being an especially frequent cause. Simple adjustment of medication or dosage usually suffices to overcome the problem.

Close follow-up is required for all patients with aortic dissection who survive hospitalization. Late complications include redissection, aortic valvular insufficiency, or localized saccular aneurysm formation, the last-mentioned being more common in medically treated patients. Routine chest films, CT scanning, and digital subtraction angiography are all useful to evaluate aortic contour or size. If the dissection extends into the abdominal aorta, the patient must be watched for the development of abdominal aortic aneurysm. Baseline measurements of the abdominal aorta with ultrasound or CT scanning are advisable in such cases.

Chronic dissection, as previously defined, is associated with a significantly better prognosis than is acute dissection. Initial therapy can be administered orally. As with acute dissection, all patients, including those who are not hypertensive, should be treated with a beta-blocking agent. An antihypertensive should added, if required. Indications for surgical intervention in patients with chronic aortic dissection include saccular aneurysm formation, progressive aortic enlargement, or significant aortic valvular insufficiency.

ABDOMINAL AORTIC ANEURYSM

FRANK J. VEITH, M.D.
ENRICO ASCER, M.D.

Most abdominal aortic aneurysms are caused by a degenerative process that is probably related in some way to atherosclerosis. The disease is associated with weakening of the aortic wall due chiefly to a breakdown in elastin fibers within the internal elastic lamina and the media. This weakening results in gradual progressive dilatation of the aortic lumen. As this process continues, it is often associated with the deposition of laminated fibrin clot lining the dilatated aortic wall. The process can cause difficulties to patients when either arterial pressure ruptures the weakened aortic wall or arterial flow dislodges a piece of the fibrin clot as an embolus, which can occlude arteries in the lower extremity and produce ischemic symptoms. Both rupture and distal embolization can be catastrophic, but both can be prevented by appropriate surgical treatment. The purpose of this chapter is to outline how and when this treatment can be applied most appropriately in afflicted patients, many of whom are elderly and have a number of other serious associated risk factors.

The obvious clinical problem is to identify those patients whose aneurysm provides significant risk to life or limb and to operate on them *before* rupture or embolization occurs. Operative treatment after embolization or rupture can be effective, but has far greater risks than it does if performed before these events occur.

The portion of the abdominal aorta particularly susceptible to aneurysm is the segment between the renal arteries and the terminal aortic bifurcation. Although aneurysmal changes can occur in the segment of the aorta that gives rise to the renal arteries, the superior mesenteric artery, and the celiac artery, such involvement is fortunately rare and occurs in less than 5 percent of cases. When this visceral segment of the aorta is involved in the aneurysm, the treatment is substantially more complicated and the operative risk greater than when the infrarenal aortic segment is involved alone. In contrast to the rarity of aneurysmal change in the renal and suprarenal segments of the abdominal aorta, aneurysmal change in the common iliac arteries is common and occurs in approximately one-third to one-half of all patients with an infrarenal abdominal aortic aneurysm. Aneurysmal dilatation of the internal iliac arteries is less common. Aneurysmal changes in the external iliac arteries are rare. Patients with infrarenal abdominal aortic aneurysms are likely to develop associated aneurysms at other sites. They include, in order of frequency, the popliteal artery, the common femoral artery, and the thoracic aorta.

Several definitions are relevant to the discussion, dealing primarily with degenerative aneurysms involving all layers of the arterial wall, the so-called *true aneurysm*. Several other lesions can involve the aorta and its main branches and produce dilatation or apparent dilatation, weakening of the aortic wall, and rupture. They include a *dissecting aneurysm*; it almost always begins within the thoracic aorta, but can advance within the aortic wall and produce either a dilatation of the abdominal aorta or an occlusion of one of its branches. A *false aneurysm* of the aorta or iliac arteries may also be the result of penetrating or nonpenetrating trauma. It represents a loss of aortic wall continuity following which the luminal continuity is maintained by surrounding structures, which for a time prevent exsanguination. Although the management of both dissecting and false aneurysms is primarily surgical, the details of this management are beyond the scope of this chapter, which is restricted to a discussion of degenerative true aneurysms of the abdominal aorta and of the common iliac arteries.

Abdominal aortic aneurysms primarily comprise a disease of later life. Most patients with the problem develop it after age 50 years, although it can occasionally be observed in men in their 40s. Between one-third and one-half of the patients have associated manifestations of arteriosclerosis. Usually, it involves the coronary arteries, but the lower extremity arteries or the carotid arteries may also have stenotic or occlusive manifestations of atherosclerosis. Any of the diseases that afflict patients in the later decades of life may coexist with abdominal aneurysms. Hypertension is probably the most common of them.

RATE OF PROGRESSION AND ESTIMATION OF RISK IN NONSURGICAL TREATMENT

Degenerative abdominal aortic or iliac aneurysms are localized dilatations of all layers of the arterial wall. They are progressive, although the rate of progression in a given patient is unknown. In many patients, particularly those with aneurysms less than twice the normal arterial diameter, the arterial dilatation will be stabilized for several years. Enlargement, however, inexorably occurs, and the average increase in aneurysmal diameter is about 0.3 cm per year. More rapid growth spurts have been observed in aneurysms of larger diameter and may signify an increased risk of rupture.

Aneurysm size itself has long been acknowledged to be an important correlative risk of rupture. Small aortic aneurysms, that is, those less than 5 cm in transverse or anteroposterior diameter, have a lower rupture rate than have aortic aneurysms more than 5 cm in diameter. On the other hand, small aneurysms can rupture, although the rate of rupture is less than 10 to 15 percent per year. When an aortic aneurysm exceeds 5 cm in diameter, the rupture risk rate approaches 50 percent in 2 to 3 years, with the greatest risk of rupture being in the largest aneurysms, particularly those occurring in relatively small aortas. The rupture risk rate for iliac artery aneurysms approaches 50 percent in 2 to 3 years for aneurysms more than 4 cm in diameter, since the iliac arteries are normally of smaller diameter than is the aorta. Arterial hypertension probably increases the risk of rupture for an aneurysm of given size in a given patient. However, this increased risk is difficult to measure. Moreover, patients with normal or low blood pressure and those with well-controlled hypertension can have aneurysms that eventually rupture.

The risk of *embolization* from aortic or iliac aneurysms is more difficult to estimate than is the risk of rupture. A rough correlation exists between embolization and aneurysm size, since the larger aneurysms are more likely to contain laminated mural thrombi. However, the overall incidence of embolization is lower than that of rupture, with highest reported incidence of embolization in abdominl aneurysms being only 15 percent. Furthermore, the difference between surgical results before and after embolization is much less than the difference in surgical results before and after rupture. Thus, it is the rupture risk rate that becomes paramount in deciding on the appropriateness and timing of operative intervention.

Since *aneurysm diameter* is such an important guide to rupture risk, assessing the size accurately is critical. Physical examination tends to overestimate aneurysm diameter by approximately 1 to 2 cm and can be notoriously inaccurate in obese patients or in those with tortuous aortas. Plain films of the abdomen, which can detect calcification in the aneurysmal wall in about 40 percent of cases, are also inaccurate in estimating aneurysmal size—either because both walls of the aneurysm cannot be clearly identified or the plain films tend to overestimate the aneurysmal dimension because of magnification distortion. The most accurate methods for estimating aneurysmal diameters are *abdominal sonography* and *computerized tomography* (CT scan). Both methods give highly accurate aneurysm diameter measurements, as long as the aneurysm occupies the normal axial position of the aorta. If the aneurysm deviates so that what would normally be a cross-sectional measurement is diagonally placed, size overestimations can occur. Such deviation of the aneurysmal aorta may be suspected if an angiogram has been performed, and highly accurate size measurements from sonography and CT scans are usually possible. Angiographic estimates of aneurysm size can also be misleading because of substantial amounts of mural thrombus, which prevent the dye from entirely filling the aneurysmal sac. Moreover, angiographic measurements are subject to the same magnification error as other radiographic studies.

DIAGNOSIS OF NONRUPTURED ABDOMINAL ANEURYSM

Abdominal aortic aneurysms can produce symptoms before they rupture. Generally, these symptoms consist of pain in the upper abdomen or back. The intensity of the pain can vary, but is often low grade and can mimic that in musculoskeletal disorders. Other aneurysms come to the patient's attention by producing a sensation of fullness or detectable pulsation in the upper abdomen; still other aneurysms produce a sensation of pressure within the abdomen. Many aneurysms can become dangerously large without producing any symptoms whatever. *Asymptomatic aneurysms* may be detected by careful routine physical examination or by plain film roentgenographic examination of the abdomen or lumbosacral spine being performed for other reasons. The aneurysm may be detected as an incidental finding of these studies as a curvilinear calcific density to the left of the lumbar spine. Similar findings may be observed as an incidental finding on intravenous pyelographic examinations. Unfortunately, 25 to 30 percent of aneurysms may be totally undetectable on physical examination, and this can be true even for large threatening aneurysms, particularly in obese or muscular persons. Furthermore, more than 50 percent of aneurysms may show no abnormal calcification on plain film abdominal examination. When back or abdominal pain produced by an aneurysm becomes severe and unrelenting, it usually reflects rapid enlargement or rupture and is an ominous sign. Another physical finding that should arouse suspicion of an aneurysm is a detectable pulsation in either lower quadrant of the abdomen above the groin. Although such pulsations may be caused by tortuous iliac vessels, they more frequently indicate a significant aortic or iliac aneurysm.

If an aneurysm is detected or suspected based on physical examination or radiographic findings, it can be confirmed and its size determined accurately by abdominal sonography. Occasionally, this test reveals that an apparently widened aorta is merely tortuous and markedly prominent. Alternatively, an obese or muscular patient with nothing more than a prominent epigastric pulsation may be shown to have a substantial and surgically significant abdominal aortic aneurysm. Computerized tomography can also document an aneurysm and accurately measure its size. However, this test is probably no better than sonography and often more difficult to obtain.

Arteriography performed by either the digital venous route or the transfemoral route is commonly regarded as an effective method for diagnosing aneurysms. Although this modality can clearly demonstrate a widened aortic lumen, aneurysmal lumens are often so full of clot that luminal widening does not exist. Moreover, for reasons already mentioned, angiographic examination is a poor way to document aneurysmal size. On the other hand, angiographic examination performed for other reasons occasionally reveals an unsuspected aortic or iliac aneurysm. Such a diagnosis is simple when luminal widening is observed. In the absence of such widening, an incidental diagnosis of aneurysm still may be made or suspected if there is sharp angulation of the aorta below the renal arteries, occlusion of the lumbar arteries for no apparent reason, or displacement of the mesenteric arteries by the aneurysmal mass.

Although arteriography is a poor method for confirming the diagnosis of an aneurysm, most vascular surgeons today believe that some form of arteriography should be performed on patients with aortic or iliac abdominal aneurysms before they undergo operation. Such angiographic studies may be helpful in assessing the degree of difficulty that the aneurysm presents from a surgical or technical point of view. Involvement of the visceral segment of the aorta should be detected preoperatively, since it may require a totally different surgical approach. Moreover, knowledge of the proximity of the aneurysm to the renal arteries may help in predicting the degree of difficulty in the surgical procedure. Similarly, preoperative knowledge of common iliac, and particularly internal iliac, aneurysms may help the surgeon in both planning his treatment and assessing the technical difficulty. In some borderline cases, the technical difficulty may fairly influence the decision whether or not a given aneurysm should be operated on in a given patient. This is certainly true for patients older than age 80 years.

Preoperative arteriography also provides a guide to the extent of stenotic or occlusive disease that may be suspected from physical examination. It is helpful to know if there is significant superior mesenteric artery, celiac, or renal artery stenosis. It is also helpful to know before operation if there are anomalous or ectopic renal arteries, if the inferior mesenteric artery is patent, and if there is a meandering mesenteric artery. In the presence of a patent inferior mesenteric artery, a meandering mesenteric artery indicates superior mesenteric artery occlusion or tight stenosis, and reimplantation of the inferior mesenteric artery may be indicated. Although some surgeons might settle for digital venous arteriography, in our opinion the ability to obtain lateral and oblique views and selective catheterizations in some patients makes direct transfemoral arteriography the route of choice. Since the risk of angiographic examination is small, we disagree with those who advocate aneurysm surgery without preoperative arteriography. Although it is true that some surprises can be dealt with effectively in the operating room, others may be more difficult to handle, and preoperative knowledge of their existence is helpful.

DIAGNOSIS OF RUPTURED ABDOMINAL ANEURYSM

The triad of a *known aneurysm* by history or physical examination, abdominal or back *pain*, and *syncope*, or other evidence of postural hypotension, is pathognomonic of a ruptured aneurysm. Depending on the site of extravasation, the pain may be localized anywhere in the abdomen or in the mid or lower back. Ocassionally, the pain may be felt in the flank and *mimic renal colic*, radiating to the groin, testicle, or labia. At other times, the pain may be in one of the lower abdominal quadrants and mimic an inflammatory process, such as *diverticulitis*. The triad of abdominal pain, a known aneurysm, and syncope is sufficient in itself to make a firm diagnosis of ruptured abdominal aneurysm and mandate surgical treatment after the briefest of evaluations. Such an evaluation should include passage of a nasogastric tube and rectal examination to rule out major gastrointestinal hemorrhage, obtaining an electrocardiogram to rule out clear-cut evidence of myocardial infarction, and a brief examination to rule out neurologic causes of syncope. In the absence of significant contraindications or other explanations for the symptom complex mentioned, an additional diagnostic work-up is unnecessary, and the patient should be routed for definitive surgical treatment. An elevated hematocrit in a patient with the triad whose condition is stable under close observation may be a reason to delay surgical treatment long enough to measure serum amylase level. In the absence of pancreatitis, it is probably better to operate on a patient with the triad than it is to delay treatment for additional observation or diagnostic evaluation. The penalty for such delay can be higher operative mortality if the patient has a ruptured aneurysm. If he does not, he almost certainly has some other surgically correctable condition within the abdomen. Patients with a ruptured aneurysm may have a normal or decreased hematocrit. They frequently have a low-grade fever and an elevated white cell blood count.

If the patient presents with severe abdominal or back pain and syncope, a ruptured aneurysm should be suspected. Evaluating such a patient should include an emergency plain film examination of the abdomen; the clinician should look for the vascular calcification that may indicate an aneurysm or for the absence of a psoas shadow, which may indicate retroperitoneal blood. Emergency evaluation may also include sonography or computerized tomography to determine if an aneurysm is present. If it is, the triad is completed, and immediate operation is usually the treatment of choice. Arteriography is rarely necessary in these circumstances and not particularly helpful in the diagnosis of ruptured abdominal aneurysm. In fact, delaying surgical treatment to perform an arteriographic study can often be fatal.

The critical element in diagnosing a ruptured abdominal aneurysm is to treat the condition surgically before a conclusive diagnosis is made. Only when the condition is surgically treated early and when only a presumptive diagnosis can be made, can mortality be reduced to less than 50 percent. The few errors that may be made when this approach is followed help to detect either other intra-abdominal conditions requiring surgical repair or an unruptured but expanding abdominal aneurysm that needs surgical management.

SURGICAL TREATMENT OF ABDOMINAL ANEURYSM

Patient Selection

As already stated, the critical element in treating unruptured abdominal aneurysm is to operate *before* it ruptures. The critical element in the treatment of *ruptured* aneurysm is to operate as soon as possible, often before the diagnosis is totally clear. Since unruptured aneurysms usually occur in older patients with various intercurrent diseases and associated risk factors, the operative risk of a major intra-abdominal operation in some patients with this condition is not inconsequential. It may range as high as 10 percent or higher in patients with serious associated cardiopulmonary disease. On the other hand, the technical aspects of aneurysm surgery have so improved that, in almost every case, the operation can be performed without technical mishap. Accordingly, the present theme should be to operate on *most* aneurysms that have any chance of rupturing in relatively healthy patients; only those aneurysms that are at high risk of rupturing in patients with serious intercurrent medical problems; and only aneurysms at very high risk of rupturing in patients who are in the most precarious condition due to their intercurrent medical problems. Examples of the latter are a patient with a cardiac ejection fraction less than 15 percent or a patient with dyspnea and orthopnea at rest from chronic lung disease. In such patients, aneurysm repair should be performed only when the aneurysm exceeds 6 to 7 cm in diameter or when the patient becomes symptomatic. On the other hand, a patient younger than age 70 years without known associated cardiopulmonary disease who has an aneurysm that exceeds 4 cm in diameter should probably be treated surgically, even though the risk of rupture in such a small aneurysm remains low. Most patients fall in between these extremes in that they have some evidence of coronary artery disese, even though it may be largely asymptomatic. Generally, if their symptomatic aneurysm is less than 5 cm in diameter, these patients should be observed closely. Abdominal ultrasonography should be performed every 4 to 6 months, and the patient should be surgically treated when the aneurysm exceeds 5 cm in any major cross-sectional diameter. If the aneurysm remains stable and less than 5 cm in diameter on ultrasound examination, continued observation is a relatively safe course, since the operative risk probably approaches the rupture risk at any given time. In the latter group of patients, medicosurgical assessment of risks is important. In addition, the patient should be allowed to influence the decision about the time of operation. Some patients may wish to accept the risk of deferring operation to avoid the small chance of an operative death or complications. Other patients may wish to have the operation carried out promptly, since in all likelihood they will have to have it eventually.

Elective Surgical Treatment of Unruptured Abdominal Aneurysm

Although a detailed description of methods for repairing abdominal aortic and iliac aneurysms is beyond the scope of this chapter, several important technical advances that have sharply reduced the morbidity of elective aneurysmectomy deserve mention. Preoperatively, patients should have a mechanical and antibiotic bowel preparation to minimize problems caused by low-grade intestinal ischemia. In addition, the preoperative placement of a balloon-tipped pulmonary artery (Swan-Ganz) catheter to monitor right- and left-sided heart pressures permits optimization of cardiac function and facilitates the administration of fluids before and during the operation.

Although aneurysm surgery in its early days was filled with technical difficulties and often associated with massive blood loss, recent improvements have minimized these problems. Paramount among these technical improvements is recognition of the fact that the entire aneurysmal wall need not be excised. Leaving all or a portion of the aneurysm in place minimizes the risk of injury to large venous structures and generally avoids the primary source of massive venous bleeding, which in the past made aneurysm resections so risky. Another technical improvement has been the avoidance of circumferential dissection of both the neck of the aneurysm and the iliac arteries beyond the aneurysmal dilatation. Such dissection was another common cause of excessive bleeding from normal or anomalous venous structures adhering to the aneurysm or to its adjacent, more normal arteries because of the associated inflammatory process. When proximal and distal control of the arterial circulation is obtained, the plastic fabric graft used to repair the aneurysm is optimally placed within the aneurysm and sutured securely without transecting the posterior aortic or iliac walls at the level of the proposed suture lines.

Following graft placement, the remaining aneurysm wall can then generally be sutured around the graft to prevent its subsequent erosion into the adjacent duodenum. This maneuver, together with either closure of the retroperitoneum or placement of omentum to separate further the graft from the duodenum, minimizes the incidence of aortoenteric fistulas. When large common or internal iliac aneurysms make arterial dissection and control difficult deep within the pelvis, no attempt to gain such control is indicated. Formerly, this was another source of major venous injury and exsanguination. With large common iliac or internal iliac aneurysms, the bifurcation graft should simply be anastomosed to the external iliac or common femoral arteries, and these arteries occluded proximally with ligatures or large clips. The proximal orifice of the common iliac artery aneurysm can then safely be oversewn from within, since this suture line will not be subjected to arterial pressure. Autotransfusion or cell-saver techniques minimize the need for homologous blood replacement and comprise another important recent technical advance in aneurysm surgery.

Because many other techincal details may be important in the safe management of abdominal aneurysms, it is wise to have these sometimes challenging operations performed by experienced surgeons. Generally, these are surgeons with specialized training and experience in vascular surgery rather than surgeons whose major commitment is to general surgery. Although some abdominal aneurysms may be simple to manage, others may be demanding and technically difficult. These latter cases can often but not always be anticipated by preoperative arteriography.

SURGICAL TREATMENT OF RUPTURED ANEURYSM

The most important consideration in the effective management of a ruptured abdominal aneurysm is the speed with which proximal aortic control can be obtained. It is one of the few surgical emergencies in which a few minutes delay can make a critical difference. The preeminent consideration in treating patients with a presumably ruptured abdominal aneurysm is to route them to the operating room as quickly as possible. Delays for confirmatory examination can be fatal.

Once in the operating room, the patient should be prepared for the induction of anesthesia as quickly as possible. If he is not profoundly hypotensive, arterial and venous lines should be placed; the bladder catheterized; a nasogastric tube inserted; and the abdomen, chest, and thighs prepped. *Anesthesia should not be induced until the surgical team is present and ready to begin the operation*; induction of anesthesia can be followed by profound circulatory collapse. On the other hand, if the patient is in cardiac arrest or suffering from profound hypotension before the entire surgical team is assembled, the senior surgical person present should rapidly open the abdomen and obtain proximal aortic control. The important step in resuscitating a patient in hypovolemic shock with a ruptured aneurysm is to control the bleeding by occluding the aorta proximal to the aneurysm. Other resuscitative measures are usually only partially effective and should not delay obtaining definitive aortic control. In most ruptured aneurysms, this is best accomplished via a supraceliac approach. An experienced vascular surgeon can usually perform this maneuver bluntly within 4 or 5 minutes in an emergency. If the rupture and the resulting hematoma are low down on the aorta or in one of the iliac arteries, the retroperitoneum may be opened safely and infrarenal control obtained, using blunt dissection in a deliberate manner. The supraceliac approach for control is critically important if the retroperitoneal hematoma is in the aorta immediately below the renal arteries. Under these circumstances, entrance into the retroperitoneum may decompress the controlling tamponade and provoke arterial hemorrhage. Furthermore, even if exsanguination does not occur, the surgeon may be driven to haste, with resulting injury to adjacent venous structures from such secondary iatrogenic bleeding. Other important technical details in the surgical management of ruptured aortic aneurysm include minimal dissection outside the aneurysm and the placement of the reparative graft within the aneurysmal lumen.

After both elective and emergency repair, a careful evaluation of the adequacy of the distal circulation is warranted. It should include a careful neurologic examination to determine tissue viability and an accurate examination of the distal pulses. The postoperative findings should be compared with the preoperative examination to detect distal embolization, thrombosis, or an intimal flap that interferes with the distal arterial perfusion. If a distal embolus or other problem is suspected, it should generally be attacked immediately in patients who are systemically stable. In systemically unstable patients, diagnostic and therapeutic maneuvers may be delayed if limb viability is not an issue. Depending on the level of loss of distal pulses and the degree of change from preoperative examination, the operative approach for these problems may be preceded by arteriography. If distal limb ischemia is associated with absent femoral pulse on one side, the abdomen may be reexplored and the problem corrected directly. Alternatively, a unilateral thrombectomy or femorofemoral bypass may be performed without reopening the abdomen. If distal limb ischemia develops in a patient with a strong femoral pulse, transfemoral embolectomy with intraoperative angiographic control may be performed. Alternatively, a preoperative arteriogram may be obtained. This is particularly useful in patients with distal limb ischemia and a popliteal pulse. The operative approach to such a problem may be difficult but should be directed at the popliteal artery at the site where the embolus seems to have lodged. After removal of the embolus, intraoperative angiographic examination should be performed to demonstrate the adequacy of the circulation and the complete removal of all clot and debris. In some patients with severe distal atheromatous disease, it may be difficult or impossible to remove all embolic material, and a distal bypass may be required to salvage the extremity. Also, the atheromatous and fibrin emboli may occasionally become lodged so far distally in arteries at the ankle or in the foot that surgical removal is impossible. Thus, although it is rare, patients occasionally lose their limb following aneurysm surgery despite the most skillful management. This is particularly true for patients who have undergone emergency surgery for a ruptured aneurysm complicated by severe distal atherosclerotic occlusive disease.

POSTOPERATIVE CARE

After repair of an abdominal aortic aneurysm, particularly a ruptured one, patients may often be critically ill. They should be cared for in an intensive care unit (ICU) with all the equipment necessary for monitoring cardiac chamber, pulmonary artery, and systemic arterial pressures. Facilities for intensive respiratory care should also be available, as should support for other organ systems since some postoperative aneurysm patients are among the sickest in any ICU. Facilities and personnel should be available to treat large fluid shifts, congestive heart failure, cardiac arrhythmias, acute renal failure, and pulmonary insufficiency.

RESULTS OF UNRUPTURED ABDOMINAL ANEURYSM REPAIR

The range of operative mortality for elective repair of aneurysm is between 2 and 5 percent. The principal cause of death is from coronary artery disease, associated as it is with myocardial infarction and congestive heart failure. Other causes of death include visceral ischemia and pulmonary insufficiency, although both these problems may be minimized by appropriate preoperative evaluation and postoperative management. Pulmonary emboli and infection are rare causes of death. Serious problems from colonic ischemia may occur after aneurysm surgery. They usually develop hypotensive patients in whom restoration of circulation to at least one internal iliac artery has not been possible.

Although the risk of aneurysmal repair increases slightly with age, it is possible to operate safely and effectively on patients in their 80s and even in their 90s. Such operations should generally be reserved for patients with larger, more threatening aneurysms. Many patients in these age groups, particularly those with smaller aneurysms, or severe heart disease, or both, should probably not have the operation.

Late complications following aneurysmal repair are unusual and restricted to incisional hernias and retroperitoneal or groin infection. The latter is a serious complication, which fortunately is rare. It carries a high mortality and usually requires removal of the graft and some form of extra-anatomic bypass.

Surgical results in *emergency aneurysmal repair* are generally poor; they are directly related to the delay in routing the patient to the operating room and the degree of hypovolemic hypotension preoperatively. Approximately 50 percent of younger patients surgically treated for ruptured aneurysm survive; this figure can be raised by prompt surgical relief, particularly of patients with well-tamponaded ruptures. But for patients who reach the operating room in profound shock and for those older than age 75 years, the chance of survival is slim. In general, the rate of complications is much higher following repair for a ruptured aneurysm than it is following elective aneurysm surgery. However, if the patient leaves the hospital in good condition, the long-term results are comparable and excellent.

THERAPEUTIC ALTERNATIVES

As already indicated, careful observation with periodic ultrasound evaluation of size changes is an acceptable alternative to operation for many small and some medium aneurysms. The importance of evaluating the relative risks of such nonsurgical observation and comparing them to the risks of operation in each patient has already been stressed.

In some patients who may be poor medical risks because of intercurrent cardiopulmonary disease and a threatening aneurysm, an alternative operative approach to aneurysmal repair has been suggested by some surgeons. It consists of the indication of thrombosis within the aneurysm followed by an axillobifemoral bypass. The thrombosis is induced by distal ligation of the external iliac arteries associated with occlusion of the internal iliac arteries and other large branches, using several radiographic approaches that include the placement of coils and surgical adhesives. These elements are placed under radiographic control by inserting an arterial catheter through an axillary artery. Although this approach has been successful in a few patients, it does not preclude the possibility of aneurysm rupture and is associated with a high rate of complication. Consequently, it is not recommended for routine use.

This work was supported in part by grants from the Manning and Brown Foundations.

COR PULMONALE

DAVID R. DANTZKER, M.D.

Cor pulmonale is defined as right ventricular hypertrophy or dilatation resulting from diseases affecting the function and/or structure of the lung except when the pulmonary alterations are the result of diseases that primarily affect the left side of the heart, or of congenital heart disease. Clinical evidence of right ventricular failure is not required for the diagnosis, although it is this occurrence that usually brings the condition to the attention of the physician. Pulmonary hypertension, a mean pulmonary artery pressure at rest greater than 25 mm Hg or a pulmonary vascular resistance greater than 2.0 mm Hg per liter per minute, is the precipitating cause of the cardiac dysfunction regardless of the underlying pulmonary disorder. The lung diseases that are associated with cor pulmonale are myriad (Table 1), and many are discussed in detail elsewhere in this book. This chapter addresses particularly the cor pulmonale that complicates chronic obstructive pulmonary disease (COPD), the most common etiology and the one with which most clinical experience has been accumulated. However, the basic principles of diagnosis and treatment can be extrapolated to patients with other chronic respiratory disorders involving the lung or chest wall. Anatomic evidence of cor pulmonale has been found in as many as 40 percent of patients dying from COPD, and a number of studies have suggested that its presence implies a poor prognosis independent of the severity of the underlying lung disease.

TABLE 1 Disease Associated with Cor Pulmonale

Pulmonary parenchymal disease
COPD
Bronchiectasis
Cystic fibrosis
Interstitial fibrosis
Sarcoidosis
Chronic hypoxia
Kyphoscoliosis
Idiopathic hypoventilation syndrome
Sleep apnea
Neuromuscular disease
Pulmonary vascular disease
Primary pulmonary hypertension
Pulmonary embolic disease
Pulmonary vasculitis
Collagen-vascular disorders

PATHOGENESIS OF PULMONARY HYPERTENSION

A reduction in the cross-sectional area of the pulmonary vascular bed is clearly responsible for the elevated pulmonary artery pressure in diseases such as recurrent pulmonary emboli, and it is often assumed that pulmonary hypertension in COPD is also due to the loss of pulmonary vessels resulting from the characteristic destruction of alveolar walls seen in emphysema. However, careful pathologic studies have failed to demonstrate a convincing correlation between the extent of emphysema and the amount of right ventricular hypertrophy. It is now accepted that vasoconstriction secondary to alveolar hypoxia, often accentuated by respiratory acidosis, is the initiating mechanism of the pulmonary hypertension. The loss of pulmonary vascular cross-sectional area plays a supporting role, as do the increased blood volume and polycythemia that often accompany the hypoxemia, magnifying the impact of the vasoconstriction on the pulmonary arterial pressure. An increased airway resistance through its effect on intrathoracic pressures may also augment the rise in pulmonary vascular resistance.

The acute reversal of hypoxemia in these patients does not cause a significant fall in pulmonary vascular resistance, and thus some factor in addition to an increase in vascular tone must be involved. Prolonged increases in pressure, regardless of the etiology, eventually lead to anatomic remodeling of the pulmonary vessels. Muscularization of the small pulmonary arteries, medial hypertrophy, and reduction in the number of small arteries occur so that vascular resistance increases further and becomes, to a great degree, independent of tone. The increased pulmonary artery pressure need not be continually present, as animal studies have shown anatomic remodeling with as little as 8 hours of hypoxia per day. The rate at which this vascular remodeling develops in the setting of COPD is uncertain, but recent studies involving repeated catheterizations of patients with mildly elevated pulmonary artery pressures have demonstrated a slow progression of the pulmonary hypertension. The degree of right ventricular dysfunction is often greater in patients with COPD than in patients with, for example, primary pulmonary hypertension, who usually have considerably higher pulmonary artery pressures. The reason for this is unclear, but it may be due to the pattern of acute changes in the degree of pulmonary hypertension that accompany the frequent exacerbations and improvements of the underlying lung disease. This, combined with the more severe hypoxemia, older age, and concurrent coronary artery disease in patients with COPD, may prevent the right heart from adapting to the high pressures.

Animal studies have demonstrated that increasing right ventricular afterload may also lead to left ventricular hypertrophy through the mechanism of ventricular interdependence. The importance of this observation to patients with cor pulmonale is unclear, although significant left-sided dysfunction resulting from pulmonary hypertension must be uncommon. Most patients with cor pulmonale and no other reason for left ventricular disease have normal indices of left-sided function. However, since patients with COPD are at risk for left ventricular disease due to coronary artery disease, left-sided failure may well complicate the clinical presentation.

DIAGNOSIS

The clinical diagnosis of cor pulmonale in patients with chronic lung disease is infrequently made prior to the elevation of systemic venous pressure and its attendant physical findings of peripheral edema, jugular venous distention and hepatomegaly, and in this setting it is often difficult to distinguish cor pulmonale from congestive heart failure secondary to left ventricular disease. The invariable complaints of dyspnea and increasing exercise limitation, which may initiate a work-up for primary or embolic pulmonary hypertension, are present in these patients due to their underlying lung disease, and there is no obvious worsening with the onset of right ventricular hypertrophy or dilatation.

Pulmonary function studies are nonspecific since all these patients have severe dysfunction prior to the onset of right heart disease. However, cor pulmonale is rarely seen with an FEV_1 greater than 1.0 liter, and the diagnosis is unlikely in the absence of significant resting oxygen desaturation. Exercise testing is of little help in patients with COPD since they are limited predominantly by their reduced ventilatory capacity.

The electrocardiogram (ECG) may suggest the diagnosis of right ventricular overload although in the presence of underlying lung disease it is often less accurate. The presence of right axis deviation, an increased amplitude of the p wave in II, III and AVF, an S_1, S_2, S_3 pattern or an R or R′ in V1 are all consistent with cor pulmonale. Perhaps the most predictive findings are the combination of an S_1Q_3 pattern along with a R:S less than 1.0 in V6. However, even this combination has a false-positive rate of 20 percent and a false-negative rate of 33 percent when validated against other clinical criteria. In autopsy studies, only about 30 percent of patients with anatomic evidence of cor pulmonale had ECG evidence of the disease.

Imaging techniques may assist in the diagnosis. The chest film is helpful when positive, but a normal cardiovascular appearance does not rule out the diagnosis. The most objective finding is the presence of a descending right pulmonary artery greater than 16 mm in diameter. In one study, this accurately predicted a mean pulmonary artery pressure of more than 20 mm Hg in 43 of 46 patients in whom it was present. Echocardiographic examination of the right side of the heart is not sensitive in these patients owing to the difficulty in visualizing the right ventricle in patients with hyperinflated lungs. Radionuclide angiocardiographic estimates of right ventricular ejection fraction are sensitive, but not specific. A value of less than 45 percent is considered abnormal, although this was also found in 35 percent of patients with COPD who were not thought to have cor pulmonale. Right ventricular performance is dependent on small changes in both preload and afterload, and thus it is often difficult to interpret changes in ejection fraction from one time to another. Examination of the left ventricle by radionuclide studies may be useful in cases of heart failure to assess the possible contribution of left heart dysfunction.

MANAGEMENT

Oxygen

Since the predominant cause of cor pulmonale in these patients is hypoxic vasoconstriction, eliminating or modulating this with supplemental oxygen should be the first priority. As already mentioned, administration of oxygen rarely leads to acute reductions in pulmonary vascular resistance, although there may be a decrease in pulmonary artery pressure secondary to a fall in cardiac output. Initial uncontrolled trials of continuous oxygen therapy did show a marked reversal of pulmonary hypertension, but two recent, large clinical studies failed to corroborate the dramatic effects of prolonged oxygen seen in the smaller trials. In a British trial, the effect of room air was compared with that of 15 hours per day of low-flow oxygen. No significant fall in the degree of pulmonary hypertension was noted, although the pressures remained stable in the treated group and continued to rise in the control patients. In an American O_2 trial, results of 11 hours of nocturnal O_2 per day were compared with those of "continuous" oxygen therapy, which averaged about 19 hours of treatment each day. There was a small, but statistically significant, difference between the nocturnal group, who had a small rise in pulmonary vascular resistance, and the "continuous" group, who had a very small decline. The failure of a more substantial improvement in pulmonary vascular resistance to take place in either trial can be explained by a number of factors. The reversal of hypoxemia was intermittent, even in the "continuous" group, and regular short periods of hypoxemia sustain hypoxia-induced pulmonary hypertension. The improvement in arterial O_2 saturation was not necessarily accompanied by similar improvements in the alveolar Po_2 of the most poorly ventilated regions of the lung. Thus the stimulus for hypoxic vasoconstriction in these regions probably persisted. Finally, it is possible that the duration of treatment over which the patients were observed, at least in the American trial, was not sufficient. The complete reversal of pulmonary hypertension in high-altitude natives who move to sea level may take more than 1 year.

Despite the failure of a dramatic reversal of the pulmonary hypertension, the oxygen-treated patients had a startlingly better survival, which directly correlated with the duration of daily oxygen administration. The mechanism of the improved survival is unclear, but it may have resulted from an improvement in oxygen delivery to the peripheral tissues at a lower cardiac output and thus a decrease in overall cardiac work. For this reason, O_2 therapy should be utilized on a continuous basis in all patients who meet the requirements of the patients in these two trials (Table 2). Although the aim of therapy should be to provide an arterial Po_2 of at least 60 to 65 mm Hg, this must often be tempered by the fact that the provision of O_2 flows higher than 4 liters per minute is neither economically nor logistically feasible. Different liter flows may be required at rest and during exercise or sleep, and the O_2 prescription for each patient should be individualized whenever possible.

For patients whose resting awake blood gases do not meet the criteria described in Table 2, but who desaturate during exercise, the decision to use O_2 is more controversial and often more difficult to justify, even though clinical studies have demonstrated an improved response to exercise with the correction of hypoxemia. Fortunately, patients with COPD who do not meet criteria for O_2 at rest do not often desaturate at the low levels of exercise they are able to sustain. A more difficult decision is whether to treat the large number of patients with COPD who only desaturate during sleep. Right now there is no clinical evidence that patients experiencing such intermittent episodes of hypoxia will develop pulmonary hypertension, although animals exposed to similar hypoxic stimuli do. At present, I prescribe nocturnal O_2 for patients in whom a significant desaturation can be documented during sleep and who are studied because they show evidence of a physiologic response to the hypoxia such as cor pulmonale or polycythemia. It is hoped that further long-term studies will clarify the need for nocturnal O_2 for the asymptomatic nocturnal desaturator.

TABLE 2 Criteria for Continuous Oxygen Therapy

British study
- FEV_1 less than 1.2 liters
- Arterial Po_2 of 40–60 mm Hg
- *and*
- Evidence of heart failure

American study
- Arterial Po_2 less than 55 mm Hg
- *or*
- Arterial Po_2 less than 59 mm Hg
- *and*
- Right heart failure or erythrocytosis

There is no evidence of significant deleterious effects associated with long-term low-flow oxygen therapy, although some subtle morphologic changes were noted in the lungs of patients who died during the nocturnal O_2 trial. Although there is always some risk of worsening CO_2 retention with the O_2, this is probably overstated. Rarely is there more than a small increase in arterial PCO_2, and this is more related to shifts in the carbon dioxide dissociation curve and slightly worsened ventilation-perfusion inequality than to further depression of respiratory drive.

Pharmacologic Therapy

Whenever possible, therapy should be directed toward the underlying lung disease. Steroids may improve gas exchange in patients with interstitial lung disease, whereas tracheostomy, weight loss, or nasal positive pressure may be curative in sleep apnea. Next to O_2, reversal of bronchospasm with bronchodilators is most important to the patient with COPD and cor pulmonale. By improving ventilation-perfusion matching and thus decreasing alveolar hypoxia, one reduces the stimulus to hypoxic vasoconstriction. By decreasing airway resistance, bronchodilators reduce the swings in transthoracic pressure, moderating the effect on pulmonary vascular resistance as well as directly reducing cardiac work as the O_2 requirements of the respiratory muscles decrease. Finally, theophylline has been shown to improve right ventricular performance in patients with COPD, and the beta agonists (even the so called selective beta-2 drugs) are known to have inotropic potential as well as being pulmonary vasodilators. Care must be taken to prevent cardiac side effects. Both families of drugs have arrhythmogenic potential, and this may further compromise cardiac function. In addition, hepatic congestion reduces the clearance of theophylline and makes the patient more prone to toxicity. Since arrhythmias and seizures may be the first manifested symptoms of theophylline toxicity, blood levels should be checked in the patient who is in overt right heart failure during acute exacerbations or prior to a change in dosage.

Digitalis

The use of digitalis in this population of patients is controversial. Its potential for improving right ventricle contractility is probably less than the propensity for digitalis toxicity, accentuated in these patients by the associated presence of hypoxemia, acidosis, and hypokalemia as well as the use of other arrhythmogenic drugs such as the xanthines and beta agonists. Its major indication in cases of cor pulmonale should be digitalis-responsive supraventricular arrhythmias or coincident left heart failure.

Diuretics

Significant peripheral edema often develops owing to the elevated right-sided pressure as well as the effect of hypoxemia and hypercapnia on renal hemodynamics and hormone function. Despite maximal therapy aimed at correcting the abnormal gas exchange, diuretics often become necessary. However, in the face of pulmonary hypertension, a high venous filling pressure is necessary to maintain right ventricular output. Since overdiuresis is often responsible for clinical deterioration due to inadequate peripheral O_2 delivery, it is useful to tolerate the presence of trace edema to ensure adequate intravascular volume.

Vasodilators

Arguing from analogies with systemic hypertension, a direct attack on the cause of the right ventricular afterload might seem appropriate. Since oxygen is not particularly effective at reducing pulmonary hypertension, at least over the period of time thus far studied, pharmacologic reduction of pulmonary vascular resistance has been attempted. Some of the many agents shown to be pulmonary vasodilators are nitroglycerine, Hydralazine, calcium-channel blockers (nifedipine, diltiazem), and prostaglandins (PGE, prostacyclin).

Although the success of vasodilation has been far from universal, it is clear that some patients with cor pulmonale do respond to vasodilators with a reduction in pulmonary artery pressure associated with an acute improvement in hemodynamic performance and, in some cases, functional ability. However, the ability to maintain this improvement for a prolonged time as well as the translation of physiologic improvement into a clear beneficial effect on survival or the quality of life has yet to be demonstrated. Since these patients are limited predominantly by their ventilatory insufficiency, it may, in fact, be difficult to demonstrate an appreciable functional gain even when significant cardiovascular improvement is accomplished. A study the size and scope of the oxygen trials, showing an improvement in survival, may be necessary to eventually prove the efficacy of vasodilators.

A major reason for proceeding cautiously is that these drugs are not without significant side effects. With successful pulmonary vasodilation often comes increased ventilation-perfusion inequality. Significant hypoxemia is less common because the increase in mixed venous Po_2 that usually accompanies the improvement in cardiac output often offsets the worsening ventilation-perfusion mismatch. Since all these drugs are also potent dilators of the systemic circulation, patients are at risk for the development of systemic hypotension and organ hypoperfusion, particularly if there is insufficient improvement in right ventricular function. Finally, the calcium-channel blockers, in cases of right ventricular failure, may have sufficient negative inotropic effect to worsen the degree of heart failure unless significant pulmonary vasodilation is achieved.

If vasodilators are to be used they should be tried only after the diagnosis of pulmonry hypertension is clearly demonstrated by right heart catheterization. Then, with the catheter in place, the acute response to one or more drugs can be assessed. I generally administer intravenous nitroglycerin (starting at 5 μg per minute) and hydralazine (starting with 0.125 mg per kilogram) and sublingual nifedipine (initial dose 10 mg) sequentially over a period of 24 hours at doses that lower the systemic arterial systolic pressure by 20 percent or increase the heart rate by 20 beats per minute. The criterion for a successful response remains controversial, although I consider it to be, as a minimum, a 20 percent fall in pulmonary vascular resistance with a concomitant fall, or certainly no rise, in pulmonary artery pressure. The usual maintenance doses are: Isordil 20 mg, hydralazine 25 to 50 mg, or nifedipine 20 mg, four times per day. Because it is common for tolerance to the drugs to occur owing to tachyphylaxis or loss of vasoreactivity, the patient should have a repeat catheterization 2 to 3 months after starting therapy.

At present, vasodilators in this setting should be considered only experimental. The empiric use of these drugs in the population of patients with COPD and cor pulmonale should be strongly discouraged until more complete clinical trials are reported.

Phlebotomy

Finally, a word on the treatment of polycythemia. Since this is a response to the body's recognition of inadequate oxygen delivery, it would seem that resorting to phlebotomy is putting the wisdom of the physician ahead of the wisdom of the body. However, as the hematocrit rises, the work of the heart also increases. Fortunately, patients treated adequately with appropriate amounts of oxygen rarely develop sufficiently high hematocrits (greater than 55) to require phlebotomy. Even when the hematocrit exceeds 55, isovolemic reduction back to a level of 50 to 55 percent should be reserved for patients with unrelenting heart failure or clear evidence of central nervous system dysfunction or thrombotic episodes.

ACUTE PULMONARY EDEMA

DAVID S. BLUMENTHAL, M.D.

Acute pulmonary edema is best defined as a circumstance in which there is an increase in total lung water. The signs and symptoms that develop relate directly to that fact. Significant disorders of gas exchange occur and further exacerbate whatever process has produced the acute pulmonary edema. Therapy is therefore aimed at relief of the pulmonary congestion.

It is essential that the clinician make an attempt to determine the etiology of pulmonary edema since therapy will not be identical in all instances. The etiology of pulmonary edema may be either cardiac or noncardiac. In the former case, an elevation of pulmonary capillary pressure leads to the increase of lung water; in the latter, damage to membranes lining alveoli leads to the problem.

Cardiac pulmonary edema may occur in the setting of euvolemia or total body fluid overload. At one extreme is the individual with chronic fluid overload and acute progression to frank pulmonary edema. In this circumstance, total body fluid overload is clearly present and needs immediate attention and prompt diuresis. At the opposite extreme is the individual with acute myocardial infarction with sudden pulmonary edema. That individual was presumably euvolemic before the infarct and remains so. There has been a redistribution of body fluid so that pulmonary vascular overload occurs. Therapy should be aimed at redistribution of the fluid rather than simple dehydration.

Finally, pulmonary edema may be either hypertensive, normotensive, or hypotensive. Fortunately, most cardiac pulmonary edema is hypertensive and permits the use of blood pressure-lowering agents in its therapy. More problematic is normotensive or hypotensive pulmonary edema. The absence of hypertension in the setting of pulmonary edema may be a clue that the etiology of the pulmonary edema is noncardiac and mandates determination of pulmonary vascular pressure. If the etiology of the pulmonary edema is cardiac, the presence of normotension or hypotension will require substantial modification in the usual measures employed.

HYPERTENSIVE PULMONARY EDEMA

Hypertensive pulmonary edema is characterized by increases in both preload and afterload. The wide variety of measures employed in its therapy are directed at their reduction.

Oxygen and Upright Posture

Individuals in acute pulmonary edema are usually relatively hypoxemic and feel extremely dyspneic. It is therefore essential that high-flow oxygen be given immediately to all such individuals. I recommend either nasal oxygen at 8 L per minute or a Venturi mask with an FIO_2 of 40 percent. The only exceptions are individuals with chronic obstructive pulmonary disease who retain CO_2. In their case, a 24 percent Venturi mask or 2 L of nasal oxygen should initially be employed.

The oxygen should be delivered to the individual while he is in a sitting position, preferably with his legs dangling over the edge of the bed. The dangling position helps to reduce preload. Conversely, it is undesirable to force an individual in pulmonary edema to lay flat since that position increases preload, dyspnea, agitation, and metabolic demand.

Nitrates

The cornerstone of therapy for pulmonary edema is the use of nitrates. I give one or two tablets of 0.4 mg nitroglycerin sublingually every 3 to 5 minutes until blood pressure begins to fall into the normal range. At the same time, I place 1 to 2 inches of topical nitroglycerin ointment on the individual's torso. The sublingual nitroglycerin will provide more immediate relief. However, there may be problems with its absorption since individuals may mouth breathe and have extremely dry mucous membranes. This problem can occasionally be circumvented by dissolving the sublingual nitroglycerin in normal saline. After several minutes, the topical nitroglycerin will begin to be absorbed and produce an additional reduction in preload.

Severe peripheral vasoconstriction may interfere with topical nitrate absorption as well. If sublingual and topical nitrates do not produce the desired effect, I quickly switch to sodium nitroprusside. This medication is a profound preload and afterload reducing agent. I mix 50 mg in 500 cc of 5 percent dextrose in water (D5W) and infuse initially at a rate of 1 μg per kilogram per minute, but will go as high as 400 μg per kilogram per minute to produce the desired reduction in blood pressure. Careful monitoring of the blood pressure is essential during nitroprusside infusion. It is most desirable that an arterial line be in place during the infusion. However, it is not necessary for an arterial line to be in place at the time of drug initiation. Frequent blood pressure monitoring by a skilled observer will suffice until an arterial line can be inserted. Alternatively, an automated blood pressure cuff can occasionally be used in place of invasive monitoring.

Morphine

Morphine sulfate is commonly employed in the treatment of acute pulmonary edema. It is useful as an agent to reduce preload and to relieve agitation. Morphine sulfate is usually given intravenously at doses of 2 to 4 mg. It may be repeated every 5 to 10 minutes as necessary. Morphine is contraindicated in individuals with chronic obstructive pulmonary disease and CO_2 retention. In addition, any individual with transiently elevated PCO_2 in the setting of acute pulmonary edema may be at risk of further deterioration should respiratory depression develop from the morphine. Since one most commonly begins the therapy of pulmonary edema before arterial blood gases are measured, I am reluctant to employ morphine sulfate routinely. Alternative measures are available for preload reduction. Although morphine is an excellent drug to reduce agitation, the most agitated patients frequently have greatly disordered blood gases and are most likely to deteriorate if respiratory depression occurs. Thus, I tend to avoid morphine except in very unusual circumstances. If morphine is given, naloxone should be readily available to counteract its effects.

Rotating Tourniquets

Rotating tourniquets are a means to reduce preload by reducing venous return. I see no role for their use at this time since there are a host of pharmacologic maneuvers that perform that function with less discomfort to the patient.

Diuretics

Diuretics are definitely indicated in the treatment of acute pulmonary edema but are most specific in individuals with total body fluid overload. I prefer furosemide. The initial effect of furosemide is acute venodilation followed by subsequent diuresis. If diuretics are to be employed in the treatment of pulmonary edema, it is essential that a Foley catheter be inserted as soon as possible to accurately measure urine output. Individuals who are being maintained on furosemide should receive double their usual maintenance dose intravenously. Individuals who have not received furosemide before should receive 40 mg intravenously. It is important to recognize the patient's prepulmonary edema fluid status. Euvolemic individuals should be managed mainly with pharmacologic preload and afterload reduction. Diuretics should be withheld or given in lower doses since important hypovolemia and hypotension may ensue once associated measures take effect and afterload has been reduced to baseline.

Phlebotomy and Ultrafiltration

Certain hypervolemic individuals are not responsive to diuretics. Although this frequently relates to abnormalities of pH, Po_2, or electrolytes, an alternative means of volume removal is required until other abnormalities can be corrected. Perhaps the simplest method is phlebotomy. The removal of 250 cc of blood can be performed either by standard phlebotomy or with special kits that enable the packed cells to be returned to the individual at a later time. Alternatively, ultrafiltration can effectively remove large volumes of fluid rapidly but requires special personnel and equipment.

Intubation

Individuals with severe disorders of gas exchange or acid-base status may require intubation. The determination that an individual in pulmonary edema requires intubation is frequently made by observing that he is beginning to tire appreciably. Alternatively, pH of less than 7.10, Pco_2 of greater than 70, or Po_2 less than 60 on maximum supplemental oxygen are indications for intubation. One should err on the side of early intubation. The vigorous use of morphine should follow to enable substantial preload reduction, elimination of the work of breathing, decrease in circulating catecholamines, and improved gas exchange. Correction of these abnormalities will rapidly bring the pulmonary edema under control.

Digitalis

Digitalis is an arteriolar constrictor and is therefore relatively contraindicated in acute pulmonary edema. I reserve digoxin for circumstances in which a digoxin-responsive arrhythmia is present. Atrial fibrillation is the most common rhythm for which digoxin is given. The goal is an adequate level of digoxin to achieve heart rate control when the pulmonary edema has cleared (some degree of increased heart rate is appropriate during pulmonary edema to maintain cardiac output). Initially I give 0.50 mg of digoxin intravenously and follow with 0.25 mg, 2 hours and 4 hours later.

Aminophylline

Aminophylline is relatively contraindicated in acute pulmonary edema. Individuals with asthma predating their pulmonary edema will surely develop an appreciable amount of bronchospasm when they are in pulmonary edema. For such individuals, bronchodilators are essential. However, the majority of individuals who wheeze in the setting of acute pulmonary edema do so on the basis of increased interstitial pulmonary pressures. Relief of the pulmonary hypertension will relieve the bronchoconstriction.

It is tempting to give aminophylline to increase contractility and provide a bit of vasodilation. However, potential negative effects far outweigh these considerations. Aminophylline may contribute to sinus tachycardia and, therefore, increase metabolic demand. It may precipitate lethal ventricular arrhythmias. In addition, it is a nonspecific vaso- and bronchodilator. It may paradoxically worsen gas exchange by increasing blood flow to poorly ventilated alveoli.

Sodium Bicarbonate

Sodium bicarbonate is relatively contraindicated in acute pulmonary edema because of its obligatory sodium load. It may occasionally be useful in the correction of metabolic acidosis. However, there is no role for sodium bicarbonate in respiratory acidosis. Individuals with acidosis because of significant hypercarbia should be intubated.

SPECIAL CIRCUMSTANCES

Mitral Stenosis

Pulmonary edema occurs in mitral stenosis because rapid heart rate disproportionately increases the transvalvular gradient and increases pulmonary vascular pressures. Major attention is therefore directed toward heart rate control to relieve pulmonary hypertension. Ventricular function is usually normal in mitral stenosis so that agents that are otherwise contraindicated in acute pulmonary edema may be employed. Specifically, verapamil is an effective means of lowering heart rate. I give a 1 mg test dose intravenously and then a total dose of 5 mg intravenously. This may be repeated every 5 to 10 minutes to achieve effective heart rate control. Alternatively, a verapamil infusion may be employed; 60 mg is mixed in 120 cc of D5W and infused initially at a rate of 20 cc per hour. Propranolol may be used as an alternative agent. I give intravenous doses of 0.5 mg every 2 minutes up to a total of 0.1 mg per kilogram. I find this to be less satisfactory than verapamil because of the tendency for individuals in acute pulmonary edema to develop a component of reactive bronchoconstriction.

Acute Regurgitant Lesions

Acute pulmonary edema may follow the abrupt development or worsening of aortic regurgitation, mitral regurgitation, or ventricular septal defect. Afterload reduction is the cornerstone here, and one should move directly to the use of nitroprusside.

Papillary Muscle Dysfunction

One occasionally encounters individuals whose pulmonary edema disappears immediately with one or two sublingual nitroglycerin tablets. This should imply significant reversible left ventricular dysfunction and, in particular, acute papillary muscle dysfunction. Such individuals should immediately receive topical application of nitroglycerin while awaiting further investigation.

Swan-Ganz Catheterization

Right-heart catheterization has little role in the acute treatment of hypertensive pulmonary edema. In such circumstances, one can infer that left ventricular and pulmonary capillary pressures are elevated, and measures directed at relief of that hypertension are the highest priority. Placing an individual flat and covering him with a drape in order to insert a right-heart catheter is contraindicated. Once the pulmonary edema has begun to resolve, right-heart catheterization can be performed if needed for diagnostic purposes or to optimize therapy while following filling pressures and cardiac output.

NORMOTENSIVE AND HYPOTENSIVE PULMONARY EDEMA

In individuals who are normotensive or, especially, hypotensive, one must insert a right-heart catheter to treat acute pulmonary edema effectively while following cardiac output. The initial purpose of catheterization at such times is to confirm the diagnosis. Noncardiogenic pulmonary edema is associated with low or normal central pressures. A cardiogenic etiology will be confirmed by the presence of hypotension, elevated central pressures, and decreased cardiac output. In such circumstances, prognosis is grave.

The therapy of hypotensive pulmonary edema is extremely difficult. Measures that exclusively reduce preload are now relatively contraindicated since profound hypoperfusion of critical organ systems may develop. Conversely, agents that increase afterload will raise blood pressure at the expense of reduced cardiac output and are relatively contraindicated as well. Correction of hypoxemia, acidosis, or electrolyte abnormalities may be followed by improvement in blood pressure and is therefore a high priority. Early intubation is frequently required.

Agents that increase contractility can be employed but rarely produce inprovement. Digitalis is relatively contraindicated because it has a delayed onset of action as an inotrope, but is an acute arteriolar constrictor and increases afterload. Intravenous dobutamine (10 μg per kilogram per minute to start) increases contractility while decreasing afterload and may increase cardiac output with no effect on blood pressure. These changes are at most modest and seldom can reverse pulmonary edema. Dopamine at intravenous doses of 10 μg per kilogram per minute will increase contractility with little effect on afterload. Higher doses of dopamine or levarterenol will increase afterload while decreasing cardiac output. In such cases, nitroprusside can be added intravenously. Amrinone can increase contractility modestly.

The best solution to the problem of hypotensive pulmonary edema is the insertion of an intra-aortic balloon pump, and this should be done as soon as possible. The purpose is to reduce afterload while improving coronary perfusion. If the pulmonary edema can be cleared, one should make the individual ready for cardiac catheterization and then look for a mechanical cause of the pulmonary edema, such as a mitral regurgitation or ventricular septal defect.

NONCARDIOGENIC PULMONARY EDEMA

Individuals with noncardiogenic pulmonary edema tend to be normotensive or hypotensive. Noncardiogenic pulmonary edema should be suspected when therapeutic measures lead to diuresis with subsequent hypotension and little or no clinical improvement. The diagnosis may be confirmed by right-heart catheterization. In addition, a clinical history that suggests an infection, toxin exposure, aspiration pneumonia, radiation pneumonitis, or other cause of adult respiratory distress syndrome may be present. Therapeutic measures are directed toward improving gas exchange via positive end expiratory pressure and treatment of the underlying condition.

NONCARDIAC SURGERY IN THE PATIENT WITH HEART DISEASE

ABRAHAM GENECIN, M.D.

Most studies of the risks of noncardiac surgery in cardiac patients have dealt with individuals already characterized as having defined cardiac conditions. The aging of the population and the expansion of surgical techniques result in the exposure of many individuals with previously unrecognized circulatory problems to the hazards of surgery. The medical physician who has responsibility for preoperative evaluation must bear in mind the high incidence of vascular disorders in older age groups. The examiner must anticipate other disorders characteristic of maturity, such as diabetes, obesity, chronic obstructive pulmonary disease, renal and urinary tract impairments, gastrointestinal disturbances, and blood dyscrasias. To ensure the success and safety of surgery in cardiac and older patients, a medical consultant is expected to take a complete medical history, perform a medical examination, and review laboratory findings. He may find it desirable, in special situations, to order additional procedures, such as echocardiograms, stress tests, or 24-hour ambulatory Holter monitoring.

The recent campaign to reduce medical costs by shortening hospital stays may have a strong impact on the quality of the evaluation of cardiac patients prior to surgery. Compressing studies into a short time may not permit adequate study, observation, consultation, and discussion, thereby resulting in enhanced risk.

The consultant who sees a patient before surgery has a complex task. He needs to be satisfied that the preoperative diagnosis is correct and that the symptoms and findings are due to a condition which can best be remedied by surgery. He should be alert to the many cardiac and medical illnesses that masquerade as acute surgical problems—for example, right-sided heart failure mimicking a surgical abdomen. A medical physician is called upon to help in both the preoperative preparation and the recognition and treatment of postoperative complications.

EVALUATION OF CARDIAC RISK

A number of excellent comprehensive studies, which are widely quoted, have helped to pinpoint and quantitate factors which contribute to risk in noncardiac surgery. Dr. Lee Goldman of Boston and his associates have been leaders in this field. In many patients the history, physical examination, chest film, and electrocardiogram may be all that are required to complete an evaluation. Some cardiac patients may need special studies, such as echocardiography or even cardiac catheterization and noninvasive vascular imaging to define risk more accurately.

Ischemic heart disease poses a higher risk for noncardiac surgery. Statistical analyses of patients undergoing surgery within various intervals after myocardial infarction have shown that there is a large potential for recurrent infarction attended by extraordinarily high death rates for operations performed within 6 months after a myocardial infarction. Recent studies on the fate of patients who have had a "non-Q-wave" infarction suggest that the prognosis for survivors in this condition is no different from those who have had infarctions characterized by the presence of Q waves.

For the individual with angina, the consultant needs to evaluate whether or not the symptoms are stable, well controlled, and of long duration or if the history suggests accelerating disease or even unstable angina. The risk of surgery in this latter group is obviously very high and postponement of elective surgery and institution of appropriate medical or surgical regimen for relief of cardiac ischemia may have a higher priority.

The detection of congestive heart failure (CHF) is of the utmost importance in preoperative evaluation, since any degree of decompensation greatly enhances the risk to the patient. Pump dysfunction may be manifested by a third-sound gallop, cardiac enlargement, rales, increased jugular venous pressure, enlargement of the liver, edema of the extremities, interstitial edema on the chest film, or, an alternating pulse. Any of these manifestations should alert the clinician to the presence of heart failure and a predictably poor outcome.

Although hypertension is common, unless severe or "malignant," there does not appear to be an undue hazard for major surgery in the well-controlled hypertensive patient.

Statistics gathered in large series suggest that almost any rhythmic abnormality represents some increased hazard. Patients with complete heart block or high degree A-V block, such as Mobitz II block, obviously require pacing to survive anesthesia and surgery. On the other hand, patients with bifascicular block do not require prophylactic pacemakers. Long-term studies have shown that only a small proportion of such patients ultimately develop complete heart block. Asymptomatic sinus bradycardia does not require special attention and does not increase risk.

Patients already equipped with permanent implanted pacemakers need to be protected from the dangers of the electric cautery during surgery, particularly if it is used within proximity of the pacemaker pulse generator. Conversion of the pacemaker to a fixed mode by the use of the external magnet protects patients during surgical procedures.

Ventricular ectopic activity tends to increase operative mortality, particularly if there are five or more ventricular ectopic beats per minute. Supraventricular arrhythmias, such as paroxysmal atrial tachycardia, atrial flutter, or atrial fibrillation likewise require assessment of the patient's underlying cardiac status because of a vastly increased risk of death, particularly in the elderly. Rapid ventricular response in the presence of supraventricular tachycardia is especially hazardous. Supraventricular tachyarrhythmias should alert the clinician to the possibility of valvular heart disease, which sometimes may be difficult to detect. Mitral valve prolapse, mitral stenosis, or aortic stenosis may be present without characteristic murmurs in patients with low cardiac outputs. Atrial myxomas, previously unrecognized atrial septal defects, hypertrophic cardiomyopathy, thyrotoxicosis, and pulmonary hypertension may likewise account for disturbances of rhythm. Ventricular arrhythmias may be a clue to unsuspected cardiomyopathy, previously unrecognized coronary artery disease, ventricular aneurysm, recent infarction, electrolyte disturbances, digitalis toxicity, hypoxia, or drug reactions.

Advanced age seems to operate as an independent risk predictor for perioperative death, and the mortality of patients over age 70 is increased tenfold compared to younger age groups.

The type and length of surgery bear some relationship to surgical risk. Whereas cardiac patients seem to tolerate some procedures, such as hernia repair and transurethral resection, with relatively few complications, cardiac problems are more common after major abdominal, thoracic, and vascular operations. Emergency surgery is particularly hazardous for the cardiac patient.

Complications may be expected more commonly in cardiac patients who are in poor medical condition due to malnutrition, basic underlying disease of other vital organs, such as chronic renal or liver disease, severe metabolic disturbances, or anemia.

Special attention must be directed to the patient with aortic stenosis, since significant obstruction of aortic outflow is associated with a high mortality during anesthesia and surgery.

After several months have elapsed, patients who have had successful bypass surgery do well, by and large, with general surgical procedures and are not at extraordinary risk.

RISK REDUCTION

If preliminary evaluation suggests that the hazards of surgery are extraordinarily high and if the operation is nonemergent, a postponement to allow for appropriate diagnostic evaluation, treatment, and cardiac surgery, such as coronary bypass or aortic valve replacement, may be appropriate. There are differences of opinion as to how extensive a preoperative evaluation is needed for patients with suspected coronary artery disease. The clinician has to use his own judgment in each instance and decide about the importance of obtaining information from preoperative exercise testing, radioisotope scanning, or coronary angiography. Limitations in specificity and sensitivity of all diagnostic procedures used in the evaluation of coronary artery disease make it difficult to know when and how to use them, particularly in the asymptomatic individual in whom coronary disease may be suspected on grounds other than classic angina pectoris or recent myocardial infarction. Routine stress tests and angiography in high-risk patients do not necessarily provide answers to the risks of cardiac complications during surgery.

For the patient with compromised ventricular function, meticulous management of CHF, including a period of preoperative preparation, is needed. Adjustment of fluid balance, the appropriate use of diuretics, attention to electrolyte imbalance and digitalis toxicity, and the provision of an adequate period of rest to allow for improvement in cardiac function may make a procedure possible that otherwise would have been out of the question. In selected cases, hemodynamic monitoring may be helpful during the perioperative period.

In a patient with a documented history of cardiac arrest, prophylactic preoperative and intraoperative antiarrhythmic agents are mandatory. Attention to the serum levels of antiarrhythmic drugs, such as procainamide and quinidine, or the use of intravenous lidocaine before and during anesthesia induction may be helpful in reducing risk to patients with high-grade ventricular arrhythmias. As already mentioned, the patient with heart block, a history of Mobitz II block, or symptomatic sinus slowing may require temporary transvenous pacing.

Preparation of patients for general surgery may require some special considerations for selected groups of cardiac diagnoses. Cardiac catheterization and elective repair of severe aortic-valve obstruction may be desirable prior to elective procedures. Other types of valvular disease, such as severe mitral stenosis may also present a clinician with a dilemma as to whether correction is desirable before general surgical procedures. In any case, all individuals with valvular disease need to be protected against the possibility of infective endocarditis by the use of appropriate antibiotics. Those who have prosthetic valves will have been on anticoagulation drug therapy, and it is necessary to discontinue anticoagulants for 4 to 7 days before surgery and to omit such medications for a time after surgery until the hazards of postoperative bleeding are no longer present. The possibility of substitution of dipyridamole during the perioperative phase should be kept in mind. Individuals who have been on aspirin therapy should stop it for a week before elective surgery to minimize the risk of intraoperative and postoperative bleeding and postoperative hematoma formation.

As a general rule, most of the commonly used medicines, which are needed for control of the cardiac disorder, should be continued up to the time of surgery. Specifically, there is no need to discontinue antihypertensive agents, digitalis preparations, antiarrhythmic drugs, or diuretics up to the time of induction of anesthesia. If oral administration is not possible, parenteral preparations of substitutes can be found.

The widespread use of diuretic therapy may lead to potassium and magnesium depletion which, although asymptomatic, may present a hazard with respect to the precipitation of cardiac arrhythmias. Whenever possible, repletion and timely substitution of potassium-sparing preparations well in advance of surgery may be desirable. Patients who have lost blood or who are anemic for other reasons obviously should have hematocrits restored to a level that minimizes circulatory stress. Those on treatment with beta-blockers or clonidine are at special risk during the perioperative period because of the hazard of dangerous hypertensive withdrawal reactions when these agents are abruptly discontinued. For this reason, it may be necessary to continue parenteral therapy throughout the perioperative interval.

There is considerable controversy with reference to digitalis therapy for the cardiac patient. Many current studies suggest that digitalis is widely used in individuals who do not really require it. It is often true that such therapy can be safely withdrawn without deterioration. Prophylactic digitalis therapy for individuals who have no definite evidence of congestive failure is not warranted. Cardiac enlargement unattended by symptoms of congestive failure is not an indication for digitalization.

Consideration may be given to digitalizing individuals who are subject to supraventricular tachycardia, particularly elderly patients who require pulmonary surgery or procedures near the mediastinum. Patients with high-grade valvular stenotic disease may not tolerate tachycardia, and digitalization may be considered for this group. Alternative methods of controlling tachycardia, such as the use of verapamil or beta-blockers, may be preferable in selected instances.

The American Heart Association has provided detailed recommendations for prophylactic therapy with antibiotics to be used for individuals with valvular heart disease. Such therapy is necessary in all procedures in which there is an infected site and for gastrointestinal, biliary, and genitourinary procedures, particularly if there is chronic urinary tract infection. The antibiotics which are chosen for genitourinary and gastrointestinal procedures should be adequate to prevent infection with the common flora of these regions, which includes gram-negative organisms and enterococci. Although gram-negative organisms are not likely to produce endocarditis on diseased valves, there is a hazard of such infection in patients who have prosthetic valves. For these patients, current recommendations include the use of large doses of aqueous crystalline penicillin G or ampicillin plus gentamicin. Alternative regimens are available for individuals who are allergic to penicillin.

As a rule, the medical consultant has little or no role to play during the operative procedure. The cardiologist should be aware of the great expertise of modern anesthesiologists in the evaluation of medical patients, particularly with respect to use of drugs, type of anesthesia, physiologic measurements, and critical care monitoring. The choice of anesthesia is best left to the surgeon and anesthesiologist.

There is no benefit to spinal anesthesia for patients with coronary heart disease, and the fall in blood pressure induced by this kind of anesthesia is potentially harmful. However, CHF is less likely to be adversely affected by spinal anesthesia, and there are situations in which, if this is possible, it may be preferred for individuals with impaired ventricular function.

POSTOPERATIVE PROBLEMS

The cardiac patient obviously has a somewhat enhanced risk of experiencing the usual postoperative complications, particularly those having to do with the lungs. Postoperative hypoventilation, atelectasis, pneumonia, pleural effusions, and pulmonary emboli may be the cause of a complicated and stormy postoperative course.

Those who have had vascular surgery may have a sudden, acute rise in blood pressure immediately postoperatively, which is usually detected and monitored in the recovery room and intensive care areas. These situations generally come to the attention of the personnel in those units. Blood pressure changes occurring later in the postoperative course may be related to fluid overload or rebound phenomena from the omission of antihypertensive drugs.

Cardiac arrhythmias occur frequently in the early postoperative period. Isolated premature ventricular contractions are best left alone and untreated unless they are related to metabolic or hypoxic problems.

Supraventricular tachyarrhythmias, such as atrial flutter or atrial fibrillation, are commonly induced by the stresses of the postoperative period, in particular pulmonary emboli, derangements of electrolytes, medication overdosage, or fever and infection. As a rule, supraventricular arrythmias respond to correction of the underlying disorder and—except for digitalis, which may be helpful in controlling ventricular response in supraventricular arrhythmias—other types of antiarrhythmic drugs are rarely called for. Electrocardioversion is seldom required.

Congestive heart failure during the early postoperative period may be precipitated by an unrecognized myocardial infarction, fluid overload, high fever, hypoxia, or anemia.

Myocardial infarction during the postoperative period is a much-dreaded complication. Over one-half of postoperative myocardial infarctions occur within the first 3 days after the surgical procedure, and the remainder sometime between the fourth and sixth postoperative days. Many such episodes are painless. Any sudden derangement in the patient's status, such as a change in the heart rate, arrhythmias, or change in the blood pressure may be clues to damage to the heart muscle. Without serial electrocardiography in the postoperative patient, infarction may be difficult to recognize. Elevation of enzymes, which are relied upon in nonsurgical patients, are not as helpful in postoperative patients because of the frequent elevation of these enzymes due to surgical trauma. However, the MB fraction of the creatine kinase isoenzyme can be a reliable guide to cardiac damage.

In summary, we should take note of the perhaps inadequately recognized accomplishments of modern surgery, anesthesiology, and cardiology, which have enabled patients with serious heart conditions to be spared suffering and death. By the cooperative effort of these specialists and many others, individuals in whom major surgery would have been unthinkable several decades ago can now safely be brought through the stresses of major surgery and restored to happy, productive lives.

ORTHOSTATIC HYPOTENSION

RONALD J. POLINSKY, M.D.

Autonomic nervous system activity is essential for circulatory and metabolic homeostasis. Although orthostatic hypotension may also result from a reduction in blood volume or exaggerated responses of circulatory reflexes, this review focuses on neurogenic orthostatic hypotension caused by disorders that directly affect autonomic nervous system function. The clinical consequences of autonomic dysfunction include numerous symptoms that may require medical attention (Table 1). Orthostatic hypotension is generally the most disabling feature of autonomic insufficiency. The objectives of treatment are to prevent syncope and to minimize the constraints on activities of daily living imposed by the low blood pressure. Successful therapy of orthostatic hypotension is facilitated by effective management of other dysautonomic symptoms. Various systemic and neurologic diseases cause autonomic dysfunction; however, a similar treatment approach can be used for all patients.

THERAPEUTIC ALTERNATIVES

The term "orthostatic hypotension" does not convey the constellation of abnormal blood pressure responses observed in patients with autonomic dysfunction. This condition causes an increased sensitivity and exaggerated response to any environmental factor, physiologic maneuver, or pharmacologic agent altering blood pressure. Thus, patients with orthostatic hypotension may experience symptoms caused by hypotension at times when they are not standing. However, they may be unaware of the low blood pressure since hypotension produces symptoms only when the perfusion of specific tissues and organs is compromised beyond tolerable limits. For example, the absolute blood pressure, the rate and magnitude of the drop in blood pressure, and the limits of cerebral autoregulation determine whether hypotension will result in syncope. Absolute blood pressure criteria have little value in the treatment of orthostatic hypotension. The frequency and severity of symptoms must be used to monitor therapeutic efficacy.

Management of orthostatic hypotension can be divided into three basic treatment modalities: practical, physiologic, and pharmacologic (Table 2). Although each modality is discussed separately in this review, it is generally necessary to employ a multifaceted approach to successfully treat orthostatic hypotension.

Practical Management

The recommendations described herein are based on a careful consideration of the abnormal blood pressure responses caused by autonomic insufficiency. Many patients become aware of their limitations through unfor-

TABLE 1 Treatment of Autonomic Insufficiency

Autonomic Dysfunction	*Clinical Symptoms*	*Management*
Orthostatic hypotension	Weakness, decreased exercise tolerance, dimming or loss of vision, dizziness, syncope	Practical suggestions, physiologic maneuvers, pharmacologic agents
Neurogenic bladder	Urinary frequency, retention	Urinary acidification
Decreased GI motility	Constipation	Bowel training program; dietary fiber, bulk agent, suppositories
Anhidrosis	Defective temperature regulation	Avoidance of extremes of ambient temperature and dressing too heavily
Decreased lacrimation	Conjunctivitis	Artificial tears
Decreased salivation	Choking	Increased fluid intake, artificial saliva
Abnormal pupillary responses	Blurry vision, diplopia	Eye patch

TABLE 2 Management of Orthostatic Hypotension

Practical suggestions
- Get up slowly
- Avoid prolonged standing
- Eat small meals
- Remain in moderate-temperature setting
- Avoid alcohol
- Establish regular bowel pattern; do not strain excessively
- Use only medications approved by physician

Physiologic methods
- Increase salt and fluid intake
- Reverse Trendelenburg position for sleeping
- Change posture frequently
- Wear compressive garments, if helpful

Pharmacologic approaches
- Volume expansion (fludrocortisone)
- Prostaglandin inhibition (ibuprofen)
- Beta-blockade (propranolol)
- Sympathomimetic
  - Direct (phenylephrine)
  - Indirect (ephedrine)
- Presynaptic receptor inhibitor (yohimbine)
- Postsynaptic receptor agonist (clonidine)
- Decreased norepinephrine catabolism
  - MAO inhibitor (tranylcypromine)
  - Block neuronal uptake (desipramine)
- Ganglionic stimulant (caffeine)
- CNS stimulant (methylphenidate)
- Promotion of norepinephrine synthesis (L-threo-DOPS)
- Venoconstriction (dihydroergotamine)

tunate experiences. A rapid change from lying or sitting to standing is not tolerated well, particularly upon arising in the morning, since an extended time in the supine position promotes pooling of body fluids. Prolonged standing should also be avoided because gravity causes approximately 500 to 700 ml of blood to pool in the lower extremities. A precipitous drop in blood pressure occurs within minutes of eating; patients often feel sleepy and are unable to walk after meals.

Hypotension is even more pronounced following ingestion of alcohol, a potent vasodilator. Heat also causes vasodilatation of skin blood vessels. Since these patients cannot dissipate body heat effectively through sweating, they should wear light clothing and remain in moderate temperature settings. Valsalva's maneuver is attended by hypotension, which is unopposed in patients with lesion(s) of the baroreflex arc. Thus, excessive straining due to bladder and bowel dysfunction can induce a syncopal attack. Urinary acidification with ascorbic acid, or mandelamine, or both, minimizes bladder infection. Neurogenic constipation responds to a bowel training program that includes increased dietary fiber and a bulk agent, such as psyllium. Patients should be advised against using nonprescription drugs without approval of their physician; eye drops and cold remedies may result in a hypertensive crisis.

Physiologic Management

One of the earliest means of treating hypotension was with compressive garments. Various styles, including tailored elastic stockings and abdominal binders, have been applied to reduce venous pooling and thereby increase venous return to the heart. Most patients, especially those with neurologic impairment, find these garments impractical for several reasons (e.g., difficulty in dressing or a neurogenic bladder). In addition, their beneficial effects have not been substantiated.

Several other physiologic approaches are of limited benefit. Increased sodium and fluid intake elevates blood pressure. A reverse Trendelenburg position during sleep helps to decrease the supine hypertension that develops as the disease progresses. Atrial tachypacing can be used to treat orthostatic hypotension, but the results are not always favorable. Constant pacing of the heart at rates sufficient to adequately elevate the standing blood pressure is probably not a safe long-term approach, particularly in elderly patients.

Pharmacologic Management

An extensive array of medications is available to treat orthostatic hypotension; an example from each class of drugs is given in Table 2. Although these drugs may have multiple, complex modes of action, their pressor effect is mediated through at least one of the following mechanisms: either increase in intravascular volume, venous return, cardiac output, or arterial tone; or decrease in circulating vasodilators. Most drugs increase arterial tone by enhancing noradrenergic neurotransmission.

PREFERRED APPROACH

Guidelines for managing orthostatic hypotension should be followed in the design of a treatment program tailored to the clinical presentation of each patient and modified in response to further progression of the illness. The "stepped-care" approach provides the maximum benefit and the fewest side effects. All patients with autonomic dysfunction should follow the practical recommendations discussed in the preceding section. In the early stages of the disorder, the minor adjustments to normal routine dictated by those principles may permit continued function without medication.

Progression of the disease is generally manifested by worsening of the hypotension and development of supine hypertension. The next step in management consists of instituting specific physiologic measures. Dietary sodium and fluid intake should be increased; salt tablets are generally not tolerated well due to gastric irritation. Elevating the head of the bed at night reduces supine hypertension and diminishes nocturnal diuresis, which may play a role in causing the low early morning blood pressure that these patients experience.

Virtually all patients require medication to maintain a functional blood pressure level as the autonomic failure becomes more advanced. Initially, fludrocortisone (0.1 mg daily) may be sufficient; the dose may be increased to 0.4 mg per day. Higher doses do not produce much additional improvement in the blood pressure, but lead to edema and bloating. A high sodium and fluid intake is important for maximal pressor effect from the mineralocorticoid. Potassium supplementation (25 mEq daily) is advisable to prevent hypokalemia. If the patient remains symptomatic on the highest recommended dose of fludrocortisone, it should be gradually discontinued so that a more potent hypertensive drug may be utilized. Ibuprofen (300 mg 3 times per day) should be given about 30 minutes before mealtime; if the pressor response is not sufficient after 3 days, the dose is increased incrementally to a maximum of 600 mg 3 times per day. Indomethacin (up to 50 mg 3 times per day) works equally well in most patients, but gastric irritation makes ibuprofen a better initial choice.

Combination therapy is necessary if neither fludrocortisone nor ibuprofen elevates the blood pressure sufficiently. These two drugs act through different mechanisms to produce an effective therapeutic regimen. In this situation, it is preferable to use ibuprofen alone initially and to increase it to the maximum dose, and then to follow it by a gradual titration with fludrocortisone. This protocol yields the maximum blood pressure improvement with the least medication.

Occasionally patients require additional medication to remain ambulatory. Although propranolol elevates blood pressure in patients with orthostatic hypotension, the improvement is generally not sufficient to allow it to be used alone. However, it can be effectively combined with either or both of the drugs just mentioned to provide additional benefit. The pressor effect is observed only during treatment with low doses (5 to 40 mg 4 times per day); hence, the dose for each patient must be carefully and gradually titrated to avoid the hypotensive effects of beta-blockade. Ephedrine (25 to 50 mg) or vasopressin (nasal spray) can provide a rapid elevation of blood pressure in acute hypotensive situations. However, neither drug should be used as a primary medication for chronic administration in patients with orthostatic hypotension.

Special consideration must be given to the treatment of those patients with autonomic insufficiency which is attended by central neurologic signs (multiple system atrophy, MSA). Antiparkinsonian drugs can improve the rigidity, bradykinesia, and tremor in patients with striatonigral involvement. Anticholinergic drugs provide substantial benefit with relatively few side effects; trihexylphenidyl is gradually increased from an initial dose of 1 mg 3 times per day. Many patients show further improvement and tolerate doses in excess of 12 mg per day. Anticholinergic drugs promote urinary retention; however, these patients regard this side effect as a benefit in view of their urinary frequency. Amantadine (100 mg 3 times per day) can be added to the maximum tolerated dose of trihexylphenidyl to achieve greater improvement. Unfortunately, patients with MSA do not respond as well as do patients with Parkinson's disease, and their response to medications wanes as the disease progresses. Levodopa, dopamine-receptor agonists (e.g., bromocriptine), and carbidopa should be avoided, since MSA patients are sensitive to the hypotensive side effects of these medications. There is no effective therapy for patients with cerebellar dysfunction.

MANAGING AUTONOMIC INSUFFICIENCY

No specific treatment is currently available for the underlying disease that causes autonomic insufficiency. Therapy is directed towards both symptomatic improvement and prevention of secondary complications due to autonomic dysfunction. Initiation and modification of treatment are guided by the clinical status of each patient and tempered by the risks and side effects of the therapeutic endeavors. As in most clinical therapeutic situations, the risk:benefit ratio must be considered. Treatment of orthostatic hypotension accompanied by supine hypertension presents a significant therapeutic dilemma, since no pressor drug affects only the standing blood pressure. As a guideline, a standing blood pressure in excess of 90 to 100/60 to 70 mm Hg with a supine blood pressure less than 160/100 mm Hg allows the patient to remain asymptomatic. Supine hypertension, a consequence of autonomic dysfunction, may be exacerbated by pressor therapy and prohibit further elevation of the standing blood pressure. Fortunately, it is sometimes possible to increase the standing blood pressure out of proportion to the supine blood pressure; in this way substantial improvement in function can be attained. Occasionally patients must sleep in a semireclining or even sitting position so that sufficient medication can be given to elevate their standing blood pressure. These compromises should be made only if there is significant benefit to patients, that is, if their functional level is improved. There is little advantage to a high standing blood pressure achieved at the risk of severe supine hypertension in those patients whose neurologic symptoms prevent them from ambulating. However, it may be necessary to increase blood pressure sufficiently to prevent syncope in other situations, such as during meals or bowel movements. More development and testing of a sympathetic neural prosthesis may resolve this dilemma; this device administers a short-acting medication only when the blood pressure falls below a preset limit.

Autonomic dysfunction causes increased sensitivity to certain side effects of many drugs. Without potassium supplementation, fludrocortisone-induced hypokalemia eventually develops as body stores of potassium become depleted. Delayed gastric emptying and elevated basal cortisol levels potentiate gastric irritation by drugs. However, ulcers are uncommon, perhaps because many of the patients are achlorhydric. Vasoconstrictor drugs cause mesenteric arterial insufficiency that can lead to bowel infarction. It is impossible to reproduce pharmacologically the dynamic sympathetic-parasympathetic balance necessary for normal bladder function; excessive stimulation of either aspect of autonomic control can lead to either painful incontinence or urinary retention. Supine hypertension may be exacerbated by therapeutic pressor agents and may also be a side effect of other medications with sympathomimetic or vasoconstrictor activity. However, there does not appear to be an increased incidence of stroke, cerebral hemorrhage, coronary insufficiency, or renal dysfunction. This is probably because blood pressure is not constantly elevated in patients with orthostatic hypotension.

Anesthetic management of patients with autonomic dysfunction poses problems that must be carefully considered prior to surgery. The fluid balance and position of the patient contribute significantly to the basal blood pressure level. In addition to the wide blood pressure swings obtained during positive pressure ventilation, these patients have exaggerated responses to pressor and hypotensive agents. Their pupillary responses cannot be used to assess the degree of anesthesia. Respiratory control may be altered in patients with central nervous system involvement. Vagal dysfunction affects the response to atropine. In the postoperative period, temperature control may be abnormal due to defective sweating, and patients may have a pronounced sensitivity to the hypotensive and respiratory suppressant effects of analgesic medications. It is best to avoid surgery, if possible. When it is essential, the choice of anesthetic is less critical than awareness, by both anesthesiologist and surgeon, of the implications of autonomic dysfunction, so that careful monitoring may prevent inappropriate and dangerous treatment.

HYPERTENSION AND RENAL DISEASES

HYPERNATREMIA IN THE ADULT

NEAL A. SNYDER, M.D.
ALLEN I. ARIEFF, M.D.

Hypernatremia is a common clinical problem with a mortality rate in excess of 60 percent in patients with serum sodium greater than 160 mEq per liter that is sustained for 48 hours or more. Reports of prevalance range from 0.5 to 2 percent, depending on the population of the institution studied.

Hypernatremia in adults usually occurs in the context of severe concomitant systemic disease, which makes precise attribution of symptoms, morbidity, and mortality difficult. However, there is little doubt that hypernatremia per se has a substantial morbidity and mortality.

Most of the damage is thought to occur in the central nervous system. In acute hypernatremia, as fluid from the intracellular space moves into the extracellular compartment to establish osmotic equilibrium, the cells initially lose volume. In the brain, this loss of volume may put mechanical traction on delicate cerebral vessels, thereby producing vascular damage (e.g., dural sinus tears). Although cerebral edema has been noted in some patients, it is more likely to be the result of overly rapid rehydration therapy than caused by hypernatremia. Findings of hemorrhage and congested cerebral vessels have also been observed in chronic hypernatremia. Animal studies in acute hypernatremia have documented an abrupt decrease in brain water and a rise in intracellular Na^+ and $C1^-$ concentration; brain osmolality increases because of concomitant loss of water and gain in solute. In chronically hypernatremic animals, brain osmolality is also elevated, but most of the increase is caused by a gain in brain solute; brain water content is similar to normal values whereas brain osmolality content is greater than control levels, mostly on account of ''idiogenic osmoles.'' This poorly characterized solute, which begins to appear after several hours of hypernatremia, is a unique adaptive mechanism that apparently serves to defend cellular volume in order to prevent abrupt shrinkage of the brain, which could lead to tearing of cerebral vessels and meninges as previously described.

CAUSES OF HYPERNATREMIA

Although there is recent evidence that some alert elderly patients may have impaired thirst, adult hypernatremia is most often associated with either depressed sensorium or the physical inability of the patient to respond to thirst and obtain water. For example, despite enormous water losses as sustained by patients with diabetes insipidus, if these individuals are able to drink freely, they maintain a normal serum sodium until they are somehow denied free access to water (or until their thirst mechanism is no longer operative). Patients with stroke, dementing illnesses, or immobility are particularly vulnerable to dehydration, as are patients with delirium. Delirium is usually associated with infection and increased insensible water loss, but may also be associated with toxic metabolic derangements.

Much adult hypernatremia is related to hospitalization or medical intervention. For example, patients given nutritional supplementation in the form of hypertonic enteral feeding can develop osmotic diarrhea or glycosuria from a large carbohydrate load, which leads to consequent dehydration. Patients on total parenteral nutrition may become hyperglycemic and glycosuric, or simply receive inadequate free water. Patients receiving intravenous solute may become hypernatremic from administration of sodium bicarbonate (for treatment of cardiac arrest, metabolic acidosis, or barbiturate overdose); administration of NaC1 (for isotonic replacement of hypotonic loss from diarrhea or ''third spacing'' of fluid in abdominal surgery); or administration of mannitol or radiologic contrast material (agents that induce an osmotic diuresis). Hypernatremia that results from diarrhea induced by lactulose or sorbital (with kayexalate), excessive water removal with dialysis, and restricted fluid intake prior to various procedures have all been described. Other causes are listed in Table 1. Adult hypernatremia is most fre-

TABLE 1 Hypernatremia in Adults

- Infirmity - Unable to Get Water
  - Stroke
  - Dementia
  - Immobility
  - Delirium
- Febrile Illness
- Nutritional Supplementation
  - Tube feeding
  - Hyperalimentation
  - Increased oral NaC1 intake
- Diabetes Mellitus
- Diarrhea
  - Lack of adequate replacement of free water
  - Sorbitol with kayexelate
  - Lactulose for therapy of hepatic encephalopathy
- Intravenous Administration of Solute
  - Sodium
    - NaHCO3
      - Cardiac arrest
      - Metabolic acidosis
      - Drug overdosage (to alkalinize urine)
    - NaC1
  - Mannitol
  - Radiologic contrast material

- Gastrointestinal Bleeding
- Dialysis Related
  - Hemodialysis
  - Peritoneal dialysis
- Increased Insensible Water Loss
  - Mechanical ventilation
  - Hyperventilation
  - Febrile illness
  - Increased ambient temperature
- Diabetes Insipidus
  - Central
  - Renal
    - Alcohol
    - Hypercalcemia
    - Postobstructive diuresis
- Mineralocorticoid Excess
- Impaired Thirst
  - Cerebral vascular disease
  - Cerebral tumors
  - Essential hypernatremia

quently attributable to a chronic process of several days rather than an acute one of several hours or less.

WATER DEFICIT ASSESSMENT

Symptoms and physical signs are unreliable for either diagnosing hypernatremic states or for assessing the severity of fluid deficits. As mentioned previously, the presence of grave underlying medical conditions usually obscures what might represent a "pure presentation of" hypernatremia. The sensation of thirst may not be verbalized because affected patients frequently have depression of sensorium. The physical signs commonly associated with dehydration, such as altered skin turgor and sunken eyes, may not be apparent because of age-related changes—most hypernatremia occurs in older adults. Additionally, there is a 20 to 30 percent prevalence of orthostatic blood pressure changes in the elderly even in the absence of dehydration or volume depletion. Clinical manifestations of hypernatremia described in animal studies and in children with gastroenteritis or salt ingestion usually involve symptoms referable to the central nervous system. There is often depression of sensorium that ranges from lethargy to coma, and although normal muscle tone is the rule, increased muscle tone, myoclonic twitches, and frank seizure activity have been described. Seizures are not commonly observed in patients with chronic hypernatremia, but after therapy is begun, up to 40 percent may exhibit seizure activity.

Hypernatremia is a laboratory diagnosis. Most texts list the range of normal serum sodium as 136 to 145 mEq per liter. We have observed a tendency for clinicians not to view hypernatremia as a significant problem until the serum Na is in excess of 150 mEq per liter. Serum sodium concentrations in excess of 145 mEq per liter often reflect significant medical illness and should be investigated.

The calculation of a patient's water deficit is based on the assumption that sodium is, in fact, distributed throughout total body water (TBW). By assuming that no sodium has been lost in achieving the hypernatremic state, one can roughly estimate the amount of water needed to correct the patient's dehydration by using the following formula: Deficit = TBW (measured Na - 140/140). It is a common error to assume that all people have a total body water that is 60 percent of body weight. Total body water is influenced by age, sex, height, weight, and the amount of body fat. Thus, an 18-year-old male may have a water content of 60 percent of body weight, and a young woman may have a water content of 55 percent; a 70-year-old-man would more likely have a water content of 51 percent, and an elderly woman would have closer to a 43 percent water content. For the calculation, body weight is the patient's weight at the time of the evaluation.

These calculations assume that serum sodium reflects osmolality. However, spuriously low values of serum sodium may be obtained in the presence of hyperlipidemia and more rarely with hyperproteinemia because the percentage of plasma water, which contains all of the sodium in serum, in an aliquot of serum is decreased. Additionally, if there are large quantities of other osmotically active substances such as urea, glucose, ethanol, methanol, mannitol, or drugs, the serum sodium determination may be accurate and yet not reflect the hyperosmolar state. In particular, since urea, ethanol, and methanol freely cross cell membranes, they do not exert an osmotic force and therefore do not cause water movement into or out of cells; hyperosmolality from these solutes in the absence of free water loss does not represent a dehydrated state. Glucose and mannitol not only do not enter cells, they in fact dehydrate them; the result is a dilutional decrement of serum Na^+. Thus, hyperosmolality may be present although there is a low serum Na^+.

THERAPY

There is a paucity of hard data available as to how hypernatremia should be treated. Hypernatremia is potentially lethal; however, overly rapid treatment of hypernatremia by infusion of hypotonic solution can cause seizures and cerebral edema, which may also be lethal.

On the basis of our present knowledge, recommendations for treatment of chronic hypernatremia, in adults, when the hyponatremia is primarily owing to water loss are, as follows:

1. If there is evidence of circulatory collapse, the patient should receive initial resuscitation with crystalloid or colloid, such as plasma or a plasma substitute, rapidly enough to correct shock and stabilize the circulatory system.
2. Severe acidosis should be treated; however, moderate acidosis (pH above 7.15) should not be corrected immediately. An arterial pH above 7.15 does not appear to depress cardiac output, and the rapid administration of sodium bicarbonate aggravates the hypernatremia.
3. Fluid deficit should be estimated and replaced over a 48-hour period so as to achieve a decrement in serum osmolality of approximately 2 mOsm per liter per hour. Maintenance fluids, which include replacement of urinary losses, are given in addition to replacement of the deficit.
4. Hypotonic fluid should be administered. In adults, there are few data that would lead to favoring one fluid over another.
5. Plasma electrolytes should be monitored at frequent intervals, usually about every 4 hours.
6. If the hypernatremia is secondary to excessive loss of other body fluids, the replacement fluid should be similar to the fluid actually lost.
7. Many patients appear to die of their underlying illnesses rather than of hypernatremia per se. Vigorous attention should be given to the therapy of associated medical conditions in order to reduce morbidity and mortality from hypernatremia as well.

HYPONATREMIA

BURTON D. ROSE, M.D.

Hyponatremia is one of the most common electrolyte disturbances. Nevertheless, several therapeutic issues concerning the method by which the plasma sodium level is raised and the optimal rate at which this should occur remain unresolved. These problems can best be understood by considering separately the management of each of the most common causes of hyponatremia (Table 1). In this regard it is important to understand that hyponatremia represents *a disorder of water, not sodium balance*. In almost all patients, the reduction in plasma sodium level results from a defect in renal water excretion, which allows ingested water to be retained.

SYMPTOMATIC HYPONATREMIA

Hyponatremia can produce a variety of neurologic symptoms, ranging from nausea and malaise to seizures and coma to irreversible neurologic damage and death. The severity of these changes is related to the degree of hyponatremia and more importantly to the *rate of reduction in the plasma sodium level*. This time-dependence is a reflection of the response of the brain to a fall in the plasma osmolality. Acutely, water moves into the brain down an osmotic gradient, leading to cerebral edema and potentially life-threatening symptoms. Within 24 to 48 hours, however, the brain volume returns toward normal because of the loss of osmoles (such as sodium, potassium, and amino acids) from the cells and/or binding of these solutes to intracellular proteins, making them osmotically inactive. The net result is that chronic hyponatremia, unless very severe, is generally well tolerated.

Patients with symptoms or a plasma sodium concentration below 110 to 115 mEq per liter represent a medical emergency. Although the hyponatremia must be corrected, the optimal rate at which this should be achieved is unresolved. It has been suggested that central pontine myelinolysis (a rare disorder characterized by paraparesis or quadriparesis, dysarthria, and dysphagia)

TABLE 1 Treatment of the Major Causes of Hyponatremia

Disorder	*Treatment*
SIADH	Water restriction Hypertonic saline (or oral salt), usually with a loop diuretic Rarely, demeclocyline, lithium, or urea
True volume depletion	Isotonic or, if severe, hypertonic saline
Edematous states	Water restriction Loop diuretic plus converting enzyme inhibitor in CHF If severe, loop diuretic plus saline, or dialysis
Primary polydipsia	Water restriction
Pseudohyponatremia	No therapy required for hyponatremia

may by induced by the overly rapid correction of hyponatremia. In humans, however, it seems likely that persistent severe hyponatremia represents the greater danger; neurologic deterioration with therapy is unusual unless there is overcorrection with the plasma sodium level being rapidly raised above 135 to 140 mEq per liter.

A reasonable compromise is to raise the plasma sodium concentration initially at a maximum rate of 2 mEq per liter per hour. Once the plasma sodium level reaches 120 to 125 mEq per liter, the patient should be out of danger and further correction of the hyponatremia can proceed slowly over 48 hours. How these goals can be achieved varies with the underlying disorder.

SYNDROME OF INAPPROPRIATE ANTIDIURETIC HORMONE SECRETION

Treatment of the syndrome of inappropriate antidiuretic hormone secretion (SIADH) varies with the severity of both the hyponatremia and the increase in urine osmolality. Asymptomatic patients with mild to moderate reductions in plasma sodium usually respond to a high-sodium diet and restricted water intake. Therapy is more complicated in symptomatic patients. In this setting, it is important to appreciate that sodium handling is normal even though there is a defect in water excretion. With this in mind, we can evaluate the effects of administering sodium in an attempt to correct the hyponatremia.

Suppose a woman with SIADH presents with lethargy and the following laboratory values: plasma sodium, 110 mEq per liter; urine osmolality, 616 mosm per kilogram of water. It is often stated that isotonic saline alone will produce only a transient rise in the plasma sodium level in this disorder. The reason for this can be illustrated by considering the steady-state effect of giving 1 L of this solution, which contains 1,000 ml of water and 308 mosm of solute (154 mEq each of sodium and chloride). The plasma sodium level will initially rise because of the higher sodium concentration in the administered fluid. With time, however, a different result is seen because the patient is euvolemic and sodium handling is normal (Table 2). Therefore, all of the salt will be excreted, but since the urine osmolity is relatively fixed at 616 mosm per kilogram, the urine volume will be only 500 ml (308 mosm in 500 ml equals 616 mosm per kilogram). The net effect is water retention (500 ml for each liter given) and a further reduction in plasma sodium.

To correct the hyponatremia with sodium, *the osmolality of the administered fluid must exceed that in the urine*. Since the urine osmolality is usually greater than 300 mosm per kilogram in patients with SIADH, there is essentially no role for the use of isotonic saline in this disorder. Even hypertonic (3 percent) saline may not be beneficial in this setting, as can be appreciated by using calculations similar to those in Table 2. Three percent saline contains 1,026 mosm of sodium chloride per liter. In the steady state, this solute will be excreted in approximately 1,670 ml of water (1,026 mosm in 1,670 ml equals 616 mosm per kilogram). The net loss of 670 ml of water will raise the plasma sodium level by only 2 to 3 mEq per liter.

TABLE 2 Effect of Isotonic Saline in a Patient with SIADH and a Urine Osmolality of 616 mOsm per Kilogram

	NaCl(mOsm)	*Water (ml)*
In	308	1,000
Out	308	500
Net	0	+500

The relative ineffectiveness of hypertonic saline in this patient is caused by the high urine osmolality. A much greater elevation in the plasma sodium level can be achieved if the urine osmolality is lowered by the administration of a loop diuretic, which impairs the establishment of medullary hypertonicity (and therefore urinary concentrating ability) by inhibiting sodium chloride reabsorption in the thick ascending limb of the loop of Henle. If, for example, 40 mg of furosemide lowers the urine osmolality to 300 mosm per kilogram in this patient, the 1,026 mosm of salt will now be excreted in 3,400 ml of water (1,026 mosm in 3,400 ml equals 300 mosm per kilogram). The associated loss of 2,400 ml of water can raise the plasma sodium level by about 10 mEq per liter.

Although frequently beneficial, a loop diuretic is not required if the urine osmolality is already near that of the plasma. In this setting, 3 percent saline alone will rapidly raise the plasma sodium level and a loop diuretic should be used only if there is some concern about possible fluid overload. In contrast, a *thiazide diuretic should never be given to a hyponatremic patient*. These drugs act in the cortex in the distal tubule; they do not impair urinary concentrating ability and therefore can further lower the plasma sodium level, since more sodium and potassium are lost in the urine, but water continues to be retained in the collecting tubules.

Sodium Deficit

The amount of sodium that should be given as hypertonic saline in patients with SIADH can be estimated by calculating the sodium deficit:

$$\text{Sodium deficit} = \text{Volume of distribution of } P_{Na} \times P_{Na} \text{ deficit per liter}$$

Although sodium itself is restricted to the extracellular fluid, changes in the plasma sodium concentration (P_{Na}) reflect changes in osmolality and therefore are distributed through the total body water (roughly 60 and 50 percent of lean body weight in men and women, respectively). Thus, if the woman under discussion weighed 50 kg, the quantity of sodium required to raise the plasma sodium level from 110 to the relatively safe level of 120 mEq per liter would be approximately 250 mEq:

$$\text{Sodium deficit} = 0.5 \times 50 \times (120 - 110) = 250 \text{ mEq}$$

This amount of sodium is contained in about 500 ml of

3 percent saline. It can be given over 5 hours (100 ml per hour) to raise the plasma sodium level at a rate of 2 mEq per liter per hour. Urinary sodium losses can be ignored in this calculation, since the urine is relatively isosmotic to plasma in the presence of a loop diuretic; these isosmotic losses will not affect the plasma osmolality or the plasma sodium.

Two points about the equation for calculating the sodium deficit deserve emphasis. First, it is only an estimate, and serial measurements of the plasma sodium concentration are necessary to assess the efficacy of treatment. Second, this formula, which can also be used in hypovolemic hyponatremic patients, estimates the amount of sodium required to return the plasma sodium to a desired value. It does not include any isosmotic losses which might also be present and which must be replaced to restore euvolemia.

In addition to the sodium deficit, therapy in patients with SIADH can also be approached by calculating the water excess, i.e., the amount of water that had to be retained to lower the plasma sodium to the current level:

$$\text{Water excess} = \text{Total body water} \times (1 - P_{Na}/140)$$

This formula, however, is of little use in treating SIADH since water excess is responsible for the fall in the plasma sodium concentration only in the initial stages. The ensuing volume expansion causes the appropriate excretion of sodium and water in the urine. The net effect is that both water retention and sodium loss contribute to the hyponatremia. The major setting in which water retention *alone* causes hyponatremia is in patients with oliguric renal failure.

Chronic SIADH

Similar considerations apply to chronic treatment of SIADH, as might be necessary in a patient with an oat cell carcinoma of the lung. Water restriction should be tried initially. This modality may be inadequate, however, if the urine osmolality is very high or if there is poor patient compliance. In this setting, treatment should be aimed at lowering the urine osmolality or at increasing the urine output by enhancing solute excretion. The former can be achieved by the administration of a loop diuretic (such as 40 to 80 mg of furosemide in divided doses) combined with salt supplementation to prevent hypovolemia. Two other drugs may also be effective by directly interfering with the effect of ADH on the collecting tubules: demeclocycline (300 to 600 mg twice a day) or lithium. In general, demeclocycline is preferred except in children, in whom this tetracycline derivative can interfere with bone development.

An infrequently used alternative to these drugs is the administration of 30 to 60 g of urea per day. In a patient in whom the urine osmolality is relatively fixed, the *urine output is determined by the rate of solute excretion.* If, as in the woman described, the urine osmolality is approximately 600 mosm per kilogram, the urine output will be 1,000 ml if 600 mosm of solute (primarily sodium and potassium salts and urea) is excreted. The urine output can be enhanced in this setting by increasing solute excretion by the administration of urea. Such treatment might be particularly useful if urea excretion is relatively low due to inadequate protein intake.

TRUE VOLUME DEPLETION

True volume depletion, usually due to gastrointestinal or renal losses, can lead to hyponatremia which is generally treated with isotonic saline or oral sodium chloride. In contrast to SIADH, both the sodium and water will be retained in hypovolemia. This fluid raises the plasma sodium level primarily by causing volume expansion, which inhibits the release of ADH, thereby allowing the excess water to be excreted. The direct effect of the exogenous saline on the plasma sodium is relatively small, as can be appreciated from a few simple calculations. Suppose that a 70-kg man has an acute episode of diarrhea associated with a fall in the plasma sodium concentration to 120 mEq per liter. At this time, his total body water (the space of distribution of the plasma sodium) is approximately 42 L (0.6 × body weight) and the total number of effective osmoles, excluding accompanying anions, is roughly 5,040 mosm (total body water × plasma sodium). If 1 L of isotonic saline is given and retained, the total body water will now be 43 L and the total effective osmoles will increase to 5,194 (5,040 plus the 154 mEq of sodium in the saline). As a result, the new plasma sodium level will rise to only 121 mEq per liter (5,194/43). Thus, the rate of rise in the plasma sodium after the administration of isotonic saline to a hyponatremic hypovolemic patient is initially slow and then more rapid once ADH secretion is shut off and the excess water is excreted.

The adequacy of volume repletion can be determined by monitoring the skin turgor, central venous pressure, and urine sodium concentration. If the initial urine sodium concentration is 2 mEq per liter, but increases to only 7 mEq per liter after the administration of 2 L of isotonic saline, then hypovolemia persists and further replacement therapy is indicated. A urine sodium level greater than 30 to 40 mEq per liter usually indicates that normovolemia has been achieved.

These considerations must be adjusted in patients with severe or symptomatic hyponatremia. Hypertonic saline should be given initially in this situation, with the quantity and the rate of administration being determined by calculating the sodium deficit as described above.

Correction of potassium depletion, if present, may be another important component of therapy. The administration of potassium will raise the plasma osmolality. As most of this potassium enters the cells to replete cellular stores, sodium (and hydrogen) leave the cells to maintain electroneutrality, thereby increasing the plasma sodium level toward normal.

EDEMATOUS STATES

Therapy is different in hyponatremic edematous patients, in whom exogenous sodium is not desirable because the extracellular volume is already expanded. As a result, treatment is aimed at removing the excess water, beginning with the restriction of water intake.

An attempt to increase the effective circulating volume (which can improve renal perfusion and decrease ADH release) should also be undertaken. In patients with congestive heart failure, for example, the cardiac output, renal blood flow, and glomerular filtration rate can be enhanced by the administration of captopril, a converting enzyme inhibitor that reduces the formation of the vasoconstrictor angiotensin II. Despite these beneficial hemodynamic actions, captopril may not raise the plasma sodium concentration when given alone, but may be very effective when combined with a loop diuretic. This synergism may result from two factors, both of which enhance urinary water excretion: captopril increases the delivery of sodium and water out of the proximal tubule, since the inhibition of angiotensin II formation may raise the glomerular filtration rate and lower proximal reabsorption; and the loop diuretic decreases water reabsorption in the medullary collecting tubule by impairing the creation of the medullary interstitial gradient.

Increasing the effective circulating volume is more difficult in the presence of severe hepatic cirrhosis. Insertion of a peritoneovenous shunt will usually be beneficial, but this procedure is generally restricted to patients with the hepatorenal syndrome or massive ascites refractory to diuretic therapy.

Demeclocycline has also been given to hyponatremic patients with cardiac or hepatic disease. Although it is frequently effective in these disorders, its use has been limited by a relatively high incidence of nephrotoxicity. This complication apparently results from elevated drug levels due to reduced hepatic metabolism.

Severe or symptomatic hyponatremia is unusual in these disorders. When it occurs, treatment with hypertonic saline alone will increase the edema, potentially inducing pulmonary edema in patients with congestive heart failure. A safer alternative is to administer a loop diuretic and to replace the urinary sodium losses (as measured from the urine sodium concentration and urine volume) with hypertonic saline. The net effect is water loss and an elevation in the plasma sodium concentration. Peritoneal dialysis or hemodialysis can also be used, if necessary.

PRIMARY POLYDIPSIA

Water excretion is normal in most patients with primary polydipsia. The most common complaints are polyuria and polydipsia; hyponatremia occurs only when the quantity of water taken in (occasionally exceeding 10 L per day) is greater than excretory capacity. In contrast to SIADH or volume depletion, the urine osmolality in primary polydipsia should be below 100 mosm per kilogram, since ADH release is appropriately suppressed. Treatment of hyponatremia in this setting is relatively simple: decreasing water intake allows the excess water to be rapidly excreted in the urine.

PSEUDOHYPONATREMIA

Pseudohyponatremia refers to disorders in which the plasma sodium concentration is reduced but the plasma osmolality is normal or increased. This problem is most often seen with hyperglycemia, but also may occur after the administration of mannitol or glycine solutions or in the presence of marked hyperlipidemia or hyperproteinemia. No therapy is required for the hyponatremia, since the plasma osmolality is not reduced and therefore the patient is not at risk for developing cerebral edema.

HYPERKALEMIA

IRA KURTZ, M.D. F.R.C.P.(C)
LEON G. FINE, M.B., Ch.B., F.R.C.P., F.A.C.P.,

POTASSIUM DISTRIBUTION

In a normal 70-kg adult there are approximately 3,500 mEq of potassium or approximately 50 mEq per kilogram of body weight. Most of the total body potassium is located intracellularly, with only 65 mEq being distributed in the extracellular fluid compartment. The intracellular concentration of potassium is about 150 mEq per liter, while in the extracellular fluid it is only 3.5 to 5 mEq per liter (the normal range depends on whether serum or plasma is measured). In addition to the extracellular–intracellular compartmentalization of potassium, there is a dynamic turnover of potassium owing to the intake and output of potassium from the extracellular compartment. In a normal adult ingesting approximately 100 mEq of potassium daily, 10 mEq are lost in the stool while 90 mEq are absorbed by the gastrointestinal tract and enter the extracellular compartment. The kidney is responsible for maintaining the constancy of total body potassium by excreting the 90 mEq of potassium which enter the extracellular compartment daily. The plasma potassium concentration is held constant by both renal and extrarenal mechanisms.

Hyperkalemia is caused by either a shift of potassium from the intracellular to the extracellular compartment or a decrease in the renal excretion of potassium. The most common causes of hyperkalemia are listed in Table 1.

TABLE 1 Etiology of Hyperkalemia

Pseudohyperkalemia
- In vitro: Hemolysis, thrombocytosis, leukocytosis
- In vivo: Tourniquet + fast exercise

Redistribution
- Acute acidemia
- Hemolysis
- Rhabdomyolysis
- Catabolic state
- Insulinopenia
- Hyperglycemia
- Hyperosmolarity
- Hypoaldosteronism
- Exercise
- Beta-adrenergic blockade
- Periodic paralysis
- Digitalis
- Succinylcholine
- Arginine hydrochloride

Impaired renal potassium excretion
- Renal failure: acute, chronic
- Impaired distal tubular flow rate
- Hypoaldosteronism, pseudohypoaldosteronism–types I and II
- Potassium secretory defect
- Spironolactone, triamterene, amiloride, digitalis

Increased intake

PSEUDOHYPERKALEMIA

When whole blood clots, potassium is released from red blood cells, white blood cells, and platelets. The normal plasma potassium level is therefore less than the normal serum level. Abnormal red cell membrane fragility, or an increase in white blood cell number or platelet number can all lead to excess release of potassium when blood clots. This effect is not seen if plasma potassium is measured concurrently. Therefore, if a large discrepancy exists between the serum and plasma levels (greater than 0.3 mEq per liter), pseudohyperkalemia should be suspected.

REDISTRIBUTION OF POTASSIUM BETWEEN INTRACELLULAR AND EXTRACELLULAR COMPARTMENTS

Acid-Base Status

An acute lowering of luminal pH in the cortical collecting tubule causes an inhibition of potassium secretion. On the other hand, chronic acidemia causes an inhibition of proximal salt and water reabsorption, thereby increasing the distal delivery of sodium and water, which increases distal potassium secretion. Therefore, acute and chronic acidemia appear to have opposing effects on renal potassium secretion. In addition, acidemia causes potassium to shift from the intracellular to extracellular space. Until recently, it has been accepted as clinical dogma that the potassium concentration changes by 0.5 to 0.6 mEq per liter for every 0.1 unit change in the opposite direction of blood pH. More recent data have suggested that the relationship between blood pH and plasma potassium is not straightforward and depends on a number of factors, such as (1) mineral versus organic acidosis, (2) respiratory versus metabolic acidosis, (3) bicarbonate concentration, and (4) duration of acid-base disturbance.

Mineral versus Organic Acidosis

Results of administration of hydrochloric acid to humans, and studies using in vitro preparations suggest that hydrochloric acid causes a greater increase in plasma potassium concentration than lactic acid or beta-hydroxybutyric acid. Since the cell membrane is less permeable to chloride than the above mentioned organic acid anions, in order to maintain electroneutrality, potassium leaves the cell as protons enter. This occurs to a lesser extent during lactic or ketoacidosis, in which the accompanying organic anions enter the cell along with a proton. The situation is further complicated by the associated abnormalities found in patients with ketoacidosis, such as osmotic diuresis, volume depletion, secondary hyperaldosteronism, insulin lack, decreased dietary intake, and renal insufficiency, all of which can independently alter the plasma potassium level by renal or extrarenal mechanisms.

Respiratory versus Metabolic Acidosis

Respiratory acidosis causes little increase in the plasma potassium concentration compared with similar degrees of metabolic acidosis. The reason for this finding is unclear.

Bicarbonate Concentration

It has been reported that when mineral acid is infused to lower the bicarbonate concentration, and blood pH is maintained constant by lowering the blood P_{CO_2}, the plasma potassium level rises. The results of these studies suggest that changes in the bicarbonate concentration per se affect the plasma potassium concentration. However, these findings have not been confirmed by all investigators.

Duration of Acid-Base Disturbance

As the duration of metabolic acidosis increases, the intracellular buffering capacity rises. As more protons move into cells to maintain blood pH, more potassium tends to leave the intracellular compartment, with the result that hyperkalemia is more severe during chronic acidemia.

Increased K^+ Influx into the Extracellular Fluid Compartment

K^+ may enter the extracellular fluid compartment from intracellular sources, i.e., rhabdomyolysis, gastrointestinal hemorrhage, and catabolic states, or from exogenous sources, such as diet or medications. It is unusual for the plasma potassium to be chronically elevated in these situations unless there is an associated decrease in the renal excretion of potassium or decreased cellular uptake of the potassium load. Normally, renal and extrarenal homeostatic mechanisms prevent the rise in plasma potassium from occurring.

There are certain circumstances under which the rise in plasma potassium is exaggerated:

Hormonal

Insulin lack, aldosterone deficiency and beta-adrenergic blockade all result in decreased potassium tolerance. All three hormonal systems appear to mediate cellular potassium uptake. Marked, sustained hyperkalemia will be present only if renal excretory mechanisms are concomitantly impaired.

Hyperkalemic Periodic Paralysis

Patients with this autosomal dominant disorder present with intermittent attacks of acute paralysis and hyperkalemia. Exercise, potassium loads, and cold can precipitate the attack. The cause of the disorder is unknown, but it appears to result from an abnormal distribution of intracellular and extracellular potassium. Recurrences are prevented prophylactically with a high carbohydrate diet, salbutamol, thiazides, and acetazolamide.

Tissue Breakdown

Release of intracellular potassium occurs in patients with tumor lysis, burns, and crush injuries. Normally the kidney would be able to excrete the increased potassium load. However, as renal failure is frequently present, marked hyperkalemia may result.

IMPAIRED RENAL POTASSIUM EXCRETION

Delivery of Fluid to the Distal Nephron

Recent microperfusion studies of the rat distal tubule have demonstrated that tubular flow rate independent of the luminal Na^+ concentration can alter distal potassium secretion. Patients with disorders causing a decrease in distal flow, such as congestive heart failure or volume depletion, can become hyperkalemic because of a decrease in distal potassium secretion in addition to decreased filtration of potassium by the glomerulus. A urinary sodium concentration of less than 20 mEq per liter and a decreased ability to excrete free water are seen clinically in these patients.

Renal Insufficiency

Patients with chronic renal failure are not hyperkalemic unless the glomerular filtration rate is less than 15 ml per minute. As nephrons are lost, there is a homeostatic increase in potassium excreted by the remaining nephrons. However, acute renal failure is commonly associated with hyperkalemia for several reasons: (1) a decreased glomerular filtration rate, (2) decreased distal flow rate, (3) direct damage to distal tubule in acute tubular necrosis, (4) the rapidity of the renal failure, which frequently precludes homeostatic mechanisms from developing, and (5) the increased release of potassium into the extracellular fluid which frequently occurs when patients with acute renal failure are catabolic.

Aldosterone Deficiency

Aldosterone stimulates potassium secretion by the cortical collecting tubule and enhances potassium uptake into cells. In the presence of a normal volume status, aldosterone deficiency results in only mild hyperkalemia, since adequate distal tubular flow maintains distal nephron potassium secretion and potassium balance.

Adrenal Enzymatic Defects

The most common enzyme defect in the aldosterone synthetic pathway is 21-hydroxylase deficiency. Patients with this disorder present in childhood with hyperkalemia, salt wasting, failure to thrive, and virilization. Both glucocorticoid and mineralocorticoid synthetic pathways are impaired.

Defects in the final two enzymatic steps in aldosterone biosynthesis have recently been described. In these disorders glucocorticoid synthesis is unimpaired.

Hyporeninemic Hypoaldosteronism. Hyporeninemia is the most common cause of hypoaldosteronism. Although the cause and pathogenesis of the syndrome are quite varied and beyond the scope of this discussion, the clinical presentation is typical. The mean age of most patients is 65 years. Patients are usually asymptomatic at presentation. Half of them have a hyperchloremic metabolic acidosis. Salt wasting is rarely present. Most patients have renal insufficiency, which is caused most commonly by diabetic glomerulosclerosis. The syndrome has also been described in patients with sickle cell disease and obstructive uropathy. Hypertension is found in more than 50 percent of the patients.

The cause of the hypoaldosteronism in these patients is probably multifactorial. All patients have a subnormal increase in plasma aldosterone concentration following volume depletion. Whether this is attributable to a primary defect in adrenal aldosterone synthesis or secretion, or is secondary to adrenal atrophy as a result of prolonged hyporeninemia, is unclear. Interestingly, hyporeninemia is present in most, but not all patients (18 to 21 percent) with this syndrome. Hyporeninemia has been attributed to decreased conversion of big renin to renin, decreased circulating catecholamine levels or autonomic neuropathy, decreased prostaglandin levels, extracellular fluid expansion, and glomerular hyperfiltration.

Potassium Secretory Defect. Some patients with hyperkalemia have normal or elevated renin and aldosterone levels and fail to respond to mineralocorticoid therapy. These patients do not develop a normal kaluresis in response to sodium sulfate, furosemide, or potassium chloride. In addition, some patients appear to have hypoaldosteronism. Clinical examples of this disorder are sickle cell trait and disease, systemic lupus erythematosus, obstructive uropathy, and renal transplantation.

Pseudohypoaldosteronism Types I and II. Pseudohypoaldosteronism type I is characterized by volume depletion, hyperkalemia, salt wasting, hyperchloremic metabolic acidosis, and failure to thrive. Most patients present in infancy. Plasma and aldosterone levels are elevated, and treatment with mineralocorticoids is not effective. The syndrome appears to diminish spontaneously in severity at about 2 years of age. In adults the syndrome is usually associated with tubulointerstitial disease.

Type II pseudohypoaldosteronism is characterized by hyperkalemia, hypertension, hyperchloremic metabolic acidosis, hypoaldosteronism, and hyporeninemia. Mineralocorticoid treatment fails to increase urinary potassium excretion normally, yet increased renal sodium reabsorption is observed in response to mineralocorticoids. Because potassium excretion increases normally in response to intravenous potassium sulfate infusions and not potassium chloride, it has been proposed that the primary defect in this disorder is enhanced electrogenic chloride reabsorption in the distal nephron. This results in a decrease in the lumen negativity which impairs potassium and proton secretion. The enhanced reabsorption of sodium and chloride results in hypertension, hyporeninemia, and hypoaldosteronism.

DRUGS THAT CAUSE HYPERKALEMIA

Captopril

An angiotensin converting enzyme inhibitor, captopril causes a rise in the serum potassium level which varies inversely with the glomerular filtration rate and is most severe in those patients with markedly impaired renal function. The mechanism is likely attributable to decreased aldosterone synthesis resulting in a decreased fractional excretion of potassium.

Beta-blocker

The beta$_2$-receptor has been shown to mediate potassium uptake into cells. Propranolol has a direct effect, blocking the influx of potassium into muscles, and also inhibits renin secretion. This results in a moderate sustained increase in the plasma potassium concentration when the drug is ingested chronically. Hyperkalemia is observed most commonly in diabetics and patients with renal insufficiency and is reversible upon discontinuation of the drug.

Prostaglandin Inhibitors

Indomethacin and other nonsteroidal anti-inflammatory agents have been reported to cause hyporeninemic hypoaldosteronism and hyperkalemia. The hyporeninemia has been attributed to decreased prostaglandin production, since prostaglandin E_2, I_2, and D_2 are stimulants of renin secretion. In a recent study of a patient with Bartter's syndrome, mepacrine (a phospholipase inhibitor) was shown to inhibit prostaglandin excretion without decreasing the plasma renin concentration. It is therefore possible that nonsteroidal anti-inflammatory agents directly inhibit renin release by a non-prostaglandin-dependent mechanism.

Heparin

Chronic heparin therapy has been reported to be associated with hyperkalemia. The hyperkalemia is attributable to a direct impairment of adrenal aldosterone synthesis and, as might be expected, these patients are hyperreninemic.

Spironolactone, Triameterene, and Amiloride

Administration of these diuretics inhibits potassium secretion by the cortical collecting tubule. These drugs should be used cautiously in those patients with diabetic or renal insufficiency.

Digitalis

Digitalis overdose results in an inhibition of sodium-potassium-adenosine triphosphatase activity which prevents cells from actively accumulating potassium, which results in a rise in plasma potassium level.

Succinylcholine

By depolarizing cells, succinylcholine causes a passive leak of potassium from the intracellular to the extracellular compartment. Hyperkalemia may result.

Arginine Hydrochloride

This drug has been reported to cause an efflux of potassium into the extracellular compartment resulting in hyperkalemia.

TREATMENT

General Considerations

In approaching the treatment of hyperkalemia, the clinician must ascertain whether the patient is symptomatic and whether the disorder is acute or chronic. Hyperkalemia should be treated aggressively if there are associated neuromuscular and cardiac abnormalities. The neuromuscular abnormalities include paresthesias and weakness of the extremities, which, in severe cases, may result in symmetric flaccid analysis. Sensory abnormalities are usually mild in comparison to the muscular findings. Cardiac toxicity is the primary reason for treating hyperkalemia. Electrocardiogram abnormalities include an increase in the amplitude of T waves, lengthening of the PR interval, and widening of the QRS complex. Severe hyperkalemia (serum concentrations greater than 8 mEq per liter) results in disappearance of P waves and a sine wave pattern resembling slow ventricular tachycardia. Any disturbance in conduction may be present, including atrioventricular (AV) nodal and fascicular conduction blocks. In patients with chronic hyperkalemia these electrocardiographic abnormalities may be absent. In addition, milder degrees of hyperkalemia may be associated with cardiac toxicity if hyponatremia, hypocalcemia, or acidemia coexists. Treatment is generally indicated in the absence of electrocardiogram abnormalities if the potassium concentration has risen above 6 mEq per liter. Patients with preexisting AV conduction abnormalities may develop Stokes-Adams episodes and complete AV block with only modest hyperkalemia.

Treatment of Acute Hyperkalemia

Treatment of an acute elevation in the plasma potassium concentration involves the following principles: (1) Oppose the effects of hyperkalemia on the cell membrane to minimize cardiac and neuromuscular toxicity; (2) increase the transport of potassium from the extracellular to the intracellular compartment; (3) increase the excretion of potassium; and (4) treat the cause of the hyperkalemia. These principles are summarized in Table 2.

TABLE 2 Treatment of Acute Hyperkalemia

	Dose
Membrane antagonism	
Calcium gluconate (10%)	10–20 ml IV
Sodium bicarbonate	50–100 mEq IV
Sodium chloride	50–100 mEq IV
Redistribution	
Insulin/glucose	20 units regular insulin plus 50 g glucose IV over 1 hour
Sodium bicarbonate	50–100 mEq IV
Increase excretion	
Furosemide	40–80 mg IV
Kayexalate	25–50 g per rectum with sorbitol, or PO
Sodium bicarbonate	50–100 mEq IV
Hemodialysis	
Peritoneal dialysis	

Membrane Antagonism

Calcium increases the threshold potential required to excite the plasma membrane of the cardiac cell. Since hyperkalemia depolarizes the cardiac cell's resting membrane potential, bringing it closer to the potential required for excitation, calcium, by increasing the difference between the resting and excitation potential, reduces the adverse effect of hyperkalemia. Calcium also reverses the decrease in conduction velocity induced by hyperkalemia by increasing the number of sodium channels in the cell membrane. Calcium is given intravenously as a bolus of 10 to 20 ml of a 10 percent solution of calcium gluconate. The dose may be repeated if no immediate effect is seen. Electrocardiographic monitoring is desirable. If the patient is also being treated with digitalis, hypercalcemia may result in digitalis toxicity, so it is preferable to give the calcium gluconate as a slow infusion over 30 minutes to prevent an acute elevation of the serum calcium concentration.

Hyponatremia may aggravate the cardiac toxicity induced by hyperkalemia, as mentioned previously. The treatment consists of administering hypertonic saline (50 to 100 mEq of sodium chloride) which may reverse the adverse effects of hyperkalemia on the cardiac cell.

Redistribution of Potassium

Insulin-Glucose. Insulin directly stimulates the uptake of potassium into cells, predominantly muscle, by depolarizing the membrane potential. Glucose is given to prevent hypoglycemia during insulin therapy. Ten to 20 units of regular insulin are added to 0.5 liters of 10 percent glucose solution and infused over 1 hour. The treatment is repeated as required. The K^+ concentration should fall 0.5 to 1.2 mEq per liter in 1 to 2 hours.

Sodium Bicarbonate. Sodium bicarbonate reduces hyperkalemia by shifting potassium into cells and by increasing renal potassium excretion. The standard dose is 50 mEq given intravenously over 10 minutes. This dose can be repeated as long as the patient can tolerate the increased sodium intake. Patients with hypocalcemia may be at increased risk of seizures and tetany as the blood pH is increased.

Increased Excretion of Potassium

Diuretics. Although not useful in an acute situation, a diuretic such as furosemide is effective in markedly enhancing the renal excretion of potassium. The usual dose is 40 to 80 mg intravenously. In the presence of renal failure, these agents are less potent.

Resins. Ion-exchange resins such as Kayexalate (Na^+ polystyrene sulfonate) bind potassium in the gastrointestinal tract in exchange for sodium. Each gram of resin binds 1 mEq of potassium in exchange for 2 to 3 mEq of Na^+. The resin may be given orally (25 to 50 g) or as a retention enema (50 g in 200 ml of 10 percent dextrose in water per rectum). Sorbitol is given to prevent the major side effect of constipation. The serum potassium level falls 0.5 to 1 mEq per liter after a 50-g dose within 1 to 2 hours. Since a sodium load is administered during this form of therapy, clinicians should be cautious in prescribing the drug for patients who cannot tolerate volume overload.

Dialysis. Potassium can be removed effectively from the body using either hemodialysis or peritoneal dialysis. The major difference between the two modes of therapy is the rapidity of potassium removal. Hemodialysis is preferred if an acute decrease in the serum potassium concentration is required. The major drawback is the time needed to set up the hemodialysis equipment and the need to have access to the circulation. Using this method, approximately 40 mEq of potassium can be removed during the first hour as opposed to approximately 5 mEq with peritoneal dialysis.

Treatment of Chronic Hyperkalemia

Chronic moderate hyperkalemia (plasma potassium concentration equal to 6 or 7 mEq per liter) is better tolerated by patients than acute hyperkalemia of a similar magnitude. For example, patients with chronic renal failure tolerate very high plasma potassium levels. In treating chronic hyperkalemia, one should be aware that many of these patients have associated diseases such as diabetes mellitus, renal failure, congestive heart failure, hypertension, and cardiovascular disease. One must be wary of the possible detrimental side effects the therapy may have on associated medical disorders.

Diet

In chronic renal failure, the plasma potassium concentration is proportional to the dietary potassium intake. Although this has not been demonstrated in all causes of chronic hyperkalemia, it is also beneficial to reduce the dietary intake in these disorders. The total daily potassium intake should be reduced to less than 60 mEq per day. Since the dietary potassium is normally exchanged for increased sodium, as in patients receiving ion exchange resins, one must be cautious when treating patients who cannot tolerate a volume load. In addition, there is a growing amount of clinical data which indicates that increasing the dietary intake of potassium may be beneficial in lowering the blood pressure in patients with hypertension. The exact mechanism involved in this blood pressure lowering effect is unknown. Whether patients with hyperkalemia and hypertension will experience an increase in their blood pressure during a decrease in dietary potassium intake is also unknown. Dietary salt substitutes containing potassium must be avoided.

Drugs

Drugs that cause an increase in the plasma potassium concentration should be avoided. These drugs include prostaglandin inhibitors, heparin, beta-blockers, angiotensin converting enzyme inhibitors, amiloride, triamterene, and spironolactone. In addition, diabetics who lack the compensatory response of an increase in insulin and aldosterone secretion during glucose infusions are susceptible to life-threatening hyperkalemia.

Acid-Base Balance

Acidemia will often result in an increased plasma potassium concentration. Bicarbonate will ameliorate the hyperkalemia both by raising the plasma pH and by directly shifting potassium intracellularly. Bicarbonate will also cause a potassium diuresis. The low plasma bicarbonate concentration can be corrected by assuming a distribution space of 40 percent of total body weight. As mentioned previously, patients with heart failure may not be able to tolerate the excess volume load associated with this form of therapy, and therefore a diuretic should be given concomitantly.

Prevention of Volume Depletion

Since potassium secretion in the distal tubule is decreased when the luminal Na^+ concentration falls and when luminal flow decreases, the volume status of the patient with chronic hyperkalemia should be adequately maintained.

HYPOKALEMIA

RICHARD L. TANNEN, M.D.

Hypokalemia is defined as a decrease in the concentration of potassium in plasma or serum. Values below the accepted lower limit of normal, i.e., 3.5 mEq per liter, clearly represent hypokalemia; however, values between 3.5 and 3.8 mEq per liter are not commonly found under normal conditions and may also reflect hypokalemia in many patients.

ETIOLOGY

Hypokalemia can result from a shift of extracellular potassium into the intracellular compartment, from depletion of total body potassium stores, or both. In the former circumstance, intracellular potassium concentration is normal, whereas the hallmark of potassium depletion is a decrease in intracellular potassium concentration.

A variety of factors can cause hypokalemia by altering the transcellular distribution of potassium. Increases in two important regulators of potassium homeostasis, insulin and epinephrine, drive potassium into cells. Hence, high levels of insulin, resulting from exogenous administration or endogenous release secondary to hyperglycemia, or from exogenous administration of epinephrine and other drugs with beta-[2] agonist properties produce hypokalemia. It has been suggested that the transient hypokalemia often detected in patients with acute stressful conditions such as myocardial infarctions, head injuries, open heart surgery, and delerium tremens may result from the endogenous release of epinephrine. Hypokalemia secondary to redistribution also results from high plasma pH or bicarbonate concentrations, from intoxication with several compounds (barium, toluene, theophylline), and in conjunction with either hereditary periodic paralysis or the acquired form associated with thyrotoxicosis.

Significant potassium depletion is almost always secondary to abnormal losses of potassium from the body by either the gastrointestinal or renal route. With gastrointestinal losses from diarrhea or, less commonly, laxative abuse or villous adenoma, the kidney typically responds by appropriately conserving potassium. Hence, urinary potassium excretion of less than 20 mEq per day can provide a clue to the source of potassium depletion in cases where the etiology is unclear.

Excessive renal potassium losses occur most frequently under either conditions which result in chloride depletion or those associated with mineralocorticoid excess states. Chloride and associated potassium depletion are typical sequelae of upper gastrointestinal tract chloride losses from vomiting or gastric drainage and of urinary chloride losses induced by diuretic therapy. Mineralocorticoid excess states such as primary aldosteronism result in potassium depletion, but inappropriate renal potassium losses sometimes can occur under conditions of secondary aldosteronism, especially when associated with hypertensive conditions such as renal artery stenosis or malignant hypertension. Other causes of renal K^+ wasting include renal tubular acidosis, diabetic ketoacidosis, high dose intravenous penicillin therapy, hereditary K^+ wasting disorders such as Bartter's syndrome, and—for reasons that remain elusive—magnesium depletion of any origin.

CLINICAL SEQUELAE OF HYPOKALEMIA

Adverse effects of hypokalemia can be either the consequence of an altered ratio between intracellular and extracellular potassium (K_i/K_e) or a result of the low intracellular potassium concentration per se. Obviously, when hypokalemia occurs owing to redistribution of potassium only the first mechanism can provoke symptoms. With potassium depletion extracellular potassium concentration decreases by a greater percentage than intracellular concentration, so K_i/K_e is increased in the same fashion as with redistribution mediated hypokalemia. Thus, potassium depletion can produce abnormalities by both mechanisms.

The litany of abnormalities produced by hypokalemia and potassium depletion is related to the severity and, in some instances, to the duration of depletion. To characterize symptomatology it is useful to arbitrarily define severity of hypokalemia (potassium depletion) as mild (serum K^+ between 3.0 and 3.5 mEq per liter, reflecting a potassium deficit ranging from 150 to 300 mEq in the depleted patient); moderate (serum K^+ between 2.5 and 3.0 mEq per liter, reflecting a deficit from 300 to 500 mEq); and severe (serum K^+ less than 2.5 mEq per liter with a deficit greater than 500 mEq).

Many patients with mild hypokalemia are entirely asymptomatic. Some exhibit nonspecific symptoms, including malaise, fatigue, muscular weakness, restless leg syndrome, cramps, and rarely myalgia. More significant effects that can be noted even in patients with mild depletion include the risk of provoking toxicity in patients treated with digitalis, an increased risk of ventricular arrhythmias especially in patients with underlying heart disease, and an increased incidence of ventricular tachycardia or fibrillation during an acute myocardial infarction. Mild glucose intolerance often accompanies this degree of K^+ depletion and blood pressure control in hypertensive patients may be impaired.

In addition to the above abnormalities, moderate potassium depletion can result in rhabdomyolysis, reduced gastrointestinal tract motility with constipation, and polyuria as a result of a renal concentrating defect, and can provoke encephalopathy in patients with underlying hepatic disease.

With severe K^+ depletion, ileus as well as frank muscular paralysis with life-threatening respiratory paralysis can occur. Metabolic alkalosis is a sequela of severe K^+ depletion regardless of cause. There are also some data to suggest that blood pressure may be lowered. Longstanding, severe K^+ depletion can result in interstitial nephritis and can lead to chronic renal failure.

THERAPY

General Concepts

Treatment of hypokalemia is dictated by its severity, the accompanying symptoms, and the underlying cause. Decisions are required concerning the type of potassium preparation to be administered, the route of replacement, and the rate and magnitude of K^+ replenishment. As a general rule, correction of hypokalemia and K^+ depletion requires the administration of potassium. The role of other treatment, such as K^+-sparing diuretics, which are either ancillary or used prophylactically, to prevent K^+ depletion, will be discussed later.

Potassium should be administered orally, unless the oral route is not feasible or an emergent clinical situation dictates prompt replacement to treat a life-threatening complication. The oral and intravenous potassium preparations available are listed in Table 1.

Three basic types of potassium salts can be given: potassium chloride, potassium phosphate, and potassium bicarbonate or the metabolic precursors of bicarbonate, such as gluconate, acetate, or citrate. The choice of anion depends on the accompanying electrolyte abnormalities that might require simultaneous therapy. For example, if the patient has an associated metabolic acidosis, as occurs when K^+ depletion results from either diarrhea or renal tubular acidosis, potassium bicarbonate or a bicarbonate precursor is indicated. Since patients with diabetic ketoacidosis usually present with both potassium and phosphate depletion, potassium phosphate therapy is a rational choice in this setting. The need for phosphate replacement in the treatment of diabetic ketoacidosis has been challenged, based on the finding that patients recover equally well without phosphate supplementation. In my view it seems appropriate, since phosphate depletion is well documented in this setting as well as potentially hazardous, and the therapy is risk free as long as phosphate replenishment is not overzealous (20 to 30 mg of elemental phosphorus per kilogram of body weight every 24 hours). Finally, if the patient is chloride depleted. e.g., because of upper gastrointestinal tract losses or diuretic therapy, potassium chloride is an absolute requirement for adequate K^+ replenishment. In fact, if there is

TABLE 1 Preparations of Potassium Salts

Preparation	*Selected Brand Names*	*Potassium Content*
Oral administration		
Potassium chloride		
10% solution	Kaochlor, Kay Ciel, K-Lor, Klorvess, others	20 mEq/15 ml
20% solution	Kaon-Cl, Klor-Con, others	40 mEq/15 ml
Dehydrated powders and packets	K-Lor, K-Lyte Cl, Kaochlor, Kato, Kay Ciel, KEEF, Klor-Con, Klorvess, others	15–25 mEq each
Wax matrix or microencapsulated tablets	Kaon-Cl, Slow K, Klotrix, Micro K, others	7–10 mEq each
Alkalinizing salts (acetate citrate, gluconate or bicarbonate)		
Solutions	Polycitra K, Kaon, Kolyum, Twin K, Potassium Triplex, Trikates	20–60 mEq/15 ml
Dehydrated powders and tablets	Kaon, K-Lyte, K-Lyte DS	5–20 mEq each
Intravenous administration		
Potassium chloride		20 mEq/20 ml
Potassium chloride		40 mEq/20 ml
Potassium acetate		40 mEq/20 ml
Potassium phosphate		66 mEq/15 ml

Adapted from Levey AS, Harrington JT. Hypokalemia. In: Glassock RJ, ed. Current therapy in nephrology and hypertension–1. Philadelphia: BC Decker Inc, 1984.

any doubt regarding the K^+ preparation to use, potassium chloride (KCl) is always an appropriate choice, since all forms of K^+ depletion can be corrected with the chloride anion.

As indicated in Table 1, a variety of KCl preparations are available for oral use. They fall into two broad categories: solutions of KCl including powdered preparations ingested as a solution, and the wax matrix or microencapsulated slow release forms of KCl. Both KCl solutions and slow-release tablets are equally effective in providing bioavailable KCl. For short-term therapy I generally recommend KCl solutions; however, for long-term K^+ replacement the slow-release forms are preferred by patients because of the unpleasant taste of KCl in solution.

In patients who are hypokalemic as a result of K^+ depletion, the magnitude of the depletion can be estimated from the serum K^+ level. A rough rule of thumb is that each 0.5 mEq per liter decrement in K^+ below 4.0 mEq per liter is equivalent to a 150 -to 175-mEq deficit in total body K^+ stores. Keep in mind, however, that factors which independently modify the transcellular distribution of K^+ can alter this relationship. Thus, a relatively acute metabolic alkalosis may not be accompanied by potassium depletion even though hypokalemia is present.

In general, unless a life-threatening complication exists one should err on the side of replenishing K^+ stores slowly. Oral medication is usually given in doses of 40 to 120 mEq per day depending on the magnitude of the potassium deficit, and also on the concurrent rate of K^+ loss, if the K+ losing abnormality persists. In nonurgent situations in which intravenous K^+ therapy is required, the concentration of K^+ in intravenous fluids should not exceed 40 mEq per liter and the rate of administration should not exceed 10 mEq per hour.

More vigorous intravenous therapy may be indicated in patients with hypokalemic-induced digitalis toxic arrhythmias, hypokalemic-induced malignant ventricular arrhythmias, or hypokalemic-induced paralysis. Under these circumstances, potassium can be administered more rapidly, but the rate should not exceed 40 mEq per hour. If concentrations of K^+ greater than 40 mEq per liter are required, it should be administered into a large vein to avoid phlebitis, but central (intracardiac) administration should be guarded against owing to the risk of K^+-induced arrhythmias. Furthermore, care should be taken to make certain that an infusion error cannot result in delivery of K^+ in life-threatening quantities. This can be accomplished in a variety of fashions. If standard delivery systems are used, the K^+ concentration in the infusion fluid should not exceed 60 mEq per liter. If less fluid administration is warranted, up to 20 mEq of potassium can be diluted to 100 ml in a Soluset with a microdrip. Ideally, an alarm-sensitive, drip-regulating infusion pump should be used as a delivery system. In those rare circumstances in which vigorous intravenous potassium therapy is indicated, cardiac monitoring in an intensive care unit is advisable.

Regardless of the route or speed of potassium replacement, the adequacy of therapy should be gauged by repeated measurements of plasma potassium levels. The frequency of measurements obviously depends on the initial degree of depletion and the clinical urgency of the situation. Although rough estimates of the rapidity and magnitude of therapy required can be made at the outset of treatment, the therapeutic plan should be adjusted based on the response as assessed from recurrent measurements of plasma K^+ levels.

The major risk of potassium replacement, either orally or intravenously, is the development of life-threatening hyperkalemia. In one large series of 4,921 hospitalized patients who received oral KCl, 3.6 percent developed hyperkalemia, which was life-threatening in 0.4 percent and fatal in an additional 0.1 percent. In this report, elderly patients and those with impaired renal function were at greatest risk of the development of hyperkalemia. In addition, extra caution should be used in other settings in which K^+ homeostasis is impaired, as for example in patients receiving K^+ sparing diuretics, in those with hypoaldosteronism, or in those with insulin-dependent diabetes mellitus.

As already noted, the other complication of intravenous KCl therapy is phlebitis, which occurs when the concentration exceeds 40 to 60 mEq per liter in solutions delivered into peripheral veins. With oral therapy, the other important risk is intestinal tract ulceration. Ulceration of the small intestine was a widely recognized complication of the early generation of enteric-coated KCl formulations, which led to their withdrawal from the market. This problem appears to have been eliminated with the current wax matrix and microencapsulated forms of KCl; however, they are not altogether risk free. Recent studies employing routine endoscopic evaluations have found a surprisingly high incidence of asymptomatic gastric ulcerations in patients treated with slow-release KCl, and this appears to be more common with the wax matrix than microencapsulated forms. Symptomatically important ulceration appears to occur infrequently; nevertheless, patients with impaired gastrointestinal tract motility are at risk of clinically important ulceration, and this may occur even with liquid KCl preparations.

Therapeutic Issues in Specific Hypokalemic Conditions

There are several hypokalemic conditions in which specific therapeutic issues different from the general approach enumerated above are applicable.

Hypokalemia Secondary to Redistribution in the Intracellular Compartment

This phenomenon is usually transient and self limited. For example, the hypokalemia secondary to insulin excess, exogenous administration of beta-adrenergic agonists, or treatment of pernicious anemia with vitamin B_{12} remits concurrently with the duration of the hormone or drug effect. Similarly, the "stress-related" hypokalemia of acute illness, which is probably secondary to release of endogenous epinephrine, is usually self limited and requires no specific therapy. On occasion, however, therapy might be appropriate, as for example in a patient receiving treatment with digitalis or one who has had an acute myocardial infarction in which hypokalemia and ventricular tachycardia and fibrillation are potentially linked in a cause and effect relationship. So long as there is no component of K^+ depletion, if treatment with K^+ is used to increase the plasma K^+ concentration, small quantities will be required. Beta-blockers that interfere with beta-2 mediated events would represent an alternative therapeutic approach. However, there are no data on the efficacy in these clinical situations of either of these treatment strategies.

Hypokalemic Periodic Paralysis

In the familial form of this illness, acetazolamide (250 to 750 mg per day) is effective in eliminating attacks and also in improving interattack weakness. The mechanism of action is not clear, although it may be related to the production of metabolic acidosis.

Magnesium Depletion

Magnesium depletion, regardless of the underlying etiology, can cause potassium depletion secondary to renal K^+ wasting. The specific mechanism whereby urinary K^+ excretion is stimulated is unresolved, but treatment in these circumstances should be directed toward replacement of the magnesium as well as the potassium deficit.

Primary Hyperaldosteronism

Medical treatment of hypokalemia is required in patients with hyperaldosteronism secondary to adrenal hyperplasia and also prior to surgical resection in patients with adenomas. Spironolactone in doses ranging from 200 to 400 mg per day is effective for both the correction of hypokalemia and the maintenance of normal K^+ homeostasis. An alternative for patients who do not tolerate spironolactone is amiloride, 20 to 40 mg per day. While amiloride effectively normalizes potassium levels, it may not be as efficacious as spironolactone in reducing blood pressure.

Bartter's Syndrome and Other Idiopathic Renal K^+ Wasting Disorders

The most difficult hypokalemic management problems are encountered in patients with Bartter's syndrome and other related primary renal K^+ wasting disorders. In these conditions, patients commonly present with severe hypokalemia and profound renal K^+ wasting. Oral potassium supplementation alone is usually inadequate either to correct the K^+ deficiency or to sustain normal K^+ balance, since urinary K^+ losses can be as high as 300 mEq per day even in the presence of hypokalemia. Although not proven conclusively, there is reason to suspect that severe, prolonged K^+ deficiency may account for the development of chronic renal insufficiency in some of these patients and it may play a role in growth retardation in affected children. Thus, there are reasons to strive vigorously for improvement in K^+ status, both for the treatment of the more acute hypokalemic symptoms these patients may manifest, as well as to prevent potential long-term serious consequences. Maintenance of serum K^+ levels at least above 3.0 mEq per liter seems to be a reasonable therapeutic objective.

Several treatment alternatives can be effective. My first recommendation is use of the K^+ sparing diuretic amiloride. Recent data suggest that 10 to 40 mg per day of amiloride in conjunction with oral KCl supplementation can be efficacious. In some instances spironolactone has been beneficial, but the results are variable and it seems to be less effective than amiloride for treatment of this patient population. The dosages of spironolactone are similar to those recommended in the treatment of primary aldosteronism. This group of diseases represents the only setting in which K^+ supplementation and K^+ sparing diuretics should be used in combination. In all other settings the risk of hyperkalemia is too great to condone it.

If adequate potassium levels are not achieved with combined amiloride and KCl treatment, the next therapeutic step worth considering is the addition of a prostaglandin synthetase inhibitor to the treatment program. Indomethacin, in doses of 100 to 200 mg per day, has been used most frequently, but other cyclo-oxygenase inhibitors appear to be equally efficacious. Data from a large number of reports indicate that prostaglandin synthetase inhibition effectively stabilizes serum potassium concentration at a level of approximately 3.0 mEq per liter. The major difficulty with use of these drugs on a chronic basis has been the inability of some patients to tolerate the gastrointestinal side effects, particularly gastritis and less frequently frank ulceration.

There have been some isolated reports of the efficacy of captopril in the treatment of Bartter's syndrome, but the data are insufficient to draw any firm conclusions. Since the mechanism of K^+ conservation might be expected to relate to a decrease in angiotensin II and aldosterone levels, it would be surprising if it were much more useful than spironolactone. Also, there is the clear potential for hypotension, as a result of the suppression of angiotensin II levels, although in some isolated reports this has not been a substantive problem. In my judgment, use of angiotensin converting inhibitors should currently be viewed as experimental.

K^+ Maintenance Therapy in the Setting of Chronic Diuretic Treatment

The most common and most controversial aspect of potassium therapy relates to the issue of whether patients chronically receiving diuretics for the treatment of hypertension or congestive heart failure should be placed on a potassium maintenance regimen. The term "K^+ maintenance" is used to imply a treatment program that sustains a normal serum K^+ level. This can be accomplished either by KCl supplementation or by the use of K^+ sparing diuretics. These two alternative approaches to K^+ maintenance therapy will be considered subsequently.

Hypokalemia is an almost universal accompaniment of therapy with either thiazide (or chlorthalidone) or loop (furosemide, ethacrynic acid, bumetanide) diuretics. With standard doses of these agents (hydrochlorothiazide, 50 to 100 mg per day; furosemide 40 to 80 mg per day), serum potassium levels decline on the average by 0.6 mEq per liter with thiazides and 0.3 mEq per liter with furosemide. A more substantial decline in K^+ concentration to values less than 3.0 mEq per liter is infrequent and is estimated to occur in less than 7 percent of patients taking thiazides and less than 1 percent of patients treated with furosemide. The degree of hypokalemia can be minimized if moderate sodium restriction (60 to 110 mEq per day) accompanies use of diuretics. Both more severe restriction and more liberal sodium intake appear to accentuate the magnitude of K^+ depletion. Potassium levels decline rapidly after the initiation of treatment with diuretics, and usually reach a stable plateau within about 1 week. Although there has been considerable debate concerning whether the hypokalemia represents actual K^+ depletion, in my view the evidence supports the development of mild K^+ depletion (approximately 150 mEq) consistent with the decrement in serum K^+ levels.

The most heated debate revolves around whether the mild K^+ depletion that accompanies diuretic use warrants therapy under the usual conditions. Since there are no appropriately controlled therapeutic trials to resolve this question, judgment currently must be based on the available data relevant to the associated risks and benefits of the two treatment options.

First, what are the potential adverse consequences of mild K^+ depletion? As noted earlier, some patients will have vague complaints of fatigue and malaise, but most will be essentially asymptomatic. The most serious potential complications are cardiovascular. Some recent studies suggest that mild, diuretic-induced hypokalemia provokes ventricular premature beats in 25 to 50 percent of patients and that these are of the complex variety (i.e., multifocal, couplets, or tachycardia) in 15 to 30 percent of patients. However, an equal number of carefully performed studies could not document any increased propensity for ventricular arrhythmias. Although there is no definite explanation for these divergent findings, there is a suggestion that patients with preexisting underlying cardiac disease may account for the group that is particularly prone to the development of K^+ induced ventricular ectopy.

The other potential cardiovascular risk of K^+ depletion is an increased incidence of ventricular tachycardia (VT) or fibrillation (VF) in patients who sustain an acute myocardial infarction. Virtually every study reported has demonstrated a twofold increase in the incidence of VT/VF in patients with a serum K^+ level less than 3.5 mEq per liter. What is unclear is whether this represents a cause and effect relationship. Does hypokalemia account for the increase in VT/VF or is it a marker of increased catecholamine levels, which induce both the hypokalemia and arrhythmia? This question has not been resolved definitively.

The other adverse consequences of mild K^+ depletion which merit consideration are glucose intolerance and blood pressure regulation. It is estimated that 30 percent of hypertensive patients treated with thiazide diuretics develop abnormal glucose tolerance. The abnormality is mild and rarely requires therapy with hypoglycemic agents, but the long-term risk for atherogenesis is undefined. A recent study also suggests that mild K^+ depletion can impair blood pressure control in hypertensive patients.

What are the adverse consequences of treatment? The most serious risk is the potential development of life-threatening hyperkalemia. Although the risk is not well defined in an ambulatory population, the 1974 Boston Collaborative Drug Surveillance Program evaluation of hospitalized patients found a 3.9 percent risk of significant hyperkalemia in patients treated with oral KCl, and a 5.7 percent risk in patients treated with the K^+ sparing diuretic spironolactone (when used without concurrent potassium supplements). In addition to this complication of drug therapy, there is the risk of gastrointestinal abnormalities with KCl preparations and drug-specific side effects, detailed below, if K^+ sparing diuretics are used. Finally, adequate K^+ maintenance therapy costs between $10 and $20 per month.

Given the impreciseness of the risk and benefit information, it is no surprise that there are divergent viewpoints regarding therapy. Most authorities agree that K^+ maintenance therapy is indicated in patients receiving concurrent therapy with digitalis, those predisposed to hepatic encephalopathy, or those in whom serum K^+ values decrease to less than 3.0 mEq per liter. I also advocate treatment in patients who develop glucose intolerance (or, alternatively, discontinue diuretics) and in any patient with defined, underlying cardiac disease. Finally, a trial of K^+ maintenance therapy seems appropriate in patients who have nonspecific symptoms that might be attributed to mild potassium depletion.

K^+ maintenance therapy can be achieved effectively with any KCl preparation or by use of K^+ sparing diuretics. The chloride salt of potassium is an absolute therapeutic requirement, because chloride depletion is a major factor in the production and maintenance of diuretic-induced K^+ depletion. It is important to recognize that 40 to 60 mEq per day of KCl is needed for adequate therapy. This can be provided as either KCl solutions or slow-release tablets. The advantages of each as well as their risks have been enumerated earlier.

Alternatively, the K^+ sparing diuretics can be used for K^+ maintenance therapy. Spironolactone inhibits renal K^+ secretion by its action as an aldosterone antagonist, while triamterene and amiloride block K^+ secretion by an aldosterone-independent mechanism. The data suggest that these agents may be more effective in sustaining normal potassium levels than potassium supplements. While all the K^+ sparing diuretics can be used effectively for K^+ maintenance therapy, I prefer amiloride because of its predictability and perhaps lower incidence of side effects. The dose and drug-specific complications of the K^+ sparing diuretics are as follow:

Spironolactone

Doses of 50 to 100 mg per day are usually needed for adequate K^+ maintenance therapy. Maximal inhibition of aldosterone's effect on the renal tubule is achieved at doses of 300 mg per day. Chronic treatment with moderate to high doses can result in estrogen-like side effects, including decreased libido, impotence, and gynecomastia in men and menstrual irregularities and painful breast enlargement in women.

Triamterene

Doses of 100 to 200 mg per day are standard, with a maximum recommended dose of 400 mg per day. Gastrointestinal side effects, including diarrhea, nausea, and vomiting, are potential complications. Megaloblastosis as a result of its folic acid antagonist properties, and renal stones containing metabolites of the drug have also been described rarely.

Amiloride

Standard doses are 5 to 10 mg per day, but up to 20 mg per day is recommended. The most common adverse effects are gastrointestinal, including nausea, vomiting, anorexia, and diarrhea.

As emphasized previously, the most important complication of K^+ sparing drugs is hyperkalemia. For this reason they should not routinely be used in conjunction with potassium supplements nor in patients with significant impairment of glomerular filtration rate (creatinine >3.0 mg per deciliter, blood urea nitrogen >45 mg per deciliter, creatinine clearance <30 ml per minute). Furthermore, these agents as well as potassium supplements should be used with extreme caution, if at all, in patients with other conditions that might increase their predisposition to hyperkalemia, e.g., insulin-dependent diabetes mellitus.

METABOLIC ALKALOSIS

ROBERT G. LUKE, M.B., Ch.B., F.R.C.P.
JOHN H. GALLA, M.D.

DIAGNOSIS

Alkalemia is the elevation of arterial blood pH above normal; alkalosis is defined as a tendency toward elevation of arterial blood pH. This difference is important diagnostically because in mixed disturbances (see the chapter *Mixed Acid-Base Disturbances*) alkalosis may conceal a more severe primary metabolic or respiratory acidosis. Metabolic alkalosis occurs when an acid-base disturbance tends to increase primarily the plasma bicarbonate concentration; the usual associated increment in arterial carbon dioxide concentration ($PaCO_2$) is a secondary compensatory phenomenon and never fully corrects arterial pH to normal in the absence of an associated primary respiratory acidosis. Patients with hypochloremia and hyperbicarbonatemia may have either respiratory acidosis and/or metabolic alkalosis; the anion gap tends to be elevated in metabolic alkalosis, but not in respiratory acidosis unless there is associated lactic acidosis due to severe hypoxia. Clearly the determination of arterial pH, $PaCO_2$, and PaO_2 is essential prior to the treatment of hypochloremic hyperbicarbonatemia in order to determine an accurate acid-base diagnosis. Respiratory compensation for chronic metabolic alkalosis averages an increase in $PaCO_2$ by 0.6 mm Hg for each milliequivalent increase in the plasma bicarbonate concentration above normal. In extreme metabolic alkalosis the $PaCO_2$ may reach 60 mm Hg or more. It is especially important to recognize that the latter situation is not a primary respiratory disorder, since treatment aimed primarily at reducing $PaCO_2$ will produce a life-threatening increase in arterial pH. In primary metabolic alkalosis, specific acid-base therapy is, in general, indicated when the plasma bicarbonate concentration is greater than 33 mEq per liter or the arterial pH is above 7.50.

The clinical manifestations of metabolic alkalosis per se are difficult to separate from those of the commonly associated pathophysiologic states such as volume or potassium depletion. However, neuromuscular irritability, cardiovascular instability and arrhythmias, and mental confusion are common when alkalosis is severe. The potential adverse effects of compensatory hypoventilation on other pulmonary functions or on the development of infections of the respiratory tract in the seriously ill patient or the immunocompromised host may be significant. Metabolic alkalosis is clearly not an innocuous condition; in one large series, patients with an arterial pH of 7.65 or greater had an 80 percent mortality. Again, associated conditions may be important, but treatment of the metabolic alkalosis per se in such circumstances is a medical emergency and requires a rapid assessment of the relevant causative mechanisms in order to prescribe corrective therapy, as discussed below.

Metabolic alkalosis can be divided into two phases: generation (loss of hydrogen ion from or gain of bicarbonate by the body) and maintenance. It is difficult to exceed the capacity of the normal kidney to excrete administered bicarbonate or its metabolic precursors such as citrate or carbonate in the absence of the conditions outlined in Table 1. Iatrogenic acute metabolic alkalosis related to oral or intravenous sodium bicarbonate administration is thus usually transient in the presence of a normal kidney. Especially when sodium bicarbonate has been given intravenously, transient metabolic alkalosis may also occur as the accumulated organic anions of diabetic ketoacidosis or lactic acidosis are metabolized to bicarbonate secondary to insulin administration and/or volume repletion. Since, in the absence of bicarbonate-retaining mechanisms, base loading alone rarely produces a sustained elevation of plasma bicarbonate concentration by more than 2 to 3 mEq per liter, the focus of this chapter is on the treatment of chronic metabolic alkalosis in which one of the sustaining causes is virtually always evident. On occasion, the pathogenesis of the generation phase of metabolic alkalosis is obscure and cannot be established by the time the physician is faced with the clinical problem. This, however, need not deter effective therapy. The paramount question to be answered by the physician prior to initiation of appropriately designed therapy is: Why is this patient's kidney not excreting the retained extracellular bicarbonate?

THERAPEUTIC OPTIONS

The answers to that question almost always lie within those listed in the first column of Table 1. In many patients multiple mechanisms may contribute and interact. In most patients the major mechanism relates to either chloride depletion or mineralocorticoid excess-potassium depletion. Associated potassium depletion is also common with chloride depletion metabolic alkalosis, but in general the alkalosis *can* be corrected in such patients without concomitant restoration of potassium balance; for the second group, in contrast, repletion of potassium is necessary for correction of metabolic alkalosis. There are, however, cogent clinical reasons to also correct the associated potassium depletion during treatment of metabolic alkalosis even when it is primarily due to chloride depletion.

In most patients the history and physical examination will be strongly suggestive of the mechanisms responsible for the maintenance of the elevated plasma bicarbonate concentration. If the cause is not obvious, determination of urinary chloride and potassium concentrations may be helpful. Patients with chloride depletion metabolic alkalosis have a urinary chloride concentration less than 10 mEq per liter except when renal chloride wasting is the cause of chloride depletion, as, for example, within the duration of therapeutic action of administered diuretics or in severe chronic potassium depletion (plasma potassium < 2.4 mEq per liter); in the latter instance chloride will not be retained until repletion of potassium is initiated. Unless these rather unusual circumstances of renal chloride wasting are present, or the patient is ingesting

TABLE 1 Causes and Treatment of Maintained Elevation of Plasma Bicarbonate on Chronic Metabolic Alkalosis

Mechanism	*Causes of Maintained Elevation of Plasma HCO_3*	*Therapeutic Options*
Chloride depletion (chronic vomiting)*	Chloride depletion Continuing H^+loss	Replace chloride as NaCl, KCl, or HCl Cimetidine
	Ineffective CBV	Improve cardiac output; acetazolamide
	Moderately depressed GFR Severely depressed GFR (at least temporarily irreversible)	NaCl; restore ECF or cardiac output HCl; dialysis against high chloride dialysate
Potassium depletion—mineralocorticoid excess (Bartter's syndrome)	Potassium depletion (depresses GFR and increases tubule reabsorption of bicarbonate)	Discontinue diuretic; KCl; amiloride, triamterene or spironolactone; indomethacin; magnesium repletion
With hypertension (primary aldosteronism)	Excess mineralo- and/or glucocorticoid activity	Low-NaCl diet—remove adenoma Spironolactone (primary aldosteronism); Treat hypertension—KCl Spironolactone (secondary aldosteronism); Pituitary surgery or irradiation Remove ACTH-producing tumor or adrenal tumor—metyrapone or aminoglutethimide (Cushing's syndrome)
Base loading (multiple blood transfusions)	Administration of $NaHCO_3$ or its precursors (e.g., citrate) *plus* bicarbonate-maintaining cause	Stop base; correct underlying cause (above)
With hypercalcemia and hypoparathyroidism (milk-alkali syndrome)	Depression of GFR and enhanced tubular reabsorption of bicarbonate	Stop high intake of base and calcium; replete chloride and ECF volume deficit

* Example of clinical cause CBV=circulating blood volume; GFR=glomerular filtration rate; ECF=extracellular fluid volume

diuretics surreptitiously, a urinary chloride concentration greater than 20 mEq per liter usually suggests that therapy other than chloride repletion is necessary.

Metabolic alkalosis is often also associated with increased urinary potassium excretion, and a urinary potassium concentration of greater than 30 mEq per liter despite hypokalemia would be anticipated unless potassium depletion is profound, i.e., greater than a 500-mEq deficit in an adult man of average weight. In such circumstances urinary potassium concentration may be less than 20 to 30 mEq per liter and yet potassium depletion may be a major contributory cause of the metabolic alkalosis. Primary potassium losses from the bowel, as in laxative abuse or villous adenoma of the colon, are also associated with low urinary potassium concentrations.

A urinary sodium concentration of greater than 20 to 30 mEq per liter is unusual in chloride depletion alkalosis, especially when urinary pH is acidic (less than 5.5) as is customary when the kidney is conserving bicarbonate. In acute-on-chronic vomiting, as the plasma bicarbonate concentration is further elevated above its chronic stable high plasma level, transient renal wasting of sodium bicarbonate may occur. This clinical state is sometimes termed disequilibrium metabolic alkalosis. In such patients urinary sodium concentration may be greater than 20 mEq per liter—even in the presence of overt clinical volume depletion—but the urine is quite alkaline, i.e., the pH is above 6.5 and contains significant amounts of bicarbonate.

If the kidney function is severely depressed and the glomerular filtration rate (GFR) cannot be improved by increasing cardiac output or improving effective circulating blood volume, some form of dialysis using a dialysate with a chloride concentration significantly above that in the patient's plasma may be necessary (see Table 1).

Patients who have alkalosis due to mineralocorticoid excess-potassium depletion can be subdivided into those with a normal or low blood pressure and plasma volume and those with extracellular fluid (ECF) volume expansion and high blood pressure (see Table 1). In the former case, mineralocorticoid excess is associated with renal wasting of sodium chloride and hence an inability to develop hypertension. In the latter case, an intact kidney responds to mineralocorticoid excess with both sodium chloride retention and potassium loss.

A particularly vexing therapeutic problem is posed by those patients who can best be described as falling into the group of the differential diagnosis of Bartter's syndrome (Table 2). Bartter's syndrome is thus important beyond its frequency of occurrence because it illustrates the pathophysiology and treatment of the several much more common conditions listed in Table 1. It further illustrates how several mechanisms may interact with one another to maintain an elevated plasma bicarbonate concentration. The syndrome is characterized by normotension; a tendency to renal sodium, chloride, and potassium wasting; and marked stimulation of the renin-aldosterone system and of renal prostaglandin (Pg) production. Some cases are familial and develop in childhood although the syndrome may also be diagnosed for the first time in adult life. One plausible explanation for the syndrome is a defect in sodium chloride reabsorption in the thick ascending limb of the loop of Henle with increased delivery of sodium and fluid to the more distal potassium secretory sites.

TABLE 2 Differential Diagnosis of Bartter's Syndrome

Diagnosis	*Comment*
Diuretic abuse	Low urine chloride when not ingesting diuretics
Bulimia	Low urine chloride; disequilibrium metabolic alkalosis may occur (see text)
Laxative abuse	Metabolic alkalosis usually not severe
Magnesium depletion	May complicate diuretic abuse or Bartter's syndrome
Bartter's syndrome	High urinary chloride

Potassium loss is accelerated by both macula densa and baroreceptor stimuli for renin release and the resultant hyperaldosteronism. Potassium depletion stimulates renal synthesis of PgE_2, which in turn further impairs sodium chloride reabsorption in the thick ascending limb and sets up a vicious circle. Diuretic abuse, which may be strenuously and continually denied by the usually female patient, mimics the syndrome by impairing sodium chloride transport in the thick ascending limb of the loop of Henle (furosemide) or in the cortical diluting segment (thiazides). Urinary chloride concentration will be high in diuretic abuse only within the therapeutic duration of action of the drug. Bulimia can also mimic the syndrome, but urinary chloride concentrations in patients with this condition will usually be low during the metabolic alkalosis. Therapy is obvious in the case of diuretic abuse or bulimia once the diagnosis is made, but expert psychiatric help may be needed.

SPECIFIC THERAPY

Chloride Repletion

For full correction of metabolic alkalosis the chloride deficit must be replaced, usually intravenously. Judicious selection of the accompanying cation—sodium, potassium, or hydrogen ion—depends on careful assessment of (1) ECF volume status and the presence or absence of cardiac failure, (2) the presence and degree of associated potassium depletion, and (3) the degree of impairment and reversibility of the depression of the GFR. If the kidney is capable of excreting sodium and/or potassium, it will excrete bicarbonate with those cations and thus rapidly correct the metabolic alkalosis as chloride is made available. When renal function is too severely depressed by acute or chronic intrinsic renal disease, however, or when there is intractable congestive cardiac failure, especially with hyperkalemia, administration of chloride with sodium or potassium may not be feasible. There are two therapeutic strategies in such situations: infuse chloride as hydrochloric acid (HCl), or provide chloride by dialysis across the peritoneal or hemodialysis membrane so that potassium status, sodium status, and plasma volume can be contemporaneously corrected. An additional indication for HCl is when speed of correction is essential and there is doubt about the capacity of the kidney to excrete bicarbonate rapidly enough. Hydrochloric acid administration is discussed further below and in Table 3.

Administration of isotonic sodium chloride is the preferred therapy if, as is most commonly the case, there is associated ECF volume depletion. This will simultaneously correct the chloride deficit, the ECF volume deficit, and the associated depression in GFR. Even though, as discussed, repletion of potassium is not essential for the correction of the alkalosis, potassium administration is usually indicated because some degree of potassium depletion is usually present and because kaliuresis may occur as plasma volume, GFR, and urinary flow rate are restored to normal. Potassium can be provided conveniently by adding potassium chloride (KCl) to isotonic saline in a concentration of 10 to 20 mEq per liter. In most patients with overt signs of volume contraction, such as hypotension (including posteral hypotension), tachycardia and diminished skin turgor, administration of 3 to 5 L of 0.15 M sodium chloride (NaCl) is necessary to correct volume deficits and metabolic alkalosis. The physician must also include replacement of ongoing losses in the fluid and electrolyte replacement schedule. As the chloride deficit is corrected a brisk alkaline diuresis should occur with a fall in plasma bicarbonate concentration. This alkaline diuresis may increase urinary potassium losses and reinforces the point of concurrently replacing potassium to avoid the effects of hypokalemia.

When the extracellular fluid volume is assessed as normal, total body chloride deficit in milliequivalents can be estimated by the formula: body weight $\times$ 0.2 $\times$ the desired increment in the plasma chloride concentration. If there is associated hypokalemia, as is customary, the deficit can be repleted conveniently by either oral or intravenous KCl.

Some recent animal studies in our laboratories suggest that chloride depletion, independent of volume depletion, may contribute not only to maintenance of chronic metabolic alkalosis, but also to reduction in GFR and stimulation of the renin-aldosterone system. This may explain the occasional patients we have seen with hypochloremic metabolic alkalosis, hypertension in the recumbent position, and a significant elevation of serum creatinine, but without overt sodium or volume depletion. In such patients—but not as yet under study conditions of metabolic balance—administration of KCI alone has not been associated with restoration of a normal serum creatinine level, amelioration of hypertension, and correction of both potassium deficits and alkalosis; potassium depletion by itself, even when quite severe, is associated with

TABLE 3 Indications for Hydrochloric Acid Administration

Arterial pH >7.55 and contraindication of NaCl or KCl administration

Need for immediate amelioration of metabolic alkalosis because of:
- Hepatic encephalopathy
- Cardiac arrhythmia
- Digitalis intoxication
- CNS effect of high arterial pH
- Arterial pH >7.60 when initial renal response to NaCl or KCl or acetazolamide is likely to be sluggish or is in doubt

only a slight to moderate depression of GFR. Our studies suggest that chloride depletion leads to depression of GFR in part via activated tubuloglomerular feedback and to stimulation of renin release from the kidney by a macula densa mechanism.

In the clinical setting of ECF volume overload and/or congestive cardiac failure in association with chloride depletion and metabolic alkalosis, administration of NaCl is clearly inadvisable. As in euvolemic patients, hypokalemia may facilitate repletion of chloride as KCl, but KCl may also be contraindicated either because of concurrent hyperkalemia or concern about the ability to deal with the potassium load in the presence of renal failure. If renal function is still reasonable in this situation (serum creatinine less than 4 mg per deciliter), the use of acetazolamide in a dosage of 250 mg two or three times daily can be considered. Such a situation is exemplified by a patient with an acute exacerbation of chronic lung disease and cor pulmonale who develops metabolic alkalosis after therapeutic reduction in $PaCO_2$ in the presence of hyperkalemia. If acetazolamide is used in a patient without hyperkalemia, KCl should be concurrently administered because the risk of developing hypokalemia during the ensuing alkaline diuresis is high. Acetazolamide should be stopped when the plasma bicarbonate concentration approaches baseline levels for that patient, and plasma electrolyte composition should be followed daily during its administration.

When the kidney is incapable of responding to chloride repletion or when dialysis is necessary for the control of renal failure, exchange of bicarbonate for chloride across the semipermeable membrane used during hemodialysis or peritoneal dialysis is an effective mechanism for correcting metabolic alkalosis. Current routine dialysate solutions for both peritoneal dialysis (including continuous ambulatory peritoneal dialysis) and hemodialysis contain concentrations of bicarbonate or its metabolic precursors, such as acetate, equivalent to 35 mEq per liter and thus must be modified in circumstances of metabolic alkalosis. In an emergency, peritoneal dialysis can be performed against solutions of 0.15 M NaCl with appropriate maintenance of plasma potassium, calcium, and magnesium concentration by intravenous infusion. Most large hospital pharmacies, however, can prepare appropriate special dialysate solutions for both hemodialysis and peritoneal dialysis in these circumstances.

The indications for the use of intravenous HCl administration are given in Table 3. Again, most hospital pharmacies are capable of making up sterile HCl as 100 or 200 mEq per liter (i.e., a 0.1 or 0.2 M solution). The amount of HCl (in milliequivalents) needed to correct alkalosis is calculated by the formula: 0.5 $\times$ body weight (kg) $\times$ desired decrement in plasma bicarbonate concentration (mEq per liter). Since the goal of such therapy is to get the patient out of the danger zone in terms of acid-base balance, it is usually prudent to plan initially to restore the plasma bicarbonate concentration halfway toward normal. The HCl must be given through a catheter placed in the vena cava or a large vein draining into it, and placement of the catheter must be confirmed radiographically, since extravasation of HCl can lead to sloughing of the mediastinal tissues. The rate of infusion should not exceed 0.2 mEq per kilogram of body weight per hour. The patient is best managed in an intensive care unit with frequent measurement of arterial blood gases and electrolytes. The formula above does not allow for ongoing loss of hydrogen ion or gain of base by the extracellular fluid. An alternative to HCI is ammonium chloride, which may be administered via a peripheral vein. The rate of nfusion should not provide more than 300 mEq NH_4 + per 24 hours, and ammonium chloride should be avoided in the presence of renal or hepatic insufficiency. We limit the use of HCI to the listed indications (see Table 3), but prefer it in such circumstances to NH_4CI. The latter is certainly contraindicated in patients with liver or renal failure. The HCI salts of cationic amino acids lysine or arginine may also be used; however, great caution should be exercised, as these compounds cause a significant shift of K^+ from intracellular to extracellular compartment and may be associated with dangerous hyperkalemia. Again, we prefer HCI.

Additional therapeutic approaches are necessary in the following clinical situations associated with chloride depletion metabolic alkalosis. In the presence of pernicious vomiting or the surgical requirement for continual removal of gastric secretions, metabolic alkalosis will continue to be generated and replacement of preexisting deficits may be complicated by these ongoing losses. In these circumstances the administration of an H_2 receptor blocker, such as cimetidine or ranitidine, will blunt acid production of the stomach and decrease gastric HCl losses. Fairly high doses of cimetidine may be required, e.g., as much as 200 to 600 mg of intravenous cimetidine every 4 hours. Because serious side effects such as acute confusion can complicate these dose levels, it is reasonable to check the pH of the gastric aspirate to determine the lowest effective dose. Even in the presence of achlorhydria, however, gastric secretions will contain significant amounts of sodium, potassium, and chloride.

While diarrhea is normally associated with metabolic acidosis, in two circumstances metabolic alkalosis can occur in association with increased fecal loss of fluid. About 20 percent of villous adenomas are associated with alkalosis; these require surgical removal after correction of the sodium chloride, potassium, and volume deficits. The second condition is the rare familial disease of chloridorrhea in which massive amounts of chloride, potassium, and fluid are secreted into the ileum because of a transport defect. This condition has been responsive only to continued repletion of these losses by supplementation of the dietary intake.

POTASSIUM DEPLETION-MINERALOCORTICOID EXCESS

Severe potassium depletion is associated with a mild to moderate metabolic alkalosis in man unless there is complicating chloride depletion or mineralocorticoid excess, in which circumstances severe metabolic alkalosis may occur. In the presence of normotension the differential diagnosis of Bartter's syndrome (see Table 2) usually will provide the cause of metabolic alkalosis. Thiazide or loop diuretics should be stopped. Oral KCl given in the liquid form diluted with fruit juice or as the slow release form can be given in doses up to 40 to 60 mEq four or five times per day. If serious effects of potassium depletion and/or metabolic alkalosis are present, such as cardiac arrhythmias or muscle paralysis, intravenous KCl may be given at rates as high as 40 mEq per hour in concentrations not to exceed 60 mEq per liter. These are high rates and should be employed only where life-threatening hypokalemia and/or metabolic alkalosis is present; the patient should be monitored by electrocardiogram and frequent determinations of plasma potassium concentration (Table 4). It is critical that the solution used to administer potassium or the solution given immediately *prior* to the administration of potassium—for example, in the emergency room—not contain glucose, since this may stimulate insulin secretion and cause hypokalemia to worsen. Once potassium repletion is clearly under way, the presence of glucose in the infusion may facilitate cellular potassium repletion, but hypokalemic nephropathy may impair free water excretion and plasma sodium concentration should also be monitored if a free water load is being administered.

Because Bartter's syndrome probably comprises several disorders with different pathophysiologies, the degree to which other solute deficiencies, such as sodium, chloride, magnesium, or calcium deficiencies, occur in or contribute to the disorder varies. Nevertheless, the principal goal of therapy is to prevent the loss of excessive potassium in the urine. Potassium-sparing diuretics (amiloride, 5 or 10 mg daily; triamterene, 100 mg twice a day; or spironolactone, 25 to 50 mg four times a day) are effective for this purpose, but dietary potassium supplementation is often also needed. Spironolactone may produce tender gynecomastia in men. Renal production of PgE_2 is increased and may contribute to sodium, chloride, and potassium wasting; Pg synthetase inhibitors such as indomethacin or ibuprofen may blunt, but usually do not completely correct, the hypokalemic alkalosis. Because magnesium depletion may increase urinary potassium wasting, an attempt should be made to correct hypomagnesemia and replete magnesium stores. However, the degree to which the correction of magnesium depletion blunts the alkalosis is uncertain, and magnesium salts usually produce an unacceptable degree of gastrointestinal irritation that may compound the patient's problems. Oral magnesium oxide can be given as 250 to 500 mg four times daily (12.5 to 25 mEq Mg). If severe hypomagnesemia is contributing to seizures or tetany, 4 ml of a 50 percent solution of magnesium sulfate (16 mEq Mg) can be given in 100 ml of 5 percent glucose over 10 to 20 minutes. Finally, there are recent preliminary reports of the possible value of the administration of captopril or enalapril to reduce the production of angiotensin II and hence the hyperaldosteronism.

TABLE 4 Estimation of Potassium Deficit

*Corrected Plasma Potassium Concentration (mEq/L)**	*Approximate Total Body Postassium Deficit*	
	%	*Total (mEq)†*
3–3.5	5	100–200
2.5–3.0	5–10	200–400
2–2.5	10–15	300–600
<2.0	15–20+	500–800+

* Increase plasma K by 0.6 mEq per 0.1 increment in arterial pH.
† For 70-kg man

In the group of alkaloses characterized by an excess of mineralocorticoid, therapy is directed at either removal of the source or blockade of the mineralocorticoid. Hypertension, often severe, may complicate many of these disorders and specific therapy for this is discussed in other chapters. Since mineralocorticoids directly and indirectly stimulate potassium and hydrogen ion secretion (equivalent to bicarbonate reabsorption) in the distal convoluted tubule and collecting duct (in part in exchange for sodium), the administration of potassium-sparing diuretics will effectively reverse the adverse effects of mineralocorticoid excess on sodium, potassium, and bicarbonate.

The stimulation of net sodium reabsorption and potassium secretion by the effect of excess mineralocorticoid on the kidney may also be ameliorated by adjustments to diet. If hypokalemia and potassium depletion develop, as is common, bicarbonate reabsorption in the proximal tubule of the kidney is stimulated and alkalosis is further intensified. In contrast, the stimulated sodium reabsorption produces volume expansion which tends to diminish fluid and HCO_3 reabsorption in the proximal tubule; however, as noted, distal bicarbonate reabsorption is stimulated by the mineralocorticoid. Thus, the restriction of sodium and the addition of potassium to the diet should aid in the control of the alkalosis as well as the hypertension that often accompanies these disorders.

Many primary disorders of mineralocorticoid excess are definitively treated by tumor ablation. Adrenocorticotropic hormone-secreting pituitary tumors may be removed by transsphenoidal resection or ablated by irradiation. With adrenal tumors, adrenalectomy, either unilateral or bilateral as appropriate, is curative. In the ectopic adrenocorticotropic hormone syndrome, the ideal treatment of the secreting tumor can rarely be accomplished. In this instance and in metastatic adrenal tumors, metyrapone, which inhibits the final step in cortisol synthesis, and aminoglutethimide, which inhibits the initial step in steroid biosynthesis, will blunt the myriad manifestations of excess cortisol. In those disorders in which curative surgery cannot be carried out, mitotane (p,p-DDD), which produces selective destruction of the zona fasciculata and reticularis and leaves aldosterone production intact, has also been used to control effectively many of the manifestations of the disease. To the extent that severe fluid and electrolyte disturbances are due to aldosterone production, this drug may not suffice. Thus, metyrapone or aminoglutethimide may be better choices when hypokalemic alkalosis is present. Cisplatin has also recently been used in the treatment of adrenal malignancies. A detailed discussion of the use of such drugs is beyond the scope of this review.

Among the alkaloses associated with excess exogenous base administration, the milk-alkali syndrome, characterized by metabolic alkalosis, hypercalcemia, and renal insufficiency, is now infrequently seen. Cessation of alkali ingestion and the calcium sources (often milk and calcium carbonate) and chloride and volume repletion for the commonly associated vomiting usually will lead to the prompt resolution of all abnormalities. Occasional occult sources of base loading are citrate in blood transfusions or release of base by metastases in bone.

METABOLIC ACIDOSIS

THOMAS D. DuBOSE Jr., M.D.

Metabolic acidosis occurs as a result of a marked increase in endogenous production of acid (such as lactic and ketoacids), loss of bicarbonate stores (diarrhea or renal tubule acidosis), or progressive accumulation of endogenous acids, the excretion of which is impaired because of renal insufficiency.

Predicting Respiratory Compensation

The most commonly encountered form of metabolic acidosis is "simple" or pure metabolic acidosis. More complicated clinical situations, especially in severely ill patients, may give rise to "mixed" forms of metabolic acidosis, that is, metabolic acidosis not in a pure or simple form, but occurring in combination with any of the other types of acid-base disorders (respiratory acidosis or alkalosis and metabolic alkalosis). To distinguish "simple" from "mixed" metabolic acidosis, the limits of predictable physiologic compensation must be appreciated.

To illustrate, metabolic acidosis as a result of gain of endogenous acids (e.g., diabetic ketoacidosis) will lower the concentration of bicarbonate in extracellular fluid and will lower extracellular pH. As a result of the prevailing acidemia, the medullary chemoreceptors will be stimulated and invoke an increase in ventilation. Thus, the ratio of HCO_3^- to $PaCO_2$ and the subsequent pH will be returned toward, but not completely to, normal. The degree of ventilatory compensation expected in simple metabolic acidosis can be predicted from the relationship:

$$PaCO_2 = (1.5 \times HCO_3^-) + 8 \pm 2$$

Therefore, a patient with metabolic acidosis attributable to ketoacidosis with a plasma bicarbonate concentration of 12 mEq per liter would be expected to have a $PaCO_2$ between 24 and 28 mm Hg. Values for $PaCO_2$ below 24 or greater than 28 mm Hg define a "mixed" disturbance (metabolic acidosis plus respiratory alkalosis, or metabolic acidosis plus respiratory acidosis, respectively). A $PaCO_2$ in or near the normal range indicates a failure of the compensatory response and defines the presence of a superimposed respiratory disturbance.

The serum potassium concentration should also be measured, but considered only in conjunction with knowledge of the bicarbonate concentration and blood pH. It is generally appreciated that the serum potassium concentration can be altered by primary acid-base disturbances as a result of shifts of K^+ into either the extracellular compartment or intracellular compartment (see also the chapter *Mixed Acid-Base Disturbances*). For each decrement in blood pH equal to 0.10 pH units, the plasma potassium concentration should increase by 0.6 mEq per liter. Thus, a patient with a pH of 7.20 would be expected to have a serum potassium level of 5.2 mEq per liter. However, considerable variation in this relationship has been reported in several conditions, especially diabetic ketoacidosis, which is often associated with potassium depletion. The lack of correlation between the degree of acidemia and the plasma potassium level is a result of several factors, including the nature of the accompanying anion, the magnitude of the osmotic diuresis, the level of renal function, the plasma osmolality, concomitant insulin deficiency, and the degree of catabolism. The failure of a patient with severe metabolic acidosis to exhibit hyperkalemia suggests a significant derangement of body potassium homeostasis.

The serum chloride concentration is often extremely useful in the evaluation of acid-base disturbances. It is helpful to compare the level of chloride with the level of sodium in plasma. The plasma sodium concentration changes only as a result of changes in hydration. The plasma chloride concentration changes for two reasons: changes in hydration, and changes in acid-base balance. Thus, changes in chloride not reflected by proportional changes in sodium suggest the presence of an acid-base disorder. For example, consider a patient with a history of vomiting, volume depletion, a plasma chloride concentration of 85 mEq and a plasma sodium concentration of 130 mEq per liter. In this case, both sodium and chloride are reduced, but the reduction in chloride is proportionally greater (15 percent versus 7 percent). A disproportional decrease in chloride suggests metabolic alkalosis or respiratory acidosis, while a disproportional increase in chloride suggest metabolic acidosis or respiratory alkalosis.

Types of Metabolic Acidosis

All evaluations of acid-base disorders should include a simple calculation of the "anion gap." The anion gap (AG) is defined as follows:

$$AG = Na^+ - (Cl^- + HCO_3^-)$$
$$AG = 10 \pm 2 \text{ mEq/L}$$

The anion gap represents those unmeasured anions normally present in plasma and is equal to 10 mEq per liter (range 8 to 12 mEq per liter). The anions normally present include anionic proteins, phosphate, sulfate, and organic anions. When acid anions, such as acetoacetate and lactate, accumulate in extracellular fluid, the anion gap increases above the normal value. This is referred to as an "anion-gap acidosis." In this form of metabolic acidosis, for each milliequivalent per liter increase in the AG, there should be an equal decrease in the plasma bicarbonate concentration.

In a pure or simple anion gap acidosis, the increase in the anion gap above the normal value (δ AG = AG of patient − 10 mEq per liter) should be approximately equal to the decrease in HCO_3^- below the normal value ($\delta\ HCO_3^-$ = 26 mEq per liter − [HCO_3^-] of patient), i.e., $\delta\ AG = \delta\ HCO_3^-$. In mixed acid-base disorders this relationship does not hold. For example, a patient with diabetic ketoacidosis and protracted vomiting may present with an elevated anion gap that exceeds the bicarbonate deficit ($\delta\ AG > \delta\ HCO_3^-$). This patient's disorder should be considered a mixed acid-base disturbance (metabolic acidosis plus metabolic alkalosis). Consideration of this problem would obviously alter the therapeutic approach to the patient, since bicarbonate therapy would be contraindicated and intravenous fluid replacement with larger quantities of isotonic saline might be necessary.

The second major type of metabolic acidosis, which is not associated with alteration of the anion gap, is referred to as a hyperchloremic acidosis. If, for example, the acid entering extracellular fluid is HCl, then one mole of Cl will be retained for each mole of HCO_3^- consumed, and the anion gap will not change while the chloride concentration will increase proportionally. Alkali may be lost from the gastrointestinal tract (diarrhea) or from the kidneys (renal tubular acidosis). In these disorders, reciprocal changes in chloride and bicarbonate leave the anion gap unchanged. In a pure form of simple hyperchloremic acidosis, therefore, the increase in chloride above the normal value ($\delta\ Cl^-$ should be equal to the arithmetic decrease in bicarbonate ($\delta\ HCO_3^-$). The absence of such a relationship suggests a mixed disturbance. For example, in a patient with classic distal renal tubular acidosis (type I) in which volume depletion and hypokalemia become severe, lactic acidosis may develop and the fall in bicarbonate will exceed the rise in chloride ($\delta\ HCO_3^- > \delta\ Cl^-$). Furthermore, in this example, lactic acidosis would result in an increase in the anion gap (mixed hyperchloremic plus high anion gap acidosis).

The increase in ventilation expected as a compensatory response in metabolic acidosis has been emphasized earlier. As mentioned previously, the failure of the patient's $PaCO_2$ to fall to the predicted level suggests a concomitant respiratory acidosis, while a value for $PaCO_2$ lower than the prediction suggests a concomitant respiratory alkalosis as indicated by equation 1.

Once these simple calculations have been performed, the clinician should be able to determine if a pure or simple anion gap or hyperchloremic acidosis exists. A knowledge of the history should allow the patient's specific disorder to be determined. Further information is obtained by demonstration of ketosis by the serum Acetest level, or by determination of the lactate level, the blood urea nitrogen or creatinine, or a toxicology screen.

General Principles of Treatment of Metabolic Acidosis

It has been emphasized in most general texts that treatment of metabolic acidosis with alkali therapy should be reserved for severe acidemia only. This dictum is clearly incorrect in the situation in which the patient has no "potential bicarbonate" in plasma. Potential bicarbonate can be estimated from the increment in the anion gap (δ AG = patient's AG minus 10). Next it must be established if the acid anion in plasma is metabolizable (i.e., beta-hydroxybutyrate, acetoacetate, lactate) or nonmetabolizable (anions that accumulate in chronic renal failure). The latter variety requires normal renal function and renal ammoniagenesis to replenish the bicarbonate deficit, a slow and often unpredictable process. Therefore, patients with no anion gap (hyperchloremic acidosis), a small anion gap (mixed hyperchloremic and anion gap acidosis), or an anion gap attributable to a nonmetabolizable anion in the face of renal insufficiency all require alkali therapy (Table 1). It has recently been reported that as many as 52 percent of patients with diabetic ketoacidosis will have a hyperchloremic component to their metabolic acidosis on admission. Moreover, after 4 to 8 hours of standard therapy, not including sodium bicarbonate, the percentage may increase to 90 percent. Thus, as emphasized by such findings, the "potential bicarbonate" (δ AG) must be assessed and alkali administered when the available potential bicarbonate is insufficient to correct the metabolic acidosis to a near normal bicarbonate (i.e., δ AG+patient's bicarbonate concentration = predicted new bicarbonate concentration). For example, a patient with diabetic ketoacidosis, a plasma bicarbonate concentration of 5.0, a pH of 7.11, an anion gap of 17, and a chloride of 110 has a mixed hyperchloremic-anion gap acidosis, insufficient potential bicarbonate to repair the bicarbonate deficit, and will therefore require sodium bicarbonate therapy.

Patients with metabolic acidosis attributable to loss of bicarbonate from the gastrointestinal tract (diarrhea) or kidney (renal tubular acidosis) and a pure hyperchloremic metabolic acidosis should obviously receive alkali therapy.

Controversy exists, however, with regard to the use of alkali therapy in patients with a pure anion gap acidosis owing to accumulation of a metabolizable organic acid anion (ketoacidosis or lactic acidosis). In general, severe acidosis ($pH < 7.15$) always warrants a small amount of sodium bicarbonate initially. The arguments against the use of bicarbonate in more modest degrees of acidosis include: (1) the potential for salt and volume overload, (2) hypokalemia, (3) central nervous system acidosis, (4)

TABLE 1 Treatment of Metabolic Acidosis

Type of Acidosis	*Treatment*	
	Specific	*Ancillary*
Anion gap acidosis		
Diabetic ketoacidosis	Volume replacement, insulin	K^+, HCO_3^-
Alcoholic ketoacidosis	Volume replacement, glucose	PO_4
Lactic acidosis	Treat underlying disease, HCO_3^-	DCA, hemodialysis
Methanol ingestion	Ethanol, HCO_3^- dialysis	HCO_3^-
Ethylene glycol ingestion	Ethanol, HCO_3^- dialysis	HCO_3^-, thiamine
Salicylate intoxication	Diuresis, HCO_3^-, charcoal	Acetazolamide
Chronic renal failure	HCO_3^-	Renal replacement therapy
Hyperchloremic acidosis		
Hypokalemia		
GI loss of bicarbonate	Volume, HCO_3^-, K^+	—
Proximal RTA (II)	HCO_3^-, volume, K^+	Thiazide diuretic, vitamin D, PO_4
Distal RTA (I)	HCO_3^-	$\pm K^+$
Hyperkalemia		
Type IV RTA	±Fludrocortisone, furosemide	HCO_3^-, Exchange resins

hypercapnia, (5) tissue hypoxia, (6) alkali stimulation of endogenous organic acid production, (7) "overshoot" alkalosis, (8) mortality data, and (9) results in experimental animals. Many of these arguments have been greatly overemphasized and overinterpreted, however. Arguments for bicarbonate therapy include: (1) knowledge of the detrimental cardiovascular effects of acidosis, (2) the frequency of mixed hyperchloremic and anion-gap acidosis, (3) the fact that severe metabolic acidosis sensitizes pH to small additional changes in bicarbonate concentration or $PaCO_2$, (4) improved response to pressor agents, and (5) restoration of more physiologic pH.

As blood pH is reduced below 7.20, the decrease in myocardial contractility predisposes patients with metabolic acidosis to congestive heart failure, so a pH of 7.20 is a reasonable therapeutic end point. Bicarbonate should be given in amounts that increase pH to this value. Elderly patients or patients receiving beta-blockers seem to be more sensitive and may require a more normal pH to prevent heart failure (pH 7.25). Thus, addition of modest amounts of alkali in the treatment of the organic acidoses seems to provide an added measure of safety that could be lifesaving. Obviously, there is no substitute for carefully monitoring the plasma electrolytes during the course of therapy for these disorders so that therapy can be modified as needed.

Lactic acidosis may be an exception to the approach endorsed above. That exogenous bicarbonate can improve the reduction in bicarbonate in many forms of lactic acidosis has been widely accepted. The massive amounts of bicarbonate that are often employed, however, have never been demonstrated to improve survival and may increase morbidity and mortality. Thus, the amount of bicarbonate administered should be the smallest that can achieve a significant increase in the plasma bicarbonate concentration—which obviously can be established only by trial and error. Isolated case reports and studies in experimental models of lactic acidosis suggest that bicarbonate therapy may *increase* rather than *decrease* lactate production. Dichloracetate, which enhances the oxidation of lactate, has been shown to reduce lactate levels in diabetic patients and to improve survival in hypoxic lactic acidosis in dogs when compared with bicarbonate alone. Clearly, these exciting findings warrant further human studies.

DIABETIC KETOACIDOSIS

Ketoacidosis develops because of insulin deficiency in conjunction with elevated glucagon levels. Metabolic acidosis from ketoacids (plasma ketones > 2.0 mmol per liter) is usually observed in conjunction with an elevated anion gap and a poorly controlled diabetic state (glucose > 300 mg per deciliter).

Treatment

A frequently updated, carefully maintained, and accurate flow sheet is essential in the treatment of diabetic ketoacidosis and allows rapid response by the physician to changes in the patient's clinical status.

Volume Therapy

Most, if not all, patients with diabetic ketoacidosis require correction of the volume depletion which almost invariably accompanies the osmotic diuresis and ketoacidosis. The serum sodium concentration may be arithmetically corrected for the degree of hyperglycemia to determine the type of intravenous fluid needed (i.e., correct Na^+ by 1.8 mEq per liter for each 100 mg per deciliter increment in plasma glucose). In general, it seems prudent to initiate therapy with isotonic saline at a rate of 1,000 ml intravenously per hour. When the pulse and blood pressure have stabilized and the corrected serum sodium concentration is in the range of 130 to 135 mEq per liter, switch to 0.45 percent NaCl. Ringer's lactate should be avoided. If the blood sugar slips below 300 mg per deciliter, 0.45 percent NaCl with 5 percent dextrose should be administered.

Insulin Therapy

Low-dose insulin therapy (0.1 units per kilogram per hour) smoothly corrects the biochemical abnormalities and minimizes hypoglycemia and hypokalemia. Regular insulin may also be administered intramuscularly (0.2 mg per kilogram initially, then 6 units every hour).

Potassium

Total body potassium depletion is usually present although the potassium level on admission may be elevated or normal. Since the plasma potassium concentration should increase 0.6 mEq per liter for each 0.1 unit decline in arterial blood pH, a normal or reduced [K^+] on admission indicates severe potassium depletion and should be approached with caution. Administration of fluid, insulin, and alkali may cause the potassium level to plummet. When the urine output has been established, 20 mEq KCl should be administered in each liter of fluid as long as the [K^+] is less than 4.0 mEq per liter. Equal caution should be exercised in the presence of hyperkalemia, especially if the patient has renal insufficiency, since the usual therapy will not always correct hyperkalemia. Never administer KCl empirically.

Alkali Therapy

The arguments for and against alkali therapy have been summarized above. The younger patient with a pure anion gap acidosis(δ AG = δ HCO_3^-) usually does not require exogenous alkali if the acidemia is not severe (< 7.15), since the metabolic acidosis should be entirely reversible. Elderly patients, patients with severe high anion gap acidosis, or patients with a hyperchloremic component should receive small amounts of sodium bicarbonate by slow intravenous infusion (2 ampules or 88 mEq over 60 minutes). Thirty minutes after this infusion is completed, arterial blood gases should be repeated. Alkali administration can be repeated if the pH is 7.15 or less, or if the patient exhibits a significant hyperchloremic component. Hypokalemia and other complications of alkali therapy dramatically increase when amounts of $NaHCO_3$ exceeding 400 mEq are administered. Therefore, the effect of alkali therapy on arterial blood pH needs to be reassessed regularly, and a total of no more than 200 mEq should be administered if possible.

Other Measures

The routine administration of phosphate (usually as potassium phosphate) is not advised because of the potential for hyperphosphatemia and hypocalcemia. Approximately 90 percent of patients with diabetic ketoacidosis will have significant hyperphosphatemia before initiation of therapy. In the volume-depleted, malnourished patient, however, a normal or elevated phosphate concentration on admission may be followed by a rapid fall in phosphate within 2 to 6 hours after initiation of therapy. I highly recommend that the serum phosphorus measurement be repeated during this interval to avoid severe hypophosphatemia. Observation of the patient in diabetic ketoacidosis cannot be left to the nursing staff. Fever is not associated with diabetic ketoacidosis unless a complication coexists, and therefore antibiotics should not be given prophylactically. Catheterize the bladder only if the patient is unable to cooperate and void spontaneously or if a large amount of residual urine is anticipated.

ALCOHOLIC KETOACIDOSIS

Chronic alcoholics may develop ketoacidosis when alcohol consumption is abruptly curtailed, usually as a result of vomiting, abdominal pain, starvation, and volume depletion. The glucose concentration is frequently low or normal, and the acidosis is frequently severe and because of elevated ketones, predominantly beta-hydroxybutyrate. Mild lactic acidosis may coexist because of alteration in the redox state. The nitroprusside ketone reaction (Acetest) can detect acetoacetic acid but not beta-hydroxybutyrate, so the initial degree of ketosis and ketonuria can be seriously underestimated. Treatment consists of intravenous volume repletion and glucose administration (5 percent dextrose in 0.9 percent NaCl, not saline alone). Hypophosphatemia, hypokalemia, and hypomagnesemia often occur. Hypophosphatemia usually emerges 12 to 24 hours after admission, so the need for therapy can be overlooked, especially if the serum phosphorus concentration on admission is normal. Profound hypophosphatemia may provoke rhabdomyolysis. Upper gastrointestinal hemorrhage, pancreatitis, and pneumonia may accompany this disorder. Recurrence is common. As the patient's general condition improves and serum ketone levels fall, the nitroprusside reaction may actually become more positive because of improvement in the redox state and a shift toward acetoacetate. This seeming worsening of the ketosis is a laboratory artifact.

LACTIC ACIDOSIS

Lactic acidosis has been classified into two types. Type A lactic acidosis is attributable to tissue hypoperfusion, shock, or hypoxia. Type B is associated with a host of diseases, drugs, toxins, and hereditary disorders. Tissue underperfusion is the most common underlying cause in hospitalized patients and prognosis is related to the degree of hyperlacticacidemia. Common causes of type B lactic acidosis include liver disease, sepsis, malignancy, and drug toxicity.

Treatment

The treatment of lactic acidosis must be directed toward reversal of the underlying pathophysiology. When the patient is extremely ill, monitoring of hemodynamics in an intensive care unit is extremely helpful to ensure aggressive fluid resuscitation. Peripheral vasodilators, such as nitroprusside, to increase oxygen delivery have been suggested, but are not recommended because of the difficulty encountered in use and the tendency to aggravate lactic acidosis at high concentrations. Methylene blue to improve the NADH/NAD^+ ratio has been generally unsuccessful. Dichloracetate, as mentioned in the section on general measures, has been shown to be beneficial in experimental lactic acidosis and in a few isolated patients. Long-term use is associated with serious neurologic disturbances. Sodium bicarbonate is frequently overused in lactic acidosis, since complete correction of the acidosis is attempted. The aggressive use of alkali carries significant risks of hypertonicity, volume overload, and even acceleration of lactate production. Sodium bicarbonate remains the mainstay of therapy when the pH is less than 7.15, however. Bicarbonate therapy alone will not improve tissue oxygenation or adenosine triphosphate generation, but protects against the harmful effects of extreme acidemia. Acute hemodialysis or peritoneal dialysis with bicarbonate dialysate is a convenient means of ensuring adequate bicarbonate delivery to the patient while avoiding volume overexpansion. Acetate or lactate dialysis is contraindicated.

TOXIN-ASSOCIATED ANION GAP ACIDOSIS

Methanol and ethanol are central nervous system depressants, but the intermediate metabolites are primarily responsible for the toxic manifestations observed after ingestion. The critical enzyme is alcohol dehydrogenase. Methanol can also be inhaled or absorbed, but is usually ingested as a cheap alternative to ethanol. Methanol ingestion results in optic nerve and central nervous system manifestations attributable to metabolism to formic acid. Lactic acid and ketoacids may also contribute to the metabolic acid. Typically the patient appears intoxicated and has an anion gap acidosis as well as an osmolar gap. The "osmolar gap" represents the difference in calculated and measured plasma osmolality and should always be obtained in cases of suspected toxin ingestion, since the assay for methanol or ethylene glycol is difficult and time consuming and may delay lifesaving measures. Ethylene glycol ingestion leads to metabolic acidosis, an osmolar gap, crystalluria (oxalate), and deposition of oxalate in brain, heart, and kidney.

Treatment

Treatment for both toxins involves the administration of ethanol to compete for alcohol dehydrogenase and thus block conversion to one of the toxic metabolites. Blood alcohol levels in excess of 100 mg per deciliter are necessary and can be achieved by either oral or intravenous loading. The oral loading dose is 0.6 g per kilogram as a 50 percent solution. When hemodialysis is initiated the ethanol maintenance dose should be increased from 154 mg per kilogram per hour to 250 mg per kilogram per hour.

Hemodialysis with bicarbonate, not acetate, as the buffer is effective and necessary in both methanol and ethylene glycol intoxication, since it corrects the acidosis and removes toxic by-products. The dialysance of toxic metabolites is not increased further by hemoperfusion. Additional measures include sodium bicarbonate (especially prior to initiation of dialysis), volume replacement, thiamine, and pyridoxine.

SALICYLATE INTOXICATION

Intoxication with salicylates in adults commonly results in an anion gap acidosis, a portion of which is owing to salicylic acid and the remainder to lactate and/or ketones. A mixed metabolic acidosis-respiratory alkalosis is observed frequently. Pulmonary edema and proteinuria may occur.

Treatment

The initial step in therapy should include vigorous gastric lavage or induced vomiting followed by activated charcoal administration. To facilitate removal of salicylate, intravenous sodium bicarbonate administration in amounts adequate to alkalinize the urine and to maintain urine output is required (urine pH > 7.5). While this form of therapy is straightforward in acidotic patients, alkalemia from a respiratory alkalosis may make this approach hazardous. Acetazolamide may be administered when an alkaline diuresis cannot be achieved, but it carries the danger of producing systemic metabolic acidosis. The systemic pH should never be allowed to fall into the acid range. Hypokalemia may occur as a result of an alkaline diuresis from sodium bicarbonate or acetazolamide and should be treated promptly. Glucose-containing fluids should be administered because of the danger of hypoglycemia. If renal failure prevents rapid clearance of salicylate, hemodialysis may be required, preferably with bicarbonate dialysate.

CHRONIC RENAL FAILURE

Renal failure may be associated with hyperchloremic metabolic acidosis or anion-gap acidosis. The latter disorder is seen only when the glomerular filtration rate is well below 20 ml per minute and is attributable to the retention of sulfate, phosphate, and other organic anions. Hyperchloremic metabolic acidosis occurs in a variety of renal diseases, more commonly tubulointerstitial disease, and the acidosis is always out of proportion to the degree of the renal insufficiency (glomerular filtration rate 20 to 70 ml per minute). The presence of hyperkalemia should suggest obstructive uropathy, sickle nephropathy, K^+-sparing diuretics, nonsteroidal anti-inflammatory drugs, beta-blockers, or captopril. With classic uremic acidosis the anion gap is rarely above 20 mEq per liter and the bicarbonate concentration rarely below 15 mEq per liter.

Treatment

Both uremic acidosis and hyperchloremic acidosis of renal insufficiency require oral alkali replacement to maintain the bicarbonate concentration near 20 mEq per liter. This can usually be accomplished with only 1.0 to 1.5 mEq per kilogram per day. Shohl's solution or sodium bicarbonate tablets are equally effective, but Shohl's solution may be better tolerated. Alternating the two on a daily or weekly basis may improve patient acceptance. Alkali therapy is necessary because bone serves as a major source of buffer in chronic stable acidosis. It is assumed that alkali replacement serves to prevent the harmful effects of prolonged positive hydrogen ion balance. When hyperkalemia is present, furosemide (60 to 80 mg per day) should be added, but fludrocortisone (0.1 to 0.2 mg per day) may be necessary on occasion. If the patient is hypertensive or volume expanded, fludrocortisone should be given only in conjunction with furosemide. An occasional patient may require chronic sodium polystyrene sulfonate (Kayexalate) therapy.

GASTROINTESTINAL LOSS OF BICARBONATE

Fecal, pancreatic, or biliary loss of bicarbonate causes hyperchloremic metabolic acidosis, volume depletion, and hypokalemia. Patients in whom ureterosigmoidostomy has been necessary may develop profound hypokalemic, hyperchloremic metabolic acidosis because of loss of Na^+, K^+, and HCO_3^- from the pouch. This occurs because of Cl^--HCO_3^- exchange in the colon which is accentuated in the face of stasis.

Treatment

Alkali, fluid, and potassium replacement are necessary, but must be appropriate for the patient's specific needs. Ureterosigmoidostomy patients who develop metabolic acidosis may require emergent therapy with volume, potassium, and bicarbonate, while mild forms of gastrointestinal bicarbonate loss can be corrected with oral Shohl's solution.

RENAL LOSS OF BICARBONATE

Renal tubular acidosis (RTA) can be defined as a clinical syndrome in which impaired acidification results in a hyperchloremic metabolic acidosis. Proximal RTA (type II) and classic distal RTA (type I are frequently associated with hypokalemia. In contrast, a unique disorder of the distal nephron associated with hypoaldosteronism or pseudoaldosteronism is recognized by the frequent occurrence of hyperkalemia (type IV RTA). Acetazolamide (Diamox) therapy always causes a mild metabolic acidosis which resembles mild proximal RTA and should be considered in the differential diagnosis.

Diagnosis and Treatment of Proximal Renal Tubular Acidosis

A patient with persistent hypokalemic-hyperchloremic metabolic acidosis should be suspected of having RTA. Patients receiving acetazolamide or Sulfamyalon may have electrolyte and urinary findings resembling those of proximal RTA and should be excluded. The presence of bicarbonate wasting with a near normal plasma bicarbonate (FE $HCO_3^- > 10$ to 15 percent), in the absence of nephrolithiasis and nephrocalcinosis strongly suggests proximal RTA. A maximally acid urine is expected in proxmial RTA during systemic acidosis, but is not present in distal RTA.

The magnitude of bicarbonate wasting serves as a rough guide to the amount of alkali therapy required. However, proximal RTA is often difficult to treat, especially if the goal is to replace the bicarbonate deficit totally. Large alkali loads, when needed, will result in additional K^+ wasting and hypokalemia. Therefore, alkali therapy ($NaHCO_3$ or Shohl's solution, 10 to 25 mEq per kilogram per day) is administered along with a thiazide diuretic and potassium supplementation. In patients with Fanconi's syndrome, oral phosphate therapy and vitamin D are required to reverse the skeletal abnormalities. These patients are in a tenuous state of acid-base and electrolyte balance and frequent monitoring is necessary.

Diagnosis and Treatment of Distal Renal Tubular Acidosis

The demonstration of a hypokalemic-hyperchloremic metabolic acidosis with a normal anion gap (10 to 12 mEq per liter) and an alkaline urine is diagnostic of distal RTA. If the urine pH is equivocal or if systemic acidosis is not present, an acid-loading test is necessary. In response to a documented fall in plasma HCO_3^- by 3 to 5 mEq per liter, the urine pH should fall below 5.5.

Patients with unrecognized distal RTA, hypokalemia, severe acidosis, and hypocalcemia may require immediate therapy. On occasion the hypokalemia is severe enough to cause paralysis and respiratory depression and should always be corrected prior to initiation of alkali therapy. Almost all patients with distal RTA (unlike proximal RTA) are able to take $NaHCO_3^-$ or bicarbonate precursors orally in amounts necessary to sustain correction of the acidosis. On average 1 to 2 mEq HCO_3^- per kilogram per day is sufficient in adults, while as much as 5 to 10 mEq per kilogram per day may be required in children. In most children with distal RTA the amount of alkali necessary will increase when growth increases, and maintenance of normal growth requires that adequate alkali therapy be provided to maintain a normal plasma HCO_3^-. In some patients, though not most, potassium supplement may be required even after the acidosis is corrected. One of the most common complications of distal RTA, especially with nephrocalcinosis, is pyelonephritis. Since the goal of therapy in distal RTA is to prevent the relentless progression of renal disease, this complication should be looked for frequently and treated as needed. Eradication of the causative organism may often be difficult, however.

The prognosis of well-managed patients is quite good, but is determined primarily by the severity of the underlying disease in acquired distal RTA. The glomerular filtration rate should be expected to stabilize and remain constant, with adequate alkali therapy even if initially reduced.

Renal Tubular Acidosis Associated With Hyperkalemia

Hyperchloremic metabolic acidosis is commonly associated with hyperkalemia in chronic diseases of the kidney that cause parenchymal damage and reduced glomerular filtration rate. In patients selected because of severe hyperkalemia (> 5.5 mEq per liter) diabetic nephropathy and tubulointerstitial disease are the most common accompanying disorders. Since the degree of hyperkalemia is far out of proportion to the reduction in glomerular filtration rate, a unique dysfunction of renal potassium and acid secretion is present and is most often attributable to selective hypoaldosteronism. Conversely, the disorder may be observed in patients with pseudohypoaldosteronism in the absence of significant renal insufficiency. In the former disorder most patients have hyporeninemic hypoaldosteronism and a marked reduction in urinary ammonium excretion. This defect appears to be a result of hyperkalemia which suppresses renal ammoniagenesis. The reduction in ammonium excretion causes metabolic acidosis. The reduced elaboration of aldosterone, or a failure of the collecting tubule to respond to normal levels of aldosterone, causes hyperkalemia by reducing K^+ secretion. Hypoaldosteronism also reduces acid secretion in the medullary collecting tubule directly. Therefore, the physiologic characteristics of this form of RTA would be predicted to occur in patients in whom aldosterone is either deficient in amount or in effect.

In hyperkalemic-hyperchloremic metabolic acidosis the underlying disease must be diagnosed. The decision to treat and the type of therapy are often based on the severity of the hyperkalemia. A reduction in serum potassium concentration often results in improvement of the metabolic acidosis. Patients with combined glucocorticoid and mineralocorticoid deficiency must receive both adrenal steroids in replacement dosages. Patients with hyporeninemic hypoaldosteronism may not require therapy. Volume depletion should be avoided unless the patient is volume overexpanded, in which case furosemide often improves the metabolic acidosis and hyperkalemia. Supraphysiologic doses of mineralocorticoids may be necessary, but should be administered only with furosemide to avoid volume overexpansion.

Infants with pseudohypoaldosteronism type 1 should receive salt supplements in sufficient amounts to correct the syndrome and allow normal growth. Adults or children with pseudohypoaldosteronism type 2 should receive thiazide diuretics.

MIXED ACID-BASE DISTURBANCES

SANDRA SABATINI, M.D., Ph.D.
NEIL A. KURTZMAN, M.D., F.A.C.P.

Mixed acid-base disturbances are defined as the coexistence of two or more simple acid-base abnormalities. The diagnosis and treatment of acid-base disorders often stress the physician needlessly. While these disorders pose some of the most challenging problems encountered in clinical medicine, the proper diagnosis should not be difficult given the state of our knowledge of acid-base physiology today. Given the many pathophysiologic processes that can alter plasma bicarbonate and arterial CO_2 tension, it is evident that the presence of one acid-base abnormality does not preclude the development of additional disturbances that have independent effects on acid-base equilibrium. Indeed, the complicated medical problems that breed one acid-base abnormality are just as likely to spawn another.

Among hospitalized patients, mixed acid-base disorders in which two components can be identified occur quite frequently. On rare occasions, three acid-base disturbances may be identified. Because the individual components of mixed acid-base disorders may be additive or counteracting as regards plasma pH, the resultant change in blood hydrogen concentration may be deceptively slight or alarmingly severe.

Table 1 summarizes the simple acid-base disturbances, indicating the primary event as well as the compensatory change (secondary event) which one expects in order to keep blood pH as close to 7.4 as possible. For example, in metabolic acidosis the maximum fall in arterial P_{CO_2} tension is approximately 1 to 1.5 mm Hg per milliequivalent (mEq) decrement in the plasma bicarbonate concentration. This requires that the patient have normal lungs, normal kidneys, and no underlying disease, and even then the arterial P_{CO_2} will rarely fall below 20 mm Hg. In such a circumstance one would expect that at an arterial pH of 7.3 the primary fall in plasma bicarbonate would be equal to 12 mEq per liter and the maximum decrement in arterial CO_2 tension in an attempt to compensate would be 25 mm Hg.

Compensation in the simple acid-base disorders is almost never complete except in chronic respiratory alkalosis. Thus, the finding of a normal plasma pH in a patient with an acid-base disorder other than chronic respiratory alkalosis immediately suggests the presence of a mixed acid-base disturbance.

The correct diagnosis of acid-base disorders can be made from a good history plus the proper interpretation of simple laboratory tests. These laboratory tests include serum electrolytes, the anion gap, arterial blood gases and pH, and occasionally urine electrolytes. The integration of these variables will assess the presence and degree of respiratory or metabolic compensation, and will thus determine whether uncomplicated or mixed acid-base disorders are present. Remember, the simple acid-base disorders may mimic mixed abnormalities if the former

TABLE 1 Primary and Secondary Changes in Arterial pH, PCO_2 Tension, and Plasma HCO_3 in the Common Acid–Base Disorders

Acid–Base Disorder	*Blood pH*	*Primary Change*	*Secondary Compensation*	*Note*
Metabolic acidosis	↓	$\downarrow HCO_3^-$	$\downarrow PCO_2$ ~1–1.5 mm Hg/mEq $\downarrow HCO_3^-$	PCO_2 rarely lower than 20 mm Hg
Metabolic alkalosis	↑	$\uparrow HCO_3^-$	$\uparrow PCO_2$ 0.2–0.9 mm Hg/mEq $\uparrow HCO_3^-$	Steady state H^+ excretion approximately equal to premorbid state
Acute respiratory acidosis	↓	$\uparrow PCO_2$	$\uparrow HCO_3^-$ (slight) 1 mEq/10 mm Hg↑	HCO_3^- should be approximately equal to 24–29 mEq/L
Acute respiratory alkalosis	↑	$\downarrow PCO_2$	$\downarrow HCO_3^-$ 2 mEq/10 mm Hg↓	Immediate cell buffering with hemoglobin, phosphate, proteins
Chronic respiratory acidosis	↓	$\uparrow\uparrow PCO_2$	$\uparrow\uparrow HCO_3^-$ 5 mEq/10 mm Hg↑	↑Net acid excretion, ↑proximal HCO_3^- reabsorption ($HCO_3^- \leq 40$ mEq/L)
Chronic respiratory alkalosis	↑,NL	$\downarrow PCO_2$	$\downarrow HCO_3^-$ 5 mEq/10 mm Hg↓	Begins in 2 hours with ↑ renal H^+ excretion (complete in 2–3 days); blood pH may be NL; hyperchloremia; profound hypophosphatemia

$pH = pKa + \log\frac{HCO_3}{(0.03)(PCO_2)}$; pKa = 6.1; 0.03 = solubility coefficient of dissolved CO_2; NL = normal

are acute in origin or are overcompensated. These "copy cats" are usually metabolic, as the time for full changes by the kidney requires 24 to 48 hours; changes in ventilation may occur in the space of a few breaths.

The most useful piece of information in unraveling the diagnosis of an acid-base disorder is the medical history. The presence of known underlying diseases should heighten the clinical suspicion that a specific acid-base disorder will be found (Table 2). In cardiopulmonary arrest, for example, both respiratory acidosis and metabolic acidosis are characteristically observed; in septic shock, mixed respiratory alkalosis and metabolic acidosis is common (lactic acidemia); in chronic obstructive pulmonary disease, respiratory alkalosis or respiratory acidosis may coexist with metabolic alkalosis, the metabolic alkalosis commonly being the consequence of diuretics or vomiting. Diarrhea is the most common cause of an acid-base abnormality—metabolic acidosis. A history of diarrhea superimposed on a patient with chronic lung disease (respiratory acidosis or respiratory alkalosis), hepatic decompensation (respiratory alkalosis), or vomiting (metabolic alkalosis) will cause a wide variation in the change of arterial pH. In the patient with severe diarrhea and respiratory acidosis, a marked decrease in arterial pH occurs; diarrhea and respiratory alkalosis will cause a slight increase in arterial pH, and diarrhea and gastric alkalosis will cause no change in arterial pH. Primary respiratory alkalosis should always be expected in the pregnant female and in patients with chronic liver disease. Chronic hypocapnia causes a low plasma bicarbonate concentration. Indeed, the finding of a normal plasma bicarbonate concentration in a patient with hepatic decompensation should immediately bring to mind the diagnosis of a mixed acid-base disorder—the cause of which should be carefully sought. The importance of the history cannot be overemphasized; it is always obtainable when one remembers that yesterday's laboratory data become today's medical history.

TABLE 2 Common Causes of Acid–Base Disorders

Metabolic acidosis
- Chloride (normal anion gap) (hyperchloremia)
  - Gastrointestinal loss of HCO_3 (e.g., diarrhea)
  - Renal loss of HCO_3 (e.g., renal tubular acidosis)
  - Hyperalimentation, NH_4Cl ingestion
  - Hypoaldosteronism
- Anion gap (normal plasma chloride concentration)
  - Ketoacidosis, lactic acidosis
  - Renal failure
  - Ingestion (salicylates, ethylene glycol, methanol, paraldehyde)

Metabolic alkalosis (normal or low plasma chloride concentration)
- Vomiting or nasogastric suction
- Mineralocorticoid excess
- Diuretics

Respiratory Acidosis (normal or low plasma chloride concentration)
- Pulmonary edema
- Acute exacerbation of underlying lung disease
- Severe asthma
- Pneumonia
- Drug overdose
- O_2 administration to a patient with chronic hypercapnia
- Sleep apnea syndrome
- Chronic obstructive pulmonary disease (COPD)*
- Pickwickian syndrome

Respiratory alkalosis (hyperchloremia)
- Hypoxemia (pulmonary embolus, congestive heart failure, high altitude, anemia)
- Pulmonary disease (interstitial fibrosis, pneumonia, COPD)*
- Stimulation of respiratory center (psychogenic, liver failure, salicylates, pregnancy, progesterone, cerebrovascular accident/infection, pontine tumors)
- Mechanical ventilation

* COPD is more commonly associated with respiratory alkalosis and is secondary to the central hypoxic drive.

RELIABILITY OF BLOOD GAS MEASUREMENTS

As mixed acid-base disorders are more likely to be disguised and are probably more common in hospitalized patients than are simple acid-base disorders, it is critical for the physician to determine the validity of blood gas measurements. At the time the arterial blood gases are drawn, virtually every patient will have a venous bicarbonate concentration measured simultaneously. Venous total CO_2 and the calculated bicarbonate concentration from the arterial blood gas should differ by no more than 1 to 2 mEq per liter. Plasma bicarbonate concentration can easily be calculated from the Henderson-Hasselbalch equation:

$$pH = pKa + \log \frac{[HCO_3^-] \quad (\text{mM per liter})}{0.03 \times \ Pco_2 \ (\text{mm Hg})}$$

where: pK_a = 6.1, the dissociation constant for the HCO_3^-/H_2CO_3 buffer system; and 0.03 = the solubility coefficient of dissolved CO_2 in whole blood at 37 °C. An alternative is:

$$[H^+] \ (\text{mM per liter}) = \frac{24 \times Pco_2 \ (\text{mm Hg})}{[HCO_3^-] \quad (\text{mM per liter})}$$

If the normal Pco_2 is 40 mm Hg and HCO_3^- concentration is 24 mEq per liter, then the normal H^+ concentration is 40 nEq per liter. Thus, to use Equation B, one must convert measured pH to H^+ concentration. A simple rule of thumb is as follows:

1. For every 0.1 *increase* in pH, multiply the H^+ concentration by 0.8 (e.g., pH = 7.5, then $H^+ = 40 \times 0.8 = 32$ nEq per liter).
2. For every 0.1 *decrease* in pH, multiply the H^+ concentration by 1.25 (e.g., pH = 7.2, then $H^+ = 40 \times 1.25 \times 1.25 = 63$ nEq per liter).

In essence, this equation can be reduced to a proportional relationship so that the blood pH is directly related to the ratio between the *metabolic* component of acid base (i.e., the blood bicarbonate concentration) and the *respiratory* component (i.e., the arterial CO_2 tension):

$$pH \propto \frac{\text{Metabolic Component}}{\text{Respiratory Component}}$$

THE PLASMA CHLORIDE CONCENTRATION

Essential to the dissection of acid-base disorders is an initial assessment of the plasma chloride concentration (normally 100 mEq per liter). The plasma chloride changes for only two reasons: a change in hydration, or a change in acid-base status. It is easy to distinguish between these by examining the plasma sodium concentration (normally 140 mEq per liter). The normal ratio of the plasma sodium to plasma chloride concentration = 140 mEq per liter over 100 mEq per liter = 1.4. If the plasma chloride concentration increases parallel and proportional to the rise in plasma sodium concentration, then a change in the state of hydration has occurred, i.e., dehydration. Dehydration should be suspected in the elderly, particularly in hot weather, or in the comatose patient who is unable to express a feeling of thirst. Hyperchloremia occurs in this instance if there is inadequate water replacement secondary to inadequate intake or large obligatory losses of free water by the skin and lungs. Dehydration can also be caused by vomiting or diarrhea, and these disorders in turn are virtually always associated with an acid-base disturbance. On the other hand, if the plasma chloride concentration falls in proportion to a decrease in plasma sodium concentration, then cellular overhydration is present. Overhydration commonly occurs from the injudicious administration of hypotonic fluids to hospitalized patients with impaired urinary diluting capacity either secondary to an inadequate circulation (heart failure) or to intrinsic renal disease.

If the plasma chloride concentration changes out of proportion to the serum sodium concentration and the ratio is not 1.4, then an acid-base disturbance is present. Of the four simple acid-base disorders, two are always associated with hyperchloremia and two are associated with a normal (or low) plasma chloride concentration (see Table 2). Hyperchloremia occurs in metabolic acidosis (nonanion gap) and compensated respiratory alkalosis. The simple disorders should be easily recognizable by the fact that the former will be associated with acidemia and the latter with either alkalemia or a near normal arterial pH. Both will be associated with a low arterial Pco_2. A low plasma chloride concentration occurs in metabolic alkalosis and compensated respiratory acidosis. While both of these will be associated with an increase in Pco_2 tension, the arterial pH will never be normal. Metabolic alkalosis will have an increase in arterial pH, whereas respiratory acidosis, regardless of the degree of compensation, will be associated with an acid blood pH. In addition to Table 2, the common causes of the simple acid-base disturbances are found in the chapters *Metabolic Acidosis, and metabolic Alkalosis.*

ANION GAP

Assessment of acid-base abnormalities includes calculation and interpretation of the anion gap and is equal to:

$$AG = \text{plasma } Na^+ + K^+ - [\text{plasma } Cl^- + HCO_3^-]$$
$$AG = 12 - 16 \text{ mEq per liter}$$

The anion gap is simply a measure of the unmeasured anions or cations present in blood. The anion gap changes as the arterial pH changes, primarily as a result of the normally negative charges on the anionic protein, albumin. Other less important anions are phosphate and sulfate. When the body makes excess endogenous anions (acetoacetic acid, lactic acid, beta-OH-butyric acid) the anion gap increases, and is exactly equal to the decrement in plasma bicarbonate concentration—anion gap acidosis (see Table 2). Plasma chloride concentration stays normal because the addition of acid is neutralized to a certain extent by the bicarbonate buffer system. If acidosis is present, but the anion gap is normal (12 to 16 mEq per liter), bicarbonate has been lost from the body, usually by the gastrointestinal tract or by the kidney. The loss of bicarbonate results in an acidosis with hyperchloremia, therefore the anion gap is normal. The anion gap increases in metabolic alkalosis as a combination of the increase in blood pH and lactate production. This may be masked, however, when one remembers that approximately one-third of hospitalized patients with metabolic alkalosis will also have an associated respiratory acidosis or respiratory alkalosis. If a mixed disorder is present, such as diabetic ketoacidosis (anion gap acidosis) and vomiting (metabolic alkalosis), the change in the gap will be much greater than the decrement of the plasma bicarbonate concentration. In this mixed abnormality both acid-base disorders will increase the anion gap; the acidosis will tend to decrease the plasma bicarbonate concentration while the alkalosis will tend to increase the bicarbonate concentration.

The anion gap is also of value to assess the unmeasured cations, such as calcium, magnesium, and certain cationic proteins. Hypercalcemia is associated with a decrease in the anion gap, as is the presence of the cationic myeloma protein.

Many nomograms have been developed to aid the clinician in the diagnosis of acid-base disorders. In general, these are of no value in mixed acid-base disorders. At pH 7.4 the normal hydrogen ion concentration of the blood is 40 nmol per liter; thus, the finding of a normal pH in the presence of an abnormal P_{CO_2} and plasma bicarbonate concentration virtually defines a mixed metabolic-respiratory disorder (P_{CO_2} tension and plasma bicarbonate concentration change in the *same* direction). Plasma pH is most affected when the P_{CO_2} and plasma bicarbonate change in the opposite direction. Remember, pH is proportional to plasma HCO_3^- concentration divided by the arterial P_{CO_2} tension.

CLINICAL EXAMPLES

Case One

A 38-year-old man with adult-onset insulin-dependent diabetes mellitus developed anorexia, nausea, and intermittent chest pain. After three days he became lightheaded, developed intractable chest pain, and was admitted to the hospital. Blood pressure on admission was 70/50 mm Hg, heart rate 120 per minute, respirations 28 per minute. He was diaphoretic and the electrocardiogram revealed anteroseptal myocardial infarction, age undetermined.

He was noted to have the following blood gases and electrolytes: pH 7.41; P_{CO_2} 14 mm Hg; P_{O_2} 50 mm Hg; Na^+128 mEq per liter; K^+5.9 mEq per liter; Cl^-92 mEq per liter; HCO_3 8 mEq per liter; glucose 522 mg per deciliter; creatinine 1.8 mg per deciliter; blood urea nitrogen 40 mg per deciliter.

The finding of a normal arterial pH in an obviously ill patient with hypotension suggests immediately that at least two acid-base abnormalities are present, and that they are counterbalancing as regards arterial pH. The presence of metabolic acidosis was established by a plasma venous bicarbonate concentration of 8 mEq per liter. The degree of hyperventilation exceeds that which would be anticipated purely as a result of this decrement in bicarbonate (P_{CO_2} 14 mm Hg). The ratio of plasma sodium to plasma chloride concentration was normal (1.4), suggesting that cell hydration was normal, but the noted acidosis however, was normochloremic (i.e., anion gap). The calculated anion gap was increased to 34 mEq per liter (plasma Na^+ + K^+ - [plasma Cl^- + HCO_3^-]). The normal anion gap varies between 12 and 16 mEq per liter and represents the anions normally present in blood which are not measured routinely (phosphate, sulfate, organic acids). Metabolic acidosis secondary to a gain of any acid other than hydrochloric acid will be associated with an increased anion gap. The likely gained acids in this patient are a combination of lactic acid and keto acid overproduction. While the acidosis of chronic renal failure is an anion gap metabolic acidosis, this possibility is excluded because renal function is only mildly impaired (serum creatinine concentration 1.8 mg per deciliter). Unless it is determined that exogenous acid was given, the most reasonable possibilities include endogenous production of keto acids in a diabetic or lactic acid secondary to circulatory shock. The longstanding diabetes mellitus suggests that diabetic ketoacidosis is present, but blood ketone measurement was found to be 2+, consequently the ketonemia is only moderate. The presence of profound hypotension makes lactic acidosis a more likely possibility, and further documentation could be achieved by measuring lactate plasma pyruvate ratio, normal being 1 mEq per liter over 0.1 mEq per liter.

Case Two

A 30-year-old woman was brought to the clinic because of weakness and malaise of three months' duration. Physical examination revealed muscle tenderness in the upper arms and thighs, and decreased deep tendon reflexes. Routine laboratory values were: Na^+140 mEq per liter; K^+1.8 mEq per liter; Cl^-118 mEq per liter; HCO_3^- 12 mEq per liter; pH was 6.90; P_{CO_2} 60 mm Hg; P_{O_2} 52 mm Hg; urine pH was 6.92; chest roentgenogram normal; routine abdominal x-ray film revealed nephrocalcinosis.

This patient had hyperchloremic metabolic acidosis with a normal anion gap of 12 mEq per liter. Were this the sole acid-base abnormality, the arterial P_{CO_2} should have been 20 mm Hg, yet this patient had a P_{CO_2} of 60 mm Hg. The profound decrease in arterial pH (6.9) demonstrates the degree of acidemia which may develop when respiratory acidosis and metabolic acidosis occur simultaneously. The finding of nephrocalcinosis on an abdominal roentgenogram in a patient with metabolic acidosis and high urine pH strongly suggests the presence of distal renal tubular acidosis, an anion gap metabolic acidosis. Hypokalemia per se is not a classic feature of all patients with distal renal tubular acidoses, as many now have been reported with hyperkalemia. Hypokalemia in this patient caused a complicating factor to occur, evidenced by marked weakness, malaise, and a second acid-base disorder, namely, respiratory acidosis. Profound potassium depletion may cause paralysis of the respiratory muscles and thus prevent the normal compensatory changes that would be expected to accompany uncomplicated metabolic acidosis, i.e., a decrease in arterial Pco_2. Shortly after potassium replacement was initiated, Kussmaul respirations began, the Pco_2 fell, and plasma pH began to rise. The patient, in the face of profound acidemia, was able to lower her arterial Pco_2 tension. The calculated pH was now in the range of approximately 7.2.

Since renal tubular acidosis of the distal type is attributable to renal retention of acid, appropriate therapy is sodium bicarbonate. Proximal renal tubular acidosis, on the other hand, is attributable to massive bicarbonate loss from the proximal tubule along with the loss of glucose and amino acids. This form of hypokalemic hyperchloremic renal tubular acidosis may be quite refractory to bicarbonate therapy, and the addition of a mild diuretic may be of value. The diuretic, usually a thiazide, causes some volume contraction, and increases proximal bicarbonate reabsorption.

Case Three

A 60-year-old man with a history of chronic obstructive pulmonary disease presented with a seven-day history of cough and dyspnea. Chest roentgenogram revealed a left lower lobe infiltrate and the following laboratory values: pH 7.33; PCO_2 75 mm Hg; Po_2 44 mm Hg; Na^+ 140 mEq per liter; K^+4 mEq per liter; Cl^-94 mEq per liter; bicarbonate 39 mEq per liter; U_{Na} 7 mEq per liter. From the outpatient clinic records he was known to have hypertension, a modest systemic acidemia, and an arterial Pco_2 greater than 50 mm Hg. Because of impending respiratory failure, he was placed on a ventilator, and the Pco_2 was rapidly brought to 40 mm Hg. While his cyanosis improved markedly, his mental status quickly deteriorated and he became somewhat combative. Since the plasma bicarbonate concentration remained 39 mEq per liter after the ventilator Pco_2 was decreased to 40 mm Hg, the calculated pH from the Henderson-Hasselbalch equation was 7.66! This is an example of a patient with overcompensated respiratory acidosis.

Because of the past history of hypertension, the patient was given thiazide diuretics, and the following morning he became extremely disoriented; his laboratory values were Pco_2 40 mm Hg, bicarbonate 38 mEq per liter, and an arterial pH of 7.66. At this point the patient had developed "post-thypercapnic metabolic alkalosis."

Chronic hypercapnia enhances the renal excretion of acid and chloride. At the same time, however, it stimulates bicarbonate reabsorption by the proximal tubule. Renal compensation does not occur immediately, but rather is a gradual process occurring over several days. Following the return of the Pco_2 to normal, renal retention of chloride occurs in parallel with an increase in bicarbonate excretion. A rapid decrease of arterial Pco_2, as can be caused by a ventilator, causes an immediate rise in arterial pH. The plasma bicarbonate concentration will remain close to that which was observed prior to use of the ventilator (e.g., approximately 39 mEq per liter), as the renal adjustment takes approximately 24 hours to occur. This alkalemia is the consequence of overcompensated respiratory acidosis.

If patients with hypercapnia are placed on a low-salt diet or are treated with diuretics as was this patient, proximal bicarbonate reabsorption will be enhanced as a consequence of volume contraction. Excretion of excess bicarbonate will not occur, and the patients are likely to develop "post-hypercapnic metabolic alkalosis." Correction of this type of metabolic alkalosis can be accomplished by salt administration. This syndrome may also occur if effective arterial volume is contracted for any reason, such as congestive heart failure. In this instance, successful treatment of the heart failure is required to correct the alkalosis, and salt administration is contraindicated.

Acetazolamide (250 to 1,000 mg daily), a carbonic anhydrase inhibitor, may be given on an acute basis to enhance the renal excretion of bicarbonate. This mild diuretic acts in the proximal tubule to prevent bicarbonate reabsorption.

Case Four

A 48-year-old man was admitted to the hospital because of protracted vomiting of 5 days' duration. On physical examination his blood pressure was 80/60 lying and in the upright position fell to 70/0. Routine laboratory values were: Na^+127 mEq per liter; K^+6.7 mEq per liter; Cl^-80 mEq per liter; pH 7.30; Pco_2 19 mm Hg; HCO_3^- 9 mEq per liter; creatinine 7.2 mg per deciliter; U_{Na} 30 mEq per liter; U_{Cl} 4 mEq per liter. He was mildly icteric.

The anion gap in this patient was 45 mEq per liter and the plasma chloride concentration was low in relationship to a plasma sodium concentration of 127 mEq per liter (calculated chloride should be 90 mEq per liter). The finding of an increased anion gap and a decreased plasma chloride concentration should immediately suggest at least two acid-base disorders. Upon examination of the arterial pH, one sees a mild acidemia in the face of a low plasma bicarbonate concentration and a low Pco_2. Thus relative normalization of the arterial pH suggests two offsetting acid-base disorders. Based on the history of vomiting and the low plasma chloride concentration, metabolic alkalosis is probably one of the disorders. Analysis of the plasma bicarbonate concentration and the arterial Pco_2 and pH suggest metabolic acidosis. The metabolic acidosis could indicate a patient with chronic renal failure, a finding further suggested by substantial quantities of sodium in the urine. Analysis of the urine chloride, however, which was vanishingly low, tells you that this is not a patient with chronic renal failure, because approximately equivalent amounts of sodium and chloride should have been present in the urine. In this setting, the urine chloride level is an index of the state of effective arterial volume and is characteristic in patients with vomiting. The anion excreted with the sodium in this instance was bicarbonate. Analysis of the urine revealed a pH of 6.8. Subsequent hydration with intravenous sodium chloride resulted in a rise in urinary chloride excretion; a fall in plasma creatinine concentration to 0.8 mg per deciliter; and arterial pH of 7.47, Pco_2 33 mm Hg, and HCO_3^- 17 mEq per liter. Abnormal liver function tests were obtained. Reanalysis of this patient revealed that he had three and not two primary acid-base disorders: metabolic alkalosis secondary to vomiting, metabolic acidosis secondary to hypotension and poor tissue perfusion, and a respiratory alkalosis that is of central origin in patients with chronic liver disease.

Case Five

An obtunded 68-year-old woman was brought to the emergency room; her laboratory values were: pH 7.15; Pco_2 15 mm Hg; Po_2 70 mm Hg; Na^+ 168 mEq per liter; K^+ 3.8 mEq per liter; Cl^-122 mEq per liter; HCO_3^- 5 mEq per liter.

The intern in the emergency room made a presumptive diagnosis of hyperchloremic metabolic acidosis. Careful analysis of the plasma electrolytes, however, revealed that the plasma sodium concentration was 168 mEq per liter and that the plasma chloride concentration had risen in direct proportion (i.e., by 20 percent) to the plasma sodium concentration. Thus, it was obvious that this was a markedly dehydrated patient as well as one with metabolic acidosis of the anion gap type (45 mEq per liter). Subsequently, blood lactate levels were found to be markedly elevated and the lactate to pyruvate ratio, normally 10:1, was increased. The cause of the profound lactic acidosis in this patient was tissue hypoxia secondary to marked dehydration, volume contraction, and pulmonary disease. Of particular note is the finding that the Po_2 was only 67 mm Hg when the Pco_2 was 15 mm Hg. While this case does not represent a mixed acid-base disorder, it does demonstrate the importance of interpreting the plasma chloride concentration pari passu with the arterial blood gases.

Case Six

A 64-year-old diabetic woman presented to the clinic with a five-day history of diarrhea. Known medications included insulin, a diuretic, phosphate binders, and oral calcium supplement. Laboratory date were: Na^+140 mEq per liter; K^+5 mEq per liter; Cl^-125 mEq per liter; pH 7.24; PCO_2 26 mm Hg; HCO_3^- 10 mEq per liter; creatinine 5 mg per deciliter; glucose 200 mg per deciliter.

Note that the plasma sodium concentration was normal, the chloride and the creatinine levels were elevated, and that metabolic acidosis was present. The calculated anion gap was 10 mEq per liter ($Na^+ + K^+ - [Cl^- + CO_2]$). Were the metabolic acidosis solely the result of chronic renal failure, inferred from the patient's known medications and confirmed by the creatinine concentration of 5 mg per deciliter, an anion gap acidosis should be present (i.e., normal plasma chloride concentration). Since hyperchloremia was present, however, the patient must have another acid-base abnormality, either respiratory alkalosis or nonanion gap acidosis. With the history of diarrhea and the laboratory data, the correct diagnosis is nonanion gap metabolic acidosis, superimposed on the anion gap acidosis of renal failure. The key clue is the finding of hyperchloremia in a patient with renal failure.

THERAPY

Once the etiologic agents of the acid-base disorders are identified, the treatment is simple. A few points are worth remembering:

First, most forms of metabolic alkalosis do not require immediate correction unless the alkalemia is severe (pH >7.55) or has occurred acutely. Attention to the state of volume (NaCl) and its replacement often causes enough bicarbonaturia that acid-base balance returns to normal. Acetazolamide (250 to 1,000 mg daily for 24 to 48 hours) will enhance bicarbonate excretion enough to decrease systemic pH toward normal. Rarely, NH_4CI, $CaCI_2$, arginine, or lysine may be necessary. Dilute infusion of HCI is a safe measure when used by those with experience. HCI (100 to 200 mmol) is given in a large vein up to a concentration of 200 to 300 mmol over a 24-hour period. The deficit is calculated according to the extracellular space (approximately 20 percent of body weight), and a portion of the deficit is given with careful monitoring of pH and PCO_2 approximately every 3 to 4 hours.

Second, acidemia requires treatment if the pH is less than 7.20. Bicarbonate is the treatment of choice if parenteral therapy is being given. Sodium lactate offers no advantage and requires conversion to bicarbonate before its potential as a base is recognized. Severe liver disease or hypotension with poor tissue perfusion further impairs the usefulness of lactate as an alkalinizing agent. Bicarbonate (or acetate) dialysis may be considered if the acidemia is severe or is worsening despite parenteral bicarbonate therapy. Using this technique, control of the patient's volume status may be easily managed. This is of particular importance in patients with severe cardiovascular disease. Oral alkali therapy may be given in the form of bicarbonate, citrate, (Shohl's solution), or gluconate, the latter two requiring conversion to base in vivo.

Third, ion shifts tend to occur simultaneously with the acid-base disorders. Hyperkalemia generally accompanies metabolic acidosis and is attributable to a shift of potassium from the intracellular space to the extracellular fluid. Patients with protracted diarrhea, renal tubular acidosis, and diabetic ketoacidosis will generally be potassium depleted despite hyperkalemia and require oral or parenteral replacement. If parenteral therapy is chosen, potassium should not be given at a rate greater than 60 mEq per hour and should not begin until urine output is ascertained. The plasma potassium concentration should be monitored carefully. Hypokalemia accompanies metabolic alkalosis and may be profound during protracted vomiting secondary to large urinary losses of potassium. Potassium supplementation may be necessary in this instance. In syndromes associated with mineralocorticoid excess, spironolactone (300 to 600 mg daily) may be of value.

Profound hypophosphatemia may also occur during the treatment of ketoacidosis. This is attributable to a shift of phosphate from the extracellular fluid to the cell interior, a phenomenon similar to that seen with potassium. Hypophosphatemia may cause myocardial dysfunction, rhabdomyolysis, leukocyte dysfunction, and decreased 2–3 diphosphoglycerate. Milk is an excellent source of phosphate (33 mmol per liter), as is Fleet Phosphoa-Soda (15 to 30 ml four times daily). If parenteral phosphate is required, sodium or potassium phosphate may be given. These preparations contain 3 mmol per mililiter of phosphate, and in most instances up to 20 mmol every 8 hours may be safely given. While hypocalcemia and metastatic calcification are the major risks of parenteral phosphate therapy, they are easily avoided if the rate of infusion is slow and plasma calcium and phosphate concentrations are monitored carefully.

A reduction in ionized fraction of total serum calcium tends to occur in alkalosis, the most dramatic instances being seen in patients with respiratory alkalosis. This is the result of increased binding of calcium to the anionic protein, albumin, and generally does not require treatment other than to correct the underlying acid-base disorder. In acidotic states plasma ionized calcium may be slightly increased; however, large quantities of calcium (and magnesium) may be lost in the urine. Some of these conditions may require supplementation (diabetic ketoacidosis, for example) and some may not (renal tubular acidosis).

OBSTRUCTIVE UROPATHY

SAULO KLAHR, M.D.
RALPH V. CLAYMAN, M.D.
ROBERT R. BAHNSON, M.D.

In humans, the effects of urinary tract obstruction on renal function are diverse. Not only are there marked reductions in renal blood flow and glomerular filtration rate, but obstructive nephropathy also can produce significant changes in renal tubular function. Partial chronic obstruction of the urinary tract can lead to progressive atrophy and destruction of nephrons and can result in chronic renal insufficiency. Unilateral complete obstruction of urine flow is well tolerated for several days; however, if the obstruction persists for more than a week, some permanent damage ensues. By the end of 3 weeks of complete obstruction, recoverable function is usually nil. On the other hand, acute complete bilateral obstruction results in renal failure. Because obstruction generally is a remediable cause of kidney failure, early and accurate diagnosis and prompt treatment are vital to the preservation and restoration of renal function.

The clinical manifestations of urinary tract obstructions vary. Bilateral complete obstruction of urine flow is manifested as anuria. Partial obstruction can cause fluctuating urine output, alternating from oliguria to polyuria; urinary tract infection, usually refractory to treatment; abdominal or flank pain; or unexplained acute or chronic renal failure. Obstruction always must be included in the differential diagnosis of acute renal failure, especially when urine output fluctuates or anuria occurs suddenly (Tables 1, 2).

GENERAL THERAPEUTIC CONSIDERATIONS

After establishing the diagnosis of urinary tract obstruction, a decision should be made whether or not to undertake surgical or instrumental procedures. High-grade or complete bilateral obstruction presenting as acute renal failure requires intervention as soon as possible. In these patients, the site of obstruction will frequently determine the approach. If the obstructive lesion is distal to the bladder, passage of a urethral catheter may suffice, although this may require the aid of a urologic surgeon. In some cases, suprapubic cystostomy may be necessary. On the other hand, if the lesion lies proximal to the bladder (upper tract lesion, e.g., malignant infiltration of the trigone by cervical or prostatic adenocarcinoma), then placement of nephrostomy tubes at the time of ultrasonography or passage of a retrograde ureteral catheter should be undertaken. Tubes should be placed in both obstructed renal calyces, since the potential for recovery of function by either kidney is not easily predicted at the time of the procedure. Such an approach may alleviate the need for dialysis and allows the physician time to determine the specific site and character of the obstructing lesion. Further, the nephrostomy tube may be useful for the local infusion of pharmacologic agents with which to treat infection, malignancy, or calculi. In patients with obstruction complicated by urinary infection and generalized sepsis, appropriate antibiotics and other supportive therapy are indicated.

In patients with low-grade acute obstruction or partial chronic obstruction, surgical intervention may be delayed for a few weeks or even months. However, prompt relief of partial obstruction is indicated when: (1) there are multiple repeated episodes of urinary tract infection; (2) the patient has significant symptoms (flank pain, dysuria, voiding dysfunction); (3) there is urinary retention; and (4) there is evidence of recurrent or progres-

TABLE 1 Causes of Upper Urinary Tract Obstruction

- Urolithiasis
- Transitional cell cancer of the pelvis/ureter
- Blood clot
- Renal papillae
- Fungus ball
- Ureteral ligation
- Primary obstruction of the ureteropelvic junction; intrinsic (congenital) vs. acquired (vessel crossing postsurgical)
- Ureteral valve
- Ureteral polyp
- Vascular lesions
  - Abdominal aortic aneurysm
  - Iliac artery aneurysm
  - Retrocaval ureter
  - Puerperal ovarian vein thrombophlebitis
  - Fibrosis following vascular reconstructive surgery
- Diseases of the female reproductive tract
  - Pregnancy
  - Mass lesions of the uterus and ovary
  - Ovarian remnants
  - Gartner's duct cyst
  - Tubo-ovarian abscess
  - Endometriosis
  - Uterine prolapse
- Diseases of the gastrointestinal tract
  - Crohn's disease
  - Diverticulitis
  - Appendiceal abscess
  - Pancreatic lesions
- Diseases of the retroperitoneum
  - Retroperitoneal fibrosis
  - Tuberculosis
  - Sarcoidosis
  - Radiation fibrosis
  - Retroperitoneal hemorrhage
  - Primary retroperitoneal tumors (lymphomas, sarcomas, etc.)
  - Secondary retroperitoneal tumors (cervix, bladder, colon, prostate, etc.)
  - Lymphocele
  - Pelvic lipomatosis

sive renal damage. The presence of post-void residual urine, urinary extravasation, ureterovesical reflux, or dilatation of the collecting system in the face of sterile urine are not indications for surgical intervention.

MANAGEMENT OF URETERAL OBSTRUCTION

Stones are by far the most common cause of ureteral obstruction. The immediate treatment for ureteral stones consists of relief of pain, elimination of obstruction, and control of infection. Relief of pain in acute renal colic is best accomplished by intramuscular injection of adequate doses of a narcotic analgesic. If the stone is less than five mm, urologic instrumentation or surgical intervention is not required, since 80 to 90 percent of these ureteral stones will pass spontaneously. Among ureteral stones in the five- to seven-mm range, however, only 40 to 50 percent will pass, and stones larger than seven mm rarely pass spontaneously. High fluid intake to produce urinary volumes of at least 1.5 to 2 L daily will help to pass the stone. The urine must be strained through a gauze sponge to recover the calculi and the stone should be sent for analysis. If a stone completely blocks a ureter and does not move, surgical treatment should be given within a few days. However, if the obstruction is partial, the urine sterile, and the pain manageable, the patient may be observed for weeks or months before surgical therapy is undertaken.

Surgical intervention for renal and/or ureteral calculi is indicated when there is unremitting colic, urinary tract infection and urosepsis, complete obstruction, calculus too large to pass (i.e., $>$ 7 mm), or a calculus that has failed to move despite a trial of time (usually months) and increased fluid intake. The surgical therapy for urolithiasis has undergone marked changes during the past 5 years.

Until 1980, the standard approach for renal or ureteral calculi *above the pelvic brim* was an open surgical procedure. This usually was accomplished by an anterior abdominal or posterior dorsal lumbotomy approach. With these procedures the usual hospital stay was 4 to 7 days with a convalescence of 2 to 6 weeks.

Because of technological advances in radiologic imaging modalities and a realization that interventional radiologic techniques could be applied to the urinary tract, a whole new branch of urologic surgery has developed: endourology. Endourology refers to the closed, controlled manipulation of the entire urinary tract. The ability of the interventional radiologist to place a percutaneous nephrostomy and dilate the tract to as large as 12 mm has provided the urologist with a direct conduit to the kidney for the removal of obstructing renal and upper ureteral calculi. The urologist can introduce a variety of rigid or flexible endoscopes through the nephrostomy tract to directly visualize and grasp calculi less than 1.5 cm in diameter. For larger stones, powerful lithotriptor probes have been devised that can use ultrasonic or electrohydraulic energy to disintegrate calculi under direct vision. From its inception in 1976, endourology has garnered rapid acceptance and development in the urologic and radiologic communities. Endourologic methods are currently successful in treating obstructing calculi in 98 percent of patients. In addition, this approach results

TABLE 2 Causes of Lower Urinary Tract Obstruction

- Phimosis
- Meatal stenosis
- Paraphimosis
- Urethral stricture
- Urethral stone
- Urethral diverticulum
- Periurethral abscess
- Posterior urethral valves
- Anterior urethral valves
- Urethral surgery
- Prostatic abscess
- Prostatic calculi
- Neurogenic bladder
- Benign prostatic hyperplasia
- Psychogenic urinary retention
- Bladder calculus
- Bladder cancer
- Ureterocele
- Trauma
  - Straddle injury
  - Pelvic fracture

in a short hospital stay (3 to 4 days) and a convalescence of only 4 to 7 days.

In 1980, another major development in the treatment of symptomatic renal and upper ureteral calculi occurred: extracorporeal shock wave lithotripsy. This technology, developed by Chaussy, Schmiedt, and co-workers in Germany, involves the focusing of extracorporeally electrohydraulically generated fluid-borne shock waves to disintegrate the calculus. The patient is given a general or spinal anesthetic and submerged in a tub of degassed water. A spark plug electrode sits in the bottom of the tub within an ellipsoid container. When fired, the electrode generates a shock wave that bounces off the sides of the ellipsoid container in such a manner that a second focal point is created above the ellipsoid where the shock waves converge. Using dual fluoroscopic control the patient can be maneuvered until the stone lies completely within the second focal point. The shock waves travel through the water and patient's body to impact upon the stone. Approximately 15,000 lb of pressure per square inch is generated by each shock wave at the second focal point. An average of 2,000 shock waves is given over the 45-minute treatment period. The method is very effective for calculi in the seven- to 15-mm range; in 90 percent of these patients the stone will be disintegrated and all particulate matter will pass within a 3-month period. In general, these patients experience little morbidity and the hospital stay is only 1 to 3 days. In selected patients, the treatment is being done on an outpatient basis. Most patients return to work within 2 to 3 days after shock wave therapy.

For obstructing calculi *below the pelvic brim*, the best approach remains transurethral. In many cases, these calculi can be removed from the ureter using a variety of stone baskets or loops. This approach is successful in upward of 70 percent of patients. When this fails, one can attempt to dilate the ureter and pass a rigid ureterorenoscope to allow for direct endoscopic manipulation of the calculus. Indeed, electrohydraulic and ultrasonic probes have been designed to enable the urologist to destroy larger distal ureteral calculi in situ through the ureterorenoscope. The ureterorenoscope can also be used for upper ureteral calculi; however, the success rate is only 70 percent owing to impaction or proximal migration of the stone. Success rates in the distal ureter with either fluoroscopic or direct endoscopic maneuvers exceed 95 percent. Thus, the need for an open surgical approach for a distal ureteral calculus is rare. Finally, for distal ureteral calculi an approach via a percutaneous nephrostomy or on the extracorporeal shock wave lithotriptor is difficult and should be attempted only when transurethral methods have failed and surgical therapy is not feasible.

Broad-spectrum antibiotics are useful when infections complicate renal calculi. The choice of drugs should be based upon the sensitivity studies of the organism isolated from the urine. However, institution of antimicrobial therapy without relief of obstruction is not effective in controlling the infection. Therefore, when primary or secondary obstruction accompanies renal calculi, temporary relief of obstruction should be instituted promptly by insertion of a retrograde ureteral catheter. If the attempted retrograde catheter diversion is unsuccessful, a percutaneous nephrostomy tube can be placed. Whenever possible, relief of obstruction and infection should be achieved prior to stone manipulation and open surgery.

In summary, a stone less than five mm in diameter is likely to be passed without surgical intervention. Even when stone removal appears necessary, this can be achieved with extracorporeal shock wave lithotripsy or via a percutaneous nephrostomy alone in 95 percent of patients regardless of the size or location of the calculus. Surgical therapy is largely reserved for the few patients in whom the aforementioned measures fail. Earlier intervention is certainly indicated for patients in whom the history, laboratory data, and radiologic studies suggest complete obstruction, for the patient with infected urine, or for the patient with partial obstruction whose stone remains in the same position in the ureter for more than a few months. The treatment and prevention of specific stones is discussed elsewhere in this book.

Obstruction of the ureter by blood clots, a fungus ball, and papillary tissue can be managed by techniques similar to those employed in the treatment of stones. Significant obstruction attributable to neoplastic, inflammatory, and neurologic disease must be treated aggressively, since it is unlikely to remit spontaneously. A decision as to whether to divert the urine in patients who have metastatic malignant disease must be made on an individual basis.

Patients with sterile hydronephrosis secondary to advanced pelvic malignancy and a short life expectancy are usually not considered for percutaneous nephrostomy, while those with a reasonable prospect for tumor response to chemotherapy and radiotherapy are strong candidates for the procedure.

THE ROLE OF NEPHROSTOMY IN THE MANAGEMENT OF UPPER URETERAL OBSTRUCTION

Nephrostomy refers to the insertion of a tube through the kidney into the renal pelvis to provide immediate renal urinary drainage. Until the 1950s, all nephrostomy tubes were placed via an open surgical approach. This resulted in a significant morbidity and mortality rate, since patients requiring emergency nephrostomy tube placement were often quite debilitated. In 1955, Goodwin reported the first case of a needle-derived nephrostomy tube placed under floroscopic guidance. The technique did not gain popularity until the 1970s, when the advent of ultrasonography and improved methods of fluoroscopy made the percutaneous approach more feasible. Currently, almost all nephrostomy tubes are placed percutaneously by an interventional radiologist or urologist. This is usually done under local anesthesia and takes less than 40 minutes.

The most common indications for placement of a nephrostomy tube are to provide a conduit to the kidney for percutaneous stone removal and to relieve ureteral obstruction secondary to neoplasia; inflammatory disease; or lower tract, extrinsic, or intrinsic obstruction in which the patient's condition will not permit a more definitive surgical procedure. Likewise, unmanageable infection behind an obstructed system is another common indication. It is not unusual to note dramatic clinical improvement within hours of percutaneous drainage in the patient with urosepsis.

The immediate complications of nephrostomy are perirenal hemorrhage and acute obstruction from clot formation. One of the more serious delayed complications is dislodgement of the nephrostomy tube. This is considered an emergency and the tube should be replaced immediately, otherwise the tract will seal off, usually within 24 hours. Another problem following nephrostomy tube removal is the exsanguinating hemorrhage from a renal pseudoaneurysm. This occurs in 0.5 to 1 percent of patients and is best managed by immediate selective embolization of the affected vessel. Long-term complications, such as infection, calculus formation, and pyelonephritis, are significant and may lead to renal failure.

Except in unusual circumstances, long-term urinary diversion by the nephrostomy tube is not recommended. However, many patients can go on for years without serious complications from their nephrostomy tubes. Also, in patients with extrinsic obstruction secondary to metastatic carcinoma, the nephrostomy tract can be used to manipulate a catheter into the bladder. A small tube can be placed through the affected flank and kidney with its pigtail end left in the bladder. The external portion of the stent can be clamped, thereby providing unobstructed flow from the affected kidney to the patient's bladder. This eliminates the need for external drainage bags and also facilitates changing the tube. In essence, all nephrostomy tubes or indwelling stents are changed every 3 months to decrease the build-up of concretions and to preclude breakage of ureteral stents within the collecting system.

In chronically obstructed kidneys, a period of percutaneous drainage may permit significant restoration of renal function. With this knowledge, and with periodic determination of split renal function studies, treatment can be planned effectively. A lack of significant improvement in function might suggest, for example, that nephrectomy rather than reparative surgery should be undertaken.

THE MANAGEMENT OF LOWER URINARY TRACT OBSTRUCTION

Bladder neck and urethral obstruction should be surgically repaired in ambulatory patients who have recurrent infections, especially when associated with reflux, evidence of renal parenchymal damage, total urinary retention, repeated bleeding, or other severe symptoms. Difficulties with voiding secondary to benign prostatic hyperplasia do not always follow a progressive course. Therefore, the man with minimal symptoms, no infection, and a normal upper urinary tract may be followed safely until he and his physician agree that surgery is desirable. Urethral stricture in men secondary to infection or trauma are frequently treated by simple dilation or direct vision internal urethrotomy. In these patients, radiographic and endoscopic follow-up care is essential to rule out recurrence. The incidence of bladder neck and urethral obstruction in women is low and has been overestimated in the past; hence urethral dilation, internal urethrotomy, meatotomy, and revision of the bladder neck are seldom indicated. In some patients, suprapubic cystostomy may be necessary for bladder drainage. It is especially indicated in patients who are unable to void after sustaining injury to the urethra or who have an impassable urethral stricture.

Again, advances in urologic instrumentation have further decreased the indications for open surgery. Almost all suprapubic cystotomies are performed using a percutaneous approach under fluoroscopic guidance. Open cystotomy is rarely performed. In addition, a closed transurethral approach is used to treat the majority of patients with prostatic hyperplasia (up to 60 or more grams of tissue), urethral strictures, bladder neck contractures, bladder calculi, and superficial bladder tumors.

When obstructive uropathy is a consequence of neuropathic bladder function, urodynamic studies are essential to establish a treatment regimen. In all cases, the main therapeutic goals are to establish the bladder as a site of urine storage without causing renal parenchymal injury, and to provide a mechanism for bladder emptying which is acceptable to the patient. In general, these patients fall into two groups: those with bladder atony secondary to lower motor neuron injury and those with unstable bladder function attributable to upper motor neuron disease. In both cases, ureteral reflux and renal parenchymal injury may occur, although it is more common with the hyperactive upper motor neuron bladder. This problem may be potentiated by sphincter-detrusor dyssynergia or by using either external compression (Credé) or increasing abdominal pressure (Valsalva) to aid voiding.

Patients with neurogenic bladder function owing to diabetes mellitus are classic examples of lower motor neuron disease. Voiding at regular intervals is one method to aid satisfactory bladder emptying in such patients. Occasionally, these individuals will respond to cholinergic medications. Recent reviews on the use of bethanechol chloride (Urecholine) 50 mg orally have seriously questioned its long-term value. In such patients, overdistention of the bladder impairs emptying, since detrusor contraction is essential to sphincter relaxation. Thus, bladder outlet obstruction may be a major problem. Alpha-adrenergic blockers such as phenoxybenzamine relax urethral sphincter tone, but have only limited success because of side effects.

Another alternative in men with a flaccid bladder is external sphincterotomy. This transurethral procedure may be successful in relieving outlet obstruction and promoting bladder emptying, but it has a disadvantage of urinary incontinence, and the need for the patient to wear an external collection device. In men, this problem can be obviated by the use of a penile clamp; however, the clamps often result in significant morbidity owing to urethral erosion and penile edema. In women, the incontinence associated with external sphincterotomy precludes its use. In addition, the implantation of newly developed artificial urinary sphincters has been partially successful.

These devices are promising; however, problems with their longevity have hindered their widespread acceptance.

The most ideal treatment for those patients with significant residual urine and recurrent bouts of urosepsis is the institution of clean intermittent catheterization (CIC) at regular intervals. The goal should be catheterization four to five times per day such that the amount of urine drained from the bladder does not exceed 300 to 400 ml. This technique has met with considerable success in almost all age groups, but requires patient acceptance and careful training.

In patients with unstable bladder function attributable to upper motor neuron lesions, the major goal is to improve the storage function of the bladder. Pharmacologic maneuvers include the use of anticholinergic agents such as, oxybutynin (Ditropan) 5 mg every 4 to 6 hours. Adjunctive therapy such as CIC is frequently necessary to ensure complete bladder emptying and prevent incontinence.

In all patients with neurogenic bladders, chronic indwelling catheters are to be avoided if at all possible. In addition to problems of external drainage, bladder stones, urosepsis, and urethral erosion, chronic indwelling catheters are associated with the occurrence of squamous cell carcinoma of the bladder. Patients managed in this fashion for more than 5 years should all undergo yearly cystoscopic examinations.

Finally, surgical diversions are indicated for (1) deterioration of renal function despite conservative measures, (2) intractable incontinence, (3) small contracted bladder, and (4) multiple bladder fistulas.Intermittent bacteriuria is seldom an indication, since it is common to all therapeutic approaches to the neurogenic bladder. The ileal conduit is the operation of choice for permanent diversion. Although many individuals do well after this procedure, operative mortality, postoperative intestinal obstruction, and stomal obstruction are complications that make the operation far from ideal. Further, recent studies have indicated that as many as 80 percent of patients will have a progressive decline in their renal function. A continent form of ileal diversion has become available, the Koch pouch. With this procedure, an ileal reservoir is made which has a 300- to 500-ml capacity. A continent stoma is placed in the right lower quadrant of the abdomen which the patient must empty by catheterization four times a day. This method of diversion alleviates the need for any external collection devices.

In patients requiring short-term indwelling urethral catheters, good care is necessary to prevent urinary tract infection. Men are instructed to cleanse the glans twice a day with an antimicrobial soap and then to apply an antibiotic ointment. Given specific indications for catheter drainage, proper patient selection, aseptic technique, closed urinary drainage, the judicious use of systemic antimicrobials, and proper catheter care, the indwelling urethral catheter is a satisfactory means of short-term diversion and in rare instances long-term urinary diversion. The principles of closed drainage are that the system is never open, that the urine in the drainage tube never comes in contact with that in the collecting bag, and that, at all times, the bag is in a dependent position. Cultures can be obtained by clamping the catheter for a few minutes and then using a small needle and syringe to aspirate urine from the lumen of the catheter. We prefer not to break the drainage system for catheter irrigation or for the use of antibiotic irrigating solutions to reduce infection, as has been advocated by some. In patients requiring long-term catheter drainage, intermittent irrigation with an acid citrate solution is useful in reducing encrustation.

In the past, there has been some concern and controversy about the possible complications of rapid decompression of a severly distended bladder. It has been advised that the grossly distended bladder be drained slowly over hours rather than all at once. It has been suggested that rapid emptying of the distended bladder may be followed by hypotension and syncope or hemorrhagic cystitis attributable to sudden decompression of stretched mucosal blood vessels. These concerns appear unjustified, since it has been found that the intravesical pressure in patients with acute urinary retention falls precipitously to near normal values after the first deciliter of urine is withdrawn, indicating that any sudden decompressive effect on blood vessels would be maximal during the removal of the initial volume of urine.

MANAGEMENT OF POSTOBSTRUCTIVE DIURESIS

Postobstructive diuresis refers to the marked polyuria that can occur after relief of urinary tract obstruction. This polyuria is usually associated with the excretion of large amounts of sodium, potassium, magnesium, and other solutes. Although self-limited (it may last several days), the losses of salt and water may be of such magnitude as to cause hypokalemia, hyponatremia or hypernatremia, hypomagnesemia and/or marked contraction of the extracellular fluid (ECF) volume, and peripheral vascular collapse. In many patients, however, a brisk diuresis after relief of urinary tract obstruction may be physiologically appropriate rather than due to inability of the postobstructed kidney to maintain volume and solute homeostasis. A postobstructive diuresis is appropriate and does not compromise the volume status of the patient when it is owing to excretion of excess salt, water, and urea retained during the period of obstruction. This diuresis is transient and usually subsides within the first day or 2 after relief of obstruction without causing depletion of the ECF volume. It is often impossible, however, to distinguish such patients from those who have a true defect in tubular reabsorption of salt and water on the basis of urine volume and composition alone. Thus, replacement therapy should be guided by clinical and laboratory evidence of the adequacy of the ECF volume and not by the volume of the urine alone.

It is well established that postobstructive diuresis could be artificially prolonged by overzealous administration of salt and water after relief of obstruction. Replacement of excreted salt and water will maintain a state of expansion of the ECF and hence result in the continuous excretion of the excess salt and water administered. Thus, fluid replacement may be justified only when excessive losses of sodium and water occur which are inappropriate for the volume status of the patient and are presumably owing to an intrinsic tubular defect in the reabsorption of sodium and water.

The appropriate fluid replacement that should be given to patients with postobstructive diuresis depends in large part on what is excreted. Intravenous fluid administration may be necessary, but urinary losses should be replaced only to the extent necessary to prevent hypovolemia, hypotension, hypokalemia, and/or hypomagnesemia. Excessive fluid administration would only prolong the duration of the postobstructive diuresis. Orthostatic hypotension and tachycardia are perhaps the best indicators of when intravenous fluid administration is needed. To distinguish between inappropriate diuresis and the excretion of fluid retained or excess fluid administration, it may be necessary to decrease the rate of intravenous fluid administration to levels below those of urinary output and observe the patient carefully for signs of volume depletion (hypotension, tachycardia, stabilization or elevation in the levels of blood urea nitrogen which were previously decreasing). In the case of inappropriate diuresis, appropriate fluid replacement requires the prompt quantitative replacement of urinary losses of water, sodium, potassium, and magnesium. This is best accomplished by frequent measurements of urine volume and serum and urine electrolytes. With massive diuresis such measurements may be required every 6 hours. Daily weighing, occasionally even more often, is necessary. Fluids administered should be tailored to match the urinary excretion of water and electrolytes.

Urinary losses of salt and water in most instances may be replaced with solutions of 0.45 percent sodium chloride to which sodium bicarbonate and potassium chloride have been added. Replacement of magnesium may be accomplished by adding magnesium sulfate (supplied as 2-ml ampules containing 4 mEq of magnesium) to the sodium chloride solution. In some instances replacement of phosphate losses may be necessary. Either 42 percent sodium phosphate (15-ml ampules containing 45 mmol of phosphate and 60 mEq of sodium) or 46 percent potassium phosphate (15-ml ampules containing 45 mmol of phosphate and 66 mEq of potassium) may be added to 5 percent dextrose or 0.45 percent sodium chloride solutions.

In summary, a persistent diuresis after relief of urinary tract obstruction is an uncommon clinical event, but one that is potentially dangerous. Its pathogenesis differs among patients, but careful assessment of the volume status, serum and urine electrolytes, and blood urea nitrogen will permit adequate evaluation leading to appropriate therapy. Routine and prolonged salt and water administration in the postobstructive period should be avoided, since it may perpetuate a diuresis through normal physiologic mechanisms.

UROLITHIASIS: CALCIUM STONES

CHARLES Y.C. PAK, M.D.

Nephrolithiasis is common, affecting 0.1 to 0.3 percent of the population yearly, and 5 to 10 percent sometime in their lifetime. Calcareous stones account for 80 to 95 percent of stones and are principally composed of calcium oxalate and calcium phosphate, usually occurring as a mixture. The progress in this field has been dramatic, resulting in pathophysiologic elucidation, diagnostic differentiation, and effective treatment of the vast majority of patients suffering from calcium stones.

PATHOPHYSIOLOGY

Causes of calcium stones include hypercalciuria, hyperuricosuria, hyperoxaluria, and hypocitraturia.

One prevailing theory considers hypercalciuria to be comprised of several entities of separate pathogenetic origin. In *absorptive hypercalciuria*, hypercalciuria results from the primary enhancement of intestinal calcium absorption. In the more severe type I presentation, hypercalciuria is found during both low and high calcium intakes, whereas in the type II presentation it occurs only during a high calcium intake. The type III presentation is believed to be secondary to a renal leak of phosphate as the primary event. The ensuing hypophosphatemia is thought to stimulate the renal synthesis of 1,25-$(OH)_2$vitamin D and intestinal calcium absorption. *Renal hypercalciuria* is the result of an impairment in the renal tubular reabsorption of calcium. It is typically accompanied by secondary stimulation of intestinal calcium absorption owing to enhanced parathyroid hormone-dependent 1,25-$(OH)_2$vitamin D synthesis. *Resorptive hypercalciuria* is characterized by primary hyperparathyroidism. Besides high skeletal resorption, intestinal calcium absorption is frequently elevated.

In contrast, the unifying theory attributes the pathogenesis of both absorptive and renal hypercalciurias to the same general defect originating in the kidney. However, considerable evidence supports the view that absorptive and renal hypercalciurias are separate and distinct entities (see Treatment section).

Among the other causes of calcareous stones, *hyperoxaluria* usually results from excessive oxalate absorption from food (enteric hyperoxaluria) and rarely is a consequence of oxalate overproduction, *hyperuricosuria* is usually attributable to high purine intake, and *hypocitraturia* is the consequence of renal tubular acidosis, acquired metabolic acidosis of excessive intestinal alkali loss, hypokalemia, or other unknown causes (idiopathic).

These causes of calcium stones often coexist in the same patient.

DIAGNOSIS

The evaluation of patients with a single stone episode without risk need not be extensive and may include blood screen (calcium, phosphorus, electrolytes, uric acid), urinalysis, stone analysis, and abdominal roentgenogram.

The "gold standard" for the diagnostic protocol is the outpatient evaluation, entailing collection of one or two random 24-hour urine sample(s) and another sample after adherence to a calcium- and sodium-restricted diet for various stone-forming risks, as well as the measurement of fasting urinary calcium (for detection of renal calcium leak) and urinary calcium following 1 g oral calcium load (for an indirect assessment of intestinal calcium absorption). As a simplified approach, one random 24-hour urine sample could be screened for stone-forming risks (stone risk profile), and further assessment could be done based on the results of this analysis. Diagnostic criteria for different causes of calcium nephrolithiasis are presented in Table 1.

TREATMENT

Patients with a single stone episode or inactive disease could be managed conservatively with high fluid intake (sufficient to produce urine output of at least 2 L per day) and avoidance of dietary excesses. More aggressive treatment involving drugs as well as conservative measures are indicated for those with active stone disease and for certain patients with a single stone episode who are at risk for developing others. Specific treatments are selected or "tailor-made" for each cause of stone disease whenever possible, to correct the underlying derangement(s).

Absorptive Hypercalciuria Type I

Sodium cellulose phosphate (5 g with lunch and dinner) may be used in patients with documented absorptive hypercalciuria type I without bone disease, especially when hypercalciuria of intestinal origin is marked (> 300 mg per day) or when alternative treatments (thiazide and orthophosphate) are ineffective or poorly tolerated. Dietary oxalate restriction and oral magnesium supplementation (0.5 g twice a day separately from sodium cellulose phosphate) are recommended, in order to avoid secondary hyperoxaluria and hypomagnesiuria. It should not be given to growing children or elderly patients at risk for osteoporosis, nor to those with normal intestinal calcium absorption or with parathyroid stimulation, because this drug reduces intestinal calcium absorption. If sodium cellulose phosphate does not produce satisfactory control of hypercalciuria, thiazide may be added. The high cost of the preparation precludes more extensive use.

Thiazide is indicated in patients with less severe hypercalciuria, as well as in those at risk for bone disease and those resistant to or intolerant of sodium cellulose phosphate therapy. If urinary citrate is adequate (> 500 mg per day), Moduretic (hydrochlorothiazide 50 mg and amiloride 5 mg), ½ tablet twice a day, may be used, since it is less likely to cause hypokalemia and hypocitraturia and it is expected to exert greater hypocalciuric action than thiazide alone. When urinary citrate is less than 500 mg per day, it would be advantageous to use thiazide alone (hydrochlorothiazide 50 mg twice a day or trichlormethiazide 4 mg a day) without a potassium-sparing agent and provide potassium supplementation (potassium citrate 15 to 20 mEq twice a day). Potassium citrate has been shown to prevent thiazide-induced hypokalemia and augment citrate excretion. Sodium intake should be kept within 150 mEq per day.

During long-term therapy, some patients may become refractory to the hypocalciuric action of thiazide, probably reflecting the failure of this treatment to restore normal intestinal calcium absorption. When this loss of hypocalciuric action occurs, sodium cellulose phosphate therapy may be offered instead. Responsiveness to thiazide usually develops after 6 to 12 months of alternative therapy.

TABLE 1 Diagnostic Criteria

	PHPT	*AH-1*	*AH-II*	*AH-III*	*RH*	*EH*	*HUCU*	*Hypocitr*
Serum calcium	↑	N	N	N	N	N/↓	N	N
Serum phosphorus	↓/N	N	N	↓	N	N/↓	N	N
Urinary calcium	↑/N	↑	N	↑/N	↑	↓	N	N
Serum PTH	↑	N/↓	N/↓	N/↓	↑	N/↑	N	N
Urinary calcium (1-g Ca load)	↑/N	↑	↑	↑	↑/N	↓	N	N
Urinary calcium (fasting)	↑/N	N	N	N	↑	↓	N	N
Urinary uric acid	N/↑	N/↑	N/↑	N/↑	N/↑	↓	↑	N
Urinary oxalate	N/↑	N/↑	N/↑	N/↑	N/↑	↑	N	N
Urinary citrate	N	N/↓	N/↓	N/↓	N/↓	↓	N/↓	↓

Fasting samples were collected for 2 hours, the morning after an overnight fast. 1-g Ca load samples were obtained over a 4-hour period after an oral ingestion of 1 g Ca.

Key: PTH = immunoreactive parathyroid hormone; ↑ = high; ↓ = low; N = normal; PHPT = primary hyperparathyroidism; AH–1 = absorptive hypercalciuria type 1; AH–II = absorptive hypercalciuria type 2; AH–III = hypophosphatemic absorptive hypercalciuria; RH = renal hypercalciuria; HUCU = hyperuricosuric calcium oxalate nephrolithiasis (pure presentation); EH = enteric hyperoxaluria; Hypocitr = hypocitraturic calcium nephrolithiasis (idiopathic) exclusive of renal tubular acidosis or acquired metabolic acidosis. Fasting urinary Ca may be high in AH, but it typically returns to normal following oral Ca restriction.

Absorptive Hypercalciuria Type II

No specific drug treatment is generally necessary, since normocalciuria may be obtained by a moderate dietary calcium restriction. A high fluid intake should be encouraged, since urinary output is often low. If hypocitraturia (< 320 mg per day) is present, potassium citrate (30 to 60 mEq per day in 2 or 3 divided doses) is advised.

Absorptive Hypercalciuria Type III

Orthophosphate (neutral or alkaline salt of sodium and potassium, 0.5 g phosphorus 3 to 4 times a day) is the treatment of choice because it is capable of reducing serum 1,25-$(OH)_2$vitamin D and urinary calcium. It is contraindicated if nephrolithiasis is complicated by urinary tract infection.

Renal Hypercalciuria

Thiazide is ideally indicated for renal hypercalciuria (same guidelines for use as in absorptive hypercalciuria type I). Potassium citrate supplementation is advised if thiazide alone (without potassium-sparing agent) is used.

Resorptive Hypercalciuria

Parathyroidectomy is the treatment of choice for nephrolithiasis of primary hyperparathyroidism. In patients who are poor surgical candidates, medical treatment alternatives include orthophosphate (0.5 g phosphorus three or four times a day) and estrogen (e.g., ethinyl estradial 0.05 to 0.1 mg per day in postmenopausal women).

Enteric Hyperoxaluria

Because of multiple causes of stone formation, the treatment program may need to be diverse. Rigid oxalate restriction is critical. A high fluid intake is necessary to overcome intestinal fluid loss. Magnesium supplementation (magnesium gluconate as tolerated) may be useful if magnesium deficiency is present. Treatment with potassium citrate (60 to 120 mEq per day) may correct the hypokalemia and metabolic acidosis and increase urinary citrate level toward normal. If there is a calcium deficiency, calcium citrate (200 to 400 mg three or four times a day) may be useful. When hypercalciuria develops, it should be controlled with thiazide.

Hyperuricosuric Calcium Oxalate Nephrolithiasis

Allopurinol (300 mg per day) is the drug of choice, especially if hyperuricemia is also present or when hyperuricosuria is marked (> 800 mg per day). A moderate sodium restriction (< 150 mEq per day) is advised to limit monosodium urate–induced crystallization of calcium oxalate.

When hyperuricosuria is not severe (< 800 mg per day) or if hypocitraturia is also present, potassium citrate (30 to 60 mEq per day in 2 or 3 divided doses) may be effective.

Hypocitraturia

In renal tubular acidosis (distal), potassium citrate (60 to 120 mEq per day in 2 or 3 divided doses) not only corrects hypokalemia and acidosis, but may augment citrate excretion. In hypocitraturia of chronic diarrheal syndrome (after gastrectomy, ileal disease, colitis), potassium citrate at a similar dosage may be required. Thiazide-induced hypocitraturia accompanied by stone relapse generally requires a lower dose of potassium citrate (30 to 60 mEq per day in 2 or 3 divided doses). A similar lower dose of potassium citrate is indicated in idiopathic hypocitraturic calcium oxalate nephrolithiasis (occurring alone or in conjuction with other derangements). If hypocitraturia accompanies absorptive hypercalciuria type I, it would be advisable to add potassium citrate to sodium cellulose phosphate or thiazide therapy. In hyperuricosuric calcium oxalate nephrolithiasis accompanied by hypocitraturia, potassium citrate may be needed unless there is hyperuricemia or marked hyperuricosuria.

Follow-up Evaluation

If a specific medical treatment has been instituted, it is imperative that the patients be evaluated within the first 6 months to make certain that they are free of side effects and that their biochemical responses are appropriate. The dose of the medication(s) may be adjusted accordingly, and the need for conservative measures reinforced.

ACUTE AND CHRONIC HYPERURICEMIC NEPHROPATHY

CATHERINE S. THOMPSON, M.D.
EDWARD J. WEINMAN, M.D.

The term "hyperuricemic nephropathy" is used to describe *three renal syndromes* associated with elevations of the plasma concentration or urinary excretion of uric acid. The first is *acute uric acid nephropathy*, which occurs as a result of a sudden and massive overproduction of uric acid. It is most commonly observed as a consequence of cancer chemotherapy for lymphoproliferative malignancies and can lead to acute renal failure. *Chronic urate nephropathy*, or gouty nephropathy, refers to a condition recognized in certain individuals with longstanding hyperuricemia and associated chronic renal insufficiency and hypertension. As will be discussed, however, there is now reason to believe that there is no definite causal relationship between chronic hyperuricemia and the development of renal insufficiency. The third disorder is *uric acid nephrolithiasis*, which is caused by the precipitation of calculi containing uric acid in the urinary collecting system. The latter disorder is discussed in a separate chapter.

Uric Acid Metabolism

Uric acid is the end product of purine metabolism in man (Fig. 1). There is a steady-state pool of uric acid of approximately 1,000 mg (Fig. 2). Input to this pool derives in large measure from de novo synthesis and to a lesser extent from the dietary intake of nucleoproteins. The major route of elimination of urate is by renal excretion. A smaller amount of urate is excreted by gastrointestinal uricolysis. The plasma concentration of uric acid, therefore, represents the balance between the rates of production and elimination. Since the contributions of dietary intake and gastrointestinal uricolysis are relatively minor, the rate of de novo synthesis and the rate of urinary excretion are the major determinants of the uric acid pool.

In normal individuals, approximately 5 to 10 percent of the filtered load of urate is excreted in the urine (Fig. 3). Urate is freely filtered at the glomerulus. In the proximal tubule, urate undergoes bidirectional transport; that is, urate is both reabsorbed from the glomerular ultrafiltrate into the blood and secreted from the peritubular capillary blood into the tubular lumen. Both the absorptive and secretory processes for urate are affected by a number of drugs and by a variety of physiologic and pathologic processes (Table 1). The ultimate urinary excretion of uric acid depends on the balance between these processes. For example, hyperuricemia may result from inhibition of urate secretion, as in patients with retention of other organic anions which compete for the organic acid secretory mechanism in the proximal renal tubule (lactate, ketoacids); enhanced tubular reabsorption, as in patients with depletion of the extracellular fluid volume; or both, as in patients treated with diuretics and a low-sodium diet.

There is little or no evidence that uric acid itself is toxic to cells. The pathophysiology of urate-related disorders, therefore, relates to the limited solubility of uric acid in acidic solution. Uric acid is a weak acid with a pK of 5.75. In solutions of pH greater than 5.75, uric acid is predominantly in its ionized and more soluble form. In acidic solution (pH <5.75), uric acid is in its unionized and less soluble form. The limited solubility of uric acid in acidic solutions results in precipitation of urate and accounts for the major pathophysiologic expressions of urate-related diseases.

ACUTE URIC ACID NEPHROPATHY

Acute uric acid nephropathy is the result of widespread precipitation of uric acid microcrystals within the distal renal tubules, collecting ducts, and pelvis of the kidney. It is caused by a sudden and massive influx of uric acid into the blood. The tremendous increase in the filtered load presented to the kidney exceeds the limits of solubility for uric acid in tubular fluid and precipitation occurs. The acute uric acid overload is most commonly recognized as a sequela of cancer chemotheraphy usually in the setting of a highly responsive lymphoproliferative malignancy such as leukemia or lymphoma. Occasionally acute uric acid nephropathy can occur

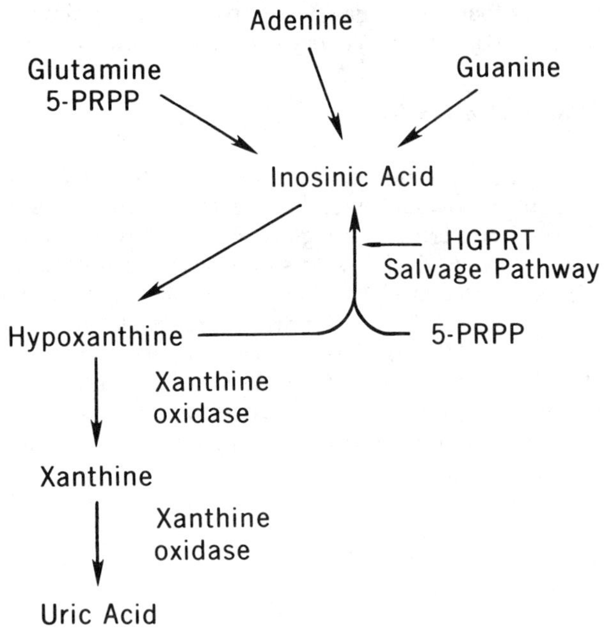

Figure 1 Simplified schema of uric acid biosynthesis. HGPRT = hypoxanthine-guanine phosphoribosyltransferase; 5-PRPP=5 phosphoribosylpyrophosphate.

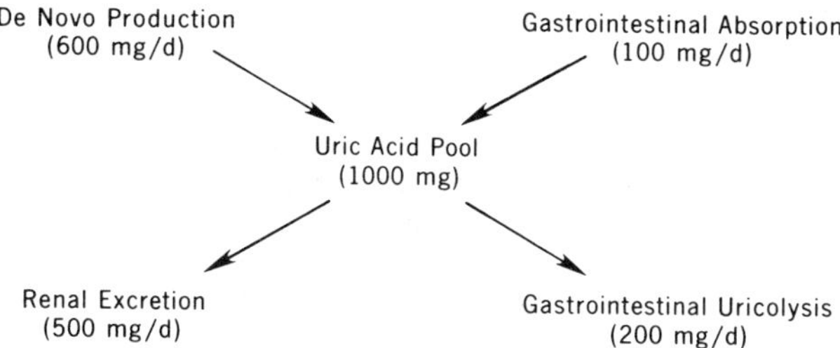

Figure 2 Daily turnover of uric acid in normal man demonstrating endogenous production, exogenous input, and disposition via kidney and gut.

after treatment of bulky solid tumors. It has also been reported to occur with radiation therapy or even as a spontaneous event in some malignancies. In the majority of cases, the condition is recognized clinically as the "tumor lysis syndrome" in which massive destruction of tumor cells leads not only to hyperuricemia, but also to hyperphosphatemia and life-threatening hyperkalemia.

The typical individual with acute uric acid nephropathy develops acute oliguric renal failure associated with marked hyperuricemia within hours to days of receiving cancer chemotherapy. Figure 4 depicts a prototypic case history of a patient with this syndrome. The uric acid level in plasma usually exceeds 15 mg per deciliter, but may be as high as 30 to 40 mg per deciliter. Other features of the "tumor lysis syndrome" such as hyperkalemia and hyperphosphatemia are often present. Although hyperuricemia is common in almost all types of acute renal failure, patients with acute uric acid nephropathy typically have hyperuricosuria as well. A useful laboratory test to distinguish individuals with acute uric acid nephropathy from those with other types of acute renal failure is a random urine uric acid to creatinine ratio. If this ratio exceeds one, acute uric acid nephropathy is suggested.

Prevention

Acute uric acid nephropathy is largely a preventable disease (Table 2). Patients at high risk of developing this syndrome should be identified prior to the initiation of cancer chemotherapy. With appropriate prophylaxis, the

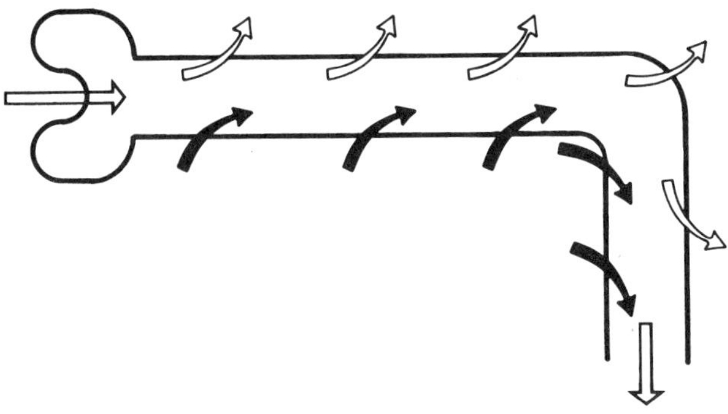

Figure 3 Simplified schema of renal uric acid excretion in the proximal tubule demonstrating glomerular filtration and tubular secretion and reabsorption.

TABLE 1 Factors Affecting the Renal Excretion of Uric Acid

Uricosuric
Ascorbic acid—high dose, >4 g/day
Glyceryl guaiacolate
Mannitol
Phenylbutazone
Probenecid
Radiocontrast agents
Salicylates—high dose, >15 mg/dl in serum
Sulfinpyrazone
Volume expansion
Antiuricosuric
Diuretics
Ethambutol
Ketoacids
Lactic acid
Salicylates—low dose, 5–10 mg/dl in serum
Volume depletion

risk of renal failure can be minimized. The goal of these interventions is twofold. The first is to decrease the production of uric acid. The second is to enhance the solubility of uric acid in the urine by instituting measures that will dilute and alkalinize the renal tubular fluid.

Patients considered at high risk for the development of acute uric acid nephropathy should be hospitalized for 48 to 72 hours prior to the initiation of chemotherapy. The production of uric acid can be reduced significantly by pretreatment with the drug allopurinol. Allopurinol is a structural analogue of hypoxanthine and a competitive inhibitor of the enzyme xanthine oxidase which catalyzes the conversion of hypoxanthine to xanthine and xanthine to uric acid. The metabolite of allopurinol, oxypurinol, is also a potent inhibitor of xanthine oxidase. Although allopurinol is usually prescribed in dosages of 200 to 300 mg per day, larger doses may be required for prophylaxis in the patient at risk for acute uric acid nephropathy because of the massive, acute overproduction of uric acid in this condition. Allopurinol should be administered orally in dosages of 600 to 900 mg per day for 3 to 5 days prior to commencing chemotherapy and should be continued throughout the course of chemotherapy. An intravenous preparation of the drug, although not universally available, should be considered in the patient who cannot take oral medications.

Adequate hydration prior to and during chemotherapy is essential. Brisk urine flow rates, in the range of 3 L per day, should be established. Oral hydration is usually not sufficient and should be supplemented with intravenous fluid, such as 0.45 percent normal saline. Alkalinization of the urine to a pH of 7 allows for enhanced solubility of filtered uric acid and lessens the risk of microcrystallization within the collecting system of the kidney. This can be accomplished by the addition of sodium bicarbonate to the intravenous fluids. One ampule of sodium bicarbonate (50 mEq) can be added to each liter of 0.45 percent saline as a simple way of providing supplemental bicarbonate. Oral bicarbonate in the form of sodium citrate (Shol's solution) can also be used. If the patient has a systemic acidosis, however, the urine will

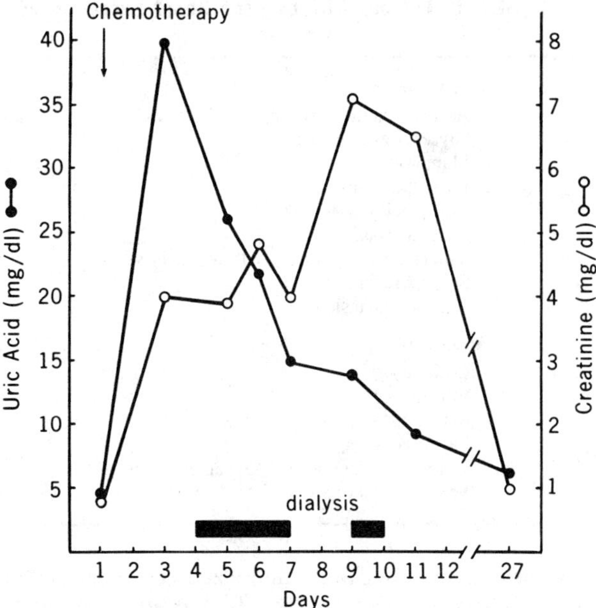

Figure 4 An example of acute uric acid nephropathy in a 24-year-old man with stage IV lymphoblastic lymphoma, treated with intravenous chemotherapy on day 1 as an outpatient. The pretreatment uric acid, creatinine, and electrolytes were normal. He was admitted on day 3 with fatigue, nausea, and oliguria. The serum uric acid was 40 mg per deciliter; blood urea nitrogen 96 mg per deciliter; potassium 8.3 mEq per liter; and phosphorus 30 mg per deciliter. Hemodialysis was performed on days 4, 5, 6, and 9. The urine output initially was less than 200 ml per day but gradually increased to 4,500 ml per day with a gradual fall in serum creatinine and blood urea nitrogen concentrations. One month later his creatinine was 1.0 mg per deciliter, blood urea nitrogen 15 mg per deciliter, and uric acid 6.0 mg per deciliter.

remain acidic despite these efforts and additional bicarbonate may be necessary. The use of the drug acetazolamide, a carbonic anhydrase inhibitor, has been advocated as a means of inducing an alkaline diuresis. The drug exerts its effect in the proximal renal tubule by inhibiting the reclamation of filtered bicarbonate. Acetazolamide is usually not necessary in most cases, but can be administered in oral or intravenous divided doses of 500 to 1,000 mg per day. The drug should be used with caution in patients with systemic acidosis as it may aggravate the condition by promoting further renal bicarbonate loss.

After the initiation of chemotherapy, the patient should be monitored closely for the development of hyperuricemia and renal dysfunction. Efforts to maintain brisk urine flow rates and an alkaline urine should be sustained. The administration of allopurinol should also be continued. On occasion, a patient may develop marked hyperuricemia and renal failure despite these interventions. In many cases the disease is mild and transient and can be managed without dialytic interventions.

Treatment

The patient with sudden cessation of renal function from acute uric acid nephropathy has micro-obstruction to urine flow due to extensive crystallization of urate within the renal collecting system. In these cases, dangerous hyperkalemia, volume overload, or systemic acidosis may be complicating features. Dialytic intervention is almost always necessary in these settings and plays a dual role in the management of the patient. Dialysis protects the patient from the immediate complications of acute renal failure and also lowers significantly the uric acid load presented to the kidney. The use of a high-efficiency hemodialysis membrane results in uric acid clearances which average 120 to 150 ml per minute, and it is therefore the preferred treatment. A single 6-hour hemodialysis treatment lowers the concentration of uric acid by about 50 percent. Peritoneal dialysis is a much less efficient method of uric acid removal, the clearances averaging only about 15 ml per minute. There is some evidence to suggest that rapid lowering of the concentration of uric acid in the plasma leads to a more rapid recovery of renal function in affected individuals, and for this reason hemodialysis should be considered early in the course of treatment for established acute uric acid nephropathy. In addition to hemodialysis, some authorities have advocated that patients with acute uric acid nephropathy be evaluated for evidence of extrarenal obstruction to urine flow. Some patients will have substantial uric acid sludge in the renal pelvis and proximal ureter. In these cases, retrograde pyelography and irrigation of the renal pelves with a solution of sodium bicarbonate may be helpful in relieving the obstruction. Such maneuvers, however, are not always feasible in the acutely ill patient.

Certain individuals prone to the development of acute uric acid nephropathy, particularly those who have received some prophylactic intervention, will develop hyperuricemia and only mild to moderate renal insufficiency as a manifestation of acute uric acid nephropathy. They are typically nonoliguric. In these settings,

TABLE 2 Prevention and Management of Acute Uric Acid Nephropathy

Decrease the production of uric acid
Pretreatment with allopurinol
600–900 mg/day in divided doses
Begin 3–5 days *before* chemotherapy is administered
Enhance the urinary excretion of uric acid
Hydration
Achieve urine flow rates of at least 3 L/day
0.45% normal saline or 0.9% normal saline intravenously
Urinary alkalinization
Bicarbonate supplements
Oral: sodium citrate (Shol's solution), 100–150 ml/day (100–150 mEq/day)
Intravenous: add 1 ampule (50 mEq) to each liter of IV fluid, preferably 0.45% saline
Carbonic anhydrase inhibition
Acetazolamide (Diamox), 500–1,000 mg/day
Avoid in patients with bicarbonate <18 mEq/L
Management of acute uric acid nephropathy
Maintain urine flow rates
Allopurinol
Urinary alkalinization
Hemodialysis
Irrigation of renal pelves with bicarbonate solutions

fluids and intravenous diuretic drugs, such as furosemide, can be used to maintain the diuresis. The prognosis for these individuals is generally good if the diuresis can be maintained.

Although acute uric acid nephropathy can be a devastating condition associated with acute renal shutdown, systemic acidosis, hyperkalemia, and volume overload, the prognosis for renal recovery is generally good if the patient does not develop complicating conditions such as sepsis or respiratory failure. The renal disease is potentially reversible, with recovery heralded by increasing urine flow rates followed by progressive improvement in the glomerular filtration rate over the course of several days. The patient who develops acute uric acid nephropathy on one occasion may well have a recurrence with subsequent courses of chemotherapy and should therefore be aggressively prepared as outlined earlier.

CHRONIC URATE NEPHROPATHY

Chronic urate nephropathy, or gouty nephropathy, has been described in the literature as a progressive form of interstitial renal disease associated with a chronic elevation of the serum concentration of uric acid. Progression to irreversible renal insufficiency has been considered a potential sequela of this disorder. Patients with this condition frequently have a long history of gouty arthritis. They may also be hypertensive and have evidence of atherosclerotic vascular disease. Histopathologically, gouty nephropathy has been characterized by the deposition of crystals of monosodium urate in the medullary interstitium of the kidney. These so-called micro-tophi are often accompanied by inflammatory reactions that are postulated to result in chronic scarring of the renal interstitium.

Although chronic urate nephropathy has been felt to represent a distinct clinical entity, there has been growing skepticism about the validity of this assumption in recent years. Evidence is now available to indicate that there is a natural age-related decline in renal function, but that the rate of decline is not accelerated in patients with chronic hyperuricemia. Moreover, the development of significant renal insufficiency in patients with chronic hyperuricemia can usually be ascribed to a coexistent renal insult. In many cases associated arterial hypertension, vascular disease, or the chronic use of analgesics or nonsteroidal anti-inflammatory drugs contribute to the renal dysfunction. Finally, therapy directed toward decreasing the plasma concentration of uric acid in patients with chronic hyperuricemia does not decrease or reverse either the age-related decline in renal function or renal insufficiency due to other independent renal processes.

Nonetheless, there remains a significant group of individuals in whom accelerated renal insufficiency in association with hyperuricemia occurs. In these patients, it has been suggested that other independent processes are operative. It has been recognized that chronic hypertension can result in interstitial renal disease and the subsequent development of hyperuricemia. The rise in the plasma concentration of uric acid, then, derives as a consequence of the primary renal insult, hypertension, rather than being the initiating factor in the development of renal insufficiency.

Recent evidence also suggests that a subset of patients with chronic hyperuricemia and renal dysfunction may have lead nephropathy as the underlying renal lesion. The association between gout and lead toxicity has been recognized for many years as *saturnine gout*, but the extension to include individuals with chronic renal disease is recent. Exposure to lead may occur in industrial settings, with the ingestion of moonshine whiskey fermented in lead-contaminated equipment, or as a result of childhood exposure to lead-based paints. The hyperuricemia identified in these patients is felt to represent an impairment in the renal excretion of uric acid, an effect that is likely induced by chronic lead nephrotoxicity. In these cases, the hyperuricemia and renal parenchymal urate deposition are the result, rather than the cause of renal functional impairment. Evidence for coexisting lead nephropathy in the patient with chronic hyperuricemia is suggested by a positive ethylenediaminetetraacetic acid (EDTA) lead mobilization test. EDTA is a chelator of lead. Individuals with the triad of hyperuricemia, hypertension, and renal insufficiency will often demonstrate increased urinary excretion of lead when administered an EDTA challenge test. This is in contrast to individuals with known causes of renal dysfunction, such as diabetic glomerulosclerosis or hypertensive nephrosclerosis, who do not demonstrate an increase in urinary lead excretion with an EDTA challenge.

Treatment

The therapy for so-called gouty nephropathy is debated. It has been proposed that treatment that effectively decreases the plasma concentration of uric acid slows or reverses the progressive development of renal insufficiency in these patients. Recent studies, however, have cast doubt on the therapeutic suggestion that treatment of these individuals with hypouricemic drugs such as allopurinol decreases or reverses the renal functional impairment. It is likely that age-related declines in renal function or coexistent renal disease account for the progressive nature of the renal disease in these patients.

In short, specific therapy directed at lowering the plasma concentration of uric acid in individuals with chronic hyperuricemia and renal insufficiency is unlikely to be effective in reversing established renal disease. Chronic lead chelation therapy with EDTA has been proposed as a treatment for those individuals with chronic lead nephropathy but its efficacy is not established. It is likely that the only effective interventions in such individuals are those directed at controlling coexistent treatable conditions such as hypertension.

Disorders of uric acid metabolism have been associated with the development of renal injury. Conversely, patients with renal dysfunction attributed to other causes commonly have alterations in the renal handling of uric acid. Acute uric acid-induced renal failure is a direct consequence of precipitation of uric acid in the renal tubules with subsequent intratubular obstruction. As already discussed, the associations between longstanding hyperuricemia and the development of chronic renal insufficiency is currently debated. In most published studies, there is little or no correlation between the plasma concentration of urate and the incidence of uric acid nephrolithiasis. Although the incidence of stones is higher in individuals with asymptomatic hyperuricemia, it is not clinically reasonable to treat such persons with drugs such as allopurinol as prophylactic therapy against uric acid stone formation. Abnormalities in urate metabolism as manifested by hyperuricemia and/or hyperuricosuria have been noted in 25 percent of patients with calcium oxalate nephrolithiasis. Based on this evidence, the plasma concentration and 24-hour urinary excretion rates of uric acid should be determined in patients with calcium oxalate stones. Treatment of such individuals with allopurinol is frequently effective in reducing the incidence of such stones. Hyperuricemia is frequently observed in patients with far advanced renal insufficiency. The degree of hyperuricemia is generally mild and attacks of gouty arthritis relatively unusual. In patients with advanced renal failure, gastrointestinal uricolysis plays a greater role in the elimination of uric acid from the body. Treatment for hyperuricemia in patients with end-stage renal disease therefore should be reserved for those with documented attacks of gouty arthritis, tophi, or uric acid renal stones.

ACUTE HYPERSENSITIVITY INTERSTITIAL NEPHRITIS

KAREN S. SERVILLA, M.D.
WAYNE A. BORDER, M.D.

Acute hypersensitivity interstitial nephritis following exposure to drugs is being increasingly recognized as a cause of acute renal failure. Since the early recognition of sulfonamide- and penicillin-induced acute interstitial nephritis (AIN) there has been a steady increase in the number of drugs incriminated as offending agents. More than 50 drugs (Table 1) have now been associated with acute hypersensitivity interstitial nephritis, and up to 8 percent of all cases of acute renal failure may be accounted for by drug-associated AIN. The clinical course and long-term outcome of renal impairment in drug-induced AIN vary. Reduction in renal function may vary from mild and transient to frank renal failure with oliguria which may require some form of chronic end-stage therapy. Unfortunately, controlled and sufficient data to support the efficacy of corticosteroids reported to have some success in anecdotal cases is not available, and their use remains controversial. It is important that the diagnosis of acute hypersensitivity interstitial nephritis due to drugs be considered in all cases of acute renal failure in which the cause remains obscure, because early recognition and withdrawal of the offending agent may avoid the not too rare renal sequelae of the disease.

DIAGNOSIS

The most established presentation of acute hypersensitivity interstitial nephritis occurs when the patient is treated for 10 to 20 days with normal doses of methicillin for infection, the drug characteristically associated with allergic AIN. The patient has an initial response to therapy with resolution of infectious symptoms. About 15 days later (range, 2 to 60 days), a high-grade fever, morbilliform rash, gross hematuria, proteinuria, and eosinophiluris (in the blood and urine) occur with azotemia. A diagnosis of methicillin-induced AIN is made. The drug is withdrawn, symptoms resolve in 2 to 3 days, and renal function usually returns to baseline. Cases in which these features occur simultaneously are readily diagnosed. It is well recognized now that this is not the usual presentation. Few or no symptoms may occur, and multiple drug regimens and multisystem diseases may add further confusion.

Other symptom complexes may also predominate which do not suggest an overt allergic reaction. One recognized agent is rifampin. Presenting symptoms are different from those of methicillin-induced AIN but quite constant in patients affected. The development of a flu-like illness, including high-grade fever with chills, myalgias, nausea, vomiting, diarrhea, headache, and lumbar pain followed by acute renal failure and sometimes anuria, is typical. On renal biopsy there is an interstitial nephritis thought to be a hypersensitivity reaction, but other factors may also be important. Some patients develop heterogeneous light chain proteinuria which results in tubular damage similar to myeloma. A variety of pathologic mechanisms may be operative in rifampin-induced renal injury, resulting in its distinct symptom complex. The disease seems to be more common with intermittent rifampin therapy.

The natural history of nonsteroidal anti-inflammatory-induced AIN is unique in that the drug has usually been taken for a prolonged period of time before the patient presents with symptoms related to the nephrotic syndrome—edema and hypertension. Allergy-related findings—rash, fever, gross hematuria and eosinophilia–have been notably lacking except in a single case report. The finding of an intense AIN is the most striking feature on renal biopsy in these patients. Discontinuing the drug has resulted in reversal of renal failure within 2 to 7 weeks. One's index of suspicion for drug-induced hypersensitivity interstitial nephritis as a cause of potentially reversible renal failure must always remain high.

TABLE 1 Drugs Implicated in Acute Hypersensitivity Interstitial Nephritis

- Antibiotics
  - Penicillin and derivatives
    - Penicillin G
    - Methicillin*
    - Ampicillin*
    - Amoxicillin
    - Carbenicillin
    - Oxacillin
    - Nafcillin
    - Mezlocillin†
  - Cephalosporins
    - Cephalothin*
    - Cephalexin
    - Caphradine
    - Cefoxitin
    - Cefotaxime
  - Others
    - Rifampicin*
    - Vancomycin†
    - Minocycline
    - Tetracycline
    - Polymyxin sulfate†
    - Ethambutol†
    - Trimethoprim-sulfamethoxazole*
    - Chloramphenicol
    - Colistin
- Sulfonamides
  - Cotrimoxazole*
  - Thiazides*
  - Salicylazosulfapyridine
  - Chlorthalidone
- Nonthiazide diuretics
  - Furosemide
  - Tienilic acid
  - Triamterene
- Analgesics and anti-inflammatory agents
  - Aminochloroquinolein derivatives
    - Glafenin*
    - Antrafenin
    - Floctafenin†
  - Nonsteroidal anti-inflammatory agents
    - Indomethacin
    - Phenylbutazone
    - Fenoprofen
    - Naproxen
    - Ibuprofen
    - Diflunisal
    - Mefenamate
    - Tolmetin
    - Niflumic acid†
    - Zomepirac
    - Diclofenac
  - Pyrazolon derivatives
    - Phenazone
    - Antipyrine
    - Noramidopyrine
    - Sulfinpyrazone
  - Para-aminophenol derivatives
    - Acetaminophen
    - Phenacetin
  - Acetylsalicylic acid
- Anticonvulsive agents
  - Phenytoin
  - Phenobarbital
  - Carbamazepine
- Others
  - Phenindione*
  - Allopurinol
  - PAS acid
  - Gold and bismuth salts
  - Azathioprine
  - Cimetidine
  - Phenylpropanolamine
  - Captopril
  - Ajmaline
  - Clofibrate
  - Cyclosporin A
  - Lithium

* Frequent cause
† Weak association

Features suggesting acute hypersensitivity interstitial nephritis are listed in Table 2. Presenting symptoms frequently include systemic manifestations of an allergic response occurring anywhere from a few hours to months after institution of drug therapy. Fever appears to be the most common clinical finding, present in 60 to 100 percent of reported series, but it is nonspecific and not of much diagnostic value. Skin rashes occur in up to 45 percent of patients. Arthralgias are less frequent and are usually not severe. The prevalence of these features occurring as a triad is between 10 and 40 percent. A note of caution is needed, however, as these findings may be fleeting, entirely absent, or difficult to differentiate from other causes of AIN, such as bacterial or viral infections and transplant rejection. Allergic symptomatology cannot be relied upon for diagnosis. Symptoms of polyuria and nocturia may also be present, reflecting the loss of the kidney's ability to concentrate early on in interstitial nephritis. Macroscopic hematuria and loin pain felt to be due to stretching of the renal parenchyma from edema may accompany the disease.

Various laboratory tests may assist in the diagnosis of acute hypersensitivity interstitial nephritis but are usually nonspecific. Mild proteinuria of the tubular type, alpha-2 or betaglobulins, and microscopic or macroscopic hematuria are common. Heavy proteinuria with nephrotic syndrome has occurred and usually is associated with the administration of a nonsteroidal anti-inflammatory agent.

The presence of eosinophils in centrifuged Wright-stained urine is a common but insensitive finding because it usually occurs late in the course, preceded by azotemia and proteinuria. The demonstration of eosinophiluria greater than 5 percent, expressed as a percentage of leukocytes in the urine, may be a good predictor of AIN from drug hypersensitivity. Significant blood eosinophilia (>700 per milliliter) is also common, and such a finding is helpful if other causes for eosinophilia are excluded. A normal eosinophil count does not exclude the diagno-

TABLE 2 Features Suggestive of Acute Hypersensitivity Interstitial Nephritis

- History—drug use
- Signs and symptoms
  - Allergic—fever, rash, arthralgia, macroscopic hematuria
  - Loss of concentrating ability—nocturia, polyuria
  - Renal stretching—loin pain
  - Uremia—malaise, nausea, vomiting, mental clouding, pruritis
  - Acute renal failure—uremic symptoms with or without oliguria
- Laboratory studies
  - Urine—mild to moderate proteinuria, leukocytosis with eosinophiluria, hematuria, occasional leukocyte casts
  - Blood—azotemia, hyperkalemia, hyperchloremic metabolic acidosis
    - eosinophilia
    - elevated IgE
    - antitubular basement membrane antibodies, immune complexes, cryoglobulins
  - X-ray—increased uptake on ^{67}Ga renal scintigraphy
  - Renal biopsy—patchy mononuclear cell infiltrate with or without eosinophils, edema, normal glomeruli by light microscopy
    - Occasional linear staining of tubules for IgG, IgM, complement, and antitubular basement membrane antibodies by immunofluorescence
    - Chaotic interstitium, damaged tubular mitochondria and enlarged tubular endoplasmic reticulum, lymphocytic infiltrate between adjacent tubular epithelial cells by electron microscopy

sis. Other findings may include a hyperkalemic-hyperchloremic metabolic acidosis and an elevated serum uric acid concentration. Detecting elevated serum IgE levels is also helpful in making the diagnosis because other than allergic phenomena, there are few causes of such a finding. Unfortunately, only about one-half of all patients with biopsy-proven hypersensitivity interstitial nephritis have elevated IgE levels. Circulating antitubular basement membrane antibodies have been found in some cases. Cryoglobulinemia or circulating immune complexes are uncommon. Serum complement levels are usually normal. Tests for cellular immunity are of questionable significance.

Drug-induced interstitial nephritis commonly presents as a sudden decline in renal function with or without oliguria. Clinical manifestations are variable. The differential diagnosis usually includes acute tubular necrosis and primary glomerular disease. The latter can frequently be excluded by the absence of hypertension and lack of significant pathologic casts in the urinary sediment. Differentiating between acute tubular necrosis and drug hypersensitivity, especially if allergic symptoms are not present, may be more difficult. It has been suggested that the urinary solute excretion indices may be of value. In contrast to the findings in acute tubular necrosis, it has been reported that the urine sodium value is relatively low and urine to plasma osmolality ratio high. These values have only been sporadically reported in studies of acute hypersensitivity interstitial nephritis and are inconsistent. In one series the excretion of sodium was low in one of the patients and indeterminate (between 20 mEq per liter and 60 mEq per liter) in the remaining patients. The urine and plasma were isosmolar in four of six patients, favoring the diagnosis of acute tubular necrosis.

Renal scintigraphy after administration of gallium citrate (^{67}Ga) may be helpful in distinguishing patients with drug-induced AIN from those with acute tubular necrosis. Renal ^{67}GA uptake is intense in AIN. It is present, but much less marked in patients with acute glomerulonephritis or acute pyelonephritis. Only in patients with nephrotic syndrome and minimal change disease is ^{67}Ga uptake by the kidney comparable to that in patients with AIN induced by drugs. Reports indicate that there is no uptake of ^{67}Ga by the kidneys in acute tubular necrosis. Further investigations of this diagnostic technique need to be completed before routine ^{67}Ga renal scintography can be recommended in patients suspected of having drug-induced interstitial nephritis.

By far the most accurate and precise method of diagnosis of hypersensitivity interstitial nephritis is the renal biopsy. It should be done especially when the diagnosis is in doubt in the setting of occult allergic symptomatology and lack of history of drug use associated with hypersensitivity interstitial nephritis.

PATHOGENESIS AND PATHOLOGY

The pathogenesis of drug-induced AIN remains poorly defined. Epidemiologic findings strongly support an immunologic mechanism for AIN associated with drugs: (1) Reactions occur in a small number of persons exposed. (2) Reactions are present after normal nontoxic doses of drug and may occur after only a small dose. (3) Reactions recur on re-exposure with a decreased latent period. (4) Reactions may be associated with other signs of allergic reaction.

The injury in AIN induced by drugs appears to be due to a hypersensitivity reaction. Hypersensitivity is the direct effect of an immune response in the host which leads to the formation of specific antibodies, sensitized lymphocytes, or a mixture of these.

The nature of the immunizing and target antigens in AIN is not clear. The antigen may be the drug, a metabolite of the drug, or even a minor immunologic contaminant. Most drugs implicated are small molecules and probably not immunogenic by themselves. Rather they most likely act as haptens, coupling to endogenous material allowing the drug to become antigenic. The endogenous component could be a plasma protein, a cellular component, or tubular basement membrane. An alternate mechanism could invoke damage to cells by the drug which promotes an autoimmune mechanism. So far no uniform model of drug-induced interstitial nephritis has been described. Most of the evidence available supports a type IV delayed hypersensitivity mechanism accounting for drug-induced AIN. This is suggested by the following observations made in cases of drug-related interstitial nephritis: (1) Delayed type hypersensitivity reaction has occurred after intercutaneous challenge with the offending drug. (2) In vitro evidence of cell-mediated immune reactivity has been described. (3) Studies identifying cell type have shown that the majority of infiltrating cells are T-lymphocytes expressing the T4+ phenotype associated with helper-inducer T cells, supporting the idea that cell-mediated reactions of the delayed hypersensitivity variety play an important part in the development of interstitial nephritis. (4) There have been pathologic findings of mononuclear cell infiltrates without immunoglobulin along with the occasional findings of noncaseating granulomas.

Antibody-mediated mechanisms have also been postulated to play a part in the development of lesions in AIN. Very rarely antitubular basement membrane antibodies have been demonstrated, especially when methicillin is incriminated. This may be a nonspecific reaction to tubular injury. The participation of a reaginic antibody has been suggested by the presence of eosinophils in blood, urine, and renal tissue, and increased levels of serum IgE and IgE-bearing cells in the interstitial infiltrates of renal tissue in some cases. These findings are inconsistent and the exact role of an immediate hypersensitivity reaction is not clear.

The weight of evidence, albeit indirect, favors the involvement of cell-mediated delayed hypersensitivity in the pathogenesis of at least some cases of drug-induced AIN. Whether this process operates alone or along with other immunologic mechanisms is not clear. It is most probable that more than one mechanism plays a role in the development of the lesion in many cases.

The morphologic changes of drug-induced interstitial nephritis have been well described and there is little if any disagreement as to what is seen. Acute hypersensitivity interstitial nephritis on light microscopy is characterized by a patchy infiltrate of plasma cells, lymphocytes, monocytes, and eosinophils in an edematous interstitium. The eosinophilic infiltrate may be very prominent, helping to distinguish a hypersensitivity etiologic agent from other causes of AIN. Polymorphonuclear cell infiltrates are seen infrequently. Variable tubular changes also occur in AIN. The tubular lumen usually contain sloughed epithelial and inflammatory cells. Small and medium-size lymphocytes are found in rows approximated in the interstitium near tubules, while other lymphocytes are insinuated between tubular epithelial cells on the other side of the tubular basement membrane. Interstitial scarring in the form of fibrosis and tubular atrophy may occur when the biopsy is performed late in the course or in the case of chronic functional impairment. The glomeruli and vessels are normal in the acute syndrome. When interstitial fibrosis is present, periglomerular fibrosis, ischemia, and other nonspecific glomerular changes may be seen.

Another pattern of injury seen in AIN caused by drug hypersensitivity is the presence of interstitial noncaseating granulomas with or without the other cellular infiltrates seen in interstitial nephritis. Giant cells may accompany the granuloma. Though this occurrence is rare, found in approximately one-third of biopsy specimens in cases diagnosed as drug-induced interstitial nephritis, the presence of granulomas is characteristic of drug hypersensitivity reactions.

Immunofluorescence studies of renal tissue are largely negative for complement, fibrin, immunoglobulins, albumin, and fibrin. With some drugs, namely allopurinol, methicillin, ampicillin, phenytoin, and nonsteroidal anti-inflammatory agents, however, antitubular basement membrane antibodies have been detected in sera of patients who on examination of renal biopsy specimens demonstrated linear deposits of methicillin antigen, IgG, IgM, and C3 along the tubular basement membrane. The significance of these findings is questionable in that they have been demonstrated in autopsy material from patients receiving penicillin class agents without evidence of AIN clinically. They may represent a nonspecific response to tubular injury.

Electron microscopic changes are numerous. The interstitial region is described as chaotic. The tubular epithelial cells contain damaged mitochondria and dilated rough endoplasmic reticulum. Vacuoles of varying size are numerous in proximal tubule cells, and inflammatory cells, usually lymphocytes, are present between tubular epithelial cells and between the tubular basement membrane and tubular cells. In AIN associated with nonsteroidal anti-inflammatory agents normal-appearing glomeruli may be seen by light microscopy, but electron microscopy reveals visceral glomerular epithelial cell foot process effacement associated with findings of AIN. As with minimal change disease, no glomerular immunoglobulin or complement deposition is detected by immunofluorescence microscopy.

PROGNOSIS

There is no doubt that the prognosis for patients who develop interstitial nephritis from drug ingestion is very good if the correct diagnosis is made and the offending drug discontinued. Early reports in the literature suggested a mortality of 10 percent usually related to complications of uremia. Death from acute hypersensitivity interstitial nephritis is very uncommon given our modern technology and knowledge. Renal impairment varies from minimal and transient to profound renal failure with oliguria requiring dialysis. The majority of patients with acute hypersensitivity interstitial nephritis follow a reversible course regardless of the initial severity. Renal function has remained impaired in some patients, and occasionally renal failure has persisted, requiring long-term dialysis. With increasing reports of drug-induced AIN it has become evident that the clinical course is very diverse. This diversity may be related to the wide variation in severity of the hypersensitivity reaction present in the renal interstitium. It is postulated that a marked initial impairment in renal function is seen in adults at onset of the disease or in any patient with a diffuse interstitial infiltrate. Recent reports have disclosed that the impaired renal function improves rapidly over the first 6 to 8 weeks—"early improvement"—followed by a slow improvement in glomerular filtration rate up to 1 year after the insult—"late improvement"—but thereafter renal function remains unchanged. One-third of patients who recover totally will do so in the first 2 weeks. Any impairment left after the phase of late improvement will remain. In this context the prognosis should be discussed only with patients with renal impairment who have been followed for at least 1 year. About 80 percent of patients will have a return of glomerular filtration rate to above 80 ml per minute; 10 percent will improve to a level of 50 ml per minute; and the remaining 10 percent will have significant impairment in renal function with a glomerular filtration rate of 15 ml per minute or less. The majority of patients whose serum creatinine level is below 2 mg per deciliter at 6 weeks will have near complete or total return of renal function. Acute renal failure for 3 weeks or more and a diffuse interstitial infiltrate which includes polymorphonuclear as well as mononuclear cell infiltrates indicate a poor prognosis. The degree of initial renal impairment and age of onset are debatable as long-term prognostic indicators. Some reports suggest that with initially severe renal dysfunction or increasing age, the outcome is worse.

Discontinuation of the responsible drug and supportive measures comprise the standard approach to the disease process. Whether or not recovery is hastened or the prognosis improved with corticosteroid therapy is uncertain. Rechallenge with the offending agent cannot be recommended. Recurrence of AIN has been noted with rechallenge, occurring with a shortened interval from time of drug institution to symptoms. Cross-reactivity of certain drugs also has been described. One should avoid all the penicillin class antibiotics and cephalosporins in cases of AIN due to one of these drugs. Likewise, the occurrence of AIN due to thiazides in a patient with a history of fuorsemide-induced interstitial nephritis has been reported. The reports of cross-reactivity among the nonsteroidal anti-inflammatory agents are sparse. The use of any of these drugs should be avoided if at all possible if one of these agents has produced AIN. If reinstitution of this type of agent is necessary, consideration should be given to one of another structural category than that responsible for the interstitial nephritis and the drug should be used with extreme caution.

THERAPY

The first and foremost step in management of the patient with drug-induced AIN is withdrawal of the drug or drugs felt to be responsible. This will often lead to reversal of renal insufficiency. We do not recommend routine steroid therapy. The literature is full of reports of steroid-responsive as well as steroid-unresponsive AIN. Besides these anecdotal accounts, there have been published series in which steroid therapy has appeared to be useful in shortening the time interval to recovery as well as increasing the number of patients who achieve complete recovery of renal function. The routine use of steroids, if based on these reports, would be very tempting. The studies available, however, are open to question. The patient populations have always been small and for the most part biased. The effects of other factors, such as infection and duration of time from drug withdrawal to institution of steroid therapy, are not clear. Corticosteroid therapy is not benign. No mortality or morbidity has been attributed to their use in the reported series, but one must always keep this possibility in mind. Because of this, we recommend that high-dose prednisone therapy, 60 mg orally for approximately 10 days, be instituted only in the setting of continued severe renal failure after drug withdrawal and where there is no contraindication to steroid use. Those patients who experience permanent moderate to severe renal insufficiency fall almost entirely into this group. If steroid therapy has a beneficial effect, this would be the population with the most to gain from its use. Low-dose prednisone is not effective. Relapses may occur during the tapering period, which respond to a higher dose of steroids.

During therapy one must always be alert to the potential complications of steroids, including infection, glucose intolerance, sodium retention, and an increase in catabolism which may result in increased potassium, blood urea nitrogen, and caloric needs in the form of high biologic value protein.

Steroid therapy is not employed in those with mild to moderate renal insufficiency. This group tends to do well with drug withdrawal alone.

The use of steroids is not influenced by the amount of proteinuria. Therapy is not complete without supportive care and dialysis when necessary to prevent unwarranted morbidity and death from renal failure and uremia.

CYSTIC DISEASES OF THE KIDNEY

PATRICIA A. GABOW, M.D.

Renal cysts are epithelial-lined cavities filled with fluid or semisolid debris. These cysts may be single or multiple, continuous with the nephron segments or isolated, inherited or acquired, clinically unimportant or capable of producing renal failure. The characteristics of the major cystic disorders are outlined in Table 1.

SIMPLE RENAL CYSTS

Simple renal cysts are the most common and least clinically significant of all renal cystic disorders. Single renal cysts occur with increasing frequency with age. Less than 0.1 percent of children have simple renal cysts, but as many as 50 percent of individuals over 50 years of age may have cysts. These cysts can be single or multiple, and they occur in the cortex more commonly than in the medulla. Simple cysts do not alter function, are not accompanied by cysts in other organs and are generally an incidental finding on renal or abdominal imaging studies. In an asymptomatic patient with characteristic imaging studies of a simple cyst, no further evaluation is required. Patients with simple cysts can present with flank pain or hematuria. If ultrasonography reveals smooth walls, good sound transmission through the cyst, and no intracystic debris, no further evaluation is needed. In selected cases of marked pain or questionable ultrasonogram, cyst puncture is recommended to address the question of malignancy. Cyst fluid should be sent to the laboratory for cell count, cytology, and cholesterol measurement. The latter appears to be elevated in cysts associated with malignancy.

Contrast media can be introduced into the cyst after fluid removal and the patient positioned to permit optimal evaluation of the cyst wall for lesions or irregularities. If abnormalities are found which are compatible with malignancy, surgery should be considered. If no abnormalities are demonstrated and flank pain and hematuria are persistent, particularly after cyst decompression with puncture, other causes for these abnormalities should be pursued, as this is not the common natural history for simple cysts.

TABLE 1 Overview of Renal Cystic Disease

	Single Cysts	*ADPKD*	*ARPKD*	*MSK*	*MCD*	*ACKD*
Hereditary	No	Yes	Yes	No	Variable	No
Prevalence	C	C	R	C	R	C
Preferred method of diagnosis	US	US	US/CT	EU	None	CT
			Complications			
Microhematuria	C	C	C	--	C	
Gross hematuria	R	C	R	R	--	+
Infection	--	+	+	+	R	+
Stone disease	--	C	--	C	--	--
Hypertension	R	C	C	R	R	Yes
Renal failure	No	C	C	R	C	Yes
Extrarenal manifestation	No	C	C	C	R	No

Key: +=occurs, R=rare, C=common, --=unknown, US=ultrasonography, CT=computer axial tomography, EU=excretory urography, ADPKD=autosomal dominant polycystic kidney disease, ARPKD=autosomal recessive polycystic kidney disease, MSK=medullary sponge kidney MCD=medullary cystic disease, ACKD=acquired cystic kidney disease, *=from underlying disease.

AUTOSOMAL DOMINANT POLYCYSTIC KIDNEY DISEASE

Autosomal dominant polycystic kidney disease (ADPKD) is common, afflicting 1 in 400 to 1 in 1,000 Americans. Patients seek medical attention either because of a known family history of ADPKD and a desire to know their clinical status or because of symptoms. In either circumstance, ultrasonography is the preferred method of diagnosis. It is sensitive and requires no radiation exposure. Computed axial tomography (CT scanning) may be slightly more sensitive, but requires radiation exposure and often contrast media. Therefore, CT scanning should be reserved for patients with nondiagnostic ultrasonographic results or complications of ADPKD as discussed below. Patients who are being screened because of a positive family history raise the question, "At what age is ADPKD accurately detected by ultrasonography?" Certainly ADPKD has been identified in utero and in the very young, but we do not have adequate data to completely answer the question of the sensitivity of ultrasonography by age group. It has been estimated that an individual with a family history of ADPKD who has normal renal imaging studies and who is over age 20 has a less than 1 in 25 chance of having ADPKD. However, this determination can be accurately made only by using a closely linked gene marker or the gene for the disease, thereby providing an alternative method for absolute diagnosis. Approximately 60 percent of patients with ADPKD will provide a positive family history. In fact, however, about 90 percent of patients have other family members with ADPKD when family members are examined by ultrasonography. Patients identified in family screening are younger and obviously have fewer symptoms than patients who are identified as having ADPKD after evaluations for symptoms.

The two most common symptoms that prompt diagnosis are pain and hematuria. Flank and/or back pain are frequent complaints. Abdominal pain appears to occur more commonly in women. The pain from ADPKD can be mild or severe and disabling; it can be intermittent or constant. In many patients, the pain prompts the use of large amounts of analgesics. Physicians need to be cautious in prescribing potentially nephrotoxic analgesics such as nonsteroidal anti-inflammatory drugs or addicting drugs. The role of percutaneous cyst puncture or surgical unroofing of cysts for pain relief is currently being investigated, but these modalities should be viewed as experimental and performed only in a study setting which permits critical evaluation of the results.

Hematuria may be microscopic or gross. About one-third of patients will have hematuria demonstrated on a random urinalysis. Proteinuria is detected by urinalysis in 34 to 95 percent of patients. However, the protein excretion is frequently less than 1 g per 24 hours and rarely requires specific attention. On the other hand, hematuria can represent a clinical problem. One-third to one-half of patients with ADPKD will have experienced at least one episode of gross hematuria by the time of initial presentation. The episode is often triggered by relatively minor trauma or strenuous exercise. These episodes appear most common in patients with large kidneys or hypertension. Thus patients with large kidneys or very large cysts should be cautioned about the risk of bleeding from contact sports such as football or wrestling. Usually the episodes are self-limited and can be treated at home with bed rest, hydration, and analgesia. Rarely is hospitalization or transfusion needed. Every effort should be made to manage hematuria conservatively without surgery. Gross hematuria accompanied by colicky pain should raise the question of obstruction by clot or by calculus. Falling hematocrit or hemodynamic instability with or without gross hematuria after abdominal trauma in a patient with ADPKD should prompt investigation for retroperitoneal hematoma with a CT scan or angiography, depending upon the urgency of the situation. Renal calculi in

ADPKD, retroperitoneal bleeding, and intracystic blood can be diagnosed by abdominal CT scan. Surgical intervention should be considered only in very unusual circumstances in which obstruction occurs, hemodynamic stability cannot be maintained, or bleeding is unremitting for weeks.

Other commonly occurring symptoms in ADPKD are headache (27 percent), gastrointestinal complaints (15 percent), nocturia (14 percent), dysuria (9 percent), frequency (9 percent), and polyuria (8 percent). Chronic headaches can often be severe. However, the headaches do not appear to be related to the presence of berry aneurysms or hypertension. The higher incidence of these two conditions complicates the approach to headaches in these patients. Berry aneurysms occur in 10 to 40 percent of patients with ADPKD. Patients should be educated about their association and instructed to seek prompt medical attention for severe headaches which differ from their usual headaches, headaches accompanied by focal neurologic signs, or headaches associated with alteration in level of consciousness. All patients with ADPKD with any signs or symptoms suggestive of berry aneurysms should undergo carotid angiography to determine if an aneurysm is present. Currently, it is not recommended that all patients with ADPKD undergo routine carotid angiography. In deciding if a patient with ADPKD should undergo angiography, the physician should also probably consider the consequences of rupture of an aneurysm in the patient. For example, a patient with ADPKD who drives a bus or flies an airplane should probably undergo angiography, because of the implications of sudden loss of consciousness.

Hypertension occurs in 60 percent of patients with ADPKD before the onset of renal insufficiency. The hypertension should be vigorously controlled in patients with headaches as well as in patients without this symptom. Patients with hypertension appear to have a more rapid deterioration of renal function than normotensive ADPKD patients. Therefore, preservation of renal function is considered to be a major reason for controlling blood pressure. Blood pressure should be monitored, with an attempt to maintain it at about 120/80 mm Hg. Currently no antihypertensive therapy appears to be preferable to another.

At the time of diagnosis, most patients with ADPKD have normal renal function, normal serum electrolytes, normal liver function tests, and normal blood counts. The urinalysis, as previously mentioned, often uncovers hematuria, proteinuria, and pyuria.

ADPKD is not a disorder affecting only the kidneys. Thirty-eight to 63 percent of patients with ADPKD have hepatic cysts. Liver function only rarely is impaired and hepatic cysts only rarely become symptomatic. Therefore the presence of hepatic cysts generally requires no special therapeutic attention. Colonic diverticuli have been reported to occur in 83 percent of patients with ADPKD undergoing chronic hemodialysis. This has led some clinicians to recommend barium enemas in all patients with ADPKD with end-stage renal disease prior to renal transplantation. Some would also suggest surgical removal of segments of the large intestine which demonstrate active or remote inflammatory involvement radiographically prior to renal transplantation. Currently there are no data to support the use of routine barium enemas in patients with ADPKD who are not preparing for transplantation. However, clinicians should be aware that diverticuli and complications of diverticuli appear to be common in this disorder. Cardiac valvular abnormalities have been seen in about one-third of patients with ADPKD involving both aortic and mitral valves, including mitral valve prolapse. Therefore, ADPKD patients with murmurs or clicks suggestive of these valvular disorders should undergo echocardiography. Pancreatic, ovarian, uterine, esophageal, and brain cysts have been seen sporadically in ADPKD. Thoracic aortic aneurysms appear to be more frequent in patients with ADPKD and thus provide an additional reason for adequate blood pressure control.

Both the renal and extrarenal involvement give rise to a wide array of complications in ADPKD. The renal complications of ADPKD include bleeding into cysts or into the retroperitoneum, cyst infection, renal calculi, and renal tumors. The frequency of urinary tract infections is not definitely known. In many older studies pyuria was equated with infection. It is clear, however, that pyuria is common without infection. Infections can occur as cystitis, pyelonephritis, or cyst infection. The latter two are difficult to separate. Cyst infections may be difficult to diagnose, but should be considered in patients with ADPKD who have fever, new or worsening flank pain, and pyuria without white cell casts. Urine cultures are not always positive, and blood cultures also may or may not be positive. Probably the clinical factor that best correlates with cyst infection is failure to respond to standard antibiotic therapy for pyelonephritis. Ultrasonography, CT scan, and gallium scan all can identify some infected cysts, but there are no adequate data regarding the sensitivity or specificity of any of these modalities in identifying infected cysts. If a cyst infection is suspected on clinical grounds, the choice of antibiotic therapy will be different from the choice in pyelonephritis. Aminoglycoside antibiotics are often given for pyelonephritis. However, aminoglycosides do not enter cyst fluids in adequate amounts. The antibiotics that appear to have the best cyst penetrance are trimethoprim and sulfamethoxazole and chloramphenicol. Therefore, one of these drugs is probably the best choice of antibiotic in suspected upper tract infection in a patient with ADPKD. One of the major antecedent events in urinary tract infections in ADPKD is instrumentation of the urinary tract. Therefore, instrumentation of any kind, including catheterization, should be done only after careful consideration of the risk-benefit ratio of the procedure.

Renal calculi occur in about 20 percent of patients with ADPKD. This complication is most easily diagnosed by CT scan. The nature of the stones in this patient population has not been well delineated, therefore, guidelines for evaluation and treatment should be the same as in any stone former.

Renal tumors (hypernephromas) occur in patients with ADPKD. These are often difficult to diagnose against the background of large kidneys, flank pain, and hematuria. The diagnosis should be considered in patients with marked discrepancy in the size of the two kidneys; patients with increasing flank pain or a new or different pattern of hematuria; and patients with weight loss and failure to thrive. CT scan and angiogram are the diagnostic tools to use in assessing the question of malignancy.

The natural history of ADPKD is variable, with renal failure occurring as early as the first decade of life or with renal function being well preserved into the seventies and eighties. A recent study indicates that 50 percent of patients with ADPKD will have normal renal function at 70 years of age. Other data have suggested that patients with ADPKD with hypertension have a worse prognosis than do normotensive ADPKD patients. Renal function should be ascertained by a yearly blood urea nitrogen or creatinine measurement until the blood urea nitrogen level exceeds 20 mg per deciliter or the creatinine level exceeds 2 mg per deciliter. At this point, patients should be monitored two to three times per year. Serum calcium, phosphorus, and alkaline phosphatase determinations should be done at these times. Although dietary protein and phosphorus restriction to 0.6 g protein per kilogram of body weight and 700 mg per 24 hours, respectively, have been suggested to ameliorate the rate of renal function decline in ADPKD, insufficient data are available to recommend this for all patients at the present time. It does seem advisable, however, to avoid protein loading and hyperphosphatemia. Patients should be referred for renal replacement therapy with dialysis or transplantation like any other patient with chronic renal failure.

Although data are not available on many issues related to ADPKD, reasonable guidelines for diagnosis and management of patients include the following:

1. Ultrasonography is the diagnostic method of choice.
2. Patients and family members should be educated about the manifestation and inheritance of the disorder.
3. Family members should be screened for ADPKD if they are participating in contact sports, have signs or symptoms suggestive of ADPKD, or are approaching childbearing age and wish the information to assist in family planning.
4. Episodes of hematuria should be managed conservatively.
5. Urinary tract instrumentation should be avoided.
6. Urinary tract infections should be treated promptly with appropriate antibiotics.
7. Hypertension should be vigorously controlled.
8. Currently it is not recommended that all patients with ADPKD should be screened for extrarenal involvement with carotid angiography, echocardiography, or barium enema.

AUTOSOMAL RECESSIVE POLYCYSTIC KIDNEY DISEASE

Autosomal recessive polycystic kidney disease (ARPKD) is a rare condition usually presenting in neonates or young children. These children often present with abdominal mass, urinary tract infection, and failure to thrive. Ultrasonography or CT scan should be used for diagnosis. The latter should probably be reserved for patients in whom ultrasonography fails to establish the diagnosis.

The major complications of this disease are hepatic fibrosis with portal hypertension, hypersplenism, hypertension, and ultimately renal failure. These children should be followed carefully for these complications. Although portocaval and splenorenal shunts have been performed in some patients with portal hypertension, there is a high surgical mortality, and this type of surgery should be performed only by teams with experience in supporting such patients. These children with chronic renal failure should be managed like other children with chronic renal failure, with attention to renal infection, growth, and renal osteodystrophy.

ACQUIRED CYSTIC DISEASE

Acquired cystic kidney disease (ACKD) is a relatively new disease initially described in 1977. Small renal cysts develop in the kidneys of patients with end-stage renal disease from noncystic underlying disease. An overwhelming majority of patients with ACKD have been maintained on dialysis for more than three years. Approximately 40 percent of dialysis patients develop this disorder. In most patients cysts are small and the kidneys remain small and shrunken. For this reason, CT scan is a more reliable diagnostic procedure than ultrasonography. However, some patients' kidneys dramatically enlarge, as in ADPKD. Most patients with ACKD are asymptomatic. The two major complications of ACKD are bleeding and renal tumor. As in ADPKD, bleeding can be into a cyst or into the retroperitoneum. Bleeding should be managed conservatively if possible. If bleeding is difficult to control, selective renal arterial embolization could be considered, as there is no need to preserve renal parenchyma. If this type of therapy is not available, nephrectomy can be considered.

Renal tumors occur in about 16 percent of patients with ACKD. This complication should be suspected in patients on hemodialysis who develop hematuria, or a rising hematocrit presumably reflecting erythropoietin production by the tumor or a metastatic lesion. Since tumors of less than 3 cm have little metastatic proclivity, tumors in this size range can be followed with yearly CT scans. Patients with large tumors or patients with any size tumors who are to receive a renal transplant should undergo nephrectomy; the latter patients are at increased risk of malignancy because of the drugs used to maintain a functional transplant. Because patients with ACKD can have bilateral tumors, it is recommended that patients with a unilateral renal tumor and ACKD undergo bilateral nephrectomy prior to transplantation.

MEDULLARY CYSTIC DISORDERS

Disorders with medullary cystic lesions should be divided into two major groups: medullary sponge kidney and medullary cystic disease.

Medullary sponge kidney is a disorder characterized by tubular dilations within the medullary collecting ducts. Patients can come to a physician's attention because of episodes of hematuria, recurrent urinary tract infections, and recurrent renal calculi with or without obstruction. The condition is diagnosed by the presence of normal sized kidneys with medullary ductal ectasia on intravenous pyelogram. A high percentage of these patients appear to have coincident hyperparathyroidism, and therefore serum calcium measurements should be obtained in every patient with medullary sponge kidney. If the serum calcium level is elevated, serum parathyroid hormone level should be determined, and renal calcium excretion should also be determined. Renal calculi in subjects without hypercalcemia and hyperparathyroidism should be evaluated and treated as in other patients with renal calculi. Although these complications may create some morbidity, renal function remains normal in this disorder in the absence of urinary tract obstruction.

Medullary cystic disease has been called many names—nephronophthisis, cystic renal medullary complex, renal-retinal dysplasia. In general, the disorder appears to be characterized by familial transmission—albeit of varying patterns, progressive renal dysfunction with shrunken kidneys, and end-stage renal disease in the third to fifth decade of life. Most people with this disease present to a physician in early childhood or adolescence with polydipsia, polyuria, enuresis, failure to thrive, weakness, and anemia. The diagnosis is not easily made because imaging techniques reveal only small shrunken kidneys. Even renal biopsy is not revealing. Approximately 20 percent of patients with this disorder may have renal sodium wasting. Therefore, it may be dangerous to reflexly limit salt intake in these subjects; severe volume depletion may ensue. With this possible exception these patients should be followed like any patient with progressive renal insufficiency.

Thus cystic disease of the kidney comprises a wide array of disorders. They should be considered in patients with a family history of renal disease, and in patients who present with flank pain, hematuria, renal calculi, or recurrent urinary tract infections.

STRATEGIES FOR PREVENTIVE TREATMENT OF RENAL FAILURE IN DIABETES MELLITUS

GIANCARLO VIBERTI, M.D., M.R.C.P.

Proteinuria exceeding 0.5 g per 24 hours is the first clinical sign of diabetic nephropathy. This complication of diabetes mellitus occurs in approximately 40 percent of insulin-dependent diabetic patients after a duration of diabetes ranging from 16 to 20 years. Non-insulin-dependent diabetics also develop persistent proteinuria and renal failure, but the prevalence and incidence of these complications in this condition are less well known. Recent evidence suggests that the incidence of renal failure differs in non-insulin-dependent diabetics of different ethnic groups, being higher in those countries in which non-insulin-dependent diabetes develops earlier in life and where the population at large demonstrates some protection from ischemic heart disease.

Clinical diabetic nephropathy is associated with increased mortality up to 100 times that of the nondiabetic population percent at age 35 to 40. The higher death rate is not only from uremia, but also from cardiovascular disease, making the development of persistent proteinuria a major life-threatening complication in patients with juvenile insulin-dependent diabetes.

MANAGEMENT OF CLINICAL NEPHROPATHY

Several years may elapse between the development of persistent proteinuria and end-stage renal failure, even though the rate of progression of the disease varies greatly in different individuals. Although this phase of renal impairment appears incurable with current therapeutic methods, this time should and can be profitably used for treating the disease process. A policy of nonintervention is nowadays unjustified. Since end-stage renal failure eventually becomes a matter for specialized intervention and renal replacement therapy, it is the diabetologist who must detect and identify the beginning of the pathologic process and plan treatment over the few years preceding terminal organ failure. The physician in charge of a diabetic patient with newly proven persistent proteinuria of diabetic origin should pose four questions: (1) When to treat? (2) What to treat? (3) How to treat? (4) Why treat?

When to Treat

The onset of proteinuria indicates a pathologic condition in which a significant loss of renal function is occurring, even though serum creatinine concentration may not become abnormal for some years. Unfortunately, when creatinine levels exceed 2.3 mg per deciliter, 50 percent or more of glomerular renal function has already been lost. The failure of therapeutic intervention in the past can almost certainly be ascribed to a wait and watch attitude until the patient developed clear signs of renal impairment.

Management should be instituted early, before serum creatinine exceeds normal levels. A patient with diabetic proteinuria has a high mortality risk, and a careful assessment of his renal functional status and systemic vascular status should be systematically and serially carried out. There are two cornerstones in this assessment. The first is to establish whether the glomerular filtration rate (GFR) is falling; this requires serial measurements, which are made approximately 4 to 6 months apart, of the GFR using a reliable indicator, such as inulin or an isotopic tracer. The second is to establish by serial determinations whether arterial pressure is rising over time, no matter whether the change is taking place within the so-called normal range. If changes in one or both of these variables develop (and usually they occur concomitantly), initiation of treatment should be considered.

What and How to Treat

Management of diabetes may become increasingly difficult as renal failure progresses, with episodes of frequent and severe hypoglycemia (of which the patient frequently has no warning) alternating with periods of extreme hyperglycemia. Ketoacidosis is an extremely rare event in renal failure, possibly due to an impairment in hepatic ketogenesis, which occurs in uremia. Even though it has been described, we have not encountered a single case in our experience of approximately 209 patient years of follow-up.

Insulin

With advancing renal failure, insulin requirements invariably decrease (in spite of a resistance to the peripheral actions of insulin which occurs in uremia), sometimes to approximately half the dose, and unusual cases have been described in which insulin was withdrawn altogether. Insulin in humans is approximately 30 to 40 percent metabolized by the kidneys; renal function is gradually lost with progressive renal failure, thereby resulting in a slower removal of insulin from the circulation and an increased half-life of the circulating hormone. Self-monitoring of blood glucose may help the patient and the doctor adjust the insulin dose to maintain adequate glycemic control.

The level of blood glucose control that should be aimed at in patients with diabetic nephropathy has become one of the most burning questions of recent years. Greatly improved levels of diabetic control can now be obtained with insulin infusion pumps combined with home blood glucose monitoring. There is, however, no convincing evidence that this significantly alters the rate of decline of the GFR or the progression of the proteinuria even when "tight" diabetic control is instituted at the time of intermittent proteinuria. Although some studies have been conducted for several years, they have used small numbers of patients, and it cannot be entirely excluded that a small effect might have been missed. There are two main shortcomings with this kind of intensified insulin treatment. Euglycemia is not achieved by the present infusion systems, and it may well be that the control obtained, though greatly improved, is not good enough to affect pathologic changes that took several years to develop. Our means of correcting hyperglycemia remain imperfect for this particular purpose. Strict blood glucose control with the existing methods is bought at the expense of an increased risk and indeed a higher rate of biochemical hypoglycemia. This is of particular concern for the patient with renal impairment who often suffers a number of other diabetic complications, including autonomic neuropathy. This may lead to loss of the adrenergic warning symptoms of hypoglycemia and may expose the patient to devastating hypoglycemic comas. The theoretical, though unproven, advantage of tight metabolic control at the stage of persistent proteinuria has to be weighed against these problems. On balance, safe, though satisfactory, levels of blood glucose control is all that should be aimed for under these circumstances. This is not to deny the role of poor control in the genesis of this complication, but is rather the realistic recognition of what can be achieved with the present means of treatment. The whole question will require reexamination when completely safe euglycemia, perhaps by the use of a portable closed loop glucose sensor feedback system or pancreatic transplantation, becomes available.

Oral Hypoglycemic Agents

Non-insulin-dependent patients who develop impairment of renal function should have their management revised. Biguanides, (e.g., phenformin), if still available on prescription, should be stopped because of risk of fatal lactic acidosis. The type of sulfonylureas to be administered should be carefully evaluated. Drugs that have long half-lives, such as chlorpropamide, and that are primarily excreted by the kidney, should be used with caution or altogether withdrawn because of the danger of profound and in some, fortunately rare cases, irreversible hypoglycemia. Sulfonylureas that are first metabolized and then excreted, such as tolazamide, glipizide and glibenclamide, or new preparations, such as gliquidone and gliclazide, which are excreted by the biliary tract, are preferred.

Raised Arterial Pressure

Blood pressure begins to climb very early in proteinuric diabetics in parallel with the decline of GFR. This increase may be apparent even at unreduced levels of GFR and certainly well before the serum creatinine becomes abnormal. A rising blood pressure, even though the actual levels are below the values for hypertension set by the World Health Organization (i.e., > 160/95 mm Hg), should be treated. Correction of rising blood pressure has been estimated to slow the rate of decline of GFR by an average of 5 to 6 ml per minute per year and to reduce proteinuria substantially. The reasons for raised blood pressure in diabetic nephropathy are not entirely clear, but intravascular fluid overload may play an important role. Thus, a reduction in fluid retention by administration of a potent loop diuretic is central to the treatment of arterial hypertension. The dose should be tailored to individual situations, and an initial dose of 40 mg of furosemide may need to be progressively increased over the years to as much as 500 mg and in rare cases 1,000 mg daily to achieve a "dry weight." The addition of a thiazide diuretic, such as chlorthalidone, is rarely necessary, but has proved useful in some patients with greatly reduced GFR (e.g., <20 ml per minute) whose response to furosemide was inadequate. Regular check of body weight is a must in the monitoring of the effect of diuretic treatment in these patients, and the patient can profitably be taught to self-monitor his weight at home, even adjusting diuretic dose by response himself.

Potassium-sparing diuretics and aldosterone antagonists as well as potassium supplements should, in principle, be avoided in patients with renal failure and GFR lower than 15 to 20 ml per minute because of the risk of acute hyperkalemia. Careful monitoring of plasma electrolytes and concomitant administration of drugs such as digoxin should guide the physician in prescribing potassium supplementation. Whenever possible, this is best obtained from food sources. For instance, 100 g of unskinned bananas contains 210 mg of potassium and 100 g of fresh orange juice gives 180 mg of potassium. A host of other hypotensive drugs are used in the treatment of arterial hypertension in diabetic renal failure and no study to date has established if, in humans, a single drug or a particular combination of drugs is especially beneficial to the kidney or the patient. Beta-blockers are often used in combination with diuretics in patients without congestive heart failure. A cardioselective blocker should be used in these cases, as nonselective drugs such as propranolol have been reported to mask the symptoms of hypoglycemia and to delay recovery from it. Among cardioselective beta-blocking drugs those with long half-lives and renal elimination, such as atenolol, should be avoided in patients with GFRs below 15 ml per minute. In advanced renal failure, the addition of a third drug is often necessary to control high blood pressure. In this case a vasodilator, such as hydralazine, prazosin, or a calcium-channel blocker, should be added in incremental doses until either the blood pressure falls or side effects preclude larger doses.

The use of angiotensin-converting enzyme (ACE) inhibitors, such as captopril and enalapril, has been rather limited in the treatment of hypertension in diabetic renal failure. There is no good theoretical argument against employing these agents, and indeed, studies in experimental animals suggest that an ACE inhibitor might be the drug of choice in normalizing the intraglomerular hypertension present in the surviving nephrons, thus preventing progression of renal lesions. Recent studies have also shown a reduction in proteinuria when an ACE inhibitor (captopril) is used to treat diabetic nephropathy. Clinical trials in humans are awaited to establish whether a particular hypotensive regimen affords better benefits to the kidney and the patient or whether it is simply the reduction of blood pressure, no matter how obtained, that is important.

Particularly difficult is the treatment of arterial hypertension in diabetic patients with nephropathy who have severe autonomic neuropathy and postural hypotension. These diabetics have elevated blood pressure in the supine position, and attempts to normalize recumbent hypertension may lead to upright blood pressure levels incompatible with standing. The physician treating these patients has to exercise common sense and find a compromise between "acceptable" levels of raised supine blood pressure and tolerable levels of upright pressure.

Diet

Regulation of diet is important in these patients. The interest in low-protein diets has been rekindled recently by a number of studies in animal models of renal disease and in nondiabetic chronic renal failure in humans. The main emphasis with these diets is to start them much earlier than was previously considered in the course of renal impairment. Prescribing low-protein diets when the patient is symptomatic has proved useful in relieving symptoms but has done little to alter the course of renal failure. Moreover, very-low-protein diets of 20 to 25 g daily are unpalatable and poorly tolerated. A less restricted diet containing 35 to 45 g of protein per day should be prescribed when the serum creatinine level reaches 2 mg per deciliter. Such a diet protects against muscle wasting, and accentuation of edema and has been shown to slow down significantly the rate of progression of renal failure in certain nondiabetic kidney diseases. No controlled clinical trials have been carried out in patients with diabetes as yet. Furthermore, the feasibility of a low-protein diet in diabetic patients needs to be worked out. There are special problems with diabetics who have been taught, perhaps erroneously, for many years to restrict their carbohydrate intake and eat more proteins. A reduction of protein intake in these patients must be accompanied by an increase in the carbohydrate intake, especially in the form of unrefined carbohydrate, in order to maintain an adequate energy intake. Failure to do this may lead to weight loss and, in extreme cases, to a catabolic state. Whether a restriction in protein comparable to that obtained in other nondiabetic patients can be achieved in diabetic subjects remains a moot point. Accordingly, these drastic dietary changes must be accompanied by readjustment of the insulin or oral agent dose.

Although acceptability and compliance as well as effect of protein-restricted diets in diabetics need to be evaluated in a proper controlled manner before general recommendations can be made, there is no reason to believe that the effect of these diets in diabetics should be different in any respect from that of patients with other renal conditions. It is therefore reasonable to expect a beneficial reduction of the rate of progression of nephropathy.

Two other important dietary-related variables must be monitored as the renal failure advances. These concern hypocalcemia and hyperphosphatemia. The former results from reduced intestinal absorption of calcium as a consequence of impaired renal synthesis of vitamin D and retention of phosphorus by the hypofunctioning kidney. Low plasma calcium levels may induce parathyroid hormone release, thereby leading to secondary hyperparathyroidism and uremic bone disease. Supplementary dietary calcium (1 to 2 g daily) and calcitriol (0.25 to 1.0 μg daily) should be given and blood levels of calcium checked at regular intervals to prevent hypercalcemia. Hyperphosphatemia should be treated by a phosphate-binding gel given with each meal, the aim being to maintain phosphate levels within the normal range. Treatment with compounds such as aluminum hydroxide or calcium carbonate may lead, in some cases, to severe constipation. Aluminum hydroxide therapy may contribute to increased total body aluminum burden if advanced renal failure is present.

Urinary Tract Infection and Papillary Necrosis

Infections of the urinary tract need special attention in diabetics, since they can rapidly escalate and result in renal papillary necrosis. This condition should be suspected in a diabetic developing a urinary tract infection with fever, loin pain, and often renal colic. Ureteric obstruction by the sloughed papillae may occur and oliguric renal failure has been described. The latter condition is associated with a high mortality rate.

Roentgenographic appearance on pyelography is characteristic, showing "moth-eaten" calyces and "ring-shadows" around the separated papillae, and in fact, the diagnosis of papillary necrosis is sometimes made during a routine intravenous pyelogram for the investigation of recurrent urinary tract infection. In these "asymptomatic" cases, renal function is well preserved in spite of extensive papillary loss and the prognosis is very good.

For these reasons, the discovery of asymptomatic bacteriuria in excess of 100,000 microorganisms per milliliter in a diabetic is an indication for treatment. Antimicrobial therapy is usually guided by in vitro sensitivity testing and clinical response. A 7- to 10-day course of the appropriate drug should lead to the production of sterile urine confirmed by reculture.

Recurrent and persistent urinary tract infection may be suppressed with long-term low-dose treatment with drugs such as amoxicillin (250 mg daily) or the combination of trimethoprin (80 mg) and sulfamethoxazole (400 mg per day).

Particular attention should be paid to patients with neuropathic bladder, as this predisposes them to repeated episodes of cystitis and the risk of pyelonephritis. Intractable urinary tract infection can be fatal in these patients. Investigations of residual urine volume and bladder function tests may help to guide treatment, which nevertheless remains very difficult. Stimulation of bladder contraction with parasympathomimetric drugs is rarely successful. A regimen of voiding every 2 hours may be attempted. Bladder neck resection is sometimes successful, but in the severely disabled patient, long-term catheterization is the only solution to interrupt the series of infections.

Retinopathy and Medium Vessel Disease

Retinopathy is always present in patients with diabetic nephropathy. Atheroma and arterial calcification are usually present, causing both ischemic heart disease and peripheral vascular disease. All these conditions are now treatable. The ophthalmologist with retinal photocoagulation and the cardiac and vascular surgeon with vascular bypass and endoarterectomy can substantially reduce the ocular and vascular morbidity in these patients.

It is very important that these conditions be treated well before severe uremia develops, so that the patient begins renal replacement therapy in the best possible general physical condition and the potential retinal and vascular sequelae of dialysis and transplantation are greatly reduced.

Why Treat

The primary aims of all therapeutic maneuvers in patients with diabetic renal disease is to delay end-stage renal disease and to prevent the complications of nephropathy. Today this is achievable by a number of interventions, the two cornerstones of which are normalization of blood pressure and, probably, reduction of total protein intake. In spite of these adjuncts, we are unable at present to arrest, let alone reverse, the progression of renal failure. By the time either intermittent or persistent proteinuria appears, the process of renal damage is so severe as to be self-perpetuating.

The question arises here as to whether the process leading to renal damage can be identified earlier, before any functional impairment is evident, and, if this is so, whether therapeutic intervention is, under these circumstances, effective in preventing clinical nephropathy.

Markers of Diabetic Nephropathy

Until recently it was thought that the increase in albumin excretion above the detection threshold of current clinical methods (e.g., dipstick test, salicylsulphonic acid) was a sudden event, preceded by years of normal protein excretion. Moreover, elevated blood pressure was believed to be an accompaniment of established clinical diabetic nephropathy. Both these notions have recently been challenged.

Albuminuria

The definition of clinical proteinuria clearly depends on the sensitivity of the methods used to detect protein in urine. At an early stage of diabetes, protein may be excreted in the urine at a rate substantially above the normal range, yet remain below the usual clinical levels of detection. This phenomenon is apparent in 30 to 45 percent of patients with insulin-dependent diabetes. Determining the degree and type of urinary protein in diabetes may therefore prove more useful than regarding it as simply present or absent.

Urinary albumin excretion rate (AER) in healthy adults ranges from 2.5 to 26.0 mg per 24 hours, and these levels are defined as normoalbuminuria. In dipstick-positive diabetic patients the AER generally exceeds 250 mg per 24 hours, and this is defined as clinical albuminuria. The wide subclinical range of albumin excretion that may occur in dipstick-negative diabetics varies between 26 and 250 mg per 24 hours (18 to 174 μg per minute) and is defined as microalbuminuria.

TABLE 1 Preventive Treatment Regimens in the Preazotemic Diabetic Patient

Disease Stage	*Therapy*	*Effect*
Prenephropathic		
Microalbuminuria (AER >30 μg/min)	Tightening of blood glucose (BG) control;	Short term: Normalization of AER, GFR, and BP in most cases
Glomerular hyperfiltration (GFR >140 ml/min/1.73m²)	hypotensive treatment (low salt intake, ? diuretics, low dose ACE inhibitors);	Long term: Unknown; possibly prevention or delay of clinical nephropathy
Microhypertension (BP ≥135/86 mm Hg)	and low protein diet	
Nephropathic		
Persistent proteinuria (>0.5 g/24 hours)	Control of BG	Uncertain
Declining GFR	Control of BP	Slows progression of nephropathy; likely to delay ESRF
Raised BP	Reduction of dietary protein	
Urinary tract infection	Antimicrobial treatment	Prevents papillary necrosis, pyelonephritis, may contribute to delay of ESRF
Proliferative retinopathy and maculopathy	Photocoagulation	Prevents blindness
Coronary and peripheral arterial disease	Surgical when indicated	Reduces morbidity and possibly mortality following renal replacement therapy

These levels of AER are usually detected by sensitive immunoassay techniques, but recently a new qualitative agglutination test for small concentrations of albumin in the urine has been developed. This method, which is specific for albumin, is ten times more sensitive than the dipstick test, reads albumin concentrations between 25 and 170 mg per liter, and is simple and quick to perform. It should allow bedside detection of microalbuminuria. This is important because insulin-dependent diabetic patients with microalbuminuria of a certain degree (in our hands, overnight AER in excess of 30 μg per minute) have approximately a twentyfold increased risk of later developing dipstick-positive proteinuria and clinical nephropathy. Moreover, microalbuminuria has also been shown to be a powerful predictor of renal disease and mortality (mainly from cardiovascular causes) in non-insulin-dependent patients. The microalbuminuria of diabetes has been shown to be associated with worse glycemic control, and the relevance of this resides in the fact that intensified diabetic treatment that achieves levels of near-normoglycemia significantly reduces and, in some cases, even normalizes the albumin excretion rate. The response to correction of hyperglycemia is not universal, however, and diabetics with persistent microalbuminuria may not lower their albumin excretion in response to improved metabolic control. This condition, which is also termed incipient nephropathy, may perhaps reflect the earlier phase of metabolically irreversible progressive diabetic nephropathy.

The fact remains that intensification of diabetic treatment and normalization of glycemia is, at this stage of microalbuminuria, a worthwhile effort that may lead to important beneficial renal effects. Prospective control trials are now needed to test this hypothesis.

Blood Pressure

Another important and novel association of microalbuminuria is that noted with higher levels of arterial pressure. Diabetic subjects with AER in excess of 30 μg per minute have systolic and diastolic blood pressures that, though still within the conventionally accepted nonhypertensive limits (<160/95 mm Hg), are higher than those of a matched group with normal AER. Whether the higher blood pressures are cause or effect of the microalbuminuria is impossible to say from the available data, but it is interesting that the vicious circle of hypertension and kidney disease characteristic of late nephropathy may be commencing at this early stage. These data pose the question of whether conventional levels of hypertension are set *too high* to detect potentially reversible kidney damage; whether lower treatment thresholds for blood pressure should be applied to microalbuminuric diabetic patients, and whether a rising blood pressure within the normal range should be recognized as an indication for intervention. Preliminary studies indicate that lowering of blood pressure reduces the microalbuminuria in these patients independently of blood glucose control.

Glomerular Filtration Rate

Whereas both increased AER and higher blood pressure are earlier signs of diabetic kidney involvement than were previously recognized, they may not be the earliest ones. Glomerular hyperfiltration, a phenomenon found in approximately 30 percent of insulin-dependent diabetic patients, has been implicated in the genesis of diabetic glomerulosclerosis.

Recent data in humans have suggested that diabetic patients who, early in the course of the disease, have high GFRs exceeding 140 to 150 ml per minute per 1.73 m² lose glomerular function over time at a faster rate than patients with lower GFRs. Although in this study high GFR was associated with microalbuminuria, a recognized independent predictor of clinical nephropathy, this finding is the first evidence that glomerular hemodynamics may influence the natural history of diabetic nephropathy in humans.

The elevated GFR is associated with moderate degrees of hyperglycemia and is normalized by long-term strict glycemic control; even moderate relaxation of control in these patients restores the hyperfiltration. Recently the amount of dietary proteins has been strongly implicated in the genesis of glomerular hyperfunction, and diabetics with persistent elevation of GFR show a prompt decrease in GFR in response to a reduction (40 g daily) in protein intake for 3 weeks. This response is independent of blood glucose and blood pressure changes.

The wealth of information accumulated about microalbuminuria and its associations allows testing of the hypothesis that diabetic nephropathy can be prevented or greatly delayed. Microalbuminuria therefore provides a powerful indicator of late renal disease that is amenable to correction by a number of therapeutic maneuvers. Our options are not restricted to blood glucose control; reduction of moderate elevation of arterial pressure, lowering of dietary protein intake, and possibly other pharmacological interventions may prove equally effective. Although correction of a marker of disease does not necessarily imply abolition of the disease itself, it is a reasonable and attractive assumption that the normalization of indices that are prognostic of renal failure may prevent its occurrence.

In preazotemic diabetic patients, one may consider tailoring treatment according to the different phases in the development of diabetic renal disease, as summarized in Table 1.

At best, our chance is that of preventing diabetic nephropathy; at worst, it is that of delaying end-stage renal failure by several years. Current preventive therapy represents a considerable advance over what only a decade ago was considered "the sad truth" about survival of patients with diabetic renal failure.

POSTSTREPTOCOCCAL GLOMERULONEPHRITIS

FRANK G. BOINEAU, M.D.
JOHN E. LEWY, M.D.

In its typical form, poststreptococcal glomerulonephritis has various manifestations, including edema, hematuria, oliguria, proteinuria, reduced glomerular filtration rate, and hypertension. Many patients do not have all of the typical features, and the symptoms and signs may be very mild. This is especially true in family contacts, in whom this disease often goes unrecognized unless the family member is examined and laboratory evidence of the disease is sought.

CLINICAL FEATURES

Epidemiology

Acute poststreptococcal glomerulonephritis (APSGN) is extremely rare before the age of 2 years. Thereafter it may occur at any age, but is most common in school-aged children. In many studies, the mean age of onset of the sporadic form of APSGN is approximately 7 years. The male to female ratio is 2:1.

Preceding Infection

APSGN has long been known to follow certain types of group A beta-hemolytic streptococcal infections of either the throat and upper respiratory tract or skin. Upper respiratory infections are associated with most cases of APSGN in the northern United States, whereas skin infections are frequently associated with cases in the South. The latent interval is usually 8 to 14 days after an upper respiratory infection, while the latent interval after skin infection is usually longer (21 to 28 days). Direct culture of streptococcal organisms from the pharynx or skin is not common, but serologic evidence of a preceding group A beta-hemolytic streptococcal infection is usually present. After an upper respiratory tract infection, the antistreptolysin O (ASO) antibody titer is elevated in about 90 percent of the patients with APSGN. After skin infections, the ASO titer is elevated in only about half of the patients, but Streptozyme (Wampole Laboratories), antihyaluronidase, or antideoxyribonuclease B antibody titers are usually elevated. If titers of antibodies to these streptococcal antigens are not elevated when APSGN is recognized, serial quantitation of the titers usually reveals a significant rise over 1 to 3 weeks after onset of the clinical illness.

Clinical Manifestations at Onset

Typically the child or adult with APSGN has a history of gross hematuria and edema. He may also have oliguria or anuria, and gastrointestinal, pulmonary, and/or central nervous system manifestations. Because neither gross hematuria nor edema may be present in an individual patient, and the predominant symptoms may be related to the gastrointestinal, central nervous system, or pulmonary system, APSGN must be considered when these symptoms are present, and the urine carefully examined. The presence of microscopic hematuria or proteinuria or both, should alert the physician to pursue the diagnosis of APSGN.

The presenting signs in patients with APSGN mirror the symptoms recorded above. Elevation in blood pressure above 140/90 is present in from 30 to 80 percent of patients. Other evidence of an expanded extracellular fluid volume is often noted. Skin infection may also be present.

Laboratory Data at Onset

Laboratory data at the time APSGN is diagnosed reflect the reduced glomerular filtration rate, serologic evidence of a preceding streptococcal infection, and consumption of complement. It is well to remember that the degree of hematuria and proteinuria may be very mild and that nephrotic range proteinuria is uncommon. Thus the diagnosis of APSGN must be considered in patients with mild degrees of hematuria and proteinuria.

PREFERRED APPROACH TO MANAGEMENT AND DRUG THERAPY

Hospitalization

Many patients with APSGN can be treated at home. The principal considerations are the severity of the clinical abnormalities and the family's and physician's ability to provide close observation and care at home. Patients with moderate to severe reduction in renal function (creatinine clearance less than 50 ml per minute per 1.73 m^2 or blood urea nitrogen greater than 50 mg per deciliter) and those with oliguria or anemia; any symptoms of hypertensive encephalopathy, including lethargy, vomiting, or ophthalmologic changes; and significant edema or pulmonary congestion should be hospitalized. If hypertension is absent or mild and responds promptly to antihypertensive measures, including bed rest and medication, hospitalization can often be avoided.

Bed rest is an extremely controversial therapeutic modality. It was once considered appropriate to maintain bed rest until all signs of nephritis were past. However, it appears that ambulation has not been associated with worsening of any variables of renal function once gross hematuria, edema, hypertension, and azotemia have resolved. Children will not comply with a regimen of complete bed rest even if the physician or parents desire it. The conflict that arises in attempting to impose complete bed rest on an unwilling child is probably not worth its questionable advantages. A reasonable guide is that patients who have gross hematuria, hypertension, edema, evidence of circulatory congestion, or moderate to severe depression of renal function be kept on bed rest as much as possible.

Nutritional Management

Alterations in diet depend on the severity of the edema, renal failure, and hypertension. If the blood urea nitrogen concentration is less than 75 mg per deciliter, dietary protein need not be restricted. If the blood urea nitrogen concentration is above this level, intake should be restricted to 0.5 g per kilogram of body weight per day of proteins of high biologic value until renal function improves and the blood urea nitrogen concentration spontaneously decreases to below 75 mg per deciliter. Calorie intake should be maintained as near to normal as possible to reduce catabolism. In patients with hypertension or edema, sodium intake should be restricted to 1 to 2 g each day. More severe degrees of sodium restriction are usually not required and lead to poor caloric intake. Fluid balance should be carefully monitored, and fluid should be restricted in the presence of severe edema, oliguria, or anuria. In these patients, fluid intake should not exceed the sum of urine output and insensible water loss minus planned weight loss. Measurement of body weight daily, or more often if needed, is an effective way to determine whether fluid intake is appropriate. Fluid and sodium restriction with a decrease in extracellular volume will assist in the management of hypertension. Once edema has resolved, fluid intake should be restricted to insensible water loss plus measured fluid output as long as oliguria persists.

Treatment of Hypertension

Hypertension may be mild or severe. There is considerable disagreement regarding levels of blood pressure in APSGN which require therapeutic intervention. Hypertension often resolves with bed rest alone. If the diastolic blood pressure is below 100 mm Hg and falls further with the patient on bed rest, sodium restriction and continued bed rest are sufficient. If the blood pressure does not decline in 2 to 4 hours, or symptoms of encephalopathy develop (headache, nausea, vomiting, seizures), treatment should be instituted promptly. Hydralazine, 0.15 mg per kilogram up to 10 mg, given intramuscularly, is usually quite effective in reducing the blood pressure in this disease. The dose may be repeated in 4 to 6 hours if needed. If hypertension responds to the above measures only transiently, hydralazine may be given orally (0.7 mg per kilogram of body weight per day) in 4 divided doses. Hydralazine can gradually be increased, if needed, to a maximum of 200 mg per day orally. An effective dose should be continued until the blood pressure has been normal for 24 to 48 hours, and then the drug may be tapered and discontinued if the blood pressure remains normal. Sustained hypertension is infrequent, but may require sustained hydralazine therapy. Occasionally the blood pressure remains moderately, but persistently elevated, and treatment with oral methyldopa or propranolol is useful. Intravenous nitroprusside or diazoxide has been used successfully to treat severe acute hypertension. Hypertension in APSGN is largely attributable to an expanded extracellular fluid volume. Renin levels at the onset of the disease are characteristically normal or suppressed. Common antihypertensive drugs used in APSGN are listed in Table 1. Diuretics can be important in lowering the blood pressure. Furosemide, 2 mg per kilogram orally or 1 mg per kilogram intravenously, is often effective in producing a diuresis and lowering of the extracellular fluid volume. An improvement in encephalopathy has been seen in patients treated with intravenous furosemide even when only minimal or no changes in blood pressure have occurred. These observations imply that edema of the central nervous system plays an important role in hypertensive encephalopathy in APSGN.

Treatment of Edema

If there is fluid overload, diuretics are indicated to reduce edema, to test renal responsiveness, and as an ad-

TABLE 1 Common Antihypertensive Drugs Used in Acute Poststreptococcal Glomerulonephritis

Drug	*Initial Dose/Route (mg/kg)*	*Dose Interval (hours)*	*Maximum Dose*	*Common Side Effects*
Direct vasodilators				
Hydralazine	0.1–0.4 IV or IM	4–6	20 mg/dose	Tachycardia, palpitations
Diazoxide	3–10 IV over 30 min	Repeat once in 0.5 hour if needed	10 mg/kg/dose	Dizziness, tachycardia, nausea, rapid fall in BP, hyperglycemia, fluid retention
Nitroprusside	0.5–8 μg/kg/min	Constant infusion		Tachycardia, fluid retention, nausea, dizziness, cyanide poisoning
Hydralazine	0.25 PO	4–6	200 mg/day	Tachycardia, palpitations
Adrenergic inhibiting drugs				
Propranolol	1–2 PO	6–12	10 mg/kg/day	Lethargy, fatigue, bradycardia
Alpha-Methyldopa	2–3 PO	6–8	40–60 mg/kg/day	Lethargy, fatigue, depression
Drugs that reduce plasma volume				
Furosemide	1–4 PO	12–24	8 mg/kg/dose	Hypokalemia, metabolic alkalosis, postural hypotension
Chlorothiazide	5 PO	12	20 mg/kg	Hypokalemia, metabolic alkalosis, postural hypotension

Adapted from Portman RJ, Robson AM. Controversies in pediatric hypertension. In: Tune BM, Mendoza SA, eds. Pediatric nephrology. New York: Churchill Livingstone, 1984:282.

junct in the treatment of hypertension. Persistent edema can be treated with oral furosemide, 2 mg per kilogram once or twice daily. Hydrochlorothiazide, 2 mg per kilogram per day, is effective when renal function is normal or nearly normal, but not when there is marked depression of the glomerular filtration rate. Pulmonary congestion in APSGN usually reflects fluid overload and not myocardial failure. It is therefore *not* responsive to administration of digitalis. Vascular congestion can usually be treated effectively with fluid and sodium restriction and the use of diuretics as outlined above.

Antibiotics

Cultures of the throat and skin lesions if present should be obtained in all patients with suspected APSGN and all immediate family members. Those with positive cultures should be treated with appropriate antibiotics. In patients with suspected APSGN, even if beta-hemolytic streptococcus is not cultured, it is probably safest to treat with a ten-day course of penicillin (or erythromycin in penicillin-sensitive patients) Additional antibiotics are not used unless infectious complications are present. Prophylactic antibiotics are not indicated in this disease, since recurrences of APSGN are very rare.

Subclinical Cases

Subclinical asymptomatic cases of APSGN have been reported by several investigators. When first-degree relatives of an index case were studied, the ratio of subclinical to clinical disease was 4 and there was documented evidence of APSGN occurring in about 33 percent of household patient contacts. Thus it seems prudent to recommend evaluation of household family members (throat or skin culture, physical examination, and urinalysis) when an index case of APSGN is identified. If symptoms of acute nephritis develop in family members, serologic and renal function tests should be performed. Serial evaluation of family members is not indicated. The prophylactic treatment of household members with antibiotics is controversial and currently, unless skin or throat cultures are positive, prophylactic treatment is not indicated.

Renal Biopsy

In a typical case of APSGN, a renal biopsy is not required to diagnose the disease. There are however, times when a renal biopsy should be considered, either because of atypical presentation or because resolution does not follow the expected course. The reasons for considering a renal biopsy are listed in Table 2. None of these is an absolute indication, but should alert the physician that APSGN may not be present and a renal biopsy should be considered for diagnostic reasons. If a renal biopsy is considered, it should be done early, since pathologic changes such as generalized proliferation tend to become focal, and subepithelial deposits of immunoglobulin G (IgG) and complement tend to resolve after the first few weeks of the illness, making the diagnosis of APSGN more difficult. It should be emphasized that there are no pathognomonic features of APSGN and the renal biopsy must be interpreted in conjunction with the clinical findings.

Immunosuppressive Therapy

Corticosteroids and other immunosuppressive drugs are not indicated in the treatment of acute poststreptococcal glomerulonephritis. Mild or moderate cases have an excellent prognosis with supportive therapy, particularly in children. Even in cases of severe APSGN, supportive therapy alone frequently results in complete recovery of renal function. Recent studies, that have compared sup-

TABLE 2 Relative Indications for Renal Biopsy in Suspected Acute Poststreptococcal Glomerulonephritis

At onset of illness
Absence of reduced serum complement
Anuria
Nephrotic syndrome
Prior history of renal disease
Retarded linear growth in children
Family history of nephritis
During period of expected resolution
Persistence of oliguria beyond 3 weeks
Low C3 or total hemolytic complement beyond 6 weeks
Gross hematuria beyond 3 weeks
Persistence of hypertension

portive care with immunosuppressive plus anticoagulant therapy in a nonrandomized fashion in crescentic glomerulonephritis of poststreptococcal origin in adults, suggest that the renal outcome is equally good in the two groups. Thus the known risks of immunosuppressive medications are not justified in APSGN even when there are diffuse crescents on the biopsy specimen.

COURSE AND PROGNOSIS

Resolution of the Acute Phase

The overt manifestations of APSGN, which include gross hematuria, edema, reduced urine output, hypertension, and central nervous system symptoms, usually resolve in the first 1 to 2 weeks of the illness in most patients. Diuresis with loss of edema is usually complete by the end of the second week or sooner. Even those with severe renal failure will begin to show an improvement in the glomerular filtration rate in the first 2 to 3 weeks after the clinical onset of the disease. Hypertension disappears in many patients once they begin bed rest or after a short course of antihypertensive treatment. An improvement in the glomerular filtration rate and renal blood flow results in diuresis with loss of edema and return of plasma volume to normal. This is one of the factors leading to a decrease in blood pressure. The total hemolytic or third component of complement (C3) usually returns to normal within 6 weeks after the clinical onset of APSGN. Failure of complement to return to normal suggests that the patient may have membranoproliferative glomerulonephritis instead of APSGN. Microscopic hematuria will persist after gross hematuria disappears, but it too will gradually resolve. Complete disappearance of hematuria may take several months to several years. Occasionally, intermittent or orthostatic proteinuria is noted. Some studies of sporadic APSGN in adults have documented persistence of abnormal proteinuria for 2 years or more. Such persistent proteinuria, especially if associated with hypertension and a reduced glomerular filtration rate, may be a manifestation of a chronic form of glomerulonephritis. If the nephrotic syndrome is present at onset, it tends to be very transient and disappears in the early phase of the illness.

Long-Term Prognosis

The long-term prognosis of APSGN is controversial and depends on the age of the patient at the onset of illness, the severity of the acute disease, and epidemiologic considerations. The prognosis of epidemic APSGN in children seems very favorable, even in those with severe acute disease. Severe oliguria and the presence of diffuse crescents on biopsy suggest a more guarded prognosis.

The long-term prognosis of the sporadic form of APSGN is less favorable in adults than in children. Severe initial disease with a creatinine clearance below 40 ml per minute per 1.73 m^2, persistent heavy proteinuria (above 2 g a day), and older age at the time of onset contribute to a guarded prognosis.

Serial renal biopsies in adult patients with APSGN have demonstrated chronic findings such as glomerulosclerosis, varying degrees of interstitial fibrosis, and arterial changes in one-third to one-half of some series. Whether these changes represent progression of disease or simply healing of the acute process and static pathologic changes is unknown. The incidence of progression to end-stage renal disease is much less than that of the chronic changes found on histopathologic examination of tissue. A review of recent literature with medium- to long-range follow-up of adults reveals that chronic renal failure develops in 3 percent of the cases of sporadic, symptomatic APSGN. Follow-up studies of longer duration will better answer the question of long-term functional outcome in APSGN.

SCHÖNLEIN-HENOCH PURPURA

GEORGE B. HAYCOCK, M.B., D.Chir., F.R.C.P., D.C.H.
J. STEWART CAMERON, M.D.

Schönlein-Henoch (anaphylactoid) purpura is a fairly common disorder of childhood, much less frequently seen in adults, characterized by a distinctive rash, colicky abdominal pain, arthropathy, and glomerulonephritis. It usually follows a respiratory infection; in a few cases, withdrawal of a specific food such as milk protein brings prompt relief, with relapse upon dietary challenge. These epidemiologic features, together with the finding of increased serum immunoglobulin A (IgA) concentration in about half the cases and the presence of deposits of Iga and the 3rd component of complement (C3) in skin and renal biopsy material, suggest an immunologic basis for the syndrome, but little is known of the mechanisms involved.

The disease is most common in winter and early spring, affects boys more often than girls, and has its highest incidence between 2 and 12 years of age. The great majority of cases are benign and self-limiting, and do not require hospital attention; most published accounts of the syndrome, being based on hospital cases, are heavily biased by patient selection toward the "bad" end of the spectrum. Exceptional patients (usually older children or rarely adults) run a chronic, relapsing course over many months or years; it is not known what causes these patients to behave differently from the majority, in whom the illness resolves completely within three months.

SIGNS AND SYMPTOMS

Rash. The rash affects the extensor surfaces of the limbs, especially the legs, and the buttocks. It is often particularly dense over the ankles. It begins as a pinkish, papular eruption resembling urticaria, but rapidly becoming obviously purpuric so that the mature rash is maculopapular in nature, with petechiae both within and between the raised lesions. Ecchymoses and even hemorrhagic bullae are occasionally seen. The lesions may be precipitated or localized by trauma. Involvement of the face and scalp is virtually confined to young patients (<2 years of age).

Arthropathy The arthropathy principally affects the large limb joints, especially knees, ankles, and wrists. Pain may be severe but joint swelling is generally slight or absent. When present, it is usually attributable to periarticular edema rather than to an intra-articular effusion. The swelling often extends diffusely over the dorsum of the carpus or tarsus without being anatomically related to any single joint.

Abdominal Pain. Abdominal pain occurs in most cases and may be the presenting symptom. It varies from mild colic to severe pain with peritoneal signs, mimicking an acute abdominal emergency. Hematemesis and melena may occur. The symptoms arise from hemorrhagic vasculitis of the intestine. Intussusception is an infrequent but serious complication. *Protein-losing enteropathy* is occasionally seen, resulting in hypoproteinemic edema even in patients without proteinuria, an important diagnostic consideration. However, edema may on occasion be seen in children with a normal serum albumin concentration; the reasons for this are not known.

Renal Involvement. Renal involvement occurs in 30 to 70 percent of patients seen in the hospital. The clinical features are those of a glomerulonephritis, ranging from minimal urinary abnormalities with no measurable alteration in renal function, through an acute nephritic syndrome with hypertension and circulatory congestion, to rapidly progressive glomerulonephritis with deterioration to end-stage renal failure in weeks or months. The nephrotic syndrome may occur, but must be carefully distinguished from protein-losing enteropathy and incidental edema.

Histologically, the appearance in involved skin are those of a leukocytoclastic vasculitis with deposition of IgA, C3, properdin, late-acting complement components (C5 through C9) and fibrin in dermal capillaries. The typical renal finding is focal and segmental lesions, often superimposed on a mesangial proliferative glomerulonephritis, with mesangial deposition of the same immune components as are seen in affected skin, IgA predominating. In severe cases, the focal, segmental lesions are so widespread that they coalesce, but they do not have the uniform homogeneity of a truly diffuse, proliferative glomerulonephritis. The lesion cannot be distinguished on histologic grounds from that of idiopathic IgA nephropathy (Berger's disease). Minor segmental extracapillary crescent formation is common, but severe, extensive, diffuse crescent formation occurs in the most severely affected patients and has the same significance as in other types of proliferative glomerulonephritis: if a majority of glomeruli are involved, prognosis for renal function is poor. However, Schönlein-Henoch purpura is a rare cause of end-stage renal failure: of 200 children aged less than 16 years treated for end-stage renal failure at Guy's Hospital up to the end of 1985, the cause was Schönlein-Henoch purpura in only eight.

MANAGEMENT

Most patients with Schönlein-Henoch purpura need no treatment, except perhaps mild analgesia for joint pain. However, abdominal pain may be severe enough to justify the use of opiate analgesics. Oral glucocorticoid therapy is claimed to be dramatically helpful in patients with severe abdominal symptoms, although this opinion is based on uncontrolled, anecdotal reports; a short trial of prednisone or prednisolone in a dosage of 1 to 2 mg per kilogram of body weight per day is worth attempting if analgesics alone are ineffective in controlling pain without excessively sedating the patient. Gastrointestinal bleeding may occasionally require blood transfusion. The possibility of intussusception should always be borne in mind in a patient with severe abdominal pain and lower gastrointestinal bleeding. Such patients should be managed in close consultation with a surgeon well acquainted with the disease and its abdominal manifestations. Investigation by abdominal ultrasonography and contrast enema may be necessary in some cases; laparotomy should not be performed without verification of the presence of an intussusception by such techniques, since patients operated on unnecessarily do not do well.

Most patients with Schönlein-Henoch purpura and glomerulonephritis recover completely without specific treatment. *Rational management depends on identification of those who are at particular risk for the development of progressive disease.* These include those who, either at presentation or during the subsequent course of the illness, show evidence of reduced renal function (elevated plasma creatinine concentration) or the nephrotic syndrome. Plasma creatinine and albumin concentrations should therefore be monitored once or twice weekly during the active phase of the disease and subsequently, while hematuria and proteinuria persist, at lengthening intervals. If one or both of these is found to be abnormal, renal biopsy should be performed. Patients should be selected

TABLE 1 Clinical and Biopsy Findings and Details of Treatment of 5 Children with Severe Schönlein-Henoch Purpura and Glomerulonephritis

Patient No.	*Age/Sex*	*Crescents (%)*	*Nephrotic Syndrome*	*Pretreatment GFR (ml/min/1.73 m)*	*Post-treatment GFR (ml/min/1.73 m)**	*Follow-up (months)*	*Methylprednisolone*	*Plasma Xch*	*Aza or Cyclo*
1	8/M	0	+	33	117	38	+	−	−
2	12/M	61	+	22	76	31	+	+	Cyclo
3	5/M	17	−	17	90	18	+	−	Aza
4	13/F	21	+	40	137	34	+	−	Aza
5†	6/M	100	+	0	35	1½	+	+	Cyclo

* These values are those obtained at latest follow-up, i.e., at the end of the follow-up period indicated in the table.
† This patient was still under treatment at the time of writing. He had required hemodialysis for 3 weeks and was anuric for most of that time.
GFR=glomerular filtration rate; Xch=exchange; Aza=azathioprine; Cyclo=cyclophosphamide.

for treatment if (1) renal function shows progressive deterioration, irrespective of the biopsy findings, or (2) the biopsy reveals extracapillary glomerulonephritis with extensive crescent formation. Patients in these two categories have universally been found to have a poor prognosis without treatment, most progressing to end-stage renal failure within months or, at most, a year or 2.

Drugs that have been used in the treatment of severe Schönlein-Henoch nephritis include oral and parenteral corticosteroids, azathioprine, alkylating agents such as cyclophosphamide, anticoagulants, and antiplatelet agents in various combinations. In the absence of controlled studies, results are hard to interpret, but have generally been disappointing. Patients with a severe nephrotic syndrome, but normal renal function, and without severe crescent formation, are best left untreated.

In our hands, a combined regimen based on high-dose parenteral steroids, plasma exchange, and azathioprine or cyclophosphamide has been more successful in the severest cases and we continue to use it. Treatment is initiated with intravenous methylprednisolone, 600 mg per square meter of body surface area, six doses being given on alternate days, followed by oral prednisolone, 60 mg per square meter on alternate days. If no improvement has occurred after the first three doses, plasma exchange is begun. Each exchange is of twice the patient's plasma volume (estimated as 50 ml per kilogram of nonedematous body weight), and the procedure is repeated ten times over a 2-week period and six times over the subsequent 2 weeks. If no improvement has been seen by the end of the first week of plasma exchange, then oral cyclophosphamide or azathioprine, 2 to 3 mg per kilogram of body weight per day, is added and is continued for 8 weeks. Prednisolone is continued at the full dosage until renal function has normalized or ceased to improve, and then slowly reduced over several months while renal function is serially measured.

In the last 6 years, since this policy was introduced, 16 children have met our criteria for renal biopsy, of whom five were considered to warrant treatment according to the protocol described above. The other 11 all recovered completely without specific therapy. The salient clinical and histologic features of the five treated patients are summarized in Table 1.

The rather rare adult patients with Schönlein-Henoch purpura do not seem to differ from their younger counterparts in any respect, although it has been alleged that their general prognosis is poorer; this probably results from greater selection of patients for hospital investigation. Many middle-aged patients given a diagnosis of Schönlein-Henoch purpura are in fact suffering from other forms of vasculitis, such as the microscopic form of polyarteritis or Wegener's granulomatosis, and the diagnosis must not be accepted without evidence of renal and/or cutaneous vascular deposition of IgA.

An unknown number of children affected with Schönlein-Henoch purpura develop hypertension 5 to 15 years later; thus an annual check of blood pressure is worthwhile for a decade or 2 following a severe attack of the disease.

GOODPASTURE'S SYNDROME

ANDREW J. REES, M.B., M.Sc., F.R.C.P.

The term Goodpasture's syndrome was originally applied to all patients who had necrotising glomerulonephritis and pulmonary hemorrhage. Nowadays it is used most frequently to describe only those patients in whom the syndrome is caused by autoantibodies to the glomerular basement membrane (anti-GBM). These autoantibodies have highly restricted specificity and probably react exclusively with determinants in the glomerular non-collagenous-1 domain of type IV collagen. Nevertheless it is important to remember that anti-GBM antibodies are the cause of disease in less than half the patients who present with pulmonary hemorrhage and nephritis; other causes include various types of systemic vasculitis, systemic lupus erythematosus, and occasionally cryoglobulinemia. These disorders differ substantially in their response to therapy. This chapter deals exclusively with the management of anti-GBM antibody-mediated disease, except to contrast differences in clinical presentation.

Two aspects of antibody-mediated Goodpasture's syndrome have ensured that its importance far exceeds its prevalence, and both have obvious consequences for therapy. First, anti-GBM disease is almost always severe and frequently life threatening and may evolve with great rapidity accompanied by complete loss of renal function within 24 hours. Up to 4 litres of blood may be lost into the lungs within a similar time. Thus the urgency of treatment should be as required for a potential medical emergency. Second, anti-GBM disease is the first type of glomerulonephritis in which the pathogenesis—autoimmunity to the GBM—is known and can be quantified by serum assay for anti-GBM antibodies. This means that it is possible to diagnose the disease noninvasively, design rational therapies to remove anti-GBM antibodies, and monitor the effectiveness of these treatments. It has also been possible to study the relation between circulating anti-GBM antibodies and the injury they cause and to show the importance of secondary factors such as intercurrent infection and cigarette smoke on the course of the disease. Thus, a better understanding of the pathogenesis has broadened the approach to management; this broader approach will be emphasized here.

CLINICAL ASPECTS

Anti-GBM disease affects people of both sexes and of all ages. Most commonly it presents during the third decade, but there is a second peak in incidence—patients over 60 years of age. Originally it was suggested that most patients were male, but this greatly exaggerates the sex difference; most current series of anti-GBM disease describe sex ratios of less than two to one. Some authors have found elderly female patients to be less severely affected than other groups, but this has not been our experience.

It is unclear what initiates anti-GBM antibody synthesis. Despite repeated claims and a few suggestions reported in anecdotes, there is no convincing evidence to generally link anti-GBM disease with exposure to hydrocarbon fumes. Equally unconvincing is the evidence that specific viral infections cause anti-GBM disease. An association with Hodgkin's disease (or its treatment) has also been noted. There is, however, strong evidence of inherited predisposition to anti-GBM disease. The frequency of the class II major histocompatability antigen (HLA-DR2) is greatly increased, and there is also an association with immunoglobulin (Gm) allotypes. Inheritance also appears to influence the severity of anti-GBM nephritis and the intensity of the autoantibody response.

Patients with anti-GBM antibodies usually present with glomerulonephritis, which is associated with hemoptysis or a past history of hemoptysis in a half to three-quarters of patients. Only rarely do patients with anti-GBM antibody-mediated nephritis have the signs or symptoms suggestive of generalized disease—rashes, arthralgia, myalgia, or fever—that are so characteristic of other types of rapidly progressive nephritis. Typically, the glomerulonephritis is severe and in untreated patients progresses to renal failure in weeks or months. Sometimes, especially in the presence of intercurrent infection, progression is much more rapid accompanied by destruction of all renal function in hours or days. Presently it is impossible to tell whether an individual who presents with comparatively little renal injury is at risk from sudden deterioration or whether they come from the subgroup of patients with truly indolent disease. Evidence from renal biopsies, including those from patients who have already developed renal failure, suggest an explosive final event in that the crescents all appear to be at a similar stage of their evolution. This is in contrast to the appearances of renal biopsies from patients with other causes of rapidly progressive nephritis in whom crescents are found in all phases of evolution from cellular to fibrous and often coexist with sclerosed glomeruli, which imply past episodes of disease.

The severity of pulmonary hemorrhage is more variable still, with none apparent in 25 to 50 percent of patients. In the remainder, pulmonary hemorrhage usually precedes evidence of nephritis, is episodic, and varies in severity from mild hemoptysis to severe respiratory failure. The presence and severity of pulmonary hemorrhage is not influenced by differences in the specificity of anti-GBM antibodies, which appears to be the same irrespective of clinical presentation; rather, it depends on external factors. The most important of these in our experience is exposure to cigarette smoke as almost all current cigarette smokers have pulmonary hemorrhage, whereas, it is rare in nonsmokers. Smoke may also precipitate acute pulmonary hemorrhage, as may intercurrent infection and fluid overload. Experimentally high concentrations of inspired oxygen have the same effect. Avoidance of circumstances known to aggravate injury caused by anti-GBM antibodies is as crucial to effective management of antibody-mediated nephritis as are attempts to control antibody levels and to suppress inflammation.

The effectiveness of therapy in anti-GBM disease is greatly influenced by the speed of diagnosis because of the rapidity with which the disease can progress. Anti-GBM disease can often be suspected clinically, even in the absence of pulmonary hemorrhage, because of the combination of nephritis, evidenced by the urinalysis and microscopy, and deteriorating renal function, which are not accompanied by the signs of generalized illness typical of other types of rapidly progressive glomerulonephritis. Glomerulonephritis is confirmed by renal biopsy and pulmonary hemorrhage is confirmed by the presence of anemia, hemoptysis, alveolar shadows on chest film, an increased diffusing capacity for carbon monoxide (kCO) after correction for lung volumes, and the patient's hemoglobin concentration. The specific diagnosis is confirmed by demonstrating anti-GBM antibodies either in the serum by radioimmunoassay (an alternative test using indirect immunofluorescence is not sensitive enough) or in kidney tissue by immunohistochemical demonstration of linear deposition of immunoglobulin along the GBM. Linear staining of the alveolar basement membrane is variable, and its absence on biopsy specimens cannot be used to exclude anti-GBM disease. Both serum and tissue diagnosis are equally effective, but the radioimmunoassay has the advantage that serial measurements can be used to follow the patient's response to treatment and to ensure the suppression of anti-GBM antibodies before renal transplantation is undertaken. Lastly, our view is that the diagnosis of anti-GBM antibody-mediated nephritis is a medical emergency, which should be confirmed or refuted within the first few hours after patient presentation.

APPROACHES TO TREATMENT

The immediate aim of treatment in anti-GBM disease is to control pulmonary hemorrhage and glomerular inflammation as swiftly as possible, thereby providing the best chance of healing and repair. Simultaneously, it may be necessary to treat infection and to support renal and pulmonary function. The longer-term objective is to suppress anti-GBM antibody synthesis permanently. Before discussing our preferred regimen, it is important to recognize the grim prognosis for untreated patients. In their 1973 survey, Wilson and Dixon reported that 25 of their 53 patients died and only seven retained useful renal function. Even now, with the general availability of dialysis and with better diagnosis of less severely affected cases, less than 15 percent of untreated patients reported in the literature in all reported series of more than five patients who presented with raised plasma creatinines, have retained useful renal function.

Immunosuppressive drugs by themselves appear to have little influence on the course of anti-GBM antibody-mediated nephritis whether prescribed singly or in combination; this observation is in contrast with their effectiveness in treating other types of rapidly progressive nephritis. It is possible that pulmonary hemorrhage is controlled by drugs more easily than is nephritis as intravenous boluses of methylprednisolone have been reported to be effective. However, this has not been our experience.

In the past, bilateral nephrectomy was advocated for treating severe pulmonary hemorrhage in patients with anti-SBM antibody mediates disease. The original rationale for bilateral nephrectomy was that removal of the GBM would minimize the stimulus to further anti-GBM synthesis. However, not surprisingly, since the autoantigen is found in lungs as well as kidneys, nephrectomy has no effect on anti-GBM antibody titres and with hindsight, the case reports that originally suggested benefit are unconvincing. This approach is strongly contradicted and should be abandoned as ineffective and potentially dangerous.

Against this background, it was argued that effective treatment should include measures to rapidly reduce the concentration of anti-GBM antibodies, as well as measures to limit their synthesis and to suppress inflammation. Thus a treatment regimen was developed that combined repeated large volume plasma exchange with cytotoxic drugs and steroids. It would be ideal to assess the effectiveness of this treatment regimen with a prospective controlled trial, but unfortunately this cannot be done because of the rarity of anti-GBM disease, the rapidity with which it progresses, and the inherited influences on its severity. Consequently, the usefulness of therapy has had to be judged by its ability to control anti-GBM antibody titres, to suppress disease activity, and by the frequency and severity of the complications.

MANAGEMENT

Specific Therapy

Our standard regimen for treating Goodpasture's syndrome is outlined in Table 1. It consists of daily whole volume (4 L for adults) plasma exchanges for albumin, combined with prednisolone 60 mg daily, cyclophosphamide (3 mg per kilogram scaled down to the nearest 50 mg), and azathioprine 1 mg per kilogram. The regimen is modified in patients over the age of 55 years who receive cyclophosphamide 2 mg per kilogram scaled down to the nearest 50 mg and no azathioprine. Plasma exchanges are performed for 14 days or longer until clinical evidence of continuing injury has subsided. Plasma exchanges are restarted if disease activity recurs or if the anti-GBM antibody titre increases rapidly after the first course of exchanges has been completed, albeit both circumstances are rare. Five plasma exchanges are routine when a second course is required. Cyclophosphamide and azathioprine are discontinued after 8 weeks, provided that anti-GBM antibody titres are no longer detectable. The prednisolone dose is also rapidly reduced. Patients receive 60 mg of prednisolone daily for 1 week, and then, the dose is reduced at weekly intervals to 45 mg daily, 30 mg daily and then 20 mg daily. Thereafter the dose of prednisolone is reduced by decrements of 5 mg weekly until it is stopped after 8 weeks.

Plasma Exchange

The development of automatic techniques for plasma separation by centrifugation or filtration opened the way for therapeutic plasma exchange. This is a technique

TABLE 1 Plasma Exchange Regimen

Plasma exchange	Daily 4 L exchanges for albumin for 2 weeks
Steroids	Prednisolone, 60 mg daily for 7 days, thereafter 45, 30, 20, 15, 10, and 5 mg for 1 week each
Cytotoxic drugs	Cyclophosphamide 3 mg/kg (down to nearest 50 mg) Azathioprine 1 mg/kg (down to nearest 50 mg) Each given concurrently for 8 weeks

in which whole blood is removed from a patient and separated into its plasma and cellular constituents before the cells are reinfused with fresh albumin instead of the patient's plasma, which is discarded. A single 4 L plasma exchange removes approximately 90 percent of an intravascular marker, such as Evans Blue injected intravenously at the start of plasma exchange, and 45 percent of IgG and is a highly effective way to remove circulating autoantibodies. Unfortunately, anti-GBM antibodies are rapidly resynthesized and repeated exchanges as well as the concurrent administration of immunosuppressive drugs are needed to reliably reduce their concentration in most patients.

Venovenous circuits can be used for plasma exchange, but the repeated exchanges needed to treat anti-GBM disease demand more effective vascular access. Arteriovenous shunts and central vein catheters are both suitable, but I prefer the latter as they are less liable to become infected. All types of cell separators are equally effective at removing IgG, and so, the choice between centrifugation and filtration is a personal one depending on the facilities available. Albumin solutions should be used as the plasma substitute and should have potassium and calcium added in sufficient amount to bring their concentrations into the physiologic range. Plasma exchange removes coagulation factors as well as immunoglobulins; these factors are returned as two units of fresh frozen plasma at the end of exchange in all patients who are at risk of bleeding, including those with fresh pulmonary hemorrhage or those who have had recent renal biopsies. The anticoagulation needed to prevent clotting in the extracorporeal circuit also poses a potential danger for these patients, but only a slight one as most of the anticoagulant is discarded with the patients plasma rather than being returned to the patient.

Plasma exchange shares the complications of all extracorporeal circuits, such as infection of vascular access sites and embolism. In addition, there is a tendency to fluid overload in patients with renal failure because the sodium concentration of most plasma substitutes is greater than that of plasma. Thus, each whole volume exchange is often associated with a sodium load of 100 to 150 mmoles. Fluid overload should be anticipated by daily measurement of body weight, and excess fluid should be removed by appropriate use of diuretics or dialysis. Acute hypervolemia associated with severe hypertension can be a problem, especially in children, because of rapid redistribution of fluid, which is caused by the sudden increase of plasma albumin concentration to normal levels in previously hypoalbuminemic patients. Finally, repeated plasma exchange can cause thrombocytopenia because of platelet destruction in the circuit. Table 2 outlines practical considerations to minimize complications.

TABLE 2 Practical Considerations to Minimize the Dangers of Plasma Exchange

Proper extracorporeal technique to prevent air embolism
Accurate volume replacement to maintain blood volume
Sterile technique to minimize the risk of infection
Use of albumin solutions not contaminated with vasoactive substances
Addition of potassium chloride (1.4 mmol) and calcium gluconate (0.45 mmol) to each 400 ml unit of albumin to prevent acute electrolyte disturbances
Diluting replacement albumin solutions given to hypoalbuminemic patients because of the risk of acute hypervolemia
Prevention of chronic fluid overload caused by sodium loading imposed by exchanges

Cytotoxic Drugs

Anti-GBM antibody titres rapidly return to preexchange values without the concomitant use of cytotoxic drugs. The main drug used is cyclophosphamide, which is an alkylating agent that is rapidly converted by hepatic microsomes to a series of active metabolites. These metabolites are incorporated into host DNA at all stages of the cell cycle, but cells are only killed during division. In man, cyclophosphamide, in daily doses over 2 mg per kilogram, suppresses primary antibody responses and, when used with plasma exchange, has been found to significantly shorten the duration of anti-GBM antibody synthesis in Goodpasture's syndrome. The principal early complication of cyclophosphamide is bone marrow suppression, which may occur at any stage and should be anticipated by daily measurement of the leucocyte count and prevented by appropriate reduction of the dosage. Later complications include hemorrhagic cystitis caused by excretion of toxic metabolites, infertility—especially in males, and a small but perceptible risk of malignancy. In the doses advocated here, short-term and long-term risks are minimal.

I use a small dose of azathioprine in conjunction with cyclophosphamide, but it is very difficult to quantify its effectiveness. Azathioprine is a purine analogue that is only incorporated during DNA synthesis, i.e., during cell division. In high doses, it is immunosuppressive, but in the dosage given here (1 mg per kilogram), azathioprine probably acts as an anti-inflammatory drug that is thought to be particularly effective at depressing monocyte-induced injury. In the dosage used here, it adds to the bone marrow suppression caused by cyclophosphamide and can occasionally cause an idiosyncratic reaction characterized by fever and diarrhea. The mechanism of this reaction is not clear.

Prednisolone

Corticosteroids are the most powerful anti-inflammatory drugs available, and they also have some immunosuppressive properties. The pharmacologic aspects of these drugs are discussed extensively in other chapters. In anti-GBM antibody-mediated injury, they are used predominantly for their anti-inflammatory properties and are prescribed in short, intensive courses to control the inflammatory response until anti-GBM antibody synthesis has been suppressed. There is no rationale for continuing their use beyond this point.

Supportive Therapy

Patients with Goodpasture's syndrome may require supportive treatment for renal or respiratory failure, as well as for anemia.

Renal Failure

Patients with Goodpasture's syndrome may progress to end-stage renal failure within 24 hours and so need to have their renal function assessed daily in the early stages of their disease. Dialysis may be needed either because of azotemia or fluid retention (exacerbated by plasma exchange or blood transfusion), which can cause new life-threatening pulmonary hemorrhage. The choice between hemodialysis and peritoneal dialysis is controversial. Hemodialysis imposes the practical risks of further heparinization as well as adding to the duration of "machine treatment." It also carries the theoretical risk that complement activation by dialysis membranes may aggravate injury, either by priming neutrophils and activating monocytes or by sequestration of neutrophils in pulmonary capillaries adjacent to the site of antibody binding. Peritoneal dialysis has neither of these problems, but does carry the risk of infection. My own preference is to use peritoneal dialysis whenever possible.

Respiratory Failure

The treatment of respiratory failure in patients with anti-GBM disease is also controversial; although a hypoxemia may need to be corrected by oxygen therapy, there are sound experimental reasons for being anxious about such therapy. Oxygen toxicity exacerbates anti-GBM antibody-mediated pulmonary injury in rats and rabbits, at least in part, by increasing alveolar-capillary-endothelial cell permeability and thus the accessibility of the GBM to circulating antibody. It is impossible to test whether high concentrations of inspired oxygen have similar effects in patients with Goodpasture's syndrome. Nevertheless, it seems prudent to limit the inspired oxygen concentration to the absolute minimum necessary to maintain safe levels of arterial oxygen concentration. Continuous positive airway pressure should be used as required.

Anemia

Some patients with Goodpasture's syndrome are anemic and may present with a hemoglobin concentration of less than 5 g per deciliter. Care must be taken to avoid hypervolemia, which exacerbates pulmonary hemorrhage, when blood transfusions are being given.

Infection

Intercurrent infection is the most powerful cause of relapse with anti-GBM disease and appears to produce the effect by enhancing the potency of inflammatory mediators rather than by changing anti-GBM antibody synthesis. Meticulous care must be taken to prevent infection during the course of treatment, especially as the risks substantially increase by the presence of indwelling catheters (intravenous, peritoneal, or urinary) and by the use of high doses of steroids.

Other Nonspecific Measures

Cigarette smoking has been identified as an important cause of pulmonary hemorrhage in patients with Goodpasture's syndrome, and resumption of smoking can precipitate relapse. These data provide exceptionally powerful reasons for stopping patients with this disease from smoking. Goodpasture's syndrome has frequently been associated with exposure to hydrocarbon fumes. Whether or not the nature of this association and its effects are analogous to those of cigarette smoke, it again seems prudent to limit such exposure as much as possible.

RESULTS OF THERAPY

We have used plasma exchange to treat antibody-mediated Goodpasture's syndrome for the past 10 years and during this time have treated 49 patients. Since 1980, we have also performed serial assays of anti-GBM antibodies and advised on the management of a further 71 patients treated in other units throughout the United Kingdom.

Control of Anti-GBM Antibody Titre

Anti-GBM antibody titres fell immediately after starting therapy in all patients treated with the combination plasma exchange and immunosuppressive drugs, and there has been little tendency for anti-GBM antibody titres to increase once the concentrations have been reduced to background values. Long-term, possibly permanent, disappearance of anti-GBM antibodies was achieved within 8 weeks in 29 of 30 patients who received a full course of the plasma-exchange regimen. A full course was defined as at least 12 plasma exchanges and 8 weeks of treatment with cyclophosphamide. In contrast, anti-GBM antibodies persisted for much longer in patients who did not receive complete treatment, and only three of 33 patients cleared of antibodies by 8 weeks; the autoantibodies persisted for more than a year in 12 of these patients. Thus it appears that cyclophosphamide and plasma exchange act synergistically to promote long-term control of anti-GBM antibody synthesis.

Renal Function

Nephrons that have been destroyed cannot regenerate, and so it comes as no surprise that the degree of improvement of renal function depends on the severity of injury at the time treatment is started. The plasma exchange regimen has been used on 58 dialysis-dependent patients with anti-GBM disease under our direct or indirect supervision, and none regained useful renal function despite control of autoantibody titres. Similarly, the results in patients whose serum creatinines exceed 600 μmoles per 1 (6.8 mg per deciliter) at the start of treatment have not been encouraging, with improvement in only one of 12 such patients. By contrast, renal function improved in 13 of 15 patients with plasma creatinines that were rapidly increasing, but were less than 600 μmoles (6.8 mg per deciliter), who were treated by us and in 2 of 5 patients monitored by us, but treated elsewhere in the United Kingdom. Improvement in these patients was evident as soon as the plasma exchange regimen was started, which argues strongly that it was a direct result of treatment. Seven patients with biopsy-proven nephritis, whose serum creatinines were within the normal range, were also treated and showed improvement when assessed, by changes of serum creatinine to within normal range or by improvement of the urine sediment. Thus the plasma exchange regimen is effective treatment for nephritis in Goodpasture's syndrome provided that it is introduced before the kidneys have been severely damaged. In a few patients, late deterioration of renal function because of progressive fibrosis has occurred without recurrence of detectable anti-GBM antibody synthesis. These patients have not been treated by reintroduction of plasma exchange or drug therapy, but have received nonspecific treatment until dialysis or transplantation was performed.

Pulmonary Hemorrhage

Pulmonary hemorrhage in anti-GBM antibody-mediated disease has a much greater tendency to be episodic than nephritis, and the lungs have a much greater capacity to recover. In all, 56 patients had evidence of pulmonary hemorrhage when treatment was started, and it improved in 51. All the remaining patients died of respiratory failure. Relapses of pulmonary hemorrhage that occurred were related to infection, fluid overload, or in one patient, resumption of cigarette smoking. None of the patients who recovered has developed pulmonary fibrosis of sufficient severity to be visible radiologically. Possibly, this is because pulmonary blood is very focal and thus even widespread pulmonary hemorrhage can be disseminated from a small lesion.

Mortality

The overall mortality at 8 weeks in patients treated at Hammersmith was 16 percent (eight of 49 patients). In three of these, mortality was unrelated to the regimen—unsuitability for long-term dialysis in two and a myocardial infarction in the third—and in the remaining five, pulmonary hemorrhage was the cause of death. All the patients who had uncontrollable pulmonary hemorrhage had concomitant infections.

MONITORING THE EFFECTS OF THERAPY

The effects of treatment should be monitored meticulously by repeated assessments of disease activity, fluid balance, and possible complications (Table 3). Routine investigations include daily measures of body weight, urine microscopy, serum creatinine, and full blood count. Chest radiographs and kCO are assessed three times weekly when clinically indicated. Cultures of urine, sputum, and vascular access sites are taken three times weekly, but antibiotics are given only when clinically indicated. Whenever possible, it is helpful to monitor anti-GBM antibody titres frequently. We measure anti-GBM antibody titres daily for the first 2 weeks and then three times weekly, but this is not essential. However, it is important to measure antibody titres initially to confirm the diagnosis, secondly at the end of therapy to assess the need for continuous immunosuppression, thirdly before transplantation in patients who develop end-stage renal failure, and fourthly in all patients with deteriorating renal function so as to distinguish active disease from progressive scarring.

TABLE 3 Routine Monitoring of Patients with Goodpasture's Syndrome

System	*Investigation*	*Frequency*
General	Weight	Daily
	Routine clinical examination	At least daily
	Blood pressure	4 hourly
Hematologic	Hemoglobin White cell count Platelets	Daily
Renal	Urine sediment Serum creatinine	Daily
Pulmonary	Chest radiography kCO	3 times weekly
Immunologic	Bacteriologic cultures of urine, throat, vascular access site	3 times weekly
	Anti-GBM antibody titres	Daily for 2 weeks; thereafter 3 times weekly until undetectable, then monthly

PATIENT SELECTION

The plasma exchange regimen described here is arduous and exposes the patient to discomfort as well as some risk. It should not be used indiscriminately, but should be reserved for those patients who are likely to benefit. Presently, we offer plasma exchange to all patients with active pulmonary hemorrhage and all those with nephritis and declining renal function. We also treat the majority of patients with nephritis and creatinines within the normal range, but who have clinical or morphologic evidence of active nephritis. Patients who are anuric, but do not have pulmonary hemorrhage, are not treated, except occasionally to limit the duration of anti-GBM antibody synthesis and allow earlier renal transplantation.

Although this plasma exchange appears to be the first consistently effective treatment for anti-GBM disease, it is clearly unsatisfactory, being cumbersome and lacking specificity. Presently, understanding of autoimmunity and the control of autoantibody responses are advancing rapidly and hopefully will result in the development of more specific ways to suppress anti-GBM antibody synthesis. It is also depressing that so many patients present after their kidneys have been destroyed, and this clearly indicates the need for earlier diagnosis.

IDIOPATHIC NEPHROTIC SYNDROME: MINIMAL CHANGE DISEASE

TYRONE R. MELVIN, M.D.
ALFRED F. MICHAEL, M.D.

Nephrotic syndrome is a consequence of proteinuria sufficiently severe to result in hypoalbuminemia, edema, and hyperlipidemia. Multiple disease entities may present with this clinical presentation. This review will deal with one of these diseases, minimal change nephrotic syndrome (MCNS). This syndrome is characterized morphologically by relatively normal appearing glomeruli, the absence of immune deposits, and epithelial foot process obliteration without other discernable change. Emphasis will be placed on the diagnosis and therapy of this disorder.

CLINICAL EVALUATION

The goal of the physician who encounters a patient with nephrotic syndrome is to determine whether it is a manifestation of a treatable disease. As a first step, systemic disease should be excluded. The list of these entities is long, but a few will serve to highlight this category. Nephrotic syndrome may occur during the course of systemic illnesses such as lupus erythematosus, hemolytic uremic syndrome, and anaphylactoid purpura—diseases readily separated from MCNS based upon historical data, clinical features, and laboratory studies. However, glomerular diseases with characteristic histologic and immunohistochemical features such as membranous nephropathy and membranoproliferative glomerulonephritis are not so easily differentiated from MCNS on clinical grounds alone and thus may require morphologic analysis of biopsy tissue.

In all of these diseases, the therapeutic response correlates well with the histologic appearance of the kidney. In general, MCNS is likely to respond completely to corticosteroid therapy, whereas other nephrotic states generally are resistant to this therapy. Since the physician's goal is to assess accurately the probability of a therapeutic response, a cogent argument can be made that a renal biopsy is indicated in all patients. However, experience has shown that certain clinical and laboratory features are good predictors of response, and these form the basis for determining who needs a renal biopsy and who does not.

During the initial evaluation it is helpful to determine whether the patient has a simple nephrotic state or a clinical picture more correctly characterized as nephritis or a combination of both. In patients with nephrotic syndrome alone, the edema is a consequence of hypoalbuminemia, whereas in nephritic states, decreased glomerular filtration often leads to fluid overload. In the latter situation, a mixed picture may be seen with fluid overload superimposed on the nephrotic syndrome. The blood pressure is usually normal in MCNS, whereas hypertension is often observed in nephritis. The urinary sediment is also a guide as MCNS has a low incidence of microscopic hematuria and is virtually never associated with gross hematuria or cellular casts. The nephritic picture is exemplified by poststreptococcal glomerulonephritis or rapidly progressive glomerulonephritis, whereas simple nephrotic syndrome is observed in MCNS and membranous nephropathy.

The clinical syndrome may be refined further by examining other parameters. Patients with nephrotic syndrome are likely to be responsive to corticosteroid therapy if they are below 10 years of age, have normal renal function, normal blood pressure, and normal levels of complement components. These parameters, in addition to those outlined above, form the basis for deciding whether to initiate a course of therapy without defining the histology by renal biopsy. The following clinical presentation illustrates the point: A 2½-year-old male child presents with a 2-week history of weight gain and puffy eyes, which progresses to generalized swelling. His medical history is remarkable only for a preceding upper respiratory illness. The physical examination reveals a normal blood pressure and generalized edema, and urinalysis demonstrates albuminuria without significant numbers of red cells or cellular casts. His renal function is normal as are the levels of serum C3 and whole complement. This child probably has a syndrome responsive to corticosteroids, and this entity, if a biopsy were performed, is most likely to be MCNS. Knowing full well that a small percentage of patients will not respond or may have abnormal glomerular histology, the institution of therapy rather than biopsy is appropriate. The expected error in this methodology can be more precisely ascertained by reviewing series of unselected patients with nephrotic syndrome and in whom all patients were subjected to kidney biopsy. Approximately 80 percent of children will have MCNS, and of these, approximately 95 percent respond to corticosteroid therapy.

If the patient has features that are suggestive or resistance to corticosteroid therapy (> 10 years of age, significant hematuria, hypertension, decreased renal function, systemic disease, or a history of nephrotoxic drugs), it is more probable that a diagnosis other than MCNS explains the nephrotic state. A biopsy to confirm the clinical suspicion is therefore indicated. This approach also defines the small number of patients with MCNS that do not fit the clinical parameters outlined above. The relatively higher incidence of glomerulonephritis in adolescents and adults with nephrotic syndrome supports the performance of renal biopsy in these patients prior to institution of corticosteroid therapy.

THERAPY

Symptomatic therapy

Symptomatic therapy generally includes dietary manipulation, the use of diuretics, and infrequently, the addition of parenteral albumin. If edema is not affecting comfort or pulmonary function and is associated with cellulitis, modest restriction in sodium intake alone is recommended. Water restriction is not recommended, and it is not necessary to modify other aspects of the diet. For edema that is causing the problems already discussed, diuretics may prove useful. Hydrochlorothiazide may be used initially in a dose of 1 to 2 mg per kilogram per day, with or without spironolactone administered in a dose of 2 mg per kilogram per day. If there is a poor response, stronger diuretics such as furosemide (orally 1 to 6 mg per kilogram per dose or intravenously 0.25 to 1 mg per kilogram per dose may be used). Two doses of furosemide per day is usually adequate. These dosages are appropriate for children. In adults, hydrochlorothiazide is usually initiated as 12.5 to 25 mg orally twice a day; furosemide 10 mg per dose orally or intravenously to be increased as required—usually no higher than 80 to 100 mg per dose; spironolactone is usually initiated at approximately 25 to 100 mg per day in 2 to 4 divided doses. The risk of diurectics in a patient with nephrotic syndrome exceeds that of the general population because the intravascular volume is not known. Some patients may be volume depleted, thereby risking further volume depletion, especially with excessive use of furosemide. Other concerns include hypokalemia, hyponatremia, and alkalosis. In rare instances, acute renal failure may be precipitated. At a minimum, it is important to monitor serum electrolytes, body weight, and renal function.

In some circumstances where rapid removal of fluid is necessary because of pulmonary compromise or a need to have the patient lie prone for a biopsy, a combination of intravenous albumin followed by furosemide has proven useful. This may be accomplished by the administration of 0.25 to 1.0 g albumin per kilogram body weight (salt poor, usually 25 percent given slowly 1 to 2 hours) followed by intravenous furosemide at 0.25 to 1 mg per kilogram body weight per dose. This usually results in prompt diuresis. However, this therapy has potential risks. The vascular volume should be assessed by clinical examination and chest X-ray films since this therapy may precipitate volume overload with concomitant congestive heart failure and/or hypertension. Further, in a patient with a pulmonary infection, this maneuver may precipitate hypoxia. In patients with severe hypocalcemia, albumin administration may lead to tetany. Because of these concerns, this therapy should be used with caution and usually not repeated more often than every 24 hours.

In nephrotic patients with hypovolemia and prerenal azotemia, albumin is of value in expanding the plasma volume.

Corticosteroid therapy

In patients with a high likelihood of response, the following regimen is recommended. Prednisone is administered in a dose of 60 mg per meter squared of body surface area per day (maximum 75 mg per day in 2 to 3 divided doses for 4 weeks). The dose is then changed to 60 mg per meter squared of body surface area as a single dose given every other morning for a period of 1 additional month. In adults who have MCNS, the dose is approximately 1 mg per kilogram body weight per day in divided doses for 1 month, and therafter, the same dose is administered every other day. For the patient with severe diarrhea that complicates nephrotic syndrome, parenteral methylprednisolone in appropriately-adjusted doses has been used with success.

Therapeutic response

Within 2 to 3 weeks more than 80 percent of patients will have responded to therapy (protein-free urine by dipstick for 3 consecutive days), and an additional 12 percent will respond over the next 5 to 6 weeks. An additional 3 to 5 percent will respond if the every other day phase is continued for 4 more months. Therefore, only 3 to 5 percent of patients are unresponsive to corticosteroids. In those that respond, the prednisone is tapered rapidly and then discontinued. In this responder group, approximately 25 percent never have a subsequent relapse, 40 percent have few relapses, and 35 percent have frequent relapses (2 or more in 6 months). For a relapse, defined as the presence of significant proteinuria (>1+ dipstick) for at least 1 week, usually with the return of edema, the following treatment is used. Prednisone is again administered as described above in a dose of 60 mg per squared meter of body surface area per day in 2 to 3 divided doses until the child is free of urinary protein (<1+

dipstick) for 1 week, at which time the dose is switched to 60 mg per meter squared of body surface area given as a single dose every other day. The time period over which the every-other-day phase is administered is arbitrary. Some clinicians discontinue therapy at this point, whereas others continue prednisone for periods that range from a few weeks to a year. The use of intermittent therapy may prevent relapses, but does not alter the natural history of the illness. Relapse therapy for adults is the same except the dose used is approximately 1 mg per kilogram. Prolonged every-other-day therapy is particularly useful in patients with frequent relapses. It is in this group that corticosteroid toxicity may become manifest. Even with the use of every-other-day therapy, patients may relapse and spend prolonged periods of time on daily prednisone. Corticosteroid toxicity may lead to poor linear growth in children, hypertension, aseptic necrosis of bones (especially in adults), and less commonly, weakness, electrolyte disturbance, gastrointestinal hemorrhage, and pseudotumor cerebri. When these manifestations make continued use of corticosteroids unacceptable or when the nephrotic syndrome persists unabated, cytotoxic drugs may be of value. All patients should have a kidney biopsy prior to cytotoxic therapy to confirm the diagnosis and to make certain that they do not have morphologic lesions that are associated with a poor prognosis and hence have little chance of response.

Cytotoxic therapy

Cyclophosphamide and chlorambucil are the two agents that have been used successfully in producing long-term remission of nephrotic syndrome. Following the successful initiation of remission in patients with frequently relapsing nephrotic syndrome using prednisone as discussed, cyclophosphamide, is given in a dose of 2 to 3 mg per kilogram per day as a single dose for 8 weeks. There is no large experience in adults with cyclophosphamide in nephrotic syndrome that has led to a concensus on dosage. This therapy leads to prolonged remission in approximately 80 percent of patients and decreases the frequency of recurrence in others. At this dose, the toxicity as manifested by cystitis, alopecia, oligospermia, and leukopenia is generally low. Although there are unknown potential threats such as oncogenicity and chromosomal damage, these risks appear to be relatively low. However, cyclophosphamide should be used with caution, with periodic evaluation of leukocyte counts and careful observation for intercurrent infections. Tuberculosis should be excluded by tuberculin testing, and children who have not had varicella should be shielded from this disease with exclusion from school if necessary. Signs of infection must be reported by the patients or their parents and evaluated by a physician. Second courses of these agents may be given. However, it is not known whether there is a cumulative risk of multiple courses of therapy with regard to the development of neoplasm, chromosomal injury, and pulmonary fibrosis.

Chlorambucil generally has been as effective as cyclophosphamide in producing long-term remissions. It is also given after a prednisone-induced remission beginning at 0.1 mg per kilogram body weight per day as a single dose, increasing to 0.2 mg per kilogram per day after 1 week. The drug is continued for 8 to 12 weeks. Experience with this drug is limited in adults with nephrotic syndrome; therefore a consensus opinion regarding dosage is unavailable. The same precautions are taken as with cyclophosphamide. Toxicity includes leukopenia, infection, focal seizures, and gastrointestinal irritation. Long-term potential risks include gonadal toxicity as well as cancer. Several patients have developed leukemia after the use of these agents, although in only one instance had the child been treated for nephrotic syndrome. Repeated courses of chlorambucil have been used, but are not recommended. Chlorambucil also leads to sustained remission for 2 to 3 years in approximately 70 to 80 percent of patients who have frequent relapses.

Steroid dependence and resistance

In a small group of patients, relapse occurs while therapy is tapered or shortly following the termination of therapy. This is termed steroid-dependence. Although it remains controversial, there is evidence that these patients have a relatively low likelihood of response to cytotoxic therapy, and in fact only 20 to 30 percent have a sustained remission at 2 to 3 years. Included within this group are patients who have MCNS, but also patients whose glomeruli show abnormalities such as focal segmental glomerulosclerosis and mesangial proliferation. Therapy should be given with the knowledge that the majority do not achieve a prolonged remission. Complete steroid resistance is uncommon with MCNS. These patients are generally treated with cytotoxic agents (as previously outlined) after causes of resistance (e.g., occult infection and poor compliance) have been ruled out. A small percentage respond partially or completely to this therapy. An occasional patient who is resistant will have a change to a steroid-dependent or to a frequently-relapsing course after cytotoxic therapy.

New agents such as cyclosporine A have been utilized in steroid-dependent patients and in the extremely uncommon steroid-resistant group (more common in adults). Reports of success have recently appeared, but further experience is required before this drug can be recommended.

COMPLICATIONS OF NEPHROTIC SYNDROME

The nephrotic state places patients at significant risk for infection and is associated with a variety of metabolic derangements. The infections tend to be caused by encapsulated organisms such as *Streptococcus pneumoniae, Escherichia coli, Haemophilus influenza, Klebsiella* species, as well as *pseudonomonas* and *serratia* species. This increased risk is thought to be a result of urinary loss of complement components (Factors B and D) and immunoglobulin. It manifests itself frequently as cellulitis, peritonitis, pneumonia, or septicemia. Efforts are aimed at decreasing the risk through use of pneumococcal vaccine, prophylactic penicillin, and the aggressive evaluation of patient complaints.

Metabolic abnormalities include symptomatic hypocalcemia attributable to hypoalbuminemia and urinary loss of vitamin D and vitamin D-binding globulin. Adequate calcium intake, and the occasional use of vitamin D taken orally, have minimized this problem. The loss of thyroglobulin virtually never necessitates thryoid replacement therapy. Electrolyte abnormalities, e.g., hyponatremia, hypokalemia are most often due to injudicious use of diuretics. Potassium supplements may be required if the serum potassium is less than 3.0 mEq per liter; however, in the nephrotic patient, sodium supplementation is almost always an incorrect response to hyponatremia. Total body sodium is usually normal or increased and significant hyponatremia (< 130 mEq per liter) is best handled through reevaluation of diurectic needs and water intake.

A more ominous complication is hypercoagulability. This is a consequence of increased synthesis of clotting factors (e.g., fibrinogen), urinary loss of antithrombin III and plasminogen, and increased platelet count and function. Serious and even life-threatening thromboses may occur including renal vein thrombosis, sagittal sinus thrombosis, and major arterial thromboses. No strategies have been specifically devised to deal with this problem, but in the unusual patient necessitating deep venous or arterial catheter placement antiplatelet therapy and systemic anticoagulation should be considered.

This work was supported in part by grants from the National Institute of Health (AI/0704, AM25518, AM26149) and the Viking Children's Fund.

FOCAL SEGMENTAL GLOMERULOSCLEROSIS

GERALD S. ARBUS, M.D., F.R.C.P.(C)
REUBEN BAUMAL, M.D., Ph.D., F.R.C.P.(C)

Focal segmental glomerulosclerosis (FSGS) is a nonspecific response of the glomeruli to injury. It may be seen in a renal biopsy specimen during the course of many diseases, such as Berger's disease, diabetic glomerulosclerosis, Alport's syndrome, reflux nephropathy, congenital nephrotic syndrome, heroin addiction, and acquired immunodeficiency syndrome (AIDS). The clinical features of these conditions, with or without the presence on a renal biopsy specimen of morphologic alterations peculiar to them, usually point to a specific diagnosis. However, when no known disease is present and the renal biopsy specimen shows only FSGS, a primary disease entity is implied, which is the subject of this chapter. FSGS is also referred to as FSGS with hyalinosis, focal sclerosing glomerulonephritis, and focal sclerosing glomerulonephropathy with segmental hyalinosis. It is most often associated with a nephrotic syndrome in children and is seen in approximately 10 percent of renal biopsies performed for investigation of nephrotic syndrome.

We have had extensive experience in managing nephrotic patients with FSGS and have found that they can be assigned to one of three groups, depending on their response to steroids and/or cyclophosphamide (Table 1). In group 1 patients, the disease follows a course similar to minimal lesion disease in that the nephrotic syndrome is brought into remission with steroids and/or cyclophosphamide and there is no progression to renal insufficiency. In group 2 patients, there is no remission of the nephrotic syndrome despite steroid and/or cyclophosphamide therapy, and progression to end-stage renal failure is common. About half of the patients in this group at our hospital have developed end-stage renal failure. Patients in group 3 respond initially to steroids and/or cyclophosphamide; the response in patients we have followed has lasted for as long as 9 years, but eventually they became nonresponsive. To date, 60 percent of our group 3 patients have gone on to end-stage renal failure, requiring dialysis and/or renal transplantation. Many of our patients in group 2 and 3 who have not yet reached end-stage renal disease have progressive renal failure.

Like others, we have found that some children who show FSGS on a renal biopsy specimen present with persistent proteinuria or hematuria and not a nephrotic syndrome. Because no current therapy appears effective in these patients, we have stressed the management of patients with FSGS who have a nephrotic syndrome.

CLINICAL FEATURES AND INVESTIGATION

Most patients with FSGS, whether children or adults, who present with a nephrotic syndrome have obvious generalized edema. However, some children with nephrotic syndrome present initially with periorbital edema and are not checked for the presence of pedal edema. Hence, they are labeled as having localized edema secondary to a cough, cold, or allergy. It is only weeks later, after the patient has returned to the physician with obvious generalized edema, that a more ominous disease process is suspected. Although an early diagnosis of nephrotic syndrome does not alter the long-term prognosis of the patient's FSGS, there is less morbidity for the patient and it is less disconcerting to the family if the physician detects the problem at the initial examination.

Many patients with FSGS and a nephrotic syndrome who progress to chronic renal failure also show evidence of a nephritic syndrome (i.e., hypertension, azotemia, and/or hematuria). However, some steroid-sensitive patients with FSGS and a nephrotic syndrome show various elements of the nephritic syndrome. A few steroid-resistant children with FSGS show glycosuria.

Routine laboratory studies on patients with FSGS and a nephrotic syndrome should include hemoglobin, routine urinalysis, 24-hour urine for protein, and serum de-

TABLE 1 Grouping of Patients with Focal Segmental Glomerulosclerosis According to Response of Nephrotic Syndrome to Drug Therapy

Group	*No. of Patients*	*Response to Steroids and/or Cyclophosphamide*	*No. (%) of Patients with Subsequent End-Stage Renal Failure*
1	36	Consistent remission	0 (0)
2	33	No remission	16 (48)
3	10	Initial remission and then permanent relapse	6 (60)
Total	79		

terminations of creatinine, urea, electrolytes, proteins by electrophoresis, cholesterol, triglycerides, total hemolytic complement, C3, and C4.

The time sequence of performing a renal biopsy and instituting drug therapy differs in adults and children. If a child who presents with nephrotic syndrome has a normal serum complement, he is usually started on a course of steroids without a renal biopsy. It is only later, if the child does not respond to steroids, that a renal biopsy should be performed and a tissue diagnosis reached. In adults, however, there are many causes of nephrotic syndrome which do not respond to steroids, and therefore they should not be given until a renal biopsy has been performed and a tissue diagnosis reached.

When a patient (adult or child) presents solely with persistent proteinuria, a biopsy is necessary. If it shows FSGS, steroids are not indicated, since there is no evidence that they will reverse the proteinuria or prevent progression to renal failure.

Interpretation of the Renal Biopsy

A diagnosis of FSGS can be made from a renal biopsy specimen when light microscopic examination shows one or more glomeruli with a sclerosed segment, often associated with obliteration of capillary lumina and hyperplastic overlying visceral epithelial cells. Hyalinosis and foam cells may be seen in the sclerosed segments but these are not essential for diagnosis. In addition to segmental sclerosis, globally sclerosed glomeruli may be present in the biopsy specimen depending on the stage of the FSGS. FSGS is known to involve the juxtamedullary glomeruli preferentially and therefore the absence of this region from a renal biopsy specimen may prevent a diagnosis of FSGS from being made. Nevertheless, FSGS should be suspected in a patient with nephrotic syndrome if the renal biopsy does not contain juxtamedullary glomeruli and instead shows only glomeruli with increases in mesangial matrix, mesangial hypercellularity, hyalinosis, and global glomerulosclerosis, as well as interstitial fibrosis and tubular atrophy. Immunofluorescence microscopy and electron microscopy are supportive of the light microscopic diagnosis, the former showing glomerular IgM and C3 in the sclerotic segments and the latter mesangial sclerosis with subendothelial electron-dense deposits due to hyalinotic masses. In addition, fusion of foot processes of visceral epithelial cells is usually present, as seen in patients with nephrotic syndrome from any cause.

MANAGEMENT

Usually patients with FSGS are admitted to the hospital for investigation when they have their first episode of nephrotic syndrome and, when indicated, for performance of a renal biopsy. Management is instituted while they are in the hospital and consists of patient and family education, drugs for control of edema and hypertension, and drugs for the treatment of nephrotic syndrome.

Education of Patient and Family

We have found two booklets to be useful for supplementing our discussions on childhood nephrotic syndrome with patients and their families: "Nephrotic Syndrome in Children," which can be obtained from both the United States National Kidney Foundation and the Kidney Foundation of Canada, and "Childhood Nephrotic Syndrome—You and Your Child," which is available from the Kidney Foundation of Canada.

Drugs for Control of Edema and Hypertension

When first seen, a patient with FSGS and edema from nephrotic syndrome should be placed on a limited sodium and water intake. If edema is mild and only a cosmetic problem, diuretic therapy may not be necessary. Should diuretics be needed, hydrochlorothiazide (2 mg per kilogram of body weight per day), either alone or in combination with spironolactone, is usually effective. Such therapy is also appropriate at home for treating mild edema. If edema is gross and symptomatic (i.e., labial or scrotal edema with the potential for breakdown of skin, or ascites causing respiratory embarrassment), a more potent regimen is necessary, consisting of intravenous albumin and furosemide in the case of steroid-sensitive FSGS. Intravenous salt-poor albumin 1 g per kilogram of body weight is administered over 1 hour, followed by furosemide, 1 mg per kilogram of body weight. The albumin draws sodium and water from the interstitial space, thereby increasing intravascular volume and allowing the furosemide to exert a more pronounced effect on the kidney. Furosemide should not be used alone, since it may produce a shock-like state by causing a sudden, drastic loss in intravascular volume.

In the case of steroid-resistant patients with FSGS, there is often concomitant poor renal function. As a consequence, the intravascular volume tends to be expanded and the response to diuretics is blunted. For these reasons, there is no need to give albumin prior to furosemide, and in fact such a step may be contraindicated, especially if severe hypertension is present. Doses as high as 2 to 5 mg of furosemide per kilogram of body weight per day may have only a mild diuretic effect. Thus, when a diuretic becomes necessary, such patients are likely to be sent home on a regular furosemide regimen to help achieve control of edema.

When hypertension sufficient to require therapy occurs in patients with FSGS, it is always associated with steroid resistance. Often it is difficult to treat, especially in the face of progressive renal failure. Triple therapy (diuretic, beta blocker, and vasodilator) may be necessary but is often ineffective, and drugs such as minoxidil or captopril may be required to control elevated blood pressure. Once the patient is started on dialysis, bilateral nephrectomy may be the only means of controlling the blood pressure.

Drugs for Treatment of Nephrotic Syndrome

Prednisone

As mentioned previously, most children who present with nephrotic syndrome do not initially undergo a renal biopsy but rather first receive a trial of steroid therapy. Approximtely 80 to 90 percent of them respond to a course of steroids, as outlined in Table 2(A). If one performed a biopsy on these steroid-sensitive children, most of them would show minimal lesion disease, some would show FSGS, and a few would show mesangial proliferative glomerulonephritis. For adults, treatment is the same except that the daily dose of prednisone is usually about 1 mg per kilogram of body weight per day. For patients with not more than one or two relapses of nephrotic syndrome per year, this treatment is ideal because they are not exposed to high doses of steroids for a prolonged period. In patients with frequent relapses, a more gradual decrease in alternate-day prednisone therapy is attempted, as shown in Table 2(B), to induce a prolonged remission. If, however, relapses occur during tapering of the alternate-day prednisone, it may be necessary to treat the patient with a decreasing daily dose of prednisone over a two to four month period. Some patients appear to develop a relapse of their nephrotic syndrome shortly after stopping medication. We and others have found that by maintaining the patient on 5 to 10 mg of prednisone daily or every second day for a prolonged period, the relapse rate is decreased. Such a protocol may be of value when the patient's susceptibility to relapses is increased, for example, during the cough/cold or allergy season.

TABLE 2 Usual Course of Prednisone for Treating a Steroid-Sensitive Patient with Focal Segmental Glomerulosclerosis and Nephrotic Syndrome

(A) To induce and maintain a remission

2 mg/kg body weight/day prednisone (maximum 80 mg/day) in 3 or 4 divided doses until the urine is protein-free for 5 days (maximum duration 28 days). Then 2 mg/kg/day prednisone as a single dose (maximum 80 mg/day) on alternate days for 28 days. The dosage is decreased to 10 mg, then 5 mg every other day over a 2 to 4 week period, then discontinued.

(B) Alternative therapy for frequently relapsing nephrotic patients

Remission is induced with daily prednisone as above, and then 2 mg/kg/day prednisone as a single dose is given on alternate days for 28 days. Prednisone is gradually reduced over 2 to 4 months by 10-mg decrements each week to 30 mg and then by 5-mg decrements weekly until discontinued.

Cyclophosphamide/Chlorambucil

Approximately 95 percent of steroid-sensitive patients with FSGS and nephrotic syndrome go into remission after four weeks of prednisone therapy and 99 percent respond after eight weeks. Therefore, if a patient with FSGS has not responded to a four to eight week course of prednisone, a trial of cyclophosphamide is indicated. One might also consider using cyclophosphamide in the steroid-dependent or steroid-toxic individual. In the past, a high dose of cyclophosphamide (5 mg per kilogram of body weight per day) was given for prolonged periods (six to twelve months). Although this succeeded in maintaining a remission that was still present one year later in all of our nephrotic patients who had previously responded to prednisone therapy, sterility developed in many of them. Therefore, cyclophosphamide is now given daily in a dose of 2.5 mg per kilogram of body weight and the course of therapy has been shortened to six to eight weeks. Cyclophosphamide is started when the patient is in remission following prednisone therapy, and is given together with prednisone, 0.5 to 2 mg per kilogram of body weight per day, on alternate days. The prednisone is gradually decreased when the course of cyclophosphamide has been completed. Unfortunately, with this lower dose of cyclophosphamide, the chance of a steroid-responsive patient with FSGS remaining in remission for at least one year after cyclophosphamide therapy has been reduced to about 70 percent. We have on occasion given a second course of cyclophosphamide to steroid-responsive patients who have become severely steroid toxic from frequent relapses.

We analyzed the clinical outcome following a course of cyclophosphamide lasting at least six weeks in 29 patients with FSGS and steroid-resistant nephrotic syndrome. None of them went into complete remission. However, the patients who developed a partial response (i.e., showed a rise in serum albumin equal to or greater than 2.5 g per deciliter with a loss or reduction of edema), despite a persistence of proteinuria, also showed an improved clinical outcome, compared with patients who were totally resistant to cyclophosphamide.

In lieu of the above mentioned protocol for administering cyclophosphamide, one might consider using cyclophosphamide intravenously, 750 mg per square meter, and repeating this dose three times at three- to four-week intervals. As a personal choice, some physicians have used chlorambucil, 0.2 mg per kilogram of body weight per day for eight to fourteen weeks, instead of cyclophosphamide. However, there is no evidence that chlorambucil provides greater benefit than cyclophosphamide in the treatment of FSGS.

Other Medications

Patients with FSGS and a nephrotic syndrome may have an abnormal platelet consumption, resulting in hemostatic abnormalities (i.e., hypercoagulability and hyperviscosity). Studies from Thailand have demonstrated that dipyridamole, combined with other antiplatelet agents and low-dose steroids, was useful in the treatment of steroid-resistant FSGS, with impovements noted in blood pressure, proteinuria, and creatinine clearance. In addition, progressive deterioration of renal function did not occur as readily. We are currently assessing this therapeutic approach in a double-blind trial on two groups of steroid-resistant FSGS patients, both of whom receive low-dose steroids. One group also receives dipyridamole, 5 mg per kilogram of body weight per day, plus acetylsalicylic acid, 10 mg per kilogram of body weight per day, while the other group receives placebo.

DIALYSIS AND TRANSPLANTATION

Patients with FSGS who have developed end-stage renal failure and undergone renal transplantation have been analyzed for long-term graft survival. There is evidence that FSGS can recur in allografts, with a rate of upwards of 30 percent documented in the literature. The incidence varies greatly among centers, however. Typically, heavy proteinuria can develop from the allograft within 24 hours after transplantation, or at times within the first few days or weeks after transplantation. When FSGS recurs in the renal transplant, there is more than a 50 percent chance that the allograft will ultimately be lost from the recurrence. Recurrent FSGS is more likely to be seen if the time from onset of the disease to terminal renal failure is less than two to three years and if the patient is a child over 6 years of age at the onset of the original diagnosis. Recurrence rates in adults over 20 years of age are said to be low. If there is a recurrence of FSGS in a first allograft, there is a greater chance of recurrence in subsequent renal grafts. In such patients, one should seriously consider whether second or further attempts at renal transplantation are warranted. Currently some centers are trying cautious administration of meclofenamate for treatment of recurrent FSGS in patients with renal allografts and heavy proteinuria.

PROGNOSIS

Patients with FSGS and nephrotic syndrome who respond to steroids do not destroy their kidneys, and any mortality or morbidity is related to infection (peritonitis), shock, or complications of steroid or immunosuppressive therapy. Patients with FSGS and steroid-resistant nephrotic syndrome have about a 50 percent ten-year kidney survival. Patients with FSGS and persistent proteinuria have been said to have a 90 percent ten-year kidney survival.

MESANGIAL PROLIFERATIVE GLOMERULONEPHRITIS

ARTHUR H. COHEN, M.D.
SHARON G. ADLER, M.D.

Glomerular lesions with mesangial IgM deposits (in this chapter to be synonymous with mesangial proliferative or injury glomerulonephritis or ''IgM nephropathy'') represent a somewhat controversial glomerulopathy. Since the initial emphasis of this immunopathologic ''entity'' in the mid-1970s, reports have both attested to, and disagreed with, the concept of it as a distinct pathologic or clinicopathologic process.

The precise categorization of this ''lesion'' is difficult. One prevailing view is that in patients with nephrotic syndrome, glomerulonephritis with mesangial IgM deposits is part of a spectrum of injury with a common pathogenesis that includes minimal change disease at the benign end and focal and segmental glomerulosclerosis at the more malignant end. The mesangial ''injury'' lesion, because of clinical and pathological similarities to each of the others, is in an intermediate position. In support of this concept is the occasional finding of transitions between these three lesions in patients who undergo serial biopsies. A polar view is that it is a distinct entity unto itself. An intermediate consideration is that, regardless of the categorization, the presence of mesangial IgM deposits in glomeruli in a patient with nephrotic syndrome might be a marker for a poor response to corticosteroids and/or progression to renal failure, despite the relatively normal appearance of glomeruli.

This ''lesion'' is defined by its immunopathologic features: IgM (and often C3) granular deposits in all mesangial regions of all glomeruli. The light microscopic appearance may vary, ranging from normal glomeruli (''mesangial injury'') to those with moderate degrees of mesangial hypercellularity. In general, all glomeruli in a biopsy are reasonably similar to one another. Capillary lumina are patent, and capillary walls and basement membranes are thin and single-contoured. Unless complicated, there are no segments of sclerosis. Ultrastructurally, there are small electron dense deposits in mesangial regions in approximately 50 percent of the cases. When heavy proteinuria is present, the foot processes of visceral epithelial cells are completely effaced. The morphologic features of mesangial proliferative glomerulonephritis may also be associated with diffuse mesangial IgA deposits (Berger's disease), isolated C3 deposits, predominant 1gG deposits, or no Ig or complement deposits. Thus "IgM nephropathy" is but one portion of a heterogenous group of disorders having mesangial proliferation or hypercellularity in common.

There are four common presentations of this form of glomerular injury: asymptomatic proteinuria, heavy proteinuria often in the nephrotic range, isolated microscopic hematuria, or heavy proteinuria with hematuria. Mild hypertension is present in up to one-third of the patients. Laboratory studies are not diagnostically helpful. Serum albumin is low and hyperlipidemia is present in association with the nephrotic syndrome. Mild to moderate azotemia may be present in 25 to 50 percent of patients at the time of diagnosis. Serum complement and immunoglobulin levels are usually normal. Antibodies to nuclear or streptococcal antigens are absent. Genetic determinants have not been identified.

The clinical course is variable and, for the most part, depends upon the initial manifestation. Patients with isolated hematuria usually maintain normal renal function for a considerable period of time, although microscopic hematuria persists, occasionally punctuated by bouts of gross hematuria. Apparently, those with low-grade proteinuria also have a good long-term prognosis. On the other hand, patients with heavy proteinuria may progress to renal insufficiency. This usually occurs within several years of the onset and is heralded by increasing proteinuria and hypertension. It is invariably in patients who are, or have been, steroid-dependent, or, more commonly steroid-resistant and who have persistent heavy proteinuria, often with hematuria. In most instances, repeat renal biopsy discloses either the same lesion or segmental glomerulosclerosis and variable presence of mesangial IgM deposits.

The approach to therapy has not been well defined. The most common indication for treatment is the nephrotic syndrome. The effects of therapy on isolated microhematuria, non-nephrotic range proteinuria, and progressive azotemia are less well appreciated. Reports from the United Kingdom in the early 1970s suggested that the prevalence of steroid-responsiveness in patients with primary mesangial proliferative glomerulonephritis was low. As a result, few patients were subsequently treated. More recently, however, many investigators have approached therapy in a manner similar to that given patients with minimal change disease. Utilizing high dose oral prednisone (i.e., 60 mg per day or 120 mg every other day in adults or equivalent in children), the nephrotic syndrome has been reported to respond in up to 65 percent of patients, although frequent relapses, steroid dependence, and partial remissions are common. Nephrotic patients with prominent hematuria are less likely to respond to steroids than those without hematuria.

The use of cytotoxic agents is more controversial than corticosteroids. However, in a few cases, agents such as chlorambucil or cyclophosphamide have been utilized for their steroid-sparing effects in patients with frequently relapsing or steroid-dependent nephrotic syndrome. An occasional report has suggested that cytotoxic agents may be useful in inducing remission in small numbers of steroid-unresponsive patients. Cyclosporine has now been utilized in patients with minimal change disease and focal and segmental glomerulosclerosis who are either steroid resistant, steroid-dependent, or frequent relapsers. The usefulness of this agent in mesangial proliferative glomerulonephritis remains to be determined. Similarly, the efficacy of nonsteroidal agents, angiotensin coverting enzyme inhibitors, and low-protein diets in inducing remission or amelioration of nephrotic syndrome has not been specifically studied.

In summary, mesangial proliferative glomerulonephritis with IgM deposits is an uncommon form of renal disease. Its pathogenesis is poorly understood, but some now believe that it may be an intermediate form in a spectrum of disorders including minimal change disease and focal and segmental glomerulosclerosis. The prognosis also appears to be intermediate, with end-stage renal disease developing in a substantial, but not a precisely quantitated number of patients over the course of many years. Patients most often present with nephrotic syndrome, but less common manifestations include non-nephrotic range proteinuria and macroscopic or microscopic hematuria. Steroid responsiveness occurs in 25 to 65 percent of patients. In a small number of patients, cytotoxic agents may be useful adjuncts in treating steroid-unresponsive, steroid-dependent, or frequently relapsing nephrotic syndrome. A prospective randomized controlled trial, although difficult to achieve for this group, would be useful to define better the natural history and responsiveness to therapy of this from glomerular injury.

IgA NEPHROPATHY (BERGER'S DISEASE)

GIUSEPPE D'AMICO, M.D.

Preponderant mesangial deposition of IgA, associated with mesangial expansion and proliferation, often focal and segmental, is the hallmark of the syndrome of IgA nephropathy, which is found in a great number of diseases, including isolated idiopathic (Berger's disease), Schönlein-Henoch purpura, chronic hepatitis, celiac disease, regional enteritis, carcinomas of the colon, carcinomas of the lung, Sjögren's syndrome, monoclonal IgA gammopathy, dermatitis herpetiformis, mycosis fungoides, leprosy, and ankylosing spondylitis. The isolated idiopathic type of IgA glomerulonephritis, which I will consider in this chapter, was first described at the end of the 1970s and subsequently became known as Berger's disease. It is increasingly recognized as the most common form of primary glomerulonephritis in many (if not in all) countries around the world.

Since clinical manifestations are often mild (there may even be none), it is possible that the disease, which is diagnosed from a renal biopsy, is unrecognized in a large number of affected individuals. In fact, the increasing awareness of its widespread distribution and high incidence has paralleled the increasing use of renal biopsy for asymptomatic patients with isolated urinary abnormalities. Where this practice is widely adopted, as in Europe, Japan, and Australia, IgA nephropathy appears to represent between 20 and 40 percent of all primary glomerular diseases. However, geographic variation in the prevalence of the disease is a possibility. Since progression to chronic renal failure is frequent, although rather slow in the majority of cases, patients with idiopathic IgA nephropathy account for an appreciable percentage of the total population of patients receiving maintenance dialysis, independently estimated to be around 10 percent in France, in Italy, and in Australia.

DIAGNOSTIC FEATURES

Prevalent mesangial deposition of IgA, which is found in all glomeruli as confluent masses or as discrete granules, is found by immunofluorescence microscopy in all cases. It is usually associated with deposition of C3 (less frequently with IgG and IgM) in a similar pattern, and is the characterizing immunohistologic feature of the disease. The histologic picture is less uniform. Mesangial enlargement, produced by various combinations of hypercellularity and excess of matrix, is the most common abnormality. It varies from minimal to very extensive, frequently differing in severity between individual glomeruli (focal and segmental mesangial proliferation), but sometimes being diffuse in all lobules of all glomeruli (diffuse mesangial proliferation). Circumscribed foci of epithelial proliferation and areas of segmental sclerosis are rather frequent.

Primary IgA nephropathy occurs at all ages but is most common in the second and third decades of life. It is two to three times more common in males than females. The syndrome of clinical presentation that is especially frequent in younger patients, in which there are recurrent episodes of macroscopic hematuria associated closely with episodes of upper respiratory tract infection or other infections involving the mucosal system, has masked the importance of other modes of clinical presentation. The most frequent of these, at least in adult patients, is incidental discovery during a chance urinalysis of asymptomatic microscopic hematuria, usually with mild proteinuria. Some laboratory signs of renal insufficiency may also be present at presentation. A minority of patients come to the physician because of a nephrotic syndrome or severe hypertension. When macroscopic hematuria is the presenting syndrome, differentiation from acute postinfectious glomerulonephritis is based on the shorter interval (24 to 48 hours) between the precipitating infection and the appearance of hematuria, on the paucity of other signs that characterize the acute nephritic syndrome (elevation of blood urea nitrogen concentration, arterial hypertension, massive proteinuria with casts), and on the absence of hypocomplementemia. However, in a minority of patients an episode of macroscopic (gross) hematuria may be associated with acute oliguric renal failure. Renal biopsies taken in this acute stage reveal the presence of cellular crescents and tubular abnormalities, including tubular necrosis and tubular obstruction with large aggregates of erythrocytes. The acute renal failure may resolve spontaneously in some cases. There is no single specific diagnostic laboratory test for IgA nephropathy apart from renal biopsy. However, increased serum concentrations of IgA, which are present in 40 to 50 percent of patients with Berger's disease, may be a useful diagnostic feature once signs of liver disease have been excluded. Idiopathic IgA nephropathy is a relentlessly chronic disease. Even though a few patients may have a rather prolonged regression of all clinical signs, including the mild urinary abnormalities, the spontaneous disappearance of IgA deposition with histologically demonstrable healing has never been described. It progresses into chronic renal failure rather frequently, but the pace of this appears to vary greatly; some patients die of renal failure quite soon after diagnosis, while others have normal renal function more than 30 years after the first episode of gross hematuria or the first accidental discovery of urinary abnormalities. The few studies of large populations suggest that actuarial renal survival is greater than 90 percent at 10 years and 75 percent at 20 years.

Some useful prognostic indicators that can help select individual patients on whom to concentrate therapeutic efforts have recently been identified. Among the clinical features that appear to be correlated with more frequent and more rapid deterioration of renal function are: male sex, older age at onset of the disease, constant proteinuria, high blood pressure, and, unexpectedly, the absence of any history of recurrent macroscopic hematuria. On the contrary, serum IgA levels have no bearing on disease severity or prognosis. As for histologic markers for unfavorable prognosis, the extent of the glomerular (segmental and global) and interstitial sclerosis appears to be the predominant factor, but the extent of intracapillary and extracapillary proliferation and of extension to the peripheral capillary walls of deposits, seen either by immunofluorescence or electron microscopy, have also been identified as prognosticators of more rapid deterioration of the renal function.

PATHOGENESIS

The association of IgA and C3 with electron-dense deposits is consistent with an immune complex (IC) pathogenesis of primary IgA nephropathy. IgA-IC have been detected transiently in some but not all patients, frequently associated with IgG-IC. Their presence was correlated with clinical evidence of disease activity but not with the high concentrations of serum IgA. In addition, glomerular IgA-IC deposits associated with histologic lesions similar to those of human IgA mesangial glomerulonephritis have been induced in laboratory animals using IgA-IC formed either in vitro or in vivo.

Since IgA is the principal immunoglobulin defense system against viral and bacterial antigens in exocrine secretions and gross hematuria and other signs of acute exacerbation of IgA nephropathy occur frequently in association with mucosal infections (respiratory, gastrointestinal, or urinary tract), it seems possible that the IgA deposited in the glomerular mesangium is an antibody to viral or bacterial antigens in the mucosa. The acute clinical exacerbations of the disease that lead to its progression to renal failure could be evoked by periodic showers of circulating immune complexes formed by union of preformed IgA antibodies with ubiquitous antigens at mucosal sites.

It is still debated whether this IgA is normal serum IgA or an abnormal IgA of mucosal origin. A large body of evidence points to this second hypothesis, suggesting the partially polymeric nature of both serum and deposited IgA.

The probably unspecific nature of the antigenic stimulation and the abnormal features of the IgA produced have suggested that some congenital or acquired impairment of the immune responsiveness may favor increased production and/or reduced clearance of normal and/or abnormal IgA. Many recent experimental data have confirmed that there is a defect in the regulation of IgA production in this disease, consisting mainly of an impairment in the generation of IgA-specific suppressor cells and an increase in IgA-specific helper Tα-cells, capable of producing after stimulation greater than normal amounts of polymeric IgA. This defect in the regulation of IgA production could be genetically mediated in at least some cases, as suggested by the increased frequencies of some HLA-related antigens (Bw 35 and DR 4) in patients with Berger's disease, described in both France and Japan (but not confirmed in many studies from several other countries), as well as by the increased frequencies of other genetic determinants (allotypes of light chains, gamma heavy chains, and complement) in some clinical subgroups of patients.

Recent evidence suggests that there may also be a defect in reticulophagocytic function in Berger's disease, leading to impairment of the immune clearance of polymeric IgA. It is difficult at this time to say whether this impairment is secondary to a chronic overload consequent to the abnormal production of mainly polymeric IgA or is favored by a subtle, latent, genetically mediated Fc-receptor dysfunction.

Many other aspects of the pathogenesis remain to be determined. One of these is the nature of the antigens responsible for the mucosal immune response. Defective exclusion of antigens by the mucosa, allowing increased antigen entry, can be postulated. In view of the infrequent association of gastrointestinal disease with IgA mesangial nephropathy, it appears improbable that this mechanism is operating in the majority of cases. However, antibodies against a certain number of food antigens, and especially antigliadin antibodies, have been found in some patients with Berger's disease.

In conclusion, the existing data suggest that idiopathic IgA mesangial nephropathy is a glomerulonephritis due to deposition of IgA immune complexes or aggregates, probably originating in the migratory lymphocytes from the secretory tissue, in response to stimulation by many common exogenous, microbic, or viral antigens or by diet-related antigens. Some abnormality of the immune system, possibly genetically mediated, responsible for increased production of circulating IgA partly polymeric in nature, probably plays an important role in the pathogenesis of the disease, possibly more important than the rather nonspecific antigenic stimulation. How important impaired or saturated removal of this polymeric IgA by the mononuclear phagocytic system and/or by the liver is, however, still to be elucidated.

It is possible that the different clinical and pathologic manifestations of Berger's disease are due to differing contributions by the three major pathogenetic factors, i.e., increased antigenic entry and stimulation of the immune system; impaired response of this immune system, with production of abnormal macromolecular IgA; and impaired or saturated removal of such macromolecular IgA. The type of antigenic stimulation may be particularly important in determining the extent and duration of the renal damage. In the subgroup of patients with recurrent bouts of macroscopic hematuria following upper respiratory tract infections, the merely intermittent entry of an exogenous microbial or viral antigen may be the preponderant factor, explaining the favorable prognosis. In contrast, in the subgroup of patients without such episodes, who progress more frequently to renal failure, a continuous injurious effect, clinically less apparent, could be due to an increased abnormal immune response to constantly available antigens (autoantigens, food antigens). Geographic differences in the immunogenetics and the clinical manifestations of the disease could be best explained by such a multifactorial pathogenesis. It is obvious that classification by the predominant pathogenetic mechanism could help to differentiate clinical and pathologic subgroups of patients with different prognoses and requiring different therapeutical approaches.

TREATMENT

Effectiveness of any therapeutic intervention in idiopathic IgA nephropathy is difficult to prove in uncontrolled trials, owing to the long, indolent natural history of the disease and to the extremely variable rate of progression to renal failure in individual patients, which is probably due to the multifactorial pathogenesis of the disease. It is therefore not surprising that no therapy has yet proven to be of long-term benefit. Controlled trials in the future are probably warranted only for the subgroup of patients with more rapid progression, who can already be identified, in our opinion, by the clinical and histologic prognostic indices that we have already discussed.

The therapeutic measures proposed, aimed at different pathogenetic mechanisms or stages of the disease, have been mainly of four types (Table 1): (1) prevention of antigen entry through the mucosa, (2) modification of the immune response to reduce the production of circulating IgA immune complexes or aggregates, (3) removal of this circulating IgA before it fixes in the mesangium, and (4) nonspecific slowing of progression to renal failure through control of hypertension and dietary manipulation.

Prevention of Antigen Entry

In the patients in whom infections of the mucosa, mainly of the upper respiratory tract, trigger macroscopic hematuria, short-term administration of antibiotics to eliminate potential microbial antigens is probably warranted, and we recommend it.

On the contrary, the validity of two other measures, aimed at preventing further exacerbations of the infections, namely, eradication of septic foci (mainly tonsillectomy) and long-term antibiotic therapy, is still

TABLE 1 Potential Therapeutic Measures in IgA Nephropathy

Proposed Therapies	*Comments*
Prevention of antigen entry:	
Antibiotic administration during episodes of gross hematuria associated with an acute infection	Probably useful
Long-term antibiotic administration to prevent recurrence of infections	Controversial
Tonsillectomy or eradication of septic foci	Controversial
Dietary manipulation to reduce food antigen load	To be evaluated in selected cases
Manipulation of an abnormal immune response:	
Short-term immunosuppression with steroids and/or cytotoxic agents during acute clinical exacerbations	Useful only when there is acute oliguric renal failure associated with severe crescentic glomerulonephritis
Long-term immunosuppression with steroids and/or cytotoxic agents for the indolent, insidiously progressive stage	Probably useless; to be evaluated with controlled trials in selected groups of patients with more rapid chronic progression
Phenytoin, d-penicillamine, antiplatelet drugs	Not effective
Selective pharmacological blockade of Tα-cells or IgA-producing B cells with monoclonal antibodies	To be evaluated when these substances become available
Removal of circulating IgA immunocomplexes:	
Short-term plasma exchange (PE) during acute clinical exacerbations	Probably useful, in association with immunosuppressive drugs, only when there is acute oliguric renal failure associated with severe crescentic glomerulonephritis
Long-term PE in patients with rapidly progressive courses (not associated with severe glomerular sclerosis) and circulating IgA-IC	To be evaluated when the harmful circulating substances have been more correctly identified and can be easily monitored in the blood longitudinally
Long-term selective PE with specific immunoadsorbents	Will probably substitute traditional PE when the harmful circulating substances have been better defined

controversial. French investigators have reported that tonsillectomy and eradication of dental foci reduce the number of recurrences of gross hematuria, the amount of proteinuria, and the serum levels of IgA. Although we have been unable to document any beneficial effects of these surgical procedures on the progression to renal failure, they can be recommended for selected patients with frequent recurrences of gross hematuria accompanied by acute nephritic syndrome and/or reversible acute renal failure.

In a controlled study from Melbourne, Australia, long-term (12 months) treatment with doxycycline, 100 mg daily, was reported very recently to reduce the urinary erythrocyte counts of patients, but this possibly beneficial effect must be confirmed, and the impact of this effect on later progression of disease is uncertain.

The possibility that gluten or other food antigens is responsible for the production of the IgA antibodies in at least some of the patients without episodes of gross hematuria associated with infections cannot be ruled out, as we have already said. If this pathogenetic mechanism is confirmed, dietary manipulation to eliminate such potential food antigens will be worth trying for selected patients. Preliminary experience with gluten-free diets in some Italian patients with primary IgA nephropathy seems to be promising.

Manipulation of the Abnormal Immune Response

We must distinguish between acute manipulation during phases of clinical activity of the disease, such as the nephritic syndrome that may follow an infectious episode, and chronic manipulation aimed at permanently reducing the production of circulating abnormal IgA antibodies and the inflammatory response that accompanies their deposition in the glomeruli.

In deciding whether and when to start immunosuppressive treatment for cases of acute clinical exacerbations, one must take into account that spontaneous resolution of the acute nephritic syndromes that may accompany the recurrences of macroscopic hematuria is the rule in Berger's disease. It is thus very difficult to evaluate the efficacy of any acutely established therapy in such circumstances. We believe that no immunosupressive treatment is warranted for the acute clinical exacerbations, with the exception of the rare case of severe acute oliguric renal failure concomitant with an episode of macroscopic hematuria. In such a situation, a renal biopsy usually reveals extensive cellular crescents in the majority of glomeruli, and we believe that treatment with intravenous steroids, immunosuppressive drugs, and perhaps also plasma exchange, which has been recommended for all types of crescentic glomerulonephritis ry. On the other hand, acutely deteriorating renal function accompanied by a predominance of tubular abnormalities, occlusive casts, and only mild crescentic involvement of glomeruli may not require such a vigorous approach.

As for long-term immunosuppressive treatment during the indolent, insidiously progressive stage of the disease, the accumulated experience suggests that it does not seem to confer any benefit, although no controlled trials have yet been reported, and would probably be warranted only for the group of patients with more rapid progression.

Steroids have been advocated, and are certainly the most correct approach, for the very few patients with the peculiar syndrome that is characterized by proteinuria in the nephrotic range associated with minimal mesangial lesions and the immunohistologic features typical of IgA nephropathy. Patients with this syndrome, which should probably be classified as "minimal change glomerulopathy" in spite of the immunohistologic features, seem to respond to corticosteroid therapy with complete disappearance of proteinuria, although a multiply relapsing steroid-sensitive course has been described for the majority of the cases reported.

Because of the probable role of IgA in this disease and the known effects of phenytoin in reducing serum IgA levels, controlled trials with this drug were carried out in Spain and in Australia. Phenytoin was able to decrease serum IgA, especially polymeric IgA levels, and to reduce the number of episodes of macroscopic hematuria and, in some patients, to decrease the IgA deposits. However, both trials failed to show any significant influence of this treatment on the clinical or histologic course. The ineffectiveness of the drug in reducing concentrations of IgA-containing circulating immune complexes might explain the therapeutic failure.

Other recently reported therapeutic approaches that have yielded disappointing results include antiplatelet drugs and dapsone, the latter given because of its known efficacy in the secondary IgA-associated disease dermatitis herpetiformis.

The recent report from Japan concerning beneficial effects on proteinuria in small numbers of patients of both the fibrinolytic agent urokinase and the heterocyclic steroid danazol, a drug that solubilizes glomerular immune complexes, awaits further confirmation.

We believe that our increasing knowledge of the pathogenetic mechanisms for the disease will lead us in the near future to more specific and successful manipulation of the immune response, based on the selective pharmacological block of Tα-cells or IgA-producing B cells with monoclonal antibodies.

Removal of Circulating IgA Immunocomplexes

I have already mentioned that plasma exchange and immunosuppression are probably useful for the infrequent case of rapidly progressive disease associated with extensive crescentic glomerulonephritis. The mechanism of possible beneficial effect of plasma exchange therapy in this, as in all types of crescentic glomerulonephritis, is as yet unknown. Many circulating substances, including immunocomplexes and chemical mediators, are probably removed by this maneuver.

Recently, plasma exchange alone or in combination with cyclophosphamide has also been advocated for treatment of clinical exacerbations not associated with severe extracapillary proliferation in patients with subacute rapidly progressive courses. Favorable results have been reported for most of the few patients treated, but we have already emphasized the difficulty of evaluating therapeutic results during the possibly spontaneously reversible episodes of clinical exacerbation of Berger's disease. A few patients have had plasma exchange therapy as long-term therapy (up to 34 consecutive thrice-weekly to weekly exchanges), and in two patients, one from Australia and another from France, disappearance of mesangial IgA deposits in the repeat biopsy after therapy was described. In a very limited number of cases, levels of circulating IgA immune complexes (IgA-IC) and reticuloendothelial system function were monitored as immunologic guidelines for plasma therapy; IgA-IC decreased and reticuloendothelial system function improved during long-term treatment, but rebound increases of IgA-IC were frequent after plasma exchange was discontinued. The many anecdotal reports suggest that plasma exchange might have a beneficial role in patients with signs of clinical activity (constantly elevated urinary erythrocyte counts, elevated circulating IgA-IC), progressive impairment of renal function, and histologic features of severe diffuse intracapillary proliferation, perhaps with some extracapillary proliferation but without severe glomerular and interstitial sclerosis. However, considering the cost and the technical difficulty of prolonged plasma exchange treatment, I think that its widespread use, even for the selected subgroup of patients with a rapidly progressive course, cannot be recommended until we know better how to monitor the immunologic activity of the disease, and until we can be confident that the levels of circulating IgA-IC or of other more reliable, measurable circulating substances that we remove with the treatment are definitely correlated with the activity of the disease and the velocity of its progression.

The identification of such circulating substances will, I hope, permit a more rational approach to plasma therapy, i.e., to selectively remove them from plasma with immunoadsorbent cartridges, thus reducing their deposition in the glomeruli and their local harmful effects.

Control of Arterial Hypertension and Dietary Manipulation

Early adequate control of arterial hypertension is undoubtedly useful for slowing down the deterioration of renal function in patients with a progressive course. More recently it has been suggested that a low-protein, low-phosphorus diet followed in the early stages of deterioration of renal function by patients with progressive renal diseases of every type could also reduce the speed of progression to severe renal failure. In my opinion, there is sufficient evidence to recommend the early prescription of such a special dietary regimen for patients with Berger's disease as soon as a functional impairment becomes evident.

Very recently, the protective effects of diets rich in eicosapentanoic acid (fish oil) against progression of the disease have also been reported from Japan.

MEMBRANOUS NEPHROPATHY

CECIL H. COGGINS, M.D.

Membranous nephropathy (which is also called idiopathic membranous, epimembranous, or extramembranous nephropathy, glomerulonephropathy, or glomerulonephritis) is the most common biopsy diagnosis in adult patients with nephrotic syndrome, accounting for about 25 to 35 percent of cases. Its clinical presentation is proteinuria, with or without the full-blown nephrotic syndrome. There are no clinical or laboratory features specific for the disease, so its identification depends on the performance of a renal biopsy.

In mild cases the biopsy findings on light microscopic examination may appear quite normal and be indistinguishable from minimal change nephropathy. More commonly, however, hematoxylin and eosin and periodic acid-Schiff stains show a diffuse and global change consisting of uniform thickening of the glomerular capillary walls. Silver stains and immunofluorescence and electron microscopic studies demonstrate the abnormalities in greater detail. Electron-dense deposits of varying sizes and shapes are present on the subepithelial surface of the capillary basement membrane. These appear to correspond to finely granular deposits containing IgG and C3 (and sometimes IgA and IgM) which are seen with fluorescence microscopy. As the deposits thicken, the normal basement membrane material appears to grow out between them. This membrane material stained with silver gives the "spiked" appearance characteristic of the disease.

Most patients with this biopsy picture have idiopathic disease, but 20 to 30 percent of cases in most series are associated with and presumably caused by systemic disease. Systemic lupus erythematosus is the most common association, but tumors, drugs, toxins, sickle cell disease, and particularly infections, including hepatitis and parasitic diseases, are also seen. In some cases cure of the associated disease leads to a remission of the membranous nephropathy; in others the renal disease persists. Membranous nephropathy occurs in patients of all ages, though its peak incidence is between ages 35 and 55. In childhood it is much less common than minimal change nephrosis and tends to occur in older children in an age distribution continuous with young adults. There is a male predominance of approximately 2:1. Perhaps as many as 30 to 50 percent of patients with membranous histologic findings have asymptomatic (less than nephrotic) proteinuria.

The cause of membranous nephropathy and the pathogenesis of its accompanying proteinuria are not well understood. Evidence from experimental models suggests that the basement membrane deposits may be the result of in situ formation of immune complexes, the result of a reaction between circulating antibodies with antigens (either endogenous or exogenous) lodged in the glomerular capillary wall.

The course of the disease is variable. After 10 years of observation perhaps a third of patients will be in renal failure, a third will have persisting proteinuria with preserved renal function, and a third will be apparently cured. Patients who have less than 2 g of proteinuria at some time during their disease course, female patients, and children appear to have relatively good prognoses.

TABLE 1 Diseases Associated with Membranous Nephropathy

Immunologic abnormalities:
- Systemic lupus erythematosus*
- Rheumatoid arthritis, Sjögren's syndrome, Hashimoto's thyroiditis, dermatitis herpetiformis, myasthenia gravis, Guillain-Barré syndrome, Weber-Christian panniculitis, dermatomyositis

Infections:
- Hepatitis B, especially in childhood*
- Quartan malaria, schistosomiasis, leprosy, congenital and acquired syphilis, hydatid disease, filariasis, and scabies may be significant causes in areas where they are prevalent

Neoplasms:
- Cancers of the lung,* breast,* colon, stomach, kidney, esophagus, carotid body, and melanoma
- Lymphoma (more frequent association with minimal change lesion in Hodgkin's disease) and leukemia

Drugs and toxins:
- Gold therapy for rheumatoid arthritis*
- Penicillamine*
- Captopril* and enalapril
- Nonsteroidal prostaglandin antagonists*
- Mercury (in skin-lightening cosmetics), other heavy metals, tri- or paramethadione, volatile hydrocarbon solvents

Other conditions:
- Diabetes mellitus, sarcoidosis, sickle cell disease

* Signifies relatively frequent causes.

MANAGEMENT OF MEMBRANOUS NEPHROPATHY

Evaluation

When a biopsy specimen in a patient with proteinuria demonstrates membranous nephropathy the physician should be alert for the possible presence of associated diseases (Table 1). A careful history and physical examination will identify many of these diseases. Laboratory investigations, including antinuclear antibodies, anti-DNA antibodies, complement, antithyroid antibodies, hepatitis B antigens and antibodies, serologic tests for syphilis, hematocrit, and blood glucose, may be useful. The importance of a search for malignancy in a patient presenting with membranous nephropathy is difficult to assess. Although some series have found neoplasms in about 10 percent of patients with membranous nephropathy, it is not clear how many of these tumors were unknown at the time of the renal biopsy. It would seem likely that approximately 5 percent of adult patients with membranous nephropathy might have an underlying malignancy that was not obvious at the time of biopsy, and that some of this 5 percent would have untreatable disease. This likelihood might be expected to vary with the patient's age, and should be interpreted in relation to the age incidence of malignancies in a population without nephrotic syndrome.

Treatment

General

Patients with membranous nephropathy will of course benefit from salt restriction, adequate dietary protein, and appropriate use of diuretics, as do patients with nephrotic syndrome from other causes. Some patients appear to achieve symptomatic benefit as well from the combination of nonsteroidal agents such as indomethacin or meclofenamate with diuretics. This may, however, reduce the glomerular filtration rate. (See also the chapter *Principles of Management of the Nephrotic Syndrome*.)

Associated Disease

When an underlying cause or associated disease is present, every effort should be made toward its successful treatment. With the removal of an underlying cause the membranous nephropathy will often, but not always, remit.

Asymptomatic Proteinuria

Although there is evidence that proteinuria in the 1 to 2 g per deciliter range will remit with prolonged low-dose steroid therapy, there is also evidence that the prognosis for such patients is good without treatment. There would seem little urgency in treating such patients and no evidence that the disease is more harmful than the treatment.

Nephrotic Syndrome with Normal Glomerular Filtration Rate

Corticosteroids. In a large collaborative trial in the United States, prednisone therapy was randomly and prospectively compared with placebo. The patients were adults with idiopathic membranous nephropathy and nephrotic syndrome. The treatment consisted of oral alternate-day prednisone in an average dose of 125 mg every other day for a period of two months with tapering over an additional 4 to 8 weeks. Treated patients had more frequent remissions of proteinuria, but the occurrence of relapses led to few long-term differences between the groups. Of greater importance was that fewer of the treated patients progressed toward renal failure during the period of observation. The steroid therapy was well tolerated with very few side effects. In some series, untreated patients have done almost as well as the treated ones in this controlled trial, while in others untreated patients have done badly. Clearly there is wide variability in the course of untreated patients with this disease. Recognized prognostic indices such as sex, age, and quantity of proteinuria account for only some of the differences. If it were possible to identify which patients would specifically benefit from steroids, then therapeutic decisions would be easy. Unfortunately this has not been possible. A number of uncontrolled observations have also suggested that corticosteroid therapy is helpful in this disease, while others failed to demonstrate benefit.

Immunosuppressive Therapy. In an Italian trial six months of alternating steroids and chlorambucil was compared with no therapy in a randomized prospective design. The initial month began with three 1-g pulses of intravenous methylprednisolone followed by daily oral methylprednisolone (0.4 mg per kilogram per day) or prednisone (0.5 mg per kilogram per day). At the end of the first month the steroid was stopped and chlorambucil (0.2 mg per kilogram per day orally) was given for a month. This two-month cycle was repeated three times for a total duration of six months of therapy. At the end of three years' follow-up, 23 of 32 of the treated patients (72 percent) were in complete or partial remission compared with 9 of 30 controls (30 percent), and there was a small but statistically significant elevation of serum creatinine in the controls as compared with the treated group. Short-term complications of this vigorous therapy were said to be few. A longer follow-up will be necessary before it is clear that the benefits of such treatment outweigh the risks. Other studies have suggested benefit from cyclophosphamide combined with prednisone or anticoagulants.

Nephrotic Syndrome with Renal Insufficiency

There is little evidence to suggest that the treatments described above will restore renal function once the serum creatinine concentration has risen to the range of 3 or 4 mg per deciliter, and it is probably safer to proceed in these patients with conservative measures for the management of chronic renal failure, including tight control of hypertension and reduction of dietary protein intake. These approaches are described in the chapters on nutritional and dialytic management of renal failure.

In light of the above information, it is my practice to treat patients with membranous nephropathy and nephrotic proteinuria with a two-month course of alternate-day steroids, as described above. In asymptomatic patients with only 1 or 2 g per deciliter of proteinuria, I am content to follow blood pressure, urine protein, and serum creatinine concentrations at intervals of a few months. In patients who remain severely symptomatic or who demonstrate rising serum creatinine levels for 2 to 3 months following steroid treatment I consider the use of cyclophosphamide, 2 mg per kilogram (if tolerated) combined with 60 mg of prednisone every other day, or a 6-month course as described in the Italian study above, though I am unconvinced so far that the long-term benefits outweigh the risks. The use of a program of intense diuresis combined with indomethacin or meclofenamate has been suggested, but the combination is a powerful one for reducing the glomerular filtration rate—sometimes profoundly—and in my hands has not produced dramatic reductions in urinary protein.

Complications of Membranous Nephropathy

General

Hypovolemia resulting from hypoproteinemia combined with overvigorous diuretic therapy may impair renal function in membranous nephropathy as it may in other forms of nephrotic syndrome. Allergic interstitial nephritis may result from the use of diuretics, antibiotics, or other drugs and be superimposed on the underlying membranous nephropathy. It is discussed further in the chapter *Acute Hypersensitivity Interstitial Nephritis* and should be considered particularly in patients in whom there is a sudden increase in the rate of decline of renal function. (See also the chapter *Principles of Management of the Nephrotic Syndrome*.)

Renal Vein Thrombosis

One complication that seems to appear quite frequently in patients with membranous nephropathy is renal vein thrombosis (see also the chapter Renal Vein Thrombosis). This complication (so common that it was formerly thought to be a major *cause* of membranous nephropathy) has been reported in up to 50 percent of patients in some series, but probably averages something like 10 to 15 percent. When this complication leads to thromboembolism it should be treated with heparin followed by long-term warfarin. Treatment usually leads to the disappearance of clot on subsequent angiographic studies and to a protection against further embolism. It is not clear when to discontinue the treatment; the tendency to thrombosis probably remains as long as the nephrotic syndrome does.

When renal vein thrombosis is present without any evidence of acute or chronic embolization, it is not clear that serious reduction in renal function or increase in proteinuria results. In patients who show no evidence of embolization then, it may not be necessary to perform routine renal vein angiograms.

Rapidly Progressive Glomerulonephritis

A clinical picture of rapidly progressive glomerulonephritis with the biopsy finding of crescentic glomerulonephritis superimposed on membranous nephropathy is occasionally seen. Antibodies directed against glomerular basement membrane antigens may or may not be present. There is no evidence to recommend any different management from that indicated in the classic form of rapidly progressive glomerulonephritis as discussed in the chapter *Idiopathic Rapidly Progressive Glomerulonephritis*.

Transplantation

In patients in whom membranous nephropathy has progressed to end-stage renal failure, transplantation is often performed. Although the membranous lesion may occasionally recur in the transplanted kidney, it frequently does not impair its function.

MEMBRANOPROLIFERATIVE GLOMERULONEPHRITIS

CLARK D. WEST, M.D.

CLINICAL AND PATHOLOGIC FEATURES

Membranoproliferative glomerulonephritis (MPGN) is a form of chronic nephritis that often first manifests itself in childhood. It has three forms, designated types I, II, and III. Proliferation of mesangial cells, found in all three types, is usually most severe in type I. In this type also, mesangial interposition is most frequently observed. However, the types are best distinguished by examination of the ultrastructure. Type I is characterized by subendothelial deposits and an intact glomerular basement membrane. Type II, also known as dense deposit disease, has a thickened basement membrane which has a lamina densa with greatly increased electron density, as if a deposit were present. In type III, the deposits, which are subepithelial and subendothelial, stimulate exuberant new basement membrane formation by contiguous endothelial and epithelial cells, resulting eventually in a basement membrane that appears disrupted and fenestrated with deposits intercollated within it. The extent to which types I and III constitute separate disease entities is not clear.

The three types are difficult to distinguish by clinical or laboratory characteristics. Those with type I disease often present with a vague systemic illness characterized by increased fatigue and anorexia, with the renal disease manifesting itself by edema and gross hematuria. Edema or red urine may also be the presenting sign in types II and III, but the patients usually have no sign of systemic disease. Among all types, the chance discovery of hematuria and proteinuria in the otherwise healthy child or young adult leads to the diagnosis in 35 to 40 percent of the patients. Approximately 75 percent of the patients are hypocomplementemic. In many of those with type II and in a few with type I disease, C3 nephritic factor (C3NeF) is demonstrable as the cause of the hypocomplementemia. In the remainder, circulating immune complexes are thought to produce the hypocomplementemia. The combination of a low C3 level and low levels of IgG, albumin, and transferrin which indicate a nephrotic syndrome is almost pathognomonic of MPGN.

The prognosis varies widely. In the 10 to 30 percent of patients who have focal or segmental lesions with the ultrastructural characteristics of MPGN I or III, the prognosis is good. A smaller number have a rapidly progressive nephritis at presentation characterized by multiple crescents and require dialysis and transplantation within 1 or 2 years. The majority of patients have all glomeruli involved in a diffusely proliferative process. These patients may remain asymptomatic and with stable renal function for periods of 3 to 20 years, but with continuing microhematuria and proteinuria. In my experience, in these patients the rate of glomerular sclerosis resulting from immunologic injury averages 3.5 percent per year in the first 2 or 3 years after clinical onset. Obviously, in some, the rate is greater than this. As sclerotic glomeruli accumulate and nonimmunologic injury is superimposed, the rate of glomerular loss can accelerate. Calculated actuarially, renal survival is 50 percent 6 to 9 years after clinical onset for all three types. Deterioration of renal function is usually heralded by the advent of a nephrotic syndrome; in fact, a nephrotic syndrome has been present at some time in all patients who deteriorate.

PROPOSED THERAPEUTIC REGIMENS

There is no consensus regarding optimum therapy for this disease and some physicians use only supportive treatment. Attempts at specific therapy have included cytotoxic agents, corticosteroids, platelet inhibitors, nonsteroidal anti-inflammatory agents, and anticoagulants, singly or in combination. Two controlled trials, each lasting 1 year, have recently been reported. One employed dipyridamole, 75 mg 3 times a day, and aspirin, 320 mg daily; the other, dipyridamole, 75 to 100 mg 4 times a day, and warfarin in a dose sufficient to keep the prothrombin time at 1½ to two times the control value. In both trials most of the patients had compromised renal function when the regimen was initiated, and in both, the decline in renal function was halted or slowed in the treatment group. With the dipyridamole-aspirin combination, hematuria and proteinuria continued unabated. With dipyridamole-warfarin, proteinuria diminished, but hypoalbuminemia was unaffected. Renal biopsies to assess changes in glomerular morphology were not performed in either trial. The severity of the renal functional deficiency in some of the patients entered in these trials raises the question of whether the regimen ameliorated or blunted immunologic or nonimmunologic injury. According to recent concepts, immunologic injury is usually considered to have ceased or to play a minor role in producing further functional deterioration after the glomerular filtration rate has fallen to 50 percent of normal or less after several years of disease, and subsequent glomerular damage is attributed to nonimmunologic injury. On this basis, it is possible that the regimens employing dipyridamole were effective, at least in some patients, because they prevented or slowed the nonimmunologic injury phase of the disease.

Alternate-Day Prednisone Regimen

Since January 1966, all patients presenting with MPGN at our institution, except those with end-stage disease, have been given prednisone in a high-dose, alternate-day regimen. The results of this experience have recently been analyzed. The regimen was given to 51 patients but six of these were omitted from the analysis because they had focal and segmental glomerular lesions which presage a good prognosis. The remaining 45 with diffuse proliferative glomerulonephritis represent a mix of all three types of the disease. Their follow-up after initiation of the regimen averaged 6.5 years (a total experience of 290 patient years on the regimen).

As currently used, the regimen is initiated with a dose of prednisone of 2.0 to 2.5 mg per kilogram of body weight, with a maximum of 80 mg, given once on alternate days. If the patient has rapidly progressive disease, as judged by clinical course and renal biopsy, a course of methylprednisolone given in a high dose intravenously, as commonly used for other rapidly progressive glomerulonephritides, can precede this regimen. We abandoned instituting the regimen by giving prednisone in divided doses daily because it appears to offer no advantage over starting immediately with the alternate-day regimen, and it has the potential of producing marked hypertension with encephalopathy. On the one hand, the alternate-day regimen does not generate hypertension, although, because of glomerular scarring, about 20 percent of the patients eventually become hypertensive while receiving the regimen. On the other hand, about 10 percent who were initially hypertensive became normotensive. In no patient has the regimen had to be discontinued because of uncontrollable hypertension. The prednisone is continued in a high dose on alternate days for at least 1 year and then the dose is slowly reduced. Our analysis suggested that disappearance of urinary occult blood, as detected by Hemastix, corresponds to cessation of immunologic glomerular injury, and it is now our practice to continue the high dose of prednisone until microhematuria ceases. Thereafter, over approximately a 4-year period, the dose is reduced to about 0.5 mg per kilogram every other day. For example, the range of dose given to six children with moderately severe disease who weighed 20 to 34 kg at the start of the regimen was initially 2.0 to 2.5 mg per kilogram; after 1 year, 1.4 to 2.4; after 2 years, 1.1 to 1.8; after 3 years, 0.8 to 1.5; after 4 years, 0.2 to 1.0; and after 5 years, 0.2 to 0.8 mg per kilogram. These decrements with time on a milligram per kilogram basis were the result not only of dose reduction, but also of weight gain. In older children and adults, assuming occult blood is no longer present in the urine, the dose is reduced after 1 year from 80 to 70 or 60 mg, with subsequent stepwise reductions over the next several years to a dose of 20 mg every other day. Recurrence of microhematuria or an increase in protein excretion is reason to increase the dose.

Since all patients we have encountered have been started on this regimen, its merits have to be judged (1) by comparing renal survivial with that in series of patients who have not been treated or treated sporadically, reported by others; (2) by its effect on glomerular morphology as observed in serial renal biopsies; and (3) by its effect on hematuria, proteinuria, hypoalbuminemia, and serum creatinine levels.

Comparison with Survival in Other Series

A number of other series have been reported in which patients have been either untreated or treated sporadically with relatively short-term courses of corticosteroids, immunosuppressive agents, antimalarials, or anticoagulants. In the eleventh year after clinical onset in our series of 45 patients, all with diffuse proliferative lesions, renal survival was 74 percent calculated actuarially, whereas over the same period, survival in three other series ranged from 30 to 48 percent. A series of 105 patients reported from France, mostly children, is the largest; survival by the ninth year in this series was 50 percent, and in ours, 88 percent. This difference has statistical significance.

Survival was found to be better when the regimen was started soon after clinical onset. Among 25 patients starting the regimen less than 1 year after clinical onset, only two (8 percent) developed end-stage renal disease (ESRD). One of the two was noncompliant with the regimen and the other had a rapidly progressive course. These 25 patients had been receiving the regimen for an average of 5 years and 11 months (range 0.5 to 14.8). Fortuitously, this observation period is very similar to that of the 105 patients reported from France, and hence renal survival of the two groups can be directly compared. Among the French patients with an observation period of 5 years and 9 months (range 1 to 18), 34 (32 percent) developed ESRD. This frequency is significantly greater than ours ($x^2 = 6.0$, $p < 0.02$). In a series of 45 children reported from England over a similar observation period, 16 (35 percent) developed ESRD.

Of the 20 patients in our series who started the regimen more than 1 year after clinical onset, five (25 percent) developed ESRD. Calculated actuarially, survival in this group in the ninth year was 88 percent and in the tenth year, 68 percent. The five who developed ESRD started the regimen 2.5 to 8 years after clinical onset (average, 5.5 years).

Effect of the Regimen on Glomerular Morphology

Aspects of glomerular morphology that were assessed were proliferation, glomerular sclerosis, and tubular atrophy. Proliferation was assessed by estimating by light microscopy both the number of open glomerular capillary lumens and the prominence of the mesangial matrix as observed with the periodic acid-Schiff (PAS) stain. Paired renal biopsies obtained before the start of the regimen and after an average of 32 months of the regimen were available for 31 patients. There was a significant increase in the number of open capillary lumens and diminution in the prominence of the PAS-positive matrix in the second biopsies. There was also a significant increase in the number of sclerotic glomeruli from 6.2 percent to 16.1 percent and a nonsignificant increase in tubular atrophy. Thus, the morphology of functioning glomeruli improved while the regimen was being given, yet glomerular sclerosis and tubular atrophy increased.

The data were also analyzed to determine more directly the effect of the regimen on glomerular morphology. The analysis was undertaken to rule out the possibility that reduction in glomerular proliferation was a normal event in the natural history of the disease. Biopsy specimens were available from 19 patients who had not been given the regimen and who were, on the average, 42 months from clinical onset. Morphologic characteristics in these specimens were compared with those in biopsy specimens from 18 patients averaging 33 months from clinical onset, but who had received the regimen for the previous 30 months. In those receiving the regimen for 30 months, the number of open capillary lumens was significantly greater, and the PAS-positive matrix was significantly less prominent. This and other observations provided evidence that reduced proloferation was the result of the regimen and not a part of the natural history of the disease. In this analysis, the extent of glomerular sclerosis and tubular atrophy was found to be approximately the same in the two groups. Again it was apparent that glomerular sclerosis was occurring as the cellularity of functioning glomeruli was diminishing.

However, the analysis further indicated that the period over which sclerosis continues after the start of the regimen is limited. Thus, third biopsies, obtained on an average of 52 months after the second biopsy, showed no further increase in sclerotic glomeruli or tubular atrophy as compared with the second biopsy. There was also further diminution in glomerular proliferation over this period, but the difference was not statistically significant.

The increased sclerosis in the first 2 or 3 years of the regimen is best explained by postulating a cohort of glomeruli present at the time the regimen starts which appear functional, but have suffered such severe immunologic injury that they become sclerotic whether the regimen is given or not. These glomeruli are indistinguishable from those that continue to function. After the regimen starts, however, no further glomeruli enter this cohort. As a result, third biopsies, obtained on an average of 4.2 years after the second and 6.5 years after the start of the regimen, showed no further increase in sclerotic glomeruli. Sclerosis, however, increases if the patient is noncompliant and/or the disease relapses.

Effect of the Regimen on Serum Chemical Values and Urinary Abnormalities

Serum creatinine levels were less than 1.5 mg per deciliter in 37 patients at the start of the regimen and remained in that range in 28 (76 percent). The level was above 1.5 mg per deciliter in eight patients at the start of the regimen. The level fell in five of these and rose in three. Thus, of the 45 patients, the renal function of 12 (27 percent) worsened while they were receiving the regimen. Seven of these 12 were those developing ESRD. Deterioration of function while receiving the regimen occurred more frequently in those starting the regimen more than 1 year after clinical onset.

The regimen tended to normalize serum albumin levels. The level was in the normal range in 13 (29 percent) at the start of the regimen and in 33 (73 percent) after the regimen had been given for an average of 6.5 years. The level remained normal or increased in 80 percent. In no patient did the level fall. The normalization of serum albumin levels gives evidence of a salutary effect of the regimen; patients who are nephrotic at presentation or who subsequently become nephrotic are said to be those eventually developing renal failure. In the patients starting the regimen without delay, the serum albumin levels rose more rapidly and became normal in a higher percentage as compared with those starting the regimen more than 1 year after clinical onset.

In parallel with the improvement in serum albumin levels, proteinuria tended to disappear while the regimen was being given. It was present in all 45 patients at the start of the regimen and disappeared in 12 (27 percent). Again, proteinuria disappeared earlier and more frequently in those starting the regimen without delay. The tendency for hypoalbuminemia and proteinuria to persist in those starting the regimen after a delay probably reflects the greater glomerular scarring in this group of patients.

Hematuria was present in 41 of the 45 patients at the start of the regimen. Seven of these developed ESRD, and of the remaining 34, hematuria disappeared in 28 (82 percent). In contrast to hypoalbuminemia and proteinuria, the rate of disappearance of hematuria was the same whether the regimen was started promptly or after a delay. This observation suggests that hematuria was not the result of scarring and that it disappeared as proliferation in functional glomeruli diminished. This was partially verified by the observation that nearly all patients who had lost their hematuria showed improvement in glomerular morphology. Thus, disappearance of occult blood from the urine is currently taken as evidence that immunologic glomerular injury has subsided.

The data were also analyzed to determine whether the rise in serum albumin level and the loss of proteinuria and hematuria were part of the natural history of the disease or the result of the regimen. Clinical and laboratory data obtained from 20 patients who were, on the average, 42 months from clinical onset and who had not received the regimen, could be compared with data obtained from 25 patients who were also 42 months from clinical onset, but had received the regimen for the last 38 of those months. Significantly fewer of those who had been receiving the regimen had hematuria, proteinuria, and reduced serum albumin levels. On the other hand, the frequency of hypertension and an elevated serum creatinine level was the same in the two groups. The persistence of the latter abnormalities probably reflects the fact noted above that after the start of the regimen, glomerular sclerosis continued for several years.

Hypocomplementemia tended to disappear after the regimen started. The level of C3 rose to the normal range most rapidly in those with type I disease, often within 4 months. On the other hand, there was no evidence that the hypocomplementemia was useful as a measure of activity of the disease; patients with continuing hypocomplementemia could show improvement both clinically and in glomerular morphology while those who remained normocomplementemic could deteriorate.

Relapses

In four patients, a febrile illness occurring 10 or more months after the start of the regimen was accompanied by an episode of gross hematuria. In all four, the dose of prednisone had been, for some time, below the usual range as defined above. No further bleeding occurred after the prednisone dose was increased. Renal biopsy specimens obtained at the time of the episode showed no improvement over the first biopsy specimen, suggesting an impending relapse. In two patients the nephrotic syndrome present when the regimen was instituted disappeared but recurred several years later after the dose of prednisone had been below the usual range for several months. In both, the nephrotic syndrome slowly resolved when the dose of prednisone was increased.

If the thesis is correct the microhematuria disappears when the disease becomes inactive, reappearance of hematuria should herald a relapse. This corollary was not satisfactorily tested in the present series. In five of the patients mentioned above with relapse or impending relapse, microhematuria had not disappeared, and the patients were, therefore, not in complete remission. However, in one of the two patients developing a nephrotic syndrome, hematuria had disappeared and did not recur until the nephrotic syndrome was severe. This experience, although limited, would indicate that patients should be monitored for both protein and occult blood excretion if a relapse is to be detected early.

Complications

The most serious side effect of the regimen was growth retardation, which in this series was more severe in the male. Several of the episodes of gross hematuria followed periods when dosage was reduced because of growth retardation. Posterior subcapsular cataracts developed in eight patients, but they were all small and did not interfere with vision. Severe hypertension with seizures was not seen.

Discontinuing the Regimen

Because of concern that a relapse might not be reversible and would increase glomerular injury, the regimen was not stopped even though the patients appeared to be in remission. However, two patients with MPGN type I became noncompliant after remission was achieved. Neither had a relapse. On the other hand, others have reported a relapse within six weeks after discontinuing the regimen in patients with type I disease. We also discontinued the regimen in two patients in remission with type II disease. They are not included in this analysis because they presented before January 1966. Both relapsed and eventually had to have renal transplants. The regimen has not been discontinued in any patient with type III.

IDIOPATHIC RAPIDLY PROGRESSIVE GLOMERULONEPHRITIS

REX F. OCHI, M.D.
WILLIAM G. COUSER, M.D.

DEFINITION

Before discussing specific therapy, it is important to clarify the definition of idiopathic rapidly progressive glomerulonephritis (RPGN) as we use it, because the term is used differently by different authors and may be applied to several glomerular diseases which are not treated in the same way. The generic diagnosis of RPGN is conventionally made in patients who demonstrate a rapid loss of renal function associated with extensive glomerular crescent formation seen on renal biopsy. Loss of renal function is considered rapid when the serum creatinine concentration doubles, or the creatinine clearance decreases by more than 50 percent, in less than 3 months. However, in many patients with RPGN this amount of renal function is lost within 1 to 2 weeks, and acute renal failure may occur. Extensive crescents usually mean the presence of cellular crescents occupying more than half the circumference of Bowman's capsule in more than 50 percent of glomeruli, but this distinction is somewhat arbitrary, since patients biopsied earlier in their disease may exhibit fewer crescents but experience a very similar clinical course. Defined in this way, RPGN may be seen in a wide variety of inflammatory glomerular diseases with quite different causes, pathogenetic mechanisms, and prognoses. These include postinfectious nephritis, several vasculitides, anti-glomerular basement membrane (GBM) antibody-induced glomerulonephritis, and a form of primary renal disease, among others. The therapeutic approach to patients with each of these entities may differ and is discussed in more detail in other chapters in this book.

In an attempt to encourage a more pathogenetic approach to the classification of RPGN, we have used the system presented in Table 1, which divides patients with RPGN into three major categories: immune complex-induced RPGN, anti-GBM antibody-induced RPGN, and RPGN without significant glomerular immune deposits. Thus, most patients with RPGN associated with granular immune complex deposits, which represent about 40 percent of the total, have a postinfectious disease or a severe form of a systemic immune complex disease, such as poststreptococcal nephritis, lupus nephritis, Schönlein-Henoch purpura, or mixed cryoglobulinemia. We would refer to such patients as having rapidly progressive poststreptococcal nephritis, rapidly progressive lupus nephritis, and so on.

A second group includes about 20 percent of all patients with RPGN as defined above who have anti-GBM antibody disease with or without pulmonary hemorrhage. Because the pathogenetic mechanism in this entity is quite well defined, we do not consider these patients examples of idiopathic RPGN but rather as cases of Goodpasture's syndrome with RPGN or rapidly progressive anti-GBM nephritis without pulmonary hemorrhage. The treatment of anti-GBM nephritis is considered in more detail in the chapter *Goodpasture's Syndrome*.

TABLE 1 Immunopathogenetic Classification of Rapidly Progressive Glomerulonephritis (RPGN)

Type of RPGN	*Frequency (%)*
RPGN associated with granular immune deposits	40
Postinfectious	
Poststreptococcal glomerulonephritis	
Visceral abscesses	
Bacterial endocarditis	
"Shunt" nephritis	
Noninfectious	
Systemic lupus erythematosus	
Schönlein-Henoch purpura	
Mixed cryoglobulinemia	
Wegener's granulomatosis	
Polyarteritis and other vasculitides	
Solid tumors	
Primary renal diseases	
IgG-IgA nephropathy	
Membranoproliferative glomerulonephritis	
Idiopathic immune complex nephritis	
Anti-GBM antibody-mediated RPGN	20
Goodpasture's syndrome	
Idiopathic anti-GBM nephritis	
Membranous nephropathy with crescents	
RPGN without glomerular immune deposits	
Idiopathic RPGN	40

The third category of patients are those with RPGN without significant glomerular immune deposits, about 40 percent of the total. Most of these patients have a primary renal disease of uncertain etiology and pathogenesis, and we apply the term idiopathic RPGN to this group of patients only. Because this histologic and immunopathologic picture may be seen in some vasculitides, such as polyarteritis and hypersensitivity vasculitis, and because some patients with idiopathic RPGN have vague systemic signs and symptoms suggestive of vasculitis, there is a growing suspicion that such patients suffer from a form of vasculitis with inflammation confined primarily to the glomerular capillaries. However, the pathogenetic mechanisms remain undefined. If one considers only patients with RPGN in the absence of a previous infection, defined collagen vascular disease, or anti-GBM antibody, the majority of such patients in our experience have idiopathic RPGN without significant glomerular immune deposits.

CLINICAL FEATURES AND PROGNOSIS

The mean age of patients with idiopathic RPGN is about 58 (range, 5 to over 80), and there is a 1.5 to 2 male predominance. Patients present episodically with some clustering in the spring and summer months. Prodromal symptoms occur in about 50 percent of patients and usually resemble a viral illness with myalgias, arthralgias, loin, back, or abdominal pain, fever and malaise. About 30 percent have pulmonary manifestations including minor hemoptysis or transient infiltrates on chest roentgenogram. As mentioned above, these constitutional signs and symptoms often resemble those seen with a vasculitis. In fact, some would categorize any patient with lung abnormalities, crescentic glomerulonephritis, and absent anti-GBM antibodies as having systemic vasculitis. Specific antecedent events have rarely been identified. Some authors have commented on an unusual frequency of hydrocarbon exposure, malignancy, and prior cardiac events including cardiac surgery and myocardial infarction.

The prognosis in idiopathic RPGN is impossible to define precisely, since most series contain patients with several types of glomerular disease. As well, all patients receive variable forms of therapy, follow-up is usually of limited duration, and the prognosis in most glomerular diseases has improved considerably in the past two decades, probably owing to factors other than improved therapy (as will be discussed). However, the best information available suggests that about 75 percent of such patients die or require dialysis within months or years if they are untreated or treated only with oral steroids and/or immunosuppressive agents.

DIAGNOSIS

RPGN should be regarded as a relative *medical emergency* because there is growing evidence that appropriate therapy benefits patients only when initiated early in the disease, usually before the serum creatinine concentration exceeds 6 mg per deciliter or oliguria develops. Irreversible loss of renal function in this disease can occur in a matter of days. Although extremely rare exceptions have been reported, virtually all patients exhibit a nephritic urinalysis with varying degrees of proteinuria, hematuria, and often red cell and other cellular casts. Thus the disease should be suspected in any patient with a nephritic urinalysis and an elevated serum creatinine concentration. If renal function was previously known to be normal or shows evidence of deteriorating in the absence of other factors such as volume depletion, nephrotoxins, infection, or obstruction, a renal biopsy should be obtained immediately. Appropriate laboratory studies such as antistreptococcal antibody titers, complement levels, antinuclear and anti-GBM antibody tests, hepatitis B surface antigen, and cryoglobulins should be done simultaneously. However, in most cases the results of light and immunofluorescence microscopy on biopsy tissue will be available first and are required to establish a definitive diagnosis. The diagnosis of idiopathic RPGN is made when the biopsy shows extensive cellular crescents in glomeruli as the predominant histologic finding, and immunofluorescence fails to detect anti-GBM antibody or significant immune complex deposits. Most severely damaged glomeruli will exhibit some focal glomerular deposits of immunoglobulin and/or complement. However, immune complex deposits sufficient to cause crescents and RPGN are not subtle findings. If extensive immune complex deposits are present, a careful clinical and laboratory search for an infectious process or evidence of collagen vascular disease should be undertaken. Infection is particularly likely if significant endocapillary proliferation is present in the biopsy as well as crescents. If no other disease is identified, such patients are treated as described below for idiopathic RPGN. If the linear staining characteristic of anti-GBM antibody-induced nephritis is seen, treatment should be as described in the chapter *"Goodpasture's Syndrome,"* even if overt pulmonary hemorrhage is absent. If extensive cellular or fibrocellular crescents without immune deposits are found, a diagnosis of idiopathic RPGN is made.

Before determining the vigor of the therapeutic approach to be employed, careful attention should also be given to the reversibility of the histologic changes observed. For example, glomerular sclerosis or necrosis, fibrous changes in the crescents, and extensive interstitial fibrosis, particularly if the serum creatinine concentration exceeds 6 mg per deciliter or kidney size is reduced, are irreversible structural alterations that suggest a more chronic process, which is unlikely to respond well to therapy. There is therefore little to be gained by subjecting such patients to any form of therapy that carries significant morbidity. However, fresh cellular crescents, regardless of how extensive, interstitial mononuclear cell infiltrates without fibrosis, tubular necrosis, and vasculitis are acute and potentially reversible findings, particularly if kidney size is normal and renal function is not yet severely compromised. In these patients the opportunity to halt progression or improve function and prognosis justifies a much more vigorous therapeutic approach.

TREATMENT

Treatment of the patient with RPGN combines the approach to the patient with acute renal failure with more specific therapeutic initiatives directed at the primary glomerular disease. One must therefore ensure that intravascular volume and renal perfusion are adequate; that the patient is not receiving potentially nephrotoxic drugs, particularly nonsteroidal anti-inflammatory agents, which can markedly reduce glomerular plasma flow in such patients; and that urinary tract obstruction is not present.

In terms of specific therapy for the glomerular disease, no good prospective therapeutic trials containing large numbers of patients have been carried out in this disease. Moreover, because of its relative rarity and the urgency of therapy, no such trials are likely to be done in the future. The clinician is thus required to sort through a mass of uncontrolled, anecdotal reports of successful treatment of RPGN with a variety of agents, including oral steroids, various immunosuppressive drugs alone or in combination with other agents, anticoagulants, antiplatelet agents, antilymphocyte serum, vasodilatory prostaglandins, pulse steroid therapy, and plasma exchange. In all cases, the results obtained are usually compared with historical controls despite the fact that the prognosis in most glomerular diseases has improved considerably over the past two decades, with very little evidence that this has resulted exclusively from improved specific therapy. This observation is also true in idiopathic RPGN, in which the 2-year renal survival rates are now 70 and 80 percent compared with about 20 percent in series published before 1970. It is also apparent from the literature that substantial differences in success rates with certain therapies have been reported from different parts of the world. Presumably this reflects either geographic differences in the severity of disease encountered or the relative experience and skill of individual centers in administering particular forms of therapy. With these limitations clearly in mind, the following summarizes the literature as we interpret it, and the approach to treating idiopathic RPGN which we feel best reflects published experience in the United States as well as our own experience in treating this group of patients.

Methylprednisolone Pulse Therapy

Application of high-dose steroid pulse therapy to glomerular disease derived from extensive experience with treating renal transplant rejection and the generally poor response encountered with other forms of drug therapy. We now regard steroid pulse therapy as the treatment of choice for idiopathic RPGN. Once the diagnosis has been firmly established by renal biopsy, relative contraindications to high-dose steroid therapy should then be excluded, including uncontrolled infection, overt psychosis, active peptic ulcer disease, or major surgery within 2 weeks. To minimize any possible side effects the patient should be normovolemic, not have received diuretic therapy within the previous 48 hours, and have a normal serum potassium concentration. Methylprednisolone is then administered in a dose of 30 mg per kilogram of body weight IV over 20 to 30 minutes diluted in 50 ml of 5 percent dextrose in water. The maximum dose is 3 g, and dosage is generally reduced by about 25 percent in patients over age 65. This treatment is given three times on alternate days, followed by oral prednisone, 2 mg per kilogram per day, also adminsitered on alternate days for about 2 months. Steroid therapy is then tapered by reducing the alternate-day dose by about 20 mg each week until therapy is discontinued at the end of 3 to 4 months.

Responses rarely occur in the first few days but are usually seen between 1 and 2 weeks. About 75 percent of patients, particularly those treated before oliguria or a serum creatinine concentration exceeding 6 mg per deciliter develop, respond with at least a 30 percent reduction in serum creatinine level or a doubling of the glomerular filtration rate within 6 weeks. However, a number of patients with severe renal failure requiring hemodialysis have also responded when treated early in their course. The clinical response indicated by an improvement in renal function has also been confirmed by repeat biopsies in several studies which have shown a marked improvement in glomerular and interstitial disease by histologic criteria. Long-term follow-up studies have shown that idiopathic RPGN is usually a self-limited disease with rare recurrences, and that patients who achieve a serum creatinine concentration of less than 3 mg per deciliter generally remain stable for many years thereafter.

The side effects of steroid pulse therapy administered as outlined above are minimal in our experience but include a metallic taste, muscle weakness, arthralgias, bright lights and other psychotropic effects, nausea, and intractable hiccups. Rare instances of seizures, severe hypertension, cardiac arrhythmias, and sudden death have been reported by others, the latter usually in patients with reductions in intravascular volume or serum potassium level. Nonetheless, pulse therapy should be administered in situations in which patients can be carefully monitored. Studies of pulse therapy in a population of more than 500 patients with acute myocardial infarction have shown no increased risk of arrhythmias in patients receiving pulse therapy compared with controls. The cost of methylprednisolone pulse therapy is also minimal, averaging about $700 for a full course in most centers. Although therapeutic benefit has not been firmly established in any controlled clinical study, the increased efficacy of pulse therapy over high-dose oral steroids has been demonstrated in studies of experimental models of crescentic glomerulonephritis. A prospective study in rapidly progressive lupus nephritis also showed a more rapid return to maximal renal function in patients treated with pulse steroids compared with oral steroids, although no significant differences in long-term levels of renal function were apparent between the two groups.

Since the pathogenetic mechanisms that induce idiopathic RPGN are not well understood, the use of this form of therapy is purely empiric, and the results observed cannot be attributed to any established underlying mechanism. However, an immune disorder is strongly suspected. We believe the apparent efficacy, low toxicity, and low cost render steroid pulse therapy the current treatment of choice for idiopathic RPGN until more data are available.

Beneficial results have also been reported with pulse steroids in patients with crescentic glomerulonephritis associated with polyarteritis nodosa and membranoproliferative glomerulonephritis. However, this regimen has been without obvious benefit in patients with anti-GBM disease, another reason for emphasizing the need for early and accurate diagnosis.

Plasma Exchange

Several centers have reported treating patients with idiopathic RPGN with plasma exchange as well as oral prednisone and an immunosuppressive agent, usually cyclophosphamide. This regimen is discussed in more detail in the chapter *"Goodpasture's Syndrome."* While only small numbers of well-characterized patients have been studied, response rates of about 75 percent, equivalent to those reported with steroid pulse therapy, have been reported. Our reason for favoring pulse therapy over plasma exchange is that it appears to produce an equivalent response at less risk and considerably less cost to the patient. A single plasma exchange is more expensive than a full course of steroid pulse therapy in most centers, and a full course of plasma exchange is 15 to 20 times more costly. There are no data which address the question of whether these two treatments might have an additive effect or whether plasma exchange might be effective when initiated after a patient has failed to respond to pulse steroids. In our experience most patients who fail to respond to steroid pulse therapy within two weeks usually have extensive structural glomerular damage which is unlikely to respond to any additional form of therapy.

Immunosuppression

Reported experience with steroid pulse therapy in idiopathic RPGN has generally not included the use of concomitant cytotoxic agents. Earlier studies have not shown oral immunosuppressive agents to be particularly effective in treating this disease. However, as mentioned earlier, it now appears increasingly likely that patients with this form of glomerulonephritis suffer from a type of vasculitis confined largely to the glomerular capillaries. Since long-term (6 months) therapy with immunosuppressive agents such as cyclophosphamide appears to be beneficial in other forms of vasculitis, it may well be rational to employ them in idiopathic RPGN. At the present time we use cyclophosphamide, 2 to 3 mg per kilogram per day, in only two groups of patients, those with established clinical or pathologic evidence of extraglomerular vascular disease or those with a focal necrotizing glomerulonephritis as the renal lesion associated with glomerular crescents, since this lesion is characteristic of glomerular involvement in vasculitis. In patients with pure idiopathic RPGN without clinical or pathologic findings suggestive of vasculitis, we employ steroid therapy alone.

Other Treatments

Response rates comparable to the 75 percent reported with steroid pulse therapy and plasma exchange have also been reported from Australia and England in patients with idiopathic RPGN treated with a quadruple regimen of steroids, immunosuppressive agents, antiplatelet agents, and anticoagulants. Experience with this approach in the United States has been limited and usually unfavorable owing to a relatively high incidence of bleeding and infectious complications. We do not feel there is any established indication for the use of currently available anticoagulant drugs in treating idiopathic RPGN. Isolated case reports of the successful use of other agents such as nirogen mustard and vasodilatory prostaglandins are too few to evaluate. These treatments appear to offer no obvious benefits over the approach described above.

PRINCIPLES OF MANAGEMENT OF NEPHROTIC SYNDROME

GABRIEL M. DANOVITCH, M.D.

The nephrotic syndrome is the consequence of the loss of one of the critical functions of the glomerular basement membrane—permselectivity—or the capacity of the basement membrane to provide an effective barrier to the passage of proteins. This chapter will focus on the consequences of this malfunction, which vary little despite the wide variety of diseases that can induce it (Table 1). Nephrotic syndrome consists of heavy proteinuria, hypoalbuminemia, and peripheral edema, frequently associated with lipidemia and lipiduria. The manifestations of heavy proteinuria are listed in Table 2 and will be discussed individually. The appropriate treatment of generalized edema, which is clearly the most important manifestation of nephrotic syndrome, requires an understanding of its pathophysiology and some of the controversy surrounding it.

MECHANISM OF EDEMA DEVELOPMENT IN NEPHROTIC SYNDROME

The "Classic" Theory of Diminished Plasma Volume

Consider a patient who develops minimal-change nephrotic syndrome with a urinary protein loss of 10 g daily (Fig.1). The protein lost is largely albumin, and as its loss exceeds the hepatic capacity of albumin synthesis, the serum albumin level falls, thereby lowering the level of oncotic pressure. The forces favoring net fluid movement from the plasma into the interstitial space will increase and plasma volume will tend to fall. In response to the threat to the volume of this critical compartment, the kidney retains sodium and the plasma volume tends to return to the original level. However, fluid continues to "leak" into the interstitium, and the kidney continues to "correct" the plasma volume. The increasing volume of the interstitial fluid eventually becomes palpable and visible as peripheral edema.

The above example represents, in abbreviated form, the standard explanations for sodium retention and edema formation in nephrosis. Several observations, however, make it clear that this sequence of events may be incorrect.

First, measurements of plasma volume made by different investigators in both human beings and experimental models of nephrosis have not produced consistent results. High values have often been reported rather than low or low normal values, as anticipated by standard teaching.

Second, following recovery from nephrotic syndrome, plasma volume does not increase as the classic theory would suggest.

Third, measurements of plasma renin activity and aldosterone levels are also variable in these conditions and are not consistently high, as would be expected if the plasma volume were low.

Fourth, in nephrosis, the standard teaching dictates that there must be a close relationship between serum albumin, plasma volume, and sodium retention. Such a relationship is frequently not observed, and clinically it is common to see patients with heavy proteinuria and low serum albumin levels but without edema. Plasmapheresis of experimental animals to lower their serum albumin levels is associated with high or normal levels of plasma volume. Patients with the rare congenital disease of analbuminemia usually are not edematous.

Finally, the response to diuretic administration in nephrosis is extremely variable. Some patients develop clinical and laboratory evidence of volume contraction with small doses of diuretics, a response that is not surprising if the plasma volume is low or low normal. Other patients, however, tolerate diuretic medications in large doses without showing evidence of volume contraction.

The "Overflow" Theory of Edema Formation

Consider a patient with acute glomerulonephritis who, together with the development of a glomerular inflamma-

TABLE 1 Causes of the Nephrotic Syndrome

Primary glomerular diseases
  Minimal-change nephrotic syndrome
  Mesangioproliferative glomerulonephritis (IgM or IgA type)
  Focal sclerosis
  Membrane nephropathy
  Membranoproliferative glomerulonephritis (types I and II)
Secondary to multisystemic disease
  Systemic lupus erythematosus
  Diabetes mellitus
  Amyloidosis
  Schönlein-Henoch purpura
  Polyarteritis (e.g., Wegener's granulomatosis)
Secondary to infections
  Bacterial: Poststreptococcal glomerulonephritis
    Infectious endocarditis
    Syphilis
  Viral: Hepatitis B
    Cytomegalovirus
    Epstein-Barr virus
    HTLV III*
  Protozoal: Malaria
  Helminthic: Schistosomiasis
    Filariasis
    Trypanosomiasis
Secondary to medications and drugs
  Organic gold
  Organic mercury
  Penicillamine
  Intravenous heroin
  Tridione
  Hydantoin
  Nonsteroidal anti-inflammatory drugs
Secondary to neoplasia
  Solid tumors: Colon, lung, breast, etc.
    Hodgkin's disease, chronic lymphatic leukemia
Secondary to allergens
  Bee sting
  Serum sickness
  Poison ivy
  Pollens
Secondary to familial and metabolic diseases
  Hypothyroidism
  Alport's syndrome
  Familial and congenital nephrotic syndromes
  Sickle cell hemoglobinopathies
Secondary to miscellaneous causes
  Preeclampsia
  Renal transplantation
  Malignant hypertension
  Congestive heart failure
  Constrictive pericarditis
  Reflux nephropathy

* Nephrotic syndrome has been associated both with AIDS and AIDS-related complex and may antedate AIDS. The frequency of AIDS-related nephrotic syndrome varies widely in reported series from occasional cases to as much as 10% of AIDS sufferers.

tory process, develops pronounced renal sodium retention and a positive sodium balance. Blood pressure rises and plasma volume expands until it cannot be accommodated within the circulation. The serum albumin level tends to fall, due to both the proteinuria and the dilution of the plasma with retained sodium and water. Eventually the expanded plasma volume compartment will "overflow" into the interstitium, and edema will result. In this case, renal sodium retention is the primary event, or at least occurs in parallel with it. It is the expansion of the plasma volume that accounts for the development of edema (Fig. 2).

It is not difficult to envision the above sequence of events in acute glomerulonephritis, in which the acute inflammatory process in the glomerulus disturbs the finely tuned balance between glomerular and tubular function, and sodium retention results. It is more difficult to explain why renal sodium retention should produce an expanded plasma volume in nephrosis. In cirrhosis there is convincing experimental evidence that sodium retention may precede an alteration in plasma volume that tends to rise rather than fall, and there is preliminary evidence in experimental nephrotic syndrome that the sodium retention may occur independently of systemic events and lead to an expansion of plasma volume. The mechanism for this sodium retention is still unclear.

The determination of the mechanism responsible for edema formation in nephrosis is not only of academic interest but has great clinical significance, particularly with respect to diuretic therapy. Clearly, vigorous direct therapy is not advisable in a patient whose plasma volume is already compromised or being maintained by a compensatory increase in renal salt and water retention (Fig. 1). Such therapy might be valuable in a patient with primary renal sodium retention and an expanded plasma volume (Fig. 2). At the present time, there is no reliable clinical test to differentiate between the traditional theory of edema formation and the overflow hypothesis, although plasma renin tends to be high in the former and low in the latter. It is becoming clear, however, that nephrotic patients are not a homogeneous group with respect to their edema-forming mechanisms, and clinical judgment regarding the use of diuretics is required.

TABLE 2 Some Consequences of Heavy Proteinuria

Loss of albumin
  Alteration of Starling forces—edema
  Enhanced hepatic lipid production—hyperlipidemia (?), accelerated atherosclerosis
  Renal tubular abnormalities consequent on heavy proteinuria (e.g., glycosuria)
  Protein-calorie malnutrition
  Meurcke's lines
Loss of other plasma proteins
  IgG and complement components ↓—increased susceptibility to infection
  Transferrin ↓—anemia
  Thyroid binding globulin ↓—chemical hypothyroidism
  Cholecalciferol binding protein ↓—osteomalacia and bone disease
  Transcortin ↓—altered tissue response to administered steroids
  Metal binding protein ↓ (e.g., Fe, Cu, Zn)—clinical consequences (?)
  Protein-calorie malnutrition
Coagulation abnormalities
  Low zymogen factors (II, V, VII, IX, X, XI, XII)
  Increase in cofactors (V, VIII)
  Decreased antithrombin level and antiplasmin activity
  Thrombocytosis and increased platelet aggregation
  Increased fibrinogen levels
  Increased beta thromboglobulin

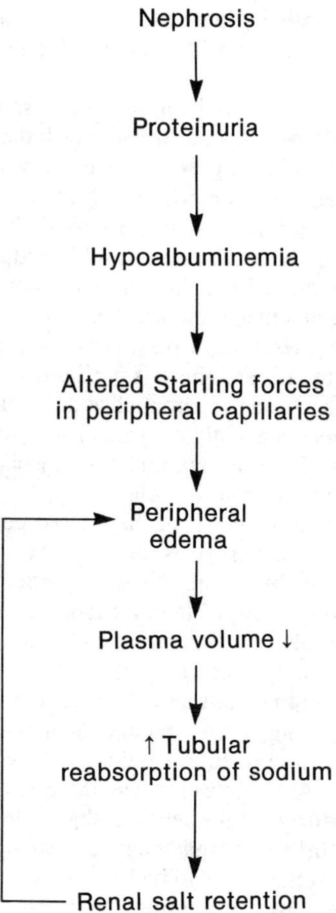

Figure 1 Schematic representation of the mechanism of edema in the nephrotic syndrome according to traditional teaching. The arrow joining the plasma volume and the tubular reabsorption of sodium is interrupted to indicate the complexity of the relationship between the two, with involvement of factors such as the renin - aldosterone axis, the volume receptors, or perhaps the atrial natriuretic factor.

CLINICAL APPROACH TO THE PATIENT WITH NEPHROTIC SYNDROME

The diagnosis and differential diagnosis of the nephrotic syndrome require confirmation of the laboratory test findings that accompany the edema: massive proteinuria, hypoalbuminemia, hyperlipidemia, and lipiduria. Accurate quantitative assessment of proteinuria is critical, and a dipstick qualitative estimate of proteinuria is inadequate. If, for some reason, a 24-hour collection of urine is impractical, it is worth measuring the specific gravity at the same time that the urine protein is estimated by dipstick. One + proteinuria is a patient with dilute urine can be equivalent to a 3+ to 4+ proteinuria in the same patient when the urine is concentrated. A given concentration of protein in the urine thus indicates a greater absolute rate of proteinuria in a dilute than a concentrated urine specimen if the rate of urine flow is the same. Careful instruction of the patient as to how to collect an accurate 24-hour urine specimen will add to its accuracy. The completeness of the specimen can be checked by simultaneous estimation of the urinary creatinine content, which should approximate 20 mg per kilogram of body weight per 24 hours. The same specimen can be used to estimate daily sodium excretion, the importance of which will be discussed later. In the event that it is impractical to collect a 24-hour sample, comparison of the urine protein and creatinine concentrations on a single voided sample may be useful. A protein;creatinine ratio of more than 3.5 (milligram;milligram) can be taken to represent "nephrotic range" proteinuria. Although, by definition, only 3.5 g of protein in the urine per day is required to make a diagnosis of nephrotic syndrome, the quantity of protein is frequently considerably greater and may reach 30 to 40 g. The quantitative estimation of proteinuria, however, is not merely valuable in making a diagnosis of nephrotic syndrome; it is also of great importance in following the course of the various conditions that produce the syndrome.

Certain caveats should be borne in mind in assessing the significance of a 24-hour protein estimation. Clearly, reduction in the amount of protein can, and most frequently does, mean improvement of the underlying disease. But this is not always the case. In patients with the nephrotic syndrome in whom the underlying disease produces gradual deterioration of renal function, the reduction in the glomerular filtration rate reduces the amount of protein filtered and excreted, and hence the disease may appear to improve when it is in fact getting worse. If proteinuria is so severe that the plasma albumin concentration has fallen further and the filtered load is reduced, urine protein excretion may also fall without alteration in the underlying lesion.

In contrast, increase in proteinuria does not necessarily mean that the underlying disease is getting worse.

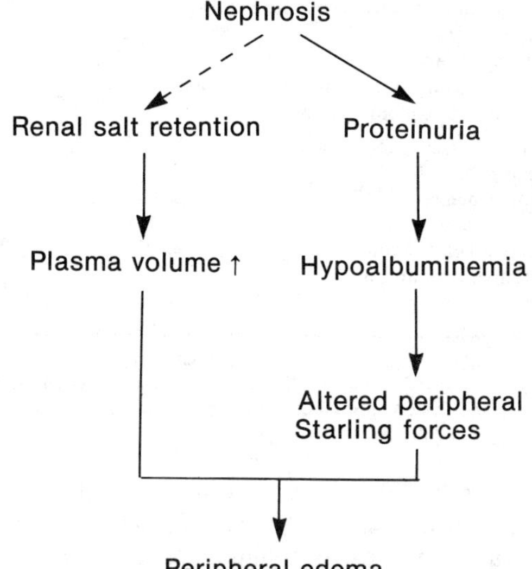

Figure 2 Schematic representation of the mechanism of edema in the nephrotic syndrome according to the "overflow" hypothesis. The interrupted lines indicate that the mechanism by which renal salt retention is produced in the absence of a systemic stimulus is unclear.

A persistent upright posture, physical exertion, high protein diets, and high fever can exaggerate proteinuria in patients with the nephrotic syndrome. When urinary protein values are compared from one follow-up visit to the next, the patient's degree of activity on the day of urine collection should always be assessed. Although deterioration of renal function in the nephrotic syndrome is most commonly accompanied by a reduction in proteinuria, as discussed, there are certain well-defined circumstances in which proteinuria will remain stable or increase. This means that the glomerular basement membrane has become more permeable to protein as the disease has progressed. This combination of heavy proteinuria and progressive renal failure most commonly occurs in the secondary renal disease associated with diabetes mellitus and amyloidosis. Of the primary nephropathies, focal glomerulosclerosis and membranous nephropathy may produce massive proteinuria despite advancing renal failure.

Measurement of the serum albumin level is also an essential part of the work-up of any edematous patient. In the nephrotic syndrome, however, it is probably less reliable for the purpose of ongoing assessment than is quantification of proteinuria. As noted earlier in this chapter, there is a poor correlation between plasma volume and serum albumin and patients may have low levels of serum albumin without edema. There is also a poor correlation between the degree of proteinuria and the level of serum albumin. The cause of these discrepancies is unclear, but they are likely to be due, at least in part, to catabolism of filtered albumin by the kidneys and a variability in the capacity of the liver to synthesize albumin. Nevertheless, in the individual patient with the nephrotic syndrome, there is an approximate correlation between the level of serum albumin and the extent of proteinuria so that the serum level does give some indication of the severity of the disease. There are, however, many other influences on the serum albumin level, such as dietary protein intake, liver function, and the state of dilution of the extracellular fluid, and it is difficult to assess the contribution of these and other factors to the serum level.

Management of Edema in the Nephrotic Syndrome

Bed Rest

Bed rest is an extremely effective way of inducing diuresis in patients with the nephrotic syndrome. Patients should exploit the diuretic potential of the horizontal position by spending as much time as possible with their legs up. If possible, an afternoon rest should be scheduled on a regular basis. Bed rest seems to work by reducing the hydrostatic pressure in the lower extremities and allowing fluid to return from the interstitial space to the plasma. The expansion of the plasma volume, in turn, signals the kidney to excrete more sodium and water. This sequence of events can be mimicked and exaggerated by immersing patients to the neck in the sitting position in a thermoneutral water bath. This so-called water immersion technique has been useful in investigating the pathophysiology of edema, but has yet to find a practical clinical application.

Diet

Patients with massive proteinuria and the nephrotic syndrome have typically been advised to eat a diet high in high-quality protein. Although the logic behind such a recommendation seems straightforward, to date there is no clear evidence that the patient's course is improved as a result. It has been suggested that high-protein diets may in fact exaggerate proteinuria, and paradoxically, in experimental models of nephrotic syndrome, there is preliminary evidence to suggest that a low-protein intake may reduce proteinuria and lead to elevation of the serum albumin level. What then should the dietary protein prescription for nephrotic patients be? Given our present state of knowledge it is probably appropriate to recommend 1 g per kilogram of body weight of high-biologic value protein daily without making extra allowance for urinary protein loss. If massive protein losses continue and induce malnutrition and profound hypoalbuminemia, consideration should be given to pharmacologic means of reducing proteinuria. In the past drastic nephron ablation techniques have been used, but it has been shown that carefully controlled administration of nonsteroidal anti-inflammatory agents may reduce proteinuria without a major reduction of glomerular filtration rate. In experimental models of nephrotic syndrome, angiotensin blockade with enalapril has had a similarly salutary affect and administration of captopril to patients with diabetic nephropathy has been reported to produce marked reduction in proteinuria. There appears to be no rationale for the repeated infusion of hyperoncotic albumin solutions, for within 24 hours most of the administered protein is excreted into the urine. The use of albumin infusion in combination with intravenous diuretic administration will be discussed later.

Dietary sodium restriction is a critical part of the therapeutic regimen of all patients with the nephrotic syndrome. It is difficult to give hard and fast rules as to how low the salt intake should be. The optimal degree of sodium restriction will vary from patient to patient at different stages in their course, but at all stages it should be clear that the goal in setting the dietary sodium intake is twofold: (1) to minimize weight gain from renal sodium retention and (2) to maintain a plasma volume as close to normal as possible. Measurement of 24-hour sodium excretion in patients whose body weight is stable is a useful way of assessing the sodium intake in the diet. A diet containing 30 to 50 mEq of sodium (2 to 3 g sodium chloride) is appropriate for most patients, and diets containing less salt are difficult to tolerate for long periods. Many patients, by dietary restriction alone, can achieve a steady state in which their edema is at an acceptable level and their body weight remains constant. Many cases of edema "resistant" to diuretic therapy will respond when sodium restriction is strict enough.

Diuretics

The decision to recommend the use of diuretics in a patient with the nephrotic syndrome should not be taken lightly. As discussed earlier, the traditional theory regarding the mechanism of edema in the nephrotic syndrome holds that sodium retention occurs in response to a diminished plasma volume. The addition of diuretics may thus negate an important adaptive mechanism and lead to potentially dangerous volume contraction. Physicians, however, may be under pressure from edematous patients to prescribe diuretics, as patients regard their edema as the primary manifestation of the disease and a marker of its severity. Nevertheless, under certain circumstances, diuretic therapy is unavoidable: (1) when edema is so severe that ambulation is impaired; (2) when trophic skin changes or intertrigo develop in edematous areas; or (3) when there is severe cosmetic deformity and the patient's difficulty in accepting the body image induces emotional trauma.

It should be understood clearly by the patient and the physician that the end point of therapy with diuretics is not an edema-free state. If this standard for the adequacy of therapy is used, many patients will suffer the consequences of severe extracellular fluid volume contraction. The rational of diuretic therapy is to reduce the edema to a level that allows free ambulation, good hygiene, and an acceptable body image. The first diuretic to be used is usually a thiazide diuretic or a more powerful loop-acting diuretic, such as furosemide in standard doses. In most patients, reduction of edema without dangerous contraction of plasma volume can be attained by the combination of a low-salt diet, adjustment of daily activities to allow for a period of bed rest, and the use of the above diuretics in standard doses. In some patients, much higher doses of furosemide ultimately may be required (200 mg or more), but before initiating such a regimen, it is important to check for dietary compliance by eliciting a careful dietary history and measuring the 24-hour urinary sodium excretion. In resistant cases it is preferable to increase the individual dose of a diuretic rather than to increase the frequency of the standard dose. A newer diuretic, metolazone, is also very effective in the management of resistant cases, particularly in combination with furosemide. However, the combination is very potent and should be given only in a hospital environment or when close outpatient follow-up is possible. There is little advantage to adding spironolactone to the diuretic regimen in nephrotic patients, although this diuretic may be of value in cirrhotic patients with ascites. When any of the potassium-losing diuretics are used, serum electrolytes should be checked at intervals and potassium supplements added when the serum potassium level falls to less than approximately 3.5 mEq per liter. Potassium supplements need not be added as a routine measure. Potassium-sparing diuretics (spironolactone, triamterene alone or in drug combinations) should be used with great care or not at all in patients with significant renal failure. All nephrotic patients receiving diuretic medication should be seen at regular intervals, with particular attention given to changes in their body weight, the presence of postural blood pressure changes, and alteration in renal function.

In occasional cases, edema is so severe, refractory, and disabling that hospital admission is necessary to administer a low-salt diet or intravenous diuretics, or to provide a combination of intravenous infusion of albumin and intravenous diuretics. Hemofiltration using a highly permeable dialysis membrane may be temporarily effective in such patients.

Acute Renal Failure

Sudden and progressive decline in renal function may be encountered in patients with the nephrotic syndrome. At times this is clearly related to an episode of profound volume depletion, secondary to administration of diuretics. Nonsteroidal anti-inflammatory drugs even in small doses may produce acute renal failure in patients with nephrotic syndrome as they may in patients with cirrhosis and ascites or heart failure. Since these drugs are now available "over the counter," patients should be questioned and warned about their use.

There are also rare but well-documented cases of minimal-change nephrotic syndrome in which acute renal failure develops which is not due to extracellular fluid volume contraction or other identifiable factors. In some of these patients renal failure can be reversed by the use of intravenous diuretics.

Hyperlipidemia

Hyperlipidemia is a common manifestation of nephrotic syndrome. The mechanisms that underlie the increased levels of triglycerides and cholesterol are not completely understood, but probably involve increased hepatic synthesis and defective peripheral utilization. The increase in hepatic lipid synthesis appears to be related quantitatively to the increased hepatic synthesis of albumin, and lipid levels have been found to be inversely correlated to both albumin concentration and oncotic pressure in adults with the nephrotic syndrome. Prolonged hypercholesterolemia, particularly when associated with a low value of high-density lipoprotein and high values of low-density lipoprotein, has the potential to accelerate atherogenesis and coronary artery disease. There is, however, considerable controversy as to how serious a problem this is, particularly since the length of time the patient is hyperlipidemic is usally limited. Treatment of the hypercholesterolemia of the nephrotic syndrome is also difficult and often unsatisfactory. Clofibrate may result in a modest diminution of total serum cholesterol levels; however, when prescribed in the usual dosage, it is often associated with unacceptable muscle tenderness and sometimes frank muscle necrosis. This is due to the fact that clofibrate is highly bound to plasma albumin, and in the presence of hypoalbuminemia, increased levels of the free drug accumulate. Dose levels one-half to one-third the usual may avoid this complication. Oral cholestyramine may reduce plasma cholesterol levels but may also lead to aggravation of vitamin D deficiency state, and it has not been used extensively. The value of a high intake of fish oils has not been tested.

Acquired Immunodeficiency

Patients with nephrotic syndrome may occasionally develop severe acquired immunoglobulin G deficiency. They may also lose complement factors for normal opsonization of bacteria in the urine and may have other associated defects of cell-mediated immunity. These abnormalities may predispose patients with nephrotic syndrome to an increased prevalence of infection. Infections with gram-positive and gram-negative encapsuled organisms appear to be most common. Spontaneous bacterial peritonitis may occur in the child with severe nephrotic syndrome, and in the preantibiotic era such infections were a major cause of death. Episodes of peritonitis are commonly related to infection with pneumococci or *Klebsiella*. Pneumococcal vaccine may be indicated in susceptible populations suffering from severe nephrotic syndrome of long duration. Viral infections are generally well tolerated in the nephrotic patient. The concomitant use of glucocorticoids and cytotoxic drugs may expose nephrotic patients to an increased incidence and severity of certain infections, particularly viral infections, such as measles, chicken pox, herpes zoster, and cytomegalovirus. Fatal cases of measles and chicken pox have been described in nephrotic children who have been treated with cyclophosphamide.

Thrombotic Tendency

The risk of thromboembolic complications in patients with nephrotic syndrome is among the highest observed in medicine. Nephrotic syndrome is a hypercoagulable state characterized by a series of alterations to the normally delicately balanced coagulation and anticoagulation mechanisms (see Table 2).

For years it was believed that renal vein thrombosis was a cause of nephrotic syndrome. This is no longer considered true; rather, it is the hypocoagulability induced by the nephrotic syndrome that predisposes to renal vein thrombosis. Deep venous thrombosis is clearly more frequent and nephrotic patients are clearly at greater risk from pulmonary infarction as a result of venous emboli from the kidneys and legs. For reasons that are yet to be adequately explained, renal vein thrombosis is particularly common when the nephrotic syndrome follows membranous nephropathy as membranoproliferative glomerulonephritis. In a patient with nephrotic syndrome the onset of flank pain, macroscopic hematuria, pleuritic chest pain, unexplained deterioration of renal function, or other evidence of thromboembolism is certainly an indication for renal venography. When a clearly defined episode of renal vein thrombosis and pulmonary embolism has occurred, long-term anticoagulation therapy with heparin followed by Coumadin is definitely indicated. In these cases anticoagulation should probably continue for as long as the patient is nephrotic. Streptokinase and urokinase have also been used successfully to lyse renal vein thrombosis; however, experience with these agents is limited.

Renal vein thrombosis may also develop in the absence of clinical symptoms. Despite the obvious potential danger of such an asymptomatic thrombosis, most nephrologists do not recommend routine venography for all patients at risk, and neither is routine anticoagulation recommended for patients with nephrotic syndrome.

ACUTE RENAL FAILURE: CONSERVATIVE NONDIALYTIC MANAGEMENT

JOEL D. KOPPLE, M.D.

Patients with acute renal failure have widely varying abnormalities in metabolic and nutritional status. Some patients show no evidence of negative nitrogen balance and have normal hydration, plasma electrolyte concentrations, and acid–base status. These patients usually have no severe catabolic underlying illnesses and they are not oliguric. The cause of their acute renal failure is typically an isolated, noncatabolic event such as the administration of radiocontrast dye or aminoglycosides. However, most patients have some degree of negative nitrogen balance and have altered fluid, electrolyte, or acid–base status. There is often overhydration, azotemia, hyperkalemia, hyperphosphatemia, hypocalcemia, hyperuricemia, and a metabolic acidosis with a large anion gap.

The net protein degradation in acute renal failure can be massive, with net losses of 150 to 200 g of protein per day or more. Patients are more likely to be catabolic when the acute renal failure is caused by shock, sepsis, or rhabdomyolysis. Enhanced net protein degradation can accelerate the rate of rise in plasma potassium, phosphorus, and nitrogenous metabolites and the fall in blood pH. In nonuremic humans, wasting and malnutrition may impair normal wound healing and immune function and increase morbidity and mortality. It is therefore likely that the profound catabolic status of many patients with acute renal failure increases their risk of delayed wound healing and infection, prolongs convalescence, and increases mortality. In my experience, patients who have acute renal failure caused by shock or sepsis and who are unable to receive adequate nutrition via the gastrointestinal tract have an 80 to 85 percent mortality rate.

A number of studies have evaluated the role of parenteral nutrition in the management of patients with acute renal failure. Patients have usually received mixtures of the nine essential amino acids, with or without nonessential amino acids, and dextrose, fat emulsions, vitamins, and minerals. The average total amino acid intake in these studies has varied from as little as 16 g per day to approximately 70 to 100 g per day. Some investigators have provided rather small quantities of calories while others have tried to match or exceed daily energy expenditure. The results of these studies have been conflicting. Some but not all reports have suggested that total parenteral nutrition (TPN) may decrease the magnitude of negative nitrogen balance and improve the survival of patients. The essential amino acid preparations are reported to decrease serum urea nitrogen (SUN) levels or the urea nitrogen appearance (UNA, net urea generation); not all studies have confirmed these results. There are also conflicting data from animal studies as to whether parenteral nutrition can accelerate the rate of recovery of renal function. The discrepant results from these studies are probably due to the following factors:

1. The clinical course of patients with acute renal failure is so complex and variable that large numbers of patients may need to be studied to show statistically significant improvement with nutritional therapy.
2. Many studies were retrospective or not randomly controlled. This may have led to unintentional biases in the results.
3. The prospective studies of parenteral nutrition in patients with acute renal failure have compared different types of nutritional therapy (e.g., hypertonic glucose with amino acids versus hypertonic glucose without amino acids; essential amino acids versus mixtures of essential and nonessential amino acids). No prospective study has compared the response in patients receiving nutritional therapy with the results in patients receiving no energy or amino acids.
4. It is probable that catabolic patients with acute renal failure may need both good nutrition and metabolic intervention to suppress catabolic processes and promote anabolism. Pharmacologic agents, not yet developed, may be necessary to improve the ability of these patients to utilize nutrients.
5. The optimal nutrient composition of the TPN infusates has not been defined, and the use of suboptimal preparations of nutrients may reduce the clinical benefits of nutritional therapy.

From the available data, it is not possible to recommend a definitive nutritional regimen for patients with acute renal failure. The following therapeutic approach is based upon my analysis of the literature and personal experience.

USE OF THE UREA NITROGEN APPEARANCE

The amount of amino acids to be prescribed for a patient with renal failure can be determined from the patient's UNA. The UNA is a simple, inexpensive, and accurate measure of net protein breakdown (degradation minus synthesis). The usefulness of the UNA is based on the fact that urea is the major nitrogenous product of protein and amino acid metabolism, and that the UNA usually correlates closely with total nitrogen output. UNA is calculated as follows:

$$\text{UNA} = \text{urinary UN} + \text{dialysate UN} + \text{change in body UN}$$

$$\text{Change in body UN} = (\text{SUN}_f - \text{SUN}_i) \times \text{BW}_i \times 0.60\ \text{L per kilogram} + (\text{BW}_f - \text{BW}_i) \times \text{SUN}_f \times 1.0\ \text{L per kilogram}$$

Where UNA and UN are given in grams per day, i and f are the initial and final values for the period of measurement, SUN is serum urea nitrogen (grams per liter), BW is body weight (kilograms), 0.60 is an estimate of the fraction of body weight that is water, and 1.0 is the volume of distribution of urea in the weight gain or loss. Usually, the period of measurement of the UNA and the change in body urea nitrogen is either 24 hours or, in patients undergoing frequent dialysis, the interdialytic interval.

The estimated proportion of body weight which is water may be increased in patients who are edematous or lean and decreased in individuals who are obese or infants. Changes in body weight during the period of measurement of UNA are assumed to be due entirely to changes in body water. In patients undergoing hemodialysis or intermittent peritoneal dialysis, the urea concentration in dialysate is low and difficult to measure accurately; hence, UNA is usually calculated during the interdialytic interval and then extrapolated to 24-hour periods.

In my experience, the relationship between UNA and total nitrogen output in chronically uremic patients not undergoing dialysis is as follows:

$$\text{Total nitrogen output} = 0.97\ \text{UNA} + 1.93$$

where total nitrogen output and UNA are expressed in grams per day. If the individual is in more or less neutral nitrogen balance, the UNA will also correlate closely with nitrogen intake; nitrogen intake may be increased by approximately 0.5 g per day to adjust for unmeasured losses through skin, respiration, and flatus. Pregnancy, large protein losses such as are found in the nephrotic syndrome or with peritoneal dialysis, and acidosis in individuals with sufficient kidney function to excrete large quantities of ammonia may cause the UNA to underestimate total nitrogen intake or output. In general, the UNA will underestimate total nitrogen output by an amount equal to the nitrogen content of the lost protein or ammonia nitrogen.

Sargent and Gotch have developed a technique for assessing UNA in hemodialysis patients which is based on the SUN and body weight at the beginning of two consecutive hemodialyses and at the end of the first dialysis. From these data—the residual renal function, the mass transfer characteristics of the dialyzer, the blood and dialysate flow rates, and the duration of the hemodialysis procedure—the net urea generation can be calculated.

Although this technique is useful, it requires a somewhat complicated computer program for calculation, and, in my preliminary experience, it does not appear to offer significant advantages over the method described here.

AMINO ACID AND PROTEIN INTAKE

A typical composition for TPN solutions in adult patients with acute renal failure is shown in Table 1. Two of the most controversial issues regarding the nutritional management of patients with acute renal failure are the quantity of nitrogen and the composition of the amino acid preparations that are administered enterally or parenterally. Some nephrologists infuse only small quantities of the nine essential amino acids, with arginine sometimes added. Others have recommended mixtures of larger amounts of essential and nonessential amino acids.

The use of essential amino acid solutions is reported to reduce the UNA, the SUN, and possibly the serum potassium or phosphorus level; to ameliorate uremic toxicity; and to reduce the need for dialysis treatments. The larger quantities of essential and nonessential amino acids may be more effective at improving nitrogen balance, but the UNA is often much greater, and the need for dialysis treatments may be increased. Some nephrologists have the impression that for the same quantity of nitrogen infused, the essential amino acids may be used more efficiently than mixtures of essential and nonessential amino acids. There is also no clear-cut evidence that TPN with the essential amino acids reduces morbidity or mortality more than does TPN with essential and nonessential amino acids; however, current data do indicate that morbidity and mortality are not greater with essential amino acid solutions.

My method for selecting the quantity and type of amino acids or protein to be given to the patient with acute renal failure is as follows: Patients are prescribed a low dietary or intravenous nitrogen intake if there is a low rate of UNA (i.e., 4 to 5 g of nitrogen per day or less), no evidence of severe protein malnutrition, and the anticipation that the patient will recover renal function within the next 1 to 2 weeks. A severely reduced glomerular filtration rate (GFR) and the desire to avoid dialysis therapy are other factors that suggest the use of a low nitrogen intake. Under these conditions, one may use 0.55 to 0.60 g of protein per kilogram per day of primarily high-quality protein, or lower quantities of protein supplemented with essential amino acids or keto acids (as will be discussed). At least 35 mg per kilogram per day of this protein should be of high biologic value. This diet may be particularly well tolerated if the patient has a residual GFR of about 4 to 15 ml per minute. Alternatively, the essential amino acids may be given, since they seem to be utilized more efficiently. In the latter case, one may prescribe a diet providing 0.04 to 0.30 g per kilogram per day of protein of miscellaneous quality (about 3 to 21 g per day) supplemented with 0.20 to 0.30 g per kilogram per day of the nine essential amino acids (approximately 14 to 20 g per day). The lowest quantities of protein are prescribed for the patients who have the most severe renal failure (i.e., GFR less than 3 to 4 ml per minute) and who are not very catabolic. Much of this small quantity of protein is provided in the high-calorie, low-protein foodstuffs that are the source of most of the energy intake. In clinically stable, chronically uremic patients who are not undergoing dialysis therapy and who have a low UNA, these diets should maintain neutral or near neutral nitrogen balance. Where available, ketoacid or hydroxyacid formulations may be substituted for the essential amino acids. This may further increase the efficiency of nitrogen utilization. Patients who are unable to receive oral or enteral nutrition may be given 0.30 to 0.50 g per kilogram (about 21 to 30 g per day) of essential amino acids intravenously, with or without arginine. No more than 40 g per day of the essential amino acids are given. These regimens should minimize the rate of accumulation of nitrogenous metabolites and, unless the patient is severely catabolic, will usually maintain neutral or only mildly negative nitrogen balance. Hence, the need for dialysis therapy may be minimized or avoided.

I prescribe a higher nitrogen intake, up to 1.0 to 1.2 g per kilogram per day of protein or amino acids, for those patients who are more catabolic and have a higher UNA (>5 g of nitrogen per day) or are severely wasted, are undergoing regular dialysis therapy, and either have or are anticipated to have acute renal failure for more than 2 weeks. When protein is administered orally or enterally, at least 50 percent should be of high biologic value. In comparison to small quantities of amino acids, these larger nitrogen intakes may improve nitrogen balance. However, the UNA will almost invariably rise, and the increased azotemia and—in those patients receiving TPN—the large volume of fluid necessary to provide this amount of amino acids may increase the requirements for dialysis. Patients with greater residual renal function, higher fluid tolerance, and a healthy cardiorespiratory system usually are more tolerant of these larger nitrogen and water intakes. With the appropriate use of dialysis or intermittent or continuous arterial-venous hemofiltration, these higher nitrogen intakes are well tolerated by most patients.

When renal failure persists for more than 2 to 3 weeks, patients undergoing regular dialysis treatment are treated, as are maintenance dialysis patients, with about 1.0 to 1.2 g per kilogram per day of protein or amino acids for maintenance intermittent hemodialysis and 1.2 to 1.5 g per kilogram per day for maintenance intermittent or continuous ambulatory peritoneal dialysis (see the chapter *Peritoneal Dialysis*). At least 50 percent of the protein should be of high biologic value.

The optimal amino acid composition for enteral or parenteral nutrition in acute renal failure has not been established. As indicated above, there is some evidence that when nitrogen intake is very low, provision of the nine essential amino acids alone (histidine, isoleucine, leucine, lysine, methionine, phenylalanine, threonine, tryptophan, and valine) may be the more efficient treatment and may result in a lower UNA and more positive nitrogen balance for any level of nitrogen intake.

The proportion of each of the essential amino acids traditionally has been designed according to the recom-

TABLE 1 Composition of Total Parenteral Nutrition for Adult Patients with Acute Renal Failure

Intake[a]	*Quantity*
Energy [b]	35–50 kcal/kg/day
70% dextrose (D-glucose)(500 ml)	350 g/L
Essential and nonessential amino acids (4.25–5.0%) [c] *or*	42.5–50 g/L
Essential amino acids (5.0%)[c]	12.5–25 g/L
Electrolytes[d]	
Sodium[e]	40–50 mEq/L
Chloride[e]	25–35 mEq/L
Potassium	≤ 35 mEq/day
Acetate[e]	35–40 mEq/L
Calcium	10 mEq/day
Phosphorus	8 mmol/day
Magnesium	8 mEq/day
Iron	1.0 mg/day
Other trace elements[f]	See text
Vitamins	
Niacin	20 mg/day
Thiamin HCl (B_1)	2 mg/day
Riboflavin (B_2)	2 mg/day
Pantothenic acid	10 mg/day
Pyridoxine HCl (B_6)	10 mg/day
Ascorbic acid (C)	60–100 mg/day
Biotin	200 mg/day
Folic acid[g]	1 mg/day
Vitamin B_{12}[g]	3 μg/day
Vitamin A	See text[h]
Vitamin D	See text[i]
Vitamin K[g]	10 mg/week
Vitamin E	10 IU/day[j]

Note: These recommendations should be considered tentative. The composition and volume of the infusate may be modified if patients are volume overloaded, very uremic, or acidotic; if serum electrolyte concentrations are not normal or relatively constant; or if dialysis therapy is not readily available.

[a] The nutrients listed below are added to each 1-L bottle containing crystalline amino acids and 70% dextrose, except for the vitamins and trace elements, which should be added to only one bottle per day. The total volume per bottle will usually be slightly greater than 1 L because of the electrolyte and vitamin additives.

[b] Energy intake (including calories derived from amino acids) is usually maintained at 35–50 kcal/kg/day; add 70% dextrose and lipids to attain this level. The dextrose in parenteral solutions is provided as dextrose monohydrate. The energy thus provided by dextrose monohydrate is approximately 3.4 kcal/g, for amino acids, it is about 3.5 kcal/g. Infuse 25–50 g/day of lipids to prevent essential fatty acid deficiency and to produce more balanced sources of fuel substrates. A 20% lipid emulsion provides the most fat calories per milliliter of water (2.0 kcal/ml). A total of 1.5–2.5 L/day of TPN solutions may be necessary to provide sufficient amino acids and energy. The fluid load necessary to provide this quantity of amino acids, lipids, and dextrose increases the need for dialysis, hemofiltration, ultrafiltration, or CAVH.

[c] Usually, when the UNA is greater than 5 g N/day, 1.0 g/kg/day of essential and nonessential amino acids is given. If the UNA is 4–5 g N/day or less, 0.30 to 0.50 g/kg/day of essential amino acids may be administered. No more than 30–40 g/day of essential amino acids (without nonessential amino acids) are given. See text for a more detailed discussion of the amounts and types of amino acid preparations administered. The prescribed amino acids often may be provided in less than 500 ml of solution, and the volume of 70% dextrose may be increased to bring the volume up to one liter and to provide additional calories.

[d] The amounts of electrolytes intrinsically present in the amino acid solutions should be considered.

[e] Refers to final concentration of electrolytes after any extra 70% dextrose has been added.

[f] Patients receiving TPN for more than 7 to 14 days may need zinc (up to 5 mg/day), copper (up to 0.5 mg/day), and other trace elements (see text).

[g] Given orally or parenterally and not in the TPN solution because of antagonisms.

[h] Vitamin A should be avoided unless TPN is continued for more than several weeks.

[i] Currently, 1,25-dihydroxycholecalciferol is not commercially available for parenteral administration.

[j] May need to be increased with use of lipid emulsions.

mended daily allowances for each of the amino acids as defined by Rose. More recently, some investigators have recommended increasing the proportion of the branched-chain amino acids and reducing the content of some of the other essential amino acids. With higher nitrogen intakes (greater than 5 to 6 g nitrogen per day) it is important to give both essential and nonessential amino acids. Patients who receive large quantities of amino acids (i.e., greater than 40 g per day) have a nutritional requirement for nonessential amino acids, particularly for the urea cycle amino acids such as arginine. The reason is that a large intake of essential amino acids with no nonessentials can lead to severe alterations in the plasma amino acid pattern and to hyperammonemia.

There is evidence, still not conclusive, that the three branched-chain amino acids (isoleucine, leucine, and valine) may have a specific anabolic effect in acutely ill patients without renal failure. If this effect is also present in acute renal failure, it may justify giving a larger proportion of the nitrogen in the form of branched-chain amino acids. The plasma concentrations of the branched-chain amino acids tend to be decreased in acute renal failure, which may be another reason for giving them in larger proportions. These observations suggest that for the essential and nonessential amino acid mixtures, it may be preferable to give a high ratio of essential to nonessential amino acids (e.g., 3:1 or 4:1). The three branched-chain amino acids may account for 40 to 50 percent of the essential amino acids in this preparation. These formulations of essential and nonessential amino acids are not currently available in the United States. More research is clearly necessary to examine the role of such preparations in patients with acute renal failute. When I administer TPN providing essential and nonessential amino acids I currently use preparations that contain essential to nonessential amino acids for uremic patients, in a ratio of 1:1 to 2:1. Mixtures of these essential and nonessential amino acids may be combined with commercially available essential amino acid solutions to obtain a higher essential: nonessential ratio; however, such preparations are costly and have not been tested in cases of acute renal failure.

ORAL OR ENTERAL VERSUS PARENTERAL NUTRITION

For patients who are able to obtain nutrition by eating or by enteral tube feeding, it is usually preferable to provide nutrition in this way rather than intravenously. Parenteral nutrition can be more hazardous, provides greater fluid loads, and is more costly. However, many patients with acute renal failure are obtunded, severely ill, or debilitated. In these patients, the risk of aspiration of food or enteral feeding preparations is very great, and parenteral nutrition may be safer. The recent development of a technique for the percutaneous insertion of a gastrostomy tube may reduce the risk of enteral feeding in some debilitated or severely ill patients.

There are liquid protein or chemically defined (elemental) preparations for patients who must be nourished by enteral tube or gastrostomy. Since amino acids seem to be utilized more efficiently than protein, I am inclined to use them rather than protein for patients in whom it is important to reduce the UNA and avoid dialysis therapy. As indicated above, experimental data indicate that when patients receive large quantities of amino acids (greater than 40 gm per day), they require nonessential as well as essential amino acids. If patients are receiving frequent dialysis therapy or if their GFR is sufficiently great that they do not need dialysis, there may be no advantage to using amino acids instead of high-quality protein.

Patients are given parenteral nutrition when they are unable to receive nutrients safely via the enteral tract. In general, TPN is started as soon as it is determined that the patient has acute renal failure and is unable to receive enteral nutrition. This treatment strategy differs from that recommended for other acutely ill patients in whom TPN usually is begun after it is determined that the patient will not be able to receive enteral nutrition for a defined number of days, usually about 7. This difference in treatment strategy is based upon suggestive evidence that parenteral nutrition may improve survival in patients with acute renal failure, if it is started early. The total quantity of nitrogen and the proportion of individual amino acids to be administered should be determined as described previously and in Table 1.

ENERGY, VITAMINS, AND MINERALS

Since patients with acute renal failure are usually in negative nitrogen balance, I tend to employ large quantities of calories to minimize net protein breakdown. There is no easy way to estimate the energy requirements for patients with acute renal failure; I therefore empirically administer 35 to 50 kcal per kilogram per day. The higher energy intakes (i.e., 50 kcal per kilogram per day) are used for patients who have a higher UNA, who tend to be severely ill, and who are not very obese. If nitrogen balance, determined by the difference between the patient's nitrogen intake and the nitrogen output calculated from the UNA, is negative, I try to provide an energy intake close to 50 kcal per kilogram per day. Recently, indirect calorimetry has been used to estimate energy expenditure in acutely ill patients with renal failure. In this case, the daily energy requirement is determined by multiplying basal energy expenditure by 1.25. Most researchers believe that there is little nutritional advantage to administering more than 50 kcal per kilogram per day to catabolic patients. Moreover, with high energy intakes, the large quantity of carbon dioxide produced from the infused carbohydrate and fat can cause hypercapnia if pulmonary function is impaired.

Since most patients with acute renal failure do not tolerate large water intakes, glucose is usually administered in a 70 percent solution. The glucose and amino acid solutions are mixed so that the amino acids and energy are provided simultaneously (see Table 1). Patients receiving TPN for more than 5 to 7 days should receive lipid emulsions. Preferably 50 to 100 gm per day of lipids should be infused daily, but no less than twice weekly to prevent essential fatty acid deficiency and to balance the energy sources. Ten percent and 20 percent lipid emulsions are available. They are approximately isotonic with plasma and provide 1.1 and 2.0 kcal per milliliter, respectively. By comparison, 70 percent dextrose (the dextrose is provided as D-glucose monohydrate) yields about 2.38 kcal per milliliter and is the parenteral solution that gives the most calories per milliliter. I rely on dextrose as the major source of calories because dextrose is the primary energy source for several tissues and is well utilized by virtually all tissues. Also, 70 percent dextrose is much less expensive per calorie than are lipid emulsions, and hyperglycemia is readily treated with insulin. For these reasons, in acutely uremic patients receiving parenteral nutrition, glucose is used as the major source of calories, and lipids are given daily, but in lesser amounts.

The vitamins and minerals recommended for TPN are shown in Table 1. For patients receiving enteral nutrition, similar quantities of minerals and vitamins can be used. The recommended intake of minerals is tentative and must be adjusted according to the clinical status of the patient. If the serum concentration of an electrolyte is increased, it may be advisable to reduce the quantity infused or not to administer it at the onset of parenteral nutrition. The patient must be monitored closely, however, because the hormonal and metabolic changes that often occur with initiation of TPN may cause the serum electrolytes to fall rapidly. This is particularly likely with serum potassium and phosphorus. On the other hand, a low concentration of a mineral may indicate that there is a need for a greater than usual intake of that element. Again, metabolic changes and the patient's low GFR can lead to a rapid rise in the serum level during repletion.

Trace element requirements in acute renal failure are not defined. At present, I add 1.0 mg per day of iron to TPN solutions. Other trace elements may be given, including zinc, up to 5 mg per day, and copper, up to 0.5 mg per day. When trace elements are given to patients with acute renal failure, blood concentrations must be carefully monitored to ensure that excess levels do not occur.

Vitamin requirements have not been well defined for patients with acute renal failure. Much of the recommended intake is based on information obtained from studies in chronically uremic patients, normal individuals, or nonuremic acutely ill patients. Vitamin A is probably best avoided because in chronic renal failure, serum vitamin A levels are elevated and small doses of vitamin A have been reported to cause toxicity in uremic patients. Also, since most patients with acute renal failure will receive TPN for only a few days or weeks, it is unlikely that a deficiency will occur for this fat-soluble vitamin.

The nutritional requirement for vitamin D in patients with acute renal failure has not been defined. Although vitamin D is fat soluble and vitamin stores should not become depleted during the few days to weeks that most patients with acute renal failure receive TPN, the turnover of its most active analogue, 1,25-dihydroxycholecalciferol, is much faster. This may indicate that there is a need for this analogue in patients with acute renal failure. At the present time, a parenteral preparation of 1,25-dihydroxycholecalciferol is not commercially available. Although vitamin K is fat-soluble, vitamin K deficiency has been reported in some nonuremic patients who were not eating and were receiving antibiotics. Vitamin K supplements are therefore given routinely to patients receiving TPN (see Table 1). Ten mg per day of pyridoxine hydrochloride (8.2 mg per day of pyridoxine) are recommended because studies in patients undergoing maintenance hemodialysis indicate that this quantity may be necessary to prevent or correct vitamin B_6 deficiency. Patients should probably not receive more than 60 to 100 mg per day of ascorbic acid because of the risk of increased serum oxalate concentrations.

It must be recognized that the nutrient intake of patients with acute renal failure must be carefully reevaluated each day and sometimes more frequently. This is particularly important for these patients because they may undergo rapid changes in their clinical and metabolic condition.

PERIPHERAL OR SUPPLEMENTAL PARENTERAL NUTRITION, ANABOLIC HORMONES

Parenteral nutrition through a peripheral vein avoids the problems of inserting a catheter into the inferior vena cava and is safer. There are several limitations to peripheral parenteral nutrition. First, the osmolality of the infusate must be restricted to about 600 mOsm per kilogram H_2O to reduce the risk of thrombophlebitis. Since the osmolality with typical TPN solutions is approximately 1,800 mOsm per kilogram H_2O, to reduce tonicity of the infusates it is necessary to use a larger volume of fluid and/or a lower intake of nutrients. Second, the needles or catheters must be changed frequently, usually every 18 to 48 hours to prevent thrombophlebitis. Heparin, 500 units per liter, and cortisol, 5 mg per liter, may reduce the risk of thrombophlebitis and allow the patient to receive somewhat more hypertonic solutions (e.g., about 900 mOsm) and to extend the duration that the catheter can be left in a peripheral vein.

Some patients with acute renal failure are able to ingest or be tube fed only part of their daily nutritional requirements. Peripheral infusions may enable these patients to receive adequate nutrition without resorting to TPN. In the latter cases it is often most practical to infuse 8.5 to 10 percent amino acids or 20 percent lipid emulsions into a peripheral vein and administer as much as possible of other essential nutrients, including carbohydrates, through the enteral tract. The peripheral vascular accesses used for hemodialysis can also be used for parenteral nutrition. However, this technique probably increases the hazard of thrombophlebitis and infection, and it should not be used in patients who will need a hemodialysis access for extended periods.

Parenteral nutrition has been administered with continuous arteriovenous hemofiltration (CAVH) to provide intravenous nutrition and, at the same time, control the water and mineral balance and reduce the accumulation of metabolic products from the infused nutrients or from endogenous substrates. Large amounts of water, minerals, urea, and other metabolites can be removed by CAVH. On the other hand, the quantity of glucose, amino acids and protein lost during CAVH is small, even when patients are receiving parenteral nutrition. Hence, it is often easier to administer adequate amino acids and energy to patients with acute renal failure when they undergo CAVH. CAVH may reduce the frequency with which hemodialysis is needed in patients with acute renal failure.

In patients who have marginally adequate intakes, supplemental amino acids and glucose may be given during hemodialysis treatment. Some nephrologists infuse 20 or 30 g of the nine essential amino acids at the end of dialysis therapy. However, since most patients who need nutritional supplements have decreased intake of energy and total nitrogen, I give 40 to 42 g of essential and nonessential amino acids and 200 g of D-glucose (150 g of D-glucose if dialysate contains glucose). This preparation is infused into the blood leaving the dialyzer at a constant rate throughout the dialysis procedure to minimize disruption of the amino acid and glucose pools which occurs with hemodialysis. Patients who have low serum concentrations of phosphorus or potassium at the start of the dialysis treatment may need supplements of these minerals. With such infusions, plasma amino acids and glucose do not fall during dialysis and over 85 percent of the infused amino acids are retained. The infusion is not stopped until the end of hemodialysis. Also, the patient should eat some carbohydrate 20 to 30 minutes before the end of the infusion. Otherwise, the infusion must be tapered or a peripheral infusion of glucose must be started to prevent reactive hypoglycemia.

Intravenous nutrition that is given only during hemodialysis is probably inadequate for stressed acutely uremic patients because their oral or enteral intake is usually very low, their nutritional needs are high, and the nutritional supplements are given only intermittently, when the patient receives hemodialysis treatment. It is possible that intravenous nutrition during hemodialysis may be of value only for patients who have a daily nutritional intake that is slightly suboptimal.

Insulin and anabolic steroids have been used to reduce the UNA and improve nitrogen balance in acutely ill patients, including those with acute renal failure. Although some studies indicate that these hormones have an anabolic effect, other studies have failed to confirm this. The therapeutic value of these hormones for promoting anabolism in catabolic patients with acute renal failure is not established.

DIALYTIC MANAGEMENT OF ACUTE RENAL FAILURE

ROBERT O. BERKSETH, M.D.
CARL M. KJELLSTRAND, M.D., F.A.C.P.

INTRODUCTION AND NEED FOR ACUTE DIALYSIS

Approximately 30 patients per million population per year require dialysis for acute renal failure (ARF). Fifty percent of them die; of the other half, almost all regain normal renal function. More than two-thirds of all cases of ARF occur in hospitals as a result of catastrophic medical or surgical disease, and thus many are iatrogenic. These patients are critically ill and require enormous personnel investment for a short time. A mean of four dialyses is necessary per patient. Less than one percent develop chronic renal failure and need continued dialysis.

INDICATIONS AND TIMING OF DIALYSIS

Dialysis can ameliorate uremia, correct acid-base and electrolyte abnormalities, and remove excess fluid. Ideally dialysis is initiated early and provided frequently. This minimizes fluctuations in serum chemistries and facilitates fluid removal obligate from intravenous antibiotics and hyperalimentation. Typically the indications for dialysis are multiple and include uremia, fluid overload and acid-base and electrolyte abnormalities. Fluid and electrolyte disturbances provide the clearest indications for dialysis. Pulmonary edema, a rapidly rising serum potassium, or a rapidly falling serum bicarbonate is easily diagnosed and treated with dialysis. The time to initiate dialysis for uremia alone is uncertain.

Although the knowledge of uremic toxins remains rudimentary, blood urea nitrogen (BUN) levels are easy to measure, available everywhere, and widely used for numerical estimates of toxicity. Predialysis BUN (pre-BUN), postdialysis (post-BUN), and mean BUN levels are governed by the following equations:

(1) BUN-production = BUN-removal (at steady state)
= (pre-BUN − post-BUN) × total body water
(2) pre-BUN − post-BUN + post-BUN
= mean BUN level 2
= BUN production × fraction time dialysis
dialyzer BUN clearance is used

Using such equations, one can at least begin to discuss when, how often, and with what efficiency dialysis should be used to effectively influence the uremic state in patients with ARF. Solving these equations by using the following example: a 70-kg patient, having a total body water of 42 L, a protein catabolic rate of 70 g per day (urea nitrogen appearance 11.5 g per day) and dialyzer clearance of urea of 150 ml per minute utilized 4 hours every other day gives the following result; mean concentration of blood of BUN = 64 mg per deciliter; pre- and post-BUN levels equal 91 and 37 mg per deciliter. The same results are obtained by using the same patients, but doubling protein catabolic rate and at the same time using dialysis 4 hours daily. Such calculations suggest that starting dialysis at a BUN level of approximately 90 ml per deciliter is reasonable. Daily or every-other-day treatment should then be used to keep the mean BUN level below 60 mg per deciliter and the fall of BUN during dialysis to less than 50 mg per deciliter.

CHOICE OF DIALYSIS METHOD

Four dialysis methods are avialable for patients who develop ARF: intermittent hemodialysis (IHD), continuous peritoneal dialysis (CPD), intermittent peritoneal dialysis (IPD), and slow continuous hemofiltration (SCHF). Several studies comparing survival between peritoneal and hemodialysis for ARF show no difference. Reliable survival statistics for SCHF are unavailable, as this method has only recently been introduced to clinical medicine.

For most patients with ARF, IHD is the treatment method of choice; it is very effective in controlling uremia and rapidly corrects the electrolyte, acid-base, and fluid imbalances. Hemodialysis facilitates patient surveillance and allows more time for other diagnostic and therapeutic procedures. For the patient with a contaminated abdominal cavity, peritoneal dialysis offers the advantages of mechanical removal of devitalized contaminated tissue and irrigation with antibiotic solutions. For patients with cardiovascular instability or severe brain trauma, CPD or SCHF is best; both minimize cardiac stress and cerebral edema from solute removal. In a given patient one method may be best at one time, but a different method best later on. An unstable patient should be started on CPD or SCHF and switched to intermittent hemodialysis when ready to be mobilized.

Hemodialysis

Blood Access

There are three blood accesses available for patients needing hemodialysis for ARF: (1) the Scribner shunt and its variations, (2) the intermittent femoral vein puncture method, and (3) the subclavian catheter.

The *Scribner shunt* has many advantages. There are no immediate life-threatening complications associated with its placement. Once in place it takes only minutes to initiate or discontinue dialysis. Between dialyses it can be used for blood sampling, and it is probably the safest route for hyperalimentation. Its main disadvantage is that it destroys a peripheral vessel site, but this is usually of little consequence for these acutely ill patients. Skilled surgeons can place this access in less than one hour. In critically ill patients it may be done at the bedside.

Intermittent femoral vein catheterization is also an excellent method of blood access. Life-threatening complications are puncture of the inferior vena cava and femoral vein thrombosis with pulmonary emboli. The first can be avoided by caution when placing the guide, the second by never leaving catheters in place more than 24 hours. It takes more physician and nursing time to place catheters repeatedly, as this should be done under sterile conditions. A trained team should be able to have a patient on dialysis 30 minutes after notification. Once the patient can be mobilized, the disadvantages of femoral catheters increase because of the need of compression at the puncture site for hours after the catheters have been removed. We prefer femoral catheters for emergency dialysis, but thereafter prefer other methods.

Catheterization of the subclavian vein is an extremely convenient method of blood access. It has the greatest number of potentially lethal complications, which include pneumothorax, hemothorax, subclavian vein thrombosis, air emboli, and sepsis. However, it can be used immediately after placement and requires little personnel time. There is no interference with mobilization or transport of the patient. It is probably the access of choice for those who have great skill in its placement.

Dialysis Equipment

There is little to distinguish between the various disposable dialyzer cartridges now available. All are small, convenient, safe, and reasonably inexpensive. A variety of membrane surface areas are available. Plate dialyzers are easiest to anticoagulate. Some of the new hollow fiber kidneys may need no anticoagulation. The hollow fibers are advantageous because there is minimal compliance, which limits variation in priming volume with negative pressure.

There is no particular advantage of one dialysate delivery system over others. Some new models provide variable sodium concentrations, which may prove effective in smoothing out osmolality shifts that may contribute to the side effects of dialysis.

The dialysate should have the same ion concentration as extracellular fluid. In particular, hyponatremic dialysate should never be used. Potassium is varied according to the patient's blood potassium. In some instances, particularly in patients with lactic acidosis, it may be necessary to use bicarbonate rather than acetate-containing dialysate. Bottle peritoneal dialysis fluid contains lactate as base source and cannot be used in these patients. Some patients who are intensely dialyzed may need phosphorus supplementation.

Side Effects of Hemodialysis and Their Treatment

The main side effects of acute hemodialysis of clinical concern are hypotension and cardiac arrhythmias. The pathogenesis, mediators, and pathophysiology are poorly understood and multifactorial, and treatment thus is unsatisfactory and controversial. Figure 1 summarizes these mechanisms and possible treatments are listed in Table 1. If significant problems are encountered with intermittent hemodialysis, it should be replaced by an alternative dialysis method.

Anticoagulation

Heparin remains the mainstay anticoagulation for intermittent hemodialysis. In the patient at risk of bleeding, such as those newly operated on, those who soon will be operated on, or patients with ongoing bleeding or pericarditis, low-dose continuous heparin infusion should be applied. It is much easier and safer than the simuataneous use of heparin and protamine regional heparinization. With low-dose heparin infusion, heparin is diluted in normal saline, an infusion of 30 units per minute is started during the first 5 minutes of dialysis, and the rate is then reduced to 15 units per minute. Repeated ac-

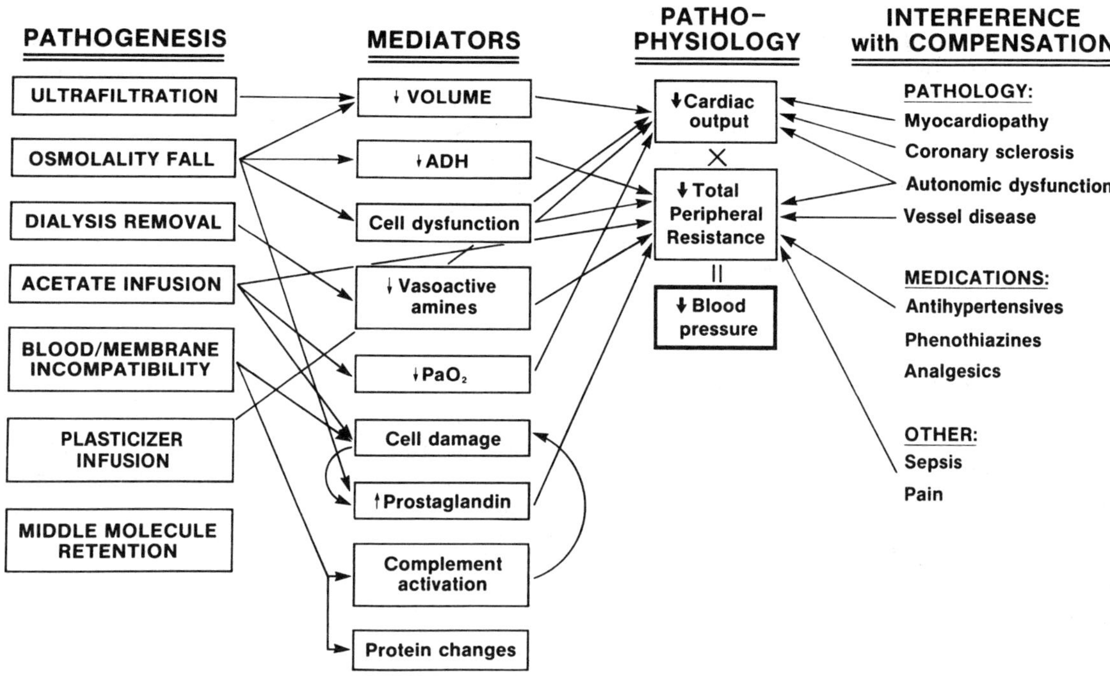

Figure 1 Known or hypothesized factors involved in dialysis hypotension. (From Kjellstrand C et al. Acute renal failure. In: Drukker W. Parson FM, and Maher JH, eds. Replacement of renal function. 2nd ed. The Netherlands: Martinus Nijhoff, 1983).

tuated clotting times, should be done and prevented from rising more than 50 percent over normal values by varying the rate of infusion. No more than 1,500 to 4,000 units of heparin should be required during dialysis.

In some of the new hollow fiber dialyzers containing cellulose acetate, dialysis can be done in bleeding patients without anticoagulation. Every 20 to 30 minutes the dialyzer is flushed with 200 ml normal saline, which is then removed by ultrafiltration.

Recently prostacyclin, sodium citrate, ticlopidine, sabexate mesilate, and heparinoids have been used for anticoagulation during dialysis. The latter methods have so far not received widespread application. The mainstay of anticoagulation for the patient at risk of bleeding remains low-dose continuous heparin infusion, as already outlined.

Immediate neutralization of remaining heparin can be achieved by giving the patient an intravenous injection of protamine sulfate slowly over 30 minutes when

TABLE 1 Treatment of Hypotension During Acute Hemodialysis

Treatment	*Dosage*
Nasal oxygen	6 L/min
Intravenous active osmols	Mannitol 1 g (5.5mOsm) per kg body weight the first two dialyses then 0.5 g per kg the next two dialyses slowly infused IV during entire dialysis. NaCI 3–5% solution infused IV entire dialysis 160 mg (5.5 mOsm) per kg body weight.
Increase dialysate calcium (if PO_4 is controlled only)	
HCO_3 instead of acetate dialysate	
Vasoactive amines	Metaraminol 1 mg IV STAT when necessary or Slow continuous intravenous infusion of approximately 1 mg per kg per dialysis
25% Albumin intravenously	Based on serum albumin level 50–200 ml
Cool blood in venous return line from dialyzer	To 35°C
Slow dialysis-efficiency	To 2–3 ml per kg per min BUN clearance
More frequent, slower dialysis	
Sequential dialysis and ultrafiltration	Each, every other day
If many problems, switch technique	Continuous slow hemofiltration technique

the dialysis is completed. The dose in milligrams of protamine is derived by dividing the total amount of heparin given during dialysis by 200.

Advantages and Disadvantages of Hemodialysis

The greatest advantage of hemodialysis is its efficiency. The patient's therapy last only 4 hours every day, or every other day. The remaining time can be used for other diagnostic and therapeutic interventions. Hemodialysis is also the method that is most readily available for such patients. The major disadvantages of hemodialysis are its negative influence on cardiovascular stability and the need for anticoagulation. Many of the problems can be avoided by tailoring the procedure's efficiency to body size and applying many of the methods already described. However, in the desperately ill patient it is not the method of choice. Once the patient stabilizes, it allows for better mobilization than other procedures. The need for heparinization is a minor problem that can be avoided by minimal infusion heparinization. In the patient with severe brain trauma, the rapidity of solute removal correlates with edema and increased brain dysfunction.

Continuous or Intermittent Peritoneal Dialysis

Studies comparing mortality rates in patients with ARF treated by peritoneal or hemodialysis have shown no difference. Peritoneal dialysis is contraindicated in patients with a contaminated abdominal wall or those with severe disruption of the peritoneal space (e.g., patients who have had operations for aortic aneurysms).

With the advent of continuous peritoneal dialysis, there is no need for intermittent peritoneal dialysis in ARF. The main risk of peritoneal dialysis, peritonitis, is probably no different between the two methods. Two-liter peritoneal dialysate exchanges every 3 hours offer approximately the same clearance as a 4-hour hemodialysis every other day. When beginning peritoneal dialysis, one may have to use more frequent exchanges to quickly regulate electrolyte abnormalities or to bring a very high BUN level down to reasonable limits in a reasonable time. Once this has been achieved and the BUN controlled, 2-liter exchanges every 3 hours will give the same mean BUN as 4-hour hemodialysis every other day.

Access

Access to peritoneal dialysis can be gained percutaneously with a stiff Teflon catheter or through a minilaparotomy using soft Silastic catheters. The first method is inferior. There is a risk of perforation of intra-abdominal organs and more problems with fluid drainage. The soft Tenckhoff-Silastic catheter is better.

Advantages and Disadvantages of Peritoneal Dialysis

The greatest advantage of peritoneal dialysis is that is does not cause, or contribute to, cardiovascular instability. For the patient in shock or with serious cardiac arrhythmias, the procedure is the best treatment, and is rivaled only by slow continuous hemofiltration. It is also the best method for patients with severe brain trauma because it does not cause or increase brain edema. In the patient with a contaminated abdominal cavity, the mechanical cleansing has a beneficial effect. The absence of any systemic heparin efects, even if heparin is added to the dialysate, is an advantage in the patient at risk of bleeding.

The main disadvantage of the procedure is its relative inefficiency in solute removal. It may not be able to control uremia in the hypercatabolic patient. It limits movement of the patient, and this problem, together with the elevation of the diaphragm, increases the risk of pulmonary complications. The patient with compromised pulmonary function is better off with other dialysis methods. It cannot be used in the patient with a contaminated abdominal wall or the patient with the disrupted retroperitoneal space (kidney operations, aortic aneurysm operations). It is difficult or impossible to do in patients who have had many previous abdominal operations.

Slow Continuous Hemofiltration

This method for treatment of ARF is under clinical investigation and has locally replaced intermittent hemodialysis as the most common method. Hemofilters are attached to the patient's blood stream through a Scribner shunt or special femoral arterial and venous catheters. The only driving force for filtration is the patient's blood pressure, to which can be added negative hydrostatic pressure by having the filtrate collection bag lower than the patient. No complicated machinery is needed. Heparin is continuously infused at the rate of 10 units per kilogram per hour on the arterial inlet side to the filter. The ultrafiltrate is replaced by sterile electrolyte-glucose fluid on the venous line to the patient. Filtration rates (and thus also BUN and creatinine clearance) are usually between 10 and 20 ml per minute. A filtration rate of 12.5 ml per minute gives the same mean BUN level as every-other-day 4-hour intermittent hemodialysis with a BUN clearance of 150 ml per minute.

Access

The arterial-venous access should be used. Thus, the only two possible accesses are the Scribner shunt or special catheters placed in the femoral artery and the femoral vein. The latter catheters are dangerous and we believe, therefore, that the only acceptable access is the Scribner shunt. If vein-to-vein hemofiltration is used, a blood pump is necessary and thus airleak detectors will be necessary.

Advantages and Disadvantages of Slow Continuous Hemofiltration

The greatest advantage of slow continuous hemofiltration is that it causes no cardiovascular embarrassment. Unlike CPD, this procedure does not cause peritonitis. Because of the large volumes removed from and replaced to the patient (21 L per day), hyperalimentation is easy to perform and fluid balance is easy to achieve in patients on slow continuous hemofiltration. No complicated equipment is necessary for the procedure. Only the shunt, the filter, the urine collection bag, and infusion apparatus for heparin and the intravenous replacement solution are necessary.

Disadvantages of the procedure are (1) the need for continuous heparinization (although the hourly heparin requirement is probably less than that for hemodialysis), (2) the need for large volumes of sterile replacement fluid (3 liters of 1.5 percent dialysate solution with additions can be used), and (3) the commitment of nursing time is considerable, as accurate intake and output record-keeping and calculations are necessary to avoid the potential catastrophe of sudden (1 L per hour) fluid imbalance. Patients on slow continuous hemofiltration are difficult to mobilize or transport for other diagnostic and therapeutic procedures. The filter, heparin infusion, and replacement fluid bag are bulky and difficult to move.

CAUSES OF DEATH AND WAYS TO IMPROVE MORTALITY

The causes of death in dialyzed patients with acute renal failure are outlined in Table 2.

Infections are the leading cause of death in 30 to 70 percent of patients with acute renal failure. They are frequently secondary to surgical complications. Patients on dialysis may not manifest the usual temperature and white blood cell response to bacterial infections. The increase in band neutrophils, however, is often preserved. Acute uremia compromises immune defenses, as do malnutrition (common in these patients) and major surgery. A high index of suspicion, frequent clinical examinations, and liberal use of x-ray studies, ultrasonography, and scanning procedures as well as often-repeated cultures, are necessary to detect the infections in time to effectively treat them. Prophylaxis consists of early mobilization and removal of all indwelling lines such as bladder, central venous pressure, and pulmonary artery catheters once they have fulfilled their mission of easing the stabilization of a patient.

As many as 30 to 90 percent of patients who experience ARF after surgery have neglected surgical complications such as abscesses, leaking suture lines, gastrointestinal perforations, or necrosis. Clinical signs are often vague or absent and are therefore difficult to diagnose. In addition, surgeons are sometimes reluctant to reoperate on these desperately ill patients, feeling that they are too sick. On the contrary, however, it has been aptly stated that "these patients are invariably too ill to be denied an operation."

In many patients, malnutrition contributes to the patient's demise. Few patients now die of gastrointestinal bleeding secondary to stress, of pulmonary emboli, or of technical dialysis complications. Possible ways to decrease mortality in these patients are clinical alertness and extensive surveillance for infections, early surgical intervention and hyperalimentation, and selected use of the three dialysis procedures already described.

TABLE 2 Causes of Death

Causes	*Percentage of Deaths*
Infections	30–70
Myocardial infarct, heart failure	5–30
Gastrointestinal hemorrhage	5–30
Pulmonary emboli	1–5
Central nervous system dysfunction	<1
Technical	<1

ROUTINE MEDICATIONS AND USE OF MEDICATION IN DIALYZED PATIENTS

Antacids and cimetidine should be used routinely in these patients. Their use has decreased the previous high incidence of stress ulcer. Aluminum hydroxide gel, 15 to 30 ml every 6 hours, should be given diluted in saline or with 20 percent sorbitol to avoid medication bezoar. With them should be mixed nystatin, 100,000 to 400,000 units, to prevent fungal opportunistic infections. Anabolic steroids, such as nandrolone phenpropionate, 100 mg IM weekly, increase protein anabolic rate at least in females. Once the patient has been stabilized hyperalimentation should be employed if the patient cannot eat. Because of the fluid load associated with the procedure, it is necessary to use one of the continuous dialysis methods or daily intermittent hemodialysis.

Before any drug is employed in patients with ARF, existing monographs and review articles must be consulted. Many drugs are metabolized through the kidneys, some are eliminated by dialysis, and both hepatic metabolism and protein binding may be changed in these patients.

SUMMARY AND CONCLUSION

Most patients who need dialysis for ARF suffer from acute tubular necrosis which is often iatrogenic. Treatment consists of early and frequent use of intermittent hemodialysis or continuous peritineal dialysis or slow continuous hemofiltration. Intermittent hemodialysis allows more time for other therapeutic and diagnostic procedures, facilitates early mobilization, and most rapidly corrects electrolytes and fluid abnormalities. The main disadvantage is cardiovascular embarrassment, particularly hypotension. The slow continuous methods (CPD, SCHF) have the advantage of the absence of hypotension or arrhythmias. Their main drawback is that they restrict patients to bed.

Infections and neglected surgical complications are the main causes of death in dialysis patients with acute renal failure. They are difficult to diagnose and require extensive clinical experience and effective surveillance. Most patients either expire or recover clinically normal renal function within 2 to 3 weeks.

CHRONIC RENAL FAILURE: NUTRITIONAL AND NONDIALYTIC MANAGEMENT

JOEL D. KOPPLE, M.D.

Nutritional therapy for patients with chronic renal failure has three major goals. These are (1) to retard the rate of progression of renal failure (in the nondialyzed patient), (2) to maintain good nutritional status, and (3) to prevent or improve the uremic syndrome. A reduction in the intake of certain nutrients may retard the progression of renal disease and, in patients with advanced renal failure, reduce uremic toxicity. However, there is much evidence that many patients undergoing maintenance dialysis have wasting and malnutrition. The wasting is usually mild or moderate, but frequently it can be severe. Since in the Western world maintenance dialysis therapy is readily available, it is more advisable to provide a diet for a patient with renal failure that maintains good nutritional status than to prescribe a nutritional therapy that may reduce uremic toxicity at the expense of inducing malnutrition. A proposed recommended intake for adult uremic patients and patients undergoing maintenance hemodialysis or continuous ambulatory peritoneal dialysis (CAPD) is shown in Table 1.

Note: When the recommended nutrient intake is given in terms of kilograms of body weight, this refers to the Metropolitan Life Insurance's desirable body weight, expressed according to the age, height, sex, and frame size of the patient.

Monitoring Nitrogen Intake: Urea Nitrogen Appearance and the Serum Urea Nitrogen to Serum Creatinine Ratio

It is important to ensure that the dietary protein intake in patients with renal failure is neither too low nor too high. Thus, it is of value to estimate accurately a patient's actual nitrogen intake. Since urea is the major nitrogenous product of protein and amino acid metabolism, the urea nitrogen appearance (UNA, net urea generation) usually correlates closely with, and can be used to estimate, total nitrogen output. UNA is calculated as follows:

UNA = urinary urea nitrogen (UN) + dialysate UN + change in body UN

Change in body UN = $(SUN_f - SUN_i) \times BW_i \times$ 0.60 L per kilogram + $(BW_f - BW_i) \times SUN_f \times$ 1.0 L per kilogram

Where UNA and UN are given in grams per day, i and f are the initial and final values for the period of measurement, SUN is serum urea nitrogen (g per liter), and BW is body weight (kg). The fraction of body weight that is water is represented by 0.60. Greater or lesser numbers may be used depending on whether the patient is lean, edematous, obese, old, or young. The assumption is made that in a uremic patient any change in BW occurring during a 1 to 3 day interval is attributable to accrual or to loss of water. Therefore, the fraction of weight change that represents gain or loss of water is taken as 1.0.

In our experience, the relationship between UNA and total nitrogen output in chronically uremic patients not undergoing dialysis is as follows:

Total nitrogen output (g per day) = 0.97 UNA (g per day) + 1.93 (g per day).

Since protein contains about 16 percent nitrogen, the relation between UNA and net protein breakdown in these patients can be estimated from the following equation:

Net protein breakdown (g per day)=6.1 UNA (g per day) + 12 (g per day)

If patients are in neutral balance, this same equation can be used to estimate protein intake; about 3.0 g per day of protein may be added to the value to adjust for unmeasured nitrogen losses.

In nondialyzed patients with chronic renal failure, there is a direct correlation between the ratio of the serum urea nitrogen (SUN) to the serum creatinine and the protein intake. This relationship can be used to estimate daily protein intake or, conversely, to select the optimal quantity of protein to be prescribed for a patient. Although this technique is easy to use and fairly accurate, several factors may reduce its usefulness. A urine flow less than 1,500 ml per day may increase the SUN:serum creatinine ratio for a given protein intake because, in contrast to the creatinine clearance, the urea clearance tends to fall progressively as urine flow decreases below this level. The SUN:serum creatinine ratio increases with catabolic stress and with reduced muscle mass, as is found in women, children, and very wasted men. Also, with a change in dietary protein, a period of 2 to 3 weeks may be necessary for the SUN to stabilize and the SUN:serum creatinine ratio to reflect the new protein intake. In clinically stable, chronically uremic men with a protein intake of 20, 40, or 60 g per day, the SUN:serum creatinine ratio should be, on an average, 3.4, 6.0, and 8.6, respectively.

Protein Intake

A number of studies in both rats and humans with renal insufficiency indicate that a diet low in protein and phosphorus may retard the rate of progression of renal failure. This effect has been observed not only in patients with advanced renal failure, but also in those with mild-to-moderate renal failure (serum creatinine values of 2 to 6 mg per deciliter). Although each of the studies carried out in humans suffers from weaknesses in experimental design, almost all reports indicate that in some patients such diets may retard progression of renal failure. The most dramatic effects have been reported with ketoacid- and hydroxyacid-supplemented diets. There are several ketoacid and hydroxyacid formulations currently in use. They usually provide four essential amino acids (histidine, lysine, threonine, and tryptophan) and the ketoacid or hydroxyacid salts of the other five essential amino acids. The ketoacids and hydroxyacids have the same structure as the respective essential amino acids except that the alpha-amino nitrogen is removed and a keto or hydroxy group is substituted.

Chronic Renal Disease with GFR Greater Than 70 ml Per Minute Per 1.73 Meters Squared

Most studies of the effects of diets low in protein and phosphorus on the rate of progression of renal failure have examined patients with moderately advanced to advanced renal failure (serum creatinine$\geq$5 mg per deciliter). Hence, there is virtually no information concerning the optimal dietary protein (or phosphorus) prescription for patients with chronic renal disease and mild impairment in renal function. Until more information is available, it is recommended that protein (and phosphorus) intake should be restricted for patients with GFR greater than 70 ml per minute per 1.73 meters squared only if there is evidence that renal function is continuing to decline. In this latter case, the patient is treated as indicated in the following paragraph.

Chronic Renal Disease with GFR 5 to 70 ml Per Minute Per 1.73 Meters Squared

It is the author's policy to discuss with the patient the evidence that low protein, low phosphorus diets may retard progression and to indicate that the data, although not conclusive, are strong enough to justify the patient ingesting a restricted protein and phosphorus diet. If the patient agrees to dietary treatment, the patient is prescribed a diet providing about 0.60 to 0.70 g protein per kilogram per day. At least 0.35 g per kilogram per day of the protein should be high biologic value (eggs, meat, fish and milk and its products, because these proteins contain a high proportion of essential amino acids that are present roughly in the proportions required by humans. Hence, these proteins are utilized more efficiently than are proteins of lower quality. On the other hand, low quality proteins, which are prevalent in foods derived from plants (e.g., grains and vegetables), are particularly valuable for increasing the palatability and acceptability of the diet. At least 12 to 16 g per day of low-quality protein seem to be necessary for a palatable diet. An intake of 0.55 to 0.60 g protein per kilogram per day provides about 30 to 35 g per day for women and small men and about 40 g per day for normal sized men. In general, we do not prescribe more than about 45 g per day of protein for any patient with a GFR below 10 ml per minute. In clinically stable patients, the SUN can almost always be maintained below 90 mg per deciliter with these low protein diets until the GFR falls below 4 to 5 ml per minute. This amount of protein should maintain neutral or positive nitrogen balance and should not be excessively burdensome for most patients.

Amino acid- and ketoacid-supplemented diets may also be offered to the patient. Currently, these diets generally provide about 0.28 g protein per kilogram per day (16 to 20 g protein per day) supplemented with about 10 to 20 g of the essential amino acids or mixtures of essential amino acids and ketoacids. Since the amino acid and ketoacid supplements provide sufficient essential amino acids, the protein derived from food does not have to be of high biologic value, thereby increasing the patient's freedom of food selection. In the author's experience, most, but not all, patients seem to prefer the 0.55 to 0.60 g protein per kilogram per day diet over the essential amino acid-supplemented diet. This former diet is less expensive than is the essential amino acid-supplemented diet.

There are several potential advantages to using amino acid or ketoacid formulations. First, with more advanced renal failure (i.e., GFR $<$ 15 to 25 ml per minute per 1.73 meters squared), potentially toxic products of nitrogen metabolism begin to accumulate in increasing quantities. Since the ketoacids and hydroxyacids lack the alpha-amino group, for the same intake of amino acid equivalents less nitrogen is provided and there is less generation of potentially toxic nitrogenous compounds. Second, because the amino acid and ketoacid preparations do not contain phosphorus (or potassium), the content of these elements in the diet can be markedly decreased (see section on recommended phosphorus intake). Third, by modifying the proportions of individual amino acids, ketoacids, or hydroxyacids in the diet, it may be possible to normalize more of the altered plasma and muscle-amino acid concentrations that develop in advanced renal failure—whether this normalization is of value to the patient is not yet established. Finally, as indicated above, these semisynthetic diets may be more effective at retarding the rate of progression of renal failure.

Given the dramatic results described with certain ketoacid formulations, it would seem reasonable that when the GFR decreases to about 25 ml per minute per 1.73 meters squared, patients should be prescribed a diet providing 0.28 protein per kilogram per day supplemented with a mixture of about 13 to 18 g of ketoacids and amino acids, if the formulation is available. Ketoacid supplements have not yet been approved for clinical use in the United States. Where ketoacids are not available, essential amino acid supplements may be substituted for the ketoacid mixture or patients may be prescribed 0.55 to 0.60 g protein per kilogram per day with at least 0.35 kg per kilogram per day of protein of high biologic value. All three of these diets generally maintain neutral or positive nitrogen balance and generate a low UNA. The protein content of each of the diets prescribed for patients with mild-to-severe renal failure should be increased by 1.0 g per day of high biologic value protein for each gram of protein excreted in the urine each day. Whether the ketoacid- or essential amino acid-supplemented very-low-protein diets should be prescribed for patients with a GFR above 25 ml per minute per 1.73 meters squared is not known.

When the GFR falls below 5 ml per minute per 1.73 meters squared, there is no conclusive evidence that patients fare as well with low nitrogen diets as with regular

TABLE 1 Recommended Daily Intakes for Nondialyzed Patients with Chronic Renal Failure and Patients Undergoing Maintenance Hemodialysis or Continuous Ambulatory Peritoneal Dialysis

	*Chronic Renal Failure**†	*Hemodialysis (HD) and Continuous Ambulatory (CAPD) or Cyclic Peritoneal Dialysis (CCPD)*
Protein‡	0.55–0.60 g/kg/day (≥35 g/kg/day high biologic value); maximum intake is 45 g/day Very-low-protein diet (about 0.28 g/kg/day of protein of any biologic value) supplemented with either a ketoacid and amino acid mixture or essential amino acid mixture	HD: 1.0–1.2 g/kg/day; ≥ 50% high biologic value protein; 1.2 g//kg/day is prescribed unless patient has normal protein status with intakes of 1.0–1.1 g protein/kg/day CAPD: CCPD: 1.2–1.3 g/kg/day; ≥50% high biologic value protein; for malnourished patients, up to 1.5 g/kg/day may be given
Calories§	≥35 Kcal/kg/day unless the patient's relative body weight is >120%	
Fat (% of total calorie intake)**††	40–55	40–55
Polyunsaturated:saturated fatty acid ration††	1.0:1.0	1.0:1.0
Carbohydrate‡‡	Rest of nonprotein calories	Rest of nonprotein calories
Total fiber intake††	20–25 g/day	20–25 g/day
Minerals		
Sodium	1,000 to 3,000 mg/day§§	750 to 1,000 mg/day§§
Potassium	40 to 70 mEq/day	40 to 70 mEq/day
Phosphorus	4 to 12 mg/kg/day***	8 to 17 mg/kg/day***
Calcium	1,400 to 1,600 mg/day†††	1,400 to 1,600 mg/day†††
Magnesium	200 to 300 mg/day	200 to 300 mg/day
Iron	10 to 18 mg/day‡‡‡	10 to 18 mg/day‡‡‡
Zinc	15 mg/day	15 mg/day
Water	Up to 3,000 ml/day as tolerated§§	Usually 750 to 1,500 ml/day§§

Vitamin supplements	Diets to be supplemented with these quantities	
Thiamin	1.5 mg/day	1.5 mg/day
Riboflavin	1.8 mg/day	1.8 mg/day
Pantothenic Acid	5 mg/day	5 mg/day
Niacin	20 mg/day	20 mg/day
Pyridoxine HCI	5 mg/day	10 mg/day
Vitamin B_{12}	3 μg/day	3 μg/day
Folic Acid	1 mg/day	1 mg/day
Vitamin A	None	None
Vitamin D	See text	See text
Vitamin E	15 IU/day	15 IU/day
Vitamin K	None§§§	None§§§

* GFR > 4–5 ml/min and ≤ 700 ml/min/1.73 meters squared.
† When recommended intake is expressed per kg body weight, this refers to the patient's desirable weight as determined from the Metropolitan Life Insurance tables.
‡ The protein intake is increased by 1.0 g/day of high biologic value protein for each g/day of urinary protein loss.
§ This includes energy intake from dialysate in CAPD and CCPD patients.
** Refers to percent of total energy intake (diet plus dialysate).
†† These dietary recommendations are considered less crucial than the others.
‡‡ Should be primarily complex carbohydrates, if tolerated by the patient.
§§ Can be higher in nondialyzed chronic renal failure or maintenance dialysis patients who have greater urinary losses or in CAPD or CCPD patients.
*** Phosphorus intake should be 4–9 mg/day for patients ingesting a very-low-protein diet supplemented with ketoacids or amino acids; with the 0.55–0.60 g protein/kg/day diet, a phosphorus intake of 8–12 mg/kg/day is more tolerable. Phosphate binders are usually needed as well (see text).
††† Dietary intake must be supplemented to provide these levels.
‡‡‡ ≥10 mg/day for males and nonmenstruating females; ≥18 mg/day for menstruating females.
§§§ Vitamin K supplements may be needed in those who are not eating and are receiving antibiotics.

dialysis therapy and higher protein intakes. Since these latter patients may be at high risk for wasting or malnutrition, it is recommended that maintenance dialysis treatment or renal transplantation should be inaugurated at this time. Patients with diabetes mellitus may develop uremic symptoms at a higher GFR; thus, such individuals are often started on maintenance dialysis or undergo renal transplantation when their GFR is between 5 and 10 ml per minute per 1.73 meters squared.

Adherence to low-protein, low-phosphorus diets requires a major change in dietary habits and even in lifestyle. Prior to beginning dietary therapy, the patient and, if possible, close family members or other participants in his or her support network must be informed of the magnitude of this undertaking and must agree to the commitment. Otherwise, there is small likelihood that the patient will adhere successfully to his dietary prescription. prescription.

Maintenance Dialysis Therapy

Patients undergoing hemodialysis 3 times per week should receive a minimum of 1.0 and preferably 1.2 g of protein per kilogram per day (Table 1). Patients undergoing CAPD should receive 1.2 to 1.3 g per kilogram per day of protein. In malnourished CAPD patients, up to 1.5 g protein per kilogram per day can be taken. At least half of their dietary protein should be of high biologic value.

Energy Intake

Studies of energy expenditure in nondialyzed chronically uremic patients and patients undergoing maintenance hemodialysis indicate that energy expenditure is normal during resting and sitting, following ingestion of a standard meal, and with graded exercise. Nitrogen balance studies in nondialyzed chronically uremic patients indicate that the amount of energy necessary to ensure neutral or positive nitrogen balance is approximately 35 Kcal per kilogram per day. However, virtually every survey of energy intake in nondialyzed chronically uremic and hemodialysis patients indicates that, on average, it is lower than this level and usually 30 Kcal per kilogram per day or less.

We currently recommend that nondialyzed chronically uremic patients and patients undergoing maintenance hemodialysis or CAPD should receive about 35 Kcal per kilogram per day. Patients who are obese with an edema-free body weight greater than 120 percent of desirable body weight may be treated with lower calorie intakes. There are many commercially available high-calorie foodstuffs that are low in protein, sodium, and potassium. A nephrology dietitian can recommend these foodstuffs as well as other low-protein high-calorie foods that can be prepared easily at home.

Hyperlipidemia

A large proportion of chronically uremic and dialysis patients have type IV hyperlipoproteinemia with elevated serum triglyceride levels and a low serum HDL cholesterol. Since in uremic patients these alterations in serum lipoproteins may contribute to the high incidence of atherosclerosis and cardiovascular disease, attention has been directed toward reducing serum triglycerides and increasing HDL cholesterol. Elevated serum triglyceride levels in uremia appear to be caused primarily by impaired clearance from blood. Also, since diets in renal failure are usually restricted in protein, sodium, potassium, and water, it is often difficult to provide sufficient energy without resorting to a large intake of purified sugars, which can increase triglyceride production. Serum triglycerides may be lowered by feeding a diet in which the carbohydrate content is reduced to supply 35 percent of calories, the fat content is increased to provide 50 to 55 percent of calories, and the polyunsaturated : saturated fatty acid ratio is raised to 1:1.

Although elevated serum triglyceride levels do not appear to be a strong risk factor for arteriosclerotic disease, this dietary treatment should be employed at least for uremic patients with markedly elevated serum triglyceride levels (e.g., greater than 1.5 to 2.0 times the upper limits of normal). L-carnitine, 1.0 g per day orally, may also decrease serum triglyceride concentrations, and patients with this magnitude of hypertriglyceridemia who have low serum carnitine should probably also be given a trial period with this compound. Low serum HDL-cholesterol levels are a strong risk factor for cardiovascular disease. Serum concentrations may increase with daily exercise.

Mineral and Water Intake

Sodium and Water

As renal failure progresses, both the glomerular filtration and fractional reabsorption of sodium fall progressively. Thus, sodium balance is usually well maintained in patients with chronic renal failure when they ingest a normal salt intake. However, there is an impaired ability to handle both a sodium load and to conserve sodium normally during intake of a low-sodium diet. Normally, only about 1 to 3 mEq per day of sodium are excreted in the feces, and in the non-sweating individual, only a few mEq per day of sodium are lost through the skin. If sodium intake exceeds the ability of the kidney to excrete sodium, sodium and water retention, hypertension, edema, and congestive heart failure may develop. Certain conditions predispose to sodium retention and may dictate earlier restriction of sodium or water intake or the use of diuretic agents. These conditions include congestive heart failure and advanced liver disease. When the GFR falls below 4 to 10 ml per minute, the ability to handle even a normal sodium intake may fall. In addition, in renal failure, hypertension may be more easily controlled with sodium restriction and may be accentuated with normal or increased sodium intakes. On the other hand, if sodium intake is not sufficient to replace obligatory renal sodium losses, sodium depletion and contraction of extracellular fluid volume may occur and may lead to reduced renal blood flow and further impairment of GFR. Hence, when evaluating patients with renal failure who do not have evidence of fluid overload or hypertension, they should be given a careful trial of sodium loading to assess whether renal function may be improved.

In general, if sodium balance is well controlled, the patient's thirst adequately controls water balance. However, when the GFR falls below 2 to 5 ml per minute, the water intake often must be controlled independently of sodium to prevent overhydration. In diabetics, hyperglycemia may increase thirst and enhance positive water balance. In patients whose total body water is at the desired level, urine excretion may be a good guide to water intake. Daily water intake should equal the urine output plus approximately 500 ml to adjust for insensible losses.

Most nondialyzed chronically uremic patients maintain sodium and water balance with an intake of 1,000 to 3,000 mg of sodium per day and 600 to 3,000 ml of fluid per day. However, the requirement for sodium and water varies markedly, and each patient must be managed individually. Usually, patients undergoing maintenance hemodialysis or peritoneal dialysis are severely oliguric or anuric. For hemodialysis patients, sodium and total fluid intake generally should be restricted to 1,000 to 1,500 mg per day and 700 to 1,500 ml per day, respectively. Patients undergoing CAPD usually tolerate a greater sodium and water intake because salt and water can be easily removed by using hypertonic dialysate. By maintaining a larger dietary sodium and water intake, the quantity of fluid removed from the CAPD patient and, hence, the daily dialysate volume can be increased. This may be advantageous since with CAPD, the daily clearance of small molecules is directly related to the volume of dialysate outflow. With this in mind, some nephrologists have recommended a larger dietary sodium and water intake for CAPD patients in order to increase the hypertonic dialysate and thus increase dialysate outflow. This treatment may be undesirable for obese or hypertriglyceridemic patients because of the greater need for hypertonic glucose exchanges that increase the glucose load. Also, there is the potential disadvantage that some patients may become hibituated to high salt and water intakes; if they are changed to hemodialysis therapy, they may have difficulty curtailing ingestion of sodium and water.

One way to monitor sodium requirements in nondialyzed patients is to follow carefully the body weight, blood pressure, and serum sodium. When sodium intake is inadequate, there is often negative water balance, a decrease in body weight, and a fall in blood pressure. Excessive sodium intake is often associated with positive water balance, a rise in body weight, and an increase in blood pressure. Serum sodium concentrations may rise, fall, or not change depending upon the water balance. On the other hand, a decrease in serum sodium in the presence of an unchanging or falling body weight usually indicates that there is a need for more sodium. The dietary sodium requirement may also be determined by decreasing or raising sodium intake for several days and monitoring body weight, blood pressure, appearance of edema, serum creatinine or clearance, serum sodium, and urinary sodium output. The optimal dietary sodium can be assessed by comparing the effects of the sodium intake on excess water gain or loss, the blood pressure, and the creatinine clearance.

In nondialyzed chronically uremic patients or patients undergoing maintenance dialysis who gain excessive sodium or water despite attempts at dietary restriction, furosemide may be used to increase urinary sodium and water excretion.

Potassium

Most patients who have nonoliguric advanced renal failure or who are undergoing maintenance dialysis can tolerate up to 70 mEq of potassium per day without hyperkalemia. Patients with hyporeninemic hypoaldosteronism, however, may be intolerant to this amount of potassium unless they are given a mineralocorticoid, such as 9-alpha-fluorohydrocortisone. In some patients who are given this mineralocorticoid, sodium retention with hypertension or congestive heart failure may occur. In susceptible patients, this usually can be prevented by administering a diuretic simultaneously with the mineralocorticoid.

Phosphorus

It is important to restrict phosphorus intake to prevent or to minimize hyperparathyroidism and possibly to retard the rate of progression of renal failure (as already discussed). The degree to which dietary phosphorus should be reduced is not well established. Clearly, phosphorus restriction should be employed to keep serum phosphorus within normal levels. However, some nephrologists have questioned whether in order to prevent or to ameliorate hyperparathyroidism, the phosphorus intake should be reduced to maintain a normal renal tubular reabsorption of phosphorus; this would require a very low phosphorus intake. The restriction of phosphorus intake that may be necessary to retard the progression of renal failure is not known. The phosphorus intake can be reduced to 300 to 500 mg per day with the essential amino acid- or ketoacid-supplemented very-low-protein diets. One small clinical trial suggests that a prescribed phosphorus intake of 6.5 mg per kilogram per day will slow progression more than an intake of 12 mg per kilogram per day.

Until more information is available, it seems prudent to use a combination of dietary phosphorus restriction and chemical binders of phosphate to maintain the morning serum phosphorus concentrations well within the normal range. Since there is a rough correlation between the protein and phosphorus content of the diet, it is easier to restrict phosphorus if protein intake is reduced. With a 0.55 to 0.60 g per kilogram per day protein diet, phosphorus intake can be decreased to 10 to 12 mg per kilogram per day and sometimes to as low as 8 mg per kilogram per day. This level of dietary phosphorus restriction usually does not maintain serum phosphorus levels within normal limits in patients with a GFR under about 15 ml per minute, and phosphate binders are therefore also employed.

Formerly, the two most commonly used phosphate binders were aluminum carbonate and aluminum hydroxide. Usually, 2 to 4 capsules are taken 3 to 4 times per day as needed. Greater doses may be used if necessary. Recent evidence that aluminum-induced osteomalacia is causally related to the total lifetime dose of aluminum phosphate binders has made many nephrologists reluctant to use them. However, the hazards of severe uncontrolled hyperparathyroidism would seem to outweigh the potential dangers of aluminum-induced osteomalacia. Thus, if serum phosphorus levels cannot be maintained within normal limits by diet alone, phosphate binders are used.

Several nonaluminum phosphate binders are now being investigated. Calcium carbonate and calcium citrate both appear to bind phosphate effectively. These calcium binders can be given in divided doses with meals and should not be given unless the serum phosphorus level is normal in order to avoid precipitation of calcium phosphate in soft tissues. Thus, hyperphosphatemic patients may be treated with an aluminum binder of phosphate until serum phosphorus falls to normal. At that time, they may be changed to calcium carbonate or calcium citrate. Normally, patients should probably not receive more than about 5.0 g per day of calcium carbonate or 8.3 g per day of calcium citrate (about 2.0 g per day of elemental calcium in soft tissues. Calcium carbonate also may counteract the metabolic acidosis frequently found in patients with renal failure. Calcium citrate may be advantageous for the same reason, since the citrate may be metabolized to generate bicarbonate.

As previously indicated, since the essential amino acid and ketoacid supplements do not contain phosphorus, one advantage to diets providing these formulations with about 0.28 g of protein per kilogram per day is the greater degree to which the phosphorus intake can be reduced, often to as low as 4 to 6 mg per kilogram per day. If future studies confirm that these very low phosphorus intakes are both safe and beneficial for patients with mild, moderate, or severe renal insufficiency, this would provide additional justification for the use of these semisynthetic diets.

Calcium

Patients with chronic renal failure have an increased dietary calcium requirement because there is often both vitamin D deficiency and resistance to the actions of vitamin D. These disorders, which lead to impaired intestinal calcium absorption, are compounded by the low calcium content of diets for uremic patients. A 40 g protein diet, for example, provides only about 300 to 400 mg per day of calcium. Dietary calcium intake is low because many foods that are high in calcium are high in phosphorus (e.g., dairy products) and are therefore restricted for uremic patients.

Chronically uremic patients usually require about 1,200 to 1,600 mg per day of calcium for neutral or positive calcium balance, and the diet, therefore, should be supplemented with elemental calcium. Probably, a good target level for total daily calcium intake (food plus supplemental calcium) is 1,400 to 1,600 mg per day. As indicated, up to 2 g of elemental calcium may be given as calcium salts to bind phosphate. Supplemental calcium therapy should not be initiated unless the serum phosphorus concentration is normal (i.e., 3.5 to 4.5 mg per deciliter) to prevent calcium phosphate deposition in soft tissues. Also, frequent monitoring of serum calcium is important since hypercalcemia may develop, particularly if serum phosphorus should fall to low or low-normal levels. Patients undergoing maintenance hemodialysis or peritoneal dialysis may also require 1.0 g per day of supplemental calcium even though there is net calcium uptake from dialysate.

Calcium comprises 40 percent of calcium carbonate, 24 percent of calcium citrate, 18 percent of calcium lactate, and 9 percent of calcium gluconate. Oral calcium chloride should be avoided in uremic patients because of its acidifying properties. As indicated above, calcium carbonate and calcium citrate have both been shown to be effective intestinal phosphate binders. Several proprietary calcium carbonate or calcium citrate tablets have been given a pleasant flavor and are well accepted.

Magnesium

In chronically uremic patients, there is net absorption from the intestinal tract of about 50 percent of ingested magnesium (net absorption is the difference between dietary intake and fecal excretion). The absorbed magnesium is excreted primarily by the kidney, and in renal failure, hypermagnesemia may occur. However, the restricted diets of uremic patients are low in magnesium (usually about 100 to 300 mg per day for a 40 g protein diet), and their serum magnesium levels are usually normal or only slightly elevated. Clinically significant hypermagnesemia usually occurs only when there are additional sources of magnesium intake such as magnesium-containing antacids and laxatives. The nondialyzed chronically uremic patient requires about 200 mg per day of magnesium to maintain neutral magnesium balance. The optimal dietary magnesium allowance for the dialysis patient has not been defined.

Trace Elements

Increased or decreased tissue levels of many trace elements are often observed in patients with chronic renal failure. Adverse clinical effects have not been identified for most of these disorders. Dietary requirements for trace elements have not been defined for uremic patients. Many trace elements are bound avidly to serum proteins, and when present in dialysate, even in small quantities, they may be taken up in the blood. It is therefore recommended that trace elements be removed routinely from the dialysate prior to use.

Since iron deficiency is common and can cause anemia, chronically uremic and dialysis patients may be given oral iron supplements. Ferrous sulfate, 300 mg 3 times a day after meals, may be used. Patients who do not tolerate this or other oral iron supplements or who have iron deficiency are usually best treated with intramuscular or intravenous iron.

The zinc content of most tissues is normal in renal failure. However, serum and hair zinc may be low, and the red cell zinc is increased. Some reports indicate that dysguesia and impaired sexual function, which occur commonly in renal failure, may be improved by giving patients zinc supplements. There is not yet sufficient evidence that routine zinc supplementation is beneficial; additional studies are clearly indicated. It is probably of value to ensure that patients ingest the recommended dietary allowance for zinc, 15 mg per day.

Increased body burden of aluminum has been implicated in dialysis patients as a cause of a progressive dementia syndrome, osteomalacia, and anemia. Current data suggest that both contamination of dialysate with aluminum and ingestion of aluminum binders of phosphate may contribute to the excess body burden of aluminum. Recent evidence that bone aluminum levels correlate with total lifetime dosage of aluminum binders of phosphate have led many nephrologists to use aluminum binders more sparingly and to rely more upon low phosphorus diets to control serum phosphorus levels. As indicated above, calcium carbonate and calcium citrate have also been used in place of aluminum hydroxide or carbonate to bind phosphate.

Acidosis

Metabolic acidosis is common in nondialyzed patients with chronic renal failure because of the impaired ability of the kidney to excrete acidic metabolites and/or the renal losses of bicarbonate. Acidosis can promote bone reabsorption and many symptoms. Ingestion of low-nitrogen diets may prevent or reduce the severity of the acidosis by decreasing the endogenous generation of acidic products of protein metabolism. Alkali supplements are usually effective for preventing or treating acidosis. Calcium carbonate or calcium citrate may correct mild acidosis and provide needed calcium. In cases of more severe acidosis, sodium bicarbonate or citrate may be administered orally or intravenously. If the nondialyzed uremic patient is not oliguric and is not particularly likely to develop edema, sodium is usually readily excreted when administered as sodium bicarbonate or citrate. Alkali therapy should probably be initiated if the arterial pH is below 7.35 or the serum bicarbonate is less than 20 mEq per liter. Before implementing alkali therapy, it must be ascertained whether the low serum bicarbonate is not a compensatory response to chronic respiratory alkalosis. If acidosis is severe and not controlled by the foregoing measures, hemodialysis or peritoneal dialysis may be employed.

Fiber Intake

A number of studies suggest that dietary fiber intake may lead to a lower incidence of constipation, irritable bowel syndrome, diverticulitis, neoplasia of the colon, and possibly greater glucose tolerance. Since the patient with renal failure also may benefit from fiber intake, we currently prescribe 20 to 25 g per day of total dietary fiber. There are so many more important nutritional restrictions on the dietary intake of the chronically uremic and dialysis patient, however, that we do not insist vigorously that the patients adhere to a high fiber diet.

Vitamin Intake

Unless supplements are given, uremic patients have a tendency to develop deficiency of the water soluble vitamins. Vitamin deficiencies are due to poor intake, altered metabolism (attributable to medicinal intake and, possibly, to uremia per se), or to losses into dialysate. Thus, deficiency of water soluble vitamins tends to occur more frequently in dialysis patients. Vitamin B_{12} deficiency is uncommon in uremia because this vitamin is protein-bound in plasma.

In renal failure, the daily requirements for most vitamins are not well defined. There is evidence that, in addition to vitamin intake from foods, the following daily supplements of vitamins can prevent or correct vitamin deficiency: pyridoxine hydrochloride, 5 mg in nondialyzed patients and 10 mg in hemodialysis or peritoneal dialysis patients; ascorbic acid, 60 mg; folic acid, 1 mg; and the recommended daily allowance for normal individuals for the other water soluble vitamins. High serum oxalate levels have been described in chronically uremic patients given large doses of ascorbic acid; therefore the recommended supplement for vitamin C has been limited to the recommended dietary allowances for healthy adults. Since serum retinol binding protein and vitamin A are elevated, supplemental vitamin A is not recommended. Additional vitamin E and K are probably not necessary. An exception is the patient who receives antibiotics for extended periods of time and who is not ingesting sufficient quantities of vitamin K; such individuals may need supplements of this vitamin. Treatment with vitamin D analogues is discussed in the chapter on renal osteodystrophy.

Some authors have reported that maintenance hemodialysis patients not receiving vitamin supplements may not develop water soluble vitamin deficiencies. They have recommended that vitamin supplements should not be prescribed routinely to maintenance dialysis patients. However, these patients were generally followed for less than 1 year and it is possible that with longer periods of time, the incidence of vitamin deficiency may increase. Poor nutrient intake is common in chronically uremic patients, and recent reports continue to show that many renal failure patients have evidence of vitamin deficiencies. Since water soluble vitamin supplements are safe, it would seem wise to use them routinely until these issues are more completely resolved.

Methods for Attaining Successful Nutritional Therapy

Successful dietary therapy usually requires that the patient make a major change in his lifestyle. The patient must procure special foods, prepare special recipes, usually must forego or severely limit his intake of many favorite foods, and is often compelled to eat foods that he may not desire. There are demands made on the time, the effort, and the emotional support system of his family or close associates.

In order to ensure successful dietary therapy, patients with renal failure must undergo extensive training concerning the principles of nutritional therapy and the design and preparation of diets. Also they need continuous encouragement regarding dietary adherence. They must receive repeated retraining regarding their nutritional therapy, and their dietary intake and nutritional status must be closely monitored. Patients who are not monitored carefully usually do not adhere closely to their diets. They may eat too little rather than too much, particularly when undergoing maintenance dialysis therapy.

A team approach to dietary management is often critical. The team should include the physician, dietitian, close family members, the nursing staff, and, when available, psychiatrists or social workers. The diet plans should be designed specifically for each patient and should take into account his or her individual tastes. At each visit, the physician should discuss dietary intake with the patient. The adequacy of energy and protein intake and nutritional status should be frequently assessed. The dietitian is often the best qualified person to perform anthropometric measurements of nutritional status because of her training, interest in nutritional therapy, and access to the patient. The physician must strongly support the efforts of the dietitian. Generally, the spouse or other close relatives or friends should work closely with the patient to provide moral support and to assist with acquisition and preparation of foods. Nurses, psychiatrists, and social workers can encourage patients and help them work through emotional conflicts that can affect dietary compliance. They are also a valuable source of information concerning the patient's attitude toward dietary therapy, his ability to adhere to the diet, and his actual dietary intake. The important lesson is that if dietary therapy is prescribed to a patient, it requires a major commitment and effort by the patient and the medical staff to attain good results.

The most sensitive, reproducible, and readily available methods for assessing nutritional status in chronically uremic and dialysis patients include the serum albumin and total protein, relative body weight (patient's weight × 100 divided by the body weight of a normal person of the same age, height, and sex), patient's weight expressed as a percentage of his weight prior to his illness, triceps and subscapular skinfold thickness, and midarm muscle circumference or cross-sectional area. Serum transferrin may also be helpful; in my experience, values are usually low even in well-nourished patients with chronic renal failure and decrease further when nalnutrition is present.

HEMODIALYSIS

THOMAS PARKER III, B.S., M.D.
ALAN HULL, M.D.

Regular hemodialysis as applied to the patient with end-stage renal disease (ESRD) seems at first glance to be in a relatively stagnant period of development, at least when compared to other medical achievements made during the period 1960 to 1980. However, whereas major breakthroughs have not been notable, a steady improvement in the understanding of the dialysis process and a commensurate improvement in technology has occurred. In discussing the current status of this therapeutic modality, we have elected to develop a selected list of topics, in no preferential order. Rather than provide a broad, but superficial, overview, selection of topics has been based largely on the impact that each has had on the care of patients in our hemodialysis program.

REHABILITATION WITH HEMODIALYSIS THERAPY

A review of the dialysis literature in 1970 would reveal great penetration of hemodialysis therapy among patients with ESRD, but a poor history of rehabilitation in the patients treated. Part of this was attributable to inadequate data collection by the Federal ESRD Medical Information System. However, it was mostly due to the failure of any group to study rehabilitation, the particular goal of our efforts. Recently such a study has been undertaken by the Batelle Institute by Dr. Roger Evans. A retrospective analyses of long-term results included 859 patients from 11 dialysis and transplant centers. This study provides the best data available to document what hemodialysis has produced for patients with ESRD. Six hundred and thirty-four of the 859 patients received either home hemodialysis or incenter hemodialysis. In this group, major important findings included the following facts:

1. With regard to "quality of life" and "patient well-being," hemodialysis patients saw themselves as being similar to people in the general population.
2. Thirty to 40 percent of patients felt that ESRD placed a strain on their marriage.
3. Sixty-two percent of home hemodialysis patients felt that the dialysis process drew the family together, compared to only 48 percent of incenter patients.
4. Fifty-six percent of home patients and 46 percent of incenter patients stated that they had essentially no physical limitation.
5. Overall rehabilitation was poor with either form of hemodialysis with only 20 percent performing any financially gainful employment.

Thus, although achieving some positive benefits for the patient over and above simple prolongation of life, hemodialysis in its present form, whether applied in the home or in the center, has many shortcomings; not the least of which is the poor prospect for true rehabilitation. This represents one of the greatest challenges for the field.

PRESCRIPTION DIALYSIS

Pressures by patients to limit time on dialysis, constraints on dialysis space and reimbursement, increased marketing by suppliers of equipment to perform shorter dialysis, and improvement in membrane technology have collectively stimulated the notion that dialysis may be shortened in a generic manner to most patients. Whereas shortening of the overall exposure time to the hemodialysis procedure is a laudable goal, we have some concern about the potential risks as compared to patient-related benefits. To date, only the National Cooperative Dialysis Study (NCDS) has meaningfully assessed the prescriptive modalities and safety parameters in a large enough population to lend validity to shortening dialysis. Two questions must be answered when prescribing dialysis to the individual patient or to broad groups of patients:

1. How does the prescribing physician determine the amount of dialysis (type of dialyzer and time on dialysis as the dominant variables) to deliver to the patient?
2. Once prescribed, how does one determine that the treatment has been safely administered and is effective?

To continue to shorten dialysis for each individual, without adequate evidence of its safety, is flirting with, at least, increasing morbidity, if not actual mortality. The NCDS provides a useful data base upon which tentative answers to these questions can be based. The NCDS was commissioned by the NIH in 1976, and the final report was published in 1984. We will not review this study in detail, but rather will describe its most important features insofar as it relates to the hemodialysis patient and allied personnel.

First, the study clearly showed that one can use the surrogate small molecule *urea* (or as it is chemically measured as urea nitrogen) to determine the *adequacy* of dialysis in the population studied. We find that a common misconception of the study is its alleged statement that only the removal of small molecules by hemodialysis is important. This is not the message. The concept of using a surrogate molecule was to design a study whereby the "safe" limits of that molecule could be determined. The very fact that the limits determined are found to be "safe" confirms that other unmeasured molecules, whether they are small or intermediate in size, must also be within acceptable limits. Thus, this was not a study to determine if small molecules are more important than "middle" ones.

The NCDS demonstrated that there is a "safe" zone for the concentration of the surrogate molecule urea (or urea nitrogen) for any given patient. This zone was termed the time-averaged concentration (TAC), the average urea level to which a patient is exposed over a week's time. This is calculated by measuring pre- and postdialysis plasma urea nitrogen for several hemodialysis sessions during a given week. Some have interpreted the study to have stated that a TAC for urea nitrogen of 50 mg per deciliter is sufficient dialysis, regardless of the amount of time of each dialysis session (range 2½ to 5 hours) or the actual removal of urea nitrogen during any given dialysis session. This is not necessarily true. The patient must eat well, as determined by protein catabolic rate (PCR) or generation rate of urea (G) (mathematically interchangeable terms). ($G=0.154$ PCR -1.7) The major contribution of the study is that it demonstrates that dialysis-related morbidity (e.g., hospitalization for complications, gastrointestinal symptoms, pericarditis), can be predicted with only the TAC of urea nitrogen and the PCR. Dialysis prescription (time, dialyzer type, blood flow rate, and dialysate flow rates) and/or diet may then be manipulated to modify morbidity, thereby *individualizing* hemodialysis for each patient.

In our center, application of the principles of dialysis prescription based on TAC and PCR has resulted in the following average parameters for 413 patients who were followed for 1 year.

Time average plasma urea nitrogen concentration (mg per deciliter -51.43 ± 10.2
PCR (g per kilogram per day) $-0.98 + 0.21$
Time on dialysis (minutes) -195 ± 25
Clearance of dialyzer (cc per minute) -209 ± 9

In our view, a major deterrent to the widespread application of prescriptive hemodialysis based on TAC and PCR measurement has been the complexity of the mathematical formulas, intrinsic to the calculations required, for "kinetic modeling" used in the NCDS. The concepts themselves are easily understood even though the math is difficult.

However, once every 2 months, the nursing staff in our center provides a peri-, post-, and predialysis plasma urea nitrogen level (for Monday-Wednesday or Tuesday-Thursday dialyses), intradialysis and interdialysis time, residual renal function (if any), weight, and dialyzer, (i.e., type, membrane surface area, blood flow and dialysate flow). Entry of these data into a preprogrammed calculator or computer provides the information that is required: this includes time on dialysis, dialyzer size, and blood and dialysate flow rates necessary to attain nominal safe dialysis based on the TAC and PCR limits. Prevailing or prescribed dietary intake of protein is not a necessary prerequisite. The benefit of this approach is twofold: to *minimize* dialysis time to the patient and to *maximize* facility and staff efficiency. Furthermore it identifies, those patients who are being "underdialyzed" and those with marginal or inadequate dietary intake of protein, which is likely to result in unnecessary future complications. The NCDS provided the data parameters that define the "safe" boundaries of dialysis. Kinetic modeling is the vehicle that assures that the prescription for hemodialysis remains within those boundaries. To shorten dialysis time *without* prescription may be harmful.

CONVENTIONAL HEMODIALYSIS

It may appear that little significant change has taken place in the technology of dialysis delivery over the last decade. This may, in part, be on account of perceived constrictions in reimbursement to facilities that prevent new technology from being applied in the clinical setting. On the other hand, perhaps the benefit of the technology has not justified the change, albeit subtle improvements have made the intradialysis and interdialysis periods more comfortable for patients with ESRD. In the *intradialysis* period, one notes the increasing use of higher dialysate sodium concentrations, bicarbonate anion replacing acetate in the dialysate, shorter dialysis (as discussed previously), higher clearance dialysis with improved vascular access, improved ultrafiltration control with conventional dialysis that includes sequential ultrafiltration, and more.

In the *interdialysis* period, little has been accomplished or changed, especially for patients undergoing dialyses in a facility setting. There seems to be little change in vocational or occupational rehabilitation. Improved antihypertensive medication has decreased the necessity for nephrectomy and has probably improved the rate of morbidity and reduced the mortality. It is difficult to find meaningful data to suggest that patients' dietary habits have been influenced in a measurable way to manage protein and phosphate intake; this seems to be a daily struggle for both dietitian and patient.

NONCONVENTIONAL HEMODIALYSIS

The principles and pragmatics of conventional hemodialysis are probably understood by all who read this chapter. Therefore, we will neither review nor add to that subject. We would, however, like to comment briefly on various techniques used by others, and which are currently being evaluated, in order to replace and improve conventional hemodialysis. Such techniques and terminology as *sequential hemodialysis, hemofiltration, "high flux" hemodialysis, diafiltration,* and *hemodiafiltration* have contributed significantly to our understanding of the various processes available to us. The sheer volume of the burdensome terminology has confused many of us who attempt to remain current. Some have suggested that these techniques should now replace *conventional* dialysis. Should they?

Technology

To oversimplify, in hemodialysis, movement of solute and water across a membrane may be achieved through osmotic, diffusive, or hydrostatic forces. *Conventional dialysis* predominantly relies on diffusive forces to drive solute transport and on hydrostatic forces to drive water transport. Other forms of dialysis depend principally on hydrostatic or hydraulic forces for solute transport (i.e., hemofiltration). Many use a combination of the two. We have become so used to conventional hemodialysis that we have almost assumed that the diffusive forces are dominant. Actually, hydraulic forces can be manipulated to create a favorable transport situation.

When hydrostatic pressure is applied to the blood side of a semipermeable membrane, water moves across the membrane at a proportionately greater rate. Depending on membrane characteristics, especially pore size in relation to solute particle size and frictional forces, solute moves with water. This is termed "solvent drag" or convective transport. (Even in conventional dialysis high hydrostatic pressures concomitant with increasing water transport mildly increases removal of "uremic solutes.") Practically speaking, pore size is sufficiently small to prevent solvent drag of proteins and cellular elements during this hydrostatically induced transport. Membranes can be constructed so that the pore size allows minimal resistance certain solutes. If this is the situation, there is less difference between the ultrafiltrate and the solution that does not traverse the membrane (a very low rejection coefficient).

So called "*high flux*" membranes that are more water permeable are now being constructed. These membranes are manufactured and engineered by various companies and may consist of polyacrylonitrile (PAN), polysulfone (PS), and polymethylmethacrylate (PMMA). (The latter has also been manufactured with properties similar to conventional cuprophane membranes.) These membranes use diffusion, but predominantly convection or solvent drage, for solute transfer.

Earlier, we mentioned the terms *hemofiltration, diafiltration,* and *hemodiafiltration*. Although these terms have been used synonymously, they vary slightly in definition. Hemofiltration is similar to ultrafiltration except that a "*high flux*" membrane is used, and consequently, some type of fluid replacement for the filtrate is needed, either before or after filtration. *Diafiltration* or *hemodiafiltration* simply means that conventional dialysis and hemofiltration occur simultaneously. *Hemofiltration* is the application of convective forces rather than diffusive forces to accomplish solute transfer. The principle advantage is purported to be removal of "middle" molecules. Hemofiltration depends on a membrane with high water (hydraulic) permeability. Small molecules appear in the ultrafiltrate in the same concentration as plasma. Larger, "middle" or intermediate molecules in the 1,000 to 9,000 dalton range are also removed convectively, depending on pore and molecule size and configuration. Because of the high convective flow, less diffusive transfer occurs, and consequently, small molecule clearance may be less with hemofiltration than hemodialysis, but the higher convective flow gives much higher "middle" molecule clearance than conventional dialysis.

The fact is that the rate of water removal (20 to 40 liters of volume per session) generated in order to remove the amount of solute in the ultrafiltrate requires simultaneous, rapid, large volume replacement at the same rate as the removal rate. Usually replacement solutions contain somewhat isosmotic concentrations of sodium, potassium, chloride, acetate, or bicarbonate, and lesser amounts of calcium, magnesium, and glucose. These solutions may be given, just before (predilution) or just after (postdilution) the hemofilter. Much has been written concerning the advantages and disadvantages of pre- versus postdilution hemofiltration. We find little difference in our reviews, except in the case of molecules greater than 5,000 daltons, which seem to be removed better with predilution. However, predilution technique does require almost twice as much replacement fluid. Some equipment is now available, which allows the replacement of regenerated filtrate; this saves significantly on the cost of replacement fluid, but adds to the complexity of design and maintenance of the machinery. Equipment is available to control precisely the amount of fluid removed, the amount returned, and consequently the net volume removed from the patient during a session.

It is unknown whether these varied techniques make a difference clinically. To date, no large studies have determined the efficacy of this procedure as compared to conventional hemodialysis, by using morbidity and mortality as outcome parameters. Some have shown better blood pressure control, but this has not been confirmed by others. Earlier studies that recorded less subjective complaints during hemofiltration as compared to conventional hemodialysis may no longer be valid with the advent of better ultrafiltration control and bicarbonate dialysate in conventional hemodialysis. The efficacy of this approach must be proven by convincing evidence that removal of large amounts of intermediate molecules affects patient well-being. Recent data germane to this notion confirms that prolonged conventional hemodialysis is associated with accumulation of beta$_2$ microglobulin and that this substance, which appears similar to amyloid, may be associated with carpal tunnel syndrome and cystic bone lesions. This seems to be the first, and perhaps only real, clinical syndrome associated with accumulation of intermediate molecules over a long course of dialysis.

A purported benefit of hemofiltration is shortened treatment time. We are not convinced that it offers any advantage over shortened conventional hemodialysis, facilitated by kinetic modeling and supplemented with bicarbonate that is substituted for acetate in the dialysate.

Hemodiafiltration. Hemodiafiltration couples hemofiltration to hemodialysis in the hope of offsetting disadvantages of inadequate-small molecule transport with hemofiltration. This requires a complex machine, and this cumbersome procedure awaits validation of the effort.

Sequential Ultrafiltration. Used in conjunction with conventional hemodialysis seems to have many of the advantages of all of the above, with the only disadvantage being a slight increase in length of each dialysis session. Usually dialysis is performed first with minimal transmembrane pressure, then dialysate flow is terminated when the ultrafiltration is performed. Evidence supports greater ease of volume removal using this technique. We use this method in the occasional patient with severe cardiovascular instability. We find that if it is used routinely, patients do not remain on dialysis long enough to attain sufficient dialysis through diffusion or develop a vicious cycle of excessive weight gains and losses that require more and more time on ultrafiltration rather than dialysis.

High Flux Dialysis. High flux dialysis uses blood flow rates in the 300 to 500 ml per minute range with conventional dialysis membranes in an attempt to shorten dialysis. If arteriovenous (AV) access allows, this seems to be an excellent alternative to many of the more sophisticated approaches. However, the problem of "adequate" shortened dialysis must again be addressed.

The technique of *spontaneous (continuous arteriovenous) hemofiltration* is primarily used in the acute setting, principally for volume removal, and we will not comment on this technique as applied to ESRD. Suffice to say, techniques other than conventional hemodialysis are becoming available. We are not convinced of their advantage over using the more simple prescriptive dialysis with kinetic modeling, plus bicarbonate dialysis to minimize vascular instability.

VASCULAR ACCESS

It is our experience that three factors are associated with long-term function of a vascular access:

1. Primary AV fistulas in the lower arm are the preferred choice when adequate vessels are available.
2. A surgeon who understands the requirements of dialysis blood flow. This usually means a surgeon with considerable experience with primary AV fistulas or forearm loop grafts.
3. Careful use of the access of both in the location of needle placement and the pressure applied after needle removal.

When these three factors are present, it is not uncommon to find primary vascular accesses functioning well at 5 to 10 years after placement. If there are not adequate vessels or someone inexperienced has done the primary access, then our second choice would be a midarm loop, using a bovine or Impra/Gortex graft; the choice of which we leave to the particular surgeon's preference.

At least one-third of our patients are diagnosed as having end-stage renal disease on admission to hospital. In such patients, the requirement for acute access becomes a major determinant of long-term graft placement. Our choices in the past have been as follows:

1. A good primary AV fistula that can be used immediately.
2. Shaldon (femoral vein) catheters in hospital until the permanent access is ready.
3. Lower limb Scribner shunt as a last resort, if the patient must be sent out of hospital while the definitive graft heals or matures.

Recently, we have been impressed with Shiley subclavian vein catheters for acute and short-term vascular access; careful placement by an experienced nephrologist or surgeon has resulted in earlier patient discharge from the hospital. This procedure is particularly helpful in patients who have inadequate vessels and require time to heal and/or develop upper limb accesses.

The technique is not without complications in placement and use. Hemothorax is the commonest serious problem. Infection may be prevented by meticulous observation of sterile dressing technique. We prefer one nephrologist or surgeon at each hospital to place all Shiley subclavian vein catheters and we utilize one outpatient center with specially trained personnel to dialyze such patients. The patient acceptance of this technique is high since it allows them freedom of movement as compared to Shaldon femoral vein catheters and lets them leave the hospital earlier. With experience and care, many patients can be dialyzed for weeks or even months using this vascular access technique.

ACQUIRED IMMUNODEFICIENCY SYNDROME (AIDS)

Any attempt to include information about AIDS in a review of this type is to flirt with outdated concepts and recommendations. However, this problem is creating increased pressure on our staff and patients and deserves comment.

Unfortunately neither the incidence nor the prevalence of AIDS or positive anti-human lymphotrophic virus type III (anti-HTLV III) is known in the ESRD population at large. The data from the Food and Drug Administration is relevant to the dialysis environment. In a survey of 1.1 million units of blood collected from 155 centers and tested throughout June 1985, 2,381 (0.25 percent) units, or about 1/400, were reported to be repeatedly reactive for antibody using the Enzyme-linked immunosorbent assay (ELISA) anti-HTLV III. The pattern varied slightly from region to region. Other studies performed by the Centers for Disease Control (CDC) and the American Red Cross suggest that about 32 percent of these would be expected to have either a positive western blot or positive culture for the virus, which is currently considered confirmatory for carrying the virus. By contrast, none had a positive culture or western blot if the ELISA anti-HTLV III was initially positive and subsequently negative. Therefore, about 1 in 1,200 donors would be expected to be potentially infectious. Less than 2 percent of reported AIDS cases have been thought to be caused by blood transfusions, and 89 percent of these found to have a positive western blot test or virus culture had identifiable risk factors. We present this data not as a review of AIDS, but in order to have a basis on which to discuss the problem in relation to ESRD and specifically hemodialysis. Perhaps it is best to start with the following questions:

1. What is the incidence and prevalence of positive anti-HTLV III, confirmed by western blot or virus culture, in the hemodialysis population and staff?
2. What isolation techniques, if any, should be used for patients? Should the technique vary for serologic or culture positivity versus clinical AIDS?
3. Should staff with positive anti-HTLV III, viral culture, or any of the AIDS complexes be restricted from the clinical areas of the facility?
4. Should patients with clinical AIDS undergo dialysis in hemodialysis facilities? What is the emotional impact of patients with AIDS on other hemodialysis patients and staff within the facility?

Few studies as of this writing address the true incidence, prevalence, or transmission of positive antibodies in patients or staff in ESRD facilities. One would expect this to vary geographically and to be influenced by urban or rural location of the facility, prevalence of drug use, and past transfusion policies.

One study among chronic hemodialysis patients showed the prevalence of positive anti-HTLV III to be approximately 1 percent higher than the normal population. There appears to be a correlation of HTLV-III positivity only with the number of blood transfusions; no evidence of transmission within the facility was noted. Noteworthy is the possibility of a higher prevalence of false positives.

Previously, guidelines had been advanced by CDC for management of positive anti-HTLV III and/or AIDS patients on hemodialysis. Essentially, the same strategy as developed for Hepatitis B surface antigen (HBsAG) positive patients had been suggested. However it should be pointed out that the HTLV-III virus is found in significantly less concentration than that of hepatitis B virus in most biological fluids. Nonetheless, isolation, a separate machine, and also designated treatment, which was based on whether the patient was positive for HBsAG in addition to anti-HTLV III, was recommended. The procedures otherwise were identical to those used for HBsAG-positive machines and included surface cleaning, proper disinfection, and no cross-use with nonpositive patients.

Recently data has confirmed the small amount of viral particles with positive anti-HTLV III antibody ($<1\times10^{1}$IU) as compared to patients with positive HBsAG ($>1\times10^{8\text{-}9}$IU). Consequent to this finding and the results of the health care workers' needle-stick study monitored by CDC, the recommendations have been revised: Patients with positive anti-HTLV III, on account of low infectivity, should not be isolated. Standard hemodialysis precautions should be followed. This revised policy, if implemented by the individual facility, of course, requires staff and patient education to overcome enormous preconception, fear, and apprehension.

From a purely medical standpoint, one could make a case for screening neither patients nor staff. The virus load in blood and consequent probability of transmission of the AIDS virus load in blood and consequent probability of transmission of the AIDS virus is vastly less than that for carriers of the hepatitis B virus. Consequently, the potential for transmission from patient to staff, patient to patient, or staff to patient is *almost* nonexistent. This statement belies the socioemotional issues of having staff or patients with positive anti-HTLV III in the facility. These are considerable and must be part of the decision to screen or not to screen. We would only recommend that the facility have a well-conceived policy as to how it will apply the information.

Current prudent recommendations might also suggest that staff with AIDS or positive anti-HTLV III should not work in a hemodialysis facility. Although we understand that the recent data of the scientific community and the regulations of varied agencies suggest otherwise, as of this writing, taking into consideration the emotional welfare of even the best-educated patient population, we cannot warrant such an approach. And, we might add, our patients' welfare is our primary objective in medicine. We will not fully answer the fourth question. The ethics are entirely too complicated for this short chapter. Hemodialysis centers in New York report their very tragic results with hemodialysis in AIDS patients, which show a 100 percent mortality in less than 2 years. The impact on patients and staff is immeasurable. In our program, we currently attempt peritoneal dialysis or home dialysis as first choice for patients with *clinical* AIDS, especially those with overt secretory or exudative lesions. Otherwise those with only positive anti HTLV III are dialyzed in the facility without isolation.

ALUMINUM OSTEODYSTROPHY AND ENCEPHALOPATHY

Recognition of the accumulation of aluminum in body tissues, especially bone and neural tissue but also the liver and spleen, has significantly changed the treatment approach to renal osteodystrophy. Since the amount of aluminum we consume in our diet is small (3 to 10 mg per day), the ESRD patient must accumulate aluminum through other sources. Certainly aluminum-containing antacids are a potential source. Absorption is greatly pH dependent and in the case of low pH aluminum may be absorbed in the stomach and duodenum. Studies in normal volunteers show a greater than tenfold increase in urinary excretion when subjects are fed 1 to 2 g of aluminum per day. The issue is, of course, how much of the absorbed aluminum is not excreted. Since the kidney is the primary excretory organ, patients with compromised renal function would be expected to be in positive balance with estimates of 2 to 3 grams total body burden being reasonable (normal, < 35 mg). Aluminum-containing phosphate binders could easily attain this.

Of course, the other major source of aluminum is dialysate, which is usually present in the domestic water supply. Since aluminum is 70 to 95 percent bound to protein in plasma, almost all aluminum in dialysate is transferred to the patient. The normal plasma aluminum concentration in humans is 10 μg per liter; consequently dialysate levels should be less than 10 μg per liter to assure minimal transfer.

Some investigators believe that encephalopathy, osteomalacia, and microcytic anemia can occur, especially in children, even with "clean" dialysate because of ingestion of large amounts of phosphate binders. A third potential source of aluminum in the dialysis population occurs in parenteral fluids.

In bone, the lesion of aluminum intoxication is osteomalacia. The exact mechanism is unknown, but probably is related to the physicochemical effect of aluminum on hydroxyapatite or calcium phosphate crystal growth at the mineralization front. New bone formation and bone marrow erythrocyte production may also be impaired.

The true incidence and prevalence of aluminum-related problems in dialysis facilities is unknown; in those units without essentially aluminum-free dialysate, the prevalence may well be in excess of 60 to 70 percent of patients. Otherwise, the prevalence is probably about 20 percent.

One must define what level of aluminum retention is acceptable and what level requires attention and treatment. The process of screening everyone following an arbitrary duration on dialysis or consumption of aluminum-containing phosphate binders may ultimately be reasonable, should future studies define the limits for us.

Currently, we use a rather mixed set of criteria to determine those patients who will be screened for aluminum osteodystrophy (osteomalacia) or encephalopathy. These are spontaneous bone fractures; bone pain; patients with hyperparathyroidism who are being considered for surgery; disporportionate hypercalcemia concomitant with calcium and vitamin D repletion; unexplained muscle wasting, muscle weakness, change in mentation, or "failure to thrive"; and unexplained progressive microcytic anemia.

Differentiation of aluminum-induced osteomalacia from osteitis fibrosa cystica due to hyperparathyroidism is absolutely crucial as subsequently noted. We depend predominantly on a desferrioxamine (DFO) challenge to make the diagnosis.

Patients within one of the above categories undergo a testing protocol that consists of the following: bone radiography, N- and C- terminal parathyroid hormone levels, serum calcium and phosphorous, alkaline phosphatase, ferritin, and DFO diagnostic challenge. DFO challenge consists of having the patient remain in the unit after dialysis, obtaining a baseline plasma aluminum level, giving DFO intravenously (40 mg per kilogram of body weight to a maximum of 2,000 mg) over a two hour period, and obtaining a plasma aluminum level 40 hours later when the patient returns for dialysis. Increases of more than 300 μg per liter are considered diagnostic, 200 to 300 equivocal and interpreted with respect to complementary studies, and less than 200 nondiagnostic. In our unit, the values of plasma aluminum for patients who are undergoing treatment have been 185 ± 160 μg per liter and 552 ± 204 μg per liter for pre- and post-DFO challenge, respectively.

DFO increases dialyzer clearance of aluminum. Since aluminum is largely protein bound, it is poorly cleared by conventional hemodialysis. The DFO-aluminum complex, aluminoxamine, has a molecular weight of 584. Aluminum clearances are approximately 30 ml per minute with the usual cellulosic membranes. This provides a removal of 1 to 5 mg of aluminum during a standard dialysis session following DFO administration and equilibration. At this rate treatment may be necessary for 1 to 2 years to significantly reduce tissue burden.

Those who require treatment undergo DFO infusion

during the last hour of dialysis with an infusion pump, twice to thrice weekly, using a DFO dosage of 40 mg per kilogram of body weight or a maximum individual dose of 2,000 mg. The following parameters are monitored: ophthamologic and auditory screening at baseline and every six months, weekly calcium and phosphorous, parathyroid hormone every three months, plasma aluminum and ferritin monthly, and multi-channel biochemical screen (SMA-12 or equivalent) monthly. When the plasma aluminum reaches 100 to 200 μg per liter, DFO infusion is stopped for 3 weeks, and the patient undergoes another DFO challenge test. Bone biopsies with tetracycline labeling are only performed in borderline or controversial situations.

A word of caution: Be absolutely certain that the laboratory is capable of giving accurate measurements of aluminum. It would be worthwhile to have them show you comparisons to reference labs. To date at our Center, we have treated 42 patients from a total pool of 295 patients. Only 2 patients have completed their course of treatment, which required 6 and 9 months and a total dose of 100 and 180 grams of DFO, respectively. Nineteen patients remained on treatment for 9.41 ± 3 months and a total dose of 136 ± 75 grams of DFO. Twenty-one no longer receive DFO, temporarily and permanently, for reasons of transfer (4), transplant (1), pruritis (1), hypocalcemia (2), abnormal liver functions (1), and death (9) (unrelated to DFO). Hypocalcemia and hypoferritinemia require close attention and interruptions of the therapy schedule.

An aluminum chelating cartridge has been used in a few patients, significantly increasing clearance, without untoward effects. This essentially doubles clearance in conjunction with DFO and a standard capillary dialyzer.

We have been unsuccessful in converting our patients from aluminum phosphate binders to those containing calcium. Calcium-phosphate products become uncomfortably elevated. We affirm the results of others who have shown that the bone lesion is refractory to 1,25$(OH)_2$D, 24,25$(OH)_2$D, and 250HD.

PARATHYROID DISEASE

Like most centers, we have used aggressive therapy to control serum phosphorous below 6 mg per deciliter (measure predialysis on 3rd day off dialysis). While this routine has undoubtedly retarded progression of parathyroid hypertrophy, we have paid a price in aluminum toxicity. We follow all dialysis patients with single-photon bone densetometry and have found this to give good supporting evidence of bone loss due to ostetitis fibrosa cystica. However, we no longer proceed with a parathyroidectomy regardless of symptoms of PTH level if the serum alkaline phosphate is not significantly elevated, rising rapidly, or the patient has not been checked for evidence of aluminum retention. Parathyroidectomy in the absence of elevated alkaline phosphatase or in the presence of aluminum retention has been universally unsuccessful.

BLOOD PRESSURE CONTROL

All patients on dialysis can and should have their blood pressure rigorously controlled. In the past, we have found that at least 50 percent of patients could be well controlled by aggressive fluid removal and adherence to restricted weight gain between dialyses. This requires continuous vigilance of staff and patients to ensure fluid removal to dry weight and restriction of interdialytic weight gain. If patients require antihypertensive medications to control their blood pressure, it is more difficult than ever to get them back to "dry weight" with blood pressure controlled by volume alone.

In our center the following has been noted:

1. Sixty to seventy percent of patients can be controlled (diastolic blood pressure below 100 mm Hg 3rd day off dialysis) by volume control.
2. Ten percent likewise can be controlled, but the effort required seems to be too great and instead physicians resort to antihypertensive medication.
3. Ten percent of patients are totally uncooperative as regards weight gain between dialyses and require antihypertensive medication.
4. We are unable to control blood pressure in 10 percent of patients, even with antihypertensives.

Recently, as greater varieties of antihypertensive drugs have become available and as we deal with more elderly or debilitated patients, only 50 percent of patients are controlled by volume depletion alone.

Regardless of the method used, control of *both* the systolic and the diastolic pressure is very important. We share the conviction that mortality is higher in the uncontrolled hypertensive group than in similar normotensive patients. Of course, this appears to be even more true in diabetic patients on dialysis.

The choice of drugs seems to vary considerably among facilities and physicians. In reviewing our charts it appears that beta-blockers (propanolol) and calcium-channel blockers have emerged as the most commonly used agents. In 10 to 15 percent of the patients who are difficult to control with any medication regimen, Minoxidil may be used. We have used less Minoxidil in females because of the problem with facial hair growth.

Finding a prescription for a fixed formulation of drugs, which allows optimal blood pressure control during the interdialytic period wherein erratic weight gains may occur, is very difficult. This, coupled with hypotension on dialysis, necessitates creative dosage schedules.

CARDIOVASCULAR DISEASE

At least 8 percent of patients present to dialysis with hypertension and almost 50 percent have an increased cardiothoracic ratio. Once extracellular volume is controlled, we are left with a smaller group who have cardiac enlargement, generally caused by hypertrophy, but occasionally by a dilated myocardiopathy. This group, while at high risk for stroke and myocardial infarction, seems to be even more at risk for sudden death presumably linked to arrhythmias.

There would appear to be two areas where treatment might lower the risk in patients with cardiac enlargement:

1. Control of blood pressure as previously outlined in order to prevent progression of arteriosclerotic heart disease.
2. Control of cholesterol and triglycerides. While the evidence to date does not show a clear cut effect in this area, we are concerned about the effect of elevated lipids. We try to control diet as a first approach, usually with limited success. Lipid lowering agents have been used with mixed success because of the side effects in the dialysis population.

HEPATITIS

The prevalence of hepatitis B has not increased in our units beyond 5 percent; we assume this is because of careful staff techniques, isolation, and blood transfusion screening. There have been no documented intrafacility transmissions of hepatitis B in the past 8 years.

Non-A, non-B viral hepatitis is definitely more common. We have used the following definition before proceeding with any work-up:

1. The serum glutamic oxaloaceric transaninase (SGOT) must be >100 (normal 45 IU) on two successive studies.

2. Such patients are then dialyzed to a lower weight to remove volume as a cause and are asked to refrain from alcohol intake. If repeat SGOT values remain over 100 IU, we assume this may be non-A, non-B hepatitis. Repeat HBsAg and antibodies for hepatitis A are performed.

3. We then follow patients to make sure that hepatitis B positively does not develop. If, as is usually the case, the disease does not progress, we continue to observe such patients without work-up until the disease remits or they are considered for transplantation.

4. We have had very little experience with hepatitis B in transplantation, but we accept that these patients do not do well as a group. In the non-A, non-B hepatitis subgroup, if elevated enzymes persist, these patients are biopsied. If an aggressive lesion is present we do not proceed. To date, patients with non-A, non-B hepatitis who have received renal transplants have not had higher-morbidity.

STAFF "BURN OUT"

In the early seventies when the great growth in dialysis units occurred, there were very imaginative concepts applied to patient care. It was exciting to see that patients possibily could be rehabilitated on dialysis, and such events were gratifying to the staff of dialysis units, both nurses and physicians. As time passed three events began to change the patient population in dialysis centers.

1. Older and sicker patients who could not be rehabilitated were accepted.
2. Many of the better motivated patients began to select CAPD and were not seen by the in-center staff.
3. Renal transplantation began to deplete dialysis units of stable younger patients and to limit the entrance of new patients, as discussed in the previous section.

These changes have had an effect on the "dialysis team" since many of the remaining dialysis patients have problems that no one can solve (e.g., What do you do for a blind diabetic, with no legs, whose only remaining joy in life is to drink water and become overloaded each weekend?). The dialysis team that was made up of problems solvers began to find no solution to the problems of most of the patients who remained in the units. The nurses seem to have handled this better than physicians.

It is very common in 1986 for a physician, who trained in nephrology in the early or mid-seventies, to suddenly realize his specialty has changed. When he or she trained, the emphasis was on acute care problems directed toward recovery. The chronic dialysis population in those early years appreciated their second chance at life and responded accordingly.

Now, 10 or 15 years later, the same nephrologist realizes that instead of dealing with acute solvable problems, where any failures died, they now face a very different future. In the current setting, the nephrologist has patients with chronic problems that often defy solution. The result is that many nephrologists either spend less time in the units or move to transplantation, if they can, or some other form of care. At least in our area, it appears that nephrologists after 10 or 15 years are moving to different endeavors and not staying in dialysis facilities. This may be a normal course because we are a very young specialty without a long track record. However, "burn-out" in chronic in-center dialysis units seems to be a major problem in the mid 1980s.

DIALYSIS TRENDS

Whereas one can argue that changes in the dialysis procedure have been slight, it has become evident over the last five years that significant changes are taking place in how patients are selected for dialysis treatment. Prior to 1980, our bias was to suggest to patients that they undergo living, related-donor transplantation. If no donor was available, we recommended dialysis. Depending on the patient's age, health, and motivation, we favored treatment selection as follows: in order of preference: (1) home hemodialysis; (2) in-center dialysis and (3) CAPD.

At that time, cadaveric transplant was encouraged once the patient was stable on dialysis. Our age cutoff during this period was generally 55 years, with special review for any older patients. In the early 1980s CAPD began to move up on the list. This was not due to doctor preference, initially, but because of patient demand. It gradually became evident to many of us that CAPD incorporated all the good things we had said about home hemodialysis in regard to patient independence. The major difference was that patients could learn and perform CAPD relatively easy as compared to home hemodialysis. Therefore, CAPD has steadily increased while home hemodialysis has slowly decreased in our population.

The second major change began in late 1983 and has accelerated since that time. This is the emphasis on transplantation mostly on account of the utilization of cyclosporine A (CyA). Up until the 1980s, cadaveric transplant results for first transplants at the end of 1 year were about

55 percent for graft survival. Patient survival was about equal to select dialysis survival in the first year (85 to 88 percent). In the early 1980s, a few groups, using a combination of matching and anti-lymphacyte globulin (ALG), began to move graft survival up toward the 70 percent survival level and reduce patient loss to less than 10 percent in primary cadaver renal transplants. In 1984, with the general use of CyA, results suddenly began to improve. By the end of 1985, many large programs had cadaveric renal transplant functional graft for first transplants (including diabetics) above 85 percent at 1 to 2 years. Patient survival in this group was approaching 95 percent at 1 year.

The marked improvement in results began to be recognized by the population on dialysis. Patients began to see a major change when their "chair-mate" went for a transplant; they returned to visit looking healthy, which was in contrast to the previous experience of one-half the transplant population either dying or returning in a very debilitated state after transplant nephrectomy. It hasn't taken our patients long to realize that transplantation is now the preferred therapy. In 1986, we are seeing the following preference expressed by patients approaching dialysis.

1. Many patients are asking for a transplant *prior* to initiating dialysis. We estimate this to be 10 percent and increasing monthly.
2. Only the very elderly and debilitated are not considered for transplant, and they often prefer CAPD over in-center dialysis.

It is now estimated in our area that 30 percent of patients who develop ESRD will receive a transplant either before going on dialysis or within 6 months of starting dialysis. Approximately 20 percent will elect CAPD from the outset; therefore, less than 50 percent will undergo in-center or home hemodialysis as a definitive form of treatment or as interum therapy pending later transplantation. The result of this change in emphasis and actual demand by patients is to leave most hemodialysis units with a *sick, aged, and/or poorly motivated* population.

Such patients require greater nursing care. This comes at a time when the government is forcing changes in staffing of dialysis units by progressive cutbacks. The result is that long-term dialysis staff are "burning out" at the very time they are needed most. This phenomenon, more than any other, is the real challenge for the future of hemodialysis.

PERITONEAL DIALYSIS

ALLEN R. NISSENSON, M.D.
EDWARD A. ROSS, M.D.

Since plastic bags of peritoneal dialysis solution became available in the United States in 1979, chronic peritoneal dialysis (CPD) has grown steadily as a treatment modality for patients with end-stage renal disease (ESRD). As of January 1985, more than 85,000 patients were on dialysis in the United States, with 14,000 currently on some form of CPD. Although initially it was thought that these numbers would stabilize by the mid-1980s, there is no indication as yet that this is happening. The continued growing popularity of CPD has broad implications to the ESRD program as well as to patients with ESRD. Frequent hospitalizations, particularly for infectious complications, remain a major problem. Overall patient survival is comparable to that seen in patients receiving hemodialysis, but CPD dropout remains high, again primarily related to infectious complications. In this chapter we will review pertinent clinical aspects of CPD.

TYPES OF CHRONIC PERITONEAL DIALYSIS AVAILABLE

Continuous ambulatory peritoneal dialysis (CAPD) is the form of CPD most widely practiced in the United States today. To perform CAPD a patient instills peritoneal dialysate into the abdomen through a permanent indwelling catheter and allows it to remain there for several hours. During this dwell-time, diffusion of solute across the peritoneal membrane is taking place, dependent on the molecular weight of the solute and its concentration gradient from blood to dialysate. At the same time water is ultrafiltered across the peritoneum because of an osmotic gradient, present because the dialysate contains a high concentration of glucose (1.5, 2.5, or 4.25 percent dextrose). After 4 to 6 hours the empty bag and tubing, still connected from the previous exchange, are unrolled and dialysate is drained into this system. The effluent is discarded and a fresh bag of dialysate is instilled. This process is usually repeated three times during the day and once before bed 7 days a week. The latter exchange remains in the abdomen until the patient awakes the next morning. Most patients use 2,000 ml of dialysate per exchange, although 1,500 ml, 2,500 ml or 3,000 ml is also used by a few patients. Small solute clearance (e.g., urea) with this technique is equal to effluent dialysate flow rate, since equilibration for these substances has occurred between blood and dialysate during the exchange period. Thus a urea clearance of approximately 10 L per day is usually seen. Patients may ultrafilter 1,000 to 3,000 ml of fluid in a 24-hour period, depending on their fluid intake, by using dialysate with varying dextrose concentrations as needed.

Similar in concept to CAPD is continuous cyclic peritoneal dialysis (CCPD). With this technique, however, a simple automated machine is used to infuse and drain dialysate at night while the patient sleeps. Usually three such exchanges of 2,000 ml each are performed over a 9- to 11-hour period. At the end of this time, when the patient awakes, the machine infuses a final exchange which dwells during the day and is drained before the patient goes to sleep the next night. Dialysate volume and use of varying dextrose concentrations in dialysate to remove fluid are similar to those used in CAPD.

Unlike CAPD and CCPD, which provide continuous dialysis 7 days a week, intermittent peritoneal dialysis (IPD) is performed only 30 to 50 hours per week, usually in 10-hour sessions. To offset the short treatment time, rapid dialysate cycling is used. Two thousand milliliters of dialysate is infused into the peritoneum, allowed to dwell for 15 to 30 minutes, and drained. A full cycle takes 30 to 40 minutes. Over a 10-hour dialysis session, therefore, 30 to 40 L of dialysate is cycled, providing adequate dialysis when this is repeated three to five times per week. An automatic cycling machine may be used to accomplish this, as in CCPD, or a reverse osmosis device that processes incoming tap water and mixes it with concentrated dialysate to provide on-line final dialysate production may be used. IPD may be performed by the patient at home or in an outpatient peritoneal dialysis center.

SELECTION OF TREATMENT

Some of the medical indications for selection of CPD over chronic hemodialysis are as follow: medical reasons include advanced age, atherosclerotic heart disease, patient being a Jehovah's Witness, severe anemia, difficulty controlling hypertension, diabetes mellitus, and failed vascular access. Patients who tolerate hemodialysis poorly because of advanced age or severe atherosclerotic heart disease would be good CPD candidates. Such individuals often poorly tolerate the rapid fluid shifts associated with hemodialysis. CPD is associated with a rise in hematocrit in most patients owing to more effective erythropoiesis coupled with hemoconcentration. For those patients with severe anemia or those unwilling to accept blood or blood products (e.g., Jehovah's Witnesses) CPD would be the modality of choice. Excellent control of hypertension, usually without the use of antihypertensive medication, is the rule when patients are on CPD. Those patients with ESRD who have resistant hypertension would thus do best on CPD. Diabetics can achieve excellent blood glucose control while on CPD with the use of intraperitoneal insulin, usually far better than when they were taking subcutaneous insulin. The combination of excellent blood pressure and blood sugar control with CPD as well as the lack of exposure to the risks of heparin make this modality highly preferable to chronic hemodialysis for such patients.

There are also a number of psychosocial considerations for use of CPD, including good motivation, good compliance, good family suport, long travel distance from a dialysis center, occupation with variable hours or location, and business and personal travel requirements. In addition, the patient is able to enjoy an overall enhanced quality of life. Though data on the latter point are scanty, a recent study we have conducted supports this possibility.

Contraindications to CPD include abdominal wall infection at the proposed site of catheter insertion, recurrent diverticulitis, and previous extensive abdominal surgery.

There are a number of potential disadvantages to selection of CPD as a treatment modality even in patients in whom it is indicated. The most important of these is the high incidence and morbidity of infectious complications, including peritonitis, and catheter exit site and tunnel infections. These will be discussed at greater length later in this chapter. In addition, CPD requires some degree of manual dexterity, particularly if CAPD is used. With CCPD, knowledge of a "machine" is necessary and a back-up person is often needed to work with the patient to perform dialysis. Metabolic complications of CPD are also common, including obesity, hyperlipidemia, and malnutrition. Our approach to these will be discussed separately. Other drawbacks to CPD include a high incidence of back pain, patient dissatisfaction with body image, and a frequently elevated muscle fraction creatine phosphokinase concentration, the significance of which is not yet clear.

Both CAPD and CCPD are gaining in popularity as treatment modalities for patients with ESRD, while IPD is being performed less frequently. The long session times, more complex equipment, and usual need for a back-up helper make it likely that the latter form of treatment will slowly disappear from use. The choice between CAPD and CCPD is an individual one based on specific patient characteristics. Some of the indications for CCPD versus CAPD are as follows: Medical reasons include recurrent peritonitis, inadequate control of chemistries or fluid balance, recurrent fluid leaks, and recurrent hernias. Psychosocial reasons include work or school setting where CAPD exchanges cannot be conveniently done, "helper" needed because patient is blind or disabled, poor body image on CAPD, and poor compliance on CAPD.

INITIATION OF CHRONIC PERITONEAL DIALYSIS

Types and Choice of Catheter

There are now several types of catheter available for use with CPD. The superiority of one over the others has not been clearly shown. Most centers use the Tenckhoff catheter, which consists of a Silastic catheter with one or two velour or felt cuffs and a straight or coiled intraperitoneal segment. The Toronto-Western catheter is similar, but has two perpendicular disks at the distal end to minimize migration of the catheter out of the pelvis as well as to prevent omental encasement and subsequent outflow obstruction. The Lifecath has a single large hole at the end flanked by a series of plastic columns to eliminate migration and outflow failure.

For catheters with cuffs, it appears that there is little difference in complications whether one cuff or two is used. The cuffs are designed to permit fibrous tissue ingrowth and thereby serve to anchor the catheter in place as well as act as a bacterial barrier. Whether the latter function is realized is unclear.

Most peritoneal catheters have a single radiopaque stripe or are completely radiopaque. It is our impression that such catheters have a tendency to crack over time, necessitating repair or replacement. We have frequently repaired such cracks using a splicing technique. This is accomplished using a Peri-Patch glue mold. The catheter is first soaked in Betadine for 5 minutes and the area to be removed is isolated by hemostats. The cracked section is removed and the indwelling catheter end is inserted into the glue mold along with the remaining distal catheter end. Sterile Silastic adhesive is infused into the mold until full, approximately 1 g. The silicone is cured for 72 hours, during which time the mold is left in place and kept absolutely dry and free of alcohol. At the end of this time the mold is removed. If the crack is in the distal half of the catheter, this end of the catheter is resected and the titanium connector is placed in the new distal end after a 5-minute Betadine soak, thus eliminating the need for the splicing procedure. Whenever catheter resection is undertaken we administer cephalexin prophylactically, 250 mg four times a day for three days.

Location of Catheter Insertion

Because of the high incidence of early leaks and hernia formation, midline catheter insertion has fallen out of favor. We insert catheters in the paramedian location through the body of the rectus muscle. The catheter tip is directed downward, preferably into the left lower quadrant where peristalsis in the descending colon helps prevent catheter migration. One-third of the deep cuff is placed in the peritoneum and two-thirds above, and the peritoneum is secured to the cuff with a purse-string suture. A curved subcutaneous tunnel is created, with care taken not to kink the catheter. The superficial cuff is placed at least 2 cm from the exit site, which is oriented as far caudad as possible. The exit site should not impinge on the belt line and should be placed laterally, particularly in sexually active patients.

Postoperative Catheter Care and "Break-In"

Immediately following placement, the catheter is irrigated with peritoneal dialysate. We use 50 percent of the anticipated maintenance volume with 1,000 units of sodium heparin per 1,000 ml of dialysate. Each irrigation consists of three sequential flushes of the solution in and out of the peritoneal cavity. At the end of each irrigation the solution should remain in the bag so that it is not absorbed and intraperitoneal pressure is minimized. Irrigation is carried out every 2 hours for the first 12 hours and every 4 hours thereafter. The irrigation bag is changed at least every 24 hours. Once the effluent is clear, the irrigation is stopped and the catheter capped until it is to be used. Even if the catheter is not used for up to 2 weeks it is not irrigated during this interval.

Whenever possible, patients requiring dialysis after catheter placement are hemodialyzed, usually through an existing vascular access or a newly placed subclavian catheter. If peritoneal dialysis must be performed, frequent, low-volume exchanges are used for 5 to 7 days (no more than 1,000 ml per exchange), and this is gradually increased over 5 to 7 days up to maintenance volume. Dialysis is performed only with the patient supine to minimize intraperitoneal pressure. We prefer to wait 10 to 14 days after catheter placement before initiating peritoneal dialysis.

CHRONIC PERITONEAL DIALYSIS MAINTENANCE

Once patients have stabilized on CPD (usually 4 weeks after completing training), maintenance care is given. In otherwise stable patients, we recommend clinic visits every 8 weeks. At these visits the patient is seen by a physician, nurse, social worker, and dietitian to review all aspects of ESRD care. At these visits routine chemistry and hematology studies are done. Every 6 months parathyroid hormone, aluminum, and ferritin are measured, while a chest roentgenogram and electrocardiogram are obtained annually. Every 6 months, at the time of the biannual tubing change, each patient undergoes a comprehensive review with all members of the health care team. Revision of the "life-plan," including discussion of renal transplantation, where appropriate, is formally carried out at this time.

All patients are followed closely by a renal nutritionist and should receive 1.2 to 1.5 g protein per kilogram of body weight per day. Protein intake is verified by performance of urea kinetic modeling and calculation of protein catabolic rate (equal to total urea output [dialysate plus urine] divided by the urea volume of distribution [roughly equal to total body water]) every quarter. Intake of sodium, potassium, and fluids is generally not limited unless hypertension, edema, or hypervolemia is present. Patients are also instructed to take folic acid, 1 mg per day, and water-soluble vitamins including B-complex and ascorbic acid (approximately 50 mg per day). Calcium carbonate is used as a phosphate binder to avoid unnecessary aluminum ingestion, and vitamin-D analogues are used in the presence of significant hypocalcemia or secondary hyperparathyroidism.

Retraining of patients is performed at least biannually, during the regular comprehensive patient review sessions. More frequent retraining is carried out if multiple episodes of peritonitis occur. On-site visits are performed for all patients on CCPD to ensure proper function of the cycling equipment and to observe the home environment. Subsequent home visits for CCPD patients are carried out on an as-needed basis.

DIALYSATE COMPOSITION

There are currently several different dialysates to choose from for CPD patients (Table 1). Most contain sodium, 132 mEq per liter, calcium 3.5 mEq per liter, chloride 96 or 102 mEq per liter, magnesium 0.5 or 1.5 mEq per liter, lactate 35 or 40 mEq per liter, and varying concentrations of glucose (1.5, 2.5, or 4.25 percent). Total osmolality varies between 347 mOsm per liter and 486 mOsm per liter and initial pH is approximately 5.5.

The majority of patients do well on the lower magnesium, higher lactate solutions. The use of acetate-containing solutions, once popular in Europe, has been associated with the progressive loss of ultrafiltration capacity and has been abandoned. Total ultrafiltration is controlled by the glucose concentration of the solutions used. For a 4- to 6-hour dwell, ultrafiltration averages 100 to 200 ml for a 1.5 percent solution and 1,000 to 1,400 ml for a 4.25 percent solution. The use of alternative osmotic agents, such as amino acids or polyglucose, remains experimental.

Transplantation in Chronic Peritoneal Dialysis Patients

Renal transplantation can be performed as successfully in the CPD patient as in those on hemodialysis. If postoperative dialysis is needed, we continue routine CAPD, performed by the patient, or CCPD using a cycler or "octopus" tubing set. There is no need to routinely perform hemodialysis rather than peritoneal dialysis in such situations. Following successful transplantation the peritoneal catheter is left in place for 3 months and then removed electively. With the increasing use of cyclosporin in renal transplantation and its excellent success, earlier removal of the catheter might eventually become reasonable. The mere presence of a peritoneal dialysis catheter, even after immunosuppressive drugs are given, does not constitute a risk to the patient. On the other hand, how soon after an episode of peritonitis has been successfully treated, a patient can be considered "safe" for transplantation, is not clear. We require a 2-month waiting period off antibiotics before putting the patient back on the active transplant list except in unusual circumstances, such as the hard-to-match, high-antibody patient.

COMPLICATIONS OF CHRONIC PERITONEAL DIALYSIS

Peritonitis

Peritonitis is the most frequent serious complication of peritoneal dialysis and is the most likely reason for discontinuing this dialytic modality. Fortunately, the rate of infections is declining with improved methodology and technology: dialysate containers have changed from glass to plastic; fewer connection procedures are required (especially with the advent of automated cyclers); and new types of connection devices and mechanical aides have simplified both the procedure and the maintenance of sterility. Fewer infections after the first 6 months of peritoneal dialysis exemplify the importance of both meticulous training and the patient's repetition of an established technique. The incidence of peritonitis in CAPD patients in large training centers has been reported as low as approximately one episode every 18 to 24 patient months. CCPD has an even smaller risk in some centers, with less than one episode every 30 patient months and a 60 percent likelihood of remaining infection-free at 18 months.

Most cases of peritonitis are caused by bacterial ("touch") contamination during bag exchanges. Less frequently the inoculum is introduced by accidental bag and/or tube disconnections or damaged tubing. The lower incidence of infection reported by some with the automated cyclers is probably attributable to fewer necessary connections; a constant environment in which to perform the sterile maneuvers; most connections being made between disposable items rather than to the permanent catheter; intrinsic peritoneal defense mechanisms during the daytime hours, if there is no dialysate dwell during that time; and the outward (rather than inward in CAPD) direction of initial dialysate flow past the new connections. These putative advantages of CCPD have not been realized in some studies and still need to be confirmed in larger groups of patients. Even when potential contamination during exchanges is essentially avoided by using ultraviolet or high temperature sterilization, peritonitis is not eliminated. The remaining infections are due to progression of exit site to tunnel infections, bowel flora (e.g., diverticulitis, ischemic bowel, or possibly bacterial migration through the intestinal wall), or hematogenous seeding of the peritoneal fluid. Uremic patients are especially susceptible to serious progression of their infections. They suffer from both cellular and humoral immune deficiencies and the peritoneal fluid itself can contribute to persistent infection. The dialysate can impair phagocytosis because of its low pH, high osmolality, large volume, urea content, intraperitoneally administered heparin or insulin, or debris and fibrin strands.

The typical circumstances of bacterial contamination are reflected in the preponderance (approximately 70 per-

TABLE 1 Available Peritoneal Dialysate Solutions

	With 1.5% Dextrose	*With 2.5% Dextrose*	*With 4.25% Dextrose*
Dextrose H_2O	15 g/L	25 g/L	42.5 g/L
Sodium	132 mEq/L	132 mEq/L	132 mEq/L
Calcium	3.5 mEq/L	3.5 mEq/L	3.5 mEq/L
Magnesium	0.5 or 1.5 mEq/L	0.5 or 1.5 mEq/L	0.5 or 1.5 mEq/L
Chloride	96 or 102 mEq/L	96 or 102 mEq/L	96 or 102 mEq/L
Lactate	35 or 40 mEq/L	35 or 40 mEq/L	35 or 40 mEq/L
Total osmolarity	347 mOsm/L	396 mOsm/L	486 mOsm/L
Approximate pH	5.5	5.5	5.5

cent) of gram-positive skin or upper airway organisms. The most likely cause is *Staphylococcus epidermidis*, which usually responds more rapidly to antibiotic treatment than the often more severe *S. aureus* infections. The latter are not infrequently complicated by sepsis or abscess formation. *Streptococcus viridans* infections are indicative of an oral or upper airway source. Approximately 25 percent of cases are owing to gram-negative enteric flora. The remaining 5 percent are caused by fungi or tuberculosis. The former are usually *Candida* species and are more common in patients with diabetes, immunosuppression, prior courses of antibiotics, or collagen vascular diseases.

The number of cases of apparently "sterile" peritonitis has steadily declined with improved culture techniques. Nevertheless, the rare "chemical" peritonitis can be caused by medications added to the dialysate, such as antibiotics. With improved preparation of the dialysate, impurities (e.g., endotoxins) have become a very unlikely cause of peritoneal inflammation. The rare entity of peritoneal eosinophilia is characterized by cloudy effluent with a high percentage of eosinophils, is usually asymptomatic, occurs shortly after beginning peritoneal dialysis, and clears spontaneously. The etiologic agent is unknown, but allergy to the plastic components and peritoneal reaction to air introduced at the time of catheter placement have been proposed.

Peritonitis is diagnosed clinically when at least two of the following are present: symptoms of peritoneal inflammation, cloudy fluid with inflammatory cells, and a positive Gram stain or culture. The clinical signs of peritonitis can occur as early as 6 hours after the bacterial inoculation, but usually take 2 to 3 days to develop. Typically, the patient presents with cloudy fluid and diffuse abdominal pain which progresses to nausea, vomiting, fever, rebound tenderness, abdominal distention, and gastrointestinal dysfunction. Poor dialysate outflow can be caused by partial obstruction of the catheter by fibrin deposits. The differential diagnosis for the CPD patient presenting with these peritoneal findings should include appendicitis, cholecystitis, pancreatitis, and perforated viscus; these disorders are often difficult to exclude. Milder degrees of abdominal pain can also be due to constipation, dialysate acidity, pressure from the catheter tip, and the force of the peritoneal fluid stream during dialysate inflow.

Since the complications of delayed treatment can be severe, including peritoneal sclerosis and catheter failure, the goal is to begin treatment rapidly—even if it means initiation by an observant patient or family member. Thus, accepting the fact that this protocol will lead to a small chance of unnecessary use of antibiotics, one should ask the patient, at the first signs of cloudy dialysate and/or abdominal symptoms, to save and bring to the clinic that effluent bag, in the meantime beginning antibiotic therapy.

Analysis of the effluent will be important, especially in the one-third of patients with atypical clinical presentations. Abdominal pain can occur before the onset of cellular peritoneal fluid abnormalities. A dialysate white cell count above 50 per cubic millimeter is abnormal, and more than 100 per cubic millimeter with a predominance of neutrophils is usually indicative of peritonitis. Most cases are associated with counts of 600 to 9,000 per cubic millimeter, and the temporal course of the cell count is important. If it does not decrease to less than 100 per cubic millimeter within 3 days, one should be suspicious of continued or recurrent sources of infections, such as perforated bowel or abscess formation. Apparent variations in the cell counts, however, can be misleading if really attributable to a different dilution in altered dialysate volume, since such counts are reported per milliliter of fluid.

The use of the Gram stain, in this era of cost containment, is controversial. Many centers reserve its use for patients with grossly cloudy peritoneal fluid, claiming that only then will the test have a positive yield of more than 50 percent. The Gram stain, however, when it does uncover organisms, is useful in guiding antibiotic treatment. If it shows polymicrobial contamination there should be an aggressive search for an abdominal viscus perforation. Discovering fungi will expedite treatment, since these organisms may otherwise take up to 5 to 6 days to grow in culture.

Cloudy peritoneal fluid with elevated cell counts may be seen under circumstances other than peritonitis. It can occur, for example, with menstruation, ovulation, diarrhea, after vaginal examination, and with pseudomembranous colitis.

The method of culturing the dialysate is important, and depends on whether or not the fluid is cloudy and whether the patient has already received antibiotics. The laboratory is asked to aerobically and anaerobically culture the specimen for 15 days and to characterize all organisms even if there are only a few colonies present. Mycobacteria are very difficult to recover from peritoneal fluid, and a biopsy of the omentum or peritoneum may be necessary for culture and histologic diagnosis.

Since there is evidence that the phagocytic activity of white blood cells and the bactericidal action of antibiotics are diminished in the setting of acid pH and high osmolarity, and since logistically simpler (and less expensive) regimens have proven effective, the routine use of continuous peritoneal lavage is no longer recommended. Instead, at the first signs of peritonitis, the patient or staff does three rapid (in/out) 2-L exchanges in hopes of mechanically clearing the abdomen of potentially inflammatory toxins and debris. The patient is then given a loading dose of antibiotics via the peritoneum. Many centers advocate both a cephalosporin and an aminoglycoside until the culture results are known. We use only a cephalosporin, adding an aminoglycoside if (1) there are clinical indications of a Gram-negative infection source (e.g., diverticulitis) or of severe infection and/or sepsis; (2) there has been gross (i.e., fecal or dirt) contamination of the tubing and/or spike system; or (3) the patient has just recovered from known gram-negative peritonitis or from an atypically prolonged episode of peritonitis treated only with cephalosporins. We use a 2-L exchange with 500 mg of cephalothin per liter to dwell for 4 to 6 hours, followed by maintenance doses of 250 mg per liter; 500 units of heparin per liter is also added to each bag. Table 2 lists the loading and maintenance doses of commonly used antibiotics. In uncomplicated cases therapy should continue for a total of 8 to 10 days, or at least 4 days after the first negative culture.

Sterile injection of the antibiotic into the dialysate bags can be a problem for some patients. Alternatively, the bags can be prepared by the nursing staff. Under logistically difficult circumstances, some authors have advocated use of oral cephalexin (0.5 g four times daily) for susceptible organisms, though the efficacy of this regimen has yet to be proven.

Continuous peritoneal lavage with fluid containing the appropriate levels of antibiotics may still be indicated in those patients with severe peritonitis (often caused by delayed treatment of *S. aureus*) not responsive to the standard regimen, and perhaps in pediatric cases using small dialysate volumes. Oral rifampin therapy may be useful for infections resistant to treatment because of sequestration of viable organisms within functionally impaired peritoneal macrophages.

Treatment plans should also include general supportive measures. By increasing the peritoneal clearances of small and large molecules, peritonitis can cause loss, for example, of up to 40 g of protein each day into the dialysate, and thus protein intake usually needs to be increased. Similarly, there may be excessive dialysance of phosphorus and potassium and patients should be monitored periodically for hypokalemia and hypophosphatemia. Increased absorption of glucose may necessitate changing to higher dialysate dextrose concentrations to maintain ultrafiltration. Peritonitis can exacerbate the constipation caused by aluminum-containing phosphate binders, necessitating more laxatives.

Eighty-five percent or more of patients have a relatively mild presentation and can be treated entirely as outpatients. The remainder require admission because they are seriously ill, often with severe nausea and vomiting, are unable to do their own exchanges, or require removal of their peritoneal catheter. In the latter circumstance it is especially helpful for the patient to already have a functioning (''back-up'') access for hemodialysis.

TABLE 2 Recommended Intraperitoneal Doses of Antibiotics

Antibiotic	*Loading Dose (mg/L)*	*Maintenance Dose (mg/L)*
Cefazolin	500	125
Cephalothin	500	125
Cefotaxime	500	125
Penicillin	1 million (U)	50,000 (U)
Ampicillin	500	50
Azlocillin	1,000	100
Cloxacillin	1,000	100
Methicillin	1,000	100
Nafcillin	1,000	100
Mezlocillin	1,000	100
Ticarcillin	1,000	100
Carbenicillin	1,000	100
Vancomycin	15 mg/kg	20–30
Clindamycin	300	50
Gentamicin	1.7 mg/kg	6–8
Tobramycin	1.7 mg/kg	6–8
Amikacin	125	25
Trimethoprim-sulfamethoxazole	400/80	25/5
Amphotericin B	...	5
5-Fluorocytosine	...	100

Patients who recognize catheter contamination can be treated prophylactically with the same intraperitoneal antibiotic regimens described above. Some centers prefer to use just oral cephalosporins (e.g., cephalexin, 250 mg every 6 hours for one week); however, that method has yet to be proven efficacious in large series of patients.

The difficulty in eradicating fungal peritonitis accounts for the usual practice of removal of the presumed infected catheter. Some centers, however, have had success in treating *Candida* using amphotericin with or without flucytosine. Since intravenous amphotericin does not reliably yield adequate peritoneal concentrations, intraperitoneal administration is recommended. Since that route can be painful, administration of the drug should begin at a dilute concentration (0.5 μg per milliliter), then gradually be increased to 2 to 4 μg per milliliter. Flucytosine can be added orally or intraperitoneally; there is less experience using this agent alone or in combination with miconazole or ketoconazole. If the patient cannot tolerate amphotericin, the catheter is removed. Our own practice, however, is to remove the catheter as soon as fungal peritonitis is diagnosed. Once that foreign body is removed and the patient undergoes interim hemodialysis, the peritoneum itself often can control the infection; hence, the controversy as to further antibiotic treatment. We suggest giving a total of 250 to 300 mg of amphotericin intravenously over 10 to 14 days. *Aspergillus* often requires more intensive treatment after catheter discontinuation. The peritoneal catheter can be replaced after 4 to 6 weeks of adequate antibiotic treatment.

Tuberculous peritonitis should be suspected in the setting of chronic or atypically relapsing peritonitis in the absence of bacterial or fungal organisms. Although there may be a predominance of mononuclear cells in the peritoneal fluid, this finding is frequently nondiagnostic and there typically is a lack of evidence of active infection in other organ systems. Effluent cultures are frequently negative or require long incubation times, and peritoneal or omental biopsy and/or culture may be necessary to make the diagnosis. Removal of the catheter is then indicated.

A dramatic improvement in the patient's symptoms and peritoneal fluid is expected within 1 to 2 days of treatment of routine bacterial peritonitis. If not, culture results will help guide changing or broadening of the antibiotic coverage. In addition, continued sources of infection need to be more seriously considered: bowel perforation, diverticulitis, abdominal abscess, abscess at the catheter site, tunnel infections (which may produce only minimal symptoms), and fungal or tuberculous infection. Abdominal computed tomography scans are often more helpful than sonograms in delineating abnormal fluid collections. Abscesses may also be detected by gallium- or indium-labeled white blood cell scans. The latter can also be useful in documenting tunnel infections. Continuing infection despite broad antibiotic coverage should lead to removal of the catheter or surgical exploration of the abdomen. Persistence of polymicrobial or anaerobic infection for more than 2 days is also a reason to explore for a bowel perforation. Note that the catheter tubing itself, or fibrin deposits attached to it, can harbor the infecting organisms. There have been reports of small series of patients in whom intraperitoneal streptokinase allegedly permitted cure of lingering infections by lysing the associated fibrin masses. Although lack of response to antibiotic therapy is one reason for catheter removal, the most common cause for its discontinuation is periluminal infection at the exit site or tunnel (see the section Exit Site and Tunnel Infections, below). If the catheter is removed, it should not be replaced until at least 10 to 14 days after there is no evidence of residual peritoneal infection.

Initial clinical improvement followed by recurrence of cloudy fluid (often without a predominance of neutrophils) suggests chemical peritonitis from the administered antibiotics.

After resolution of the peritonitis, efforts should be made to retrain the patient in proper sterile technique. Since depression is associated with errors in the aseptic procedure, psychological assessment is often indicated. Those patients with inadequate exchange technique can be switched to systems with simplified connection procedures, mechanical spike aides, ultraviolet or heat sterilization ("hot blade") devices, or they can have insertion of an in-line microbial filter. Barium enema examination can be done to detect diverticular disease. Women who have vaginal leak and thus contamination of dialysate should be considered for tubal ligation. Those patients who have had severe or recurrent peritonitis may ultimately have long-term deleterious effects on their peritoneal membrane (see the section Diminished Peritoneal Membrane Function).

Exit Site and Tunnel Infections

Some centers have reported a greater than 30 percent incidence of infections at the catheter skin exit site within the first year of use, with up to one-half of these patients requiring catheter removal. Despite the frequency of this problem, there is no consensus as to the best method of prevention. Mechanical irritation of the exit site should be avoided by instructing the patient not to be overly compulsive about cleaning and manipulation. The surgeon should locate the exit site away from the beltline and caudad, and attach the outer cuff at least 2 cm from the skin surface. Although some centers advocate leaving the healed exit site uncovered, we suggest daily cleaning with hydrogen peroxide and then use of a light bandage to prevent local friction. Experience helps differentiate the acceptable postoperative erythema and serous crusting from the lesions that become purulent. A majority of the latter lesions, if they persist for several months, have periluminal progression to tunnel infection and peritonitis. Uncomplicated infections should be cultured and oral antibiotics given to cover skin flora while culture results are pending. Although the frequent occurrence of exit site infections has at times been attributed to extrusion of the distal cuff through the exit site when two-cuff catheters are used, the incidence of infection has not been greatly altered by the use of single-cuff catheters. Severe or nonhealing lesions suggest extension of the infection into the outer cuff, which may then require extrusion and removal by shaving. This can be done using a scalpel, but great care must be exercised to avoid damaging the catheter. Unless all of the glue can be removed along with the cuff, such shaving is generally ineffective in relieving exit site irritation.

Catheter Complications

A number of mechanical and infectious complications of peritoneal catheters lead to significant morbidity in CPD patients.

Dissection of dialysate into the tunnel or the abdominal wall and extending to the genitalia and thighs can occur in the early postoperative period. This is particularly a problem for elderly or multiparous patients or those receiving corticosteroids. The leakage site will usually heal adequately if peritoneal dialysis is discontinued for at least 2 days and the patient rests to avoid abdominal muscle straining or activity. Dialysis should then resume, at first with small volumes (i.e., 1.5 L). Approximately 2 to 10 percent of patients will develop late leakage, months or years after catheter insertion. In these cases, peritoneal dialysis should be stopped for approximately two weeks and then resumed, initially with low volumes. Use of CCPD with an empty abdomen during the day will also minimize intra-abdominal pressure. Experience has shown that the peritoneal opening for the catheter will form a stronger scar if placed by a paramedian approach through the rectus muscle rather than the linea alba, thus decreasing the incidence of leakage and herniation.

Approximately 10 percent of CPD patients will develop incisional, inguinal, ventral, or umbilical hernias. This again emphasizes the importance of good surgical technique and location in placement of the catheter. Up to two-thirds of those patients who develop incisional hernias reportedly initially suffered from a temporary leak at the time of catheter insertion. Ideally, the incisions should be allowed to heal for 10 to 14 days before peritoneal dialysis is begun. The risk of herniation is proportional to the volume used, particularly for those using 3 L. Because of the danger of bowel incarceration, every patient should be fully examined for hernias before commencing peritoneal dialysis and should undergo surgical correction then or immediately upon development of that complication. After hernia repair peritoneal dialysis should, when possible, be discontinued for at least 3 days and then restarted at small (i.e., 1 L) volumes initially. CCPD may be most appropriate in this situation as well, as discussed.

Slow dialysate outflow may be seen when the catheter tip has migrated cephalad out of the lower quadrant. Enemas or repositioning the patient may return the catheter to its proper location or this may occur spontaneously, usually within two days. The catheter can be redirected manually by peritoneoscopy, but open surgical correction or replacement (suturing it in that direction) is often necessary.

Dialysate flow can also become impaired if the catheter ports become obstructed by the omentum, a problem that is reported less frequently with the Toronto-Western-Hospital device. If the openings are obstructed by fibrin, approximately 250,000 to 750,000 IU of streptokinase infused into the catheter has reportedly been successful in restoring patency.

Diminished Peritoneal Membrane Function

Decreased peritoneal clearance is a major concern after severe peritonitis. There can be peritoneal sclerosis, compartmentalization of the abdomen by adhesions, or inadequate flow through the catheter because of fibrin deposits. There are also fears that dialysate fluid itself may injure the peritoneum by virtue of the repeated physical trauma of the exchanges, acid pH, hyperosmolarity, or chemical impurities (i.e., plasticizers and particulate matter). It has been suggested that hyperparathyroidism may be associated with decreased peritoneal clearances. Clinically, the syndrome of ultrafiltration failure is often more of a problem than loss of solute clearance. Enhanced glucose absorption causes a rapid loss of the osmotic gradient, and necessitates using shorter exchange cycles or dialysate solutions with higher dextrose concentrations.

Documenting diminished mass transfer coefficients is too laborious and impractical for clinical use. To test the peritoneum crudely, even before a permanent catheter is placed, one can instill 2 L of 2.5 percent dialysate and measure both blood and dialysate urea and creatinine at 4 hours. The dialysate urea nitrogen should be at least 85 percent and the creatinine at least 65 percent of the respective plasma levels if the peritoneum is functioning well.

Peritoneoscopy can be used to demonstrate and possibly lyse adhesions. Peritoneal air-contrast studies are done by first introducing the water-soluble contrast media and then instilling nitrous oxide. This technique may visualize fibrous bands, adhesions, and abscesses.

Other Complications

Hydrothorax. Pleural accumulation of dialysate fluid is thought to be secondary to congenital or acquired small pleuroperitoneal channels. It usually occurs on the right side and may become massive. Early diagnosis can be established by the elevated glucose levels in the pleural fluid. If, however, enough time has elapsed to allow systemic equilibration of the dialysate, then one can attempt to scintigraphically image the pleural accumulation of intraperitoneally injected ^{99m}Tc-albumin. Patients can be managed by 2 to 4 weeks off peritoneal dialysis, followed by slow reinstitution with increasing volumes. If this approach fails, the patient should subsequently be maintained on hemodialysis. If CPD is still deemed necessary, however, an attempt at pleurodesis should be made before peritoneal dialysis is reinstituted.

Hyperlipidemia. Lipid abnormalities develop in at least 50 percent of CPD patients and are especially worrisome because of the already high incidence of cardiovascular disease in individuals with ESRD. Hypertriglyceridemia usually occurs within the first 3 months of CPD and is in large part secondary to the approximately 160- to 200-g of glucose absorbed daily from the dialysate. Obesity is not an infrequent complication from the additional calories of hypertonic solutions. Initial low levels of high-density lipoprotein cholesterol may improve in some patients with initiation of peritoneal dialysis. Considering the lack of effective pharmacologic therapy (including the potential toxicity of clofibrate even at reduced doses), diet and weight control remain the most important treatment modalities for the lipid disorders.

Back Pain. Patients compensate for the weight of the dialysate by increasing their lumbar lordosis, thereby changing the center of gravity. This frequently causes or exacerbates the low back pain from preexisting (i.e., degenerative or metabolic) spine disease. Patients should avoid activities that cause further stress, be instructed on exercises to strengthen that musculature, and may benefit from abdominal binders.

Dialysis-associated Osteomalacia. As in hemodialysis, there has been a growing awareness of aluminum-related bone disease in CPD patients. The dignostic criteria are the same and as controversial as those for hemodialysis patients (i.e., bone biopsy or elevated serum aluminum levels after deferoxamine infusion). Intravenous deferoxamine is currently recommended for chelation therapy, but studies are under way examining the efficacy of intramuscular or intraperitoneal administration. When possible, aluminum-containing phosphate binders should be replaced with calcium carbonate. Commercially available dialysate is not a significant source of aluminum.

Malnutrition. As noted above, peritoneal protein loss can be considerable. Most of the approximately 6 to 12 g lost each day is albumin, with about 2 g as amino acids. Adequate protein supplementation can be complicated by the sense of abdominal fullness or early satiety caused by the weight and volume of dialysate. Dialysate solutions containing amino acids rather than dextrose are currently under investigation.

Hypotension. Hypotension is frequently more eas-

TABLE 3 Long-term Outcome of Chronic Peritoneal Dialysis in Southern California and Southern Nevada*

Patients followed	1,061
Peritonitis episodes per patient year	1.3
Catheter replacements per patient year	0.3
Hospital days per patient year (total)	16.2
Peritonitis	5.3
Other CAPD complications	4.8
Actuarial 3-year patient survival	
Nondiabetic	72%
Diabetic	36%
Actuarial 3-year technique success	48%

* January 1, 1979, to December 31, 1984

ily controlled on CPD than on hemodialysis. Some patients become hypotensive, seemingly because of excessive ultrafiltration. They may be managed with dialysate solutions of low tonicity, but they may also require oral salt and water repletion.

Lower Extremity Ischemia. Since patients with vascular disease may suffer from peripheral ischemia during episodes of hypotension, excessive ultrafiltration should be avoided.

LONG-TERM RESULTS

Table 3 summarizes the long-term outcome of patients placed on CAPD in southern California and southern Nevada between January 1, 1979, and December 31, 1984. Infectious complications remain a major source of morbidity, though a solvable one. Continued expansion of CPD probably depends on further control of these serious complications.

RENAL OSTEODYSTROPHY

SHAUL G. MASSRY, M.D.
ELAINE M. KAPTEIN, M.D., F.A.C.P.

Disturbances in divalent ion metabolism are common in patients with renal failure. The major features of these abnormalities are summarized in Table 1.

The processes causing disordered divalent ion metabolism and osteodystrophy begin in the early stages of renal insufficiency, continue throughout the life of the patient, and may be influenced beneficially or adversely by the various therapeutic approaches employed. The goals of the therapy of these disorders are (1) to maintain the blood concentrations of calcium and phosphorus as near normal as possible; (2) to prevent the development of secondary hyperparathyroidism, and if the latter already exists, to suppress the activity of the parathyroid glands; (3) to prevent and reverse soft tissue calcification; and (4) to ameliorate or reverse the proximal myopathy, bone pain, pruritis, and soft tissue necrosis.

Despite our increased knowledge of the pathogenesis of the deranged divalent ion metabolism in patients with renal failure, there is still no unified approach to optimal therapy. The various therapeutic modalities currently in use are neither completely effective nor without hazards. The overall management includes the use of one or more of the following therapeutic approaches: (1) control of phosphate retention and hyperphosphatemia; (2) supplementation of calcium; (3) treatment with vitamin D or one or more of its metabolites; (4) adjustment of dialysate composition; (5) chelation of aluminum in those with increased aluminum burden; and (6) parathyroidectomy.

CONTROL OF PHOSPHATE RETENTION AND HYPERPHOSPHATEMIA

Phosphate retention and hyperphosphatemia play an important role in the pathogenesis of the disorders of divalent ion metabolism of renal failure. The prevention of phosphate retention in patients with mild or moderate renal insufficiency and the control of hyperphosphatemia in those with advanced renal failure are major factors in the management of these patients. The hyperphosphatemia of uremia may be reduced by dietary restriction of phosphate, by the use of phosphate binding antacids, by increased frequency of hemodialysis, and by the inhibition of parathormone (PTH)- mediated bone resorption.

The dietary intake of phosphate is a function of the meat and dairy products ingested by the patient. The usual phosphate intake of a normal adult in the United States ranges between 1.0 and 1.8 g per day. One can reduce dietary intake of phosphate by 40 percent (600 to 900 g per day) by the elimination of dairy products and the restriction of protein intake. Further reduction may be difficult to achieve without jeopardizing adequate protein intake or compromising the palatability of the food. Thus, restriction of dietary phosphate intake in proportion to the decrease in glomerular filtration rate (GFR) as the sole measure for the prevention of phosphate retention is feasible only in patients with moderate renal failure (GFR 60 to 30 ml per minute). Indeed, this approach has been successful in reversing many of the abnormalities in divalent ion metabolism in such patients.

In patients with advanced renal failure, dietary phosphate restriction alone is not adequate to control hyperphosphatemia. In a group of patients with creatinine clearances of 2 to 10 ml per minute who were treated with rigid protein restriction (20 or 40 g per day) for 30 to 60 days, serum phosphorus levels remained elevated, with mean levels of 7.2 $\pm$ 0.86 and 7.3 $\pm$ 0.72 mg per deciliter respectively, despite continued negative phosphorus balance in some of the patients. It is evident that in patients with advanced renal failure other measures are needed to maintain serum phosphorus levels within the normal range. This could be achieved with the use of phosphate binding antacids, which would render the ingested phosphate and the phosphate contained in the saliva (12 mM per liter), bile (5 mM per liter), and intestinal juices (1 mM per liter) unabsorbable.

Several compounds that bind phosphate in the intestinal tract are available in liquid, tablet, and capsule forms (Table 2). The capsules are less effective than liquid gels in binding phosphate, but patient compliance is easier to achieve with capsules than with either the liquid or the tablets. The most frequently used compounds are Alucaps, Amphogel, and Basaljel concentrate. The latter is tasteless and only a small volume is necessary per dose; hence the patients more readily follow the prescribed regimen. The goal of treatment is to reduce the level of serum phos-

TABLE 1 Major Features of Disordered Divalent Ion Metabolism in Renal Failure

Hyperphosphatemia
Hypocalcemia
Elevated serum levels of alkaline phosphatase
Secondary hyperparathyroidism
Defective intestinal absorption of calcium and phosphate
Altered vitamin D metabolism resulting in relative or absolute deficiency of 1,25 dihydroxyvitamin D
Bone disease
  Enhanced bone resorption
  Increased endosteal fibrosis
  Defective mineralization (rickets or osteomalacia)
Soft tissue calcification
  Vascular
  Visceral
  Periarticular
  Cutaneous
  Occular
Alterations in renal handing of phosphate (increased fractional excretion), calcium (hypocalciuria), and magnesium (increased fractional excretion)
Pruritus
Proximal myopathy
Skin ulcerations and soft tissue necrosis

phorus to near normal. With these agents, care should be exercised to avoid both a fall in serum phosphorus to a very low level and phosphate depletion. Phosphate depletion per se may aggravate bone disease and even cause osteomalacia. Therapy may be started with 2 to 3 tablets of Amphogel or capsules of Alucaps, or 5 to 10 ml of Basaljel with each meal. The levels of serum phosphorus should be monitored at least twice per month and the dosage of the phosphate binders adjusted accordingly. Continued coaxing and emphasis on the importance of this treatment are essential to obtain adherence to this therapy by the patients. These compounds are ineffective in controlling the concentration of serum phosphorus if phosphate intake exceeds 2.0 g per day.

The fall in serum phosphorus concentration during therapy with dietary phosphate restriction and the use of phosphate binding antacids is usually associated with a rise in the level of serum calcium; if the magnitude of the latter is adequate, a fall in the blood levels of parathormone (PTH) may occur, and this in turn contributes to the maintenance of the concentration of serum phosphorus at lower levels.

The aluminum in the phosphate binding antacids is absorbed by the intestine and may accumulate in various tissues of the body, such as brain and bone. Increased aluminum burden of the brain has been incriminated in the pathogenesis of dialysis encephalopathy, and accumulation of aluminum in bone may be responsible for the low turnover osteomalacia that is refractory to therapy. Despite these potential hazards, these compounds are still recommended to control hyperphosphatemia in patients with advanced renal failure and in dialysis patients. The use of magnesium containing compounds should be avoided because of the risks of hypermagnesemia.

CALCIUM SUPPLEMENTATION

The low dietary intake of calcium and the defect in intestinal calcium absorption, which is more evident at low intake, put patients with renal failure in double jeopardy regarding their calcium metabolism. Evidence exists that indicates normal amounts of calcium could be absorbed by the gut of these patients when their calcium intake is high. Indeed, long-term calcium supplementation has been associated with beneficial effects, such as a rise in the concentration of serum calcium, a fall in the serum levels of alkaline phosphatase and PTH, and a reduction in bone resorption and the number and incidence of fractures; such therapy, however, did not result in normal mineralization of osteoid. Thus, there is a good rationale for calcium supplementation, but the time in the course of renal insufficiency at which such therapy should be initiated is not clear. It is reasonable to suggest that patients with GFRs between 40 and 10 ml per minute should receive 1.2 to 1.5 g of elemental calcium per day. Calcium supplements may be given to these patients to bring their total daily intake to this level. Patients with advanced renal failure (GRF $<$10 ml per minute) may need a supplement of 1.0 to 2.0 g of calcium per day.

Treatment with calcium salts is not without hazards. It is dangerous to administer large quantities of oral calcium compounds in the face of marked hyperphosphatemia

TABLE 2 Partial List of Available Phosphate Binding Compounds

Generic Name	*Proprietary Name*	*Manufacturer*	*Form Available*
Aluminum hydroxide gel	Amphogel	Wyeth	Tablets (0.3 and 0.6 g)
Aluminum hydroxide gel	Alu-Cap	Ricker	Capsules (0.6 g)
Aluminum carbonate	Basaljel	Wyeth	Solution (3.6 g/30 ml) Tablets (0.5 g) Capsules (0.5 g)
Aluminum hydroxide and magnesium hydroxide	Aludrox	Wyeth	Tablets
Aluminum hydroxide and magnesium hydroxide	Maalox	Roter	Tablets
Aluminum hydroxide, magnesium hydroxide, and simethicone	Gelusil	Parke-Davis	Tablets
Aluminum hydroxide, magnesium hydroxide, and simethicone	Mylanta	Stuart	Tablets

because of the danger of an elevation in calcium-phosphorus product, which predisposes to soft tissue calcification. It is thus imperative that hyperphosphatemia be controlled and the level of serum phosphorus be less than 5.5 mg per deciliter prior to treatment with calcium salts. Hypercalcemia may also appear during therapy with large doses of oral calcium, especially in patients with advanced renal failure; this is particularly true when there has been a concomitant reduction in the levels of serum phosphorus to less than 2.0 mg per deciliter. A variety of symptoms may accompany even mild hypercalcemia in uremic patients. Nausea, vomiting, mental confusion, lethargy, pruritus, dysesthesias, and severe hypertension have been encountered. Therefore, weekly or bimonthly monitoring of the concentration of serum calcium and phosphorus is advisable. If the serum concentration of calcium exceeds 10.5 mg per deciliter, calcium supplements may be cut in half or may even be discontinued temporarily.

Elemental calcium consitiutes 40 percent of calcium carbonate, 12 percent of calcium lactate, and 8 percent of calcium gluconate. Calcium chloride should be avoided in uremic patients because of its acidifying properties. Calcium carbonate is inexpensive, tasteless, and relatively well tolerated. Calcium carbonate is available in several proprietary preparations, such as Titralac, Tums, or Os-cal. Titralac provides 0.42 g of calcium carbonate and 0.18 g of glycine per tablet (160 mg of elemental calcium per tablet). Neo-Calglucon syrup is another preparation well accepted by patients, but it is costly; each 4 ml contains 92 mg of calcium ion. To maximize calcium absorption, the amount prescribed should be ingested in several small doses divided throughout the day rather than in one or two large doses.

USE OF VITAMIN D COMPOUNDS

Since many of the features of abnormal calcium metabolism in uremia resemble those of vitamin D deficiency, this compound and its related steroids have been used in the management of renal osteodystrophy. The forms of vitamin D metabolites currently available for clinical use in the United States are vitamin D_2 (ergocalciferol); vitamin D_3 (cholecalciferol), which is the naturally occurring form of the steroid in mammals; dihydrotachysterol (DHT); $250HD_3$; and $1,25(OH)_2D_3$. Another vitamin D analogue, 1 alpha-OHD_3, is available for clinical use outside the United States.

Because of its low cost, vitamin D_2, a steroid obtained from plant sources, has been most widely used in medicine. Vitamin D_3 can now be prepared inexpensively but it does not enjoy widespread use. Moreover, there is little evidence to indicate that vitamin D_2 differs in activity from vitamin D_3 in man.

Vitamin D_2 and D_3

The amount of vitamin D required by patients with advanced renal failure varies greatly. Doses as high as 50,000 to 200,000 IU per day (1.25 to 5.0 mg) may be needed to achieve beneficial effects. Long-term therapy with large doses of vitamin D causes a rise in serum calcium level and may be followed by a fall in serum levels of alkaline phosphatase and PTH, reduced bone resorption, and amelioration or healing of rickets in uremic children or of osteomalacia in uremic adults. Because of the need for large doses of vitamin D, hypercalcemia is a real and frequent hazard. *Such hypercalcemia may persist for weeks* after the discontinuation of therapy. In addition to the clinical side effects of hypercalcemia, the elevation in the serum levels of calcium in a hyperphosphatemic patient would cause a marked rise in calcium-phosphorus product, predisposing to soft tissue calcification. Therapy with vitamin D sould not be started prior to the normalization of the serum levels of phosphorus. Frequent monitoring of the levels of serum calcium and phosphorus during such therapy is advisable.

25 Hydroxyvitamin D_3

Despite the block in the conversion of 250HD to $1,25(OH)_2D$, therapy with 50 to 100μg of $250HD_3$ per day has been shown to be beneficial. Treatment with this metabolite was associated with amelioration of bone pain and proximal myopathy, a rise in serum calcium concentration, and a fall in serum levels of alkaline phosphatase and PTH. A decrease in the degree of osteitis fibrosa and even improvement in bone mineralization have been noted.

1,25 Dihydroxyvitamin D_3

A relative deficiency of this active metabolite exists in patients with mild and moderate renal failure, and absolute deficiency exists in those with advanced renal failure. Furthermore, the kidney is required to convert the parent vitamin D to this active metabolite. Therefore, it is rational to treat renal failure patients with this metabolite to correct the vitamin D–deficient state. Indeed, such therapy has proven beneficial. It is important to emphasize at this point that some or most of the beneficial effects of $1,25(OH)_2D_3$ in the management of renal osteodystrophy could be produced by other vitamin D compounds. The small dose of $1,25(OH)_2D_3$ that is needed to achieve beneficial effects and its shorter half-life make it a better and safer agent than other vitamin D compounds. On the other hand, the high biologic potency of $1,25(OH)_2D_3$ is mandatory.

Dosage Schedule. The suggested initial dose is 0.5 μg per day, although it may be safer to begin therapy with 0.25 μg per day. Although the limited data suggest that 0.5 μg per day of $1,25(OH)_2D_3$ is beneficial and safe in patients with GFRs of 30 to 50 ml per minute and normophosphatemia, it is possible that smaller or larger dosages may be required by patients with higher or lower GFRs, respectively. Caution should be exercised in the use of $1,25(OH)_2D_3$ in patients with GFRs less than 25 ml per minute. These patients may be hyperphosphatemic, and a rise in blood calcium concentration in the presence of elevated blood phosphorus concentration would result in an increase in the calcium-phosphorus product to a hazardous level. In such an eventuality, calcium deposition may occur in various tissues, including the renal parenchyma. The latter effect could be associated with deterioration in renal function. Intravenous $1,25(OH)_2D_3$ given in doses of 1.0 to 1.5μg 3 times weekly has been well tolerated and has proven remarkably effective. Serum calcium levels return to normal and secondary hyperparathyroidism is completely suppressed. Ultimately, this approach to Vitamin D therapy may become the preferred therapy for hypocalcemia and secondary hyperparathyroidism in patients with advanced renal failure.

The changes in the concentrations of serum calcium provide the best clinical guide for modification of the dosage. Failure of the level of serum calcium to rise by at least 0.5 mg per deciliter with any particular dosage given for 4 to 6 weeks justifies increasing the dose by 0.25 to 0.5μg per day. Such an approach may be used until the serum calcium level reaches the upper normal range (10.0 to 10.5 mg per deciliter). When this is achieved, frequent monitoring of serum calcium is needed, and if the latter approaches hypercalcemic range, a reduction of the dosage or temporary discontinuation of therapy should be considered. It is our experience and that of others that the requirement of and the tolerance for $1,25(OH)_2D_3$ may decrease progressively during treatment in many patients; therefore, reduction of the maintenance dosage after a prolonged period of therapy may be needed.

Effect on Serum Calcium. The most consistent effect of $1,25(OH)_2D_3$ in uremic and dialysis patients is elevation in the serum concentration of calcium. Although it is reasonable to assume that the higher the dosage of the metabolite the greater the rise in serum calcium concentration, many variables in addition to the dosage may modify the calcemic response to therapy with $1,25(OH)_2D_3$. These may include duration of treatment, dietary calcium intake, changes in intestinal absorption of calcium, type of bone disease and its response to treatment, and the severity of the state of secondary hyperparathyroidism. Occasionally, serum calcium concentration may fall during the first 1 to 2 weeks of therapy, probably owing to rapid remineralization of the skeleton.

Hypercalcemia is a frequent complication of treatment with $1,25(OH)_2D_3$. It has been reported that 30 to 67 percent of the patients treated with this metabolite developed one or more hypercalcemic episodes during the course of their therapy. The overall incidence of one episode was 42 percent. Hypercalcemia occurred with a dosage of 0.5 to 3.0 μg per day of $1,25(OH)_2D_3$ and was more frequent with a dosage of 1.0 to 3.0 μg per day. Certain patients are more prone to develop hypercalcemia: (1) patients with osteitis fibrosa and pre-treatment serum calcium concentration greater than 10.5 mg per day, and (2) patients with low turnover osteomalacia, low serum concentration of PTH, and absent bone marrow fibrosis. Hypercalcemia may appear at any time during therapy with $1,25(OH)_2D_3$. It usually occurs after 2 to 3 months of therapy but has been encountered as early as 5 days and as late as 6 to 18 months after treatment. A high starting dose may be the cause for the early appearance of hypercalcemia. In patients with severe osteitis fibrosa and pre-treatment serum calcium concentration of 10.5 mg per deciliter, early hypercalcemia within 1 to 4 weeks of therapy may also occur. Extreme caution should be exercised in the management of such patients with $1,25(OH)_2D_3$. It has been noted that the incidence of hypercalcemia increases as serum alkaline phosphatase activity returns to normal, and it is recommended that the dose of $1,25(OH)_2D_3$ be reduced when serum levels of alkaline phosphatase normalize. The hypercalcemia is usually mild and asymptomatic, but serum calcium concentrations greater than 13.0 mg per deciliter and occasionally even higher than 15.0 mg per deciliter have been encountered during therapy with $1,25(OH)_2D_3$. The elevated levels of serum calcium usually return to normal shortly after reduction of the dose or discontinuation of therapy. The hypercalcemia may occasionally persist for several weeks. It is advisable to stop treatment completely rather than to reduce the dose when hypercalcemia appears and to reinstitute therapy with a smaller dose as serum calcium concentrations return to normal.

Effect on Serum Phosphorus. The effect of $1,25(OH)_2D_3$ treatment on the concentration of serum phosphorus in uremic or dialysis patients is not consistent. Increases, decreases, and no change have been reported. This variability among patient populations may be related to differences in dietary intake of phosphate and/or the ingestion of phosphate binding antacids, the dosage of $1,25(OH)_2D_3$, the effect of the metabolite on intestinal absorption of phosphate, the degree of suppression of the parathyroid gland activity, and the status of the remineralizion of bone. Monitoring of serum phosphorus concentrations during therapy with $1,25(OH)_2D_3$ is mandatory because the development of hyperphosphatemia, especially in the face of rising serum calcium concentration, would result in elevation of calcium-phosphorus product and augment the hazards of soft tissue calcification. If hyperphosphatemia occurs and calcium-phosphorus product approaches 55, every effort should be made to control the levels of serum phosphorus with phosphate binding antacids. If this procedure is not successful, the dose of $1,25(OH)_2D_3$ should be reduced or temporary cessation of therapy should be considered. Under no circumstances should the calcium-phosphorus product be allowed to exceed 55.

Effect on Alkaline Phosphatase, PTH, and Calcium Absorption. Serum alkaline phosphatase activity usually decreases during therapy with $1,25(OH)_2D_3$, but several months may elapse before levels return to normal. Occasionally, serum alkaline phosphatase may rise during the critical phase of therapy. Monitoring the serum alkaline phosphatase could provide an additional guide for the adjustment of the dosage of $1,25(OH)_2D_3$ for two reasons. First, normalization of serum levels of alkaline phosphatase reflects improvement in bone disease, and second, the occurrence of hypercalcemia increases as serum alkaline phosphatase returns to normal.

Long-term therapy with $1,25(OH)_2D_3$ may be associated with a marked fall in or even normalization of the serum levels of PTH. No change, or even an increase in serum levels of the hormone has also been encountered during therapy with this metabolite. The reduction in the serum levels of PTH during therapy with $1,25(OH)_2D_3$ is probably due to the rise in the concentration of serum calcium. We have found an inverse correlation between the percentage change in serum calcium concentrations and PTH levels.

Intestinal absorption of calcium is usually increased in uremic patients during therapy with $1,25(OH)_2D_3$. The increment in calcium absorption is most evident during the first 2 hours after calcium ingestion, which suggests that the metabolite exerts its effect in the duodenum and proximal part of the small intestine. This metabolite may also affect calcium absorption in the jejunum, since this segment of the intestine has receptors for $1,25(OH)_2D_3$. There is a dose-response relationship between $1,25(OH)_2D_3$ and intestinal absorption of calcium. Finally, the quantity of the sterol required to elicit an increase in intestinal calcium absorption in the uremic patients is greater than in normal subjects, which indicates that uremia, per se, may interfere with the action of the sterol on the gut. $1,25(OH)_2D_3$ also augments intestinal absorption of phosphate. The metabolite may produce a modest rise in urinary calcium in uremic patients.

Clinical Response. Among the most disturbing clinical symptoms of renal osteodystrophy are muscle weakness and bone pain. The muscle weakness is a clinical manifestation of uremic myopathy, which is probably due to vitamin D deficiency. The exact cause of bone pain is not known but may be related to the presence of osteomalacia, osteitis fibrosa, or both. These disturbances may interfere seriously with the daily activity of the patients and may even render them totally disabled. Improvement in these symptoms appears rapidly after initiation of therapy with $1,25(OH)_2D_3$. The improvement in muscle strength may become noticeable within 2 to 5 weeks of treatment. A significant amelioration or complete disappearance of bone pain may also occur in some patients within 1 to 3 weeks of treatment, while in others it may take 6 to 28 weeks before a decrease in bone pain becomes evident. This clinical improvement produces a remarkable change in the physical disability of the patients; many of them become symptom free and are able to perform their daily activity without limitation (Fig. 1). Similar observations have been made in children. For example, three children who had ceased to walk for several months prior to therapy began walking within 1 month and were running after 4 months of treatment. Treatment of uremic children with $1,25(OH)_2D_3$ may also increase growth velocity; this effect is extremely important, since retarded growth in uremic children is a very common and serious problem.

Therapy with $1,25(OH)_2D_3$ for several months can be associated with a decrease in bone resorption, and treatment for 2 to 3 years may result in complete healing of bone resorption. The effect on bone resorption reflects the degree of success in suppressing the activity of the parathyroid glands. Endosteal fibrosis is either markedly reduced or completely reversed after several months of treatment irrespective of whether serum levels of PTH are decreased or not. This observation raises the possibility that endosteal fibrosis is not entirely the result of excess PTH, but could also be related to vitamin D deficiency as well. The osteomalacia in patients with mixed bone disease (osteomalacia and osteitis fibrosa) responds well to therapy with $1,25(OH)_2D_3$. Long-term treatment usually results in marked improvement or healing of the osteomalacia. In patients with pure low-turnover osteomalacia, the response to $1,25(OH)_2D_3$ is poor; these patients may respond better to long-term therapy (4 to 6 months) with both $1,25(OH)_2D_3$ and $24,25(OH)_2D_3$ (2.5 to 10μg per day). The healing of the bone lesions during treatment with $1,25(OH)_2D_3$ may also be evidenced by improvement in the radiographic findings of the skeleton.

Failure of therapy with $1,25(OH)_2D_3$ to improve clinical signs and symptoms has been reported. The treatment-failure group appears to be heterogeneous and does not display a specific biochemical pattern of bone disease. Although such patients had higher serum calcium concentration than those who responded to treatment, the serum levels of PTH were normal, moderately elevated, or very high, and the bone lesions varied from pure osteomalacia in some to marked osteitis fibrosa in others. Further analysis of the data, however, indicates that there are two distinct subgroups among these patients. The first group consists of patients with severe osteitis fibrosa and marked elevation of serum PTH. In the second group, the patients had normal serum levels of PTH and pure osteomalacia without evidence of hyperparathyroid bone disease. Both of these groups rapidly developed hypercalcemia. As this complication requires cessation of treatment, it would preclude long-term therapy and result in failure to improve the clinical and histologic abnormalities of renal osteodystrophy.

Effect on Renal Function. Data on the effect of $1,25(OH)_2D_3$ on the derangements of divalent ion metabolism in patients with moderate renal failure are

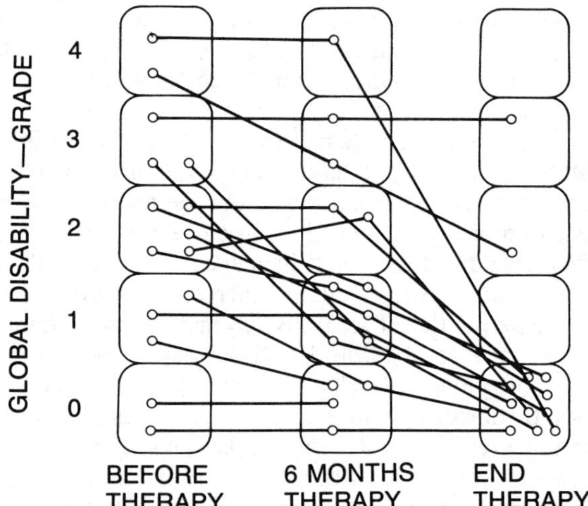

Figure 1 Global disability scoring of the patients before and during therapy with $1,25(OH)_2D_3$. Grade 4, totally disabled, restricted to bed or wheelchair; grade 3, marked disability, pain or weakness restricts activity, walks with aid; grade 2, symptoms reduce activity moderately, walks with aid; grade 1, symptoms only with strenous activity; grade 0, asymptomatic and no activity restriction. Reprinted with permission from Goldstein DA, Malluche HH, Massry SG. Management of renal osteodystrophy with $1,25(OH)_2D_3$. Min Elect Metab 1979; 2:35.

limited. Treatment of patients with GFR of 32 to 51 ml per min with 0.5 μg per day of $1,25(OH)_2D_3$ for 6 months raised serum calcium levels, reversed the defect in intestinal calcium absorption, normalized the serum levels of PTH, and healed the bone disease. These observations suggest that initiation of therapy with $1,25(OH)_2D_3$ early in the course of renal failure could be beneficial for the prevention of the progression of renal osteodystrophy. Such an approach could be justified, however, if treatment with this metabolite has no harmful effect on renal function.

Theoretically, a deleterious effect of $1,25(OH)_2D_3$ on renal function could be caused by action of the metabolite on the structure or function of the kidneys or by other metabolic consequences of the treatment, such as hypercalcemia. It has been claimed that the administration of $1,25(OH)_2D_3$ to patients with moderate renal failure produced a significant reduction in GFR due to direct adverse effect. Analysis of all available and pertinent data does not support the contention that $1,25(OH)_2D_3$ has a direct deleterious effect on renal function. The metabolite could produce a reversible or permanent fall in GFR, however, if sustained hypercalcemia develops during its administration. The use of the proper dosage, the frequent monitoring of serum calcium and creatinine concentrations, and the discontinuation of therapy as hypercalcemia develops are are precautionary measures that should be followed to reduce the likelihood of a harmful effect on renal function.

DIALYSATE AND ITS COMPOSITION

There is evidence for numerous geographic variations in the incidence of skeletal disease in patients undergoing hemodialysis. Various impurities and trace elements, such as fluoride or aluminum, may be responsible for these variations. It is now accepted that water treatment and purification should be employed prior to the preparation of the dialysate.

Variations in the concentration of calcium in dialysate may affect the course of renal osteodystrophy. It should be emphasized that all the calcium present in dialysate is ionized and diffuses freely across the membrane of the dialyzer. This contrasts to calcium in blood; only 60 percent of the total amount is not bound to protein and is able to move across the membrane. Depending upon the gradient, the dialysate calcium level, and the concentration of diffusible calcium in blood, there will be either a loss or a gain of this ion by the patient. The use of dialysate containing 5.0 to 5.5 mg of calcium per deciliter is associated with a high incidence of radiographic evidence of bone disease, progressively rising serum levels of alkaline phosphatase, loss of calcium from bones, and persistently elevated serum levels of PTH. For these reasons, dialysate containing such a low concentration of calcium should be abandoned. The use of dialysate containing 8.0 mg of calcium per deciliter may be hazardous in that it may cause hypercalcemia and enhance soft tissue calcification. Most authorities recommend a calcium concentration of 7.0 mg per deciliter.

Most centers have used dialysate containing magnesium in a concentration varying between 0.6 and 1.8 mg per deciliter (0.5 to 1.5 mEq per Liter). With the lower dialysate magnesium concentration, predialysis levels of magnesium are usually normal and are slightly below normal immediately after dialysis. Patients treated with dialysate containing the higher concentration of magnesium have moderate hypermagnesemia all the time. There is no evidence that variations in dialysate magnesium concentration *within this range* have an effect on the incidence, course, or severity of skeletal disease, soft tissue calcification, or symptoms related to altered divalent ion metabolism.

ALUMINUM CHELATION

It is now widely accepted that a major factor in the pathogensis of low-turnover osteomalacia in renal failure is the accumulation of aluminum in bone at the mineralization front. Such deposition may also be involved in depressed bone marrow response to chronic anemia of renal failure, and brain accumulation of aluminum is probably involved in the pathogenesis of dialysis encephalopathy.

Thus, chelation of aluminum from tissue stores may be very helpful. Desferrioxamine (DFO) is a potent chelator of aluminum (and iron) and has been successfully used in the therapy of low-turnover osteomalacia (and dialysis encephalopathy). The aluminum - DFO complex is easily removed by hemodialysis, hemofiltration, peritoneal dialysis, and charcoal hemoperfusion. After confirming the diagnosis of increased body aluminum burden by appropriate study of plasma aluminum concentration (before and after DFO) and bone biopsy, the DFO should be infused post-dialyzer in a dose of 40 to 80 mg per kilogram once weekly. Although post-DFO, the serum aluminum concentration rises dramatically in those patients with greatly increased body aluminum burden, this is not usually associated with toxic symptoms.

Removal of 600 mg or more of aluminum can be accomplished over several months of treatment with DFO. Bone lesions heal promptly, weakness and bone pain often improve dramatically, and anemia may abate significantly. The recurrence of osteitis fibrosa cystica responsive to $1,25(OH)_2D_3$ has been observed following DFO therapy. Side effects of DFO include anaphylaxis, posterior cataract, and visual impairment. Regular ophthamologic examinations are desirable.

PARATHYROIDECTOMY

The various medical therapeutic modalities detailed earlier can result in suppression of the hyperplastic parathyroid glands in uremic patients. However, these measures may not be successful and parathyroidectomy may be the only way to treat the clinical, biochemical, and skeletal manifestations of secondary hyperparathyroidism. Subtotal parathyroidectomy should be considered (1) when persistent hypercalcemia develops; (2) when severe intractable pruritus unresponsive to dialysis is present, especially when the blood levels of PTH are markedly elevated; (3) when marked soft tissue calcification (especially vascular) and radiographic evidence of marked osteitis fibrosa are present, and they cannot be adequately controlled with conservative therapy; and (4) when ischemic lesions of soft tissue with ulcerations and necrosis develop.

The amount of parathyroid tissue to be removed at surgery depends on the size of the parathyroid glands in any particular patient. We recommend that all four glands be identified first; three glands are then removed and weighed. By comparing the size of the fourth gland with those removed, one can roughly estimate the weight of the fourth gland. The surgeon should leave only 150 to 200 mg of this remaining gland. Since the residual parathyroid tissue may undergo further hyperplasia and a second operation may be required, it is recommended that the residual tissue be marked by a metal clip. An alternative approach is to remove all four glands and transplant part of a gland in the forearm. If fewer than four glands are identified in the neck, they should all be removed. Rarely does removal of three identified glands result in a state of permanent hypoparathyroidism. Total parathyroidectomy may be considered in patients who are to be maintained with hemodialysis and who are not candidates for renal transplantation. The medical and/or surgical treatment of uremic secondary hyperparathyroidism assumes greater significance with the accumulation of evidence indicating that excess PTH in blood may play a major role in uremic toxicity.

The technical problems during the surgical procedure are few. The glands are grossly enlarged and easily identifiable. In the hands of an experienced surgeon the operation is not hazardous, and the patient leaves the hospital within a week. The patients should be treated with dialysis one day prior to surgery.

A major problem during the postoperative period is the control of serum calcium concentration. Its level invariably falls after the removal of three or more parathyroid glands. The magnitude and duration of the hypocalcemia vary from one patient to another. Those with marked periarticular calcification usually maintain the serum levels of calcium between 8.0 and 9.0 mg per deciliter until the ectopic calcifications disappear. Also, the use of dialysate containing 7.0 mg of calcium per deciliter causes a rise in serum calcium concentration during dialysis and may alleviate the hypocalcemia during the interdialytic intervals. Profound hypocalcemia may develop in certain patients, especially in those with radiographic evidence of bone resorption; treatment of such patients with $1,25(OH)_2D_3$ may reduce the severity of the postoperative hypocalcemia. Tetany may occur in those who develop severe hypocalcemia. When the level of serum calcium falls below 7.5 mg per deciliter, oral calcium supplementation may prevent a further decrease. The amount of oral calcium needed is usually quite large. The initial treatment should provide at least 2.0 g of calcium and the dose can be increased at intervals of 3 to 7 days until adequate rise in serum calcium concentration is achieved. If the concentration of serum calcium falls to lower levels and if tetany appears, intravenous calcium should be given in addition to the oral supplements of calcium. In patients with profound and sustained hypocalcemia, $1,25(OH)_2D_3$ may be needed; careful monitoring of serum calcium and phosphorus levels should be undertaken with this therapy. Serum levels of phosphorus almost always fall after parathyroidectomy. Therefore, phosphate binding antacids should be withheld if serum levels of phosphorus decrease to less than 3.0 mg per deciliter. Also, serum levels of phosphorus should not be allowed to rise above 4.0 mg per deciliter, because the hyperphosphatemia may aggravate the hypocalcemia in the parathyroidectomized patients.

OTHER THERAPEUTIC MEASURES

The use of beta-adrenergic blocking agents (such as propranolol) may cause a decrease in the serum levels of PTH, but this action is variable and does not completely reverse secondary hyperparathyroidism. Claims that cimetidine may be effective in controlling secondary hyperparathyroidism in uremic patients have not been convincingly substantiated. Occasionally, treatment with diphosphonate (disodium-ethane-1-hydroxy-1, 1-diphosphonate, or DHDP) may cause regression of ectopic calcification resistant to the usual therapy (control of the hyperphosphatemia, suppression of parathyroid gland activity, or parathyroidectomy). Treatment with DHDP by itself may produce osteomalacia.

MILD HYPERTENSION: NEW STRATEGIES IN THERAPY

NORMAN M. KAPLAN, M.D.

As millions more patients with mild hypertension, defined as a diastolic blood pressure (DBP) between 90 and 104 mm Hg, are being identified and treated, increasing attention is being directed to the initial choice of their therapy. Today the majority of practitioners in the United States choose a diuretic as the first drug in the "stepped-care" approach to therapy. However, the wisdom of the routine use of this approach has been questioned for two reasons: first, doubts about the long-term efficacy of the diuretic-first stepped-care approach in the prevention of coronary disease; second, the availability of a number of other drugs that provide equal or even better antihypertensive potency while they also promise to protect better against coronary disease. This chapter will examine the rationale for and results of current practices and make specific recommendations for future changes.

Before any therapy is begun, the diagnosis should be firmly established and the decision as to whether the patient needs active drug therapy made according to the guidelines shown in Table 1. These guidelines are based on the premise that there is little immediate risk from mild hypertension and that non-drug therapies may be effective in reducing the pressure to safer levels, precluding the need for drugs.

Some would disagree with these guidelines. On one hand there are those, mainly in the United States, who argue that even those with DBP above 85 are at increased risk and certainly that all with DBP above 90 should be treated. On the other hand, other experts, mainly outside the United States, argue that even 95 mm Hg is too low a level and that only those with sustained DBP above 100 mm Hg should be given antihypertensive drugs. The 95 mm Hg figure seems to be a reasonable compromise and will likely become the consensus.

INITIAL CHOICE OF THERAPY

Once the decision to treat is made, an equally important decision must be addressed: which drug to use. The decision is important for two interrelated reasons. First, if that initial drug is successful, as it likely will be, it may be taken for the rest of the patient's life, for as long as 40 years or more; second, the long-term side effects of antihypertensive drugs may not be easily recognized, either because we are not aware of them or because our patients do not call them to our attention. Remember that the cholesterol-raising effect of diuretics was not identified until these drugs were widely used for almost 20 years, and the problem would likely not have been identified if hypercholesterolemia was not being independently looked for.

Diuretic As First Choice

As noted, diuretics are now chosen by most practitioners as the first drug. The practice arose empirically: diuretics were among the earliest orally effective drugs made available, they were effective, relatively well accepted by patients, and capable of sustaining their antihypertensive action indefinitely. Other types of drugs were tried as initial agents, but a tendency for fluid retention to blunt their effectiveness was often noted. The increase in plasma volume reflects a tendency by the kidneys of hypertensive patients to retain sodium and water whenever the blood pressure is lowered by nondiuretic agents. Such fluid retention is a natural reaction to the lowering of the blood pressure by the kidneys of hypertensive patients, which have their pressure-sodium excretion relationship reset at a higher level. With direct vasodilators, an additional mechanism is involved, the activation of the renin-angiotensin system with secondary increases in aldosterone.

The use of a diuretic as initial therapy therefore seemed logical: up to half the patients could be controlled on it alone and, if another drug were needed, the diuretic was usually required to obtain maximal effectiveness. However, concerns about the routine use of diuretics as the initial choice of therapy have been raised in the past few years.

TABLE 1 Guidelines for Therapy of Mild Hypertension

Recheck blood pressure 3–6 months while using nondrug therapy:
- Weight reduction, if obese
- Moderate sodium restriction (2 g sodium = 88 mmol/day)
- Relaxation
- Isotonic exercise
- Moderate alcohol intake (1 ounce ethanol/day = 2 drinks)

If diastolic blood pressure remains above 95, start drug therapy

If diastolic blood pressure is 90 to 95:
- Low-risk patients: continue on nondrug therapy
- High-risk patients: start drug therapy

Side Effects of Diuretics

Numerous side effects have been known to follow the continuous use of diuretics in the treatment of hypertension (Fig. 1). Some, such as postural hypotension, hyponatremia, and prerenal azotemia, are unusual or of little apparent consequence. Others, such as hyperuricemia and transient hypercalcemia, are common but seldom harmful. Still others may be a cause of increased risk of cardiovascular complications, reducing or blunting the protection provided by the lowering of the blood pressure. These include hypokalemia, worsening of glucose tolerance, and rises in plasma cholesterol—a complication that should be shown in Figure 1 with a question mark as to its mechanism, since its relationship to hypokalemia has not been proved.

Hypokalemia appears in about 30 percent of patients given long-term diuretic therapy. The average fall in plasma potassium with sustained use of diuretics is about 0.7 mmol per liter. The primary hazard of diuretic-induced hypokalemia is its tendency to increase myocardial irritability, inciting ventricular ectopic activity. This may become clinically apparent only when the myocardium suffers acute ischemia, as after an acute myocardial infarction. The higher frequency of ventricular fibrillation after an infarction in those who have diuretic-induced hypokalemia is of concern because coronary artery disease is far and away the most common cause of death among hypertensives. The danger is known to be greater in those who are taking digitalis and in those with left ventricular hypertrophy, a significant portion of hypertensive patients.

The hazards of diuretic-induced hypokalemia may be exposed only after acute stress. With severe stress, plasma catecholamine levels rise to concentrations which have themselves been shown to reduce plasma potassium levels by 0.5 to 1.0 mmol per liter by accelerating the movement of potassium into cells. When added to the effects of stress, the usual diuretic-induced fall in plasma potassium concentration of 0.7 mmol per liter may be more hazardous than previously assumed. At minimum, these potential risks should justify steps to reduce diuretic

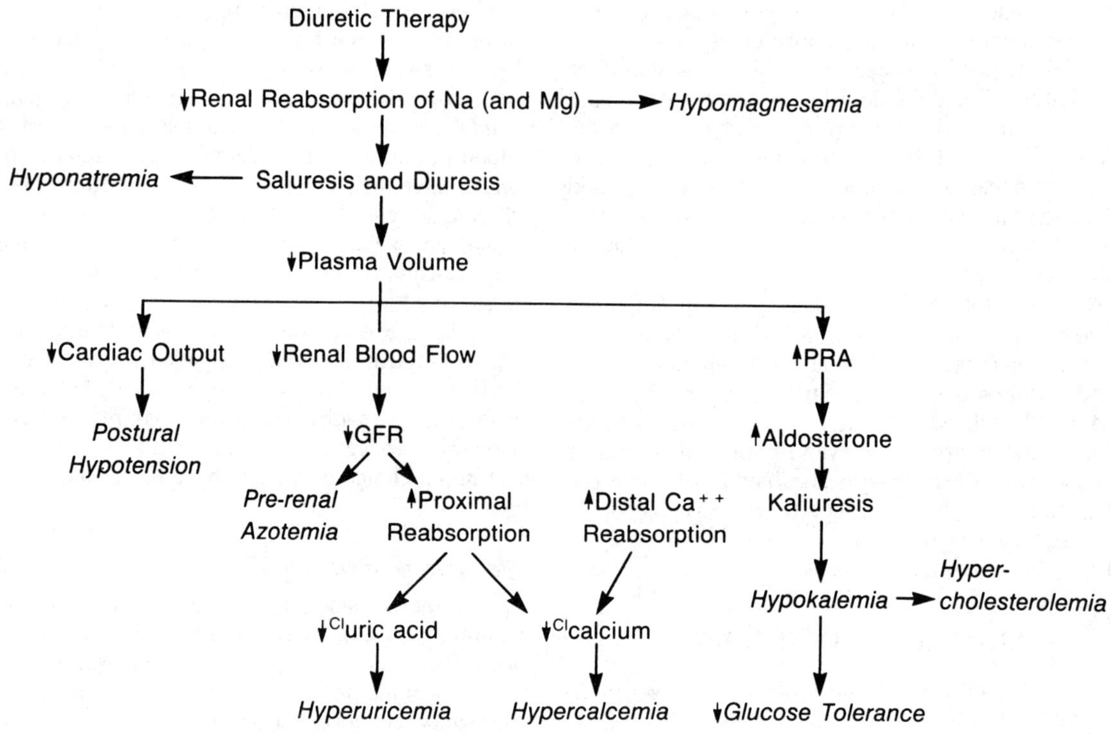

Figure 1 Schema for the various complications seen with diuretic therapy. The mechanism for hypercholesterolemia is uncertain.

wastage of potassium: the use of the smallest effective dose of diuretic, a reduced dietary sodium intake, and the concomitant use of potassium-sparing agents.

Glucose intolerance may accompany prolonged diuretic therapy. In the first three years of the recently completed Medical Research Council of England trial, the incidence of impaired glucose tolerance was significantly higher in both men and women taking bendrofluazide than in those taking either a placebo or propranolol. The atherogenic potential of such changes in glucose tolerance is unknown, but it poses another concern about the long-term safety of diuretic therapy.

As shown in Figure 1, the decrease in glucose tolerance is thought to be caused by hypokalemia. Insulin resistance may also play a role, since the elevations in blood glucose have been found to be closely correlated to higher plasma insulin levels.

Elevations of plasma cholesterol of 10 to 20 mg per deciliter usually occur with diuretic therapy and are also correlated to higher plasma-insulin levels. The atherogenic potential of a 20 mg per deciliter rise in plasma cholesterol can, by use of the Framingham data on the risks for coronary heart disease, be shown to reverse completely the reduction in risk provided by the 10 to 15 mm Hg fall in systolic blood pressure that might be expected with chronic diuretic therapy.

Protection Against Coronary Disease

These three biochemical aberrations may be responsible for a worsening of cardiovascular risk. Separately or collectively they may be factors in the failure to find protection from coronary artery disease in three of the six trials of treatment of hypertension which have been completed, all of which used a diuretic as the first step (Table 2). In all of these trials, antihypertensive therapy has been found to be effective in reducing mortality from strokes, and likely has reduced the frequency of congestive heart failure, aortic dissection, and progression of renal damage. In the Oslo study, however, more myocardial infarctions occurred in the treated patients. A higher rate of coronary mortality was noted in the diuretic-treated patients in the Medical Research Council (MRC) trial. And in the Multiple Risk Factor Intervention Trial (MRFIT), those hypertensives whose initial resting electrocardiogram was abnormal and who were given more intensive diuretic-first stepped-care therapy had significantly more coronary deaths. The possibility that those hypertensives who start with an abnormal electrocardiogram would be even more susceptible to mischief from diuretic-induced hypokalemia seems to be borne out by these data.

Furthermore, hypokalemia was effectively prevent-

TABLE 2 Mortality Rates per 1,000 Person-Years

Trials	*Cerebrovascular Disease*			*Coronary Heart Disease*		
Drugs vs. Placebo	*No Rx*	*Rx*	*Difference (%)*	*No Rx*	*Rx*	*Difference (%)*
Australian, 1980	0.9	0.4	−56	1.6	0.7	−56
Oslo, 1980	1.0	0	−100	1.0	2.7	+170
Elderly, 1985	16.0	11.0	−32	24.0	15.0	−38
MRC, 1985	0.6	0.4	−33	2.3	2.5	+9
More vs. Less Drugs	*Less*	*More*	*Difference (%)*	*Less*	*More*	*Difference (%)*
HDFP, 1979	1.6	0.9	−41	5.6	4.5	−20
MRFIT, 1982						
Normal ECG		Not reported		3.4	2.6	−24
Abnormal ECG		Not reported		2.9	4.9	+70

ed in the European Trial in the Elderly by concomitant use of a potassium-sparing agent. In that trial, protection against coronary disease was equal to that against stroke. These data, overall, suggest that diuretics provide less protection from the progression of coronary artery disease than their antihypertensive potency should offer. Since antihypertensive potency of usual doses of a diuretic is comparable to that of moderate doses of a beta-blocker or other adrenergic inhibitors, the biochemical aberrations that accompany the diuretic may reduce or ablate the protection they provide by their reduction in blood pressure.

These concerns about the side effects and potential dangers of diuretics should not detract from their proven antihypertensive potency and the overall protection from cardiovascular diseases they have been shown to provide along with other antihypertensive drugs in patients with DBP above 100 mm Hg. Recall, however, that we are treating more and more patients with less elevated pressures, including a larger proportion of those with a diastolic blood pressure in the 90 to 100 range, who make up more than half of all hypertensive patients. Such patients are at less risk from their hypertension; therefore they can be provided less protection by a reduction of their blood pressure than patients with higher pressures. Thus, any additional risk, be it ever so small, from the therapy used to lower their blood pressure must be weighed on a balance with correspondingly less counterweight. For example, among those with a level of blood pressure high enough to impose a 50 percent excess risk of premature cardiovascular disease, the use of a therapy that removes that excess risk while in itself adding a 10 percent risk can easily be defended as beneficial. But for those with a lower level of blood pressure which in itself increases risk by only 10 percent, the use of such a therapy cannot be defended.

In the presence of even a small degree of risk from long-term use of diuretics, the administration of such therapy to the 25 to 30 million Americans with diastolic pressures in the 90 to 100 mm Hg range must obviously be reconsidered. As stated earlier, a reasonable course might be to withhold drugs from those with diastolic pressures in the 90 to 100 range who are otherwise at relatively low risk for at least six months while they are encouraged to follow non-drug therapies, including weight reduction for the obese, moderate sodium restriction for all, isotonic exercise and relaxation therapy for those who are willing, and moderation of alcohol intake. According to this view, only if the diastolic pressure remains above 95 mm Hg is there a definite indication for drug therapy.

THE AVAILABILITY OF OTHER DRUGS

The second major issue relates to the considerations discussed above: If diuretics pose various problems, are other drugs available which pose fewer potential risks and which therefore are alternative choices for the initial treatment of hypertension. One point made previously should be reiterated: There is little to choose between the various available antihypertensive drugs with regard to their efficacy in lowering the blood pressure in the majority of hypertensives. Therefore, the choice of initial drug should be based mainly upon safety and side effects (Table 3). Unfortunately, there is only one controlled study, the MRC trial, which compared two choices, a diuretic and a beta-blocker. Among the patients in the MRC trial, overall mortality was similar with the two drugs, with only nonsmoking men showing a lower rate of coronary mortality if they were given a beta-blocker than if they were given a diuretic.

The Use of Beta-Blockers

If a diuretic is not chosen, the alternative approach recommended by the Third Joint National Committee is to start therapy with a beta-blocker. There are now seven available in the United States and probably more on the way. These drugs, as a class, offer numerous advantages.

On the other hand, beta-blockers pose numerous disadvantages. Some, such as bronchospasm, are immediate and obvious and therefore not much of a long-term problem. But, similar to the biochemical changes seen with diuretics, beta-blockers may adversely affect blood lipids and, to a lesser extent, carbohydrate metabolism. In many studies, rises in triglycerides and falls in cardioprotective high-density lipoprotein cholesterol levels

TABLE 3 Characteristics of Nondiuretic Antihypertensive Drugs for Initial Therapy

	Advantages	*Disadvantages*
Central agonists	Little decrease in cardiac output Reduce lipids (guanabenz)	Sedation Dry mouth "Autoimmune" reactions (Aldomet)
Alpha-blockers	Vasodilate Reduce lipids	Hypotension (rare)
Beta-blockers		
No intrinsic sympathomimetic activity	Relieve concomitant problems (angina, migraine, etc.)	$Beta_2$-blockade (bronchospasm, etc.) Vasoconstrictor (cold extremities) Reduce cardiac output (fatigue, loss of exercise ability) Raise triglycerides Lower high-density lipoprotein cholesterol
Intrinsic sympathomimetic activity	No decrease in cardiac output No alteration of lipids	
Converting enzyme inhibitors	Vasodilate No central nervous system effects No decrease in cardiac output	Rare but serious toxicity (renal, neutropenia) Rash Loss of taste
Calcium antagonists	Vasodilate No central nervous system effects Relieve angina	Variable types of bothersome but rarely serious side effects

have been observed. Though this is less of a problem with those beta-blockers having high intrinsic sympathomimetic activity, lipid levels should be monitored in all patients given any beta-blocker. For various reasons, those with intrinsic sympathomimetic activity (pindolol and acebutolol) seem to be more attractive than those without.

Alpha-Blockers

In contrast to the adverse effects on lipids seen with beta-blockers, alpha-blockers appear to be either neutral or beneficial. Though the manner by which they may improve lipid levels—or the manner by which beta-blockers may worsen them—remains unknown, numerous studies with prazosin and preliminary data on other alpha-blockers have shown beneficial effects.

Beyond the beneficial effects upon lipids, alpha-blockers lower the blood pressure in a hemodynamically more favorable manner. Whereas much of the antihypertensive effect of beta-blockers resides in their reduction of cardiac output, alpha-blockers primarily reduce peripheral resistance and tend to have little effect on cardiac output. This may translate clinically into little beyond a lesser frequency of fatigue and cold extremities, but, since the hemodynamic abnormality of established hypertension is an increased peripheral resistance, drugs that lower resistance should provide even more ''physiologic'' reduction in the blood pressure.

Converting Enzyme Inhibitors

The first of the converting enzyme inhibitors (CEI), captopril, has recently been approved for use in the treatment of patients with mild hypertension. Among such patients, smaller doses of the drug than used to treat more severe hypertension appear to cause relatively few side effects and fewer of the more common problems that interfere with the quality of life, such as sedation, fatigue, and perhaps impotence. The second of these to be approved, enalapril, may provide all of the advantages with somewhat fewer side effects.

Clinical research conducted over the past 15 years by Drs. Norman Hollenberg, Gordon Williams, and their colleagues suggests that as many as 40 percent of all hypertensive patients will be particularly responsive to CEI therapy. These patients appear unable to modulate their adrenal or vascular responses to variations in sodium intake, apparently because of high, fixed levels of angiotensin II within the target tissues. These ''nonmodulators'' therefore are unable to increase aldosterone secretion normally in response to sodium restriction, which in turn decreases the degree of sodium retention and fails to dampen the further release of renin. More angiotensin II is thereby generated when sodium intake is low, leading to more vasoconstriction and hypertension.

On the other hand, under the more usual circumstance

of high sodium intake, these nonmodulators fail to increase renal blood flow and therefore do not excrete the sodium load. Body fluid volume expands and the blood pressure rises.

Beyond the demonstration that half of hypertensive patients with normal to high plasma renin levels are nonmodulators, these investigators have shown that even short-term therapy with CEI corrects the problems within both the adrenals and the renal vasculature. As a result, the majority of such patients have a significant fall in blood pressure with CEI monotherapy.

The results of this research need to be confirmed and extended to a larger population. If they hold up, the data strongly support the use of a CEI to correct an underlying defect that is responsible for hypertension in a considerable portion of the population. The prospect of using such specific therapy, rather than the empirical approaches that lower blood pressure because they happen to alter one or another mechanisms that sustain the blood pressure, is an exciting one. Even if the relationship turns out to be less common, or if it is impractical to identify the individual patients who have it, a CEI will likely be increasingly used as initial therapy, since, when one is used in unselected populations, about half the patients have a significant fall in blood pressure.

Calcium Antagonists

This class of drugs lowers the level of free calcium within vascular smooth muscle cells, mainly by blocking its entry from the extracellular fluid. With lower levels of free calcium, vessels relax, lowering tone and vascular resistance, thereby reducing blood pressure.

These drugs may also be acting to correct a fundamental mechanism responsible for hypertension. Increased concentrations of free intracellular calcium have been measured within tissues of hypertensive animals and people, perhaps as a consequence of defects in cell membrane transport mechanisms. The use of calcium antagonists may correct the cause for increased vascular tone and resistance.

Whether or not they too are specific "corrective" therapies, calcium antagonists are potent antihypertensive agents. All three currently available in the United States—diltiazem, nifedipine, and verapamil—have been shown to lower blood pressure comparably to other antihypertensive drugs with relatively few side effects. When they are approved for use in hypertension and when longer-lasting formulations become available so that they may be used on a once- or twice-a-day basis, they will likely be widely used early in the course of therapy.

Central Alpha Agonists and Others

Although alpha-blockers, CEIs, and calcium antagonists seem to be likely replacements for the current widespread use of diuretics and beta-blockers, some of the old standbys still have a valid place among the available choices.

Reserpine is still an appropriate choice—inexpensive, once-a-day, relatively free of side effects if used in the small doses (0.05 to 0.25 mg per day, shown to be as effective as larger doses). However, it has a bad reputation for causing severe depression and cancer, neither probably true, but hard to dispel.

Methyldopa, clonidine, and guanabenz share many features as centrally acting alpha-agonists. Clonidine may cause more sedation and dry mouth, but neither it nor guanabenz is associated with the multiple "autoimmune" reactions reported with methyldopa. Both clonidine and quanabenz drugs may not cause as much fluid retention as other nondiuretic antihypertensive agents. Guanabenz has been found to lower total serum cholesterol levels. Clonidine may be used in a transdermal patch in the hope of a smoother antihypertensive effect and fewer side effects.

SUBSTITUTION RATHER THAN STEPPED-CARE

The preceding sections described a number of choices that can be made as initial (and often sole) therapy for patients with mild hypertension. In addition to using one of them rather than a diuretic, another change in the present common practice of stepped-care is probably in the offing: Rather than adding a second drug if the first is not enough, stop the first and substitute another as sole therapy.

The approach using substitution rather than addition is based on the premise that some patients respond better to one class of drugs than to another. Despite the generalization made earlier that all of the drugs have comparable antihypertensive potency, there are some patients who respond better to one or another. Elderly people and blacks, for example, seem to respond less well to beta-blockers and perhaps CEIs and better to diuretics and calcium antagonists. Without having ways to predetermine the likelihood of a good response, the clinician may logically try a different type of drug if the first is inadequate.

Differences in response may be caused by differences in adherence to therapy with different drugs. If a patient develops such intolerable side effects as to stop therapy, the problem is usually obvious and a second agent would routinely be substituted. However, patients may not volunteer or admit problems with their drugs, and instead just not take them. For whatever reason, if a patient does not have the desired effect from the initial drug, a logical next step might be to stop it and try a drug from another category. The patient may thereby be more successfully treated with fewer medications.

This approach differs in specifics, but not in principle, from that advocated for many years by Dr. John Laragh. His approach is based upon a renin profile, with a beta-blocker or CEI to be given to those with high or normal renins and a diuretic or calcium antagonist to those with low renin. The problems of renin profiling seem to be so great as to preclude its routine use. Moreover the responses to either a diuretic or a beta-blocker have not uniformly been found to be predicted by the preexisting plasma renin level. The decision as to which drug to choose can be made on the basis of the age and race of the patient.

In the future, the choice may be made on the basis of the potential for reversal of cardiac and arterial smooth muscle hypertrophy. Most, if not all, of the adrenergic inhibitors and both CEIs and calcium antagonists have been shown experimentally to reverse left ventricular hypertrophy. Whether that will be included in the decision to treat and the choice of therapy remains to be seen.

Beyond the First Drug

If one drug is well tolerated, but is only partially effective, the addition of a second of another class, in keeping with the stepped-care approach, is rational. Half or more of the patients in various trials require a second drug and about 10 percent require three.

There is little comparative evidence upon which to base a decision as to which drugs should be chosen second or third. The tradition has been to include a diuretic if there are two and to include a direct vasodilator if there are three. Other combinations may work as well. In particular, CEIs or calcium antagonists may increasingly be chosen as the vasodilator, rather than the ''direct'' acting hydralazine or minoxidil. Since they do not induce as much reflex sympathetic activity as the direct vasodilators, CEIs or calcium antagonists can likely be used as first, second, or third choices, as can the various adrenergic inhibitors.

INDIVIDUALIZED CARE IN MILD ESSENTIAL HYPERTENSION

VITO M. CAMPESE, M.D.

A substantial number of epidemiologic studies have definitively demonstrated that hypertension is associated with increased risk of cardiovascular morbidity and mortality. Therefore, one might conclude that any reduction in blood pressure should result in improved cardiovascular morbidity and mortality. However, although large cooperative studies have demonstrated that management of hypertension in patients with moderate or severe hypertensions (i.e. with diastolic blood pressure greater than 104 mm Hg) improves morbidity and mortality arising from cardiovascular complications, controversies still remain, especially regarding the efficacy of drug therapy in reducing cardiovascular complications in patients with mild hypertension (i.e., with diastolic blood pressure between 90 and 104 mm Hg). These controversies persist despite of, and at times because of, the findings of several major multicenter studies on the effect of drug therapy in the management of mild essential hypertension.

The first of these large multicenter studies was the Veterans Administration Cooperative study, which was conducted in patients with diastolic blood pressure ranging between 90 and 114 mm Hg. This study, which included a placebo-treated group, showed that drug therapy reduced the incidence of morbid cardiovascular events. Unfortunately, this study included only a small number of patients with diastolic blood pressure (DBP) between 90 and 104 mm Hg. Therefore, the generally optimistic conclusions of this study could not be extrapolated to patients with mild hypertension (i.e., diastolic blood pressure between 90 and 104 mm Hg). Subsequently, the Hypertension Detection and Follow-up Program (HDFP) attempted to address this issue more specifically. Unfortunately, this study did not include a placebo-treated group, but comprised approximately 11,000 patients with DBP greater than 90 mm Hg. Patients were randomly divided into two groups. In the first group, patients were followed in specialized centers and given a more intense stepped-care therapy (SC group), whereas patients in the second group were referred back to their usual care (RC group). At the end of 5 years of follow-up, the mean DBP was significantly lower in the SC than in the RC group, thereby indicating a better adherence to and/or a more aggressive management of hypertension. This was associated with a 28.6 percent reduction in mortality from all causes in the SC group and in a significant reduction in cardiovascular events: 30 myocardial infarctions and 17 strokes occurred in the SC group compared to 56 and 31, respectively, in the RC group. This study, however, owing to pitfalls in its experimental design, has not resolved the basic issue of if and when to treat patients with mild essential hypertension.

A study, better designed than the HDFP, was performed in Australia at almost the same time. The Australian trial included a placebo-treated group and dealt with patients with DBP ranging between 95 and 109 mm Hg. This trial demonstrated several important points. First, the group of patients receiving drug therapy displayed 30 percent less morbidity and mortality than the placebo-treated group. *Second*, this study showed that *two-thirds* of patients with initial DBP between 95 to 99 mm Hg and *one-half* of the patients with initial DBP between 95 and 104 mm Hg achieved DBP below 95 mm Hg while on placebo, thus suggesting that early drug therapy may be *unnecessary* in a large proportion of patients. *Third,* this study failed to demonstrate a significant improvement in coronary heart events in the drug-treated group when compared with the placebo-treated group. Finally, this study showed that the incidence of cardiovascular complications was greater in those patients in whom a certain level of blood pressure was achieved with drugs rather than with placebo. This latter finding, on one hand, could indicate that long range antihypertensive drug therapy may introduce some degree of cardiovascular risk that offsets the benefit of lowering blood pressure. On the other hand, this could simply indicate that those patients, whose blood pressure reached a certain level with drug therapy, may have had higher blood pressure and, consequently, greater cardiovascular complications prior to the onset of the study.

The notion that antihypertensive drugs, particularly the diuretics, may introduce an element of cardiovascular risk is not unique to the Australian study. Two other studies have added further support to this contention. The first study, the Multiple Risk Factor Interventional Trial (MRFIT) was designed to determine if "special intervention" (SI) aimed at reducing a variety of risk factors could reduce cardiovascular morbidity and mortality in comparison to usual care (UC). This study showed that SI did not improve morbidity from coronary artery disease in patients with DBP less than 100 mm Hg and, actually, that it increased the number of coronary events in patients with DBP between 90 and 94 mm Hg. The second of these studies (the OSLO study), also failed to demonstrate a reduction in deaths from myocardial infarction in the drug-treated group. All these studies have raised the suspicion that antihypertensive drug therapy performed in accordance to the stepped-care approach (i.e., use of a diuretic as first line of therapy) may be responsible for the failure to achieve improvement in coronary heart events despite the reduction in blood pressure. Further support to this notion came from the Swedish study. This study for the first time utilized as beta-adrenergic blocking agent as first line of therapy in the treatment of mild hypertension, and it showed a reduction in the incidence of coronary heart events. Unfortunately, this study has been criticized for the many flaws in its experimental design.

The most recent findings of the Medical Research Working Party further substantiate the notion that the modality of drug intervention not only affects the degree of reduction in blood pressure, but also the incidence of cardiovascular events. This was a single-blind placebo-controlled study of 17,354 patients with essential hypertension with 85,572 patient years of observation. Patients were randomly divided in three groups: one was treated with placebo, the second with a thiazide diuretic, and the third with propranolol. The study showed that propranolol, but not Bendrofluazide, reduced the overall cardiovascular events in nonsmokers. Propranolol did not influence the incidence of coronary events in smokers, thereby suggesting that smoking may offset any benefit from drug treatment in hypertension. This study also showed that both thiazide and propranolol reduced the incidence of strokes; however, thiazide did not reduce the rate of coronary heart events, whereas propranol showed a trend toward reduction which did not achieve statistical significance. Finally this study showed that the all-cause mortality decreased in men, but it increased in women on active treatment.

The following conclusions can be drawn from the analysis of these studies:

1. Attempts should be made to lower blood pressure in every patient with sustained DBP greater than 90 mm Hg.
2. Drug interventions in the management of mild essential hypertension, if performed according to the stepped-care approach, reduced the rate of strokes, but not of coronary heart events.
3. Alternative forms of drug therapy, such as beta-adrenergic blocking agents may possibly result in improved incidence of coronary heart events, but further studies are needed to substantiate this concept.
4. Spontaneous normalization of blood pressure can be achieved in a substantial number of patients with DBP less than 104 mm Hg.
5. The elimination of other risk factors, particularly smoking may be as, or more, important than antihypertensive therapy for the prevention of cardiovascular complications. Concerted efforts to reduce, simultaneously, all these risk factors are important to achieve a significant impact on the risk of cardiovascular complications in hypertensive subjects.
6. Early pharmacologic therapy may possibly be deleterious and, therefore, unjustified in women with mild uncomplicated essential hypertension.

STRATEGIES IN MANAGEMENT

Before deciding if to treat and which form of treatment to apply to an individual patient, it is essential to compile a complete risk profile (Table 1). If the total risk score is equal to, or exceeds, three, pharmacologic as well as nonpharamacologic intervention should be started without delay. Alternatively, if the total risk score is less than three, normalization of blood pressure exclusively, with nonpharmacologic interventions, should be attempted for a period of 6 to 12 months and followed by drug therapy only if normalization of blood pressure is not accomplished with these therapeutic interventions.

NONPHARMACOLOGIC THERAPY

A large number of nonpharmacologic interventions can be applied effectively in the management of hypertension. The measures must be individualized according to age, sex, race, body weight, dietary and other habits, use of drugs, lifestyle, compliance etc. These aspects of management of the patient with hypertension are covered in detail elsewhere in this book and are only summarized here to serve as an introduction to pharmacologic therapy.

Smoking

Pharmacologic therapy of hypertension may be ineffective in reducing the risk of cardiovascular complications in smokers despite adequate control of blood pressure. Stopping smoking may be more important than antihypertensive drug therapy for the prevention of cardiovascular complications in patients with mild essential hypertension. Thus, all patients with hypertension should be adequately counseled about the risks of smoking.

Sodium Restriction

There is a clear relationship between dietary sodium intake and hypertension. However, not all patients with hypertension manifest a sensitivity to salt. Salt restriction

TABLE 1 Risk Factors in Mild Essential Hypertension

	Diastolic Blood Pressure		
Factor	*90-94*	*94-99*	*>100*
No other risks	1	2	3
Age > 50 years	1	1	1
Male sex	1	1	1
Obesity	1	1	1
Cigarette smoking	2	2	2
LVH by voltage	1	1	1
LVH by strain	2	2	2
Diabetes	1	1	1
Renal disease	2	2	2
Coronary heart disease	2	2	2
Hypercholesterolemia	1	1	1
Strong family history of premature cardiovascular events	1	1	1
Blacks	1	1	1

Adapted by Freis ED. Kaplan NM. The case for nondrug treatment. In: Narins G. ed. Controversies in nephrology and hypertension. New York: Churchill Livingstone. 1984: 75.

or diuretics result in blood pressure reduction only in approximately 60 percent of patients with hypertension. Metabolic balance studies performed in our laboratory have indicated that severe sodium restriction, 10 mEq per day, results in a decrease in blood pressure in only 60 percent of the patients. However, increased dietary intake of potassium appears to counteract the pressor effect of sodium in both humans and in experimental animals. The patients more likely to be salt-sensitive are Blacks and those with low plasma renin activity (PRA). A moderate sodium restriction (70 to 80 mEq per day) should be initially emphasized in most patients with essential hypertension, probably with the exception of young Caucasians. If 2 months of sodium restriction (adequately monitored with two measurements of 24 hours urinary sodium excretion to ascertain compliance) does not result in improvement of blood pressure control, the patients can be labeled as salt-resistant and rigorous control of his or her dietary sodium intake should not be further pursued. If on the other hand, salt restriction results in improved blood pressure control, it should be continuously pursued in subsequent follow-up.

Calcium Supplementation

Several abnormalities in calcium metabolism have been shown in rats as well as in patients with essential hypertension. These include decreased serum ionized calcium, hypercalciuria and increased serum levels of parathyroid horomone. In one study, these abnormalities were shown to be limited to patients with low PRA. A double-blinded placebo-controlled crossover study has demonstrated a modest reduction in blood pressure (3.8 mm Hg in systolic and 2.3 mm Hg in DBP) in patients with essential hypertension. However, owing to the inconclusive nature of such studies, no generalized recommendations for calcium supplementations can be given to hypertensive patients. However, in patients in whom PRA is determined to be low, and in elderly patients in whom calcium supplementations may be warranted for other medical reasons, oral administration of calcium may be used as an additive form of therapy in the management of hypertension.

Weight Loss

Several lines of evidence clearly indicate that obesity is an important factor in the genesis of hypertension and that a clear association exists between excessive body weight and blood pressure. Thus, hypertensive patients, with body weight greater than 115 percent of ideal body weight, should be counseled to reduce body weight.

Alcohol Consumption

Chronic excessive alcohol consumption (> 2 ounces per day) may result in increased blood pressure and should be discouraged in every hypertensive subject.

Caffeine

Acute, but not chronic, administration of caffeine appears to increase blood pressure probably by activation of the sympathetic nervous system. However, in subjects sensitive to caffeine, the ingestion of beverages containing this drug should be discouraged and limited.

Behavioral Modifications

Biofeedback and relaxation therapies can result in modest reduction in blood pressure. However, these modalities of treatment can only be applied to a small number of highly motivated patients and are not a suitable form of therapy for the majority of hypertensive subjects.

Exercise

Regular *isotonic* exercise may result in body weight and blood pressure reduction and should be encouraged in most hypertensive patients. However, isometric exercise should be avoided.

PHARMACOLOGIC THERAPY

Nonpharmacologic therapies frequently fail to normalize blood pressure because of poor compliance of patients and inadequate counseling by physicians and allied health professionals. When nonpharmacologic therapies have been used for a period of 6 to 12 months and fail to control blood pressure or when patients have a risk score of three or more (see Table 1), drug therapy should be initiated. Major controversies presently exist about which drug to select as first line of therapy. The Joint National Committee on Detection, Evaluation, and Treatment of High Blood Pressure has set up certain guidelines (the stepped-care approach) for the pharmacologic management of hypertension. According to those guide-lines, in step 1 patients should receive a thiazide diuretic; in step 2 an antiadrenergic agent or a beta-aderenergic blocker and in step 3 patients should receive a vasodilator. Unfortunately, this highly schematized approach disregards the multiplicity of pathophysiologic mechanisms involved in human hypertension, ignores the recent notion that the failure of most large cooperative studies to demonstrate reduced incidence of coronary heart disease could be the result of the unfavorable effect of diuretics on plasma lipids, and finally, does not take into account the potential advantages for the cardiovascular system of some newer antihypertensive agents, such as the calcium channel blockers.

A different approach to the management of mild essential hypertension is proposed in Figure 1. First a risk profile is established for each patient, and this is followed by attempts to determine sensitivity to salt with moderate salt restriction; patients are then characterized as *Salt-sensitive* or *Salt-resistant* depending on whether DBP decreased more or less than 10 percent from baseline. In salt-sensitive patients we continue salt restriction alone, if DBP normalizes with dietary interventions. If DBP remains greater than 90 mm Hg, simple observation of the patient is continued for 6 to 12 months if the risk score is less than 3, and oral calcium supplementation is encouraged (1 g orally per day)-if there are not contraindications. If a patient has a risk score of 3 or greater, a calcium-channel blocker is started. In salt-resistant patients with a risk score of less than 3, observation is continued with non-pharmacologic intervention for a period of 6 to 12 months. Thereafter, if DBP remains greater than 90 mm Hg, drug therapy, is initiated. Antihypertensive agents are started sooner in patients with a risk score of 3 or greater. In these patients, beta-adrenergic blocking agents or sympatholytic drugs are preferred as first line of therapy. Since most nonselective beta-adrenergic blocking agents increase plasma triglycerides and very low-density lipoproteins while decreasing high-density lipoproteins, it is preferable to use cardioselective beta-blockers (atenolol, metoprolol), those with intrinsic sympathomimetic activity (such as pindolol), or those with combined

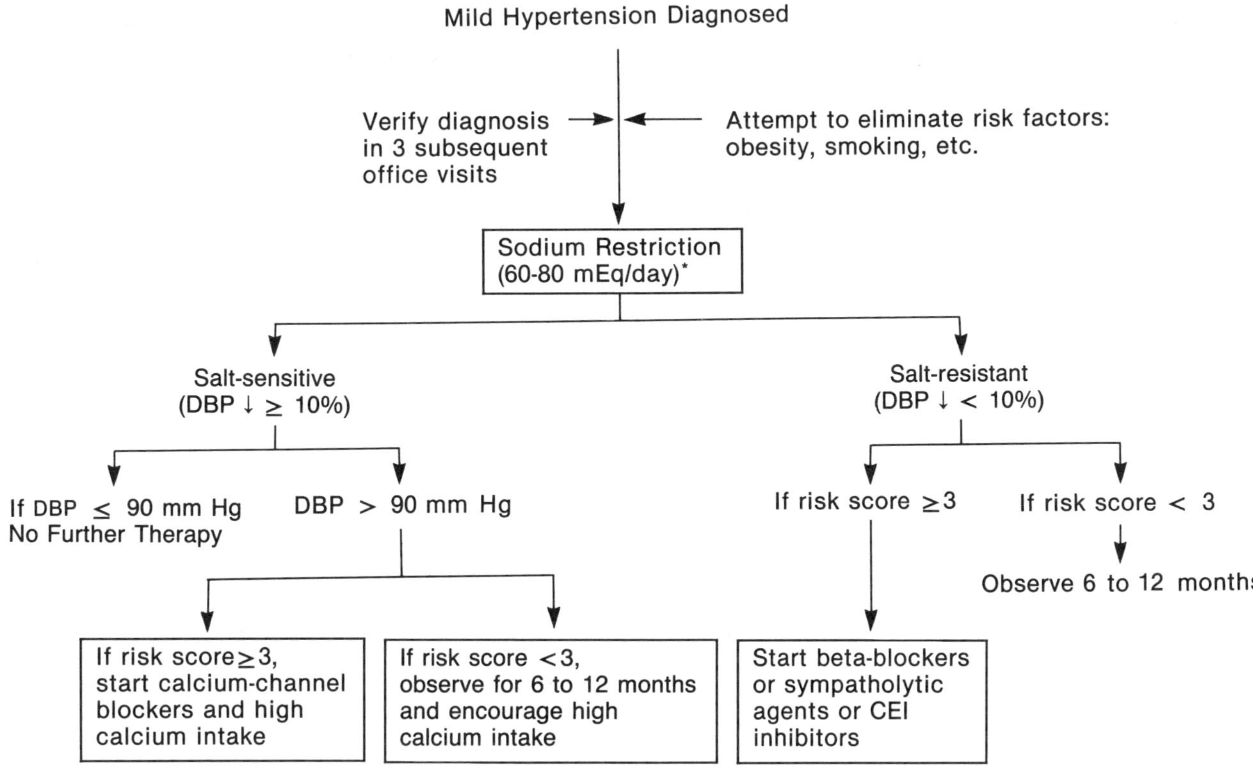

Figure 1 Algorithm for the management of mild hypertension (DBP 90-104 mm Hg)

alpha and beta-antiadrenergic blocking properties (such as labetalol) since these agents appear to have less pronounced effects on lipid metabolism.

Other sympatholytic agents, such as clonidine and prazosin, or converting enzyme inhibitors can also be used as first-line therapy in salt-resistant patients. The latter agents are less prone to cause side-effects and to affect the lifestyle of the patients. If these agents alone do not result in normalization of blood pressure, small doses of thiazide can be added to the salt-sensitive patients and calcium-channel blockers to the salt-resistant. The combination of beta-blockers and calcium-channel blockers may have additive antihypertensive effects, but should be used with caution in patients with borderline congestive heart failure. Therefore, all patients with DBP greater than 100 mm Hg would have a risk score of at least 3 and should be treated with drug therapy earlier according to our schema detailed in Table 1.

Therefore, mild essential hypertension should not be universally treated with drug therapy immediately after the original diagnosis. Instead, therapy should be *individualized* according to age, sex, race, life-style, and risk profile. More intense emphasis should be placed on nonpharmacologic interventions. When pharmacologic therapy is deemed necessary, drugs with less effect on the lipid profile are preferable as a first line of therapy.

The stepped-care approach to the management of hypertension has served its time; the management of hypertension should not be simply aimed at numerically reducing blood pressure values, but rather should be intended to reduce the risk of cardiovascular morbidity and mortality. The concerted effort of physicians and patients towards a more individualized approach is essential to achieve this goal.

NONPHARMACOLOGIC TREATMENT OF ESSENTIAL HYPERTENSION

DAVID A. McCARRON, M.D.

Approximately 25 million Americans have essential hypertension, which is defined as a systolic blood pressure of greater than 160 mm Hg and/or a diastolic blood pressure of greater than 95 mm Hg on repeated observations. An additional 20 to 30 million Americans have transient elevations of either their systolic or diastolic pressure and are considered labile or borderline hypertensives. The definition of hypertension based upon a level of blood pressure is arbitrary, as the risk, in terms of morbidity and mortality associated with the level of blood pressure, is a continuous one. Consequently, to assign individuals to a category of either hypertensive or nonhypertensive, based upon an arbitrarily chosen value of either the systolic, diastolic, or mean arterial pressure is misleading for both the physician and the patient. It is in the patient's best interest to maintain a blood pressure that is as low as is possible and that is also compatible with a sense of well-being.

Consequently, many of the principles reviewed in this chapter, which relate to nonpharmacologic interventions in the management of essential hypertension, are applicable not only to those who are categorized as hypertensive, but to all individuals, who are under the care of a physician and who are interested in lowering their blood pressure. The reemergence of nonpharmacologic measures to lower blood pressure in patients with essential hypertension is based upon several recent phenomena. First, during the past 30 years, medicine has witnessed a logarithmic expansion of pharmacologic agents to manage hypertension. In spite of this remarkable increase in therapeutic agents, it is still unknown whether drug intervention in the treatment of mild hypertension, that is, diastolic blood pressure below 100 mm Hg and systolic blood pressures below 160 mm Hg, will yield, on the average, an increase in life expectancy. The results of several large trials done outside the United States (the Oslo study, the Medical Research Council Trial, and the Australian Hypertension Trial) have all indicated that life expectancy and prevention of premature cardiac events are not significantly reduced by the use of antihypertensive medication in individuals who have either borderline or minimally elevated arterial pressure. In the United States, the results of the Hypertension Detection Follow-up Program, the Multiple Risk Factor Intervention Trial, and the VA Cooperative Trial have been invoked as primary evidence that treating mild hypertension is beneficial, though authorities have disagreed with that interpretation. The current best assessment would lead the practicing physician to conclude that if it were possible to introduce a lifestyle or nutritional adjustment, which would lower blood pressure to a level equal to that accomplished with an antihypertensive agent, then the former would be the treatment of choice. This chapter reviews a number of such nonpharmacologic options from this latter category.

COMPLICATIONS OF DRUG THERAPY

In electing to manage some, if not many, hypertensives, with nonpharmacologic intervention, it is important to identify, prospectively, those individuals who might benefit from such a therapeutic approach. Obese subjects have significantly greater cardiovascular complications if they are hypertensive than do their lean counterparts. Also, an intervention which lowers body weight is extremely likely to lower blood pressure in parallel. However, the long-term use of selected antihypertensive medications are associated with an increase in body mass. The physiologic mechanisms underlying the weight gain associated with these antihypertensive drugs are unknown.

It is obvious, then, that an intervention designed to lower weight may be the optimal choice in an obese, mildly hypertensive subject.

A second category of patients, who appear to be at greater risk from fatal or morbid cardiovascular events resulting from high blood pressure, are those who comsume alcohol excessively. These individuals frequently experience wide fluctuations in their blood pressure, as well as the debilitating effects of alcohol. The use of antihypertensive medications in these patients if frequently doomed because of failure to comply with drug regimens. The use of nonpharmacologic interventions may have great benefits for this group. Complete elimination or a significant reduction in alcohol consumption to a maximum of 1 to 2 drinks per day may yield remarkable reductions in blood pressure. This response will be sustained if the patient is capable of abstaining from alcohol.

Older hypertensive patients (> 60 years of age), who must confront the reality that morbid and/or fatal cardiovascular events will prematurely shorten or impair the quality of their lives, are individuals in whom drug therapy would appear to hold the greatest benefits. However, that hypothesis has not been substantiated by all studies. The older hypertensive, although apparently at some greater risk of short-term complications of hypertension, is also at greater risk of complications from long-term antihypertensive medication use. On the basis of side-effects alone, the older patient is much more likely to develop significant and limiting adverse responses from many current antihypertensive medications. Because of the older patient's sensitivity to the antihypertensives, it is critical that nonpharmacologic measures be used wherever possible. This would prevent many of the complications of drug therapy, which reduce the quality of life and, which, tragically, in some patient's actually limit their life expectancy.

PATHOPHYSIOLOGY

Essential hypertension represents a disorder whose final pathophysiologic expression is through the vasculature. Over the decades, a great deal of interest has been focused on the regulation of cardiac output and the role of the heart in the development of high blood pressure. Nevertheless, at this juncture, our understanding of the principal mechanisms underlying abnormal elevations of arterial pressure dictate that we focus on altered vascular smooth muscle function of the arteriolar resistance vessels.

The postulated and established mechanisms that precede the development of altered regulation of the resistance vasculature are multiple. The multifactorial genesis of altered smooth muscle function reflects the heterogeneity of essential hypertension. In acknowledging the primacy of vascular resistance, one should not assume that all essential hypertension is strictly mediated through this alteration. In a given patient, changes in central nervous system regulation, baroreceptor sensitivity, circulating vasoconstrictors, endogenous vasodilating substances, or altered regulation of volume by the kidney may be of primary importance in the development of high blood pressure.

As an example to demonstrate that nonvascular mechanisms can be involved, is the fact that it is possible to lower blood pressure by changing cardiac output. The beta-adrenergic blockers, now widely used in the management of hypertension, are the principal therapeutic modality that attacks elevated arterial pressure through nonvascular pathways.

Since a wide variety of pharmacologic and nonpharmacologic interventions, which do not appear to share common mechanisms in their lowering blood pressure, are effective, one must conclude that a variety of mechanistic pathways exist for the down regulation of blood pressure in humans. Consequently, in both the nonpharmacologic, as well as in the pharmacologic management of hypertension, it is essential that patients be identified who have a greater likelihood of responding to one form of therapy versus another based upon clinical and laboratory observations.

CLINICAL EVALUATION

In the outpatient evaluation of mild essential hypertension, the documentation and verification of the presence of increased arterial pressure is the essential step. Considering how common is the diagnosis of essential hypertension, it is remarkable how poorly the presence of increased arterial pressure is documented in many patients who are ultimately subjected to therapy. In our practice, a patient referred for the continued management of hypertension, or for a new evaluation of suspected hypertension, has a minimum of four separate blood pressure determinations before any therapeutic decisions are made. The blood pressure recordings are made over a 4 to 6 week period by the same observer. Typically, the patients are seen at the same time for each visit and blood pressures are recorded using a cuff that is appropriate for the individual's arm size. Blood pressures are taken after a discussion that permits the patient to express his sense of well-being and any concerns she or he might have since the previous visit. Blood pressures are taken in the recumbent position, after 1 minute sitting, 3 minutes sitting, and then after 3 minutes of standing. In extensive experience in the nonpharmacologic treatment of essential hypertension under research protocols, we have observed that less than 40 percent of individuals who demonstrate elevated readings on the first visit (using a criteria of a diastolic blood pressure of > 95 mm Hg) persist in having abnormal values on the fourth visit. This experience from our research clinics has prompted us to be even more cautious in the labelling of individuals as being hypertensive until a careful longitudinal assessment of the blood pressure profile is established. Similarly, in obtaining the medical history, past evidence that increased arterial pressure had been noted is sought. The medical history of parents and siblings is also carefully reviewed. Current occupation, level of physical activity, leisure-time pursuits, and stressful situations in the patient's life are also solicited in detail. Any complicating medical or surgical problems for which the patient is currently being treated, or has been treated in the past, are assessed in terms of their relationship to increased arterial pressure. Individuals who have established problems with known vascular disorders, particularly, are reviewed in detail. Once a diagnosis of increased arterial pressure is confirmed (diastolic pressure > 90 mm Hg or systolic pressure > 150 mm Hg) based upon the four readings and a stable baseline blood pressure is established, active consideration of an intervention is undertaken. Prior to any therapeutic intervention, a routine biochemistry screen, hemoglobin, hematocrit, and urinalysis are obtained. If the patient has had an electrocardiogram and a chest film within the previous 5 years, additional x-ray films and electrocardiagrams are not done at that time.

Laboratory studies provide insights into possible secondary causes of hypertension. The most common ones encountered in our society are those of renal-vascular hypertension and drug-induced hypertension (oral contraceptives, combination analgesics, sympathomimetics, steroids, and nonsteroidal, anti-inflammatory agents). A history of renal disease or an endocrine disorder is pursued in detail, and the appropriate diagnostic studies for the specific entities under consideration are utilized. The ECG and chest X-ray films are reviewed for evidence of cardiac hypertrophy and coronary artery disease. In patients whom I suspect of having significant pulmonary dysfunctions from smoking, I obtain pulmonary function studies. This is done to assess their pulmonary reserve in anticipation of possible complications from either pharmacologic therapy (beta-blockers) or nonpharmacologic treatment (exercise). On the physical examination, particular attention is paid to the anthropomorphic characteristics of the individual (height, weight, skinfold thickness, and maximum chest circumference on deep inspiration and deep expiration). A careful assessment of resting heart rate and the heart rate after 3 minutes of stepping exercises are also recorded. Physical signs of secondary forms of hypertension, including those of vascular disease and endocrine disorders, such as thyroid disease, Cushing's syndrome, or pheochomocytoma are sought. Whereas the latter two are extremely rare, as correctable disorders, they need to be identified. Each patient is evaluated for evidence of orthopaedic problems that might limit their level of physical activity.

Following the completion of the laboratory and physical examination, we carefully review the patient's data, relate the individual's blood pressure to her or his overall cardiovascular risk profile (smoking history, weight, cholesterol, etc.) and compare it to that found in other individuals in their age group. Our assessment of whether or not to treat their hypertension with drugs focuses on what the reduction in cardiovascular risk would be if their weight were near normal, if they did not smoke, if their serum cholesterol was below 220 mg per deciliter, and if they exercised on a regular basis. Our assessment is discussed with the patient in a positive fashion, thereby reinforcing the conviction that the patient can largely determine whether she or he must take medications or employ a nonpharmacologic treatment to control her or his blood pressure. As is noted above, whereas many patients are not hypertensive by the fourth visit, typically these individuals still require lifestyle counselling, as they remain at some greater risk of ultimately developing hypertension in later years based upon their having transient elevations of their pressure.

NONPHARMACOLOGIC THERAPY

General Considerations. All individuals with diastolic pressures of less than 100 mm Hg and systolic blood pressures of less than 165 mm Hg are encouraged to employ nonpharmacologic interventions for the first 3 months, that is unless an overriding medical condition (Table 1) dictates an immediate reduction in blood presssure by pharmacologic agents. These criteria for diastolic and systolic pressure cutoffs are based upon the fact that conclusive evidence does not yet exist to indicate that pharmacological interventions for the treatment of blood pressures in that range are effective in lowering cardiovascular risk. Some individuals, whose diastolic pressures may be as high as 105 to 110 mm Hg and/or whose systolic pressures are between 160 and 180 mm Hg, we may also encourage to begin a nonpharmacologic intervention based upon specific indications. Such indications are listed in Table 2.

NONPHARMACOLOGIC INTERVENTION

Table 3 lists the types of nonpharmacologic interventions that we utilize. It is, however, artificial to consider these as separate and distinct, as there is functional overlap amongst them. As an example, it is unlikely that weight reduction will be achieved unless the patient also increases her or his daily exercise. Dietary adjustments will not be successful in the setting of a patient who is not exercising and endeavoring to maintain her or his weight. Consequently, a multifaceted intervention is prescribed for most patients. Such intervention emphasizes the incorporation of multiple changes in lifestyle, all of which, individually and collectively, will contribute to the control of blood pressure.

Since body mass index, as a measure of obesity, is the single best predictor of blood pressure status in Western countries, our nonpharmacologic intervention emphasizes weight control. For better than 50 percent of hypertensive patients we care for, weight loss is indicated. We initiate weight loss primarily through an exercise regimen and the ingestion of a nutritionally balanced diet. Patients are encouraged to initiate a graded dynamic exercise program utilizing fast walking, jogging, swimming,

TABLE 1 Contraindication to Use of Nonpharmacologic Intervention as Sole Therapy in Essential Hypertension

Unstable angina
Left ventricular dysfunction
Progressive renal dysfunction
Advanced diabetes
Peripheral vascular disease (functionally significant)
Aortic aneurysm

TABLE 2 Specific Indications for Nonpharmacologic Therapy in Moderate Essential Hypertension

Morbid obestiy (>50% above ideal weight)
Alcohol abuse
Aberrant dietary patterns
Pregnancy

or cycling. Patients are told to exercise a minimum of 5 days per week for at least 35 to 40 minutes. Initially, we advise individuals not to seek a group activity where they would be dependent upon a group's effort and schedule to meet their exercise requirements. They are counselled to select a program that fits their lifestyle and living conditions. Besides formal exercise periods, we also encourage our patients to reduce their reliance on automobiles in their daily activities. They are also asked to use stairs when moving between floors in buildings instead of elevators—a simple adjustment which increases caloric utilization. Although it is possible in some clinical settings to put the patients through sophisticated testing procedures in order to devise individual weight loss and exercise programs, we have found these endeavors to be less useful in many patients. Our initial efforts are now directed at a detailed personal discussion with the patient. In this discussion, we emphasize the need for them to make the personal decision to increase their level of exercise in order to control their weight. By reviewing the health consequences of failing to control their blood pressure and the universal complications of long-term drug therapy, we position nondrug therapy, appropriately, in a positive light. The exercise regimen that the patient chooses to adopt is discussed at each return visit. Some documentation by the patient of a commitment to this program, such as a record of times they have walked or days that they have swam, is encouraged.

Cigarette smoking does not appear to increase arterial pressure directly. In the later stages of mild hypertension, however, smoking may accentuate the progressive rise in arterial pressure through its direct contribution to the pathogenesis of atherosclerosis and the attendant increases in vascular resistance that accompany this process. In addition, routine smoking is virtually incompatible with regular physical exercise and inhibits the patient's efforts to reintroduce this into their lifestyle. Whereas behavior modification programs can be successful for some patients as a means of successfully stopping smoking, an alternative approach is for the patient to begin a graded exercise program. Most individuals, if committed to the exercise program, will eventually discontinue smoking voluntarily.

We do not typically use relaxation therapy, but have relied upon exercise as an effective means to induce relaxation and lower stress levels. In our experience, most individuals do not have the time to exercise and to participate in relaxation exercises both. Our experience has suggested that exercise, although providing some improvement in stress management, is the more useful and more acceptable intervention in the vast majority of our patients. As noted above, we do not advise individuals to seek professional advice in terms of the exercise program. When indicated, they are encouraged to obtain specific recommendations about equipment needed for the exercise programs, they choose, i.e. the type of shoe for walking or running or the bicycle, stationary or otherwise, for those choosing that form of exercise.

Nutritional Advice

It is critical that individuals adopt good nutritional habits as part of any endeavor to control weight. In the past, a remarkable degree of energy has been devoted to restriction of key nutritional elements in the control of blood pressure. This has been motivated principally to achieve a reduction in sodium intake. Secondarily, many patients have been advised to ingest fewer calories and lower the saturated fats in the diet. Our clinical research experience has sensitized us to the fact that the majority of patients with essential hypertension do not exhibit patterns of dietary excesses, but typically demonstrate one or more nutritional deficiencies in their diet. Statistically, the two most common deficiencies are calcium and potassium.

It is an unusual finding for one of our hypertensives to be consuming more than the United States average of 140 to 160 mEq of sodium per day. We make an effort to educate individuals as to the source of selected essential nutrients, calcium, magnesium, and potassium, which we consider cardioprotective. We then instruct them in ways in which they can moderate their sodium intake (100 to 150 mEq per day) without drastically changing their diet in a way that might expose them to deficiencies of other critical nutrients. A similar tack is employed in an attempt to reduce total and saturated fat intake. As an example of our approach, a patient would not be advised to reduce her or his cheese consumption as a means of lowering either total or saturated fat intake. Such a recommendation would reduce the exposure to the principal source of dietary calcium other than fluid milk. Instead, although emphasizing the need to maintain 1,000 to 1,200 mg of calcium per day, we provide the patient with dietary options that maintain daily intake of cheese while lowering excessive saturated fats from other parts of the diet. In our research experience we have found it possible to increase the intake of such nutritional factors as calcium and potassium without imposing an increase in total calorie, fat, or sodium intake. Potassium intake (70 to 80 mEq per day) will be achieved automatically if individu-

TABLE 3 Nonpharmacologic Interventions for Mild Essential Hypertension

Weight Control
Dynamic physical exercise
Alcohol moderation and abstention
Diet modification
Increase Ca_2^+
Increase K^+
Reduce fats
Moderate Na^+
Moderate caffeine
Cessation of Cigarettes
Relaxation Therapy

als maintain their dietary calcium consumption. It is not appreciated by most clinicians or many nutritionists that dairy products represent the principal dietary source of potassium in the human diet.

We do not rigorously monitor sodium intake. If the patient experiences a therapeutic response (normalization of arterial pressure) to the regimen outlined above (exercise, weight reduction, and increases in calcium and potassium intake), then no effort is made to reduce sodium intake. Individuals who freely describe themselves as using excessive amounts of sodium are encouraged to moderate their intake to 100 to 150 mEq per day.

Individuals who consume more than three caffeine-containing beverages per day are advised to limit themselves to no more than three. Although, caffeine's direct role in the pathogenesis of essential hypertension remains controversial, the negative effects of excessive caffeine on net calcium balance in the average patient warrants moderation in hypertensives.

Patients who are consuming more than two alcoholic drinks per day are counselled either to discontinue all alcohol consumption or to have no more than one or two drinks each day. Many moderate drinkers will readily adapt to this lifestyle change. Subjects who are consuming more than four or five drinks per day, however, typically have had tremendous difficulty in making this adjustment. Our experience suggests that couselling from the physician is of limited value in these situations. The patient is advised to seek professional counselling in order to gain an in-depth understanding as to why she or he drinks and how to modify her or his lifestyle to reduce or discontinue all alcohol use.

HYPERTENSIVE EMERGENCIES AND URGENCIES

STANLEY S. FRANKLIN, M.D.

Over the past 30 years, with the development and increasing use of effective antihypertensive agents in the therapy of hypertension, there has been an associated steady decline in the incidence of accelerated and malignant hypertension. Therefore, high blood pressure rarely constitutes a medical emergency; this is despite the large number of patients with chronic hypertension. Indeed, the hypertensive crisis probably occurs in less than 1 percent of the hypertensive population. In the majority of these cases, the hypertensive emergency represents a failure of early diagnosis or inadequate drug therapy.

Not all patients who present with severe hypertension have true hypertensive emergencies. In their 1984 report, The Joint National Committee on Detection, Evaluation, and Treatment of High Blood Pressure proposed an operational classification of hypertensive emergencies and urgencies. On the one hand, *emergencies* were defined as situations in which greatly elevated blood pressure must be lowered within 1 hour to reduce actual patient risk and on the other, *urgencies* were defined as situations in which severe elevations in blood pressure were not causing immediate end organ damage but which should be controlled within 24 hours in order to reduce potential patient risk.

A physician's first task is to diagnose accurately if a patient's severe hypertension represents (1) a true hypertensive emergency, (2) urgent hypertension, or (3) labile hypertension without evidence of an immediate threat to the vasculature or vital organs. If a true hypertensive emergency exists, the physician must choose the proper antihypertensive agent, or agents, and make a decision with regard to how rapidly and to what extent blood pressure should be lowered. The question of the desirability of a rapid lowering of blood pressure must necessarily take into account the risk of excessive delay in lowering the pressure versus the risk of neurologic or cardiac damage brought about by excessive reduction.

DIFFERENTIAL DIAGNOSIS OF A POTENTIAL HYPERTENSIVE CRISIS

A true hypertensive emergency is a life-threatening condition that requires the immediate lowering of blood pressure; both idiopathic and secondary hypertension can lead to a hypertensive emergency. The diagnosis is not based on any specific level of blood pressure, but rather on numerous factors that include the rapidity in rise of blood pressure, the duration of the hypertension, and the clinical determination of the immediate direct threat to the patient. For example, a young woman with eclampsia could develop a hypertensive emergency with a blood pressure of only 170/110 mm Hg, whereas a patient with long-standing hypertension may not be in a crisis situation with a blood pressure of 250/150 mm Hg.

Conditions that can be classified as a true hypertensive emergencies are shown in Table 1. Hypertensive encephalopathy represents an emergency characterized by markedly elevated blood pressure with symptoms and signs of increased intracranial pressure or cerebral edema. Frequent symptoms are severe headache, altered mental status (e.g., irritability, lethargy, or confusion), nausea or vomiting, seizures, or focal neurologic signs. The hypertensive crises of toxemia of pregnancy, pheochromocytoma, or of drug-induced catecholamine excess syndromes frequently are associated with an extremely rapid rise in blood pressure to crisis level, which can cause an acute intracranial bleed, even in the absence of hypertensive encephalopathy. In contrast, malignant hypertension, which can be defined as severe hypertension with hemorrhages,

TABLE 1 Hypertensive Emergencies

Hypertensive encephalopathy
Eclampsia
Pheochromocytoma crisis
Drug-induced catecholamine excess syndromes
Accelerated malignant hypertension with decreasing vision, acute renal failure, mesenteric insufficiency, acute GI hemorrhage, or acute pancreatitis
Intracranial or subarachnoid hemorrhage
Dissecting aneurysm or leaking abdominal aortic aneurysm
Refractory crescendo angina or myocardial infarction
Refractory pulmonary edema
Postoperative bleeding at vascular suture lines

exudates, and papilledema of the optic fundi, may not represent a true hypertensive emergency unless it is also associated with encephalopathy. Other life-threatening presentations that demand immediate lowering of malignant hypertension are decreasing visual acuity, the onset of acute renal failure, mesenteric insufficiency, acute gastrointestinal hemorrhage, or acute pancreatitis.

Moderate to severe elevations in blood pressure, without features of accelerated malignant hypertension, may constitute a true hypertensive emergency when complicated by refractory pulmonary edema, crescendo angina or recent myocardial infarction, dissecting or leaking aneurysms, intracranial hemorrhage, or postoperative bleeding at vascular suture lines.

In contrast to the true hypertensive emergency, Table 2 lists urgent hypertension, which requires a slower reduction in blood pressure. A review of the clinical manifestations and of the differential diagnostic features of each of the entities listed in Tables 1 and 2 is clearly beyond the scope of this presentation. However, accurate clinical diagnosis represents the keystone to successful therapeutic management of these high-risk patients.

POTENTIAL DANGERS OF RAPID LOWERING OF BLOOD PRESSURE

Whenever arterial blood pressure rises too high or falls too low, the cerebral arteries constrict or dilate as required to ensure a constant cerebral blood flow. This phenomenon, referred to as autoregulation, occurs primarily in the small resistance arterioles of the cerebral arteries. In normotensive subjects, cerebral blood flow is autoregulated down to a mean blood pressure of 60 mm Hg. As the blood pressure decreases below this critical level, no further dilation of the vascular bed of the brain can compensate for the decreased perfusion pressure and, thus, cerebral blood flow decreases. Early symptoms of hypoxia follow such as lightheadedness, confusion, and dimming of vision. If mean blood pressure decreases below 35 to 40 mm Hg, somnolence and loss of consciousness ensue. On the other hand, if blood pressure exceeds the upper limit of autoregulation (150 to 200 mm Hg of mean blood pressure), cerebral blood flow increases and hypertensive encephalopathy may develop. In chronically hypertensive patients, there is a shift of the autoregulatory cerebral blood flow curve to the right; this implies that a chronically hypertensive patient has a greater resistance to autoregulatory breakthrough of cerebral blood flow than his normotensive counterpart. Thus, these chronically hypertensive patients reach the lower limit of autoregulation and subsequently suffer a decrease in cerebral blood flow at a mean arteriolar pressure easily tolerated by normotensive patients. This is not an argument to be used against the treatment of severe hypertension, but it does illustrate the necessity for careful, gradual, and not excessive reduction in blood pressure, which can prevent ischemia to the vital organs of the body. Over a period of months, with successful treatment of hypertension, there appears to be a readaptation of cerebral blood flow autoregulation to a more normal curve.

Hypertensive encephalopathy is best explained as a severe hypertensive state in which there is a decompensation of the normal cerebral autoregulation of blood flow that results in breakthrough hyperperfusion, damage to the blood brain barrier with the subsequent development of increased permeability, petechial hemorrhage, infarction, and necrosis. Cerebral edema is not a necessary or obligatory component of hypertensive encephalopathy. The autoregulation of cerebral blood flow may be lost in the presence of cerebral ischemia or edema as well as from local tissue acidosis that results from an acute intracerebral hemorrhage or thrombosis. In the presence of a completed cerebral thrombosis, minimal reduction in systemic arterial blood pressure may lead to further ischemia to the compromised area of the brain, which may cause an enlargement of the original infarct with worsening of neurologic symptoms. Deterioration in cerebral blood flow during reduction in systemic blood pressure may result in part from a steal syndrome, in which the normal surrounding areas of the brain maintain normal cerebral blood flow at the expense of the injured area. Disturbed autoregulation of cerebral blood flow has recently been observed in patients with accelerated malignant hypertension who develop acute neurologic signs and symptoms in association with rapid and excessive lowering of blood pressure.

From the preceding discussion, it is obvious that blood pressure ought not be reduced to values below the autoregulatory range for cerebral or myocardial blood flow. Numerous studies have shown that critical blood flow is maintained in the normal range if hypertensive pressures are not reduced to mean values below 120 mm Hg. Therefore, an initial blood pressure reduction to a mean value of 130 to 120 mm Hg, which translates into a blood pressure of 170/110 to 160/100, respectively, would appear to be a safe level for initial blood pressure reduction.

TABLE 2 Hypertensive Urgencies

Accelerated and malignant hypertension (uncomplicated)
Hypertension associated with coronary disease
Hypertension associated with incipient congestive heart failure
Severe hypertension in a kidney transplant patient
Moderate to severe elevations in blood pressure ($\geq$ 120 mm mercury diastolic) with minimal end-organ damage and no impending complications

However, there may be the rare patient who develops deteriorating neurologic symptoms at this level, especially if there is an unrecognized completed stroke in association with accelerated malignant hypertension. The prevention of both neurologic and myocardial damage in these high-risk hypertensive emergency situations would argue strongly for the selection of an antihypertensive agent with both a short onset and a brief duration of action; thus, if disturbing cerebral or myocardial symptoms develop with the lowering of blood pressure, the infusion of medication could be discontinued in order to allow for a rapid return of blood pressures towards previous baseline levels and, hopefully, prevention of irreversible tissue damage.

CLINICAL STRATEGIES IN REGARD TO DIAGNOSIS AND THERAPY

During the initial evaluation of the severely hypertensive patient, an effort should be made to triage the patient into one of several categories: a *pseudohypertensive crisis* patient, i.e., one with labile hypertension without evidence of an immediate threat to the vasculature or vital organs, can be treated with sedation and reassurance and sent home; a *true hypertensive emergency* state that frequently requires parenteral therapy and intensive care unit observation; and finally, the *intermediate state of urgent hypertension* which depending on the circumstances, can be treated with rapidly acting oral antihypertensive agents either inside or outside the hospital.

A brief but concise history and physical examination are necessary to establish an accurate etiologic diagnosis and to determine the status of the cerebral, cardiac, and renal function (Table 3). This has an important clinical bearing on the safety of subsequent reduction of blood pressure values. Of special note is the onset of hypertension and knowledge about past and more recent use of antihypertensive drug therapy. The majority of patients have chronic hypertension, and although it may be severe, they do not necessarily have resistant hypertension. Clinical assessment, often accompanied by screening laboratory tests, electrocardiograms, and chest films are of paramount importance in answering the following questions: How rapidly should the blood pressure be lowered?; What is the first end point in blood pressure reduction?; What agent or agents should be used?; What should be the route of administration?; and finally is there a need for intensive care unit monitoring?

TABLE 3 Check List of Useful Information for the Assessment of Hypertensive Urgencies and Emergencies

Date of onset of hypertension and when it become severe or accelerated.
Recent and past antihypertensive drug history
Status of circulatory blood volume and possible presence of congestive heart failure
Optic fundi evidence of hemorrhages, exudates, and/or papilledema
Clinical picture compatible with hypertensive encephalopathy
Neurologic findings compatible with an evolving or completed stroke
History or ECG evidence of coronary artery disease
Proteinuria, active urinary sediment and/or elevated serum creatinine suggestive of acute or chronic hypertensive renal disease
History compatible with a high catecholamine state
Clinical and laboratory evidence of a potential high renin-angiotensin state

STRATEGY FOR PROPER DRUG SELECTION

The ideal medication for *hypertensive emergencies* should have a rapid onset and a brief duration of action, be easy to administer and monitor and not adversely to affect critical organs such as the brain, heart, or kidneys, and have few side effects. Such an ideal drug is not available. Drugs recommended for use in hypertensive emergencies and urgencies are shown in Table 4.

Sodium Nitroprusside

Sodium nitroprusside is predictably the most effective drug used in the treatment of hypertensive emergencies. The mechanism of action is that of direct peripheral vasodilatation with a balanced effect on both capacitance and resistance blood vessels. When administered by intravenous infusion, the antihypertensive effect of nitroprusside is apparent within seconds and is highly dose-dependent. After discontinuation of therapy, blood pressure rises rapidly to previous levels within 1 to 5 minutes. In many centers, nitroprusside has become the drug of choice for maintaining hypotension during surgery because of its ease of administration and its sparing of sympathetic reflexes. Serious toxicity and death from cyanide accumulation have rarely occurred, and then only with a total dose that exceeds 300 mg per hour. Safe maximum doses recommended for short-term use have ranged from 0.5 to 1.5 mg per kilogram per hour. Since nitroprusside reduces both venous return and afterload, it can be used safely and effectively in the presence of cardiac failure. It may be used in cases of dissecting aneurysm, but should be combined with intravenous propranolol in order to reduce effectively the myocardiac contractility. In patients who have become refractory to phentolamine, it may even be the drug of choice in the treatment of pheochromocytoma.

The suggested protocol for nitroprusside use, that follows appears efficacious. Sodium nitroprusside is supplied as a 50 mg lyophilized powder, which can be dissolved in 500 ml of 5 percent dextrose in water, thereby yielding a final concentration of 100 μg per ml. Infusions are started at a rate of approximately 0.5 μg per kilogram of body weight per minute by means of infusion pump (IVAC, Holter, or Harvard). There are three phases to nitroprusside administration as follows:

1. Initial titration phase. In this phase, infusion rates are doubled every 3 to 5 minutes until blood pressure falls. When this occurs, the infusion can be turned off until the blood pressure begins to turn upward once again.
2. Stabilization phase. In this phase, the nitroprusside infusion is restarted at rates half way between the last two values of the titration phase. If there is a fluctuation in blood pressure, the rate is adjusted until the pressure is stabilized.

Table 4 Drugs Recommended for Hypertensive Emergencies and Urgencies

Hypertensive emergencies treated with parenteral drug therapy
Sodium nitroprusside
Diazoxide
Trimethaphan camsylate
Nitroglycerin
Hydralazine
Phentolamine
Hypertensive urgencies treated with oral antihypertensive agents
Clonidine
Nifedipine
Labetalol
Minoxidil
Angiotensin-coverting enzyme inhibitors (captopril, enalapril)

3. Discontinuation phase. At this point, oral antihypertensive agents are used concurrently with the nitroprusside. The nitroprusside infusion can be discontinued at 4 to 6 hour intervals to determine new baseline blood pressures and to assess the need for continuation of parenteral therapy.

The use of nitroprusside requires careful monitoring of the patient in an intensive care unit and the use of an arterial line to monitor blood pressure accurately. Experienced nursing care for assessment of blood pressure and cardiac and neurologic status is necessary to ensure safe management.

Nitroprusside crosses the placenta, and its metabolites may accumulate in the fetus; therefore, in eclampsia it is not the drug of choice.

Diazoxide

Diazoxide is a benzothiadiazine derivative that is closely related chemically to thiazide diuretics. Diazoxide exerts its hypotensive effect by reducing arteriolar vascular resistance through direct relaxation of arteriolar smooth muscle. It has little effect on capacitance vessels and no direct effect on the heart or autonomic reflexes. Consequently, when the drug decreases arterial pressure, baroreceptor reflexes are activated, thereby leading to an increase in heart rate, myocardial contractility, stroke volume, and cardiac output. In addition to increased sympathetic reflex activity, diazoxide has several other recognized disadvantages. With the bolus administration of 300 mg of diazoxide, blood pressure may rapidly decrease to normal or even to subnormal levels. An alternate method of multiple small intravenous injections of 50 to 100 mg of diazoxide at 10 minute intervals would appear to produce a more controlled reduction in blood pressure. However, the duration of action of diazoxide is from 2 to 12 hours or more, thereby preventing rapid return of blood pressure to baseline levels in the presence of any deterioration in neurologic or cardiac function. Therefore, it would appear that diazoxide is not the drug of choice in treating (1) hypertensive encephalopathy, (2) eclampsia, (3) dissecting or leaking aneurysms, (4) refractory hypertension in association with angina or myocardial infarction, and (5) impending or completed strokes that are either hemorrhagic or thrombotic in nature.

Trimethaphan Camsylate

Trimethaphan camsylate is a short-acting ganglionic blocking drug which has long been in use. The advantages of trimethaphan are that it is potent, acts rapidly, and has a hypotensive action that can be reversed rapidly by stopping the infusion and placing the patient in a Trendelenburg position. However, its adverse effects are many and result from its ganglionic blockade action. These include paralytic ileus, urinary retention, and the development of tachyphylaxis. Because of the availability of newer drugs with fewer side effects, trimethaphan is seldom used today. However, it can be used as a substitute when nitroprusside is not available.

Nitroglycerin

Nitroglycerin has recently been released for intravenous administration. In a manner similar to that of sodium nitroprusside, its features are rapid onset and offset of action with the ability to titrate blood pressures by careful control infusion rates. At low infusion rates, venodilatation is the predominant effect, whereas at higher doses arteriolar dilatation also occurs. Thus, nitroglycerin infusions reduce both preload and afterload without appreciable changes in heart rate.

When, hypertension has not responded to analgesia and sedation, intravenous nitroglycerin would appear to be the drug of choice in the management of hypertensive patients who present with crescendo angina or myocardial infarctions in evolution. There is evidence that intravenous nitroglycerin may dilate collateral blood vessels and improve perfusion to ischemic areas of the myocardium, whereas sodium nitroprusside may decrease perfusion to ischemic myocardium in patients with severe coronary artery disease. Moreover, cardiac output is improved to a greater extent with nitroglycerin than with nitroprusside when pre-treatment pulmonary capillary wedge pressures are increased.

The method of administration is similar to that recommended for sodium nitroprusside. Since nitroglycerin is rapidly absorbed into plastic from solution, glass containers and special intravenous tubing should be utilized for its administration. Headache, nausea, and vomiting are the most frequent side effects.

Hydralazine

Hydralazine, like diazoxide, reduces arterial blood pressure by direct relaxation of arteriolar smooth muscle without much effect on venous capacitance. Thus, sympathetic overactivity is frequently noted with the same contraindications to its use as were described for diazoxide. Hydralazine is still considered the drug of choice for the treatment of eclampsia. Reflex tachycardia and palpitations may occur, but the risk of myocardial ischemia is minimal in young women with freedom from significant coronary atherosclerosis.

Phentolamine

Phentolamine is a short-acting alpha-adrenergic blocker that is specifically indicated in patients with disorders associated with high circulating levels of catecholamines. This would include (1) pheochromocytoma; (2) hypertensive crisis associated with monoamine oxidase inhibitors; (3) drug overdoses with phencyclidine, cocaine, or LSD; and (4) hypertensive rebound following sudden discontinuation of agents such as clonidine or guanabenz. Intravenous administration of phentolamine is associated with tachycardia and frequently with symptoms of abdominal pain, cramps, nausea, vomiting, and diarrhea. Because of these symptoms and the drug's tendency towards tachyphylaxis, nitroprusside infusions represent an alternative mode of therapy for the described clinical emergencies.

For the urgent hypertensive patient (see Table 2), the administration of antihypertensive therapy by intravenous infusion is most often not necessary. However, several oral agents have been shown to be effective and relatively safe in treating urgent hypertension (see Table 4). Currently, it is difficult to choose between these agents on the basis of efficacy and safety because no randomized comparative studies have yet been published.

Clonidine

Oral clonidine loading has been used successfully in a large percentage of patients with hypertensive urgencies. Clonidine is absorbed rapidly, and its antihypertensive effects are noted within 30 minutes with peak levels being achieved within 2 to 4 hours. An initial dose of 0.2 mg of clonidine is given orally, followed by 0.1 mg hourly for several hours, or until blood pressure has reached the desired level. Because clonidine is a central $alpha_2$–agonist, there is no interference with normal baroreceptor reflex control of blood pressure. The average total dose of clonidine required to control hypertension initially is 0.45 mg, the range being between 0.2 to 0.7 mg. For chronic use, approximately one-half of the total loading dose is given daily in split doses—in the morning and at bedtime. The main contraindication to use is second or third degree heart block or sick sinus syndrome.

Nifedipine

When given either sublingually or orally, nifedipine can promptly reduce blood pressure. There is no evidence for more rapid absorption of oral nifedipine when the soft capsule is chewed and swallowed. The blood pressure lowering effect peaks within 15 to 30 minutes and remains effective for up to 3 to 5 hours.

The hemodynamic effects of nifedipine are variable, but in general, an increase in heart rate and cardiac output are noted, along with a reduction in left ventricular end-diastolic pressure in patients with impaired left ventricular function. In the absence of significant cerebrovascular disease, the acute oral administration of nifedipine has been associated with preservation or improvement of cerebral blood flow; however, in the presence of significant cerebrovascular disease, nifedipine, which penetrates the blood-brain barrier, can dilate the cerebral vessels and lead to an uneven cerebral perfusion attributable to an intracranial "steal" effect. Furthermore, the calcium antagonist effect of nifedipine on the coronary vessels can lead to generalized vasodilatation, but in the presence of significant coronary artery disease, can produce a "steal" effect from a segment of fixed, obstructed coronary artery. This may explain the occasional occurrence of the paradoxical worsening of angina pectoris or the appearance of ischemic ECG changes with or without the associated angina that follows the oral administration of nifedipine.

Oral or sublingual nifedipine would appear to be an effective and safe agent in the control of hypertensive urgencies, with the possible exception of patients with cerebrovascular or coronary disease. Furthermore, a drug such as nifedipine, which dilates cerebral vessels and increases cerebral blood flow, may cause an immediate increase in intracranial pressure; therefore, this agent should be used with extreme caution in patients with malignant hypertension because of its potential for cerebral herniation.

Labetalol

Labetalol is a combination alpha– and beta–adrenergic blocker, which in an oral dose of 200 to 400 mg, results in a gradual decrease in blood pressure that begins within 2 hours. Large, single doses of intravenous labetalol appear to be less effective than diazoxide in controlling blood pressure, but may lead to severe prolonged hypotension. Because labetalol is lipid-soluble and has a considerable first pass hepatic metabolism, the oral dosage range to produce controlled hypotension varies considerably. For this reason, the antihypertensive effect of labetalol is not nearly as predictable as it is with oral clonidine or nifedipine. Also, Labetalol is contraindicated in patients with congestive heart failure, asthma, sinus bradycardia, or atrial ventricular block graded in first degree.

Minoxidil

Minoxidil is a potent, oral active vasodilator that works predominantly at the arteriolar level. This drug is usually reserved for patients who are refractory to conventional therapy. The reason for this is that minoxidil is usually given as triple therapy along with a beta-blocker or clonidine and vigorous diuretic therapy. The rationale for this type of triple therapy is to overcome severe reflex sympathetic overactivity and marked sodium and fluid retention. Because of the effectiveness of this regimen, minoxidil will undoubtedly continue to be used in the role of a last-resort antihypertensive agent. Chronic use in women is also made difficult by its tendency to cause hypertrichosis.

Angiotensin-Converting Enzyme Inhibitors

Angiotensin-converting enzyme inhibitors (captopril and enalapril) are frequently effective in acutely lowering blood pressure in hypertensive urgencies, especially when in association with accelerated malignant hypertension and renal insufficiency. The major problem with the use of these agents is that the urgent hypertensive patient is in need of close observation to detect a possible first-dose hypotensive response; this tends to occur frequently in salt-depleted vasoconstricted patients. Significant hyperkalemia may also be a problem when these agents are used in patients with renal insufficiency, and one must also be aware of a precipitous deterioration in renal function when these agents are administered to patients with bilateral renal artery stenosis. Although angiotensin-converting enzyme inhibitors are undoubtedly important antihypertensive agents in severe and resistant hypertension, one must be extremely cautious when they are used in the urgent hypertensive patient.

In summary, therefore, the physician must use clinical judgment in deciding which patient has a true hypertensive emergency and which has a less severe, urgent hypertension that can be lowered more slowly and with oral agents. Thus, accurate diagnosis determines (1) selection of the route of administration, (2) selection of a specific agent, (3) the need for special monitoring, and (4) determination of how rapid the initial blood pressure should be lowered.

In the true hypertensive emergency, blood pressure should be lowered in a controlled manner in order to intermediate blood pressure levels below the danger level of hypertensive catastrophe, but above the level of impaired or autoregulatory control of cerebral and myocardial blood flow. This is best achieved by using parenteral drugs that can be given via slow infusion in a controlled manner, by using a drug that has a rapid onset and offset of action, and by using it in a setting where optimal monitoring of myocardial and cerebral function can be achieved—in an intensive care unit with specially trained nurses in attendance. Sodium nitroprusside would appear to be the drug of choice in a variety, but not in all, hypertensive emergency states. In contrast, in the urgent hypertensive state, several oral antihypertensive agents have been shown to be effective and relatively safe, the need for hospitalization depending on individual circumstances.

RENOVASCULAR HYPERTENSION

MORTON H. MAXWELL, M.D.
ABRAHAM U. WAKS, M.D.

Renovascular hypertension (RVH) is defined as high blood pressure caused by occlusive disease of a main renal artery or of a primary branch that is potentially curable by reconstitution of vessel patency. Since renal artery stenosis may be present without causing hypertension, the diagnosis of RVH must be made retrospectively after correction of the occlusive disease. However, a tentative diagnosis may be suspected by certain anatomic findings and functional tests. The incidence of RVH varies widely depending on methods of patient selection. Several studies have shown a prevalence of RVH of 3 to 6 percent in hospital referral populations with the remaining patients mainly having essential hypertension.

TYPES OF LESIONS

Although there are multiple etiologies of RVH, 90 to 95 percent of cases present with two principal lesions: atherosclerosis and fibrous dysplasia. In the national Cooperative Study of Renovascular Hypertension, patients with atherosclerotic lesions constituted 60 percent of cases of renovascular disease; the lesions had a striking predilection for the osteum and proximal one-third of the main renal artery. The left side was more frequently involved than the right, and approximately one-third of patients had bilateral lesions. Fibrous dysplasia was present in 35 percent of patients with renovascular disease mainly involving the middle and distal third of the renal artery, and commonly extending into the primary branches. The right side was more commonly affected than the left. When bilateral disease was present from either major disease entity, one side usually predominated.

PATHOPHYSIOLOGY

The pathophysiology of RVH involves the release of renin from the ischemic kidney. However, RVH may be divided into two-kidney and one-kidney models. In the two-kidney model, the ischemic (ipsilateral) kidney secretes an excess of renin and retains sodium and water; whereas the opposite (contralateral) intact kidney loses sodium and water. In this model, there is an overall negative sodium balance, a persistence of elevated plasma renin activity, and a continual blood pressure responsiveness to inhibitors of the renin-angiotensin systems. Clinical variants of the two-kidney model are unilateral main or segmental stenosis and a solitary kidney with segmental renal artery stenosis.

In contrast, the one-kidney model secretes renin and conserves sodium—the absence of a contralateral kidney thereby preventing sodium loss and leading to eventual expansion of total body sodium and extracellular fluid volume. Fluid volume expansion suppresses renin; hence, hypertension in the one-kidney model is relatively insensitive to the inhibitors of the renin-angiotensin system. Clinical variants of the one-kidney model are bilateral, high grade, main renal artery stenosis; solitary kidney with main renal artery stenosis; and unilateral main renal artery stenosis with contralateral loss of excretory function secondary to nephrosclerosis or parenchymal renal disease.

CLINICAL CHARACTERISTICS

The natural history of renovascular disease depends on the etiology. In terms of clinical characteristics, two prototypical patterns of RVH are recognized. First, there is the young or middle–aged woman with fibrous dysplasia who has hypertension of brief duration that is moderate to severe in intensity, minimal evidence of target organ damage, and a systolic–diastolic epigastric bruit that lateralizes from the midline to the right upper quadrant. Second there is the elderly male with atherosclerotic renovascular disease who has had mild hypertension for many months that has recently accelerated to severe values and has demonstrated grade III or IV optic fundi, cardiomegaly, and azotemia. An abdominal bruit may or may not be present. More common than either of the two prototypical patterns is RVH that cannot be clearly separated from the clinical picture of essential hypertension.

Fibrous Dysplasia

Diffuse medial fibroplasia accounts for 70 to 80 percent of fibrous dysplasia, is often bilateral, and shows slow progression. Dissection, thrombosis, or rupture are unusual. Studies from the Cleveland and the Mayo Clinic, which utilized serial arteriography, revealed progression in 33 percent of patients during a 3-year follow-up period. No patient progressed to total occlusion during follow-up of up to 11 years. In contrast, patients with localized, intimal, medial, or adventitial hyperplasia often demonstrate rapid progression.

Atherosclerosis

Atherosclerotic lesions are part of a systemic disease that involves different segments of the vascular system. Mortality is higher because of cardiovascular events and target organ disfunction. Renal lesions tend to progress in 44 to 50 percent of the patients, as reflected by impairment of renal function and loss of renal mass. Total occlusion was observed in 16 percent of the patients followed by the Cleveland Clinic.

THERAPY

The therapeutic goals are (1) reversal of hypertension, and (2) restoration of renal blood flow, preservation of renal tissue, and improvement of renal function. Medical therapy with antihypertensive drugs may control the hypertension, but has no effect on the progression of the disease. Therefore, every effort should be made to find patients that can benefit from angioplastic or operative procedures.

The diagnosis of RVH involves careful risk-benefit and cost-benefit analysis when one is evaluating individual patients. The availability of newer antihypertensive drugs that are usually successful in lowering blood pressure in patients with RVH and the development of percutaneous transluminal angioplasty (PTA) as an alternative to operative treatment drastically change the decision matrix.

DIAGNOSTIC STRATEGIES

With regard to the need for aggressive work-up, the hypertensive population can be classified into three subgroups.

Patients in Whom Intervention with Possible Cure or Improvement of Hypertension is Preferable to Long-Term Drug Therapy

"This group includes: children; patients with severe or accelerated hypertension; hypertension that is uncontrollable (poor blood pressure response, adverse side effects, lack of compliance) with antihypertensive drug therapy; progressive diminution of kidney function; and progressive hypertension after kidney transplantation." Angiography should be used here as the initial diagnostic procedure and PTA may be attempted during the same procedure. Blood pressure response as well as reductions in plasma renin levels after successful dilation confirm the diagnosis of RVH. Thus, PTA is used as a definitive diagnostic test as well as a therapeutic modality.

Patients Suspected of Having RVH

Patients with inappropriate age of onset, abrupt worsening of hypertension, or systolic–diastolic epigastric bruits should be screened for RVH with digital subtraction intravenous angiography, rapid sequence intravenous urography, or radioisotope studies, which are followed by arteriography only if screening tests are positive.

Patients with Moderate Hypertension who are not Suspected of Having RVH

This group of asymptomatic patients represents the majority of the hypertensive population and are usually treated medically. Patients with marked response to angiotensin–converting enzyme (ACE) inhibitors or patients who do not respond to diuretics are more likely to have renin dependent hypertension, which includes RVH, thereby representing the best group for further diagnostic work-up.

MEDICAL THERAPY

Since the introduction of the oral converting enzyme inhibitor, captopril, which is often used concomitantly with a diuretic, successful control of hypertension has been reported in 85 to 90 percent of renovascular hypertensive patients. Similar results will likely occur with the use of the other ACE inhibitor, enalapril.

The greater effect of captopril is undoubtedly related to the specificity of action on underlying pathophysiological mechanisms of RVH. The acute depressor response to captopril correlates with the pre-treatment plasma renin activity; in contrast, the long-term response correlates poorly with renin levels. Although the vasodilatory action of captopril is not accompanied by significant sodium or volume retention, the addition of a diuretic greatly enhances its activity. Since many patients with RVH are extremely sensitive to the blood pressure lowering effect of captopril, a test dose of 6.25 mg (¼ tablet) should be given initially, followed by a dose of 12.5 mg, then increased to 25 mg 2 times per day or 3 times per day as necessary to obtain an optimal blood pressure response. By maintaining the total daily dose of captopril at no greater than 100 mg daily, serious side effects, such as leukopenia and membranous glomerulopathy, can be largely avoided. Captopril must be used with caution and in substantially lower doses in patients with renal insufficiency.

In patients with high-grade bilateral renal artery stenosis, effective control of blood pressure may contribute to slow progressive reduction in renal function by lowering perfusion pressure. In addition, several reports have described reversible acute renal failure after treatment with converting enzyme inhibitors such as captropril or enalapril in patients with bilateral renal artery stenosis, unilateral stenosis with contralateral renal dysfunction, or a single kidney with renal artery stenosis. Renal failure may occur even when there is no significant reduction in blood pressure from the converting enzyme inhibitor.

The complication of renal failure is best understood by considering the role of angiotensin II in the control of glomerular filtration. Angiotensin II, by preferentially constricting the efferent arteriole, maintains the glomerular filtration rate during hypoperfusion. Converting enzyme inhibitors therefore cause a selective dilation of the efferent arteriole by blocking angiotensin II, with a resulting decrease in renal perfusion and glomerular filtration. The overall incidence of converting enzyme-inhibitor-induced renal failure in the treatment of RVH is not known. Considering that bilateral, hemodynamically significant renal artery stenosis occurs in less than 10 percent of all renovascular patients, the majority of patients with RVH can be given converting enzyme inhibitors without the danger of renal failure.

The question of medical versus operative therapy for RVH continues to be a subject of controversy. The 1973 report of Hunt and Strong from the Mayo Clinic is the most extensive study that compares medical and operative therapy. Two hundred and fourteen patients with RVH were placed on drug therapy. From this initial group, 100 patients were selected for operative therapy after 3 months of unsuccessful medical treatment. Over the 7- to 14- year follow-up period of the atherosclerotic group, 30 percent of operatively treated patients died, as compared to 70 percent of the medically treated group. There was no significant difference in mortality for medical versus operative therapy in patients with fibrous dysplasia. Because the patients in this study were not selected randomly, one must use caution in the interpretation of results. Moreover, with newer, more effective drug therapy, the long-term prognosis of RVH may be improved.

A prospective, randomized study of RVH at Vanderbilt University, which compared medical versus operative therapy, has been ongoing for more than 12 years. Although this study has not been reported in detail, Dean has reported a 41 percent incidence of progression of renal artery stenosis in medically treated patients, demonstrated either by a significant decrease in renal length, and hence functioning renal mass, or by a decrease in creatinine clearance. Of great significance was the presence of continued good blood pressure control with medical therapy in 15 of 17 (88 percent) patients who showed deterioration of renal function. Thus, drug therapy cannot stop the progression of renal artery stenosis, despite good blood pressure control. In as many as 40 percent of cases, progressive renal artery stenosis may eventually impair renal function in the affected kidney.

With the use of currently available antihypertensive medication, good blood pressure control can probably be obtained in 85 to 90 percent of patients with RVH. Medical failures probably represent high-grade stenoses with extremely elevated, autonomous production of renin or severe bilateral renal artery stenosis with superimposed salt and water retention. Because of possible progression of renal artery stenosis, monitoring of kidney function is mandatory in patients receiving medical treatment. This monitoring is vital because blood pressure may continue to be well controlled with medications despite progressive loss of renal function. Moreover, serum creatinine or creatinine clearances may not change in the presence of progressive unilateral renal artery stenosis because of a counterbalancing improvement in renal function in the contralateral kidney without arterial stenosis. Thus, both creatinine clearance and renal size are important signs to follow. Renal size can be assessed by computed tomography, ultrasonography, or intravenous urography. It is important to note that a 10 percent loss in renal length is equivalent to a 30 percent loss in functioning renal mass since the kidney is shaped like an ovoid ellipsoid.

PERCUTANEOUS TRANSLUMINAL ANGIOPLASTY

The development by Gruentzig and associates of catheters fitted with an expansible balloon to dilate vascular obstructive lesions has stimulated interest in the possibility of correcting occlusive renal artery disease and benefitting RVH without the risks of surgery. The efficacy of renal PTA is difficult to determine because most early reports are relatively small in sample size, are largely retrospective and nonrandomized, and consist primarily of short-term (12 months or less) clinical follow-up. In general, success rates appear to be higher in (1) fibrous dysplasia as compared to atherosclerotic disease; (2) vessels with only one or two short stenoses, rather than more extensive disease; and (3) in stenoses located completely within the renal artery, rather than lesions that include the aortic wall or renal artery orifice. Only occasional success has been reported in occluded renal arteries.

The most comprehensive series to date is that of Sos and associates, reported in 1983 (Table 1). In this study, 89 patients with RVH, 51 with atheromatous stenosis, and 31 with fibrous dysplasia were followed for an average of 16 months (range 4 to 40 months) after angioplasty therapy. Angioplasty was technically successful in 87 percent of patients with fibrous dysplasia, but in only 57 percent of those with unilateral atherosclerotic lesions. Technical failure in atherosclerotic lesions resulted from both ostial

TABLE 1 Success Rate of Angioplasty in Renovascular Hypertension

Type of Lesion	*Number of Patients*	*Technical (%) Success*	*Improved (%) Hypertension*	*Overall (%) Benefited*	*Major (%) Complications*
Fibrous Dysplasia					
Combined lesions	31	87	93	81	6
Atherosclerosis					
Combined lesions	51	37	84	31	8
Unilateral lesions	31	57	82	47	

(By permission of Sos, et al. N Engl J Med 1983; 309:274.)

lesions, which could not be successfully dilated, and total occlusion of the vessels, which rarely allowed passage of a catheter. After successful angioplasty, blood pressure was reduced to normal or was improved in 93 percent of patients with fibrous dysplasia and in 82 percent of those with unilateral atheromatous disease.

Therefore, the overall benefit rate (percent technically successful multiplied by percent improved) was 81 percent in fibrous dysplastic disease and only 47 percent in unilateral atherosclerotic lesions. Much poorer results were obtained in bilateral atherosclerotic lesions, largely attributable to a high rate of technical failures. In a later report by Sos and associates, angiographic follow-up in 14 patients at 1 year and 13 patients at 2 years showed no evidence of restenosis or deterioration in blood pressure control, thereby suggesting that restenosis is unusual when full technical success has been obtained. In contrast, other investigators have noted a restenosis rate of 10 to 17 percent.

In addition to improved blood pressure control, successful angioplasty may stabilize or improve renal function. In the Sos series, there was a 12 percent increase in kidney size in patients who had technically successful angioplasties. Others have noted improved renal function in approximately 50 percent of azotemic patients after successful angioplasty.

The morbidity and mortality from angioplasty for both atheromatous and fibrous dysplastic disease of the renal arteries appear to be less than that from operative therapy. However, emergency operative repair of renal artery dissections was necessary in 6 percent of patients treated by Sos; this is higher than the usual 1 to 2 percent dissections reported by others and is perhaps explainable by more advanced atheromatous disease and the participation of many angiographers with varying experiences. Also to be considered is that follow-up operative therapy would have been necessary in those patients with technical failures. Other potential complications are massive hematoma, subsegmental infarcts, distal embolization, and acute deterioration in renal function. Most of these latter complications are self-limited and reversible. Randomized clinical trials of angioplasty versus surgery are needed to establish the long-term rate of complications and patency of arteries.

Informed consent of the patient requires explanation of the potential need for emergency operative correction of possible renal artery dissections. Thus the patient should be judged a good operative risk, and a surgical support team should be available prior to undertaking angioplasty therapy. Blood pressure should be monitored for at least 24 hours after the procedure, and if hypotension develops, the patient should be treated with short-term volume or vasopressor support. Because PTA may be done under local anesthesia, patients generally can be discharged from the hospital within several days of their procedure as compared to 1 to 2 weeks of hospitalization after surgery.

OPERATIVE INTERVENTION

In 1974, the National Cooperative Study on Renovascular Hypertension summarized operative results as follows. In 300 patients with atherosclerotic renal artery disease who underwent operative intervention, there were cure, improvement, failure, and mortality rates of 41, 15, 32, and 12 percent, respectively. In contrast, in 179 patients with fibrous dysplasia, there were cure, improvement, failure, and mortality rates of 64, 11, 25, and 3 percent, respectively. The unacceptably high mortality rate in individuals with atherosclerotic lesions reflected a high prevalence of generalized atherosclerosis, angina pectoris, previous myocardial infarctions, left ventricular hypertrophy, and impaired renal function.

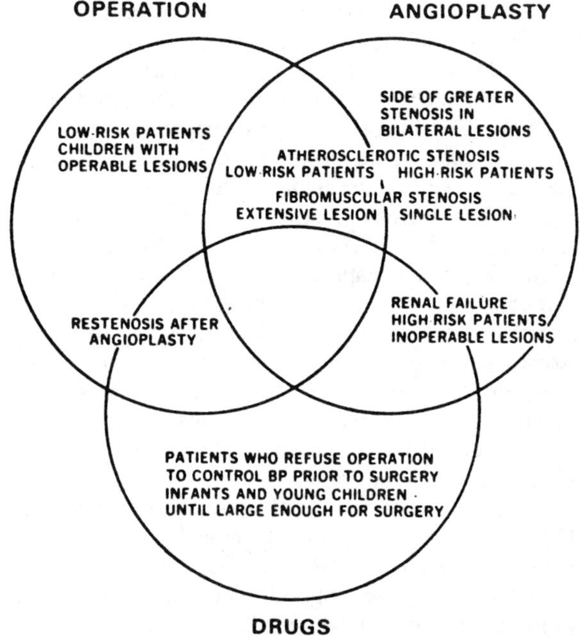

Figure 1 Treatment modalities in patients with renovascular hypertension.

When cardiovascular risk factors are considered in order to optimize patient selection, and only patients operated on by experienced personnel in specialized centers are included in the series, overall operative results are more impressive. Tables 2 and 3 summarize the more recent operative results in atherosclerotic and fibrous dysplastic RVH, respectively. Operative mortality has been reduced to 3 percent in patients with underlying atherosclerotic disease and to 1 percent or less in those with fibrous dysplastic RVH. Whereas one-third of atherosclerotic patients are cured by successful reconstructive surgery, as compared to two-thirds with underlying fibrous dysplastic disease, the overall benefit rate (improvement or cure of hypertension) was 85 percent versus 96 percent, thus supporting the efficacy of operative intervention in selected cases, regardless of underlying etiology of the renal artery stenosis or age of the patient.'

Frequently omitted from a discussion of the management of RVH is the long-term adverse effects of uncorrected renal artery occlusive disease on renal function. As discussed earlier, as many as 40 percent of patients with atherosclerotic renal artery stenosis show deterioration of renal function over a period of several years while on medical therapy. Recent studies (Table 4) have shown that 68 percent of patients have a marked improvement in renal function, as well as significant improvement in blood pressure when successful reconstructive surgery was performed. Indeed, the presence of a complete renal artery stenosis may still be compatible with operative improvement in renal function.

The most dependable predictors of improvement in renal function and blood pressure control after operative correction of occluded renal arteries are (1) renal length of 9 cm or greater; (2) arteriographic demonstration of a patent distal vessel, without evidence of severe intrarenal stenosis; (3) demonstration of an early nephrogram phase during arteriography; and (4) demonstration of an abundant collateral circulation, frequently with retrograde flow through the occluded vessel.

Because RVH is frequently a bilateral disease, which is progressive, one should avoid ablative treatment of RVH whenever possible. However, there are occasions when reconstructive surgery has a minimal chance of success, thereby making it necessary for either partial or total nephrectomy to be the operative treatment of choice. Such indications are as follows (1) renal atrophy, with length less than 9 cm; (2) main renal artery occlusion with renal infarction; (3) unilateral parenchymal disease; (4) segmental renal infarction; (5) segmental renal hypoplasia (Ask-Upmark kidney); and (6) noncorrectable renovascular disease such as intrarenal aneurysm or arteriovenous malformation.

Of the many operative procedures used to treat RVH, aortorenal bypass has emerged as the single most preferred operative treatment. In the past, satisfactory results have been obtained by using saphenous veins, although more recently a higher success rate has been reported by means of autogenous arterial grafts. Technical success rates in experienced hands now range between 95 and 97 percent.

Particularly challenging are renovascular lesions that extend into the renal arterial branches. Previously, these patients would have been candidates for nephrectomy. With the advent of microvascular extracorporeal operative techniques, renal revascularization may be the treatment of choice. However, it has been the experience of many surgeons that the main renal artery and its branches frequently can be repaired in situ, particularly when disease-free branches occur outside the renal hilus, by means of aortorenal bypass, which is the preferred technique.

There are occasions when other reconstructive techniques are preferable to aortorenal bypass. A splenorenal bypass may be the operation of choice when the stenosis is on the left side and when mobilization and use of the aorta may be hazardous owing to previous aortorenal operations, severe degenerative atherosclerosis, or complete aortic thrombosis. Since a splenorenal bypass involves only a single vascular anastomosis without the need for cross-

TABLE 2 Operative Results in Atherosclerotic Renovascular Hypertension

Reference	*Number of Patients*	*Cured (%) No.*	*Improved (%) No.*	*Failures (%) No.*	*Died (%) No.*
Dean et al (1977)	78	29 (36%)	39 (50%)	11 (14%)	1 (1%)
Stanley & Fry (1977)	105	29 (28%)	55 (52%)	18 (18%)	3 (3%)
Lankford (1979)	52	15 (29%)	30 (58%)	4 (8%)	3 (6%)
Novick et al (1981)	100	39 (40%)	50 (51%)	9 (0%)	2 (2%)
Totals	335	111 (33%)	174 (52%)	42 (13%)	9 (3%)

TABLE 3 Operative Results in Fibrous Dysplastic Renovascular Hypertension

Reference	*Number of Patients*	*Cured (%) No.*	*Improved (%) No.*	*Failures (%) No.*	*Died (%) No.*
Korobkin (1976)	19	14 (81%)	1 (5%)	2 14%)	1 (5%)
Stanley & Fry (1977)	159	101 (63%)	53 (33%)	6 (4%)	0 (0%)
Lankford (1979)	25	14 (56%)	20 (40%)	0 (0%)	1 (4%)
Totals	203	129 (64%)	64 (32%)	8 (4%)	2 (1%)

TABLE 4 Operative Results in Renovascular Hypertensive Patients with Azotemia

Reference	Number of Patients	Cure (%) No.	BP Results Improved (%) No.	Failure (%) No.	Improved Renal Function (%) No.
Dean (1979)	25	9 (36%)	15 (60%)	1 (4%)	16 (60%)
Libertino (1980)	15	10 (67%)	5 (33%)		13 (87%)
Novick (1983)	51				34 (67%)
Totals	91	19 (47%)	20 (50%)	1 (3%)	91 (68%)

clamping of the aorta, less operating time is required than for many of the more conventional reconstructive procedures, and thus may be indicated in the poor surgical risk patient. An aortorenal reimplantation procedure may be used to treat renovascular disease caused by a short, fibrous lesion, such as intimal fibroplasia or true fibromuscular hyperplasia, that involves the proximal one-third of the renal artery. This operation is particularly well suited to the anatomical variant of an anomalous high origin of the renal artery since an adequate amount of disease-free distal renal artery is a prerequisite for successful surgery.

The transfer of a kidney from one site to another in the same patient is termed renal autotransplantation. Autotransplantation has been used in patients with renovascular disease secondary to renal trauma, staghorn renal calculus, extensive ureteral loss, or tumors occurring in a solitary kidney. Other candidates for renal autotransplantation in the operative treatment of RVH are patients with a surgically difficult aorta, in whom relatively disease-free iliac arteries are present and in patients with extensive branch renal artery lesions that cannot be repaired by conventional revascularization techniques in situ. However, whenever possible, conventional in situ renal revascularization techniques should be used for the above indications because these techniques are associated with significantly reduced operative time and postoperative morbidity.

Certain general precautions can be taken to minimize renovascular operative morbidity and mortality. Atherosclerotic lesions of the renal artery are frequently associated with generalized vascular disease. When indicated, prophylactic coronary or carotid bypass surgery should be performed in patients with associated renal artery stenosis; these lesions should be corrected prior to operative repair of renal arteries—otherwise a high incidence of stroke and myocardial infarction occurs during routine renal artery bypass. In the presence of significant impairment in cardiac function, a Swan-Ganz flow catheter should be used to monitor the patient during renovascular surgery. Refractory hypertension should be treated with parenteral sodium nitroprusside infusions before, during, and after operative procedures.

CHOICE OF THERAPY AND CLINICAL MANAGEMENT

Reconstruction of vessel patency by operation or by PTA is preferable to medical therapy for the following reasons:

1. Patient can discontinue antihypertensive drugs, which results in substantial reduction of cost as well as avoidance of side effects.
2. Renal artery lesions, especially atherosclerotic, may worsen and thereby cause an increase in hypertension and reduction of renal function.
3. Operative techniques have been improved.
4. The introduction of transluminal angioplasty helps to avoid complicated and risky operative procedures.

Medical therapy should be favored for the following subgroups:

1. Patients with extensive bilateral and/or segmental lesions that are both inoperable and nondilatable.
2. Infants and young children who are not large enough for surgery.
3. Patients who refuse invasive procedures.
4. High-risk patients with nondilatable lesions.

All other patients, including high–risk patients, should be considered for invasive procedures.

PTA should be attempted as the initial procedure in all patients with RVH, unless technically unfeasible. PTA may be attempted at the time of initial arteriography when stenosis is demonstrated, regardless of its type or degree. If initial dilation by PTA is successful, as judgbed by the radiologic appearance and confirmed by a decreased pressure gradient, then the short-term blood pressure response offers the most accurate and practical diagnosis of RVH; if the blood pressure falls significantly the diagnosis of RVH is established, even if the blood pressure should subsequently increase because of restenosis. When PTA is not technically feasible or is initially unsuccessful in dilating a stenotic lesion, then diagnostic confirmation of RVH should be obtained and surgery is recommended unless contraindicated.

Specific indications for surgery are (1) progressive fibrous dysplasia lesions, usually associated with intimal fibroplasia and subadventitial fibroplasia; (2) atherosclerotic-ostial lesions in patients with progressive decrease in renal function despite good response to medical management; and (3) patients whose hypertension or azotemia responds only transiently to successful angioplasty (PTA might be reattempted in such cases prior to operative procedures).

To conclude, the choice of treatment depends on two principal considerations: control of blood pressure and preservation of renal function. The outcome of PTA or surgery depends on (1) accurate diagnosis of renin mediated hypertension, (2) technically successful procedure, and (3) type of renal artery disease (with more favorable results in patients with fibromuscular hyperplasia).

The introduction of PTA has modified the decision matrix (Figure 1) in the management of renal artery stenosis and should be attempted in amost every patient with an arteriographically demonstrable lesion, regardless of its severity. Immediate blood pressure response may then be used as the "ultimate" diagnostic test. The introduction of ACE inhibitors has increased the success rate of medical therapy, and they are also useful in patients with poor blood pressure response to surgery. However, their use involves the risk of renal failure in the patient with high-grade stenosis.

PHEOCHROMOCYTOMA

MICHAEL D. CRESSMAN, D.O.
RAY W. GIFFORD Jr., M.D.

The treatment of pheochromocytoma is surgical extirpation of the tumor whenever possible. Since the disease is life-threatening, but usually curable, it is essential for the practicing physician to be familiar with the varied clinical manifestations of this fascinating neoplastic endocrinopathy. Inherent in the proper management of patients with pheochromocytoma is accurate diagnosis and localization of the tumor, careful preoperative preparation of the patient, and meticulous postoperative care. Medical therapy may be required for patients with a hypertensive crisis secondary to pheochromocytoma or for patients with metastatic disease. The purpose of this chapter is to provide the clinician with a rational approach to the diagnosis, localization, and management of pheochromocytoma.

CLINICAL MANIFESTATIONS

Hypertension is the most consistent manifestation of pheochromocytoma, although rare cases have occurred in normotensive patients. The hypertension is continuous in about 50 percent of patients, but marked lability of the blood pressure is present even in patients with sustained hypertension. Symptoms related to the catecholamine release generally correlate with the paroxysms of hypertension and may be present for minutes to days. Pregnancy may aggravate the symptoms and increase the frequency of paroxysms. An unexplained rise in blood pressure during the induction or maintenance of anesthesia should also alert the clinician to the possibility of pheochromocytoma.

Approximately 80 clinical manifestations of pheochromocytoma have been described, but headache, diaphoresis, and palpitations are particularly common. At least one of these three cardinal symptoms is present in over 95 percent of patients, and approximatey 70 percent report at least two of them. The headaches usually occur in discrete episodes. Typically, they are severe, pounding, and frontal or occipital in location. Patients with sustained hypertension may complain of only mild generalized headaches that are indistinguishable from tension headaches or those experienced by patients with essential hypertension. Two-thirds of the patients note excessive sweating, sometimes drenching, usually generalized, and particularly prominent in the upper part of the body. The most profuse sweating usually occurs during a paroxysm of hypertension, but occasionally appears after the blood pressure has returned to normal. Palpitations, the third most common symptom, are usually, but not always, accompanied by tachycardia.

Symptomatic paroxysms have been noted to occur as seldom as every few months or as often as 25 times per day. About 75 percent of the patients experience one or more attacks per week. Attacks may persist for minutes to days, but last less than 1 hour in 80 percent of the patients. With time, they often become more frequent, but not necessarily more severe. The symptoms and their order of occurrence remain remarkably similar during each episode in an individual patient, but their duration may vary considerably.

Several conditions occur in patients with pheochromocytoma more frequently than in the general population. The identification of familial multiple endocrine neoplasia (MEN) syndromes makes it of utmost importance for the physician to inquire about a family history of endocrine disease and exclude associated endocrinopathies in patiients with pheochromocytoma. This tumor may be associated with medullary carcinoma of the thyroid and hyperparathyroidism in MEN II or Sipple's syndrome. Pheochromocytomas, medullary carcinoma of the thyroid, multiple mucosal neuromas, thickened corneal nerves, alimentary tract ganglioneuromas, marfanoid habitus, and, rarely, hyperparathyroidism may coexist in varying combinations in patients with MEN III. The pheochromocytomas are nearly always intra-adrenal and usually bilateral in these familial syndromes.

Neurofibromatosis (von Recklinghausen's disease) occurs in about 5 percent of patients with pheochromocytoma, and approximately 1 percent of patients with neurofibromatosis have pheochromocytoma. Pheochromocytoma occurs in some patients with von Hippel-Lindau syndrome (cerebellar hemangioblastoma and retinal angiomata), acromegaly, or Addison's disease. Ectopic ACTH production by pheochromocytoma may produce Cushing's syndrome. Hyperglycemia, which abates after removal of the tumor, has also been described. Up to 30 percent of patients with pheochromocytoma have cholelithiasis for reasons that are not clear.

DIFFERENTIAL DIAGNOSIS

A number of clinical entities may mimic pheochromocytoma (Table 1); increased excretion of catecholamines or their metabolites in urine has been observed in a few of these conditions. Acute anxiety attacks, hyperthyroidism, and a hyper-beta-adrenergic state cause the greatest diagnostic confusion. The last-mentioned condition, a variant of the hyperdynamic heart syndrome, is characterized by labile hypertension, tachycardia, anxiety, and occasionally diaphoresis. Symptoms are precipitated by isoproterenol infusion and often abate after the administration of beta-blocking drugs. Less frequently, the menopausal syndrome, migraine headache, and coronary insufficiency with severe hypertension can be mistaken for pheochromocytoma. Plasma catecholamines or urinary catecholamines (vanillylmandelic acid [VMA], metanephrines) are normal or only minimally increased in these conditions.

Symptomatic hypertension with strikingly elevated levels of plasma and urinary catecholamines and their metabolites may occur after the abrupt withdrawal of clonidine or when patients receiving monoamine oxidase inhibitors ingest tyramine-containing foods or beverages, ephedrine, or amphetamines. This condition is characterized by acute hypertensive crisis, headache, tremor, tachycardia, anxiety, or diaphoresis, and closely resembles pheochromocytoma crises. The hypertension is rapidly controlled by the intravenous injection of phentolamine as it is in pheochromocytoma. Reinstitution of clonidine with gradual withdrawal is indicated in patients with the clonidine discontinuation syndrome.

TABLE 1 Differential Diagnosis

Anxiety, tension states, psychoneurosis
Hyper β-adrenergic circulatory state
Hyperthyroidism
Paroxysmal tachycardia
Vasodilating headache (migraine and cluster headache)
Menopause
Acute coronary insufficiency
Hypovolemia
Diabetes mellitus
Intracranial lesions (with or without intracranial pressure)
Renal artery or renal parenchymal disease
Focal arterial insufficiency of the brain
Autonomic hyperreflexia*
Diencephalic seizure syndrome
Toxemia of pregnancy
Clonidine withdrawal*
Food and drug interactions with MAO inhibitors*
Carcinoid*
Hypoglycemia*
Mastocytosis
Familial dysautonomia
Acrodynia*
Tetanus*
Porphyria*
Lead poisoning
Guillain-Barré syndrome
Tabetic crisis
Encephalitis
Hypothalamic dysregulation
Pulmonary artery fibrosarcoma
Pork hypersensitivity

* Conditions in which circulating catecholamines or the urinary excretion of catecholamines and their metabolites may be increased.

SCREENING AND DIAGNOSIS OF PHEOCHROMOCYTOMA

Any patient with a history of hypertension associated with clinical symptoms even remotely suggestive of pheochromocytoma should be carefully evaluated. The diagnosis depends on the demonstration of increased levels of catecholamines in the plasma or elevated levels of catecholamines or their metabolites in the urine. In our experience, determination of plasma catecholamines using a radioenzymatic assay is the most reliable method of diagnosis. Others feel that determination of urinary metanephrines remains the preferred biochemical method of establishing the diagnosis.

Blood for catecholamine determination, is collected after an overnight fast or, when possible, during a paroxysmal episode. When samples are obtained while the patient is hypertensive or symptomatic there is nearly always a clear elevation in plasma catecholamine levels (>2,000 ng per liter) if a tumor is present. However, catecholamine levels may be normal or only minimally increased in patients suspected to harbor a pheochromocytoma, particularly when catecholamine release from the tumor is episodic.

We perform a clonidine suppression test when the clinical history suggests pheochromocytoma but the plasma catecholamine levels are only minimally increased. This test relies on the observation that circulating catecholamine levels are reduced after oral administration of clonidine in patients with essential hypertension, but not in those with pheochromocytoma. When possible, prior antihypertensive medications should be discontinued at least 48 hours before performing a clonidine suppression test, since these medications may interfere with interpretation of plasma catecholamine levels or contribute to a significant hypotensive response to the drug. Plasma catecholamine levels are obtained prior to, and 180 minutes after, the oral administration of 0.3 mg of clonidine. The patient remains supine in a quiet room throughout the test, and blood pressure and heart rate are monitored at no greater than 30-minute intervals. Plasma catecholamine levels fall to within a clearly normal range in patients with essential hypertension, but do not change in patients with pheochromocytoma (Fig. 1). The antihypertensive effect of clonidine does not differentiate these two groups of patients.

A provocative test may be required to establish a diagnosis of pheochromocytoma in patients whose baseline catecholamine levels are well within the normal range. This is most likely to occur in patients with intermittently functioning tumors. A number of pharmacologic agents have been shown to stimulate catecholamine release from pheochromocytoma, but glucagon and histamine are the most useful diagnostic aids for this purpose. Certain patients will respond to one of these agents, but not to the other. It is advisable to administer glucagon first, since

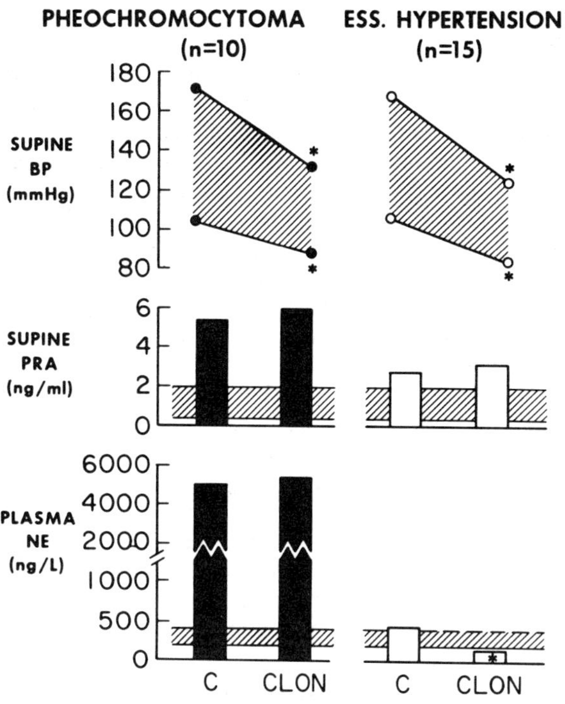

Figure 1 The clonidine suppression test. Catecholamine levels fall to within a normal range when patients with essential hypertension are given 0.3 mg of clonidine hydrochloride orally. In contrast, catecholamine levels do not change in patients with pheochromocytoma during the clonidine suppression test. Reprinted with permission from the American Heart Association. Hypertension 1983; 4:Suppl. 2:193–199.

this agent produces fewer side-effects than does histamine. Phentolamine should always be available during a glucagon or histamine stimulation test because of the risk of inducing a hypertensive crisis.

LOCALIZATION

The increasing availability of high resolution CT scanners has allowed for noninvasive localization of pheochromocytoma in the majority of instances. The adrenal glands are initially imaged, since 90 percent of pheochromocytomas are found in this location. If a mass is not visualized in the adrenal glands, attention is directed to the para-aortic areas and the organ of Zukerkandl at the aortic bifurcation. Occasionally, an intrathoracic tumor may be localized by CT. Noninvasive localization may also be accomplished using radiolabeled ^{131}I-metaiodobenzylguanadine (^{131}I-MIGB). In molecular structure, this agent resembles norepinephrine and probably enters adrenergic tissue by the same mechanism as the neurotransmitter substance. Benign and malignant adrenal and extra-adrenal tumors have been identified using this agent, even when CT has failed to localize a tumor.

If the tumor cannot be localized noninvasively, abdominal aortography, caval sampling for catecholamines, or both of these procedures may be required. The radiologist must be aware of the suspicion of pheochromocytoma, since a hypertensive crisis may occur when contrast material is injected into the area of the tumor. Phentolamine or sodium nitroprusside must be available during these invasive radiographic procedures, and it may be advisable to administer phenoxybenzamine or prazosin orally for 24 to 48 hours before arteriography in an effort to blunt a pressor response. Surgical exploration for pheochromocytoma is indefensible unless every attempt to localize the tumor preoperatively has been made.

Management of Hypertensive Crisis

Several drugs are effective in controlling the acute hypertensive crisis of pheochromocytoma. Alpha-adrenergic receptor blocking agents are attractive from a pharmacologic standpoint, since the major mechanism of the hypertension in pheochromocytoma is norepinephrine-induced vasoconstriction. Phentolamine, a nonselective alpha-receptor blocking agent, was formerly advocated as a diagnostic test for pheochromocytoma, but false-positive responses are often observed in patients with accelerated or malignant hypertension. Blood pressure is rapidly reduced after bolus injections of 5 to 20 mg of this agent, usually administered in 5-mg increments. The duration of action of phentolamine is so brief that a continuous infusion of the drug is required if the paroxysm is prolonged.

Labetalol, a combined alpha- and beta-adrenergic receptor blocking agent, has also been successfully utilized in the management of hypertensive patients with pheochromocytoma. This agent may be given as a single intravenous injection of 1 to 2 mg per kilogram, by graded continuous incremental infusion of 20 to 160 mg per hour, or by a method of repeat intravenous injections of 20 to 80 mg of the drug at 10-minute intervals. The beta-blocking properties of this agent are theoretically desirable since beta-blockade may blunt the effects of catecholamines on the myocardium and decrease the tachycardia and myocardial irritability that may accompany the hypertension. However, paradoxical hypertension has been observed after the intravenous administration of labetalol in patients with pheochromocytoma. Presumably, this occurs because of the disproportionate beta- to alpha-blocking effects of the drug, which could lead to a relative state of unopposed alpha stimulation.

Sodium nitroprusside remains the drug of choice for the management of hypertensive crises associated with pheochromocytoma. It is also the hypotensive agent of choice during intraoperative management of these patients. The recommended dose is 0.5 to 10.0 μg per kilogram per minute by continuous intravenous infusion, but higher doses can generally be given for brief periods in patients with normal hepatic and renal function.

PREOPERATIVE CARE

Controversy continues to revolve around the preoperative management of patients with pheochromocytoma, particularly as regards the routine use of alpha-adrenergic blockade with oral phenoxybenzamine or prazosin argue that this controls hypertension, reverses the hypovolemia that is frequently present in these patients, and promotes smooth induction and maintenance of anesthesia. Those who oppose routine preoperative alpha-blockade believe that complete blockade may reduce the surgeon's ability to locate unsuspected tumors, since the hypertensive response to tumor manipulation may be blunted.

Oral phenoxybenzamine or prazosin is generally used to induce preoperative alpha-blockade. Phenoxybenzamine is given in doses ranging from 10 to 40 mg every 8 to 12 hours. More recently, prazosin, a selective postsynaptic alpha-receptor blocker has been employed for the preoperative management of patients with pheochromocytoma. A significant hypotensive response occurs within an hour of the administration of a 1-mg oral dose of the drug. The antihypertensive response persists for up to 8 hours and may be associated with symptomatic orthostatic hypotension. Beta-blocking agents may be necessary to control tachycardia and/or palpitations, but these agents should only be utilized after alpha-blockade has been established, since beta-blockers may exacerbate the hypertension by producing unopposed alpha-stimulation. We do not use alpha-blockers preoperatively unless the patient is precariously ill or the paroxysmal attacks are unusually severe.

Preoperative expansion of the plasma volume is highly advisable, particularly in patients who have not received alpha-blocking agents. Preoperative volume expansion reduces the incidence of postoperative hypotension. In our institution, 2 units of whole blood are given 12 hours before the operative procedure.

SURGICAL TECHNIQUE

We strongly recommend a transabdominal (transperitoneal) approach to surgery for pheochromocytoma. This allows for inspection and palpation of the entire contents of the abdomen for extra-adrenal or unsuspected tumors and recognition of associated intra-abdominal disease (such as cholelithiasis). A bilateral subcostal incision is usually made; however, in thin patients, a long midline incision may provide better exposure. After the peritoneal cavity is entered, most surgeons examine the intra-abdominal viscera, the para-aortic and lumbar ganglia, the perirenal area, the organ of Zuckerkandl, the pelvic area, the bladder, and the uninvolved adrenal gland. After this, the presumably involved adrenal gland is inspected, since palpation of the tumor may precipitate a hypertensive crisis. Ligation of the adrenal veins from an obvious tumor before manipulation minimizes the risk of hypertension.

It is advisable to continue intra-arterial blood pressure monitoring early in the postoperative period because of the risk of hypotension. The goal of volume replacement is the maintenance of an adequate urine volume and a blood pressure of 90 to 100 mm Hg systolic. Hypotension despite adequate volume replacement should suggest intra-abdominal bleeding, which may result from persistent oozing in the area of the tumor. Continued hypertension after the removal of the involved adrenal gland should suggest the presence of pain, an unsuspected residual pheochromocytoma, or inadvertent ligation of the renal artery.

Operative mortality is less than 2 percent in experienced hands and 5-year survival has been roughly 95 percent in patients with benign tumors and 44 percent in those with malignant tumors. Paroxysmal hypertension is nearly always cured after resection of the tumor, but persistent hypertension may be present in up to 20 to 25 percent of patients who have sustained hypertension preoperatively. Recurrence of paroxysmal attacks suggests the presence of another tumor. This is most likely to occur in patients with familial pheochromocytoma if a unilateral adrenalectomy had been performed. Occasionally, the recurrence of "spells" with paroxysms of hypertension may signify the presence of metastatic tumor.

METASTATIC PHEOCHROMOCYTOMA

Approximately 10 percent of patients with pheochromocytoma have metastatic disease. These tumors are usually resistant to radiation and chemotherapy, but preliminary reports suggest that the radioisotope ^{131}I-MIBG may be effective in the management of patients with malignant pheochromocytoma.

Pharmacologic agents that decrease catecholamine production or antagonize the action of these vasoactive amines may also be useful in the palliative treatment of these patients. Alpha-methyl-p-tyrosine inhibits tyrosine hydroxylase activity, which catalyzes the rate-limiting step in norepinephrine production and decreases circulating catecholamine levels in patients with pheochromocytoma. Treatment is generally initiated with 250 mg of the drug given 3 to 4 times daily increased to as much as 4,000 mg per day in an attempt to control the paroxysmal symptoms. However, CNS depression frequently occurs when high doses of the drug are given. Crystalluria and renal dysfunction may also complicate treatment.

Adrenergic inhibitors are also useful in the management of patients with metastatic disease. Alpha-receptor antagonists are the mainstays of therapy, but beta-receptor blocking agents are often required to control the tachycardia and palpitations that frequently occur in these patients. Prazosin is probably the alpha-blocking agent of choice, since it is as effective as and better tolerated than the older, nonselective alpha-blockers such as phentolamine or phenoxybenzamine. Initially, small doses (1 to 2 mg every 8 hours) of prazosin controls hypertension, but larger doses of the drug are generally required with long-term treatment. Expansion of the extracellular fluid volume may occur after the hypertension is controlled, and the addition of a thiazide diuretic may be of benefit during chronic treatment.

Oral labetalol (a combined alpha- and beta-blocking agent) would seem to be an attractive agent for chronic treatment, but there is little experience with this agent in the management of patients with metastatic disease. The risk of paradoxical hypertension from the disportionate beta- to alpha-blocking effects of this drug must be kept in mind. Perhaps this will be the beta-blocker of choice to add when tachycardia develops in a patient treated with prazosin.

MINERALOCORTICOID HYPERTENSION

GAIL K. ADLER, M.D., Ph.D.
GORDON H. WILLIAMS, M.D.

Mineralocorticoids promote renal tubular reabsorption of sodium, chloride, and bicarbonate and excretion of potassium and hydrogen ions. Aldosterone, the preeminent mineralocorticoid in humans, is produced in the adrenal zona glomerulosa cells and is regulated by the renin-angiotensin system, ACTH, and the potassium concentration and perhaps by plasma sodium and atriopeptin levels. Biosynthetic precursors to aldosterone, deoxycorticosterone, and corticosterone, which are also produced in the zona fasciculata, usually are present in insufficient concentrations to exert clinically relevant mineralocorticoid activity. Under conditions of mineralocorticoid excess, there is retention of sodium, chloride, and water, which results in expansion of extracellular fluid and blood volume and thus hypertension. Hypokalemia and metabolic alkalosis occur as sodium is exchanged for potassium and hydrogen ions in the renal distal tubules and collection ducts.

Whereas a variety of conditions can cause mineralocorticoid hypertension, the most common cause is primary aldosteronism i.e., hypersecretion of aldosterone in the absence of a definable stimulus. This is most frequently caused by an adrenal adenoma although bilateral adrenal hyperplasia is also common. Rarely, primary aldosteronism results from an adrenal carcinoma, glucocorticoid-suppressible adrenal hyperplasia, or ectopic production. Infrequently, mineralocorticoid hypertension occurs secondary to (1) adrenocortical tumors that produce non-aldosterone mineralocorticoids, (2) adrenal enzyme deficiency, either 11β-hydroxylase and/or 17α-hydroxylase, or (3) the excess ingestion of exogenous mineralocorticoids, i.e., synthetic mineralocorticoids, carbenoxolone, and glycyrrhizinic acid which is found in black licorice and aniseed-derived aperitifs. Rarely a form of mineralocorticoid hypertension can be evoked secondary to excess elaboration of renin from a hemangiopericytomia (Reninoma) of the kidney.

PRIMARY ALDOSTERONISM

Approximately 1 percent of all patients with hypertension have primary aldosteronism. Since primary aldosteronism is potentially curable, it is important to have a relatively simple, cost-effective, screening method for its detection. Unfortunately, hypertension owing to hyperaldosteronism cannot be distinguished from essential hypertension on the basis of clinical symptoms. Even symptoms that can be attributed to hypokalemia, such as polyuria, fatigue, muscle weakness, and muscle cramps, often are vague and inconsistent.

Thus, we feel that the most reliable and cost-effective way of screening for hyperaldosteronism is not through the history or physical examination, but by a common laboratory test—a serum potassium. Spontaneous hypokalemia in a hypertensive patient is a reliable indicator of excess mineralocorticoid activity. However, the physician must be aware of the conditions under which the serum potassium is drawn. A potassium-sparing diuretic, a low sodium intake, an excessive potassium intake, or renal impairment can mask the kaliuretic effect of excess mineralocorticoid acitivity, whereas a potassium-wasting diuretic can cause hypokalemia in a patient with normal mineralocorticoid acitivity.

We recommend the following steps in order to obtain an accurate measure of a patient's spontaneous potassium balance (Fig. 1). If the serum potassium is normal, patients are instructed to stop ingesting potassium-sparing diuretics and/or potassium supplements and to follow a normal (100 to 200 mEq daily) sodium diet for 1 week. In our experience, if a repeat serum potassium is normal, the patient does not have mineralocorticoid hypertension. If the serum potassium is low on either the first or second measurement, all potassium-wasting diuretics should be stopped for 10 to 14 days and a serum potassium obtained. Again a normal sodium and potassium intake should be maintained during this 2 week period. A low serum potassium is suggestive of mineralocorticoid excess, and the plasma renin activity (PRA) should be measured. A low PRA is consistent with primary mineralocorticoid excess, and the patient should be hospitalized for a definitive work-up. A high plasma renin indicates a secondary hyperaldosteronemic disorder such as renovascular hypertension or a reninoma.

There are several cautionary points regarding assessment on an outpatient basis. First, if mineralocorticoid excess is suspected, a hypokalemic patient's sodium intake should not be increased until the potassium has been normalized because severe hypokalemia could result. Second, sodium intake should be increased cautiously in patients with severe hypertension or congestive heart failure. Third, some patients are unable to tolerate discontinuation of their diuretics for 2 weeks because of severe hypertension that is uncontrolled by other medications. If the hypokalemia in these patients is secondary to administration of diuretics, discontinuation of the diuretic(s) should result in a reduction in potassium excretion to less than 40 mEq per day. In patients with excess mineralocorticoid activity, a urinary potassium of greater than 50 mEq per 24 hours usually is found, despite concomitant hypokalemia.

Some investigators have reported that an elevated plasma aldosterone to plasma renin activity ratio that occurs 2 hours after a 50 mg dose of captopril may also be a reliable screening test for primary aldosteronism. We have had limited experience with this test, but it occasionally may be useful because it can be used in patients with relatively severe hypertension. However, it is our opinion that the cost of approximately $100 for the hormone and enzyme determinations makes this procedure too expensive to be used as a screening test.

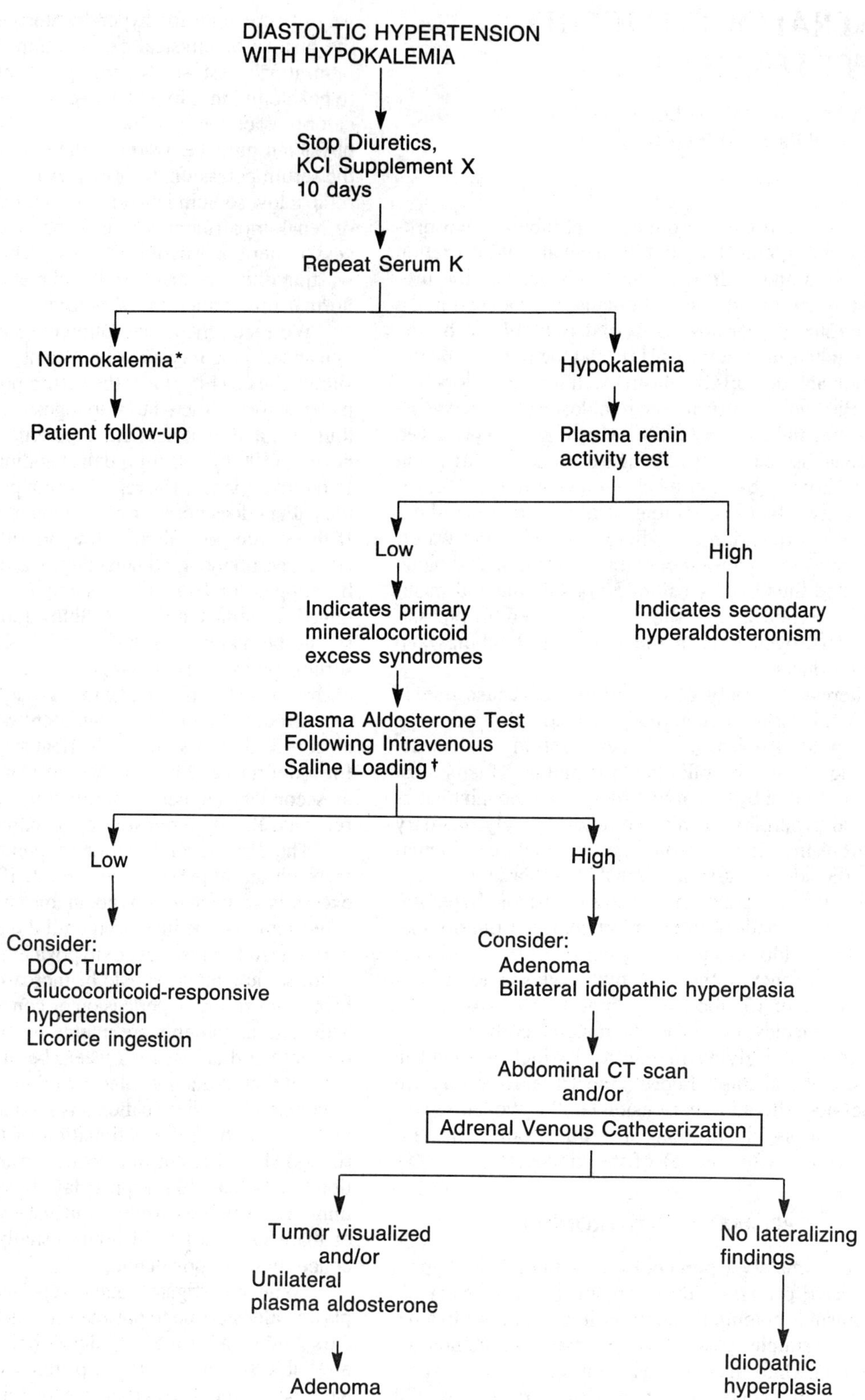

Figure 1 Flow chart for assessing whether hypertensive patients have primary aldosteronism.

* Some patients with primary aldosteronism may have normal serum potassium levels if they are taking potassium-sparing diuretics or ingesting a low-sodium: high-potassium diet.

† If cardiac failure is present or hypertension severe, this step should not be taken. Additionally, saline should not be given until the patient's hypokalemia is corrected. (Reprinted with permission from Williams GH, Dluhy RG. Diseases of the adrenal cortex. In: Petersdorf RG, et al, eds. Harrison's principles of internal medicine. 10th ed. New York: McGraw-Hill, 1983:647.)

Definitive Diagnosis

A definitive diagnosis of primary aldosteronism is made if the following criteria are met:

1. With sodium restriction, hypokalemia is corrected; with salt loading, renal potassium wasting occurs.
2. PRA levels are suppressed on a low-sodium diet and do not rise with upright posture.
3. Plasma or urinary aldosterone levels are not suppressed by a salt load.

If the first two criteria for mineralocorticoid excess are met, but plasma aldosterone levels are low, then a search should be initiated for other forms of mineralocorticoid excess, e.g., a deoxycorticosterone-producing adrenal tumor, congenital adrenal hyperplasia, or an exogenous source of mineralocorticoid (licorice or synthetic mineralocorticoid abuse).

Our standard in-patient evaluation of a patient we suspect has mineralocorticoid excess consists of the following: Patients are tapered off their antihypertensive medications, admitted to a metabolic unit, and placed on a 10 mEq sodium, 100 mEq potassium diet. After approximately 5 to 7 days, when 24 hour urinary sodium excretion matches dietary sodium intake, blood is sampled for plasma aldosterone and PRA. The sampling is carried out at 8 am when the patient has been supine overnight and again after 2 hours of upright posture. Patients with mineralocorticoid excess do not show the normal rise in PRA and plasma aldosterone associated with upright posture. We have found that upright PRA levels are less than 2 ng AI per milliliter per hour. The patient then receives an intravenous infusion of 3 liters of normal saline over 6 hours. Plasma aldosterone and cortisol levels are measured prior to and after the saline infusion. During the infusion blood pressure and serum potassium levels are monitored frequently. The study is terminated if significant hypokalemia or hypertension develop. In patients without hyperaldosteronism, plasma aldosterone levels suppress to less than 5 ng per deciliter. In patients with elevated aldosterone levels, we then assess the plasma cortisol level to make sure that the elevation is not secondary to stress-induced ACTH release. We feel that it is prudent to place patients on a low-sodium diet prior to the administration of a saline load since the low sodium intake usually results in correction of the hypokalemia and an amelioration of the hypertension. We prefer a 6-hour saline infusion instead of a 4-hour infusion since approximately 40 percent of patients with essential hypertension take longer than 4 hours to fully suppress their PRA and plasma aldosterone levels. It is important to check the serum potassium the next day since the sodium load can result in significant kaluriesis that may not be immediately apparent. Saline infusions are not performed in subjects with congestive heart failure, recent history of a myocardial infarction, or severe hypertension. We have recently modified this procedure in compliant patients. They are placed on a low-salt diet for several days prior to admission, daily blood pressure measurements are taken. The patient is admitted to hospital the day prior to the posture study. This results in considerable cost savings, but is only possible with the compliant patient.

Etiology

If a diagnosis of mineralocorticoid excess secondary to primary aldosteronism is made, it is therapeutically important to determine the source of the excess aldosterone. Between 60 percent and 80 percent of patients with hyperaldosteronism have an aldosterone-producing adenoma, and the remainder have bilateral adrenal hyperplasia. To distinguish between these two, we've found a high-resolution computed tomography (CT) scan of the abdomen particularly useful. CT scan detects greater than 80 percent of adenomas with a less than 1 percent false-positive rate. Adenomas that are less than 1 cm in diameter and isodense with the surrounding tissue are difficult to detect and account for most of the false-negative results. If both adrenals are adequately visualized by CT scan and an adenoma is found, the patient can be assumed to have an aldosterone-producing adenoma, and therapy is instituted. This work-up does not differentiate between an adenoma and a carcinoma. However, carcinomas are quite rare, and in any case, surgery is the treatment of choice for both. If both adrenals are not visualized or if they are of equal size, we believe adrenal vein sampling should be performed. The adrenal veins should be sampled for cortisol and aldosterone. Cortisol levels are obtained to indicate adequate sampling to detect any episodic changes in ACTH. Lateralization of aldosterone production is indicative of an adenoma, whereas equal aldosterone production suggests hyperplasia. When adequate venous samples are obtained, the sensitivity is greater than 90 percent. Adrenal vein sampling should only be performed by an experienced radiologist as significant complications, e.g., adrenal vein thrombosis, adrenal infarction, and adrenal vein rupture, can occur. There is a relatively high frequency of adrenal masses that are noted on abdominal CT scans; this is indicated by the 2 to 9 percent incidence of adrenal tumors that has been reported in several autopsy series. However, adrenal tumors detected incidentally by abdominal CT scan are nonfunctional in greater than 90 percent of cases. Because benign nonfunctioning adrenal masses are relatively common, we do not recommend obtaining a CT scan unless there is biochemical evidence that suggests an adrenal disorder.

It is our opinion that both adrenal venography and iodocholesterol scanning are less useful than the previously mentioned approach because of increased risk, less sensitivity and specificity, and greater cost. We also have found that the use of nonradiologic tests to distinguish between bilateral adrenal hyperplasia and an aldosterone-producing adenoma is less reliable. For example, supine 18-hydroxycorticosterone levels are thought to be greater than 100 ng per deciliter in patients with adenomas and less than 100 ng per deciliter in patients with adrenal hyperplasia, but we have experienced false-positives and negatives with this test. After 2 hours of upright posture, plasma aldosterone levels tend to fall in about 80 percent of patients with aldosterone-producing adenomas. However, we have found that up to 30 percent of patients with adrenal hyperplasia also show this decline in plasma aldosterone.

If the diagnosis of adrenal hyperplasia is made, one should consider the relatively rare diagnosis of glucocorticoid-suppressible hyperplasia. Patients with a family history of hyperaldosteronism should be placed on prednisone, 5 mg orally twice a day. After 4 to 6 weeks, blood pressure, serum potassium plasma renin activity, and plasma aldosterone levels should have normalized in patients with glucocorticoid-suppressible hyperaldosteronism. Transient decline in aldosterone production can occur in nonglucocorticoid-suppressible hyperaldosteronism.

Management

Initial medical management of primary aldosteronism consists of a low-sodium diet (60 mEq) coupled with administration of a potassium-sparing diuretic. The low-sodium diet decreases the amount of potassium being lost in the distal tubule and may result in a mild decrease in blood volume, which leads to an improvement in blood pressure. The potassium-sparing diuretic promotes a further reduction in blood pressure as well as an increase in potassium retention. Often spironolactone, a competitive antagonist of aldosterone, increases serum potassium levels and normalizes blood pressure within 1 to 2 months. We usually start with spironolactone, 50 mg twice a day. The dose may be increased by 100 mg increments every 1 to 2 weeks up to 300 to 400 mg a day. Initially, blood pressure and serum potassium should be monitored weekly. We have found that patients sometimes are unable to tolerate the side effects of spironolactone—gynecomastia, impotence, decreased libido, lassitude, and gastrointestinal discomfort—particularly if the dose required is greater than 100 mg per day.

An alternative potassium-sparing diuretic is amiloride, which promotes sodium excretion by blocking sodium channels in the renal distal tubule. Amiloride is also effective in normalizing blood pressure and serum potassium in the majority of patients with an aldosterone-producing adenoma. Patients with bilateral adrenal hyperplasia usually are less responsive. The initial dose of amiloride is 10 mg once a day. This dose can be increased at 10 mg increments up to 40 mg a day. The side effects are relatively mild and include headaches, lassitude, muscle cramps, gastrointestinal disturbances, and, occasionally, impotence. Blood urea nitrogen and uric acid may increase slightly.

In our opinion, a combination of triamterene and thiazide is less effective in reducing blood pressure and normalizing serum potassium than either spironolactone or amiloride. The maximum dose of triamterene: thiazide (50 mg:25 mg) is two tablets twice a day. Side effects include blood dyscrasias, weakness, headaches, liver damage, gastrointestinal and potential renal disturbances, and anaphylaxis.

Occasionally, a patient on a low-sodium diet and a potassium-sparing diuretic remains hypokalemic. Potassium supplementation may be initiated with careful monitoring. Potassium supplementation should not be started concurrently with the initiation of a low-sodium diet and a potassium-sparing diuretic because of the potential risk of hyperkalemia.

Adequate blood pressure control is often more difficult to achieve in patients with adrenal hyperplasia than in those with an adenoma. When necessary we have added either a beta-blocker or a converting-enzyme inhibitor to the diet and diuretic regimen, which usually further lowers the blood pressure. Recently, it has been demonstrated that nifedipine, a calcium-channel blocker, reduces plasma aldosterone levels and normalizes blood pressure and serum potassium in patients with primary aldosteronism. While we have not treated patients with primary aldosteronism with calcium-channel blockers, a combination of a calcium-channel blocker and a potassium-sparing diuretic may be especially helpful in patients whose hypertension and/or hypokalemia are not controlled by diet and a potassium-sparing diuretic alone.

Because serotonin is known to have aldosterone-stimulating properties in humans, a variety of antiserotoninergic agents, which include cyproheptadine, metergoline, and ketanserin, have been given to these patients with mixed success in reducing plasma aldosterone levels, lowering blood pressure, and raising serum potassium levels. Since dopamine inhibits aldosterone secretion, bromocriptine, a dopamine agonist, also has been given to patients with primary aldosteronism. Unfortunately, it has proven to be ineffective.

If the radiologic procedures demonstrate an aldosterone-producing adenoma, surgical removal of the adenoma is recommended. Patients should be treated medically as described, so that they are normotensive and normokalemic at the time of operation. This reduces the incidence of intra- and postoperative complications, especially cardiac arrythmia and paralytic ileus. A posterior rather than a transabdominal surgical approach is usually preferred because of fewer complications and a more rapid recovery. Because the remaining adrenal gland may not function normally, we recommend that patients receive steroid coverage intraoperatively—intravenous hydrocortisone at a rate of 10 mg per hour. Postoperatively, patients can be switched to oral hydrocortisone and the dose tapered to zero over the subsequent 2 to 4 weeks. The administration of high doses of hydrocortisone in the immediate postoperative period prevents rebound mineralocorticoid deficiency as well as glucocorticoid deficiency. The remaining adrenal may take 3 to 6 months to recover normal aldosterone responsiveness. During this period, patients should ingest a high-sodium diet, monitor daily weight, and be alert for symptoms of hypokalemia. We do not recommend giving fluorohydrocortisone as this further retards adrenal recovery. We have found that approximately 95 percent of our patients become normokalemic and normotensive postoperatively. Over the next few years, roughly 20 percent of these again require antihypertensive therapy although they remain normokalemic. Very rarely a second adrenal adenoma is found in the remaining adrenal.

Patients who have bilateral adrenal hyperplasia should be continued on medical therapy. We avoid bilateral adrenalectomy because it is generally ineffective in correcting the hypertension despite correction of the biochemical abnormalities and adds the problem of dealing with the resulting adrenal insufficiency to the patients overall treatment program.

CONGENITAL ADRENAL HYPERPLASIA

Hypertension and hypokalemia caused by excess mineralocorticoid production can also be associated with two types of congenital adrenal hyperplasia, 11β-hydroxylase deficiency and 17α-hydroxylase deficiency (Fig. 2). In these disorders, a defect in an enzyme essential for cortisol production results in low cortisol production and activation of the hypothalamic-pituitary-adrenal axis. The increased ACTH levels stimulate steroidogenesis, which results in a build-up of those steroids proximal to the block and an overproduction of steroids that do not require the defective enzymatic step.

Deficiency of 11β-hydroxylase results in the accumulation of the preblock steroids, 11-deoxycortisol and 11-deoxycorticosterone, as well as overproduction of androgens. Thus, infants with 11 β-hydroxylase deficiency present with virilization, hypokalemia, and hypertension. The enzyme deficiency is diagnosed by demonstrating elevated plasma levels of 11-deoxycortisol, 11-deoxycorticosterone, and 17-hydroxyprogesterone, as well as urinary metabolites of these compounds—tetrahydro-11-deoxycortisol, pregnanetriol, 17-hydroxysteroids, and 17-ketosteroids. Plasma aldosterone and PRA may be suppressed secondary to 11-deoxycorticosterone-induced volume expansion. Therapy consists of glucocorticoid replacement to supress ACTH secretion and, occasionally, fluorohydrocortisone to provide mineralocorticoid coverage.

17α-hydroxylase deficiency affects both adrenals and gonads. The 17-hydroxylation of pregnenolone and progesterone is blocked, preventing the normal production of androgens, estrogens, and cortisol and resulting in the overproduction of mineralocorticoids. Initially, 11-deoxycorticosterone, corticosterone, 8-hydroxycorticosterone, and aldosterone are all overproduced, but the resulting expansion in extracellular fluid and blood volume suppresses PRA. With the fall in PRA, plasma aldosterone levels drop. Patients with 17α-hydroxylase deficien-

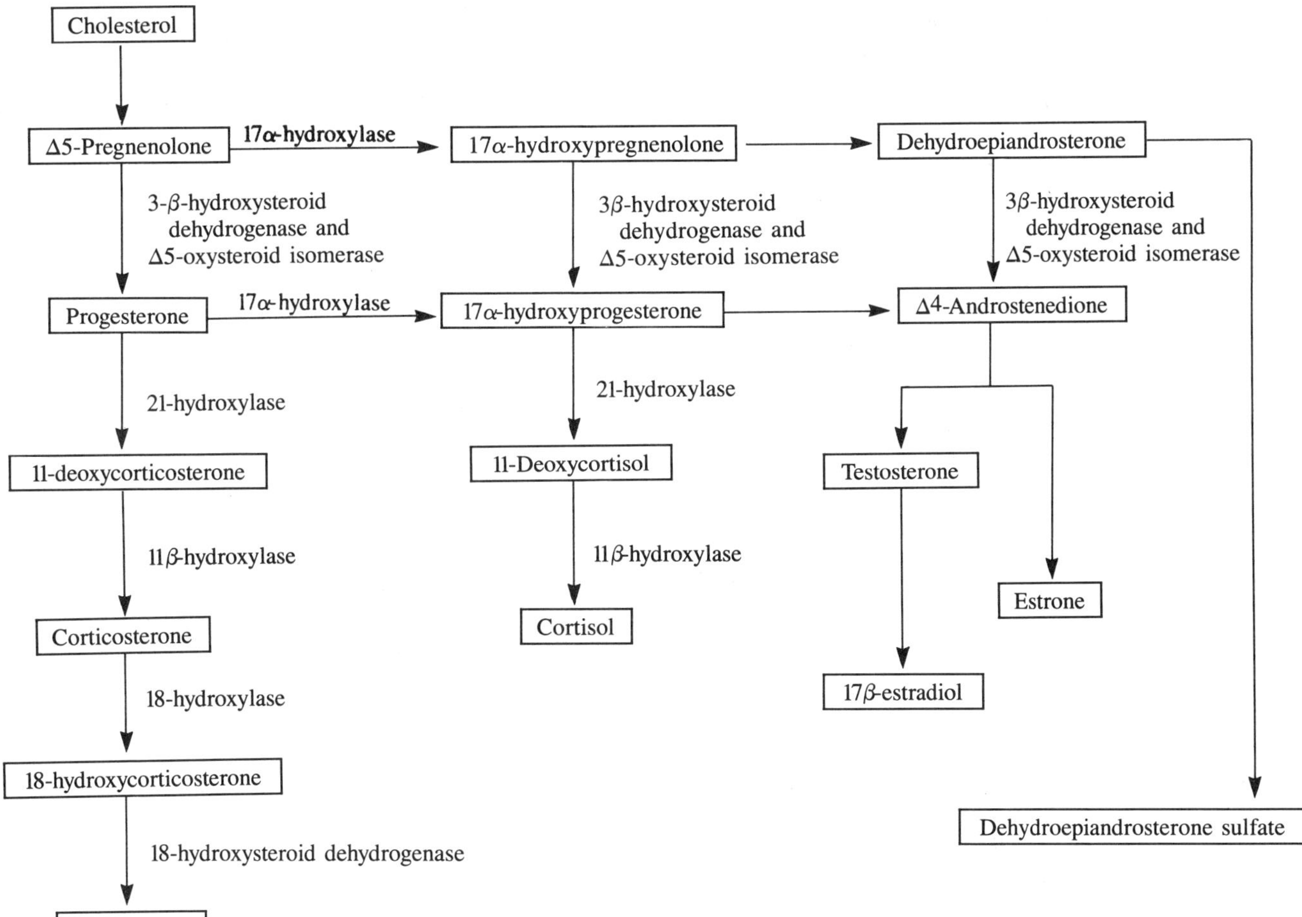

Figure 2 Pathways of adrenal steroid biosynthesis. Major pathways to mineralocorticoids, glucocorticoids, and androgens.

cy usually present at the time of puberty with hypertension, hypokalemia, and primary amenorrhea in females and hypertension, hypokalemia, and pseudohermaphroditism in males. The normal increase in steroidogenesis at the time of puberty exacerbates the hypertension and hypokalemia. 17α-hydroxylase deficiency can usually be diagnosed by the elevated plasma 11-deoxycorticosterone levels and the extremely low levels of plasma 17α-hydroxyprogesterone, urinary pregnanetriols, and urinary 17-ketosteroids. Treatment with glucocorticoids to suppress ACTH is similar to that described for 11β-hydroxylase deficiency. Again the minimum dose of prednisone required to suppress ACTH should be employed. With the administration of glucocorticoids, ACTH levels and, thus, 11-deoxycorticosterone levels fall, which results in a natriuresis and diuresis. Because the renin-aldosterone system has been suppressed by excesss 11-deoxycorticosterone production, patients are in danger of developing hypovolemia when the 11-deoxycorticosterone levels drop. Thus, patients should follow a high-salt diet, record their daily weight and be alert for signs of hypovolemia until aldosterone secretion returns to normal; this can take months. Patients should also be treated with estrogens and androgens as necessary in order to induce normal sexual development.

HYPERTENSION IN PREGNANCY

MARSHALL D. LINDHEIMER, M.D., F.A.C.P.
ADRIAN I. KATZ, M.D., F.A.C.P.

High blood pressure complicates approximately 10 percent of all gestations; in nulliparas the incidence is almost 20 percent, and 40 to 50 percent of women carrying twins develop hypertension. Furthermore, high blood pressure in pregnancy remains an important cause of fetal loss and maternal morbidity. Nevertheless, hypertension associated with pregnancy remains an understudied area of reproductive medicine beset by considerable controversy. Thus, current textbooks and reviews may advise diametrically opposite approaches to management: the reader of the previous edition of this text, for example, will find in it contrasting opinions to those expressed below. Our contribution, a brief survey of hypertension in pregnancy, focuses on preeclampsia as well as on the results of recent drug trials of agents used to treat chronic hypertension in pregnancy.

BLOOD PRESSURE IN NORMAL PREGNANCY

Mean blood pressure decreases early in pregnancy and by midtrimester diastolic levels are often 10 mm Hg less than before conception. Blood pressure then increases gradually, approaching prepregnancy values near term. Cardiac output also changes in pregnancy, increasing by 40 to 60 percent above the nongravid state during the first trimester and remaining relatively constant thereafter. Thus the decrement in pressure during gestation is due to a marked decrease in peripheral vascular resistance.

The physiologic changes described above mean that norms for pregnancy must be lowered: Diastolic levels exceeding 75 mm Hg in the second trimester and 85 mm Hg in the third trimester are abnormal. Perinatal mortality rates increase significantly when mean arterial pressures exceed 90 mm Hg in midtrimester and 95 mm Hg in late pregnancy—all values that would not be of great concern in nonpregnant patients. Another interesting aspect of the cardiovascular alterations in pregnancy is the slow pressure rise that follows the midtrimester nadir, because it demonstrates that increasing vasoconstrictor tone is a feature of late pregnancy in normal women as well as in those who develop preeclampsia .

CLASSIFICATION OF HYPERTENSION IN PREGNANCY

There are many classifications of the hypertensive disorders of gestation, which is a source of confusion to the reader. We recommend the classification suggested by The American College of Obstetricians and Gynecologists, which is both sound and concise. It considers pregnancy-associated hypertension in only four categories: preeclampsia and eclampsia, chronic hypertension (of whatever cause), chronic hypertension with superimposed preeclampsia, and late transient hypertension.

Preeclampsia—Eclampsia

Category 1 accounts for more than 50 percent of the hypertensive disorders complicating gestation. In preeclampsia the high blood pressure is associated with proteinuria, edema, and at times coagulation or liver functon abnormalities or both. This disease occurs primarily in nulliparas, usually after the 20th gestational week, and most frequently near term. Preeclampsia can progress rapidly to a convulsive phase termed eclampsia, a dramatic and life-threatening event. The eclamptic convulsion is usually preceded by a number of premonitory symptoms and signs, including headache, severe epigastric pain, hyperreflexia, and hemoconcentration, but it can also appear suddenly and without warning in a seemingly stable patient, with only minimal blood pressure elevations. This is why attempts to categorize preeclampsia as "mild" or "severe" (in the latter case, increases in diastolic and systolic levels to 110 and 160 mm Hg or higher, heavy proteinuria, and neurologic signs and symptoms) can be misleading. *Therefore, the appearance of de novo third trimester hypertension in a nullipara whether or not other signs are present is sufficient reason to hospitalize her.*

One form of preeclampsia whose clinical appearance may be misleadingly benign affects patients presenting with minimal changes in platelet counts and/or liver function tests and almost no evidence of hypertension. While most preeclamptic women with coagulation abnormalities and/or hepatic involvement have other markers of severe disease, an occasional gravida has only a borderline elevation in blood pressure, little or no proteinuria, a small decrement in platelet count, and minimal elevations of liver enzyme values. Such patients, however, can rapidly progress to a syndrome characterized by hemolysis and marked signs of both liver dysfunction and coagulation changes. The bilirubin level may become elevated; transaminase values often exceed 1,000 to 2,000 IU, circulating platelet counts frequently decrease to below 40,000 per cubic millimeter, and evidence of microangiopathic hemolysis appears on the blood smear. (In the literature this is called the HELLP syndrome, an acronym for Hemolysis, Elevated Liver enzymes, and Low Platelet count.) This uncommon form of preeclampsia is life-threatening and constitutes a medical emergency. Fortunately, most patients survive with supportive care, the abnormalities abating two days to one week after evacuation of the uterus. There have been maternal deaths associated with this syndrome, however, which in some instances were due to a failure to appreciate the severity of the situation at an early stage.

Chronic Hypertension (of Whatever Cause)

Category 2 includes approximately one-third of all cases of high blood pressure in pregnancy, and in most cases the underlying pathologic factor is essential hypertension. In some, however, the hypertension is secondary to such conditions as kidney disease, renal artery stenosis, coarctation of the aorta, pheochromocytoma, primary aldosteronism, and in very rare instances a renin-secreting tumor. These patients, whose hypertension predates the gestatin, are more prone to superimposed preeclampsia (the third category, as will be discussed), but otherwise pregnancy seems to have little influence on the course of their underlying disease: fetal outcome appears related to the extent of end-organ damage before conception, and to the severity of the preeclamptic complication. In fact, some hypertensive diseases may be ameliorated by gestation; normalization of blood pressure has been described during pregnancy in a woman with renal artery stenosis; gestation has ameliorated the tendency to lose potassium in some patients with primary aldosteronism; and gestational increases in circulating free cortisol may ameliorate certain uncommon forms of high blood pressure characterized by overproduction of desoxycorticosterone or other mineralocorticoids (categorized in the literature as dexamethasone suppressible hypertension).

There are exceptions to the generally favorable outcome for category 2 patients. Certain women with systemic renal diseases, mainly scleroderma and periarteritis nodosa, do poorly during gestation, and both entities have been associated with maternal deaths. Thus, one should advise against conception or continuing gestation in women with these collagen diseases. Another hypertensive disorder with catastrophic potential is pheochromocytoma. In the past, pheochromocytoma was associated with maternal mortality rates in excess of 40 percent. Most of these deaths were due to fulminating disease at times mistaken for preeclampsia, and the true nature of the tumor remained unsuspected and was found only at autopsy. More recently, a greater percentage of these cases are being diagnosed prenatally, and because the tumor is resected or managed medically through term (using alpha-adrenoceptor inhibiting drugs), a successful outcome for both mother and fetus is achieved. Thus screening for pheochromocytoma is indicated when hypertension has predated conception or was discovered during early pregnancy.

Chronic Hypertension with Superimposed Preeclampsia

Women in category 2 have a high propensity to develop superimposed preeclampsia. (This complication may occur in 20 to 40 percent of women with hypertensive disorders predating conception, and the combination represented by category 3 affects 10 to 15 percent of all women with hypertension in pregnancy.) In our experience hypertensive gravidas with superimposed preeclampsia are most often multiparas whose disease accelerates during the early and middle parts of the third trimester. If their gestation is allowed to continue, they often manifest extremes of hypertension, heavy proteinuria, decreasing renal function, and a susceptibility to hepatic and coagulation-type syndromes, and the fetus often succumbs. In essence, the combination of another hypertensive disorder and superimposed preeclampsia may produce an acute medical emergency, and the women with this condition have the poorest fetal outcome. Furthermore, there is a good probability that this dangerous complication will recur in subsequent pregnancies.

Late or Transient Hypertension

Category 4, which includes a number of women who are otherwise difficult to classify, is characterized by the appearance of hypertension only (*without proteinuria*) late in pregnancy or in the immediate puerperium, and the blood pressure returns to normal by the 10th postpartum day. Among such patients may be nulliparas who may have early preeclampsia but have manifested no other signs of the disease, and it is prudent to manage them as if preeclampsia were present. Another group develops hypertension during two or more pregnancies and again become normotensive soon after delivery (manifesting an entity once erroneously labeled "recurrent toxemia"). The outcome of such pregnancies, however, is usually good compared with the more reserved prognosis in patients with preeclampsia. There is evidence that transient hypertension in such gravidas is a forerunner of essential hypertension later in life, analogous to the situation of women with gestational diabetes who eventually become frank diabetics.

It should be noted that the classification scheme above avoids a number of terms in the current literature that we find misleading. For example, "gestational," "pregnancy-induced," and "pregnancy-associated" hypertension do not differentiate between the more serious preeclampsia and the rather benign transient hypertension of pregnancy. The term "toxemia" is archaic (no one has ever identified a toxin in the blood of such women), and its use in the older literature covers a variety of different forms of hypertension and is thus especially confusing. Another classification "EPH gestosis," which mainly appears in European publications, categorizes patients on the basis of symptomatology such as E for edema, P for proteinuria, and H for hypertension, the individual being defined as mono- or polysymptomatic. We see little value in such a schema, because edema alone occurs in 80 percent of normal gestations, proteinuria may be observed in gravidas with renal disease who have no hypertension, and high blood pressure is a manifestation of all the etiologic entities described above.

Finally, one should be aware of two uncommon conditions: "late postpartum eclampsia" (hypertension and convulsions occurring days to weeks after delivery), the existence of which is debated, and "postpartum hypertension" (in women who were normotensive during gestation), which is characterized by abnormal increments in blood pressure 2 weeks to 6 months after delivery. The latter, about which little is known, is rather benign, the blood pressure becoming normal within one year of delivery.

DIAGNOSIS, CLINICAL COURSE, AND PATHOPHYSIOLOGY

It can be very difficult to distinguish clinically among preeclampsia, essential or secondary hypertension, renal disease, and combinations of these entities. For example, certain women with undiagnosed hypertension experience the physiologic decrement in mean blood pressure early in gestation and have normal levels when first examined near midpregnancy. Later, when frankly elevated pressures are recorded near term, they are erroneously labeled as preeclamptics. Also, an accelerated phase of essential hypertension (albeit a rare event during gestation), pheochromocytoma, and certain renal diseases (e.g., glomerulonephritis, lupus erythematosus) occurring late in pregnancy may all mimic preeclampsia. Such diagnostic problems are illustrated best in reports of cases in which the cause of hypertension complicating pregnancy has been determined by renal biopsy. These studies reveal that the clinical impression of preeclampsia could be erroneous in more than 15 percent of nulliparas and in 50 percent or more of multiparas, and that unsuspected renal disease was uncovered in 10 to 20 percent of the cases. In one of these reports, in which an academic obstetrician and a nephrologist recorded their impressions prior to biopsy, a correct diagnosis was made on clinical grounds in only 58 percent of the patients. However, renal biopsy is rarely indicated prepartum; in the absence of a morphologic diagnosis, a nullipara developing high blood pressure in late pregnancy and manifesting proteinuria, elevated plasma urate levels, and decrements in platelet counts is the patient in whom the diagnosis of preeclampsia is most secure. Some suggest that the presence of a low circulating antithrombin III level also increases the sensitivity of this diagnosis. In any event, it is always better to *overdiagnose* preeclampsia. The pathophysiology is such that when this disease is neglected, fetal and occasionally maternal prognosis is poor, while early intervention often results in a successful outcome for both mother and child.

Pathophysiology of Preeclampsia

Women with preeclampsia may have a reversal of the normal diurnal blood pressure rhythm (morning peaks and nighttime nadirs), so that the highest levels occur during the night. Thus one may be unaware of dangerous pressure elevations if only daytime values are recorded.

Hypertension in preeclampsia is characteristically labile, reflecting the intense sensitivity of the vasculature to endogenous pressor peptides and catecholamines. Whereas normal pregnant women are extremely resistant to the pressor effects of infused angiotensin, those in whom preeclampsia is destined to develop have increased pressor responsiveness to this peptide weeks before the appearance of clinical manifestations. Similar alterations occur in women with chronic hypertension who develop superimposed preeclampsia. The vasculature of preeclamptics is also quite sensitive to infused norepinephrine and vasopressin. These alterations in vascular sensitivity may be due to decreased production of vasodilating prostaglandins (E and I), which has also been linked to coagulopathies associated with preeclampsia.

Glomerular filtration rate (GFR) decreases in preeclampsia partly due to a characteristic renal lesion that consists mainly of intracapillary cell swelling ("glomerular endotheliosis"). The drop in GFR is approximately 25 percent in mild cases. Because renal hemodynamics increase 30 to 50 percent in normal pregnancy, the filtration rate in preeclamptic women often remain above prepregnancy values. Levels of serum creatinine and urea nitrogen of 0.9 mg and 15 mg per deciliter respectively, considered normal in nonpregnant subjects, indicate decreased function in gravidas and should concern the clinician. This is because renal function in preeclamptics with plasma creatinine concentrations between 1 and 1.5 mg per deciliter (which are seemingly benign but already represent a 50 percent loss of GFR for pregnancy) has been known to deteriorate suddenly and progress to acute tubular (and rarely cortical) necrosis.

Uric acid clearance is also increased in normal gestation but reduced in preeclampsia. These decrements may occur earlier and be more profound than those in GFR, and uric acid levels above 4.5 mg per deciliter are already suspect in gravidas. The level of hyperuricemia correlates with the extent of the renal lesion in preeclampsia, as well as with fetal outcome.

Salt handling and volume homeostasis are also altered in preeclampsia. The ability to excrete sodium is decreased, but the degree of impairment varies and severe disease can occur in the absence of edema (the so-called dry preeclamptic). It is important to recognize that even when interstitial edema is present, plasma volume is decreased and hemoconcentration occurs. In most instances central venous and pulmonary capillary wedge pressures are low, and when studied prior to any therapeutic intervention cardiac output is decreased compared with normal gestation. Uteroplacental blood flow is also impaired in preeclampsia, this being one reason for the increased incidence of fetal loss and intrauterine growth retardation. The combination of low plasma volume and cardiac output, decreased central venous and pulmonary wedge pressures, and suboptimal uterine blood flow are the major reasons why most experts avoid the use of diuretics in preeclampsia.

MANAGEMENT

Preeclampsia

Women in whom preeclampsia is suspected should be hospitalized, an approach which diminishes the frequency of convulsions (and other consequences of diagnostic error), and enhances fetal survival. Such "prophylactic" hospitalization may appear overly expensive, but it delays termination of the pregnancy and reduces the higher costs incurred by very premature infants in intensive care nurseries. If blood pressure decreases to less than 120/80 mm Hg, and renal and hepatic function as well as coagulation indices remain normal over a period of several days, an occasional informed and trustworthy patient may be allowed to return to a quiet home environment, but in this case she should be evaluated twice weekly until delivery.

In general, induction is the therapy of choice near term, whereas attempts can be made to postpone action if pregnancy is at an early stage (mainly before 34 weeks). If a decision is made to temporize, several antihypertensive agents considered safe and effective in pregnancy are available (Tables 1 and 2). However, if severe hypertension (diastolic levels above 105 mm Hg in most women, above 100 mm Hg in teenage gravidas, or above 110 mm Hg in chronic hypertensives with superimposed disease) persists after 24 to 48 hours of treatment, delivery is indicated regardless of the stage of gestation, since the mother is at risk and further delay rarely saves the fetus. Advances in neonatology have been such that most infants weighing 1,500 g or more survive better in a premature nursery than in the womb of a woman with preeclampsia. The appearance of clotting abnormalities, decreasing renal function, and signs of impending convulsions (headache, epigastric pain, and hyperreflexia) are indications for termination of pregnancy. Persistence of hemoconcentration, increasing hyperuricemia, and proteinuria may be signs that the fetus is in jeopardy. Obstetricians have an armamentarium of tests to evaluate fetal well-being, certain patterns of fetal heart rhythm recordings being among the most reliable indication of fetal jeopardy.

Treatment of the Acute Hypertensive Crisis

There is controversy concerning how aggressively acute hypertension near term should be treated. Some authorities believe that reductions in maternal blood pressure tend to decrease uteroplacental perfusion, and caution against large or precipitous decrements in mean arterial pressure, because placental blood flow is already compromised in preeclampsia. Others believe that uteroplacental blood flow autoregulates appropriately and prefer a more aggressive approach in treating the hypertension. Data from studies in human beings are scarce, but there are documented instances in which precipitous reductions in blood pressure were accompanied by signs of fetal distress, even when diastolic levels remained at or above 80 mm Hg. Thus, when treating acute elevations of blood pressure in late pregnancy or during labor, we recommend an intermediate approach (see Table 1) in which antihypertensive agents are withheld as long as maternal pressure is only mildly elevated. When diastolic pressure is 105 mm Hg or higher, parenteral hydralazine is given cautiously and is successful in most instances. Diazoxide is restricted to the occasional resistant case and should be administered in small doses (30 mg boluses). Preliminary successes have been recorded when calcium-channel blockers (e.g., sublingual nifedipine) have been used, and in 1985 this group of drugs was undergoing extensive testing. Despite anecdotal reports of the usefulness of sodium nitroprusside, this agent should be avoided because cyanide poisoning and fetal death have been observed in laboratory animals. In the last analysis, however, the mother's well-being should take precedence even if the therapy necessary to control pressure may potentially harm the fetus.

TABLE 1 Guidelines for Treating Severe Hypertension Near Term or During Labor

The degree to which blood pressure should be decreased is disputed. Levels between 90 and 105 mm Hg diastolic are recommended (see text):

Drug therapy

- Parenteral hydralazine is the drug of choice. Use low doses (start with 5 mg, then give 5 to 10 mg every 20 to 30 minutes) in order to avoid precipitous decreases. Side effects include tachycardia and headache. Neonatal thrombocytopenia has been reported.
- Diazoxide is recommended for the occasional patient whose hypertension is refractory to hydralazine. Use 30-mg miniboluses, since maternal vascular collapse and death have been associated with the customary 300-mg dose. Side effects include arrest of labor and neonatal hyperglycemia.
- Do not use sodium nitroprusside (fetal cyanide poisoning has been reported in animals), ganglion-blocking agents (meconium ileus has been reported), or loop diuretics (e.g., furosemide) (see text). (However, in the final analysis, maternal well-being will dictate the choice of therapy.)

Parenteral magnesium sulfate is the drug of choice for preventing impending eclamptic convulsions. Therapy should continue for 12 (and sometimes 24) hours into the puerperium, since one-third of patients with preeclampsia have convulsions after childbirth.

Reprinted with permission from Lindheimer MD, Katz AI. Hypertension in pregnancy. N Engl J Med 1985; 313:675–680.

Magnesium sulfate is the drug of choice in North America for impending convulsions or frank eclampsia, although its use evokes controversy. The mode of action of magnesium sulfate is poorly understood, but the empiric success of this drug documented in the obstetric liter-

TABLE 2 Antihypertensive Drugs in Pregnancy

α_2-Receptor agonists	Methyldopa (0.5 to 3 g per day) is the most extensively used drug of this group in the United States; its safety and efficacy have been supported in randomized trials. Neonatal tremors have been reported; other side effects are the same as in the nongravid population. Trials with clonidine are in progress; embryopathy has been described in animals, and this drug is not currently recommended.
β-Receptor antagonists	These agents, currently undergoing extensive testing, appear to be safe and efficacious. Atenolol (50 to 100 mg per day), metoprolol (50 to 225 mg per day), and propranolol (40 to 240 mg per day) are used most frequently to date. Fetal and neonatal bradycardia and hypoglycemia have been reported, and animal data suggest the possibility of a decreased ability of the fetus to tolerate hypoxic stress.
α- and β-Receptor antagonists	Labetalol, for example—currently undergoing extensive testing—appears to be as effective as methyldopa. A possible association with retroplacental hemorrhage is under investigation.
Arteriolar vasodilators	Hydralazine (50 to 200 mg per day) is used frequently as adjunctive therapy with methyldopa and β-receptor antagonists. There has only been fragmentary experience with minoxidil, which is thus not recommended at present.
Converting-enzyme inhibitors	Captopril is associated with fetal death in several animal species. Do not use in pregnancy.
Diuretics	Most authorities discourage their use, though some continue these medications if they were prescribed before gestation. We would prescribe diuretics when blood-pressure control was poor despite the use of other agents, the fetus was immature, and pregnancy termination was the only alternative.
Miscellaneous	Calcium-channel blockers and serotonin antagonists (e.g., ketanserin) are currently under investigation. Do not use ganglion-blocking agents or nitroprusside.

Reprinted with permission from Lindheimer MD, Katz AI. Hypertension in pregnancy. N Engl J Med 1985; 313:675–680.

ature makes it the standard by which all others must be assessed.

Magnesium sulfate is administered parenterally either by intramuscular or intravenous injections. In the former regimen, a loading injection of 20 ml of 20 percent magnesium sulfate solution (4 g) is first given intravenously at the rate of 1 g per minute, immediately followed by 20 ml of 50 percent magnesium sulfate solution, half (5 g) of which is injected into each buttock through a 3-inch-long, 20-gauge needle. Every 4 hours thereafter, 10 ml of a 50 percent solution (5 g) is similarly injected intramuscularly into alternate buttocks, after ascertaining that the patellar reflex is present, respirations are not depressed, and urine flow was above 100 ml during the preceding 4 hours.

An intravenous regimen is used at the University of Chicago's Lying-in Hospital. A loading dose of 4 tgo 6 g of magnesium sulfate in a 10 percent solution is infused over a 10-minute period (it must never be given as a bolus), after which a sustaining solution of 24 g of magnesium sulfate in 1 liter of 5 percent dextrose solution is delivered at a rate of 1 g per hour. Blood levels of magnesium and deep tendon reflexes are monitored, and the infusion rate may be increased to 2 g per hour if the patient remains hyperreflexic or if plasma magnesium levels remain below 5 mg per deciliter. Once levels exceed 9.5 mg per deciliter, however, the drug is more likely to lead to respiratory and cardiac depression. In such instances the infusion should be decreased or temporarily stopped with the aim of maintaining levels between 5 and 9.5 mg per deciliter throughout labor. Following delivery magnesium sulfate treatment is usually continued for 12 to 24 hours, depending on the clinical severity of the preeclampsia. A vial of calcium gluconate should be kept at the bedside as an antidote for the sudden appearance of magnesium toxicity.

Volume Expansion

The literature contains claims that volume expansion may reduce blood pressure during preeclampsia and currently there are advocates for the use of such therapy in selected patients. This approach has been prompted by repeated observations that many preeclamptics present with decreased cardiac output, central venous and pulmonary capillary wedge pressures, and occasionally have postpartum vascular collapse. It has also been noted that hemodilution precedes the occasional improvement in hospitalized patients before delivery. In one well-documented study the rapid replenishment of intravascular volume with a commercial stable-protein substitute decreased blood pressure for periods of 24 hours or more in third trimester hypertensives. The authors further demonstrated that the decrement in pressure coincided with an increase in plasma volume. While the results appear impressive, most of the patients under study had only mild disease, and a review of available documentation by other authors who have used volume expansion reveals equivocal or unconvincing results.

Currently we recommend against "volume expansion" in preeclampsia for the following reasons: Myocardial performance may be compromised in severe cases, and volume expansion (especially with saline) may enhance vascular reactivity. Furthermore, the infusion of crystalloids alone decreases oncotic pressure (which is already markedly decreased in preeclampsia) and this can lead to pulmonary and cerebral edema, especially after childbirth when plasma oncotic levels decrease further (Fig. 1) while central volume and pressures tend to rise. Our current recommendations therefore are to minimize crystalloid infusions into preeclamptic women in labor (goal should be <75 ml per hour). Most problems of apparent poor renal perfusion will resolve quickly postpartum, and if fluid therapy does seem necessary, a colloid infusion is preferable and should be given concurrently with hemodynamic monitoring (i.e., a central venous pressure line).

Anticoagulation and Antiplatelet Therapy

Past reports on the use of heparin or aspirin in the management of preeclampsia have been contradictory, the majority showing these drugs to have limited efficacy at best. Also, administration of anticoagulants to patients with frank hypertension and a disease sometimes complicated by cerebral bleeding or subcapsular liver hematomas appears to us too hazardous, especially when other approaches succeed. In one instance, the latter complication occurred insidiously in a gravida under our care who received anticoagulants for thrombophlebitis and had begun to manifest minimal signs of preeclampsia.

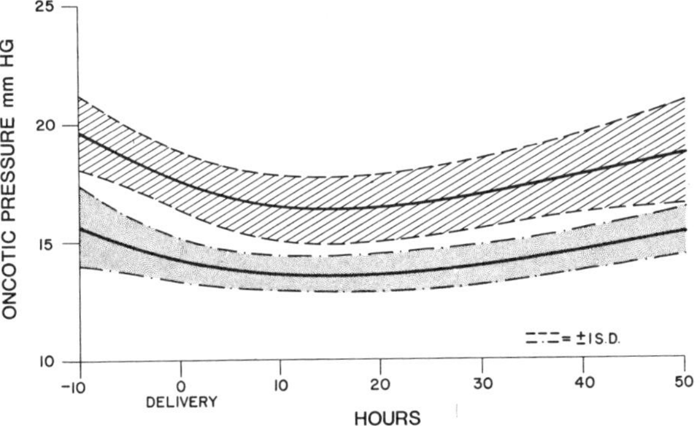

Figure 1 Intrapartum and postpartum plasma colloid oncotic pressure in nine normotensive gravidas (upper curve) and nine severe preeclamptics (lower curve). (From Zinaman M, Rubin J, Lindheimer MD. : Lancet 1985; 1:1245–1247. Reprinted with permission.)

It has been recently suggested that a combination of antiplatelet agents (dipyridamole and aspirin) can prevent preeclampsia if started early in pregnancy. At present, several investigators are evaluating the use of low-dose antiprostaglandin drugs or specific thromboxane inhibitors to prevent or reverse the manifestations of preeclampsia. This approach, which shows promise on theoretical grounds, is interesting but cannot be recommended until a great deal more is known concerning its efficacy as well as its safety during gestation.

Special Considerations

Monitoring of central venous or pulmonary capillary wedge pressures may be required in severe or complicated cases, especially during operative procedures. It is our experience, however, that the need for Swan-Ganz catheterization (a procedure that causes a certain morbidity) during preeclampsia is uncommon, and virtually all cases of preeclampsia can be managed using clinical acumen and an occasional central venous catheter. Patients with marked coagulation changes and severe right upper quadrant pain should be considered for ultrasonographic or (postpartum) computed tomographic scanning of the liver which may reveal subcapsular hemorrhages that can rupture and produce an acute emergency.

CHRONIC HYPERTENSION IN THE ABSENCE OF PREECLAMPSIA

There is a great deal of literature documenting the increased risk associated with pregnancy in women with chronic hypertension. Complications include superimposed preeclampsia, accelerated rise of pressure to a malignant phase, placental abruption, acute renal tubular and cortical necrosis, intrauterine growth retardation, and midtrimester fetal death. Such events seem to correlate with the age of the gravida and the duration of her high blood pressure. Thus the majority of these complications occur in women 30 years of age or over, or in those whose preexistent hypertension has caused end organ damage (primarily nephrosclerosis). On the other hand, more than 85 percent of patients with essential hypertension have uncomplicated gestations.

Women with chronic essential hypertension often manifest reductions in blood pressure by midpregnancy which may exceed those observed in normotensive gravidas. In fact, failure of this decrement to occur or increments in blood pressure in early pregnancy or midtrimester portends a reserved prognosis.

Fetal outcome is poorer in hypertensive women with superimposed preeclampsia than in previously normotensive women with this complication, and it is the combination of chronic hypertension and preeclampsia that seems responsible for most cases of cerebral hemorrhage in pregnancy. As was the case for previously normotensive patients, the marked increase in morbid events is due primarily to the specific pathophysiology of preeclampsia. This includes marked increments in pressor responsiveness to infused angiotensin weeks before the appearance of clinical manifestations of superimposed disease such as coagulation changes, liver function abnormalities, or both.

As was the case for women with pure preeclampsia, the gravida with chronic hypertension and superimposed disease must be hospitalized and her hypertension controlled. A substantial number of these patients present between the 25th and 30th gestational weeks and the wish to temporize may be strong. However, the fetal prognosis of chronic hypertensives with early third trimester superimposed preeclampsia is quite poor, and many clinicians consider delaying actions too risky for maternal well-being thus most terminate the gestation.

There is controversy about whether women with mild blood pressure elevations should be treated during pregnancy. Most authorities withhold therapy unless diastolic blood pressure is more than 15 mm Hg above what they consider "borderline" (in our clinic 75 to 80 mm Hg in the second and 85 to 90 mm Hg in the third trimester, taking into consideration the age of the gravida).

The use of antihypertensive agents in pregnancy is summarized in Table 2. It is only in the past decade that efforts have been made to determine the efficacy and safety of these drugs in pregnant women. Many of the published studies are limited in scope and often were performed at the request and with the support of pharmaceutical companies. There is a critical need for large, multicenter clinical trials using the combined services of obstetricians, hypertension specialists, epidemiologists, and statisticians. Currently methyldopa, on occasion combined with hydralazine, is the drug most often used in the United States. This medication has been administered to gravidas for several decades and is thus considered "safe" in pregnancy, and it has been demonstrated to be effective in a meticulously performed controlled trial. Several beta-adrenoceptor antagonists, and the combined alpha- and beta-blocking agent labetalol (see Table 2) are undergoing protracted testing and gaining increasing acceptance. These drugs have the advantage of being administered but once or twice daily, which facilitates patient compliance. However, beta-blocking agents cross the placenta and cause fetal bradycardia, thus restricting the value of alterations in fetal heart rate in evaluating the course of labor. Experimental studies suggest that beta-blocking agents may compromise the ability of the fetus to tolerate hypoxic stress, and one investigator has suggested that labetalol may be associated with retroplacental bleeding. It is for reasons such as these that we continue to use methyldopa as our primary drug in treating chronic hypertension in pregnancy.

Diuretics

There is controversy concerning the use of diuretics during gestation, and currently most obstetricians avoid their use in pregnant women. Ironically, it was once suggested that these drugs should be given prophylactically to high-risk populations to avoid preeclampsia, a claim subsequently disproved in controlled trials. Furthermore, there is a suggestion from one large epidemiological survey that diuretics increase fetal and maternal morbidity when used to treat edema in normotensive gravidas.

Saluretic drugs are successful in mobilizing edema fluid, but it is unclear whether such therapy influences favorably the course of pure or superimposed preeclampsia. It remains to be established whether the normal increments in maternal extracellular volume are required for optimal uteroplacental perfusion, but some investigators claim that diuretics limit the "physiological hypervolemia" of pregnancy and are associated with decreased weight of the neonate. As already noted, cardiac output, intravascular volume, and central venous as well as pulmonary capillary wedge pressures are low in many hypertensive gravidas. For these reasons saluretic agents should not be used as the initial treatment of these patients, because mobilization of the intravascular fluid may conceivably decrease cardiac output further and compromise placental perfusion. Also, diuretics are not without risk; their complications can affect both mother and fetus.

In essence, we do not recommend the use of diuretics during gestation, with two exceptions. First, they should be used in gravid women with heart disease, for the same indications as in nonpregnant women. Second, we occasionally prescribe diuretics for women with chronic hypertension refractory to antiadrenergic agents and vasodilators (especially if the refractoriness appears due to excessive sodium retention secondary to the antihypertensive agent's action), in particular when the fetus is immature and termination of the pregnancy is the only alternative.

Supported by Grants (HD 5572, AM 13601, RR 55) from the National Institutes of Health and by the American Heart Association.

DIURETIC USE IN EDEMATOUS AND NONEDEMATOUS STATES

GABRIEL M. DANOVITCH, M.D.

Broadly speaking, the term *diuretic* refers to any agent that increases the flow of urine. In clinical medicine, however, a diuretic is presumed to lead to a net negative balance of sodium from the body. Agents such as lithium and demeclochlortetracycline, which increase urine flow by increasing free water clearance, will not be discussed here and are included in the chapter on Hyponatremia.

Diuretics were initially introduced into clinical medicine approximately 30 years ago for the management of heart failure. The first compounds to be widely used, the organic mercurials, have been superseded by much less toxic compounds. A wide variety of compounds are now available, and the differences in their action and degree of potency are currently exploited in a variety of clinical situations. Table 1 classifies the diuretics most commonly used in clinical practice according to their primary sites of actions.

DIURETICS IN EDEMATOUS STATES

Nephrotic Syndrome

Currently there is considerable controversy regarding the mechanism of edema formation in nephrotic syndrome, and a brief understanding of the disputed mechanisms makes for a more rational use of diuretics in this condition. Traditionally it has been taught that the edema results from the loss of protein in the urine, which lowers the plasma albumin. The reduction in plasma onocotic pressure then leads to loss of plasma volume into the interstitium, thus producing edema at the expense of the plasma volume. The kidney responds by reabsorbing sodium avidly in an attempt to keep plasma volume close to the normal level. The dispute over this mechanism centers around the observation that the measured plasma volume in nephrotic syndrome frequently is not low. It has been suggested that the renal sodium retention, rather than being a response to a low plasma volume, is a primary phenomenon that expands the plasma volume, which then overflows into the interstitium under the influence of the low plasma oncotic pressure. It is probable that both these mechanisms apply in different populations of patients with nephrotic syndrome, and it would be rational to use diuretics when plasma volume is high and sodium retention is primary and to avoid diuretics when plasma volume is low and sodium retention compensatory. Unfortunately, there is at present no clinically reliable way of differentiating between these two mechanisms, and until there is, it is wise to avoid use of diuretics in nephrotic syndrome except under specific circumstances. Excessive use of diuretics can unquestionably lead to deterioration of renal function and circulatory compromise if an already diminished plasma volume is further reduced.

TABLE 1 Classification of Commonly Used Diuretics by Sites of Action

Osmotic diuretics
Mannitol, urea
Proximal tubular diuretics
Acetazolamide
Loop of Henle diuretics
Furosemide
Ethacrymic acid
Bumetanide
Distal tubule diuretics
Thiazide
Chlorthalidone
Metalozone
Distal tubule diuretics (potassium "sparing")
Triamterene
Spironolactone
Amiloride

With this warning constantly in mind, diuretics can be used with care in patients in whom edema formation limits ambulation, impairs respiration or cardiac function, excessively stretches the skin over the extremities, or produces disabling psychologic suffering because of the deformity of the patient's body image. It is important that the end-point in the use of diuretics not be the total removal of edema, but rather its reduction to a tolerable level. In many patients compulsive salt restriction alone with bed rest is adequate to control edema, but if this is inadequate and diuretics are employed, patients must be warned to stop them if postural symptoms, develop. A strict record must be kept of body weight, and supine and upright blood pressure must be measured at each clinic visit together with frequent assessment of renal function.

The intense sodium retention of nephrotic syndrome usually requires that the diuretic that is used be a loop diuretic, and furosemide is most frequently employed in doses that may need to be increased from standard dosage levels to 400 to 600 mg daily in intractable cases. Spironolactone may sometimes be added to enhance the diuretic effect and limit hypokalemia. The thiazide diuretic metolazone, has proved to be particularly effective when used alone or with furosemide. In patients with anasarca, intravenous diuretics may safely induce diuresis when followed by an infusion of hyperoncotic albumin, administered to maintain the plasma volume. This procedure, however, should be reserved for inpatients whose volume status can be carefully monitored.

Ascites

Many of the comments on diuretic use in nephrotic syndrome are applicable to ascites, around which a similar controversy exists regarding the pathophysiology of the fluid retention. Traditionally it has been taught that protal hypotension and hypoabuminemia from hepatic parenchymal dysfunction lead to fluid seepage into the peritoneum at the expense of the plasma volume and that the avid renal sodium retention is a compensatory renal response. More recently, however, it has been suggested that the renal sodium retention is a primary phenomenon that leads to expansion of the plasma volume, which then overflows into the peritioneal space under the influence of the altered Starling forces at the peritoneal membrane. Once again, rational use of diuretics could potentially be determined by defining the mechanism of edema formation in the individual patient. Such a determination is not available clinically, but it is clear that many cirrhotic patients manifest deterioration of renal and hepatic function after diuretic use. It is interesting to note that the hepatorenal syndrome typically occurs in patients with cirrhosis and ascites 10 to 14 days after admission to the hospital, at which time dietary manipulation and diuretic therapy were instituted.

Certain specific issues must be considered before diuretic therapy is started in ascitic cirrhotic patients. As mentioned earlier, the predisposition to renal failure that may occur in any edematous patient treated with diuretics may be irreverisible in cirrhotic patients, particularly when therapy is excessively vigorous. For reasons described in the chapter *"Hyponatremia"*, many patients develop hyponatremia during diuretic therapy, and this can lead to deterioration in mental function. Hypokalemia, which may be induced by any of the kaliuretic diuretics, may exaggerate the reduction in the already depleted body potassium stores. It has frequently been observed that there is a temporal relationship between diuretic therapy and the induction of hepatic encephalopathy. The enhanced renal ammonia production in hypokalemia has been suggested to account for this. Many patients with advanced cirrhosis have acid-base abnormalities, most frequently respiratory alkalosis, and since thiazides and loop diuretics frequently induce metabolic alkalosis, a dangerous mixed acid-base disturbance may be induced that may exaggerate or induce encephalopathy.

The presence of ascites in a patient with cirrhosis is not an indication for diuretic therapy, just as the presence of edema in a nephrotic patient is not an indication for diuretics. Diuretics should be used only when ascites is massive and uncomfortable or when ambulation and respiratory function are compromised. Many patients with ascites can be managed adequately by bed rest and salt restriction alone. The first diuretic to be employed is usually spironolactone. If diuresis is inadequate, furosemide is added, starting at 20 mg twice a day and reaching a maximum of 80 mg twice a day. The massive doses of diuretics sometimes applied in nephrotic syndrome and heart failure should not be used in ascites, nor should diuretics be employed at a time of deteriorating hepatic and renal function. There remains a group of patients who do not respond to the foregoing regimen, and the most frequent cause for this is inadequately compulsive dietary sodium restriction. The observation that ascitic fluid appears frequently to be compartmentalized, and thus represents a relatively nonmobile segment of the extracellular fluid, might well account for some of the difficulties in managing ascitic patients and the rapidity with which they can develop renal and circulatory compromise.

Heart Failure

The avid renal sodium reabsorption of heart failure has typically been regarded as a compensatory response to diminished effective circulatory volume. Sodium retention leads to increased venous return, thereby increasing preload, stretching the myocardium, and increasing cardiac output. Sodium retention, however, occurs at the expense of an increased absolute level of circulatory volume, and this frequently expresses itself as pulmonary and/or peripheral edema. Thus, as in other edematous states, diuretics can be a two-edged sword. By decreasing preload they can improve congestive symptoms and exercise tolerance, but this may occur at the expense of a reduced cardiac output. Thus, although diuretics are frequently effective in the management of congestive heart failure, they must be used with caution. It must not be forgotten, however, that it is the heart and not the kidney that fails in this condition, and the most effective treatment is to increase the contractile force of the heart with digitalis or other inotropic agents. In severe heart failure, diuretics need to be combined with cardiac glycosides or vasodilator therapy.

Edema in Pregnancy

Most women experience asymptomatic edema at some time during pregnancy, and in the majority, the issue of diuretic use does not arise. During the frequently severe hypertension and edema of full-blown pre-eclampsia, however, diuretics are often considered. There has been considerable vacillation among nephrologists and obstetricians regarding the indications for their use, and the controversy has revolved around the observation that in pre-eclampsia and essential hypertension in pregnancy, intravascular volume is decreased and placental blood flow is compromised. For fear of further diminishing placental perfusion, diuretics and strict salt restriction are used only in those gravidas with heart disease and when hypertension is severe and fluid retention massive.

Idiopathic Edema

Idiopathic edema is used to describe the not infrequent complaint of intractable or recurrent edema and fluctuating body weight in women in whom none of the usually recognized causes of edema can be recognized. It is discussed at this point because of the possible role of diuretics in both its induction and treatment. Physicians frequently use diuretics to manage the edema in this condition, and indeed, short-term benefit may follow. It has been suggested, however, that the condition is a manifestation of diuretic abuse, and there is little question that intermittent use of diuretics, particularly when combined with drastic swings in sodium and caloric intake, can lead to very large changes in body weight with sodium retention and edema. Although it is not clear whether diuretic abuse is responsible for all of these cases, every attempt should be made to manage the edema with salt restriction, a stable diet, and excercise. Amphetamines and dopamine agonists may be useful, and many patients benefit from psychotherapy. Diuretics should be avoided whenever possible.

DIURETICS IN NONEDEMATOUS STATES

Disorders of Calcium Metabolism

Hypercalcemia and hypercalciuria are excellent examples of how the different mechanisms by which diuretics lead to increased sodium excretion can be exploited in the management of a variety of nonedematous states. Furosemide and other loop diuretics increase calcium excretion by virtue of the fact that their action is largely on the thick ascending link of Henle's loop, where calcium is reabsorbed. Calcium and sodium excretion thus tend to increase in parallel. Thiazide diuretics, however, decrease sodium reabsorption more distally at a site where calcium is not absorbed. The volume contraction that the thiazides induce leads to avid sodium reabsorption at other nephron sites (mainly the proximal tubule), where calcium and sodium reabsorption are linked. Sodium excretion therefore increases at a time when calcium excretion decreases. The hypocalciuric action of thiazides thus depends on the presence of simulataneous volume contraction, and their effects can be largely mimicked by a low-sodium-diet and be overcome by a salt-replete diet.

The calciuric effect of furosemide is exploited in the treatment of hypercalcemia. Therapy consists of the administration of the drug together with the replacement of urinary losses of sodium and potassium, so that extracellular fluid volume is maintained at a somewhat expanded level. In most cases, useful reduction of plasma calcium can be obtained and further therapy will be determined by the nature of the underlying illness. The hypocalciuric effect of thiazides has become the backbone of the management of idiopathic hypercalciuria.

Pituitary and Nephrogenic Diabetes Insipidus

It seems paradoxical to treat diabetes insipidus with a diuretic, but thiazide diuretics, used alone or in combination with vasopressin and a low-salt-diet, can lead to reduction of urine flow and amelioration of the social and psychologic impact of massive urine output. The mechanism of the effect relates to the natriuresis and volume contraction induced by the diuretic, which in turn leads to decreased glomerular filtration rate and increased proximal tubular reabsorption of isotonic filtrate. With lesser amounts of filtrate reaching the distal nephron to free water, excretion and urine volume will be decreased, even though sodium excretion may have been increased by the diuretics.

The use of a diuretic in both central and nephrogenic diabetes insipidus can produce up to a 50 percent reduction in the 24-hour urine volume and thus provide useful adjunctive therapy for patients whose urine output is massive. It is important, however, to clearly define the cause of the polyuria before starting such therapy, since patients suffering from primary polydipsia may devlop dangerous hyponatremia when treated with diuretics.

Acute Renal Failure

There has been fluctuating enthusiasm regarding the use of diuretics in acute renal failure, and in the absence of carefully controlled clinical trials, policy regarding their use as depended largely on clinical judgment and experience.

There is evidence that diuretics can prevent certain forms of acute renal fialure. Mannitol administered during intravenous administration of radiocontrast materials may reduce the incidence of nephrotoxicity in patient at high risk from this complication. In patients susceptible to rhabdomyolytic acute tubular necrosis, the maintenance of a high urine output with intravenous fluids and furosemide may protect the kidney by preventing intratubular obstruction with pigmented casts. A similar beneficial effect may be seen in the prevention of acute urate nephropathy. It is probable that diuretics (usually furosemide and mannitol) administered in the early stages of other forms of acute tubular necrosis (e.g. with sepsis or hypotension) may serve to change the course from an oliguric one to a nonoliguric one. Therefore diuretics should be tried, since nonoliguric acute tubular necrosis is typically easier to manage and has a better prognosis. However, whenever diuretics are used in acute renal failure, great care must be taken to prevent dehydration, which may add a further prerenal element to the renal failure. Repeated doses of diuretics should not be used, and there is no place for their use in established oliguric acute tubular necrosis. In these circumstances, diuretics may further reduce renal blood flow. Potassium-sparing diuretics should not be used in acute or chronic renal failure because of the frequency of dangerous hypercalcemia.

Renal Tubular Acidosis

Proximal renal tubular acidosis is a defect in acidification resulting from inadequate reabsorption of bicarbonate in the proximal tubule. Bicarbonate then floods the distal tubule and is lost in the urine, leading to systemic acidosis. When thiazides are administered in this condition, a degree of systemic volume contraction develops which leads to increased avidity for sodium and hence bicarbonate reabsorption in the proximal tubule. The mechanism for the beneficial effect of thiazides is thus similar to that in diabetes insipidus and hypercalciuria.

Urinary Alkalinization

There are several situations in which diuretic-induced urinary alkalinization may be of therapeutic benefit, and the drug most frequently used to achieve this is the carbonic anhydrase inhibitor, acetazolamide. The solubility of both uric acid and cystine is greater at alkaline pH. During massive uric acid production, as is seen during treatment of myelo- and lymphoproliferative diseases, urine alkalinization with acetazolamide, together with the maintenance of a high urine output, may serve to prevent uric acid nephropathy. Urine alkalinization is usually inadequate as the sole treatment of cystinuria. A urine pH persistently higher than 7.5 is necessary to dissolve cystine stones, and penicillamine therapy is usually required. When promoting urine alkalinization, it should be remembered that a high urine pH may decrease the solubility of calcium salts and promote calcium stone formation in susceptible patients.

RENAL ALLOGRAFT REJECTION

WILLIAM E. BRAUN, M.D.

DIAGNOSIS

The diagnosis of renal allograft rejection is based on reasonable, though usually not absolutely definitive, information identifying the deterioration of renal allograft function as being due to an immunologic rejection. The typical finding that triggers the suspicion of rejection is a significant rise in the serum creatinine level. In a few cases, however, the sudden and dramatic fall in urine output, the onset of pain in the area of the allograft indicating its rupture, or the poorer uptake, excretion, and clearance of ^{123} I-orthoiodohippurate on the renal scan may indicate rejection before a significant rise in serum creatinine has occurred.

The degree of rise in the serum creatinine level used to determine rejection will vary somewhat from center to center, and possibly even from one rejection episode to another. In children, in whom the serum creatinine level following a successful transplant may be as low as 0.5 mg per deciliter, a rise in the creatinine of just 0.2 mg per deciliter represents a 40 percent decrement in renal function and must raise serious question of rejection. On the other hand, in an adult whose serum creatinine level rises 0.2 mg per deciliter from 2.0 to 2.2 mg per deciliter there is just a 10 percent decrement. Such a small change, if confirmed by repeat laboratory measurement, would need further documentation for the diagnosis of rejection to be sustained. Unfortunately, the mental translation of serum creatinine values to glomerular filtration rates (GFR) is usually ignored and is complicated by the nature of the relationship between serum creatinine and GFR. The flat portion of this relationship shows that at high levels of GFR large decreases can occur with only relatively small rises in serum creatinine, whereas the steep portion of the curve shows that at low GFRs only small decreases occur despite greater numerical increases in the serum creatinine level. Laboratory variability in the serum creatinine determinations must also be taken into account. In addition, the influence of drugs such as trimethoprim-sulfamethoxazole and cimetidine, which can cause an elevation in the serum creatinine level because of interference with the tubular secretion of creatinine without alteration of the GFR, must be considered. Increases and decreases in muscle mass and body weight also can have positive correlations with rises and falls, respectively, in the serum creatinine level without any necessary alteration in the GFR. Because many patients gain weight following a successful renal transplant, a baseline ^{123}I-iothalamate GFR is obtained near the time of a patient's discharge following transplantation for later comparisons when rejection is suspected because of a rising serum creatinine level.

Although any rise in the serum creatinine level should alert one to the possibility of rejection, a rise of approximately 15 to 25 percent, depending on the initial creatinine level, is usually the threshhold for considering therapy. Just as with the evaluation of any deterioration of renal function, one should consider, in a focused way, the differential diagnosis of allograft rejection (Table 1).

Among patients receiving cyclosporine for prophylaxis of rejection, the most common differential diagnosis will be cyclosporine nephrotoxicity, but one must thoughtfully consider the other possibilities outlined in Table 1. Prerenal causes are often contributory factors in serum creatinine elevations and usually result from overenthusiastic use of diuretics or unnoticed hyperglycemia-induced diuresis in diabetics whose insulin requirements are climbing with their newly functioning kidneys and steroid medication. The total cessation of urinary output should make one acutely aware of postrenal causes, including both obstruction and extravasation. In considering obstruction early after transplantation one can mentally work right up the urinary tract from the Foley catheter backward to exclude intrinsic causes, such as a stricture, clot, stone, or stenosis, and extrinsic causes such as a large lymphocele, hematoma, or a subtle form of obstruction produced by idiopathic perureteral fibrosis occurring many years after transplantation and leading to an insidious rise in serum creatinine that has traditionally been confused with chronic rejection. This problem, however, is not associated with significant increases in urinary protein excretion. Extravasation of urine, on the other hand, seems to be a much rarer event since the introduction of techniques that allow the ureteroneocystostomy to be done without a large central cystotomy incision. Typically fever and occasionally pain accompany extravasated urine, although these findings may be diminished if a patient is receiving large doses of methylprednisolone. Extravasation can also be extremely subtle and may be intermittent from one 8-hour nursing shift to another. Consequently, what appears to be an adequate 24-hour urine output may mask a significant period of time in which there was no urine output because of an intermittent leak.

Renal vascular disease may occur in either the renal artery or the renal vein, although the former is the more likely culprit. The occurrence of significant renal allograft arterial occlusions will depend on a variety of factors, including the discrepancy in size between donor and recipient vessels, intimal injury or atherosclerosis, hyperacute rejections due to unsuspected ABO incompatibilities or positive T-lymphocyte crossmatches, and surgical technique. There have also been situations in which patients with high-grade renal artery stenosis not yet causing a rise in serum creatinine level have had a rapid and significant rise in the serum creatinine and, in at least one instance, total occlusion of the artery when an angiotensin II converting enzyme inhibitor (captopril) was used in high doses. In fact, low doses of captopril have been used in the hospital to determine the physiologic significance of stenotic lesions. Angiotensin converting enzyme inhibitors (e.g., captopril and enalapril) relax the

TABLE 1 Differential Diagnosis of Allograft Rejection

Prerenal	In addition to the usual cardiac and hypotensive causes, look for volume depletion due to excessive diuretics and hyperglycemia-induced diuresis.
Postrenal Obstruction	Consider all sites from the Foley catheter back up the urinary tract and both intrinsic (e.g., stricture, clot, stone, and stenosis) and extrinsic causes (e.g., spermatic cord lymphocele, and hematoma). Note the subtle occurrence of idiopathic periureteral fibrosis and progressive obstruction years after transplant.
Extravasation	This occurs more commonly in ureteropelvic anastomosis, but also arises from the cystotomy incision and ureteroneocystotomy site; newer "extravesical" anastomoses without a separate cystotomy incision are more leak-proof.
Renal Vascular Renal artery	The frequency of thrombosis and stenosis will depend on factors that include discrepancy in size between donor and recipient vessels, intimal injury, atherosclerosis, hypotension, hyperacute rejections, and surgical technique. Angiotensin coverting enzyme inhibitors (e.g. captopril, enalapril) may prevent the autoregulation, that preserves GFR in patients with significant renal artery stenosis.
Renal vein	Occlusion is an uncommon event with an acute early form that may cause graft failure and should be suspected with ipsilateral lower extremity thrombophlebitis; a subacute or partial form that may permit protective collaterals to develop; and a late form. Thrombotic events, once rare with conventional therapy, are becoming more frequent in those receiving cyclosporine and in patients who are hemodynamically unstable, or volume contracted while receiving OKT3 monoclonal antibody, or both cyclosporine and OKT3.
Renal Parenchymal	
Rejection	(See text)
Cyclosporine nephrotoxicity	(See text and Tables 2 and 3)
Recurrent disease	(See Table 4.)
De Novo Disease	Although almost any disease can occur in an allograft, in the appropriate situation consider pyelonephritis with obstruction from late periureteral fibrosis, interstitial nephritis or other non-cyclosporine drug nephrotoxicity (e.g., furosemide, aminoglycosides, amphotericin, and IV acyclovir), CMV nephropathy, syndromes with non-steroidal anti-inflammatory agents, captopril or enalapril usage in unsuspected renal artery stenosis, and hypercalcemia with autonomous hyperparathyroidism.
Miscellaneous	Laboratory error, drugs that interfere with tubular secretion of creatinine (e.g., trimethoprim-sulfamethoxazole cimetidine), and increased muscle mass.

autoregulatory efferent arteriolar constriction that preserves GFR in patients with significant renal artery stenosis already compromising afferent arteriolar flow. Two other significant sites of vascular disease, often overlooked, but causing hypertension, are iliac occlusive disease proximal to the allograft artery and intrarenal vascular occlusions. Renal venous occlusion has really been an uncommon event in the past, appearing either as an early acute problem associated with ipsilateral thrombophlebitis of the leg, a subacute or partial form that may allow protective collaterals to develop, or a very rare late type associated with chronic rejection. However, the two newest immunosuppressants, cyclosporine and OKT3 monoclonal antibody, both appear to have a propensity for causing thrombotic events and may be particularly worrisome together. The risk is accentuated in patients who become volume depleted, as may happen in those who develop very high fevers and continuing diarrhea after receiving OKT3.

Renal parenchymal causes create the most difficult differential diagnoses for rejection. Primary among these differential possibilities is cyclosporine nephrotoxicity (Tables 2 and 3). Although there are helpful guidelines to identify cyclosporine nephrotoxicity, the rules are not absolute. Within the first few weeks after transplantation, when gastrointestinal absorption is relatively poor, cyclosporine doses as low as 6 mg per kilogram of body weight (used in triple drug prophylaxis protocols with low-dose prednisone and azathioprine) may not cause any nephrotoxicity, whereas 6 weeks after transplant they certainly may do so. Cyclosporine levels greater than 200 ng per milliliter by the high performance liquid chromatography assay are considered nephrotoxic and require decreases in the cyclosporine dose usually by 50 to 100 mg per day. When abnormally high blood levels are returned from the laboratory in the afternoon for a patient receiving his doses twice a day, I omit the second dose entirely and start the next day on the reduced level of cyclosporine. This will quickly bring the cyclosporine level back into a normal range. At the other end of the spectrum, however, and especially beyond the first month after transplantation, cyclosporine levels less than the "therapeutic" lower limits of 50 to 75 ng per milliliter may still cause nephrotoxicity. It is at this point that a slow rate of rise of the serum creatinine level, the intermediate height of that serum creatinine elevation, the lack of any significant decrease in urinary output, and the timing more than one month after transplant make the likelihood of cyclosporine nephrotoxicity great enough to empirically decrease or withdraw cyclosporine altogether. This can usually be done under close observation on an outpatient basis while azathioprine is substituted. Patients can decrease their serum creatinine levels substantially within 10 days off cyclosporine and continue to improve them even beyond that. Although it is not an entirely pure approach, if there is any question of concurrent rejection while the cyclosporine is reduced or tapered, increasing low oral prednisone dosage to about 30 mg per day is useful. If the serum creatinine level begins to rise rapidly during this period, however, one should rework the

TABLE 2 Cyclosporine Nephrotoxicity versus Rejection

	Toxicity	*Rejection*
Serum creatinine rise >50%		+
Urine output decrease >50%		+
Slow rise of serum creatinine	+	
Time >1 month post-transplant	+	
Cyclosporine level >200 ng/ml	+	
Initial ATN	+	
Second transplant (early rejection of 1st)		+
Physical signs of rejection		+
Decreased radionuclide scan		+

differential diagnosis of rejection, since problems as common as prerenal volume contraction or as uncommon as an obstructing lymphocele may have entered the picture.

Awareness of drugs that increase the nephrotoxicity of cyclosporine or elevate its blood level (see Table 3) is very important. Elevated blood levels have been reported after cimetidine, erythromycin, ketoconazole, and high-dose prednisolone therapy. These are usually easy enough to detect, but the rapidly expanding list of agents that have additional nephrotoxicity in conjunction with cyclosporine makes this the area to be watched for especially. Acyclovir, which is being used more commonly intravenously for severe herpetic infections, can augment the nephrotoxicity of cyclosporine, as can the aminoglycosides and amphotericin that has a vasoconstrictor effect as well. Mannitol, which in high doses in animals causes vacuolization of proximal tubular epithelial cells, has been found to augment cyclosporine nephrotoxicity which itself has provoked similar morphologic lesions not only in animals but also in man. Other antimicrobial agents that increase the nephrotoxicity of cyclosporine include cotrimoxazole, trimethoprim, and vancomycin. Prolonged ischemia following cadaver organ harvesting and transplantation or nonsteroidal anti-inflammatory drugs may also set the stage for augmentation of cyclosporine nephrotoxicity. On the other hand, drugs such as isoniazid, phenylhydantoin, rifampin, and intravenous sulfadimidine with trimethoprim can reduce the blood levels of cyclosporine and increase the prospects for rejection despite what appear to be adequate dosage levels.

Many diseases can recur in the transplanted kidney (Table 4). Although some have a high frequency of recurrence (e.g., membranoproliferative glomerulonephritis type II, diabetes, and cystinosis), the affected allograft will usually not be seriously compromised for years by these causes. On the other hand, diseases such as the malignant form of focal segmental glomerulosclerosis, hemolytic uremic syndrome, and oxalosis may cause severe and early dysfunction. Systemic lupus erythematosus has had a surprisingly low rate of recurrence, with just four cases reported.

To summarize, the key tests to be considered for the differential diagnoses of rejection include: (1)serial serum creatinine determinations; (2)cyclosporine blood levels in those receiving it; (3) a review of the patient's medication for drugs that may be mephrotoxic or that alter renal hemodynamics; (4)a visual test of renal parenchymal function (e.g., ^{123}I-orthoiodohippurate renal scan); (5) a test for mechanical problems such as obstruction, extravasation, or a fluid collection (e.g., ultrasound, computed tomography, intravenous pyelogram, if the level of renal function permits, or with laminograms, if the serum creatinine level is 3 to 5 mg per deciliter; percutaneous antegrade pyelogram, or cystogram); (6) a test for arterial lesions (e.g., technetium^{99m} glucoheptonate scan to pick up renal infarcts, intra-arterial digital subtraction or standard angiogram for iliac, allograft arterial, and intrarenal arterial lesions); (7) a renal venogram for thrombosis or compression; (8) bacterial, viral, and fungal cultures and/or serology; (9) a urinalysis with careful examination of the sediment for evidence of new or recurrent glomerulonephritis; (10) quantitative protein excretion; (11) serologic tests that may indicate recurrent disease (e.g., anti-GBM antibody, decreased C3 and C4); and (12) a renal biopsy. The only tests that require hospitalization are a renal biopsy, a formal angiogram to definitely rule out significant iliac artery, renal artery, or intrarenal arterial disease, and an antegrade pyelogram for those patients in whom significant obstruction is suspected and the placement of a nephrostomy tube and stent catheter are contemplated. From a practical point of view, when starting to treat for rejection, one should know that the change in creatinine is significant; the cyclosporine dose has already been adjusted, and no other nephrotoxins are involved; the ultrasound is negative; the orthoiodohippurate scan is compatible with rejection; the urine sediment shows no infection (but a culture is obtained too); and based on history and physical examination there are no prerenal causes for the rise in creatinine level (e.g., volume contraction with orthostatic hypotension in a nondiabetic), no renal arterial or iliac stenosis when auscultating the area medial to the graft (e.g., systolic and diastolic bruits), and no abnormalities when inspecting or palpating the graft (e.g., extensive wound infection or pneumonia) that would exaggerate the risk. Fever early after transplantation may be due to rejection as well as

TABLE 3 Cyclosporine Drug Interactions

Elevated blood levels	Increased nephrotoxicity
Cimetidine	Acyclovir
Erythromycin	Aminoglycosides
Ketoconazole	Amphotericin
High-dose prednisolone	Co-trimoxazole
	Mannitol
Increased functional effect	Melphalan
Verapamil (in vitro)	Ranitidine
	Trimethoprim
	Vancomycin
Reduced blood levels	Prolonged ischemia
Isoniazid	Nonsteroidal anti-inflammatory drugs
Phenylhydantoin	
Rifampin	No change
Intravenous sulfadimidine with trimethoprim	Captopril
	Theophylline

infection, drug fever and other causes, but late after transplant fever is rarely, if ever, due to rejection. Acute rejection does not often have nephrotic range proteinuria, but nephrotic range proteinuria is most often caused by chronic rejection.

OVERVIEW OF TREATMENT

When acute rejection is present, it should be treated if it is the sole or dominant factor responsible for allograft dysfunction and only when there is an acceptable benefit-to-risk ratio for the specific patient being treated. One does not treat when there is substantial doubt about the presence of rejection, a significant contribution of other factors to deteriorating renal function, or an unacceptable benefit-to-risk ratio for the patient. In circumstances in which there is little or no chance of reversing a rejection, aggressive treatment with immunosuppressants should be withheld because of the unacceptable benefit-to-risk ratio. Such irreversible rejections may need documentation by a biopsy that would typically show changes such as substantial cortical necrosis, diffuse intravascular or glomerular thromboses, widespread interstitial hemorrhage, extensive fibrosis, generalized and diffuse sclerosing glomerular changes, and severe thickening of vascular walls with virtual occlusion of the lumina.

The treatment of rejection is most effective in uncomplicated acute *cellular* rejections, especially within the first 3 to 6 months after transplant. Cellular rejection at this time is typically characterized by large lymphoblastoid cells that have not yet destroyed the basement membrane of the tubules or caused a vasculitis. Acute rejections at a later time, particularly beyond one year, may be cellular in type, but are usually comprised of smaller lymphocytes and more plasma cells and macrophages. This type of acute cellular rejection has a lower incidence of complete reversal even with first-line drugs.

If a serious infection (e.g., severe pneumonia, septicemia, meningitis, deep wound abscess, cytomegalovirus pancreatitis, or perforated viscus with peritonitis) occurs in the course of rejection therapy, the safest course is to stop all other immunosuppression and support the patient with an adequate prednisone dose (e.g. approximately 15 mg per day).

In conjunction with initiating the primary therapy for rejection it is also important to try to reduce or eliminate, whenever possible, drugs that either stimulate cell-mediated immunity (cimetidine, propranolol, and alpha methyldopa), accelerate hepatic microsomal enzyme metabolism of prednisone (phenobarbital and diphenylhydantoin), compromise renal vascular responses (nonsteroidal anti-inflammatory agents) or are potentially serious nephrotoxins (amino glycosides).

The *first-line* treatment of acute cellular allograft rejection involves three agents: *intravenous methylprednisolone, Minnesota antilymphocyte globulin (ALG),* and *possibly OKT3 monoclonal antibody.* As *second-line* therapy there is high-dose *oral prednisone* and *cyclosporine* for those who have not received it. As adjunctive therapy one can consider the use of *low-dose heparin* in the hospital, and coumadin and dipyridamole for outpatients. *Plasma pheresis* may, in exceptional circumstances, be useful.

TABLE 4 Recurrent Diseases

Antiglomerular basement membrane nephritis
Membranoproliferative types I and II
Focal segmental glomerulosclerosis
Minimal change disease
Membranous glomerulonephritis
Extracapillary (crescentic) glomerulonephritis
IgA nephropathy
Anaphylactoid purpura Schönlein-Henoch
Thrombotic microangiopathy
Hemolytic—uremic syndrome
Wegener's granulomatosis
Progressive systemic sclerosis
Systemic lupus erythematosus
Familial glomerulonephritis
Diabetic glomerulopathy
Amyloid
Multiple myeloma
Oxalosis
Cystinosis

First-Line Treatment of Allograft Rejection

Intravenous Methylprednisolone

Intravenous methylprednisolone (IVMP) has been used in doses of a gram per day for the treatment of acute allograft rejection for about 15 years. It is given in daily doses of 1 g divided into 250-mg portions that are administered every 6 hours in 50 to 100 ml of normal saline infused over at least 30 minutes. The IVMP is given in 250-mg doses at 6-hour intervals for the possible advantage of affecting different populations of macrophages and lymphocytes in susceptible periods of their cell cycle as well as to allow the gram dosage to be interrupted at an earlier point in time should any complications be detected in the course of a day's therapy. The doses are clustered in 3 day sets (a total of 12 doses of 250 mg every 6 hours) with at least one full ''skip'' day in between. The IVMP should be given relatively slowly, as noted above, to avoid acute, and at times fatal, arrhythmias and anaphylaxis. If a patient does not respond to the first set of 3 g given over 3 days, then, after a skip day, another set of 3 g may be used with continual evaluation of the patient's condition. If the patient has not responded to these 6 g of IVMP, another set of 3 g may cautiously be given if no contraindications have arisen. However, one should be aware of the fact that the euphoria that the IVMP imparts to the patient should not be overinterpreted and allowed to prevent withholding of further treatment if it does not seem to be fully justified.

The chance of reversing a first rejection with a full set of 6 to 9 g of IVMP with intervening skip days is about 85 percent. The likelihood of IVMP reversing an acute cellular rejection seems greatest within the first 3 to 6 months after transplant and then gradually diminishes thereafter as the characteristics of the cellular infiltrates change and evidence of chronicity increases. It does not take a long time for early fibrosis to appear in rejecting allografts, and I have seen it as early as 6 to 8 weeks after transplantation. In the uncommon situation of a rejection beginning while a prophylactic course of ALG is being given, the ALG is stopped and IVMP begun.

Early rejections are likely to have early responses, and later rejections have longer response times. Whereas early acute rejections, sometimes producing swelling of the allograft and fever, will begin to show a response to IVMP within 24 to 48 hours, later rejections occurring 6 months or more after transplantation usually have slower and slower response times. In such late rejections it is often possible to admit the patient to the hospital, treat with 3 g of IVMP in divided doses as described above, and then discharge the patient for follow-up of the response and possible complications.

The complications of IVMP include, most prominently, an increased susceptibility to infection, which is particularly deceptive because IVMP obliterates virtually any semblance of fever and imparts a sense of well-being to the patient that makes the toxicity of infection difficult to suspect. The mechanism by which IVMP obliterates a febrile response appears to be related to one of its primary immunologic functions, namely, interfering with the production by macrophages of interleukin-1, which is the same as endogenous pyrogen. We have found it useful in patients who have undergone treatment with more than 3 g of IVMP to draw blood cultures, even while they are afebrile, during the subsequent 4 to 9 g of an extended IVMP course. Although some infections may occur in the course of IVMP therapy, there is frequently a lag period between the completion of IVMP and the development of infection. Consequently, if the patient has been discharged from the hospital immediately after such therapy, he should be alerted to the possible occurrence of any delayed infection, instructed to report fever of localizing symptoms, and be examined in the clinic within a week following such therapy.

A second problem is the development of hyperglycemia, possibly resulting from a steroid-provoked cytomegalovirus infection of the pancreas, which is usually sustained and often requires chronic insulin therapy. Rarely, the hyperglycemia may be so high (> 1,000 mg per deciliter) that nonketotic hyperosmolar coma may ensue. Ever since my first, and only, case of this 15 years ago, blood glucose levels are monitored twice weekly and urine specimens checked for glucose in the course of IVMP therapy.

Third, the fluid retention, weight gain, and hypertension that may occur in the course of IVMP, particularly in the presence of renal allograft dysfunction, are often sufficient to necessitate using diuretics daily. One should not ignore the possibilities of overdoing it and causing a prerenal component to the elevated serum creatinine level, or superimposing a drug-induced interstitial nephritis. In patients with severe renal dysfunction in the course of their rejection, IVMP has been associated with hyperkalemia that may be due to a transient decrease in GFR. The use of potassium-losing diuretics may be helpful at these times, although they are often ineffective in severe rejection. Conversely, potassium-sparing diuretics may be particularly hazardous at this time. Arrhythmias, at times fatal, have been reported with rapid bolus injections of IVMP (particularly in patients receiving diuretics), so our regular policy is to infuse the 250 mg of IVMP, over at least 30 minutes. Actue steroid psychosis may also develop with IVMP, but one should be careful not to overlook central nervous system infections masquerading as psychiatric problems which may develop behind the mask of IVMP. Impairment of wound healing can be a serious complication of high-dose steroid therapy, especially if dehiscence or infection complicates it. However, improved dialysis and nutritional management before transplantation as well as better wound management with transplantation have made this much less of a problem in the last 10 years.

More remote consequences of steroid therapy include the occurrence of avascular necrosis, typically of the femoral head. This most often occurs between 6 and 18 months after transplantation and has some relation to the overall steroid dose. The frequency of this complication, in my experience, has been 5 percent, both in the period preceding the use of IVMP and during the height of that period. When the patient develops the lesion in the femoral head(s), it usually presents as pain with weight bearing, often anteriorly and laterally or referred to the knee. The patient can benefit from a few weeks on crutches to allow the acute inflammatory process to subside, but if this is not successful and the condition deteriorates, total hip replacement may eventually be required. However, two new approaches have become available for patients with this disease: magnetic resonance imaging can detect abnormalities compatible with the disease even before bone scans and certainly before standard roentgenograms, and surgical intervention with decompression of the femoral head at an early stage may avert the need for total hip replacement. Some patients who are relieved of weight bearing by using crutches very early after the onset of the lesion may also not show deterioration or require hip replacements. Avascular necrosis is usually bilateral and occurs most often in the hips and knees. I have not seen it occur in the shoulder joints for nearly 20 years. Another steroid bone complication of great importance in children is inhibition of long bone growth. Consequently, IVMP and daily oral prednisone doses should be carefully weighed for their risks in this group of patients. Long-term steroid dosage has also been associated with osteoporosis and fractures.

Posterior subcapsular cataracts are a delayed complication of steroid therapy, and may progress rapidly; some patients have required cataract surgery within a year or two after their transplantation. In younger patients, with a stable course, the posterior subcapsular cataracts often develop only as minute deposits that do not seem to progress as they do in the older patients, but all patients are examined by an ophthalmologist at least by one year after transplantation. The development of malignancies after renal transplantation may also be caused, in part, by steroid therapy, though these patients are generally receiving at least one other immunosuppressant with the same type of risk. The development of a cushingoid appearance is sometimes an unavoidable problem with prolonged high-dose steroid therapy and may have a certain genetic background. However, the limitation of total caloric intake may significantly ameliorate this problem. Whether steroids are a prime cause of peptic ulcer is still being debated, but with aggressive endoscopy, cimetidine or ranitidine usage, and antacid therapy at the first signs or symptoms of this problem, I have rarely encountered a serious complication. The involvement of the cytomegalovirus in such gastrointestinal lesions makes their cause even more difficult to specify. Steroid myopathy is sometimes present in the aftermath of treatment with large doses of IVMP, and its diagnosis can be confirmed, by finding, on muscle biopsy, predominant and diffuse atrophy of the type II muscle fibers stained darkly by enzyme histochemistry (adenosine triphosphatase at pH 9.8).

The termination of a course of IVMP at a total of 3, 6, or 9 g is obviously an arbitrary one designed to reduce morbidity and mortality, particularly due to infections. Some individuals may not tolerate even this dosage of IVMP, whereas others may be able to benefit from higher doses. With each higher plateau of therapy there are usually steadily rising risks of serious infections, cataracts, avascular necrosis, myopathy, and de novo diabetes in the susceptible patient. As a result, most of us settle for a total of 3 to 6 g of IVMP for treatment of acute cellular rejection. Perhaps the mistake that we make in using it, however, is that we are not patient enough to wait for its effect in rejections occurring beyond 3 months after transplant when the response time becomes longer.

When one switches rejection therapy from IVMP to ALG or vice versa, one must appreciate that the patient is acquiring a cumulative risk from the combined immunosuppressants. There are no crisp equivalency tables available to compare the amount of ALG that would equal a certain amount of IVMP in terms of immunosuppression or risk. However, I do not give a full 10–day course of ALG and then immediately, if there is no response, embark on a full 9–g course of IVMP, because that usually creates an excessive risk of infection that may not occur immediately, but is very likely to turn up within roughly 10 to 14 days from the onset of treatment. A crude guideline equates one full daily dose of ALG to 1 g of IVMP and to one full dose of OKT3 monoclonal antibody. For example, if a patient were able to tolerate only 5 days of a projected 10–day course of ALG therapy and had to be switched to IVMP, he would receive about 5 additional g of IVMP for the rejection. In terms of infection risk, one dose of OKT3 monoclonal antibody might have a similar equivalency to one full dose of ALG.

Antilymphocyte Globulin

ALG produced at the University of Minnesota by immunizing horses or goats with cultured human lymphoblasts has been about 90 to 95 percent effective in treating first rejections. The success of ALG treatment of allograft rejection may be influenced by the intensity of prior prophylactic immunosuppression. For example, when a 14-day course of prophylactic ALG was used along with azathioprine as well as a 2 mg per kilogram dose of oral prednisone, the ability of ALG to reverse the first allograft rejection in cadaveric recipients was nearly 100 percent, but with a protocol of low-dose predisone (30 mg per day), there has been a tendency for first rejections to occur earlier and to be somewhat more resistant to ALG. Now with the use of triple low-dose prophylactic protocols, including cyclosporine at 6 mg per kilogram in divided doses per day, azathioprine at 50 to 100 mg per day, and prednisone at 30 mg per day, the occurrence of rejection has been pushed back and the response to ALG improved again.

The protocol for treatment of a first transplant rejection with ALG involves placement of a central venous catheter either through the subclavian or the jugular route. In patients with no immediate possibility of such access the arteriovenous fistula used for dialysis may be used carefully as a temporary solution. The value of skin testing for horse sensitivity is uncertain. If the patient already has documented sensitivity to horse serum, then it is possible to use goat or rabbit ALG. If the patient has had ALG before, it may be necessary to test for existing antibody to horse serum. If antibodies to horse serum are present, the readministration of horse ALG would be expected to result in complexing of the ALG by the preexisting antibody and exceptionally rapid elimination from the circulation with little or no immunosuppressant effect and possibly a hypersensitivity reaction.

The ALG is administered through the central line in a dose of 15 to 20 mg per kilogram over a period of 4 to 6 hours for 10 days. If the patient has a febrile response to the ALG infusion, pretreatment can be tried with 100 mg of hydrocortisone IV, 50 mg of diphenhydramine IM, and 650 mg of acetaminophen PO 30 to 60 minutes before administration of the ALG. The ALG itself is given piggyback into a constant infusion of saline, which is running at 30 ml per hour, to ensure a slow continuous rate and avoid clotting the central line or overloading the patient with fluid.

Because of variability in the potency of certain batches of ALG, the milligram per kilogram dosage must be established with the University of Minnesota. Full-dose therapy has ranged from as high as 30 mg per kilogram to as low as 15 mg per kilogram. With this regimen, approximately 90 to 95 percent of first cadaver allograft rejections can be either reversed or substantially improved. Usually the rejection begins to respond within the first 3 days of therapy, but in a small percentage of cases the serum creatinine concentration continues to rise through the fifth to seventh day, suggesting that no effect is taking place, until suddenly the serum creatinine level begins to fall, so that by 10 days there is a clear indication that the rejection has begun to reverse.

The early complications with ALG include the frequent development of fever and chills, thrombocytopenia, and leukopenia—the severity of which will depend upon the batch and dosage; the occasional development of serum sickness (with arthralgias, arthritis, and skin rash); the rare development of renal function impairment due either to immune complex deposition involving horse protein or antiglomerular basement membrane antibody; and very rarely anaphylaxis. Later complications of ALG include an increased susceptibility to infections, particularly viral infections of the herpes-cytomegalovirus group, that may develop within a few weeks of therapy. A remote risk is the possible increased susceptibility to malignancy. Although it does not bother the patient, it is worthwhile to remember that circulating horse ALG can interfere with red cell crossmatching as well as with the determination of lymphocytotoxic antibodies in a histocompatibility laboratory.

Batches of ALG can vary not only in their immunosuppressant potency but also in their capacity to diminish the platelet count and/or white cell count. Usually leukopenia and thrombocytopenia require only a temporary cessation of ALG or a downward adjustment of the dose. If the platelet count is reduced to a range between 75,000 and 100,000 per cubic millimeter, the ALG dose is reduced to one-half; if the platelet count is reduced to a range between 50,000 and 75,000 per cubic millimeter, the ALG dose is reduced to one-fourth; if the platelet count is reduced below 50,000 ALG is usually not given. If the white cell count is reduced to a level between 3,500 and 5,000, azathioprine is the first drug to be reduced or eliminated; if the white blood cell count drops below 3,500 when ALG is the only leukopenia-producing drug being given, then ALG is omitted until the white count has risen to a near normal range. Some clinicians will follow a more aggressive course with ALG and use it even with white counts below 2,000 as long as the absolute granulocyte count is between 500 and 1,000. Following the daily trend in platelet and leukocyte counts can usually lead one to identify serious potential problems ahead of time. One should check the patient's medications for other drugs that may also depress the white cell count, such as allopurinol, trimethoprim-sulfamethoxazole, cimetidine, and cephalosporin, to mention a few. If azathioprine was being used during ALG therapy and had to be reduced or discontinued because of severe leukopenia near the end of the 10-day ALG rejection course, it is worthwhile covering the immediate post-ALG transition with 100 mg of prednisone a day for the few days it usually takes the white count to recover and permit the reinstitution of azathioprine. This has reduced rebound rejections.

If serious toxicities are encountered with ALG, one may be able to change immediately to IVMP, as described above, or to an ALG made in goats.

If the patient had been receiving cyclosporine at the time of ALG therapy, it is usually decreased or discontinued.

*Anti-T3 Monoclonal Antibody**

Just recently approved by the Food and Drug Administration for general use, monoclonal antibody to the T3 molecular complex on T-lymphocytes (OKT3) offers promise of being a first-line reagent for treating allograft rejection. It is an IgG_{2a} monoclonal antibody secreted by a murine hybridoma cell line. Its mechanism of action has not been definitely established, but presumably includes blocking the function of sessile killer cells in the transplanted organ, opsonizing (coating) circulating T-lymphocytes that are then removed by the reticuloendothelial cells, and modulating the T3-antigen recognition complex from the surface of T cells.

The OKT3 monoclonal antibody can be used either as initial treatment for rejection or as rescue treatment. A recent collaborative study has reported that OKT3 reversed 94 percent of first rejections in cadaver allograft recipients being treated with conventional therapy. Because this murine antibody, after a 10-day course, evokes an antibody to itself in about 75 percent of patients (described below), it may be effective only in its first use. Similar statements were made about ALG at the beginning of its use, and it has been used more than once, and successfully too, in many patients. If the prevailing attitude is correct, however, one must decide whether to use

---

This section is based in part on information presented at the Monoclonal Antibody Symposium by Drs. JF. Burdick, AB Cosimi, G. Goldstein, R. Gordon, L. Kahana, DJ. Norman, CF. Shield, III and T.E. Starzl through the sponsorship of the Ortho Pharmaceutical Corporation in Miami, Florida, February 7, 1986.

this "silver bullet" as the very first treatment of rejection or to try traditional first-line agents beforehand. Currently, a brief course of IVMP (about 3 g total in 3 days) is usually used first to reverse as many rejections as possible before committing to the use of OKT3. If ALG has been used beforehand, there is a tendency to a higher frequency of antibody production. Whether the use of ALG after OKT3 will reduce the sensitization rate remains to be seen.

The use of OKT3 will often be considered in a patient who has been receiving cyclosporine (with or without prednisone and azathioprine). If the rejection does not respond to 3 g of IVMP, then OKT3 may be appropriate. When OKT3 is started, the question is whether to leave the cyclosporine dose as is, lower it, or stop it. Because cyclosporine nephrotoxicity can be so subtle (as discussed) and because the serum creatinine level remains higher and reversal rates lower when it is not reduced, it is usually wise to stop the cyclosporine altogether for the first 8 days of the 10-day course of OKT3 and to substitute azathioprine during that time in low doses of less than 1 mg per kilogram, as permitted by the white blood cell count. This approach still begs the question of whether presumed rejection is really cyclosporine nephrotoxicity. If the patient can be followed daily, and if one is more suspicious of cyclosporine nephrotoxicity, then the first step would be to stop cyclosporine, and in the event of no effect, either try 3 g of IVMP or go directly to OKT3 treatment. Short delays in the use of OKT3 do not seem to impair significantly its ability to reverse a cellular rejection.

After starting OKT3, the serum creatinine level initially may rise at a faster rate for unknown reasons, peak at about 4 days of treatment, and then begin to decline. T-lymphocytes virtually all disappear from the circulation with the first 1 or 2 doses, begin within 4 days and return quickly but with phenotypes devoid of T3 (e.g., T4, T8, T11), and finally show with the termination of therapy a full return of even T3-lymphocytes.

The standard dose is 5 mg (concentration 1 mg per milliliter) given rapidly over 1 to 3 minutes intravenous through a heparin lock in a peripheral vein, although some hospital policies necessitate giving it over a longer period of time. Protracted infusions seem to have caused protraction of the acute symptoms noted below.

Three of the very frequent or major early side effects of OKT3 are: (1) chills, to the point of rigors and high fever, occurring within 30 to 60 minutes, most prominently after the first 1 or 2 doses (75 percent); (2) diarrhea that persists for several days (30 percent); and, (3) a pulmonary syndrome with dyspnea and wheezing that may progress to pulmonary edema or an anaphylactoid reaction requiring immediate intubation and ventilatory support. Thus far there is worldwide experience with five instances of pulmonary edema and two deaths in the initial cases, but with none in the last 500 cases. Complications are so prominent with the first dose in particular that these features are referred to as the "first dose syndrome." Premedication with 100 mg of methylprednisolone sodium succinate IV, 50 mg of diphenhydramine hydrochloride IM, and 650 mg of acetaminophen PO 1 hour before the first dose of OKT3 can diminish the fever and chills and may lessen the chance of a pulmonary syndrome. The primary caveat, however, in avoiding pulmonary edema or an anaphylactoid reaction that seem to be due to increased pulmonary capillary permeability is not to use OKT3 in patients who are more than 3 percnet over their dry weight (ideally euvolemic as confirmed with a chest roentgenogram if necessary) or in those who are hemodynamically unstable. At the other extreme of excessive diuresis and volume contraction, there may be an increased risk of renal vein thrombosis which has already been reported with OKT3. Unitl the cause of the diarrhea is known, the most important part of its treatment is to maintain fluid, electrolyte, and acid-base balance while using conventional therapy for symptomatic relief. Accurate body weights are especially important before, during, and after this therapy. The serious potential side effects of the first few doses have made it necessary to have a physician and epinephrine immediately available as well as to have a nurse in attendance monitoring vital signs every 15 minutes for the first 2 hours, every 30 minutes for the next 2 hours, and hourly until the patient is stable. An emergency cart and anesthesia notification may be necessary until the transplant team has experience with selecting patients for OKT3 therapy and in administering it to them. In any event, the first 3 doses are given in the hospital with appropriate precautions, and subsequent doses might be given in an outpatient setting to stable patients by an experienced team with appropriate back-up.

Other early side effects seen in association with OKT3 therapy have included headache, anorexia, nausea, vomiting, tremor, seizure, chest pain, rash, pruritus, arthritis, thrombocytopenia, transient ischemic attack, myocardial infarction, renal vein and renal artery thrombosis, liver enzyme elevation, and leukopenia that may be worsened with azathioprine, viral infection, and the need for dialysis. If a patient receiving OKT3 is being dialyzed, the dose is best given afterward to minimize the leukopenia.

Late complications have included serum sickness, shedding of cytomegalovirus in those with prior infection, severe viral infections in those whose treatment with OKT3 lasts more than 30 days or who are receiving high doses of corticosteroids concomitantly, and the development of antibodies against the mouse monoclonal antibody in the form of anti-isotype and anti-idiotype. After completion of a 10-day course, the antibodies peak at 2 to 4 weeks. These antibodies may disappear over a period of months, and whether rechallenge with OKT3 would cause anamnestic response or simply be rendered ineffective is uncertain. The frequency of such antibodies developing has been reduced by some clinicians who add 3 daily doses of 400 mg of cyclophosphamide and 1 dose of 500 mg of IVMP on the last 3 days and last day, respectively, of OKT3 therapy.

Rebound rejections, after completion of OKT3 therapy, have tended to diminish when the patient has been receiving cyclosporine before and has had it reinstituted on the last 2 days of the 10-day course of OKT3.

However, as many as two-thirds of conventionally treated patients have rebound rejections.

Overall, when OKT3 has been used as the primary treatment for a first transplant rejection, only a rare case of nonreversal has been reported in living-related transplants and only a 5 percent nonreversal in cadaver recipients. When used as rescue therapy for steroid-resistant or ALG-resistant rejections, there has been approximately a 15 percent failure of reversal in recipients of living-related transplants and a 21 percent failure of reversal in cadaver recipients. The effectiveness of OKT3 therapy appears to depend on how long after transplantation the rejection being treated occurred, since less than 10 percent of rejections occurring within 90 days after transplant failed to reverse whereas nearly half of those beyond 90 days failed to reverse. Because of the high failure rate after 90 days and the likelihood that features of chronic rejection have become dominant, an allograft biopsy in those cases would seem important to avoid wasting this one-time therapy in a low-benefit situation.

Second-Line Treatment of Allograft Rejection

Increased Oral Prednisone

Mild acute rejections can be managed effectively in about two-thirds of cases with increases of oral prednisone in the range of 2 mg per kilogram initially and then a rapidly tapered dose. The course begins with 150 mg daily for 3 days, then 125 mg daily for 3 days, 100 mg daily for 3 days, 75 mg daily for 5 days, 50 mg daily for 5 days; 40 mg daily for 5 days, 35 mg daily for 1 week, 30 mg daily for 1 week, and 25 mg daily for 2 weeks as the maintenance dose of approximately 15 mg per day is approached. A few practical pointers on giving the prednisone dose may be helpful: (1) The dose is given in the morning as a single dose to simulate the diurnal variation in ACTH–triggered corticosteroid secretion as well as to approach the benefits that may accrue from alternate-day therapy; (2) the prednisone is prescribed in a 5-mg dose so that the patient, doctor, and anyone else involved are always talking about the same number of pills having the same 5-mg dose and can discuss dosage changes in terms of number of pills which translates into the same number of milligrams in all cases; (3) the pills are packed in #/00 plain gelatin capsules that make dosage simpler and may protect the upper gastrointestinal tract from any local effects of large amounts of the drug.

One of the most distressing features of this type of treatment is the fact, that despite the appearance of a reversal of rejection, as soon as the prednisone dose enters the tapering range of less than 0.5 mg per kilogram a rebound rejection too often appears. If one were to continue with higher doses for a much longer period of time, then the excessive risks of high sustained levels of oral prednisone of bygone days would reappear. Consequently, this shortcoming of the drug needs to be recognized and rebound rejections handled with a first-line drug or possibly cyclosporine, if it had not already been in use.

When a late rise in the serum creatinine level is encountered against a background of chronic rejection, for example, 5 to 10 years after transplant, the slow functional deterioration can sometimes be interrupted for 6 months or so with a brief course of modestly increased oral prednisone. In this situation, a maintenance dose of what might be 10 to 15 mg of prednisone is increased to 50 mg for 5 days, 40 mg for 5 days, 35 mg for 1 week, 30 mg for 1 week, 25 mg for 2 weeks, and so on, and then reduced to the maintenance level thereafter. However, if the baseline value from which the serum creatinine level rose a year or more after transplant was 1.5 mg per deciliter or less and proteinuria was less than 300 mg per 24 hours, such an acute change in the serum creatinine level with the usual differential diagnoses excluded may be best evaluated with an open renal biopsy. If the biopsy shows predominantly a mononuclear type of interstitial infiltrate with very few plasma cells and little in the way of interstitial fibrosis, interstitial hemorrhage, vascular or glomerular changes, then this type of delayed acute rejection could be approached more aggresively with ALG or IVMP as already outlined. In contrast before embarking on a full ALG or IVMP antirejection treatment in a late rejection with elements of chronic rejection, or, on the other hand before giving up all forms of antirejection therapy, it is often wise to document the status of the transplant by open renal biopsy.

Cyclosporine

For acute allograft rejection cyclosporine must be considered a second-line drug, although it is certainly a first-line drug for prophylaxis of rejection. When used in conventionally treated patients as initial therapy for first rejection it has only about a 50 percent chance of reversing the rejection. Even in the responsive patients the decrease in serum creatinine level is slow. This corresponds well with evidence from experimental animal models showing that after sensitization to donor antigen has occurred, cyclosporine is not very effective.

Treatment is initiated at 14 mg per kilogram with adjustments to keep the blood level between 75 and 200 mg per milliliter, as measured by high performance liquid chromatography. Depending on the response, treatment is continued for 10 to 14 days. If the patient has a remarkably responsive rejection, consideration should obviously be given to making cyclosporine a longer maintenance treatment, but in reduced dosages. When it has been used for rejection more than 6 weeks after transplant in a recipient who had achieved good renal function beforehand, excessively high blood levels seem to occur more frequently with standard doses, suggesting much better absorption. As with any other treatment for rejection, when chronic changes predominate on the renal biopsy, its use is not worth the risk.

The toxicities of cyclosporine include its well-known nephrotoxicity (as discussed) as well as increased susceptibility to infection and neoplasia, a hemolytic-uremic—like syndrome, hepatotoxicity, gynecomastia, tremor, seizures, paresthesias, gingival hyperplasia, hypertrichosis, hypertension, hiccups, cramps, diarrhea, nausea, vomiting, flushing, hyperkalemia, hypomagnesemia, and anaphylaxis.

Adjuntive Therapies for Allograft Rejection

Anticoagulants and Antithrombotics

In some acute rejections associated with a clinical suspicion of or biopsy evidence for intravascular coagulation as a secondary feature, I have used low-dose continuous intravenous heparin as adjunctive therapy. This circumstance may be suspected in early allograft rejection of the accelerated type or when there is considerable allograft swelling with interstitial edema that may well compress and stagnate intrarenal flow with secondary thrombosis. The dosage levels used here are not designed to create any additional hazards in the early post-transplant period, but rather are in the conservative range of 750 units per hour. Obviously, one does not use heparin in patients who have recently undergone or will immediately be undergoing biopsies or surgical procedures, or in patients with contraindications including active peptic ulcer disease, fresh hemorrhagic diabetic retinopathy, and uncontrolled hypertension. However, I have used it safely about 24 hours after open allograft biopsies. If anticoagulants are clearly indicated by the biopsy, after heparin therapy has bene used in the hospital, long-term low-dose Coumadin has been continued in conjunction with dipyridamole. The reports suggesting a greater number of thrombotic events with cyclosporine and OKT3 monoclonal antibody may make it worthwhile to keep this option in mind.

Several other approaches to treating allograft rejection have been used by other centers, but we have either not used them or not found them to be helpful. These approaches include plasmapheresis, leukapheresis, and local graft irradiation.

NEUROLOGIC DISEASES

COMA

MICHAEL P. EARNEST, M.D.
STEPHEN V. CANTRILL, M.D., F.A.C.E.P.

Coma denotes a state of unawareness and unresponsiveness to environmental stimuli. However, coma is only one level in a full spectrum of depression of consciousness ranging from slight drowsiness to brain death. A patient with any degree of depression of alertness is at risk for permanent neurologic injury or death from respiratory arrest, cardiac arrhythmia, brain herniation, or progressive structural brain injury. Thus, every patient with depression of consciousness having no obvious cause should be treated as an urgent emergency until an etiology is determined and the condition is treated.

Hereafter, the term "coma" will be used but will imply any significant depression of consciousness. Also, the following management scheme should be viewed as a conceptual framework that must be altered to fit each patient's situation. However, a systematic approach to the patient with coma of unknown etiology assures that all reasonable diagnostic and therapeutic steps are taken in an efficient manner (Fig. 1).

IMMEDIATE HISTORY

The patient in coma often has an important history. The immediately available history should be quickly obtained from whomever found the patient in coma—a family member, friend, landlord, policeman, fireman, paramedic, or nurse. This brief history should inquire about how the patient was found (e.g., in bed, with empty pill bottles nearby) and any known medical or psychiatric illnesses, medications, alcoholism, or drug abuse. Also, details of recent trauma, fever, or headaches and the onset of the coma should be sought. The sudden onset of nontraumatic coma (i.e., instantaneous or within a few minutes) is usually due to a cardiac or cerebrovascular event. This early history may guide the immediate management (e.g., the known diabetic patient on insulin is presumed to have hypoglycemia; the heroin addict probably has an opiate overdose).

PRINCIPLES OF EARLY MANAGEMENT

The early management of the comatose patient is guided by four principles: (1) save the whole patient; (2) preserve the brain; (3) make a diagnosis and begin therapy; and (4) closely follow the patient's course for signs of deterioration or until full alertness has returned.

Save the Whole Patient

The ABCs of emergency medical care (Airway, Breathing, and Circulation) guide the first steps of management. First, place an intravenous (IV) line, start nasal oxygen, begin cardiac monitoring, and have the patient fully undressed. The pulse, respirations, blood pressure, and rectal temperature are then obtained. Any severe abnormality of vital signs must be immediately treated. Hypotension and signs of shock demand vigorous treatment with intravenous fluids, volume-expanding agents, or drugs (e.g., dopamine) appropriate for the cause of shock. If the vital signs do not demand immediate treatment, one must assess the airway.

A patient in coma often has a compromised airway. In deep coma or bulbar paralysis the tongue may fall back into the pharynx, partially obstructing it. An oral airway device may be placed to keep the passage open. Secretions or vomitus should be suctioned from the pharynx to prevent aspiration into the trachea. Large boluses of solid food may be removed manually or by forceps under direct visualization. The patient should be placed in a lateral decubitus position to prevent aspiration of secretions or vomitus. Vigorous suctioning of the oropharynx should be repeated as often as is necessary.

The physician should *always consider intubation* once the airway has been cleared. Tracheal intubation protects the patient from aspiration of secretions or vomitus, ensures immediate treatment if respirations fail, and allows prompt hyperventilation if brain herniation occurs. Our practice is to intubate any patient with depressed consciousness if we believe the patient will not become agitated or combative because of intubation. However, orotracheal intubation should not be done if there is any suspicion of a fractured cervical spine.

If the choice is made not to intubate, equipment for intubation should be obtained and should be kept close to the patient. The equipment must accompany the patient at all times. Comatose patients have a disturbing propensity to stop breathing or develop brain herniation while in the radiology department!

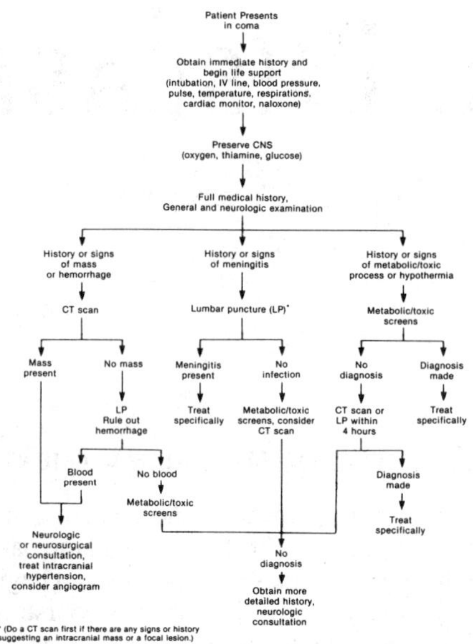

Figure 1 Early management of a patient in nontraumatic coma.

If the patient has obvious hypoventilation, cyanosis, or respiratory distress, ventilation should be begun, initially by hand and then by mechanical ventilation. Arterial blood gases are then drawn. If the patient is breathing adequately, mechanical ventilation may be deferred, but the patient should be continuously observed and an Ambu bag or other means of ventilation must be at the bedside.

Naloxone (Narcan) should be given to comatose patients with a history of known drug abuse, multiple needle tracks on the extremities, or suspected oral overdose of narcotic pain medications and to those with the clinical syndrome of coma, small pupils, and respiratory depression. The initial dose is 0.8 to 1.0 mg IV followed at 2-minute intervals by two additional doses, to a maximum of 2.0 mg.

Preserve the Brain

After the basic life support measures, treatment should begin for potentially lethal or brain-damaging, but easily reversed, causes of coma.

Intravenous glucose, as a bolus of 50 ml of 50 percent dextrose in water, should be given to any adult who does not have a clearly evident etiology for depression of consciousness. (Children should receive 25 percent dextrose, 2 to 4 ml per kilogram weight.) A blood sample for glucose should be drawn prior to administration.

Thiamine, as a 100-mg IV bolus, should be given to patients who appear to be malnourished, emaciated, or alcoholic. Wernicke's encephalopathy may complicate the course of a thiamine-deficient person given large amounts of glucose.

If the patient improves with these measures, the physician usually knows which step in the management was effective and so can make presumptive diagnosis and give further treatment. However, if the patient has not improved dramatically, the next phase begins.

Make a Definitive Diagnosis

At this point multiple laboratory studies must be obtained (Table 1), including a complete blood count, electrolytes, biochemical screen, arterial gases, routine urinalysis, blood and urine toxicology screens, and an electrocardiogram. Occasionally, determination of a quantitative blood level of a specifically suspected drug is helpful. Blood and other cultures, serum osmolality studies, carboxyhemoglobin and cyanide determinations, endocrine function tests, and coagulation studies should be done when indicated.

The physician should then turn to the detailed bedside evaluation of the patient with the specific goal of distingiuishing between a toxic or metabolic etiology or a structural lesion/mass etiology (e.g., brain abscess, tumor, traumatic intracranial hematoma, cerebrovascular disease, or acute hydrocephalus). The three steps toward that goal are the history, general medical examination, and neurologic examination.

A full medical history should be obtained from any possible source, including any available medical records and the patient's primary physician. Specific data sought are those listed previously (see Immediate History), but in more detail. Clues suggesting a structural lesion are a known systemic tumor (possible metastasis), history of focal neurologic symptoms, recent ear or sinus infection (possible brain abscess), trauma or alcoholism (possible subdural hematoma), and bleeding disorder, anticoagulant use, or sudden onset of coma (all three suggest intracranial hemorrhage).

The general examination may suggest a metabolic process (e.g., icterus), sepsis, or meningitis. However, specific clues for a structural lesion must be sought, including signs of tumor, ear or sinus infection, trauma, alcoholism, or bleeding disorder. The vital signs may also be helpful. Hypertension in a comatose patient, especially when combined with bradycardia, is often due to increased intracranial pressure from a structural brain lesion.

The neurologic examination is focused on three key issues: (1) carefully defining the level of consciousness, (2) looking for signs of either increased intracranial pressure or intracranial hemorrhage, and (3) seeking any significant asymmetry of the neurologic signs.

Carefully defining the state of consciousness helps to gauge the severity of illness and also documents a baseline from which the patient's course is followed. The physician should observe the best levels of eye opening, verbal response, and motor response. The level of each is carefully recorded in one's memory and the patient's chart. The best level is obtained by progressively stronger stimuli (e.g., do the eyes open spontaneously, or with calling the patient's name, or with shaking, or with a painful stimulus, or do they never open?). Both verbal and motor

TABLE 1 Initial Laboratory Tests for Patients with Coma of Unknown Etiology

Routine tests
- Complete blood count
- Urinalysis
- Serum glucose
- Serum electrolytes
- Biochemical panel, including calcium, hepatic and renal function tests
- Blood and urine toxicologic screens
- Arterial blood gases
- Electrocardiogram

When clinical history or signs are appropriate
- Quantitative serum level of specific drug
- Carboxyhemoglobin level
- Cyanide level
- Coagulation profile
- Thyroid and other appropriate endocrine tests
- Serum osmolality
- Blood and other appropriate cultures

responsiveness are similarly tested.

The signs of increased pressure or intracranial hemorrhage are papilledema, large retinal hemorrhages, increased muscle tone, and increased deep tendon reflexes.

Significant asymmetry of neurologic signs is sought by examining the position and movement of the eyes (either spontaneous movement or that induced by the "doll's eyes" or caloric reflexes), corneal reflexes, facial movement, limb position and tone, limb movement (spontaneous or induced by painful stimulation), deep tendon reflexes, and toe responses to plantar stimulation. Any clear differences between the signs on the right side of the body versus the left indicate a possible structural intracranial lesion.

The presence of clues of a structural lesion based on the history, general examination, or neurologic examination requires that the patient has a computed tomography (CT) or magnetic resonance (MR) scan of the head to confirm or rule out such a lesion. In contrast, the patient who is comatose, hypotensive, and hypotonic; who has depressed reflexes and reactive pupils; and whose neurologic signs are symmetrical probably has a metabolic or toxic process and probably does not need an immediate CT scan.

DIAGNOSTIC PROCEDURES

The next step requires a decision to admit the patient to a medical intensive care unit (ICU) for management of the presumed toxic/metabolic process or to obtain a CT or MR scan to rule out or confirm a structural lesion of the brain. If any of the preceding clues indicating structural lesion are present, a CT scan should be done immediately. If a structural lesion is demonstrated, neurologic or neurosurgical consultation is requested to assist in further diagnosis and management. If a structural lesion is not seen but there are clinical clues suggesting one, one must be aware of several lesions that may cause coma but may not be easily seen on a CT scan: (1) posterior fossa lesions, especially brain stem infarction or hemorrhage and inferiorly located cerebellar hemorrhage or tumor; (2) bilateral isodense subdural hematomas; (3) herpes simplex encephalitis; or (4) large middle cerebral artery distribution infarctions (when the CT scan is done in the first 8 hours). The clinician should carefully review the CT scan and should inform the radiologist of what is suspected. Usually such lesions produce some CT scan signs that are visible to the suspicious eye searching for specific lesions. An MR scan more effectively demonstrates these lesions. MR imaging is more sensitive than CT scanning for many processes, but its use in the acute evaluation of the comatose patient is limited by the extended time to do the required scan.

If the CT or MR scan is unequivocally normal, the physician should probably proceed to a lumbar puncture, especially if the initial chemical and toxicologic laboratory results are nondiagnostic. Examination of the cerebrospinal fluid (CSF) may show red blood cells (suggesting subarachnoid hemorrhage), white blood cells (meningitis or encephalitis), xanthochromia (intracranial hemorrhage or subdural hematoma), or elevated opening pressure (elevated intracranial pressure) that indicate the need for further diagnostic tests.

Cranial angiography has a limited role in evaluation of the comatose patient. If the clinical evaluation and CT or MR scan suggest but do not prove a vascular occlusion, cerebellar lesion, or bilateral subdural hematomas, an angiogram may be diagnostic. Also, if a CT or MR scan cannot be obtained and if 4 hours after admission the etiology of the coma is still unknown, an angiogram or a lumbar puncture should be done. This practice assures that the physician makes a commitment to a diagnosis of structural or nonstructural etiology and then proceeds with an aggressive work-up.

Skull films may show fractures in trauma patients. Isotope brain scanning has been replaced by CT scanning.

One strong reminder—any patient in coma with suspected or known trauma *must have cervical spine films* to rule out a fracture or subluxation.

SUSPECTED DRUG OVERDOSE

If, based on the history and clinical findings, an oral drug overdose is suspected, the patient should be lavaged with body temperature tap water or saline via a large-bore orogastric tube in the left lateral decubitus Trendelenburg position after the airway has been secured by endotracheal intubation. Adults and children over 5 years of age should receive 150 to 200 ml per wash and children under 5 years, 50 to 100 ml. After lavage, the adult patient should receive 1 to 2 g per kilogram of activated charcoal through the tube. The charcoal should be mixed with 30 g of magnesium sulfate. Children should receive the same dose of charcoal but 250 mg per kilogram of magnesium sulfate.

The results of the toxicology screens may help to determine the cause of the overdose, but the physician must be aware of the substances screened for by the laboratory because the overdose may be caused by a drug not detected by the laboratory's methods.

HERNIATION

Patients with focal mass lesions of the brain causing coma often progress to herniation of the brain. Herniation must be identified early and treated immediately to prevent irreversible brain injury or death.

The signs of herniation are best considered in two groups: (1) the general signs of impending herniation, and (2) the specific signs of progressing herniation. Impending herniation should be suspected whenever the patient's clinical condition is deteriorating, especially if the vital signs change, the state of consciousness declines, or any focal signs increase. Such changes should prompt the physician to watch closely for the first specific signs of herniation and to prepare to treat the herniation.

Treatment should begin the moment the specific signs appear. The easiest specific sign to recognize is the third nerve palsy of mesial temporal lobe (uncal) herniation. This palsy first appears when one pupil becomes slightly larger and less reactive to light than the opposite one. Often the pupil quickly enlarges and becomes unreactive, and the eye deviates laterally and down. The more difficult herniation syndrome to recognize is the central herniation syndrome in which both mesial temporal lobes and the hypothalamus herniate through the tentorial notch. Often the earliest sign is merely that previously normal pupils become small, remain symmetrical, and still react to light. The next stage is midposition pupils that are unreactive to light. Other herniation syndromes occur but are more rare or are less critical to recognize or treat.

Treatment of brain herniation begins with vigorous hyperventilation, as fast and deep as possible for at least 2 minutes. An arterial P_{CO_2} of 28 to 30 mm Hg should be maintained if hyperventilation is continued. The best route for hyperventilation is via an endotracheal tube, so one should be placed.

A bolus of dexamethasone (Decadron) 10 mg IV also should be given. This reduces brain edema in and around many mass lesions. Some clinicians also give furosemide (Lasix) 20 to 40 mg IV as a bolus. We do not routinely use this drug unless we believe the patient has a systemic fluid overload.

The next step is to give a rapid infusion of mannitol, 0.5 to 1.0 g per kilogram. If the patient's weight is unknown, a bolus of 75 g for a smaller patient and 100 g for a larger person can be used.

Using these measures, herniation usually can be reversed and the intracranial process stabilized for 4 to 8 hours, long enough to obtain a CT scan and a neurologic or neurosurgical consultation. During the subsequent hours, repeated boluses of mannitol may be given to reverse recurrent herniation. Other intravenous fluids should be maintained at "keep open" rates and the patient's head elevated to 30 degrees.

OBSERVING FOR PROGRESSION

Patients with significant depression of consciousness should be observed almost constantly until a diagnosis is made and definitive treatment begun. Unobserved patients too often are later found to have respiratory or cardiac arrest, herniation, seizures, vomiting with aspiration, or other major complications.

The important serial observations are vital signs (including temperature), level of consciousness, pupil size and reaction to light, extraocular movements, and limb movements and reflexes. A bedside chart of vital signs and neurologic observations should be kept. Such a chart can be maintained by the nurse or other attendant and is an extremely valuable, easily scanned summary of the patient's course.

SYNCOPE

PERITZ SCHEINBERG, M.D.

Syncope is a brief, temporary loss of consciousness caused by decreased cerebral perfusion. The term syncope is derived from the Greek word *synkope*, which means "a cutting short" or "pause." Indeed, it is a brief pause in the stream of consciousness. Synonyms include "faint" or "swoon," and incomplete faints with incomplete loss of consciousness (the state of presynocope) have the same qualitative physiologic basis as a complete faint. Syncope is associated with complete recovery, usually shortly after the patient assumes the recumbent posture, and the period of unconsciousness is brief, usually no more than 5 to 30 seconds. This definition excludes such rare metabolic causes of unconsciousness as hypoglycemia or hypoxia, but does include very brief episodes of cardiac arrest. Although we are far from having a convincing explanation of the physiologic mechanism involved in every instance of syncope, the key mechanistic words are *decreased cerebral perfusion*; "reflex" syncope, as in the reflex form of carotid sinus syncope, probably does not exist.

MANAGEMENT

There are two general principles that must be observed in the management of a patient with a history of brief spontaneous loss of consciousness. The first is to be certain that the episode was truly syncope and not epilepsy. The second is to discover the specific mechanism responsible for the faint because, as is the case in many symptoms caused by various etiologies, treatment is directed at the underlying cause while also protecting the patient from the consequences of the faint.

Akinetic epilepsy may resemble syncope, but it is usually more abrupt in onset and without the typical presyncopal feelings of weakness, giddiness, nausea, and dimness of vision and hearing. It may occur in any position, whereas syncope almost invariably begins with the patient upright. The return of consciousness is usually much slower in epilepsy, and the patients are often confused and drowsy, whereas the patient with syncope feels weak, appears pale, and has cool, moist skin. A detailed history from an observer is essential in this distinction, as is the clinical skill of the physician in interpreting the signs and symptoms of the episode (Table 1).

The underlying cause of the syncope must be sought and established. Unfortunately, such a quest is not always successful; no cause can be identified in about 50 percent of cases. If no cause can be found after a careful search, it is unlikely that the patient has a serious or life-threatening underlying cardiac or vascular disorder, and the patient can therefore be so informed. He should also be advised to take certain common-sense precautions at the onset of presyncopal symptoms in order to avoid loss of consciousness. These include either lying down or placing one's head in the dependent posture. Such maneuvers will almost invariably abort the attack if the etiology of the syncope is benign. The patient should also remove himself from a situation or posture in which loss of consciousness would cause significant trauma or danger. Extremely anxious and sensitive individuals will require reassurance, counseling and, occasionally, mild sedation in order to deal with some of the threatening circumstances that seem to provoke syncope. If the syncopal attacks are repetitive, the physician must continue to look for the underlying cause (Table 2).

MANAGEMENT OF INDIVIDUAL TYPES OF SYNCOPE

Vasodepressor syncope is usually a benign disorder, probably caused by subversion of the "fight or flight" phenomenon in circumstances of threat or stress. The usual stimuli are those that provoke fear (such as having blood drawn or being stuck by a needle) or anxiety (such as before public speaking) or anxiety compounded by physiologic stress (such as standing rigidly in a group). In circumstances in which the individual anticipated a problem, I have tried propranolol 20 to 30 mg or atropine 0.4 to 0.6 mg prophylactically with considerable, but not invariable, success. The patients require reassurance and common-sense counseling about the need to avoid provocative stimuli and to react at once to the sensations of presyncope by putting the head in the dependent posture. Beta-adrenergic blockers, such as propranolol, have been used successfully to combat or inhibit stage fright, which may lead to syncope. Their effect appears to be to counter the vascular and cortical effects of the catecholamine surge, which is common to circumstances that induce anxiety, and to inhibit peripheral vasodilatation. Atropine acts by inhibiting the parasympathetic action of the vagus, thereby preventing the bradycardia and reduced cardiac output that occur in patients with vasodepressor syncope.

Patients who complain of faintness on assuming the upright posture must be questioned carefully about medications they may be taking or examined carefully for one of the other potential causes (see Table 2), and the etiologic factor must be treated appropriately. Such patients must be warned to get up from a lying or sitting position slowly and to maintain support for a few seconds before moving. They should wear snug elastic stockings and, particularly if there is a protuberant abdomen, an abdominal binder or girdle. If the problem is chronic and there are no contraindications, expansion of blood volume by increasing Na^+ intake and/or use of fludrocortisone acetate (Florinef) 0.1 mg three times a day is often helpful. Ephedrine sulfate (40 mg) or dextroamphetamine (10 mg) is also of supplemental value, presumably by promoting peripheral vasoconstriction and helping to maintain an effective blood pressure. Elevating the head of the bed by 10 to 12 inches improves postural adjustment. In persistent cases, the patient's surroundings should be modified by use of heavy carpeting and by placing rubber mats or pads on tile floors and the bathtub or shower.

Patients with tussive syncope must be warned to sit or lie down during coughing paroxysms, because the prolonged Valsalva maneuver induced by coughing inhibits venous return to the heart and eventually reduces cardiac output severely. Severe venous insufficiency in the lower extremities can be successfully treated surgically or, more conservatively, by elastic stockings. There is some evidence that micturition syncope may be associated with hypokalemia and atrial fibrillation; therefore, patients who complain of this rare phenomenon should have a careful medical evaluation, including a 24-hour Holter monitor electrocardiogram.

Syncope associated with one of the cardiac arrhythmias requires sophisticated cardiologic management. The most frequent and serious of these arrhythmias are type II atrioventricular block and the sick-sinus syndrome. The former causes Stokes-Adams attacks, a form of syncope produced by temporary circulatory cessation. The attacks occur suddenly, without warning, and with the patient in either the recumbent or the upright posture. Presyncopal symptoms rarely occur. Such patients almost invariably have severe heart disease. The syndrome may actually be precipitated by acute myocardial infarction. The treatment of choice is implantation of a permanent cardiac pacemaker. Atropine or isoproterenol may be used to accelerate ventricular rate acutely and temporarily as a substitute for more definitive therapy. Since patients with Stokes-Adams

TABLE 1 Differential Between Syncope and Seizures

	Syncope	*Seizures*
Rapidity of onset	Usually slow	Abrupt
Upright position	Practically always	Any position
Prodromal symptoms	Giddiness, nausea, weakness, sweating, pallor, yawning, sighing, deep breathing, dimness of vision	May be a brief aura
Posture	Usually lies motionless, mild clonic jerks (rarely)	Tonic and clonic jerks or motionless
Loss of sphincter control	Very rare	Frequent
Vital functions	Depressed	Tachycardia, elevated blood pressure
Recovery	Rapid	Delayed
Sequel	Weakness	Confusion, drowsiness

TABLE 2 Types and Causes of Syncope

- Orthostatic syncope
  - Vasodepressor syncope (vasovagal syncope)
  - Defective vasopressor mechanisms
    - Drug-induced: ganglionic blocking agents, diuretics, salt restriction, phenothiazines, antidepressants, particularly tricyclics, LDopa
    - Poor postural adjustment
    - Decreased blood volume: hemorrhage, dehydration, Addison's disease
    - Diseases of the nervous system: diabetic neuropathy, other neuropathies, acquired dysautonomia (Shy-Drager syndrome)
    - Sympathectomy
    - Impaired venous return to heart: venous insufficiency in the legs, tussive syncope, micturition syncope, valsalva maneuver
- Syncope due to heart disease
  - Cardiac arrhythmias
    - Bradyarrhythmias: type II atrioventricular block with Stokes-Adams attacks, sick-sinus syndrome, ventricular asystole
    - Tachyarrhythmias: episodic ventricular fibrillation or tachycardia, supraventricular tachycardia
  - Aortic or hypertrophic subaortic stenosis
  - Miscellaneous: myocardial infarction, primary pulmonary hypertension, pulmonary embolism, left atrial or ventricular myxoma, tetralogy of Fallot
- Carotid sinus syncope
  - Due to hypersensitive carotid sinus
  - Due to severe carotid stenosis
- Extracerebral carotid artery disease
  - Bilateral carotid artery occlusion or severe stenosis
  - Pulseless (Takayasu's) disease
- Vagovagal syncope and vagoglossopharyngeal neuralgia
- Hyperventilation
- Hysterical syncope

attacks may faint without warning, special precautions should be taken to prevent injury while they await proper treatment of the underlying cardiac disorder. A lightweight padded protective helmet may prevent serious head injury to these patients.

Sick-sinus syndrome usually results from severe myocardial disease and is characterized by profound bradycardia with poor ventricular response to exercise. Syncope is a common complication. Such patients require permanent cardiac pacing. Both atropine and isoproterenol may provide temporary improvement.

Tachyarrhythmias are less frequently responsible for syncope and are usually easily identified. Patients with paroxysmal atrial tachycardia may require vasopressors to inhibit syncope during an attack. Propranolol, quinidine, or procainamide are useful in preventing recurrences. and are usually easily identified. Patients with paroxysmal atrial tachycardia may require vasopressors to inhibit syncope during an attack. Propranolol, quinidine, or procainamide is useful in preventing recurrences.

Syncope from aortic stenosis usually follows exercise and is often abrupt in onset. Diagnosis can frequently be made by the history of prior dyspnea and angina pectoris and by auscultation of an appropriate systolic ejection murmur. When prolonged, the syncopal attack is accompanied by convulsions. Such patients must avoid strenuous activity. The only effective treatment is surgical, usually aortic valve replacement.

Unexplained syncope may be caused by atrial or ventricular myxoma, which may act as a ball valve, temporarily stopping effective cardiac ejection of blood. Myxomas also produce cerebral emboli. Diagnosis can be made by echocardiography; treatment is by surgical excision. Medication is not useful.

Syncope from a sensitive carotid sinus is rare. The patient should be instructed to wear a loose collar if the diagnosis is suspected. Atropine may inhibit the attacks, but when it is ineffective, a demand pacemaker may be used or the carotid sinus can be denervated by surgery or radiation. In the presence of severe bilateral carotid stenosis, manual manipulation or compression of the carotid sinus region may provoke syncope due to cerebral ischemia. Carotid sinus massage as a diagnostic test should be avoided or conducted with extreme caution in elderly patients. Patients with bilateral carotid thrombosis or severe stenosis may develop global cerebral ischemia with faintness or syncope when they assume the upright position. Such patients may be candidates for endarterectomy (if stenosis is present) or extracranial-intracranial bypass surgery, although the efficacy of these procedures for this purpose is not universally accepted. Takayasu's disease may respond to steroid therapy, or a surgical bypass procedure may be considered.

Vagovagal or swallow syncope probably has the same mechanism as vagoglossopharyngeal neuralgia and syncope, such as pain or esophageal traction (i.e., some stimulus provokes a profound vagal discharge, resulting in bradycardia, hypotension, and syncope). Anticholinergic drugs (atropine, propantheline, trihexyphenidyl) may inhibit the vagal effect and resultant syncope.

Patients who hyperventilate to the point of syncope should be instructed to breathe into a paper bag when the sense of air hunger begins. Patients with hysterical fainting may require psychiatric evaluation and counseling. Fortunately, these patients never injure themselves.

VERTIGO

ROBERT W. BALOH, M.D.

An illusion of movement (vertigo) is specific for vestibular system disease. The most common illusion is that of rotation, although patients occasionally complain of linear displacement or tilt. The otoliths and semicircular canals of each inner ear maintain a balanced tonic rate of firing into the vestibular nuclei via their afferent nerves. Vertigo results from asymmetrical involvement of this balanced baseline activity. For example, damage to a semicircular canal or its afferent nerve produces a sensation of angular rotation in the plane of that canal. More commonly, lesions involve all the canals and otoliths of one inner ear; such lesions produce sensation of rotation in a plane determined by the balance of afferent signals from the opposite inner ear (usually near the horizontal, since the vertical canal and otolith signals partially cancel). If a patient with vertigo attempts to fixate on an object, it will appear blurred and seem to move in the opposite direction of the slow phase of his spontaneous nystagmus (i.e., away from the side of the lesion). This illusion of movement occurs because the brain lacks eye proprioceptive information and interprets the target displacement on the retina as object movement rather than eye movement. By contrast, if the patient closes his eyes, he senses that his body is turning toward the side of the lesion owing to the imbalance of tonic vestibular signals arriving at the subjective sensation centers in the cortex. An illusion of linear movement alone suggests isolated involvement of an otolith or its central connections.

Symptoms of autonomic overactivity (sweating, pallor, nausea, and vomiting) nearly always accompany vertigo. Occasionally, vegetative symptoms are the most prominent feature of a vestibular lesion. Numerous interconnecting pathways between brain-stem vestibular and autonomic centers account for this close association of vestibular and vegetative symptoms.

Unfortunately, the patient's description of vertigo does not clarify whether it is coming from a peripheral or a central vestibular lesion. For this, one must rely on the associated symptoms. Lesions of the inner ear or the vestibulocochlear nerve usually produce auditory symptoms such as hearing loss, tinnitus, and a sensation of pressure or fullness in the ear. In addition to hearing loss and tinnitus, lesions of the internal auditory canal are often associated with ipsilateral facial weakness, whereas those in the cerebellopontine angle may cause ipsilateral facial numbness and weakness and ipsilateral extremity ataxia. Because of the close approximation of neural centers and fiber tracts in the brain stem and cerebellum, lesions in these areas invariably produce many other symptoms along with the vertigo. As a general rule, repeated episodes of vertigo without associated symptoms suggest a peripheral vestibular lesion.

The first step toward successful treatment of vertigo is to make a specific diagnosis whenever possible. For example, specific therapies include antibiotics for bacterial or luetic labyrinthitis, salt restriction plus diuretics for Meniere's disease, anticoagulants for some varieties of vertebrobasilar insufficiency, and surgery for a tumor of the vestibulocochlear nerve. In many cases, however, specific therapy is not available and the clinician must rely on symptomatic treatment.

SYMPTOMATIC TREATMENT

General Considerations

Vertigo is a disturbing symptom that is invariably associated with some degree of fear and anxiety. Regardless of the cause of vertigo, the physician can help by being supportive and reassuring. Often the patient becomes involved in a "vicious circle" in which the patient's fear and anxiety result in hyperventilation that, in turn, produces dizziness and presyncope from cerebral vasoconstriction and pooling of blood in the lower extremities. Patients with vertigo often suspect that they have a brain tumor or another life-threatening neurologic disorder. In most cases these possibilities can be ruled out after the history and physical examination have been completed. The physician can then inform the patient that the condition is not life-threatening and that it can be treated.

Patients with acute vertigo prefer to lie still in bed in a darkened, quiet room. An explanation to the patient of how head movements and changes in position exacerbate the vertigo during this acute stage can often help relieve the stress and anxiety. The CNS has a remarkable ability to adapt to most types of vestibular imbalance, and therefore, regardless of its cause, acute vertigo usually resolves within a few days. Rehabilitation should begin as soon as possible, sometimes even during the first day. Since, as noted above, vertigo is aggravated by head movements, patients typically hold themselves stiffly when turning and moving about. They also tire easily during physical activity. Patients must realize that a gradual return to normal physical activity is vital to recovery. For the nervous system to recalibrate the relationship between visual, proprioceptive, and vestibular signals, repeated head, eye, and body movements are essential. Patients may drift into a state of chronic invalidism if they are unaware of this requirement.

Antivertiginous Drugs

Commonly used antivertiginous drugs and their dosages are listed in Table 1. The effectiveness of these drugs has been determined empirically, and it is difficult to predict which drug or combination of drugs will be most effective in any given patient. These drugs apparently act by suppressing the spontaneous firing rate of primary afferent neurons and decreasing the transmission from primary to secondary vestibular neurons, thereby decreasing the imbalance resulting from a vestibular lesion. As the complexities of the neuropharmacology of vestibular neurotransmission are worked out, more reliable antivertiginous drugs will most likely be developed.

I choose a drug or drug combination based on the known effects of each drug (Table 1) and on the severity and time course of the patient's symptoms. Acute severe vertigo is an extremely distressing symptom, and I find sedation useful during this phase of treatment (i.e., those drugs listed toward the bottom of Table 1). Each of these drugs has important side effects, however, and must be used with caution. Parenteral diazepam can cause respiratory depression and hypotension and therefore should be used in a hospital setting with emergency resuscitation equipment available. When nausea and vomiting are prominent, I combine the antiemetic prochlorperazine with an antivertiginous medication.

Chronic recurrent vertigo is a different therapeutic problem, since the patient is trying to carry on normal activities and sedation is undesirable. Of the antihistamines, promethazine has the most sedating effect and is therefore useful in situations in which moderate sedation is desirable. The combination of promethazine and the sympathomimetic agent ephedrine (25 mg of each) produces less sedation than promethazine alone and is more effective for relieving the vegetative symptoms associated with vertigo. Meclizine, cyclizine, dimenhydrinate, and scopolamine are all effective in treating mild episodes of vertigo. Transdermal application of scopolamine results in fewer side effects than oral use and is effective for relief of chronic recurrent vertigo. However, scopolamine does have significant side effects, particularly in elderly patients (e.g., mental confusion, memory loss). With a transdermal delivery system, scopolamine is gradually released through a microporous polypropylene membrane contained in a patch that is placed on the skin behind the ear. A small dose (0.5 mg) is slowly released and absorbed over a 3-day period. Transdermal scopolamine has been shown to be particularly effective in the prophylaxis of motion sickness. To be effective the patch must be in place several hours before exposure to motion.

Treatment of positional vertigo is difficult because, although the vertigo is very severe, it usually lasts only a few seconds. In order to suppress these brief episodes completely, the patient would have to be heavily sedated

TABLE 1 Dosage and Important Effects of Commonly Used Antivertiginous Medications

Class	Drug	Dosage	Actions: Sedation	Actions: Antiemetic	Potential Major Side Effects
Antihistamine	Meclizine	25 mg orally q4–6h	±	+	–
	Cyclizine	50 mg orally or IM q4–6h or 100-mg suppository q8h IM	+	+	–
	Dimenhydrinate	50 mg orally or IM q4–6h or 100-mg suppository q8h	+	+	–
	Promethazine	25 or 50 mg orally or IM or as suppository q4–6h	++	+	–
	Trimethobenzamide	250 mg orally or IM q6–8h	±	+++	–
Anticholinergic	Scopolamine	0.6 mg orally q4–6h or 0.5 mg transdermally q3d	±	+	Mental status changes
Phenothiazine	Prochlorperazine	5 or 10 mg orally or IM q6h or 25-mg suppository q12h	+	+++	Extrapyramidal
Benzodiazepine	Diazepam	5 or 10 mg orally IM or IV q4–6h	+++	+	Respiratory depression
Butyrophenone	Haloperidol	1 or 2 mg orally or IM q8–12h	+++	++	Extrapyramidal
	Droperidol	2.5 or 5 mg IM q12h	+++	++	Extrapyramidal

throughout the day, usually an unacceptable circumstance. The most common type, so-called benign paroxysmal positional vertigo, is characterized by short duration (usually less than 30 seconds) and decreasing severity with repeated positioning (fatigability). As the name implies, it is usually a benign disorder and is not associated with other symptoms. Most patients have a spontaneous remission within 6 months, although the vertigo recurs in a large percentage of patients. Once the diagnosis is clear, a simple explanation of the nature of this disorder and its favorable prognosis provides much relief for the patient.

Vestibular Exercises

As noted, the inner ears maintain a toxic rate of firing into the vestibular nuclei; this tonic activity, in turn, is passed on to motor neurons of ocular and skeletal musculature via the vestibulo-ocular and vestibulospinal pathways. Lesions that produce asymmetry in this tonic vestibular activity result in vertigo, nystagmus, and imbalance. Immediately after an acute unilateral peripheral vestibular lesion, the ipsilateral vestibular nucleus loses its spontaneous activity and becomes unresponsive to ipsilateral rotation. Animal studies have shown that the nervous system compensates for this abnormality in a predictable systematic fashion. Initially, the tonic activity of the normal contralateral vestibular nucleus is suppressed so that the asymmetry is diminished. Gradually, new intrinsic activity is generated in the depressed vestibular nuclei, and the nucleus on the damaged side again responds to angular rotation in both directions. The latter results from activity carried in commissural pathways between the vestibular nuclei, so that the remaining intact labyrinth can drive secondary vestibular neurons on both sides.

Clinicians have long been aware that vestibular compensation occurs more rapidly and is more complete if the patient begins exercising as soon as possible after a vestibular lesion. Controlled studies in primates support this clinical observation. Baboons whose hind limbs are restrained by plaster casts after a unilateral vestibular neurectomy show markedly delayed ataxia compensation compared with animals who are allowed normal motor exploration after an identical neurectomy. Squirrel monkeys given daily exercises in a motor-driven rotating cage compensate for unilateral labyrinthectomy faster than animals given no exercise. Whether vestibular exercises improve compensation for central causes of vertigo is unknown. If key structures in the compensation process are involved, little benefit from an exercise program might be expected. In fact, I have found that patients with central lesions often show minimal or no compensation.

The vestibular exercises that we use in our neurotology clinic are outlined in Table 2. These exercises have been adapted from those originally proposed in 1946 by Cooksey and Cawthorne. We attempt to retrain the patient's eye and body musculature to use vision and proprioceptive signals to compensate for the loss of vestibular signals. The eye and head movements listed under A are started as soon as possible after the acute vertigo, nausea, and vomiting subside. The exercises under B through D are then gradually introduced as the patient recovers. Three exercise sessions per day for at least 5 minutes are recommended. Patients should seek the head positions and movements that cause vertigo as much as can be tolerated, since the more frequently vertigo is induced, the more quickly compensation occurs. The antivertiginous medications listed at the top of Table 1 are used regularly during the course of exercises to make the vertigo more tolerable.

Grouping patients together for their vestibular exercises is ideal, since members of the group encourage each other and beginners are able to witness progress of long-term members. The rationale for the exercises should be explained to each patient, and each should be given written instructions outlining the exercise regimen. The exercises are usually continued for 1 to 3 months, and during this time the patient is encouraged to return to a normal work schedule and sports activities as soon as possible.

As noted previously, the natural history of benign

TABLE 2 Vestibular Exercises

A.	In bed
	Eye movements at first slow, then quick
	  Gazing up and down
	  Gazing from side to side
	  Focusing on finger moving from 30 to 10 cm away from face
	Head movements at first slow, then quick
	  Bending forward and backward
	  Turning from side to side

B.	Sitting Head movements as above Shoulder shrugging and circling Bending forward and picking up objects from ground
C.	Standing Eye and head movements, shoulder shrugging and circling as above Changing from sitting to standing position with eyes open and closed Throwing small ball from hand to hand (above eye level) Throwing ball from hand to hand under knee Changing from sitting to standing position, turning around in between
D.	Moving about Walking across room with eyes open and then closed Walking up and down slope with eyes open and then closed Performing any game involving stooping and stretching and aiming

paroxysmal positional vertigo is spontaneous recovery within months, although rarely the condition persists for years. Positional exercises can accelerate remissions of benign paroxysmal positional vertigo. For positional exercising the patient sits on the edge of the bed with eyes closed and tilts laterally to the precipitating position with the lateral aspect of the occiput resting on the bed. The patient remains in this position until the positional vertigo subsides and then returns to the sitting position for 30 seconds before assuming the opposite head-down position. This sequence of positions is repeated until the positional vertigo fatigues. The positional exercises are carried out by the patient every 3 hours while awake and are terminated after 2 consecutive vertigo-free days.

SURGICAL TREATMENT

The rationale for ablative surgical treatment of vertigo is that the nervous system compensates better for unilateral complete loss of vestibular function than for partial loss that fluctuates in degree. Surgical treatment is most effective in patients with unilateral vestibular lesions who have no functional hearing on the damaged side. Surgical therapy should not be considered if the abnormal side is not well defined or if the nature of the disease is unclear.

Severe vertigo occurs during the immediate postoperative period because the imbalance in tonic activity is increased, but most patients who follow the exercise program outlined in Table 2 can return to normal activity within 1 to 3 months. Ablative surgical procedures generally should be avoided in elderly patients because they have difficulty adjusting to the postoperative ataxia. The two main types of destructive surgery for vertigo are labyrinthectomy and vestibular nerve section.

Labyrinthectomy is useful in those situations in which no functional hearing remains on that side. The goal of a labyrinthectomy is to remove the neuroepithelium of the vestibular end organ. Trans-oval-window or trans-round-window exterpodions are simple procedures, but parts of the neuroepithelium are often left intact, which may lead to return of episodic vertigo. For total removal of the vestibular neuroepithelium a translabyrinthine labyrinthectomy is required. With this procedure the surgeon first performs a simple mastoidectomy to outline the three semicircular canals. Next the canals are opened, their neuroepithelium is removed, and the dissection is carried into the vestibule where the remaining neuroepithelium is identified and removed. The operation can be extended at this point to include section of the superior and inferior divisions of the vestibular nerve in the internal auditory canal. Major complications with this procedure are infrequent, since preservation of hearing is not a factor, the subarachnoid space is not violated, and the facial nerve is usually not exposed in areas where it is not covered by a thick sheath.

Vestibular neurectomy offers the possibility of preserving hearing, but the risks of complications are greater. The middle cranial fossa approach to the vestibular nerve is most popular. Complications of this procedure include trauma to the facial and cochlear nerves (hearing loss on the side of operation in 5 to 10 percent of patients), CSF leak, and subdural or epidural hematoma.

SLEEP DISORDERS

DAVID BUCHHOLZ, M.D., A.C.P.

In order to treat a sleep disorder effectively it must first be properly diagnosed. The initial step in diagnosis is to identify which of the four major categories of sleep disorders best fits the patient's symptoms (Table 1).

Disorders of excessive waketime sleepiness (EWS) present as difficulty staying awake during routine activities such as driving (causing swerving and motor vehicle accidents) and working (leading to reprimands and unemployment). Simple fatigue and lack of energy without an increased tendency to fall asleep do not signify true EWS. Depending on the cause, the patient with EWS may have no complaints regarding nocturnal sleep, or he may describe disruptions of nocturnal sleep that reduce its restorative effect, thereby leading to EWS.

Disorders of initiating and maintaining sleep (insomnias) are characterized by delayed sleep onset, frequent nocturnal awakenings, and/or premature final awakening. Despite these disturbances of sleep duration and continuity, patients with insomnia typically do *not* describe true EWS, although daytime fatigue and lack of energy are common complaints.

Disorders of the sleep-wake schedule (circadian rhythm disturbances) vary from minor shift of an orderly sleep-wake schedule (such as with "jet lag") to severe fragmentation of sleeping and waking (as in a bedridden patient without day-night cues). Patients with these disorders often complain of *both* EWS *and* insomnia because of the asynchrony between their sleep-wake schedule and the clock on the wall, which social pressure dictates that they follow.

Parasomnias are miscellaneous abnormal behaviors in sleep such as bruxism (tooth grinding), sleep-related seizures, and somnambulism (sleepwalking). Usually, the behavior is confined to sleep, and wakefulness is normal.

DISORDERS OF EXCESSIVE WAKETIME SLEEPINESS

General medical evaluation is essential to screen for conditions causing EWS, such as hypothyroidism, pulmonary insufficiency, uremia, and hepatic failure (Table 2). Medication side effects should be considered, especially with anxiolytic, hypnotic, antidepressant, beta-adrenergic antagonist, narcotic, antihistaminic, and antihypertensive medications. Chronic alcohol abuse and illicit drug use (such as marijuana smoking) may lead to EWS, and toxicologic examination of blood and urine may be indicated.

TABLE 1 Four Major Categories of Sleep Disorders

Disorders of excessive waketime sleepiness (EWS)
Disorders of initiating and maintaining sleep (insomnia)
Disorders of the sleep-wake schedule (circadian rhythm disturbances)
Parasomnias

Insufficient duration of nocturnal sleep is a common but often overlooked cause of EWS. Individual sleep needs vary widely over a range of 4 to 10 hours daily, so that a person obtaining 7 hours of sleep daily may or may not be getting enough sleep. A several-week trial of sleep extension (adding 1 to 2 hours of sleep per night) may resolve EWS, thereby efficiently achieving both diagnosis and treatment.

If EWS remains unexplained at this point, a formal sleep disorder evaluation should come next. In addition to a thorough sleep history, nocturnal polysomnography and daytime sleep latency testing may be indicated. Polysomnography simultaneously records cerebral, pulmonary, cardiovascular, and other functions during nocturnal sleep, and it is the only way to accurately diagnose and precisely characterize sleep disorders such as sleep apnea and sleep-related myoclonus. Daytime sleep latency testing measures the tendency to fall asleep during the day and provides objective confirmation or refutation of the patient's complaint of EWS. Normal, refreshed individuals take 10 or more minutes to fall asleep in bed in a dark, quiet room during the day, whereas patients with EWS fall asleep within 5 minutes or less. In addition, patients with narcolepsy usually have premature onset of rapid eye movement (REM) sleep during these brief daytime naps.

All patients with true EWS that is unexplained by known medical disease, medication, alcohol or drug abuse, or insufficient sleep should have these nocturnal and daytime sleep studies. Conditions such as sleep apnea have many varieties and many potential treatments; the best treatment can be determined only by detailed information obtained from polysomnography. Even classic narcolepsy with cataplexy is only an historical diagnosis without the confirmation provided by sleep latency testing, and the symptoms may be convincingly reported by a clever drug-seeking individual. Sleep disorders causing EWS *co*-exist with more than coincidental frequency, and a dual diagnosis of sleep apnea and narcolepsy is virtually impossible to make without sleep studies. Finally, assessment of therapeutic efficacy may be difficult when based on patient reports alone, whereas follow-up sleep studies can document improvement of EWS which may be essential in determining whether the patient can safely drive and operate machinery.

TABLE 2 Approach to Excessive Waketime Sleepiness (EWS)

Is the complaint true EWS, not simply fatigue?
Consider medical conditions such as hypothyroidism.
Consider medication side effects.
Is there alcohol/drug abuse?
Is nocturnal sleep too short?
Consider a trial of sleep extension.
If no cause for EWS is yet found, request formal sleep disorders evaluation, including nocturnal and daytime sleep studies.
Caution patients with EWS about driving, operating machinery, and using alcohol, CNS depressant medications, and drugs.

Patients with confirmed EWS should be cautioned about driving and operating machinery, and the physician should be familiar with local motor vehicle regulations pertaining to driving privileges for patients with narcolepsy and other causes of EWS. It is wise to encourage patients to pull over and take a roadside nap if they become excessively sleepy while driving. Alcohol, illicit drugs, and medications adding to the effects of EWS should be avoided.

The major sleep disorders causing EWS are narcolepsy, sleep apnea, and sleep-related myoclonus, and the specific treatments will now be discussed.

Narcolepsy

Narcolepsy is a partly genetically determined CNS disorder causing EWS beginning in adolescence or early adulthood. The EWS may be constant, or it may suddenly overcome the patient in the form of "sleep attacks." Half or more of patients with narcolepsy report cataplexy, which is sudden weakness without loss of consciousness, precipitated by emotional stimuli. A minority of patients describe sleep paralysis (a form of cataplexy occurring at sleep onset) and nocturnal hallucinations. The symptoms of narcolepsy are due to inappropriate intrusions of REM sleep phenomena into periods of wakefulness. Sleep attacks represent complete REM sleep episodes; cataplexy and sleep paralysis represent REM sleep–related limb muscle inhibition; and nocturnal hallucinations are dreams of REM sleep occurring during nocturnal wakefulness. Disturbed nocturnal sleep is common in narcolepsy, but it is an effect rather than a cause of the disorder.

The goal of narcoleptic management is near normalization of patient functioning with minimal dependence on medications (Table 3). A consistent sleep-wake schedule with sufficient nocturnal sleep and preventive daytime naps is important. The value of one to several brief daytime naps cannot be overemphasized. These naps "recharge the batteries" and should be obtained before overwhelming sleepiness develops. Ideally, a patient should routinely nap for 15 minutes or so during morning and afternoon work breaks and at lunch.

TABLE 3 Treatment of Narcolepsy

Maintain a consistent sleep-wake schedule, including preventive daytime naps.
Use lowest possible dosage of stimulant medication to treat EWS.
Encourage "drug holidays" to avoid drug tolerance.
Begin with pemoline 18.75 mg b.i.d., increasing as needed/tolerated to 112.5 mg daily in divided doses.
If pemoline fails, try methylphenidate 5 mg b.i.d., increasing as needed/tolerated to 80 mg daily in divided doses, and consider switching to a sustained-release preparation.
If necessary, treat cataplexy with protriptyline 10 to 60 mg daily in divided doses or imipramine 50 to 150 mg daily.
Consider the use of protriptyline alone for both EWS and cataplexy.
Avoid amphetamines.

The EWS of narcolepsy responds to stimulant medication. Such medication should be given at the lowest effective dosage in order to reduce risks of side effects and eventual drug tolerance. Side effects of stimulant medications include anxiety, restlessness, palpitations, and anorexia. Medication given too close to bedtime may increase nocturnal sleep disruption and thereby aggravate EWS. The likelihood of drug tolerance is reduced with "drug holidays," usually 1 or 2 weekend days each week during which the patient does not take stimulant medication. The patient needs to be especially careful about driving during drug holidays.

Pemoline (Cylert) is the best stimulant with which to initiate treatment. Dosage starts at one-half of a 37.5-mg tablet at awakening and at mid-day. Increments of one-half tablet per day should be added every several weeks until EWS is controlled or until a maximum of three tablets (112.5 mg) daily is reached. Reliable patients may be allowed to modify the timing of dosage depending on their schedule for the day, such as deferring the mid-day dose until mid-afternoon if a long evening of activities requiring alertness is planned.

Methylphenidate (Ritalin) is the second-line stimulant for narcolepsy. Dosage begins at 5 mg at awakening and again at mid-day, preferably one-half hour before mealtimes. Depending on response, dosage may be increased every few weeks by 5-mg or 10-mg increments daily to a maximum dose of 60-mg to 80-mg daily. The duration of action of methylphenidate is only several hours, and a sustained release preparation lasting about 8 hours can be substituted once the daily dosage requirement has been established.

Cataplexy and the other "accessory symptoms" of narcolepsy do not require drug treatment in most patients. Injury as a result of cataplectic falls is infrequent, and most patients learn to control the symptoms by a combination of avoiding provocative situations and stabilizing themselves at the onset of an attack. Disabling cataplexy is not usually helped much from stimulant medication, even if the medication controls the patient's EWS. However, tricyclic antidepressant medications such as protriptyline (Vivactil) and imipramine (Tofranil) are quite effective for cataplexy.

Protriptyline is a relatively stimulating tricyclic antidepressant, and some patients achieve control of both EWS and cataplexy with protriptyline alone. Because of this activating effect, protriptyline should be avoided close to bedtime so as not to increase nocturnal sleep disruption. Anticholinergic side effects are considerable and may limit the usefulness of protriptyline. The starting dose is 5 mg 2 or 3 times daily, increasing as needed and tolerated to a maximum of 60 mg daily. Imipramine is a more sedating drug and may be useful when given close to bedtime in order to relieve nocturnal restlessness. The dose begins at 25 mg twice a day and may be increased to a total of 150 mg a day.

No mention has been made of amphetamines in the treatment of narcolepsy because there is rarely, if ever, a need for these potentially dangerous drugs. Caffeine is also not an effective stimulant for most patients with narcolepsy.

Many patients with narcolepsy are undiagnosed for years and decades, and their EWS is misinterpreted as laziness and dullness. While some patients quickly acquire a new attitude and image following proper diagnosis and treatment, other patients need individual, family, and career counseling in order to overcome their "sleepy" past. Contact with other individuals with narcolepsy may help greatly, and this can be accomplished by writing the American Narcolepsy Association, Inc., Box 5846, Stanford, California, 94305.

Sleep Apnea

Sleep apnea is abnormal breathing during sleep characterized by breathing pauses longer than 10 seconds occurring more than 5 times per hour. Central sleep apnea is due to intermittent lack of breathing effort, and obstructive sleep apnea (the more common type) is due to intermittent upper airway obstruction. Both sexes and all ages may be affected, and the source of the problem is sometimes evident, e.g., a child with large tonsils or an elderly person with a brain-stem stroke. More often, sleep apnea is found in middle-aged men without apparent cause. Onset of EWS in middle age is more likely to represent sleep apnea than narcolepsy, that usually presents earlier in life.

The EWS of sleep apnea occurs because of nocturnal sleep fragmentation and hypoxemia. Other symptoms are loud snoring, gasping and snorting noises, witnessed breathing pauses, abnormal movements in sleep, and morning headache. Complications include hypertension, right heart failure, cardiac arrhythmias, sudden nocturnal death, and motor vehicle accidents due to EWS.

Complete polysomnography is essential in diagnosing sleep apnea and determining optimal treatment for each individual patient. If the patient is overweight, weight loss may be the only treatment necessary (Table 4). The benefits of weight loss in sleep apnea are not fully understood, and it may not be necessary to achieve "normal" weight in order to obtain substantial therapeutic effects.

Medication has a limited role in the treatment of sleep apnea. Protriptyline 10 to 60 mg daily suppresses REM sleep and may be useful in cases of sleep apnea occurring mainly during REM sleep. Progesterone and other central respiratory stimulants do not benefit most patients with sleep apnea. Low-flow oxygen delivered by nasal prongs at night may help in two situations: (1) central sleep apnea, in which improved oxygenation may lead to improved function of brain-stem neurons controlling respiration; and (2) sleep apnea with low baseline oxygenation, in which elevation of the baseline attenuates oxygen desaturation during apnea. Continuous positive airway pressure (CPAP) is a promising new approach to the treatment of sleep apnea. CPAP is administered through a tight-fitting facial mask and acts as a "pneumatic splint" to maintain upper airway patency during sleep.

Severe sleep apnea that is unresponsive to the therapies discussed above may require surgical correction. The conventional procedure has been tracheostomy with a valve for daytime closure. The tracheostomy creates a passage for air exchange below the site of nocturnal upper airway obstruction. A newer surgical approach is uvulopalatopharyngoplasty (UPPP), which involves removal of excessive soft palate and oropharyngeal tissue, thereby creating a more spacious and less easily obstructed upper airway. Surgery for sleep apnea should only be considered in consultation with a sleep disorders specialist.

TABLE 4 Treatment of Sleep Apnea

Weight loss.
Consider protriptyline, especially for primarily REM sleep apnea.
Consider low-flow oxygen at night in cases of central sleep apnea and low baseline oxygenation.
Consider continuous positive airway pressure (CPAP).
Consider uvulopalatopharyngoplasty (UPPP) or tracheostomy for severe sleep apnea unresponsive to other measures.

Sleep-Related Myoclonus

Sleep-related myoclonus is characterized by repetitive leg jerks during sleep. They take place in clusters lasting 5 to 60 minutes, during which the leg jerks occur about every 30 seconds. The recurrent nature of these leg jerks is very different from the occasional leg jerks that normal individuals experience while falling asleep. Sleep-related myoclonus is often associated with *restless legs syndrome*, that involves feelings of cramping and restlessness in the legs while relaxing in bed just prior to sleep. Sleep-related myoclonus may cause EWS as a result of arousal from sleep associated with leg jerks, leading to sleep fragmentation. Alternatively, sleep-related myoclonus and restless legs syndrome may present as insomnia with difficulty initiating and maintaining sleep.

Sleep-related myoclonus and restless legs syndrome have been associated with a variety of underlying causes, some of which are potentially reversible. Calcium and potassium deficiency, anemia due to iron and folate deficiency, uremia, diabetes, use of tricyclic antidepressant medication, withdrawal from sedative/hypnotic medication, abuse of alcohol and caffeine, and pregnancy may provoke sleep-related myoclonus. It also occurs in patients with neurologic disorders such as polyneuropathy, lumbar radiculopathy, neuronopathy, and myelopathy. Sleep-related myoclonus seems to have increased prevalance in patients with other sleep disorders such as sleep apnea and narcolepsy. In many cases of sleep-related myoclonus there is no identifiable underlying cause.

The diagnosis and optimal management of sleep-related myoclonus can be properly determined only by polysomnography. Evaluation should include a search for the associated problems mentioned previously. Any underlying cause should be treated, if possible (Table 5).

Medication for sleep-related myoclonus is indicated only if the disorder is causing substantial EWS or nocturnal sleep disruption. An ideal medication would directly suppress the leg jerks, but most available medications seem to suppress the arousal from sleep caused by the

TABLE 5 Treatment of Sleep-related Myoclonus

Look for and, if possible, treat any underlying cause.
Use medication only for patients with substantial EWS and/or nocturnal sleep disruptions.
Begin with triazolam 0.125–0.5 mg or temazepam 15–30 mg at bedtime.
If benzodiazepines fail, consider codeine 30–60 mg O.S.C. or propoxyphene 65 mg at bedtime.
Carbamazepine and baclofen in standard dosage may help.
Beware of drug tolerance and dependence, that may be avoided by use of "drug holidays."
For restless legs syndrome, consider light exercise before bedtime and quinine sulfate 325 mg at bedtime.

leg jerks rather than the leg jerks themselves. The medications are sedating, and as a result they sometimes exacerbate EWS (because of "hangover" effect), even though the nocturnal arousals are reduced. "Drug holidays" should be employed to avoid problems of drug tolerance and dependence.

A benzodiazepine is the drug of choice for sleep-related myoclonus. In the past, clonazepam (Clonopin) 0.5 to 1.0 mg at bedtime has been advocated, but newer, shorter-acting benzodiazepines such as triazolam (Halcion) 0.125 to 0.5 mg or temazepam (Restoril) 15 to 30 mg at bedtime are less likely to cause sedation the following day. Codeine 30 to 60 mg and propoxyphene (Darvon) 65 mg may be useful, and carbamazepine (Tegretol) and baclofen (Lioresal) in standard dosages have helped some patients. Quinine sulfate 325 mg at bedtime and light exercise before bedtime may benefit restless legs syndrome but probably not sleep-related myoclonus.

DISORDERS OF INITIATING AND MAINTAINING SLEEP

Unlike excessive sleepiness, which usually has a physical basis, insomnia usually has a psychological basis. Before concluding that insomia is due to psychological factors, however, other possible physical causes must be considered (Table 6). Use of medications such as corticosteroids and theophylline, withdrawal from medications such as anxiolytics and narcotics, and abuse of caffeine, alcohol, and illicit drugs may lead to disturbed sleep. Medical illnesses such as gastroesophageal reflux and carpal tunnel syndrome are often most symptomatic at night, and other medical disorders such as nocturia, paroxysmal nocturnal dyspnea, and pain may cause sleep-disrupting symptoms. Sleep apenia and sleep-related myoclonus, although typically producing EWS, may also cause complaints of insomnia.

Transient insomnia due to acute life stress is normal, but persistent insomnia lasting more than 1 month is not. Insomnia cannot be defined simply on the basis of sleep duration, because sleep needs vary from 4 to 10 hours among normal individuals. Insomnia, like pain, is a subjective perception that may be difficult to confirm by objective means. It is reasonable to define adequate sleep as that which restores daytime alertness. However, many chronic insomniacs are fully alert during the day despite

TABLE 6 Approach to Insomnia

Look for physical causes such as medications/alcohol/drugs, medical illnesses, and sleep disorders such as sleep apnea and sleep-related myoclonus.
Give sleep hygiene advice (see Table 7).
Consider a trial of sleep restriction.
Consider psychotherapy.
Use sedative/hypnotic medication only cautiously and briefly.
Consider antidepressant medication if depression is suspected.
Polysomnography is generally not necessary to diagnose and manage insomnia unless a physical cause of insomnia such as sleep apnea is suspected.

their complaints about disturbed nocturnal sleep. Some insomniacs have normal sleep studies despite the patient's claim of poor sleep while being studied. Other insomniacs have abnormal sleep studies that document difficulty initiating and/or maintaining sleep, although the cause of the problem may not be apparent, especially if psychological.

The most common form of psychologically based insomnia is a combination of personality and learned factors. For example, an individual who is by nature tense and anxious may develop acute insomnia due to a stressful life event. Even after the stress subsides, insomnia may persist indefinitely because the individual has learned to anticipate (and dread) difficulty sleeping, which is a self-fulfilling prophecy. Depression is strongly associated with insomnia and insomia may in fact be the primary presenting symptoms of depression. Some insomiacs require psychotherapy in order to resolve their underlying psychological problems, and others respond readily to sleep hygiene advice (Table 7).

A new approach known as "sleep restriction" is an attempt to alter the insomniac's attitude about sleep. If an insomniac ordinarily goes to bed at 11 PM but does not fall asleep until 2 AM, the individual is instructed to stay awake and out of bed until 2 AM. Instead of worrying about not being able to fall asleep at 11 PM, the individual tends to worry about not being able to stay awake

TABLE 7 Sleep Hygiene

Sleep in a comfortable place (quiet, proper temperature, etc.)
Keep a regular sleep-wake schedule. Get out of bed at the same time each morning.
Avoid naps. Substitute light exercise for naps.
Don't consume excessive alcohol or food close to bedtime. A light snack may help to induce sleep.
Avoid caffeine, which may have a very prolonged stimulant effect.
Put mental concerns "to sleep" by writing them down and setting them aside.
Don't lie in bed unable to sleep for more than 30 minutes. Get out of bed, do something relaxing, and return to bed only when sleepy.
Don't worry about the impact of missing sleep. In most cases, the mind and body will eventually get the rest that they need, and there seems to be little harm in the waiting.

until 2 AM. The bedtime is then gradually shifted to the desired hour of 11 PM as the patient's anticipation of difficulty initiating sleep is extinguished.

Sedative and hypnotic medication is intended for transient, not persistent, insomnia. Long-term use of these drugs leads to drug accumulation, tolerance, and dependence, and withdrawal can be very difficult. Nonprescription hypnotic medication is usually an antihistamine that causes drowsiness. L-Tryptophan is converted into serotonin, one of the neurotransmitters involved in sleep control; therefore, doses of 500 to 2000 mg at bedtime may induce sleep.

Benzodiazepines are the safest and most effective prescription medications for transient insomnia. New shorter-acting agents such as triazolam (Halcion) 0.125 to 0.5 mg and temazepam (Restoril) 15 to 30 mg at bedtime are superior to longer-acting compounds such as flurazepam (Dalmane) because of their relative lack of daytime sedation. A tricyclic antidepressant such as amitriptyline (Elavil) or nortriptyline (Pamelor, Aventyl), even at the low dose of 25 to 50 mg at bedtime, can be very effective, especially if depression is playing a role in the patient's sleep disturbance.

DISORDERS OF THE SLEEP-WAKE SCHEDULE

Transient sleep-wake schedule disturbances include jet lag and rotating work shifts. Jet lag is more troublesome with west-to-east than east-to-west travel. Moving east to west, one can fairly easily postpone bedtime the appropriate number of hours. Moving west to east, one must go to sleep prematurely, which is difficult, or reduce sleep duration, which leads to EWS. A short-acting benzodiazepine may help to induce sleep prematurely following west-to-east travel.

Rotating work shifts are a major public health problem. Shift workers may be chronically "out of synch" with respect to both their endogenous body rhythms and society's schedule. The disruption can be alleviated by allowing maximal time (at least several weeks) between rotations and by rotating forward; i.e., a worker on a 7 AM to 3 PM shift should next be on a 3 PM to 11 PM shift. If possible, the worker should maintain the same sleep-wake schedule for the full duration of each rotation rather than switching back and forth in order to synchronize with family and society on days off.

Sleep-wake schedule disorders often develop in hospitalized patients who lose day-night distinction. These patients should be kept awake and active during daytime hours in order to enhance nocturnal sleep needs, and hypnotic medication should be used cautiously, if at all.

Some otherwise healthy individuals have persistent sleep-wake schedule disruption because they are unable to reset their "internal clocks" in accordance with the clock on the wall. Most individuals have an endogenous sleep-wake cycle of *25* hours duration. This requires that a daily adjustment be made by each individual in order to conform to the 24-hour day. An individual who cannot do this becomes chronically out of synch with the clock on the wall, as he is relentlessly driven by his internal clock. Chronotherapy is a method of achieving synchrony of endogenous and exogenous sleep-wake schedules, and its long-term success depends on rigid adherence to the newly established bedtimes and waketimes. Chronotherapy is available at many sleep disorders centers.

PARASOMNIAS

This miscellaneous category of sleep disorders includes many unrelated abnormal behaviors in sleep such as bruxism and sleep-related seizures. However, three of these disorders are related, familial, and common: sleepwalking, night terrors, and enuresis. These conditions occur in children who have profoundly deep slow-wave sleep (non-REM sleep stages 3 and 4). During an arousal from slow-wave sleep, the patient enters an unusual state between sleeping and waking, and these behaviors take place in that state. Spontaneous resolution of the problem usually occurs by adolescence, and persistence or recurrence after childhood suggests underlying psychopathology.

Treatment in children should be conservative, such as avoiding sleep deprivation and protecting sleepwalkers from injury by locking windows and gating stairs. Benzodiazepines such as triazolam may be useful in difficult cases; these drugs probably function by suppressing both deep slow-wave sleep and arousals from sleep.

PATIENT RESOURCES

The Association of Sleep Disorders Centers (ASDC) is an organization devoted to the clinical study of sleep and its disorders. For information, the ASDC can be contacted at P.O. Box 2604, DelMar, California 92014 (619) 755-6556

FOCAL AND GENERALIZED SEIZURES

TIMOTHY A. PEDLEY, M.D.

There can be little argument that the majority of patients with epilepsy benefit from treatment with antiepileptic drugs. However, growing knowledge of the natural history of epilepsy, delineation of relatively homogenous epileptic syndromes, and an increased awareness of the often insidious long-term side effects of antiepileptic drugs require that therapy be introduced critically and individually in each patient. While this discussion is limited to pharmacologic aspects of treatment, it must be emphasized that this is only a part of what must be a comprehensive therapeutic approach to patients with epilepsy. Other, and at times equally important, components of treatment include recognition of environmental or physiologic circumstances that may precipitate seizures and attention to the psychosocial consequences of epilepsy.

Is It Epilepsy?

Not every paroxysmal behavioral event is an epileptic seizure. Other conditions, nonepileptic in nature, may cause episodic symptoms. A thorough and accurate history is the single most important part of the diagnostic process; the physician must elicit details that not only support a diagnosis of epilepsy but also actively exclude other diagnostic possibilities. Table 1 lists some of the disorders that may, depending on the age of the patient and the circumstances of the attacks, be confused with seizures. Review of an alternative diagnosis may also be necessary in the setting of intractable seizures, since apparent lack of therapeutic success using antiepileptic drugs is sometimes due to a faulty original diagnosis. In our video monitoring unit, for example, about 30 percent of patients referred for "intractable epilepsy" have been misdiagnosed. The vast majority of these patients have psychogenic seizures, but we regularly encounter patients with movement disorders, cataplexy, various forms of syncope, and transient cerebral ischemia as well.

THE SINGLE SEIZURE

Patients who have had a single seizure constitute a special group and one, I believe, that must be considered separately. In making a decision to treat patients with seizures, important factors include estimates of the probability and frequency of recurrence. Recurrence rates for single seizures are different in adults and children.

In adults, the recurrence rate varies from about 25 to 60 percent at 3 years. Recurrence rate is strongly influenced by the presence of a prior neurologic insult that may be reasonably considered causative for the seizures, a family history of epilepsy, and generalized spike-wave discharges on the EEG. In an individual with a normal neurologic examination, normal EEG, and no relevant past or family history of seizures, the risk for a recurrent seizure is probably less than 15 percent in the first year following the initial episode, rising steadily to about 25 percent at 3 years. Given these considerations, I prefer to defer treatment following a single ictal event unless the individual's circumstances are such that even one additional attack will result in consequences more serious than the estimated adverse effects of antiepileptic drugs.

In children, the overall recurrence rate for nonfebrile seizures is higher, approaching 60 percent with 90 percent of these occurring within the first 12 months after the initial attack. Recurrence risk is increased if the seizures are unprovoked (i.e., not occurring as part of an acute medical or neurologic illness) and if there is a history of neonatal convulsions. An exception is benign focal epilepsy of childhood, most commonly associated with a central-midtemporal EEG focus, or less often with an occipital EEG spike focus. Virtually all children with this syndrome do well, becoming seizure-free with or without treatment by middle to late adolescence. Since some of these children have only one or an isolated cluster of such seizures, pediatric neurologists are increasingly asking whether one or two benign focal seizures require treatment at all. Most physicians would still agree that when these seizures are recurrent, drug prophylaxis should be instituted.

CLASSIFICATION OF SEIZURES AND OF EPILEPTIC SYNDROMES

If a patient has had more than a single seizure, the recurrence risk rises sharply, to over 75 percent, irrespective of other considerations. In these circumstances, I virtually always recommend treatment, as I do following single seizures when adverse risk factors exist. Once the decision is made to treat, correct classification of the seizures is essential, since some drugs are *relatively* more effective for some seizure types than for others. A working classification is presented in Table 2. The most important distinction is between seizures of focal, or partial, onset and those that seem to involve the brain diffusely from the outset (primary generalized seizures). A care-

TABLE 1 Differential Diagnosis of Epilepsy and Episodic Symptoms

Gastroesophageal reflux
Breath-holding spells
Pallid infantile syncope
Sleep disorders (especially parasomnias)
Migraine (including confusional and basilar forms)
Panic attacks and hyperventilation
Transient ischemic attacks
Syncope and cardiac arrhythmias
Movement disorders (especially myoclonus and paroxysmal choreoathetosis)
Psychogenic seizures

TABLE 2 Classification of Seizures and Epileptic Syndromes

Epileptic seizures

Partial (focal) seizures
- Simple partial seizures (consciousness preserved)
  - With motor signs (Jacksonian, adversive)
  - With somatosensory or special sensory symptoms
  - With autonomic symptoms or signs
  - With psychic symptoms
- Complex partial seizures (with loss or impairment of consciousness)
  - Simple partial onset followed by impairment of consciousness
  - With impairment of consciousness at onset
- Secondarily generalized seizures
  - Simple partial seizures evolving to generalized tonic-clonic seizures
  - Complex partial seizures evolving to generalized tonic-clonic seizures
  - Simple partial seizures evolving to complex partial seizures evolving to tonic-clonic seizures

Primary generalized seizures
- Absence seizures
- Atypical absence seizures
- Myoclonic seizures
- Tonic seizures
- Tonic-clonic seizures (primary grand mal)
- Atonic seizures

Epileptic syndromes
- Neonatal seizures
- West's syndrome (infantile spasms)
- Lennox-Gastaut syndrome (childhood epileptic encephalopathy)
- Benign focal epilepsy of childhood
- Infantile hemiplegia syndrome
- Juvenile myoclonic epilepsy
- Idiopathic epilepsy, otherwise unclassified
- Symptomatic (or lesional) epilepsy, otherwise unclassified

ful history will usually provide clues to this differentiation, especially if attention is paid to the initial ictal symptoms and any localizing postictal deficits. Neurologic symptoms between attacks or findings on neurologic examination may also indicate localized brain disease. On the other hand, behavioral manifestations of the seizure reflect seizure spread as much as the actual site of seizure origin. Thus, a seizure that originates in a clinically "silent" area of the brain (e.g., rostral frontal lobe) may not be behaviorally evident until it has spread to other brain areas. Many clinical grand mal seizures are actually secondarily generalized partial seizures, a fact that has implications for treatment. Similarly, absence seizures may be a manifestation either of generalized epilepsy or of partial epilepsy. The practical consequence is that while carbamazepine may be quite effective in treating partial disturbances, including secondarily generalized seizures, it may actually exacerbate absence or complex absence seizures that result from a generalized disturbance. Therefore, final classification may require EEG data to supplement other clinical information.

In some instances, the seizures and their electrical manifestations are so distinctive that relatively stereotyped electro-clinical syndromes can be defined. Common examples of these are given in Table 2. Recognition that a particular epileptic syndrome exists in a given patient is important for both treatment and prognosis. One of the most commonly overlooked syndromes, in my experience, is so-called juvenile myoclonic epilepsy in which tonic-clonic seizures occur exclusively or most often shortly after awakening. Preceding the grand mal seizures, or more often occurring independently of them, are early morning myoclonic jerks that cause shaving cuts, falls in the shower, or coffee spills. The tell-tale myoclonic jerks are often overlooked without specific questioning, and carbamazepine or phenytoin is therefore prescribed for the grand mal convulsions. There may be no therapeutic response or an unsatisfactory response, and the patient is then either considered "refractory" or subjected to higher doses of multiple drugs. Correct identification of this epileptic syndrome should lead to treatment with valproate, which is typically of extraordinary effectiveness.

CHOICE OF ANTIEPILEPTIC DRUGS

Partial and Secondarily Generalized Seizures

The most common partial seizures, those with complex symptomatology, are discussed in the chapter on *Complex Partial Epilepsy*. Several antiepileptic drugs are potentially useful in treating partial and secondarily generalized seizures (Table 3). Carbamazepine, phenytoin, primidone, and phenobarbital appear to be equally effective in terms of antiepileptic potency, but differ substantially in terms of toxicity (and to a lesser extent in cost and ease of dosage schedules). I prefer to begin treatment with carbamazepine because of the lower incidence of side

TABLE 3 Drugs for Different Seizure Types

Seizure Type	Drugs
Simple and complex partial seizures	Carbamazepine, phenytoin, primidone, phenobarbital
Secondarily generalized seizures	Carbamazepine, phenytoin, primidone, phenobarbital, ? valproate
Primary generalized seizures	
Tonic-clonic	Carbamazepine, phenytoin, valproate, phenobarbital
Myoclonic	Valproate, clonazepam
Atonic	Valproate, clonazepam, carbamazepine
Absence	Ethosuximide, valproate

effects with chronic use compared with phenytoin and the barbiturates. At the least, carbamazepine avoids the hirsutism, coarsening of facial features, and acneiform eruptions that are so distressing to women, especially adolescent girls. I have also noted, however, that patients have fewer complaints of memory loss, a common symptom with chronic phenytoin use, especially after several years of therapy. In recent years, I have used less and less phenobarbital or primidone and now almost never prescribe these drugs as first agents in ambulatory outpatients. This is because of the high incidence of sedative and cognitive side effects of these drugs at therapeutic dosages and plasma concentrations, even in the absence of overt clinical toxicity. Careful questioning of patients on phenobarbital or primidone almost always reveals symptoms of morning or early afternoon sleepiness, times of being moody or depressed, some loss of mental sharpness at school or work, and occasinal inattention or forgetfulness.

Primary Generalized Seizures

Information as to the relative effectiveness of different anticonvulsant drugs is less clear for primary grand mal (tonic-clonic) seizures. The results of an ongoing comparative study may provide a more objective basis for making recommendations in the future. At this time, I use carbamazepine or phenytoin as drugs of first choice in patients who have mainly tonic-clonic seizures. Valproate is equally (or, according to many European authors, more) effective, but it also has potentially more serious side effects. Nonetheless, if there are mixed absence and tonic-clonic seizures or myoclonic and tonic-clonic seizures, I prefer valproate because it can often be used successfully as monotherapy in such cases.

General Pharmacologic Considerations

Monotherapy should be strived for, as two-thirds of patients can be optimally controlled on a single drug and only about 30 percent of the remainder will benefit from the addition of a second agent. Except for phenytoin and phenobarbital, most patients tolerate an antiepileptic drug best if it is introduced slowly, with gradual increments in dosage to produce a satisfactory clinical response or a high therapeutic plasma concentration. In adult outpatients, I start carbamazepine at a dose of only 100 mg twice daily and valproate at 250 mg 2 or 3 times daily. Although most patients will tolerate greater dosages, I believe it is important in building confidence to avoid side effects whenever possible at initiation of treatment. These drugs may be increased, as tolerated, every 3 to 5 days. Dosage intervals should be less than one-third the drug's half-life at steady state. Compliance is a problem for many patients, and it is the physician's obligation to provide education about the need for stable blood levels to achieve the best seizure control.

The widespread availability of reliable plasma concentrations of antiepileptic drugs has been a great benefit to management of patients with epilepsy. However, published therapeutic ranges are only guidelines, and some patients develop adverse reactions at low or "therapeutic" concentrations. Others benefit from "toxic" levels without developing side effects. As a rule of thumb, I advocate pushing the dose of a drug until toxicity appears if seizures remain uncontrolled. This is preferable, in my view, to substituting another drug prematurely or adding a second one to the regimen.

Antiepileptic drug levels should be measured when control is achieved or when side effects appear as a guide to future management. Levels should also be obtained to document compliance and a satisfactory concentration when seizures remain unresponsive to reasonable drug dosages at a presumed steady state. Levels must be monitored more frequently when two or more drugs are used concurrently, since interactions cannot be reliably predicted. I advise obtaining blood levels at the same time of day in each patient so that serial levels over time can be compared. It is usually most convenient to arrange for morning "trough" levels before the first dose of the day is taken.

Specific Drug Considerations

Carbamazepine. Patients, and many physicians, are concerned about hematologic and hepatic toxicity caused by carbamazepine. Both aplastic anemia and toxic hepatitis are extremely rare, and I have seen far fewer of these types of complications from carbamazepine than from phenytoin. Indeed, I do not believe that there is convincing information to indicate that either hepatic or bone marrow toxicity occurs sufficiently more frequently with carbamazepine than with other anticonvulsants (phenytoin in particular) to warrant regular blood tests on this basis alone. Furthermore, such side effects are idiosyncratic, and the usual monthly blood testing schedule is as likely to miss a significant alteration as to detect it. What does occur commonly in most patients treated with carbamazepine is a benign leukopenia. The white cell count drops after starting treatment, reaches its nadir about the third to sixth week, and then recovers (although often not fully) to pretreatment levels. The total white cell count rarely falls below 3,000, and the absolute neutrophil count, even at total levels lower than this, remains within a safe range.

Often overlooked are reactions due to carbamazepine's antidiuretic effect. Hyponatremia and lowered serum osmolality probably account for some transient symptoms such as weight gain, edema, postural dizziness, and, perhaps, some intermittent mental symptoms. Increased antidiuretic hormone (ADH) activity may pose a cardiovascular risk in some elderly patients, and pulmonary edema has been attributed to the drug. Awareness of this complication is necessary when the drug is used in patients with cardiovascular disease.

The most common dose-related side effect encountered with carbamazepine is diplopia.

Valproate. The major concern with valproate is hepatic toxicity, which may be fatal. The risk is greatest in children under 10, when valproate is used with other drugs, and in the first 6 months of treatment. Whenever possible, therefore, valproate should be used as monotherapy, especially in children. Hepatic toxicity does not correlate with plasma concentration, and thus maintaining low drug levels does not provide protection against this life-threatening side effect. I obtain liver function tests weekly for the first month of therapy, every 2 weeks for the second month, and monthly thereafter for the next 6 months. I warn patients to call the office immediately if they have symptoms of unexplained malaise or fatigability, vomiting, jaundice, or edema (especially of the face).

Other and unusual side effects with valproate, which should be discussed with each patient before initiating treatment, include weight gain, hair loss, and essential tremor. If unexpected sedation ensues or if frank encephalopathy develops, hyperammonemia should be suspected. Sometimes this occurs as a manifestation of an acute metabolic stress without other evidence of hepatic failure. Secondary amenorrhea occurs in a few young women, but is reversible. Nausea may be disabling with the valproic acid formulation (Depakene), but is substantially decreased with the enteric-coated preparation (Depakote).

Diurnal valproate levels are notoriously variable, and many patients have random levels of 150 μg per milliliter or even higher without problems. In the absence of dose-related toxicity, dosage need not be adjusted.

MEDICAL ALTERNATIVES WHEN FIRST TREATMENT FAILS

If optimal monotherapy with the drug of first choice fails, it is preferable to substitute another drug than to add a second one immediately. For partial and secondarily generalized seizures, phenytoin is a reasonable alternative to carbamazepine. For primary grand mal seizures, phenytoin or valproate may be used if carbamazepine is ineffective. If monotherapy with these drugs is still unsuccessful, I add methsuximide (up to 1,200 mg daily), clorazepate (up to 0.5 mg per kilogram daily), or phenobarbital to carbamazepine in cases of partial seizures, and phenobarbital or primidone to carbamazepine for secondarily generalized convulsions. For uncontrolled primary grand mal seizures, I add valproate or primidone to carbamazepine. Contrary to some authors, I do not believe that the combination of phenytoin and carbamazepine has any additional benefit compared with optimal use of either drug alone, and I rarely use the two together. Atonic seizures, often associated with evidence of a static encephalopathy, respond poorly to all treatment efforts. Valproate is probably the drug of choice, with clonazepam and carbamazepine typical necessary adjuncts.

Beyond these general guidelines, success with refractory seizures requires patients, frequent monitoring of antiepileptic drug plasma levels, and realistic treatment goals (e.g., suppression of major convulsive seizures but with the possibility of occasional partial attacks). Partial seizures associated with demonstrable brain pathology are always difficult to suppress entirely without unacceptable drug toxicity, and atonic generalized seizures are often refractory to the best efforts. Finally, when faced with seizures unresponsive to reasonable treatment, it is always useful to reevaluate the patient to ensure that the diagnosis is, in fact, correct.

SURGICAL OPTIONS

Intractable partial seizures may be amenable to surgical therapy even when the epileptogenic focus is outside the temporal lobe. The development of electrophysiologic monitoring techniques that permit delineation of functionally vital brain areas in relation to sites of ictal generation now allows tailored excisions to be performed in patients previously considered inoperable. In patients with generalized seizures, corpus callosotomy may be helpful in treating refractory atonic seizures or intractable seizures associated with an atrophic cerebral hemisphere (so-called infantile hemiplegia syndrome).

POST-TRAUMATIC SEIZURES

Depending on the type and severity of the head injury, clinically evident seizures are usually partial, secondarily generalized, or tonic-clonic mal without a clear focal origin ("symptomatic grand mal"). When a patient presents with post-traumatic seizures, the general approach to treatment follows the previously discussed pharmacologic guidelines.

The most controversial issue, and the one that generates the greatest variability in approach among practicing physicians, is the use of prophylactic antiepileptic drugs following head trauma to retard or abort subsequent seizure development. It is now clear that routine use of phenytoin or phenobarbital without controlling for plasma concentration has no effect on the frequency of post-traumatic epilepsy. Although there are animal data suggesting that early use of phenytoin suppresses development of an epileptogenic focus following experimental localized brain injury, this beneficial effect has never been demonstrated in controlled investigations in humans. Both civilian and military studies indicate that the risk of developing post-traumatic epilepsy is directly related to the severity of the head injury, that seizures occurring on impact are not correlated with later epilepsy, and that frequent seizures within the first few months after moderate to severe trauma are a good predictor of continuing seizures in the future.

In the absence of more definitive information, I believe that use of a prophylactic antiepileptic drug should be limited to patients with severe trauma in whom the risk of seizures at 1 year following injury ranges from 10 to 30 percent (or higher). Such patients would include those with persistent focal neurologic deficits, intracranial hematoma, and coma for more than 24 hours. In other patients with head injuries, I wait until seizures become overt before initiating drug therapy.

DISCONTINUING ANTICONVULSANT DRUGS

In someone who has become seizure free, the main reasons to consider drug withdrawal relate to actual or potential adverse effects. It is clear that some drugs produce subtle systemic toxicity that may take years to become apparent (e.g., the effects of phenytoin on connective tissue, the peripheral nervous system, and the immune system). Others (e.g., barbiturates) may produce insidious depression of cognition or alter behavior. The principal argument against discontinuing antiepileptic drugs, of course, is the very real risk of seizure relapse, which may have devastating consequences for some patients.

Only limited reliable data are available based on methodologically sound studies that provide guidance for physicians and patients about risk factors for seizure recurrence when drug withdrawal is considered. The best information comes from investigations of children, but because of the relatively small size of the study groups, the prevalence of "benign" epileptic syndromes in the pediatric population, and the discrepancies in EEG and seizure classifications between the two best reports, it is difficult to extrapolate these results to adults.

The issue is further complicated by longitudinal epidemiologic studies demonstrating that nearly two-thirds of patients followed for more than 5 years become seizure-free, apparently independent of drug treatment, for at least 5 consecutive years within 10 years of diagnosis. Once in remission, however, there is a steady attrition in the seizure-free group due to relapses. There is also complete lack of information about whether continued drug treatment guarantees continued freedom from seizures and whether "subtherapeutic" drug levels in seizure-free patients have any role to play in this regard.

At this time, the best one can say is that drug withdrawal can be accomplished safely in many patients after 2 or more years of being seizure-free; however, there is clearly a substantial risk of seizure recurrence, and the factors that would allow this risk to be estimated precisely are now incompletely understood. I do not aggressively attempt to withdraw drugs at any specific time, especially if there is no clear reason to do so. I do try to avoid long-term use of phenytoin and barbiturates, especially in children, and I scrutinize each patient carefully for evidence of subtle toxicity, seeking supplemental information from teachers, family, and work colleagues as necessary. I am more apt to attempt drug withdrawal in children than in adults, in patients with "idiopathic" epilepsy than in those with symptomatic epilepsy, and in patients in whom seizure control had been achieved easily to begin with. I use the EEG as one factor to be considered in making the decision; it is never decisive. I pay particular attention to disturbances of background rhythms and nongenetic epileptiform patterns, but this too is never decisive.

SOURCES FOR PATIENTS

Epilepsy Foundation of America
4351 Garden City Drive #406
Landover, Maryland 20785
(301) 459-3700.

COMPLEX PARTIAL EPILEPSY

ROBERT FISHER, M.D., Ph.D.

Complex partial epilepsy (CPE), previously called temporal lobe epilepsy, psychomotor epilepsy, or limbic epilepsy, is the most common form of epilepsy in adults. Approximately 60 to 70 percent of people with CPE can be managed satisfactorily by good medical therapy. An unknown fraction of the remainder can be treated by surgical ablation of a seizure focus. In practice, this success rate may not be achieved because of suboptimal management. Principles governing successful management of CPE are listed in Table 1.

SECURE THE CORRECT DIAGNOSIS

Conditions that may lead to a mistaken diagnosis of epilepsy have been discussed in the preceding chapter. Those most commonly confused with CPE are complicated migraine, functional disturbances including psychogenic seizures, hyperventilation spells and panic attacks, and occasionally presyncopal episodes.

The most useful diagnostic maneuver for CPE remains obtaining a detailed description of the spell. CPE consists of recurrent, stereotyped episodes of blunted awareness and either arrest of ongoing activity or substitution of normal behavior with repetitive automatisms such as lip smacking, vocalizations, slow limb movements, or other "robot-like" fragments of behavior. About 50 percent of seizures are preceded by an aura. Most commonly, this is a sense of visceral distress, nausea, and bodily tingling; sometimes the aura presents with distorted feelings, memories, or sensory misperceptions. Complex partial seizures last from 15 seconds to 2 minutes and are followed by a longer period of confusion. There may or may not be secondary generalization to a tonic-clonic seizure.

The EEG is a useful adjunct to diagnosis, especially if it shows interictal or, more definitively, ictal activity originating over the temporal lobes. If a routine EEG is negative, epileptiform EEG events may be observed by repeat studies, by use of special recording electrodes, by recording after 24 hours of sleep deprivation, or by extending the recording period with a 24-hour ambulatory EEG study. In the presence of a good history, negative EEG findings do not rule out CPE. Conversely, positive EEG findings in the absence of a consistent clinical history for seizures should never be grounds for treatment.

The distinction between seizures and functional pseudoseizures generally presents the most difficult challenge. Awareness of the psychiatric history may help, as may induction of a seizure-like event by suggestion, usually while videorecording the patient's behavior and EEG for analysis.

TABLE 1 Principles of Management of CPE

Secure the correct diagnosis
Investigate etiology
Instigate monotherapy
Start drugs slowly to avoid side effects
Aim for therapeutic effect or toxicity
Follow serum levels
Add another drug if monotherapy fails
Consider surgery if medications fail

INVESTIGATE ETIOLOGY

Complex partial epilepsy may be caused by a variety of etiologies: mesial temporal scerosis, hematomas, arteriovenous malformations, tumors, infarcts, encephalitis, meningitis, or granulomas. The most common finding in patients coming to surgical resection is mesial temporal sclerosis, but a search for underlying curable lesions with a contrast computed tomography (CT) scan is usually justified. If negative, repeat CT scans should be done when the clinical condition changes or the seizure control suddenly deteriorates. Magnetic resonance imaging (MRI) may prove more sensitive than CT scanning in identification of lesions. A lumbar puncture may be warranted, although its yield in chronic CPE is low. Other special studies, such as arteriography, positron emission tomographic (PET) scanning, and depth electroencephalography, are reserved for special clinical and research indications.

INSTIGATE MONOTHERAPY

People vary widely in the degree to which they are disturbed by complex partial seizures. Infrequent and mild episodes may not require treatment; however, the majority of recurrent seizures should be treated, especially if they are severe, frequent, secondarily generalized, or socially disabling. Once initiated, treatment should be continued until the patient has been seizure-free for several years and the EEG has normalized.

As discussed in the preceding chapter, initial treatment should be with a single medication. Often, a practitioner is presented with a patient already taking multiple anticonvulsants. In such instances it is usually more effective to simplify the regimen in the direction of monotherapy, rather than to add a new drug. Choice of particular agents depends very much upon side effects, convenience, cost, and familiarity of the drug to the prescriber.

In our seizure clinic the drug of choice for CPE is carbamazepine (CBZ). Before taking the first pill, patients should be aware of potential side effects. These are detailed in a prior chapter. A common error with CBZ is initiation of therapy at too high a starting dose. Dose-related side effects can be minimized by starting with 100 to 200 mg orally twice a day. Every 3 days, as tolerated, the dose is increased by 200 mg to 200 mg three times a day, then 200 mg four times a day. At this point, the serum level is measured, and hematocrit, WBC, platelet count, and SGOT are assayed. If the medication is tolerated, the regimen is usually shifted to 400 mg twice a day for convenience and compliance. Occurrence of side effects 1 to 2 hours after taking the pill (peak levels) or breakthrough seizures at the time of the dose (trough levels) may require more frequent dosing. Blood tests are regularly obtained briefly for 2 weeks, biweekly for 2 months, and thereafter every 1 to 4 months, depending upon the individual case. Therapeutic levels of CBZ are 4 to 12 μg per milliliter. The dose to achieve this level is adjusted upward or downward and may range between 10 and 30 mg per kilogram per day.

As with patients with other types of partial seizures, patients with CPE who cannot tolerate CBZ are started on monotherapy with phenytoin or a barbiturate such as phenobarbital or primidone. Dosages, serum levels, and major side effects of the commonly used anticonvulsants are given in Table 2. Special note should be made of the cosmetic side effects of chronically administered phenytoin and the sedative-behavioral side effects of the barbiturates.

The most common cause of treatment failure is poor compliance. Nevertheless, some patients continue to experience seizures with high-range therapeutic levels of a first-line anticonvulsant. Occasionally, supratherapeutic drug levels are effective and tolerated. In other instances, addition of a second or third drug is required. Our main second-line agents for CPE are valproic acid and lorazepam. Valproic acid is active against the broad spectrum of seizure types, including complex partial seizures. There is some feeling that its effectiveness in this seizure type may wane after 4 to 6 months of use. About 20 percent of our patients develop significant gastrointestinal side effects on valproic acid, even when taking the enteric-coated form of the drug. Valproic acid will regularly increase serum levels of concurrently administered barbiturates approximately 30 percent. Lorazepam is FDA approved for parenteral use in status epilepticus, but not for oral use in chronic therapy. Its action is similar to clonazepam, but sleepiness is less severe. In adults, we begin lorazepam at 1 mg orally twice a day and increase this by 1 mg per day every 3 days as tolerated to effect or to a maximum daily dose of 10 mg.

Other drugs, such as acetazolamide and methsuximide, are used in rare instances. With 20 available anticonvulsants there are over 1,000 three-drug combinations. Obviously, only a small fraction of these are useful in practice. In choosing the precise combination, it is helpful to ask patients and family which drugs have been most effective in the past. Flow charts should be made of prior anticonvulsants, available serum levels, monthly seizure frequencies, and major side effects. This practice is far more than an academic exercise. A reportedly "ineffective drug" may actually have been quite effective or inadequately tested.

In drug-naive patients we usually start with CBZ, and then add phenobarbital or primidone to the regimen. If this fails, we try CBZ and phenobarbital, and, if necessary, three-drug combinations such as CBZ + primidone + valproic acid or CBZ + primidone + lorazepam. Each combination requires a 2- to 6-month trial, depending upon the underlying seizure frequency. Patients often exhibit the "honeymoon" phenomenon, with dramatic efficacy of a new agent for a few months, followed by progressive deterioration in seizure control. If seizure control is obtained, attempts are made to taper the previously ineffective components of the combination. I never use four or more anticonvulsants; addition of the fourth drug mandates tapering of the presumed least effective of the prior three. In our experience, most patients who continue to have seizures on a two-drug combination that includes adequate dosages of CBZ are unlikely to be fully controlled on any currently available regimen.

Special problems are raised by a woman with epilepsy who is, or wishes to become, pregnant. Antiepileptic medications are believed to be teratogenic, but we do not know the relative contribution of medication and of epilepsy itself to the increased incidence of birth defects. We ask our female patients to plan their pregnancies and to alert us a year in advance. We then make efforts to taper medications or to switch to CBZ, which may be less teratogenic than phenytoin, phenobarbital, or valproic acid. If pregnancy is unexpected, an ongoing successful regimen of anticonvulsants should probably be continued in order to avoid the possibility of fulminant withdrawal seizures during a critical obstetrical stage. Actual decisions are made after discussion with the patient, family, and obstetricians. Mothers may breastfeed while taking anticonvulsants, because the amount of medication excreted in breast milk is small.

Patients who are not helped by the medical management detailed above are offered three options: continuation, with limited control of seizures; enrollment in protocols for experimental anticonvulsant drug therapy; or evaluation for possible surgery.

SURGICAL THERAPY

Surgical extirpation of a seizure focus is standard therapy and is highly effective in selected cases. This type of therapy is underutilized, but it should only be done at centers experienced in treatment of intractable epilepsy. It is always elective surgery, except when done to treat an underlying epileptogenic structural lesion.

The ideal surgical candidates are adults who have not improved with good medical management and who continue to suffer from seizures frequent enough to disrupt their life routine; there is no absolute number of seizures used as a criterion for surgery. Futhermore, a well-localized, unilateral, anterior temporal lobe seizure focus must be present, preferably in the nondominant hemisphere. Unilaterality of the seizure focus is documented by multiple surface EEG recordings showing one-sided seizure origin or by prolonged monitoring of implanted frontotemporal depth electrodes. Hemispheric dominance is ascertained by the Wada test, with speech and memory testing during transient inactivation of a cerebral hemisphere by intracarotid sodium amytal. MRI and PET scans are used more and more to localize

TABLE 2 Medications Useful for Complex Partial Seizures

Medication	*Typical Adult Dose and Range*	*Half-life (hr)*	*Blood Levels (μg/ml)*	*Major Side Effects*
Carbamazepine	200 mg q.i.d. (400–2000 mg)	10–25	4–12	Gastrointestinal distress, ataxia, blurred vision, blood changes, hepatotoxicity
Phenytoin	300 mg q.d. (200–500 mg)	22	10–20	Ataxia, cosmetic changes, rash, rare blood changes, osteomalacia
Phenobarbital	100 mg q.d. (64–200 mg)	72	15–40	Sedation, hyperactivity, confusion, mood changes
Primidone	250 mg q.i.d. (500–1,500 mg)	3–12	15–40	Sedation, hyperactivity, mood changes
Valproic acid	250 mg q.i.d. (500–4,000 mg)	8–12	500–100	Gastrointestinal distress, drowsiness, ataxia, alopecia, tremor, blood changes, rare liver toxicity, rare pancreatitis
Lorazepam	2 mg t.i.d.	10–13	?	Drowsiness, dizziness, behavior changes

seizure foci, but the ultimate role of these tests remains to be determined.

Different seizure centers employ widely varying surgical techniques. We use a modification of the Falconer en bloc resection of the anterior temporal lobe to a length of 4 to 5 cm in the dominant hemisphere and 6 to 8 cm in the nondominant hemisphere. We believe it important to extirpate the amygdala and the mesial temporal cortex. The importance of removing the hippocampus is less clear. Operative mortality and morbidity generally range between 2 and 5 percent. Properly selected individuals according to the preceding criteria can expect a chance for cure of 50 percent and for major improvement in another 25 percent.

SOCIAL ISSUES

Epilepsy is most often a medically benign and socially malignant condition. It is part of the physician's task to enlighten patient and family about the nature of epilepsy and to assist people with epilepsy in obtaining jobs, housing, and normal social status. Whereas a single seizure should not be labeled "epilepsy," definite epilepsy should not be mislabeled. Patients should be told that individual seizures do not lead to intellectual deterioration, insanity, or death. The prognosis of epilepsy is good.

Family members should be instructed about how to behave when the patient has a seizure. Panic is unnecessary. There is nothing they can do to shorten the seizure, and unless it progresses to a prolonged (e.g., 10 minute) tonic-clonic convulsion, they need not call an ambulance. The patient should be protected from falls, sharp corners, and tight collars. The mouth should not be forced open for insertion of matchbooks, pencils, fingers, or other objects. The tongue may be bitten, but never swallowed. Forcible restraint during the automatisms of partial complex seizures may increase agitation. There is little need to fear behavior during automatisms, because directed violence is extremely rare. After a seizure the physician should be contacted for an evaluation.

Patients and family often solicit advice about permitted activities. The goal should be maximal activity consistent with avoidance of personal injury. Contact sports and strenuous exercise are safe for people with seizures. Swimming is acceptable if provisions can be made for proper supervision. Common sense dictates limits on activities during which a seizure could be fatal, e.g., flying, rock climbing, or scuba diving. Moderate alcohol consumption is permitted.

People with epilepsy must be seizure-free for periods ranging from 3 months to 3 years in different states before they are allowed to drive. State regulations may or may not require physician reporting of seizures to motor vehicle administrations; however, physicians should always give their opinion on the safety of driving to the patient and document the discussion in the medical record. We believe that a 3 month seizure-free period is a fairly good (although not perfect) predictor of ability to drive safely.

Too many physicians assume that people with epilepsy cannot work. There have been athletes, physicians, writers, congressmen, and emperors with epilepsy. Employment should be encouraged. Discrimination in the job market because of epilepsy is illegal. We refer unemployed people with epilepsy to the Epilepsy Foundation of America (address below) for vocational evaluation, job training, or legal actions.

SOURCES FOR PATIENTS

Epilepsy Foundation of America
4351 Garden City Drive #406
Landover, Maryland 20785
(301) 459-3700

PRINCIPLES OF PAIN MANAGEMENT

RAYMOND MACIEWICZ, M.D, Ph. D.
LENNART MUCKE, M.D.

Approximately half of all patients who seek medical help have a primary complaint of pain. In general neurology practices, this figure is even higher and can exceed 60 percent of cases referred for evaluation. In most patients with acute pain, the correct treatment of a self-evident, limited disease process alleviates the pain. However, many patients are referred to a neurologist only after an initial trial of conservative therapy has failed. In these instances the symptom of pain itself must be carefully assessed and evaluated to interpret its significance and to establish an approach for its treatment.

SOMATIC PAIN

Pain can be a symptom of either somatic or neuropathic disease. Somatic pain results when a disease process activates nociceptive afferents in the skin or viscera. Somatic pain is usually easily localized and characterized when it involves the skin or subcutaneous tissues; on the other hand, pain of visceral origin is often poorly localized and may be referred to an area of skin supplied by the same sensory roots that innervate the diseased organ.

Somatic pain is a common experience and is not always associated with disease; the somatic pain that results from a new injury or illness is therefore generally familiar to the patient and described in the context of prior similar pains. Acute somatic pain is usually effectively relieved by a brief course of an appropriate analgesic.

Many acute somatic pains can be effectively treated with oral nonnarcotic analgesics such as aspirin 650 mg or acetaminophen 650 mg orally every 4 hours. These drugs have few side effects, do not cause sedation, and are not associated with tolerance or dependence. Other nonsteroidal anti-inflammatory drugs (NSAIDs), such as naproxen, indomethacin, ibuprofen, or suprofen, are also often effective for minor or moderately severe somatic pain; however, there is little evidence that these agents are clearly better than aspirin, and, in addition, aspirin is much less expensive. Acetaminophen and suprofen have little anti-inflammatory action compared with aspirin and indomethacin. Pain associated with inflammatory disease is therefore better managed with the latter drugs. However, the side effects of NSAIDs and aspirin, particularly dyspepsia, gastrointestinal bleeding, and inhibition of platelet aggregation, can limit their usefulness in certain patients; these side effects are not observed with acetaminophen.

Narcotic analgesics are usually required for relief of severe pain. We do not use low-strength narcotic analgesics such as propoxyphene or mixed agonist and antagonist drugs such as pentazocine. The analgesic effectiveness of these drugs is little better than aspirin, and the frequency of side effects is much greater. Mixed agonist and antagonist drugs can also precipitate withdrawal symptoms in patients habituated to stronger narcotics.

We begin narcotic therapy with an intermediate-strength narcotic such as codeine 30 mg or oxycodone 5 mg every 4 to 6 hours. In oral doses, codeine is relatively safe, potent, and well tolerated. Aspirin or acetaminophen potentiates the analgesic effect of codeine; therefore, the two drugs can be used together. Oxycodone 5 mg is commonly available only in tablet form combined with aspirin or acetaminophen. However, if codeine 60 mg (or oxycodone 10 mg) orally every 4 hours fails to provide relief, it should be discontinued, as larger doses of codeine increase the frequency of side effects without clearly adding to analgesic effectiveness. In these situations codeine should be stopped and a higher potency narcotic used, such as intramuscular morphine 10 mg every 4 hours or oral hydromorphone 4 mg every 3 to 4 hours. There is substantial variation in the effective analgesic dose and the duration of action of narcotics in individual patients. Dosages should therefore be individualized according to the patient's needs.

Constipation is the most common side effect of narcotics. This can be a significant problem and should be anticipated with an appropriate bowel regimen. Other side effects of narcotics include nausea, urinary retention, respiratory depression, and sedation. In patients with severe hepatobiliary disease, it may be wise to recheck amylase and lipase levels 24 hours after the start of narcotics or to avoid narcotics altogether if possible. Frequent monitoring of vital signs, pulmonary vital capacity, and arterial blood gases should be carried out in patients on high doses of narcotics who have underlying cardiovascular or respiratory problems. Routine use of incentive spirometry and chest physical therapy can help prevent atelectasis.

A more common problem is underutilization of analgesics. Hospitalized patients, including postoperative and cancer patients, frequently receive inadequate doses of narcotics. The reasons that underlie inadequate narcotic use in patients with evident painful disease are unclear. Concerns about inducing dependence and addiction in a medically ill population are largely unfounded. Similarly, concerns about respiratory depression and delayed recovery in patients on narcotics are often overstated. More often, *inadequate* analgesia in postoperative patients produces a reduction in tidal volume due to splinting and delays mobilization of the patient. When indicated, therefore, narcotic analgesics should be given frequently enough and in high enough doses to alleviate pain. A single narcotic medication should be offered the patient on a routine rather than an "as needed" basis, with the understanding that the patient can refuse the drug if the level of analgesia is sufficient. Changes in analgesic dosages and the need to taper narcotics as the acute phase of pain passes should be understood by the patient.

The pharmacokinetics of narcotics are greatly influenced by disease. Hepatic cirrhosis or renal failure can enhance the bioavailability and decrease the elimination of narcotics. This is a particular problem with meperidine. In debilitated patients receiving high doses of meperidine, the active metabolite normeperidine can accumulate, resulting in symptoms of tremor, confusion, and seizures. Morphine may be a superior drug to use when long-term large doses of narcotics are required in debilitated patients. The pharmacokinetics of morphine do not appear to be altered in patients with cirrhosis.

A variety of drugs, including antihistamines, amphetamines, and antidepressants, may enchance the analgesic effects of narcotics and can be useful in certain situations. Oral hydroxyzine 25 mg 4 times daily can potentiate narcotic analgesia and decrease associated nausea without adding to the sedative effects. In aptients who are excessively sedated by narcotics, oral dextroamphetamine (Dexedrine) 5 mg twice daily can make the patient more alert while enhancing analgesia. Benzodiazepines and phenothiazines have numerous side effects and do not enhance analgesia; they should not be used as narcotic adjuvants.

The various types of analgesics, including doses and intervals, are listed in Table 1.

Chronic diseases usually cause recurrent episodes of acute pain rather than continuous discomfort. The management of acute painful exacerbations should be the same as the treatment of any new acute pain. Analgesics should be available to the patient when pain is present, with the understanding between patient and physician that the drugs will be discontinued as the acute episode subsides. In a small group of patients, however, psychological and social factors significantly contribute to pain complaints, making evaluation and management difficult. The approach to such patients with chronic pain is considered below.

CANCER PAIN

Patients with terminal diseases such as metastatic cancer often suffer from continuous or recurrent acute pain. In such patients, tolerance to medications can become an important factor. Although the underlying disease process remains essentially unchanged, increasing doses of narcotic analgesics may be necessary in such patients to maintain satisfactory analgesia. The rate at which patients clinically develop tolerance to narcotics is variable; some patients require a doubling of their dose as often as every 1 to 2 weeks. There is no absolute tolerance barrier, however, and patients who develop tolerance to even very high doses of narcotics can still achieve analgesia by doubling or tripling their medication dosage. Although tolerance is an important issue, it should also be emphasized that most cancer patients develop tolerance only gradually and remain responsive to relatively low doses of narcotics throughout the course of their disease.

In outpatients with somatic pain due to cancer, we usually begin with oral oxycodone 5 mg and acetaminophen 325 mg as needed to control pain. Patients with bony metastases often benefit from the addition of an NSAID, such as oral naproxen 500 mg twice daily. When a patient's pain is unrelieved by a total daily dose of 30 to 40 mg of oxycodone, the oxycodone is stopped and the patient is given either oral hydromorphone 4 mg or levorphanol 2 mg as needed; levorphanol has a longer duration of action than hydromorphone. Methadone has a very long half-life and may therefore be more useful in individual patients; however, the cumulative effects of methadone over many days require careful follow-up monitoring of patients.

As narcotic doses are increased, the frequency of other side effects, including sedation and dysphoric reactions, may also increase. When these side effects limit the use of analgesics or require administration of continuous intravenous narcotics, other approaches to pain relief are worth considering. For example, morphine injections through spinal epidural or intrathecal catheters can provide substantial analgesia, potentially minimizing some of the side effects of large systemic doses of narcotics. Several systems are now available that allow patients to continue administering their own intrathecal morphine injections at home. The success rate and long-term effects of this treatment are currently under evaluation at many centers. An anterolateral cordotomy can also provide effective relief in patients with pain that is isolated to a single leg or hip. Touch sensation, motor power, and bladder control are all usually spared by the procedure. Cordotomy is less effective in patients with pain involving an upper extremity or both sides of the trunk. In evaluating patients for this procedure, the extent of disease may be as important as the location of pain. A patient with unilateral pain but evidence of bilateral or midline disease (such as extensive vertebral metastases) is not likely to get substantial relief from a cordotomy.

For most cancer patients, however, surgical pain-relieving procedures are unnecessary. Usually a change in drug or dosage or the addition of an adjuvant analgesic can improve pain releif while minimizing adverse reactions.

NEUROPATHIC PAIN

Pain can result not only from somatic disease, but also from injury to or chronic changes in peripheral or central somatosensory pathways. Damage to a peripheral nerve by trauma or disease can result in neuroma formation or chronic neuralgia, with associated pain in the distribution of the affected nerve. The pain is often (but not always) accompanied by signs of nerve dysfunction. The quality of the pain can be highly variable. In some forms of neuralgia (such as trigeminal neuralgia) ''electric,'' lancinating pain predominates; in other conditions (such as causalgia) the pain is constant, dull, and burning.

Pain may also be a debilitating symptom following damage to central somatosensory pathways. Lesions of the ascending somatosensory pathways at the level of the cord, brain stem, thalamus, or cortex can result in a syndrome of continuous spontaneous pain that is referred to the periphery, often with superimposed sensory abnormalities.

TABLE 1 Classification of Drugs Indicating Usual Doses and Intervals

Non-narcotic Analgesics

Generic Name	*p.o. Dose (mg)*	*Interval*	*Comments*
Acetylsalicylic acid	650	q4h	Enteric-coated preparations available
Acetaminophen	650	q4h	Side effects uncommon
Ibuprofen	400	q4–6h	
Naproxen	250–500	q12h	Delayed effects may be due to long half-life
Suprofen	200	q6h	Little anti-inflammatory effect
Indomethacin	25–50	q8h	Gastrointestinal side effects common

Narcotic Analgesics

Generic name	*Parenteral Dose and Interval (mg)*	*p.o. Dose and Interval (mg)*	*Comments*
Codeine	30–60 q4h	30–60 q4h	Nausea common
Oxycodone	—	5–10 q4–6h	Usually available only combined with acetaminophen or aspirin
Morphine	10 q4h	60 q4h	
Hydromorphone	1–2 q4h	2–4 q4h	Shorter acting than morphine sulfate
Levorphanol	2 q6–8h	4 q6–8h	Longer acting than morphine sulfate; absorbed well p.o.
Methadone	10 q6–8h	20 q6–8h	Delayed sedation due to long half-life
Meperidine	75–100 q3–4h	300 q4h	Poorly absorbed p.o.; normeperidine is a toxic metabolite

Anticonvulsants

Generic Name	*p.o. Dose (mg)*	*Interval*
Phenytoin	100	q6–8h
Carbamazepine	200–300	q6h
Clonazepam	1	q6h

Tricyclic Antidepressants

Generic Name	*Uptake Blockade*		*Sedative Potency*	*Anticholinergic Potency*	*Orthostatic Hypotension*	*Cardiac Arrhythmia*	*Dose (mg/day)*	*Range (ng/100 ml)*
	*5HT**	*NE†*						
Doxepin	++	+	High	Moderate	Moderate	Less	200	75–400
Amitriptyline	++++	++	High	Highest	Moderate	Yes	150	75–300
Imipramine	++++	++	Moderate	Moderate	High	Yes	200	75–400
Nortriptyline	+++	++	Moderate	Moderate	Low	Yes	100	40–150
Desipramine	+++	++++	Low	Low	Low	Yes	150	75–300

* 5 = Hydroxytryptamine (serotonin).
† Norepinephrine.

The medical management of neuropathic pain is disappointing; patients rarely achieve substantial, lasting improvement with any single therapy. Standard narcotic and non-narcotic analgesics are often only minimally effective and should be avoided when possible. In this setting, patients frequently use narcotics for their sedative effects rather than their analgesic properties and request higher doses of medication in the hope of achieving analgesia. Patients with neuropathic pain are usually better managed with anticonvulsant and antidepressant medications than with narcotics.

Anticonvulsants

Anticonvulsants such as phenytoin, carbamazepine, and clonazepam are often effective in treating the sharp, lancinating pain associated with focal neuralgias, such as trigeminal neuralgia. They are less effective for the more constant, dull, burning sensations that are a major component of conditions such as postherpetic neuralgia or diabetic neuropathy. We usually begin patients on oral phenytoin 100 mg 3 to 4 times daily, since this drug is well tolerated and inexpensive. Gingival hypertrophy, adenopathy, and skin rashes are side effects that should be watched for.

If patients are not helped by phenytoin, we switch them to carbamazepine, which may more effectively control neuropathic pain. Carbamazepine can be associated with numerous side effects. The most common ones (gastrointestinal upset and sedation) may be diminished by gradually increasing the dose, beginning gradually with 100 mg daily and increasing the amount until patients are taking 800 to 1,200 mg daily. Since bone marrow suppression and hepatic damage may occur with carbamazepine and phenytoin, we check blood counts and liver function tests at the beginning of treatment and periodically thereafter. Patients should be warned about the signs of agranulocytosis, and drug levels should be kept under 12 ng per milliliter for carbamazepine and 20 ng per milliliter for phenytoin.

Patients who are not helped by or cannot tolerate carbamazepine are switched to oral clonazepam in gradually increasing doses until they are taking a total of 4 mg daily. The major side effect of clonazepam is sedation, although a variety of other adverse reactions occur rarely. We check blood counts and liver function tests periodically in patients taking clonazepam.

Tricyclic Antidepressants

Antidepressant drugs are frequently used to treat pain following peripheral nerve injury. Although their site of action for pain relief is not clear, it is not simply due to relief of coexisting clinical depression. Antidepressants may be superior to anticonvulsants for management of the spontaneous, dull, burning pain that characterizes many neuropathies. We usually use oral doxepin 50 mg daily in gradually increasing doses until the patient is taking 150 to 200 mg. Since the medication can be sedating, we give the full dose at bedtime. When patients are taking the full dose, we usually obtain a serum doxepin level. If the combined level of doxepin and desmethyldoxepin is less than 150 ng per 100 milliliters, we will increase the doxepin dose if the patient is free of side effects.

At the present time, there is no strong evidence that one antidepressant is superior to another in pain management. The choice of drug should be dictated by the physician's clinical experience and the profile of side effects of the different tricyclics.

Antisympathetic Agents

In some patients, injury to a nerve can result in "causalgia," a syndrome of spontaneous burning pain associated with sympathetic dysfunction in the affected limb. Causalgia may be a distinct form of sympathetic dystrophy, and the pain in this disorder may be induced by sympathetic hyperactivity in the affected limb. Sympathectomy by either surgery or local anesthetic block frequently relieves the pain in causalgia, and, in the opinion of a number of authors, pain relief by sympathetic block is an essential part of the diagnosis.

Since the clinical presentation in causalgia is often highly variable, we routinely use stellate or lumbar local anesthetic sympathetic blocks to evaluate patients with burning neuropathic pain confined to a limb. Such blocks should be performed by an anesthesiologist or other specialist skilled in these techniques. Patients who have pain relief associated with this "test" sympathetic block are then given a course of sympathetic blocks coordinated with a program of physical therapy. Oral antisympathetic agents such as guanethidine 10 mg twice daily or phenoxybenzamine 10 mg 4 times daily may also be helpful. Since these drugs can induce postural hypotension, they should be instituted slowly and monitored carefully. The use of sympathetic blocks, physical therapy, and oral antisympathetic agents often results in a prolonged reduction in pain with an associated increase in functional ability.

In patients who clearly respond to sympathetic blocks but then quickly relapse, a regional intravenous guanethidine block may provide extended relief. This procedure depletes sympathetic terminals in the painful limb, producing an extended "chemical sympathectomy." Intravenous guanethindine is an investigational drug at present and is only available at pain treatment centers. Even in this group, however, a small number of patients remain who require surgical sympathectomy to maintain a good response.

Transcutaneous Electrical Nerve Stimulation (TENS)

Electrical stimulation with a TENS unit applied to the painful region or over the proximal nerve may provide substantial pain relief in patients with painful nerve injuries. TENS may also be useful in a variety of somatic pain problems, such as low back pain or surgical incisional pain. However, the duration of the effect is usually limited to the period of stimulation. After a period of days to months, the analgesic response to TENS habituates in many patients, and electrical stimulation may actually increase the patient's pain.

CHRONIC PAIN

Unrelieved pain that continues to be a major, disabling condition for more than 6 months is usually referred to as "chronic" pain. Patients with chronic pain often present special problems in evaluation and management.

Psychological Aspects of Chronic Pain

In patients with chronic pain there is often little correlation between the severity of disease (as determined by objective tests) and the amount of pain behavior. Social and psychological factors may exacerbate pain complaints in such patients. An evaluation by a psychiatrist is therefore part of the full work-up of most patients with chronic pain whom we see. Psycological tests, including the Minnesota Multiphasic Personality Profile, can form an important part of this evaluation.

Although there are a variety of studies of psychological profiles of patients with chronic pain, there is little agreement about the frequency or nature of psychological diagnoses associated with chronic pain syndromes. Depressive symptoms are common, however, in patients with chronic pain, and a diagnosis of clinical depression can be made in approximately one-third of patients. The relationship between pain and depression in such patients is complex. The pain threshold is lowered in clinically depressed patients, and pain is a common complaint in patients who have primary depression. Patients with pain associated with chronic somatic disease also frequently develop depressive symptoms, however, and the incidence of depression, as defined by strict clinical criteria, is not clearly different in chronic pain patients when compared with medically ill patients without pain. Therefore, although patients with chronic pain often have symptoms of depression, it is not clear if these symptoms are due to, or the result of, their pain problem.

For the initial clinical management, this distinction may be unimportant. Antidepressant drugs can stabilize the sleep pattern and improve the dysphoric symptoms of patients with chronic pain. There is often a reduction in the intensity of reported pain that may be associated with a decrease in the requirement for analgesics. Antidepressants therefore have an important role in the management of chronic pain, although it is still uncertain whether these drugs act primarily to potentiate analgegsics or to relieve depressive symtpoms in individual patients.

A separate group of patients with chronic pain can be identified who have repeated, variable complaints of pain with no evidence of a physical disorder that might explain these symptoms on repeated testing. Such patients seek out physicians and undergo repeated tests to evaluate vague complaints. A variety of analgesics, anxiolytics, and muscle relaxants are usually prescribed for such patients with little or no benefit. Surgical procedures are often performed for pain relief without success. Some of these patients fit the psychiatric diagnostic criteria of a "somatoform disorder." Although symptoms of chronic pain are often part of the presentation of a somatoform disorder, patients with this diagnosis often do not have depressive symptoms and do not usually respond to antidepressants. Such patients need frequent reassurance that their pain is benign; the management of these conditions is therefore primarily supportive. These patients should have careful follow-up from a small number of care-givers to minimize unnecessary tests and reduce the amount of medication prescribed. In this group of patients, diagnosing new pains that signal true organic pathology can be a clinical challenge.

Multidisciplinary Approach to Chronic Pain Problems

When patients with longstanding chronic pain are seen for a new evaluation, they often have unrealistic expectations of the physician. Frequently they state that none of their prior physicians were competent and that this is their last hope for relief from their suffering. A detailed medical history will often reveal poor compliance with previous treatment recommendations made by other physicians.

To avoid another treatment failure, the patient with chronic pain should be evaluated by a multidisciplinary group of specialists skilled in managing chronic pain complaints. The specialists composing this group may vary, depending on the nature of the pain complaint and the resources available at an institution. At a minimum, however, a patient should receive a medical, psychological, neurologic, and physical therapy evaluation. Patients with particular pain problems, such as facial pain or low back pain, may also benefit from a dental or an orthopedic evaluation. A group approach avoids potential confrontation between patient and physician that may stall progress; it also enhances the credibility of the treatment group, increasing the likelihood of patient compliance. The goal of this evaluation is to establish a treatment plan with specific objectives. Each objective should be accomplished according to a timetable mutually agreed on by the patient and the treatment team.

In general, there are three main treatment goals with chronic pain patients. The first goal of therapy is to simplify and minimize drug treatment. In many patients with chronic pain, common analgesics and muscle relaxants are only minimally effective. Our patients almost universally comment that such drugs "only take the edge off" their pain. They tend to increase their dosage of medication in the hope of enhancing pain relief and fear that stopping medication will be associated with an exacerbation of pain symptoms.

With the patient's understanding, the number of medications should be reduced by eliminating redundant or ineffective drugs. The dosages of the remaining medications should then be decreased systematically to a point where the patient is taking only drugs that have a definite beneficial effect with minimal side effects.

The second goal of therapy is to help the patient develop a better understanding of the pain and the factors that exacerbate it. A patient's physical activities and work environment may have a direct, although often subtle, effect on his pain. More difficult to assess is the psychological significance of the pain and its relationship to developmental or interpersonal factors. These issues may be worth exploring with individual patients.

The third goal of therapy is to increase mobilization and functional ability. With the assistance of a physical therapist or a specialist in rehabilitation medicine, a program of physical treatment for pain relief (TENS, massage, etc.) should be coupled with an exercise program to increase range of motion and endurance. The therapy should encourage patients to meet realistic functional goals and to continue with the program despite a transient increase in their level of pain. Patients should understand that pain relief is not necessarily the objective of therapy; instead, increased functional ability for a given level of pain is the goal. At the conclusion of such a program, patients frequently comment that their pain is unchanged, although their range of motion, functional ability, and endurance are greatly enhanced.

Certain patients with chronic pain are refractory to treatment on an outpatient basis. For some, an inpatient multidisciplinary pain treatment facility can provide an opportunity for an intensive program of evaluation and therapy. Treatment standards for such inpatient units have been set by the Committee on Standards of Pain Treatment Facilities of the American Pain Society. Many patients who complete such a program require few analgesic medications and have increased functional ability. Such patients need encouragement and careful follow-up to ensure that these improvements are sustained.

ACUTE BACK PAIN AND DISC HERNIATION

JOHN D. RYBOCK, M.D.

Episodic back pain, with or without sciatica, is extremely common, accounting for about one-quarter of the time lost from work in the United States and affecting the majority of the population at one time or another. Prompt and appropriate initial care must be instituted to minimize the impact of such episodes, both upon the individual patient and upon society. The physician providing early evaluation in such cases must remain aware that acute back pain, with or without leg pain, is usually not attributable to disc herniation and that, even when the symptoms result from disc herniation, spontaneous resolution usually occurs. The failure to recognize these two points has led to a several-fold excess in lumbar spine operations with a poor overall success rate.

INITIAL DIAGNOSIS

The first step in treating the patient with acute back pain is to decide whether the symptoms are due to back strain and soft tissue injury (which we will refer to as mechanical back pain) or to disc herniation. Although initial treatment in both cases is similar, patient education should be started immediately, and the approach taken depends upon the probable cause of the patient's symptoms. In the case of mechanical back pain, early remobilization with the patient making an aggressive effort to return to a normal level of functioning is the goal, whereas in the case of probable disc herniation, a prolonged period of reduced activity with the recognition that surgery is not a quick and easy cure is essential.

The classic history, symptoms, and signs of disc herniation are well described in textbooks. As a basic rule, unless the leg pain is at least as severe as the back pain, radiates below the knee, and is reproduced by the straight leg-raising test, the patient probably has mechanical pain. Particularly with a negative straight leg-raising test or one that produces mostly back pain, it is best to tentatively treat the patient as having mechanical back pain. With acute disc herniation, the leg pain and positive straight leg-raising test usually appear within hours of the onset of symptoms.

INITIAL THERAPY—MECHANICAL BACK PAIN

Several days of bedrest are generally recommended for any significant acute back strain. There are no good data to show that bedrest acutally helps, and continuing a moderate level of functioning may help reduce the overall period of disability. However, it is almost impossible to convince most patients to keep functioning; everyone "knows" that a strained area needs to be rested and suggesting otherwise often leads to loss of patient trust and poorer compliance in the long run. The patient must be helped to understand, however, that after a short period of rest, the back muscles must be "reactivated" and "built back up" before they weaken from disuse. The physician should explain clearly that recovery is largely dependent upon stretching and strengthening the back muscles by the patient in order to reverse the tightening and weakening effect of the injury and that this process will of necessity cause some back discomfort. It is important for the patient to understand that it is not beneficial in the long run to wait until he is fully pain free to resume normal activities. These points cannot be overstressed, especially in the case of work-related injuries, in which the usual assumption is that the "victim" is entitled to rest until he feels completely normal; however, the resulting back muscle deconditioning virtually guarantees prolonged disability.

Specific instructions include bedrest for several days, gradual easing into a back exercise program as will be described, gradual increase in the overall activity level, and a tentative return-to-work date. A few days may be adequate for recovery from a minor injury in a sedentary worker, ubt up to 3 or 4 weeks may be necessary for a physical laborer with a significant amount of muscle spasm. An open-ended off-work determination generally leads to much longer disability periods.

In most cases, the pain can be adequately controlled by non-narcotic medications, such as ibuprofen or acetaminophen. If such agents are ineffective, a brief course of mid-range narcotics such as codeine with acetaminophen or oxycodone compounds may be necessary. Their use should be strictly limited; use on a regular basis beyond a week or 10 days is seldom warranted.

INITIAL THERAPY—PROBABLE DISC HERNIATION

Whereas a clearly limited period of rest and prompt increase in activity level are needed in the majority of patients with back pain, the small percentage with probable disc herniation need an open-ended period of bedrest. However, the indefinite length of time as well as the unpredictability of the outcome (including the possible need for surgery) makes it difficult to obtain full compliance in many cases. Best long-term results are obtained only through careful patient education that makes the patient an active informed participant in his own treatment. Three points should be explained to the patient. The first is that, given appropriate care and time, at least two-thirds of disc herniations will resolve without surgery and the patient will be able to return to a normal, unlimited lifestyle. The second point is that surgery has a limited success rate and that the patient is more likely to end up with permanent limitations if surgical, rather than nonsurgical, therapy is required. The final point is that each patient is different, and activity limitations have to be made on the basis of individual progress. Arbitrary schedules won't work well, and despite the disruption caused by open-ended "conservative" treatment, the alternatives are much less desirable. A patient who understands these points will be more compliant and less impatient with what can seem like slow progress at times.

After explaining the basic disease process and the goals of therapy, I advise patients with possible disc herniation to begin a period of restricted activity for a minimum of 1 week. It is unnecessary to insist upon complete bedrest. I suggest resting or reclining in a comfortable position and getting up for bathroom use only. The basic rule is that activities and positions that aggravate the leg pain must be absolutely avoided, but otherwise no specific maneuvers are required or even helpful. Traction specifically is of no added benefit. I also warn the patient that some increase in the discomfort is common during the first 2 or 3 days of bedrest and that this is not a bad prognostic sign.

The pain level in acute disc herniation can be extremely high and often requires narcotic medication. In most cases, codeine with acetaminophen or an oxycodone compound is adequate. To help reduce any muscle spasm and to help the patient tolerate prolonged bedrest, diazepam may be given.

Since nerve root tension signs, most commonly the straight leg-raising sign, are the most useful indices of the degree of nerve root compression, I use them as the primary means of assessing progress of "conservative" therapy. To minimize physical stress, especially walking and automobile riding, I often monitor initial progress by telephone. It is therefore useful at the initial evaluation to have the patient demonstrate his ability to raise his leg with the knee extended and to describe how far he can lift it before he experiences radicular-type leg pain. This gives a baseline to which subsequent reports can be compared.

Using both degree of pain and amount of tolerated straight leg-raising as criteria, the patient's status is reconsidered after 1 week of rest. If no significant improvement has been noted, plans are made either for referral to a surgeon or for neuroradiologic testing within the next week, since the likelihood of spontaneous improvement has decreased. If any improvement has been noted, the patient is encouraged to continue his current regimen; he may want to become more active, but, if there is still any significant limitation of leg raising, he should be discouraged from "undoing his progress."

Once the patient is pain free with limited walking and can raise his leg without producing sciatica, a gradual increase in activity can be permitted. If pain recurrence is noted, a reduction in activity is necessary, but otherwise progressive return to normal functioning can be attempted. Once the patient can function reasonably well around the house, he should begin a back exercise program before returning to work or other strenuous activities.

EVALUATION FOR SURGERY

Patients are surgical candidates if they fall into one of the following groups:

1. Impaired bowel or bladder control: Disc herniation causing impairment of sphincter control raises the possibility of a massive midline disc herniation. This should be considered a medical emergency, and prompt referral for evaluation and possible surgery should be carried out to salvage some sphincter control.
2. Major neurologic deficit: The presence of a complete foot drop or loss of ankle plantar flexion warrants early care by a surgical specialist. If prompt improvement in function does not occur, surgery is undertaken without a full trial of bedrest.
3. Failure of "conservative" therapy: To be considered a surgical candidate, the patient should demonstrate persistent nerve root tension signs despite a minimum of 10 days of true restriction of activity. If there is any suggestion of improvement, a longer period, 3 to 4 weeks, should pass before surgery is actively considered.

If the patient has persistent pain without definitely positive nerve root tension signs, if the back pain is greater than the leg pain, or if the leg pain has a diffuse pattern, it is unlikely that surgery will be indicated. The move toward surgery should be based upon a definite selection process rather than upon the desire to have something to offer the patient who continues to suffer despite a trial of bedrest. Unless the patient clearly falls into one of the specific surgical groups, the physical therapy and rehabilitation approach should be taken.

If surgery is a consideration, neuroradiologic studies should be undertaken. Water-soluble contrast myelography, perferably followed by computed tomography (CT) scanning, remains the most complete means of evaluating disc and nerve root lesions. With the improved resolution of newer CT scanners, plain scanning is rapidly becoming the preferred study, since it can be done quickly on an outpatient basis with minimal patient discomfort and no morbidity.

Electromyography is rarely needed to make or confirm the diagnosis of disc herniation and should be carried out only when an alternative diagnosis must be confirmed or excluded.

INTERVENTIONAL TREATMENT OF THE HERNIATED DISC

If neuroradiologic studies demonstrate an abnormality that correlates well with the patient's complaint and findings, surgery is indicated; an abnormality that does not correlate well or normal studies indicate that surgery should be avoided. Exploratory surgery in presumed disc disease is unjustifiable.

The actual surgical technique is dependent upon the surgeon's training and experience and is beyond the scope of this book. The minor variations employed, including using a microscope, probably make less difference in outcome than do the surgeon's basic skill and judgement.

Some surgeons use chemonucleolysis (the injection of chymopapain into the disc) as an alternative to surgery. The indications for this procedure must be as stringent as for surgery, and the risks are significant. I find that chymopapain injection is less successful than surgery and that, when failure occurs, subsequent treatment is less effective. I therefore do not recommend this treatment.

PHYSICAL THERAPY AND REHABILITATION

The single most valuable therapy for the majority of patients with back and leg pain, including those recovering spontaneously or postsurgically from disc herniation, is an active back exercise program. The patient must understand that most back and nonradicular leg pain is the result of chronic back muscle strain and that his own hard work to build up the back muscles is the only solution. Although back supports reduce the stress on strained muscles, they also promote back muscle deconditioning, making rehabilitation more difficult. I therefore usually discourage their use.

A variety of exercise programs exist, each with its own rationale and group of supporters, but in my experience, the basic set of flexion exercises remains the most effective. Such exercises are referred to as Williams exercises and feature pelvic tilts, knee-to-chest stretches, and partial sit-ups. These exercises reduce the lumbar lordosis, taking stress off the posterior portion of the intervertebral disc and widening the spinal canal by stretching out the ligamentum flavum. Additionally, they strengthen the abdominal muscles, which increases the ability of the abdominal cavity to provide support of the upper body. Instruction sheets and booklets are available that explain the basic exercises to the patient and should be stocked by any physician who treats back pain with any regularity. Alternatively, the patient may be referred to a back school or a physical therapist for exercise instruction. This will ensure that the patient does the exercises correctly, but it must be stressed that the only long-term benefit comes from active exercises, not passive modalities such as diathermy or massage. The patient should be made aware that the investment of 5 to 10 minutes twice a day to do a simple exercise program is the surest way to prevent future back problems.

A patient who has recovered from an episode of mechanical back pain, from a spontaneously resolved disc herniation, or from surgical excision of a herniated disc should generally be able to return to his previous level of activity. I view any pain episode as a warning that the patient's usual activity is capable of producing further back injuries, and I advise the patient accordingly. In most cases future problems will be prevented if the patient continues his back exercise program on a regular basis to keep his back stronger than before. In patients whose usual occupation involves frequent lifting, bending, or stooping, a careful review of proper body mechanics is also important. Finally, despite the best conditioning and use of good body mechanics, many activities will place stresses on the lower back that approach its physical limits. Therefore, one severe episode or several minor episodes of back strain warrant consideration of vocational rehabilitation in individuals with physically demanding jobs.

IF ALL ELSE FAILS

The approach just discussed will adequately treat the vast majority of patients with acute back pain and sciatica. However, some patients will continue to report disabling pain. Although some cases represent malingering or compensation neurosis, there are poorly defined causes of such pain that do not respond well to the basic program. In patients who have had an adequate trial of rest and who have conscientiously carried out an exercise program, referral to a pain clinic or a physiatrist, orthopedist, or neurosurgeon with an interest in back problems is appropriate. A variety of alternative treatments, including facet joint blocks, trigger-point injections, biofeedback, and stimulation techniques, are being continually refined in an attempt to treat such patients.

CERVICAL SPONDYLOSIS

SIMON HORENSTEIN, M.D.

Cervical spondylosis is a degenerative disorder of the neck that affects the vertebrae, intervertebral disks, apophyseal joints, and related ligaments. Loss of intervertebral disk integrity is usually the first sign and ordinarily begins at the disk between the fifth and sixth cervical vertebrae. This is commonly followed by hypertrophic changes affecting the opposing intervertebral joint surfaces and demineralization of the adjacent vertebral bodies. Motion becomes reduced at the affected level, and a similar process slowly involves the intervertebral disk spaces and later the vertebral bodies immediately above and below. The vertebrae lose bone mass and undergo partial collapse, usually anteriorly. As this occurs, the vertebral bodies assume a wedged appearance and develop "traction spurs." Osteoarthritic changes appear in the apophyseal joints, and spur formation forms on the uncinate processes. Bulging of one or more intervertebral disks commonly occurs, accompanied by thickening of the ligaments which line the vertebral canal anteriorly and posteriorly. The latter (ligamenta flava) appear to undergo a greater degree of hypertrophy than the former (posterior longitudinal ligament). The net result of the process is shortening of the cervical spine, narrowing of the vertebral canal at one or more levels, stenosis of lateral recesses and intervertebral foramina which bear the vertebral artery. Symptom formation appears dependent upon the manner in which the disease affects the spine, the motor and sensory roots, and the spinal cord and its blood supply, as well as that of the brain stem, cerebellum, diencephalon, occipital lobes, and portions of the basal and medial temporal lobes.

SYMPTOMS AND SIGNS

Symptoms attributed to the spine are frequently mild relative to extensive radiologic changes. It is not unusual to find that except in those patients who display the changes of true arthritis of the apophyseal joints, the condition gives rise to no neck symptoms whatsoever. The patient who is symptomatic and behaves like any other with hypertrophic osteoarthritis in any body part, exhibiting stiffening proportional to immobility and thus particularly severe in the morning. An occasional individual is wakened from sleep for this reason. Crepitus is often reported, and the range of comfortable turning or tilting may be diminished. The patient frequently reports increased pain or stiffness upon exposure to cold or damp weather. Apparently minor trauma associated with rapid movement of the neck may give rise to long-lasting discomfort.

Symptoms pertaining to arterial insufficiency in the territory of the vertebral artery or its branches are quite uncommon. An occasional patient will report spontaneous numbness about the mouth and tongue or dizziness. It is not unusual, however, to hear reports of dizziness, double vision, and, rarely, graver indications of ischemia within the territory of the vertebrobasilar vessels following manipulation of the neck incidental to the performance of certain diagnostic procedures such as myelography.

Symptoms pertaining to disorders of motor and sensory cervical roots occur commonly. Involvement of the former may have become quite extensive before the patient notices weakness or atrophy of the muscles of the hand or forearm. Since the disease process usually begins adjacent to the sixth cervical root, it is common that the initial symptoms involve the thumb and index finger, though any other location may be affected. For the most part, all patients who suffer cervical root disorders secondary to spondylosis will manifest some disturbance of use of the hand. More proximal muscle weakness and wasting (especially of the long head of the triceps) are common, though frequently overlooked by examiners who do not make a special effort to study the brachial or periscapular muscles. The symptoms which indicate involvement of sensory roots consist chiefly of numbness and tingling and, less often, burning. The symptoms ordinarily exceed the signs of sensory loss discovered at physical examination. Patterns of sensory loss may be found which correspond to known root distributions. Patterns which indicate involvement of overlapping or adjacent roots suggest affection of the decussating spinothalamic fibers in the central portion of the spinal cord.

Any type of spinal cord decompensation may be observed. The commonest is spastic paraparesis with minimal or no involvement of the bladder or bowel and preservation of sexual function. The reason is that when the spinal cord is subjected to ventrally applied forces which displace it posteriorly, an oblique ischemic fracture plane results owing to tension of the dentate ligaments. This extends across the anterior horn to the corticospinal tracts but spares the spinothalamic tracts and descending bulbar projections to the lumbosacral segments which innervate the genitourinary organs. The posterior columns are involved less often and almost always in association with corticospinal disturbance. As a general rule, patients suffering myelopathy secondary to cervical spondylosis retain the ability to walk unless they have been injured, operated, or otherwise manipulated. Diabetes mellitus appears to impose a special liability, presumably secondary to involvement of small spinal arteries. Studies of the arterial supply of the spinal cord in cases of spondylosis indicate frequent impingement upon the anterior median sulcal artery. In adult men, regardless of occupational status the leading cause of slowly evolving spastic paraparesis, is the myelopathy of cervical spondylosis.

RADIOLOGIC EVALUATION

Since the bony changes of cervical spondylosis occur more frequently than do its neurologic manifestations, it is important to be certain that the patient's neurologic disorder has been caused by the spinal pathology. Characteristic radiologic changes must be present along with evidence of narrowing of the cervical canal. Those patients in whom the sagittal diameter of the cervical canal, as measured from the base of a spinous process to the nearest vertebral body, is less than 12 mm will always have some neurologic symptoms. When the dimensions are larger, it is still possible that neurologic symptoms arise from such radiolucent structures as thickened or plicated ligaments.

A necessary second step is demonstration that compression of the nervous system has occurred in relation to the bony disorder. This is ordinarily most effectively displayed by myelography, but owing to the risks and complications of that procedure one or two safer alternatives may be chosen. The first is the instillation of a small amount of metrizamide into the lumbar canal followed by a computed tomography (CT) scan of the neck. Images displaying bone detail must be obtained in addition to the usual soft tissue ones which demonstrate the nervous system. CT scan of the neck without metrizamide usually is useless owing to artifacts originating from the shoulders and the lack of a distinct epidural fat pattern. The scan may be reconstructed or "reformatted" to display the relationship between the spinal cord and the vertebral canal.

Another useful method is that of magnetic resonance imaging (MRI). This procedure has the advantage of requiring no metrizamide but does not show bone detail. MRI does provide increasingly high resolution images of the spinal cord and spinal roots in multiple planes and is becoming the leading method of delineating the pathologic process.

Myelography is employed either when patients have been selected for surgery or the other procedures have failed. Selection for surgery is discussed below. Electromyography, nerve conduction studies, and somatosensory evoked potentials are not particularly helpful in establishing the diagnosis, and one generally does better with a reflex hammer and tuning fork. A general medical survey is essential. A search for diabetes mellitus or for vitamin B_{12} deficiency in patients with predominant loss of position sense is often rewarding.

GENERAL MANAGEMENT

The most important information derived from assessment of the patient is that derived from the physical examination, as it not only defines the locus of disease but leads to understanding of the mechanisms of symptom formation. Three steps of critical importance include establishing the range of active neck motion, defining the sensory and motor status of the upper limbs, and identifying spasticity and impairment of position and vibration to the lower limbs. The neck should not be manipulated, but the active range can easily be recorded. Movements including flexion, extension, tilting, and turning. Owing to nerve root or central spinal cord disease, one or more of the branchial reflexes will be found absent or diminished. Other reflexes, especially the finger jerks, may be exaggerated. Spasticity of the lower limbs is marked by exaggeration of the reflexes frequently accompanied by clonus. Extensor plantar responses occur so variably that they cannot be depended upon to mark spinal cord dysfunction. Testing vibration sense, especially with a 256-Hz tuning fork, is a most effective way of discovering involvement of the posterior columns. The information obtained in this fashion is equivalent to that afforded by somatosensory evoked potentials. Vibration sense is best tested by seeking its threshold, starting with a fork vibrating below threshold. The strength of the stimulus is increased until the patient reports having felt it.

Management is entirely opportunistic and is directed toward relief of those symptoms and signs which appear responsible for the complaints and neurologic deficits. The articular symptoms are generally quite mild and usually require little more than commonly available analgesic drugs, which should be chosen for their safety, effectiveness, and freedom from side effects. Aspirin or acetaminophen is usually sufficient. The patient should be encouraged to combine heat, massage, and medication empirically until he has secured relief from pain. Most patients report some morning stiffness and aching. This ordinarily responds to natural movement, the application of a warm towel, and analgesic drugs. Exercises directed toward the neck are not likely to be beneficial and may in fact evoke complaints pertaining to nerve roots. Neck traction often helps reduce night pain. The use of a small pillow to support the head when lying on the side is often helpful as well.

The symptoms secondary to compression of the vertebral artery occur infrequently, ordinarily in relation to injury or manipulation. These are best dealt with anticipation. During myelography, for example, one should be alert to complaints of dizziness, facial numbness, thickness of the tongue, or lower limb numbness or weakness. When these occur, the neck, which is likely to have been placed in extension, should be restored to an upright position and the contrast material allowed to run to the lumbar region.

Weakness, atrophy, fasciculation, and cramping in the arms are common manifestations of motor root compression and frequently cannot be reversed. Muscular weakness and atrophy are not likely to recover or even improve. Some use of the hand is usually retained, though a rare patient loses complete use of it. Many, however, suffer impairment of skilled acts, such as playing a musical instrument. Occasinally, severe local weakness of the thumb or a finger requires splinting or other support. Cramping is not likely to respond to such medication as diazepam, baclofen, or dantrolene. Many patients report massage helpful, especially after the limb has been warmed. Contracture of the weakened parts of the limb is not seen with any degree of frequency. Persistent postural deformity may be corrected by means of a self-applied program of passive movement, which maintains the range of motion. The movement patterns are simple, as the wrist, metacarpophalangeal, and interphalangeal joint extensors are most likely to be affected. The hand, thus, is put through a range which replicates the lost motion. This can be done by the patient several times daily and is usually all that is required as long as a consistent effort is made to increase the range of motion.

Sensory symptoms, however, are frequently annoying, particularly at night, and are especially agonizing when a causalgic component is present. The latter is usually described as burning, searing, hot, stinging, or electrical. Pinprick and thermal stimuli are usually much better perceived than light touch. Relief may be obtained either from medication or traction. Drugs which inhibit sensory spinal reflexes are preferred. Baclofen, carbamazepine, and diazepam are the most useful. I begin with carbamazepine, starting with small doses of 100 mg at bedtime. As induction of this drug frequently causes drowsiness, especially in older patients, it should be started slowly and initial medication and increments concentrated at bedtime. The ordinary individual is relieved by doses between 250 and 600 mg per day. The level is achieved over 10 to 14 days. Long-term use of carbamazepine has an important limitation; i.e., autoinduction of hepatic microsomal enzymes which make the maintenance of an effective drug level difficult. Drug "vacations" or increasing the dose may help surmount this complication. Fortunately, causalgia is usually not long lasting. Thus, many patients have limited need for medication. Precautions regarding inhibition of the maturation of granulocyte should be observed, though nearly all patients who use carbamazepine suffer slight granulocytopenia, which is well tolerated.

Baclofen may be used instead of or in combination with carbamazepine. This drug, too, is occasionally associated with drowsiness, especially in the elderly. It is thus prudent to begin administration at bedtime, using 5- or 10-mg doses which may be increased in number every few days (until spaced at 4- to 6-hour intervals) until satisfactory relief of the symptom has been achieved. The drowsiness usually disappears with habituation. Dantrolene is used for only short-term administration owing to unresolved doubts about its long-term safety. It is administered in 25- or 50-mg doses. The maximum safe dose is 400 mg daily.

NECK TRACTION

The mainstay of management of the painful disorder associated with sensory radiculopathy is neck traction. Traction may also be used to relieve skeletal complaints. It is not likely to help sensory symptoms unless the patient reports that neck movement causes radiating electrical pain into the forearm, hand, or fingers. The traction can be applied at home using commercially available kits which may be obtained at surgical supply houses or drug stores. The most satisfactory kits deliver traction from a plastic bag of 1 gallon capacity. When water is used, the net weight of the apparatus is approximately 10 pounds, as the total load includes the weight of the bag, rope, and other parts of the traction kit. In most women, 4½ or 5 pounds of water are adequate to start. In a brawny man, 6½ to 7 pounds are satisfactory at the beginning. The patient may then increase the load until relief has been obtained. Relief usually comes slowly over the course of days or weeks.

As the traction is delivered to a halter which embraces the chin, the patient's teeth may ache. False teeth should be removed. The jaws or teeth may then be protected by having the patient bite on a small rubber wedge on each side during the period of traction. These can easily be cut from foam rubber or a doorstop.

Traction may be applied either with the patient sitting or lying, as he chooses. It is most commonly used upright. If the cantilever which holds the traction is placed over a door, bracing with a doorstop is usually required. The precise position is determined by the patient's comfort. Generally, the axis of traction is directly perpendicular in the sagittal plane, but is angled slightly forward, putting the head ever so slightly into flexion. The timing and duration of traction depend upon the taste and comfort of the patient. Those who have difficulty sleeping commonly benefit most from traction applied before bedtime. Some prefer several continuous hours, while others are better relieved by several briefer episodes distributed through the day. Many find that pain relief is more effective when analgesic medication is used simultaneously or a warm towel is applied to the neck ("muscle-relaxing" agents seem not particularly effective beyond their sedative effects). With the use of a program of medication and traction, nearly all patients will become comfortable over the course of a few weeks. Relapses, which are to be expected, may be treated in the same fashion.

SPINAL CORD COMPRESSION

Spinal symptoms require first that the structural relationship between the spinal cord and the cervical canal be established. The noninvasive diagnostic procedures mentioned previously (enchanced CT scan and MRI) enable the physician to decide whether a subarachnoid space exists around the spinal cord and to estimate with reasonable accuracy the sagittal diameter of the latter. Surgical procedures in the presence of intact and continuous subarachnoid space are of no proved benefit. Approximation of the dimension of the spinal cord, using either form of imaging, enables one to identify atrophy, the inevitable consequence of longstanding intermittent compression. When the latter is present, management is totally symptomatic.

If the patient has difficulty walking as a result of spasticity, baclofen is the drug of choice owing to its flexibility and ease of tolerance. It may be administered as described above for painful states. The end-point is patient satisfaction, and may be as high as 80 to 100 mg daily. Some patients depend upon the enhanced quadriceps and gluteus tone of extensor spasticity to assist them when standing or walking. Its inhibition may actually impair the patient's ability to walk. This is readily reversed by reducing or discontinuing the dose of medication. Many patients learn to secure an end-point which reduces the spasticity with little loss of strength. Weakness may be managed with the use of a cane or, in some instances, a walker. Many patients with spasticity complain of severe lumbar pain, as the spinal extensor muscles participate in the extensor posture. Frequently, medication relieves this pain at moderate doses. "Central pain," a diffuse burning sensation in limbs and trunk, is uncommon in patients with spondylosis. Painless paresthesias (prickling and tingling) in the feet are usually not improved by medication at all. Happily, this is an annoyance to which most patients adapt.

Surgical Management

If diagnostic studies disclose obliteration of the cervical subarachnoid space, a decision must be made concerning the probability that relief can be obtained by surgical means. It is usually possible to predict functional stenosis of the canal by inference from symptoms and deduction from image-derived data. The patient who reports electrical paresthesias in his trunk or lower limbs (Lhermitte's phenomenon) on neck motion (usually flexion) will ordinarily be found with obliteration of the subarachnoid space. Disappearance of this symptom commonly means that for one or another reason the relationship between the spinal cord and the canal has altered, usually owing to atrophy. Thus, some information in the history usually allows identification of present or past compression and prediction of the size of the spinal cord. Bilateral symmetrical paresthesias involving the same parts of the same fingers of both hands suggest functional vertebral canal stenosis at the level of the intervertebral disk appropriate to the root zone of which the patient complains. This is occasionally associated with bilateral symmetrical sensory loss. It is most often found when there is a large midline bony bar or prolapsed disk with or without calcification at one segment. Anterior diskectomy with or without interbody fusion is usually indicated for the latter state. When canal stenosis involves multiple segments, and hence is more widespread, the surgical procedures are of much less certain value. In the latter case, posterior decompression and bilateral laminectomy to facets are often recommended. In the event that a surgical procedure is chosen, it is wise to remind the patient that the goal of surgery is preventing the condition from worsening and that only the most recently acquired features are likely to improve. There is no unequivocal evidence that surgical treatment is beneficial, except in the presence of monostotic disease. Some experienced neurologists and neurosurgeons prefer not to offer operation unless this condition is met.

Nonsurgical Management

If nonoperative management is selected, a cervical supporting collar may be employed. Its principal function appears to be inhibition of neck flexion, but it has little effect on extension, turning, or tilting. If the former movement produces the Lhermitte phenomenon, indicating postural compression of the spinal cord, a collar is likely to be helpful. No currently used collar is strong or snug enough to prevent the patient bending, though it does remind him not to and may affort deceleration of motion when he forgets. The goal of treatment is to teach the patient to avoid neck flexion. On the other hand, when neck extension is the offending movement, its inhibition is quite difficult, if not impossible, to accomplish.

Cervical collars may be fashioned from orthopaedic felt and stockinette, shaped and trimmed to a comfortable height, and fastened with clips or pins. Alternatively, a commercial collar may be purchased. A collar may be useful when the patient is being transported or even walking, as it appears to help restrain sudden flexion, which may result from rapid acceleration or deceleration of a vehicle. It may be worn at any other time the patient chooses, but there should be no expectation that the collar will cure anything.

The management program requires prophylaxis against injury owing to falls. The patient who suffers spasticity is particularly prone to this complication, as hopping reactions are usually impaired, making him particularly likely to fall on slippery, smooth, or uneven surfaces. In doing so, he is subject to forceful displacement of the neck and secondary injury to the spinal cord. He may at the same time suffer injuries to his limbs or their joints, which will add to his disability. Patterns, (devices of metal worn on the sole of the shoe to improve grip), are extremely useful when patients must walk on hazardous surfaces. Those commercially available are light and consist of devices resembling rubbers with studs in the bottom. These can easily be removed from the shoe and folded into small packages, which may be carried in a pocket or purse.

The home should be modified to accommodate the needs of the patient with spasticity. Friction stripping should be placed in the bathtub. If the patient is severely impaired he should bathe or shower from a tub bench made of plastic. The stationary shower head may be replaced by one attached to a flexible hose. Rails may be placed on the tub or the wall around it. Other portions of the bathroom should be so provided. Rails should be placed in studs rather than plaster or dry wall. The spastic patient is less likely to fall when rising from the toilet if an elevated seat is added. This can be used as well by other members of the family. Firmly seated balustrades and bannisters should be available in all exposed locations. Many homes have no rails on basement or external staircases. These, too, should be protected.

For the patient with a weakened hand grip which interferes with eating or shaving thickened utensil handles may be employed. Some may be purchased in medical supply stores or shops operated by local Arthritis Foundations. Others can be made, often to greater patient satisfaction. A simple method is to find the thickness of a wooden dowel which the patient can grasp securely and cut a length slightly longer than the breadth of the hand. This is then slit longitudinally with an ordinary ripsaw, and a channel is grooved wide and deep enough to hold the handle of a fork, spoon, toothbrush, or razor. The halves of the dowel are then placed about the utensil, and two or more holes are drilled through the entire assembly and countersunk. A stove bolt of appropriate size holds the apparatus together. The advantage of this homemade equipment is that it is possible to choose and shape a handle which uniquely fits the individual. Some patients prefer to use a large spoon which has been modified by tines cut into one side. A runcible spoon such as this is very helpful for patients with extreme degrees of hand and forearm weakness.

The patient who has difficulty with pronation and supination may benefit from a swivel spoon that may be purchased or fabricated by bending the shortened handle of a spoon 1½ inches from the bowl to approximately 90 degrees. A hole is then drilled through the bent portion and fastened with a wood screw to the end of the intact dowel. By leaving a small length of the smooth portion of the shaft of the wood screw exposed, the spoon will swivel with gravity, thus compensating for inability to pronate and supinate the forearm. A fork may be made in the same fashion.

The ordinary hairbrush and electric razor are thick enough to be used by most patients. If the fingers of both hands are so weak that buttons cannot be fastened, the buttonholes may be closed and a button sewn on for facing. Swatches of adhesive nylon may then be used as fastenings. This can also be used on trousers if slide fasteners cannot be operated. Slide fasteners may be made easier to handle by slipping a lanyard through a hole in the tab and fastening the ends to a round button sufficiently large to permit a firm grip by the patient. Clip-on neckties can also be used as substitutes for those which require tying.

Special attention should be paid to areas of digital anesthesia which occur from time to time and are especially likely to be found in the patient who has acquired a cyst in the center of the spinal cord. These individuals are prone to injuries acquired as the result of anesthesia. They should be instructed to inspect the anesthetic areas, reminded of their presence, and shown how to protect them from injury. The insensitive portions of the body should never be used to estimate temperature. Neuropathic or Charcot's joints are rare in patients with cervical spondylosis, as the lesions necessary for their development are usually more extensive than those ordinarily encountered.

Lower extremity bracing is rarely necessary. An occasional patient has such severe extensor spasticity that equinovarus posture complicates walking. This may be treated with a corrective appliance if the patient cannot tolerate doses of baclofen large enough to accomplish the same purpose. Upper limb appliances are rarely necessary. An occasional patient with severe intrinsic hand muscle weakness will require an opponens splint, and a rare patient with global paralysis of intrinsic hand muscles but preservation of wrist extension benefits by a tenodesis or flexor hinge splint.

MIGRAINE AND CLUSTER HEADACHE

JAMES W. LANCE, M.D., F.R.C.P. (Lond), F.R.A.C.P., F.A.A.

Migraine may be defined as episodic headache and/or cerebral disturbance with intervening periods of relative freedom from headache and without evidence of primary structural abnormally. Migraines are differentiated by the presence or absence and nature of neurologic symptoms (Table 1). Most attacks are accompanied by gastrointestinal disturbance and hyperacuity of the special senses, while some are preceded for 24 hours or more by premonitory changes in mood or appetite that may guide the timing of therapy.

Cluster headache commonly recurs in bouts and is therefore termed episodic cluster headache. Fewer than 20 percent of patients experience regular attacks without remission when the condition is known as chronic cluster headache or chronic migrainous neuralgia. A rare variant, in which brief attacks recur six or more times daily, has been named chronic paroxysmal hemicrania. Each of these three forms of cluster headache requires different management.

MIGRAINE

Individual Attacks

Some children and adults respond rapidly to aspirin or a similar analgesic administered at the first sign of an attack, particularly if 10 mg of metoclopramide is given orally or intramuscularly at the same time to promote gastric absorption and reduce nausea. Some patients try to induce vomiting, since they have found that the headache subsides shortly afterwards. If patients are able to lie down in a darkened room and go to sleep, they often awaken free from headache. A cold pack applied to the forehead, temples, and upper neck is usually comforting. Unfortunately, most attacks do not succumb to such simple measures.

Ergotamine tartrate is some form remains the most satisfactory means of managing acute attacks, aborting or shortening the attack in about 50 percent of patients and proving of some benefit in another 30 percent. Ergotamine has a biphasic vascular action, constricting dilated vessels and dilating constricted vessels, but it may well have a central action of greater importance. It should be given at the first indication of prodromal symptoms or headache. One to 2 mg can be taken orally alone, in combination with caffeine (Cafergot), or with caffeine and

TABLE 1 Varieties of Migraine

Headache associated with neurologic symptoms
- Prodromal symptoms: classic migraine
- Symptoms at height of headache
  - Vertebrobasilar migraine
  - Migraine stupor
  - Periodic confusional states of childhood
  - Hemiplegic migraine
  - Ophthalmoplegic migraine

Headache without neurologic symptoms
- Common migraine
- Facial migraine ("lower half headache")

Neurologic symptoms without headache
- Migraine equivalents
- Transient migrainous accompaniments (TMAs) of middle age

Neurologic symptoms and signs outlasting headache
- Complicated migraine

Periodic syndromes that may be allied to migraine
- Childhood vomiting (bilious) attacks
- Episodic abdominal pain (abdominal migraine)
- Episodic chest pain (cardiac migraine)
- Episodic vertigo (benign recurrent vertigo)
- Alternating hemiplegia of childhood

an antiemetic in various proprietary preparations. Since gastric absorption is often impaired in migraine, the gastric route may be bypassed with a pressure-pack inhaler, parenteral injection, or suppository. The usual intramuscular (IM) dose is 0.25 to 0.5 mg of ergotamine tartrate or 1 to 2 mg of dihydroergotamine. The most commonly available suppository is Cafergot, which contains 2 mg of ergotamine tartrate and may cause nausea and aching in the legs. This can be avoided by instructing the patient to place the suppositories in a refrigerator to harden, and then to slice them in half lengthwise. One-half suppository can be inserted at the onset of an attack and the other half later if the headache does not abate. It is said that no more than 10 mg of ergotamine should be taken in one week, but individual tolerance varies and vascular side effects are not common. Patients who use ergotamine frequently may suffer daily rebound headaches and feel generally unwell, in which case the drug should be discontinued, at least until the previous intermittent pattern of headache has reestablished itself. Whenever patients are able to predict the onset of migraine by premonitory feelings of elation or hunger, ergotamine may be given at night to anticipate and abort the next day's headache. Its oxytoxic effect is slight and it may be used with caution in pregnancy.

As an alternative to ergotamine (and said to be as effective), the fenemates (mefenamic, tolfenamic, and flufenamic acid) may be given at the onset of an acute migraine attack. I have given patients who were resistant to ergotamine 100 mg of flufenamic acid (2 capsules at the onset of symptoms and again in half an hour) with modest success. Fenemates should be taken with food as they are gastric irritants. Isometheptene mucate is said to be effective in relieving acute migrane, but I have no personal experience of this.

Severe Continuing Attack

Initial treatment for a severe episode is usually intramuscular injection of 0.5 mg of ergotamine tartrate or 1.0 mg of dihydroergotamine with an antiemetic phenothiazine derivative such as metoclopramide (10 mg), prochlorperazine (12.5 mg), or chlorpromazine (50 to 100 mg). (Injectable ergotamine has been withdrawn from use in most countries in favor of dihydroergotamine). Diazepam, 10 mg IM, may be injected in place of a phenothiazine. If this first step is ineffective, intramuscular injection of 50 to 100 mg of pethidine (meperidine) must be considered, providing that the patient shows obvious signs of distress and is not known to be habituated to narcotics. Morphine is less effective in migranous patients than pethidine, and pentazocine may cause hallucinations. If headache continues despite these measures, short-term use of high-dose corticosteroids (prednisone, 75 mg daily or dexamethasone, 8 mg daily for 5 days) may terminate the attack. If not, a lignocaine (lidocaine) drip may be given intravenously in hospital as for coronary care, 1 g per 500 ml of 5 percent glucose in 5–N saline, at the rate of 1 ml per minute (2 mg lignocaine per minute) with observation of blood pressure. The drip can be continued for about 3 days if necessary. Once the headache has ceased, interval therapy can be prescribed in an attempt to prevent recurrence.

Increasing Frequency of Migraine

It is not uncommon for patients to suffer from classic migraine once or twice a year in childhood, from common migraine once or twice a month in their 20's, and from daily tension-vascular headaches in their 30s and 40s. Although a change in character of the patient's headache must alert the physician to the possibility of cerebral tumor or other organic disability, the cause is much more often mental than physical.

Factors commonly underlying a progressive increase in frequency of headache include: a "trapped" situation arising in the patient's work or social life, the onset of a depressive state, development of systemic hypertension, use of oral contraceptive pills, and excessive intake of ergotamine, analgesics, or caffeine. These possibilities are assessed during history-taking and physical examination. Although 10 percent of women with migraine improve when their headaches are restricted to the premenstrual phase by taking an oral contraceptive, about one-third suffer more severe and frequent attacks. Low-estrogen pills may be tried, or other forms of contraception advised. Manipulating hormone levels in women rarely improves migraine and may cause unacceptable menstrual irregularities. If the blood pressure is elevated, it should be controlled, preferably by a beta-blocking drug with no intrinsic sympathomimetic activity.

The majority of patients with frequent headaches are in a state of anxiety or depression and require counseling by a sympathetic neurologist or family physician, although referral to a psychologist or psychiatrist may prove necessary. Admission to a hospital may be advisable to wean the patient from ergotamine and analgesics if daily intake has become habitual and excessive. The judicious use of tricyclic antidepressants, particularly amitriptyline, can be helpful in overcoming daily headaches. My custom is to prescribe amitriptyline as a single noctural dose, starting with a 10-mg tablet or half of a 25-mg tablet, then increasing progressively to a maintenance dose of 75 mg if the patient tolerates the medication well. Common side effects are morning drowsiness or confusion and dry mouth. Glaucoma and prostatism are relative contraindications because of atrophine-like side effects. Relaxation therapy, with or without biofeedback, is an important adjuvant to psychological counseling.

Interval Therapy for Frequent Migrainous Attacks

If the patient suffers three or more migraine attacks per month, and particularly if ergotamine is ineffective, regular daily use of prophylactic drugs (interval therapy) should be considered. At the same time, any known trigger factors should be eliminated and attention paid to imbalance of the bite, painful cervical spondylosis, or other disabilities that could aggravate muscle contraction or mental tension. Relaxation therapy and tricyclic antidepressants are helpful for patients whose headaches recur almost daily. Some patients may improve after dietary restriction, cervical manipulation, acupuncture, hypnosis, histamine desensitization, or other more dubious maneuvers, but such response is regrettably capricious.

Most agents used in the prophylaxis of migraine work by simulating or blocking various actions of serotonin and the catecholamines (Table 2), but, at present, it is not possible to state precisely how they work or even whether their action is primarily central or peripheral, neural or vascular.

Interval therapy is usually initiated with one of the antiserotonin antihistamine group (pizotyline, ceproheptadine), or a beta-blocker without intrinsic sympathomimetic activity, such as propranolol. Since the former group promotes appetite, I tend to select from it for the initial treatment of the anorectic patient with migraine. Pizotyline (pizotifen, Sandomigran) in 0.5-mg tablets is best given in the evening because of its soporific effect, increasing steadily to 3 or even 6 tablets nightly. Cyproheptadine in 4-mg tablets may be used similarly, increasing to 3 tablets each night. Drowsiness and a tendency to gain weight are the only common side effects.

Drugs that block beta-adrenoceptors without exerting any agonist effect (intrinsic sympathomimetic activity or ISA) are beneficial in the prophylaxis of migraine, whereas those with ISA are not. The first group includes propranolol, atenolol, metoprolol, and timolol. Propranolol (Inderal) is most commonly used because of many favorable double-blind trials, but must be avoided if there is a history of asthma or if the patient is on the brink of congestive cardiac failure. In children or susceptible adults, the dosage may be as low as 10 mg twice daily, but most adults require 40 mg twice daily, and the dose may be increased slowly to 80 mg 3 times daily if necessary. Asthenia, postural hypotension, and vivid dreams may limit dosage.

The next line of defense, and probably the most effective antimigrainous agent, is the serotonin-blocking drug, methysergide (Sansert, Deseril). In the external carotid circulation, methysergide acts as a serotonin agonist by potentiating vasoconstrictor agents. I advise patients to halve a tablet (1 or 1.4 mg depending on the country of manufacture) for the initial test dose. The reason for this is that about 40 percent of patients experience side effects such as abdominal discomfort, muscle cramps, vasoconstrictive phenomena, or mood changes if the full dosage of 1 to 2 mg 3 times daily is started immediately. Methysergide suppresses migraine completely in about 25 percent of patients and reduces the frequency of headaches by half or more in another 40 to 50 percent.

If the patient improves substantially, methysergide should be continued for 4 to 6 months and then slowly withdrawn, allowing 1 month without the drug, to minimize the possibility of fibrotic complications. These, which include retroperitoneal, pleural, and pulmonary valvular fibrosis, are probably idiosyncratic reactions and are fortunately rare. I have maintained many patients for years on continuous methysergide therapy (because they were not prepared to suffer a severe recrudescence of headache during withdrawal); and they have remained clinically well and have shown no abnormality on precautionary intravenous pyelography. Nevertheless, patients on methysergide should be examined every 3 months.

Those patients who do not respond to regular medication with amitriptyline, pizotyline, cyproheptadine, propranolol, or methysergide present a difficult management problem. Certain agents, listed in Table 2, have been advocated for the treatment of migraine, many on shaky grounds. Calcium-channel blocking agents, such as verapamil, nifedipine, and nimodipine, are still under investigation.

I employ the monoamine oxidase (MAO) inhibitor phenelzine (Nardil) to permit the accumulation of serotonin and norepinephrine, since this has benefited 80 percent of otherwise refractory patients in my experience. Phenelzine is prescribed initially in a dose of 15 mg 3 times daily, with the usual cautionary list of foods and drugs to be avoided by anyone taking MAO inhibitors being given to the patient. Particular emphasis should be placed on tablets, nose drops, and inhalants for nasal congestion or sinusitis, since most contain vasoconstrictor amines.

Migraine Equivalents

Since the prodrome of classic migraine (and presumably migraine equivalent) is associated with low regional cerebral blood flow, vasodilators are employed in the management of migraine equivalent and its counterpart in middle-aged patients, *transient migrainous accompaniment* (TMA). An isoprenaline spray may be administered by pressure-pack inhaler, or the patient can inhale 6 percent carbon dioxide in oxygen if a cylinder is available (or breathe repeatedly into a paper bag if it is not). The calcium-channel blocking agents may help prevent migraine equivalents. My policy is to prescribe aspirin, 300 mg daily, as well as interval therapy (described previously).

CLUSTER HEADACHE

Episodic Cluster Headache

In the first few bouts, the headaches can usually be prevented by administration of ergotamine 1 to 2 hours before the predicted onset of pain. For example, if the patient is usually awakened by cluster headache at 1 AM, 2 mg of ergotamine tartrate is taken on retiring, preferably with 600 mg of aspirin or a similar analgesic. If the characteristic pain recurs more than once in 24 hours, ergotamine can be given twice daily or 1 to 2 mg of methysergide 3 times daily. In some patients, the bouts become progressively more severe and may cease to respond to ergotamine or methysergide. Other drugs for interval therapy of migraine may then be tried, but I have not found them particularly helpful. My preference is for prednisone, 60 to 75 mg, given at night for 3 nights and

TABLE 2 Drugs Acting on Various Receptors and Their Effects on Migraine

Class	*Agent*	*Effect**
Serotonin		
Releasing agents	Reserpine	XX
	Fenfluramine	XX
Uptake inhibitors	Zemelidine	XX
	Femoxetine	XX
	Amitriptyline	✓
Antagonists	Methysergide	✓
	Pizotifen	✓
	Cyproheptadine	✓
Catecholamines		
Alpha adrenoceptor		
Agonist	Clonidine	X
Antagonists		
Alpha 1, alpha 2	Phenoxybenzamine	X
	Phentolamine	X
Alpha 1	Indoramin	?
	Prazosin	?
Beta adrenoceptor		
Agonist	Isoproterenol (migraine equivalent only)	✓
Antagonists		
NO ISA†		
Beta 1, beta 2	Propranolol	✓
	Timolol	✓
Beta 1	Atenolol	✓
	Metoprolol	✓
ISA		
Beta 1, beta 2	Pindolol	X
	Alprenolol	X
	Oxyprenolol	X
Histamine		
Antagonists H1	Chlorpheniramine	X
H2	Cimetidine	X
Prostaglandins		
Agonists	PGE 1	XX
	Prostacyclin	X
Antagonists	Aspirin	✓
	Fenemates	✓
	Indomethacin	?
Miscellaneous		
Calcium-channel blocking agents		?
Anticonvulsants		?
Platelet deaggregants		?
Bradykinin antagonists		X
Lithium carbonate		X

* A beneficial effect is indicated by ✓, precipitation or aggravation of headache by XX, lack of effect by X, and uncertain effect by ?.

† Intrinsic sympathomimetic activity.

reduced progressively to the minimum dose that is effective in controlling the cluster pains. This minimum dose is then continued for the duration of the bout. This regimen suppresses cluster headache in about 80 percent of patients. Should the pains continue despite these measures, a trial of oxygen inhalation is worthwhile. Most patients respond to oxygen inhalation within 10 minutes. For such patients, an oxygen cylinder, valve, and mask can be installed in the home. The application of a hot towel or hot water bottle to the painful areas also gives some relief. Chlorpromazine has been advocated for resistant cases of cluster headache, but I have not had the opportunity to evaluate its effectiveness. Alcohol commonly precipitates cluster pains and should be avoided.

Chronic Cluster Headache

All the preceding measures may be applied in the management of chronic cluster headache. If they fail, as they often do, the headaches may be controlled with lithium carbonate in a dose of 250 to 300 mg 2 to 3 times daily, to provide a blood level within the therapeutic range (0.7 to 1.0 mEq/L). Side effects, sometimes experienced within conventional therapeutic blood levels, include tremor, abdominal pain, weight loss, and confusion. Blood levels should be obtained weekly at first, then, once equilibrium is achieved, at less frequent intervals. Recently, the calcium-channel blocking agents verapamil, nifedipine, and nimodipine have been reported as controlling chronic cluster headache in the majority of patients, but only after some months. Medication must be instituted gradually since the vasodilator effect of these drugs may precipitate cluster pains if the initial dose is overzealous. Verapamil, for example, may be slowly increased from 20 mg twice daily to 320 mg daily if necessary. Caution must be exercised if the patient is already taking beta-blocking agents, and verapamil should not be given by injection to such patients, since the combination may cause cardiac arrest. The dose of nifedipine used ranges from 30 to 120 mg per day, and the dose of nimodipine up to 240 mg per day. Side effects of calcium-channel blockers include flushing, postural hypotension, tachycardia, fatigue, and headache if the dose is elevated too rapidly.

Chronic Paroxysmal Hemicrania

This rare variant of cluster headache responds specifically to indomethacin (Indocid), 25 mg 3 times daily, given after meals to avoid gastric irritation. Postural hypotension and a dull daily headache may be side effects. Indomethacin is worth a trial in any patient with brief attacks of cluster headache recurring more than three times in 24 hours.

TRIGEMINAL AND GLOSSOPHARYNGEAL NEURALGIA

DONALD J. DALESSIO, M.D.

TRIGEMINAL NEURALGIA

Trigeminal neuralgia is a terrifying disease to the patient, but one for which the treatment is excellent. I make it a point to *tell the patient this* as soon as the diagnosis is made. Many of these patients are frantic, and they need reassurance that you and your colleagues can manage their problem successfully, one way or another.

Clinical Features

Trigeminal neuralgia is usually a disease of later adult life, but may affect the young, including a rare teenager. There is a tendency to look for multiple sclerosis when trigeminal neuralgia occurs in the young, but in my experience trigeminal neuralgia associated with multiple sclerosis usually appears when multiple sclerosis is far advanced. Thus, most of the young patients with facial pain for whom I have cared have had typical trigeminal neuralgia, not associated with multiple sclerosis.

The pain is of high intensity and usually occurs in association with trigger zones (which are areas of increased sensitivity on the face). These zones are often about the nares and mouth and set off the attack when they are stimulated — often by trivial sensations. Thus, the behavioral characteristics of patients with trigeminal neuralgia are to avoid touching the face, washing, shaving, biting, chewing, or any other maneuvers that stimulate the trigger zones and produce the pain. This avoidance technique is an invaluable clue to the diagnosis. In almost every other facial pain syndrome, patients will be found massaging the painful area, abrading it, or applying heat or cold, but in trigeminal neuralgia exactly the opposite occurs; the patient goes to great lengths to avoid any stimulation of the face or mouth whatsoever.

The pain paroxysm is usually a high-intensity jab lasting less than 20 to 30 seconds, followed at times by a period of relief lasting a few seconds to a minute, again followed by another jab of pain. Repeated episodes of pain may occur, but the pain is not long-lived, as is usually the case in other chronic facial pains.

Medical Treatment

Medical treatment is indicated first, if for no other reason than its use constitutes a therapeutic challenge to the diagnosis. If a patient presumed to have trigeminal neuralgia does not rapidly respond to carbamazepine in 24 to 48 hours, the diagnosis is seriously in doubt. After all, the diagnosis is made on the basis of history alone, and, in general, patients are not good observers of their own pains or sensations — unless by a billion-to-one chance your patient is Proust.

If the patient does respond to carbamazepine, then clearly this is the treatment of choice. Those clinicians who have followed patients with trigeminal neuralgia for more than a decade realize that the disease is often remitting. Using drugs, it may be possible to nudge the patient into another remission, following which medication can sometimes be stopped. If this is not the case, and the response to carbamazepine is only partial, other drugs may also be useful, including phenytoin, baclofen, and chlorphenesin. Some neurosurgeons suggest that unpleasant side effects occur frequently with carbamazepine and that up to 20 to 30 percent of patients need to stop taking this drug, which is surprising, since the drug seems better tolerated when used in treatment of epilepsy.

Specifics of Drug Use

Generally, treatment is begun with carbamazepine, 100 to 200 mg 2 or 3 times daily (Table 1). If this is well tolerated and if the pain is rapidly relieved, this dosage may be continued for several weeks or months, depending upon the course of the disease. One should titrate the medication to the severity of the patient's pain. It may be necessary to continue carbamazepine at a maintenance level, such as 200 mg per day, in order to keep the patient pain-free.

If symptoms persist I increase carbamazepine up to 1,000 mg per day, depending upon the tolerance of each patient to the drug. If pain relief is incomplete, I add baclofen, 10 mg, to the regimen. Baclofen can be increased to 10 mg 3 times a day, depending on pain relief. Rarely, it may be necessary to increase the drug to 60 to 80 mg per day.

If there is no response, discontinue medications over a week and start phenytoin, 100 mg 4 times a day. A fourth drug, chlorphenesin, 400 mg daily, can be used as a supplementary medication with either carbamazepine or phenytoin.

I no longer use three drugs for pain relief, as such combinations are not well tolerated. If the patient's pain is not responding to two drugs in adequate dosage, consider referring the patient to a neurosurgeon. Generally, parenteral doses of medications are not employed.

Monitoring Serum Levels. Serum levels of anticonvulsants are a useful way of monitoring treatment. For carbamazepine, at least initially, levels of 6 to 12 μg per ml (25 to 50 mmol per liter) are usually required to relieve the pain. For phenytoin, therapeutic levels are 10 to 20 μg per ml (40 to 80 mmol per liter).

Side Effects of Medical Treatment

Carbamazepine. The side effects of carbamazepine that most frequently limit therapy include ataxia, drowsiness, and fatigue. Older patients may note confusion while taking the drug. Idiosyncratic side effects include leukopenia, agranulocytosis, and, rarely, aplastic anemia. It is therefore advisable to obtain pretreatment baseline values of whole blood serum and platelets and to repeat these tests at regular intervals (e.g., monthly) during treatment.

Phenytoin. The most common side effects of this drug are drowsiness, dizziness, and diplopia, which can be reduced by appropriate dosage modification. More severe central nervous system (CNS) effects such as ataxia, nystagmus, and slurred speech are an indication for immediate reduction of the dosage. Idiosyncratic side effects of phenytoin include gum hypertrophy and occasionally megaloblastic anemia.

Chlorphenesin and Baclofen. The most common side effect noted with chlorphenesin is drowsiness. Similarly, drowsiness, weakness, nausea, and vomiting may occur with baclofen.

Surgical Treatment

Between 25 and 50 percent of patients will eventually fail on drug therapy and need some form of neurosurgical treatment (Table 2). The type of operation performed varies widely from center to center. Patients need to be completely and clearly apprised of the nature of the operations proposed, procedures to be undertaken, possible side effects, costs, and morbidity and mortality. Informed consent regarding these neurosurgical procedures, given their many differences, is mandatory.

Selective lesions of the trigeminal root using a radiofrequency electrode placed in the root under radiologic control (radiofrequency rhizotomy) is an operative procedure that has gained wide acceptance. It has the advantages of safety and simplicity. The anesthesia used is light, and the patient is awake during some of the procedure, recovers rapidly, and is often found eating supper a few hours after the operation has been completed. Almost always the patient can be discharged the next day.

However, there is a recurrence rate of about 25 percent, occasional corneal anesthesia occurs, and rarely, uncomfortable dysesthesias or facial or jaw weakness develops. Altered sensation in the face is reported by many patients, but only a few are bothered by it. To the present, there has been no mortality associated with this operation.

A variation on this procedure has been proposed by Hakanson. He injects 0.2 to 0.4 ml of glycerol by the anterior percutaneous route into the trigeminal cistern (Meckel's cavity), which is visualized by aid of contrast medium (metrizamide). Hakanson reports excellent

TABLE 1 Drug Therapy of Trigeminal Neuralgia

Generic Drug	*Brand Name*	*Dosage*	*Precautions*	*Preparations*
Carbamazepine	Tegretol	200–600 mg/day	Monitor for blood disorders weekly, monthly	Oral
Phenytoin	Dilantin	200–400 mg/day	CNS, hematopoietic, gingival hyperplasia	Oral
Chlorphenesin	Maolate	800–2,400 mg/day	Drowsiness	Oral
Baclofen	Lioresal	30–80	Drowsiness, weakness, nausea, vomiting	

TABLE 2 Comparisons of Operative Procedures in Trigeminal Neuralgia

Procedure	*Advantages*	*Disadvantages*
Radiofrequency rhizotomy	90% effective Minor procedure Brief hospital stay No craniotomy	Facial sensory loss Facial weakness Corneal hypesthesia (10 – 15%) Masseter weakness
Glycerol injection	85% effective Minor procedure	Facial sensory loss
Microvascular decompression	90% effective	±4% serious postoperative complications 1% mortality Long hospital stay Major craniotomy

response to his procedure, with only minimal disturbance of facial sensitivity. Sweet and his colleagues have also reported their experience with this procedure. They describe greater pain on injection and more sensory loss. The presumption is made that glycerol is neurotoxic, acts on partially demyelinated nerve fibers, and eliminates the compound action potential in the trigeminal rootlets associated with pain. We now use the glycerol procedure *preferentially* in patients who request a quick, effective surgical procedure but who wish to avoid a formal craniotomy.

A third procedure is microvascular decompression of the trigeminal root. Here, the neurosurgeon assumes that a lesion (usually an arterial loop) will be found compressing the trigeminal root close by the brainstem. So, in effect, the operation is exploratory, for *none* of our current sophisticated neurodiagnostic studies, including arteriography, computed tomography (CT) of the head, or other special views, will in fact allow the surgeon to predict with certainty before the operation that such a lesion will be found. If and when it is found, the compressing lesion is removed from the trigeminal root, often by interposing a sponge. By deduction, it is suggested that in most cases trigeminal neuralgia is a compressive cranial mononeuropathy.

There is a significant difference in cost between these various operations. Radiofrequency lesions and glycerol injections are done rapidly, and almost always the patient is quickly discharged. With microsurgical decompression of the trigeminal root, a formal craniotomy is required, and the patient frequently spends 7 to 10 days in the hospital and a similar period of time convalescing.

To summarize, both medical and surgical therapies may be used in the individual patient with trigeminal neuralgia (Table 3). Ordinarily, the treatment is medical. If response to drugs is not forthcoming, or if the patient becomes toxic while taking medications or refuses to follow an appropriate medical program, then surgical consultation and appropriate operation should be obtained. The form and type of the neurosurgical procedure to be done will probably depend to a considerable extent on the expertise of the neurosurgeon and his own training. Generally, in the elderly, the simplest procedures should be attempted first. It may be necessary to employ both medical and surgical procedures in the individual patient. I have followed a group of patients who were managed with drugs initially and who gradually became unresponsive to therapy, required surgical procedures of one sort or another, eventually also had recurrences of pain, and who are now finally being managed medically once more. Thus, treatment is not an either/or matter in this disease and cooperation between physician and surgeon is essential (Figure 1).

GLOSSOPHARYNGEAL NEURALGIA

Glossopharyngeal neuralgia (tic) is characterized by severe pain in the region of the tonsil and ear. It has timing and features similar to those of trigeminal neuralgia and may be initiated by yawning and swallowing or contact of food with the tonsillar region. Rarely, the patient may become unconscious during a paroxysm of pain (probably due to asystole). Examination reveals no evidence of reduction in perception of pinprick or touch or of motility function in the nasopharynx.

Often the pain of glossopharyngeal neuralgia can be relieved by temporary cocainization of the involved side of the throat. Extracranial block of the glossopharyngeal nerve with alcohol is not recommended, since the injection of alcohol in the region of the jugular foramen might well cause paralysis of the tenth, eleventh, and twelfth cranial nerves and could conceivably also involve the sympathetic trunk.

In treating glossopharyngeal neuralgia one employs the same regimen used in trigeminal neuralgia (see Table 1). Carbamazepine is the drug of choice. If the patient does not respond to carbamazepine, the treatment of choice is intracranial section of the nerve. Usually the exposure is through a unilateral suboccipital craniectomy. The nerve can be identified as it passes along the floor of the posterior fossa to emerge through the jugular foramen.

TABLE 3 Summary of the Management of Trigeminal Neuralgia

Use of carbamazepine
1. Establish diagnosis
2. Carbamazepine, 100–200 mg t.i.d., increase to 1,000 mg/day if indicated
3. Obtain serum levels in 1 week
4. Follow CBC monthly
5. If pain control is insufficient, add baclofen, 10 mg t.i.d.; increase if indicated

Ancillary drugs
1. Phenytoin, 100 mg q.i.d.; stop other medications first
2. Chlorphenesin, 400 mg t.i.d.; can use in combination with other drugs

Surgery Considered
1. If pain is unresponsive to drugs, or if there are
2. Toxic reactions to drugs, or as an
3. Alternative to medical therapy

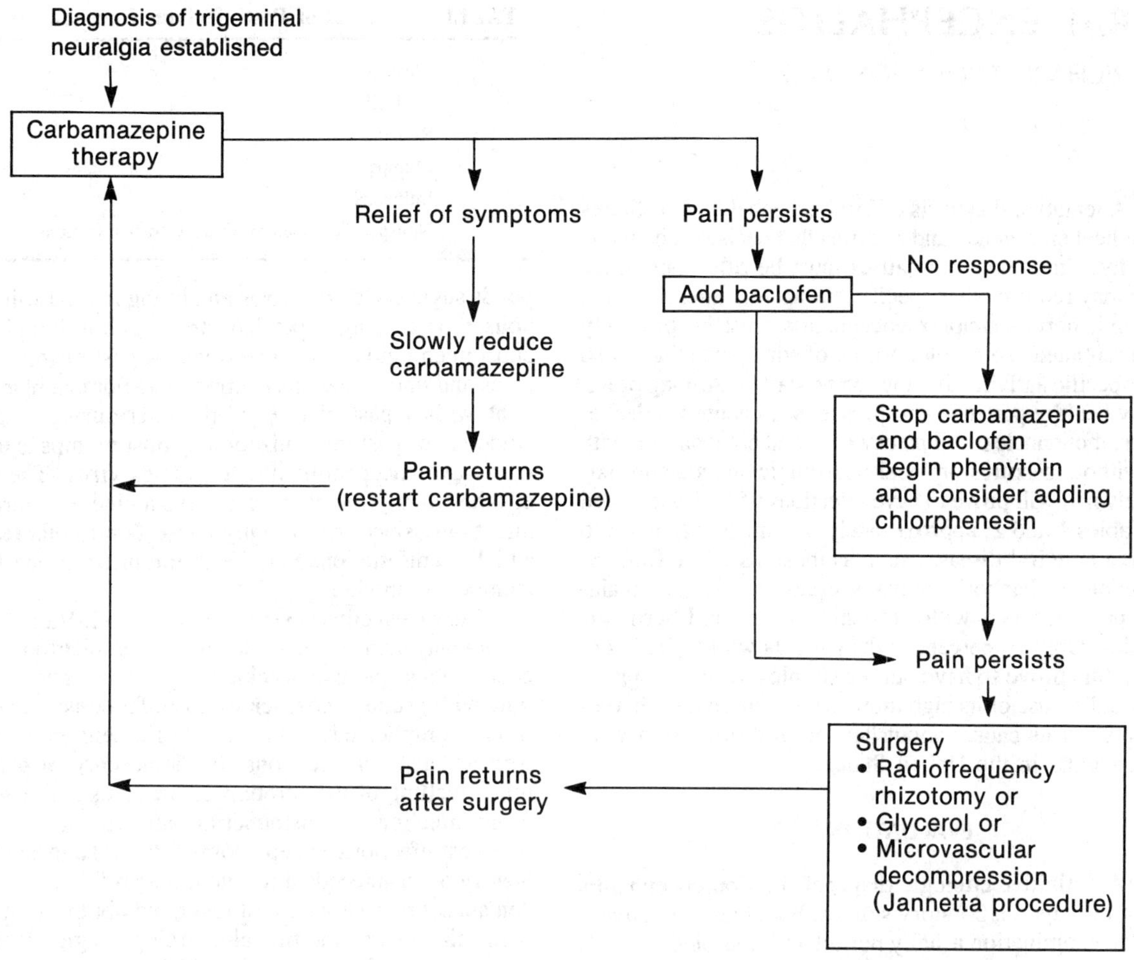

Figure 1 Schematic representation of management of trigeminal neuralgia.

Some authors use the term ''glossopharyngeal and vagal neuralgia'' or ''vagoglossopharyngeal neuraglia'' instead of glossopharyngeal neuralgia, implying that the pain can radiate into the distribution of the vagus nerve as well as that of the glossopharyngeal nerve. The original term ''glossopharyngeal neuralgia'' is recognized by most neurologists and is more commonly used.

Since the ear and its adjacent structures are supplied by pain fibers from the fifth, seventh, ninth, and tenth cranial nerves, neuralgias of these structures often closely resemble each other and sometimes become indistinguishable. It is therefore not surprising that there has been controversy concerning the existence of separate neuralgias of these nerves and conflict as to the best surgical procedures. However, the mechanism of the pain in all forms is likely the same.

PATIENT RESOURCES

National Migraine Foundation
5252 N. Western Avenue
Chicago, Illinois 60625

VIRAL ENCEPHALITIS

RICHARD T. JOHNSON, M.D.

A tentative diagnosis of viral encephalitis constitutes a medical emergency and requires that decisions be made rapidly. First, nonviral causes must be ruled out, since they may require other specific therapeutic interventions. Second, herpes simplex encephalitis must be promptly differentiated from other forms of viral encephalitis so that specific antiviral therapy can be started. Among previously healthy patients who present with acute headache, fever, mononuclear cell pleocytosis, and obtundation (with or without seizures or focal neurologic signs), approximately half will prove to have infections with viruses listed in Tables 1 and 2; approximately one-third will prove to have a nonviral disease, such as those listed in Table 3. An etiologic diagnosis cannot be established in the remaining patients even with optimal cultures and serologic studies. Only 10 percent of the patients with ''viral'' encephalitis prove to have herpes simplex virus encephalitis, but because of its high mortality and morbidity, herpes simplex virus causes about half of all deaths from viral encephalitis in the United States.

EVALUATION

A definitive etiologic diagnosis in viral encephalitis must rely upon laboratory studies, but clues in the history and examination usually permit an ''educated guess.'' A careful history of immunizations, past exposure to insect bites, place of residence, contacts with animals, areas of recent travel, and health of family members is needed. The season is of primary consideration, since mumps virus infections occur predominantly in the spring and arbovirus and enterovirus infections in the late summer and early fall. Indeed, arboviruses need not be considered in the winter unless the patient has returned in the past week or two from the tropics. Public health information is usually available on viruses circulating in the community at a particular time. A history of animal contact is relevant not only for rabies, as a history of swimming in farm ponds suggests leptospirosis and living in mouse-infected houses or owning a pet hamster suggests lymphocytic choriomeningitis virus infections. A past history of diseases and immunizations is important. For example, a patient with a past history of parotitis during a mumps epidemic or past immunization against mumps is unlikely to have encephalitis due to mumps virus. The health of other family members may give a clue to enterovirus infections, since they usually cause family outbreaks in which manifestations may be different from one family member to another.

TABLE 1 Causes of Acute Viral Encephalitis*

Mumps virus
Arboviruses (Eastern, Western, St. Louis, California, Venezuelan equine, and Colorado tick fever viruses)
Herpes simplex viruses
Lymphocytic choriomeningitis virus
Enteroviruses (coxsackie and echoviruses)
Cytomegalovirus
Adenoviruses
Rabies virus

* In approximate order of frequency

TABLE 2 Causes of Postinfectious Encephalomyelitis

Measles
Varicella
Rubella
Mumps
Influenza
Nonspecific upper respiratory tract infections

Associated clinical signs can be helpful. Varied rashes accompany some enterovirus infections; pleurodynia can occur with group B coxsackievirus infections and herpangina with group A coxsackievirus infections; pneumonitis can complicate lymphocytic choriomeningitis virus as well as bacterial infections. In the absence of parotitis, mild swelling of the scrotum or breasts suggest mumps virus infections in postpubertal patients.

Postinfectious encephalomyelitis is suggested by a history of an antecedent febrile illness followed by a sudden abrupt recrudescence of fever and obtundation, often with seizures and multifocal neurologic signs. If the antecedent infection is measles, this diagnosis is straightforward, but if it is a nonspecific respiratory disease, the differential diagnosis of direct viral invasion of the central nervous system (CNS) and postinfectious perivenular demyelinating disease may be possible only by histologic examination.

In contrast, herpes simplex encephalitis has no seasonal variation. A past history of herpes labialis, exposure to herpes simplex, or even the presence of herpes labialis at the time of examination is of essentially no value in implicating herpes simplex virus in encephalitis when it occurs after the newborn period. A history of personality changes (such as episodes of terror, hallucinations, or bizarre behavior) in addition to fever and headache and the presence of focal seizures, hemiparesis, aphasia, and superior quadrant visual field defects all implicate herpes simplex virus, since this viral encephalitis usually is localized to the medial temporal and orbital frontal areas and is often unilateral or asymmetrical. Other viral infections can cause these signs and symptoms by chance, but only herpes simplex virus shows uniform localization.

Routine laboratory studies are of less value in differential diagnosis. A marked leukocytosis may suggest a bacterial infection; an elevated amylase may suggest mumps. Evidence of immune deficiency diseases should be sought, since immunodeficient patients present with a different spectrum of CNS infections.

TABLE 3 Diseases That Stimulate Viral Encephalitis

Infectious Diseases
- Rickettsiae
  - Rocky Mountain spotted fever
  - Typhus
- Bacteria
  - *Mycoplasma pneumoniae*
  - Leptospirosis
  - Lyme disease
  - Syphilis (secondary or meningovascular)
  - Listeriosis
  - Brucellosis (particularly *Brucella melitensis*)
  - Tuberculosis
  - Typhoid fever
  - Parameningeal infections (epidural, petrositis)
  - Partially treated bacterial meningitis
  - Subacute bacterial endocarditis
  - Brain abscess
- Fungi
  - Cryptococcosis
  - Coccidioidomycosis
  - Histoplasmosis
  - North American blastomycosis
  - Candidiasis
- Parasites
  - Toxoplasmosis
  - Cysticercosis
  - Echinococcosis
  - Trypanosomiasis
  - *Plasmodium falciparum*
  - Amebiasis (*Naegleria* and *Acanthamoeba*)

Noninfectious Diseases
- Neoplasms
  - Carcinomatous meningitis
  - Gliomatosis cerebri
  - Ruptured cysts
- Vascular disease
  - Granulomatous angiitis
  - Systemic lupus erythematosus
  - Rheumatoid meningitis
- Others
  - Neurosarcoidosis
  - Behçet's syndrome
  - Oculocephalic syndromes

Cerebrospinal fluid (CSF) is critical in establishing the diagnosis. If the patient has focal signs or evidence of increased intracranial pressure, a computed tomography (CT) scan with contrast should precede the lumbar puncture. If there are no focal abnormalities or shift of midline structures, proceed with the lumbar puncture. In viral encephalitis there are typically modest numbers of mononuclear cells, although large numbers of polymorphonuclear cells can be present in the first day or two of disease. In 3 percent of patients with herpes simplex encephalitis no pleocytosis is found on the initial CSF examination. Red blood cells in the CSF are suggestive of herpes simplex encephalitis, but their presence does not clearly implicate herpetic encephalitis, nor does their absence exclude it. Protein content is usually elevated. In most cases of encephalitis, the CSF sugar shows a normal ratio with blood sugar, although it may be mildly depressed, particularly in mumps or lymphocytic choriomeningitis virus infections. When there is an absence of cells or a preponderance of polymorphonuclear cells, a repeat examination in 12 to 24 hours usually shows transition to typical findings if the diagnosis of viral encephalitis is correct. Virus cultures of CSF for enteroviruses, mumps, and occasionally arboviruses may be positive, but herpes simplex virus is only rarely found in CSF. Assays of CSF virus-specific IgM can be useful for the rapid diagnosis of arbovirus infections, but not for herpes simplex virus encephalitis.

TREATMENT OF SUSPECTED HERPETIC ENCEPHALITIS

Herpes simplex virus encephalitis must be suspected if there is a history of behavioral abnormalities or focal seizures or if there are focal signs on examination (Figure 1). In these circumstances a CT scan is usually obtained first to exclude a mass effect. If the CT signs and symptoms are consistent and the scan shows an edematous temporal lobe lesion with mass effect, I recommend going directly to biopsy without a CSF examination. Otherwise, spinal fluid is examined to establish a diagnosis of encephalitis. If the CT scan is normal or equivocal, it is important to rapidly determine if there is a localized abnormality and to determine its localization by other methods. The most sensitive test early in disease is the electroencephalogram (EEG); suspicion of herpes simplex encephalitis is one of the few indications for an emergency EEG. The EEG may show only diffuse slowing, but often there are unilateral or bilateral periodic discharges in the temporal leads. In some patients a characteristic slow wave complex seen at regular intervals of 2 to 3 per second is highly suggestive of the diagnosis. The second choice of tests is a radionucleotide scan that may show increased isotope uptake in one or both temporal lobes, and this finding may be evident earlier than the low-density temporal lobe abnormality later seen on CT scans. In addition to the low-density abnormalities, the CT scan may document bilaterality and the scan with contrast may show an enhancement pattern along the sylvian fissure and the opercular areas as well as the temporal lobe. Magnetic resonance imaging has shown sharply defined lesions in the temporal lobes, but as yet this imaging method has not been evaluated for its specificity or early sensitivity in diagnosing herpes simplex encephalitis.

If there is not clear localization by history or clinical examination, or if the EEG, radionucleotide scan, and CT scan fail to show temporal localization, institute supportive care (as will be discussed), watch the patient carefully, and repeat tests as indicated. For example, if the history is consistent with herpes encephalitis and the EEG and scans fail to lateralize a lesion, repeat studies in 24 hours or sooner if there is any deterioration of clinical status. Rapid deterioration with clear-cut focal signs on examination probably justifies a biopsy even without clear-cut localization on EEG or scans.

Biopsy

Brain biopsy is the only reliably method of diagnosis. If localization suggests herpes simplex encephalitis,

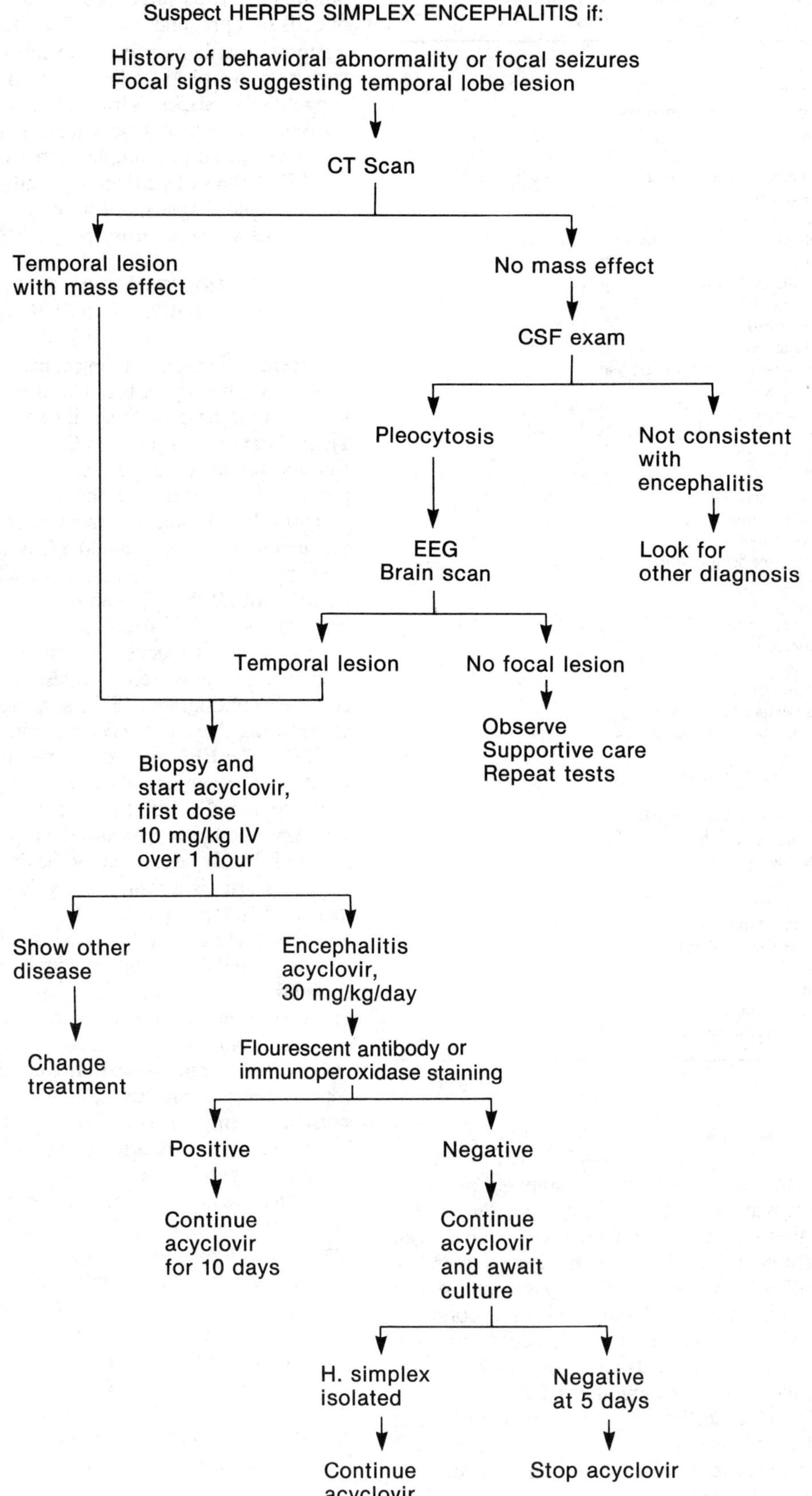

Figure 1 Steps in management of suspected herpes simplex encephalitis.

a biopsy should be arranged and acyclovir should be started. Acyclovir is given at a dose of 30 mg per kilogram per day, divided into three doses. The doses are diluted in at least 100 ml of standard intravenous solution and administered over 1 hour. In the protocol for the experimental trial of efficacy, acyclovir was not begun until after the biopsy was performed. However, early treatment, before the patient is comatose, is a critical determinant of quality of outcome and patients can deteriorate rapidly. Therefore, it seems advisable to start acyclovir as the biopsy is being organized. The administration of one of the doses immediately prior to biopsy will not interfere with histologic biopsy results and is unlikely to affect culture results.

The argument is often made that a relatively nontoxic drug such as acyclovir should be given without biopsy diagnosis. There are, however, compelling reasons to do a biopsy: (1) Only one-third of the patients suspected of having early herpes simplex encephalitis will prove to have this disorder, and one-third of the nonherpes group have diseases for which other specific therapeutic modalities are appropriate and urgent. (2) The efficacy of acyclovir and vidarabine has been established only in patients with biopsies. Since open biopsy provides decompression of the swollen temporal lobe, it may also have therapeutic benefit and may be a significant part of the efficacy of these therapies. (3) If there is a failure to respond, later deterioration, or relapse, knowledge of the initial pathology and virology is critical.

Biopsy should be made in the area of maximal disease. False-negative biopsies have been due most frequently to the arbitrary surgical decision to biopsy the frontal convexity or the nondominant temporal lobe when disease is in the dominant temporal lobe. Virus is found where the pathology is located. Biopsy should be done via a craniotomy, not a needle biopsy (CT directed or otherwise). First, the complication rate of open biopsy in our institution has been nil, but bleeding may complicate needle biopsies. Second, an open biopsy allows decompression of the swollen temporal lobe, and this in itself may offer therapeutic benefit. Third, direct visualization of the temporal lobe may reveal an alternative diagnosis and allows delineation of an area of maximal encephalitic involvement for precise localization of the biopsy (an area of cortical petechiae) and avoidance of the speech area if biopsy is in the left temporal lobe. The biopsy specimen should be of adequate size so that a segment can be frozen for fluorescent antibody or immunoperoxidase staining. A portion should also be put in formalin for routine histologic staining, and homogenates should be prepared for inoculation onto cell cultures for virus isolation.

Frozen sections rarely show inclusions, but in herpes simplex encephalitis sections usually show inflammatory reactions and rule out tumor or other noninfectious diseases. Frozen sections stained for viral antigen are highly reliable in experienced hands, with a low number of false-positive or false-negative results. If staining is positive, continue acyclovir therapy for 10 days. If this is negative, the paraffin-embedded material can be examined on the next day. Intranuclear inclusions are highly suggestive of the diagnosis, but are found in only about half of the early biopsies, and they may result from Epstein-Barr virus and other infections. Cultures are observed daily for cytopathic effects of herpes simplex virus. If at the end of 5 days the cultures are negative and other studies indicative of herpes infections are absent, acyclovir should be discontinued. It is continued for 10 days if the cultures are positive.

Treatment Failure

Failure to improve or deterioration after stabilization or improvement presents a difficult problem in management of patients with suspected herpes encephalitis. If herpes simplex virus has not been established as the etiologic agent, an alternative diagnosis must be sought, since other etiologies are likely under these circumstances. In biopsy-proved cases with late deterioration or relapse, EEG, radionucleotide scan, and CT scan should be repeated to rule out hemorrhage, subdural hematoma, herniation, or other noninfectious complications. Rare patients have relapsed after vidarabine treatment, with progressive deterioration accompanied by striking contrast enhancement of the cortical ribbon. In such cases, rebiopsy is indicated. Although not yet observed in encephalitis, acyclovir treatment can lead to selection of drug-resistant mutants. If it appears that the patient has ongoing or reactivated herpes simplex encephalitis, attempts should be made to recover virus to establish this, and the patient should be started on a course of vidarabine, 15 mg per kilogram per day IV, given continuously rather than intermittently as with acyclovir.

GENERAL SUPPORTIVE CARE

Bedrest is indicated. Strict isolation procedures are not essential, since most of the viruses that cause meningitis and encephalitis are common in our environment. If an enterovirus infection is suspected, precautions in handling stools and careful handwashing should be instituted. If measles, chickenpox, rubella, or mumps virus infections are evident, the usual isolation from susceptible persons is recommended.

The headache and fever of aseptic meningitis can usually be managed with judicious doses of aspirin or acetaminophen. Severe hyperthermia may develop in encephalitis, necessitating use of more vigorous therapy, but it should be remembered that viruses are thermolabile. Therefore, modest temperature elevations may serve as a natural defense mechanism, and attempts to reduce mild temperature elevations to normal or subnormal levels may be ill-advised.

Patients with severe encephalitis are often in coma. Since these patients may make remarkable recoveries even after prolonged periods of coma, vigorous supportive therapy and avoidance of complications are essential. The airway often must be maintained by intubation or tracheotomy, and mechanical respiration may be necessary. Although intravenous fluids may suffice for brief periods, prolonged coma necessitates feeding with a nasogastric tube. Blood glucose and electrolytes should be checked frequently, since water, glucose, and salt control are not infrequently compromised during encephalitis. Paradoxical antidiuretic hormone secretion is particularly frequent during St. Louis encephalitis. The respiratory tract, urinary tract, intravenous site, and skin are common sites of infection in comatose patients, and infection should be checked assiduously, treated vigorously, and avoided by skillful nursing, maintenance of bronchial drainage, frequent turning to avoid decubitus ulcers, and meticulous catheter care.

Continuous pressure monitoring has not usually proved helpful. In cases of herpes encephalitis in which herniation is of greatest danger, the surgical decompression is a major aid in controlling pressure. Steroids are not used routinely, but are indicated for increased pressure or signs of pending herniation. Dexamethasone (Decadron) is given with a loading dose of 0.6 mg per kilogram IV, followed by 0.2 mg per kilogram every 6 hours. Despite the theoretical adverse effects of corticosteroids in infections, they have been widely used in herpes simplex, even before the advent of antiviral chemotherapy, without evidence of exacerbating the disease. A study of the routine use of steroids in arbovirus encephalitis has shown neither efficacious nor adverse effects. Corticosteroids in postinfectious encephalomyelitis have similarly shown no effect in modifying the course of disease. Corticosteroids are used only to reduce edema.

Anticonvulsants are not given routinely. In patients with suspected herpes encephalitis who have had a biopsy, I do give prophylactic anticonvulsants for several months. In other patients, when seizures occur, they should be treated with intravenous diazepam, phenobarbital, or phenytoin. Once fever has abated, anticonvulsants are discontinued and are reinstated only if recurrent seizures develop after the patient is afebrile.

HERPES ZOSTER

DIANE E. GRIFFIN, M.D., Ph.D.

Herpes zoster is a common inflammatory vesicular skin eruption that is characteristically dermatomal in distribution. This eruption is a manifestation of the reactivation of a latent infection of sensory ganglia with the varicella-zoster virus. The primary infection with this virus produces the systemic disease varicella, or chickenpox, which commonly occurs during childhood. During the primary infection the varicella-zoster virus travels from the generalized skin lesions by way of the sensory nerve retrograde axonal transport to the sensory ganglion cells. The virus establishes a latent infection in the ganglion cells that may be reactivated at any time. Reactivation occurs most commonly in elderly individuals or those who are immunocompromised either by diseases such as leukemia, lymphoma, or acquired immunodeficiency syndrome (AIDS) or by immunosuppressive therapy. Like the primary infection, the reactivated infection is usually benign. However, in immunocompromised patients the virus may disseminate to skin sites outside of the originally involved dermatome and to other organs such as the brain, heart, lungs, or liver. In severe cases of dermatomal disease, particularly in individuals who are over the age of 60, a debilitating pain syndrome, termed postherpetic neuralgia, may develop.

The treatment of herpes zoster is in a state of evolution at the current time with both the development of new effective antiviral agents and the promise of drug formulations that are effective when given orally offering new possibilities for therapeutic intervention. The mortality from this common disease is extraordinarily low. Therefore, the objectives of treatment are to relieve the local discomfort in the involved skin area, prevent dissemination of the virus to other organ systems, and prevent postherpetic neuralgia. The potential for the development of these various problems differs significantly according to the type of patient experiencing reactivated infection.

TREATMENT

Normal Host

In the immunologically normal individual under the age of 60, both disseminated infection and postherpetic neuralgia are uncommon. The usual sequence of lesion development involves a period of prodromal pain that may last up to 7 days. The pain may be severe, is felt in the dermatome that will eventually have lesions, and, depending on the location, may be mistaken for appendicitis, pleurisy, cholecystitis, or myocardial infarction. The skin lesions begin as erythematous papules and progress to clear vesicles on an erythematous base within 12 to 24 hours. With the onset of the cellular immune response and influx of leukocytes from the peripheral blood, the vesicles become pustular. As recovery continues, the vesicles crust over and begin to heal. Treatment of these lesions requires only symptomatic relief with the application of a soothing drying substance such as calamine lotion. Pain relievers such as acetylsalicylic acid (aspirin) or acetaminophen (Tylenol) are usually sufficient. Healing is usually complete within 10 to 14 days. The development of herpes zoster in an otherwise healthy individual should not prompt a search for underlying disease.

If the lesions are kept dry, secondary bacterial infections are unusual. Mild infection can be treated locally with an ointment containing an antibiotic such as neomycin. If there is evidence of significant cellulitis with local skin induration and fever, appropriate cultures should be obtained. Oral therapy with an antistaphylococcal antibiotic such as cephalexin (500 mg 4 times a day) or dicloxacillin (500 mg 4 times a day) for 5 to 7 days may be indicated.

Approximately 20 percent of individuals with herpes zoster involving the ophthalmic portion of the trigeminal ganglion will develop ocular viral infection (keratoconjunctivitis, iridocyclitis). This complication is thought to be more likely with involvement of the nasociliary branch of the ophthalmic nerve, which is indicated by vesicles on the side and tip of the nose. If the eye is infected, local application of the specific antiviral agent acyclovir may be necessary, and referral to an ophthalmologist is recommended. In addition to a small number of patients with ophthalmic herpes zoster have been described who developed contralateral hemiparesis 3 to 5 weeks later. This appears to be caused by a virus-induced granulomatous angiitis that may become associated with even more widespread neurologic deficits. Systemic antiviral therapy (see below) is indicated for these individuals.

Elderly Patients

If the patient is elderly, has had severe prodromal pain, and/or has persistent or confluent painful lesions, he or she is at greater risk for the development of postherpetic neuralgia. Even in these patients pain resolves steadily with time and lasts less than 8 weeks in almost half and less than a year in 80 percent. Prolonged pain is least frequent in patients with lumbar involvement. There is some evidence that treatment with systemic steroids (45 to 60 mg of prednisone for 7 days, tapered over the subsequent 2 weeks) during the acute eruption decreases the incidence of postherpetic neuralgia in patients over 60 years of age, but does not affect the rate of healing or shorten the period of acute pain. This regimen entails a small, but significant, risk of dissemination of the infection, and its usefulness is currently being re-evaluated in a much larger controlled trial that is also analyzing the effect of specific antiviral treatment with oral acyclovir (Zovirax), 800 mg 5 times per day, on the length of time that pain persists. Several studies have suggested that antiviral therapy may be useful in preventing postherpetic neuralgia.

In some patients pain may persist for months after the eruption has healed. This pain is usually refractory to conventional analgesics, and many regimens for control of it have been suggested. Treatment with narcotics should be avoided. Transcutaneous nerve stimulation may benefit some patients. The best results have been obtained with phenytoin (Dilantin), 200 to 500 mg per day, or carbamazepine (Tegretol), 400 to 800 mg per day, combined with tricyclic antidepressants (e.g., amitriptyline, 25 to 150 mg per day). Therapy should be initiated with a low dose of drug, which is then gradually increased over 4 to 6 weeks while monitoring side effects and efficacy in pain reduction. Blood levels of the drug, white blood cell counts, and liver function tests should also be followed, since full therapeutic doses of these agents are usually necessary for successful pain control. Surgical intervention, such as proximal root destruction or cordotomy, needs to be considered as a last resort in only rare instances.

Immunocompromised Patients

Recovery from herpes zoster and containment of the virus to the initially involved skin area depend on a specific cell-mediated immune response to the virus. Antibody does not appear to be significantly involved in recovery, and use of zoster immune globulin is not indicated for this disease. Disseminated infection occurs in less than 2 percent of the general population, but persons who are immunocompromised, because of either chemotherapy or an underlying condition that compromises immune function, have diminished cellular immunity to the virus and are at increased risk for developing disseminated disease. Cutaneous dissemination is the most common form of disseminated infection and often begins as the original dermatomal lesion is healing. A few lesions may appear outside the involved dermatome by direct spread of the virus in normal individuals, but in patients with true dissemination, virus is spread by the bloodstream, and large numbers of skin lesions appear outside the dermatome in an order and distribution similar to that seen in chickenpox. Skin dissemination increases morbidity, but is not associated with significantly increased mortality. Vesicles continue to appear outside the original dermatomal area for 3 to 8 days and then heal naturally. In a few patients with profound and prolonged immunosuppression, these lesions may persist for weeks to months. In addition to cutaneous spread, virus may also spread to involve internal organs such as the liver, myocardium, lung, and/or central nervous system (CNS). In addition to the contralateral hemiplegia described with ophthalmic zoster, CNS complications also include local paralysis due to motor neuron development myelitis, meningitis, and diffuse encephalitis with confusion and hallucinations. Cerebrospinal fluid (CSF) pleocytosis occurs in many individuals with uncomplicated disease and alone should not be considered an indication of CNS involvement. Visceral complications are seen almost exclusively in immunocompromised patients (approximately 10 percent of these patients will be affected) and may be life-threatening.

A number of antiviral agents have been shown to decrease the incidence of disseminated cutaneous and visceral infection when initiated within 72 hours of the onset of the rash. Treatment is indicated for those most at risk for dissemination (e.g., patients with transplanted organs or lymphoreticular malignancies) and those with demonstrated visceral involvement. No topical therapy has demonstrated efficacy for shortening the course of the dermatomal lesions or for decreasing the incidence of disseminated disease. Although human leukocyte interferon, 5×10^5 U per kilogram per day for 7 days, and adenine arabinoside (vidarabine), 10 mg per kilogram per day IV over 12 hours for 5 days, have been demonstrated to be efficacious, acyclovir (Zovirax), 500 mg per M^2 or 10 mg per kilogram every 8 hours IV for 7 days, is an easier drug to administer and is equally efficacious. Intravenous acyclovir decreases the incidence of dissemination in immunocompromised patients with isolated dermatomal lesions and visceral dissemination when given within 72 hours of the onset of cutaneous dissemination. There are few complications associated with acyclovir treatment, but in patients with compromised renal function the drug or a metabolite of the drug appears to accumulate and cause neurologic toxicity. Therefore, the dose should be altered by increasing the dosing interval from every 8 hours to every 12 hours with a creatinine clearance of 25 to 50 ml per minute and to every 24 hours with a creatinine clearance of less than 25 ml per minute. In addition, the dose should be halved (5 mg per kilogram every 24 hours) for individuals with a creatinine clearance of less than 10 ml per minute. The drug is removed by dialysis, so the dosing schedule for patients on hemodialysis should be adjusted so that a dose is administered after each dialysis.

Hospitalized patients should be placed in respiratory isolation to prevent secondary cases of chickenpox in nonimmune patients and hospital workers. The lesions of herpes zoster are infectious until all are crusted over. Prior to that time virus can be transmitted to the respiratory mucosa of a nonimmune individual who will get chickenpox (not herpes zoster).

Although intravenous acyclovir shortens the course of disease in the immunologically normal, as well as the immunocompromised, patient with herpes zoster and may decrease the incidence of postherpetic neuralgia, hospitalization for parenteral therapy is not usually indicated for these otherwise normal patients who are most likely to recover without incidence if left untreated. Oral therapy with acyclovir, 800 mg 5 times per day, is currently being evaluated and if found to be efficacious would simplify therapy and probably extend the number of patients for whom antiviral treatment would be indicated.

NEUROLOGICAL DYSFUNCTION IN ACQUIRED IMMUNODEFICIENCY SYNDROME

BRADFORD A. NAVIA, M.D.
RICHARD W. PRICE, M.D.

The acquired immunodeficiency syndrome (AIDS) is often complicated by central nervous system (CNS) or peripheral nervous system (PNS) dysfunction. In approaching diagnosis and therapy, CNS complications can be divided into two general types: (1) those causing predominantly focal symptoms and signs, and (2) those generally presenting with more diffuse dysfunction. PNS disorders are pathogenetically less well defined, but also can be segregated into more than one clinical type. Although AIDS is a progressive lethal disease, careful neurologic management, including accurate diagnosis and, when possible, prompt therapy, can alleviate some of the morbidity of the disease and prolong meaningful survival in certain patients. Even when specific therapy is not available, supportive management can do much to relieve the suffering of AIDS victims.

FOCAL CNS DISEASES

While a broad variety of opportunistic conditions causing focal neurologic dysfunction have been described in AIDS patients, most important with respect to both incidence and therapeutic response are cerebral toxoplasmosis and primary CNS lymphoma. Less common are progressive multifocal leukoencephalopathy (PML), focal encephalitis and cerebral vasculitis caused by varicella-zoster virus (VZV) infections, and infections by herpes simplex virus types 1 and 2 (HSV-1 and HSV-2). A number of other conditions have been described, but either occur in an agonal setting or are sufficiently rare that discussion of therapy is not justified in the present context.

Cerebral Toxoplasmosis

Cerebral toxoplasmosis is the most frequent treatable CNS disorder complicating AIDS and develops in about 10 to 15 percent of patients. It characteristically presents as a subacute illness in which aspects of both focal and nonfocal cerebral dysfunction are often combined. Focal manifestations usually relate to hemispheric lesions, but less commonly cerebellar or even brainstem signs may be prominent. The nonfocal aspects include general confusion or altered consciousness with lethargy and at times coma. Headache and fever are common.

In approaching AIDS patients with suspected toxoplasmosis or other focal disorders, we rely strongly on neuro-imaging techniques, particularly computerized tomography (CT) and, more recently, magnetic resonance imaging (MRI), this is in order to confirm both the presence of macroscopic focal disease and to determine the nature of the lesions. Multiple lesions involving the cortex or deep nuclei surrounded by edema strongly favor cerebral toxoplasmosis. In most cases *Toxoplasma* abscesses exhibit ring-like contrast enhancement on CT scan, but either homogeneous contrast enhancement or nonenhancing hypodense lesions may be noted in some cases.

Double-dose contrast CT studies, or preferably MRI, may help in more clearly defining or showing additional spherical lesions characteristic of the disease. The major differential diagnosis in such patients is cerebral lymphoma, which may have a similar CT appearance, although lymphoma commonly exhibits more diffuse or vague contrast enhancement, and the lesions tend to be single and more often located in the white matter. *Toxoplasma* serology is of additional help in separating these two disorders. Only very rarely do patients with cerebral toxoplasmosis have negative serum IgG antibody titers, although it is important to emphasize that these titers may be low and characteristically do not rise during the course of the disease.

To establish the diagnosis of cerebral toxoplasmosis, we now rely principally on therapeutic trial and reserve brain biopsy for treatment failures or clinically atypical patients, including those who are sero-negative. When treated promptly, patients with toxoplasmosis characteristically respond with clear clinical and CT improvement within 1 to 2 weeks. Many patients, in fact, improve clinically within 24 to 48 hours.

Treatment of toxoplasmosis is initiated with a loading dose of 50 mg of pyrimethamine followed by a single oral daily dose of 25 mg thereafter, together with a sulfa drug, usually sulfadiazine, 2 to 6 g daily in four divided doses. Patients also receive folinic acid, 10 mg daily as a single oral dose. Adverse reactions to sulfa, including allergy and bone marrow depression, are frequent in AIDS patients and may necessitate substitution of clindamycin at an oral dose of 600 mg four times a day. In our own experience this has not resulted in adverse consequences, but the efficacy of clindamycin has not yet been established by controlled study. If possible, treatment should be continued indefinitely, since stopping combined therapy or lowering the dose will often lead to relapse. In our experience, one-half of patients tried on chronic treatment with pyrimethamine alone relapsed.

In patients with cerebral toxoplasmosis, and indeed in all AIDS patients, corticosteroids should be avoided when possible. This is particularly important when treatment is instituted in the context of a therapeutic trial to differentiate between toxoplasmosis and CNS lymphoma. Since the latter may respond symptomatically to corticosteroids alone, clinical or CT improvement on combination antibiotic and steroid treatment will be difficult to interpret. More generally, corticosteroids increase the impairment of immune defenses in AIDS patients, potentially exacerbating not only toxoplasmosis but other systemic opportunistic infections as well. On the other hand, if cerebral edema related to brain lesions threatens brain herniation, then judicious short-term corticosteroids should be instituted along with appropriate specific therapy and subsequently tapered rapidly once the patient improves.

Primary CNS Lymphoma

Primary CNS lymphomas are opportunistic neoplasms that develop in about 5 percent of AIDS patients, although in perhaps one-half of these the lymphoma represents only an incidental autopsy finding. When symptomatic, these tumors present with progressive neurologic deficit similar to toxoplasmosis. Brain biopsy is necessary for diagnosis. Following our approach, this is usually undertaken when anti-*Toxoplasma* therapy has failed to relieve a focal CNS lesion. We have now seen several patients with CNS toxoplasmosis who had good response to therapy, but while on treatment developed a new lesion that proved to be a lymphoma. Although controlled trials have not yet determined the optimal therapy for this tumor in AIDS patients, a standard approach includes whole-brain radiation (dose equivalent to 3,000 rads delivered in 10 fractions over 10 to 14 days). More recently, we have begun to explore the effect of systemic chemotherapy, but its impact is presently uncertain. In general, AIDS patients suffering primary CNS lymphoma have fared poorly.

Progressive Multifocal Leukoencephalopathy

PML is an opportunistic viral infection causing selective white matter destruction. The tempo of its presentation is usually more protracted than that of toxoplasmosis or lymphoma, and altered consciousness related to brain swelling is not a feature of the disease. Diagnosis is made only by brain biopsy, but suspicion is aroused by the clinical history and an examination suggesting more than one cerebral focus, along with a CT scan or MRI demonstrating white matter lesions, usually without mass effect or contrast enhancement and most often located subcortically.

There is no proven effective therapy for the disease. Individual reports involving non-AIDS patients suggest that the antineoplastic drug cytosine arabinoside may be helpful in some cases, although there has been no controlled trial, and favorable experience has not yet accumulated with AIDS patients. In vitro, cytosine arabinoside has antiviral activity against the responsible agent, JC virus, which is a human papovavirus causing little or no discernible disease in the normal host. However, this drug is cytotoxic and potentially immunosuppressive and was previously noted to have a deleterious effect on the course of herpes zoster in immunosuppressed patients.

Herpesviruses

Although unusual, VZV and, to a lesser extent, HSV-1 and HSV-2 have been reported to cause CNS disease in AIDS patients. VZV infections are of two types: (1) multifocal direct brain infection affecting principally the white matter and partially mimicking PML, and (2) cerebral vasculitis, which characteristically occurs in the setting of ophthalmic herpes zoster and presents with contralateral hemiplegia. VZV can also cause a myelopathy complicating herepes zoster. HSV-2 has been reported to cause myelopathy, either alone or in concert with CMV, and HSV-1 has been identified in the brain of some AIDS patients, although the clinical correlates of this infection have not been well delineated.

Because of the rarity of these conditions and the difficulty in their diagnosis, the effects of therapy generally have been unclear. Moreover, experience with antiviral therapy in VZV vasculitis has been disappointing. Nonetheless, when these disorders are clinically recognized and documented by biopsy or viral culture, attempting therapy with established antiherpetic drugs is justified. Acyclovir is a potent, generally safe antiviral agent with selective activity against HSV-1 and HSV-2, and, at a higher dosage, against VZV. This drug is now the treatment of choice for herpes encephalitis in the nonimmunosuppressed patient at a dose of approximately 10 mg per kilogram by intravenous infusion every 8 hours for 7 to 14 days. This dose must be reduced in patients with renal insufficiency, while in some AIDS patients therapy for a more prolonged period may be needed.

NONFOCAL CNS DISORDERS

Among the predominantly nonfocal CNS disorders noted in AIDS patients are cryptococcal meningitis, CMV encephalitis, and the most frequent neurologic complication of AIDS, the AIDS dementia complex. In addition, some patients with cerebral toxoplasmosis may present with a generalized subacute encephalitis. Also, systemically ill AIDS patients are susceptible to more common bacterial infections and metabolic encephalopathies, which present in a manner similar to that of nonimmunosuppressed patients; however, since therapy for these conditions is not specific to AIDS patients, they will not be discussed further.

Cryptococcal Meningitis

Cryptococcal meningitis is the most common CNS fungal infection in AIDS patients. It most frequently presents as a subacute meningitis or meningoencephalitis with headache, nausea, vomiting, confusion, and lethargy. However, in some patients the symptomatology may be relatively mild, and similarly, the CSF formula in many cases is remarkably bland, with few or no cells and little or no perturbation in glucose or protein levels. For this reason it is important to obtain CSF cryptococcal antigen titers and fungal cultures routinely on all AIDS patients at lumbar puncture.

Treatment of cryptococcal meningitis in AIDS patients follows the guidelines used in other patients and relies on intravenous amphotericin B along with 5-flucytosine, although AIDS patients may be vulnerable to the bone marrow suppression associated with the latter. In patients who fail systemic therapy, intrathecal amphotericin B can also be added. Unfortunately, AIDS patients with cryptococcal meningitis generally do poorly. Although some exhibit an initial response, frequently they relapse and subsequently fail to clear the CSF of organisms.

CMV Encephalitis

Systemic CMV infection is common in AIDS patients, and evidence of minor brain CMV infection can be found in approximately one-third of such patients at autopsy in the form of single inclusion-bearing cells within an occasional microglial nodule. Although some uncertainty remains regarding the contribution of CMV infection to neurologic symptoms and signs in AIDS patients, in most patients its effect is far more likely to be overshadowed by the AIDS dementia complex. Severe CMV brain infection more clearly contributes to clinical symptomatology in only an occasional AIDS patient. CMV can be isolated from the brain or CSF in some of these patients who present with ventricular ependymitis with local contrast enhancement on CT scan, cortical infection with seizures, or radiculomyelitis.

In patients in whom CMV is highly suspected clinically or demonstrated by biopsy or culture, specific antiviral therapy can be considered. Unfortunately, acyclovir has relatively low activity against CMV compared wth HSV-1, HSV-2, and VZV. However, two newer drugs with superior activity, an acyclic nucleoside structurally related to acyclovir (9-[2-hydroxyl-1-(hydroxymethyl)ethoxymethyl]guanine) and phosphonoformate, are now being evaluated.

AIDS Dementia Complex

The AIDS dementia complex, characterized by a triad of cognitive, motor, and behavioral dysfunction, eventually affects the majority of AIDS patients, in whom it is a major source of morbidity. Early in its course, the disease is characterized by impaired concentration and recent memory, which then progresses in some to devastating global dementia. Motor dysfunction may begin with tremor or ataxia and in its severe form eventuate in paraplegia with fecal and urinary incontinence. Behavioral disturbances most commonly include social withdrawal and apathy, but a minority of patients exhibit more florid organic psychosis with paranoia, hallucinations, agitation, or mania. Pathologically, the white matter and subcortical nuclei, as well as the spinal cord, bear the brunt of the disease. Accumulating evidence suggests that direct brain infection by human immunodeficiency virus (HIV) underlies this disorder.

At present, management is largely focused on symptom control and supportive therapy. Thus, early cognitive impairment requires psychosocial support provided by friends, relatives, or professionals. Later, as the condition progresses, assistance is required to manage patients' home and business affairs, while rehabilitative services can help to maintain activities of daily living. Preterminally, institutionalization or full-time care at home is often necessary. Appropriate medications should be administered to alleviate behavioral disturbances. For example, alprazolam may reduce anxiety associated with early dementia in some patients, while haloperidol, phenothiazines, or lithium may be required in psychotic patients. Unfortunately, butyrophenones and phenothiazines can increase the immobility of these patients, who are characteristically slow and hypokinetic owing to their underlying disease. Tricyclics can be tried to alleviate depression, although our experience with patients misdiagnosed as suffering reactive depression rather than early dementia suggests that these agents are often of little benefit. Clearly, further study is needed to define the indications, efficacy, and particular toxicities of the various psychotropic drugs in AIDS patients.

Considerable effort is now underway to develop specific antiviral therapy for HIV infections, and several compounds have already been introduced in limited clinical trials. Unfortunately, there is as yet no evidence that they can impact on the course of the AIDS dementia complex. At the time that this chapter was prepared, interest was most intense in a nucleoside analogue of thymidine, azidothymidine, which inhibits the reverse transcriptase of HIV and appears to penetrate relatively well into the CNS.

PERIPHERAL NEUROPATHIES

Patients with HIV infection frequently develop peripheral neuropathies. At least three clinically separate syndromes have been noted: (1) a predominantly sensory distal polyneuropathy that produces relatively minor neurologic deficit but may be painful to the point of severe disability; (2) a predominantly motor polyneuropathy resembling chronic Guillain-Barré syndrome; and (3) a mononeuritis multiplex. These neuropathies can antecede overt AIDS and thus strike HIV-infected patients when they are otherwise well or are suffering only the relatively benign complications of the AIDS-related complex; they can also complicate full-blown AIDS. Their pathogenesis is uncertain. HIV has been isolated from nerve biopsies in some patients, and autoimmune phenomena have been speculated to operate in some patients.

At present, treatment of these neuropathies is largely symptomatic. Patients with distal painful paresthesias can sometimes be helped with amitriptyline or, if there is a tic-like component, with carbamazepine or phenytoin. In the case of the Guillain-Barré-like polyneuropathy, reports have begun to appear that plasmapheresis may be helpful in some patients. Patients in whom this therapy is considered should be referred to one of the centers investigating this issue so that efficacy can be more accurately and rapidly evaluated. In a small number of patients, CMV infection can produce a polyradiculopathy with or without myelopathy. In such cases, antiviral therapy as previously outlined may be tried.

MULTIPLE SCLEROSIS

JUSTIN C. MCARTHUR, M.B., B.S.

Multiple sclerosis (MS) is a common neurologic disorder caused by an immunologically mediated attack on myelin. The disease is characterized by the unpredictable and episodic involvement of discrete areas of the central nervous system (CNS). It is the third most common cause of disability between the ages of 15 and 50 years, affecting 250,000 persons in the United States, with an annual incidence of 8,800 persons. Ninety percent of patients are between the ages of 20 and 40 years. The case fatality rate is extremely low, and on aggregate there is little or no effect on expected life span. Although the disease is unpredictable and prognostication is uncertain, there are several clinical pointers that can be helpful:

1. Age of onset: Persons between the ages of 20 and 35 years at onset have a better outcome in terms of disability than patients under 20 and over 50.
2. Presentation: Patients with cerebellar, cognitive, or severe motor symptoms fare worse than those with visual or sensory complaints.
3. Remission: Patients who achieve a complete remission with resolution of neurologic symptoms and signs after each relapse have a better prognosis than those accumulating neurologic deficits after each exacerbation.
4. Course: A steadily progressive course from onset implies little chance of remission. Subsequent handicap and disability also occurs sooner.

The natural history of MS is variable, although most patients can be categorized as having either relapsing-remitting or progressive MS. Ninety percent of patients will present initially with the relapsing-remitting form, but each year between 5 and 10 percent will go on to develop the steadily progressive form. Table 1 gives some indication of the prognosis for the two different groups.

DIAGNOSIS

The comprehensive treatment of the patient with MS involves far more than simply recruitment for research protocols. The first and obvious step must be to confirm the diagnosis unequivocally. The disclosure of any chronic illness, and particularly one such as MS, with its emo-

TABLE 1 Prognosis in Multiple Sclerosis

	% of Patients	
	Relapsing-Remitting	*Progressive*
At diagnosis	90	10
At 10 years	50	50
Not disabled	80	40
Moderately disabled	20	30
Severely disabled/dead		30

tional and economic implications and the possibility of handicap and disability, must never be made casually. Despite the plethora of neurodiagnostic studies available, the diagnosis of MS remains based on clinical criteria. Laboratory, immunologic, and imaging studies can be corroborative and helpful in excluding other conditions, but should not supplant detailed historical information and clinical examination. For a diagnosis of *definite* MS, the patient should have a history of two episodes of neurologic symptoms affecting discrete areas of the CNS and should have evidence on examination of white matter involvement in at least one area. Laboratory evidence (e.g., the presence of oligoclonal banding in the cerebrospinal fluid) may substantiate the clinical criteria. The impact of magnetic resonance imaging (MRI) in aiding the diagnosis of MS has not been fully defined. The sensitivity of this technique for detection of demyelination in the brain and spinal cord may aid in earlier and more confident diagnosis, but specificity is limited so that MRI cannot replace clinical corroboration.

COUNSELING

An interdisciplinary approach, with input from a neurologist, nurse-specialist, rehabilitation specialist, urologist, psychologist, and psychiatrist, is essential to optimize care for such a multifaceted disease. The patient should be honestly and directly advised that he or she has MS, when this is definite. Patients will need to receive this information in an individualized manner, sometimes even in stages over the course of several visits. We feel that it is important for the patient and family to be told "this is MS," rather than to use obscure and ambiguous terms such as "viral illness" or "demyelinating disease." The spouse and family should be included in counseling sessions with the patient's permission.

A direct and straightforward explanation of the condition may dissuade the patient from "hospital hopping" and perhaps receiving unnecessary tests or harmful treatments. The disclosure of MS should be accompanied by a realistic yet optimistic assessment of the individual's prognosis, as well as encouragement, empathy, and education. It is important to explain to the patient that to many people the first image of MS that springs to mind is of a person who is wheelchair- or bed-bound. However, this unfortunate group of patients constitutes "only the tip of the iceberg," and the far larger proportion of MS patients are not disabled or significantly handicapped.

Certain questions arise frequently and predictably in the treatment of MS.

1. Course: While the unpredictability of the disease should be emphasized, it is often possible to give some prognosis, using the clinical predictors discussed above. Assessment of handicap and disability at 5 years after diagnosis can often provide a functional forecast. Since the disease often remains relatively static after this point, this "5-year rule" is often helpful.
2. Work: Unless medically contraindicated, employment should be maintained for as long as possible. Fifty percent of patients are still working 10 years after diagnosis, and 30 percent are still working after 20 years. Use of Vocational Rehabilitation and other employment services should be encouraged and facilitated for the unemployed person who can work.
3. Diet: Obesity will compound problems of gait difficulty and weakness. Vitamin supplements are not indicated for the person eating a well-balanced diet. There is some potential for neuropathic damage in patients using large doses of pyridoxine (vitamin B_6), and megavitamin regimens should be avoided.
4. Pregnancy and contraception: Since MS frequently strikes during the reproductive years, questions pertaining to sex and pregnancy are frequent. For the MS patient with mild or moderate disability, there is no increased risk for complications in pregnancy or labor and no increased frequency of birth defects, but offspring will have a 10- to 15-fold greater risk of developing MS. Epidural anesthesia and breast feeding are usually tolerated well. The effect of pregnancy on MS is intriguing. Presumably because of the natural immunosuppression afforded by alpha-fetoprotein and other pregnancy hormones, the risk of a relapse is reduced during the 9 months of pregnancy, whereas a rebound in frequency of relapse occurs during the puerperium. Overall, the 9 months of pregnancy and the 3 months of the puerperium have little net effect on the course of the disease. There is no evidence that oral contraceptives are harmful in the MS patient, although concomitant use of corticosteroids may stimulate their metabolism and reduce their contraceptive efficacy. The patient with severe MS should be counseled to avoid pregnancy because of the physical and emotional strains this might generate.
5. Exercise: Strenuous exercise should be discontinued, particularly if fatigue and heat intolerance are troublesome symptoms. Swimming is probably the best exercise, as the water can provide anti-gravity support for weak muscles. Patients should be cautioned against swimming in pools that are too warm, as this may provoke transient neurologic symptoms (Uthoff's phenomenon). Ideally, the water temperature should not exceed 82 °F. Exercise within the patient's capability often increases self-esteem and helps create a generalized feeling of well-being.
6. Sex: Sexual dysfunction can affect both men and women and is easily overlooked in the review of symptoms. Sexual performance in the MS age group is important for self-esteem, and an aggressive diagnostic approach should be undertaken to identify remediable causes. Combined consultation with a psychologist, sexual counselor, and urologist will be helpful. In the man with erectile impotence, measurement of nocturnal penile tumescence can help differentiate psychogenic from organic causes. A mixed pattern of sexual dysfunction may be present. To provide a usable erection, penile prostheses can be considered, or techniques such as self-injection of papaverine into the corpus callosum can be tried. Sexual dysfunction in women includes vaginal anesthesia and vaginismus, which may

benefit from antispasticity agents. Joint sexual counseling with both partners is necessary to address these issues.

7. Research protocols: Many patients have a fear of being used as a "guinea pig" or of being coerced into experimental treatments. Other patients will literally volunteer for anything without objectively weighing the pro's and con's of treatment. Any treatment protocols must be explained in detail, encompassing both what will be expected of the patient and the potential short- and long-term side effects.

TREATMENT

Symptomatic Treatment

Tremor. Cerebellar outflow or intention tremor can be both embarrassing and incapacitating. Medical treatment is empirical and too often is ineffective, making use of a number of different medications tried sequentially. Clonazepam (Clonopin) is most helpful, starting with 0.5 mg twice a day and increasing the dose gradually to 2 to 4 mg daily in divided doses. Sedation is the limiting side effect, but often improves after a period of time on the drug. Propranolol (Inderal) 40 mg three times a day, may be helpful in some patients, and isoniazid (with vitamin B_6 supplementation) may be worth trying for a 4- to 6-week trial in a dose of 300 mg daily. Unless there are clearly demonstrable functional benefits, these drugs should not be used indefinitely.

With recent advances in neuroradiology and computer technology, stereotactic thalamotomy may be effective in the patient with severe and functionally limiting tremor who is refractory to medications. In several centers, computed tomography (CT) guided lesioning of thalamic nuclear groups can now be performed to suppress contralateral tremor without damage to the adjacent internal capsule. Bilateral thalamotomies carry a higher risk of complications, including hypophonia or production of a pseudobulbar state. The danger of provoking new lesions along the needle track remains a major concern.

Spasticity. Flexor spasms and spontaneous clonus respond quite well to judicious use of antispasticity agents. A spastic paraparesis can, however, be negatively affected by overmedication. For example, the paraparetic patient may make use of spastic tone for pivoting and independent transfer. Baclofen (Lioresal) and diazepam (Valium) are the most useful agents, and self-titration of these agents within prescribed limits is possible. High doses of baclofen are well tolerated if the maxim "start low and go slow" is followed. The starting dose is 5 mg three times a day with increments of 5 mg every 3 days. Severely spastic patients may require 80 to 120 mg daily. At higher doses or with rapid increments, sedation and delirium can occur. The drug should never be stopped abruptly, as a hallucinatory withdrawal state may result. Diazepam may also be useful, particularly at night if spasms interrupt sleep. The starting dose is 2 to 5 mg three times a day, to a maximum of 10 mg three times daily. Sedation and daytime "hangover" effect are common initially, but usually improve. Dantrolene (Dantrium) has more potential for side effects, mainly hepatotoxicity, but can be helpful when spasticity is refractory to other agents, particularly in the bed- or chair-bound patient with painful spasms. The medication is started at 25 mg three times a day and increased to a maximum of 300 mg daily in divided doses. With careful attention, use of antispasticity agents, and implementation of range of motion and stretching exercises, most patients with MS will be spared the development of fixed joint contractures or shortened tendons. Once these occur, neither medications nor physical therapy is of much use, and surgical release may be required to bring the limb into a more comfortable position. For the occasional patient with painful spasms or spasticity, phenol neurectomy may be used; however, the effect may persist for only 6 months. Rhizotomy or myelotomy is rarely performed, but can reduce spasticity by interrupting the reflex arc.

Decubitus Ulceration. The malnourished patient, the patient with fixed contractures or limb posturing, and the immobile, bed-bound patient are all at risk for decubitus ulcer formation over the sacrum, trochanters, heels, and knees. Prevention is infinitely easier than cure, and all efforts must be made to prevent the initial skin breakdown. Measures include:

1. Temporary use of an indwelling catheter or intermittent catheterization in the incontinent patient to avoid perineal soaking.
2. Frequent turning and use of flotation mattresses for the immobile, bed-bound patient.
3. Use of gel flotation cushions for the patient in a wheelchair.
4. Massage to pressure-point areas to increase circulation.
5. Correction of fixed contractures and relief of spastic posturing.
6. Discontinuation of steroids, which may inhibit wound healing.

If a decubitus ulcer develops, aggressive debridement and dressing will often permit healing of even deep ulcers. Special air flotation beds for bed-bound patients, although expensive and cumbersome, will promote more rapid healing. Occasionally, plastic surgery with muscle flap implants will be necessary.

Fatigue. Patients with MS may experience excessive fatigue or a general lack of stamina and endurance independent of their degree of disability. Fatigue is now recognized as an important contributory symptom when disability from MS is assessed. This symptom can often be an additional limitation and is not helped by most medications, although amantadine (Symmetrel) in doses of 100 mg twice a day may be worth a trial.

Sensory Disturbances. Radicular or localized positive sensations such as trigeminal neuralgia are distracting and painful, and paresthesias can be annoying. Agents such as carbamazepine (Tegretol), amitriptyline (Elavil), and phenytoin (Dilantin) are often helpful, although each of these can have troublesome side effects.

Dementia and Depression. These may coexist or occur separately, and appropriate management depends on correct differentiation. Early recognition of depression, psychiatric consultation, treatment with antidepressants, and psychotherapy may be indicated. Similarly, in the patient who manifests subtle changes in personality and memory or language deficits, the possibility of dementia should be considered. Detailed neuropsychological testing can help define the specific cognitive problems and help focus the attention of physican, patient, and family on measures to compensate for them.

Rehabilitation. The role of rehabilitation services (physical and occupational therapy) has been a controversial and often understated one. We work extremely closely with rehabilitation specialists and find their services invaluable. A joint approach with discussion between patient, rehabilitation specialist, and neurologist is most useful in defining an individual patient's needs. The areas of greatest benefit include:

1. Provision and adjustment of assistive devices, such as canes, walkers, and wheelchairs.
2. Assessment of the home and work place for installation of safety or assistive devices.
3. Teaching range of movement, strengthening, and stretching exercises to the patient and/or family.
4. Involvement in general exercise programs, e.g., swimming.
5. Assessment for provision of mobility devices such as electric wheelchairs, scooters (Amigo, Rascal, Portascoot), or car adaptations.

Swallowing Dysfunction. This may occur without obvious symptoms such as choking or regurgitation and is common in the MS patient with brainstem involvement. Repeated episodes of nocturnal aspiration may cause "fever of unknown origin" and lead to chronic lung infection, abscess, or empyema. Liquids are usually more difficult to swallow than solids, and dysphagia may, over a period of months or years, lead to malnourishment or dehydration. Cine-esophagrams are helpful in detailing the swallowing mechanisms, both normal and abnormal, and can demonstrate whether there is tracheal penetration and hence a risk of aspiration. In the patient who aspirates or has severe dysphagia, we consider either intensive swallowing rehabilitation or placement of a soft nasogastric feeding tube. The tube is well tolerated without discomfort and can remain in place for several weeks or months. For the patient with longstanding swallowing problems, a feeding gastrostomy should be placed. This can be performed as an endoscopic outpatient procedure.

Specific Treatment

Acute Relapses. Current evidence suggests that corticotropin (ACTH) and corticosteroids may be useful in shortening relapses. These agents have no effect on the overall course of the disease, and there is no indication for their long-term use. Both the total dose and the duration of use must be limited because both ACTH and corticosteroids are potent agents with numerous side effects. Certain broad guidelines should be followed:

1. These agents are contraindicated in patients with poorly controlled diabetes mellitus or electrolyte imbalance, active peptic ulceration or psychiatric disturbance, severe hypertension or heart failure, or infections.
2. A tuberculin skin test should be placed and read *before* initiation of therapy.Isoniazid prophylaxis is unnecessary during a short course of ACTH or a corticosteroid; however, careful monitoring for reactivation of tuberculosis is mandatory.
3. Dosing schedules must be explicit, and patients must be followed carefully for side effects, including oral candidiasis, hypertension, or fluid retention. Electrolytes should be checked regularly.
4. Patients who have recently received ACTH/corticosteroids develop suppression of the hypothalamic-pituitary-adrenal (HPA) axis and may require supplemental corticosteroids during stresses such as infection, trauma, or surgery.
5. There is no definite causal link between ACTH/corticosteroid use and peptic ulceration. Prophylactic antacids/antihistaminics (ranitidine, cimetidine) are not suggested.

The beneficial effects of both ACTH and corticosteroids are apparently mediated via anti-inflammatory and immunosuppressive actions. The synthetic corticosteroids used in treatment of MS (prednisone, prednisolone, and methylprednisolone) are glucocorticoids with minimal mineralocorticoid activity. ACTH, however, stimulates adrenal release not only of glucocorticoids, but also of mineralocorticoids and androgens. Thus, while the side effects of both ACTH and glucocorticoids are similar, there are predictable differences.

Both have anti-inflammatory and immunosuppressive properties and increase protein catabolism with impairment of wound healing and an increased incidence of osteoporosis. Physical changes are similar, with development of moon-facies, buffalo bump, striae, and central obesity. If used during pregnancy, both agents may cause cleft palate in the newborn. Posterior subcapsular cataract is common, particularly in children. Mental disturbances ranging from euphoria to frank psychosis can occur with use of both ACTH and glucocorticoids.

Because of additional mineralocorticoid actions, ACTH tends to produce electolyte imbalance, fluid retention, and hypertension more frequently. Its androgenic actions provoke acne and hirsutism. With glucocorticoids there may be more suppression of the HPA axis than with ACTH; and, these agents cause dyspepsia and skin thinning more often. Glucocorticoids can also interfere with hepatic metabolism of drugs, e.g., cyclophosphamide alkylation.

ACTH is much more expensive than the synthetic glucocorticoids. ACTH costs 5 to 10 dollars per day, not including the injection cost, compared with 15 cents per day for prednisone tablets.

For the ambulatory patient with an acute, mild and/or moderate relapse, one daily dose has less effect on the HPA axis. The schedule for prednisone is: 60 mg every day × 5 days, 40 mg every day × 5 days, 30 mg every day ×4 days, 20 mg every day × 3 days, 10 mg every × 3 days, and 10 mg every other day × 3 doses.

In the nonambulatory patient with a severe relapse, methylprednisolone (Solu-Medrol), 1 g IV every day ×3 to 7 days, is given, depending on clinical response. This is followed by the above tapering course of prednisone.

Chronic Progressive MS. This group of patients is the most difficult to manage because the level of disability is generally higher than in the relapsing and/or remitting group and remissions are uncommon. There are no definitively proven treatments as yet; however, some of the experimental immunosuppressive regimens have shown promise. We *do not* suggest use of potent immunosuppressants outside of established protocols. An ongoing cyclophosphamide-ACTH protocol (under the auspices of the Northeastern Multiple Sclerosis Cooperative Treatment Group) includes patients showing definite deterioration in ambulatory functioning. Randomization is made to groups of patients receiving one of two "induction" regimens with cyclophosphamide doses of 70 to 100 mg per kilogram IV. Patients are also randomized to receive either "maintenance" cyclophosphamide, 700 mg per square meter IV every 2 months, or no maintenance. Short-term effects of transient bone marrow suppression and alopecia are predictable, but serious infections or hemorrhagic cystitis is very uncommon. Long-term effects, including leukemia risk, infertility, and teratogenicity, are not known.

Results to date suggest that up to 75 percent of selected patients may show stabilization of their progressive disease. It is hoped that "maintenance" therapy will prolong this stabilization.

Other Treatments. Many other treatments are in use across the United States, both for relapsing-remitting and for progressive forms of MS. Some, such as interferon and cyclosporine, have some rationale for their use in this disease. Others, such as apheresis and hyperbaric oxygen, have little or no rationale.

PATIENT RESOURCES

Wolf JK, ed. Mastering multiple sclerosis, a handbook for MSers and families. Chicago: Academy Books, 1984.

Therapeutic claims in multiple sclerosis. By the International Federation of Multiple Sclerosis Societies (IFMSS). Available from the National Multiple Sclerosis Society.

Scheinberg LS. Multiple sclerosis: a guide for patients and their families. New York: Raven Press, 1983.

National Multiple Sclerosis Society; 205 East 42 Street; New York, NY 10017, (212) 986-3240. Local chapters throughout the United States are listed in telephone directories.

TRANSIENT ISCHEMIC ATTACK

CATHY A. SILA, M.D.
ANTHONY J. FURLAN, M.D.

A transient ischemic attack (TIA) is an acute, focal, painless episode of neurologic dysfunction referrable to a specific vascular territory of the brain. By convention a TIA lasts less than 24 hours, but more commonly resolves in less than 20 minutes without residua. TIAs are classified as either carotid or vertebral-basilar and are presumed to be of vascular origin. The clinical manifestations depend upon the vascular distribution of the ischemia (Table 1). Carotid distribution TIAs can be classified as either monocular or hemispheric. Nonfocal symptomatology such as lightheadedness, dizziness, confusion, mental deterioration, or syncope should not be called a TIA. Symptoms such as vertigo, diplopia, dysarthria, and dysphagia occurring in isolation should also not be included in the definition of a posterior circulation TIA ("VBI").

The differential diagnosis of sudden transient focal neurologic events is given in Table 2. Initially a distinction must be made between TIAs, migraine, and focal seizures. A *marching evolution* over a period of seconds of positive sensory or motor phenomena suggests partial epilepsy. Migraine may manifest as homonymous or central visual loss usually accompanied by *positive visual phenomena* such as flashes of light, scintillating scotomas, fortification spectra, or the appearance of heat waves. Sensory or motor disturbances may also occur as a result of migraine in the absence of headache, and there is often a marching evolution over a period of minutes. Rarely, demyelinating disease, such as multiple sclerosis, may mimic TIAs. These patients are usually younger and without evidence of widespread vascular disease, and examination often discloses evidence of neurologic dysfunction that is not easily classified within a single arterial distribution. Hypoglycemia may very occasionally result in episodes of focal neurologic dysfunction, but is usually accompanied by impaired consciousness, hunger, pallor, and sweating associated with a known history of diabetes treated with oral hypoglycemic agents or insulin. Brain tumors can produce transient focal symptoms through seizure activity, hemorrhage into the tumor, and tumor emboli. Subdural hematomas can also cause episodes of focal dysfunction, often in the presence of impaired consciousness and headache. Arteriovenous malformations may produce focal seizures as well as focal ischemia by shunting blood away from normal brain tissue. Psychogenic factors such as conversion reactions, hyperventilation, and other stress-related phenomena may also mimic TIAs.

TABLE 1 Vascular Distribution of TIAs

Distribution of Ischemia	*Neurologic Manifestations*
Carotid System	
Ophthalmic artery	"Amaurosis fugax," total or partial; monocular blindness, usually altitudinal
Anterior cerebral artery	Contralateral hemiparesis, maximal for leg and proximal arm
Middle cerebral artery	
Anterior branches	Contralateral motor and sensory loss, maximal for face, hand, and arm; if dominant hemisphere, nonfluent aphasia
Posterior branches	Contralateral hemisensory loss and homonymous hemianopsia; if dominant hemisphere, fluent aphasia
Deep perforating arteries: lenticulostriate, anterior choroidal	Contralateral hemiparesis and hemisensory loss, affecting face, arm, and leg about equally
Vertebral-Basilar System	
Combined symptoms	Dysarthria, diplopia, vertigo, ataxia, vomiting, etc.
Crossed symptoms	Ipsilateral cranial nerve/contralateral limbs
Bilateral symptoms	Binocular visual loss, quadriparesis

Transient ischemic attacks are a major risk factor for subsequent stroke, although less than 50 percent of patients with cerebral infarction have prior warning TIAs. About 33 percent of patients who are alive 5 years after the occurrence of their first TIA will have suffered a stroke. Of these, 20 percent will do so within the first month and 50 percent within a year. After the first 6 months there is a 5 percent per year incidence of stroke in patients with TIAs.

PATHOGENESIS

Probably the most common cause of TIAs is embolism of platelet fibrin or other debris from atherosclerotic plaques in proximal conducting vessels. Hemodynamic disturbances may also play a role when superimposed upon a severe arterial stenosis or occlusion. Atherosclerotic disease is usually most severe at the extracranial carotid bifurcation, but can also occur intracranially in the region of the carotid siphon or the stem of the middle cerebral artery. Atherosclerosis may produce symptoms by a variety of mechanisms, including embolization, progressive stenosis from enlargement of the plaque, or local thrombosis.

Embolism may also occur from a cardiac source. A potential cardiac source is present in about one-third of patients with TIAs. The most common source of cardiac embolism is chronic nonvalvular atrial fibrillation. Other common cardiac sources include acute myocardial infarction, rheumatic valve disease, and mitral valve prolapse (Table 3). Cardiac embolism should be suspected in patients under age 45 who present with TIAs and stroke, especially if there are cardiac symptoms or signs.

EVALUATION

Risk Factors

The major risk factors for cerebral vascular disease include increasing age, hypertension, atherosclerotic heart disease, cardiac valvular disease, diabetes, cigarette smoking, and lipid abnormalities. A stroke risk profile that includes these variables should be developed for each patient. A review of systems should also be directed to other possible causes, including systemic illnesses, hematologic abnormalities, coagulopathies, and neck trauma or cervical manipulation, as well as a drug history, including intravenous drug abuse, amphetamines, over-the-counter diet aids, oral contraceptives, and other hormonal agents.

Physical Examination

The general physical status of the patient should be ascertained. Particular attention should be paid to the cardiovascular system. A detailed neurologic examination should be performed to establish the presence and severity of any neurologic deficit. TIAs resolve over a 24-hour period, and any deficit remaining after that time classifies the episode as a stroke or raises the possibility of nonvascular diagnosis.

The *neurovascular examination* consists of determination of brachial blood pressure bilaterally and the rhythm and rate of the pulse. Blood pressure measurements should be done in the supine, sitting, and standing positions. After auscultating the heart, listen for bruits in the supraclavicular fossa, over the carotid artery from the level of the clavicle to the jaw angle, and also over the orbits and cranium. We have found that neck and orbital bruits are heard best with a pediatric bell fitted with a rubber rim. Orbital bruits can be normal in infants and children, but in adults are often indicative of occlusive

TABLE 2 Differential Diagnosis of Sudden Transient Focal Neurologic Events

TIAs
Partial seizures
Migraine
Multiple sclerosis
Hypoglycemia
Structural lesions
Brain tumors — especially meningioma
Subdural hematoma
Arteriovenous malformation
Psychogenic

TABLE 3 Pathogenesis of TIAs

- Atherosclerosis
  - Embolization
    - Platelet-fibrin material
    - Atheromatous debris
  - Local thrombosis
  - Hemodynamic disturbances
- Cardiac and other embolic sources
  - Disorders of the heart wall
    - Myocardial infarction
    - Primary myocardial disease
    - Congestive heart failure
    - Congenital heart disease
    - Intracardiac myxoma
    - Ventricular aneurysm
  - Disorders of heart valves
    - Rheumatic valvular disease
    - Mitral valve prolapse
    - Prosthetic heart valves
    - Infective endocarditis
    - Nonbacterial thrombotic endocarditis
    - Calcific aortic stenosis
    - ? Mitral annulus calcification
    - ? Bicuspid aortic valve
  - Cardiac rhythm disturbances
    - Atrial fibrillation — chronic, paroxysmal, valvular, nonvalvular
  - Complications of cardiac manipulation
    - Open heart surgery
    - Cardiac catheterization
    - Percutaneous angioplasty
  - Pulmonary sources
    - Patent foramen ovale
    - Intracardiac right to left shunt
  - Other
    - Fat embolism
    - Tumor embolism
- Hematologic
  - Polycythemia vera
  - Myeloproliferative disorders
  - Thrombotic thrombocytopenic purpura
  - Disseminated intravascular coagulation
  - Dysproteinemias
  - Essential thrombocytosis
  - Sickle cell anemia
  - Antithrombin-III deficiency
  - Protein C, protein S deficiency
- Arteriopathies
  - Inflammatory
    - Granulomatous arteritis
    - Infective — tuberculosis, herpes zoster virus, syphilis, malaria, mucor
    - Associated with systemic disease — systemic lupus erythematosus, polyarteritis nodosa, rheumatoid arthritis, Wegener's granulomatosis, inflammatory bowel disease
    - Takayasu's aortitis
    - Allergic arteritis
  - Noninflammatory
    - Arterial dissection
    - Fibromuscular dysplasia
    - Radiation arteritis
    - Homocystinuria
    - Fabry's disease
    - Angioendotheliosis
- Miscellaneous
  - Drug related — oral contraceptives, diet aids, amphetamines
  - Peripartum and postpartum — arterial or venous occlusion

disease in the carotid siphon or tight stenosis or occlusion of the extracranial internal carotid arteries. The cervical bruit best correlated with internal carotid artery stenosis is loudest at the angle of the jaw. High-pitched bruits with a diastolic component suggest a greater degree of stenosis. Bruit intensity peaks at approximately 90 percent stenosis, then declines with more severe compromise of blood flow. Murmurs that are transmitted from the heart or the aortic arch will decrease in intensity as one approaches the angle of the jaw. Venous hums vary in intensity, are continuous, and are position dependent.

Palpation of the carotid pulses is seldom helpful and potentially dangerous in that vigorous manipulation may result in embolization of atheromatous material. Palpation of the superficial temporal, supraorbital, and facial arteries may suggest collateral flow through the external carotid artery or provide evidence of cranial arteritis.

The *neuro-ophthalmologic examination* may disclose retinal vascular changes from diabetes and hypertension. Retinal emboli may suggest the etiology of the TIA. Platelet-fibrin emboli originate from the carotid arteries or the heart, appear grayish-white with indistinct margins, and are often seen at the bifurcations of peripheral arterioles. Cholesterol emboli (Hollenhorst plaques) are yellowish-white, refractile, and needle-shaped and may not impede blood flow. Their presence implies carotid atherosclerosis. Calcific emboli from degenerated heart valves are chalky-white with sharp edges and are usually found at the bifurcations of arterioles on or near the optic disc with obstruction of distal blood flow.

Laboratory Evaluation

The following screening studies should be performed routinely in any patient with TIAs: complete blood count with quantitative platelet count, serum chemistries, lipid profile, urinalysis, prothrombin time, activated partial thromboplastine time, serologic test for syphilis, sedimentation rate, electrocardiogram, and chest radiograph. A computed tomography (CT) scan of the head without contrast should be performed to exclude a small hemorrhage, and contrast medium is administered to exclude a tumor or arteriovenous malformation. An unsuspected infarct may be demonstrated on either a nonenhanced or an enhanced CT scan, depending upon the timing of the study.

Echocardiography and Holter monitoring are of low yield when performed routinely in patients with TIAs. Cardiac tests should be reserved for patients with historical and clinical evidence of underlying heart disease, evidence of systemic embolism or multiple ischemic events in different vascular distributions, and in younger patients.

Selected patients are tested for vasculitis, rare hematologic disorders, and other uncommon causes of TIA and stroke.

Angiography and Noninvasive Tests

In otherwise healthy patients who are acceptable surgical risks and who have had clear-cut carotid distribution TIAs, angiographic imaging of the extracranial and intracranial circulation is usually indicated. This is accomplished with either intra-arterial digital subtraction angiography (IA-DSA) or film screen angiography (FSA). The advantages of IA-DSA include smaller volumes of contrast material, less risk, and lower cost. FSA is superior for assessing changes in smaller-caliber intracranial arteries or complex collateral flow patterns. Angiography entails some risk of neurologic deficit, often due to dislodging of atheromatous material during catheter manipulation; an acceptable risk is 1 percent.

Noninvasive tests (NITs) and intravenous digital subtraction angiography (IV-DSA) are sometimes used in the evaluation of patients with TIAs. Direct NITs give information regarding the anatomy and flow characteristics within the extracranial internal carotid artery, and real-time Doppler ultrasound imaging is currently the preferred technique. IV-DSA is less time consuming and less costly than conventional angiography, can be done in the outpatient setting, and is not as operator dependent as the noninvasive studies. However, IV-DSA carries slight risks, including contrast reactions, renal failure, and angina and is subject to motion and other artifacts. Doppler ultrasound imaging is performed without contrast material, but is highly operator dependent and produces images that are not easily interpreted by clinicians who lack special training in this technique. As with IV-DSA, Doppler ultrasound cannot differentiate total occlusion from tight carotid stenosis with certainty. The image is limited to a few centimeters of the carotid artery in the neck, and in patients with high bifurcations the probe may not be able to visualize the area of interest.

Indirect NITs such as oculoplethysmography or ophthalmodynamometry monitor pressure and flow changes within the orbital branches of the ophthalmic and posterior ciliary arteries to reflect stenosis occurring in more proximal portions of the internal carotid artery. The major disadvantage of indirect tests is poor localization, as carotid stenosis may occur anywhere from the common carotid artery through the region of the carotid siphon.

When a battery of both direct and indirect NITs is used, accuracy should be 85 to 90 percent for detecting greater than 50 percent internal carotid stenosis. Accuracy is about the same for IV-DSA. NITs should be reserved for patients who are poor surgical risks, patients with a good alternative explanation for their TIAs, those with symptoms that are only equivocal for carotid disease, or to follow nonsurgical carotid lesions in patients who are treated medically.

Arteriographic imaging in patients with vertebral-basilar TIAs is usually reserved for those who continue to have TIAs despite optimal medical therapy. In this instance IA-DSA is the procedure of choice to image the aortic arch, both vertebral arteries, the basilar artery, and collateral flow patterns derived from the carotid circulation.

Ancillary Investigations

Myocardial infarction is the leading cause of death among patients with TIAs, accounting for a mortality rate of 5 percent per year. This compares with a cardiac mortality rate of about 4 percent per year in patients with angina pectoris. Concomitant symptomatic coronary artery disease also increases the operative risk of carotid endarterectomy. It is important to note that although classic angina is highly correlated with coronary artery disease, less than one-third of patients with severe coronary atherosclerosis have classic symptoms, and one-half of patients suffering sudden cardiac death have no prior symptoms of heart disease. Recent studies of various populations with cerebrovascular disorders suggest that nearly 60 percent harbor significant coronary atherosclerosis, only 50 percent of which are symptomatic.

In TIA patients with symptomatic coronary artery disease, coronary angiography should be considered in order to define the location and severity of coronary artery stenoses. In TIA patients without cardiac symptoms, screening procedures such as exercise electrocardiography, exercise radionuclide ventriculography, and exercise or dipyridamole radionuclide angiography can be employed followed by coronary angiography if the noninvasive studies suggest significant coronary artery disease.

MEDICAL THERAPY

Antiplatelet Agents

Aspirin is the drug of choice for lowering stroke risk in patients with TIAs. Aggregate data from randomized trials of long-term aspirin treatment after TIA or minor stroke demonstrate a 25 percent reduction in risk of stroke and death. Most of the trials employed doses of about 1200 mg per day (i.e., 4 adult aspirin tablets). The optimum daily dosage of aspirin is controversial. It has been shown in vitro that inhibition of platelet thromboxane A_2 production (which causes platelet aggregation) may be accomplished at lower dosages, thus sparing vessel wall prostacyclin synthesis (which promotes platelet disaggregation). Although the optimum dosage of aspirin for stroke prophylaxis is not clear, we employ 650 mg orally twice a day. For patients with gastric intolerance to aspirin, coated aspirin or aspirin combined with antacids may be used. We reserve so-called "mini-dose" aspirin (325 mg daily or a pediatric aspirin tablet) for patients unable to tolerate higher doses.

Dipyridamole and sulfinpyrazone have not been shown to provide additional benefit compared with aspirin alone in stroke prophylaxis, and we no longer use these agents. Newer agents such as ticlopidine and selective thromboxane inhibitors are under investigation.

Anticoagulants

Studies of long-term oral anticoagulation after TIAs suffer many methodologic flaws, and there is no consensus regarding the effects of anticoagulants on stroke risk. There is a suggestion that whatever benefit is achieved occurs within the first few months of therapy. Hence, warfarin is sometimes used for a 3- to 6-month period after the onset of TIAs, and then the patient is switched to aspirin. Alternatively, the patient is started on aspirin and switched to a brief course of warfarin if the attacks continue.

If a clear cardiac source of embolization is diagnosed, anticoagulation with warfarin should begin to maintain the prothrombin time at 1½ to 2 times control. The duration of warfarin anticoagulation is dependent upon the nature of the cardiac source. In the setting of an acute myocardial infarction, warfarin is continued for 6 months, but other sources such as rheumatic valvular disease or chronic atrial fibrillation may require lifetime anticoagulation. For certain cardioembolic sources (e.g., mitral prolapse) antiplatelet therapy is preferred.

Risk Factor Reduction

Hypertension is the most critical risk factor affecting stroke. Even moderate or low levels of hypertension should be aggressively monitored and treated. However, certain patients require a higher than normal blood pressure to maintain cerebral blood flow. These are usually patients with diffuse cerebral atherosclerosis and/or multiple large vessel disease. In such cases the blood pressure should be managed less aggressively. Other risk factors such as diabetes, hyperlipidemia, cigarette smoking, and cardiovascular disease should be identified and treated appropriately.

SURGICAL THERAPY

Carotid Endarterectomy

Carotid endarterectomy is the most common vascular procedure performed in the United States and is one of the most common surgical procedures overall. Carotid endarterectomy does not eliminate stroke risk, but probably reduces it in well-selected patients with carotid system TIAs. The major thrust of any stroke prevention plan is to initiate treatment(s) with the greatest probability of benefit at the lowest possible risk and cost. The surgical risk of carotid endarterectomy is highly dependent upon the skill of the available surgeon and the medical and neurologic condition of the patient. In stable patients with carotid TIAs the risk of endarterectomy should not exceed 3 percent. Some series have reported a surgical risk as high as 20 percent, and a recent metropolitan survey found an average risk of 9.5 percent.

It is not clear from the literature what degree of stenosis and/or ulceration determines a "surgical lesion." We recommend endarterectomy for patients with clear carotid distribution TIAs and an ipsilateral carotid stenosis of greater than 70 percent. In general, we do not recommend surgical therapy for patients with ulceration alone or stenosis of lesser severity unless they have initially failed medical therapy. A prospective randomized trial of carotid endarterectomy is now underway in Europe.

Extracranial-Intracranial Bypass Surgery

A recent extracranial-intracranial bypass study showed that this procedure does not reduce stroke risk in patients who have carotid lesions inaccessible to conventional carotid endarterectomy. A small subset of patients may exist for whom this procedure may be of benefit, but until such time as this group can be clarified we do not recommend this operation.

Surgery for Vertebral-Basilar Insufficiency

Surgical therapy for patients with recurrent VB-TIAs should be restricted to those patients who have failed maximal medical therapy. Carotid endarterectomy is of unproven benefit in patients with VB ischemia. Surgical options in selected cases include vertebral artery transposition or posterior fossa bypass procedures.

ATHEROTHROMBOTIC CEREBRAL VASCULAR DISEASE

J. PHILIP KISTLER, M.D.
JAE KYU ROH, M.D.

Atherothrombotic cerebral vascular disease is the most common cause of transient cerebral ischemia and stroke and is among the most lethal and disabling of the neurologic diseases. It is not a diffuse process, but one with a predilection for certain sites in the cerebral vasculature. Because the brain cannot repair itself by forming new tissue, therapy in atherothrombotic cerebral vascular disease is primarily preventive; however, protecting ischemic brain tissue from the secondary effects of stroke is sometimes successful. The prelude to proper therapy is a precise diagnosis that includes not only characterization and localization of the atherothrombotic lesion causing the stroke or transient ischemic attack (TIA) and the size and location of the resulting ischemic or infarcted brain, but also knowledge of the spared collateral circulation. Based on pathophysiologic reasons that suggest different therapeutic interventions, atherothrombotic cerebral vascular disease is divided into two broad categories: large and small vessel disease. Large vessel disease affects both the carotid and the vertebral-basilar systems. Small vessel disease affects the penetrating vessels arising from the stem of the middle cerebral artery (lenticulostriate arteries), the vertebral and basilar arteries, and the arteries of the circle of Willis.

Broadly, preventive therapy of atherothrombotic ischemic stroke has three goals: (1) to prevent stroke by reducing risk factors, thus preventing the pathologic process; (2) to prevent initial or recurrent stroke by removing the underlying pathologic process, e.g., by performing a carotid endarterectomy; and (3) to ameliorate secondary brain damage by maintaining adequate perfusion to marginally ischemic areas and perhaps by reducing edema formation. Except for the elimination of risk factors, all aspects of therapy are controversial. Published proof of any given therapeutic approach is lacking; hence, current therapy is largely empirical and based on each institution's knowledge of the risks associated with its own diagnostic procedures and therapies.

RISK FACTORS

Hypertension is the most important risk factor associated with stroke. It promotes the formation of atherosclerosis in the extracranial and intracranial arteries and damages the small penetrating blood vessels of the brain by causing deposition of lipid (lipohyalinosis). Lipohyalinotic lesions result in small lacunar infarctions and, some believe, in hypertensive hemorrhages as well. Systolic blood pressure is as important as diastolic, for both cause large vessel and small vessel disease. Furthermore, effective long-term control of high blood pressure decreases the incidence of both ischemic stroke and hemorrhage. Smoking, obesity, and hyperlipidemia increase risk, particularly of carotid atherosclerosis.

ATHEROTHROMBOTIC DISEASE OF THE INTERNAL CAROTID AND ITS BRANCHES

Symptomatic Disease

In the carotid artery system, atherosclerosis and superimposed atherothrombosis that lead to TIA or stroke most commonly occur at the origin of the internal carotid artery and less often at the siphon (S-shaped portion of the internal carotid artery in the cavernous sinus) or at the proximal segment (stem) of the middle or anterior cerebral arteries. Rarely, atherothrombotic disease occurs at the origin of the common carotid artery. In the internal carotid artery, a lesion becomes symptomatic when it produces emboli that lodge in the stem or distal branches of the middle or anterior cerebral artery or when it causes reduced flow in the watershed territories between the middle and anterior or posterior cerebral arteries. Low flow stroke or TIAs tend to occur when the collateral flow around the circle of Willis or through the external carotid artery (ophthalmic distal internal carotid artery anastomotic channels) is inadequate. The usual symptom of an atherothrombotic lesion of the stem of the middle cerebral artery or anterior cerebral artery is "low flow." The lesion being distal to the circle of Willis, the only chance for collaterol flow is through the tenuous cortical surface border zone collateral channels between the anterior, posterior, and middle cerebral arteries. The natural history of atherothrombotic stenosis or ulcerated lesions at any of these locations that have not yet become symptomatic is also unknown. In most instances, presumably, the disease is progressive.

Minor Stroke. If a patient presents with a minor stroke or TIA in the territory of the internal carotid artery, preventing the further progression of the minor stroke or a subsequent stroke is vital. After clinical assessment and an electrocardiogram have excluded the heart as a source of embolism, noninvasive evaluation of the bifurcation of the common carotid artery is suggested.If auscultation of the neck over the bifurcation of the common carotid artery discloses a high-pitched bruit that fades into diastole, a tightly stenotic lesion (1.5-mm residual lumen diameter or less) at the origin of the internal carotid artery is suspected. In experienced hands, noninvasive testing that includes CW Doppler or range-gated pulsed-Doppler assessment of flow in the proximal internal carotid artery, external carotid artery, and distal common carotid artery can often suggest a tightly stenotic lesion. When Doppler assessment of flow at the bifurcation of the common carotid artery, B-mode imaging, oculoplethysmography, and quantitative bruit analysis are combined, the noninvasive evaluation can diagnose atherothrombotic disease accurately and distinguish tightly stenotic lesions at the origin of the internal carotid artery from less severe lesions.

If a tightly stenotic lesion is suspected, most physicians proceed to angiography to confirm the lesion visually. Intravenous digital subtraction angiography circumvents the need for arterial injection and its inherent risks, but it offers poor resolution of the lesion and may exacerbate angina, congestive heart failure, or renal insufficiency. It cannot demonstrate a thread-like lumen when noninvasive tests suggest occlusion of the internal carotid artery. Only arteriography can detect such a lesion or reliably demonstrate a tightly stenotic lesion with ulceration. If a tightly stenotic or thread-like lumen lesion is found at the origin of the internal carotid artery and the patient has no medical or cardiac contraindications, carotid endarterectomy is the treatment of choice, provided the combined risk of angiography and surgery is less than 3 percent. However, it must be pointed out that this has not been subjected to the scrutiny of an adequate randomized clinical trial. While some physicians delay surgery for 3 weeks, this need not be done. Prompt surgery with careful control of the blood pressure in the postoperative period can be advised.

If the internal carotid artery is occluded and there is only a minor stroke, anticoagulation with heparin followed by coumadin (prothrombin time no greater than 1½ times control) for 6 months is suggested. Although without proven efficacy, anticoagulation is given with the assumption that it prevents further embolism. Most physicians resort to antiplatelet therapy (½ of a 300-mg aspirin tablet per day) when carotid siphon stenosis results in symptoms of stroke or TIA, although no study exists as to the efficacy of this treatment. If embolism rather than low flow is the suspected cause of stroke when siphon stenosis is the source, coumadin anticoagulation for 6 months is also considered. When middle cerebral stem stenosis results in a TIA or minor stroke, coumadin anticoagulation is recommended. Thus, in symptomatic acute carotid occlusion, siphon stenosis, or middle cerebral stem stenosis, either antiplatelet or anticoagulant therapy is recommended. However, no study exists establishing the efficacy of either therapy in these specific pathophysiologic settings. The only controlled, randomized therapeutic study in each of these three clinical settings that exists failed to show the efficacy of extracranial–intracranial bypass surgery. Antiplatelet versus anticoagulant therapy, however, was not evaluated in that study.

Major Stroke. In the event that the stroke is large, occupying the major portion of the middle cerebral artery territory or the territory of the upper or lower division of the middle cerebral artery, early endarterectomy is not beneficial. It can be considered later if the atherothrombotic lesion threatens further infarction and a worsening neurologic status. Intravenous heparin is considered in the interim. These major carotid territory strokes are usually due to an artery-to-artery embolus causing occlusion in the stem of the middle cerebral artery. Cerebral edema often follows. In most cases the ensuing edema is aggravated by lysis and dispersion of the occluding embolus that allows recirculation to the infarcted tissue. In such cases, early institution of hyperosmotic therapy becomes critical. Mannitol has become the mainstay of hyperosmotic therapy. It is given as 100 ml of 25 percent mannitol every 4 hours to raise the serum osmolality to between 300 and 310 mOsm per liter.

Asymptomatic Carotid Bifurcation Stenosis that Causes Bruit

The natural history of a bruit resulting from an atherosclerotic lesion of the carotid bifurcation that has not yet caused a TIA or stroke is unknown. The available studies have examined small populations, and most failed to localize and quantitate the severity of the stenotic lesion. The studies of asymptomatic patients with cervical bruits who are about to undergo major surgical procedures have the same deficiencies. In most studies, patients with cervical bruits were found to be at increased risk of heart disease, stroke, and death. The strokes, however, did not necessarily occur in the vascular territory of the carotid bruit. Given these facts, there is little reason to operate on the carotid artery, either routinely or before surgery, in patients with asymptomatic carotid stenosis.

However, patients with a tightly stenotic lesion at the origin of the internal carotid artery (1.5 mm or less) that reduces flow in the distal internal carotid artery may be at higher risk of thrombotic occlusion. Even though these patients have reduced flow in the distal internal carotid artery, they are asymptomatic probably because of adequate collateral flow across the anterior circle of Willis to the ipsilateral middle and anterior cerebral arteries. Stroke, therefore, should occur only by subsequent artery-to-artery embolism. The bruit associated with such a tightly stenotic carotid bifurcation lesion is high-pitched and prolonged, often fading into diastole. The bruit becomes fainter as the stenosis progresses and flow is further slowed and finally disappears when occlusion is imminent. Noninvasive carotid testing that includes B-mode ultrasound imagery, Doppler analysis of flow immediately distal to the stenosis, quantitative spectral analysis of the bruit itself, and measurement of the oculosystolic pressure by oculoplethysmography can identify these tightly stenotic lesions. In the absence of a randomized trial of the efficacy of endarterectomy versus antiplatelet therapy for this type of lesion, the physician has an option for either. In most cases, antiplatelet therapy is recommended. Only when signs of progressive narrowing are documented and the residual lumen diameter is 1.5 mm or less is surgery considered an option by some physicians. In their institutions, the surgical morbidity should be less than 2 percent. Even then, there is no evidence to suggest that surgery is more efficacious than medical therapy, and there is great need for a randomized clinical trial.

Posterior Cerebral Territory Ischemic Stroke

A stroke in the territory of the posterior cerebral artery most often signals an embolus up the basilar artery from the heart or, rarely, from the vertebral-basilar junction. Also rarely, the posterior cerebral artery can be an extension of the internal carotid artery via a large posterior communicating artery. In that case, the posterior cerebral artery can be embolized from an atherothrombotic lesion that exists at the bifurcation of the common carotid artery. In any event, embolic infarction in the territory of the posterior cerebral artery requires no specific therapy. Anticoagulation with coumadin is recommended to prevent further embolic infarction. Rarely, atheroma produces thrombosis in the posterior cerebral artery with subsequent infarction. This also requires no specific therapy.

Atherothrombotic Disease of the Vertebral and Basilar Arteries

As it does in the carotid artery, atherosclerosis has a predilection for certain parts of the posterior circulation — most frequently the distal vertebral artery and the lower or middle basilar artery. An occlusion of the distal vertebral artery and its major branch, the posterior inferior cerebellar artery, is most often caused by atherothrombosis, but sometimes by an embolus. An occlusion of either artery produces infarction in the lateral medulla, which often causes a TIA or a minor stroke before the complete stroke. The symptoms and signs vary. The posterior inferior cerebellar artery also supplies the posterior inferior cerebellum, which may become infarcted if collateral circulation from the anterior inferior cerebellar artery is inadequate. Then, edema formation in the infarcted cerebellum may increase the pressure in the posterior fossa enough to result in progressive obtundation, respiratory arrest, and death. Although cerebellar edema can be treated with osmotic agents such as mannitol, surgical decompression may be necessary. When a lateral medullary infarction occurs, short-term anticoagulation therapy with heparin has been used with the justification that a clot in the distal vertebral artery may propagate into the proximal basilar artery. However, the value of this therapy is unknown, and computed tomography (CT) scanning should be performed before anticoagulation is started. There is little justification for long-term use of warfarin sodium, although occasional instances of delayed artery-to-artery embolus (vertebral to basilar or posterior cerebral) can occur.

A TIA may herald atherothrombotic basilar artery occlusion and devastating brainstem infarction. The symptoms of a TIA in the territory of the vertebral-basilar artery are more varied than in the carotid territory because many different neuronal structures are involved. Moreover, brainstem TIAs may be caused by disease either of the small penetrating branches of the basilar or vetrebral arteries or of the basilar or vertebral arteries themselves. The disease process may be atherothrombotic, involving the proximal origins of these small branch vessels, or lipohyalinotic, involving the small vessels deeper in the brainstem. In general, small vessel disease is less threatening than disease of the basilar trunk. Therefore, when brainstem TIAs or acute stroke occurs, it is important to determine whether the basilar artery or one of its branches is occluded. Disease of a basilar branch usually produces unilateral symptoms, whereas disease of the basilar artery itself usually produces bilateral symptoms. In both instances, the neurologic deficit may fluctuate. When fluctuation occurs, the prudent course is to postpone angiography in favor of short-term anticoagulation with heparin, provided that a CT scan has already excluded hemorrhage. When the patient's condition is stable, one should consider angiography again. If basilar artery stenosis or occlusion is associated with a minor or improving stroke, long-term anticoagulation with warfarin sodium is recommended. If the basilar artery branch is diseased, the rationale for using warfarin sodium is less clear. The difference between using long-term anticoagulation and using antiplatelet therapy to treat TIAs caused by basilar branch disease has not been studied. Antiplatelet therapy would seem to carry less risk and have some rationale on theoretical grounds. One-half a 300-mg aspirin tablet or its equivalent is recommended.

LACUNAR DISEASE

Atherothrombotic and Lipohyalinotic Occlusive Disease of the Penetrating Branches of the Circle of Willis, Middle Cerebral Stem, Vertebral and Basilar Arteries

The middle cerebral artery stem, the arteries comprising the Circle of Willis (A-1 segment of the anterior cerebral artery, anterior and posterior communicating arteries, and precommunal segment of the posterior cerebral arteries) and the basilar and vertebral arteries all give rise to 100- to 400-μ branches that penetrate the deep gray and white matter of the cerebrum or brainstem. Each of these small branches can be thrombosed either by atherothrombotic disease at its origin (basilar or middle cerebral stem branch disease) or by the development of lipohyalinotic thickening of its wall more distally. When they become thrombosed, small (less than 2 cm) infarcts occur and are referred to as lacunes. Many may be as small as 3 to 4 mm. Hypertension is invariably a risk factor for such small vessel disease. These infarcts represent 10 percent of strokes.

The clinical picture resulting from lacunes are called lacunar syndromes. Often transient symptoms (lacunar TIAs) herald a lacunar infarct. Such TIAs may occur many times a day, but last only a few minutes. When infarction occurs, it may present with a sudden deficit or evolve in a progressive fashion over a few days. Recovery often begins within hours or days after the infarction, although in some cases significant disability persists. Recovery over weeks or months may be complete or result in minimal residual deficit. Many lacunar syndromes have been described, and many more await documenation.

The CT scan can document many supratentorial lacunar infarctions, and magnetic resonance imaging (MRI) successfully documents both supratentorial and infratentorial infarctions when the lacunes are 7 mm or greater. MRI can also reliably document whether a small infarct in the white matter extends into the gray matter of the cortical surface. Such an extension implies cortical surface branch embolism rather than small penetrating vessel occlusion, and lacunar infarction should not be diagnosed. The electroencephalogram (EEG) is usually normal in white matter lacunar infarction in contrast to cortical surface infarction.

The best therapy for small vessel disease is prevention, i.e., careful control of hypertension. However, during stroke evolution, a reduction in blood pressure may increase the symptoms. Antihypertensive therapy is begun after the patient's symptoms become stable. The value of anticoagulant or antiplatelet agents in patients with lacunar TIAs and fluctuating stroke is unknown. Some suggest that thalamic lacunes secondary to lipohyalinosis may be associated with minor hemorrhage. Hemosiderin-laden macrophages are sometimes seen at autopsy in such infarctions. This condition precludes use of heparin. On the other hand, some patients with fluctuating hemiparesis from atherothrombotic disease of a basilar branch or of the middle cerebral stem lenticulostriate arteries may improve coincident with heparin administration. Lacunar stroke does not require long-term anticoagulant therapy; instead, it requires careful control of hypertension to prevent progression of the underlying vascular disease.

EMBOLIC STROKES OF CARDIAC ORIGIN

FRANK M. YATSU, M.D.
JAMES GROTTA, M.D.
L. CREED PETTIGREW, M.D.

Embolic strokes of cardiac origin are becoming more frequent, which necessitates their accurate diagnosis and optimum management. This review will summarize the diagnostic criteria for embolic strokes of cardiac origin, but will also provide guidelines for therapeutic intervention, i.e., anticoagulation, to minimize the occurrence of re-embolization while minimizing the dread of hemorrhagic transformation.

EPIDEMIOLOGY

Embolic strokes of cardiac origin, hereafter termed embolic strokes, must be differentiated from artery-to-artery emboli such as those originating from extracranial occlusive disease at the carotid bifurcation. Although formation of a platelet-fibrin thrombus is the underlying pathologic process accounting for the emboli, the distinction between cardiac and artery-to-artery emboli is not trivial, since therapeutic approaches and outcome vary. Emboli of cardiac origin warrant consideration of anticoagulation, while those of artery-to-artery origin require considerations of antiplatelet aggregation therapy, such as aspirin, or of carotid endarterectomy.

Embolic stroke occurs in both the elderly and the young and accounts for one-fifth of all strokes, but is becoming more prominent in the elderly. One explanation for an apparent increase in the diagnosis of embolic strokes of cardiac origin may be the use and availability of more accurate diagnostic methods such as 2-D echocardiography and Holter monitoring. Another explanation is the increasing life expectancy, which is accompanied by cardiac diseases that lead to thromboemboli. These include atrial fibrillation due to coronary heart disease but unassociated with valvular disease and postmyocardial infarction states, particularly anterior and septal infarcts with akinetic ventricular segments.

In addition to these more common causes, the following should be excluded: atrial fibrillation due to rheumatic heart disease and associated with mitral valve pathology, prosthetic valves replacement, mitral valve prolapse, and bacterial endocarditis. Rare causes for embolic strokes include left atrial myxoma, nonbacterial thrombotic endocarditis or marantic endocarditis due to occult carcinoma, Libman-Sacks disease associated with lupus erythematosus, cardiomyopathy, and paradoxical venous emboli resulting from a functionally patent foramen ovale. In this review, consideration will be given only to (1) atrial fibrillation, (2) postmyocardial infarction states, and (3) mitral valve prolapse.

PATHOPHYSIOLOGY

For atrial fibrillation, myocardial infarction, and mitral valve prolapse, the pathophysiologic basis for thromboemboli formation involves two of Virchow's triad for thrombus formation (stasis, vascular damage, and abnormal coagulation). In atrial fibrillation, blood stasis in the left atrium may lead to coagulation, while in akinetic segments associated with myocardial infarction and collagen defects associated with mitral valve prolapse, vascular damage sets the stage for thrombus formation.

For the latter process of exposing differing vascular surfaces to the circulating blood, platelets play a crucial role in initiating thrombus formation. Platelets will "stick" either to abnormal collagen or to basement membrane by a complex process called "adhesion," which is mediated by platelet surface receptors such as the glycoproteins (Ib, IIb, and IIIa), by von Willebrand factor, and by factor VIII. The process of adhesion quickly triggers the "release reaction" and the secretion of compounds such as adenosine diphosphate (ADP) and thromboxane A_2, which recruit additional platelets to form a "platelet plug." The rapid mobilization of a platelet plug can assist in preventing exsanguination due to an arterial tear, but its occurrence intra-arterially is a perversion of this normal life-saving process. Aggravating this occurrence is the "pro-coagulant" activity of platelets in recruiting the coagulation cascade to form a solid interlacing thrombus.

On the basis of this known pathophysiology of platelet adhesion–release reaction and procoagulant activity, studies assessing either platelet or coagulation functions might be expected to yield insights into both definitive diagnosis of patients with presumed embolic strokes of cardiac origin and the effects of therapy. Unfortunately, studies of both have failed. For example, during the release reaction, platelets not only secrete the above-noted ADP and thromboxane A_2, but also platelet factor 4 (PF4) and beta-thromboglobulin (beta-TG). The precise functions for each are not known, but they provide convenient markers for platelet adhesion/aggregation activity. In addition, measurement of platelet aggregates by the Wu-Hoak technique can complement these studies as a determination of platelet hyperaggregatility. While these studies show an increase in these parameters of platelet function, they remain insensitive as a means of precisely identifying strokes of cardiac origin and separating those from other causes of thrombosis, such as the so-called thrombotic strokes or emboli of artery-to-artery origin. Furthermore, assessment of platelet adhesion following radioactive labeling with ^{111}chromium and quantitating its accumulation by external radioactive counting has identified increased activity over areas of recent myocardial infarction, but is insensitive in identifying those patients who are prone to develop emboli.

The increased sensitivity and predictability of these diagnostic tools should increase in the future in order to identify more precisely those individuals who have already or are prone to develop emboli. On the basis of current investigations, more precise therapeutic interventions should be forthcoming, particularly for agents that will block the platelet adhesion reaction. Similarly, better and more reliable agents that affect the coagulation process, such as the use of low-molecular-weight heparin by gene cloning techniques, will provide measurable means of limiting the coagulation process and the deposition of fibrin without risking exsanguination or undue hemorrhaging.

ATRIAL FIBRILLATION

As with the other causes of embolic stroke, three issues are raised with atrial fibrillation (AF): (1) does the natural history of embolic strokes with AF warrant consideration of prophylactic therapy with antiplatelet therapy or with anticoagulation? (2) Will interventional therapy with these agents after embolization significantly minimize re-embolization? (3) How can the dreaded complications of hemorrhage, particularly intracerebral hemorrhage, be minimized? Each of these will be discussed after a brief overview of the demographic characteristics of AF.

AF occurs in less than 0.5 percent of the general population, and as might be expected on the basis of pathophysiology, its incidence increases with advancing age. For example, in the Framingham Study, of the 5184 patients between ages 30 and 60 followed biennially since 1950, 169 cases of AF were identified. Of these patients with AF, 59 (35 percent) developed strokes attributable to the AF. Of interest, the greatest percentage of embolic strokes occurred during the first year after AF detection and declined to an incidence of approximately 5 percent per year. Complicating the analysis of these patients was the bimodal distribution of AF among the younger patients with rheumatic heart disease and valvular pathology and the older patients with arteriosclerotic heart disease and without valvular pathology. As expected, the former had a nearly three-fold increase in emboli risk.

Although no diagnostic technique nor data exist that can accurately predict embolic stroke occurrence in a single patient with AF, the data can be reduced to the following: (1) AF of any cause is associated with an increased incidence of embolization; (2) the incidence of embolization is roughly 5 percent per year; (3) the majority of the embolization events occur within the first year after AF detection; and (4) the majority of emboli are cerebral and therefore potentially devastating. While any individual with AF is likely to develop emboli if he lives long enough, i.e., a 5 percent per year incidence over 20 years will account for all of the patients at risk, only one-third of patients with AF coming to autopsy will demonstrate evidence of embolization. Thus, the implications of findings from autopsy, a biased sampling, must be balanced with theoretical extrapolations of short-term observations. The practical translation of these data is that a roughly 5 percent per year risk of embolization exists with AF, greater during the first year, but that other diseases or complications will likely affect the patient's morbidity and mortality.

Prophylactic Anticoagulation or Antiplatelet Therapy to Prevent Embolization

Normal sinus rhythm should be restored when possible as this is optimal therapy to minimize the future risk of embolization. The issue of prophylactic anticoagulation or antiplatelet therapy for chronic AF remains disputed, since no prospective study has clarified their value. Nonetheless, until these data are forthcoming, a strong argument can be made for utilizing either agent to reduce the incidence of embolic strokes. However, Starkey and Warlow make an equally persuasive argument that without definitive data from prospective studies, treatment with anticoagulation (and its attendant hazards) is ethically unsound; other relative contraindications to prophylactic anticoagulation are the unreliability of patients, since improper dosing and tendencies to injury present major hazards, and uncontrolled hypertension because of the greater risk for intracerebral hemorrhage.

Anticoagulation or Antiplatelet Therapy After Embolization

In a patient with AF and a presumed embolic stroke, the possibility of re-embolization, particularly during the subsequent 2 weeks, is a threatening reality. Collectively, in patients with AF associated with either arteriosclerotic heart disease (ASHD) or rheumatic heart disease (RHD) or that of a paroxysmal nature, the average rate of re-embolization is roughly 1 percent per day over that first 2-week period. The occurrence of re-embolization is not related to either duration of AF or other demographic features, such as age, or other comorbid diseases, such as hypertension, or to the presence or absence of a definable thrombus in the left atrium by 2-D echocardiography. With anticoagulation, the re-embolization rate can be reduced to one-third or one-quarter. For example, in the only prospective study on this subject (the Cerebral Embolism Study Group, headed by Robert G. Hart) immediate and sustained anticoagulation was associated with a statistical trend toward significantly reduced re-embolization. In the Cerebral Embolism Study Group, 2 of 22 patients who were not anticoagulated developed re-embolizations over the first 2 weeks, while none of the 20 anticoagulated patients re-embolized. Furthermore, two of the nonanticoagulated patients inexplicably developed hemorrhagic infarctions. Although the numbers on first analysis seem impressive, they do not reach statistical significance because they are too small. Nonetheless, this study encourages the judicious use of anticoagulation and provides the basis for larger prospective investigations.

The issue of preventing re-embolization is complicated by the tendency of anticoagulation to trigger or aggravate bleeding, particularly intracerebral hemorrhage. This latter concern is a small but not negligible complication even in patients without strokes or transient ischemic attacks (TIAs) not of cardiac embolic origin. The rate is close to 1 percent per year. However, the problem is exaggerated with cardiogenic emboli, perhaps related to the trail of proximally ischemic vessels left by a temporarily occluding embolus that travels distally. In aggregate, the complication rate of hemorrhagic infarction approaches 5 percent, which begins to approach the point at which any purported benefit in minimizing re-embolization is "washed."

Specific Recommendations for Anticoagulation

The issue of identifying those individuals who are prone to develop hemorrhagic infarction remains unsettled, but clearly that risk should be minimized. Despite its controversial nature, which remains prospective, randomized studies for clarification, we recommend the following approach to reduce hemorrhagic infarction from cardiac emboli:

1. Intravenous heparin followed by coumadin should be utilized immediately in all patients with AF who develop emboli and who do not meet the disqualifications listed below. The objective of therapy is to reduce the nearly 14 percent incidence of re-embolization over the first 2 weeks to approximately 5 percent or less while conveying no hemorrhagic tendencies.
2. The heparin and coumarin treatment should prolong the partial thromboplastin time (PTT) and prothrombin time (PT) respectively, approximately 1½ to 2 times control. An increased level of anticoagulation is associated with bleeding tendencies, while lower levels do not affect re-embolization rates.
3. Heparin should be started as a continuous infusion without bolusing, i.e., at 1000 units per hour, since bolusing appears to be associated with an increased incidence of hemorrhagic brain infarction. It is prudent to treat with heparin alone for 48 hours, since the anticoagulation achieved can be quickly reversed in the event of hemorrhage. If no such complications occur, coumadin can then be started, but with heparin continuing until the PT time reaches 1½ to 2 times the control values.
4. Patients with large infarcts on CT or major neurologic deficits, such as hemiplegia, should not be anticoagulated immediately, since the hazards of hemorrhagic transformation are greater during the 2 to 3 days after the stroke. Following a period of 3 to 5 days, a repeat CT scan should be obtained to exlude hemorrhagic transformation before anticoagulation is initiated.
5. Patients who are demented or unreliable, e.g., alcoholics, should not be anticoagulated long term because of the hazards of improper dosing and of body injury.
6. Patients who are medically fragile, by virtue of other co-morbid diseases or senescence, should not be anticoagulated because of the increased risks of bleeding. While the distinction between fragility and aging may be argued as one without practical meaning, "medical judgment" by the patient's attending physician must be relied upon.
7. With third- and fourth-generation CT scanners, lumbar puncture is not needed to exclude definitively the presence of bleeding not detected by CT scans. Furthermore, complications from bleeding at the lumbar puncture site, even when heparinization is delayed for more than 2 to 3 hours, makes it prudent to avoid lumbar punctures.
8. When hypertension is associated with the acute embolic event to brain, immediate heparinization is in general contraindicated. Since we believe it prudent not to lower the elevated blood pressure during the acute stroke period, anticoagulation can be deferred until the 2- to 3-day period when the blood pressure customarily falls or hypotensive measures can be instituted without risk of aggravating the stroke.
9. The duration of anticoagulation for chronic AF is indefinite, but the 1 percent per year risk for hemorrhagic complications requires semiannual assessment. For older individuals for whom hemorrhagic tendencies are a worry, conversion to antiplatelet drugs such as aspirin after 1 year is practical.
10. For patients who are not candidates for anticoagulation, antiplatelet drugs such as aspirin should be utilized to minimize re-embolization.

MYOCARDIAL INFARCTION

Re-embolization following myocardial infarction (MI) is a problem similar to that of AF, but the magnitude differs, perhaps reflecting the underlying pathophysiologic mechanisms, i.e., sizable thrombi may develop more readily in the left atrium as opposed to the more turbulent and forcefully contracting left ventricle. Thus, the frequency of both embolization with MI and the re-embolization rate is considerably lower than in AF. For example, in one series of 740 acute MIs, 18 or 2.4 percent of patients had strokes that were predominantly embolic.

While various series differ on the relationship of potential risk factors for embolization with MI, the size, location, and associated complications generally correlate with acute embolization. For example, larger MIs, which are through-and-through or subendocardial and are correlated with higher creatine phosphokinase values (particularly over 1500 units) and akinetic segments by 2-D echocardiography, predispose to embolization. Anterior, anterolateral, and septal MIs are also at greater risk than inferior wall MIs. Aggravating the likelihood of embolization are pump failure and arrhythmias. For the latter, atrial arrhythmias are inexplicably more predisposing than ventricular arrhythmias.

In the presence of these predisposing factors for embolization, particularly with a demonstrable thrombus by 2-D echocardiography, acute anticoagulation with heparin is justified, although a prospective study assessing risk/benefit of this approach is greatly needed. Since the risk for embolization is greatest over the acute 1- to 2-month period, anticoagulation could be discontinued after a period of 3 months, particularly if the 2-D echocardiogram is free of thrombus. For patients with a large akinetic segment, consideration should be given to long-term anticoagulation. Although no large series of re-embolization in patients with MIs and embolic strokes have been evaluated, the incidence remains low in the absence of akinetic segments or ventricular aneurysms, which precludes recommending routine, long-term prophylactic anticoagulation.

MITRAL VALVE PROLAPSE

Mitral valve prolapse (MVP) detected by 2-D echocardiography or cardiac angiography is a frequent, coincidental, and asymptomatic finding among young people, particularly women. The incidence may exceed 5 to 10 percent. However, in younger patients less than 40 to 50 years of age who have experienced a stroke, particularly of an embolic type with apoplectic onset in association with severe throbbing headache, nearly one-half may demonstrate MVP. These high figures are disputed, but, nonetheless, raise the issue of whether treatment of asymptomatic MVP to avert embolization should be considered or whether a subset of MVP patients are particularly vulnerable. Finally, the problem of re-embolization with MVP provokes consideration of long-term anticoagulation or antiplatelet therapy.

Although MVP is a common finding and these patients are at risk for arrhythmias, congestive heart failure, and endocarditis, no reliable risk factor identifies those prone to embolic strokes. A recent review found only two cerebral embolic events attributable to MVP in 237 patients followed for up to 10 years, but did identify redundant mitral valve leaflets as a variable associated with severe cardiovascular complications.

Since the incidence of strokes is low, no justification can be made for prophylactic therapy for asymptomatic MVP patients. For those who have developed emboli, the occurrence of re-embolization is similarly low, and the hazards of anticoagulation to minimize embolization outweigh any purported benefits. As a result, the conventional approach is to treat these patients with antiplatelet drugs, such as aspirin, uninfluenced by the appearance of the leaflets on 2-D echocardiography. However, should a second episode of embolization occur, long-term anticoagulation is warranted.

Acknowledgment: This work was supported in part by the Cullen Trust for Health Care, Houston, Texas.

CEREBRAL HEMORRHAGE

ALLAN H. ROPPER, M.D.

CLINICAL AND COMPUTED TOMOGRAPHY CONSIDERATIONS

Most cerebral hemorrhages present suddenly as strokes with a focal neurologic syndrome reflecting the location of the clot. Large hemorrhages occasionally cause an intracerebral catastrophe syndrome with dilated pupils, coma, and a lack of focal signs, and are indistinguishable from the neurologic state caused by global ischemia, massive subarachnoid hemorrhage, etc. The focal syndrome usually evolves over minutes, but the incidence of exacerbation from rebleeding in the first few hours has been underestimated. Several clinical problems arise regularly in unresponsive patients unable to give a history. There may be difficulty in distinguishing spontaneous hematomas (related to hypertension, bleeding diathesis, or arteriovenous malformation) from (1) single traumatic hemorrhages, (2) aneurysmal bleeding, or (3) frank hemorrhage into an infarction in patients on warfarin sodium (Coumadin). Traumatic hemorrhages may be deep and spherical or oval shaped, thus simulating spontaneous bleeding. Their favored sites are the low frontal lobes and anterolateral temporal areas, but clots in the putamen are not uncommon. There is often an associated overlying contusion or sometimes a small subdural hematoma, and patients tend to be drowsier or have a more severe focal neurologic deficit than expected from the computed tomography (CT) scan appearance. The presence of many red blood cells in the cerebrospinal fluid (CSF) soon after the ictus also suggests trauma when the hemorrhage is deeply situated, but lumbar puncture is not recommended as a means of diagnosis. Bleeding from a saccular aneurysm of the circle of Willis sometimes projects upwards into the frontal temporal parenchyma ("jet bleeding"), with little associated subarachnoid blood. Apoplectic headache or stiff neck, or the CT appearance of a teardrop-shaped clot pointing basally, suggests aneurysmal bleeding. Early angiography is recommended to define the aneurysm in these patients. A stroke evolving subacutely after an abrupt onset in patients on warfarin sodium, especially with atrial fibrillation, often indicates hemorrhage into an infarction. This represents a greater risk than simple hemorrhagic infarction.

Cerebral vascular amyloid deposition is probably an underappreciated cause of lobar hemorrhage in the elderly. There is often preceding minor trauma. Amyloid hemorrhages should not be operated on, except in extreme circumstances, because of the difficulty in stopping bleeding in the hemorrhage cavity and the occurrence of postoperative hemorrhages at a second site. Multiple cerebral hemorrhages suggest trauma, amyloid, or sagittal sinus thrombosis.

The major features guiding therapy are the level of consciousness; size, depth, and location of the hematoma; amount of horizontal displacement of the pineal gland; and the presence of hydrocephalus. The last is prone to occur with hemorrhages close to the third ventricle or aqueduct. Hemorrhages uncomplicated by ventricular blood or hydrocephalus, in the absence of direct destruction of the reticular activating system structures in the subthalamic region, cause a decrease in the level of consciousness in a graded fashion depending on the extent of pineal shift. Patients with less than 3 mm of horizontal pineal displacement are awake; 4 to 6 mm, drowsy; 6 to 8.5 mm, stuporous; and above 8 or 9 mm, comatose. If the level of consciousness is not commensurate with the expected pineal shift, hydrocephalus, subarachnoid or intraventricular blood, or hypoxia at the onset of the ictus is probably playing a role. Pupillary enlargement on the side of the hemorrhage is usually associated with stupor or coma and a large horizontal pineal shift. Pupillary enlargement with only drowsiness accompanies aneurysms near the bifurcation of the internal carotid artery.

THERAPY AND MONITORING

The First Hour

Acute treatment is chiefly medical, with surgical evacuation considered only with clinical worsening or if the size of the hemorrhage on CT scan and the clinical state indicate that medical therapy is unlikely to be successful in saving the patient's life. Immediate therapy for a stuporous or a comatose patient includes the administration of 0.5 to 1 g per kilogram of mannitol intravenously followed rapidly by intubation and hyperventilation to attain a P_{CO_2} of 28 to 34 mm Hg. Vomiting and drowsiness also justify immediate intubation, but not necessarily mechanical ventilation. The effect of corticosteroids is not evident for several hours, so they play a minor role in acute management. Phenytoin (Dilantin) administration is generally favored, but is not a high priority unless there have been recent seizures. If there are ecchymoses or known anticoagulant use, vitamin K, 5 mg, is administered intramuscularly. If an emergent operation is considered (to be discussed), fresh-frozen plasma is used in anticoagulated patients. Hydrocephalus is judged significant if the cortical sulci or basal cisterns are compressed to any degree; treatment is with a ventricular drain in patients who are stuporous or comatose. Bilateral ventricular drains are required if there is a clot in the third ventricle. If time permits, blood samples for prothrombin time, partial thromboplastin time, and platelet count are drawn as the first intravenous access line is inserted.

Intracranial Pressure Monitoring. Managing patients who remain stuporous or comatose after immediate medical therapy is greatly aided by intracranial pressure (ICP) monitoring. We use a modified subarachnoid screw because of our familiarity with this device and its ease of handling and safety, but any device that has been used repeatedly by the ICU staff is satisfactory. Patients with ventricular drains for hydrocephalus should have ICP monitored through a three-way stopcock, allowing intermittent ventricular drainage, but otherwise keeping the system closed and free of infection. The drain is opened when the ICP exceeds 15 to 20 mm Hg; more aggressive or rapid drainage has led to rebleeding of AVMs and aneurysms in a few cases.

Blood Pressure and Fluids. Hypotension after cerebral hemorrhage is always, with the exception of brain death, due to a separate medical complication such as sepsis, myocardial infarction, overzealous, osmatic, dehydration with mannitol, or retroperitoneal bleeding associated with anticoagulants or trauma. Resuscitation is best accomplished with colloid (5 percent albumin), normal saline (0.9 percent), or red blood cells if there is systemic bleeding. Dextrose and water (250 mOsm per L), 2.5 percent dextrose–0.5 percent sodium chloride (280 mOsm per L), lactated Ringer's solution (275 mOsm per L), and particularly 0.5 percent sodium chloride (155 mOsm per L) should be avoided because the excess water will exaggerate cerebral edema surrounding the hemorrhage.

The treatment of hypertension, extremely common in the several hours after cerebral hemorrhage, is controversial. Many patients have been chronically hypertensive and will return to their outpatient blood pressure levels over 2 days. The risk of causing hypotension should temper an aggressive approach to acutely raised blood pressure because cerebral perfusion pressure can be critically lowered by even mild hypotension. On the other hand, unchecked hypertension raises cerebral blood flow and blood volume, particularly in areas around the hemorrhage, thus exaggerating cerebral edema. This edema cannot be removed from the brain acutely; rather, *medical therapy depends on shrinking remaining normal brain tissue.* In a previously hypertensive patient, blood pressure is left untreated up to 165/95 mm Hg; in patients without previous hypertension, or in whom the history is unknown, approximately 160/90 mm Hg is the acceptable upper limit. Systolic pressures between approximately 160 and 200 mm Hg are treated with propranolol (0.5-mg bolus at 5-minute intervals IV up to 4 mg), and furosemide (Lasix), 20 to 60 mg IV. These drugs do not have the potentially adverse effects on ICP shared by many other antihypertensive agents, and furosemide may also be beneficial in reducing brain water volume. If these are unsuccessful after 40 minutes, or if systolic blood pressure is above 200 mm Hg, nitroprusside, intravenous methyldopate (Aldomet), or (less preferably) hydralazine or trimethaphan camsylate (Arfonad) is used. It is not necessary to lower the systolic blood pressure below 150 to 160 mm Hg; care must be taken to reduce the doses of antihypertensive medications on the second and third days, compensating for the expected natural decline in blood pressure. In previously hypertensive patients the tolerated limits for systolic blood pressure are 10 to 20 mm Hg higher.

Medical Therapy After the First Hour

Intracranial pressure monitoring makes possible anticipation and treatment of exacerbations related to edema around the hemorrhage. Mannitol and hyperventilation therapy are adjusted to keep the ICP below 15 to 20 mm Hg and systolic blood pressure between 120 and 150 mm Hg. If ICP monitoring is not used, desirable serum osmolarities are 280 to 290 (Na, 140) for awake patients, 290 to 305 (Na, 145) for drowsy patients, and 305 to 315 (Na, 150) for stuporous and comatose patients. Mannitol, 0.25 g per kilogram administered IV every 2 to 3 hours, or 0.5 to 0.75 g per kilogram every 4 hours, will usually achieve these target osmolarities. Fully awake patients are managed with fluid restriction alone (approximately 1.5 L per day) without the use of osmotic agents. All other drugs (such as cimetidine, antibiotics) should be mixed in small volumes of normal saline. The risk of a nonketotic hyperosmolar state in susceptible elderly individuals is considered when the combination of dehydration, steroids, and phenytoin is used. Diabetes insipidus is rare until brain death occurs; it drives serum osmolarity and sodium very high and can cause precipitous hypotension. Even in healthy individuals, serum osmolarity above 330 may have a direct negative inotropic effect on the myocardium that, in conjunction with osmotic dehydration, hyperventilation, or barbiturates, also causes hypotension. Peripheral vascular dilation is likely the major cause of acute hypotension after mannitol administration. Fever is treated aggressively with acetaminophen and a cooling blanket if necessary.

Because most hemorrhages are surgically accessible to varying degrees, we infrequently resort to high-dose barbiturate therapy when ICP persists above 20 mm Hg despite maximal medical therapy. In an emergency, as one pupil dilates and the patient becomes comatose, a single dose of pentobarbital, 150 mg IV given over several minutes, affords time to transport the patient safely to the operating room. Intermittent injections of pentobarbital, 100 mg IV, are used liberally before suctioning, chest physical therapy, or moving the patient off and on beds for CT scanning. Barbiturates have been more effective in this situation than intravenous lidocaine (Xylocaine). The limiting factor for barbiturate use is hypotension.

SURGICAL EVACUATION OF HEMORRHAGES

Surgery is viewed as a life-saving procedure, but is not delayed until the patient is moribund. Hemorrhages into the putamen extending into both limbs of the internal capsule or extensively into the corona radiata are appropriate for acute surgical evacuation. Surgery is also considered if the ICP remains persistently above 20 mm Hg despite maximal medical therapy (excluding barbiturates) or if the patient is clinically deteriorating, but this is not due to fever, excess fluid administration, etc.

Stereotactic procedures have generally not been as satisfactory as direct corticectomy. We have evacuated large amounts of liquefied clot on several occasions as a temporizing maneuver in acutely deteriorating patients between the fourth and eighth day. This is done by placing a ventricular needle through the burr hole used for the subarachnoid screw or ventricular catheter. Patients with thalamic hemorrhages extending laterally, involving a large portion of the internal capsule, or damaging the midbrain have poor outcomes with surgical or medical therapy. Ventricular drainage in appropriate circumstances and aggressive medical therapy for raised ICP are therefore preferred. Lobar hemorrhages, accessible surgically, are less likely to cause raised ICP or compression of the subthalamic region leading to coma; they uncommonly require surgical evacuation, and we have used the clinical state more than ICP to guide therapy. However, if a lobar hemorrhage is extremely large or the edema surrounding it produces progressively elevated ICP, surgical evacuation is undertaken as early as possible to prevent secondary damage to reticular activating structures. With the basal cisterns open and the patient drowsy or better, medical therapy is usually successful.

Operative evacuation is accomplished through an incision at a point where the lesion is closest to the surface. Speech areas are generally avoided; occasionally an incision through the insula is used. For temporal lobe and putaminal clots, an approach through the anterior temporal gyrus is used. Hemostasis must be meticulous to prevent reaccumulation of the clot.

Cerebellar hemorrhages greater than 3 cm diameter, with compression or shift of the fourth ventricle, are evacuated immediately, almost regardless of the clinical state. They may cause rapid deterioration, probably from hydrocephalus, and quickly exceed surgical redemption. Smaller cerebellar hemorrhages with hydrocephalus are sometimes followed clinically with a ventricular drain alone. Once bilateral posturing occurs it is often too late to benefit the patient surgically. Patients with cerebellar hemorrhages are initially treated with corticosteroids 0.5 g per kilogram of mannitol. We have not found a role for surgical evacuation of brainstem hemorrhages.

Signs of brainstem damage, such as pupillary dilation or bilateral extensor limb posturing for more than several hours, generally lead to poor outcome with any type of hemorrhage, regardless of whether medical or surgical therapy is undertaken. Younger patients may still benefit from surgical evacuation in the first day after the ictus. Alcoholics with coagulation defects and patients over 70 years of age who may have cerebrovascular amyloid are high-risk surgical candidates and benefit from aggressive medical therapy with ICP monitoring.

MANAGEMENT OF MEDICAL COMPLICATIONS

Aspiration Pneumonia. Vomiting at the onset of cerebral hemorrhage is common, often leading to severe respiratory problems. To prevent passive regurgitation the "Sellick maneuver" is useful. This consists of manual compression of the cricothyroid cartilage, occluding the esophagus while waiting for intubation. Single doses of lidocaine, 100 mg IV, or pentobarbital, 100 to 150 mg IV, are useful in preventing the reflex rise in ICP associated with endotracheal manipulation. Penicillin is given for out-of-hospital or emergency room pulmonary aspirations. Nosocomial pneumonias, acquired after the first 4 hours in the hospital, with or without aspiration, are usually penicillin resistant and should be treated based on culture results and predominant organism on a Gram stain of the sputum.

Seizures. Seizures occur with about 10 percent of cerebral hemorrhage at the onset or during the first 3 days. Because they may cause devastating rises in ICP and deleterious cardiovascular effects, the prophylactic administration of phenytoin is reasonable. Intractable seizures are rarely a problem, sometimes indicating hemorrhage into a metastasis, but are best handled with the rapid induction of general anesthesia by pentobarbital. Time lost in controlling convulsions with conventional anticonvulsants may lead to a severely raised ICP and cerebral edema.

MANAGEMENT OF THE STABILIZED AND IMPROVING PATIENT

Hyperventilation and mannitol are withdrawn gradually, beginning on the fourth to tenth day, depending on alertness. Patients with hemorrhages in unusual locations, with configurations suggesting aneurysmal rupture, or young individuals are considered for angiography. As deep hemorrhages are absorbed, CT scans often show contrast enhancement at the rim of the clot, giving the misleading appearance of an AVM. Anticonvulsants are continued for 6 months, or longer if there were seizures early in the illness. I have generally resumed warfarin sodium in reduced doses after 6 months in patients with atrial fibrillation who have had hemorrhagic embolic strokes or lobar hemorrhage into an embolic stroke.

HYPERTENSIVE ENCEPHALOPATHY

HENRY B. DINSDALE, M.D., F.R.C.P. (C), F.A.C.P.

Hypertensive encephalopathy (HTE) refers to a cerebral syndrome caused by a sudden sustained elevation of systemic blood pressure. It should not be confused with the various cerebrovascular complications of chronic hypertension or uremic encephalopathy. HTE is an uncommon medical emergency that clinicians must recognize because it responds to prompt and vigorous treatment, but, if unrecognized, can lead to an otherwise avoidable fatal conclusion.

HTE may present at any age, but is most common in the second to fourth decades, particularly in patients with a history of acute nephritis or toxemia. It may develop in patients with accelerated hypertension from any cause, including chronic renal disease, eclampsia, vasculitis (especially polyarteritis nodosa), acute nephritis, Cushing's disease, and pheochromocytoma. HTE may develop during the hypertensive crises of phencyclidine poisoning or after tyramine ingestion in patients taking monoamine oxidase inhibiting drugs.

Acute hypertensive disorders presenting in pregnancy include pre-eclampsia, eclampsia (HTE occurring in pregnancy), and exacerbations of essential hypertension during the last trimester. Careful management is necessary to prevent patients with pre-eclampsia (hypertension, proteinuria, and persistent edema) from entering the eclamptic phase.

Symptoms of HTE are caused by cerebral swelling, alterations of regional cerebral blood flow (CBF), and focal ischemia or hemorrhage in the brain. Headache, nausea, and vomiting may develop rapidly with increased intracranial pressure (ICP). There may be a variety of visual symptoms, including dimness of vision, scintillating scotomata, or visual field defects. Transient visual loss after changes in head position, particularly when adopting the upright posture, is a symptom of papilledema. Diplopia may result from third or sixth cranial nerve compression. Anxiety, agitation, and headache characterize the early stages of encephalopathy, followed by slowness of mentation, drowsiness, confusion, and disorientation. Generalized or focal seizures may be the first event bringing the patient to medical attention.

The blood pressure is elevated to high levels. Fundus examination may reveal papilledema, subhyaloid hemorrhage, retinal detachment, fibrinoid necrosis of vessels, focal hemorrhages, and cotton-wool spots. Areas of narrowing of retinal arteries are usually due to structural change in the vessels, not to "spasm." Focal or lateralizing motor and sensory signs may be present. The patient's condition may deteriorate within a few hours in the absence of treatment, with stupor progressing to coma and death.

Clinical judgment is particularly important because laboratory investigation may not be diagnostic. Investigations to rule out intracranial mass lesions, meningitis, seizures from other causes, or intoxications such as lead poisoning may be indicated.

TREATMENT

Hypertension

The first objective in treating HTE is to lower blood pressure adequately in the hospital, where systemic blood pressure, airway patency, seizures, level of consciousness, and ICP (when indicated) can be monitored.

The Extent of Blood Pressure Reduction

The question is often asked "How rapidly and how severely should blood pressure be lowered?" Arriving at an appropriate answer requires an awareness of factors affecting CBF. Under normal circumstances the most important factors controlling the intracranial blood volume are the Pa_{CO_2} and the local metabolic requirements of the brain. Cerebral perfusion pressure varies with changes in systemic arterial pressure or ICP. The effective perfusion pressure is approximately the difference between arterial pressure and ICP. Ideally, we should know the metabolic rate and CBF of all patients in coma and with increased ICP.

CBF normally remains constant in spite of wide variations in systemic blood pressure. This quality of autoregulation results from a myogenic response in arterial resistance vessels and is largely independent of autonomic control under normal conditions, although sympathetic nerves may exert important tonic influences in the presence of acute hypertension.

Chronic hypertension causes the CBF curve to shift to the right owing to thickening of vessel walls and decreased responsiveness of resistance vessels. Therefore, high elevations of blood pressure are required to produce HTE in a patient with chronic hypertension compared with a normotensive patient. Adults rarely develop HTE at levels less than 250/150 mm Hg. The higher and faster the development of hypertension, the more likely the production of a "breakthrough of autoregulation" with forced dilation of arterial resistance vessels, abnormal permeability, and subsequent brain swelling co-existent with areas of excessive vascular constriction (spasm).

Cerebral autoregulation maintains CBF within the normal range in hypertensive and normotensive patients until the resting level of mean arterial pressure is reduced by more than 25 or 30 percent. At that level and below, the frequency of the electroencephalogram (EEG) decreases and the brain metabolic rate declines, but without clinical evidence of frank ischemia. Symptoms of general or focal cerebral hypoperfusion develop when the mean arterial pressure declines to 40 percent of baseline level. For example, a patient with a blood pressure of 225/150 mm Hg will have diminished CBF if the blood pressure is lowered to 140/100 mm Hg and will develop clinical symptoms if it drops to 110/70 mm Hg. CBF may be particularly jeopardized in hypertensive patients by lowering blood pressure too rapidly, because their lower limit of autoregulation is higher than in normotensive patients. Cerebral infarction may then occur in the distal territory of supply of major cerebral arteries (boundary zones) in such circumstances.

Clinical experience indicates that rapid but prudent lowering of blood pressure is the key initial step in the treatment of HTE. Final target values of blood pressure will depend on the patient's history, with slightly higher levels appropriate for patients with chronic hypertension. Some patients respond promptly to blood pressure lowering, whereas symptoms resolve less rapidly in patients with a longer duration of encephalopathic symptoms or concomitant uremia.

The Choice of Antihypertensive Drug

The second question asked about treatment is "Which is the best drug to use to lower blood pressure?" The ideal drug would have predictable and easily controlled action, a low toxic-to-therapeutic ratio, rapidly reversible effects, and be free of depressant effects upon the central nervous system. Such an ideal drug does not yet exist. Drugs currently in favor come mainly from the group of vasodilators (Table 1).

Because vasodilating or ganglionic blocking drugs can cause sodium and water retention, furosemide, 40 to 120 mg, should usually be administered initially and at appropriate intervals throughout the time that hypotensive agents are used, unless the patient is initially volume-depleted.

Sodium nitroprusside (SNP) given by infusion pump is the most effective way to reduce blood pressure in a hypertensive crisis, but it requires careful titration and constant monitoring. The immediate effect of SNP results from its ability to increase venous capacitance by venous relaxation without a change in cardiac output despite a slight increase in heart rate. SNP does not impair myocardial blood flow and therefore is a preferred drug to use in patients with ischemic heart disease. Within 30 seconds of starting the infusion, blood pressure begins to fall and may drop to hypotensive levels within another 30 seconds. The duration of the effect is so transient that slowing the infusion will permit blood pressure to rise within 1 or 2 minutes.

SNP is metabolized to cyanide and thiocyanate. Cyanide toxicity (manifested by metabolic acidosis) or thiocyanate toxicity (characterized by muscle weakness, confusion, hyperreflexia, and coma) may occur with prolonged use, especially in patients with renal insufficiency. A criticism of SNP is that it may dilate cerebral vessels and therefore theoretically elevate pressure in the cerebral microvascular bed. This, in turn, increases cerebral edema and blood volume, both of which increase intracranial pressure.

Diazoxide also is a potent vasodilator, but its effect is less predictable and controllable than SNP. It is avidly bound by plasma protein and quickly inactivated. Therefore, it requires rapid intravenous administration to guarantee a hypotensive effect. The pressure drop may be greater than desired, especially in patients who receive other nondiuretic antihypertensive drugs, and may last for periods ranging as long as 18 hours. The recommended dose is 150 mg given over 15 to 30 seconds, which usually produces a dramatic lowering of blood pressure within 2 minutes. Constant blood pressure monitoring usually is not required. The side effect of fluid retention can be counteracted by a loop diuretic. Diazoxide produces reflex stimulation of the heart rate and may precipitate angina pectoris or myocardial infarction and exacerbate pulmonary edema. It is contraindicated in patients with coronary artery disease. Because diazoxide increases cardiac output and stroke volume, it increases shear forces of ejected blood, which may extend the tear in patients with a dissecting aortic aneurysm.

Hydralazine is less effective than SNP or diazoxide in treating HTE. It may be given intravenously or intramuscularly, but must be used cautiously in patients with coronary artery disease because it increases cardiac work. For reasons that remain unclear, hydralazine appears less

TABLE 1 Antihypertensive Drugs

Drug	*Administration*	*Onset of Action*	*Duration*	*Side Effects*	*Comments*
Sodium nitroprusside (SNP) (Nipride) (vasodilator)	Prepare 50-150 mg/500 ml 5% dextrose in water; infuse at rate of 0.5-1.5 mg/kg/min. Titrate with constant monitoring; usual range 0.5-0.8 mg/kg/min.	Immediate	2-3 min after infusion stopped	Nausea, vomiting, sweating, muscle twitching, thiocyanate intoxication	Useful in patients with ischemic heart disease. Monitor blood thiocyanate levels; discontinue if level exceeds 10 mg/dl. May aggravate intracranial hypertension due to cerebral arterial dilation.
Diazoxide (Hyperstat IV) (vasodilator)	50-150 mg rapid IV push or 150 mg IV every 5 min. To minimize overshoot hypotension, use 30 mg/min constant IV infusion.	2-4 min	1-18 hr	Nausea, flushing, tachycardia, chest pain, hyperglycemia, hyperuricemia	Avoid in patients with ischemic heart disease intracranial hemorrhage. Determine blood glucose regularly.
Hydralazine (Apresoline) (vasodilatory)	10-20 mg IV or 10-50 mg IM; repeat q4-6 hr prn	IV 10 min, IM 20-30 min	4-6 hr	Vomiting, flushing, tachycardia, anginal pain	Generally less effective than SNP or diazoxide except possibly in patients with acute glomerulonephritis or toxemia. Avoid in patients with congestive heart failure, angina, dissecting aneurysm.
Trimethaphan (Arfonad) (ganglion blockade)	Prepare 500 mg/500 ml 5% dextrose in water; administer 1 mg/min and titrate with constant monitoring	5-10 min	5-10 min after infusion stopped	Blurred vision, dry mouth, bowel and bladder paresis, pupillary dilation	Not to be used postoperatively because of intestinal atony. Head up position of patients augments antihypertensive effect. May be used in patients with ischemic heart disease. Contraindicated in patients with glaucoma or pyloric stenosis.
Nifedipine (Procardia) (vasodilator and calcium entry blocker)	10-20 mg, chewed and swallowed, constant monitoring required	10-15 min		Headache, flushing	Overshoot hypotension a problem in hypovolemic patients
Labetalol (alpha and beta blocker, vasodilator)	20-80 mg IV bolus; 2 mg/min IV infusion	5-10 min		Nausea, vomiting, scalp tingling, burning in throat and groin	Useful in patients with coronary artery disease or impaired hemodynamic function

effective in managing hypertensive emergencies when renal function is normal than when it is impaired. The decrease in blood pressure produced by hydralazine is not accompanied by a commensurate decrease in renal blood flow. Therefore, this drug may be more effective in managing HTE associated with acute glomerulonephritis or toxemia of pregnancy than HTE complicating preexisting essential hypertension. Unfortunately, observations in animals and man suggest that hydralazine may increase ICP.

Trimethaphan is a rapidly acting, powerful ganglionic blocking agent. It is difficult to use because tachyphylaxis interferes with a prolonged effect and creates problems with titration, resulting in severe hypotension. However, its combination of hypotensive and negative inotropic properties makes trimethaphan an appropriate alternative drug for the treatment of HTE when SNP is ineffective or poorly tolerated.

Nifedipine, a calcium entry blocker, is a potent peripheral and coronary vasodilator and has been released for the treatment of angina. Preliminary experience with this drug in hypertensive emergencies, when given sublingually or orally as a broken capsule, indicates that it lowers blood pressure effectively within minutes. Overshoot hypotension may occur in hypovolemic patients. Nifedipine dilates coronary vessels and therefore may be used in patients with coronary insufficiency. It may prove to be the drug of choice for rapid lowering of blood pressure when constant monitoring is unavailable, but further clinical studies are required.

Labetalol is a parenteral and oral antihypertensive agent that competitively blocks alpha- and beta-adrenergic receptors and, in addition, has a direct systemic vasodilator action. It lowers total peripheral vascular resistance with little, if any, effect on cardiac output. It does not alter CBF. Early experience suggests that labetalol may be a useful drug when patients fail to respond to conventional therapy with SNP or "pulse" diazoxide. The decrease in heart rate and attendant lack of reflex tachycardia (presumably with preserved cardiac output) make labetalol a suitable antihypertensive drug in patients with atherosclerotic cardiovascular disease and hypertensive heart disease.

Whichever drug is used, blood pressure may on occasion fall too low. Elevation of the foot of the bed by 30 degrees will improve systemic arterial pressure by increasing venous return.

Increased Intracranial Pressure

Patients may present at different stages of mental impairment, ranging from agitation to confusion, drowsiness, or coma. When consciousness is seriously impaired, there are no visible clinical signs to indicate further variations in ICP or its resting level. Changes in respiration, heart rate, and blood pressure may occur as a result of intracranial hypertension, but they do not provide an accurate reflection of changing ICP. Some patients will have a very elevated ICP without any alteration in vital signs. Respiratory arrest occurs when ICP approximates systemic arterial pressure.

The diagnosis of HTE should be made early enough in most patients to institute effective treatment and prevent the development of coma. Unfortunately, some patients proceed to the comatose state. Therefore, it is necessary for clinicians to understand the general principles underlying the current approach to the management of unconscious patients with raised ICP.

Unconscious patients require an adequate Pa_{O_2} (80 to 100 mm Hg) and a Pa_{CO_2} less than 40 mm Hg. Ventilatory support is often required. Excessive rotation of the head, which might occlude one of the jugular veins, is to be avoided. In the unconscious patient with HTE, monitoring the ICP is desirable and can be achieved using an intraventricular catheter, subarachnoid bolt, solid state or implantable transducer, or fontanelle transducer. The choice will depend upon the experience of the neurosurgical staff and the age of the patient.

The normal maximum level of ICP is 15 mm Hg accompanied by a low-amplitude trace that has few fluctuations. Treatment is indicated with a continuously rising ICP above 25 mm Hg, pressure waves more frequent than once an hour and exceeding 20 to 25 mm Hg, or single waves if they exceed 30 mm Hg. Efforts should be made to keep the baseline pressure below 20 mm Hg.

It may be necessary to attempt to decrease cerebral edema coincidentally with lowering blood pressure during the acute phase of HTE. Dexamethasone, 4 to 6 mg IM every 4 to 6 hours, may reduce cerebral edema and improve CNS function by decreasing the permeability of cerebral vessels or influencing neurotransmitter systems.

Mannitol is a preferred hyperosmolar agent to lower cerebral edema by providing an osmotic gradient to move water from brain to blood. It is given in a 20 percent solution in doses from 0.5 to 1.5 g per kilogram. When ICP constantly rises or cannot be controlled, it is necessary to infuse mannitol continuously to maintain a serum osmolality of 315 to 320 mOsm. During large infusions of mannitol, it is necessary to check serum and urine electrolytes and osmolality frequently to ensure correct electrolyte and volume replacement. Mannitol can reduce ICP within 5 to 10 minutes.

Seizures

Patients with a diagnosis of HTE, whether or not they have experienced clinical seizures, should be given a loading dose of phenytoin by intravenous infusion at a rate no greater than 50 mg per minute to a total of 18 mg per kilogram. Phenytoin, 50 mg per milliliter in propylene glycol, may be placed in a 100-ml volume control set and diluted with normal saline. The anticonvulsant effect is evident 10 to 20 minutes after the start of phenytoin infusion. Status epilepticus is controlled in 30 percent of patients after approximately 400 mg of phenytoin has been administered. Maximal anticonvulsant effects appear only after the full dose of phenytoin is administered, about 20 to 30 minutes after the start of the infusion. To terminate convulsions rapidly, diazepam is administered simultaneously with phenytoin. Diazepam should be given intravenously no faster than 2 mg per minute until seizures stop, the total dose not to exceed 20 mg.

Phenytoin should be continued until the patient has passed well through the period of acute encephalopathy, ICP has returned to normal, and blood pressure is under satisfactory control.

Eclampsia

The ultimate goals of therapy for eclampsia are the safety of the mother and consideration of optimal perinatal outcome. Initial treatment in eclampsia should stabilize vital signs, control convulsions, lower blood pressure, and maintain renal output. Pregnancy can then be terminated with anticipation of possible complications such as hypovolemia, disseminated intravascular coagulation, and the cumulative effects of various medications. Hydralazine may be the preferred drug to lower blood pressure in eclampsia. There have been reports of maternal hyperglycemia, fetal hypoglycemia, and interruption of uterine contractions with diazoxide use. SNP may cause fetal cyanide poisoning.

Magnesium sulfate, IV loading dose of 2 to 4 g followed by continuous infusion of 1 to 2 g per hour, is effective in controlling eclamptic seizures.

OUTCOME

The patient usually makes a complete functional neurologic recovery when HTE is treated promptly and adequately. CT findings compatible with diffuse white matter edema, such as white matter hypodensity with sulcal and ventricular compression, have been documented during the acute phase. These CT signs improve within 6 days of treatment and usually resolve completely in several weeks. Occipital lobe infarction, other large or medium-sized focal lesions, or the cumulative effects of microinfarctions remain as permanent CNS defects in some patients.

FOLLOW-UP

Patients who have recovered from HTE need careful follow-up, especially those with malignant hypertension. Unfortunately, the quality of follow-up care and management of blood pressure in patients with HTE have been documented to be as unsatisfactory as the management of hypertension in the general population. Adequate treatment of hypertension is essential to prevent not only the uncommon situation of a recurrence of HTE in the same patient, but also the more usual cerebrovascular complications of chronic, untreated hypertension.

PATIENT RESOURCES

American Heart Association
732 Greenville Ave.
Dallas, Texas 75231

American Society for Hypertension
c/o Slack Inc.
6900 Grove Road
Thorofare, New Jersey 08086

Council for High Blood Pressure
c/o Cleveland Clinic Foundation
9500 Euclid Ave.
Cleveland, Ohio 44106

TEMPORAL ARTERITIS AND CEREBRAL VASCULITIS

RICHARD J. BURNS, M.B., F.R.A.C.P., F.R.C.P. (Lond)

Temporal arteritis is a distinct vasculitis that is readily diagnosed and easily treated. The remaining diseases described under the rubric of cerebral vasculitis are often difficult to diagnose with certainty, their prognosis is hard to predict, and their treatment is usually empirical. In contradistinction to temporal arteritis, in which biopsy is used to establish the diagnosis, biopsy is rarely a feasible option with cerebral vasculitis, and indirect means of diagnosis, such as evidence of systemic vasculitis or arteriographic features of segmental narrowing, are usually relied upon. Cerebral vasculitis includes the systemic necrotizing vasculitides (polyarteritis nodosa, allergic angiitis and granulomatosis, and an overlap syndrome), hypersensitivity vasculitis, lymphomatoid granulomatosis, Wegener's granulomatosis, Behçet's disease, isolated angiitis of the central nervous system (CNS) (granulomatous angiitis), and vasculitis secondary to other conditions, including systemic lupus erythematosus.

The typical symptoms of temporal arteritis are headache and visual impairment. Cerebral infarction is seen only occasionally. In cerebral vasculitis, symptoms are commonly produced by vascular occlusion with infarction. However, the spectrum of symptoms and signs is quite diverse and can include cranial nerve palsies, a diffuse encephalopathy, seizures, venous infarction, intracranial and subarachnoid hemorrhage, and occasionally even symptoms produced by a mass effect. It is assumed that the development of CNS symptoms against a background of a systemic or known vasculitis indicates that the disease is active, but this is not necessarily so.

SPECIFIC THERAPY

General Principles

In general the drugs most commonly used for all these cerebral vasculitides are steroids and cyclophosphamide, both as anti-inflammatory and as immunosuppressive agents. Only on rare occasions are other drugs such as azathioprine considered. As artery-to-artery embolism does not occur, and as hemorrhagic lesions are seen with vasculitis, anticoagulants and platelet inhibitory drugs are generally not prescribed. Carotid endarterectomy is not a therapeutic option with cerebral vasculitis, and extracranial-intracranial bypass surgery has now been largely discredited. In patients with systemic vasculitis, one needs to enlist the help of appropriate specialists when necessary.

Corticosteroids. I normally use a single oral daily dose of 50 mg of prednisolone or equivalent. Most patients seem to comply better when steroids are given daily than on alternate days, and this form of administration is more effective, especially with giant cell arteritis. As a routine precaution, a careful history regarding the possibility of recent or past peptic ulceration is taken, a fasting blood glucose determination is performed to exclude diabetes, and radiographs of the chest are obtained to exclude active or past tuberculosis. Antacids are rarely required and treatment with histamine H_2 antagonists are used only if there is a recent history of peptic ulceration or the patient develops dyspeptic symptoms not responsive to antacids. Treatment with isoniazid and pyridoxine is added in patients who have a positive Mantoux skin test and Ghon complex or who are thought to be at risk for other reasons. I aim to reduce the corticosteroid dose to the minimum necessary to control symptoms, and I am guided also by the various parameters of disease activity. In most patients I aim for a daily maintenance dose of 10 to 15 mg of prednisolone. With some forms of cerebral vasculitis it is possible to discontinue treatment eventually.

The short-term side effects of corticosteroid therapy rarely present major problems, except the development of an acute psychosis, which is more prevalent in elderly patients. Weight gain, fluid retention, and acne are rarely severe enough to necessitate withdrawal of therapy. In the majority of patients, long-term treatment is necessary, and the development of some of the features of iatrogenic Cushing's syndrome can be expected.

Cyclophosphamide. I usually begin treatment with 100 mg of cyclophosphamide daily, 150 mg might be used in a very large patient. The recommended dose is 2 mg per kilogram per day, but cyclophosphamide comes in 50-mg tablets and multiples of 50 mg are convenient. Considerable care is needed when this drug is being used. Young male patients who express a wish to have a family later are informed of the availability of sperm storage. Women of child-bearing age are informed of the effects on fertility. In this group of patients who do express a desire to have a family, I attempt to treat the vasculitis with steroids alone and I make sure that patients are part of the decision-making process. Both renal and hepatic function are assessed before treatment is initiated, because if either is impaired, one needs to be even more cautious with therapy.

The two other major side effects are bone marrow depression and hemorrhagic cystitis. I obtain twice-weekly complete blood profiles for the first 4 weeks of therapy, looking for leukopenia and thrombocytopenia. Thereafter, this is done on a weekly basis and then less frequently; however, studies are done regularly, depending on the clinical indications and progress of the patient. If the white blood cell count falls below 5.0×10^9/L and the platelet count is below 150×10^9/L, the dose is reduced to 50 mg daily. If the white blood cell levels reach 3.0×10^9/L or the platelets fall to 100×10^9/L, cyclophosphamide is discontinued. Patients are asked to look for any signs of macroscopic haematuria, which might be the first manifestation of hemorrhagic cystitis, and their urine is tested for blood twice weekly and at every office visit. I also give the daily dose in the mornings to help overcome nocturnal concentration of the drug metabolites in the bladder, and patients are also advised to drink plenty of fluids.

The long-term complications of hematologic and bladder malignancies are borne in mind, but are discussed with patients only in exceptional circumstances. However, they are warned about alopecia.

Cyclophosphamide is frequently used in conjunction with steroids, and the same general principles of treatment apply in all cases, i.e., attempts are made to reduce the dose of both drugs to the minimum maintenance levels as judged by the clinical progress of the patients and the return to normal of studies that indicate activity of the vasculitis. It must be emphasized that the role of cyclophosphamide in the treatment of cerebral vasculitis has not been proved and that such aggressive treatment is adopted only because of the high morbidity and mortality.

Supportive Care

Those patients who occasionally have seizures will require anticonvulsant therapy. Simple analgesics are used for headache, which can be a problem. Parenteral codeine phosphate, 60 mg, is useful if the headache is very severe. Sedation may be required for those who develop an acute encephalopathy. The usual principles of treatment apply for patients who develop fixed neurologic deficits, and the help of physiotherapists, speech therapists, and occupational therapists is enlisted, depending on the nature of the deficit and the age of the patient. For those patients with deficits so severe that they are confined to bed, subcutaneous heparin, 5,000 units twice daily, is given unless there is some complication such as computed tomography (CT) scan evidence of intracerebral hemorrhage or a history of gastrointestinal hemorrhage.

SPECIFIC TYPES OF VASCULITIS

Temporal Arteritis

The aim of treatment is to relieve headache and polymyalgia, if present, and to prevent visual loss. Cerebral infarction occurs uncommonly. I begin with 50 to 75 mg of oral prednisolone per day, depending on the size of the patient. Treatment is started immediately if the diagnostic suspicion is high or if there are symptoms and signs to suggest retinal or optic nerve involvement. The treatment will not influence the biopsy findings, providing biopsy is performed within a few days. Relief of headache and other pain can be expected within 24 to 48 hours. The rate of reduction of steroids will depend on the resolution of symptoms and the erythrocyte sedimentation rate (ESR). It is usually possible to reach a maintenance dose of 7.5 to 10 mg of prednisolone per day after 6 to 8 weeks.

Maintenance therapy is required for at least 1 to 2 years, and in some patients indefinite treatment will be necessary. In those patients with a history of visual impairment, an attempt to discontinue steroids must be undertaken very cautiously and with very close supervision. Headache relief can be confidently predicted, but in those patients with visual impairment prior to treatment, steroids cannot guarantee any significant return of vision.

A temporal artery biopsy is obtained routinely as soon as the diagnosis is suspected. If there is some doubt, an angiogram may reveal areas of segmental narrowing of the superficial temporal artery to indicate the best site for biopsy, although areas of localized tenderness will often enable one to direct the surgeon appropriately. Very occasionally the temporal arteries seem to be spared and the occipital arteries involved, and in these cases occipital artery biopsy is done. In the very elderly patient, particularly when the diagnosis seems clinically obvious, I occasionally forgo biopsy.

Takayasu's Disease

It would seem logical to give corticosteroids for the early cases of Takayasu's arteritis when an active vasculitis is present. However, neurologic complications tend to occur later in the course of the disease and are due to infarction as a result of major vessel occlusion. The efficacy of corticosteroids in these later cases is not proved. I give prednisolone, 50 mg per day, reducing to a maintenance dose of 7.5 to 10 mg per day, but I do not use cytotoxic agents because their long-term efficacy in this disease has not been properly evaluated. Hypertension occurs in more than 50 percent of patients and may require treatment, and headache is also common. There is often an associated anemia and elevated ESR, which can be used as markers of disease activity. Arteriography will often show symmetrical narrowing and/or complete occlusion, and arteriographic changes can also be used as a guide to disease progress to help with steroid dosage adjustment.

Behçet's Disease

Neurologic complications occur in approximately one-third of patients with Behçet's disease. Headache is common and focal neurologic signs frequently indicate a brainstem lesion. Elevation of cerebrospinal fluid (CSF) protein and CSF pleocytosis, together with a CT scan of areas of focal hypodensity, can all be used as parameters of response to therapy. I use corticosteroids in those patients with neurologic deficits, even though these agents have no beneficial effect on the cutaneous and genital lesions. I use cyclophosphamide only if there is no response to corticosteroids.

Isolated CNS Vasculitis

This rare vasculitis can present with signs of either a diffuse encephalopathy or focal lesions. Visual signs are frequent. The CSF often shows a lymphocytic pleocytosis with a raised protein concentration, while the CT scan may show multiple hypodense areas and occasionally a mass lesion. Angiography is not diagnostic, but reveals small-vessel segmental narrowing. Signs of systemic disease are singularly absent, and the diagnosis can only be made with certainty by leptomeningeal biopsy. All biopsy tissue should be cultured for infectious agents. There are insufficient data available to recommend definitive treatment, but I begin with corticosteroids and add cyclophosphamide if there is no response. This aggressive approach is taken because the disease is fatal if left untreated.

Vasculitis Secondary to Other Conditions

Vasculitis can occur secondary to infection (viral, fungal, and bacterial, including tuberculosis and syphilis), in association with malignancy (e.g., Hodgkin's disease can precede the diagnosis), and in patients with systemic lupus erythematosus. It is less common in patients with rheumatoid arthritis, systemic sclerosis, and Sjögren's syndrome. Drug abuse, particularly amphetamines, may also be associated with a cerebral vasculitis, and management consists of removing the offending agent and treating the underlying cause when possible. CNS involvement is common in systemic lupus erythematosus and can occur in the early stages of the disease. While not all manifestations are due to cerebral vasculitis, I use corticosteroids on a trial basis, being prepared to discontinue these agents if there is no response.

Lymphomatoid Granulomatosis

This rare disease affects predominantly the lungs, skin, and nervous system. CNS involvement occurs in only about 20 percent of patients, often early in the course of the disease. There can be widespread focal deficits and sometimes granuloma formation. The CSF shows a mildly elevated protein concentration and pleocytosis in about 50 percent of those with CNS signs. While the disease may remain indolent in some patients, treatment with a combination of corticosteroids and cyclophosphamide is advised. Some patients may go into remission, at which time all therapy can be discontinued.

Wegener's Granulomatosis

Although the lungs and kidneys are the organs commonly affected in Wegener's granulomatosis, the CNS can be involved with cranial neuropathy, aseptic meningitis, focal lesions, and diabetes insipidus. A CT scan might detect an occasional granuloma requiring surgical decompression. The treatment of choice is cyclophosphamide.

Hypersensitivity Vasculitis

This mixed group of disorders includes cutaneous vasculitis, drug-induced allergic vasculitis, postinfectious vasculitis, serum sickness, Schönlein-Henoch purpura, and cryoglobulinemia. Cutaneous manifestations are common, while involvement of the CNS is uncommon. Treatment consists of the identification and removal of the sensitizing agent when known and administration of corticosteroids. Very rarely the addition of cyclophosphamide is necessary.

Systemic Necrotizing Vasculitis

Although involvement of the peripheral nervous system is more frequent, the CNS can be involved in up to one-third of patients with systemic necrotizing vasculitis, although this usually occurs later in the disease. As with other forms of cerebral vasculitis, the manifestations can be diffuse or focal. An elevated ESR with anemia, leukocytosis, and thrombocytosis; red cells, casts, and protein in the urine, and circulating immune complexes are all ways of measuring disease activity. A CT scan may show areas of focal infarction or hemorrhage. Biopsy of other tissues, such as the kidneys or sural nerve, may establish the diagnosis. Patients with polyarteritis nodosa are treated with corticosteroids and cyclophosphamide, which can usually prevent development of new neurologic lesions. I give azathioprine, 150 mg daily, if side effects prevent the use of cyclophosphamide or in young patients who wish to have children. Often it is possible to discontinue the steroids and maintain the patient on cyclophosphamide alone. Hypertension and seizures are seen frequently and will require specific treatment.

GLIOMA

HENRY BREM, M.D.

Primary brain tumors need to be considered in the differential diagnosis of patients who present with seizures, focal neurologic deficits, and mental status changes. Of the primary brain tumors in adults, approximately 30 percent are low-grade astrocytomas (grades I and II), and over 50 percent are malignant astrocytomas (grades III and IV). The peak incidence for low-grade astrocytomas occurs between ages 20 and 50. The survival with a low-grade astrocytoma is highly variable. There is an 87 percent 15-year survival in "good" patients, i.e., those who are young, present with a seizure, do not have a pre- or postoperative deficit or headache, and do not have an altered level of consciousness. In contrast, the 15-year survival is 16 percent in those who do not have these characteristics, i.e., present at an older age, initially have neurologic deficits or change in mental status, or have tumors that cannot be totally resected.

The high-grade astrocytomas (anaplastic glioma and glioblastoma) have a peak incidence in the sixth decade. Factors that improve prognosis are age of the patient being less than 45 years, lack of personality change at presentation, symptoms that are present more than 6 months, presentation with seizures, and a functional postoperative performance status. Nonetheless, the survival with malignant gliomas is generally less than 2 years.

DIAGNOSIS

As with most intracranial lesions, the symptoms of astrocytomas are caused either by focal neurologic deficits due to the mass or by diffuse increased intracranial pressure. Signs and symptoms of increased intracranial pressure include headache (the presenting symptom of approximately one-third of the patients with a glioma), nausea, vomiting, diplopia due to palsy of the trochlear or abducens nerves, and papilledema. The premier sign of increased intracranial pressure is altered mental status, lethargy, and obtundation. The headaches are characteristically worse in the morning because of differences in cerebrospinal fluid (CSF) circulation between the supine and upright positions. There is often a regional correlation to the headache, especially with frontal astrocytomas causing frontal headaches and occipital lesions causing occipital or posterior cervical pain. This may be due to local stretching of pain fibers in the dura. There is an urgent need to begin treating patients who present with increased intracranial pressure.

A far better prognostic sign is a presentation with local symptoms, e.g. seizures. Almost half the patients have experienced a seizure at the time of first presentation. The seizure may be the focal jacksonian type, which aids in localization, or the generalized grand mal type. Often, the first seizure is a momentary loss of alertness and may be ignored by the patient. Other focal signs observed in patients with supratentorial hemispheric gliomas include personality changes, weakness, sensory loss, visual deficits, hearing loss, anosmia, speech deficits, memory deficits, and other defects in mental functions.

An important characteristic of the symptom complex in the patient with a glioma is the *relentless progression* of the symptoms and signs, which correlates with continued tumor growth.

The evaluation of a patient with a suspected glioma begins with a detailed history and neurologic examination. Approximately 50 percent of the patients with a glioma have one of the following findings at the time of presentation: hemiparesis, cranial nerve palsy, mental deterioration, or papilledema. It is the *level of consciousness* that determines the urgency of work-up and treatment. The disoriented patient or one with a declining level of consciousness requires immediate evaluation and treatment to lower intracranial pressure. Hyperactive reflexes, a Babinski sign, and papilledema are also indicative of an intracranial lesion.

Adjuncts to the physical examination include visual field testing. This is useful in that the visual fibers can be specifically affected by local lesions in each of the cerebral lobes. Electroencephalography (EEG) is useful in managing patients who have seizures. In general, brain tumors produce a regional slowing of electrical activity. However, a specific epileptogenic focus may produce spikes or spike and wave foci. Examination of the CSF by lumbar puncture carries significant risk and should only be performed when intracranial mass effect or increased intracranial pressure has been definitively ruled out by neurologic examination and CT scan. The primary indication for examination of CSF is to rule out meningitis or for evaluation of subarachnoid hemorrhage. CSF protein above 40 mg per dl is highly suggestive of a tumor, although it can be a consequence of bleeding or infection. Tumors may lower CSF sugar, as do infections or viral encephalitis. CSF Millipore filtration for cytology, as well as tissue culture, is specifically indicated for the diagnosis of tumors in the CSF. Tumor markers, such as alpha-fetoprotein, human chorionic gonadotropin (hCG), polyamines, and angiogenesis factor, are useful for following tumor response to treatment.

Radiographic evaluation of the patient with a suspected glioma may begin with a plain skull film. Approximately 20 percent of astrocytomas have calcifications, which generally are suggestive of slow tumor growth. Chronic increased intracranial pressure is demonstrated by erosion of the clinoid processes of the sella turcica. In children, chronic pressure erosion of the inner table can lead to a "hammered metal" appearance.

Computed tomography (CT) scanning is the most definitive diagnostic measure for evaluating the patient with a possible glioma. The CT scan demonstrates the configuration of the lesion, its relative vascularity and calcification, and its effects on surrounding structures. The edema and consequent mass effect can also be evaluated. The presence of increased intracranial pressure and hydrocephalus is also apparent.

CT scans can be obtained in axial and coronal directions in order to better localize the tumor for surgical intervention. Dynamic CT scanning, whereby a pulse of contrast dye is injected with rapid sequential scanning, is useful for determining the vasculature of the tumor and for ruling out the presence of vascular lesions mimicking a tumor. A low-grade, well-differentiated astrocytoma occasionally may not be apparent on routine CT scanning. It is therefore necessary to follow some patients with sequential CT scans if their symptoms continue to develop. Vascular lesions such as stroke often mimic the mass effect seen with brain tumors. These can be differentiated by sequential CT scans. Strokes tend to resolve within a few weeks, whereas tumors progressively worsen.

Magnetic resonance imaging (MRI) is playing an increasing role in the evaluation of astrocytomas. MRI is frequently more accurate than CT scanning in defining distinct borders of lower-grade astrocytomas. This has led to an improvement in our ability to surgically resect low-grade astrocytomas. Spread of edema to the opposite hemisphere appears to signify a poorer prognosis. Positron emission tomography (PET) scanning, while still experimental, holds the additional promise of using radioisotope-labeled, metabolically active substances (e.g., glucose of methionine) to evaluate the functional activity of a tumor.

Cerebral angiography is only occasionally necessary. Its major role is to outline the detailed vascular supply to a tumor as an aid to surgical intervention. Occasionally, a tumor that is not seen on CT scan may be visualized with angiography. For example, with hemorrhage into a tumor, the angiogram may demonstrate the presence of tumor vessels, whereas the CT scan may not differentiate tumor from clot.

SURGERY

Despite the advances in diagnostic techniques, the definitive diagnosis of glioma cannot be made without pathologic examination of the tissue. The surgical goals are to remove as much tumor as is safely possible without creating a new neurologic deficit. In addition, if the tumor infiltrates through the frontal, temporal, or occipital lobes, a partial lobectomy may be necessary for decompression. Hydrocephalus can be relieved by either ventricular drainage or an internal shunt. For tumors located in a critical area of the brain (e.g., the speech area or motor strip) or for deep-seated lesions, an open biopsy may be done through a small craniotomy with direct observation of the tissue to be examined. A useful adjunct to surgical biopsy is intraoperative ultrasound. With this technique, a cyst or mass can be identified, and the biopsy needle can be observed directly. A further refinement in biopsy technique is the stereotactic CT-guided biopsy. This approach is useful for deep-seated lesions located in critical areas. The techniques are now so refined that a specific area of CT enhancement can be identified for biopsy.

All surgical patients are prophylactically treated with antiseizure medication, usually phenytoin or phenobarbital, as well as with a corticosteroid, usually dexamethasone, 4 mg every 6 hours. If there is significant mass effect, the dose of steroid is increased. One week after the operation, the steroid doses are slowly tapered and eventually discontinued, whereas the antiseizure medication is continued indefinitely. The operative mortality is less than 1 percent. Surgery alone prolongs survival in patients with malignant gliomas by an average of 14 weeks.

ADJUVANT THERAPY

The role of postoperative radiation therapy has not been definitively proved for low-grade gliomas. Patients who undergo a subtotal resection generally receive postoperative radiation with apparent benefit. Patients who undergo a gross total resection of a grade I astrocytoma and have no further CT evidence of disease may be followed closely clinically for evidence of recurrence before radiation therapy is given. At present, there is no indication for chemotherapy in the treatment of low-grade astrocytomas.

Ten percent of patients with pathologically proved grade I or II gliomas later present with evidence of a malignant glioma. A variety of explanations have been proposed for this "malignant degeneration." It is possible that the benign astrocytoma represents a time point on the continuum of development of a malignant astrocytoma. In these cases, there would appear to be a steady progression toward malignancy. It is possible that the acquisition of an important biologic function, such as the production of tumor angiogenesis factor, may be responsible for allowing a tumor to express its malignant growth potential. It is also possible that cases in which "malignant degeneration" occurs may be misdiagnosed initially owing to sampling errors. For example, a glioblastoma may have sections that appear more benign or a specimen adjacent to the actual tumor nodule may be interpreted as being a low-grade glioma. With the refinement of CT-guided biopsies, this problem should be reduced. Finally, it is conceivable that the radiation therapy itself may contribute to further malignant transformation of tissue that is already defective.

Low-grade astrocytomas generally have a more

favorable outlook when compared with the poorer course of the glioblastoma and because there is such variability in results of treatment. Indeed, a certain percentage of patients are "cured" of a low-grade glioma. However, the overall outlook is still grim, with an average survival of 4 years for all grade I astrocytomas and 2½ years for all grade II astrocytomas.

For high-grade gliomas, surgical therapy is followed by 6,000 cGy of radiation therapy. Surgery plus radiation therapy improves the median survival from 14 weeks with surgery alone to 36 weeks. At our institution, 5100 cGy are administered with the last 2,100 cGy being coned down to the specific region of the tumor. The addition of intravenous chemotherapy with either 1,3-*bis*-(2-chloroethyl)-1-nitrosourea (BCNU) or methyl-1-(2-chloroethyl)-3-cyclohexyl-1-nitrosourea (methyl-CCNU) does not significantly change median survival, but does dramatically increase the proportion of patients surviving more than 18 months (27.2 percent with surgery, radiation therapy, and BCNU versus 4 percent for surgery and radiation therapy or BCNU alone).

A variety of experimental protocols are available for malignant gliomas. The efficacy remains to be determined. Interstitial radiation and hyperfractionation of external beam radiation are being used to treat tumor recurrences. These therapies are associated with a high percentage of patients suffering radiation necrosis to the surrounding brain. Re-operation is commonly required. This complication is partially offset by the increased survival in these patients. Other protocols involve intra-arterial chemotherapy, immunotherapy, hyperthermia, and manipulation of the blood-brain barrier. Re-operation is reserved for patients who have benefited significantly from their prior surgery, are in good neurologic condition, have a local recurrence, and are not easily managed with steroids alone. Chemotherapy with nitrosoureas is effective in about 40 percent of patients with late relapse. Chemotherapy may help such patients either after re-operation or instead of re-operation.

Progress needs to be made in a number of areas. Diagnostically, stereotactic CT scan biopsies and MRI scanning techniques need to be further utilized. Further progress is needed to expand the role of the PET scan in determining metabolic activity of a tumor and thereby its grade and aggressiveness as well as in differentiating between tumor recurrence and radiation necrosis. The role and methods of radiation therapy need further investigation. The role of interstitial radiation in the poor-risk groups needs to be defined. Finally, newer approaches, such as the development of new chemotherapeutic agents or drugs that could inhibit neovascularization of tumors, or better methods of drug delivery need to be developed and tested. With an increased understanding of the fundamental biologic characteristics of the gliomas, we should be able to improve the outlook for these patients.

METASTASIS TO THE BRAIN

NICHOLAS A. VICK, M.D.

Computed tomography (CT) has made the diagnosis of brain metastasis relatively easy. Some metastases still may remain invisible without augmented contrast dosage or delayed scanning, but this is relatively uncommon. There seem to be fewer instances of false-negative scans associated with diagnosis of metastases to brain than with primary brain tumors. If a patient with cancer presents with new and consequential headache, localizing neurologic signs, or a convulsive seizure, the causative brain metastasis (or multiple metastases) probably will be seen with accuracy on the first try. The CT appearance of a metastasis gives no information whatsoever as to its histologic type. While most metastatic lesions incite considerable peritumoral edema, some do not. Some have a ring configuration that may look very much like a malignant glioma, and some abscesses cannot be distinguished from a metastasis by radiologic methods. Nevertheless, if a patient has a known systemic cancer, a new mass lesion within the brain is almost certainly a metastasis, whatever its radiologic appearance.

One occasionally sees a patient with a systemic cancer that so rarely metastasizes to the brain that an alternative diagnosis immediately seems reasonable. A good example is Hodgkin's disease in which a brain mass is more likely to be a fungal abscess than intracerebral spread of the tumor. In any event, before the nature of the metastasis can be defined or at least carefully considered, and before other treatment options can be considered, several important general management measures must be initiated.

THERAPEUTIC MEASURES AT THE TIME OF DIAGNOSIS

Dexamethasone should be given with a 50-mg loading dose, either intravenously or by mouth. Smaller doses are less effective for relieving symptoms and reducing peritumoral edema. There is absolutely no evidence that large doses cause greater side effects. In the acute situation, short half-life oral corticosteroids such as prednisone are not adequate, despite their considerable role in long-term management. Phenytoin should be given to all patients with brain metastasis, whether or not they have had a convulsive seizure. The incidence of seizures is simply too high to play the odds and wait until an attack occurs. Obviously, if the patient presented with a convulsive seizure, phenytoin will be appropriately given intravenously. In other circumstances, the loading dose can be given by mouth over an 8- to 12-hour period. The total daily dosage is thereafter adjusted, with the assistance of blood levels, to a range of 13 to 20 μg per milliliter, The long half-life of phenytoin permits once daily doses.

Because of the concern that dexamethasone may cause stomach ulceration or, at least, gastrointestinal upset, it seems prudent to divide the daily dose of dexamethasone in half and instruct the patient to take the medication with breakfast and dinner. It may be more convenient for patients to split their phenytoin dosage in half in the same manner in order to ease compliance with instructions. The gastrointestinal difficulties with dexamethasone may be one of the minor fallacies of medicine. They virtually never occur, and only those patients who have a history of ulcer disease or stomach difficulties should be advised to take antacids. There is no role for drugs such as cimetidine or ranitidine, although their efficacy for patients with true peptic ulcer disease has led to their use in virtually all other possible disorders of the upper gastrointestinal tract, including the specious quest to prevent such problems in individuals taking corticosteroids.

SURGERY

Once treated with dexamethasone and phenytoin, the patient with a known systemic cancer with brain metastasis should always be considered as a candidate for a neurosurgical procedure. This is a complicated matter. For each patient a series of factors need to be considered. It is usually stated that multiple metastases preclude surgery in any circumstance; this is not strictly true. If the patient is not known to have a systemic primary tumor and none is detected, one of the tumors must be biopsied to establish a diagnosis before proceeding to radiotherapy. No patient should be started on radiotherapy without a tissue diagnosis. A stereotactic biopsy can be done with 1 percent or less morbidity and mortality and requires no more than 2 days in the hospital and only local anesthesia. If the patient has a known primary tumor and has multiple metastases with a neurologic deficit, surgery is not appropriate. There are, however, patients with known primaries with metastases elsewhere, such as to bone, who may benefit greatly by resection of a solitary brain metastasis prior to radiotherapy.

Metastatic brain tumors are remarkably well-circumscribed in most instances and are neither invasive to the adjacent brain tissue nor difficult for the surgeon to demarcate. Patients who undergo surgery with a considerable neurologic deficit often improve afterwards, sometimes within only a few days. This is often unexpected, especially when dexamethasone at adequate dosage for several days may not, alone, have reversed the neurologic abnormalities. The idea that response to dexamethasone may be a useful guide to the advisability of resection is quite unreliable. The relative safety of neurosurgery and its low morbidity with associated quick postoperative recovery are not as widely appreciated by all concerned in the decision-making process.

The evidence that it is preferable to first resect a solitary brain metastasis before proceeding to radiotherapy is somewhat limited and unfortunately more anecdotal than statistical in nature. Attempts to resolve the matter definitively have not been entirely satisfactory. This is because of the remarkable number of variables that must be dealt with, including factors such as histologic type of the tumor, location within the brain, general medical status of patients with metastatic cancer, the clinical course of cancer, the role of chemotherapy, and the variations in neurosurgical skill.

RADIOTHERAPY

After surgery, or if surgery is not possible, the next step is radiotherapy. This treatment has been demonstrated to be useful, and no type of metastasis should be considered to be radioresistant, although the variability of response from one tumor type to another is considerable. The problem is how much radiotherapy to give and whether it should be directed to the whole brain as well as to the site of the metastasis. Patients with multiple metastases obviously must be given whole-brain irradiation. Those with a single metastasis from common primary tumors, such as lung, breast, and melanoma, are so vulnerable to multiple metastases that it is appropriate to use wide-field irradiation in a preventative fashion with a total dosage, at least initially, in the range of 3000 to 4000 rads. The remaining several thousand rads that can be tolerated by the brain are best withheld. In certain well-documented instances, a metastasis will respond a second time to additional radiotherapy, which may maintain (sometimes for many months) a high quality of neurologic function and life.

CHEMOTHERAPY

Chemotherapy, either in conjunction with or after radiotherapy, remains a limited treatment modality for brain metastasis. In many patients it is completely ineffective for brain metastasis, while at the same time having some effect on the same cancer elsewhere in the body. The problematic factor of drug delivery, chiefly in the form of blood-to-tumor transport, has not been solved. Lipid-soluble drugs have been most widely used because of the assumption that brain tumor capillaries have permeability characteristics similar to those of normal brain. In most instances, they do not; these capillaries are fenestrated and permit access of substances in the blood to the tumor that are impeded by normal brain capillaries. The obvious examples are the radioiodinated contrast agents used in CT scanning. Unfortunately, the degree of increased permeability of brain tumors, which permits their detection by CT, does not mean that the permeability advantage over normal brain will have therapeutic consequence. Brain tumor chemotherapy remains experimental and empirical at the present time, although there is increasing interest in developing knowledge about drug concentrations, time of access to the tumor, and the biologic fate of what drug is actually delivered, including speed of degradation and efflux.

SUPPORTIVE CARE

Supportive care, in addition to the judicious use of corticosteroids and anticonvulsants, is extremely important. Patients with metastatic brain tumors often benefit considerably from physical and occupational therapy, especially when it can be given at home rather than in the hospital setting. A frank personal approach on the part of the physician, combined with a willingness to spend time with the patient, cannot be overemphasized.

Patients with brain metastasis know their lives are limited. They nevertheless can be assisted by the physician if there is a clearly stated and obvious effort to maintain the highest quality of life possible. When this fails, terminal care should be directed toward measures of comfort with liberal use of narcotic drugs in conjunction with withdrawal of corticosteroids. Life support measures that prolong the process of dying and promote suffering must be avoided. Decision-making at this juncture of care should depend upon the patient's previously stated wishes. These, when solicited, invariably include a desire for aggressive care while quality of life remains and prompt withdrawal of treatment when personal dignity is lost. These are difficult matters to discuss in any context. Only the most general of principles can be considered in the abstract. In the particular, however, the decisions are more often than not exceedingly clear, especially when the physician is capable of managing a patient in the same manner that he would wish for himself.

RESOURCES

The Association for Brain Tumor Research has a well-conceived patient education and referral program and has available clearly-written brochures suitable for both physicians and patients.

The Association for Brain Tumor Research
6232 North Pulaski Road
Chicago, Illinois 60646
Telephone: (312) 286-5571

NEOPLASTIC SPINAL CORD COMPRESSION AND CARCINOMATOUS MENINGITIS

RONALD G. WILEY, M.D., Ph.D.
KARL E. MISULIS, M.D., Ph.D.

EDIPURAL SPINAL CORD COMPRESSION

Compression of the spinal cord and nerve roots by extradural tumor is the second most common neurologic complication of systemic cancer. The majority of cases result from a vertebral metastasis encroaching upon the spinal canal. Lymphomas frequently enter the spinal canal by extension of a paravertebral mass through an intervertebral (neural) foramen. Rarely, a metastasis arises in the epidural space without an antecedent bony metastasis or paravertebral mass. Virtually all patients (95 percent) initially develop back pain that becomes progressively more severe, often with the addition of radicular pain radiating along the corresponding dematome. Spinal cord dysfunction, initially manifest as a gait disturbance, develops late in the course. If inadequately or unsuccessfully treated, a complete transverse myelopathy ensues with paraplegia, sensory level, and loss of sphincter control that results in a severely disabled patient who requires high level nursing care for the rest of his life.

The principal objective in the care of patients with epidural tumor is to establish the diagnosis and initiate therapy before significant spinal cord damage occurs. Paraplegia is rarely reversible regardless of treatment. Consequently, the clinical management challenge is to identify patients and initiate therapy at a time when spinal cord function is normal or nearly normal. The single most useful test in this regard is the complete Pantopaque myelogram. Recently, we have also been favorably impressed with the usefulness of magnetic resonance imaging (MRI). However, success with MRI depends on imaging the entire spine and use of a surface coil to obtain high-resolution images. Regardless of MRI findings, lumbar puncture is still generally required to obtain cerebrospinal fluid (CSF) cytology specimens. Major concerns in the patient without epidural tumor are carcinomatous meningitis, intramedullary tumor, or radiation myelopathy.

The principal therapeutic modalities available include glucocorticoids, radiation therapy, surgery, and chemotherapy. Figure 1 shows our approach to the patient with known cancer.

Glucocorticoids

In epidural spinal cord compression from solid tumor metastases, glucocorticoids are used to decrease vasogenic edema within the substance of the spinal cord, thereby protecting it from irreversible ischemic infarction. Experimental data indicate that such edema is relatively resistant to gluococorticoids. Also, the anti-edema effect of glucocorticoids has a substantial lag time to onset (18 to 24 hours). Because of these considerations and because

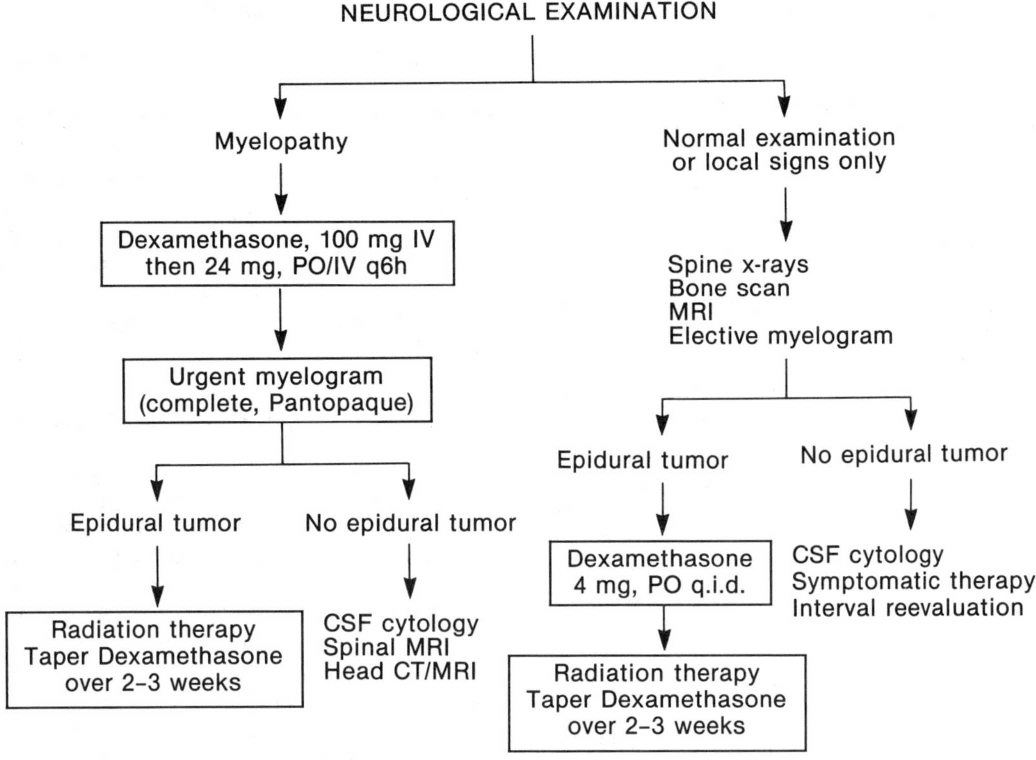

Figure 1 Approach to management of cancer patient with persistent, progressive back pain with or without radicular symptoms or signs.

some patients may unpredictably experience rapid progression of their myelopathy (within hours), we routinely give 100 mg of dexamethasone as an intravenous push as soon as we detect evidence of spinal cord dysfunction. If the subsequent emergency myelogram reveals epidural spinal cord compression, the dexamethasone is continued at 24 mg orally or IV every 6 hours for 3 days and then tapered, as tolerated, by halving the dose every third day. If recrudenscence of symptoms occurs during the taper, the dose can be increased back to the previous level and tapering attempted again in a few days.

Surgery

Without doubt the most compelling indication for surgery is epidural spinal cord compression in a patient without known cancer. In this situation surgery is required for tissue diagnosis. Similarly, we favor surgery when there is substantial diagnostic uncertainty, such as a patient with no detectable bony lesions or paravertebral masses, a cancer patient who is thought to be disease-free without any other known metastases, or whenever an epidural abscess is a serious concern on the basis of the patient's condition and the radiographic data. Surgery in these situations is followed by radiation therapy, preferably allowing 7 to 10 days for wound healing if the patient's condition permits. Wound dehiscence and wound infection are relatively common in debilitated cancer patients treated with glucocorticoids and radiation therapy. Also, spinal instability may ensue after a posterior decompression.

Surgery can be useful in other special situations, including (1) isolated single vertebral/epidural metastasis of a radioresistant tumor in a patient with otherwise limited disease; (2) severe pain due to compression fracture or spinal instability after successful radiotherapy for metastasis; and (3) occasionally in the patient who fails to respond to radiotherapy or relapses after maximally tolerable radiation (about 4,500 rads, cord dose).

The most promising approach to the patient with a single involved vertebra is an anterolateral procedure with resection of all involved bone and all visible tumor followed by placement of a methacrylate prosthesis and extra-spinal stabilizing hardware as needed. Preservation of the anterior longitudinal spinal ligament seems important in maintaining stability. Obviously, patients selected for this type of therapy should have an expectation of extended survival, be a good general anesthesia risk, and have vertebrae on either side of the metastasis that are free of tumor or significant osteoporosis. Radiation is routinely administered postoperatively, after a delay to permit wound healing. Properly selected, these patients can do extremely well, but the requirement for thoracotomy or laparotomy to obtain surgical exposure limits the applicability of this approach to otherwise healthy patients.

Patients with persistent severe pain due to bony deformity and/or spinal instability, usually with compression fracture, may benefit from surgical stabilization and relief of the associated neural compression. In this situation, we favor methacrylate and wire fusion with the placement of distraction rods (Harrington rods). Relatively small ''mini''-distraction rods have been recently developed. Direct attempts to resect these bone deformities are rarely feasible and are associated with a high risk of complications such as postoperative instability.

Failure to respond to radiotherapy and recurrence of spinal cord compression after maximally tolerable radiation are extremely difficult problems; no form of therapy is reliably useful in this situation. However, it is extremely difficult not to operate on such patients if they are otherwise reasonably functional and not imminently terminal. The surgical risk is high (20 percent or more combined mortality and major morbidity), and control of the neoplastic neural compression is likely to be transient unless an anterolateral resection and prosthesis can be undertaken.

Radiation Therapy

The cornerstone of managing most cancer patients with epidural metastases is radiotherapy. Because spinal cord tolerance of irradiation is limited, it is crucial to be precise in the design of ports and dosimetry. Correct port design requires complete definition of the location and extent of all epidural metastases. It is dangerous to attempt to approximate portal margins because of possible overlap at the edges delivering toxic radiation doses to the spinal cord. Consequently, we attempt to include all the epidural tumor within the radiation field along with generous margins (generally two vertebral bodies above and below the limits of radiographically demonstrable tumor). Also, we prefer to treat multiple discrete lesions all at the same time. An additional consideration is irradiation of adjacent vertebrae containing metastases even without epidural extension. In general, we favor radiotherapy to these adjacent ''asymptomatic'' vertebrae at the same time as that to the epidural tumor unless effective systemic chemotherapy is available for specific tumors (e.g., germ cell tumors, lymphoma). Similarly, we utilize radiotherapy for *all* epidural metastases that are symptomatic at the time of diagnosis *regardless of tumor type* and for all epidural tumors, even asymptomatic lesions, except for the most chemosensitive types. Clearly, the radiation port must entirely encompass any paraspinal tumor associated with epidural cord compression.

Even though recovery from paraplegia is rare, we strongly favor irradiating such patients for two reasons: (1) a high percentage of these patients obtain pain relief from radiotherapy, and (2) a small percentage obtain some recovery of neurologic function. For example, quality of life is far superior if sphincter control can be preserved or recovered, even if paraplegia persists. Survival may also be prolonged somewhat by radiotherapy in these patients.

Chemotherapy

Systemic chemotherapy has a major role in management of patients with epidural spinal cord compression when the underlying malignancy is drug sensitive, e.g., lymphoma, germ cell tumor. In patients with drug-responsive tumors, we use radiation therapy only for bulky, symptomatic epidural massses and avoid irradiating metastases confined to bone or small asymptomatic epidural deposits unless they fail to respond to chemotherapy. This approach spares as much bone marrow as possible from ablation by radiotherapy, thus permitting maximal doses of cytotoxic drugs.

CARCINOMATOUS MENINGITIS

Seeding of the leptomeninges with tumor cells of distant origin is an uncommon complication of solid tumors and has traditionally signified a poor prognosis for long-term survival. Treatment of meningeal involvement by solid tumors is less successful than that due to leukemia and lymphoma. Meningeal involvement may be the first manifestation of systemic carcinoma in up to 50 percent of patients who develop this complication. Solid tumors likely to cause meningeal involvement include lung, breast, and gastrointestinal (especially stomach) tumors and melanoma. Of the nonadenomatous lung tumors, small cell neoplasms are much more likely to have meningeal involvement than squamous cell neoplasms. Meningeal involvement is very common with acute lymphoblastic leukemia and transformed cell lymphomas. Indeed these latter neoplasms are generally treated prophylactically for prevention of overt meningeal involvement.

The clinical features include those that would be expected from meningeal irritation, hydrocephalus, and nerve root infiltration. Headache is the most common presenting symptom, although frank meningeal signs are rare. Other common symptoms are weakness, radicular sensory symptoms, back or neck pain, diplopia, cognitive changes, gait difficulty, and nausea and vomiting. Signs include reflex asymmetry, focal motor weakness, sensory deficits, diffuse encephalopathy, and cranial nerve palsies, with the most common being extraocular motor and facial nerve palsies. Diagnosis depends primarily upon clincal suspicion. The first CSF sample may yield negative or equivocal cytologic findings; consequently, if clinical suspicion is high, we routinely obtain at least three CSF samples of 10 to 20 ml for cytology and frequently include a cisternal or lateral cervical sample. CSF findings include increased protein, pleocytosis, and raised pressure. A low glucose level is seen in a minority of patients. The definitive diagnosis rests on positive cytologic findings, which are present in up to 80 percent of patients if multiple CSF samplings are performed.

Radiation Therapy

Radiation therapy was the first treatment used for carcinomatous meningitis and has resulted in improved survival. It can be delivered to the entire neuraxis, but the risk of serious myelosuppression is greatest with this regimen. We favor limiting radiation to the sites of symptomatic involvement, in conjunction with intrathecal chemotherapy. The potential benefits from local irradiation are reduced myelosuppression, as a result of limited spinal column irradiation, and prompt control of local symptoms. Response rates for meningeal involvement by lung and breast cancer are approximately 40 percent, with an improvement in median survival to 5 months with radiation therapy alone compared with 2 to 3 months without any treatment. Of course, limited field radiotherapy cannot be expected to provide sustained control of neoplastic meningitis when the tumor cells are free to infiltrate throughout the ventricles and subarachnoid space.

The complications of radiation therapy include myelosuppression, especially with irradiation of the entire neuraxis, which may limit the total amount of radiation that may be administered as well as make the optimal use of systemic chemotherapeutic agents impossible. As patient survival has increased, leukoencephalopathy has become more frequently recognized as a complication of cranial irradiation and methotrexate therapy. This is characterized clinically by confusion progressing to somnolence and coma in some patients; in others, it may be manifested as only a diffuse encephalopathy.

Chemotherapy

Although radiotherapy is appropriate for most patients to provide symptomatic relief of local symptoms or hydrocephalus, intrathecal chemotherapy is generally reserved for patients with lymphoreticular neoplasms or limited-extent solid tumors and good performance status.

Methotrexate (MTX) is the most commonly used chemotherapeutic agent for treatment of carcinomatous meningitis. Administration must be intrathecal since this drug has poor penetration of the blood-brain barrier due to lipid insolubility and high protein binding in the blood. Early studies of intrathecal administration employed injection into the lumbar sac during lumbar puncture, and this is still used to a limited extent. However, we favor intraventricular administration of MTX, which is accomplished by means of an intraventricular catheter connected to a subcutaneous reservoir (Ommaya reservoir). Careful use of the Ommaya reservoir has a low complication rate and is much more convenient for both patient and physician. Distribution of drug throughout the subarachnoid space is generally more consistent with intraventricular injection, except in patients with increased intracranial pressure and/or hydrocephalus. When in doubt concerning drug distribution, we obtain interval CSF samples from the ventricle and from the lumbar sac for drug concentration measurements. If distribution is not uniform, we alternate giving MTX by intraventricular injection and lumbar puncture.

The regimen of administration may have a marked effect on the incidence of side effects of treatment. This has been shown especially for meningeal leukemia. Administration of a single large dose into the reservoir is associated with much greater toxicity than administration of smaller doses over a longer period of time; there is no significant difference in efficacy of treatment with either method. When possible, we favor an initial dose of 12 mg of MTX intraventricularly followed by daily ventricular CSF MTX determinations and daily doses of MTX, 1 to 3 mg, to maintain the CSF MTX concentration between 10^{-5}M and 10^{-6}M. Oral citrovorum factor, 9 mg twice a day, *must* be given concurrently. Daily MTX is continued for 2 weeks or until cytologic findings are negative from intraventricular and lumbar CSF samples, whichever comes first, and then switched to 12 mg twice weekly, gradually decreasing to every other week. Citrovorum factor must be given for 3 to 4 days after each intrathecal dose of MTX.

If rapid, reliable determinations of CSF MTX concentration are not available, the initial 12-mg dose of MTX can be followed by 1 mg every 12 hours for 6 doses repeated every 4 to 8 days with concurrent citrovorum factor orally. The interval between treatments is gradually lengthened to every month. This regimen is equally applicable to lymphoreticular or solid tumor meningitis.

At each administration, CSF should be removed for cytology studies as well as for determination of glucose, protein, and cell count with differential. The MTX should be withheld if the peripheral white cell count is less than 3,000 mm^3, the platelet count less than 100,000 mm^3, or the blood urea nitrogen (BUN) greater than 25 mg per deciliter.

Complications of intrathecal chemotherapy include hemorrhage or infection associated with the intraventricular catheter and a subacute to chronic leukoencephalopathy, characterized clinically by cognitive changes and gait disturbance. Computed tomography (CT) shows decreased density in the white matter. Most of these patients initially received radiation therapy; therefore, the etiology is probably multifactorial. Also, an acute meningoencephalitis has been described that is not associated with bacterial contamination of the CSF, resolves in 24 to 72 hours, and does not recur with further chemotherapy. Intrathecal MTX produces severe mucositis and/or myelosuppression, which can be prevented by oral administration of citrovorum factor. This procedure does not significantly increase the concentration of "rescue" folate in the CSF; therefore, it does not compromise therapeutic benefit.

Intrathecal MTX in conjunction with radiation therapy has produced the greatest improvement in outcome of carcinomatous meningitis, with the proportion of improved patients approaching 50 percent, and a median survival time increased from 5 months with radiation alone to 7 months with combined radiotherapy and chemotherapy.

Other possible chemotherapeutic agents include cytosine arabinoside, 20 mg per m^2 twice weekly, but this drug is primarily of benefit in leukemic meningitis and should not be used unless MTX administration is contraindicated or ineffective. There is no convincing evidence for a beneficial effect of cytosine arabinoside in combination with MTX. Thio-TEPA, 10 mg per m^2 twice weekly, can be used if MTX and cytosine arabinoside are contraindicated or initially ineffective.

With optimal therapy, survival from neoplastic meningitis is greater than without therapy, although the response is still less than would be desired. Patients with lymphoreticular neoplasms often experience complete responses, only to relapse if control of systemic disease is unsuccessful; whereas the most common positive response in patients with solid tumors is clinical stabilization. With combined radiation and chemotherapy the overall stabilization rate in patients with solid tumors is approximately 50 percent, with the best prognosis being with breast cancer and the worst with melanoma. Cytology may become negative in less than 25 percent of patients with solid tumors.

One common complication of carcinomatous meningitis is hydrocephalus. If this requires ventriculoperitoneal shunting, the peritoneal tubing may be attached to the Ommaya reservoir with an on-off valve to prevent passage of the instilled drug into the peritoneal tubing for 30 minutes after MTX injection. Levels of MTX obtained using this technique have been therapeutic, even in the lumbar sac CSF, although this should be checked and lumbar MTX injections given if distribution is inadequate after ventricular instillation.

PSEUDOTUMOR CEREBRI

JAMES J. CORBETT, M.D.

Pseudotumor cerebri is a common neurologic problem occurring primarily in obese women of childbearing age. Of unknown cause and tenuously associated with many conditions, the major symptoms are headache, brief visual obscurations in one or both eyes, and horizontal double vision. Less common symptoms include pain in the neck, shoulders, back, and arms and pulsatile tinnitus. Consciousness is never altered. Spinal fluid pressure is elevated, protein is normal or low (frequently less than 20 mg per deciliter), and glucose and cell count are normal. The spinal fluid pressure is almost invariably greater than 200 mm H_2O. If cerebrospinal fluid (CSF) pressure is not elevated at a first spinal tap, a repeat tap should be done to establish that the pressure is truly increased. Troughs of normal CSF pressure in patients with pseudotumor cerebri are extremely rare. Papilledema is usually bilateral, but occasionally may be unilateral. Visual loss is the only serious and potentially permanent complication of pseudotumor cerebri. Papilledema may cause serious visual loss in 10 to 25 percent of patients with pseudotumor cerebri. Thus the alternative name "benign intracranial hypertension" is a misnomer.

The first problem in management of these patients is to clearly establish that they have pseudotumor cerebri and not some other condition. Since pseudotumor is overwhelmingly a problem of obese women of childbearing age, one should be especially careful when making this diagnosis in men, women who are not obese, and children (see Table 1).

Children can have pseudotumor cerebri, but the frequency of occurrence is lower than in adults and the sex incidence is equal. Pseudotumor precipitated by antibiotic use (tetracyclines and nalidixic acid) and steroid withdrawal is seen almost exclusively in children.

Probably the most common reason for a mistaken diagnosis of pseudotumor cerebri is the patient who has headaches and pseudopapilledema. Table 2 includes the important conditions mistaken for pseudotumor cerebri.

DIAGNOSTIC IMAGING

Computed tomography (CT) scanning has supplanted earlier studies, including arteriography and pneumoencephalography. The CT scan shows normal or small ventricles, and an empty sella occurs about 15 to 20 percent of the time. While CT is very useful, the occasional sagittal sinus or lateral sinus thrombosis may not be detected. The addition of digital subtraction angiography to detect occult venous occlusions increases individual case cost with a relatively low overall yield.

In the future, when it is more widely available, magnetic resonance imaging (MRI) will provide the single best tool for detecting occult venous occlusions and identifying underlying masses without radiation risk. The typical overweight patient with pseudotumor is a problem because of MRI weight limitations and claustrophobia. At this time, CT scan, with and without contrast, is the preferred imaging procedure.

LABORATORY STUDIES

Most of the reputed assocations listed with pseudotumor are casual or occur with no greater frequency in patients with pseudotumor than in age- and sex-matched controls. Extensive laboratory studies are not helpful in most patients. The most important studies to perform include serum calcium to rule out hypoparathyroidism, antinuclear antibody (ANA), venereal disease reasearch laboratory test (FDRL), and fluoresent treponeal antibody (FTA). Further endocrine studies are useful only if there is serious reason to believe the patient is cushingoid, addisonian, or is suffering from hypoparathyroidism.

TABLE 1 Patients with "Symptomatic"Pseudotumor Cerebri

Vitamin A intoxication: "liver lover's headache" and patients taking large daily quantities of vitamin A (also cod liver oil, fish liver oil)
Phlebothrombosis of the sagittal or lateral sinuses, post-traumatic or puerperal
Radical neck dissection, unilateral or bilateral
Treated cases of deprivation dwarfism or occasional cases of newly treated hypothyroidism in children
Guillain-Barré syndrome and elevated CSF protein
Systemic lupus erythematosus

A lumbar puncture is a crucial study in all patients with suspected pseudotumor. Not only does one need an elevated opening pressure to make the diagnosis, but the CSF must be carefully studied to exclude tumor and infection.

Once imaging studies (CT or MRI) and lumbar puncture have been done and the diagnosis is firmly established, an ophthalmologist should examine the patient.

VISION ASSESSMENT

Since visual loss is the only proven serious complication of pseudotumor cerebri, proper assessment of visual function using modern kinetic perimetry (Goldmann or Aimark), visual acuity testing, and fundus photography should be undertaken. The need for repeated accurate observations of best corrected visual acuity, careful perimetric examination, and observation for afferent pupil defects cannot be overstressed.

Perimetry by the standard kinetic Goldmann technique utilizing an Armaly-Drance testing strategy is able to detect visual defects when about 30 percent of the fibers are lost. Static perimetry is more sensitive than this method, but is not always available. Tangent screen testing and measurement of the blind spot size are inadequate and may lull the examiner into complacency, since serious peripheral field loss, a harbinger of rapid visual field collapse, may not be detected on a 30-degree tangent screen.

Examination for a *relative afferent pupil defect* (RAPD) may reveal asymmetries in pupil function suggesting visual loss that is frequently unrecognized by the patient. The presence of an RAPD is objective evidence of loss of visual field and is proportional to the amount of field lost.

Visual acuity should be measured in good light at 20 feet with best eyeglass correction or using a pinhole. Anything less than 20/20 is evidence of visual loss unless the patient is known to have a "lazy" amblyopic eye. Hand-held Shellen visual acuity is second best.

Visual evoked potential (VEP) unfortunately gives little information about impending visual loss in pseudotumor. It confirms that central vision (visual acuity) is usually the last thing to go when vision is being lost in association with papilledema. When central vision is affected, latencies become prolonged. Do not fall into the trap of believing that VEP is helpful — it is not.

Fundus photographs provide graphic evidence of improvement or deterioration. Today, with fundus photography abundantly available, it is possible to have photographs done that permit the clinician to accurately assess the efficacy of any particular treatment regimen. Memory serves everyone poorly when trying to recollect fundus appearances, and most drawings are too crude to be useful. The sudden appearance of multiple nerve fiber layer infarcts, hemorrhages, or new optociliary collateral veins may be forerunners of visual deterioration and should be documented.

TREATMENT

Once the preliminary radiographic, laboratory, CSF, and visual studies have been done, treatment depends on the patient's symptoms, the severity of visual loss, and the presence of other underlying conditions such as glaucoma, systemic hypertension, episodic hypotension, renal disease, pregnancy, or other medical conditions. Characteristic treatment settings include the following:

1. The *asymptomatic patient* who has no visual loss and in whom the condition was accidentally discovered needs no treatment and should be followed at 1- to 3-month intervals with ophthalmologic studies. If visual loss occurs, treat with acetazolamide or furosemide; if it progresses, consider surgery.
2. When the patient has only *headache* and visual loss is trivial or nil, he or she should be treated with standard headache medications. Severe, persistent headache frequently responds to spinal tap. Paradoxically, while headaches are frequently relieved with lumbar puncture, long-term intracranial pressure (ICP) monitoring in patients with pseudotumor has shown no direct correlation between the height of CSF pressure and the severity of headaches. Severe chronic headache as a major symptom of pseudotumor may, on rare occasion, require a lumbar peritoneal (LP) shunt. I have had to resort to LP shunt infrequently and encourage the vigorous use of prophylactic migraine medication to control headache before using shunts. If headaches are postural and remit when recumbent, consider a blood patch, since patients with pseudotumor may also develop post-lumbar puncture headaches.
3. The patient with *serious loss of visual fields* or *loss of visual acuity* should not undergo multiple trials of

TABLE 2 Conditions Mistaken for Pseudotumor Cerebri

The combination of anomalously elevated optic discs and headache (most common)
Unrecognized brain tumors (rare when careful CT scan is done)
Glioma
Gliomatosis cerebri
Metastatic tumors, especially pelvic tumors, breast and lung cancer to venous sinuses
Meningeal carcinomatosis
Spinal cord or peripheral nerve (cauda equina) tumors with high protein in the CSF
Arteriovenous malformation with high intracranial venous sinus pressure
Infectious diseases
Viral encephalitis
CNS syphilis with optic papillitis
Sarcoidosis

different medications before surgery is contemplated. LP shunt or preferably optic nerve sheath fenestration, should be done early rather than late if the patient reports visual loss as a major complaint, especially if visual fields and visual acuities corroborate the symptom. Multiple medications and medication changes have not been effective in preventing progressive visual loss. Surgery may not always prevent blindness, especially when visual loss is severe or rapidly progressive or has been present for a long time (many days or weeks).

Careful documentation of visual acuity, visual fields, and photographic appearance of the fundus is crucial, since patients with serious visual loss may actually believe that the *treatment* caused the problem.

4. *Rapidly progressive visual loss with pseudotumor cerebri* is seen rarely, but the patient may lose vision to the point of total blindness within a few days. These patients are, paradoxically, almost all men, usually black, and have high blood pressure. None qualifies for a diagnosis of hypertensive encephalopathy, but the management of their high blood pressure and their increased intracranial pressure poses a serious treatment challenge. To date, all patients with this constellation of severe hypertension, pseudotumor cerebri, and rapid visual failure have gone blind despite LP shunt, optic nerve sheath fenestration, and multiple medications. The concomitant attempts to regulate systemic blood pressure should be cautious; a rapid drop in blood pressure may well decrease blood flow at the optic disc and result in ischemic infarction.
5. The *pregnant patient with severe headache* is probably best treated with repeat lumbar punctures or with beta blockers. These methods are relatively safe during pregnancy and should provide headache relief. If headache is incapacitating, bed rest and, as a last resort, LP shunt could be considered. If *visual loss* ensues while the patient is pregnant, optic nerve sheath fenestration is the safest way to preserve vision. Pregnancy is not a contraindication to any treatment. Pseudotumor is not an indication for therapeutic abortion.
6. If the patient has *renal disease* requiring hemodialysis, recurrent drops in blood pressure with volume shifts are common. Hypotension is poorly tolerated by a swollen optic disc and may result in compound visual loss due to papilledema and to ischemic infarction. Visual loss can be safely prevented with optic nerve sheath fenestration.

Specific Treatment Modalities

Diet is recommended for all obese patients with pseudotumor. For the asymptomatic obese patient, diet may be the only therapeutic recommendation. Diet should be recommended with encouragement and not with threats of blindness. If the patient is sent for dietary instruction, avoid obese dietitians; they give a double message. Use of commercial weight reduction programs such as Weight Watchers is also helpful.

Diuretics have been used for years, and the diuretics most commonly used are acetazolamide 1000 to 1500 mg daily in the sequel form (500 mg two or three times per day) and furosemide (Lasix). Both drugs are capable of reducing headache frequency and severity and decreasing transient visual obscurations, but none of the diuretics has ever been subjected to a randomized prospective trial of therapy. Side effects of acetazolamide are numbness of the hands and feet and circumoral numbness. Rarely, patients taking acetazolamide will develop renal stones. They all develop a mild metabolic acidosis, which is never serious, and the bicarbonate of 14 to 18 mEq per L is objective evidence of compliance. In addition to the somatosensory symptoms, these patients complain that carbonated beverages taste metallic. Patients may rarely become anorectic or depressed. It is unusual for these symptoms to cause a patient to stop taking the medication. Potassium wasting occurs and may require substantial potassium chloride replacement, either in elixir or sustained relase form.

Furosemide may be used in 40- to 160-mg doses divided to a twice daily dose of 20 to 80 mg. The problem of potassium wasting is even greater here, but can be controlled. The diuresis may present a practical problem. One secretary lost her job because the furosemide caused her to go to the bathroom too frequently. These drugs may be used for many months to over a year.

Steroids are commonly used and are usually initially effective, but when given for 2 to 6 weeks and discontinued (a regimen commonly advocated), recurrence of papilledema is the rule. The temptation to prolong steroid administration takes the patient into 6- to 12-month bouts of steroid use with all of the attendant complications. I avoid the use of steroids. Their administration adds new problems to patient management, and results are ordinarily no better than using acetazolamide or furosemide. Hair loss, further weight gain, abdominal striae, and acne further detract from the patient's already low self-esteem.

Frequent lumbar punctures are advocated by some, but I have had the most success when the objective of the therapy was headache relief. Repeated lumbar taps frequently are difficult and painful in obese patients and reduce patient compliance. Occasional patients will develop post-lumbar puncture headaches. It is likely that patients who improve with frequent spinal taps do so because of the leak of CSF from the multiple fenestrations in the lumbar theca. These holes may act like an LP shunt.

Surgery

Surgery is considered when the patient is losing vision or has severe, unremitting headaches, unresponsive to medical management. The use of surgery to relieve headache is self-explanatory. However, before surgery is recommended, every effort should be made to relieve headache with standard prophylactic medications such as beta-blockers, calcium channel blockers, and tricyclics. An LP shunt is effective in relieving headache, but is fraught with problems.

An LP shunt is not a recommended technique for relief of CSF pressure in any patient who will subsequently require abdominal surgery, e.g., renal transplantation. The frequency with which LP shunts require revision and their propensity to fail make them treacherous at best. Failure of an LP shunt may precipitate rapid visual failure. LP shunts require careful long-term follow-up, since shunt failure even 5 years after placement may result in abrupt return of papilledema.

Optic nerve sheath fenestration, usually performed by an ophthalmic plastic surgeon, is an effective way of preserving or restoring vision, but is unreliable for the relief of headache. By making a hole in the bulbous anterior dural covering of the optic nerve, the nerve sheath collapses around the nerve. The sheath no longer fills with CSF under pressure, and development of axoplasmic stasis and papilledema is prevented.

When a patient loses visual acuity, develops a visual field defect, or has enlargement of a pre-existing visual field abnormality, surgery should be undertaken immediately — early rather than late. Surgical intervention usually reverses or arrests visual loss.

PROGNOSIS

Visual loss is a feature of about one-half of all patients with pseudotumor cerebri, although serious visual loss is seen in only about 10 to 25 percent. Most patients have a course that lasts 6 to 12 months once the condition is discovered. Recurrence occurs in about 10 percent of patients and may develop from weeks to many years later. Spinal fluid pressure remains elevated in 75 to 80 percent of patients with pseudotumor, even when papilledema is no longer present. Late progression of visual loss without papilledema is very unusual and may be evidence of some other disease progress such as glaucoma.

PARKINSON'S DISEASE

ABRAHAM N. LIEBERMAN, M.D.

Parkinson's disease (PD) is characterized by five main features: rigidity, tremor, bradykinesia, postural instability, and a gait disorder. Other signs may include depression, dementia, postural deformity, speech impairment, and autonomic insufficiency, including dysphagia, sialorrhea, orthostasis, impotence, and constipation.

The pathology of PD is characterized by degeneration of the pigmented neurons in the substantia nigra. The neurons in the substantia nigra synapse with neurons in the caudate nucleus. The nigral neurons synapse with at least two different populations of striatal dopamine receptors. One population of dopamine receptors is linked to the enzyme adenyl cyclase; the other population of dopamine receptors is not linked to adenyl cyclase. There are also dopamine receptors on the axons of the nigral neurons (autoreceptors). Stimulation of these dopamine autoreceptors results in feedback inhibition of dopamine synthesis. The histologic marker of PD is the Lewy body, an eosinophilic inclusion body in the affected neurons of the nigra. The nigral neuronal degeneration and the striatal dopamine loss parallel the disease's severity. As the nigral neurons degenerate, the remaining neurons compensate for the loss by increasing their own activity. In addition, the striatal receptors also compensate for the nigral neuronal loss by becoming more sensitive to dopamine. The first PD symptoms appear when these compensatory mechanisms fail. Compensation fails after 80 percent loss of the nigral neurons and 80 percent loss of the striatal dopamine content.

WHEN TO TREAT

The first decision I make when I see a new patient with PD is whether the patient should be treated. This decision will vary from patient to patient. I question both the patient and the spouse about the patient's symptoms and the impact the symptoms have on the patient's life. I question the patient's spouse because I often find there is a discrepancy between what the patient says and what the spouse says. I question the patient about those activities of daily living that may be affected early in PD. These activities include speaking, salivating, swallowing, writing, feeding, dressing, shaving, turning in bed, and walking. I also ask the patient about the occurrence of tremor, "freezing" spells, or falls. Some patients may have special difficulty with one particular activity. This activity may then serve as a sensitive marker for following the course of treatment in that patient. Thus, one patient may have difficulty in buttoning his collar or shirt sleeves, while another patient may have difficulty in putting on her stockings, and a third patient may have difficulty in cutting meat with a knife. During the course of treatment, I ask the patient about those activities that they were unable to perform before starting treatment. I often find this type of information more valuable than the examination I conduct on the patient in my office.

INITIAL THERAPY

If I have decided that a patient needs treatment, the next decision is which drug to use. This is not a difficult decision because I start all of my patients whose symptoms need treatment on levodopa combined with an extracerebral dopa-decarboxylase inhibitor.

There is much controversy about whether levodopa should be used early in the treatment of PD. This controversy centers on whether the proven benefits of levodopa are commensurate with the possible development of certain adverse effects that may occur with chronic treatment. These adverse effects include dyskinesias, which consist of a combination of dystonia, chorea, and athetosis. The dyskinesias occur in approximately one-third of patients treated with levodopa. The adverse effects also include diurnal oscillations in performance, which consists of " wearing off " phenomena (a gradual loss of the effectiveness of a given dose of levodopa) and the rarer " on-off " phenomena (an abrupt loss of the effectiveness of a given dose of levodopa). Both "wearing off" and " on-off " phenomena may occur in the same patient. Diurnal oscillations in performance may eventually occur in more than one-half of patients treated with levodopa. Because patients with PD treated with other antiparkinson drugs (anticholinergics, amantadine, dopamine agonists) without levodopa do not develop dyskinesias or diurnal oscillations in performance during the course of treatment with these drugs, it is reasonable to assume that the development of dyskinesias and diurnal oscillations in performance are somehow related to levodopa. However, the underlying disease process is as important in the development of dyskinesias and diurnal oscillations in performance as is the administration of levodopa. Thus, when levodopa is given to nonparkinson patients, they do not develop dyskinesias or diurnal oscillations in performance.

Although there is evidence relating the dyskinesias and diurnal oscillations in performance in part to the duration of levodopa treatment, the evidence is not compelling. Indeed, there is now evidence that it is the severity of the disease and not the duration of levodopa treatment that is crucial for the development of these findings. The new evidence comes from the study of patients who develop marked symptoms of PD after injecting themselves with a synthetic street drug, a byproduct of meperidine synthesis, 1-methyl-4-phenyl 1,2,5,6-tetrahydropyridine (MPTP), which is a neurotoxin. These patients respond to levodopa, but shortly after starting treatment they develop dyskinesias and diurnal oscillations in performance. Although there may be a relationship between the development of dyskinesias and diurnal oscillations in performance and the duration of treatment with levodopa, the relationship is not compelling enough to delay treatment with levodopa. The development of these findings must be weighed against the greater antiparkinson effect achieved with levodopa.

My rationale for beginning treatment with levodopa relates to PD's biochemistry. The main problem in PD is the striatal dopamine deficiency. Before symptoms appear, the striatal dopamine content has to be 80 percent depleted. This implies that early clinical disease is already advanced biochemical disease. The association of early clinical disease with advanced biochemical disease has been re-emphasized by recent work with positron emission tomography (PET). From these studies, it appears that the most logical treatment for patients with early PD is to use levodopa and restore the advanced striatal dopamine deficiency. Because the disease is already advanced when the first symptoms appear, little useful time will be gained for the patient by using a drug that is not as effective as levodopa and that may have more adverse effects (mental changes, difficulty urinating, orthostatic hypotension) than levodopa. I use as low a dose of levodopa as is necessary to control the patient's major symptoms. Some neurologists advocate using levodopa in arbitrarily low doses without achieving a satisfactory antiparkinson effect. The studies supporting such low-dose levodopa treatment are not impressive. Thus, in one study in which low-dose levodopa, less than 500 mg per day (combined with carbidopa) was compared with high-dose levodopa treatment, low-dose levodopa resulted in less improvement than high-dose levodopa, but initially was associated with fewer dyskinesias and diurnal oscillations in performance. However, after 6 years both the low-dose and the high-dose levodopa groups had the same number and severity of dyskinesias and diurnal oscillations. Thus,

I use enough levodopa to achieve a satisfactory antiparkinson effect. I do not strive for complete resolution of all symptoms.

Levodopa is combined with an extracerebral dopa-decarboxylase inhibitor. The inhibitor blocks the conversion of levodopa to dopamine outside the brain, thus allowing more levodopa to enter the brain. Because the decarboxylase inhibitor itself does not enter the brain, the inhibitor does not block levodopa's conversion to dopamine inside the brain. There are two decarboxylase inhibitors, carbidopa and benserazide, but only carbidopa is available in the United States. For most patients, between 75 and 200 mg of carbidopa is needed to completely block the conversion of levodopa to dopamine outside the brain. Carbidopa is combined with levodopa (Sinemet) in a ratio of 10 mg of levodopa to 1 mg of carbidopa (10:1) or in a ratio of 4 mg of levodopa to 1 mg of carbidopa (4:1). The 4:1 Sinemet tablet contains the same amount of inhibitor as the 10:1 Sinemet tablet and blocks extracerebral dopa-decarboxylase to the same degree as the 10:1 tablet. However, since the 4:1 tablet contains less levodopa than the 10:1 tablet, the 4:1 tablet delivers a smaller amount of levodopa to the brain. Using the 4:1 tablet, I can determine the minimum amount of levodopa needed to treat the patient's symptoms and spare the patient some of the symptoms of too much levodopa.

I begin treatment with Sinemet 25/100, using one-half a tablet twice a day. I recommend taking Sinemet with meals for the first 3 days so as to minimize nausea, which may occur at this time. After 3 days, I ask the patient to take Sinemet 1 hour before meals. After a week, if the patient is tolerating Sinemet, I increase the dose to one tablet twice a day. After 2 weeks I increase Sinemet to 3 times a day. I see the patient 1 month after starting treatment. If both the patient and I are satisfied, I make no further changes and see the patient in 3 months. I try not to exceed four tablets of Sinemet 25/100 per day. Occasionally, I will substitute up to two Sinemet 25/250 tablets for two of the Sinemet 25/100 tablets.

I tell patients that there are certain foods that may block levodopa's absorption from the gut and its passage from the blood through the capillaries into the brain. These foods contain large amounts of the neutral amino acids phenylalanine, leucine, and isoleucine. These amino acids compete with levodopa for transport through the gut and through the capillaries. This competition is not important early in the course of levodopa treatment. However, the competition between the neutral amino acids and levodopa may be later responsible, in part, for some of the diurnal oscillations in performance. Foods that are high in phenylalanine, leucine, and isoleucine and whose use should be minimized include milk, milk products, lentils, meats, split peas, nuts, and seeds. These dietary restrictions may be difficult to follow. Thus, I will educate patients about their diet, but will only insist they follow it if they are having diurnal oscillations in performance.

Tremor

Patients with tremor as a prominent early symptom may be particularly difficult to treat. In these patients I often combine levodopa with an anticholinergic drug because tremor does not always respond to levodopa alone. The reason for this is that tremor may develop not because of the striatal dopamine deficiency but because of an imbalance between levodopa and acetylcholine. Among patients with tremor, decreasing the activity of striatal acetylcholine with an anticholinergic drug may be more useful than increasing the content of striatal dopamine. The anticholinergic drugs are much less useful than levodopa for treating the symptoms of bradykinesia and the disordered gait. Anticholinergic drugs may also cause dry mouth, blurred vision, mental changes, and urinary difficulty. These side effects are more disturbing than the side effects of levodopa. There are two classes of anticholinergic drugs: (1) the piperidyl derivatives, which include trihexyphenidyl (Artane), biperiden (Akineton), and procyclidine (Kemadrin); and (2) the tropanol derivatives, which include benztropine (Cogentin). A poor response with one class of drugs should not exclude a trial with the other class. Other drugs that may be useful in patients with tremor are the dopamine agonist bromocriptine (Parlodel), the antihistamine orphenadrine (Disipal), the phenothiazine ethopropazine (Parsidol), and occasionally the beta blockers.

Depression

About half of patients with PD are depressed. In some, the depression may be a reaction to their disease, while in others it may be part of the disease, i.e., related to a dopamine deficiency in the mesolimbic cortex. I find that in many depressed patients with PD, treatment with both an antidepressant and levodopa is necessary. I can seldom treat a depressed PD patient with only an antidepressant or only with levodopa. Two antidepressants are especially useful. Nomifensine is an antidepressant that blocks the reuptake of dopamine and also has a mild antiparkinson effect. I begin treatment with 50 mg per day and build up to a maximum of 150 mg per day. Nomifensine does not result in drowsiness. Among patients who are depressed and are also having difficulty sleeping, I use amitriptyline. Patients require between 25 and 75 mg of amitriptyline given as a single bedtime dose. Few patients with PD can tolerate more than 75 mg per day of this drug. In addition to being a sedative, amitriptyline also has anticholinergic activity. Such anticholinergic activity may be desirable in patients with tremor, but may not be desirable in patients with dementia or difficulty urinating.

SUBSEQUENT THERAPY

I use several approaches in patients whose response to levodopa begins to decline, usually 6 months to 1 year after starting the drug. These include increasing the dose of levodopa or changing the ratio of levodopa to carbidopa. However, I have found that the most useful approach is to leave patients on a relatively low dose of levodopa (four tablets per day) and then add the dopamine agonist bromocriptine (Parlodel). Bromocriptine in low doses (less than 30 mg per day) combined with levodopa is effective in patients whose response to levodopa begins to decline. Indeed many neurologists even add bromocriptine to levodopa before the response to levodopa begins to decline. Bromocriptine is begun at a dose of 1.0 to 2.5 mg per day and built up gradually (in increments of 1.0 to 2.5 mg per day each week) to a maximum of 10 to 30 mg per day. It is thought that such combined treatment may prolong the period of the optimal levodopa response, the "levodopa honeymoon." Combination therapy using the two drugs levodopa and bromocriptine, each with a different antiparkinson effect, is, in my opinion, as important in PD as combination therapy is in conditions such as hypertension, infectious diseases, and cancer. Bromocriptine's half-life (3 hours) is longer than the half-life of levodopa (2 hours), and this is why bromocriptine may be effective in patients who are experiencing " wearing off " phenomena on levodopa. Bromocriptine alone, in low doses, 5 to 30 mg per day, is also effective in patients with mild or moderate disease who have never been on levodopa or who cannot tolerate levodopa. However, it takes a longer time for bromocriptine to exert its antiparkinson effect, and eventually the patient will require levodopa as well.

There is debate about the dose of bromocriptine that is needed to treat PD. The debate is unnecessary because the dose of bromocriptine used depends on the patient. In most patients with mild to moderate disease, a good effect (with few adverse reactions) is achieved on a low dose of bromocriptine. Bromocriptine's peak effect occurs within 3 to 6 months of starting treatment. After a year the effect of bromocriptine may decline. The declining efficacy, like that of levodopa, is more pronounced in patients with advanced disease. Such patients then require a higher dose of bromocriptine. In these patients it may also be useful to add amantadine (Symmetrel). Amantadine releases dopamine from nerve terminals and is effective in many patients. However, its benefits are temporary, and some patients develop adverse effects such as confusion, urinary retention, or livedo reticularis.

Drug Holidays

Among those patients whose response to levodopa has greatly declined and who are experiencing dyskinesias and diurnal oscillations in performance the question of a levodopa drug holiday arises. I seldom use levodopa drug holidays because I find that their benefits are not commensurate with their risks. The basis of the levodopa drug holiday is the assumption that chronic levodopa treatment itself may lead to the accumulation of toxins and that these toxins may be responsible, in part, for the declining response, the dyskinesias, and the diurnal oscillations in performance. Some credence is lent to this view by the temporary benefits that may follow the 3- to 14-day period of levodopa withdrawal. Thus, after completion of the levodopa drug holiday, improvement may occur on a lower dose of levodopa than before the drug was stopped. Many patients also have fewer dyskinesias and diurnal oscillations. The improvement after the holiday may last days to months. However, many patients do not respond to the drug holiday, and it must be stressed that this maneuver is not benign. During the drug holiday, the patient's baseline PD state emerges, the state the patient would have been in were it not for levodopa. The patient may become bed-bound, depressed, have difficulty swallowing, and aspirate. Drug holidays should be done only in a hospital.

Poor Response in Advanced Disease

Among patients with advanced PD who are doing poorly despite levodopa and low-dose bromocriptine, I increase the dose of levodopa, the dose of bromocriptine, or use an experimental agonist. The dopamine agonists stimulate the striatal dopamine receptors directly, bypassing the degenerating nigral neurons. These nigral neurons are no longer able to generate enough dopamine to stimulate the striatal receptors directly. Bromocriptine in high doses, between 30 and 50 mg per day, results in clinical improvement and often permits a 10 to 25 percent reduction in the dose of levodopa. This reduction results in fewer dyskinesias.

Two experimental agonists are now undergoing clinical trials. Pergolide is a semisynthetic ergot that is longer acting than bromocriptine. When added to levodopa in patients with advanced disease, pergolide reduces disability. The mean daily dose of pergolide is 2.5 mg (0.2 to 10.0 mg per day). Maximum improvement occurs within 2 months, and improvement begins to decline within 6 months to 1 year. Adverse effects are dyskinesias, mental changes, and orthostatic hypotension.

Lisuride is also a semisynthetic ergot alkaloid. This drug is more potent than bromocriptine, but has a shorter duration of action. Lisuride, like pergolide and bromocriptine, also reduces PD disability. Adverse effects are similar to those of bromocriptine and pergolide.

POSSIBLE FUTURE PREVENTION

PD is thought of as an idiopathic degenerative disorder. However, recent work suggests that PD might result from a neurotoxin. Thus, MPTP caused marked parkinson symptoms in several young drug addicts. All of the patients subsequently responded to levodopa. However, some of them are now showing disease progression. A postmortem examination on one of these patients revealed nigral neuronal loss comparable to, but not identical with, that seen in idiopathic PD.

Subsequent studies with monkeys have shown that MPTP results in destruction of the nigral neurons with loss of striatal dopamine. Pretreatment of the monkeys with a monoamine oxidase (MAO) inhibitor, either pargyline (a nonspecific Type A and Type B inhibitor) or deprenyl (a specific Type B inhibitor) protects the nigral dopamine neurons from the effects of MPTP. Speculation now centers on the possibility that human PD might result from an environmental MPTP-like substance or from an endogenous MPTP-like substance produced in the brain. Identification of such an exogenous or endogenous MPTP-like substance and the prevention of its destructive ability by pretreatment with an MAO inhibitor are two of the more exciting ideas in PD.

ESSENTIAL TREMOR

GEORGE W. PAULSON, M.D.
STEVEN J. HUBER, Ph.D.

Benign tremor, idiopathic tremor, familial tremor, or essential tremor (ET) is a chronic and often slowly progressive neurologic disorder. The typical tremor is absent at rest and becomes noticeable with postural changes or with actions such as eating or writing. The tremor increases in amplitude with stress or anxiety. ET most often affects one or both of the upper limbs, is maximal distally in the hands, but also is often seen in the neck and head. ET is usually less conspicuous in the lower extremities. While the disorder is rarely as disabling as Parkinson's disease (PD), the adjective "benign" can be misleading. The level of disability and the appropriate treatment depend on many factors. For example, even a slight tremor can be totally disabling for an ophthalmologist or an artist, but may be well tolerated by a psychiatrist or a housewife. As in all of medicine, both the disease and the patient's reaction to the disease affect therapy, and the patient's emotional reactions may take more physician time than does the diagnosis. Concerned patients are more likely to be given therapy; all need education.

DIAGNOSIS

Correct therapy for ET is unlikely without a correct diagnosis. Diagnosis of ET can often be uncertain because there are many patients, particularly elderly ones, in whom it is difficult to be sure whether the tremor is largely due to PD, caused by ET, related to both, or whether it reflects some other and more rare process. Some authors have suggested that there is an increased incidence of PD in patients who earlier had ET, and certainly both conditions are common in the later years of life. In addition, there are patients with PD who complain of increased tremor whenever they exert effort or as they become excited, just as there also are elderly individuals with ET who develop striking extrapyramidal features of aging. There may be, of course, an unexplained biochemical predisposition for PD to develop in patients who already have ET. It has been suggested that patients with ET are taller and healthier than siblings or the population at large and are remarkably vigorous and long-lived. This opinion may only reflect the fact that tremor increases with age; therefore, older patients are likely to shake more, and the sample is biased toward longevity. Even if patients with ET are no healthier than the unaffected population, the possibility of vigor and long life may comfort the patient who feels heavily burdened by ET and who is often fearful of PD.

The main reason to emphasize the characteristics of ET is that therapies that are useful for PD rarely help ET. Many clinical differences exist between PD and ET, including the high incidence of a positive family history, present in perhaps 40 percent of patients with ET. ET is probably transmitted as an autosomal dominant trait with remarkably varied penetrance. One family member develops the disease in youth, whereas another displays no tremor until advanced age. In rare instances, the tremor may be present in youth, improve, and then worsen again in later decades. Tremor in PD is classically present at rest, but can be present during exertion. Parkinsonian tremor is often slower and may shift rhythmically from one muscle group to another: wrist, arm, finger, etc. ET is more prominent with effort and action or with postural changes. The more severe cases are associated with a larger amplitude of tremor, and when patients say they are worse, they mean amplitude rather than frequency. Tremor in ET, although usually faster than in PD, may vary more from patient to patient than is true of PD. Another characteristic difference between ET and PD is that tremor is more likely to be seen in the head and heard in the voice in ET. Patients with PD often do have tremor of the protruded tongue or of the chin, but rarely as much in the voice, head, and neck as in patients with ET. More significant for the distinction between ET and PD, ET is traditionally *not* associated with significant akinesia, truncal rigidity, hypomimia in facial expression, or any overall decline in mental function.

There are subvariants of ET such as writing tremor, position tremor, or senile tremor, but for the purposes of this chapter all these are considered the same as ET. ET is not always benign, is usually embarrassing, and occasionally does lead to major disability, particularly for skilled motor performance. Furthermore, it should be recognized that a similar tremor may be seen with other conditions such as dystonia, cerebellar disease, torticollis, or multiple sclerosis, but tremor in these conditions usually responds poorly to therapy aimed at ET.

THERAPY

Alcohol

One of the oldest therapeutic regimens is the use of small amounts of alcohol. This has been successfully employed by cautious patients for many years, often just prior to a special occasion, e.g., before a social event in which eating soup would be hazardous to clothes, tranquility, and neighbors at the table. Some patients notice remarkable improvement in the tremor a few minutes after even part of one glass of wine or following one can of beer. The frequency of the tremor in ET, usually faster than that of PD, is very similar to the tremor seen in withdrawal states, e.g., in patients with "the shakes" after a binge with alcohol or following a barbiturate overdose. This fact has not elucidated the cause for either withdrawal tremor or ET, although it is tantalizing to assume that measures that truly assist patients with ET might also assist those who are in a phase of severe withdrawal tremor and agitation. Despite temporary benefit by alcohol for patients with ET, the amplitude of the tremor may be worse the day after excessive alcohol intake. Perhaps because alcohol is so seductive for all, or perhaps because receptors are different in people with ET, or perhaps simply because alcohol briefly is effective in patients with ET, it has been suggested that the use of alcohol by patients with ET predisposes these patients to significant alcoholism. We feel this threat is no more true for the patient with ET than for anyone else in the population who drinks, particularly after patients with ET discover that withdrawal from alcohol actually leads to accentuation of tremor. By transient accentuation we mean, of course, increased amplitude, not necessarily a change in location or frequency of the tremor. As mentioned earlier, there are occasional patients who, despite real or theoretical hazards, find alcohol useful to reduce the tremor during social occasions.

Sedatives

For decades sedatives of all types have been usefully employed for patients with ET, including in particular varieties of barbiturates. There is no evidence that any one compound is better than phenobarbital, and if patients are not unduly disturbed by the sedative effect, phenobarbital at 30 mg twice a day can be valuable. Benzodiazepines, particularly diazepam, have been utilized from about 1970 on, but probably are best used as intermittent or adjunctive therapy, e.g., in patients who display a marked increase in tremor at times of stress or excitement. We have used alprazolam at 0.5 mg 3 times a day in more than 25 patients, and it also has a moderately useful effect, generally apparent within 1 hour after the drug is taken. If patients tolerate these agents well, they should be employed just prior to the time when the tremor is anticipated or when apprehension will be greatest.

Propranolol

The most useful and accepted single drug for ET is probably propranolol. There are now dozens of reports that indicate relief of ET by use of this beta-adrenergic agent. The effective dose, as reported, varies widely, but many patients require larger doses. We prefer to start at a lower level, perhaps 30 to 60 mg per day and then cautiously raise the level to as high as 320 mg per day in divided doses, depending on the results. It is unlikely that higher doses add much additional benefit, but a few clinicians have felt otherwise. The use of propranolol, particularly in very high doses, requires that the drug not be abruptly stopped, since sudden changes may accentuate any tendency toward cardiac irregularities and could cause cardiac arrest. The long-acting slow-release form of propranolol (Inderal LA) may be the best approach. There is great variability in response in different patients. Other forms of medications also used in cardiac or vascular disorders, such as atenolol, are sometimes effective in ET, but are probably not superior to propranolol. As with propranolol, these drugs must be used more cautiously in the elderly. So far, the fact that medications that affect the catecholamine systems can influence ET has not explained the pathophysiology of ET.

Anticholinergics

Although anticholinergics such as trihexyphenidyl (Artane) can be quite useful for PD, they are not usually effective for ET. In fact, according to some, the levodopa that is so successful for parkinsonism, may even accentuate ET. There are, however, scattered reports suggesting that anticholinergics, levodopa, or amantadine help individual patients. In any condition for which there is no definitive therapy and in which psychological factors are major contributors, there is certain to be a scattering of enthusiastic case reports with variable credibility. The effectiveness of anticholinergics for most patients with ET is usually not striking—if beneficial at all—and there is no indication for steadily increasing the doses of anticholinergics, as is now commonly done to treat childhood dystonia.

Primidone

Recently, primidone has been found to be effective at a level of up to as high as 1000 mg per day. It is suggested by some researchers who studied this drug in controlled trials that primidone is as useful as is propranolol and definitely more useful than barbiturates alone. It has also been suggested that the effectiveness of primidone is not due to barbiturates but to derived compounds such as phenylethylmalonamide. A percentage of primidone is converted into barbiturates, but there is more than just an isolated barbiturate effect at work when primidone is used. Much clinical work needs to be done utilizing varied metabolites of the compounds that are potentially useful in ET. Primidone can be used jointly with propranolol, if required.

When primidone is used, it must be given cautiously, employing a very slow increase in dosage, and it may take several months to approach 1000 mg per day. Administration of 250 mg at bedtime may be as effective as high doses. Even patients with seizures often have poor initial tolerance for primidone, and those with ET are at least as vulnerable to the sedative and emotional lability that are side effects of this drug. Some patients are totally unable to tolerate the drug owing to extreme lethargy, confusion, ataxia, and slurred speech. With time, most of these side effects generally dissipate, and with slow administration most patients can tolerate primidone.

Surgery

Stereotactic surgery can relieve ET and has been presented as a "cure." In most cases, the destructive lesions are made in the ventral lateral nucleus of the thalamus and utilize a procedure similar to that traditionally done in patients with PD. Earlier literature suggested that the success rate was as high as 80 percent, but potential complications of surgery were numerous, including difficulty with gait, speech, and motor power. Surgical procedures should be reserved for exceptionally severe cases and then done only by surgeons who are both skillful and experienced.

Supportive Treatment

There are several approaches in addition to medication or surgery. Some (perhaps most) patients simply learn to tolerate the tremor. For some it is important to internalize the concept that tremor does not imply "nervousness" or psychological weakness. It may be necessary to explain to family members what the shaking seems to mean and that tremor can affect a person's body image. Some patients still feel "shaking inside" even if medication is overtly useful and tremor greatly dissipated. Detailed work-up, with the exception of thyroid tests, is rarely of value, but certainly more than one visit may be required to educate the patient in how to live with the handicap. Some effective medications, such as primidone and propranolol, may cause sufficient side effects that a follow-up visit is desirable.

Counseling should be done with empathy and skill and with particular awareness of occupational and cosmetic considerations. There are features in life-style that are important for the individual with ET. Internal and external tranquility is, of course, desirable, but even without becoming phlegmatic the patient can obtain understanding of potential sources of stress. The tremor may be worse in the morning, and patients may modify their behavior accordingly. Tremors can be accentuated by caffeine in all its myriad forms, and some choose to abstain from coffee or cola beverages. There are patients who are able to force a diminution of the tremor by will, as when sewing or writing. More patients seem to learn to work "around or through" the tremor rather than to harness it. A few note that certain hand postures, such as the vertical position, accentuate tremor, and they thus avoid these postures. Some patients feel more in control the day after physical exertion.

Selection of occupational and recreational activities should include awareness that ET may worsen as the individual ages. Empathy, education, and symptomatic management are more likely to be helpful than prolonged or intensive psychotherapy, which fortunately is rarely required for patients with ET. There are no data to suggest that biofeedback or physical therapy is of great value.

GENERAL APPROACH TO THERAPY

The therapist must remember the patient, not the tremor. The obtainable goal may not be total elimination of tremor, but enough reduction in amplitude to soften the burden. Optimal doses of all medications, including propranolol, may vary from patient to patient. Older patients may be less responsive to this drug. All the therapies have side effects, some of which may be more troublesome for the elderly. Management can include both a chronically administered agent and short-acting or temporary therapy such as diazepam or alprazolam. Sedatives, including phenobarbital, which has a long half-life (72 hours), can also be administered intermittently.

At this time we prefer propranolol, which helps over 50 percent of patients, but cures none. Primidone is a reasonable second-line drug, to be added slowly. We employ diazepam or alprazolam in some patients, often when emotional tension is particularly obvious. These agents can be used as primary or adjunctive medications. Alprazolam may be helpful for patients who seek intermittent relief, such as during work hours, but who are not sufficiently bothered by tremor at other times to require medication. We do not recommend surgery.

Patients with this common disorder deserve more effective and newer treatments and increased attention by therapists. The disorder is as common as PD, and research may lead to exciting advances that may be useful even beyond the rather broad confines of ET.

NORMAL PRESSURE HYDROCEPHALUS

HAMILTON MOSES III, M.D.

The diagnosis of normal pressure hydrocephalus (NPH) is a conundrum; decisions about appropriate therapy are vexing. Although it is clear that many patients who present with the constellation of gait disturbance, dementia, and incontinence benefit from measures to relieve increased intracranial pressure, predicting which patients will improve is an art, not a science. Likewise, because morbidity caused by the currently available surgical procedures is substantial, treatment of NPH has a narrow therapeutic index.

CLINICAL PRESENTATIONS

Patients rarely present with all aspects of the clinical triad being equally evident. Unfortunately, those who do have all three features usually have passed the time when therapy would have been most beneficial.

History

Patients and their families describe difficulty with walking, balance, athletics, or coordination, and many describe stiffness in the legs. The usual symptoms of dementia may have been recognized, but a general slowness of thinking is particularly characteristic. Frank incontinence is an unusual symptom initially; nocturia, urgency, frequency, and dribbling with stress are usual and often have been misattributed to prostatism or bladder prolapse. Although some patients do have a history of repeated head trauma (boxing, football), subarachnoid hemorrhage, meningeal inflammation, etc., most patients have had no such occurrences. Those who do usually present at an earlier age, e.g., the forties or fifties, whereas patients with idiopathic NPH present in the sixties or seventies and may have a better prognosis. The sequence of symptoms is especially important in predicting outcome, as it is generally held that those who have prominent gait disturbance and bladder symptoms early, with dementia later, respond more predictably to shunting, whereas those who have early dementia rarely improve. I concur with this view.

Physical Findings

The patient with the gait disturbance of NPH walks with small, short steps, as if his feet are stuck to the ground. Foot placement is defective, which may be tested by rapid tapping of the toe and heel alternately. Peculiarly, this feature is evident when the patient is standing, but rarely so when he is seated. He also demonstrates compass turning (pivoting around a planted foot). In addition to these apractic features, spasticity of the legs is often present and becomes more prominent as the disease progresses, eventually with upgoing toes. When pyramidal features are prominent, the differential diagnosis becomes more difficult, and exclusion of cervical spondylosis, other cord lesions, the lacunar state, etc., is imperative.

The dementia of NPH is evidenced by general slowing of cognition, impairment of memory, and often by a great degree of variability from day to day. It cannot be easily distinguished from senile dementia of Alzheimer's type on clinical grounds, although patients with NPH rarely have the focal signs that are so characteristic of Alzheimer's disease, e.g., aphasia or agnosia. Hakim and Adams recognized two additional features: hypersomnolence (thought to be due to enlargement of the third ventricle) and nystagmus (due to enlargement of the fourth ventricle). I have been struck by mild parkinsonian features, especially microphagia, cogwheel rigidity of the legs, and occasionally tremor.

PATHOPHYSIOLOGY

Intracranial pressure (ICP) is most probably truly "normal" only in later phases of the illness. It is generally assumed that ICP is intermittently elevated in early phases of the illness, often nocturnally coincident with rapid eye movement (REM) sleep, when plateau waves can be measured. During this phase of intermittently increased ICP, progressive enlargement of the ventricles occurs, followed by cortical loss, leading (according to Pascal's law) to "normal" pressure eventually. Although this progression has never been proved unambiguously, it explains the clinical features of the condition, the importance of early treatment, and the likelihood of failure with late treatment. The underlying defect leading to these changes in pressure and volume has never been discerned. Impaired absorption of cerebrospinal fluid (CSF), overproduction of CSF, altered permeability of the periventricular parenchyma, and altered cerebral venous pressure have all been implicated, and each may apply in certain circumstances. The first of these theories is generally held to be most important, however.

DIAGNOSTIC INTERVENTIONS

I use all of the diagnostic tools presently reviewed in patients with the characteristic clinical syndrome. As the number of positive studies increases, the likelihood of improvement with therapy likewise increases.

Computed Tomography (CT). Ventricular enlargement (especially lateral and third ventricle) without concomitant cortical atrophy is the hallmark, although interpretation of the latter is often difficult. Atrophy is not uniformly a poor prognostic sign, although prominent frontal and perisylvian atrophy generally is. I have not found the various measurements of mantle thickness or ventricular volume to be of prognostic value. Periventricular edema is usually evident in CTs of high quality, especially in the early intermittent high-pressure phase of the illness.

Magnetic Resonance Imaging (MRI). Periventricular edema is usually very obvious, without other evidence of involvement of white matter. MRI distinguishes NPH from Binswanger's disease, a condition that may present in a very similar fashion, although usually less insidiously, and may be more common than has generally been recognized.

Radioisotope Cisternography. Cisternography demonstrates ventricular entry of isotope, stasis within the ventricles for more than 24 hours, retarded uptake over the convexities, and delay in disappearance of total isotope from the intracranial cavity. However, these features (especially ventricular entry and stasis) may be seen in up to one-half of patients with Alzheimer's disease. Therefore, we do not feel that cisternography should be heavily weighed in isolation when recommending surgery.

Psychometric Testing. Detailed testing generally confirms the clinical suspicion of a mild generalized dementia without focal features. In confirmation of the impression of generalized psychomotor slowing, cognitive tests that are not scored by performance time may reveal surprisingly normal mental acuity. This pattern is particularly helpful, as those patients may greatly improve with therapy.

Cystometrography. Bladder spasticity is usually evident, although obstruction may also be found at the time of urologic evaluation. Post-void residuals are rarely impressive, however, unless spasticity is marked. Frequency with small volumes is most characteristic.

Monitoring of Intracranial Pressure. Direct measurement of ICP via a subarachnoid bolt is a safe and valuable procedure when applied by an experienced team using standardized techniques. Morbidity of the procedure should be less than 0.5 percent in experienced hands. Testing is performed over a 2- to 3-day session in an intensive care unit. Monitoring of the electroencephalogram (EEG) is a useful adjunct, although surface eletromyography (EMG) of the eyelid may suffice. Patients in the early stages of the illness show intermittent bursts of raised

ICP lasting from 1 to 10 minutes, frequently only in the early morning hours. Although they may occur during the time of REM sleep, this is not uniform. Baseline pressures are not usually increased, but they may be unusually sensitive to postural changes, falling disproportionately with change to the upright position. Analysis of the waveform of the intravascular pulse as it is transmitted to the CSF has been advocated by some, although I have not found it of value. Determination of intracranial compliance (by measurement of pressure before and after an injection of a small amount of artificial CSF) has likewise been advocated, but I find the test technically difficult to perform and its results difficult to interpret. Therefore, I do not use it.

Therapeutic Lumbar Puncture. Routine CSF studies (protein, cell count, VDRL, etc.) should be performed at the time of cisternography. Routine lumbar puncture is rarely of diagnostic value. However, many patients improve following even a single diagnostic lumbar puncture, presumably as a result of removal of a small amount of CSF or subsequent leakage. Gait is especially likely to improve immediately. When this occurs, it is highly predictive of therapeutic success of a shunt procedure. I perform three sequential lumbar punctures at an interval of every day or every other day during an inpatient hospital stay. The time required to walk 30 feet, tap the foot 20 times, and perform a set series of mental tasks is sequentially followed. Patients who develop symptoms of low pressure (postural headache, nausea, or dizziness) are more likely to note improvement in gait and to benefit from shunting. Therapeutic lumbar punctures should not be performed before measurement of ICP, as punctures adversely bias pressure measurements. An interval of at least 1 week after cisternography or lumbar puncture should pass before measurement of ICP occurs. Unfortunately, repeated lumbar puncture is relatively contraindicated in those patients who may undergo lumbar-peritoneal shunting procedures and, as the lumbar shunt may be preferable to ventricular shunting, I now reserve sequential lumbar punctures for those patients who have ambiguous cisternography or ICP measurements.

OUTCOME

Procedures to divert CSF outflow will be most successful if performed during the stage of intermittently increased ICP. Patients with prominent gait disturbance, with or without urinary symptoms, and with mild dementia are most likely to improve, especially if the characteristic psychometric findings, CT appearance, cisternography, and increased ICP have been found (see Table 1). In this group, improvement following surgery occurs in about three-quarters of patients, although unfortunately at a price of a 10 to 30 percent surgical morbidity. Improvement may indeed be striking, with the patient virtually coming out of the anesthetic with remarkable improvement in the speed of his thinking, the ability of his memory, and the facility of his feet. While immediate improvement is the rule, some patients require considerably longer to improve, especially in the mental sphere, where improvement over several months is reliably observed. I counsel that 6 months should elapse before reaching a verdict on whether improvement has or has not occurred.

Some patients have substantial initial improvement, but deteriorate later, usually several months after shunt placement. Late subdural hematomas, infections of the shunt with an indolent organism (*Staphylococcus epidermidis*), or shunt malfunction due to obstruction in either the central or the terminal end should all be considered and properly evaluated in patients with late deterioration. Unfortunately, however, a large number of patients have late deterioration without evidence of a proven cause. Some of these patients are aided by replacement of the high-pressure valve with a lower-pressure valve, although this is often not of convincing benefit. Sometimes late deterioration occurs in the cognitive and memory sphere, while improvement in gait may be sustained. This group of patients is a particularly vexing one, and the changes most probably occur owing to secondary changes in the cortex, as reflected in the progressively slowed EEG that is often seen.

I advocate open discussion and counseling of the patient about the rationale for therapy. If the patient is significantly demented, it is imperative that a member of the family also be made aware of the diagnosis, rationale for therapy, risk, and likely therapeutic response. I openly discuss with the patient and the family the 50 to 75 percent likelihood of success, which must be balanced against the 10 to 30 percent risk of morbidity. This has proved to be an extremely beneficial and well-received technique for counseling. It prepares everyone concerned for the long-term observation that is required and the likely complications of shunts and discourages expectations of a magical and immediate solution to an illness that may not improve.

TABLE 1 Clinical Predictors of Prognosis in NPH

Favorable	*Unfavorable*
Symptoms of short duration	Atrophy by CT
Young age	Early dementia
Predisposing conditions (subarachnoid hemorrhage, trauma, infection)	Long duration of symptoms (> 3 years)
Early gait disturbance	Generalized dementia without disproportionate psychomotor slowing
Early incontinence	Apraxia other than gait, aphasia
Variability of symptoms day to day	
Improvement after lumbar puncture	
Spasticity in legs	
Periventricular edema	
Demonstrably raised ICP	

THERAPY

Surgical. Shunts are of three types: ventricular-atrial, ventricular-peritoneal, and lumbar-peritoneal. A variety of shunt tubes are available, and a number of valves with several different pressure and flow characteristics have been advocated to minimize morbidity, especially from subdural hematoma. Surgical fashion has changed over the past two decades, with ventricular procedures used initially, followed by lumbar procedures in the early and mid-1970s, with ventricular procedures replacing these, although the lumbar procedures have again become more fashionable. Ventricular-atrial shunts with high-pressure valves have been preferred by most surgeons for technical ease, despite the somewhat greater incidence of shunt failure due to obstruction of the atrial end. Ventricular-peritoneal shunts are less likely to become obstructed at the peritoneal end, but they are slightly more difficult to insert or change. Lumbar-peritoneal shunts are also prone to obstruction and are somewhat more difficult to insert, especially in older patients with spondylosis. Advocates point out, however, that the risk of subdural hematoma may be less with lumbar shunts. It has been our practice to use ventricular-atrial shunts because of the ease of insertion. Placement can be done under local anesthesia, thereby avoiding the additional risk of a general anesthetic. An anticonvulsant (usually phenytoin) is given for the first 3 months after placement of a ventricular shunt; I discontinue it thereafter if no seizures have occurred.

Risks of surgery occur with relatively predictable frequency. Ranges from the largest published series include: subdural hematoma, 5 to 40 percent; acute infection, 5 to 20 percent; late infection, 2 to 5 percent; seizures, 3 to 5 percent; and chronic low pressure symptoms, 5 to 10 percent. The aggregate risk is in the range of 20 to 30 percent for all patients. Unfortunately, meticulous surgical technique cannot avoid the production of subdural hematoma, which is the greatest cause of postoperative morbidity. Even if substantial cortical atrophy has not occurred, the patient who is most likely to benefit from a shunt is also the one in whom subdural hematoma is most likely to occur. Undoubtedly the mechanism is a combination of "settling" of the brain causing stretching of the subdural veins. To minimize the risk of subdural hematoma, I raise the head of the bed in small increments over 5 days, mobilize the patient slowly thereafter, proscribe strenuous physical activity (especially bending or straining), counsel against airplane flights and diving, and, of course, restrict activities that are likely to result in direct blows to the head. Routine CT scans to follow ventricular size and to guard against the appearance of asymptomatic subdural hematomas should be performed at the time of hospital discharge, at monthly intervals for the first 3 months, at 6-month intervals thereafter, or at any time that clinical deterioration is observed.

Medical Therapy. Furosemide (Lasix) and acetazolamide (Diamox) have been advocated for normal pressure hydrocephalus, although there was no convincing evidence of their efficacy. This medical regimen may well be of value in both childhood obstructive and nonobstructive hydrocephalus. I have tried it in adult hydrocephalus without therapeutic effect.

Rehabilitation. The gait disturbance of NPH rarely improves with gait training, probably because of the striking difficulty with foot placement. Canes, walkers, or other devices rarely help, and the provision of additional visual cues is similarly rarely helpful. A conscious strategy for walking (left-right, one-two) has been advocated, but is rarely helpful in NPH, in contrast to Parkinson's disease in which it is often useful.

Urinary Precautions. Prophylaxis of infections with urinary antisepsis and intermittent catheterization may be required even after clinical improvement following shunting or if no improvement has ensued. This is especially needed, since urinary features may not improve as much as other manifestations of the condition following therapy. Prophylactic measures may need to be continued indefinitely.

ALZHEIMER'S DISEASE

MAREK-MARSEL MESULAM, M.D.
SANDRA WEINTRAUB, Ph.D.
LISSA KAPUST, M.S.W.

Alzheimer's disease is a relentlessly progressive, eventually terminal, and relatively common condition of unknown cause that has not yet lent itself to effective treatment or prevention. Although it can occur at any time during adulthood, its prevalence increases with age. In sharp contrast to the practices of the recent past, there is now a tendency for Alzheimer's disease to be overdiagnosed. There are no pathognomonic clinical or laboratory signs and even brain biopsy can be quite misleading. Definitive diagnosis can be established only through careful microscopic examination of the brain following an autopsy. The presumptive clinical diagnosis of Alzheimer's disease is reached by excluding other dementing diseases. Many clinicians make this diagnosis whenever dementia (without major sensory-motor deficits) is seen in association with negative results in a series of laboratory tests. While some of the alternative diagnostic entities (e.g., hydrocephalus, hypothyroidism) are associated with specific laboratory findings, others (e.g., depression, amyloid angiopathy, Pick's disease) are not. Since conditions that belong to the latter group cannot be excluded in any definitive fashion by commonly available laboratory tests, the diagnosis of Alzheimer's disease during the patient's lifetime always carries a degree of uncertainty. This is an important consideration, since it influences what the patient and the family are told and also encourages flexibility for midcourse alterations in management and further diagnostic investigations.

Although there is no definitive treatment, patients with the presumptive diagnosis of Alzheimer's disease require long-term management. These patients and their families have special needs that range from legal advice to psychiatric support, cognitive training, and the pharmacologic treatment of aberrant or obstreperous behaviors. A multidisciplinary team comprised of neurologists, neuropsychologists, psychiatrists, and social workers is usually necessary for addressing these needs.

NEUROPSYCHOLOGICAL ASSESSMENT

The salient feature of Alzheimer's disease is an alteration in mental state. The formal neurologic examination of cranial nerves and sensory-motor function is usually normal until the very advanced stages. Therefore, a proper evaluation of severity and temporal course can be achieved only by careful neuropsychological evaluation. There are standardized tests that take from 10 to 45 minutes to administer and offer a composite score of severity. The most commonly used are the Mini-Mental State Test, the Blessed Scale, and the Mattis Dementia Rating Scale. These are useful for monitoring change over time, but they are broad screening measures and may lack sensitivity, particularly in the early stages of the disease.

More extensive neuropsychological evaluation is often desirable in the early stages in order to differentiate the effects of aging from the presence of a dementing disease. This may be especially relevant in patients with high premorbid levels of achievement or education in whom subtle alterations may escape detection on broad screening tests of mental state. Sometimes even a very careful initial examination is not sufficient to make this distinction. In those instances, repeat examinations at 6-month intervals are the most helpful. If relatively modest deficits remain static over a year or more, the likelihood of a progressive disease such as Alzheimer's dementia is reduced. Detailed neuropsychological examination also gives a more precise indication of the patient's major cognitive weaknesses and of those areas that are relatively preserved. This contributes to the formulation of management strategies.

The patient comes to medical attention for dementia not because of difficulties in drawing a cube or memorizing a word list, but because of difficulties in daily living activities such as driving, keeping a checkbook, and maintaining hygiene. Therefore, these activities also need to be assessed quantitatively in parallel to the neuropsychological evaluation. Quantitative questionnaires of activities of daily living, some of which can be completed by family members, are available. Sometimes even this is not sufficient to provide a clear picture of the behavioral difficulties experienced by the patient. In those instances, we have found it useful to assess selected daily living activities in the patient's own home. Such behavioral observations assist in the management of the patient and also provide additional information for differential diagnosis, especially in differentiating psychiatric from neurologic disease.

WHAT TO TELL THE PATIENT AND THE FAMILY

Because of the publicity that Alzheimer's disease has recently attracted, many families and sometimes even patients will directly ask if what they have is Alzheimer's disease. Since the physician can only reach a tentative diagnosis of this incurable disease of unknown cause, communicating with the family is a delicate matter. While the patient and family require a realistic understanding of the diagnosis in order to plan for the future, individual differences need to be considered. Some families are relieved to learn that there is a neurologic rather than a psychiatric explanation for the troubling behavioral alterations. Others may be thrown into emotional crisis. In most instances, it is desirable to meet with the family alone, both in taking the history and in discussing the findings of the examination. This provides the family with the opportunity to candidly discuss their observations and concerns.

When a presumptive diagnosis of Alzheimer's disease has been reached, we usually tell patients that the examination does show difficulties with language, memory, and other areas of mental state beyond those changes that we might expect as a normal consequence of aging. If the work-up has been completed at the time, we state that no treatable cause has been discovered and that there are no specific medications that we can recommend to improve memory or language. We also point out that the extent of impairment and rate of progression cannot be predicted and that it is therefore desirable to have follow-up assessments at approximately 6-month intervals. To the family, we will emphasize that while some patients may show a precipitous progression, others with mild deficits may remain essentially unchanged for many years. We will also point out that Alzheimer's disease is only one of several possibilities. Although more definitive diagnosis can be reached by brain biopsy, we emphasize that this is rarely justified. If questioned about the remaining diagnostic possibilities, we will explain that their implications are not very different from those of Alzheimer's disease. If questioned about cause, we will admit the absence of definite information about etiology and explain that certain parts of the brain seem to be aging too rapidly. We also add that we keep abreast of developments in the field and that we will contact the patient if new treatment strategies become available.

The question of heredity is often raised. In rare instances, Alzheimer's disease is transmitted as an autosomal dominant trait. More often, there is no definite evidence for Mendelian inheritance as a dominant or recessive trait even though some investigators have made such suggestions. Since the incidence of Alzheimer's disease increases with age, many individuals will have a positive history of late-life dementia in a parent or a grandparent. This does not necessarily mean that they have a familial type of Alzheimer's disease. This explanation can allay unnecessary apprehension. The physician can also direct families to one of several publications that address educational needs and questions of practical management.

BEHAVIORAL-COGNITIVE STRATEGIES

Few environmental or cognitive manipulations are effective in improving the functional level of patients with late-stage Alzheimer's disease. However, in earlier stages some intervention is possible. For patients who have a memory disturbance (and especially if this is primarily at the level of retrieval), clearly marked calendars and lists or notes may be useful. For patients who have trouble retrieving facts concerning numbers, a calculator may help to balance checkbooks. Marking emergency telephone numbers clearly and specifically labeling hot and cold water faucets and "on" and "off" dials on the stove may provide assistance. Switching to a digital clock with large numbers and leaving a light on in the bedroom and in the bathroom may facilitate temporal and spatial orientation, especially at night.

DRIVING

The ability to drive is critical for many patients' independence. In early stages of dementia, the patient may be quite resistant to relinquish driving. Moreover, the spouse may not be able to drive, so that limiting the patient's access to a car may jeopardize the mobility of the entire household. Family members often request that the physician impose this restriction, thus exonerating themselves from the difficult task of depriving the patient in a critical area. Decisions about driving require a great deal of judicious consideration. In early stages, if the problem is limited to memory and language and if the patient has reasonably preserved reflexes, then driving to familiar places need not be curtailed. However, when judgment begins to falter and when mental reflexes are no longer reliable, the physician must take a strong stand against continued driving.

INCONTINENCE

Strategies used for other causes of incontinence (e.g., multiple sclerosis or spinal cord diseases) are rarely effective in Alzheimer's disease. The approach to this type of incontinence is merely practical. The urine has to be monitored frequently for infection, since this would increase incontinence. The intake of liquids, especially coffee and caffeine-containing sodas, should be limited in the evenings. The patient should be taken to the bathroom at regular intervals. Adult diapers at bedtime help to contain the wetness. Incontinence is a major emotional issue for caregivers and often is the impetus for initiating nursing home placement.

LEGAL ISSUES

As the dementia progresses, the stage is reached where appropriate financial decisions can no longer be made by the patient. Allowing the patient control of finances may jeopardize the welfare of spouse and children. In these circumstances, the physician must raise the issue of mental competence and suggest that power of attorney be assumed by another family member.

Sometimes, patients with early dementia may continue to maintain responsible positions in business, medicine, or government. In these instances, gentle persuasion and, if necessary, a firmer attitude must be taken to encourage early retirement or a major shift in the pattern of authority and responsibility.

ABERRANT BEHAVIOR AND MEDICATIONS

In addition to a decline in mental abilities, patients with dementia also display a number of aberrant behaviors that complicate management. Some patients have delusions, hallucinations, and paranoid ideas of reference. Some have an incessant outpouring of speech that cannot be stopped and keep repeating the same story or the same question. Others hoard items ranging from money to food in the most inaccessible or unpredictable places. Still others keep wandering out of the house and are brought back by the police.

Some of these behaviors respond to pharmacologic treatment. We begin by using oxazepam (start at 10 mg once a day and increase to 10 mg four times a day over 2 to 3 weeks). If this does not work, then neuroleptic agents (haloperidol or thiothixene) may become necessary. Since patients are exquisitely sensitive to these medications, dosages have to be increased very gradually. Usually results are obtained at doses that are lower than the customary effective dose. Although neuroleptics can decrease some driven and psychotic behaviors, they can also increase the likelihood of falls and incontinence. Parkinsonian symptoms and dyskinesias are common nueroleptic side effects in this group. In some patients, the cognitive deficits are worsened by introducing these medications.

Occasionally, dementia occurs together with severe depression. In those instances, antidepressants may be useful. In such patients the antidepressants will alleviate the depression, but not the dementia. In fact, sometimes treating the depression will give rise to increased aberrant behaviors. Antidepressants with the least amount of anticholinergic activity(e.g., desipramine or trazodone) are advisable. Ergot derivatives (e.g., ergoloid mesylates [Hydergine]), vasodilators (e.g., cyclandelate), and analeptics (e.g., methylphenidate) may provide partial benefit for the occasional patient. However, there is no consistent evidence that these substances are effective in treating Alzheimer's disease. Cholinergic agonists such as lecithin and physostigmine are being investigated for treating memory disturbances. However, most of the relevant studies show no lasting beneficial effect.

BECLOUDED DEMENTIA

Patients with dementia are particularly sensitive to toxic-metabolic encephalopathies. An upper respiratory tract infection, a moderately elevated temperature, a slightly excessive blood level of a medication, or a mild head injury may give rise to a severe exacerbation of the symptoms in the form of a beclouded dementia. When such a clinical turn of events occurs, the physician should not automatically attribute it to a worsening in the natural course of the disease. In fact, a relatively abrupt exacerbation should always raise the possibility of an added toxic or metabolic insult and should lead to the appropriate work-up. Treatment of the superimposed toxic-metabolic condition can re-establish the baseline condition even though there may be considerable delay between improvement and the removal of the contributing factor.

FAMILY SUPPORT NEEDS, COMMUNITY RESOURCES, AND NURSING HOME PLACEMENT

Spouses, adult children, and other caretakers of patients with dementia bear formidable burdens. In later stages, they have to provide round-the-clock assistance for even the most rudimentary daily living activities. They have to manage aberrant behaviors such as leaving the stove on, wandering out of the house, and incontinence. The patient's behavior may be interpreted as a deliberate attempt at retaliation or a display of hostility. Roles become reversed. For example, a wife who has been shielded by her husband from all practical and financial responsibilities may have to act as the head of the family. A husband who has relied on his wife for managing the home may be unprepared for such chores as laundry and meal preparation. Adult children assume parental roles for their aging parents. Parenting one's parents often leads to anxiety, guilt, resentment, and sadness. The stress of caring for a family member with dementia sometimes leads to physical abuse, a condition that is rarely spontaneously reported to the physician but that needs to be specifically inquired about at regular intervals.

Caretakers of patients with dementia are a vulnerable population. While they themselves are not identified as primary patients, the physician should consider them potentially "hidden patients." The most common problem within this group is depression. Stress-related medical problems (e.g., headache, hypertension, gastric disorders) frequently appear or are exacerbated in this group. The problems are further compounded by a tendency to neglect or postpone their own health care needs until a crisis arises.

The expertise of a clinical social worker can be called upon to help families deal with emotional adjustment, plan for the patient's current and future care, and identify resources that can contribute to keeping the patient in the community. These include adult day health programs, homemaker services, hot meal programs, and respite care. When care at home is no longer feasible, the social worker can assist the family in the complex and emotionally demanding task of nursing home placement. Families appreciate the active involvement of the physician at this point to sanction their decision at this difficult crossroad.

Support groups organized by the Alzheimer's Disease and Related Disorders Association or by other institutions allow family members to share stresses and experiences and also to discuss management. Sometimes, however, individual psychotherapy and even medication for depression and anxiety become necessary for the caregivers.

PATIENT RESOURCES

The organization devoted to education, family support, and research in Alzheimer's disease that can be contacted for information is:

Alzheimer's Disease and Related
Disorders Association (ADRDA)
National Headquarters
70 East Lake Street
Chicago, Illinois 60601

A practical guide to patient management that is useful for physicians, but especially for families is: The 36-Hour Day. By Mace, N. L., and Rabins, P. V. Baltimore: The Johns Hopkins University Press, 1981.

MOTOR NEURON DISEASE

MEHRSHEED SINAKI, M.D.
WILLIAM J. LITCHY, M.D.
DONALD W. MULDER, M.D.

Amyotrophic lateral sclerosis (ALS), the most common form of motor neuron disease, is the focus of this chapter. Therapies for the more chronic forms of motor neuron disease (e.g., Kugelberg-Welander disease and postpolio weakness) are similar.

ALS is an adult-onset, chronic, progressive disorder causing wasting and atrophy due to the death of anterior horn cells. Characteristically, when upper motor neurons are involved, these findings are also accompanied by hyperactive deep reflexes and spasticity. The disease is often asymmetric and focal in onset and has various initial clinical manifestations. In most patients, ALS is a rapidly progressive, untreatable disorder. Many physicians and also patients and their families equate this diagnosis with a loss of hope for the future, an attitude that results in a nihilistic approach to therapy.

Specific therapy, although the focus of much research, has eluded our grasp. The goal of the treating physician is to provide access to aids that will allow the patient to maintain an optimal quality of life. In some patients, such therapy permits continuation of a productive and satisfying life for many years. Physicians should initiate and provide supportive therapy for patients who choose to combat this malignant neurologic disease. Patients who are provided access to supportive therapy are able to make decisions that often allow them to adapt far better than expected.

Before diagnosis, patients with ALS often report that they are well. Many patients state that their disability began with the hopelessness engendered by the diagnosing physician. Thus, the initial discussion of the diagnosis must be carefully planned. This discussion often permanently influences a patient's understanding of the disorder, and he or she may ask questions that may not be asked again during the course of the disease. Many patients and their families interpret the frequently brief and often noninformative discussion that accompanies the diagnosis as a rejection of the patient by the medical system.

Before the discussion, the physician, the patient, and the patient's family must believe that the diagnosis is accurate. A second opinion is often expedient. We begin discussion of the illness when the diagnosis has been established. Significant members of a patient's family or friends should be included in the discussion. Whenever possible, other members of the evaluation team who have been involved in the evaluation may be included in the discussion.

We begin the discussion with a description of ALS and our knowledge and lack of knowledge of the disorder. We stress the lack of major involvement of the intellect, of the sensory system, of bladder control, and of sexual dysfunction in this disease. The discussion is unhurried, and the patient regulates the speed with which new information is provided by asking questions. Usually, a patient, if given sufficient time, will ask the necessary questions with the family present. In the rare instances in which a patient has not asked questions about essential information and when it is apparent that the patient does not wish to address the problem, we suggest that we discuss it further with his or her family. In no instance have we found it necessary to discuss the disease with only members of the family. We often observe that the patient is more aware of the seriousness of the diagnosis than the physician assumes. The physician's anxiety, which often accompanies this discussion, may interfere with his or her ability to discuss ALS adequately. This lack of discussion often adds to a patient's fears. A patient's memory of this discussion may reflect this anxiety and account for his or her feeling of helplessness. We have found that giving the patient a brochure about the illness (e.g., one from the ALS Society) during the interview is a useful way to clarify the information for patients and their families. Finally, whenever possible, the patient and his or her family should be given a follow-up appointment for further discussion of questions that may arise.

A neurologist usually makes the initial diagnosis, but advice regarding care is a responsibility shared by several specialists, including physiatrists, nutritionists, internists, respiratory care specialists, paramedical personnel, nurses, and others. The physician should encourage the patient to use all available resources, including religious counselors, friends, relatives, social workers, and support organizations. ALS is a disease that involves the whole family, and the individual who is affected will need the help of a support group, ideally his or her family. One physician should coordinate the care of a patient. Usually, this physician is a neurologist, preferably one who has had experience with other patients who have ALS and one who has ready access to necessary consultation. For some patients, clinics such as those supported by the Muscular Dystrophy Association or other support groups are ideal. If the diagnosing physician is unable to provide or is uninterested in the further care of a patient, he or she must arrange a referral of the patient and family to a physician or medical center equipped to give such care.

SPECIFIC MEDICAL TRIALS

Many physicians and their patients need the reassurance of clinical trials of medication. However, physicians have conducted ALS clinics with great success without the use of such trials or placebos. If patients are to be given medication, and many wish to receive medication, the physician must meet certain obligations. He or she must be completely honest with the patient, the family, and him- or herself. Any medication used will initially be reported by the patient, the family, and often the physician as being of *some* help. These reports often lead to the inadvertent reports of "cures," which may necessitate the expenditure of effort and monies by patients and society before their repudiation. No treatment should be used in casual trials if it is unduly expensive or dangerous.

SYMPTOMATIC TREATMENT

Variability in the distribution of weakness among patients with ALS requires that rehabilitation techniques be individualized. The progression of the illness will require continuous modification of treatment for each patient. We have found it useful to classify patients according to the rapidity of their illness, the site of onset of their disease, and the stage of their disability. Patients with long clinical courses have a remarkable capacity to compensate for motor unit loss, which may enable them to continue daily activities for several years. Patients with a slow clinical course will continue to have such a course throughout their illness, whereas those in whom the illness has been rapidly progressive can be expected to continue to deteriorate rapidly. Differentiation of patients according to whether the symptoms began in the bulbar or in the axioappendicular musculature is helpful. In the axioappendicular group, we have found it particularly useful to "stage" the severity of the illness when outlining a therapeutic program (Table 1).

TABLE 1 Exercise and Rehabilitation Programs for Patients With ALS, According to Stage of Disease

Stage, Characteristics	*Treatment*
Stage I:	
Patient is ambulatory, independent ADL* Mild weakness, clumsiness	Encourage ROM* exercises, normal activities Encourage strengthening of unaffected muscles to compensate for weakened muscles Discourage strenuous exercise to strengthen already weakened muscles because it leads to increased fatigue and disability Psychological support is very important†
Stage II:	
Patient is ambulatory Moderate selective weakness Slightly decreased independence in ADL (e.g., difficulty climbing stairs, raising arms, or buttoning clothing)	Substitute Velcro closures for buttons Encourage ankle-foot orthoses, wrist and thumb splints Encourage cautious, selective strengthening for unaffected muscles and stretching exercises to avoid contractures; advise to avoid overuse and fatigue
Stage III:	
Patient is ambulatory Moderately decreased independence in ADL Easily fatigued with long-distance ambulation Severe selective weakness in ankles, wrists, and hands	Goal is to keep patient physically independent as long as possible Encourage deep-breathing exercises to strengthen auxiliary muscles of respiration Prescribe wheelchair—standard or battery operated with proper modifications
Stage IV:	
Patient is confined to wheelchair Able to perform ADL Severe lower extremity weakness (± spasticity)‡ Moderate upper extremity weakness Hanging-arm syndrome with shoulder pain and sometimes edema in the hand	Heat, massage, and application of shoulder splint Preventive anti-edema measures Passive ROM exercises to the weakly supported joints Encourage isometric strengthening of the few remaining uninvolved muscles
Stage V:	
Patient is in wheelchair Increasingly dependent in ADL Severe lower extremity weakness,§ moderate to severe upper extremity weakness Possible skin breakdown	Encourage family to learn proper transfer and positioning principles Encourage modifications at home to aid patient's mobility and independence Water mattress or waterbed is helpful
Stage VI:	
Patient is bedridden Completely dependent in ADL	For dysphagia, use soft diet, long spoons, or tube feeding For accumulated saliva, use suction, medications, surgery to decrease flow For dysarthria, use palatal lifts, electronic speech amplification For breathing difficulty, clear airway, tracheostomy, or respirator

* ADL, activities of daily living; ROM, range of motion.

† Sedatives or tranquilizers (e.g., diazepam) may cause depression.

‡ Spasticity may serve as a splinting effect for ambulation; if it is severe, try the smallest dose of baclofen that is effective.

§ Thrombophlebitis in flaccid lower extremities can be prevented by avoiding trauma; applying passive ROM (twice a day), elastic stockings, dorsal and plantar flexion q2–3h, and thromboguards; or using a trial of subcutaneous heparin (5,000 U q12h) in selected cases.

Bulbar Symptoms

Although the earlier discussion has focused on the treatment of symptoms and signs related to the involvement of the extremities in patients with ALS, the most life-threatening problems and anxiety-provoking symptoms are due to dysfunction of the bulbar nerves and muscles. Although only about 20 percent of patients with ALS present with prominent bulbar abnormalities, virtually all will have significant problems caused by bulbar dysfunction as the disease progresses. The most prominent problems include dysphagia, sialorrhea, and dysarthria. Symptomatic treatment of these problems may lead to not only a longer but also a more comfortable life for patients.

Dysphagia

Swallowing is a complex physiologic process that involves several muscle groups working in synchrony. Abnormalities of the muscles of mastication, the tongue, pharyngeal constrictor muscles, and also the esophagus can produce difficulty with swallowing (dysphagia).

The treatment of these symptoms depends on the severity of the abnormality (Table 2). At some stage a patient may have to use a feeding tube. For patients with severe dysphagia, a percutaneous feeding gastrostomy is the method of choice for maintaining caloric intake. Placement of the feeding tube can be done without general anesthesia and is associated with extremely low morbidity. Patients tolerate it well and it is not cosmetically unsightly. We believe that when patients lose weight, have a recent history of aspiration, or have a very strong potential for aspiration, placement of a feeding percutaneous gastrostomy should be discussed with the patient and family. After the feeding gastrostomy is placed, a program of feeding is arranged with a nutritionist to ensure adequate caloric intake with appropriate supplemental nutrients.

TABLE 2 Treatment of Common Symptoms of Motor Neuron Disease*

Symptom	*Treatment*
Constipation	Hydration High-fiber diet Stool softener (e.g., Colace) Suppositories (e.g., Dulcolax, glycerol)
Cramps	Quinine (200 mg at bedtime)† Phenytoin (Dilantin)†
Spasticity	Baclofen (Lioresal)
Sialorrhea	Amitriptyline (10 mg four times daily)† Hyoscyamine sulfate (0.125 mg four times daily)† Trihexyphenidyl hydrochloride†
Dysphagia	Slow eating Food that is easy to swallow Frequent meals Caloric supplementation (e.g., Ensure, Isocal) Pureed food Percutaneous gastrostomy
Dysarthria	Speech therapy Writing (e.g., Magic Slate) Alphabet cards Typewriters (Canon Communicator) Computerized communication devices

* For patients with motor neuron disease, we use medications cautiously because of untoward side effects.
† Titrate to effective dose.

Sialorrhea

Even though there is no known change in the rate of salivary secretion in patients with ALS, those with impaired swallowing or facial muscle weakness or both will often complain of drooling or difficulty controlling their saliva. This problem not only is embarrassing for the patient but also can be life-threatening if secretions are aspirated. The approaches to this problem have been numerous, but our general approach is to use the tricyclic antidepressant amitriptyline to control secretions initially (Table 2).

In severe cases, transtympanic chorda tympani neurectomy may be used. This approach is not always successful because of variation in the innervation of the salivary glands; some patients may experience denervation hypersensitivity with excess salivation, and reinnervation of the glands may occur.

Dysarthria

Management of speech problems is difficult and frustrating. The goal is to maintain communication skills, and several aids have proved effective in many patients (Table 2).

Respiratory Complications

Most patients with ALS will die of complications due to dysfunction of the respiratory system. These problems can arise for different reasons: (1) weakness of the muscles of breathing results in hypoxemia and respiratory failure; (2) bulbar muscle weakness and incoordination result in poor cough, difficulty keeping the lower airway clear, and aspiration; and (3) sleep apnea can be a result of all of these problems. The strength of the respiratory muscles should be monitored with pulmonary function studies. Maximal inspiratory and expiratory pressures are good indicators of respiratory muscle strength. When pulmonary problems are present, they should be discussed with the patient and family, and the alternatives for treatment should also be discussed at that time.

Therapy to avoid respiratory complications is important, and this should be stressed to the patient. Breathing exercises such as inhaling deeply, holding the breath for 1 or 2 seconds, and exhaling should be repeated frequently. Although the exercises can be done in any position, they are best done when the patient is on his or her back. Assisted coughing after a deep breath and chest physiotherapy for postural drainage are also beneficial.

The critical question is if and when a patient should have a tracheostomy and assisted ventilation with a respirator. There is rarely a simple answer to this question, and it must be thoroughly discussed with the patient and family. Although there are no hard-and-fast rules, when signs of severe respiratory compromise (e.g., nocturnal hypoxemia) or significant difficulties with aspiration are present, a tracheostomy should be strongly considered. When respiratory muscle weakness is the main problem, a Pneumobelt or a Cutress ventilator may be a consideration. We do not believe that either of these is particularly helpful for any period, and both may be unreliable. For this reason, we recommend a tracheostomy when intervention is indicated. The patient and family must be part of these decisions. Thus, the discussion should take place before any catastrophe that requires emergency intervention.

For patients who need only nighttime ventilatory assistance, a fenestrated tracheostomy tube can be used so that talking is possible. A cannula can be placed when it is necessary to assist the patient with mechanical ventilation. Many people live happy and productive lives for long periods after the need for ventilatory assistance arises. Portable respirators are available, and patients with these are often able to travel and continue with their occupations—often to their physicians' amazement. In our experience, the decisions about life-prolonging measures such as the use of respirators are least difficult when the problem has been discussed with the patient and family before the need arises.

EMOTIONAL SUPPORT

Emotional support of the patients and their families must be addressed at any stage of the disease. Reactive depression is not uncommon, but suicide is rare. Counseling and planning for the future must begin at the early stages. Chapters of the ALS Society and the Muscular Dystrophy Association are helpful not only for providing emotional support but also for extending specific help to both the patient and the physician.

PATIENT RESOURCES

The ALS Association
15300 Ventura Boulevard
Suite 315, P.O. Box 5951
Sherman Oaks, California 91403

Muscular Dystrophy Association
810 Seventh Avenue
New York, New York 91403

ALS of Canada
250 Rogers Road
Toronto, Ontario, Canada, M6E 1R1

ALCOHOL INTOXICATION AND WITHDRAWAL

ELLIOTT L. MANCALL, M.D.
PAUL A. SILVER, M.D.

ACUTE INTOXICATION

Although ethyl alcohol is readily absorbed in the gastrointestinal tract and quickly distributed throughout most tissues, initial clinical effects are on the central nervous system (CNS). Ethanol is fundamentally a CNS depressant; at low concentrations it inhibits cortical activity with paradoxical behavioral stimulation characterized by gregariousness, emotional lability, and expansiveness of mood. Autonomic changes include a rise in cardiac output and systolic and pulse pressures, dilatation of cutaneous vessels with hyperhydrosis and heat loss along with compensatory splanchnic vasoconstriction, and gastric mucosal hyperemia. Diuresis reflects transient inhibition of the release of antidiuretic hormone, and there is increased urinary excretion of phosphate and magnesium.

Impairment of motor and intellectual performance parallels the rise in blood alcohol level. At 50 mg per deciliter there is mild incoordination of the limbs, progressing to frank ataxia at 100 mg per deciliter. When the level reaches 200 mg per deciliter, drowsiness, mental confusion, and slurring of speech appear. Stupor generally develops at levels of 300 mg per deciliter. A concentration of 400 mg per deciliter is usually considered fatal. At high ethanol concentrations, reflex pylorospasm develops, which prolongs the period of intoxication, as the alcohol is only slowly released into the small intestine.

Factors that influence the severity of the state of inebriation in any given individual at any point in time include not only the precise alcohol level per se, but also by the rapidity of ingestion of alcohol and, thus, the rapidity of rise of the blood alcohol level; the concomitant use or avoidance of food; the degree of tolerance in the accustomed drinker; and perhaps familial predisposition and psychological attitude and expectations. The accustomed alcoholic tolerates alcohol better than the occasional drinker, although the metabolic events responsible for this discrepancy are not well understood. It should be emphasized, however, that the chronic alcoholic is not immune to the acute effects of alcohol, provided a sufficient amount of the drug is ingested. Although the chronic user of alcohol tolerates lower levels with relative ease as compared with the sporadic drinker, the alcoholic may still succumb to levels ordinarily fatal to others.

Treatment

Appropriate management is initially determined by evaluation of the level of consciousness and of respiratory function. Stuporous patients require attention to the airway and, of course, a search for other life-threatening causes of impairment of consciousness such as an intracranial hematoma. Prompt venous access is essential. Determinations of blood glucose concentration, blood urea nitrogen level, ethanol level, electrolytes, magnesium and phosphate levels, PT and PTT, arterial blood gases, and screening for other drugs are all helpful in selected cases. When dextrose and saline solutions are infused, parenteral thiamine must be given simultaneously to avoid exhaustion of marginal thiamine stores and precipitation of acute Wernicke's encephalopathy; immediate thiamine doses of 100 mg IM or 50 mg IV and 50 mg IM should be employed, with subsequent parenteral and/or oral doses of 100 mg daily in all alcoholic patients.

There is, unfortunately, no effective way to hasten the metabolism of ethanol itself. The administration of glucose and insulin has been advocated in the past, but appears to have no real value. The use of caffeine or other CNS stimulants is nonspecific and generally ineffective. Gastric lavage may be helpful if the patient is seen almost immediately after the ingestion of a large amount of ethanol, but is otherwise of very limited value. In patients with potentially lethal blood alcohol levels (400 mg per deciliter or more), or who have ingested other more toxic substances such as methanol, prompt hemodialysis may be life-saving. For the less critically ill patient, a quiet and protective environment should be provided. Monitoring for the development of early withdrawal symptoms is necessary.

Idiosyncratic Intoxication

Also referred to as "pathologic intoxication," this disorder is characterized by the abrupt emergence of aggressive, often violent, behavior following the ingestion of alcohol in an amount insufficient to induce intoxication in a normal individual. When faced with a patient in such a situation, other causes for violent behavior, such as intoxication causing disinhibition in a usually aggressive individual, must be considered. The period of agitation tends to be short-lived and usually ends in deep sleep within a few hours. One must be alert to the possibility of attempted suicide. Provision of a quiet environment may be sufficient for management. If violence is a prominent feature, restraints may be necessary. High-potency antipsychotic agents such as haloperidol (Haldol) in a dose of 5 mg IM repeated every 30 to 60 minutes may be helpful. Vital signs must be closely monitored and the possible development of extrapyramidal side effects borne in mind.

ALCOHOL WITHDRAWAL

Physical dependence on alcohol develops rapidly. The dependent individual is at risk for development of withdrawal symptoms whenever the blood alcohol level falls appreciably. The critical alcohol level is not known, but appears to vary from patient to patient. Withdrawal symptoms may be precipitated by a relative reduction in intake without complete abstinence.

There are four distinct stages that can be identified in the full-blown withdrawal syndrome, although relatively few patients, even when untreated, actually proceed to the final and most serious phase, i.e., delirium tremens. Each of these stages may appear independently in any given patient, but do tend to occur in chronologic sequence in the majority. Since delirium tremens is a life-threatening disorder, prompt recognition of the earlier manifestations of withdrawal and their appropriate management are essential.

Within as few as 6 to 8 hours of reduction in intake of alcohol the first symptoms of withdrawal appear, so-called alcoholic tremulousness. The patient becomes anxious, nauseated, and irritable and commonly has an increase in pulse and blood pressure. Coarse tremors of the limbs, face, and tongue are characteristic. Abstinence due to an overnight sleep may be sufficient to precipitate this disorder; as a result, many alcoholics consume an "eye opener" on arising to "steady the nerves," in an attempt to avoid this complication. Most clinical manifestations decrease gradually within several days; however, the tremor itself often lingers for several weeks.

In 12 to 24 hours after withdrawal, patients may develop hallucinations, which are usually auditory, but may be visual or mixed. These ordinarily subside within days to weeks, but a small proportion of these patients continue to experience hallucinations indefinitely in a state of chronic auditory hallucinosis. The relationship between this chronic hallucinatory state and other psychoses, in particular schizophrenia, is unclear; it is possible in some cases that alcohol withdrawal has in some way triggered or unmasked a preexisting but perhaps not clinically manifest psychotic disorder in the susceptible individual. On occasion the development of hallucinations has been observed in the absence of abstinence.

Within a period of 36 to 48 hours following withdrawal, a number of patients develop withdrawal *seizures*, commonly referred to as "rum fits" or "alcoholic epilepsy." Seizures are typically generalized and grand mal in type, appearing in isolation or in a flurry of at most two to three attacks; status epilepticus only rarely occurs. Focal seizures are distinctly uncommon, and their appearance under these circumstances must always alert the physician to the need to search for other causes of seizure activity. It is probable that alcohol withdrawal may itself potentiate the development of seizures in an individual harboring a preexisting epileptogenic focus.

Finally, about 5 percent of patients in withdrawal develop frank delirium tremens, characterized by autonomic dysfunction, fever, insomnia, agitation and psychomotor overactivity, anorexia, confusion, perceptual distortions, and hallucinations, usually visual in type. Delirium usually develops within 3 days of abstinence, but onset may be delayed for up to a week following general anesthesia. Tremulousness, hallucinations, and seizures may all precede the development of the full-blown syndrome. The potential gravity of the state of delirium here is reflected by the fact that most series report a fatality rate of approximately 10 percent.

Treatment

As in the treatment of intoxication, therapy for concurrent illnesses, metabolic alterations, and nutritional deficiency is vital. The benzodiazepines are the pharmacologic cornerstone for management of at least the milder withdrawal symptoms, although the adjunctive use of beta blockers has recently been suggested as well. Cross tolerance of benzodiazepines with alcohol provides the rationale for their use. Chlordiazepoxide (Librium) has been the agent most widely used under these circumstances. There are, however, advantages to the use of a shorter-acting agent such as oxazepam (Serax). Since it has no active metabolites, this drug is easier to titrate without risking accumulation and resultant oversedation, a factor particularly important in patients with severe liver disease. However, since the half-life of oxazepam is short, doses must be frequent enough to prevent the reemergence of the withdrawal symptoms, and the medication must be tapered slowly. Oxazepam is utilized in an initial dose of 15 to 30 mg as early signs of withdrawal emerge; the subsequent dosage schedule is then determined by the degree of control of symptoms. Initially, 15 mg every 6 hours may be adequate, but up to 120 mg per day may be required. When a maintenance dose is established, it should be continued for 24 hours; if no further signs of withdrawal appear, medication may be tapered over several days, but increased if symptoms recur. If chlordiazepoxide is utilized, the initial dose is 25 to 100 mg, with additional doses administered as necessary until the symptoms are controlled, up to a maximum daily dose of 300 mg. The preferred route of the administration of all benzodiazepines is oral. Of this class of drugs, only lorazepam (Ativan) is reliably absorbed intramuscularly; for parenteral use the other drugs must be given intravenously. Rectal paraldehyde may be utilized if necessary.

Treatment of withdrawal seizures per se is rarely necessary, since by definition this disorder is self-limited. Particularly in individuals with a prior history of seizures, it is often advocated that an intravenous loading dose of phenytoin, 1000 mg, should be given promptly on arrival at the hospital, followed by oral doses of 300 mg daily until the period of withdrawal is past. When status epilepticus appears, it must of course be treated, as under other circumstances. Since patients with typical withdrawal seizures are not liable to have further seizures when abstinent, they do not require ongoing management with anticonvulsants. In any case, noncompliance poses a serious problem in any attempt to continue medication of this sort over the long term.

Full-blown delirium tremens must be considered a medical emergency, often requiring management in an intensive care unit. The patient may require sedation with intravenous diazepam in an initial dose of 5 to 10 mg in a slow IV push, followed by 5-mg doses every 5 minutes until the patient becomes calm, and must be monitored closely for respiratory depression and hypotension. A maintenance dose of diazepam, 5 mg orally or IV, may be given every few hours thereafter, the size of the dose gradually being decreased and the interval increased, to avoid oversedation. Every effort should be made to orient the patient and to provide constant reassurance. Physical restraints should be employed only as a last resort to prevent the patient from injuring himself or others. The use of neuroleptics should be avoided, since these agents may lower the seizure threshold and impair hypothalamic temperature regulatory mechanisms. Furthermore, they may actually worsen the delirium because of their anticholinergic action. Aggressive management of concomitant fluid loss, electrolyte imbalance, and hypoglycemia is essential. Treatment with vitamins, particularly with thiamine, must accompany the use of parenteral carbohydrate supplementation. Cardiovascular collapse poses a major risk in these individuals and must be dealt with promptly if it appears.

It is essential that the physician address the problems of chronic alcohol abuse when the given episode of intoxication and/or withdrawal has been satisfactorily managed. Referral to inpatient or outpatient rehabilitation programs, or to lay organizations such as Alcoholics Anonymous, can be helpful. Patients are frequently more receptive to such a referral following a severe episode of intoxication or withdrawal than at other times, and every effort should be made to take advantage of their willingness to accede to such therapeutic recommendations.

PATIENT RESOURCES

For Alcoholics:
Alcoholics Anonymous World Service
Box 459 Grand Central Station
New York, New York 10163
(212) 686-1100

For Family Members:
Al-Anon
P.O. Box 862 Mid-Town Station
New York, New York 10018-0862
(212) 302-7240

In addition, listings for local chapters of Alcoholics Anonymous and Al-Anon can often be found in the White Pages of the phone book.

WERNICKE'S ENCEPHALOPATHY AND OTHER ALCOHOLIC NUTRITIONAL DISORDERS

MAURICE VICTOR, M.D.

A certain number of nutritional diseases occur regularly as a complication of alcoholism. These include Wernicke's disease, Korsakoff's psychosis, "alcoholic" cerebellar degeneration, and peripheral neuropathy. Pellagra and so-called alcohol amblyopia, better termed nutritional amblyopia or optic neuropathy, occur much less frequently. The role of alcohol in the genesis of these disorders is purely secondary. Alcohol acts mainly by displacing food in the diet, but also by increasing the demand for B vitamins, which are necessary to metabolize the carbohydrate furnished by alcohol itself. Also, alcoholics may have a decreased capacity to absorb thiamine and folic acid, among other nutrients, and to digest fat, because of impaired pancreatic function. These defects in absorption and digestion are probably due to disturbances of nutrition rather than to the action of alcohol itself and, once established, serve to exaggerate the deficiencies that result from dietary deprivation.

In the United States nutritional diseases of the nervous system are observed almost exclusively among alcoholics. Other causes—dietary faddism, impaired absorption of dietary nutrients (sprue, pernicious anemia, resection of portions of the gastrointestinal tract), the use of vitamin antagonists (e.g., isoniazid, hydralazine), and certain iatrogenic disorders (prolonged treatment iwth intravenous fluids and hyperalimentation, plication or partitioning of the stomach for treatment of obesity)—account for a relatively small proportion of cases. All of the nutritional disorders that are observed in alcoholics have occurred as well under conditions in which alcohol plays no part (e.g., in prisoner-of-war camps and communities in which polished rice is the staple of the diet). There is no fundamental difference, clinically or pathologically, between the nutritional disorders that are observed in alcoholics and those in nonalcoholics.

The treatment of nutritional diseases of the nervous system is a relatively simple matter, once the patient's illness is recognized for what it is. In other words, the problem is not so much one of treatment as of recognition of the deficiency disease, failure of which may lead to severe destructive changes in both the peripheral and the central nervous systems and often to irreversible changes in the mental state. A requisite for intelligent treatment, therefore, is a high index of suspicion of the presence of deficiency diseases and a knowledge of the clinical circumstances in which such diseases tend to occur. These features will be mentioned briefly as a prelude to the discussion of treatment.

WERNICKE'S DISEASE

Wernicke's disease is a common disorder, seen most frequently, but not exclusively, in the alcoholic population. It is characterized by nystagmus, abducens and conjugate gaze palsies, ataxia of gait, and mental confusion. These symptoms have an acute or subacute onset and may occur singly or, more often, in various combinations. When all the symptoms are present, there is no difficulty in diagnosis. Patients frequently present with only fragments of the syndrome, however. The ocular paralyses are so sensitive to the administration of thiamine that they may be obliterated by a meal or two and then the patient's only ocular abnormalities may consist of a horizontal nystagmus on lateral gaze; unless this sign is specifically sought, it will be missed. Similarly, the ataxia of Wernicke's disease may be quite subtle and elicited only when the patient is asked to walk tandem. Since most of the patients are alcoholics, the mental confusion is often incorrectly ascribed to alcohol withdrawal. If the ocular signs, ataxia, and a confusional state are not recognized for what they are, or if specific treatment is delayed for other reasons, the patient may slip into a stupor or coma, making recognition even more difficult and recovery less likely.

Finally, one must be aware of the special danger associated with treating severely depleted alcoholic patients with glucose solutions. Usually these individuals have subsisted on a diet low in thiamine and disproportionately high in carbohydrate, to which is added the carbohydrate calories of alcohol itself. Often, gastroenteritis and diarrhea have been present as well. Under the circumstances the body's available thiamine may be exhausted after 7 to 8 weeks. The administration of intravenous glucose (without vitamin supplements) at this point may actually precipitate Wernicke's disease or cause an early form of the disease to deteriorate rapidly. For this reason it is good practice to administer B vitamins to all alcoholic patients requiring parenteral glucose, even though the complication under treatment, e.g., delirium tremens, is not due to vitamin deficiency.

Treatment

Wernicke's disease represents a medical emergency and its recognition demands the immediate administration of thiamine. Although a few milligrams of this vitamin are sufficient to modify the ocular signs, much larger doses need to be employed in order to replenish the exhausted thiamine stores. It is our practice to administer 50 mg IV and 10 mg IM, the latter dose being repeated each day until the patient resumes a normal diet. The prompt use of thiamine prevents the progression of the nervous system disease and actually reverses those lesions or portions thereof in which permanent damage has not occurred (the "biochemical lesion"). The remarkable sensitivity of the ocular palsies to the administration of thiamine (improvement may *begin* in several hours) constitutes an important diagnostic as well as therapeutic measure. In patients who show only ocular and ataxic signs, the prompt administration of thiamine is crucial in preventing the development of irreversible and incapacitating amnesic psychosis.

Although the frank signs of beriberi heart disease are unusual in Wernicke's disease, a resting tachycardia and marked dyspnea on effort are practically universal findings, and sudden cardiovascular collapse and death may occasionally follow even mild exertion. For this reason bed rest is mandatory in patients with this disease, even if they do appear acutely ill. If the signs of beriberi heart disease appear (peripheral edema, pulmonary congestion, faint heart sounds, rapid circulation time, etc), rapid digitalization should be undertaken in addition to the administration of thiamine.

The further management of Wernicke's disease involves the use of a balanced diet and all the B vitamins, since the patient is usually deficient in more than thiamine. If the patient cannot or will not eat the prescribed diet, parenteral feeding and administration of vitamins becomes necessary.

Another important aspect of treatment consists of the search for and treatment of complicating medical and neurologic illnesses, e.g., liver disease, polyneuropathy, gastroenteritis, and other infections (particularly pneumonia and tuberculosis). Because of the high incidence of associated medical disorders, these patients must be supervised continually on a medical rather than a psychiatric ward.

KORSAKOFF'S PSYCHOSIS

(Amnesic Confabulatory Psychosis; Psychosis Polyneuritica)

Korsakoff's psychosis refers to a unique mental disorder in which retentive memory is impaired out of all proportion to other cognitive functions in an otherwise alert and responsive patient. In the nutritionally deficient alcoholic patient, Korsakoff's psychosis is usually associated with Wernicke's disease. Stated in another way, Korsakoff's psychosis is the psychic manifestation of Wernicke's disease. Most instances of Korsakoff's psychosis begin with the signs of Wernicke's disease. In the initial stages of the disease the amnesic state is often obscured by the profound general confusion, apathy, drowsiness, and so forth. However, in a small proportion of patients, the amnesic state arises de novo, without the other manifestations of Wernicke's disease.

Treatment

The treatment of Korsakoff's psychosis is the same as for Wernicke's disease, although one cannot be sanguine about the possibility of recovery of the amnesic symptoms. In some patients (less than 20 percent in our experience), memory function is restored completely, and in the majority, partial recovery is the rule. The extent to which the patient will recover is rarely predictable when he is first seen. Moreover, the onset of recovery of mental function may be delayed for several weeks or even months, and then it proceeds slowly. Failure to appreciate these facts may result in the premature commitment of the patient to a mental hospital. The eventual disposition of the patient to his family, a nursing home, or a mental institution is undertaken on the basis of the severity of the amnesic psychosis as well as existing family and social circumstances, but only after one is certain that no further improvement in memory function is possible.

"ALCOHOLIC" CEREBELLAR DEGENERATION

This is a highly stereotyped disorder, characterized by an ataxia of gait and of the legs, with relatively less involvement of the arms, speech, and ocular motility. The symptoms may arise acutely or subacutely; in either event, the symptoms tend to stabilize after a short period of progression. The lesions also are remarkably uniform, taking the form of a degeneration of the neurocellular elements of the cerebellar cortex, particularly of the Purkinje cells, and affecting predominantly the midline vermain structures. This form of cerebellar degeneration does not differ fundamentally from the cerebellar manifestations of Wernicke's disease, either clinically or pathologically. In other words, the cerebellar ataxia of Wernicke's disease and that which is referred to as alcoholic cerebellar degeneration probably represent the same disease process, the former term being used when the cerebellar abnormalities are associated with ocular and mental signs and the latter when the cerebellar syndrome occurs alone.

It follows that the treatment of alcoholic cerebellar degeneration is the same as for the other manifestations of the Wernicke-Korsakoff syndrome. If thiamine, in large doses, is given soon after the onset of cerebellar symptoms, considerable or complete recovery may be anticipated. Most patients only seek help long after onset. In these patients improvement is slight at best and is the result of abstinence from alcohol, improvement in general health, and recovery from polyneuropathy, which is often conjoined.

ALCOHOLIC POLYNEUROPATHY

The symptomatology of alcoholic polyneuropathy varies considerably. Some patients are virtually asymptomatic, the signs of disease becoming evident only on examination. Most patients complain of weakness, paresthesias, and pain, and in them examination discloses varying degress of motor, sensory and reflex loss. The legs are involved earlier and more severely than the arms, and with rare exceptions, the trunk and face are unaffected. Usually, the distal segments of the limbs are involved more than the proximal ones, but in virtually all patients with discernible weakness, proximal muscles are significantly affected. In some patients the weakness may seemingly be greater in proximal parts than in distal ones. These latter cases are often loosely referred to as "alcoholic myopathy,'' but almost invariably, on careful examination, they prove to be instances of polyneuropathy.

Unlike the ocular and ataxia manifestations of Wernicke's disease, which are due to a specific deficiency of thiamine, the precise nutritional factor responsible for polyneuropathy has not been established. It would appear that polyneuropathy may result from a deficiency of pyridoxine, pantothenic acid, thiamine, or vitamine B_{12} or possibly from a deficiency of more than one of the B vitamins.

Treatment

Maintence of Proper Nutrition. This is an important factor in all neuropathies, not only those that are due to a dietary deficiency. The patient must consume a diet high in calories (3000 calories daily for the average adult male) and high in proteins and carbohydrates. Supplemental B vitamins should be given in the following minimal daily dosages: thiamine 25 mg, niacin 100 mg, riboflavin 10 mg, pantothenic acid 10 mg, and pyridoxine 5 mg. In patients with persistent vomiting or other gastrointestinal complications, the vitamins may be given intramuscularly or added to intravenous fluids. A suitable parenteral preparation is Berroca-C, one ampule daily.

Relief of Pain. In some patients, pain, rather than impairment of motor-sensory function, is the outstanding manifestation of the neuropathy. The feet may be so sensitive to tactile stimulation and light pressure that the patient literally cannot bear the contact of bedclothes. In cases of severe weakness or paralysis, aching of the limbs may be related to their immobility. Pressure of the bedclothes may be avoided by placing a cradle support over the legs. Moist hot packs may give some relief. The aching due to immobility is best managed by gently massaging the affected limbs and passively manipulating them through a full range of motion on frequent occasions. Acetylsalicylic acid, 0.3 to 1.0 g (5 to 15 grains) every 4 hours, is usually sufficient to control hypertathia, but occasionally codeine in doses of 15 to 30 mg has to be added for a short period. Opiates or addicting synthetic analgesics should be avoided, particularly if the pain is chronic in nature.

Maintenance of Muscle Tone. The process of nerve regeneration may take many months and frequently longer than a year. The successful regeneration of peripheral nerves will be of no avail if the muscles that they innervate have been allowed to undergo contracture and the joints to become fixed. During the day, the patient's legs should be positioned so that the soles of the feet rest firmly against a footboard, in order to prevent shortening of the heel cords. In cases of severe paralysis, molded splints should be applied to the arms, hands, legs, and feet during periods of rest. Pressure on the heels, and elbows can be avoided by padding the splints and by turning the patient frequently if he is unable to do so alone. As soon as the patient's general condition permits, the limbs must be passively manipulated through a full range of motion several times daily. Gentle massage is also useful. Attention to these procedures should be as routine a matter as the inspection of the temepratury chart of a febrile patient. As function returns, more vigorous physiotherapeutic measures can be undertaken.

When it comes time for the patient to leave the hospital, the great danger to continued recovery is the resumption of alcoholic habits; suitable arrangements must therefore be made for complete supervision during the long and tedious convalescence.

ALCOHOL (TOBACCO-ALCOHOL) AMBLYOPIA

These terms refer to a relatively uncommon but characterisitic disorder of vision in alcoholic patients. The usual complaint is a blurring of vision for near and distant objects, evolving gradually over a period of several weeks. Examination discloses a reduction of visual acuity and the presence of central or centrocecal scotomata and occasionally a mild papillitis and retinal hemorrhages. These changes are always bilateral and more or less symmetrical. Untreated, the disease may progress to irreversible optic atrophy. With a nutritious diet and vitamin supplements, improvement occurs in all instances, although the degree of improvement may vary, depending upon the duration of symptoms before treatment is started. The few cases studied pathologically have shown a symmetrical degeneration of the optic nerves, chiasm, and tracts, occupying a zone that coresponds roughly to the region of the papillomacular bundle. The evidence is overwhelming that this disorder is due not to the toxic effects of tobacco or alcohol, but to nutritional deficiency, so that the continued use of the term ''tobacco-alcohol amblyopia'' and its classification as a toxic amblyopia are hardly justified. The terms "deficiency amblyopia" or "nutritional optic neuropathy" are preferable.

Rarely, amblyopia is the initial manifestation of vitamin B_{12} deficiency, in which case treatment consists of the prompt intramuscular administration of this vitamin, in doses of 1000 μg repeated daily at first and then at monthly intervals. In most alcoholic patients, a specific deficiency cannot be identified, and in these patients one depends on the interdiction of alcohol and the administration of a balanced diet and supplementary B vitamins.

ALCOHOLIC PELLAGRA

In the United States, the endemic form of pellagra has been virtually abolished because of the widespread practice of enriching bread with niacin. Sporadic cases of pellagra are still encountered in the alcoholic population and are often overlooked, a failure that is due no doubt to the rarity of the disease.

In its fully developed form, pellagra is characterized by mental and nervous symptoms, diarrhea, mouth lesions, and dermatitis. All parts of the nervous system may be affected. In the early stages, the symptoms may be mistaken for those of psychoneurosis. Sometimes an acute confusional psychosis dominates the clinical picture. The manifestations of spinal cord involvement have not been clearly delineated, perhaps because the patient's mental state often preculdes accurate testing. In genral, the signs are referable to both posterior and lateral columns of the cord, predominantly the former. Peripheral nerve involvement is the least common of the neurologic manifestations and from the descriptions is indistinguishable from neuropathic beriberi.

Although pellagra is generally equated with a deficiency of nicotinic acid, a deficiency of other B vitamins and the amino acid tryptophan is undoubtedly important in the genesis of this disorder. For this reason treatment should consist of the administration of a balanced diet and all the B vitamins.

DRUG ABUSE: OVERDOSE AND WITHDRAWAL

JOHN C. M. BRUST, M.D.

The term "drug abuse" is an arbitrary social judgment, variably applied to agents that are illegal in any setting (e.g., heroin or marijuana), illegal when used without prescription (e.g., amphetamines or barbiturates), legal but dangerous in any dosage (e.g., tobacco), or legal but dangerous when used excessively (e.g., ethanol). "Psychic dependence" is the compulsion to continue administration of a drug to produce pleasure or avoid discomfort; it corresponds to what is loosely termed "addiction." "Physical dependence" is the adaptive state that leads to physical disturbance when use of a drug is stopped or its effects are countered by an antagonist. "Tolerance" refers to diminished response to the same amount of a drug, such that ever higher doses are required to achieve the desired effect.

Drugs of course differ in the type and degree of dependence and tolerance they produce, and symptoms of intoxication and withdrawal vary accordingly. The popularity of various drugs also varies among cultural or socioeconomic groups, and in any emergency room some syndromes are common, whereas others are seen seldom, if at all. In this chapter I will address the management of overdose and withdrawal from drugs currently abused in the United States, excluding ethanol and tobacco and focusing mainly on those agents encountered at my own institution, Harlem Hospital Center in New York City. Not described here are complications of drug abuse such as infection (e.g. abscesses, hepatitis, endocarditis, tetanus, or the acquired immunodeficiency syndrome), trauma, heroin nephropathy, amphetamine vasculitis, pentazocine myopathy, parkinsonism secondary to methylphenyl-tetrahydropyridine (MPTP), meperidine-induced myoclonus, glue-sniffer's neuropathy, or cocaine-induced myocardial infarction, although such problems may complicate intoxication or withdrawal. Also not addressed here are approaches to long-term management, such as methadone maintenance for heroin addicts.

OPIATES

Among the various opiates abused in the United States (Table 1), heroin constitutes the bulk of most urban street trafficking. The drug has enormous addiction liability, and tolerance in daily users leads to the need for huge doses. Many take it only occasionally however (e.g., on weekends), and street mixtures vary greatly in potency. Even someone with considerable tolerance may, therefore, take too much.

Overdose causes coma, pinpoint but reactive pupils, and respiratory depression. If brain anoxia-ischemia or hypothermia occurs, however, the pupils may be large and unreactive. Moreover, although it would be very unusual for opiates to cause coma without respiratory depression, multiple substance abuse can produce confusing combinations of symptoms and signs. Heroin is frequently taken with cocaine or amphetamine ("speedball") and many heroin addicts also abuse ethanol. Signs of overdose from one agent may coexist with signs of withdrawal from another. Seizures in heroin users may be the combined result of other drug effects, of brain anoxia, and of heroin's own capacity to lower seizure threshold.

Treatment of overdose begins with attention to apnea or shock. Opiate depression of brainstem carbon di-

TABLE 1 Opiates Available in the United States

Agonist
Powdered opium
Tincture of opium (laudanum)
Camphorated tinture of opium (paregoric)
Purified opium alkaloids (Pantopon)
Morphine
Heroin (legally available only for investigational use)
Methadone (Dolophine, etc.)
Fentanyl (Sublimaze)
Oxymorphone (Numorphan)
Hydromorphone (Dilaudid)
Codeine
Oxycodone (in mixtures, e.g., Percodan)
Levorphanol (Levo-Dromoran)
Meperidine (pethidine, Demerol, etc.)
Alphaprodine (Nisentil)
Anileridine (Leritine)
Diphenoxylate (in Lomotil)
Loperamide (Imodium)
Ethoheptazine (Zactane, and in Zactirin)
Propoxyphene (Darvon)
Ethorphine (for animal use)
Apomorphine
Mixed agonist-antagonist
Levallorphan (Lorfan)
Nalorphine (Nalline)
Pentazocine (Talwin)
Butorphanol (Stadol)
Nalbuphine (Nubain)
Cyclazocine (for investigational use only)

oxide sensitivity mandates caution in using oxygen. Hypotension is usually responsive to correction of hypoxia and administration of fluids, use of which may, however, be limited by the presence of heroin-induced pulmonary edema. Vasopressors or plasma expanders are seldom needed. Naloxone is given in boluses of 0.4 mg (1 ml) IV, IM, or subcutaneously every few minutes. A patient not responding to 10 mg is unlikely to respond to more; the great majority respond to 2 mg or less. (Higher doses have been reported necessary to reverse propoxyphene overdose.) Naloxone's very high margin of safety, the fact that opiates can exacerbate the symptoms of other diseases or intoxicants, and reports that naloxone can at least partially reverse signs of ethanol intoxication justify not only occasionally using high doses of naloxone, but giving it to patients whose examinations are atypical for opiate overdose. (On the other hand, some patients who become comatose following parenteral heroin fail to respond to naloxone or die suddenly before it can be given. Speculations on the nature of these "nonoverdose sudden heroin deaths" include allergy and quinine cardiotoxicity.)

Giving too much naloxone can produce abstinence symptoms. Maximal effects occur 2 to 3 minutes after intravenous naloxone, but only about 15 minutes after intramuscular or subcutaneous administration. Because of vomiting, endotracheal intubation has been recommended before giving naloxone; at Harlem Hospital the potential hazard of performing this procedure on so many emergency room patients is felt to outweigh its benefits. Moreover, many patients have already received naloxone from the Emergency Medical Service by the time they reach the hospital.

Naloxone is shorter-acting than most opiate agonists, especially methadone, and a patient who seems to have recovered fully may slip back into coma and apnea. Hospital admission and close observation are required for at least 24 hours with heroin and 72 hours with methadone, and it may be necessary during that time to give more naloxone in repeated small boluses or even by prolonged infusion.

Daily heroin users rapidly develop physical dependence, and signs and symptoms of abstinence begin within a few hours of withdrawal. By 8 to 12 hours there is pronounced drug-craving, irritability, anxiety, weakness, lacrimation, rhinorrhea, sweating, and yawning, followed by (sometimes after a few hours of restless sleep), achiness, mydriasis, piloerection, anorexia, nausea, vomiting, diarrhea, abdominal cramps, hot flashes, fever, tachypnea, tachycardia, hypertension, sweating alternating with chills, rales, rhonchi, and coughing. Leukocytosis is common. Except for rare instances of dehydration, ketosis, and hypotension, the syndrome is not life-threatening, and seizures, hallucinations, or delirium tremens do not occur, at least in adults. With heroin, symptoms peak at 24 to 72 hours and last 7 to 10 days. Methadone's abstinence symptoms begin 8 to 24 hours after the last dose, peak at 6 days, and last up to 3 weeks. (With either drug "protracted abstinence," consisting of a variety of mild autonomic disturbances, can last for months; the relationship of these abnormalities to persistent drug-craving is uncertain.)

Opiate abstinence symptoms can usually be relieved by oral methadone, 20 mg once or twice in the first 24 hours, with subsequent tapering of dosage titrated to symptoms. One-fourth of the previous day's dose is likely to suffice. (It is a violation of federal law, however, to prescribe opiates to relieve abstinence symptoms except as "emergency" treatment for hospitalized patients or in federally approved drug-treatment programs.) Claims that clonidine suppresses opiate withdrawal symptoms are intriguing, but its use at the present time should be considered experimental.

Withdrawal symptoms in newborns of opiate-dependent mothers (including those receiving methadone maintenance) can be severe or even fatal, with irritability, tremor, jitteriness, muscle hypertonia, hyperreflexia, screaming, sneezing, yawning, lacrimation, tachypnea, tachycardia, poor food intake but frantic fist-sucking, vomiting, diarrhea, and myoclonus or convulsions (although seizures may be secondary to other agents such as barbiturates). Mortality is as high as 90 percent without treatment, and symptoms resemble those associated with neonatal hypoglycemia, hypocalcemia, intracranial hemorrhage, sepsis, or meningitis, any of which may coexist. Data are lacking that would enable one to select confidently among currently recommended treatments, which include barbiturates, benzodiazepines, phenothiazines, paregoric, and methadone, but the clinical experience at Harlem Hospital, as well as considerations of cross-tolerance, have made opiates our agents of choice. Phenobarbital is most useful when there has been prenatal exposure to multiple drugs.

AMPHETAMINES

Oral amphetamine abusers include truck drivers, students, and housewives; street preparations may be used orally or parenterally (Table 2). Either route can produce marked psychic dependence and tolerance, and intravenous amphetamine users may take hundreds of milligrams daily. During "runs"—several days of repeated parenteral administration—subjects are continuously awake and may experience a variety of mental effects, including a sense of profundity, rapid mood changes, paranoia, and frank psychosis with auditory and visual hallucinations. Violent behavior can lead to homicide. Abnormal movements include bruxism, stereotypic activity (e.g. stringing beads), tremor, dystonia, and choreoathetosis. More acute overdose causes excitement, confusion, chest pain, hypertension, tachycardia, sweating, and mydriasis, and then delirium, hallucinations, tachypnea, cardiac arrhythmia, fever (sometimes over 109°F), seizures, coma, shock, and death. Myoglobinuria, disseminated intravascular coagulation, and intracranial hemorrhage can occur.

Treatment of acute amphetamine overdose includes temperature control and fluid replacement. Urinary acidification enhances drug excretion, which is markedly reduced when the urine is alkaline. Alpha-adrenergic blockers or nitrites may be necessary for severe hypertension. If both mental disturbance and seizures are present, treatment should be directed at whichever is con-

TABLE 2 Amphetamines and Related Agents

Amphetamine (Benzedrine)
Dextroamphetamine (Dexedrine)
Methamphetamine (Methedrine, Desoxyn, Fetamin, "speed")
Ephedrine
Phenmetrazine (Preludin)
Methylphenidate (Ritalin)
Pemoline (Cylert)
Diethylpropion (Tenuate, Tepanil)
Benzphetamine (Didrex)
Chlorphentermine (Pre-Sate)
Phendimetrazine (Plegine)
Phentermine (Ionamin, Wilpo)
Phenylpropanolamine (Propadrine, and in decongestants, e.g., Ornade, Comtrex, and in diet pills, e.g., Dex-a-Diet, Dexatrim, Maxi-Slim, Vita-Slim)
Propylhexedrine (Benzedrex)
Tuaminoheptane (Tuamine)
Naphazoline (Privine)
Tetrahydrozoline (Tyzine)
Oxymetazoline (Afrin)
Xylometazoline (Otrivin)
Cyclopentamine (Clopane)
Fenfluramine (Pondimin)

sidered the major problem. Phenothiazines and haloperidol dampen psychosis or delirium, but lower seizure threshold. Barbiturates, however, can aggravate delirium.

Amphetamines produce physical as well as psychic dependence. "Runs" of parenteral use are followed by sleep, sometimes lasting several days, and on awakening there is hunger, lethargy, and depression. Withdrawal from more prolonged use is followed by similar symptoms. Although they are not directly life-threatening, suicidal depression can last for weeks, necessitating hospitalization and treatment with tricyclic antidepressants. It is unusual for the toxic paranoid psychosis to persist after the drug is stopped.

COCAINE

Although active orally, cocaine (as hydrochloride) is usually administered nasally or parenterally; as "free base" it can be smoked, with considerable potential for addiction. Low doses of cocaine slow the heart rate; higher doses can cause tachycardia, tachypnea, fever, hypertension, skin pallor, mydriasis, headache, vomiting, vertigo, cold sweats, tremor, bruxism, stereotypic movements, hyperreflexia, myoclonus, convulsions, cardiac arrhythmia, and pulmonary edema. Seizures can occur without other signs of toxicity. Anxiety, confusion, paranoia, and hallucinatory psychosis are common. Death may follow coma and respiratory arrest and has occurred within minutes of administration, probably from cardiac arrhythmia or anaphylaxis. Psychosis can cause accidental death or suicide.

Treatment of overdose may require ventilatory or blood pressure support and cardiac monitoring. Dangerous hypertension is less common than with amphetamines, but may require attention. Urinary acidification accelerates drug excretion, but metabolic acidosis may already be severe enough to warrant bicarbonate. Data are limited on the relative merits of phenothiazines, (which are antidopaminergic, sedative, and antihyperthermic) and benzodiazepines (which are sedative and anticonvulsant). If seizures occur, diazepam would be preferred; if psy chosis, delirium, abnormal movements, or fever are present, chlorpromazine could be given. Claims for the efficacy of propranolol have not been confirmed in clinical trials. Reports of benefit from tricyclic antidepressants and calcium channel blockers are promising, but these agents should be considered experimental at this time. Recovery from cocaine intoxication usually occurs within a few hours and is complete unless there has been hypoxic-ischemic brain damage.

As with amphetamines, there seems to be tolerance for cocaine's euphoriant and cardiovascular effects (including lethality); however, "reverse tolerance" may exist for psychosis. Whether physical dependence occurs is controversial; in any case, depression appears to be the only withdrawal symptom requiring medical attention.

BARBITURATES AND OTHER SEDATIVES

Sedative drugs can be divided into the barbiturates, the nonbarbiturate hypnotics, and the benzodiazepines (Tables 3 and 4). Differing in many of their properties, they nonetheless resemble ethanol (with which they are partially cross-tolerant) in their sedative effects and withdrawal symptoms.

Barbiturate poisoning is most often from a suicide attempt or from accidental ingestion by children. Addicts usually take short-acting agents orally or parenterally. Although tolerance develops rapidly, in contrast to opiates or amphetamines, there is less increase in the lethal dose, and severe symptoms can therefore follow small increments in dosage. Ethanol, moreover, can greatly aggravate the effects of barbiturates.

Overdose causes coma and altered respirations, which may be rapid and shallow, of the Cheyne-Stokes type, or

TABLE 3 Barbiturates Commercially Available in the United States

Amobarbital (Amytal, and in Tuinal)
Aprobarbital (Alurate)
Barbital (in Plexonal)
Butabarbital (Butisol)
Butalbital (Sandoptal, and in mixtures, e.g., Amaphen, Fiorinal, Plexonal, Repan)
Hexobarbital (Sombulex)
Mephobarbital (Mebaral)
Metharbital (Gemonil)
Methohexital (Brevital)
Pentobarbital (Nembutal, and in Carbrital)
Phenobarbital (Luminal, etc., and in mixtures, e.g., Donnatal)
Secobarbital (Seconal, and in Tuinal)
Talbutal (Lotusate)
Thiamylal (Surital)
Thiopental (Pentolhal)

TABLE 4 Nonbarbiturate Sedatives and Tranquilizers

Benzodiazepines
- Alprazolam (Xanax)
- Bromazepam (Lectopam)
- Chlorazepate (Tranxene)
- Chlordiazepoxide (Librium)
- Diazepam (Valium)
- Flunitriazepam (Rohypnol)
- Flurazepam (Dalmane)
- Halazepam (Paxipam)
- Lorazepam (Ativan)
- Nitrazepam (Mogadon)
- Oxazepam (Serax)
- Oxazolam (Serenal)
- Prazepam (Verstran, Centrax)
- Temazepam (Cerepax, Levanxol)
- Triazolam (Halcion)

Others
- Bromide
- Carisoprodal (Soma)
- Chloral betaine (Beta-Chlor)
- Chloral hydrate (Noctec)
- Chlormezanone (Trancopal)
- Ethchlorvynol (Placidyl)
- Ethinamate (Valmid)
- Glutethimide (Doriden)
- Hydroxyzine (Atarax, Vistaril)
- Meprobamate (Miltown, Equanil)
- Methaqualone (Quaalude, Sopor)
- Methyprylon (Noludar)
- Paraldehyde
- Triclofos (Triclos)

slow, progressing to apnea. Hypotension may be secondary to hypoxia or, less often, medullary depression and peripheral drug effect. Treatment begins with respiratory support, including an oropharyngeal airway or endotracheal intubation and oxygen. If only a few hours have elapsed since ingestion, emesis is induced in patients still awake (syrup of ipecac or apomorphine followed by naloxone), and gastric lavage is performed in those who are comatose. (When bowel hypotonicity is present, considerable drug may remain in the stomach.) Activated charcoal and a cathartic are then given. Hypotension usually responds to artificial ventilation and oxygen, but sometimes blood pressure support with volume expansion or pressors (e.g., dopamine) and correction of metabolic acidosis are necessary. For long-acting barbiturates (e.g., phenobarbital) forced diuresis with mannitol (8 to 14 liters daily) and urinary alkalinization are of benefit. If shock has caused anuria, dialysis can be employed. Hemodialysis works faster than peritoneal dialysis and is more effective for long-acting agents. Central nervous system (CNS) stimulant drugs are contraindicated.

Physical dependence on barbiturates produces a severe, sometimes lethal, withdrawal syndrome that resembles withdrawal from ethanol. Within hours of stopping short-acting agents, the following occur: insomnia, anxiety, tremor, hyperreflexia, weakness, anorexia, nausea, vomiting, abdominal cramps, mydriasis, postural hypotension, tachypnea, and tachycardia. Hallucinations occur, more often auditory than visual, and last days or weeks. Seizures are most likely to occur on the second or third day. Beginning on the second to the fifth day there may be symptoms resembling delirium tremens, with confusion, disorientation, agitation, delusions, hallucinations, hyperthermia, and cardiovascular collapse. Severe symptoms can last weeks.

Mild barbiturate withdrawal symptoms can be prevented or treated with short-acting barbiturates (e.g., pentobarbital), 200 to 400 mg orally every 4 to 6 hours, until there are signs of mild intoxication (nystagmus, ataxia, or dysarthria). After 2 to 3 days at this dose, the drug is tapered by 100 mg daily or less, with resumption of a higher dosage should abstinence symptoms occur. If the initial 200-mg dose produces gross signs of intoxication, physical dependence is unlikely.

Seizures (which may be single, clustered, or status epilepticus) are treated with phenobarbital; higher than usual dosage may be required. As with ethanol-related seizures, additional epileptogenic pathology (e.g., meningitis or cerebral trauma), may be present. Hallucinations can be treated with pentobarbital; phenothiazines or haloperidol, which lower seizure threshold, should be avoided.

Delirium tremens is a medical emergency, and symptoms are not rapidly reversed simply by giving barbiturates. Either short-acting agents or phenobarbital, often in very high dosage, are appropriate sedatives. Fever, either from infection or as a sign of withdrawal itself, may require antipyretics, sponging, or a cooling blanket. Strict attention must be paid to fluid and electrolyte balance, and there may be considerable cardiovascular instability. An intensive care unit is the appropriate setting for such patients.

A neonatal barbiturate withdrawal syndrome resembles that of opiate abstinence, but usually occurs several days after delivery and can last months. It is treated with titrated doses of phenobarbital.

The abuse potential of benzodiazepines is less than that of barbiturates, but illicit use does occur, and emergency room treatment for overdose, especially involving diazepam, is common. Symptoms, which are often aggravated by other agents (especially ethanol), are infrequently severe, and treatment is similar to that of barbiturate overdose. Mild abstinence symptoms can sometimes follow even standard therapeutic doses of benzodiazepines. We have not encountered a severe withdrawal syndrome at Harlem Hospital from these agents.

Nonbarbiturate sedatives also produce coma and respiratory depression in overdose and anxiety, tremor, seizures, or delirium on withdrawal. In addition, they can produce a variety of symptoms not encountered with barbiturates. Methaqualone poisoning causes delirium, hallucinations, myoclonus, seizures, papilledema, congestive heart failure, and elevated prothrombin time with bleeding. Glutethimide and methyprylon are less likely than barbiturates to produce severe respiratory depression, but they sometimes cause more severe circulatory failure. Glutethimide poisoning causes fever, muscle spasms, seizures, dilated unreactive pupils, ileus, atonic bladder, and prolonged coma of fluctuating depth. Ethchlorvynol overdose can cause deep and prolonged coma, hypotension, and pulmonary edema. With meprobamate poisoning there is a tendency to relapse after apparent reversal from coma. Paraldehyde causes metabolic acidosis, hemorrhagic gastritis, and pulmonary damage. Acute chloral hydrate intoxication can cause pinpoint pupils. Bromide salts cause a skin rash in one-third of intoxicated subjects; to be remembered is that if laboratory "chloride" determinations actually measure total halide, serum levels may seem normal in patients poisoned by bromides.

Treatment of overdose by these agents follows the same principles as with barbiturates. Recent literature has recommended exchange transfusion and hemoperfusion with activated charcoal or Amberlite resin for ethchlorvynol poisoning. We have not encountered such patients. Treatment of bromide intoxication includes sodium chloride, 2 g three times daily, plus diuresis.

PHENCYCLIDINE

By the mid-1970s abuse of phencyclidine ("PCP," "angel dust") had become epidemic across the United States. It can be eaten, snorted, or injected but is most often smoked (sprinkled on tobacco or marijuana), and it is commonly misrepresented as or mixed with other drugs such as marijuana, amphetamine, or LSD. Most users take other drugs as well, including ethanol.

Low doses cause euphoria or dysphoria, emotional lability, a sense of numbness, and sensory distortions. At moderate doses there is often confusion, agitation, bizarre behavior, synesthesias, and analgesia. Higher doses produce psychosis, often resembling stuporous or excited catatonia or paranoid schizophrenia with auditory hallucinations. There is also fever, flushing, sweating, hypertension, miosis, hypersalivation, vertigo, ataxia, myoclonus, burstlike horizontal and vertical nystagmus, and, at anesthetic doses, seizures (including status epilepticus), coma with extensor posturing, respiratory depression, and hypotension. Myoglobin can cause anuria, and liver necrosis has followed malignant hyperthermia. Death may be the result of direct overdose, accidents, violence, or suicide. Recovery can take days, during which time mild stimuli can provoke agitated or psychotic behavior.

Treatment includes diuresis and urinary acidification (unless myoglobinuria is present.) Gastroenteric recirculation makes continuous gastric suctioning particularly useful. Frequent oropharyngeal suctioning is needed for hypersalivation, and there may be need for treatment of respiratory depression or hyperthermia. Hypertension (which can appear days after phencyclidine intake and has caused intracerebral hemorrhage) may require powerful agents such as diazoxide. Seizures can be treated with diazepam or phenytoin.

Delirium and psychosis may be present from the outset or emerge as a patient awakens from coma. "Talking down" is ineffectual, and the use of sedatives or antipsychotics poses dilemmas. Intramuscular chlordiazepoxide and diazepam are unreliably absorbed, and it is difficult to give intravenous drugs to a violent patient. Diazepam, moreover, may prolong phencyclidine's half-life, and sedatives can aggravate phencyclidine's depressant actions, including respiratory depression. On the other hand, phenothiazines and haloperidol lower seizure threshold and can potentiate hypotension or cause a malignant neuroleptic syndrome with exacerbation of myoglobinuria. The anticholinergic action of some phenothiazines can aggravate delirium. It is our practice to give diazepam intramuscularly and to use haloperidol for patients who fail to respond and in whom neither myoglobinuria, hypotension, nor seizures are present. On theoretical grounds, lorazepam, with its more reliable intramuscular absorption, would be a preferred benzodiazepine, but this drug lacks FDA approval for this purpose. We have not had occasion to try propranolol, which has been recommended for signs of "adrenergic crisis."

Symptoms of phencyclidine overdose usually last hours to days, but in some patients psychosis requiring neuroleptics (or psychosis resistant to these agents) can last several weeks.

Tolerance develops to phencyclidine's effects, but although craving occurs with abstinence, physical dependence and withdrawal symptoms have not been reported. Newborns of phencyclidine-abusing mothers have had jitteriness, hypertonicity, vomiting, and diarrhea.

MARIJUANA

Despite the diverse effects of marijuana's cannabinoid compounds—euphoriant, sedative, bronchodilator, convulsant, anticonvulsant, hyperthermic, hypothermic, analgesic—and the fact that it is the most widely used illicit drug in the United States, acute adverse effects are infrequent, and fatal overdose has never been convincingly described. (Marijuana users are, to be sure, overrepresented in traffic fatalities.) High doses cause auditory or visual illusions or hallucinations, confusion, anxiety, and psychotic depression or excitement, and conventional doses can cause confusion, paranoia, delusions, depression, or panic ("freaking out"). There are also "flashbacks," the spontaneous experience weeks or months after using marijuana of hallucinations or other feelings associated with the original use. These adverse reactions usually last a few hours and can be managed with calm reassurance. When they are severe, diazepam or a short-acting barbiturate may be beneficial. Unusual reactions to marijuana may result from contamination of the street product with other agents (e.g. phencyclidine,) or from additive or synergistic effects with another agent such as ethanol.

Tolerance develops to marijuana's cardiovascular, motor, and perhaps depressant behavioral effects; there may be "reverse tolerance" for excitement or psychosis. Psychological dependence to the point of addiction is common, but whether or not physical dependence occurs is uncertain. The symptoms that follow abrupt withdrawal—jitteriness, anorexia, headache, and mild gastrointestinal upset—are unlikely to require medical attention.

HALLUCINOGENS

Although the popularity of *d*-lysergic acid diethylamide (LSD) has waned in the United States, extensive use of this and other hallucinogens continues (Table 5). Most

TABLE 5 Hallucinogens Abused in the United States

Mescaline (peyote cactus)
Psilocybin and psilocin (*Psilocybe mexicana* mushroom)
d-Lysergic acid diethylamide (LSD)
Dimethyltryptamine (DMT)
Diethyltryptamine (DET)
Dimethoxymethylamphetamine (DOM, "STP")
Dimethoxyethylamphetamine (DOET)
Methylenedioxyamphetamine
d-Lysergic acid amide (morning glory seeds)
Myristicin (nutmeg)
Nepetalactone (catnip)

of these agents produce indistinguishable symptoms and are cross-tolerant with one another.

LSD's effects are dose-related and include, in addition to often gaudy illusions and hallucinations, autonomic signs (hyperthermia, piloerection, pupillary dilatation with preserved light reflex, hypertension, and tachycardia), but it is the psychiatric symptoms that pose potential danger. Derealization, depersonalization, autism, or mystical elation can lead to accidents or self-injury, and "bad trips," with marked paranoia or panic, can cause homicide or suicide. Such symptoms usually clear within 24 hours and can be managed with "talking down." Benzodiazepines can be given to unmanageable patients; phenothiazines, which can paradoxically exacerbate symptoms, should be avoided. LSD "flashbacks," the spontaneous recurrence of LSD symptoms without taking the drug, may cause considerable anxiety, which is managed in a similar fashion as treatment of acute overdose or adverse reactions. Death directly attributable to LSD had not been described. Although tolerance develops to LSD's effects, there seems to be no physical dependence or abstinence syndrome.

INHALANTS

Sniffing volatile substances to achieve euphoria is very common among American children. Although a wide variety of agents are used, many with multiple constituents (Table 6), their acute effects, including toxicity, are remarkably similar. Substances are usually sniffed from a saturated rag, a plastic bag, directly from a container, or from a heated frying pan, sometimes for hours at a time daily over years. Moderate doses produce euphoria and ataxia resembling ethanol intoxication, with a similar propensity to accidents or violence. Higher doses cause psychosis with delusions and hallucinations, as well as cyanosis, seizures, and coma. Death has followed aspiration of vomitus and suffocation by plastic bags; death has also occurred suddenly without apparent cause, perhaps secondary to cardiac arrhythmia. Respiratory depression can also occur. Acute lead encephalopathy has followed gasoline sniffing, and fatal brain anoxia has occurred in nitrous oxide abusers. Butyl nitrite sniffing causes methemoglobinemia, but syncope tends to prevent inhalation of a life-threatening amount.

TABLE 6 Substances Commonly Abused as Inhalants

Aerosols (refrigerants, frying pan sprays, antitussives, bronchodilators, deodorants, hair sprays, shampoos, antiseptics)
Lacquers, paints, enamels, and lacquer and paint thinners
Lighter fluids
Fingernail polish removers
Cleaning fluids (spots, shoes, wigs)
Airplane model cements
Furniture polishes
Household cements
Plastic (polystyrene) cements
Rubber, tire-patching, or tube repair cements
Gasoline
Anesthetics (ether, nitrous oxide, halothane, trichlorethylene)
"Room fresheners" (nitrites)

Acute effects of inhalants usually last minutes to hours. Treatment in most instances is simply supportive. Although tolerance develops, a withdrawal syndrome has not been described.

ANTICHOLINERGICS

Anticholinergic abuse in the United States includes ingestion of seeds of *Datura stramoni* ("jimson week," a plant found in most states), antiasthmatic inhalators (e.g., "Asthmador"), antiparkinsonian anticholinergics, and tricyclic antidepressants, especially amitriptyline. Symptoms and signs include suphoria, excitement, delirium, hallucinations, dilated unreactive pupils, dysphagia, urinary retention, dry flushed skin, high fever, hypertension, tachypnea, and tachycardia. There may be nystagmus, hyperreflexia, myoclonus, convulsions, extensor posturing, coma, respiratory failure, circulatory collapse, and death. Delusions and hallucinations, which may be prominent during recovery, can lead to fatal accidents.

Symptoms last hours to days. Gastric lavage is given even if ingestion occurred many hours earlier, as anticholinergics decrease gastrointestinal motility. Physostigmine, 1 to 3 mg IV, is given as needed at 30-minute to 2-hour intervals. Fever may require aspirin, sponging, a cooling blanket, or bypass cooling. Further treatment includes fluid administration, bladder catheterization, and, as needed, anticonvulsants. Phenothiazines, which have anticholinergic actions, are contraindicated. Sedatives, if given at all, should be used with caution.

ACUTE INFLAMMATORY POLYNEUROPATHY

JERRY S. WOLINSKY, M.D.

GUILLAIN-BARRÉ SYNDROME

Acute inflammatory polyneuropathy, or as it is more commonly called, the Guillain-Barré syndrome (GBS), is an acutely or subacutely evolving symmetrical demyelinative polyneuropathy of unknown but presumed autoimmune etiology. Although uncommon, it is presently the most frequent cause of rapid-onset generalized motor paralysis in industrialized nations. The majority of cases progress from first neurologic symptoms to maximum weakness within 4 weeks and are usually readily differentiated from other illnesses with similar features on the basis of both clinical and laboratory findings. Cases that evolve more slowly are likely to have a different etiology or to represent initial presentations of the closely related chronic relapsing inflammatory demyelinative polyneuropathy (CRIDP). The potential for precipitous progression of weakness to respiratory failure, the propensity for complete resolution of the neurologic deficit, and the recent advances in therapy have converged to make accurate diagnosis and early institution of treatment mandatory.

When considering management, it may be useful to construct an idealized representation of the natural history of acute GBS. The majority of patients recall symptoms of upper respiratory tract infection or gastrointestinal illness 2 or 3 weeks prior to the onset of the first neurologic symptoms. Distal paresthesia or musculoskeletal pain, especially low back pain, are prominent harbingers, soon overshadowed by early symptoms of motor weakness. Symptoms increase in severity, causing the patient to seek medical attention within the initial week of symptoms of the neurologic disease.

The proportion of GBS victims whose disorder proves severe enough to require hospitalization is difficult to estimate from the literature, but is likely to include the majority of all cases that meet ad hoc NINCDS committee diagnostic criteria. Most patients reach the greatest degree of weakness within 2 or 3 weeks of hospitalization, and about 30 percent of all hospitalized patients will develop respiratory compromise sufficient to require ventilatory support. The duration of maximal disability varies remarkably among cases, but generally is most prolonged for the elderly and those who progress to bulbar involvement or respiratory compromise. On average, patients who progress to require respiratory support will be ventilator dependent for 3 to 7 weeks.

Once improvement begins, it is usually sustained; only rare GBS patients experience relapse in the absence of another intercurrent illness. When substantial fluctuation in neurologic status occurs, the diagnosis is probably CRIDP. The recovery phase can be prolonged, but half of all patients can be expected to regain the ability to walk unassisted within 3 months. Less than 5 percent of hospitalized patients die of GBS or its complications, and 85 percent or more of survivors will have a satisfactory return of function.

Symptomatic Management

The idealized outcome described above presupposes optimal symptomatic management by an experienced multidisciplinary team. When confronted with a possible GBS patient, decision-making should err on the side of a worst case analysis until the sequence of evolving events proves otherwise. The first critical care decision arises when the diagnosis of GBS is initially considered. Most patients require hospital admission for monitoring on a general care unit until the tempo of their individual disease progression is fully apparent. The rapidity with which motor weakness, including respiratory failure, can ensue must never be underestimated. Furthermore, the facility chosen for initial admission of any patient with probable GBS should as a minimum have a fully staffed intensive care unit. When this is unavailable, arrangements for transfer of the patient with progressing GBS should be completed as soon as feasible, with due precaution to provide for mechanical respiratory support in transit.

The next issues confronted are the level of care to be assigned and development of an initial data base. This problem is simplified for the patient whose weakness is progressing and whose vital capacity is at or below 25 ml per kilogram; an intensive care unit is mandatory. Most hospitals make placement of GBS patients whose respiratory status is not yet significantly impaired more problematic. Until progressing weakness has been clearly documented to have been arrested for at least 72 hours, patients should not be assigned to private or semi-private rooms, where they receive infrequent direct monitoring by the nursing and medical staff. Intermediate care units, where more frequent monitoring is assured, are preferable in this setting. Baseline studies must include a chest radiograph, electrolytes, electrocardiogram, and accurate vital capacity determination in addition to other studies deemed necessary based on the appropriate differential diagnosis for a given patient and his particular medical history. Early electrodiagnostic studies are likely to be nonsupportive of the diagnosis during the first 7 to 10 days of hospitalization, although somatosensory evoked potentials may confirm the presence of proximal conduction delays somewhat sooner. Similarly, early examination of the cerebrospinal fluid is more helpful in excluding other conditions than in directly supporting the diagnosis of GBS. The remaining initial approach to the GBS patient will vary, depending on the extent of weakness on presentation.

Monitoring the patient requires at least daily or more frequent neurologic examinations combined with accurate vital capacity or, alternatively, maximum negative inspiratory pressure measurements obtained at least every 4 to 6 hours. The patient must be informed about the possible extent of weakness that may ensue and be appropriately limited in unaided ambulation, since he may injure himself in attempting to move without help, even though he was able to do this only a few hours previously. Furthermore, educating the patient and his family about GBS, its usual course, treatment plans and favorable expected long-term outcome facilitates patient management.

Once the patient becomes bedbound, additional prophylactic measures should be instituted to minimize potential complications. These include elastic hose and subcutaneous administration of 5,000 units of heparin twice daily to reduce the incidence of deep vein thrombosis and pulmonary embolism. As motor movement is further restricted, every attempt should be made to prevent pressure injury to the skin or already compromised peripheral nerves. Appropriate measures include the use of alternating air mattress beds, frequent repositioning of the patient, egg crate footwear, and protective padding at other bony prominences. Passive physical therapy and splints to maintain position of function and prevent contractures should be initiated early.

As the patient becomes increasingly dependent on nursing personnel for his every need, it becomes important to provide some form of signaling device that utilizes his remaining motor functions. This allows the patient some residual sense of control and is an important psychological support. An unchanging medical care team, particularly primary nursing personnel, will ease some of the patient's anxiety and generally provides more empathic and effective care. The fully conscious patient who requires extended high-level attention in a critical care unit is unusual and presents additional challenges to unit personnel.

Because of the parallel between autonomic nervous system dysfunction and motor and especially bulbar weakness, continuous cardiac monitoring should be established at this junction, if not previously. Autonomic dysfunction is common, especially among more severely affected patients. Substantial fluctuation of heart rate or rhythm may require pharmacologic intervention and rarely the temporary insertion of a transvenous cardiac pacemaker. Management of hypertension should be judicious and preferably with short-acting agents, as spontaneous alteration of blood pressure can be both marked and unpredictable. Hypotension can often be managed with positional changes or the judicious use of volume expansion.

Pain can complicate any phase of GBS. When simple analgesic agents fail, morphine or synthetic analogs of morphine given on a fixed dosage schedule may be indicated. During the recovery phase some patients will experience prolonged painful dysesthesia that may respond to carbamazepine.

Respiratory Assistance

When to intubate often engenders considerable debate. Ideally, intubation should be performed electively rather than emergently. Intubation performed when blood gas status is deteriorating reflects inappropriate patient management. Recent series show a reduction in the frequency of basal atelectasis, pulmonary collapse or consolidation, and severe bronchopneumonia if intubation and assisted respiration are initiated when the vital capacity remains above 20 to 25 ml per kilogram. Even earlier intubation is indicated when an inadequate cough or aspiration pneumonia develops.

Respiratory failure with GBS can be sudden. Fatigue frequently compounds motor weakness. Thus, the slope of the prior gradual decline in vital capacity often fails to predict the sudden need for assisted respiration. Increased anxiety unexplained by clinical events or arterial carbon dioxide retention often precedes respiratory failure. These factors argue for early intubation to assure that the procedure can be done by an expert. Using an aggressive approach, a few patients will be intubated for a short interval of several days. In retrospect for some of these patients the procedure may not have been needed. However, overall morbidity for most GBS patients should be reduced if early intubation is performed.

With an appropriately sized and placed nasotracheal or endotracheal tube, tracheotomy can be safely deferred for 2 to 3 weeks. Many patients are thus spared tracheostomy. When necessary, tracheostomy should be performed as an elective procedure under optimal conditions on a fully prepared patient. Frequent clinical pulmonary evaluation supplemented by arterial blood gas determinations and chest radiographs should be used for the detection and treatment of pneumonia and mucous plugs. When to extubate should be a joint decision of the medical care team. Patients should show sustained arrest of progression of weakness, an improved ventilatory profile, and documented tolerance to increasing intervals on a Briggs adapter (T-piece) prior to extubation. Intermittent position pressure therapy may be useful in weaning selected patients from mechanical ventilation.

Specific Therapy

Until recently no clearly established therapy existed to modify the natural course of GBS. Various preparations of corticosteroids have been used, but several studies strongly suggest that prednisone or other corticosteroids are associated with a prolonged hospital course and possibly greater residual neurologic deficit. While this form of therapy finds support in cases of CRIDP, its use in acute inflammatory polyneuropathies appears contraindicated.

At least three controlled studies have now shown that the course of GBS is substantially shortened by early plasma exchange therapy. Initiation of plasma exchange within the first 2 to 3 weeks of neurologic symptoms reduces the time required to achieve functionally important motor recovery, shortens the duration of ventilator dependence, and substantially reduces the duration of acute hospital care. Patients in these studies had weakness severe enough to impair walking markedly by the time plasmapheresis was started. However, it is likely that exchange therapy would be preferable for rapidly evolving GBS at even earlier stages. The procedure is not without risk and is therefore inappropriate for patients with modest involvement. If considered, facilities to administer plasma exchange must be available within the intensive care unit to allow careful monitoring of the patient throughout the exchange.

The details of the exchange vary with the equipment used and the choice of replacement fluids. Each plasmapheresis should target on an exchange of 40 to 50 ml per kilogram, with sessions scheduled not more frequently than every other day to achieve a cumulative plasma exchange of 200 to 250 ml per kilogram. Salt-poor albumin and crystalloid are expensive, although perhaps somewhat preferable replacement solutions, compared with solutions that use plasma as a source of colloid. A major problem associated with this approach is continued venous access. Placement of indwelling catheters into the subclavian or femoral veins is almost always required to maintain adequate flow rates during exchanges. A significant portion of the morbidity of plasma exchange can be ascribed to the placement and maintenance of these lines.

Pregnancy

GBS occurs with increased frequency during pregnancy. While GBS has no clear adverse effects on the fetus, the pregnant state may complicate treatment. In the later stages of pregnancy the bulk of the fetus and placenta can lead to more rapid respiratory failure than might otherwise be anticipated. Similarly, considerable care must be given to positioning and frequent repositioning of the mother to prevent compression of the lumbar plexus and deep venous return. Plasma exchange can be carried out safely when indicated, but carries the additional risk of inducing labor. Monitoring of the fetal heart rate is probably indicated during such therapy, especially as inadvertent volume contraction of the mother during the exchange could potentially jeopardize the fetus. Early termination of pregnancy does not appear to alter the matural history of GBS.

CHRONIC RELAPSING INFLAMMATORY DEMYELINATIVE POLYNEUROPATHY

CRIDP is much more readily diagnosed when the patient has had a prior documented episode of motor weakness or sensory impairment reasonably attributable to peripheral nerve dysfunction. However, certain features may help to distinguish acute from chronic forms of GBS during the later phases of the initial episode. CRIDP is more likely to have a slower and less predictable mode of onset, to progress less often to respiratory compromise, and to be associated with greater fluctuations in functional impairment. That is, any improvement in function is less likely to be sustained.

The distinction between GBS and CRIDP becomes important at the time when treatment of these related syndromes begins to diverge. Half to three-quarters of all patients with CRIDP initially appear to respond favorably to plasma exchange, but this improvement often proves to be plasmapheresis dependent. Immunosuppression is usually then required to control the process. Chronic administration of oral prednisone, azathioprine, or cyclophosphamide can be started, and all three agents have their proponents. Whichever of these agents is used, withdrawal of immunosuppressive therapy following clinical arrest of the process must be done gradually to avoid the return of symptoms.

CHRONIC NONINFLAMMATORY POLYNEUROPATHY

JAMES G. McLEOD, M.D.

Chronic noninflammatory polyneuropathy is defined here as a condition that includes all patients with chronic polyneuropathy with symptoms for more than 1 year, but excludes patients with leprosy or chronic inflammatory demyelinating polyradiculoneuropathy. There are a wide range of etiologic factors to be considered in chronic noninflammatory polyneuropathy, including genetically determined disorders, alcohol and nutritional deficiencies, diabetes and other metabolic and endocrine disorders, malignancy, paraproteinemias and dysproteinemias, drugs, heavy metals and industrial agents, connective tissue disorders, and vasculitis. The clinical features of the neuropathy may suggest an underlying cause. Laboratory investigations for all patients should include urinalysis, complete blood count, erythrocyte sedimentation rate, fasting blood glucose, serum electrolytes, serum creatinine,serum proteins and plasma electrophoresis, liver function tests, and chest radiographs. Other investigations may be indicated when specific disorders are suspected, including determination of urinary porphyrins, of heavy metals, and cryoglobulins, radiologic skeletal survey and bone scan, fecal fats and other tests of malabsorption, thyroid function studies, serum vitamin B_{12} and folate levels, urinary Bence-Jones protein, bone marrow biopsy, and radiologic and endoscopic investigation of the upper and lower gastrointestinal tract. Biopsies of enlarged lymph nodes and liver may be indicated, as may rectal and renal biopsy for amyloidosis. Nerve conduction studies should be performed to confirm the neuropathic nature of the symptoms. Marked slowing of conduction, suggestive of demyelination, may be seen in genetically determined neuropathies, diabetes, and some cases of neuropathy secondary to carcinoma, lymphoma, and paraproteinemias and dysproteinemias. When all other investigations have been performed, sural nerve biopsy is indicated to establish a diagnosis in some patients.

The treatment of chronic noninflammatory polyneuropathy consists of *general measures* and *specific therapy* for the underlying disease.

GENERAL MEASURES

The diagnosis should be explained to the patient and the likely course of the illness and its prognosis discussed taking into account its effect on the patient's career, social activities, and family.

Motor Disability

Physiotherapy. This is an important part of treatment and should be commenced early in the course of the illness. It is valuable in preserving the range of motion of joints, preventing contractures, maintaining optimal motor function, assisting in the re-education of muscles, and developing muscle strength and endurance.

Occupational Therapy. Use of occupational therapy may help the patient adapt to the disability by developing new skills and, if necessary, new occupations. In more severely disabled patients assistance will be required with the tasks of daily living, and a visit from the occupational therapist will facilitate the installation of appropriate aids in the home. Patients should be referred for occupational therapy if their disease is likely to affect their lifestyle or occupation.

Orthoses. Foot drop is a common problem that can be helped with a light plastic splint. When there is weakness of wrist extension, a light plastic splint to maintain the wrists in a position of extension for optimal function may be necessary. Dynamic assistance in the form of springs or rubber bands to maintain extension of the fingers is sometimes helpful.

Surgery. Tendon transfers and other orthopaedic reconstructive procedures may be considered when there is severe distal muscle wasting and weakness in the upper and lower limbs. In generalized peripheral neuropathies, surgical treatment is rarely indicated, but an orthopaedic opinion should be sought in patients with severe irreversible distal muscle wasting.

Sensory Disturbances

Distal Sensory Loss. In severe sensory neuropathies (particularly the hereditary sensory neuropathies, diabetes, and amyloidosis), the prevention of burns, trauma, and ulceration of anesthetic areas of skin is of major importance. Careful attention to footwear and meticulous care of the feet and toes are essential. Patients should not walk barefoot, and should inspect their shoes daily for foreign bodies and protrusions. If foot ulcers develop, weight bearing should cease until healing occurs, and the ulcer will need to be cleaned and dressed and, if necessary, debrided. Antibiotic therapy is indicated if infections occur.

Pain and Dysesthesias. Pain may be a feature of sensory neuropathies due to different causes, including alcohol abuse and nutritional deficiencies, diabetes, hereditary sensory neuropathy, carcinomatous sensory neuropathy, amyloidosis, cryoglobulinemia, uremia, and multiple myeloma. Treatment is difficult. Some patients obtain relief from bathing the feet and hands in warm or cold water. Drug therapy is generally unsatisfactory. Analgesics such as salicylates and paracetamol (acetaminophen) should be tried initially. Sedation at night, e.g., nitrazepam, 5 to 10 mg may be helpful. Minor tranquilizers, e.g. diazepam, 5 to 10 mg at night and during the day, may sometimes provide relief. Anticonvulsant therapy in doses sufficient to achieve therapeutic blood levels is worthy of trial, particularly for paroxysmal pain. Carbamazepine, commencing at a small dose, e.g. 100 mg daily, and gradually increasing the dosage, is the most effective of these drugs; however, the results are often disappointing and the side effects of drowsiness, ataxia, and nausea usually discourage the patient from continuing. Phenytoin is less effective than carbamazepine. The best relief is usually obtained from the use of tricyclic antidepressants, e.g. amitriptyline, 25 mg at night and 10 mg three times a day, increasing if necessary during the day. A combination of phenothiazines and tricyclic drugs, e.g. fluphenazine, 1 to 2.5 mg and amitriptyline, 10 to 25 mg at bedtime, may be helpful.

Transcutaneous electrical nerve stimulation is worthy of trial in some painful neuropathies. When lower limb pain is intractable, lumbar sympathectomy should be considered.

Autonomic Dysfunction

Postural hypotension may accompany chronic polyneuropathy, particularly that resulting from diabetes and amyloidosis. Treatment with elastic stockings and lower abdominal support and sleeping with the head of the bed raised on 6- to 9-inch blocks are physical measures worthy of trial.

The most effective drug therapy is fludrocortisone, 0.1 mg a day, increasing as required to prevent symptoms of postural hypotension or until the side effects of fluid retention or supine hypertension limit its use.

Restless Legs

In addition to the drugs used in the treatment of painful neuropathy, baclofen may also be helpful occasionally. Treatment should commence with a small dose, e.g., 5 mg daily, and gradually increase with increments of 5 mg every 3 to 4 days.

Tremor

Tremor may be a feature of some peripheral neuropathies, such as Roussy-Lévy syndrome, neuropathy associated with IgM kappa paraproteinemia, diabetes, and uremia. Some patients respond to propranolol, 40 mg three times a day.

SPECIFIC THERAPY

Specific therapy is available for many causes of chronic noninflammatory polyneuropathy (Table 1).

Genetically Determined Neuropathies

Genetically determined neuropathies represent about 30 to 40 percent of cases of chronic polyneuropathy. They include Charcot-Marie-Tooth disease (hereditary motor and sensory neuropathies [HMSN] types I and II), Dejerine-Sottas disease (HMSN type III), Refsum's disease (HMSN type IV), the leukodystrophies, hereditary amyloid neuropathy, porphyria, analphalipoproteinemia, abetalipoproteinemia, giant axonal neuropathy, and ataxia-telangiectasia. Peripheral neuropathy is also associated with the spinocerebellar degenerations, especially Friedreich's ataxia.

Patients with Refsum's disease should be treated with a low phytanic acid diet, and plasma exchange may sometimes be helpful if rapid deterioration occurs. In patients with porphyria the administration of drugs known to precipitate attacks, e.g., barbiturates, must be avoided. Chlorpromazine may be helpful in controlling pain during acute attacks. Abetalipoproteinemia should be treated with large doses of oral or parenteral vitamin E (100

TABLE 1 Specific Therapy of Chronic Noninflammatory Polyneuropathy

Cause	*Predominant Type of Neuropathy*	*Treatment*
Genetically determined		
Refsum's disease	Mixed sensorimotor	Low phytanic acid diet
Abetalipoproteinemia	Mixed sensorimotor	Vitamin E
Porphyria	Motor and autonomic	Avoid barbiturates and drugs precipitating attacks
Alcohol, nutritional		
Alcoholism	Sensorimotor	Thiamine, avoid alcohol
Vitamin B_{12}	Sensory	Vitamin B_{12}
Folic acid	Sensory	Folic acid
Vitamin E	Sensory	Vitamin E
Endocrine, metabolic		
Diabetes	Mixed sensorimotor	Maintain normal blood glucose levels
Acromegaly	Sensory	Treat pituitary tumor
Hypothyroidism	Sensory	Thyroxine
Uremia	Sensory, sensorimotor	Increase duration of dialysis, renal transplantation
Malignancies		
Carcinoma	Sensory, sensorimotor	Specific treatment for malignancy—surgery, radiotherapy or chemotherapy
Lymphoma	Sensorimotor	
Chronic lymphatic leukemia	Sensorimotor	
Polycythemia vera	Sensory	Venesection (phlebotomy), ^{32}P
Paraproteinemias and dysproteinemias		
Multiple myeloma	Sensorimotor	Chemotherapy, radiotherapy
Macroglobulinemia	Sensorimotor	Cytotoxic drugs, steroids, plasmapheresis
Cryoglobulinemia	Sensorimotor	Avoid cold, cytotoxic drugs, steroids, plasmapheresis
Monoclonal gammopathy	Sensorimotor	Immunosuppressive therapy, plasmapheresis
Vasculitis		
Polyarteritis nodosa, systemic lupus erythematosus, rheumatoid arthritis, Sjögren's syndrome, mixed connective tissue disease	Mononeuritis multiplex, sensorimotor	Steroids, immunosuppressive drugs

mg per kilogram per day), since this has been shown to prevent or reduce the neurologic complications.

Although there is no specific treatment for many of these conditions, an important part of management is exact diagnosis, determination of the type of inheritance, genetic counseling, and discussion of the prognosis and natural course of the disease.

Alcoholic And Nutritional Neuropathies

Alcoholic neuropathy is one of the most common causes of neuropathy in Western countries and is associated with nutritional deficiencies. Specific treatment consists of giving vitamin supplements, especially thiamine and other B vitamins, expert counseling and avoidance of alcohol. Administration of excessive doses of vitamins (megavitamin therapy) should, however, be avoided, as toxicity can occur; pyridoxine overdose may itself cause peripheral neuropathy. Sensory symptoms of nutritional neuropathies may persist in spite of adequate replacement therapy.

Vitamin B_{12}, thiamine, riboflavin, pyridoxine, pantothenic acid, folic acid, and vitamin E deficiencies may be the cause of peripheral neuropathy and sensory symptoms in malabsorption syndromes. Adequate vitamin replacement is essential in these cases.

Endocrine And Metabolic Disorders

Diabetes. Diabetes is one of the most common causes of peripheral neuropathy. Meticulous diabetic control with maintenance of normal blood glucose levels is the most important part of management. Careful foot care is essential. In addition to the general measures for the treatment of painful neuropathy (as discussed), aldose reductase inhibitors may prove effective in some cases.

Acromegaly. A predominantly sensory chronic polyneuropathy may be associated with acromegaly. Some improvement follows specific treatment of the pituitary tumour.

Hypothyroidism. A painful sensory neuropathy may precede the diagnosis of hypothyroidism by many years. Improvement usually follows treatment with thyroxine.

Uremia. A mixed sensorimotor neuropathy, frequently with pain and burning sensations in the feet, occurs commonly in patients undergoing hemodialysis. Increasing the frequency and duration of dialysis may result in improvement, although this is not a universal finding. Rapid improvement, even in patients with long-standing neuropathy, usually follows successful renal transplantation.

Vitamin B_{12} Deficiency. The predominantly sensory neuropathy of vitamin B_{12} deficiency does not always respond to treatment sufficient to cause hematologic remission. Treatment with 1000 μg of vitamin B_{12} every 2 to 4 weeks is recommended, but symptoms of sensory neuropathy frequently respond poorly to treatment and may persist indefinitely.

Malignancy

The peripheral neuropathy of carcinoma, lymphoma, leukemia, and polycythemia vera may sometimes remit following removal of the primary malignancy or chemotherapy for the condition.

Paraproteinemias And Dysproteinemias

Clinical peripheral neuropathy occurs in about 13 percent of patients with multiple myeloma, and there is a high incidence (about 50 percent) in the osteosclerotic type of myeloma. The peripheral neuropathy usually progresses in spite of treatment of the myeloma, although in some patients with a single lesion, improvement has followed radiation therapy.

Macroglobulinemia. Chlorambucil and other cytotoxic drugs, corticosteroids, and plasmapheresis are used in the treatment of macroglobulinemia, but remission of the peripheral neuropathy is unusual.

Cryoglobulinemia. Patients should be advised to avoid cold. There is little evidence that the treatment of the underlying disease with cytotoxic agents, corticosteroids, and plasmapheresis improves the neuropathy.

Monoclonal Gammopathy. Peripheral neuropathy may be associated with IgG, IgA, and IgM paraproteinemias. Improvement may follow the use of plasma exchange and immunosuppressive therapy in some patients.

Vasculitis

Peripheral neuropathy, both mononeuritis multiplex and a chronic symmetrical polyneuropathy, may be associated with the vasculitis of polyarteritis nodosa, systemic lupus erythematosus, rheumatoid arthritis, Sjögren's syndrome, and mixed connective tissue diseases. Treatment with corticosteroid therapy, and if necessary the addition of cytotoxic agents such as azathioprine or cyclophosphamide, is recommended.

Heavy Metals, Drugs, And Other Toxic Agents

The most important part of treatment is diagnosis of the cause and removal of the toxic agent. Specific therapy is not available in most cases. There is little evidence that chelating agents are effective in the treatment of lead, arsenic, mercury, thallium, and gold neuropathy.

Chronic Polyneuropathy Of Undertermined Cause

After intensive investigation the cause of about 20 percent of chronic polyneuropathies remains undetermined. However it is important to follow up and reinvestigate such cases, since a probable etiologic factor may subsequently be revealed in about 20 to 30 percent. These etiologic factors include alcohol, paraproteinemia, malignancy, and connective tissue diseases.

BELL'S PALSY

DAVID A. CHAD, M.D.
DAVID A. DRACHMAN, M.D.

When Sir Charles Bell first described paralysis of the facial nerve, he was concerned with facial nerve mononeuropathy due to any cause. Bell's original description even included facial paralysis due to goring by an ox. Subsequently, the term "Bell's palsy" has been restricted to indicate an *idiopathic* facial nerve paralysis, or at least one in which the cause is not immediately apparent. Although we still do not know the etiology of idiopathic Bell's palsy, a number of other disease processes, both central and peripheral, may mimic this condition. The first step in management is accurate differential diagnosis; only when other known causes have been considered and eliminated can the patient with facial paralysis be regarded as having Bell's palsy and treated accordingly. Second, those patients with a poorer prognosis for complete recovery must be identified and given further treatment as indicated below.

ANATOMIC FEATURES

The facial nerve is comprised of two components, the motor division and the nervus intermedius, which join together in the internal auditory canal. Because Bell's palsy involves the peripheral facial nerve, it is often characterized by clinical features reflecting disturbances in the functions of both components of this nerve. The motor division of the facial nerve supplies all the muscles of facial expression as well as the stapedius, the scalp muscles and platysma, and the buccinator, among others. The neruvs intermedius contains three functionally different types of axons: taste fibers for the anterior two-thirds of the tongue, secretory fibers for salivation and lacrimation, and sensory fibers supplying part of the ear. Clinical tests often try to "localize" lesions along the length of the facial nerve, from the internal auditory canal to the stylomastoid foramen, by the exact combination of visceral and motor findings. We do not believe that this is a reliable observation, since cranial nerve lesions may be incomplete and often occur over some length of the nerve. Nonetheless, the mnemonic "Hear, Tear, Taste, Face" describes the adjacent or integral functions associated with the facial nerve from proximal to distal. Regardless, the finding of combined motor and visceral abnormalities clearly identifies a facial paralysis as being of *peripheral* rather than central origin.

CLINICAL FEATURES

Bell's palsy is the most common disorder of the facial nerve, affecting all age groups. It has an annual incidence of 20 per 100,000 persons and increases in each decade to reach 35 per 100,000 persons after age 60. The onset of Bell's palsy is usually rapid, occurring over hours to (at most) several days. The severity of the paralysis may vary from mild to complete. In some patients weakness may be mild for the first day or so and then progress to total paralysis over the next 48 to 72 hours. In about 60 percent of patients, pain occurs at the onset of paralysis in or around the ear on the paretic side. Other symptoms include diminished taste (in 30 to 50 percent of patients), phonophobia (in 30 percent), disturbed hearing (either increasd or decreased), facial numbness, xerostomia, and xerophthalmia or (more commonly) *increased* tearing. Paralysis is rarely bilateral (in only 0.3 percent of cases), but almost 10 percent of patients have had an episode of previous paralysis. Diabetics and pregnant women are three to four times more likely to develop facial paralysis than the general population. Some 10 to 20 percent of patients give a history of recent upper respiratory tract illness, and 25 percent of patients note that onset of facial weakness was preceded by exposure to cold or drafts.

On *physical examination* the main tasks are:

1. To exclude central disorders, including upper motor neuron and pontine lesions, since strokes and brainstem plaques of multiple sclerosis may be difficult to distinguish.
2. To look for signs of a more generalized radicular or neuropathic process liable to produce facial neuropathy, such as the Guillain-Barré syndrome or diabetes and to search for herpes zoster vesicles.
3. To assess the extent and severity of facial nerve dysfunction, including tearing, taste, and modulation of sound. The degree of facial paralysis is of great importance; almost all patients with *incomplete* paralysis achieve satisfactory recovery, whereas *some* of those with complete paralysis may not.

In many patients with Bell's palsy, careful evaluation discloses hypesthesia or dysesthesia in the territories of the trigenimal nerve, the glossopharyngeal nerve, or both. In about 20 percent of patients, decreased appreciation of light touch is found in the territory of the second cervical dermatome. Weakness of muscles supplied by the vagus nerve is found in approximately 20 percent of patients (deviation of the uvula, rotation of the larynx, vocal cord shortening).

LABORATORY STUDIES

The main purpose of laboratory studies is to make certain that there is no underlying systemic disturbance that might predispose to or cause facial neuropathy. Unless there is concern that facial paralysis is secondary to a cerebellopontine angle or pontine tumor, we do not perform a computerized tomographic (CT) scan of the head. A cerebrospinal fluid examination may be useful to evaluate the possibilities of herpes zoster, chronic meningitis, or leptomeningeal carcinomatosis. Mild protein elevation and slight lymphocytic pleocytosis have been found in patients with otherwise uncomplicated Bell's palsy. We generally order fasting and 2-hour postprandial glucose levels, serum thyroxine determination, complete blood count, and sedimentation rate. A Schirmer test often confirms the observation of excessive (or diminished) tearing with Bell's palsy. If the blink reflex has been impaired, an ophthalmologic examination with fluorescein can reveal any corneal abrasion.

Electrodiagnostic Studies

Electrodiagnostic tests are helpful in assessing the degree of damage to the facial nerve. They are valuable both in determining prognosis and in assessing progression or improvement in the neuropathy. This is especially true for patients with *complete* facial paralysis, since some of these patients will not recover full function spontaneously. A valuable test early in the course of Bell's palsy is the facial nerve conduction study: measurement of the amplitude of the evoked motor response (direct response) 5 to 7 days after onset of Bell's palsy will allow reliable prediction of outcome. If the amplitude on the affected side is 30 percent of normal or greater (normal being the amplitude evoked on the contralateral side), full recovery can be expected within 2 months. If the amplitude is 10 percent of normal or less, recovery, if it occurs, will be prolonged (taking as long as 6 months to 1 year), with a high incidence of sequelae such as contracture and synkinesis. If the amplitude lies somewhere in between (10 to 30 percent of normal), recovery will take from 2 to 8 months and some degree of synkinesis and contracture usually will occur.

The blink reflex can identify conduction block in proximal portions of the facial nerve not otherwise studied by routine methods of conduction. During the first week of Bell's palsy, almost all patients show delay or absence of the blink response (R1) on the paretic side. When serial testing discloses return of the previously absent R1, this demonstrates that recovery of conduction is taking place across the involved facial nerve segment and there is no distal degeneration. Clinical recovery will be good in such circumstances. In a small percentage of patients the direct response is severely diminished in amplitude and the blink response cannot be elicited. This indicates distal nerve degeneration and the likelihood of incomplete recovery.

NATURAL HISTORY

Eighty to 90 percent of patients with Bell's palsy regain good power of the muscles of facial expression. Typically, recovery begins within 8 weeks and reaches its maximum in 9 months to a year; it may begin as early as the second week in patients with incomplete paralysis. Fewer than 15 percent of patients have obvious residual weakness. Almost 80 percent of patients rate their own recovery as 95 percent or better. Factors predicting *good* prognosis are incomplete facial palsy, relative youth (age less than 60), short interval between onset and initial improvement (within 2 weeks), and favorable electrodiagnostic studies. Factors predicting *poor* prognosis are complete paralysis, older age (age greater than 60), long interval between onset and improvement (about 2 months), and unfavorable electrodiagnostic studies. The predictive value of features associated with facial palsies (such as ear pain, phonophobia, absent taste, reduced or increased tearing, and reduced or increased salivary flow) is not clear, but impairment in these functions could indicate more extensive degeneration of motor axons than when these functions are spared.

Many patients with previous Bell's palsy with good functional recovery may show subtle evidence of residual abnormalities, including slight facial weakness, facial synkinesis, "crocodile" tears, and facial muscle contracture.

MANAGEMENT

Since about 85 percent of patients with Bell's palsy will recover satisfactorily without treatment, it is important that any treatment have a lower morbidity than the natural history of the disease. Prednisone clearly decreases the pain of Bell's palsy as well as the frequency of "crocodile" tears. While there is some debate over the degree of its effectiveness in reducing the duration and severity of paresis, we feel that a 14-day course of prednisone is advisable if there is no strong medical contraindication to the use of corticosteroids (i.e., poorly controlled diabetes, hypertension, or active peptic ulcer disease). If the palsy is moderate to severe and has been present for less than 4 days, we feel that a course of prednisone is strongly indicated. We recommend 60 mg per day in divided doses for 1 week with gradual tapering over the next 7 days. A similar course should be employed in patients with facial paralysis due to herpes zoster, in whom progression (untreated) may last for a week of more. In addition, we tentatively suggest the use of oral acyclovir, 5 mg per kilogram every 8 hours (in patients with normal renal function), although its value in this specific circumstance has not yet been proved.

Management of Bell's palsy by surgical decompression of the facial nerve in its bony canal was proposed first in the 1930s. At that time the ischemic hypothesis held sway; relief of presumed elevated intraneural pressure by surgical means to prevent nerve damage seemed logical. After almost 5 decades and numerous studies there is no valid evidence that surgical decompression is of any benefit. At present we recommend consideration of surgical management *only* for the minority of patients who have severe muscle weakness a year or more after onset of Bell's palsy. In these patients microsurgical procedures can anastomose the distal end of the hypoglossal nerve with the facial nerve trunk distal to the stylomastoid foramen and eventually relieve some of the facial asymmmetry.

When there is paralysis of the orbicularis oculi, the eye loses its protective lid cover and eye protection becomes essential. Protective glasses during the day—especially the light-sensitive sunglass type with a protective side-shield over the temple—and artificial tears are helpful. We have found that at night a large patch of plastic wrap (such as Saran wrap) sealed around the forehead, temple, and cheek with Scotch tape affords reliable, safe protection and maintains moisture.

Some patients with severe lower facial weakness speak more clearly and feel better if the sagging lip is elevated with Scotch "Magic tape" applied with tension and attached to the cheek above.

There is no evidence that electrical stimulation of the facial muscles or other physical therapy measures hasten the recovery from paralysis or decrease any residual sequelae. The benefits of such treatment, if any, are psychological—both for the patient and for the physician.

Fortunately, the patient with Bell's palsy can often be reassured that the outcome will be satisfactory, since no more than 10 to 15 percent of patients are left with significant degrees of residual abnormality, and possibly even fewer will have incomplete recovery with early steroid treatment.

MYASTHENIA GRAVIS

MARJORIE E. SEYBOLD, M.D.

Myasthenia gravis (MG) is an organ-specific autoimmune disorder directed at the acetylcholine receptor (AChR) of skeletal muscle. It may afflict patients of either sex at almost any age, but occurs most commonly in young adult women and older men. Children born to mothers with MG may display transient weakness at birth (neonatal MG), which characteristically disappears within 1 to 2 months.

Clinically, MG is characterized by skeletal muscle weakness and fatigability that are usually fluctuating and asymmetric. In approximately 20 percent of patients the disease is symptomatic only in the ocular muscles (ocular MG). In the remainder of patients, any skeletal muscle may be involved (generalized MG). Bulbar muscle weakness is particularly common and may produce nasal regurgitation, dysphagia, or dysarthria. Bulbar weakness, along with respiratory muscle involvement, represents the most dangerous manifestation of MG.

The symptoms of MG result from a loss of AChRs on the postsynaptic membrane of the neuromuscular junction. More than 80 percent of patients have detectable circulating antibody to AChR (AChR-ab). The antibody is thought to interfere with acetylcholine receptor function in a variety of ways, including enhancement of its normal degradation, complement-mediated destruction of the postsynaptic membrane, and direct and indirect blockade of the receptor. Absolute serum levels of AChR-ab do not correspond to clinical severity, although clinical improvement is often accompanied by decreasing levels of antibody in the individual patient.

The diagnosis of MG can at times be made on clinical grounds alone. More often supplementary tests are used. These include the observation of objective improvement with cholinesterase inhibitors such as edrophonium chloride (Tensilon), the presence of characteristic electromyographic abnormalities, and the finding of AChR-ab in the sera.

MG may occur in association with other autoimmune diseases, the most common of which is thyroid disease. Recognition and correction of thyroid imbalance or any other coexisting disorder are mandatory to achieve good control of MG as well as to aid in the selection of the therapeutic approach.

THERAPEUTIC ALTERNATIVES

Therapy in MG must be tailored to the needs of the individual patient. Clinical severity of the disease, patient tolerance of symptoms, and age all influence the therapies employed and their sequence. The commonly employed measures are cholinesterase inhibitors, thymectomy, corticosteroids, azathioprine, and plasmapheresis. These are generally used in the sequences and circumstances indicated in Table 1.

MG patients may experience worsening of symptoms caused by many factors, including infection, metabolic or endocrine imbalance, menses, surgery, emotional upset, or the action of many different drugs. Neuromuscular blocking agents must be used with extreme caution,

TABLE 1 Sequence of Therapies in Myasthenia Gravis

Ocular myasthenia gravis
Anti-ChE
Symptomatic Rx, e.g., eye patch
Prednisone q.o.d., if necessary
Generalized myasthenia gravis (<50–60 year-old patient)
Anti-ChE
Thymectomy
Prednisone q.o.d., if necessary
Azathioprine, if necessary
Plasmapheresis, if necessary
Generalized myasthenia gravis (>60 year-old patient)
Anti-ChE
Prednisone q.o.d., if necessary
Azathioprine, if necessary
Plasmapheresis, if necessary
Crisis
Respiratory support
Stop anti-ChE 24–72 hours
Restart anti-ChE
Prednisone, if necessary
Plasmapheresis, if necessary

if at all. Other drugs, including aminoglycoside antibiotics, antiarrhythmic and local anesthetic agents, morphine and other central nervous system depressants, and d-penicillamine, should all be used with caution in MG patients.

Cholinesterase Inhibitors

Cholinesterase inhibitors (anti-ChE) are used first in virtually all patients with MG. These medications increase the synaptic concentration of acetylcholine(ACh) by decreasing its degradation rate, thereby enhancing the likelihood that available AChRs will become activated. The three available anti-ChE preparations are pyridostigmine (Mestinon), neostigmine (Prostigmin), and ambenonium (Mytelase). Pyridostigmine is the most frequently used and is available in 60-mg tablets, 180-mg sustained release tablets (timespan), syrup, and injectable form. Neostigmine is available in tablets and injectable form and ambenonium is available in tablet form only. Pyridostigmine taken orally has its onset of action within 10 to 30 minutes and a duration of 3 to 4.5 hours. A similar onset and duration are reported for neostigmine and ambenonium.

Pyridostigmine therapy is usually initiated with 60 mg three times a day taken with meals if chewing and swallowing are not affected or 45 minutes before meals (with a small amount of food) if they are. The patient is asked to keep a record of symptoms at the peak of medication effectiveness (usually about 2 hours) and at the time immediately preceding the next dose. If the medication is noted to "wear off" before the next dose, the interval between medications is gradually shortened. If an individual dose results in only partial relief of symptoms, a larger amount may be tried (in 30- to 60-mg increments). When an increase in medication no longer produces a definite improvement in symptoms, the previous lower amount of medication is resumed. Patients rarely benefit from more than 120 mg of pyridostigmine every 3 hours. Some patients require larger amounts of medication at certain times of day (for example, late afternoon) and thus each dose need not be the same. In patients with dysphagia or jaw fatigue, meal times should be adjusted to correspond to medication peaks.

Pyridostigmine timespan may be used by the patient who experiences weakness during the night or on awakening in the morning. It is not generally used during the day because of its somewhat uneven release. The pyridostigmine syrup is not commonly used, but may be easier to administer in small children or in adults with marked dysphagia. However, careful observation should be made to assure that the salivation induced by the muscarinic effect of pyridostigmine, and enhanced by the sweet syrup vehicle of this form of the drug, does not lead to excessive secretions. Parenteral anti-ChE is reserved for those occasions when oral intake is not possible or for diagnostic testing.

Many patients experience gastrointestinal discomfort and diarrhea with anti-ChE medications. These symptoms often lessen with time and are diminished by taking the medication with a small amount of food. When needed, diphenoxylate with atropine (Lomotil) may be taken once or twice a day for control of diarrhea. Excessive amounts of anti-ChE flood the neuromuscular junction with ACh, thereby resulting in blockade and increased weakness. Thus, any increase in medication that does not produce a clear improvement should not be continued.

Most patients benefit significantly from anti-ChE medication and some have relief of symptoms from this medication alone. Often some symptoms, especially diplopia, persist. In this case the physician and patient must decide if the symptoms are sufficiently severe or distressful to warrant other forms of therapy. Diplopia, for instance, may be adequately relieved by patching one eye. However, many patients find a patch disfiguring or occupationally threatening and request further treatment.

Thymectomy

The thymus gland is abnormal in most patients with MG. Ten to 15 percent of MG patients have a thymoma, while most others demonstrate thymic hyperplasia. Hyperplasia is particularly common in younger patients with MG and is less frequent in the elderly.

The presence of a thymoma as suggested by chest films, tomography, or computed tomography (CT) scan is considered an indication for its removal. These tumors are often locally invasive, but rarely metastasize outside of the chest. When a thymoma has been incompletely removed, radiation therapy is administered postoperatively. Following thymomectomy, the patient may temporarily show clinical improvement in MG symptoms, and postoperative care should be as described for thymectomy in general. Long-term improvement in MG after thymoma removal does occur, but is unpredictable for the individual patient. Should symptoms worsen postoperatively, corticosteroids should be added to the therapeutic regimen.

Thymectomy in the absence of suspected thymoma is more controversial. The theoretical basis of thymectomy in MG is the suspicion that the thymus harbors a cell or cell-bound material that acts in the propagation of MG. Well-controlled studies are difficult to obtain, but most investigations suggest that thymectomy in the young MG patient increases the chances of remission or improvement of the disease for at least the first 3 years after the surgery. Best results appear to occur if the surgery is done within a year after onset of MG symptoms.

I favor the use of thymectomy in all patients with generalized MG above the age of puberty and below the age of 50. Children below the age of puberty would be considered candidates for thymectomy if they were not well controlled on anti-ChE medication. Adults between 50 and 60 who were otherwise in good health but not responding well to anti-ChEs would also be considered. At some institutions MG patients over the age of 60 years are advised to have thymectomy. I have found these patients to be very responsive to corticosteroid therapy and prefer to use this medication in older MG patients, rather than thymectomy, unless there is evidence of thymoma.

Thymectomy requires a skilled surgeon and

anesthesiologist, with postoperative intensive care in an experienced unit, and careful attention to medication needs. It is most often done through a trans-sternal approach with removal of all thymic tissue and adjacent fat. The transcervical approach is more controversial because of the possibility of incomplete removal of thymic tissue. While almost all of my patients have been operated on by the trans-sternal approach, I feel the transcervical approach could be considered if a surgeon skilled in this procedure is available and the patient, for reasons of better cosmetic appearance or faster recovery, requests this approach.

The medication needs of the MG patient usually decrease immediately postoperatively. This may occur following any operative procedure, but is especially true following thymectomy. I advise that anti-ChEs be discontinued postoperatively and be restarted as needed, either because of recurrence of symptoms or following a positive response to parenteral anti-ChE. The latter can be given in the short-acting form edrophonium (Tensilon) in increments of 2 mg, 3 mg, and 5 mg spaced at 1- to 2-minute intervals. Improvement can be expected within 20 to 40 seconds after injection with a duration of 2 to 3 minutes. If improvement occurs with 2 or 3 mg, the test is discontinued. It is highly unlikely that a response will be obtained from a large (for example, 10 mg) edrophonium bolus if no response is obtained from a smaller injection. Additionally, muscarinic side effects are much more distressing with the larger injections.

Often anti-ChE medications do not have to be resumed until the patient is able to take oral medications. If so, they are restarted on a 60 mg three times a day basis to be increased as necessary on a program similar to that used for the initiation of anti-ChEs. When parenteral therapy is necessary postoperatively, it may be administered either intramuscularly, subcutaneously, or intravenously (0.5 mg of neostigmine methylsulfate every 4 hours by continuous infusion). If the patient was taking alternate-day prednisone prior to surgery, he should receive an equivalent dose of daily parenteral corticosteroids until oral medications can be resumed. Occasionally a patient is difficult to wean from the ventilator postoperatively. In this circumstance a short course of plasmapheresis may be helpful.

Corticosteroids

Corticosteroids are widely accepted as a treatment for MG, although the mechanism of action is incompletely understood. Steroids decrease AChR-ab in some MG patients, usually those showing the most definite improvement. Whether there are additional immunosuppressive actions and/or direct effects on the neuromuscular junction that are significant is not known at present. Older male patients in particular seem to benefit greatly from prednisone therapy and can often be maintained for years in a relatively asymptomatic state. Patients with only ocular symptoms often benefit more from steroids than from anti-ChE drugs. In these patients the risk-benefit ratio must be considered carefully by the physician and patient before steroids are begun. If the benefits seem significant (for example, job preservation), steroids may be warranted in some patients with ocular MG.

The method of commencing steroid administration varies with the severity of the patient's disease. For the patient with only ocular symptoms or with mild generalized MG, I begin with low-dose (20 mg), alternate-day prednisone on an outpatient basis. The prednisone is increased by 5 mg to 10 mg every 2 weeks to a level at which a good result is obtained. For some patients this may be as low as 25 or 30 mg. If a good result is not obtained by the time a level of 40 mg is reached, the prednisone is increased in 20-mg increments at 2-week intervals until 100 mg every other day is reached. The patient is maintained at 100 mg every other day until a satisfactory response is obtained or for 3 to 6 months, after which a slow tapering (5 to 10 mg per month) is attempted. Early in their treatment, patients usually feel better during the day "on" prednisone. Generally a more balanced effect is achieved as time goes on. The maintenance level selected is whatever amount of prednisone is required to allow the patient an acceptable relief of symptoms. Rarely, a patient may have no improvement with prednisone. When no improvement is observed in 3 months, a slightly more rapid tapering seems justified in anticipation of alternative therapy.

The method described probably results in a slower improvement than obtained from daily prednisone or higher initial doses. It has advantages, however, that seem to me to outweigh this disadvantage: patients may be treated as outpatients and continue to work while beginning therapy; exacerbations of symptoms (a common occurrence with prednisone when initiated in high daily doses) can be avoided; side effects such as cushingoid appearance, mood change, and sleeplessness are rare; and some patients respond while on a low dose, thus avoiding the need to take higher doses. Most patients show a definite response within 3 to 6 weeks after beginning prednisone by this method, and improvement may continue over several months.

When the patient has more severe symptoms, more rapid introduction of prednisone is necessary. Patients with rapidly evolving disease, or with difficulties with food intake or respiratory symptoms or signs, should be hospitalized for the initiation of steroids. Patients with respiratory difficulties should be placed in an intensive care unit. The initial dose and rapidity of increase must be determined by the patient's clinical status. Elderly patients with bulbar symptoms often tolerate increments of 10 mg of prednisone every 5 days from an initial dose of 20 mg without exacerbation. Only in the most desperate of circumstances would I start a patient on high-dose daily prednisone (60 to 100 mg), as this requires admission to the intensive care unit and has a high probability of inducing an exacerbation requiring respiratory support.

Long-term maintenance on prednisone, as previously mentioned, should be at the lowest dosage that controls symptoms. For most patients this is from 15 to 40 mg every other day. Few patients can be tapered from prednisone completely, and if exacerbation occurs during tapering, the dose must often be raised substantially to obtain the same level of improvement seen previously. While on prednisone, patients may benefit from vitamin D (400 IU per day) and calcium gluconate or carbonate (1,000 mg per day).

The side effects of prednisone therapy include osteoporosis, aseptic necrosis of bone, increased risk of infection, ulcers, cataracts, hypertension, exacerbation of diabetes, fluid retention, and so on. Periodic examination of the blood count, blood glucose, and electrolytes, and yearly chest films and eye examination are recommended.

Azathioprine and Other Immunosuppressive Drugs

Azathioprine should be considered for the patient who has disabling symptoms despite careful regulation of anti-ChE and steroid medications, or for the patient who is unable or unwilling to take steroids. Like steroids, azathioprine often results in a lowering of AChR-ab in the sera. Whether this depletion of AChR-ab is responsible for its therapeutic effectiveness is not known.

Azathioprine is given orally. The usual recommended dosage is 2.0 to 2.5 mg per kilogram per day (125 to 200 mg per day for most patients). I have found it effective to start with 50 mg per day and to increase to 100 mg after 2 weeks. As with prednisone, some patients improve with small amounts of azathioprine, thus obviating the need for higher dosages and diminishing the risks of the drug. Incremental increases to 2.5 mg per kilogram per day may be given over the following month if necessary and as tolerated by the patient. Improvement may be seen as early as 1 month after starting treatment, but often several months are required for maximal effect.

Side effects from azathioprine include leukopenia, thrombocytopenia, increased hazard of infection, nausea and vomiting, hepatic toxicity, and alopecia. Reduction in dosage or discontinuation of the drug usually results in improvement in the side effects. Blood counts and liver function studies should be carefully monitored for the patient on azathioprine, weekly for the first month and biweekly or monthly thereafter. Whether long-term azathioprine treatment in MG is associated with the development of neoplasia, as it is in transplant patients, remains to be seen. As yet, no such association has been recognized for MG.

I have found azathioprine particularly helpful for the patient who requires large amounts of prednisone to control MG. In these patients, the addition of azathioprine often results in improvement and allows the prednisone to be tapered to a lower maintenance level.

Other immunosuppressive medications, such as cyclophosphamide (Cytoxan), have been employed in MG patients. While effective in some cases, the high toxicity of these drugs limits their use to the most severely ill patients.

Plasmapheresis

Plasmapheresis is well accepted as a method to induce improvement in MG patients. Usually a series of 4 to 8 plasmaphereses are administered over a 5- to 10-day period. This treatment decreases the amount of circulating AChR-ab, but whether this is the cause of the improvement is not known. The effects of plasmapheresis often last only 2 to 4 weeks and the patient may revert back to the previous level of disease. This appears less likely to happen if prednisone and/or azathioprine are given concomitantly.

Indications for plasmapheresis in MG include ventilatory dependency, life-threatening exacerbation of disease, and chronic severe MG despite high doses of prednisone and azathioprine. It may also be used prior to thymectomy in the moderately severe MG patient in an attempt to obtain improved strength during the perioperative period.

The complications of plasmapheresis include infection, hypotension, thrombocytopenia, and hypocalcemia. It is also expensive. It should only be employed when other methods for control of MG have not been successful; fortunately, this is uncommon.

CRISIS

Rarely, a patient with MG may experience an abrupt increase in symptoms that appears refractory to medication. This may be caused by excessive anti-ChE medications (cholinergic crisis) or by an actual deterioration in MG responsiveness (myasthenic crisis). In either case, the patient should be hospitalized immediately and placed in an intensive care unit if ventilatory inadequacy is suspected or has occurred in the past. Patients in crisis may deteriorate extremely rapidly and precautionary support of ventilation is judicious. Once adequate ventilation is assured, assessment of cholinergic versus myasthenic crisis can be made. Treatment of cholinergic crisis usually requires that all anti-ChE medications be discontinued for 24 to 72 hours and then restarted as at the beginning of anti-ChE therapy. If the patient is receiving steroid therapy, this is not altered. For myasthenic crisis, anti-ChE medications are also withheld for 24 to 72 hours and then restarted in the standard manner. In addition, a source for the induction of the crisis should be sought. This is often an infection, but may be attributable to medications, emotional upset, surgery, or other factors. When necessary, prednisone may be started or increased and/or patients may undergo plasmapheresis. With ventilatory assistance already being provided, the danger from prednisone-induced exacerbation is reduced and high doses (60 to 100 mg of prednisone) may be used. My preference has been to use 100 mg every other day, although a daily dose is employed in most centers.

NEONATAL MG

Twelve to 15 percent of infants born to mothers with MG experience transient weakness. Symptoms are usually present on the first day of life and persist for an average of 18 days. Feeding difficulties are the most common evidence of the disorder. The child should also be carefully observed for respiratory difficulty and support given if necessary. Medications such as pyridostigmine syrup (4 to 10 mg) may be given orally or by nasogastric tube if necessary, preferably 45 minutes before feedings. Decreasing doses of anti-ChE are needed as the disorder spontaneously improves, and care should be taken to avoid overmedication.

POLYMYOSITIS

CHRISTOPHER M. CLARK, M.D.

Polymyositis is a syndrome with the predominant clinical manifestation of proximal muscle weakness due to destruction of skeletal muscle tissue. Affected muscles have histopathologic changes of a nonsuppurative inflammatory reaction associated with muscle fiber necrosis and regeneration. The clinical spectrum runs the gamut from an acute (possibly self-limited) viral-like illness to a chronic progressive disorder. A growing body of evidence suggests that immune responses play an important role and that the syndrome may fall under the general category of an autoimmune disorder. Diagnostic criteria include: (1) progressive bilateral proximal limb weakness, (2) myopathic changes on electromyography (EMG), (3) elevated muscle enzymes (usually creatine kinase), (4) inflammatory changes on muscle biopsy with fiber necrosis and regeneration, and (5) absence of an alternative explanation for the weakness.

Polymyositis is divided into the following clinical categories: (1) polymyositis, (2) dermatomyositis, (3) myositis associated with cancer, (4) childhood myositis, and (5) myositis with associated collagen vascular disease. Inclusion body myositis may represent a sixth category.

The presence of clinically identifiable subgroups does not imply the existence of well-established or distinct pathophysiologic mechanisms. The subgroups do not predict the clinical course or the response to a particular therapy. There are three possible exceptions to this:

1. Patients with polymyositis and cancer are more likely to have a skin rash than those without cancer. However, there are too many exceptions to ignore the possibility of cancer in patients without a rash.
2. In childhood dermatomyositis with calcinosis, the basic pathologic change may involve a vasculitis rather than a primary inflammatory disorder of the muscle fiber.

TABLE 1 Adult Onset Muscle Disease

Genetic	Endocrine
Dystrophy	Thyroid
Facioscapulohumeral	Parathyroid
Limb-girdle	Adrenal
Myotonic	Carcinoid
Metabolic deficiencies	Periodic Paralysis
Acid maltase	Hypokalemic (with or without thyroid disease)
Phosphorylase	Hyperkalemic
Phosphofructokinase	Drugs
Carintine	Alcohol
Carintine transferase	Heroin
Inflammatory	Amphetamine
Polymyositis	Epsilon-Aminocaproic acid
Dermatomyositis	Emetin
Childhood dermatomyositis with calcinosis	D-Penicillamine
Myositis with malignancy	Clofibrate
Myositis with collagen vascular disease	Steroids
Inclusion body myositis	Chloroquine
Infectious	Diuretics
Viral	Quinidine
Trichinosis	Lithium
Toxoplasmosis	Phencyclidine
Cysticercosis	Cromolyn
Malignant	Vincristine
Eaton-Lambert syndrome	Other
Paraneoplastic syndrome	Myasthenia Gravis
Rhabdomyosarcoma	Sarcoid
Lipoma	Amyloid
	Psoriasis

TABLE 2 Laboratory Evaluation

Complete blood count
Erythrocyte sedimentation rate
Electrolytes
Thyroid studies
Blood chemistry screen
Creatine kinase level
Antinuclear antibody titer
Serum protein electrophoresis
Urinalysis for myoglobin
Chest x-ray
Electromyography
Muscle biopsy with following analysis:
  Hematoxylon and eosin
  Histochemistry for oxidative enzymes
  Stain for glycogen
  Stain for lipids
  Electron microscopy for inclusion bodies

Therapy and prognosis for this group of patients may differ from those in the other categories.

3. Patients with vacuoles in their muscles biopsy (inclusion body myositis) may have a less favorable outcome.

The presence of a skin rash or a malignancy cannot be used to predict the effect of therapy on the muscle weakness. The ultimate outcome for those patients with cancer is usually dictated by the type of malignancy and its response to treatment.

It is not known whether polymyositis in association with a well-defined collagen vascular disorder represents a different disease from "pure polymyositis" or simply a broader manifestation of the same basic problem. In any event, the treatment of the muscle disorder remains the same.

EVALUATION

The diagnosis of polymyositis is established by a history of progressive proximal muscle weakness with an elevated creatine kinase, myopathic changes on electrolmyopgraphy, and a muscle biopsy demonstrating characteristic features of inflammation, fiber necrosis, and regeneration. Muscle disorders such as myasthenia gravis, Eaton–Lambert syndrome, and the others listed in Table 1 should be excluded by the appropriate laboratory procedures (Table 2). All adult patients should have a general screen for malignancy. This includes a detailed history and physical examination, routine hematologic studies including blood chemistries, chest radiograph, stool guaiac determination, and intravenous pyelogram. Additional studies for cancer detection are done only if they are indicated.

TREATMENT

Treatment is directed at the following goals:

1. Suppression of the inflammatory response.
2. Reduction of any immunologically mediated attack against muscle.
3. Preservation of current muscle function.
4. Prevention of complications due to weakness.
5. Avoidance of complications due to therapy.

None of the therapies currently used to treat polymyositis has been evaluated in a prospective randomized controlled trial. There is an incomplete understanding of the pathophysiology and natural course of the disease and no real proof that the current standard therapy (high dose steroids) is beneficial. On occasion improvement may occur despite treatment rather than because of it. Some patients with polymyositis may respond to a therapy that is ineffective in other patients. Although some investigators feel that the presence of inclusion bodies in the muscle carries a poor prognosis, there are no *proven* clinical or laboratory parameters that will predict the therapeutic response. This should be kept in mind when considering the risk of treatment-related complications (Tables 3 and 4).

Prednisone remains the accepted first-line treatment.

TABLE 3 Percent of Patients With Polymyositis and Treatment-Associated Side Effects (N=65)

	Treatment	
Side Effects	*Prednisone Only*	*Prednisone and Immunosuppressant*
Skin changes	52	50
Personality change	52	60
Cushingoid changes	37	57
Insomnia	30	50
Weight gain	30	60
Vertebral collapse	22	3
Infection	22	27
Hyperglycemia	22	27
Cataracts	22	27
Hair loss	0	10
Aseptic bone necrosis	7	7
Psychosis	0	7
Peptic ulcer	0	7
Required treatment change	30	37

TABLE 4 Side Effects of Immunosuppressant Medications

Drug	*Side Effects*
Methotrexate	Nausea and vomiting
	Diarrhea
	Fever
	Oral and gastrointestinal ulceration and perforation
	Bone marrow suppression
	Hepatic toxicity (cirrhosis and acute necrosis)
	Renal toxicity
	Pulmonary infiltrates
	Osteoporosis
	Chills, fever
	Alopecia
	Depigmentation and other cutaneous reactions
	Infertility
	Menstrual dysfunction
Azathioprine	Nausea and vomiting
	Thrombocytopenia
	Leukopenia
	Increased risk of infection
	Alopecia
	Pancreatitis
	Increased risk of leukemia and lymphoma
Cyclophosphamide	Nausea and vomiting
	Bone marrow suppression
	Alopecia
	Hemorrhagic cystitis
	Sterility
	Pulmonary fibrosis
	Hyperpigmentation
	Secondary malignancies
	Nonspecific dermatitis
	Hyponatremia
Cyclosporine	Nephrotoxicity
	Increased incidence of infection, including reactivation of Epstein-Barr virus
	Hypertension
	Hepatotoxicity
	Gingival hypertrophy
	Hirsutism
	Nausea
	Tremor
	Fluid retention

Nowhere is the dilemma of when to initiate treatment and how long to persist more clearly posed than when considering prednisone therapy. If the drug had a high degree of efficacy, the ideal regimen would be to begin treatment as early as possible with high doses until the muscle weakness improved or the patient developed unacceptable side effects. On the other hand, if the therapeutic benefits were questionable or, at best, only marginal, delaying treatment as long as possible, would be beneficial because one would avoid exposing patients, who showed spontaneous improvement to prednisone. If the drug was used at all, the dosage would be kept as small as possible, consistent with the clinical situation, and would be discontinued at the first sign of a significant complication unless there was a clear-cut response to treatment.

Since it is not known which of these two extremes represents the correct approach, I explain the dilemma to each patient, outlining the important complications associated with steroid use and the possible results if the problem remains untreated. I feel that it is very important that patients participate in the therapeutic decisions, to the fullest extent possible as they must bear the consequences of whatever action is taken.

If the weakness is minimal and does not interfere with the patient's ability to function, I suggest either no treatment or a nonsteroidal anti-inflammatory drug such as ibuprofen (300 mg 3 times a day). If the weakness is severe enough to interfere with function and if there are no medical contraindications, I begin treatment with 60 mg of prednisone per day. That dose is maintained until there is a clear-cut improvement in muscle strength or development of an unacceptable side effect. I routinely prescribe ancillary therapy in an attempt to reduce the possibility of prednisone-associated problems. All patients take either a specific H_2 histamine blocker (such as cimetidine, 300 mg 3 to 4 times per day) or a standard antacid (such as Maalox, one tablespoon with the prednisone and an additional tablespoon at bedtime). All women take calcium (1,500 mg per day) and vitamin D (50,000 units weekly). Everyone is placed on a low-salt diet and warned about the importance of monitoring their blood pressure. Fasting blood sugars are obtained at every office visit, and the patients check their morning urine for glucose once a week. If there is a family history of diabetes mellitus, monitoring is done more frequently. I do not treat insulin-dependent diabetic patients with prednisone, but, would begin medical therapy with an immunosuppressant, if the clinical situation warrants it.

As soon as there is clear improvement in muscle strength, the patient is changed to alternate-day therapy by decreasing the "off" day dose by 10 mg and increasing the "on" day by an equal amount every week. If improvement continues once the conversion has been completed (a process that usually takes 5 weeks), I begin to taper the "on" day dose by no more than 5 mg per week. Patients who will have a good recovery usually show considerable improvement within the first 4 to 6 months of treatment.

There is a natural tendency to follow a patient's creatine kinase level throughout treatment with the hope that it will reflect disease activity and provide an objective marker of the response to therapy. This should be avoided. Therapeutic decisions must be based on meaningful improvement in muscle strength, and it is on this clinical sign that the physician must focus (Fig. 1).

If there is no response after 4 to 6 weeks of 60 mg per day of prednisone (or 1 mg per kilogram), I add methotrexate, starting at 0.04 mg per kilogram orally giving three doses per week, with a 12-hour interval between each dose. If after an additional 4 weeks there is still no response, the dose is increased to 0.08 mg per kilogram, using the same schedule of three doses per week spaced 12 hours apart. This is continued for an additional 2 months before making a final judgment regarding efficacy.

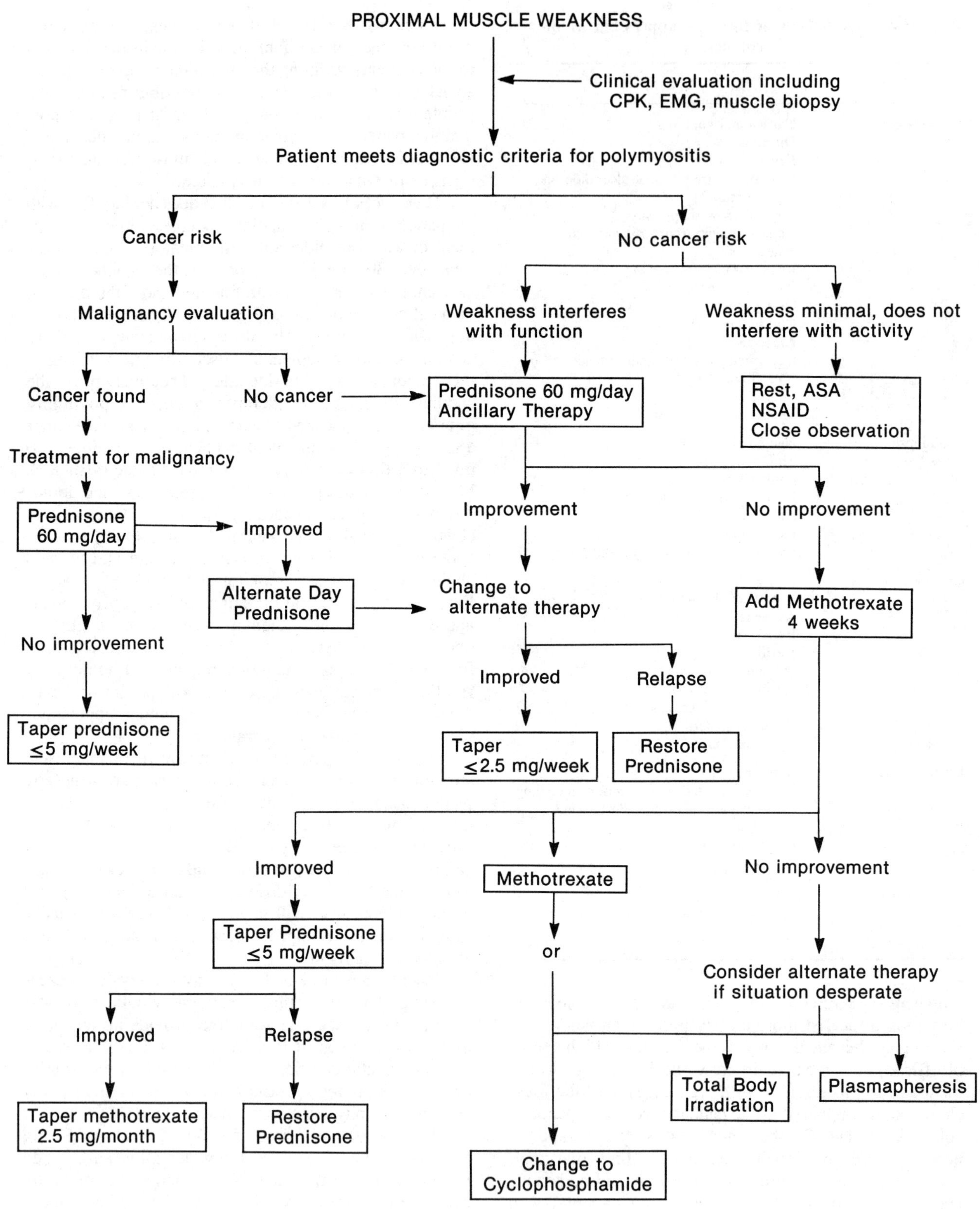

Figure 1 Management protocol in polymyositis.

TABLE 5 Treatments Used in Polymyositis

Drug	*Dose*	*Schedule*	*Maximum*	*Monitor*
Prednisone*	60 mg PO	Once daily	Unknown	Blood pressure Blood sugar Stool quiac
Methotrexate*	0.04 mg/kg PO	q12h×3/wk	0.08 mg/kg ×3/wk	Liver function WBC >3,500
Azathioprine*	75 mg PO	Once daily	2.5 mg/kg	WBC >3,500 Lymphocytes >1,000 Liver function
Cyclophosphamide*	50 mg PO (2.5 mg/kg)	t.i.d.	Unknown	WBC >3,500
Cyclosporine†	6 mg/kg PO	Once daily	Unknown	Renal function
Plasmapheresis†	Exchange volume equal to 5% body weight	Once weekly	Unknown	
Total body irradiation†	15 rads	Twice weekly	150 rads	Platelet count WBC

* Of unproven value.
† Of unproven value and experimental in nature.

Alternatives to methotrexate include azathioprine (starting at 75 mg orally per day and increasing every 4 to 7 days to a maximum of 2.5 mg per kilogram) or cyclophosphamide (50 mg orally 3 times a day or 2.5 mg per kilogram). The choice of which immunosuppressant to use is usually based on the physician's experience with the medication, the patient's tolerance for the drug, and the risks of side effects, primarily organ toxicity and the subsequent development of a malignancy (Table 2). Azathioprine may require a long time before demonstrating an effect, and thus it may not be the best choice if a rapid response is needed.

With all immunosuppressant medication, it is important to monitor the white blood count and reduce or discontinue the drug if this falls below 3,500 or if the lymphocyte count drops below 1,000. Liver function tests should be obtained every 3 months. There are no randomized controlled trials demonstrating that one immunosuppressant is more beneficial than another or that any of the agents in current use are beneficial at all.

When using methotrexate, I do not obtain a liver biopsy before treatment unless there is some suggestion of pre-existing liver disease. During treatment, liver function is monitored by measurement of hepatic enzymes levels, and total bilirubin.

I have not used any of the other therapeutic modalities that have been suggested as possibly beneficial (Table 5). These include plasmapheresis (exchanging a volume of plasma equal to 5 percent of body weight weekly for up to 10 weeks and then increasing the interval to a maximum of every 4 weeks for a total of 4 to 33 exchanges in a manner outlined by Dau); total body irradiation, giving two 15-rad treatments per week for 5 weeks for a total of 150 rads; or cyclosporine (6 to 10 mg per kilogram per day for a maximum of 6 months). The latter drug is currently being evaluated using a randomized double-blind placebo controlled protocol, so information regarding its efficacy and safety may be available soon.

I do not routinely ask patients to become involved in a formal physical therapy program, but feel there is a definite benefit for severely weak patients to do passive range of motion exercises in order to avoid complications of inactivity. A physical therapist can also help patients with weakness to learn to walk safely. In addition, information is available concerning aids to help with activities of daily living. Such information may be of considerable benefit to patients with muscle weakness. Good nutrition is always important. Some diet modification may be necessary in those patients who have trouble swallowing.

PATIENT RESOURCES

Polymyositis is covered by the Muscular Dystrophy Association (MDA), and patients who are registered with the local MDA office are entitled to receive authorized services from any of the 240 clinics nationwide at no direct cost to them or their families. The local MDA office is usually listed in the phone directory. Information may also be obtained by calling Patient Services at the national office (212) 586–0808.

PERIODIC PARALYSIS

JACK E. RIGGS, M.D.

The periodic paralyses are an extraordinarily rare group of disorders. Their clinical presentation is so dramatic that few physicians, once having encountered such a patient during an attack, will forget the experience. Although generally regarded as disorders of potassium metabolism, many patients with episodic muscle weakness and laboratory evidence of altered potassium metabolism do not have one of the primary periodic paralyses (Table 1), but rather another disorder that secondarily affects potassium homeostatis and may present with a clinical picture of periodic muscle weakness (Table 2).

The treatment of the periodic paralyses cannot and should not be separated from their diagnosis. Effective treatment necessitates accurate diagnosis. Screening of patients for disorders that may mimic one of the primary periodic paralyses often requires hospitalization and detailed laboratory testing. If a disorder other than one of the primary periodic paralyses is identified, appropriate treatment for that particular disorder should be rendered.

This chapter is limited to treatment of the primary periodic paralyses. With regards to the management of acute attacks of weakness in this group of disorders, a safe clinical dictum to follow is "when in doubt, do nothing," but provide supportive care. Death during acute attacks of weakness was not uncommon 50 years ago. Today, death during an acute attack of weakness associated with one of the primary periodic paralyses must be essentially nonexistent since it is not reported. Fifty years ago, the only treatment was administration of potassium salts. If the patient had hyperkalemic periodic paralysis, this treatment could have resulted in increased weakness, perhaps to the point of respiratory failure and death.

TABLE 1 Classification of the Primary Periodic Paralyses

- Hypokalemic
  - Familial
  - Sporadic
  - Thyrotoxic
- Hyperkalemic (potassium sensitive)
  - With myotonia
    - Familial
    - Sporadic
  - Without myotonia
    - Familial
    - Sporadic
- Normokalemic (usually potassium sensitive)
- Paramyotonia with periodic paralysis
  - Paramyotonia congenita
  - Paralysis periodica paramyotonia

TABLE 2 Disorders With Altered Potassium Metabolism and Episodic Weakness

- Disorders with hypokalemia
  - Primary hyperaldosteronism (Conn's syndrome)
  - Renal tubular acidosis
  - Bartter's syndrome (juxtaglomerular apparatus hyperplasia)
  - Villous adenoma
  - Alcoholism
  - Drugs and other agents
    - Diuretics
    - Corticosteroids
    - Licorice
    - *p*-Aminosalicylic acid
    - Barium
- Disorders with hyperkalemia
  - Addison's disease
  - Chronic renal failure
  - Chronic heparin administration
  - Hyporeninemic hypoaldosteronism

HYPOKALEMIC PERIODIC PARALYSIS

Familial and Sporadic

The management of acute attacks and preventive therapy in familial and sporadic forms of hypokalemic periodic paralysis are identical.

Treatment of Acute Attacks. Administration of potassium salts is the primary treatment for acute attacks of weakness. If the patient is known to the treating physician, potassium can be administered immediately after the initial blood samples for potassium, BUN, and creatinine have been drawn and sent to the laboratory STAT. However, if the patient is not known to the treating physician, it is important to know that renal function is normal prior to the administration of potassium. I use a sugar-free 10 percent solution of potassium chloride (KCl) in the treatment of acute attacks. The 10 percent KCl solution produces less gastric irritation than the 20 percent KCl solution. A sugar-free KCl solution is preferable to a sweetened solution, which may "paradoxically" produce initial lowering of potassium. A 20-mEq KCl dose (15 ml using a 10 percent solution) is administered orally and repeated at 30- to 60-minute intervals until the patient's strength returns to near normal. Typically the patient will require three to five doses of KCl. I draw a potassium level prior to administration of each KCl dose, although it is not necessary to wait for the result in a patient with normal renal function.

In reality, most acute attacks of weakness are treated at home by the patient with repeated self-administered oral doses of KCl. Patients with periodic paralysis are often reluctant to go to an emergency room to be treated by physicians unfamiliar with their disorder. The situation is quite understandable. A healthy appearing, nonanxious individual is brought to the emergency room quadriplegic and tries to tell the staff that he or she will get better if just given potassium. Not infrequently the net result for the patient is a psychiatric consultation and a label of conversion reaction.

In the unusual situation in which the patient cannot take oral potassium, intravenous administration of KCl is an acceptable, although less desirable, alternative route. Forty mEq of KCl per liter of 5 percent mannitol or half-normal saline can be infused at 250 ml per hour in the patient with normal renal and cardiac function.

Preventive Therapy. Although potassium salts abort acute attacks of weakness in hypokalemic periodic paralysis, they are not effective preventive therapy, even in large doses.

Acetazolamide (125 to 1,500 mg per day) is effective prophylactic treatment in most patients with hypokalemic periodic paralysis. In adults, an initial dose is 125 mg twice a day, whereas in children less than 12 years old, an initial dose is 62.5 mg either once or twice a day. The dose is increased in adults by 125-mg increments and in children by 62.5-mg increments. The pretreatment frequency of attacks is the primary determinant in deciding how often the dosage should be adjusted. In the patient with only one or two attacks per month, it might take several months to determine the efficacy of a particular dosage. When adjusting the dosage, the increase should be added to the evening dose first, since many attacks are nocturnal. There is little benefit in increasing the total daily dose of acetazolamide above 1,500 mg in adults and 750 mg in children. If patients do not improve at these dosages, the medication should be discontinued.

Administration of acetazolamide is often accompanied by paresthesias, dysgeusia for carbonated beverages, nausea, and anorexia. Long-term administration has been associated with the development of renal calculi. Thus, it is important to keep the acetazolamide dosage as low as possible, ensure adequate fluid intake, avoid concomitant sulfonamide administration, and periodically screen for signs of renal calculi.

Triamterene is also effective in preventing attacks of weakness in hypokalemic periodic paralysis and is particularly useful in patients who cannot tolerate the side effects of acetazolamide. A typical initial dose is 50 mg one to three times per day. The dose is increased by 50-mg increments, with the frequency of attacks determining how often the dosage should be adjusted. There is no benefit in increasing the total daily dose of triamterene above 300 mg. If patients do not improve at this dosage, the medication should be discontinued.

The most serious toxic effect of triamterene is hyperkalemia. This is particularly worrisome, since most patients with hypokalemic periodic paralysis often have oral potassium available for self-administration during acute attacks of weakness. Therefore, patients taking triamterene should have periodic electrolyte determinations to check for the development of hyperkalemia.

In some patients dietary manipulation may be helpful. Patients should be advised to avoid heavy carbohydrate meals, particularly in the evening. Excessive alcohol intake should be avoided. A low-sodium diet is effective adjuvant therapy in some patients. Additionally, patients should avoid unusually exhausting and heavy exercise, particularly prior to eating or sleeping.

Thyrotoxic

Preventive therapy in thyrotoxic periodic paralysis is quite different from that used in the familial and sporadic forms of hypokalemic periodic paralysis.

Treatment of Acute Attacks. The therapeutic approach to shortening an acute attack of weakness in thyrotoxic periodic paralysis is identical to that used in familial and sporadic forms of hypokalemic periodic paralysis.

Preventive Therapy. The primary and essential aspect of preventive therapy in thyrotoxic periodic paralysis is rendering the patient euthyroid. Once the euthyroid state is achieved and maintained, paralytic attacks cease to occur. However, if the patient becomes hypothyroid following treatment and requires exogenous thyroid hormone, episodes of weakness can recur if the patient is overtreated. If the attacks of weakness require additional preventive therapy until the patient has been rendered euthyroid, propranolol, 20 to 40 mg four times per day, is often effective.

The use of acetazolamide in thyrotoxic periodic paralysis is contraindicated. Patients with this disorder receiving acetazolamide have experienced increased frequency and severity in their attacks of weakness, some to the point that ventilatory assistance is required.

HYPERKALEMIC PERIODIC PARALYSIS

With and Without Myotonia

The treatment of acute attacks and preventive therapy in myotonic and nonmyotonic forms of hyperkalemic periodic paralysis are identical.

Treatment of Acute Attacks. Acute attacks of weakness in hyperkalemic periodic paralysis are often so brief that medical intervention is unnecessary. Prompt ingestion of high-carbohydrate beverages at the onset of weakness will usually abort or abbreviate an attack. Many patients will eat or drink something sweet at times when attacks are most likely to occur. Measures used to treat hyperkalemia have proved useful in the management of unusually severe attacks of weakness in hyperkalemic periodic paralysis. Thus, glucose, epinephrine, calcium gluconate, insulin, and glucagon have all been shown to be effective in aborting attacks, although these measures are seldom necessary.

Preventive Therapy. Acetazolamide is effective prophylaxis in many patients with hyperkalemic periodic paralysis. Administration follows the same guidelines as that described above for hypokalemic periodic paralysis. An additional benefit of acetazolamide in patients with hyperkalemic periodic paralysis and myotonia is that this drug is very effective in alleviating myotonia. Patients with hyperkalemic periodic paralysis and myotonia is that this drug is very effective in alleviating myotonia. Patients with hyperkalemic periodic paralysis receiving acetazolamide often experience prominent paresthesias, which may limit therapy. Consequently, thiazides are often better tolerated. Hydrochlorothiazide, 25 mg once a day, or chlorothiazide, 250 mg once a day, are typical starting doses in adults. In children, starting doses are hydrochlorothiazide, 2 mg per kilogram per day, or chlorothiazide, 20 mg per kilogram per day. The frequent side effects of thiazide diuretics are well known and necessitate serial monitoring of blood glucose and electrolytes.

NORMOKALEMIC PERIODIC PARALYSIS

The existence of normokalemic periodic paralysis as a distinct and separate clinical entity remains unconfirmed and is doubted by many authorities. Since most patients described as having this entity are potassium sensitive, i.e., attacks can be provoked by the oral administration of potassium, there appears to be little practical distinction between normokalemic periodic paralysis and hyperkalemic periodic paralysis. Patients with normokalemic periodic paralysis who are potassium sensitive should be treated in the same manner as patients with hyperkalemic periodic paralysis.

PARAMYOTONIA WITH PERIODIC PARALYSIS

Paramyotonia is a prominent feature in two distinct disorders with associated periodic paralysis, i.e., paramyotonia congenita and paralysis periodica paramyotonia. The optimal treatment of periodic paralysis in paramyotonia remains ill-defined because of a failure to distinguish between these two separate disorders.

Paramyotonia Congenita

Spontaneous attacks of weakness unrelated to cold exposure are generally infrequent in paramyotonia congenita. Attacks of weakness in this disorder are associated with hypokalemia and may be provoked by glucose-insulin challenges. Acute attacks of weakness in paramyotonia may be treated with potassium administration, similar to treatment in hypokalemic periodic paralysis. However, one must take into consideration that potassium will exacerbate the patient's myotonic symptoms. Unlike treatment in hypokalemic periodic paralysis, acetazolamide is contraindicated in paramyotonia congenita, since it precipitates weakness in this disorder. If attacks of weakness in paramyotonia congenita are sufficiently frequent, a potassium-sparing diuretic such as spironolactone may be useful, but again this may exacerbate the myotonic symtoms.

Paralysis Periodica Paramyotonia

Spontaneous attacks of weakness in this disorder are more frequent than in paramyotonia congenita, are associated with hyperkalemia, and may be induced by potassium administration. Attacks are generally brief in duration and medical intervention is rarely required. Thiazide diuretics, as in hyperkalemic periodic paralysis, are useful in preventing attacks of weakness unrelated to cold exposure and have the additional benefit of alleviating the myotonic symptoms.

INDEX

Page numbers followed by "f" indicate figures; those followed by "t" indicate tables.

D

H

J

K

L

N

Q

R